Diagnostic Surgical Pathology

———— Third Edition ————

Diagnostic Surgical Pathology

Third Edition

VOLUME 2

Editor

Stephen S. Sternberg, M.D.
*Attending Pathologist
Memorial Sloan-Kettering Cancer Center
New York, New York*

Associate Editors

Donald A. Antonioli, M.D.
*Professor of Pathology
Harvard Medical School
Senior Pathologist
Department of Pathology
Beth Israel Deaconess Medical Center
Boston, Massachusetts*

Darryl Carter, M.D.
*Professor
Department of Pathology
Yale University School of Medicine
New Haven, Connecticut*

Stacey E. Mills, M.D.
*Associate Chair and Professor
Department of Pathology
University of Virginia Health Sciences Center
Charlottesville, Virginia*

Harold A. Oberman, M.D.
*Professor
Department of Pathology
University of Michigan Health Sciences Center
Ann Arbor, Michigan*

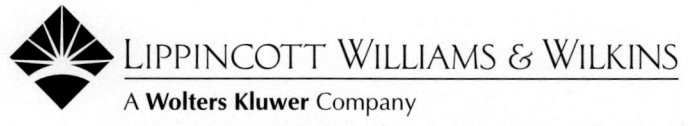

LIPPINCOTT WILLIAMS & WILKINS
A **Wolters Kluwer** Company
Philadelphia · Baltimore · New York · London
Buenos Aires · Hong Kong · Sydney · Tokyo

SOUTH UNIVERSITY
709 MALL BLVD.
SAVANNAH, GA 31406

Acquisitions Editor: Anne S. Patterson
Developmental Editor: Maureen Iannuzzi
Manufacturing Manager: Timothy Reynolds
Production Manager: Jodi Borgenicht
Production Editor: Karen G. Edmonson
Indexer: Nancy Newman
Compositor: Maryland Composition

© 1999, by Lippincott Williams & Wilkins. All rights reserved. This book is protected by copyright. No part of it may be reproduced, stored in a retrieval system, or transmitted, in any form or by any means—electronic, mechanical, photocopy, recording, or otherwise—without the prior written consent of the publisher, except for brief quotations embodied in critical articles and reviews. For information write **Lippincott Williams & Wilkins, 227 East Washington Square, Philadelphia, PA 19106-3780.**
Materials appearing in this book prepared by individuals as part of their official duties as U.S. Government employees are not covered by the above-mentioned copyright.

Printed and bound in China

9 8 7 6 5 4 3 2

Library of Congress Cataloging-in-Publication Data

Diagnostic surgical pathology /   editor, Stephen S. Sternberg :
   Associate editors, Donald A. Antonioli . . . [et al.]. — 3rd ed.
      p.   cm.
   Includes bibliographical references and index.
   ISBN 0-397-58792-9 (set)
   1. Pathology, Surgical.   I. Sternberg, Stephen S.
   [DNLM: 1. Pathology, Surgical.   2. Diagnostic Techniques,
Surgical.   WO 142 D536 1999]
   RD57.D53   1999
   617'.075—dc21
   DNLM/DLC
   for Library of Congress   98-49375
                                                  CIP

Care has been taken to confirm the accuracy of the information presented and to describe generally accepted practices. However, the authors, editors, and publisher are not responsible for errors or omissions or for any consequences from application of the information in this book and make no warranty, expressed or implied, with respect to the contents of the publication.

The authors, editors, and publisher have exerted every effort to ensure that drug selection and dosage set forth in this text are in accordance with current recommendations and practice at the time of publication. However, in view of ongoing research, changes in government regulations, and the constant flow of information relating to drug therapy and drug reactions, the reader is urged to check the package insert for each drug for any change in indications and dosage and for added warnings and precautions. This is particularly important when the recommended agent is a new or infrequently employed drug.

Some drugs and medical devices presented in this publication have Food and Drug Administration (FDA) clearance for limited use in restricted research settings. It is the responsibility of the health care provider to ascertain the FDA status of each drug or device planned for use in their clinical practice.

Contents

Contributing Authors ix
Preface to the First Edition xvii
Preface xix

VOLUME 1

I. Skin, Soft Tissue, Bone, and Joints

1. Nonneoplastic Diseases of the Skin 3
   Hemella L. Sweatt, William J. Hardman III, and Alvin R. Solomon

2. Nonmelanocytic Cutaneous Tumors 49
   Daniel J. Santa Cruz and Mark A. Hurt

3. Melanocytic Lesions 89
   Michael J. Imber and Martin C. Mihm, Jr.

4. Muscle Biopsy in Neuromuscular Diseases 109
   Reid R. Heffner, Jr.

5. Disorders of Soft Tissue 131
   John S. J. Brooks

6. Joint Diseases 223
   Peter G. Bullough

7. Nonneoplastic Disease of Bone 243
   Peter G. Bullough

8. Bone Tumors 263
   Carrie Y. Inwards and K. Krishnan Unni

II. Breast

9. The Breast 319
   Andrew M. Hanby, Rosemary R. Millis, and Harold A. Oberman

III. Central Nervous System

10. The Brain, Spinal Cord, and Meninges 389
    Paul E. McKeever

IV. Endocrine System

11. The Neuroendocrine and Paracrine Systems 483
    Ricardo V. Lloyd

12. The Pituitary and Sellar Region 495
    Bernd W. Scheithauer

13. Thyroid Disease 529
    Virginia A. LiVolsi, Kathleen T. Montone, and Martha Sack

14. The Adrenal Glands 589
    Ronald A. DeLellis

15. Paragangliomas 625
    Ernest E. Lack

V. Hematopoietic and Lymphatic Systems

16. Disorders of Bone Marrow 651
    Robert W. McKenna, Russell L. Maiese, and Steven H. Kroft

17. The Lymph Nodes 709
    John B. Cousar, Terence T. Casey, William R. Macon,
    Thomas L. McCurley, and Steven H. Swerdlow

18. The Spleen 779
    Jerome S. Burke

VI. Head and Neck

19. The Jaws and Oral Cavity 805
    Kenneth D. McClatchey and Richard J. Zarbo

20. The Salivary Glands 853
    Andrew G. Huvos and Augusto F. G. Paulino

21. The Nose, Paranasal Sinuses, and Nasopharynx 885
    Stacey E. Mills and Robert E. Fechner

22. The Larynx 925
    John A. Kirchner and Darryl Carter

23. The Ear 949
    Leslie Michaels

24. The Eye and Ocular Adnexa 975
    Gordon K. Klintworth and Mark W. Scroggs

VII. Intra-Thoracic Organs and Blood Vessels

25. Nonneoplastic Pulmonary Disease 1011
    Arthur S. Patchefsky

26. Pulmonary Neoplasms 1069
    Yukio Shimosato

27. The Pleura 1117
    Hector Battifora

28. The Mediastinum 1147
    Mark R. Wick

29. The Heart 1209
    H. Thomas Aretz

30. Blood Vessels 1253
    Patrick J. Gallagher

VOLUME 2

VIII. Alimentary Canal and Associated Organs

31. The Esophagus 1283
Randall G. Lee

32. The Stomach 1311
David A. Owen

33. Nonneoplastic Intestinal Diseases 1349
Robert E. Petras

34. Intestinal Neoplasms 1413
Harry S. Cooper

35. The Pancreas 1469
James E. Oertel, Yolanda C. Oertel, and Clara S. Heffess

36. Nonneoplastic Liver Disease 1509
Dale C. Snover

37. Masses of the Liver 1553
Scott H. Saul

38. The Gallbladder and Extrahepatic Biliary Tree 1629
Scott H. Saul

39. The Anus and Perianal Area 1671
Donald A. Antonioli and Henry D. Appelman

IX. Urinary Tract and Male Genital System

40. Developmental Abnormalities of the Kidney 1685
Jay Bernstein and Enid Gilbert-Barness

41. Nonneoplastic Adult Renal Diseases 1701
Tibor Nadasdy and Fred G. Silva

42. Adult Renal Tumors 1785
Victor Reuter and Paul B. Gaudin

43. Renal Neoplasms of Childhood 1825
J. Bruce Beckwith

44. The Urothelial Tract 1853
Victor E. Reuter and Myron R. Melamed

45. The Prostate and Seminal Vesicles 1893
Jonathan I. Epstein and Kirk J. Wojno

46. Nonneoplastic Diseases of the Testis 1943
Howard S. Levin

47. Testicular and Paratesticular Tumors 1973
Thomas M. Ulbright and Lawrence M. Roth

48. The Penis 2035
Antonio L. Cubilla, Jose E. Barreto, and Gustavo Ayala

X. Female Reproductive System and Peritoneum

49. Gestational Trophoblastic Disease 2067
Ie-Ming Shih, Michael T. Mazur, and Robert J. Kurman

50. The Placenta 2087
Geoffrey Altshuler

51. The Vulva and Vagina 2111
Henry F. Frierson, Jr. and Stacey E. Mills

52. The Cervix 2155
Christopher P. Crum, Gerard J. Nuovo, and Kenneth R. Lee

53. The Uterine Corpus 2203
Michael R. Hendrickson, Teri A. Longacre, and Richard L. Kempson

54. The Ovary 2307
Robert H. Young, Philip B. Clement, and Robert E. Scully

55. The Fallopian Tube and Broad Ligament 2395
Robert H. Young, Robert E. Scully, and Philip B. Clement

56. The Peritoneum 2415
Philip B. Clement, Robert H. Young, and Robert E. Scully

Subject Index I-1

Contributing Authors

Geoffrey Altshuler, M.D.
Clinical Professor
Department of Pathology and Pediatrics
University of Oklahoma
Oklahoma City, Oklahoma
Staff Pathologist
Department of Pathology
Children's Hospital of Oklahoma
940 Northeast 13th Street
Oklahoma City, Oklahoma 73104

Donald A. Antonioli, M.D.
Professor of Pathology
Harvard Medical School
Senior Pathologist
Department of Pathology
Beth Israel Deaconess Medical Center
330 Brookline Avenue
Boston, Massachusetts 02215

Henry D. Appelman, M.D.
Professor of Pathology
Department of Pathology
University of Michigan Hospital
1500 E. Medical Center Drive
Ann Arbor, Michigan 48109-0054

H. Thomas Aretz, M.D.
Associate Professor of Pathology
Harvard Medical School
Director, Cardiovascular Pathology
Massachusetts General Hospital
55 Fruit Street
Boston, Massachusetts 02114-2696

Gustavo Ayala, M.D.
Assistant Professor
Department of Pathology
Baylor College of Medicine
Houston, Texas 77000

Enid Gilbert-Barness, M.D.
Professor
Departments of Pathology, Pediatrics and Obstetrics-Gynecology
Director of Pediatric Pathology
Tampa General Hospital
P.O. Box 1289
Tampa, Florida 33601

Jose E. Barreto, M.D.
Professor
Department of Pathology
Universidad Católica
Villarica, Paraguay
Chairman
Department of Pathology
Hospital del Cancer
Capiatá, Paraguay

Hector Battifora, M.D.
Clinical Professor
Department of Pathology
University of Southern California
Los Angeles, California
Medical Director
Pacific Coast Reference Laboratories
11215 Knott Avenue
Cypress, California 90630

J. Bruce Beckwith, M.D.
Professor
Department of Pathology and Human Anatomy
Loma Linda University
AH 327
Loma Linda, California 92354

Jay Bernstein, M.D.
Clinical Professor
Department of Pathology
Wayne State University School of Medicine
Detroit, Michigan
Associate Medical Director for Research
Research Institute
William Beaumont Hospital
3601 West Thirteenth Mile Road
Royal Oak, Michigan 48073

Mila Blaivas, M.D., Ph.D.
Clinical Assistant Professor
Department of Pathology
University of Michigan Medical Center
1301 Catherine Road
Ann Arbor, Michigan 48109

John S. J. Brooks, M.D.
Professor and Vice Chairman
Department of Pathology
State University of New York at Buffalo
Buffalo, New York
Chairman and Professor
Department of Pathology and Laboratory
 Medicine
Roswell Park Cancer Institute
Elm and Carlton Streets
Buffalo, New York 14263

Peter G. Bullough, M.B., Ch.B.
Professor of Pathology
Cornell University Medical College
Director of Laboratory Medicine
The Hospital for Special Surgery
535 East 70th Street
New York, New York 10021

Jerome S. Burke, M.D.
Director of Anatomic Pathology
Department of Pathology
Alta Bates Medical Center
2450 Ashby Avenue
Berkeley, California 94705
Clinical Professor
Department of Pathology
Stanford University Medical Center
Stanford, California 94305

Darryl Carter, M.D.
Professor of Pathology
Department of Pathology
Yale University School of Medicine
333 Cedar Street
New Haven, Connecticut 06520

Terence T. Casey, M.D.
Attending Staff
Associated Pathologists, PLC
Columbia Centennial Medical Center
2300 Patterson Street
Nashville, Tennessee 37203

Philip Clement, M.D.
Professor
Department of Pathology
University of British Columbia
Consultant Pathologist
Department of Anatomic Pathology
Vancouver General Hospital
910 West 10th Avenue
Vancouver, British Columbia V5Z 1M9
Canada

Harry S. Cooper, M.D.
Senior Member and Director of Clinical
 Laboratories
Department of Pathology
Fox Chase Cancer Center
7701 Burholme Avenue
Philadelphia, Pennsylvania 19111

John B. Cousar, M.D.
Professor and Vice-Chairman
Director of Hematopathology
Department of Pathology
Vanderbilt University Medical Center
1161 21st Avenue South
Nashville, Tennessee 37232

Christopher P. Crum, M.D.
Professor of Pathology
Harvard Medical School
Director, Women's and Perinatal Pathology
Brigham & Women's Hospital
75 Francis Street
Boston, Massachusetts 02115

Antonio L. Cubilla, M.D.
Director
Instituto de Patología e Investigación
Martín Brizuela 323 c/Ayala Velazquez
Asunción, Paraguay
Professor
Catedra de Anatomia Patologica
Instituto de Anatomia Patologica
Facultad de Ciencias Medicas
Asuncion, Paraguay

Ronald A. DeLellis, M.D.
Professor
Department of Pathology
Joan and Sanford I. Weill Medical College of
 Cornell University
Vice Chairman for Anatomic Pathology
Department of Pathology
The New York Presbyterian Hospital
525 East 68th Street
New York, New York 10021

Jonathan I. Epstein, M.D.
Professor
Departments of Pathology, Urology, and Oncology
Associate Director of Surgical Pathology
Department of Pathology
The Johns Hopkins Hospital
600 North Wolfe Street
Baltimore, Maryland 21287

Robert E. Fechner, M.D.
Professor
Department of Pathology
University of Virginia Health Sciences Center
Box 214
Charlottesville, Virginia 22908

Henry F. Frierson, Jr., M.D.
Professor of Pathology
Department of Pathology
University of Virginia Health Sciences Center
Box 214
Charlottesville, Virginia 22908

Patrick J. Gallagher, M.D., Ph.D.
Reader in Pathology,
University of Southhampton and
Consultant Pathologist
Department of Pathology
Southampton University Hospitals
Southampton, S016 6YD
England

Paul B. Gaudin, M.D.
Assistant Attending Pathologist
Memorial Sloan-Kettering Cancer Center
Assistant Professor of Pathology
Cornell University Medical College
1275 York Avenue
New York, New York 10021

Andrew M. Hanby, B.M.
Senior Lecturer and Honorary Consultant
Hedley Atkins/Imperial Cancer Research Fund
  Breast Pathology Laboratory
GKT School of Medicine and Dentistry
King's College and Guy's Hospital Campus
St. Thomas Street
London SE1 9RT
England

William J. Hardman III, M.D.
Clinical Assistant Professor
Department of Dermatology
Emory University School of Medicine
Atlanta, Georgia
Department of Pathology
St. Mary's Hospital
1230 Baxter Street
Athens, Georgia 30606

Clara S. Heffess, M.D.
Chief, Endocrine Division
Department of Endocrine and Otorhinolaryngic-
  Head and Neck Pathology
Armed Forces Institute of Pathology
Washington, District of Columbia
9112 Falls Bridge Lane
Potomac, Maryland 20854

Reid R. Heffner, Jr., M.D.
Chairman
Department of Pathology
State University of New York at Buffalo
  School of Medicine
Farber Hall
3435 Main Street
Buffalo, New York 14214-3000

Michael R. Hendrickson, M.D.
Professor
Co-Director of Surgical Pathology
Department of Pathology
Stanford Health Services
300 Pasteur Drive
Stanford, California 94305

Mark A. Hurt, M.D.
Associate Dermatopathologist
Department of Cutaneous Pathology
American Pathology Resources
2320 Schuetz Road
St. Louis, Missouri 63146

Andrew G. Huvos, M.D.
Professor of Pathology
Cornell University Medical College
Attending Pathologist
Department of Pathology
Memorial Sloan-Kettering Cancer Center
1275 York Avenue
New York, New York 10021

Michael J. Imber, M.D., Ph.D.
Director
Dermatopathology Services
Palm Beach Pathology
2013 Ponce de Leon Avenue
West Palm Beach, Florida 33407

Carrie Y. Inwards, M.D.
Assistant Professor of Pathology
Mayo Medical School
Consultant
Division of Anatomic Pathology
Mayo Clinic and Mayo Foundation
200 First Street, Southwest
Rochester, Minnesota 55905

Richard L. Kempson, M.D.
Professor
Department of Pathology
Stanford Health Services
300 Pasteur Drive
Stanford, California 94305

John A. Kirchner, M.D.
Honorary Staff
Department of Surgery (Otolaryngology)
Yale-New Haven Hospital
Professor Emeritus, Otolaryngology
Department of Surgery (Otolaryngology)
Yale University School of Medicine
333 Cedar Street
New Haven, Connecticut 06520

Gordon K. Klintworth, M.D., Ph.D.
Professor of Pathology
Joseph A.C. Wadsworth Research Professor of Ophthalmology
Duke University Medical Center
Durham, North Carolina 27710

Steven H. Kroft, M.D.
Medical Director
Hematology Laboratory
Department of Pathology
Parkland Memorial Hospital
Assistant Professor of Pathology
University of Texas Southwestern Medical Center
5323 Harry Hines Boulevard
Dallas, Texas 75235

Robert J. Kurman, M.D.
Professor
Departments of Pathology and Gynecology
Johns Hopkins Hospital
600 North Wolfe Street
Baltimore, Maryland 21212

Ernest E. Lack, M.D.
Professor and Director of Anatomic Pathology
Department of Pathology
Georgetown University School of Medicine
3900 Reservoir Road, Northwest
Washington, District of Columbia 20007

Kenneth R. Lee, M.D.
Associate Professor of Pathology
Harvard Medical School
Pathologist
Divisions of Cytology and Pathology
Brigham & Women's Hospital
75 Francis Street
Boston, Massachusetts 02115

Randall G. Lee, M.D.
Director
Department of Pathology
Providence Portland Medical Center
4805 Northeast Glisan Street
Portland, Oregon 97213-2970

Howard S. Levin, M.D.
Staff Pathologist
Department of Anatomic Pathology
The Cleveland Clinic Foundation
9500 Euclid Avenue
Cleveland, Ohio 44195

Virginia A. LiVolsi, M.D.
Professor
Department of Pathology and Laboratory Medicine
Vice Chair
Department of Anatomic Pathology
Hospital of the University of Pennsylvania
3400 Spruce Street
Philadelphia, Pennsylvania 19104

Ricardo V. Lloyd, M.D.
Professor and Consultant
Departments of Laboratory Medicine and Pathology
Mayo Foundation and Mayo Clinic
200 First Street, Southwest
Rochester, Minnesota 55905

Teri A. Longacre, M.D.
Associate Professor of Pathology
Department of Surgical Pathology
Stanford Health Services
300 Pasteur Drive
Stanford, California 94304

William R. Macon, M.D.
Associate Professor
Department of Pathology
Vanderbilt University Medical Center
11621 21st Avenue South
Nashville, Tennessee 37232

Russell L. Maiese, M.D.
Staff Pathologist
Division of Hematopathology
Dianon Systems, Inc.
200 Watson Boulevard
Stratford, Connecticut 06497

Michael T. Mazur, M.D.
Clinical Professor of Pathology
Department of Pathology
Crouse Irving Memorial Hospital
736 Irving Avenue
Syracuse, New York 13210

Kenneth D. McClatchey, D.D.S., M.D.
Director of Clinical Laboratories
Department of Pathology
Foster G. McGaw Hospital
Professor and Chairman of Pathology
Department of Pathology
Helen M. & Raymond M. Galvin Professor
Loyola University Medical Center
2160 South First Avenue
Maywood, Illinois 60153

Thomas L. McCurley, M.D.
Associate Professor and Director of
  Immunopathology
Department of Pathology
Vanderbilt University Medical Center
1161 21st Avenue South
Nashville, Tennessee 37232

Paul E. McKeever, M.D., Ph.D.
Chief, Section of Neuropathology
University of Michigan Medical School
Associate Professor
Department of Pathology
The University of Michigan
1301 Catherine Road, Box 0602
Ann Arbor, Michigan 48109

Robert W. McKenna, M.D.
Professor
Department of Pathology
University of Texas Southwestern Medical Center
5323 Harry Hines Boulevard
Dallas, Texas 75235

Myron R. Melamed, M.D.
Professor and Chairman
Department of Pathology
New York Medical College
Valhalla, New York 10595

Leslie Michaels, M.D.
Consultant Pathologist
Department of Pathology
Royal National Throat, Nose, and Ear Hospital
Professor Emeritus
Department of Histopathology
University College London Medical School
University Street
London WC1E 6JJ
England

Martin C. Mihm, Jr., M.D.
Senior Dermatopathologist
Departments of Pathology and Dermatology
Massachusetts General Hospital
Clinical Professor
Department of Pathology
Harvard Medical School
25 Shattuck Street
Boston, Massachusetts 02115

Rosemary R. Millis, M.B., B.S.
Honorary Consultant Histopathologist
Hedley Atkins/Imperial Cancer Research Fund
  Breast Pathology Laboratory
Guy's Hospital
Third Floor Thomas Guy House
St. Thomas Street
London SEI 9RT
England

Stacey E. Mills, M.D.
Professor and Associate Chair
Department of Pathology
University of Virginia Medical Center
Jefferson Park Avenue
Charlottesville, Virginia 22908

Kathleen T. Montone, M.D.
Physician Pathologist
Department of Pathology
Abington Memorial Hospital
1200 Old York Road
Abington, Pennsylvania 19001

Tibor Nadasdy, M.D.
Assistant Professor
Department of Pathology
The Johns Hopkins Hospital
720 Rutland Avenue
Baltimore, Maryland 21205

Gerard J. Nuovo, M.D.
Director
MGN Medical Research Laboratories
Setauket, New York
Pathologist
Enzo Clinical Laboratories
60 Executive Boulevard
Farmingdale, New York 11735

Harold A. Oberman, M.D.
Professor
Department of Pathology
University of Michigan Health Sciences Center
1500 East Medical Center Drive
Ann Arbor, Michigan 48109

James E. Oertel, M.D.
Chairman Emeritus
Department of Endocrine Pathology
Armed Forces Institute of Pathology
Washington, District of Columbia 20306

Yolanda C. Oertel, M.D.
Professor Emerita
Department of Pathology
George Washington University Medical Center
Staff Pathologist
Department of Pathology
Washington Hospital Center
110 Irving Street, Northwest
Washington, District of Columbia 20010

David A. Owen, M.B., B.Ch.
Professor
Department of Pathology and Laboratory
  Medicine
University of British Columbia
Vancouver, British Columbia, Canada
Consultant Pathologist
Department of Pathology
Vancouver General Hospital
855 West 12th Avenue
Vancouver, British Columbia V5Z 1M9
Canada

Arthur S. Patchefsky, M.D.
Chairman and Senior Member
Department of Pathology
Fox Chase Cancer Center
7701 Burholme Avenue
Philadelphia, Pennsylvania 19111

Augusto F. G. Paulino, M.D.
Assistant Professor
Department of Pathology
University of Michigan Hospitals
1500 E. Medical Center Drive
Ann Arbor, Michigan 48109-0054

Robert E. Petras, M.D.
Chairman
Department of Anatomic Pathology
Cleveland Clinic Foundation
9500 Euclid Avenue, L25
Cleveland, Ohio 44195

Victor E. Reuter, M.D.
Associate Professor of Pathology
Cornell University Medical College
Attending Pathologist
Department of Pathology
Memorial Sloan-Kettering Cancer Center
1275 York Avenue
New York, New York 10021

Lawrence M. Roth, M.D.
Professor of Pathology
Director of Surgical Pathology
Indiana University School of Medicine
Indiana University Hospital
550 North University Boulevard
Indianapolis, Indiana 46202

Martha J. Sack, M.D.
Assistant Physician
Department of Pathology
Abington Memorial Hospital
1200 Old York Road
Abington, Pennsylvania 19001

Daniel J. Santa Cruz, M.D.
Associate Professor (Visiting Staff)
Department of Pathology
Washington University School of Medicine
Department of Cutaneous Pathology
American Pathology Resources
2320 Schuetz Road
St. Louis, Missouri 63146

Scott H. Saul, M.D.
Adjunct Associate Professor
Department of Pathology and Laboratory
  Medicine
University of Pennsylvania School of Medicine
34th and Spruce Streets
Philadelphia, Pennsylvania
Director, Surgical Pathology
Department of Pathology
Chester County Hospital
701 East Marshall Street
West Chester, Pennsylvania 19380

Bernd W. Scheithauer, M.D.
Professor
Department of Anatomic Pathology
Mayo Medical Center
200 First Street, Southwest
Rochester, Minnesota 55905

Mark W. Scroggs, M.D.
Washington Eye Clinic
211 North Market Street
Washington, North Carolina 27889

Robert E. Scully, M.D.
Professor Emeritus
Department of Pathology
Massachusetts General Hospital
Harvard Medical School
32 Fruit Street
Boston, Massachusetts 02114

Ie-Ming Shih, M.D., Ph.D.
*Fellow
Department of Pathology
Johns Hopkins University School of Medicine
Clinical Fellow
Department of Pathology
The Johns Hopkins Hospital
600 North Wolfe Street
Baltimore, Maryland 21287-6917*

Yukio Shimosato, M.D.
*Former Chief
Clinical Laboratory Division
National Cancer Center Hospital
Tokyo, Japan
Visiting Professor
Department of Pathology
Keio University School of Medicine
35 Shinanomachi
Shinjukuku, Tokyo 160
Japan*

Fred G. Silva, M.D.
*Lloyd E. Rader Professor and Chairman
Department of Pathology
University of Oklahoma Health Sciences Center
940 Stanton L. Young Boulevard
Oklahoma City, Oklahoma 73104*

Dale C. Snover, M.D.
*Pathologist
Department of Pathology
Fairview Southdale Hospital
Clinical Professor
Department of Laboratory Medicine and Pathology
University of Minnesota Medical School
420 Delaware Street, Southwest
Minneapolis, Minnesota 55455*

Alvin R. Solomon, M.D.
*Director of Dermatopathology
Departments of Dermatology and Pathology
Emory University Hospital and Emory Clinic
Professor
Departments of Dermatology and Pathology
Emory University School of Medicine
5001 WMB, Box SS
Atlanta, Georgia 30322*

Stephen S. Sternberg, M.D.
*Attending Pathologist
Memorial Sloan-Kettering Cancer Center
1275 York Avenue
New York, New York 10021*

Hemella L. Sweatt, M.D.
*The Richfield Laboratory of Dermatopathology
Ameripath Incorporated
9670 Kennwood Road
Cincinnati, Ohio 45242*

Steven H. Swerdlow, M.D.
*Director of Hematopathology
Department of Pathology
UPMC–Presbyterian Hospital
Pittsburgh, Pennsylvania
Professor
Department of Pathology
University of Pittsburgh School of Medicine
Montefiore University Hospital
200 Lothrop Street
Pittsburgh, Pennsylvania 15213*

Thomas M. Ulbright, M.D.
*Professor of Pathology
Department of Pathology and Laboratory
 Medicine
Indiana University School of Medicine
Director of Anatomic Pathology
Department of Pathology and Laboratory
 Medicine
Indiana University Hospital
550 North University Boulevard
Indianapolis, Indiana 46202*

K. Krishnan Unni, M.B., B.S.
*Consultant
Section of Surgical Pathology
Department of Pathology
Mayo Clinic
200 First Street, Southwest
Rochester, Minnesota 55905*

Mark R. Wick, M.D.
*Director of Surgical Pathology
Department of Pathology
Barnes-Jewish Hospital
Professor
Department of Pathology
Washington University Medical Center
One Barnes Hospital Plaza
Peters Building, Suite 300
St. Louis, Missouri 63110*

Kirk J. Wojno, M.D.
*Associate Pathologist
Department of Pathology
St. John's Hospital and Medical Center
22101 Moross Road
Detroit, Michigan 48236*

Robert H. Young, M.D.
Professor
Department of Pathology
Massachusetts General Hospital
Harvard Medical School
32 Fruit Street
Boston, Massachusetts 02114

Richard J. Zarbo, M.D., D.M.D.
Vice Chairman and Director of Surgical Pathology
Henry Ford Hospital
Professor of Pathology
Henry Ford Health System/Case Western Reserve University
2799 West Grand Boulevard
Detroit, Michigan 48202

Preface to the First Edition

We speak of the loneliness of the long-distance runner, but there may be no one lonelier than a surgical pathologist working solo. Those working in large hospitals have the luxury of being able to consult ad lib with one or more pathologists about a given case, and may even have an associate who is a specialist in the area of difficulty. Easy access to consultation is a prerequisite for accurate diagnosis, and, accordingly, for optimal patient care. It is especially critical in those instances when the busy pathologist has a low level of diagnostic doubt, but this is tempered by the need to sign out the case without consultation because of the press of time. Very difficult cases, those readily recognizable as problem cases, are in a sense less troublesome, as the need for a diagnostic consultation is self-evident. Therefore, knowing when and what one doesn't know is of singular importance.

A pathology reference library is the other information source for the working pathologist. Textbook consultation and human consultation go hand-in-hand. In this text we have attempted to emphasize differential diagnosis of the surgical specimen, and to keep to a minimum discussion of the natural history of disease, treatment and autopsy findings. Although no textbook can take the place of a face-to-face discussion of a diagnostic problem (especially over a multi-headed microscope) between two or more pathologists, we have asked our authors to provide the reader with their reasoning in approaching differential evaluation of a biopsy specimen, thereby giving the flavor of a personal consultation. Moreover, the authors for the various chapters have been chosen based not only upon their recognized knowledge of the specific area, but also upon their skill in written communication. Since surgical pathologic diagnosis is a visual exercise, the book is generously illustrated with color and black-and-white photographs. In addition, the chapter authors have been liberal in their use of references, thereby enhancing the value of their presentations for the reader who wishes additional information.

The Section Editors have worked closely with the chapter authors to ensure that the objectives of the text are met; namely, that it is a treatise on the diagnosis of conditions which confront the surgical pathologist. In summary, the goal of the Editors is that this book will be a working companion, and thereby be accorded a place adjacent to the microscope of the reader.

Stephen S. Sternberg
Donald A. Antonioli
Darryl Carter
Joseph C. Eggleston
Stacey E. Mills
Harold A. Oberman

Preface

In reviewing the preface to the Second Edition of *Diagnostic Surgical Pathology* (as good editors should), we discovered that we could (rhetorically, of course) repeat the first paragraph of that preface for this Third Edition and remain quite modern. We noted then that, "pathologists are inundated by ever increasing immunologic stains for lymphocytes, leading to new ways to classify lymphomas and, of course, raising questions about where to put the 'nouveau riche' lymphomas, if indeed they belong in a separate category." In the intervening years, of course, new lymphomas have continued to be described at a feverish pace.

Progress in pathology is also reflected by the startling advances in immunohistochemistry and molecular biology. In fact, new journals have appeared to cover both these highly active subjects, and existing journals have expanded to include this subject matter. Our authors have updated and rewritten much of the content of *Diagnostic Surgical Pathology* to reflect these advances.

Nevertheless, let us not forget that the basis for all diagnostic surgical pathology remains to be paraffin sections and hematoxylin and eosin stains—they are the cornerstones of our profession. Therefore, we continue to stress the importance of routine light microscopy in daily practice. Our authors have succeeded in presenting to the reader the latest information on both old and new entities for all organ systems. We trust that the reader will find the Third Edition to be an even more valuable diagnostic tool than the two previous editions.

Among the many new additions is the REAL classification of the lymphomas with a review of the equivalents according to earlier classifications. In addition, there is an introduction to the proposed WHO classification of lymphoma. There is an update of gut lymphomas, as well as an expanded discussion of cutaneous lymphomas. The new classification of papillary urothelial neoplasms has been added based on a meeting of the International Society of Urological Pathology. Newer aspects of kidney tumors are also represented in a new classification.

Other gastrointestinal topics include details of gastric and other intestinal tract stromal tumors, and, especially noteworthy, the relation of these tumors to the interstitial cells of Cajal. A major new addition to the non-neoplastic intestinal chapter is the discussion of inflammatory lesions of the mesentery and retroperitoneum.

In the breast chapter, among many other items, there is an updated discussion of ductal carcinoma *in situ*. The sections on medullary carcinoma and cystosarcomas are also expanded. Newer techniques in handling breast specimens, as well as prognostic markers are summarized. In the genitourinary area, the updated classifications are presented, both for the kidney and the urinary bladder. In the non-neoplastic kidney chapter there are greatly expanded discussions of glomerulonephritis, basement membrane abnormalities, and Alport's syndrome. In the Wilm's tumor area, there is an added discussion on focal and diffuse anaplasia and, of course, the latest on PMET's. The recent advances in regard to prostate cancer, in particular the early stage of the disease, are well presented.

In the thoracic section, the latest on immunohistochemical differentiation of pleural lesions is presented, which should be of great practical value. There is now a better understanding of the testicular germ cell tumors and their response to chemotherapy. A complete update on the status of intersex problems, reflected by the advances in clinical cytogenetics, has been added.

The almost exclusive use of color photography has greatly enhanced most chapters. This is most notably reflected in the chapters on neoplastic and non-neoplastic pulmonary disease and salivary gland lesions. Finally, the list of references for most of the chapters has been divided by subject matter to facilitate use.

Stephen S. Sternberg
Donald A. Antonioli
Darryl Carter
Stacey E. Mills
Harold A. Oberman

Diagnostic Surgical Pathology

Third Edition

VIII
Alimentary Canal and Associated Organs

CHAPTER 31

Esophagus

Randall G. Lee

NORMAL FEATURES

Anatomy

The esophagus is among the simplest of organs: a hollow muscular conduit lacking significant secretory or absorptive function that serves to connect the pharynx and stomach. Beginning at the cricopharyngeus muscle, it extends through the posterior mediastinum, passing the trachea, left main bronchus, aorta, and left atrium en route, and terminates at the gastric cardia a few centimeters beneath the diaphragm. The total length varies with the height of the individual, but averages about 25 cm in adults. By the common endoscopic method of mensuration, this corresponds to an esophagus beginning at 15 to 18 cm from the incisor teeth and extending to approximately 40 cm (range 30 to 43 cm) (1,2).

The arterial blood supply derives from several primary sources. The cervical esophagus is supplied primarily by the inferior thyroid artery; the upper thoracic esophagus by the bronchial and intercostal arteries; the lower thoracic esophagus by branches directly from the aorta; and the abdominal esophagus by left gastric and inferior phrenic arteries. Numerous anastomoses connect the various arterial supplies. The venous drainage forms an extensive submucosal plexus that communicates with longitudinally oriented periesophageal veins and eventually flows into the inferior thyroid, azygos, and gastric veins. In this manner, the caval and portal venous systems are connected, so that portal hypertension can result in the development of esophageal varices.

The esophagus is also richly endowed with lymphatic vessels that form freely anastomosing networks within the submucosa and with connecting longitudinal channels in the muscularis propria. Lymphatic flow thus tends to run longitudinally, coursing cephalad in the upper two-thirds and caudad in the lower third of the esophagus, an arrangement that facilitates length-wise intramural tumor dissemination. The cervical esophagus eventually drains primarily into the internal jugular and paratracheal nodes; the thoracic esophagus into the mediastinal and bronchial nodes; and the abdominal esophagus into a variety of subdiaphragmatic nodes. Because of the plentiful lymphatic interconnections, however, esophageal carcinomas can show widely and unpredictably distributed nodal metastases.

Histology

Similar to the rest of the gastrointestinal tract, the esophagus is assembled from four microscopic layers: mucosa, submucosa, muscularis propria, and serosa.

The mucosa comprises nonkeratinizing stratified squamous epithelium, a supporting lamina propria, and a thick, longitudinally oriented band of muscularis mucosae. The epithelium, in turn, is formed by two basic zones (Fig. 1). The basal zone consists of a three-cell thick proliferative layer of basophilic cells with little cytoplasm. Normally this zone occupies less than 15% of the epithelial thickness, although it may be slightly thicker in the distal 2 to 3 cm of the esophagus, perhaps reflecting the transient episodes of gastroesophageal reflux that occur in most healthy people. Overlying the basal zone is a superficial layer of maturing glycogen-rich squamous cells that progressively flatten as they mature and approach the lumen. Scattered within the epithelium are melanocytes, endocrine cells, T lymphocytes (which may have irregularly shaped nuclei and be mistaken for neutrophils), and Langerhans cells (3).

The underlying lamina propria consists of fibrovascular tissue folded into slender papillae that project into the epithelium. These papillae generally extend to less than two-thirds of the epithelial thickness, except in the distal 2 to 3 cm of the esophagus where mild elongation may normally be found. The lamina propria contains capillaries, lymphatic vessels, elastic fibers, and scattered mononuclear cells and lymphoid aggregates; these should not be interpreted as evidence of esophagitis. Indigenous mucus-secreting glands known as "cardiac or superficial glands" are also found

---

R. G. Lee: Department of Pathology and Nuclear Medicine, Providence Portland Medical Center, Portland, Oregon 97213-2970.

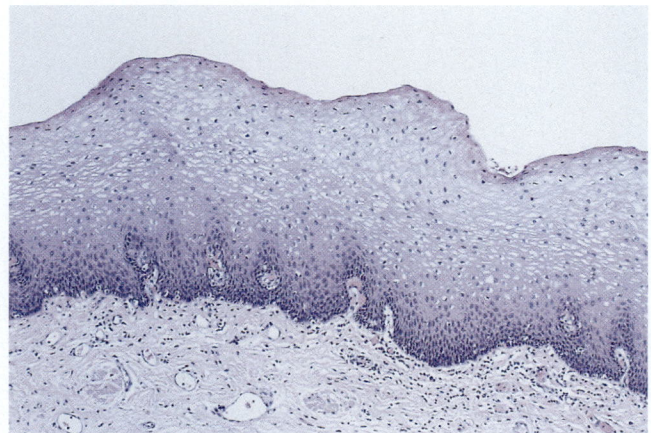

FIG. 1. Normal esophageal mucosa with a thin basal epithelial zone and lamina propria papillae that, in this field, are less than about 20% of the total epithelial thickness.

within the lamina propria, particularly along the distal esophagus. These glands, which produce neutral mucins, resemble the mucous glands of the stomach and may contain a few parietal or chief cells.

The junction between squamous and columnar mucosa in the distal esophagus is often referred to as the "Z-line or ora serrata" because of its irregular, serrated profile. This junction does not necessarily coincide with the anatomic gastroesophageal junction (the site at which the tubular esophagus joins the saccular stomach) but is instead typically located up to 2 to 3 cm proximally, within the region of the lower esophageal sphincter (4). Consequently, the distal-most few centimeters of the esophagus can be normally lined by gastric-type cardiac or fundic mucosa. Some investigators suggest that this native esophageal columnar mucosa is, in fact, a metaplastic response to gastroesophageal reflux (4,5), and it thus may be analogous to the basal zone hyperplasia and elongation of lamina propria papillae that also commonly occur in the lower esophagus. Foci of pancreatic acinar tissue can also be seen in the area of the gastroesophageal junction, although this represents an incidental, presumably congenital, occurrence without clinical significance (6).

The submucosa is represented by a wide layer of loose connective tissue bearing blood vessels, lymphatics, nerve fibers, and scattered lymphocytes and lymphoid aggregates. In addition, there is a population of tubuloalveolar mucous glands that are dispersed throughout the esophagus. These submucosal glands, which secrete acidic mucins and are analogous to the minor salivary glands of the oropharynx, drain through cuboidal or squamous cell–lined ducts that obliquely penetrate the mucosa.

The muscularis propria is distinguished by a screw-like arrangement of both smooth and striated muscle fibers fashioned into inner circular and outer longitudinal layers. Striated muscle predominates in the uppermost esophagus, but it soon yields to smooth muscle, which alone forms the distal half of the musculature (2). Each end of the esophagus is demarcated by a sphincter. The upper esophageal sphincter is an anatomically distinct structure composed of fibers of the cricopharyngeus and inferior pharyngeal constrictor muscles. The lower esophageal sphincter, on the other hand, lacks a single anatomic counterpart and is instead formed from the intrinsic muscles of the distal esophagus, the sling fibers of the proximal stomach, and the crural diaphragm. Together these structures create a functional zone of increased intraluminal pressure (1). A serosal lining covers short segments of the thoracic and abdominal esophagus, but most of the organ is instead ensheathed by an adventitia of loose connective tissue.

SPECIMEN HANDLING

Surgical pathologists most often encounter the esophagus through mucosal biopsy specimens. The typical endoscopic biopsy is obtained with cupped cylindrical forceps that grasp and avulse a fragment of the mucosa. The resulting specimen, usually 1 to 5 mm in diameter, includes the epithelium with a variable amount of lamina propria and occasionally a slip of muscularis mucosae. In some situations, an aspiration technique may instead be used, yielding specimens that are larger and deeper, typically including part of the submucosa.

The biopsy specimens ideally should be mounted at the time of procurement by placing them, submucosal side down, on a supporting medium such as filter paper, nylon mesh, or Gelfoam, and then placing them immediately in fixative, thus facilitating proper orientation during embedding and sectioning. When mounting procedures are not available, the specimen can be promptly dropped unmounted into fixative, although the orientation may be less than optimal. Standard formalin fixation generally suffices, although picric acid fixatives or mercury-based fixatives are preferred by some pathologists. Multiple sections at several levels in the paraffin block are necessary because of the focal nature of many lesions; this can also help obviate the lack of precise orientation in unmounted specimens. Serial sectioning is not necessary or practical, but retaining extra sections from each level for possible special stains or other procedures can be helpful.

Esophagectomy specimens are best handled by opening longitudinally, preferably in the fresh state, and then pinning them flat and fixing overnight. Directed attention can then be given to the size, appearance, and anatomic relationships of any lesions, and appropriate blocks obtained to evaluate their nature and extent. The status of the resection margins, including the radial or adventitial margin deep to tumors, must be established, lymph nodes in the periesophageal adipose tissue should also be carefully searched for and submitted, and involvement of any adjacent structures should be documented.

The handling and reporting of esophageal biopsy and resection specimens have been comprehensively reviewed elsewhere (7–9).

ESOPHAGITIS

The most common diagnostic problems encountered with esophageal biopsy specimens involve the evaluation of esophagitis and its consequences. A general approach to examining these biopsies entails identifying the histologic features of esophagitis, searching for clues to the cause, and appraising possible complications.

In a broad sense, esophagitis is recognized by the presence of epithelial damage and inflammation. Although this recognition is straightforward when mucosal exudation, erosion, or ulceration is present, these findings denote more severe degrees of esophagitis. They can be absent in low-grade epithelial injury, including that caused by gastroesophageal reflux, so that attention also needs to be given to other less conspicuous indicators of epithelial injury and repair. The term *acute esophagitis* is often employed to indicate this spectrum of changes, but because it ambiguously carries both temporal and morphologic connotations, the term *active esophagitis* is employed here instead.

Esophagitis can be caused by diverse agents—physical, chemical, and biologic—but by far the most common culprit is gastroesophageal reflux, with infectious organisms holding a distant second place. The precise cause, however, may not be apparent from biopsy examination; correlation with clinical, radiologic, and endoscopic details is necessary before a final diagnosis can be rendered. Occasionally, however, the biopsy reveals features diagnostic or suggestive of a specific cause (Table 1). These findings should be carefully sought, particularly when warranted by a pertinent clinical setting.

Other reasons for examining esophageal specimens are to investigate the long-term consequences of persistent or recurrent esophagitis: fibrosis (with the possibility for stricture formation), chronic ulceration, Barrett's esophagus, and carcinoma.

Gastroesophageal Reflux Disease

Reflux of gastric contents into the esophagus is the preeminent cause of esophagitis. Although reflux episodes occur in normal individuals, abnormal gastroesophageal reflux can cause clinical and pathologic manifestations that are described under the generic label of gastroesophageal reflux disease (GERD). (The term *reflux esophagitis* is often used to specifically designate the GERD subgroup with histopathologic alterations.) Exactly how physiologic reflux becomes the pathologic process of GERD is incompletely understood, but numerous complex factors are likely involved, including the volume and potency of the refluxate, the duration of esophageal exposure, and the efficiency of esophageal defense mechanisms.

Epidemiologic studies suggest a 3% to 4% prevalence of GERD in the general population, with the preponderance of individuals having mild or moderate disease. There are four different approaches to establishing the diagnosis: reflux-related clinical symptoms (primarily heartburn and regurgitation), abnormal esophageal acid exposure (as measured by intraesophageal pH monitoring), mucosal sensitivity to acid (as assessed with the Bernstein acid infusion test), and mucosal damage (as determined by endoscopic and histologic examination). However, there is only a rough correspondence among these features: symptoms may occur without other positive diagnostic tests, and, conversely, abnormal endoscopic and pathologic findings may be found in asymptomatic patients (10,11). Consequently, there is no completely sensitive and specific gold standard for the diagnosis of GERD.

Endoscopic examination is commonly used to evaluate patients with suspected GERD. The appearances may be clearly diagnostic: linear or punctate erosions or ulcerations, often with attendant inflammatory exudation, that occur predominantly in the distal esophagus (12). Other, less dramatic changes such as mucosal erythema or edema can also be seen, but these are subject to greater observer variation, and thus are diagnostically less conclusive. Moreover, up to 50% of patients with documented symptomatic GERD can display normal or only minimally abnormal endoscopic findings (13). Mucosal biopsy in these cases can aid in establishing the diagnosis.

The histologic abnormalities of GERD encompass a range of features denoting epithelial injury and repair (Table 2). These changes, although not specific, are characteristic of GERD, and have been most extensively studied in that setting. As diagnostic criteria, each feature is limited to some degree by practical utility or diagnostic sensitivity (14–16). Although these numerous features, alone or in combination, can contribute to establishing the diagnosis of GERD, none is an absolutely reliable criterion. Multiple biopsy specimens sectioned at several levels provide the best diagnostic oppor-

TABLE 1. *Esophagitis: histologic clues to etiology*

Etiology	Histologic features
Gastroesophageal reflux	Range of possible findings; see Table 2
Candida	Budding yeast forms (3–4 μm in diameter) and pseudohyphae
Herpes simplex virus	Cowdry A intranuclear inclusions, ground-glass intranuclear inclusions, multinucleation
Cytomegalovirus	Cytomegaly, large intranuclear inclusions, cytoplasmic inclusions
Bacteria	Invasive cocci and bacilli
Corrosive agents	No specific features
Pill-induced	No specific features
Irradiation	± Atypical fibroblasts, homogenized collagen
Eosinophilic gastroenteritis	Marked intraepithelial eosinophilia
Crohn's disease	Aphthoid ulcers, granulomas
Graft-vs.-host disease	Apoptosis of individual squamous cells
Primary skin disorders	Similar to cutaneous histopathology

TABLE 2. *Histologic features in gastroesophageal reflux disease (GERD)*

Feature	Diagnostic sensitivity	Comments	Differential considerations
Epithelial hyperplasia Basal zone hyperplasia (>15%) Papillary elongation (>67%)	45–85%	Can be found normally in distal 2–3 cm of esophagus	Other causes of low-grade epithelial insult
Ballooned squamous cells	~65%	PAS-negative cytoplasm; positive immunostains for plasma proteins	Glycogenic acanthosis, normal glycogen-rich squamous cells
Vascular dilatation	60–80%	Most characteristic when noted in superficial papillae	Exclude procedural artefact
Intraepithelial eosinophils	25–55%	Rare eosinophils can be found in normal adult esophagus	Infectious esophagitis; drug-contact esophagitis; eosinophilic esophagitis
Intraepithelial lymphocytes	20–30%	Can be confused with neutrophils because of irregular nuclear contours	Normal specimens (usually <10/HPF; >20/HPF more indicative of GERD)
Neutrophil infiltration	15–30%	Associated with intercellular edema and ultimately mucosal erosion	Infectious esophagitis; drug-contact esophagitis
Mucosal erosion/ulceration	10–30%	Indicative of severe esophagitis	Other causes of high-grade epithelial injury
Cardiac mucosa inflammation	75%(?)	Diagnostic role needs further definition	Exclude *H. pylori* gastritis

HPF, high-power field.

tunity. Because the changes seen are not specific, the differential diagnosis includes the other causes of esophagitis (Table 1). Again, clinical correlation is the keystone.

Epithelial hyperplasia is manifest by expansion of the basal zone and elongation of lamina propria papillae (Fig. 2).

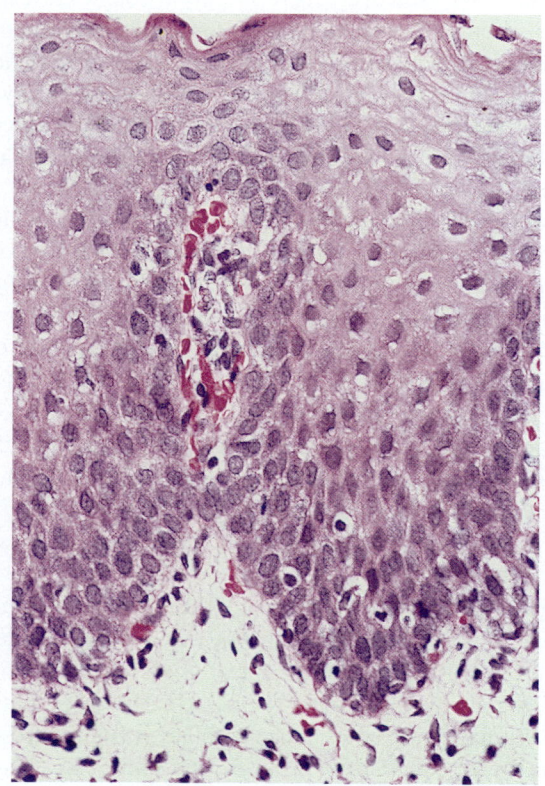

FIG. 2. Epithelial hyperplasia denoted by lengthening of the lamina propria papillae and expansion of the basal zone in an example of gastroesophageal reflux disease. Intraepithelial lymphocytes are focally prominent.

Basal-zone expansion is typically specified as a basal zone exceeding 15% of the total epithelial thickness; papillary elongation is defined as lengthening greater than two-thirds of the epithelial thickness. These findings are indicative of increased epithelial proliferation and turnover, and, since their description in 1970, have garnered much attention as manifestations of mild reflux-induced injury (17,18).

Most studies confirm that epithelial hyperplasia serves as a marker of reflux, but the sensitivity of this feature is debated, with reported values averaging 60% to 70%. Difficulties in interpretation arise for several reasons. One problem is that the changes can be noted in normal subjects in the distal 2 to 3 cm of the esophagus, and may be a manifestation of the transient episodes of reflux that most healthy people undergo (19). Biopsies should therefore be procured from above this region and, because the changes are irregularly distributed, multiple specimens should be obtained.

An additional issue is that accurate evaluation of epithelial hyperplasia requires precisely oriented biopsies sectioned perpendicularly to the mucosal surface. In practical terms, this means that the "jumbo" or suction-type biopsy specimens, which are larger, deeper, and more readily oriented, are preferable to the usual grasp specimens, which are often superficial and thus less satisfactory (13,19).

Judging the basal-zone thickness may also present problems since this layer is not obviously demarcated. Periodic acid-Schiff (PAS) stains, by accentuating the overlying glycogen-rich squamous cells, help define the nonstaining basal zone, but the exact measurement is still prone to observer variation (17).

Another proposed indicator of epithelial injury is the presence of *balloon cells*—swollen, rounded squamous cells with pale staining cytoplasm (20). This appearance derives from the leakage of extracellular fluid and proteins into the damaged cells. These cells are PAS-negative (unlike normal mature squamous cells), but contain immunoreactive intracytoplasmic plasma proteins such as albumin or immunoglobulins. Balloon cells may be seen in active esophagitis of many causes and, in one study, were identified in about two-thirds of GERD cases (20); additional studies of their diagnostic utility are needed. An association has also been suggested between GERD and glycogenic acanthosis (21), which, as noted below, is characterized by enlarged, glycogen-laden squamous cells, but this has not been generally accepted.

Part of the response of the lamina propria in GERD includes marked *dilatation and congestion of capillaries,* forming vascular "lakes" or hemorrhages in the superficial papillae (Fig. 3) (22). This feature corresponds to the red streaks noted at endoscopy, and has been proffered as an early sign of esophagitis. Unfortunately, it is commonly accompanied by other markers of esophagitis and may therefore be of little use as an independent indicator. In addition, it is found in 10% to 30% of normal controls, further limiting its diagnostic reliability (17,22). In some cases, dilatation probably represents an artifact of the biopsy procedure, but these affected vessels tend to be located in the basal rather than superficial mucosa. Dilated mucosal vessels are also consistently noted in patients with esophageal varices.

Intraepithelial eosinophils are an additional indicator of GERD (Fig. 4) (18,23,24). Because specimen orientation is not crucial to its interpretation, this feature is particularly useful when evaluating endoscopic grasp biopsies. The number of eosinophils noted may vary, but their distinctive appearance makes identification easy. However, use of solutions that contain picric acid, such as Bouin's fixative or some eosin dyes, hampers the staining of the eosinophil granules. In GERD, eosinophils also accumulate within the lamina propria, but because they can normally reside there, this finding is not as diagnostically useful (18).

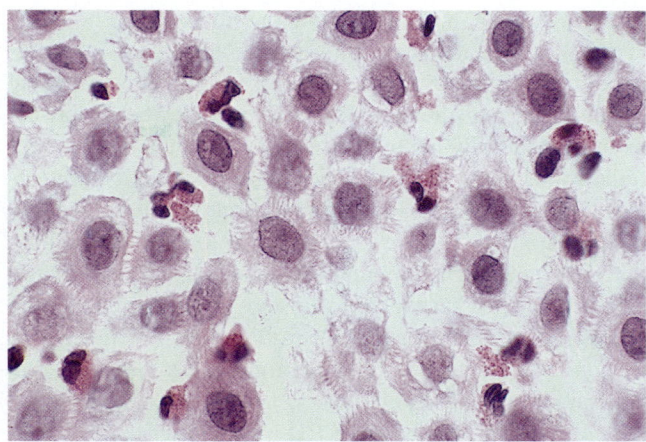

FIG. 4. Numerous eosinophils with their distinctive bilobate nuclei are scattered among squamous cells.

The diagnostic value of intraepithelial eosinophils is limited by poor sensitivity; they are found in only 30% to 50% of cases of GERD, despite being the only histologic abnormality in some 10% to 25% of patients (23,24). In addition, a rare isolated eosinophil may appear in the epithelium of occasional normal subjects (24). Although their presence is characteristic of GERD, intraepithelial eosinophils are not specific but can be found in other circumstances, including infectious esophagitis, pill-induced esophagitis, and forms of eosinophilic esophagitis (25,26).

Intraepithelial lymphocytes are a normal attribute of the esophageal mucosa, but the number can be increased, sometimes conspicuously, as part of the inflammatory reaction in GERD (27). As a rule, normal specimens demonstrate fewer than about ten lymphocytes per high power field; with GERD, this value can exceed 20 (15). An increase in intraepithelial lymphocytes correlates with the presence of intraepithelial eosinophils and thus is not an independent (nor a sensitive) histologic indicator of GERD.

Neutrophil infiltration denotes more severe degrees of epithelial injury and is consequently an insensitive diagnostic marker, being noted in only 15% to 30% of cases (13,14,17). This infiltration is associated with varying degrees of intercellular edema, in addition to other features of GERD, and is especially prominent in and around epithelial erosions and ulcerations. Other causes of active esophagitis, including infectious and pill-induced, thereby enter the differential diagnosis.

Mucosal erosion and *ulceration* represent the extreme end of the GERD spectrum. Biopsy specimens show the expected fibrinopurulent inflammatory exudate, necrotic slough, and active granulation tissue. Identification of these

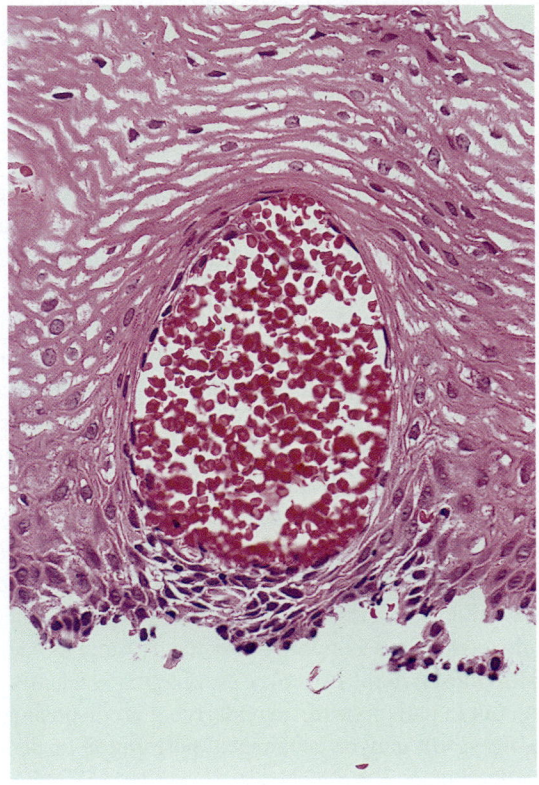

FIG. 3. Dilated and congested vascular channel at the tip of a lamina propria papilla in a mucosal biopsy specimen.

changes is not a diagnostic problem, but sections should be carefully examined to exclude infectious agents or malignancy. In particular, the presence of inflammatory exudate strongly suggests mucosal destruction, even when it has not been directly sampled by the biopsy specimen, and the sections should then be studied for possible infectious organisms. The granulation tissue composing the ulcer bed can contain large, atypical mesenchymal cells that can be mistaken for carcinoma; immunohistochemical stains for cytokeratins are helpful in excluding this possibility. Similarly, the squamous epithelium adjacent to the erosion or ulcer may demonstrate reactive atypia and prominent hyperplasia that can mimic invasive carcinoma.

A recognized feature of GERD is the presence of inflammatory changes in the cardiac mucosa located at the gastroesophageal junction region (5,15). Specifically, this *cardiac mucosa inflammation* is characterized by neutrophil, eosinophil, or plasma cell infiltration of the lamina propria (Fig. 5). The changes are similar to *Helicobacter pylori*-associated gastritis (28), but are distinguished by being limited to the cardiac region. In preliminary studies, this feature was a more sensitive marker of GERD than intraepithelial eosinophil or neutrophil infiltration (29), but additional investigations are need to examine this issue.

Infectious Esophagitis

The esophagus is host to few infections. Numerous organisms may involve the esophagus as part of a disseminated illness; in practice, however, most infectious esophagitis is caused by *Candida* species, herpes simplex virus, or cytomegalovirus. Affected patients often have some reason for impaired host response: immunosuppression (caused by congenital conditions, infection with human immunodeficiency virus, or cytotoxic and immunosuppressive therapy), malignant neoplasms, chronic debilitating disease, diabetes mellitus, or antibiotic therapy (30). Normal hosts, however, are not exempt from infectious esophagitis (31,32). Because effective therapy is often available, careful scrutiny for infectious agents is indicated, especially when biopsies show ulceration or exudate, and the possibility of multiple infections needs to be kept in mind. By sampling wide areas of the esophagus, brush cytology can be an effective adjunct in identifying the causative organisms (33).

Candida Esophagitis

Candida species are the best-known cause of infectious esophagitis. The usual culprit is *Candida albicans,* although sometimes *C. tropicalis, C. krusei,* or *C. glabrata* is implicated. The gross appearances at endoscopy classically entail white plaques, discrete to confluent, issuing from erythematous, edematous, ulcerated, or diffusely friable mucosa of the mid- or distal esophagus (34). These plaques are composed of the diagnostic fungal pseudohyphae and budding spores embedded in keratinous squamous material, fibrinous exudate, and necrotic debris (Fig. 6A). Special stains for fungi such as PAS or methenamine silver facilitate detection of the organism (Fig. 6B). The plaques overshadow the underlying epithelial changes of active esophagitis with variable neutrophilic inflammation, mucosal erosion, or ulceration with inflamed granulation tissue. Because *Candida* is a ubiquitous commensal of the gastrointestinal tract, fungal invasion into tissue or ulcer slough is required for a definite diagnosis. In severe instances, the organism can invade deeply into the esophageal wall, rarely resulting in perforation, and can lead to disseminated candidiasis. Chronic infection has been associated with esophageal strictures and intramural pseudodiverticulosis.

Herpes Esophagitis

Esophagitis due to herpes simplex virus is usually seen as an opportunistic infection in immunosuppressed patients, but it also can occur in otherwise healthy children and adults (32). Grossly, the mucosa exhibits small vesicles that evolve into discrete shallow ulcers; in severe cases these coalesce into extensive zones of mucosal denudation (35). The ulcer bed is histologically undistinguished, consisting of necrotic debris and neutrophil-rich inflammatory exudate. The diagnostic herpetic inclusions are located in discohesive or multinucleated squamous cells at the margins of the ulcers (Fig. 7A). The characteristic inclusions include dense eosinophilic intranuclear (Cowdry type A) bodies, which are separated from a thickened nuclear membrane by a clear halo, and homogeneous ground-glass inclusions that fill the nuclei. Herpetic ulcers may be secondarily infected by fungi or bacteria. In healthy hosts, herpes simplex esophagitis is usually self-limited, but in patients with an underlying predisposing condition, the result may be esophageal perforation or disseminated infection.

Documenting herpes simplex esophagitis can be difficult. Biopsy sampling may miss the ulcer edges where the diag-

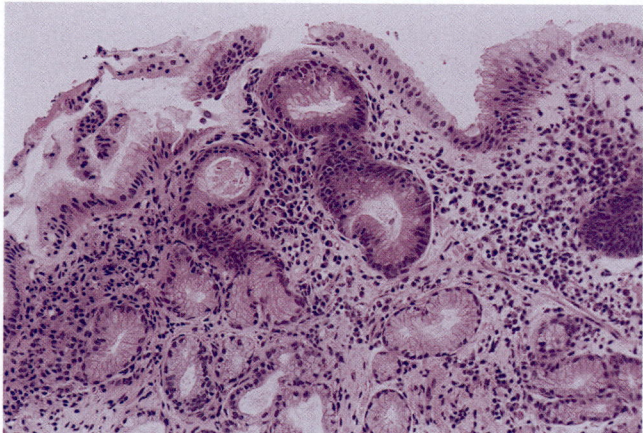

FIG. 5. Inflammation of cardiac mucosa in gastroesophageal reflux disease, characterized primarily by plasma cell infiltration of the lamina propria. Stains for *Helicobacter pylori* were negative.

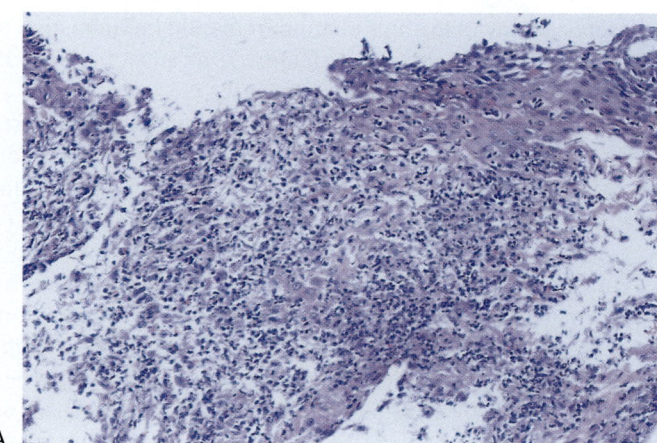 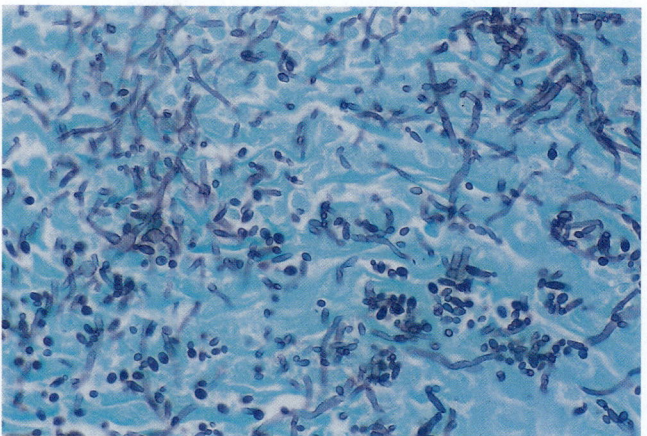

FIG. 6. *Candida* esophagitis. **A:** Luminal fibrinopurulent exudate attached to inflamed, reactive, and degenerating squamous epithelium; the fungal organisms can barely be discerned on this hematoxylin and eosin stain. **B:** The Grocott stain clearly demonstrates the characteristic budding yeast-like cells and pseudohyphae of *Candida*.

nostic changes reside, or these changes may be obscured by necrosis and inflammation. The presence of ulceration in biopsies from susceptible patients should always raise suspicion, especially when prominent aggregates of large mononuclear cells are noted in the exudate (36). Immunohistochemical methods can be helpful in confirming the presence of herpesvirus antigens in suspect or questionable cases (Fig. 7B), and may demonstrate infected cells before cytopathic effects are histologically recognizable.

Cytomegalovirus Esophagitis

Cytomegalovirus (CMV) can infect the esophagus of immunocompromised patients [and only rarely normal individuals (31)], producing ulcers similar to those of herpes simplex esophagitis (37). The ulcer bed is the diagnostic focus: enlarged mesenchymal cells of the granulation tissue contain the heralded cytomegalovirus inclusions—conspicuous intranuclear bodies surrounded by a clear halo together with, in many infected cells, coarse intracytoplasmic granules. In patients under antiviral therapy, however, the inclusions may be less distinctive and the appearances mistaken for enlarged and reactive, but noninfected, cells. The presence of macrophage aggregates within the granulation tissue, particularly in a perivascular distribution, may be a diagnostic clue to CMV esophagitis (38). Immunostains are valuable in establishing the diagnosis when definitive inclusions are not seen.

Other Infections

Rare examples of fungal esophagitis caused by *Aspergillus* and the Phycomycetes are reported. In addition, histoplasmosis, blastomycosis, and cryptococcosis may involve the esophagus, usually in association with either disseminated or mediastinal disease (39). Unusual examples of varicella-zoster virus esophageal infections are also seen.

Bacterial colonization of esophageal ulcers is a frequent

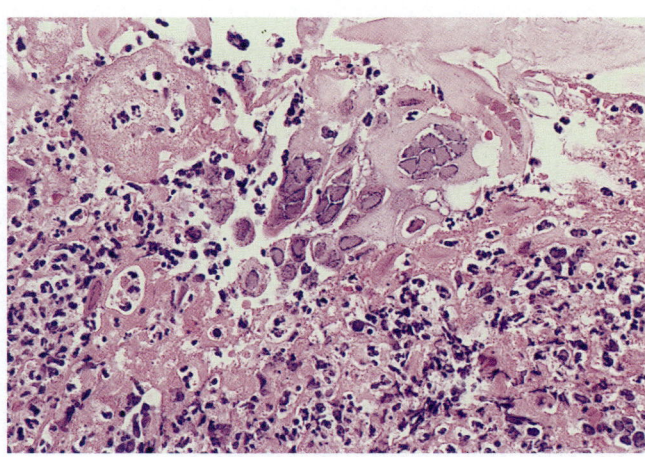 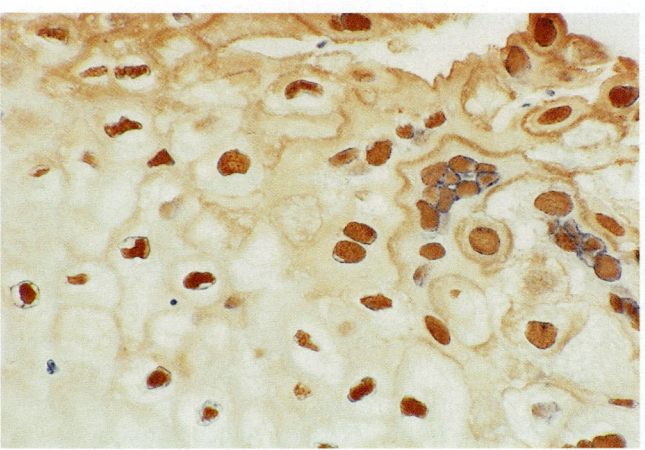

FIG. 7. Herpes esophagitis. **A:** The distinctive intranuclear inclusions are found in multinucleated squamous cells present within an inflammatory and necrotic background. **B:** Immunoreactivity for herpes simplex virus antigens confirms the diagnosis of herpes esophagus.

observation, but in severely immunocompromised patients, bacteria can also become a primary opportunistic pathogen (40,41). Implicated bacteria include a range of gram-positive and gram-negative organisms, with a mixed population (chiefly representing oropharyngeal flora) being commonly noted. Histologically, bacterial esophagitis is characterized by clusters of bacteria invading the esophageal wall and involving blood vessels with associated necrosis. Other unusual esophageal infections include bacillary angiomatosis, tuberculosis, actinomycosis, syphilis, Whipple's disease, and Chagas' disease (39,42).

Idiopathic esophageal ulcers are sometimes found in patients infected with human immunodeficiency virus (HIV) (43). Although HIV has been identified in these ulcers by immunohistochemical and electron microscopic studies, its presence probably does not reflect a pathogenetic role, and other, as yet unidentified, agents may instead be responsible (44). The ulcers may heal with empiric therapy using corticosteroids.

Miscellaneous Causes of Esophagitis

Additional types of esophagitis are biopsied primarily to exclude infection and malignancy. Although histologic features may suggest the cause, the microscopic appearances are typically not specific, and the location of the lesions and the clinical data are the diagnostic attributes.

Corrosive esophagitis is caused by the ingestion of caustic agents, including strong alkalis, acids, and nonphosphate detergents, either accidentally or with suicidal intent (45). These agents produce varying degrees of esophageal damage, ranging from mucosal erythema and edema to extensive mural ulceration, hemorrhage, and necrosis with thrombosis and secondary bacterial invasion. Potential complications include stricture formation, Barrett's esophagus, and squamous carcinoma, although the overall risk of the latter is low. Biopsy specimens are seldom obtained from the acute phase of injury, but they may be employed to assess any complications.

Pill-induced esophagitis refers to the esophageal injury resulting from direct contact of medication with mucosa. A wide range of drugs have been implicated; frequently cited agents include doxycycline and other antibiotics, aspirin and other nonsteroidal antiinflammatory agents, slow-release potassium preparations, ferrous salts, and alendronate (46,47). The local caustic action of these agents leads to discrete erosions or ulcers without distinguishing histologic features. This injury is commonly located at the mid-esophagus, the site of anatomic narrowing produced by the aortic arch or by an enlarged left atrium. Another cause of iatrogenic esophageal ulceration is the injection of sclerosing agents for treatment of esophageal varices. Varying degrees of localized necrosis and vascular thrombosis leading to ulceration and fibrosis are described, although biopsy specimens are seldom obtained (48). Other drugs can produce active esophageal injury through mechanisms other than direct mucosal contact. The best examples are cytotoxic chemotherapeutic agents, which can cause an active esophagitis with features ranging from mild inflammation to erosions, ulcerations, and strictures. Care must be taken in this setting to exclude infectious causes.

Irradiation esophagitis develops as a complication of radiation therapy directed at neoplasms of the lung, the mediastinum, or the esophagus itself. This radiation-induced injury can be potentiated by concurrent administration of cytotoxic chemotherapy. Acute radiation damage, which occurs during the first few weeks after treatment, is manifest by mucosal necrosis and submucosal edema, but is seldom biopsied. Chronic radiation injury develops weeks to months after irradiation, usually when fractionated doses exceed about 60 Gy. The histologic changes are characterized by progressive submucosal fibrosis, capillary telangiectasia, thick-walled hyalinized arterioles, and atrophy of mucous glands, leading to persistent ulceration, strictures, or fistulas (49). Although mucosal biopsies usually show only nonspecific changes of active esophagitis, granulation tissue, and fibrosis, the presence of atypical fibroblasts and "smudged" hyalinized collagen may suggest the correct diagnosis.

Eosinophilic esophagitis denotes esophageal involvement occurring as part of the spectrum of eosinophilic gastroenteritis. Even in the absence of esophageal symptoms, eosinophil infiltration of the esophagus is a regular feature of eosinophilic gastroenteritis (25). Numerous eosinophils infiltrate the epithelium, occasionally forming large clusters near the luminal surface. GERD-related intraepithelial eosinophilia must be excluded. In some cases, esophageal involvement represents a major manifestation of the disease. These patients may present with dysphagia or esophageal strictures, commonly display other allergic disorders or peripheral eosinophilia, and often have concurrent gastric or small intestinal involvement (26,50).

Crohn's disease rarely affects the esophagus. The pathologic features mirror those found elsewhere in the gastrointestinal tract: discrete ulcers, granulomas, fistulas, and transmural inflammation (51). A definitive diagnosis requires a resected specimen, but aphthoid ulcers and granulomas on mucosal biopsy may be suggestive in the proper setting.

Chronic *graft-versus-host disease* may be accompanied by a necrotizing and desquamative esophagitis of the proximal esophagus (52). Apoptosis of individual squamous cells in an uninflamed epithelium is the diagnostic finding, just as in cutaneous graft-versus-host disease. Diverse *skin disorders,* including lichen planus, pemphigus, bullous pemphigoid, epidermolysis bullosa, and Behçet's syndrome, can also involve the esophagus (53).

Rarely, examples of severe necrotizing esophagitis or esophageal ulceration are recognized that lack a clearly defined cause despite extensive diagnostic evaluation (54).

BARRETT'S ESOPHAGUS (COLUMNAR EPITHELIUM-LINED ESOPHAGUS)

Barrett's esophagus is the eponymous designation for replacement of the squamous epithelium of the distal esophagus by glandular mucosa. It represents an acquired metaplastic condition that most commonly develops as an aftermath of chronic gastroesophageal reflux, but may also follow other causes of esophageal mucosal injury such as lye ingestion, chemotherapy, and reflux of bile-pancreatic fluid (55,56). Other features of GERD, including hiatal hernia, peptic ulceration, and esophageal stricture, often occur together with Barrett's esophagus, but its major significance is that, as a premalignant condition, it confers an increased risk for esophageal adenocarcinoma.

The general concept is that destruction of the normal squamous epithelium produced by chronic reflux is followed by reepithelialization by a columnar epithelium more resistant to acid, pepsin, and bile. The source of this metaplastic epithelium is not known, but recent studies point to a multipotential stem cell of esophageal origin (57). Some evidence suggests that the process develops to its full length rapidly, but then the extent of Barrett's esophagus remains static over many years (58). In general, Barrett's esophagus is considered an irreversible condition, although a few cases of partial posttreatment regression have been reported (59).

Barrett's esophagus is noted in 3% to 12% of patients with symptomatic reflux, and is estimated to affect 376 per 100,000 individuals in the general population, but is identified clinically in only a minority of these cases (60). Its prevalence increases with age, and thus it is primarily a disorder of adults; the average age at diagnosis is in the seventh decade, although cases in children are also clearly recognized (58,61). Men are affected about twice as often as women.

In the past, Barrett's esophagus was commonly defined by the presence of at least 2 to 3 cm of columnar epithelium in the lower esophagus. This requirement avoided the diagnostic difficulties posed by the normal occurrence of gastric-type epithelium in the distal-most esophagus, but it was an arbitrary criterion and did not reflect the difficulties in determining the exact location of the gastroesophageal junction at endoscopy (56). The current tendency is, instead, to define Barrett's esophagus on histologic criteria, specifically by the presence of goblet cell–containing intestinal metaplasia (15,62). Because it is not based on precise biopsy localization, this definition avoids the problems associated with endoscopic localization, particularly in the Barrett's-related setting of active esophagitis, mucosal erosion, and hiatal hernia (63). It also permits the recognition of so-called short-segment Barrett's esophagus, designated as less than a 2- to 3-cm length of involvement (64,65). The importance is that even short segments of esophageal intestinal metaplasia have been associated with epithelial dysplasia and adenocarcinoma (66–68).

Pathologic Features

Grossly, Barrett's esophagus appears as velvety, orange-red mucosa involving the distal esophagus, either as a circumferential sleeve or as one or more tongues extending from the gastroesophageal junction. Within this field of Barrett's mucosa, islands of squamous mucosa may be retained. The Barrett's mucosa displaces the native pink-tan squamous epithelium proximally so that the new squamocolumnar junction lies above its normal site near the esophageal terminus.

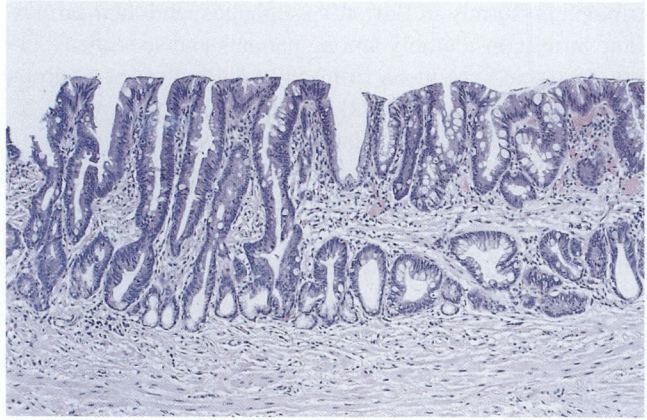

FIG. 8. Barrett's esophagus composed of a superficial foveolar-like component (with a villiform surface) and underlying mucous glands, which have focally split the muscularis mucosae. The diagnostic goblet cells are evident even at low power.

The mucosa of Barrett's esophagus includes a heterogeneous population of epithelial cell types similar to those found in the stomach, small bowel, and large bowel, organized into a superficial component composed of surface epithelium and gastric-like pits and an underlying component of mucous glands (69,70). A villiform configuration is sometimes adopted (Fig. 8).

The characteristic and diagnostic feature is the *intestinal metaplastic epithelium* characterized by goblet cells interspersed among columnar mucous cells (Fig. 9) (62,71). This epithelium, also referred to as "*specialized epithelium*," "*distinctive epithelium*," and "*Barrett's mucosa*," is indistinguishable from incomplete intestinal metaplasia of the stomach. The goblet cells contain acid mucins, usually with sialomucins predominating, and thus are strongly positive with Alcian blue stains at pH 2.5 (Fig. 10). They are not dis-

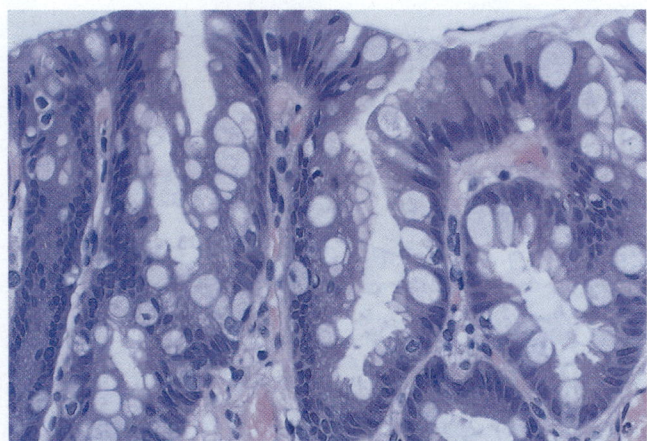

FIG. 9. Intestinal metaplastic epithelium of Barrett's esophagus. Numerous goblet cells are dispersed among columnar cells, some of which show apical mucin.

tributed uniformly in Barrett's esophagus, and their proportion varies considerably among patients and specimens, being sparse in specimens from children and more common with advancing age (61,72). The columnar cells often resemble gastric foveolar cells, but can also display features of intestinal absorptive cells, and hybrid attributes of both cell types are often noted ultrastructurally (73). Characteristically, these cells produce PAS-positive neutral mucins, but, unlike normal gastric foveolar cells, they can also contain Alcian blue-positive acidic mucins, either sialomucins, sulfomucins, or both (Fig. 10).

The glandular component contains a variable numbers of goblet cells, neuroendocrine cells, and Paneth cells. The latter are especially conspicuous in the unusual cases with well-developed intestinal absorptive cells (so-called complete intestinal metaplasia). Pancreatic acini have also been described (74). Typically the lamina propria demonstrates mild chronic inflammation and fibrosis; the muscularis mucosae can be thickened, splayed, or duplicated.

Intestinal metaplasia is variably admixed with foci of gastric cardiac-type epithelium, in which mucus-containing epithelial cells are the predominant element of both surface and glandular epithelium (Fig. 11). This epithelium lacks goblet cells and, as its name implies, resembles the gastric cardia, but the architecture tends to be disorganized with atrophic glands, a variable inflammatory component, and disrupted muscularis mucosae. Cardiac-type epithelium in patients with *Helicobacter pylori* gastritis can be secondarily colonized by the organism, which may then provoke an active inflammatory reaction (75). Fundic-type epithelium with parietal and chief cells has also been noted, almost exclusively in the extreme distal region of the affected esophagus.

Barrett's esophagus can be complicated by mucosal erosions or ulcerations, which demonstrate the expected fibrinopurulent inflammatory exudate and underlying granula-

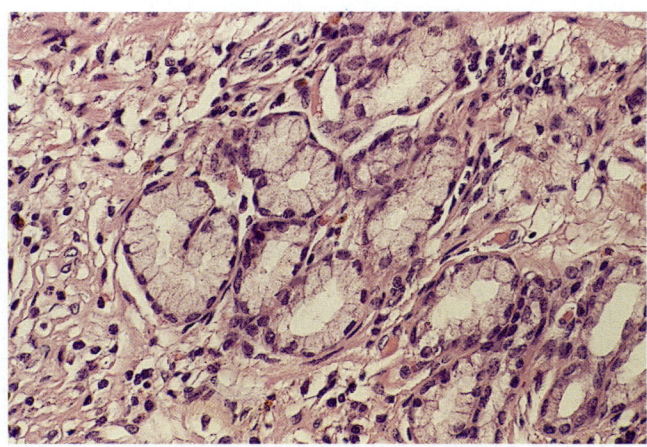

FIG. 11. Cardiac-type glands in Barrett's esophagus. A cluster of loosely packed mucous glands is noted within a mildly inflamed lamina propria. These glands are composed purely of mucous cells, but a few scattered parietal cells are sometimes seen.

tion tissue. When exuberant, the granulation tissue can be mistaken for carcinoma and, in some cases, can form a pyogenic granuloma-like polypoid mass (76).

Diagnosis and Differential Considerations

Intestinal metaplasia is not found in the normal esophagus, and its presence in an esophageal biopsy specimen is, for all practical purposes, diagnostic of Barrett's esophagus. Typically the requisite goblet cells are readily identified on routine sections, but Alcian blue stains (pH 2.5) are helpful in highlighting scarce goblet cells and in distinguishing them from potentially confusing mucus-distended columnar cells, which are either negative or only modestly alcinophilic. Some investigators have considered Alcian blue-positive columnar cells to represent transitional forms between gastric-like columnar cells and goblet cells, and therefore have regarded their presence in the surface epithelium to be indicative of Barrett's esophagus (77). However, similar cells can be seen in reactive gastric mucosa (62), and thus it is not clear that their presence in the absence of goblet cells is indeed diagnostic of Barrett's esophagus.

Biopsy specimens from patients with endoscopically convincing Barrett's esophagus may show only cardiac-type epithelium without intestinal metaplasia. In adults this is an unusual occurrence that generally suggests inadequate sampling, but in children it may reflect an early stage in the evolution of Barrett's esophagus (61). In such cases, a tentative diagnosis of Barrett's esophagus can be rendered, but only with careful evaluation of the endoscopic findings. The more common problem is misinterpreting a hiatal hernia as Barrett's esophagus. The true gastroesophageal junction can typically be recognized as the site at which the tubular esophagus joins the saccular hiatal hernia at the proximal margin of the gastric folds, but this identification may be problematic in the face of a patulous sphincter or active

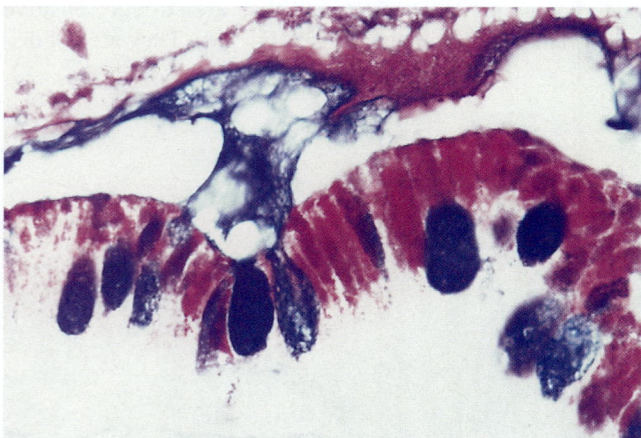

FIG. 10. The goblet cells with their globular profiles and alcian blue-positive acid mucins contrast with the columnar cells, which largely contain magenta-colored (periodic acid-Schiff positive) neutral mucins. Note, however, that acid mucins can also be found in some columnar cells (alcian blue pH 2.5/periodic acid-Schiff stain).

esophagitis (56). If the hiatal hernia is not recognized, gastric mucosa may mistakenly be sampled; biopsy specimens that consist of completely unremarkable gastric-type mucosa have, in fact, probably been obtained from the stomach.

One area of unsettled controversy is the significance of intestinal metaplasia found in the region of the gastroesophageal junction and gastric cardia, which has been described in up to 18% of patients, either with or without reflux symptoms, who undergo endoscopy (5,78–80). The relationship between this metaplastic epithelium and short segment Barrett's esophagus is not clear: Although the two processes are conceptually separable by their respective locations above or below the gastroesophageal junction, the inaccuracies in precisely localizing this landmark suggest that the distinction may not always be possible or practical; in fact, some studies have not attempted to distinguish them.

One view of junctional/cardiac intestinal metaplasia considers it part of a GERD-Barrett's esophagus continuum and emphasizes its association with adenocarcinomas of the gastroesophageal junction and gastric cardia (5,15,81). Others, however, dispute this, pointing to the inconsistent correlation with gastroesophageal reflux, the relatively high prevalence, and the uncertain, but probably low, absolute risk of malignancy (56,79). The issue is as yet unresolved and awaits further investigation. For the practicing pathologist, the best approach is to render a descriptive diagnosis of intestinal metaplasia and then to correlate this finding with the endoscopic features and sites of biopsy (if provided), reserving the term *Barrett's esophagus* for those instances in which the specimen has definitely been noted as being from the esophagus.

The presence of intestinal metaplasia distinguishes Barrett's esophagus from several other types of glandular epithelium that may occur in the esophagus (Table 3).

Dysplasia in Barrett's Esophagus

Barrett's esophagus would remain an intriguing pathologic novelty except that it represents a premalignant condition predisposing to esophageal adenocarcinoma. The magnitude of the risk is not clearly established, but the incidence is estimated from prospective studies at 1/52 to 1/98 patient-years, corresponding to a 30- to 50-fold excess risk compared to the general population (82–84). Some studies have related the risk of carcinoma to the duration of disease or the length of affected esophagus, but other investigations have discounted these associations (85,86).

Considerable evidence supports the concept that the adenocarcinomas develop through a stepwise progression from intestinal metaplastic epithelium to epithelial dysplasia to malignancy. This concept provides the basis for endoscopic surveillance of patients with Barrett's esophagus: regular examination and biopsy is recommended, usually at 1- to 2-year intervals, to detect dysplasia and thus identify those patients at particularly high risk of carcinoma (87,88). Although the efficacy and value of surveillance are debated, adenocarcinomas discovered during surveillance are more likely to be resectable and to have a better outcome than cancers detected outside of such a program (89,90). [Note that rare examples of squamous cell and adenosquamous carcinoma have also been reported to arise in Barrett's esophagus (91).]

Dysplasia is defined histologically as unequivocally neoplastic epithelium that does not invade the lamina propria, and is characterized by various degrees and combinations of cytologic atypia and architectural disarray (62,92). Most often dysplasia occurs with a patchy, irregular distribution in flat and unexceptional mucosa (93,94), but occasionally it appears as thickened velvety mucosa or a polypoid mass; the presence of endoscopic mass lesions raises the possibility of an invasive carcinoma.

Histologically, dysplastic epithelium is crowded and variably stratified with progressive loss of cellular orientation (Figs. 12 and 13). Cells within the epithelium are characterized by enlarged hyperchromatic nuclei with irregular nuclear membranes, clumped and erratic chromatin, and often prominent nucleoli. Cytoplasmic mucin is diminished, but residual goblet cells, occasionally dystrophic in appearance, can be found. Affected glands are distorted and irregular in contour with budding, branching, and luminal infoldings, and a villous configuration may be adopted. Following the schema proposed for dysplasia in inflammatory bowel disease, these abnormalities are generally classified into low and high grades (95). In low-grade dysplasia, architectural changes are modest; nuclear stratification is limited and does not involve the entire epithelial thickness; and the nuclear changes are less pronounced (Fig. 12). In high-grade dysplasia, on the other hand, there is more evident distortion and complexity of the crypt architecture; nuclear stratification is more pronounced and reaches to the luminal surface; and nuclear aberrations are greater (Fig. 13). Changes that would be classified as carcinoma *in situ* are, by convention, included in the high-grade category.

The major problem in interpretation is distinguishing dysplasia, especially low-grade dysplasia, from reactive epithelial changes. The inflammatory, metaplastic, and regenerative processes that give rise to Barrett's esophagus can also generate morphologic alterations that simulate neoplastic features. Reactive nuclei are often enlarged and stratified with conspicuous nucleoli, but, in general, lack the hyper-

TABLE 3. *Differential diagnosis of esophageal glandular epithelium*

Inadvertently sampled gastric mucosa
Esophageal junctional mucosa
Cardiac-like mucosa located in distal 1–2 cm
Esophageal superficial cardiac glands
Often located in upper esophagus
Heterotopic gastric fundic mucosa
Noted in upper esophagus of 4–10% of normal subjects
Ciliated columnar epithelium
Embryologic remnant found in infants
Sebaceous glands
Present endoscopically as small yellow papules

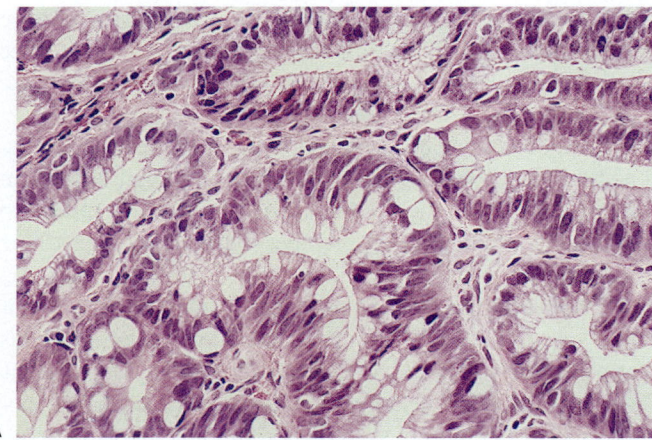
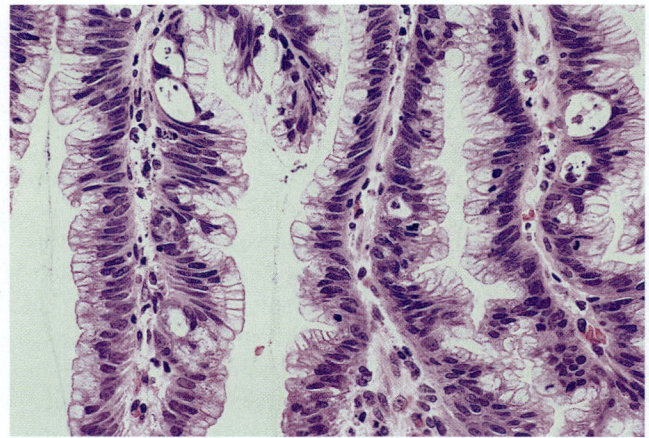

FIG. 12. Low-grade dysplasia in Barrett's esophagus. **A:** The glands are crowded, display focal branching, and are lined by dysplastic epithelium with enlarged, hyperchromatic, and partially stratified nuclei. Dystrophic goblet cells can be seen, but they are not specific for dysplasia. **B:** In another example, a villiform configuration is present. The epithelium again shows dysplastic features including densely clumped chromatin, irregular nuclear profiles, and occasional nucleoli.

chromasia, crowding, and sharply defined nuclear membranes of dysplastic nuclei. The reactive changes often tend to be more evident at the proliferative zone at the base of the pit-like structures with evidence of maturation toward the luminal surface, whereas dysplastic features commonly involve the superficial aspects of the mucosa.

Discrimination between the two processes may not, however, always be straightforward (62,63,96). In these cases a diagnosis of "indefinite for dysplasia" is appropriate, signifying that the histologic changes are neither unequivocally neoplastic ("positive for dysplasia") nor clearly reactive ("negative for dysplasia"). The indefinite category is typically employed when dysplastic-like epithelial atypia is noted in a background of active neutrophilic inflammation and mucosal erosion; because the abnormalities could possibly represent florid regeneration, an express diagnosis of dysplasia is unsuitable. Obtaining additional specimens after successful antireflux treatment is often helpful in resolving these problems. In general, the diagnosis of dysplasia should be confirmed by an experienced pathologist before aggressive therapy is contemplated.

The natural history of dysplastic Barrett's esophagus is not well understood, leading to uncertainties and controversies over appropriate patient management (88,97). Many studies are retrospective in nature and have included relatively few patients, although prospective investigations are becoming increasingly available (83,98,99). Several tentative conclusions can be drawn. High-grade dysplasia is as-

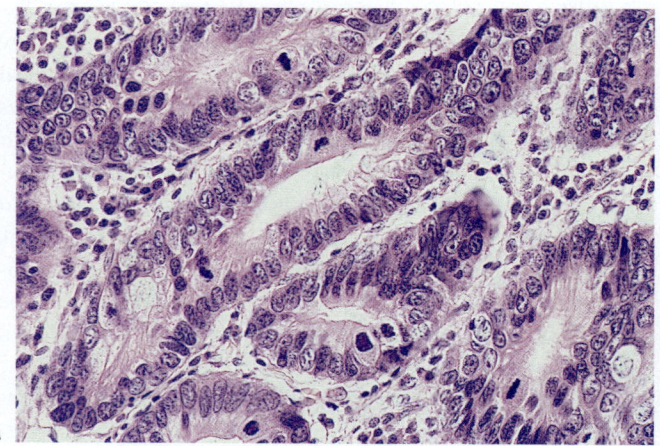
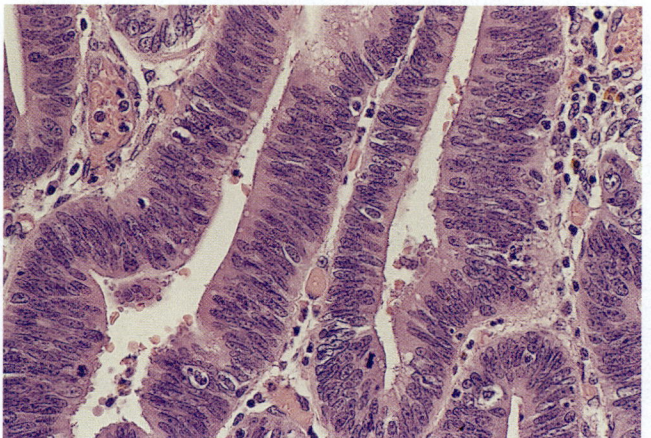

FIG. 13. High-grade dysplasia in Barrett's esophagus. **A:** Cytologic atypia is pronounced with an irregular chromatin distribution and loss of polarity. Mitoses are conspicuous, but they can also be noted in reactive epithelium. **B:** Another example demonstrates an adenomatous appearance with prominent hypercellularity and full-thickness stratification.

sociated with concurrent invasive adenocarcinoma in up to 50% of patients (100), although intensive sampling of the Barrett's epithelium can reduce this rate (101,102). In the absence of carcinoma, approximately 50% of patients with high-grade dysplasia will progress to malignancy, but in some cases it can persist without progression for months to years (83,93,98). Therefore, after the presence of high-grade dysplasia is confirmed, common recommendations are for immediate rebiopsy (to exclude missed carcinoma) followed by an individualized consideration of surgical resection in good-risk patients (87,88,97). Low-grade dysplasia has an even less predictable natural history, reflecting in part the problems in reliably distinguishing it from reactive atypia, but progression to high-grade dysplasia or carcinoma has been documented in a few patients after a time period ranging up to 10 years (83,98). Again, the usual recommendation for biopsies showing confirmed low-grade dysplasia (or changes indefinite for dysplasia) is for intensive antireflux therapy, followed by an accelerated program of surveillance (87,88,97).

Other Premalignant Markers

Neoplastic progression in Barrett's esophagus is thought to result from the accumulation of genetic and phenotypic abnormalities, genomic instability, and proliferative abnormalities (103,104). Much of the work in this area, while increasing our understanding of the process, has little current application in the clinical setting, but some of these features have been considered as practical indicators of malignant risk. The presence of DNA aneuploidy and an increased 4N (G2/tetraploid) phase fraction by flow cytometry or DNA image analysis has been associated with the development of high-grade dysplasia and adenocarcinoma (105,106). In cross-sectional immunohistochemical analyses, overexpression of p53 protein and expansion of the Ki-67 proliferative compartment have correlated with neoplastic progression (107–109). Similar results have been found with immunohistochemical detection of overexpressed *c-erb* B-2 (110) and transforming growth factor-α (111). Further studies are required to assess whether these markers have a role in supplementing or supplanting epithelial dysplasia as a risk factor.

NEUROMUSCULAR DISORDERS

Assorted disorders of the esophagus are manifest by abnormalities in motility and sphincter function and are diagnosed by clinical, radiographic, and manometric findings. Pathologic correlates have generally been studied only in end-stage autopsy specimens; consequently, the nature and evolution of the relatively inaccessible early changes are poorly understood. The surgical pathologist is therefore largely limited to evaluating the complications of disordered motility, notably reflux-associated esophagitis, Barrett's esophagus, and carcinoma. The morphologic features of these conditions are only briefly sketched; details can be found elsewhere (1).

Idiopathic muscular hypertrophy is characterized by marked thickening of the muscularis propria, particularly the inner circular layer of the distal esophagus (112). This is the pathologic counterpart of diffuse esophageal spasm, a rare condition of older men manifesting with dysphagia and angina-like chest pain. Functional evidence suggests that the primary abnormality is in the neural control of muscular contraction, but a neuropathologic lesion is not well documented; however, lymphocytic infiltration of the myenteric plexus is sometimes noted.

This condition should be differentiated from *leiomyomatosis,* in which multiple confluent nodules of disorganized smooth muscle expand the lower esophageal and proximal gastric musculature. Leiomyomatosis primarily affects young adults and adolescents, usually women, and may be associated with vulvar leiomyomas (113).

Systemic sclerosis (scleroderma) commonly involves the esophagus, resulting in atrophy and replacement fibrosis of the smooth muscle of the muscularis propria, chiefly the inner circular layer. Varying degrees of submucosal fibrosis, nonspecific inflammatory infiltration, and proliferative changes of smaller arteries can also be noted. These changes can lead to gastroesophageal reflux with the subsequent development of esophagitis, Barrett's esophagus, and an increased risk of adenocarcinoma. Atrophy and fibrosis of the muscularis can also be seen in other conditions, including systemic lupus erythematosus, Sjögren's syndrome, primary visceral myopathies, and cricopharyngeal dysphagia.

Achalasia is characterized by marked depletion or absence of ganglion cells in Auerbach's plexus, apparently the end result of a primary inflammatory process affecting the myenteric region (114,115). This leads to the characteristic functional impairments of incomplete relaxation of the lower esophageal sphincter and aperistalsis. Achalasia also predisposes to squamous cell carcinoma, although the degree of risk is debated, and endoscopic surveillance is therefore sometimes recommended (116). Treatment of achalasia by esophagomyotomy decreases the sphincter tone; achalasia can thereby be complicated by gastroesophageal reflux, peptic ulceration, fibrous stricture, and, in some cases, Barrett's esophagus and adenocarcinoma (117).

Loss of ganglion cells is also recognized in Chagas' disease, in a variety of visceral neuropathies, and in normal aging, but identification usually depends on use of specialized silver impregnation techniques not routine in the surgical pathology laboratory.

BENIGN TUMORS AND TUMOR-LIKE LESIONS

A diversity of benign tumors and nonneoplastic masses can be seen in the esophagus (92). They are, however, mostly uncommon lesions, small and asymptomatic, whose importance lies in their distinction from malignant tumors.

TABLE 4. *Differential diagnosis of polypoid esophageal tumors*

Lesion	Distinguishing features
Benign	
Squamous papilloma	Bland epithelium covering fibrovascular cores
Fibrovascular polyp	Pedunculated mass of fibrous (+/− adipose) tissue; found in upper esophagus
Inflammatory fibroid polyp	Vascular fibroblastic tissue with mixed inflammation
Submucosal tumors	Leiomyoma and granular cell tumor most common
Malignant	
Squamous cell carcinoma	Especially verrucous variant
Adenocarcinoma	Infrequently polypoid
Sarcomatoid carcinoma	Atypical spindle cell stroma predominates
Malignant melanoma	Melanin pigmentation; junctional changes
Sarcomas	Rare, distinguish from carcinoma with spindle cell component
Metastatic tumors	Occasionally produce polypoid mass

Most clinically apparent tumors grow or protrude into the lumen, and thus appear as polyps at endoscopy. The differential diagnosis of polypoid esophageal lesions is summarized in Table 4.

Squamous Papilloma

Squamous papillomas are small (≤0.5 cm) sessile masses, usually solitary, composed of mature acanthotic squamous epithelium arranged along branched fibrovascular stalks (Fig. 14). They are rare lesions noted in fewer than 0.04% of endoscopic examinations, and typically represent an incidental finding in the lower esophagus of men over the age of 40 years. In some cases, condylomatous features such as koilocytosis, parakeratosis, and binucleated cells are noted, suggesting human papillomavirus (HPV) infection. Indeed, several studies have identified HPV DNA in some squamous papillomas, but other lesions may instead represent a response to chronic mucosal irritation (118,119). Although in biopsy specimens verrucous carcinomas may be mistaken for squamous papillomas because they share a papillary architecture and bland cytology, the carcinomas are typically much larger lesions.

Adenoma

Rare esophageal tumors are reported that fall under the general heading of benign glandular neoplasms, but the pathologic details in these reports are often sparse. These lesions include mucous gland adenomas similar to those of the bronchus, salivary gland-like pleomorphic adenomas, parathyroid and thyroid adenomas, serous cystadenomas, and papillotubular adenomas apparently originating in the ducts of submucosal glands (120). Lesions with the same dysplastic histology as adenomas elsewhere in the gastrointestinal tract can also develop in Barrett's esophagus, but these are best considered polypoid examples of dysplastic Barrett's mucosa (121).

Leiomyoma

Although it is the most common benign tumor of the esophagus, the leiomyoma seldom poses a clinical problem. In general these tumors appear as circumscribed mural masses, usually solitary and 2 to 5 cm in diameter, that bulge into the lumen and may even form pedunculated polyps. Minute "seedling" leiomyomas of 1- to 2-mm diameter can be commonly identified in the vicinity of the gastroesophageal junction (122). The morphologic features mirror those of other classic leiomyomas: interlacing fascicles of bland spindle cells with variable fibrosis produce the traditional circumscribed, white-gray whorled appearance on gross examination.

Mesenchymal Polyps

A polypoid configuration is the most memorable feature of several benign esophageal lesions of unsettled pathogenesis. *Fibrovascular polyps* are characterized by a core of mature fibrous tissue, occasionally myxoid, with scattered thin-walled vessels and a variable admixture of adipose tissue. The overlying mucosa is generally intact, but may be secondarily eroded. The histologic variety explains this polyp's numerous synonyms, which include fibroma, fibrolipoma, fibromyxoma, and lipoma. Typically these polyps arise in the upper esophagus from the cricopharyngeal region, and

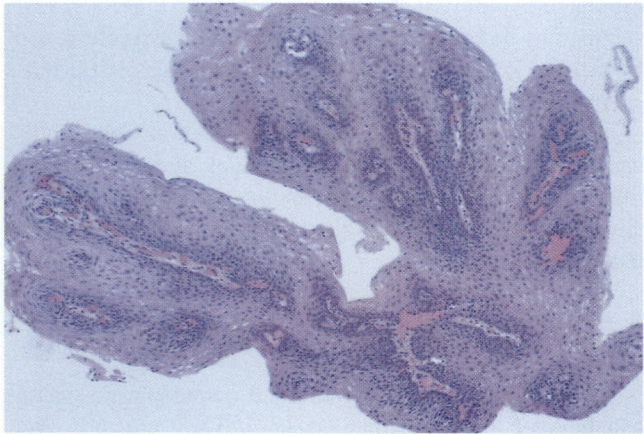

FIG. 14. Squamous papilloma showing benign squamous epithelium lining delicate connective tissue stalks.

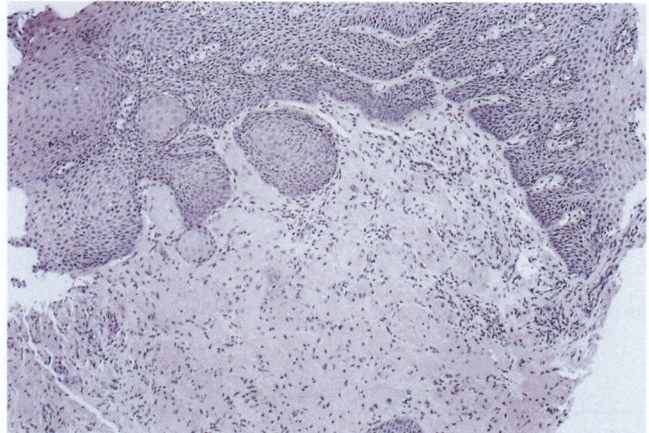

FIG. 15. Granular cell tumor in an endoscopic biopsy specimen from an incidentally discovered 1-cm mass. The lamina propria contains the uniform rounded cells with coarsely granular cytoplasm, and the overlying epithelium shows acanthotic, pseudoepitheliomatous changes.

they present as elongated pedunculated masses that may range up to 20 cm in length (123).

Inflammatory fibroid polyps similar to those elsewhere in the gastrointestinal tract have also been described in the esophagus. They comprise a submucosal proliferation of reactive fibroblasts and small vessels bestrewn with inflammatory cells including eosinophils. Unlike fibrovascular polyps, inflammatory fibroid polyps are located in the mid- or lower esophagus and harbor a more diffuse inflammatory component, although the distinction between the two is without great clinical importance.

Inflammatory esophagogastric polyps are composed of granulation tissue and edematous lamina propria with inflammation. They occur near the gastroesophageal junction and probably result from reflux-associated ulceration and repair.

Granular Cell Tumor

The esophagus is one of the favored gastrointestinal sites for granular cell tumors. Usually solitary, incidental lesions of the lower esophagus, they may present with obstruction when large. Multiple tumors are found in about 10% of cases. Grossly they appear as intramural nodules, poorly circumscribed and generally less than 2 cm in diameter. Histologically identical to granular cells tumors elsewhere, they comprise sheets of uniform cells with small nuclei and abundant PAS-positive cytoplasm that exhibits S-100 protein immunoreactivity (Fig. 15). The overlying squamous epithelium may undergo pseudoepitheliomatous hyperplasia that can be mistaken for squamous cell carcinoma. Most esophageal granular cell tumors are stable or slowly growing lesions, but rare examples with malignant behavior have been reported (124).

Miscellaneous

Case reports describe all manner of benign soft tissue tumors occurring in the esophagus: hemangiomas, lymphangiomas, glomus tumors, osteochondromas, and neurofibromas. Hamartomas fashioned from a mixture of fibrous, muscular, cartilaginous, and glandular tissues are found in infants (1).

MALIGNANT NEOPLASMS

Esophageal cancer poses several general diagnostic tasks for the surgical pathologist: establishing the diagnosis of malignancy, classifying the histologic type, and assessing prognostic factors. The recognition of esophageal malignancies in mucosal biopsy specimens is usually straightforward, although the diagnostic features may be hidden by more abundant inflamed, fibrotic, or necrotic tissue. Cytologic examination is an effective and valuable adjunct; the diagnostic yield of combined endoscopic biopsy and brush cytology approaches 100% (125).

The features that should be evaluated in biopsy and resection specimens are listed in Table 5 (9). The most important prognostic indicators include the tumor stage, depth of invasion, presence of nodal or distant metastases, and status of resection margins. These features form the basis of the widely used TNM staging classification (Table 6).

TABLE 5. *Pathologic evaluation of esophageal tumors*

Biopsy specimens
  Gross evaluation
    Number and size of pieces
    Portion of tissue submitted
  Microscopic evaluation
    Tumor type
    Histologic grade
    Depth of invasion (as approriate)
    Additional findings (esophagitis, Barrett's esophagus, squamous or glandular dysplasia, etc.)
Resection specimens
  Gross evaluation
    Overall dimensions; organs and tissue received
    Location, size, and configuration of lesions
    Assessment of depth of invasion
    Assessment of proximal, distal, and radial margins
    Other esophageal lesions
    Lymph nodes
  Microscopic evaluation
    Tumor type
    Histologic grade
    Depth and extent of invasion
    Blood/lymphatic vessel invasion; perineural invasion
    Proximal, distal, and radial margins
    Number of lymph nodes (total and positive)
    Additional findings (esophagitis, Barrett's esophagus, squamous or glandular dysplasia, etc.)
    Pathologic stage (see Table 6)

TABLE 6. *TNM staging of esophageal carcinoma*

Stage	Primary tumor (T)	Regional lymph nodes (N)	Distant metastasis (M)	Approximate 5-year survival
	TX: cannot be assessed	NX: cannot be assessed	MX: cannot be assessed	
	T0: no primary tumor	N0: no nodal metastases	M0: no distant metastases	
0	Tis: carcinoma *in situ*	N0	M0	100%
I	T1: invades lamina propria or submucosa	N0	M0	80–90%
IIA	T2: invades muscularis propria	N0	M0	40–50%
	T3: invades adventitia	N0	M0	
IIB	T1 or T2	N1: regional nodal metastases	M0	25–40%
III	T3	N1	M0	
	T4: invades adjacent structures	Any N	M0	15–25%
IV	Any T	Any N	M1: distant metastases	<5%

Adapted from *American Joint Committee on Cancer Staging Manual.* Philadelphia: Lippincott-Raven, 1997:67–69.

SQUAMOUS CELL CARCINOMA

Squamous cell carcinoma accounts for most esophageal cancer worldwide. Its incidence differs dramatically, however, in different countries, with smoking, alcohol abuse, dietary exposure, genetic factors, and human papillomavirus all suspected of playing an etiologic role. A fraction of cases are associated with other predisposing conditions: achalasia, corrosive strictures, squamous cell carcinoma of other aerodigestive tract sites, and tylosis palmaris et plantaris (an exotic genetic disorder characterized by hyperkeratosis of the palms and soles) (126–128). In low-risk areas including North American and much of Western Europe, the tumor occurs primarily in men over the age of 50 years. Blacks are disproportionately affected. Most tumors in these regions are discovered at an advanced stage, and thus dysphagia, anorexia, and weight loss are common presenting symptoms.

Pathologic Features

Squamous cell carcinomas are usually located in the mid- and lower esophagus; only about 10% are found in the cervical and upper thoracic regions. At the time of diagnosis, most are advanced lesions with invasion into or beyond the muscularis propria. Grossly they can present as deep irregular ulcers with nodular margins (Fig. 16), as fungating exophytic masses, or as plaque-like mural thickenings, but mixtures of these types are common (92). Infiltration along the submucosa can undermine adjacent intact mucosa, narrowing the lumen and mimicking a benign stricture; in some cases, this submucosal spread is not apparent on gross examination.

The microscopic features are the same as in other squamous cell carcinomas. Any degree of differentiation may occur, and variation within a single tumor is common. In better differentiated lesions, mild nuclear atypia and cellular pleomorphism are accompanied by readily identified keratinization (Fig. 17A), whereas in poorly differentiated tumors keratinization is sparse and cytologic abnormalities more pronounced (Fig. 17B). Small foci of glandular or small cell differentiation are sometimes found, and a prominent lymphoid stroma may be present.

As the carcinoma grows from its intraepithelial origin, it progressively invades deeper layers of the esophageal wall and eventually infiltrates into and through the muscularis propria. (Tumors confined to the mucosa and submucosa are designated as superficial carcinomas, and are discussed in more detail below.) The tumor can also extend peripherally, undermining the adjacent mucosa. Extension through to the adventitial tissues can lead, perhaps abetted by the lack of a serosal barrier, to invasion of contiguous organs. Indeed, involvement of mediastinal structures is noted in 30% to 40% of surgically resected specimens (129), and provides the potential for malignant fistula formation.

The carcinomas also disseminate via lymphatics, blood vessels, and perineural spaces (130). Once the submucosa is breached, longitudinal intramural spread can occur via the profuse lymphatic networks (131), and submucosal foci of tumor can consequently be found many centimeters away from the gross lesion. Attention to the surgical margins of resected specimens is therefore imperative. Lymph node metastases are observed in 50% to 60% of resected specimens, but given

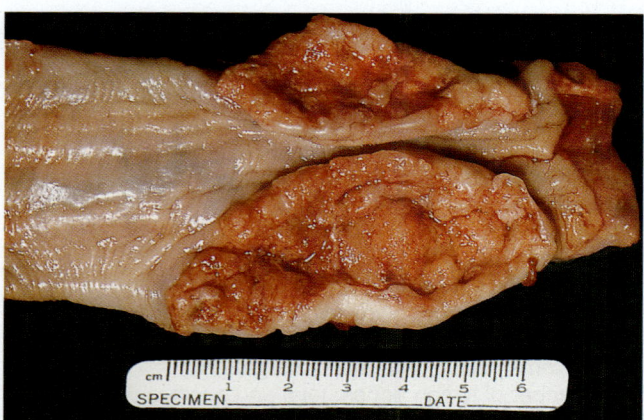

FIG. 16. Squamous cell carcinoma. A large ulcerated mass demonstrates nodular, heaped-up edges and invasion into the underlying esophageal wall.

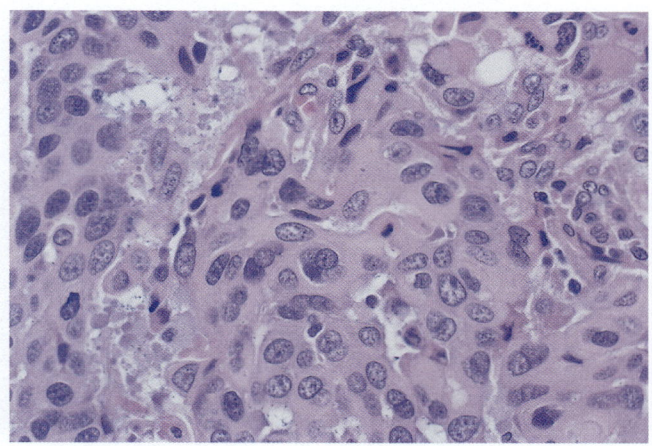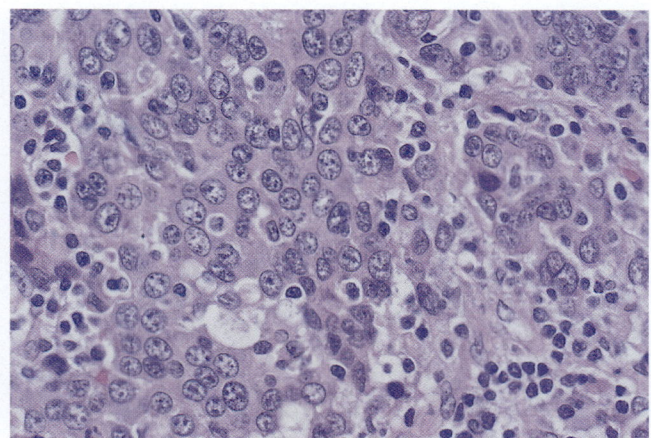

FIG. 17. Squamous cell carcinoma. Two microscopic fields from the same tumor, showing a moderately differentiated area with large differentiated squamous cells **(A)** and a poorly differentiated area with sheets of malignant cells that lack obvious squamous features and are accompanied by a brisk lymphocytic response **(B)**.

the complex anastomosing of esophageal lymphatics, they are widely and unpredictably distributed among cervical, mediastinal, and upper abdominal chains (132,133). Carcinomas of the lower esophagus, for example, expectedly involve the lower mediastinal and abdominal nodes but also metastasize to cervical and superior mediastinal nodes in about 10% of cases. Distant metastases are usually a minor clinical feature as compared with local and regional spread, but they are noted at autopsy in many cases, with frequently involved sites being lungs, liver, and bone (134).

Differential Diagnosis

Generally the diagnosis of esophageal squamous cell carcinoma is straightforward (Table 7), although up to five to six biopsy specimens from an endoscopically suspicious lesion are, as a rule, necessary to ensure diagnostic material (135). The major differential consideration is benign reactive or reparative processes. Large atypical mesenchymal cells may be encountered in the granulation tissue of ulcer beds and be mistaken, particularly in biopsy specimens, for malignancy. Although these cells are pleomorphic and hyperchromatic, they have only sparse mitoses, tend to "mature" in the deeper stroma, and, in contrast to carcinomas, are negative by cytokeratin immunostains. In addition, reactive or regenerative epithelium associated with benign ulcerations or with injury induced by radiotherapy or chemotherapy may be misinterpreted. These cells can have enlarged, hyperchromatic nuclei and prominent mitoses, but their relatively monomorphic appearance and the inflammatory or granulation tissue context are clues to their true nature. Rebiopsy and cytologic examination are appropriate in problem cases.

Prognosis

The advanced stage of most squamous cell carcinomas heralds a dismal prognosis: the 5-year survival rate for all patients is less than 10%. The single best predictor of outcome is the pathologic stage, which is largely based on the depth of tumor invasion. The 5-year survival rate among tumors limited to the esophageal wall is in the 40% to 50% range, whereas invasion into or beyond the adventitia is associated

TABLE 7. Differential diagnosis of esophageal cancer

Histologic type	Peak age (years)	Male/female ratio	Location	Distinguishing features
Squamous cell carcinoma	55–65	3–7:1	60% mid 30% lower	Keratinization; intercellular bridges
Sarcomatoid carcinoma	55–65	5:1	60% mid 30% lower	Polypoid; biphasic
Basaloid squamous carcinoma	60–70	3:1	60% mid	Basaloid nests with high-grade cytology
Verrucous carcinoma	55–65	4:1	60% mid or lower	Low grade with pushing invasion
Adenocarcinoma	55–65	5:1	80% lower	Gland formation; mucin production
Small cell carcinoma	55–65	2:1	90% mid or lower	Similar to lung counterpart
Adenosquamous carcinoma	55–65	3:1	90% mid or lower	High-grade intermingling of glandular and squamous elements
Malignant melanoma	55–65	2:1	90% mid or lower	Melanin, appropriate immunostains, exclude metastatic origin

with only a 5% to 15% survival (133,136,137). The status of regional lymph nodes is also of crucial prognostic importance; survival at 5-years is approximately 40% to 50% when nodal metastases are absent, but drops to less than 10% in their presence. This poor outcome is seen even when the metastatic involvement consists only of isolated, immunohistochemically detected tumor cells (138). The number of positive nodes also shows some correlation with prognosis, with the best outcome being noted when three or fewer nodes are involved (139,140).

Many other histologic features, including histologic grade, tumor growth pattern, vascular invasion, and host response, have been assessed for their prognostic power, but their utility as independent indicators of outcome is controversial (92). The presence of DNA aneuploidy, mutations or overexpression of p53 protein, a high proliferative rate, overexpression of transforming growth factor-α, epidermal growth factor and epidermal growth factor receptor, and low-level expression of bcl-2 have all been associated with more aggressive biologic behavior (141–144); whether these markers provide prognostic information in addition to the pathologic stage is not certain.

Superficial Squamous Cell Carcinoma

Squamous cell carcinomas that are confined to the mucosa and submucosa, regardless of nodal status, are referred to as superficial carcinomas (92,145). First identified in screening programs for esophageal cancers in China and Japan, superficial carcinomas account for up to 22% of resected esophageal squamous cancer in series from the United States and Western Europe (146,147). The clinical features and tumor locations are similar to those of the more typical advanced carcinoma.

Superficial carcinomas arise as thin plaques, eroded mucosal depressions, or polypoid masses, but may also be subtle or inapparent on gross examination. Histologically they consist of invasive nests, often with irregular borders, within the lamina propria or submucosa; the degree of tumor differentiation is variable. Superficial carcinomas are potentially curable and carry a more favorable prognosis than advanced cancers, with overall 5-year survival rates of 65% to 90%. Those tumors limited to the lamina propria have a low rate of nodal metastasis (approximately 5%), and the 5-year survival is accordingly in the 90% to 100% range (148). However, when the cancer invades the submucosa, the risk of node involvement is about 35% to 45%. In those cases without positive lymph nodes, the 5-year survival rate is about 85%, but falls to the 40% range when nodes are involved (148).

Squamous Dysplasia

Squamous cell carcinoma is generally thought to evolve through a dysplasia-carcinoma pathogenetic sequence (149). Dysplastic squamous epithelium is frequently found adjacent to the cancers, and prospective follow-up studies, particularly among individuals in areas of high incidence, have documented the progression to carcinoma (150,151). Endoscopically, squamous dysplasia may appear as normal mucosa, as focal areas of erythema and friability, or as plaques or nodules (152). Applying Lugol's solution or toluidine blue on the mucosal surface can help highlight potentially dysplastic areas.

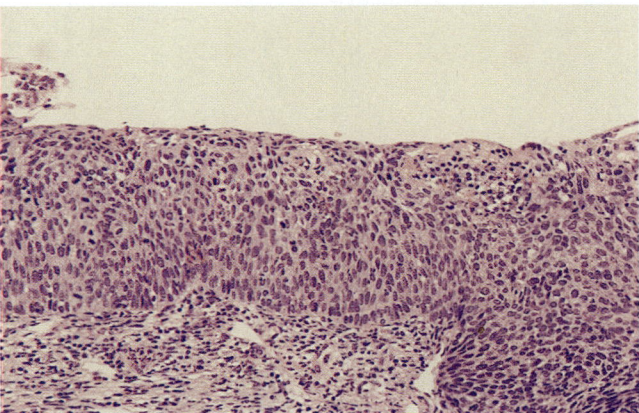

FIG. 18. High-grade squamous dysplasia (carcinoma *in situ*) noted adjacent to an advanced squamous cell carcinoma.

Squamous dysplasia is characterized by nuclear enlargement, pleomorphism and hyperchromasia, irregularly clumped chromatin, and abnormal mitoses with varying degrees of altered maturation and cytoplasmic differentiation (Fig. 18). These changes are often categorized as low grade (mild to moderate dysplasia) when the abnormal cells are limited to the basal half of the mucosa, and as high grade (severe dysplasia to carcinoma *in situ*) when they extend to the upper half (150). By definition, there is no invasion into the lamina propria, although sometimes the distinction between dysplasia and microinvasive superficial carcinoma is a difficult one; one clue is that invasion is frequently associated with a morphologic switch to larger keratinized cells with greater atypia and pleomorphism.

VARIANTS OF SQUAMOUS CELL CARCINOMA

Sarcomatoid Carcinoma

This neoplasm is an unusual and controversial polypoid cancer characterized by biphasic histology with both carcinomatous and spindle cell components (153,154). The assortment of names applied to this tumor—carcinosarcoma, pseudosarcoma, pseudosarcomatous squamous cell carcinoma, and polypoid tumor—testifies to the differing views of its histogenesis and biology. The dispute focuses on whether the spindle cell component is epithelial or mesenchymal in nature; the predominant concept is that it originates by sarcomatous metaplasia of malignant epithelial cells (155).

The tumors typically occur in the mid- or lower esophagus of middle-aged men, and present as bulky exophytic masses averaging about 6 cm in diameter. Microscopically they comprise a mixture of carcinoma and malignant-appearing sarcoma-like elements (Fig. 19). The latter typically form the bulk of the tumor and consist of atypical spindled or stellate cells in fascicular, storiform, or random assemblage. Bizarre giant cells, osseous and cartilaginous differentiation, and rhabdomyoblastic-like strap cells have all been reported. The carcinoma complement is usually squamous in nature and ranges from a minor *in situ* or minimally invasive component confined to the base of the polyp to obvious infiltrating nests intermixed with the spindle cells. Adenocarcinoma or undifferentiated carcinoma elements have also been described (156).

Overall, the prognosis of sarcomatoid carcinoma is more favorable than the usual esophageal carcinoma, largely because they tend to grow into the lumen and, despite their size, often show limited intramural invasion. Stage for stage, their behavior is probably similar to the usual squamous cell carcinoma. The presence of nodal metastases, noted in about 30% of cases, correlates with the depth of invasion; the metastatic foci may be composed of either carcinomatous or spindle-cell elements (92).

The differential diagnosis centers on the other polypoid esophageal masses (Table 4). Biphasic histology is the key diagnostic feature, but the carcinomatous element may not always be obvious and the tumor may be mistaken for a primary sarcoma.

Basaloid Squamous Carcinoma

In the past this carcinoma has been referred to as adenoid cystic carcinoma, but rather than representing an esophageal version of the salivary gland namesake, it instead corresponds to the aggressive basaloid squamous carcinoma recognized elsewhere in the upper aerodigestive tract (157). The clinical profile and features are similar to those of the usual squamous cell carcinoma. Histologically, the characteristic findings include invasive lobules of basaloid cells that demonstrate nuclear crowding and pleomorphism, areas

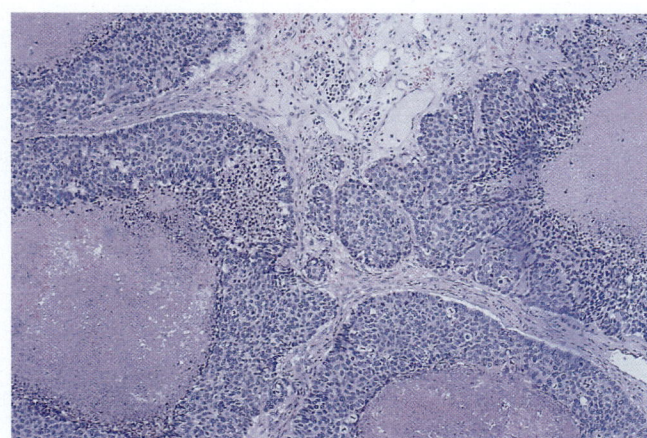

FIG. 20. Basaloid squamous carcinoma characterized by large rounded nests with small dark cells and central necrosis. Foci of basophilic myxoid matrix are additionally seen.

of necrosis, and conspicuous mitoses together with foci of squamous differentiation and deposits of hyalinized basal lamina stroma (Fig. 20) (157,158). Squamous dysplasia can be present in the overlying or adjacent mucosa. These tumors tend to be deeply invasive, frequently with widespread metastases at the time of diagnosis, and the prognosis is accordingly poor.

Verrucous Squamous Cell Carcinoma

Verrucous carcinoma, a rare but distinctive variant of squamous cell carcinoma, warrants special note (159). The tumor resembles verrucous carcinomas occurring at other sites in the upper aerodigestive tract, and is thus characterized by a large exophytic mass composed of papillary fronds covered by exuberant and highly differentiated squamous epithelium. The cytologic features are deceptively bland, with only slight and focal nuclear atypia; varying degrees of parakeratosis and hyperkeratosis are seen. At the base, the tumor demonstrates blunt epithelial projections and a pushing mode of invasion. An origin from squamous papillary hyperplasia was suggested in one reported case (160). Although the natural history of this tumor in the esophagus is not well defined, it tends to be slowly growing and only locally invasive, with infrequent lymph node involvement. Superficial biopsies are apt to be underdiagnosed as benign or squamous papilloma unless attention is paid to the endoscopic findings.

ADENOCARCINOMA

Esophageal adenocarcinoma is an uncommon malignancy, but it accounts for approximately 30% to 40% of primary esophageal cancers (92). In the vast majority of cases (85–95%), the tumor originates from Barrett's esophagus, although rare examples deriving from ectopic gastric mucosa in the upper esophagus or from submucosal glands are also reported. The incidence of esophageal adenocarcinoma

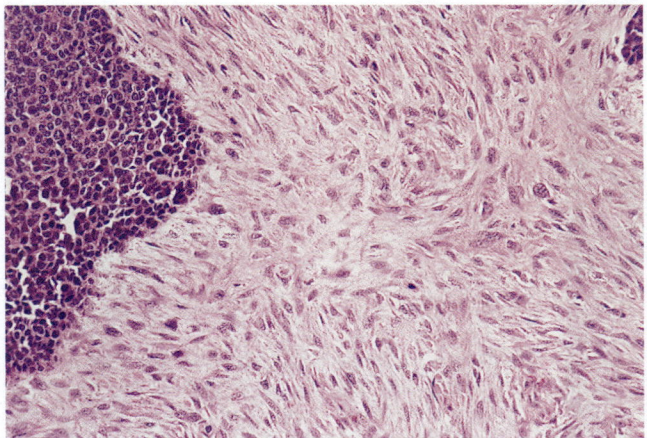

FIG. 19. Sarcomatoid carcinoma. An island of poorly differentiated carcinoma is present within the more abundant sarcoma-like proliferation of malignant spindle and stellate cells.

has increased dramatically over the past 20 years (161,162). The reason for this rise is not known, but it likely reflects some combination of improvements in diagnostic techniques, growing recognition of the entity, and perhaps a true increase in occurrence. It is predominantly a tumor of white men, usually in their sixth or seventh decades, who may be asymptomatic or have a clinical history suggesting gastroesophageal reflux disease; heavy tobacco or alcohol usage may be predisposing factors.

Pathologic Features

Most adenocarcinomas (up to 80%) develop in the lower third of the esophagus, where they rival squamous cell carcinoma in frequency; some may extend into the proximal stomach. The gross appearances are similar to squamous cell carcinoma, ranging from flat irregular plaques or slightly depressed lesions to advanced ulcerating or fungating masses (Fig. 21). The size can vary from a few millimeters to 10 cm, and multiple tumors are occasionally seen (163–165).

A range of histologic patterns similar to those of gastric adenocarcinoma are seen, but most are well or moderately differentiated. Intestinal-type glandular formation is common (Fig. 22A), but papillary structures, irregular invasive sheets of cells, and occasionally signet ring cell infiltration or abundant extracellular mucin production are seen (Fig. 22B) (164). Focal squamous or endocrine differentiation may be evident, and rare examples with germ cell differentiation have also been reported (166). Some tumors are sufficiently well differentiated that they can be recognized only by their invasion into the submucosa, and thus the diagnosis may be difficult to establish with endoscopic biopsy specimens (62). The manner of growth and spread are the same as in squamous cell carcinoma. Because esophageal adenocarcinomas have a propensity for proximal spread via the submucosal lymphatics, close attention must be paid to this surgical margin, especially at frozen section.

The intestinal metaplastic epithelium of Barrett's esophagus can be identified adjacent to the tumor in most cases, and epithelial dysplasia, usually high grade, is a common coexisting feature (163–165). In some tumors, however, no residual Barrett's esophagus is seen, presumably because it has been overgrown by the carcinoma.

Differential Diagnosis

In general, adenocarcinoma can be readily distinguished from other esophageal cancers (Table 7), and stains for epithelial mucins (PAS or alcian blue) can be of occasional aid in less well differentiated lesions. A greater problem is differentiating adenocarcinoma from high-grade dysplasia in cases where the atypical glands are distorted or tightly packed within the lamina propria; finding invasion by single cells or definite involvement of the muscularis mucosae or submucosa can help establish a malignant diagnosis, but often additional biopsy specimens are required. An additional issue, which is discussed below, is the relationship among adenocarcinomas of the esophagus, gastroesophageal junction, and gastric cardia.

Prognosis

Adenocarcinoma shares the disheartening natural history and poor prognosis of squamous cell carcinoma. Depth of invasion, occurrence of lymph node metastases, and status of resection margins are of similar prognostic importance. Most patients present at an advanced stage, with invasion through the esophageal wall noted in 60% to 80% and nodal involvement in 30% to 60% of cases. The overall 5-year survival rate is in the 15% to 25% range (165,167,168).

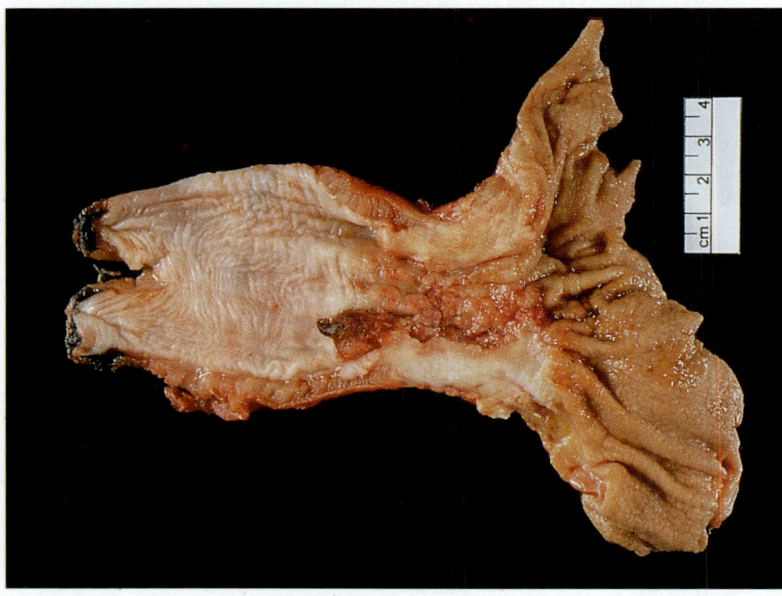

FIG. 21. Adenocarcinoma. The irregular granular tumor is situated just above the gastroesophageal junction and has deeply invaded the esophageal wall. Barrett's esophagus was recognized microscopically, but is difficult to appreciate grossly.

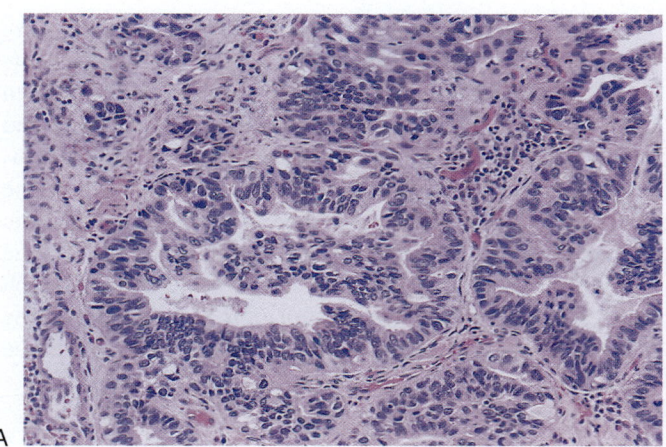 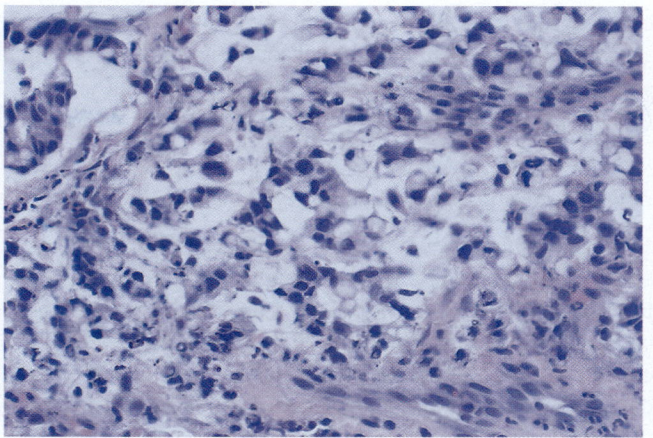

FIG. 22. Esophageal adenocarcinomas can range from well or moderately differentiated (A) to poorly differentiated tumors with abundant mucus and signet-ring cells (B).

Most reported series are too small to provide accurate survival data stratified by stage, but prognosis on a stage-by-stage basis likely approximates that for squamous cell carcinoma (Table 6) (167,169). Tumors limited to the mucosa and submucosa analogous to superficial squamous cell carcinoma have the best patient outcome, with 5-year survival rates of up to 85% (170). This rate decreases to about 45% when the muscularis propria is involved, to 15% to 25% with transmural invasion, and to approximately 0% with invasion of adjacent organs (167). Several other markers have been examined as prognostic indicators in esophageal adenocarcinoma, including DNA aneuploidy and overexpression of p53 protein or epidermal growth factor receptor, but their status as independent predictive factors has not been widely studied (171–173).

Adenocarcinoma Unassociated with Barrett's Esophagus

Rare tumors are derived from heterotopic gastric mucosa located in the upper esophagus (the so-called inlet patch). This patch is noted at endoscopy in up to 4% of individuals, although microscopic foci may be even more common (174). The complicating adenocarcinomas resemble the usual esophageal adenocarcinoma in their histologic appearance and biologic behavior, but are distinguished by their location and lack of accompanying Barrett's esophagus (175). In addition, rare adenocarcinomas of the esophagus have been considered to arise from mucosal or submucosal glands, but this derivation is difficult to prove (92).

Adenocarcinoma of the Gastroesophageal Junction

Adenocarcinomas that straddle the gastroesophageal junction are about twice as common as esophageal adenocarcinomas (161,162). Attempts have been made historically to assign them to a primary site in either the esophagus or cardia, with an esophageal origin being suggested when the bulk of the tumor is located in the esophagus or when its epicenter is more than 2 to 3 cm above the junction. In addition, many of these junctional tumors are accompanied by Barrett's esophagus, often of the short segment type, providing further evidence of an esophageal derivation. In other cases, progressive tumor growth is suspected to have obliterated the antecedent mucosa (66,67).

Distinguishing between an esophageal and cardiac origin is not always possible, however, and it is becoming increasingly clear that it may be more an academic than a practical or biologic categorization. Adenocarcinomas occurring in the vicinity of the gastroesophageal junctional, whether designated as esophageal, junction, or cardiac, all share similar clinicopathologic features, including a striking increase in incidence, predominance in white men, association with reflux symptoms, parallel histopathologic characteristics, and comparable tumor spread and prognosis (67,176–178). These tumors likely have a shared pathogenesis and biology and may therefore represent a single disease entity.

OTHER MALIGNANT NEOPLASMS

Small Cell Carcinoma

This cancer is an uncommon, but rapidly lethal, esophageal malignancy that occurs primarily in men in their sixth decade. The average survival is less than 1 year. The tumor is usually found in the lower half of the esophagus and displays the same range of macroscopic appearances seen with squamous cell carcinoma. Characteristic is the histology, comprising sheets and nests of small round to oval cells with densely hyperchromatic nuclei and sparse cytoplasm, similar to the pulmonary counterpart. Rosettes and carcinoid-like features may be seen, and focal squamous or glandular components are occasionally found. Some tumors express endocrine differentiation manifested by cytoplasmic argyrophilia, dense-core neuroendocrine granules on ultrastructural examination, and immunoreactivity for synaptophysin, chromogranin, and in some instances, gastrin, serotonin, or calcitonin. Differential considerations include metastatic small cell carcinoma of the lung, malignant lymphoma, and the rare esophageal carcinoid tumor (179,180).

Adenosquamous and Mucoepidermoid Carcinomas

Mixed squamous and glandular differentiation is noted in some esophageal carcinomas. Usually the mixture is morphologically and diagnostically insignificant: a squamous cell carcinoma may contain a negligible glandular or mucus-secreting element; or, conversely, an adenocarcinoma can incorporate small bland squamous foci (adenoacanthoma) (181). *Adenosquamous carcinomas* are rare aggressive neoplasms in which both malignant components coexist in more equal proportions. These tumors have commonly been reported in association with Barrett's esophagus, but can also occur de novo (182,183). They should be distinguished from the rare *mucoepidermoid carcinoma,* which is also composed of both squamous and glandular elements, but displays a more intimate admixture, with islands of squamous carcinoma containing central well-formed glands or mucus-secreting cells. An origin from submucosal glands is often suggested. These tumors have generally demonstrated extensive local invasion and metastases at the time of diagnosis (184,185).

Malignant Melanoma

Primary malignant melanoma, which accounts for only about 0.1% of esophageal malignancies, is noted principally in men over the age of 50 years (186,187). The prognosis is very poor, with most patients dying within 2 years of diagnosis. Grossly, the tumor presents as a pigmented polypoid mass, usually in the lower esophagus, but amelanotic lesions are also seen. Microscopically the tumor duplicates its cutaneous counterpart and is composed variably of epithelioid and spindled cells in sheets or nests. Immunohistochemistry for S-100 protein or HMB45, or electron microscopy, can be helpful in diagnostically difficult cases. The adjacent epithelium occasionally demonstrates an *in situ* junctional component or a basal proliferation of benign melanocytes (melanosis) (188,189), features that help establish the esophagus as the primary site, but in their absence the possibility of metastatic melanoma should be kept in mind.

Miscellaneous

Other unusual carcinomas reported in the esophagus include choriocarcinoma, carcinoid tumor, and Epstein-Barr virus-associated lymphoepithelioma (190,191). There are also rare instances of intramural tumors that probably correspond to adenoid cystic carcinoma or mucoepidermoid carcinomas of the salivary gland, but these have not been clearly delineated (92). Leiomyosarcomas are the most common esophageal sarcoma, but singular examples of many other mesenchymal malignancies (including synovial sarcoma, osteosarcoma, and Kaposi's sarcoma) have also been described (192,193). Examples of primary Hodgkin's and non-Hodgkin's lymphoma, plasmacytoma, and pseudolymphoma are recognized, but secondary involvement of the esophagus is clearly more common (194). Finally, metastatic tumors can involve the esophagus by direct spread from the stomach, larynx, lungs, or pharynx or via mediastinal lymph nodes, as with breast or lung primaries. Rarely, blood-borne metastases occur from distant primary sites as diverse as the endometrium, prostate, testis, and kidney.

MISCELLANEOUS ESOPHAGEAL LESIONS

Glycogenic acanthosis refers to white mucosal plaques produced by localized epithelial thickening with unusually enlarged, glycogen-packed squamous cells (195). This is a common endoscopic finding, considered by some to be a normal variant, particularly in the lower esophagus. Glycogenic acanthosis is of little consequence and notable largely for its lack of inflammatory or dysplastic qualities. The appearances may not be clearly distinguishable from normal mucosa in biopsy specimens.

Esophageal cysts are unusual lesions that may assume several morphologic patterns (196,197). Developmental cysts occur within or attached to the esophageal wall; they are typically unilocular, lined by ciliated or squamous epithelium, and contain smooth muscle in their walls. Some cysts also demonstrate mucous glands and cartilage and are designated as bronchogenic cysts. Another group of cysts, referred to as duplication cysts or gastroenteric cysts, are formed by mucosal, submucosal, and muscular layers that mimic those of the normal gastrointestinal tract. Retention cysts, usually small and located in the lower esophagus, derive from obstructed submucosal gland ducts. Occasionally, this ductal dilatation can give rise to the condition known as *intramural pseudodiverticulosis,* characterized by multiple flask-shaped invaginations into the esophageal wall (198,199). These changes can be recognized radiographically, but the complicating esophagitis (often due to *Candida*) may be documented by mucosal biopsy.

Esophageal atresia (with or without tracheoesophageal fistula) is the dominant congenital anomaly of the esophagus but is uncommonly the purview of the surgical pathologist. Current surgical techniques have increased survival to over 90%, but a late complication of successful repair is development of gastroesophageal reflux and esophagitis (200). Congenital *esophageal stenosis* is unusual, since most stenosis appears to be acquired as a postinflammatory sequel, but it may be caused by esophageal webs, remnants of tracheobronchial cartilage and glands, or muscular hypertrophy and disorganization (201).

Esophageal webs and rings describe thin mucosal membranes that project into the esophageal lumen. Microscopically they consist of normal mucosa, sometimes with acanthosis or hyperkeratosis, covering a thin layer of fibrous tissue. They may occur at the upper esophagus and be associated with the now-disappearing Plummer-Vinson syndrome, but are much more common in the lower esophagus (Schatzki's rings), where they may be related to gastroesophageal reflux (202). Webs may also form as a consequence of epithelial injury due to radiotherapy or graft-versus-host disease.

Esophageal diverticula, defined as outpouchings of one or more layers of the esophageal wall, are divided into three general types based on their location: Zenker's diverticula are found along the posterior wall of the pharyngoesophageal region, epiphrenic diverticula just above the diaphragm, and mid-esophageal diverticula at the level of the tracheal bifurcation (203). The first two are generally considered to be pulsion-type diverticula resulting from motility disturbances affecting the upper or lower esophageal sphincter, respectively. Mid-esophageal diverticula have traditionally be ascribed to traction on the esophageal wall produced by external inflammatory processes, but abnormalities in esophageal motility may also play a role. Of greatest interest for the surgical pathologist are the occasional examples of squamous cell carcinoma arising in diverticula, usually Zenker's type.

REFERENCES

Normal Features

1. Enterline H, Thompson J. *Pathology of the esophagus.* New York: Springer-Verlag, 1984.
2. DeNardi FG, Riddell RH. The normal esophagus. *Am J Surg Pathol* 1991;15:296–309.
3. Mangano MM, Antonioli DA, Schnitt SJ, Wang HH. Nature and significance of cells with irregular nuclear contours in esophageal mucosal biopsies. *Mod Pathol* 1992;5:191–196.
4. Csendes A, Maluenda F, Braghetto I, Csendes P, Henriquez A, Quesada MS. Location of the lower oesophageal sphincter and the squamous columnar mucosal junction in 109 healthy controls and 778 patients with different degrees of endoscopic oesophagitis. *Gut* 1993;34:21–27.
5. Öberg S, Peters JH, DeMeester TR, et al. Inflammation and specialized intestinal metaplasia of cardiac mucosa is a manifestation of gastroesophageal reflux disease. *Ann Surg* 1997;226:522–532.
6. Wang HH, Zeroogian JM, Spechler SJ, Goyal RK, Antonioli DA. Prevalence and significance of pancreatic acinar metaplasia at the gastroesophageal junction. *Am J Surg Pathol* 1996;20:1507–1510.

Specimen Handling

7. Haggitt RC, Rubin CE. Endoscopy and endoscopic biopsy. In: Ming S-C, Goldman H, eds. *Pathology of the gastrointestinal tract.* Philadelphia: WB Saunders, 1992:37–47.
8. Lewin KJ, Appelman HD. *Handling of esophageal and gastric biopsy and resection specimens. Tumors of the esophagus and stomach.* (Atlas of tumor pathology; 3rd series, fascicle 18). Washington, DC: Armed Forces Institute of Pathology, 1996:3–16.
9. Lee RG, Compton CC. Protocol for the examination of specimens removed from patients with esophageal carcinoma. A basis for checklists. *Arch Pathol Lab Med* 1997;121:925–929.

Esophagitis

10. Howard PJ, Maher L, Pryde A, Heading RC. Symptomatic gastro-oesophageal reflux, abnormal oesophageal acid exposure, and mucosal acid sensitivity are three separate, through related, aspects of gastro-oesophageal reflux disease. *Gut* 1991;32:128–132.
11. Pace F, Santalucia F, Bianchi Porro G. Natural history of gastro-oesophageal reflux disease without oesophagitis. *Gut* 1991;32:845–848.
12. Armstrong D, Bennett JR, Blum AL, et al. The endoscopic assessment of esophagitis: a progress report on observer agreement. *Gastroenterology* 1996;111:85–92.
13. Knuff TE, Benjamin SB, Worsham GF, Hancock JE, Castell DO. Histologic evaluation of chronic gastroesophageal reflux. An evaluation of biopsy methods and diagnostic criteria. *Dig Dis Sci* 1984;29:194–201.
14. Frierson HF Jr. Histological criteria for the diagnosis of reflux esophagitis. *Pathol Annu* 1992;27(pt 1):87–104.
15. Riddell RH. The biopsy diagnosis of gastroesophageal reflux disease, "carditis," and Barrett's esophagus, and sequelae of therapy. *Am J Surg Pathol* 1996;20(suppl 1):S31–S51.
16. Schindlbeck NE, Wiebecke B, Klauser AG, Voderholzer WA, Müller-Lissner SA. Diagnostic value of histology in non-erosive gastro-oesophageal reflux disease. *Gut* 1996;39:151–154.
17. Collins BJ, Elliott H, Sloan JM, McFarland RJ, Love AHG. Oesophageal histology in reflux oesophagitis. *J Clin Pathol* 1985;38:1265–1272.
18. Black DD, Haggitt RC, Orenstein SR, Whitington PF. Esophagitis in infants. Morphometric histological diagnosis and correlation with measures of gastroesophageal reflux. *Gastroenterology* 1990;98:1408–1414.
19. Fink SM, Barwick KW, Winchenbach CL, DeLuca V, McCallum RW. Reassessment of esophageal histology in normal subjects: a comparison of suction and endoscopic techniques. *J Clin Gastroenterol* 1983;5:177–183.
20. Jessurun J, Yardley JH, Giardiello FM, Hamilton SR. Intracytoplasmic plasma proteins in distended esophageal squamous cells (balloon cells). *Mod Pathol* 1988;1:175–181.
21. Vadva MD, Triadafilopoulous G. Glycogenic acanthosis of the esophagus and gastroesophageal reflux. *J Clin Gastroenterol* 1993;17:79–83.
22. Geboes K, Desmet V, Vantrappen G, Mebis J. Vascular changes in the esophageal mucosa. An early histologic sign of esophagitis. *Gastrointest Endosc* 1980;26:29–32.
23. Brown LF, Goldman H, Antonioli DA. Intraepithelial eosinophils in endoscopic biopsies of adults with reflux esophagitis. *Am J Surg Pathol* 1984;8:899–905.
24. Tummala V, Barwick KW, Sontag SJ, Vlahcevic RZ, McCallum RW. The significance of intraepithelial eosinophils in the histologic diagnosis of gastroesophageal reflux. *Am J Clin Pathol* 1987;87:43–48.
25. Goldman H, Proujansky R. Allergic proctitis and gastroenteritis in children. Clinical and mucosal biopsy features in 53 cases. *Am J Surg Pathol* 1986;10:75–86.
26. Attwood SEA, Smyrk TC, DeMeester TR, Jones JB. Esophageal eosinophilia with dysphagia. A distinct clinicopathologic syndrome. *Dig Dis Sci* 1993;38:109–116.
27. Wang HH, Mangano MM, Antonioli DA. Evaluation of T-lymphocytes in esophageal mucosal biopsies. *Mod Pathol* 1994;7:55–58.
28. Genta RM, Huberman RM, Graham DY. The gastric cardia in *Helicobacter pylori* infection. *Hum Pathol* 1994;25:915–919.
29. Clark GWB, Ireland AP, Chandrasoma P, DeMeester TR, Peters JH, Bremner CG. Inflammation and metaplasia in the transitional epithelium of the gastroesophageal junction: a new marker for gastroesophageal reflux disease. *Gastroenterology* 1994;106:A63.
30. Sutton FM, Graham DY, Goodgame RW. Infectious esophagitis. *Gastrointest Endosc Clin North* 1994;4:713–729.
31. Altman C, Bedossa P, Dussaix E, Buffet C. Cytomegalovirus infection of the esophagus in an immunocompetent adult. *Dig Dis Sci* 1995;40:606–608.
32. Galbraith JC, Shafran SD. Herpes simplex esophagitis in the immunocompetent patient: report of four cases and review. *Clin Infect Dis* 1992;14:894–901.
33. Teot LA, Ducatman BS, Geisinger KR. Cytologic diagnosis of cytomegaloviral esophagitis. A report of three acquired immunodeficiency syndrome-related cases. *Acta Cytol* 1993;37:93–96.
34. Haulk AA, Sugar AM. Candida esophagitis. *Adv Intern Med* 1991;36:307–318.
35. McBane RD, Gross JB Jr. Herpes esophagitis: clinical symptoms, endoscopic appearance, and diagnosis in 23 patients. *Gastrointest Endosc* 1991;37:600–603.

36. Greenson JK, Beschorner WE, Boitnott JK, Yardley JH. Prominent mononuclear cell infiltrate is characteristic of herpes esophagitis. *Hum Pathol* 1991;22:541–549.
37. Wilcox CM, Straub RF, Schwartz DA. Prospective endoscopic characterization of cytomegalovirus esophagitis in AIDS. *Gastrointest Endosc* 1994;40:481–484.
38. Greenson JK. Macrophage aggregates in cytomegalovirus esophagitis. *Hum Pathol* 1997;28:375–378.
39. Hamilton SR. Esophagitis. In: Ming S-C, Goldman H, eds. *Pathology of the gastrointestinal tract*. Philadelphia: WB Saunders, 1992:383–438.
40. Walsh TJ, Belitsos NJ, Hamilton SR. Bacterial esophagitis in immunocompromised patients. *Arch Intern Med* 1986;146:1345–1348.
41. Richert SM, Orchard JL. Bacterial esophagitis associated with CD4+ T-lymphocytopenia without HIV infection. Possible role of corticosteroid treatment. *Dig Dis Sci* 1995;40:183–185.
42. Chang AD, Drachenberg CI, James JP. Bacillary angiomatosis associated with extensive esophageal polyposis: a new mucocutaneous manifestation of acquired immunodeficiency disease (AIDS). *Am J Gastroenterol* 1996;91:2220–2223.
43. Rabeneck L, Popovic M, Gartner S, et al. Acute HIV infection presenting with painful swallowing and esophageal ulcers. *JAMA* 1990;263:2318–2322.
44. Wilcox CM, Zaki SR, Coffield LM, Greer PW, Schwartz DA. Evaluation of idiopathic esophageal ulceration for human immunodeficiency virus. *Mod Pathol* 1995;8:568–572.
45. Moore WR. Caustic ingestions. Pathophysiology, diagnosis, and treatment. *Clin Pediatr* 1996;25:192–196.
46. Kikendall JW. Pill-induced esophageal injury. *Gastroenterol Clin North Am* 1991;20:835–846.
47. deGroen PC, Lubbe DF, Hirsch LJ, et al. Esophagitis associated with the use of alendronate. *N Engl J Med* 1996;356:1016–1021.
48. Papadimos D, Kerlin P, Harris OD. Endoscopic sclerotherapy: lessons from a necropsy study. *Gastrointest Endosc* 1986;32:269–273.
49. Soffer EE, Mitros F, Doornbos JF, Friedland J, Launspach J, Summers RW. Morphology and pathology of radiation-induced esophagitis. Double-blind study of naproxen vs placebo for prevention of radiation injury. *Dig Dis Sci* 1994;39:655–660.
50. Vitellas KM, Bennett WF, Bova JG, Johnston JC, Caldwell JH, Mayle JE. Idiopathic eosinophilic esophagitis. *Radiology* 1993;186:789–793.
51. Howden FM, Mills LR, Rubin JW. Crohn's disease of the esophagus. *Am Surg* 1994;60:656–660.
52. McDonald GB, Sullivan KM, Schuffler MD, Shulman HM, Thomas ED. Esophageal abnormalities in chronic graft-versus-host disease in humans. *Gastroenterology* 1981;80:914–921.
53. Souto P, Sofia C, Cabral JP, et al. Oesophageal lichen planus. *Eur J Gastroenterol Hepatol* 1997;9:725–727.
54. Goldenberg SP, Wain SL, Marignani P. Acute necrotizing esophagitis. *Gastroenterology* 1990;98:493–496.

Barrett's Esophagus (Columnar Epithelium-Lined Esophagus)

55. Stein HJ, Siewert JR. Barrett's esophagus: pathogenesis, epidemiology, functional abnormalities, malignant degeneration, and surgical management. *Dysphagia* 1993;8:276–288.
56. Spechler SJ, Goyal RK. The columnar-lined esophagus, intestinal metaplasia, and Norman Barrett. *Gastroenterology* 1996;110:614–621.
57. Boch JA, Shields HM, Antonioli DA, Zwas F, Sawhney RA, Trier JS. Distribution of cytokeratin markers in Barrett's specialized columnar epithelium. *Gastroenterology* 1997;112:760–765.
58. Cameron AJ, Lomboy CT. Barrett's esophagus: age, prevalence, and extent of columnar epithelium. *Gastroenterology* 1992;103:1241–1245.
59. Barham CP, Jones RL, Biddlestone LF, Hardwick RH, Shepherd NA, Barr H. Photothermal laser ablation of Barrett's oesophagus: endoscopic and histological evidence of squamous re-epithelialisation. *Gut* 1997;41:281–284.
60. Cameron AJ, Zinsmeister AR, Ballard DJ, Carney JA. Prevalence of columnar-lined (Barrett's) esophagus. Comparison of population-based clinical and autopsy findings. *Gastroenterology* 1990;99:918–922.
61. Hassall E. Columnar-lined esophagus in children. *Gastroenterol Clin North Am* 1997;26:533–548.
62. Haggitt RC. Barrett's esophagus, dysplasia, and adenocarcinoma. *Hum Pathol* 1994;25:982–993.
63. Petras RE, Sivak MV Jr, Rice TW. Barrett's esophagus. A review of the pathologist's role in diagnosis and management. *Pathol Annu* 1991;26(pt 2):1–32.
64. Weston AP, Krmpotich P, Makdisi WF, et al. Short segment Barrett's esophagus: clinical and histological features, associated endoscopic findings, and association with gastric metaplasia. *Am J Gastroenterol* 1996;91:981–986.
65. Nandurkar S, Talley NJ, Martin CJ, Ng THK, Adams S. Short segment Barrett's oesophagus: prevalence, diagnosis and associations. *Gut* 1997;40:710–715.
66. Hamilton SR, Smith RRL, Cameron JL. Prevalence and characteristics of Barrett esophagus in patients with adenocarcinoma of the esophagus or esophagogastric junction. *Hum Pathol* 1988;19:942–948.
67. Cameron AJ, Lomboy CT, Pera M, Carpenter HA. Adenocarcinoma of the esophagogastric junction and Barrett's esophagus. *Gastroenterology* 1995;109:1541–1546.
68. Sharma P, Morales TG, Bhattacharyya A, Garewal HS, Sampliner RE. Dysplasia in short-segment Barrett's esophagus: a prospective 3-year follow-up. *Am J Gastroenterol* 1997;92:2012–2016.
69. Paull A, Trier JS, Dalton MD, Camp RC, Loeb P, Goyal RK. The histologic spectrum of Barrett's esophagus. *N Engl J Med* 1976;295:476–480.
70. Rothery GA, Patterson JE, Stoddard CJ, Day DW. Histological and histochemical changes in the columnar lined (Barrett's) oesophagus. *Gut* 1986;27:1062–1068.
71. Gottfried MR, McClave SA, Boyce HW. Incomplete intestinal metaplasia in the diagnosis of columnar lined esophagus (Barrett's esophagus). *Am J Clin Pathol* 1989;92:741–746.
72. Qualman SJ, Murray RD, McClung HJ, Lucas J. Intestinal metaplasia is age related in Barrett's esophagus. *Arch Pathol Lab Med* 1990;114:1236–1240.
73. Zwas F, Shields HM, Doos WG, et al. Scanning electron microscopy of Barrett's epithelium and its correlation with light microscopy and mucin stains. *Gastroenterology* 1986;90:1932–1941.
74. Krishnamurthy S, Dayal Y. Pancreatic metaplasia in Barrett's esophagus. An immunohistochemical study. *Am J Surg Pathol* 1995;19:12172–1180.
75. Loffeld RJ, Ten Tije BJ, Arends JW. Prevalence and significance of Helicobacter pylori in patients with Barrett's esophagus. *Am J Gastroenterol* 1992;87:1598–1600.
76. Craig RM, Carlson S, Nordbrock HA, Yokoo H. Pyogenic granuloma in Barrett's esophagus mimicking esophageal carcinoma. *Gastroenterology* 1995;108:1894–1896.
77. Offner FA, Lewin KJ, Weinstein WM. Metaplastic columnar cells in Barrett's esophagus: a common and neglected cell type. *Hum Pathol* 1996;27:885–889.
78. Spechler SJ, Zeroogian JM, Antonioli DA, Wang HH, Goyal RK. Prevalence of metaplasia at the gastro-oesophageal junction. *Lancet* 1994;344:1533–1536.
79. Trudgill NJ, Suvarna SK, Kapur KC, Riley SA. Intestinal metaplasia at the squamocolumnar junction in patients attending for diagnostic gastroscopy. *Gut* 1997;41:585–589.
80. Weston AP, Krmpotich PT, Cherian R, Dixon A, Topalovski M. Prospective evaluation of intestinal metaplasia and dysplasia within the cardia of patients with Barrett's esophagus. *Dig Dis Sci* 1997;42:597–602.
81. Chandrasoma P. Pathophysiology of Barrett's esophagus. *Sem Thorac Cardiovasc Surg* 1997;9:270–278.
82. Cameron AJ, Ott BJ, Payne WS. The incidence of adenocarcinoma in columnar-lined (Barrett's) esophagus. *N Engl J Med* 1985;313:857–859.
83. Hameeteman W, Tytgat GNJ, Houthoff HJ, van den Tweel JG. Barrett's esophagus: development of dysplasia and adenocarcinoma. *Gastroenterology* 1989;96:1249–1256.
84. Drewitz DJ, Sampliner RE, Garewell HS. The incidence of adenocarcinoma in Barrett's esophagus: a prospective study of 170 patients followed 4.8 years. *Am J Gastroenterol* 1997;92:212–215.
85. Iftikhar SY, James PD, Steele RJC, Hardcastle JD, Atkinson M. Length of Barrett's oesophagus: an important factor in the development of dysplasia and adenocarcinoma. *Gut* 1992;33:1155–1158.
86. Menke-Pluymers MBE, Hop WCJ, Dees J, van Blankenstein M,

Tilanus HW. Risk factors for the development of an adenocarcinoma in columnar-lined (Barrett) esophagus. *Cancer* 1993;72:1155–1158.
87. Tytgat GNJ. Does endoscopic surveillance in esophageal columnar metaplasia (Barrett's esophagus) have any real value? *Endoscopy* 1995;27:19–26.
88. Clark GWB, Ireland AP, DeMeester TR. Dysplasia in Barrett's esophagus: diagnosis, surveillance and treatment. *Dig Dis* 1996;14: 213–227.
89. van der Burgh A, Dees J, Hop WCJ, van Blankenstein M. Oesophageal cancer is an uncommon cause of death in patients with Barrett's oesophagus. *Gut* 1996;39:5–8.
90. Wright TA, Gray MR, Morris AI, et al. Cost effectiveness of detecting Barrett's oesophagus. *Gut* 1996;39:574–579.
91. Paraf F, Fléjou JF, Potet F, Molas G, Fékété F. Esophageal squamous carcinoma in five patients with Barrett's esophagus. *Am J Gastroenterol* 1992;87:746–750.
92. Lewin KJ, Appelman HD. *Tumors of the esophagus and stomach.* (Atlas of tumor pathology; 3rd series, fascicle 18). Washington, DC: Armed Forces Institute of Pathology, 1996.
93. Reid BJ, Weinstein WM, Lewin KJ, et al. Endoscopic biopsy can detect high-grade dysplasia or early adenocarcinoma in Barrett's esophagus without grossly recognizable neoplastic lesions. *Gastroenterology* 1988;94:81–90.
94. McArdle JE, Lewin KJ, Randall G, Weinstein W. Distribution of dysplasias and early invasive carcinoma in Barrett's esophagus. *Hum Pathol* 1992;23:479–482.
95. Riddell RH. Premalignant and early malignant lesions in the gastrointestinal tract: definitions, terminology, and problems. *Am J Gastroenterol* 1996;91:864–872.
96. Reid BJ, Haggitt RC, Rubin CE, et al. Observer variation in the diagnosis of dysplasia in Barrett's esophagus. *Hum Pathol* 1988;19: 166–178.
97. Levine DS. Management of dysplasia in the columnar-lined esophagus. *Gastroenterol Clin North Am* 1997;26:613–634.
98. Robertson CS, Mayberry JF, Nicholson DA, James PD, Atkinson M. Value of endoscopic surveillance in the detection of neoplastic change in Barrett oesophagus. *Br J Surg* 1988;75:760–763.
99. Reid BJ, Blount PL, Rubin CE, Levine DS, Haggitt RC, Rabinovitch PS. Predictors of progression to malignancy in Barrett's esophagus: endoscopic, histologic, and flow cytometric follow-up of a cohort. *Gastroenterology* 1992;102:1212–1219.
100. Wright TA. High-grade dysplasia in Barrett's oesophagus. *Br J Surg* 1997;84:760–766.
101. Levine DS, Haggitt RC, Blount PL, Rabinovitch PS, Rusch VW, Reid BJ. An endoscopic biopsy protocol can differentiate high-grade dysplasia from early adenocarcinoma in Barrett's esophagus. *Gastroenterology* 1993;105:40–50.
102. Cameron AJ, Carpenter HA. Barrett's esophagus, high-grade dysplasia, and early adenocarcinoma: a pathological study. *Am J Gastroenterol* 1997;92:586–591.
103. Reid BJ, Barrett MT, Galipeau PC, et al. Barrett's esophagus: ordering the events that lead to cancer. *Eur J Cancer Prev* 1996;5(suppl 2):57–65.
104. Souza RF, Meltzer SJ. The molecular basis for carcinogenesis in metaplastic columnar-lined esophagus. *Gastroenterol Clin North Am* 1997;26:583–597.
105. Reid BJ, Blount PL, Rubin CE, Levine DS, Haggitt RC, Rabinovitch PS. Flow-cytometric and histological progression to malignancy in Barrett's esophagus: prospective endoscopic surveillance of a cohort. *Gastroenterology* 1992;102:1212–1219.
106. Montgomery EA, Hartmann DP, Carr NJ, Holterman DA, Sobin LH, Azumi N. Barrett esophagus with dysplasia. Flow cytometric DNA analysis of routine, paraffin-embedded mucosal biopsies. *Am J Clin Pathol* 1996;106:298–304.
107. Hardwick RH, Shepard NA, Moorghen M, Newcomb PV, Alderson D. Adenocarcinoma arising in Barrett's oesophagus: evidence for the participation of p53 dysfunction in the dysplasia/carcinoma sequence. *Gut* 1994;35:764–768.
108. Polkowski W, van Lanschot JJ, Ten Kate FJ, et al. The value of p53 and Ki67 as markers for tumour progression in the Barrett's dysplasia-carcinoma sequence. *Surg Oncol* 1995;4:163–171.
109. Hong MK, Laskin WB, Herman BE, et al. Expansion of the Ki-67 proliferative compartment correlates with the degree of dysplasia in Barrett's esophagus. *Cancer* 1995;75:423–429.
110. Hardwick RH, Shepard NA, Moorghen M, Newcomb PV, Alderson D. c-erbB-2 overexpression in the dysplasia/carcinoma sequence of Barrett's oesophagus. *J Clin Pathol* 1995;48:129–132.
111. Brito MJ, Filipe MI, Linehan J, Jankowski J. Association of transforming growth factor alpha (TGFA) and its precursors with malignant change in Barrett's epithelium: biological and clinical variables. *Int J Cancer* 1995;60:27–32.

Neuromuscular Disorders

112. Iver SK, Chandrasekhara KL, Sutton A. Diffuse muscular hypertrophy of esophagus. *Am J Med* 1986;80:840–849.
113. Heald J, Moussalli H, Hasleton PS. Diffuse leiomyomatosis of the oesophagus. *Histopathology* 1986;10:755–759.
114. Goldblum JR, Whyte RI, Orringer MB, Appelman HD. Achalasia: a morphologic study of 42 resected specimens. *Am J Surg Pathol* 1994;18:327–337.
115. Goldblum JR, Rice TW, Richter JE. Histopathologic features in esophagomyotomy specimens from patients with achalasia. *Gastroenterology* 1996;111:648–654.
116. Sandler RS, Nyren O, Okborn A, Eisen GM, Yuen J, Josefsson S. The risk of esophageal cancer in patients with achalasia: a population-based study. *JAMA* 1995;274:1359–1362.
117. Ellis FH Jr, Gibb SP, Balogh K, Schwaber JR. Esophageal achalasia and adenocarcinoma in Barrett's esophagus: a report of two cases and a review of the literature. *Dis Esophagus* 1997;10:55–60.

Benign Tumors and Tumor-like Lesions

118. Odze R, Antonioli D, Shocket D, Noble-Topham S, Goldman H, Upton M. Esophageal squamous papillomas: a clinicopathologic study of 38 lesions and analysis for human papillomavirus by the polymerase chain reaction. *Am J Surg Pathol* 1993;17:803–812.
119. Carr NJ, Bratthauer GL, Lichy JH, Taubenberger JK, Monihan JM, Sobin LH. Squamous cell papillomas of the esophagus: a study of 23 lesions for human papillomavirus by in situ hybridization and the polymerase chain reaction. *Hum Pathol* 1994;25:536–540.
120. Takubo K, Esaki Y, Watanabe A, Umehara M, Sasajima K. Adenoma accompanied by superficial squamous cell carcinoma of the esophagus. *Cancer* 1993;71:2435–2438.
121. Paraf F, Fléjou JF, Potet F, Molas G, Fékété F. Adenomas arising in Barrett's esophagus with adenocarcinoma. Report of three cases. *Pathol Res Pract* 1992;188:1028–1032.
122. Takubo K, Nakagawa H, Tsuchiya S, Mitomo Y, Sasajima K, Shirota A. Seedling leiomyoma of the esophagus and esophagogastric junction. *Hum Pathol* 1981;12:1006–1010.
123. Avezzano EA, Fleischer DE, Merida MA, Anderson DL. Giant fibrovascular polyps of the esophagus. *Am J Gastroenterol* 1990; 85:299–302.
124. Brady PG, Nord HJ, Connar RG. Granular cell tumor of the esophagus: natural history, diagnosis, and therapy. *Dig Dis Sci* 1988; 33:1329–1333.

Squamous Cell Carcinoma

125. Geisinger KR. Endoscopic biopsies and cytologic brushings of the esophagus are diagnostically complementary. *Am J Clin Pathol* 1995;103:290–295.
126. Tavani A, Negri E, Franceschi S, LaVecchia C. Risk factors for esophageal cancer in women in Northern Italy. *Cancer* 1993; 72:2531–2536.
127. Chang F, Syrjänen S, Shen Q, Wang L, Syrjänen K. Screening for human papillomavirus infections in esophageal squamous cell carcinomas by in situ hybridization. *Cancer* 1993;72:2525–2530.
128. Ashworth MT, Nash JRG, Ellis A, Day DW. Abnormalities of differentiation and maturation in the oesophageal squamous epithelium of patients with tylosis: morphologic features. *Histopathology* 1991;19:303–310.
129. Galandiuk S, Hermann RE, Cosgrove DM, Gassman JJ. Cancer of the esophagus. The Cleveland Clinic experience. *Ann Surg* 1986; 203:101–108.
130. Sarbia M, Porschen P, Borchard F, Horstmann O, Willers R, Gabbert HE. Incidence and prognostic significance of vascular and neural in-

vasion in squamous cell carcinomas of the esophagus. *Int J Cancer* 1995;61:333–336.
131. Kato H, Tachimori Y, Watanabe H, et al. Intramural metastases of thoracic esophageal carcinoma. *Int J Cancer* 1992;50:49–52.
132. Akiyama H, Tsurumaru M, Kawamura T, Ono Y. Principles of surgical treatment for carcinoma of the esophagus. Analysis of lymph node involvement. *Ann Surg* 1981;194:438–445.
133. Ide H, Nakamura T, Hayashi K, et al. Esophageal squamous cell carcinoma: pathology and prognosis. *World J Surg* 1994;18:321–330.
134. Sons HU, Borchard F. Esophageal cancer. Autopsy findings in 171 cases. *Arch Pathol Lab Med* 1984;108:983–988.
135. Lal N, Bhasin DK, Malik AK, Gupta NM, Singh K, Mehta SK. Optimal number of biopsy specimens in the diagnosis of carcinoma of the oesophagus. *Gut* 1992;33:724–726.
136. Sugimachi K, Matsuura H, Kai H, Kanematsu T, Inokuchi K, Jingu K. Prognostic factors of esophageal carcinoma: univariate and multivariate analyses. *J Surg Oncol* 1986;31:108–112.
137. Ellis FH Jr, Heatley GJ, Krasna MJ, Williamson WA, Balogh K. Esophagogastrectomy for carcinoma of the esophagus and cardia: a comparison of findings and results after standard resection in three consecutive eight-year intervals with improved staging criteria. *J Thorac Cardiovasc Surg* 1997;113:836–846.
138. Izbicki JR, Hosch SB, Pichlmeier U, et al. Prognostic value of immunohistochemically identifiable tumor cells in lymph nodes of patients with completely resected esophageal cancer. *N Engl J Med* 1997;337:1188–1194.
139. Robey-Cafferty SS, El-Naggar AK, Sahin AA, Bruner JM, Ro JY, Cleary KR. Prognostic factors in esophageal squamous carcinoma. A study of histologic features, blood group expression, and DNA ploicy. *Am J Clin Pathol* 1991;95:844–849.
140. Kato H, Tachimori Y, Watanabe H, Iizuka T. Evaluation of the new (1987) TNM classification for thoracic esophageal tumors. *Int J Cancer* 1993;53:220–223.
141. Doki Y, Shiozaki H, Tahara H, et al. Prognostic value of DNA ploidy in squamous cell carcinoma of esophagus. Analyzed with improved flow cytometric measurement. *Cancer* 1993;72:1813–1818.
142. Shimaya K, Shiozaki H, Inoue M, et al. Significance of p53 expression as a prognostic factor in oesophageal squamous cell carcinoma. *Virchows Arch [A]* 1993;422:271–276.
143. Youssef EM, Matsuda T, Takada N, et al. Prognostic significance of the MIB-1 proliferation index for patients with squamous cell carcinoma of the esophagus. *Cancer* 1995;76:358–366.
144. Coggi G, Bosari S, Roncalli M, et al. p53 protein accumulation and p53 gene mutation in esophageal carcinoma. A molecular and immunohistochemical study with clinicopathologic correlation. *Cancer* 1997;79:425–432.
145. Tachibana M, Yoshimura H, Kinugasa S, et al. Clinicopathological features of superficial squamous cell carcinoma of the esophagus. *Am J Surg* 1997;174:49–53.
146. Schmidt LW, Dean PJ, Wilson RT. Superficially invasive squamous cell carcinoma of the esophagus. A study of seven cases in Memphis, Tennessee. *Gastroenterology* 1986;91:1456–1461.
147. Bogomoletz WV, Molas G, Gayet B, Potet F. Superficial squamous cell carcinoma of the esophagus. A report of 76 cases and review of the literature. *Am J Surg Pathol* 1989;13:535–546.
148. Yoshinaka H, Shimazu H, Fukumoto T, Baba M. Superficial esophageal carcinoma: a clinicopathological review of 59 cases. *Gastroenterology* 1991;86:1413–1418.
149. Dawsey SM, Lewin KJ. Histologic precursors of squamous esophageal cancer. *Pathol Annu* 1995;30(pt 1):209–226.
150. Mandard AM, Marnay J, Gignoux M, et al. Cancer of the esophagus and associated lesions: detailed pathologic study of 100 esophagectomy specimens. *Hum Pathol* 1984;15:660–669.
151. Jacob P, Kahrilas PJ, Desai T, et al. Natural history and significance of esophageal squamous cell dysplasia. *Cancer* 1990;65:2731–2739.
152. Dawsey SM, Wang GQ, Weinstein WM, et al. Squamous dysplasia and early esophageal cancer in the Linxian region of China: distinctive endoscopic lesions. *Gastroenterology* 1993;105:1333–1340.

Variants of Squamous Cell Carcinoma

153. Gall AA, Martin SE, Kernen JA, Patterson MJ. Esophageal carcinoma with prominent spindle cells. *Cancer* 1987;60:2244–2250.
154. Linder J, Stein RB, Roggli VL, et al. Polypoid tumor of the esophagus. *Hum Pathol* 1987;18:692–700.
155. Guarino M, Tricomi P, Giodano F, Cristofori E. Sarcomatoid carcinomas: pathological and histopathogenetic considerations. *Pathology* 1996;28:298–305.
156. Orsatti G, Corvalan AH, Sakurai H, Chai HSH. Polypoid adenosquamous carcinoma of the esophagus with prominent spindle cells. *Arch Pathol Lab Med* 1993;117:544–547.
157. Tsang WYW, Chan JKC, Lee KC, Leung AKF, Fu YT. Basaloid-squamous carcinoma of the upper aerodigestive tract and so-called adenoid cystic carcinoma of the oesophagus: the same tumour type? *Histopathology* 1991;19:35–46.
158. Epstein JI, Sears DL, Tucker RS, Eagan JW Jr. Carcinoma of the esophagus with adenoid cystic differentiation. *Cancer* 1984;53:1131–1136.
159. Agha FP, Weatherbee L, Sams JS. Verrucous carcinoma of the esophagus. *Am J Gastroenterol* 1984;79:844–849.
160. Kavin H, Yaremko L, Valaitis J, Chowdhury L. Chronic esophagitis evolving to verrucous squamous cell carcinoma: possible role of exogenous chemical carcinogens. *Gastroenterology* 1996;110:904–914.

Adenocarcinoma

161. Blot WJ, Devesa SS, Kneller RW, Fraumeni JF Jr. Rising incidence of adenocarcinoma of the esophagus and gastric cardia. *JAMA* 1991;265:1287–1289.
162. Pera M, Cameron AJ, Trastek VF, Carpenter HA, Zinsmeister AR. Increasing incidence of adenocarcinoma of the esophagus and esophagogastric junction. *Gastroenterology* 1993;104:510–513.
163. Haggitt RC, Tryzelaar J, Ellis FH Jr, Colcher H. Adenocarcinoma complicating columnar epithelium-lined (Barrett's) esophagus. *Am J Clin Pathol* 1978;70:1–5.
164. Smith RRL, Hamilton SR, Boitnott JK, Rogers EL. The spectrum of carcinoma arising in Barrett's esophagus. A clinicopathologic study of 26 patients. *Am J Surg Pathol* 1984;8:563–573.
165. Paraf F, Fléjou JF, Pignon J-P, Fékété F, Potet F. Surgical pathology of adenocarcinoma arising in Barrett's esophagus. Analysis of 67 cases. *Am J Surg Pathol* 1995;19:183–191.
166. Wasan HS, Schofield JB, Krausz T, Sikora K, Waxman J. Combined choriocarcinoma and yolk sac tumor arising in Barrett's esophagus. *Cancer* 1994;73:514–517.
167. Streitz JM Jr, Ellis FH Jr, Gibb SP, Balogh K, Watkins E Jr. Adenocarcinoma in Barrett's esophagus. A clinicopathologic study of 65 cases. *Ann Surg* 1991;213:122–125.
168. Menke-Pluymers MBE, Schoute NW, Mulder AH, Hop WCJ, van Blankenstein M, Tilanus HW. Outcome of surgical treatment of adenocarcinoma in Barrett's oesophagus. *Gut* 1992;33:1454–1458.
169. Lieberman MD, Shriver C, Bleckner S, et al. Carcinoma of the esophagus: prognostic significance of histologic type. *J Thorac Cardiovasc Surg* 1995;109:130–139.
170. de Baecque C, Potet F, Molas G, Flejou JF, Barbier P, Martignon C. Superficial adenocarcinoma of the oesophagus arising in Barrett's mucosa with dysplasia: a clinico-pathological study of 12 patients. *Histopathology* 1990;16:213–220.
171. Menke-Pluymers MB, Hop WC, Mulder AH, Tilanus HW. DNA ploidy as a prognostic factor for patients with an adenocarcinoma in Barrett's esophagus. *Hepatogastroenterology* 1995;42:786–788.
172. Moskaluk CA, Heitmiller R, Zahurak M, Schwab D, Sidransky D, Hamilton SR. p53 and p21 (WAF1/CIP1/SDI1) gene products in Barrett esophagus and adenocarcinoma of the esophagus and esophagogastric junction. *Hum Pathol* 1996;27:1211–1220.
173. Yacoub L, Goldman H, Odze RD. Transforming growth factor-alpha, epidermal growth factor receptor, and MIB-1 expression in Barrett's-associated neoplasia: correlation with prognosis. *Mod Pathol* 1997;10:105–112.
174. Borhan-Manesh F, Farnum JB. Incidence of heterotopic gastric mucosa in the upper oesophagus. *Gut* 1991;32:968–972.
175. Christensen WN, Sternberg SS. Adenocarcinoma of the upper esophagus arising in ectopic gastric mucosa. Two case reports and review of the literature. *Am J Surg Pathol* 1987;11:397–402.
176. Kalish RJ, Clancy PE, Orringer MB, Appleman HD. Clinical, epidemiologic, and morphologic comparison between adenocarcinomas arising in Barrett's esophageal mucosa and in the gastric cardia. *Gastroenterology* 1984;86:461–467.
177. Wang HH, Antonioli DA, Goldman H. Comparative features of esophageal and gastric adenocarcinoma: recent changes in type and frequency. *Hum Pathol* 1986;17:482–487.

178. Clark GWB, Smyrk TC, Burdiles P, et al. Is Barrett's metaplasia the source of adenocarcinoma of the cardia? *Arch Surg* 1994;129:609–614.

Other Malignant Neoplasms

179. Briggs JC, Ibrahim NBN. Oat cell carcinoma of the oesophagus: a clinicopathological study of 23 cases. *Histopathology* 1983;7:261–277.
180. Casas F, Ferrer F, Farrus B, Casals J, Biete A. Primary small cell carcinoma of the esophagus: a review of the literature with emphasis on therapy and prognosis. *Cancer* 1997;80:1366–1372.
181. Kuwano H, Ueo H, Sugimachi K, Inokuchi K, Toyoshima S, Enjoji M. Glandular or mucus-secreting components in squamous cell carcinoma of the esophagus. *Cancer* 1985;56:514–518.
182. Pascal RR, Clearfield HR. Mucoepidermoid (adenosquamous) carcinoma arising in Barrett's esophagus. *Dig Dis Sci* 1987;32:428–432.
183. Bombi JA, Riverola A, Bordas JM, Cardesa A. Adenosquamous carcinoma of the esophagus. A case report. *Pathol Res Pract* 1991;187:514–519.
184. Bell-Thomson J, Haggitt RC, Ellis FH Jr. Mucoepidermoid and adenoid cystic carcinomas of the esophagus. *J Thorac Cardiovasc Surg* 1980;79:438–446.
185. Sasajima K, Watanabe M, Takubo K, Takai A, Yamashita K, Onda M. Mucoepidermoid carcinoma of the esophagus: report of two cases and review of the literature. *Endoscopy* 1990;22:140–143.
186. De Mik JI, Kooijman CD, Hoekstra JB, Tytgat GN. Primary malignant melanoma of the oesophagus. *Histopathology* 1992;20:77–79.
187. DeMatos P, Wolfe WG, Shea CR, Prieto VG, Seigler HF. Primary malignant melanoma of the esophagus. *J Surg Oncol* 1997;66:201–206.
188. Guzman RP, Wightman R, Ravinsky E, Unruh HW. Primary malignant melanoma of the esophagus with diffuse melanocytic atypia and melanoma in situ. *Am J Clin Pathol* 1989;92:802–804.
189. Sharma SS, Venkateswaran S, Chacko A, Mathan M. Melanosis of the esophagus. An endoscopic, histochemical, and ultrastructural study. *Gastroenterology* 1991;100:13–16.
190. Siegal A, Swartz A. Malignant carcinoid of oesophagus. *Histopathology* 1986;10:761–765.
191. Mori M, Watanabe M, Tanaka S, Mimori K, Kuwano H, Sugimachi K. Epstein-Barr virus-associated carcinomas of the esophagus and stomach. *Arch Pathol Lab Med* 1994;118:998–1001.
192. Bloch MJ, Iozzo RV, Edmunds LH Jr, Brooks JJ. Polypoid synovial sarcoma of the esophagus. *Gastroenterology* 1987;92:229–232.
193. McIntyre M, Webb JN, Browning GCP. Osteosarcoma of the esophagus. *Hum Pathol* 1982;13:680–682.
194. Gelb AB, Medeiros LJ, Chen YY, Weiss LM, Weidner N. Hodgkin's disease of the esophagus. *Am J Clin Pathol* 1997;108:593–598.

Miscellaneous Esophageal Lesions

195. Bender MD, Allison J, Cuaratas F, Montgomery C. Glycogenic acanthosis of the esophagus: a form of benign epithelial hyperplasia. *Gastroenterology* 1973;65:373–380.
196. Arbona JL, Fazzi JG, Mayoral J. Congenital esophageal cysts: case report and review of the literature. *Am J Gastroenterol* 1984;79:177–182.
197. Nobuhara KK, Gorski YC, La Quaglia MP, Shamberger RC. Bronchogenic cysts and esophageal duplications: common origins and treatment. *J Pediatr Surg* 1997;32:1408–1413.
198. Medeiros LJ, Doos WG, Balogh K. Esophageal intramural pseudodiverticulosis: a report of two cases with analysis of similar, less extensive changes in "normal" autopsy esophagi. *Hum Pathol* 1988;19:928–931.
199. Herter B, Dittler HJ, Wuttge-Hannig A, Siewert JR. Intramural pseudodiverticulosis of the esophagus: a case series. *Endoscopy* 1997;29:109–113.
200. Spitz L. Esophageal atresia: past, present, and future. *J Pediatr Surg* 1996;31:19–25.
201. Groote AD, Laurini RN, Polman HA. A case of congenital esophageal stenosis. *Hum Pathol* 1985;16:1170–1171.
202. DeVault KR. Lower esophageal (Schatzki's) ring: pathogenesis, diagnosis and therapy. *Dig Dis* 1996;14:323–329.
203. Watemberg S, Landau O, Avrahami R. Zenker's diverticulum: reappraisal. *Am J Gastroenterol* 1996;91:1494–1498.

CHAPTER 32

The Stomach

David A. Owen

NORMAL APPEARANCES

The normal stomach (1) is lined by a complex mucosa. This consists of surface epithelium, below which are the pits and the more deeply located gastric glands (Fig. 1). The epithelium lining the surface and pits is similar throughout the stomach and consists of a single layer of columnar cells, all of which contain mucus in the superficial cytoplasm (Fig. 1). The histologic appearance of the mucus varies depending on which type of hematoxylin and eosin (H&E) staining is used. With alcoholic eosin, the mucus is either completely clear or stains a very pale pink. In contrast, aqueous eosin stains the mucus a deep pinkish or reddish color.

The glands vary in the different mucosal zones. The cardiac zone, which extends for 1 to 2 cm distal to the lower end of the esophagus, has loosely packed mucus-secreting glands, some of which may be cystic. It appears that, in some individuals, this zone may be small and irregular, so that biopsies from the "cardia" fail to reveal cardiac mucosa. This has led to speculation that cardiac mucosa is really not a normal histologic feature but is the result of metaplasia, resulting from acid reflux. Autopsy studies on neonates and small babies appear to have disproved this suggestion and confirmed that cardiac mucosa is a normal finding. The pyloric region, which corresponds roughly to the gastric antrum, occupies the distal 3 to 4 cm of the stomach. However, this zone is irregular, and pyloric mucosa is found more proximally along the lesser curvature than along the greater curvature. Pyloric glands are similar to cardiac glands, although cysts are not a feature. The glands are mucus secreting, loosely packed, and occupy about half of the mucosal thickness. On H&E sections, the cytoplasm is lightly eosinophilic with a bubbly appearance.

The remainder of the stomach is occupied by fundic or corpus-type mucosa, which is thicker than other types because of the presence of glands specialized to produce acid and pepsin. These glands occupy 75% of the mucosal thickness and are tightly packed, with little intervening lamina propria. The parietal cells (acid producing) have a light eosinophilic cytoplasm, and the chief cells (enzyme producing) have a bluish or amphophilic cytoplasm (Fig. 2). Throughout the stomach, the epithelial cell nuclei are basally located within the cell and have a rounded or oval contour with an even distribution of chromatin and small, fine nucleoli.

None of these mucosal zones has distinct boundaries; a gradual transition between them is seen, particularly in the pyloric mucosa, where isolated parietal cells are often found within the mucous glands. Also, with age, there tends to be a shrinkage of the fundic mucosa, which is replaced by pyloric mucosa, thus moving the fundopyloric border proximally (2). This change has been referred to as pseudopyloric metaplasia. A similar gradual merging of the mucosal types is seen at the gastroduodenal junction. In biopsy diagnosis, it is important to avoid overinterpreting patches of normal small bowel mucosa in the pyloric canal as intestinal metaplasia.

Endocrine cells of the gastric mucosa are located in the gastric glands, particularly in the antrum. On routine sections (Fig. 3), they are inconspicuous, with clear, rather than granular, cytoplasm. A minority are argentaffinic, but most will stain with an argyrophilic technique, such as Grimelius or Churukian–Schenck. In the antrum, 50% of endocrine cells are gastrin-producing G cells, 30% are serotonin-producing EC (enterochromaffin) cells, and 15% are the somatostatin-producing D cells. In the fundic mucosa, the majority of endocrine cells are enterochromaffinlike (ECL) and are histamine-producing (3), with smaller numbers of X cells (secretion product unknown) and EC cells (1).

Lymphoid tissue is sparse in the normal stomach. The superficial lamina propria between the gastric pits contains only small numbers of lymphocytes and mature plasma cells. These are predominately of B-cell origin, although small numbers of T lymphocytes also may be found. Intraepithelial lymphocytes are absent in the normal stomach. Lymphoid follicles with germinal centers are also not found in the nor-

---

D. A. Owen: Department of Pathology, Vancouver General Hospital, Vancouver, British Columbia V5Z 1M9.

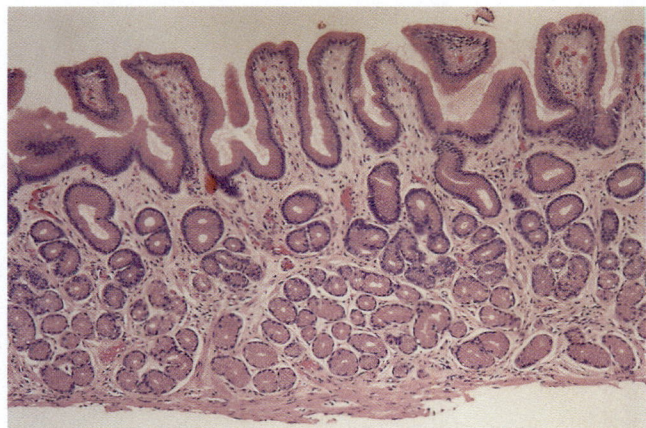

FIG. 1. Normal gastric antrum. The glands are loosely packed and occupy approximately half the mucosal thickness.

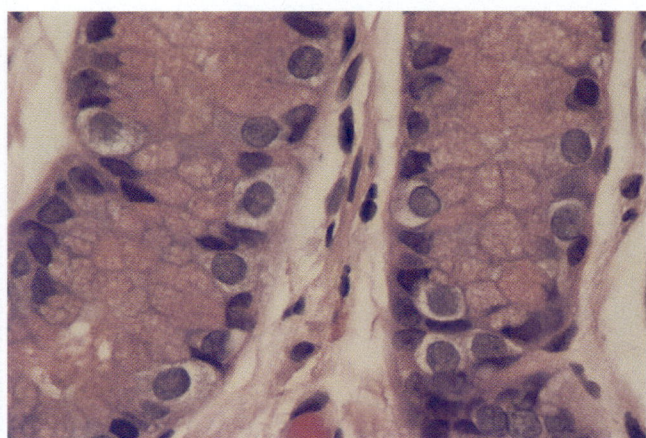

FIG. 3. Neck region of gland, showing endocrine cells with a clear cytoplasm.

mal stomach and, if present, are almost invariably indicative of *Helicobacter pylori* infection. However, the normal gastric antrum and corpus may contain small aggregates of lymphocytes without germinal centers located immediately above the muscularis mucosae (4).

Recent studies (5,6) disproved the previously held view that lymphatic channels extend to all levels of the gastric mucosa. By using careful techniques, it has been shown that lymphatics are found only in that portion of the lamina propria immediately superficial to the muscularis mucosae. This fact may well explain the observed low incidence of lymph node metastases in early gastric cancer.

BIOPSY SPECIMEN HANDLING

All gastrointestinal (GI) mucosal biopsies are delicate tissue that should be handled with care. The material should be removed gently from the biopsy forceps and fixed immediately. Ideally, the tissue should be oriented and attached to a supportive mesh, filter paper, or card before being placed into fixative. However, the success of this step is usually dependent on the clinic nurse, so that variable results might be predicted. Formalin is an adequate fixative for most purposes, although some pathologists prefer Bouin's fluid. Each biopsy specimen should be sectioned at 3 to 5 µm, and 20 to 30 serial sections should be prepared. These may be mounted on one to three slides, depending on the size of the biopsies. H&E staining is satisfactory for routine purposes; special stains are generally not required in the first instance. The ideal number of biopsies to be taken will vary with the disease present, but two should be a minimum from each area of the stomach under study.

HETEROTOPIAS, DUPLICATIONS, AND CYSTS

Ectopic pancreas (pancreatic heterotopia) in the wall of the stomach is a relatively common finding, both at surgery and at autopsy. The exact prevalence is unknown, but is of the order of 1% to 2% (7). It rarely gives rise to symptoms, but occasionally has been associated with ulceration (8), obstruction (9), and intussusception (10). Grossly, it appears typically as a firm intramural mass, 1 to 2 cm in diameter, located in the prepyloric region. The mass is spherical or hemispherical, with a nipplelike projection into the gastric lumen, at which point the ectopic ducts enter the gastric lumen. In 75% of cases, the mass is located in the submucosa, but it may be present also within the muscularis propria or subserosa. Histologically, it consists of well-differentiated ductlike structures, some of which may be dilated, and smaller ducts intimately adjacent to muscle bundles. Acinar tissue is almost invariably present to a greater or lesser degree, although islets are found in only 30% of cases (Fig. 4).

Rare histologic variants of ectopic pancreas may be encountered. Cases in which only ducts and ductular elements are present have been referred to as adenomyomas (11). Cases with mucus inspissation and duct rupture may give rise to an erroneous clinical and histologic impression of mucinous carcinoma (12). Examples in which the deep intramuscular and serosal portions of the lesion consist exclusively of islet cells may, on biopsy at the time of surgery, be difficult to distinguish from a carcinoid tumor (13).

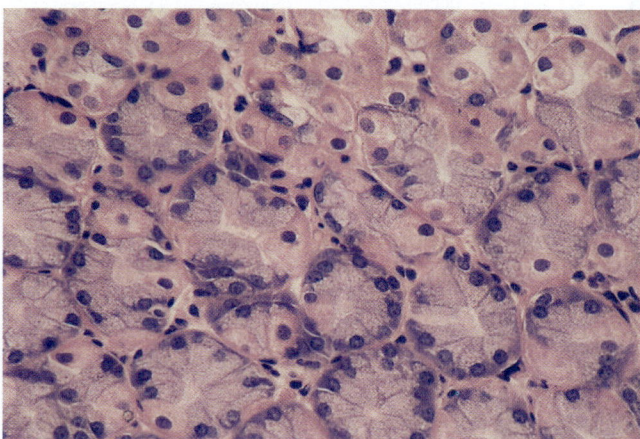

FIG. 2. Gastric fundic mucosa. The chief cells have a basophilic cytoplasm, and the parietal cells have an eosinophilic cytoplasm.

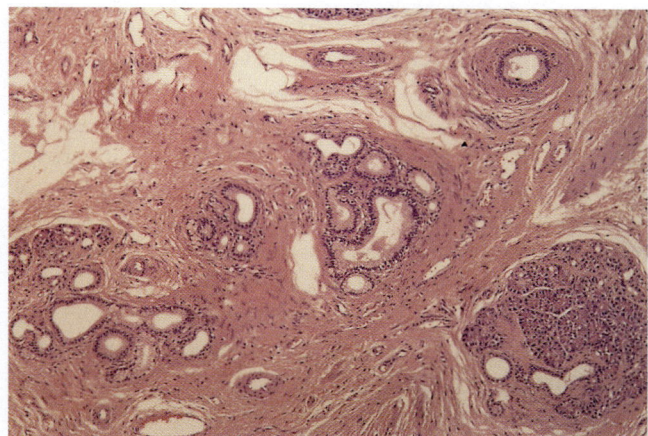

FIG. 4. Heterotopic pancreas. There is a predominance of dilated irregular ducts with a small island of acinar tissue.

The presence of heterotopic mucous glands in the gastric submucosa has been described (14). It is relatively common and occurs in 1% to 2% of the general population. These collections, which resemble Brunner's glands, may be focal or diffuse, but probably have no clinical significance.

Duplications of the stomach are distinctly uncommon. They are seen mainly in the pediatric age group and are more common in girls. There is usually a cystic mass located within the abdomen, but not necessarily attached or intimately related to the stomach (15–20). The lining consists of normal gastric mucosa with the usual muscle layers in the wall (18). Occasionally, the duplication can impinge on the gastric wall, producing overlying ulceration (19). Gastric diverticula (21) are probably an incomplete variant of duplication. In contrast, pyloric duplication is most commonly acquired and is usually the result of extensive peptic ulceration (22). True congenital pyloric duplication accounts for only 10% of cases (23).

In neonates, an accessory juxtagastric lung may occasionally be present (24). This arises from a foregut bud in the fundus, with the main mass lying alongside the stomach. Histologically, it is made up of tubular structures lined by a ciliated epithelium. The arterial supply is generally directly from the aorta.

Cysts of the stomach are an integral component of a variety of diseases, such as Ménétrier's disease and gastritis cystica profunda. Lesions of this type are discussed elsewhere. Primary cystic lesions appear to be of three types. Intramural cysts (25) are usually solitary masses, several centimeters in diameter, that are lined by respiratory epithelium. They are thought to be developmental in origin. Diffuse cystic disease of the mucosa and submucosa (26–28) is a rare condition that may be seen with a gross polypoid enlargement of the mucosa. These cysts are usually only a few millimeters in diameter and are lined by normal gastric mucosal epithelium. These, too, are considered congenital in origin, probably a form of heterotopia. Last, a variety of gastric intramucosal cysts appear to be of diverse etiologies; however, most are acquired and are metaplastic in origin (29).

XANTHELASMA

These lesions, also called xanthomas or lipid islands, have been reported in up to 53% of autopsy stomachs and in up to 4% of endoscopy biopsies (30,31). Grossly, they appear as cream-colored plaques, less than 5 mm in diameter, mostly occurring along the lesser curvature in the region of the antrum, where they may be single or multiple (32). Histologically, they consist of loosely organized aggregates of foamy histiocytes in the upper lamina propria (Fig. 5). The nuclei are bland and the cytoplasm contains lipid, which is periodic acid–Schiff (PAS) negative. These features serve to distinguish xanthelasma cells from a mucin-secreting adenocarcinoma.

The pathogenesis of xanthelasmas is unknown; they are not directly related to chronic gastritis. They are commonly found in the gastric remnant after a partial gastrectomy, and it has been postulated that bile reflux is the etiologic factor (30). Xanthelasmas have also developed in patients with cholestasis and have regressed with relief of the cholestasis (31). Biochemical analysis reveals that xanthelasmas consist of cholesterol, neutral fat, low-density lipoproteins, and oxidized low-density lipoproteins but are not linked to any type of inherited hypercholesterolemia (30,32–34).

HYPERTROPHIC PYLORIC STENOSIS

This is predominantly a disease of infants (35,36), but also may rarely affect adults (37). The infantile form is usually manifest at about age 3 weeks. It has a predilection for first-born male infants and has an inheritance pattern that is polygenetically determined. The macroscopic appearance is of a fusiform mass 3 to 5 cm in diameter, involving the pyloric sphincter in a circular fashion. The overlying mucosa may contain secondary edema and ulceration. Microscopically, the thickening involves mainly the circular muscle and has a very abrupt termination distally. The lesion is thought now to be a primary muscle disorder, and any neuronal changes present are secondary.

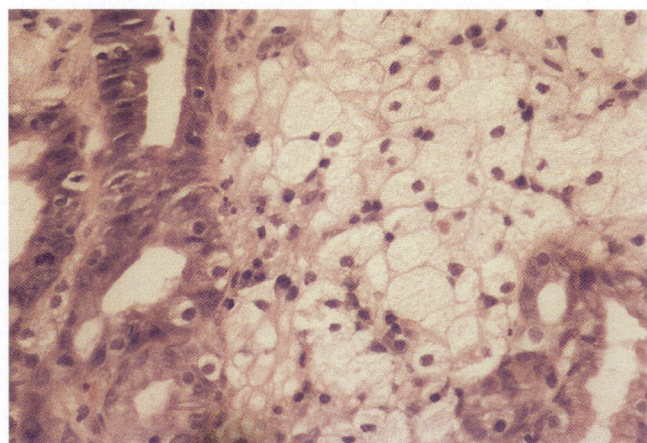

FIG. 5. Gastric xanthelasma. The lamina propria is expanded by foam cells. Note the regular inconspicuous nuclei.

Primary hypertrophic pyloric stenosis of adults is excessively rare. In addition to the circular form of hypertrophy seen in children, there are also focal and multinodular variants (37).

METAPLASIA

Pyloric Metaplasia

Pyloric metaplasia is an age-related change, in which the fundic gland mass of acid- and enzyme-secreting cells is gradually replaced by mucus-secreting pyloric-type glands (2). Presumably this change accounts for a reduction in maximal gastric acid output that may be encountered in some older people.

Ciliated Metaplasia

This type of metaplasia was recently described in North American, European, and Japanese patients. Most examples have been found incidentally in gastrectomy specimens removed for neoplasms or peptic ulcers. Ciliated cells may be found lining dilated antral glands (38,39). The cause and significance of this change are unknown.

Subnuclear Vacuolated Cells

This change in the gastric mucosa is not strictly a form of metaplasia, because it does not simulate the appearances of any other type of normal cell. Nevertheless, although it probably represents a degenerative reaction to cell injury, a discussion is included here because of possible confusion with true intestinal metaplasia. Subnuclear vacuolation may affect the antral gastric glands, Brunner's glands, and the antral pit epithelium (40,41). The vacuoles are clear with H&E stains and are PAS negative. On ultrastructural examination, they consist of a membrane-lined space, derived from either endoplasmic reticulum or Golgi, that probably contains an abnormal accumulation of nonglycoconjugated mucus core protein (40). Subnuclear vacuolated cells have been found in stomachs showing chronic gastritis and in patients with probable duodenogastric reflux.

Pancreatic Acinar Metaplasia

In this condition, single or multiple cell nests and lobules of acinar tissue are encountered among or at the base of gastric glands (42,43). These nests are surrounded by thin fibrous and smooth-muscle septa. Islets of Langerhans are not present. Initially, pancreatic acinar differentiation of the gastric mucosa was considered to be a true metaplasia, resulting from the effects of chronic gastritis (42). More recently, however, it was identified in 24% of unselected biopsies from the gastric cardia. Its lack of correlation with other biopsy abnormalities suggests that it may, in fact, be congenital in origin (43).

Intestinal Metaplasia

Stomachs with atrophic gastritis may also show intestinal metaplasia. This is a complex process, in which the superficial and pit-lining epithelium changes, both morphologically and histochemically. There are two major types of metaplasia: small-bowel metaplasia and large-bowel metaplasia. Both may be either complete or incomplete, or there may be a mixture of the two (Table 1). In incomplete metaplasia, the mucin content of the columnar cells is reduced and changes from the normal gastric neutral mucin to acidic mucin. In the case of small-bowel metaplasia, only sialomucin is produced; in large-bowel metaplasia, however, sialo- and sulfomucin are found (Fig. 6). Because there is no change in cell structure, special staining is necessary to demonstrate these changes. Neutral mucin is PAS positive and alcian blue negative at both pH 2.5 and pH 0.5. Sialomucin is PAS positive, alcian blue positive at pH 2.5, but alcian blue negative at pH 0.5. Sulfomucin is weakly PAS positive but is alcian blue positive at pH 2.5 and pH 0.5. It is also high iron diamine positive (44).

Complete intestinal metaplasia may be identified morphologically as loss of columnar mucus-secreting cells and their replacement by an epithelium that contains goblet cells and absorptive cells (Fig. 7). In the histochemical identification of intestinal metaplasia of all types, it is convenient to use a combined alcian blue, pH 2.5, and high iron diamine stain. This is a relatively simple technical procedure and will stain

TABLE 1. Histochemical identification of intestinal metaplasia

	Incomplete metaplasia		Complete metaplasia	
	Small-bowel type	Large-bowel type	Small-bowel type	Large-bowel type
Cell type	Columnar	Columnar	Goblet	Goblet
Mucin type	Sialomucin	Sulfomucin	Sialomucin	Sulfomucin
PAS/diastase	+	Weakly +	+	Weakly +
Alcian blue pH 2.5	+	+	+	+
Alcian blue pH 0.5	—	+	—	+
High iron diamine	—	+	—	+

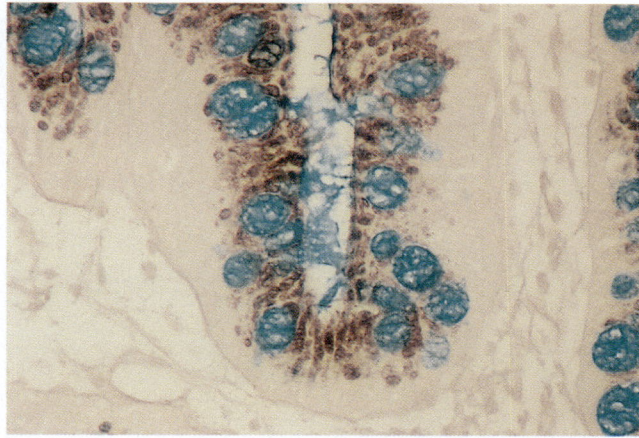

FIG. 6. Incomplete intestinal metaplasia (high iron diamine and alcian blue). The goblet cells contain sialomucin and the columnar cells contain sulphomucin.

sulfomucin brown–black and sialomucin aqua blue. In the most advanced forms of intestinal metaplasia, small villi may form, and there may be Paneth cells at the base of the glands. The significance of finding intestinal metaplasia in gastric biopsies is discussed later.

INFLAMMATORY CONDITIONS

A classification of gastritis is given in Table 2. The scheme presented is not completely satisfactory, because some entities are defined morphologically and some etiologically. This difficulty is inevitable, given the current state of knowledge; the classification may be expected to change as more information becomes available.

The term "chronic nonspecific gastritis" can no longer be regarded as a clinically useful diagnosis and has been displaced in favor of more precise terminology. This does not mean, however, that every gastric biopsy can be definitively assigned to one of the listed categories. Particularly when the

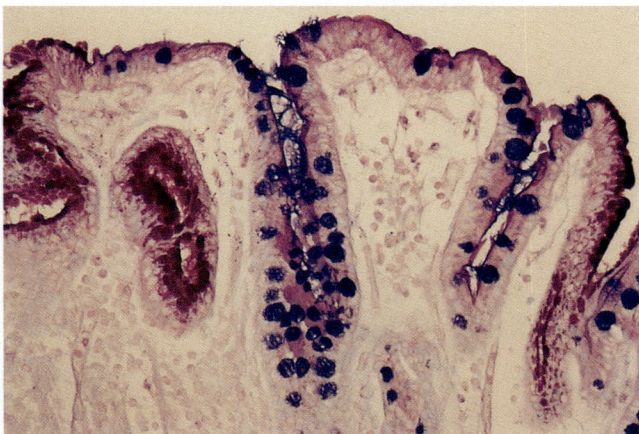

FIG. 7. Complete intestinal metaplasia [periodic acid–Schiff (PAS) and alcian blue]. The normal neutral gastric mucus stains magenta. The goblet cells, which contain acidic and neutral mucin, stain purple.

TABLE 2. *Inflammatory disease of the stomach*

Acute erosive gastritis
Suppurative gastritis
Helicobacter pylori gastritis
Autoimmune gastritis
Multifocal atrophic gastritis
Granulomatous gastritis
    Isolated granulomatous gastritis
    Crohn's disease
    Sarcoidosis
    Infectious: tuberculosis, fungal, etc.
Eosinophilic gastritis
Lymphocytic gastritis
Reactive gastropathy (chemical gastritis)
Radiation gastritis
Ischemic gastritis
Gastritis secondary to drug therapy
Gastritis in immunosuppressed patients
    Cytomegalovirus
    Herpes simplex
    Mycobacterium avium-intracellulare
    Cryptosporidiosis
    Epstein–Barr virus
Graft-versus-host disease

tissue supplied is insufficient, or shows biopsy artifact, it is still reasonable to issue a report indicating that only nonspecific inflammation is present.

Strickland and MacKay (45) originally divided chronic nonspecific gastritis into type A (associated with pernicious anemia) and type B (not associated with pernicious anemia). Other authors (46) later added a type C (chemical gastritis, related to drug therapy or bile reflux). Although these concepts are still valid, the discovery of *H. pylori* as an important cause of gastritis means that type B gastritis is now too broad a category to be clinically useful. This alphabetic terminology should now be abandoned.

The terms "superficial gastritis," "atrophic gastritis," and "gastric atrophy" are still useful for descriptive purposes and may be retained. In superficial gastritis (Fig. 8), inflammation is largely confined to the portion of mucosa occupied by the gastric pits. In atrophic gastritis (Fig. 9), inflammation involves the whole thickness of the mucosa and is accompanied by a loss of gastric glands. In gastric atrophy (Fig. 10), there is widespread, if not complete, gland loss. At this stage, inflammation is relatively scanty, and extensive complete intestinal metaplasia is frequently encountered.

A system of classification and description of gastritis, referred to as the Sydney system, has been devised by a group of pathologists and gastroenterologists (47). It was recently modified and updated (48). This is a rather complicated scheme in which there are several components, some of which are graded in a semiquantitative fashion. Full application of the system requires that a minimum of five biopsies be taken, two from antral mucosa, two from fundic mucosa, and one from the incisura. Involvement of these areas by the inflammatory process is assessed and recorded separately. The morphologic features of inflammation are evaluated by

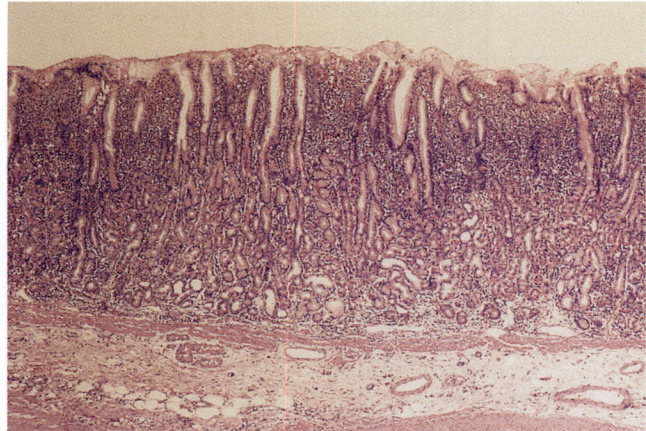

FIG. 8. Gastric antral mucosa showing a superficial gastritis.

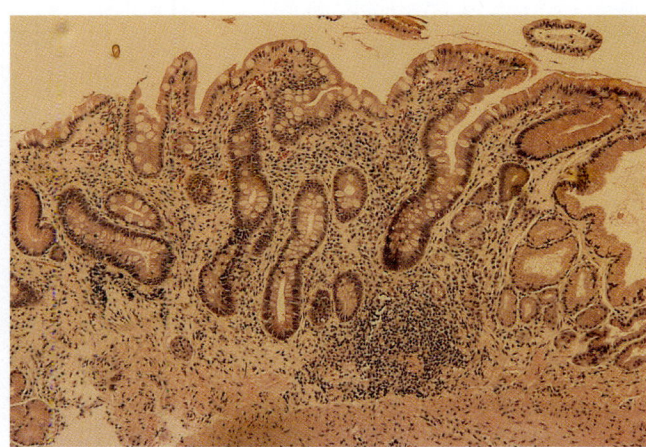

FIG. 10. Advanced intestinal metaplasia characteristic of gastric atrophy in pernicious anemia.

a series of graded (mild, moderate, or marked) or ungraded variables. The graded variables are atrophy, chronic inflammation, activity, intestinal metaplasia, and *H. pylori* density. The system provides a diagrammatic visual scale for grading (48). Ungraded variables include granulomas, eosinophils, and intraepithelial lymphocytes.

The classification of gastritis adopted in the revised Sydney system is similar to the one listed in Table 2. The system may be used to generate detailed morphologic descriptions that will imply a diagnosis. For example, a diffuse corpus-restricted chronic atrophic gastritis with intestinal metaplasia, but without *H. pylori* organisms present, is probably an example of autoimmune gastritis. The Sydney system has much to recommend it, but may be of more value in an academic institution than a community hospital. Its weakness is that it uses results in complex descriptions rather than true diagnoses. It is also questionable whether grading has much clinical utility.

Acute Erosive Gastritis

A gastric erosion may be defined as an ulcer that has not penetrated the muscularis mucosae. Erosions are a relatively common finding at gastroscopy, but biopsies of them are performed less frequently, probably because of the possibility of provoking bleeding.

There is a rather wide spectrum of severity in erosive gastritis. At one end is acute hemorrhagic gastritis, in which multiple erosions are found in a gastric mucosa that is diffusely hemorrhagic. This condition may be responsible for up to 25% of hospital admissions with acute upper GI bleeding (49). Occasionally the bleeding may be so massive that an emergency gastrectomy is required to save the patient's life. Histologic examination of these specimens reveals erosions with a base consisting of slough and necrotic tissue, beneath which is viable basal epithelium (Fig. 11), so that when healing occurs, there is regeneration of the normal mucosa with a minimum of architectural disturbance. At the edge of the erosions, the lamina propria shows intense capillary congestion, with extravasation of blood. Recently it was suggested that, in the early stages of hemorrhagic gastritis, subepithelial hemorrhage may exist without actual erosions (50).

At the other end of the spectrum of acute erosive gastritis, the disease consists only of small numbers of localized ero-

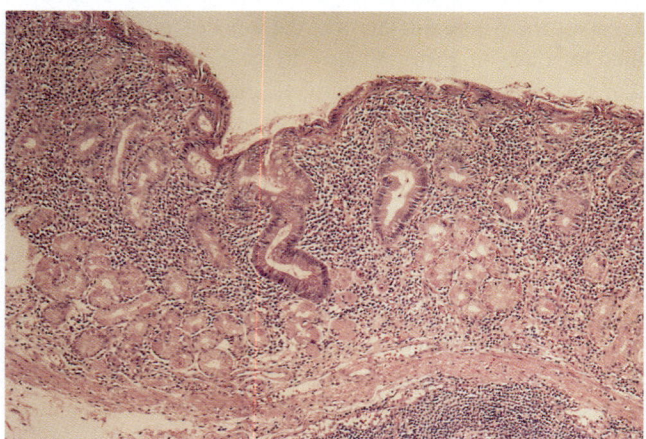

FIG. 9. Antral mucosa showing an atrophic gastritis with loss of glands.

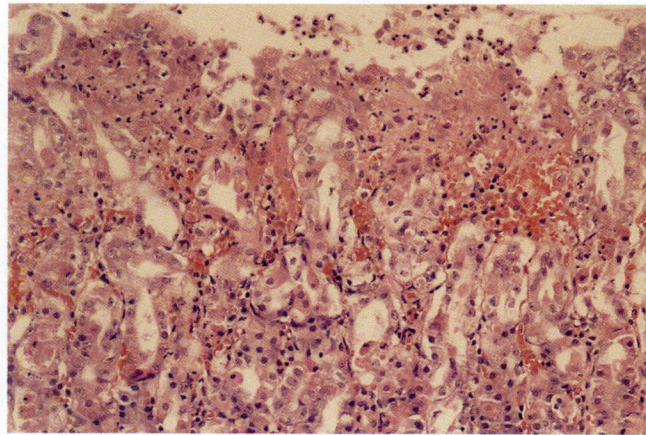

FIG. 11. Gastric erosion from a case of acute erosive gastritis.

sions present in an otherwise normal mucosa. These may ooze blood, resulting in anemia, but rarely give rise to acute symptoms. The pathology of erosive gastritis (51,52) in its various clinical forms is incompletely studied, although there is extensive literature on the etiology and pathogenesis. Recognized causes include alcohol (49), aspirin (53), other nonsteroidal antiinflammatory drugs (NSAIDs) (54), stress (shock, sepsis, and hypoxia) (55), and the presence of nasogastric tubes.

Suppurative Gastritis

Suppurative (phlegmonous) gastritis is a bacterial cellulitis, predominantly affecting the submucosal layer of the stomach. *Streptococcus* type A is the organism most commonly isolated, with occasional cases due to *Staphylococci*, *Escherichia coli*, or *Haemophilus influenzae*. Gas-forming organisms may produce submucosal bubbles (so-called emphysematous gastritis). The route of infection is presumed to be via a breach in the mucosa; predisposing factors include alcoholism, chronic renal failure, immunodeficiency, hypochlorhydria, and endoscopic polypectomy. The clinical picture is one of rigors, fever, and rapid prostration (56–58), with a high mortality rate. Grossly, the stomach shows distention, with marked thickening of the wall due to submucosal edema. Histologically, there is submucosal edema, congestion, and hemorrhage, with a massive neutrophil exudation, among which bacterial organisms can be demonstrated. Typically, the overlying mucosa may be relatively unremarkable, making the diagnosis difficult on endoscopic biopsy.

Helicobacter Gastritis

There is an enormous volume of literature describing the epidemiology, clinical features, pathology, and significance of chronic *Helicobacter* gastritis. Excellent review articles concisely summarize the current knowledge (59,60). It is generally accepted that *H. pylori* is the cause of most cases of chronic gastritis. However, there is controversy as to its natural history and outcome. In North America and Western Europe, most individuals with *H. pylori* infection have an active superficial gastritis, largely confined to the antrum, in which organisms are easily identified (diffuse antral gastritis or DAG). This type of gastritis may result in duodenal ulcer formation, probably as a result of increased basal acid output and a heightened parietal cell response to stimulation (61). It may also cause nonulcer dyspepsia, although this association is controversial. In contrast, individuals in underdeveloped countries typically have an atrophic gastritis (multifocal atrophic gastritis or MAG), which is patchy in distribution and involves both pyloric and fundal mucosa (62). *Helicobacter pylori* organisms may be more sparse in this form of gastritis, which is associated with gastric peptic ulcer and gastric carcinoma (62–64). The reasons for this geographic difference are unclear. Virulence differences among various strains of the organism cannot explain the phenomenon (65). One possibility is that individuals in Third World countries acquire the infection at an earlier age: progression from nonatrophic superficial gastritis to an atrophic gastritis simply relates to the duration of infection or the increased susceptibility of children's stomachs to sustain damage. This too, however, seems unlikely (66). The most plausible explanation is that additional, but as yet unspecified, dietary factors may be required to mediate damage leading to atrophy and intestinal metaplasia (62,63).

Acute gastritis due to *H. pylori* is rarely seen in biopsy material because the infection is usually either asymptomatic or accompanied by minor GI discomfort. The histologic features include conspicuous pit abscesses and exudation of neutrophils into the surface epithelium. This is accompanied by marked epithelial degeneration and regeneration, which may be syncytial in type (67,68). Initially, the changes affect all mucosal zones of the stomach, but later the fundal inflammation subsides, leaving only an antral gastritis.

Diffuse chronic *H. pylori* gastritis predominantly affects the pyloric mucosa, and although inflammatory changes are generally scanty in the fundus, organisms may be found in the surface mucus in all areas. The mucosa shows a dense infiltrate of chronic inflammatory cells, in which plasma cells are especially prominent. In the fundus, any inflammation present is confined to the superficial portion of the mucosa, but in the antrum, it is commonly full thickness and may surround and separate the glands without causing atrophy. Lymphoid follicles with germinal centers are usually seen, particularly in the deeper portion of the mucosa (Fig. 12). This finding, which is easy to identify on low-power microscopic examination of biopsies, is virtually pathognomonic for the presence of *H. pylori* (4). The surface and pit-lining epithelium is infiltrated by neutrophils, which may be so prominent that pit abscesses are formed (Fig. 13). This neutrophil infiltration is termed "active gastritis" and is seen predominantly in areas where the *Helicobacter* organisms are most abundant and most readily identified (Fig. 14).

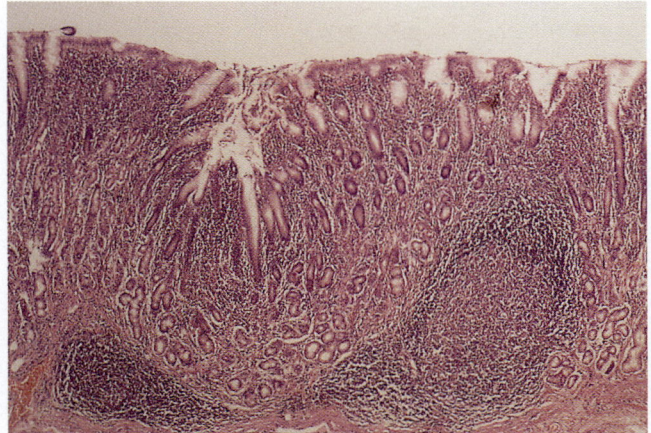

FIG. 12. Follicular gastritis. This appearance is almost invariably associated with the presence of *Helicobacter pylori* organisms.

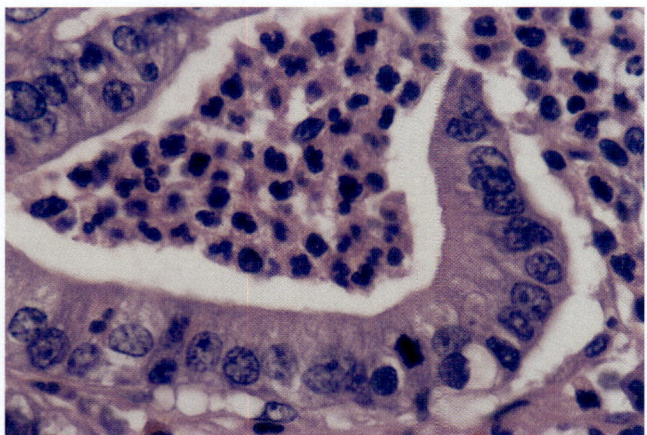

FIG. 13. Pit abscess from a case of *Helicobacter pylori* gastritis.

Usually, the bacteria are easily seen on well-differentiated H&E sections, and it is not necessary to use Giemsa, Modified Steiner, or Leung (69) stains for routine diagnosis (70). The organisms are slender, curved spirals in the superficial mucous layer, where they tend to be attached to the epithelium at the site of intercellular junctions. This location provides protection from the acid gastric contents, but permits enzymes (urease and catalase) produced by the *Helicobacter* to damage the gastric epithelium. Occasionally, *H. pylori* can be present in the stomach as coccoid forms (71). These are solid, round, basophilic, dotlike structures on routine histology. Ultrastructurally, they are U-shaped with the ends of the two arms joined by a membranous structure. Coccoid forms invariably coexist with spiral forms but can be reliably identified only by specific immunohistochemical staining (72). It is important not to confuse coccoid forms of the organism with nonpathogenic cocci or cryptosporidia.

Treatment of *H. pylori* gastritis with appropriate antibiotics will usually result in rapid elimination of organisms and abolition of the neutrophilic infiltrate. Chronic inflammation, however, may persist for several years before disappearing (73,74).

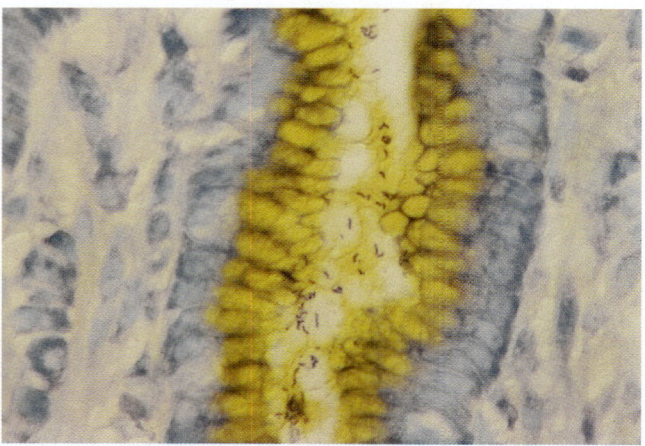

FIG. 14. *Helicobacter pylori* organisms, which are easily recognized on hematoxylin and eosin staining.

Other intragastric organisms have been rarely identified as a cause of gastritis histologically similar to *H. pylori* gastritis. These organisms, recently renamed *Helicobacter heilmanii*, have a tight corkscrew appearance that is most easily recognized on special stains (75,76).

Reactive epithelial changes accompany active gastritis and consist of cytoplasmic mucin loss with nuclear enlargement and prominent nucleoli (Fig. 13). On occasion, these reactive changes may be so prominent that difficulty is experienced in distinguishing them from dysplasia. The problem is similar to that encountered in distinguishing reactive changes in ulcerative colitis from colonic dysplasia (77). The single most useful criterion for the identification of inflammatory atypia is the presence of an associated neutrophilic infiltrate. It is, therefore, recommended that in acutely inflamed mucosa, a positive diagnosis of dysplasia should be made with extreme reluctance. It is better to issue a noncommittal report and request that repeated biopsies be taken after an interval of antibiotic therapy.

Multifocal Atrophic Gastritis

Multifocal atrophic gastritis (MAG) affects both the pyloric and fundic mucosa in a patchy fashion. The characteristic histologic feature is atrophy of the glands, which is accompanied by varying degrees of full-thickness chronic inflammation. Intestinal metaplasia is invariably present in the later stages, but may not be found with minor degrees of atrophy. Early atrophy may be difficult to recognize in situations in which there is an intense full-thickness infiltrate in the lamina propria that pushes apart adjacent glands. Because minor degrees of atrophy do not seem to be clinically important, it is recommended, therefore, that MAG should be diagnosed only when there is unequivocal evidence of mucosal atrophy. For practical purposes, this means the presence of intestinal metaplasia. Intestinal metaplasia is typically present as small patches of goblet cells and Paneth cells without the formation of villi. Adjacent to these patches, the mucosa may show active inflammation with pit abscess formation and *Helicobacter* infection (78). However, as intestinal metaplasia progresses, the gastric microenvironment changes, so that inflammation lessens and *H. pylori* organisms are eliminated (79). MAG is the commonest pattern of chronic gastritis in the Third World (80), whereas DAG is the commonest pattern in westernized countries.

The generally held opinion now is that most, but not necessarily all, examples of multifocal atrophic gastritis represent the end stage of *H. pylori* gastritis, in which the organisms have damaged the mucosa so severely that the intragastric environment is altered and conditions become inhibitory to further bacterial growth (64,79,81). Longitudinal studies suggest that, in all patients with gastritis, the severity of the disease and extent of atrophy increase with advancing age (82). However, this does not exclude the possibility that multifocal atrophic gastritis has other causes. Factors promoting atrophy and metaplasia in *H. pylori* gastritis are ill understood. However, there are theoretic grounds for believing that a lack of dietary vitamin C (83,84), intragastric nitrosamine formation (84), and salt consumption (85) may be responsible. Recent studies (86) demonstrated that patients with *H. pylori*–induced atrophic gastritis have autoantibodies that cross-react with gastric antigens. It appears possible, therefore, that autoimmunity may play a role in disease progression. Because of epidemiologic and prognostic differences, it now seems reasonable to identify separately nonatrophic and atrophic forms of *H. pylori* gastritis, as DAG and MAG, respectively. In advanced MAG, there may be hypochlorhydria, but, in contrast to autoimmune gastritis, achlorhydria and pernicious anemia do not occur.

Autoimmune Gastritis

This condition accounts for less than 5% of cases of chronic gastritis. There are usually no symptoms referable to the stomach, so biopsies are often obtained incidentally. The pathogenesis of autoimmune gastritis is, as yet, not fully elucidated; both humoral and cell-mediated reactions may be important. Parietal cell antibodies are present in the serum of 60% of patients with autoimmune gastritis who have not yet developed pernicious anemia and in 80% to 90% of patients with established pernicious anemia (62). They may rarely occur in patients with a normal mucosa. In contrast, intrinsic factor antibodies are found in only 50% to 70% of patients with pernicious anemia but are virtually specific for this condition. It is becoming apparent that a link may exist between *H. pylori* and autoimmune gastritis, through the presence of cross-reacting antibodies (86). Further work currently in progress will assess the strength of this association (87).

The early stages of autoimmune gastritis have only recently been described (88). These include a chronic inflammatory infiltrate in the lamina propria around the glands of the gastric fundus and a destruction of individual glands by infiltrating lymphocytes. The superficial mucosa is free of inflammation. In the advanced stages, when pernicious anemia may be present, the histology is that of a severe atrophic gastritis or gastric atrophy, largely confined to the fundic mucosa (45). There is a diffuse mucosal thinning, with partial or complete loss of acid- and enzyme-secreting cells of the fundic glands, and a variable increase of chronic inflammatory cells within the lamina propria; however, lymphoid follicles and an active gastritis are not usually present (Fig. 10). The surface and pit-lining epithelium generally shows patchy complete intestinal metaplasia with goblet cell formation. Less commonly, villi and Paneth cells may be encountered (89).

Because patients with autoimmune gastritis have hypochlorhydria or achlorhydria, they also develop a compensatory hyperplasia of antral G cells with hypergastrinemia. In the fundus, there can also be ECL cell hyperplasia. In the early stages of hyperplasia, increased numbers of endocrine cells line the lower pit and glandular portion of the mucosa in a linear fashion. These cells may be recognized by their clear cytoplasm and are present as a single layer. In the later stages, nodular hyperplasia of fundic ECL cells and microcarcinoid tumors can develop (see later section on endocrine tumors).

Carditis

Inflammation of the cardia of the stomach (carditis) is a recently described condition that is of particular interest, because of a possible relation to gastroesophageal reflux, short-segment Barrett's esophagus, and gastric cardiac cancer. Discussion of this topic is, however, hampered by certain practical considerations, revolving around the definition and delineation of the normal gastroesophageal junction. By strict anatomic criteria, this junction occurs where the tubular esophagus becomes the saccular stomach. The squamocolumnar junction may coincide with the anatomic junction, but may also be found as much as 3.0 cm proximal to this point. The intervening lower end of the esophagus is lined by cardiac-type mucosa. By endoscopic examination, the squamocolumnar junction is generally easily recognized, but it is frequently difficult to define the anatomic esophagogastric junction. By histologic examination, it is impossible to tell whether a biopsy containing columnar epithelium is taken from the cardia or from the lower end of the esophagus.

The biopsy appearances of carditis may vary from a superficial gastritis resembling DAG, characterized by the presence of neutrophil infiltration of the pit and surface epithelium, to an atrophic gastritis resembling MAG, which shows foci of intestinal metaplasia (89a). These appearances can be identical to those found in biopsies from "long-segment" Barrett's esophagus.

This diagnosis of carditis is not controversial, but its significance is. Two schools of thought exist: one considers carditis the result of gastroesophageal reflux (89b); the other, that it is caused by *H. pylori* infection (89a,89c,89d). Data exist to justify both opinions. Studies of individuals with clinical features of gastroesophageal reflux disease (GERD) have shown that carditis is present in 98% (89b). Furthermore, carditis may be present when the squamous esophageal mucosa is histologically normal (89e). These studies did not look for *H. pylori* in cardiac biopsies, probably because it was considered that the organism had no role in the causation and perpetuation of Barrett's esophagus. On the other hand, a study comparing the prevalence of carditis in individuals with and without GERD concluded that it was similar in both groups (89a). In all individuals with carditis, *H. pylori* organisms were detected in the areas of cardiac inflammation, as well as in more distal gastric locations (89a).

Reconciling these two theories and sets of data is now difficult. Part of the solution may revolve around the definition of carditis. It is conceivable that inflammation in intragastric cardiac mucosa is caused by *H. pylori* infection, but that inflammation of the intraesophageal cardiac-type mucosa is the result of reflux. It remains to be seen how reflux and infection are related to the development of cardiac cancer. From the practical point of view, it is suggested that, for the present, biopsies from these sites be diagnosed descriptively, noting the type of epithelium and the presence or absence of inflammation, *H. pylori*, and metaplasia. As only the endoscopists can determine the exact site of the biopsy, they should determine whether the patient has carditis or distal esophagitis.

Granulomatous Gastritis

Although granulomatous gastritis is rare, a wide variety of infectious and noninfectious diseases have to be considered in the differential diagnosis. The extent of the disease is variable, although typically the antrum is the major site of involvement. In the early stages, the only finding may be isolated granulomas in mucosal and submucosal tissue. In advanced disease, inflammation spreads to the muscularis propria, producing thickening, fibrosis and, often, pyloric stenosis (90).

Tuberculosis is still an important consideration in the differential diagnosis, particularly if the granulomas are caseating. In some of these cases, especially in malnourished, alcoholic, and immunosuppressed individuals, the diagnosis may be unsuspected and there may be no obvious lung disease. When patients have obvious pulmonary tuberculosis, the frequency of gastric involvement has been estimated as 0.57% (91,92).

Fungal granulomas, occurring as a result of a fungemia in immunosuppressed patients, may also produce caseation and necrosis; however, in most cases, the cause will usually be obvious from the clinical picture. The organisms responsible include *Candida*, *Histoplasma*, and *Phycomycetes* (93–96). In patients without fungemia, organisms, usually *Candida*, may grow on the surface of the gastric mucosa as yellowish plaques. These lesions usually occur in association with esophageal candidiasis and are not characterized by a granulomatous reaction. In nonimmunosuppressed individuals, fungi may be found growing in the craters of peptic ulcers among inflammatory debris. These are of little clinical significance and do not influence the rate of ulcer healing (97,98).

Rarely cases of syphilis of the stomach have been described (99–101). In the tertiary stage of the disease, the stomach wall becomes fibrotic, with widespread endarteritis and poorly formed granulomas (gummas) present. Secondary syphilis of the stomach is nonspecific histologically and is characterized by submucosal edema, early fibrosis, and large numbers of plasma cells in the lamina propria. Rarely an endarteritis with lymphocytic cuffing is present.

There are isolated case reports describing gastric granulomas in patients with Whipple's disease (102,103). However, in most instances, the organisms of Whipple's disease (*Tropheryma whippelii*) are present within histiocytes that are not organized into granulomas.

Noninfectious diseases are the usual causes of gastric non- caseating granulomas, and five major differentials should be considered: Crohn's disease (104,105), foreign-body reaction (102), tumor-associated granulomas, sarcoidosis, and isolated granulomatous gastritis (102,106,107). Crohn's disease of the stomach is the most common cause for gastric granulomas, accounting for more than 50% of cases (104,105) (Fig. 15). Histologically, it is entirely similar to Crohn's disease elsewhere in the bowel. Microgranulomas are a typical feature; the likelihood of finding them increases with the number of biopsies examined (105). The dominant appearance is a patchy acute and chronic inflammation, with or without erosions. Even when granulomas are absent, the focal nature of the inflammation may suggest the correct diagnosis. Attention should be paid to the presence of localized collections of chronic inflammatory cells surrounding single gastric pits at the level of the isthmus or around more deeply located glands (107a). These lesions may be encountered in both pyloric and fundal mucosa (106). Only in a minority of cases are aphthoid ulcers (erosions), or fissurelike ulcers seen. Because gastric involvement is almost invariably synchronous with Crohn's disease of the ileum or colon, exclusion of disease at these sites will eliminate Crohn's disease as a cause of unexplained gastric granulomas.

"Isolated granulomatous gastritis" is the term applied to granulomatous inflammation confined to the stomach for which no obvious cause can be found (102,106). In some series, it accounted for about 25% of all gastric granulomas (102,106), but in others, it was rare (107). Before making a diagnosis of idiopathic granulomatous inflammation, it is important to exclude Crohn's disease and some of the less common causes of granuloma formation. These include sarcoidosis (108,109) and granulomas associated with neoplasms, particularly lymphoma (110), and ingested foreign material (102). Exceptionally, gastric granulomas have also been associated with vasculitis (111), Wegener's disease (112), and as xanthogranulomas extending from an adjacent chronic cholecystitis (113).

Gastric sarcoidosis (108) and isolated granulomatous gastritis (102,106) are similar histologically: both have bland granulomas with little associated nonspecific inflammation.

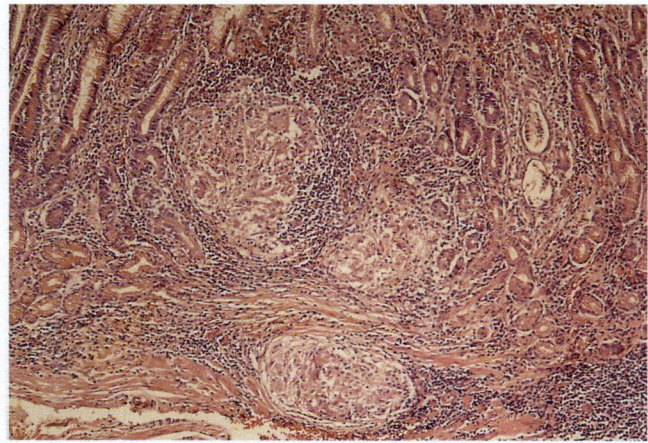

FIG. 15. Gastric granulomas from a case of Crohn's disease.

However, they tend to affect significantly different groups of patients. Sarcoidosis is more common in young black patients, whereas isolated granulomatous gastritis is more common in the older white male population. Sarcoid of the stomach is very frequently associated with granulomatous inflammation elsewhere, usually lungs, hilar lymph nodes, skin, or salivary glands. As its name implies, isolated granulomatous gastritis has histologic findings confined to the stomach. Its cause is unknown, and it is essentially a diagnosis of exclusion.

Eosinophilic Gastritis

It is important to remember that eosinophils may be present in gastric mucosal biopsies in a wide variety of conditions. Small numbers may be found, for example, in multifocal atrophic gastritis, allergic granulomatosis (Churg–Strauss syndrome) (114), Löffler's syndrome (115), inflammatory fibroid polyps (116), and Crohn's disease. Large numbers of eosinophils may accompany invasion of the gastric wall by parasitic worms, such as *Eustoma rotundatum* (117) and anisakiasis (118). In many instances, particularly in children, eosinophilic infiltration of the stomach is due to a food allergy, usually to milk or soy protein (119,120). Some individuals will respond to removal of these items from the diet; however, in other cases, especially where there is gastric involvement, corticosteroids may be required. Eosinophils in the gastric mucosa may also be encountered in some patients with connective tissue disorders (scleroderma, polymyositis, and dermatomyositis). These conditions may have a bandlike eosinophil infiltrate in the lower lamina propria, just superficial to the muscularis mucosae (121).

When all known causes of eosinophilic infiltration have been excluded, the diagnosis of idiopathic eosinophilic gastroenteritis may be considered (122–124). This condition may involve any part of the GI tract but is most common in the antrum. In a particular patient, as well as being segmental, the inflammation tends to maximally affect a single layer of the gut wall. Mucosal involvement will, therefore, result in nausea, vomiting, and abdominal pain, characteristically provoked by certain foods. Involvement of the muscularis propria will produce thickening and scarring, often with pyloric stenosis. Serosal involvement, which is the rarest pattern, will produce a localized peritonitis with ascites. Specimens from either endoscopic biopsy or partial gastrectomy show an intense, but patchy, infiltration by sheets of eosinophils (Fig. 16), which displace and distort the mucosal pits, producing occasional pit abscesses. Mucosal edema and vascular congestion are present, sometimes with necrosis of the surface epithelium and small erosions. Deep ulcers are uncommon, however. Unless the eosinophilic infiltration is massive and sheetlike, it is usually not possible to establish a diagnosis of eosinophilic gastritis. Eosinophils in small numbers are a normal component of the lamina propria of the stomach; however, their distribution is quite variable, making it difficult to give an exact value for the upper limit of normal (125). A useful ancillary finding is the presence of a peripheral blood eosinophilia, noted in up to 75% of patients with eosinophilic gastroenteritis (122).

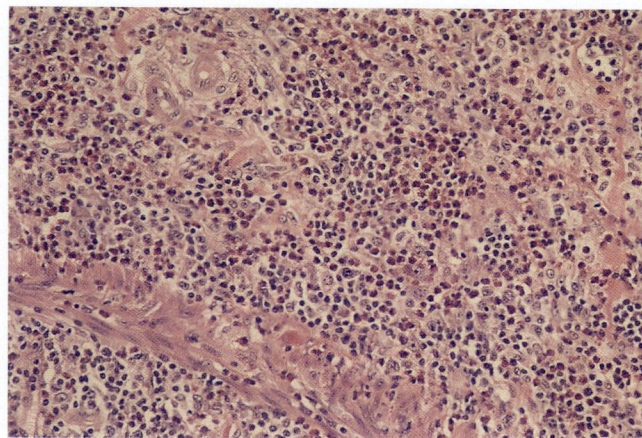

FIG. 16. A dense sheetlike infiltrate of eosinophils typical of eosinophilic gastroenteritis.

Lymphocytic Gastritis

Lymphocytic gastritis predominantly affects the fundic mucosa. The lamina propria, surface epithelium, and pit epithelium are infiltrated by large numbers of small, mature lymphocytes (126). The glandular portion of the mucosa is usually uninvolved. The epithelial lymphocytes are usually so abundant (more than 25 per 100 epithelial cells) that they are readily identified as a characteristic low-power feature (Fig. 17). In comparison, *H. pylori* gastritis may have four to seven lymphocytes per 100 epithelial cells. At high power, these lymphocytes are often surrounded by a clear halo (a fixation artifact). Immunostains reveal that they are of T-cell origin.

Mild cases of lymphocytic gastritis may appear normal endoscopically, or resemble *Helicobacter* gastritis. More advanced cases may be characterized by mucosal nodules, sur-

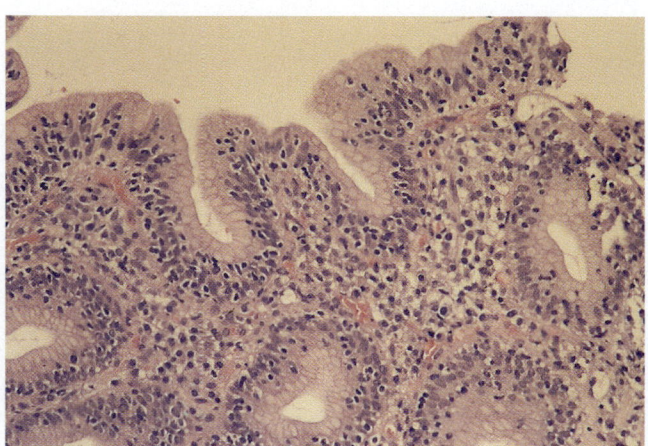

FIG. 17. Lymphocyte infiltration of superficial and pit-lining epithelium from a case of lymphocytic gastritis.

mounted by shallow aphthoid erosions. The term varioliform gastritis (chronic erosive gastritis) has been applied to this endoscopic appearance. However, it is not clear whether all cases of varioliform gastritis are the result of lymphocytic gastritis, or whether this endoscopic lesion can be the result of other diseases (127). Rarely lymphocytic gastritis may present with prominent mucosal folds, epithelial protein loss, and bleeding. This situation has been termed *hypertrophic lymphocytic gastritis* and has some clinical similarities to Ménétrier's disease (128,129).

It is presumed that lymphocytic gastritis represents a T-cell response to an intraluminal antigen. Some cases may represent an unusual reaction to *Helicobacter* infection (130,131). In other examples, there is gluten sensitivity with the typical lesion of celiac disease present in small-bowel biopsies (132–135). Patients have also been described who have an associated lymphocytic duodenitis (epithelial lymphocyte infiltration without villous atrophy) (135). Other recently described associations of lymphocytic gastritis include collagenous gastritis (136), malignant lymphoma (137,138), and gastric carcinoma (137).

Reactive Gastropathy

Reactive gastropathy, also known as reflux gastritis and chemical gastritis (46), is now the second commonest diagnosis made on gastric biopsies performed in North America (139). As originally described in postgastrectomy stomachs (140), the mucosa shows edema, congestion, pit hyperplasia often producing a corkscrew appearance, and paucity of mucosal inflammatory cells (Fig. 18). Individual pit-lining cells show mucin depletion with enlargement and diffuse hyperchromasia of nuclei. These are unlike the nuclei in active *Helicobacter* gastritis, which are vesicular with prominent nucleoli. The glandular portion of the mucosa is unaffected. Identical findings have also been described in the prepyloric region of intact stomachs with demonstrated bile reflux (141). These changes are considered to represent the results of increased surface cell exfoliation; thus they are not specific for reflux and are also commonly encountered in patients taking NSAIDs (140,142). The changes of reactive gastropathy should be looked for carefully in cases in which there is an endoscopic diagnosis of gastritis, but inflammatory cell infiltrates are not seen on low-power examination of biopsy fragments. Reactive gastropathy is a diffuse process and is generally present in more than one biopsy. The minimal criteria required for diagnosis are pit-cell mucin depletion and nuclear hyperchromasia. Marginal changes may be reported as suggestive, but nondiagnostic, of reactive gastropathy.

Of interest, not all authors have encountered these findings in gastric reflux. Niemela et al. (143) observed that some cases of reflux were associated with mucosal infiltration by mononuclear cells, neutrophils, and eosinophils, as well as with pit hyperplasia. This observation supports the suggestion that gastroduodenal reflux may be the cause of prepyloric ulcers in a mucosa already damaged by *Helicobacter* gastritis (144). In this clinical situation, it is hardly surprising that biopsies might show a mixed picture.

Radiation and Chemotherapy Gastritis

Assessment of radiation changes in the stomach is sometimes difficult because of the complicating effects of the underlying disease for which treatment was given. However, generally speaking, the lesions will be similar to those produced by radiation elsewhere in the body. Small doses (up to 1,500 R) will cause degenerative changes in epithelial cells and a nonspecific chronic inflammatory infiltrate in the lamina propria. This phase is followed, after a period of about 4 months, by recovery with restoration of the normal structure. Intermediate doses of radiation (1,500 to 4,000 R) will produce permanent mucosal damage, usually in the form of atrophy of the fundic glands. Above 4,000 R, more serious damage is likely. Initially there may be surface epithelial loss, resulting in mucosal erosions, which expose a lamina propria containing dilated bleeding capillaries. Later the erosions heal, producing a profound atrophic gastritis. At this stage, deep nonhealing ulcers may form that are not responsive to peptic ulcer therapy and may require surgical excision. These are caused by localized mucosal ischemia, resulting from a submucosal obliterative endarteritis (Fig. 19).

In the early stages of regeneration after radiotherapy, the gastric mucosa may show atypical changes that are not always easy to distinguish from true dysplasia and superficial carcinoma (Fig. 20). Criteria that favor a diagnosis of radiotherapy atypia include the following: atypia maximal in the deeper portions of the mucosa; very bizarre nuclear changes, but preservation of a normal nuclear/cytoplasmic ratio; few mitotic figures; cytoplasmic degenerative changes consisting of eosinophilia and vacuolation; atypical changes within fibroblasts and endothelial cells; and absence of adjacent intestinal metaplasia.

Distinguishing a peptic ulcer from a radiation-induced ul-

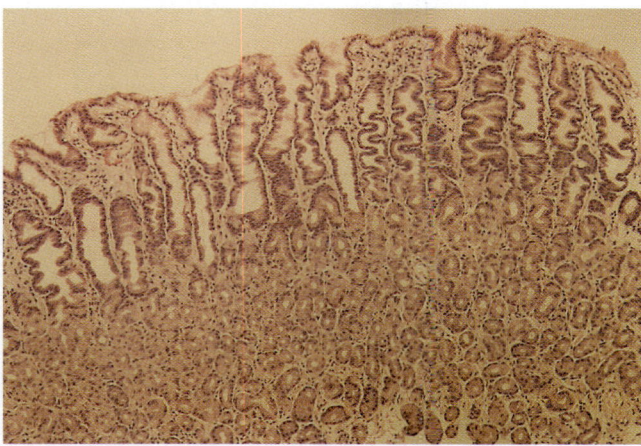

FIG. 18. Antral gastric mucosa showing reflux gastritis. Note the extreme hyperplasia of pits, some of which have a "corkscrew" appearance.

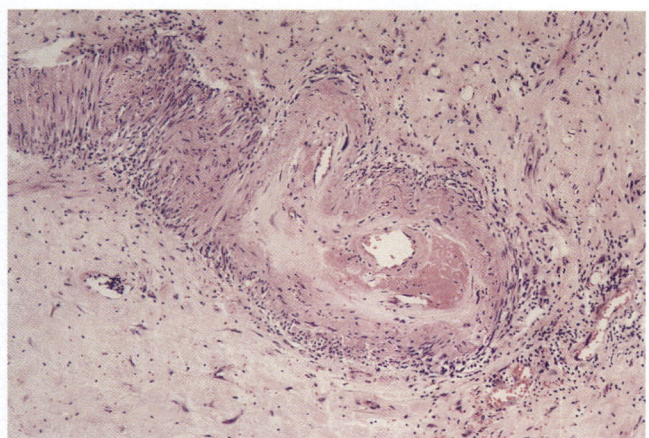

FIG. 19. Endarteritis obliterans from a case of radiation gastritis.

cer by mucosal biopsy is likely to be difficult, if not impossible. A similar diagnostic problem will be encountered also in gastrectomy specimens because peptic ulcers may also have extensive endarteritis at their base. However, examination of gastric vessels at some distance from the ulcer is likely to be more helpful in defining radiation as the cause, because these, too, will show radiation changes consisting of neovascularization, telangiectasia, and intimal obliterative lesions (145,146).

Gastric epithelial atypia was recently described in individuals who have received chemotherapy for malignant disease (147,148). 5-Fluorouracil, administered by hepatic artery infusion for treatment of liver metastases, has been particularly incriminated. High concentrations of the drug may reach the stomach via collaterals or catheter displacement. Gastric ulceration may follow 10 to 45 days later (149). Grossly, the lesions resemble typical peptic ulcers, but biopsy reveals marked cytologic atypia of the adjoining epithelium. The features of atypia are essentially similar to those encountered after radiotherapy (Fig. 20).

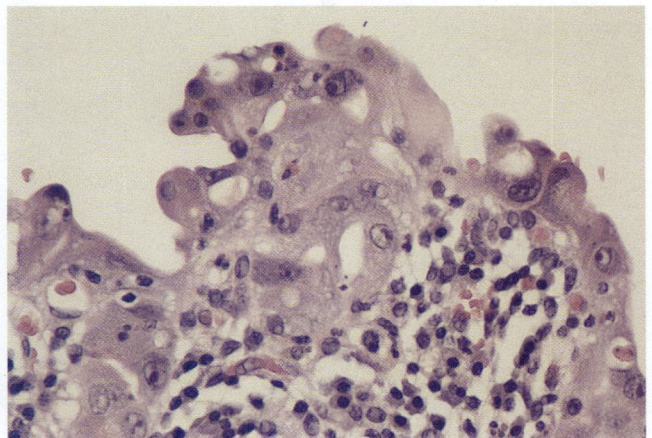

FIG. 20. Epithelial atypia associated with chemotherapy. Note the syncytial growth pattern of the cells.

Ischemic Gastritis

Lesions of the stomach resulting from vascular disease are uncommon, probably because of the richness and diversity of the gastric blood supply and the presence of abundant vascular anastomoses. However, in some circumstances, ischemia may produce superficial erosions (150,151) and even deep ulcers (152). Occasionally biopsies may reveal the ghost outlines of glands and pits containing columns of necrotic epithelial cells with pyknotic nuclei (152a). Ischemic ulcers are difficult to distinguish from peptic ulcers but are typically antral in location and irregular in shape with sloping edges and a sclerotic white base. The adjacent mucosa frequently contains multiple erosions (152). In most cases, the underlying cause appears to be showers of atherosclerotic emboli, arising from the celiac and superior mesenteric arteries.

It seems that a specific ischemic gastritis analogous to ischemic colitis or necrotizing enterocolitis does not occur in the stomach. Acute ischemia, due to shock or poor cardiac output, results in a hemorrhagic and erosive gastritis that may bleed profusely, but heals rapidly when gastric perfusion is restored.

Gastritis Resulting from Drug Therapy

Drug therapy is an extremely common cause of gastritis and may produce a variety of morphologic appearances. Alcohol (49,50), aspirin (53,153), and NSAIDs (53,54,153) are well-recognized causes of acute erosive gastritis and may produce a hemorrhagic or nonhemorrhagic lesion. Chronic use of these drugs may lead to more extensive ulceration. When compared with the usual type of gastric peptic ulcer, drug-induced ulcers are deeper and larger. They have little associated chronic gastritis and intestinal metaplasia (154) and are not accompanied by *Helicobacter*.

NSAIDs may also result in reactive gastropathy (140,142). It seems probable that this arises from a direct irritative effect of the drugs on the mucosa, rather than being the result of a drug-induced increase in bile reflux. Reactive gastropathy is not seen in all patients taking NSAIDs (155) and is particularly difficult to diagnose in biopsies where there is a concurrent *H. pylori* gastritis (156). Interestingly, in patients taking concurrent NSAIDs and prostaglandins (mistoprostol), the prevalence of reactive gastropathy but not *H. pylori*–associated inflammation is reduced (157).

A number of other drugs may produce alterations in the gastric mucosal histology. Most of these involve agents administered for the treatment of peptic ulcer disease. Long-term treatment by protein-pump inhibitors can produce a worsening of *H. pylori* gastritis, which spreads to the fundic mucosa, resulting in accelerated atrophy. The associated hypergastrinemia causes linear or nodular endocrine cell hyperplasia of the ECL cells and linear hyperplasia of G cells (158). To date, no actual carcinoid neoplasms have resulted (159). Aluminum-containing antacids may precipitate in the stomach, resulting in mucosal calcinosis (160).

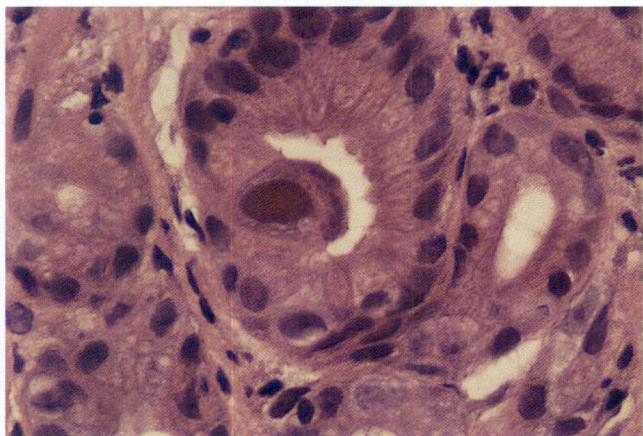

FIG. 21. Cytomegalovirus inclusions in gastric epithelial cells.

Gastritis in Immunosuppressed Patients

A common clinical situation in which this problem is encountered is in patients with the acquired immune deficiency syndrome (AIDS), but it also occurs in other types of immunosuppression, such as in organ-transplant recipients, patients receiving anticancer chemotherapy, or in inherited immunologic defects.

Cytomegalovirus (CMV) infection is one of the most common problems in immunosuppression (161). The disease is more frequent and more severe in the small bowel and colon, but can affect the stomach. In the early stages, GI symptoms may be relatively minor, and the endoscopic appearances can be normal; the main findings on biopsy are the typical eosinophilic intranuclear inclusions (Fig. 21), which may or may not be accompanied by smaller purple-staining granular cytoplasmic inclusions and a patchy nonspecific infiltrate in the lamina propria. Initially, the inclusions are located in epithelial cells of the lower portion of the pit or in the upper part of the glands. In the more advanced stages of disease, when ulceration is present, the inclusions become more frequent in mesenchymal cells, usually endothelium. Severe CMV gastritis is manifested by necrosis of epithelium with ulceration (162,163), which can lead to severe hemorrhage or even perforation (164). It has been postulated that mucosal ischemia, caused by a viral endothelialitis, is the pathogenetic mechanism leading to ulceration (162). Rarely, mucosal nodules may occur (165), and in children, a hypertrophic gastritis similar to Ménétrier's disease has been described (166).

Changes of herpes simplex virus (HSV) are rarely described in the stomach but are common in the esophagus and, to a lesser extent, in the small bowel (167). In the stomach, they consist of basophilic, ground-glass intranuclear inclusions in epithelial cells. If these are suspected, but not confidently identified, on H&E sections, *in situ* hybridization, with biotinylated DNA probes, may be used to prove the presence of viral infection (167).

The protozoal organism cryptosporidium is now recognized as an uncommon cause of self-limited diarrhea in immunocompetent patients. In AIDS patients, however, it can produce persistent watery diarrhea, with vomiting and colicky abdominal pain (168). The organism, which may be found in the stomach as well as in other parts of the GI tract, is usually recognized easily in routine H&E-stained sections as rounded basophilic objects 2 to 4 μm in diameter, adherent to surface epithelial cells. Penetration into the lamina propria is not seen, although there may be underlying mucosal edema (168). If there is uncertainty as to correct identification, histochemical stains may be helpful. Cryptosporidia stain positively with PAS, Giemsa, and gram, but stain negatively with Gomori's methanamine silver. They are also readily identified by a Leung stain (69). Rare examples of gastric involvement by leishmaniasis (169), toxoplasmosis (170), and giardiasis (171) have also been described.

Another organism, often encountered in gastric biopsies from AIDS patients, is *Mycobacterium avium-intracellulare*. On histologic examination, the appearances resemble Whipple's disease, because the lamina propria is filled with a monotonous infiltrate of foamy histiocytes. These histiocytes rarely form aggregates recognizable as granulomas; caseation is also rare, although ulceration may occur (172). If suspicious cells of this type are seen on biopsies, a Ziehl-Neelsen (ZN) stain should be performed. Unlike tubercle bacilli, these atypical mycobacteria are usually present in large numbers, so identification is easy. On rare occasions, *M. avium-intracellulare* may be present in the lamina propria without a conspicuous histologic response. Thus a ZN stain should be performed routinely on GI biopsies from AIDS patients.

The changes seen in gastric graft-versus-host disease (GVHD) are similar to those encountered in GVHD at other locations in the GI tract. However, the stomach is usually the least severely affected site. Early changes (grade I) consist of isolated epithelial cell necrosis (Fig. 22), with associated karyorrhexic debris and pit or gland dilatation (173). This characteristic lesion, called "an exploding crypt cell," is only rarely seen in other conditions but can occur in CMV infec-

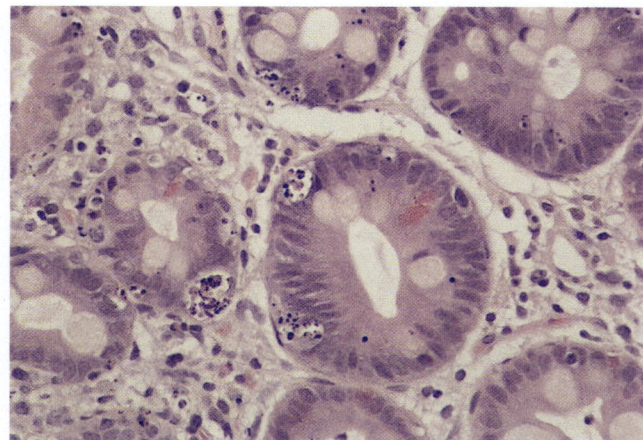

FIG. 22. Graft-versus-host disease of the stomach in a patient who had received a bone marrow transplant. Note the "exploding crypt cells" (karyorrhexic debris).

tions of the gut (174). In more severe disease (grade II), there may be pit and gland atrophy with mucosal simplification and intestinal metaplasia. Ultimately, mucosal denudation will occur (grade III) (175).

Chronic granulomatous disease may involve the gastric antrum, where it is seen with outlet obstruction (176). Resection specimens show inflammatory lesions in the mucosa, submucosa, or muscularis propria. Distinct granulomas with necrosis may be present, or there may simply be a poorly organized mass of histiocytes, multinuclear giant cells, lymphocytes, and eosinophils. The presence of pigment-containing macrophages is highly suggestive of the diagnosis.

PEPTIC ULCER DISEASE

By definition, a peptic ulcer results from the effects of acid on the mucosa and may be acute or chronic. A chronic ulcer is defined clinically as one that does not heal over a reasonable period and is defined histologically as one that has fibrosis in the base and walls. An acute gastric ulcer is merely a large erosion that has penetrated through the muscularis mucosae into the wall of the stomach. Sectioning a chronic ulcer reveals three distinct zones: a superficial zone of necrotic slough and fibrin, infiltrated by polymorphs; a middle zone consisting of chronically inflamed granulation tissue; and a deep zone consisting of fibrous tissue with vessels showing endarteritis obliterans.

All gastric ulcers, except those that are the result of treatment by NSAIDs (154), are surrounded by areas of acute and chronic inflammation (177). The pattern of gastritis will differ, depending on the location of the ulcer. Ulcers in the pyloric canal and in the immediate prepyloric area are accompanied by a diffuse antral gastritis and by the presence of *Helicobacter*. They have the same clinical and epidemiologic features as duodenal ulcers. More proximal ulcers, usually in the region of the incisura, are typically accompanied by multifocal atrophic gastritis and intestinal metaplasia. In these ulcers, *H. pylori* are found in smaller numbers. The presence of *H. pylori* in mucosa adjacent to ulcers can often be inferred by finding evidence of superficial mucosal damage. *Helicobacter* infection produces loss of apical cytoplasmic mucus, erosions, and cell tufting (178).

At the edge of ulcers of all types, reactive epithelial changes can occasionally be confused with dysplasia or a carcinoma. It is important to diagnose these as accurately as possible. A vague report indicating the presence of "atypia" and changes "somewhat suggestive of early malignancy" is not much use to the gastroenterologist, who likely would not have performed the biopsy in the first place if there were no clinical suspicion. Examples of reactive changes are shown in Figs. 9 and 13. Examples of dysplasia are shown in Figs. 34 and 35. Some useful points to aid in the distinction are as follows:

1. Biopsies fixed in Bouin's fluid or other nonformalin fixatives have very sharply defined basophilic nuclei in which the nucleoli are more prominent than those in biopsies fixed in formalin. Allowance should be made for this.
2. In examples of intestinal metaplasia, the base of the gland can show nuclear crowding and increased mitotic activity similar to normal small bowel. Toward the surface, however, fully mature epithelial cells are identified.
3. Inflammatory epithelial changes will be of varying severity, with a gradual transition from normal to atypical. The transition between malignant and normal epithelium tends to be abrupt.
4. Reactive nuclei are vesicular and rounded, with single or double enlarged nucleoli. Neoplastic nuclei are enlarged, crowded, and compressed, and tend to have overall hyperchromacity (179). The appearances of gastric dysplasia are similar to those encountered in colonic adenomas.
5. In peptic ulcers, inflammation is most severe in the areas of severe atypia. Carcinomas may show focal inflammation, but the uninflamed areas are equally atypical.

It must be admitted, however, that on occasion a clear-cut diagnosis is impossible, and the biopsy must be repeated after antiinflammatory therapy. Examination of a brush cytology specimen from the lesion may aid in distinguishing reactive from dysplastic cellular changes.

Gastric hyalinization is a rare condition that may be a consequence of ulceration or perimortem damage to the stomach mucosa (180). It is hypothesized that luminal acid leaks into the submucosa, producing thickening by an amorphous hyaline material.

THE POSTGASTRECTOMY STOMACH

It is well recognized that any form of gastric surgery may ultimately result in gastritis, and that the changes are usually most marked after partial gastrectomy. A variety of histologic lesions have been described. The most obvious is a multifocal atrophic gastritis with intestinal metaplasia (181,182). *Helicobacter* typically is not found. This type of gastritis may take 10 to 20 years to develop fully. Reactive gastropathy (140,143) is a recently recognized condition, which may also involve the gastric remnant after surgery. The characteristic histologic appearance is mucosal congestion and edema with pit hyperplasia, often resulting in a corkscrew appearance. Inflammatory polyps may occur in postgastrectomy stomachs, particularly in the region of the stoma. These are discussed fully in the section on gastric polyps.

The risk of developing cancer in patients who have had a subtotal gastrectomy is still in dispute. Some studies (183) have been unable to demonstrate any increased risk over a control population. Other investigators (184) have shown an excess of gastric cancer incidence that is not significant 20 years after gastrectomy, but increases to 7% after 40 years. In Norway, 9.5% of all stomach cancer patients have had a previous partial gastrectomy (184). The cancer that develops is an intestinal-type adenocarcinoma located in the distal gastric remnant (185). In many instances, these carcinomas are preceded by dysplasia of the gastric mucosa (181,186).

POLYPS

A classification of gastric polyps is given in Table 3. Enlarged mucosal folds are included because there may be some clinical overlap between prominent folds and polyposis. Although histologic examination is the key to differential diagnosis, much practical diagnostic help can also be obtained by determining (a) if a biopsy comes from a discrete polyp or from a prominent mucosal fold; (b) whether a polyp is sessile or pedunculated; (c) whether polyps are present in other parts of the GI tract; and (d) whether the surrounding mucosa is normal.

Peutz–Jeghers Syndrome

Peutz–Jeghers polyps most commonly present in childhood or adolescence and are usually regarded as hamartomatous in type. Most are 1 to 3 cm in size, with a coarsely lobulated surface and a short broad stalk. Histologically, the most useful diagnostic feature is the presence of a core of finely arborizing branches of smooth muscle from the muscularis mucosae (187,188). The core is covered by abundant mucosa, histologically identical with the normal stomach, but often disorganized. It consists predominately of surface and pit-type epithelium, although occasional antral glands and small cysts may be found. Inflammation is usually not prominent. Rarely, Peutz–Jeghers polyps have been found in association with carcinomas of the gastric antrum (189).

Juvenile Polyp

Juvenile polyps, sometimes called retention polyps, are rounded smooth-surfaced lesions, averaging 1 to 2 cm in diameter, with a short narrow stalk. They consist principally of lamina propria that contains irregularly shaped cysts lined by normal gastric surface epithelium (187,190). Repeated episodes of torsion may produce stromal hemorrhage, surface ulceration, and secondary chronic inflammation. The appearances of juvenile polyps may mimic those of hyperplastic polyps; however, differential diagnosis is aided by consideration of the clinical setting. In rare instances (190), juvenile polyps may be confined to the stomach. There is a small, but definite, risk of colorectal carcinoma developing in patients with juvenile polyposis (187), and recent evidence of an increased risk for gastric cancer, also (191).

Cowden Disease

Cowden disease is an extremely rare syndrome, in which there is an association between skin lesions on the face (typically tricholemmomas) and GI polyps. There is also an increased incidence of breast and thyroid carcinomas in these patients. The gastric lesions are generally sessile polyps, a few millimeters in diameter. The histology is poorly documented, and there is some diversity between different polyps. Generally, they contain excess lamina propria splayed and dissected into lobules by disorganized fascicles of muscularis mucosae running upward from the base of the mucosa (187,192).

Hyperplastic Polyp

Hyperplastic polyps, also called regenerative polyps or hyperplaseogenous polyps, are the most common polyps in the stomach, amounting to 85% to 90% of cases (193,194). In contrast to hamartomas, they tend to occur in older adults, typically at the junction of pyloric and fundic mucosa. Often multiple, hyperplastic polyps generally vary from 0.5 to 2.5 cm in diameter, with an average size of 1.4 cm (195), and have a coarsely lobulated surface. Small polyps tend to be sessile, but the larger ones may have a short broad stalk (Fig. 23). The presumed histogenesis is an exaggerated regenerative response to mucosal damage; in many cases, the adjacent nonpolypoid mucosa shows chronic atrophic gastritis. A recent report suggests that some polyps have a clonal origin (196). Hyperplastic polyps of the stomach are structurally similar to inflammatory colonic polyps (pseudopolyps) but are not related to hyperplastic colonic polyps. In contrast to gastric adenomas, hyperplastic polyps rarely (2% to 3.5%) undergo malignant change (194,195), with the risk of malignancy largely being confined to polyps more than 2 cm in diameter. For this reason, and to avoid diagnostic confusion, it

TABLE 3. *Classification of gastric polyps and enlarged mucosal folds*

Hamartomas
    Peutz–Jeghers syndrome
    Juvenile polyp
    Cowden disease
Hyperplastic and inflammatory polyps
    Hyperplastic polyp
    Polypoid mucosal prolapse
    Fundic gland polyp
    Inflammatory fibroid polyp
    Cronkhite–Canada polyp
    Lymphoid hyperplasia
Neoplastic polyps
    Adenoma
    Carcinoma
    Carcinoid
    Lymphomatous polyposis
    Stromal tumors
Mucosal folds
    Giant folds (normal variant)
    Zollinger–Ellison syndrome
    Ménétrier's disease
    Hypertrophic hypersecretory gastropathy
    Malignant infiltration (carcinoma or lymphoma)
    Giant folds caused by inflammation

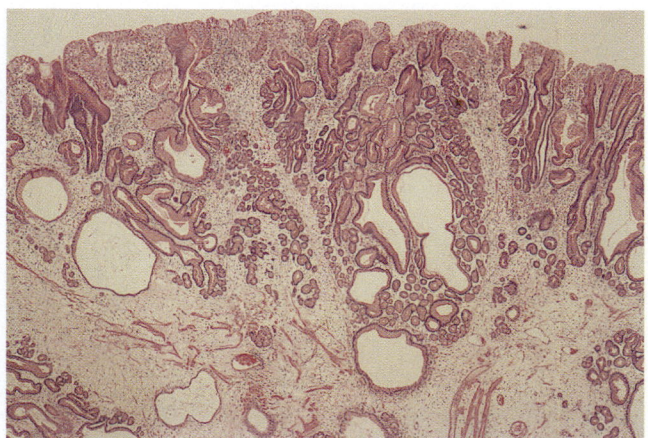

FIG. 23. Hyperplastic polyp of the stomach. Note the irregular epithelial proliferation, cyst formation, and excess of lamina propria.

is strongly recommended that the older terminology of "hyperplastic adenomatous polyp" not be used.

The histology of gastric hyperplastic polyps is variable, but basically they consist of elongated, distorted, and branched gastric pits (Fig. 23). There is often abundant lamina propria, which may be inflamed and edematous. The pit-lining cells are frequently hypertrophic with excess superficial cytoplasm, with or without intestinal metaplasia. The nuclei are typically bland and resemble normal gastric pit nuclei; however, in heavily inflamed areas, regeneration can produce nuclear enlargement with prominent nucleoli (197).

Polypoid Mucosal Prolapse

This condition has a variety of other names, including gastritis cystica polyposa, polypoid cystic gastritis, polypoid hypertrophic gastritis, and stomal polypoid hyperplasia (198,199). Typically, lesions occur on the gastric side of gastroenterostomy stomas, commonly producing a large sessile polyp. Histologically, these polyps resemble gastric hyperplastic polyps with various combinations of pit hyperplasia, distortion, and dilatation, with or without associated edema and nonspecific inflammation. The mucosal changes are identical with those of reflux gastritis. Occasionally, excessive regeneration may occur, resulting in epithelium extending downward through the muscularis mucosae, producing cysts in the submucosa. This lesion has been called gastritis cystica profunda (200) and is analogous to colitis cystica profunda and to misplaced glands in the tip of colonic adenomas.

Fundic Gland Polyp

The pathogenesis of these common gastric lesions is not clear; they have variously been considered examples of either hyperplasia or hamartomas (201–203). Recent studies pointed to a proliferation and differentiation of aberrantly located proliferative cells (204). Macroscopically, they appear as minute mucosal bumps 1 to 5 mm in diameter. Microscopically, they consist of single or small groups of cystically dilated fundic glands, lined by an attenuated, but otherwise normal, layer of chief and parietal cells (Fig. 24). The overlying pit-containing portion of the mucosa is normal. As the name implies, these polyps occur predominantly in the fundic mucosa; however, occasionally polyps of similar type, but lined by mucus-secreting cells, may occur in the antral mucosa. Most fundic gland polyps occur in small numbers (one to 20); however, occasionally they are part of a diffuse fundic gland polyposis (202,203). Polyposis of this type is characterized by many hundreds of polyps.

The initial descriptions of fundic gland polyposis were in patients with familial adenomatosis coli (202), or Gardner's syndrome (205), in which it was present in 27% of patients and was considered to be a specifically associated entity. Later, however, fundic gland polyposis was found in patients who did not have colonic polyposis. Fundic gland polyposis generally becomes manifest in middle adulthood, at a time when any associated colonic polyps are already evident, so that there is unlikely to be clinical confusion between sporadic and familial types. However, it should also be noted that in 67% of individuals with familial adenomatosis coli and Gardner's syndrome, there are also small numbers of gastric adenomas (202,205,206). Carpeting of the mucosa by many hundreds of adenomas does not occur in the stomach as it does in the colon. These adenomas have an appreciable risk of malignant change, such that endoscopic surveillance and polypectomy are warranted. Fundic gland polyps, occurring either with or without colonic adenomas, have no malignant potential and do not require surgery.

Inflammatory Fibroid Polyp

Inflammatory fibroid polyps may occur anywhere in the GI tract (116,207), but about 75% of recorded cases have been in the stomach, particularly the antrum. The sex incidence is similar, and the mean age at presentation is 53 years.

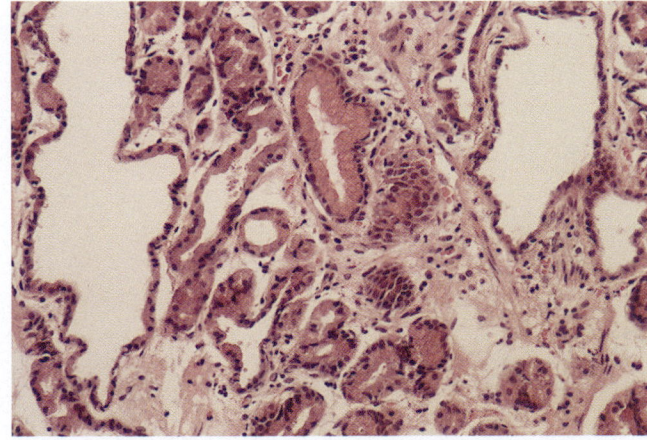

FIG. 24. A fundic gland polyp of the stomach consisting of dilated glands lined by an attenuated, but otherwise normal, epithelium.

They generally are first seen with colicky abdominal pain and pyloric obstruction; vomiting, diarrhea, and bleeding are uncommon. In the stomach, these polyps are sessile rather than pedunculated. As would be expected, asymptomatic polyps discovered incidentally are small, whereas symptomatic lesions may be several centimeters in diameter. One recorded polyp measured 9 cm in length and 6 cm in diameter. The pathogenesis is unknown but is widely assumed to be related to minor trauma. Earlier suggestions that they are benign neurogenic neoplasms have been discounted, and a myofibroblastic origin has been proposed (208).

Histologically (Fig. 25), they consist of an overgrowth of loose connective tissue in the submucosa that initially stretches and later ulcerates mucosa at the polyp tip. This tissue may also infiltrate and partly replace the muscularis propria. Numerous small-caliber thin-walled vessels are present, which are commonly surrounded by a hypocellular zone of stroma (Fig. 26). Also present is a light scattering of inflammatory cells, including lymphocytes, plasma cells, and eosinophils. Mitotic activity is usually not a feature, and giant cells are not found. In some polyps, eosinophils are particularly abundant, but it is now clear that this feature is not associated with a blood eosinophilia. There is no connection between inflammatory fibroid polyps and eosinophilic enteritis (122) or eosinophilic granulomatosis.

Cronkhite–Canada Syndrome

This extremely rare condition is characterized by diffuse GI polyposis, alopecia, hyperpigmentation, and dystrophic changes in fingernails and toenails. Morphologically, the polyps are sessile, consisting of hyperplastic, edematous mucosa with epithelial cysts (209). They resemble hyperplastic polyps and juvenile polyps.

Neoplastic Polyps

Adenomas compose approximately 10% of all gastric polyps (194). Most are sessile and grow in a tubulovillous or pure villous pattern; pure pedunculated tubular lesions are rare. Histologically, they are identical with adenomas of the colon and show epithelial dysplasia, ranging from low to high grade (Fig. 27). Larger polyps (larger than 2.0 cm) are considered to have a significant chance of becoming malignant. Although the magnitude of risk has not been precisely defined, it is generally considered to be in the range of 5% to 10% (193,194,210). In patients with gastric adenoma, there also is a risk of finding a coexistent carcinoma elsewhere in the stomach. The magnitude of this risk is also difficult to assess, but is probably in the range of 10% to 15% (193, 194,210). It is strongly recommended that gastric adenomas be removed entirely and that, when they are present, the remainder of the stomach be carefully scrutinized for additional lesions.

A recently described variant of gastric adenoma is the depressed (flat) adenoma. These constitute 11% of all adenomas and appear to have a higher rate of malignant change than do polypoid adenomas. These tumors are recognized

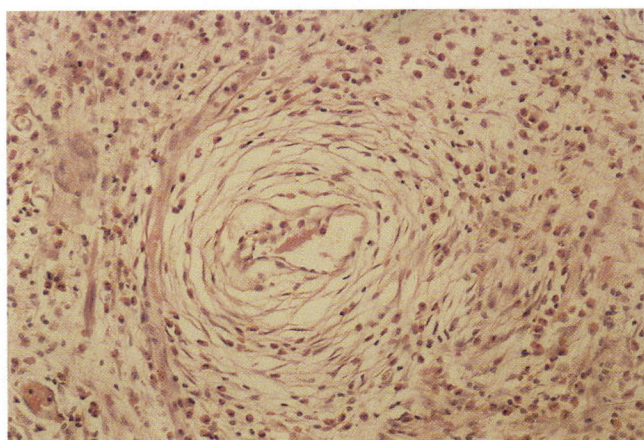

FIG. 26. Inflammatory fibroid polyp demonstrating a perivascular hypocellular zone and an infiltration by eosinophils.

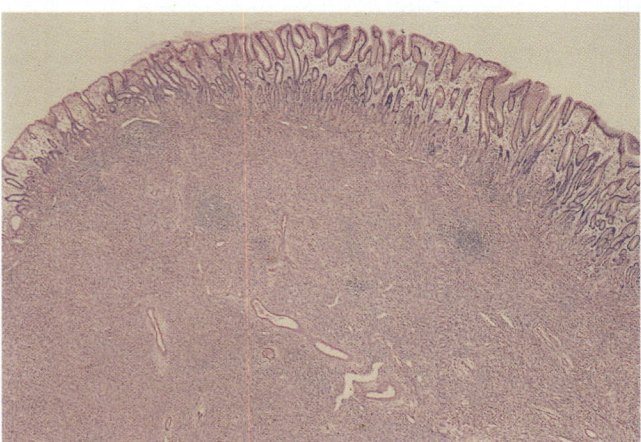

FIG. 25. Inflammatory fibroid polyp consisting of cellular connective tissue with a variable inflammatory component.

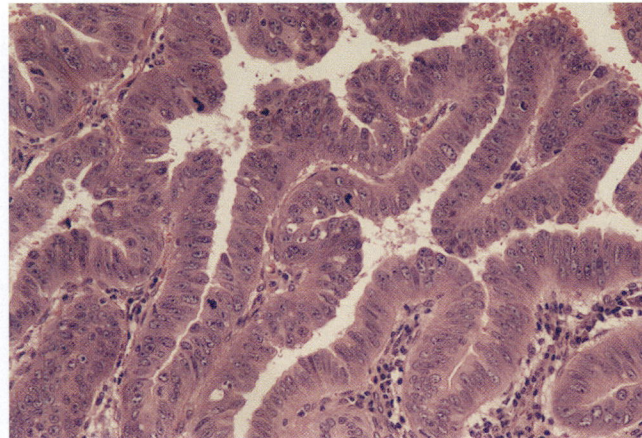

FIG. 27. Villous adenoma of stomach. The appearances are very similar to adenomas elsewhere in the gastrointestinal tract.

grossly with difficulty as shallow depressions, averaging 1.3 cm in diameter (2- to 39-mm range) (211).

It is rare to find polypoid lymphoid tissue within the stomach. Examples of focal lymphoid hyperplasia have been described (212), and rarely, lymphoreticular neoplasms are polypoid (213). Gastric adenocarcinomas, carcinoids, and stromal tumors may rarely be polypoid. The features of these lesions are described later.

ENLARGED MUCOSAL FOLDS

The most common cause of giant gastric folds is a variant of normal (214). Apart from causing diagnostic confusion, this finding has no clinical significance. The folds result from excessively long cores of submucosa and are covered by entirely normal gastric mucosa.

The diagnosis of abnormally enlarged gastric folds may be difficult on a standard-sized biopsy. However, I have found that the use of "jumbo forceps" will, in most cases, produce satisfactory tissue and obviate the need for an open full-thickness biopsy. The classification of gastric-fold diseases is given in Table 3. In the majority of cases, the cause is inflammatory disease, either *Helicobacter* gastritis or lymphocytic gastritis (215). Neoplastic infiltrates, such as diffuse carcinoma or lymphoma, also can produce enlarged folds, although this is not their normal presentation. More rarely, giant folds are due to mucosal hyperplasia, with various possible permutations, depending on whether the pits, the glands, or both are hyperplastic.

Zollinger–Ellison Syndrome

In the Zollinger–Ellison (ZE) syndrome, there is an increase in the mass of fundic glands with normal-sized antral glands and gastric pits (214–216). This is the result of excess production of gastrin, usually by a pancreatic or duodenal neoplasm, but less commonly by a primary hyperplasia of G cells within the antral gastric mucosa (217). In about 20% of cases, the pancreatic neoplasm is part of the type I multiple endocrine neoplasia syndrome (MEN I). The excess gastrin has a trophic effect on parietal cells, causing them to enlarge and proliferate. The resulting increase in hydrochloric acid production contributes to the clinical symptoms and signs, which include recurrent duodenal ulceration and diarrhea.

Grossly, the fundic mucosal folds are enlarged and thrown into a cerebriform pattern. Histologically, the fundic gland thickness is expanded 1.5 to 2 times normal. The glands contain hypertrophied and hyperplastic parietal cells that appear to crowd out chief cells and mucus neck cells. The gland lumen is of normal size, and no cysts are present. Hyperplastic endocrine cells may also be present in fundic glands; however, these are ECL cells, rather than G cells. This hyperplasia is considered to be the result of a direct trophic action of gastrin on ECL cells. These cells respond by producing histamine, which further stimulates acid production by parietal cells.

Hypertrophic Hypersecretory Gastropathy

This condition is closely related to the ZE syndrome (214). There are two clinical variants: One is accompanied by protein loss (218) and the other is not (219). In cases without protein loss, the gastric structure and symptoms are similar to those of the ZE syndrome. However, these patients do not have pancreatic tumors, G-cell hyperplasia, or hypergastrinemia. Possibly the excess acid output results from an exquisite sensitivity of parietal cells to normal serum gastrin levels. The protein-losing variant has much in common with Ménétrier's disease, but also has features of ZE syndrome, including hypergastrinemia. Both conditions are exceedingly rare, and the pathology is not well described.

Ménétrier's Disease

This is still a poorly defined entity. The confusion started with Ménétrier himself and has continued in numerous publications ever since. These articles typically describe the clinical features of one or two cases, with no satisfactory description of gastric histology. Some authors continue to regard Ménétrier's disease as a syndrome, characterized by prominent gastric folds and mucosal protein loss, for which no other primary cause can be diagnosed (e.g., ZE syndrome, linitis plastica, or gastric lymphoma). However, this approach included diverse conditions with different morphologies and different clinical outcomes under the umbrella term of Ménétrier's disease. This usage is particularly apt to occur in children, where cases of "Ménétrier's disease" have been described in association with cytomegalovirus infection (166,220). To avoid this problem, Appelman (214) suggested that the diagnosis of Ménétrier's disease be restricted to cases fulfilling the following criteria: (a) giant mucosal folds involving the fundus and possibly antrum; (b) low acid production, even after stimulation; (c) mucosal protein loss; and (d) histologic findings of gastric pit hyperplasia and glandular atrophy. I endorse this practical suggestion. However, it should be recognized that early and incomplete forms of the disease exist, in which it may be difficult to establish a definite diagnosis. These variants may be focal and affect only occasional mucosal folds, or there may be a mild generalized form, in which fundic gland atrophy has not yet developed and the acid output is normal.

The histologic features of Ménétrier's disease, as defined, are constant (Fig. 28). On the surface of the folds, the gastric pits are enormously elongated and may have a corkscrew appearance. Often they are cystically dilated with mucus accumulation. Cysts extend into the deeper mucosal layers and even occasionally the submucosa, producing gland atrophy. There is frequently nonspecific inflammation in the superficial mucosa, but this is not an essential component of the disease.

In adults, the fully developed disease is progressive, so that most patients eventually require a subtotal gastrectomy. Cases in which there is spontaneous regression are probably

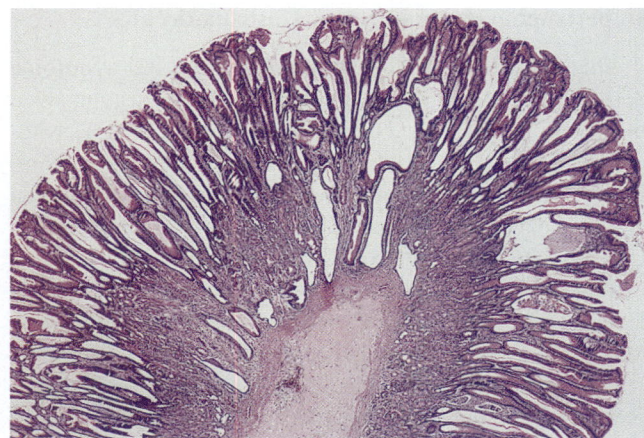

FIG. 28. Ménétrier's disease, showing the pit hyperplasia and cyst formation.

inflammatory in nature and not Ménétrier's disease as rigidly defined here. Pediatric cases of so-called Ménétrier's disease are of the type that spontaneously resolve.

Giant Folds Caused by Inflammation

Inflammation is a common cause of giant folds (215). Most cases are associated with *H. pylori* gastritis (221) and peptic ulcer disease. In these instances, the folds may be localized, rather than generalized, and are the result of mucosal edema and inflammatory cell infiltration. Lymphocytic gastritis is also recognized as a cause of giant gastric folds, with mucosal protein loss (222,223).

CARCINOMA OF THE STOMACH

Unusual Variants

The vast majority of gastric cancers are adenocarcinomas. Occasionally, however, adenosquamous carcinomas (224, 225) or pure squamous carcinomas (226,227) are encountered. Recently a hepatoid variant of adenocarcinoma was described (228–230), in which some portions of the tumor are typical adenocarcinoma, whereas others resemble hepatocellular carcinoma, even to the extent of secreting bile and being α-fetoprotein positive on immunostaining. Other rare gastric carcinomas include parietal cell carcinomas (231,232), choriocarcinomas (233), and rhabdoid tumors (234). Metastatic tumors to the stomach are relatively uncommon, with lung cancer being the most frequent source (235). Occasional examples of gastric carcinosarcoma have also been reported (236,237), as have spindle cell carcinomas (238).

Classification and Histopathology

There is no entirely satisfactory histologic subclassification of gastric adenocarcinoma. The World Health Organization (WHO) classification lists papillary, tubular, mucinous, and signet-ring types. This system is easy to apply and is reproducible, but unfortunately is not much value in studies of pathogenesis or etiology. More useful is the system of Lauren (239), who recognized two histologic types: intestinal and diffuse. For epidemiologic purposes, the intestinal type should be subdivided into those occurring in the distal stomach and those occurring at the cardia (240).

Intestinal adenocarcinomas of the stomach closely resemble typical colon cancers (Fig. 29). Grossly, they tend to be nodular, polypoid, or ulcerated and are well demarcated. Histologically, they are characterized predominantly by a well-formed glandular pattern, which may have solid or papillary areas. The individual cells are columnar or cuboidal, with a basally located nucleus. Cells with intracytoplasmic mucin are uncommon, although moderate quantities of mucin are present within gland lumens.

In contrast, diffuse carcinoma (Fig. 30) is more likely to have a plaquelike surface component and an ill-defined, widely infiltrating growth, which is composed of individual cells or small groups and cords of cells. Between these is a fibrous or mucoid stroma. Many cells of diffuse carcinoma contain mucin droplets, sometimes producing a signet-ring configuration (Fig. 31). Most cases of linitis plastica (leather-bottle stomach) will be classified as diffuse carcinomas. Mucinous carcinomas can be intestinal or diffuse, depending on the gross configuration (241).

As with all schemes, Lauren's classification is not perfect; about 16% of cases will be unclassifiable or of mixed type. Some authors tended to equate the terms intestinal and diffuse with well differentiated and poorly differentiated. However, this is misleading, as some poorly differentiated carcinomas may be sharply circumscribed and intestinal in type. Most diffuse carcinomas are, however, also poorly differentiated.

Epidemiology of Gastric Cancer and Precursor Lesions

In most parts of the world, adenocarcinoma of the stomach is primarily a disease of older individuals and is rare under the age of 40 years. Intestinal carcinoma involving the distal stomach is now seen much less frequently in persons

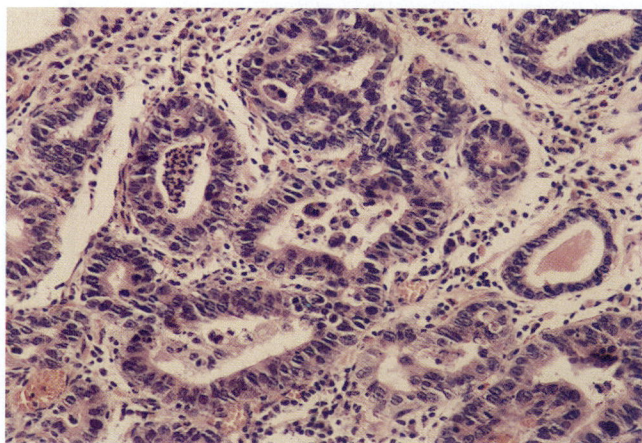

FIG. 29. Intestinal adenocarcinoma of the stomach. Note the well-formed glands and lack of cytoplasmic mucin.

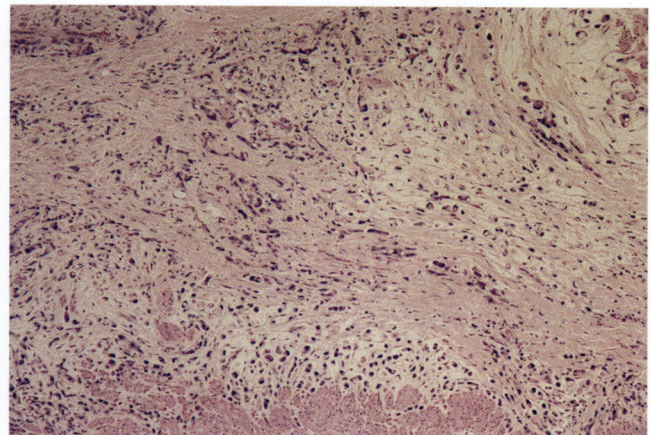

FIG. 30. Diffuse carcinoma of the stomach showing submucosal infiltration by single cells and small strings of cells.

born in North America or Western Europe than it is in persons born in Third World countries. There is a statistical association between this type of cancer and the intestinal metaplasia seen in multifocal atrophic gastritis, particularly incomplete metaplasia with sulfomucin production (also known as type III metaplasia) (242,243). Unfortunately, however, this association is weak, so the presence of metaplasia with sulfomucin production cannot be used as a marker for screening populations at risk for this type of cancer. There is only a weak association between diffuse cancer and intestinal metaplasia (244). Both types of cancer are, however, strongly associated with *H. pylori* infection (63, 245), but the mechanism of carcinogenesis may differ (246). Diffuse cancer is not confined to the elderly and may occur in adults of all ages (247), as well as occasionally affecting children (248).

Intestinal carcinoma involving the gastric cardia is now becoming much more common in North America (249,250). It is not associated with *H. pylori*. It shares many clinical, histologic, and epidemiologic features with carcinomas arising in Barrett's esophagus (251), particularly a strong male predominance (M/F, 6:1). It is probable that cardiac cancers arise in the small zone of cardiac mucosa, but the precursor lesion is not yet defined.

A major risk for the development of gastric carcinoma is a prior partial gastrectomy that has been present for 20 years or more (184,252). Such individuals are 3 to 5 times more likely to develop cancer than are age-matched controls. The mechanisms underlying this neoplastic potential are now poorly understood; patients who had a peptic duodenal ulcer without gastrectomy are not at an increased cancer risk. Rarer and less profound risk factors include the presence of pernicious anemia (253) and Ménétrier's disease (254).

Prognostic Factors

The overall prognosis of gastric cancer is poor, with an average of only 10% to 15% 5-year survival, even in patients who receive a "curative" resection. Adverse prognostic factors include age older than 70 years, carcinoembryonic antigen (CEA) more than 10 ng/ml, and CA19-9 more than 37 µg/ml (255). Survival is highest in individuals with intestinal-type carcinoma, because they generally are seen earlier with less advanced disease. When matched stage for stage, there is no difference in survival between the tumor types (255). Three modes of tumor spread may occur: via lymphatics, via the bloodstream, or via the transperitoneal route. Lymphatic metastases to lymph nodes along the greater and lesser curvatures are present in more than 70% of resection specimens. Later, there is spread to porta hepatis and paraaortic nodes. Occasionally, there may be early spread via the thoracic duct to a left supraclavicular node (the node of Virchow). Spread via the bloodstream results initially in liver metastases. Later, the lungs and other distant sites are affected. Spread transperitoneally may involve any intraabdominal site, but particularly the pelvis, the ovary being a favored location. Krukenberg's tumor is ovarian metastases of a signet-ring carcinoma, which in most cases originates in the stomach.

The most powerful determinant of prognosis is the pathologic stage. The TNM system (256) is widely used, and it is recommended that staging be included in all surgical pathology reports of resection specimens (Table 4). More than 15 lymph nodes should be sampled for adequate staging.

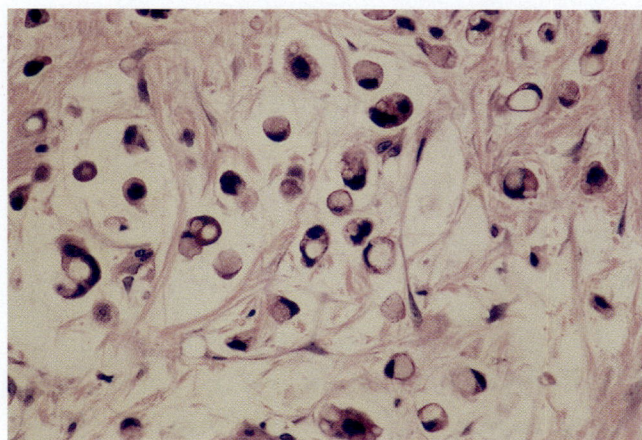

FIG. 31. Diffuse carcinoma showing multiple signet-ring cells.

TABLE 4. *TNM Staging of gastric carcinoma*

Tis	Carcinoma *in situ*
T1	Tumor invades lamina propria or submucosa
T2	Tumor invades muscularis propria or subserosa
T3	Tumor penetrates visceral peritoneum
T4	Tumor invades adjacent structures
N0	No regional nodes involved
N1	Tumor involves 1–6 regional nodes
N2	Tumor involves 7–15 regional nodes
N3	Tumor involves more than 15 regional nodes
M0	No distant metastases
M1	Distant metastases present

DNA ploidy studies now appear to be of limited value in the diagnosis and assessment of gastric cancer (255). Overall, 50% to 75% of tumors are aneuploid, although early carcinomas may be diploid. Tumors of the gastric cardia and distally located intestinal carcinomas are more likely to be aneuploid than are diffuse carcinomas. Aneuploidy also has been reported in gastric dysplasia and gastritis.

Gross Appearance, Biopsy, and Cytologic Diagnosis

Distal gastric and cardiac intestinal carcinomas may show a variety of gross appearances and can be described as superficial, polypoid, fungating, or ulcerated. Diffuse cancers are generally infiltrative in type (257). These appearances carry no prognostic significance independent of stage. Ulcerated carcinomas may be distinguished from gastric peptic ulcer by being bigger, more irregular, and having a heaped-up or rolled edge. Any endoscopically suggestive lesion in the stomach should have multiple biopsies taken for full pathologic evaluation. Eight is not an unreasonable number, and these should be taken from the edge of an ulcer, rather than the base; otherwise, only necrotic debris may be obtained.

Special problems may arise in some cases of diffuse carcinoma, because occasionally, the intramucosal component may be small in comparison to an extensive submucosal and mural involvement. In this clinical situation, the biopsies must be examined carefully, as commonly the only tumor present is in the form of inconspicuous "histiocyte"-like cells in the lamina propria or superficial submucosa. On closer examination, the "histiocytes" turn out to be tumor cells, often with a signet-ring appearance. Signet-ring cells may have nuclei that, on first examination, appear deceptively bland (Fig. 31). If a diagnostic problem is encountered, it is recommended that, first, the presence of cytoplasmic mucus be confirmed by an alcian blue with PAS stain, and second, that the nuclei of the signet-ring cells be compared with the nuclei of typical lamina propria histiocytes. The nuclei of signet-ring cells will be much larger.

With adequate biopsy material, the diagnostic accuracy of gastric biopsies performed for a suspicion of cancer is 83%. Brush cytology of these lesions, when used by itself, is 85% accurate; however, when used in conjunction with biopsy, a combined accuracy of 96% is achieved (258,259). Normal gastric surface epithelial cells appear in clumps in brush cytology specimens. The clumps are regular with a honeycomb appearance, and the individual cells have rounded nuclei containing an even distribution of chromatin. Occasional individual cells can be seen to be columnar (tapered at one end, squat at the other). The cytology of inflamed gastric mucosa is similar, but the cells become more cuboidal and have reduced amounts of cytoplasm. They also have mildly enlarged nuclei, with prominent single or double nucleoli. Cells showing intestinal metaplasia can be confused with signet-ring cancer. They have a globule of cytoplasmic mucus displacing (and sometimes indenting) the nucleus, but the nuclei themselves are bland and show inflammatory features only (Fig. 32). Carcinoma cells are usually present singly or in small irregular groups. They are large with distorted hyperchromatic nuclei that contain multiple or giant nucleoli (Fig. 33).

Gastric Carcinoma with Lymphoid Stroma

Attention has recently been drawn to a subset of gastric carcinomas that are poorly differentiated and have a prominent lymphocytic stromal infiltrate (260,261). These tumors bear a striking resemblance to the so-called lymphoepithelioma of the upper respiratory tract, which are thought to be related to Epstein–Barr virus (EBV) infection. With *in situ* hybridization techniques, many gastric tumors are also found to contain EBV RNA, but it is not clear what role, if any, the virus has in carcinogenesis (262).

Early Gastric Cancer

This term was originally used in the Japanese literature to describe infiltrating adenocarcinomas in which the primary growth is confined to the mucosa or submucosa of the stomach. Early gastric cancer is not the same as carcinoma *in situ* or gastric dysplasia, conditions in which tumor cells have not penetrated the basement membrane and have no metastatic potential. Some cases of early gastric cancer may have isolated local lymph node metastases, or even hepatic metastases, but most cases are still potentially curable by surgery.

A sophisticated subclassification of the gross appearances of early gastric cancer was devised by the Japanese Gastroenterological Endoscopic Society. The lesions can be categorized as flat, elevated, protruded, depressed, excavated, or combined forms (263). Although this terminology may be useful for the accurate gross descriptions of lesions, it correlates weakly with microscopic appearances and prognosis

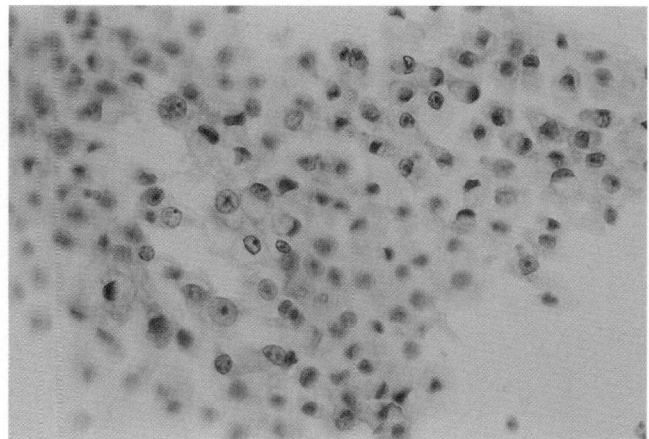

FIG. 32. Brush cytology specimen of stomach showing intestinal metaplasia (goblet cells) and cells with inflammatory changes (nuclear enlargement and prominent nucleoli). Papanicolaou stain.

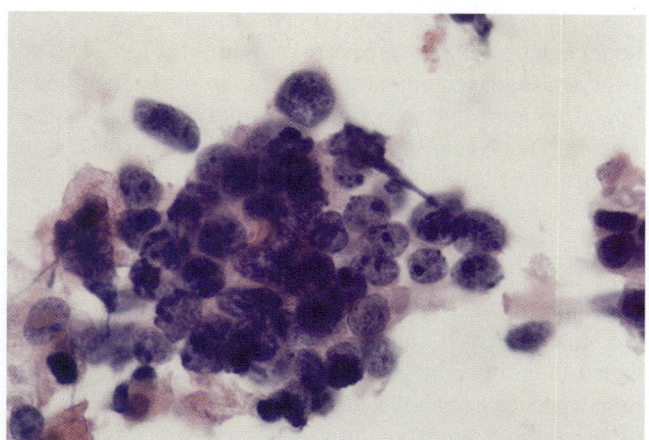

FIG. 33. Brush cytology specimen of intestinal carcinoma. Note the high nuclear/cytoplasmic ratio, the irregular nuclear outlines, and the uneven distribution of chromatin.

(264,265). Its chief value is as an aid to the endoscopist in detecting the often subtle surface features of early cancer.

As would be expected, early gastric cancer is mainly identified in the distal stomach, particularly along the lesser curve (264). The incidence of multicentricity has been estimated at 10%. Most tumors are 2.0 cm or less in diameter, although cases as large as 8.0 cm have been described (264,266). The histology of early gastric cancer is similar to that of advanced cancer, with intestinal, diffuse, and mixed forms described.

The importance of correctly identifying early gastric cancer lies in the excellent results of surgical treatment. For intramucosal cancer, the cure rate is quoted as 93% when no regional lymph-node metastases are present and 91% when they are present. For early cancers with submucosal involvement, the cure rate is 89%, which decreases to 80% in cases with lymph-node metastases (266).

Gastric Dysplasia

Several recent publications on this subject clarified many previously controversial issues (267–269). There is general agreement that the term *dysplasia* implies a neoplastic, but noninvasive, process in the gastric mucosa (270). Dysplasia now incorporates the term *carcinoma in situ*. By definition, therefore, an adenoma also consists of dysplastic epithelium. By convention, however, the term *adenoma* is reserved for circumscribed polypoid or sessile lesions and the term *dysplasia* is used for flat diffuse lesions that are grossly difficult to distinguish from the surrounding mucosa. Theoretically, dysplasia is quite distinct from regenerative atypia, although practically, there is morphologic overlap, especially in inflamed mucosa. It is recommended that only two grades of dysplasia be diagnosed: high grade and low grade. This simplifies the diagnostic problem and permits a two-tiered management decision (269).

The two most lucid accounts of gastric dysplasia each describe morphologically distinct variants (271,272). The first of these, variously called type I dysplasia or adenomatous dysplasia, closely resembles the epithelium of an adenoma and can be observed with both villous and flat configurations (Fig. 34). The dysplastic cells are crowded, with pseudostratified cigar-shaped nuclei and abundant amphophilic cytoplasm; only small amounts of intracytoplasmic mucin are present. The adjacent epithelium may be normal or may show intestinal metaplasia. In low-grade dysplasia of this type, the changes are generally superficial and consist of simple tubules with no complex branching. The nuclei are confined to the basal half of the cell and show only scanty mitotic activity. Conversely, in high-grade dysplasia, the tubules often have a profound architectural irregularity, resulting in a complex budding or cribriform pattern. The nuclei occupy more than 50% of the cell volume and display abundant mitotic activity. This type of dysplasia is considered to give rise to well-differentiated intestinal carcinomas.

The second type of dysplasia is called type II, or hyperplastic dysplasia (Fig. 35). Both goblet and columnar cells are present. The cytoplasm of the columnar cells is pale and inconspicuous, and the nuclei are enlarged, rounded, and vesicular with prominent nucleoli. Loss of polarity is not a prominent feature. The distinction between high- and low-grade dysplasia of this type is more subjective, but relies on the complexity of the architectural pattern and the increased irregularity of cell shape and chromatin distribution. This type of dysplasia arises against a background of incomplete metaplasia and is associated with poorly differentiated intestinal adenocarcinoma (206). Type II dysplasia is the most difficult to separate from regenerative changes. The nuclear morphology is basically similar in both regeneration and dysplasia, but is more severely abnormal in dysplasia. Regenerative changes are frequently accompanied by inflammation, with the severity of inflammation paralleling the severity of nuclear abnormality.

Interobserver variation may be considerable in the diagnosis of gastric dysplasia. With cases preselected as difficult

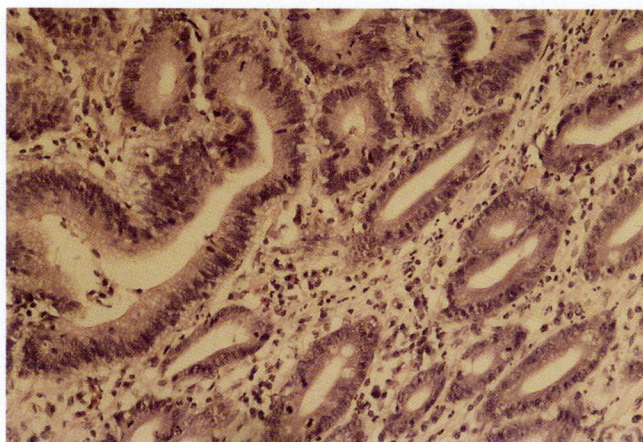

FIG. 34. Low-grade gastric dysplasia (type I). The nuclei are elongated and crowded with some loss of polarity.

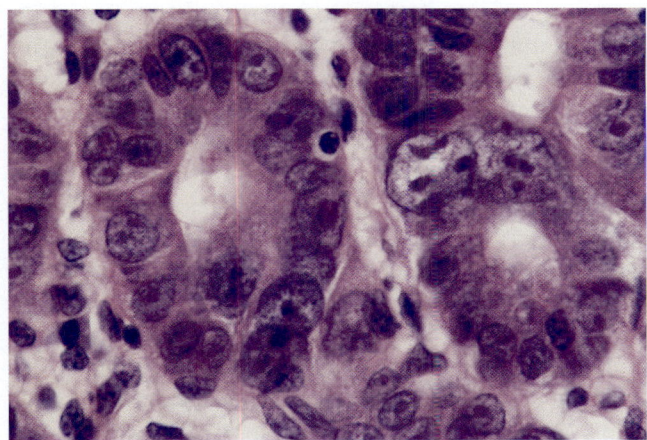

FIG. 35. High-grade gastric dysplasia (type II). There is considerable nuclear pleomorphism, but the nuclei are rounded and have prominent nucleoli.

diagnostic problems, experienced observers agree in only 66% to 75% of instances (273). Between inexperienced and experienced observers, the discrepancy may be as high as 50% (267). In unselected cases, discrepancy is not nearly so great, although inexperienced observers tend to underdiagnose advanced cancer in favor of early gastric cancer or dysplasia (265). These differences in interpretation were recently highlighted by a publication comparing the opinions of Japanese and Western pathologists (273). It is apparent that considerable differences exist, with agreement obtained in only 11 of 35 cases. Japanese pathologists' diagnosis of gastric cancer is based purely on nuclear features and structural complexity. Western pathologists require invasion of the lamina propria before rendering a diagnosis of intramucosal carcinoma.

From various publications (267,271,272,274,275), a general picture of the significance of gastric dysplasia is beginning to emerge. Low-grade dysplasia is generally a lesion that does not progress or progresses slowly. It may even regress. It seems likely that some of these cases are not true dysplasia, but misdiagnosed regenerative atypia. Follow-up with repeated biopsy is probably adequate treatment. On the other hand, high-grade dysplasia is a significant finding. Up to 60% of cases have a coincident cancer, and a further 25% will develop cancer within 15 months (267). The risk of cancer being present is particularly high in individuals with an associated gross lesion, such as a polyp or ulcer. Once a diagnosis of high-grade dysplasia is confirmed, endoscopic resection or a gastrectomy is usually indicated (267,269). There is increasing evidence that gastric dysplasia is one step on a sequence that leads from *H. pylori* infection, through chronic atrophic gastritis and large bowel–type incomplete metaplasia, to dysplasia and carcinoma (276).

ENDOCRINE TUMORS

At one time, it was thought that gastric endocrine tumors were rare, but it is now apparent that they account for between 11% and 41% of all GI endocrine neoplasms (277). Four clinicopathologic types are recognized (277,278). Type 1 tumors are the commonest. These arise in a background of fundal atrophic gastritis, usually resulting from pernicious anemia. They occur in association with achlorhydria, antral G-cell hyperplasia, and hypergastrinemia (279–281). Gastrin is trophic for fundic ECL cells, which proliferate, resulting initially in simple hyperplasia and later in nodular hyperplasia, and then neoplasia (282). Tumor development, which occurs very slowly, results in the formation of multiple small mucosal and submucosal nodules seldom more than 1.0 cm in diameter. Histologically, these carcinoid tumors appear as small clusters or ribbons of cells at the base of the lamina propria. Individual cells are regular with rounded nuclei having a diffuse chromatin pattern. The cytoplasm is greyish and not obviously granular (Fig. 36). They are strongly immunopositive for chromogranin. Metastatic spread to lymph nodes is exceedingly rare and generally occurs only in tumors greater than 1.0 cm in diameter. Interestingly, removing the gastrin stimulation by antrectomy may cause tumor regression (283). No systemic hormonal effects are attributable to type 1 tumors.

Type 2 gastric endocrine tumors are second in order of frequency. They are sporadic, solitary, and comparable in morphology and behavior to carcinoids arising in the small bowel. Type 2 tumors may occur anywhere in the stomach and are not associated with atrophic gastritis or pernicious anemia (277,284). They may be derived from EC or G cells. EC tumors may produce serotonin or histamine; they occasionally give rise to a carcinoid syndrome. G-cell tumors are generally located in the antrum and may give rise to gastrin production (285). Type 2 tumors may behave in a malignant fashion if they are larger than 2.0 cm in diameter or show angio- or deep-muscle invasion (285). Histologically, they have a trabecular pattern.

Type 3 tumors arise in individuals with the MEN-I syndrome, who also have the ZE syndrome (ZES). They arise from ECL cells in the fundus in a background of ECL hy-

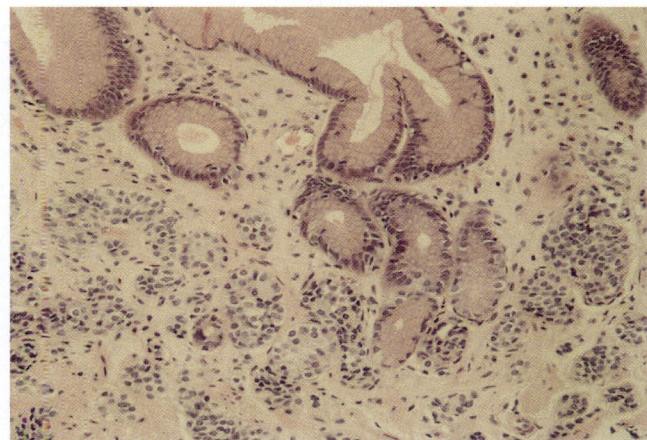

FIG. 36. Extreme endocrine cell hyperplasia is present, resulting in microcarcinoid nodules in the gastric mucosa.

perplasia and occur in association with a gastrin-producing duodenal carcinoid (286,287). In contrast to type 1 carcinoids, however, hypergastrinemia does not appear to be the growth trigger for type 3 carcinoids, because they do not occur in the ZES caused by sporadic (i.e., non–MEN-I) duodenal carcinoids. Morphologically, they are generally similar to type 1 tumors, but may occasionally become large and metastasize to regional nodes (287).

Type 4 endocrine tumors are poorly differentiated malignancies. Morphologically, they are generally typical small-cell carcinomas or may show a mixture of small and intermediate cells (288). The prognosis is uniformly poor.

GASTRIC LYMPHOMAS

The stomach is one of the most common sites of extranodal lymphomas, with primary lymphomas accounting for approximately 5% of malignancies at this site and apparently increasing in frequency (289). They occur with equal sex incidence, most commonly in the over-50 age group. Grossly, lesions in the fundus and antrum appear as ulcerated or plaquelike growths indistinguishable from adenocarcinoma (290). It is very important to distinguish between primary gastric lymphomas and nodal lymphomas that are disseminated with secondary involvement of the stomach. A primary GI lymphoma is defined as a neoplasm of the GI tract that at the time of presentation has no evidence of involvement of liver, spleen, bone marrow, or extramesenteric lymph nodes. Positive mesenteric lymph nodes are regarded as localized metastases when they occur at the time of diagnosis and do not invalidate a diagnosis of primary GI lymphoma (291).

Although occasionally we may encounter examples of Hodgkin's disease (292), T-cell non-Hodgkin's lymphoma (293), and true histiocytic lymphoma(294), the vast majority of gastric lymphomas are of B-cell origin. The term "pseudolymphoma" is obsolete. It is now realized that most of the cases previously described as pseudolymphoma are, in fact, examples of low-grade lymphoma (295). Nevertheless, lymphoid hyperplasia may occasionally involve the stomach, particularly in association with peptic ulcers. On light-microscopic appearances alone, it may be impossible to separate hyperplasia from low-grade lymphoma. It is, therefore, strongly recommended that, to facilitate this distinction, unfixed tissue should be obtained for immunohistochemical analysis and gene-rearrangement studies.

A recent study (296) of 145 cases of gastric lymphoma revealed that 49% were low grade, 34% were pure high grade, and 17% had low- and high-grade components. The patients' survival was strongly correlated with lymphoma grade, but not with treatment (by gastrectomy alone or by gastrectomy plus radiotherapy, chemotherapy, or both). Five-year survival with low-grade lymphoma was 91%; with high-grade lymphoma, it was 56%; and for mixed high- and low-grade lymphoma, it was 73%.

Large-Cell Lymphoma

Most high-grade lymphomas of the stomach are classified as either diffuse large cell or immunoblastic in the Working Classification. There is good evidence that many of them arise from a preexistent low-grade mucosa-associated lymphoid tissue (MALT) lymphoma (296a). The major diagnostic challenge with biopsy material from this type of case is to separate lymphoma from a poorly differentiated carcinoma. Lymphoma cells tend to infiltrate widely in the lamina propria in a sheetlike fashion, but they generally spare existing gastric pits and glands (Fig. 37). In contrast to low-grade lymphoma, epithelial infiltration (lymphoepithelial lesion) is not a common finding (297). Carcinomas tend to destroy mucosal structures as they infiltrate. The cells of a lymphoma are totally noncohesive, with no tendency to form clumps and cords. The nuclei of large-cell lymphomas are characteristically vesicular, with prominent nucleoli and nuclear membranes (Fig. 38). Further help in separating lymphoma from carcinoma can be obtained by special staining. Obviously, the presence of intracytoplasmic mucus virtually confirms the diagnosis of adenocarcinoma, although negative stains do not exclude it. A combined PAS with alcian blue at pH 2.5 stain is strongly recommended here, as not all tumor mucin is PAS positive. Immunohistochemistry for BER H2 and cytokeratin may be performed on fixed tissue and for Ki-1 on frozen tissue. Gastric large-cell lymphomas are characteristically negative for cytokeratin and positive with BER H2 and Ki-1. Signet-ring cells have been identified rarely in gastric lymphomas, where the appearance is usually considered to be the result of retained immunoglobulin (298). It should be noted, however, that rarely "reactive" signet-ring epithelial cells may occur as a degenerative feature in low-grade lymphoma when pits are destroyed by extensive lymphocyte infiltration (299).

Small-Cell Lymphoma

The majority of primary low-grade gastric lymphomas now are thought to arise from MALT. These lymphomas

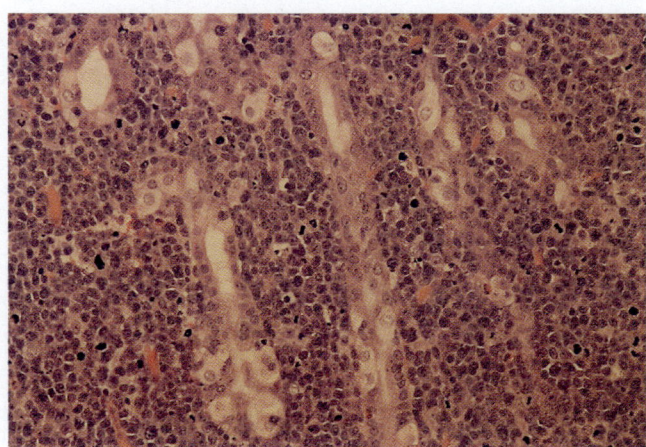

FIG. 37. Gastric lymphoma infiltrating the mucosa in a sheetlike fashion with relative sparing of epithelial elements.

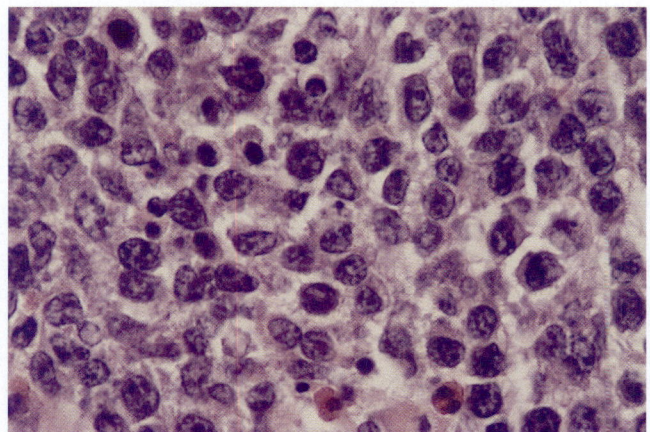

FIG. 38. Large-cell lymphoma of the stomach.

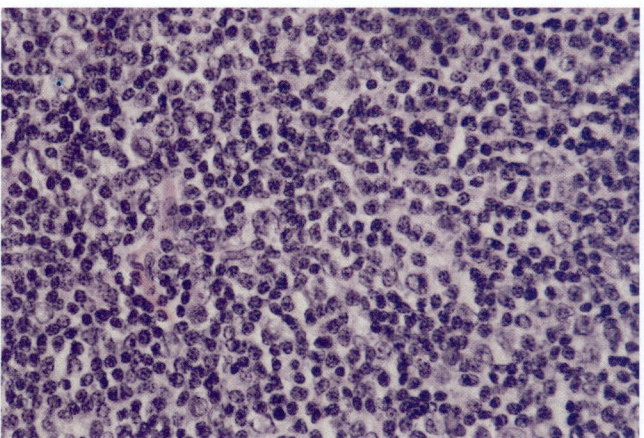

FIG. 40. Mucosa-associated lymphoid tissue (MALT) lymphoma consisting predominantly of intermediate-sized cells (small cleaved), with smaller numbers of larger cells.

have a unique appearance (Fig. 39) and behavior. Because of this, they have been designated as a special class of lymphoma called MALT lymphoma (300). There are four cardinal histologic features characteristic of low-grade MALT lymphomas: (a) an infiltrate of small lymphocytes and small cleaved follicle center (centrocytelike or CCL) cells (Fig. 40), (b) lymphoid follicles, (c) neoplastic plasma cells, and (d) lymphoepithelial lesions (Fig. 41). The CCL cells may have a variety of cytologic appearances. In most instances, they are of intermediate size (slightly bigger than a small lymphocyte), with an irregular dense nucleus. The cytoplasm is clear and there is a well-defined nuclear membrane (Fig. 40). In some cases, a few, or even many, larger cells may be present. These resemble noncleaved small lymphocytes (centroblasts). In other cases, the neoplastic cells can be extremely inconspicuous and show only subtle differences from small lymphocytes. Most MALT lymphomas contain mixtures of these cell types.

Typically, the clear CCL cells are present in a perifollicular location, where they are thought to arise from the marginal zone. As the disease progresses, these cells may begin to infiltrate the follicles themselves (follicular colonization). Frequently MALT lymphoma cells appear reactive in nature, but by specific immunostaining demonstrate light-chain restriction (301). In about one third of MALT lymphomas, plasma cell differentiation is present, particularly in the zone of lamina propria immediately beneath the surface epithelium. Rarely are these cells bizarre and easily recognizable as neoplastic, so that, again, immunohistochemical demonstration of light-chain restriction is required to prove their neoplastic nature.

Lymphocytes infiltrating the epithelium of the stomach are highly characteristic of MALT lymphomas (302) but can also be present in lymphocytic gastritis. To be suggestive of lymphoma, the infiltrate must be present as a lymphoepithelial lesion (a discrete cluster of three or more lymphocytes; Fig. 41). These distort or displace adjacent epithelial cells, partially destroying the gland. In lymphocytic gastritis, the lymphocytes, which are T cells rather than B cells, are usually present as single cells within the epithelium.

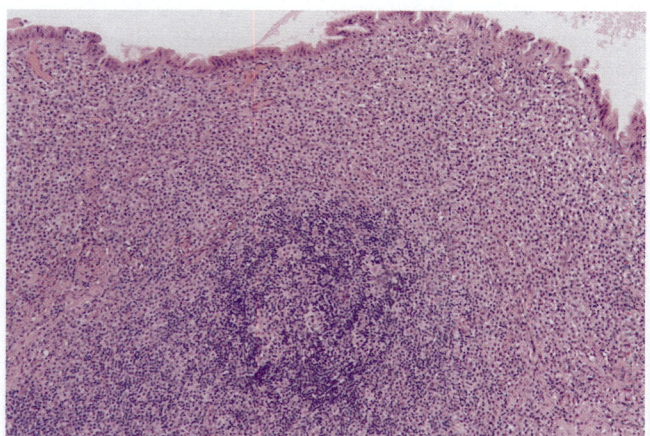

FIG. 39. Mucosa-associated lymphoid tissue (MALT) lymphoma producing expansion of the submucosa in an ill-defined nodular pattern.

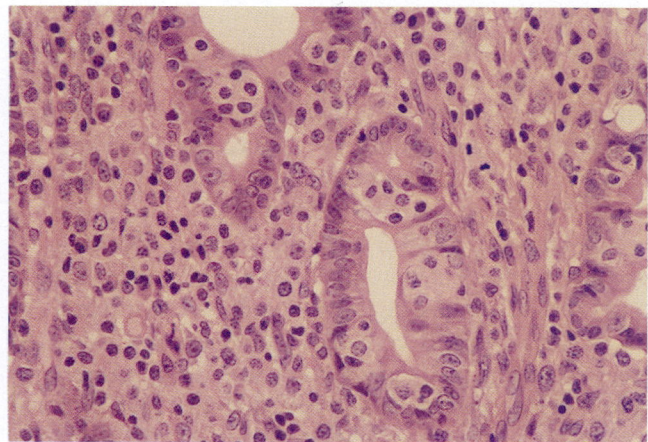

FIG. 41. Lymphoepithelial lesion from a case of mucosa-associated lymphoid tissue (MALT) lymphoma.

A characteristic immunophenotype has been detected in MALT lymphomas that is constant for tumors with different proportions of cells types. They are usually CD5⁻, CD10⁻, CD21⁺, CD35⁺, immunoglobulin M (IgM⁺), and express bcl-2 protein. In particular, CD5 negativity is considered very useful in separating MALT lymphomas from other small-cell lymphomas (303). Genotypic investigations show Ig gene rearrangements, but not bcl-2 gene rearrangements or bcl-1 translocation. About 60% of MALT lymphomas show trisomy 3 (300).

The purpose in specifically identifying MALT lymphomas is that they generally have an excellent prognosis and tend to remain localized to the stomach for many years. They may, however, ultimately convert to a large-cell lymphoma with a corresponding deterioration in prognosis (296). Recently there have been several reports that low-grade MALT lymphomas may respond to antibiotic therapy directed against *H. pylori* (300,304). *Helicobacter pylori* antigens do not directly stimulate MALT lymphoma cells, but produce secretion of interleukin-2 (IL-2) from adjacent T cells and induce IL-2 receptors on the tumor cells themselves (305). Whether these clinical responses represent "cure" or suppression remains unclear at present. It does seem, however, that *H. pylori* has a pivotal role in the causation and progression of MALT lymphoma (300).

Other primary gastric lymphomas (non-MALT type) include diffuse small cleaved cell lymphoma (intermediate cell lymphoma, mantle cell lymphoma, or centrocytic lymphoma), follicular lymphoma (small cleaved and large cell noncleaved lymphoma, also called centrocytic–centroblastic follicular lymphoma), and Burkitt's lymphoma. Mantle cell lymphomas are multicentric and commonly are seen with polyposis involving multiple sites in the GI tract (306). Histologically, they contain uniform small or medium-sized lymphocytes with round or cleaved nuclei and no admixture of blast cells. The immunophenotype is typically IgM, IgD, CD5, and CD43 positive and CD23 negative. Most cases are also CD10-negative and have bcl-1 rearrangements. The course of this lymphoma is very aggressive, with few patients surviving longer than 4 years. Other types of lymphoma involving the stomach are extremely rare (307). The coincidental occurrence of MALT lymphoma with intestinal gastric carcinoma has been noted by several authors (308), and perhaps this is not surprising considering that both diseases are related to *H. pylori* infection.

STROMAL TUMORS

The classification of gastric stromal tumors is given in Table 5. Determining the exact histologic type is considered less important than assessing their malignant potential, and it is common to refer to these tumors collectively as GI stromal tumors (GISTs). Previously, the vast majority were considered to be of smooth-muscle origin, although only 50% to 60% are desmin positive and 60% to 70% are muscle actin positive by immunohistochemistry (309,310). Moreover,

TABLE 5. *Gastric stromal neoplasms*

Benign
  Spindle-cell stromal tumor
  Epithelioid stromal tumor
  Leiomyoma
  Schwannoma
  Glomus tumor
  Lipoma
  Mesenchymoma
Malignant
  Spindle-cell stromal tumor
  Epithelioid stromal tumor
  Leiomyosarcoma
  Pleomorphic sarcoma
  Rhabdomyosarcoma
  Malignant fibrous histiocytoma
  Liposarcoma
  Gastrointestinal autonomic nerve tumor

typical smooth-muscle tumors are CD34 negative, whereas most stromal tumors are CD34 positive (311). Some tumors have ultrastructural features of smooth muscle, but these features are scanty and particularly difficult to demonstrate in neoplasms with epithelioid differentiation (312).

The enigma of GI stromal tumor origin appears now to have been solved by work suggesting that most stromal tumors are derived from GI pacemaker cells (interstitial cells of Cajal) (312a). These cells, which are intercalated between the autonomic nerves and smooth-muscle cells, control the peristaltic action of the intestinal tract. Ultrastructurally, Cajal cells show features similar to GI stromal tumors. These include incomplete myoid differentiation with interdigitating cytoplasmic processes, desmosomelike gap junctions, and synapselike cell contacts. By immunohistochemical analysis, normal Cajal cells are positive for the *kit* protooncogene, which encodes for a transmembrane tyrosine-kinase receptor (CD117). When 78 stromal tumors were tested using C-19 *kit* antibody, all 78 were positive. Similarly, 77 of 78 stromal tumors tested by using KO89-kit antibody were also positive (312a).

It appears, therefore, that the immunohistochemical testing of stromal tumors for C-*kit* activity can reliably differentiate tumors arising from Cajal cells (the vast majority) from the small numbers of smooth-muscle and nerve sheath neoplasms. It has been suggested that tumors arising from Cajal cells be renamed GI pacemaker cell tumors (GIPACTs) (312a). Although there is considerable justification for this change, it appears that it will not alter the previously established data relating to clinical management and biologic behavior of stromal tumors.

Spindle Cell Tumors

The traditional spindle cell type of GIST accounts for only 20% of all clinically significant gastric stromal neoplasms. Eighty percent are found in the fundic area, 13% at the cardia, and only 8% in the antrum. Histologically, they are composed of interlacing fascicles and whorls of elongated cells, with cigar-shaped nuclei (Fig. 42). Occasionally, a palisading pattern may be so prominent that there is a close resemblance to a schwannoma. Most gastric spindle cell tumors are benign, with only occasional malignancies. Small spindle cell leiomyomas are extremely common incidental findings, with lesions less than 5 mm in diameter being present in 16% of all resected stomachs (313).

Epithelioid Tumors

Epithelioid stromal tumors involve the fundus and antrum in approximately equal numbers (314). Histologically, they are composed of rounded cells, frequently with a clear cytoplasm (Fig. 43). Cytoplasmic clearing appears to be the result of a fixation artifact, because frozen sections do not show this feature. Close examination of formalin-fixed sections reveals condensed, retracted eosinophilic cytoplasm surrounding the nuclei. Sometimes the vacuolation is eccentric, giving a false impression of a fat-containing neoplasm or signet-ring cells (315). The growth pattern of epithelioid tumors is sheetlike, often with some arrangement around blood vessels. Mixed tumors may occur, with spindle and epithelioid differentiation present in adjacent lobules, rather than as an intimate admixture.

Carney's syndrome (316) consists of gastric epithelioid stromal tumor, pulmonary chondroma, and functioning extraadrenal paraganglioma. Patients with this condition tend to be young females (average age at presentation, 16.5 years; M/F ratio, 1:12), and the gastric neoplasms tend to be multicentric.

Other Benign Stromal Tumors

By far the most common of these is the schwannoma, which accounts for about 5% of all stromal tumors. Histologically, they are similar to schwannomas at other sites. Un-

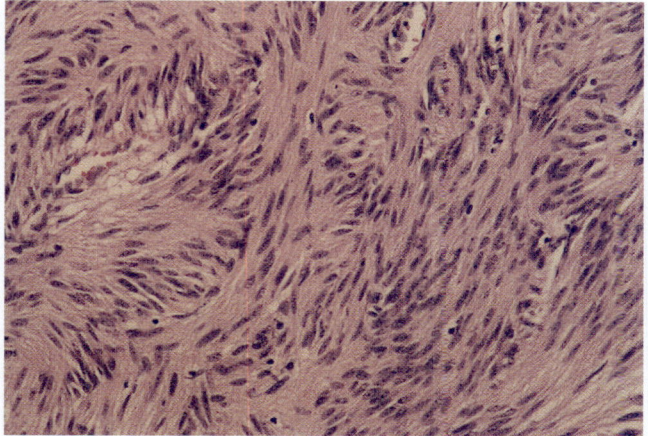

FIG. 42. Typical low-grade spindle cell gastric stromal tumor composed of interlacing fascicles of cells with cigar-shaped nuclei.

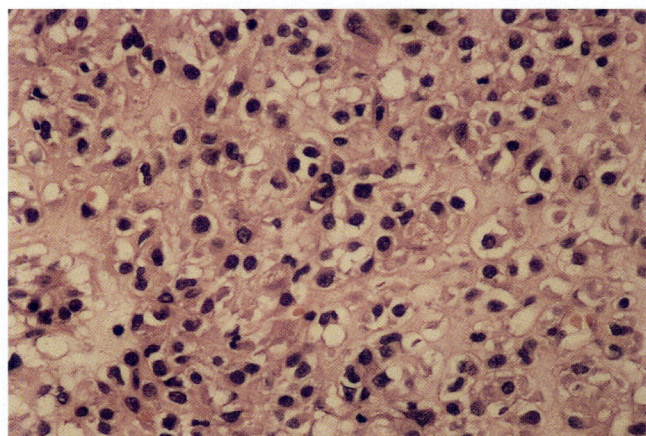

FIG. 43. Epithelioid stromal tumor of the stomach with rounded nuclei and a clear cytoplasm.

less the immunoprofile of a stromal tumor shows strong diffuse positivity for S-100 and negative results for desmin and muscle actin staining, it is probably not a schwannoma, because focal S-100 positivity may be caused by staining of normal neural elements trapped within another type of stromal tumor. Other benign stromal tumors of the stomach include lipomas (317), mesenchymomas (318), and glomus tumors (319).

Gastrointestinal Autonomic Nerve Tumors

These are uncommon GISTs that may occasionally involve the stomach (320). On light microscopy, they show a fascicular, storiform, palisaded, or lobular pattern. Most tumors consist of spindle cells, but some may be epithelioid in type (320). The distinction from the usual type of GIST can only be made ultrastructurally, where neuronlike cells with long cytoplasmic processes containing dense core neurosecretory granules and clear vesicles may be identified. These appearances resemble those of autonomic ganglia. The clinical behavior is variable, although most behave in a malignant fashion. Predictors of malignant behavior include size greater than 10 cm diameter and more than five mitoses per 10 high-power fields (320).

Sarcomas

This category includes obvious sarcomas and comprises tumors that are so undifferentiated that they cannot be readily assigned to a more specific histologic category (321). These are composed of spindle or round cells displaying considerable pleomorphism and mitotic activity. In addition, the stomach may occasionally develop sarcomas that are recognizable as specific entities. These include rhabdomyosarcoma (322), malignant fibrous histiocytoma (323), and liposarcoma (324).

Malignancy in Stromal Tumors

Predicting the biologic behavior of gastric stromal tumors is not straightforward, and a number of practical points should be considered (322,325,326). First, it is misleading to combine GI stromal tumors occurring at a variety of locations and devise a single set of rules for predicting malignant behavior. It is, however, acceptable to consider gastric spindle cell and epithelioid neoplasms as a single category. Second, it is never possible to give an absolute guarantee of behavior, because on rare occasions, even benign-appearing tumors will metastasize. Third, it must be recognized that small "malignant" tumors may be cured by excision. For these reasons, therefore, it is more useful clinically that tumors be classified according to their biologic potential, rather than their light-microscopic appearance.

Three major factors enter into the determination of malignant potential: size, cellularity, and mitotic activity. To these may also be added aneuploid DNA pattern, if this information is available (327). Gastric GISTs smaller than 6 cm in diameter rarely metastasize, although occasional neoplasms behave in an unexpected malignant fashion. For larger tumors, 30% of those measuring between 6 and 10 cm in diameter will metastasize, and 60% measuring more than 10 cm in diameter will metastasize (328). Mitotic rates for 50 high-power fields (HPF) should be determined. The usual precautions should be observed in mitosis counting (329). Up to 50% of tumors with mitotic rates of four per 50 HPF will metastasize, whereas 95% of tumors with five or more mitoses per 50 HPF will metastasize. Most benign tumors have only exceedingly rare mitoses. Mitotic rate and size are not completely independent variables, however, and it is unusual to find that small tumors are mitotically active. Conversely, larger tumors that may initially be assessed as benign will have occasional mitotic figures present when multiple areas of the lesion are sampled. For tumors in an intermediate category, tumor cellularity should be assessed. The greater the cellularity, the greater the risk of malignant behavior (328). Tumors that invade adjacent organs are obviously malignant and have a zero 5-year survival. Flow-cytometry measurements do not appear to offer significant prognostic advantages over these traditional methods (329).

VASCULAR LESIONS

The most important vascular lesion of the stomach is gastric antral vascular ectasia (GAVE), also called the "watermelon stomach" (330–332). This lesion, which is first seen with severe and persistent blood loss, is identified endoscopically by the presence of prominent parallel mucosal red stripes that radiate from the pylorus. A biopsy of the reddened area shows dilated capillaries in the superficial lamina propria immediately below the surface epithelium. These may contain fibrin thrombi (Fig. 44) and may be surrounded by eosinophilic homogeneous material (fibrohyalinosis). There may also be fibromuscular hyperplasia of the lamina propria. The cause of GAVE is unknown, but some cases are related to mucosal trauma or mucosal prolapse through the pylorus (330).

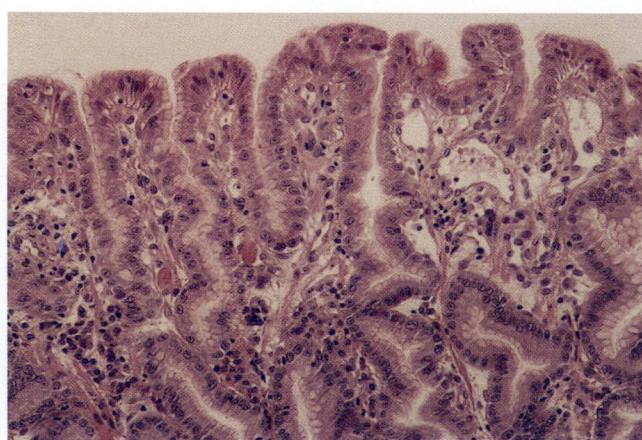

FIG. 44. Gastric antral vascular ectasia (GAVE) characterized by dilated capillaries beneath the surface epithelium.

Vascular ectasia also may occur in the stomach of patients with portal hypertension (333). Endoscopically, this may appear as flat red spots 2 to 5 mm in diameter, or as larger areas of erythema. Generally the changes involve the gastric fundus rather than the antrum. Inflammation of the mucosa is not associated with these lesions, which should be distinguished from GAVE and the acute erosions characteristic of alcoholics (334). The gastric mucosa in portal hypertension shows a relatively mild degree of capillary dilatation that is not accompanied by fibrin thrombi, fibrohyalinosis, or fibromuscular hyperplasia of the lamina propria (334).

Dieulafoy's lesion (caliber persistent artery of the stomach) is an uncommon lesion, but one that has a high mortality (60%) (335,336). It is characterized by the presence of an unusually large-diameter artery in the gastric submucosa, generally located on the lesser curvature within a few centimeters of the pylorus. The vessel is normal histologically, but is attached to the deep surface of the muscularis mucosae. As this vessel compresses the mucosa, there is gradual erosion, ultimately resulting in bleeding both from the artery and its accompanying vein (335).

Other vascular lesions of the stomach include arteriovenous malformations, which consist of tortuous vessels distributed through all layers of the gastric wall. Isolated hemangiomas and lymphangiomas are uncommon, although angiomatosis may occur as part of the Osler–Weber–Rendu, Mafucci's, and Klippel–Trenaunay syndromes. Vascular neoplasms of the stomach include Kaposi's sarcoma (337) and, rarely, angiosarcoma. These tumors have the same histologic features in the stomach as they do at other sites.

METABOLIC DISEASES INVOLVING THE STOMACH

Gastrointestinal involvement is common in amyloidosis. In the stomach, amyloid deposits may be present in the walls of submucosal arteries and within the muscularis mucosae and muscularis propria (338). Rarely amyloidosis is more widely distributed in the lamina propria and is a cause of enlarged gastric folds.

Uremia may produce gastric petechial hemorrhages, or even large areas of extravasated blood. Slow oozing, rather than rapid loss, is usual. This is presumed to occur because of a functional platelet abnormality. Gastric erosions and ulcers may also be present (339), probably produced by a direct toxic effect of urea on the mucosa.

Diabetes mellitus may result in gastroparesis (dilatation and delayed emptying). This disturbed motility is likely the result of an autonomic neuropathy (340).

REFERENCES

Normal Appearances

1. Owen DA. Stomach. In: Sternberg SS, ed. *Histology for pathologists*. 2nd ed. Philadelphia: Lippincott-Raven, 1997:481–493.
2. Kimura K. Chronological transition of the fundic-pyloric border determined by stepwise biopsy of the lesser and greater curvatures of the stomach. *Gastroenterology* 1972;63:584–592.
3. Lonroth H, Hakanson R, Lundell L, Sundler F. Histamine containing endocrine cells in the human stomach. *Gut* 1990;31:383–388.
4. Genta RM, Hamner HW, Graham DY. Gastric lymphoid follicles in *Helicobacter pylori* infection: frequency, distribution and response to triple therapy. *Hum Pathol* 1993;24:577–583.
5. Lehnert T, Erlandson DA, Decosse JJ. Lymph and blood capillaries of the human gastric mucosa. *Gastroenterology* 1985;89:939–950.
6. Listrom MM, Fenoglio-Preiser CM. Lymphatic distribution of the stomach in normal, inflammatory, hyperplastic and neoplastic tissue. *Gastroenterology* 1987;93:506–514.

Heterotopias, Duplications, and Cysts

7. Barbosa JJ, Dockerty MM, Waugh JM. Pancreatic heterotopia: review of the literature and report of 41 authenticated surgical cases, of which 25 were clinically significant. *Surg Gynecol Obstet* 1946;82:527–542.
8. Busard JM, Walters W. Heterotopic pancreatic tissue: report of a case presenting with ulcer symptoms and review of the recent literature. *Arch Surg* 1950;60:674–682.
9. Krieg EG. Heterotopic pancreatic tissue producing pyloric obstruction. *Ann Surg* 1941;113:364–370.
10. Keeley JL. Intussusception associated with aberrant pancreatic tissue: report of a case and review of the literature. *Arch Surg* 1950;60:691–698.
11. Stewart MJ, Taylor AL. Adenomyoma of the stomach. *J Pathol Bacteriol* 1925;28:195–202.
12. Nopajaroonsri C. Mucus retention in heterotopic pancreas of the gastric antrum. *Am J Surg Pathol* 1994;18:953–957.
13. Padberg BC, Schroder S. Mucus retention in heterotopic pancreas of the gastric antrum: a lesion mimicking mucinous carcinoma. *Am J Surg Pathol* 1995;19:1445–1446.
14. Yamigiwa H, Matsuzaki O, Ishiara A, Yoshimura H. Heterotopic gastric glands in the submucosa of the stomach. *Acta Pathol Jpn* 1979;29:347–350.
15. Parker BC, Guthrie J, France NE, Atwell JD. Gastric duplications in infancy. *J Pediatr Surg* 1972;7:294–298.
16. Seidman JD, Yale-Loehr AJ, Beaver B, Sun C-CJ. Alimentary duplication presenting as a hepatic cyst in a neonate. *Am J Surg Pathol* 1991;15:695–698.
17. Abrami G, Dennison WM. Duplication of the stomach. *Surgery* 1961;49:794–801.
18. Lewis PL, Holder T, Feldman M. Duplication of the stomach: report of a case and review of the English literature. *Arch Surg* 1961;82:634–640.
19. Tabrisky J, Szalay GC, Meade WS. Duplication of the stomach: a cause of anemia. *Am J Gastroenterol* 1973;59:327–331.
20. Wieczorek RL, Siedman I, Ranson JH, Ruoff M. Congenital duplication of the stomach: case report and review of the English literature. *Am J Gastroenterol* 1984;79:597–602.
21. Meeroff M, Gollan JR, Meeroff JC. Gastric diverticulum. *Am J Gastroenterol* 1967;47:189–203.
22. Farack UM, Goresky CA, Jabbari M, Kinnear DG. Double pylorus: A hypothesis concerning its pathogenesis. *Gastroenterology* 1974;66:596–600.
23. Sulfian S, Ominsky S, Matsumoto T. Congenital double pylorus. *Gastroenterology* 1977;73:154–157.
24. Pai SH, Cameron CT, Lev R. Accessory lung presenting as a juxtagastric mass. *Arch Pathol Lab Med* 1971;91:569–572.
25. Shireman PK: Intramural cyst of the stomach. *Hum Pathol* 1987;18:857–858.
26. Oberman HA, Lodmell JG, Sower ND. Diffuse heterotopic cystic malformation of the stomach. *N Engl J Med* 1963;269:909–911.
27. Ignatius JA, Armstrong CD, Eversole SL. Multiple diffuse cystic disease of the stomach in association with carcinoma. *Gastroenterology* 1970;59:610–614.
28. Pillay I, Petrelli M. Diffuse cystic glandular malformation of the stomach associated with adenocarcinoma: case report and review of the literature. *Cancer* 1976;38:915–920.
29. Kato Y, Sugano H, Rubio CA. Classification of intramucosal cysts of the stomach. *Histopathology* 1983;7:931–938.

Xanthelasma

30. Domellof L, Eriksson S, Helander HF, Januger KG. Lipid islands in the gastric mucosa after resection for benign ulcer disease. *Gastroenterology* 1977;72:14–18.
31. Coates AG, Nostrant TT, Wilson JA, Dobbins WO, Agha FP. Gastric xanthomatosis and cholestasis: a causal relationship. *Dig Dis Sci* 1986;31:925–928.
32. Kimura K, Hiramoto T, Buncher CR. Gastric xanthelasma. *Arch Pathol Lab Med* 1969;87:110–117.
33. Pieterse AS, Rowland R, Labrooy JT. Gastric xanthomas. *Pathology* 1985;17:455–457.
34. Kaiserling E, Heinle H, Itabe H, et al. Lipid islands in the human gastric mucosa: morphological and immunohistochemical findings. *Gastroenterology* 1996;110:369–374.

Pyloric Stenosis

35. Benson DC. Infantile pyloric stenosis. *Prog Pediatr Surg* 1970;1:63–89.
36. Batcup G, Spitz L. A histopathological study of gastric mucosal biopsies in infantile hypertrophic stenosis. *J Clin Pathol* 1979;32:625–628.
37. Wellman IKF, Kagan A, Fang H. Hypertrophic pyloric stenosis in adults: survey of the literature and report of a case of localized form. *Gastroenterology* 1964;46:601–608.

Metaplasia

38. Rubio CA, Antonioli D. Ciliated metaplasia in the gastric mucosa. *Am J Surg Pathol* 1988;12:786–789.
39. Rubio CA, Hayashi T, Stemmerman G. Ciliated gastric cells: a study of their phenotypic characteristics. *Mod Pathol* 1990;3:720–723.
40. Thompson IW, Day DW, Wright NA. Subnuclear vacuolated cells: a novel abnormality of simple mucin-secreting cells of non-specialized gastric mucosa and Brunner's glands. *Histopathology* 1987;11:1067–1081.
41. Rubio CA, Slezak P. Foveolar cell vacuolization in operated stomachs. *Am J Surg Pathol* 1988;12:773–776.
42. Doglioni C, Laurino L, Dei Tos AP, et al. Pancreatic (acinar) metaplasia of the gastric mucosa: histology, ultrastructure, immunocytochemistry and clinicopathologic correlations of 101 cases. *Am J Surg Pathol* 1993;17:1134–1143.
43. Wang HH, Zeroogian JM, Spechler SJ, et al. Prevalence and significance of pancreatic acinar metaplasia at the gastro-esophageal junction. *Am J Surg Pathol* 1996;20:1507–1510.
44. Spicer SS. Diamine methods for differentiating mucosubstances histochemically. *J Histochem Cytochem* 1965;13:211–234.

Gastritis

45. Strickland RG, MacKay IR. A re-appraisal of the nature and significance of chronic atrophic gastritis. *Am J Dig Dis* 1973;18:426–440.
46. Wyatt JI, Dixon MF. Chronic gastritis: a pathogenetic approach. *J Pathol* 1988;154:944–951.
47. Price AB. The Sydney system: histological division. *J Gastroenterol Hepatol* 1991;6:209–222.
48. Dixon MF, Genta RM, Yardley JH, et al. Classification and grading of gastritis: an updated Sydney system. *Am J Surg Pathol* 1996;20:1161–1181.
49. Amir-Ahmadi H, McCray RS, Martin F, Mitch W, Kantrowitz PA, Zamcheck N. Reassessment of massive upper gastrointestinal hemorrhage on the wards of the Boston City Hospital. *Surg Clin North Am* 1969;49:715–726.
50. Laine L, Weinstein WM. Histology of alcoholic hemorrhagic 'gastritis': a prospective evaluation. *Gastroenterology* 1988;94:1254–1262.
51. Goldman H, Antonioli DA. Mucosal biopsy of the esophagus, stomach and proximal duodenum. *Hum Pathol* 1982;13:423–448.
52. Laine L, Weinstein WM. Subepithelial hemorrhages and erosions of human stomach. *Dig Dis Sci* 1988;33:490–503.
53. Holvoet J, Terriere L, Van Hee W, Verbist L, Fierens E, Hautekeete ML. Relation of upper gastrointestinal bleeding to non-steroidal anti-inflammatory drugs and aspirin: a case control study. *Gut* 1991;32:730–734.
54. Aabakken L. NSAIDs and the gastrointestinal tract: case closed? *Scand J Gastroenterol* 1991;26:801–805.
55. Cheung LY. Pathogenesis, prophylaxis and treatment of stress gastritis. *Am J Surg* 1988;156:437–440.
56. Miller AI, Smith B, Rogers AI. Phlegmonous gastritis. *Gastroenterology* 1975;68:231–238.
57. Bron BA, Deyhle P, Pelloni S, Krejs GJ, Siebenmann RE, Blum AL. Phlegmonous gastritis diagnosed by endoscopic snare biopsy. *Am J Dig Dis* 1977;22:729–733.
58. O'Toole PA, Morris JA. Acute phlegmonous gastritis. *Postgrad Med J* 1988;64:315–316.
59. Blaser MJ. Hypothesis on the pathogenesis and natural history of *Helicobacter pylori*-induced inflammation. *Gastroenterology* 1992;102:720–727.
60. McGowan CC, Cover TL, Blaser MJ. *Helicobacter pylori* and gastric acid: biological and therapeutic implications. *Gastroenterology* 1996;110:926–938.
61. El Omar EM, Penman ID, Ardill JE, et al. *Helicobacter pylori* infection and abnormalities of acid secretion in patients with duodenal ulcer disease. *Gastroenterology* 1995;109:681–691.
62. Correa P, Yardley JH. Grading and classification of chronic gastritis: one American response to the Sydney system. *Gastroenterology* 1992;102:355–359.
63. Correa P. *Helicobacter pylori* and gastric carcinogenesis. *Am J Surg Pathol* 1995;19(suppl 1):S37–S43.
64. Parsonnet J, Freidman GD, Vandersteen DP, et al. *Helicobacter pylori* infection and the risk of gastric carcinoma. *N Engl J Med* 1991;325:1127–1131.
65. Blaser MJ. Intrastrain differences in *Helicobacter pylori*: a key question in mucosal damage. *Ann Intern Med* 1995;27:559–563.
66. Hu PJ, Li YY, Lin HL, et al. Gastric atrophy and regional variation in upper gastrointestinal disease. *Am J Gastroenterol* 1995;90:1102–1106.
67. Rocha GA, Queiroz DM, Mendes EN, et al. *Helicobacter pylori* acute gastritis: histological, endoscopical, clinical and therapeutic features. *Am J Gastroenterol* 1991;86:1592–1595.
68. Sobala GM, Crabtree JE, Dixon MF, et al. Acute *Helicobacter pylori* infection: clinical features, local and systemic immune response, gastric mucosal histology and gastric juice ascorbic acid concentrations. *Gut* 1991;32:1415–1418.
69. Vartanian RK, Leung JK, Davis JE, et al. A novel alcian yellow-toluidine blue (Leung) stain for *Helicobacter* species: comparison with standard stains, a cost-effectiveness analysis and supplemental utilities. *Mod Pathol* 1998;11:72–78.
70. Guy CD, Giltman LI, Varman VA. Comparison of histochemical stains for the diagnosis of *Helicobacter pylori*. *Am J Clin Pathol* 1997;107:473.
71. Chan WY, Hui PK, Leung KM, et al. Coccoid forms of *Helicobacter pylori* in the human stomach. *Am J Clin Pathol* 1994;102:503–507.
72. Cartun RW, Kryzmowski GA, Pederson CA, et al. Immunocytochemical identification of *Helicobacter pylori* in formalin-fixed gastric biopsies. *Mod Pathol* 1991;4:498–502.
73. Genta RM, Lew GM, Graham DY. Changes in the gastric mucosa following eradication of *Helicobacter pylori*. *Mod Pathol* 1993;6:281–289.
74. Witteman EM, Mravunac M, Becx MJ, et al. Improvement of gastric inflammation and resolution of epithelial damage one year after eradication of *Helicobacter pylori*. *J Clin Pathol* 1995;48:250–256.
75. Yang H, Dixon MF, Li X, et al. Acute gastritis associated with infection of large spiral-shaped bacteria. *Am J Gastroenterol* 1995;90:307–309.
76. Hilzenrat N, Lamoureux E, Weintrub I, et al. *Helicobacter heilmannii*-like spiral bacteria in gastric mucosal biopsies: prevalence and clinical significance. *Arch Pathol Lab Med* 1995;119:1149–1153.
77. Riddell RH, Goldman H, Ransohoff DF, et al. Dysplasia in inflammatory bowel disease. *Hum Pathol* 1983;14:931–966.
78. Craanen ME, Dekker W, Block P, Ferwerda J, Tytgat GN. Intestinal metaplasia and *Helicobacter pylori*: an endoscopic bioptic study of the gastric antrum. *Gut* 1992;33:16–20.
79. Karnes WE, Samloff IM, Siurala M, et al. Positive serum antibody and negative tissue staining for *Helicobacter pylori* in subjects with atrophic body gastritis. *Gastroenterology* 1991;101:167–174.
80. Correa P. Chronic gastritis: a clinico-pathological classification. *Am J Gastroenterol* 1988;83:504–509.
81. Recavarren Arce S, Leon Barua R, Cok J, et al. *Helicobacter* and progressive gastric pathology that predisposes to gastric cancer. *Scand J Gastroenterol* 1991;181(suppl):S1–S7.
82. Villako K, Kekki M, Tamm A, Savisaar E. Development and progression of chronic gastritis in the antrum and body mucosa: results of long term follow-up examinations. *Ann Clin Res* 1986;18:121–123.
83. Caygill CP. Epidemiology relating N-nitroso compounds to human cancer. *Eur J Cancer Prev* 1996;5(suppl 1):125–130.
84. Xu GP, SO PJ, Reed PI. Hypothesis on the relationship between gastric cancer and intragastric nitrosonation: N-nitrosamines in gastric juice of subjects from a high risk area for gastric cancer and the inhibition of N-nitrosamine formation by fruit juices. *Eur J Cancer Prev* 1993;2:25–36.
85. Chen VW, Abu-Elyazeed RR, Zavala DE, et al. Risk factors of gastric precancerous lesions in a high-risk Columbian population: II. nitrate and nitrite. *Nutr Cancer* 1990;13:67–72.
86. Negrini R, Savio A, Poiesi C, et al. Antigenic mimicry between *Helicobacter pylori* and gastric mucosa in the pathogenesis of body atrophic gastritis. *Gastroenterology* 1996;111:655–665.
87. Fong T-L, Dooley CP, Dehesa M, et al. *Helicobacter pylori* infection in pernicious anemia: a prospective controlled study. *Gastroenterology* 1991;100:328–332.
88. Stolte M, Bauman K, Bethke B, et al. Active autoimmune gastritis without total atrophy of the glands. *Z Gastroenterol* 1992;30:729–735.
89. Appelman HD. Gastritis: terminology, etiology and clinicopathologic correlations. *Hum Pathol* 1994;25:1006–1019.

Carditis

89a. Goldblum JR, Vicari JJ, Falk GW, et al. Inflammation and intestinal metaplasia of the gastric cardia: the role of gastroesophageal reflux and *H. pylori* infection. *Gastroenterology* 1998;114:633–639.
89b. Oberg S, Peters JH, DeMeester TR, et al. Inflammation and specialized intestinal metaplasia of the cardiac mucosa is a manifestation of gastroesophageal reflux disease. *Ann Surg* 1997;226:522–532.
89c. Genta RM, Huberman RM, Graham DY. The gastric cardia in *Helicobacter pylori* infection. *Hum Pathol* 1994;25:915–919.
89d. Hackelsberger A, Gunther T, Schultze V, et al. Prevalence and pattern of *Helicobacter pylori* gastritis in the gastric cardia. *Am J Gastroenterol* 1997;92:2220–2224.
89e. Riddell RH. The biopsy diagnosis of gastroesophageal reflux disease, 'carditis,' and Barrett's esophagus and sequelae of therapy. *Am J Surg Pathol* 1996;20(suppl 1):S31–S51.

Infectious Granulomatous Gastritis

90. Tromba JL, Inglese R, Rieders B, et al. Primary gastric tuberculosis presenting as pyloric outlet obstruction. *Am J Gastroenterol* 1991;86:1820–1822.

91. Chazan B, Aitchison J. Gastric tuberculosis. *Br Med J* 1960;2:1288–1290.
92. Subei I, Attar B, Schmitt G, Levendoglu H. Primary gastric tuberculosis: a case report and literature review. *Am J Gastroenterol* 1987;82:769–772.
93. Pedraza MA. Mycotic infections at autopsy: a comparative study in two university hospitals. *Am J Clin Pathol* 1969;51:470–476.
94. Eras P, Goldstein MJ, Sherlock P. *Candida* infection of the gastrointestinal tract. *Medicine (Baltimore)* 1972;51:367–379.
95. Fisher JR, Sanowski RA. Disseminated histoplasmosis producing hypertrophic gastric folds. *Dig Dis Sci* 1978;23:282–285.
96. Lawson H, Schmaman A. Gastric phycomycosis. *Br J Surg* 1974;61:743–746.
97. Katzenstein AL, Maksem J. Candidal infection of gastric ulcers. *Am J Clin Pathol* 1979;71:137–141.
98. Gotlieb-Jensen K, Andersen J. Occurrence of *Candida* in gastric ulcers: significance for the healing process. *Gastroenterology* 1983;85:535–537.
99. Inagaki H, Kawai T, Miyata M, et al. Gastric syphilis: polymerase chain reaction detection of treponemal DNA in pseudolymphomatous lesions. *Hum Pathol* 1996;27:761–765.
100. Greenstein DB, Wilcox CM, Schwartz DA. Gastric syphilis: report of seven cases and review of the literature. *J Clin Gastroenterol* 1994;18:4–9.
101. Kasmin F, Reddy S, Mathur-Wagh U, et al. Syphilitic gastritis in a HIV infected individual. *Am J Gastroenterol* 1992;87:1820–1822.
102. Ectors NL, Dixon MF, Geboes KJ, et al. Granulomatous gastritis a morphological and diagnostic approach. *Histopathology* 1993;23:55–61.
103. Ectors N, Geboes K, Wynants P, et al. Granulomatous gastritis and Whipple's disease. *Am J Gastroenterol* 1992;87:509–513.

NonInfectious Granulomatous Gastritis

104. Korelitz BI, Waye JD, Kreuning J, et al. Crohn's disease in endoscopic biopsies of the gastric antrum and duodenum. *Am J Gastroenterology* 1981;76:103–109.
105. Kreuning J, Meijer CJ. Morphological and immunohistochemical findings in upper gastrointestinal biopsies of patients with Crohn's disease of the colon and ileum. *J Clin Pathol* 1982;35:934–940.
106. Fahimi HD, Deren JJ, Gottlieb MD, Zamcheck N. Isolated granulomatous gastritis: its relationship to disseminated sarcoidosis and regional enteritis. *Gastroenterology* 1963;45:161–175.
107. Shapiro JL, Goldblum JR, Petras RE. A clinicopathologic study of 42 patients with granulomatous gastritis: is there really an 'idiopathic' granulomatous gastritis? *Am J Surg Pathol* 1996;20:462–470.
107a. Wright CL, Riddell RH. Histology of the stomach and duodenum in Crohn's disease. *Am J Surg Pathol* 1998;22 383–390.
108. Chinitz MA, Brandt LJ, Frank MS, Frager D, Sablay L. Symptomatic sarcoidosis of the stomach. *Dig Dis Sci* 1985;30:682–688.
109. Fireman Z, Sternberg A, Yarchovsky Y, et al. Multiple antral ulcers in gastric sarcoid. *J Clin Gastroenterol* 1997;24:97–99.
110. Leach IH, Maclennan KAS. Gastric lymphoma associated with mucosal and nodal granulomas: a new differential diagnosis in granulomatous gastritis. *Histopathology* 1990;17:87–88.
111. O'Donovan C, Murray J, Staunton H, et al. Granulomatous gastritis: part of a vasculitic syndrome. *Hum Pathol* 1991;22:1057–1059.
112. Temmesfeld-Wollbrueck B, Heinrichs C, Szelay A, et al. Granulomatous gastritis in Wegener's disease: differentiation from Crohn's disease supported by a positive test for antineutrophil antibodies. *Gut* 1997;40:550–553.
113. Guarino M, Reale D, Micoli G, et al. Xanthogranulomatous gastritis: association with xanthogranulomatous cholecystitis. *J Clin Pathol* 1993;46:88–90.

Eosinophilic Gastritis

114. Abell MR, Limond RV, Blamey WE, Marzel W. Allergic granulomatosis with massive gastric involvement. *N Engl J Med* 1970;282:665–668.
115. Ruzic JP, Dorsey JM, Huber HL, Armstrong EH. Gastric lesion of Loeffler's syndrome: report of a case with inflammatory lesion simulating carcinoma. *JAMA* 1952;149:534–537.
116. Johnstone JM, Morson BC. Inflammatory fibroid polyp of the gastrointestinal tract. *Histopathology* 1978;2:349–361.
117. Ashby BS, Appleton PJ, Dawson J. Eosinophilic granuloma of gastrointestinal tract caused by herring parasite *Eustoma rotundatum*. *Br Med J (Clin Res Ed)* 1964;1:1141–1145.
118. Ikeda K, Kumashiro R, Kifune T. Nine cases of acute gastric anisakiasis. *Gastrointest Endosc* 1989;35:304–308.
119. Goldman H, Pronjansky R. Allergic proctitis and gastroenteritis in children: clinical and mucosal biopsy features in 53 cases. *Am J Surg Pathol* 1986;10:75–86.
120. El Mouzan MI, Al Quorain AA, Anim JT. Cow's milk induced erosive gastritis in an infant. *J Pediatr Gastroenterol Nutr* 1990;10:1111–1113.
121. DeSchryver-Kecskemeti K, Clouse RE. A previously unrecognized sub-group of 'eosinophilic gastroenteritis': association with connective tissue diseases. *Am J Surg Pathol* 1984;8:171–180.
122. Johnstone JM, Morson BC. Eosinophilic gastroenteritis. *Histopathology* 1978;2:349–361.
123. Blackshaw AJ, Levison DA. Eosinophilic infiltrates of the gastrointestinal tract. *J Clin Pathol* 1986;39:1–7.
124. Talley NJ, Shorter RG, Phillips SF, Zinsmeister AR. Eosinophilic gastroenteritis: a clinicopathological study of patients with disease of the mucosa, muscle layer and subserosal tissues. *Gut* 1990;31:54–58.
125. Lowichik A, Weinberg AG. A quantitative evaluation of mucosal eosinophils in the pediatric gastrointestinal tract. *Mod Pathol* 1996;9:110–114.

Lymphocytic Gastritis

126. Haot J, Hamichi L, Wallez L, Mainguet P. Lymphocytic gastritis: a newly described entity: a retrospective endoscopic and histologic study. *Gut* 1988;29:1258–1264.
127. Haot J, Jouret A, Willette M, Gossuin A, Mainguet P. Lymphocytic gastritis: prospective study of its relationship to varioliform gastritis. *Gut* 1990;31:283–285.
128. Wolber R, Owen DA, Freeman H, et al. Lymphocytic gastritis and giant gastric folds: a cause of gastrointestinal protein loss. *Mod Pathol* 1991;4:13–15.
129. Groisman GM, George J, Berman D, et al. Resolution of protein-losing hypertrophic lymphocytic gastritis with therapeutic eradication of *Helicobacter pylori*. *Am J Gastroenterol* 1994;89:1548–1551.
130. Dixon M, Wyatt J, Burke D, Rathbone B. Lymphocytic gastritis: relationship to *Campylobacter pylori* infection. *J Pathol* 1988;154:125–132.
131. Niemela S, Karttunen T, Kerola T, et al. Ten year follow up study of lymphocytic gastritis: further evidence on *Helicobacter pylori* as a cause of lymphocytic gastritis and corpus gastritis. *J Clin Pathol* 1995;48:1111–1116.
132. Wolber R, Owen D, DelBuono L, Appelman H, Freeman H. Lymphocytic gastritis in patients with celiac sprue or sprue-like intestinal disease. *Gastroenterology* 1990;98:310–315.
133. De Giacomo C, Gianetti A, Negrini R, et al. Lymphocytic gastritis: a positive relationship with celiac disease. *J Pediatr* 1994;124:57–62.
134. Alsaigh N, Odze R, Goldman H, et al. Gastric and esophageal intraepithelial lymphocytes in pediatric celiac disease. *Am J Surg Pathol* 1996;20:865–870.
135. Lynch DA, Sobala GM, Dixon MF, et al. Lymphocytic gastritis and associated small bowel disease: a diffuse lymphocytic gastroenteropathy? *J Clin Pathol* 1995;48:939–945.
136. Groisman GM, Meyers S, Harpaz N. Collagenous gastritis associated with lymphocytic colitis. *J Clin Gastroenterol* 1996;22:134–137.
137. Griffiths AP, Wyatt J, Jack AS, et al. Lymphocytic gastritis, gastric adenocarcinoma and primary gastric lymphoma. *J Clin Pathol* 1994;47:1123–1124.
138. Miettenen A, Karttunen TJ, Alavaikko M. Lymphocytic gastritis and *Helicobacter pylori* infection in gastric lymphoma. *Gut* 1995;37:471–476.

Reactive Gastropathy

139. Carpenter HA, Talley NJ. Gastroscopy is incomplete without biopsy: clinical relevance of distinguishing gastropathy from gastritis. *Gastroenterology* 1995;108:917–924.

140. Dixon MF, O'Connor HJ, Axon AT, et al. Reflux gastritis: a distinct histopathological entity? *J Clin Pathol* 1986;39:524–530.
141. Sobala GM, King RF, Axon AT, Dixon MF. Reflux gastritis in the intact stomach. *J Clin Pathol* 1990;43:303–306.
142. Quinn CM, Bjarnson I, Price AB. Gastritis in patients on non-steroidal anti-inflammatory drugs. *Histopathology* 1993;23:341–348.
143. Niemela S, Karttunen T, Heikkila J, Lehtola J. Characteristics of reflux gastritis. *Scand J Gastroenterol* 1987;22:349–354.
144. Karttunen T, Niemela S. *Campylobacter pylori* and duodenogastric reflux in peptic ulcer disease and gastritis. *Lancet* 1988;I:118.

Radiation and Chemotherapy Changes

145. Berthrong M, Fajardo LF. Radiation injury in surgical pathology: part II. alimentary tract. *Am J Surg Pathol* 1984;8:171–180.
146. Coia LR, Myerson RJ, Tepper JE. Late effects of radiation therapy on the gastrointestinal tract. *Int J Radiat Oncol Biol Physics* 1995;31:1213–1236.
147. Petras RE, Hart WR, Bukowski RM. Gastric epithelial atypia associated with hepatic arterial infusion chemotherapy; its distinction from early gastric cancer. *Cancer* 1985;56:745–750.
148. Becker SN, Sass MA, Petras RE, Hart WR. Bizarre atypia in gastric brushings associated with hepatic arterial infusion chemotherapy. *Acta Cytol* 1986;30:347–355.
149. Weidner N, Smith JG, LaVanway JM. Peptic ulceration with marked epithelial atypia following hepatic arterial infusion chemotherapy. *Am J Surg Pathol* 1983;7:261–268.

Ischemic Gastritis

150. Force T, MacDonald D, Eade OE, Doane C, Krawitt EL. Ischemic gastritis and duodenitis. *Dig Dis Sci* 1980;25:307–310.
151. Allende H, Ona F. Celiac artery and superior mesenteric artery insufficiency: unusual cause of erosive gastroenteritis. *Gastroenterology* 1982;82:763–766.
152. Cherry RD, Jabbari M, Goresky CA, Herba M, Reich D, Blundell PE. Chronic mesenteric vascular insufficiency with gastric ulceration. *Gastroenterology* 1986;91:1548–1522.
152a. Trowell JE, Bell GD. Biopsy specimen appearances of ischemic gastritis in splanchnic arterial insufficiency. *J Clin Pathol* 1998;51:255–256.

Drug-Induced Gastritis

153. Oren R, Ligumsky M, Lysy J, et al. Gastro-duodenal injury associated with intake of 100-325 mg aspirin daily. *Postgrad Med J* 1993;69:712–714.
154. MacDonald WC. Correlation of mucosal histology and aspirin intake in chronic gastric ulcer. *Gastroenterology* 1973;65:381–389.
155. El-Zimaity HM, Genta RM, Graham DY. Histological features do not define NSAID-induced gastritis. *Hum Pathol* 1996;27:1348–1354.
156. McCarthy CJ, McDermott M, Hourihane D, O'Morain C. Chemical gastritis induced by naproxen in the absence of *Helicobacter pylori* infection. *J Clin Pathol* 1995;48:61–63.
157. Shah K, Price AB, Talbot IC, Bardhan KD, Fenn CG, Bjarnson I. Effect of long term mistoprostol coadministration with non-steroidal anti-inflammatory drugs: a histological study. *Gut* 1995;37:195–198.
158. Lamberts R, Creutzfeld W, Struber AG, Brunner G, Solcia E. Long-term omeprazole therapy in peptic ulcer disease: gastrin, endocrine cell growth and gastritis. *Gastroenterology* 1993;104:1356–1370.
159. Solcia E, Fiocca R, Villani L, Luinetti O, Capella C. Hyperplastic, dysplastic and neoplastic enterochromaffin-like cell proliferations of the gastric mucosa: classification and histogenesis. *Am J Surg Pathol* 1995;19(suppl 1):S51–S57.
160. Greenson JK, Trinidad SB, Pfeil SA, et al. Gastric mucosal calcinosis: calcified aluminum phosphate deposits secondary to aluminum-containing antacids or sucralfate therapy in organ transplant recipients. *Am J Surg Pathol* 1993;17:45–50.

Gastritis in Immunodeficiency

161. Niedt GW, Schinella RA. Acquired immunodeficiency syndrome: clinicopathologic studies of 56 autopsies. *Arch Pathol Lab Med* 1985;109:727–734.
162. Hinnant KL, Rotterdam HZ, Bell ET, Tapper ML. Cytomegalovirus infection of the alimentary tract: a clinicopathological correlation. *Am J Gastroenterol* 1986;81:944–950.
163. Strayer DS, Phillips GS, Barker KH, Winokur T, DeSchryver-Kecskemeti K. Gastric cytomegalovirus infection in bone marrow transplant patients: an indication of generalized disease. *Cancer* 1981;48:1478–1483.
164. Aqel NM, Tanner P, Drury A, Francis ND, Henry K. Cytomegalovirus gastritis with perforation and gastrocolic fistula formation. *Histopathology* 1991;18:165–168.
165. Shuster LD, Cox G, Bhatia P, Miner PB Jr. Gastric mucosal nodules due to cytomegalovirus infection. *Dig Dis Sci* 1989;34:103–107.
166. Kovacs AA, Churchill MA, Wood D, Mascola L, Zaia JA. Molecular and epidemiologic evaluations of a cluster of cases of Menetrier's disease associated with cytomegalovirus. *Pediatr Infect Dis J* 1993;12:1011–1014.
167. Corey L, Spear PG. Infections with herpes simplex. *N Engl J Med* 1986;314:749–757.
168. Guarda LA, Stem SA, Cleary KA, Ordonez NG. Human cryptosporidiosis in the acquired immunodeficiency syndrome. *Arch Pathol Lab Med* 1983;107:562–566.
169. Delsedime F, Coppola F, Mazzucco G. Gastric localization of systemic leishmaniasis in a patient with AIDS. *Histopathology* 1991;19:83–95.
170. Alpert L, Miller M, Alpert E, Satin R, Lamoureux E, Trudel L. Gastric toxoplasmosis in acquired immunodeficiency syndrome: antemortem diagnosis with histopathologic characterization. *Gastroenterology* 1996;110:258–264.
171. Quincey C, James PD, Steele RJ. Chronic giardiasis of the stomach. *J Clin Pathol* 1992;45:1039–1041.
172. Roth RI, Owen RZ, Keren DF, Volberding PA. Intestinal infection with *Mycobacterium avium* in acquired immune deficiency syndrome (AIDS): histological and clinical comparison with Whipple's disease. *Dig Dis Sci* 1985;30:497–504.
173. McGlave P. A histopathologic study of gastric and small intestinal graft-versus-host disease following allogenic bone marrow transplantation. *Hum Pathol* 1985;16:387–392.
174. Snover DC. Mucosal damage simulating graft-versus-host reaction in cytomegalovirus colitis. *Transplantation* 1985;39:667–670.
175. Thorning D, Howard JD. Epithelial denudement in the gastrointestinal tracts of two bone marrow transplant recipients. *Hum Pathol* 1986;17:560–566.
176. Dickerman JD, Colleti RB, Tampas JD. Gastric outlet obstruction in chronic granulomatous disease. *Am J Dis Child* 1986;140:567–570.

Peptic Ulcer

177. Gear MWL, Truelove SC, Whitehead R. Gastric ulcer and gastritis. *Gut* 1971;12:639–645.
178. Chan WY, Hui PK, Chan JKC, et al. Epithelial damage by *Helicobacter pylori* in gastric ulcers. *Histopathology* 1991;19:47–53.
179. Jarvis LR, Whitehead R. Morphometric analysis of gastric dysplasia. *J Pathol* 1985;147:133–138.
180. McGregor DH, Haque AU. Gastric hyalinization associated with peptic ulceration. *Arch Pathol Lab Med* 1982;106:472–475.

Postgastrectomy Stomach

181. Geboes K, Rutgeerts P, Broeckaert L, Vantrappen G, Desmet V. Histologic appearances of endoscopic mucosal biopsies 10-20 years after partial gastrectomy. *Ann Surg* 1980;192:179–182.
182. Bedossa P, Lemaigre G, Martin ED. Histochemical study of mucosubstances in carcinoma of the gastric remnant. *Cancer* 1987;60:2224–2227.
183. Ross AH, Smith MA, Anderson JR, Small WP. Late mortality after surgery for peptic ulcer. *N Engl J Med* 1982;307:519–522.
184. Viste A, Bjornstad E, Opheim P. Risk of carcinoma following gastric operations for benign disease: a historical cohort study of 3470 patients. *Lancet* 1986;ii:502–504.
185. Picton TD, Owen DA, MacDonald WC. Comparison of esophagocardia and more distal gastric cancer in patients with prior ulcer surgery. *Cancer* 1993;71:5–8.
186. Offerhaus GJ, Stadt JVD, Huibregtse K, Tytgat GN. Endoscopic

screening for malignancy in the gastric remnant: the clinical significance of dysplasia in gastric mucosa. *J Clin Pathol* 1984;37:748–754.

Polyps

187. Haggitt RC, Reid BJ. Hereditary gastrointestinal polyposis syndromes. *Am J Surg Pathol* 1986;10:871–887.
188. Estrada R, Spjut HJ. Hamartomatous polyps in Peutz-Jeghers syndrome: a light, histochemical and electron-microscope study. *Am J Surg Pathol* 1983;7:747–754.
189. Reid JD. Intestinal carcinoma in the Peutz-Jeghers syndrome. *JAMA* 1974;229:833–834.
190. Watanabe A, Nagashima H, Motoi M, Ogawa K. Familial juvenile polyposis of the stomach. *Gastroenterology* 1979;77:148–151.
191. Sassatelli R, Bertoni G, Serra L, Bedogni G, Ponz de Leon M. Generalized juvenile polyposis with mixed pattern and gastric cancer. *Gastroenterology* 1993;104:910–915.
192. Carlson GH, Nivatongs S, Snover DC. Colorectal polyps in Cowden's disease (multiple hamartoma syndrome). *Am J Surg Pathol* 1984;8:763–770.
193. Tomasulo J. Gastric polyps: histologic types and their relationship to gastric carcinoma. *Cancer* 1971;27:1346–1355.
194. Orlowska J, Jarosz D, Pachlewski J, Butruk E. Malignant transformation of benign epithelial gastric polyps. *Am J Gastroenterol* 1995;90:2152–2159.
195. Zea-Iriarte WL, Sekine I, Itsuno M, et al. Carcinoma in gastric hyperplastic polyps: a phenotypic study. *Dig Dis Sci* 1996;41:377–386.
196. Dijkhuizen SM, Entius MM, Clement MJ, et al. Multiple hyperplastic polyps in the stomach: evidence for clonality and neoplastic potential. *Gastroenterology* 1997;112:561–566.
197. Dirschmid K, Walser J, Hugel H. Pseudomalignant erosion in hyperplastic gastric polyps. *Cancer* 1984;54:2290–2293.
198. Koga S, Watanabe H, Enjoji M. Stomal polypoid hypertrophic gastritis: a polypoid lesion at gastroenterostomy site. *Cancer* 1979;43:647–657.
199. Stemmerman GN, Hayashi T. Hyperplastic polyps of the gastric mucosa adjacent to gastroenterostomy stomas. *Am J Clin Pathol* 1979;71:341–345.
200. Franzin G, Novelli P. Gastritis cystica profunda. *Histopathology* 1981;5:535–547.
201. Lee RG, Burt RW. The histopathology of fundic gland polyps of the stomach. *Am J Clin Pathol* 1986;86:498–503.
202. Watanabe H, Enjoji M, Yao T, Ohsato K. Gastric lesions in familial adenomatosis coli. *Hum Pathol* 1979;9:269–283.
203. Iida M, Yao T, Watanabe H, Itoh K, Isawhita A. Fundic gland polyposis in patients without familial adenomatosis coli: its incidence and clinical features. *Gastroenterology* 1984;86:1437–1442.
204. Odze RD, Marcial MA, Antonioli D. Fundic gland polyps: a morphological study including mucin histochemistry, stereometry and MIB-1 immunohistochemistry. *Hum Pathol* 1996;27:896–903.
205. Burt RW, Berenson MM, Lee RG, Tolman KG, Freston JW, Gardner EJ. Upper gastrointestinal polyps in Gardner's syndrome. *Gastroenterology* 1984;86:295–301.
206. Domizio P, Talbot IC, Spigelman AD, Williams CB, Philips RK. Upper gastrointestinal pathology in familial adenomatous polyposis: results from a prospective study of 102 patients. *J Clin Pathol* 1990;43:738–743.
207. Shimer GR, Helwig EB. Inflammatory fibroid polyps of the intestine. *Am J Clin Pathol* 1984;81:708–714.
208. Navas-Palacios JJ, Colina-Ruizdelgada F, Sanchez-Larrea MD, Cortez-Cansino J. Inflammatory fibroid polyps of the gastrointestinal tract: an immunohistochemical and electron microscopic study. *Cancer* 1983;51:1682–1690.
209. Burke AP, Sobin LH. The pathology of Cronkhite-Canada polyps: a comparison to juvenile polyps. *Am J Surg Pathol* 1989;13:940–946.
210. Laxen P, Sipponen P, Ihamaki T, Dortschera Z. Gastric polyps: their morphological characteristics and relation to gastric carcinoma. *Acta Pathol Microbiol Immunol Scand [A]* 1982;90:221–228.
211. Nakamura K, Sakaguchi H, Enjoji M. Depressed adenoma of the stomach. *Cancer* 1988;62:2197–2202.
212. Ranchod M, Lewin KJ, Dorfman RF. Lymphoid hyperplasia of the gastrointestinal tract: a study of 26 cases and a review of the literature. *Am J Surg Pathol* 1978;2:383–400.
213. Fishbach W, Kestel W, Kirchner T, Mossner J, Wilms K. Malignant lymphomas of the upper gastrointestinal tract. *Cancer* 1992;70:1075–1080.

Enlarged Mucosal Folds

214. Appelman HD. Localized and extensive expansions of the gastric mucosa: mucosal polyps and giant folds. In: Appelman HD, ed. *Pathology of the esophagus, stomach and duodenum: contemporary issues in surgical pathology,* Vol 4. New York: Churchill-Livingstone, 1984: 79–119.
215. Komorowski RA, Caya JG. Hyperplastic gastropathy: clinicopathologic correlation. *Am J Surg Pathol* 1991;15:577–585.
216. Hirschowitz BI. Zollinger-Ellison syndrome: pathogenesis, diagnosis and management. *Am J Gastroenterol* 1997;92(suppl):445–485.
217. Lewin KJ, Yang K, Ulich T, Elashoff JD, Walsh J. Primary gastrin cell hyperplasia: report of five cases and a review of the literature. *Am J Surg Pathol* 1984;8:821–832.
218. Tan DT, Stempien SJ, Dagradi AE. The clinical spectrum of hypertrophic hypersecretory gastropathy. *Gastrointest Endosc* 1971;18:69–73.
219. Overhold BF, Jeffries GH. Hypertrophic, hypersecretory protein-losing gastropathy. *Gastroenterology* 1970;58:73–77.
220. Eisenstat DD, Griffiths AM, Cutz E, Petric M, Drumm B. Acute cytomegalovirus infection in a child with Menetrier's disease. *Gastroenterology* 1995;109:592–595.
221. Groisman GM, George J, Berman D, Harpaz N. Resolution of protein-losing hypertrophic lymphocytic gastritis with therapeutic eradication of *Helicobacter pylori*. *Am J Gastroenterol* 1994;89:1548–1551.
222. Wolber RA, Owen DA, Anderson FH, Freeman HJ. Lymphocytic gastritis and giant gastric folds associated with gastrointestinal protein loss. *Mod Pathol* 1991;4:13–15.
223. Wolfson HC, Carpenter HA, Talley NJ. Menetrier's disease: a form of hypertrophic gastropathy or gastritis. *Gastroenterology* 1993;104:1310–1319.

Carcinoma of the Stomach

224. Mori M, Iwashita A, Enjoji M. Adenosquamous carcinoma of the stomach. *Cancer* 1986;57:333–339.
225. Mori M, Fukuda T, Enjoji M. Adenosquamous carcinoma of the stomach: histogenetic and ultrastructural studies. *Gastroenterology* 1987;92:1078–1082.
226. Hee Won OK, Farman J, Krishnan MN, Iyer S, Vuletin JC. Squamous cell carcinoma of the stomach. *Am J Gastroenterol* 1978;69:594–598.
227. Ruck P, Wehrman M, Campbell M, Horny HP, Breucha G, Kaiserling E. Squamous carcinoma of the gastric stump: a case report and review of the literature. *Am J Surg Pathol* 1989;13:317–324.
228. Ishikura H, Kirimoto K, Shamoto M, et al. Hepatoid adenocarcinoma of the stomach. *Cancer* 1986;58:119–126.
229. de Lorimer A, Park F, Aranha GV, Reyes C. Hepatoid carcinoma of the stomach. *Cancer* 1993;71:293–296.
230. Petrella T, Montagnon J, Roignot P, et al. Alphafetoprotein-producing gastric adenocarcinoma. *Histopathology* 1995;26:171–175.
231. Capella C, Frigerio B, Cornaggia M, Solcia E, Pinzon-Trujillo Y, Chejfec G. Gastric parietal cell carcinoma: a newly recognized entity: light microscopic and ultrastructural features. *Histopathology* 1984;8:813–824.
232. Robey-Cafferty SS, Ro JY, McKee EG. Gastric parietal cell carcinoma with an unusual, lymphoma-like histologic appearance: report of a case. *Mod Pathol* 1989;2:536–540.
233. Saigo PE, Brigati DJ, Sternberg SS, Rosen PP, Turnbull AD. Primary gastric choriocarcinoma: an immunohistological study. *Am J Surg Pathol* 1981;5:333–342.
234. Ueyama T, Nagai E, Yao T, Tsuneyoshi M. Vimentin-positive gastric carcinomas with rhabdoid features. *Am J Surg Pathol* 1993;17:813–819.
235. Green LK. Hematogenous metastases to the stomach: a review of 67 cases. *Cancer* 1990;65:1596–1600.
236. Aiba M, Hirayama A, Suzuki T, Hamano K, Nomura K. Carcinosarcoma of the stomach: report of a case with review of the literature of gastrectomized patients. *Surg Pathol* 1991;4:75–83.
237. Siegal A, Freund U, Gal R. Carcinosarcoma of the stomach. *Histopathology* 1988;13:350–353.

238. Robey-Cafferty SS, Grignon DJ, Ro JY, et al. Sarcomatoid carcinoma of the stomach: a report of three cases with immunohistochemical and ultrastructural observations. *Cancer* 1990;65:1601–1606.
239. Lauren P. The two histologica main types of gastric carcinoma: diffuse and so-called intestinal type. *Acta Pathol Microbiol Immunol Scand [A]* 1965;64:31–49.
240. Locke GR, Talley NJ, Carpenter HA, Harmsen WS, Zinsmeister AR, Melton J. Changes in site and histology-specific incidence of gastric cancer during a 50-year period. *Gastroenterology* 1995;109: 1750–1756.
241. Adachi Y, Mori M, Kido A, Shimono R, Maehara Y, Sugimachi K. A clinicopathologic study of mucinous gastric carcinoma. *Cancer* 1992;69:866–871.
242. Jass JR. Role of intestinal metaplasia in the histogenesis of gastric cancer. *J Clin Pathol* 1980;33:801–810.
243. Segura DI, Montero C. Histochemical characterization of different types of intestinal metaplasia in gastric mucosa. *Cancer* 1983;52: 498–503.
244. Yamishina M. A variant of early gastric carcinoma: histologic and histochemical studies of early signet ring cell carcinomas discovered beneath preserved surface epithelium. *Cancer* 1986;56:1333–1339.
245. Hansson L-E, Engstrand L, Nyren O, Lindgren A. Prevalence of *Helicobacter pylori* infection in subtypes of gastric cancer. *Gastroenterology* 1995;109:885–888.
246. Solcia E, Fiocca R, Luinetti O, et al. Intestinal and diffuse gastric cancers arise in a different background of *Helicobacter pylori* gastritis through different gene involvement. *Am J Surg Pathol* 1996;20(suppl 1):S8–S22.
247. Grabiec J, Owen DA. Carcinoma of the stomach in young persons. *Cancer* 1985;56:388–396.
248. Nottingham J. Signet ring carcinoma of stomach in a child. *Histopathology* 1994;24:490–491.
249. Fuchs CS, Mayer RJ. Gastric carcinoma. *N Engl J Med* 1995;333: 32–40.
250. MacDonald WC, MacDonald JB. Adenocarcinoma of the esophagus and/or gastric cardia. *Cancer* 1987;60:1094–1098.
251. Kalish RJ, Clancy PE, Orringer MB, Appelman HD. Clinical, epidemiologic and morphologic comparison between carcinomas arising in Barrett's esophageal mucosa and in the gastric cardia. *Gastroenterology* 1984;86:461–467.
252. Tersmette AC, Giardello FM, Tytgat GN, et al. Carcinogenesis after remote peptic ulcer surgery: the long term prognosis of partial gastrectomy. *Scand J Gastroenterol* 1995;212(suppl):109–116.
253. Borch K. Epidemiologic, clinicopathological and economic aspects of gastroscopic screening of patients with pernicious anemia. *Scand J Gastroenterol* 1986;21:21–30.
254. Wood GM, Bates C, Brown RC, Losowsky MS. Intramucosal carcinoma of the gastric antrum complicating Menetrier's disease. *J Clin Pathol* 1983;36:1071–1075.
255. Kirkwood KS, Khitin LM, Barwick KW. Prognostic indicators for cancer. *Surg Oncol Clin North Am* 1997;6:495–514.
256. Hermanek P, Hutter RVP, Sobin LH, et al. TNM atlas: illustrated guide to the TNM/pTNM classification of malignant tumors. 4th ed. Berlin: Springer Verlag, 1997:81–92.
257. Ming SC. Gastric carcinoma: a pathobiological classification. *Cancer* 1977;39:2475–2485.
258. Witzel L, Halter F, Gretillat PA, Scheurer U, Keller M. Evaluation of specific value of endoscopic biopsies and brush cytology for malignancies of the esophagus and stomach. *Gut* 1976;17:375–377.
259. Qizilbash AH, Castelli M, Kowalski MA, Churby A. Endoscopic brush cytology and biopsy in the diagnosis of cancer of the upper gastrointestinal tract. *Acta Cytol* 1980;24:313–318.
260. Tokunaga M, Oland E, Uemura Y, et al. Epstein-Barr virus in gastric carcinoma. *Am J Pathol* 1993;143:1250–1254.
261. Yuen ST, Chung LP, Leung SY, et al. In situ detection of Epstein-Barr virus in gastric and colorectal adenocarcinomas. *Am J Surg Pathol* 1994;18:1158–1163.
262. Ott G, Kirchner TH, Mulcer-Hermelink HK. Monoclonal Epstein-Barr virus genomes, but lack of EBV-related protein expression in different types of gastric carcinoma. *Histopathology* 1994;25:323–329.
263. Green PH, O'Toole KM, Weinberg LM, Goldfarb JP. Early gastric cancer. *Gastroenterology* 1981;81:247–256.
264. Bogomoletz WV. Early gastric cancer. *Am J Surg Pathol* 1984;8: 381–391.
265. Qizilbash AH, Stevenson GW. Early gastric cancer. *Pathol Annu* 1979;14:317–351.
266. Johansen AA. Early gastric cancer. In: Morson BC, ed. *Current topics in pathology: pathology of the gastrointestinal tract*. Vol 63. Berlin: Springer Verlag, 1976:1–48.

Dysplasia

267. Lansdown M, Quirke P, Dixon MF, Axon ATR, Johnston D. High grade dysplasia of the gastric mucosa: a marker for gastric carcinoma. *Gut* 1990;31:977–983.
268. DeDombal FT, Price AB, Thompson H, et al. The British Society of Gastroenterology early gastric cancer/dysplasia survey: an interim report. *Gut* 1990;31:115–120.
269. Goldstein NS, Lewin KJ. Gastric epithelial dysplasia and adenoma: historical review and histological criteria for grading. *Hum Pathol* 1997;28:127–133.
270. Jass JR. A classification of gastric dysplasia. *Histopathology* 1983;7:181–193.
271. Cuello C, Correa P, Zarama G, Lopez J, Murray J, Gordillo G. Histopathology of gastric dysplasias: correlations with gastric juice chemistry. *Am J Surg Pathol* 1979;3:491–500.
272. Falck VG, Novelli MR, Wright NA, Alexander N. Gastric dysplasia: interobserver variation, sulphomucin staining and nucleolar organizer region counting. *Histopathology* 1990;16:141–149.
273. Schlemper RJ, Itabashi M, Kato Y, et al. Differences in diagnostic criteria for gastric carcinoma between Japanese and Western pathologists. *Lancet* 1997;349:1725–1729.
274. Kokkola A, Haapiainen R, Laxen F, et al. Risk of gastric carcinoma in patients with mucosal dysplasia associated with atrophic gastritis: a follow-up study. *J Clin Pathol* 1996;49:979–984.
275. Rugge M, Farinati F, Baffa R, et al. Gastric epithelial dysplasia in the natural history of gastric cancer: a multicentre prospective follow-up study. *Gastroenterology* 1994;107:1288–1296.
276. Antonioli DA. Precursors of gastric carcinoma: a critical review with a brief description of early (curable) gastric carcinoma. *Hum Pathol* 1994;25:994–1005.

Endocrine Tumors

277. Kloppel G, Clemens A. The biological relevance of gastric neuroendocrine tumors. *Yale J Biol Med* 1996;69:69–74.
278. Rindi G. Clinicopathologic aspects of gastric neuroendocrine tumors. *Am J Surg Pathol* 1995;19(suppl 1):S20–S29.
279. Borch K, Renvall H, Liedberg G. Gastric endocrine cell hyperplasia and carcinoid tumors in pernicious anemia. *Gastroenterology* 1985;88:638–648.
280. Borch K, Renvall H, Kullman E, Willander E. Gastric carcinoid tumor associated with a syndrome of hypergastrinemic atrophic gastritis: a prospective study of 11 cases. *Am J Surg Pathol* 1987;11:435–444.
281. Muller J, Kirchner T, Muller-Hermelink HK. Gastric endocrine cell hyperplasia and carcinoid tumors in atrophic gastritis: type A. *Am J Surg Pathol* 1987;11:909–917.
282. Solcia E, Fiocca R, Villani L, et al. Hyperplastic, dysplastic and neoplastic enterochromaffin-like cell proliferations of the gastric mucosa: classification and histogenesis. *Am J Surg Pathol* 1995;19(suppl 1):S1–S7.
283. Hirschowitz BI, Griffith J, Pellegrin D, Cummings OW. Rapid regression of enterochromaffin-like cell gastric carcinoids in pernicious anemia after antrectomy. *Gastroenterology* 1992;102:1409–1418.
284. Thompson NW, Vinik AI, Ekhauser FE, Strodel WE. Extrapancreatic gastrinomas. *Surgery* 1985;98:1113–1120.
285. Rindi G, Luinetti O, Cornaggia M, Capella C, Solcia E. Three subtypes of gastric argyrophil carcinoid and the gastric neuroendocrine carcinoma: a clinicopathology study. *Gastroenterology* 1993;104: 991–1006.
286. Pipeleers-Marichal MA, Somers G, Willems G, et al. Gastrinomas in the duodenums of patients with multiple endocrine neoplasia type I and the Zollinger-Ellison syndrome. *N Engl J Med* 1990;322: 723–727.
287. Padberg B, Schroder S, Capella C, et al. Multiple endocrine neoplasia type I (MEN-I) revisited. *Virchows Arch* 1995;426:541–548.
288. Chejfec G, Gould VE. Malignant gastric neuroendocrineomas. Ultra-

Gastric Lymphomas

289. Severson RK, Davis S. Increasing incidence of primary gastric lymphoma. *Cancer* 1990;66:1283–1287.
290. Dragosics B, Bauer P, Radaszikiewicz T. Primary gastrointestinal non-Hodgkin's lymphomas: a retrospective clinicopathologic study of 150 cases. *Cancer* 1985;55:1060–1073.
291. Lewin KJ, Ranchod M, Dorfman RF. Lymphomas of the gastrointestinal tract: a study of 117 cases presenting with gastrointestinal disease. *Cancer* 1978;42:693–707.
292. Soderstrom KO, Joensuu H. Primary Hodgkin's disease of the stomach. *Am J Clin Pathol* 1988;89:806–809.
293. Shepherd NA, Blackshaw AJ, Hall PA, et al. Malignant lymphoma with eosinophilia of the gastrointestinal tract. *Histopathology* 1987;11:115–130.
294. Alvaro T, Bosch R, Salvado HT, Piris MA. True histiocytic lymphoma of the stomach associated with low-grade B-cell mucosa-associated lymphoid tissue (MALT)-type lymphoma. *Am J Surg Pathol* 1996;20:1406–1411.
295. Abbondanzo SL, Sobin LH. Gastric 'pseudolymphoma': a retrospective morphologic and immunophenotypic study of 97 cases. *Cancer* 1997;79:1656–1663.
296. Cogliatti SB, Schmid U, Schumacher U, et al. Primary B-cell gastric lymphoma: a clinicopathologic study of 145 patients. *Gastroenterology* 1991;101:1159–1170.
296a. Peng H, Du M, Diss TC, Isaacson PG, Pan L. Genetic evidence for a clonal link between low and high grade components in gastric MALT B-cell lymphoma. *Histopathology* 1997;30:425–429.
297. Zukerberg LR, Ferry JA, Southern JF, Harris NL. Lymphoid infiltrates of the stomach: evaluation of histologic criteria for the diagnosis of low-grade gastric lymphoma on endoscopic biopsy specimens. *Am J Surg Pathol* 1990;14:1087–1099.
298. Tungekar MF. Gastric signet-cell lymphoma with alpha heavy chains. *Histopathology* 1986;10:725–734.
299. Zamboni G, Franzin G, Scarpa A, et al. Carcinoma-like signet-ring cells in gastric mucosa-associated lymphoid tissue (MALT) lymphoma. *Am J Surg Pathol* 1996;20:588–598.
300. Isaacson PG. Recent developments in our understanding of gastric lymphoma. *Am J Surg Pathol* 1996;20(suppl 1):S1–S7.
301. Isaacson PG, Wotherspoon AC, Diss T, Laxing P. Follicular colonization in B-cell lymphoma of mucosa-associated lymphoid tissue. *Am J Surg Pathol* 1991;15:819–828.
302. Harris NL. Extranodal lymphoid infiltrates and mucosa-associated lymphoid tissue (MALT): a unifying concept. *Am J Surg Pathol* 1991;15:879–884.
303. Sundeen JT, Longo DL, Jaffe ES. CD5 expression in B-cell small lymphocytic malignancies: correlations with clinical presentations in sites of disease. *Am J Surg Pathol* 1992;16:130–137.
304. Weber DM, Dimopoulos MA, Anandu DP, et al. Regression of gastric lymphoma of mucosa-associated lymphoid tissue with antibiotic therapy for *Helicobacter pylori*. *Gastroenterology* 1994;107:1835–1838.
305. Hussell T, Isaacson PG, Crabtree JE, Spencer J. *Helicobacter pylori* specific infiltrating T cells provide contact dependent help for the growth of malignant B cells in low-grade gastric lymphoma of mucosal associated lymphoid tissue. *J Pathol* 1996;178:122–127.
306. Ruskoná-Fourmestraux A, Delmer A, Lavergne A, et al. Multiple lymphomatous polyposis of the gastrointestinal tract: prospective clinicopathologic study of 31 cases. *Gastroenterology* 1997;112:7–16.
307. Isaacson PG. Gastrointestinal lymphoma. *Hum Pathol* 1994;25:1020–1029.
308. Goteri G, Ranaldi R, Rezai B, et al. Synchronous mucosa-associated lymphoid tissue lymphoma and adenocarcinoma of the stomach. *Am J Surg Pathol* 1997;21:505–509.

Stromal Tumors

309. Saul SH, Rast ML, Brooks JJ. The immunocytochemistry of gastrointestinal stromal tumors: evidence supporting an origin from smooth muscle. *Am J Surg Pathol* 1987;11:464–473.
310. Hjermstad BM, Sobin LH, Helwig EB. Stromal tumors of the gastrointestinal tract: myogenic or neurogenic? *Am J Surg Pathol* 1987;11:383–386.
311. Meittinen M, Virolainen M, Rikala MS. Gastrointestinal stromal tumors: value of CD34 antigen and their identification and separation from true leiomyomas and true schwannomas. *Am J Surg Pathol* 1995;19:207–216.
312. Weiss RA, Mackay B. Malignant smooth muscle tumors of the gastrointestinal tract: an ultrastructural study of 20 cases. *Ultrastruct Pathol* 1981;2:231–240.
312a. Kindblom L-G, Remotti HE, Aldenberg F, Meis-Kindblom JM. Gastrointestinal pacemaker cell tumors (GIPACT): gastrointestinal stromal tumors show phenotypic characteristics of the interstitial cells of Cajal. *Am J Pathol* 1998;152:1259–1269.
313. Yamada Y, Kato Y, Yanagisawa A, Sugano H, Kitagawa T. Microleiomyomas of the human stomach. *Hum Pathol* 1988;19:569–572.
314. Appelman HD, Helwig EB. Gastric epithelioid leiomyoma and leiomyosarcoma (leiomyoblastoma). *Cancer* 1976;38:708–728.
315. Suster S, Fletcher CD. Gastrointestinal stromal tumors with prominent signet-ring features. *Mod Pathol* 1996;9:609–613.
316. Carney JA. The triad of gastric epithelioid leiomyosarcoma, pulmonary chondroma and functioning extra-adrenal paraganglioma: a five year review. *Medicine (Baltimore)* 1983;62:159–169.
317. Turkington RW. Gastric lipoma: report of a case and review of the literature. *Am J Dig Dis* 1965;10:719–726.
318. Haqqani MT, Krasner N, Ashworth M. Benign mesenchymoma of the stomach. *J Clin Pathol* 1983;36:504–507.
319. Appelman HD, Helwig EB. Glomus tumors of the stomach. *Cancer* 1969;23:203–213.
320. Lauwers GY, Erlandson RA, Casper ES, et al. Gastrointestinal autonomic nerve tumors: a clinicopathological, immunohistochemical and ultrastructural study of 12 cases. *Am J Surg Pathol* 1993;17:887–897.
321. Appelman HD, Helwig EB. Sarcomas of the stomach. *Am J Clin Pathol* 1977;67:2–10.
322. Fox KR, Moussa SM, Mitre RJ, Zidar BL, Raves JJ. Clinical and pathologic features of primary gastric rhabdomyosarcoma. *Cancer* 1990;66:772–778.
323. Wright JR, Kyriakos M, DeSchryver-Kecskemeti K. Malignant fibrous histiocytoma of the stomach: a report and review of malignant fibrohistiocytic tumors of the alimentary tract. *Arch Pathol Lab Med* 1988;112:251–258.
324. Hawkins PE, Terrell GH. Liposarcoma of the stomach: a case report. *JAMA* 1965;191:758–759.
325. Appelman HD. Mesenchymal tumors of the gut: historical perspectives, new approaches, new results, and does it make any difference? In: Goldman H, Appelman HD, Kaufman N, eds. *Gastrointestinal pathology*, Baltimore: Williams & Wilkins, 1990:220–246.
326. Shiu MH, Farr GH, Parachristu DN, Hajdu SI. Myosarcomas of the stomach: natural history, prognostic factors and management. *Cancer* 1982;49:177–187.
327. El-Naggar AK, Ro JY, McLemore D, Garnsey L, Ordonez N, Mackay B. Gastrointestinal stromal tumors: DNA flow-cytometric study of 58 patients with at least 5 years of follow-up. *Mod Pathol* 1989;2:511–515.
328. Appelman HD. Stromal tumors of the esophagus, stomach and duodenum. In: Appelman HD, ed. *Pathology of the esophagus, stomach and duodenum: contemporary issues in surgical pathology*. Vol 4. New York: Churchill Livingstone, 1984:192–242.
329. Baak JP. Mitosis counting in tumors. *Hum Pathol* 1990;21:683–685.

Vascular Lesions

330. Jabbari M, Cherry R, Lough JO, Daly DS, Kinnear DG, Goresky CA. Gastric antral vascular ectasia: the watermelon stomach. *Gastroenterology* 1984;87:1165–1170.
331. Suit PF, Petras RE, Bauer TW, Petrini JL. Gastric antral vascular ectasia: a histologic and morphometric study of 'the watermelon stomach.' *Am J Surg Pathol* 1987;11:750–757.
332. Gilliam JH, Geisinger KR, Wu WC, et al. Endoscopic biopsy is diagnostic in gastric antral vascular ectasia: the watermelon stomach. *Dig Dis Sci* 1989;34:885–888.
333. McCormack TT, Sims J, Eyre-Brook I, et al. Gastric lesions in portal hypertension: inflammatory gastritis or congestive gastropathy. *Gut* 1985;26:1226–1232.

334. Payen J-L, Cates P, Voigt J-J, et al. Severe portal hypertensive gastropathy and gastric antral vascular ectasia are distinct entities in patients with cirrhosis. *Gastroenterology* 1995;108:138–144.
335. Miko T, Thomazy VA. The caliber persistent artery of the stomach: a unifying approach to gastric aneurysm, Dieulafoy's lesion and submucosal arterial malformation. *Hum Pathol* 1988;19:914–921.
336. Reilly HF, Al-Kawas FH. Dieulafoy's lesion: diagnosis and management. *Dig Dis Sci* 1991;36:1702–1707.
337. Friedman SL, Wright TL, Altman DF. Gastrointestinal Kaposi's sarcoma in patients with acquired immunodeficiency syndrome. *Gastroenterology* 1985;89:102–108.

Metabolic Diseases

338. Shousha S, Lowdell CP, Bull TB, Parkins A. Secondary amyloidosis of the gastrointestinal tract: an electron microscopic study. *Hum Pathol* 1985;16:596–601.
339. Franzin G, Musola R, Mencarelli R. Morphological changes in the gastroduodenal mucosa in regular dialysis uremic patients. *Histopathology* 1982;6:429–437.
340. Moscoso GH, Driver M, Guy RJC. A form of necrobiosis and atrophy of smooth muscle in diabetic gastric autonomic neuropathy. *Pathol Res Pract* 1986;181:188–194.

CHAPTER 33

Nonneoplastic Intestinal Diseases

Robert E. Petras

EVALUATION OF SMALL INTESTINAL MUCOSAL BIOPSY SPECIMENS IN PATIENTS WITH MALABSORPTION

Specimen Procurement and Processing

Small bowel mucosal biopsy examination remains one of the most important steps in evaluating patients with malabsorption (1). A standard gastroscope may be used to obtain duodenal specimens as distally as possible (2,3). The specimen size is adequate to evaluate mucosal disease, and, because the procedure is performed under direct vision, many specimens can safely be obtained.

The most critical part of the procedure is the proper orientation of the specimen in the endoscopy suite. Ideally, specimens are immediately mounted, mucosal side up, on a solid substance, such as filter paper, and then placed into Hollande's (or other) fixative. After processing, the histotechnologist embeds the tissue perpendicular to the mounting material. Proper specimen evaluation requires examination of optimally oriented intestinal villi obtained from the central region of the biopsy specimen. Although serial sectioning is advocated by some (4), step sectioning (obtaining ribbons of sections from at least three levels) is a reasonable alternative. Our standard small bowel biopsy procedure consists of obtaining four to six endoscopic biopsy specimens. These tissue samples are fixed in Hollande's solution and routinely processed. Five step-section slides are obtained; three are stained with hematoxylin and eosin (H&E), one with periodic acid-Schiff (PAS), and one with trichrome stain. The PAS stain is a useful screen for Whipple's disease and *Mycobacterium avium-intracellulare* complex (MAIC) infection and can be used to detect foveolar metaplasia in villous epithelium. The trichrome stain confirms collagen deposition seen in ischemia or collagenous sprue. In addition, the iron hematoxylin counterstain used in the trichrome technique makes identification of *Giardia lamblia* easier.

R. E. Petras: Department of Anatomic Pathology, The Cleveland Clinic Foundation, Cleveland, Ohio 44195

Normal Small Intestinal Histology

The ratio of villus to crypt length approximates 3:1 to 5:1 (Fig. 1) (5). Inflammatory cells, including plasma cells, are normally present in the lamina propria. Intraepithelial lymphocytes are present in a ratio of approximately one lymphocyte per five enterocytes (4,5). A brush border is often discernible on the enterocyte. The enterocyte nuclei should be basilar in location and evenly aligned (Fig. 2).

Brunner's glands in proximal duodenal specimens have an inconsistent effect on villous architecture (5). In some circumstances, normal length villi may be encountered overlying Brunner's glands, but usually the villi are distorted and appear short. Similarly, villi are often short and distorted next to or overlying lymphoid aggregates. Such shortened villi should not be misinterpreted as evidence of celiac sprue (CS). The muscularis mucosae tends to hold the mucosa together, resulting in the elegantly normal villi illustrated in Fig. 1. When muscularis mucosae is not included in the biopsy specimen, the mucosa can spread laterally, giving the impression of shortened villi (5).

In general, identification of four normal villi in a row indicates that the villous architecture of the whole biopsy specimen is probably normal (4–6). This does not mean that biopsy specimens with less than four aligned normal villi should be considered inadequate for evaluation, because even one normal villus in a proximal small bowel biopsy specimen rules out CS. Conversely, finding four normal villi in a row does not necessarily rule out focal lesions, although it almost always does.

Accumulations of various pigments are frequently seen in the small intestines of apparently normal individuals. The term *pseudomelanosis duodeni* has been used to describe the accumulation of brown-black pigment in the lamina propria macrophages of the proximal duodenum (5,7). Iron and sulfur are the principal components of these apparently acquired deposits. The etiology and significance of pseudomelanosis duodeni remain uncertain. Irregularly distributed granular brown-black pigment is commonly encountered in the deep portion of Peyer's patches in adults (5,8). The pigment prob-

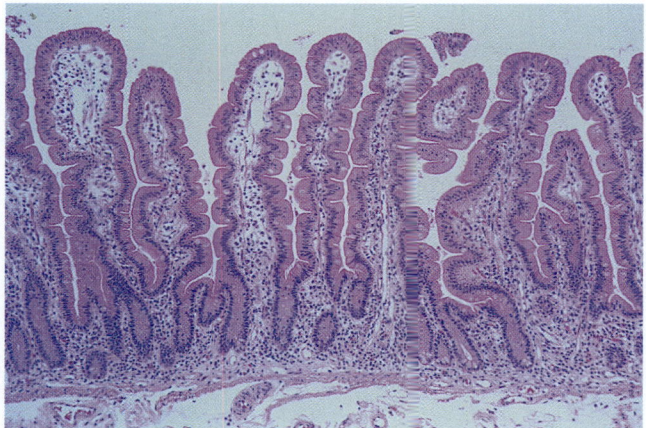

FIG. 1. Section of small bowel mucosa obtained near the center of the biopsy specimen. The villi are long and slender, and the ratio of the villus to crypt length is approximately 5:1. Inflammatory cells are present within the lamina propria.

ably originates in the atmosphere or diet (8,9). Accumulating principally within macrophages, this pigment has been shown by x-ray spectroscopy to contain a distinct mineral composition that includes silicates, aluminum, and titanium (8,9). The pigment is inert and has no known clinicopathologic significance.

Patterns of Abnormal Small Bowel Architecture

The small bowel mucosal responses to injury are limited, and recognition of a response pattern can be useful in differential diagnosis (Table 1). In this chapter, the term *severe villus abnormality* describes a flat intestinal mucosa in which no villi are seen. Usually this change is diffuse, accompanied by epithelial lymphocytosis and associated with crypt hyperplasia, evidenced by numerous mitotic figures. The terms *se-*

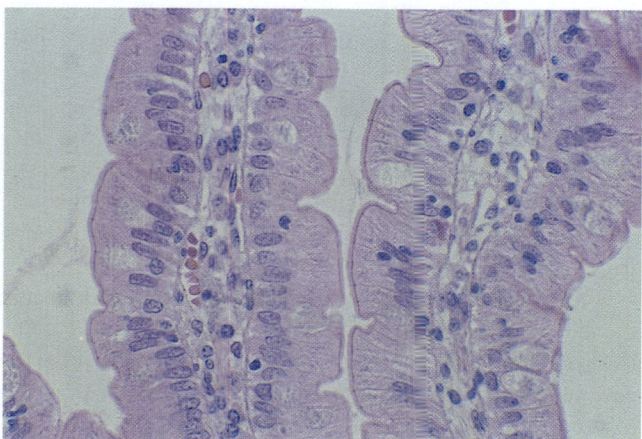

FIG. 2. Normal small intestine. The brush border is discernible, and inflammatory cells (including plasma cells) are seen within the lamina propria. Enterocyte nuclei are basilar in location and are evenly aligned. An occasional intraepithelial lymphocyte is present.

TABLE 1. *Patterns of abnormal small bowel architecture*

I. Entities usually associated with a diffuse severe villus abnormality and crypt hyperplasia
  A. Celiac sprue
  B. Refractory or unclassified sprue
  C. Other protein allergies
  D. Lymphocytic enterocolitis
II. Entities usually associated with a variable villus abnormality and crypt hypoplasia
  A. Kwashiorkor, malnutrition
  B. Megaloblastic anemia
  C. Radiation and chemotherapeutic effect
  D. Microvillus inclusion disease
III. Entities usually associated with a nonspecific variable villus abnormality, usually not flat
  A. Changes associated with dermatitis herpetiformis
  B. Partially treated or clinically latent celiac sprue
  C. Infection
  D. Stasis
  E. Tropical sprue
  F. Zollinger-Ellison syndrome
  G. Mastocytosis
  H. Nonspecific duodenitis
  I. Autoimmune enteropathy
  J. Torkelson syndrome
IV. Entities associated with variable villus abnormalities illustrating specific diagnostic changes
  A. Collagenous sprue
  B. Common variable immunodeficiency
  C. Whipple's disease
  D. *Mycobacterium avium-intracellulare* complex infection
  E. Eosinophilic gastroenteritis
  F. Intestinal lymphoma
  G. Parasitic infestation
  H. Waldenström's macroglobulinemia
  I. Lymphangiectasia
  J. Enteropathy-associated T-cell lymphoma
  K. Abetalipoproteinemia
  L. Acrodermatitis enteropathica
  M. Tufting enteropathy

vere villus abnormality and *flat intestinal mucosa* are preferred to villus atrophy because the mucosa in the forms associated with crypt hyperplasia is actually of normal thickness. The term *variable villus abnormality* describes specimens in which the villi are either only focally flat or are less than flat (mild or moderate villus shortening) (4). Many specimens in this category also show increased intraepithelial lymphocytes. These changes may be associated with features that suggest a specific diagnosis (i.e., numerous eosinophils, granulomas, parasites) or may be nonspecific.

Entities Associated with a Diffuse Severe Villus Abnormality and Crypt Hyperplasia

Celiac Sprue (CS)

CS, also known as *gluten-induced enteropathy, gluten-sensitive enteropathy,* and *nontropical sprue,* is a major cause of malabsorption. Although it is true that "all that flattens is not sprue" (10), the fact remains that almost all adult

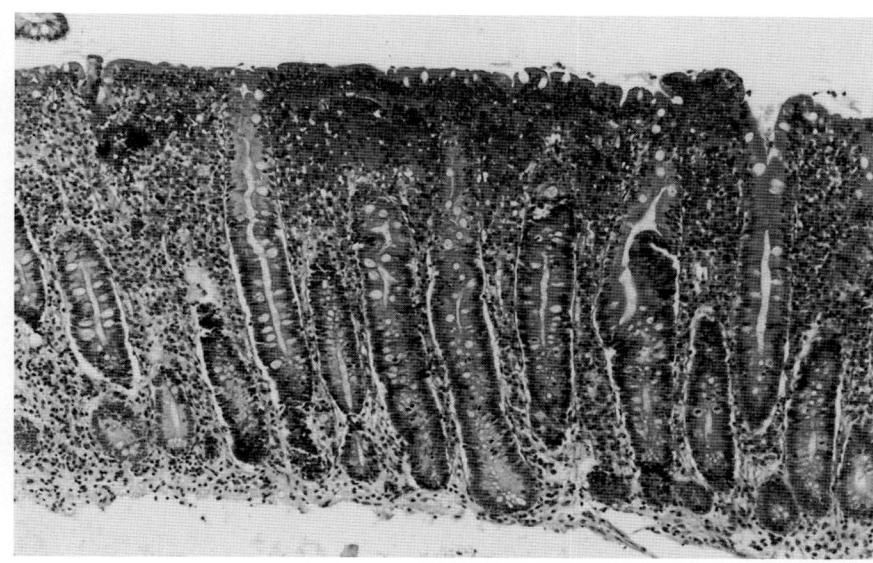

FIG. 3. Severe villous abnormality typical of celiac sprue. The mucosa is flat with no villi discernible. Inflammatory cells are increased in the lamina propria and within the epithelium.

patients in North America with a severe villus abnormality and crypt hyperplasia have CS (4). The pathogenesis of CS involves immunologic injury to the enterocyte associated with the ingestion of the protein gluten, which is found in cereal grains such as wheat, rye, and barley. Infection with type 12 adenovirus may play a role in acquiring this gluten sensitivity (11). Patients with CS usually show a quick and dramatic clinical and histologic improvement upon removal of gluten from the diet and quickly relapse following its reintroduction (12–14).

The flat mucosa of CS is associated with increased lymphocytes and plasma cells in the lamina propria and increased intraepithelial lymphocytes (Figs. 3 and 4). The enterocyte nuclei lose their basilar alignment and become stratified. Neutrophils may be present but are usually not prominent. The histologic abnormality is most severe in the proximal intestinal mucosa and gradually lessens distally.

With gluten withdrawal, the abnormalities recede from distal to cephalad in the small intestinal mucosa. Thus, proximal small bowel biopsy specimens may remain abnormal for quite some time, even in patients showing marked clinical improvement. A pathologist does not make the diagnosis of CS. All that can be said is that the specimens contain a severe villus abnormality that is consistent with CS. Definitive diagnosis depends on demonstration of a suitable clinical presentation, compatible serologic tests (15) (e.g., IgA-endomesial antibodies, IgG- and IgA-antigliadin antibodies) and small bowel histology (16), clinical and, ideally, histologic response to a gluten-free diet, and relapse following gluten challenge.

The histologic differential diagnosis includes all entities that may cause at least a focal severe villus abnormality: common variable immunodeficiency, protein allergies other than gluten, some cases of infectious gastroenteritis (17),

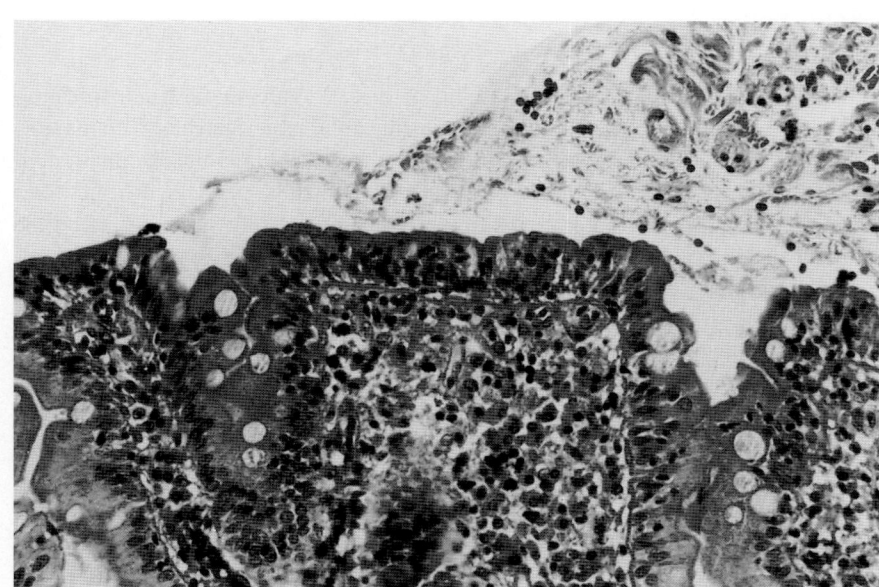

FIG. 4. High magnification view of small bowel mucosa in celiac sprue. In addition to the expansion of the lamina propria by inflammatory cells, there are numerous intraepithelial lymphocytes.

rare cases of tropical sprue (18), stasis (19), the Zollinger-Ellison syndrome (4,6), Crohn's disease (CD), and nonspecific duodenitis. Clinicopathologic correlation is essential for proper diagnosis. All biopsy specimens should be carefully evaluated for plasma cells, because their absence in common variable immunodeficiency syndrome (CVID) is easy to overlook. Numerous neutrophils, cryptitis, and crypt abscess formation are usually not part of CS, and entities such as infectious gastroenteritis, Zollinger-Ellison syndrome, CD, nonspecific duodenitis, and stasis syndromes, therefore, should be considered.

The most common cause of unresponsiveness after implementing a gluten-free diet is that the diet is not really gluten free (6). Furthermore, wheat is commonly used as an extender in processed foods and can occasionally be present in seemingly non–cereal-grain products, such as ice cream, cocoa mixes, instant coffee, and salad dressings. If dietary indiscretions are ruled out, patients may have refractory or unclassified sprue (4), which may respond to the administration of corticosteroids. Refractory sprue can also be associated with cavitation of mesenteric lymph nodes and hyposplenism (20). Lymphoma must also be considered in nonresponsive patients (21) and should prompt re-review of biopsy specimens or rebiopsy.

Other Protein Allergies

Patients with allergic reactions to chicken, soy protein, milk, eggs, and tuna fish have been reported to show a flat small bowel mucosa similar to that seen in CS (22–25). Definitive diagnosis depends on identifying the offending protein, showing a response to its withdrawal from the diet, and demonstrating recrudescence of symptoms and pathology with its reintroduction.

Lymphocytic Enterocolitis

CS and other sprue-like lesions may be associated with a colonic epithelial lymphocytosis (26,27), with or without gastric epithelial lymphocytosis (28). Approximately 25% of patients with CS who have also had colonic biopsy have demonstrated this form of lymphocytic colitis. Colonic microscopic abnormalities in patients with CS occur after experimental exposure to wheat or gliadin enemas (29,30), suggesting that the entire intestinal tract may be susceptible to gluten-induced injury. It is possible that, in some patients with true CS (responsive to gluten withdrawal), occult dietary gluten actually reaches the colon and induces the histologic changes of lymphocytic colitis. However, approximately one half of the patients with sprue-like small bowel lesions and lymphocytic colitis have not responded to gluten withdrawal. The term *lymphocytic enterocolitis* has been coined to describe this refractory sprue-like condition associated with colonic mucosal abnormalities (26).

Entities Associated with a Variable Villus Abnormality and Crypt Hypoplasia

Marasmus/Kwashiorkor

Biopsy specimens from malnourished patients with marasmus (severe calorie and protein deficiency) may be normal, but patchy areas of decreased villus height associated with markedly decreased mitotic activity have been reported. In kwashiorkor (low protein but adequate caloric intake), six of ten patients reported by Brunser and colleagues (31) showed lesions indistinguishable from those of CS. Some cases have shown a variable villus abnormality associated with increased intraepithelial lymphocytes (32). The mitotic rates in crypts are decreased in kwashiorkor but not as profoundly as in marasmus.

Megaloblastic Anemia

Nutritional deficiency of folate and vitamin B_{12} may result in impaired epithelial cell replacement because of decreased DNA synthesis. Consequently, a variable villus abnormality with or without megaloblastic epithelial changes can be seen. Evaluation of mucosal biopsy specimens usually allows differentiation from CS because, in folate and vitamin B_{12} deficiency, (a) the villus abnormality is not severe and is associated with decreased mitoses in the crypts and (b) increased inflammatory cells are not present (33,34).

Radiation and Chemotherapy Effect

Because radiation therapy and chemotherapeutic agents inhibit DNA synthesis, the intestinal mucosal changes are similar to those in folate and vitamin B_{12} deficiency and are associated with decreased mitotic activity in the crypts. Chemotherapy and irradiation may also cause focal necrosis of epithelial cells and increased numbers of chronic inflammatory cells within the mucosa and submucosa (35–37).

Microvillus Inclusion Disease

Microvillus inclusion disease is an inherited autosomal recessive condition causing intractable diarrhea with steatorrhea in infants. It was first reported under the designation *familial enteropathy* (38). Diarrhea persists despite total parenteral nutrition, and patients rarely survive beyond the age of 2 years. Successful treatment with small bowel transplantation has been reported (39). The entity should be recognized so that genetic counseling can be offered (40). Small bowel biopsy specimens show a severe villus abnormality with crypt hypoplasia. In general, the mucosal specimen may resemble CS, but intraepithelial lymphocytes are usually not increased. Transmission electron microscopy establishes the diagnosis by identifying abnormal microvillus structures at the luminal border of the enterocyte and apical intracytoplasmic inclusions lined by microvilli in the same cells (40,41). The intracytoplasmic vacuoles can also be detected with PAS stain or with carcinoembryonic antigen (CEA) immunostaining (42).

Entities Associated with a Nonspecific Variable Villus Abnormality

Many diseases are associated with nonspecific variable villus abnormalities that are usually not flat. Although most biopsy specimens showing this change are from patients with partially treated CS (Fig. 5), other conditions enter the differential diagnosis (see Table 1).

Dermatitis Herpetiformis

The similarities between dermatitis herpetiformis and CS are numerous and include response to a gluten-free diet, a high prevalence of HLA-B8 and HLA-DR3 phenotypes, and predisposition to malignant lymphoma (43). Approximately 60% to 80% of patients with dermatitis herpetiformis show a villus abnormality of the proximal small intestine (44–47). Although severe lesions similar to those of CS are reported, many patients show a distinctly patchy lesion with a variable villus abnormality. Approximately 75% of patients with dermatitis herpetiformis show clinical improvement of their skin lesions while on a gluten-free diet (43,44).

Tropical Sprue

Tropical sprue is a chronic diarrheal process associated with steatorrhea that is seen in patients from Southeast Asia, the Caribbean islands, and some areas of Central and South America (6,18,48–50). Affected patients have usually lived in these regions for years, but symptoms may be seen in people who have been there for as little as a few months. Patients usually respond dramatically to the administration of folate, vitamin B_{12}, and tetracycline (or other broad-spectrum antibiotics), implying that an infectious agent may be important in the etiology.

Small bowel biopsy specimens show a variable villus abnormality. The usual histologic appearance includes a mild to moderate villus shortening, increased numbers of chronic inflammatory cells in the lamina propria and epithelium, and crypt hyperplasia (Fig. 6). On occasion, a severe histologic lesion indistinguishable from CS may be seen.

Infectious Gastroenteritis

Jejunal mucosal lesions in infectious gastroenteritis are typically patchy with a variable villus abnormality; rarely,

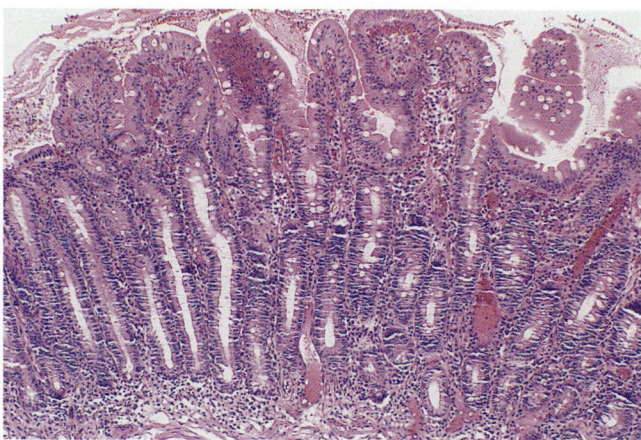

FIG. 5. Small bowel biopsy obtained from a patient with celiac sprue several weeks after gluten withdrawal. The specimen demonstrates a variable villous abnormality. Although some areas show a severe villous abnormality with a flat mucosa (*left*), the majority of the specimen shows some return of intestinal villi. Increased chronic inflammatory cells are still present within the lamina propria and within the epithelium.

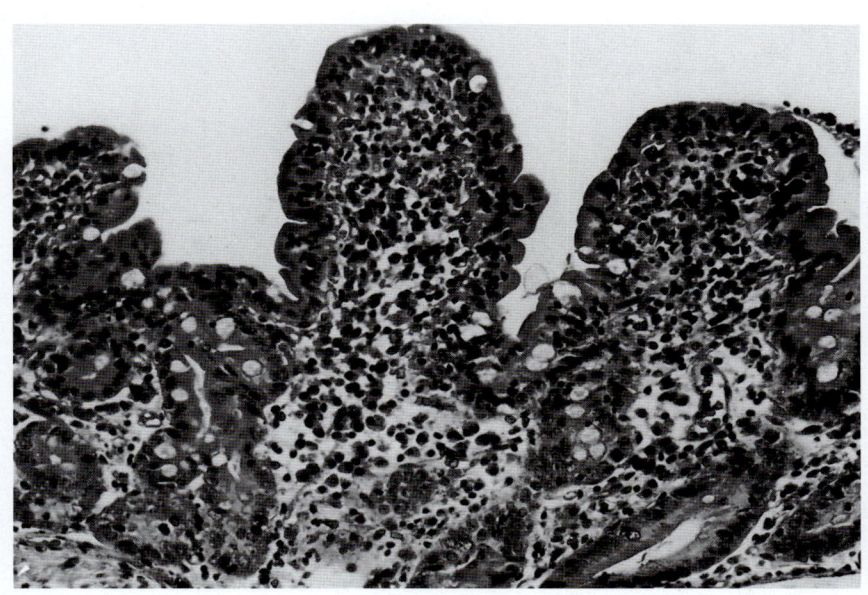

FIG. 6. Variable villous abnormality from a patient with tropical sprue. This specimen demonstrates moderate villous shortening associated with increased inflammatory cells within the epithelium and lamina propria.

the villus abnormality can be severe and closely mimic CS (6,17,51,52). In addition to increased chronic inflammatory cells, acute inflammatory cells are often seen both within epithelial cells and in the lamina propria (51). The acute onset and temporary nature of the symptoms, coupled with the acute inflammatory changes in biopsy specimens, usually help in the distinction from CS. However, the inflammatory changes can persist for months (4).

Stasis Syndromes

Stasis of small intestinal contents may occur in surgical blind loops, bowel obstruction, small intestinal diverticulosis, and intestinal pseudo-obstruction. With stasis, bacteria multiply and may be associated with malabsorption of fat and, on occasion, vitamin B_{12}, owing primarily to bacterial degradation of bile salts and intestinal mucosal injury (6,19).

Morphologic changes are typically patchy and composed of a variable villus abnormality associated with increased chronic inflammatory cells in the lamina propria and epithelium (10,53). Occasional neutrophils may be seen within the lamina propria and epithelium.

Small Bowel Histology in the Zollinger-Ellison Syndrome

Three patterns of focal structural injury are described in small bowel biopsy specimens from patients with Zollinger-Ellison syndrome. First, in the inflammatory response, there is a patchy variable villus abnormality associated with increased mononuclear cells and neutrophils in the lamina propria; erosions can occur. In the second pattern, gastric foveolar metaplasia is seen. In the third pattern, the histology is normal by light microscopy but abnormal by electron microscopy (54).

Mastocytosis

Systemic mastocytosis is a rare disorder characterized by the infiltration of mast cells in the skin (urticaria pigmentosa), bones, lymph nodes, and other parenchymal organs (55). The gut is affected in almost one half of patients; malabsorption may occur (56,57). Histologic features in small bowel biopsy specimens are inconsistent. Some specimens show a variable villus abnormality associated with increased numbers of mast cells, whereas others show no increase in mast cells but, instead, increased numbers of eosinophils. Rare patients have had the histologic features and clinical syndrome of CS (57,58).

Systemic mast cell disease can, on occasion, involve the intestinal tract without skin involvement (57,58). Some authors think that a gastrointestinal biopsy specimen showing more than six mast cells per high-magnification field should at least suggest the diagnosis of systemic mast cell disease (58).

Duodenitis and Peptic Ulcer Disease

The normal duodenal mucosa often shows a mild decrease in villus height and increased mitotic activity when compared to normal jejunum. This is thought to be the normal physiologic response of the mucosa to the presence of acid in the gut lumen (59). Duodenitis may represent an exaggeration of this response and probably has the same pathogenesis as peptic ulcer disease (60), representing a milder preulcer form. Active duodenitis is generally limited to the first part of the duodenum (61) and demonstrates a variable villus abnormality associated with increased acute and chronic inflammatory cells and, with hyperacidity, gastric foveolar metaplasia of villous epithelium (54,60) (Fig. 7). CS should be considered if acute inflammatory changes occur more distally in the duodenum, especially if associated with increased intraepithelial lymphocytes (61,62). Nodular or diffuse hyperplasia of Brunner's glands within the lamina

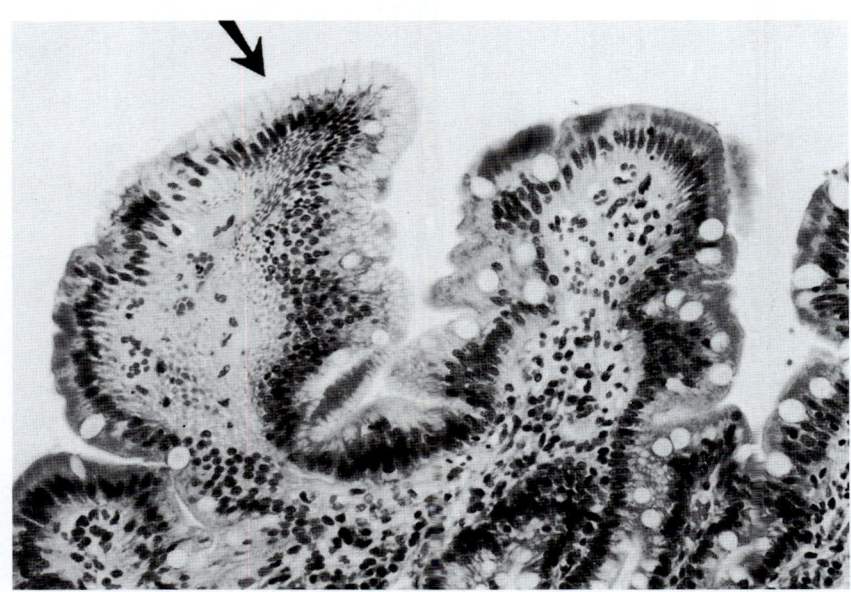

FIG. 7. Gastric foveolar metaplasia of the duodenum. The metaplastic epithelium (*arrow*), composed of columnar cells with basilar-placed nuclei and clear cytoplasm, contrasts with the absorptive and goblet cells of the normal duodenum.

propria may also be present in peptic duodenitis. A close association between peptic ulcer disease and gastric infection with *Helicobacter pylori* has been reported (63–66). Some authors think that gastric heterotopia or metaplasia is an important predisposing factor for the effect of *H. pylori* because the organism is found in these ectopic gastric tissues by H&E, silver, or modified Giemsa stain techniques. The organism is not usually found on normal small intestinal epithelium or on gastric mucosa in which intestinal metaplasia has occurred.

The histologic differential diagnosis of gastric metaplasia in duodenal villi includes gastric heterotopia (67). This usually appears as a mural nodule or mucosal polyp (67,68) on the anterior wall of the proximal duodenum. Histologic distinction between gastric metaplasia and heterotopia is made by recognition of the specialized gastric gland cells in the latter. Gastric heterotopia, which is usually of no clinical significance, has been described throughout the gastrointestinal tract, including the rectum (69).

Autoimmune Enteropathy

The term *autoimmune enteropathy* has been applied to an intractable watery diarrhea syndrome occurring in infants that has been associated with circulating autoantibodies against intestinal epithelial cells (70,71). A similar condition may also present as a refractory spruelike syndrome in adults (72). The patients often have variable immunodeficiency and autoimmune phenomena such as juvenile-onset diabetes mellitus, rheumatoid arthritis, and hemolytic anemia (73–75). The small bowel mucosa shows a variable villus abnormality that is often severe and resembles CS. Surface and crypt epithelial degenerative and regenerative changes occur, but many illustrated cases show few intraepithelial lymphocytes, a feature that may distinguish autoimmune enteropathy from CS. Some patients with autoimmune enteropathy have also had colitis. In some cases, the associated colitis has resembled lymphocytic colitis, whereas in others, the endoscopic and histologic picture is similar to ulcerative colitis (UC) (76,77). Autoimmune enteropathy is usually severe and intractable, often requiring total parenteral nutrition. There have been scattered reports of favorable responses to immunosuppressive agents such as cyclosporine (78,79) or tacrolimus (77,80).

Torkelson Syndrome

Torkelson syndrome has been described in Mennonite kindred in Canada and is inherited as an autosomal dominant trait (81). In symptomatic individuals, diarrhea and rapid dehydration develop early in childhood and can lead to death. Many affected individuals show evidence of common variable immunodeficiency but no overt malabsorption. Histologic changes in the small bowel consist of edema of the lamina propria, shortening and broadening of intestinal villi, and focal acute inflammatory changes.

Entities Associated with Variable Villus Abnormalities Illustrating Specific Diagnostic Changes

Collagenous Sprue

The term *collagenous sprue* describes the excessive subepithelial deposition of collagen associated with a severe villus abnormality noted in small bowel biopsy specimens from some patients with malabsorption unresponsive to gluten-free diet (82). Although some patients with this finding have ultimately responded to a gluten-free diet (83), many have followed a fulminant and generally fatal course (4,82). The collagen distribution is typically patchy and may not present early in the disease; multiple biopsies may be necessary to establish the diagnosis (4,82). Collagenous sprue should be considered in patients with refractory or unclassified sprue unresponsive to a gluten-free diet.

Immunodeficiency Syndromes (Excluding Acquired Immunodeficiency Syndrome)

Normal small bowel morphology seen on routine light microscopy is the rule in selective IgA deficiency, although nodular lymphoid hyperplasia may be present. Decreased numbers of IgA-containing plasma cells can be demonstrated by immunocytochemical techniques. Selectively IgA-deficient patients reportedly do not show a predisposition to *G. lamblia* infection (4).

Patients with common variable immunodeficiency syndrome (CVID) may have chronic diarrhea, malabsorption, and recurrent gastrointestinal giardiasis (84). The morphology of small intestinal biopsy specimens may vary from normal to a severe abnormality mimicking CS. In contrast to CS, plasma cells in CVID are decreased and IgA-containing plasma cells are absent (85). Occasionally in CVID, the mucosa demonstrates nodular lymphoid hyperplasia associated with absent or markedly reduced numbers of plasma cells (4,84). Giardiasis commonly is found with either histology. Nodular lymphoid hyperplasia without plasma cell changes may also be seen in asymptomatic patients without an immunodeficiency syndrome, especially in children, in whom it may be considered a normal finding. An injury pattern resembling acute graft-versus-host disease, with numerous apoptotic bodies deep in crypts, can also be seen in CVID (86).

With routine light microscopy, nodular lymphoid hyperplasia of the gastrointestinal tract can be difficult to distinguish from non-Hodgkin's lymphoma. Furthermore, non-Hodgkin's lymphoma associated with nodular lymphoid hyperplasia has been described in patients with CVID (86). Immunocytochemistry or molecular analysis can aid in proper diagnosis and classification of gut lymphoid proliferations. When confronted with an atypical gut lymphoid proliferation, I recommend rebiopsy to obtain fresh tissue for flow cytometric immunotyping or molecular studies (gene rearrangement studies by Southern blot hybridization analysis or polymerase chain reaction [PCR]) if required to establish or refute clonality. If rebiopsy is not possible, PCR for immunoglobulin or T-cell gene rearrangements can often be successful in formalin-fixed paraffin-embedded tissue.

Whipple's Disease

Whipple's disease, a chronic systemic illness with numerous gastrointestinal features such as diarrhea and malabsorption, is caused by the Whipple's bacillus, an as yet uncultured rod-shaped microorganism (87–90). PCR amplification studies of the Whipple's bacillus and sequencing of the bacterial 16s ribosomal RNA gene (91) have confirmed the uniqueness of the organism, and the name *Tropheryma whippelii* has been proposed (92). Whipple's disease responds dramatically to antibiotic therapy; without treatment, it is fatal. The characteristic histopathology of Whipple's disease is infiltration of various organs with macrophages containing the Whipple's bacillus. This infiltration has a predilection for the lamina propria of the small intestine, mesenteric lymph nodes, cardiac valves, and the central nervous system (4,89).

Positive gut mucosal biopsy specimens demonstrate infiltration of the lamina propria, muscularis mucosae, and, in some cases, submucosa by macrophages with a foamy gray-blue cytoplasm (Fig. 8). The number of intraepithelial lymphocytes is not increased. In addition, fat vacuoles are seen in the lamina propria, although many illustrated as such are clearly dilated lymphatic vessels. The diagnostic changes of Whipple's disease are easily seen on H&E; the PAS stain, although dramatic, is probably not necessary to make the diagnosis. The macrophage cytoplasm contains intensely PAS-positive material that is coarsely granular and not bacillary in shape (Fig. 9). With antibiotic treatment, the pattern of mucosal infiltration can become patchy (93). The macrophages recede to the muscularis mucosae, submucosa, and basilar portions of the lamina propria, and the cytoplasmic inclusions become "tissue-paper-like" with PAS stain—reminiscent of the inclusions of Gaucher's cells. PAS-positive macrophages can persist for years after treatment.

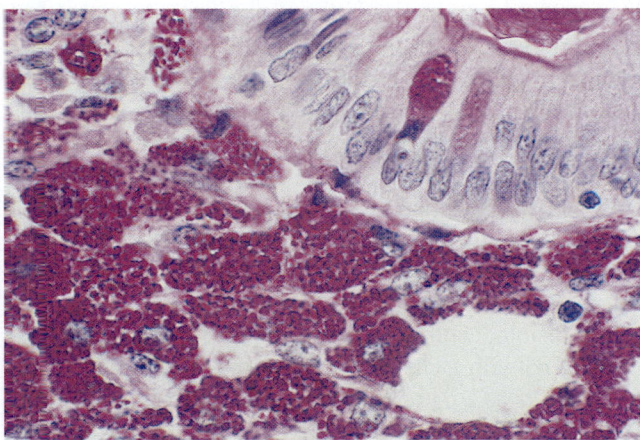

FIG. 9. The cytoplasm of the macrophages in Whipple's disease contains intensely periodic acid-Schiff (PAS)-positive material that is coarsely granular. PAS stain.

The histologic differential diagnosis of Whipple's disease includes disseminated histoplasmosis (94) and MAIC infection (95,96). The macrophages in disseminated histoplasmosis contain faintly blue dotlike inclusions usually surrounded by a clear halo. PAS and silver stains demonstrate budding yeast forms. The similarity of Whipple's disease to MAIC infection has perhaps been overemphasized in the literature. The H&E appearance may be similar, but MAIC involvement of the small bowel tends to be patchy, whereas Whipple's disease is diffuse, and the lipid vacuoles of Whipple's disease are not seen in MAIC. PAS-positive inclusions are present within macrophages in both Whipple's disease and MAIC; however, the shapes are different. In Whipple's disease the inclusion is bright-staining and coarsely granular; in MAIC, the PAS stain reveals a faintly positive bacillary form. Distinction of the two entities is made by use of the acid-fast stain that is positive in MAIC but negative in Whipple's disease.

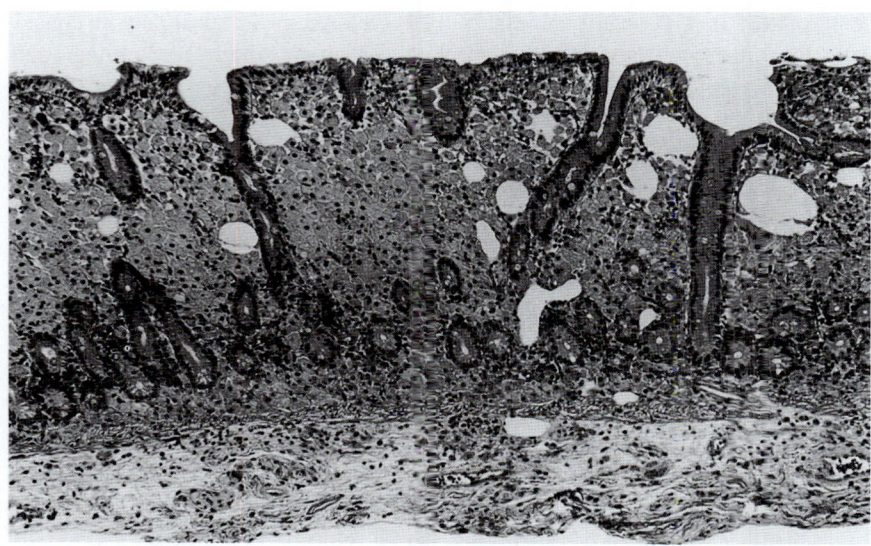

FIG. 8. Whipple's disease. The lamina propria is infiltrated by macrophages that broaden and flatten the intestinal villi. Note the scattered "fat vacuoles."

Eosinophilic Gastroenteritis

The term *eosinophilic gastroenteritis* has been used to describe a collection of clinical syndromes that are usually seen in children or young adults and that have in common infiltration of the gastrointestinal tract by large numbers of eosinophilic leukocytes (97–99). Infiltration primarily in the mucosa of the stomach and small intestine is associated with diarrhea and malabsorption, whereas eosinophils predominantly in the submucosa and muscularis propria are associated with intestinal obstruction. Ascites is a major manifestation when the eosinophils infiltrate chiefly the subserosa (97–103).

The histologic diagnosis of eosinophilic gastroenteritis may be difficult. Infiltration of the submucosa, muscularis propria, and subserosal connective tissue by eosinophils is always abnormal and, when corroborated clinically, is diagnostic of eosinophilic gastroenteritis; however, this type of evaluation does, in general, require a resection specimen. The diagnosis of the mucosal pattern of eosinophilic gastroenteritis in biopsy specimens can be particularly challenging to the pathologist. Scattered intramucosal eosinophils are normal in the gastrointestinal tract, and their mere presence should not prompt a diagnosis of eosinophilic gastroenteritis. However, collections of eosinophils not associated with other inflammatory cells, groups of eosinophils associated with focal mucosal architectural distortion or injury (cryptitis, crypt abscesses), and infiltration of the muscularis mucosae by eosinophils are all abnormal and, in a corroborative clinical setting, are diagnostic of eosinophilic gastroenteritis. The mucosal involvement in eosinophilic gastroenteritis is notoriously patchy; therefore, if the clinical suspicion is great, multiple or additional biopsy specimens should be obtained.

Numerous intramucosal eosinophils can be seen in other conditions. A search for parasites should always be done when eosinophils are prominent, but particularly for obstructive eosinophilic enteritis (ileitis), which is sometimes caused by *Sarcocystis* species (104) or *Ancylostoma caninum* (105). Eosinophils may occasionally be a major component of primary inflammatory bowel disease (IBD) and non-Hodgkin's lymphoma involving the gut. Additional histopathologic features and clinical findings distinguish these entities from eosinophilic gastroenteritis; also, eosinophilic gastroenteritis is essentially never associated with the architectural or metaplastic changes of chronicity.

Enteropathy-Associated T-cell Lymphoma (So-Called Ulcerative Jejunoileitis)

Ulcerative jejunoileitis is a rare and poorly understood condition characterized by mucosal ulcers associated with a severe small-intestinal villus abnormality. Patients have abdominal pain, fever, intestinal obstruction, perforation, or hemorrhage, usually in association with malabsorption (106–109). Examples of ulcerative jejunoileitis have been reported under a number of synonyms, including diffuse ulceration of the jejunum and ileum, chronic ulcerative nongranulomatous jejunoileitis (110), idiopathic chronic ulcerative enteritis (107), malignant histiocytosis (111), enteropathy-associated T-cell lymphoma (112), and epitheliotropic lymphoma of the small bowel (113). Although some researchers exclude patients who have had clinical CS (i.e., malabsorption initially responsive to dietary gluten withdrawal) (108,109), in my opinion, patients with ulcers and a severe villus abnormality share a common clinical course and histologic appearance regardless of an initial response to gluten withdrawal. Both patient groups demonstrate clinical malabsorption, a similar histologic appearance (ulcer associated with a flat small bowel mucosa and atypical lymphoid cells), poor prognosis (75% dead within 2 years), and close association with concomitant or subsequent malignant lymphoma (108,111–115).

The striking association with lymphoma has prompted some investigators to conclude that all cases of ulcerative jejunoileitis probably represent intestinal non-Hodgkin's lymphoma (synonyms include malignant histiocytosis and enteropathy-associated T-cell lymphoma) (111,115). Isaacson and Wright chose the term *malignant histiocytosis* to describe this lymphoma because the morphology, erythrophagocytosis, ultrastructural appearance, and immunocytochemical reaction for alpha$_1$-antitrypsin in the "atypical cells" favored origin from tissue macrophages (111, 116–118). The same investigators later demonstrated T-cell immunophenotype and T-cell receptor beta chain gene rearrangements (115,119). T-cell lineage has been confirmed (120–122), thus accounting for the popularity of the alternative term *enteropathy-associated T-cell lymphoma*. There may well be "benign" ulcer complications of malabsorption, but I have been impressed with the focality of lymphoma and with the difficulty in making that diagnosis with certainty. Any ulcer in patients with CS or an unclassified malabsorption syndrome associated with a flat mucosa must be viewed as a potential harbinger of intestinal lymphoma. Therefore, I recommend extensive sampling of the lesion (including frozen tissue samples) and careful clinical follow-up.

Another controversial point concerns whether the villus abnormality in ulcerative jejunoileitis is, in fact, CS, a low-grade intramucosal T-cell lymphoma, mucosal injury resulting from cytokines released by abnormal T cells, or some other, as yet unrecognized, small intestinal disorder (123–126). Demonstration of T-cell receptor gene rearrangement in the mucosa not involved by lymphoma provides a compelling argument that the "enteropathy" may not be CS but could represent *de novo* low-grade epitheliotropic/mucosatropic T-cell lymphoma (113,124–128). This concept may revolutionize the current perception and treatment of adult-onset unclassified sprue and CS that has become nonresponsive to dietary gluten withdrawal. If T-cell receptor gene rearrangements are confirmed in these patients, then they could potentially benefit from lymphoma-directed chemotherapeutic regimens rather than the standard malabsorption treatments.

Parasitic Infestations

Although a large number of parasites may infect the gastrointestinal tract, this discussion concentrates on those that are typically associated with intestinal malabsorption. *Cryptosporidium* species, *Microsporidia* species, and *Isospora* species infection are discussed in Interpretation of Endoscopic Biopsy Specimens from Patients with the Acquired Immunodeficiency Syndrome.

Giardiasis (*Giardia lamblia* Infection). Infection by *G. lamblia* is common, especially in underdeveloped countries or in areas where the water supply has become contaminated by feces (129–131). Symptomatic patients demonstrate a spectrum of complaints, from mild abdominal discomfort with intermittent diarrhea to frank intestinal malabsorption (131).

Although giardiasis is usually identified in duodenal biopsy specimens, the organism has been found in the gastric antrum, ileal specimens, and even colonic biopsy specimens (132). The small bowel mucosal histology in biopsy specimens is usually normal; however, a patchy villus abnormality of variable severity can be observed (132–136) (Fig. 10). The histologic diagnosis rests upon demonstration of trophozoites either along the surface of epithelial cells in biopsy specimens or in touch preparations (Fig. 11). The organism is approximately the same size as the enterocyte nucleus. In profile, the trophozoite of *G. lamblia* is sickle shaped; seen *en face*, it has a characteristic pear shape with a tapered posterior region. It has prominent paired nuclei, paired median rods, a curved median body, and four pairs of flagellae. These morphologic features are most easily recognized on Giemsa- or trichrome-stained touch preparations. In tissue sections, fragments of mucus may closely mimic the appearance of *G. lamblia* trophozoites.

Although trophozoites are readily seen on H&E staining, I routinely stain one small bowel biopsy slide with the trichrome technique. The counterstain in most trichrome stains is iron hematoxylin, a stain that makes the organism

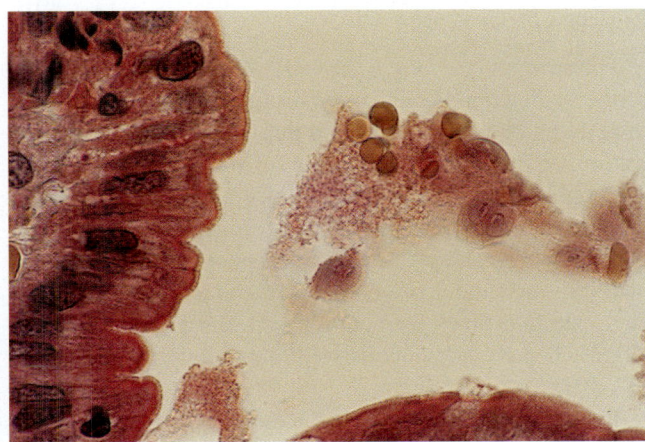

FIG. 11. Small bowel biopsy specimen in giardiasis. The diagnosis rests on demonstration of trophozoites in tissue section. Seen *en face*, *Giardia lamblia* is pear shaped and demonstrates prominent paired nuclei. Trichrome stain.

more conspicuous. Furthermore, the red staining easily distinguishes it from blue-staining mucus. Because giardiasis is also associated with the CVID, biopsy specimens may show absent or decreased numbers of plasma cells, with or without nodular lymphoid hyperplasia. The diagnosis of giardiasis can usually be made by detecting cysts, trophozoites, or *Giardia* antigens in stool specimens (131,136).

Strongyloidiasis (*Strongyloides stercoralis* Infection). Several species of *Strongyloides* infect humans (131). Intestinal infection, usually the result of infestation with the nematode *Strongyloides stercoralis*, develops when the worms bury themselves within the mucosa of the duodenum and jejunum. Within the mucosa, females then lay their eggs, which develop into rhabditiform larvae that pass in the stool. In most cases, these larvae mature into the infective form in the soil and then can penetrate intact skin, thus completing the life cycle. In some patients, the rhabditiform larvae may develop into infective filariform larvae before they are

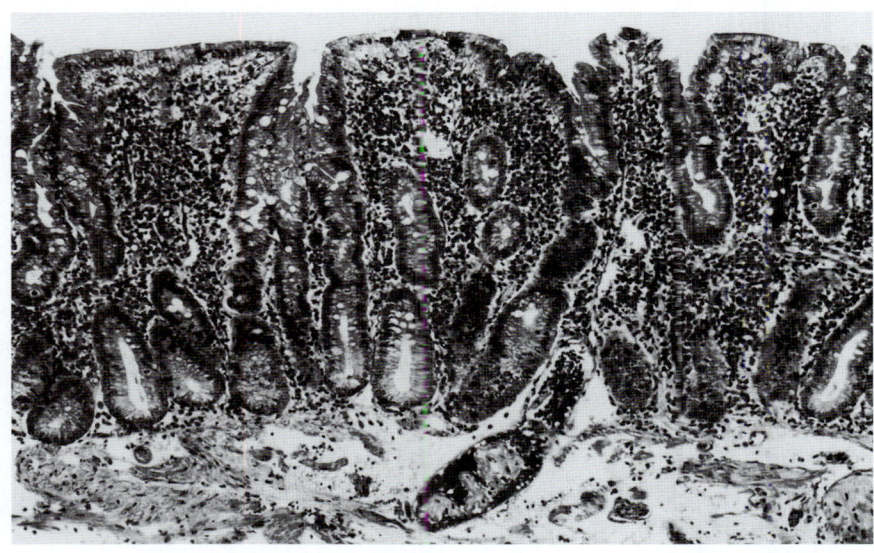

FIG. 10. Mucosal histology in giardiasis is variable; in this case, it shows a severe villous abnormality similar to that seen in celiac sprue.

passed. These infective larvae may invade the intestinal mucosa or the perianal skin and set up a cycle referred to as "autoinfection" (137).

Although many infected patients have no gastrointestinal symptoms, some may have diarrhea or malabsorption (138), and in the immunocompromised patient, autoinfection occurs. Such infections are severe and often fatal (137–140). The diagnosis is usually made by demonstrating larvae in the stools; the pathologist is unlikely to see the organism in biopsy material. In autopsy or surgical specimens, the adult female and the eggs can be seen in the small bowel mucosa. With autoinfection, the filariform larvae may also be identified in fresh stool or in the bowel wall where they are sometimes accompanied by an eosinophilic granulomatous inflammatory reaction (131,139–141).

Capillariasis (*Capillaria philippinensis* Infection). Nematodes of the species *Capillaria philippinensis* can infect humans and cause a protein-losing enteropathy that can be fatal (142). Infections have been described in patients from the Philippines, Thailand, Iran, Korea, and Egypt (131,143). The worms infest the jejunum and upper ileum and have only rarely been described in biopsy specimens (143,144). The adult worm and eggs bear a morphologic resemblance to those of trichuriasis. The diagnosis is usually made by identifying eggs, larvae, or adult worms in the stool.

Waldenström's Macroglobulinemia

Intestinal involvement by Waldenström's macroglobulinemia is rare but distinctive (145–147). Grossly, the small bowel serosa shows small white nodules and, occasionally, distended serosal lymphatics. The mucosal surface of the bowel may be white, nodular, granular, or mottled. Microscopically, biopsy specimens have shown marked mucosal and submucosal lymphangiectasia associated with short, broad villi. A coarse and sometimes fragmented eosinophilic material is present in the dilated lymphatics, in the lamina propria, and in macrophages. Immunocytochemistry can be used to confirm that the eosinophilic material is, in fact, the macroglobulin.

Intestinal Lymphangiectasia

Intestinal lymphangiectasia is characterized by focal or diffuse dilatation of the mucosal, submucosal, and subserosal lymphatics that may be associated with protein-losing enteropathy, hypoalbuminemia, hypoproteinemic edema, and lymphocytopenia (148,149). It can occur in a primary or secondary form. The primary form has a predilection for children and is caused by a congenital obstructive defect of the lymphatics (4,149). Secondary lymphangiectasia is associated with many diseases, including retroperitoneal fibrosis, pancreatitis, constrictive pericarditis, primary myocardial disease, intestinal Behcet's disease, intestinal malignancy, Waldenström's macroglobulinemia, and sarcoidosis (4,6,149,150). In both forms, the histology in mucosal biopsy specimens is identical: dilated lymphatics located in otherwise normal tissue (Fig. 12). Therapy includes treatment of underlying conditions, dietary manipulation, and, in some localized forms of lymphangiectasia, resection (148).

Abetalipoproteinemia

In abetalipoproteinemia, a condition inherited as an autosomal recessive trait (151), patients are unable to synthesize apoprotein B (4). Therefore, fatty acids within intestinal absorptive cells can be re-esterified to triglyceride but cannot be changed into chylomicrons for transport. As a result, fat accumulates in the absorptive cells. Biopsy specimens have a normal villus architecture. Enterocytes, however, have cytoplasm packed with droplets of lipid that appear optically clear or foamy with H&E staining. The changes are most prominent at the tips of the villi. This enterocyte vacuolization, although characteristic, is not pathognomonic, because similar vacuolar change has been described in megaloblastic anemia, CS, and tropical sprue (152). I have occasionally observed it in patients without any apparent disease process.

Acrodermatitis Enteropathica

Acrodermatitis enteropathica is inherited as an autosomal recessive trait, manifests itself in children, and has been linked to zinc deficiency. Patients are typically afflicted by cutaneous lesions (perioral and extremity skin lesions, alopecia, nail dystrophy), diarrhea, and malabsorption; they usually respond favorably to the administration of zinc sulfate

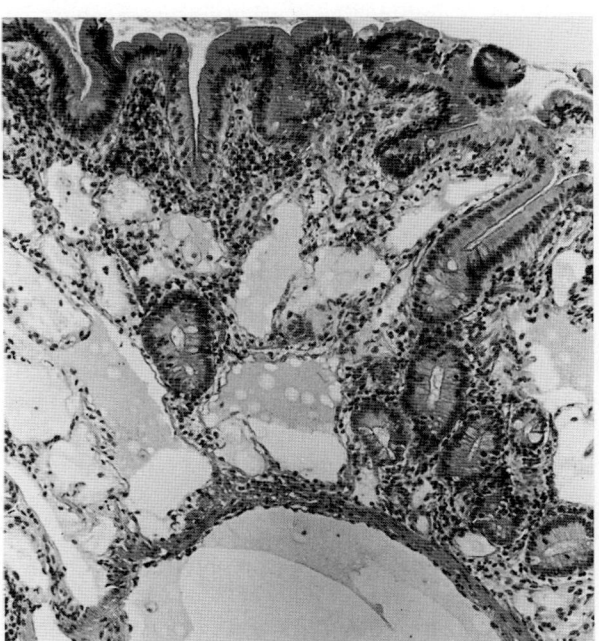

FIG. 12. Intestinal lymphangiectasia. The primary and secondary forms appear identical in mucosal biopsy specimens and demonstrate dilated lymphatics located in otherwise normal mucosa and submucosa.

(153–155). Small bowel morphology varies, with some workers reporting a severe villus abnormality similar to that in CS and which improved with zinc therapy (153) and others reporting normal or only minimally abnormal small intestinal mucosa by routine light microscopy (153–155). Ultrastructural changes in Paneth cells consisting of rodlike fibrillar inclusions are considered diagnostic for acrodermatitis enteropathica (154,155).

Tufting Enteropathy

The term *tufting enteropathy* has been applied to a sometimes familial intractable diarrhea syndrome in children (156–158). Symptoms usually begin in the neonatal period with the patient requiring total parenteral nutrition. Small bowel biopsy specimens have demonstrated a variable villus abnormality that is usually not associated with epithelial lymphocytosis as well as a distinctive surface epithelial change consisting of epithelial crowding, disorganization, and focal tufting. Abnormalities of basement membrane structure have been described.

NONNEOPLASTIC POLYPS AND NODULES OF THE SMALL BOWEL

Pancreatic Heterotopia, Adenomyoma, and Myoepithelial Hamartoma

Pancreatic heterotopia, adenomyoma, and myoepithelial hamartoma are variants of the same process. Pancreatic heterotopia is characterized by the presence of pancreatic acinar, islet, and/or ductular elements, usually associated with smooth muscle proliferation, outside the topographic boundaries of the pancreas. Adenomyoma and myoepithelial hamartoma are synonymous terms and differ from pancreatic heterotopia in that acinar and islet-like tissue are not present. In my experience, the distribution of acinar and islet elements in heterotopic pancreas has been quite variable, and some areas of a pancreatic heterotopia may be indistinguishable from adenomyoma.

The prevalence of heterotopic pancreas in different series has varied from 0.55% to 13.7% (159,160). The common sites are the stomach, duodenum, and jejunum, but ectopic pancreatic tissue may also be encountered in Meckel's diverticulum, the ampulla of Vater, gallbladder, umbilicus, fallopian tube, and mediastinum (161). Most examples are encountered incidentally at surgery, and the pathologist is often asked to identify these lesions on a frozen section. On rare occasions, epigastric pain, weight loss, hemorrhage, gastric outlet obstruction, and intussusception have been attributable directly to the presence of the heterotopic pancreas (159,160). Malignancy arising in association with pancreatic heterotopia has been reported (161).

Pancreatic heterotopia presents grossly as a submucosal nodule, as an intramural mass, or as a nodular lesion involving the serosa. The color is typically yellow or yellow-white; on cut section the surface is lobulated. Size ranges from 0.2 to 4.0 cm (160,161). Occasionally, it contains a central mucosal dimple, which is an important diagnostic clue radiologically, endoscopically, and grossly (161–163). Histologically, those cases of pancreatic heterotopia associated with acinar elements or islet cells pose little problem in differential diagnosis. Those composed purely of ducts and smooth muscle may be difficult to diagnose and are often confused with metastatic adenocarcinoma. However, the adenomyomatous pattern shows an orderly arrangement or lobular pattern of benign ducts set in a background of proliferating smooth muscle (Fig. 13). In those cases showing a gross central mucosal dimple, the pattern of ducts recapitulates the major duodenal papilla.

Hyperplasia of Brunner's Glands

Brunner's glands are branched tubuloalveolar glands confined predominantly to the duodenum in humans. Most Brunner's glands are submucosal, but about one third of their volume can be found above the muscularis mucosae, where the glands empty into the crypts of Lieberkuhn (164).

Hyperplasias of Brunner's glands exist in three forms (164–168): (a) diffuse glandular proliferation, imparting a coarse nodularity to most of the duodenum, (b) limited discrete nodules in the proximal duodenum, and (c) solitary nodules, often referred to as "adenoma" of Brunner's glands. Most are encountered as incidental findings during investigation of the upper gastrointestinal tract. Histologically, these Brunner's gland proliferations suggest a hamartoma or reactive hyperplasia in that they consist of increased numbers of normal-appearing Brunner's glands accompanied by variable proliferations of smooth muscle. Inflammatory cells are often present, and some larger lesions may ulcerate.

Differentiating normal Brunner's glands from hyperplasia is difficult. If a gross nodule or polyp is present and is composed solely of Brunner's-type glands, then it is probably correct to refer to it as a hyperplasia. The distinction between

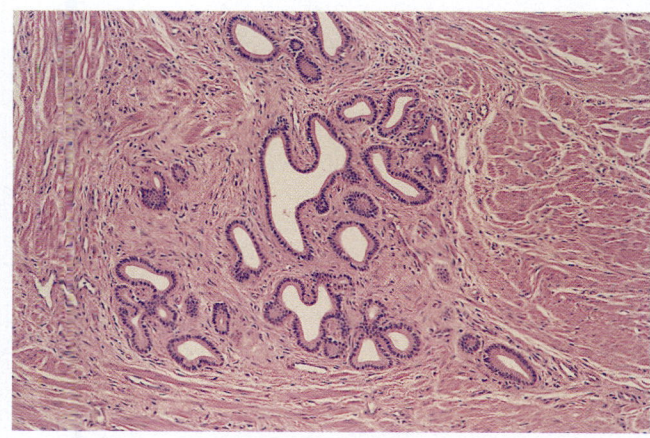

FIG. 13. Adenomyoma involving duodenal wall demonstrating an orderly arrangement of benign ducts in a background of proliferating smooth muscle.

adenoma and hyperplasia is arbitrary, and no substantial evidence exists to suggest that any of these proliferations are truly neoplastic (165); thus, the term *Brunner's gland nodule* is preferred. There is no convincing evidence of carcinoma having arisen either from normal Brunner's glands or Brunner's gland nodules.

INTERPRETATION OF COLONIC MUCOSAL BIOPSY SPECIMENS IN THE EVALUATION OF PATIENTS WITH SUSPECTED INFLAMMATORY BOWEL DISEASE

With increased availability of total colonoscopy and flexible sigmoidoscopy, pathologists can expect an increasing number of colorectal biopsy specimens. The pathologist plays an increasingly important role in the diagnosis and management of patients with colitis. The numerous uses of mucosal biopsy to evaluate these conditions are summarized in Table 2.

Colonic Biopsy Specimen Processing and Normal Colonic Histology

Colonic biopsy specimen orientation is not as critical as in small bowel samples; however, the interpretation is still facilitated by good orientation. A procedure similar to that used in small intestinal biopsy specimen procurement and processing can be used. Colonic mucosal biopsy specimens are oriented immediately in the endoscopy suite, mucosa side up, on a solid substance such as filter paper, and then placed into Hollande's (or other) fixative. Two to three step-section slides stained with H&E are examined.

Normal colonic histology is illustrated in Fig. 14 (169). The luminal surface is straight. Colonic tubules are tightly packed, parallel, nonbranching, and all closely approximate the muscularis mucosae. The appearance is similar to test tubes in a rack. Goblet cells are numerous. The lamina propria contains a modest amount of mixed inflammatory cell infiltrate, including plasma cells, lymphocytes, eosinophils, and macrophages. An occasional intraepithelial lymphocyte can be seen. The muscularis mucosae is thin and regular. The submucosa is generally devoid of inflammation. Scattered intramucosal lymphoid follicles are normally encountered, especially in younger individuals. In areas of lymphoid follicles, the architecture may be mildly distorted, the muscu-

TABLE 2. *Uses of colonic mucosal biopsies in the evaluation of colitis*

1. Documentation of colitis
2. Identification of specific forms of colitis (e.g., collagenous colitis, ischemic colitis)
3. Documentation of the severity, extent, and nature (focal versus diffuse) of inflammatory bowel disease
4. To follow the clinical course of disease
5. Surveillance for dysplasia and carcinoma
6. Detection of conditions that mimic inflammatory bowel disease (e.g., solitary rectal ulcer syndrome)

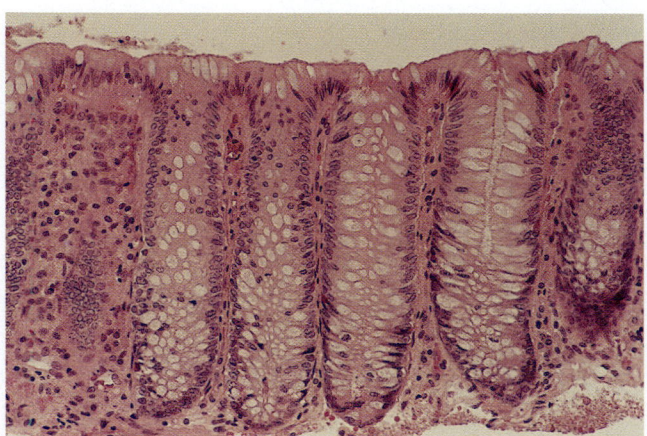

FIG. 14. Normal colonic mucosal biopsy specimen. Normal colonic tubules are tightly packed, parallel, and nonbranching. The luminal surface is straight.

laris mucosae may be incomplete, and some of the lymphoid follicles may spill over into the submucosa. Overlying the lymphoid aggregates are flattened surface cells termed *M cells*. In this M-cell region, the epithelium normally contains more mononuclear inflammatory cells and the amount of intraepithelial mucin is decreased (169,170). Paneth cells can be seen in the base of colonic crypts but are considered a normal finding only in the cecum and proximal ascending colon (169,170).

Changes associated with bowel preparation or the trauma of biopsy itself can be expected. Bowel preparation decreases the amount of intracellular mucin, causes a mild increase in the number of mitotic figures, causes surface degeneration in the form of apoptosis, and can even be associated with rare neutrophils in the surface epithelium and crypts (169–172). Edema and recent hemorrhage into tissue not associated with other degenerative or inflammatory changes are best attributed to biopsy trauma.

Muciphages (macrophages containing PAS-positive material) are often present within the lamina propria of the large intestine, especially in the distal rectum. I do not consider their presence abnormal because they do not correlate with any inflammatory or infiltrative disorder (173), whereas other authors think that they represent a nonspecific response to mucosal injury (174). Muciphages have been confused with Whipple's disease and with MAIC infection. The macrophages in Whipple's disease are mucicarmine-negative, and acid-fast stains are positive in mycobacterial infection.

Chronic Colitis—Differential Diagnosis

The pattern of abnormality in chronic ulcerative colitis (UC) in remission (quiescent UC) is probably the easiest to identify in biopsy specimens. The predominant features are mucosal atrophy and mucosal architectural distortion (175,176) (Fig. 15). The luminal border is irregular. The

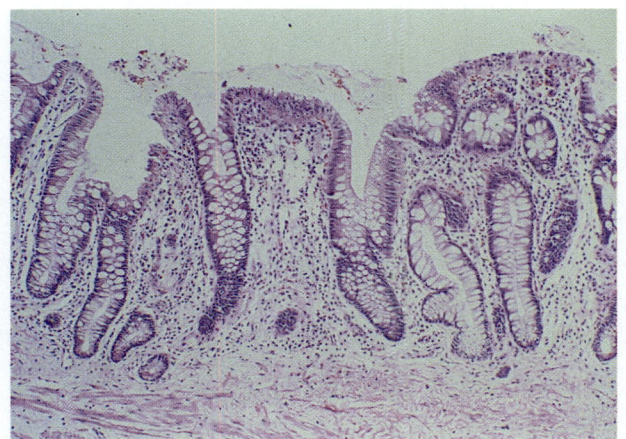

FIG. 15. Chronic ulcerative colitis in remission. There is a decreased number of colonic tubules associated with mucosal architectural distortion. The luminal border is irregular; the colonic crypts have lost their parallel arrangement and are branched and budded. The muscularis mucosae is hypertrophied.

number of crypts decreases; in addition, the remaining crypts appear short (i.e., they do not touch the muscularis mucosae), lose their parallel arrangement, and become branched and budded. The goblet cell population is usually preserved. Chronic inflammatory cells are only mildly increased in the lamina propria. Paneth cells may be present. The muscularis mucosae, if present in the specimen, is usually hypertrophied. These changes, although consistent with a diagnosis of chronic UC, must be interpreted in light of the clinical and endoscopic findings because identical changes can be seen in focal healed or healing areas of other chronic colitides such as Crohn's disease (CD), ischemia (including chronic irradiation injury), tuberculosis, and schistosomiasis.

Care must be taken when interpreting biopsy specimens obtained from normal mucosa adjacent to lymphoid follicles, from normal mucosa containing the innominate groove, and from the lower portion of the rectum near the anorectal transition zone. These areas may normally show some crypt shortening and loss of crypt parallelism and should not be interpreted as chronic colitis (172). Likewise, histologically normal biopsy specimens must not be reported as showing chronic nonspecific inflammation consistent with chronic UC. Unless one or more of the features discussed in the preceding paragraph are also present, it is a good rule not to diagnose chronic UC based only on an evaluation of inflammatory cells in the lamina propria.

Active Colitis—Differential Diagnosis

The term *active colitis* is used to describe an inflammatory condition in which neutrophils are present in the lamina propria, within epithelial cells (cryptitis), or within crypt lumens (crypt abscesses). Included under this heading are (a) UC in an active phase, (b) most examples of Crohn's colitis, and (c) infectious colitis/acute self-limited colitis (177,178). Recognition of an inflammatory pattern coupled with clinical and endoscopic correlation allows a fairly specific diagnosis to be made in many biopsy specimens.

Diffuse Active Colitis

Untreated UC in an active phase represents the prototypic diffuse active colitis. Biopsy specimens usually demonstrate a diffuse abnormality, meaning that changes are of approximately the same intensity in all areas of the tissue (Fig. 16). The luminal border of the mucosa is irregular (176,179,180). Increased numbers of chronic inflammatory cells are present in the lamina propria and may spill over into the superficial portion of the submucosa. Intracellular mucin in the goblet cells is depleted (181). Cryptitis and crypt abscess formation are often prominent (180). It is surprising that even in UC of

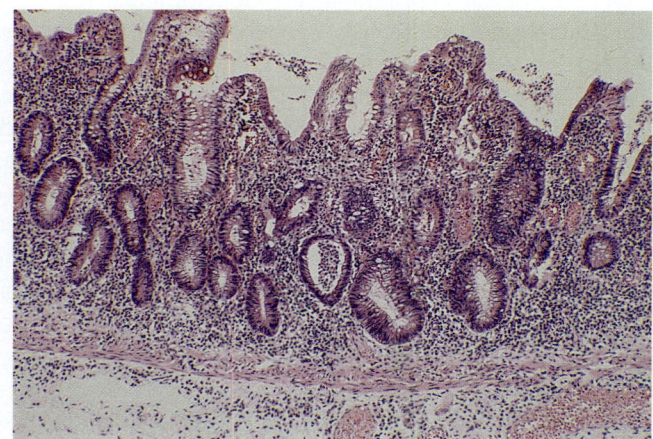
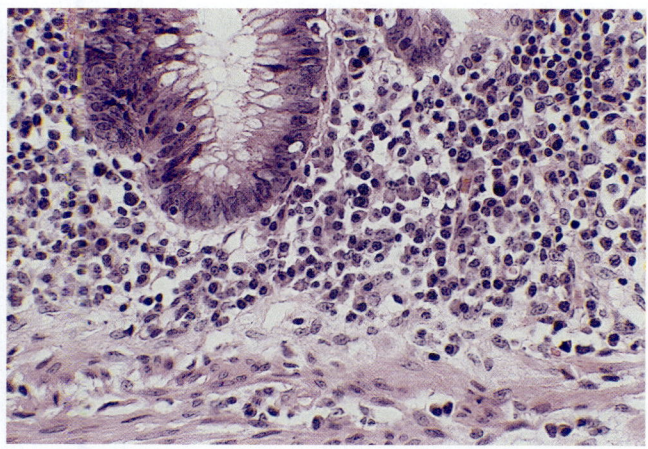

FIG. 16. *A:* Ulcerative colitis in an active phase demonstrating the "diffuse active colitis" pattern of injury. The changes are of approximately the same degree in all areas of the tissue. The luminal border is irregular. Increased inflammatory cells are present within the lamina propria. The mucosal architecture is distorted with scattered crypt abscesses. Intraepithelial mucin is diffusely depleted. *B:* Ulcerative colitis in an active phase highlighting basal plasmacytosis, a major histologic criterion that is useful in distinguishing ulcerative colitis from acute infectious-type colitis.

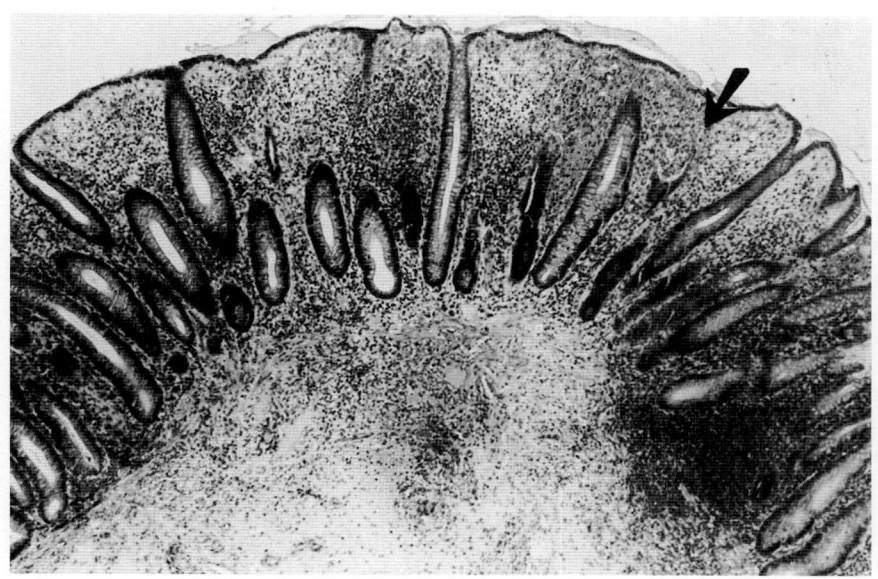

FIG. 17. Mucosal biopsy specimen from a patient with Crohn's colitis demonstrating the "focal active colitis" pattern of injury. Infiltration of chronic inflammatory cells in the lamina propria is patchy, and the inflammation involves the submucosa. Crypt abscesses (*arrow*) are found adjacent to almost normally straight colonic crypts that show preservation of the goblet-cell population.

extremely short overt clinical duration, some atrophy, branching, and budding of crypts are already apparent in many specimens (172,177,178,180). This crypt distortion, coupled with basal plasmacytosis (increased numbers of plasma cells in the lower fifth of the mucosa), has been proposed as the most useful criterion to differentiate UC from infectious colitis/acute self-limited colitis (176–179). The most a pathologist can conclude from a biopsy specimen showing this pattern is that the changes are consistent with UC in an active phase because the diffuse active colitis pattern can also be seen in some examples of Crohn's colitis (179) and in some cases of documented infectious colitis (182). The diffuse active colitis pattern can also be seen in a form of colitis associated with diverticular disease (183); this entity is distinguished from classic UC by its rectal sparing and its presence exclusively in areas of diverticula.

Focal Active Colitis

Focal active colitis refers to the patchy distribution of combined architectural change and inflammation in a mucosal biopsy specimen. Chronic colitis showing diffuse chronic changes, as described earlier, coupled with patchy acute inflammation is not considered focal active colitis. The focal active colitis pattern consists of limited areas of increased inflammatory cells associated with focal architectural distortion; characteristically, some areas of the biopsy specimen maintain an essentially normal appearance (Fig. 17). The focal active colitis pattern is usually not seen with UC, and, when present, suggests Crohn's colitis (172,184) or infectious colitis/acute self-limited colitis (172,176–179,181, 185). However, the focal active colitis pattern can be seen in resolving UC under medical treatment (181,186), and areas of previously inflamed colon and rectum in UC can return, with therapy, to an almost normal histologic appearance.

The major differential diagnostic features in biopsy specimens containing the diffuse and focal active colitis patterns are summarized in Table 3. Granulomas, typically found in CD, should be sought in all biopsy specimens, and some authors advocate serial sectioning for their detection (187) (Fig. 18). In my experience, granulomas are rarely missed; however, germinal centers, tangential cuts of blood vessels, tangential cuts of the pericryptal fibroblastic sheath, and inflammatory reactions to extravasated mucin are often misin-

TABLE 3. *Differential features in biopsy specimens demonstrating the active colitis pattern*

	Ulcerative colitis	Resolving ulcerative colitis	Crohn's disease	Infectious colitis/acute self-limited colitis
Diffuse change	Yes	Yes	Sometimes	Sometimes
Focal change	Never	Sometimes	Usually	Usually
Irregular luminal surface	Yes	Yes	Sometimes; may be focal	Sometimes; may be focal
Crypt abscesses and cryptitis	Yes	Yes; focal	Yes; focal	Yes; luminal accentuation
Mucin depletion	Diffuse	Focal	Usually focal	Usually focal
Architectural abnormality	Diffuse	Usually diffuse	Usually focal	Usually focal
Basal plasmacytosis	Yes	Yes	Usually absent	Usually absent
Neutrophils in the lamina propria	No	No	No	Usually yes
Granulomas	No	No	Yes, up to 28%	Usually no
Submucosal inflammation	Usually no	Usually no	Sometimes	Usually no

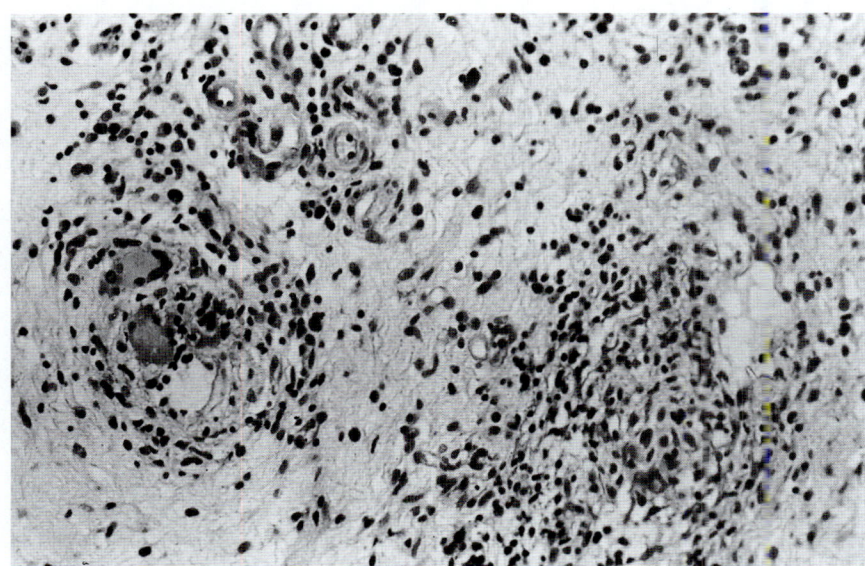

FIG. 18. Submucosal non-necrotizing granulomas in a biopsy specimen from a patient with Crohn's disease. The granulomas are often poorly formed and tend to aggregate adjacent to blood or lymphatic vessels.

terpreted as the granulomas of CD. In the absence of true granulomas, biopsy specimens from patients with CD often show the focal active colitis pattern without neutrophils in the lamina propria. However, some examples of CD may be indistinguishable from resolving UC in biopsy specimens (176,179).

A fibrinopurulent exudate in the specimen overlying, but separate from, the mucosa is always abnormal; the clinician must be informed that ulceration is likely in a more proximal location of the bowel. All inflammatory exudates should be examined under high magnification for trophozoites of *Entamoeba histolytica*, because this is their preferred hiding place.

The definitive classification of IBD rests on clinicopathologic correlation. The pathologist should convey the histologic pattern of injury to the clinician, who then collates that information with the clinical history and data obtained from endoscopic and radiologic examination. Through consideration of all this information, an accurate diagnosis can be rendered.

Infectious Colitis

Common Bacterial Agents

Colitis can be caused by a host of bacteria, including *Campylobacter* species, *Salmonella* species, *Shigella* species, *Staphylococcus aureus*, *Neisseria gonorrhoeae*, *Escherichia coli*, *Treponema pallidum*, *Yersinia* species, and *Mycobacterium* species. Although the colonic mucosal biopsy appearance in these infections can vary greatly (from essentially normal to lesions like those of idiopathic UC), a large number of specimens demonstrate the focal active pattern of injury outlined earlier that strongly suggests infectious colitis/acute self-limited colitis (171,177,178, 188–193). The definitive diagnosis of infectious colitis requires recovery of the offending organism or demonstration of a fourfold increase in specific antibody titer. In general, invasive organisms cause greater changes in morphology than those producing their effect by toxins (171).

Histologic evaluation, although helpful in suggesting an infectious etiology, can only rarely suggest a specific agent. True granulomas can be seen in tuberculosis, syphilis, *Chlamydia* species infection, and *Yersinia pseudotuberculosis* infection. Microgranulomas are described in infection with *Salmonella* species, *Campylobacter* species, and *Yersinia enterocolitica*. Isolated mucosal giant cells, although nonspecific, have been described in *Chlamydia trachomatis* infection (177,194).

There remains, even after extensive microbiologic workup, a subset of patients presumed clinically to have infectious colitis, who experience spontaneous recovery in less than 5 months, in whom biopsy specimens demonstrate focal active colitis, and in whom no infectious etiology can be identified. The term *acute self-limited colitis* has been used to describe such patients (177–179,181). I prefer the term *infectious-type colitis* because some examples of acute self-limited colitis may not be self-limited (172). Others prefer the term *nonrelapsing colitis* (179,180).

Hemorrhagic Colitis Syndrome

The clinical syndrome of hemorrhagic colitis is characterized by abdominal cramping, bloody diarrhea, and no or low-grade fever (195,196). Patients typically demonstrate right-sided colonic edema, erosions, and hemorrhage (195–197). Investigations of epidemic outbreaks have confirmed the association between hemorrhagic colitis and enterohemorrhagic *E. coli*, the most important of which is *E. coli* O157:H7 (195–202).

Symptoms in patients with hemorrhagic colitis characteristically present several days after ingestion of contaminated food, usually undercooked hamburger. In almost all patients, the disease resolves spontaneously, but severe cases can be complicated by the hemolytic uremic syndrome (HUS) and thrombotic thrombocytopenic purpura (200,202–204). In some geographic areas, the majority of HUS cases can be linked to *E. coli* O157:H7 (205–208).

Most investigators have reported hemorrhage and edema within the lamina propria as major histologic findings (195,209). Most patients also demonstrate focal necrosis of the superficial mucosa, associated with hemorrhage and acute inflammation, and preservation of the deep portion of the colonic crypts, an appearance similar to the pattern of injury described with acute ischemic colitis. Some specimens have shown the focal active colitis pattern of injury (see Focal Active Colitis). Specimens from patients with hemorrhagic colitis may also demonstrate inflammatory pseudomembranes similar to those seen in *Clostridium difficile*-associated colitis (195,210). Because routine stool culture media do not distinguish *E. coli* O157:H7 from other strains of *E. coli* normally present in the stool, physicians suspecting hemorrhagic colitis caused by enterohemorrhagic *E. coli* should specifically request that stools be screened for these organisms.

Because options for treating enterohemorrhagic *E. coli* disease are limited, emphasis must be placed on public health and prevention. Enterohemorrhagic *E. coli* infection is reportable to state health departments in most of the United States. Rapid identification of outbreaks is important because it can reduce morbidity and mortality by allowing for recall of tainted foods, closing of contaminated swimming pools, and initiation of educational programs to reduce person to person spread (211).

Antibiotic-Associated Colitis and Pseudomembranous Colitis

Toxin-producing *C. difficile* may cause some antibiotic-associated diarrheas but is more strongly associated with pseudomembranous colitis. Administration of any antibiotic that favors the growth of *C. difficile* can lead to pseudomembranous colitis. Usually, symptoms develop during therapy but occasionally they are delayed (212–215). Characteristic lesions only occur early in the disease. Grossly, the surface of the mucosa contains focal plaquelike cream to yellow pseudomembranes (216); some early lesions resemble aphthoid ulcers of CD (217). Histologically, there is patchy necrosis of the superficial portions of the colonic crypts, not unlike that seen in ischemia. The affected crypts become dilated, and an inflammatory pseudomembrane exudes from the superficial aspects of the degenerating crypt in an eruptive or mushroom-like configuration (Fig. 19). This pseudomembrane extends laterally to overlie adjacent virtually normal colonic mucosa. The karyorrhectic debris and neutrophils within the pseudomembrane often align in a curious linear configuration within the mucin. Very early lesions (as well as the mucosa between diagnostic lesions) can, on occasion, show the focal active colitis pattern of inflammation

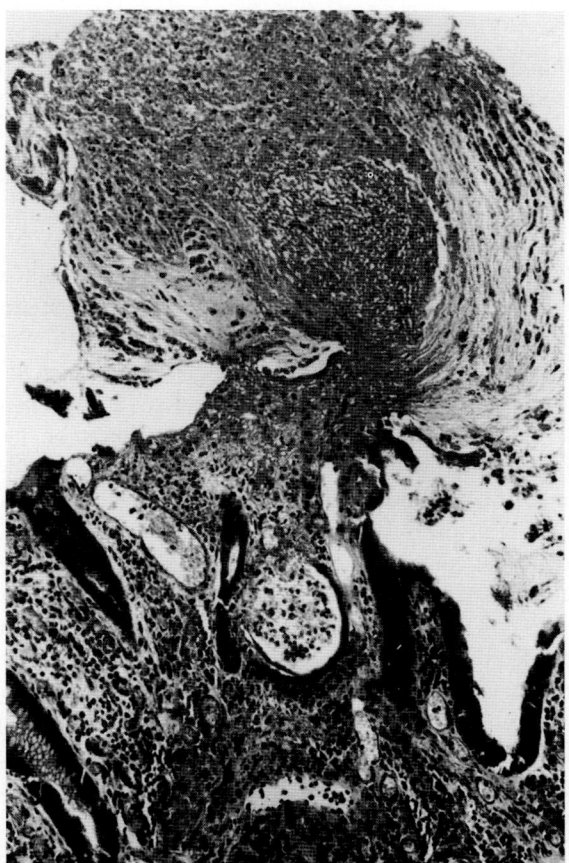

FIG. 19. Pseudomembranous colitis. An inflammatory pseudomembrane exudes from the dilated degenerating crypt in an eruptive fashion. The karyorrhectic debris and neutrophils within the pseudomembrane tend to align in a linear configuration within the mucin.

associated with infectious colitis/acute self-limited colitis (216). With progression of disease, the plaques become confluent and the crypt necrosis becomes complete. At this point, pseudomembranous colitis becomes indistinguishable from ischemic colitis. Toxic megacolon and perforation can occur (212).

Spontaneous recovery has been reported, but most patients are given vancomycin or metronidazole. *C. difficile* has been linked to exacerbations of IBD (218,219). These patients have not shown the characteristic gross features of pseudomembranous colitis, and cases examined histologically have revealed only the features of the underlying primary IBD (171).

Viral Agents

Norwalk agent and rotavirus, common causes of viral gastroenteritis, are not known to cause morphologic changes in the colon (171). Cytomegalovirus (CMV) and herpes simplex virus (HSV) may cause proctitis and colitis; they are described in more detail in Interpretation of Endoscopic Biopsy Specimens from Patients with the Acquired Immunodeficiency Syndrome.

Other Infectious Agents

Fungi, parasites, and *Mycobacterium* species are discussed elsewhere in this chapter.

Specific Forms of Colitis

Collagenous Colitis and Lymphocytic Colitis

Collagenous colitis is a distinct clinicopathologic syndrome consisting of watery diarrhea occurring predominantly in middle-aged or older (mean age, 59 years) women (male:female ratio = 1:7.5) (220,221). Colonoscopic and barium enema examinations in these patients are usually normal. Therefore, diagnosis depends on recognition of characteristic changes in biopsy specimens. The primary histologic change of collagenous colitis consists of a patchy increase in thickness of the subepithelial collagenous plate (220,222). The normal colonic subepithelial collagen layer is approximately 5 μm in thickness, but in collagenous colitis it may increase to 10 μm or more (Fig. 20). The lamina propria is expanded by a mild to moderate chronic inflammatory infiltrate. Patchy injury to the surface epithelium, characterized by increased numbers of intraepithelial lymphocytes, epithelial degeneration, and sloughing, may also occur. Atrophy, mucosal architectural distortion, and acute inflammation are usually not present or are minimal (220,222,223).

Differential diagnostic considerations include nonspecific changes, primary IBD, acute colitis, mucosal prolapse syndrome (solitary rectal ulcer syndrome), ischemic bowel disease, amyloidosis, and lymphocytic ("microscopic") colitis. Features comparing and contrasting these conditions are listed in Table 4.

Read and colleagues introduced the term *microscopic colitis* to describe chronic watery diarrhea of unknown origin occurring in middle-aged (mean = 54 years) patients (224). As in collagenous colitis, the colonoscopic appearance and the barium enema are usually normal. Biopsy specimens demonstrated increased inflammatory cells in a pattern not specific for any established entity (224). Since this initial report, several additional investigators have refined the clinical, and especially the histologic, diagnostic criteria (223,225,226). The histologic changes include increased chronic inflammatory cells in the lamina propria and surface epithelium, degenerative changes of the surface epithelium, minimal architectural changes, and minimal acute inflammation (Fig. 21).

The changes of microscopic colitis resemble the surface epithelial and lamina proprial changes of collagenous colitis; indeed, changes identical to microscopic colitis may be seen in biopsy specimens from patients with collagenous colitis if areas in which the collagen plate is not thickened are sampled. Because of the lymphocyte predominance in the inflammatory infiltrate, Lazenby and colleagues proposed the term *lymphocytic colitis* to describe this entity (223). They noted that the term *microscopic colitis* could be confused with other diseases that may have a normal gross appearance but histologic abnormalities (e.g., CD and acute self-limited colitis). *Lymphocytic colitis,* therefore, has emerged as the preferred term for this entity.

The histologic differential diagnosis of lymphocytic colitis includes changes caused by enema (bowel preparation), the mucosal M-cell zone, acute colitis, primary IBD, and collagenous colitis. Features comparing and contrasting these various conditions are included in Table 4.

The similarities between lymphocytic colitis and collagenous colitis are dramatic. They share a common symptomatology and endoscopic findings. The histologic similarities include increased intraepithelial lymphocytes, surface epithelial damage, and increased chronic inflammatory cells within the lamina propria (222,223,227). Both collagenous and lymphocytic colitis may be associated with autoimmune phenomena such as thyroid disease, rheumatoid arthritis, myasthenia gravis, and celiac sprue (228,229). Progression of lymphocytic colitis to collagenous colitis has been de-

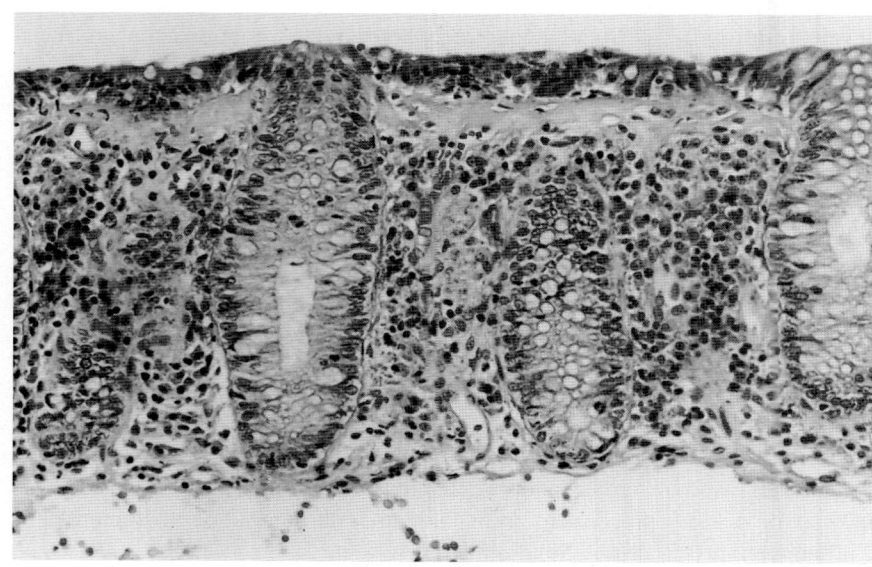

FIG. 20. Collagenous colitis. The markedly thickened subepithelial collagen layer is accompanied by an increased number of chronic inflammatory cells in the lamina propria and within the surface epithelium. The surface epithelial degenerative changes are accompanied by epithelial lymphocytosis.

TABLE 4. *Collagenous and lymphocytic colitis; differential diagnosis*

	Lymphocytic colitis	Collagenous colitis	IBD	Acute colitis	SRUS	Ischemia	Amyloid	Enema	M-cell zone
Intraepithelial lymphocytes	+++	+++	0	0	0	0	0	0	+++[a]
Lamina propria chronic inflammation	++	++	+++	±	0	±	0	0	+++[a]
Surface PMNs	0	0	+	+	0	+	0	±	0
Apoptosis	0	0	+	+	0	+	0	+[b]	0
Lamina propria PMNs	±	±	0	++	0	+	0	0	0
Cryptitis/crypt abscesses	±	±	+++	++	0	+	0	0	0
Surface epithelial degeneration	++	+++	0	++	±	++	0	±	0
Mucosal architectural distortion	±	±	+++	±	++	++	+	0	+
Collagen deposits	0	Yes[c]	0	0	Yes[d]	Yes[d]	0	0	0
Positive amyloid stain	0	0	±	0	0	0	+++	0	0

[a] Over lymphoid aggregate only.
[b] Surface only.
[c] Subepithelial.
[d] Throughout lamina propria.
IBD, primary inflammatory bowel disease; SRUS, solitary rectal ulcer syndrome; PMN, neutrophil.

scribed (223). Although there is still some controversy about the subject, it appears likely that lymphocytic colitis and collagenous colitis are either the same or very similar entities, perhaps representing different morphologic phases of one disease state (223,227,228).

Spontaneous resolutions of collagenous colitis and lymphocytic colitis have occurred, thus rendering evaluation of therapeutic regimens difficult (230). A minority of patients with these colitides has been seen with relatively minor diarrhea, and medical control has been achieved with dietary restriction, bulking agents, and antimotility drugs (230,231). This type of "symptomatic" therapy has failed, however, in the vast majority of patients, thus necessitating the addition of anti-inflammatory agents. Approximately 80% to 90% of patients eventually respond to therapy with sulfasalazine and corticosteroids (227,231,232). Treatment of the often-associated thyroid problems can also improve bowel function. There are also case reports of improvement after treatment with Pepto-bismol, mepacrine hydrochloride, steroid enemas, metronidazole, and 5-aminosalicylate (227,230,231).

Although nonsteroidal anti-inflammatory drugs have been reportedly linked to some occurrences of collagenous colitis (233), and lymphocytic colitis has been reported in patients receiving the drugs Cyclo 3 Fort (234) and ranitidine (235), the bulk of evidence suggests that lymphocytic colitis and collagenous colitis share a common immune-mediated etiology and pathogenesis. Both conditions have a striking histologic similarity to celiac sprue, a condition known to be autoimmune, possibly having a viral or infectious trigger (223). In addition, both lymphocytic and collagenous colitis have been linked to other conditions thought to have an autoimmune pathogenesis such as hypothyroidism, hyperthyroidism, inflammatory arthropathies, pernicious anemia, small bowel villous atrophy, iritis, and myasthenia gravis. Finally, both conditions respond dramatically to anti-inflammatory agents (230,231). Recently, a lymphocytic colitis-

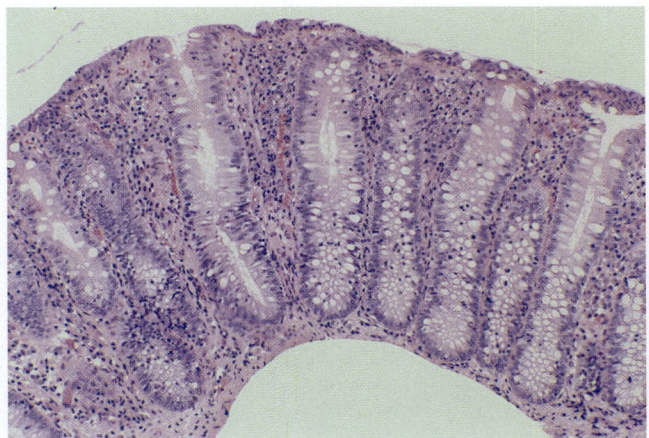
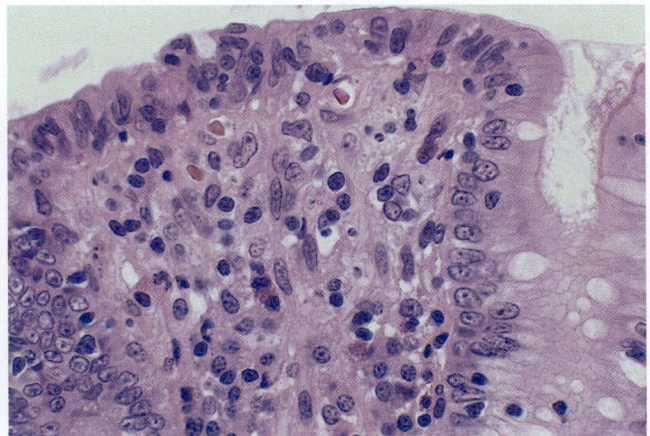

FIG. 21. Lymphocytic colitis. **A:** Chronic inflammatory cells are increased within the lamina propria and are not associated with architectural distortion. **B:** Higher magnification reveals a striking epithelial lymphocytosis.

like histology was reported in an epidemic outbreak of Brainerd diarrhea linked to a water tank aboard a cruise ship, supporting the idea of an infectious trigger for some cases of lymphocytic colitis.

Brainerd Diarrhea

The term *Brainerd diarrhea* has been applied to outbreaks of diarrhea of unknown etiology characterized by acute onset and prolonged duration (236). The clinical and epidemiologic characteristics of these outbreaks were typical for a point-source epidemic infectious diarrhea. However, unlike typical infectious diarrhea, a chronic watery diarrhea syndrome developed with symptoms lasting longer than 6 months and often lasting for years.

In general, the small bowel biopsy specimens are histologically normal in Brainerd diarrhea. Colonic biopsy specimens reveal surface epithelial lymphocytosis without distortion of mucosal architecture, surface degenerative changes, or a thickened subepithelial collagen plate. The degree of surface epithelial lymphocytosis is similar to that seen in collagenous colitis and lymphocytic colitis (236).

Patients with the clinical syndrome of chronic watery diarrhea of unknown etiology and patients reported as having lymphocytic colitis represent a heterogeneous group that may contain persons with unrecognized Brainerd diarrhea. With longer term follow-up, the Brainerd diarrhea cases appear to be self-limited, with patients recovering in 3 years or less. Surface epithelial lymphocyte counts should be performed on all colonic biopsy specimens from patients with chronic diarrhea, especially chronic watery diarrhea. Somewhat lower lymphocyte counts and a lesser degree of surface degeneration may distinguish Brainerd diarrhea from other types of lymphocytic colitis, but more study is required. Currently, Brainerd diarrhea cannot be recognized outside the setting of an epidemic.

Eosinophilic Colitis/Proctitis

Infiltration of the large intestine by large numbers of eosinophils correlates with a variety of clinical syndromes. One variant is probably an extension of the eosinophilic gastroenteritis discussed earlier. Peripheral eosinophilia is marked, and a history of atopy is common (237–240). A second type, termed *allergic proctitis,* is, in my opinion, a form of UC (241). Whenever large numbers of eosinophils are encountered in colonic biopsy specimens, this should prompt a thorough search for parasites, especially *Strongyloides* species.

The most common type of primary colorectal eosinophilic infiltrate is confined to the mucosa and occurs in infants and young children as a result of dietary-related (protein) allergy (allergic proctitis/colitis) (242,243). These children typically have rectal bleeding with or without diarrhea, and many show peripheral blood eosinophilia. Colonic biopsy specimens may show increased numbers of eosinophils within the lamina propria, often accompanied by a mild focal active colitis. Precise biopsy classification may be difficult. In general, however, more than 60 eosinophils per ten high-magnification fields and eosinophils in the muscularis mucosae or as the predominant cell in crypt abscesses are features suggestive of an allergic etiology (243).

Graft-Versus-Host Disease

Allogenic bone marrow transplantation, which has been used effectively for treatment of hematologic malignancies, aplastic anemia, various immunodeficiency states, and genetic disorders, can be complicated by GVHD (244–247). GVHD can occur in an acute or chronic form. The changes of acute GVHD in mucosal biopsy specimens have been described (Fig. 22), and a grading system proposed (244,248), which is summarized in Table 5. Biopsy specimens should be carefully examined for the presence of CMV inclusions, because CMV infection may cause changes that mimic acute GVHD. Also, both conditions may coexist.

A change similar to that seen in grade I GVHD is encountered in chemotherapy and irradiation damage. Because patients receiving bone marrow transplantation for malignant conditions are prepared with chemotherapy and irradiation, distinction of effects of therapy from GVHD may be impossible. However, changes of chemotherapy or irradiation resolve in 7 to 20 days (4,171,246,248); therefore, with knowledge of the clinical setting, an accurate diagnosis is possible. Lesions identical with grade I GVHD have been seen in patients with severe immunodeficiencies and T-cell defects (85,249–252) as well as in patients with acquired immunodeficiency syndrome (AIDS), in whom it may represent a primary AIDS-related enterocolitis (253). Grade IV GVHD cannot be distinguished from typhlitis or ischemic bowel disease without knowledge of the clinical picture.

Chronic GVHD usually spares the small bowel and colon; however, rare cases of presumed chronic GVHD involving

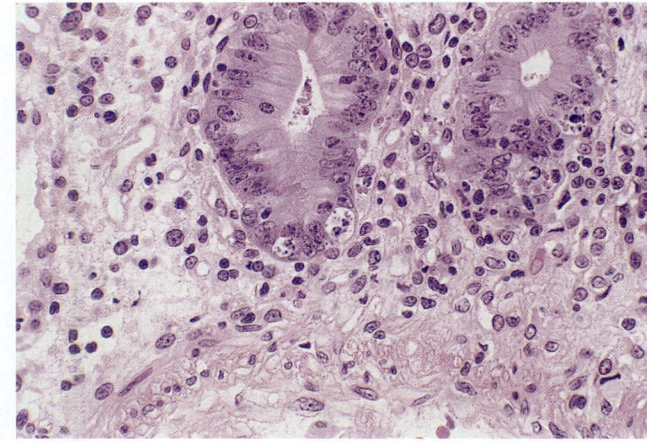

FIG. 22. Acute graft-versus-host disease. Numerous apoptotic bodies (eosinophilic globules and nuclear debris) are present.

TABLE 5. *Grading system for acute graft-versus-host disease*

Grade	Histologic features
I	Apoptosis (single-cell necrosis characterized by formation of apoptotic body, a collection of eosinophilic globules and nuclear debris)
II	Apoptosis accompanied by crypt abscesses
III	Total necrosis of individual crypts
IV	Total denudation of areas of bowel

Modified from ref. 244.

these organs have been described. The pathologic changes have included colonic submucosal fibrosis, mucosal calcification, and focal fibrosis of the lamina propria (244,246). Chronic colitis-type changes can be seen in a subset of patients with GVHD; however, the relationship between this histologic alteration and the clinical diagnosis of chronic GVHD requires more study (254).

Acute Ischemic Colitis

Ischemic bowel disease can closely mimic IBD, especially CD, because the bowel involvement is typically patchy, ulcers may be discrete or serpiginous, and healing ischemic damage may form strictures. This section deals with changes of early ischemic bowel disease in biopsy specimens. Ischemic bowel disease is discussed in more detail in a later section.

Acute ischemic damage may be focal or diffuse. The characteristic pattern of injury consists of hemorrhage into the lamina propria associated with superficial epithelial necrosis, usually sparing the deep portion of the colonic crypt (255). This may be associated with an inflammatory pseudomembrane (Fig. 23); however, associated inflammatory changes are typically mild. Depending on the duration of ischemia, these early changes may progress to full-thickness mucosal ulceration, at which point the histology becomes nonspecific (170). Although infection with enterohemorrhagic *E. coli* such as *E. coli* O157:H7 can produce the injury pattern of acute self-limited colitis, in my experience, many cases look identical with early ischemic colitis (195). Clusters of "ischemic colitis" cases, especially if they occur in younger patients and are associated with a right-sided colonic distribution, should be investigated for the presence of these bacteria.

Lesions that Mimic Inflammatory Bowel Disease

Colorectal Mucosal Prolapse Syndromes

The solitary rectal ulcer syndrome, localized colitis cystica profunda, prolapsing mucosal fold in diverticular disease, and inflammatory cloacogenic polyp are closely allied conditions that have been linked to mucosal prolapse (256–264). Affected patients often demonstrate abnormal function of the anal and pelvic floor musculature during defecation that leads to rectal mucosal prolapse or even intussusception (257,265,266). The resulting trauma is thought to cause the clinical symptoms and the pathologic changes. The term *solitary rectal ulcer syndrome* is a misnomer because the ulcers are often multiple, there is a preulcer polypoid phase, and similar lesions can also occur in the anal canal and sigmoid colon (256,258,264). Furthermore, colitis cystica profunda and inflammatory cloacogenic polyp are also misnomers. Because these conditions share a common histologic appearance, clinical presentation, clinical course, and pathogenesis, I prefer to consider them together under the heading *mucosal prolapse syndromes*.

Symptoms usually present in the third and fourth decades of life, with constipation and other difficulties in defecation (256,267). Rectal bleeding occurs commonly (256,267). The ulcer, when present, typically occurs on the anterior or anterolateral wall of the rectum, is irregular in shape, and often

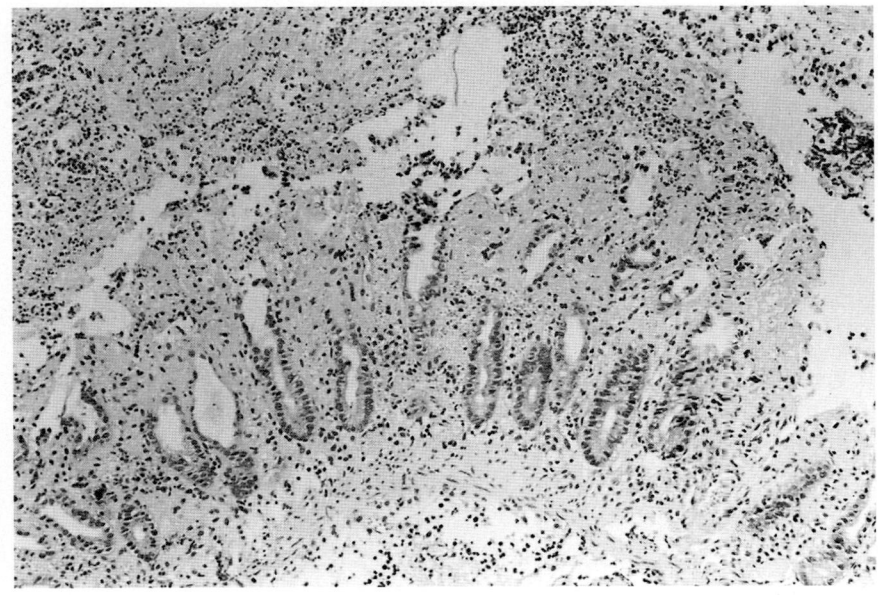

FIG. 23. Acute ischemic colitis. There is necrosis of the superficial epithelium associated with hemorrhage into the lamina propria. The base of the colonic crypts tends to be preserved.

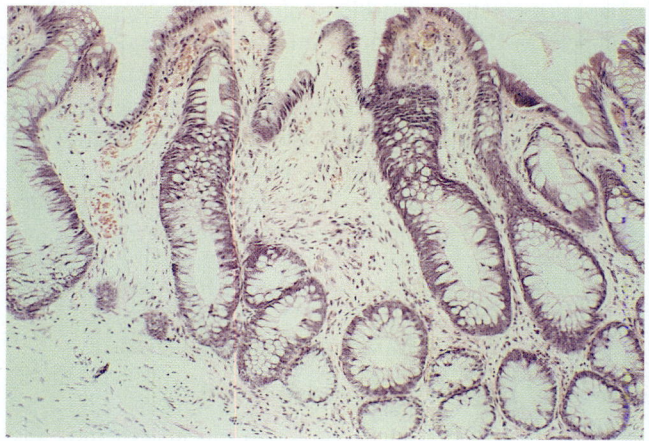

FIG. 24. Biopsy specimen of the mucosa adjacent to an ulcer from a patient with solitary rectal ulcer syndrome. The normal lamina propria has been replaced by fibrosis and smooth muscle. Mucosal capillaries are ectatic.

appears well demarcated. In patients without ulceration, the mucosa may be rough, red, and polypoid. Inflammatory cloacogenic polyp involves the lower rectum and anal transition zone (259,260). The clinical impression in patients with mucosal prolapse syndromes is often incorrect and includes ulcer, CD, nonspecific proctitis, carcinoma, or villous adenoma (268).

The characteristic histopathologic changes, found in the mucosa adjacent to ulcers or in the polypoid areas, consist of fibromuscular obliteration of the lamina propria associated with mucosal architectural distortion (Fig. 24), often with a hyperplastic or villiform appearance (257,258,261,263,268). Inflammation is typically mild or absent, and mucosal capillaries may be ectatic. Superficial erosions occur and can be associated with acute inflammation and the formation of inflammatory "pseudomembranes." On occasion, colonic glands may be misplaced into muscularis mucosae or submucosa, a histology often referred to as localized colitis cystica profunda. Submucosal blood vessels may also be ectatic and hyalinized. The histology of specimens obtained from ulcerated areas is usually nonspecific, consisting of fibrinopurulent debris and granulation tissue (268).

Differential diagnostic considerations include mucinous carcinoma, chronic UC, Cowden's disease, and ulcers resulting from ergotamine suppositories. The misplaced glands of mucosal prolapse syndrome (colitis cystica profunda) may be associated with dissecting mucous pools and can be easily mistaken for invasive mucinous adenocarcinoma (269–271). Table 6 lists histologic features that aid in this distinction.

The mucosal abnormalities of mucosal prolapse syndromes also mimic chronic UC. Knowledge of the clinical picture and recognition of the characteristic fibromuscular obliteration of the lamina propria aid in this distinction. The histologic appearance of colorectal polyps from patients with Cowden's disease (multiple hamartoma syndrome) is identical to that of the mucosal prolapse syndrome (272). Mucosal prolapse syndrome and Cowden's disease must be separated on clinical grounds. Rectal ulcers associated with the use of ergotamine suppositories may be grossly and microscopically identical to mucosal prolapse syndrome (273).

INTERPRETATION OF ENDOSCOPIC BIOPSY SPECIMENS FROM PATIENTS WITH THE ACQUIRED IMMUNODEFICIENCY SYNDROME

Interpretation of intestinal biopsy specimens from patients with AIDS is one of the premier challenges in surgical pathology. These patients are afflicted by a virtual smorgasbord of traumatic, infectious, and neoplastic conditions, and many of these lesions are subtle and easily missed unless specifically and systematically sought. Furthermore, multiple lesions characteristically coexist in the same biopsy specimen.

Traumatic lesions in AIDS are usually recognized by the clinician and biopsy is not performed. The neoplastic diseases associated with AIDS, such as anal and perianal squamous carcinoma and malignant lymphoma, are covered in more detail elsewhere in this text. This section concentrates specifically on the infectious and inflammatory-like processes affecting the small bowel and colon in AIDS patients.

TABLE 6. Differential features between dissecting mucus of mucosal prolapse syndrome (colitis cystica profunda) and invasive mucinous adenocarcinoma

Feature	Mucosal prolapse syndrome (colitis cystica profunda)	Invasive mucinous adenocarcinoma
Shape of mucous pools	Rounded	Irregular, infiltrating
Location of epithelium	Periphery of pool	Floating in pool
Configuration of epithelium	Single, often discontinuous, layer; basal polarity of nuclei	Cellular piling up, complex glandular proliferation, gland in gland configuration
Cytologic features	No dysplasia	Atypia sometimes pronounced
Tumor desmoplasia	Absent	Usually present
Hemorrhage and hemosiderin deposits	Sometimes present	Usually absent
Supporting lamina propria	Sometimes present	Absent

Modified from refs. 269–271.

Common Infectious Agents

Bacterial Infection

Infection with the usual bacterial intestinal pathogens is common in the homosexual community and in patients with AIDS (194,274–276). The diagnosis is made by identification of the organism in stool culture. Biopsy specimens often illustrate the spectrum of changes associated with infectious colitis/acute self-limited colitis as discussed earlier (194).

Parasitic Infestations

G. lamblia infects about one third of homosexual men in the urban community and can be seen in patients with AIDS (276–278). *E. histolytica* shows an increased prevalence in the homosexual community and in AIDS patients. It often represents a nonpathogenic commensal in homosexual men; in patients with AIDS, it can rarely cause fulminant colitis (275,276,279). The pathologic changes noted with each parasite are similar to those seen in the non-AIDS patient.

Viral Infections

CMV infection is extraordinarily common in AIDS patients and is often present in biopsy specimens (276,280). CMV inclusions are usually encountered in endothelial cells, fibroblasts, and smooth-muscle cells and are only rarely seen in epithelial cells. CMV inclusions in the gut usually reflect disseminated CMV infection; the precise role of CMV in the pathogenesis of intestinal disease is unknown and difficult to assess (280,281). However, marked endothelial CMV infection with "vasculitis" and luminal thrombosis is the probable cause of severe necrotizing gut injury and perforation, typically in the ileocecal area.

HSV is associated with painful discrete ulcers, vesicles, or pustular lesions in the distal rectum or perianal skin (276,282,283). It is easily cultured. The inflammatory pattern in the rectum shows (a) ulceration with neutrophils within the lamina propria, (b) cryptitis, and (c) crypt abscess formation. In my experience, HSV inclusions are not seen in the colon but are found in the anal transition zone epithelium or perianal skin.

Adenovirus-associated colitis has also been described in patients with AIDS (276). The mucosa shows moderate architectural changes and chronic inflammation. Infected colonic epithelial cells can be seen at the surface and have the appearance of dystrophic goblet cells with a crescent- or sickle-shaped amphophilic nucleus that occasionally contains inclusion bodies (284). Adenovirus can be verified by immunohistochemistry or electron microscopy.

Fungal Infections

Although oral and esophageal candidiasis is common in AIDS (276,285–287), it is unusual to see this organism in biopsy specimens from the small intestine or colon unless disseminated candidiasis has occurred.

Unusual Infectious Agents Commonly Found in AIDS Patients

Bacterial Infections

Although intestinal spirochetosis is common in patients with AIDS (288,289), its significance as a cause of colitis and appendicitis is controversial (288,290–292). The microscopic appearance is subtle—a thickening or accentuation of the colonic brush border, deeply stained with hematoxylin, caused by the spirochetes aligned in parallel, embedding themselves into the luminal border of the absorptive cells (Fig. 25). They apparently do not attach to goblet cells. Identification of intestinal spirochetosis can be enhanced by use of the Warthin-Starry or Dieterle stain, or by electron microscopy.

Gastrointestinal tract involvement by MAIC is usually part of disseminated infection (293,294). The organism is

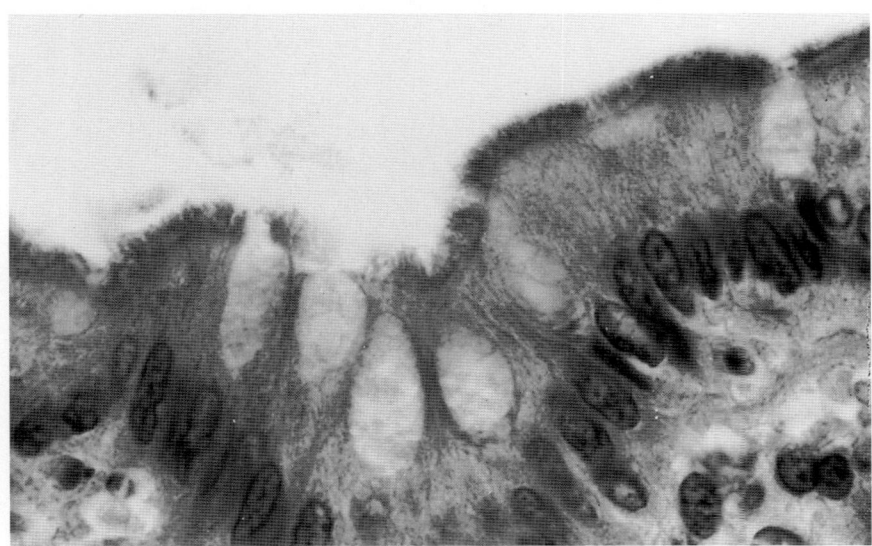

FIG. 25. Intestinal spirochetosis from a patient with acquired immunodeficiency syndrome. The spirochetes appear as a thickening or accentuation of the colonic brush border that stains deeply with hematoxylin. The organism appears not to attach to goblet cells.

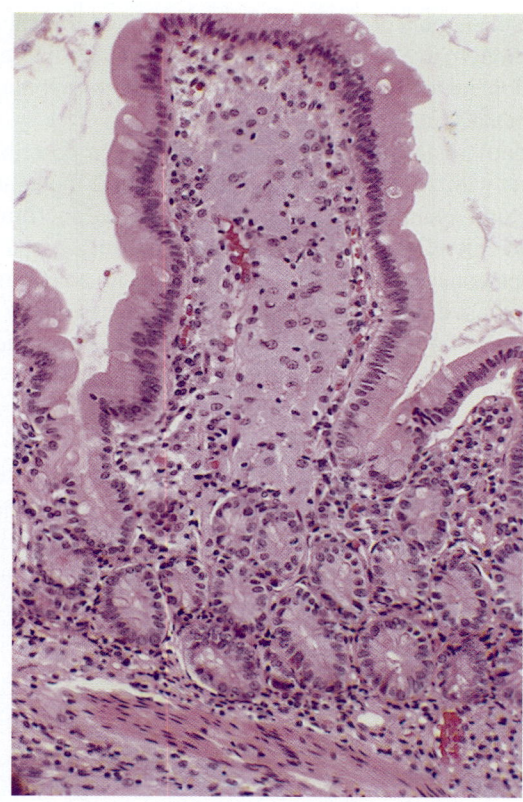

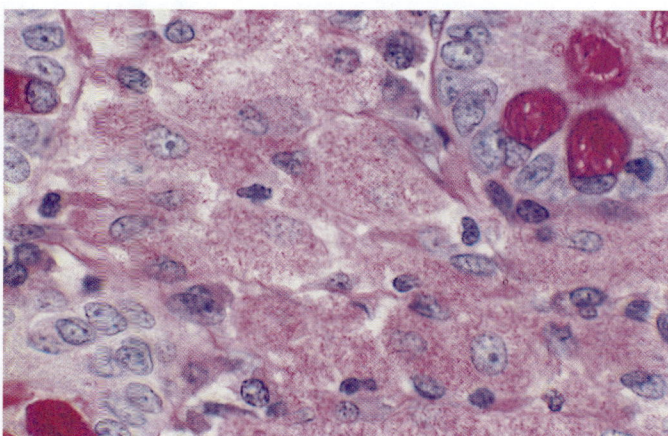

FIG. 26. A: Typical appearance of *Mycobacterium avium-intracellulare* complex (MAIC) infection in a colonic biopsy specimen. The lamina propria is infiltrated by foamy macrophages, and the appearance closely mimics Whipple's disease (see Fig. 8). In contrast to Whipple's disease, the "fat vacuoles" are absent. **B:** The periodic acid-Schiff (PAS) stain in MAIC reveals faintly positive bacillary forms, in contrast to the coarsely granular, intensely PAS-positive inclusions of Whipple's disease (see Fig. 9).

readily cultured from stool and even from blood. MAIC may affect any part of the gastrointestinal tract. The characteristic histology is infiltration of the lamina propria by foamy macrophages that can closely mimic Whipple's disease (95,96,293,295) (Fig. 26A). In addition, MAIC is also PAS-positive, further adding to the possibility of a misdiagnosis. MAIC is easily distinguished from Whipple's disease in that MAIC is characteristically patchy, the fat vacuoles of Whipple's disease are absent, the PAS stain shows faintly staining bacillary forms (Fig. 26B), and the acid-fast stain is positive. The infiltrative macrophages may be subtle, and it is recommended that an acid-fast stain be done on all mucosal biopsy specimens from AIDS patients.

Diarrheogenic bacterial enterocolitis has been described in AIDS patients (296). Colonic biopsy specimens demonstrate surface epithelial inflammation and degeneration associated with gram-negative bacteria adherent to the surface colonocytes (Fig. 27). The histology resembles that seen in enteropathogenic *E. coli* infection (297).

Parasitic Infestations

Although cases of cryptosporidiosis have been reported in immunocompetent humans in whom the disease runs a self-limited clinical course (131,276,298–302), *Cryptosporidium parvum* infection in patients with AIDS and other immunodeficiencies causes severe, explosive, watery diarrhea that is resistant to most forms of therapy (131,276,300,303–305). The organism usually infects the small intestine, where it is associated with a variable villus abnormality (306), and, rarely, infiltration of the mucosa by eosinophils (298). *C. parvum* can occasionally be seen in the colon, stomach, bile ducts, pancreatic ducts, and gallbladder (307). The diagnosis is readily made by identifying the acid-fast infective oocyst in stool specimens; concentration techniques such as Sheather's sugar flotation method or the zinc sulfate technique may enhance identification (131,302). In biopsy specimens, the cryptosporidia are identified as basophilic dots, measuring approximately 3 μm, attached to the luminal border of the ep-

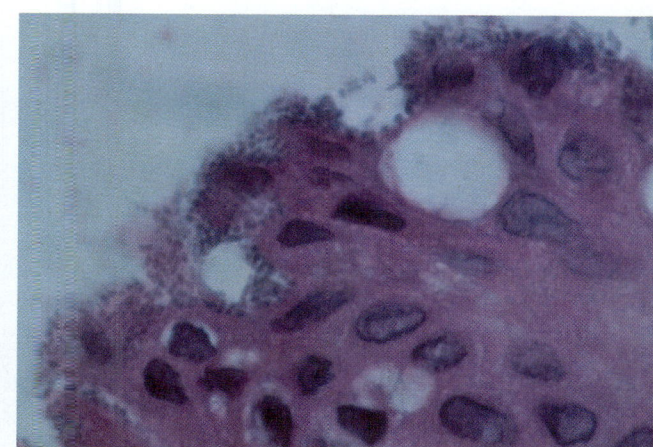

FIG. 27. Diarrheogenic bacterial colitis in acquired immunodeficiency syndrome. Note the surface epithelial changes and adherent rod-shaped bacteria. (Courtesy of Mary P. Bronner, M.D.)

ithelial cells in small bowel or deep colonic crypts (Fig. 28). Although easily seen on H&E-stained sections, Giemsa stain does enhance its appearance. The organism is not acid fast in biopsy specimens. Immunocytochemical methods for identification have also been described (308).

Infection with *Isospora belli* is usually diagnosed by identification of cysts in stool specimens (131,276,309,310). It is characteristically a small bowel pathogen that causes a variable villus abnormality. In biopsy specimens, the organism is identified by recognizing the ovoid developmental forms of the coccidia in and beneath epithelial cells (Fig. 29) (309–313). The developmental forms are small and easily missed (4,131); they can be highlighted with the Giemsa stain.

Several members of the order Microsporida may cause human infection in immunocompromised individuals or in "immune-privileged" sites such as the cornea. The two major microspordia seen in the gastrointestinal tract are *Enterocytozoon bieneusi* and *Encephalitozoon intestinalis* (formerly known as *Septata intestinalis*). They have been recognized in up to 50% of AIDS patients with chronic unexplained diarrhea (314–317). Early reports stressed the importance of electron microscopy in establishing the diagnosis (316,318); however, microsporidia can be recognized by conventional light microscopy (276,316). The organism is associated with a variable villus abnormality and, like *Isospora* species, developmental forms are found in enterocytes (Fig. 30). Mature spores measuring 1.5 μm are an inconsistent finding, stain gram-positive, and can be seen as a cluster of small dots in the apical cytoplasm of the enterocyte (316,319). The nucleated sporont is a larger (3 to 5 μm), rounded, basophilic structure often surrounded by a halo and is found in surface enterocytes near the villus tips or in degenerating cells. This form frequently causes a cup-shaped indentation of the enterocyte nucleus that can be an important clue in identification on H&E-stained sections.

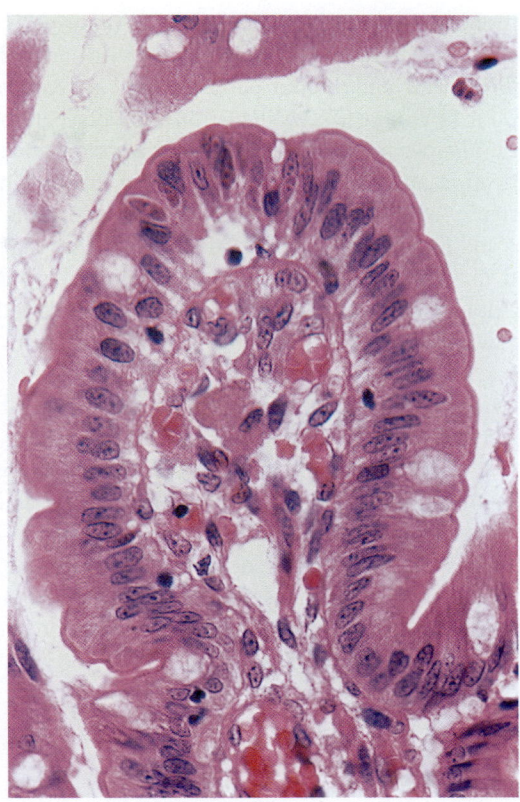

FIG. 29. *Isospora* species infection in proximal small bowel. Note the ovoid developmental forms within the enterocyte cytoplasm near the villus tip. (Courtesy of Audrey J. Lazenby, M.D.)

The diagnosis of microsporidia is usually made on the basis of stool examination using stains that chemofluoresce or by using a modified trichrome stain (320). Genus and species identification has become important because albendazole is effective against *E. intestinalis* whereas no effective specific therapy for *E. bieneusi* is currently known (321). One impor-

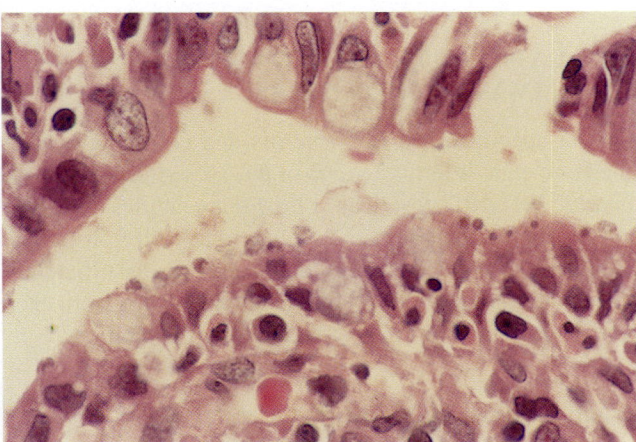

FIG. 28. Cryptosporidiosis in small bowel biopsy specimen. The organism appears as basophilic dots (measuring approximately 3 μm) that attach to the luminal border of epithelial cells.

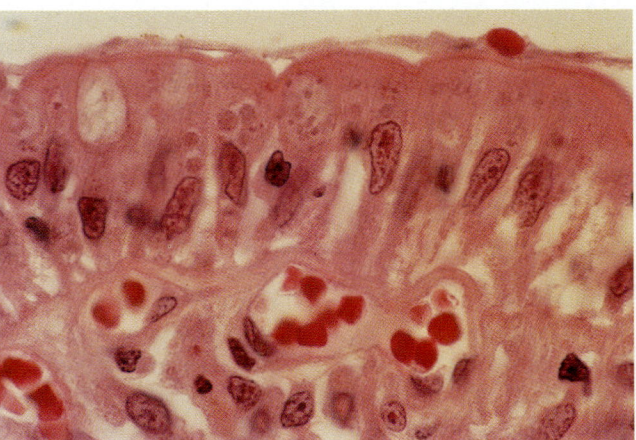

FIG. 30. *Enterocytozoon bieneusi* infection of small bowel. Mature spores appear as tiny (1.5 mm) dots, whereas the larger nucleated sporont are rounded basophilic structures often surrounded by a halo within the enterocyte cytoplasm.

tant difference between *E. bieneusi* and *E. intestinalis* is the propensity for the latter to infect lamina propria macrophages, fibroblasts, and endothelial cells, as well as enterocytes (322,323). In contrast, *E. bieneusi* infects only enterocytes. Electron microscopy is still considered the gold standard for identification and can be done on stool or mucosal biopsy specimens. Monoclonal antibodies to encephalitozoan species and *E. intestinalis* have been produced that can be exploited in immunofluorescent and enzyme-linked assays (324). Molecular diagnosis by PCR has been developed.

A newly recognized coccidia, initially referred to as cyanobacterium, has been linked to enteric infection in patients with AIDS. It has been assigned to the genus *Cyclospora* and the name *Cyclospora cayetanensis* has been proposed. Cases are usually diagnosed on stool examination by recognizing the oocysts (325) with modified acid-fast stains. The organism can be seen with difficulty in small bowel biopsy specimens and demonstrates intraenterocyte developmental forms that resemble those seen in *Isospora* species infection (326). Transmission electron microscopy is usually required for verification.

Other Lesions in AIDS

Primary AIDS-Related Enterocolitis

A common problem in AIDS patients is severe debilitating diarrhea for which no infectious agent can be found. Although it is possible that normal flora become pathogenic in AIDS, there may also be an immune-mediated enterocolitis associated with AIDS, or the human immunodeficiency virus itself infects the gut and causes the diarrhea (253,276,315,327–329). For example, a variable villus abnormality is frequently found in AIDS patients even in the absence of intestinal pathogens (276,315,328,329). Furthermore, many AIDS patients with diarrhea demonstrate apoptosis deep in colonic crypts (Fig. 31). Although apoptosis is associated with a variety of injurious agents, it is also the characteristic form of cell death associated with cell-mediated immune cytotoxicity. Indeed, the apoptosis in colonic biopsy specimens in AIDS is identical with the grade I lesion of GVHD (244) and other immunodeficiency syndromes (86,251). Apoptosis may thus reflect immune damage to colonic epithelium as the cause for the diarrhea and wasting seen in many AIDS patients.

Kaposi's Sarcoma

Kaposi's sarcoma is highly prevalent in the intestinal tract of AIDS patients (330–332), and because this type of involvement is usually a sign of a more severe immunologic impairment, gastrointestinal Kaposi's sarcoma has been linked to poor prognosis in AIDS (333). Grossly, Kaposi's sarcoma appears as red macules or nodules measuring 5.0 to 15 mm; they bleed surprisingly little after biopsy. The diagnostic yield in biopsy specimens is low and may be due to both the preferential submucosal location of Kaposi's sar-

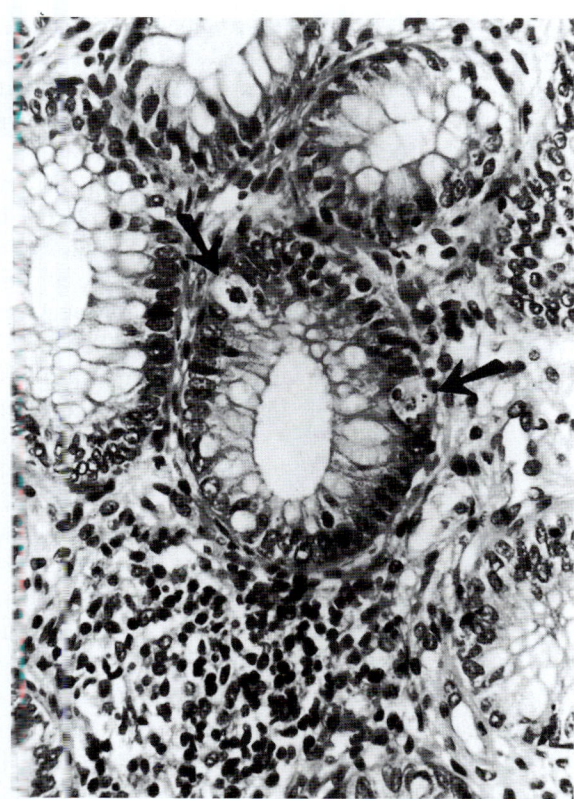

FIG. 31. Apoptotic bodies (*arrows*) deep in colonic crypts in a patient with acquired immunodeficiency syndrome. Although the significance is unknown, this change may reflect immune damage to the colonic epithelium. The changes are identical with the grade I lesion of graft-versus-host disease.

coma and the subtlety of the histologic change. In contrast to the normal delicate lamina propria with scattered inflammatory cells, Kaposi's sarcoma causes an expansion of the lamina propria by a spindle cell proliferation that may not be very atypical (Fig. 32). Recognizing slits that contain red blood cells is an important clue, as is the tendency for the neoplasm to overrun or obliterate the muscularis mucosae.

EVALUATION OF RESECTION SPECIMENS IN INFLAMMATORY BOWEL DISEASE

After specific causes of enteritis and colitis have been ruled out, what is left is a group of diseases referred to as *idiopathic IBD*. IBD describes at least three entities: CD, UC, and colitis of indeterminate type. Despite their nonspecific nature, the pathologic features of CD and UC are sufficiently distinctive that they can usually be distinguished from each other and from other kinds of bowel inflammation.

Crohn's Disease and Ulcerative Colitis

The distributional features, gross appearance, and histologic characteristics of typical cases of CD and UC have been well described (334–341). The distinguishing features of CD and UC are summarized in Tables 7 and 8. In the

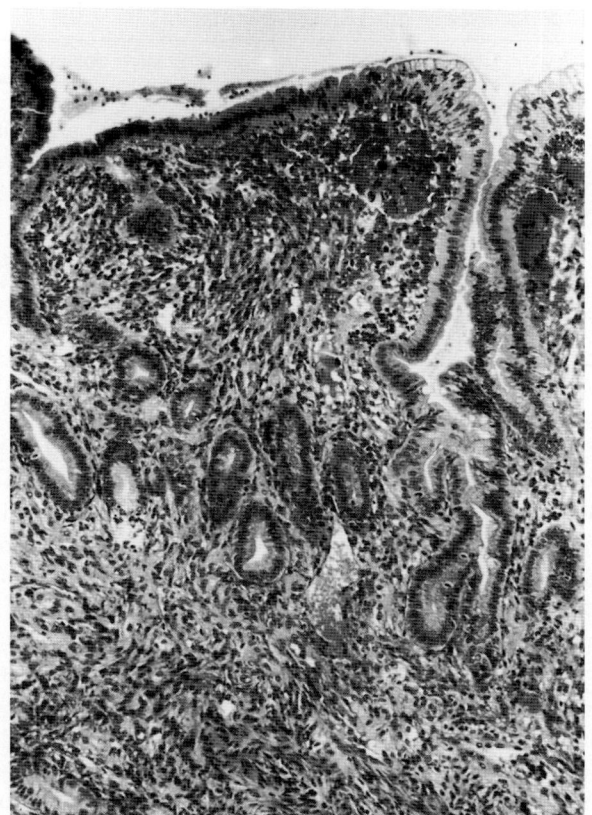

FIG. 32. Kaposi's sarcoma in a duodenal biopsy specimen. The neoplasm, composed of spindle cells, replaces and expands the lamina propria. The spindle cells overrun and obliterate the muscularis mucosae, an important clue to the proper diagnosis.

colon, rectal sparing, skip areas of involvement, and preferential right-sided localization are gross features favoring CD over UC. Discriminating microscopic features of CD include nonnecrotizing granulomas, fissuring ulcers, and transmural inflammation. The granulomas, noted in 50% to 70% of cases, are generally poorly formed, few in number, and are more often seen in Crohn's enteritis. The fissuring ulcers are lined by granulation tissue rather than neutrophils and extend into the deep submucosa, muscularis propria, or beyond.

Transmural inflammation is usually in the form of lymphoid aggregates having a propensity to localize around lymphatic vessels and small blood vessels. The inflammatory infiltrate may extend into the wall of adjacent vessels creating the so-called Crohn's "vasculitis," which, on occasion, may be a prominent feature (339). Although it is still customary to sample resection margins in CD, it is clear that microscopic abnormalities at these margins do not correlate with anastomotic recurrence (342). The principal differential diagnostic considerations in CD are ischemic bowel disease and tuberculosis. Features helpful in distinguishing among these three conditions are summarized in Table 9.

Colitis—Type Indeterminate

The term *colitis—type indeterminate* describes approximately 5% to 10% of operative specimens, almost always cases of acute or severe clinical disease requiring urgent or emergent colectomy (fulminant colitis), in which pathologic features are ambiguous and do not permit precise separation of CD from UC (174,343). In fulminant colitis, fissuring ulcers and transmural inflammation (normally major criteria of CD) may be seen in otherwise typical cases of UC. Although fulminant colitis with toxic megacolon is strongly associated with UC, many of such patients do, in fact, follow a clinical course indicative of CD (174,334,343,344). A four-tiered classification system for primary IBD in colectomy specimens is listed in Table 10 (345). The definitive diagnosis of UC requires all of the following features (345): diffuse disease limited to the large intestine, involvement of the rectum, more proximal colonic disease occurring in continuity with an involved rectum (i.e., no gross or histologic skip lesions), no deep fissural ulcers, no mural sinus tracts, and no transmural lymphoid aggregates or granulomas. The definitive diagnosis of CD requires histologic verification, with the demonstration of transmural lymphoid aggregates in areas not deeply ulcerated or the presence of nonnecrotizing granulomas (345,346). In cases in which the gross and clinical features suggest CD (e.g., skip lesions, linear ulcers, cobblestoning, fat wrapping, terminal ileal inflammation), extensive histologic sampling should be done to find definitive histologic features of CD.

TABLE 7. *Distinguishing gross features of Crohn's disease and ulcerative colitis*

Feature	Crohn's enteritis	Crohn's colitis	Ulcerative colitis
Serositis	Yes	Yes	No, except in fulminant colitis
Thick bowel wall	Yes	Yes	No, except when complicated by carcinoma
Stricture	Often	Sometimes	No, except when complicated by carcinoma
Mucosal edema	Yes	Yes	Usually no
Discrete mucosal ulcers	Yes	Yes	Usually no, except in fulminant colitis
Fat wrapping	Often present	Often present	Usually no
Fistula	Common	Sometimes	No
Distribution	Focal	Usually focal	Diffuse
Rectal involvement	No	Sometimes	Yes
Inflammatory polyps	Rare	Sometimes	Sometimes

TABLE 8. Distinguishing histologic features of Crohn's disease and ulcerative colitis

Feature	Crohn's enteritis	Crohn's colitis	Ulcerative colitis
Granulomas	Common	Sometimes	No
Fissuring ulcer	Common	Common	No, except in fulminant colitis
Transmural inflammation	Yes	Yes	No, except in fulminant colitis
Submucosal edema	Yes	Yes	Usually no
Submucosal inflammation	Yes	Yes	Usually no
Neuronal hyperplasia	Yes	Sometimes	Usually no
Thickening of muscularis mucosae	Yes, patchy	Yes, patchy	Yes, diffuse (in chronic MUC)
Pyloric gland metaplasia	Common	Rare	Rare
Mucosal inflammation and architectural distortion	Focal	Usually focal	Diffuse
Paneth-cell metaplasia	No	Sometimes	Sometimes

MUC, mucosal ulcerative colitis.

The term *indeterminate colitis* is used for cases of idiopathic colonic IBD that have ambiguous pathologic features inconclusive for a diagnosis of UC or CD (343,345–347). Indeterminate colitis can be further classified into cases that are probably UC and those that are probably CD. Indeterminate colitis, probably UC, usually shows mucosal involvement that resembles UC. However, the specimen has atypical features such as deep linear fissural ulcers associated with transmural lymphoid aggregates, skip lesions, or terminal ileal involvement. Indeterminate colitis, probably CD, often shows prominent gross or histologic skip lesions, deep linear ulcers associated with transmural lymphoid aggregates, submucosal edema with lymphoid aggregates extending deep into the submucosa, or terminal ileal involvement. However, cases in this "probably CD" category lack the definitive histologic features of CD, such as granulomas and transmural lymphoid aggregates in areas not deeply ulcerated, even after extensive sampling. Following our institutional policy, patients without clinical, endoscopic, or radiologic evidence suggestive of CD in whom the final pathology is indeterminate are, in general, considered suitable for ileal pouch-anal anastomosis (345).

Several studies have apparently concluded that indeterminate colitis clinically acts like UC. Several limitations surround these current analyses of indeterminate colitis, making such firm conclusions premature. The limitations include the retrospective nature of the studies, the undefined criteria for indeterminate colitis, and the unknown influence of patient selection. A report by Pezim and colleagues included 25 patients with a pathologic diagnosis of indeterminate colitis (348). After careful clinical evaluation, all were thought to have UC. Two patients were lost to follow-up, and, in two of the remaining 23 (9%), abdominal wall and perianal fistulas developed and the patients eventually lost their pouches (versus 4% in the UC group) within a relatively short follow-up period (38 months ± 18 months). In an update of this cohort, two additional patients had pouch failure requiring pouch removal; three other patients, including one originally lost to follow-up, are thought to have CD (349). Wells and coworkers (350) reported on 46 patients with a pathologic diagnosis of indeterminate colitis. After clinical, endoscopic, and radiologic features were taken into account, the patients were reclassified as probably CD (19 patients), probably UC (11 patients), and indeterminate colitis (16 patients). Although the patients ultimately categorized as having indeterminate colitis were clinically similar to the patients with UC, of the original 46 with the pathologic diagnosis of indeterminate colitis, 19 (41%) were reclassified clinically as having CD.

Ulcerative Proctitis

A localized form of UC with a good prognosis has been described as mucosal proctosigmoiditis, follicular proctitis, or ulcerative proctitis (351,352). The gross mucosal appearance resembles that observed in more extensive forms of UC. Mucosal biopsy specimens show typical changes of UC,

TABLE 9. Differential diagnosis of Crohn's disease

Feature	Crohn's disease	Ischemic bowel disease	Tuberculosis
Discrete ulcers	Yes	Yes	Yes
Longitudinally running ulcers	Yes	Yes	Usually no
Stricture	Yes	Yes	Yes
Lymphoid aggregates	Yes	No	Usually no
Hemorrhage and necrosis	No	Yes (acute)	No
Granulation tissue and fibrosis	No	Yes (late)	Sometimes
Hemosiderin deposition	Usually no	Often	Usually no
Preferred location	Ileum and cecum	Splenic flexure	Ileum and cecum
Granulomas	Often	No	Yes
Confluence of granulomas	No	Not applicable	Sometimes
Necrotizing granulomas	No	Not applicable	Sometimes
Fibrosis of muscularis propria	Usually no	Yes	Yes

TABLE 10. *Primary colonic inflammatory bowel disease: pathologic classification*

Ulcerative colitis
Crohn's disease
Indeterminate colitis, probably ulcerative colitis
Indeterminate colitis, probably Crohn's disease

From ref. 345.

but some may also show prominent mucosal lymphoid follicles (follicular proctitis) (Fig. 33) (334,353). Most patients respond dramatically to the local administration of corticosteroids, but approximately 10% of patients progress to pancolitis (351,352). There is some evidence to suggest that patients with prominent lymphoid follicles are less likely to respond to treatment (353).

Inflammatory Bowel Disease and Diverticular Disease

IBD and diverticular disease are both common and can occasionally coexist. UC-like mucosal inflammation associated with diverticular disease has been described (183,354). Both CD and diverticular disease may show focal mucosal inflammation, stricture, and fistula formation. Not infrequently, pathologists attribute all the changes to one disease (usually diverticular disease) and overlook the coexisting IBD (usually CD). Features suggesting CD complicating diverticular disease are the presence of fissuring ulcers, ulcers outside areas of active diverticulitis, and internal fistulas other than colovesicle or colovaginal fistula (334,355).

Lesions Associated with Surgical Procedures

Diversion Colitis/Defunctionalized Bowel

A rectum surgically placed out of circuit acquires histologic changes associated with defunctioning alone, regardless of the original reason for diversion (356–359). The changes probably reflect a physiologic response to stasis and the loss of trophic factors in the feces, most notably short-chain fatty acids (360). However, the patient is usually asymptomatic. The mucosa of the diverted segment appears erythematous, granular, and friable. Histologic changes include marked lymphoid hyperplasia with germinal center formation, usually accompanied by mild colitis with crypt abscess formation (Fig. 34). The changes may be indistinguishable from follicular proctitis (ulcerative proctitis or localized UC). With time, the muscularis mucosae hypertrophies, the submucosa shows fatty and fibrous tissue infiltration, the muscularis propria thickens, and the lumen becomes progressively smaller (345). The mucosal lymphoid hyperplasia may be accompanied by lymphoid aggregates scattered in the deep submucosa, muscular wall, and perirectal adipose tissue (361,362). Because these changes may occur in diverted segments in patients without IBD, care must be taken not to base a diagnosis of primary IBD, especially CD, solely on histologic changes seen in such specimens. In many patients, the rectum is placed out of circuit during an operation for IBD. In these instances, the rectum can show changes of both primary IBD and diversion colitis. The histologic changes in defunctioned rectums do not, in general, correlate with the original diagnosis or clinical outcome (361,362).

Ileal Reservoirs (Pouches) and Pouchitis

For patients requiring total colectomy, several surgical operations have been developed that either create continence in an ileostomy (Kock's ileostomy) or preserve anal sphincter function and restore the continuity to the bowel (ileal pouch-anal anastomosis) (363,364). These operations have in common the creation of a reservoir (pouch), which is formed by connecting loops of terminal ileum. These pouch procedures are contraindicated in patients with CD because of increased morbidity (e.g., fistula and abscess) (365,366). Furthermore,

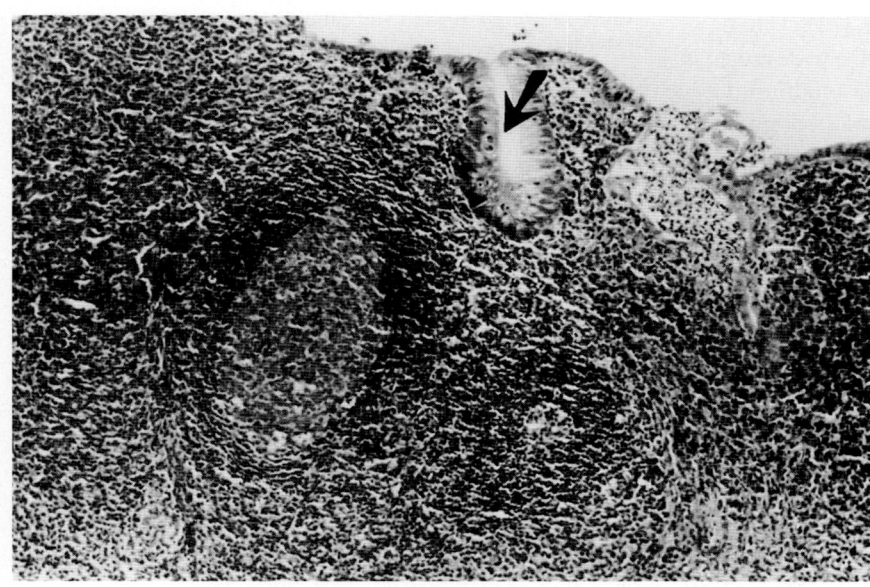

FIG. 33. Follicular proctitis demonstrating prominent lymphoid follicle formation associated with cryptitis (*arrow*) and superficial erosion.

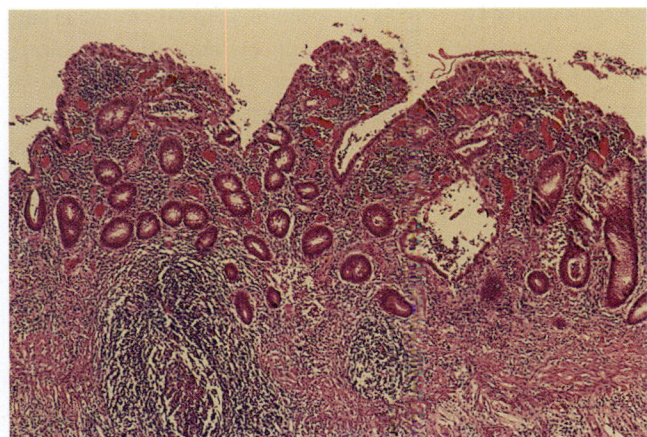

FIG. 34. Typical appearance of a mucosal biopsy specimen from a defunctionalized rectum. Lymphoid follicle formation is accompanied by cryptitis and crypt abscess formation and appears similar to follicular proctitis (see Fig. 33).

complications requiring pouch removal can result in the loss of considerable lengths of small bowel, sometimes enough to cause short-bowel syndrome. In our experience, there is nothing quite like a pouch to bring out the CD in a patient!

Pouch complications include fistula, obstruction, incontinence, and anastomotic leaks (363). Although many complications result from surgical and mechanical difficulties, and others relate to the development of primary inflammation in the pouch ("pouchitis"), some of these complicated cases likely represent pouch recurrence of initially undiagnosed CD. These cases illustrate the pathologist's inability to reliably differentiate UC from CD in severe colitis, even after examination of the colectomy specimen (367) (see Colitis—Type Indeterminate). Virtually all reports of surgical experiences with ileal pouch-anal anastomosis for presumed UC contain approximately 2% to 7% of patients in whom the actual diagnosis proved to be CD (366–371).

A late complication of pouch construction is the development of primary inflammation in the pouch with its associated clinical syndrome termed *pouchitis* (372,373). The reported incidence varies from 8% to 46%, with the wide range likely because of the lack of an accepted case definition (374). Nausea, vomiting, malaise, fever, and abdominal cramping develop. There is increased effluent and stool from the ileum that may be watery, foul smelling, or grossly bloody; patients often become incontinent. Pouch bacterial ecology is often altered, and patients usually respond to antibiotics, suggesting a bacterial etiology. However, some patients require sulfasalazine, corticosteroids, or even pouch excision for management of pouchitis (363,373–379).

Pouch biopsy may be performed to confirm the presence of inflammation or to evaluate the possibility of CD. Biopsy specimens obtained from nondysfunctional pouches may show mild villous shortening and increased chronic inflammation with increased crypt mitoses, but, in my experience, most specimens appear similar to the normal terminal ileum. A few neutrophils in surface epithelium and in the lamina propria are commonly seen (376,380). In contrast, pouches with classic pouchitis often have decreased epithelial cell mucin and decreased or absent lymphoid follicles. The most consistent findings in pouchitis have been ulcers with granulation tissue and patchy accumulations of neutrophils in the lamina propria, with cryptitis and crypt abscess formation (373,376,380–382).

Many investigators report an inconsistent relationship between endoscopic and histologic changes in the pouch and patient symptoms (368,375,383,384). Therefore, many clinicians diagnose pouchitis solely on clinical grounds and reserve endoscopic examination with biopsy for those patients with refractory pouchitis or possible CD (378,379). There are no reliable endoscopic or histologic criteria to differentiate most examples of pouchitis from new onset or recurrence of CD in the pouch.

The clinical syndrome of pouchitis probably represents at least five different conditions (345) (Table 11). There are two variants of antibiotic-responsive pouchitis: classic pouchitis and jejunal bacterial overgrowth (345,375,383). Classic pouchitis demonstrates endoscopic and histologic findings that support the pouch as the source for the clinical symptoms (345,373,374,377,378). Patients with classic pouchitis usually respond dramatically to antibiotics. Rarely, patients with the clinical symptoms of pouchitis have endoscopically and histologically negative pouches but still respond to antibiotics (373). Some of these patients have had proximal jejunal bacterial overgrowth (376,383–386), probably as a result of pouch distention, causing an "ileal brake" that decreases motility in the proximal small intestine (385,386,387). This decreased motility may predispose some individuals to bacterial overgrowth.

Pouchitis syndromes refractory to antibiotic therapy include short-strip pouchitis, CD, and primary refractory pouchitis (345) (see Table 11). To obtain a more functional pouch, many surgeons have abandoned the rectal mucosectomy in ileal pouch-anal anastomoses (388,389). In short-strip pouchitis, clinical symptoms may, in fact, be caused by exacerbation of UC in the small retained rectal segments (377,378). Many patients with this form of pouchitis respond to topical corticosteroids (378).

Although debated (390), I believe that missed CD is much more likely to present as a late pouch fistula than as refractory pouchitis. However, on rare occasions, refractory pouchitis has been seen in which pouch biopsy specimens con-

TABLE 11. *Pouchitis syndromes: proposed clinicopathologic classification*

Antibiotic-responsive pouchitis syndromes
Classic pouchitis
Proximal jejunal bacterial overgrowth
Chronic and refractory pouchitis syndromes
Short-strip pouchitis
Crohn's disease
Chronic primary refractory pouchitis

Modified from ref. 345.

tained granulomas or in which the excised pouch has shown major histologic criteria for CD (377). Invariably, the original pathology of the colectomy specimen was either missed Crohn's colitis or indeterminate colitis. I believe these cases represent CD (345,391).

Other cases of refractory pouchitis have required surgical removal of the pouch. After careful pathologic evaluation, no criteria for CD were found in either the excised pouch or in the original colectomy specimen (377). Several other similar cases have been reported (372,379). These cases may represent primary refractory pouchitis (345). The causes of classic pouchitis and primary refractory pouchitis are unknown, but are probably related to a combination of stasis, bacterial overgrowth, the abnormal immune response of patients with primary IBD, and colonic-type metaplasia occurring in some pouches (345,374,375,392).

With long-term follow-up and surveillance, it appears that dysplasia in the pouch can occasionally develop in patients with ileal pouch-anal anastomosis. This complication seems to be limited to a subgroup (<10%) of patients in whom refractory pouchitis and colonic-type metaplasia develop (393–395).

Ileostomies and Colostomies

Specimens from ileostomy or colostomy revisions show changes associated with trauma and mucosal prolapse, such as superficial erosions, hemorrhages, acute and chronic inflammation, and fibromuscular obliteration of the lamina propria. Rarely, an ulcerative process of the ileum called *postcolectomy ileitis* or *prestomal ileitis* may develop (396,397). Patients have profuse watery ileostomy drainage, pyrexia, tachycardia, and anemia; perforation of the ileostomy can occur. Resection specimens contain superficial and deep ulcers of nonspecific nature; the cases I have reviewed resemble ischemic damage.

INFLAMMATORY BOWEL DISEASE, DYSPLASIA, AND CARCINOMA

Ulcerative Colitis and Carcinoma

Patients with long-standing UC are at increased risk for colorectal adenocarcinoma (175,398). Because colitis-associated carcinomas are often flat, infiltrative, and difficult to visualize by standard radiographic techniques, most gastroenterologists recommend regular surveillance for cancer or dysplasia, using total colonoscopy with biopsy, in patients with long-standing extensive colitis (399–401).

Dysplasia, the presumed precancerous epithelial lesion, has been regularly recognized in colons both adjacent to and distant from colitis-associated carcinomas. Circumstantial evidence suggests that dysplasia may not only be a marker for carcinoma but may itself progress to invasive carcinoma (175).

Dysplastic epithelium can occur in a grossly flat mucosa, in a mucosa with a villous configuration, or in a nodular

TABLE 12. *Dysplasia versus repair: comparison of histologic features*

	Dysplasia	Repair
1. Nuclear enlargement	+ to +++	+
2. Nuclear hyperchromasia	++	+
3. Nuclear pleomorphism	+ to +++	0 to +
4. Irregular nuclear contour	+ to +++	0 to +
5. Chromocenters/nucleoli	0 to +	++ to +++
6. Nuclear stratification	0 to +++	+
7. Loss of nuclear polarity	0 to ++	0
8. Increased mitoses	+ to +++	++
9. Inflammatory millieu	+ to ++	++
10. Decreased intracellular mucin	0 to +++	++
11. High nuclear to cytoplasmic ratio	++ to +++	0 to +
12. Cytoplasmic eosinophilia	0	+
13. Distortion of mucosal architecture	0 to +++	+ to ++
14. Villous configuration	0 to +++	0

0, none; +, mild; ++, moderate; +++, severe.

growth resembling adenoma. Dysplasia is recognized by means of well-defined cytologic criteria (175), and the pathologist should use the term only as a synonym for intraepithelial neoplasia. It should not be used in reference to reactive or reparative epithelial changes seen with active inflammation. The histologic features of dysplasia and epithelial repair are compared in Table 12 and are illustrated in Figures 35 through 38.

Both dysplasia and repair are associated with nuclear enlargement and hyperchromasia, increased mitotic figures, and decreased intracellular mucin. However, some histologic features favor repair over dysplasia. The nuclei in repair are often round to oval with a smooth external contour, are evenly spaced, contain granular chromatin with single or multiple chromocenters or nucleoli, and are remarkably sim-

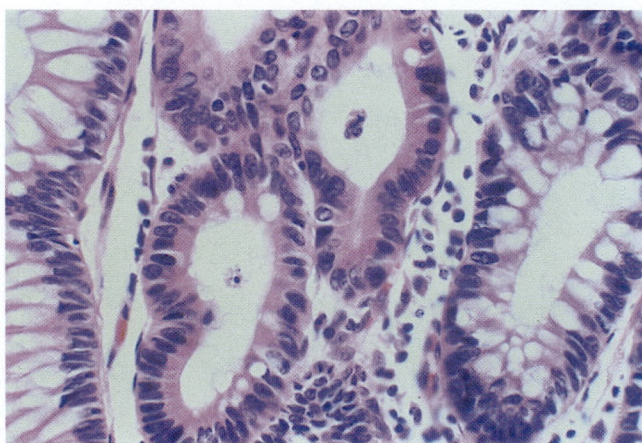

FIG. 35. Low-grade dysplasia in a patient with chronic ulcerative colitis. In contrast to the more normal epithelium (*left*), the dysplastic epithelium (*right*) demonstrates deceased intracellular mucin and nuclear enlargement with nuclear crowding and hyperchromasia. Nuclei, for the most part, maintain a basilar orientation.

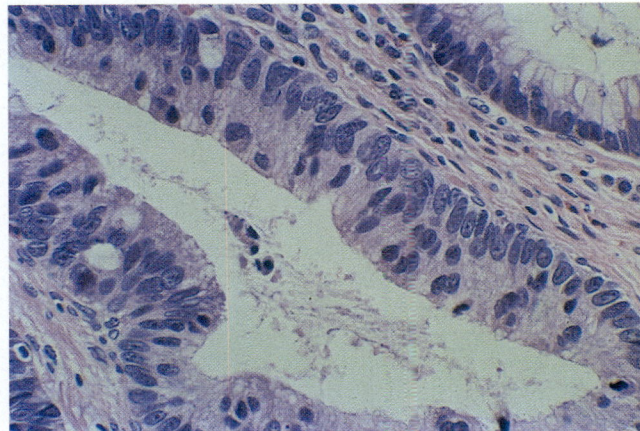

FIG. 36. High-grade dysplasia in chronic ulcerative colitis. The nuclei are hyperchromatic and pleomorphic. In contrast to low-grade dysplasia, there is increased nuclear stratification with many nuclei located in the luminal half of the cell.

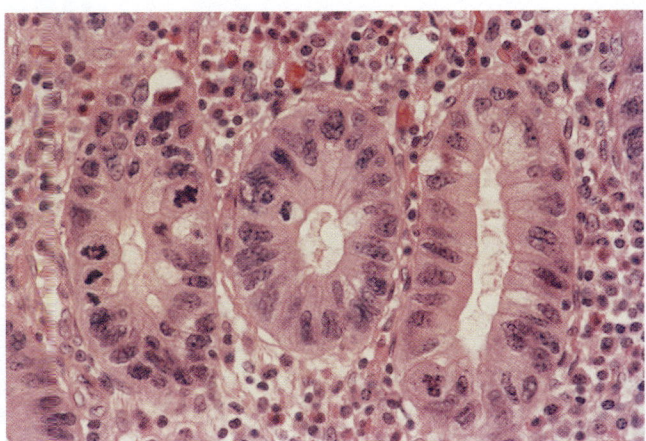

FIG. 38. Nonadenomatous type high-grade dysplasia in a patient with ulcerative colitis. Note the irregular nuclear crowding, the variable nuclear hyperchromasia, and the markedly irregular external nuclear contours.

ilar in size and appearance. In contrast to dysplasia, the nuclear to cytoplasmic size ratio of regenerative cells is often actually decreased (especially in cells adjacent to ulcerated areas), and the cell cytoplasm is often intensely eosinophilic. Nearby crypt abscesses and cryptitis help to confirm the diagnosis of repair. Features that favor dysplasia over repair are (a) nuclear hyperchromasia associated with pleomorphism, (b) irregular nuclear contours, (c) marked nuclear stratification with crowding, and (d) loss of nuclear polarity. Intracellular mucin is usually decreased in dysplastic epithelium, but on occasion it may be increased. Dystrophic or signet ring–type goblet cells are common in dysplasia but are not pathognomonic. Major distortions of mucosal architecture also favor dysplasia.

The Inflammatory Bowel Disease-Dysplasia Morphology Study Group has proposed the following three-tiered classification for biopsy interpretation in IBD: positive, negative, and indefinite for dysplasia (175). This classification is useful and reasonably reproducible (402). Biopsy specimens negative for dysplasia include normal colon, changes of UC in an active phase, or changes of UC in remission. Positive biopsy specimens are reported as containing either high-grade dysplasia or low-grade dysplasia.

The distinction between low-grade dysplasia and high-grade dysplasia is made largely by the degree of cytologic change present. In low-grade dysplasia, the abnormal nuclei are limited to the basal half of the cell (see Fig. 35). In high-grade dysplasia, hyperchromasia and pleomorphism are more marked (see Fig. 36). Stratification with loss of nuclear polarity is often present. Nuclei may be found in the luminal half of the cells. High-grade dysplasia is often associated with distortion of mucosal architecture, most commonly taking the form of a villous or nodular growth resembling an adenoma in the noncolitic patient. High-grade dysplasia also encompasses lesions with cribriform glands that formerly were classified as adenocarcinoma *in situ*.

It is correct to classify biopsy specimens as indefinite for dysplasia when unusual epithelial changes are present that are insufficient to warrant a diagnosis of dysplasia. Indefinite changes are usually seen in a background of active inflammation with regeneration. Specimens indefinite for dysplasia also include odd mucosal patterns or epithelial changes that have not yet been observed to give rise to carcinoma (e.g., a hyperplastic polyp-like change). The category *indefinite for dysplasia* should not be considered a wastebasket. It is a legitimate diagnosis alerting the treating physician that worrisome changes are present and that the patient requires more frequent surveillance.

The Inflammatory Bowel Disease-Dysplasia Morphology Study Group subdivides indefinite dysplasia into three groups: probably inflammatory, probably dysplastic, and unknown (175). This subcategorization is cumbersome, subjective, and associated with marked interobserver and intraobserver variation. Therefore, at the Cleveland Clinic, we do not subcategorize biopsy specimens in the indefinite category (402).

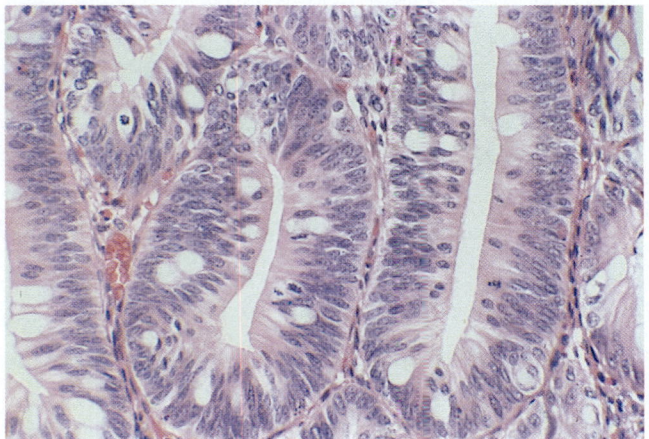

FIG. 37. High-grade dysplasia in a patient with ulcerative colitis. In general, the histologic change resembles adenoma as might be seen in a noncolitic patient.

The utility of endoscopic surveillance in chronic UC seems well established (400–402). There is a high association of carcinoma with dysplasia, especially high-grade dysplasia. Conversely, there is a low incidence of carcinoma in patients whose surveillance biopsies have been negative for dysplasia. Management recommendations based on surveillance biopsy are summarized in Table 13.

Patients whose biopsy specimens are negative for dysplasia probably can safely continue regular surveillance. Most authorities recommend annual total colonoscopy for patients with extensive colitis who have had their disease more than 7 to 10 years (175,402). In patients whose biopsies show changes indefinite for dysplasia, shorter-term follow-up and vigorous treatment of active colitis are indicated (403). For low-grade dysplasia, short-term follow-up may be reasonable, but if this dysplasia is associated with any suspicious gross lesion or stricture, colectomy should be considered (175,402,404). Some workers advocate immediate colectomy for low-grade dysplasia (405,406). If high-grade dysplasia is identified, colectomy should be recommended. Our experience with surveillance biopsy interpretation has shown that true negative results are rarely interpreted as dysplasia and true dysplasias are rarely missed (402,407).

Variations in interpretations do occur (408), and, in general, confirmation of the biopsy diagnosis is desirable before colectomy. The Inflammatory Bowel Disease-Dysplasia Morphology Study Group considered any one or more of the following as adequate confirmation: the finding of dysplasia in a repeat biopsy from the same site; unequivocal dysplasia in one or more additional sites during the same endoscopic examination; review and confirmation of the interpretation by another experienced pathologist (175).

Surveillance endoscopy with biopsy has significant limitations. Dysplasia is a rather unusual phenomenon; therefore, it is difficult for any one pathologist to acquire significant experience in its interpretation. Dysplasia is extremely focal and therefore subject to tremendous sampling errors. Because dysplasia is considered a neoplastic change, it is unlikely that it ever resolves spontaneously. Thus, a clinician should never be lulled into a false sense of security by negative follow-up biopsies once true dysplasia has been identified.

TABLE 13. *Mucosal ulcerative colitis and dysplasia: management recommendations based on surveillance biopsy*

Biopsy interpretation	Recommendation
Negative for dysplasia	Continue regular follow-up
Indefinite for dysplasia	Short-term follow-up
Positive; low-grade dysplasia	Short-term follow-up; consider colectomy if associated with suspicious gross lesion[a]
Positive; high-grade dysplasia	Consider colectomy[a]

[a] Dysplasia must be confirmed (see text).

Although not proven scientifically, it seems likely that some patients benefit from a surveillance program, because many carcinomas are detected in early curable phases (403,409–411). In addition, there is a low incidence of carcinoma in patients in whom biopsy specimens have remained negative for dysplasia (403,411). It is unclear whether this benefit justifies the large cost of surveillance endoscopy. Finally, surveillance programs are pointless unless the patient complies with the regular surveillance and agrees to colectomy when the end point (dysplasia) has been reached.

Many groups have searched for other specific markers for precancer in UC. Sialomucins predominate in cancer and dysplasia in UC (412,413), but mucin staining is generally not considered useful in cancer surveillance (414–416). Similarly, the results of lectin-binding studies, CEA immunocytochemistry, and immunocytochemical analysis for oncogene products have produced variable results and cannot be used to differentiate dysplastic from reparative epithelium in UC (415–419).

Several investigators have described significant correlations between DNA aneuploidy and dysplasia and carcinoma in UC (420–422). However, only 80% to 90% of invasive carcinomas and 50% of dysplasias demonstrate DNA abnormalities by flow cytometry. This finding indicates that DNA analysis by flow cytometry could not be used alone in a cancer surveillance program. These studies also found that many specimens (6% or more) interpreted as negative or indefinite for dysplasia showed DNA aneuploidy. This finding could be interpreted in a number of ways. These DNA results could represent false-positive results. Technical problems linked to false-positive results include failure to disaggregate nuclear clumps, prolonged exposure of the sample to high temperature, and debris in the sample (423). Alternatively, this test may identify a subgroup of patients, different from the group identified by dysplasia, that show objective chromosomal abnormalities in the absence of recognizable histologic dysplasia.

It is tempting to speculate that DNA aneuploidy could be used as a marker for some of the carcinomas complicating UC, but it is premature to make this conclusion because follow-up studies have not yet been concluded. It is currently unknown whether carcinoma will develop in this "DNA aneuploid-histology negative" group or whether histologic dysplasia will develop before carcinoma. Other workers have concluded that detection of DNA aneuploidy is not useful as a predictor of the presence of concurrent carcinoma in UC (420). Until large prospective studies determine the usefulness of DNA aneuploidy as a marker for malignancy in UC, dysplasia, recognized histologically, remains the only reliable marker for cancer in a surveillance program (407,424). DNA analysis may have a role in cancer surveillance, in that patients with a normal DNA content and no signs of histologic dysplasia probably could be examined at longer intervals (422).

A special problem concerns the occurrence of adenoma in the colitic patient. Because both disorders are common, there is probably no theoretic reason why they could not coexist. Because most colitis-associated dysplasias resemble adenomas (see Fig. 37), the distinction in practice is impossible. In general, a diagnosis of "adenoma" in a colitic patient must be viewed with skepticism because the changes probably represent IBD-associated dysplasia, an ominous change that implies a substantial risk either for the development of carcinoma or for coexisting carcinoma (175,425). IBD patients with adenomas in areas not involved by colitis can be treated by polypectomy alone (425–427). Adenomas occurring in areas of endoscopically involved colitis should probably be considered IBD-associated dysplasia; however, that designation may not necessarily require colectomy. Occasionally, an "adenoma" in a colitic may be treated by local excision, but only if all the following criteria are met: the patient is in an adenoma age group (older than 40 years old), the polyp is pedunculated, excision is complete, the patient is endoscopically easy to survey (e.g., without inflammatory polyposis), and the mucosa of the stalk and mucosa away from the "adenoma" lack dysplasia (175,403,425–427). This type of patient must receive careful short-term follow-up.

The differential diagnosis of adenomas and dysplastic lesions in colitis has been the focus of several publications. Distinction based on pathomorphologic features has been proposed (427,428). Studies of APC gene mutations using *in vitro* synthesized protein assays in UC-associated dysplasia versus sporadic adenoma/adenocarcinoma have yielded conflicting results. Tarmin and colleagues reported significantly lower (6%) rates of APC mutation in UC-associated dysplasia and carcinoma as compared to sporadic neoplasia (74%) (429). However, Redson and coworkers reported a prevalence of APC gene mutations in UC-associated dysplasia and carcinoma (50%) that was much closer to that seen in sporadic colorectal neoplasia (430). Fogt and associates suggested that the low frequency of loss of heterozygosity (LOH) in the p16 gene (9p) in adenomas compared with dysplasia in UC, combined with infrequent LOH in APC gene loci in cases of pure dysplasia in UC, may be used to differentiate polypoid dysplasia from adenoma in UC (431). These molecular approaches remain to be tested clinically.

Dysplasia and Cancer in Crohn's Disease

Patients with CD seem to be at increased risk for intestinal carcinoma (432–436). Small bowel carcinoma in CD occurs in younger patients and tends to occur, on average, 20 years after onset of CD. They most often occur in the ileum, almost always in areas of intestine actively involved by CD. The carcinomas are grossly subtle, mostly occurring in strictured areas and usually not associated with intraluminal lesions. The carcinomas tend to be poorly differentiated and have been associated with a poor prognosis (432,435). Approximately 25% of reported small bowel carcinomas associated with CD have been in bypassed or out-of-circuit segments (432,435,437).

The colon carcinomas in CD occur in patients who, on average, are 10 years younger than those with colonic cancer in the general population; these carcinomas generally develop after 20 years of disease (433,434,438,439). The diagnosis of carcinoma is made preoperatively more often in the colon than in the small bowel because the colonic cancers are more easily visualized by standard radiologic and endoscopic techniques, and there is usually a gross intraluminal lesion. The carcinomas tend to be better differentiated than their small bowel counterparts; they are rarely multifocal, but approximately 20% have occurred in out-of-circuit rectums. The prognosis is much better than for CD-associated small bowel carcinoma and seems to be approximately the same, stage for stage, as for colonic carcinoma in the general population.

Reports using current histologic criteria almost invariably note dysplasia in the epithelium adjacent to carcinoma in CD (433,434,436–438). In addition, dysplasia in areas distant from carcinoma has commonly been encountered in specimens exhibiting both colonic carcinoma and CD. These features provide evidence that a dysplasia-carcinoma sequence similar to that proposed for UC exists in CD, but the extent of dysplasia seems to be less than that encountered in UC.

ISCHEMIC BOWEL DISEASE

Ischemic bowel injury occurs whenever the oxygen or vascular supply is insufficient to meet the metabolic demands of the tissue. Ischemia and damage can result from arterial or venous occlusion or, most frequently, from reduced blood flow associated with shunting of blood from the splanchnic bed. Ischemia can result in little or no damage or in a variety of pathologic abnormalities that depend upon the etiology, severity, and duration of the hypoxia. Thus, ischemic bowel disease may present as hemorrhagic infarction, discrete or serpiginous ulcers that mimic CD, a mucosal plaque with pseudomembrane, or as a stricture. Any part or length of bowel can be affected, but lesions associated with reduced blood flow show a propensity to affect the watershed zones such as the splenic flexure (170).

Early, organizing, and healed phases of ischemia can be recognized histologically (255,440). Acute ischemic change may be patchy or diffuse and characteristically consists of hemorrhage into the lamina propria associated with superficial epithelial necrosis with preservation of the deep portion of the intestinal crypts (170). Depending on the extent and duration of hypoxia, the changes may be reversible or they may proceed to ulcer or full-thickness infarct (441). In its organizing phase, ischemic damage becomes somewhat nonspecific in appearance. An ischemic origin should be suspected when an ulcer and organizing inflammation appear bland and unassociated with the marked chronic inflammation and lymphoid aggregates typical of primary IBD. The presence of hemorrhage or hemosiderin deposits, although not pathognomonic, suggests ischemic damage. In the healing phase, the colonic mucosa may assume an architectural appearance reminiscent of UC in remission (255), whereas

TABLE 14. *Distinguishing features of syndromes having an ischemic component*

Syndrome	Clinical features	Preferred location of bowel lesions	Other pathologic features	References
Necrotizing enterocolitis of the neonate	Affects premature or low-birth-weight Infants Onset within 10 days of birth Bacterial infection may be important in pathogenesis	Stomach, terminal ileum, and right colon	Pneumatosis cystoides intestinalis Fibrous stricture late if patient survives	440,442,443
Hemorrhagic necrosis of the gastrointestinal tract (synonyms: typhlitis; neutropenic enterocolitis; necrotizing enterocolitis; ileocecal syndrome)	Occurs clinically in patients with leukemia or lymphoma who are receiving immunosuppressive therapy Poor prognosis	Terminal ileum, cecum, right colon	Secondary bacterial and fungal overgrowth prominent Paucity of active inflammation	440,444
Nonspecific ulcer syndromes				
Colon	Association with (a) patients with end-stage renal disease, (b) patients on hemodialysis, or (c) patients with renal transplants	Cecum and right colon	Sometimes associated with right-sided diverticula High frequency of CMV inclusions in ulcers	445–448
Small intestine	Associated with ingestion of enteric-coated potassium and hydrochlorothiazide pills, NSAIDs No known etiology in many cases	Mid- to distal small intestine	Strictures and diaphragms	440,449–451
Behcet's disease	Aphthous stomatitis, genital ulcers, and relapsing iritis M:F ratio 2:1 Gastrointestinal involvement in 10%–15% of patients	Ileum, cecum	"Punched-out" ulcers, may be deep with perforation Perivascular inflammation and necrotizing vasculitis may be seen	452–455
Late radiation enterocolitis	Occurs a few weeks to years after therapy May be associated with enterocolitis, stricture, ulcer, or fistula	Bowel within radiation field	Atrophic mucosa; ectatic blood vessels; fibrosis, often hyalinized; "radiation" fibroblasts; vascular wall thickening and vascular luminal stenosis	334,456
Stercoral ulcer associated with bowel obstruction	Result of pressure of feces May be seen with intractable constipation	Colon and rectum	Sharply demarcated Secondary bacterial overgrowth may be seen	57, 334
Pseudomembranous enterocolitis	Onset of symptoms after antibiotic therapy Cream-to-yellow plaques on endoscopy	Colon	Prominent pseudomembranes May have infectious pattern of injury in colon biopsy specimens	216,217

NSAIDs, nonsteroidal anti-inflammatory drugs; CMV, cytomegalovirus.

in the small bowel, villous distortion and pyloric gland metaplasia are common. Healed phases of ischemia are usually accompanied by fibrous stricture. The fibrosis in an ischemic stricture tends to affect all bowel layers, including the muscularis propria. In contrast, fibrosis of the muscularis propria is not common in primary IBD. Again, hemosiderin deposition is a helpful clue to the ischemic nature of the injury.

In resected specimens, the blood vessels should be carefully dissected and many sections obtained to detect vascular lesions such as thrombosis and inflammation. The significance of vascular inflammation in areas of ulcer and infarct is dubious, because this "vasculitis" is most likely secondary in nature. However, acute inflammation in vascular walls associated with fibrinoid necrosis found in areas that are apparently viable may indicate systemic vasculitis.

Other Entities Having an Ischemic Component

Other entities considered part of the spectrum of ischemic bowel disease include necrotizing enterocolitis of the premature infant, hemorrhagic necrosis of the gastrointestinal tract (typhlitis), intestinal Behcet's disease, pseudomembranous enterocolitis, late radiation enterocolitis, uremic colitis, stercoral ulcer associated with bowel obstruction, potassium chloride–induced ulcer, nonsteroidal anti-inflammatory drug-related injury, and stress ulcer (334,440,442–457). The pathologic features of these lesions resemble ischemic bowel disease as previously described and are indistinguishable without corroborative clinical and laboratory information.

Their major clinical, distributional, and other distinguishing characteristics are summarized in Table 14.

SPECIFIC ENTERIC INFECTIONS THAT MAY BE ENCOUNTERED IN RESECTION SPECIMENS

Most of the infections reviewed in this section are typically diagnosed by evaluation of a combination of clinical features, laboratory studies, and enteric mucosal biopsy specimens (see Evaluation of Small Intestinal Mucosal Biopsy Specimens in Patients with Malabsorption). However, they may occasionally be detected in resection specimens performed either because of a severe or fulminant clinical course, development of a complication, or confusion with IBD (either UC or CD). The major bacterial infections in this category are yersiniosis, tuberculosis, and salmonellosis, whereas the parasitic diseases include amebiasis, schistosomiasis, balantidiasis, and trichuriasis. The salient diagnostic and differential diagnostic features of these infections are summarized in Tables 15 and 16, and selected examples are illustrated in Figures 39 and 40 (131,171, 458–470).

DIVERTICULAR DISEASE

Left-Sided Colonic Diverticular Disease

Left-sided diverticular disease is a common lesion in middle-aged and older individuals (471) and is associated with a characteristic muscular abnormality of the bowel wall (472).

TABLE 15. *Bacterial infections that may be encountered in resection specimens*

Infection	Clinical features	Pathology	References
Yersiniosis			
Y. enterocolitica	Variable from mild self-limited disease to typhoid fever-like picture; may mimic appendicitis	Preferred sites: ileum, right colon, and appendix; discrete ulcers typically overlying lymphoid nodules; variable mural thickening; enlarged mesenteric lymph nodes showing follicular hyperplasia with microabscesses; gram-negative rods on stain of lesion	171,458–460
Y. pseudotuberculosis	Similar to *Y. enterocolitica*	Similar to *Y. enterocolitica* plus the characteristic suppurative granuloma (central acute inflammation with fibrin surrounded by epithelioid histiocytes)	171,461
Tuberculosis	Gastrointestinal symptoms that may mimic Crohn's disease	Preferred sites: terminal ileum, cecum, and appendix; ulceration and stricture; granulomatous inflammation that may be necrotizing and confluent; mural fibrosis; granulomatous inflammation in mesenteric lymph nodes; positive acid-fast stain	462
Salmonellosis	Variable from mild self-limited "food poisoning" to enteric fevers (typhoid) Enteric fevers often associated with neutropenia	Preferred site: terminal ileum; ulcers over Peyer's patches; paucity of acute inflammatory cells in ulcers; collections of histiocytes showing erythrophagocytosis are common	463,464

TABLE 16. *Parasitic infections that may be encountered in resection specimens*

Infection	Clinical features	Pathology	References
Amoebiasis	Prevalent in tropics and in homosexual population; variable symptoms ranging from asymptomatic to fulminant colitis; majority of patients have dysentery	Preferred site; colon, cecum Flask-shaped ulcers Trophozoites in ulcer base or in adherent inflammatory exudate and mucus	131,465,466
Schistosomiasis	Colitis or bowel obstruction	Focal ulcers; stricture; inflammatory polyps; eggs identified in lesion	131,467,468
Balantidiasis	Like amoebiasis	Preferred sites: cecum, rectosigmoid colon; flask-shaped ulcers; trophozoites in lesion	131,469
Trichuriasis	Variable from asymptomatic to bloody diarrhea; rectal prolapse in children; may mimic acute appendicitis	Focal ulcers; adult worm identified in histologic sections	131,470

The abnormality is a marked thickening of the inner circular muscle coat of the muscularis propria that results in a narrowed lumen and a mucosa thrown into prominent accordion-like folds. The muscular abnormality and associated diverticula are most prominent in the sigmoid colon; they may extend for a variable distance proximally, but they never involve the rectum. The diverticula are usually still enveloped by an intact, albeit attenuated, longitudinal muscle layer and are typically present in two rows, situated between the mesenteric and the two antimesenteric tinea. In severe cases, small diverticula can also be found between the antimesenteric tinea. Similar clinical signs and symptoms occur regardless of whether objective inflammatory changes are present in the diverticula; therefore, I prefer the term *diverticular disease* rather than making the distinction routinely between diverticulosis and diverticulitis.

Diverticula are sometimes difficult to demonstrate in resected specimens. Resected fresh bowel loses muscle tone and intraluminal pressure; as a result, the diverticula often evert and are mistaken for polyps. The best way to demonstrate diverticula is to fix an intact specimen with formalin under pressure for 24 hours before the dissection.

Complications of diverticular disease include inflammation of the diverticula (diverticulitis), perforation, adhesion, fistula formation, inflammatory mass formation, hemorrhage, and obstruction (473). Although colovesicle or colovaginal fistula can occur in diverticular disease, other fistula combinations must raise the suspicion of CD, because both diseases can and do coexist. Any granularity or ulceration of the luminal mucosa, accompanied by microscopic findings of crypt abscesses or lymphoid aggregates away from inflamed diverticula, must raise the possibility of coexisting CD (334). Likewise, features of colitis distal to the zone of diverticula (e.g., at the distal resection margin) raise the question of coexisting CD.

Right-Sided Colonic Diverticular Disease

Diverticula of the right colon are often isolated, are usually not associated with left-sided diverticular disease, occur

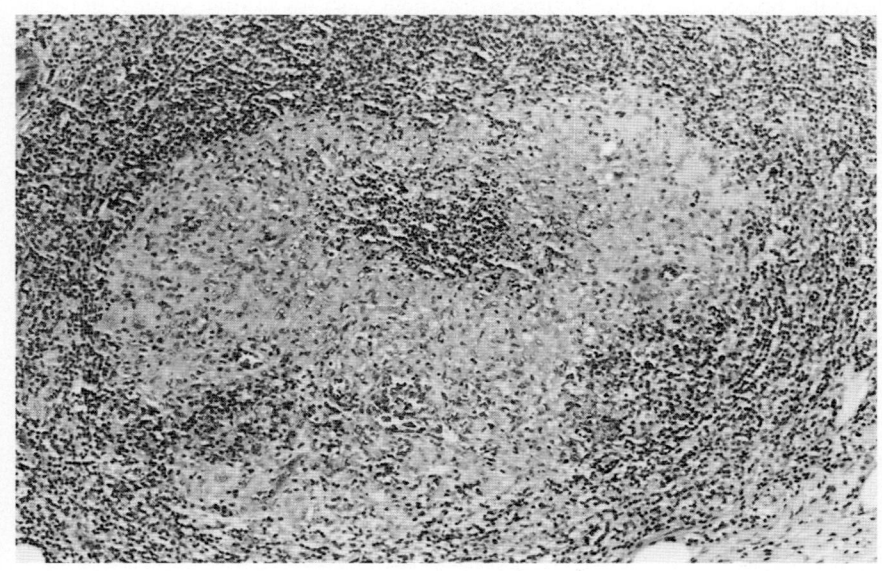

FIG. 39. The suppurative granuloma of *Yersinia pseudotuberculosis* infection. The central acute inflammatory cells are surrounded by epithelioid histiocytes.

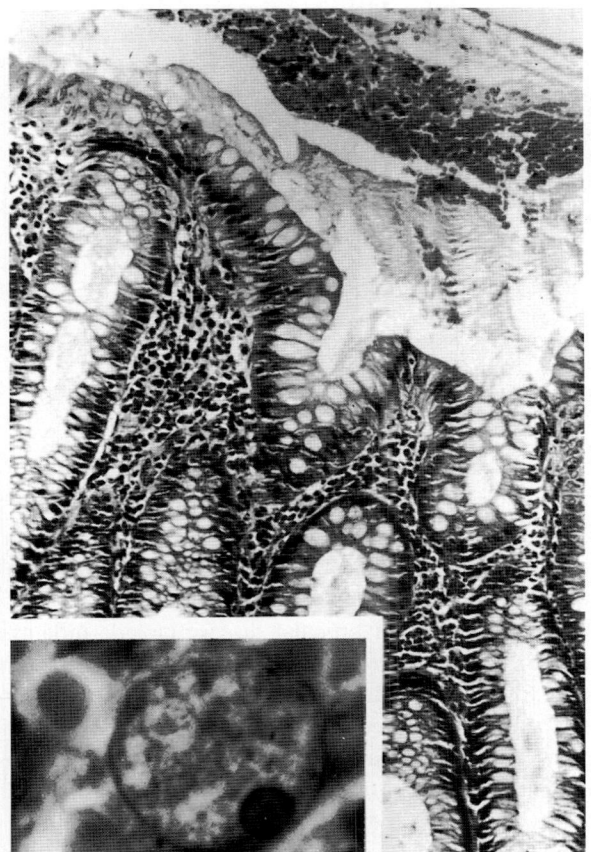

FIG. 40. Colonic biopsy specimen in a patient with amoebiasis. There are increased chronic inflammatory cells within the lamina propria and an inflammatory exudate overlying the mucosa. High-magnification examination of the inflammatory exudate (*inset*) reveals typical trophozoites of *Entamoeba histolytica*.

in younger patients (often in the third and fourth decade), and are frequent in Asians (474–478). Clinically, right-sided diverticular disease mimics acute appendicitis (479). Some authors classify these diverticula as either *congenital* (or "true") if the outpouching contains all layers of the bowel wall or as *acquired* if they resemble those seen in left-sided diverticular disease (334). Complications include inflammation, hemorrhage, pericolonic abscess, and peritonitis; these diverticula may be the cause of some solitary ulcers of the cecum or ascending colon (334).

VASCULAR LESIONS OF THE INTESTINAL TRACT

A number of classifications for intestinal vascular lesions have been proposed (480,481), but none is totally satisfactory. Recently, my approach has been to divide them into two groups: those forms confined to the gastrointestinal tract and those associated with a recognized systemic syndrome (Tables 17 and 18) (480–495).

TABLE 17. *Isolated intestinal vascular abnormalities*

A. Vascular ectasia of right colon
B. Hemangiomas
   1. Capillary hemangioma
   2. Cavernous hemangioma
      a. Localized
      b. Diffuse
   3. Arteriovenous hemangioma
C. Phlebectasia

Isolated Intestinal Vascular Abnormalities

Vascular Ectasia of Right Colon

Vascular ectasia of the right colon, the type I lesion described by Moore and colleagues (480), has several synonyms such as angiodysplasia and arteriovenous malformation (482,483). Patients with right colonic vascular ectasia are typically elderly and have episodes of recurrent low-grade lower gastrointestinal bleeding; however, approximately 15% have massive gastrointestinal hemorrhage. The lesions, which are generally confined to the cecum or ascending colon and are often multiple, are not associated with other abnormalities except for an increased frequency in patients with aortic valvular stenosis.

Demonstration of vascular ectasia in resection specimens is notoriously difficult by standard pathologic techniques, and usually requires vascular injection. Boley and Brandt's technique uses injection of the fresh specimen vasculature with a silicone rubber compound. The specimen is then fixed in formalin, dehydrated in graded alcohols, and cleared with methyl salicylate (482). This method produces a transparent specimen in which the vasculature can be examined by transillumination under the dissecting microscope. With this technique, the vascular ectasias stand out as a 1 mm to a 1 cm in diameter coral reef–like arrangement of vessels that contrast with the honeycomb pattern of the normal colonic mucosal vasculature. Histologic examination reveals abnormal thin-walled ectatic veins, venules, and capillaries in the mucosa and submucosa. The lesions are thought to result from repetitive partial obstruction to venous drainage caused by contraction of the muscularis propria (482).

Vascular injection techniques require some preparation in terms of materials on the part of the pathologist. If the pathologist does not have such materials ready, the larger ectasias may still be demonstrated by carefully and gently washing off the mucosal surface of the specimen with water. Sometimes a blood clot adheres to the lesion, and this may direct one's histologic sections. I have been disappointed with injection of contrast media and specimen radiography, but I have had success in demonstrating right-sided vascular ectasia by injecting brightly colored ink into the ileocolic artery.

TABLE 18. *Intestinal vascular abnormalities associated with systemic syndromes*

Syndrome	Inheritance	Histologic type of lesion	Preferred location in the gestrointestinal tract	Other manifestations	References
Hereditary hemorrhagic telangiectasia	AD	Telangiectasia	Anywhere	Telangiectasias of skin, mucous membrane, and internal organs	489
Progressive systemic sclerosis	—	Telangiectasia	Stomach	Calcinosis; Raynaud's phenomenon; sclerodactaly; telangiectasias of skin, lips, and tongue	481,490
Blue rubber bleb nevus syndrome	AD or sporadic	Hemangioma	Small intestine	Skin and visceral hemangiomas	491
Turner's syndrome	—	Telangiectasia	Small intestine, large intestine	XO karyotype; short stature; webbed neck; shield chest; streak gonads	492
Klippel-Trenaunay-Weber syndrome	—	Hemangioma	Anywhere	Somatic and bony hypertrophy; port wine stain; urinary bladder hemangioma	481
Pseudoxanthoma elasticum	Variable	Arteriovenous hemangioma	Stomach	"Plucked chicken" skin; angioid streaks in the retina	493
Ehlers-Danlos syndrome	Variable	Spontaneous vascular rupture	Anywhere	Hyperelasticity of skin and joints	481,494,495

AD, autosomal dominant.

Hemangiomas

Hemangiomas unassociated with systemic syndromes may be classified on the basis of the predominant vessel type into capillary, cavernous, or arteriovenous hemangioma. Capillary hemangiomas are usually asymptomatic, are typically small, are rarely multiple, and are composed of small closely packed capillaries. They may be found in the colon but are usually encountered in the small intestine, appendix, and perianal skin (481–484). Cavernous hemangiomas may occur in a localized or diffuse form (484–487). Histologically, they are composed of blood-filled sinus-like spaces supported by scant connective tissue that occasionally contains smooth muscle (481,484). They can occur in the small bowel but have a predilection for the colon and rectum. Patients may have symptoms of a mass or have rectal bleeding. A lesion composed of abnormal veins and arteries is an arteriovenous hemangioma. It has the same distribution and implications as the cavernous hemangioma.

Phlebectasia

Phlebectasia is a nonneoplastic venous varicosity (481) that occasionally causes severe gastrointestinal bleeding. The most frequent site of bleeding caused by phlebectasias associated with portal hypertension is the lower esophagus. Other sites of phlebectasia with hemorrhage are the rectosigmoid colon (488) and, rarely, the small intestine (481).

Intestinal Vascular Lesions Associated with Systemic Syndromes

Intestinal vascular lesions have been described in association with hereditary hemorrhagic telangiectasia, scleroderma, blue rubber bleb nevus syndrome, Turner's syndrome, Klippel-Trenaunay-Weber syndrome, pseudoxanthoma elasticum, and the Ehlers-Danlos syndrome (481,489–495). The salient clinical and pathologic features are summarized in Table 18.

DISORDERS OF INTESTINAL MOTILITY

Intestinal Pseudo-obstruction

Intestinal pseudo-obstruction is the term used to describe patients with signs and symptoms of intestinal obstruction in whom no mechanical obstructive lesion can be demonstrated (496). Intestinal pseudo-obstruction may be caused by a heterogeneous group of lesions. A classification of the causes of intestinal pseudo-obstruction, along with what is known about their pathology, is summarized in Tables 19 through 21 (496–502). In some cases, intestinal pseudo-obstruction is associated with a familiar disease or drug (see Table 19). The bowel obstruction is considered a local manifestation of the more generalized disease process or drug effect, and, in general, the intestinal pathology is either unknown or nonspecific. In other cases, pseudo-obstruction is associated with a familiar disease in which pathologic changes can be

TABLE 19. *Secondary intestinal pseudo-obstruction with unknown or nonspecific pathologic changes*

Diabetes
Hypoparathyroidism
Pheochromocytoma
Parkinson's disease
Systemic lupus erythematosis
Drugs
    Amanita (mushroom poisoning)
    Antiparkinsonian drugs
    Clonidine
    Ganglionic blockers
    Tricyclic antidepressants
    Phenothiazines
Psychosis

Modified from ref. 496.

TABLE 21. *"Primary" intestinal pseudo-obstruction: pathologic changes primarily affecting the gastrointestinal tract*

Disease	Pathologic change
Ceroidosis	Lipofuscin deposition in smooth muscle of muscularis propria and muscularis mucosae
Cathartic colon	Melanosis coli; evidence of neuron damage by silver stain techniques
Hirschsprung's disease	Absence of ganglion cells
Visceral myopathies	Vacuolar degeneration of muscle cells with fibrosis of muscularis propria; predilection for outer longitudinal layer
Visceral neuropathies	Variable changes: some with eosinophilic intranuclear inclusion bodies, some with evidence of neuron or axon damage by silver stains; some inflammatory neuropathies

seen in the intestine (see Table 20). Finally, there are several intestinal motility disorders in which the primary pathologic changes and clinical manifestations are gastrointestinal (see Table 21).

Visceral Myopathies

There are multiple variants of familial visceral myopathy that demonstrate differences in the mode of inheritance (autosomal dominant versus recessive), sites of involvement in the gut, clinical symptoms, and extraintestinal manifestations. Visceral myopathies also occur in a sporadic form (498).

The intestinal pathologic changes in familial and sporadic hollow visceral myopathies are identical and consist of muscle-cell degeneration, muscle-cell loss, and fibrosis of the muscularis propria. The degenerative fibers appear swollen and rarefied. Collagen may encircle the residual muscle fibers in areas of muscle-fiber dropout and impart a vacuolated appearance (498,503). These changes are limited to, or more severe in, the external layer of the muscularis propria. The small intestinal mucosa may show changes associated with stasis; these include a variable villus abnormality with increased chronic inflammatory cells, occasionally mixed with acute inflammatory cells.

The differential diagnosis of the visceral myopathies includes other entities that cause fibrosis of the muscularis propria, and it encompasses ischemia, tuberculosis, and scleroderma. Ischemia usually is associated with a fibrous stricture and hemosiderin deposits. Tuberculosis also causes strictures, and granulomas (often with central necrosis) are seen histologically. Progressive systemic sclerosis shows more patchy bowel involvement than the visceral myopathies. The fibrosis tends to be denser, and the fibrosis either replaces all of the muscle of the muscularis propria or is accentuated in the inner layer. Vacuolar change is not seen in progressive systemic sclerosis (502).

Desmin myopathy has been described in a single patient with intestinal pseudo-obstruction (504). The authors reported eosinophilic perinuclear cytoplasmic inclusions within intestinal smooth muscle cells that were immunoreactive for desmin and ubiquitin. A complicated classifica-

TABLE 20. *Secondary intestinal pseudo-obstruction with demonstrable intestinal pathology*

Disease	Pathologic change	References
Myxedema	Mucopolysaccharide infiltration of stroma	496
Dermatomyositis/polymyositis	Fibrosis in muscularis propria	496
Amyloidosis	Amyloid deposits in bowel wall	497
Chagas' disease	Decreased or absent ganglion cells; thickening of muscularis propria; and lymphoplasmocytic infiltrate of the myenteric plexus	496,498
Myotonic dystrophy	Fatty infiltration of muscularis propria with atrophy and fibrosis	496,499
Duchenne's muscular dystrophy	Fatty infiltration of muscularis propria; focal necrosis of smooth muscle; fatty infiltration of ganglionic plexi	498,500,501
Scleroderma	Fibrosis in muscularis propria with predilection for inner circular layer	502

tion for enteric smooth muscle disease in children using electron microscopy, histochemistry, and immunohistochemistry appears too cumbersome for routine application (505).

Visceral Neuropathies

The visceral neuropathies form a complex group of unusual entities that vary in their pattern of inheritance (familial versus sporadic), the extent of intestinal and extraintestinal involvement, and the nature of the histopathologic changes in the intramural neural plexi of the gut (Table 22). Many of the neuronal and axonal changes are subtle; with the exception of inflammatory neuropathies or, perhaps, familial neuropathies associated with intranuclear inclusions, they cannot be recognized in routine H&E-stained sections, and they require special silver-staining techniques for their demonstration (506). Difficult and unusual cases should probably be referred for consultation to pathology departments with particular expertise in evaluating visceral neuropathies. Some sporadic cases demonstrate mononuclear inflammation in the myenteric plexus, and these cases can be identified by routine light microscopy alone (507,508).

An increasing role for the interstitial cells of Cajal as gut pacemakers and as mediators of neurotransmission has been proposed (509–511). Interstitial cells of Cajal stain specifically with the tyrosine kinase receptor, c-kit (511). Immunohistochemistry for c-kit (CD117) and for CD34 (which reacts with many c-kit receptors) represents a relatively easy way (easier than Smith's Silver Stain) to study severe constipation and intestinal pseudo-obstruction. Campbell and coworkers have described completely absent or markedly reduced numbers of interstitial cells of Cajal in intestinal pseudo-obstruction (511). Although these observations could be an epiphenomenon, they could form the basis of an alternate classification system for pseudo-obstruction.

Jejunal Diverticulosis

Jejunal diverticulosis has traditionally been considered an acquired condition, often (50% of cases) associated with colonic diverticula (512). However, several groups have recently presented evidence to suggest that jejunal diverticulosis is often a reflection of an underlying gut motility disorder because, in many cases, lesions identical with progressive systemic sclerosis, hollow visceral myopathy, or forms of visceral neuropathy have been demonstrated (498). Symptomatic patients usually have chronic intestinal pseudo-obstruction. Complications include hemorrhage, diverticulitis, perforation, vitamin B_{12} deficiency, and steatorrhea.

Ceroidosis: "The Brown Bowel Syndrome"

Severe intestinal malabsorption for whatever reason can be associated with dark brown or orange-brown discoloration of the bowel wall (513,514), owing to deposition of a granular material that has the characteristics of lipofuscin in the smooth muscle of the muscularis propria and, to a lesser degree, the muscularis mucosae. This excessive accumulation of lipofuscin is termed *ceroidosis,* or the "brown bowel syndrome." Whether this pigment deposition adversely affects muscle function is debated; however, damage to smooth muscle mitochondria has been described, and several reports have linked ceroidosis to intestinal pseudo-obstruction (515). Because of the name "brown bowel syndrome," ceroidosis may be confused with melanosis coli.

Melanosis Coli, Cathartic Colon, and Severe Idiopathic Constipation

Melanosis coli is a condition in which macrophages filled with lipofuscin-like pigment are found within the lamina propria or deeper in the wall of the colon (516,517). They may be of such numbers as to impart a brown or black color to the colon. Melanosis coli has been associated with the ingestion of purgatives of the anthracene group (cascera, sagrada, aloe, rhubarb, senna, frangula).

There exists a group of patients with severe and persistent constipation for which no cause is evident (idiopathic constipation). These patients, usually women, may have as little as one stool every 1 to 4 weeks (498) and many are so uncomfortable that they require colectomy for relief (518). Because these patients almost invariably take laxatives, melanosis coli is consistently found. What is so frustrating to the pathologist is that, by H&E staining, the neuronal plexi and smooth muscle in these patients appear normal. Distinctive abnormalities of the myenteric plexus (such as loss of argyrophilic neurons) have been reported using special silver-staining techniques (498,516,519,520). Perhaps staining of these cases with antibodies to CD34 and CD117 will shed light on their pathogenesis (see Visceral Neuropathies).

Cathartic colon is thought to be the end stage of idiopathic constipation, in which the bowel no longer can contract effectively. The mucosa has the gross appearance of snake skin and histologically shows melanosis coli. The muscularis propria is thin and atrophic, and neurons are decreased in Auerbach's plexus (520).

TABLE 22. *Classification of visceral neuropathies*

I. Familial visceral neuropathies
  A. Recessive trait associated with intranuclear eosinophilic inclusions
  B. Recessive trait associated with steatorrhea, mental retardation, and cerebral calcification
  C. Dominant trait
II. Sporadic visceral neuropathies
  A. Degenerative, noninflammatory
  B. Degenerative, inflammatory

Modified from ref. 498.

Hirschsprung's Disease and Allied Conditions

Hirschsprung's Disease

Hirschsprung's disease (aganglionic megacolon) demonstrates a predilection for male patients. Approximately 90% of patients are first seen in infancy, usually with constipation, abdominal distention, vomiting, and delay of meconium stool; diarrhea may occur (521,522) and some may even be affected by life-threatening enterocolitis. Hirschsprung's disease has been linked to inactivating mutations of the RET proto-oncogene (523). In the typical clinical picture, the anus is normal; the anal canal and rectum are usually small and devoid of stool. In classic cases, these physical findings are confirmed with barium enema: The contrast material flows into an unexpanded distal segment, then passes through a cone-shaped area, and finally into the dilated proximal bowel. The pathologic change is aganglionosis. The narrowed distal segment shows complete absence of ganglion cells from both the submucosal and myenteric plexi, usually accompanied by hypertrophy of the muscularis mucosae and increased numbers and size of nerves in the submucosa and between the muscle layers of the muscularis propria (524). In the tapered or cone-shaped region, the number of ganglion cells may be decreased.

Historically, histologic diagnosis was made on full-thickness rectal biopsy specimens. However, this procedure requires general anesthesia and risks the development of stricture and perforation. Because the submucosal and myenteric plexi stop at about the same level in Hirschsprung's disease (525), suction biopsy sampling the mucosa and submucosa is considered the method of choice for the diagnosis. All rectal biopsy specimens for suspected Hirschsprung's disease should be serially sectioned throughout the block, and each section examined. If no ganglion cells are found, then some comment should be made concerning the adequacy of the specimen. Biopsy specimens devoid of ganglion cells, but in which the amount of submucosa is less than the thickness of the mucosa, should be considered as insufficient to diagnose Hirschsprung's disease (524). If biopsy specimens contain epithelium of the anal canal, this specimen should be considered inadequate, because the anal canal and distal 2 cm of rectum typically are relatively hypoganglionated or aganglionated.

Many pathologists prefer to examine a frozen-section slide stained for acetylcholinesterase in addition to standard H&E sections (526). In Hirschsprung's disease, the acetylcholinesterase stain demonstrates a marked increase in the acetylcholinesterase-positive nerve fibers in the lamina propria and muscularis mucosae. The utility of this technique as an adjunct to diagnosis is debated. False-positive and false-negative reactions have been reported, and its use is a matter of personal preference (524,527–529).

Occasionally, ganglion cells may be difficult to identify using light microscopy alone, especially in the neonate (524). In such cases, a positive immunocytochemical reaction for neuron-specific enolase can be invaluable in documenting ganglion cells (530). In our laboratory, we have been successful in performing immunohistochemistry tests for neuron-specific enolase on sections after they have been stained with H&E and examined. Other immunostains such as cathepsin D and PGP 9.5 can also decorate ganglion cells (531).

Long-Segment Hirschsprung's Disease

In 90% of patients with Hirschsprung's disease, the aganglionosis involves segments of colon less than 40 cm in length. The remaining cases demonstrate a longer aganglionic segment that may extend even into the small intestine (498). Microscopically, the hypertrophied nerve trunks of short segment Hirschsprung's disease are absent, but the increased number of acetylcholinesterase-positive mucosal nerve fibers can be seen (526).

Ultrashort-Segment Hirschsprung's Disease

Ultrashort-segment Hirschsprung's disease (segment is smaller than 2 cm) reportedly exists but is probably impossible for a pathologist to document by routine H&E stains of rectal mucosa and submucosa alone because this segment of rectum is relatively hypoganlionated or aganglionated even in normal individuals. Rectal manometry plays a premier role in the diagnosis of this lesion. Acetylcholinesterase nerve abnormalities similar to Hirschsprung's disease may complement that study.

Hypoganglionosis

Hypoganglionosis is regularly observed in the cone-shaped transition zone between normal and aganglionic bowel in Hirschsprung's disease (498). Some authors believe that diffuse hypoganglionosis of the colon may give rise to megacolon similar to that observed in Hirschsprung's disease (524,532). There is no accepted definition of hypoganglionosis; however, guidelines are offered by Meier-Ruge, suggesting that a decrease by a factor of 10 in the number of ganglion cells per centimeter of bowel as compared to normal (40 to 80 myenteric plexus neurons per 100 mm bowel) is diagnostic of hypoganglionosis (526). In general, the condition has not been well characterized, and many reports lack quantitation (498). Some cases of hypoganglionosis may be similar to cases reported as severe idiopathic constipation or cathartic colon.

Intestinal Neuronal Dysplasia (Hyperganglionosis)

Intestinal neuronal dysplasia is characterized by hyperplasia of myenteric plexi, increased acetylcholinesterase activity in nerves of the lamina propria and submucosa, and increased numbers of ganglion cells with formation of giant ganglions (533,534). These giant ganglions typically contain more than 7 to 10 neurons (normal: 3 to 5), make up only 3% to 5% of all ganglions in a given case, and are usually not seen in the distal rectum. Occasionally, ganglion cells may be found within the lamina propria (532). The condition may give rise to signs and symptoms similar to Hirschsprung's disease. It may occur in a localized or disseminated form. Similar lesions, sometimes referred to as ganglioneuromatosis, may be observed in patients with von Recklinghausen's disease or the multiple endocrine neoplasia syndrome, type IIB (498,534). Although some investigators diagnose intestinal neuronal dysplasia based on abnormal acetylcholinesterase staining in specimens containing ganglion cells, others believe that one cannot rely on acetylcholinesterase staining alone for the diagnosis (535). Diagnostic criteria for intestinal neuronal dysplasia and even its existence are challenged (536) because 95% of infants so diagnosed experience normalization of gut motility within 1 year. Therefore, many of the observed abnormalities could be within normal range and, in general, the diagnosis should be reserved for florid pathologic cases (537).

Other Related Conditions

In zonal aganglionosis or "skip-segment" Hirschsprung's disease, ganglion cells are found distal to one or more aganglionic segments (537–539). The problem here is that a rectal biopsy specimen may yield ganglion cells despite an authentic, more proximal Hirschsprung's-like aganglionic lesion. Immaturity of ganglion cells (398,526,530) and hypogenesis of the myenteric plexus (520,526) have also been reported to cause signs and symptoms similar to Hirschsprung's disease.

Amyloidosis

The gastrointestinal tract is commonly involved in systemic amyloidosis, with the prevalence estimated to be 70% in primary cases and 50% in secondary cases (540,541). Secondary (AA-type) amyloidosis preferentially deposits in the lamina propria and the walls of blood vessels, whereas primary or myeloma-associated amyloidosis (AL-type) accumulates in blood vessel walls and in the muscularis propria (497,542). Although subcutaneous abdominal fat biopsy or aspiration stained with Congo red is the simplest way to obtain a sample (543), rectal biopsy is still widely used to demonstrate amyloid (544). I have seen cases of amyloidosis closely mimic the increased subepithelial collagen deposition of collagenous colitis; usually, however, amyloidosis lacks the surface epithelial damage and epithelial lymphocytosis. Amyloid stains should be performed in difficult cases.

DEVELOPMENTAL ABNORMALITIES OF THE INTESTINE

Congenital Diverticula, Duplications, and Enteric Cysts

Meckel's Diverticulum

Meckel's diverticulum, an outpouching on the antimesenteric border of the terminal ileum approximately 20 cm from the ileocecal valve, represents the persistence of the embryologic omphalomesenteric duct. It is the most common intestinal congenital anomaly (found in 1% to 2% of the general population) and is usually an incidental finding. The rare symptomatic patient may have (1) intestinal obstruction, (2) ulcer with hemorrhage, (3) perforation, or (4) diverticulitis (545–547). Microscopic examination reveals small intestinal mucosa alone lining the diverticulum in about 50% to 70% of cases. Ectopic gastric or pancreatic tissues are found in the remainder and are usually encountered in the distal portion of the diverticulum (546,548).

Other Small Intestinal Diverticula and Enterogenous Cysts

Most small bowel diverticula are multiple and are believed to be acquired (512). Isolated intestinal diverticula have much in common with enteric or enterogenous cysts and are probably developmental anomalies (334). Diverticula or simple outpouchings of the mucosa into or through the muscularis propria are usually lined by small intestinal–type epithelium, but heterotopic gastric epithelium can occasionally be found. Enterogenous cysts may be found in the wall of the small bowel, in the mesentery, in the posterior mediastinum, or in the retrorectal space. The walls of such cysts are usually composed of irregularly oriented smooth muscle, and the cyst is lined by respiratory, small intestinal, or gastric epithelium. Diverticula and enterogenous cysts of foregut origin are almost invariably associated with vertebral body abnormalities, an association not noted with more distal cysts. Enterogenous cysts and diverticula associated with vertebral abnormalities are thought to be caused by failure of the notochord or ingrowing mesoderm to separate the ectoderm from the endoderm. This mechanism would account for (1) the failure of the vertebrae to form properly and (2) the adherence of these developing gut remnants to the vertebrae (334).

Intestinal Duplications

The rare duplications of the small intestine or colon consist of partial or complete doubling of a variable length of bowel. The duplicated segments usually lie within the mesentery of the normal bowel and may or may not communicate with the lumen (334). Duplications differ from enteric cysts and congenital diverticula by demonstrating more organized smooth muscle, often with nerve plexi, within the wall, and are not associated with vertebral body abnormalities. Hindgut duplications may be associated with complex genital and urinary tract abnormalities.

Developmental Cysts of the Retrorectal Space

The major types of retrorectal developmental cysts are epidermoid (dermoid) cysts, rectal duplication cysts, and the cystic hamartomas (tailgut cysts) (549–551). Their main distinguishing features are summarized in Table 23.

Developmental cysts in the retrorectal space are susceptible to infection and fistula, and there have been rare reports of associated malignancy (550). Therefore, total excision is recommended.

MISCELLANEOUS CONDITIONS AFFECTING THE INTESTINE

Pneumatosis Cystoides Intestinalis

Pneumatosis cystoides intestinalis (PCI) is the occurrence of multiple gas-filled cysts in the gastrointestinal tract. It occurs in benign and fulminant forms (552,553). The fulminant form is most often seen in infants, in whom it complicates ischemic bowel injury, and is probably due to mural invasion and overgrowth by gas-forming bacteria with subsequent formation of gas cysts. The fulminant form occurs rarely in adults, in whom it is associated with drugs or chemotherapy or with ischemic or pseudomembranous enterocolitis (553). Microscopic analysis of fulminant PCI demonstrates gas cysts in the submucosa, compounding a picture of ischemic bowel infarct with secondary bacterial overgrowth. The pathologist often ignores the gas cysts or mistakes them for cutting artifact. Occasionally, an endothelial or histiocytic lining may be seen, but this is far more common in the benign form of the disease.

Adults more often demonstrate the benign form of PCI. Although benign PCI involving segments of bowel proximal to the terminal ileum is usually asymptomatic (552), PCI involving the terminal ileum or colon may cause diarrhea, constipation, rectal bleeding, or other symptoms (552,554). It is often associated with conditions that either increase intraluminal pressure or provide a break in mucosal integrity by which gas may enter the bowel wall. These diseases include chronic obstructive pulmonary disease, emphysema, diverticulitis, appendicitis, cholelithiasis, peptic ulcer, trauma, CD, or complications resulting from previous gastrointestinal tract surgery (552,553). Histologically, there may be tears in the submucosal connective tissue in the benign form of PCI, but more usually one encounters dilated spaces lined totally or partially by endothelium, chronic inflammatory cells, histiocytes, and foreign-body giant cells.

The differential diagnosis includes consideration of an entity termed *pseudolipomatosis* (555,556) (Fig. 41). Pseudolipomatosis resembles fatty infiltration of the lamina propria, and, indeed, reports of cases showing such fatty infiltration as a sign of chronic IBD are probably describing and illustrating pseudolipomatosis. Ultrastructural study has convincingly shown that the lipid-like spaces are, in reality, gas cysts. Their presence in the lamina propria may be related to excessive air inflation used to distend the bowel during colonoscopy, or to cleaning agents used to disinfect the colonoscopes.

Radiation and Antineoplastic Chemotherapy Injury

Acute Changes

The histology of acute enteritis or colitis associated with radiation and antineoplastic chemotherapeutic agents is similar. Necrosis, ulcer, and acute and chronic inflammation involving the mucosa may be seen, usually within 2 weeks after cessation of therapy (456,557–561). The epithelium lining crypts often shows marked cellular enlargement, with large atypical nuclei and mucin depletion (Fig. 42). Apoptotic bodies similar to those seen in the "exploding crypt lesion" of GVHD may be prominent (562,563). Typically, the abnormalities subside in 1 to 2 months (558,559).

The epithelial atypia associated with radiation and chemotherapy can be alarming because it may simulate the appearance of metastatic or primary carcinoma. Features that favor the presence of acute chemotherapy or radiation effect rather than carcinoma include (1) general preservation of mucosal architecture, (2) bizarre atypia beyond that seen in carcinoma, (3) preservation of a relatively low nuclear-cytoplasmic ratio despite the presence of atypia, (4) lack of mitotic figures, (5) recognition of similar atypical changes in nearby fibroblasts and endothelium, and (6) lack of an infiltrative pattern or tumor desmoplasia (564).

Late Effects

Late complications of radiation, which may occur from a few weeks to many years after therapy (557), include enterocolitis, stricture, ulcer, and fistula (565). Histologically, the mucosa is atrophic. Blood vessels in the lamina propria

TABLE 23. *Developmental cysts of the retrorectal space*

Feature	Epidermoid (demoid) cysts	Rectal duplication cysts	Retrorectal cystic hamartoma (tailgut cysts)
Gross features	Unilocular	Unilocular	Multilocular; ± solid areas
Cyst lining	Squamous epithelium ± skin adnexa	Colonic, gastric, or respiratory	Squamous, transitional, and glandular
Smooth-muscle wall	No	Yes; organized; recapitulates muscularis propria	Yes; disorganized bundles
Other findings	—	—	Foreign-body giant-cell granulomatous inflammation occasionally noted

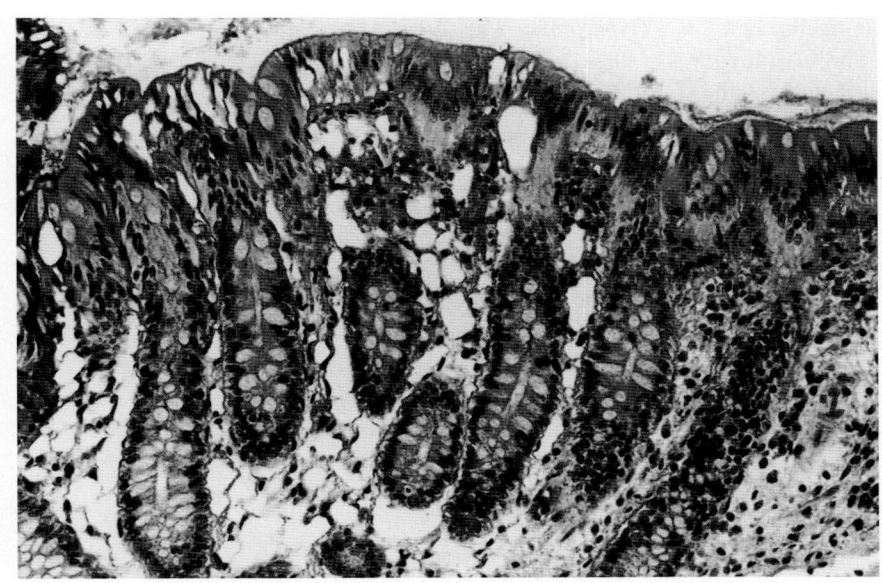

FIG. 41. Pseudolipomatosis. The tiny gas cysts characteristically involve the lamina propria and resemble fat infiltration.

and submucosa may be ectatic, and patchy fibrosis is noted in the submucosa, muscularis propria, and serosa. The fibrosis can be quite extensive, have a "hyalinized" quality, and contain larger, atypical "radiation" fibroblasts, although their presence is not pathognomonic for radiation injury. Vascular changes include intimal fibroplasia, accumulations of foamy macrophages, and hyalin thickening of the walls, all of which result in luminal stenosis. Indeed, many of the late complications of radiation exposure may, in fact, be due to ischemia related to vascular changes.

Small Bowel Transplantation and Rejection

Human small bowel transplantation has been attempted at several centers in the United States and Europe. The original efforts were unsuccessful because the complex immunologic reactions (rejection and GVHD) could not be controlled (566). Introduction of immunosuppressive agents such as cyclosporin A and tacrolimus has resulted in a new era of clinical small bowel transplantation, with reports of modest successes (566,567).

Endoscopic mucosal biopsy is used to monitor rejection episodes (566,568). In general, the histologic changes of small bowel rejection are similar in humans and in animal models (566–571). Damage caused by cold ischemic time associated with graft transportation and surgery (epithelial denudation, regenerative crypt epithelium, mild acute inflammation) usually resolves in 3 days (572). Acute cellular rejection occurs in weeks to months after transplantation, and consists of focal increases in transformed lymphocytes in the gut-associated lymphoid tissues accompanied by crypt epithelial damage and apoptosis (572,573), increased

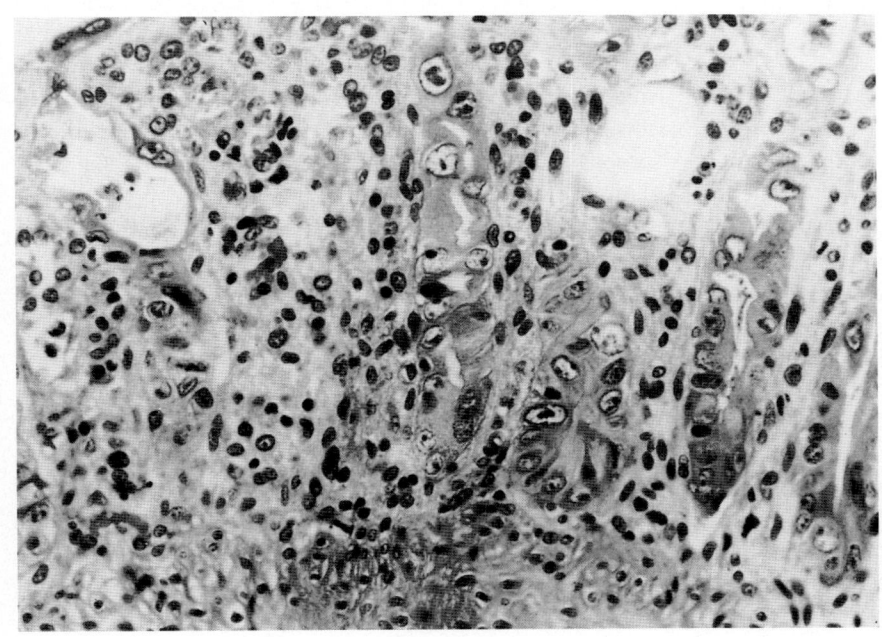

FIG. 42. Colonic biopsy specimen demonstrating antineoplastic chemotherapy effect. The enlarged cells with large atypical nuclei are alarming. However, the cells do not exhibit an infiltrative pattern of growth and maintain a relatively low nuclear to cytoplasmic size ratio.

chronic inflammation in the lamina propria, epithelial lymphocytosis, and lymphocytic "vasculitis." The histology closely mimics GVHD, which also occurs in patients with small bowel transplantation; indeed, the distinction sometimes cannot be made histologically unless the location of the biopsy (i.e., graft versus native bowel) is known with certainty (569). Fibrosis of the bowel wall and vascular sclerosis characterize chronic rejection. The histologic picture in patients with small bowel transplants can be compounded by coexisting Epstein-Barr virus infection and the related development of posttransplant lymphoproliferative disorders and spindle cell nodules (573).

Fibrosing Colonopathy in Cystic Fibrosis

The term *fibrosing colonopathy* has been applied to fusiform strictures of the colon found in some children with cystic fibrosis (574,575). The pathologic change is severe submucosal fibrosis that has been linked to the administration of high-strength pancreatic supplements.

Nonneoplastic Tumors of the Intestine

Infarcted Epiploic Appendices

Epiploic appendices are pedunculated, mesothelial-covered accumulations of fat located on the lateral aspects of the colon. The pedicles of these collections of fat are thin and tenuous; occasionally they may twist, leading to infarct or even amputation. Infarcted epiploic appendices are firm, gray-white nodules that, at surgery, may grossly mimic metastatic carcinoma. The subsequent biopsy specimen is often the source of confusion to the pathologist who is asked to identify it at frozen section. Microscopically, infarcted epiploic appendices usually show zonation, with infarcted, mummified adipose tissue in the central portion. More peripherally, variable amounts of fat necrosis and calcification are seen. The outermost portion is usually fibrotic and inflamed (334,576).

Barium Granuloma

Extravasation of barium sulfate outside the confines of the gut lumen may elicit a granulomatous response referred to as *barium granuloma*. It is usually encountered as an incidental finding in resection specimens for IBD or other conditions; however, rarely it can produce a polypoid or ulcerative lesion that mimics neoplasm (334,577). Microscopically, barium sulfate appears olive green and crystalline. The small granular crystals are found in clusters within connective tissue or macrophages. Although barium sulfate does not bend polarized light, it is dramatically refractile and is best demonstrated with the microscope condenser lowered. Water-soluble contrast media such as Gastrografin tend not to elicit inflammatory responses and morphologically are composed of large rectangular or rhomboid-like light tan to yellow crystals.

Hyperplastic Pacinian Corpuscle

Pacinian corpuscles occur in many parts of the body, including the mesentery of the gut around the pancreas (578). For unknown reasons, these intraabdominal pacinian corpuscles may occasionally enlarge up to 1 cm or more in diameter and grossly simulate tumor implants or carcinomatosis (578–580). They may be a source of confusion and embarrassment to the pathologist who is asked to identify them at frozen section. Histologically, this specialized end-organ resembles its cutaneous counterpart. There is usually a central blood vessel and nerve ending in the inner core, surrounded by 14 to 45 tortuous, roughly concentric, lamellae. Hyperplastic pacinian corpuscle is usually confused with a nematode; however, pacinian corpuscles lack a cuticle or internal structures.

THE VERMIFORM APPENDIX

Specimen Processing and Normal Histology

The vermiform appendix, the slender tubular extension of the posterior medial cecum, can vary remarkably in length. The four layers of the appendiceal wall (mucosa, submucosa, muscularis externa, and serosa) are similar to the remainder of the gut. Generally, the histologic composition of the appendix is similar to that of the colon (581).

Gross dissection and processing are generally straightforward. Descriptions should include the size and appearance of the appendix. Luminal patency should be assessed. The focality and regional distribution of any unusual lesion or change should be recorded. The distal tip should be closely inspected for carcinoid tumors because they commonly occur in this region (582,583). Routine sections of the tip are standard at most institutions. A longitudinal section of the distal tip is often difficult to orient and cut; therefore, we prefer a cross section of the distal end of the appendix. In the usual specimen, 1-cm serial cross-sections are performed along the entire length of the appendix. In addition to the section of the tip, two additional cross sections, one from the middle and one from the proximal line of resection, should always be examined histologically. Because appendiceal neoplasia is often discovered only during microscopic evaluation of an otherwise typical appendicitis specimen, we routinely sample the margin of resection. Otherwise, it could be difficult to reconstruct the gross specimen to assess the adequacy of the excision (581).

Developmental Abnormalities

The appendix rarely is congenitally absent or hypoplastic. These changes may be associated with either a normal or malformed cecum (334). Duplication of the appendix may occur with a normal-appearing cecum or may be associated with cecal duplication (584). Diverticula infrequently involve the appendix. Most are acquired, either from obstruction of the appendiceal orifice by neoplasm or from other conditions associated with increased intraluminal pressure (e.g., cystic fibrosis) (585).

Inflammatory Conditions

Acute Appendicitis

Acute appendicitis results from a combination of bacterial proliferation and ischemic damage, often precipitated by luminal obstruction by fecalith (586). Resection specimens usually demonstrate serosal erythema, adhesion, or exudate. Areas of perforation may be present; on cross section, the lumen often contains blood-tinged pus.

Histologic changes of early acute appendicitis can be quite minimal and consist of focal collections of neutrophils within the lumen and lamina propria (334,581,587). Focal erosions, cryptitis, and crypt abscess formation occur somewhat later. Most specimens, however, show extensive suppuration extending deep into or through the appendiceal wall.

Complications of acute appendicitis include perforation, peritonitis, and periappendiceal abscess. Although *Actinomyces israelii* may occasionally be present in the lumen of an appendix as a commensal, in the milieu of appendicitis and chronic appendiceal abscess, *Actinomyces* species should also be considered pathogens. Actinomycosis should also be considered in any patient in whom a fistula or sinus tract develops following appendectomy (334).

Whether acute appendicitis becomes chronic or whether it can be recognized in a chronic state has been long debated (334). Fibrous obliteration of the appendix is probably not a consequence of acute appendicitis (588), because fibrous obliteration shows no association with signs or symptoms of appendicitis (586,588). However, prominent fibrosis, a marked chronic inflammatory cell infiltrate within the wall, and granulation tissue are abnormal and support a diagnosis of organizing appendicitis (582). In occasional specimens, the appendiceal wall is infiltrated by eosinophilic leukocytes with no other apparent abnormality (586). This change may reflect the presence of appendicitis elsewhere in the specimen that was not sampled, but the possibility remains that it may represent appendicitis in a resolving phase or a manifestation of eosinophilic gastroenteritis (581).

Other Infections

Infection by the nematode *Enterobius vermicularis* (pinworm) is common in temperate and cold climates (589). The adult worms usually inhabit the colon; they may be associated with minute ulcers of the colonic mucosa but rarely cause symptoms. In appendectomy specimens, the worm is most frequently encountered as an incidental finding within the lumen (131). The adult worm is identified in cross section by its characteristic narrow lateral cuticular alae. Whether *E. vermicularis* causes appendicitis is debatable.

Infection with *Yersinia* species may demonstrate predominant appendiceal involvement. The pathologic changes are described earlier. Parasitic infestation of the appendix by *Schistosoma* species, although common, usually is not associated with signs or symptoms of acute appendicitis.

Fibrous Obliteration (Appendiceal Neuroma)

Fibrous obliteration/appendiceal neuroma of the vermiform appendix is a common finding in resection specimens, with a reported prevalence of nearly 30% (582,588). The process characteristically involves the distal tip, may progress for a variable length along the appendiceal lumen, and in some instance may obliterate the entire organ. Microscopically, the lumen is replaced by fibrous tissue and chronic inflammatory cells, usually accompanied by a nerve- and neuroendocrine-cell proliferation (588,590,591). Immunostaining for neuron-specific enolase and S-100 protein can be done to highlight this neural tissue proliferation (588,590).

The pathogenesis of the process remains unknown. Some authors believe that fibrous obliteration may be secondary to the hyperplasia of neuroendocrine cells (588,592). "Appendiceal carcinoids" are often reported in association with fibrous obliteration; perhaps the excellent prognosis of appendiceal carcinoid, when compared to other gut carcinoid tumors, relates to the fact that many reported cases may be exaggerated neuroendocrine cell hyperplasias seen in otherwise typical fibrous obliteration/appendiceal neuromas. I have strict criteria for the diagnosis of carcinoid tumors in the vermiform appendix. I require (1) collections of cells demonstrating a definite insular pattern of growth with extension of cells into or through the appendiceal muscular wall or (2) proliferations of neuroendocrine cells associated with a gross nodule or an expansion of the appendix.

Crohn's Disease of the Appendix

In patients with CD, the vermiform appendix is involved in approximately 25% of cases; however, CD first diagnosed in, and isolated to, the appendix is rare. Criteria for diagnosis are similar to those used elsewhere in the gastrointestinal tract and include granulomatous inflammation, transmural lymphoid aggregates, and fissuring-type ulcers. Infection with *Yersinia* species, *Mycobacterium* species, and *Actinomyces* species must be excluded. CD develops elsewhere in the gastrointestinal tract in less than 10% of patients with CD initially isolated to the appendix (593–597).

INFLAMMATORY LESIONS OF THE MESENTERY AND RETROPERITONEUM

Study of mesenteric and retroperitoneal inflammatory and fibrosing processes and analysis of cases falling into this category are hampered by the rarity of such lesions and the lack of standardized nomenclature. The differential diagnosis of fat necrotizing and fibrosing lesions of the mesentery and retroperitoneum is listed in Table 24 (334,598–601). Inflammatory processes of the kidney (e.g., xanthogranulomatous pyelonephritis), bowel (e.g., diverticulitis, ischemic bowel disease), appendix (e.g., perforating suppurative appendicitis, chronic periappendiceal abscess), and pancreas (e.g., pancreatitis with fat necrosis) can spread to involve the retroperitoneum and mesentery. The precise classification of these lesions depends on relative localization, demonstration of continuity with an involved organ, and clinical history. Surgical and other trauma can lead to fibrosis of the mesentery and retroperitoneum. Diagnosis in these cases is based mostly on history; the histology can suggest trauma when it contains hemosiderin deposits, capillary hemorrhage, postnecrotic pseudocysts, and cholesterol clefts (598,599). Malakoplakia, an abnormal immune response to gram-negative bacilli, can cause tumors at any site. Malakoplakia is characterized by xanthogranulomatous inflammation accompanied by the pathognomonic Michaelis-Gutman bodies.

Metastatic carcinomas can cause retroperitoneal and mesenteric fibrosis, inflammation, and fat necrosis, but should at least be suspected upon examination of H&E stained sections. The diagnosis of metastatic carcinoma can usually be confirmed with clinical history, mucin stains, or cytokeratin immunocytochemistry.

The sarcomas that enter into the differential diagnosis of mesenteric and retroperitoneal fibrosis and inflammation do so either by mimicking fat necrosis (liposarcoma) (602,603), or because of the associated inflammatory component (inflammatory malignant fibrous histiocytoma and inflammatory fibrosarcoma) (600). These sarcomas can usually be recognized by their distinctive vascularity, increased cellularity, nuclear atypism, and mitosis figures. In the case of inflammatory malignant fibrous histiocytoma, these atypical cells may be exceedingly rare and require close inspection of the inflammatory milieu.

TABLE 24. *Mesenteric/retroperitoneal inflammatory lesions: differential diagnosis*

Idiopathic retractile (sclerosing) mesenteritis
Trauma
Inflammation involving kidneys, bowel, appendix, pancreas
Malakoplakia
Retroperitoneal fibrosis (idiopathic and those associated with trauma or drugs)
Malignant lymphoma with sclerosis
Metastatic carcinoma (lobular breast carcinoma, signet ring carcinoma)
Retroperitoneal and mesenteric fibromatosis
Weber-Christian disease
Sclerosing peritonitis
Inflammatory myofibroblastic tumor
Liposarcoma
Retroperitoneal xanthogranulomatosis (with or without associated Erdheim–Chester disease)
Inflammatory malignant fibrous histiocytoma
Inflammatory fibrosarcoma
Whipple's disease

Non-Hodgkin's lymphoma involving the retroperitoneum and mesentery frequently is seen with dense fibrosis (604). Therefore, sclerosing lymphoma represents one of the most important differential diagnostic considerations in patients suspected of having idiopathic retroperitoneal fibrosis (IRF) or idiopathic retractile mesenteritis (IRM), mainly because lymphoma is more treatable. There may actually be an association between IRF and lymphoma. In one study, malignant lymphoma occurred in or developed in 15% of 53 patients with IRF (605). Even though IRF could be a premalignant condition, this high association could be explained by sampling error or the problems inherent in recognizing lymphoma in extranodal sites with only routine stains. Usually, retroperitoneal and mesenteric lymphomas demonstrate at least some areas of follicular or nodular growth in which the follicles closely approximate one another (in contrast to the widely scattered germinal centers of IRF and IRM). With a well-prepared H&E stain, one can frequently see the cytologic features of lymphomas (606). Demonstration of light chain restriction by immunocytochemistry or flow cytometry, or the identification of gene rearrangements by molecular techniques, should improve diagnostic accuracy.

Whipple's disease must be considered in the differential diagnosis of mesenteric and retroperitoneal fibrosis and panniculitis (599,607,608). The diagnosis is important to make because Whipple's disease is serious (causing irreversible central nervous system damage), easily curable (by appropriate antibiotic therapy), and fatal if left untreated. I routinely obtain a digested PAS stain on all biopsy specimens of mesentery or retroperitoneum that contain fat necrosis and foamy macrophages. The characteristic appearance of Whipple's disease in mesentery or retroperitoneal lymph nodes is lipogranulomatous inflammation associated with large round empty spaces. The diagnosis of Whipple's disease outside of the gut requires PAS positive staining plus electron microscopic or PCR verification of the bacillus.

After the exclusion of neoplasms and specific inflammatory and traumatic processes, one is still left with a long list of exotic idiopathic inflammatory and fibrosing processes of the mesentery and retroperitoneum that are not well understood (Table 24).

Idiopathic Retractile (Sclerosing) Mesenteritis

IRM is identified by a variety of names including mesenteric panniculitis, mesenteric lipodystrophy, lipogranuloma of mesentery, sclerosing lipogranulomatosis, primary liposclerosis of the mesentery, and multifocal subperitoneal sclerosis (598–601). IRM is a rare idiopathic nonneoplastic condition that leads to thickening and shortening of the small intestinal mesentery (Fig. 43). This process can fix and kink loops of small bowel, producing obstruction or a mass. Patients, usually middle-aged or elderly men, are typically seen with signs and symptoms of intestinal obstruction (598). A similar process can affect the colonic mesentery (609) and the retroperitoneum (retroperitoneal xanthogranulomatosis)

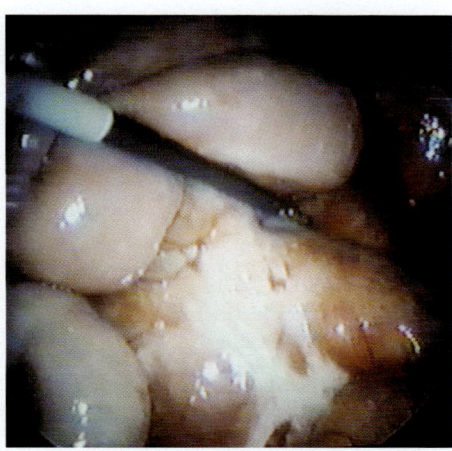

FIG. 43. Laparoscopic view of idiopathic retractile mesenteritis. The small bowel has been retracted to demonstrate a fibrosing process that has thickened and shortened the mesentery.

(600). Retroperitoneal xanthogranulomatosis can occur in an isolated form or can be associated with Erdheim-Chester disease (600) (multisystem fibroxanthomas usually presenting with bone pain and symmetric sclerotic lesions of long bones).

Histologic features of IRM include sclerosing fibrosis, fat necrosis with numerous lipid-laden macrophages, chronic inflammation with scattered germinal centers, and occasionally focal calcification (598,599) (Fig. 44). Polymorphonuclear leukocytes are rare, the vascularity meager, and the spindle cells lack nuclear atypism. Only rare mitotic figures are seen.

Weber-Christian Disease

Weber-Christian disease represents an inflammatory disorder of fat, often occurring in young women, that is usually characterized by multiple tender skin nodules. Patients have a relapsing clinical picture accompanied by fever and other systemic signs and symptoms (610). The histologic changes in the skin are those of panniculitis. Panniculitis of Weber-Christian disease can sometimes be seen in the pericardium, bone marrow (599,610), and retroperitoneum and mesentery where the histologic descriptions appear identical to IRM. Therefore, the diagnosis of Weber-Christian disease depends on an appropriate clinical picture with nodules of fat necrosis at multiple sites including the subcutaneous tissues.

Inflammatory Myofibroblastic Tumor (Inflammatory Pseudotumor)

Inflammatory myofibroblastic tumor has many clinical and histologic overlaps with IRM and may actually be a form of IRM (611). However, in the classic descriptions, there are several differences. Inflammatory myofibroblastic tumors are more typically described as grossly circumscribed tumors in contrast to the diffuse thickening of IRM. Patients with inflammatory myofibroblastic tumors are frequently children who often have fever, weight loss, anemia, leukocytosis, high sedimentation rate, thrombocytosis, and hypergammaglobulinemia. In contradistinction, IRM occurs in adults and systemic symptoms are rare. There is much histologic overlap between IRM and inflammatory myofibroblastic tumors, but the latter typically contain many more plasma cells and the associated fibrosis is more often laminated or whorled (598,612,613). A histologic variant of inflammatory myofibroblastic tumor that contains psammoma bodies can occur in the peritoneum (614).

Fibromatosis

Fibromatosis affecting the mesentery or retroperitoneum is sometimes referred to as fibrous dysplasia of the mesentery or intraabdominal desmoid. Fibromatosis is best thought of as neoplastic (598,599). It can be associated with the Gardner's syndrome variant of familial adenomatous polyposis, or can occur outside of that setting (602). Distinction from fibrosis related to trauma and from IRM can be difficult. Some keys to the diagnosis of fibromatosis include recognition of a uniform fibroblastic proliferation with areas of increased cellularity, an arrangement of spindle cells in interlacing bundles, a tendency for the spindle cells to infiltrate the muscularis externa of the intestines and adipose tissue, and a paucity of inflammatory and foam cells (598,599).

Idiopathic Retroperitoneal Fibrosis

IRF describes a condition in which fibrosis develops in the retroperitoneum and is frequently centered on the aortic bifurcation, anterior to the L4-5 vertebrae. The fibrotic process spreads to involve various portions of the retroperitoneum and mesentery (598–600). IRF, like IRM, is usually not well circumscribed. The fibrosis is frequently associated with prominent plasma cells, scattered germinal centers, and occasionally a mononuclear cell "vasculitis" (598). Typically,

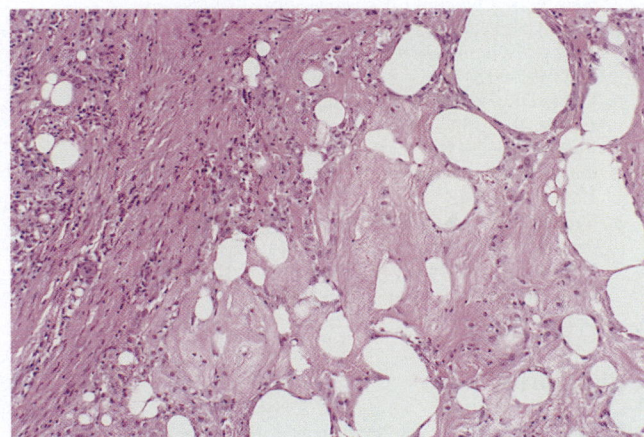

FIG. 44. Histologic appearance of idiopathic retractile mesenteritis illustrating fat necrosis, fibrosis, and chronic inflammation.

neutrophils and foamy macrophages are sparse. Some cases of retroperitoneal fibrosis have been associated with drugs such as methysergide. Others have been associated with a syndrome of multifocal fibrosclerosis (inflammatory sclerosing lesions of the mediastinum, sclerosis of major bile ducts, Riedel's thyroiditis, inflammatory pseudotumor of the orbit). Some investigators believe that the idiopathic form of retroperitoneal fibrosis may be caused by an autoimmune response to antigens associated with atherosclerotic plaque (600).

Sclerosing Peritonitis

Sclerosing peritonitis is an inflammatory and fibrosing process affecting the visceral peritoneum that can cause a dramatic clinical appearance referred to as *abdominal cocooning* or *peritonitis fibroplastica encapsulatum* (598,599). A fibrous membrane encases the small bowel. In addition, some patients have an oculocutaneous syndrome of dry eyes with itchy, scaly skin lesions (598). Some cases are idiopathic, but most have been associated with chronic peritoneal dialysis, or with use of beta-adrenergic blocking agents such as propranolol and practolol. As the name implies, the sclerosing peritonitis principally involves the peritoneum and only infiltrates the mesentery at its attachment site, usually without involvement of the retroperitoneum.

REFERENCES

Small Bowel Biopsy

1. Trier JS. Diagnostic value of per oral biopsy of the proximal small intestine. *N Engl J Med* 1971;285:1470–1473.
2. Achkar E, Carey WD, Petras R, Sivak MV, Revta R. Comparison of suction capsule and endoscopic biopsy of small bowel mucosa. *Gastrointest Endosc* 1986;32:278–281.
3. Dandalides WM, Carey WD, Petras RE, Achkar E. Endoscopic small bowel mucosal biopsy: a controlled trial evaluating forcep size and biopsy location in the diagnosis of normal and abnormal mucosal architecture. *Gastrointest Endosc* 1989;35:197–200.
4. Dobbins WO III. Small bowel biopsy in malabsorptive states. In: Norris HT, ed. *Pathology of the colon, small intestine, and anus,* 2nd ed. New York: Churchill Livingstone, 1991:137–188.
5. Segal GH, Petras RE. The small intestine. In: Sternberg SS, ed. *Histology for pathologists,* 2nd ed. Philadelphia: Lippincott-Raven, 1997:495–518.
6. Perera DR, Weinstein WM, Rubin CE. Small intestinal biopsy. *Hum Pathol* 1975;6:157–217.
7. Rex DK, Jersild RA. Further characterization of the pigment in pseudomelanosis duodeni in three patients. *Gastroenterology* 1988;95:177–182.
8. Shepherd NA, Crocker PR, Smith AP, Levison DA. Exogenous pigment in Peyer's patches. *Hum Pathol* 1987;18:50–54.
9. Urbanski SJ, Arsenault AL, Green FHY, Haber G. Pigment resembling atmospheric dust in Peyer's patches. *Mod Pathol* 1989;2:222–226.

Celiac Sprue

10. Katz AJ, Grand RJ. All that flattens is not "sprue." *Gastroenterology* 1979;76:375–377.
11. Kagroff MF, Paterson YJ, Kumar PJ, et al. Evidence for the role of human intestinal adenovirus in the pathogenesis of coeliac disease. *Gut* 1987;28:995–1001.
12. Rubin CE, Brandborg LL, Phelps PC, et al. Studies of celiac disease. The apparent identical and specific nature of the duodenal and proximal jejunal lesions in celiac diseases and idiopathic sprue. *Gastroenterology* 1960;38:28–49.
13. Rubin CE, Eidelman S, Weinstein WM. Sprue by any other name. *Gastroenterology* 1970;58:409–413.
14. Walker-Smith JA, Guardlini S, Schmitz J, Shmerling PH, Visakorpi JK. Revised criteria for diagnosis of coeliac disease. *Arch Dis Child* 1990;65:909–911.
15. Vogelsang H, Genser O, Wyatt J, et al. Screening for celiac disease: a prospective study on the value of noninvasive tests. *Am J Gastroenterol* 1995;90:394–398.
16. Valdimarsson T, Fransen L, Grodzinsky E, Skogh T, Strom M. Is small bowel biopsy necessary in adults with suspected celiac disease and IgA anti-endomesial antibodies? 100% positive predictive value for celiac disease in adults. *Dig Dis Sci* 1996;41:83–87.
17. Barnes GL, Townley RRW. Duodenal mucosal damage in 31 infants with gastroenteritis. *Arch Dis Child* 1973;48:343–349.
18. Swanson VL, Thomasson RW. Pathology the jejunal mucosa in tropical sprue. *Am J Pathol* 1965;46:511–551.
19. Ament ME, Shimoda SS, Saunders DR, Rubin CE. Pathogenesis of steatorrhea in three cases of small intestinal stasis syndrome. *Gastroenterology* 1972;63:728–747.
20. Matucharski C, Colin R, Hemet J, et al. Cavitation of mesenteric lymph nodes, splenic atrophy, and a flat small intestinal mucosa. *Gastroenterology* 1984;87:606–614.
21. Barry RE, Read AE. Coeliac disease and malignancy. *Q J Med* 1973;42:665–675.

Protein Allergies

22. Baker AL, Rosenberg IH. Refractory sprue: recovery after removal of nongluten dietary proteins. *Ann Intern Med* 1978;89:505–508.
23. Kuitenen P, Visakorpi JK, Savilahti E, et al. Malabsorption syndromes with cow's milk intolerance. *Arch Dis Child* 1975;50:351–356.
24. Ament ME, Rubin CE. Soy protein—another cause of the flat intestinal lesion. *Gastroenterology* 1972;62:227–234.
25. Nagata S, Yamashiro Y, Ohtsuka Y, et al. Quantitative analysis and immunohistochemical studies on small intestinal mucosa of food-sensitive enteropathy. *J Pediatr Gastroenterol Nutr* 1995;20:44–48.

Lymphocytic Enterocolitis

26. DuBois RN, Lazenby AJ, Yardley JH, Hendrix TR, Bayless TM, Giardiello FM. Lymphocytic enterocolitis in patients with "refractory sprue." *JAMA* 1989;262:935–937.
27. Wolber R, Owen D, Freeman H. Colonic lymphocytosis in patients with celiac sprue. *Hum Pathol* 1990;21:1092–1096.
28. Wolber R, Owen D, DelBuono L, Appelman H, Freeman H. Lymphocytic gastritis in patients with celiac sprue or spruelike intestinal disease. *Gastroenterology* 1990;98:310–315.
29. Dobbins WO, Rubin CE. Studies of rectal mucosa in celiac sprue. *Gastroenterology* 1964;47:471–478.
30. Austin LA, Dobbins WO. Studies of the rectal mucosa in coelic sprue: the intraepithelial lymphocyte. *Gut* 1988;29:200–205.

Entities Associated with Variable Villus Abnormality and Crypt Hypoplasia

31. Brunser O, Reid A, Monckeberg F, Maccioni A, Contreres I. Jejunal biopsies in infant malnutrition: with special reference to mitotic index. *Pediatrics* 1966;38:605–611.
32. Barbezat GO, Bowie MD, Kaschula ROC, Hansen JDL. Studies on the small intestinal mucosa of children with protein-calorie malnutrition. *S Afr Med J* 1967;41:1031–1036.
33. Foroozan P, Trier JS. Mucosa of the small intestine in pernicious anemia. *N Engl J Med* 1967;277:553–559.
34. Bianchi A, Chipman DW, Dreskin A, Rosensweig NS. Nutritional folic acid deficiency with megaloblastic changes in the small-bowel epithelium. *N Engl J Med* 1970;282:859–861.
35. Smith FP, Kisner DL, Widerlite L, Schein PS. Chemotherapeutic al-

teration of small intestinal morphology and function: a progress report. *Clin Gastroenterol* 1979;1:203–207.
36. Trier JS, Browning TH. Morphologic response of the mucosa of the human small intestine to x-ray exposure. *J Clin Invest* 1966;45:194–204.
37. Houtman PM, Hofstra SS, Spoelstra P. Non-celiac sprue possibly related to methotrexate in a rheumatoid arthritis patient. *Netherlands J Med* 1995;47:113–116.

Microvillus Inclusion Disease

38. Davidson GP, Cutz E, Hamilton JR, et al. Familial enteropathy: a syndrome of protracted diarrhea from birth, failure to thrive, and hypoplastic villus atrophy. *Gastroenterology* 1978;75:783–790.
39. Oliva MM, Perman JA, Saavedra JM, Young-Ramsaran J, Schwartz KB. Successful intestinal transplantation for microvillus inclusion disease. *Gastroenterology* 1994;106:771–774.
40. Bell SW, Kerner JA Jr, Sibley RK. Microvillus inclusion disease. The importance of electron microscopy for diagnosis. *Am J Surg Pathol* 1991;15:1157–1164.
41. Cutz E, Rhoades JM, Drumm B, Sherman PN, Durie PR, Forstner GG. Microvillus inclusion disease; an inherited defect of brush-border assembly and differentiation. *N Engl J Med* 1989;320:646–651.
42. Groisman GM, Ben-Izhak O, Schwersenz A, Berant M, Fyfe B. The value of polyclonal carcinoembryonic antigen immunostaining in the diagnosis of microvillus inclusion disease. *Hum Pathol* 1993;24:1232–1237.

Dermatitis Herpetiformis

43. Gawkrodger DJ, Blackwell JN, Gilmour HM, Rifkind EA, Heading RC, Barnetson St RC. Dermatitis herpetiformis: diagnosis, diet and demography. *Gut* 1984;25:151–157.
44. Garioch JJ, Lewis HM, Sargent SA, Leonard JN, Fry L. 25 years' experience of gluten-free diet in the treatment of dermatitis herpetiformis. *Br J Dermatol* 1994;131:541–545.
45. Brow JR, Parker F, Weinstein WM, Rubin CE. The small intestinal mucosa in dermatitis herpetiformis I. Severity and distribution of the small intestinal lesion and associated malabsorption. *Gastroenterology* 1971;60:355–361.
46. Weinstein WM, Brow JR, Parker F, Rubin CE. The small intestinal mucosa in dermatitis herpetiformis: II. Relationship of the small intestinal lesion to gluten. *Gastroenterology* 1971;60:362–368.
47. Scott BB, Losowsky MS. Patchiness and duodenal-jejunal variation of the mucosal abnormality in coeliac disease and dermatitis herpetiformis. *Gut* 1976;17:984–992.

Tropical Sprue

48. Brunser O, Eidelman S, Klipstein FA. Intestinal morphology of rural Haitians: a comparison between overt tropical sprue and asymptomatic subjects. *Gastroenterology* 1970;58:655–668.
49. Klipstein FA, Schenk EA. Enterotoxigenic intestinal bacteria in tropical sprue II. Effects of the bacteria and their enterotoxins on intestinal structure. *Gastroenterology* 1975;68:642–655.
50. Haghighi P, Wolf PL. Tropical sprue and subclinical enteropathy: a vision for the nineties. *Crit Rev Clin Lab Sci* 1997;34:313–341.

Infectious Gastroenteritis

51. Schreiber BS, Blacklow NR, Trier JS. The mucosal lesion of the proximal small intestine in acute infectious nonbacterial gastroenteritis. *N Engl J Med* 1973;288:1318–1323.
52. Agus SG, Dolin R, Wyatt RG, Tousimis AJ, Northrup RS. Acute infectious nonbacterial gastroenteritis: intestinal histopathology. *Ann Intern Med* 1973;79:18–25.

Stasis Syndromes

53. King CE, Toskes PP. Small intestinal bacterial overgrowth. *Gastroenterology* 1979;76:1035–1055.

Zollinger-Ellison Syndrome

54. Fang M, Ginsburg AL, Glassman L, et al. Zollinger-Ellison syndrome with diarrhea as the predominant clinical feature. *Gastroenterology* 1979;76:378–387.

Mastocytosis

55. Ammann RW, Vetter D, Deyhle P, Tschen H, Sulser H, Schmid M. Gastrointestinal involvement in systemic mastocytosis. *Gut* 1976;17:107–112.
56. Mutter RD, Tannenbaum M, Ultmann JE. Systemic mast cell disease. *Ann Intern Med* 1963;59:887–906.
57. Fishman RS, Flemming CR, Li C. Systemic mastocytosis with review of gastrointestinal manifestations. *Mayo Clin Proc* 1979;54:51–54.
58. Scott BB, Hardy GJ, Losowsky MS. Involvement of the small intestine in systemic mast cell disease. *Gut* 1975;16:918–924.

Duodenitis and Peptic Ulcer Disease

59. Kreuning J, Bossman FT, Kuiper G, van der Wal AM, Lindeman J. Gastric and duodenal mucosa in "healthy" individuals: an endoscopic and histopathological study of 50 volunteers. *J Clin Pathol* 1978;31:69–77.
60. Goldman H, Antonioli DA. Mucosal biopsy of the esophagus, stomach, and proximal duodenum. *Hum Pathol* 1982;13:423–448.
61. Leonard N, Feighery CF, Hourihane DO. Peptic duodenitis—does it exist in the second part of the duodenum? *J Clin Pathol* 1997;50:54–58.
62. Jeffers MD, Hourihane DO. Coeliac disease with histological features of peptic duodenitis: value of assessment of intraepithelial lymphocytes. *J Clin Pathol* 1993;46:420–424.
63. Graham DY, Klein PD. *Campylobacter pyloridis* in, gastritis: the past, the present, and speculations about the future. *Am J Gastroenterol* 1987;82:283–286.
64. Goodwin CS, Armstrong JA, Marshall BJ. *Campylobacter pyloridis*, gastritis, and peptic ulceration. *J Clin Pathol* 1986;39:353–365.
65. Khulusi S, Badve S, Patel P, et al. Pathogenesis of gastric metaplasia of the human duodenum: role of *Helicobacter pylori*, gastric acid and ulceration. *Gastroenterology* 1996;110:452–458.
66. Gormally SM, Kierce BM, Daly LE, et al. Gastric metaplasia and duodenal ulcer disease in children infected by *Helicobacter pylori*. *Gut* 1996;38:513–517.
67. Lessels AM, Martin DF. Heterotopic gastric mucosa in the duodenum. *J Clin Pathol* 1982;35:591–595.
68. Nowak M, Deppisch L. Giant heterotopic gastric polyp in the jejunum. *Arch Pathol Lab Med* 1998;122:90–93.
69. Wolff M. Heterotopic gastric epithelium in the rectum. A report of three new cases with a review of 87 cases of gastric heterotopia in the alimentary canal. *Am J Clin Pathol* 1971;55:604–616.

Autoimmune Enteropathy

70. Unsworth J, Hutchins P, Mitchell J, et al. Flat small intestinal mucosa and auto-antibodies against the gut epithelium. *J Pediatr Gastroenterol Nutr* 1982;1:503–513.
71. Mirakian R, Richardson A, Milla PJ, et al. Protracted diarrhoea of infancy: evidence in support of an autoimmune variant. *BMJ* 1986;293:1132–1136.
72. Corazza GR, Biagi F, Volta U, Andreani ML, DeFranceschi L, Gasbarrini G. Autoimmune enteropathy and villous atrophy in adults. *Lancet* 1997;350:106–109.
73. Pearson RD, Swebsib I, Schaenk EA, Klish WJ, Brown MR. Fatal multisystem disease with immune enteropathy heralded by juvenile rheumatoid arthritis. *J Pediatr Gastroenterol Nutr* 1989;8:259–265.
74. Catassi C, Mirakian R, Natalini G, et al. Unresponsive enteropathy associated with circulating enterocyte autoantibodies in a boy with common variable hypogammaglobulinemia and type I diabetes. *J Pediatr Gastroenterol Nutr* 1988;7:608–613.
75. Martino-Villa JM, Rugueiro JR, De Juan D, et al. T-lymphocyte dysfunctions occurring together with apical gut epithelial cell autoantibodies. *Gastroenterology* 1991;101:390–397.

76. Hill SM, Milla PJ, Bottazzo GF, Mirakian R. Autoimmune enteropathy and colitis: is there a generalised autoimmune gut disorder? *Gut* 1991;32:36–42.
77. Steffen R, Wyllie R, Kay M, Kyllonen K, Gramlich T, Petras R. Autoimmune enteropathy in a pediatric patient: partial response to tacrolimus therapy. *Clin Pediatr* 1997;36:295–299.
78. Seidman EG, Lucaille F, Russo P, Galeano N, Murphy G, Roy CC. Successful treatment of autoimmune enteropathy with cyclosporine. *J Pediatr* 1990;117:929–932.
79. Sanderson IR, Phillips AD, Spencer J, Walker-Smith JA. Response of autoimmune enteropathy to cyclosporin A therapy. *Gut* 1991;32:1421–1425.
80. Bousvaros A, Leichtner AM, Book L, et al. Treatment of pediatric autoimmune enteropathy with tacrolimus. *Gastroenterology* 1996;111:237–243.

Torkelson Syndrome

81. Smith LJ, Szymanski W, Foulston C, Jewell L, Pabst H. Torkelson syndrome: life-threatening secretory diarrhea, distinctive small bowel morphology and variable immunodeficiency. *Gastroenterology* 1992;102:A698.

Collagenous Sprue

82. Weinstein WM, Saunders DR, Tytgat GN, Rubin CE. Collagenous sprue—an unrecognized type of malabsorption. *N Engl J Med* 1970;283:1297–1301.
83. Bossart R, Henry K, Booth CC, Doe WF. Subepithelial collagen in intestinal malabsorption. *Gut* 1975;16:18–22.

Immunodeficiency Syndromes (Excluding AIDS)

84. Eidelman S. Intestinal lesions in immune deficiency. *Hum Pathol* 1976;7:427–434.
85. Eidelman S, Davis SD, Rubin CE. Immunologic studies in "hypogammaglobulinemic sprue." *Clin Res* 1968;16:117.
86. Washington K, Stenzel TT, Buckley RE, Gottfried MR. Gastrointestinal pathology in patients with common variable immunodeficiency and X-linked agammaglobulinemia. *Am J Surg Pathol* 1996;20:1240–1252.

Whipple's Disease

87. Comer GM, Brandt LJ, Abissi CJ. Whipple's disease: a review. *Am J Gastroenterol* 1983;78:107–114.
88. Dobbins WO III, Kawanishi H. Bacillary characteristics in Whipple's disease: an electron microscopic study. *Gastroenterology* 1981;80:1468–1475.
89. Maizel H, Ruffin JM, Dobbins WO III. Whipple's disease: a review of 19 patients from one hospital and a review of the literature since 1950. *Medicine* 1979;49:175–201.
90. Keinath RD, Vlietstra MR, Dobbins WO III. Antibiotic treatment and relapse in Whipple's disease: long-term follow up of 88 patients. *Gastroenterology* 1985;88:1867–1873.
91. von Herbay A, Ditton HJ, Maiwald M. Diagnostic application of a polymerase chain reaction assay for the Whipple's disease bacterium to intestinal biopsies. *Gastroenterology* 1996;110:1735–1743.
92. Relman DA, Schmidt TM, MacDermott RP, Falkow S. Identification of the uncultured bacillus of Whipple's disease. *N Engl J Med* 1992;327:293–301.
93. von Herbay A, Maiwald M, Ditton HJ, Otto HF. Histology of intestinal Whipple's disease revisited. A study of 48 patients. *Virchows Arch* 1996;429:335–343.
94. Bank S, Trey C, Gaus I, et al. Histoplasmosis of the small bowel with "giant" intestinal villi and secondary protein-losing enteropathy. *Am J Med* 1965;39:492–501.
95. Strom RL, Gruninger RP. AIDS with *Mycobacterium avium-intracellulare* lesions resembling those of Whipple's disease. *N Engl J Med* 1983;309:1323–1324.
96. Roth RJ, Owen RL, Keren DF. AIDS with *Mycobacterium avium-intracellulare* lesions resembling those of Whipple's disease. *N Engl J Med* 1983;309:1324.

Eosinophilic Gastroenteritis

97. Klein NC, Hargroove RL, Sleisenger MH, Jeffries GH. Eosinophilic gastroenteritis. *Medicine* 1970;49:299–319.
98. Johnstone JM, Morson BC. Eosinophilic gastroenteritis. *Histopathology* 1978;2:335–348.
99. Steffen RM, Wyllie R, Petras RE, et al. The spectrum of eosinophilic gastroenteritis: report of six pediatric cases and review of the literature. *Clin Pediatr* 1991;30:404–411.
100. Goldman H, Proujansky R. Allergic proctitis and gastroenteritis in children. *Am J Surg Pathol* 1986;10:75–86.
101. DeSchryver-Kecskemeti K, Clouse RE. A previously unrecognized subgroup of "eosinophilic gastroenteritis." Association with connective tissue diseases. *Am J Surg Pathol* 1984;8:171–180.
102. McNabb PC, Fleming CR, Higgins JA, Davis GL. Transmural eosinophilic gastroenteritis with ascites. *Mayo Clin Proc* 1979;54:119–122.
103. Lee M, Hodges WG, Huggins TL. Eosinophilic gastroenteritis. *South Med J* 1996;89:189–194.
104. Bunyaratrej S, Bunyawongwiroj P, Nitiyanant P. Human intestinal sarcosporidiosis: report of six cases. *Am J Trop Med Hygiene* 1982;31:36–41.
105. Walker NI, Croese J, Clouston AD, et al. Eosinophilic enteritis in Northeastern Australia. Pathology, association with *Ancylostoma caninum*, and implications. *Am J Surg Pathol* 1995;19:328–337.

Enteropathy-Associated T-cell Lymphoma

106. Klaeveman HL, Gebhard RL, Sessoms S, Strober W. In vitro studies of ulcerative ileojejunitis. *Gastroenterology* 1985;68:572–582.
107. Armstrong BK, Ammon RK, Finlay-Jones LR, Joske RA, Vivain AB. A further case of chronic ulcerative enteritis. *Gut* 1973;14:649–652.
108. Baer AN, Bayless TM, Yardley JH. Intestinal ulceration and malabsorption syndromes. *Gastroenterology* 1980;79:754–765.
109. Bayless TM, Kapelowitz RF, Shelley WM, Ballinger WF, Hendrix TR. Intestinal ulceration—a complication of celiac disease. *N Engl J Med* 1967;276:996–1002.
110. Jeffries GH, Steinberg H, Sleisenger WH. Chronic ulcerative (nongranulomatous) jejunitis. *Am J Med* 1968;44:47–59.
111. Isaacson P, Wright DH. Malignant histiocytosis of the intestine: its relationship to malabsorption and ulcerative jejunitis. *Hum Pathol* 1978;9:661–677.
112. Spencer J, Cerf-Bemsissan N, Jarry A, et al. Enteropathy-associated T-cell lymphoma (malignant histiocytosis of the intestine) is recognized by a monoclonal antibody (HML-1) that defines a membrane molecule on human mucosal lymphocytes. *Am J Pathol* 1988;132:1–5.
113. Foucar K, Foucar E, Mitros F, Clamon G, Goeken J, Crossett J. Epitheliotropic lymphoma of the small bowel: report of a fatal case with cytotoxic/suppressor T-cell immunotype. *Cancer* 1984;54:54–60.
114. Robertson DAF, Dixon MF, Scott BB, Simpson FG, Losowsky MS. Small intestinal ulceration: diagnostic difficulties in relationship to coeliac disease. *Gut* 1983;24:565–574.
115. Isaacson PG, O'Connor NTJ, Spencer J, et al. Malignant histiocytosis of the intestine: a T-cell lymphoma. *Lancet* 1985;ii:688–691.
116. Isaacson PG, Wright DH. Intestinal lymphoma associated with malabsorption. *Lancet* 1978;i:67–70.
117. Isaacson P, Wright DH, Judd MA, Mepham BL. Primary gastrointestinal lymphomas: a classifications of 66 cases. *Cancer* 1979;43:1805–1819.
118. Isaacson PG, Jones DB, Sworn MJ, Wright DH. Malignant histiocytosis of the intestine: report of three cases with immunologic and cytochemical analysis. *J Clin Pathol* 1982;35:510–516.
119. Ashton-Key M, Diss TC, Pan L, Du MQ, Isaacson G. Molecular analysis of T-cell clonality in ulcerative jejunitis and enteropathy-associated T-cell lymphoma. *Am J Pathol* 1997;151:493–498.
120. Loughran TP Jr, Kadin ME, Deeg HJ. T-cell intestinal lymphoma associated with celiac sprue. *Ann Intern Med* 1986;104:44–47.
121. Salter DM, Krajewski AS, Dewar AE. Immunophenotypic analysis of malignant histiocytosis of the intestine. *J Clin Pathol* 1986;39:8–15.
122. Salter DM, Krajewski AS. Histogenesis of malignant histiocytosis of the intestine. *Gastroenterology* 1987;92:2050–2051.
123. Spencer J, MacDonald TT, Diss TC, Walker-Smith JA, Ciclitira PJ, Isaacson PG. Changes in intraepithelial lymphocyte subpopulation in

celiac disease and enteropathy-associated T-cell lymphoma (malignant histiocytosis) of the intestine. *Gut* 1989;30:339–346.
124. Alfsen GC, Beiske K, Bell H, Marton PF. Low grade intestinal lymphoma of intraepithelial T-lymphocytes with concomitant enteropathy-associated T-cell lymphoma: case report suggesting possible histogenic relationship. *Hum Pathol* 1989;20:909–913.
125. Wright DH, Jones DB, Clark H, Mead GM, Hodges E, Howell WM. Is adult-onset coeliac disease due to low-grade lymphoma of intraepithelial T lymphocytes? *Lancet* 1991;337:1373–1374.
126. Murray A, Cuevas EC, Jones DB, Wright DH. Study of the immunohistochemistry and T-cell clonality of enteropathy-associated T-cell lymphoma. *Am J Pathol* 1995;146:509–519.
127. Cellier C, Patey N, Mauvieux L, et al. Abnormal intestinal intraepithelial lymphocytes in refractory sprue. *Gastroenterology* 1998;114:471–481.
128. DeBruin PC, Connolly CE, Oudejans JJ, et al. Enteropathy-associated T-cell lymphomas have a cytotoxic T-cell phenotype. *Histopathology* 1997;31:313–317.

Parasitic Infestations

129. Smith JW. Identification of fecal parasites in the special parasitology survey of the College of American Pathologists. *Am J Clin Pathol* 1979;72:371–373.
130. Mahmoud AAF, Warren KS. Algorithms in the diagnosis and management of exotic diseases. II. Giardiasis. *J Infect Dis* 1975;131:621–624.
131. Gutierrez Y. *Diagnostic pathology of parasitic infections with clinical correlations.* Philadelphia: Lea & Febiger, 1990.
132. Oberhuber G, Kastner N, Stolte M. Giardiasis: a histologic analysis of 567 cases. *Scand J Gastroenterol* 1997;32:48–51.
133. Hartong WA, Gourley WK, Arvanitakis C. Giardiasis: clinical spectrum and functional-structural abnormalities of the small intestinal mucosa. *Gastroenterology* 1979;77:61–69.
134. Levinson JD, Nastro LJ. Giardiasis with total villus atrophy. *Gastroenterology* 1978;74:271–275.
135. Yardley JH. Giardiasis. In: Binford CH, Connor DH, eds. *Pathology of tropical and extraordinary diseases.* Washington, DC: Armed Forces Institute of Pathology, 1976:328–331.
136. Ament ME, Rubin CE. Relationship of giardiasis to abnormal intestinal structure and function in gastrointestinal immunodeficiency syndrome. *Gastroenterology* 1972;62:216–226.
137. Eveland LK, Kenney M, Yermakov V. Laboratory diagnosis of autoinfection with strongyloidiasis. *Am J Clin Pathol* 1975;63:421–425.
138. Milder JE, Walzer PD, Kilgore G, Rutherford I, Klein M. Clinical features of *Strongyloides stercoralis* infection in an endemic area of the United States. *Gastroenterology* 1981;80:1481–1488.
139. Igra-Siegman Y, Kapila R, Sen P, Kaminski ZC, Louria DB. Syndrome of hyperinfection with *Strongyloides stercoralis*. *Rev Infect Dis* 1981;3:397–407.
140. Meyers WM, Connor DH, Neafie RC. Strongyloidiasis. In: Binford CH, Connor DH, eds. *Pathology of tropical and extraordinary diseases.* Washington, DC: Armed Forces Institute of Pathology, 1976:428–432.
141. Gutierrez Y, Bhatia P, Garbadawala ST, Dobson JR, Wallace TM, Carey TE. Strongyloides stercoralis eosinophilic granulomatous enterocolitis. *Am J Surg Pathol* 1996;20:603–612.
142. Neafie RC, Connor DH, Cross JH. Capillariasis (intestinal and hepatic). In: Binford CH, Connor DH, eds. *Pathology of tropical and extraordinary diseases.* Washington, DC: Armed Forces Institute of Pathology, 1976:402–408.
143. Lee S, Hong S, Chai J, et al. A case of intestinal capillariasis in the Republic of Korea. *Am J Trop Med Hygiene* 1993;48:542–546.
144. Whalen GE, Rosenberg EB, Strickland GT, et al. Intestinal capillariasis, a new disease in man. *Lancet* 1969;I:13–16.

Waldenström's Macroglobulinemia

145. Bedine MS, Yardley JH, Elliott HL, Banwell JG, Hendricks TR. Intestinal involvement in Waldenström's macroglobulinemia. *Gastroenterology* 1973;65:308–315.
146. Harris M, Burton IE, Scarffe JH. Macroglobulinaemia and intestinal lymphangiectasia: a rare association. *J Clin Pathol* 1983;36:30–36.
147. Brandt LJ, Davidoff A, Bernstein LH, Biempica L, Rindleisch B, Goldstein ML. Small-intestinal involvement in Waldenström's macroglobulinemia. Case report and review of the literature. *Dig Dis Sci* 1981:26;174–180.

Intestinal Lymphangiectasia

148. Vardy PA, Lebenthal E, Shwachman H. Intestinal lymphangiectasia: a reappraisal. *Pediatrics* 1975;55:842–851.
149. Waldmann TA. Protein-losing enteropathy. *Gastroenterology* 1966;50:422–443.
150. Popovic OS, Brkic S, Bojic P, et al. Sarcoidosis and protein-losing enteropathy. *Gastroenterology* 1980;78:119–125.

Abetalipoproteinemia

151. Greenwood N. The jejunal mucosa in two cases of A-beta-lipoproteinemia. *Am J Gastroenterol* 1976;65:160–162.
152. Joshi M, Hyams J, Treem W, Ricci AJ. Cytoplasmic vacuolization of enterocytes: an unusual histopathologic finding in juvenile nutritional megaloblastic anemia. *Mod Pathol* 1991;4:62–65.

Acrodermatitis Enteropathica

153. Kelly R, Davidson GP, Townley RRW, Campbell PE. Reversible intestinal mucosal abnormality in acrodermatitis enteropathica. *Arch Dis Child* 1976;51:219–222.
154. Longbeck I, von Bassewitz DB, Becker K, Tinschmann P, Kastner H. Ultrastructural finding in acrodermatitis enteropathica. *Pediatr Res* 1974;8:82–88.
155. Mack D, Koletzko B, Cunnane S, Cutz E, Griffiths A. Acrodermatitis enteropathica with normal serum zinc levels: diagnostic value of small bowel biopsy and essential fatty acid determination. *Gut* 1989;30:1426–1429.
156. Reifen RM, Cutz E, Griffiths AM, Ngan BY, Sherman PM. Tufting enteropathy: a newly recognized clinicopathological entity associated with refractory diarrhea in infants. *J Pediatr Gastroenterol Nutr* 1994;18:379–385.
157. Goulet O, Kedinger M, Brousse N, et al. Intractable diarrhea of infancy with epithelial and basement membrane abnormalities. *J Pediatr* 1995;127:212–219.
158. Goulet OJ, Brousse N, Canioni D, et al. Syndrome of intractable diarrhea with persistent villous atrophy in early childhood: a clinicopathological survey of 47 cases. *J Pediatr Gastroenterol Nutr* 1998;26:151–161.

Pancreatic Heterotopia, Adenomyoma, and Myoepithelial Hamartoma

159. Armstrong LP, King PM, Dickson JM, et al. The significance of heterotopic pancreas in the gastrointestinal tract. *Br J Surg* 1981;68:384–387.
160. Barbosa J, Dockerty MB, Waugh JM. Pancreatic heterotopia: review of the literature and report of 41 authenticated surgical cases of which 25 were clinically significant. *Surg Gynecol Obstet* 1946;82:527–542.
161. Lai ECS, Thompkins RK. Heterotopic pancreas: review of a 26 year experience. *Am J Surg* 1986;151:697–700.
162. Dolan RV, ReMine WH, Dockerty MB. The fate of heterotopic pancreatic tissue. *Arch Surg* 1974;109:762–765.
163. Littner M, Kirsch I. Aberrent pancreatic tissue in the gastric antrum. *Radiology* 1952;59:201–211.

Hyperplasia of Brunner's Glands

164. Robertson HE. The pathology of Brunner's glands. *Arch Pathol Lab Med* 1941;31:112–130.
165. Silverman L, Waugh JM, Huizenga KA, Harrison EG. Large adenomatous polyp of Brunner's glands. *Am J Clin Pathol* 1961;36:438–443.
166. Goldman RL. Hamartomatous polyp of Brunner's glands. *Gastroenterology* 1963;44:57–62.

167. Buchanan EB. Nodular hyperplasia of Brunner's glands of the duodenum. *Am J Surg* 1961;101:253–257.
168. Franzin G, Musola R, Ghidini O, Manfrini C, Fratton A. Nodular hyperplasia of Brunner's glands. *Gastrointest Endosc* 1985;31:374–378.

Colonic Mucosal Biopsy in Patients with Suspected Inflammatory Bowel Disease

169. Levine DS, Haggitt RC. Colon. In: Sternberg SS, ed. *Histology for pathologists*, 2nd ed. Philadelphia: Lippincott-Raven, 1997:519–537.
170. Goldman H, Antonioli DA. Mucosal biopsy of the rectum, colon, and distal ileum. *Hum Pathol* 1982;13:981–1012.
171. Haggitt RC. The differential diagnosis of inflammatory bowel disease. In: Norris HT, ed. *Pathology of the colon, small intestine, and anus*, 2nd ed. New York: Churchill Livingstone, 1991:23–60.
172. Jenkins D, Balsitis M, Gallivan S, et al. Guidelines for the initial biopsy diagnosis of suspected chronic idiopathic inflammatory bowel disease. The British Society of Gastroenterology Initiative. *J Clin Pathol* 1997;50:93–105.
173. Azzopardi JG, Evans DJ. Muciprotein-containing histiocytes (muciphages) in the rectum. *J Clin Pathol* 1966;19:368–374.
174. Dawson IMP. *Atlas of gastrointestinal pathology as seen on biopsy*. Philadelphia: JB Lippincott, 1983.
175. Riddell RH, Goldman H, Ransohoff DF, et al. Dysplasia in inflammatory bowel disease: standardized classification with provisional clinical applications. *Hum Pathol* 1983;11:931–968.
176. Seldenrijk CA, Morson BC, Meuwissen SGM, Schipper NW, Lindermand J, Meijer CJLM. Histopathological evaluation of colonic mucosal biopsy specimens in chronic inflammatory bowel disease: diagnostic implications. *Gut* 1991;32:1514–1520.

Infectious Colitis

177. Surawicz CM, Belic L. Rectal biopsy helps to distinguish acute self-limited colitis from idiopathic inflammatory bowel disease. *Gastroenterology* 1984;86:104–113.
178. Norstrant TT, Kumar NB, Appelman HD. Histopathology differentiates acute self-limited colitis from ulcerative colitis. *Gastroenterology* 1987;92:318–328.
179. Schumacher G. First attack of inflammatory bowel disease and infectious colitis. *Scand J Gastroenterol* 1993;28:1–24.
180. LeBerre N, Heresback O, Kerbaol M, et al. Histological discrimination of idiopathic inflammatory bowel disease from other types of colitis. *J Clin Pathol* 1995;48:749–753.
181. Surawicz CM. Mucosal biopsy diagnosis of colitis. *Semin Colon Rectal Surg* 1992;3:154–159.
182. Anand BS, Malhotra V, Bhattacharya SK, et al. Rectal histology in acute bacillary dysentery. *Gastroenterology* 1986;90:654–660.
183. Makapugay LM, Dean PJ. Diverticular disease-associated chronic colitis. *Am J Surg Pathol* 1996;20:94–102.
184. Volk EE, Shapiro BD, Easley KA, Goldblum JR. The clinical significance of a biopsy-based diagnosis of focal active colitis: a clinicopathologic study of 31 cases. *Mod Pathol* 1998;11:789–794.
185. Greenson JK, Stern RA, Carpenter SL, Barnett JL. The clinical significance of focal active colitis. *Hum Pathol* 1997;28:729–733.
186. Odze R, Antonioli D, Peppercorn M, Goldman H. Effect of topical 5-aminosalicylic acid (5-ASA) therapy on rectal mucosal biopsy morphology in chronic ulcerative colitis. *Am J Surg Pathol* 1993;17:869–875.
187. Surawicz CM, Meisel JH, Ylvisaker T, Saunders DR, Rubin CE. Rectal biopsy in the diagnosis of Crohn's disease: value of multiple biopsies and serial sectioning. *Gastroenterology* 1981;81:66–71.
188. Kelly JK, Pai CH, Jadusingh IH, Macinnis ML, Shaffer EA, Hershfield NB. The histopathology of rectosigmoid biopsies from adults with bloody diarrhea due to verotoxin-producing *Escherichia coli*. *Am J Clin Pathol* 1987;88:78–82.
189. McGovern VJ, Slavutin LJ. Pathology of salmonella colitis. *Am J Surg Pathol* 1979;3:483–490.
190. Akdamar K, Martin RJ, Ichinose H. Syphilitic proctitis. *Dig Dis* 1977;22:701–704.
191. Elavathil LJ, Qizilbash AH, Ciok J, Mahoney JB, Chernesky MA. *Chlamydia trachomatis* proctitis. *Arch Pathol Lab Med* 1984;108:5–6.
192. Price AB, Jewkes J, Sanderson PJ. Acute diarrhoea: *Campylobacter* colitis and the role of rectal biopsy. *J Clin Pathol* 1979;32:990–997.
193. Dickinson RJ, Gilmour HM, McClelland DBL. Rectal biopsy in patients presenting to an infectious disease unit with diarrhoeal disease. *Gut* 1979;20:141–148.
194. Surawicz CM, Goodell SE, Quinn TC, et al. Spectrum of rectal biopsy abnormalities in homosexual men with intestinal symptoms. *Gastroenterology* 1986;91:651–659.

Hemorrhagic Colitis Syndrome

195. Griffin PM, Olmstead LC, Petras RE. *Escherichia coli* O157:H7-associated colitis: a clinical and histologic study of 11 cases. *Gastroenterology* 1990;99:142–149.
196. Riley LW. The epidemiologic, clinical, and microbiologic features of hemorrhagic colitis. *Annu Rev Microbiol* 1987;41:383–407.
197. Remis RS, MacDonald KL, Reily LW, et al. Sporadic cases of hemorrhagic colitis associated with *Escherichia coli* O157:H7. *Ann Intern Med* 1984;101:624–626.
198. Riley LW, Remis RS, Helgerson SD. Hemorrhagic colitis associated with a rare *Escherichia coli* serotype. *N Engl J Med* 1983;308:681–685.
199. Brotman M, Giannella RA, Alm PF, et al. Consensus conference statement: *Escherichia coli* O157:H7 infection—an emerging national health crisis. July 11–13, 1994. *Gastroenterology* 1995;108:1923–1934.
200. Griffin PM, Tauxe RV. The epidemiology of infections caused by *Escherichia coli* O157:H7, other enterohemorrhagic *E. coli* and the associated hemolytic uremic syndrome. *Epidemiol Rev* 1991;13:60–68.
201. CDC Update: Multistate outbreak of *Escherichia coli* O157:H7 infection from hamburgers—Western United States, 1992—1993 MMWR 1993;42:258–263.
202. Griffin PM, Ostroff SM, Tauxe RV, et al. Illness associated with *Escherichia coli* O157:H7 infections: A broad clinical spectrum. *Ann Intern Med* 1988;109:705–712.
203. Ryan CA, Tauxe RV, Hosek GW, et al. *Escherichia coli* O157:H7 diarrhea in a nursing home: clinical, epidemiologic, and pathologic findings. *J Infect Dis* 1986;154:631–638.
204. Carter AO, Borczyk AA, Carlson JAK, et al. A severe outbreak of *Escherichia coli* O157:H7-associated hemorrhagic colitis in a nursing home. *N Engl J Med* 1987;317:1496–1500.
205. Neill MA, Tarr PI, Clausen CR, et al. *Escherichia coli* O157:H7 as the predominant pathogen associated with the hemolytic uremic syndrome: a prospective study in the Pacific Northwest. *Pediatrics* 1987;80:37–40.
206. Laboratory Centres for Disease Control. Enterohemorrhagic *Escherichia coli* and the hemolytic uremic syndrome—the Alberta experience. *Can Dis Wkly Rep* 1989;15:9–12.
207. Karmali MA, Petric M, Lim C, Fleming PC, Arbus GS, Lior H. The association between idiopathic hemolytic uremic syndrome and infection by verotoxin-producing *Escherichia coli*. *J Infect Dis* 1985;151:775–782.
208. Pai CH, Ahmed N, Lior H, Sims HV, Johnson WM, Woods DE. Epidemiology of sporadic diarrhea due to verocytotoxin-producing *Escherichia coli* (VTEC): a two year prospective study. *J Infect Dis* 1988;157:1054–1057.
209. Kelly J, Oryshak A, Wenetsek M, Grabiec J, Handy S. The colonic pathology of *Escherichia coli* O157:H7 infection. *Am J Surg Pathol* 1990;14:87–92.
210. Eidus LB, Guindi M, Drovin J, Gregoire S, Barr JR. Colitis caused *Escherichia coli* O157:H7: A study of six cases. *Can J Gastroenterol* 1990;4:141–146.
211. Petras RE. Enterohemorrhagic *Escherichia coli*-associated colitis. *Pathol Case Rev* 1997;2:66–70.

Antibiotic-Associated Colitis and Pseudomembranous Colitis

212. Talbot RW, Walker RC, Beart RW Jr. Changing epidemiology, diagnosis, and treatment of *Clostridium difficile* toxin-associated colitis. *Br J Surg* 1986;73:457–460.
213. Bartlett JG, Chang TW, Gurwith M, Gorbach SL, Onderdonk AB. Antibiotic-associated pseudomembranous colitis due to toxin-producing clostridia. *N Engl J Med* 1978;298:531–534.

214. Lishman AH, Al-Jumaili IJ, Record CO. Spectrum of antibiotic-associated diarrhoea. *Gut* 1981;22:34–37.
215. Viscidi R, Wiley S, Bartlett JG. Isolation rates and toxigenic potential of *Clostridium difficile* isolates from various patient populations. *Gastroenterology* 1981;81:5–9.
216. Price AB, Davies DR. Pseudomembranous colitis. *J Clin Pathol* 1977;30:1–12.
217. Gephard RL, Gerding DN, Olson MM, et al. Clinical and endoscopic findings in patients early in the course of *Clostridium difficile*-associated pseudomembranous colitis. *Am J Med* 1985;78:45–48.
218. Lamont JT, Trnka YM. Therapeutic implications of *Clostridium difficile* toxin during relapse of chronic inflammatory bowel disease. *Lancet* 1980;I:381–383.
219. Bolton RP, Sherriff RJ, Read AE. *Clostridium difficile*-associated diarrhoea: a role in inflammatory bowel disease? *Lancet* 1980;i:383–384.

Collagenous and Lymphocytic Colitis

220. Giardiello FM, Bayless TM, Jessurun J, Hamilton SR, Yardley JH. Collagenous colitis: physiologic and histopathologic studies in 7 patients. *Ann Intern Med* 1987;106:46–49.
221. Rams H, Rogers AI, Ghandur-Mnaymneh L. Collagenous colitis. *Ann Intern Med* 1987;106:108–113.
222. Jessurun J, Yardley JH, Giardiello FM, Hamilton SR, Bayless TM. Chronic colitis with thickening of the subepithelial collagen layer (collagenous colitis): histopathologic findings in 15 patients. *Hum Pathol* 1987;18:839–848.
223. Lazenby AJ, Yardley JH, Giardiello FM, Jessurun J, Bayless TM. Lymphocytic ("microscopic") colitis: a comparative histopathologic study with particular reference to collagenous colitis. *Hum Pathol* 1989;20:18–28.
224. Read NW, Krejs GJ, Read MG, et al. Chronic diarrhea of unknown origin. *Gastroenterology* 1980;78:264–271.
225. Bo-Linn GW, Vemdrell DD, Lee E, Fordtran JS. An evaluation of the significance of microscopic colitis in patients with chronic diarrhea. *J Clin Invest* 1985;75:1559–1569.
226. Mill LR, Schuman BM, Thompson WD. Lymphocytic colitis: a definable clinical and histological diagnosis. *Dig Dis Sci* 1993;38:1147–1151.
227. Jessurun J, Yardley JH, Lee EL, Vendrell DD, Schiller LR, Fordtran JS. Microscopic and collagenous colitis: different names for the same condition? [letter]. *Gastroenterology* 1986;91:1583–1584.
228. Bayless TM, Giardiello FM, Lazenby A, Yardley JH. Collagenous colitis. *Mayo Clin Proc* 1987;62:740–741.
229. Wang KK, Perrault J, Carpenter HA, Schroeder KW, Tremaine WJ. Collagenous colitis: a clinical pathologic correlation. *Mayo Clin Proc* 1987;62:665–671.
230. Pimental RR, Achkar E, Bedford R. Collagenous colitis: a treatable disease with an elusive diagnosis. *Dig Dis Sci* 1995;40:1400–1404.
231. Giardiello FM. Collagenous and lymphocytic (microscopic) colitis. In: Bayless TM, ed. *Current therapy in gastroenterology and liver disease,* 3rd ed. Toronto: BC Decker, 1990:360–362.
232. Weidner N, Smith J, Pittee B. Sulfasalazine in treatment of collagenous colitis. Case report and review of the literature. *Am J Med* 1984;77:162–166.
233. Giardiello FM, Hansen FC II, Lazenby AJ, et al. Collagenous colitis in the setting of nonsteroidal anti-inflammatory drugs and antibiotics. *Dig Dis Sci* 1990;35:257–260.
234. Beaugerie L, Lubionski J, Brousse N, et al. Drug induced lymphocytic colitis. *Gut* 1994;35:426–428.
235. Beaugerie L, Patey N, Brousse N. Ranitidine, diarrhea, and lymphocytic colitis. *Gut* 1995;37:708–711.
236. Bryant DA, Mintz ED, Puhr ND, Griffin PM, Petras RE. Colonic epithelial lymphocytosis associated with an epidemic of chronic diarrhea. *Am J Surg Pathol* 1996;20:1102–1109.

Eosinophilic Colitis/Proctitis

237. Schulze K, Mitros FA. Eosinophilic gastroenteritis involving the ileocecal area. *Dis Colon Rectum* 1979;22:47–50.
238. Tedesco FJ, Huckaby CB, Hamby-Allen M, Ewing GC. Eosinophilic ileocolitis: expanding spectrum of eosinophilic gastroenteritis. *Dig Dis Sci* 1981;26:943–948.
239. Haberkern CM, Christie DL, Haas JE. Eosinophilic gastroenteritis presenting as ileocolitis. *Gastroenterology* 1978;74:896–899.
240. Partyka EK, Sanowski RA, Kozarek RA. Colonoscopic features of eosinophilic gastroenteritis. *Dis Colon Rectum* 1980;23:353–356.
241. Rosekrans PCM, Meijer CJLM, Van Der Wal AM, Lindeman J. Allergic proctitis, a clinical and immunopathologic entity. *Gut* 1980;21:1017–1023.
242. Jenkins HR, Pincott JR, Soothill JF, Milla PJ, Harries JT. Food allergy: the major cause of infantile colitis. *Arch Dis Child* 1984;59:326–329.
243. Winter HS, Antonioli DA, Fukaguwa N, Marcial M, Goldman H. Allergy-related proctocolitis in infants: diagnostic usefulness of rectal biopsy. *Mod Pathol* 1990;3:5–10.

Graft-Versus-Host Disease

244. Sale GE, Shulman HM. *The pathology of bone marrow transplantation.* New York: Masson, 1984.
245. Slavin RE, Woodruff JM. The pathology of bone marrow transplantation. In: Sommers SD, ed. *Pathology annual,* vol 9. New York: Appleton-Century-Crofts, 1974:291–344.
246. McDonal GB, Shulman HM, Sullivan KM, Spencer GD. Intestinal and hepatic complications of human bone marrow transplantation. Part I. *Gastroenterology* 1986;90:460–477. Part II. *Gastroenterology* 1986;90:770–784.
247. Sloane JP, Norton J. The pathology of bone marrow transplantation. *Histopathology* 1993;22:201–209.
248. Sale GE, Shulman HM, McDonald GB, Thomas ED. Gastrointestinal graft-versus-host disease in man. A clinical pathological study of the rectal biopsy. *Am J Surg Pathol* 1979;3:291–299.
249. Snover DC, Filipovich AH, Ramsay NK, Weisdorf SA, Kersey JH. Graft-versus-host-disease-like histopathologic findings in pre-bone-marrow transplantation biopsies of patient with severe T-cell deficiency. *Transplantation* 1985;39:95–97.
250. Wirt DP, Brooks EG, Vaidya S, Klimpel GR, Waldmann TA, Goldblum RM. T-lymphocyte population in combined immunodeficiency with features of graft-vs-host disease. *N Engl J Med* 1989;321:370–374.
251. Lee EY, Clouse RE, Aliperti G, DeSchryver-Kacskemeti K. Small intestinal lesion resembling graft-vs-host disease: a case report in immunodeficiency and review of the literature. *Arch Pathol Lab Med* 1991;115:529–522.
252. Kornacki S, Hansen FC 3rd, Lasenby A. Graft-versus-host-like colitis associated with malignant thymoma. *Am J Surg Pathol* 1995;19:224–228.
253. Kotler DP, Gaetz HP, Lang M, et al. Enteropathy associated with the acquired immunodeficiency syndrome. *Ann Intern Med* 1984;101:421–428.
254. Asplund S, Gramlich TL. Chronic mucosal changes of the colon in graft-versus-host disease. *Mod Pathol* 1998;11:513–515.

Acute Ischemic Colitis

255. Whitehead R. The pathology of intestinal ischemia. *Clin Gastroenterol* 1972;1:613–637.

Rectal Mucosal Prolapse Syndromes

256. Madigan MR, Morson BC. Solitary ulcer of the rectum. *Gut* 1969;10:871–881.
257. Levine DS. "Solitary" rectal ulcer syndrome: are "solitary" rectal ulcer syndrome and "localized" colitis cystica profunda analogous syndromes caused by rectal prolapse? *Gastroenterology* 1987;92:243–253.
258. Rutter KRP, Riddell RH. The solitary ulcer syndrome of the rectum. *Clin Gastroenterol* 1975;4:505–530.
259. Lobert PF, Appelman HD. Inflammatory cloacogenic polyp. A unique inflammatory lesion of the anal transtion zone. *Am J Surg Pathol* 1981;5:761–766.
260. Saul SH. Inflammatory cloacogenic polyp: relationship to solitary rectal ulcer syndrome/mucosal prolapse and other bowel disorders. *Hum Pathol* 1987;18:1120–1125.
261. DuBoulay CE, Fairbrother J, Isaacson PG. Mucosal prolapse syn-

261. drome—a unifying concept for solitary ulcer syndrome and related disorders. *J Clin Pathol* 1983;36:1264–1268.
262. Guest CB, Reznick RK. Colitis cystica profunda: review of the literature. *Dis Colon Rectum* 1989;32:983–988.
263. Saul SH, Christie Sollenberger L. Solitary rectal ulcer syndrome: its clinical and pathological underdiagnosis. *Am J Surg Pathol* 1985;9:411–421.
264. Kelly JK. Polypoid prolapsing mucosal folds in diverticular disease. *Am J Surg Pathol* 1991;15:871–878.
265. Womack NR, Williams NS, Holmfield JH, Morrison JF. Anorectal function in the solitary rectal ulcer syndrome. *Dis Colon Rectum* 1987;30:319–323.
266. Sun WM, Read NW, Carmel Donnelly C, Bannister JJ, Shorthouse AJ. A common pathophysiology for full thickness rectal prolapse, anterior mucosal prolapse, and solitary rectal ulcer. *Br J Surg* 1989;76:290–295.
267. Mackle EJ, Manton Mills JO, Parks TG. The investigation of anorectal dysfunction in the solitary rectal ulcer syndrome. *Int J Colorectal Dis* 1990;5:21–24.
268. Tjandra JJ, Fazio VW, Petras RE, Lavery IC, Milsom JW, Church JM. Clinical and pathological factors associated with delayed diagnosis in solitary rectal ulcer syndrome. *Dis Colon Rectum* 1993;36:146–153.
269. Silver H, Stolar J. Distinguishing features of well-differentiated mucinous adenocarcinoma of the rectum and colitis cystica profunda. *Am J Clin Pathol* 1969;51:493–500.
270. Petras RE. Adenomas and malignant polyps of the colon and rectum: invasive carcinoma versus pseudocarcinomatous invasion. *Mod Pathol* 1989;2:250–251.
271. Wayte DM, Helwig EB. Colitis cystica profunda. *Am J Clin Pathol* 1967;48:159–169.
272. Carlson GJ, Nivatvongs S, Snover DC. Colorectal polyps in Cowden's disease (multiple hamartoma syndrome). *Am J Surg Pathol* 1984;3:763–770.
273. Eckardt VF, Kanzler G, Remmele W. Anorectal ergotism: another cause of solitary rectal ulcers. *Gastroenterology* 1986;91:1123–1127.

Interpretation of Biopsy Specimens from Patients with AIDS

274. Quinn TC, Stamm WE, Goodell SE, et al. The polymicrobial origin of intestinal infections in homosexual men. *N Engl J Med* 1983;309:576–582.
275. Baker RW, Peppercorn MA. Gastrointestinal ailments of homosexual men. *Medicine (Baltimore)* 1982;61:390–405.
276. Smith PD, Quinn TC, Strober W, Janoffer EN, Masur H. Gastrointestinal infections in AIDS. *Ann Intern Med* 1992;116:63–77.
277. Kean BH, William DC, Luminais SK. Epidemic of amoebiasis and giardiasis in a biased population. *Br J Vener Dis* 1979;55:375–378.
278. Schmerin MJ, Jones TC, Klein H. Giardiasis associated with homosexuality. *Ann Intern Med* 1978;88:801–803.
279. Schmerin MJ, Gelston A, Jones TC. Amebiasis: an increasing problem among homosexuals in New York City. *JAMA* 1977;238:1386–1387.
280. Rotterdam H, Sommers SC. Alimentary tract biopsy lesions in the acquired immune deficiency syndrome. *Pathology* 1985;17:181–192.
281. Chachoua A, Dieterich D, Krasinski K, et al. 9-(1,3, Dihydroxy-2-propoxymethyl) guanine (ganciclovir) in the treatment of cytomegalovirus gastrointestinal disease with the acquired immunodeficiency syndrome. *Ann Intern Med* 1987;107:133–137.
282. Goodell SE, Quinn TC, Mkrtichian E, Schuffler MD, Holmes KK, Carey L. Herpes simplex virus proctitis in homosexual men: clinical, sigmoidoscopic, and histopathological features. *N Engl J Med* 1983;308:868–871.
283. Siegal FP, Lopez C, Hammer GS, et al. Severe acquired immunodeficiency in male homosexuals, manifested by chronic perianal ulcerative herpes simplex lesions. *N Engl J Med* 1981;305:1439–1444.
284. Maddox A, Francis N, Moss J, Blanshard C, Gazzard B. Adenovirus infections of the large bowel in HIV positive patients. *J Clin Pathol* 1992;45:684–688.
285. Tavitian A, Raufman JP, Rosenthal LE. Oral candidiasis as a marker for esophageal candidiasis in the acquired immunodeficiency syndrome. *Ann Intern Med* 1986;104:54–55.
286. Tavitian A, Raufman JP, Rosenthal LE, et al. Ketaconazole-resistant *Candida* esophagitis in patients with acquired immunodeficiency syndrome. *Gastroenterology* 1986;90:443–445.
287. Levine MS, Macones AJ Jr, Laufer I. *Candida* esophagitis: accuracy of radiographic diagnosis. *Radiology* 1985;154:581–587.
288. Kirkham N, Cotton DWK. Intestinal spirochetosis in homosexual men. *N Engl J Med* 1984;310:392–393.
289. Tompkins DS, Foulkes SJ, Godwin PGR, West AP. Isolation and characterization of intestinal spirochaetes. *J Clin Pathol* 1986;39:535–541.
290. Rodgers FG, Rodgers C, Shelton AP, Hawley CJ. Proposed pathogenic mechanism for the diarrhea associated with human intestinal spirochetes. *Am J Clin Pathol* 1986;86:679–682.
291. Henrik-Nielsen R, Lundbeck FA, Teglbjaerg PS, Ginnerup P, Hovind-Hougen K. Intestinal spirochetosis of the vermiform appendix. *Gastroenterology* 1985;88:971–977.
292. Henrik-Nielsen R, Orholm M, Pedersen JO, Hovind-Hougen K, Teglbjaerg PS, Thaysen EH. Colorectal spirochetosis: clinical significance of the infection. *Gastroenterology* 1983;85:62–67.
293. Hawkins CC, Gold KWM, Whimbey E, et al. *Mycobacterium avium* complex infections in patients with the acquired immunodeficiency syndrome. *Ann Intern Med* 1986;105:184–188.
294. Wong B, Edward FF, Kiehn TE, et al. Continuous high grade *Mycobacterium avium intracellulare* bacteremia in patients with the acquired immune deficiency syndrome. *Am J Med* 1985;78:35–40.
295. Roth RI, Owen RL, Keren DF, Volberding PA. Intestinal infection with *Mycobacterium avium* in acquired immune deficiency syndrome (AIDS). Histological and clinical comparison with Whipple's disease. *Dig Dis Sci* 1985;30:497–504.
296. Orenstein JM, Kotler DP. Diarrheogenic bacterial enteritis in acquired immune deficiency syndrome: a light and electron microscopy study of 52 cases. *Hum Pathol* 1995;26:481–492.
297. Levine MM. *Escherichia coli* that cause diarrhea: enterotoxigenic, enteropathogenic, enteroinvasive, enterohemorrhagic and enteroadherent *J Infect Dis* 1987;155:377–389.
298. Petras RE, Carey WD, Alanis A. Cryptosporidial enteritis in a homosexual male with an acquired immunodeficiency syndrome. *Cleve Clin Q* 1983;50:41–45.
299. Soave R, Armstrong D. Cryptosporidium and cryptosporidiosis. *Rev Infect Dis* 1986;8:1012–1023.
300. Current WL, Reese NC, Ernst JV, Bailey WS, Heyman MB, Weinstein WM. Human cryptosporidiosis in immunocompetent and immunodeficient persons: studies of an outbreak and experimental transmission. *N Engl J Med* 1983;308:1253–1257.
301. Wolfson JS, Richter JM, Waldron MA, Weber DJ, McCarthy DM, Hopkins CC. Cryptosporidiosis in immunocompetent patients. *N Engl J Med* 1985;312:1278–1282.
302. Current W, Reese N, Ernst J, Bailey W. Human Cryptosporidiosis—Alabama. *Morb Mortal Wkly Rep* 1982;31:252–254.
303. Centers for Disease Control. Cryptosporidiosis: assessment of chemotherapy of males with acquired immune deficiency syndrome (AIDS). *Morb Mortal Wkly Rep* 1982;31:589–592.
304. Portnoy D, Whiteside ME, Buckley E, MacLeod CL. Treatment of intestinal cryptosporidiosis with spiramycin. *Ann Intern Med* 1984;101:202–204.
305. Centers for Disease Control. Update: treatment of cryptosporidiosis in patients with the acquired immunodeficiency syndrome (AIDS). *Morb Mortal Wkly Rep* 1984;33:117–119.
306. Lefkowitch JH, Krumholz S, Feng-Chen K, et al. Cryptosporidiosis of the human small intestine: a light and electronmicroscopic study. *Hum Pathol* 1984;15:746–752.
307. Greenberg PD, Koch J, Cello JP. Diagnosis of *Cryptosporidium parvum* in patients with severe diarrhea and AIDS. *Dig Dis Sci* 1996;41:2286–2290.
308. Loose JF, Sedergram DJ, Cooper HS. Identification of cryptosporidium in paraffin-embedded tissue sections with the use of a monoclonal antibody. *Am J Clin Pathol* 1989;91:206–209.
309. Dehovitz JA, Pape JW, Concy M, Johnson WD. Clinical manifestations and therapy of *Isospora belli* infection in patients with the acquired immunodeficiency syndrome. *N Engl J Med* 1986;315:87–90.
310. Soave R, Johnson WD Jr. Cryptosporidiosis and *Isospora belli* infections. *J Infect Dis* 1988;157:225–229.
311. Brandborg LL, Goldberg SB, Breidenbach WC. Human coccidiosis—a possible cause of malabsorption: the life cycle in small bowel mu-

cosal biopsies as a diagnostic feature. *N Engl J Med* 1970;23: 1306–1313.
312. Trier JS, Moxey PC, Schimmel EM, Robles E. Chronic intestinal coccidiosis in man: intestinal morphology and response to treatment. *Gastroenterology* 1974;66:923–935.
313. Liebman WM, Thaler MM, DeLorimier A, Brandborg LL. Goodman J. Intractable diarrhea of infancy due to intestinal coccidiosis. *Gastroenterology* 1980;78:579–584.
314. Modigliani R, Bories L, LeCharpentier Y, et al. Diarrhoea and malabsorption in acquired immune deficiency syndrome: a study of four cases with special emphasis on opportunistic protozoan infections. *Gut* 1985;26:179–187.
315. Greenson JK, Belitsos PC, Yardley JH, Barlett JG. AIDS enteropathy: occult enteric infections and duodenal mucosal alterations in chronic diarrhea. *Ann Intern Med* 1991;114:366–372.
316. Orenstein JM, Chlang J, Steinberg W, Smith PD, Rotterdam H, Kotler DP. Intestinal microsporidiosis as a cause of diarrhea in human immunodeficiency virus-infected patients. *Hum Pathol* 1990;21: 475–481.
317. Simon D, Weiss LM, Tanowitz HB, Call A, Jones J, Wittner M. Light microscopic diagnosis of human microsporidiosis and variable response to octreotide. *Gastroenterology* 1991;100:271–273.
318. Call A, Owen RL. Intracellular development of Enterocytozoon, a unique microsporidian found in the intestines of AIDS patients. *J Protozool* 1990;37:145–155.
319. Lucas SB, Papadakl L, Conlon C, Sewankambo N, Goodgame R, Serwadda D. Diagnosis of intestinal microsporidiosis in patients with AIDS. *J Clin Pathol* 1989;42:885–890.
320. Didier ES, Orenstein JM, Aldras A, Bertucci D, Rogers LB, Janney FA. Comparison of three staining methods of detecting microsporidia in fluids. *J Clin Microbiol* 1995;33:3138–3145.
321. Molina JM, Oksenhendler E, Beauvais B, et al. Disseminated microsporidiosis due to Septata intestinalis in patients with AIDS: clinical features and response to albendazole therapy. *J Infect Dis* 1994;171:245–249.
322. Croft SL, Williams J, McGowan I. Intestinal microsporidicsis. *Semin Gastrointest Dis* 1997;8:45–55.
323. Schwartz DA, Sobottka I, Leitch GJ, Cali A, Visvesvara GS. Pathology of microsporidiosis. Emerging parasitic infections in patients with acquired immunodeficiency syndrome. *Arch Pathol Lab Med* 1996;120:173–188.
324. Beckers PJA, Derks GJMM, van Gool T, Rietveld FJR, Sauerwein RW. Encephalitozoon intestinalis-specific monoclonal antibodies for laboratory diagnosis of microsporidiosis. *J Clin Microbiol* 1996; 34:282–285.
325. Eberhard ML, Pieniazek NJ, Arrowood MJ. Laboratory diagnosis of Cyclospora infections. *Arch Pathol Lab Med* 1997;121:792–797.
326. Tran van Nhieu J, Nin F, Fleury-Feith J, Chaumette MT, Schaeffer A, Bretagne S. Identification of intracellular stages of cyclospora species by light microscopy of thick sections using hematoxylin. *Hum Pathol* 1996;27:1107–1109.
327. Kotler DP, Weaver SC, Terzakis JA. Ultrastructural features of epithelial cell degeneration in rectal crypts of patients with AIDS. *Am J Surg Pathol* 1986;10:531–538.
328. Ullrich R, Zeitz M, Heise W, L'age M, Hoffker G, Riecker EO. Small intestinal structure and function in patients infected with human immunodeficiency virus (HIV): evidence for HIV-induced enteropathy. *Ann Intern Med* 1989;111:15–21.
329. Ullrich R, Heise W, Bergs C, L'age M, Riecker EO, Zeitz M. Gastrointestinal symptoms in patients infected with human immunodeficiency virus: relevance of infectious agents isolated from the gastrointestinal tract. *Gut* 1992;33:1080–1084.
330. Friedman SL, Wright TL, Altman DF. Gastrointestinal Kaposi's sarcoma in patients with acquired immunodeficiency syndrome: endoscopic and autopsy findings. *Gastroenterology* 1985;89:102–108.
331. Friedman SL. Gastrointestinal and hepatobiliary neoplasms in AIDS. *Gastroenterol Clin North Am* 1988;17:465–486.
332. Ioachim HL, Adsay V, Giancotti FR, Dorsett B, Melamed J. Kaposi's sarcoma of internal organs: a multiparameter study of 86 cases. *Cancer* 1995;75:1376–1385.
333. Parente F, Cernuschi M, Orlando G, Rizzardini G, Lazzariln A, Bianchi-Porro G. Kaposi's sarcoma in AIDS. Frequency of gastrointestinal involvement and its effects on survival. A prospective study in a heterogeneous population. *Scand J Gastroenterol* 1991;26: 1007–1012.

Crohn's Disease and Ulcerative Colitis

334. Morson BC, Dawson IMP, Day DW, Jass JR, Price AB, Williams GT. *Morson and Dawson's gastrointestinal pathology.* Oxford: Blackwell, 1990.
335. Warren S, Sommers SC. Pathology of regional ileitis and ulcerative colitis. *JAMA* 1954;154:189–193.
336. Farmer RG, Hawk WA, Turnbull RB Jr. Regional enteritis of the colon: a clinical and pathologic comparison with ulcerative colitis *Am J Dig Dis* 1968;13:501–514.
337. Price AB, Morson BC. Inflammatory bowel disease. The surgical pathology of Crohn's disease and ulcerative colitis. *Hum Pathol* 1975;6:7–29.
338. Hamilton SR. Diagnosis and comparison of ulcerative colitis and Crohn's disease involving the colon. In: Norris HT, ed. *Pathology of the colon, small intestine, and anus,* 2nd ed. New York: Churchill Livingstone, 1991:1–20.
339. McGovern VJ, Goulston SJM. Crohn's disease of the colon. *Gut* 1968;9:164–176.
340. Rowland R, Pounder DJ. Crohn's colitis. In: Sommers SC, Rosen PP, eds. *Pathology annual,* vol 17. Norwalk, CT: Appleton-Century-Crofts, 1982:267–290.
341. vanPatter WN, Bargen JA, Dockerty MB. Regional enteritis. *Gastroenterology* 1954;26:347.
342. Kotanagi H, Kramer K, Fazio WV, Petras RE. Do microscopic abnormalities at resection margins correlate with increased anastomotic recurrences in Crohn's disease? *Dis Colon Rectum* 1991;34:909–916.

Colitis—Type Indeterminate

343. Price AB. Overlap in the spectrum of nonspecific inflammatory bowel disease—"colitis indeterminate." *J Clin Pathol* 1978;31:567–577
344. Price AB. Difficulties in the differential diagnosis of ulcerative colitis in Crohn's disease. In: Yardley JH, Morson BC, Abell MR, eds. *The gastrointestinal tract. International Academy of Pathology Monograph No. 18.* Baltimore: Williams & Wilkins, 1977:1–14.
345. Petras RE, Oakley JR. Intestinal complications of inflammatory bowel disease: pathologic aspects. *Semin Colon Rectal Surg* 1992;3: 160–172.
346. Lee KS, Medline A, Shockey S. Indeterminate colitis in the spectrum of inflammatory bowel disease. *Arch Pathol Lab Med* 1979;103: 173–176.
347. Glotzer DJ, Gardner RC, Goldman H, et al. Comparative features and course of ulcerative and granulomatous colitis. *N Engl J Med* 1970;282:582–589.
348. Pezim ME, Pemberton JH, Beart RW Jr, et al. Outcome of "indeterminant" colitis following ileal pouch-anal anastomosis. *Dis Colon Rectum* 1989;32:653–658.
349. McIntyre PB, Pemberton JH, Wolff BG, Dozois RR, Beart RG Jr. Indeterminate colitis: Long-term outcome in patients after ileal pouch-anal anastomosis. *Dis Colon Rectum* 1995;38:51–54.
350. Wells AD, McMillian I, Price AB, et al. Natural history of indeterminate colitis. *Br J Surg* 1991;78:179–181.

Ulcerative Proctitis

351. Farmer RG, Brown CH. Emerging concepts of proctosigmoiditis. *Dis Colon Rectum* 1972;15:142–146.
352. Lennard-Jones JE, Cooper GW, Newell CW, Wilson CWE, Jones EA. Observations on idiopathic proctitis. *Gut* 1962;3:201–206.
353. Flejou JF, Potet F, Bogomoletz WV, et al. Lymphoid follicular proctitis: a condition different from ulcerative proctitis? *Histopathology* 1991;19:55–61.

Inflammatory Bowel Disease and Diverticular Disease

354. Shepherd NA. Diverticular disease and chronic idiopathic inflammatory bowel disease: associations and masquerades. *Gut* 1996;38: 801–802.
355. Schmidt GT, Lennard-Jones JE, Morson BC, Young AL. Crohn's disease of the colon and its distinction from diverticulitis. *Gut* 1968; 9:7–16.

Diversion Colitis/Defunctionalized Bowel

356. Glotzer DJ, Glick ME, Goldman H. Proctitis and colitis following diversion of the fecal stream. *Gastroenterology* 1981;80:438–441.
357. Murray FE, O'Brien MJ, Birkett DH, et al. Diversion colitis: pathologic findings in a resected sigmoid colon and rectum. *Gastroenterology* 1987;93:1404–1408.
358. Ma CK, Gottlieb C, Hass DA. Diversion colitis: a clinicopathologic study of 21 cases. *Hum Pathol* 1990;21:429–436.
359. Geraghty JM, Talbot IC. Diversion colitis: histologic features in the colon and rectum after defunctioning colostomy. *Gut* 1991;32:1020–1023.
360. Harig JM, Soergel KH, Komorowski RA, et al. Treatment of diversion colitis with short chain fatty acid irrigation. *N Engl J Med* 1989;320:23–28.
361. Warren BF, Shepherd NA, Bartolo DC, Bradfield JW. Pathology of the defunctioned rectum in ulcerative colitis. *Gut* 1993;34:514–516.
362. Asplund S, Gramlich T, Navarro G, Fazio V, Petras R. The histology of defunctioned rectum: correlation with original diagnosis and clinical outcome. *Lab Invest* 1996;73:54A.

Ileal Reservoirs (Pouches) and Pouchitis

363. Cranley B. The Kock reservoir ileostomy: a review of its development, problems and role in modern surgical practice. *Br J Surg* 1983;70:94–99.
364. Parks AG, Nicholls RJ. Proctocolectomy without ileostomy for ulcerative colitis. *BMJ* 1978;2:85–88.
365. Schrock TR. Surgery for Crohn's colitis. In: Bayless TM, ed. *Current management of inflammatory bowel disease*. Philadelphia: Decker, 1989;290–294.
366. Hyman NH, Fazio VW, Tuckson WB, et al. Consequences of ileal pouch-anal anastomosis for Crohn's colitis. *Dis Colon Rectum* 1991;34:653–657.
367. Koltun WA, Schoetz DJ Jr, Roberts PK, et al. Indeterminate colitis predisposes to perineal complications after ileal pouch-anal anastomosis. *Dis Colon Rectum* 1991;34:857–860.
368. Dozois RR, Kelly KA, Welling DR, et al. Ileal pouch-anal anastomosis: comparison of results in familial adenomatous polyposis and chronic ulcerative colitis. *Ann Surg* 1989;210:268–273.
369. Galandiuk S, Scott NA, Dozois RR, et al. Ileal pouch-anal anastomosis: reoperation for pouch-related complications. *Ann Surg* 1990;212:446–454.
370. Deutsch AA, McLeod RS, Cullen J, et al. Results of the pelvic-pouch procedure in patients with Crohn's disease. *Dis Colon Rectum* 1991;34:475–477.
371. Poppen B, Svenberg T, Bark T, et al. Colectomy-proctomucosectomy with S-pouch: operative procedures, complications, and functional outcome in 69 consecutive patients. *Dis Colon Rectum* 1992;35:40–47.
372. Bonella JC, Thow GB, Manson RR. Mucosal enteritis: a complication of the continent ileostomy. *Dis Colon Rectum* 1981;24:37–41.
373. Madden MV, Farthing MJG, Nicholls RJ. Inflammation in ileal reservoirs; "Pouchitis". *Gut* 1990;31:247–249.
374. Sandborn WJ. Pouchitis following ileal pouch-anal anastomosis: definition, pathogenesis, and treatment. *Gastroenterology* 1994;107:1856–1860.
375. Klein K, Stenzel P, Katon RM. Pouch ileitis: report of a case with severe systemic manifestations. *J Clin Gastroenterol* 1983;5:149–153.
376. Moskowitz RL, Shepherd NA, Nicholls RJ. An assessment of inflammation in the reservoir after restorative procto-colectomy with ileal reservoir. *Int J Colorectal Dis* 1986;1:161–174.
377. Zuccaro G, Fazio VW, Church JM, et al. Pouch ileitis. *Dig Dis Sci* 1989;34:1505–1510.
378. Rauh SM, Schoetz DJ Jr, Roberts PL, et al. Pouchitis—is it a waste basket diagnosis? *Dis Colon Rectum* 1991;34:685–689.
379. Lohmuller JL, Pemberton JH, Dozois RR, et al. Pouchitis and extraintestinal manifestations of inflammatory bowel disease after ileal pouch-anal anastomosis. *Ann Surg* 1990;211:622–629.
380. Shepherd NA, Jass JR, Duval I, et al. Restorative proctocolectomy with ileal reservoir: pathologic and histochemical study of mucosal biopsy specimens. *J Clin Pathol* 1987;40:601–607.
381. Bona SJ, Petras RE, McGonagle B, et al. The histopathology of pouchitis. *Lab Invest* 1988;58:11A.
382. Setti Carraro P, Talbot IC, Nicholls RJ. Longterm appraisal of the histological appearances of the ileal reservoir mucosa after restorative proctocolectomy for ulcerative colitis. *Gut* 1994;35:1721–1727.
383. Kelly DG, Phillips SF, Kelly KA, et al. Dysfunction of the continent ileostomy: clinical features and bacteriology. *Gut* 1983;24:193–201.
384. Di Febo G, Miglioli M, Lauri A, et al. Endoscopic assessment of acute inflammation of the ileal reservoir after restorative ileo-anal anastomosis. *Gastrointest Endosc* 1990;36:6–9.
385. Nasmyth GD, Godwin PGR, Dixon MF, et al. Ileal ecology after pouch-anal anastomosis or ileostomy: a study of mucosal morphology, fecal bacteriology, fecal volatile fatty acids, and their inter-relationship. *Gastroenterology* 1989;96:817–824.
386. O'Connell PR, Rankin DR, Weiland LH, et al. Enteric bacteriology, absorption, morphology, and emptying after ileal pouch-anal anastomosis. *Br J Surg* 1986;73:909–914.
387. Soper NJ, Chapman NJ, Kelly KA, et al. The "ileal brake" after ileal pouch-anal anastomosis. *Gastroenterology* 1990;98:111–116.
388. Levitt MD, Lewis AAM. Determinants of ileoanal pouch function. *Gut* 1991;32:126–127.
389. Tuckson W, Lavery I, Fazio V, et al. Manometric and functional comparison of ileal pouch-anal anastomosis with and without anal manipulation. *Am J Surg* 1991;161:90–96.
390. Goldstein NS, Sandford WW, Bodzin JH. Crohn's-like complications in patients with ulcerative colitis after total proctocolectomy and ileal pouch-anal anastomosis. *Am J Surg Pathol* 1997;21:1343–1353.
391. Fazio VW, Church JM. Complications and function of the continent ileostomy at the Cleveland Clinic. *World J Surg* 1988;12:148–154.
392. Scott AD, Phillips RKS. Ileitis and pouchitis after colectomy for ulcerative colitis. *Br J Surg* 1989;76:668–669.
393. Setti Carraro P, Talbot JC, Nicholls RJ. Longterm appraisal of the histological appearances of the ileal reservoir mucosa after restorative proctocolectomy for ulcerative colitis. *Gut* 1994;35:1721–1727.
394. Veress B, Reinholt FP, Lindquist K, et al. Long-term histomorphological surveillance of the pelvic ileal pouch: dysplasia develops in a subgroup of patients. *Gastroenterology* 1995;109:1090–1097.
395. Gullberg K, Stahlberg D, Liljeqvist L, et al. Neoplastic transformation of the pelvic pouch mucosa in patients with ulcerative colitis. *Gastroenterology* 1997;112:1487–1492.
396. Hawk WA, Petras RE. The pathology of mucosal ulcerative colitis. In: Jagelman DG, ed. *Mucosal ulcerative colitis*. Mount Kisco, NY: Futura, 1986:37–55.
397. Knill-Jones RP, Morson B, Williams R. Prestomal ileitis: clinical and pathologic findings in five cases. *Q J Med* 1970;39:287–297.

Inflammatory Bowel Disease, Dysplasia, and Carcinoma

398. Ekbom A, Helmick C, Zack M, Adami H. Ulcerative colitis and colorectal cancer: a population-based study. *N Engl J Med* 1990;323:1229–1233.
399. Collins RH Jr, Feldman M, Fordtran JS. Colon cancer, dysplasia, and surveillance in patients with ulcerative colitis. *N Engl J Med* 1987;316:1654–1658.
400. Lennard-Jones JE, Morson BC, Ritchie JK, Williams CB. Cancer surveillance in ulcerative colitis; experience over 15 years. *Lancet* 1983;2:149–152.
401. Lennard-Jones JE, Melville DM, Morson BC, et al. Precancer and cancer in extensive ulcerative colitis: findings among 401 patients over 22 years. *Gut* 1990;31:800–806.
402. Rosenstock E, Farmer RG, Petras R, Sivak MV Jr, Rankin GB, Sullivan BH. Surveillance for colonic carcinoma in ulcerative colitis. *Gastroenterology* 1985;89:1342–1346.
403. Nugent FW, Haggitt RC, Gilpin PA. Cancer surveillance and ulcerative colitis. *Gastroenterology* 1991;100:1241–1248.
404. Woolrich AJ, DaSilva MD, Korelitz B. Surveillance in the routine management of ulcerative colitis: the predictive value of low-grade dysplasia. *Gastroenterology* 1992;103:431–438.
405. Choi PM, Nugent FW, Schoetz DJ Jr, Silverman JL, Haggitt RC. Colonoscopic surveillance reduces mortality from colorectal cancer in ulcerative colitis. *Gastroenterology* 1993;105:418–424.
406. Bernstein CN, Chanahan F, Weinstein WM. Are we telling patients the truth about surveillance colonoscopy in ulcerative colitis? *Lancet* 1994;343:71–74.

407. Petras RE, Farmer RG, Rankin GB, Sivak MV Jr. Dysplasia in ulcerative colitis: aneuploidy versus morphology. *Gastroenterology* 1989;97:243–245.
408. Melville DM, Jass JR, Morson BC, et al. Observer study of the grading of dysplasia in ulcerative colitis: comparison with clinical outcome. *Hum Pathol* 1989;20:1008–1014.
409. Morson BC, Pang LSC. Rectal biopsy as an aid to cancer control in ulcerative colitis. *Gut* 1967;8:423–434.
410. Gyde S. Screening for colorectal cancer in ulcerative colitis: dubious benefits and high costs. *Gut* 1990;31:1089–1092.
411. Cornell WR, Lennard-Jones JE, Williams CB, Talbot JC, Price AB, Wilkinson KH. Factors affecting the outcome of endoscopic surveillance for cancer in ulcerative colitis. *Gastroenterology* 1994;107:934–944.
412. Ehsanullah M, Filipe MI, Gazzard B. Mucin secretion in inflammatory bowel disease: correlation with disease activity and dysplasia. *Gut* 1982;23:485–489.
413. Ehsanullah M, Morgan MN, Filipe MI, Gazzard B. Sialomucins in the assessment of dysplasia and cancer risk in patients with ulcerative colitis treated with colectomy and ileorectal anastomosis. *Histopathology* 1985;9:223–235.
414. Jass JR, England J, Miller K. Value of mucin histochemistry and follow-up surveillance of patients with long-standing ulcerative colitis. *J Clin Pathol* 1986;39:393–398.
415. Fozard JBJ, Dixon MF, Axon ATR, Giles GR. Lectin and mucin histochemistry as an aid to cancer surveillance in ulcerative colitis. *Histopathology* 1987;11:385–394.
416. Ahnen DJ, Warren GH, Greene LJ, Singleton JW, Brown WR. Search for a specific marker of mucosal dysplasia in chronic ulcerative colitis. *Gastroenterology* 1987;93:1346–1355.
417. Cooper HS, Farano P, Coapman RA. Peanut lectin binding sites in colon of patients with ulcerative colitis. *Arch Pathol Lab Med* 1987;111:270–275.
418. Ciclitira PJ, McCartney JC, Evan G. Expression of C-myc in non-malignant and pre-malignant gastrointestinal disorders. *J Pathol* 1987;151:293–296.
419. McKenzie JK, Purnell DS, Shamsuddin AM. Expression of CEA, T-antigen, and oncogene products as markers of neoplastic and preneoplastic colonic mucosa. *Hum Pathol* 1987;18:1282–1286.
420. Fozard JBJ, Quirke P, Dixon MF, Giles GR, Bird CC. DNA aneuploidy in ulcerative colitis. *Gut* 1987;28:1414–1418.
421. Melville DM, Jass JR, Shepherd NA, et al. Dysplasia and deoxyribonucleic acid aneuploidy in the assessment of precancerous changes in chronic ulcerative colitis. *Gastroenterology* 1988;95:668–675.
422. Lofberg R, Brostrom O, Karlen P, Ost A, Tribukait B. DNA aneuploidy in ulcerative colitis: reproducibility, topographic distribution, and relation to dysplasia. *Gastroenterology* 1992;102:1149–1154.
423. Reid BJ, Blount PL, Rubin CE, Levine DS, Haggitt RC, Rabinovitch PS. Flow cytometric and histological progression to malignancy in Barrett's esophagus: prospective endoscopic surveillance of a cohort. *Gastroenterology* 1992;102:1212–1219.
424. Lennard-Jones JE. Colonoscopic surveillance for cancer in patients with chronic ulcerative colitis: is it working? *Gastroenterology* 1991;100:571–572.
425. Bennett RC, Bozdech JM, Farmer RG, Petras RE. "Adenomas" (polyps containing adenomatous dysplasia) in ulcerative colitis: a report of 27 cases. *Am J Clin Pathol* 1990;94:500.
426. Cornell WR, Lennard-Jones JE, Williams CB, Talbot JC, Price AB, Wilkinson KH. Factors affecting the outcome of endoscopic surveillance for cancer in ulcerative colitis. *Gastroenterology* 1994;107:934–944.
427. Torres C, Antonioli D, Odze RD. Polypoid dysplasia and adenomas in inflammatory bowel disease: a clinical, pathologic and follow-up study of 89 polyps from 59 patients. *Am J Surg Pathol* 1998;22:275–284.
428. Schneider A, Stole M. Differential diagnosis of adenomas and dysplastic lesions in patients with ulcerative colitis. *Z Gastroenterol* 1993;31:653–656.
429. Tarmin L, Yin J, Harpaz N, et al. Adenomatous polyposis coli gene mutations in ulcerative colitis-associated dysplasia and carcinoma versus sporadic colon neoplasms. *Cancer Res* 1995;55:2035–2038.
430. Redson MS, Papadopoulos N, Caldas C, Kinzler KW, Kern SE. Common occurrence of APC and K-ras gene mutations in the spectrum of colitis-associated neoplasias. *Gastroenterology* 1995;108:383–392.
431. Fogt F, Alexander O, Vortmeyer AO, Goldman H, Giordano TJ, Merino MJ, Zhuang Z. Comparison of genetic alterations in colonic adenoma and ulcerative colitis-associated dysplasia and carcinoma. *Hum Pathol* 1998;29:131–136.
432. Collier PE, Turowski P, Diamond DL. Small intestinal adenocarcinoma complicating regional enteritis. *Cancer* 1985;55:516–521.
433. Hamilton SR. Colorectal carcinoma in patients with Crohn's disease. *Gastroenterology* 1985;89:398–407.
434. Petras RE, Mir-Madjlessi SH, Farmer RG. Crohn's disease and intestinal carcinoma: a report of 11 cases with emphasis on associated epithelial dysplasia. *Gastroenterology* 1987;93:1307–1314.
435. Glotzer DJ. The risk of cancer in Crohn's disease. *Gastroenterology* 1985;89:438–441.
436. Cuvelier C, Bekaert E, DePotter C, Pauwels C, DeVos M, Roels H. Crohn's disease with adenocarcinoma and dysplasia: macroscopical, histological, and immunohistochemical aspects of two cases. *Am J Surg Pathol* 1989;13:187–196.
437. Cornell WR, Sheffield JP, Kamm MA, Ritchie JK, Hawley PR, Lennard-Jones JE. Lower gastrointestinal malignancy in Crohn's disease. *Gut* 1994;35:347–352.
438. Choi PM, Zelig MP. Similarity of colorectal cancer in Crohn's disease and ulcerative colitis: implication for carcinogenesis and prevention. *Gut* 1994;35:950–954.
439. Ribeiro MB, Greenstein AJ, Sachar DB, et al. Colorectal adenocarcinoma in Crohn's disease. *Ann Surg* 1996;223:186–193.

Ischemic Bowel Disease

440. Norris HT. Re-examination of the spectrum of ischemic bowel disease. In: Norris HT, ed. *Pathology of the small intestine, colon, and anus*, 2nd ed. New York: Churchill Livingstone, 1991;121–136.
441. Robinson JWL, Mirkovitch V, Winistorfer B, Saegesser F. Response of the intestinal mucosa to ischaemia. *Gut* 1981;22:512–527.
442. Kleigman RM, Fanaroff AA. Necrotizing enterocolitis. *N Engl J Med* 1984;310:1093–1103.
443. Tait RA, Kealy WF. Neonatal necrotizing enterocolitis. *J Clin Pathol* 1979;32:1090–1099.
444. Shamberger RC, Weinstein HJ, Delorey MJ, Levey RH. The medical and surgical management of typhlitis in children with acute nonlymphocytic (myelogenous) leukemia. *Cancer* 1986;57:603–607.
445. Shallman RW, Kuehner M, Williams GH, Sajjad S, Sauter R. Benign cecal ulcers: spectrum of disease and selective management. *Dis Colon Rectum* 1985;28:732–737.
446. Jablonski M, Putzki H, Hemann H. Necrosis of the ascending colon in chronic hemodialysis patients: report of three cases. *Dis Colon Rectum* 1987;30:623–625.
447. Mahoney TJ, Bubrick MP, Hitchcock CR. Nonspecific ulcers of the colon. *Dis Colon Rectum* 1978;21:623–626.
448. Sutherland DE, Chan FY, Foucar E, Simmons RL, Howard RJ, Najarian JS. The bleeding cecal ulcer in transplant patients. *Surgery* 1979;86:386–398.
449. Borsch G, Jahnke A, Bergbauer M, Nebel W. Solitary nonspecific ileal ulcer: diagnosis by coloileoscopy in a patient with previously assumed irritable bowel syndrome. *Dis Colon Rectum* 1983;26:734–737.
450. Kiser JL. Focal lesions of the small intestine. *Am J Surg* 1966;112:48–51.
451. Bjarnason I, Hayllar J, Macpherson AJ, Russell AS. Side effects of nonsteroidal anti-inflammatory drugs on the small and large intestines in humans. *Gastroenterology* 1993;104:1832–1847.
452. Chajek T, Fainaru M. Behcet's disease. Report of 41 cases and a review of the literature. *Medicine* 1975;54:179–196.
453. Baba S, Maruta M, Ando K, Teramoto T, Endo I. Intestinal Behcet's disease: report of 5 cases. *Dis Colon Rectum* 1976;19:428–440.
454. Kasahara Y, Tanaka S, Nishino M, Umemura H, Shiraha S, Kuyama T. Intestinal involvement in Behcet's disease: review of 136 surgical cases in the Japanese literature. *Dis Colon Rectum* 1981;24:103–106.
455. O'Duffy JD, Carney JA, Deodhar S. Behcet's disease. Report of 10 cases, three with new manifestations. *Ann Intern Med* 1971;75:561–570.
456. Berthrong M, Fajardo LF. Radiation injury in surgical pathology. *Am J Surg Pathol* 1981;5:153–178.
457. Gratama S, Smedts F, Whitehead R. Obstructive colitis: an analysis of 50 cases and a review of the literature. *Pathology* 1995;27:324–329.

Enteric Infections Encountered in Resection Specimens

458. Gleason TH, Patterson SD. The pathology of *Yersinia enterocolitica* ileocolitis. *Am J Surg* 1982;6:37–355.
459. Vantrappen G, Agg HO, Ponette E, Geboes K, Bertrand P. Yersinia enteritis and enterocolitis: gastroenterological aspects. *Gastroenterology* 1977;72:220–227.
460. Bradford WD, Noce PS, Gutman LT. Pathologic features of enteric infection with *Yersinia enterocolitica*. *Arch Pathol Lab Med* 1974;98:17–22.
461. El-Maraghi NRH, Mair NS. The histopathology of enteric infection with *Yersinia pseudotuberculosis*. *Am J Clin Pathol* 1979;71:631–639.
462. Tandon HD, Prakash A. Pathology of intestinal tuberculosis and its distinction from Crohn's disease. *Gut* 1972;13:260–269.
463. Smith JH. Typhoid fever. In: Binford CH, Connor DH, eds. *Pathology of tropical and extraordinary disease*. Washington, DC: Armed Forces Institute of Pathology, 1976:123–129.
464. Sprinz H, Gangarosa EJ, Williams M, Hornick RB, Woodward TE. Histopathology of the upper small intestines in typhoid fever. Biopsy study of experimental disease in man. *Am J Dig Dis* 1966;11:615–624.
465. Connor DH, Neafie RC, Meyers WM. Amebiasis. In: Binford CH, Connor DH, eds. *Pathology of tropical and extraordinary disease*. Washington, DC: Armed Forces Institute of Pathology, 1976:308–316.
466. Brant H, Perez Tamayo R. Pathology of human amebiasis. *Hum Pathol* 1970;1:351–385.
467. McCully RM, Barron CN, Cheever AW. Schistosomiasis (bilharziasis). In: Binford CH, Connor DH, eds. *Pathology of tropical and extraordinary disease*. Washington, DC: Armed Forces Institute of Pathology, 1976:482–508.
468. Smith JH, Christie JD. The pathobiology of *Schistosoma haematobium* infection in humans. *Hum Pathol* 1986;17:333–345.
469. Neafie RC. Balantidiasis. In: Binford CH, Connor DH, eds. *Pathology of tropical and extraordinary disease*. Washington, DC: Armed Forces Institute of Pathology, 1976:325–327.
470. Neafie RC, Connor DH. Trichuriasis. In: Binford CH, Connor DH, eds. *Pathology of tropical and extraordinary disease*. Washington, DC: Armed Forces Institute of Pathology, 1976:415–420.

Diverticular Disease

471. Connell AM. Pathogenesis of diverticular disease of the colon. *Adv Intern Med* 1977;22:377–395.
472. Whiteway J, Morson BC. Elastosis in diverticular disease of the sigmoid colon. *Gut* 1985;26:258–266.
473. Almy TP, Howell DA. Diverticular disease of the colon. *N Engl J Med* 1980;302:324–332.
474. Bova JG, Hopens TA, Goldstein HM. Diverticulitis of the right colon. *Dig Dis Sci* 1984;29:150–156.
475. Sugihara K, Muto T, Morioka Y, Asano A, Yamamoto T. Diverticular disease of the colon in Japan: a review of 615 cases. *Dis Colon Rectum* 1984;27:531–537.
476. Magness LJ, Sanfelipo PM, van Heerden JA, Judd ES. Diverticular disease of the right colon. *Surg Gynecol Obstet* 1975;140:30–32.
477. Markham N, Li AKC. Diverticulitis of the right colon—experience from Hong Kong. *Gut* 1991;33:547–549.
478. Lo CY, Chu KW. Acute diverticulitis of the right colon. *Am J Surg* 1996;171:244–246.
479. Nirula R, Greaney G. Right-sided diverticulitis: a difficult diagnosis. *Am Surg* 1997;63:871–873.

Vascular Lesions of the Intestinal Tract

480. Moore JD, Thompson NW, Appelman HD, Foley D. Arteriovenous malformation of the gastrointestinal tract. *Arch Surg* 1976;11:381–389.
481. Camilleri M, Chadwick VS, Hodgson HJF. Vascular anomalies of the gastrointestinal tract. *Hepatogastroenterology* 1984;31:149–153.
482. Boley SJ, Brandt LJ. Vascular ectasias of the colon—1986. *Dig Dis Sci* 1986;31:26S–42S.
483. Wolff WI, Grossman MB, Shinya H. Angiodysplasia of the colon: diagnosis and treatment. *Gastroenterology* 1977;72:329–333.
484. Lyon DT, Mantia AG. Large-bowel hemangiomas. *Dis Colon Rectum* 1984;27:404–414.
485. Allred HW, Spencer RJ. Hemangiomas of the colon, rectum, and anus. *Mayo Clin Proc* 1974;49:739–741.
486. Coppa GF, Eng K, Localio SA. Surgical management of diffuse cavernous hemangioma of the colon, rectum, and anus. *Surg Gynecol Obstet* 1984;159:17–21.
487. Stening SG, Heptinstall DP. Diffuse cavernous hemangioma of the rectum and sigmoid colon. *Br J Surg* 1970;57:186–189.
488. Waxman JS, Tarkin N, Dave P, Waxman M. Fatal hemorrhage from rectal varices: report of two cases. *Dis Colon Rectum* 1984;27:749–750.
489. Smith CR Jr, Bartholomew LG, Cain JC. Hereditary hemorrhagic telangiectasia and gastrointestinal hemorrhage. *Gastroenterology* 1963;44:1–6.
490. Rosekrans PCM, de Rooy DJ, Bosman FT, Eulderink F, Cats A. Gastrointestinal telangiectasia as a cause of severe blood loss in systemic sclerosis. *Endoscopy* 1980;12:200–204.
491. Sandhu KS, Cohen H, Radin R, Buck FS. Blue rubber bleb nevus syndrome presenting with recurrences. *Dig Dis Sci* 1987;32:214–219.
492. Rutlin E, Wisloff F, Myron J, Serck-Hanssen A. Intestinal telangiectasia in Turner's syndrome. *Endoscopy* 1981;13:86–87.
493. Cunningham JP, Lippman SM, Renie WA, Francomano CA, Maumenee IH, Pyeritz RE. Pseudoxanthoma elasticum: treatment of gastrointestinal hemorrhage by arterial embolization and observations on autosomal dominant inheritance. *Johns Hopkins Med J* 1980;147:168–173.
494. Krane SM. Understanding genetic disorders of collagen. *N Engl J Med* 1980;303:101–102.
495. Harris RD. Small bowel dilatation in Ehlers-Danlos syndrome—an unreported gastrointestinal manifestation. *Br J Radiol* 1974;47:623–627.

Intestinal Pseudo-obstruction

496. Faulk DL, Anuras S, Christensen J. Chronic intestinal pseudoobstruction. *Gastroenterology* 1978;74:922–932.
497. Yamada M, Hatakeyama S, Tsukagoshi H. Gastrointestinal amyloid deposition in AL (primary or myeloma associated) and AA (secondary) amyloidosis: diagnostic value of gastric biopsy. *Hum Pathol* 1985;16:1206–1211.

Visceral Myopathies

498. Krishnamurthy S, Schuffler MD. Pathology of neuromuscular disorders of the small intestine and colon. *Gastroenterology* 1987;93:610–639.
499. Pruzanski W, Huvos AG. Smooth muscle involvement in primary muscle disease I. Myotonic dystrophy. *Arch Pathol Lab Med* 1967;83:229–233.
500. Huvos AG, Pruzanski W. Smooth muscle involvement in primary muscle disease II. Progressive muscular dystrophy. *Arch Pathol Lab Med* 1967;83:234–240.
501. Leon SH, Schuffler MD, Kettler M, Rohrmann CA. Chronic intestinal pseudo-obstruction as a complication of Duchenne's muscular dystrophy. *Gastroenterology* 1986;90:455–459.
502. Schuffler MD, Beegle RG. Progressive systemic sclerosis of the gastrointestinal tract and hereditary visceral myopathy: two distinguishable disorders of intestinal smooth muscle. *Gastroenterology* 1979;77:664–671.
503. Mitros FA, Schuffler MD, Teja K, Anuras S. Pathologic features of familial visceral myopathy. *Hum Pathol* 1982;13:825–833.
504. Ariza A, Coll J, Fernandez-Figueras MT, et al. Desmin myopathy: A multi-system disorder involving skeletal, cardiac and smooth muscle. *Hum Pathol* 1995;26:1032–1037.
505. Smith VV, Milla PJ. Histological phenotype of enteric smooth muscle disease causing functional intestinal obstruction in childhood. *Histopathology* 1997;31:112–122.

Visceral Neuropathies

506. Schuffler MD, Jonak Z. Chronic idiopathic intestinal pseudo-obstruction caused by a degenerative disorder of the myenteric plexus: the use

of Smith's method to define neuropathology. *Gastroenterology* 1982;82:476–486.
507. Schuffler MD, Baird HW, Fleming CR, et al. Intestinal pseudo-obstruction as the presenting manifestations of small-cell carcinoma of the lung: a paraneoplastic neuropathy of the gastrointestinal tract. *Ann Intern Med* 1983;98:129–134.
508. Krishnamurthy S, Schuffler MD, Belic L, Schweid AI. An inflammatory axonopathy of the myenteric plexus producing a rapidly progressive pseudo-obstruction. *Gastroenterology* 1986;90:754–758.
509. Sanders KM. A case for interstitial cells of Cajal as pacemakers and mediators of neurotransmission in the gastrointestinal tract. *Gastroenterology* 1996;111:492–515.
510. Der-Silaphet T, Malysz J, Hagel S, Arsenault AI, Huizinga JD. Interstitial cells of Cajal direct normal propulsive contractile activity in the mouse small intestine. *Gastroenterology* 1998;114:724–736.
511. Campbell F, Hewlett B, Ho J, Huizinga J, Riddell RH. Interstitial cells of Cajal (ICC) are absent or deranged in intestinal pseudo-obstruction. *Lab Invest* 1998;75:61A.
512. Forse RA, Tabah EJ. Jejunal diverticulosis. *Can J Surg* 1980;23: 291–303.
513. Gallager RL. Intestinal ceroid deposition—"brown bowel syndrome": a light and electron microscopic study. *Virchows Arch [A] Pathol Anat Histopathol* 1980;389:143–151.
514. Hitzman JL, Weiland LH, Oftedahl GL, Lie JT. Ceroidosis in the "brown bowel syndrome." *Mayo Clin Proc* 1979;54:251–257.
515. Foster CS. The brown bowel syndrome: a possible smooth muscle mitochondrial myopathy. *Histopathology* 1979;3:1–17.
516. Smith B. Pathologic changes in the colon produced by anthroquinone purgatives. *Dis Colon Rectum* 1973;16:455–458.
517. Badiali D, Marcheggino A, Pallone F, et al. Melanosis of the rectum in patients with chronic constipation. *Dis Colon Rectum* 1985;28: 241–245.
518. Preston DM, Hawley PR, Lennard-Jones, Todd IP. Results of colectomy for severe idiopathic constipation in women (Arbuthnot Lane's disease). *Br J Surg* 1984;71:547–552.
519. Krishnamurthy S, Schuffler MD, Rohrmann CA, Pope CE II. Severe idiopathic constipation is associated with a distinctive abnormality of the colonic myenteric plexus. *Gastroenterology* 1985;88:26–34.
520. Smith B. Pathology of cathartic colon. *Proc R Soc Med* 1972;65:288.

Hirschsprung's Disease and Allied Conditions

521. Nixon HH. Hirschsprung's disease in the newborn. In: Holschneider AM, ed. *Hirschsprung's disease*. New York: Thieme-Stratton, 1982:103–113.
522. Molenaar JC. Pathogenetic aspects of Hirschsprung's disease. *Br J Surg* 1995;82:145–147.
523. Eng C. The RET proto-oncogene in multiple endocrine neoplasia type 2 and Hirschsprung's disease. *N Engl J Med* 1996;335:943–951.
524. Yunis EJJ, Dibbins AW, Sherman FE. Rectal suction biopsy in the diagnosis of Hirschsprung's disease in infants. *Arch Pathol Lab Med* 1976;100:329–333.
525. Aldrige RT, Campbell PE. Ganglion cell distribution in the normal rectum and anal canal: a basis for the diagnosis of Hirschsprung's disease by anorectal biopsy. *J Pediatr Surg* 1968;3:475–490.
526. Meier-Ruge W. Morphological diagnosis of Hirschsprung's disease. In: Holschneider AM, ed. *Hirschsprung's disease*. New York: Thieme-Stratton, 1982:62–71.
527. Hamoudi AB, Reiner CB, Boles ET Jr, McClung HJ, Kerzner B. Acetylthiocholinesterase staining activity of rectal mucosa. Its use in the diagnosis of Hirschsprung's disease. *Arch Pathol Lab Med* 1982;106:670–672.
528. Ariel I, Vinograd I, Lernav OZ, Nissan S, Rosenmann E. Rectal mucosal biopsy in aganglionosis and allied conditions. *Hum Pathol* 1983;14:991–995.
529. Doody DP, Kim SH. Pathology of Hirschsprung's disease and related neuroenteric disorders. *Semin Colon Rectal Surg* 1992;3:207–212.
530. Vinores SA, May E. Neuron-specific enolase as an immunohistochemical tool for the diagnosis of Hirschsprung's disease. *Am J Surg Pathol* 1985;9:281–285.
531. Abu-Alfa AK, Kuan S, West AB, Reyes-Mugica M. Cathepsin D in intestinal ganglion cells: a potential aid to diagnosis in suspected Hirschsprung's disease. *Am J Surg Pathol* 1997;21:201–205.
532. Munakata K, Okabe I, Morita K. Histologic studies of rectocolic aganglionosis and allied disease. *J Pediatr Surg* 1978;13:67–75.

533. Scharli AF, Meier-Ruge W. Localized and disseminated forms of neuronal intestinal dysplasia mimicking Hirschsprung's disease. *J Pediatr Surg* 1981;16:164–170.
534. Reiffersheid P, Flach A. Particular forms of Hirschsprung's disease. In: Holschneider AM, ed. *Hirschsprung's disease*. New York: Thieme-Stratton, 1982:133–142.
535. Meier-Ruge WA, Bronnimann PB, Gambazzi F, Schmid PC, Schmidt CP, Stoss F. Histopathological criteria for intestinal neuronal dysplasia of the submucosal plexus (type B). *Virchows Arch* 1995;426:549–556.
536. Lake BD. Intestinal neuronal dysplasia: why does it only occur in parts of Europe? *Virchows Arch* 1995;426:537–539.
537. Qualman SJ, Murray R. Aganglionosis and related disorders. *Hum Pathol* 1994;25:1141–1149.
538. Yunis E, Sieber WK, Ackers DR. Does zonal aganglionosis really exist? Report of a rare variety of Hirschsprung's disease and review of the literature. *Pediatr Pathol* 1983;1:33–49.
539. Seldenrijk CA, van der Harten HJ, Kluck P, Tibboel D, Moorman-Voestermans K, Meijer CJLM. Zonal aganglionosis: an enzyme and immunohistochemical study of two cases. *Virchows Arch [A] Pathol Anat Histopathol* 1986;410:75–81.
540. Symmers WStC. Primary amyloidosis: a review. *J Clin Pathol* 1956;9:187.
541. Dahlin DC. Secondary amyloidosis. *Ann Intern Med* 1949;31: 105–119.
542. Gilat T, Revach M, Sohar E. Deposition of amyloid in the gastrointestinal tract. *Gut* 1969;10:98–104.
543. Falk RH, Comenzo RL, Skinner M. The systemic amyloidoses. *N Eng J Med* 1997;337:898–909.
544. Kyle RA, Spencer RJ, Dahlin DC. Value of rectal biopsy in the diagnosis of primary systemic amyloidosis. *Am J Med Sci* 1966;25: 501–506.

Congenital Diverticula, Duplications, and Enteric Cysts

545. Mackey WC, Dineen P. A 50-year experience with Meckel's diverticulum. *Surg Gynecol Obstet* 1983;156:56–64.
546. Artigas V, Calabuig R, Badia F, Rius X, Allende L, Jover J. Meckel's diverticulum: value of ectopic tissue. *Am J Surg* 1986;151:631–634.
547. DiGiacomo JC, Gottone FJ. Surgical treatment of Meckel's diverticulum. *South Med J* 1993;86:671–675.
548. Cserni G. Gastric pathology in Meckel's diverticulum. Review of cases resected between 1965 and 1995. *Am J Clin Pathol* 1996; 106:782–785.
549. Hjermstad BM, Helwig EB. Tailgut cysts: report of 53 cases. *Am J Clin Pathol* 1988;89:139–147.
550. Marco V, Fernandez-Layos M, Autonell J, Doncel F, Farre J. Retrorectal cyst-hamartomas: report of two cases with adenocarcinoma developing in one. *Am J Surg Pathol* 1982;6:707–714.
551. Mills SE, Walker AN, Stallings RG, Allen MS Jr. Retrorectal cystic hamartoma: report of three cases, including one with a perirenal component. *Arch Pathol Lab Med* 1984;108:737–740.

Pneumatosis Cystoides Intestinalis

552. Galandiuk S, Fazio VW. Pneumatosis cystoides intestinalis: a review of the literature. *Dis Colon Rectum* 1986;29:358–363.
553. Heng Y, Schuffler MD, Haggitt RC, Rohrmann CA. Pneumatosis intestinalis: a review. *Am J Gastroenterol* 1995;90:1747–1758.
554. Pieterse AS, Leong ASY, Rowland R. The mucosal changes and pathogenesis of pneumatosis cystoides intestinalis. *Hum Pathol* 1975;16:683–688.
555. Snover DC, Sandstad J, Houtton S. Mucosal pseudolipomatosis of the colon. *Am J Clin Pathol* 1985;84:575–580.
556. Kaassis M, Croue A, Carpentier S, Burtin P, Boyer J. A case of colonic pseudolipomatosis: a rare complication of colonoscopy? *Endoscopy* 1997;29:325–327.

Radiation and Antineoplastic Chemotherapy Injury

557. Novak JM, Collins JT, Donowitz M, Farman J, Sheahan DG, Spiro HM. Effects of radiation on the human gastrointestinal tract. *J Clin Gastroenterol* 1979;1:9–39.
558. Weisbort IM, Liber AF, Gordon BS. The effects of therapeutic radiation on colonic mucosa. *Cancer* 1975;36:931–940.

559. Gelfand MD, Tepper M, Katz L, et al. Acute irradiation proctitis in man. Development of eosinophilic crypt abscesses. *Gastroenterology* 1975;54:401.
560. Miles S, Muggia A, Spiro H. Colonic histologic changes induced by 5-fluorouracil on rectal mucosa. *Gastroenterology* 1962;43:391–399.
561. Floch M, Hellman L. The effects of 5-fluorouracil on rectal mucosa. *Gastroenterology* 1965;48:430–437.
562. Searle J, Kerr JFR, Bishop CJ. Necrosis and apoptosis: distinct modes of cell death with fundamentally different significance. *Pathol Annu* 1982;17:229–259.
563. Bennet RE, Harrison MW, Bishop CJ, et al. The role of apoptosis in atrophy of the small gut mucosa produced by repeated administration of cytosine arabinoside. *J Pathol* 1984;142:259–263.
564. Petras RE, Hart WR, Bukowski RM. Gastric epithelial atypia associated with hepatic arterial infusion chemotherapy: its distinction from early gastric carcinoma. *Cancer* 1985;56:745–750.
565. DeCosse JJ, Rhodes RS, Wentz WB, Regan JW, Dworken HJ, Holden WD. The natural history and management of radiation induced injury of the gastrointestinal tract. *Ann Surg* 1969;170:369–384.

Small Bowel Transplantation and Rejection

566. Deltz E. Current status of small bowel transplantation. *Ann Med* 1991;23:507–508.
567. Frezza EE, Tzakis A, Fung JJ, van Thiel DH. Small bowel transplantation: current progress and clinical application. *Hepatogastroenterol* 1996;43:363–376.
568. Banner B, Hoffman A, Cai X, Starzl TE, Sheehan DG. Transplantation of the small intestine: the pathologists's perspective. *Am J Surg Pathol* 1990;14[Suppl]:109–116.
569. Hoffman AL, Makowka L, Banner B, et al. The use of FK-506 for small intestinal allotransplantation. *Transplantation* 1990;49:483–490.
570. Murase N, Demetris AJ, Matsuzaki T, et al. Long survival in rats after multivisceral versus isolated small-bowel allotransplantation under FK-506. *Surgery* 1991;110:87–98.
571. Murase N, Demetris AJ, Kim DG, Todo S, Fung JJ, Starzl TE. Rejection of multivisceral allografts in rats: a sequential analysis with comparison to isolated orthotopic small-bowel and liver grafts. *Surgery* 1990;108:880–889.
572. Lee RG, Nakamura K, Tsamandas C, et al. Pathology of human intestinal transplantation. *Gastroenterology* 1996;110:1820–1834.
573. White FV, Reyes J, Jaffe R, Yunis EJ. Pathology of intestinal transplantation in children. *Am J Surg Pathol* 1995;19:687–698.

Fibrosing Colonopathy

574. Pawel BR, de Chandarevian J, Franco ME. The pathology of fibrosing colonopathy of cystic fibrosis: a study of 12 cases and review of the literature. *Hum Pathol* 1997;28:395–399.
575. Smyth RL, Ashby D, O'Hea U, et al. Fibrosing colonopathy in cystic fibrosis: results of a case-control study. *Gastroenterology* 1996;111:260–264.

Nonneoplastic "Tumors" of the Intestines

576. Vuang PN, Gujot H, Moulin G, Houissa-Vuang S, Berrod J. Pseudotumoral organization of a twisted epiploic fringe or "hard-boiled egg" in the peritoneal cavity. *Arch Pathol Lab Med* 1990;114:531–533.
577. Phelps JE, Sanowski RA, Kazarek RA. Barium ulceration of the rectum resembling carcinoma. *Gastrointest Endosc* 1980;26:74.
578. Stouder DJ, McDonald LW. Enlarged intra-abdominal pacinian corpuscles simulating tumor implants. *Am J Clin Pathol* 1968;49:79–83.
579. Warthin AS. The pathology of the pacinian corpuscles. *Philadelphia Monthly Med J* 1899;February:1–20.
580. Dembinski AS, Jones JW. Intra-abdominal pacinian neuroma: a rare lesion in an unusual location. *Histopathology* 1991;19:89–90.

Vermiform Appendix and Appendicitis

581. Segal G, Petras R. The Vermiform Appendix. In: Sternberg SS, ed. *Histology for pathologists*, 2nd ed. Philadelphia: Lippincott-Raven, 1997:539–550.
582. Gray GF Jr, Wackym PA. Surgical pathology of the vermiform appendix. In: Sommers SC, Rosen PP, Fechner RE, eds. *Pathology annual.* Norwalk, CT: Appleton-Century-Croft, 1986:111–144.
583. Glasser CM, Bhagavan BS. Carcinoid tumors of the appendix. *Arch Pathol Lab Med* 1980;104:272–285.
584. Bluett MK, Halter SA, Salhany KEW, O'Leary JP. Duplication of the appendix mimicking adenocarcinoma of the colon. *Ann Surg* 1987;122:817–820.
585. George DH. Diverticulosis of the vermiform appendix in patients with cystic fibrosis. *Hum Pathol* 1987;18:75–79.
586. Butler C. Surgical pathology of acute appendicitis. *Hum Pathol* 1981;12:870–878.
587. Schenken JR, Anderson TR, Coleman FC. Acute focal appendicitis. *Am J Clin Pathol* 1959;26:352–359.
588. Stanley MW, Cherwitz D, Hagen K, Snover DC. Neuromas of the appendix. A light-microscopic, immunohistochemical and electron microscopic study of 20 cases. *Am J Surg Pathol* 1986;10:801–815.
589. Neafi RC, Connor DH, Meyers WM. Enterobiasis. In: Binford CH, Connor DH, eds. *Pathology of tropical and extraordinary disease.* Washington, DC: Armed Forces Institute of Pathology, 1976:455–459.
590. Hofler H, Kasper M, Heitz PU. The neuroendocrine system of normal human appendix, ileum, and colon and in neurogenic appendicopathy. *Virchow Arch [A] Pathol Anat Histopathol* 1983;399:127–140.
591. Aubock L, Ratzenhofer M. "Extraepithelial enterochromaffin cell-nerve-fibre complexes" in the normal human appendix and in neurogenic appendicopathy. *J Pathol* 1982;136:217–226.
592. Olsen BS, Holck S. Neurogenous hyperplasia leading to appendiceal obliteration: an immunohistochemical study of 237 cases. *Histopathology* 1987;11:843–849.

Crohn's Disease of the Appendix

593. Ariel I, Vinograd I, Hershlag A, et al. Crohn's disease isolated to the appendix: truths and fallacies. *Hum Pathol* 1986;17:1116–1121.
594. Timmcke AE. Granulomatous appendicitis: is it Crohn's disease? Report of a case and review of the literature. *Am J Gastroenterol* 1986;81:283–287.
595. Wettergren A, Munkholm P, Larson LG, et al. Granulomas of the appendix: is it Crohn's disease? *Scand J Gastroenterol* 1991;26:961–964.
596. Dudley Jr TH, Dean PJ. Idiopathic granulomatous appendicitis, or Crohn's disease of the appendix revisited. *Hum Pathol* 1993;24:595–601.
597. Huang JC, Appelman HD. Another look at chronic appendicitis resembling Crohn's disease. *Mod Pathol* 1996;9:975–981.

Inflammatory Lesions of the Mesentery and Retroperitoneum

598. Kelly JK, Wei-Sek H. Idiopathic retractile (sclerosing) mesenteritis and its differential diagnosis. *Am J Surg Pathol* 1989;13:513–521.
599. Remmele W, Müller-Lobeck H, Paulus W. Primary mesenteritis, mesenteric fibrosis and mesenteric fibromatosis. Report of four cases, pathology, and classification. *Pathol Res Pract* 1989;184:77–85.
600. Eble JN, Rosenberg AE, Young RH. Retroperitoneal xanthogranulomatosis in a patient with Erdheim-Chester Disease. *Am J Surg Pathol* 1994;18:843–848.
601. Emory TS, Monihan JM, Carr NJ, Sobin LH. Sclerosing mesenteritis, mesenteric panniculitis and mesenteric lipodystrophy: a single entity? *Am J Surg Pathol* 1997;21:392–398.
602. Enzinger FM, Weiss SW. *Soft tissue tumors,* 2nd ed. St. Louis: CV Mosby, 1988.
603. Kraus MD, Guillou L, Fletcher CDM. Well-differentiated inflammatory liposarcoma: an uncommon and easily overlooked variant of a common sarcoma. *Am J Surg Pathol* 1997;21:518–527.
604. Waldron JA, Newcomer LN, Katz ME, Cadman E. Sclerosing variants of follicular center cell lymphomas presenting in the retroperitoneum. *Cancer* 1983;52:712–720.
605. Kipfer RE, Moetel CG, Dahlin DC. Mesenteric lipodystrophy. *Ann Intern Med* 1974;80:582–588.
606. Osborne BM, Butler JJ, Bloustein P, Sumner G. Idiopathic retroperi-

toneal fibrosis (sclerosing retroperitonitis). *Hum Pathol* 1987; 18:735–739.
607. Dobbins WO III. Whipple's disease. Springfield, IL: Thomas, 1987.
608. Scherrer P, Gonvers JJ, Ruzicka J, Schnyder P, Godat A. Un cas de maladie de Whipple a presentation pseudotumorale: diagnostic deifferential avec une panniculite mesenterique. *Schweiz Med Wochr* 1984;114:272–276.
609. Steely WM, Gooden SM. Sclerosing mesocolitis. *Dis Colon Rectum* 1986;29:266–268.
610. Panush RS, Yonker RA, Delesk A, Longley S, Caldwell JR. Weber-Christian disease, analysis of 15 cases and review of the literature. *Medicine* 1985;64:181–191.
611. Coffin CM, Watterson J, Priest JR, et al. Extrapulmonary inflammatory myofibroblastic tumor (inflammatory pseudotumor). A clinco-pathological and immunohistochemical study of 84 cases. *Am J Surg Pathol* 1992;19:859–872.
612. Day DL, Sane S, Dehner LP. Inflammatory pseudotumor of the mesentery and small intestine. *Pediatr Radiol* 1986;16:210–215.
613. Wu JP, Yunis EJ, Fetterman G, Jaeschke WF, Gilbert EF. Inflammatory pseudo-tumors of the abdomen, plasma cell granulomas. *J Clin Pathol* 1973;26:735–738.
614. Kocova L, Michal M, Sulc M, Zamecnik M. Calcifying fibrous pseudotumor of visceral peritoneum. *Histopathology* 1997;31:182–184.

CHAPTER 34

Intestinal Neoplasms

Harry S. Cooper

POLYPS

Polyp is a clinical term or gross description of any circumscribed tumor or growth that projects above the surrounding mucosa. The term *polyp* by itself has no clinical significance. Polyps may be neoplastic, inflammatory, or hamartomatous in nature; only by histologic examination can one be certain of their nature and clinical significance.

Nonneoplastic Polyps

Hyperplastic Polyp

Clinical Features

Hyperplastic polyps are benign epithelial proliferations located predominantly in the rectum (1). They are also commonly found in the sigmoid colon but are less common in the more proximal large intestine (2). In the Western world, they may be found in approximately 85% of the adult population, whereas in Third World countries the incidence may be 2% to 3% (3). The incidence of hyperplastic polyps is age related, increasing after age 40.

The vast majority of hyperplastic polyps are 3 to 6 mm in size. Earlier studies indicated that 80% to 90% of colonic polyps <5 mm in size were of the hyperplastic type (4); however, more recent reports have shown that small polyps (<6 mm) in the proximal colon are more likely to be adenomas than hyperplastic polyps, whereas small polyps in the sigmoid colon and rectum are more likely to be of the hyperplastic type (2,5,6). In large series of hyperplastic polyps, approximately 1% to 4% are greater than 1 cm in size (7,8); however, these may actually be serrated adenomas rather than hyperplastic polyps. Because of their small size, hyperplastic polyps rarely cause symptoms and are usually detected incidentally at proctoscopic or colonoscopic examination. Nevertheless, there are reports of large or multiple hyperplastic polyps responsible for gastrointestinal symptoms (9–12).

Hyperplastic polyps are not considered to be premalignant, although there have been reports of adenomatous or carcinomatous transformation in hyperplastic polyps, a feature usually associated with large polyp size or with patients having multiple polyps (7,8,11–16). Results are conflicting as to whether hyperplastic polyps of the rectosigmoid colon are "markers" for the presence of more proximal adenomas (2,17–19). A position paper by the American College of Gastroenterology states that a hyperplastic polyp found during sigmoidoscopy is not an indication for colonoscopy (20).

As with other polyps of the large intestine, multiple hyperplastic polyposis has been reported. The number of polyps have varied from numerous to hundreds; there is a marked male predominance. Intestinal cancers have arisen in some of these patients (7,9,11,12,15,16,21). All the studies report no familial history, except for one series that reports a family fulfilling the Amsterdam criteria for hereditary nonpolyposis colon cancer syndrome in the presence of giant hyperplastic polyposis (21). However, in this family the polyps were not all reported as hyperplastic but as a mixture of hyperplastic polyps, admixed hyperplastic-adenomatous polyps, and serrated adenomas. Some reported cases may not truly be hyperplastic polyposis but rather serrated adenomatous polyposis (see below). Classification can be difficult because in many reports the illustrations preclude one from differentiating between serrated adenomas and hyperplastic polyps. However, Burt and Samowitz (22) have noted cases of true hyperplastic polyposis. It should also be noted that there is no definition as to the minimum number of polyps needed for a case to qualify as hyperplastic polyposis.

Pathologic Features

Grossly, hyperplastic polyps tend to be small, dome (convex)-shaped structures that are the same color as, or paler than, the surrounding mucosa. They often sit on the crest of the mucosal folds (Fig. 1). Occasionally, hyperplastic polyps may be pedunculated and grossly mimic adenomas.

H. S. Cooper: Department of Pathology, Fox Chase Cancer Center, Philadelphia, Pennsylvania 19111.

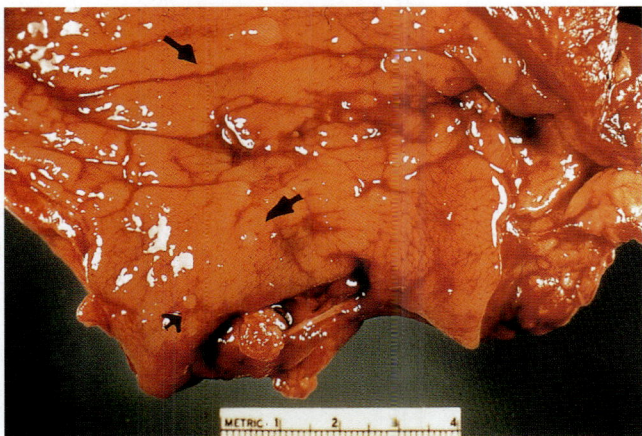

FIG. 1. Gross appearance of hyperplastic polyp. *Arrows* point to hyperplastic polyps. These lesions are small, convex, and the same color as the background mucosa. (From ref. 302.)

Microscopically, they are quite characteristic (1,7,23). At low power, well-oriented specimens tend to have a serrated or sawtooth appearance not unlike a secretory endometrium (Fig. 2). When biopsy material is cut tangentially, the crypts assume a star-shaped appearance (Fig. 3). Hyperplastic polyps consist of mixtures of goblet and absorptive cells, with the latter usually predominating. In both cell types the nuclei are basally located and bland in appearance (Fig. 2). Occasionally, the nuclei may be stratified. The columnar cells have a distinct eosinophilic cytoplasm with well-defined brush borders. These cells may also have apical mucin vacuoles. Paneth cells may be seen at the base of the crypts. There is usually a thickening of the subepithelial collagen layer. Mitotic figures are limited to the lower two-thirds of the crypt and are never seen at the surface. In well-oriented material, the cells at the basal portion of the crypt tend to show nuclear elongation, crowding, and increased mitotic rate compared to

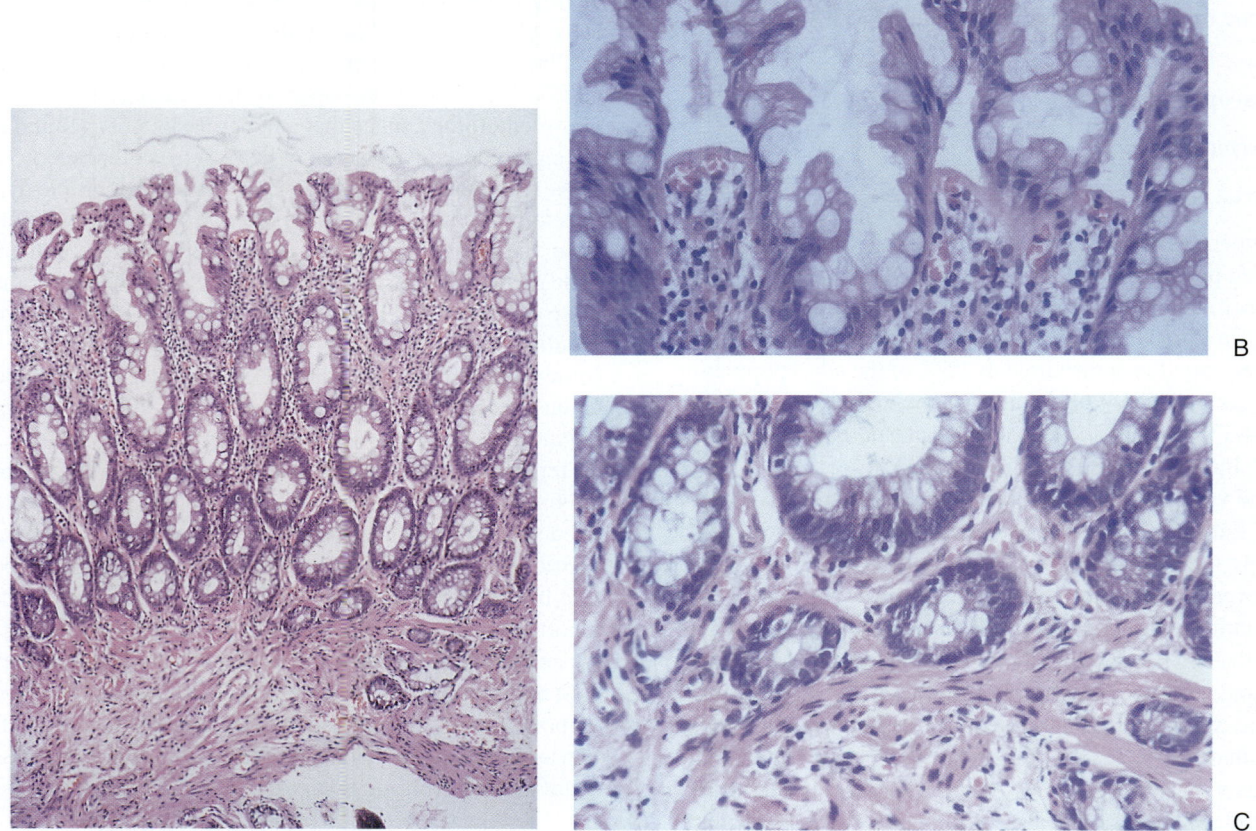

FIG. 2. A: Low-power microscopic view of a well-oriented hyperplastic polyp. Note that toward the surface the epithelium is serrated or has papillary infoldings. **B:** High-power view of the surface epithelium showing bland basally placed nuclei. The epithelial cells are an admixture of goblet cells and eosinophilic absorptive cells. **C:** Base of the crypt showing mild splaying of the muscularis mucosae around crypts. Note that the cells at the crypt base appear crowded with somewhat hyperchromatic nuclei (not to be confused with those of an adenoma).

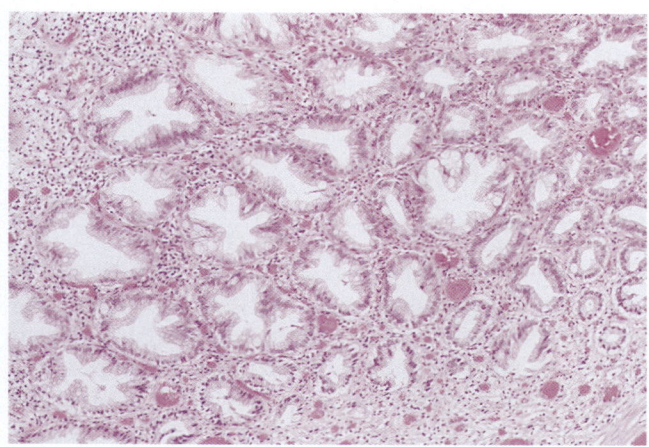

FIG. 3. Low-power view of a poorly oriented biopsy of a hyperplastic polyp. One can see star-shaped crypts, which should alert the observer that this may be a hyperplastic polyp.

the normal surrounding mucosa. These findings can be impressive and should not be interpreted as adenomatous change in a hyperplastic polyp. The muscularis mucosae often show a characteristic splaying, with muscle fibers extending into the mucosa and surrounding individual crypts (Fig. 2). This splaying can be so extensive as to give the false impression of invasion of glands into the submucosa. One should be cognizant of this pseudoinvasion and not diagnose it as cancer (7,24). In routine practice, special studies (e.g., mucin histochemistry, immunohistochemistry, molecular markers) play no role in diagnosing hyperplastic polyps.

Variants of hyperplastic polyps are (a) large size and (b) admixed hyperplastic polyp-adenoma. Larger hyperplastic polyps (>1 cm) may grossly be pedunculated or sessile. At low power they may have a villous pattern or may superficially resemble Peutz-Jeghers polyps. In large hyperplastic polyps columnar cells having eosinophilic cytoplasm predominate, with few goblet cells. The nuclei may be stratified and show nucleoli (7). However, in light of the recent characterization of the serrated adenoma, one must query whether these lesions represent large hyperplastic polyps or serrated adenomas. In the author's personal experience, cases that in the past I had considered to be large hyperplastic polyps on re-review I now believe to be serrated adenomas. (See below for further discussion and differential diagnosis.) Adenomatous foci admixed with hyperplastic epithelium occur (Fig. 4) with a reported prevalence of 0.6% to 9.6%. (7,8). This feature is seen most commonly in large hyperplastic polyps.

Hyperplastic polyp-type epithelium can be seen in juvenile polyps, Peutz-Jeghers polyps, and inflammatory polyps, especially inflammatory cloacogenic polyps of the anal region. That these latter lesions can be easily misdiagnosed as hyperplastic polyps is evidenced by the fact that retrospective review of cases recorded as hyperplastic polyps in our institution revealed a large number of inflammatory cloacogenic polyps misdiagnosed as hyperplastic polyps.

Villous adenomas may occasionally mimic hyperplastic polyps. At low-power microscopy, some villous adenomas have a serrated appearance and eosinophilic cytoplasm. However, on closer inspection at high power, the finding of obvious adenomatous epithelium rules out hyperplastic polyp and confirms the diagnosis of villous adenoma.

Serrated Adenoma (Mixed Hyperplastic/Adenomatous Polyp)

Serrated adenomas are discussed in the section on hyperplastic polyp because of their morphologic similarity to and confusion with hyperplastic polyps.

Clinical Features

Serrated adenomas are uncommon; 101 were found in one series of 18,000 polyps (0.6%) (25). They are found most commonly in the rectosigmoid colon and range in size from 0.2 to 7.5 cm; 60% are 0.1 to 0.6 cm and 21% are greater than 1.0 cm in diameter. Sixty-five percent and 35% of serrated adenomas are sessile and pedunculated, respectively; 24% have foci of traditional adenoma, whereas 10% have foci of intramucosal cancer (25).

Pathology

At low power, these polyps have a serrated pattern similar to that of the traditional hyperplastic polyp (Fig. 5). However, serrated adenomas tend to have elongated and dilated crypts. Compared to hyperplastic polyps, they are more villiform and have more complex branching. Columnar cells predominate over goblet cells, with the former having very eosinophilic

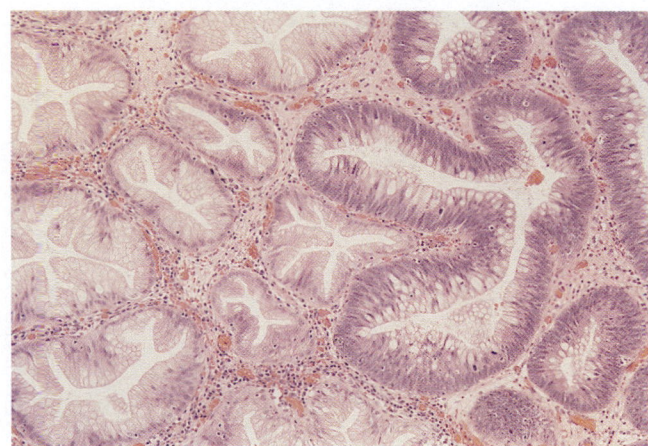

FIG. 4. Admixed hyperplastic adenomatous polyp. At low power one can appreciate hyperplastic polyp *(left)* compared to adenoma *(right)*.

cytoplasm. Serrated adenomas lack the thickened subepithelial collagen layer seen in hyperplastic polyps.

However, the most discriminating feature is the nuclei, which show atypia that is greater than that in hyperplastic polyps but less than that in traditional adenomas. In hyperplastic polyps, the nuclei are ovoid or round, basophilic with occasional faint nucleoli, and basally placed with little pseudostratification. By contrast, the nuclei of the serrated adenoma, are longer, more ovoid, exhibit focal pseudostratification and are often vesicular with more prominent nucleoli (Figs. 5 and 6). Mitoses can be seen occasionally in the upper crypt and at the surface (25,26). Torlakovic and Snover (26) suggest that hyperplastic polyps can be distinguished from serrated adenomas by the following features of serrated adenomas: (a) dilatation of the crypts that is most prominent at the base; (b) horizontally oriented crypts just above the muscularis mucosae; (c) nuclear atypia, with vesicular round nuclei with nucleoli; (d) focal mucin overproduction (resembling mucinous cystadenoma of the appendix); and (e) eosinophilia of columnar cell cytoplasm.

Patients with multiple serrated adenomas (polyposis) are described in the literature. As noted above, many of the reported cases of large hyperplastic polyposis most likely are serrated adenomas. Torlakovic and Snover (26) reported six cases of serrated adenomatous polyposis. Five of the six cases were males, four had associated cancers, and two had associated adenomas. In four cases polyps were described as >100 in number and in two cases as >50 in number. There were no reported familial cases.

Peutz-Jeghers Polyp

Clinical Features

The Peutz-Jeghers polyp is a hamartomatous lesion that can occur in the stomach, small intestine, and colon. They are most often identified in patients with the Peutz-Jeghers syndrome; however, solitary Peutz-Jeghers polyps in patients without the syndrome do occur with some frequency (27–30). The Peutz-Jeghers syndrome (31,32) is an autosomal dominant disorder consisting of gastrointestinal hamartomatous polyps associated with mucocutaneous pigmentation, and, in female patients, with ovarian sex cord tumors with annular tubules, breast cancer, and adenocarcinoma of the uterine cervix. In males it has been associated with testicular Sertoli cell tumors (Table 1). Most patients are diagnosed in their twenties. The presenting clinical symptoms depend on the location of the polyps. Patients with small-intestinal polyps present with symptoms of obstruction and abdominal pain, whereas those with large-intestinal and rectal lesions present with bloody stools and protrusion or prolapse of the polyps.

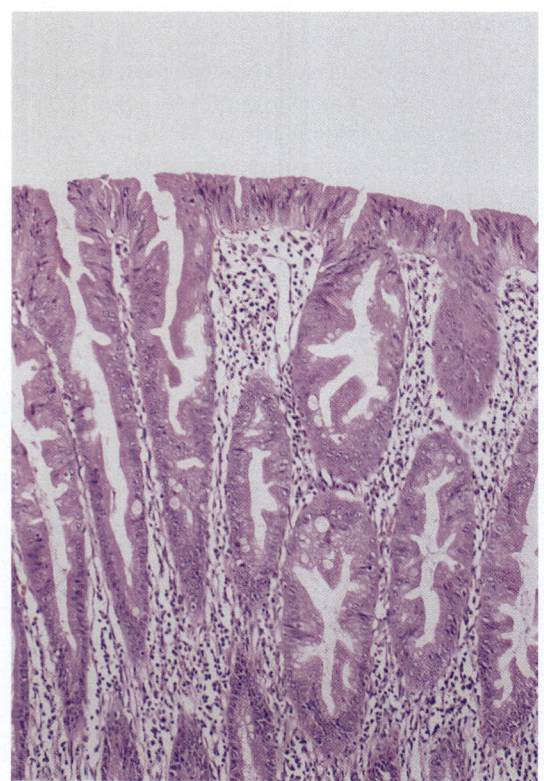
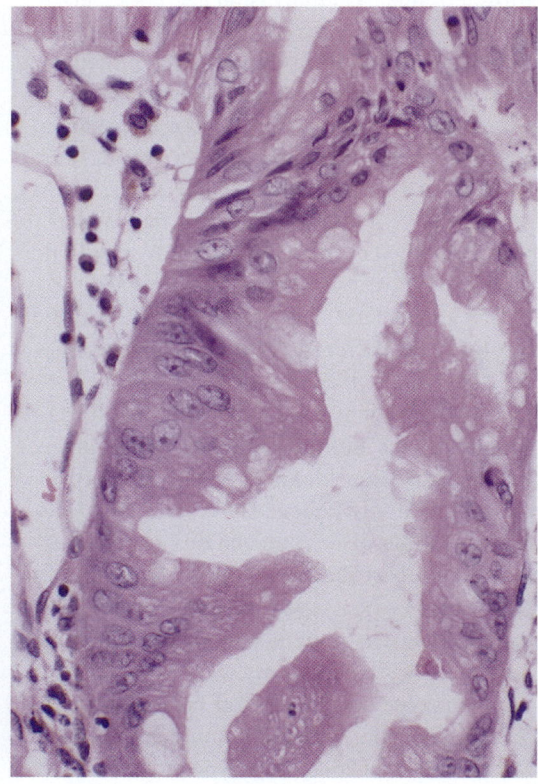

FIG. 5. A: Low-power microscopic view of serrated adenoma showing a saw-toothed or serrated appearance. At this power one can also appreciate the eosinophilia of the lesion. **B:** High-power view showing occasional goblet cells admixed with eosinophilic columnar cells. Note that the nuclei are vesicular and have nucleoli. Compare to Figs. 2B and 6.

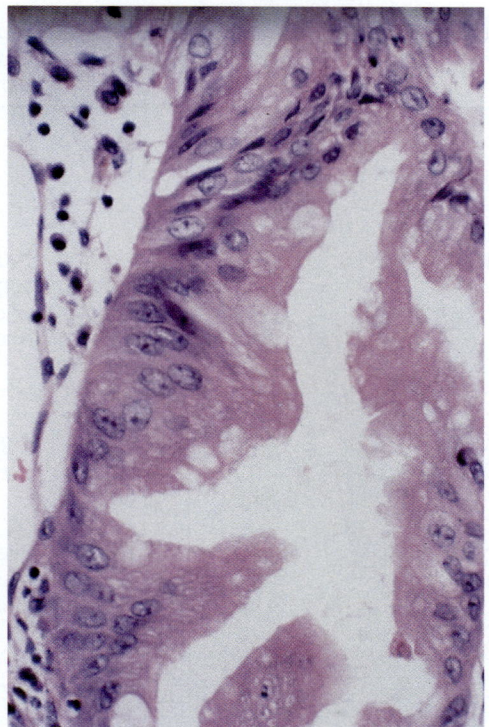 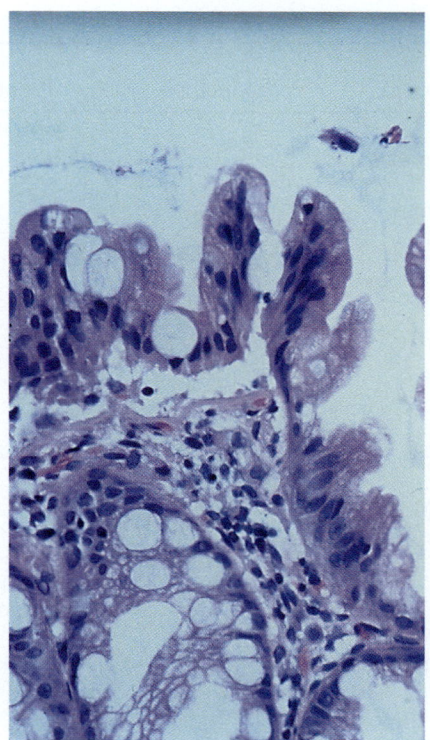

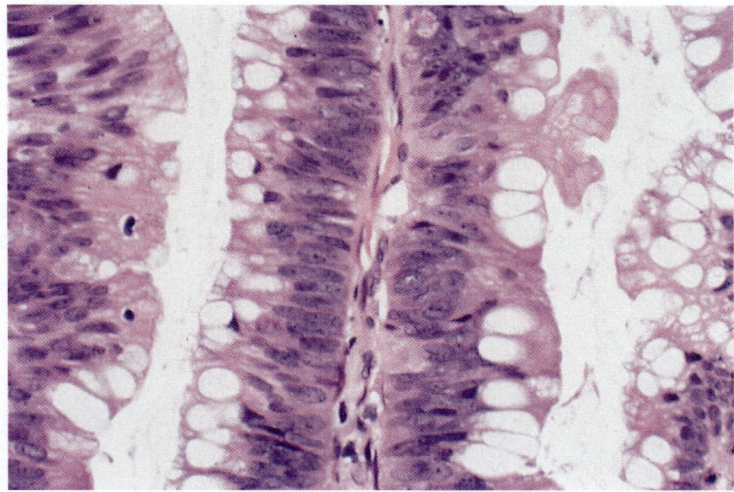

FIG. 6. High-power view comparing nuclear features of serrated adenoma *(upper left)*, hyperplastic polyp *(upper right)*, and adenoma *(bottom)*. One can readily see how these can be differentiated by nuclear detail. The serrated adenoma has open vesicular nuclei with nucleoli. The hyperplastic polyp has ovoid basally-placed bland nuclei and the adenoma has elongated, palisading dysplastic nuclei.

Studies have shown a prevalence of cancer ranging from 22% to 50% in patients with the Peutz-Jeghers syndrome, a rate significantly greater than expected for a control population. The cancers have been divided between gastrointestinal and nongastrointestinal types, with pancreas, gut, lung, breast, ovary, cervix, uterus, and thyroid being the major sites of primary neoplasms. In some instances the gastrointestinal cancers arose from the Peutz-Jeghers polyp (33–35).

Pathology

The Peutz-Jeghers polyp varies in size from <1 to >3.5 cm in diameter, and may be sessile or pedunculated. The basic architecture is that of glandular epithelium resting on a branching smooth muscle framework that arises from the muscularis mucosae. This framework, essential in making the proper diagnosis, is easily recognized at low power: the

TABLE 1. *Intestinal polyposis syndromes*

Syndrome	Inheritance	Type(s) of polyp	Location of polyp	Location of GI cancer	Location of extraintestinal tumors
Familial polyposis coli (familial adenomatous polyposis)	AD	Adenoma, FGP	C,SI,ST	C,SI	None
Gardner's	AD	Adenoma; FGP, lymphoid	C,SI,ST	C,SI	Lipoma; fibroma; desmoid tumor; dental cysts; osteoma; carcinoma of thyroid and adrenal glands
Turcot's*	AD	Adenoma	C	C	Central nervous system tumors
Peutz-Jeghers	AD	Hamartoma	C,SI,ST	C,SI,ST	Cancers of the breast, ovary, uterus, and testis
Juvenile polyposis (one-third of cases)	AD	Juvenile	C,SI,ST	C,SI,ST	None
Cowden's	AD	Hamartoma; inflammatory; ganglioneuroma; lipoma; lymphoid	C,SI	None	Facial trichilemomas; oral mucosal papillomas; carcinoma of thyroid gland and breast
Cronkite-Canada	None	Juvenile-like	C,SI,ST	Colon (rare)	None
Attenuated familial polyposis coli**	AD	Adenoma; FGP	C,SI,ST	C,SI,ST	None
Hereditary flat Adenoma syndrome**	AD	Adenoma; FGP	C,SI,ST	C,SI,ST	None
Muir Torre syndrome	AD	Adenoma	C	C	Skin cancer: basal cell; squamous cell; sebaceous carcinoma
Hereditary mixed polyposis syndrome	AD	Adenoma; juvenile; hyperplastic	C	C	None

GI, gastrointestinal, AD, autosomal dominant, FGP, fundic gland polyp; C, colon; SI, small intestine; ST, stomach.

*Some cases of Turcot's syndrome have mutations in APC gene. Some cases of Turcot's syndrome have germline mutations in mismatch repair genes (hMLH1 and hPMS2).

**Attenuated familial polyposis coli and hereditary flat adenoma syndrome most likely are the same disorder, but they are listed separately in this table. Attenuated familial polyposis coli and hereditary flat adenoma syndrome are considered variants of familial polyposis coli.

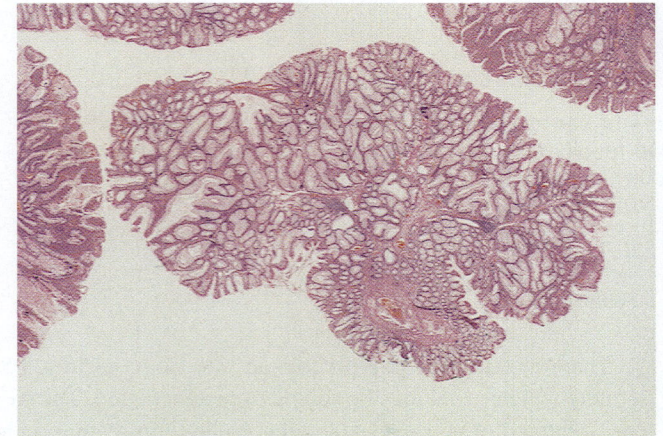 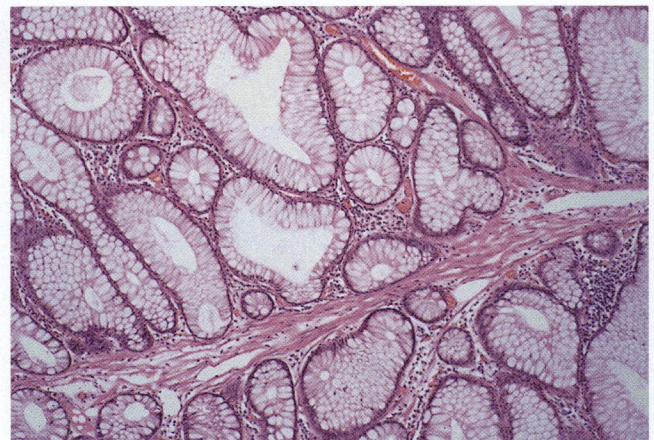

FIG. 7. A: Whole mount of colonic Peutz-Jegher polyp. At this power one can appreciate the intricate "Christmas tree" or racemose appearance. **B:** Higher power showing smooth muscle bundles between benign nonneoplastic epithelium.

polyp has a "Christmas tree" or arborescent-like appearance.

The epithelial component resembles the normal epithelium of the intestinal area from which the polyp arises. In the small intestine, the epithelium consists of goblet and absorptive cells with a normal component of endocrine and Paneth cells. In the large intestine, the epithelium is predominantly of the goblet-cell type, often with branching crypts lined by hypertrophic goblet cells (Figs. 7 and 8). Areas of hyperplastic polyp-type epithelium may be noted.

Areas of adenomatous and carcinomatous transformation within Peutz-Jeghers polyps have been reported (35–41), with a prevalence ranging from 6% to 12% (35,41). Importantly, one should not be misled into making a diagnosis of cancer based simply on the finding of epithelial structures admixed with smooth-muscle fibers, since this is the basic histology of this lesion. Occasionally, there is herniation of cystically dilated epithelial structures into the bowel wall, even extending into the serosa and forming true tumor masses, analogous to colitis cystica and/or jejunitis cystica profunda (Fig. 9) (42–44). In these instances, the herniated epithelium is nonneoplastic in nature and may be accompanied by smooth muscle fibers, lamina propria, and mucin pools, important findings that help distinguish epithelial misplacement from neoplasia. This pseudoinvasive pattern has been reported in approximately 10% of small-intestinal Peutz-Jeghers polyps (44). There has also been a report of a leiomyosarcoma arising in a small-intestinal Peutz-Jeghers polyp (45).

Hamartomatous Polyp; Cowden's Disease

Cowden's disease is an autosomal dominant disorder associated with colonic and small-intestinal polyps, breast and

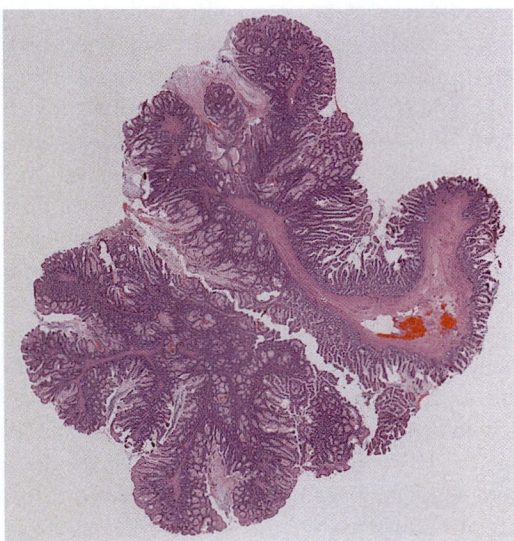

FIG. 8. Whole mount view of small-intestinal Peutz-Jegher polyp. At this power the tree-like branching with central smooth muscle bundles can be appreciated.

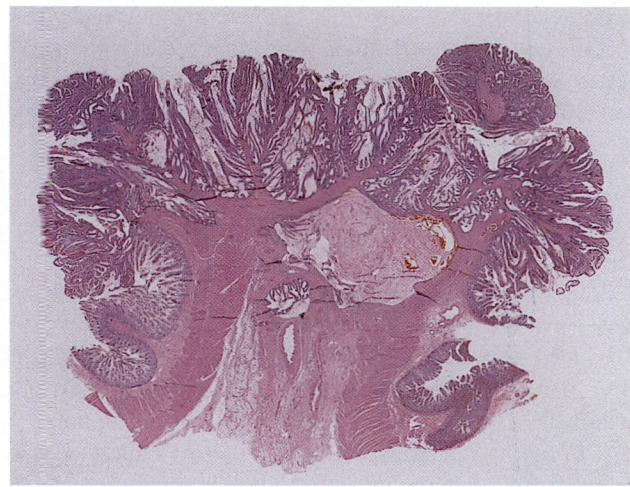

FIG. 9. Whole mount view of small-intestinal Peutz-Jegher polyp showing pseudoinvasion. There is transmural herniation of mucosa. This pattern is often best appreciated at low power. At higher power one would also note the benign nature of the epithelial cells.

thyroid cancer, facial trichilemomas, acral keratoses, and oral mucosal papillomatosis. Gastrointestinal polyps are seen in 35% of cases (31,32) (Table 1).

The pathology of the gastrointestinal polyps is varied, but they have been grouped as hamartomas. The most common lesion is a polyp showing a mildly fibrotic and disorganized mucosa with extensive splaying of the muscularis mucosae. These lesions are morphologically similar to the nonulcerated mucosa in the solitary rectal ulcer syndrome. Other polyps have been described as inflammatory, lipoma, ganglioneuroma, or nodular lymphoid hyperplasia. The gastrointestinal polyps of Cowden's disease have no malignant potential (31,32,46,47).

Ganglioneuroma

Ganglioneuromas may occur in the small and large intestine as either solitary lesions (48) or, more commonly, as multiple lesions (ganglioneuromatosis). The former are very rare, whereas ganglioneuromatosis may be associated with von Recklinhausen's disease and multiple endocrine neoplasia (MEN) type IIB (49). The lesions may be polypoid; histologically, they consist of a proliferation of ganglion cells and Schwann cells in the mucosa or deeper in the wall. In MEN type IIB, the ganglioneuromatosis may consist of a marked accentuation of both the submucosal and myenteric nerve plexuses. There have been reports of patients with polyposis in which the polyps showed features of both a juvenile polyp and ganglioneuroma (50). Also reported is a diffuse mucosal ganglioneuromatosis of a nonpolypoid nature (51). The pathologist can, at times, make the diagnosis from biopsy material simply by identifying ganglion and Schwann cells in the mucosa.

Immunohistochemistry (e.g., use of antibodies for neuron-specific enolase for detection of neurons and Schwann cells and of S-100 protein for the detection of Schwann cells) can be helpful.

Juvenile Polyp

Clinical Features

Although juvenile polyps occur mainly in the first two decades of life, they are not uncommonly seen in adults (52). They are localized chiefly in the rectum and are usually solitary. Bleeding is the most common sign, with anal protrusion of polyps seen in 20% and autoamputation of the polyp in 10% of cases. A polyposis syndrome exists (Table 1); it may be limited to the colon (juvenile polyposis coli) or may be associated with polyps in the small intestine and stomach (31,53–56). In the polyposis cases, the polyps are counted in the dozens to hundreds; however, they are not as numerous as in familial adenomatous polyposis coli. One-third of these cases have a genetic, probably autosomal dominant, etiology. Associated intestinal and extraintestinal congenital defects (such as malrotation of the gut, mesenteric lymphangioma, hypertelorism, hydrocephalus, tetrology of Fallot, and coarctation of the aorta) have been reported.

There is an increased risk of colon cancer in patients with juvenile polyposis. Colon cancer has been reported in 15% to 21% of patients with juvenile polyposis (53,57,58). In some of the familial cases, intestinal and gastric cancers have been seen in family members without juvenile polyps (53,54,55,59). However, it should be stated emphatically that solitary juvenile polyps are not markers for subsequent colorectal cancer and do not require further follow-up investigation (60).

Pathology

Grossly, juvenile polyps are mainly pedunculated, rarely sessile, and usually under 3.0 cm in diameter. They have a smooth glistening surface and are red-tan to red in color. On cut section, one can often appreciate cystic fluid-filled spaces (Fig. 10). Microscopically, fully developed juvenile polyps consist of cystically dilated and tortuous glands in an inflamed stroma (Fig. 10). This classic pattern is readily appreciated at low power and should alert the pathologist to the diagnosis. The glands are made up of well-formed mucus-secreting cells that may become flattened and attenuated. In approximately 45% of cases, one can appreciate pink regenerative epithelial cells similar to those seen in hyperplastic polyps. The stroma usually contains acute and chronic inflammatory cells and granulation tissue. When dilated glands rupture into the stroma, there may be a foreign-body giant cell reaction. Occasionally, one can identify areas of osseous metaplasia.

The juvenile polyp is nonneoplastic. Nevertheless, in patients with solitary juvenile polyps (nonsyndromic), there are rare cases of polyps with areas of adenomatous transformation and even carcinoma (61–64). However, adenomatous change (dysplasia) has been reported in 15% to 30% of juvenile polyps from patients with juvenile polyposis (57,58,65). It should be noted that there is interobserver variation in diagnosing dysplasia in juvenile polyps (65). Some studies have reported separate adenomas and hyperplastic polyps (57,58,61). A large study of juvenile polyposis cases reported that 9% of typical juvenile polyps and 47% of atypical juvenile polyps showed foci of dysplasia. These atypical juvenile polyps grossly formed lobular or multilobular masses (appearance of closely packed juvenile polyps attached to a single stalk), rather than the typical smooth and spherical polyp. The atypical juvenile polyps revealed relatively less lamina propria and more epithelium than the typical juvenile polyp and often had a villous or papillary configuration (57).

Small or "early" juvenile polyps may be histologically indistinguishable from inflammatory polyps, since both have a cap of granulation tissue above cystically dilated glands. In this instance, it is judicious to comment that the lesion in question may be either a juvenile polyp or an inflammatory polyp. Also reported are rare cases of juvenile polyposis in which the polyps show classic features of both a juvenile polyp and ganglioneuroma (50).

Inflammatory Polyp

These lesions may be secondary to inflammatory disorders of the intestine. They are seen in 10% to 20% of cases of ulcerative colitis and may also be noted in Crohn's disease, ischemic disease, amebiasis, and schistosomiasis; in addition, they are seen adjacent to ulcers and at surgical anastomotic sites.

In ulcerative colitis and Crohn's disease, the polyps are simply raised tags of mucosa and/or submucosa. The mucosa may show changes of inactive inflammatory bowel disease, or the epithelial crypts may show abscesses and an inflamed stroma (Fig. 11). Inflammatory polyps may also be rounded nodules or caps of granulation tissue overlying epithelial structures (Fig. 12), or they may closely resemble early juvenile polyps. In young children with no history or pathology of inflammatory bowel disease, one must be careful not to misdiagnose an early juvenile polyp as an inflammatory polyp.

Occasionally, inflammatory polyps can have bizarre stromal changes that mimic a sarcoma (66,67). The vast majority of these patients have inflammatory bowel disease. These polyps with bizarre stroma are usually solitary and less than 2 cm in size. Histologically one sees bizarre spindle, epithelioid, and large ganglion-like or multinucleated cells in a fibroblastic or granulation tissue stroma. Mitoses are rare and atypical mitoses are absent. Often there is a zonation effect separating the bizarre cells from the more characteristic spindle cells; however, this appearance is often not evident in small biopsies (Fig. 13). In distinguishing this reaction from

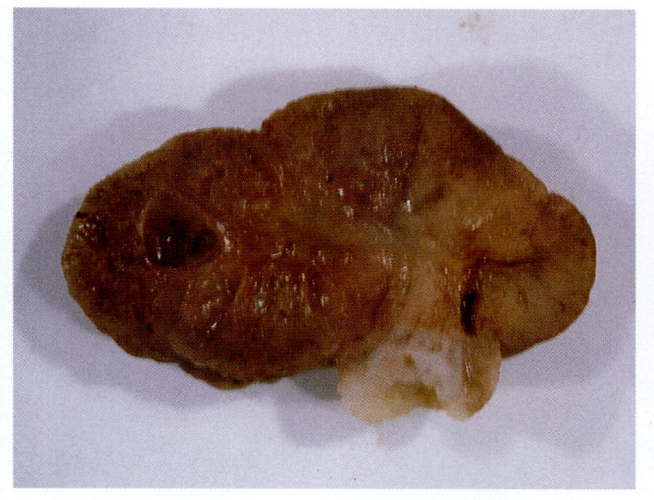
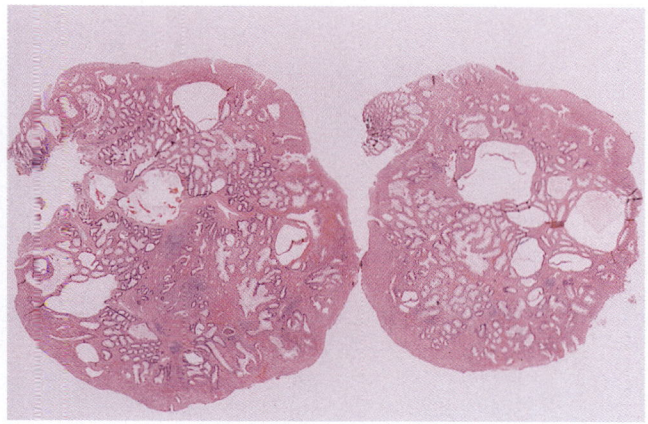
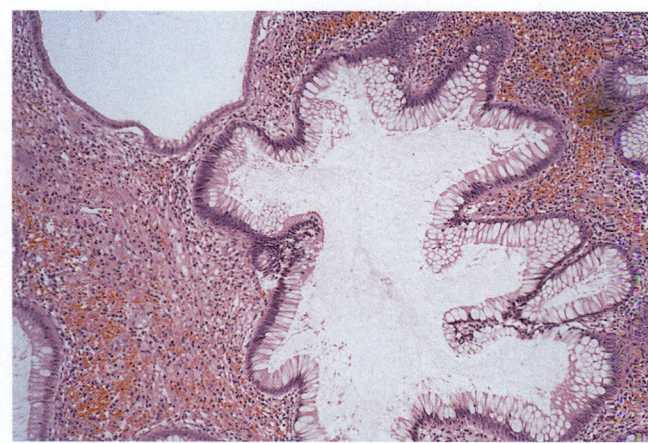
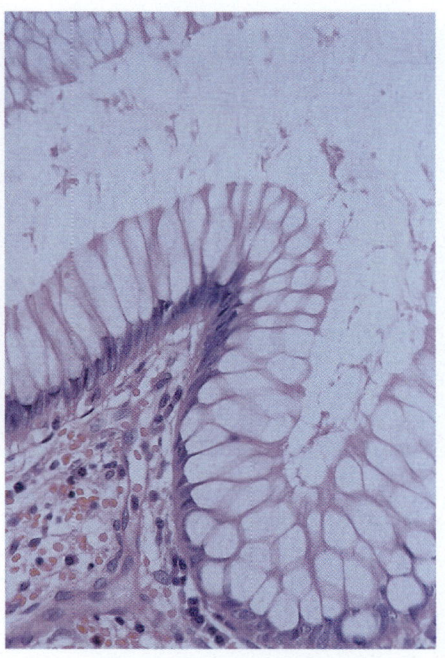

FIG. 10. A: Gross view of juvenile polyp. Note smooth surface and numerous cystically dilated spaces within the head of the polyp. **B:** Whole mount view of juvenile polyp. At this power one can appreciate cystically dilated glands and an expanded lamina propria (from ref. 302). **C:** Medium-power view showing dilated and irregularly shaped glands. **D:** Benign epithelium in juvenile polyps.

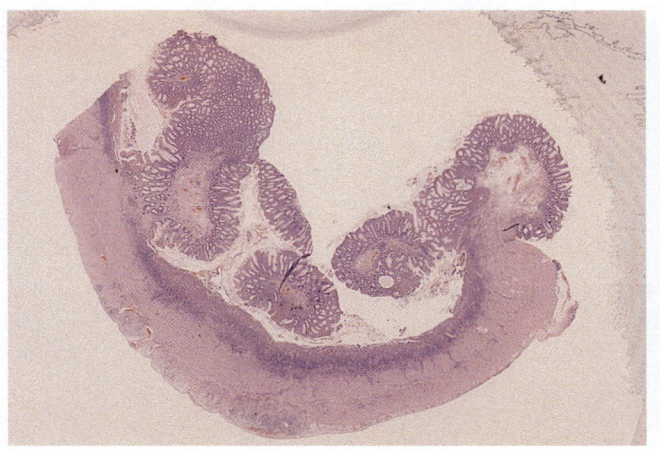
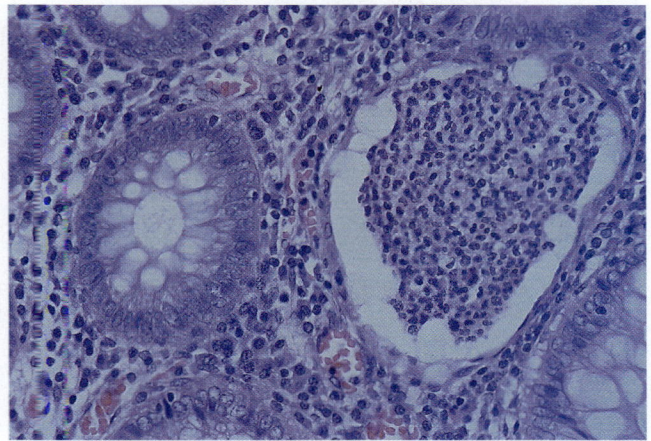

FIG. 11. A: Inflammatory polyps from a patient with ulcerative colitis. Whole mount view shows that polyps are formed by residual inflamed islands of mucosa adjacent to ulceration (from ref. 302). **B:** High-power view showing benign mucosa with crypt abscess

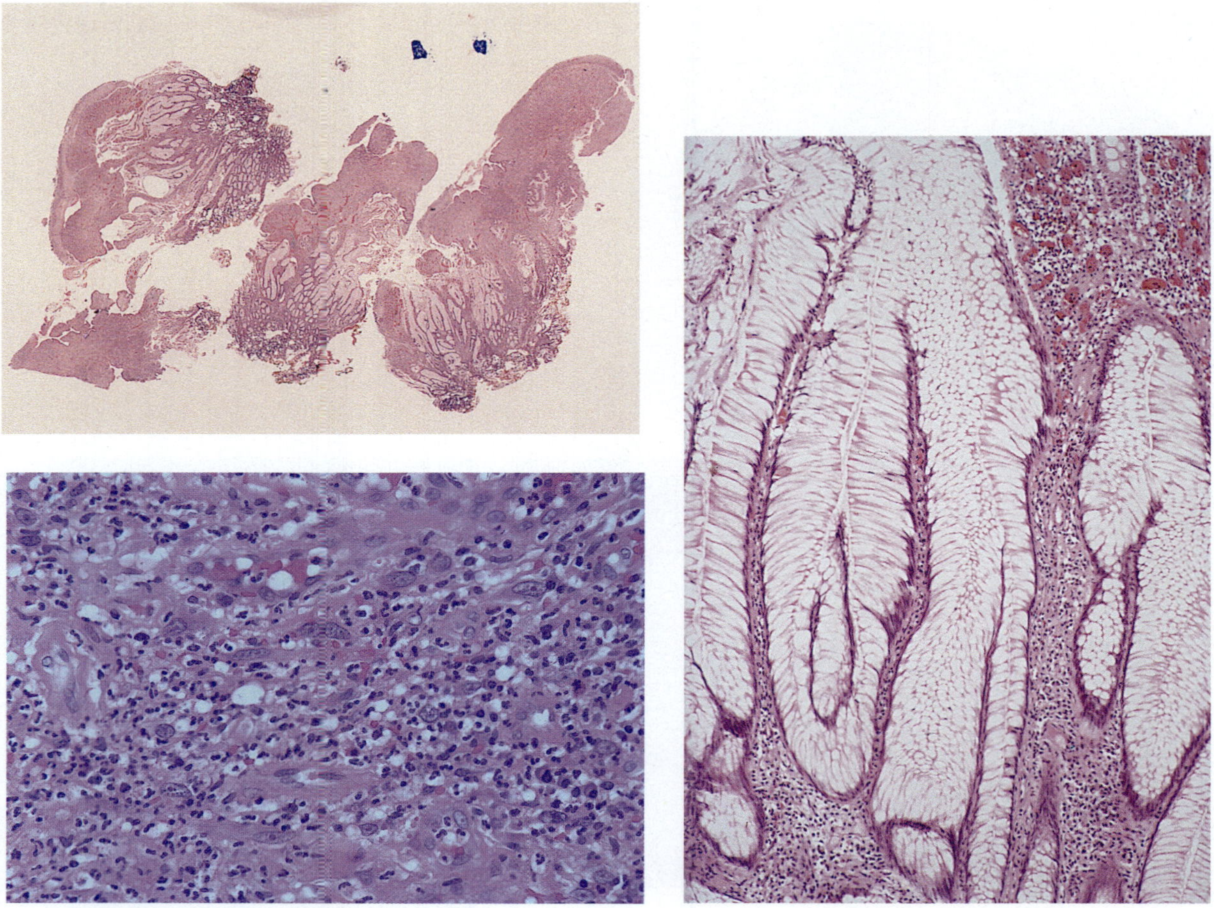

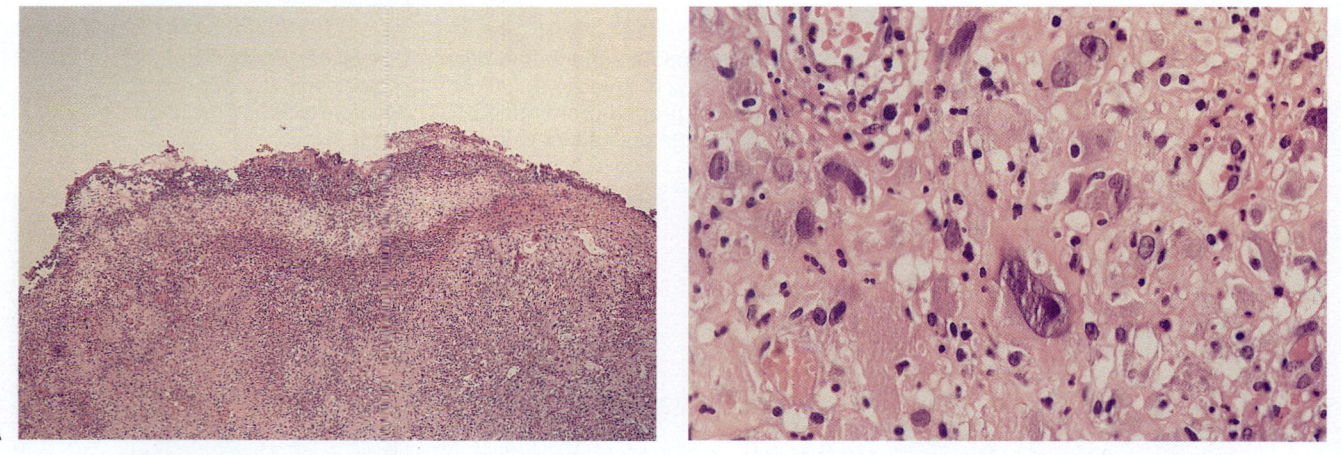

FIG. 12. A: Whole mount view of inflammatory polyp. **B:** Inflammatory fibrin cap. **C:** The cap overlies distorted benign glands.

FIG. 13. A: Inflammatory polyp with bizarre stroma. **B:** Higher power showing cells with enlarged bizarre nuclei. This appearance is benign. See text for details.

a malignant process, one should take into consideration the pattern of zonation of bizarre cells, scanty mitoses, lack of atypical mitoses, solitary occurrence, small size, and association with inflammatory bowel disease.

Inflammatory Polyps Secondary to Mucosal Prolapse

The entities of inflammatory cap polyposis, inflammatory myoglandular polyp, and diverticular polyp are thought to be different spectrums/stages in mucosal prolapse (68).

Inflammatory cap polyps are limited to the rectosigmoid/distal colon. They are sessile, and can be solitary or numerous. Histologically, one sees an eroded surface with a fibrinopurulent inflammatory cap. The body of the polyp consists of acute and chronic inflammation, proliferation of the muscularis mucosae, and fibromuscular obliteration of the lamina propria. The epithelial component shows hyperplastic changes, goblet cell hyperplasia, and tortuosity of glands (69–71).

Inflammatory myoglandular polyps, mainly located in the distal colon, can rarely be found in the ileum, where they can cause intussusception. They are solitary and usually pedunculated. Histologically, one sees branching and dilated glands within a background of radially proliferating smooth muscle, an appearance not unlike that of the Peutz-Jeghers polyp. The surface is often eroded with a fibrinopurulent cap (72).

Diverticular polyps are those that arise in the background of diverticular disease. Grossly these lesions may be confused with an adenoma. The early lesions have mucosal hemorrhage and congestion, whereas advanced lesions show changes resembling that of mucosal prolapse: mucosal edema, fibromuscular obliteration of the lamina propria, epithelial hyperplasia and branching, dilated crypts, and occasional misplaced glands in the submucosa. Pseudosarcomatous changes in the stroma have been noted (73).

Inflammatory Fibroid Polyp

Inflammatory fibroid polyps are benign tumor masses occurring in the small intestine, stomach, and, less commonly, in the large intestine (74–76). They occur at any age and are not associated with any medical conditions or syndromes. Other terms used to describe this entity are eosinophilic granuloma, submucosal fibroma, hemangiopericytoma, inflammatory pseudotumor, and fibroma.

These polyps range from 1.5 to 13 cm in size (mean size, 3.0–4.0 cm) and are polypoid with a broad base. Most often they are limited to the submucosa, but they can infiltrate the musoca or the muscularis propria and extend to the serosa. Grossly, they are tan, gray, or yellow; the overlying mucosa may be ulcerated (Fig. 14). Microscopically, they are mesenchymal lesions with an inflammatory infiltrate and a vari-

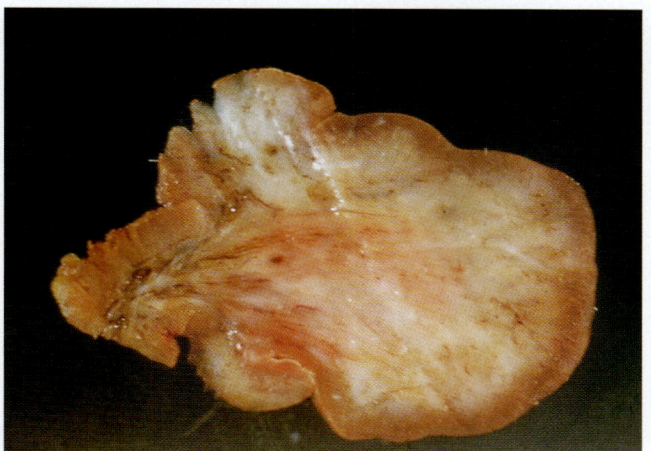
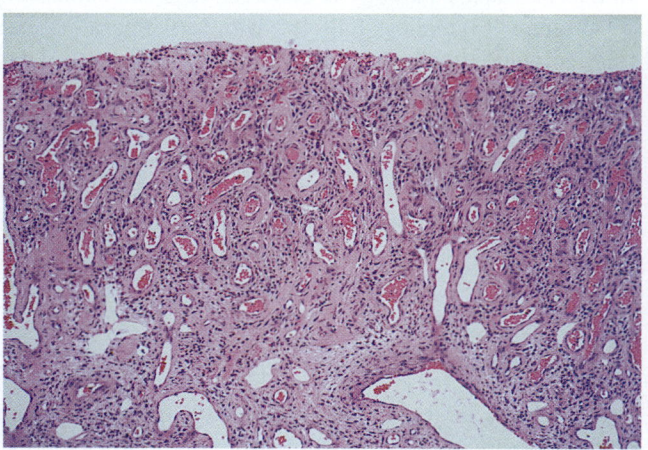
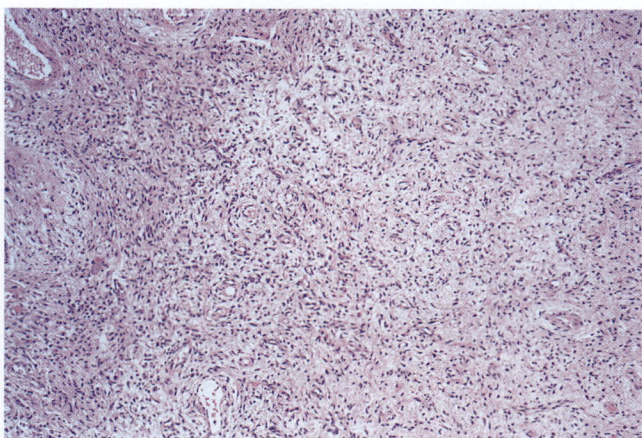

FIG. 14. A: Gross appearance of inflammatory fibroid polyp from small intestine. **B:** Surface is eroded with granulation tissue. **C:** Low-power view of polyp with loose, edematous, myxoid stroma.

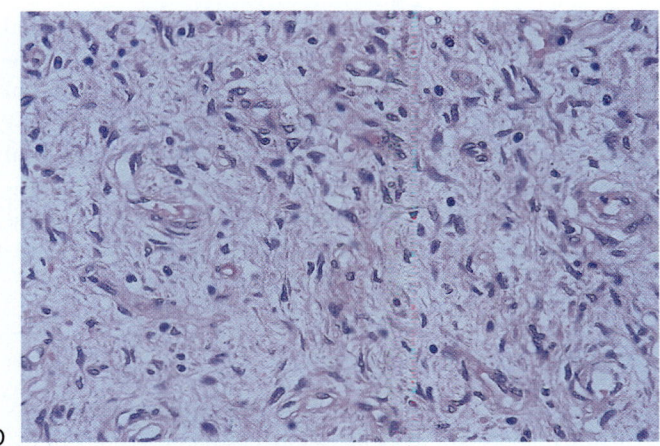 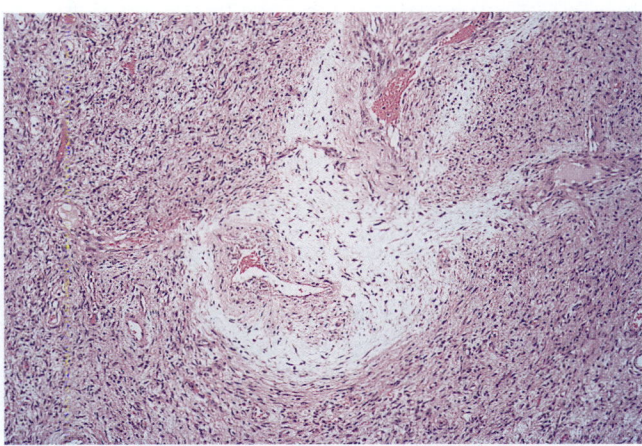

FIG. 14. *Continued.* **D:** Higher-power view showing bland spindled wavy cells in loose stroma. **E:** Characteristic rarefaction around muscular-walled blood vessels.

able vascular component. The fibroblasts may be spindle-shaped or stellate with indistinct basophilic cytoplasm. In some areas, the lesions may be sparsely cellular with a prominent myxoid component (Fig. 14). Cellular fields may show cells with mitotic figures, with some lesions showing up to two mitoses per high power field. The inflammatory infiltrate consists of eosinophils, lymphocytes, plasma cells, macrophages, and mast cells. The eosinophils may vary in number from few to many. The vascular component may be prominent, with many lesions containing a distinctive zone of loose connective tissue around larger blood vessels (Fig. 14). It is very difficult, if not impossible, to diagnose these lesions from endoscopic biopsies, as biopsies may show only granulation tissue from the eroded surface.

Inflammatory fibroid polyp is a benign lesion. The spindle cell component expresses vimentin, muscle specific actin, and smooth muscle actin but is negative for S-100 protein and desmin. Other lesions to consider in the differential diagnosis are neurogenic tumors, desmoid tumors, and malignant mesenchymal tumors. Neurogenic tumors will express S-100 protein and often are associated with von Recklinhausen's disease. Desmoid tumors are made up of fibroblasts (desmoid type of fibromatosis), but tend to arise outside of the bowel and invade the bowel secondarily. Malignant mesenchymal tumors, in addition to their cellular characteristics, tend to infiltrate the bowel wall by pushing aside the muscular layer, while the inflammatory fibroid polyp may penetrate the bowel wall with a pattern of dissection between the muscle fibers, causing a splaying or splitting of the muscularis propria.

Cronkite-Canada Syndrome

This syndrome is a nonhereditary gastrointestinal polyposis associated with alopecia, nail atrophy, and hyperpigmentation of the skin (77). Unlike most polyposis disorders in which the onset is noted earlier in life, in this disorder 80% of cases present initially at or after 50 years of age (Table 1). Clinical features are diarrhea, weight loss, abdominal pain, anorexia, and weakness. Physical findings include nail changes (dystrophy, thinning, splitting), hair loss, and hyperpigmentation of the skin. Fifty percent of these patients die secondary to cachexia. The polyps occur in the stomach, small intestine, colon, and rectum.

Histologically, these polyps are identical to juvenile polyps, with tortuous and cystically dilated glands. However, in the Cronkite-Canada syndrome, the nonpolypoid intervening mucosa contains cystically dilated glands, whereas in patients with juvenile polyps, the intervening mucosa is histologically normal (Fig. 15). Similarly, the clinical setting and symptoms of juvenile polyps and Cronkite-Canada syndrome are entirely different. Adenomatous change in Cronkite-Canada polyps has been reported (78), and occasional cases of colorectal adenocarcinoma have been reported in patients with this syndrome (78,79).

Lymphoid Polyp

Lymphoid polyps are benign lesions that occur mainly in the rectum. They occur in all age groups and may be found incidentally or may cause symptoms such as bleeding, discomfort, or prolapse. Eighty percent are sessile and solitary; the remainder are pedunculated and/or multiple (two to six in number). Their pathology is quite characteristic, consisting of prominent lymphoid follicles, with active germinal centers, located in the mucosa and submucosa (Fig. 16). Local excision is curative; occasionally, spontaneous remission of these lesions has been noted (80). Cases of multiple lymphoid polyposis have been reported. They occur mainly in children; some have been associated with a family history, whereas other cases represent lymphoid polyposis of the terminal ileum in patients with familial adenomatous polyposis coli and Gardner's syndrome (81–84).

Neoplastic Polyps (Adenoma)

Adenomas are traditionally divided into three types: tubular, tubulovillous, and villous. However, classification may

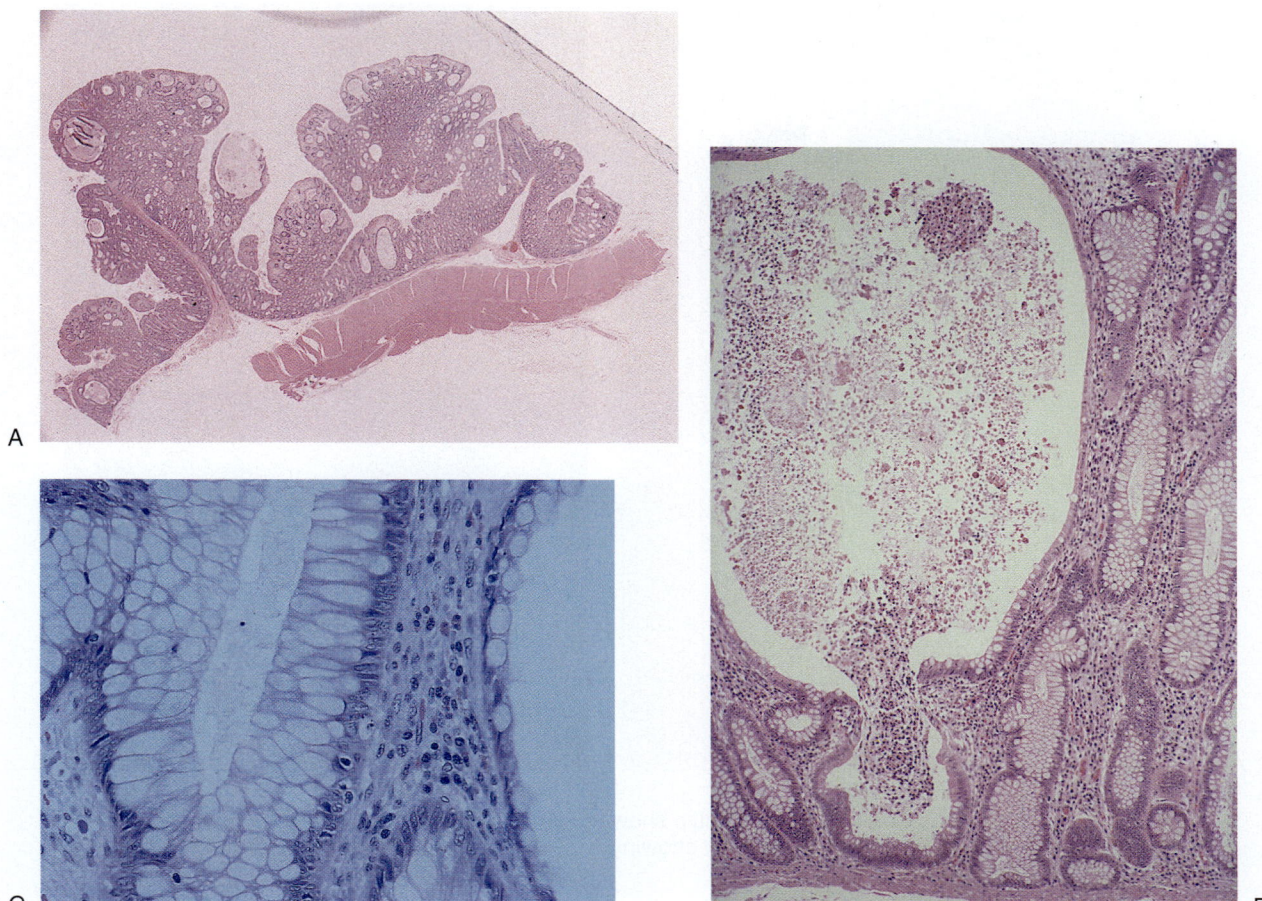

FIG. 15. A: Whole mount of Cronkite-Canada polyp. There are polypoid structures with cystically dilated spaces. Note that the flat nonpolypoid mucosa has dilated glands. **B:** Dilated glands from flat nonpolypoid mucosa. **C:** High-power view showing that the epithelium is nonneoplastic in nature. The gland *(right)* is dilated (from ref. 302).

also be based on gross appearance (e.g., polypoid versus flat adenoma). Adenomas are important clinically because they are premalignant lesions. Adenomas are very common in the large intestine, but are rare in the small intestine.

Small Intestine

Small-intestinal adenomas are tubular or villous and are usually sessile. Microscopically, they resemble adenomas of the colon. All degrees of dysplasia can occur, as can *in situ* and invasive cancer (Fig. 17). Patients with familial adenomatous polyposis coli and Gardner's syndrome often have small-intestinal adenomas, many of which are only evident microscopically (85,86).

Large Intestine

Prevalence of Adenomas

The prevalence of large-intestinal adenomas varies in different parts of the world. Adenomas are common in Westernized cultures and uncommon in developing countries, with autopsy studies showing a prevalence as high as 60% in the former and as low as 5.5% in the latter (87,88). Most adenomas less than 1.0 cm in size tend to show an even distribution throughout the large intestine, whereas those greater than 1.0 cm tend to be localized in the distal colon. The prevalence of tubular adenomas, tubulovillous adenomas, and villous adenomas is 95%, 2% to 4%, and 1% to 3%, respectively, in autopsy studies (87,88), whereas the prevalence is 65% to 85%, 16% to 27%, and 3% to 9%, respectively, in colonoscopic studies (89–91).

Polyp (Adenoma)-Cancer Sequence

Adenomas are of clinical importance because they may develop into cancer. The data to support this polyp (adenoma)-cancer sequence are derived from both epidemiologic and morphologic studies.

The epidemiologic facts are simple: The incidence of adenomas parallels the incidence of large-intestinal cancer. Countries with low rates of large-intestinal cancer also have low rates of adenomas, whereas countries with high rates of cancer have a high incidence of adenomas (3).

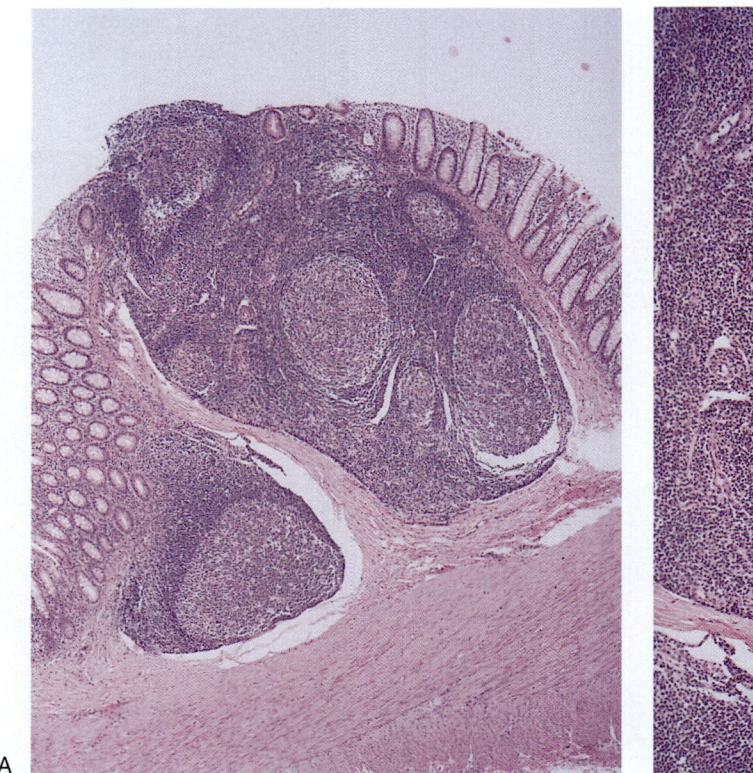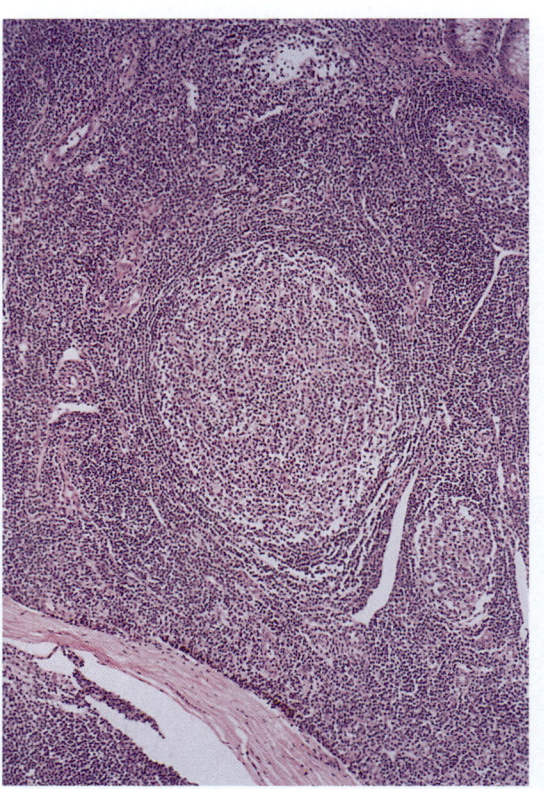

FIG. 16. A: Low-power view of lymphoid polyp showing that the polyp is secondary to lymphoid tissue with germinal centers. **B:** Higher power view showing lymphoid nodule with reactive germinal center.

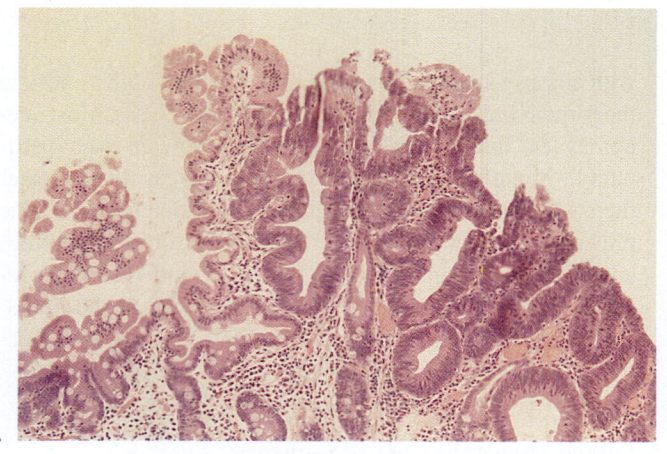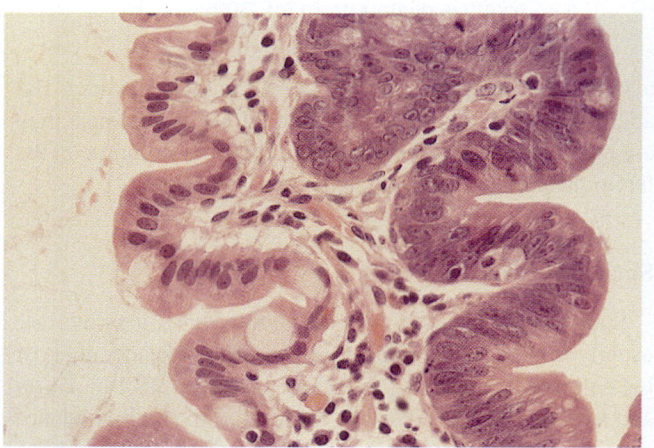

FIG. 17. A: Medium-power view of small intestine adenoma from a patient with FAP: adenoma *(right)*; nonneoplastic small intestine *(left)*. **B:** Higher power view showing a villus, one-half of which has adenomatous change.

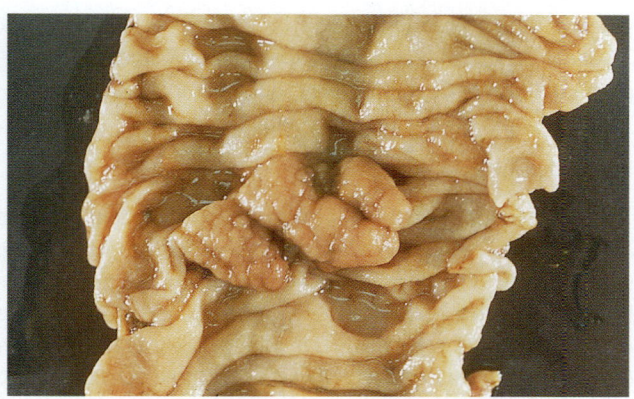

FIG. 18. Tubular adenoma from a resection specimen. The head of the polyp is divided into lobules.

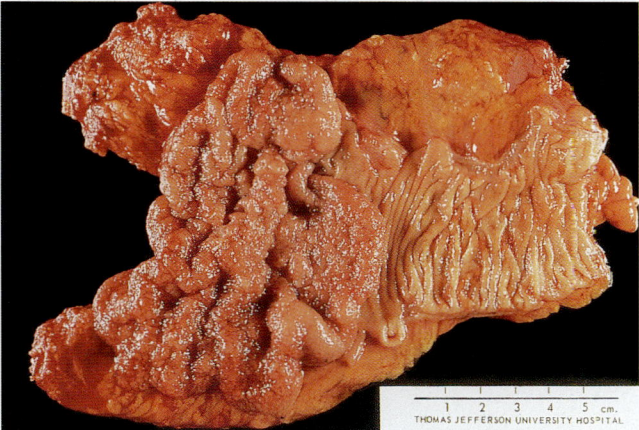

FIG. 19. Gross photograph of a large villous adenoma. The lesion is spreading and sessile (from ref. 302).

The morphologic evidence relates to size, adenoma type, and dysplasia. Invasive adenocarcinoma is found in approximately 5% of all adenomas; however, this relationship is size dependent. Invasive cancer is found in 0.5% of adenomas <1.0 cm, 5.0% of adenomas 1 to 1.9 cm, and 10% of adenomas >2.0 cm in size. Adenoma type also is related to cancer, with invasive cancer found in 2% to 3%, 6% to 8%, and 10% to 18% of tubular, tubulovillous, and villous adenomas, respectively. Most large-intestinal cancers arise in the distal colon, the location in which adenomas with marked dysplasia have their highest prevalence (89,91).

Pathology

Grossly, adenomas may be pedunculated (stalked), sessile, or flat (see below for discussion of flat adenomas). Classically, tubular adenomas have been described as pedunculated. In general, this is probably true; however, tubular adenomas may be sessile, and villous adenomas may be pedunculated. Tubular adenomas tend to be spherical, with a relatively smooth surface that is often divided into lobules secondary to intercommunicating clefts in the head of the adenoma. The adenoma is reddish or darker in color when compared to the surrounding mucosa (Fig. 18). Villous adenomas tend to have a shaggy surface with obvious papillary fronds (Fig. 19). In general, the size of the adenoma correlates with the histologic type. Ninety-one percent of adenomas <1.0 cm in size are tubular adenomas, 7% are tubulovillous adenomas, and 2% are villous adenomas. When adenomas are >2.0 cm in size, 50%, 38%, and 12% are tubular, tubulovillous, and villous adenomas, respectively (89).

Adenomas, irrespective of type, consist of similar adenomatous epithelium. The overall growth pattern determines whether an adenoma is tubular, tubulovillous, or villous. Tubular adenomas have a proliferation of adenomatous epithelium showing gland or tubule formation. These tubules are separated from each other by normal lamina propria (Fig. 20). In villous adenomas, one sees similar epithelium; how-

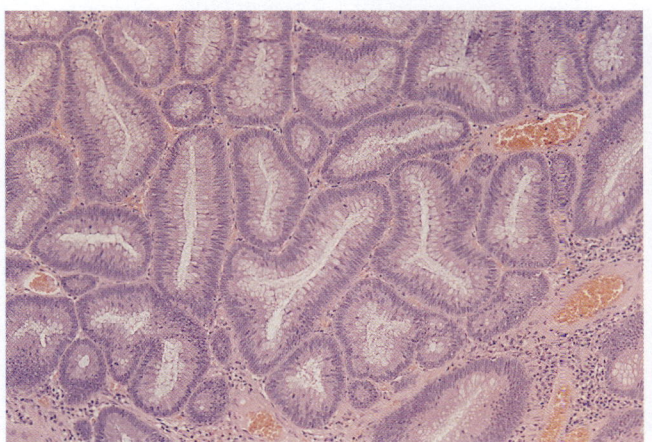 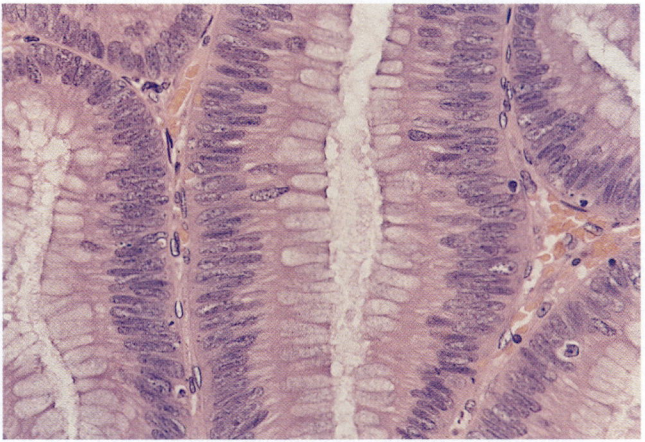

FIG. 20. A: Low-power view of tubular adenoma. The neoplastic glands form tubules. **B:** Higher power view. The nuclei are elongated and dysplastic. Some nuclear palisading is noted. The nuclei do not reach the cell surface. The apical portion of the cell shows mucin production. These adenomatous changes are considered low-grade dysplasia.

ever, the overall growth pattern or configuration is fine fingerlets or villi that project perpendicularly from the muscularis mucosae to the outer tip of the adenoma (Fig. 21). Since many lesions show mixed tubular and villous features, how is each specific type defined? Various authors have said that if 75% to 80% of the lesion is tubular or villous in nature, then it is classified as tubular adenoma or villous adenoma, respectively, with all lesions falling in between being classified as tubulovillous adenomas (89–92). In adenomas of all types, the epithelial cells show enlarged, elongated, hyperchromatic nuclei that are stratified within the cell. Mucin may be absent or, when present, may vary in amount from well-formed goblets to small apical vacuoles.

By definition, adenomas consist of dysplastic epithelium. The World Health Organization (92) and the National Polyp Study (93) both use a classification of mild, moderate, and severe dysplasia and/or a classification of low-grade (mild and moderate) and high-grade (severe) dysplasia. In today's practice, most pathologists use the high-grade/low-grade system (92–94). The usual/common adenoma is considered to show low-grade dysplasia (Figs. 20 and 21). High-grade dysplasia encompasses changes that in the past were considered *in situ* cancer and is replacing that term in practice. In high-grade dysplasia one sees both architectural and cytologic changes. Architecturally, the crypts show irregular branching, budding, or cribriform configurations. Cytologically, the nuclei are enlarged, hyperchromatic, or vesicular with prominent nucleoli. The nuclei are stratified within the cell and reach the luminal border of the cell. Mitotic figures are prominent. Areas of necrosis may be present, and cytoplasmic mucin production may be reduced or absent (Figs. 22 and 23). Adenomas may contain foci of Paneth-cell metaplasia, melanocytic metaplasia, and squamous metaplasia.

Flat Adenomas

Flat adenomas may be a subtype of colonic adenoma with a propensity for high-grade dysplasia when the lesions are small (95,96). They may be precursors of small malignancies that rapidly grow into deep penetrating cancers. Many of the reported studies regarding flat adenomas are from Japan (97–99); some believe that these aggressive adenomas are rare in Western societies (100). In prospective screening studies, the incidence of flat adenoma has varied from 2.8% to 24% (99,101).

Grossly, these lesions are flat, or slightly raised, plaques that often have a central depression (which can easily be missed on colonoscopy), and are usually small (<1 cm in size). Histologically, they lack a polypoid or exophytic growth pattern, and appear to be plaque-like. In vertical extent these lesions are never greater than twice the thickness of the adjacent nonneoplastic epithelium. Characteristically, they are tubular adenomas, with the adenomatous or dysplastic epithelium limited to the luminal surface of the crypt, associated with underlying nonneoplastic epithelium. Adenomatous transformation can develop throughout the full thickness of the crypt; however, this feature is usually limited to the center of the lesion, with the radial portion showing the characteristic histology (Fig. 24). However, it must be noted that this histologic finding of dysplastic glands lim-

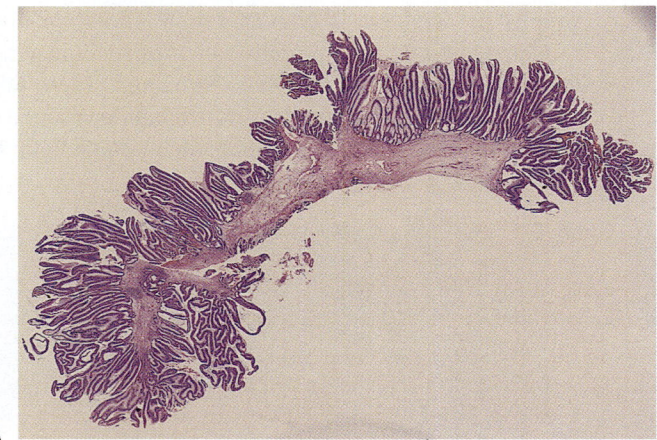

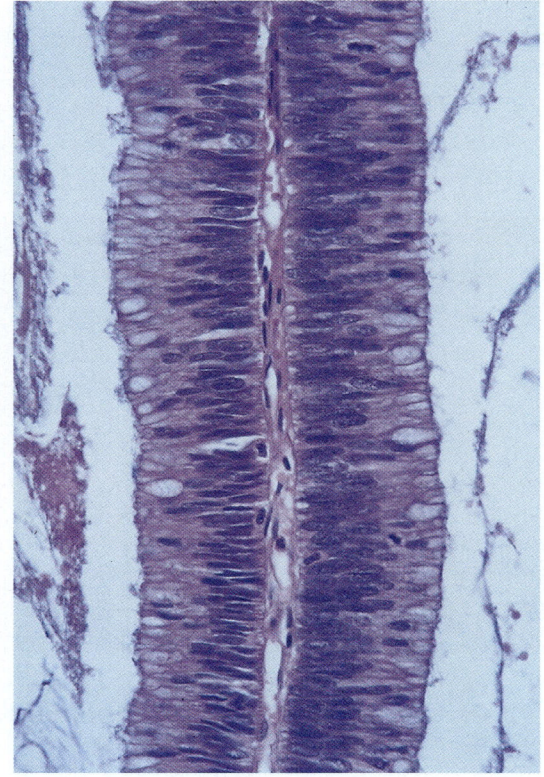

FIG. 21. A: Whole mount of villous adenoma showing adenomatous epithelium growing in a villous or finger-like arrangement. **B:** High-power view showing elongated nuclei with some palisading. Nuclei do not reach the cell surface and the apical portion of cells shows mucin production. This is low-grade dysplasia.

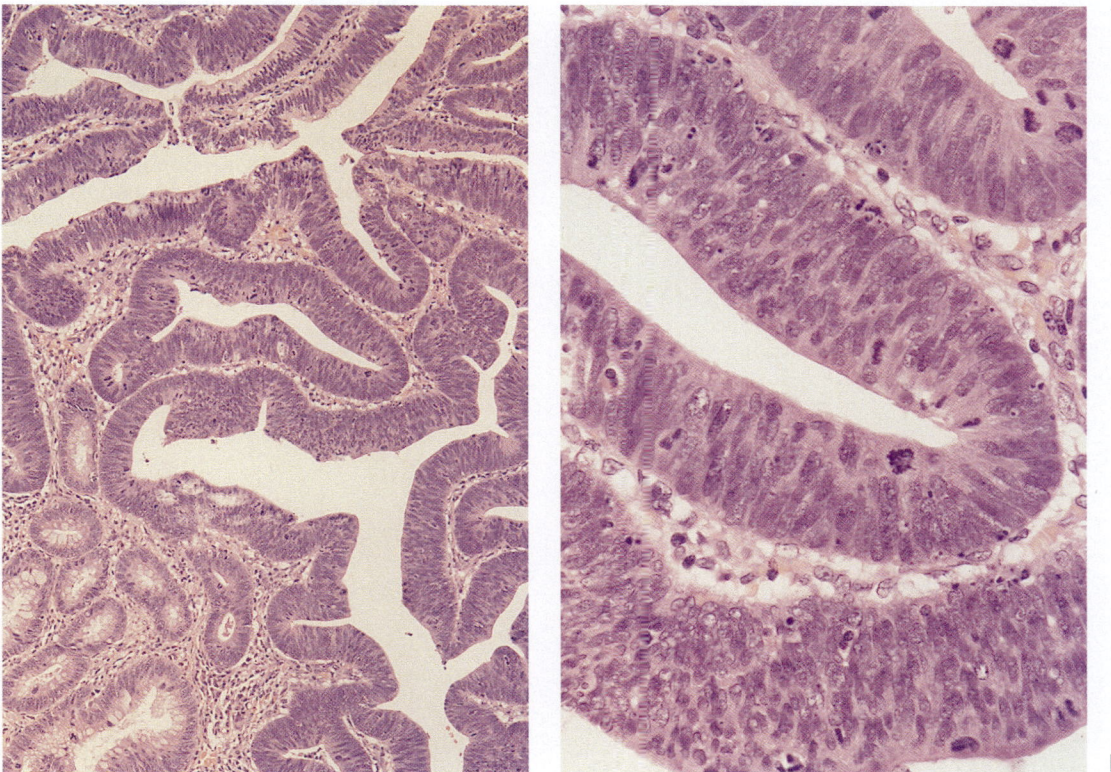

FIG. 22. A: Adenoma with high-grade dysplasia. Low-power view shows architectural changes of glandular buckling. **B:** Higher power shows dysplastic nuclei extending to the cell surface. There is also a mitosis at the surface. The changes in this lesion are those of high-grade dysplasia.

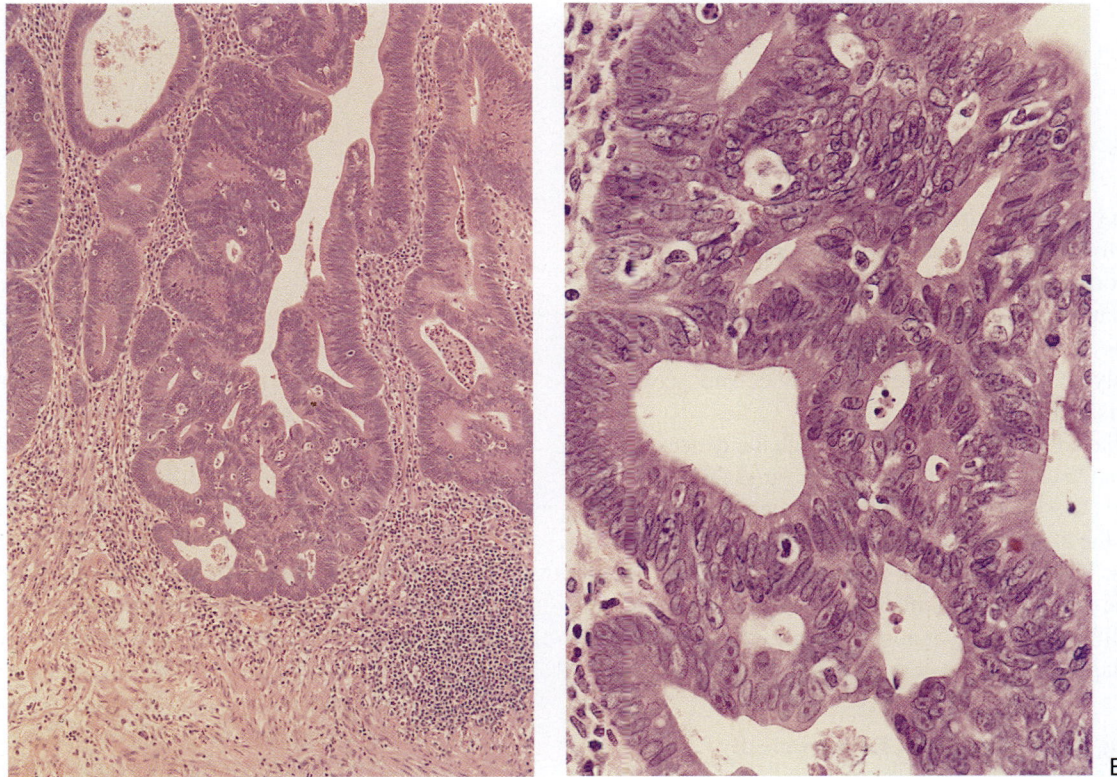

FIG. 23. A: Adenoma with high-grade dysplasia. Low-power view of a cribriform (gland in gland) pattern. **B:** Higher power view. These changes represent high-grade dysplasia.

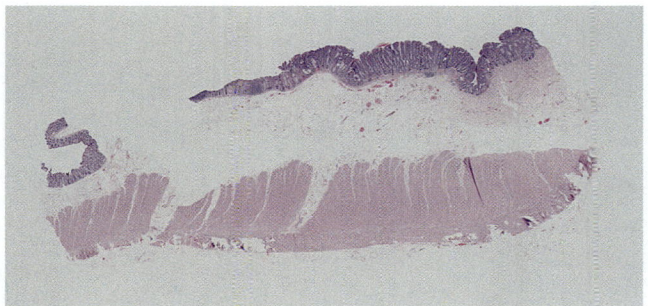
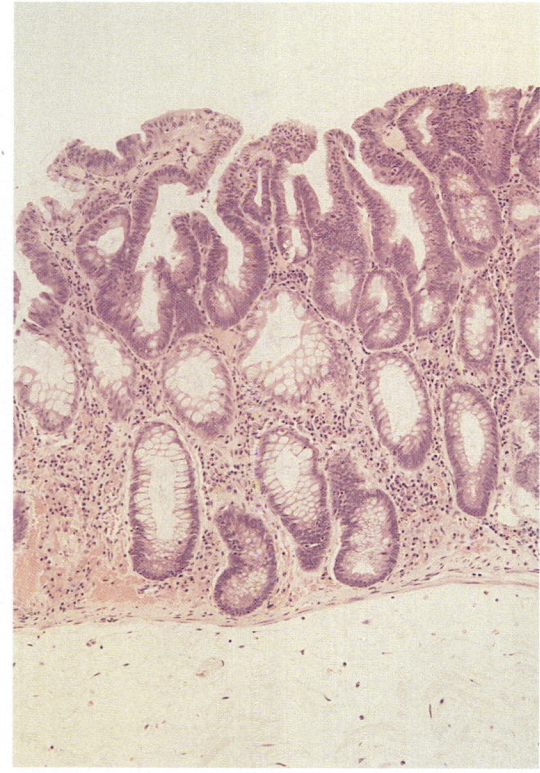
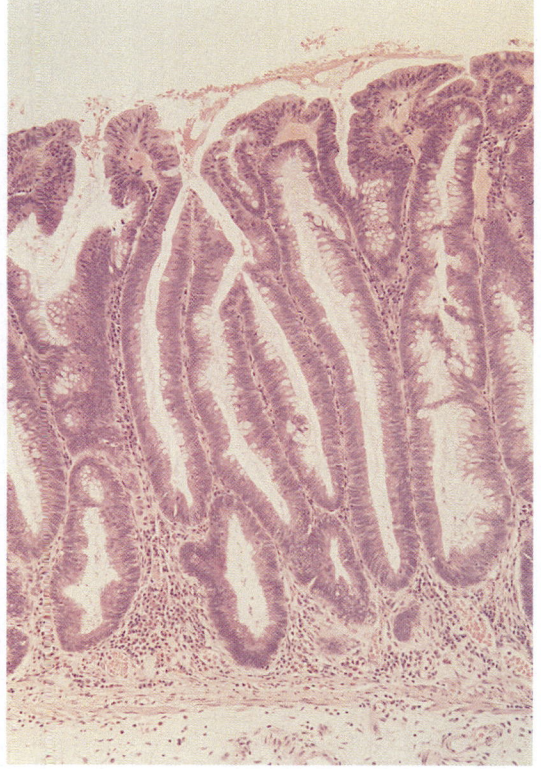

FIG. 24. A: Flat adenoma (whole mount). To the *left* is normal mucosa. The adenoma is less than two times the height of the normal mucosa. **B:** The junction of the normal mucosa with adenoma shows that the surface of the glands is adenomatous while the deeper parts are nonneoplastic. **C:** The center of the flat adenoma shows dysplastic (adenomatous) changes throughout the full length of the mucosa (from ref. 302).

ited to the luminal surface is not diagnostically pathognomonic for flat adenoma. One study reported that in a review of consecutive adenomas, 25% showed the above histologic features, none were flat endoscopically, and none had high-grade dysplasia (102). The diagnosis of flat adenoma should only be made when the characteristic endoscopic appearance is present.

These flat adenomas tend to have a high incidence of high-grade dysplasia (carcinoma *in situ*) ranging from 10% (97,99,101) to 41% (95,96), which are much higher percentages than the 4% incidence seen in comparable-sized classic adenomas. The discrepancies in the reported incidence of high-grade dysplasia and small early cancers could be related to differences in diagnostic criteria (103), especially between Japanese and Western pathologists (98).

Processing and Reporting of Endoscopically Removed Material

The endoscopically removed material that the pathologist receives is usually excised by either snare cautery (including polypectomy) or forceps biopsy. Forceps biopsy material should be submitted in its entirety, and levels (usually three) should be cut. Ideally, the tissue should be blocked so that multiple ribbons can be placed on a slide. When a polypectomy specimen is received, the pathologist must carefully inspect the gross specimen and look for the stalk or transection point. The polyp should be cut so that all the proper landmarks become evident on the glass slide (Fig. 25). The entire specimen should be submitted. In order for the polyp to be properly cut, it must be well fixed. Polyps <1.5 cm in diameter may require 2 to 3 hours of fixation of the entire lesion prior to gross sectioning, whereas those larger in size may require longer or possibly overnight fixation.

The report that the pathologist renders from forceps biopsy material usually can provide only limited information (e.g., adenoma present or cancer present). Attempts to classify an adenoma precisely as to type from this kind of material can be futile. A diagnosis of cancer can be rendered; however, if no submucosa is present, the pathologist cannot absolutely make a diagnosis of invasive cancer. At times forceps biopsy material will provide nondiagnostic material

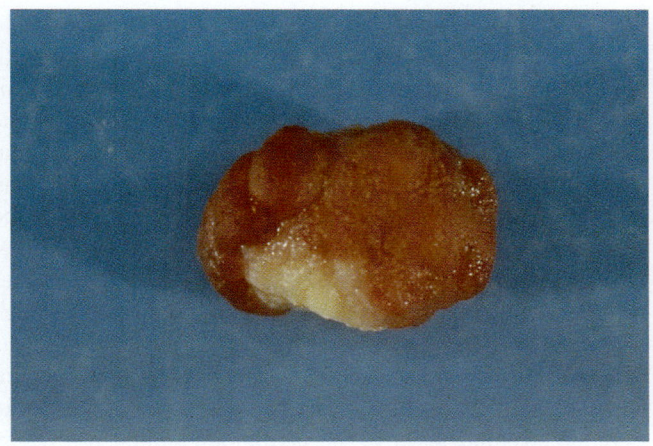 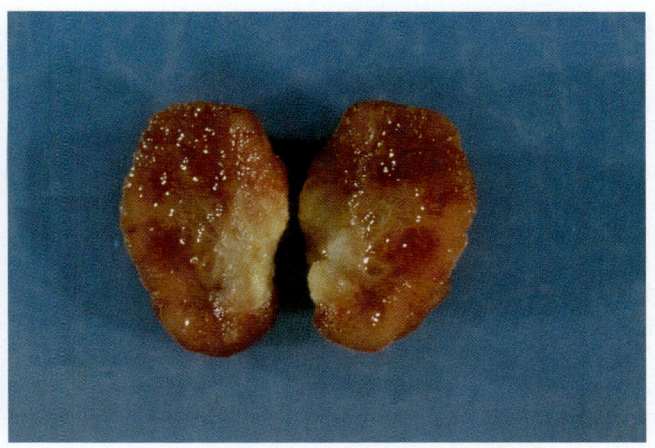

FIG. 25. A: Endoscopically removed polyp without obvious stalk. Note whitish ashened area that is the transection point. **B:** Polyp after orientation and proper sectioning through the transection point. All important landmarks will be microscopically present (from ref. 104).

(e.g., the eroded surface of an inflammatory fibroid polyp) and resection or polypectomy is required for diagnosis. Obviously, polypectomy material enables the pathologist to categorize lesions exactly and, if cancer is present, to determine (a) whether or not it is invasive, (b) its grade, (c) its relationship to the margin of transection, and (d) if lymphatic or venous invasion is present. (See example of the pathology report in the section on malignant polyps, below.)

Adenomas with Cancer—Definitions

The incidence of high-grade dysplasia (formerly called *in situ* cancer) and invasive cancer arising in adenomas is approximately 12.3% and 5.0%, respectively (89,91). It is important to differentiate between invasive cancer and high-grade dysplasia, because the former has the biologic potential to metastasize, whereas the latter does not. The term *invasive adenocarcinoma* should be restricted to the situation in which cancer has invaded through the muscularis mucosae and into the submucosa.

High-grade dysplasia is a pathologic process that is limited to the mucosa, and more precisely, is confined within its crypt or gland basement membrane. The diagnosis of high-grade dysplasia is made on architectural and cytologic changes. At low and medium power the glands show irregular complex branching, budding, or cribriform pattern. Cytologically, the individual cells usually show loss of mucin, severe nuclear atypia (hyperchromasia or vesicular pattern with enlarged nucleoli) and stratification reaching the luminal surface of the cell, increased mitoses, and, occasionally, necrosis (Figs. 22 and 23). The term *intramucosal cancer* is often used by pathologists. It is defined as cancer limited to the mucosa, wherein the cancer actually invades the lamina propria within the mucosa, eliciting a desmoplastic tissue response (Fig. 26). Intramucosal carcinoma has no biologic potential for metastases (94).

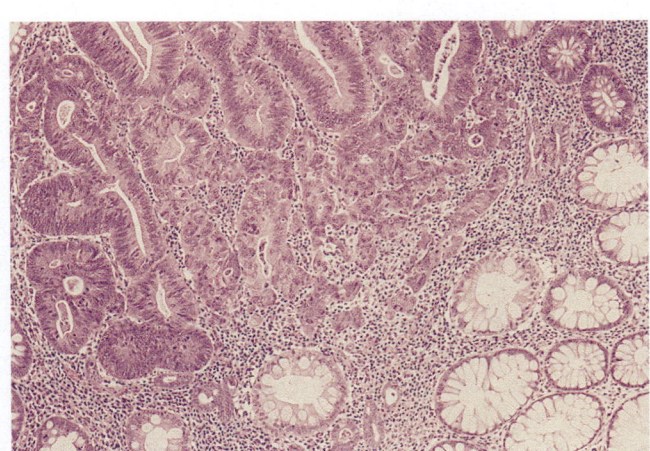 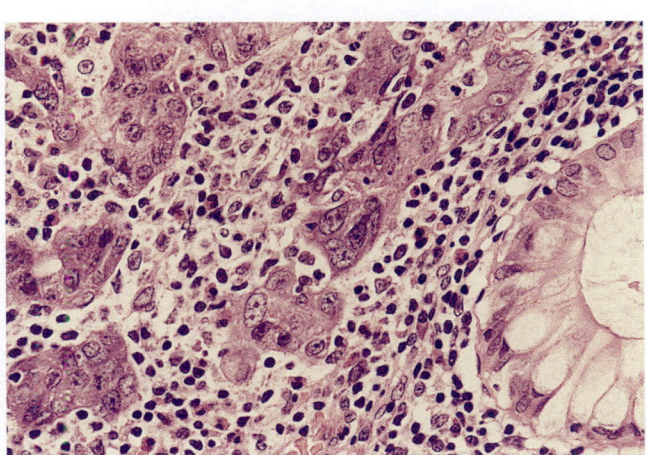

FIG. 26 A: Intramucosal adenocarcinoma. At low power one can see small buds of malignant glands invading into the lamina propria. **B:** Higher power view showing buds of malignant cells in the lamina propria (from ref. 302).

The Endoscopically Removed Malignant Polyp

A malignant polyp is one in which cancer has invaded into the submucosa. Cancer limited to the mucosa or only into the muscularis mucosae is not a malignant polyp and has no metastatic potential.

The evaluation of an endoscopically removed malignant polyp is a stepwise process that involves (a) adequate fixation, (b) sectioning, (c) knowledge of the type of removal, (d) examination of slides, and (e) pathologist-clinician interaction.

Fixation and sectioning are discussed in the section on processing of polyps, above. If the polyp is not properly fixed, sectioning may be difficult and result in a less than optimum specimen that may preclude the pathologist from properly evaluating the lesion. The pathologist should be informed as to whether the polyp was removed piecemeal or in one piece. Piecemeal polypectomy results in multiple fragments of tissue showing diathermy and may preclude one from properly evaluating the true margin of resection. The pathologist should be informed about this so as to make a true and accurate statement about the margin of resection.

When examining the slides, one should evaluate and report on the following: (a) status of resection margin, (b) grade of cancer, and (c) presence or absence of lymphatic or venous invasion (Figs. 27–30). Most investigators believe that if cancer is at or near the resection margin, and/or is grade III, and/or is in lymphatics or veins, then the polypectomy should be followed by a definitive surgical resection. However, if the margin is negative, the cancer is grade I or II, and no lymphatic or venous invasion is noted, then polypectomy should be curative (104–113). The definition of cancer at the margin is tumor cells in the actual free edge of the submucosal transection point that contains diathermy. Tumor close to the margin has been defined as cancer within the actual diathermy, one high power field from the diathermy, less than 1 mm from the transected margin, or less than 2 mm from the transected margin. The grading is similar to that for colorectal adenocarcinoma. The detection of lymphatic invasion requires tumor emboli in true endothelial lined channels, which should be differentiated from retraction artifact, which is commonly present. Retraction artifact is most often present within the tumor itself, while true lymphatic invasion is more confidently diagnosed in the pertumoral submucosa (away from the tumor) (104,105,114). There is great interobserver variation in diagnosing lymphatic invasion (105); because of this, some investigators do not even bother evaluating such invasion (107,108).

In a large interinstitutional study (105), the adverse outcome rate (recurrent disease in those treated by polypectomy only, or lymph node metastases or residual local disease in those treated by resection post polypectomy) was 19.7% in those patients with cancer at or near the margin, and/or grade III cancer, and/or lymphatic or venous invasion. Analyzed further, the adverse outcome rate was 21.4% for cancer at or near the margin, 16.6% for lymphatic invasion, and 37.5% for grade III cancer (Tables 2 and 3). Polypoid carcinoma (cancers with no residual adenoma) are treated in a similar fashion to cancers with background adenoma.

Examples of Reporting Malignant Polyps

Example 1. Sigmoid colon, polypectomy: grade III adenocarcinoma arising within an adenoma. The cancer extends to the transected margin of resection. No evidence of lymphatic or venous invasion.

Example 2. Rectum, polypectomy: grade II adenocarcinoma arising within an adenoma. Cancer is 2.5 mm from the transected margin (the margin is negative for cancer). No evidence of lymphatic or venous invasion.

Adenoma with Pseudoinvasion/Misplaced Epithelium

Pseudoinvasion is defined as the situation in which, possibly as a result of torsion or other trauma (e.g., biopsy), the mucosa (or epithelium) of the polyp has been "misplaced" into the submucosa, mimicking invasive carcinoma (115–117). Other terms to describe this entity are *epithelial misplacement* and *hamartomatous inverted polyp*. It is important for the pathologist to recognize this entity so that a mistaken diagnosis of cancer is not rendered and unnecessary surgery is not performed. The prevalence of pseudoinvasion varies from 2.5% to 3.5% of all adenomas. The male-to-female ratio is 3:1. Most of these lesions are located in the sigmoid colon and occur in adenomas with well-defined stalks. The diagnosis of pseudoinvasion is best appreciated

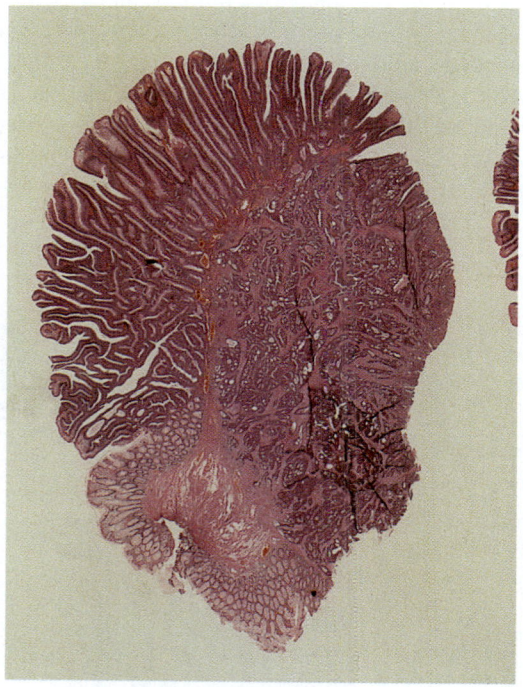

FIG. 27. Whole mount of endoscopically removed malignant polyp with obvious stalk. One can appreciate the transected margin of resection (diathermy). The cancer is >1 mm from the resection margin.

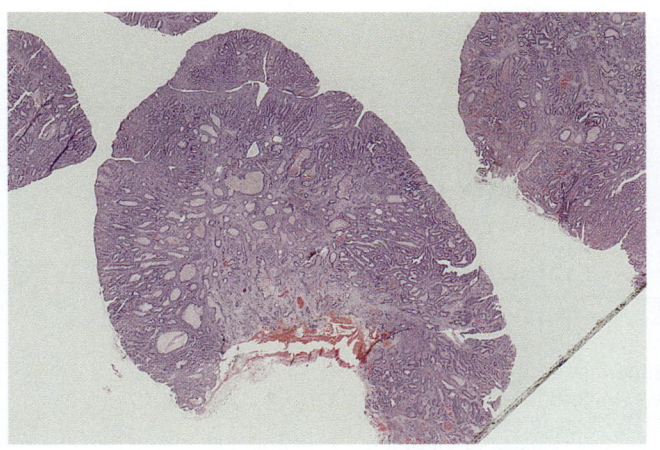 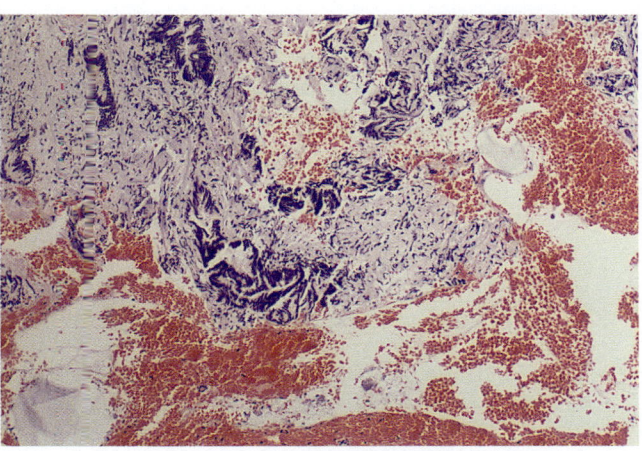

FIG. 28. A: Whole mount of endoscopically removed malignant polyp with cancer extending to the transected margin of resection. **B:** High-power view of cancer at margin. Note diathermy effect on the cancer.

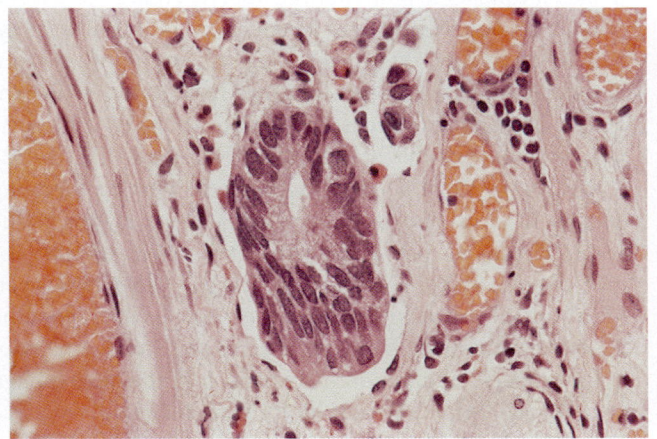 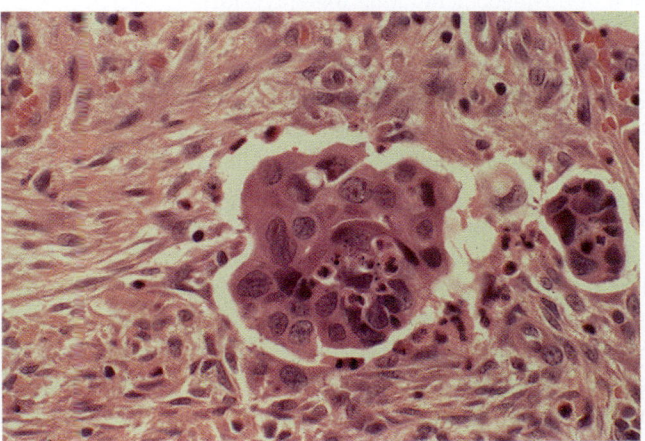

FIG. 29 A: High-power view of cancer in a lymphatic vessel. One can readily appreciate tumor cells within an endothelial lined channel. **B:** Retraction artifact mimicking lymphatic invasion. One can appreciate retraction of cancer from surrounding tissue. No endothelial lining can be appreciated; rather, the tumor cells are surrounded by fibroblasts.

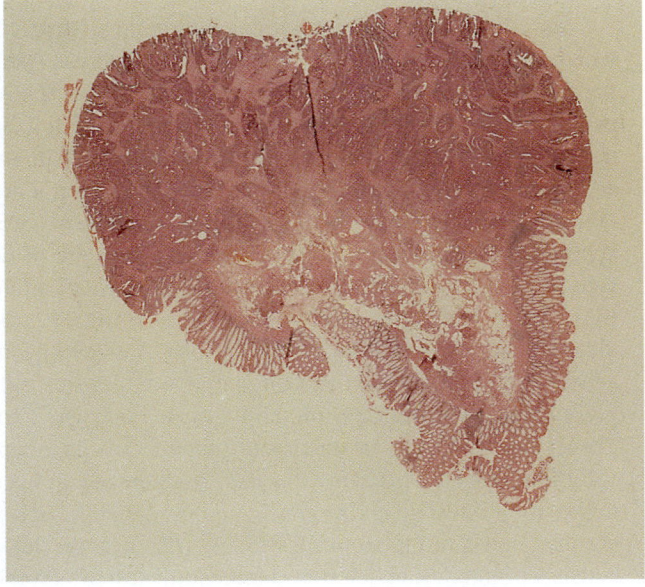 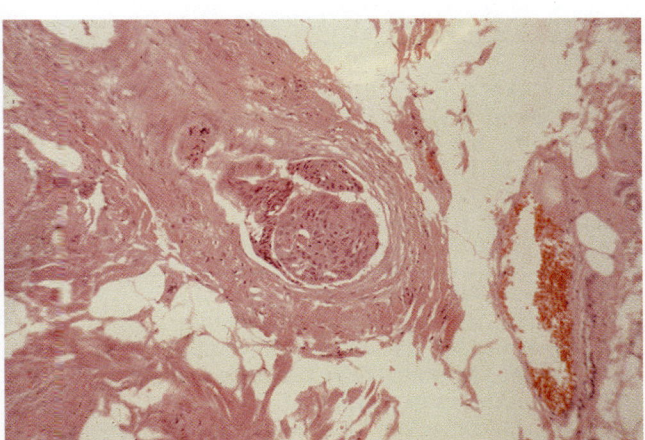

FIG. 30. A: Whole mount of malignant polyp with cancer invading a vein. **B:** High-power view of tumor in a vein (from ref. 104).

TABLE 2. *Malignant polyps: outcome related to histologic parameters*

Unfavorable histology	Adverse outcome	No adverse outcome	Total
Present	14/71 (19.7%)	57/71 (80.3%)**	71/140 (50.7%)
Indefinite	2/23 (8.7%)*	21/23 (91.3%)***	23/140 (16.4%)
Absent	0/46 (0.0%)	46/46 (100%)	46/140 (32.9%)
Total	16/140 (11.4%)†	124/140 (88.6%)	140/140 (100%)

Present vs. absent, $p < .0005$, p only 2/36 (5.6%) vs. P + R 14/104 (13.5%) = NS.
* ($1LI_I$ $1LI_I$).
** Three patients, negative resection, later metastases.
*** One patient, negative resection, later metastases (LI_I and III_I).
†13 lymph nodes metastases (P + R), 1 local (P + R), 2 distant metastases (P).
P, polypectomy only, P + R, polypectomy followed by resection; LI_I, indefinite for lymphatic invasion; III_I, indefinite for grade III. Data from ref. 105.

at low-power magnification, which reinforces the impression of misplacement rather than invasion.

The pathology is characterized by the presence of epithelial structures misplaced into the submucosa. In invasive cancer, malignant epithelial glands infiltrate into the submucosa and cause a desmoplastic reaction. In pseudoinvasion, the misplaced structures consist of both epithelium and surrounding lamina propria. The finding of lamina propria surrounding these misplaced glands is extremely helpful in differentiating pseudoinvasion from invasive cancer (Fig. 31). This situation is somewhat analogous to adenomyosis of the uterus. The misplaced glands can show histologically normal epithelium, adenomatous changes, or even high-grade dysplasia (118). The submucosal glands can show cystic dilatation, with rupture and secondary inflammation. The submucosa often contains fresh hemorrhage and/or hemosiderin deposition. In these cases with possibly misplaced glands, it is important to determine if cancer is present in the mucosa. Without the presence of cancer in the mucosa, one should consider pseudoinvasion as the correct diagnosis rather than invasive carcinoma.

TABLE 3. *Malignant polyps: Status of margins, lymphatic invasion, grade, and venous invasion related to outcome*

	Adverse outcome	No adverse outcome
Margin		
and/or <1 mm ($n = 56$, 40.5%)	21.4%	78.0%
>1 mm ($n = 82$, 59.4%)	4.9%*	95.1% $p < .003$
LI^+ ($n = 17$, 12.1%)	17.6%**	82.3% $p < .025$
LI_I ($n = 22$, 15.7%)	18.1%***	81.8% $p < .04$
Grade III ($n = 8$, 5.7%)†	37.5%	62.5% $p < .05$
VI ($n = 5$, 3.5%)	40.0%††	60.0%

* Two cases with LI^+ and 2 cases with LI_I.
** Two of 3 cases with absent unfavorable.
*** Two of 4 cases with absent unfavorable.
†All 8 cases had unfavorable histology present.
††Unfavorable histology present.
LI^+, lymphatic invasion; LI_I, indefinite for lymphatic invasion; VI, venous invasion.
Data from ref. 105.

Epithelial misplacement can also occur in colorectal adenomas secondary to biopsy prior to polypectomy and it is important for the pathologist to be cognizant of this possibility. Within the first few days following forceps biopsy, ulceration develops at the biopsy site. As a result, there is an exudate with admixed mucus and small groups of dysplastic (adenomatous) epithelial cells in the lamina propria. By day 7 one can see small pools of mucus-containing proliferating dysplastic cells embedded in abundant granulation tissue within the submucosa. These changes are different from the type of epithelial misplacement described above. However, the history of a recent biopsy and the presence of granulation tissue, ulceration, re-epithelialization, and small groups of dysplastic epithelium in mucin pools are distinctive enough to diagnose epithelial misplacement rather than invasive cancer (117).

Adenomatous Polyposis Syndromes

Familial Polyposis Coli (Familial Adenomatous Polyposis, FAP)

This condition is an autosomal dominant disorder in which the large intestine is carpeted with adenomas (ranging from hundreds to 3,000) (Fig. 32; Table 1) (31,32). All patients will develop colonic adenocarcinoma if left untreated. The incidence of this disorder has been estimated at 1 in 8,000 births, with 20% of cases representing a new mutation. The average age of detection in patients with symptoms is 36.5 years; however, the average age of detection is 23.5 years in patients screened because of a family history. Adenomas rarely appear prior to age 10, and there are no extraintestinal manifestations. A clue to the diagnosis of familial polyposis coli in mucosal biopsies is the presence of adenomatous epithelium in single crypts (single-crypt adenomas) in specimens taken from endoscopically flat, normal-appearing mucosa. Adenomas can occur in the small intestine and stomach, and fundic gland polyps are also noted in the stomach (85,86). The genetic defect consists of interstitial deletions on the long arm of chromosome 5 (31).

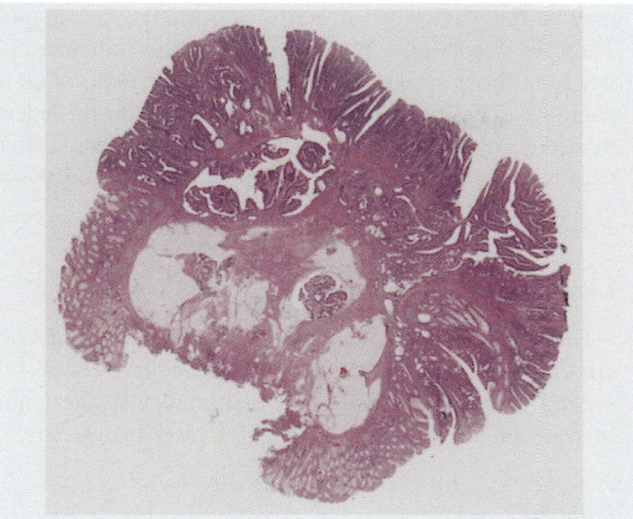
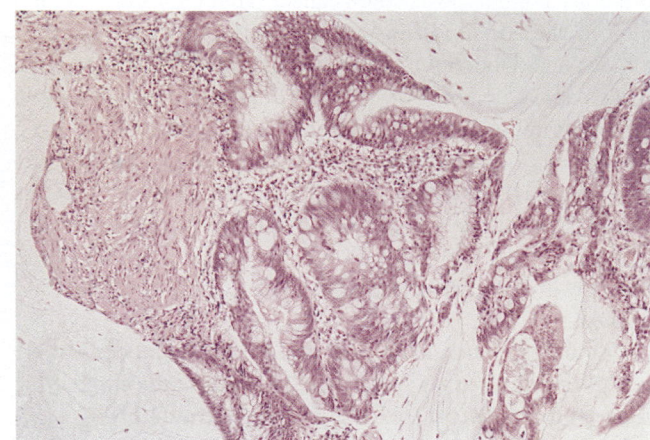

FIG. 31. A: Whole mount of adenoma with pseudoinvasion. At this power one can appreciate that the mucin pools with epithelium are misplaced into, rather than invading, the submucosa. **B:** Higher power view of mucosa (in mucin pool) in submucosa. Here one can appreciate lamina propria surrounding the adenomatous glands. This indicates pseudoinvasion, not invasive cancer.

Gardner's Syndrome (Table 1)

This syndrome is an autosomal dominant disorder consisting of intestinal polyposis (adenomas), soft tissue abnormalities, and bony abnormalities (31,32). The colonic adenomas are similar to those seen in familial polyposis coli. Adenomas are also present in the small intestine and stomach, along with gastric fundic gland polyps and, occasionally, lymphoid polyps of the ileum (82–86). The soft tissue abnormalities can be lipomas, fibromas, epidermal cysts, and desmoid tumors. The latter mainly occur in areas of previous surgery and can be quite aggressive and cause death. The bony abnormalities are cortical thickening of long bones and ribs, impacted teeth, supernumerary teeth, and dental cysts. The patients have an increased incidence of periampullary adenocarcinoma and cancer of the thyroid and adrenal glands.

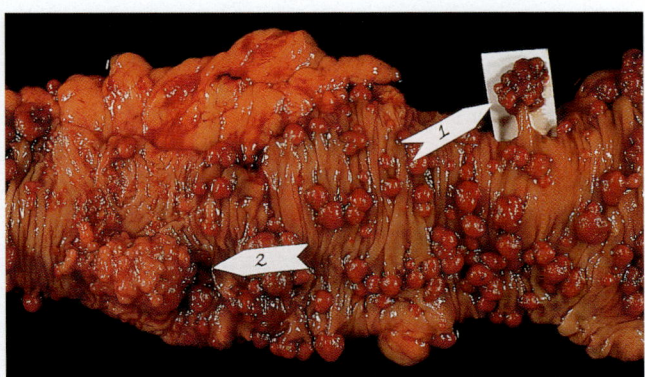

FIG. 32. Gross photograph of colon from a patient with FAP. Note the numerous polyps that carpet the mucosa.

Turcot's Syndrome (Table 1)

Turcot's syndrome was originally described in two siblings with polyposis coli who developed malignant brain tumors. This is a rare disorder that is probably autosomal dominant. The true frequency of Turcot's syndrome is difficult to assess, as brain tumors are associated with a high mortality and may precede the detection of colonic polyps. Studies indicate that there may be two forms of Turcot's syndrome: one group consists of patients with gliomas and colorectal adenomas (nonpolyposis patients), and the other group consists of patients with brain tumors (which are predominately medulloblastomas) associated with adenomatous polyposis. Molecular studies have shown that the former group has germline mutations of mismatch repair genes (hMLH 1 and hPMS2) whereas the latter group is associated with germline mutations of the APC gene (31,119,120).

Attenuated FAP (Table 1)

This is a less severe form of polyposis with a low number of polyps (adenomas), usually less than 100, yet patients sustain a high risk for colorectal cancer. The cancers usually develop 15 years later than in the classic FAP patient, but 10 years earlier than sporadic cancer. The genetic defect in this disorder is linked to 5q21, similar to FAP (31).

Hereditary Flat Adenoma Syndrome (Table 1)

Hereditary flat adenoma syndrome (HFAS) is presently thought to be a variant of FAP, with the genetic defect linked to 5q21-22. These individuals have multiple colorectal adenomas, but usually less than 100. The adenomas tend to occur at a later age than in classic FAP and tend to show a proximal location. The onset of colorectal cancer is later than in hereditary nonpolyposis colon cancer (HNPCC) and FAP. In addition, these individuals have adenomas and cancers of the stomach and duodenum. Fundic gland polyps of the stomach are also noted, and in some patients fundic gland polyps may be present in the absence of colorectal adenomas (121,122). The majority of adenomas are of the flat type (see section on flat adenomas). However, Lynch et al. (121) report that in their experience, only 3 of 235 flat adenomas (1.3%) in the familial setting showed high-grade dysplasia, which is a much lower rate than reported in patients with sporadic flat adenoma.

Although the attenuated FAP and HFAS have been listed and described separately, they may in fact be the same disorder, with *attenuated FAP* the preferred term (123).

Muir Torre Syndrome (Table 1)

The Muir Torre syndrome was originally subclassified as a form of hereditary adenomatous polyposis (FAP) syndrome. The Muir Torre syndrome is a rare autosomal dominant disorder with fewer than 100 adenomas, typically in the proximal colon. This syndrome is associated with skin lesions such as basal cell carcinoma, sebaceous carcinoma, and squamous carcinoma. The genetics of this syndrome are as yet unknown (31).

Hereditary Mixed Polyposis Syndrome (Table 1)

This is an autosomal dominant disorder involving a single family that has been mapped to chromosome 6q. Five types of polyps have been described in individuals with this disorder: (a) tubular adenomas, (b) villous adenomas, (c) flat adenomas, (d) hyperplastic polyps, and (e) atypical juvenile polyps. The number of polyps is usually less than 15 per patient. Colorectal cancer is seen in this disorder. The characteristic lesion appears to be atypical juvenile polyps. This disorder might be a variant of juvenile polyposis; however, in juvenile polyposis, adenomas are uncommon, while in hereditary mixed polyposis the majority of polyps are adenomas. In hereditary mixed polyposis the number of polyps is lower than that seen in juvenile polyposis. Juvenile polyposis usually presents one decade earlier than hereditary mixed polyposis (124).

CARCINOMA

Small Intestine

Small-intestinal adenocarcinomas account for approximately 40% of small-intestinal malignant tumors; however, compared to colonic adenocarcinoma they are uncommon. The distribution along the small bowel varies, depending on whether the series includes ampullary cancers. In one series, 48.4%, 32.5%, and 19.2% were located in the duodenum, jejunum, and ileum, respectively (125). Grossly, the cancers may be flat, stenosing, ulcerative, infiltrative, or polypoid. They are morphologically similar to adenocarcinomas elsewhere in the gastrointestinal tract, but they more often are papillary. These cancers are often associated with adenomas; their diagnosis by endoscopic biopsy may be difficult because they are frequently interpreted as adenomas with dysplasia.

Large Intestine and Rectum

Carcinoma of the colon and rectum is a disease of Western-world lifestyle. Among both males and females, it is the second most common visceral malignancy in the United States, with an expected 185,000 new cases each year.

Pathology

Macroscopically, most colorectal cancers are either polypoid or of the ulcerative-infiltrating type. Generally, polypoid cancers have a better prognosis than ulcerative lesions; however, this association is most probably directly related to the fact that polypoid cancers are usually of a lower clinicopathologic stage than ulcerative lesions at the time of diagnosis. Rarely (0.3% of cases), colorectal cancer may have a gross appearance similar to linitis plastica of the stomach. However, many cases with a gross linitis plastica appearance may not be primary colorectal lesions but are, instead, metastases from other sites (126,127).

Table 4 lists the histopathologic classification of colorectal cancer according to the World Health Organization.

Adenocarcinoma

Adenocarcinoma can be divided into three grades based primarily on an overview of the arrangement of cells in regard to the degree of tubular (acinar) formation. Fifteen percent to 20% of colorectal adenocarcinomas are grade I (low grade or well differentiated), 60% to 70% are grade II (average grade or moderately differentiated), and 15% to 20% are grade III (poorly differentiated). Grade I cancers are composed mainly of simple tubules, in which nuclear polarity is easily discerned and nuclei are of uniform size. There is a distinct resemblance to adenomatous epithelium (Fig. 33). Grade II cancers are composed of tubules that may be simple, complex, or slightly irregular, in which nuclear polarity

TABLE 4. *Histopathologic types of colorectal carcinoma—World Health Organization (92)*

Adenocarcinoma
Mucinous adenocarcinoma
Signet-ring cell carcinoma
Small-cell carcinoma (oat cell)
Adenosquamous carcinoma
Squamous cell carcinoma
Undifferentiated carcinoma

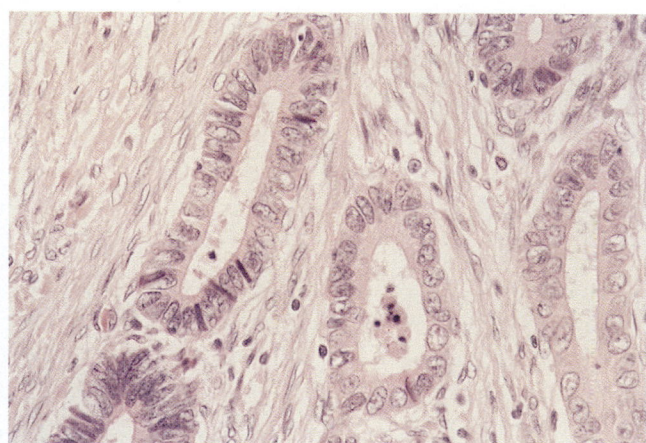

FIG. 33. Grade I colorectal adenocarcinoma. Note orderly, well-formed glands and basally placed nuclei without stratification.

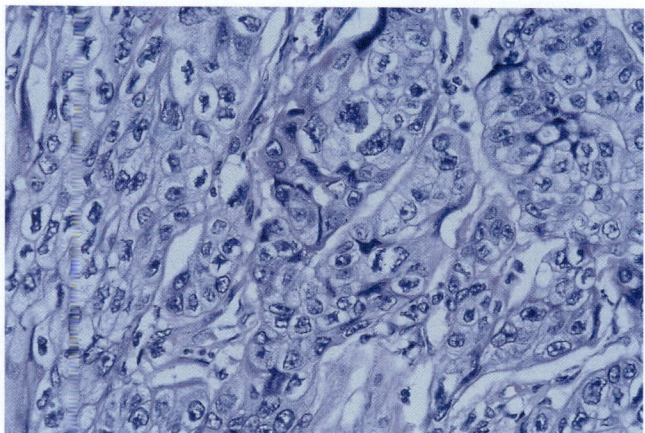

FIG. 35. Grade III cancer. Cancer grows in solid sheets; gland formation is not evident.

is barely discernible or is lost (Fig. 34). Grade III tumors are characterized by an absence of glandular differentiation as well as by loss of nuclear polarity (Fig. 35). Grade III cancers have a significantly poorer prognosis than grade I and II lesions (128–130). To define a colorectal carcinoma as a grade III lesion, the poorly differentiated component should form the vast majority of the tumor rather than only small rare foci of the neoplasm. The disorganized glands commonly seen at the advancing edge of the cancer should not be construed as high-grade malignancy and should not be assessed in grading (92).

Mucinous Adenocarcinoma

Mucinous adenocarcinomas (including signet cell cancers) account for approximately 10% of colorectal cancers. The definition of mucinous carcinoma is variable: some authors state that at least 50% of the lesion must be mucinous (92), whereas others claim that at least 75% of the lesion must be mucinous (131,132). Mucinous cancers are associated with young adults and children, villous adenomas, cancers arising secondary to therapeutic irradiation, ulcerative colitis, and colorectal cancers in low-incidence developing countries. Compared to nonmucinous colorectal cancers, mucinous carcinomas usually present at a more advanced stage, have more extensive perirectal spread, show a greater incidence of lymph node involvement, and tend to have an overall poorer prognosis (131,132). However, studies of rectal cancers have shown that stage for stage, there is no difference in survival between mucinous and nonmucinous cancers (131).

Multivariate analysis has shown that stage is important in prognosis and that mucinous histology itself is not an independent prognostic factor in colorectal cancer (133). Among the mucinous tumors, the extracellular type is much more common than the intracellular, or signet cell, type. The extracellular type is characterized by tumor cells floating freely in large pools of mucin. The cells that are floating in the mucin often have a bland histologic appearance (Fig. 36). The intracellular type is morphologically identical to signet cell cancer seen in the stomach. The signet cell variant behaves very aggressively, and has a poor prognosis.

Small Cell Cancer

A rare variant is small cell cancer, which composes <1% of colorectal cancers (134–137). Histologically, these cancers are identical to small cell carcinoma of the lung (oat cell type and intermediate type) (Fig. 37). They have an extremely poor prognosis, with almost all cases having lymph node and liver metastases. One-third of these cancers have arisen within typical adenomas. These small cell cancers may also show areas of squamous differentiation and intimate association with the usual type of adenocarcinoma. Immunopathology may be helpful in making a diagnosis of small cell cancer. These neoplasms express neuron-specific enolase (84% of cases), Leu-7 (18%), synaptophysin (50%),

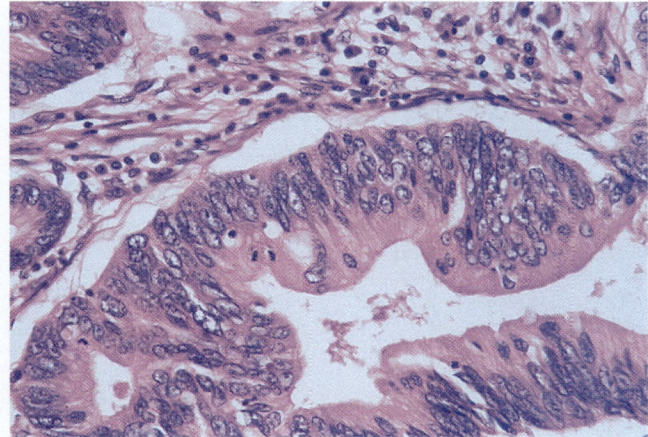

FIG. 34. Grade II colorectal adenocarcinoma. Note gland formation with focal cribriform areas. Nuclei are elongated and stratified.

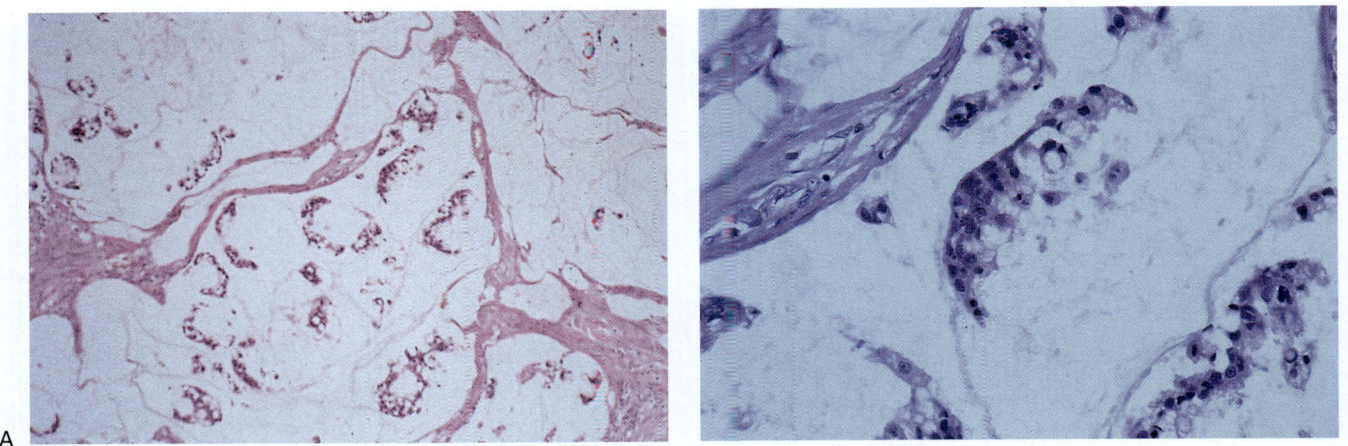

FIG. 36. A: Low-power view of mucinous adenocarcinoma. Tumor cells are floating in a sea of mucin. **B:** Higher power view.

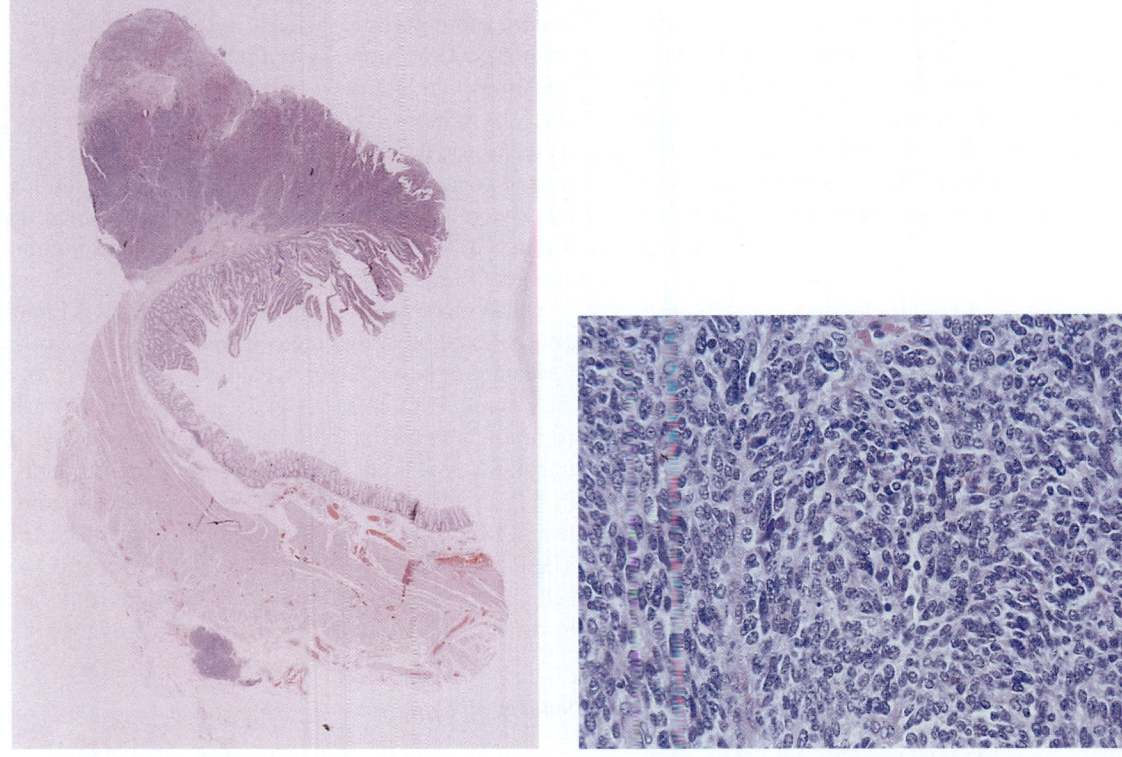

FIG. 37. A: Whole mount section of small cell carcinoma. The upper half is the small cell cancer component *(dark blue)*, while a villous adenoma component is evident below. **B:** Higher power view showing proliferation of small cells similar to anaplastic small cell cancer of the lung.

and chromogranin (37%). However, the histopathology is so characteristic that the diagnosis can readily be made by examination of routine hematoxylin and eosin (H&E)-stained slides in most instances.

Undifferentiated Cancer

Undifferentiated cancer is uncommon, accounting for approximately 1% of colorectal neoplasms (138). They are malignant epithelial tumors that have no glandular structures or other features to indicate definite differentiation. The absence of intracytoplasmic mucin helps to differentiate these tumors from poorly differentiated adenocarcinoma (92). Histologically, these tumors at low power show well-circumscribed masses, with pushing borders having a so-called medullary pattern. At higher power the cells are uniform and round, have small to medium-sized nuclei with prominent nucleoli, and exhibit numerous mitoses. Often they have a peritumoral brisk lymphocytic infiltrate. They have a close resemblance to neuroendocrine tumors but lack neuroendocrine markers by immunohistochemistry (139,140).

Surprisingly, these undifferentiated carcinomas have a good prognosis and show less frequent lymph node metastasis than other variants (138–141). The undifferentiated tumors with a medullary pattern are often diploid (85%), lack expression of p53, and show microsatellite instability (141). This medullary pattern has been described in cancers associated with hereditary nonpolyposis colorectal cancer (142,143).

Squamous/Adenosquamous Cancers

Squamous cancers or adenoacanthomas of the colon are very rare. They have been associated with ulcerative colitis, schistosomiasis, and pelvic irradiation. To make a diagnosis of primary colorectal squamous cancer or adenoacanthoma, certain criteria must be met: there must be no other sites of squamous cancer in the body and no involvement of cloacogenic or squamous-lined mucosa. Survival correlates with Dukes's staging, similar to garden variety adenocarcinoma (144).

Unusual Forms of Colorectal Cancer

Carcinosarcoma has been reported in both the large and small intestine; however, it is very rare (145,146). The cancers have areas of typical adenocarcinoma merging with sarcoma (spindle cells, and sarcoma with osseous and cartilaginous differentiation). Cytokeratin reactivity of the sarcomatous element is helpful in making the diagnosis.

Rare cases of adenocarcinoma with areas of choriocarcinoma have been reported (147–149), as have cases of adenocarcinoma with tumor cells producing human chorionic gonadotropin (HCG) and having features of mucinous cystadenocarcinoma (150).

Occasionally, colorectal adenocarcinoma can be predominantly of the clear cell type. This pattern greatly resembles renal clear cell adenocarcinoma. Primary clear cell colonic cancers produce glycogen and are negative for mucin production; however, the majority strongly express carcinoembryonic antigen (CEA), which is helpful in differentiating these lesions from metastatic renal carcinoma (151,152).

Hepatoid adenocarcinoma is rare and has combined features of classic adenocarcinoma and tumor indistinguishable from hepatocellular carcinoma. Mucin production is noted in the glandular component. Polyclonal CEA shows cytoplasmic staining for the glandular component and canalicular staining for the hepatoid component. Serum AFP is markedly elevated (153).

Small Early Flat Carcinoma

Small flat carcinomas are a topic of controversy. They are commonly seen in Japan and reported mainly in the Japanese literature, where they compose between 6% and 10% of all colonic cancers. However, they are considered uncommon in Western societies (100,154,155), although one report from the West has detected them with some frequency (101). Grossly, they are flat plaque-like lesions, often with a central depression, and are usually no larger than 10 mm. They are difficult to detect grossly; techniques using dye spraying of the mucosa greatly facilitate their detection. By definition these lesions are limited to the mucosa or are invasive only to the submucosa. Cases with submucosal invasion and lymph node metastases have been reported, thus validating them as true cancers. In one series 65% were intramucosal and 35% were invasive to the submucosa.

Part of the difference in the reported frequency of these lesions as cancers might be due to differences in diagnostic criteria between Western and Japanese pathologists (98). Many of the lesions diagnosed as intramucosal cancer by Japanese pathologists would be diagnosed as high-grade dysplasia by Western pathologists. However, this difference in interpretation has been shown to exist even between Japanese pathologists (154). These lesions are often described as de novo cancers (without associated adenoma) even when quite small. Small flat cancers may also develop from flat adenomas. Histologically, the height of the lesion is usually not more than twice the height of the adjacent normal mucosa. The glands show cytologic features of high-grade dysplasia with mild architectural changes. The diagnosis of cancer is obvious when submucosal invasion is noted. Some believe that these small flat cancers may be the precursors for rapidly growing, deeply penetrating, ulcerating cancers. However, follow-up studies from the National Polyp Study indicate that in the United States flat adenomas and small flat cancers are not common and are not precursors of rapidly growing deeply penetrating cancers (156). In a report from Germany (157) of 155 small submucosally invasive cancers with a maximum diameter of 10 mm, 59% were grossly polypoid while 41% were flat.

Hereditary Nonpolyposis Colon Cancer (HNPCC)

Cancers arising in patients with HNPCC have a characteristic profile. They tend to be proximal in location, 18% are multiple at presentation, and there is a 40% metachronous rate for new cancers. No histologic feature or set of features infallibly identifies a cancer as belonging to HNPCC; however, certain histologic types are more frequently found than in control populations: (a) poorly differentiated carcinoma, (b) mucinous cancer, (c) signet ring cell cancer, and (d) medullary (undifferentiated) cancer.

The medullary type is composed of solid sheets of tumor cells without tubule formation. These sheets consist of cells with fairly round and regular nuclei and abundant eosinophilic cytoplasm, features somewhat suggestive of neuroendocrine differentiation; however, immunohistochemical stains for neuron specific enolase, synaptophysin, and chromogranin are negative. The medullary type grows in sheets with well-circumscribed rounded or pushing borders, with the presence of a marked peritumoral lymphocytic response. Another finding in HNPCC cancers is the presence of a prominent peritumoral Crohn's-like reaction.

Despite the higher incidence of poorly differentiated cancers, HNPCC patients have a statistically significant better prognosis (stage for stage) compared to non-HPNCC patients (142,143,158). Poorly differentiated medullary cancers in patients without HNPCC have been statistically significantly associated with the presence of microsatellite instability (141) as have the dense peritumoral lymphoid infiltrate, Crohn's-like reaction, and plexiform growth pattern (159).

Staging

One major role the pathologist plays is in the proper staging of colorectal cancer, which provides the clinician with important information regarding the patient's prognosis and the need for adjuvant therapy. For many years, pathologists have used the classic Dukes's classification, devised in 1932 (160) (Table 5), and the Astler-Coller classification, devised in 1954 (161) (Table 6). However, the TNM system, as advocated by (AJCC/UICC) American Joint Committee on Cancer/Union Internationale Centre Le Cancer, is becoming more frequently used (162) (Table 7). Another staging system is that of Jass (163,164); however, it has not gained wide acceptance in the United States.

TABLE 5. Dukes' classification of rectal carcinoma

Stage A:	Growth limited to wall of rectum
Stage B:	Extension of growth to extrarectal tissues, but no metastasis to regional lymph nodes
Stage C:	Metastases in regional lymph nodes
	Modification of Stage C (1935):
Stage C_1:	Metastases to regional lymph nodes
Stage C_2:	Metastases to lymph nodes at point of mesenteric blood vessel ligature

From ref. 160.

TABLE 6. Astler-Coller classification for colorectal carcinoma

Stage A:	Lesion limited to the mucosa
Stage B_1:	Lesion involves muscularis propria but does not penetrate through it
Stage B_2:	Lesion penetrates through the muscularis propria
Stage C_1:	Metastatic tumor in lymph nodes but the tumor itself is still confined to the bowel wall
Stage C_2:	Metastatic tumor in lymph nodes and tumor itself has penetrated through the entire bowel wall

From ref. 161.

The reader should be acutely aware that both the Dukes and Astler-Coller systems have stages C1 and C2, but they are defined differently in the two systems. In the Astler-Coller classification, there is no mention of cancer limited to submucosal invasion. It should also be noted that the number of lymph nodes containing metastatic cancer is not taken into consideration in either the Dukes or the Astler-Coller classification. In Table 8 comparisons of survival data among various staging systems are presented (165,166). It becomes quite obvious that the number of lymph nodes involved is an important factor in determining prognosis. Similarly, the depth of tumor penetration in patients with positive lymph nodes is also important in prognosis. A study by the National Surgical Adjuvant Breast and Colon Cancer Project has given us data showing that colorectal cancers limited to the bowel wall and with one to four positive lymph nodes have the same 5-year survival as classic Dukes's B cancers (167).

Fisher et al. (168), using data from the National Surgical Adjuvant Breast and Bowel Project, compared the Dukes, Astler-Coller, and TNM systems, and found all three systems to be highly interrelated; however, consistency and prognostic discrimination were best demonstrated by the Dukes and TNM classifications. They failed to find an advantage for the

TABLE 7. AJCC and UICC staging for colorectal cancer

Stage 0:	T_{is}, N_0, M_0
Stage I:	T_1, N_0, M_0 or T_2, N_0, M_0
Stage II:	T_3, N_0, M_0 or T_4, N_0, M_0
Stage III:	T_{any}, N_1, M_0 or T_{any}, N_2, N_3, M_0
Stage IV:	T_{any}, N_{any}, M_1

AJCC, American Joint Committee on Cancer; UICC, T_{is}, carcinoma in situ T_1, tumor invades into submucosa; T_2, tumor invades into muscularis propria; T_3, tumor invades through the muscularis propria into the subserosa or into non-peritonealized pericolonic or perirectal tissue; T_4, tumor perforates the visceral peritoneum or invades directly into other organs or tissues; N_0, no lymph-node metastases; N_1, metastatic tumor in one to three pericolic or perirectal lymph nodes; N_2, metastatic tumor in four or more pericolic or perirectal lymph nodes; N_3, metastases in any lymph node along the course of a major named blood vessel; M_0, no distant metastases; M_1, distant metastases present.

From ref. 162.

TABLE 8. *Colorectal carcinoma: survival comparing staging systems*

AJCC/UICC (%)			Dukes' (%)	Astler-Coller (%)
Stage 0		(100)		A (100)
Stage I	(T_1)	(100)	A (92–99)[a]	B_1 (67)
	(T_2)	(85)		
Stage II	(T_3)	(70)		
	(T_4)	(30)	B (72–78)[a]	B_2 (54)
Stage III	(N_1)	(60)	C (30–37)[a]	
	(N_2)	(30)	C_1 (45)[b]	C_1 (43)
			C_2 (12)[b]	C_2 (22)
Stage IV		(3)		

[a] Data from refs. 165 and 166.
[b] Data from ref. 131.

TNM system. Considering the independent prognostic value of depth of tumor penetration in patients with lymph node metastases, they recommended the use of the Dukes' staging system, but with subclassification of stage C according to the Astler-Coller system. However, it is the author's personal experience that the TNM system is becoming more acceptable and widely used, especially for protocols, adjuvant therapy, and intergroup comparisons (Table 8).

Proper Handling and Reporting of Colorectal Cancer Specimens

When the pathologist receives a colon or rectal resection for examination, the following tumor parameters should be examined and reported (169):

1. Location of tumor.
2. Size and configuration of the cancer.
3. Direct extension to other organs (if present).
4. Status of resection margins (see note below).
5. Grade of the cancer, as well as the type of cancer (typical, mucinous, small cell, etc.).
6. Status of lymph nodes (see note below):
   a. Number of lymph nodes involved.
   b. Level of lymph nodes involved (level I = nodes proximal to cancer, level II = nodes at level of cancer, level III = nodes distal to cancer, level IV = nodes at the vascular margin of resection).
7. Depth of penetration
8. Status of veins in regards to tumor invasion:
   a. Intramural veins.
   b. Extramural veins (thick-walled or thin-walled).
9. Presence or absence of lymphatic invasion.
10. Other lesions present.

Note: The resection margins (item 4) are proximal, distal, radial and peritoneal margins. One should comment if they are positive or negative for cancer, and if the tumor is close, the actual distance of cancer from the margin. The radial margin is important in rectal cancers: if tumor is at or near the radial margin, postoperative adjuvant therapy is indicated (170–172). The rectal radial margin is the distance from the outermost part of the tumor to the lateral margin of resection along a radius drawn from the center of the lumen through the deepest penetration of the carcinoma and continued through the bowel wall. It is suggested that the specimen be inked in order to best evaluate the radial and peritoneal margin of resection. If tumor is at the peritoneal margin, it should be reported, because cancer at the peritoneal margin is an independent pathologic prognosticor that signals a high incidence of intraperitoneal recurrence (173).

Note: Status of lymph nodes (item 6)—The number of lymph nodes varies with the individual and the extent of the resection. Cases treated with preoperative radiation and/or chemotherapy usually have fewer retrievable lymph nodes. The pathologist should attempt to find as many nodes as possible. In colorectal cancer, the majority of lymph nodes with metastases are <5 mm in size. Some studies have reported that one must find at least 13 to 17 lymph nodes in order to accurately stage a tumor (174,175). If the surgeon marks the apical node, it should be examined and separately reported. In the pericolorectal fat, a tumor nodule >3 mm in size without histologic evidence of remaining lymph node is classified as a regional lymph node metastasis. A similar tumor nodule <3 mm in size in the pericolorectal fat is classified as a discontinuous tumor nodule (T3) (169) (AJCC/UICC).

An example of a report is as follows:

Rectum (resection): Grade II adenocarcinoma extending through the entire bowel wall thickness and into pericolonic fat. Metastatic cancer in two of eight (2/8) level II lymph nodes. Five level I lymph nodes (0/5), five level III lymph nodes (0/5), and one level IV lymph node (0/1), all negative for tumor. Proximal, distal, and radial margins of resections are negative for tumor. Negative for venous invasion. Two separate tubular adenomas and two separate hyperplastic polyps are identified.

When examining a local excision of rectal cancer, the pathologist should apply the same protocol as above with modifications. The specimen should be inked and oriented, then placed flat and fixed on a surface. Once the specimen is firm, sections should be taken from the circumferential margins (12 o'clock, 3 o'clock, 6 o'clock, 9 o'clock) and the deep (radial) margin. These specimens do not have lymph nodes

An example of a report would be:

Rectum (local excision): Grade II rectal adenocarcinoma extending into the submucosa. Negative deep margin of resection. Negative circumferential margin of resection. Lymphatic invasion present. No evidence of venous invasion.

Other Histopathologic Prognostic Features

The following histopathologic features have been shown to be prognostic indicators in multivariate analysis: (a) microacinar (worse prognosis) versus macroacinar growth pattern (176), (b) endocrine cells detected by chromogranin immunohistochemistry (chromogranin positive tumors have a worse prognosis) (177), (c) Crohn's-like reaction (those tumors with a predominant Crohn's-like reaction have a significantly better prognosis) (178,179), (d) tumor budding (cancers with tumor budding have a significantly worse prognosis) (180).

Biologic Markers of Prognostic Significance

A voluminous literature relates to biologic and molecular markers as prognostic indicators in colorectal cancer. These can be broadly divided into differentiation markers (CEA, CA19-9, Sial Tn, E-cadherins, integrins, type IV collagen, gelatinase, gastrin receptors, epidermal growth factor receptor [EGFR], etc.); ploidy and proliferation markers (ploidy/DNA index, S-phase fraction, proliferating cell nuclear antigen [PCNA], Ki 67, silver staining nucleolar organizing regions [AgNORS]); and molecular markers (c-*myc*, K-*ras*, CD44, NM 23, P53, DCC, etc.). Many of these markers appear promising; however, more studies and standardization of methods are needed before they can be considered for routine use in clinical practice. The review of each of these is beyond the scope of this chapter. Recent references for all of the above can be found in ref. 181.

Workup of Undifferentiated Neoplasms

Occasionally, an intestinal lesion will be histologically undifferentiated by light microscopy so that the pathologist cannot be certain if it is a carcinoma, lymphoma, mesenchymal lesion, metastatic tumor, or malignant carcinoid tumor. Electron microscopy and immunohistochemistry may be helpful. The potential value of immunohistochemistry in differentiating among the above-mentioned tumors is summarized in Table 9. This table is not all inclusive but rather a brief summary/overview of how immunohistochemistry can help in everyday practice. Citations for immunohistochemical markers that are useful in the diagnostic surgical pathology of these tumors are given elsewhere (182–195).

VERMIFORM APPENDIX

Mucocele

Mucocele of the appendix is the term for a macroscopically dilated, usually thin-walled, and mainly unilocular (occasionally multilocular) cyst filled with thick tenacious mucus (196). Although mucoceles may be either nonneoplastic or neoplastic in origin, most mucoceles are secondary to mucinous cystadenomas or cystadenocarcinomas (Fig. 38). If the neoplastic process dissects through the appendiceal wall and reaches the peritoneum, pseudomyxoma peritonei may develop. In the neoplastic mucocele, histologically one finds a mucus-filled lumen lined by dysplastic epithelium. As the lesion increases in size, the epithelium may become flattened and even ulcerated, with contact between mucin and the appendiceal wall leading to a granulomatous reaction. Occasionally, mucin can dissect into the appendiceal wall, or adenomatous epithelium can herniate into the appendiceal wall. In these situations, distinction from carcinoma may be a difficult diagnostic problem (see below).

The nonneoplastic mucocele is secondary to sterile obstruction of appendiceal outflow, with accumulation of mucin in the lumen. These nonneoplastic mucoceles are rarely >1.0 cm in size. Histologically, there is a mucus-filled lumen with flattening of the mucosa; there is no evidence of neoplastic epithelium.

Hyperplastic Lesions

Mucosal hyperplasia or hyperplastic polyps of the appendix occur (197–200). Younes et al. (197) found mucosal hyperplasia of the appendix in 18.8% of ileocolectomies and 8.3% of appendectomies; they also noted that 25% of consecutive appendices with mucosal hyperplasia were associated with colonic adenocarcinoma. Most cases of epithelial hyperplasia are "diffuse nonpolypoid"; however, rarely a solitary polyp will occur.

Histologically, the changes are identical to colonic hyperplastic polyps with one possible difference. Some workers report that mucosal hyperplasia of the appendix lacks the characteristic thickening of the subepithelial collagen layer noted in colorectal hyperplastic polyps (196,197); however, other studies report its presence (200). Villous adenomas coexisting in appendices with mucosal hyperplasia have been reported (198). The differential diagnosis of mucosal hyperplasia is a villous adenoma, which may often mimic hyperplasia. However, adenomas have true neoplastic nuclei (although they are relatively bland) compared to those of hyperplasias.

Adenomas

Localized and pedunculated adenomas as seen in the colon are rare in the appendix (196). More commonly, appendiceal adenomas are diffuse or circumscribed sessile villous adenomas. Most of the epithelial cells are mucin producing. When the lesions become dilated, the term *cystadenoma* (or *mucocele*) is appropriate. As mentioned earlier, these lesions may dissect through the appendiceal wall, forming large pools of mucin and mimicking invasive cancer. In these instances, the morphologic distinction between cystadenoma and carcinoma may be extremely difficult; however, conclusive evidence of tissue invasion must be found before a diagnosis of cancer can be made. The entire lesion, as well as the margin of resection, should be examined histologically to determine whether or not cancer is present (Fig. 39).

Mucinous Tumor of Undetermined Malignant Potential

Because of the difficulty in differentiating adenomas that dissect into and through the muscularis propria from adeno-

TABLE 9. Immunohistochemistry in evaluation of undifferentiated intestinal tumors

Markers	Lymphoma	Primary carcinoma	Primary mesenchymal	Metastasis	Endocrine
Leukocyte common antigen CD45	+	−	−	−	−
Vimentin	+	− or +	+	− or +	−
Cytokeratin	−[1]	+	−[2]	+ or −[3]	+
Epithelial membrane antigen	−[4]	+	−	+ or −[5]	+
Carcinoembryonic antigen	−	+	−	+ or −[6]	+
BER-EP4	−	+	−	+ or −[7]	NA
Chromogranin	−	−[8]	−	−	+
Synaptophysin	−	−	−	−	+
Leu-7	−[9]	−	−	+ or −[10]	+
S-100	−	−	+ or −[11]	+ or −[12]	−
HMB-45	−	−	−	+ or −[13]	−
CD30	+	−	−	−	−
CD34	−	−	+ or −[14]	−	−
CD31	−	−	+ or −[15]	−	−
CK7	−	−[16]	−	+[16] or −	NA
CK20	−	+[16]	−	+[16] or −	NA
Villin	−	+[17]	−	+ or −[17]	+
Prostate specific antigen	−	−	−	+[18]	−
Prostatic specific acid phosphatase	−	−	−	+[19]	+[19]
Muscle specific actin	−	−	+ or −[20]	+ or −[20]	−

[1] CD30 (+) large cell anaplastic lymphomas can rarely express cytokeratin (182, 183).
[2] "Smooth muscle" sarcomas can occasionally express cytokeratin (184, 185).
[3] Epithelial neoplasms express cytokeratin; sarcomas most often negative for cytokeratin, melanomas are usually negative for cytokeratin (however, they can rarely be positive for cytokeratin) (186, 187).
[4] Plasmacytomas and CD30+ large cell anaplastic lymphomas can express epithelial membrane antigen (188).
[5] Epithelial neoplasms express epithelial membrane antigen (189).
[6] Most epithelial neoplasms express CEA. Renal cell cancer is negative for CEA as are mesenchymal lesions (186).
[7] Epithelial neoplasms express BER-EP4 (190).
[8] Primary colon cancers can focally express chromogranin (177).
[9] T cell natural killer like lymphomas can express Leu 7 (CD57) and CD56 (191,192,251,252).
[10] Prostate cancer expresses Leu 7 (193).
[11] Gastrointestinal stroma tumors can express S-100 protein (265, 266).
[12] Metastatic melanoma expresses S-100.
[13] Metastatic melanoma expresses HMB45.
[14] Most gastrointestinal stromal tumors and vascular neoplasms (Kaposi's sarcoma) express CD34 (267,269,270).
[15] Vascular tumors (Kaposi's sarcoma) express CD31 (267).
[16] Breast, nonmucinous ovarian cancers, adenocarcinoma of the lung and endometrial cancers are most often CK7 (+) and CK20 (−). Colorectal cancers are CK7 (−) and CK20 (+). Transitional cell carcinoma of the bladder and mucinous ovarian tumors are most often CK7 (+) and CK20 (+) (194).
[17] Primary colorectal cancers have a characteristic diagnostic pattern of villin expression along the apical brush border. Breast cancers, lung adenocarcinoma, renal clear cell cancer, and endometrial cancers show focal villin positivity. Melanomas are negative for villin (195).
[18] Prostate carcinoma.
[19] Rectal carcinoid tumors and prostate cancers are positive for prostatic specific acid phosphatase (220).
[20] Some gastrointestinal stromal tumors express muscle specific actin, as will some metastatic sarcomas (265,266).
CEA, carcinoembryonic antigen.

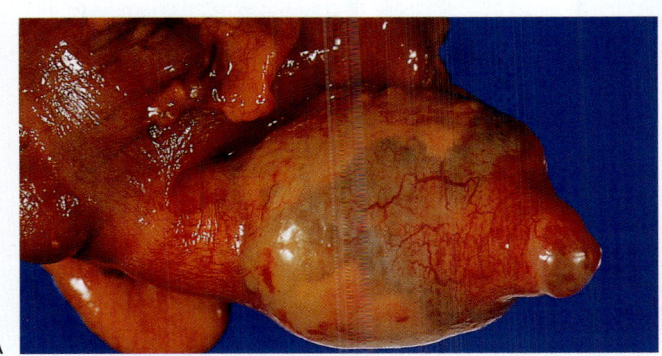
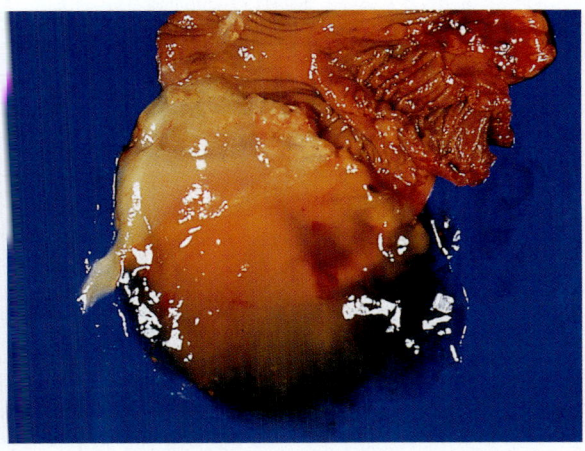

FIG. 38. A: Gross photograph of mucinous cystadenoma of the appendix. The lesion produces a markedly dilated appendix. **B:** Opened lesion showing mucinous contents.

carcinomas, the (AFIP) Armed Forces Institute of Pathology has offered the term *mucinous tumors of undetermined malignant potential* (UMP) for these cases (201). This UMP group reflects the poorly defined criteria for invasion in appendiceal mucinous tumors. The degree of dysplasia is not helpful in differentiating adenomas from adenocarcinomas as both can be extremely well differentiated.

Acellular mucin dissecting through the wall may be seen with adenomas, but it poses problems in excluding malignancy. Acellular mucin in the appendiceal wall with an intact muscularis mucosae and without features of true invasion is diagnosed as an adenoma. The criteria for UMP tumors are well-differentiated mucinous epithelium pushing deeply into underlying tissue without clear-cut invasion, or mucin present in the wall or outside of the appendix in the absence of clear-cut invasion, provided there is also loss of the muscularis mucosae. These UMP lesions behave as low-grade neoplasms and seem to have a better prognosis than adenocarcinoma (201).

Adenocarcinoma

Seventy-five percent of appendiceal adenocarcinomas present with clinical symptoms (appendicitis, mass, carcinomatosis of the abdomen), while 25% are incidental findings (196). Grossly, low-stage lesions (tumor confined to the appendix wall) present as thickening of the appendix, whereas lesions that have spread beyond the wall present as masses, often inflammatory in appearance. The appendix is often buried within the mass, and numerous tissue sections may have to be taken before the appendix itself is identified.

One-quarter of cancers are described as cystadenocarcinoma typically presenting as mucoceles. This type is grossly indistinguishable from a cystadenoma. The most common histology is a fairly well-differentiated mucinous adenocarcinoma. Appendiceal cancers tend to produce dilated mucus-filled structures as they invade through the wall of the appendix; single-cell invasion and desmoplasia may be

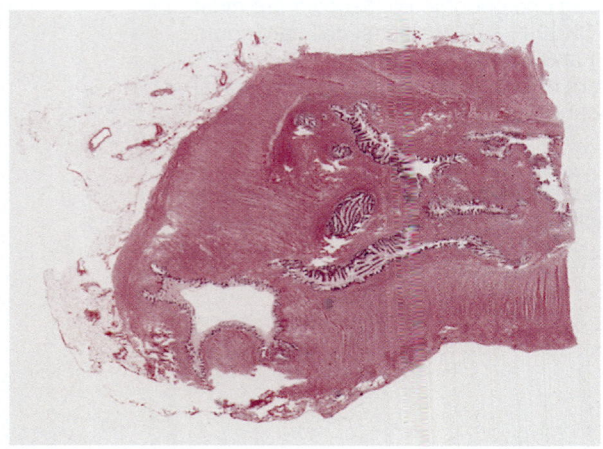
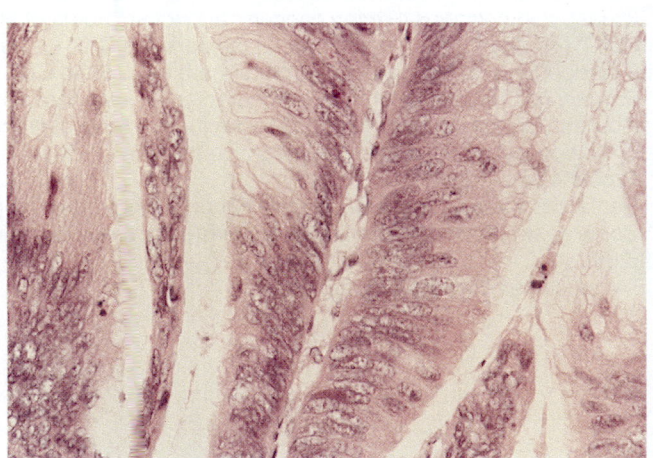

FIG. 39. A: Whole mount view of cystadenoma of the appendix. At this power one can appreciate dissection, rather than invasion of the adenoma through the appendix. This is not invasive cancer. **B:** Higher power showing obvious dysplastic (adenomatous) epithelium.

difficult to identify, so multiple sections of the tumor should be obtained (Fig. 40).

Carcinoid Tumor

This tumor accounts for 85% of all appendiceal neoplasms (196). Most patients with carcinoid tumors are operated on for acute appendicitis. Carcinoids are classically yellow when grossly visible; however, the vast majority are found only incidentally on microscopic examination of the appendix. Microscopically, carcinoids have solid and trabecular growth patterns; transmural spread and invasion of the mesoappendix are frequent.

The frequency of metastasis from carcinoids of the appendix is reported to be between 1.4% and 8.8% (202). The vast majority of biologically malignant cases have metastases present at the time of initial presentation, making a diagnosis of malignancy easy. Only rare cases of metastasis after initial appendectomy have been reported (202). In general, size greater or equal to 2 cm significantly correlates with metastatic potential (202,203). A long-term follow-up study from the Mayo Clinic found no metastases in carcinoid tumors less than 2 cm in size (203). Metastases do occur in carcinoids less than 2 cm but are uncommon (202). In those tumors less than 2 cm with metastases, the presence of invasion of the mesoappendix significantly correlates with metastases. However, in benign nonmetastasizing carcinoids, invasion of the serosal surface or periappendiceal fat is quite common (203). Perineural, vascular, and lymphatic invasion do not correlate with metastatic potential.

Adenocarcinoid (Goblet Cell Carcinoid) Tumor

This distinctive neoplasm of the appendix has acquired a variety of names: adenocarcinoid, goblet-cell carcinoid, crypt-cell carcinoma, and mucous carcinoma (204–206). This tumor, considered to be a variant of carcinoid tumor, has two major histologic subtypes, goblet-cell and tubular. The goblet-cell type is composed mainly of goblet cell or signet ring-like cells arranged in clusters (Fig. 41), with a bland infiltrative pattern like that typical of carcinoid tumor. The individual glands are separated by smooth muscle or stroma. Paneth cells and endocrine cells are readily recognized. Mucin lakes within the wall of the appendix may be present. However, unlike mucinous carcinoma, the glands of adenocarcinoid within mucinous lakes have central lumens, resembling normal crypts, and remain separated from each other, with no solid or cribriform areas. The tubular type consists of small discrete glands or tubules, some with inspissated mucin in the lumen. The cells have pale eosinophilic cytoplasm and round to oval nuclei with small nucleoli. Paneth cells and classic carcinoid are also present.

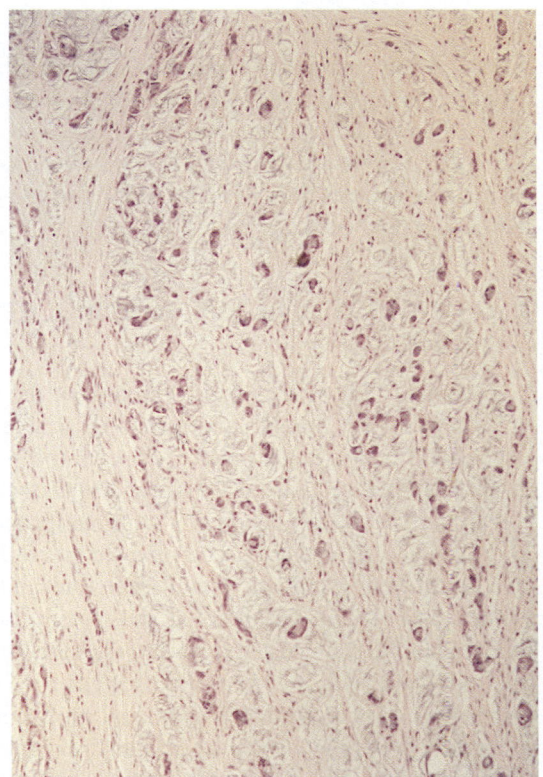 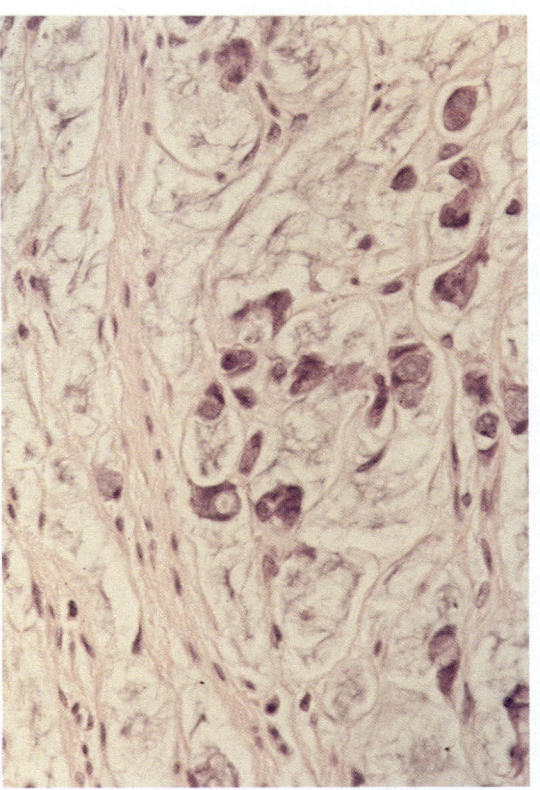

FIG. 40. A: Mucinous adenocarcinoma of the appendix. The photograph shows destructive mucinous tumor in the appendix wall. **B:** Higher power view showing signet ring cells. Compare to adenocarcinoid (Fig. 41). In the cancer, large pools of mucin/cells are infiltrating and destroying the muscularis propria.

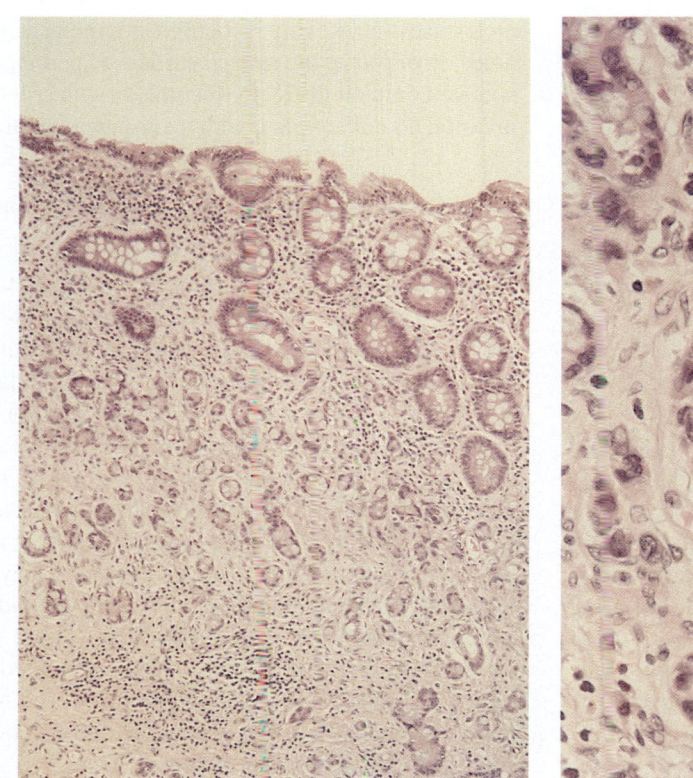 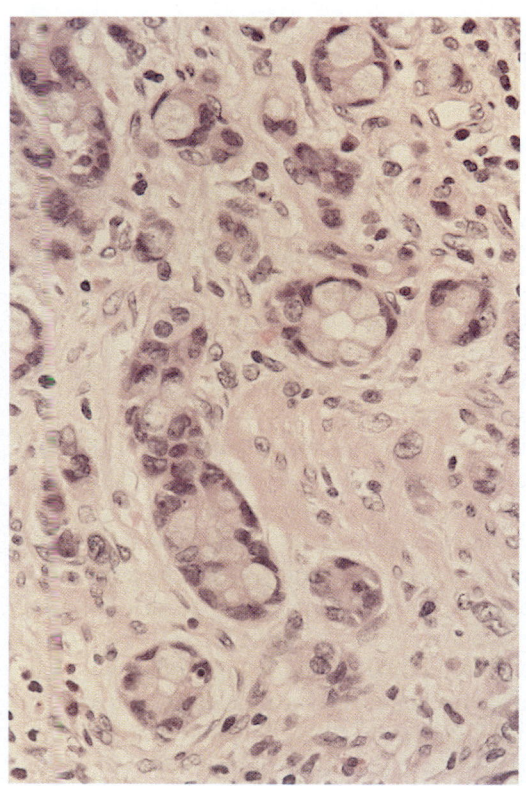

FIG. 41. A: Low-power view of goblet cell carcinoid (adenocarcinoid) of the appendix. At this power one can appreciate the infiltrative pattern of tumor at the base of the crypts, through the muscularis mucosae and in the submucosa. **B:** Higher power view showing bland, benign-appearing glands with prominent goblet cells.

One can occasionally see transitions between the tubular and goblet-cell types. The pure tubular variants do not show any metastatic potential (205).

Mixed Carcinoid-Adenocarcinoma

A third variant, mixed carcinoid-adenocarcinoma, has been described (207). Recognition of this new variant may help to explain and clarify the controversy regarding the biologic behavior of adenocarcinoids. Follow-up of a group of pure goblet-cell carcinoids for a mean of 97 months showed that all patients were free of disease; however, all patients with mixed carcinoid-adenocarcinoma were dead of disease (these data were obtained from reclassification of the original patients in the report of Warkel and colleagues [205,207]).

All cases of mixed carcinoid-adenocarcinoma grossly showed diffuse infiltrating masses, often growing into the cecum. Microscopically, these tumors contain areas typical of goblet-cell carcinoid, but greater than 50% of the growth resembles carcinoma. The carcinomatous component may have any of the following patterns: (a) glands with signet cells and little intervening stroma, (b) linear single file growth, (c) mucinous appearance, (d) glandular formations, and (e) poorly differentiated tumor with signet ring cells. The mitotic rate averaged 10/10 high power fields (HPF) in the study by Burke et al. (207). Importantly, most, if not all, of the mixed carcinoid-adenocarcinomas and those goblet cell carcinoids with malignant behavior show gross evidence of malignant disease (metastases) at the time of surgery (207–209). However, there have been rare documented cases of metastases years after initial appendectomy in cases diagnosed as goblet cell carcinoid (204,210).

CARCINOID TUMORS (NEUROENDOCRINE TUMORS)

Carcinoid tumors are located throughout the entire gastrointestinal tract. Initially thought to be benign, it is now recognized that with the possible exception of appendiceal carcinoids (see section on the appendix, above) all others should be considered neoplasms with malignant potential. Classically, carcinoids have been divided into foregut (stomach, duodenum), midgut (small intestine and proximal colon), and hindgut (distal colon and rectum) types. Some individuals have suggested replacing the term *carcinoid tumor* with *neuroendocrine tumor* to designate the total spectrum from classic carcinoids with slow growth and a good prognosis to poorly differentiated highly malignant tumors.

The classic carcinoid tumor is composed of uniform round or polygonal cells having monotonous, round, centrally located nuclei with finely stippled chromatin and small nucleoli, infrequent mitoses, and no necrosis. The tumor may show a variety of patterns, such as solid, trabecular or ribbon-like, and acinar (Figs. 42 and 43). Along the histologic spectrum of these neuroendocrine tumors, one can occasionally see cases with malignant histology showing marked cellular pleomorphism, large irregular hyperchromatic nuclei, prominent nucleoli, tumor necrosis, and mitoses. These latter lesions are often reminiscent of what has been called atypical carcinoids of the lung and are uniformly fatal. Variants such as combined adenoma-carcinoid tumor or adenocarcinoma-carcinoid tumor have been reported (211–213).

The vast majority of intestinal carcinoid tumors arise in the small intestine; the remainder develop in the rectum, and, uncommonly, in the colon. The frequency of small intestinal tumors increases as one moves distally, with 40% located within 2 feet of the ileocecal valve. In the small intestine 35% of patients have multicentric (two or more) tumors (214).

Duodenal Carcinoid

Carcinoids of the duodenum are the least frequent of small intestinal carcinoids. Two-thirds of duodenal carcinoids express gastrin and one-third of these are associated with the Zollinger-Ellison syndrome; the latter tumors are almost always metastatic. They may also be associated with the MEN-1 syndrome (215,216). Somatostatin-producing tumors make up 15% to 20% of duodenal carcinoids. They are almost exclusively in the region of the ampulla of Vater and are usually malignant. These tumors are often associated with von Recklinhausen's disease. Histologically, they characteristically have glandular structures and psammoma bodies. While producing somatostatin immunohistochemically, they rarely produce the somatostatin syndrome of diabetes mellitus, cholelithiasis, and diarrhea.

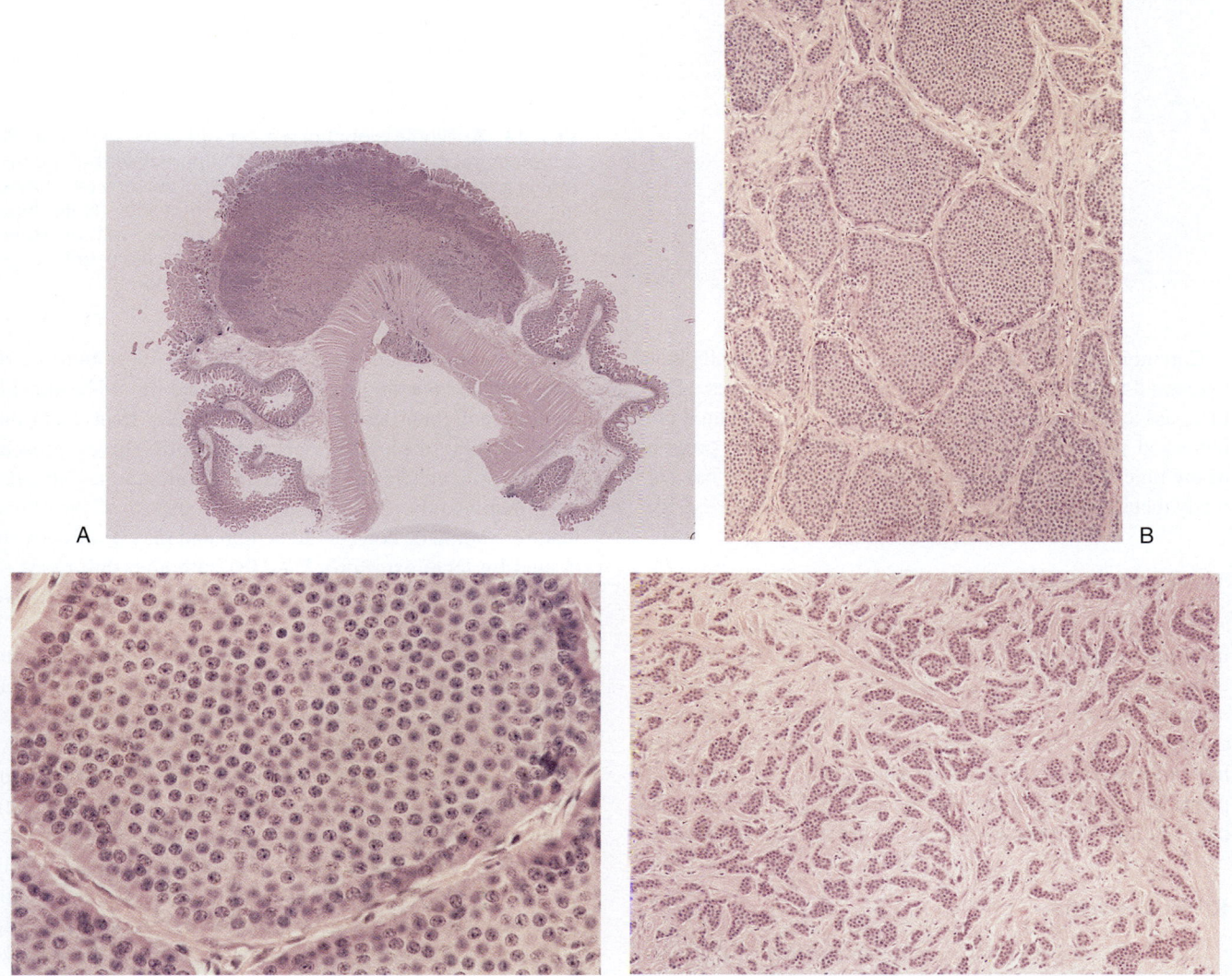

FIG. 42. A: Whole mount view of small intestinal carcinoid tumor. There is no neoplastic change of the surface epithelium The tumor involves the submucosa extensively, with focal transmural involvement. **B:** Tumor grows in a solid pattern. **C:** Higher power view of **B** showing round regular nuclei and faint indistinct cell borders. Note the uniformity from one cell to the next. **D:** Another area of tumor shows an infiltrative pattern.

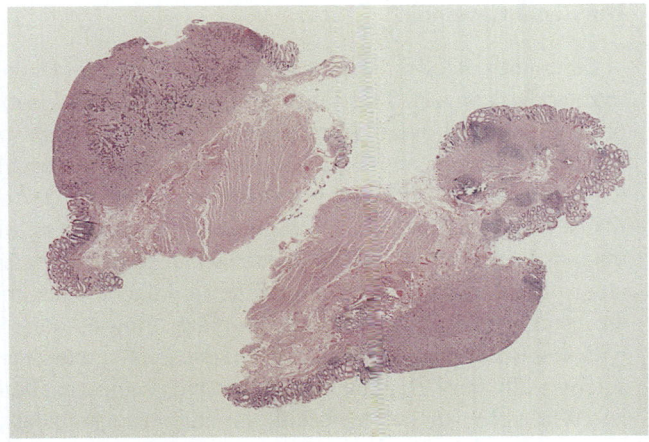
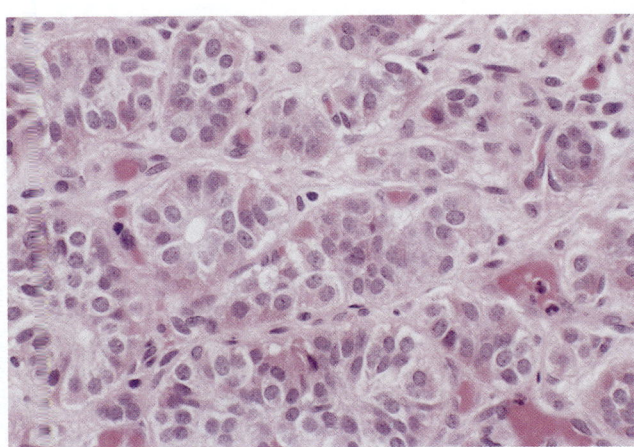
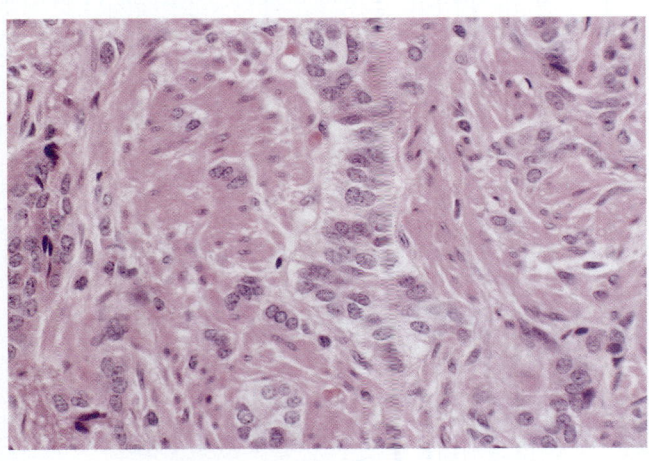

FIG. 43. A: Whole mount of a carcinoid of the rectum from a transmural local excision. One can appreciate that the tumor is limited to the submucosa. **B:** High-power view showing tight small glands with bland uniform nuclei. (Note: In a male patient this could very well be confused with prostate cancer. See text for differentiation of carcinoid from prostatic carcinoma.) **C:** Ribbon pattern of tumor.

Carcinoids that behave in a malignant fashion usually have expressed such behavior at the time of initial surgery. Features associated with malignancy are size greater than 2 cm, increased mitoses, and invasion of the muscularis propria. Many functioning tumors less than 1 cm in diameter have already metastasized at the time of first presentation (215,216).

Small Intestinal Carcinoids

In surgical series that encompass the symptomatic cases, most tumors are larger than 1 cm; those larger than 2 cm are almost always malignant, presenting with regional lymph node metastases. Up to 40% are multiple and 20% are associated with the carcinoid syndrome (215). These tumors often have widespread intraabdominal disease with relatively small primary tumors. Although having metastatic disease, these patients may experience survivals of greater than 10 years.

Rectal Carcinoids

The pathologist plays a very important role in the management of the patient with a rectal carcinoid. Whereas small intestinal and colonic carcinoids are usually received as resection specimens, rectal carcinoids are often received in the laboratory as biopsy specimens (Fig. 43). Most investigators report that rectal carcinoids >2 cm in size and/or with invasion of the muscularis propria and/or 2 or more mitoses/10 HPF have the potential to metastasize and should be considered as malignant lesions. Tumors smaller than 2 cm but with invasion of blood vessels, lymphatics, nerves, muscularis propria, anaplasia, and increased mitoses may also behave malignantly (217). Lesions without any of the above features should be considered benign and may be effectively treated by local excision (217,218), although rare cases of metastases of lesions with apparently benign features have been reported (219).

In biopsy material of rectal carcinoids, one often sees tumor cells limited to the submucosa; in the male, these carcinoids can histologically mimic prostate cancer. Immunohistochemical staining with prostatic-specific antigen (PSA) and prostatic-specific acid phosphatase (PSAP) may be helpful; however, 80% of rectal carcinoids express PSAP (220). The pathologist should be cognizant of this fact and not misdiagnose a carcinoid tumor as prostate cancer based solely on positive staining for PSAP. Addition of PSA to the immunohistochemical profile along with classic carcinoid markers should clarify any diagnostic problems. The markers most commonly used are neuron-specific enolase, chromogranin, synaptophysin, and Leu-7. By electron microscopy, intracytoplasmic dense-core granules are noted. Saving preoperative sera for future analysis in those patients with functional tumors is suggested.

LYMPHOMA

Small Intestine and Large Intestine

Primary malignant lymphomas of the intestinal tract account for approximately 17% of primary small-intestinal malignancies and <5% of colorectal malignancies. Two major classifications of GI lymphoma (Isaacson and Kiel) (221–223) are listed in Tables 10 and 11. The major categories are discussed below and summarized in Table 12.

Small intestinal lymphomas account for 20% to 40% of primary gut lymphomas in Western populations and are among the most common malignant tumors of the small intestine. Tumors occur more commonly in males and peak in the seventh decade. Presenting features are abdominal pain, weight loss, small intestinal obstruction, and acute abdomen. Two-thirds are B cell and one-third are T cell lesions. Primary colorectal lymphomas are uncommon (224), accounting for 0.2% of large intestinal malignancies and 10% to 15% of primary gut lymphomas. The clinical presenting features are no different from those of primary colorectal cancer. Associated conditions are ulcerative colitis (224) and AIDS (225). Colorectal lymphomas (exclusive of multiple lymphomatous polyposis) are diffuse and polymorphic in appearance, showing mixed populations of centrocyte-like, plasmacytoid, centroblast-like, and immunoblast-like cells; they are difficult to categorize using standard classifications (224).

Lymphoma of Mucosa-Associated Lymphoid Tissue (MALT) (Western Type)

Most intestinal B cell lymphomas are of the MALT type (221,223,226) and of these the vast majority are of the Western type (227). High-grade neoplasms of this type account for 40% to 60% of all intestinal lymphomas (228). They are often advanced at presentation and have an aggressive clinical course. A high percentage of these high-grade lymphomas show evidence of transformation from low-grade MALT lymphomas (221,224,226).

The high-grade lymphomas have sheets of noncleaved cells with round vesicular nuclei and nucleoli. Immunoblasts are present. These lymphomas may also be polymorphic, with large bizarre atypical lymphocytes (Reed Sternberg–like) and admixed mature lymphocytes, plasma cells, histiocytes, and eosinophils. In low-grade MALT lymphomas, the histology shows an infiltrate of centrocyte-like cells that often show plasma cell differentiation. Lymphoepithelial lesions are noted, but are less common than in the stomach. Follicular colonization is present and can cause confusion with follicular lymphoma. These MALT lymphomas are CD20+, CD10-, CD5-, CD23-, and bcl-1 (-).

MALT Immunoproliferative Small-Intestinal Disease (Mediterranean Type)

This variant, which has been classified as immunoproliferative small-intestinal disease (IPSID) (Table 12), is a disorder commonly manifested by diarrhea, malabsorption, weight loss, abdominal pain, and clubbing of the digits (229). These manifestations, which typically become manifest in the second and third decades of life, are attributed to a diffuse plasma-cell infiltrate of the mucosa (227,230–232). This entity is restricted mainly to Third World countries, where low socioeconomic status and poor hygiene lead to a high incidence of gastrointestinal infection. However, in endemic areas the incidence of IPSID-related lymphoma is now decreasing, probably due to better hygiene. In more recent publications from Middle Eastern areas, gut lymphomas are more closely following the distribution seen in Western

TABLE 10. *Primary gastrointestinal non-Hodgkin's lymphoma (Isaacson) (221)*

B cell
  I. MALT type
    a. Low grade
    b. High grade with or without low-grade component
    c. Immunoproliferative small intestinal disease
      1. Low grade
      2. High grade with or without low-grade component
  II. Mantle cell (lymphomatous polyposis)
  III. Burkitt's and Burkitt's-like
  IV. Other—nodal equivalent
T cell
  I. Enteropathy associated
  II. Other types unassociated with enteropathy
  III. Rare types

MALT, mucosa-associated lymphoid tissue.

TABLE 11. *Classification of gut lymphomas, updated—Kiel (modified from the European Association for Hematopathology) (222,223)*

B cell	T cell
Low grade	Low grade
Low-grade lymphoma of MALT	Pleomorphic small cell
Immunocytoma	
Alpha-chain disease	
Centroblastic/centrocytic	
Centrocytic with MLP	
Plasmacytic	
High grade[a]	High grade[b]
Centroblastic	Pleomorphic medium and large cell
Classical	immunoblastic
Polymorphic	Large cell anaplastic
Centrocytoid	(Ki − 1 positive)
Multilobated	Unclassifiable
Burkitt's lymphoma	
Lymphoblastic	
Immunoblastic	
Large cell anaplastic	
(Ki − 1 positive)	
Unclassifiable	

MALT, mucosa-associated lymphoid tissue, MLP, malignant lymphomatous polyposis.
[a] With or without a low-grade component.
[b] Any of which can be with enteropathy or eosinophilia

TABLE 12. Intestinal lymphomas

Feature	MALT (Western type)	MALT (IPSID)	EATCL	MLP	Burkitt's
M:F (ratio)	1.5–2.0	1:1	1:1	9:1	1:1
Age (decades)	5th and 6th	2nd and 3rd	5th and 6th	5th	1st and 2nd
Associated conditions	None	Developing countries	Celiac disease	None	Africa, Middle East
Site	Ileum, (most common) colon (less common)	Jejunum and duodenum	Jejunum and duodenum	Multiple stomach Small intestine, colon polyps— ileal mass	Ileocecal
Gross appearance	Nodular, polypoid	Diffuse bowel wall thickening, later tumor	Ulcers	Polyps—multiple ileal mass	Mass
Mucosal histology	Normal	Plasma cell infiltrate	Villous atrophy, ulcers	Tumor cells in deep mucosa	Normal
Histology of tumor	Low grade: centrocyte-like cells with plasma cells and lympho-epithelial lesions; follicular colonization High grade: centroblastic (classical, polymorphic, multilobated); can occasionally see low-grade background	Immunoblastic Polymorphous Small cleaved, plasmacytoid Reed-Sternberg–like, lympho-epithelial lesions; follicular colonization	Polymorphic Immunoblast and Reed-Sternberg–like cells Occasionally eosinophils	Centrocyte Mantle cell	Small Noncleaved
Markers	$CD20^+$ $CD10^-$ $CD5^-$ bcl-1^- $CD23^-$	$CD20^+$ $CD10^-$ $CD5^-$ bcl-1^- $CD23^-$	$CD30^+$ $CD3^+$ $CD7^+$ $CD8^-$ $CD4^-$ HML-1^+	$CD20^+$ $CD5^+$ $CD10^-$ bcl-1^+ $CD23^-$ $CD43^+$	$CD20^+$ $CD10^+$ $CD5^-$ $CD23^-$

EATCL, enteropathy T-cell lymphoma; IPSID, immunoproliferative small-intestinal disease.

societies (233,234). In 20% to 90% of cases, the serum contains an abnormal immunoglobulin A (IgA) molecule devoid of light chains (229), a condition that is often called alpha chain disease.

The disease process is usually limited to the jejunum and duodenum; however, the colon rarely may also be involved. Grossly, the early lesion consists of a diffuse thickening of the small-intestinal wall; only when frank lymphoma develops does any gross tumor mass occur. The early pathology is a diffuse plasma cell infiltrate of the mucosa without areas of intervening normal mucosa. As the disease progresses, the plasma cell infiltrate may invade the bowel wall proper and may involve the regional lymph nodes (Fig. 44). Lympho-epithelial lesions and colonization of follicles by centrocyte-like cells may also be seen (221). Lymphoma may also develop, which has been variously described as immunoblastic, mixed non-Hodgkin's, lymphoplasmacytic, and nodular lymphocytic lymphoma. Immunohistochemical studies show that the plasma cells and lymphoma express cytoplasmic and surface alpha chain (IgA heavy chain) (231) (Fig. 45). Variants with monoclonal and polyclonal light chains have also been described. Staging systems have been devised for IPSID (230,235).

Enteropathy-Associated T cell Lymphoma (EATCL)

For many years, it was noted that some patients with malabsorption would develop small-intestinal lymphoma. Long-term follow-up studies of patients with celiac disease report a 14% incidence of small-intestinal lymphoma. Also included in this group are patients with malabsorption unresponsive to gluten withdrawal and associated with multiple intestinal ulcers (ulcerative jejunitis) (236,237). These two entities may be considered together, since their clinical picture and lymphoma pathology are identical. The clinical manifestations may be malabsorption for years and then the development of lymphoma; or patients may present with abdominal pain, at which time multiple small-bowel ulcers and/or lymphoma may be found. The prognosis is very poor.

By routine light microscopy, one sees a flat sprue-like mucosa with areas of malignant histiocytic-like cells (medium to large blast-like cells with ample cytoplasm, vesicular nuclei with enlarged nucleoli) involving the bowel wall and lymph nodes. Most often the tumor cells are at the base of ulcers and may be quite focal (Fig. 46). The tumor cells are often obscured by benign inflammatory cells, especially eosinophils. It is not uncommon for these lesions to be passed over as nonspecific ulcers, thereby missing the diagnosis of lymphoma (236,238,239). In some cases, the lymphoma is so focal as to require 10 to 20 tissue sections to make a diagnosis of malignancy.

Besides finding pleomorphic malignant histiocytic-like cells, one may also see a gradation to mature-appearing histiocytes or macrophages, often with erythrophagocytosis. It was this finding, along with tumor cells expressing intracytoplasmic alpha$_1$-antitrypsin, that led investigators to ini-

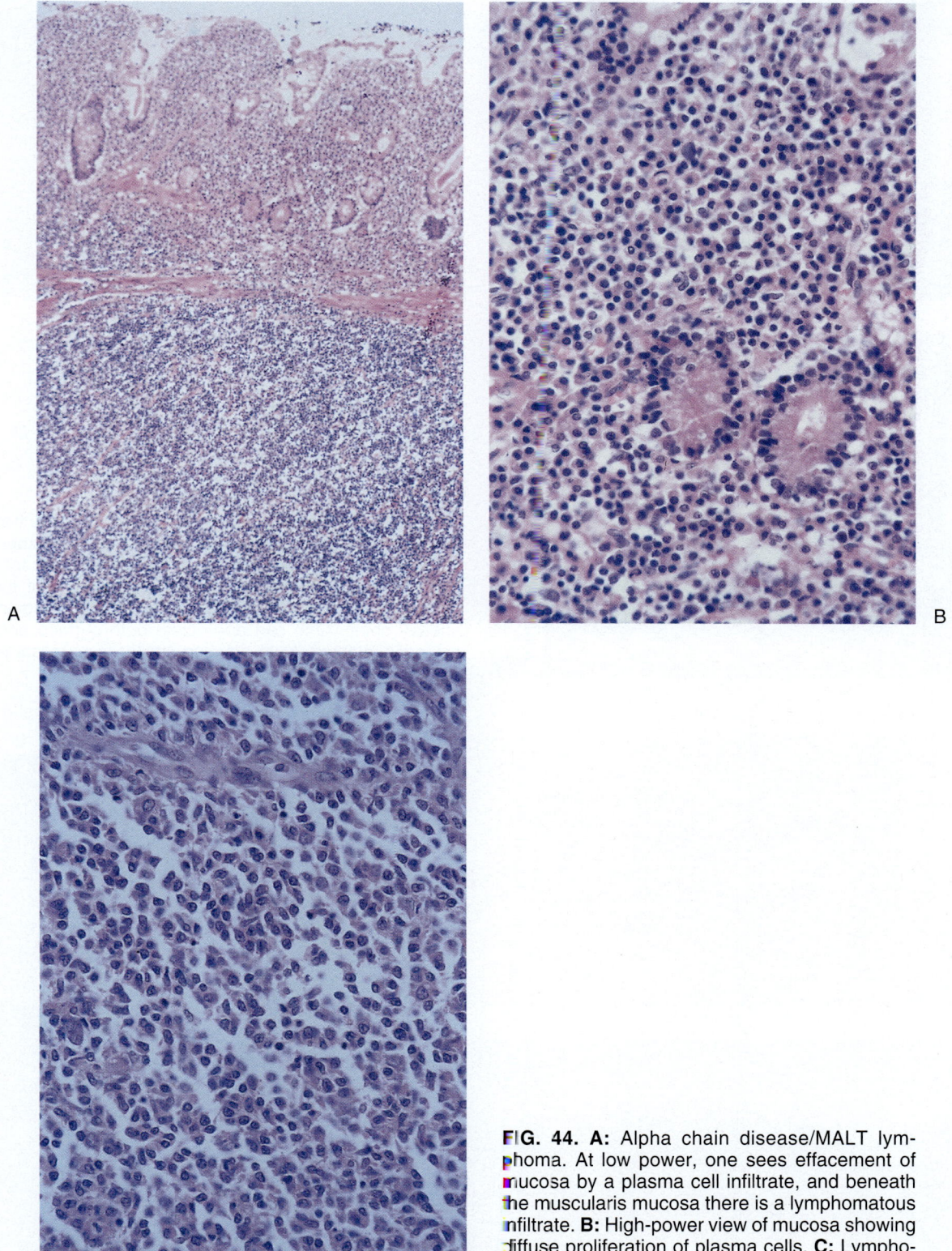

FIG. 44. A: Alpha chain disease/MALT lymphoma. At low power, one sees effacement of mucosa by a plasma cell infiltrate, and beneath the muscularis mucosa there is a lymphomatous infiltrate. **B:** High-power view of mucosa showing diffuse proliferation of plasma cells. **C:** Lymphoplasmacytoid lymphoma.

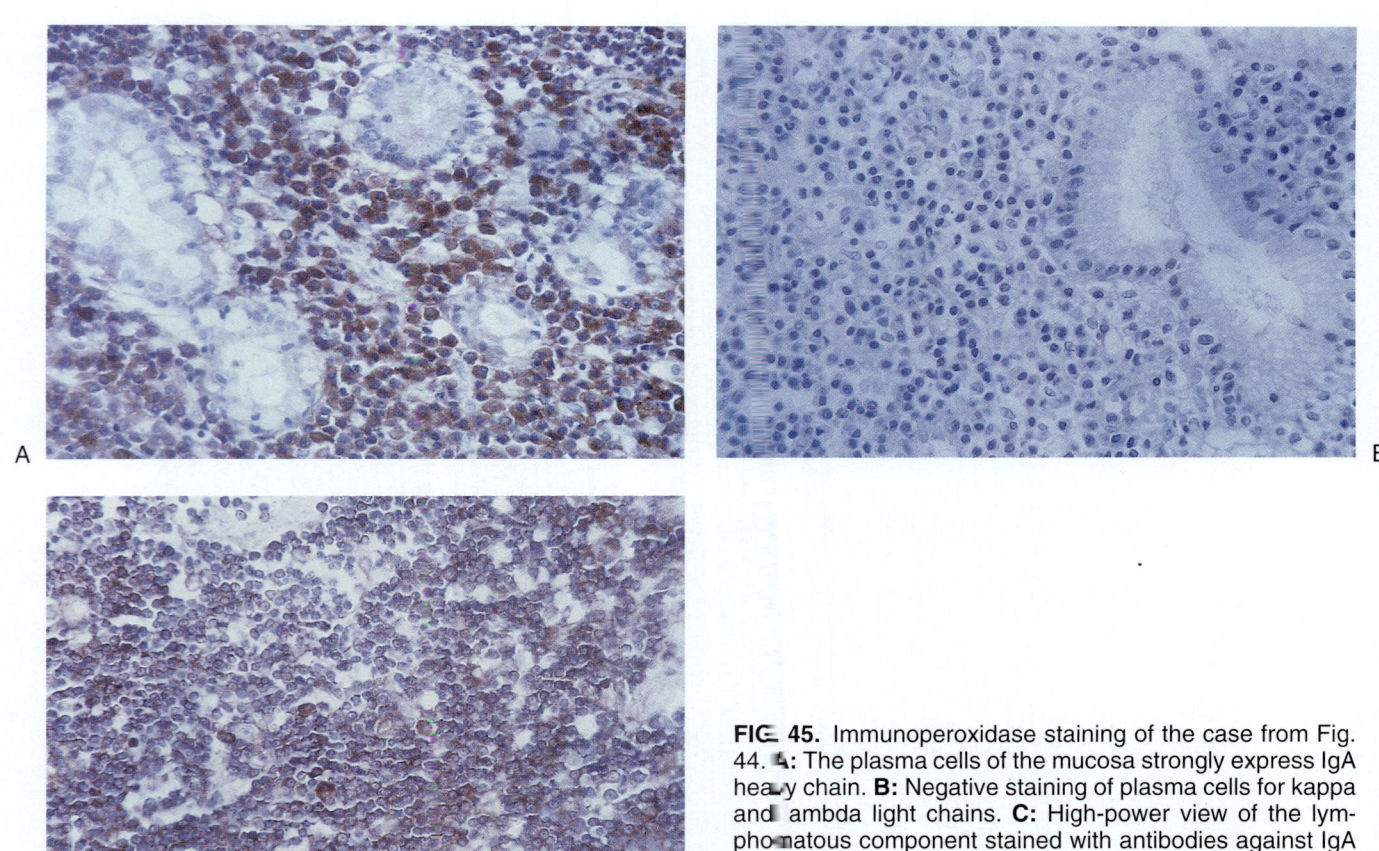

FIG. 45. Immunoperoxidase staining of the case from Fig. 44. **A:** The plasma cells of the mucosa strongly express IgA heavy chain. **B:** Negative staining of plasma cells for kappa and lambda light chains. **C:** High-power view of the lymphomatous component stained with antibodies against IgA heavy chain. One can appreciate both surface and cytoplasmic staining. Note staining similar to mucosal plasma cells.

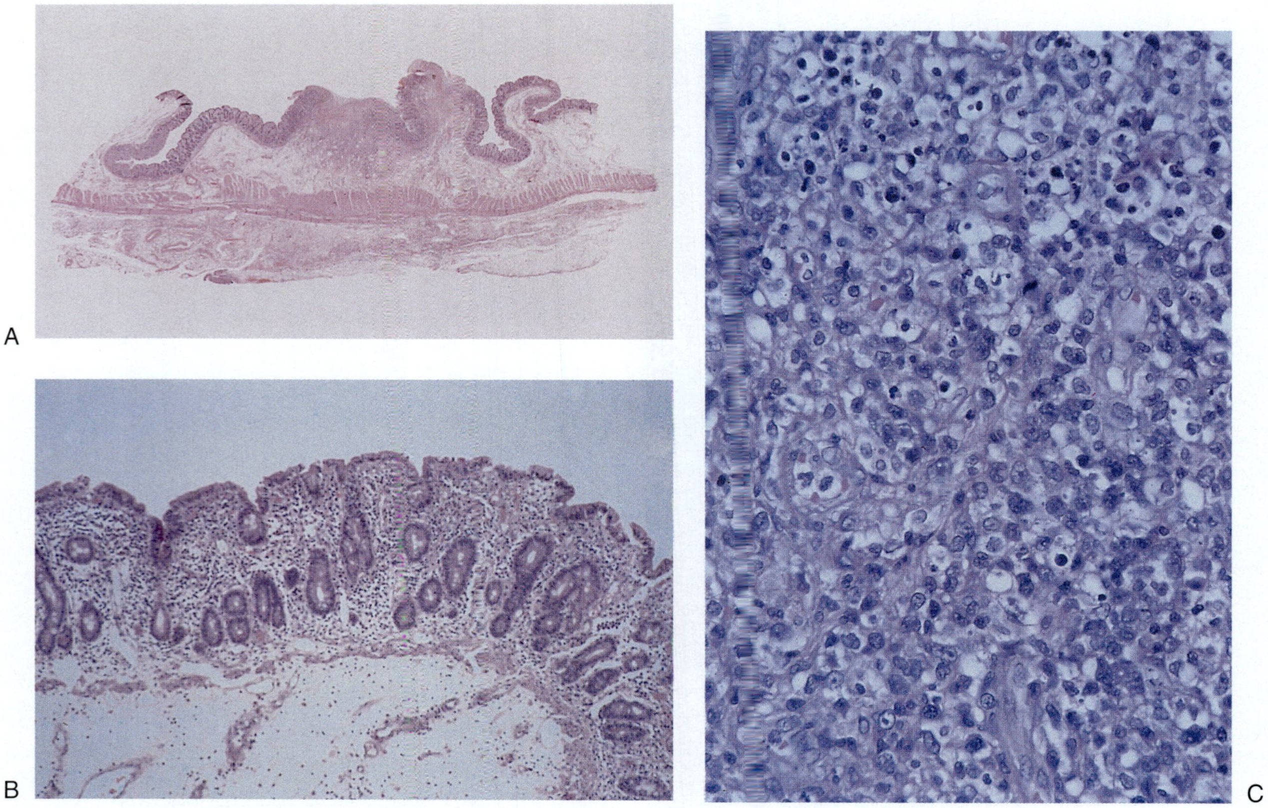

FIG. 46. A: Whole mount of enteropathy-associated T-cell lymphoma. At this power one can appreciate focal ulceration. Also, the nonulcerated mucosa is flattened. **B:** Low power of nonulcerated mucosa. The mucosa is flat like that in celiac disease. **C:** High-power view of the ulcer showing malignant cells admixed with inflammatory cells.

tially classify these tumors as malignant histiocytosis (238). However, more sophisticated marker studies indicate that these lymphomas are of T-cell origin (240); the malignant cells react with the monoclonal antibody HML-1 and have an immunophenotype of CD3+, CD7+, CD30+, CD4-, CD8-, and CD22- (241). Since the malignant lesions may be quite focal, a very careful and extensive search for malignant lymphoma should be undertaken whenever a segment of small intestine with multiple ulcers is received for evaluation.

Multiple Lymphomatous Polyposis

Multiple lymphomatous polyposis of the gastrointestinal tract is a distinct clinicopathologic entity (242–245) (Table 12). This disorder is quite uncommon; its prevalence in large series of gastrointestinal lymphomas is 3% to 9% (228,242,244). It affects primarily males (88% of reported cases), with a mean age of 61 years. The lymphomatous process can involve the stomach, small intestine, and large intestine. The mean survival is usually less than 3 years.

Grossly, the mucosal neoplastic lesions may be nodular, sessile, or polypoid. When enumerating these polyps, terms such as *myriad*, *multiple*, or *innumerable* have been used. The polyps may produce a confluent studded or cobblestone-like appearance, or they may be widely spaced, with intervening normal mucosa. The polyps range in size from 2 to 3 mm to several centimeters (Fig. 47). In about 50% of cases, there is also a dominant tumor mass that is most often ileocecal in location. Histologically, one sees a nodular or diffuse proliferation of small lymphocytes that produces the polyps. Cytologically, these cells have small cleaved nuclei and pale cytoplasm; they represent what has been called intermediate lymphocytic lymphoma or mantle zone lymphoma. These cells are of the centrocytic type in the Kiel classification. The early tumor nodules tend to straddle the muscularis mucosae, involving the deep mucosa and submucosa with sparing of the superficial mucosa. There is no epithelial invasion by tumor cells in early lesions. As lesions progress, focal epithelial invasion and ulceration may develop. Also noted is a pattern of proliferation of neoplastic cells around germinal centers, as has been described in mantle zone lymphoma. Immunohistochemical studies have shown that these lesions are B cell lymphomas that are CD5+, CD10-, CD23-, and bcl-1+; most are mantle zone lymphomas. A rare case of primary T cell

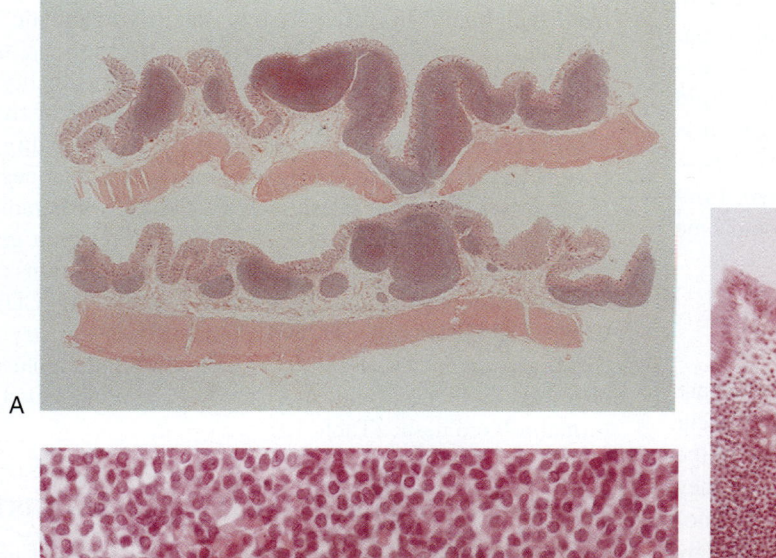
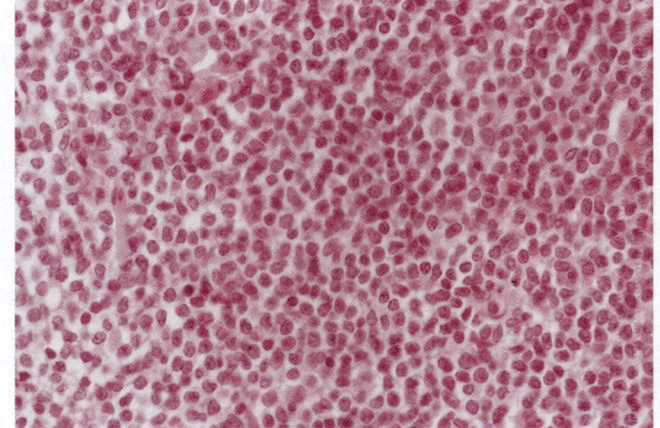
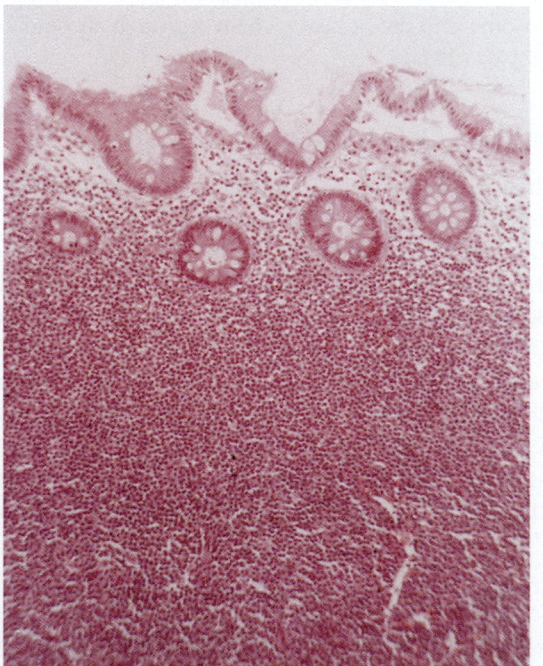

FIG. 47. A: Whole mount view of malignant lymphomatous polyposis. Note numerous tumor nodules that form polyps. **B:** Low-power photomicrograph showing tumor nodules straddling the muscularis mucosae and involving deep mucosa and upper submucosa. No lymphoepithelial lesions are present. **C:** High-power view of lymphoma showing small lymphocytes with cleaved irregular nuclei.

lymphoma resembling multiple lymphomatous polyposis has been reported (246).

Multiple lymphomatous polyposis must be differentiated from other lymphoid lesions with multifocal gastrointestinal involvement, namely, nodular lymphoid hyperplasia and lymphoid polyposis. In nodular lymphoid hyperplasia, one sees benign lymphoid nodules of the small intestine, usually in patients with the common variable immunodeficiency syndrome. Multiple lymphoid polyps are benign lesions with well-formed germinal centers, usually seen in children and also in patients with Gardner's syndrome. The clinical picture and histopathologic findings of these two disorders should easily enable the pathologist to differentiate them from multiple lymphomatous polyposis. Marker studies are helpful in differentiating multiple lymphomatous polyposis from other small cell lymphomas (Table 12).

Burkitt's Lymphoma

Endemic Burkitt's lymphoma rarely presents with gastrointestinal disease; however, in contrast, sporadic Burkitt's lymphoma in the Western world and the Middle East often presents with abdominal pain and obstructive features caused by ileocecal involvement (221). The tumor cells are small, noncleaved, monomorphic medium-sized cells with round nuclei, multiple (2–5) nucleoli, and abundant basophilic cytoplasm that may give the cells a cohesive appearance. On touch imprints or smears cytoplasmic lipid vacuoles are often noted. A classic "starry-sky" pattern is present (247). The tumor cells are CD 20+, CD 10+, CD5-, and CD23-. Most cases have translocation of C-*myc* from chromosome 8 to the Ig heavy chain region in chromosome 14 [t (8;14)] (247).

Other Primary B Cell Lymphomas

Follicular (centrocytic/centroblastic) lymphomas are rarely seen in the gastrointestinal tract (221,248). They occur most frequently in the small intestine (55%), mainly in the terminal ileum, and in the colon (22%). In the colon they have been reported as mucosal polyps; however, the diagnosis of follicular lymphoma was based on light microscopy only and not on molecular markers or CD analysis (244,248). AIDS-associated lymphomas occur frequently in the GI tract. They occur in the stomach, colon, and ileum in decreasing order of frequency. Most are B cell lymphomas of the large cell immunoblastic or Burkitt-like type (249).

Other Primary T-Cell Lymphomas

Angiocentric T-cell lymphoma of the intestine is an uncommon disorder. The lesions present as ulcerated or transmurally necrotic small and/or large intestine masses. The tumor cells are large and pleomorphic, permeate the bowel wall, and invade blood vessels in an angiocentric, angiodestructive pattern. These tumors are highly aggressive and fatal. The T cells also express Epstein-Barr virus transcripts (250). Many of these lesions may be natural killer cell phenotype with or without azure granules (seen on Wright's stained imprints). Other natural killer–like T-cell lymphomas of the small intestine with immunoblastic and centrocyte-like morphology have been reported (251,252).

Peripheral T-cell lymphomas unassociated with enteropathy may involve the intestines. Most commonly they involve the small intestine, but colonic disease can also be seen. These lesions tend to be ulcerated; the vast majority are histologically high grade. According to the Kiel classification, they are pleomorphic medium and large cell, pleomorphic small cell, immunoblastic, and large cell anaplastic lymphomas. The small cell lesions may show lymphoepithelial lesions. These lymphomas are highly aggressive with high mortality (223,253).

Immunohistochemical and Molecular Techniques in Lymphoid Lesions

The diagnosis of lymphoma of the intestines can usually be made on routine H&E-stained sections. However, small biopsies of small-lymphocytic lesions can present diagnostic difficulty in differentiating reactive from neoplastic lesions, and small biopsies of highly anaplastic lymphomas may present difficulties in differentiating carcinoma and sarcoma from lymphoma. In differentiating small-lymphocytic lesions into reactive or neoplastic processes, fresh tissue may be helpful. This tissue can be used for detecting clonality of B cells by flow cytometry (kappa and/or lambda light chain restriction) or by immunohistochemistry. Monoclonality of B cells can also be detected by the molecular techniques of Ig gene rearrangement (fresh or fixed tissue), while monoclonality of T cells can be detected by T-cell receptor gene rearrangement (fresh or fixed tissue). Anaplastic lesions can be diagnosed as lymphoma by reactivity with CD45, CD30, CD20, CD45RO, and CD3 by immunohistochemistry on fixed tissue. For classifying the lymphomas, immunohistochemistry is helpful, with most markers being detected in formalin-fixed tissue (Table 12).

GASTROINTESTINAL STROMAL TUMORS (GIST)

Gastrointestinal stromal tumors are mesenchymal neoplasms of the gastrointestinal tract that formerly were often designated "smooth muscle tumors." Two-thirds of GIST arise from the stomach and 25% from the small intestine, of which one-third arise in the duodenum. Colorectal lesions account for approximately 10% of gastrointestinal stromal tumors. These tumors present clinically with pain, obstruction, and bleeding or as a mass (254,255).

Pathology

Grossly, GISTs usually produce a mass that may involve all layers of the gut, grow extramurally, and extend intraluminally to cause mucosal ulceration. Most benign and malignant GISTs are circumscribed, solitary, rounded or ovoid masses. On cross section, GISTs are not whorled or bulging;

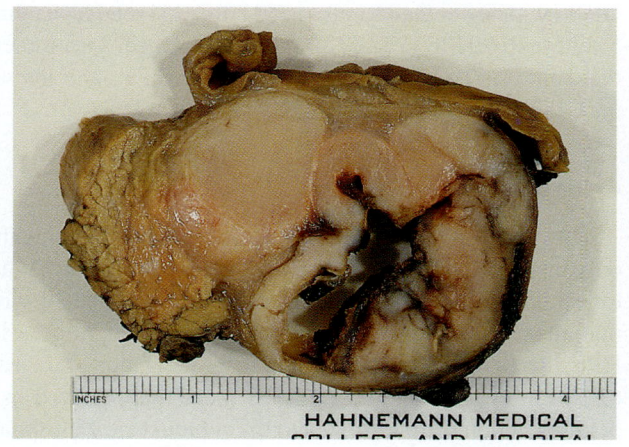 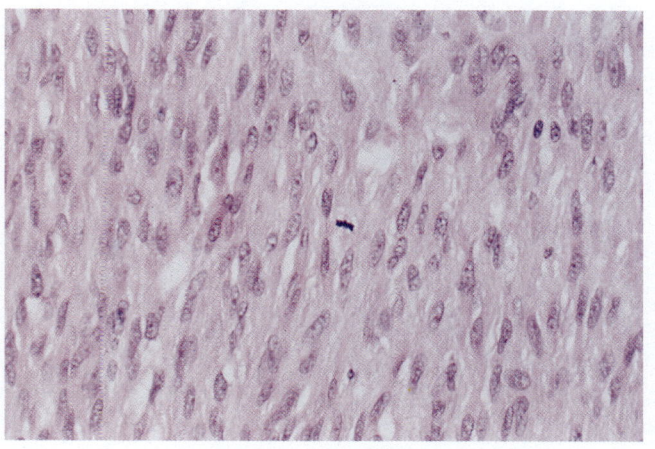

FIG. 48. A: Gross photograph of malignant gastrointestinal stromal tumor (GIST) of the small intestine. It has a fish-flesh appearance and central degeneration. **B:** High-power photomicrograph showing spindle cells with atypical nuclei. A mitotic figure can be appreciated.

rather, they have a relatively nondescript pinkish-white appearance, often with areas of hemorrhage, necrosis, myxoid change, or cavitary degeneration. Both benign and malignant GISTs have similar macroscopic appearances, thus preventing categorization as to biologic behavior based on gross configuration (Fig. 48).

Microscopically, the majority of GISTs of the small and large intestine are composed of spindle cells forming fascicles. The spindle cells may vary in size, mitotic rate, and density; these features may have biologic predictive value (Fig. 49) (see below). Fibrovascular septa may be present that at times impart an organoid pattern (Fig. 49). Epithelioid patterns are less common, but in the duodenum may signal aggressive behavior (Fig. 50) (256). In addition, some tumors have eosinophilic PAS-positive extracellular deposits called skenoid fibers (257). Occasionally, these tumors have a prominent myxoid stromal background (258) and, rarely, signet cell ring features due to accumulation of glycogen rather than mucin (259). Some colorectal tumors have the appearance of classic esophageal leiomyomas or gastric cellular leiomyomas (254,260–262). Rectal lesions can also present as small polyps originating from the muscularis mucosae (254–262).

Immunohistochemistry

There have been a multitude of articles regarding the cell of origin of GISTs or its cell of differentiation using immunohistochemical techniques. These studies have shown conflicting results for expression of some markers such as S-100 and desmin, but more consistent results for expression of vimentin, muscle-specific actin, and CD34 (263–270). A recently published study has shown that the majority of GIST originate from gastrointestinal pacemaker cells (interstitial cells of Cajal) which can be detected immunohistochemically with antibodies C-kit (CD117) (270a). The vast

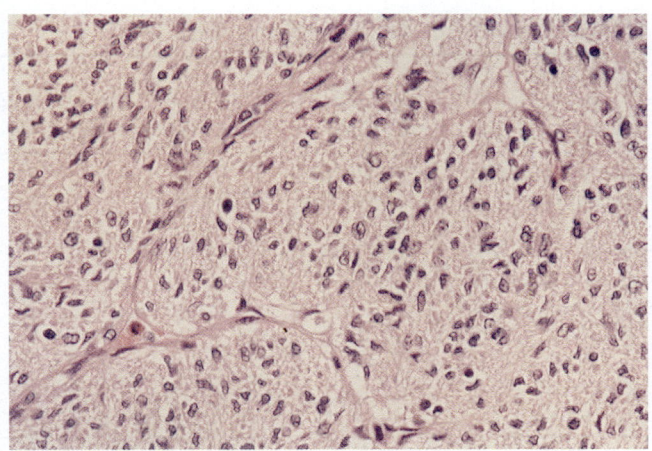 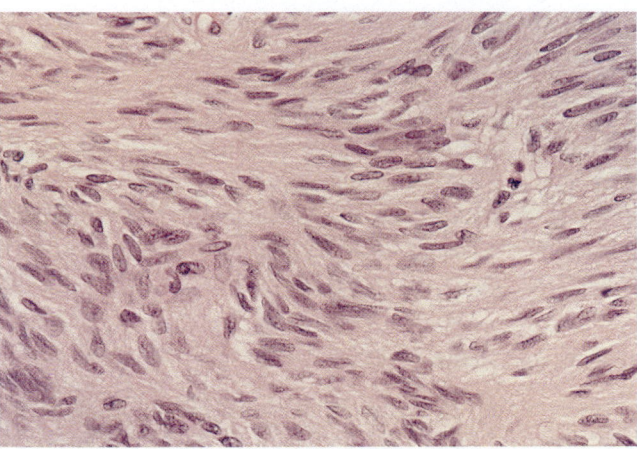

FIG. 49. A: Benign GIST showing an organoid pattern. Capillaries separate the tumor cells into groups. **B:** Another view, showing spindle cells with bland nuclei. This lesion does not show increased cellularity. No mitotic figures were noted. These features are associated with benign GIST.

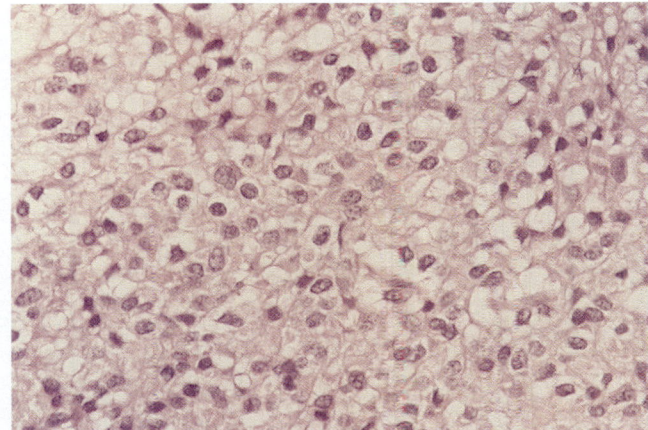

FIG. 50. Epithelioid malignant GIST. The tumor cells have centrally placed nuclei and rounded distinct cell membranes.

majority of GISTs can be diagnosed with routine H&E-stained slides. Immunohistochemistry plays no role in the everyday diagnosis of GISTs; however, it can be helpful in differentiating a GIST from an epithelial neoplasm or other spindle cell neoplasms (e.g., metastatic melanoma).

Biologic Behavior

The pathologist is asked to determined whether a GIST is benign or malignant and to grade the malignant GIST. The criteria for determining benign versus malignant are site-specific throughout the GI tract (i.e., the criteria for the stomach are different from those for the small intestine or the colon/rectum). One helpful major criterion is clinical presentation. Asymptomatic incidentally discovered GISTs almost always behave in a benign fashion (254,268).

Duodenal GIST

The only article specifically addressing duodenal GIST is that of Goldblum and Appleman (256). They found that benign GISTs had uniform spindle cells, low cellularity, an organoid growth pattern, skenoid fibers, were 4.5 cm or smaller in size, and had 2 or fewer mitoses/50 HPF. Malignant tumors were highly cellular, had 2 or more mitoses/50 HPF, and were 4.5 cm or larger in size. GISTs with a predominant epithelioid pattern behaved in a malignant fashion. In benign cases, the spindle cells were bland with abundant pink cytoplasm and low cellularity. Fibrovascular septa conferred an organoid pattern. The malignant tumors had smaller spindle cells with less cytoplasm, and little or no organoid pattern.

Jejunum and Ileum GIST

Criteria for differentiating benign versus malignant GISTs are presented in Table 13. However, it should be emphasized that while mitotic activity of 5 or greater mitoses/50 HPF statistically could separate out benign from malignant tumors in some series (268–271), other authors have reported malignant GISTs with fewer than 5 mitoses/50 HPF (254) and fewer than 5 mitoses/10 HPF (272,273). Akwari et al. (272) comment that 1 mitosis/10 HPF if found consistently in a small intestinal GIST is evidence of potentially malignant behavior.

Colon and Rectum

Moyana et al. (261) report that a size of >5 cm was the only important parameter for diagnosing malignancy. A mitotic rate of 5 or greater mitoses/10 HPF correlated with malignancy, but some tumors with 2 or fewer mitoses/10 HPF also behaved in a malignant fashion. Haque and Dean (262) reported on anorectal GIST; those that behaved in a benign fashion were localized to the submucosa, were small (mean size: 2.1 cm), sparsely cellular, and had no more than 1 mitosis/50 HPF. Malignant tumors were larger (mean 4.5 cm), involved the muscularis propria, had necrosis, and exhibited 5 to 58 mitoses/50 HPF. Morgan et al. (254) noted that benign colorectal GISTs were all <2 cm and had rare mitoses (1/50 HPF).

Grading GIST

Malignant GISTs can be separated into high and low-grade lesions based solely on mitotic rate. Evans (260) noted that low-grade malignant GISTs (1–5 mitoses/10 HPF) had a median survival of 98 months, while high-grade tumors (>10 mitoses/10 HPF) had a median survival of 25 months. Dougherty et al. (255) reported an 80% disease free survival for low-grade malignant tumors (<10 mitoses/50 HPF) at 8 years, whereas high-grade tumors (>10 mitoses/50 HPF) had an approximately 10% disease-free survival at 8 years.

Frozen Sections

What is the role of frozen section in GIST? The pathologist need only diagnose a lesion as a GIST (versus carcinoma, lymphoma, etc.) since most small intestinal and colonic lesions are resected with adequate margins. The pathologist

TABLE 13. *Jejunal and ileal GIST*

Features associated with malignancy	Brainard* (257)	Tworek* (254)	Multivariate analysis
High cellularity	+	+	+
High mitotic count	>5/50 HPF	5/50 HPF	+
Size	>5 cm	≥ 7 cm	
Epithelioid cells	+	+	
Mucosal invasion	+	+	
Ischemic necrosis	+	−	
Pleomorphic histology	+	−	

HPF, high-power filed.
*Univariate analysis.
Modified from Appleman HA—Presentation at Fall 1997 ASCP meeting, Philadelphia, PA

making a diagnosis of GIST should tell the surgeon if margins are grossly free, as it has been shown that there is no survival benefit for radical extended resection versus lesser resections encompassing the entire lesion (255).

Proliferation Markers and DNA Ploidy

Numerous studies have attempted to determine if proliferation markers or DNA ploidy can be used to predict the biologic behavior of GISTs. Some studies have evaluated GISTs by site, whereas others have combined all sites. Some studies using PCNA have reported that the proliferation index can act as an independent prognostic indicator in multivariate analysis (274,275), while others have claimed that PCNA is not an independent prognosticator in multivariate analysis (256,271,276). Similar findings have been reported for Ki 67 (MIB-1) (256,277). These proliferation markers cannot separate benign from malignant GISTs because, although there are often significant differences in mean values, there is great overlap in range of values between benign and malignant groups. Some authors have found them useful in the borderline GIST lesions. Franquemont et al. (274), using a system consisting of size, mitoses, and PCNA proliferative index, were able to develop an algorithm that significantly correlated with clinical behavior and showed 95% sensitivity, 75% specificity, 83% positive predictive value, and 92% negative predictive value (Table 14). Regarding DNA ploidy analysis, some studies have shown its independent prognostic value in multivariate analysis (278,279), but others failed to verify these findings (277). At present, more studies, refinement and uniformity of techniques, and longer follow-up are needed before proliferation markers and DNA ploidy can be considered part of the routine workup of GIST.

NEUROGENIC TUMORS

Gastrointestinal Autonomic Nerve Tumor (GANT)

Gastrointestinal autonomic nerve tumors are a type of GIST in which the tumor shows ultrastructural differentiation toward myenteric plexus elements. They can only be diagnosed by ultrastructural analysis as their light microscopic and immunohistochemical features are nondiagnostic (280–283). GANTs are more commonly seen in males than

TABLE 14. *Risk of aggressive behavior in GIST (259,260)*

High risk
  a. Size ≥5 cm *and* mitotic rate ≥2/10 HPF
  b. Size ≥5 cm *or* mitotic rate ≥ 2/10 HPF, PCNA index > 10%
Low risk
  a. Size <5 cm *and* mitotic rate <2/10 HPF
  b. Size ≥5 cm *or* mitotic rate ≥2/10 HPF, PCNA index ≤10%

18/21 (86%) High risk showed aggressive behavior.
1/12 (8%) Low risk showed aggressive behavior.
GIST, gastrointestinal stromal tumor; PCNA, proliferating cell nuclear antigen.

females, with a mean age of 55 years. Abdominal pain or a mass is the characteristic clinical presentation.

These tumors occur in the stomach, small intestine, mesentery, and retroperitoneum. The vast majority are large (>10 cm). Grossly, they tend to be well-circumscribed masses; when involving the bowel wall they often show extramural extension. On cut surface, they are lobulated and tan to light pink. Areas of hemorrhage, necrosis, and cystic degeneration are common. Fresh tumors have been described as soft, and their softness and color have been likened to that of brain tissue.

By light microscopy, GANTs are predominantly spindle cell tumors with little pleomorphism. The cells form storiform, palisading, or whorled patterns or grow as diffuse cellular sheets. Lobulation and compartmentalization are often appreciated. Skenoid fibers and myxoid changes are common. Some tumors have an epithelioid appearance, with cells having eosinophilic cytoplasm or cytoplasmic clear vacuoles reminiscent of leiomyoblastoma. Fifty percent of tumors have >5 mitoses/10 HPF.

By electron microscopy, the tumors contain neuron-like cells with large thick or thin axonic cytoplasmic processes joined by scattered rudimentary cell junctions. All cases show bulbous synapse-like structures that are joined to adjacent cells by rudimentary cell junctions. Most GANTs fail to express muscle-specific actin or desmin, but do show variable immunohistochemical expression of neuron-specific enolase, synaptophysin, chromogranin, and S-100 protein. All GANTs express vimentin (280–283).

The vast majority of GANTs behave in a malignant fashion. However, Lauwers et al. (280) noted that 85% of GANTs that recurred or metastasized were >10 cm in size and had >5 mitoses/10 HPF.

Schwannomas

Neurogenic tumors (schwannomas) have been reported with a frequency of 11% of all GISTs (284). Most schwannomas occur in the stomach (267,284,285). Twenty-five percent of people with von Recklinghausen's disease have gastrointestinal involvement. Grossly, schwannomas present as ovoid tumor nodules that may occasionally cause mucosal ulceration. Microscopically, they consist of woven nests or bundles of spindle cells in a myxoid matrix with vague palisading and compact bundles. Occasionally the cells exhibit perivascular swirling or have a whorl-like neuroid arrangement reminiscent of nerve bundles or tactoid corpuscles. Nuclei are bland with rare to absent mitoses. A peripheral cuff of lymphoid aggregates formed around the tumor tissue produces an impressive and unique pathognomonic feature of these lesions. However, they differ from conventional soft tissue schwannomas in that they have regular whorls or storiform pattern and lack distinct palisading; also, the prominent lymphoid cuffing is rare in soft tissue schwannomas. Most gastrointestinal mesenchymal tumors that microscopically have prominent nuclear palisading are not schwannomas but rather are GISTs. Schwannomas express S-100 protein, leu7

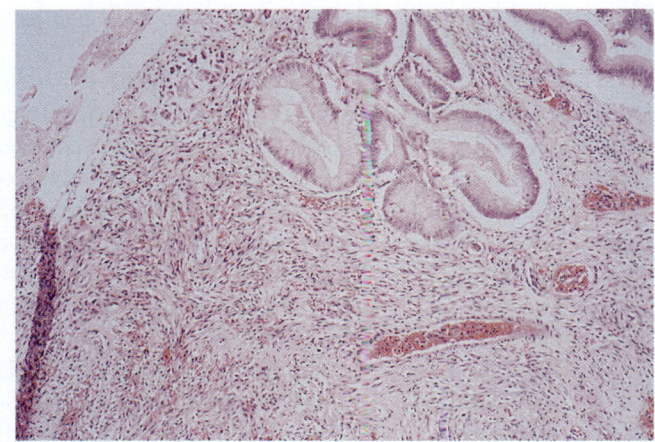 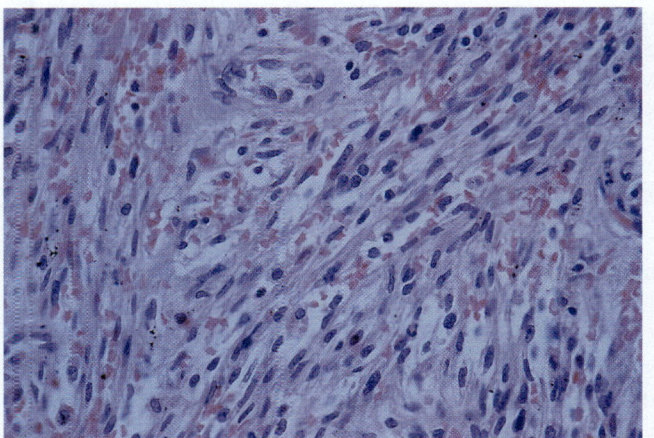

FIG. 51. A: Low-power view showing Kaposi's sarcoma infiltrating the mucosa. The tumor cells infiltrate between as well as replace the epithelium. **B:** High-power view showing malignant spindle cells with extravasated red blood cells.

(HNK-1), and glial fibrillary acidic protein (GFAP). They are negative for CD34, desmin, and muscle-specific actin.

VASCULAR TUMORS

Kaposi's Sarcoma

Prior to the AIDS epidemic, Kaposi's sarcoma of the gastrointestinal tract was a disorder rarely seen in the United States. However, in endemic areas of Africa, gastrointestinal involvement by Kaposi's sarcoma has been noted in approximately 80% of patients with visceral disease (286). In the AIDS population, the incidence of gastrointestinal involvement is 50% (287). Gastrointestinal involvement may either precede, be synchronous with, or develop without the appearance of skin lesions. Symptoms referable to the gastrointestinal tract are rare, being noted in only 10% of AIDS cases (287). When symptoms do occur, they include diarrhea, protein-losing enteropathy, and abdominal pain; these symptoms clinically mimic colitis (288–291).

Grossly, one sees multiple reddish-brown to purple nodules or a single tumor mass involving any level of the gastrointestinal tract. Histologically, these tumors are identical to the classic vascular spindle pattern seen in cutaneous Kaposi's sarcoma (Fig. 51). Other spindle cell neoplasms (e.g., melanoma, GIST, etc.) may be considered in the differential diagnosis; however, electron microscopy and immunohistochemistry (Kaposi's sarcoma expresses CD34 and CD31, and is negative for S-100 protein, desmin, and muscle-specific actin) are helpful in arriving at the correct diagnosis.

Angiomas

Angiomas of the gastrointestinal tract occur, but they are rare. They may cause obstruction or intussusception or, more commonly, melena and anemia. These angiomas may present as diffuse infiltrating lesions, circumscribed tumors, or polypoid growths. The histology is usually that of either cavernous or capillary hemangioma.

Gangliocytic Paraganglioma

Gangliocytic paragangliomas are uncommon lesions of the gastrointestinal tract that are found almost exclusively in

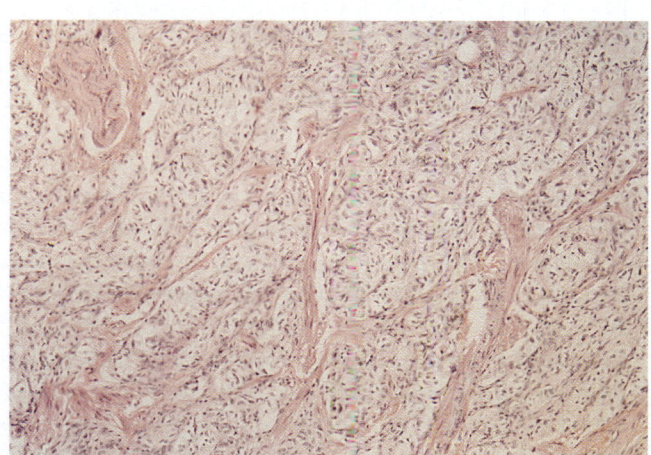 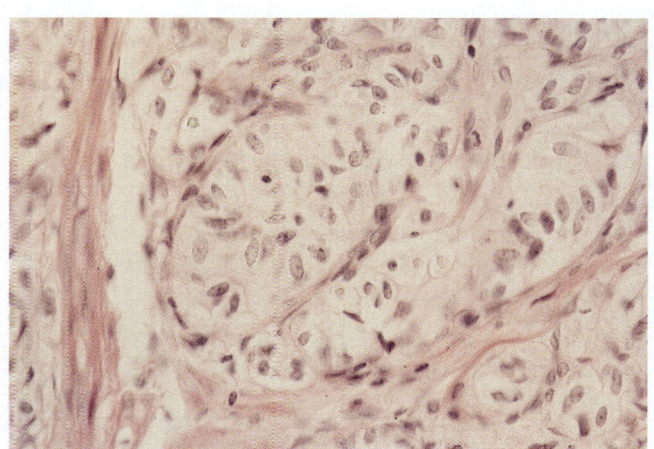

FIG. 52. A: Gangliocytic paraganglioma at medium power. The tumor cells are separated into nests. **B:** High-power view showing characteristic cells in nests.

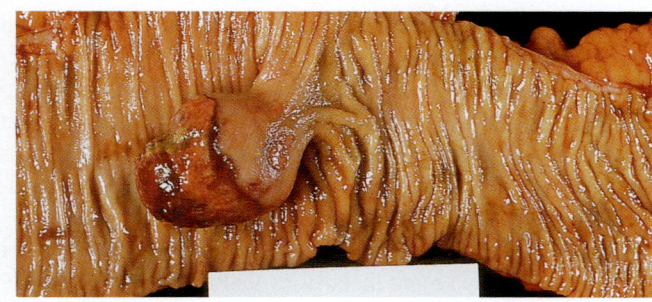 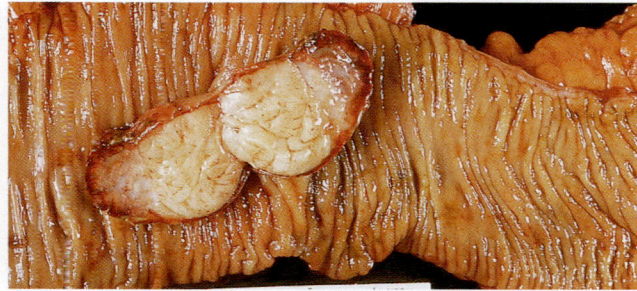

FIG. 53. A: Gross view of polypoid colonic lipoma. **B:** Gross view after dissection. The characteristic fatty nature of the lesion is apparent.

the second part of the duodenum (292–294). Although gangliocytic paragangliomas are typically benign, rare cases with documented metastases have been reported (295,296). They are either sessile or polypoid, and may present as gastrointestinal hemorrhage secondary to mucosal erosion. Histologically, these lesions are typically submucosal and are very characteristic, with a pattern of paraganglioma, ganglioneuroma, and/or carcinoid tumor in various mixtures (Fig. 52). Stromal amyloid has also been reported. These lesions express S-100 protein (sustentacular cells and Schwann cells), neuron-specific enolase (ganglia and paraganglioma cells), somatostatin, serotonin, and human pancreatic polypeptide (ganglion cells and neuroendocrine cells) (293,294).

Lipoma

Lipomas are rare, but well-recognized, tumors of the small and large intestine. They are more commonly seen in the large intestine than the small intestine, and are more common in the right than in the left colon. Lipomas usually arise from the submucosa and may occasionally protrude into the lumen, thus causing symptoms (Fig. 53). Ulceration of the mucosa with secondary hemorrhage may also be noted. By light microscopy, these lesions consist of mature adipose tissue mixed with various amounts of fibrous tissue. Larger lesions may also show areas of necrosis and hemorrhage. The vast majority of cases are diagnosed only after resection; however, occasionally the diagnosis can be made from a deep biopsy

Lipohyperplasia of the ileocecal valve is a fairly common entity usually found in operative specimens removed for other conditions. It consists of an excess of adipose tissue in the submucosa of the ileocecal valve. The ileocecal valve is thickened and protrudes into the lumen. The lesion rarely causes symptoms but may, on occasion, be confused clinically with an adenoma or carcinoma at radiologic or endoscopic examination.

BENIGN CONDITIONS MIMICKING NEOPLASMS

Endometriosis

Involvement of the colon and rectum by endometriosis is quite common (15–20% of cases of endometriosis), but the small intestine is less frequently involved (297). Most cases are noted as incidental findings in specimens removed for other surgical indications. Symptoms are rare; however, when they occur, they may mimic those of cancer. Most endometriomas are ill-defined tumors, rarely larger than 5.0 cm in size. These lesions tend to involve the subserosa and muscle coats but may project into the lumen. The overlying mu-

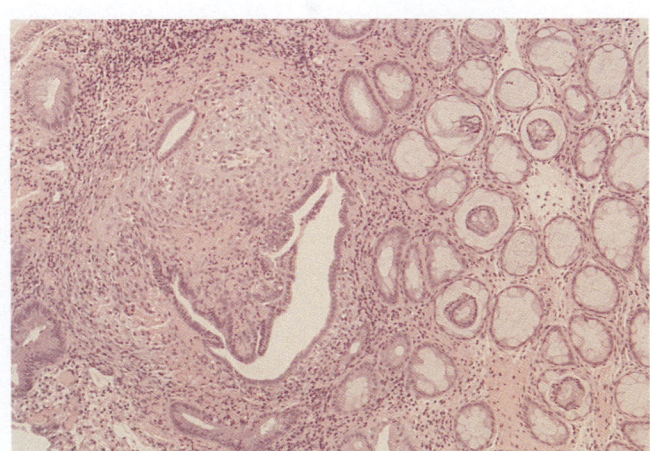 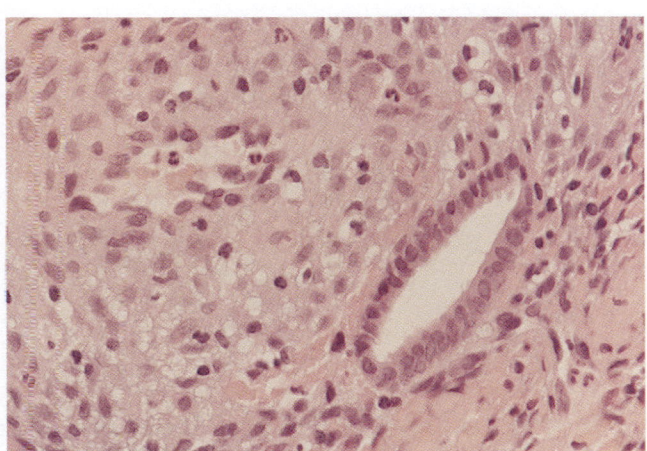

FIG. 54. A: Endometriosis of the rectum detected on mucosal biopsy—low-power view: rectal mucosa *(right)*, endometrial glands and stroma *(left)*. **B:** Higher power view showing inactive endometrial gland with decidualized stroma.

cosa is usually intact unless repeated biopsies have damaged this layer. On cut surface, endometriomas are often gray with tiny areas of hemorrhage within the substance of the tumor. Histologically, they consist of endometrial glands and stroma, often accompanied by fibrosis in the adjacent bowel wall. Mucosal biopsy material will show normal mucosa until a time when endometrial tissue has extended through a defect in the mucosa. When this situation occurs, biopsies can be mistaken for adenocarcinoma, because the endometrial tubules tend to become separated from their stroma secondary to trauma from the biopsy procedure (Fig. 54).

Malakoplakia

This disorder, which is most likely secondary to a defective inflammatory reaction to bacteria, may occur in the large intestine as a tumor or polypoid lesion (298). It often occurs as a pericolonic mass, with a fistula between the bowel lumen and the serosal mass. This lesion may present diagnostic problems on frozen sections, because the calculospherule-bearing histiocytes characteristic of malakoplakia may mimic signet cell adenocarcinoma. A helpful hint in arriving at the correct diagnosis is to lower the microscope condenser, which makes the calculospherules (Michaelis-Gutmann bodies) appear refractile, thus differentiating them from mucin vacuoles.

TUMORS METASTATIC TO THE INTESTINES

Tumors metastatic to the intestines may present as intestinal primaries. By careful gross and histologic examination, the pathologist should arrive at the correct diagnosis. However, obtaining a complete clinical history is imperative.

Prostate Cancer

Not infrequently, evaluation of a biopsy specimen labeled as rectal tumor reveals cancer metastatic from a primary in the prostate. Grossly, these tumors rarely are polypoid but are usually infiltrative into the submucosa. One key in making the correct diagnosis is the lack of *in situ* or intramucosal cancer. Prostate cancers have a characteristic histology that is usually different from routine rectal adenocarcinoma. As mentioned above, prostatic cancer may mimic rectal carcinoid tumor (see section on carcinoid tumors, above).

Occasionally in male patients, resections for rectal cancer will reveal lymph node metastases that are morphologically different from the rectal primary. In our laboratory, we see approximately one such case per year, in which regional lymph nodes reveal metastatic prostate cancer. The pathologist should be cognizant of this phenomenon in order to perform proper staging and to inform the clinician that the patient also has a prostate cancer. In some instances these prostate cancers are occult (unknown to the clinician) and are detected for the first time in the rectal resection. Routine light microscopy is usually sufficient to make the correct diagnosis; however, adjunctive immunohistochemistry (PSAP, PSA, and Leu-7) is confirmatory.

Melanoma

The propensity of melanomas to metastasize to the intestines is a treacherous feature, since the time interval between primary melanoma and metastasis may be years (299). Characteristically, the metastases are multiple and submucosal, with normal overlying mucosa (Fig. 55). These findings are helpful in reaching the correct diagnosis. However, the metastases may be solitary and, like a primary tumor, may involve the mucosa. By routine light microscopy, the pathologist is initially struck by the fact that the tumor is unusual for an intestinal primary (Fig. 55). The presence of an undifferentiated epithelial neoplasm with nesting of discohesive cells with pink cytoplasm, nuclei with large nucleoli, spindle cells, or a mixture of spindle and epithelial cells are features characteristic of melanoma. Electron microscopy

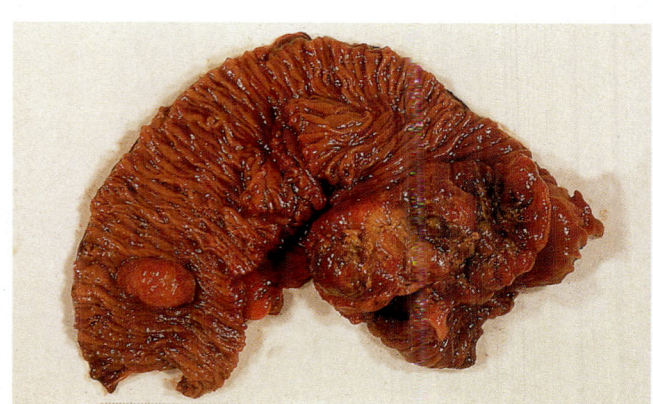
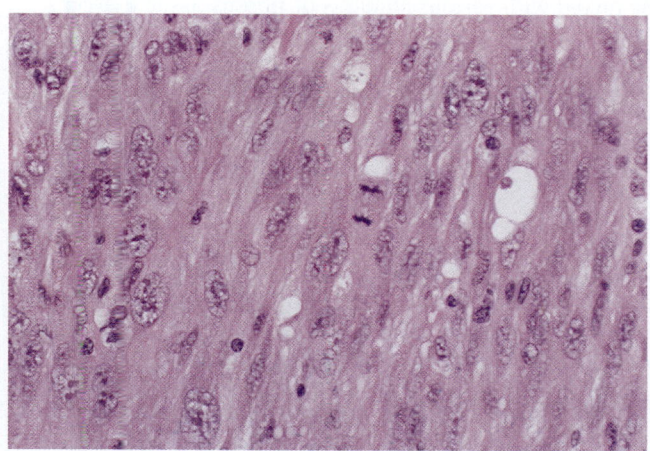

FIG. 55. A: Gross photograph of melanoma metastatic to the small intestine. There are two large polypoid tumor nodules. **B:** High-power photomicrograph of the lesion, showing spindle cells with a mitotic figure. Histologically, this tumor could be confused with a GIST (see Fig. 48B). Immunohistochemistry (S-100+, HMB 45+, CD34-, and HHF 35-) helps diagnose this lesion as a melanoma.

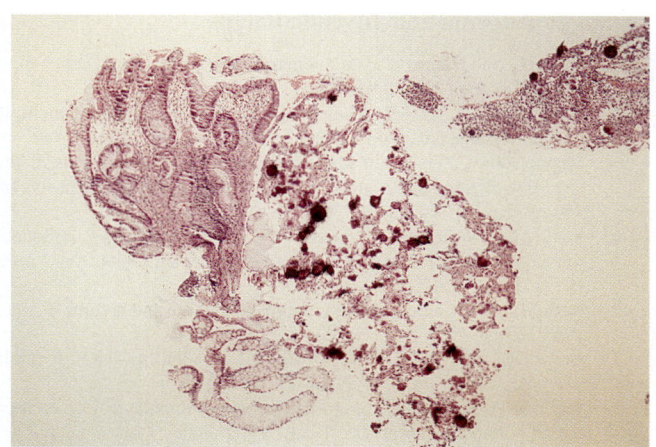 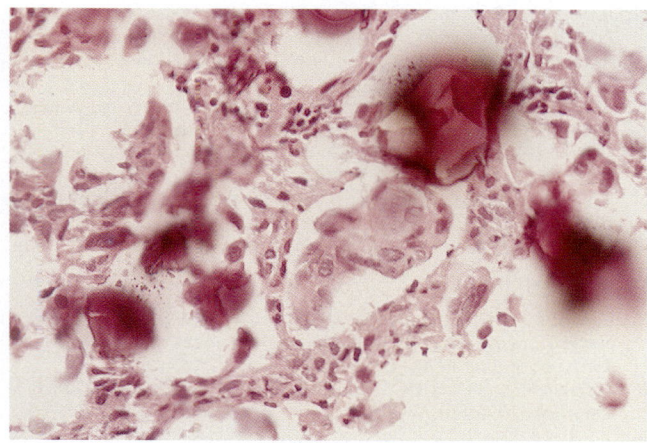

FIG. 56. A: Biopsy specimen from the sigmoid colon. Low-power view of ovarian papillary serous tumor of low malignant potential metastatic to the sigmoid colon. At this power one can see the colonic mucosa *(left)* and juxtaposed papillary serous tumor *(right)*. Psammoma bodies are obvious at this magnification. **B:** High-power view showing characteristic papillary serous tumor of low malignant potential with psammoma bodies.

and immunohistochemistry (S-100 protein, HMB-45, and vimentin) are also helpful.

Leukemia

The lesions caused by leukemia can be single or multiple and most commonly involve the right colon and terminal ileum (300,301). They may present as polyps or may diffusely involve the bowel wall. Histologically, the infiltrate is characteristic for a hematopoietic malignancy. Clinical history is helpful in arriving at the correct diagnosis.

Carcinoma

Carcinomas of other primary sites may metastasize to the intestines, the most common being breast, stomach, and ovary (Fig. 56). These lesions are usually multiple and extend from the serosal surface inward. The lack of *in situ* or mucosal cancer, combined with the characteristic gross and histologic picture, should be diagnostic. Occasionally, one may encounter a linitis plastica type of cancer involving the intestines that grossly and histologically may mimic a primary poorly differentiated intestinal cancer. However, in most instances the lesion represents metastasis from a gastric primary site.

REFERENCES

Hyperplastic Polyp

1. Arthur JF. Structure and significance of metaplastic nodules in the rectal mucosa. *J Clin Pathol* 1968;21:735–743.
2. Waye JD, Lewis BS, Frankel A, Geller SA. Small colon polyps. *Am J Gastroenterol* 1988;83:120–122.
3. Correa P. Epidemiology of polyps in cancer. In: Morson BC, ed. *Pathogenesis of colorectal cancer*. Philadelphia: WB Saunders, 1978;126–152.
4. Lane N, Kaplan H, Pascal RR. Minute adenomatous and hyperplastic polyps of the colon: divergent patterns of epithelial growth with specific associated mesenchymal changes; contrasting roles in the pathogenesis of carcinoma. *Gastroenterology* 1971;60:537–551.
5. Achkar E, Carey W. Small polyps found during fiberoptic sigmoidoscopy in asymptomatic patients. *Ann Intern Med* 1988;109:880–887.
6. Estrada RG, Spjut HJ. Hyperplastic polyps of the large bowel. *Am J Surg Pathol* 1980;4:127–133.
7. Williams GT, Arthur JF, Bussey HJR, Morson BC. Metaplastic polyps and polyposis of the colorectum. *Histopathology* 1980;4:155–170.
8. Franzin G, Zamboni G, Scarpa A, Dina R, Iannucci A, Novelli P. Hyperplastic (metaplastic) polyps of the colon. A histological and histochemical study. *Am J Surg Pathol* 1984;8:687–698.
9. Sumner HW, Wasserman NF, McClain CJ. Giant hyperplastic polyposis of the colon. *Dig Dis Sci* 1981;26:85–89.
10. Whittle TS, Varner W, Brown FM. Giant hyperplastic polyp of the colon simulating adenocarcinoma. *Am J Gastroenterol* 1978;69:105–107.
11. Warner AS, Glick ME, Fogt T. Multiple large hyperplastic polyps of the colon with adenocarcinoma. *Am J Gastroenterol* 1984;89:123–125.
12. Bengoechea O, Martinez-Penula JM, Larrinaga B, Valerdi J, Borda F. Hyperplastic polyposis of the colorectum and adenocarcinoma in a 24 year old man. *Am J Surg Pathol* 1987;11:323–327.
13. Urbanski SJ, Kossakowska AE, Marcou NN, Bruce WR. Mixed hyperplastic-adenomatous polyps. An underdiagnosed entity. Report of a case of adenocarcinoma arising with a mixed hyperplastic adenomatous polyp. *Am J Surg Pathol* 1984;8:551–556.
14. Cooper AS, Patchefsky AP, Marks G. Adenomatous and carcinomatous changes within hyperplastic colonic epithelium. *Dis Colon Rectum* 1979;22:152–156.
15. Teoh HH, Delahunt B, Isbister WH. Dysplastic malignant areas in hyperplastic polyps of the large intestine. *Pathology* 1989;21:138–142.
16. Jorgensen H, Morgensen AM, Svendsen LB. Hyperplastic polyposis of the large bowel. Three cases and a review of the literature. *Scand J Gastroenterology* 1996;31:825–830.
17. Provenzale D, Garrett JW, Condon SE, Sandler RS. Risk for colon adenomas in patients with rectosigmoid hyperplastic polyps. *Ann Intern Med* 1990;113:760–763.
18. Blue MG, Sivak MV, Achkai E, Matzen R, Stahl RR. Hyperplastic polyps seen at sigmoidoscopy are markers for additional adenomas seen at colonoscopy. *Gastroenterology* 1991;100:564–566.
19. Brady PG, Straker RJ, McClave SA, Nord HJ, Pinkas M, Robinson BE. Are hyperplastic rectosigmoid polyps associated with an increased risk of colonic neoplasms? *Gastrointest Endosc* 1993;39:481–485.
20. Bond JH and the Practice Parameters Committee of the American College of Gastroenterology. Polyp guideline: diagnosis, treatment, and surveillance for patients with non-familial colorectal polyps. *Ann Intern Med* 1993;119:836–843.

21. Jeeveratnam P, Cottier DS, Browett PJ, Van De Water NS, Pokos V, Jass JR. Familial giant hyperplastic polyposis predisposing to colorectal cancer: a new hereditary bowel cancer syndrome. *J Pathol* 1990;179:20–25.
22. Burt RW, Samowitz WS. Serrated adenomatous polyposis. A new syndrome? *Gastroenterology* 1996;110:950–952.
23. Morson BC. Some peculiarities in the histology of intestinal polyps. *Dis Colon Rectum* 1962;5:337–344.
24. Sobin LH. Inverted hyperplastic polyps of the colon. *Am J Surg Pathol* 1985;9:265–272.

Serrated Adenoma

25. Longacre TA, Fenoglio-Preiser CM. Mixed hyperplastic adenomatous polyps/serrated adenoma. A distinctive form of colorectal neoplasia. *Am J Surg Pathol* 1990;14:524–537.
26. Torlakovic E, Snover DC. Serrated adenomatous polyposis. *Gastroenterology* 1996;110:748–755.

Peutz-Jegher's Polyp

27. Gibbs NM. Juvenile and Peutz-Jeghers polyps. In: Morson BC, ed. *Pathogenesis of colorectal cancer.* Philadelphia. WB Saunders, 1978:33–42.
28. Lewin KJ, Riddell R, Weinstein W. *Gastrointestinal pathology and its clinical implications.* New York: Igaku-Shoin. 1992:1215.
29. Talbot IC, Price A. *Biopsy pathology in colorectal disease.* London: Chapman and Hall, 1987:254.
30. Nakayama H, Fuji M, Kimura A, Kajihara H. A solitary Peutz-Jegher type hamartomatous polyp of the rectum: report of a case and review of the literature. *J Clin Oncol* 1996;26:273–276.
31. Rustgi AK. Hereditary gastrointestinal polyposis and nonpolyposis syndrome. *N Engl J Med* 1994;331:1694–1702.
32. Haggitt RC, Reid BJ. Hereditary gastrointestinal polyposis syndromes. *Am J Surg Pathol* 1986;10:871–887.
33. Spigelman AD, Murday V, Phillips RKS. Cancer and the Peutz-Jeghers syndrome. *Gut* 1989;30:1588–1590.
34. Giardiello TM, Welsh SB, Hamilton SR, Offerhaus JH, Luk GD. Increased risk of cancer in the Peutz-Jeghers syndrome. *N Engl J Med* 1987;316:1511–1514.
35. Hizawa K, Iida M. Matsumoto T, Kohrogi N, Kinoshita H, Yao T, Fujishima M. Cancer in Peutz-Jeghers syndrome. *Cancer* 1993;72:2777–2781.
36. Williams JP, Knudsen A. Peutz-Jeghers syndrome with metastasizing duodenal carcinoma. *Gut* 1965;6:179–184.
37. Perzin KH, Bridge MF. Adenomatous and carcinomatous changes in hamartomatous polyps of the small intestine (Peutz-Jeghers syndrome). Report of a case and review of the literature. *Cancer* 1982;49:971–983.
38. Miller LJ, Bartholomew LG, Dozois RR, Dahlin DC. Adenocarcinoma of the rectum arising in a hamartomatous polyp in a patient with Peutz-Jeghers syndrome. *Dig Dis Sci* 1983; 28:1047–1051.
39. Matuchanuky C, Babin P, Costrot S, Druart P, Barbier J, Marie P. Peutz-Jeghers syndrome with metastasizing carcinoma arising from a jejunal hamartoma. *Gastroenterology* 1979;77 1311–1315.
40. Narita T, Eto T, Ito T. Peutz-Jeghers syndrome with adenomas and adenocarcinomas in colonic polyps. *Am J Surg Pathol* 1987;11:76–81.
41. Hizawa K, Iida M, Matsumoto T, Kohrigi N, Hay T, Fugishima M. Neoplastic transformation arising in Peutz-Jeghers polyposis. *Dis Colon Rectum* 1993;36:953–957.
42. Bolwel JS, James PD. Peutz-Jeghers syndrome with pseudoinvasion of hamartomatous polyps and multiple epithelial neoplasms. *Histopathology* 1979;3:39–50.
43. Spjut HJ, Helgason AH, Trabinino JG. Jejunitis cystica profunda in a hamartomatous polyp. Report of case. *Am J Surg Pathol* 1987;11:328–332.
44. Shepherd NA, Bussey HJR, Jass JR. Epithelial misplacement in Peutz-Jeghers polyps. A diagnostic pitfall. *Am J Surg Pathol* 1987;11:743–749.
44. Patterson MJ, Kernen JA. Epithelioid leiomyosarcoma originating in a hamartomatous polyp from a patient with Peutz-Jeghers syndrome. *Gastroenterology* 1985;88:1060–1064.
46. Carlson GJ, Nivatvongs S, Snover DC. Colorectal polyps in Cowden's disease (multiple hamartomatous syndrome). *Am J Surg Pathol* 1984;8:763–770.
47. Weary PE, Gorlin RJ, Gentry WC Jr, Comer JE, Greer KE. Multiple hamartoma syndrome. Cowden's disease. *Arch Dermatol* 1972;106:682–690.

Ganglioneuroma and Juvenile Polyps

48. Hoff RC, San Diego AC. Ganglioneuroma of the ileocecal valve. *Arch Pathol Lab Med* 1972;93:549–551.
49. Carney JA, Hayles AB. Alimentary tract manifestations of multiple endocrine neoplasia, type IIB. *Mayo Clin Proc* 1977;52:543–548.
50. Mendelsohn G, Diamond MP. Familial ganglioneuromatosis of the large bowel. Report of a family with associated juvenile polyposis. *Am J Surg Pathol* 1984;8:515–520.
51. Snover DC, Weigent CE, Sumner HW. Diffuse mucosal ganglioneuromatosis of the colon associated with adenocarcinoma. *Am J Surg Pathol* 1981;75:225–229.
52. Roth SI, Helwig EB. Juvenile polyps of the colon and rectum. *Cancer* 1963;16:468–479.
53. Desai DC, Neale KF, Talbot IC, Hodgon SV, Phillips RKS. Juvenile polyposis. *Br J Surg* 1995;82:14–17.
54. Jarvinen H, Fransila KO. Familial juvenile polyposis coli: increased risk of colorectal cancer. *Gut* 1984;25:792–800.
55. Stemper EJ, Kents TA, Summers RW. Juvenile polyposis and gastrointestinal carcinoma. A study of a kindred. *Ann Intern Med* 1975;183:639–646.
56. Rozen P, Baratz M. Familial juvenile polyposis with associated colon cancer. *Cancer* 1982;49:1500–1503.
57. Jass JR, Williams CB, Bussey HJR, Morson BC. Juvenile polyposis a precancerous condition. *Histopathology* 1988;13:619–630.
58. Giardiello FM, Hamilton SR, Kern SE, et al. Colorectal neoplasia in juvenile polyposis or juvenile polyps. *Arch Dis Child* 1991;66:971–975.
59. Rozen P, Baratz M. Familial juvenile polyposis with associated colon cancer. *Cancer* 1982;49:1500–1503.
60. Nugent KP, Talbot IZ, Hodgson SV, Phillips RKS. Solitary juvenile polyp: not a marker for subsequent malignancy. *Gastroenterology* 1993;105:698–700.
61. Goodman ZD, Yardley J, Miligan FD. Pathogenesis of colonic polyps in multiple juvenile polyposis. Report of a case associated with gastric polyps and carcinoma of the rectum. *Cancer* 1979;43:1906–1913.
62. Lipper S, Kahn LB, Sandler RS, Varma V. Multiple juvenile polyposis. The study of the pathogenesis of juvenile polyps and their relationship to colonic adenomas. *Hum Pathol* 1981;12:804–813.
63. Girgioni WF, Alampi O, Martinelli G, Piccaulga A. Atypical juvenile polyposis. *Histopathology* 1981;5:361–376.
64. Tung-hua L, Min-chang C, Hsien-Chiu T, Lan C, Chieh L. Malignant change of juvenile polyp of the colon. A case report. *Chin Med J (Engl)* 1978;4:434–439.
65. Wu TT, Rezal B, Rashid A, et al. Genetic alterations and epithelial dysplasia in juvenile polyposis syndromes and sporadic juvenile polyps. *Am J Pathol* 1997;150:939–997.

Inflammatory Polyps

66. Shekitka KM, Helwig EB. Deceptive bizarre stromal cells in polyps and ulcers and of the gastrointestinal tract. *Cancer* 1991;67:2111–2117.
67. Jessurun J, Paplanus SH, Nagle RB, Hamilton SR, Yardley JH, Tripp M. Pseudosarcomatous changes in inflammatory polyps of the colon. *Arch Pathol Lab Med* 1986;110:883–836.

Inflammatory Polyps Secondary to Prolapse

68. Chetty R, Bhathel PS, Slavin JL. Prolapsed induced inflammatory polyps of the colorectum and anal transitional zone. *Histopathology* 1993;23:63–67.
69. Williams GT, Bussey HJR, Morson BC. Inflammatory cap polyps of the large intetine. *Br J Surg* 1985;72:5133.
70. Gehenot M, Colombel JF, Wolschies E, et al. Inflammatory cap polyposis occurring in the post operative course of pelvic surgery. *Gut* 1994;35:1670–1672.
71. Campbell AP, Cobb CA, Chapman RWG, et al. Cap polyposis, an unusual cause of diarrhea. *Gut* 1993;34:562–564.
72. Nakamura SI, Kino I, Akagi T. Inflammatory myoglandular polyps of the colon and rectum. A clinicopathological study of 32 pedunculated polyps distinct from other types of polyps. *Am J Surg Pathol* 1992;16:772–779.
73. Kelly JK. Polypoid prolapse in mucosal folds in diverticular disease. *Am J Surg Pathol* 1991;15:871–878.

Inflammatory Fibroid Polyp

74. Shimer GR, Helwig EB. Inflammatory fibroid polyps of the intestine. *Am J Clin Pathol* 1984;81:708–714.
75. Benjamin SP, Hawk WA, Turnbull RB. Fibrous inflammatory polyps of the ileum and cecum. Review of five cases with emphasis on differentiation from mesenchymal neoplasms. *Cancer* 1977;39:1300–1305.
76. LiVolsi VA, Perzin KH. Inflammatory pseudotumors (inflammatory fibrous polyps) of the small intestine: a clinicopathological study. *Am J Dig Dis* 1975;20:325–336.

Cronkite-Canada Syndrome

77. Daniel ES, Ludwig SL, Lewin KJ, Ruprecht RM, Rajacich GM, Schwab AD. The Cronkite-Canada syndrome. An analysis of clinical and pathological features and therapy in 55 patients. *Medicine (Baltimore)* 1982;61:293–309.
78. Katayama Y, Kimura M, Konn M. Cronkite-Canada syndrome associated with rectal cancer and adenomatous changes in colonic polyps. *Am J Surg Pathol* 1985;9:65–71.
79. Nomoura A, Ohta G, Ihata T, Shinozaki K, Nishino T. Cronkite Canada syndrome associated with sigmoid cancer. *Acta Pathol Jpn* 1980;30:825–845.

Lymphoid Polyps

80. Corres JS, Wallace MH, Morson BC. Benign lymphomas of the rectum and anal canal; a study of 100 cases. *J Pathol Bacteriol* 1961;82:371–382.
81. Louw JH. Polypoid lesions of the large bowel in children with particular reference to benign lymphoid polyposis. *J Pediatr Surg* 1968;3:195–209.
82. Venkitachalam PS, Hirsch E, Elguezabal A, Littman L. Multiple lymphoid polyposis and familial polyposis of the colon: a genetic relationship. *Dis Colon Rectum* 1978;21:336–341.
83. Dorazio RA, Whelan TJ Jr. Lymphoid hyperplasia of the terminal ileum associated with familial polyposis coli. *Ann Surg* 1970;171:300–302.
84. Thomford NR, Greenberger NG. Lymphoid polyps of the ileum associated with Gardner's syndrome. *Arch Surg* 1968;96:289–291.

Adenomas—Small Intestine

85. Sarre RG, Frost AG, Jagelman DG, Petras RE, Sivak MV, McGannun E. Gastric and duodenal polyps in familial adenomatosis polyposis: a prospective study of the nature and prevalence of upper gastrointestinal polyps. *Gut* 1987;28:306–314.
86. Domizio P, Talbot IC. Spiegelmann AD, Williams CB, Phillips RKS. Upper gastrointestinal pathology in familial adenomatous polyposis: results from a prospective study of 102 patients. *J Clin Pathol* 1990;43:738–743.

Adenomas—Large Intestine

87. Rickert RR, Auerbach O, Garfinkle L, Hammond EC, Frasca JM. Adenomatous lesions of the large bowel. An autopsy survey. *Cancer* 1979;43:1847–1857.
88. Correa P, Duque E, Cuello C, Haenszel W. Polyps of the colon and rectum in Cali, Columbia. *Int J Cancer* 1972;9:86–96.
89. Shinya H, Wolff WI. Morphology, anatomic distribution and cancer potential of polyps. An analysis of 7000 polyps endoscopically removed. *Ann Surg* 1979;190:679–683.
90. Konishi F, Morson BC. Pathology of colorectal adenomas: a colonoscopic survey. *J Clin Pathol* 1982;35:830–841.
91. Gillepsie PE, Chambers TJ, Chan KW, Doronzo F, Morson BC, Williams CB. Colonic adenomas—colonoscopic survey. *Gut* 1979;20:240–245.
92. Jass JR, Sobin LH. *Histological typing of intestinal tumors. World Health Organization International Histological Classification of Tumors,* 2nd ed. New York: Springer-Verlag, 1989.
93. O'Brien MJ, Winawer SJ, Zauber AG, et al. The National Polyp Study Works Group: patient and polyp characteristics associated with high grade dysplasia—colorectal adenomas. *Gastroenterology* 1990;98:371–379.
94. Pascal RR. Dysplasia in early carcinoma in inflammatory bowel disease and colorectal adenomas. *Hum Pathol* 1994;25:1160–1171.

Flat Adenomas

95. Wolber RA, Owen DA. Flat adenomas of the colon. *Hum Pathol* 1991;22:70–74.
96. Muto K, Kamiya J, Sawada T, et al. Small "flat adenoma" of the large bowel with special reference to its clinicopathological features. *Dis Colon Rectum* 1985;28:847–851.
97. Adechi M Muto T, Okinaga K, Morioka Y. Clinicopathological features of the flat adenoma. *Dis Colon Rectum* 1991;34:981–986.
98. Minamoto T, Sawaguchi K, Ohta T, Ito HT, Mai M. Superficial type adenoma in adenocarcinoma of the colon and rectum. A comparative morphological study. *Gastroenterology* 1994;106(2):1436–1443.
99. Mitooka F, Fujimori T, Moeda S, Nagasuko K. Minute flat neoplastic lesions of the colon detected by chromoscopy using an indigo carmine capsule. *Gastrointest Endosc* 1995;41:453–459.
100. Bond JH. Small flat adenomas appear to have little clinical importance in Western countries. *Gastrointest Endosc* 1995;42:184–186.
101. Jaramillo E, Watanabe EM, Slezak P, Rubio C. Flat neoplastic lesions of the colon and rectum detected by high resolution video endoscopy and chromoscopy. *Gastrointest Endosc* 1995;42:114–122.
102. Samowitz WS, Burt RL. The nonspecificity of histological findings reported for flat adenoma. *Hum Pathol* 1995;26:571–573.
103. Uno Y, Munakata A, Tanaka M. The discrepancy of histological diagnosis between flat early colon cancers and flat adenomas. *Gastrointest Endosc* 1994;40:1–6.

Endoscopically Removed Malignant Polyp

104. Cooper HS, Deppisch LM, Kahn EI, et al. Pathology of the malignant colorectal polyp. *Hum Pathol* 1998;29:15–26.
105. Cooper HS, Deppisch LM, Gourley WK, et al. Endoscopically removed malignant colorectal polyps: clinicopathological correlations. *Gastroenterology* 1995;108:1657–1665.
106. Muller S, Chesner IM, Egan MJ, et al. Significance of venous and lymphatic invasion in malignant polyps of the colon and rectum. *Gut* 1989;30:1385–1391.
107. Geraghty MJ, Williams CB, Talbot IC. Malignant colorectal polyps: venous invasion and successful treatment by endoscopic polypectomy. *Gut* 1991;32:774–778.
108. Morson BC, Whiteway JF, Jones EA, Macrae FA, Williams CB. Histopathology and prognosis of malignant colorectal polyps treated by endoscopic polypectomy. *Gut* 1985;25:437–444.
109. Cranley JF, Petras RE, Carey WD, Paradis K, Sivak MV. When is endoscopic polypectomy adequate therapy for colonic polyps containing invasive carcinoma? *Gastroenterology* 1986;91:419–427.
110. Cooper HS. Surgical pathology of endoscopically removed malignant polyps of the colon and rectum. *Am J Surg Pathol* 1983;7:613–623.
111. Wolff WI, Shinya H. Definitive treatment of malignant polyps of the colon. *Ann Surg* 1975;182:516–525.
112. Haggitt RC, Golzbach RE, Soffer EE, Wruble LD. Prognostic factors in colorectal carcinomas arising in adenomas: implications for lesions removed by endoscopic polypectomy. *Gastroenterology* 1985;89:326–328.
113. Cooper HS. The role of the pathologist in the management of patients with an endoscopically removed malignant polyp of the colon and rectum. In: Rosen PP, Levine RE, eds. *Pathology annual,* vol 23, part 1. Norwalk, CT: Appleton and Lange, 1988:24–43.
114. Jass JR. Malignant colorectal polyps. *Gastroenterology* 1995;109:2034–2035.

Adenoma with Pseudoinvasion

115. Greene FL. Epithelial misplacement in adenomatous polyps of the colon and rectum. *Cancer* 1974;33:206–217.
116. Muto T, Bussey HJR, Morson BC. Pseudocarcinomatous invasion in adenomatous polyps of the colon and rectum. *J Clin Pathol* 1973;26:25–31.
117. Qirschmic K, Kiesler J, Mathis G, Beller S, Stoss F, Schobel B. Epithelial misplacement after biopsy of colorectal adenomas. *Am J Surg Pathol* 1993;17:1262–1265.
118. Pascal RR, Hertzler G, Hunter S. Goldschmid S. Pseudoinvasion with high grade dysplasia in a colonic adenoma. Distinction from adenocarcinoma. *Am J Surg Pathol* 1990;14:694–607.

Polyposis Disorders

119. Paraf F, Jothy S, Van Meir EG. Brain tumor polyposis syndrome: two genetic diseases? *J Clin Oncol* 1977;15:2744–2758.
120. Hamilton SR, Liu B, Parsons RE, et al. The molecular basis of Turcot's syndrome. *N Engl J Med* 1995;332:839–847.
121. Lynch HT, Smyrk R, Watson P, et al. Hereditary flat adenoma syndrome. A variant of familial adenomatous polyposis. *Dis Colon Rectum* 1992;35:411–421.
122. Lynch HT, Smyrk TZ, Lanspa SJ, et al. Upper gastrointestinal manifestations in families with hereditary flat adenoma syndrome. *Cancer* 1993;71:2709–14.
123. Lynch HT, Smyrk T, McGinn T, et al. Attenuated familial adenomatous polyposis (AFAP). A phenotypically and genetically distinctive variant of FAP. *Cancer* 1995;76:2427–2433.
124. Whitelaw SC, Murday VA, Tomlinson PM, et al. Clinical and molecular features of the hereditary mixed polyposis syndrome. *Gastroenterology* 1997;112:327–334.

Small Intestinal Carcinoma

125. Weiss NS, Yang GP. Incidence of histologic types of cancer of the small intestine. *J Natl Cancer Inst* 1987;78:653–656.

Large Intestinal Carcinoma

126. Nikahara H, Ishikawa T, Itobashi M, Hirota T. Diffusely infiltrating primary colorectal carcinoma of the linitis plastica and lymphangiosis types. *Cancer* 1992;69:901–906.
127. Chowdhuny JR, Das K, Das KM. Primary linitis plastic of the colon: report of a case and review of the literature. *Dis Colon Rectum* 1975;18:332–338.
128. Dukes CE, Bussey HJR. The spread of rectal cancer and its effect on prognosis. *Br J Cancer* 1958;12:309–320.
129. Murray D, Hoeno A, Dalton J, Hampson LG. Prognosis in colon cancer. A pathologic assessment. *Arch Surg* 1975;110:908–913.
130. Newland RC, Chapiris PH, Pheils MT, MacPherson JG. The relationship of survival to staging and grading of colorectal carcinoma: a prospective study of 503 cases. *Cancer* 1981;47:1424–1429.

Mucinous Adenocarcinoma

131. Saski O, Atkin WS, Jass Jr. Mucinous carcinoma of the rectum. *Histopathology* 1987;11:259–272.
132. Symonds DA, Vickery AL. Mucinous carcinoma of the colon and rectum. *Cancer* 1976;37:1891–1900.
133. Wu CS, Tong, SY, Chen PC, Kuo YC. Clinicopathological study of colorectal mucinous carcinoma in Taiwan: a multivariate analysis. *J Gastroenterol Hepatol* 1996;11:77–81.

Small Cell Carcinoma

134. Mills SE, Allen MS, Cohen AR. Small cell undifferentiated carcinoma of the colon. A clinicopathological study of 5 cases and their association with colonic adenomas. *Am J Surg Pathol* 1983;7:643–651.
135. Schwartz AM, Orenstein JM. Small cell undifferentiated carcinoma of the rectosigmoid colon. *Arch Pathol Lab Med* 1985;109:629–632.
136. Wick MR, Weatherby RP, Weiland LH. Small cell neuroendocrine carcinoma of the colon and rectum: clinical, histological, and ultrastructural comparison with cloacogenic cancer. *Hum Pathol* 1987;18:9–21.
137. Burke AB, Shekita KM, Sobin LH. Small cell carcinoma of the large intestine. *Am J Clin Pathol* 1991;95:315–321.

Undifferentiated Carcinoma

138. Gibbs NM. Undifferentiated carcinoma of the large intestine. *Histopathology* 1977;1:77–84.
139. Morson BC, Dawson IM, Day DW, Jass JR, Price AB, Williams GT, eds. *Morson and Dawson's Gastrointestinal Pathology*, 3rd ed. Oxford: Blackwell Scientific, 1990.
140. Jass JR. In: Fletcher CDM, ed. *Diagnostic histopathology of tumors*. New York: Churchill Livingstone, 1995:243–274.
141. Ruschoff J, Dietmaier W, Luttges J, et al. Poorly differentiated colonic adenocarcinoma medullary type. *Am J Pathol* 1997;150:1815–1825.

Hereditary Non-Polyposis Colon Cancer (see also 158, 159)

142. Lynch HT, Smyrk T. Hereditary nonpolyposis colorectal cancer (Lynch Syndrome). An updated review. *Cancer* 1996;78:1149–67.
143. Smyrk TC. Colon cancer connections. Cancer syndrome meets molecular biology meets histopathology. *Am J Pathol* 1994;145:1–6.
144. Comer TP, Beahrs OH, Dockerty MD. Primary squamous cell carcinoma and adenoacanthoma of the colon. *Cancer* 1971;28:1111–1117.
145. Weidner N, Zekan P. Carcinosarcoma of the colon. Report of a unique case with light and immunohistochemical studies. *Cancer* 1986;58:1126–1130.
146. Radi MF, Gray GF Jr, Scott HW Jr. Carcinoma of the ileum in regional ileitis. *Hum Pathol* 1984;15:385–387.
147. Nguyen GK. Adenocarcinoma of the sigmoid colon with focal choriocarcinoma metaplasia. *Dis Colon Rectum* 1982;25:230–234.
148. Park CH, Reid JD. Adenocarcinoma of the colon with choriocarcinoma in its metastases. *Cancer* 1980;46:570–575.
149. Hainsworty JD, Greco TA. Human chorionic gonadotropin production by colon cancer. *Cancer* 1985;56:1337–1340.
150. Nakqyama H, Akikusa B, Kondo Y, Saito Norio, Sarashina H, Okui K. Mucinous cystadenocarcinoma of the colon. Report of a case. *Dis Colon Rectum* 1989;32:243–246.
151. Jewell LD, Barr JR, McCaugher WTE, Nguyen G-K, Owen DA. Clear cell epithelial neoplasms of the large intestine. *Arch Pathol Lab Med* 1988;112:197–199.
152. Rubio CA. Clear cell adenocarcinoma of the colon. *J Clin Pathol* 1995;48:1142–1144.
153. Ishikura H, Kishimoto T, Andachi H, Kakuta Y, Yoshiki T. Gastrointestinal hepatoid adenocarcinoma; venous permeation and mimicry of hepatocellular carcinoma, a report of four cases. *Histopathology* 1997;31:47–54.

Small Early Flat Carcinoma

154. Kuramoto S, Oohara T. Flat early cancers of the large intestine. *Cancer* 1989;64:950–955.
155. Tada S, Iida M, Matsumoto Y, Yao T, Aoyagi K, Koga H. Small flat cancer of the rectum. Clinicopathological and endoscopic features. *Gastrointest Endosc* 1995;42:109–113.
156. Winawer SJ, Zauber AG, Ho MN, et al. Prevention of colorectal cancer by colonoscopic polypectomy. *N Engl J Med* 1993;329:1977–1981.
157. Stolte M, Bethke B. Colorectal mini de novo carcinoma: a reality in Germany too. *Endoscopy* 1995;27:286–290.
158. Sankila R, Aaltonen LA, Jarvinen HJ, Meeklin J-P. Better survival rates in patients with MLH-1 associated hereditary colon cancer. *Gastroenterology* 1996;110:682–687.
159. Risio M, Reato G, De Celle PF, Fizzotti M, Rossini FP, Foa R. Microsatellite instability is associated with the histological features of tumors in non-familial colorectal cancer. *Cancer Res* 1996;56:5470–574.

Staging, Reporting, and Histological Prognosticators

160. Dukes CE. The classification of cancer of the rectum. *J Pathol Bacteriol* 1932;35:323–332.
161. Astler VB, Coller FA. The prognostic significance of direct extension of carcinoma of the colon and rectum. *Ann Surg* 1954;139:846–851.
162. Hutter RVP, Sobin LH. A universal staging for cancer of the colon and rectum. *Arch Pathol Lab Med* 1986;110:367–368.
163. Jass JR, Atkin WS, Cuzick J, et al. The grading of rectal cancer: historic perspectives and multivariate analysis of 447 cases. *Histopathology* 1986;10:437–459.
164. Jass JR, Love SB, Northover JMA. A new prognostic classification of rectal cancer. *Lancet* 1987;1:1303–1306.
165. Cohen JR, Theile DE, Evans ER, Quinn RL, Davis MK. Colorectal cancer at the Princess Alexandria Hospital: a prospective study of 729 cases. *Aust N Z J Surg* 1987;53:113–119.
166. Whittaker M, Goligher JC. The prognosis after surgical treatment for carcinoma of the rectum. *Br J Surg* 1976;63:384–388.

167. Wolmark N, Fisher B, Wieand HS. The prognostic value of the modification of the Dukes' C class of colorectal cancer. *Ann Surg* 1986;203:115–122.
168. Fisher ER, Sass R, Palekar A, Fisher B, Wolmark N. Contributing National Surgical Adjuvant Breast and Bowel Project Investigators. Dukes' classification revisited. Findings from the National Surgical Adjuvant Breast and Bowel Projects (Protocol R-01). *Cancer* 1989;64:2354–2360.
169. Henson DE, Hutter RVP, Sobin LH, Bowman HE. Protocol for the examination of specimens removed from patients with colorectal carcinoma. *Arch Pathol Lab Med* 1994;118:122–125.
170. Chan KW, Boey J, Wong SKC. A method of reporting radial invasion and surgical clearance of rectal cancer. *Histopathology* 1985;9:1319–1327.
171. Quirke P, Dixon MF, Durdey P, Williams NS. Local recurrence of rectal adenocarcinoma due to inadequate surgical resection. *Lancet* 1986;2:996–998.
172. De Haas-Koch DFM, Baeten GMI, Jager JJ, et al. Prognostic significant of radial margins of clearance in rectal cancer. *Br J Surg* 1996;83:781–785.
173. Shepherd NA, Baxter KJ, Love SE. The prognostic importance of peritoneal involvement in colonic carcinoma. A prognostic evaluation. *Gastroenterology* 1997;112:1090–1102.
174. Scot KWM, Grace RLT. Detection of lymph node metastases before and after fat clearance. *Br J Surg* 1989;1165–1167.
175. Goldstein NS, Sanford W, Coffey M, Layfield LJ. Lymph node recovery from colorectal resections removed for adenocarcinoma. Trends over time and a recommendation for a minimum number of nodes to be recovered. *Am J Clin Pathol* 1996;106:209–216.
176. Gagliardi G, Stepeniewska KA, Hirshman MJ, Hawley PR, Talbot IC. New grade-related prognostic variable for rectal cancer. *Br J Surg* 1995;82:599–602.
177. Hamada Y, Oishi A, Shoji T, et al. Endocrine cells and prognosis in patients with colorectal cancer. *Cancer* 1992;69:2641–2646.
178. Graham DM, Appleman HD. Crohn's like lymphoid reaction and colorectal carcinoma: a potential histological prognosticator. *Modern Pathology* 1990;3:332–335.
179. Harrison JC, Dean PJ, El-Zeky F, Vander Zwang R. From Dukes through Jass pathological prognostic indicators in rectal cancer. *Hum Pathol* 1994;25:498–505.
180. Hase K, Shatney C, Johnson D, Trollope M, Vierra M. Prognostic value of tumor budding in patients with colorectal cancer. *Dis Colon Rectum* 1993;36:627–635.

Biological Markers

181. Hermanek P, Sobin LH. Colorectal carcinoma. In: Hermanek P, Gospodarowicz MIC, Henson DE, Hutten RVP, Sobin LH, eds. *Prognostic factors in cancer. International Union Against Cancer.* New York: Springer-Verlag, 1995.

Immunohistochemical Markers

182. Frierson HF Jr, Bellafinore FJ, Gaffey MJ, McCary WS, Innes DJ Jr, Williams ME. Cytokeratin in anaplastic large cell lymphoma. *Mod Pathol* 1994;7:317–321.
183. Losota J, Hyjek E, Koo CH, Blonski J, Miettinen M. Cytokeratin positive large-cell lymphomas of B cell lineage. *Am J Surg Pathol* 1996;20:346–354.
184. Norton AJ, Thomas JA, Isaacson PG. Cytokeratin specific antibodies are reactive with tumors of smooth muscle derivation. An immunocytochemical and biochemical study using antibodies to intermediate filament cytoskeletal proteins. *Histopathology* 1987;11:487–499.
185. Miettinen M. Immunoreactivity for cytokeratin and epithelial membrane antigen in leiomyosarcoma. *Arch Pathol Lab Med* 1988;112:637–640.
186. Taylor CR, Cote RJ. Immunomicroscopy: a diagnostic tool for the surgical pathologist. *Major Problems in Pathology,* 2nd ed. Philadelphia: WB Saunders, 1994.
187. Zarbo RJ, Gown AM, Nagle RB, Visscher DW, Crissman JD. Anomalous cytokeratin expression in malignant melanoma: one and two-dimensional Western blot analysis and immunohistochemical survey of 100 melanomas. *Mod Pathol* 1990;3:494–501.
188. Chittal S, Al Saati T, Delsol G. Epithelial membrane antigen in hematolymphoid neoplasms. A review. *Appl Immunohistochem* 1997;5:203–215.
189. Pinkus GS, Kurtin PJ. Epithelial membrane antigen—a diagnostic discriminant in surgical pathology. Immunohistochemical profile in epithelial, mesenchymal, and hematopoietic neoplasms using paraffin section and monoclonal antibodies. *Hum Pathol* 1985;16:929–940.
190. Sheihani K, Shin SS, Kezirian J, Weiss LM. Ber-EP4. Antibody as a discriminant in the differential diagnosis of malignant mesothelioma vs adenocarcinoma. *Am J Surg Pathol* 1991;15:779–784.
191. Arber DA, Weiss LM. CD 57. A review. *Appl Immunohistochem* 1995;3:137–152.
192. Shipley WR, Hammer RD, Lennington WJ, Macon WR. Paraffin immunohistochemical detection of CD 56, a useful marker for neural cell adhesion molecule (NCAM), in normal and neoplastic fixed tissue. *Appl Immunohistochem* 1997;5:87–93.
193. May EE, Perentes E. Anti-Leu 7 immunoreactivity with human tumors. Its value in the diagnosis of prostate cancer. *Histopathology* 1987;11:295–304.
194. Wang NP, Zee S, Zarbo RJ, Bacchi CE, Gowan AM. Coordinate expression of cytokeratins 7 and 20 defines unique subsets of carcinoma. *Appl Immunohistochem* 1995;3:99–107.
195. Savera A, Torres FX, Linden MD, Bacchi CE, Gown AM, Zarbo RJ. Primary vs metastatic primary adenocarcinoma. An immunohistochemical study using villin and cytokeratins 7 and 20. *Appl Immunohistochem* 1996;4:86–94.

Appendix

196. Appelman HD. Epithelial neoplasia of the appendix. In: Norris HT, ed. *Pathology of the colon, small intestine, and anus,* 2nd ed. New York: Churchill Livingstone, 1991:263–303.
197. Younes M, Katikaneni PR, Lechago J. Association between mucosal hyperplasia of the appendix and adenocarcinoma of the colon. *Histopathology* 1995;26:33–37.
198. Qizilbash AH. Hyperplastic (metaplastic) polyps of the appendix. *Arch Pathol Lab Med* 1974;97:385–388.
199. MacGillivray JB. Mucosal hyperplasia of the appendix. *J Clin Pathol* 1972;25:809–811.
200. Higa E, Rosai J, Pizzimbono CA, Wise L. Mucosal hyperplasia, mucinous cystadenoma, and mucinous cystadenocarcinoma of the appendix. A re-evaluation of appendiceal mucocele. *Cancer* 1973;32:1525–1541.
201. Carr NJ, McCarthy WF, Sobin LH. Epithelial noncarcinoid tumors and tumor-like lesions of the appendix. A clinicopathological study of 184 patients with a multivariate analysis of prognostic factors. *Cancer* 1995;75:757–68.
202. MacGillivary DC, Heaton RB, Rushin JM, Cruess DF. Distant metastasis from a carcinoid of the appendix less than 1 cm in size. *Surgery* 1992;111:466–71.
203. Moertel CG, Weiland LH, Nagorney DM, Dockerty MB. Carcinoid tumor of the appendix: treatment and prognosis. *N Engl J Med* 1987;317:1699–1701.
204. Subbuswamy SG, Gibbs NM, Ross CF, Morson BC. Goblet cell carcinoid of the appendix. *Cancer* 1974;34:338–344.
205. Warkel RL, Cooper PH, Helwig EB. Adenocarcinoid, a mucin producing carcinoid tumor of the appendix. *Cancer* 1978;42:2781–2793.
206. Isaacson P. Crypt cell carcinoma of the appendix (so-called adenocarcinoid tumor). *Am J Surg Pathol* 1981;5:213–244.
207. Burke AP, Sobin LH, Federspiel BH, Shikitka KM, Helwig EB. Goblet cell carcinoid and related tumors of the vermiform appendix. *Am J Clin Pathol* 1990;94:27–35.
208. Butler JA, Houshiar A, Lin F, Wilson SE. Goblet cell carcinoid of the appendix. *Am J Surg* 1994;168:685–687.
209. Edmunds P, Merino MJ, LiVolsi VA, Duray PH. Adenocarcinoid (mucinous carcinoid) of the appendix. *Gastroenterology* 1984;86:302–309.
210. Park K, Blessing K, Kerr K, Chetty U, Gilmour H. Goblet cell carcinoid of the appendix. *Gut* 1990;31:322–324.

Carcinoid Tumors

211. Klappenboch RS, Kurman RJ, Sinclair CF, Jones LPL. Composite carcinoma-carcinoid tumors of the gastrointestinal tract. A morphologic, histochemical, and immunocytochemical study. *Am J Clin Pathol* 1985;84:137–143.
212. Lewin K. Carcinoid tumors and the mixed (composite)—glandular endocrine cell carcinomas. *Am J Surg Pathol* 1987;11(suppl 1):71–86.

213. Moyana TN, Qizilbash AH, Murphy F. Composite glandular and carcinoid tumors of the rectum. *Am J Surg Pathol* 1988;12:607–611.
214. Moretel CG. An odyssey in the land of small tumors. *J Clin Oncol* 1987:5:1503–1522.
215. Capella C, Heitz PU, Hofler H, Solcia E, Kloppel G. Revised classification of neuroendocrine tumors of the lung, pancreas, and gut. *Virchows Arch* 1995;425:547–560.
216. Burke AP, Sobin LH, Federspiel BH, Shekitka KM, Helwig EB. Carcinoid tumors of the duodenum. A clinicopathological study of 99 cases. *Arch Pathol Lab Med* 1990;114:700–704.
217. Koura AN, Giacco CG, Curley SA, Skibber JM, Feig BW, Ellis LM. Carcinoid tumors of the rectum. Effect of size, histopathology, and surgical treatment on metastases-free survival. *Cancer* 1997;79:1294–1298.
218. Federspiel BH, Burke AP, Sobin LH, Shekitka KM. Rectal and colonic carcinoids. A clinicopathological study of 84 cases. *Cancer* 1990;65:135–140.
219. Genre CF, Roth LM, Reed RJ. Benign rectal carcinoids. A report of two cases with metastases to regional lymph nodes. *Am J Clin Pathol* 1971;56:750–757.
220. Kimura N, Sasno N. Prostatic specific acid phosphatase in carcinoid tumors. *Virchows Arch [A]* 1986;410:247–251.

Lymphoma

221. Isaacson PG. Gastrointestinal lymphoma. *Hum Pathol* 1994;25:1020–1029.
222. Stansfield AG, Diebold J, Yapanci Y et al. Updated Kiel classification for lymphoma. *Lancet* 1988;1:292.
223. Domizio P, Owen RA, Shepherd NA, Talbot IC, Norton AJ. Primary lymphoma of the small intestine. A clinicopathological study of 119 cases. *Am J Surg Pathol* 1993;17:429–442.
224. Shepherd NA, Hall PA, Coates PJ, Levison DA. Primary malignant lymphoma of the colon and rectum. A histopathological and immunohistochemical analysis of 45 cases with clinicopathological correlations. *Histopathology* 1988;12:235–252.
225. Ioachim HC, Antonescu C, Giancolt F, Dorsett B, Weinstein MA. EBV-associated anorectal lymphomas in patients with acquired immunodeficiency syndrome. *Am J Surg Pathol* 1997;21:997–1006.
226. Radasziewicz T, Dragosics B, Bauer P. Gastrointestinal malignant lymphomas of the mucosa associated lymphoid tissue. Factors relevant to prognosis. *Gastroenterology* 1992;102:1628–1638.
227. Lewin KJ, Kahn LB, Novis BA. Primary intestinal lymphoma of Western and Mediterranean type, alpha chain disease and massive plasma cell infiltration. A comparative study of 37 cases. *Cancer* 1976;38:2511–2528.
228. Lewin K, Ranchod M, Dorfman RF. Lymphoma of the gastrointestinal tract. A study of 117 cases presenting with gastrointestinal disease. *Cancer* 1978;42:693–707.
229. Gilinsky NH, Novis BH, Wright JP, Dent DM, King H, Marks IN. Immunoproliferative small intestine disease: clinical features and outcome in 20 cases. *Medicine* 1987;66:438–446.
230. Khojasteh A, Haghshenass M, Haghighi P. Immunoproliferative small intestinal disease. A third world lesion. *N Engl J Med* 1983;308:1401–1405.
231. Asselah R, Slavin G, Soeter G, Asselah H. Immunoproliferative small intestinal disease in Algerians. I. Light microscopic and immunochemical studies. *Cancer* 1983;52:227–237.
232. Nassar VH, Salem PA, Shahid MJ, et al. Mediterranean abdominal lymphoma or immunoproliferative small intestinal disease. Part II. Pathological aspects. *Cancer* 1983;52:1340–1354.
233. Almasri NM, Al-Abbadi M, Rewaily E, et al. Primary gastrointestinal lymphomas in Jordan are similar to those in Western countries. *Mod Pathol* 1997;10:137–141.
234. Amer MH, El-Akkad S. Gastrointestinal lymphoma in adults: clinical features and management of 300 cases. *Gastroenterology* 1994;106:846–858.
235. Galian A, Lecestre MJ, Scotto J, Bognel C, Matuchansky C, Rambaud JC. Pathological study of alpha chain disease with special emphasis on evolution. *Cancer* 1977;39:2081–2111.
236. Baer AN, Bayless TN, Yardley JH. Intestinal ulceration and malabsorption syndromes. *Gastroenterology* 1980;79:654–665.
237. Robertson DAF, Dixon MF, Scott BB, Simpson FG, Lowisky MS. Small intestinal ulceration: diagnostic difficulties in relation to celiac disease. *Gut* 1983;24:565–574.
238. Isaacson P, Wright DH. Malignant histiocytosis of the intestine. Its relationship to malabsorption and ulcerative jejunitis. *Hum Pathol* 1978;9:661–667.
239. Shepherd NAA, Blackshaw AJ, Hall PA, et al. Malignant lymphoma with eosinophilia of the gastrointestinal tract. *Histopathology* 1987;11:115–130.
240. Isaacson PG, Spencer JO, Connelly CE, et al. Malignant histiocytes of the intestine: a T cell lymphoma. *Lancet* 1985;2:688–691.
241. Spencer J, Bensussan NC, Jarry A, et al. Enteropathy-associated T cell lymphoma (malignant histiocytosis of the intestine) is recognized by a monoclonal antibody (HML-1) that defines a membrane molecule on human mucosal lymphocytes. *Am J Pathol* 1988;132:1–5.
242. Ruskone-Fourmestraux A, Delmer A, Lavergne A, et al. Groupe d'etude des lymphomes digestifs. *Gastroenterology* 1997;112:7–16.
243. Lavergne A, Brouland JP, Lanuay E, Nemeth J, Ruskonee-Fourmestraux A, Galian A. Malignant lymphomatous polyposis of the gastrointestinal tract. *Cancer* 1994;74:3042–50.
244. Moynihan MJ, Bast MA, Chan WC, Delabie J, Wickert RS, Wu Guanqing Weisenberger DD. Lymphomatous polyposis. A neoplasm of either follicular mantel or germinal center origin. *Am J Surg Pathol* 1996;20:442–452.
245. O'Brian DS, Kennedy MJ, Daly PA, et al. Multiple lymphomatous polyposis of the gastrointestinal tract. A clinicopathologically distinctive form of non-Hodgkin's lymphoma of B cell centrocytic type. *Am J Surg Pathol* 1989;13:691–699.
246. Hirakawa K, Fuchigomi T, Nakamura S, et al. Primary gastrointestinal T cell lymphoma resembling multiple lymphomatous polyposis. *Gastroenterology* 1996;111:778–782.
247. Harris NL, Jaffe ES, Stein H, et al. A revised European-American classification of lymphoid neoplasms: a proposal from the International Lymphoma Study Group. *Blood* 1994;85:1361–1392.
248. Le Brun DP, Kamel OW, Cleary ML, Dorfman RF, Warnke RA. Follicular lymphomas of the gastrointestinal tract. Pathological features in 31 cases and bcl-2 oncogenic protein expression. *Am J Pathol* 1992;140:1327–1335.
249. Coppell MS, Botros N. Predominately GI symptoms and signs in 11 consecutive AIDS patients with gastrointestinal lymphoma. A multicenter, multiyear study including 763 HIV seropositive patients. *Am J Gastroenterol* 1994;89:545–549.
250. Hsiao CH, Lee WI, Chang SL, Ih-Jen S. Angiocentric T cell lymphoma of the intestine. A distinct etiology of ischemic bowel disease. *Gastroenterology* 1996;110:985–990.
251. Weiss RC, Lazarus KH, Macon WR, Gulley ML, Kjeldsberg CR. Natural killer like T cell lymphoma in the small intestine of a child without evidence of enteropathy. *Am J Surg Pathol* 1997;21:964–969.
252. Longacre TA, Listrom MB, Spigel JH, Willman CL, Dressler C, Clark D. Aggressive jejunal lymphoma of large granular lymphocytes. *Am J Clin Pathol* 1990;93:124–132.
253. Chott A, Dragosics B, Radaszkiewicz T. Peripheral T cell lymphomas of the intestine. *Am J Pathol* 1992;141:1361–1371.

Gastrointestinal Stromal Tumors

254. Morgan BK, Compton C, Talbert M, Gallagher WJ, Wood WE. Benign smooth muscle tumors of the gastrointestinal tract. A 24-year experience. *Ann Surg* 1990;211:63–66.
255. Dougherty MJ, Compton C, Talbert M, Wood WC. Sarcomas of the gastrointestinal tract. Separation into favorable and unfavorable prognostic groups by mitotic count. *Ann Surg* 1991;214:569–574.
256. Goldblum JR, Appleman HA. Stromal tumors of the duodenum. A histological study and immunohistochemical study of 20 cases. *Am J Surg Pathol* 1995;19:71–80.
257. Min KW. Small intestinal stromal tumors with skenoid fibers. *Am J Surg Pathol* 1992;16:145–155.
258. Suster S, Sorace D, Moran CA. Gastrointestinal stromal tumors with prominent myxoid matrix. Clinicopathologic, immunohistochemical, and ultrastructural study of nine cases of a distinctive morphological variant of myogenic stromal tumor. *Am J Surg Pathol* 1995;19:59–70.
259. Suster S, Fletcher CDM. Gastrointestinal stromal tumors with prominent signet ring features. *Mod Pathol* 1996;9:609–613.
260. Evans HL. Smooth muscle tumors of the gastrointestinal tract. A study of 56 cases followed for a minimum of 10 years. *Cancer* 1985;56:2242–2250.

261. Moyana TN, Friesen R, Tan LK. Colorectal smooth muscle tumors. A pathological study with immunohistochemistry and histomorphometry. *Arch Pathol Lab Med* 1991;115:1016–1021.
262. Haque S, Dean PJ. Stromal neoplasms of the rectum and anal canal. *Hum Pathol* 1992;23:762–767.
263. Saul SH, Rast ML, Brooks JJ. Immunohistochemistry of gastrointestinal stromal tumors. Evidence supporting an origin from smooth muscle. *Am J Surg Pathol* 1987;11:464–473.
264. Appleman HD. Smooth muscle tumors of the gastrointestinal tract. What we know now that Stout didn't know. *Am J Surg Pathol* 1986;10(suppl 1):83–99.
265. Miettinen M. Gastrointestinal stromal tumors. An immunohistochemical study of cellular differentiation. *Am J Clin Pathol* 1989;89:601–610.
266. Pike AM, Lloyd RV, Appleman HD. Cell markers in gastrointestinal stromal tumors. *Hum Pathol* 1988;19:830–834.
267. Miettinen M, Viralainen M, Rikala MS. Gastrointestinal stromal tumors—value of CD 34 antigen in their identification and separation of true leiomyomas amd schwannoma. *Am J Surg Pathol* 1995;19:207–216.
268. Tworek JA, Appleman HA, Singleton TP, Greenson JK. Stromal tumors of the jejunum and ileum. *Mod Pathol* 1997;10:200–209.
269. Van De Rijw M, Hendrickson MR, Rouse RV. CD 34 expression by gastrointestinal tract stromal tumors. *Hum Pathol* 1994;25:766–771.
270. Mikhael AI, Bacchi CE, Zarbo RJ, Ma CK, Gown AM. CD 34 expression in stromal tumors of the gastrointestinal tract. *Appl Immunohistochem* 1994;2:89–93.
270a. Kindblom L-G, Remotti HE, Aldenborg F and Meis-Kindblom JM. Gastrointestinal pacemaker cell tumor (GIPACT). Gastrointestinal stromal tumors show phenotypic characteristics of the interstitial cells of Cajal. *Am J Pathol* 1998;152:1259–1269.
271. Brainard JA, Goldblum JR. Stromal tumors of the jejunum and ileum. *Am J Surg Pathol* 1997;21:407–416.
272. Akwari OE, Dozois RR, Weiland LH, Beahrs OH. Leiomyosarcoma of the small and large bowel. *Cancer* 1978;42:1375–1384.
273. Franquemont DW. Differentiation and risk assessment of gastrointestinal stromal tumors. *Am J Clin Pathol* 1995;103:41–47.
274. Franquemont DW, Frierson HF. Proliferating cell nuclear antigen immunoreactivity and prognosis of gastrointestinal stromal tumors. *Mod Pathol* 1995;8:473–477.
275. Amin MB, Ma CK, Linden MD, Kuhns JJ, Zarbo RJ. Prognostic value of proliferating cell nuclear antigen in gastric stromal tumors. *Am J Clin Pathol* 1993;100:428–432.
276. Sbasching RJ, Cunningham RE, Sobin LH, O'Leary TJ. Proliferating-cell nuclear antigen immunocytochemistry in the evaluation of gastrointestinal smooth muscle tumors. *Mod Pathol* 1994;7:780–783.
277. Carrillo R, Candia A, Rodriguez-Peralto JL, Caz V. Prognostic significance of DNA ploidy and proliferative index (MIB-1 index) in gastrointestinal stromal tumors. *Hum Pathol* 1997;28:160–165.
278. El-Naggar AK, Ro JY, McLemore D, Garnsey L, Ordonez N, McKay B. Gastrointestinal stromal tumors: DNA flow-cytometric study of 58 patients with at least 5 years follow-up. *Mod Pathol* 1989;2:511–515.
279. Cooper PN, Quirke P, Hardy GJ. Dixon MF. A flow cytometric, clinical, and histological study of stromal neoplasms of the gastrointestinal tract. *Am J Surg Pathol* 1992;16:163–170.

Gastrointestinal Autonomic Nerve Tumors

280. Lauwers GY, Erlandson RA, Casper ES, Brennan MF, Woodruff JM. Gastrointestinal autonomic nerve tumors. A clinicopathological, immunohistochemical, and ultrastructural study of 12 cases. *Am J Surg Pathol* 1993;17:887–897.
281. Shanks JH, Harris M, Banerjee SS, Eyden BP. Gastrointestinal autonomic nerve tumors: a report of 9 cases. *Histopathology* 1996;29:111–121.
282. Ojanguren I, Ariza A, Navas-Palacious JJ. Gastrointestinal autonomic nerve tumor: further observations regarding an ultrastructural and immunohistochemical analysis of six cases. *Hum Pathol* 1996;27:1311–1318.
283. Herrera GA, Cevezo L, Jones JE, et al. Gastrointestinal autonomic nerve tumors: plexosarcomas. *Arch Pathol Lab Med* 1989;113:846–853.

Neurogenic Tumors

284. Daimaru Y, Kido H, Hashimoto H, Enjoji M. Benign schwannoma of the gastrointestinal tract. A clinicopathologic and immunohistochemical study. *Hum Pathol* 1988;19:257–264.
285. Sivak M, Sullivan BH, Farmer RG. Neurogenic tumors of the small intestine. Review of the literature and report of a case with endoscopic removal. *Gastroenterology* 1975;68:374–380.

Vascular Tumors

286. Taylor FJ, Templeton AC, Vogel CL, Ziegler JL, Kyalwazi SK. Kaposi's sarcoma in Uganda. A clinicopathological study. *Int J Cancer* 1971;8:122–135.
287. Liebman SL, Wright TL, Altman DF. Gastrointestinal Kaposi's sarcoma in patients with acquired immunodeficiency syndrome. Endoscopic and autopsy findings. *Gastroenterology* 1985;89:102–108.
288. Roth JA, Schell S, Panzarino S, Coronato A. Visceral Kaposi's sarcoma presenting as colitis. *Am J Surg Pathol* 1978;2:209–214.
289. Novis BH, King H, Bank S. Kaposi's sarcoma presenting with diarrhea and protein-losing enteropathy. *Gastroenterology* 1974;57:996–1000.
290. Thompson GB, Pemberton JH, Morri S, et al. Kaposi's sarcoma of the colon in a young HIV negative man with chronic ulcerative colitis. Report of a case. *Dis Colon Rectum* 1989;32:73–76.
291. Weber JN, Carmichael DJ, Boylston A, Monroe A, Whitear WP, Pinching AJ. Kaposi's sarcoma of the bowel presenting as apparent ulcerative colitis. *Gut* 1985;26:295–300.

Gangliocytic Paraganglioma

292. Reed RJ, Daroca PJ, Harkin JC. Gangliocytic paraganglioma. *Am J Surg Pathol* 1977;1:207–216.
293. Scheithauer BW, Nora FE, Lechago J, et al. Duodenal gangliocytic paraganglioma. Clinicopathologic and immunohistochemical study of 11 cases. *Am J Clin Pathol* 1986;86:559–565.
294. Burke AP, Helwig EB. Gangliocytic paraganglioma. *Am J Clin Pathol* 1989;92:1–9.
295. Dookhan DB, Miettinen M, Finkel G, Gibas Z. Recurrent duodenal gangliocytic paraganglioma with lymph node metastases. *Histopathology* 1993;22:399–401.
296. Inai K, Kobulce T, Yonehura S, Tokooka S. Duodenal gangliocytic paraganglioma with lymph node metastases. *Cancer* 1989;15:2540–2545.

Benign Conditions Mimicking Neoplasms

297. Spjut HJ, Perkins DE. Endometriosis of the sigmoid colon and rectum. *Am J Roentgenol* 1969;82:1070–1077.
298. Damjanov I, Katz SM. Malakoplakia. In: Sommers SC, Rosen PP, eds. *Pathology annual*, part 2. New York: Appleton-Century-Crofts, 1981:103–126.

Tumors Metastatic to the Intestines

299. Sachs B, Joffe N, Antonioli DA. Metastatic melanoma presenting clinically as multiple colonic polyps. *Am J Roentgenol* 1977;129:511–513.
300. Cornes JS, Jones TG. Leukemic lesions of the gastrointestinal tract. *J Clin Pathol* 1962;15:305–313.
301. Prolla JC, Kirsner JB. The gastrointestinal lesions and complications of the leukemics. *Ann Intern Med* 1964;61:1084–1103.

General Reference

302. Cooper HS. Benign polyps of the intestines. In: Ming SC, Goldman H, eds. *Pathology of the gastrointestinal tract,* 2nd ed. Baltimore: Williams & Wilkins, 1998.

CHAPTER 35

Pancreas

James E. Oertel, Yolanda C. Oertel, and Clara S. Heffess

ANATOMY AND ANOMALIES

Pancreatic primordia develop as outpouchings of the foregut (in close association with cells that will form the bile ducts and liver) designated as dorsal and ventral anlagen. As the gut rotates and becomes fixed, about the seventh week of gestation, the dorsal and ventral anlagen normally fuse to become a single gland (1–3). The ventral anlage becomes part of the head and the uncinate process; the dorsal anlage becomes the tail, body, and anterior part of the head. The principal pancreatic duct (Wirsung) is formed by fusion of the main dorsal duct in the body and tail with the segment of the ventral duct close to the duodenum. The accessory duct (Santorini) represents the persistence of the segment of the dorsal duct that lies next to the duodenum. Sometimes the dorsal duct does not fuse with the ventral duct, and pancreas divisum results (see below). The principal pancreatic duct and the common bile duct join in the papilla of Vater.

The pancreatic lobules are complex and composed principally of the exocrine elements (2–5). Acini occur alongside and at the ends of the smallest ducts; these ducts may run entirely through acini or end in acini. Therefore, an intercalated duct may lie between an acinus and an intralobular duct or between acini. Anastomoses between ducts are common. Consequently, many acini have several pathways for drainage. Although acini appear uniform in routine histologic preparations, animal studies suggest that they are heterogeneous (6).

In a manner similar to the acini, the developing islet cells arise from the embryonic ducts, beginning at about gestational age 9 weeks (7). In the newborn, the islets, individual islet cells, and mesenchyme constitute a larger part of the organ than in the adult; the acinar tissue continues to increase its relative proportion after birth (2). In the adult, most islets are round or ovoid with regular contours, except those in the posterior part of the head (from the ventral anlage), which are rich in cells producing pancreatic polypeptide. These islets are irregular in outline, and their cells tend to be arranged in trabecular patterns that are more conspicuous than in the islets of the rest of the gland (7,8). In adults, most islets of Langerhans are composed principally of insulin cells (about 70% of the total), except for those of the posterior part of the head. The glucagon cells (about 20%) are arranged around the outside of the islet and along sinusoids in the islet. Somatostatin cells constitute less than 10% of the islet cells. Pancreatic polypeptide cells are rare (except in the special islets of the head) and are found within islets and along the ducts. Serotonin cells are occasionally found along the ducts and rarely in islets.

Pancreatic anomalies include congenital cysts, abnormalities of the ducts, abnormal positions of pancreatic tissue, and accessory spleen in the organ (3,9). An anomaly can be confused with a neoplasm when it presents as an obstruction, pain, or a mass. Total agenesis of the pancreas has been reported in stillborn fetuses with multiple anomalies (9). Partial agenesis (short pancreas) is extremely rare.

Annular Pancreas

Annular pancreas is a rare congenital anomaly that can present (in adults as well as in children) with complete or partial obstruction of the duodenum (3,9,10). Presumably, it represents a failure of migration or rotation of the ventral pancreatic anlage combined with a relative overgrowth of part of the pancreas. Morphologically normal pancreatic tissue encircles the duodenum. It may be associated with other anomalies, such as malformation of other abdominal viscera and Down syndrome. Complications may occur, such as peptic ulceration, acute or chronic pancreatitis, and common duct obstruction.

J. E. Oertel and C. S. Heffess: Armed Forces Institute of Pathology, Washington, DC 20306.

Y. C. Oertel: Department of Pathology, George Washington University School of Medicine and Health Sciences, Washington, DC 20037.

Heterotopic Pancreas

Ectopic pancreatic tissue may occur from displacement of small amounts of pancreas during embryologic development, resulting in the formation of a nodule independent of the pancreas but with a proper ductal system and circulation (3,9). It may be symptomatic (obstruction, ulceration), but the majority of cases are incidental findings. The tissue is found most frequently in the stomach, duodenum, and jejunum (usually in the submucosa), but other locations are possible, such as Meckel's diverticulum, the umbilicus, and the mediastinum. If the ectopic tissue is large enough to be seen upon gross inspection, it appears as a firm, pale, nodular mass. The classical example is composed of acini, islets, and ductal structures with the usual lobular architecture, but either ducts or acini may predominate in an abnormal fashion.

Pancreatic acini may be found in the gastric mucosa, and have been studied particularly at the gastroesophageal junction (11). Occasionally, pancreatic tissue occurs as part of a teratoma.

Pancreas Divisum

A congenital anomaly of uncertain significance, pancreas divisum occurs in 3% to 10% of the population (3,9,12). The major ducts of the dorsal and ventral components fail to fuse. The tail, the body, and the superior-anterior part of the head are drained by the dorsal duct (Santorini) through the accessory or minor papilla. The posterior-inferior part of the head is drained by a short, narrow Wirsung duct that joins the bile duct at the papilla of Vater. A few patients with pancreas divisum have recurrent attacks of pain and bouts of acute pancreatitis, which can lead (although rarely) to chronic fibrosing pancreatitis (13). The diagnosis of pancreas divisum is usually made by imaging studies undertaken because of abdominal pain or bouts of acute pancreatitis.

Anomalous junction of the pancreatic and common bile ducts and choledochal cysts are discussed in the chapter by Saul, "Gallbladder and Extrahepatic Biliary Tree."

COMMON MINOR ABNORMALITIES

The adult pancreas decreases in weight with advancing age (3,14,15). Fatty replacement (lipomatosis) is a common phenomenon with increasing age, but this process tends to increase the weight of the gland (16). Marked fatty replacement is associated with severe generalized atherosclerosis and type II diabetes mellitus.

Focal fibrosis, usually of unknown etiology, is another finding that may increase with age (14) and accompanies diabetes mellitus (17). The pancreata of elderly individuals often contain focal or relatively diffuse fibrosis. Minor focal chronic inflammation is another common occurrence and is often present in regions of fibrosis. Diffuse inflammatory infiltrates tend to be associated with major bacterial infections elsewhere in the body (14).

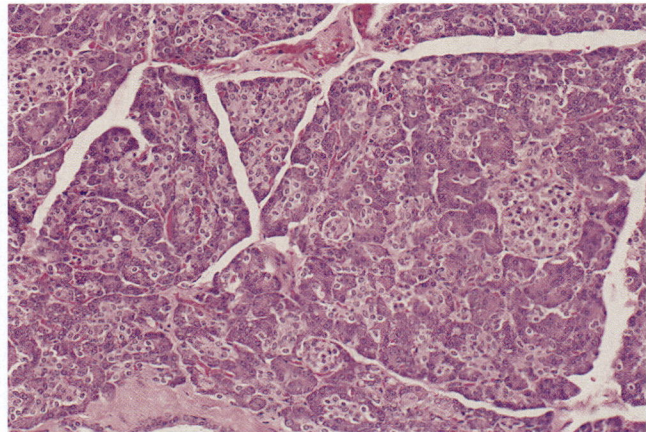

FIG. 1. Proliferation of centroacinar cells and intercalated duct cells with some reduction in the number of acinar cells.

Centroacinar cells and intercalated ductal cells may be increased in numbers (8), either because of proliferation of these cells or transformation of acinar cells into these cells (Fig. 1). Such changes may be found (a) in some cases of recent ductal obstruction, (b) in instances of acute ethanol abuse, (c) sometimes in chronic pancreatitis (18), and (d) in association with hyperinsulinemia and hypergastrinemia (19,20).

Altered acinar cells are found with moderate frequency when multiple sections of pancreas are evaluated (Fig. 2). Acinar dilatation (acinar ectasia) is rare in surgical specimens (21) and has been related to uremia, dehydration, and severe bacterial infections (14,22). *Eosinophilic degeneration of acini, focal acinar cell dysplasia,* and *localized acinar cytopathology* are terms used by various authors to describe a variety of abnormalities apparently having various causes. (a) The most common change consists of small

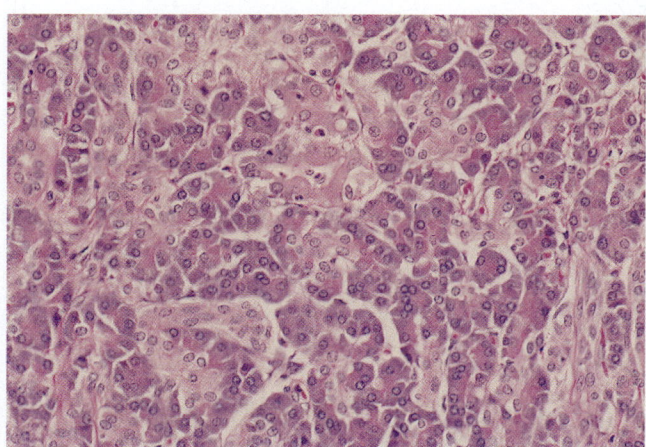

FIG. 2. Pancreatic parenchyma near a neoplasm with partial obstruction. In the superior central part of the figure several acini appear dilated with general loss of zymogen granules.

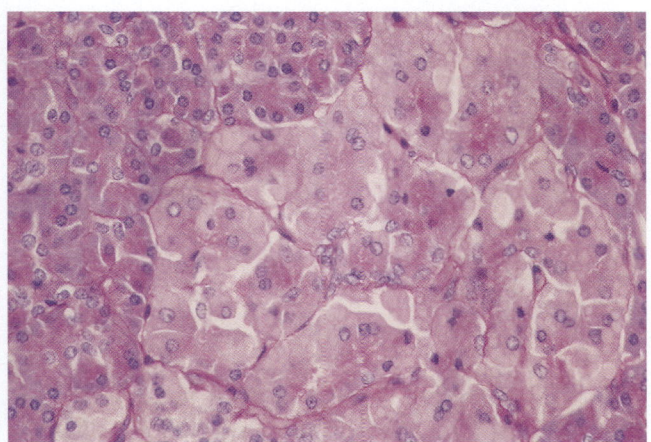

FIG. 3. A group of altered acinar cells with reduction in the zymogen granules and central location of the nuclei. Several pyknotic nuclei are present.

groups of cells having less cytoplasm than normal, with variably reduced basophilia (ribosomes) and zymogen granules. Nuclei are variably placed (often central), often smaller, and appear condensed (even pyknotic in some cells) (Fig. 3). Cytoplasmic vacuolation (dilated endoplasmic reticulum) may occur and occasionally is marked (23). Depending on the cytoplasmic contents, cells are slightly basophilic or slightly eosinophilic. The pallor of the cytoplasm may cause the groups of altered acinar cells to be mistaken for islets of Langerhans (14,23). These changes are probably retrogressive, but may be reversible. (b) Less commonly, there are groups of slightly enlarged acinar cells filled with zymogen granules and with virtually no cytoplasmic basophilia. Rare vacuoles occur in the cytoplasm. Nuclei appear normal and are basal (8,24). This alteration could represent an abnormal acinar secretory mechanism. (c) Cells vary in size with some cells smaller than usual, but they have nuclei that are normal to slightly enlarged (Fig. 4). Occasional nuclei are considerably larger or irregular in shape. The number of zymogen granules and the degree of cytoplasmic basophilia are variable. These findings might represent abnormal proliferations (25,26).

Altered acini have been noted incidentally in a wide variety of disorders, both intrapancreatic and extrapancreatic, including alcoholism and pancreatic endocrine excess (19,24). Heavy cigarette smoking and chemotherapy have been associated with the acinar changes just discussed, especially the dysplastic nuclear alterations (25,27,28).

Dilatation of the major ducts and of tiny peripheral ducts (with inspissated secretions common in the latter) occurs fairly frequently in older individuals (14). Dilated minor ducts tend to be associated with fibrosis. Enlargement of ductal epithelial cells (29,30) may occur by acquiring large amounts of lightly eosinophilic cytoplasm (extra-tall epithelial cells).

Multilayered ductal epithelial metaplasia, focal or widespread (including characteristic squamous metaplasia) (Fig. 5) (1,30) may be present in medium-sized and large ducts in normal pancreata (occasionally) and in chronic pancreatitis. This change may include focal epithelial hyperplasia. There does not appear to be any significant association with carcinoma (1).

Tubular complexes are probably the same as tubular accumulation, ductular or tubular hyperplasia, ductular metaplasia, adenomatous hyperplasia of small ducts, and focal pseudoproliferation of small ducts, with or without mucous cell hypertrophy (or pyloric gland metaplasia). They probably represent metaplastic acini (31). The change is noted most often in chronic pancreatitis and in acute pancreatitis undergoing healing.

Columnar cells with increased amounts of supranuclear mucus-rich cytoplasm (mucinous cell hyperplasia, goblet-cell metaplasia) (Fig. 6) (25,32) may occur with increased age, in chronic pancreatitis, after large doses of adrenal steroids, and in association with pancreatic ductal carcinomas; they are found most often in ducts of the head, rarely in

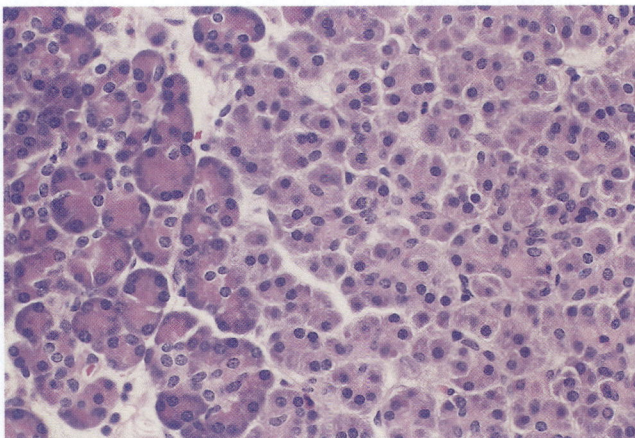

FIG. 4. Acinar cells have less cytoplasm than normal, do not have many zymogen granules, and have hyperchromatic nuclei.

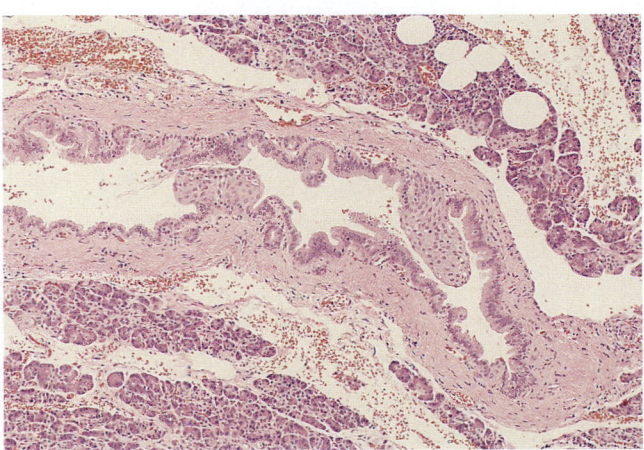

FIG. 5. Focal squamous metaplasia in an interlobular duct.

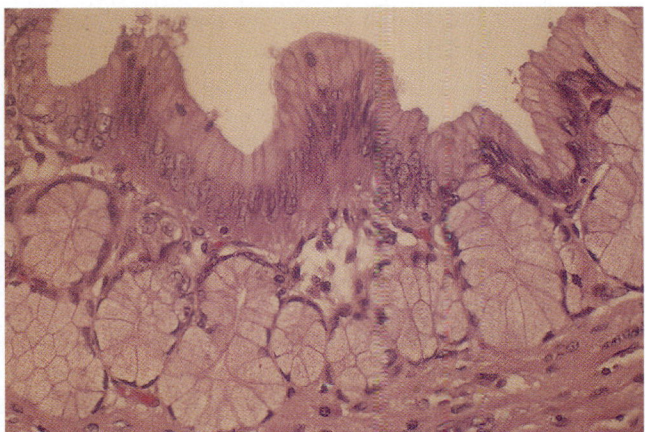

FIG. 6. The columnar cells have undergone mucinous metaplasia. Goblet cells have replaced the normal cells in the pouches along this large duct.

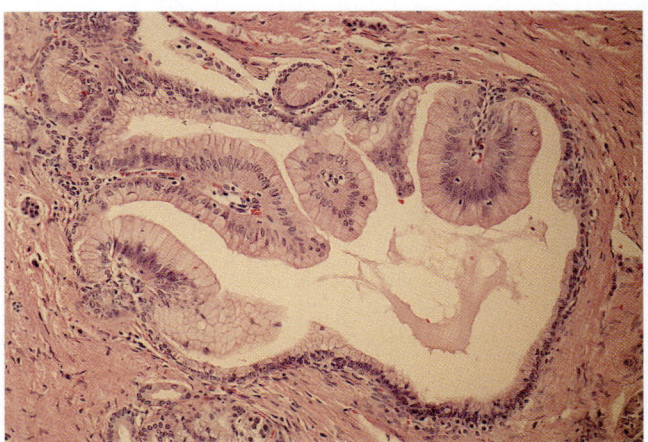

FIG. 8. Papillary hyperplasia with mucinous metaplasia.

acini (Fig. 7). This change may be called pyloric gland metaplasia, having mucus that is periodic acid-Schiff (PAS) positive and alcian blue negative at pH 2.5 (i.e., neutral mucin) (33). A considerable proportion of these cells may contain the K-*ras* oncogene (34,35).

Pseudopapillary and papillary hyperplasia (30,33) of the ductal epithelium occurs in medium-sized and large ducts, and is variably reported with aging, chronic pancreatitis, diabetes mellitus, and ductal carcinoma (Fig. 8). Ductal obstruction for any reason seems to predispose to these alterations (33). Mucinous cell hyperplasia usually accompanies the papillary formations. Atypical epithelium (33) and especially atypical papillary epithelial hyperplasia (Figs. 9 and 10) are uncommon in the normal pancreas and in chronic pancreatitis (30), except for minor degrees of atypia. When these alterations occur, they may represent first steps in the hyperplasia-dysplasia–carcinoma *in situ* sequence. The K-*ras* mutation is common in such cells.

Large islets may occur in the pancreata of middle-aged and elderly persons; the authors believe they are more common in the body and tail. The largest islets tend to have a

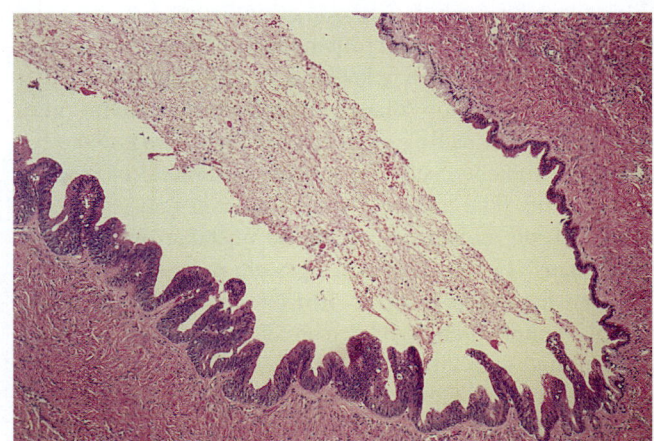

FIG. 9. Atypical pseudopapillary and papillary hyperplasia. Note abrupt transition from normal ductal epithelium.

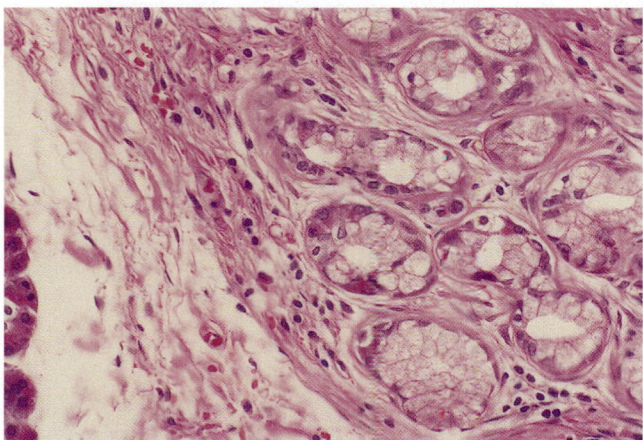

FIG. 7. Goblet cells have replaced a majority of acinar cells.

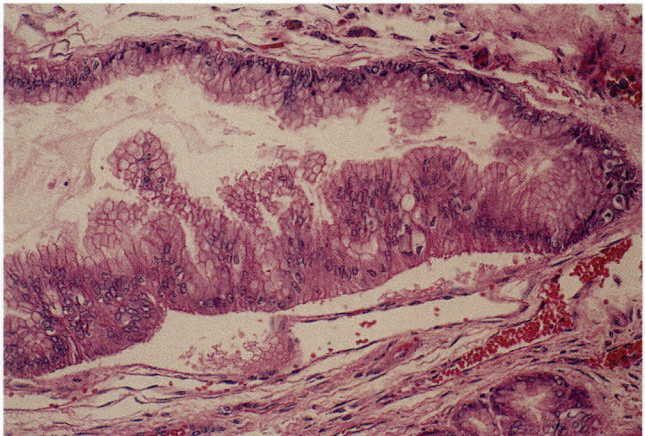

FIG. 10. Atypical pseudopapillary and papillary hyperplasia. The transition from the normal epithelium is more gradual.

greater proportion of noninsulin cells than do normal islets. Another change occasionally evident is selective congestion and dilatation (peliosis) of the vessels of the islets without marked congestion of the vessels elsewhere in the lobules.

DIAGNOSTIC TECHNIQUES

Fine-needle aspiration (FNA) is the diagnostic method of choice at any institution where an experienced cytopathologist is available. It is more likely to provide an accurate diagnosis than core-needle biopsy or wedge biopsy of abnormal pancreatic tissue (36). Thin needles can penetrate deeply into the organ with relative ease and allow multiple samples to be obtained (37). Most core-needle biopsies are performed at laparotomy, whereas many FNAs are performed percutaneously with guidance by imaging techniques (38–40). Recently, endoscopic ultrasound-guided FNA is advocated as safer than percutaneous aspiration (41–43). FNAs under direct visualization at surgery (44,45) (regardless of the reason for the abdominal operation) have the advantages of considerable accuracy (44–47), very rare complications (44,45), and faster diagnosis. Hence, we advocate their use rather than frozen sections of wedge biopsies or needle biopsies. In cachectic patients with a palpable mass, a direct aspiration through the abdominal wall without imaging guidance is possible.

Inadequate samples result from failure to master these deceptively simple techniques. Common problems in wedge biopsies and in core-needle biopsies are crushing or otherwise distorting the tissues, failure to obtain enough tissue for adequate interpretation, and the frequent presence of chronic pancreatitis obscuring the ductal carcinoma. Difficulties with FNA result from missing the lesion because of improper localization and/or incorrect placement of the needle (44,46), applying too much suction (which causes bleeding, dilutes the sample, and interferes with further sampling), using too long a needle (which bends, misses the target, and makes the procedure awkward), and utilizing a needle larger than 22-gauge.

The interpretation of aspirates requires that the pathologist be acquainted with the appearance of the following normal cells:

- Acinar cells (Fig. 11) are arranged in small groups or clusters, resembling rosettes, and sometimes may show a central lumen but otherwise indistinct cellular borders. They have a moderate amount of cytoplasm (finely granular and with few vacuoles) and small, round, regular nuclei with visible nucleoli.
- Ductal cells (Fig. 12) are arranged in monolayers of over 50 nuclei. These nuclei are smaller and have denser chromatin than those of acinar cells; nucleoli are not evident, and the cytoplasm is scanty. The cells appear tightly packed and in a honeycomb arrangement.
- Mesothelial cells (Fig. 13) may be a source of false-positive diagnosis. They have a distinctive pattern at low magnification, appearing as large sheets or monolayers of cells

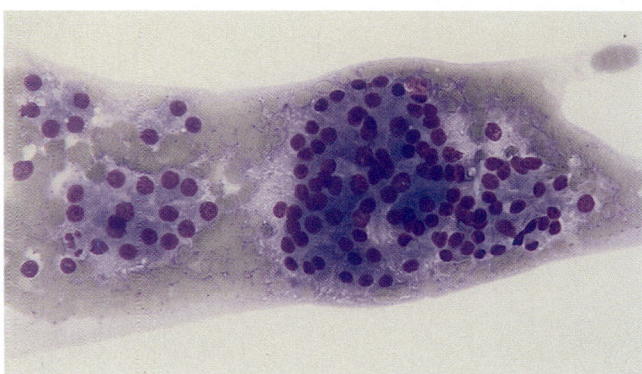

FIG. 11. Fine-needle aspiration (FNA): acinar cells and many red blood cells (RBCs) in the background. Note glandular arrangement (rosettes).

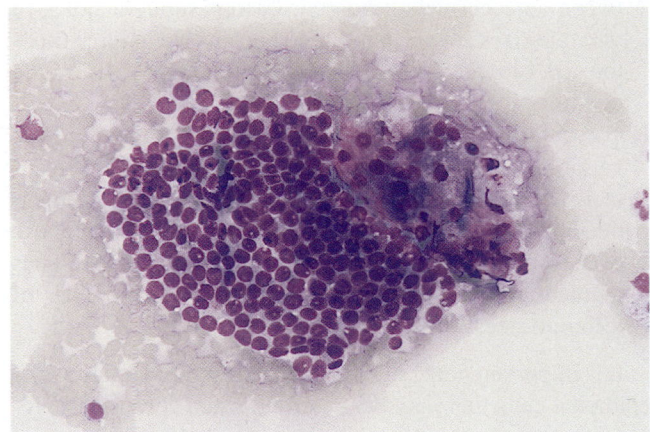

FIG. 12. FNA: Large sheet of ductal cells and small clusters of acinar cells on the right.

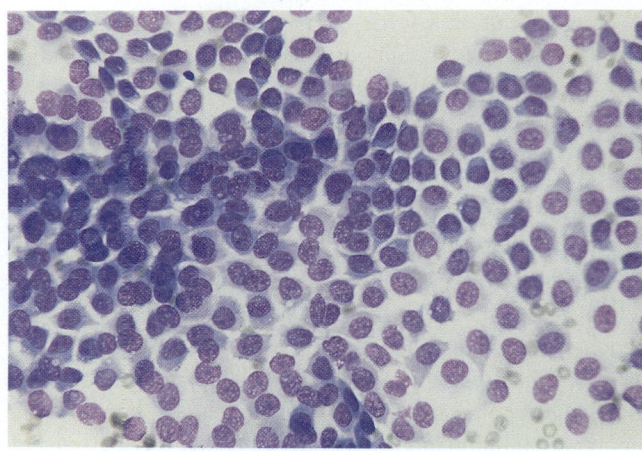

FIG. 13. FNA: Sheet of loosely cohesive mesothelial cells.

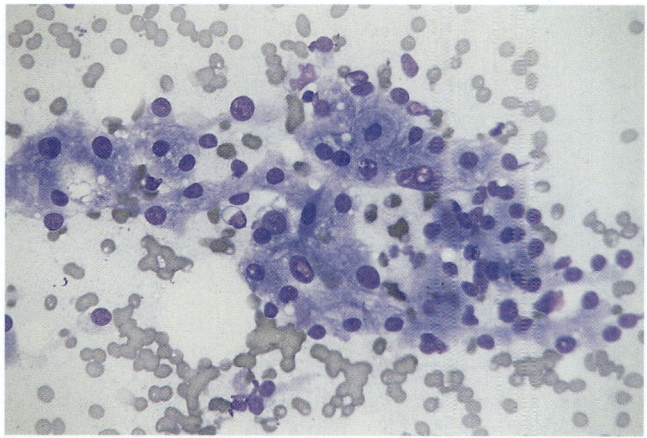

FIG. 14. FNA: Hepatocytes with some variation in nuclear size and cytoplasmic vacuoles.

with moderate amounts of bluish cytoplasm and well-demarcated cell borders. Frequently, slits or separations between adjacent cells are seen. Cytoplasmic vacuoles of variable sizes are present. Large nuclei (two to three times the size of ductal-cell nuclei) and prominent nucleoli are common.

Hepatocytes (Fig. 14) are arranged in groups and cords of variable sizes and also are seen as single cells or naked nuclei. There is more variation in nuclear size than in acinar, ductal, or mesothelial cells. Nucleoli are larger than those of mesothelial cells. The abundant cytoplasm usually has pigment granules (either bile or iron) and/or vacuoles of different sizes.

It is important not to overdiagnose the minor alterations of epithelial cells that may be identified when chronic pancreatitis is present (46). In addition to its considerable success in separating ductal carcinomas from benign lesions, aspiration cytology has allowed the recognition of other pancreatic neoplasms and has provided cells for histochemical, ultrastructural, and DNA studies (48).

PANCREATIC TRANSPLANTATIONS

Transplantation of the pancreas has been attempted mostly in young to middle-aged adults afflicted with insulin-dependent diabetes mellitus (49). Needle biopsies of the graft (50,51) and cytologic studies of pancreatic juice drained from the graft (52) have been utilized to evaluate the transplanted tissue. Immediately after surgery, grafts are altered by interstitial edema, mild acinar cell injury, and a slight infiltrate of neutrophils and lymphocytes. Later, even in syngeneic grafts, there are frequent sparse inflammatory cell infiltrates (mostly lymphocytes) of the acinar tissue, loss of acinar cells, fibrosis, and slight ductal alterations (inflammation, dilatation, and some cellular atypia). In allogeneic grafts undergoing rejection, there are patchy lymphocytic and mixed inflammatory infiltrates in acinar tissue, frequent ductal inflammation and cellular atypia, acinar cell loss, in-

terstitial fibrosis, and vascular changes. The latter consist of endothelialitis of capillaries and venules and occasional fibrinoid necrosis in vessels. In chronic rejection, endarteritis, fibrointimal proliferation, and accumulations of foam cells may narrow or occlude vessels. Acute pancreatitis, which may occur early or late in the graft (53), has neutrophilic infiltrates, necrosis of acinar cells, and fat necrosis. As time passes, a successful graft may be affected by the process leading to type I diabetes mellitus. The islets are infiltrated by mononuclear cells (predominantly T lymphocytes), insulin cells decrease in number, and there is a substantial relative increase in glucagon cells.

INFLAMMATORY CONDITIONS

Acute Pancreatitis

Acute pancreatitis has been associated with biliary tract disease (especially gallstones), abuse of ethanol, ischemia, systemic shock, various drugs, pancreatic trauma, hypercalcemia, hyperlipidemia, infections, and hereditary factors, to name several recognized conditions (3). Dynamic contrast-enhanced computed tomography for detection of necrosis, the use of percutaneous needle aspiration, and the development of more precise terminology of each patient's status have enhanced the understanding and management of acute pancreatitis (54). Nevertheless, the process may be difficult to separate from chronic pancreatitis. The surgical pathologist rarely receives tissue, but an occasional pancreatic biopsy or partial resection of damaged tissue is performed. The gross appearance ranges from a slightly swollen, wet, firm organ to hemorrhagic and/or necrotic tissue. Fat necrosis is manifested as grayish-yellow plaques and nodules in extrapancreatic and intrapancreatic adipose tissue.

Histologic features vary with the severity of the process (55). In relatively common, mild pancreatitis (56), the interstitial fibrous tissue, adipose tissue, and pancreatic parenchyma are edematous and contain scattered acute inflammatory cells. Limited fat necrosis may be present in and around the gland (Fig. 15). The pancreatic acini adjacent to the fat necrosis often are dilated, and some acinar cells are necrotic. Because changes in edematous (or interstitial) pancreatitis are most marked in the fibrous and adipose tissues, and much of the pancreatic parenchyma is preserved (although altered), a substantial reconstitution of normal structure and function is possible, provided the acute attack is only minimally destructive.

Interstitial pancreatitis has been detected without any known symptoms or signs of pancreatic inflammation during the patient's life (57–59). Edema and neutrophils and/or lymphocytes are present in the connective tissue. Focal fat necrosis is occasionally present.

When severe pancreatitis is present, marked hemorrhage, panlobular coagulative necrosis, and extensive fat necrosis occur (55,60,61). A layer of neutrophilic leukocytes lies in the region between the intact tissues and the necrosis, and thrombi are common in capillaries and venules in this same

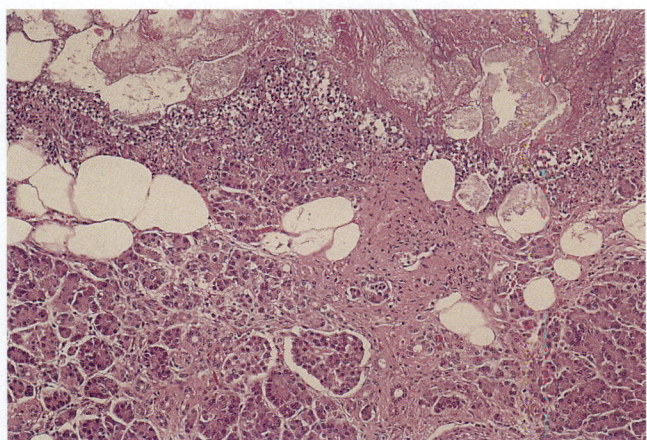

FIG. 15. Acute pancreatitis. Necrotic adipose tissue and damaged pancreatic parenchyma contain inflammatory cells. Intact pancreas lies in the lower part of the figure.

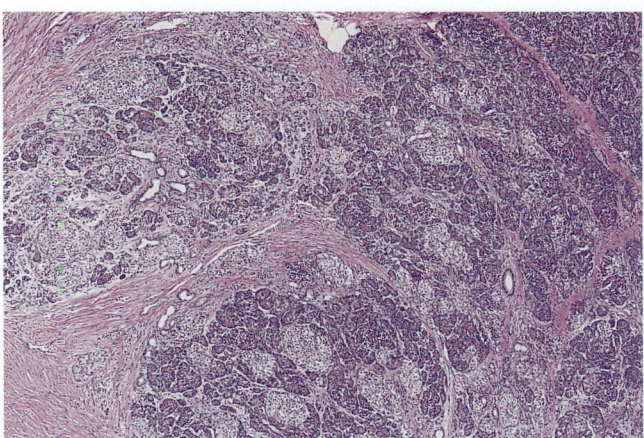

FIG. 17. Chronic pancreatitis. Considerable loss of acinar tissue has caused islets to lie close together.

region. Some of the intact pancreatic acini adjacent to the necrotic tissues are dilated, contain inspissated secretions, and have flattened cells with smaller and fewer zymogen granules (62).

Intraductal and periductal inflammation, ductal dilatation, and ductal disruption have been described, but many ducts are intact. It is possible that these changes occur more often in cases of acute exacerbation of chronic pancreatitis than in acute pancreatitis. Viral or bacterial pancreatitis may be manifest by necrosis of individual acinar cells (55).

Major anatomic complications of acute pancreatitis are acute fluid collections lacking a wall, acute pseudocysts (possess a wall of granulation tissue and occur after 4 weeks), abscesses near the pancreas, extensive hemorrhages, thrombi in large vessels near the pancreas, and fat necrosis in distant sites.

Chronic Pancreatitis

Chronic pancreatitis, whether predominantly focal, segmental, or diffuse, is difficult to define but is of interest to the surgical pathologist because it simulates a pancreatic neoplasm on gross examination or because a neoplasm often is accompanied by chronic pancreatitis. Ingestion of ethanol and ductal obstruction by calculi are the most common etiologies in much of the world (Fig. 16) (55). Malnutrition and environmental factors probably cause the disorder in some tropical countries (63,64). All larger series of patients with chronic pancreatitis include those with idiopathic pancreatitis, which indicates the need for more research. Other uncommon types include hereditary familial pancreatitis (65) and primary sclerosing cholangitis with pancreatic involvement (66). Continuing exposure to ethanol probably leads from acute pancreatitis to progressive chronic pancreatitis (67); this process does not occur in all patients.

In chronic nonobstructive pancreatitis, fibrosis, inflammation, and acinar atrophy are unevenly distributed, with some lobules almost untouched and others more markedly involved (Figs. 17 and 18) (55). Even in advanced disease, the lobular pattern of the organ tends to be visible. The extent of the chronic inflammatory infiltrates is variable, and such in-

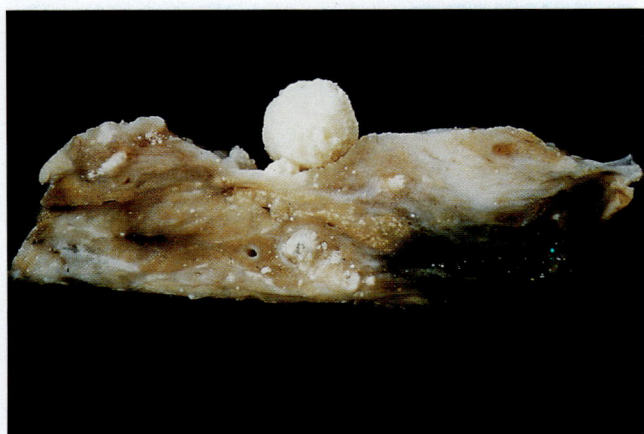

FIG. 16. Chronic pancreatitis. A calculus lies in a fibrotic duct.

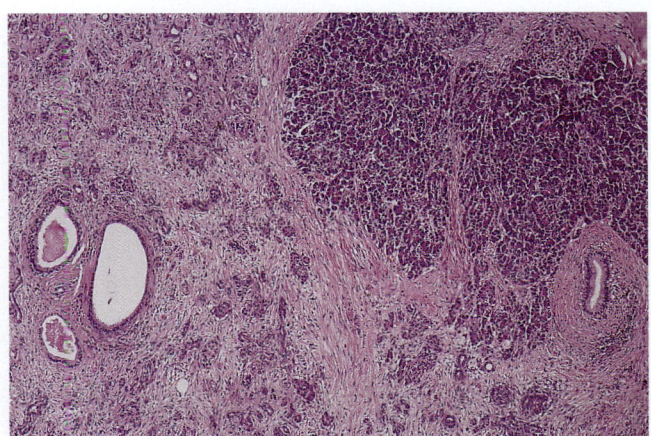

FIG. 18. Chronic pancreatitis. Acinar atrophy and fibrosis are unevenly distributed. Two of the dilated ducts contain inspissated secretions.

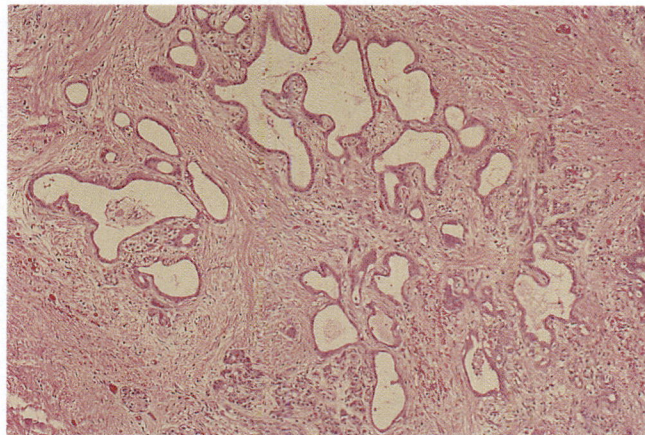

FIG. 19. Chronic pancreatitis. There is marked loss of acini; fibrosis is extensive; and remaining ducts are irregularly dilated and distorted.

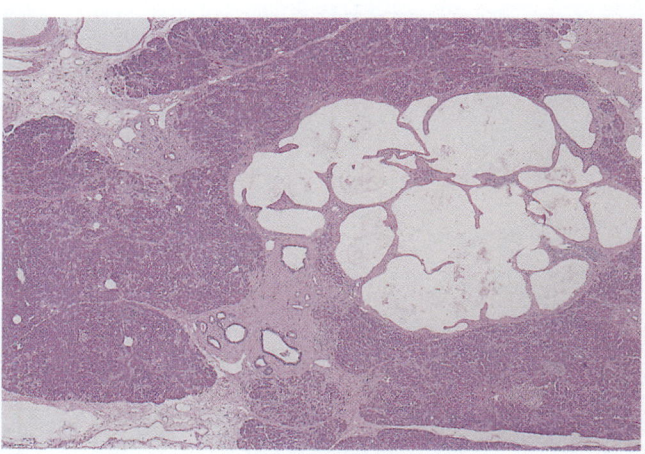

FIG. 21. Chronic pancreatitis. Dilated ducts have flattened epithelium and contain some inspissated secretions.

filtrates can be minor. Intrapancreatic nerves are increased in number and diameter. Fibrosis (periductal, intralobular, and interlobular) is a major feature but is variable in amount and distribution (Figs. 19 and 20) (68). Part or all of the organ is enlarged and hard. In late stages of the disease, the pancreas is shrunken and distorted.

The normal ductal pattern is altered variably by deletion, stricture, and dilatation (Figs. 18–21) (55,69). In alcoholic and idiopathic pancreatitis, protein-rich secretions (often calcified) plug many small ducts and ductules; well-developed calculi of various sizes frequently occur; and the adjacent ductal epithelium undergoes metaplasia, atrophies, or disappears (Fig. 21). Many small ducts are dilated; marked ectasia of even the smallest ducts is evident in some lobules. Groups of tiny ducts may be present (30) and probably are the result of several factors: the loss of zymogen granules and reduction in the height of acinar cells (formation of tubular complexes) (31); possible loss of acinar cells; the persistence of ductular-ductular and ductular-acinar anastomoses; and possible proliferation of cells of the smallest ducts. Saccular dilatations of larger ducts are common and are visible upon radiologic examination or gross inspection. Pseudocysts are identified in and adjacent to the pancreas (70).

Alterations in the ductal epithelium are frequent: epithelial hyperplasia (including pseudopapillary and papillary hyperplasia) (Figs. 8 and 9), mucus-cell metaplasia (pyloric gland metaplasia), squamous metaplasia (Fig. 5), atrophy, and local ulcerations. Epithelial atypia, when present, is usually minor (Figs. 9 and 10). Nuclei usually are small. Mitotic figures in ducts are rare.

Aspirates from pancreatitis (acute and/or chronic) show many acinar cells, a mixture of inflammatory cells (neutrophilic leukocytes, lymphocytes, plasma cells, and histiocytes), and a few sheets of ductal cells (71).

The islets of Langerhans are relatively resistant to chronic pancreatitis in comparison with the pancreatic acini (72,73). As acini disappear and fibrosis and fatty infiltration occur, the lobules collapse; the islets tend to be concentrated together, thereby causing them to be more conspicuous (Fig. 17). Some islet-cell proliferation can occur (Fig. 22). Many

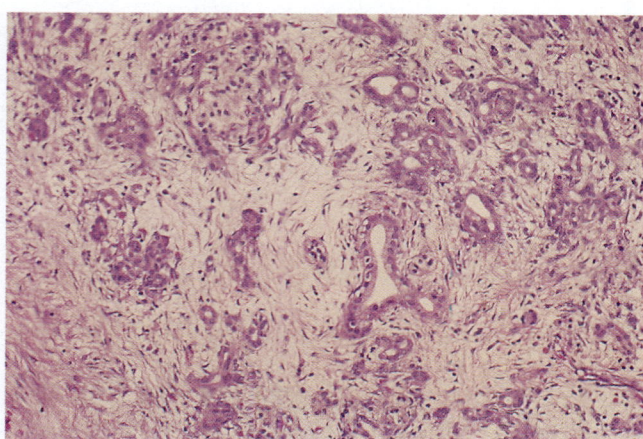

FIG. 20. Chronic pancreatitis. Marked loss of acini and abundant loose connective tissue with scattered inflammatory cells.

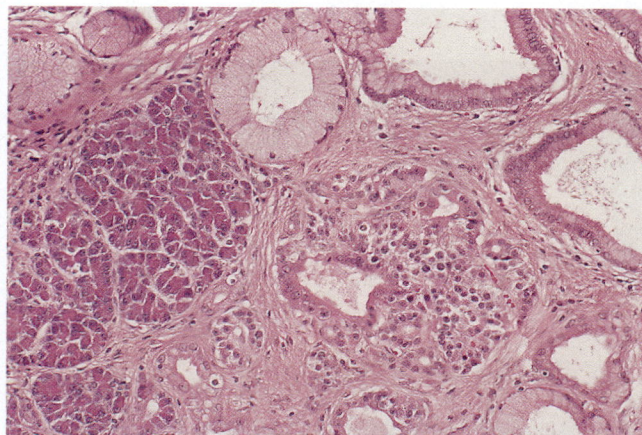

FIG. 22. Chronic pancreatitis. Islet cells are closely related to several tiny ducts (neo-islet formation). Fibrosis and goblet cell metaplasia are also evident.

islets are surrounded by fibroadipose tissue and become atrophic. As the process progresses, the insulin cells are reduced in number, and glucagon cells are proportionately increased. A larger number of pancreatic polypeptide cells has been reported in chronic pancreatitis (72,74). Eventually there is a substantial loss of the endocrine elements.

When chronic pancreatitis results from obstruction of a major pancreatic duct, the affected tissue is evenly involved, the process typically is less severe, and the ductal epithelium is less altered than in chronic calcifying pancreatitis. Intraductal proteinaceous plugs and small calculi are rare (often absent). The process may be more marked in the head than elsewhere in the gland or may involve only one group of lobules, depending on the location of the obstruction.

Any pancreatic neoplasm can obstruct ducts, thereby favoring the development of pancreatitis in part of the gland, and this inflammation and fibrosis in turn make recognition of the neoplasm more difficult. The fibrosis and calculi that occur in many cases of chronic pancreatitis not only obstruct the ducts of the pancreas but may block the biliary tree. If the resultant jaundice is accompanied by marked fibrosis of the pancreatic head, both the surgeon and the pathologist find it difficult to exclude the presence of carcinoma.

Other Inflammatory Diseases

Specific infectious and parasitic diseases sometimes involve the pancreas (3), and these have the pathologic features expected for the particular organism. In the immunosuppressed patient, opportunistic infections can involve the pancreas. Vasculitis of various etiologies sometimes occurs, causing pain and enlargement, which might lead to a segmental resection of the part that appears most abnormal.

Nonspecific granulomata of chronic pancreatitis should not be mistaken for sarcoidosis or mycobacterial or fungal disease (75).

EXOCRINE NEOPLASMS

Ductal Adenocarcinoma

Clinical Features

Most cancers of the pancreas are ductal adenocarcinomas (1,3,76), of which about two-thirds involve the head, with the remainder in the body and tail (Fig. 23) (77,78). In a few instances the entire gland appears to be involved (79). Usually there is only a single focus, but in a few patients there are multiple foci (either multicentric origin or intraglandular spread). The patients are usually over 50 years of age; the disease occurs somewhat more often in men. Rarely, the patient is under 40 years. Pain, jaundice, and loss of weight are the most common manifestations. Carcinoma in the head commonly causes painless obstructive jaundice. Carcinoma of the body and tail tends to extend to the peritoneum, the spleen, the stomach, and the left adrenal; pain and weight loss are common (77). A few patients with pancreatic cancer

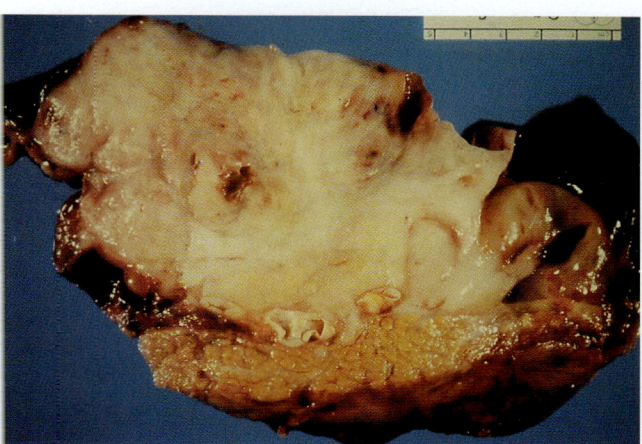

FIG. 23. Ductal adenocarcinoma. A pale, fleshy mass protrudes from the tail of the pancreas.

have a recent onset of diabetes mellitus. Metastases to lymph nodes and the liver are common, regardless of the location of the primary focus or the size of the neoplasm (76).

Pathologic Features

Ductal carcinomas usually grow rapidly and are discovered after they have already spread beyond the pancreas. Cures are rare. For the pathologist, the principal problems relate to distinguishing ductal adenocarcinoma from chronic pancreatitis and from other pancreatic neoplasms that have a less grave prognosis. Chronic inflammation and fibrosis accompany ductal adenocarcinoma (79,80), and any pancreatic neoplasm that obstructs a principal duct may cause ductal dilatation, parenchymal atrophy, and fibrosis, thereby confusing the gross anatomical findings and, possibly, the microscopic features (3) (Table 1).

On gross examination, ductal carcinoma usually appears as a poorly defined, pale, hard mass (Fig. 23), often accompanied by enlarged lymph nodes and/or metastatic masses in the liver (1,3). Occasionally the cancer presents as a scar.

When tissue sections are examined at low magnification, the pathologist can appreciate that the neoplastic structures are arranged with little regard to the lobular architecture of the gland (Fig. 24). This finding contrasts with chronic pancreatitis, in which partial preservation of the lobular architecture is common. Ductal carcinoma is characterized by atypical cells forming irregular, often incomplete, often complex, tubular or glandular structures, usually accompanied by dense stroma (Figs. 24 and 25) (1,3,76). Many cells and their nuclei are much larger than those of normal ducts, and the nuclear-cytoplasmic ratio is biased toward the nuclei. Variation in the shape and size of the nuclei is common (Figs. 26–28). Conspicuous nucleoli are frequently present, and mitotic figures are usually easy to find. The cellular arrangement is often haphazard (the cells' polarity is disturbed), no definite basement membrane is present around the epithelial structures, and isolated atypical cells (presumably neoplastic) are visible in the stroma. Sometimes the

TABLE 1. *Comparison between chronic pancreatitis and ductal adenocarcinoma*

	Chronic pancreatitis	Ductal adenocarcinoma
Distribution of lesions	Focal, segmental, or diffuse	Most common in head
Gross appearance	Irregular scarring; ductal cysts; stones	Hard, poorly demarcated solitary mass
Light-microscopic features	Irregular atrophy; fibrosis; chronic inflammation of variable degree, with preservation of basic lobular architecture	Neoplastic tubules or glands formed by atypical columnar or cuboidal cells, with dense fibrous stroma
	Ductal dilatation; protein plugs and intraductal calcifications in some cases	Variable mucin production
	Atrophy, hyperplasia, and metaplasia of ductal epithelium with minimal atypia	Large, irregular nuclei; conspicuous nucleoli; frequent mitoses
		Necrotic cells in some glands or tubules
Islets of Langerhans	No alterations (early stages)	Minor abnormalities
	Abnormal (late stages)	
Associated lesions	Pseudocysts	Chronic obstructive pancreatitis

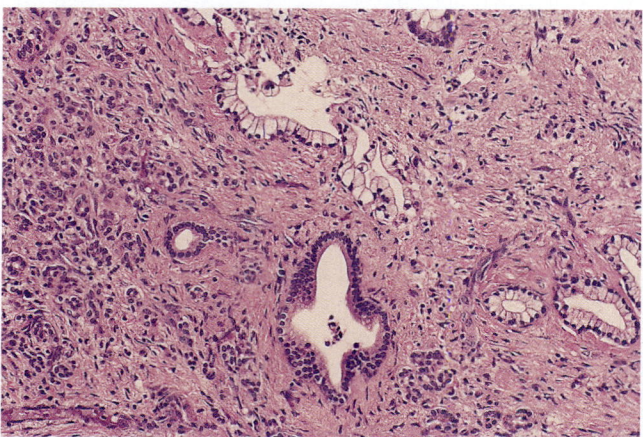

FIG. 24. Ductal adenocarcinoma and chronic pancreatitis. The well-differentiated clear cell ductal adenocarcinoma contrasts with the nonneoplastic tissue *(inferior and to the left)*.

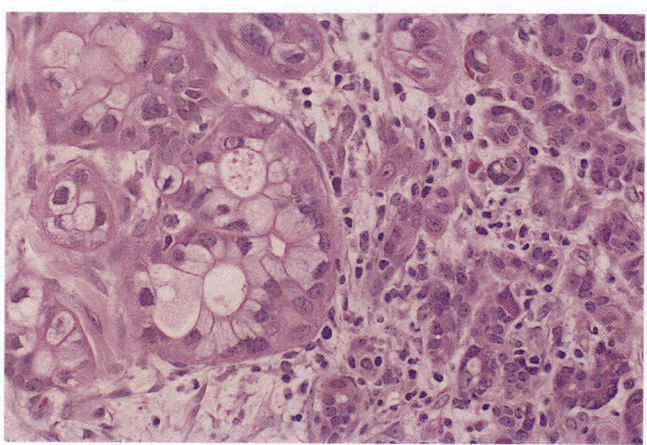

FIG. 26. Ductal adenocarcinoma, well differentiated. The cancer occupies the *left* side of the field.

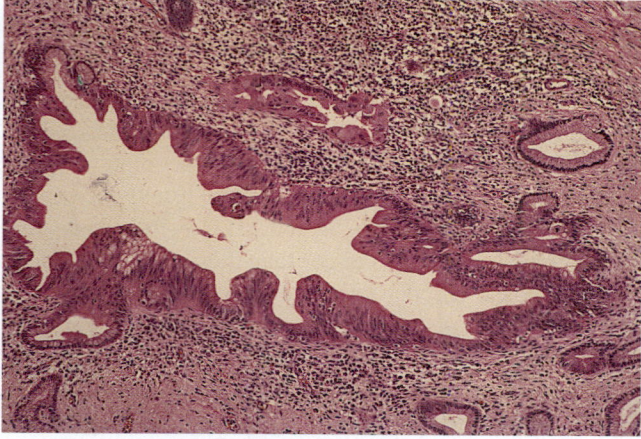

FIG. 25. Ductal adenocarcinoma and chronic pancreatitis. A focus of cancer lies above the major duct lined by atypical epithelium.

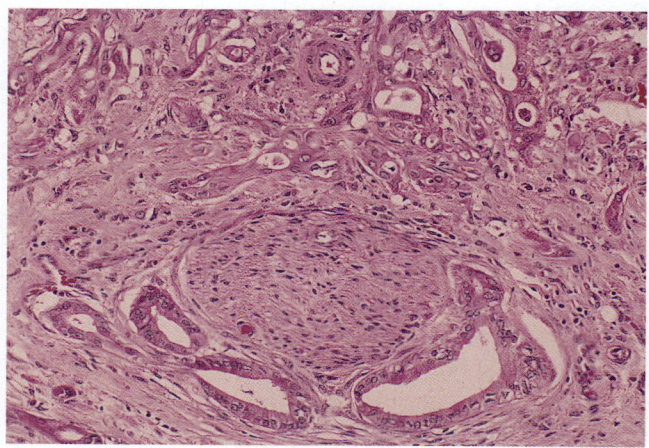

FIG. 27. Ductal adenocarcinoma surrounds a small nerve.

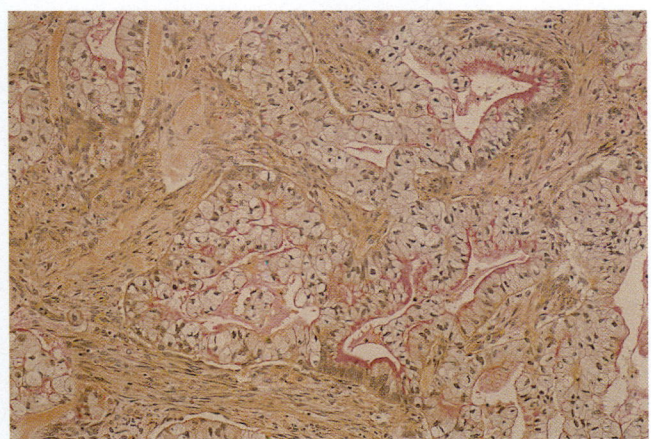

FIG. 28. Ductal adenocarcinoma. Clear cells with apical mucus (mucicarmine stain).

cancer is well differentiated; in these instances, the arrangement of the cells and the neoplastic structures is of special importance in allowing the carcinoma to be recognized (1). It is important not to confuse tiny accessory pancreatic ducts with cancer (81).

Necrotic cellular debris is common in the neoplastic ductal lumens. Invasion into tiny vessels, the islets, and around nerves almost always can be found at the time of diagnosis (Fig. 27). Inappropriately large droplets of mucus may be seen in the cytoplasm of individual carcinoma cells, and pools of mucus may occur in the stroma, sometimes without visible neoplastic cells in a given section. Cancer can extend through the ducts beyond the grossly evident tumor (82). Thromboembolic phenomena in the patients are moderately common and may be more likely when the tumor involves the tail (79).

Most ductal carcinomas are classified as well- to poorly differentiated adenocarcinomas (Figs. 24–29) (1,83–85). The degree of differentiation may vary within the same neoplasm, and occasional anaplastic foci may occur in an otherwise well-differentiated cancer. Phenotypic (86) and genetic (87) heterogeneity has been demonstrated in single cancers. Although relating the grade of histologic differentiation to prognosis is attractive (84,88), so far it has not been very helpful in practice (89). Likewise, staging has been difficult, and a large proportion of the neoplasms have reached an advanced stage by the time of diagnosis. Small size (2.5 cm in diameter or less) is somewhat favorable (90–92), but very few cancers are discovered when they are small, and even some of these have metastatic foci (79,92).

Chromosomal abnormalities are common (93,94). Cytometry usually has shown that a majority of ductal carcinomas are nondiploid; these are less likely to be resectable, and patients with such tumors have considerably shorter survivals (95,96).

Lymph nodes around the pancreas nearly always contain metastatic foci, but the groups of nodes involved vary depending on the location of the cancer in the organ. Even cancers smaller than 2 cm in diameter may spread outside the organ (97).

Invasion of intrapancreatic nerves is frequent, and spread into the nerves outside the pancreas is correlated with the intrapancreatic neural invasion and with shorter postoperative survival (98). Benign groups of epithelial cells in close association with pancreatic nerves must be differentiated from cancer (99).

Cytologic Features

Aspirates from ductal adenocarcinoma are extremely cellular (so-called tumor cellularity) (Fig. 30). Consistent features are the lack of acinar cells and increased number of atypical ductal cells arranged in sheets, clusters, and singly. The groups of neoplastic cells vary in size, shape, and degree of cohesiveness (37,71). The cell borders are usually evident; the cytoplasm may be scant to abundant and clear or

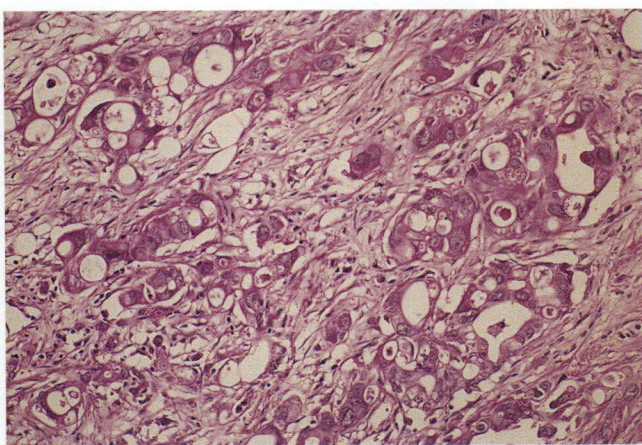

FIG. 29. Ductal adenocarcinoma, poorly differentiated. The ductular structures are not as well formed as those in the previous figures.

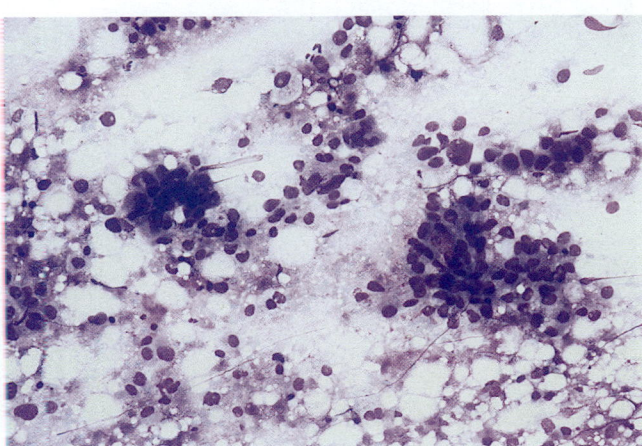

FIG. 30. Ductal adenocarcinoma, FNA. Tumor cellularity. Many atypical epithelial cells are present in loosely cohesive groups and as scattered single cells.

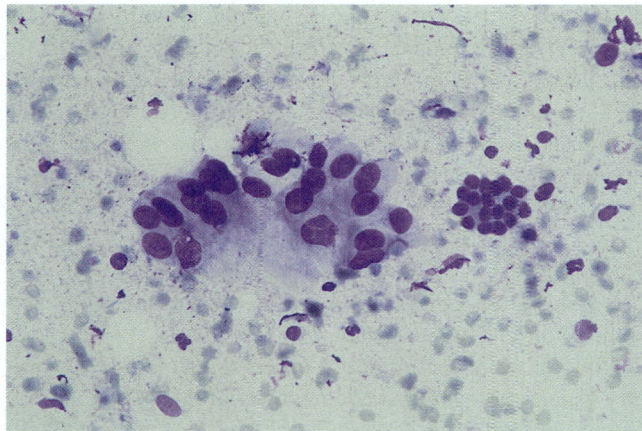

FIG. 31. Ductal adenocarcinoma, moderately well differentiated. FNA. Neoplastic cells have larger and more irregular nuclei than the benign ductal cells.

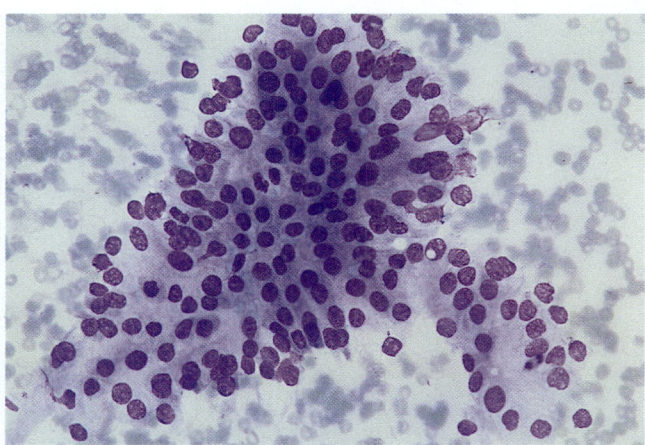

FIG. 33. Ductal adenocarcinoma, well differentiated. FNA. Note slight variation in nuclear size and shape and a suggestion of a glandular arrangement.

pale; the nuclei are enlarged and may show palisading, overlapping, or a disorderly arrangement. Frequently, groups of benign ductal cells are seen adjacent to groups of malignant epithelial cells (Fig. 31), a feature that is quite helpful in the diagnosis. The degree of nuclear atypia and cellular cohesiveness varies according to the degree of differentiation of the carcinoma (Figs. 31–35) (37,71). The less differentiated the neoplasm, the greater the number of bizarre cells and single cells. Fragments of thick-walled blood vessels, sometimes in close proximity to the neoplastic cells, are frequently observed. Abnormal mitoses are common, and necrosis is variable. Foci of pancreatitis can be present in the same aspirate as carcinoma.

Uncommon Types of Pancreatic Ductal Carcinoma

Various uncommon types of pancreatic carcinoma have been described: adenosquamous carcinoma (sometimes nearly all squamous), mucinous adenocarcinoma (either with large pools of mucus or, rarely, with clear cells filled with mucus), papillary adenocarcinoma (some of these are probably intraductal papillary-mucinous neoplasms), the microglandular adenocarcinoma (a controversial entity difficult to distinguish from some endocrine carcinomas; see below), and the rare oncocytic carcinoma and clear cell carcinoma.

Adenosquamous Carcinoma

Two distinct malignant epithelial elements are found in adenosquamous carcinoma (Fig. 36) (1,100). Their proportions vary, and transitional zones are evident. In the authors' experience, the two major cellular types are so intermingled that this pattern is unlikely to be overlooked if several sections are taken from different parts of the neoplasm. Although the squamous elements may be extensive in the primary neoplasm, the adenocarcinomatous element may predominate or may be the only pattern in the metastatic foci.

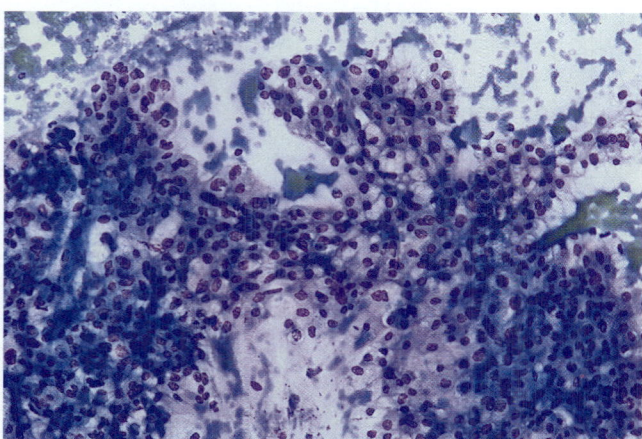

FIG. 32. Ductal adenocarcinoma, well differentiated. FNA. Large sheets of neoplastic cells with abundant clear to dense cytoplasm, distinct cellular borders, and slight variation in nuclear size and shape.

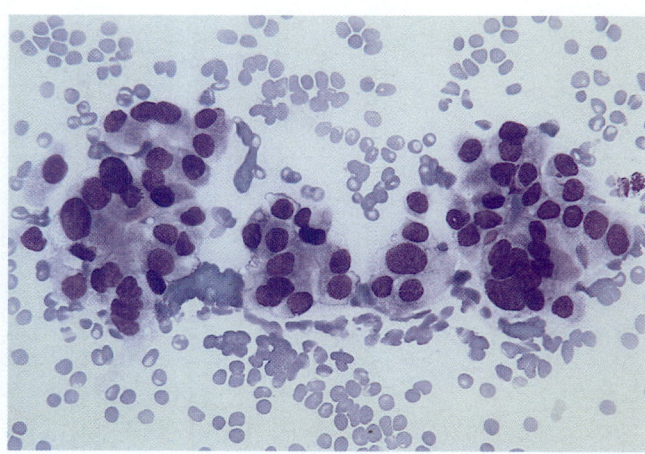

FIG. 34. Ductal adenocarcinoma, moderately differentiated. FNA. Cells show moderate variation in nuclear size and shape.

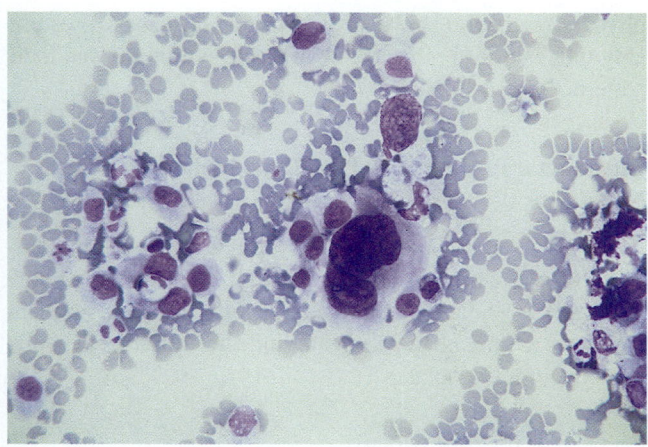

FIG. 35. Ductal adenocarcinoma, poorly differentiated. Markedly atypical neoplastic cells lacking cohesiveness are present.

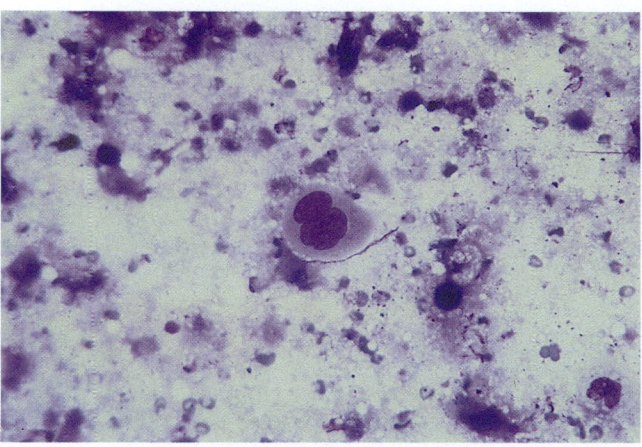

FIG. 37. Adenosquamous carcinoma. FNA. One atypical binucleated cell with dense cytoplasm lies in a necrotic background.

Aspirates from adenosquamous carcinoma show a distinctive necrotic background (Fig. 37). In the granular amorphous debris are dense blue globules, ghosts of squamous cells with angular borders, and anucleate squames. Atypical single cells with dense cytoplasm and enlarged pyknotic nuclei are present. Also seen are sheets and clusters of atypical cells with moderate to abundant cytoplasm (that varies from dense to vacuolated) and nuclei of variable sizes and shapes in a disorderly arrangement (Fig. 38).

Pure squamous-cell carcinoma of the pancreas is very rare, if it exists at all. Exposure of the pancreas to ionizing radiation might predispose to the occurrence of adenosquamous carcinoma.

Mucinous Adenocarcinoma

Mucinous adenocarcinomas (1,83) may occur in two forms: (a) In colloid adenocarcinoma, pools of mucus are conspicuous upon gross and microscopic examination (Fig. 39). The tumor is soft. Signet-ring cells may be present. In

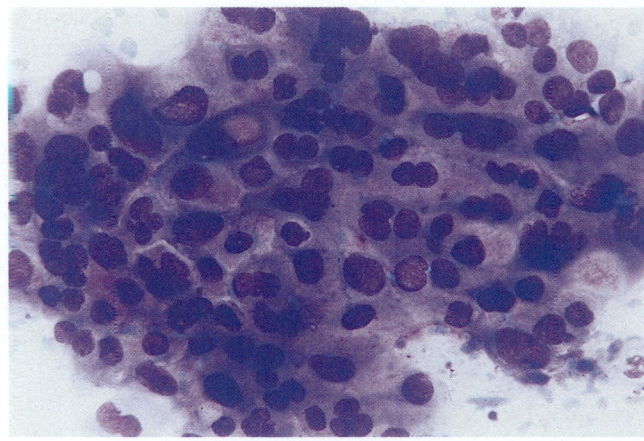

FIG. 38. Adenosquamous carcinoma. FNA. Cluster of atypical cells with well-demarcated cell borders, mostly dense cytoplasm, and occasional vacuoles.

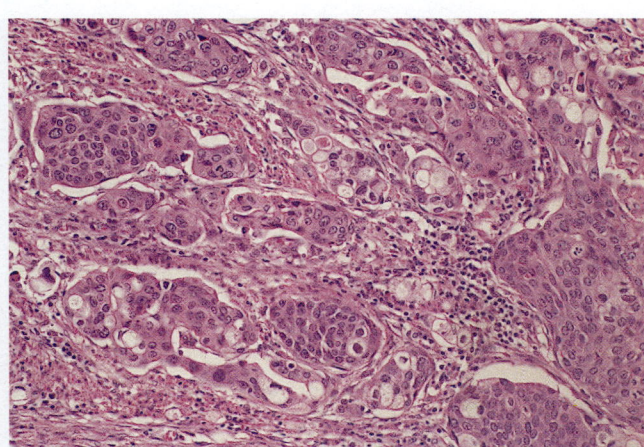

FIG. 36. Adenosquamous carcinoma. Gland-like structures are mixed with the squamous nests.

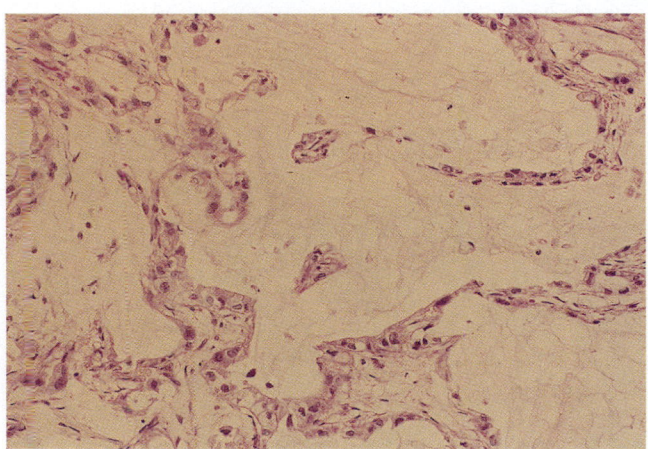

FIG. 39. Mucinous adenocarcinoma. Large pools of mucus are surrounded by atypical epithelial cells.

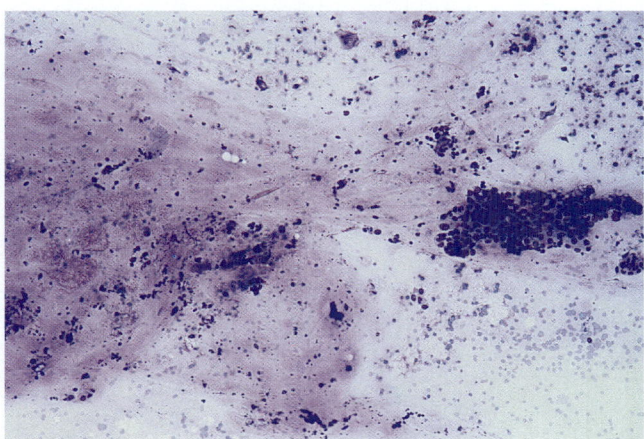

FIG. 40. Mucinous adenocarcinoma. FNA. A large amount of mucus covers most of the slide. A large cluster of neoplastic cells is present.

some of the collections of mucus, only rare malignant cells may be found after a careful search. (b) In the other type of mucinous adenocarcinoma, the cells have clear cytoplasm (a form of clear-cell carcinoma), and appropriate stains are required to recognize that the cytoplasm contains mucus. Some (or most) of both these mucous neoplasms may originate as intraductal papillary-mucinous neoplasms and are not the usual ductal adenocarcinomas.

Aspirates from mucous adenocarcinomas are difficult to smear thinly on the slides because of abundant mucus (Figs. 40 and 41). On microscopic examination, the mucous pools are large and may be acellular in some smears. However, other smears show the groups of malignant epithelial cells.

Papillary Adenocarcinoma

Rare ductal adenocarcinomas have a somewhat papillary structure, but are otherwise similar to the usual ductal cancers. The intraductal papillary-mucinous neoplasms are discussed later in this chapter. Carcinomas of the ampulla of Vater and of the distal common duct have papillary, exophytic growth with a relatively favorable prognosis, presumably the result of both early obstructive symptoms and their patterns of growth.

Intraductal Proliferative Processes, Including Neoplasms

Intraductal epithelial processes include the apparently benign ones already described (see Common Minor Abnormalities), atypia associated with cigarette smoking, atypical papillary epithelial hyperplasia, and the intraductal papillary-mucinous neoplasms.

Atypical Papillary Hyperplasia

This is an intraductal lesion, usually segmental, that is believed to be premalignant and is closely related to (or may be the same as) carcinoma *in situ* (29,32). It is characterized by (a) large cells; (b) enlarged, irregular nuclei; (c) deviations from the normal cellular polarity; (d) a local piling-up of the epithelium; and (e) mitotic activity. An important attempt has been made to quantitate such changes and to reduce the subjectivity of the interpretation (101). The proliferation may obstruct a duct (102). Atypical papillary hyperplasia has often occurred near a ductal adenocarcinoma, which suggests that the changes might represent intraductal spread of the cancer in some instances. The linkage with carcinoma might be coincidental, however. Other examples reported may represent the early stages of the intraductal papillary-mucinous neoplasms described below.

Intraductal Papillary-Mucinous Neoplasms (IPMN)

This neoplasm presents as a principal pancreatic duct that is often dilated, filled with mucus, and contains papillary structures (103,104). The papillae in the duct are soft to firm, may appear as irregularly nodular fungating masses (Fig. 42), or may be of microscopic size. Major branches are often mucus-filled and dilated, with papillary tumor also evident.

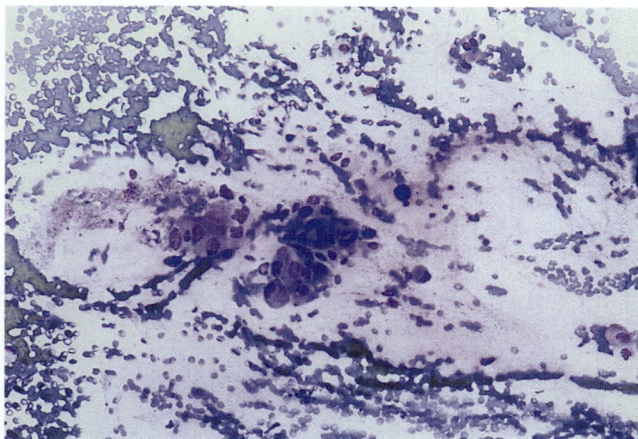

FIG. 41. Mucinous adenocarcinoma. FNA. Atypical epithelial cells lie in a mucoid and hemorrhagic background.

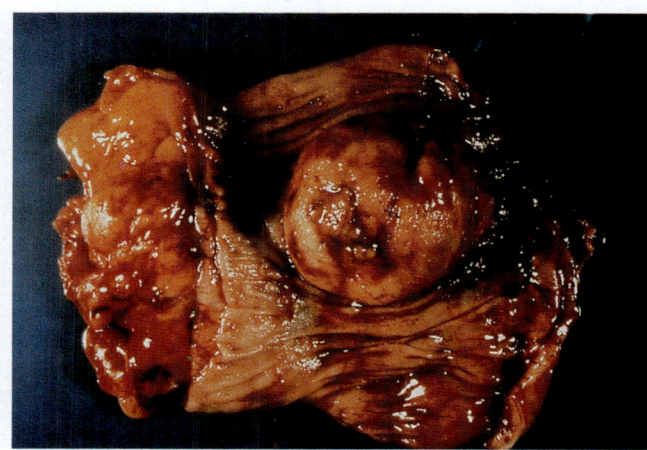

FIG. 42. Intraductal papillary-mucinous neoplasm protrudes through the ampulla of Vater into the duodenum.

When the gland is sectioned and multiple ducts are involved, the lesions appear as multilocular cysts. Rarely, only a small duct is affected.

Most of these tumors lie in the head or in the head and body together. The majority occur in middle-aged and elderly men. Symptoms are often vague abdominal complaints related to ductal obstruction and low-grade pancreatitis. A moderate number of patients present with episodes of acute pancreatitis, but lack gallstones or a history of alcohol abuse. Remaining pancreatic parenchyma is either normal or altered by chronic pancreatitis and/or atrophy secondary to the ductal obstruction.

On microscopic examination the neoplasm consists of dilated ducts within which there are numerous papillae composed of columnar cells with clear to eosinophilic cytoplasm (Figs. 43–45). The papillae vary greatly in size. Many cells contain apical mucus, and there usually is a large amount of extracellular mucus. A few of these tumors have little mucus present. The fibrovascular stroma of the larger papillae may contain some neoplastic glands, but these are usually a minor feature. The epithelium is extremely variable (Fig. 44) (105): regular tall columnar cells with round to ovoid basal nuclei (consistent with hyperplastic epithelium), to less uniform columnar cells having elongated, hyperchromatic nuclei with occasional mitotic figures (consistent with atypical adenomatous epithelium), to markedly abnormal cells having irregular nuclei, conspicuous nucleoli, stratification of nuclei, and easily detected mitotic figures (consistent with severe dysplasia/carcinoma *in situ*). Transitions from hyperplasia to carcinoma may be found in a single neoplasm. Some of the epithelial cells may invade the stroma—as infiltrating glands and tubules (resembling the usual ductal adenocarcinoma) or as tiny mucous pools in which the neoplastic cells are floating (the so-called muconodular invasion) (105). Thus the lesions range from a benign appearance to atypia to invasive cancer. A variant with a predominance of oncocytic epithelium has been reported (106); this feature has been noted by others (Fig. 45) (105).

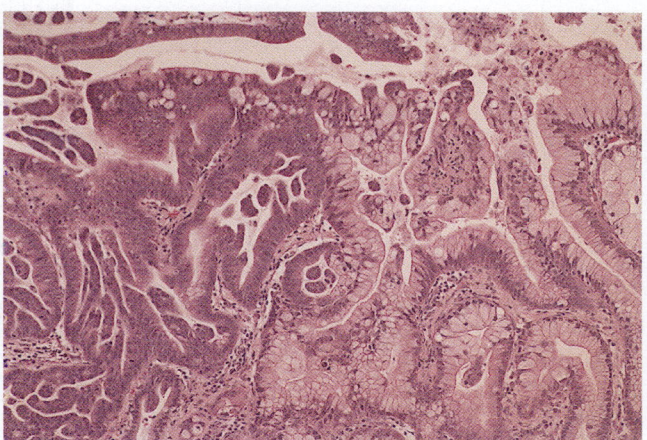

FIG. 44. Intraductal papillary-mucinous neoplasm. The mucous cells are generally regular. The columnar cells in the other half of the field have little mucus and are atypical.

Resections are often successful because the tumors grow slowly and tend to be confined to the ducts. These peculiar neoplasms, especially those that are invasive, probably have been misclassified as ductal carcinomas with extensive papillary patterns or as mucinous ductal adenocarcinomas (colloid carcinomas). Predominantly intraductal adenocarcinoma (107), sometimes with an extensive solid component, is presumably the most malignant end of the spectrum of these intraductal proliferative processes.

Differential Diagnosis

The differential diagnosis of pancreatic carcinoma, IPMN, and chronic pancreatitis is challenging (Fig. 46). In addition to the frequent presence of chronic pancreatitis adjacent to the carcinomas, which can confuse the diagnosis, other aspects of the pathologic process must be considered. The pancreatic islets and isolated endocrine cells may be altered by the cancer-associated pancreatitis (72,73) and can be trapped in the neoplasm. Endocrine cells may proliferate

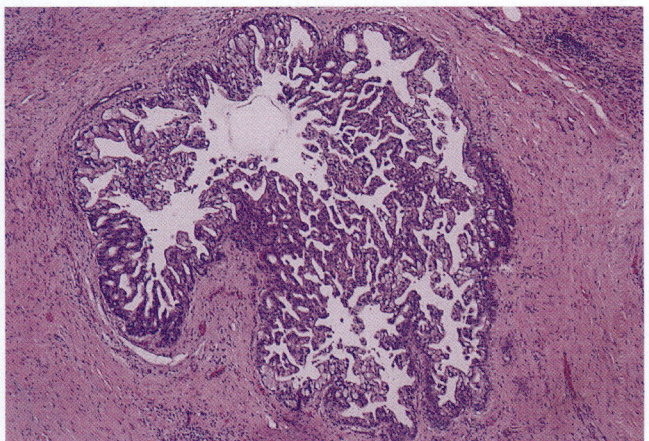

FIG. 43. Intraductal papillary-mucinous neoplasm. A major duct is filled with papillary fronds. Note the fibrosis surrounding the duct.

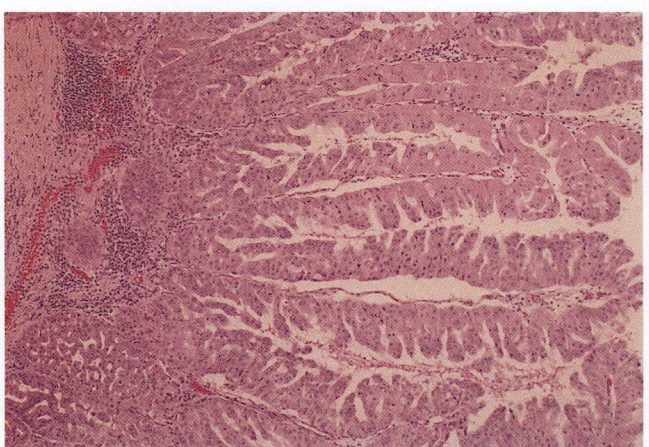

FIG. 45. Intraductal papillary-mucinous neoplasm. This example is composed of oncocytic cells.

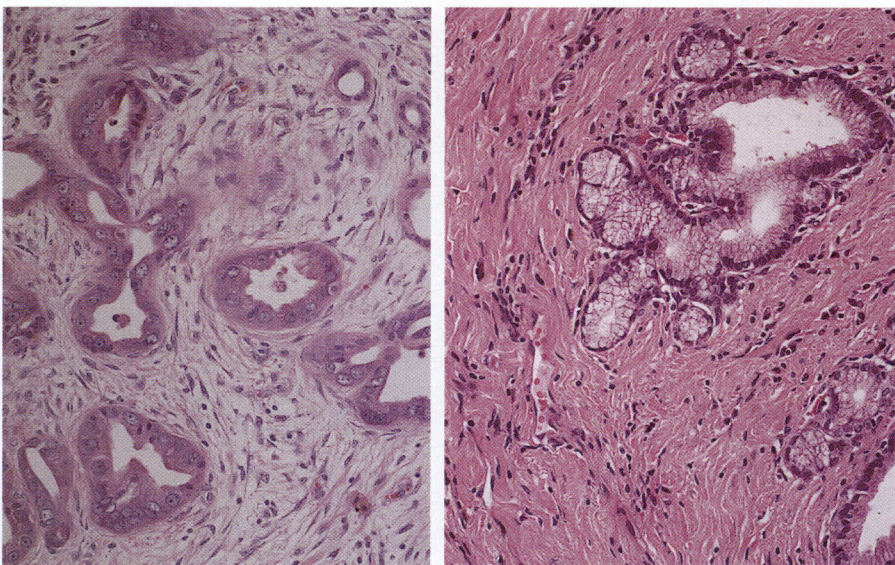

FIG. 46. Comparison of well-differentiated adenocarcinoma and chronic pancreatitis.

in the nonneoplastic pancreas, and they also grow as a part of the exocrine carcinoma (108,109).

The part of the pancreas believed most likely to represent the presumed neoplasm should be selected for aspiration or biopsy. More than one sample should be obtained. Attempts to diagnose cancer without actually entering the pancreatic parenchyma often fail. For example, fat necrosis with inflammation may simulate carcinoma to the naked eye, but a biopsy or an aspiration will not show cancer. Peripancreatic lymph nodes can be enlarged because of reactive changes, but might not contain carcinoma. Focal alterations in the liver unrelated to the pancreas may be mistaken for metastatic disease.

Segmental chronic pancreatitis can be densely fibrotic, thereby suggesting carcinoma. Tissue from chronic pancreatitis shows distortion and atrophy of the ducts and acini associated with inflammation and fibrosis of variable density. However, the relationship of the epithelium and the stroma is essentially that of the normal gland, although these components differ in quantity. In ductal adenocarcinoma there are abnormal epithelial cells, loss of cellular polarity, presence of complex patterns of the epithelium, frequent mitotic figures, disruption and loss of basement membranes around tubular and glandular structures, and the dense (desmoplastic) stroma usually present lacks an orderly relationship to the epithelium.

Ductal dilatation and/or atrophy may be caused by calculi, inflammation, scarring, and neoplasms; thus, these changes are nonspecific and should neither be regarded as necessarily caused by carcinoma nor mistaken for carcinoma. The tiny accessory ducts in the duodenal wall must not be confused with adenocarcinoma (81). Pancreatic lobular collapse and the proliferation and distortion of islet cells (or other epithelium) that may occur in chronic pancreatitis may cause epithelial cells to lie close to nerves; this phenomenon must be differentiated from perineural invasion by carcinoma (99,110). Finally, the pathologist may note the presence of a neoplasm in the sections, but the uniformity of its cells and its architecture may suggest an endocrine neoplasm or a Gruber-Frantz tumor (solid-cystic-papillary epithelial neoplasm) rather than ductal carcinoma.

Acinar Cell Carcinoma

Carcinomas with substantial acinar cell differentiation are rare, constituting less than 5% of all pancreatic malignant neoplasms (1,111). They are more common in men and present with abdominal pain and loss of weight. Most patients are middle-aged or elderly. Some tumors are essentially pure acinar cell types. When ductal or endocrine elements form a considerable proportion of the tumor, the neoplasm probably should be considered as having dual differentiation. Acinar cell cancers are of interest because the secretion of lipase and other digestive enzymes by the neoplasm sometimes causes polyarthropathy, nonbacterial thrombotic endocarditis, and multifocal fat necrosis in the subcutaneous tissues, bone marrow, and abdomen (112).

The carcinoma may occur anywhere in the organ, but the majority occur in the head. Rarely, more than one focus of carcinoma has been described in the organ. The tumors are usually large and fairly well circumscribed, even partly encapsulated. The external surface is bosselated; the cut surfaces are pink to tan, homogeneous, and fleshy, with thin fibrous bands separating the tumor into lobules (Fig. 47). There is not much stroma. Necrosis and/or hemorrhage may be conspicuous.

The most common histologic patterns are acinar and solid (Figs. 48–50). The acinar pattern consists of small lumina surrounded by cells of various sizes with eosinophilic granular cytoplasm and basal nuclei. In the solid regions, most cells

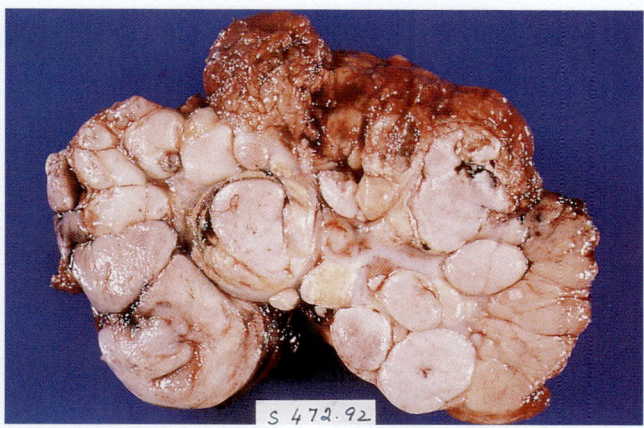

FIG. 47. Acinar cell carcinoma. The cut surface is pale, fleshy, and lobulated.

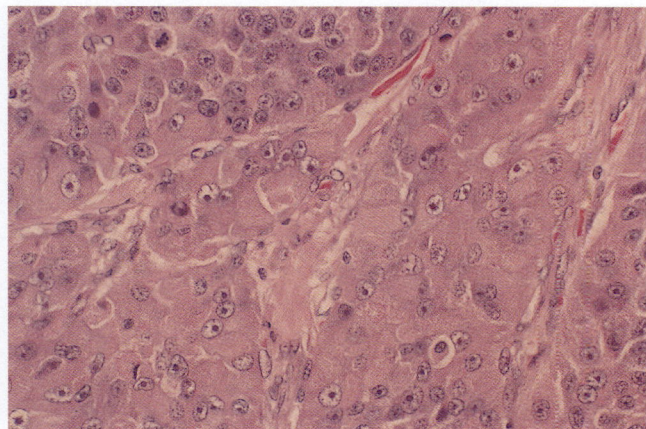

FIG. 48. Acinar cell carcinoma, solid pattern. The cells vary in size, and some have large amounts of eosinophilic, granular cytoplasm.

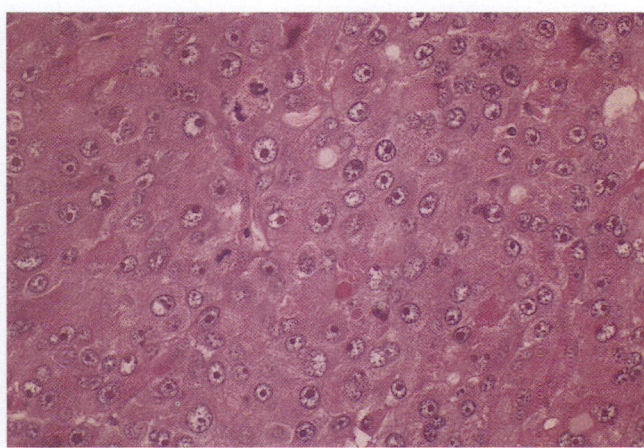

FIG. 49. Acinar cell carcinoma, solid pattern. Nuclei are round and have conspicuous nucleoli. Note the mitotic figures.

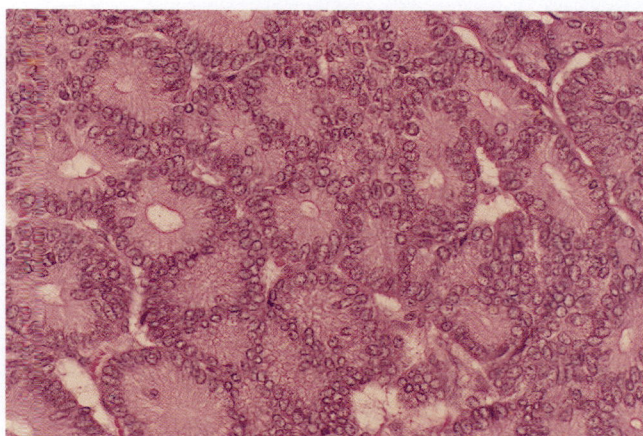

FIG. 50. Acinar cell carcinoma, acinar pattern. The cells are columnar.

have central nuclei and little cytoplasm. The tendency to have basal nuclei may be evident in cells adjacent to stroma or to the capsule. Because of the small amount of cytoplasm in the solid regions, such a tumor initially may be considered poorly differentiated. Additional sections and special studies may be needed to demonstrate more typical acinar cell features. Less common patterns include the glandular pattern (large and often irregular lumina—the result of dilated acini), and the trabecular pattern, which consists of long strands of rather regular cells with double rows of nuclei close to the accompanying stroma and capillaries. These other patterns are accompanied by acinar or solid regions. Delicate vessels course through the cancers; sometimes there is extensive hemorrhage. When perivascular spaces are large, they cause a gyriform pattern of the epithelial elements.

The neoplastic cells have nuclei that are round or oval, rather uniform, and medium-sized. Clumps of chromatin often lie next to the nuclear membrane. Strongly eosinophilic nucleoli may be central or peripheral and may be conspicuous. Mitotic figures vary greatly in numbers from case to case.

The PAS technique applied after diastase digestion demonstrates the zymogen granules. It is therefore useful in assisting the pathologist's search for the acinar structures, which are the most characteristic features of these cancers. The butyrate esterase stain demonstrates lipase activity in about three-fourths of the cases (Fig. 51). Immunohistochemical techniques for demonstrating trypsin, chymotrypsin, salivary amylase, and lipases are frequently positive. Careful evaluation of these procedures on a neoplasm and on normal control pancreas is essential for interpreting the results. When the neoplastic cells exhibit polarity, the products of these special procedures are usually localized in the apical portions of the cells. Ultrastructural studies have demonstrated a resemblance to normal acinar tissue with zymogen granules, ample amounts of rough endoplasmic reticulum, and membrane-bound inclusions of filaments (113).

A minor population of endocrine cells can be scattered through a tumor. Their detection depends on staining the

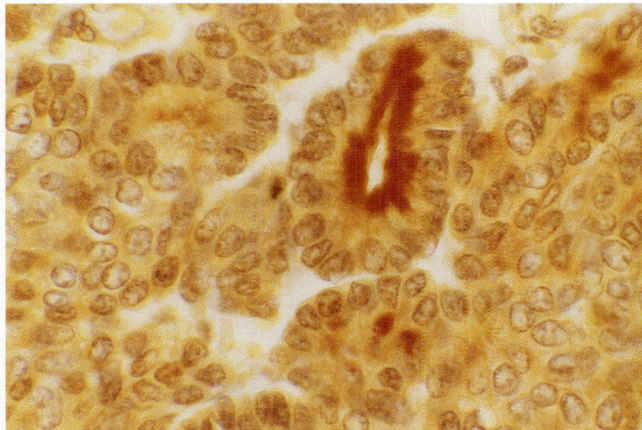

FIG. 51. Acinar cell carcinoma. A butyrate-esterase procedure demonstrates the reaction product in the apical parts of the cells, probably the result of lipase activity.

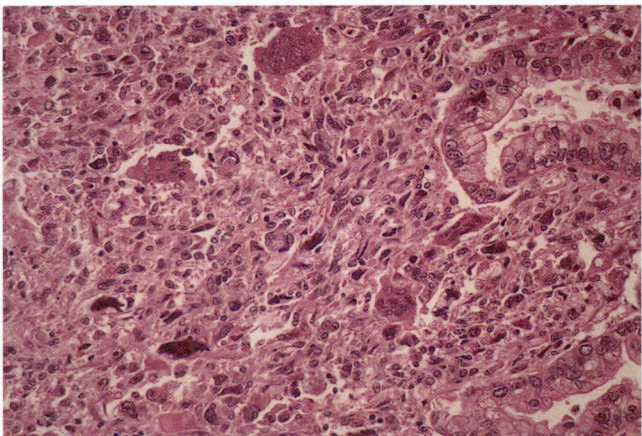

FIG. 52. Anaplastic carcinoma. Moderately differentiated ductal adenocarcinoma is mixed with the anaplastic carcinoma. Pleomorphic tumor giant cells and osteoclast-like giant cells are present.

neoplasm with appropriate antibodies, such as antichromogranin. Rarely, a substantial component of endocrine cells is present (25% or more), either scattered through the neoplasm or evident as large numbers of endocrine cells in specific regions (114). In the latter situation, the endocrine cells may resemble normal islet cells sufficiently to be recognizable in routine histologic preparations.

No special pattern of metastases has been noted, and most patients have died in a few months. The patients have included a few children (115). A few of these neoplasms are probably less malignant than the usual ductal carcinomas, especially in children.

Rare acinar-cell cystadenocarcinomas have been reported. (See Pancreatic Cysts, Pseudocysts, and Cystic Neoplasms, below.)

Anaplastic Carcinoma

Anaplastic, pleomorphic, sarcomatoid, and *undifferentiated carcinoma* are the terms applied to those neoplasms that are not readily recognizable as exocrine or endocrine carcinomas, but that are believed to be epithelial in type rather than lymphoma or sarcoma (1,116–118). Although occasional examples (especially the small cell types) have been suspected to be endocrine neoplasms, most have been regarded as variants of ductal adenocarcinomas.

The distribution by age and sex is similar to the usual ductal cancers. They can be located anywhere in the pancreas, are distributed approximately equally in the head and tail, present with the usual signs and symptoms of a nonendocrine pancreatic neoplasm, and are often large. Hemorrhage, necrosis, and cystic degeneration often are conspicuous, and the tumor may be soft. Extensive nodal metastases are usually present.

The majority of these rare neoplasms are composed of spindled cells, pleomorphic large cells, and scanty supporting stroma (Figs. 52–54). The proportions of these components vary; in a few examples, spindle cells constitute virtu-

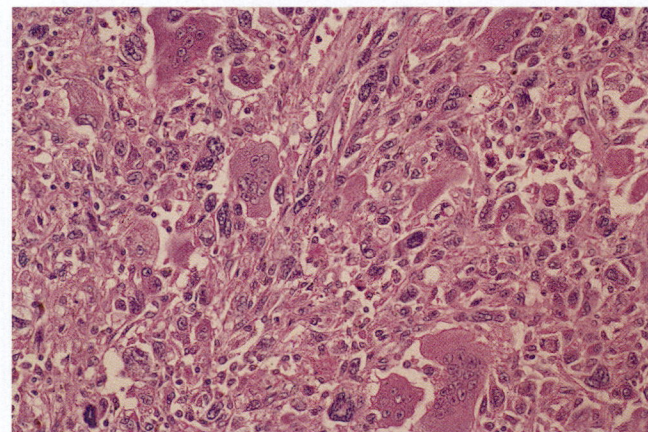

FIG. 53. Anaplastic carcinoma. Bizarre neoplastic cells are accompanied by osteoclast-like giant cells.

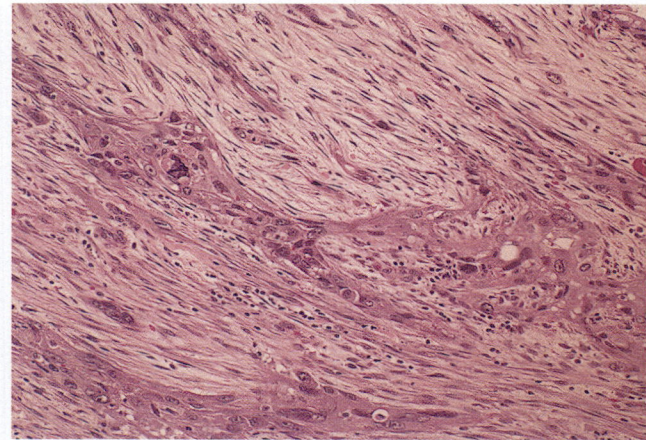

FIG. 54. Anaplastic carcinoma. Neoplastic spindle cells lie in the fibrous stroma.

ally all of the mass (Fig. 54). Medium-sized to giant neoplastic cells often have oddly shaped, hyperchromatic, or bizarre nuclei, which can be very large and may be multiple (Figs. 52 and 53). Nucleoli frequently are large, mitoses are frequent, and phagocytosis by the giant cells is common. When multiple sections of an anaplastic carcinoma are examined, regions of usual ductal adenocarcinoma may be found in the mass (Fig. 52) (117), or the anaplastic carcinoma may appear to arise from abnormal epithelium of a medium-sized or large duct. A few neoplastic cells may contain intracytoplasmic mucin droplets; some of the spindled cells and large pleomorphic cells of anaplastic carcinomas contain immunoreactive keratin (Fig. 55). Well-differentiated ductal adenocarcinomas occasionally contain small regions of anaplastic carcinoma; this finding provides additional support for the epithelial nature of these anaplastic neoplasms.

In a small number of anaplastic carcinomas, osteoclast-like, multinucleated giant cells are numerous (Figs. 52 and 53). Their nuclei are regular. They may occur in a carcinoma composed predominantly of spindle cells or, occasionally, in a carcinoma composed of spindle cells and pleomorphic giant cells. Some of these osteoclast-like giant cells are rich in acid phosphatase and the markers for histiocytes. They may be concentrated near regions of hemorrhage or near foci of osseous metaplasia or calcification, features also suggesting that these giant cells are reactive and not essentially neoplastic.

An occasional anaplastic carcinoma is composed largely or entirely of rounded or polygonal, medium-sized cells. There is a vaguely epithelial appearance because of a minor degree of cellular coherence.

Small Cell Carcinoma

A rare microscopic pattern is the small cell type, in which very little cytoplasm surrounds the nucleus of each cell (119,120). When only a single mass in the pancreas is present and there is no convincing clinical or pathologic evidence that the neoplasm began in the lung or in another site, then a pancreatic origin is reasonable. The authors have seen several possible examples in which a pulmonary origin could not be excluded, so an especially critical evaluation is needed before proposing pancreatic origin for a small cell carcinoma. A few are small cell neuroectodermal tumors similar to other examples in the lungs, soft tissue, and bone (121).

Distinguishing small cell carcinoma from lymphoma may be accomplished by making good histologic preparations; taking multiple sections of tissue; using antibodies to keratin proteins, leukocyte common antigen, and lymphoid antigens; and sometimes performing electron microscopy.

In general, the pancreatic anaplastic and small cell carcinomas must be distinguished from metastatic carcinoma, malignant fibrous histiocytoma, leiomyosarcoma, lymphoma, and other retroperitoneal neoplasms of the soft tissues that involve the pancreas secondarily.

PANCREATIC CYSTS, PSEUDOCYSTS, AND CYSTIC NEOPLASMS

Cysts

Cysts can be congenital or acquired (122). Although their origins differ, the clinical manifestations, some imaging characteristics, and surgical treatment have similarities. Imaging techniques now detect many small cystic lesions.

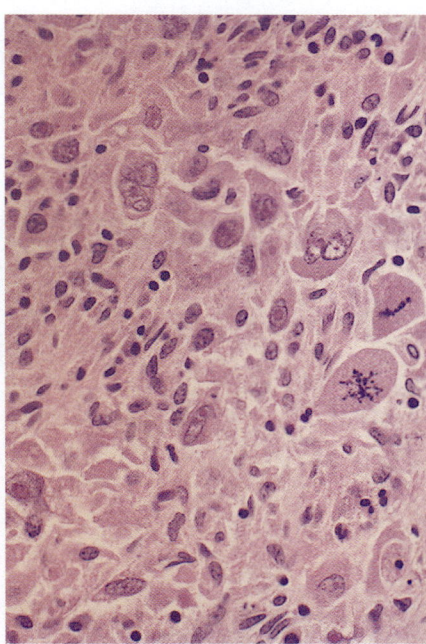
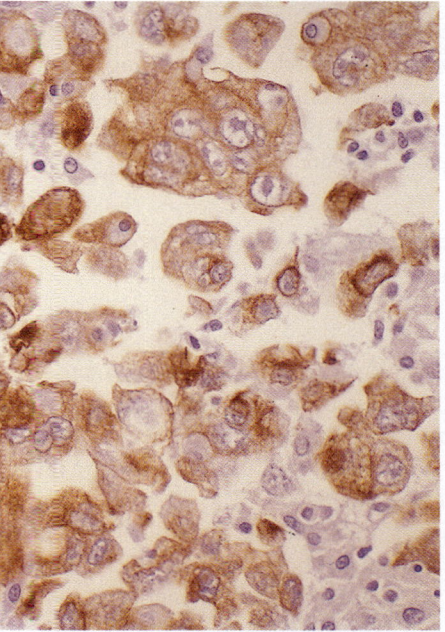

FIG. 55. Anaplastic carcinoma. Immunoreactive keratin is demonstrated in the tumor. Note the abnormal mitotic figures.

The intraductal papillary-mucinous neoplasm may present as a cyst. Also, the usual ductal adenocarcinoma, a sarcoma (such as leiomyosarcoma), and the Gruber-Frantz tumor may undergo substantial cavitary necrosis.

A true solitary cyst is unilocular and characterized by the presence of an epithelial lining of cuboidal to flattened cells devoid of glycogen and mucin (123). The epithelial retention cysts are lined by ductal epithelium.

Congenital cysts are rare and include: (a) the simple, or solitary, cyst apparently resulting from abnormal development of a duct; (b) multiple cysts associated with inherited polycystic diseases; (c) pancreatic and parapancreatic lymphoepithelial cysts; and (d) dermoid cysts. Cystic fibrosis is a genetic disorder, but the small cysts that develop are the result of the viscid secretions, obstruction, and fibrosis. Acquired cysts consist of epithelial retention cysts, parasitic cysts, pseudocysts, and cystic neoplasms.

Pseudocysts

Acute fluid collections (in early acute pancreatitis) and the pseudocysts account for about 80% of all cystic lesions related to the pancreas (54,124). Pancreatitis, trauma, ductal calculi, and obstructing neoplasms are the common causes. The lesions result from autodigestion of tissues or from retention of fluid by ductal obstruction. The acute fluid collection lacks epithelium and a well-defined wall (54). A pseudocyst has a wall composed of granulation tissue, adipose tissue, or part of the pancreas; it contains an inflammatory infiltrate and lacks an epithelial lining (70). These lesions nearly always are unilocular. The usual contents are watery fluid containing necrotic debris, fibrin thrombi, serum, and blood. The fluid may be rich in amylase (125). The pseudocyst often lies outside the pancreas (usually between the stomach and transverse colon), may become infected (an abscess is a dangerous complication), and may erode into blood vessels, resulting in massive intraabdominal bleeding. Perforation into a hollow viscus and compression of adjacent organs are other complications. A pseudocyst may or may not be connected with a pancreatic duct.

Mucinous Cystic Neoplasms, Including Mucinous Cystadenocarcinoma

Clinical Features

Mucinous cystic neoplasms occur most often in young to middle-aged women, and less frequently are found in middle-aged or elderly men. In the authors' experience (126), the age at diagnosis ranged between 20 and 82 years; in another series (127), ages extended from 32 to 85 years. Many patients have intermittent or continuous abdominal pain or discomfort and an enlarging abdominal mass (124,126). Weakness, anorexia, and weight loss are moderately common. Occasionally, the mass is found during a routine physical examination or abdominal imaging study.

The duration of signs and symptoms varies from a few days to many years, but is usually only a few months. When the mass is palpable, it frequently occupies the left upper abdomen, because the majority of the neoplasms occur in the body and tail of the pancreas. Imaging techniques reveal multilocularity in some cases and solid foci in occasional tumors. Some are hypovascular, and others contain focal calcifications, especially in their capsules.

Pathologic Features

The neoplasms may be irregular in shape, have well-developed capsules with smooth, glistening (sometimes translucent) external surfaces, and are usually multilocular (Fig. 56). They range from 2 to 20 cm in diameter (average 10–11 cm). The tumor can be adherent to adjacent organs and may be surrounded by dense fibrosis (similar to a pseudocyst). Part of the surface may be irregular and dense because of this fibrosis or because malignant epithelium has extended through the capsule. Large blood vessels may extend over the exterior surfaces of the tumor. Sectioning demonstrates the dense collagenous capsule of variable thickness, cavities of different sizes (the largest often several centimeters in diameter), thick mucoid contents, and (if present) papillary excrescences on the interior surfaces. Hemorrhage, degenerative changes, and loss of epithelium occasionally are extensive and therefore suggest a pseudocyst (124). The adjacent pancreatic parenchyma may be somewhat atrophic.

The neoplasms have columnar epithelium similar to that of the large pancreatic ducts and the intestine, especially the colon, and have characteristic stroma composed of plump spindle cells similar to those of ovarian stroma (Figs. 57 and 58) (126,128). The lining cells include nonciliated mucous columnar cells, goblet cells, absorptive-type cells, cuboidal cells, and (rarely) Paneth cells. Papillary formations are common and range from microscopic in size to large, complex structures visible to the naked eye. Careful search of multiple sections frequently reveals atypical epithelium (Fig.

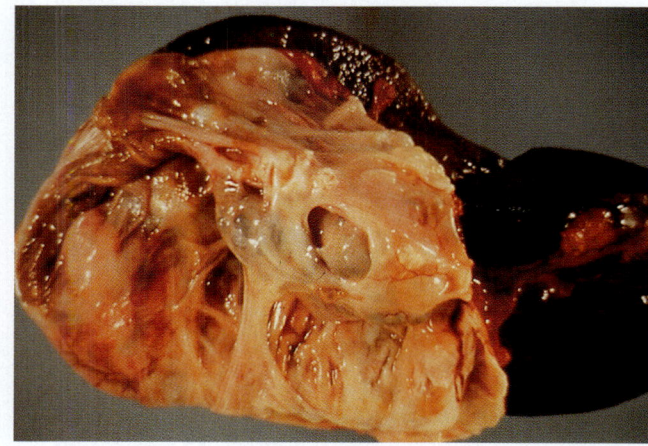

FIG. 56. Mucinous cystic neoplasm. Several locules are visible in this tumor located in the tail.

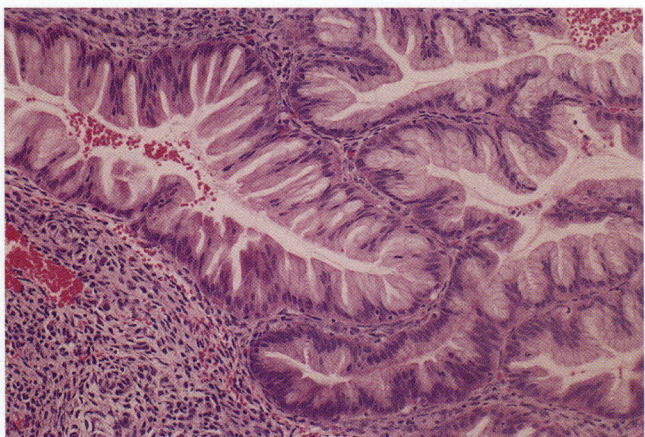

FIG. 57. Mucinous cystic neoplasm. The epithelium is generally regular. The characteristic stroma is hypercellular.

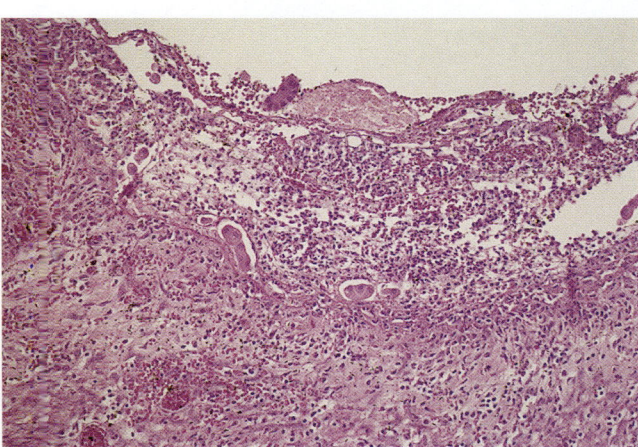

FIG. 59. Mucinous cystic neoplasm. Part of the lining is ulcerated. Atypical epithelial cells, presumably carcinoma, lie in tiny vessels at the base of the ulcer.

58), often pseudostratified (with or without the suggestion of invasion into the stroma or the presence of atypical cells in tiny vessels) (Fig. 59). Obvious regions of invasive adenocarcinoma may be apparent (Fig. 60). These findings combine with cases in which clinical carcinoma arose from mucinous "cystadenoma" to suggest that most or all of these neoplasms have malignant potential (124,126). Also, the bland epithelial cells typical of mucinous cystadenoma have been found in lymph node metastases (1). Failure to remove the entire tumor can result in the death of the patient from carcinoma, even if the resected tissue has only the regular epithelium of a mucinous cystadenoma. Conversely, when carcinoma is present within the mass, complete resection can result in cure because the tumor seems to spread less readily than the usual ductal adenocarcinoma. Studies suggest that aneuploidy in the cystadenocarcinomas indicates a bad prognosis (129). Classifying the neoplasms as carcinomas, borderline tumors, and adenomas has been suggested, but we doubt that we can make a reliable benign or borderline diagnosis with confidence for the reasons just mentioned.

Considerable portions of the neoplasm may not have a well-preserved epithelial lining, and parts of the epithelium may be cuboidal (rather than columnar), so a limited sample of the lesion may be misleading and an incorrect diagnosis may be made (124). The principal epithelial cells express immunoreactive carcinoembryonic antigen, carbohydrate antigens 19-9 and 72-4, keratins, and epithelial membrane antigen.

Several localized neoplastic processes have occurred within the cystic tumors, reported as a malignant fibrous histiocytoma (130), a mesenchymal giant cell tumor (131), sarcomatous stroma of the tumors (Fig. 61) (132), a pseudosarcomatous carcinoma (133), and an anaplastic carcinoma (134). Although these associated lesions are rare, they suggest that the mucinous cystic neoplasms have a special capacity for behaving aggressively. The pathologist should search for such lesions as well as the characteristic mucinous epithelium.

The notable ovarian-type stroma is quite different from other pancreatic tumors. Similar neoplasms have been found

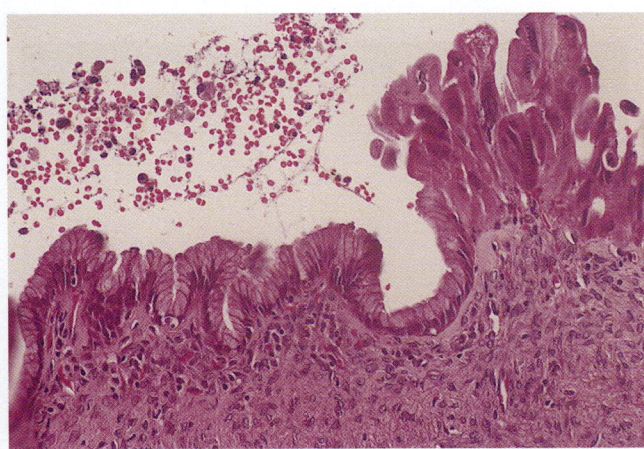

FIG. 58. Mucinous cystic neoplasm. Contrast the markedly atypical epithelium with the adjacent regular cells. Note the hypercellular stroma.

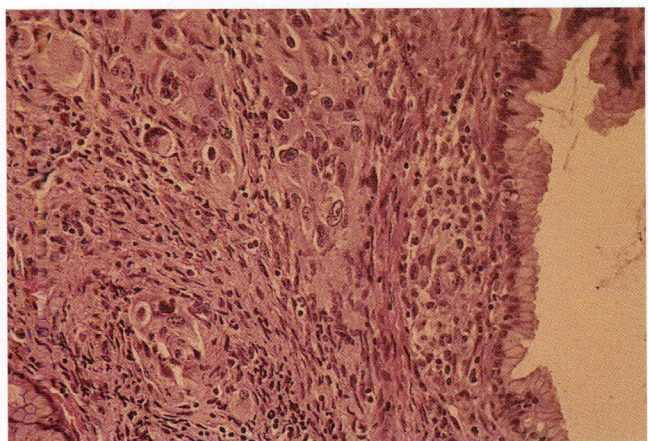

FIG. 60. Mucinous cystic neoplasm. Although the lining epithelium is bland, carcinoma has infiltrated the stroma.

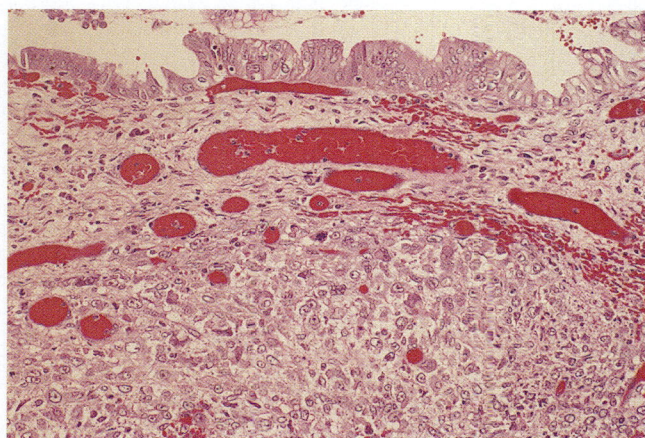

FIG. 61. Mucinous cystic neoplasm. The edge of a sarcoma is visible in the stroma.

in liver and spleen. Occasionally the stroma contains foci of dense, hyalinized tissue resembling the corpora albicantia of the ovary. Other notable aspects of these tumors are the predominance in women, the occasional presence in relatively youthful patients, their rare occurrence in the retroperitoneum unattached to the pancreas (135), and the frequent presence of scattered endocrine cells among the columnar lining cells (Fig. 62) (136). Such endocrine cells are often argyrophilic and contain amines or regulatory peptides: serotonin, somatostatin, gastrin, and pancreatic polypeptide.

Serous Neoplasms

Clinical Features

Most pancreatic serous neoplasms are microcystic, glycogen-rich adenomas (also known as serous cystadenomas) and occur in elderly patients, with only a moderate predominance of women (122,137). One may be found incidentally during physical examination or at autopsy. The tumor can present as an abdominal mass, with or without associated pain or discomfort, usually of several months' duration. If the mass is located in the pancreatic head, it can obstruct the biliary tract or the gastrointestinal tract. Sometimes a large hemorrhage originates from one of these tumors. Rarely, the lesions are multiple, especially when associated with von Hippel–Lindau syndrome. Other pancreatic neoplasms and various nonpancreatic neoplasms are also present in a few patients, possibly as a result of their advanced ages.

Pathologic Features

The mean diameter of the benign tumors in the authors' experience was about 11 cm (range, 1–25 cm) (137), but now many smaller ones are found using modern imaging techniques. They occur anywhere in the organ and appear as partly encapsulated, lobulated masses typically composed of innumerable tiny cysts (occasionally with a few larger ones), and having a sponge-like appearance on sectioning (Fig. 63). The smaller tumors are likely to be soft and spongy. Irregular central scars, frequently calcified, occur with moderate frequency in the larger tumors. The fluid in the cysts is clear and watery, appearing colorless, yellow, or blood-stained. Foci of hemorrhage are common. Conspicuous blood vessels may be noted on the outer surfaces of the tumors.

Occasional examples are macrocystic or oligocystic, largely or completely composed of much larger cysts and devoid of central fibrosis or calcification (138–140). Obviously, such a tumor lacks the internal vascularity of the microcystic examples. Only a single cyst may be evident, thus simulating some mucinous cystic neoplasms and pseudocysts. Such a cyst may be missing much of its lining (138), therefore requiring multiple sections to find the epithelium. The border of the tumor may be irregular and rather poorly defined (139).

Microscopic examination of most serous tumors reveals two principal patterns: (a) groups of minute, regular cysts (a honeycomb pattern resembling immature pulmonary tissue) formed by cuboidal epithelium; and (b) larger, more irregular cysts (up to several centimeters in diameter) lined by low cuboidal to flat cells. The two patterns are usually mixed (141).

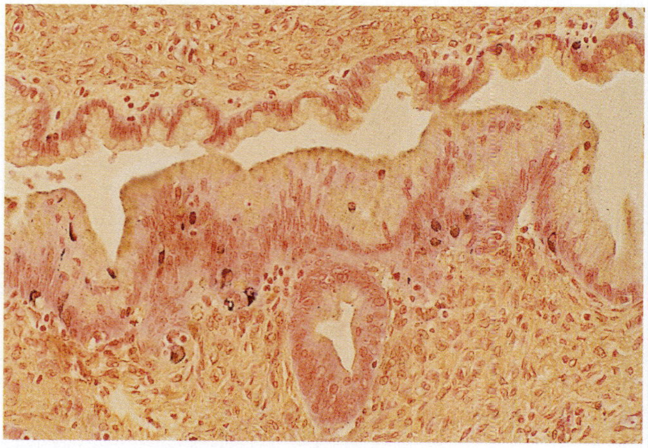

FIG. 62. Mucinous cystic neoplasm. Argyrophilic endocrine cells lie among the mucinous cells.

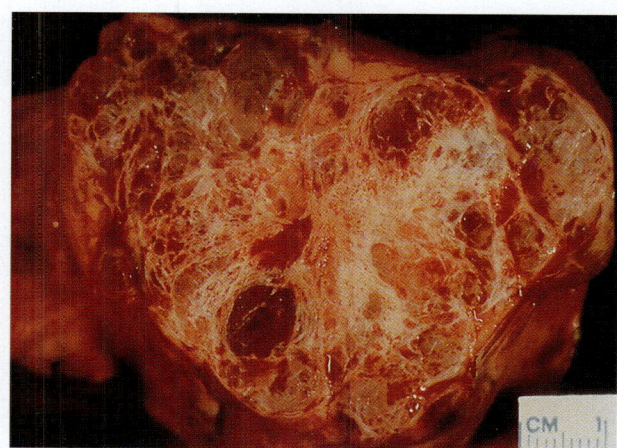

FIG. 63. Serous neoplasm, microcystic type. Many cysts of various sizes are visible on the cut surface.

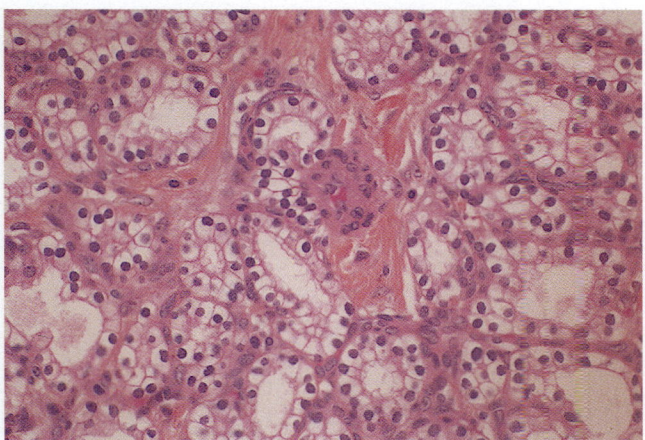

FIG. 64. Serous neoplasm, microcystic type. The tiny cysts are lined by regular, cuboidal cells with uniform nuclei and clear cytoplasm.

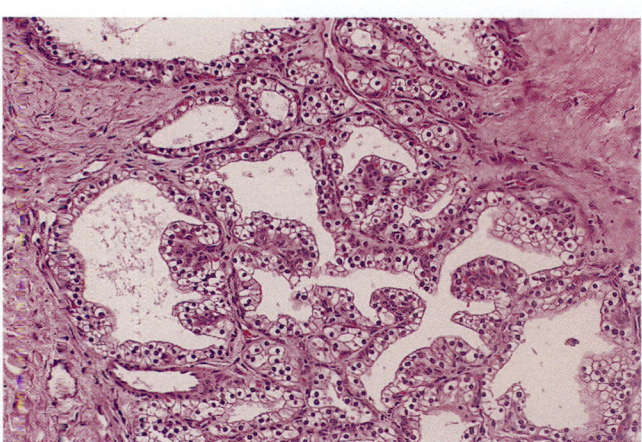

FIG. 66. Serous neoplasm. Tiny papillae are present.

The cytoplasm is clear (Fig. 64) to occasionally eosinophilic, is rich in glycogen (Fig. 65), and contains keratin and epithelial membrane antigen (141). Rare tiny papillae, even with branching, are formed by the regular cuboidal cells (Fig. 66). Nuclei are small, round, compact, and uniform, with inconspicuous nucleoli. On rare occasions, groups of cells have larger and/or irregular nuclei. Nearly all serous neoplasms are diploid.

Electron microscopy (141) demonstrates simple cells attached to one another by desmosomes and containing generous collections of glycogen, with scattered mitochondria and profiles of endoplasmic reticulum. Sparse, short microvilli are present on the apical surfaces. Bundles of filaments lie in the apical and basal parts of the cells. Myoepithelial cells have been reported to lie beneath some of the epithelial cells (142).

Dense fibrous trabeculae run through the microcystic tumors, and, in addition to the central scars commonly present, small irregular nodules of fibrous tissue may be encountered.

These scars can be calcified. Dense stroma can occur in the lesions with large cysts. Some of the stroma may be hyalinized or myxoid. Rarely, lymphocytes are present in part of the stroma. Trapped islets, ducts, and segments of acinar tissue may lie near the periphery. Imaging studies and histologic examination demonstrate large numbers of vessels in the microcystic tumors. Although these neoplasms often have irregular margins because of their lobulations, they almost never are truly invasive. Rarely, they lie mostly outside the pancreas or in the liver, but typically lack metastatic foci.

A solid serous tumor has been described, composed of nests and tiny acini formed by the typical glycogen-laden cells of serous tumors (143).

Serous Microcystic Carcinoma

One example reported had invaded the spleen and had metastases in liver and stomach (144). Another report described focal nuclear atypia and two hepatic metastases (145). In general, these were otherwise similar to the adenomas. In one patient (146) there were multiple serous tumors in the pancreas; they had enlarged, atypical nuclei with coarse nuclear chromatin, and they were aneuploid. The one in the head invaded nerves.

Acinar Cell Cystadenocarcinoma

Two large, multilocular, cystic, malignant tumors of the body and tail of the pancreas have been reported in men 42 and 64 years old (147,148). The individual cysts of the tumors varied markedly in size and were lined by neoplastic acinar cells (Fig. 67). Metastases occurred.

Rare Cystic Neoplasms

A multicystic tumor of the body and tail in a 4-year-old boy was believed to be benign (149). The epithelium consisted of bland, cuboidal and columnar cells devoid of glycogen and mucus.

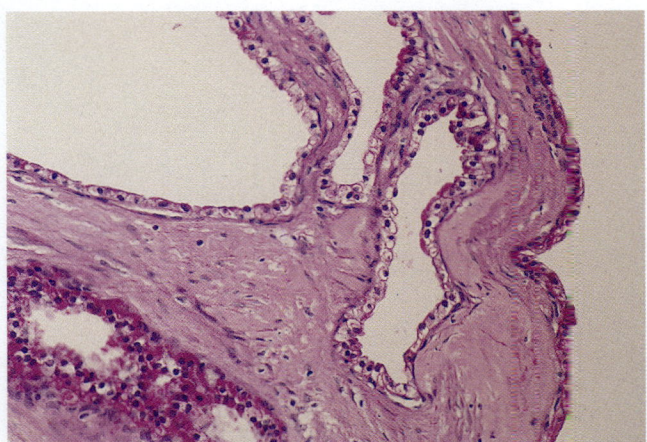

FIG. 65. Serous neoplasm. The PAS stain shows that the amount of glycogen present varies in different parts of the tumor.

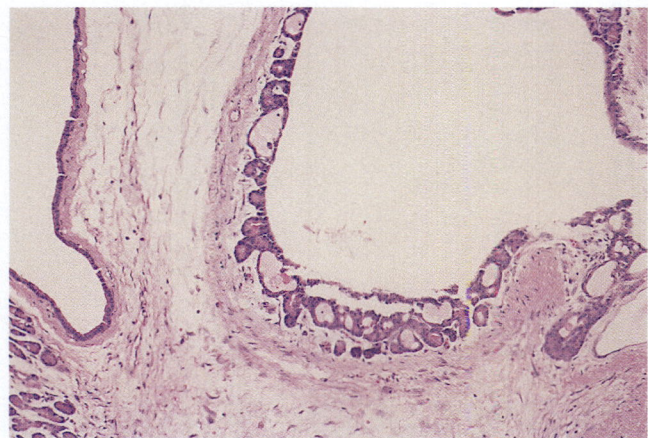

FIG. 67. Acinar cell cystadenocarcinoma. There is striking variation in the sizes of the locules, which are lined by acinar cells.

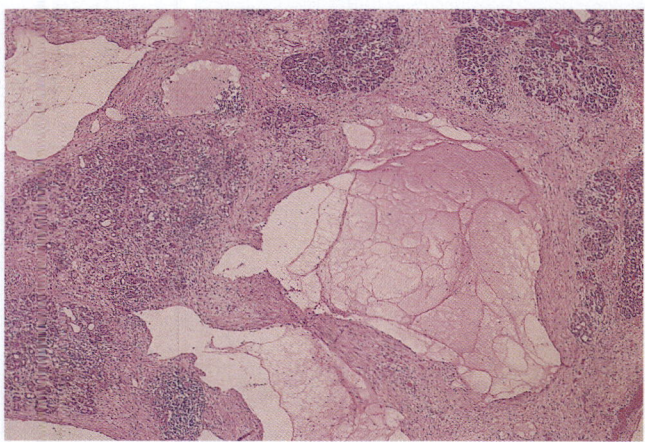

FIG. 68. Lymphangioma. Parenchymal atrophy, fibrosis, and lymphoid infiltration contrast with the spaces filled with coagulated lymph.

A multilocular neoplasm protruded from the pancreatic head in a 74-year-old woman (150). There was great variation in the size of the cysts and the contents were watery. The lining epithelium ranged from flat to columnar to pseudostratified and papillary with pleomorphic cells. The cytoplasm was finely granular and eosinophilic. Antibodies to synaptophysin and carcinoembryonic antigen were positive. Ultrastructural studies revealed many swollen mitochondria and lipid droplets, but no endocrine granules. No mucus and only a trace of glycogen could be found. Metastases were present.

Lymphangiomas

Lymphangioma may present as an abdominal mass or may be discovered incidentally during abdominal imaging studies or during abdominal surgery (151). The mass may closely resemble the other cystic neoplasms, especially if cavernous or cystic in type. The capillary lymphangioma might be mistaken for a solid tumor. Clear or hemorrhagic fluid occupies the spaces in the lesions. The endothelial cells lining the spaces are flat and do not contain glycogen, keratin, or epithelial membrane antigen. Factor VIII–related antigen and other markers for endothelial cells can be demonstrated. Lymphoid tissue, fibrous stroma with scattered smooth muscle fibers, and tiny capillaries in the stroma are present (Fig. 68).

Hemangiomas in the pancreas are similar to these lesions elsewhere and are extremely rare.

Lymphoepithelial Cysts

Lymphoepithelial cysts (152) are typically unilocular or multilocular cystic masses that lie within or protrude from the pancreas. The patients are mostly male, usually middle-aged. Some lesions are asymptomatic, found incidentally or at autopsy. Gross examination shows an encapsulated cystic lesion. Contents may be watery fluid or keratinous material. Microscopic examination reveals a fibrous capsule, lymphoid tissue with lymphoid follicles, and a cyst lining of stratified squamous epithelium (Fig. 69). The lesion is distinct from a dermoid cyst because of the large amount of organized lymphoid tissue present.

Differential Diagnosis of Cystic Lesions

Alcoholism, biliary tract disease, or former abdominal trauma suggest a pseudocyst; most patients are young to middle-aged men. The pseudocyst is usually unilocular and may communicate with the ductal system. The absence of an epithelial lining and of specialized cellular stroma favors pseudocyst over mucinous cystic neoplasm. Fluid in pseudocysts typically is thin, contains necrotic debris or blood, and is rich in pancreatic enzymes.

Fluid of the mucinous tumors usually is viscid, low in enzymes, and rich in carcinoembryonic antigen, CA 19-9, and CA 72-4 (125). There are exceptions (153). Imaging studies usually show multiple locules.

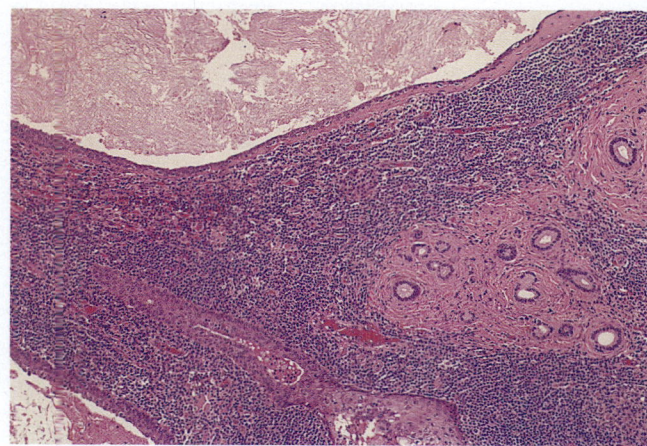

FIG. 69. Lymphoepithelial cyst. Keratinous material fills the cysts lined by squamous epithelium. Lymphoid tissue is closely associated wih the epithelium, and atrophic pancreatic tissue is visible.

Hemorrhage, necrosis, and loss of epithelium may occur in any cystic neoplasm, thereby obscuring portions of its characteristic architecture. Critical evaluation of the history, the imaging and clinical laboratory data, and the pathologic specimen is essential with all cystic lesions (124). Needle aspiration or surgical biopsy may be insufficient for diagnosis. Close follow-up is needed; if a supposed pseudocyst does not disappear a few weeks after drainage, then a neoplasm must be considered likely.

Ductal carcinoma sometimes has a cystic component (cavitary necrosis) or is associated with a retention cyst or a pseudocyst. The same is true for endocrine tumors.

Serous neoplasms should be differentiated from the mucinous cystic neoplasms (Table 2), lymphangiomas, the pseudomicrocystic pattern sometimes present in the Gruber-Frantz tumors, renal cell carcinoma with clear cells, and clear cell endocrine tumors. In lymphangioma, the cells lining the spaces are positive for the factor VIII–related antigen and other endothelial markers; lymphoid follicles and occasional bundles of smooth muscle are present in the stroma. Renal cell carcinomas typically have larger cells with less regular nuclei and are not organized into a microcystic pattern. In the Gruber-Frantz tumors, the cells lack glycogen, the nuclei are usually ovoid (some with a groove), and the pseudomicrocysts are actually multiple small foci of loose connective tissue; these tumors are usually invasive at their borders.

NEOPLASMS OF INDETERMINATE TYPE OR MIXED EXOCRINE-ENDOCRINE TYPE

Neoplasms in Children, Including Pancreatoblastoma

Pancreatic neoplasms in infants and children are rare and consist of endocrine neoplasms, ductal adenocarcinomas,

TABLE 2. *Pancreatic cystic masses*

	Pseudocysts	Mucinous cystic neoplasms	Serous neoplasms	Intraductal papillary mucinous neoplasms (IPMN)
Incidence	More common	Rare	Rare	Rare
Nature of lesions	Postnecrotic; posttraumatic	Neoplastic	Neoplastic	Neoplastic dilated ducts
Clinical setting	Alcoholism; biliary tract disease; abdominal trauma	Nonspecific	Nonspecific	Bouts of pancreatitis
Age	Youth to middle age	Mostly 40–60 years	Middle-aged and elderly	Middle-aged to elderly
Sex	Men predominate	Mostly women	Moderate majority of women	Majority are men
Location in pancreas	In pancreas and adjacent tissues	More in tail	Evenly distributed	Head, head and body
Gross appearance	Thick-walled; adherent to surrounding tissues	Encapsulated, rounded or bosselated masses with smooth surfaces; unilocular or multilocular; internal papillary excrescences common; occasional focal calcification	Round to ovoid, may be delicately encapsulated; honeycombed cut surfaces; rarely one or two large locules; stellate scar common and often calcified	Elongated, irregular, dilated ducts; occasional nodular or papillary mass in duct
Contents	Hemorrhage (old and/or recent); necrotic debris; fluid rich in pancreatic enzymes	Thick, mucoid, or gelatinous turbid fluid; occasional necrotic foci and hemorrhage	Thin, clear, watery fluid; occasional hemorrhage	Usually copious thick mucus
Light-microscopic features	Fibrous wall with chronic inflammation and necrotic debris; no epithelial lining or mucus production	Columnar, mucus-producing cells in a single row or forming papillae; hypercellular ("ovarian type") stroma; atypical epithelium common; carcinoma may be found	Cysts (usually tiny), with cuboidal to flattened cells; nuclei round and regular; cytoplasm rich in glycogen; scattered small papillae may be present; hypocellular stroma	Columnar mucinous cells or cuboidal eosinophilic cells; cells regular to markedly atypical; forming papillae
Adjacent pancreas	Healing pancreatitis common	Normal pancreas or occasional atrophy secondary to obstruction; some surrounded by dense fibrosis	Normal pancreas; rare atrophy secondary to obstruction	Atrophy or scarring common

and acinar cell carcinoma, generally morphologically similar to those of adults.

A group of rather pleomorphic tumors called pancreatoblastomas present as generally encapsulated masses, often large, that may extend outside the pancreas (154,155). About three-fifths occur in males, mostly during infancy and early childhood. The cut surfaces are described as yellow, white, gray, or tan, firm, and sometimes lobulated (Fig. 70). Hemorrhage, necrosis, and focal cystic change are rather frequent and may be extensive.

The tumors are composed of polygonal epithelial cells and variable amounts of stroma, usually quite cellular, which in turn divides the epithelial masses into irregular islands and trabeculae. The cells form solid islands and structures resembling acini and short tubules (Fig. 71). Cells are medium-sized and polygonal, have central round or ovoid nuclei with generally central nucleoli, and possess amphophilic to eosinophilic cytoplasm. When the cells form structures resembling acini and tubules, nuclei are basal, and usually these cells contain zymogen granules. Lipase, trypsin, and chymotrypsin have been detected. The amount of cytoplasm and the size and characteristics of the nuclei may vary in different parts of the neoplasm. Foci of necrosis may occur. Usually there are multiple groups of cells forming squamoid nests or corpuscles (whorls of plump elongated cells with variably eosinophilic cytoplasm) (Figs. 71 and 72). Some of these cells are keratinized, and occasional keratin pearls are present. Eosinophilic cytoplasm and keratinization of cells along the strands of stroma are sometimes evident also (Fig. 73). When distinct ductular structures are present, the apical surfaces of the cells are positive for mucin; in occasional ducts there are mucinous columnar cells.

Endocrine differentiation in the solid parts is commonly detected with immunohistochemical stains, but is less likely to be found with electron microscopy. Carcinoembryonic antigen occurs in scattered cells and in some squamoid corpuscles. Myxoid, collagenous, cartilagenous, and osteoid elements in the stroma occasionally are evident.

Several patients have had successful resections; others have died because of recurrence and metastases (especially to the liver). The authors and others have seen a few pancreatoblastomas in adults.

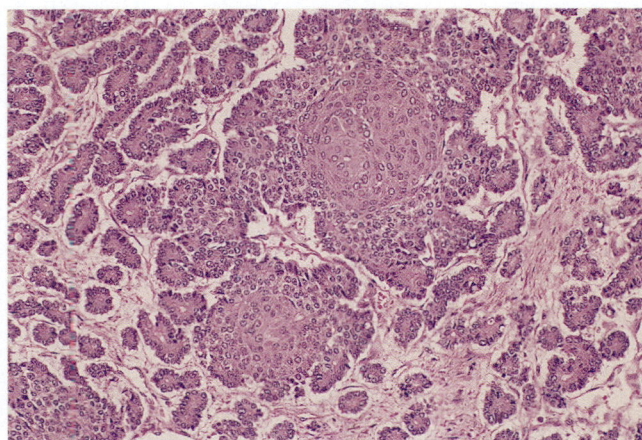

FIG. 71. Pancreatoblastoma. The cells are arranged in solid islands, acini, and short tubules. In the solid part the squamoid corpuscles are evident.

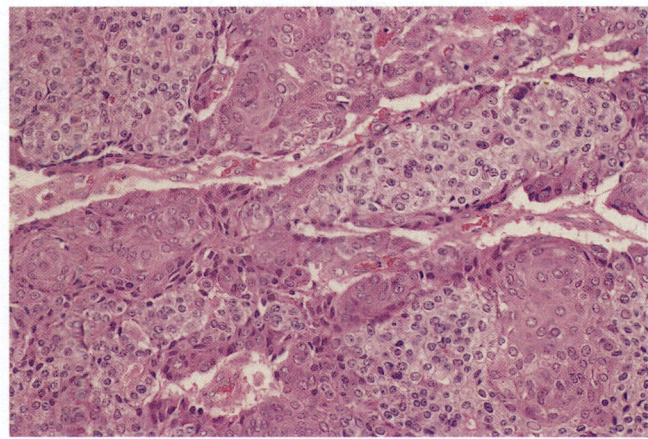

FIG. 72. Pancreatoblastoma. The epithelial cells alongside the stroma have eosinophilic cytoplasm and a tendency to form squamoid corpuscles.

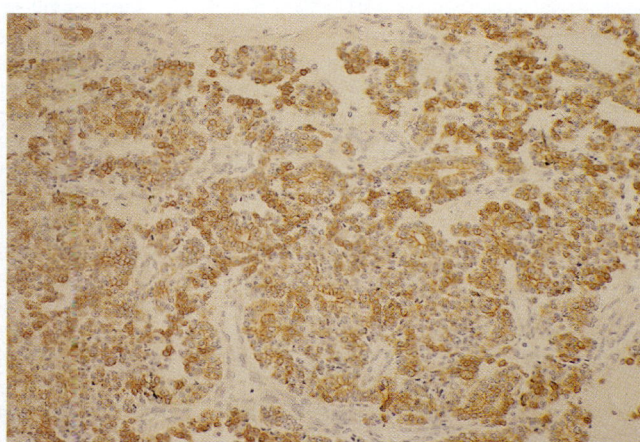

FIG. 73. Pancreatoblastoma. A generous amount of immunoreactive keratin is visible, but note that some cells are negative for keratin.

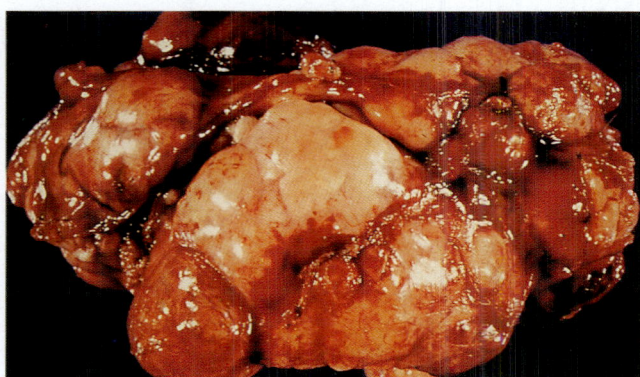

FIG. 70. Pancreatoblastoma. Note the lobulation.

Neoplasms of Mixed Endocrine and Exocrine Elements

Foci with endocrine characteristics have been demonstrated within several pancreatoblastomas (154); this has occurred also in the usual ductal adenocarcinomas (108,109) and in acinar cell carcinomas (111). Furthermore, ductular structures have been described often in the endocrine tumors. Beyond these examples, there are rare neoplasms in which extensive exocrine and endocrine differentiation have been represented (114,156–158).

Another related issue is the existence of cells with both exocrine and endocrine features, the existence of which has been affirmed (159–161) or denied (162). The authors have not recognized this phenomenon in their materials.

Gruber-Frantz Tumor (Solid-Cystic-Papillary Epithelial Neoplasm)

This neoplasm occurs often in adolescent girls and young women and has been mistaken for an endocrine neoplasm or a cystic tumor (154). It is rare in childhood, in older women, and in men; rarely it may be parapancreatic in location (163). It occurs in all races. Some have been found on routine physical examination or imaging study, others after abdominal trauma caused hemorrhage in the neoplasms, and some have presented with abdominal discomfort or pain accompanied by an enlarging mass. Some tumors are large (10 cm or greater diameter). Many are encapsulated. The cut surfaces are typically soft, with cystic foci, hemorrhage, and necrosis (Fig. 74) (164,165).

The neoplasms appear to begin as solid masses in which there are many poorly supported tiny vessels; then the cells farthest from the small vessels undergo swelling and degenerative changes, whereas the cells next to the vessels remain intact (Fig. 75) (166). The result is a pseudopapillary pattern and cystic spaces. Groups of foamy macrophages accumulate, and there are clusters of lipid crystals surrounded by foreign-body giant cells (Fig. 76). Myxoid connective tissue proliferates around the tiny blood vessels, and these regions of loose, hypocellular connective tissue may be mistaken for microcysts (a pseudomicrocystic pattern) (Fig. 77). As collagen is deposited in the tumor along the blood vessels, a trabecular pattern of epithelial cells may emerge. Consequently, microscopic examination reveals a variety of patterns (solid, pseudopapillary, cystic, pseudomicrocystic, trabecular). Confusion may result because of the resemblance to other pancreatic neoplasms.

The cells are small to medium-sized and polygonal to elongated (Fig. 75), with ovoid nuclei that often are grooved or indented. Rarely, a few cells have nuclei that are large or irregular in shape (Fig. 78). Nucleoli are inconspicuous. Mitotic figures are rare. The cytoplasm ranges from clear to eosinophilic and lacks glycogen and mucin. Vimentin is common. Immunoreactive keratin is occasionally expressed in patchy fashion. Alpha$_1$-antitrypsin and alpha$_1$-chymotrypsin are frequently demonstrated in small, eosinophilic (Fig. 79), PAS-positive cytoplasmic globules. Most cells are nonde-

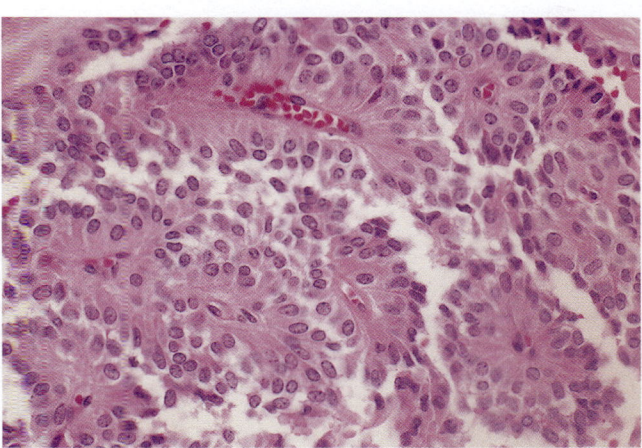

FIG. 75. Gruber-Frantz tumor. The cells adjacent to the tiny blood vessels are attached to the stroma and to one another, but those that are farther away are detached from each other. Tiny slits separate the pseudopapillae.

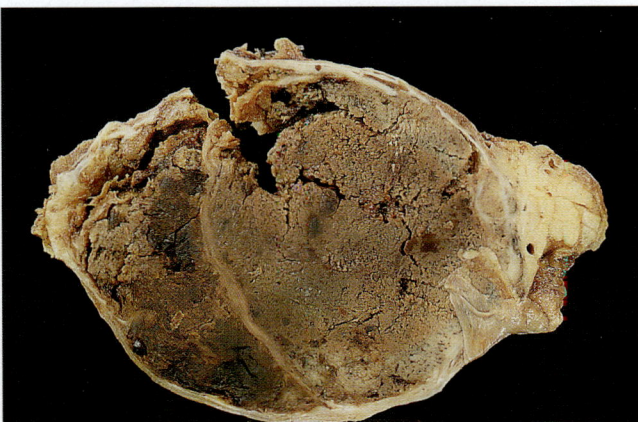

FIG. 74. Gruber-Frantz tumor (solid-cystic-papillary epithelial neoplasm). Focal cystic change and extensive hemorrhage are visible in this neoplasm. The cut surface appears granular.

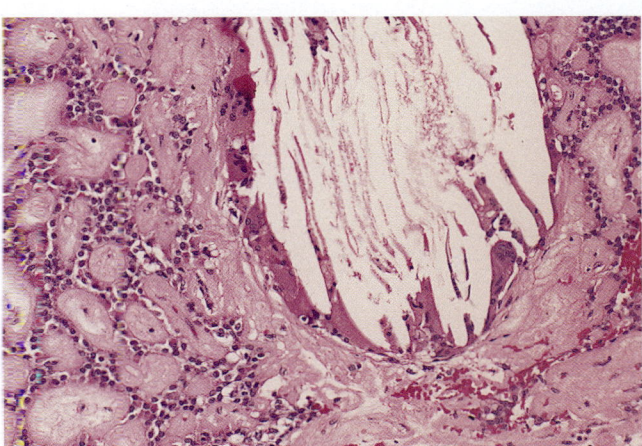

FIG. 76. Gruber-Frantz tumor. Lipid crystals are surrounded by foreign-body giant cells.

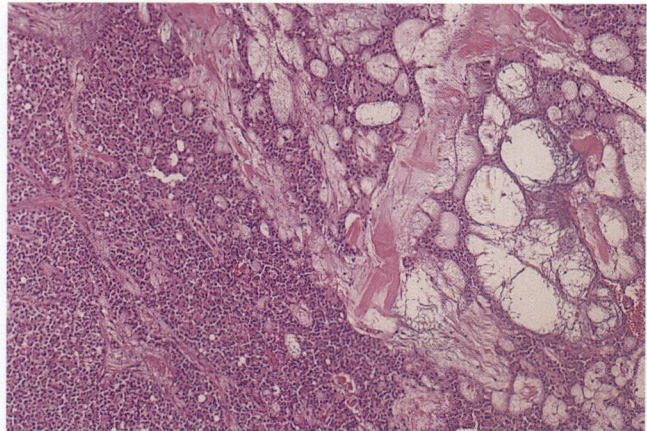

FIG. 77. Gruber-Frantz tumor. Part of the tumor is solid. The remainder contains myxoid connective tissue producing the pseudomicrocystic pattern.

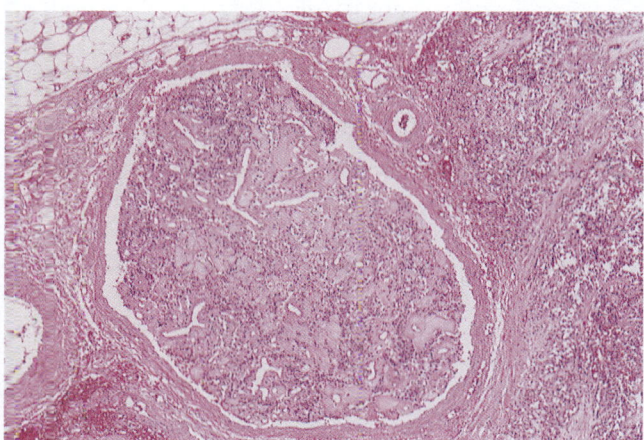

FIG. 80. Gruber-Frantz tumor. The tumor lies in a blood vessel in adjacent pancreatic parenchyma.

script by electron microscopic examination (167). When they have numerous mitochondria, the tumor cells may be considered oncocytic (168). In a few cases either zymogen-type granules or endocrine-type granules have been reported. It is probably a neoplasm of uncommitted cells, with most cells similar to intercalated duct cells or centroacinar cells (164,165). Its infiltrative tendencies can trap acinar or islet cells within the tumor, so such cells should not be regarded as evidence of specific differentiation by the neoplasm.

The neoplasm can invade vessels in the surrounding capsule or extend into adjacent normal pancreas (Fig. 80) (164). Some lack capsules. Metastases to the liver and peritoneum are uncommon, and most patients have fared well after limited resections because of its indolent growth (164,165,169,170).

Microglandular Adenocarcinoma

Microglandular adenocarcinoma was described as a solid mass (a variant of ductal carcinoma), formed of small to medium-sized cells, that contained small glands (Fig. 81)

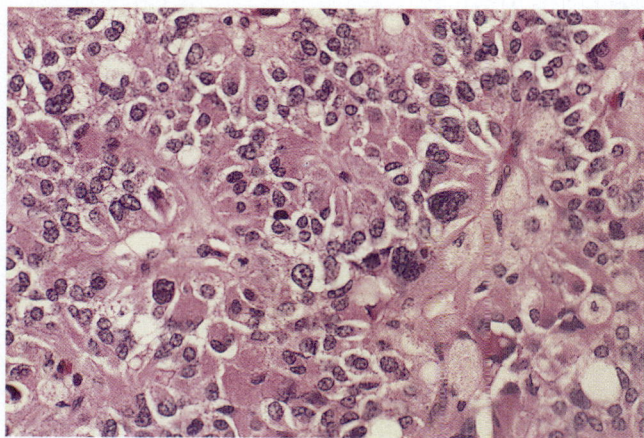

FIG. 78. Gruber-Frantz tumor. The large atypical nuclei present in this case are unusual.

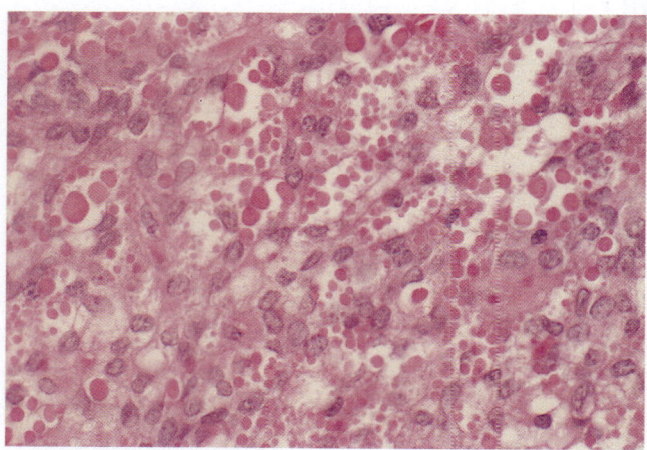

FIG. 79. Gruber-Frantz tumor. Large numbers of eosinophilic globules are sometimes present.

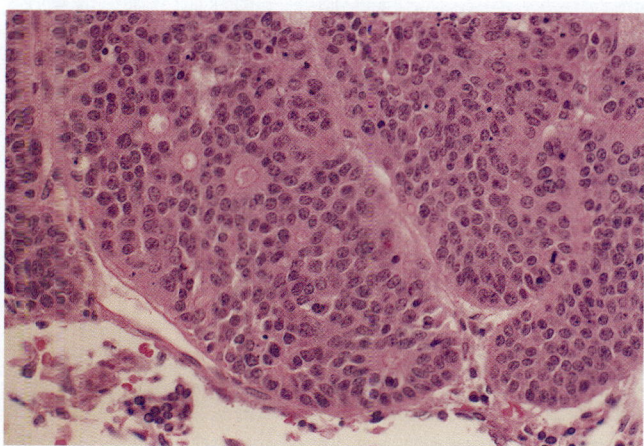

FIG. 81. Microglandular adenocarcinoma. This pattern has been reported in ductal adenocarcinoma, in acinar cell carcinoma, and in pancreatic endocrine neoplasms.

(1,171). The neoplasms were large; they contained less fibrosis and more necrotic tissue than the usual adenocarcinomas; some were extremely aggressive. Subsequently it was suggested that these were variants of either endocrine or acinar cell carcinomas, not a clinicopathologic entity (172). Others continue to believe that the category is a valid subdivision of ductal adenocarcinoma, as well as agreeing that the pattern may occur in neoplasms with endocrine or acinar differentiation.

Oncocytic Carcinoma

This rare neoplasm has been described as an invasive solid carcinoma with pale cut surfaces and without much stroma (173,174). It consists of large cells having eosinophilic granular cytoplasm (caused by innumerable mitochondria). A few glandular structures have been detected, but most cells form a solid mass. It was considered a variant of ductal adenocarcinoma.

Rare tumors of islet cells (175), the Gruber-Frantz tumors (168), and occasional intraductal papillary neoplasms (106) are composed of oncocytes

Clear Cell Carcinoma

Only a few of these neoplasms occur. The alteration sometimes is the result of mucus in the cytoplasm (176). A pancreatic endocrine tumor with clear cells has been described (177).

A single solid neoplasm with clear cells and eosinophilic granular cells has been reported as a clear cell "sugar" tumor because of its glycogen content (178).

ENDOCRINE NEOPLASMS

The neoplasms resembling the endocrine elements of the pancreas are most commonly called islet-cell adenomas and carcinomas, but because of their unpredictable behavior and frequent resemblance to intestinal carcinoid tumors, a variety of names have been utilized. *Pancreatic endocrine neoplasm* may be the least confusing term and perhaps the most accurate.

The pathologist should remember that about 1% of pancreata examined at autopsy contain these rare neoplasms, usually small ones that have caused no signs or symptoms (179).

Syndromes occur related to the excessive production of a normal pancreatic hormone (insulin, for example) or an ectopic hormone (gastrin, vasoactive intestinal peptide), or the neoplasm may present as an abdominal mass, as pain in the abdomen or back, or with obstructive phenomena (180). Therefore, endocrine neoplasms must be included in the surgical pathologist's differential diagnosis of masses in the pancreas. In particular, the large tumors may not be associated with a clinical endocrine syndrome. The functional capacity of the neoplasms is not related to their sizes; as a result, those of clinical significance range from less than 1 cm to 15 cm or more in diameter (181). Most are solitary, but more than one tumor is common in multiple endocrine neoplasia (MEN) type I (180,182). Peptic ulcer may be associated with multiple pancreatic tumors in which gastrin has not been detected; instead, small gastrinomas are present outside the pancreas, usually in the duodenum (183).

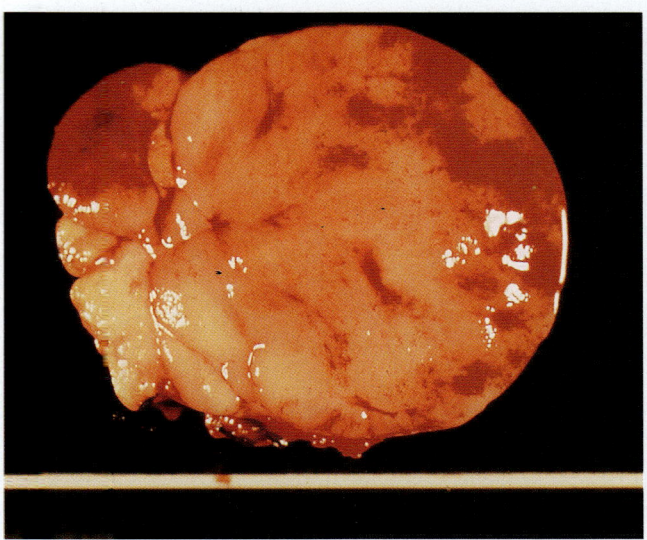

FIG. 82. Endocrine neoplasm. The yellowish cut surface of this well-circumscribed mass contains multiple hemorrhagic foci.

Gross Findings

On gross examination, most endocrine neoplasms are discrete masses, often partly or completely encapsulated. The color depends on the amount of stroma, the degree of vascularity, and whether or not a considerable amount of lipid is present; thus, it ranges from pale gray or tan, to pink or red, to yellow (181). Fibrosis is sometimes marked. Cystic degeneration rarely occurs (124). Hemorrhage into and from the tumor is occasionally notable (Figs. 82 and 83).

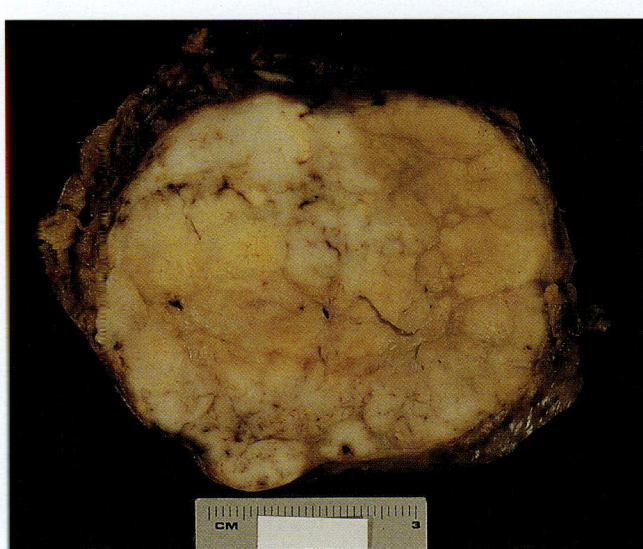

FIG. 83. Endocrine neoplasm. Although generally well circumscribed, there is a protrusion along the inferior border.

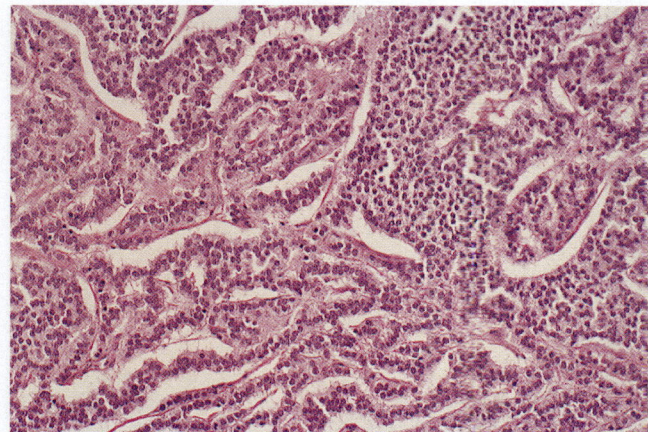

FIG. 84. Endocrine neoplasm. There is a mixture of solid and ribbon-like patterns.

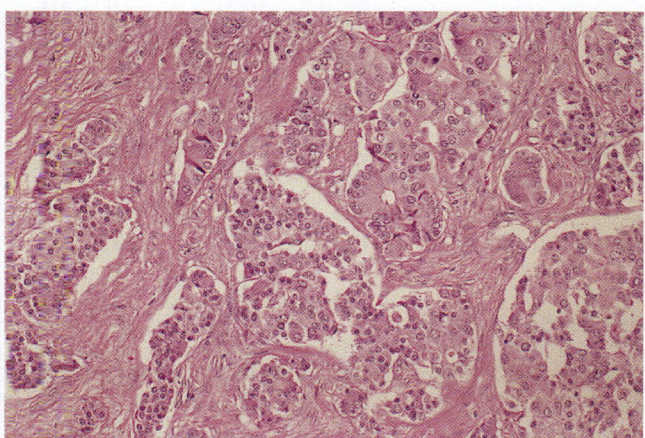

FIG. 86. Endocrine neoplasm. The neoplastic cells are present in irregular islands and as a well-formed glandular structure (center).

The tumors are evenly distributed throughout the pancreas. Many gastrin-producing neoplasms occur in the duodenum, the gastric antrum, along the common bile duct, and in the peripancreatic soft tissues (182).

Microscopic Features

Patterns suggesting an endocrine neoplasm are the result of a well-organized relationship of the neoplastic cells to numerous small blood vessels and the tendency of most cells to be rather uniform in appearance. Three principal microscopic patterns may occur, singly or in combination: (a) the ribbon-like, trabecular, or gyriform pattern (Figs. 84 and 85); (b) acinar or duct-like formations (Fig. 86); and (c) the solid, diffuse, or medullary pattern (Fig. 84) (180,181). Other patterns have been described (180). Striking differences in the architecture may be present within the same neoplasm, and generally there is no constant relationship of the architecture to the functional capacity, if any, of the neoplasms. Exceptions exist. Insulinomas usually have ribbon-like patterns and deposits of amyloid. The tumors producing somatostatin often contain psammoma bodies.

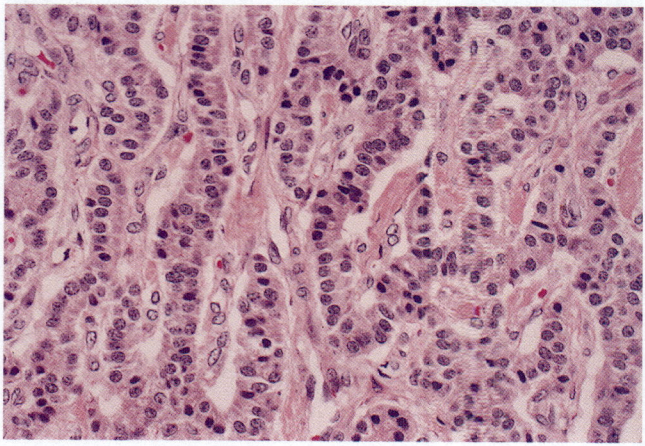

FIG. 85. Endocrine neoplasm. An irregular trabecular pattern is present. Many nuclei are elongated.

The cells are usually rounded or polygonal, and in the majority of cases they are similar to one another in size and shape. The cells are sometimes elongated, especially when the ribbon or trabecular pattern is present (Fig. 85). In this instance, the long axis of the cells tends to be perpendicular to the long axis of the ribbon. Nuclei tend to be round when the cells are round and elongated when the cells are elongated (Fig. 85). Frequently, most of the cells are small to medium-sized; rarely, all or most of the cells are large. A minority of cells may be large to very large, sometimes irregular in shape, with large, or even giant, nuclei (184). These large, irregular, or bizarre cells tend to be superimposed on a relatively uniform population of cells, which contrasts these neoplasms with the usual ductal carcinomas.

The nuclei often resemble those of normal islet cells (with tiny clumps of dense heterochromatin scattered through the nuclei), the nucleoli range from relatively inconspicuous to prominent, and the cytoplasm varies from pale to moderately eosinophilic. Typical oncocytes can occur (175). Rarely, the cytoplasm is clear (177). Usually little or no glycogen can be demonstrated with the PAS technique; exceptions occur (177). Argyrophilic cytoplasmic granules frequently can be demonstrated. Occasional neoplasms are rich in neutral lipid (185) and therefore may have foamy cytoplasm; in the authors' experience, these are not insulin-producing but, instead, produce other substances or are apparently nonfunctional. PAS-positive globules may occur in the cytoplasm or in extracellular locations; these contain alpha$_1$-antitrypsin (185). Trapped normal exocrine structures and islets (Fig. 87) may be present; ductal elements may form within the tumors. Many tumors are devoid of mucus, but when droplets of mucus are present, they often are evident in the centers of glandular or ductal structures. Typical goblet cells can occur. Dense stroma may be a conspicuous feature (Fig. 88). Deposits of amyloid may be seen, and the islet amyloid polypeptide may be detected in blood and the tissues (186).

Aspirates from pancreatic endocrine neoplasms are extremely cellular ("tumor cellularity") (Fig. 89). At low mag-

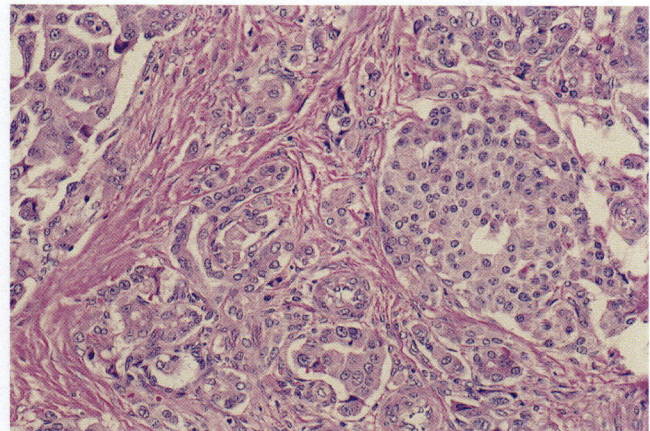

FIG. 87. Endocrine neoplasm. Note poorly formed glands and the trapped islet.

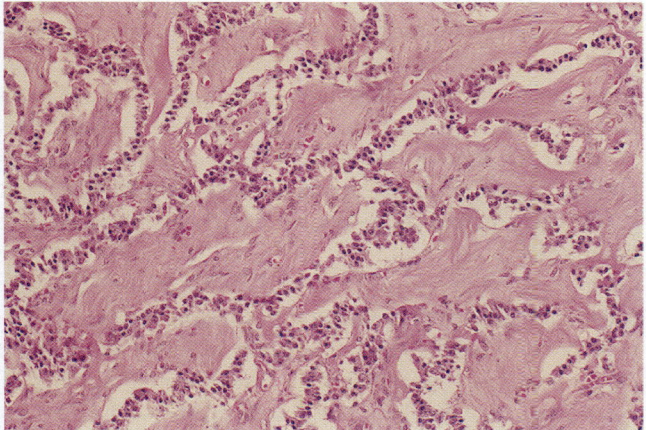

FIG. 88. Endocrine neoplasm. A large amount of dense stroma separates the ribbons of neoplastic cells.

nification, loosely cohesive cells predominate (187). However, some cellular clusters (consisting of a few cells to over a hundred cells) are scattered throughout the smears. Although the single-cell pattern has been emphasized in the literature, this clumping has been observed in the authors' cases. The cells are uniform, are relatively small, and have small round nuclei, usually eccentric; the nucleoli are not evident with hematologic stains. The cytoplasm of these cells is often scanty, grayish-pink, and varies from thin to dense. The eccentric location of the nuclei and the character of the cytoplasm may give the cells a plasmacytoid appearance (Fig. 90) (187). In one case, most of the cells (singly and in clusters) had finely vacuolated cytoplasm. Although the cells tend to be uniform, occasional moderately large, atypical single cells are present.

The amount of stroma in endocrine neoplasms is extremely variable. Some may be dense and hyalinized (Fig. 83). Calcification may be present and has two principal forms: (a) irregular masses in the stroma, and (b) tiny calcospherites (psammoma bodies). Probably because of the slow growth of some of the endocrine tumors, the irregular stromal calcifications may be extensive, even in metastatic foci.

Routine morphologic examination may not allow the pathologist to predict which tumor will spread outside the pancreas. Larger size of the tumor and considerable mitotic activity usually indicate a poorer prognosis. The pathologist should search for local invasion. Nuclear ploidy does not discriminate between benign and malignant neoplasms, but aneuploidy has been reported as associated with greater aggressiveness in the malignant examples. Cells expressing Ki-67 antigen and increased numbers of nuclei demonstrating the proliferating cell nuclear antigen (PCNA) have been claimed to be indicators of malignancy (188,189). Insulin-producing tumors often behave in a benign fashion, with successful surgical resections. Neoplasms producing hormones other than insulin and the nonfunctional ones frequently have metastatic foci, and the chance of cure is less (181,190).

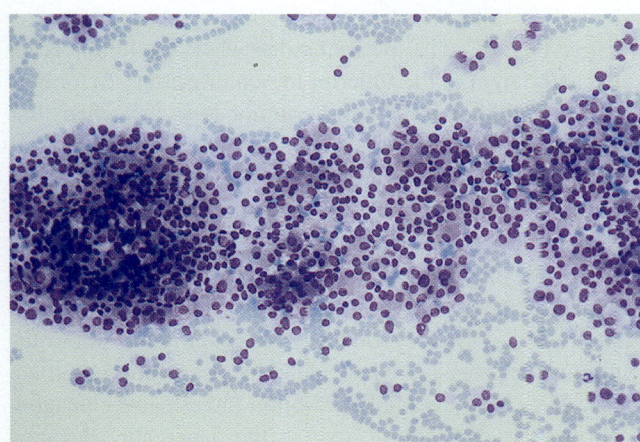

FIG. 89. Endocrine neoplasm. FNA. Tumor cellularity. Neoplastic cells in clumps of different sizes and also scattered singly.

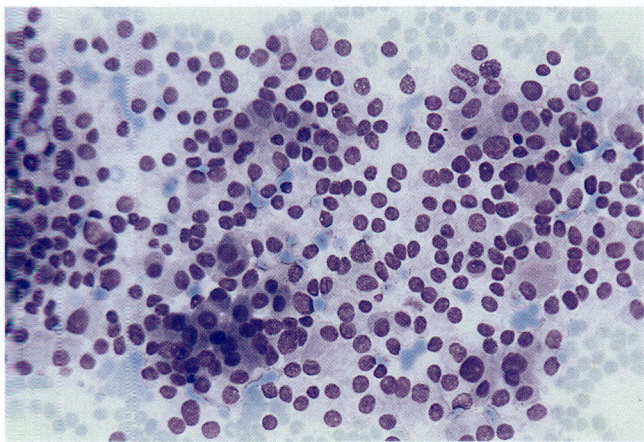

FIG. 90. Endocrine neoplasm. FNA. Loosely cohesive cells with some variation in nuclear size. Note resemblance to plasma cells.

We believe that all the tumors should be regarded as potentially malignant, and the term *adenoma* should be avoided.

Because the endocrine tumors frequently grow slowly and trap various normal pancreatic elements within them (Fig. 87), these normal structures should not be mistaken for part of the tumor when special staining procedures or ultrastructural studies are performed.

The pathologist must remember that defining a small endocrine neoplasm versus a localized hyperplasia of endocrine elements (and possible associated ductal structures) sometimes may be difficult or impossible.

Pleomorphic endocrine neoplasms sometimes resemble solid ductal adenocarcinoma (184). When evaluating a neoplasm of uncertain type, the following ancillary studies may be useful: (a) additional sections from the tumor; (b) silver procedures for demonstrating argyrophilic granules; (c) immunohistochemical techniques (for carcinoembryonic antigen, synaptophysin, the chromogranins, and specific pancreatic and gastroenteric hormones); and (d) electron microscopy. The rarity of mitotic figures in most endocrine neoplasms is also helpful in making this distinction.

Associated Clinical Syndromes

Pancreatic endocrine neoplasms are of special interest because of the consequences of hormonal hypersecretion when it occurs. The hormones produced may not be secreted by normal pancreatic islet cells: gastrin, vasoactive intestinal peptide, adrenocorticotropic hormone (ACTH), parathyroid-like hormone, calcitonin, and growth hormone-releasing hormone. Serotonin normally is present in extremely limited amounts in the pancreas, but rarely a pancreatic endocrine tumor is the source of the carcinoid syndrome (191). Immunohistochemical techniques are invaluable in demonstrating the hormones and prohormones present. Often, a minor population of hormone-producing cells is present in addition to the principal cellular type (for example, somatostatin cells in a tumor producing insulin). Electron microscopic examination is useful in demonstrating the secretory granules, but the neoplastic granules may differ from those of normal cells; they may be nonspecific in appearance. Also, in a particular tumor, only a small proportion of the cells may have demonstrable hormone by the various special techniques applied. Characteristically, some of the neoplastic cells are devoid of any demonstrable hormones, the intensity of immunochemical staining (or the number of granules demonstrable by electron microscopy) varies from cell to cell, and the patterns of immunochemical staining are variable within the same tumor (Fig. 91). Also, within an individual cell the hormone may be diffusely present throughout the cytoplasm, may be concentrated at the capillary pole of the cell, or may be present as a localized focus (180). If the staining is quite uniform in the tumor, the possibility of an artifact must be considered. When multiple hormones are produced (Fig. 92), different metastatic deposits may release different hormones.

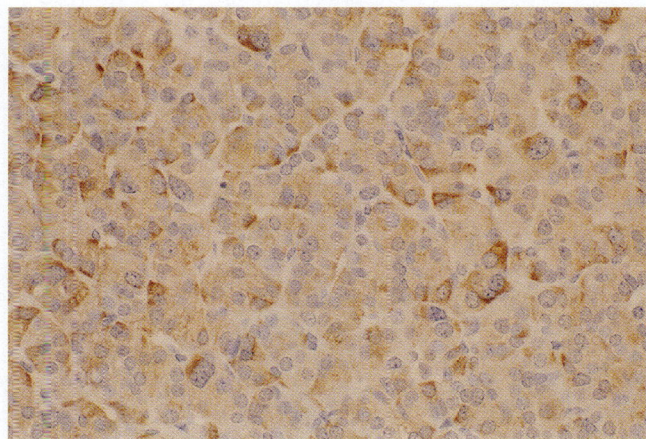

FIG. 91. Endocrine neoplasm producing insulin. Note the marked irregularity of the distribution of the immunoreactive insulin.

The insulin-producing neoplasms constitute a majority of those tumors that develop clinical manifestations as a result of their hormonal production (180,192,193). Most are solitary, occur in adults, and are small. Insulin can be demonstrated in nearly all of those producing hypoglycemia; about half are multihormonal (192). Proinsulin in varying amounts is commonly present, and defects in the production and secretion of insulin are believed to be present in nearly all cases. Islet amyloid polypeptide is usually produced in these tumors (186).

Approximately one-fifth to one-fourth of the clinically functional pancreatic tumors are gastrin-producing; a moderate proportion behave in a malignant fashion (although the progression may be indolent). A considerable number of these tumors are multiple, most occur in adults, and their locations often are extrapancreatic (duodenum, for example) (182,183,194). In patients with the Zollinger-Ellison syndrome, occasionally no primary tumor can be found in the pancreas or duodenum, but the cancer is present in lymph nodes. Hyperplasia of pancreatic polypeptide cells has been reported in the nonneoplastic pancreas when a gastrinoma is present (195). In sporadic gastrinomas, intratumoral pancreatic polypeptide cells are numerous when the tumor is located to the right of the superior mesenteric artery (in or near the pancreatic head). When the tumor is to the left of this artery, such cells are rare (196).

The other endocrine neoplasms with clinical syndromes are quite rare. Those producing glucagon with clinical manifestations of the hormonal excess are usually aggressive and large; often, only a relatively few cells can be demonstrated to contain glucagon by the usual immunohistochemical techniques (197). Tumors producing glucagon, but without the syndrome, are discovered accidentally at operation or at autopsy. They may be small and often have many glucagon-positive cells. Nesidioblastosis of the pancreatic glucagon cells may accompany such a tumor (198).

Pancreatic polypeptide frequently has been found as a second hormone in the glucagon-producing tumors and the gas-

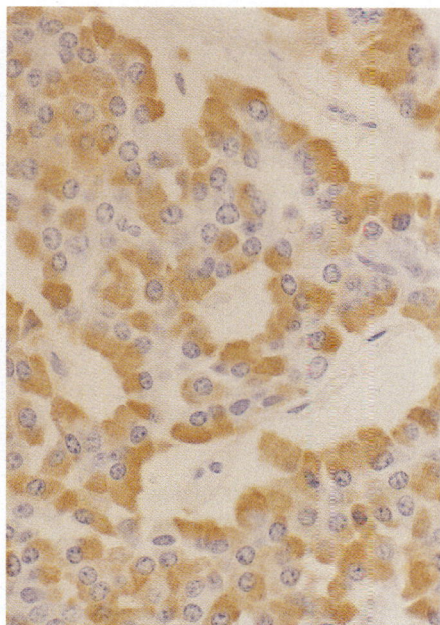 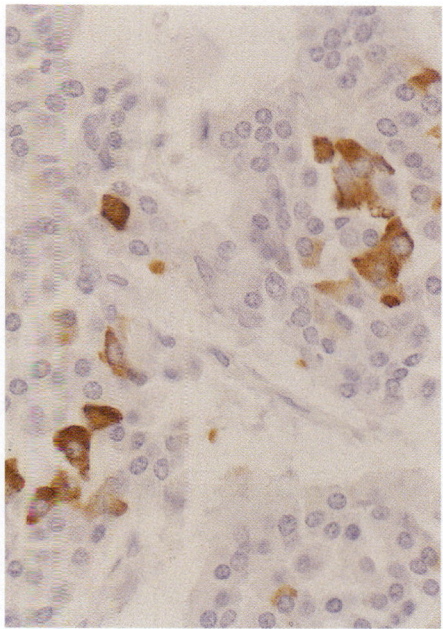

FIG. 92. Endocrine neoplasm (glucagonoma). Immunoreactive studies show glucagon in most of the cells and (left) pancreatic polypeptide in a minority of the cells (right).

trinomas. The somatostatin-producing tumors are usually solitary and malignant (199). The serotonin-producing neoplasms (pancreatic carcinoid tumors) have included several malignant examples (191). The tumors composed largely of cells containing pancreatic polypeptide usually have not been associated with a distinct clinical syndrome, although some patients have had diarrhea or a variety of other nonspecific problems such as weight loss, abdominal pain, or gastrointestinal bleeding. Tumors producing vasoactive intestinal peptide have caused intractable diarrhea and metabolic disturbances and are often aggressive (200). Rarely, ACTH has been the principal hormone liberated by a pancreatic tumor; these tumors have been malignant (181).

The nonfunctional pancreatic endocrine neoplasms discovered accidentally at surgery or autopsy may be devoid of hormones or may contain variable numbers of cells producing hormones (190,201). Rarely, a hormonal syndrome has occurred from a nonendocrine pancreatic neoplasm because of a population of endocrine cells within the predominantly exocrine neoplasm. Multiple pancreatic endocrine tumors typically represent a part of MEN type I, and each pancreatic tumor may produce different hormones (182,194).

Abnormal islets of Langerhans, proliferation of islet cells associated with ducts, and enlargement of islets may accompany the pancreatic endocrine neoplasms (180,202–204). All types of islet cells are represented in both enlarged islets and in the neoislets. A shift in the islet cell population may occur; the authors and others have seen a glucagon-producing tumor accompanied by islets in which the islet glucagon cells were smaller than usual and sparse (205). In the pancreas outside an insulin-producing tumor, the insulin cells may be altered in number and the proportion of glucagon cells and somatostatin cells increased (203,204). Likewise, proliferation of islet cells, the presence of abnormal islets,

and various changes in exocrine elements have been noted in instances of the Zollinger-Ellison syndrome (19,206). Groups of degranulated acinar cells occur with moderate frequency when islet cell tumors are present (8,203).

HYPOGLYCEMIA AND OTHER SYNDROMES WITHOUT A DETECTABLE ENDOCRINE NEOPLASM

Hyperinsulinemic Hypoglycemia

Hyperinsulinemic hypoglycemia in adults is usually the result of an endocrine neoplasm releasing insulin in abnormal amounts or at inappropriate times. The syndrome in infants and children is almost never caused by an endocrine neoplasm. Instead, the endocrine cells of the pancreas apparently function abnormally. There may be deviations from the normal histologic pattern of the pancreas expected for the age of the child, but often morphologic alterations are absent or minimal (162,207). When changes are present, they consist of (a) relatively large localized collections of islet cells displacing acinar tissue and containing neoproliferation of islet cells from ducts (focal adenomatosis); (b) the very rare, but similar, diffuse proliferation of islet cells (generalized adenomatosis); (c) endocrine-cell dysplasia or nesidiodysplasia (loss of the usual centrilobular concentration of larger islets, increased numbers of small aggregates of islet cells distributed irregularly in the lobules, irregularity of the contour of the islets) (Fig. 93); and (d) the presence of scattered islet cells (mostly insulin cells) with hypertrophic nuclei (Fig. 94). When evidence of islet cell proliferation occurs, insulin cells predominate. Also reported, but less well documented, is a possible decrease in the volume density of somatostatin cells.

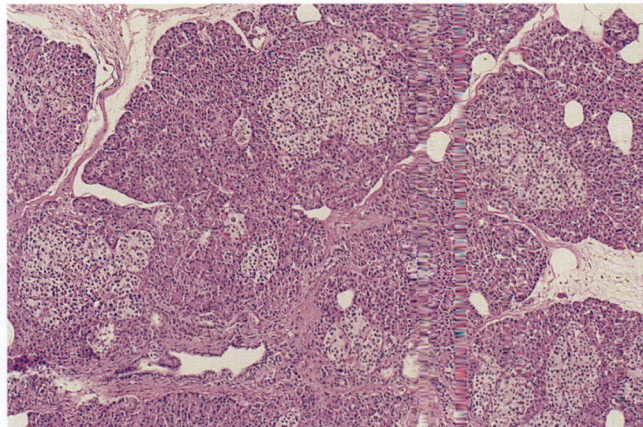

FIG. 93. Nesidiodysplasia. Large islets of irregular shape are present as well as small groups of islet cells.

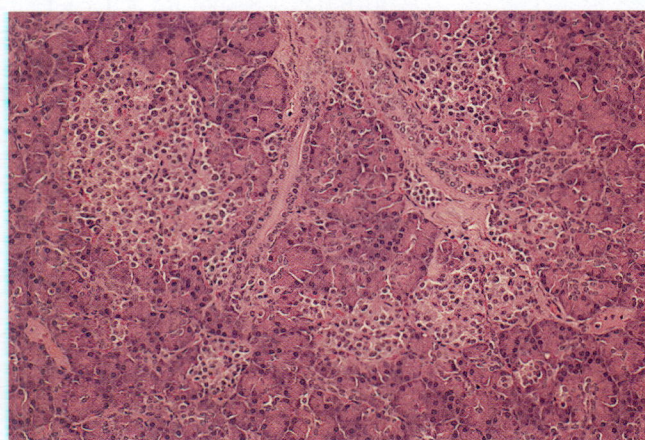

FIG. 95. Nesidioblastosis. Islet cells have proliferated in close association with pancreatic ducts.

In a small number of adult patients with hyperinsulinemic hypoglycemia or other evidence of endocrine hyperfunction, no neoplasm has been detected (208). Instead, other features have been described, such as: (a) numerous islet cells (singly or in clusters, with or without cytologic abnormalities), apparently arising from ducts (usually called nesidioblastosis) (Fig. 95); (b) increase in the size and number of otherwise normal islets; (c) irregularly shaped large islets unevenly distributed through the lobules; (d) numerous septal islets; (e) localized extraordinary increases in the amount of islet tissue (focal adenomatosis); and (f) abnormal characteristics of hyperplastic islets in cell cultures in vitro.

Many of the reported cases have not been carefully compared with controls, however. Critical reviews have demonstrated some of the same features in control pancreata, but have also suggested that when notable abnormalities of the endocrine pancreas are evident, an associated pancreatic endocrine tumor is usually present, but has been overlooked (203). The frequent presence of an endocrine neoplasm, perhaps as the principal cause of the syndrome, is suggested by another report (202). A diligent search for an endocrine neoplasm in any pancreatic tissue removed because of an endocrine hyperfunction is essential. The surgeon should be warned that if no tumor is found in the resected specimen, one may have been left in the patient.

Hypergastrinemia and Watery Diarrhea, Hypokalemia

Hypergastrinemia has been reported without a pancreatic neoplasm being found, but the tumor may have been overlooked in the pancreas or duodenum. The pancreas may be abnormal in various respects, but gastrin-producing cells have not been found in the organ, suggesting that the changes may be secondary (directly or indirectly) to gastrin excess. On the other hand, in some cases of the watery diarrhea–achlorhydria syndrome the pancreas has contained a notable diffuse proliferation of endocrine cells producing vasoactive intestinal peptide without a neoplasm being present (209).

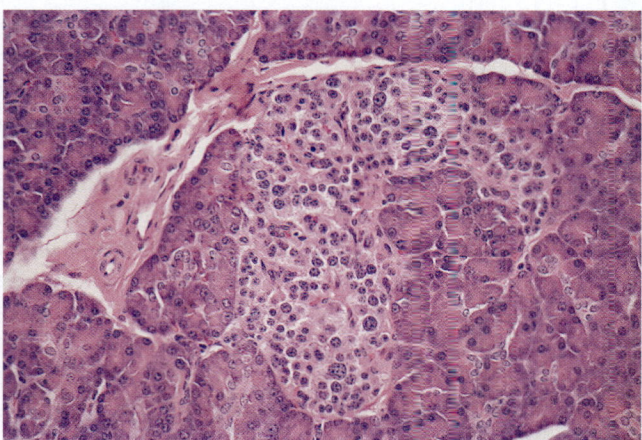

FIG. 94. Nesidiodysplasia. Hypertrophic nuclei are evident in an irregularly shaped islet.

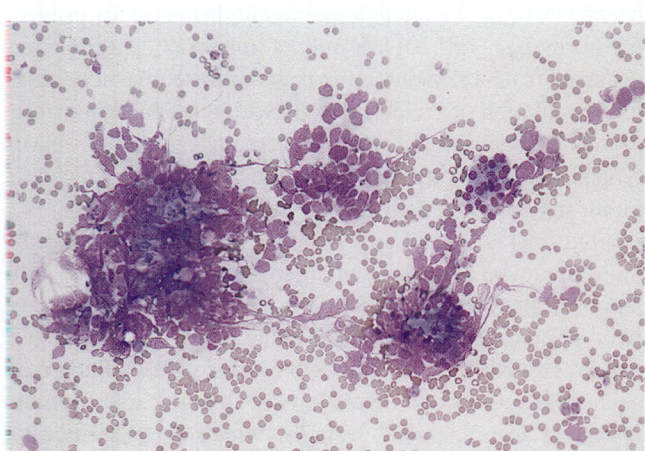

FIG. 96. Metastatic oat cell carcinoma from the lung. Loosely cohesive clusters of neoplastic cells with fragile nuclei and no visible cytoplasm are seen in a hemorrhagic background. A group of pancreatic acinar cells with bluish cytoplasm and small, regular nuclei is present.

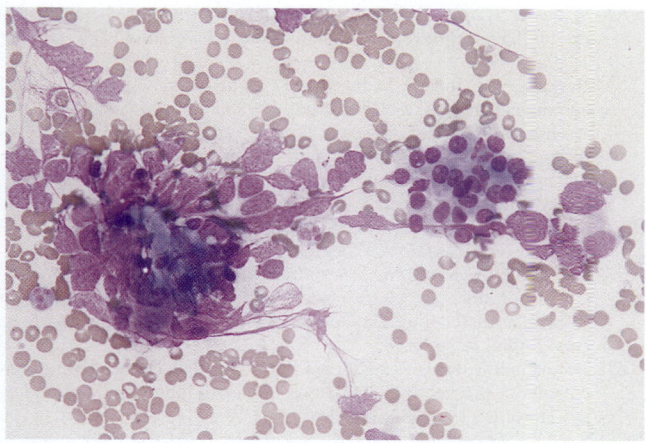

FIG. 97. Metastatic oat cell carcinoma from the lung. This higher magnification of Fig. 96 allows easier comparison of the acinar cells and the neoplastic cells.

OTHER NEOPLASMS

Inflammatory pseudotumor has been reported in the pancreas (210).

Malignant lymphomas rarely may appear to be primary in the pancreas, and a similar situation occurs for neoplasms of soft tissue origin, such as leiomyosarcoma or malignant fibrous histiocytoma. In most instances, these neoplasms arise in the retroperitoneal tissue, nearby lymph nodes, or adjacent gastrointestinal tract, and they involve the pancreas secondarily.

Metastatic neoplasms occur in the pancreas. They are often multifocal and lack the fibrosis so common in primary pancreatic adenocarcinoma. Carcinoma of the lung (Figs. 96 and 97) and renal cell carcinoma are among the most common.

REFERENCES

1. Cubilla AL, Fitzgerald PJ. Tumors of the exocrine pancreas. In: Hartmann WH, Sobin LH, eds. *Atlas of tumor pathology*, vol 19, 1st ed. Washington, DC: AFIP, 1984.
2. Lee PC, Lebenthal E. Prenatal and postnatal development of the human exocrine pancreas. In: Go VLW, Lebenthal E, DiMagno EP, Reber HA, Gardner JD, Scheele GA, eds. *The pancreas. Biology, pathobiology, and disease*, vol 1, 2nd ed. New York: Raven Press, 1993:57–73.
3. Cruickshank AH, Benbow EW. *Pathology of the pancreas*, 2nd ed. Berlin: Springer-Verlag, 1995.
4. Akao S, Bockman DE, Lechene de la Porte P, Sarles H. Three-dimensional pattern of ductuloacinar associations in normal and pathological human pancreas. *Gastroenterology* 1986;90:661–668.
5. Watanabe T, Yaegashi H, Koizumi M, Toyota T, Takahashi T. The lobular architecture of the normal human pancreas: a computer-assisted three-dimensional reconstruction study. *Pancreas* 1997;15:48–52.
6. Jeraldo TL, Coutu JA, Verdier PA, McMillan PN, Adelson JW. Fundamental cellular heterogeneity of the exocrine pancreas. *J Histochem Cytochem* 1996;44:215–220.
7. Klöppel G, Lenzen S. Anatomy and physiology of the endocrine pancreas. In: Klöppel G, Heitz PU, eds. *Pancreatic pathology*, 1st ed. Edinburgh: Churchill Livingstone, 1984:133–153.
8. Oertel JE. The pancreas. Nonneoplastic alterations. *Am J Surg Pathol Suppl* 1989;13(1):50–65.
9. Seifert G. Congenital anomalies. In: Klöppel G, Heitz PU, eds. *Pancreatic pathology*, 1st ed. Edinburgh: Churchill-Livingstone, 1984:22–26.
10. Kiernan PD, ReMine SG, Kiernan PC, ReMine WH. Annular pancreas. Mayo Clinic experience from 1957 to 1976 with review of the literature. *Arch Surg* 1980;115:46–50.
11. Wang HH, Zeroogian JM, Spechler SJ, Goyal RK, Antonioli DA. Prevalence and significance of pancreatic acinar metaplasia at the gastroesophageal junction. *Am J Surg Pathol* 1996;20:1507–1510.
12. Uomo G, Manes G, D'Anna L, Laccetti M, Di Gaeta S, Rabitti PG. Fusion and duplication variants of pancreatic duct system. Clinical and pancreatographic evaluation. *Int J Pancreatol* 1995;17:23–28.
13. Bernard JP, Sahel J, Giovannini M, Sarles H. Pancreas divisum is a probable cause of acute pancreatitis: a report of 137 cases. *Pancreas* 1990;5:248–254.
14. Stamm BH. Incidence and diagnostic significance of minor pathologic changes in the adult pancreas at autopsy: a systematic study of 112 autopsies in patients without known pancreatic disease. *Hum Pathol* 1984;15:677–683.
15. Seifert G. Lipomatous atrophy and other forms. In: Klöppel G, Heitz PU, eds. *Pancreatic pathology*, 1st ed. Edinburgh: Churchill-Livingstone, 1984:27–31.
16. Robson HN, Scott GBD. Lipomatous pseudohypertrophy of the pancreas. *Gastroenterology* 1953;23:74–81.
17. Shimizu M, Hayashi T, Saitoh Y, Itoh H. Interstitial fibrosis in the pancreas. *Am J Clin Pathol* 1989;91:531–534.
18. Brubaker R, Ray MB. Hyperplasia of centroacinar cells (CAC) and ductular proliferation in pancreas adjacent to islet cell tumors (ICT) and in chronic pancreatitis (CP). *Mod Pathol* 1990;3:12A(abst).
19. Brown RE, Still WJS. Nesidioblastosis and the Zollinger-Ellison syndrome. *Am J Dig Dis* 1968;13:656–663.
20. Bani D, Magnani L, Bani Sacchi T, Biliotti G. The exocrine pancreas in patients with hyperinsulinemic hypoglycemia. A morphometrical and ultrastructural study. *Int J Pancreatol* 1989;5:239–248.
21. Osborne BM, Butler JJ. Pancreatic acinar ectasia and intraoperative needle biopsy. *Hum Pathol* 1988;19:480–483.
22. Walters MN-I. Studies on the exocrine pancreas. I. Nonspecific pancreatic ductular ectasia. *Am J Pathol* 1964;44:973–981.
23. Kishi K, Nakamura K, Yoshimori M, et al. Morphology and pathological significance of focal acinar cell dysplasia of the human pancreas. *Pancreas* 1992;7:177–182.
24. Weidenheim KM, Hinchey WW, Campbell Jr WG. Hyperinsulinemic hypoglycemia in adults with islet-cell hyperplasia and degranulation of exocrine cells of the pancreas. *Am J Clin Pathol* 1983;79:14–24.
25. Longnecker DS, Shinozuka H, Dekker A. Focal acinar cell dysplasia in human pancreas. *Cancer* 1980;45:534–540.
26. Pour PM, Konishi Y, Klöppel G, Longnecker DS. Preneoplastic lesions of the exocrine pancreas. In: Pour PM, Konishi Y, Klöppel G, Longnecker DS, eds. *Atlas of exocrine pancreatic tumors. Morphology, biology, and diagnosis with an international guide for tumor classification*, vol 1, 1st ed. Tokyo: Springer-Verlag, 1994:211–219.
27. Longnecker DS, Hashida Y, Shinozuka H. Relationship of age to prevalence of focal acinar cell dysplasia in the human pancreas. *J Natl Cancer Inst* 1980;65:63–66.
28. Auerbach O, Garfinkel L. Histologic changes in pancreas in relation to smoking and coffee-drinking habits. *Dig Dis Sci* 1986;31:1014–1020.
29. Kozuka S, Sassa R, Taki T, et al. Relation of pancreatic duct hyperplasia to carcinoma. *Cancer* 1979;43:1418–1428.
30. Volkholz H, Stolte M, Becker V. Epithelial dysplasias in chronic pancreatitis. *Virchows Arch [A]* 1982;396:331–349.
31. Bockman DE, Boydston WR, Anderson MC. Origin of tubular complexes in human chronic pancreatitis. *Am J Surg* 1982;144:243–249.
32. Pour PM, Sayed S, Sayed G. Hyperplastic, preneoplastic and neoplastic lesions found in 83 human pancreases. *Am J Clin Pathol* 1982;77:137–152.
33. Klöppel G, Bommer G, Rückert K, Seifert G. Intraductal proliferation in the pancreas and its relationship to human and experimental carcinogenesis. *Virchows Arch [A]* 1980;387:221–233.
34. Yanagisawa A, Ohtake K, Ohashi K, et al. Frequent c-Ki-ras oncogene activation in mucous cell hyperplasias of pancreas suffering from chronic inflammation. *Cancer Res* 1993;53:953–956.
35. Rivera JA, Rall CJN, Graeme-Cook F, et al. Analysis of K-ras oncogene mutations in chronic pancreatitis with ductal hyperplasia. *Surgery* 1997;121:42–49.

36. Moossa AR, Altorki N. Pancreatic biopsy. *Surg Clin North Am* 1983;63:1205–1214.
37. Al-Kaisi N, Siegler EE. Fine needle aspiration cytology of the pancreas. *Acta Cytol* 1989;33:145–152.
38. Paksoy N, Lilleng R, Hagmar B, Wetteland J. Diagnostic accuracy of fine needle aspiration cytology in pancreatic lesions. A review of 77 cases. *Acta Cytol* 1993;37:889–893.
39. Brandt KR, Charboneau JW, Stephens DH, Welch TJ, Goellner JR. CT- and US-guided biopsy of the pancreas. *Radiology* 1993;187:99–104.
40. Linder S, Blåsjö M, Sundelin P, von Rosen A. Aspects of percutaneous fine-needle aspiration biopsy in the diagnosis of pancreatic carcinoma. *Am J Surg* 1997;174:303–306.
41. Faigel DO, Ginsberg GG, Bentz JS, Gupta PK, Smith DB, Kochman ML. Endoscopic ultrasound-guided real-time fine-needle aspiration biopsy of the pancreas in cancer patients with pancreatic lesions. *J Clin Oncol* 1997;15:1439–1443.
42. Chang KJ, Nguyen P, Erickson RA, Durbin TE, Katz KD. The clinical utility of endoscopic ultrasound-guided fine-needle aspiration in the diagnosis and staging of pancreatic carcinoma. *Gastrointest Endosc* 1997;45:387–393.
43. Reading CC. Percutaneous needle biopsy. *Abdom Imaging* 1997;22:311–312.
44. Alpern GA, Dekker A. Fine needle aspiration cytology of the pancreas. An analysis of its use in 52 patients. *Acta Cytol* 1985;29:873–878.
45. Edoute Y, Lemberg S, Malberger E. Preoperative and intraoperative fine needle aspiration cytology of pancreatic lesions. *Am J Gastroenterol* 1991;86:1015–1019.
46. Soudah B, Fritsch RS, Wittekind C, Hilka B, Spindler B. Value of the cytologic analysis of fine needle aspiration biopsy specimens in the diagnosis of pancreatic carcinomas. *Acta Cytol* 1989;33:875–880.
47. Sáez A, Català I, Brossa R, Funes A, Jaurrieta E, Ferrer JE. Intraoperative fine needle aspiration cytology of pancreatic lesions. A study of 90 cases. *Acta Cytol* 1995;39:485–488.
48. Weger AR, Glaser KS, Schwab G, et al. Quantitative nuclear DNA content in fine needle aspirates of pancreatic cancer. *Gut* 1991;32:325–328.
49. Nakhleh RE, Gruessner RWG, Swanson PE, et al. Pancreas transplant pathology. A morphologic, immunohistochemical, and electron microscopic comparison of allogeneic grafts with rejection, syngeneic grafts, and chronic pancreatitis. *Am J Surg Pathol* 1991;15:246–256.
50. Drachenberg C, Klassen D, Bartlett S, et al. Histologic grading of pancreas acute allograft rejection in percutaneous needle biopsies. *Transplant Proc* 1996;28:512–513.
51. Kuo PC, Johnson LB, Schweitzer EJ, et al. Solitary pancreas allografts. The role of percutaneous biopsy and standardized histologic grading of rejection. *Arch Surg* 1997;132:52–57.
52. Kubota K, Reinholt FP, Tydén G, Bohman S-O, Groth CG. Cytologic patterns in juice from human pancreatic transplants: correlation with histologic findings in the graft. *Surgery* 1991;109:507–5014.
53. Linder R, Tydén G, Tibell A, Groth C-G. Late graft pancreatitis. *Transplantation* 1990;50:257–261.
54. Bradley III EL. A clinically based classification system for acute pancreatitis. Summary of the international symposium on acute pancreatitis, Atlanta, Ga, September 11 through 13, 1992. *Arch Surg* 1993;128:586–590.
55. Klöppel G, Maillet B. Pathology of acute and chronic pancreatitis. *Pancreas* 1993;8:659–670.
56. Bockman DE. Pathology of edematous (interstitial) pancreatitis. In: Bradley EL III, ed. *Acute pancreatitis: diagnosis and therapy*, 1st ed. New York: Raven Press, 1994:241–247.
57. Evans HW, Gross JB, Baggenstoss AH. Acute and subacute interstitial pancreatitis: a clinicopathologic study. *Gastroenterology* 1958;35:457–464.
58. Czernobilsky B, Mikat KW. The diagnostic significance of interstitial pancreatitis found at autopsy. *Am J Clin Pathol* 1964;41:33–43.
59. Lankisch PG, Schirren CA, Kunze E. Undetected acute pancreatitis. *Digestion* 1989;43:155.
60. Seligson U, Cho J-W, Ihre T, Lundh G. Clinical course and autopsy findings in acute and chronic pancreatitis. *Acta Chir Scand* 1982;148:269–274.
61. Renner IG, Savage III WT, Pantoja JL, Renner VJ. Death due to acute pancreatitis. A retrospective analysis of 405 autopsy cases. *Dig Dis Sci* 1985;30:1005–1018.
62. Willemer S, Adler G. Histochemical and ultrastructural characteristics of tubular complexes in human acute pancreatitis. *Dig Dis Sci* 1989;34:46–55.
63. Braganza JM, John S, Padmalayam I, et al. Xenobiotics and tropical chronic pancreatitis. *Int J Pancreatol* 1990;7:231–245.
64. Azad Khan AK, Ali L. Tropical calcific pancreatitis and fibrocalculous pancreatic diabetes in Bangladesh. *J Gastroenterol Hepatol* 1997;12(suppl):S48–52.
65. Gorry MC, Gabbaizedeh D, Furey W, et al. Mutations in the cationic trypsinogen gene are associated with recurrent acute and chronic pancreatitis. *Gastroenterology* 1997;113:1063–1068.
66. Kawaguchi K, Koike M, Tsuruta K, Okamoto A, Tabata I, Fujita N. Lymphoplasmacytic sclerosing pancreatitis with cholangitis: a variant of primary sclerosing cholangitis extensively involving pancreas. *Hum Pathol* 1991;22:387–395.
67. Ammann RW, Heitz PU, Klöppel G. Course of alcoholic chronic pancreatitis: a prospective clinicomorphological long-term study. *Gastroenterology* 1996;111:224–231.
68. Suda K, Takase M, Takei K, Nakamura T, Akai J, Nakamura T. Histopathologic study of coexistent pathologic states in pancreatic fibrosis in patients with chronic alcohol abuse: two distinct pathologic fibrosis entities with different mechanisms. *Pancreas* 1996;12:369–372.
69. Grodsinsky C, Schuman BM, Block MA. Absence of pancreatic duct dilation in chronic pancreatitis. Surgical significance. *Arch Surg* 1977;112:444–449.
70. Klöppel G, Maillet B. Pseudocysts in chronic pancreatitis: a morphological analysis of 57 resection specimens and 9 autopsy pancreata. *Pancreas* 1991;6:266–274.
71. Stormby N. Pancreas. In: Zajicek J, ed. *Aspiration biopsy cytology. Part 2: Cytology of infradiaphragmatic organs*, vol 7, 1st ed. Basel: S. Karger, 1979:194–211. (Wied GL, ed. *Monographs in Clinical Cytology*.)
72. Klöppel G, Bommer G, Commandeur G, Heitz P. The endocrine pancreas in chronic pancreatitis. Immunocytochemical and ultrastructural studies. *Virchows Arch [A]* 1978;377:157–174.
73. Lászik Z, Pap A, Farkas G, Ormos J. Endocrine pancreas in chronic pancreatitis. A qualitative and quantitative study. *Arch Pathol Lab Med* 1989;113:47–51.
74. Bommer G, Friedl U, Heitz PU, Klöppel G. Pancreatic PP cell distribution and hyperplasia. Immunocytochemical morphology in the normal human pancreas, in chronic pancreatitis and pancreatic carcinoma. *Virchows Arch [A]* 1980;387:319–331.
75. Stürmer J, Becker V. Granulomatous pancreatitis—granulomas in chronic pancreatitis. *Virchows Arch [A]* 1987;410:327–338.
76. Klöppel G. Pancreatic, non-endocrine tumours. In: Klöppel G, Heitz PU, eds. *Pancreatic pathology*, 1st ed. Edinburgh: Churchill-Livingstone, 1984:79–113.
77. Duff GL. The clinical and pathological features of carcinoma of the body and tail of the pancreas. *Johns Hopkins Med J* 1939;65:69–100.
78. Allen-Mersh TG. Significance of the site of origin of pancreatic exocrine adenocarcinoma. *J Clin Pathol* 1982;35:544–546.
79. Mao C, Domenico DR, Kim K, Hanson DJ, Howard JM. Observations on the developmental patterns and the consequences of pancreatic exocrine adenocarcinoma. Findings of 154 autopsies. *Arch Surg* 1995;130:125–134.
80. Gambill EE. Pancreatitis associated with pancreatic carcinoma: a study of 26 cases. *Mayo Clin Proc* 1971;46:174–177.
81. Loquvam GS, Russell WO. Accessory pancreatic ducts of the major duodenal papilla. Normal structures to be differentiated from cancer. *Am J Clin Pathol* 1950;20:305–313.
82. Klöppel G, Lohse T, Bosslet K, Rückert K. Ductal adenocarcinoma of the head of the pancreas: incidence of tumor involvement beyond the Whipple resection line. Histological and immunocytochemical analysis of 37 total pancreatectomy specimens. *Pancreas* 1987;2:170–175.
83. Morohoshi T, Held G, Klöppel G. Exocrine pancreatic tumours and their histological classification. A study based on 167 autopsy and 97 surgical cases. *Histopathology* 1983;7:645–661.
84. Klöppel G, Lingenthal G, von Bülow M, Kern HF. Histological and fine structural features of pancreatic ductal adenocarcinomas in relation to growth and prognosis: studies in xenografted tumours and clinico-histopathological correlation in a series of 75 cases. *Histopathology* 1985;9:841–856.
85. Kern HF, Röher HD, von Bülow M, Klöppel G. Fine structure of three major grades of malignancy of human pancreatic adenocarcinoma. *Pancreas* 1987;2:2–13.

86. Elsässer H-P, Lehr U, Agricola B, Kern HF. Establishment and characterisation of two cell lines with different grade of differentiation derived from one primary human pancreatic adenocarcinoma. *Virchows Arch [B]* 1992;61:295–306.
87. Suto T, Sasaki K, Sugai T, Kanno S, Saito K. Heterogeneity in the nuclear DNA content of cells in carcinomas of the biliary tract and pancreas. *Cancer* 1993;72:2920–2928.
88. Miller JR, Baggenstoss AH, Comfort MW. Carcinoma of the pancreas. Effect of histological type and grade of malignancy on its behavior. *Cancer* 1951;4:233–241.
89. Giulianotti PC, Boggi U, Fornaciari G, et al. Prognostic value of histological grading in ductal adenocarcinoma of the pancreas vs TNM grading. *Int J Pancreatol* 1995;17:279–289.
90. Manabe T, Miyashita T, Ohshio G, et al. Small carcinoma of the pancreas. Clinical and pathologic evaluation of 17 patients. *Cancer* 1988;62:135–141.
91. Tsuchiya R, Tsunoda T. Tumor size as a predictive factor. *Int J Pancreatol* 1990;7:117–123.
92. Fortner JG, Klimstra DS, Senie RT, Maclean BJ. Tumor size is the primary prognosticator for pancreatic cancer after regional pancreatectomy. *Ann Surg* 1996;223:147–153.
93. Bardi G, Johansson B, Pandis N, et al. Karyotypic abnormalities in tumours of the pancreas. *Br J Cancer* 1993;67:1106–1112.
94. Bratt DJ, Hahn SA, Griffin CA, Yeo CJ, Kern SE, Hruban RH. The structural basis of molecular genetic deletions. An integration of classical cytogenetic and molecular analyses in pancreatic adenocarcinoma. *Am J Pathol* 1997;150:383–391.
95. Böttger TC, Störkel S, Wellek S, Stöckle M, Junginger T. Factors influencing survival after resection of pancreatic cancer. A DNA analysis and a histomorphologic study. *Cancer* 1994;73:63–73.
96. Rugge M, Sonego F, Sessa F, et al. Nuclear DNA content and pathology in radically treated pancreatic carcinoma. The prognostic significance of DNA ploidy, histology and nuclear grade. *Cancer* 1996;77:459–466.
97. Hosch SB, Knoefel WT, Metz S, et al. Early lymphatic tumor cell dissemination in pancreatic cancer: frequency and prognostic significance. *Pancreas* 1997;15:154–159.
98. Nakao A, Harada A, Nonami T, Kaneko T, Takagi H. Clinical significance of carcinoma invasion of the extrapancreatic nerve plexus in pancreatic cancer. *Pancreas* 1996;12:357–361.
99. Costa J. Benign epithelial inclusions in pancreatic nerves. *Am J Clin Pathol* 1977;67:306–307.
100. Yamaguchi K, Enjoji M. Adenosquamous carcinoma of the pancreas: a clinicopathologic study. *J Surg Oncol* 1991;47:109–116.
101. Furukawa T, Chiba R, Kobari M, Matsuno S, Nagura H, Takahashi T. Varying grades of epithelial atypia in the pancreatic ducts of humans. Classification based on morphometry and multivariate analysis and correlated with positive reactions of carcinoembryonic antigen. *Arch Pathol Lab Med* 1994;118:227–234.
102. Ferrari BT, O'Halloran RL, Longmire Jr WP, Lewin KJ. Atypical papillary hyperplasia of the pancreatic duct mimicking obstructing pancreatic carcinoma. *N Engl J Med* 1979;301:531–532.
103. Sessa F, Solcia E, Capella C, et al. Intraductal papillary-mucinous tumours represent a distinct group of pancreatic neoplasms: an investigation of tumour cell differentiation and K-ras, p53, and c-erbB-2 abnormalities in 26 patients. *Virchows Arch* 1994;425:357–367.
104. Nagai E, Ueki T, Chijiiwa K, Tanaka M, Tsuneyoshi M. Intraductal papillary mucinous neoplasms of the pancreas associated with so-called "mucinous ductal ectasia." Histochemical and immunohistochemical analysis of 29 cases. *Am J Surg Pathol* 1995;19:576–589.
105. Fukushima N, Mukai K, Kanai Y, et al. Intraductal papillary tumors and mucinous cystic tumors of the pancreas: clinicopathologic study of 38 cases. *Hum Pathol* 1997;28:1010–1017.
106. Adsay NV, Adair CF, Heffess CS, Klimstra DS. Intraductal oncocytic papillary neoplasms of the pancreas. *Am J Surg Pathol* 1996;20:980–994.
107. Milchgrub S, Campuzano M, Casillas J, Albores-Saavedra J. Intraductal carcinoma of the pancreas. *Cancer* 1992;69:651–656.
108. Kodama T, Mori W. Morphological behavior of carcinoma of the pancreas. 2. Argyrophil cells and Langerhans' islets in the carcinomatous tissues. *Acta Pathol Jpn* 1983;33:483–493.
109. Pour PM, Permert J, Mogaki M, Fujii H, Kazakoff K. Endocrine aspects of exocrine cancer of the pancreas. Their patterns and suggested biologic significance. *Am J Clin Pathol* 1993;100:223–230.
110. Bartow SA, Mukai K, Rosai J. Pseudoneoplastic proliferation of endocrine cells in pancreatic fibrosis. *Cancer* 1981;47:2627–2633.
111. Klimstra DS, Heffess CS, Oertel JE, Rosai J. Acinar cell carcinoma of the pancreas. A clinicopathologic study of 28 cases. *Am J Surg Pathol* 1992;16:815–837.
112. Burns WA, Matthews MJ, Hamosh M, Vander Weide G, Blum R, Johnson FB. Lipase-secreting acinar cell carcinoma of the pancreas with polyarthropathy. A light and electron microscopic, histochemical, and biochemical study. *Cancer* 1974;33:1002–1009.
113. Tucker JA, Shelburne JD, Benning TL, Yacoub L, Federman M. Filamentous inclusions in acinar cell carcinoma of the pancreas. *Ultrastruct Pathol* 1994;18:279–286.
114. Klimstra DS, Rosai J, Heffess CS. Mixed acinar-endocrine carcinomas of the pancreas. *Am J Surg Pathol* 1994;18:765–778.
115. Osborne BM, Culbert SJ, Cangir A, Mackay B. Acinar cell carcinoma of the pancreas in a 9-year-old child: case report with electron microscopic observations. *South Med J* 1977;70:370–372.
116. Manci EA, Gardner LL, Pollock WJ, Dowling EA. Osteoclastic giant cell tumor of the pancreas. Aspiration cytology, light microscopy, and ultrastructure with review of the literature. *Diagn Cytopathol* 1985;1:105–110.
117. Nojima T, Nakamura F, Ishikura M, Inoue K, Nagashima K, Kato H. Pleomorphic carcinoma of the pancreas with osteoclast-like giant cells. *Int J Pancreatol* 1993;14:275–281.
118. Gatteschi B, Saccomanno S, Bartoli FG, Salvi S, Liu G, Pugliese V. Mixed pleomorphic-osteoclast-like tumor of the pancreas. Light microscopical, immunohistochemical, and molecular biological studies. *Int J Pancreatol* 1995;18:169–175.
119. O'Connor TP, Wade TP, Sunwoo YC, et al. Small cell undifferentiated carcinoma of the pancreas. Report of a patient with tumor marker studies. *Cancer* 1992;70:1414–1519.
120. Ordóñez NG, Cleary KR, Mackay B. Small cell undifferentiated carcinoma of the pancreas. *Ultrastruct Pathol* 1997;21:467–474.
121. Danner DB, Hruban RH, Pitt HA, Hayashi R, Griffin CA, Perlman EJ. Primitive neuroectodermal tumor arising in the pancreas. *Mod Pathol* 1994;7:200–204.
122. Pyke CM, van Heerden JA, Colby TV, Sarr MG, Weaver AL. The spectrum of serous cystadenoma of the pancreas. Clinical, pathologic, and surgical aspects. *Ann Surg* 1992;215:132–139.
123. Sperti C, Pasquali C, Costantino V, Perasole A, Liessi G, Pedrazzoli S. Solitary true cyst of the pancreas in adults. Report of three cases and review of the literature. *Int J Pancreatol* 1995;18:161–167.
124. Warshaw AL, Compton CC, Lewandrowski KB, Cardenosa G, Mueller PR. Cystic tumors of the pancreas. New clinical, radiologic, and pathological observations in 67 patients. *Ann Surg* 1990;212:432–445.
125. Sperti C, Pasquali C, Guolo P, Polverosi R, Liessi G, Pedrazzoli S. Serum tumor markers and cyst fluid analysis are useful for the diagnosis of pancreatic cystic tumors. *Cancer* 1996;78:237–243.
126. Compagno J, Oertel JE. Mucinous cystic neoplasms of the pancreas with overt and latent malignancy (cystadenocarcinoma and cystadenoma). A clinicopathologic study of 41 cases. *Am J Clin Pathol* 1978;69:573–580.
127. Albores-Saavedra J, Gould EW, Angeles-Angeles A, Henson DE. Cystic tumors of the pancreas. *Pathol Annu* 1990;25(pt 2):19–50.
128. Albores-Saavedra J, Angeles-Angeles A, Nadji M, Henson DE, Alvarez L. Mucinous cystadenocarcinoma of the pancreas. Morphologic and immunocytochemical observations. *Am J Surg Pathol* 1987;11:11–20.
129. Southern JF, Warshaw AL, Lewandrowski KB. DNA ploidy analysis of mucinous cystic tumors of the pancreas. Correlation of aneuploidy with malignancy and poor prognosis. *Cancer* 1996;77:58–62.
130. Tsujimura T, Kawano K, Taniguchi M, Yoshikawa K, Tsukaguchi I. Malignant fibrous histiocytoma coexistent with mucinous cystadenoma of the pancreas. *Cancer* 1992;70:2792–2796.
131. Bergman S, Medeiros LJ, Radr T, Mangham DC, Lewandrowski KB. Giant cell tumor of the pancreas arising in the ovarian-like stroma of a mucinous cystadenocarcinoma. *Int J Pancreatol* 1995;18:71–75.
132. Wenig BM, Albores-Saavedra J, Buetow PC, Heffess CS. Pancreatic mucinous cystic neoplasm with sarcomatous stroma. A report of three cases. *Am J Surg Pathol* 1997;21:70–80.
133. Garcia Rego JA, Valbuena Ruvira L, Alvarez Garcia A, Santiago Freijanes MP, Suarez Peñaranda JM, Rois Soto JM. Pancreatic mucinous cystadenocarcinoma with pseudosarcomatous mural nodules. A report of a case with immunohistochemical study. *Cancer* 1991;67:494–498.
134. Marinho A, Nogueira R, Schmitt F, Sobrinho-Simoes M. Pancreatic mucinous cystadenocarcinoma with a mural nodule of anaplastic carcinoma. *Histopathology* 1995;26:284–287.

135. Fetisoff F, Dubois MP, Legue E, de Calan L, Jobard P. Tumeurs mucineuses rétropéritonéales et pancréatique. Etude immunohistochimique. *Ann Pathol* 1985;5:53–57.
136. Albores-Saavedra J, Nadji M, Henson DE, Angeles-Angeles A. Entero-endocrine cell differentiation in carcinomas of the gallbladder and mucinous cystadenocarcinomas of the pancreas. *Pathol Res Pract* 1988;183:169–175.
137. Compagno J, Oertel JE. Microcystic adenomas of the pancreas (glycogen-rich cystadenomas). A clinicopathologic study of 34 cases. *Am J Clin Pathol* 1978;69:289–298.
138. Lewandrowski K, Warshaw A, Compton C. Macrocystic serous cystadenoma of the pancreas: a morphologic variant differing from microcystic adenoma. *Hum Pathol* 1992;23:871–875
139. Egawa N, Maillet B, Schröder S, Mukai K, Klöppel G. Serous oligocystic and ill-demarcated adenoma of the pancreas: a variant of serous cystic adenoma. *Virchows Arch* 1994;424:1–17.
140. Mori K, Takeyama S, Hirosawa H, et al. A case of macrocystic serous cystadenoma of the pancreas. *Int J Pancreatol* 1995;17:91–93.
141. Alpert LC, Truong LD, Bossart MI, Spjut HJ. Microcystic adenoma (serous cystadenoma) of the pancreas. A study of 14 cases with immunohistochemical and electron-microscopic correlation. *Am J Surg Pathol* 1988;12:251–263.
142. Nyongo A, Huntrakoon M. Microcystic adenoma of the pancreas with myoepithelial cells. A hitherto undescribed morphologic feature. *Am J Clin Pathol* 1985;84:114–120.
143. Perez-Ordonez B, Naseem A, Lieberman PH, Klimstra DS. Solid serous adenoma of the pancreas. The solid variant of serous cystadenoma? *Am J Surg Pathol* 1996;20:1401–1405.
144. George DH, Murphy F, Michalski R, Ulmer BG. Serous cystadenocarcinoma of the pancreas: a new entity? *Am J Surg Pathol* 1989;13:61–66.
145. Yoshimi N, Sugie S, Tanaka T, et al. A rare case of serous cystadenocarcinoma of the pancreas. *Cancer* 1992;69:2449–2453.
146. Kamei K, Funabiki T, Ochiai M, et al. Some considerations on the biology of pancreatic serous cystadenoma. *Int J Pancreatol* 1992;11:97–104.
147. Cantrell BB, Cubilla AL, Erlandson RA, Fortner J, Fitzgerald PJ. Acinar cell cystadenocarcinoma of human pancreas. *Cancer* 1981;47:410–416.
148. Stamm B, Burger H, Hollinger A. Acinar cell cystadenoma of the pancreas. *Cancer* 1987;60:2542–2547.
149. Warfel KA, Faught PR, Hull MT. Pancreatic cystadenoma in an infant: ultrastructural study. *Pediatr Pathol* 1988;8:559–565.
150. Friedman HD. Nonmucinous, glycogen-poor cystadenocarcinoma of the pancreas. *Arch Pathol Lab Med* 1990;114:888–891.
151. Viola G, Frontera D, Bellantone R, Doglietto GB, Crucitti F. Lymphangiomas of the pancreas: a case report. *Pancreas* 1997;14:207–210.
152. Iacono C, Cracco N, Zamboni G, et al. Lymphoepithelial cyst of the pancreas. Report of two cases and review of the literature. *Int J Pancreatol* 1996;19:71–76.
153. Sachs JR, Deren JJ, Sohn M, Nusbaum M. Mucinous cystadenoma: pitfalls of differential diagnosis. *Am J Gastroenterol* 1989;84:811–816.
154. Kissane JM. Pancreatoblastoma and solid and cystic papillary tumor: two tumors related to pancreatic ontogeny. *Semin Diagn Pathol* 1994;11:152–164.
155. Klimstra DS, Wenig BM, Adair CF, Heffess CS. Pancreatoblastoma. A clinicopathologic study and review of the literature. *Am J Surg Pathol* 1995;19:1371–1389.
156. Schron DS, Mendelsohn G. Pancreatic carcinoma with duct, endocrine, and acinar differentiation. A histologic, immunocytochemical, and ultrastructural study. *Cancer* 1984;54:1766–1770.
157. Nonomura A, Kono N, Mizukami Y, Nakanuma Y, Matsubara F. Duct-acinar-islet cell tumor of the pancreas. *Ultrastruct Pathol* 1992;16:317–329.
158. Hassan MO, Gogate PA. Malignant mixed exocrine-endocrine tumor of the pancreas with unusual intracytoplasmic inclusions. *Ultrastruct Pathol* 1993;17:483–493.
159. Bani D, Bani Sacchi T, Biliotti G. Nesidioblastosis and intermediate cells in the pancreas of patients with hyperinsulinemic hypoglycemia. *Virchows Arch [B]* 1985;48:19–32.
160. Cossel L. Electron microscopic demonstration of intermediate cells in the healthy adult human pancreas. *Virchows Arch [B]* 1986;52:283–287.
161. Laine VJO, Ekfors TO, Gullichsen R, Nevalainen TJ. Immunohistochemical characterization of an amphicrine mucinous islet-cell carcinoma of the pancreas. Case report. *APMIS* 1992;100:335–340.
162. Vitte DP, Greider MH, DeSchryver-Kecskemeti K, Kissane JM, White NH. The juvenile human endocrine pancreas. Normal v. idiopathic hyperinsulinemic hypoglycemia. *Semin Diagn Pathol* 1984;1:30–42.
163. Klöppel G, Maurer R, Hofmann E, et al. Solid-cystic (papillary-cystic) tumours within and outside the pancreas in men: report of two patients. *Virchows Arch [A]* 1991;418:179–183.
164. Yamaguchi K, Miyagahara T, Tsuneyoshi M, et al. Papillary cystic tumor of the pancreas: an immunohistochemical and ultrastructural study of 14 patients. *Jpn J Clin Oncol* 1989;19:102–111.
165. Pettinato G, Manivel JC, Ravetto C, et al. Papillary cystic tumor of the pancreas. A clinicopathologic study of 20 cases with cytologic, immunohistochemical, ultrastructural, and flow cytometric observations, and a review of the literature. *Am J Clin Pathol* 1992;98:478–488.
166. Friedman AC, Lichtenstein JE, Fishman EK, Oertel JE, Dachman AH, Siegelman SS. Solid and papillary epithelial neoplasm of the pancreas. *Radiology* 1985;154:333–337.
167. Balercia G, Zamboni G, Bogina G, Mariuzzi GM. Solid-cystic tumor of the pancreas. An extensive ultrastructural study of fourteen cases. *J Submicrosc Cytol Pathol* 1995;27:331–340.
168. Lee W-Y, Tzeng C-C, Jin Y-T, Chow N-H, Yip C-M, Lee J-C. Papillary cystic tumor of the pancreas: a case indistinguishable from oncocytic carcinoma. *Pancreas* 1993;8:127–132.
169. Sclafani LM, Reuter VE, Coit DG, Brennan MF. The malignant nature of papillary and cystic neoplasm of the pancreas. *Cancer* 1991;68:153–158.
170. Horisawa M, Niinomi N, Sato T, et al. Frantz's tumor (solid and cystic tumor of the pancreas) with liver metastasis: successful treatment and long-term follow-up. *J Pediatr Surg* 1995;30:724–726.
171. Eerho M, Blaustein A, Willis I, Sorace D, Suster S. Microglandular carcinoma of the pancreas. Immunohistochemical and ultrastructural study of an unusual variant of pancreatic carcinoma that may closely resemble a neuroendocrine neoplasm. *Am J Clin Pathol* 1996;105:727–732.
172. Leonardo F, Cubilla AL, Klimstra DS. Microadenocarcinoma of the pancreas—Morphologic pattern or pathologic entity? A reevaluation of the original series. *Am J Surg Pathol* 1996;20:1385–1393.
173. Huntrakoon M. Oncocytic carcinoma of the pancreas. *Cancer* 1983;51:332–336.
174. Nozawa Y, Abe M, Sakuma H, et al. A case of pancreatic oncocytic tumor. *Acta Pathol Jpn* 1990;40:367–370.
175. Kadi MJ, Fenoglio-Preiser CM, Chiffelle T. Functioning oncocytic islet-cell carcinoma. Report of a case with electron-microscopic and immunohistochemical confirmation. *Am J Surg Pathol* 1985;9:517–524.
176. Kanai N, Nagaki S, Tanaka T. Clear cell carcinoma of the pancreas. *Acta Pathol Jpn* 1987;37:1521–1526.
177. Guarda LA, Silva EG, Ordoñez NG, Mackay B, Ibanez ML. Clear cell islet cell tumor. *Am J Clin Pathol* 1983;79:512–517.
178. Zamboni G, Pea M, Martignoni G, et al. Clear cell "sugar" tumor of the pancreas. A novel member of the family of lesions characterized by the presence of perivascular epithelioid cells. *Am J Surg Pathol* 1996;20:722–730.
179. Fukada T, Yamada S. Dysplasia and carcinoma in situ of the exocrine pancreas. *Tohoku J Exp Med* 1982;137:115–124.
180. Mukai K, Grotting JC, Greider MH, Rosai J. Retrospective study of 77 pancreatic endocrine tumors using the immunoperoxidase method. *Am J Surg Pathol* 1982;6:387–399.
181. Solcia E, Capella C, Klöppel G. *Tumors of the pancreas*, vol 1, 1st ed. Washington, DC: Armed Forces Institute of Pathology, 1997.
182. Donow C, Pipeleers-Marichal M, Schröder S, Stamm B, Heitz PU, Klöppel G. Surgical pathology of gastrinoma. Site, size, multicentricity, association with multiple endocrine neoplasia type 1, and malignancy. *Cancer* 1991;68:1329–1334.
183. MacFarlane MP, Fraker DL, Alexander HR, Norton JA, Lubensky I, Jensen RT. Prospective study of surgical resection of duodenal and pancreatic gastrinomas in multiple endocrine neoplasia type 1. *Surgery* 1995;118:973–980.
184. Taniguchi K, Tomioka T, Komuta K, et al. Pleomorphic nonfunctioning islet cell tumor of the pancreas. *Int J Pancreatol* 1995;17:83–89.
185. Ordóñez NG, Silva EG. Islet cell tumour with vacuolated lipid-rich cytoplasm: a new histological variant of islet cell tumour. *Histopathology* 1997;31:157–160.

186. Williams AJK, Coates PJ, Lowe DG, McLean C, Gale EAM. Immunochemical investigation of insulinomas for islet amyloid polypeptide and insulin: evidence for differential synthesis and storage. *Histopathology* 1992;21:215–223.
187. Al-Kaisi N, Weaver MG, Abdul-Karim FW, Siegler E. Fine needle aspiration cytology of neuroendocrine tumors of the pancreas. A cytologic, immunocytochemical and electron microscopic study. *Acta Cytol* 1992;36:655–660.
188. Tomita T. DNA ploidy and proliferating cell nuclear antigen in islet cell tumors. *Pancreas* 1996;12:36–47.
189. Pelosi G, Bresaola E, Bogina G, et al. Endocrine tumors of the pancreas: Ki-67 immunoreactivity on paraffin sections is an independent predictor for malignancy: a comparative study with proliferating-cell nuclear antigen and progesterone receptor protein immunostaining, mitotic index, and other clinicopathologic variables. *Hum Pathol* 1996;27:1124–1134.
190. Liu T-H, Zhu Y, Cui Q-C, et al. Nonfunctioning pancreatic endocrine tumors. An immunohistochemical and electron microscopic analysis of 26 cases. *Pathol Res Pract* 1992;188:191–198.
191. Wilson RW, Gal AA, Cohen C, DeRose PB, Millikan WJ. Serotonin immunoreactivity in pancreatic endocrine neoplasms (carcinoid tumors). *Mod Pathol* 1991;4:727–732.
192. Liu T-H, Tseng H-C, Zhu Y, Zhong S-X, Chen J, Cui C-C. Insulinoma. An immunocytochemical and morphologic analysis of 95 cases. *Cancer* 1985;56:1420–1429.
193. Ooi A, Nakanishi I, Kameya T, Funaki Y, Kobayashi K. Calcitonin-producing insulinoma. An immunohistochemical and electron microscopic study. *Acta Pathol Jpn* 1986;36:1897–1903.
194. Shepherd JJ, Challis DR, Davies PF, McArdle JP, Teh BT, Wilkinson S. Multiple endocrine neoplasm, type 1. Gastrinomas, pancreatic neoplasms, microcarcinoids, the Zollinger-Ellison syndrome, lymph nodes, and hepatic metastases. *Arch Surg* 1993;128:1133–1142.
195. Martella EM, Ferraro G, Azzoni C, Marignani M, Bordi C. Pancreatic-polypeptide cell hyperplasia associated with pancreatic or duodenal gastrinomas. *Hum Pathol* 1997;28:149–153.
196. Howard TJ, Sawicki M, Lewin KJ, et al. Pancreatic polypeptide immunoreactivity in sporadic gastrinoma: relationship to intraabdominal location. *Pancreas* 1995;11:350–356.
197. Ruttman E, Klöppel G, Bommer G, Kiehn M, Heitz PU. Pancreatic glucagonoma with and without syndrome. Immunocytochemical study of 5 tumour cases and review of the literature. *Virchows Arch [A]* 1980;388:51–67.
198. Balas D, Senegas-Balas F, Delvaux M, et al. Silent human pancreatic glucagonoma and "A" nesidioblastosis. *Pancreas* 1988;3:734–739.
199. Krejs GJ, Orci L, Conlon JM, et al. Somatostatinoma syndrome. Biochemical, morphologic and clinical features. *N Engl J Med* 1979;301:285–292.
200. Ooi A, Kameya T, Tsumuraya M, et al. Pancreatic endocrine tumours associated with WDHA syndrome. An immunohistochemical and electron microscopic study. *Virchows Arch [A]* 1985;405:311–323.
201. Capella C, Heitz PU, Höfler H, Solcia E, Klöppel G. Revised classification of neuroendocrine tumours of the lung, pancreas and gut. *Virchows Arch* 1995;425:547–560.
202. Campbell IL, Harrison LC, Ley CJ, Colman PG, Ellis DW. Nesidioblastosis and multifocal pancreatic islet cell hyperplasia in an adult. Clinicopathologic features and in vitro pancreatic studies. *Am J Clin Pathol* 1985;84:534–541.
203. Goudswaard WB, Houthoff HJ, Koudstaal J, Zwierstra RP. Nesidioblastosis and endocrine hyperplasia of the pancreas: a secondary phenomenon. *Hum Pathol* 1986;17:46–54.
204. Bani Sacchi T, Bani D, Biliotti G. The endocrine pancreas in patients with insulinomas. An immunocytochemical and ultrastructural study of the nontumoral tissue with morphometrical evaluations. *Int J Pancreatol* 1989;5:11–28.
205. Bani D, Biliotti G, Bani Sacchi T. Morphological changes in the human endocrine pancreas induced by chronic excess of endogenous glucagon. *Virchows Arch [B]* 1991;60:199–206.
206. Bani Sacchi T, Bani D, Biliotti G. Nesidioblastosis and islet cell changes related to endogenous hypergastrinemia. *Virchows Arch [B]* 1985;48:251–276.
207. Jaffe R, Hashida Y, Yunis EJ. Pancreatic pathology in hyperinsulinemic hypoglycemia of infancy. *Lab Invest* 1980;42:356–365.
208. Farley DR, van Heerden JA, Myers JL. Adult pancreatic nesidioblastosis. Unusual presentations of a rare entity. *Arch Surg* 1994;129:329–332.
209. Gould VE, Chejfec G, Shah K, Paloyan E, Lawrence AM. Adult nesidiodysplasia. *Semin Diagn Pathol* 1984;1:43–53.
210. Kroft SH, Stryker SJ, Winter JN, Ergun G, Rao MS. Inflammatory pseudotumor of the pancreas. *Int J Pancreatol* 1995;18:277–283.

CHAPTER 36

Nonneoplastic Liver Disease

Dale C. Snover

The first part of this chapter provides a brief introduction to technical aspects of the preparation and evaluation of the liver biopsy and a tabular guide to the interpretation of liver biopsies based on the most prominent histologic finding. This approach is intended to direct the general pathologist to the correct differential diagnosis for the large number of liver biopsies that arrive in the surgical pathology laboratory with a "history of elevated liver function tests (LFTs)" without further information. The second part discusses narrowing the differential diagnosis for specific diseases based on the data presented.

TECHNICAL ASPECTS OF THE EVALUATION OF LIVER BIOPSIES

As with any biopsy material, adequate size of the biopsy and good technical preparation are essential to interpretation. Adequacy of size depends in large part on the process being evaluated. If one is looking for metastatic carcinoma and there is tumor present, the size is adequate, no matter how small. On the other hand, to rule out some diseases such as chronic hepatitis, more tissue is needed; a minimum of 2.5 cm is said to be necessary, but for many processes it is really the number of portal tracts that indicates adequacy (1,2). Although not scientifically codified, caution in interpretation is indicated with less than four portal tracts for evaluation. This would be a reasonable estimate for the diagnosis of most types of chronic hepatitis. Similarly, what constitutes adequate technical preparation may vary. What is most important, however, is for the pathologist to realize the limitation of the tissue being evaluated. If the biopsy is inadequate in size or preparation, it should be so stated in the report.

The use of special stains varies with the situation and with the particular bias of the pathologist. Our routine consists of hematoxylin and eosin (H&E) (three step levels), trichrome, and reticulin preparations. The trichrome stain is useful in evaluating portal tract structures (e.g., bile ducts) in inflamed livers in addition to its traditional use as a stain for assessing degree of fibrosis. The reticulin preparation is most useful for assessing regeneration and focal necrosis, and for detecting early fibrosis. Many laboratories perform an iron stain routinely to screen for possible hemochromatosis. In my experience, if the biopsy is assessed carefully on H&E staining, significant iron deposition is visible without the iron stain. If pigment is identified, an iron stain stain can then be performed as a confirmatory test. Other stains are ordered as needed to assess specific diseases (see below).

Our recommended approach to interpretation of a biopsy obtained for diagnostic purposes is to review the slide first, without any knowledge of clinical aspects of the patient. A systematic evaluation of the portal tracts, lobules, and central veins should be undertaken, assessing features such as degree and type of inflammation, necrosis, and fibrosis (Table 1). After recording these data, a differential diagnosis should be generated. Only after this evaluation should the clinical situation be incorporated into the diagnosis. After considering the clinical situation, the correct diagnosis may be apparent or further review of the biopsy may be necessary. Although this exercise may seem time-consuming, it ensures that unsuspected pathology is not overlooked. It also prevents the bias of the clinician from unduly affecting the interpretation of the case.

The final diagnosis should take into account all information available, both clinical and pathologic. In most cases of nonneoplastic liver disease, a definitive etiologic diagnosis is not possible based on biopsy findings alone. The liver biopsy in these circumstances plays two major roles: first, to limit the differential diagnosis and rule out some considerations; and second, to provide prognostic information, as in the case of staging primary biliary cirrhosis. On rare occasions, a definitive diagnosis such as cytomegalovirus inclusion disease can be made. In the case of biopsies taken to as-

---

D. C. Snover: Department of Pathology, Fairview Southdale Hospital; Department of Laboratory Medicine and Pathology, University of Minnesota Medical School, Edina, Minnesota 55435.

TABLE 1. *Histopathologic features to evaluate in liver biopsies*

Overall (low power)
    Quality of biopsy (size, technical preparation, staining)
    Presence or absence of normal structures (portal tracts, central vein, capsule)
    Relationship of portal tracts to central veins ("overall architecture")
    Fibrosis and/or gross areas of necrosis
    General pattern of involvement with abnormal processes such as inflammation (portal, lobular, both; patchy, diffuse)
    Other features such as congestion and nodularity
Portal tracts (medium and high power)
    Presence of all normal structures (vein, artery, and, especially important, bile duct)
    Inflammation—type, intensity, relationship to structures such as bile ducts
    Bile duct changes—inflammation, proliferation, necrosis, atypia, cholestasis, loss
    Arterial changes—arteritis, thrombosis
    Venous changes—inflammation, thrombosis, thickening
    Fibrosis
    Edema
    Bile ductular (cholangiolar) proliferation
Lobule (medium and high power)
    Inflammation—type, intensity, location (e.g., zonality, sinusoidal vs. involving cell plates)
    Necrosis—type (e.g., focal, confluent, piecemeal), intensity, location (e.g., zonality)
    Status of cell plates—regeneration, atrophy
    Status of sinusoids—dilated, congested
    Other changes—inclusions, infiltrates (e.g., amyloid), fibrosis
Central veins (medium and high power)
    Character—size, shape (e.g., round, compressed)
    Inflammation
    Fibrosis

sess efficacy of therapy, comparison with previous biopsies is mandatory.

One major problem often encountered in liver pathology is that of definition of terms (3,4). To avoid confusion, definitions of some common terms are given in Table 2.

DIFFERENTIAL DIAGNOSIS BASED ON MAJOR HISTOLOGIC FINDINGS

This section provides a starting point for the diagnosis of liver disease based on the predominant histologic findings. After review of the biopsy, major features should be evaluated in the context of the suggestions given in Tables 3 to 18. Often, many of the possible diagnoses can be eliminated by the absence of more specific histologic features. In other cases, clinical information is necessary, as is usually the case in primary biliary cirrhosis, for example. In some cases, such as medication reactions, final diagnosis may require clinical manipulation of the patient (e.g., withdrawal of the medication). While not totally inclusive, this approach should provide diagnoses in the majority of cases seen on a daily basis.

Tables 3 and 4 refer to lobular inflammation with or without hepatocellular degeneration and with or without a portal infiltrate, although for practical purposes there is almost always a portal infiltrate if there is a lobular one. Note that in the liver, as in most organs, the terms *acute* and *chronic* have little to do with the type of inflammatory cell present; that is, lymphocytes do not equate with chronic inflammation as they do in the traditional teaching example of wound healing. Rather, the cell type present is in large part a reflection of the nature of the insult. For example, virally infected cells are eliminated from the body by a process of cell-mediated immunity involving lymphocytes. These cells are a reflection of the type of immunity and not duration of process. Therefore, acute processes involving this type of immunity (e.g., acute viral hepatitis) are characterized by a lymphocytic infiltrate. Conversely, irritants such as bile or chemotactants like Mallory hyalin will elicit a polymorphonuclear response in the acute phase.

Tables 6 to 8 refer to portal inflammation in excess of lobular inflammation. In some cases there is a lobular component to the process, but it should be much less prominent than the portal component.

Table 9 presents the differential diagnosis of granulomas of the liver. While in general a definitive etiology of granu-

TABLE 2. *Definition of commonly used terms*

Term	Definition
Acidophil body	A particular type of focal necrosis in which the dead hepatocyte is still identifiable as a shrunken, eosinophilic round body, with or without a nucleus; not specific for any disease
Ballooning degeneration	Swelling of individual hepatocytes with subsequent enlargement and pallor of the cytoplasm, nonspecific
Ductule	Synonym: cholangiole; small ductal structure usually without an evident lumen found at the edge of portal tracts or fibrous bands
Interlobular bile duct	Bile duct of a medium-sized portal tract that is more or less centrally located in the tract and accompanies an arteriole of similar diameter
Necrosis, piecemeal	Necrosis of the limiting plate (the layer of hepatocytes that abuts directly upon the portal tract); may be identified by actual necrosis of cells or by irregularity of the limiting plate caused by loss of hepatocytes and replacement with inflammatory cells and/or fibrosis
Necrosis, focal	Synonym: spotty necrosis; necrosis of individual hepatocytes
Necrosis, zonal	Necrosis of hepatocytes involving a specific zone of the lobule (e.g., centrilobular necrosis)
Necrosis, confluent	Necrosis of clusters of adjacent hepatocytes; confluent necrosis may be random or zonal
Necrosis, massive	Essentially total necrosis of the hepatocytes in a biopsy
Necrosis, bridging	Necrosis that joins ("bridges") between identifiable structures, such as portal tract to portal tract

TABLE 3. *Lobular lymphocytic infiltrate with or without hepatocellular degeneration/necrosis*

Diagnosis	Additional features
Acute medication-induced hepatitis	Eosinophils, granulomas or mixed macro- and microvesicular fat may suggest this etiology, but are present only in a minority of cases
Acute viral hepatitis: hepatitis A, B, C, cytomegalovirus (CMV), Epstein-Barr virus (EBV), delta virus, others	No absolute distinguishing features among the various viruses exist in the immunocompetent host, although increased plasma cells are seen in hepatitis A and a predominantly sinusoidal infiltrate and minimal necrosis are characteristic of hepatitis C, CMV, and EBV; in immunocompromised hosts inclusions are typical of CMV but the infiltrate tends to be neutrophilic rather than lymphocytic
Autoimmune hepatitis	Abundance of plasma cells, centra-portal bridging necrosis and central necrosis with plasma cells are characteristic but not universal
Carcinoma	Rarely, small cell carcinomas will simulate lymphocytes in the sinusoids
Extramedullary hematopoiesis	Erythroid precursors in the sinusoids may simulate lymphocytes, particularly in neonatal livers
Leukemia/lymphoma	The infiltrating cells are usually somewhat atypical; T-cell leukemia has a particular propensity to simulate mononucleosis; mastocytosis may also cause differential diagnostic difficulties
Primary biliary cirrhosis	Usually a predominantly portal process but may have a sinusoidal lymphocytic infiltrate, particularly early

TABLE 4. *Lobular polymorphonuclear infiltrate with or without hepatocellular degeneration/necrosis*

Disease	Additional features
Alcoholic hepatitis	Fatty change and Mallory hyalin should be present
Bacterial or fungal infection with direct hepatic involvement	Special stains define the infection; this condition is extremely rare
Medication reactions	A rare manifestation of medications simulating alcoholic liver disease
Sepsis	Often accompanied by cholestasis; organisms usually absent; diagnosis by exclusion
"Surgical" hepatitis	Often has a centrilobular and/or subcapsular predominance and may be associated with necrosis; most important clue is the clinical history of biopsy taken during surgery; biopsy is usually a wedge biopsy; one of the most common causes of neutrophils in the lobule
Viral infections (CMV, rarely herpes) in the immunocompromised host	Inclusions present; immunohistochemical staining may be definitive

TABLE 5. *Hepatocellular necrosis with minimal inflammation*

Disease	Additional features
Acute viral infection in immunocompromised hosts	Random areas of band coagulative necrosis; inclusions may be present with herpes or adenovirus; this pattern of necrosis is uncommon with CMV
Hepatic venous outflow obstruction including veno-occlusive disease, Budd-Chiari syndrome, congestive heart failure	More congested than necrotic, but some degree of necrosis may be present; centrilobular
Ischemia, including secondary to intrahepatic arteritis	Usually centrilobular, but may be mid-zonal in heart failure or random with arteritis; may be coagulative necrosis or ballooning degeneration with dropout of hepatocytes
Massive necrosis associated with hepatotrophic viral infections or medications	Diagnosis by serology (viral) or history (medication)
Medication or toxin reaction	Zonation dependent on particular agent, e.g., centrilobular necrosis with acetaminophen toxicity
Trauma	This includes trauma of a long surgical procedure
Tumors replacing portions of liver	Epithelioid hemangioendothelioma may simulate hepatic venous outflow obstruction

TABLE 6. Portal lymphocytic and/or plasmacellular infiltrate: lobular inflammation or degeneration/necrosis minimal (note: small numbers of lymphocytes in the portal tract is normal)

Disease	Additional features
Acute viral hepatitis, resolving	History of less than 6 months of viral hepatitis; randomly scattered lipofuscin and/or iron in Kupffer cells indicating recent necrosis
Autoimmune hepatitis	May be difficult to distinguish from chronic viral hepatitis and some medication reactions; plasma cells, extensive piecemeal necrosis, central necrosis with plasma cells and central-portal bridging favor autoimmune
Biliary tract obstruction, chronic low-grade or intermittent	Generally mild inflammation, diffuse bile ductular proliferation, Mallory hyalin late
Graft-versus-host disease	Look for bile duct damage, endothelialitis
Lymphoma/leukemia	Some lymphomas, particularly the small cell types, may simulate inflammatory lesions of the liver; diagnosis by atypia of the cells and history
Mass lesion (granuloma, neoplasm)	Found adjacent to any mass lesion, often accompanied by cholestasis and sinusoidal congestion
Primary biliary cirrhosis	Most helpful are loss of small interlobular bile ducts, portal granulomas, a mixed infiltrate with eosinophils and plasma cells; Mallory hyalin and copper accumulation seen late
Primary sclerosing cholangitis	Generally mild inflammation, diffuse bile ductular proliferation, Mallory hyalin late
Rejection	Look for bile duct damage in acute and chronic rejection, endothelialitis in acute rejection, loss of ducts and ischemic change in chronic rejection
Viral hepatitis B or C, chronic	Longer than 6 months' duration; plasma cells may be present with hepatitis C and fibrosis may be seen; hepatitis B may show ground glass cells; both may have lymphoid aggregates
Wilson's disease	Infiltrate mainly lymphocytes; glycogenated nuclei and fatty change early, Mallory hyalin late; copper stains only moderately useful

TABLE 7. Portal polymorphonuclear infiltrate: lobular inflammation or degeneration/necrosis minimal

Disease	Additional features
Ascending cholangitis	Distinguished from uncomplicated biliary tract obstruction by neutrophils within lumen of ducts
Biliary tract obstruction, acute	Portal edema, bile ductular proliferation (nearly always present), cholestasis (variable)
Hyperalimentation	Simulates biliary obstruction, may also have centrilobular ballooning, PAS-positive material in Kupffer cells, fatty change
Medication reactions	Caused by a limited number of drugs, e.g., phenothiazines; diagnosis by history
Viral hepatitis, "cholangiolytic"	May have more lobular damage that other diseases in this table

PAS, periodic acid-Schiff.

TABLE 8. Portal eosinophilic infiltrate: not necessarily predominant but easily identifiable

Disease	Additional features
Autoimmune hepatitis	Usually accompanied by plasma cells, lobular infiltrate, may also see central-portal bridging or central necrosis with plasma cells
Extramedullary hematopoiesis	Immature myeloid elements may be mistaken for eosinophils, especially in neonates
Medication reaction	Granulomas, mixed fatty change may be present
Parasitic infestation	Organisms may be seen, e.g., schistosomes
Primary biliary cirrhosis	Loss of bile ducts, granulomas helpful, Mallory hyalin, copper accumulation late
Primary sclerosing cholangitis	Diffuse bile ductular proliferation
Rejection	Bile duct damage, endothelialitis

TABLE 9. Granulomatous inflammation (note: granulomas may be incidental and not related to the liver disease that led to the biopsy)

Disease	Additional features
Chronic granulomatous disease of childhood	Necrotizing poorly formed granulomas with lipofuscin in histiocytes
Crohn's disease	May be accompanied by fatty change; rare
Foreign material	Includes talc in IV drug users, silicone in dialysis patients (portal in both cases), ingested lipid (lipogranulomas), and reaction to amyloid; polarization useful to visualize
Idiopathic hepatic granulomatosis	Many granulomas, usually lobular, diagnosis by exclusion; may be forme fruste of sarcoidosis
Immunocholangitis	May simulate PBC histologically; proper diagnosis needs serologic study and clinical correlation with treatment
Infection, bacterial	*Brucella, Listeria*: finding organisms is uncommon
Infection, fungal	Histoplasma is only common fungus with well-formed granulomas; fungi common in immunocompromised hosts (e.g., *Aspergillus, Candida*) tend to cause necrosis and abscess formation
Infection, mycobacterial	Caseation may be seen with *M. tuberculosis* but is uncommon in atypical mycobacteriosis; acid-fast stain needed to identify organisms; infectious granulomas tend to be in lobule, not portal tract
Infection, rickettsial	Q-fever characterized by doughnut-hole granulomas with hyalin ring
Infection, viral	Poorly formed granulomas may be seen with CMV and EBV infections
Lipogranulomas	Usually centrilobular but may be portal; always contain lipid; may or may not be accompanied by steatosis in adjacent liver
Malignancy	Epithelioid granulomas, seen most commonly with Hodgkin's disease but also other malignancies; granulomas do not imply involvement of liver by the tumor
Medication reaction	Eosinophils and fatty change common and suggestive of this etiology
Primary biliary cirrhosis	Granulomas usually poorly formed epithelioid type, but may have giant cells; mainly portal and associated with bile duct damage; other features include mixed infiltrate, bile duct loss; Mallory hyalin and copper accumulation late.
Sarcoidosis	Need clinical confirmation; granulomas tend to be both portal and lobular; may simulate PBC if granulomas are portal

PBC, primary biliary cirrhosis.

TABLE 10. Fibrosis

Process	Additional features
Amyloid	May simulate pericellular fibrosis; special stains needed.
Bridging fibrosis, noncirrhotic	Complete nodules and regeneration cannot be demonstrated; biopsy may be cirrhotic or precirrhotic but nondiagnostic; other processes such as congenital hepatic fibrosis or hepatoportal sclerosis should be considered as well
Central hyaline sclerosis	Centrilobular stellate fibrosis characteristic of alcoholic liver disease
Cirrhosis	Must see complete abnormal hepatocellular nodules, usually with regenerative activity
Congenital hepatic fibrosis	Complete nodules of hepatocytes are present but have normal architecture (i.e., central veins, no regeneration); characteristic serpiginous duct-like structures (ductal plate malformation)
Congenital syphilis	Pericellular fibrosis
Cystic fibrosis	Stellate scarring with eosinophilic inspissated material in ducts; fatty change common
Focal nodular hyperplasia	An inadvertent biopsy may resemble cirrhosis; diagnosis made by knowing there is a mass present and being biopsied
Hepatoportal sclerosis	May have bridging and regenerative activity, but not complete regenerative nodules; sclerosed portal veins diagnostic
Hepatic venous outflow obstruction, chronic	Central stellate fibrosis seen usually with congestion in chronic veno-occlusive disease, congestive heart failure, Budd-Chiari syndrome
Metabolic disease	Many metabolic diseases will develop pericellular fibrosis with a stellate appearance
Pericentral sclerosis	Dense band of fibrosis around central vein, significance uncertain
Tumor	Sclerosis may be part of several tumors including sclerosing hepatocellular carcinoma, fibrolamellar hepatoma, cholangiocellular carcinoma, epithelioid hemangioendothelioma, and others; neoplastic cells diagnostic

TABLE 11. *Cholestasis in relative isolation*

Etiology	Additional features
Benign familial recurrent cholestasis	History, clinical and family; may be portal infiltrate, but usually not
Cholestasis of pregnancy	Clinical data
Medications	May be an isolated finding; need history of medication
Postoperative cholestasis	History of surgery
Sepsis	May have clusters of PMNs in sinusoids, cholangiolar cholestasis very characteristic

PMN, polymorphonuclear leukocytes.

lomatous disease is not possible based on histology alone, attention to the type of granuloma and other features of the biopsy helps to narrow the differential diagnosis (see Common Problems in Biopsy Diagnosis, below).

Tables 17 and 18 refer to biopsies taken from patients in whom definite liver function abnormalities exist but that on cursory examination appear nearly normal or are missing certain structures. The differential diagnosis generated may solve this apparent paradox. The other tables are self-explanatory.

A COMMENT ON LABORATORY STUDIES IN LIVER DISEASE

The pathologist should always be aware of the results of laboratory testing prior to rendering a diagnosis on a liver

TABLE 12. *Congestion or hemorrhage, often in association with sinusoidal dilatation*

Diagnosis	Additional features

Hepatic venous outflow obstruction
  Budd-Chiari syndrome
  Veno-occlusive disease
  Heart failure
	Centrilobular congestion and atrophy in all cases; clinical and radiologic information necessary for diagnosis

Mass lesion (granuloma, neoplasm)	Cholestasis, portal lymphocytic infiltrate may be present adjacent to mass
Medication reaction	Often associated with or a precursor to peliosis
Neoplasm	Some neoplasms, particularly angiosarcoma and epithelioid hemangioendothelioma, may appear as congestion at low power
Nodular regenerative hyperplasia	Congestion occurs in areas of atrophy at the edge of regenerative nodules; confirmed by reticulin stain to see alternating areas of atrophy and regeneration
Peliosis hepatis	Random blood filled lakes
Portal vein obstruction	Central atrophy with secondary congestion

TABLE 13. *Pigments*

Type	Identifying features
Bile	Green to greenish brown; can be positively identified when found in bile ducts or, more commonly, bile canaliculi; predominantly centrilobular; intrahepatocellular bile cannot be distinguished without special stains from iron or lipofuscin
Iron	Brown to golden brown; most commonly periportal except in cases with congestive liver disease, when it is centrilobular; found predominantly in hepatocytes in primary hemochromatosis, in Kupffer cells with hemolysis, iron overload or in cases of recent hepatocellular necrosis, in which case the distribution tends to be random; stains with several techniques (Perl's, Prussian blue).
Lipofuscin	Brown; located predominantly within centrilobular hepatocytes, secondarily in Kupffer cells in cases of recent hepatocellular necrosis; almost never predominantly in periportal cells; stains with acid-fast stain (Fite).
Other exogenous pigments	Rare, including gold (patents treated for arthritis; black to brown Kupffer cell or portal macrophages), thorium dioxide (used for scanning in the 1940s; gray to gray blue, in Kupffer cells)

biopsy. It is remarkable how often these results are not available (except for the ubiquitous "abnormal LFTs"), and how often little attention is paid to them in diagnosis. Routine testing is usually available for serum enzymes including the transaminases and alkaline phosphatase, bilirubin, viral serologies, antimitochondrial antibody, and antinuclear antibody or anti–smooth muscle antibody. Occasionally when the findings on biopsy are equivocal or suggest somewhat differing diagnoses, these values pin down the final diagnosis. The viral serologies and the antimitochondrial antibody are specific tests (although the presence of one diagnosis does not always rule out secondary diseases), but the other antibodies are not. It is a relatively common finding, for example, to find an elevated antinuclear antibody associated with nonalcoholic steatohepatitis in an obese individual. This does not imply that the patient has autoimmune hepatitis.

The less specific tests may lead to a limitation of the differential diagnosis. Elevation of the transaminases is indicative of hepatocellular damage and is consistent with various forms of hepatitis including viral and medication-induced hepatitis, autoimmune hepatitis, steatohepatitis, and alcoholic liver disease. Elevation of alkaline phosphatase with normal transaminases and bilirubin is characteristic of focal or low-grade bile duct damage and is very suggestive of the diagnoses of primary biliary cirrhosis, primary sclerosing

TABLE 14. Intracellular inclusions

Type of inclusion	Description and significance
Adenovirus	Basophilic, dark homogeneous nuclear inclusion in hepatocyte, often associated with confluent necrosis
Alpha$_1$-antitrypsin	Eosinophilic round intracytoplasmic droplets with a predelection for periportal hepatocytes; PAS positive and can be stained with immunohistochemical staining. Similar in appearance to alpha$_1$-antichymotrypsin droplets and occasional droplets of alpha-fetoprotein and albumin
Amylopectin	Intracytoplasmic basophilic inclusion-like accumulation of diastase-resistant unbranched glycogen found in glycogen storage disease type IV
Cytomegalovirus	Large nuclear inclusion in an enlarged cell; basophilic to brick red with surround clearing of chromatin; may be associated with small amphophilic cytoplasmic inclusions; found in all cell types
Fat, macrovesicular	Large, usually single intracytoplasmic fat droplets; exquisitely nonspecific; present in abundance in alcoholic hepatitis, nonalcoholic steatohepatitis, drug reactions, cystic fibrosis
Fat, microvesicular	Multiple tiny intracytoplasmic droplets of fat, sometimes so small as to simulate ballooning degeneration rather than fatty change; seen in a variety of storage, metabolic and toxic processes including drug reactions, fatty liver of pregnancy, Reye's syndrome and acute foamy degeneration associated with alcohol
Glycogen nuclei	Homogeneous clearing of the nuclei of hepatocytes, usually with enlargement, predominantly periportal; a few seen in most biopsies; abundant in hyperglycemia, glycogen storage disease, Wilson's disease, and nonalcoholic steatohepatitis
Giant mitochondria	Round to needle-shaped intracytoplasmic structures, PAS negative; need EM for definitive diagnosis; common in alcoholic liver disease
Ground glass cells	Eosinophilic granularity to the cytoplasm of hepatocytes; usually caused by proliferation of endoplasmic reticulum (ER) or mitochondria (oncocytic change), accumulation of excess hepatitis B surface antigen, less commonly by accumulation of other proteins (e.g., fibrinogen); distinction possible based on diffuseness of process (proliferation of ER by drugs tends to be diffuse, all others tend to be focal), and by special staining for HBsAg
Herpes simplex or Varicella zoster	Eosinophilic homogeneous nuclear inclusion in hepatocytes, often associated with confluent hepatocyte necrosis
Mallory hyalin	Rope-like, irregular intracytoplasmic eosinophilic deposits of prekeratin; cells often also demonstrate ballooning; found in alcoholic and nonalcoholic steatohepatitis as well as many cholestatic states and Wilson's disease

EM, electron microscopy; HBsAg, hepatitis B surface antigen.

TABLE 15. Fatty change predominant with no or mild necrosis

Disease	Additional features
Alcoholic steatohepatitis	Fat usually more macrovesicular except in acute foamy degeneration; Mallory hyalin, if present, is centrolobular and associated with neutrophils; pericellular fibrosis common around central vein
Fatty liver of pregnancy	Microvesicular fatty change, often associated with cholestasis
Focal fatty change	Clinical history of a "mass" lesion being biopsied
Hepatocellular adenoma or carcinoma	Occasionally these tumors contain abundant fat
Medication or toxin reaction	Usually mixed or predominantly microvesicular; may or may not have associated inflammation or other features of inflammatory liver disease
Metabolic disease	Location within hepatocytes and/or Kupffer cells defined by the specific metabolic disease
Nonalcoholic steatohepatitis	Fat usually mixed micro- and macrovesicular, has patchy portal and lobular infiltrate, usually lymphocytes and/or plasma cells, delicate pericellular fibrosis and glycogenated nuclei common; Mallory hyalin, if present, is not well formed and not centrilobular
Nonspecific steatosis	Minimal inflammation or other change, usually mainly macrovesicular
Wilson's disease	An early finding, usually associated with portal infiltrate and glycogenated nuclei, but not always

TABLE 16. *Unusual cells in the liver*

Cell type	Distinguishing features
Extramedullary hematopoiesis	Erythroid precursors tend to be located in sinusoids and simulate lymphocytic infiltration; myeloid precursors tend to be located in the portal tracts and may be confused with a mixed cell portal infiltrate
Megakaryocytes	Very atypical sinusoidal cells, often but not always accompanied by other cells of extramedullary hematopoiesis
Metastatic tumor	
Storage cells	May be hepatocellular, Kupffer cell or Ito cell in origin; appearance depends on nature of storage disease

cholangitis, or other forms of extrahepatic biliary tract obstruction, and other focal intrahepatic lesions such as tumors or granulomas. Pure elevations of bilirubin are very suggestive of medication reactions, sepsis, or familial cholestatic syndromes.

HISTOLOGIC FEATURES OF SPECIFIC LIVER DISEASES

Developmental Anomalies

The major developmental anomalies likely to be encountered by the surgical pathologist are extrahepatic biliary atresia, intrahepatic biliary atresia [paucity of the intrahepatic bile ducts, either syndromic (arteriohepatic dysplasia; Alagille's syndrome) or nonsyndromic], choledochal cysts, and lesions associated with polycystic hepatorenal disease. The latter two processes are discussed in detail in the chapter by Sau, "Gallbladder and Extrahepatic Biliary Tree," and are discussed only briefly here. The first three of these pro-

TABLE 17. *The "nearly normal" biopsy*

Diagnosis	Additional features
Hepatoportal sclerosis	Absence or sclerosis of portal veins diagnostic but patchy and difficult to identify in needle biopsy; nodular hyperplasia usually present
Medication reactions	Clinical history
Missed lesion	In some cases, the lesion causing the disease may be missed on biopsy, e.g., granulomatous inflammation causing elevated alkaline phosphatase
Nodular regenerative hyperplasia	Central veins often compressed; areas of congestion surround nodules; reticulin stain confirms atrophy and regeneration
Storage/metabolic disease	Clinical information usually suggestive; ultrastructural examination may be useful

TABLE 18. *Absence of normal structures*

Structure missing from biopsy	Cause of absence
Bile ducts	Long-standing biliary tract obstruction Primary biliary cirrhosis Primary sclerosing cholangitis Paucity of intrahepatic bile ducts in the neonate Idiopathic adulthood ductopenia Medication reactions (e.g., Augmentin) Arterial ischemia Chronic graft versus host disease Chronic allograft rejection
Central veins	Sampling error Cirrhosis Adenoma or carcinoma Nodular regenerative hyperplasia (central veins are present but difficult to see on routine staining because of compression; can be seen with trichrome stain)
Hepatocytes	Massive necrosis due to Viruses Medications Ischemia
Portal tracts	Sampling error Cirrhosis Adenoma or carcinoma
Portal veins (in the presence of portal tracts)	Hepatoportal sclerosis
Sinusoids	Storage disease with compression of sinusoids by enlarged hepatocytes (e.g., glycogen storage disease) Cirrhosis

cesses, as well as many metabolic diseases and neonatal hepatitis, constitute the differential diagnosis for biopsies taken to evaluate cholestasis in the neonatal period (5). Although these conditions are traditionally considered developmental anomalies, there is considerable data to suggest that in at least some cases perinatal viral infections may play a role in their development.

In *extrahepatic biliary atresia* (EBA), portions of the extrahepatic biliary tree are stenotic or atretic, leading to chronic extrahepatic large-duct obstruction (LDO) (5,6). Although usually listed as developmental, this process may have an infectious etiology (7). The basic pathology consists of cholestasis, a portal polymorphonuclear infiltrate, bile ductular proliferation, and eventual fibrosis and cirrhosis (6) (Fig. 1). EBA cannot be distinguished histologically from choledochal cysts or other causes of LDO. EBA can usually be distinguished from neonatal hepatitis, which is characterized by lobular disarray with giant cell transformation, cholestasis, and extramedullary hematopoiesis without portal fibrosis or ductular proliferation (6,8) (Fig. 2). Giant cell transformation and extramedullary hematopoiesis may be seen in EBA, but if present are less extensive; also, the giant

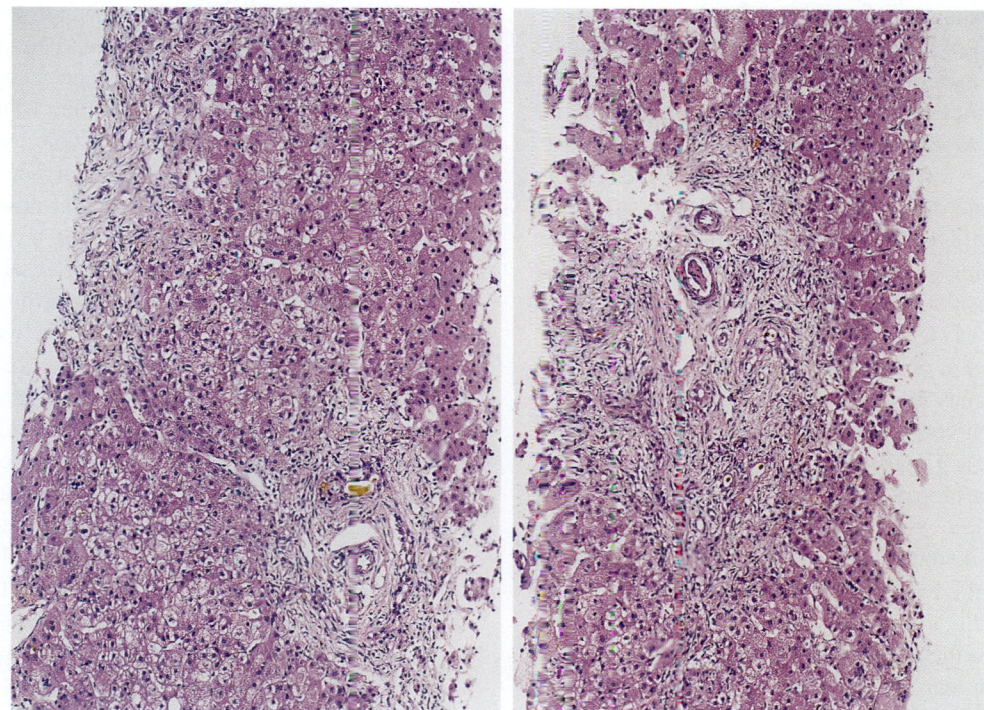

FIG. 1. Extrahepatic biliary atresia. Two different portal tracts from a single biopsy demonstrating diffuse bile ductular proliferation. The hepatocellular parenchyma is relatively unremarkable, without significant giant cell transformation.

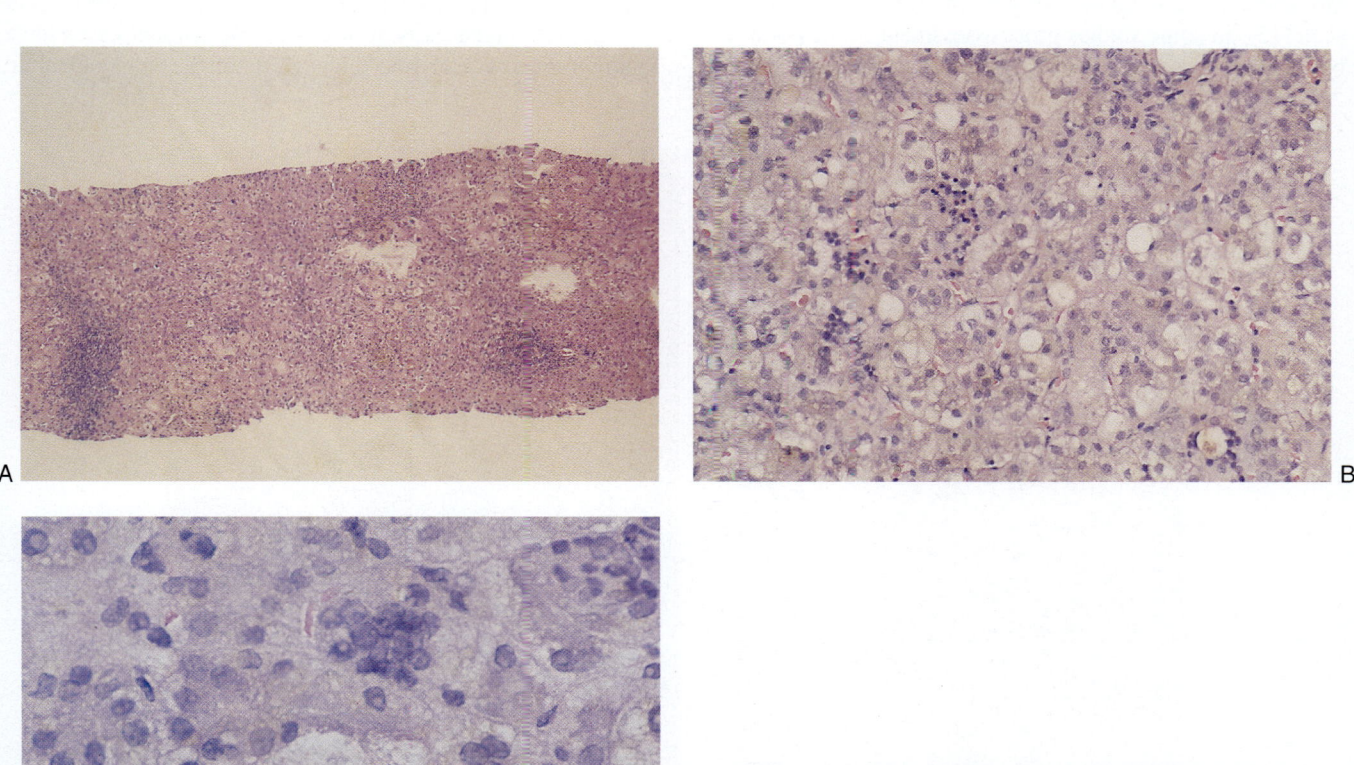

FIG. 2. Neonatal hepatitis. **A:** At low power, generalized lobular disarray is notable and the portal tracts are inflamed but only mildly expanded and do not demonstrate marked bile ductular proliferation. **B:** The lobule shows generalized hepatocellular unrest and extramedullary hematopoiesis. **C:** Giant cell transformation characterized by an hepatocyte with six or more nuclei.

cell transformation tends to be periporal rather than diffuse. Alpha$_1$-antitrypsin (AAT) deficiency occasionally simulates EBA, as do rare cases of congenital cytomegalovirus infection (9,10). Distinction of surgically treatable causes of cholestasis such as EBA from medical diseases such as neonatal hepatitis is very important since the former are potentially correctable if operated on early enough. Although one may strongly favor a diagnosis of biliary atresia on biopsy, radiographic studies are always warranted because there is a false-positive diagnosis rate of approximately 7% on biopsy alone (6,11).

Once the diagnosis of EBA has been established, the surgical pathologist may be asked to assess the probability of success of surgical correction by hepatic portoenterostomy (Kasai procedure). To do this, the surgeon provides the pathologist with a biopsy of the porta hepatis taken at the time of the operation. Assessment of the biopsy to reveal the presence of real bile ducts versus blind saccules adjacent to a scar where the old duct was destroyed has been suggested to be prognostically important (12). Attempts have been made to quantitate the size of bile ducts for this purpose as well, but this technique is rife with technical problems such as deciding exactly how to measure the duct and how to distinguish the duct from periductal glands (13,14). Recent studies have questioned the value of assessing duct size, in that prognosis appears to correlate only with the absence of any ducts in the remnant, not with the size of the remnants seen (15). In some studies gross assessment of the porta has been found to be as effective as microscopic examination (16). Given the ambiguity of the data, the most practical way to address this circumstance may be to provide the surgeons with the facts (e.g., "there are ducts present up to x cm in diameter") and let them decide what they want to do with this information.

Intrahepatic biliary atresia (paucity of the intrahepatic bile ducts) occurs in a syndromic and nonsyndromic form (17–20). The syndromic form (Alagille's syndrome) is associated with a characteristic facies, vertebral arch anomalies, and supravalvular pulmonic stenosis (thus the alternative name of "arteriohepatic dysplasia"), as well as other less common or characteristic anomalies. In both forms of paucity, the characteristic pathology consists of loss of interlobular bile ducts, usually with little ductular proliferation, although the latter may occur to a limited extent. The diagnosis rests on an assessment of the percentage of missing interlobular bile ducts (Fig. 3). Alagille has suggested that less than 0.5 ducts per portal tract (vs. a normal of 0.9 to 1.8) is diagnostic. It is important to count only true interlobular ducts (i.e., those accompanying hepatic arterioles located in the center of the portal tracts), since there may be some focal ductular proliferation that grossly alters the average number of ducts per tract. Immunoperoxidase staining for cytokeratin may be useful in assessing absence of ducts, although caution is necessary to avoid misinterpreting proliferating ductules as interlobular ducts. In the syndromic form, the bile duct loss appears to be progressive; ducts may be present in biopsies taken early in life (21). Occasional cases have shown regrowth of bile ducts (22). In the nonsyndromic

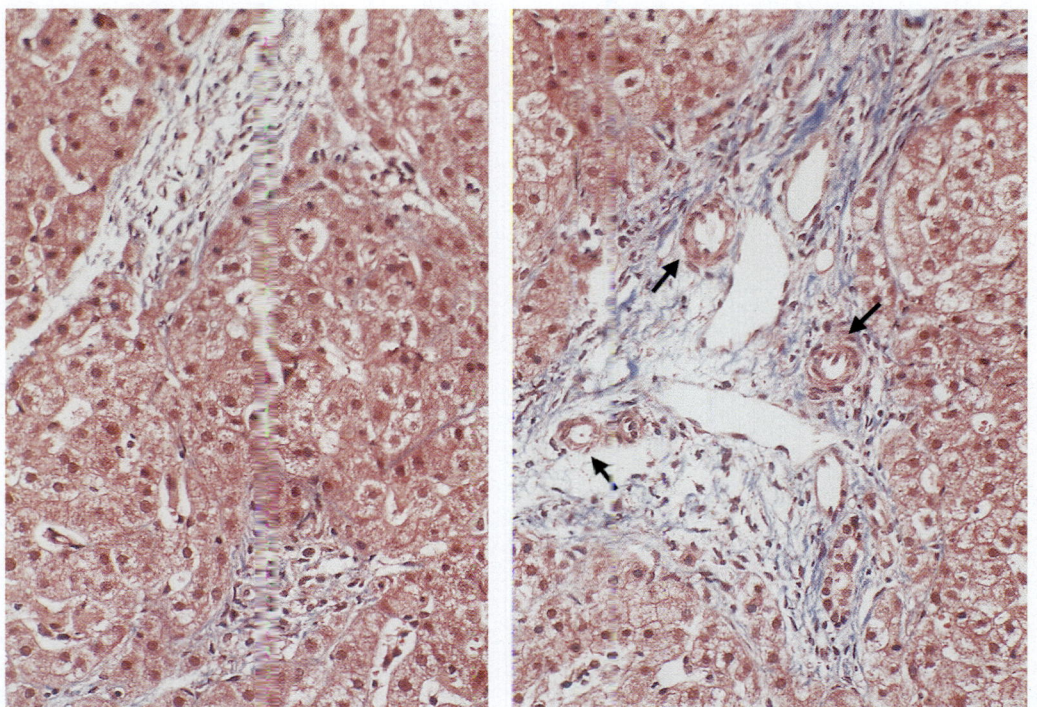

FIG. 3. Intrahepatic biliary atresia. The portal tracts are small and the hepatocellular parenchyma is unremarkable **(A)**. The portal area shows a minimal lymphocytic infiltrate. Several arterioles are identifiable *(arrows)*, but their accompanying interlobular bile ducts are absent **(B)**.

form, the paucity appears to exist at birth (23). The nonsyndromic form in actuality represents many diseases including cystic fibrosis, AAT deficiency, trihydroxycoprostanic acidemia, and others; the prognosis is to a large extent driven by the underlying etiology (19). In some cases bile ducts recover, whereas in others the prognosis is poor.

The liver lesions of *polycystic hepatorenal disease* may be encountered in several settings. Often they represent incidental findings, particularly the Meyenberg complex (bile duct hamartoma), which may be associated with the adult type of polycystic hepatorenal disease (24). The Meyenberg complex consists of a periportal collection of bile-filled ductal structures in a fibrous stroma (Fig. 4). Although Meyenberg complexes may be associated with hepatorenal disease, most cases are incidental and of no clinical significance.

The lesion associated with infantile polycystic disease, termed *congenital hepatic fibrosis,* may be discovered in a biopsy taken because of evidence of portal hypertension in an adolescent. Congenital hepatic fibrosis is characterized by anastomosing biliary channels embedded in a fibrous matrix (Fig. 5). The lesion may not be present at birth, and progresses from minimal fibrosis to diffuse bridging fibrosis (25). Congenital hepatic fibrosis can be distinguished from inflammatory bridging fibrosis or cirrhosis by lack of inflammation, lack of regenerative nodules, and presence of anastomosing biliary channels rather than proliferating bile ductules.

Metabolic Diseases

Metabolic diseases fall into several categories from a surgical pathology perspective (Tables 19–21). Some diseases are diagnosable by routine light microscopy alone, e.g., glycogen storage disease type IV (Fig. 6). A second category may or may not show typical light microscopic changes but requires special stains for diagnosis, e.g., AAT deficiency (Fig. 7) and the mucopolysaccharidoses (Fig. 8). Diseases in a third category have nonspecific light microscopy but diagnostic ultrastructure, e.g., Zellweger's syndrome, whereas those in a fourth category have abnormal biopsies that suggest a range of possible diagnoses but are not diagnostic, e.g., tyrosinemia. Finally, some diseases show no or very nonspecific changes by light or electron microscopic examination. In most cases, the purpose of the biopsy is to obtain tissue for biochemical examination, as well as to examine histologically.

Metabolic diseases can be divided into congenital inborn errors of metabolism, including the storage diseases, and acquired metabolic diseases such as amyloidosis. Limitation of space does not allow a discussion of most forms of metabolic disease in this chapter. Features of some of the more common genetic diseases are described in Tables 19–21 (Figs. 6–11). The more common diseases are reviewed in some detail. The reader is referred to standard works in the field for more complete information (3,26,27).

Alpha₁-antitrypsin (AAT) deficiency is one of the more common causes of neonatal cholestasis. By routine light microscopy, the AAT-deficient liver may have the appearance of a normal liver, or may show features of neonatal hepatitis, intrahepatic biliary atresia, or extrahepatic biliary atresia. The liver will eventually develop cirrhosis in many cases (9,28). Therefore, AAT deficiency must be considered in the differential diagnosis of virtually any histologic pattern in the proper clinical setting and must be ruled out by review of the serum protein electrophoresis and by staining for AAT accumulation in the liver with the diastase-treated periodic acid-Schiff (PAS) stain and/or immunoperoxidase staining for AAT (Fig. 7).

It should be noted that AAT accumulation may not be present in early life, becoming more reliably visible after 3 months of age. Conversely, accumulation of AAT is not diagnostic of AAT deficiency since it has been shown that regenerating hepatocytes, and perhaps damaged cells as well,

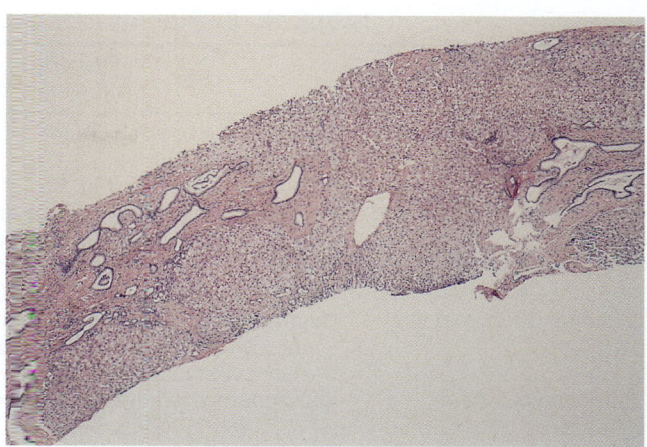

FIG. 5. Congenital hepatic fibrosis. Fully developed lesion with fibrous bands subdividing the liver into nodules of essentially normal hepatic parenchyma. The fibrous bands have serpiginous biliary channels concentrated at the periphery that are lined by cuboidal biliary epithelium.

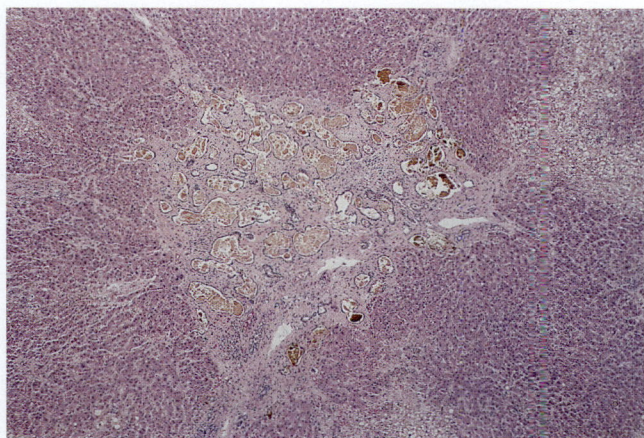

FIG. 4. Meyenberg complex (bile duct hamartoma). Irregular bile-filled spaces are surrounded by fibrous stroma in continuity with adjacent portal tract. The spaces are lined with cuboidal biliary epithelium.

TABLE 19. *Examples of metabolic disease diagnosable by light microscopy*

Disease	Diagnostic light microscopic findings	Diagnostic electron microscopic findings
Alpha$_1$-antitrypsin deficiency	PAS-positive hyalin globules in periportal distribution (Fig. 7)	Granular material in dilated endoplasmic reticulum
Cystic fibrosis	Focal biliary fibrosis (Fig. 9)	Filamentous material in bile ducts
Gaucher's disease	Enlarged Kupffer cells and portal macrophages with "crinkled paper" cytoplasm (Fig. 10)	Intralysosomal tubular inclusions
Glycogen storage disease type IV	Basophilic intracytoplasmic inclusion; PAS positive partially digestable (Fig. 6)	Filamentous nonbranching cytoplasmic aggregates
Mucopolysaccharidosis	Usually normal by H&E but staining of Kupffer cells and hepatocytes by colloidal iron for mucosubstance (Fig. 8)	Lysosomes of all cell types contain characteristic flocculent material
Porphyria cutanea tarda	Intrahepatocellular needle-shaped inclusions	Intrahepatocellular needle-shaped inclusions
Erythropoietic protoporphyria	Deep brown pigmented bile in canaliculi, ducts, and Kupffer cells displaying red "Maltese cross" with polarization (Fig. 11)	"Star-burst" crystalline array

H&E, hematoxylin and eosin.

TABLE 20. *Examples of metabolic disease with diagnostic ultrastructure and nonspecific light microscopy*

Disease	Light microscopy	Electron microscopy
Glycogen storage disease type II	Increased intrahepatocellular glycogen	Lysosomally bound glycogen
GM$_2$ gangliosidosis	Normal	Membrane-bound laminated inclusions ("zebra bodies")
Niemann-Pick disease	Foamy Kupffer cells and hepatocytes	Intralysosomal myelin-like inclusions
Wolman disease	Foamy Kupffer cells and hepatocytes	Lipid droplets in hepatocytes and Kupffer cells; cholesterol clefts in Kupffer cells
Zellweger syndrome	Nonspecific hepatocellular changes	Absence of peroxisomes

TABLE 21. *Metabolic diseases with characteristic but not diagnostic light and electron microscopy*

Disease	Light microscopy	Electron microscopy
Galactosemia	Same as tyrosinemia	Same as tyrosinemia
Glycogen storage disease types I and III	Enlarged hepatocytes compressing sinusoids leading to "mosaic" pattern; fatty change; hyperglycogenated nuclei	Increased cytoplasmic glycogen separating other organelles; lipid droplets; glycogenated nuclei
Hereditary fructose intolerance	Same as tyrosinemia	Lucent partially membrane bound areas of cytoplasm ("fructose holes") and concentric arrays of endoplasmic reticulum and glycogen
Tyrosinemia	Hepatocellular degeneration with focal fatty change, particularly in regenerative nodules: pseudorosette formation; cholestasis; fibrosis; cirrhosis	Cholestasis; lipid droplets; increased endoplasmic reticulum; abnormal mitochondria

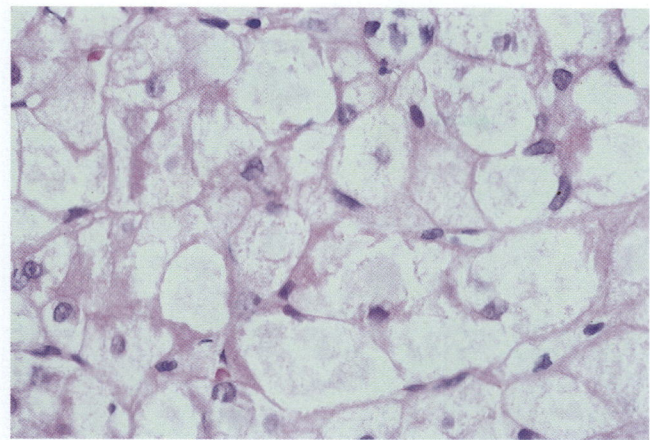

FIG. 6. Glycogen storage disease type IV (amylopectinosis) is recognizable by the intracytoplasmic inclusions, which are basophilic by H&E stain and are PAS positive and incompletely diastase digestible.

may accumulate AAT (29). This nonspecific accumulation can usually be distinguished from that of AAT deficiency by its diffuse granular character rather than formation of hyaline globules. This difference results in a PAS-negative cell that is diffusely stained by immunoperoxidase staining for AAT. In addition, in AAT deficiency the globules are located in a periportal location rather than in the random distribution of damaged hepatocytes.

On rare occasions, AAT deficiency presents in an adult as rapidly progressive liver disease occurring after a relatively minor insult such as biliary obstruction by a stone. The adult cases have a massive accumulation of AAT. Although most cases of liver disease associated with AAT deficiency occur in homozygous PiZZ patients, there is evidence that individuals who are heterozygous for some abnormal alleles (e.g., PiMZ) may have an increased incidence of chronic liver disease (30).

Cystic fibrosis is the most common lethal genetic disease of Caucasians in the United States and may present as neonatal cholestasis. The liver may show marked fatty change with cholestasis, both nonspecific changes. The most diagnostic feature of the liver is focal biliary fibrosis, an area of stellate scarring with proliferating bile ducts filled with inspissated eosinophilic material (Fig. 9) (31,32). This lesion, which is diagnostic, is rarely seen on biopsy because of its focal nature.

Idiopathic hemochromatosis refers to a genetic defect in iron storage that results in increased stores and damage to the heart and liver as well as other organs (33). A disease of similar name seen in the neonate (neonatal hemochromatosis) bears little resemblance to its adult namesake aside from the accumulation of iron (34,35). The biopsy diagnosis of idiopathic hemochromatosis rests on the identification of iron

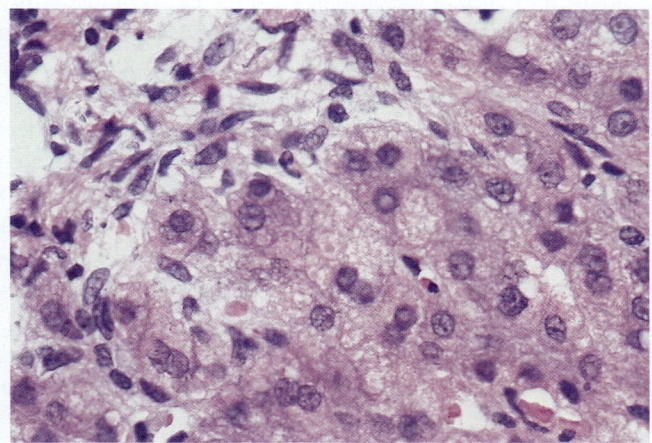

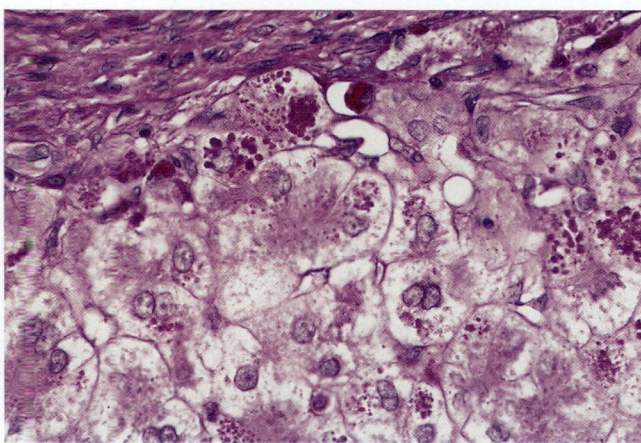

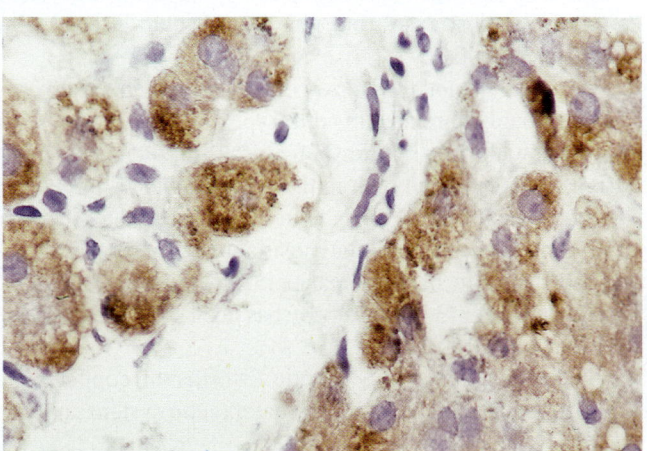

FIG. 7. Alpha$_1$-antitrypsin (AAT) deficiency. **A:** Characteristic hyaline globules are barely discernible by H&E. **B:** The inclusions are PAS positive and diastase resistant. PAS with diastase. **C:** The identity of the globules can be confirmed by using the immunoperoxidase method with antisera against AAT. Note that the amount of AAT is greater by this method than by PAS and that much of the AAT is not in the form of visible globules. Peroxidase-antiperoxidase method.

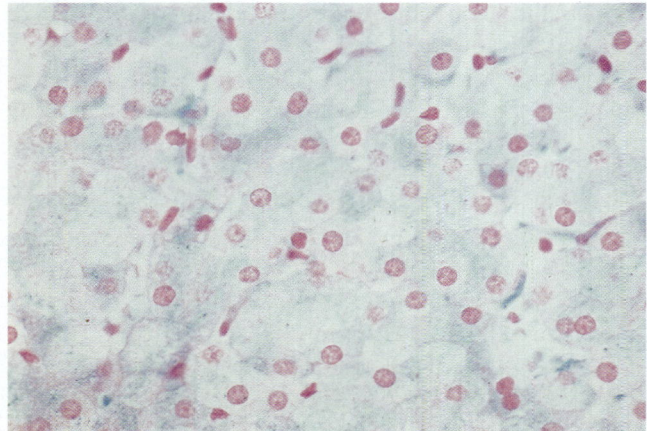

FIG. 8. Colloidal iron stain in Hurler's disease (mucopolysaccharidosis type 1) showing the presence of mucopolysaccharide in Kupffer cells and hepatocytes. Other stains for mucopolysaccharide (such as alcian blue) are less sensitive and do not demonstrate the mucopolysaccharide. By hematoxylin and eosin, the liver looks essentially normal. Colloidal iron.

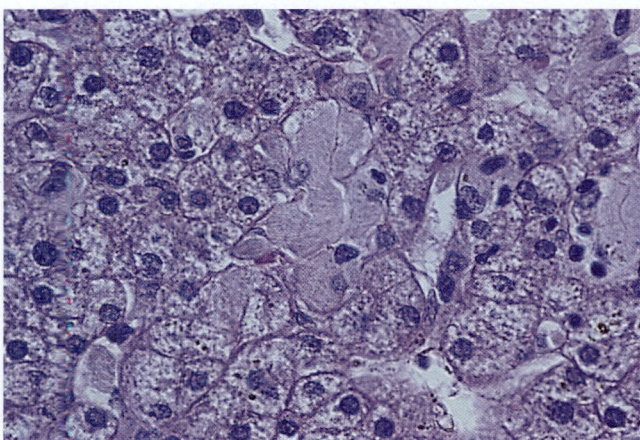

FIG. 10. Gaucher's disease showing enlarged Kupffer cells with a "crinkled" appearance to the cytoplasm.

confined to the hepatocytes, usually in a periportal distribution (Fig. 12). The major differential diagnosis is secondary hemosiderosis in which the iron is located primarily in Kupffer cells (Fig. 13). Unfortunately, the distinction may not be clear unless the biopsy is taken early because, with time, both processes will show mixed hepatocellular and Kupffer cell iron. In such a case, the relative distribution may be useful in favoring one etiology over the other, but a definite diagnosis cannot be made. It should be noted that anemias with ineffective erythropoiesis may show iron deposition in the liver identical to that of hemochromatosis (36).

Quantitation of hepatocellular iron and the calculation of the hepatic iron index (HII) have become a semi–gold standard for the diagnosis of hemochromatosis (37). Quantita-

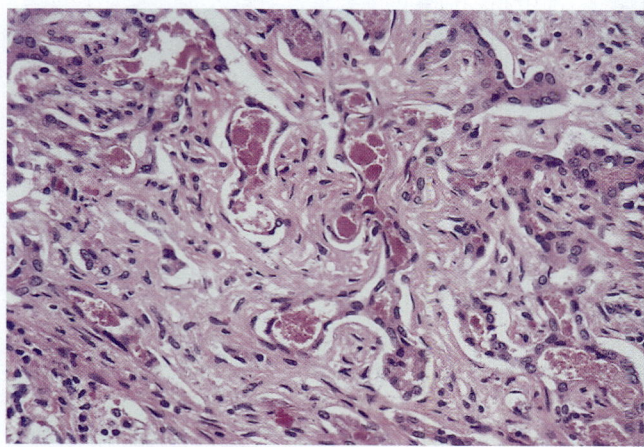

FIG. 9. The most characteristic features of cystic fibrosis are stellate scars containing bile ducts filled with eosinophilic inspissated material. Extensive fatty change and cholestasis may be present as well.

tion can be performed on a paraffin-embedded specimen. As a cost-effective measure it is recommended that tissue not be sent for quantitation until the tissue is examined; if there is no iron present on iron stain, then there is no utility in quantitation (37). Although an HII of greater than 2 has been considered diagnostic of hemochromatosis, this is true only in noncirrhotic livers and livers with no other reason for excess iron accumulation (38,39). A problem occurs when a cirrhotic liver contains excess iron since the iron may or may not be the cause of the cirrhosis and the HII is of less utility. If iron is found only in the regenerative nodules and not in the fibrous bands, one can be relatively confident that the iron is a secondary phenomenon because if it were present at the time of the formation of the cirrhosis, it should have been trapped in the bands. Conversely, if there is abundant iron in the bands and bile ducts, then the iron may be responsible for the cirrhosis; however, this is not definitive, since the accumulation could be a secondary event occurring simultaneously with another insult that led to the cirrhosis. In questionable cases, molecular testing for the altered allele of hemochromatosis may be used to diagnose the disease, although this test does have false negatives since there appear to be multiple mutations that can cause the disease (40). Molecular testing is not necessary to diagnose hemochromatosis in most cases, but may be of value in counseling family members.

Neonatal hemochromatosis is a disease of uncertain etiology, probably unrelated to adult-type hemochromatosis, that presents with liver failure soon after birth; the name derives from the excess iron seen in the liver. However, in neonatal hemochromatosis, identification of iron in tissue other than the liver is necessary for diagnosis since most causes of massive necrosis in the neonatal period demonstrate abundant iron in the liver (34). Lip biopsy has been suggested as a useful diagnostic tool (41).

Wilson's disease is a genetic disorder of copper metabolism that affects the liver, hematopoietic system, and cen-

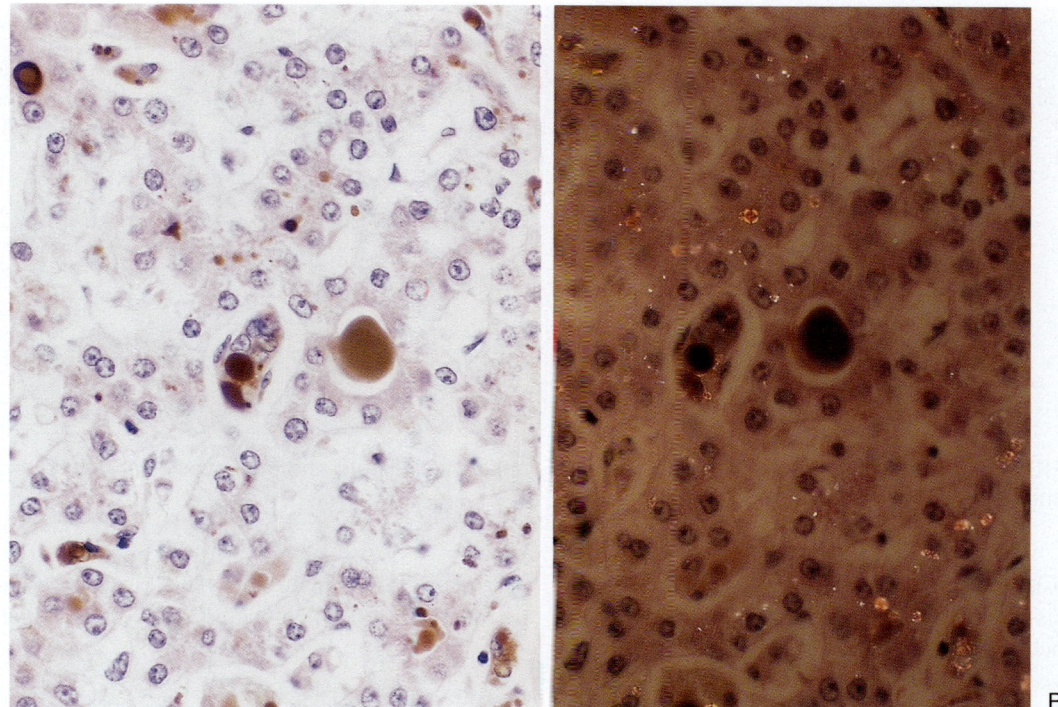

FIG. 11. A: Erythropoietic protoporphyria typically shows abundant brown-stained canalicular cholestasis in addition to hepatocellular damage and fibrosis. **B:** The porphyrins in the liver in erythropoietic protoporphyria show red cross-shaped birefringence when polarized.

tral nervous system (42–46). Age at clinical onset may vary widely, but it usually occurs after 6 years of age. Presentation may be neurologic, although this is often presaged by hemolytic anemia or liver dysfunction. The liver shows a variable picture with portal lymphocytic infiltration with or without piecemeal necrosis, abundant glycogen nuclei, Mallory hyalin, and copper accumulation (43) (Fig. 14). Patients presenting with indolent hepatic disease show a histologic picture of chronic hepatitis with a portal lymphocytic infiltrate, often associated with fatty change and glycogenated nuclei. Wilson's disease should be considered in any young patient presenting with such a picture, and the appropriate clinical evaluation should be performed (46). Patients presenting with hemolytic crisis and fulminant hepatitis demonstrate areas of liver collapse with abundant lipofuscin accumulation from degraded membrane fragments (Fig. 15). Since fulminant hepatitis typically is superimposed on a liver that has had ongoing low-grade liver disease with develop-

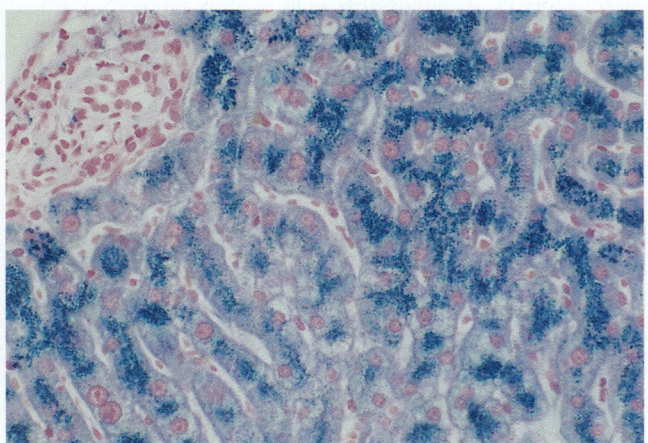

FIG. 12. Idiopathic hemochromatosis showing the characteristic hepatocellular distribution of iron with sparing of the Kupffer cells.

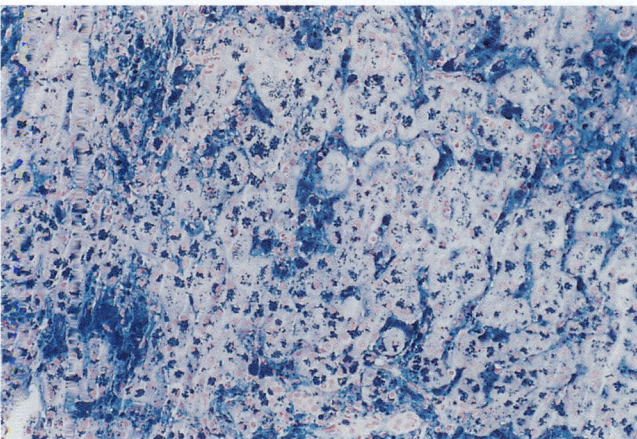

FIG. 13. Hemosiderosis secondary to hemolysis shows a predominately Kupffer-cell distribution of iron. Eventually both hepatocytes and Kupffer cells will contain iron in both primary and secondary iron overload. Prussian blue.

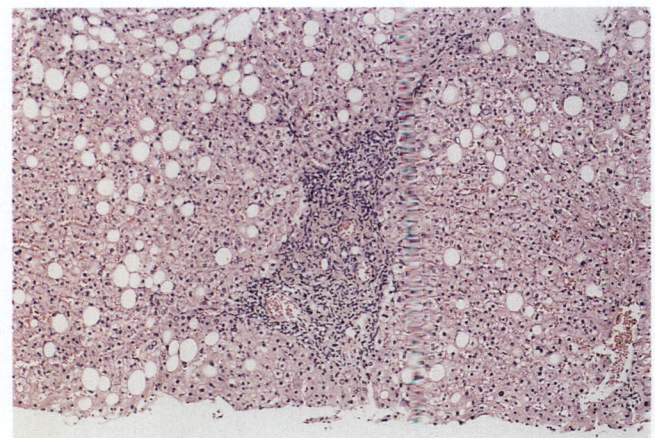
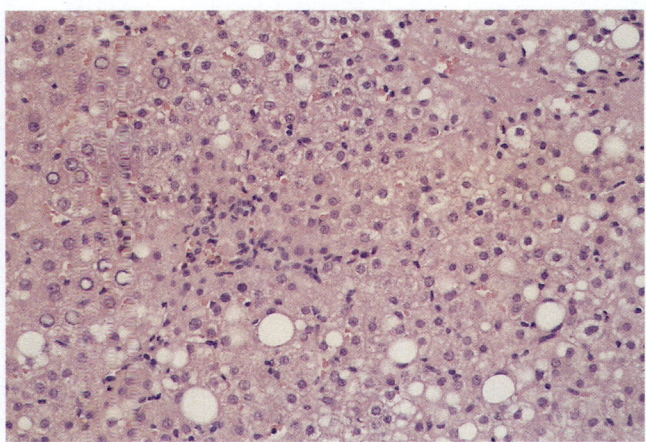

FIG. 14. Wilson's disease showing **(A)** a portal lymphocytic infiltrate and macrovesicular fatty change and **(B)** abundant nuclear glycogenation.

ment of fibrosis, the finding on trichrome staining of well-formed fibrous bands with collapse of the adjacent hepatocellular parenchyma is highly suggestive of the disease.

Quantitative copper determinations can be performed on paraffin-embedded liver tissue; therefore, submitting a separate specimen for quantitation is considered unnecessary (44). Unfortunately, although excess copper is invariably present by tissue assay, it is rather infrequently seen histochemically. Copper accumulation is also nonspecific, being found in many cholestatic states, including primary biliary cirrhosis. Similarly, Mallory hyalin if present is a useful clue to the diagnosis but is nonspecific. It is rarely present prior to the development of cirrhosis. Ultrastructurally, the liver is characterized by microvesicular steatosis, glycogen nuclei, copper deposits, and highly characteristic mitochondrial changes (45). The latter consist of enlargement with increased size of matrical bodies, increased density of matrix, and crystalline inclusions. The cristae are swollen and separated with flocculent material in cyst-like dilatations.

Biliary Tract Disease

This section discusses acquired diseases of the biliary tract that may affect the liver. Extrahepatic biliary atresia was dealt with previously and is not considered here.

Obstructive Liver Disease

When one speaks of acquired biliary tract disease affecting the liver, the usual manifestation is obstructive liver disease, which may take two forms: acute and chronic. Complications of biliary tract obstruction, such as biliary tract bacterial infection (ascending cholangitis), may add superimposed histologic findings.

Acute large-duct destruction (LDO) most commonly results from the passage of gallstones into the common bile duct, although in exceptional circumstances other etiologies such as bile plugs or surgical ligation may be the proximate cause. The earliest change seen in LDO is centrilobular canalicular cholestasis, followed by edema of the portal tracts. This edema is accompanied by proliferation of bile ductules at the periphery of the portal tracts and the accumulation of polymorphonuclear cells, probably in response to extravasated bile (Fig. 16) (47). The peripheral ductular proliferation is one of the most diagnostic changes of LDO. Note that polymorphonuclear neutrophil leukocytes (PMNs) are not observed within the lumen of the bile ducts, although occasionally a cell is seen in the wall of a duct. The term *cholangitis* has been used by some for this stage of LDO, and it is favored by clinicians. However, we reserve the term for the process of ascending cholangitis, which implies an infection of the biliary tree. The proliferating ductules are characterized by their small size, lack of a lumen, and peripheral location.

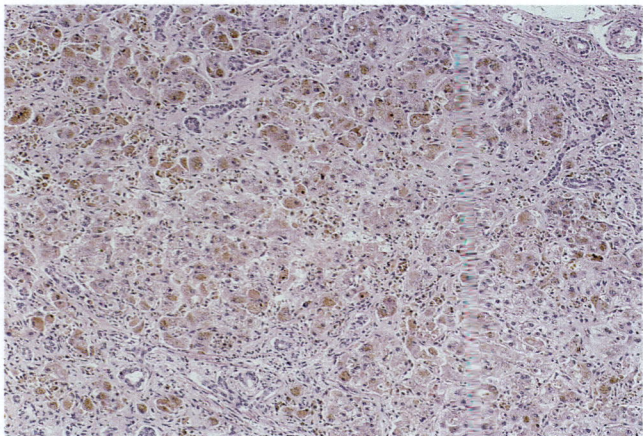

FIG. 15. A case of Wilson's disease that presented as fulminant hepatitis in association with a hemolytic crisis. There is massive necrosis with extensive loss of hepatocytes. Many of the residual hepatocytes contain pigment that is a combination of bile and lipofuscin.

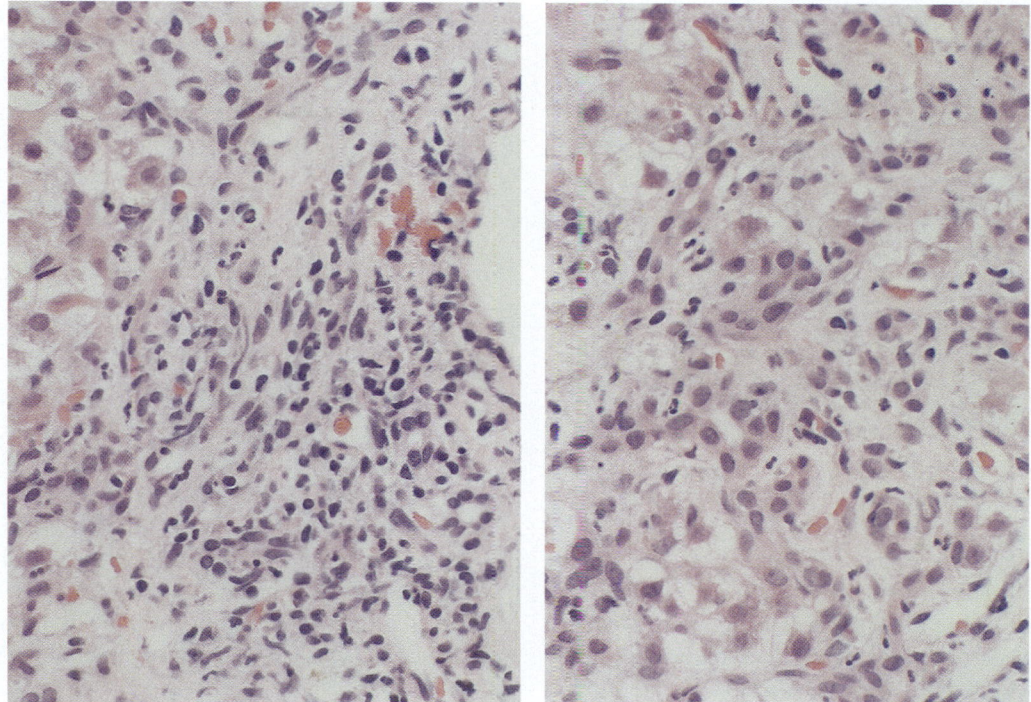

FIG. 16. Extrahepatic biliary obstruction. Two different portal areas from the same biopsy demonstrating bile ductular proliferation and a polymorphonuclear infiltrate.

With the passage of time in severe unresolved LDO, bile may accumulate in bile ducts, in ductules, and even in the parenchyma in the form of bile "lakes." Accumulation in hepatocytes may lead to so-called feathery degeneration, in which the hepatocellular cytoplasm becomes lucent and the cells somewhat swollen. Accumulation of foamy, bile-laden Kupffer cells may also be seen with long-standing cholestasis. Bile lakes are considered almost pathognomonic of LDO; the specificity of ductal bile is considerably less. Ductal bile accumulation may be seen in sepsis, some drug reactions, and treated liver transplant rejection.

The fully developed picture of acute LDO, therefore, consists of portal edema, cholestasis (canalicular and/or ductal), bile ductular proliferation, and portal accumulation of PMNs. Without treatment, portal fibrosis may develop and lead eventually to biliary cirrhosis. With long-standing obstruction (see chronic LDO, below), bile ducts may disappear, as with primary biliary cirrhosis (PBC). With the exception of the hepatocellular bile accumulation described earlier, the lobule is not affected by LDO. This is what one would expect since the injury is occurring via the portal tracts.

The differential diagnosis of acute LDO depends on which features are present. If the entire histologic picture is present, then considerations are drug reactions, sepsis, hyperalimentation toxicity, and treated acute liver transplant rejection. Alcoholic hepatitis may have PMNs in portal areas with cholestasis and bile ductular proliferation, but can be distinguished by the presence of hepatocellular necrosis and fatty change and lack of portal edema. Although sepsis may cause cholestasis (including ductular cholestasis) and PMN accumulation, PMNs are often in the lobule as well as portal areas, and there is little edema. Other processes with PMNs, such as bacterial and fungal infections (excluding ascending cholangitis) and surgical hepatitis, are so predominantly lobular that LDO is not a consideration. Hyperalimentation in the neonate and some drugs cannot always be accurately distinguished by histologic criteria alone (48).

Many processes, particularly those resulting in fibrosis of the liver, have some degree of ductular proliferation. For this reason, this feature is of little diagnostic importance in isolation, although absence of such proliferation makes the diagnosis of obstruction very unlikely. Similarly, cholestasis in and of itself is nonspecific.

If biliary tract infection is superimposed on obstruction, a diagnosis of ascending cholangitis is warranted. This diagnosis is made if PMNs are seen within the lumen of the interlobular bile ducts (Fig. 17). The other features of acute LDO are usually present.

Chronic LDO may result from impacted stones, recurrent passed stones, biliary fibrosis secondary to previous surgery or low-grade cholangiocarcinoma, and idiopathic chronic destructive biliary lesions such as primary sclerosing cholangitis (49,50). The histologic features of chronic LDO have some similarity to those of acute LDO in that there is bile ductular proliferation and there may be cholestasis, including canalicular and ductal variants. However, there is more fibrosis, and the portal infiltrate, while it may still contain a few

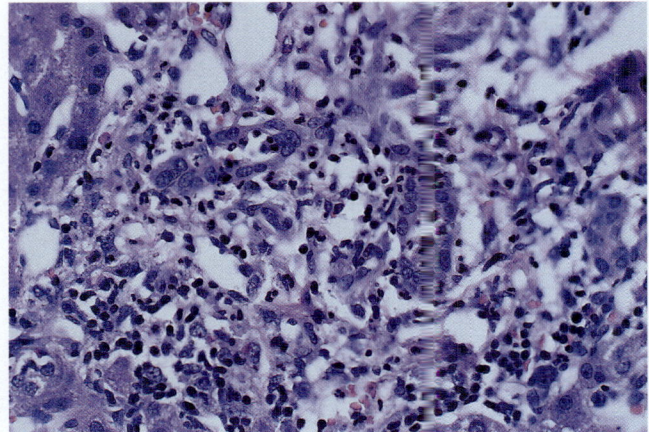

FIG. 17. Ascending cholangitis with a cluster of polymorphonuclear cells in the lumen of an interlobular bile duct.

PMNs, has a significant number of lymphocytes, but in general is quite mild. The lymphocytes may form lymphoid aggregates similar to those of hepatitis C. In addition, edema is generally not present. Interlobular bile ducts may disappear in long-standing obstructive disease, leading to a picture similar to that of PBC. In addition, there may be an "onion-skin" cuffing of fibroblasts around larger bile ducts, a feature that also occurs commonly in primary sclerosing cholangitis (50). Mallory hyalin in liver cells may be seen in the periportal area along with intrahepatocellular copper accumulation, although Mallory hyalin tends to be a late feature. The Mallory hyalin brings alcoholic liver disease into the differential; however, its periportal location and lack of associated PMN infiltrate and fatty change should allow distinction.

The differential diagnosis of chronic LDO is long and if cirrhosis has developed, the diagnosis is often impossible to make. Included are PBC, primary sclerosing cholangitis (PSC), and essentially any cause of micronodular cirrhosis. If relatively specific features such as granulomas are present, one may favor a diagnosis of PBC; however, an absolute diagnosis can essentially never be made on biopsy alone.

Primary Sclerosing Cholangitis

Primary sclerosing cholangitis is a disease associated with chronic ulcerative colitis in about 70% of cases, although it may occur in isolation or precede the onset of the inflammatory bowel disease (50–53). It occurs more commonly in males. The pathology consists of progressive inflammatory destruction of the extrahepatic biliary tree, although the intrahepatic tree may be involved as well. It needs to be distinguished clinically from sclerosis of the biliary tree due to other causes such as previous surgery or impacted stones that are termed secondary sclerosing cholangitis.

If one has a large bile duct available for examination, one sees necrosis and ulceration of the biliary epithelium with an associated lymphoplasmacellular infiltrate. However, the major bile ducts are not generally available for examination. On needle biopsy the liver demonstrates histologic features of chronic large bile duct obstruction as described above (50). In addition, there may be lymphocytic damage to the

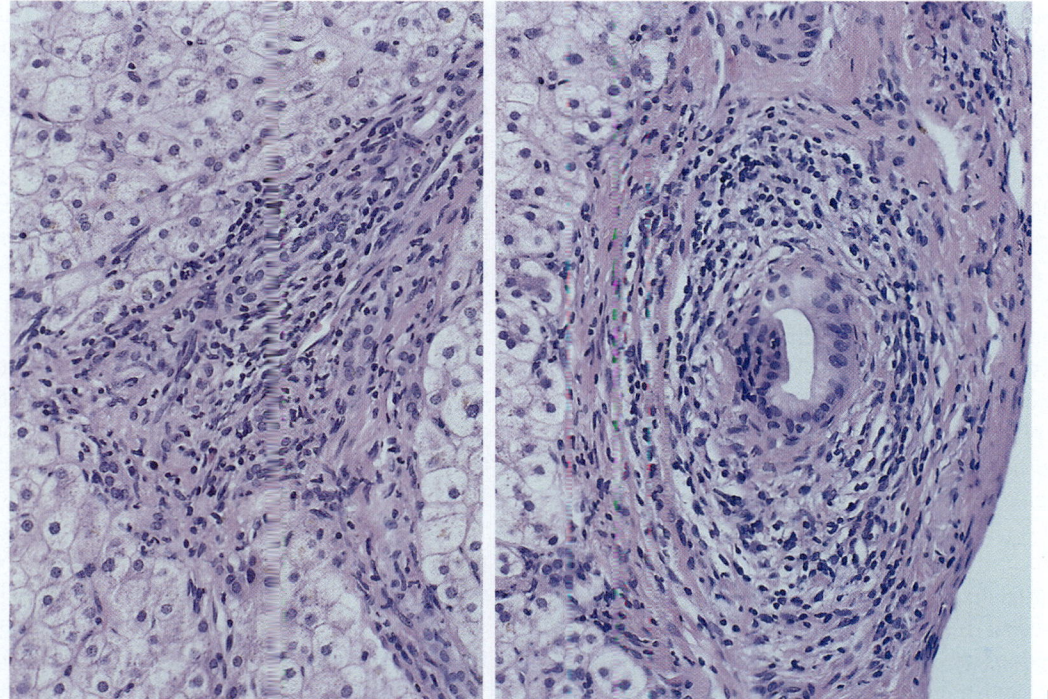

FIG. 18. Primary sclerosing cholangitis (PSC) associated with ulcerative colitis. **A:** A typical portal tract is expanded with bile ductular proliferation, and there is a mild lymphocytic infiltrate. **B:** Typical damaged duct with pleomorphism and loss of nuclei as well as infiltration by lymphocytes and concentric fibroblasts.

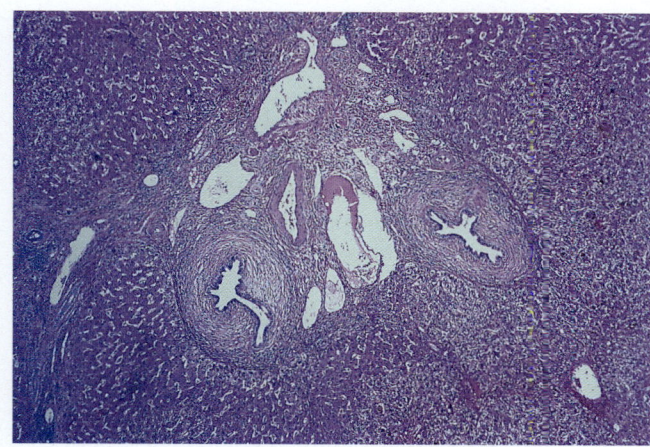

FIG. 19. A large portal tract in a case of primary sclerosing cholangitis demonstrating circumferential fibrosis around bile ducts, so-called onion-skinning. This feature, while characteristic of PSC, can be seen in other obstructive processes as well.

interlobular bile ducts ("pericholangitis") (Fig. 18) (53). Eventually the interlobular duct may disappear, leaving a scar in its place. Concentric periductal fibrosis ("onion skinning") is a common but nonspecific finding (Fig. 19). A staging system for PSC is based on the degree of fibrosis of the liver (54) (Table 22). In most cases of PSC the biopsy can only suggest the diagnosis; the final diagnosis is made by endoscopic retrograde cholangiopancreatography, which demonstrates multifocal stenoses of the extrahepatic biliary tree, often with intervening dilated segments. Since the bile ductular proliferation of PSC can be very subtle in early disease, it is a commonly overlooked diagnostic finding in liver pathology.

Primary Biliary Cirrhosis

Primary biliary cirrhosis is a disease that affects primarily middle-aged women and is usually accompanied by the presence of antimitochondrial antibodies (in approximately 95% of cases) (55–58). It is included in the differential diagnosis of granulomatous hepatitis since granulomas are present in 40% to 70% of cases (57,59).

The pathology of PBC involves the progressive destruction of the intrahepatic biliary tree by a lymphoplasmacellular infiltrate (56,58). The disease progresses through the four histologic stages detailed by Scheuer (56). The first stage, the florid duct lesion, is characterized by a portal lymphocytic infiltrate centered on interlobular bile ducts (Fig. 20). The bile ducts often demonstrate histologic abnormalities including, in addition to lymphocytic infiltration, increased eosinophilia of the cytoplasm, loss of individual cells, nuclear pseudostratification, duct dilatation, and eventual loss of ducts. The medium-sized ducts are the most commonly affected, so a small needle biopsy may miss the most characteristic lesions. However, often there is loss of the smaller ducts (particularly notable in tracts without inflammation) so that absence of ducts in a significant number of portal tracts favors PBC over other inflammatory diseases, such as viral hepatitis or autoimmune hepatitis, that may enter into the differential diagnosis (60). In addition to lymphocytes, one usually sees eosinophils, plasma cells, and even neutrophils in the portal tracts. Eosinophils and/or plasma cells may be particularly prominent; neutrophils tend to be located at the periphery of portal tracts in areas with proliferating bile ducts. The infiltrate may spill over into the periportal parenchyma with an appearance of piecemeal necrosis. There may also be a sinusoidal infiltrate of lymphocytes in the parenchyma, usually without hepatocellular necrosis (Fig. 21). It is at this early stage that granulomas are most often seen. If the granuloma, which is usually of the epithelioid type without giant cells, is surrounding a damaged bile duct, PBC is nearly always the correct diagnosis. Only sarcoidosis and rarely a drug reaction may simulate this pattern.

Granulomas may also be seen in the lobule; however, since lobular granulomas can occur in many conditions and

TABLE 22. *Staging of primary biliary cirrhosis (PBC) and primary sclerosing cholangitis (PSC)*

Stage	Scheuer system for PBC (56)	Ludwig (Mayo) system for PBC/PSC (54)
1	Florid duct lesion: portal inflammation with damage to septal or interlobular bile ducts	Portal stage: inflammation without expansion of portal tracts or piecemeal necrosis
2	Ductular proliferation: expansion of portal tracts with piecemeal necrosis and ductular proliferation	Periportal stage: piecemeal necrosis or fibrosis without bridging
3	Scarring: decreased inflammation with fibrous septum formation	Septal stage: bridging necrosis or fibrosis
4	Cirrhosis	Cirrhosis

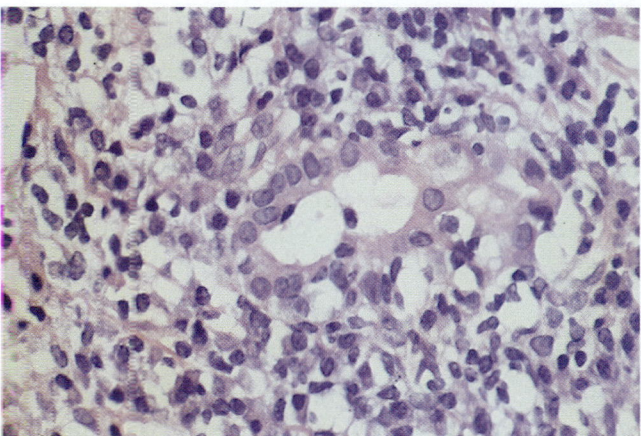

FIG. 20. The florid duct lesion of primary biliary cirrhosis. This interlobular bile duct is surrounded by lymphocytes, some of which are invading the epithelium leading to necrosis and stratification of the epithelial cells.

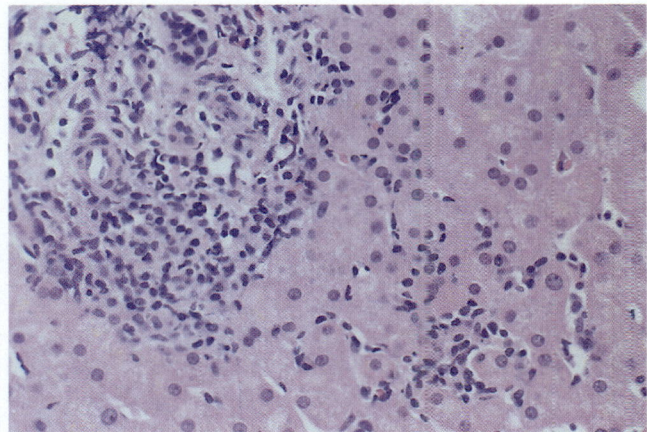

FIG. 21. A sinusoidal lymphocytic infiltrate is often seen in early primary biliary cirrhosis.

may represent incidental findings unrelated to the underlying liver disease, they are not as diagnostically useful as portal tract granulomas.

Over time, the portal tracts begin to widen and ductules proliferate, possibly due to focal obstruction caused by loss of ducts. This is the second stage of disease, the ductular proliferation stage. The disease then progresses through scarring (stage 3) to full-fledged cirrhosis (stage 4). Other features sometimes useful in the differential diagnosis are hepatocellular Mallory hyalin and copper accumulation as seen with the rubeanic acid or rhodamine stains. The Mallory hyalin of PBC differs from that of alcoholic hepatitis by its periportal location and lack of polymorphonuclear infiltrate. The other features of the disease are such that alcoholic hepatitis is generally not a consideration in diagnosis. Once the liver has reached the cirrhotic stage, it is difficult to distinguish PBC from any other cause of cirrhosis. However, features suggestive of PBC, in decreasing order of specificity, are granulomas, absence of bile ducts, Mallory hyalin, ill-defined margins to the fibrous bands, and a patchy character to the infiltrate.

Although the histologic stages of disease are useful descriptors and have been used to stage the extent of disease, they lead to some confusion since there is nothing to prevent a liver from showing features of several stages at the same time. To alleviate this problem, we prefer to use the staging system proposed at the Mayo Clinic, a system that can be used in PSC as well as PBC (54). This system is shown in Table 22 and is contrasted with the Scheuer system (56).

Medication-Induced Liver Disease

Medication-induced liver disease can only be touched on in this chapter. Detailed descriptions and tabulations are available in several reviews (3,61–64). Since so many drugs are capable of affecting the liver, the only reliable source of information ultimately remains the library and the literature, because no reference source is completely up to date.

Before determining that a drug is the probable offending agent, a complete medication history (including nonprescription items) must be obtained and made available to the pathologist.

Classically, liver disease due to medications can be subdivided by presumed pathogenesis (e.g., toxic or idiosyncratic) and by biochemical and histologic expression of location of damage (i.e., hepatocellular, biliary, etc.). It is important to try to assign both categories to a case since this may help in determining the most likely candidate drug. It should be kept in mind that although many drugs show biopsy features that suggest a drug etiology, almost any histologic pattern can be produced by a drug and, therefore, any biopsy finding may theoretically be caused by a drug. Drugs as a cause of specific histologic findings are discussed in the sections of this chapter that review those findings.

Pathogenetically, drug reactions are divided into idiosyncratic and toxic reactions. The former group is so named because the reaction to the drug is unpredictable. Some patients suffer with a small dose, whereas others may tolerate a large dose without ill effect. This category is often thought of as resulting from an allergic reaction to the drug, but other idiosyncracies, such as familial lack of an enzyme necessary for metabolism of a drug, may lead to similar clinical features. Drugs that act as haptens and set up an autoimmune destructive reaction against liver tissue may also fall into this category. If the reaction is of the allergic type, it is usually characterized histologically by an eosinophilic infiltrate typical of an allergic response. The autoimmune type of reactions is characterized by a lymphocytic infiltrate.

Toxic reactions are characterized as such because the drug involved affects virtually everyone taking it if enough drug is given and because the risk of damage is directly related to the dosage. It is presumed that the agent is directly toxic to some component of the liver. The target of attack most often involves the hepatocyte, although the biliary system may be preferentially involved with certain drugs, such as paraquat. These reactions do not show an eosinophilia and, indeed, inflammation of any type may be sparse. The specific type of damage as well as such features as location of damage and typical associated histologic features may allow a more or less specific diagnosis.

Drug reactions may also be characterized as hepatocellular, cholestatic, or mixed in type, reflecting the laboratory and histologic findings in a case. Usually the clinical categorization reflects the histology. The histology may provide specific features that allow some narrowing of the differential diagnosis. In the purely cholestatic drug reactions, the centrilobular canaliculi are the site of earliest cholestasis. It has been postulated that some drugs may act by paralyzing the contractile mechanism of the canaliculi. Hepatocellular reactions may be characterized by relatively bland hepatocellular necrosis as in acetaminophen toxicity (Fig. 22) or by a more hepatitic picture with inflammation as in acute isoniazid reaction. Although it may seem logical that most toxic agents cause extensive bland hepatocellular necrosis, not all

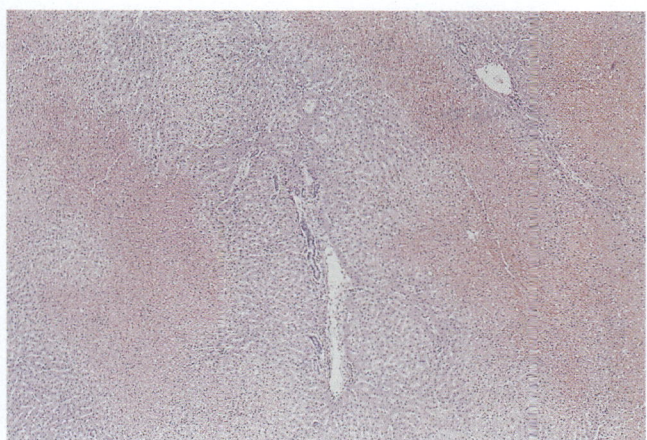

FIG. 22. Acute acetaminophen toxicity characterized by discrete centrilobular coagulative necrosis.

necrosis of this type is toxic, as exemplified by the idiosyncratic reaction to halothane.

Although virtually any histologic picture may be caused by a drug, certain features should alert one specifically to the possibility. Eosinophilia is a characteristic (but extremely nonspecific) change seen in a number of hypersensitivity-type drug reactions. Another important diagnostic feature is granulomatous inflammation. Drug reactions are a relatively common cause of granulomatous hepatitis (65). When granulomas are present they are usually epithelioid in type and are often accompanied by an acute hepatitic picture. A less specific feature of hepatitis caused by drugs is mixed micro- and macrovesicular fatty change. This type of fatty reaction is particularly uncommon in most viral infections (except hepatitis C) and, therefore, may be useful in the differential diagnosis of drug versus viral hepatitis. Isolated canalicular cholestasis is also characteristic of a number of medication reactions.

In addition to the more common hepatitic, granulomatous, and cholestatic drug reactions, there are many less common reactions that occur with a much smaller number of drugs. Included among these are vascular changes, hepatocellular proliferative changes, pseudobiliary tract obstruction, and neoplasms, all of which are discussed elsewhere in this chapter and in the chapter by Saul on hepatocellular neoplasms.

Included among vascular changes due to drugs are the Budd-Chiari syndrome (associated with oral contraceptives), peliosis hepatitis (associated with steroids, particularly of the androgenic type), veno-occlusive disease (VOD) (associated with a number of chemotherapeutic agents), and nonspecific sinusoidal dilatation, which may be caused by contraceptive steroids and many chemotherapeutic drugs (66). VOD has also been associated with radiation therapy.

Hepatocellular proliferative changes include nodular regenerative hyperplasia have been associated with corticosteroids and other drugs, as have hepatocellular neoplasms, including hepatocellular adenoma and carcinoma. Pseudobiliary tract obstruction may be caused by total parenteral alimentation (hyperalimentation) and by phenothiazines and related drugs.

Alcoholic Liver Disease

Alcohol constitutes the single largest cause of liver failure in the United States today. The degree of damage to the liver is affected by the duration of consumption, the quantity of consumption, and the genetic makeup of the drinker (67).

Pathologically, the liver may show changes ranging from simple fatty change to cirrhosis (68–70). The earliest and commonest manifestation is reversible macrovesicular fatty change. This change is nonspecific and may persist for several months after drinking is discontinued. More significant is the presence of Mallory hyalin and a portal and lobular infiltrate of polymorphonuclear cells, usually with concomitant hepatocellular necrosis (Figs. 23 and 24). The Mallory hyalin is usually found in ballooned hepatocytes in the centrilobular region. This constellation has been termed *alcoholic hepatitis*. All of the features of alcoholic hepatitis are nonspecific in isolation but are nearly diagnostic if seen together with fatty change.

Other etiologies for these findings are liver disease following jejunoileal bypass, drug reactions, and other forms of nonalcoholic steatohepatitis (NASH) (71–76). NASH is defined by the exclusion of alcohol as a possible etiologic factor; it occurs most often in obese diabetic patients but may also be seen in association with a number of medications (e.g., tamoxifen and amiodarone) and toxins, and is occasionally seen in nonobese patients without other risk factors (see The Liver in Systemic Disease, below). Mallory hyalin in isolation can be seen in numerous conditions, many of which are cholestatic, but it differs from that of alcoholic liver disease both in distribution and associated findings. In alcoholic liver disease, the Mallory hyalin tends to be centrilobular, as opposed to a periportal location in cholestatic processes such as PBC or biliary obstruction. In addition, alcoholic Mallory hyalin is characteristically chemotactic for

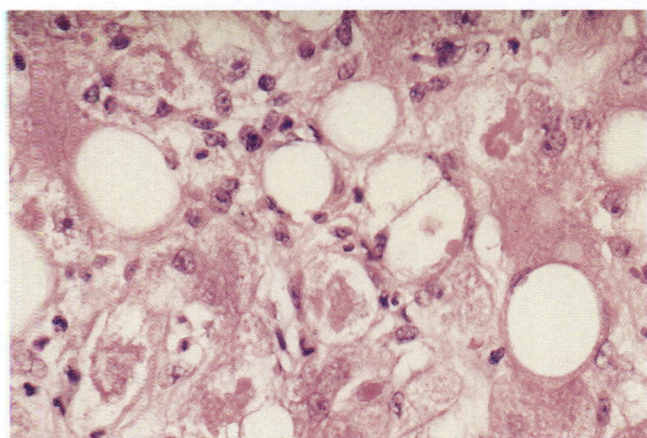

FIG. 23. Mallory hyalin in alcoholic liver disease is characterized by its irregular "rope-like" shape and marked eosinophilia.

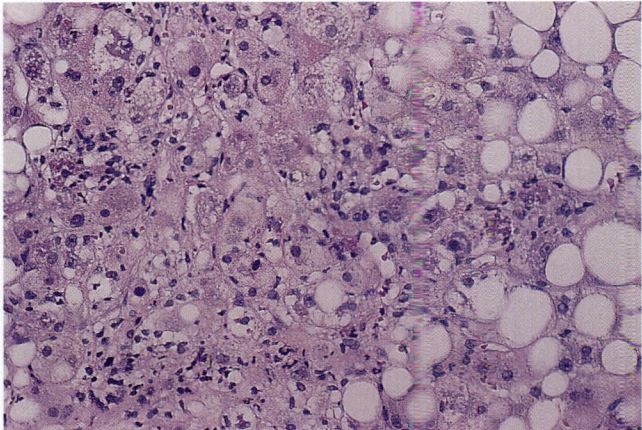

FIG. 24. Acute alcoholic hepatitis consisting of macrovesicular fatty change, Mallory hyalin and a polymorphonuclear infiltrate. These changes are often most prominent in the centrilobular region.

polymorphonuclear cells. Alcoholic Mallory hyalin may persist for up to 1 year after drinking is discontinued (77).

The central predominance of the hepatocellular damage in alcoholic liver disease leads to centrilobular fibrosis, the lesion known as sclerosing hyaline necrosis (Fig. 25) (78). In this condition, stellate fibrosis extends from the central vein into surrounding parenchyma in a pericellular fashion. This lesion is characteristic but not diagnostic since it can be seen in metabolic diseases, long-standing congestive heart failure, and NASH. This fibrosis itself may lead to portal hypertension, but more commonly leads to cirrhosis by the formation of central to portal bridges, resulting in classic micronodular cirrhosis. Once cirrhosis develops, it may become impossible to establish an etiology, although if the patient continues to consume ethanol, alcoholic hepatitis may remain.

Chronic hepatitis has been reported as a sequel to alcohol consumption (79,80). In this condition, a histologic picture of chronic active hepatitis that persists following cessation of alcohol consumption develops in former heavy alcohol consumers. Although it was previously suggested that alcohol-induced damage leads to the development of an autoimmune response to the liver, a more probable explanation is that the patient had contracted other causes of chronic active hepatitis such as hepatitis C (80,81). It must always be remembered that alcoholic patients may develop liver disease from agents other than alcohol. In one study as many as 20% of alcoholic patients with newly developed liver abnormalities had pathology other than alcoholic liver disease (82). The temptation to blame all problems on the alcohol must be avoided. This is especially true for the pathologist, who must not be swayed by the opinion of clinical colleagues if the pathology does not fit the history.

Viral Hepatitis

Although bacteria, fungi, and viruses may infect the liver, the most common and unique of these causes are viral infections. Most notable are the hepatotrophic viruses: hepatitis A, B, and C viruses (HAV, HBV, and HCV) delta agent virus (HDV); epidemic hepatitis virus (HEV); and possibly other non-A, non-B viruses. When the term *viral hepatitis* is used without qualification, usually one of these agents is assumed. A large number of other viruses may cause liver disease, however, including those that may affect both the immunocompetent and immunocompromised host, such as Epstein-Barr virus (EBV) and cytomegalovirus (CMV), as well as those that preferentially affect the immunocompromised liver, such as herpes simplex virus and adenovirus. Most of these latter viruses have features that allow some distinction from the hepatotrophic viruses. Infections in immunocompromised hosts often differ clinically and histologically from those in immunocompetent individuals.

Infection with hepatotrophic viruses may have several outcomes (83). In the case of HAV there is usually a self-limiting acute hepatitis, although a small number of patients suffer from massive hepatic necrosis and acute liver failure. Any of the hepatotrophic viruses may, in fact, cause massive necrosis and acute liver failure, although this outcome is most rare with hepatitis C. HBV and HCV infection may lead to chronic liver disease and cirrhosis. Hepatitis A does not produce chronic disease in the immunocompetent host. HDV infection can only occur in conjunction with HBV, and may cause any of the clinical syndromes and histologic patterns of HBV alone. Hepatitis E, which is rare in the United States, has a particular predilection for a poor outcome in pregnant women (84). Infection with CMV or EBV usually leads to acute self-limited disease, although there are some poorly documented reports of chronic hepatitis due to these agents. Rare cases of hepatic failure have been reported with both of these agents.

Histologic Features of Viral Hepatitis in the Immunocompetent Host

Acute Viral Hepatitis

Acute viral hepatitis in the immunocompetent host is characterized by hepatocellular necrosis, a portal and lobular

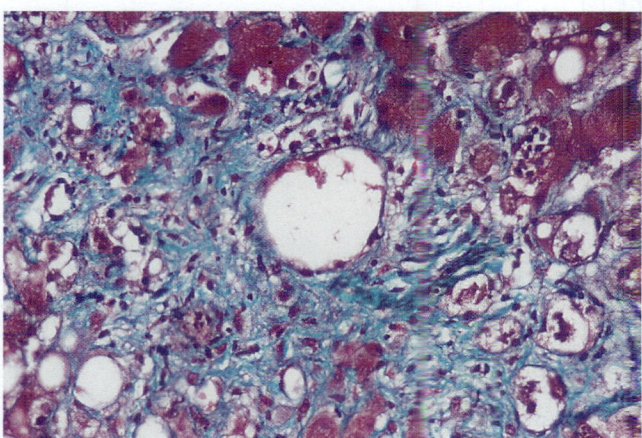

FIG. 25. Sclerosing hyaline necrosis characteristic of alcoholic liver disease. Note the central vein that is surrounded by an area of fibrosis that extends into the surrounding parenchyma between hepatocytes.

lymphocytic infiltrate, and regenerative activity (85–91). The hepatocellular necrosis may take the form of ballooning degeneration, acidophil body formation, or simple dropout of single cells, as documented by a small area of collapse seen on the reticulin stain (Fig. 26). The type, location, and degree of degeneration may be influenced to some extent by the virus causing the disease.

The infiltrate of viral hepatitis is predominantly composed of small lymphocytes, although there may be rare intermixed eosinophils, neutrophils, and plasma cells. The infiltrate is most prominent in the portal tracts and may spill over into the periportal parenchyma. In the lobule, the infiltrate usually is found in areas of hepatocellular necrosis, although with some agents such as HCV, CMV, and EBV it has a more sinusoidal location (90–94).

There are some special features that may aid in the differential diagnosis of the specific agent of a viral infection. Hepatitis A infection is often characterized by an abundance of plasma cells and cholestasis, two features that distinguish it from other acute viral hepatitides (87,88). Predominant central ballooning degeneration favors HBV over HCV or HAV. Conversely, the presence of dense portal lymphoid aggregates, bile duct damage, and a predominantly sinusoidal infiltrate are characteristic of HCV (Figs. 27–29) (87,88,95). CMV and EBV are considered below. While these features are characteristic of the specific viral types, none is pathog-

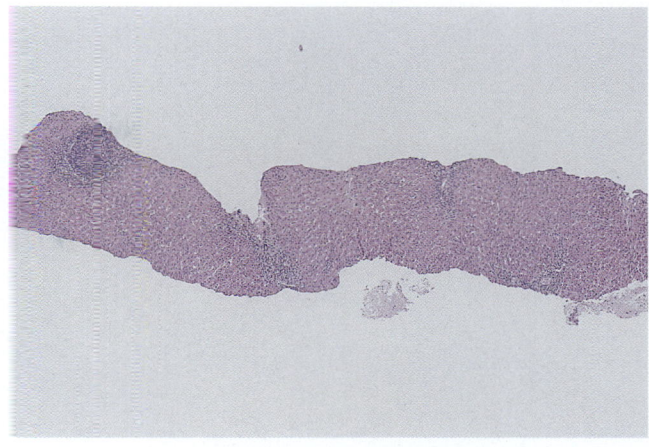

FIG. 27. Chronic hepatitis C with several mildly inflamed portal tracts as well as one showing a dense aggregate of lymphocytes *(left)*.

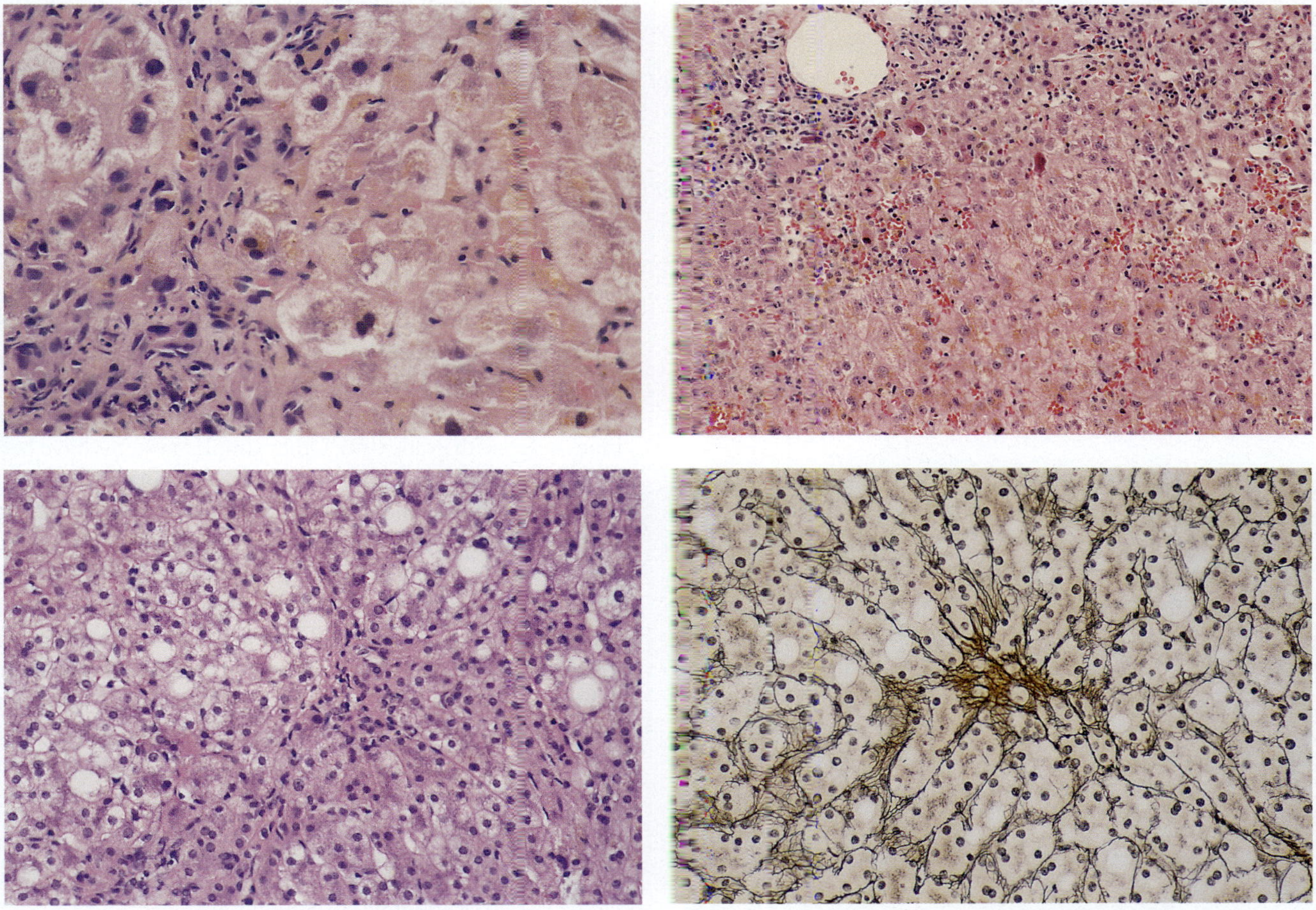

FIG. 26. Types of necrosis that may be seen in viral hepatitis. **A:** Ballooning degeneration characterized by enlargement of hepatocytes with rarefaction of cytoplasm in a case of acute hepatitis A. **B:** Acidophilic body, a round to oval, eosinophilic dead hepatocyte with or without nuclear remnants, usually located in a sinusoid, accompanied by ballooning in this specimen of acute hepatitis A. **C:** Focal necrosis characterized by collapse and a small focus of lymphocytes. **D:** Reticulin stain demonstrating the "collapse" of the reticulin framework in the area of focal necrosis seen in C.

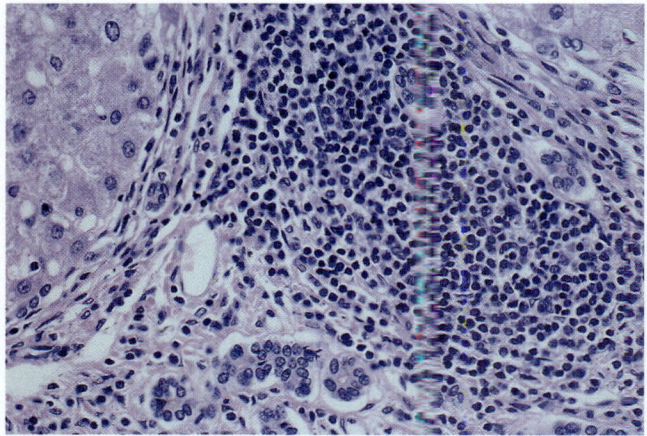

FIG. 28. Portal tract of chronic hepatitis C showing the purely lymphocytic infiltrate surrounding an interlobular bile duct.

nomonic, and many variations occur. In general a biopsy is not expected to provide an etiologic diagnosis given the accuracy of serologic methods, and biopsy is rarely obtained during acute viral hepatitis if serologic findings indicate an infection (96). Special stains are rarely of value in diagnosing any of the viral infections in immunocompetent patients in the acute phase, with the possible exception of delta hepatitis (97). In acute viral hepatitis, the infected cells are destroyed as soon as viral antigens are expressed on the cell surface; thus, staining is possible only in the preclinical late incubation period.

Massive hepatic necrosis following viral infection is characterized by extensive to total loss of hepatocytes with collapse of the reticulin framework (Fig. 30). In these cases there is often proliferation of residual cells, including bile ducts. In the central areas, a lymphocytic endophlebitis may be seen. Inflammation in general is modest.

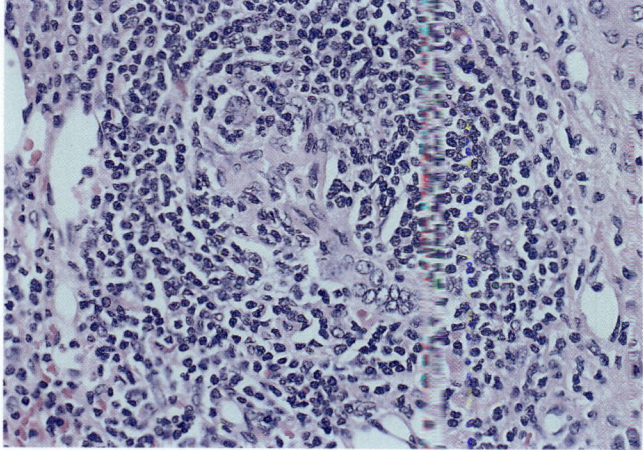

FIG. 29. The damaged bile ducts of hepatitis C are infiltrated with lymphocytes and have pseudostratified nuclei in eosinophilic cytoplasm, thus resembling the damaged bile ducts of primary biliary cirrhosis.

Chronic Viral Hepatitis B and C

As stated above, HBV and HCV infection may lead to the development of chronic hepatitis, defined by the persistence of abnormal liver function studies for greater than 6 months. Although this 6-month figure has been used as a landmark for chronic hepatitis, it is now apparent that it has no value outside of the context of viral hepatitis, and may even be inaccurate for hepatitis C. In particular, for patients with acute hepatitis with negative viral markers, biopsy should not be delayed since several diseases such as autoimmune hepatitis and Wilson's disease are adversely affected by delay in diagnosis. Biopsy is often performed in chronic viral hepatitis to confirm the diagnosis and to assess the inflammatory grade and fibrotic stage of disease.

Chronic viral hepatitis is characterized by a predominantly lymphocytic portal infiltrate with much less lobular involvement than is seen in acute hepatitis. Piecemeal necrosis and fibrosis may be present. Traditionally, chronic hepatitis has been divided on histologic grounds into chronic active hepatitis (CAH) and chronic persistent hepatitis (CPH), based on the presence or absence of piecemeal necrosis (Fig. 31) (83). Although such a classification was useful in providing prognostic information prior to the recognition of multiple causes of chronic hepatitis, it now appears that the prognostic information provided was a reflection of etiology more than different expressions of the same disease process. Several issues have been raised that render these terms of limited usefulness (98). Therefore, current recommendations are to diagnose chronic hepatitis by etiology, with the biopsy providing an assessment of degree of necroinflammatory activity (the grade) and fibrosis (the stage) (90,91,99–102). The terms *chronic persistent* and *chronic active hepatitis* should be avoided.

Several systems have been suggested for grading these diseases, and unfortunately none has received general acceptance. The Knodell Hepatitis Activity Index (HAI) has been widely used for research but is rather complicated and combines stage with grade (99). Other simpler systems have been proposed by several authors (98,101). A recent consensus document recommended using descriptive terms, although without specific definition of those terms (102). The assignment of grade can be numeric or descriptive, and should include an assessment of portal inflammation, piecemeal necrosis, lobular activity, and fibrosis. Some authors recommend providing an overall inflammatory grade that includes the portal, lobular, and piecemeal portions, although some have used only the degree of lobular/periportal inflammation and have not counted portal activity (101). Several systems have also been proposed for fibrotic stage, using a four-tiered system. One relatively simple grading system proposed by Scheuer provides a useful model for daily use (98):

Grade 0—no or minimal inflammation
Grade 1—portal inflammation or lobular inflammation with no necrosis
Grade 2—mild piecemeal necrosis or focal hepatocellular necrosis

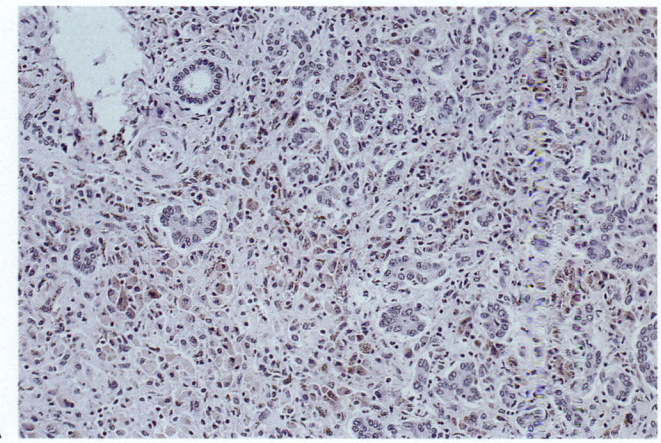
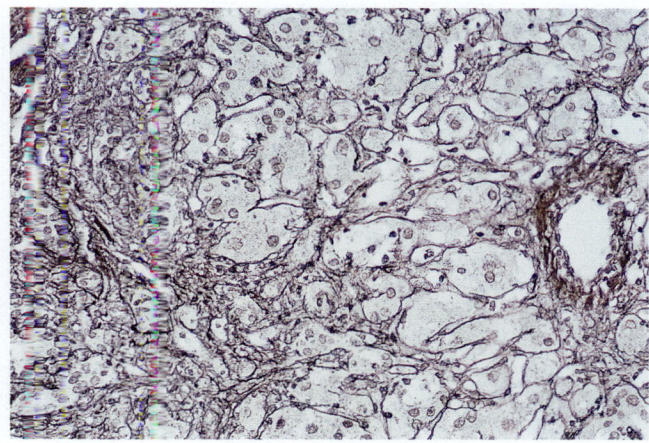

FIG. 30. Massive hepatic necrosis. **A:** The biopsy demonstrates a residual portal tract *(left)* surrounded by collapsed parenchyma with pseudoductular transformation. There is minimal inflammation but extensive hemosiderin deposition. **B:** Reticulin stain emphasizes the collapsed nature of the parenchyma and a very close approximation of the portal tract *(left)* and central vein *(right)*.

Grade 3—moderate piecemeal necrosis or severe focal cell damage

Grade 4—severe piecemeal necrosis or bridging necrosis

The overall grade is based on the most severe degree of portal or lobular injury. The corresponding staging system is as follows:

Stage 0—no fibrosis
Stage 1—enlarged fibrotic portal tracts
Stage 2—periportal or portal to portal septa
Stage 3—bridging fibrosis with architectural distortion, no obvious cirrhosis
Stage 4—cirrhosis

A typical diagnosis might read as follows: "Chronic hepatitis C with moderate portal infiltrate and moderate piecemeal necrosis (grade 3) with bridging fibrosis (stage 3)." This quantitative approach emphasizes the continuum of the process and does not force cases into unrealistic categories. The assessment of grade and stage not only provides some prognostic information, but also is sometimes used to determine the feasibility of treating the hepatitis with interferon (95).

In addition to grade and stage, it has been suggested that iron content in the liver plays a role in predicting efficacy of therapy for hepatitis C (103–105). Specifically, iron observed in portal tract macrophages has been suggested as a marker for poor response to interferon (103,104). Unfortunately, other studies have either contradicted the effect of iron or have suggested that other forms of iron accumulation, such as hepatocellular iron content, are the true predictors (105). The reported prevalence of stainable iron in the liver of hepatitis C patients is only about 10%, which is in keeping with personal observations. Since there is controversy regarding this aspect of the pathology of hepatitis C, it may be worth reporting iron content and location if hepatologists wish to use this information in patient management.

The histologic features of the various types of chronic hepatitis are different enough to allow some degree of distinction based on histology alone. The characteristic and diagnostic feature of chronic hepatitis B is the expression of hepatitis B surface (HBsAg) or core (HBcAg) antigen in hepatocytes (97). The HBsAg is usually expressed in the cytoplasm and correlated with the presence of "ground-glass" hepatocytes, although many cases with demonstrable HBsAg in hepatocytes do not manifest ground glass cells (Fig. 32). HBsAg expression carries no particularly useful clinical information. Expression of HBcAg may be cytoplasmic, membranous, or nuclear. If present, it infers active replication of the virus and hence is indicative of infectivity (106). Since both of these antigens are detected by serologic studies, however, it is rarely useful to stain for them.

Chronic hepatitis C infection is characterized by a patchy portal infiltrate with dense aggregates of small lymphocytes devoid of plasma cells or eosinophils (Figs. 27 and 28). These aggregates often surround damaged bile ducts, but ducts are

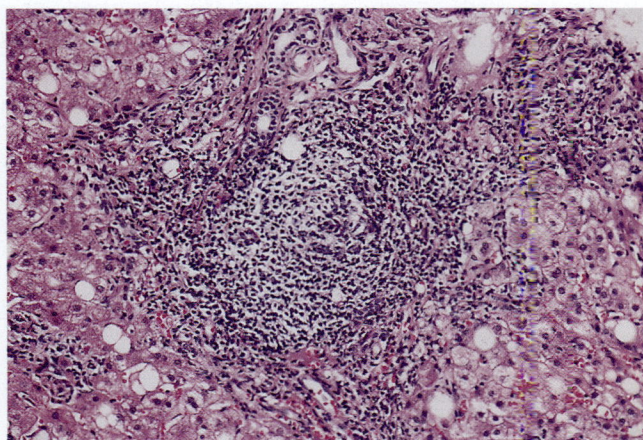

FIG. 31. Portal tract from a case of autoimmune hepatitis showing piecemeal necrosis. Note how the portal tract lymphocytes penetrate into the limiting plate to entrap and destroy hepatocytes.

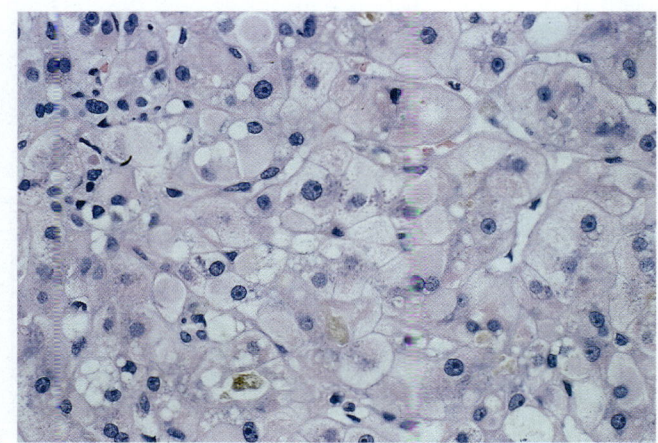 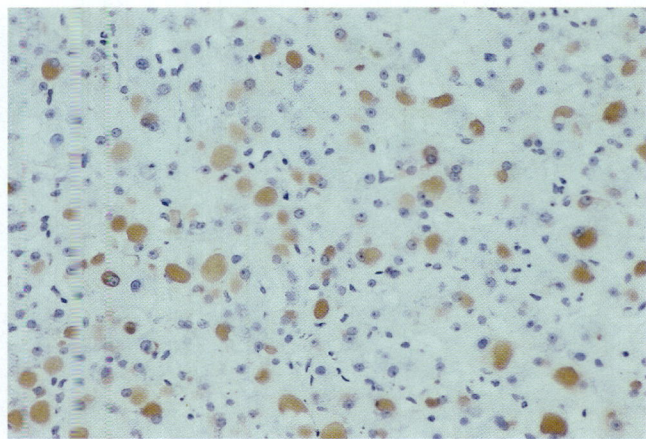

FIG. 32. Chronic hepatitis B infection. **A:** By hematoxylin and eosin, hepatocytes containing excess hepatitis B surface antigen (HBsAg) are recognizable as ground-glass cells. The cytoplasm has a uniform eosinophilic appearance that is distinguishable from ground-glass change associated with simple proliferation of endoplasmic reticulum secondary to drug administration by its eccentric character. **B:** Specific staining for HBsAg by the immunoperoxidase method will also provide specific confirmation of the identity of ground-glass cells.

not destroyed. The area around the aggregates is often devoid of inflammation or contains a few scattered lymphocytes and occasional plasma cells or eosinophils. Piecemeal necrosis is uncommon. These aggregates are characteristic enough to allow a presumptive diagnosis of HCV in the appropriate clinical setting. However, only about 50% of cases of chronic hepatitis C have the aggregates, with the other cases showing variable degrees of nonspecific portal infiltrate. Although fatty change has been reported as a common feature of hepatitis C, in my experience the degree of fatty changes is usually minimal and its absence not unusual. As a practical matter, biopsies taken in hepatitis B and C are generally done for the purpose of grading and staging disease, not for diagnosis.

The Delta Agent

The delta agent is a defective virus that can replicate only in the presence of concurrent active hepatitis B viral replication (107–110). If the hepatitis B and delta infections occur simultaneously, they may lead to typical acute hepatitis that resolves, acute hepatitis with an atypical biphasic pattern ("recurrent" acute hepatitis), or fulminant hepatitis (107). If the delta agent is superimposed on a chronic hepatitis B–infected liver, it may result in fulminant hepatic failure, acute hepatitis, or histologic chronic hepatitis that may progress rapidly to cirrhosis in 15% of such patients (109). In none of these cases is there usually anything histologically different between the delta-infected liver and the hepatitis B–infected liver alone. However, delta infection should be considered in any case of recurrent acute hepatitis or the sudden development of fulminant hepatitis in a carrier of hepatitis B. Occasionally, acute delta infection shows a characteristic pattern of vacuolar change in the infected hepatocytes, resulting in a multivesicular cell that has been termed the *morule cell*. This pattern has been seen most commonly in the Amazon basin (Santa Marta hepatitis) but has also been described in the United States (110). Delta hepatitis can be diagnosed by serologic evaluation or by the identification of delta antigen in the nuclei of infected hepatocytes (97).

Epstein-Barr Virus and Cytomegalovirus Infection

The other main viruses affecting the immunocompetent individual are EBV and CMV, both in the context of an infectious mononucleosis-like syndrome. These viruses both produce a mild acute hepatitis with nearly identical histologic features (92–94). There is a predominantly portal and sinusoidal infiltrate of atypical lymphocytes with relatively little necrosis (Fig. 33). Mitoses may be abundant in the hepatocytes, and small epithelioid granulomas may also be seen. Although these features are suggestive of EBV or CMV mononucleosis hepatitis, they are not diagnostic; the diagnosis must be made by serologic criteria. Similar histology is seen in some cases of HCV and some drug reactions such as with diphenylhydantoin (111). CMV inclusions as seen in the immunocompromised host (see below) are not found in mononucleosis in immunocompetent individuals, presumably due to destruction of the infected cell prior to accumulation of large quantities of viral products. Immunohistochemical staining is also not diagnostically useful for CMV mononucleosis.

Differential Diagnosis

The histologic differential diagnosis of acute viral hepatitis in the immunocompetent patient encompasses any of the causes of acute hepatitis, including drug and autoimmune etiology. While these various causes may be distinguishable only by serology or clinical features, acute medication-induced hepatitis may show granulomas, mixed micro-

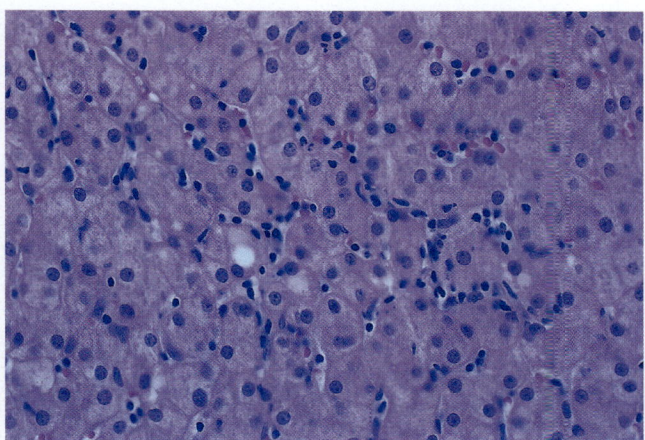

FIG. 33. Cytomegalovirus mononucleosis hepatitis characterized by, in addition to a portal lymphocytic infiltrate, a predominantly sinusoidal lobular lymphocytic infiltrate with minimal hepatocellular necrosis or ballooning. Despite this, hepatocellular mitoses may be abundant.

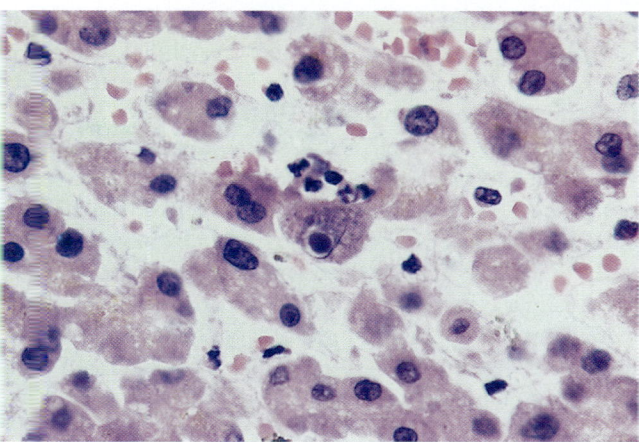

FIG. 34. Cytomegalic inclusion disease. This hepatocyte contains a typical large, basophilic to brick red nuclear inclusion with surrounding halo and peripheral condensation of chromatin. Cytoplasmic amphophilic inclusions are commonly present as well.

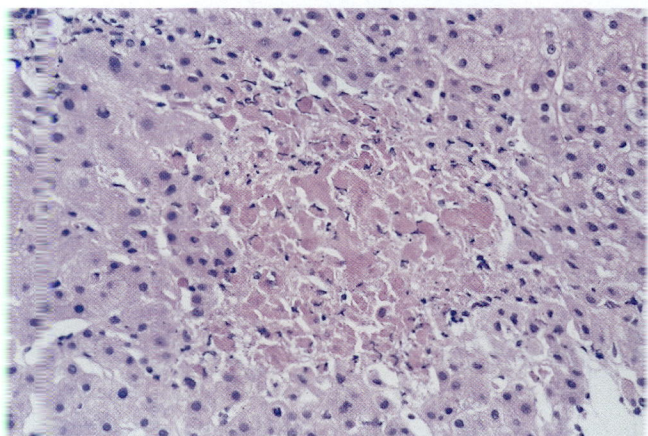

FIG. 35. Herpes simplex hepatitis characterized by randomly scattered foci of coagulative necrosis. Typical nuclear inclusions are found in hepatocytes at the periphery of the necrosis.

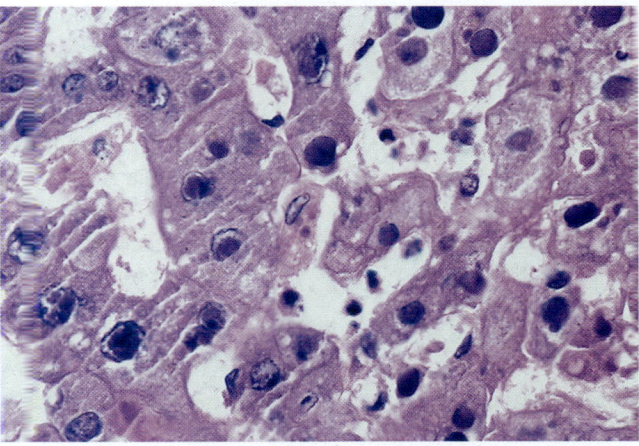

FIG. 36. Typical herpes simplex hepatitis has eosinophilic homogeneous nuclear inclusions in hepatocytes.

macrovesicular fat, or eosinophils. Acute autoimmune hepatitis is characterized by abundant plasma cells, periportal areas of collapse, and bridging necrosis (60).

The differential diagnosis of chronic viral hepatitis includes drug reactions, autoimmune hepatitis, Wilson's disease, sclerosing cholangitis, and resolving acute hepatitis (60). Distinction from autoimmune hepatitis is based on the degree of plasma cell infiltrate in the latter, although absolute distinction may require clinical studies. Drug reactions also need clinical history for absolute diagnosis, although granulomas favor drugs. Wilson's disease generally lacks plasma cells or eosinophils and should always be considered, particularly in young patients presenting with chronic hepatitis of unknown etiology. Distinction from resolving acute hepatitis may be difficult without a history unless abundant lipofuscin pigment from degradation of dead hepatocytes is identifiable in Kupffer cells.

Viral Hepatitis in the Immunocompromised Host

In the immunocompromised host, CMV, herpes simplex, varicella, and adenovirus are major problems. In CMV infection, intranuclear and cytoplasmic inclusions may be seen in all cell types, with hepatocytes being affected most often (112,113) (Fig. 34). The nuclear inclusion is variably colored but usually eosinophilic to amphophilic and is surrounded by a clear halo. The cytoplasmic inclusions are basophilic dots. The infected cells are frequently surrounded by a cluster of neutrophils (microabscess), thus providing a clue that should lead one to search carefully for inclusions.

Both herpes and adenovirus infections are characterized by randomly scattered foci of confluent necrosis (Fig. 35). Inclusions are seen at the periphery of the necrotic areas. In the case of the herpes infections, these consist of eosinophilic ground-glass nuclei (Fig. 36). The infected hepatocytes in herpes infections are mainly mononuclear rather than multinucleate. In adenovirus, the inclusion is less distinctive. In some cases the nuclei are large and basophilic, whereas in others the nuclei have a bubbly, vesicular appearance (114). In these infections, immunoperoxidase staining or in situ hybridization may assist in the positive identification of the virus if the inclusions are not well formed. Occasional cases of massive hepatic necrosis have been reported with all three of these viruses as well as by echovirus in the neonate.

Epstein-Barr virus may also affect the liver in a variety of patterns in the immunocompromised patient. These include a predominantly portal infiltrate of large lymphocytes (polymorphic B-cell hyperplasia or lymphoma) in addition to an infectious mononucleosis-like pattern (115). Immunostaining for EBV antigen or Epstein-Barr-encoded-RNA (EBER) is often useful in diagnosis.

In addition to direct viral hepatic infection, the liver may be involved as part of the viral-associated hemophagocytic syndrome (VAHS). This process, which often is accompanied by EBV and CMV infections, is characterized by prominent erythrophagocytosis by sinusoidal Kupffer cells and by histiocytes in the portal tracts (116). Similar histologic features are seen in the liver in sinus histiocytosis with massive lymphadenopathy (SHML), although in the latter case the accumulated Kupffer cells have a nodular configuration and portal areas tend not to be involved (117). In addition, it has been suggested that the presence of lipofuscin and fat may distinguish SHML from VAHS. VAHS has on occasion been misdiagnosed as malignant histiocytosis, although the lack of atypicality and prominent erythrophagocytosis should allow the distinction to be made.

Bacterial Infections

Bacterial infections may involve the liver in three ways: cholestasis of sepsis, ascending cholangitis, and direct bacterial infection of the liver itself. Ascending cholangitis has been discussed under biliary tract disease.

Cholestasis of sepsis can occur in association with a variety of infectious agents, although it has been most frequently described with gram-negative sepsis. The changes consist of canalicular cholestasis, with or without cholangiolar cholestasis, and accumulation of polymorphonuclear cells in sinusoids (118–120). Cholangiolar cholestasis is the most diagnostic feature if present (Fig. 37). The major differential diagnoses are cholestatic drug reaction, early biliary obstruction, postoperative cholestasis, and familial cholestatic syndromes. Biliary obstruction can sometimes be ruled out by a lack of portal involvement as well as by the clinical history; the other differential items must be ruled out clinically, so cholestasis of sepsis often becomes a diagnosis of exclusion.

Direct bacterial infection of the liver can result from any number of species. In many cases the findings consist of nonspecific abscess formation, although a few bacteria have characteristic features. These include Brucella and Listeria, which have poorly formed sinusoidal granulomata, and the mycobacteria, including Mycobacterium tuberculosis,

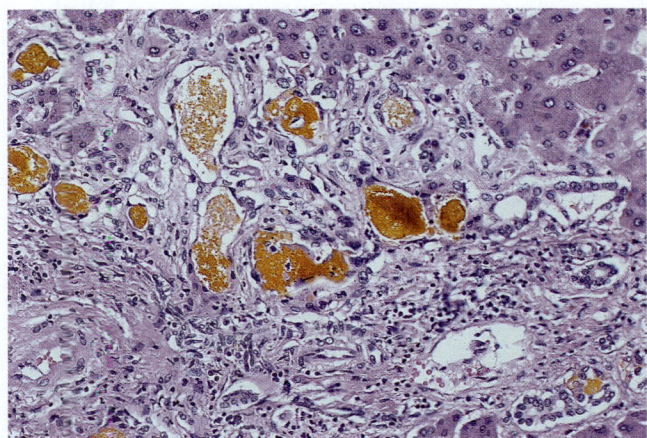

FIG. 37. Portal tract from a patient with sepsis. Note the dilated, bile filled cholangioles (cholangiolar cholestasis).

which have giant cell granulomas with or without necrosis; atypical mycobacterial infections display smaller, more epithelioid granulomas (121). Appropriate special stains may reveal an organism in these cases, but a negative stain does not exclude the diagnosis of any of these infections. Congenital syphilis shows a characteristic pericellular fibrosis. Recently, infection of the liver with the organism that causes bacillary epithelioid angiomatosis in the skin of immunosuppressed patients has been described. The histologic significance of the infection rests in the vascular proliferation that accompanies the infection and may simulate Kaposi's sarcoma or peliosis (122,123).

Fungal Infections

Fungal infections are seen most commonly in the immunosuppressed population, although occasionally an immunocompetent individual is also infected, particularly with Histoplasma. Histoplasma granulomas are not uncommon in biopsies taken in areas where the fungus is endemic, such as the Ohio River valley, and tend to be necrotizing or hyalinized granulomas (124). Silver stain is necessary to reveal the organism. The immunocompromised host may harbor any of a variety of species, including those of Candida, Aspergillus, and Mucor. Although not commonly identified in needle biopsies, these organisms are often found in the liver at autopsy. Candida typically causes abscess formation, and the characteristic combination of yeast forms and pseudohyphae can frequently be detected by silver stain, although there may be few organisms within each abscess (Fig. 38) (125). Aspergillus and Mucor species often produce areas of hemorrhagic infarction, since both tend to be vasoinvasive. Aspergillus is characterized by straight septate hyphal forms with acute angle branching. Mucor has irregular nonseptate hyphae with right-angle branching. Because of the irregular growth pattern of Mucor, only small fragments of the hyphae are seen in tissue sections. They may stain poorly with silver stains, especially if refrigerated, so the PAS stain is recom-

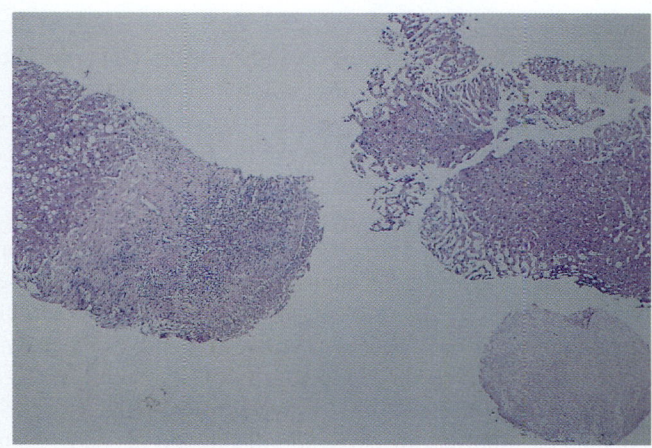 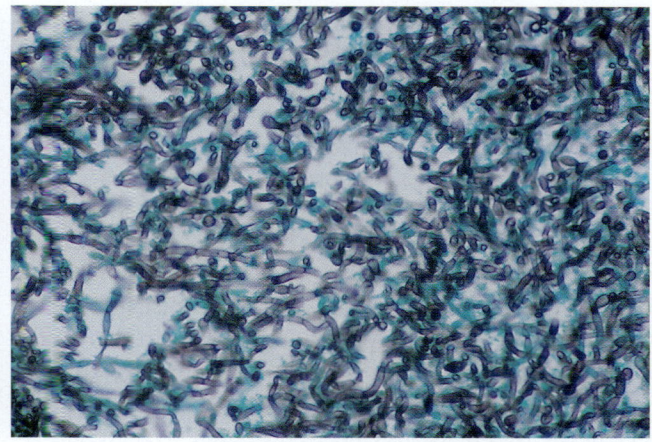

FIG. 38. *Candida* hepatitis in a needle biopsy. **A:** In this relatively unusual case, an area of necrosis is noted at the end of a needle biopsy. **B:** Silver stain reveals the typical pseudohyphae of *Candida*.

mended if *Mucor* is suspected. All diagnoses of fungal infections should be confirmed as to species by culture since histologic identification is imprecise, particularly in immunosuppressed patients, who are developing with increasing frequency infections with agents previously thought to be nonpathogenic.

Protozoa and Helminths

Although they constitute a major problem in some developing countries, protozoa and helminth infections are rare in the United States. Among the most common are *Entamoeba, Schistosoma,* and *Clonorchis* infections. The reader is referred to standard texts on parasitic infections for descriptions of these organisms and their life cycles (124). *Toxoplasma* hepatitis has been described in bone marrow transplant patients, and the biliary tree has been involved with *Cryptosporidium* and *Giardia* infections in patients with the acquired immunodeficiency syndrome, creating a sclerosing cholangitis-like pattern in the liver (126). *Pneumocystis carinii* has been described in the liver as well as other organs in severely immunocompromised individuals (127).

Other Infectious Agents

Q fever, caused by the rickettsia *Coxiella burnetii,* may involve the liver as well as respiratory tract (128,129). Histologically, Q-fever hepatitis is characterized by the presence of granulomas with a central vacuole surrounded by a hyalin ring (Fig. 39). Other features include a nonspecific portal and lobular lymphohistiocytic infiltrate, hepatocellular necrosis, and mild to moderate fatty change. The necrosis can be extensive and may lead to scarring of the liver, although cirrhosis is not a sequel. The "doughnut-hole" granulomas are not absolutely diagnostic of Q fever, having been described also in Hodgkin's disease, allopurinol toxicity, and other infectious diseases including CMV hepatitis and staphylococcal infection (129–131). Not all granulomas of Q fever have the characteristic hole, so a search for the hole with serial sections may be necessary if Q fever is in the differential diagnosis.

Vascular Disorders

Vascular damage to the liver may be caused by obstruction to hepatic inflow (either the portal vein or the hepatic artery) or outflow. The latter phenomenon occurs with obstruction to the central veins (terminal hepatic veins; VOD), major hepatic veins or inferior vena cava (Budd-Chiari syndrome), or congestive heart failure. Severe hypotension may also result in ischemic damage to the liver, although this is most commonly seen as an agonal event at autopsy. Also included among the nonneoplastic vascular lesions is peliosis hepatis, the formation of blood-filled pools in the liver.

The normal liver is unusually resistant to obstruction of either the hepatic artery or portal vein, in part due to the dual nature of the blood supply and, possibly, to collateral circu-

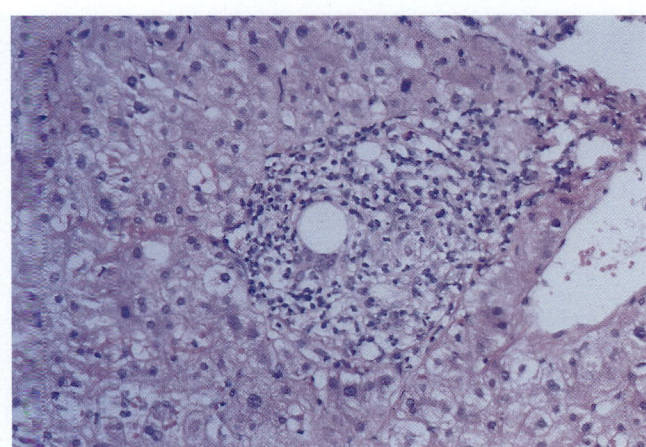

FIG. 39. Q fever is characterized by hepatitis with granulomas showing a central clearing surrounded by a fine hyaline ring. However, not all granulomas in Q fever will show this feature; conversely, other processes such as allopurinol toxicity and CMV mononucleosis may also have such "doughnut-hole" granulomas.

lation. Sudden hepatic artery obstruction may lead to infarction, although this is most uncommon. Arterial obstruction may also lead to loss of interlobular bile ducts. Obstruction to the portal vein may lead to hemorrhagic infarction or to central atrophy or necrosis. In addition, extrahepatic as well as intrahepatic portal venous obstruction may lead to a condition known variously as hepatoportal sclerosis in the United States, portal venopathy or noncirrhotic portal fibrosis in India, and idiopathic portal hypertension in Japan (132–135). This condition is characterized clinically by portal hypertension, with or without a variety of other liver function and hematologic abnormalities, but usually without overt liver failure. Histologic studies show mural thickening or complete fibrotic obstruction of the portal veins; frequent portal vein thromboses; mild, delicate portal fibrosis that may bridge but does not form complete regenerative nodules, as in cirrhosis; multiple channels in the portal areas with spaces resembling portal veins directly abutting the hepatic parenchyma; and hepatocellular regenerative activity (Fig. 40). The regenerative activity may lead to noncirrhotic nodule formation identical to that of nodular regenerative hyperplasia (NRH), and indeed this is one of the causes of the biopsy finding of NRH (see below).

Although the portal vein changes in hepatoportal sclerosis are characteristic, they are patchy and therefore difficult to identify on needle biopsy. For this reason, the best one can usually diagnose is "consistent with" or "suggestive of" hepatoportal sclerosis. In this context, it is best to know the clinical features of the case before rendering a diagnosis since the subtlety of the findings may lead one to report the biopsy as "normal" even in the face of known portal hypertension. Hepatoportal sclerosis may develop secondary to exposure to vinyl chloride and arsenic (136,137).

Obstruction of the hepatic outflow at any level leads to nonspecific central passive congestion and eventually hepatocellular atrophy and fibrosis. The fibrosis is centrilobular and may narrow or obliterate the lumen of central veins. The various causes of outflow obstruction may be apparent clinically, as in the case of congestive heart failure; in other cases radiologic studies may be necessary to ascertain the final cause. History may be helpful since some of these conditions are caused by fairly specific agents. Budd-Chiari syndrome is often associated with contraceptive steroids or tumors, and may be associated with other conditions causing sluggish blood flow such as paroxysmal nocturnal hemoglobulinuria (138,139). VOD is associated with radiation or the use of chemotherapeutic agents, particularly alkylating agents. Cases are also associated with herbal teas, particularly Compfrey tea. Absolute distinction of VOD from other causes of central congestion is impossible without clinical assistance (140). The congestion of VOD may be patchy, however, as opposed to the generalized central congestion of other types of obstruction, and the lumen of the veins may contain reticulin fibers and fibrin prior to development of fibrosis (Fig. 41).

Peliosis hepatis is defined as pools of blood in the liver or spleen (141). It is most commonly associated with the use of androgenic steroids, although estrogens have also been implicated, and occasional cases appear to be sporadic (66). Histologically, the pools of blood have no zonal distribution and are not lined by endothelium but rather by hepatocytes (Fig. 42). The parenchyma away from the pools almost invariably shows sinusoidal dilatation; herniation of hepatocytes into the central veins is common.

Nonneoplastic Hepatocellular Proliferative Disease

Although tumefactive hepatocellular proliferations are discussed in the chapter by Saul, "Masses of the Liver," two nontumorous proliferative processes, nodular regenerative

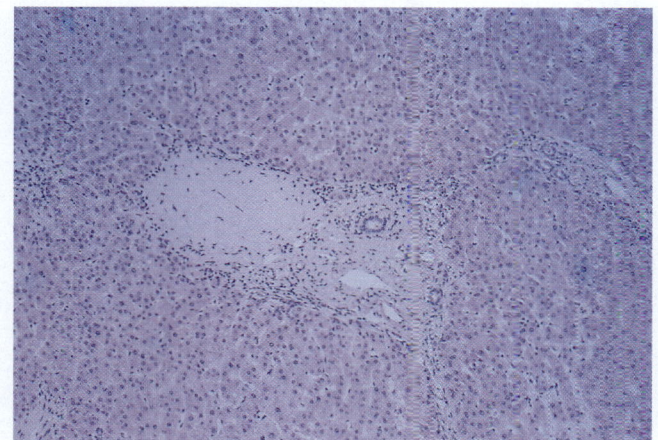
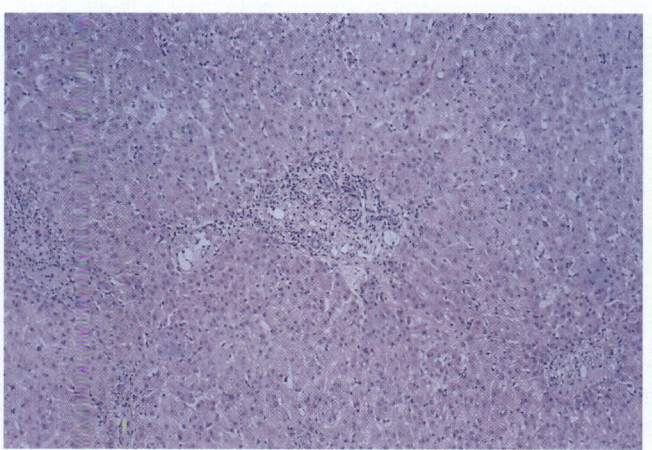

FIG. 40. Hepatoportal sclerosis. **A:** This biopsy demonstrates a portal tract with a large hyalinized scar representing a totally obliterated portal vein, as well as a second portal area with thickening of the portal vein wall. **B:** A second portal tract from the same liver demonstrating bile ductular proliferation and multiple portal-vein like vascular spaces, one abutting directly upon the hepatocellular parenchyma, a characteristic feature of these cases.

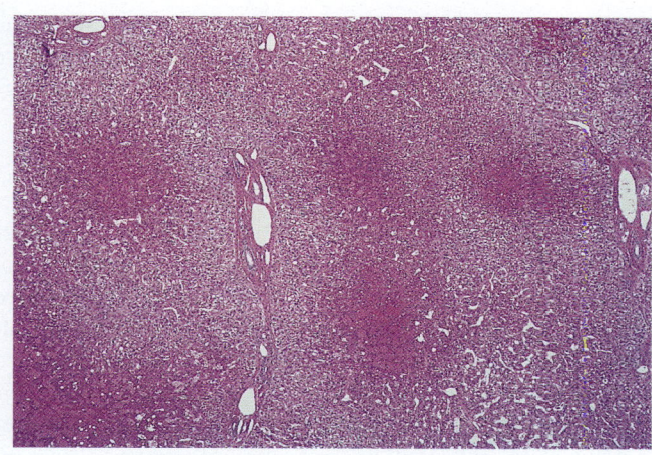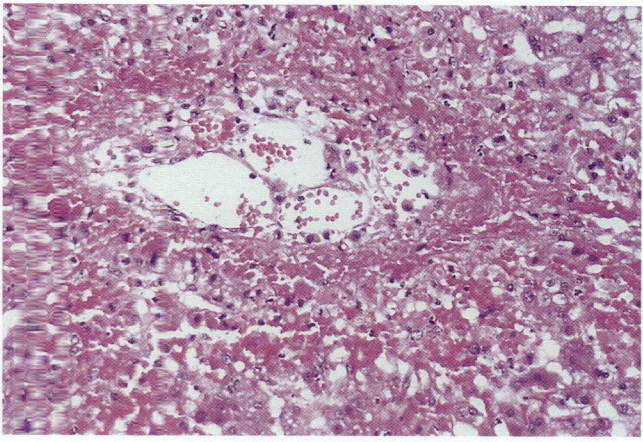

FIG. 41. Veno-occlusive disease. **A:** The central areas are markedly congested. **B:** Central veins may be difficult to identify without using the trichrome stain. However, when identified, they often are partially or totally occluded by fibrinous material.

hyperplasia (NRH) and partial nodular transformation (PNT), may be encountered in biopsies taken to evaluate portal hypertension or mild liver function abnormalities. These processes are often not diagnosed on biopsy, in the case of NRH because the abnormalities are subtle and the biopsy is misinterpreted as normal, and in the case of PNT because the process is focal and not amenable to biopsy recognition.

Nodular regenerative hyperplasia is a diffuse nonfibrotic nodulation of the liver that has been associated with a variety of etiologic factors, including collagen-vascular diseases, use of corticosteroid drugs, and abnormalities of intrahepatic portal veins (see earlier discussion of hepatoportal sclerosis) (142,143). Most cases in the literature are diagnosed at autopsy because the nodules are then visible grossly as discrete white spheres and are completely present on large microscopic sections (Fig. 43). In such specimens, one sees ill-defined nodularity of the liver caused by areas of hepatocellular atrophy (usually centrilobular) surrounding areas of hepatocellular regeneration. In these latter areas, the hepatocytes are generally plump with paler cytoplasm than the hepatocytes of the atrophic areas. On reticulin stain, which is necessary to make this diagnosis, the regenerating compartment is characterized by cell plates that are two or more cells thick (Fig. 44), in contrast to the thin plates seen in the atrophic areas. Other common features are congestion in the atrophic areas and difficulty in finding central veins, which are often compressed by the regenerating nodules.

On needle biopsy, it is these latter two features that suggest a diagnosis of NRH. If one carefully evaluates all structures in the biopsy, the apparent lack of central veins and/or the presence of randomly located, somewhat curvilinear, areas of congestion are noted. Closer inspection reveals atrophy in association with the congestion, and the periportal

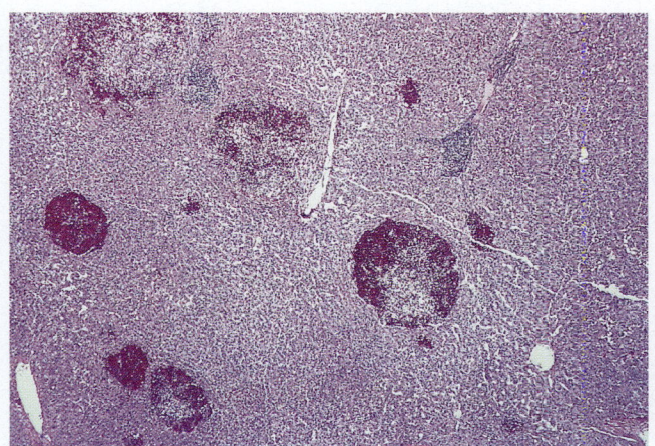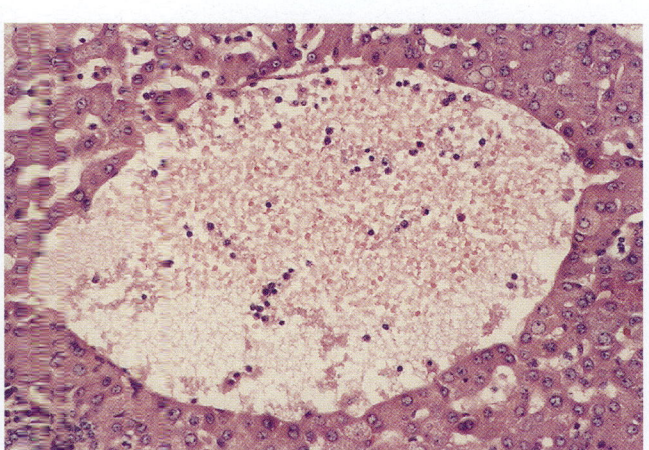

FIG. 42. A: Peliosis hepatis with multiple blood-filled spaces randomly scattered throughout the parenchyma, usually in association with sinusoidal dilatation. **B:** Note that the spaces are unlined, although they are in continuity with the sinusoids.

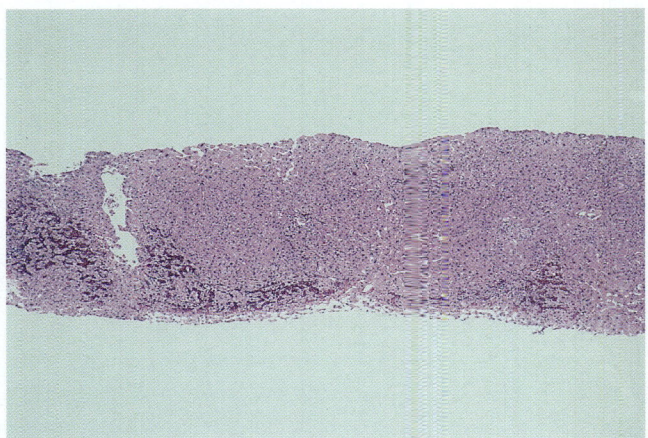

FIG. 43. Nodular regenerative hyperplasia, with areas of congestion corresponding to atrophy, alternating with areas of hepatocellular enlargement, corresponding to regeneration. The congested areas are frequently curvilinear, outlining the regenerative nodules, and the hepatocytes in the atrophic areas are more eosinophilic than elsewhere. Conversely, the regenerating hepatocytes have pale cytoplasm.

hepatocytes appear clear and plump. The reticulin stain reveals alternating areas of regeneration and atrophy, although complete nodules are not seen because of the size of the biopsy. The reticulin stain or trichrome stain also confirms the presence of compressed central veins. In the final analysis, the diagnosis rendered in these cases is usually "consistent with" NRH, with suggestion for correlation with clinical features and associated factors such as medication usage.

Partial nodular transformation is thought to represent a focal form of NRH. The process is characterized by nonfibrotic nodulation of the liver confined to the area near the porta hepatis (144). Because of this location, needle biopsy diagnosis is nearly impossible.

Cirrhosis

Cirrhosis is defined as: (a) a diffuse nodulation of the liver resulting from (b) fibrous bands subdividing the liver into (c) regenerative nodules (145). From a purist viewpoint, all three features must be present for a diagnosis to be rendered, although the diffuse nature of the process cannot be confirmed on biopsy of a small portion of the liver. As a corollary to this definition, there are well-defined processes in which the liver shows some, but not all, of the features of cirrhosis. These include congenital hepatic fibrosis in which the liver is diffusely subdivided by fibrosis into nodules that are not regenerative, focal nodular hyperplasia in which the liver is focally rather than diffusely subdivided by fibrous bands into regenerative nodules, and nodular regenerative hyperplasia in which the liver is diffusely converted into regenerative nodules but is not cirrhotic because of the lack of fibrosis.

Possible cirrhosis on needle biopsy entails two issues: the problem of accurate diagnosis, and the prognostic and etiologic significance of the biopsy. The problem of diagnosis stems from the fact that the needle is often smaller than the size of the regenerative nodules. Thus, the diagnosis becomes tentative since one sees definite fibrous bands crossing the biopsy, but one cannot be certain of the distinction of cirrhosis from bridging fibrosis. The reticulin stain is useful in this setting since it may confirm the presence of regenerative ac-

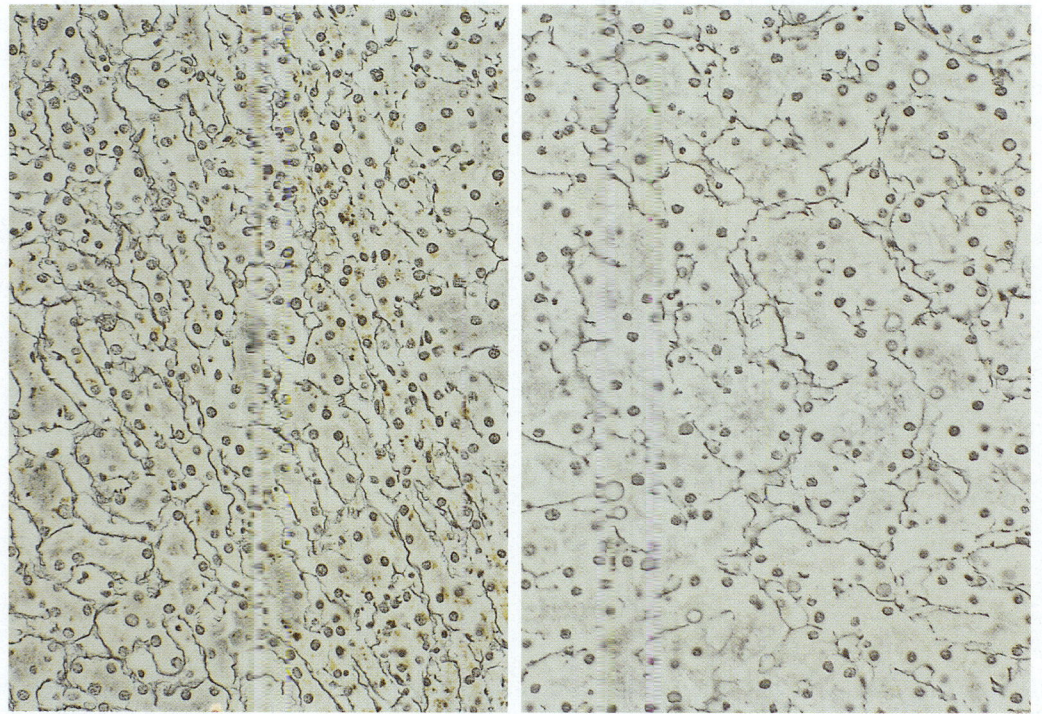

FIG. 44. Reticulin stain of nodular regenerative hyperplasia showing atrophy and collapse **(A)** alternating with regeneration characterized by thickened cell plates **(B)**.

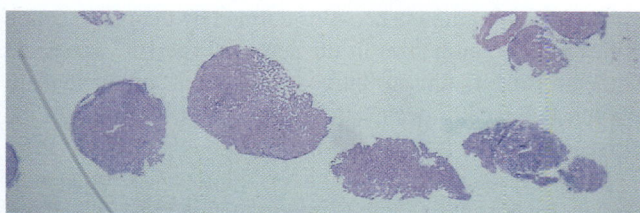
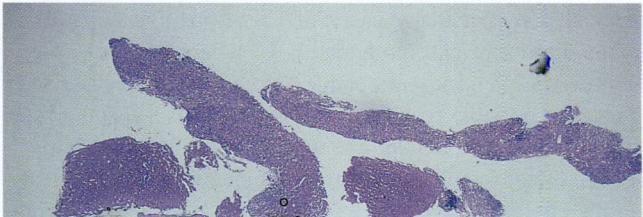

FIG. 45. Fragmented biopsy of a cirrhotic liver compared to a normal liver. Note the rounded contour of the cirrhotic fragments **(A)**, as opposed to the more angular nature usually seen in a fragmented biopsy of normal liver **(B)**.

tivity as evidenced by cell plates greater than two cells thick in the cirrhotic liver. Although some regenerative activity may be seen in the noncirrhotic liver (e.g., in hepatoportal sclerosis), absence of regenerative activity argues against the diagnosis of cirrhosis. Also, the presence of normally arranged portal tracts and central veins in the biopsy argues against the diagnosis of cirrhosis, although abnormally arranged portal tracts or central veins may be seen occasionally in regenerative nodules. When in doubt, it is prudent to diagnose a biopsy with fibrosis and some regenerative activity as "consistent with" rather than absolutely as cirrhosis. The latter diagnosis is reserved for those biopsies in which at least one complete regenerative nodule can be identified (146).

An occasional finding on biopsy of the cirrhotic liver is the fragmented biopsy (Fig. 45), in which the needle retrieves only parenchyma and leaves the fibrous tissue behind. The tissue obtained consists of multiple small fragments of hepatocytes with a smooth, rounded appearance. While this fragmented appearance strongly suggests cirrhosis, fragmentation can be seen in biopsies from normal livers as well. The reticulin stain helps here, both by demonstrating regenerative activity if the liver is cirrhotic and by identifying a delicate layer of reticulin surrounding the nodule (Fig. 46). Under these circumstances, the biopsy may be diagnosed as "consistent with" cirrhosis, even without seeing good fibrosis. If the fragments are of normal liver, their edges consist of hepatocytes without the rim of collagen.

Once the diagnosis of cirrhosis is made, the problem of classification remains. Cirrhosis can be classified on the basis of the size of the nodules as micronodular (nodules <0.3 cm, with delicate narrow fibrous bands), macronodular (nodules >0.3 cm, fibrous bands wide), and mixed. This classification gives some idea as to the etiology. The second feature to classify is activity as identified by continued damage to the liver parenchyma. For example, the presence of contin-

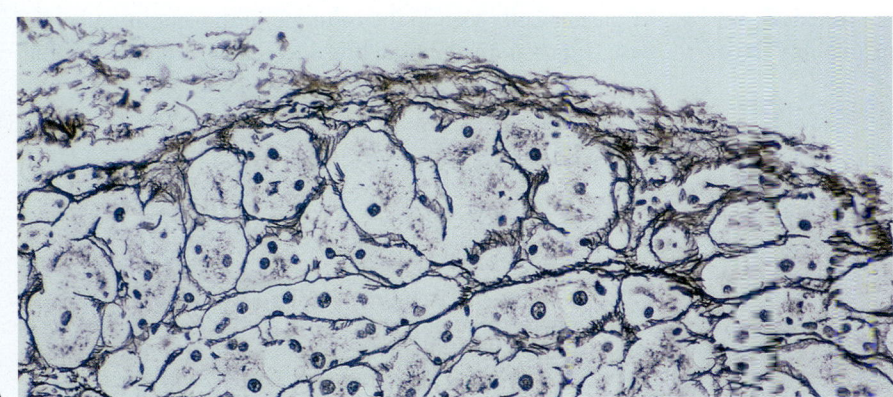
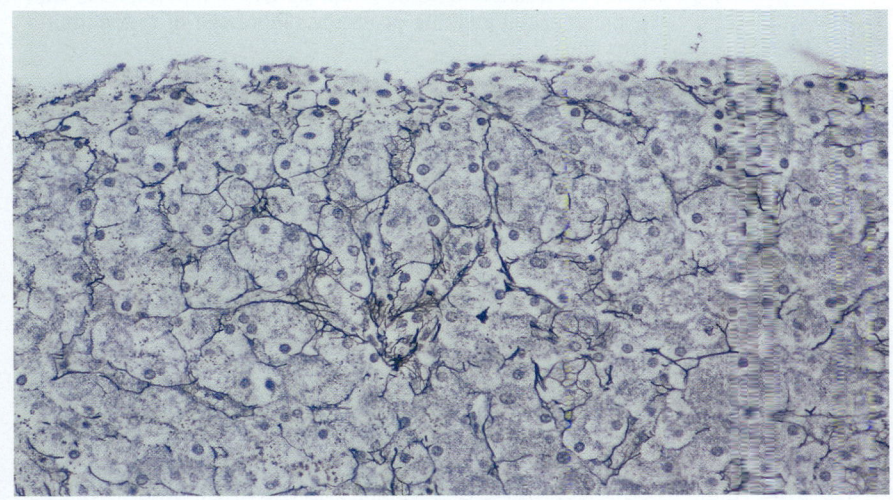

FIG. 46. Reticulin stain of the cirrhotic liver **(A)** shows thick regenerative cell plates and a condensed band of reticulin at the edge of the specimen. Compare this with the lack of condensation at the edge of a fragment of normal liver **(B)**.

ued inflammation and necrosis in a viral cirrhosis would be evidence of an active cirrhosis; absence of these features would lead to a classification of inactive. The most difficult classification is that of etiology, which can be done histologically in only a minority of cases. Features that suggest one etiology over another are those that allow the diagnosis of the underlying disease, such as granulomas for PBC or the combination of Mallory hyalin, fatty change, and polymorphonuclear infiltrate for alcoholic liver disease. Unfortunately, many of these features disappear in the end stage of the disease, and the determination of etiology becomes impossible on histologic grounds.

Diseases of Uncertain Etiology

There are several well-recognized diseases for which etiologic agents have not been identified. These include PBC (chronic nonsuppurative destructive cholangitis), PSC, and autoimmune hepatitis. All three of these diseases are suspected to have an underlying autoimmune pathogenesis, and all are characterized histologically by some degree of bile duct destruction, albeit involving different parts of the biliary tree. Primary biliary cirrhosis and PSC have been described previously under biliary tract disease.

Autoimmune hepatitis is a disease of presumed autoimmune pathogenesis that may simulate viral hepatitis on presentation (147,148). Although often termed chronic, the disease not uncommonly presents in an acute form that is important to recognize since many cases are amenable to treatment with steroids. There are now two and possibly three variants of autoimmune hepatitis defined by their association with different antibodies in the serum. Type I is associated with anti–smooth muscle antibody and, often, antinuclear antibody. It typically occurs in adolescent girls, although the clinical spectrum is wide and the disease is not rare in men. Type II is associated with anti–liver-kidney microsomal antibodies (LKM) and is more common in children (147). It appears likely that many cases of LKM-positive hepatitis in adults represent chronic hepatitis C, whereas the disease in children is often truly idiopathic autoimmune hepatitis (149). The third possible type, not yet designated as a specific type, is associated with antisoluble liver protein (SLP) antibody.

The histology of type I is the best characterized and is described below. The other two types have not been well characterized histologically to date, although there is evidence that type II may resemble type I. Anti–smooth muscle and antinuclear antibodies are nonspecific, and are not uncommonly found in a number of disease states. Their presence does not imply that a patient has autoimmune hepatitis; other diagnostic features are necessary.

In the acute phase of autoimmune hepatitis type I, the liver demonstrates a dense uniform portal infiltrate, often with extensive piecemeal necrosis and abundant plasma cells, and hepatocellular ballooning and necrosis, which is often discretely centrilobular and associated with a lymphoplasmacellular infiltrate. There may be portal to central bridging necrosis. The main difference between autoimmune hepatitis and acute viral hepatitis with bridging is the large number of plasma cells seen in the infiltrate of the autoimmune disease (Fig. 47). In addition, bile duct damage may be present,

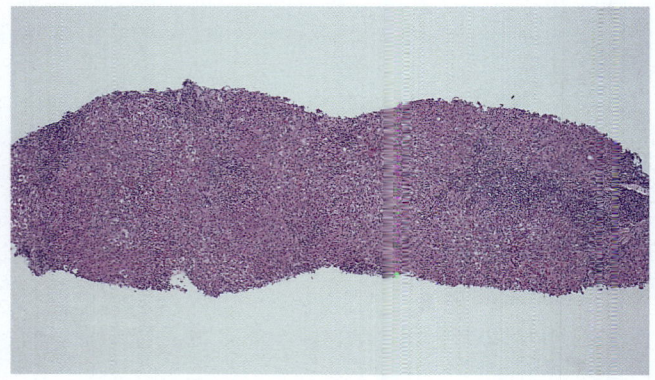

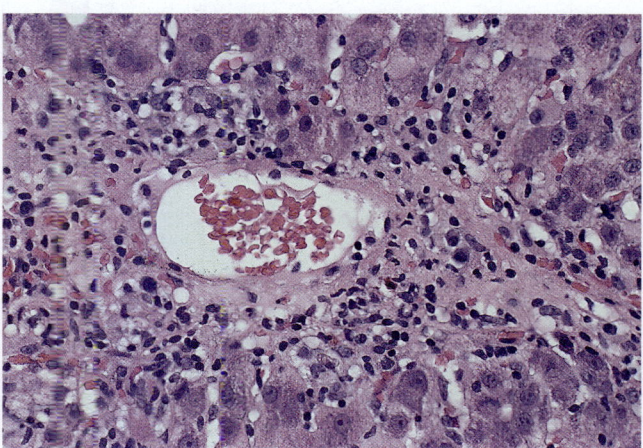

FIG. 47. Acute autoimmune hepatitis. **A:** There is a diffuse mixed inflammatory infiltrate of the portal tracts with piecemeal necrosis. **B:** The infiltrate, both in the portal areas and lobule, contains an easily identifiable component of plasma cells, as well as some eosinophils. **C:** Central necrosis with a plasma cell infiltrate is nearly diagnostic of autoimmune hepatitis.

although this is also a feature of hepatitis C and thus is of minimal diagnostic help. The only acute viral hepatitis manifesting abundant plasma cells is hepatitis A, which should always be ruled out serologically in suspected cases of autoimmune hepatitis.

If not detected until the chronic phase, the histologic picture of autoimmune hepatitis is that of chronic hepatitis with fibrosis and piecemeal necrosis. Since plasma cells can be part of chronic hepatitis B, they are less useful diagnostically and are also less prominent than in acute disease. In the chronic context, the differential diagnosis includes hepatitis C, PBC, PSC, and medication-induced chronic liver disease. The differential diagnosis of autoimmune hepatitis is discussed below (see Common Problems in Biopsy Diagnosis).

Recently a possible variant of autoimmune hepatitis resembling primary biliary cirrhosis clinically and histopathologically has been described under the designation of immunocholangitis or autoimmune cholangitis (150–153). In this condition the biopsy and clinical features suggest primary biliary cirrhosis; however, the serologic studies reveal negative antimitochondrial antibodies but a high titre of antinuclear antibody. A defining feature of these cases is their response to low-dose steroids. As opposed to typical PBC, these cases respond quickly, as expected for autoimmune hepatitis, hence the name. The existence of this disease as an entity has been disputed, in part because not all cases of anti-mitochondrial antibody-negative PBC respond to steroid therapy. In this author's opinion, this condition exists but needs to be defined in part by its response. True cases of AMA-negative PBC exist and should not be placed in this category. As a practical matter, in cases where there is a doubt about the diagnosis, a short trial of immunosuppression is worthwhile to rule out this possibility.

Reye's syndrome is an encephalopathy associated with characteristic liver findings that occurs primarily in children, often following a febrile viral-like illness treated with aspirin (154). Liver biopsy is used to diagnose the disease, although in recent years the disease has essentially disappeared. Characteristically, the liver shows microvesicular fatty change with minimal or no necrosis or inflammation. If the diagnosis is suspected, frozen section with fat stain aids in assessing the presence of the fat. The changes are identical to those seen in Jamaican vomiting sickness and valproic acid toxicity (155).

The Liver in Systemic Disease

The liver may be affected as a secondary event in many systemic diseases. Some of the more prominent of these are summarized in Table 23. Most of the liver pathology associated with these conditions is described elsewhere in the chapter. Nonalcoholic steatohepatitis, liver disease associated with pregnancy, and amyloidosis are addressed here.

Nonalcoholic steatohepatitis (NASH), as introduced in the section on alcoholic liver disease, refers to livers characterized by the accumulation of fat associated with inflammation and evidence of hepatocellular damage. The fatty change is usually mixed macro- and microvesicular, associated with a

TABLE 23. *Systemic conditions with associated liver disease*

Condition	Liver pathology
Amyloidosis	Amyloid deposition
Crohn's disease	Fatty change; granulomas; primary sclerosing cholangitis
Diabetes mellitus	Glycogenated nuclei; steatohepatitis
Metastatic carcinoma	Sinusoidal dilatation; cholestasis; portal lymphocytic infiltrate; tumor
Myeloproliferative disorders	Nodular regenerative hyperplasia
Obesity	Steatohepatitis
Pregnancy	Recurrent cholestasis; fatty liver of pregnancy; toxemia; viral hepatitis
Rheumatoid arthritis	Nodular regenerative hyperplasia
Sarcoidosis	Granulomatous hepatitis
Sickle cell and hemolytic anemia	Hemosiderosis
Ulcerative colitis	Primary sclerosing cholangitis; pericholangitis; fatty change; bile duct carcinoma

mild to moderate lymphoplasmacellular infiltrate involving the portal tracts and/or the lobule. Fibrosis, especially delicate pericellular fibrosis, is common; fibrosis may on occasion progress to cirrhosis. Mallory hyalin may be present but, in distinction from the Mallory hyalin of alcoholic liver disease, tends to be poorly formed, more randomly distributed (rather than centrilobular) and not associated with either a neutrophilic reaction or much ballooning degeneration (73,74). Prominent glycogenated nuclei are also more common in NASH than in alcoholic liver disease. Although alcohol abuse should be considered clinically in all cases of steatohepatitis, in many cases the histologic features allow the pathologist to favor either an alcoholic or nonalcoholic etiology. Nonalcoholic etiologies include obesity, diabetes, medications (e.g., methotrexate, tamoxifen, amiodarone), and organic solvents. Some putative cases have occurred in nonobese individuals without known risk factors; it has been suggested that these cases may have a better prognosis than cases occurring in the obese individual (156).

Liver disease in pregnancy includes (a) benign cholestasis of pregnancy, characterized by bland canalicular cholestasis; (b) jaundice associated with toxemia, in which the liver biopsy may be relatively normal or may show periportal hemorrhage associated with fibrin thrombi; and (c) fatty liver of pregnancy, characterized by microvesicular steatosis and, occasionally, central necrosis (157). While the first condition is relatively indolent as far as the liver is concerned, toxemia and the associated HELLP syndrome (*h*emolysis, *e*levated *l*iver tests, *l*ow *p*latelets) may result in hepatic rupture, and fatty liver of pregnancy often leads to liver failure (157). The major diagnostic problem in these diseases occurs with fatty liver of pregnancy in which the droplets of fat may be so tiny as to simulate ballooning degeneration rather than fatty liver. In this situation a misdiagnosis of cholestatic hepatitis may be made. In addition to these diseases that are specific for pregnancy, pregnant patients also may develop viral hepatitis and medication-induced disease.

The liver may be involved in both primary and secondary amyloidosis (158,159). Deposits of characteristic homogeneous eosinophilic material are seen in blood vessels and in the sinusoids (Fig. 48). In the early stage of the disease the findings may be very subtle, but as the amyloid accumulates the hepatocyte cell plates become atrophic and are eventually replaced. The major differential diagnosis of amyloid is pericellular fibrosis. The distinction can usually be made by a battery of amyloid stains, including Congo red with polarization showing apple-green birefringence, and metachromatic stains. On rare occasions, amyloid does not stain by these methods, and ultrastructural examination will be necessary to reveal the characteristic nonbranching filaments. Trichrome stain is not reliable to differentiate between collagen and amyloid since amyloid sometimes stains with trichrome.

The Liver and Transplantation

The pathology of the liver following transplantation can be thought of as consisting of two different classes of disease processes. First are those that are not unique to the transplant patient but are found in increased frequency in this population due to technical aspects of the transplant procedure. These include infectious diseases, especially due to so-called opportunistic organisms, diseases related to drugs or radiation therapy, and disease related to surgical manipulation of the liver. The second group of diseases are those uniquely related to transplantation, namely graft-versus-host disease (GVHD) in the bone marrow transplant (BMT) patient and rejection in the liver transplant patient (160).

In the BMT patient, the types of diseases encountered vary depending on the time after transplantation (161,162). Early after bone marrow transplantation (in the first 30 days), many problems are related to opportunistic infections, especially with fungi and CMV, and to drugs used in cytoreductive therapy, which may cause VOD or nodular regenerative hyperplasia. The diagnosis of these diseases is discussed in the relevant sections. After about 20 days of transplantation, acute GVHD becomes an issue in addition to infectious and drug-related problems.

Acute GVHD results from an attack by donated cells against the host. The skin, gastrointestinal tract, and liver are the most commonly affected organs. In the liver biopsy, diagnosis relies on finding bile duct damage in association with a lymphocytic infiltrate of the portal tracts and venous endothelium ("endothelialitis") (162,163). This latter feature, while nearly diagnostic if identified, is uncommonly encountered in GVHD compared to its frequency in liver rejection (see below).

The usual bile duct damage consists of vacuolation of the cytoplasm, loss of individual cells, pleomorphism of duct cell nuclei, and eventual loss of ducts, all in association with lymphocytes within the epithelial layer (Fig. 49). The portal infiltrate in acute GVHD is usually minimal due to the profound leukopenia present in the early posttransplant period and to prior immunosuppressive therapy. The degree of bile duct damage varies. Bile duct damage is not specific for GVHD, being found to some degree in many inflammatory conditions. In most of these latter conditions less than 50% of bile ducts are damaged; therefore, more than 50% bile duct damage is good evidence of GVHD. A grading system for GVHD has been proposed based on degree of biliary damage, although in our experience the grade bears not on prognosis but on certainty of the diagnosis of GVHD. Endothelialitis consists of lymphocytic infiltration of the portal or central vein endothelium with evidence of damage to the endothelium (Fig. 50). The damage takes the form of lifting

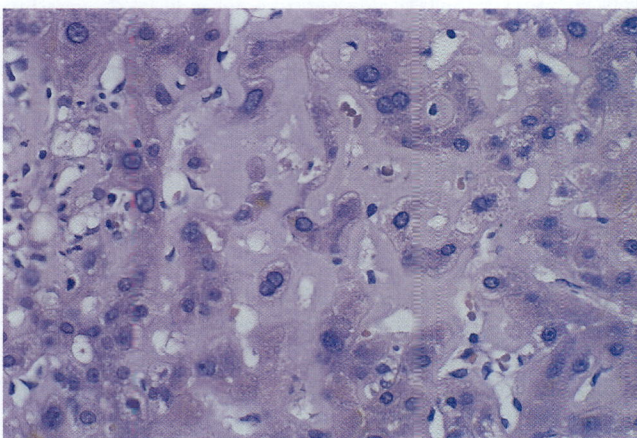

FIG. 48. Amyloidosis of the liver is characterized by homogeneous eosinophilic material in the sinusoids. Confirmation of the amyloid nature of the material is done with the Congo red or metachromatic stains.

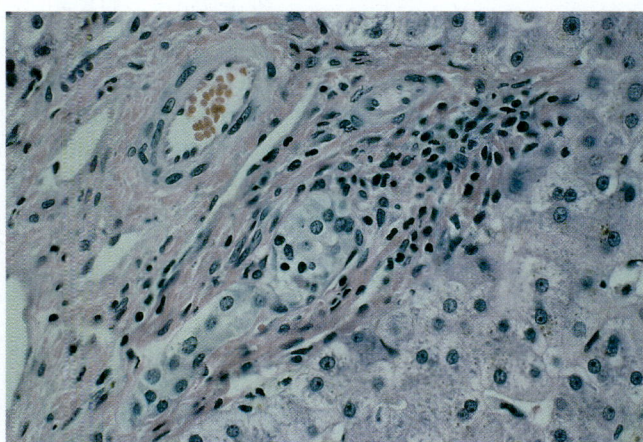

FIG. 49. Acute graft-versus-host disease is characterized by damage to the interlobular bile ducts, which usually takes the form of vacuolation of the cytoplasm, pleomorphism of nuclei, and/or necrosis of individual cells. The bile duct just to the right of the arteriole in this portal tract is infiltrated by lymphocytes, and demonstrates obliteration of its lumen caused by reactive proliferation of the bile duct epithelial cells.

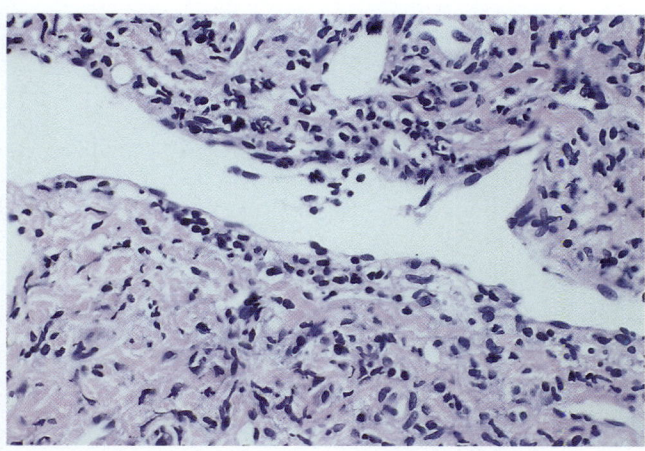

FIG. 50. The most diagnostic feature of graft-versus-host disease is endothelialitis, i.e., damage to the venous endothelium associated with a lymphocytic infiltrate seen in the portal vein in this portal tract.

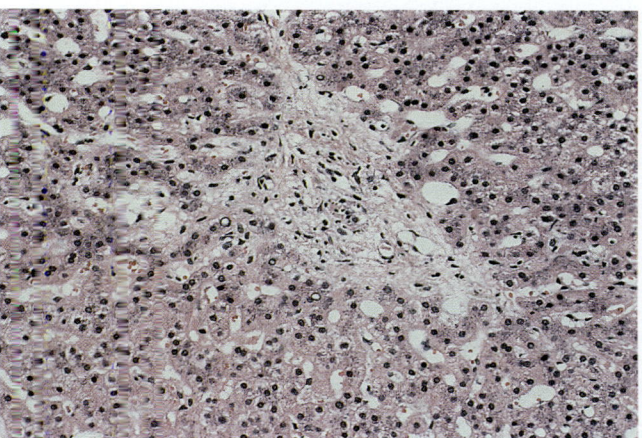

FIG. 51. Vanishing bile duct syndrome secondary to chronic graft-versus-host disease. Note the absence of a bile duct accompanying the arteriole in this portal tract.

of the endothelium from its basement membrane, and an attachment is usually present between the endothelium and lymphocyte.

Although the diagnosis of GVHD is not exceptionally difficult if only the above features are present, a common problem is the associated presence of hepatocellular damage in acute GVHD. In early acute GVHD, the predominant finding may be hepatocellular damage in the form of ballooning degeneration or focal necrosis with acidophil bodies. In these cases, distinction from viral or medication-induced hepatitis may be impossible. As a general rule, the degree of bile duct damage still holds the key, since those biopsies with extensive hepatocellular damage and little bile duct damage are probably not GVHD, those with much bile duct damage and little hepatocellular damage are probably GVHD, and those with equal bile duct and hepatocellular damage could be either.

After day 100, the main problem encountered is that of chronic GVHD (164). In chronic GVHD, the biopsy is used not only to make the diagnosis of GVHD but also to provide prognostic information, since piecemeal necrosis, fibrosis, or cirrhosis places the patient in a bad prognostic category of "extensive" disease (164). As in the acute disease, the bile duct is the primary target of attack. However, hepatocellular damage (with the exception of piecemeal necrosis) is not a feature of chronic GVHD; if hepatocellular damage is present, the diagnosis of viral or drug hepatitis is much more likely. The lymphocytic infiltrate of chronic GVHD is more brisk than that of acute disease, in keeping with the reconstituted nature of the patient's bone marrow by this time. One other relatively unique complication of chronic GVHD is the total loss of interlobular bile ducts, the vanishing bile duct syndrome (Fig. 51). This process can happen quite quickly following transplantation. There are other conditions that lead to loss of bile ducts as listed in Table 18; however, the only one likely to be relevant in a bone marrow transplant patient is medication reaction.

The liver pathology following liver transplantation is in many ways similar to that following BMT. One major difference is that the transplantation procedure is surgical rather than chemotherapeutic. Hence, problems with the surgical anastomoses, such as Budd-Chiari syndrome, portal vein thrombosis, and arterial thrombosis, replace VOD and NRH in importance early after transplantation.

Rejection of the liver can be hyperacute, acute, or chronic. Hyperacute rejection is an antibody-mediated process characterized by necrotizing arteritis, a polymorphonuclear infiltrate, and ischemic damage to the organ. It requires preformed antibodies against the donated organ and results from antibody-complement–mediated damage to endothelium. It is a rare event in the liver (165–167).

Acute rejection is a cell-mediated, potentially reversible process. It is characterized by a mixed portal infiltrate predominantly composed of lymphocytes with intermixed neutrophils and eosinophils (165,166). The major targets of attack are bile duct epithelium and venous endothelium, much as in GVHD (Fig. 52). The hepatocytes are not a major target of attack in acute disease. Other features seen in rejection include loss of bile ducts, arteritis, and/or central ischemic damage in the form of hepatocellular ballooning and dropout of clusters of hepatocytes. These changes are all associated with a poor outcome and progression to chronic rejection. Although there are several grading systems in the literature, none has been universally accepted. A recent proposal by an international group provides a reasonable basis for grading (168). Once treated, acute rejection may resolve or progress to chronic rejection.

Chronic rejection may be defined as an irreversible sequel of acute rejection. Two forms have been recognized: chronic vascular rejection with ischemic damage to hepatocellular parenchyma and chronic biliary rejection with total loss of bile ducts, the vanishing bile duct syndrome (VBDS) (169). The hallmark of chronic vascular rejection is obliterative endarteritis, the obstruction of arteries by subintimal fibrosis, or the accumulation of foamy histiocytes (Fig. 53). The vas-

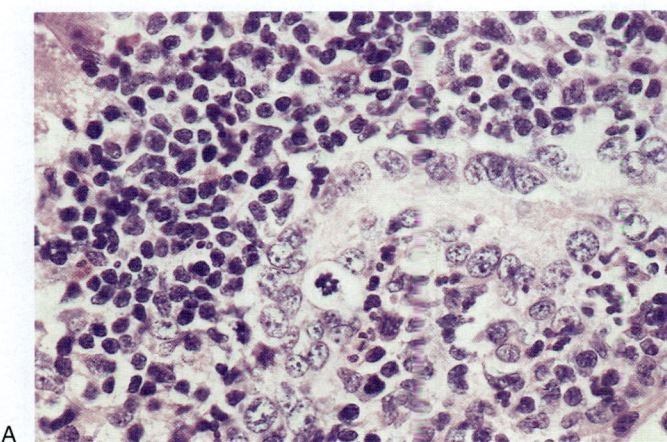 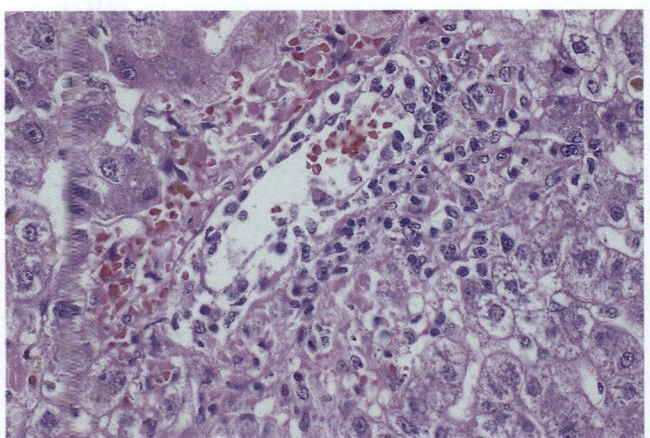

FIG. 52. Acute liver allograft rejection. **A:** Portal area showing bile duct damage in association with a mixed inflammatory infiltrate. **B:** Central vein endothelialitis with accumulation of lymphocytes damaging and elevating the endothelium.

cular obstruction leads to ischemic changes that are seen on needle biopsy (the arteritis rarely is), including centrilobular ballooning degeneration and pericellular fibrosis and eventual cirrhosis. Note that these findings are the same as those used to diagnose severe acute rejection and, indeed, the distinction of severe reversible acute from irreversible chronic rejection is not always feasible on biopsy alone. The findings on needle biopsy are rarely diagnostic of chronic rejection. In most cases, the biopsy is described as consistent with chronic rejection, with the final diagnosis resting on the combined clinicopathologic findings.

In VBDS, the interlobular bile ducts disappear as in chronic GVHD. With the disappearance of the ducts, the portal inflammation disappears as well, leaving the tract with an empty appearance. Loss of bile ducts may accompany typical chronic vascular rejection. The irreversibility of "pure" VBDS has recently been questioned, with several groups reporting apparent regrowth of bile ducts (169,170).

Our experience has been that liver disease following transplantation should be considered irreversible only if there is evidence of synthetic liver failure in conjunction with appropriate histologic evidence of hepatocellular necrosis, in addition to loss of bile ducts. As with VBDS in bone marrow transplantation, other causes of bile duct loss (Table 18) are unlikely with the exception of medication reactions and arterial ischemia (which is probably a contributing factor to loss of ducts in chronic vascular rejection).

The Liver in the Acquired Immunodeficiency Syndrome

In the absence of infection, the liver in AIDS is characterized by the absence of the small number of lymphocytes normally found in the portal areas (171), a reflection of the generalized leukopenia found in these patients. The most common findings in the liver in AIDS patients are the result of the numerous opportunistic infections that such patients suffer (123,171–173). These include atypical mycobacteria, CMV, various fungi (*Histoplasma, Cryptococcus, Coccidioides,* and others), and hepatitis B. Interestingly, although many AIDS patients are positive for markers of hepatitis B, the incidence of significant liver disease due to HBV is small. The severe immune suppression of the patients may account for this discrepancy. This severe immune suppression is also reflected in the fact that some patients with *Mycobacterium* cultured from their livers at autopsy show no evidence of granulomas in the liver; the same is not true of biopsy specimens, which usually do have granulomas or "granulomatoid" collections of foamy cells in the sinusoids if the patients have mycobacterium. CMV infection takes the form of CMV inclusion disease as seen in other immunosuppressed populations. *Cryptosporidium* can affect the biliary tree of these individuals, and there are reports of *Pneumocystis* infecting lymph nodes, skin, and liver as well (127). Bacillary angiomatosis has also been reported in the liver of these patients, somewhat simulating peliosis hepatis (121,123).

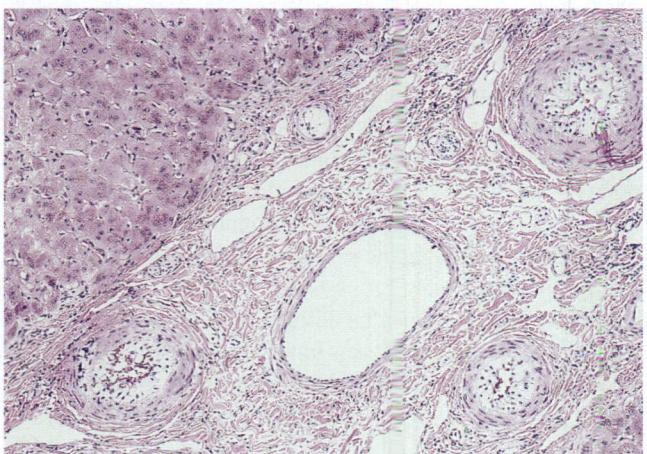

FIG. 53. Chronic liver allograft rejection with subintimal accumulation of foamy histiocytes in arteries in this large portal tract.

In addition to direct identification of infective agents, nonspecific changes including canalicular cholestasis reflecting cholestasis of sepsis, may be seen. In patients who are drug abusers, polarizable material may be identified in the portal areas (174). One report of AIDS in children has identified bile duct damage and endothelialitis in conjunction with portal and lobular lymphocytic infiltration (175). These features are suggestive of an autoimmune phenomenon resembling GVHD, a consideration of some interest in view of the suggestion that these patients may manifest GVHD-like changes in their large intestine and skin as well. The liver can also be affected with lymphoma and Kaposi's sarcoma (171,174). Peliosis hepatitis has also been described both with and without Kaposi's sarcoma. The significance of this peliosis in isolation is unknown, but, as noted earlier, it may be related to infection with the agent of bacillary angiomatosis (123,176).

COMMON PROBLEMS IN BIOPSY DIAGNOSIS

In day-to-day practice there are several disease processes that present recurrent problems in differential diagnosis. Although the diseases constituting these problems have been discussed earlier in the chapter, a brief summary of the differential diagnosis is given here. These problems include histologic chronic liver disease, with particular regard to primary biliary cirrhosis, and autoimmune hepatitis, granulomatous disease, and the fatty liver.

The term *histologic chronic liver disease* refers to those biopsies taken from patients presenting with either acute or chronic liver disease in whom the biopsy shows a predominantly mononuclear, predominantly portal infiltrate. The differential diagnosis consists of chronic viral hepatitis B or C, autoimmune hepatitis, PBC, PSC, steatohepatitis, Wilson's disease, and drug reaction (60). Acute hepatitis A infection may produce similar histologic findings, although usually a biopsy is not taken in these cases, which are diagnosed serologically; the disease tends to be acute. Hepatitis B and C infections are usually diagnosed serologically as well, but biopsy is still performed to evaluate prognosis rather than for diagnosis. Since medication reactions can show virtually any histologic feature including that of chronic hepatitis, it is imperative to consider medication reactions regardless of pattern.

Evaluation of these biopsies begins with an overall assessment of the pattern of involvement. If the infiltrate varies significantly between portal tracts, with some tracts spared while others are affected, the favored diagnoses are PBC, chronic hepatitis C, and steatohepatitis. Autoimmune hepatitis, PSC, and Wilson's disease tend to be more diffuse in their involvement. Piecemeal necrosis may be seen in any of these processes but tends to be most prominent in autoimmune hepatitis, as does bridging necrosis.

The cell types within the portal infiltrate should be assessed next. The presence of easily identified plasma cells or eosinophils, especially if present in relatively equal distribution throughout the infiltrate, makes the diagnosis of chronic hepatitis C or Wilson's disease unlikely. The diagnosis of PBC or autoimmune hepatitis should be considered less likely if these cell types are not present, although occasional cases of these diseases do have a nearly purely lymphocytic infiltrate. The infiltrate of steatohepatitis usually contains a few plasma cells, as does the infiltrate of hepatitis B. Conversely, an exclusively lymphocytic infiltrate, especially if located in dense aggregates or follicles, favors chronic hepatitis C. Without the aggregates, Wilson's disease is still a prime consideration.

The status of the bile ducts should also be assessed. Bile duct damage is a relatively nonspecific finding, since all of these processes, with the possible exception of Wilson's disease, show focal bile duct damage. Loss of ducts is a much more important finding. PBC and PSC lead to loss of interlobular bile ducts. Both processes may also show considerable bile ductular proliferation, although it is much more prominent and diffuse in PSC. Ducts are rarely, if ever, lost in chronic hepatitis B or C, Wilson's disease, autoimmune hepatitis, or steatohepatitis.

Lobular changes also offer some differential features. PBC may have a sinusoidal lymphocytic infiltrate, but hepatocyte necrosis is a rare occurrence, as are lobular plasma cells. Hepatitis C also may have a sinusoidal infiltrate, although the degree of necrosis may be slightly more than that seen in PBC. The presence of considerable necrosis, especially if bridging and if accompanied by lobular plasma cells, strongly favors autoimmune hepatitis. Wilson's disease presenting as chronic hepatitis usually shows little lobular involvement, although cases presenting with a fulminant picture have significant lobular necrosis and collapse. The lobule is generally unremarkable in PSC except for cholestasis. Steatohepatitis is defined by the presence of fatty change, although some degree of fatty change may be seen in essentially all of these diseases. Moderate to marked fatty change, however, is unusual in any of these diseases except steatohepatitis.

Finally, special features may allow a more specific diagnosis. Copper staining is occasionally useful since copper may be demonstrable in Wilson's disease, PBC, and PSC but not in early autoimmune hepatitis or hepatitis C. Mallory hyalin, if present, favors these same diseases, although it is a relatively uncommon finding except late in the course, usually after the liver is cirrhotic. The presence of granulomas strongly favors the diagnosis of PBC, especially if they are epithelioid granulomas located in portal regions with bile duct damage. A summary of the differential diagnosis of chronic hepatitis is found in Table 24.

The diagnosis of granulomatous disease requires an assessment of the type and location of granulomas as well as evaluation of features of the biopsy in addition to the granulomas (177) (see Table 9). Granulomas can be categorized as epithelioid, giant cell, necrotizing, fibrin-ring, and lipogranulomas. The latter, which consist of collections of histiocytes containing intracytoplasmic lipid, are generally thought to be

TABLE 24. Histologic differential diagnosis of "chronic hepatitis"

Feature	Hepatitis B	Hepatitis C	Autoimmune hepatitis	Primary biliary cirrhosis	Primary sclerosing cholangitis	Steatohepatitis	Wilson's disease	Medication reaction
Portal change distribution								
Diffuse	+	−	++	−	−+ (ductular proliferation)	−	++	+
Patchy	+	+−	−	++	−	+	−	+
Portal infiltrate type								
Lymphocytes	++	+− (aggregates)	++	++	++	++	++	++
Plasma cells	+	−	++	++	+	+	−	+
Eosinophils	−	−	+	+	+	−	−	+
Piecemeal necrosis	+	+	++	+	−	−	−	+
Lobular necrosis	−	−	+	−	−	+	−	+
Lobular infiltrate type/location	−	+ (lymphs) (sinusoidal)	+ (plasma cells) (with necrosis)	+ (lymphs) (sinusoidal)	−	+ (lymphs plasma cell's) (patchy)	−	+
Bile duct damage	+	+	+	++	+	−	−	+
Bile duct loss	−	−	−	++	+	−	−	+
Bile ductular proliferation*	−	−	−	++ (patchy)	++ (diffuse)	+	−	+
Mallory hyalin	−	−	−	+ (late)	+ (late)	+	+ (late)	+
Copper accumulation*	−	−	−	+	+	−	+	−
Granulomas	−	−	−	+	−	−	−	+
Ground glass cells	+	−	−	−	−	−	−	+**

++, almost always true; +, sometimes true; −, never or very rare.
*In precirrhotic state.
**Due to induced endoplasmic reticulum (negative by orcein or immunohistochemical stains).

of little clinical significance, although occasional cases of VOD have been ascribed to them (175). Necrotizing granulomas are most suspicious for infectious disease, and special stains for acid-fast organisms and fungi are always indicated. Epithelioid granulomas and those containing significant numbers of giant cells constitute the most generic and difficult category.

Granulomas found exclusively in the portal tracts are more likely to be due to PBC, sarcoidosis, or foreign material than those found exclusively in the lobule, although most granulomatous processes may involve the portal tract from time to time. If the granulomas surround the interlobular bile duct with damage to the duct, PBC is the most likely diagnosis, although occasionally sarcoidosis and medication reactions produce an identical pattern (179). In general, granulomas of malignancy, sarcoidosis, fungal and acid-fast infections, and idiopathic granulomatosis are not associated with other inflammatory changes, while the granulomas of many other infectious diseases (e.g., viral and rickettsial organisms) and PBC are found in association with other inflammatory changes typical of those diseases. The granulomas of drug reactions are often also accompanied by an inflammatory infiltrate, frequently containing eosinophils. It should always be kept in mind that the mere presence of a granuloma does not necessarily imply that the granuloma is a result of the same process causing the other changes. Occasionally, incidental granulomas have other processes superimposed on them. These granulomas are almost invariably lobular in location.

The histologically fatty liver is also a common problem. Many liver biopsies contain a mild degree of fatty change, which can usually be ascribed to nutritional status or drug use. A common cause of moderate to severe fatty change significant enough to lead to biopsy in the United States is alcoholic liver disease, in which case the fatty change is often accompanied by centrilobular Mallory hyalin, a neutrophilic or mixed inflammatory infiltrate, and fibrosis, particularly stellate fibrosis around the central vein. However, one should in general not make a diagnosis of alcoholism on biopsy alone since obesity-related nonalcoholic steatohepatitis, drug reactions, and fatty change related to jejunoileal bypass may produce a very similar picture. Jejunoileal bypass and nonalcoholic drug-related steatohepatitis should be diagnosable by clinical history. Some degree of distinction of alcoholic from nonalcoholic steatohepatitis can also be made by observing the type of fatty change and character and location of Mallory hyalin; the type of inflammatory infiltrate; and presence of glycogenated nuclei. A cause other than alcohol should be suspected if there is mixed micro- and macrovesicular fatty change, a prominent lymphocytic and/or plasma cell (rather than neutrophilic) infiltrate, prominent glycogenated nuclei, and a distribution of the Mallory hyalin other than the usual centrilobular one. Lipogranulomas are commonly found in steatohepatitis of any cause.

REFERENCES

Introduction and Developmental Abnormalities

1. Holund B, Poulsen H, Schlichting P. Reproducibility of liver biopsy diagnosis in relation to the size of the specimen. *Scand J Gastroenterol* 1968;15:329–335.
2. Soloway RD, Baggenstoss AH, Schoenfield LJ, et al. Observer error and sampling variability tested in evaluation of hepatitis and cirrhosis by liver biopsy. *Am J Dig Dis* 1971;16:1082–1086.
3. Snover DC. *Biopsy diagnosis of liver disease.* Baltimore: Williams & Wilkins, 1992.
4. Bianchi L. Liver biopsy interpretation in hepatitis. Part I: presentation of critical morphological features used in diagnosis (glossary). *Pathol Res Pract* 1983;178:2–19.
5. Balistreri WF. Neonatal cholestasis. *J Pediatr* 1985;106:171–184.
6. Brough AJ, Bernstein J. Conjugated hyperbilirubinemia in early infancy: a reassessment of liver biopsy. *Hum Pathol* 1974;5:507–516.
7. Balistreri WF, Grand R, Hoofnagle JH, et al. Biliary atresia: current concepts and research directions. Summary of a symposium. *Hepatology* 1996;23:1682–1692.
8. Montgomery CK, Ruebner BH. Neonatal hepatocellular giant cell transformation: a review. *Perspect Pediatr Pathol* 1976;3:85–101.
9. Hadchouel M, Gautier M. Histopathologic study of the liver in the early cholestatic phase of -1-antitrypsin deficiency. *J Pediatr* 1976;89:211–215.
10. Lurie M, Elmalach I, Schuger L, Weintraub Z. Liver findings in infantile cytomegalovirus infection: similarity to extrahepatic biliary obstruction. *Histopathology* 1987;11:1171–1180.
11. Tolia V, Dubois RS, Kagalwalla A, Fleming S, Dua V. Comparison of radionuclear scintigraphy and liver biopsy in the evaluation of neonatal cholestasis. *J Pediatr Gastroenterol Nutr* 1986;5:30–34.
12. Ohi R, Shikes RH, Stellin GP, Lilly JR. Biliary atresia duct histology correlates with bile flow. *J Pediatr Surg* 1984;19:467–470.
13. Chandra RS, Altman RP. Ductal remnants in extrahepatic biliary atresia: a histopathologic study with clinical correlation. *J Pediatr* 1978;93:196–200.
14. Gautier M, Jehan P, Odievre M. Histologic study of biliary fibrous remnants in 48 cases of extrahepatic biliary atresia: correlation with postoperative bile flow restoration. *J Pediatr* 1976;89:704–709.
15. Tan CE, Davenport M, Driver M, Howard ER. Does the morphology of the extrahepatic biliary remnants in biliary atresia influence survival? A review of 205 cases. *J Pediatr Surg* 1994;29(11):1459–1464.
16. Davenport M, Howard ER. Macroscopic appearance at portoenterostomy—a prognostic variable in biliary atresia. *J Pediatr Surg* 1996;31:1387–1390.
17. Kahn E. Paucity of interlobular bile ducts. Arteriohepatic dysplasia and nonsyndromic duct paucity. *Perspect Pediatr Pathol* 1991;14:168–215.
18. Hadchouel M. Paucity of interlobular bile ducts. *Semin Diagn Pathol* 1992;9:24–30.
19. Woolf GM, Vierling JM. Disappearing intrahepatic bile ducts: the syndromes and their mechanisms. *Semin Liver Dis* 1993;13:261–275.
20. Alagille D, Estrada A, Hadchouel M, Gautier M, Odievre M, Dommergues JP. Syndromic paucity of interlobular bile ducts (Alagille syndrome or arteriohepatic dysplasia): review of 80 cases. *J Pediatr* 1987;110:195–200.
21. Dahms BB, Petrelli M, Wyllie R, et al. Arteriohepatic dysplasia in infancy and childhood: a longitudinal study of six patients. *Hepatology* 1982;2:350–358.
22. Fujisawa T, Kage M, Ushijima K, Kimura A, Ono E, Kato H. Alagille syndrome with a spontaneous appearance of the interlobular bile ducts. *Acta Paediatr Jpn* 1994;36:506–509.
23. Kahn E, Daum F, Markowitz J, et al. Nonsyndromic paucity of interlobular bile ducts: light and electron microscopic evaluation of sequential liver biopsies in early childhood. *Hepatology* 1986;6:890–901.
24. Thommesen N. Biliary hamartomas (von Meyenberg complexes) in liver needle biopsies. *Acta Pathol Microbiol Scand* 1978;86A:93–99.
25. Bernstein J, Stickler GB, Neel IV. Congenital hepatic fibrosis: evolving morphology. *Acta Pathol Microbiol Immunol Scand* 1988;4(suppl):17–26.

Metabolic Diseases

26. Scriver CR, Beaudet AL, Sly WS, Valle D, eds. *The metabolic basis of inherited disease,* 7th ed. New York: McGraw-Hill Information Services, 1995.
27. MacSween RNM, Anthony PP, Scheuer PJ, Burt AD, Portmann BC eds. *Pathology of the liver,* 3rd ed. Edinburgh: Churchill Livingstone, 1995.
28. Qu D, Teckman JH, Perlmutter DH. Review: alpha-1-antitrypsin deficiency associated liver disease. *J Gastroenterol Hepatol* 1997;12:404–416.
29. Gerber MA, Thung SN, Shen S, Stromeyer FW, Ishak KG. Phenotypic characterization of hepatic proliferation: antigenic expression by proliferating epithelial cells in fetal liver, massive hepatic necrosis and nodular transformation of the liver. *Am J Pathol* 1983;110:70–74.
30. Rakela J, Goldschmiedt M, Ludwig J. Late manifestation of chronic liver disease in adults with alpha-1-antitrypsin deficiency. *Dig Dis Sci* 1987;32:1358–1362.
31. Oppenheimer EH, Esterly JR. Pathology of cystic fibrosis: review of the literature and comparison with 146 autopsied cases. *Perspect Pediatr Pathol* 1975;2:241–278.
32. Roy CC, Weber AM, Morin CL, et al. Hepatobiliary disease in cystic fibrosis: a survey of current issues and concepts. *J Pediatr Gastroenterol Nutr* 1982;1:469–478.
33. Gordeuk VR, Bacon BR, Brittenham GM. Iron overload: causes and consequences. *Annu Rev Nutr* 1987;7:485–508.
34. Witzleben CL, Uri A. Perinatal hemochromatosis: entity or end result? *Hum Pathol* 1989;20:335–340.
35. Silver MM, Beverley DW, Valberg LS, Cutz E, Phillips MJ, Shaheed WA. Perinatal hemochromatosis: clinical, morphologic and quantitative iron studies. *Am J Pathol* 1987;128:538–554.
36. Kent G, Popper H. Secondary hemochromatosis; its association with anemia. *Arch Pathol* 1960;70:623–639.
37. Ludwig J, Batts KP, Moyer TP, Baldus WP, Fairbanks VF. Liver biopsy diagnosis of homozygous hemochromatosis: a diagnostic algorithm. *Mayo Clin Proc* 1993;68:263–267.
38. Deugnier Y, Turlin B, le Quilleuc D, et al. A reappraisal of hepatic siderosis in patients with end-stage cirrhosis: practical implications for the diagnosis of hemochromatosis. *Am J Surg Pathol* 1997;21:669–675.
39. Ludwig J, Hashimoto E, Porayko MK, Moyer TP, Baldus WP. Hemosiderosis in cirrhosis: a study of 447 native livers. *Gastroenterology* 1997;112:882–888.
40. Camaschella C, Piperno A. Hereditary hemochromatosis: recent advances in molecular genetics and clinical management. *Haematologica* 1997;82:77–84.
41. Knisely AS, O'Shea PA, Stocks JF, Dimmick JE. Oropharyngeal and upper respiratory tract mucosal-gland siderosis in neonatal hemochromatosis: an approach to biopsy diagnosis. *J Pediatr* 1988;113:371–374.
42. Sternlieb I. Perspectives on Wilson's disease. *Hepatology* 1990;12:1234–1239.
43. Stromeyer FW, Ishak KG. Histology of the liver in Wilson's disease; a study of 34 cases. *Am J Clin Pathol* 1980;73:12–24.
44. Ludwig J, Moyer TP, Rakela J. The liver biopsy diagnosis of Wilson's disease. Methods in pathology. *Am J Clin Pathol* 1994;102:443–446.
45. Phillips MJ, Poucell S, Patterson J, Valencia P. *The liver: an atlas and text of ultrastructural pathology.* New York: Raven Press, 1987.
46. Scott J, Gollan JL, Samourian S, Sherlock S. Wilson's disease, presenting as chronic active hepatitis. *Gastroenterology* 1978;74:645–651.

Biliary Tract Disease

47. Poulsen H, Christoffersen P. Histological changes in liver biopsies from patients with surgical bile duct disorders. *Acta Pathol Microbiol Scand* 1970;78A:571–579.
48. Dahms BB, Halpin TC. Serial liver biopsies in parenteral nutrition-associated cholestasis of early infancy. *Gastroenterology* 1981;81:136–144.
49. Afroudakis A, Kaplowitz N. Liver histopathology in chronic common bile duct stenosis due to chronic alcoholic pancreatitis. *Hepatology* 1981;1:65–72.

50. Ludwig J, Barham SS, LaRusso NF, Elveback LR, Weisner RH, McCall JT. Morphological features of chronic hepatitis associated with primary sclerosing cholangitis and chronic ulcerative colitis. *Hepatology* 1981;1:632–640.
51. Desmet VJ, Geboes K. Liver lesions in inflammatory bowel disorders. *J Pathol* 1987;151:247–255.
52. Farrant JM, Hayllar KM, Wilkinson ML, et al. Natural history and prognostic variables in primary sclerosing cholangitis. *Gastroenterology* 1991;100:1710–1717.
53. Wee A, Ludwig J. Pericholangitis in chronic ulcerative colitis; primary sclerosing cholangitis of the small bile ducts? *Ann Intern Med* 1985;102:581–587.
54. Ludwig J, Dickson ER, McDonald GSA. Staging of chronic non-suppurative destructive cholangitis (syndrome of primary biliary cirrhosis). *Virchows Arch [A]* 1978;379:103–112.
55. Kaplan MM. Primary biliary cirrhosis. *N Engl J Med* 1996;335:1570–1580.
56. Scheuer PJ. Primary biliary cirrhosis. *Proc R Soc Med* 1967;60:1257–1260.
57. Portmann B, Popper H, Neuberger J, Williams R. Sequential and diagnostic features in primary biliary cirrhosis based on serial histologic study in 209 patients. *Gastroenterology* 1985;88:1777–1790.
58. Nakanuma Y, Tsuneyama K, Gershwin ME, Yasoshima M. Pathology and immunopathology of primary biliary cirrhosis with emphasis on bile duct lesions: recent progress. *Semin Liver Dis* 1995;15:313–328.
59. Nakanuma Y, Ohta G. Quantitation of hepatic granulomas and epithelioid cells in primary biliary cirrhosis. *Hepatology* 1983;3:423–427.
60. Snover DC. The histological differential diagnosis of chronic hepatitis. *Adv Pathol Lab Med* 1992;5:333–355.

Medication-Induced Liver Disease

61. Cameron RG, Feuer G, de la Iglesia FA. *Drug-induced hepatotoxicity.* Berlin: Springer-Verlag, 1996.
62. Stricker BHC. *Drug-induced hepatic injury.* Amsterdam: Elsevier Science, 1992.
63. Ishak KG. The liver. In: Riddell RH, ed. *Pathology of drug-induced and toxic diseases.* New York: Churchill Livingstone, 1982.
64. Ludwig J, Axelsen R. Drug effects on the liver: an updated tabular compilation of drugs and drug-related hepatic diseases. *Dig Dis Sci* 1983;28:651–666.
65. Ishak KG, Zimmerman HJ. Drug-induced and toxic granulomatous hepatitis. *Bailliere Clin Gastroenterol* 1988;2:463–480.
66. Zafrani ES, Pinaudeau Y, Dhumeaux D. Drug-induced vascular lesions of the liver. *Arch Intern Med* 1983;143:495–502.

Alcoholic Liver Disease

67. Hills KS, Westaby D. Alcohol and the liver. *Br J Hosp Med* 1997;57:517–521.
68. Hall P de la M, Mackinnon AM, Cooksley WGE, Williams DR. Alcoholic liver disease: a review. *Pathology* 1979;11:677–687.
69. Review by an international group. Alcoholic liver disease: morphological manifestations. *Lancet* 1981;1:707–711.
70. Ishak KG, Zimmerman HJ, Ray MB. Alcoholic liver disease: pathologic, pathogenetic and clinical aspects. *Alcohol Clin Exp Res* 1991;15:45–66.
71. Neuschwander-Tetri BA, Bacon BR. Nonalcoholic steatohepatitis. *Med Clin North Am* 1996;80:1147–1166.
72. Powell EE, Cooksley WGE, Hanson R, Searle J, Halliday JW, Powell LW. The natural history of nonalcoholic steatohepatitis: a follow-up study of forty-two patients for up to 21 years. *Hepatology* 1990;11:74–80.
73. Diehl AM, Goodman Z, Ishak KG. Alcohol-like liver disease in nonalcoholics. *Gastroenterology* 1988;95:1056–1062.
74. Pinto HC, Baptista A, Camilo ME, Valente A, Saragoca A, de Moura MC. Nonalcoholic steatohepatitis. Clinicopathological comparison with alcoholic hepatitis in ambulatory and hospitalized patients. *Dig Dis Sci* 1996;41:172–179.
75. Peters RL, Gay T, Reynolds TB. Post jejuno-ileal bypass hepatic disease: its similarity to alcoholic hepatic disease. *Am J Clin Pathol* 1975;63:318–331.
76. Lewis JH, Mullick F, Ishak KG, et al. Histopathologic analysis of suspected amiodarone hepatotoxicity. *Hum Pathol* 1990;21:59–67.
77. Galambos JT. Natural history of alcoholic hepatitis III: histological changes. *Gastroenterology* 1972;63:1026–1035.
78. Edmondson HA, Peters RL, Reynolds TB, Kuzma OT. Sclerosing hyaline necrosis of the liver in the chronic alcoholic: a recognizable clinical syndrome. *Ann Intern Med* 1963;59:646–673.
79. Takase S, Takada N, Enomoto N, Yasuhara M, Takada A. Different types of chronic hepatitis in alcoholic patients: does chronic hepatitis induced by alcohol exist? *Hepatology* 1991;13:876–881.
80. Sawabe M, Okayasu I, Izumi N, et al. Focal hepatocellular necrosis and portal lymphocytic infiltration of the liver in chronic alcoholics: histopathological study of 40 liver biopsies. *Pathol Int* 1994;44:511–617.
81. Pares A, Barrera JM, Caballeria J, et al. Hepatitis C virus antibodies in chronic alcoholic patients: association with severity of liver injury. *Hepatology* 1990;12:1295–1299.
82. Levin DM, Baker AL, Riddell RH, Rochman H, Boyer JL. Nonalcoholic liver disease: overlooked causes of liver injury in patients with heavy alcohol consumption. *Am J Med* 1979;66:429–434.

Viral Hepatitis

83. Bianchi L, De Groote J, Desmet VJ, et al. Acute and chronic hepatitis revisited. *Lancet* 1977;2:914–919.
84. Krawczynski K. Hepatitis E. *Hepatology* 1993;17:932–941.
85. Peters RL. Viral hepatitis: a pathologic spectrum. *Am J Med Sci* 1975;270:17–31.
86. Bianchi L. Liver biopsy interpretation in hepatitis. Part II: Histopathology and classification of acute and chronic viral hepatitis/differential diagnosis. *Pathol Res Pract* 1983;178:180–213.
87. Teixeira MR, Weller IVD, Murray A, et al. The pathology of hepatitis A in man. *Liver* 1982;2:53–60.
88. Okuno T, Sano A, Deguchi T, et al. Pathology of acute hepatitis A in humans: comparison with hepatitis B. *Am J Clin Pathol* 1984;81:162–169.
89. Scheuer PJ, Ashrafzadeh P, Sherlock S, Brown D, Dusheiko GM. The pathology of hepatitis C. *Hepatology* 1992;15:567–571.
90. Goodman ZD, Ishak KG. Histopathology of hepatitis C virus infection. *Semin Liver Dis* 1995;15:70–81.
91. Dhillon AP, Dusheiko GM. Pathology of hepatitis C virus infection. *Histopathology* 1995;26:297–309.
92. Gowing NFC. Infectious mononucleosis; histopathologic aspects. *Pathol Annu* 1975;10:1–20.
93. Snover DC, Horwitz CA. Liver disease in cytomegalovirus mononucleosis: a light microscopic and immunohistochemical study of six cases. *Hepatology* 1984;4:408–412.
94. Kunno A, Abe M, Yamada M, Murakami K. Clinical and histological features of cytomegalovirus hepatitis in previously healthy adults. *Liver* 1997;17:129–132.
95. Perrillo RP. The role of liver biopsy in hepatitis C. *Hepatology* 1997;26(3 suppl 1):57S–61S.
96. McPherson RA. Laboratory diagnosis of human hepatitis viruses. *J Clin Lab Anal* 1994;8:369–377.
97. Gerber MA, Thung SW. The diagnostic value of immunohistochemical demonstration of hepatitis viral antigens in the liver. *Hum Pathol* 1987;18:771–774.
98. Scheuer PJ. Classification of chronic viral hepatitis: a need for reassessment. *J Hepatol* 1991;13:372–374.
99. Knodell RG, Ishak KG, Black WC, et al. Formulation and application of a numerical scoring system for assessing histological activity in asymptomatic chronic active hepatitis. *Hepatology* 1981;1:431–435.
100. Desmet VJ, Gerber M, Hoofnagle JH, Manns M, Scheuer PJ. Classification of chronic hepatitis: diagnosis, grading and staging. *Hepatology* 1994;19:1513–1520.
101. Batts KP, Ludwig J. Chronic hepatitis. An update on terminology and reporting. *Am J Surg Pathol* 1995;19:1409–1417.
102. International Working Party. Terminology of chronic hepatitis. *Am J Gastroenterol* 1995;90:181–189.
103. Bonkovsky HL. Therapy of hepatitis C: other options. *Hepatology* 1997;26(3 suppl 1):143S–151S.
104. Kaji K, Nakanuma Y, Harada K, Sakai A, Kaneko S, Kobayashi K. Hemosiderin deposition in portal endothelial cells is a histologic marker predicting poor response to interferon-alpha therapy in chronic hepatitis C. *Pathol Int* 1997;47(6):347–352.
105. Fargion S, Fracanzani AL, Sampietro M, et al. Liver iron influences

the response to interferon alpha therapy in chronic hepatitis C. *Eur J Gastroenterol Hepatol* 1997;9:497–503.
106. Suzuki K, Uchida T, Shikata T. Histopathological analysis of chronic hepatitis B virus (HBV) infection in relation to HBV replication. *Liver* 1987;7:260–270.
107. Craig JR, Govindarajan S, DeCock KM. Delta viral hepatitis: histopathology and course. *Pathol Annu* 1986;21:1–21.
108. Verme G, Amoroso P, Lettieri G, et al. A histological study of hepatitis delta virus liver disease. *Hepatology* 1986;6:1303–1307.
109. DeCock KM, Govindarajan S, Redeker AG. HDV infection in the Los Angeles area. *Prog Clin Biol Res* 1987;234:167–179.
110. Lefkowitch JH, Goldstein H, Yatto R, Gerber MA. Cytopathic liver injury in acute delta virus hepatitis. *Gastroenterology* 1987;92:1262–1266.
111. Mullick FG, Ishak KG. Hepatic injury associated with diphenylhydantoin therapy: a clinicopathologic study of 20 cases. *Am J Clin Pathol* 1980;74:442–452.
112. Snover DC, Hutton S, Balfour HH, Bloomer JR. Cytomegalovirus infection of the liver in transplant recipients. *J Clin Gastroenterol* 1987;9:659–665.
113. Colina F, Juca NT, Moreno E, et al. Histological diagnosis of cytomegalovirus hepatitis in liver allografts. *J Clin Pathol* 1995;48:351–357.
114. Koneru B, Jaffe R, Esquivel CO, et al. Adenoviral infections in pediatric liver transplant recipients. *JAMA* 1987;258:489–492.
115. Randhawa PS, Markin RS, Starzl TE, Demetris AJ. Epstein-Barr virus-associated syndromes in immunosuppressed liver transplant recipients. Clinical profile and recognition on routine allograft biopsy. *Am J Surg Pathol* 1990;14:538–547.
116. Reiner AP, Spivak JL. Hematophagic histiocytosis: a report of 23 new patients and a review of the literature. *Medicine* 1988;67:369–388.
117. Brown RE, d'Cruz CA. Sinus histiocytosis with massive lymphadenopathy syndrome: histopathogenesis of the hepatic lesion. *Ann Clin Lab Sci* 1987;17:162–170.
118. Franson TR, Hierholzer WJ Jr, LaBrecque DR. Frequency and characteristics of hyperbilirubinemia associated with bacteremia. *Rev Infect Dis* 1985;7:1–9.
119. Lefkowitch JH. Bile ductular cholestasis: an ominous histopathological sign related to sepsis and 'cholangitis lenta.' *Hum Pathol* 1982;13:19–24.
120. Ishak KG, Rogers WA. Cryptogenic acute cholangitis—association with toxic shock syndrome. *Am J Clin Pathol* 1981;76:619–625.
121. Simson IW, Gear JHS. Other viral and infectious diseases. In: MacSween RNM, Anthony PP, Scheuer PJ, eds. *Pathology of the liver*, 2nd ed. Edinburgh: Churchill Livingstone, 1987.
122. Kemper CA, Lombard CM, Deresinski SC, Tompkins LS. Visceral bacillary epithelioid angiomatosis—possible manifestations of disseminated cat scratch disease in the immunocompromised host—a report of two cases. *Am J Med* 1990;89:216–222.
123. Steeper T, Snover DC. Bacillary epithelioid angiomatosis involving liver, spleen and skin in an AIDS patient. *Am J Clin Pathol* 1992;97:713–718.
124. Binford CH, Connor DH, eds. *Pathology of tropical and extraordinary diseases*. Washington, DC: Armed Forces Institute of Pathology, 1976.
125. Johnson TL, Barnett JL, Appelman HD, Nostrant T. Candida hepatitis. Histopathologic diagnosis. *Am J Surg Pathol* 1988;12:716–720.

Other Infectious Agents

126. Lerner CW, Tapper ML. Opportunistic infection complicating acquired immune deficiency syndrome: clinical features of 25 cases. *Medicine* 1984;63:155–164.
127. Poblete RB, Rodriguez K, Foust RT, Reddy R, Saldana MJ. Pneumocystis carinii hepatitis in the acquired immunodeficiency syndrome (AIDS). *Ann Intern Med* 1989;110:737–738.
128. Srigley JR, Vellend H, Palmer N, et al. Q-fever. The liver and bone marrow pathology. *Am J Surg Pathol* 1985;9:752–758.
129. Vanderstigel M, Zafrani ES, Lejonc JL, Schaeffer A, Portos JL. Allopurinol hypersensitivity syndrome as a cause of hepatic fibrin-ring granulomas. *Gastroenterology* 1986;90:188–190.
130. Nenert M, Mavier P, Dubuc N, Deforges L, Zafrani ES. Epstein-Barr virus infection and hepatic fibrin-ring granulomas. *Hum Pathol* 1988;19:608–610.
131. Lobdell DH. 'Ring' granulomas in cytomegalovirus hepatitis. *Arch Pathol Lab Med* 1987;111:881–882.

Vascular Disorders

132. Mikkelsen WP, Edmondson HA, Peters RL, Redeker AG, Reynolds TB. Extra-and intrahepatic portal hypertension without cirrhosis (hepatoportal sclerosis). *Ann Surg* 1965;162:602–620.
133. Okuda K, Takashima T, Okudaira M, et al. Liver pathology of idiopathic portal hypertension: comparison with non-cirrhotic portal fibrosis of India. *Liver* 1982;2:176–192.
134. Sarin SK. Non-cirrhotic portal fibrosis. *Gut* 1989;30:406–415.
135. Nakanuma Y, Hoso M, Sasaki M, et al. Histopathology of the liver in non-cirrhotic portal hypertension of unknown aetiology. *Histopathology* 1996;28:195–204.
136. Thomas LB, Popper H, Berk PD, Selikoff I, Falk H. Vinyl-chloride-induced liver disease. From idiopathic portal hypertension (Banti's syndrome) to angiosarcomas. *N Engl J Med* 1975;292:17–22.
137. Morris JS, Schmid M, Newman S, Scheuer PJ, Sherlock S. Arsenic and noncirrhotic portal hypertension. *Gastroenterology* 1974;66:86–94.
138. Mitchell MC, Boitnott JK, Kaufman S, Cameron JL, Maddrey WC. Budd-Chiari syndrome: etiology, diagnosis and management. *Medicine* 1982;61:199–218.
139. Dilawari JB, Bambery P, Chawla Y, et al. Hepatic outflow obstruction (Budd-Chiari syndrome). Experience with 177 patients and a review of the literature. *Medicine* 1994;73:21–36.
140. Shulman HM, McDonald GB, Mathews D. An analysis of hepatic veno-occlusive disease and centrilobular hepatic degeneration following bone marrow transplantation. *Gastroenterology* 1980;79:1178–1191.
141. Taxy JB. Peliosis: a morphologic curiosity becomes an iatrogenic problem. *Hum Pathol* 1978;9:331–340.

Non-Neoplastic Hepatocellular Proliferative Disease

142. Stromeyer FW, Ishak KG. Nodular transformation (nodular "regenerative" hyperplasia) of the liver: a clinicopathologic study of 30 cases. *Hum Pathol* 1981;12:60–71.
143. Wanless IR. Micronodular transformation (nodular regenerative hyperplasia) of the liver: a report of 64 cases among 2,500 autopsies and a new classification of benign hepatocellular nodules. *Hepatology* 1990;11:787–797.
144. Wanless IR, Lentz JS, Roberts EA. Partial nodular transformation of liver in an adult with persistent ductus venosus. Review with hypothesis on pathogenesis. *Arch Pathol Lab Med* 1985;109:427–432.

Cirrhosis

145. Anthony PP, Ishak KG, Nayak NC, Poulsen HE, Scheuer PJ, Sobin LH. The morphology of cirrhosis: recommendations on definition, nomenclature and classification by a working group sponsored by the World Health Organization. *J Clin Pathol* 1978;31:395–414.
146. Schlichting P, Fauerholdt L, Christensen E, et al. Clinical relevance of restrictive morphological criteria for the diagnosis of cirrhosis in liver biopsies. *Liver* 1981;1:56–61.

Diseases of Uncertain Etiology

147. Meyer zum Buschenfelde K, Lohse AW, Manns M, Poralla T. Autoimmunity and liver disease. *Hepatology* 1990;12:354–363.
148. Czaja AJ. Diagnosis and therapy of autoimmune liver disease. *Med Clin North Am* 1996;80:973–994.
149. Lunel F, Abuaf N, Frangeul L, et al. Liver/kidney microsome antibody type 1 and hepatitis C virus infection. *Hepatology* 1992;16(3):630–636.
150. Brunner G, Klinge O. A chronic destructive non-suppurative cholangitis-like disease picture with antinuclear antibodies. *Dtsch Med Wochenschr* 1987;112:1454–1458.
151. Sanchez-Pobre P, Castellano G, Colina F, et al. Antimitochondrial antibody-negative chronic nonsuppurative destructive cholangitis. Atypical primary biliary cirrhosis or autoimmune cholangitis? *J Clin Gastroenterol* 1996;23:191–198.

152. Goodman ZD, McNally PR, Davis DF, Ishak KG. Autoimmune cholangitis: a variant of primary biliary cirrhosis. Clinicopathologic and serologic correlations in 200 cases. *Dig Dis Sci* 1995;40:1232–1242.
153. Taylor SL, Dean PJ, Riely CA. Primary autoimmune cholangitis. An alternative to antimitochondrial antibody–negative primary biliary cirrhosis. *Am J Surg Pathol* 1994;18:91–99.
154. Heubi JE, Partin JC, Partin JS, Schubert JK. Reye's syndrome: current concepts. *Hepatology* 1987;7:155–164.
155. Zimmerman HJ, Ishak KG. Valproate-induced hepatic injury: analyses of 23 fatal cases. *Hepatology* 1982;2:591–597.

The Liver in Systemic Disease

156. Bacon BR, Farahvash MJ, Janney CG, Neuschwander-Tetri BA. Nonalcoholic steatohepatitis: an expanded clinical entity. *Gastroenterology* 1994;107(4):1103–1109.
157. Rolfes DB, Ishak KG. Liver disease in pregnancy. *Histopathology* 1986;10:555–570.
158. Chopra S, Rubinow A, Koff RS, Cohen AS. Hepatic amyloidosis: a histopathologic analysis of primary (AL) and secondary (AA) forms. *Am J Pathol* 1984;115:186–193.
159. Gertz MA, Kyle RA. Hepatic amyloidosis (primary [AL], immunoglobulin light chain): the natural history in 80 patients. *Am J Med* 1988;85:73–80.

The Liver and Transplantation

160. Sale GE, Shulman HM, eds. *The pathology of bone marrow transplantation.* New York: Masson USA, 198–;104–135.
161. Snover DC. Biopsy interpretation in bone marrow transplantation. *Pathol Annu* 1989;24:63–101.
162. Snover DC, Weisdorf SA, Ramsay NK, McGlave P, Kersey JH. Hepatic graft-versus-host disease: a study of the predictive value of liver biopsy in diagnosis. *Hepatology* 1984;4:123–130.
163. Shulman HM, Sharma P, Amos D, Fenster LF, McDonald GB. A coded histologic study of hepatic graft-versus-host disease after human bone marrow transplantation. *Hepatology* 1988;8:463–470.
164. Shulman HM, Sullivan KM, Weiden PL et al. Chronic graft-versus-host syndrome in man: a long term clinicopathologic study of 20 Seattle patients. *Am J Med* 1980;69:204–217.
165. Snover DC. The pathology of liver transplantation. In: Sale GE, ed. *The pathology of organ transplantation.* Boston: Butterworths, 1990.
166. Hubscher SG. Pathology of liver allograft rejection. *Transplant Immunol* 1994;2:118–123.
167. Hanto DW, Snover DC, Noreen HJ, et al. Hyperacute rejection of a human orthotopic liver allograft in a presensitized recipient. *Clin Transplant* 1987;1:304–310.
168. Anonymous. Banff schema for grading liver allograft rejection: an international consensus document. *Hepatology* 1997;25:658–663.
169. Freese DK, Snover DC, Sharp H, Gross CR, Savick SK, Payne WD. Chronic rejection after liver transplant: a study of clinical, histopathologic, and immunologic features. *Hepatology* 1991;13:882–891.
170. Hubscher SG, Buckels JAC, Elias E, McMaster P, Neuberger J. Vanishing bile duct syndrome following liver transplantation—is it reversible? *Transplantation* 1991;51:1004–010.

The Liver in the Acquired Immunodeficiency Syndrome

171. Schneiderman DJ, Arenson DM, Cello JP, Margaretten W, Weber TE. Hepatic disease in patients with the acquired immunodeficiency syndrome (AIDS). *Hepatology* 1987;7:925–930.
172. Schaffner F. The liver in HIV infection. *Prog Liver Dis* 1990;9:505–522.
173. Lefkowitch JH. Pathology of AIDS-related liver disease. *Dig Dis* 1994;12:321–330.
174. Glasgow BJ, Anders K, Layfield LT, et al. Clinical and pathologic findings in the liver in the acquired immunodeficiency syndrome (AIDS). *Am J Clin Pathol* 1985;83:582–588.
175. Duffy LF, Daum F, Kahn E, et al. Hepatitis in children with acquired immune deficiency syndrome; histological and immunocytologic features. *Gastroenterology* 1986;90:173–181.
176. Perkocha LA, Geaghan SM, Yen TS, et al. Clinical and pathological features of bacillary peliosis hepatis in association with human immunodeficiency virus infection. *N Engl J Med* 1990;323:1581–1586.
177. Ferrell LD. Hepatic granulomas: a morphologic approach to diagnosis. *Surg Pathol* 1990;3:87–106.
178. Keen ME, Engstrand DA, Hafez GR. Hepatic lipogranulomatosis simulating veno-occlusive disease of the liver. *Arch Pathol Lab Med* 1985;109:70–72.
179. Devaney K, Goodman ZD, Epstein MS, Zimmerman HJ, Ishak KG. Hepatic sarcoidosis. Clinicopathologic features in 100 patients. *Am J Surg Pathol* 1993;17:1272–1280.

Most Important References

1. Ludwig J, Batts KP, Moyer TP, Baldus WO, Fairbanks VF. Liver biopsy diagnosis of homozygous hemochromatosis: a diagnostic algorithm. *Mayo Clinic Proceedings.* 1993;68:263–267.
2. Portmann B, Popper H, Neuberger J, Williams R. Sequential and diagnostic features in primary biliary cirrhosis based on serial histologic study in 209 patients. *Gastroenterology.* 1985;88;1777–1790.
3. Stricker BHC. Drug-induced hepatic injury. Amsterdam: Elsevier Science Publishers, 1992.
4. Neuschwander-Tetri BA, Bacon BR. Nonalcoholic steatohepatitis. *Medical Clinics of North America.* 1996;80:1147–1166.
5. Dhillon AP, Dusheiko GM. Pathology of hepatitis C virus infection. *Histopathology.* 1995;26:297–309.
6. Desmet VJ, Gerber M, Hoofnagle JH, Manns M, Scheuer PJ. Classification of chronic hepatitis: diagnosis, grading and staging. *Hepatology.* 1994;19:1513–1520.
7. Okuda K, Nakashima T, Okudaira M, et al. Liver pathology of idiopathic portal hypertension: comparison with non-cirrhotic portal fibrosis of India. *Liver.* 1982;2:176–192.
8. Stromeyer FW, Ishak KG. Nodular transformation (nodular "regenerative" hyperplasia) of the liver: a clinicopathologic study of 30 cases. *Hum Pathol.* 1981;12:60–71.
9. Czaja, AJ. Diagnosis and therapy of autoimmune liver disease. *Medical Clinics of North America.* 1996;80:973–994.
10. Anonymous. Banff schema for grading liver allograft rejection: an international consensus document. *Hepatology.* 1997;25:658–63.

CHAPTER 37

Masses of the Liver

Scott H. Saul

Hepatic masses are increasingly being detected on radiography—albeit most commonly as incidental findings as small as 1 cm or less—with the use of sophisticated abdominal imaging studies (1). Specific diagnoses can often be suspected based on sensitive radiographic imaging techniques (computed tomography, magnetic resonance imaging) coupled with clinical data and blood studies. Except for hemangiomas, however, biopsy diagnoses remains the gold standard in determining tumor classification and appropriate clinical treatment.

The varied array of primary benign and malignant masses (Table 1) and the high rates of metastases to the liver account for much of the diagnostic difficulty encountered by the pathologist. Primary tumors can be solid or cystic and can arise from epithelium (hepatocyte, bile duct epithelium, neuroendocrine cells), mesenchymal cells (principally endothelium), or (rarely) heterotopic tissues (2–4). The age of the patient can be an important discriminating feature in the evaluation of hepatic masses because several tumors, such as hepatoblastoma (HBL), mesenchymal hamartoma, and infantile hemangioendothelioma (IHE), are usually found in the pediatric population, whereas others, such as cholangiocarcinoma, are virtually unheard of in childhood (3,5,6a) (Table 2). The appearance of the surrounding nonneoplastic liver and/or the clinical history of chronic liver disease/cirrhosis can be of great importance. The majority of malignant hepatic neoplasms represent metastatic carcinoma derived from virtually any primary site, whereas in patients with cirrhosis, hepatocellular carcinoma (HCC) is more common.

Many pathologists have little experience in the diagnosis of primary hepatic tumors, and they are much more familiar with metastatic lesions. Although diagnosis of the former is often straightforward in resection specimens, definitive classification of a biopsy specimen (core or fine-needle aspiration) showing evidence of benign-appearing hepatocytes can be quite difficult; great care is required in writing the surgical pathology report. Criteria for distinguishing macroregenerative and borderline (dysplastic) nodules from differentiated HCC (WD-HCC) in the cirrhotic liver have evolved, but definitive evaluation of such nodules in biopsy specimens still remains challenging. Making the distinction between HCC and metastatic carcinoma, the most common problem encountered in biopsy specimens, occasionally can be difficult even for the most seasoned hepatopathologist. The selective use of immunohistochemistry can be quite useful in this situation. One can virtually never distinguish primary (intrahepatic) cholangiocarcinoma from metastatic adenocarcinoma in biopsy specimens.

The goal of this chapter is to provide a framework for understanding the important clinicopathologic features of hepatic tumors, particularly stressing histopathologic differential diagnosis and pitfalls in biopsy interpretation. Since fine-needle aspiration (FNA) biopsy has assumed a primary diagnostic role in the evaluation of hepatic masses, the appearance of specimens obtained using this technique is described where appropriate.

SPECIMEN HANDLING

The salient macroscopic features of neoplasms in hepatic resection specimens should be described, including tumor appearance (color, consistency, cysts, necrosis, etc.), number and size (smallest, largest, average) of nodules, presence or absence of encapsulation and venous tumor thrombi, and distance of the tumor from the inked margins of resection (5a). As with tumors from other sites, the degree of differentiation of hepatic tumors may vary in a given specimen. Therefore, the preparation of one paraffin block for every 1 to 2 cm of tumor diameter in surgical specimens is a reasonable guide to adequate sampling of primary tumors; tumors 2 cm or smaller should be entirely submitted. Known metastatic tumors can be less vigorously sampled.

S. H. Saul: Department of Pathology, Chester County Hospital, West Chester, Pennsylvania 19380.

TABLE 1. *Classification of primary hepatic neoplasms and nonneoplastic masses*

Benign	Malignant
Epithelial	Epithelial
Hepatocellular	Hepatocellular
Hepatocellular adenoma	Hepatocellular carcinoma (HCC)[a]
Focal nodular hyperplasia	HCC, fibrolamellar variant
Nodular regenerative hyperplasia	Combined HCC-cholangiocacarcinoma
Macroregenerative nodule	Hepatoblastoma, epithelial type
Borderline (dysplastic) nodule[b]	
Compensatory lobar hyperplasia	
Accessory lobe	
Cholangiocellular	Cholangiocellular
Bile duct hamartoma (von Meyenburg complex)	Cholangiocarcinoma (CC)[a]
Bile duct adenoma	Intraductal variant ("biliary papillomatosis")
Biliary cysts (nonneoplastic)	Cholangiocellular carcinoma[a]
Solitary	Adenosquamous carcinoma
Polycystic disease (noncommunicating)	Mucoepidermoid carcinoma
Caroli's disease	Squamous cell carcinoma
Multiple hilar cysts	Combined CC-neuroendocrine tumor
Biliary cystadenoma	Biliary cystadenocarcinoma
Mucinous (+/− mesenchymal stroma)	
Serous	
Mesenchymal	Mesenchymal
Vascular	Vascular
Hemangioma	Angiosarcoma
Infantile hemangioendothelioma	Epithelioid hemangioendothelioma
Hemangiomatosis	Kaposi's sarcoma
Lymphangioma (-tosis)	
Hereditary hemorrhagic telangiectasia	
Peliosis hepatis	
Fatty tumors	Fatty tumors
Angiomyolipoma (and related tumors)	Liposarcoma
Pseudolipoma	
Focal (hepatocellular) fatty change[c]	
Other	Other
Solitary (localized) fibrous tumor	Undifferentiated (embryonal) sarcoma
Inflammatory myofibroblastic tumor (pseudotumor)	Rhabdomyosarcoma
Leiomyoma	Fibrosarcoma, malignant fibrous histiocytoma
	Leiomyosarcoma
	Osteosarcoma
Mixed epithelial and mesenchymal	Mixed epithelial and mesenchymal
Mesenchymal hamartoma	Mixed hepatoblastoma
	Sarcomatoid carcinoma (carcinosarcoma)
Other	Other
Necrotic/fibrous nodule	Malignant schwannoma
Heterotopia (adrenal, pancreas, spleen)	Germ cell tumors (teratoma, yolk sac tumor)
Endometrial cyst (endometrioma)[d]	Malignant rhabdoid tumor
Benign nerve sheath tumors	Primary lymphoma
Sarcoid pseudotumor ("sarcoidoma")	Primary neuroendocrine neoplasm
Abscesses	Pheochromocytoma
Parasitic cysts	Solid and cystic tumor
Ciliated foregut cyst	
Alimentary duplication cysts	
Pseudocysts (pancreatic, traumatic)	

[a] Scirrhous variants (diffuse hyalinized fibrous stroma) that may be associated with hypercalcemia have been termed "sclerosing hepatic carcinoma."
[b] For convenience, placed in the benign category rather than listing in its own borderline category.
[c] Placed here for convenience.
[d] Cases reported as such most probably represent biliary cystadenomas.

TABLE 2. *The relative prevalence rates of primary hepatic tumors in the general and pediatric populations in the United States*

	General population (%)[a]	Pediatric population (%)[b]
Malignant (total)	(94)	(55–68)
Hepatocellular carcinoma	82	19–20
Hepatoblastoma	1	26–36
Cholangiocarcinoma	10	—
Angiosarcoma	<1	≤2
Undifferentiated sarcoma	<1	7–9
Other malignant tumors	<1	≤1
Benign (total)	(6)	(32–45)
Infantile hemangioendothelioma	—	18
Hepatocellular adenoma	1	2–4
Focal nodular hyperplasia	3	3–10
Nodular regenerative hyperplasia	—	0–5
Mesenchymal hamartoma	—	8
Other benign tumors	2	—

[a] Adapted from ref. 3. Hemangiomas and bile duct hamartomas were excluded from the calculations in this series. They are by far the most common hepatic tumors in adults.
[b] Adapted from refs. 5, 6, and 6a.

Histologic sections should include tissue from the tumor center and periphery as well as adjacent and distant nontumorous hepatic parenchyma and surgical resection margins. To preserve biopsy tissue, unstained levels between routinely stained sections should be saved on slides (poly-L-lysine coated or sialinized) for potential application of immunohistochemical stains. Although other techniques, such as flow cytometric DNA analysis, in situ hybridization, clonality studies, and chromosome/oncogene analysis, are not performed in the routine evaluation of hepatic tumors, studies are ongoing to determine if they can be of any help in the diagnosis, classification, and prognostic assessment of hepatic tumors.

INTRAOPERATIVE CONSULTATION

In the best of circumstances the pathologist should have available before operation any pertinent clinical data (history of previous malignancy, presence of a mass elsewhere, results of imaging studies and serum tumor markers such as alpha-fetoprotein (AFP), history of chronic hepatitis/cirrhosis, etc.). He or she should also review any previous biopsies of the mass and discuss the case *a priori* with the surgeon (7). In the real world, however, we have to deal with much less information; in addition, hepatic masses are often incidental findings at the time of abdominal surgery for another condition. In this situation the appropriate clinical questions should be asked at the time of surgery. The pathologist should always determine whether any specimen submitted for intraoperative consultation is from a mass, so as not to misinterpret, for example, chronic liver disease/cirrhosis as focal nodular hyperplasia (FNH). The distance of the tumor from the surgical margins should be reported. For malignant lesions, if it is closer than 1 cm, re-excision can be suggested.

Problematic areas that may alter operative intervention must be distinguished at the time of frozen section. For example, one may be asked to differentiate: (a) bile duct hamartoma or adenoma from metastatic adenocarcinoma at the time of a Whipple procedure for pancreatic adenocarcinoma, (b) macroregenerative/borderline nodules from HCC in the cirrhotic liver, and (c) hepatocellular adenoma (HCA) from FNH. If, after employing the diagnostic criteria enumerated elsewhere in this chapter, a definitive diagnosis cannot be made even after requesting more tissue, the pathologist should defer the diagnosis.

THE UTILITY OF LIVER BIOPSY FOR TUMOR DIAGNOSIS

Is the Specimen from the Liver?

Whether or not the specimen is from the liver is answered affirmatively by finding both hepatic parenchyma and tumor within the biopsy material. If the former is not present, then the source of the tumor cannot be definitively confirmed, because the biopsy needle can penetrate other abdominal viscera, particularly the right kidney and gallbladder, leading to an erroneous diagnosis (Fig. 1). Close collaboration with the radiologist in cases of biopsies guided by radiography should help resolve the location of the biopsy site in most cases.

Biopsy Types (Fine-needle Aspiration and Thick-needle Core Biopsies)

Radiographically guided (ultrasound and computed tomography) biopsies of hepatic mass lesions have become the standard; unguided biopsies generally are performed only in the context of diffuse disease (8,9). Guided biopsies allow previously inaccessible portions of the right lobe, as well as the left lobe, to be sampled. FNA (20- to 23-gauge needle) biopsy has become a well-established method in the diagnosis of malignant hepatic neoplasms in adults (8–12); occasionally, this technique has been used in the pediatric population (13,14).

FNA has several advantages over thick-needle biopsies: (a) Multiple aspirations can be performed to ensure an adequate specimen, with only rare cases of morbidity (less than 0.1–0.5%) and exceptional instances of mortality (0.01%) (15). (b) Biopsies can be obtained from patients with ascites, portal hypertension, or obstructive jaundice; (c) Immediate interpretation of the material is possible, and specimen adequacy can be checked, thus affording the possibility of obtaining additional material; and (d) implantation of malignant cells along the needle track appears to be less common than with thick-needle biopsy, although more than 15 such cases have been reported with hepatic FNA (16,17).

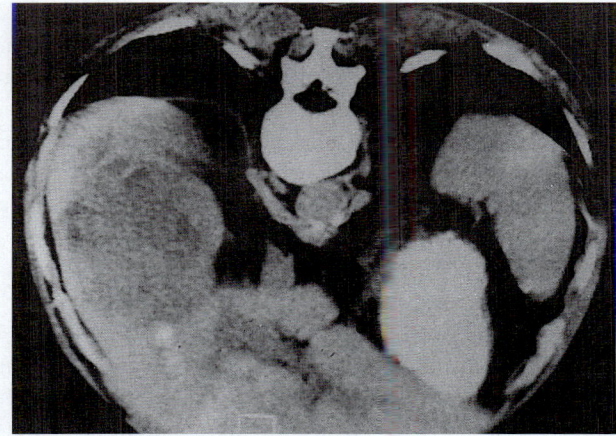 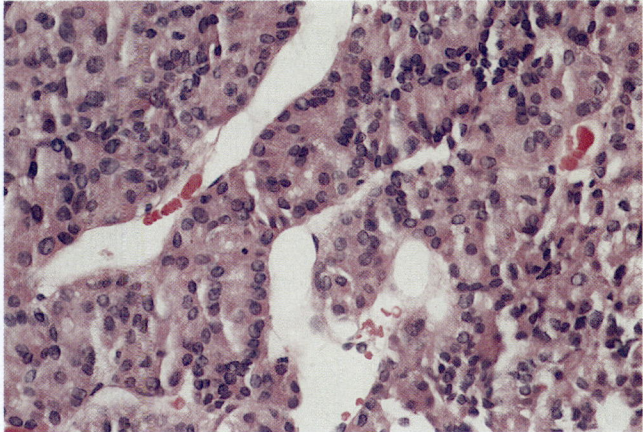

FIG. 1. Always ask yourself, "Is the biopsy sample really from the liver?" **A:** Computed tomography scan shows a large mass originally interpreted as hepatic in origin. **B:** Percutaneous "liver biopsy" of the mass first interpreted as hepatocellular carcinoma (HCC) or combined HCC-cholangiocarcinoma by referring pathologist and his consultants. Note that no normal hepatic parenchymal elements are evident. The patient was referred for liver transplantation. At the time of surgery, the mass was found to be in the right kidney, while the liver was normal. Histologic examination of the kidney revealed renal cell carcinoma with foci identical to those seen in the original "liver" biopsy.

The sensitivity of guided FNA for a diagnosis of hepatic malignancy ranges in most recent series from 90% to 96%, with a specificity of 90% to 100% (8,12,18). Similar figures for sensitivity and specificity have been reported for spring-loaded cutting thick-needle biopsies (18). Laparoscopic (thick and fine needle, ultrasound guided or unguided) biopsy, which allows direct visualization, may be useful for initial diagnosis or as a secondary technique to help classify and stage a malignant neoplasm. Its successful use may help avoid laparotomy (19).

With FNA, good cytologic specimens with optimal preservation are essential for accurate diagnosis. False positives are most often a reflection of the examiner's lack of experience. The yield of diagnostic information is maximized by the preparation of cell blocks (microhistology), which can be obtained in 70% to 85% of cases (20–22). Cell blocks increase by 10% to 20% the sensitivity of a malignant diagnosis based on smears alone, and allow the pathologist to perform special stains as well as immunohistochemical analysis, thereby increasing his or her ability to classify the tumor precisely. In one review, 80% of 200 primary and secondary hepatic malignancies were easily classified based only on FNA-derived cytomorphologic features and clinical/radiographic correlation (12). Immunohistochemistry helped in assigning a specific diagnosis in one-half of the remaining diagnostically challenging cases.

One of the most common and difficult problems encountered by the pathologist in hepatic FNA is attempting to make a specific diagnosis of HCC. The HCCs that go undiagnosed as malignancy are often very well differentiated and, thus, may be difficult to identify on cytologic evidence as neoplastic, whereas poorly differentiated HCC is easily recognized as malignant but is difficult to identify as being hepatocellular in origin (8,10–12). Obtaining a second specimen from the nontumorous liver for comparison with the mass biopsy and the combination of both FNA and core biopsy techniques can aid in definitive diagnosis (18,23,24). The well-recognized histologic patterns of HCC have their correlates in smear preparations, and cell blocks often assist in definitive histologic characterization (25–27). Reactive hepatocytes or those demonstrating large- or small-cell change (dysplasia) can lead to false-positive diagnoses.

Although guided FNA has intentionally or inadvertently been used to diagnose cavernous hemangiomas (CHs), occasionally with untoward consequences, the smears are often dominated by blood and are considered inadequate (8,10,11,28). Diagnosis of a benign hepatocellular tumor is generally not possible by FNA and should be made only with great caution and careful clinicopathologic correlation (10,11). Similar caveats apply when attempting to make a definitive diagnosis of benign hepatocellular lesions using thick-needle biopsies. Specific details on the FNA appearance of selected hepatic tumors, particularly HCC, are found in later sections of this chapter.

Histologic Findings Adjacent to Liver Tumors

The nonneoplastic liver adjacent to a tumor mass typically shows nonspecific changes presumably related to local interruption of blood and bile flow. The portal tracts are edematous and contain more inflammatory cells, particularly neutrophils, in association with bile ductule proliferation. Sometimes the latter feature may appear atypical and resemble adenocarcinoma involving the portal tract. Within the lobule, focal sinusoidal dilatation and congestion, compression and distortion of hepatocyte plates with focal hepatocyte necrosis, and a pattern of nonspecific reactive hepatitis can be seen. When tumor is suspected by clinical examination, but only the cited constellation of findings is present in the biopsy (even after sampling deeper levels), the search should continue for a hepatic space-occupying lesion (29). Arterialized zones of nodular hepatocytic hyperplasia, histologically simulating FNH, have been described adjacent to the fibrolamellar variant of HCC (FL-HCC) (30,31) and presumably could be seen adjacent to any hypervascular mass. This should be kept in mind when evaluating needle biopsies of hepatic masses.

CYSTIC MASSES

Confusion and controversy surround the derivation and precise classification of hepatic cysts (32). Table 3 is an attempt to classify these lesions for the surgical pathologist. In this section, the term cyst is used to denote a tissue-enclosed space that is abnormal in location or size; it may contain liquids or solids (32). This definition, therefore, includes cysts that both have (true cyst) and lack (pseudocyst) an epithelial lining. Infectious agents (parasites and bacteria) can appear

TABLE 3. *Cystic masses of the liver*

Classification	Diagnostic findings
Abcesses	
Amebic	Cavities filled with odorless necrotic hepatic tissue ("anchovy sauce"); neutrophils rare or absent; trophozoites at periphery, don't mistake for histiocytes; reactive hepatocytes may be present; PAS and iron hematoxylin stains may be helpful
Pyogenic	Cavities filled with foul-smelling necrotic hepatic tissue containing many neutrophils; often polymicrobial; *E. coli* most common; anaerobes frequently isolated
Parasitic (echinococcal) cysts	*Echinococcus granulosus*—unilocular cysts (three layers) often with daughter cysts; brood capsules; protoscolices with attached or detached acid-fast, birefringent hooklets
Nonparasitic (nonneoplastic) cysts	
Solitary (unilocular)	Typically, cuboidal flattened, biliary type epithelial lining; rarely squamous; thin fibrous wall; found in <1% of routinely performed autopsies
Polycystic liver disease	
Adult polycystic disease; (ADPKD; non communicating ductal cysts)	Typically multiple cysts with autosomal dominant inheritance; prevalence of 0.15% at autopsy; associated with adult polycystic kidney disease in 71% to 93% of cases; rarely, liver is massively enlarged; histologically similar to solitary type
Communicating ductal cysts	Typically autosomal recessive inheritance
Caroli's disease	Ectatic intrahepatic bile ducts, inspissated bile ± hepatolithiasis, cholangitis
Caroli's syndrome	Caroli's disease plus congenital hepatic fibrosis
Congenital hepatic fibrosis/ ARPKD	Angulated bile ducts often with inspissated bile in fibrotic portal tracts with portal-portal bridging fibrosis; only rarely macroscopic hepatic cysts
Multiple hilar cysts	Noncommunicating cysts arising from dilatation of peribiliary glands typically in hilum; often associated with cirrhosis, portal vein thrombosis. Common in patients with ADPKD
Mesenchymal hamartoma	Solid and cystic mass, 75% ≤1 yr of age; admixture of nonneoplastic tissue types (myxoid stroma, hepatocytes, bile ducts, blood vessels); association with translocation involving chromosome 19q; rare association with undifferentiated sarcoma
Alimentary tract–related cysts	Intrahepatic ileal and duodenal duplications and ciliated foregut cyst described
Pseudocysts (trauma, ischemia, pancreatic origin)	Fibrous lining; may contain blood (hematoma), bile (biloma))
Neoplastic cysts	
Biliary cystadenoma/cystadenocarcinoma	
Mucinous type	Most common type of multilocular cyst, but only 5% of all solitary cysts; 95% occur in women; lined by columnar-cuboidal mucin containing epithelium; spindle-cell stroma (85%) only in women; search carefully for dysplasia (borderline lesion), cystadenocarcinoma; rule out metastasis from other primary site (pancreas, ovary, appendix)
Serous (microcystic, glycogen rich) type	Very rare; multilocular; bland, flattened to cuboidal cell lining; clear, glycogen-rich, mucin-negative cytoplasm; no spindle-cell stroma; rule out metastasis from pancreas
Teratoma	Derivatives from three germ layers; problem of "teratoid hepatoblastoma"
Other	Cystic degeneration of various neoplasms

ADPKD, autosomal dominant polycystic kidney disease; ARPKD, autosomal recessive polycystic kidney disease; PAS, periodic acid–Schiff.

as cystic masses and are therefore considered briefly in this section. Sonography and computed tomography (CT) are excellent imaging methods for the diagnosis of cystic hepatic lesions, some of which may show signs of calcification (1,9,32). The precise role of magnetic resonance imaging (MRI) in the workup of cystic lesions remains to be established.

Abscesses

Amebic Abscesses

Hepatic abscess complicates amebiasis in 3% to 9% of cases (33). The earliest lesions are well circumscribed, firm, yellow, and demonstrate coagulative necrosis. They are preferentially found in the right lobe. Subsequently, as the lesions presumably coalesce, one or more cavities containing the classic orange-brown, pasty, blood-stained necrotic hepatic tissue (often described as "anchovy sauce") are formed. This material is odorless, bacteriologically sterile, and contains virtually no neutrophils (the term abscess is a misnomer) unless it is secondarily infected, an uncommon occurrence in previously unaspirated cases (33–36). The organisms are most likely to be found in the periphery of the so-called abscess, which possesses a shaggy necrotic fibrinous zone and a layer of granulation tissue. A zone of compressed liver, often with nonspecific chronic inflammation and fibrosis, gives support to the abscess wall.

The trophozoites of *Entamoeba histolytica* are oval and usually 10 to 60 μm in diameter. They contain a small, single, round nucleus with a distinctive central karyosome; a thick, beaded nuclear membrane; and bubbly cytoplasm that often contains phagocytosed red blood cells. Although readily identified on hematoxylin and eosin–stained sections, the organisms can be also demonstrated with the periodic acid–Schiff (PAS) stain, iron hematoxylin preparations, or the Diff-Quick stain. Aspirate fluid should be examined in both saline wet mounts and stained preparations. Direct microscopy of aspirated material from the center of the cyst reveals necrotic debris with few cells and only rare amebic trophozoites, whereas if material is obtained specifically from the periphery, trophozoites are seen in approximately 50% of cases. Trophozoites should be distinguished from macrophages, which have a more bean-shaped nucleus, finer chromatin, a more delicate nuclear membrane, and a small nucleolus. Moreover, reactive hepatocytes in the adjacent liver should not be misconstrued as a neoplastic process (10).

The availability of highly sensitive and specific serologic tests for the diagnosis of invasive amebiasis, which give positive results in more than 90% of cases, has eliminated the need for diagnostic aspiration in most cases. Metronidazole is the drug of choice, and surgery is indicated only for complicated cases. In uncomplicated cases, the fatality rate should be less than 1%.

Pyogenic Abscesses

Pyogenic abscesses most commonly result from seeding of bacteria from the biliary tract (30% to 70%; patients with benign or malignant biliary tract disease). Other major sources of bacteria include portal blood (15%; intraabdominal sepsis, appendicitis, diverticulitis, etc.), arterial blood (6% to 15%; generalized septicemia), and direct extension from a contiguous infection (3% to 15%; subphrenic abscess, perforated cholecystitis) (36–38). Hepatic trauma and cannulation of umbilical vessels in the neonate are also causes of pyogenic hepatic abscesses. In up to 40% of cases no obvious source is found (37).

The abscesses are most frequently in the right lobe, may be single or multiple, and are variable in size. Their coalescence can impart a honeycomb appearance to the liver. They consist of creamy yellow, foul-smelling pus that contains necrotic liver tissue and numerous neutrophils. A fibrous capsule may be present. Reactive hepatocytes from the adjacent liver should not be misinterpreted as neoplastic in aspiration specimens (10).

Bacteria can be recovered in 85% to 100% of cases by using aerobic, microaerophilic and strict anaerobic techniques. *Escherichia coli* represents the single most frequently recovered bacterium (35% to 45% of cases), although infections are often polymicrobial. If *Yersinia enterocolitica* is isolated, the patient should be evaluated for hereditary hemochromatosis or other disorders of iron overload (38a).

Most cases of pyogenic abscess can be treated with antibiotics, either alone or in combination with percutaneous drainage. Therapy must also be directed at the underlying cause of the abscess. Overall mortality, which has dropped as low as 10% in some series, is related to the patient's age, severity of the underlying disease, and number of abscesses.

Echinococcosis (Hydatidosis)

Echinococcosis is perhaps the most common cause of hepatic cysts worldwide, particularly in the Middle East, Greece, Australia, North Africa, and some parts of South America. In the United States, it is principally seen in immigrants from these countries (34,39,40). It is caused most typically by *Echinococcus granulosis*, the agent of cystic hydatid disease. Much less often, *E. multilocularis* (alveolar hydatid disease) or *E. vogeli* (polycystic hydatid disease, not discussed) are the causal species. Immunodiagnostic serum assays are about 90% sensitive for liver cysts of *E. granulosis*; however, false positives do occur. Serum assays for *E. multilocularis* have a higher sensitivity and specificity.

The hepatic cysts of *E. granulosis* are unilocular, white, fluid filled and enlarge at the rate of about 1 to 5 cm per year. They are single in 75% of cases and are asymptomatic until they become at least 10 cm in diameter. Fertile cysts may coexist with sterile cysts. The cysts can arise deep within the liver or superficially, just underneath Glisson's capsule, where they can become pedunculated. The cyst wall contains three layers (Fig. 2). The germinal layer (innermost) is 10 to

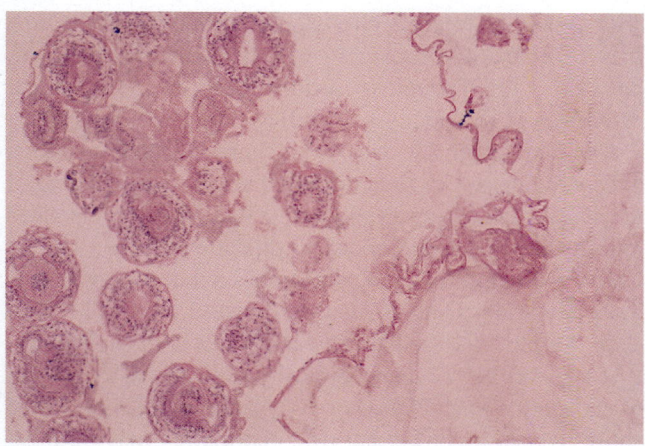

FIG. 2. Echinococcal cyst contents. Multiple protoscolices of *Echinococcus granulosus* within daughter cysts (left). Note the cyst wall (right) with innermost thin, germinal layer and adjacent avascular, refractile, chitinous, laminated membrane. The adventitial layer is not shown.

25 μm thick and possesses nuclei. In fertile cysts it gives rise to brood capsules, which are attached by a short stalk. Protoscolices (future heads of the adult tapeworm) develop within the brood capsules. Each protoscolex has a double row of refractile, birefringent, and acid-fast hooklets that are each 22 to 40 μm in length, as well as four round suckers. When the brood capsules detach, they are called "daughter cysts." These secondary cysts are of varying sizes, may merge into a multivesicular conglomerate, and are responsible for the internal septations seen on imaging studies of the mother cyst in 25% to 50% of cases. The cyst fluid or "hydatid sand" obtained in aspirated specimens consists of daughter cysts and protoscolices, freed by brood capsule rupture, as well as loose hooklets. Inflammation is absent.

The second layer, the laminated membrane, located immediately beneath the germinal layer, is avascular, eosinophilic, refractile, and chitinous. It is 1 mm thick and nonnucleated, and it stains strongly with PAS, Gomori methenamine silver, and Best's carmine. The outer, adventitial layer (pericyst) consists of dense fibrovascular tissue with a varying number of mononuclear inflammatory cells, depending on the age of the cyst. Ringlike (eggshell) calcification of this layer is seen in up to 25% of cases, usually in older cysts, and may take 5 to 10 years to develop. In terms of radiologic evaluation, its presence is helpful in differential diagnosis, because nonparasitic cysts less often calcify.

The hepatic lesions caused by the less common, more slowly growing, more geographically restricted (limited to the Northern Hemisphere), and more tissue-invasive *E. multilocularis* may simulate a malignant neoplasm or cirrhosis on macroscopic examination. Typically they demonstrate an alveolar structure composed of numerous irregular cysts, each with a diameter from less than 1 mm up to 20 mm. The border with the adjacent liver has an infiltrative appearance. The inner part of the lesion may become necrotic; calcifica-

tion (70%) is often present. At the microscopic level, a thin, laminated layer is evident, but brood capsules and protoscolices are seen in less than 10% of cases. The germinal layer is frequently absent or attenuated.

Treatment of cystic hydatid disease has generally been surgery, but the PAIR method (PAIR stands for "Puncture of cysts percutaneously, Aspiration of fluid, Introduction of protoscolicidal agent, and Reaspiration") in conjunction with medical therapy has been suggested as a suitable alternative, since it carries little risk of adverse reactions (anaphylaxis, peritoneal spread) (39,41). In light of the fact that pathologists may expectedly or unexpectedly encounter FNA biopsy–derived hydatid cyst fluid, a diligent search of all hepatic cyst fluid for hooklets, intact protoscolices, or laminated membrane is advisable (10). Radical surgery is the treatment of choice for *E. multilocularis*.

Nonparasitic Nonneoplastic Cysts

Solitary (Unilocular, Simple, Congenital) Cyst

The term solitary cyst refers to unilocular cysts that are typically single and unassociated with cysts in other organs (32). While they may be congenital, they are not hereditary. These cysts are far more common (95%) than the multilocular type (5%), a term that is often used interchangeably for cystadenoma in the literature (42). Solitary cysts are found in less than 1% of routinely performed autopsies, but they have been identified in up to 14% of autopsies when specifically sought (43,44). They demonstrate a predominance among women and are usually asymptomatic (3,32,42). Although their origin is still debated, a likely source of many of these cysts is the persistence of small remnants of ductal plate malformation (von Meyenburg complexes) that separate from the biliary tree and become dilated (44,45).

Most cysts are superficially located just under the liver capsule, although they may be found now and then in the falciform ligament (46). They vary in diameter from a few centimeters up to 40 cm and have a flat, glistening lining. They may contain up to 17 L of fluid, which is usually clear amber, although it may occasionally be bloody, bile-tinged, mucoid, or purulent (3,32,42). Only rarely do these cysts connect with the biliary tree. On microscopic examination, the cysts are frequently lined by a single layer of biliary-type epithelium that is typically cuboidal but may be flattened, or simply columnar and even ciliated (*ciliated hepatic foregut cyst*) or squamous (*epidermoid cyst*) epithelium (3,32,42, 47–49). The epithelium sits on a thin collagenous wall that lacks the dense spindle-cell stroma often found in biliary cystadenomas. Ciliated hepatic foregut cysts are less than 4 cm in diameter and, in contrast to other unilocular cysts, demonstrate bundles of smooth muscle in the cyst wall (47,48).

Secondary degenerative changes of unilocular cysts may lead to epithelial desquamation, a multilocular appearance, and infrequently, calcification. Old collapsed cysts with central fibrosis and a hyalinized wall reminiscent of ovarian corpora albicans may be found (42). Complications include torsion, hemorrhage, rupture or extrinsic compression of the biliary tree. Partial or complete surgical excision is often performed in symptomatic cases; cyst fenestration or sclerotherapy are alternative therapies. Although it is uncommon, adenocarcinoma or squamous cell carcinoma can arise in a solitary unilocular cyst (49–51).

Polycystic Liver Disease (Multiple, Heritable Cysts)

According to Witzleben, the term polycystic liver disease designates a group of heritable disorders in which there is actual or potential cystic dilatation of elements of the bile ducts and actual or potential development of renal lesions, especially cysts of tubular origin (32). Each appears to represent a ductal plate malformation at different levels of the biliary tree. Controversies and overlap in the classification of polycystic liver disease notwithstanding (32,43,45,52–55), the condition may be divided into two basic groups. Autosomal dominant polycystic kidney disease (ADPKD) (also termed adult polycystic liver disease) is a disorder inherited in an autosomal dominant fashion in which the cysts lack communication with the biliary tree (noncommunicating ductal cysts) and thus generally lack bile. The prevalence of adult polycystic liver disease is about 0.15% at autopsy, with 71% to 93% of patients having associated polycystic kidneys (44,55). About 85% to 95% of ADPKD cases are linked to a defect on chromosome 16 (ADPKD1), and a few cases are linked to a defect on chromosome 4 (ADPKD2) or currently unmapped foci. Caroli's disease/syndrome, autosomal recessive polycystic kidney disease (ARPKD), and congenital hepatic fibrosis (CHF) make up a group of autosomal recessively inherited disorders in which hepatic cysts, if present, communicate with the biliary tree (communicating ductal cysts) and therefore contain bile.

In adult polycystic disease, the cysts are unilocular, of variable size, and may diffusely involve the liver. They may also, however, be limited to one lobe, and they rarely calcify. Massive hepatomegaly, up to nearly 10 kg, has been reported (55). A markedly elevated serum AFP level was reported in one unusual case (56). At the microscopic level and in developmental terms, they are similar to solitary cysts (44,45); von Meyenburg complexes can be found in the overwhelming majority of cases. The number and size of hepatic cysts in patients with adult polycystic liver disease have a strong correlation with older age, increased severity of renal cystic disease, decreased creatinine clearance, female gender, oral contraceptive use or estrogen replacement therapy, and pregnancy (57). Whereas cysts are seen in less than 5% of patients in the second decade of life, they are present in 75% to 90% of patients older than age 70 years (52,57,58).

Previously reported as uncommon, hepatic complications (such as cyst infection and cholangiocarcinoma) (50,51,58) have been associated with 10.5% of the overall deaths in one series (58), presumably related to longer survival of patients with end-stage renal failure. Common bile duct dilatation may be noted, and squamous cell carcinoma has been reported (58,59). Treatments include those mentioned in the discussion of solitary cyst, as well as transplantation (60).

Communicating ductal cysts are found in Caroli's disease, a disorder caused by total or partial arrest of remodeling of the ductal plate of larger intrahepatic bile ducts (45). Isolated multifocal intrahepatic bile duct dilatation is often termed Caroli's disease, whereas in Caroli's syndrome, which is more common, CHF is also present (32,42,45,52). Like CHF, Caroli's disease has been associated with choledochal cyst and ADPKD. Patients typically show initial symptoms of cholangitis in childhood or early adult life. Generally the entire liver is involved, but cyst distribution may be lobar (particularly the left lobe) or segmental. The cysts are 1 to 4.5 cm in diameter and are separated by portions of relatively normal bile duct. The dilated ducts are lined by cuboidal or columnar epithelium, which may be ulcerated or focally hyperplastic; gallstones may be found in the duct lumen. The duct wall is usually fibrotic, with varying degrees of acute and chronic inflammation. Occasionally, distinguishing this condition from primary sclerosing cholangitis (PSC) may be difficult. Cholangiocarcinoma, preceded by epithelial dysplasia, may complicate this disorder in 7% to 14% of cases (50,61,62).

CHF and the hepatic lesion of ARPKD are also classified as communicating ductal cysts, although macroscopic cysts are rare (32,45,52). The entire liver is typically affected, but involvement may be lobar or segmental. The hepatic lesions arise as the result of ductal plate malformation at the level of the interlobular bile ducts, leading to a distinctive noninflamed (unless complicated by cholangits) fibrous enlargement and bridging of portal tracts that contain abnormally shaped bile ducts, often with inspissated bile (identical to those in bile duct hamartoma), an increased number of arterial vessels, and a paucity of portal vein structures (45). Whether these two entities are distinct or represent different clinical presentations of the same disorder is unclear. Cholangiocarcinoma has been reported (50,63).

Multiple Hilar Cysts (Peribiliary Gland Cysts)

Extrahepatic and large intrahepatic bile ducts in the region of the hilum contain peribiliary glands (64). Although about 20% of autopsies demonstrate noncommunicating cystic dilatation of these glands, it is generally an incidental microscopic finding. The cysts may be as large as 2 cm, however, and detectable on radiography. From time to time, symptoms result from compression of the adjacent bile duct, resulting in obstructive jaundice. The cysts are unilocular and frequently multiple, often imparting a spongy appearance to the parenchyma. They are lined by columnar to cuboidal epithelium and contain clear serous fluid. The regions surrounding the cysts often demonstrate mild chronic inflammation, fibrosis, and fibrous obliteration of small veins. The cyst lining may become hyperplastic. The most commonly associated conditions include chronic advanced liver disease (typically cirrhosis), portal vein thrombosis, and ADPKD (adult polycystic liver disease). Some mucinous cystadenomas and hilar cholangiocarcinomas may arise from peribiliary glands (64).

Other Nonparasitic Cysts

Pseudocysts are often delimited by fibrous tissue but do not have an epithelial lining. They may be quite large, often contain blood and/or bile (biloma), and can become secondarily infected. Trauma (traumatic cysts), either extrinsic or iatrogenic (such as stems from endoscopic retrograde cholangiopancreatography), ischemia, and hepatic involvement by a pancreatic pseudocyst are possible causes (2,32,65). Definitive histologic distinction of these pseudocysts from unilocular biliary-derived cysts with degenerative changes generally is not possible. *Intrahepatic ileal and duodenal duplication cysts have been described (66), and ciliated hepatic foregut cysts have been discussed previously (47). The few cases reported as hepatic endometrioma most likely represent biliary cystadenomas (67).*

Neoplastic Cysts

Biliary (Hepatobiliary) Cystadenoma and Cystadenocarcinoma

Mucinous Type

Nearly all biliary cystadenomas are of the mucinous type; this is the lesion referred to when the term biliary cystadenoma is used in an unqualified fashion (2,3,42,68,69). This type makes up 5% of all solitary cysts; they are multilocular and lined by cuboidal or columnar, mucin-secreting epithelium (similar to bile duct or gastric foveolar epithelium) and are analogous to mucinous cystadenomas of the pancreas (70). About 95% of cases develop in women (69), and the distinctive dense, spindle-cell or "ovarian-like" stroma is found only in this sex. The mean age at initial diagnosis is 45 years (range, 2 to 87 years). Patients show initial symptoms of abdominal pain, an abdominal mass, and, occasionally, jaundice. Mucinous cystadenomas are intrahepatic in 84% of cases; the remainder are found in the common bile duct (6%), hepatic ducts (4%), cystic duct (4%), and gallbladder (2%) (69).

Calcification is visible on CT scan in about 20% of cases, sometimes leading to diagnostic confusion with echinococcal cysts (71). Elevated levels in cyst fluid and serum of CA 19-9, as well as carcinoembryonic antigen (CEA) in mucinous cystadenoma/cystadenocarcinoma may aid in distinguishing these cysts from nonmucinous cystic lesions and serve as adjuncts to FNA cytology diagnosis (72,73). Elevated CA 19-9 levels to date have been detected only in cases with an ovarian-like stroma (73).

Intrahepatic mucinous biliary cystadenomas are encapsulated and solitary (Fig. 3). They are 2.5 to 28 cm in diameter (mean, 15 cm) and contain fluid (up to several liters), which is usually clear and mucinous but is sometimes described as brown, serous, bilious, gelatinous, or frankly hemorrhagic. The internal surface is customarily smooth, with a few trabeculations or polypoid cystic projections. Rarely, intracystic gallstones are noted. Individual locules vary from a few millimeters to 18 cm in diameter. The multilocular nature of the cyst may be identified only microscopically in about 25% of cases (3). Superimposed malignancy should be suspected if there are nodules of solid tissue.

On microscopic examination, these mucinous biliary cystadenomas have characteristic features. The lining epithelium contains basally oriented nuclei and, often, apical mucin. The epithelium may be focally flattened, denuded, or pseudostratified, and may manifest squamous cells on occasion. Intestinal metaplasia (goblet cells, occasionally with Paneth cells) can be found in about 20% of cases, and neuroendocrine cells (chromogranin immunoreactivity) can be

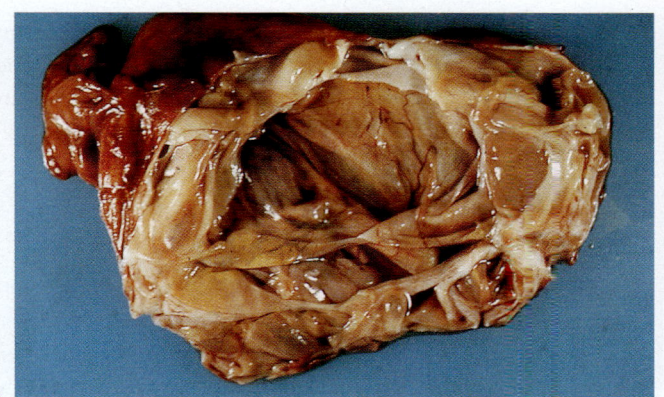
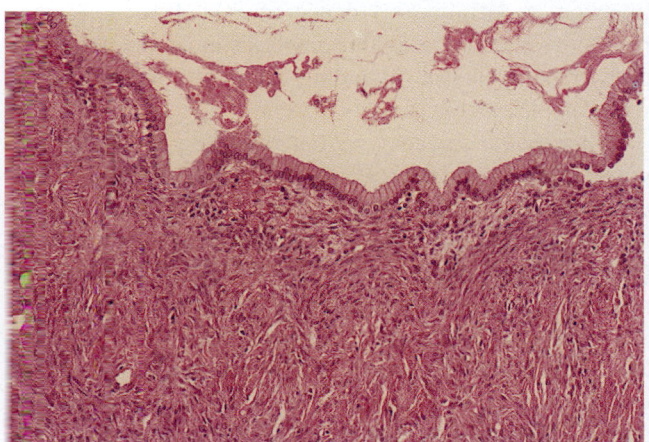

FIG. 3. Biliary cystadenoma. **A:** Biliary cystadenomas are multilocular by definition. **B:** Photomicrograph demonstrates a columnar mucin-containing epithelial lining with a dense spindle-cell (mesenchymal or ovarian-like) stroma. The epithelial lining may be cuboidal or flattened, without mucin or focally denuded.

identified in about one-third of cases (59). In one series (69), 10% of cases showed signs of dysplasia (low grade) and in some classifications would be called borderline malignancy (69,70). In regions of ulceration, lipofuscin- or hemosiderin-laden macrophages, cholesterol clefts with foreign body giant-cell reaction, or focal calcification can be noted.

The dense subepithelial spindle-cell stroma (85% of cases), while resembling normal ovarian stroma, is likely related to recapitulation of the primordial biliary tree, perhaps with the female hormonal milieu serving as a promoter. The spindle-cell stroma can be quite focal and may contain areas of smooth muscle and mature adipose tissue (3,68,69,74). Immunoreactivity for muscle-specific actin is usually present; less often desmin can be detected. A focal, linear, subepithelial, hyalinized, collagenous zone (similar to that seen in collagenous colitis) is often seen just above the dense stroma. The adventitial or capsular layer, which may be incomplete, is composed of dense collagen and separates the cystadenoma from the surrounding liver. It often contains many blood vessels. Anomalous bile ducts may be evident.

Cystadenocarcinomas are rare hepatic malignancies, accounting for 1% of primary hepatic carcinomas (75). They are encountered with nearly equal frequency in men and women, almost two decades later than cystadenomas. About 30% of cases have a spindle-cell stroma (always in women), while one-half (nearly all women) have benign foci identical to cystadenoma. The available data suggest that an intestinal metaplasia-dysplasia-carcinoma sequence may be operative in many cases, similar to that seen elsewhere in the biliary tract (69).

Although solid foci on macroscopic evaluation are the best clue of possible malignant change in a cystadenoma and should guide sectioning, appropriate processing requires extensive sectioning (about one section per centimeter). The cystadenocarcinomas most often demonstrate a tubulopapillary intracystic component with invasive glands, although solid foci may be present (Fig. 4). Adenosquamous, pure squamous, hepatoid, oncocyte-like, and spindle-cell features may infrequently be identified (3,69,76–78). While stromal invasion is definitive evidence of cystadenocarcinoma, many investigators make this diagnosis in its absence when high-grade dysplasia (including carcinoma *in situ*), often with complex architecture, is present.

A borderline category, as noted earlier, has been proposed. Akin to the pancreas, some researchers might regard all hepatic mucinous cystic neoplasms to be of uncertain malignant potential, particularly incompletely resected lesions. Given these nosologic problems, the surgical pathology report should state the criteria used by the pathologist to arrive at a given diagnostic rubric. The possibility that the hepatic lesion represents a metastasis from similar neoplasms arising in the pancreas, ovary, or appendix should always be considered when evaluating these lesions.

Complete excision of a cystadenoma, the treatment of choice, is nearly always curative, but delayed recurrence after 32 years has been reported (79). Subtotal excision often

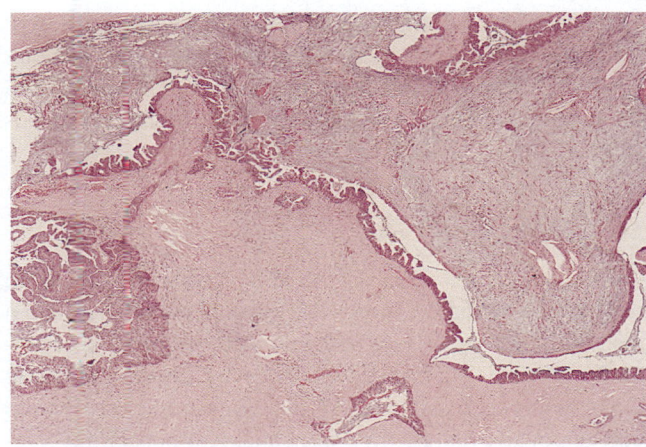

FIG. 4. Biliary cystadenocarcinoma. Complex, often papillary intraluminal architecture is often noted with high-grade dysplasia. In the absence of definitive stromal invasion (which may be difficult to detect), some investigators might classify this tumor as "borderline" or "of uncertain malignant potential."

results in persistent disease. About 50% of patients with cystadenocarcinoma survive up to four years; the presence of a spindle-cell stroma appears to identify a group with a good prognosis (69).

Serous (Microcystic or Glycogen-rich) Type

Serous cystadenomas, consisting of small cystic spaces lined by flattened, bland cells with clear, glycogen-rich, mucin-negative cytoplasm identical to their pancreatic counterparts, have infrequently been described as primary hepatic tumors (2,69). The dense spindle-cell stroma characteristic of most biliary (mucinous) cystadenomas is absent. Histopathologic distinction from a hepatic metastasis of the extremely rare pancreatic serous cystadenocarcinoma (only two reported cases) is impossible; therefore, clinical correlation is suggested (80).

Papillary and Cystic Tumor

A single case of a primary hepatic tumor identical in terms of histologic and ultrastructural evidence to papillary and cystic tumor of the pancreas has been reported in a 41-year-old woman in the absence of tumor in the pancreas or elsewhere (81).

Teratoma (And Other Germ Cell Tumors)

Hepatic teratomas are uncommon (2,3). Women and girls are more frequently affected than men and boys, and most patients have been less than 1 year old. The tumors are often large, cystic, and calcified. At the microscopic level, one finds derivatives of all three germ layers; the cyst lining is either ectodermal, with skin appendages, or endodermal. Outcomes are variable, although long-term survival has been reported. Primary yolk sac tumor and choriocarcinoma as well as cases of combined hepatoblastoma (HBL) or hepatocellular carcinoma (HCC) with germ cell tumors have been reported (82–84). Occasionally, distinguishing germ cell tumors from HBL may be difficult (5,85,86).

Mesenchymal Hamartoma

Clinical Features

Mesenchymal hamartoma makes up about 8% of all pediatric tumors and is the second most common benign pediatric tumor (5,6,87,88) (Table 24). Seventy percent of patients are male, and three-quarters of the patients show symptoms by 1 year of age. Rare cases in adults have been described (89). Although typically within the normal range or minimally elevated, the serum AFP level can be markedly increased (87,90). While the exact pathogenesis of this tumor is unknown, theories include aberrant development of primitive mesenchyme in portal tracts associated with ductal plate malformation (2,45), an ischemic source (91), and a neoplastic process (92). Reports of a specific translocation involving chromosome 19q, the presence of aneuploidy in a minority of cases, and association with undifferentiated (embryonal) sarcoma in two cases give some support to the latter theory (90,92).

Pathologic Findings

The tumor is solitary and well circumscribed, varies in size from 5 to 23 cm, and is most frequently found in the right lobe (3,5,6,88). About 20% of cases are pedunculated. Multiple grossly visible cysts, ranging in size from a few millimeters to 14 cm, are present in more than 90% of cases. The tumors become fibrotic with age and may be multilocular, simulating a biliary cystadenoma. The cysts, which contain clear or mucoid fluid, alternate with solid, pink-white areas. On microscopic examination, one sees an admixture of different cell types. Primitive mesenchymal tissue consists of bland stellate and spindle cells embedded in a myxoid matrix with a variable amount of collagen. Electron microscopic and immunohistochemical analysis of the spindle-cell stroma (vimentin, desmin, and actin positive) reveals features suggestive of myofibroblasts (93). Fluid accumulation may lead to an alveolar pattern, simulating a lymphangioma (Fig. 5). Foci of extramedullary hematopoiesis are found in nearly 90% of cases. Proliferation of thick-walled veins may focally resemble a vascular malformation.

Hepatocytes are often found in small plates at the periphery of the lesion or as small nodules or single cells more centrally. Bile ducts, often with unusual contours and a branching pattern reminiscent of ductal plate malformation, are found within the stroma. Frequently they have a mesenchymal "collar" when they are located at the tumor periphery, where they may form satellite extensions into the uninvolved parenchyma. The biliary epithelium may show atrophic or degenerative changes, and a periductal neutrophilic infiltrate

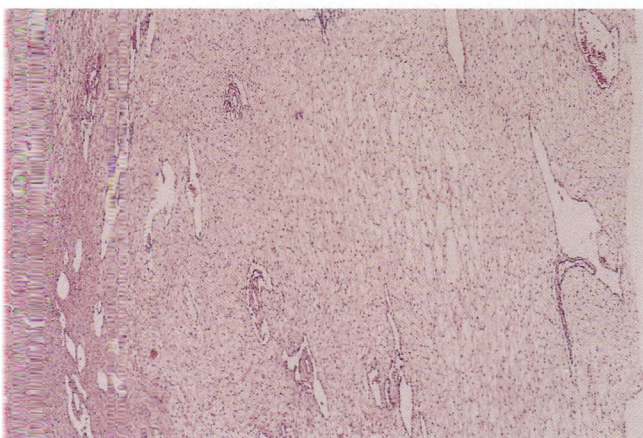

FIG. 5. Mesenchymal hamartoma. The bland stellate and spindle cells are present in a myxoid matrix. Pools of fluid impart an alveolar pattern that has been confused with lymphangioma.

may be present. The cysts, on microscopic inspection, represent microscopically either dilated bile ducts with a flattened epithelial lining or pools of fluid in regions of degenerating mesenchyme.

FNA cytologic findings include an abundant mucoid basophilic background with scattered individual cells or loose cell clusters. Most of the cells are oval to spindle-shaped, with round to oval nuclei demonstrating evenly distributed chromatin and inconspicuous nucleoli (89). Because myxoid foci may occasionally be abundant in IHE, this tumor must also be considered in the differential diagnosis (3,6,88). Features helpful in differentiating mesenchymal hamartoma from undifferentiated (embryonal) sarcoma are summarized in Table 24.

Total excision is curative, although the mortality rate at operation can be high (7% to 17%). While recurrence of incompletely resected lesions has not been reported (88), the coexistence of mesenchymal hamartoma and undifferentiated sarcoma in two adolescents (92) makes one hesitant about the practice of performing incomplete excision or marsupialization in surgically difficult cases (87).

EPITHELIAL TUMORS

Benign and Borderline Hepatocellular Tumors

These masses are best separated into those that arise in livers which are normal or near normal and those that are associated with chronic liver disease (generally cirrhosis) (4). Needle biopsies obtained from any of these lesions may simply demonstrate bland hepatocytes and therefore may be indistinguishable from one another and from normal liver. In the normal liver, FNH and HCA are most common; nodular regenerative hyperplasia (NRH) is encountered less frequently as a mass in clinical practice. In the cirrhotic liver, macroregenerative nodules (MRNs) and those nodules that appear to have acquired some, but not all of the histologic features of HCC (borderline or dysplastic nodules) are the important diagnostic considerations. While in resection specimens precise classification of each of these nodules is usually straightforward, in biopsy specimens their specific classification and distinction from WD-HCC can be challenging. Pinpointing a specific diagnosis of benign hepatocellular tumors by FNA is generally not feasible (11). The possibility of clinically occult chronic liver disease must be always considered by the pathologist thus emphasizing the importance of open dialogue with the involved clinicians. Major points of differential diagnosis are summarized in Table 4.

Compensatory segmental or *lobar hyperplasia* is usually associated with disproportionate atrophy (collapse), necrosis, or fibrosis of other lobes where there has been venous or major bile duct occlusion. Caudate lobe enlargement in the Budd-Chiari syndrome is one example that occurs because of independent venous drainage (2,4,42,94). *Accessory lobes*, which are a developmental anomaly, may appear as hepatic masses, but they rarely cause difficulty in diagnosis.

Hepatocellular Adenoma

Clinical Features

HCA (Table 4) is a benign hepatocellular neoplasm that arises in a normal or nearly normal liver, almost always in the context of an abnormal hormonal or metabolic milieu. Diagnosis of so-called spontaneous HCA should be made only with great caution, since these neoplasms may represent WD-HCC (3,4). Ninety-five percent of HCAs develop in women, usually in their child-bearing years (peak, third and fourth decades). HCAs are quite rare in children, in whom they account for 2% to 4% of all hepatic tumors (5–6a). Oral contraceptive steroid (OCS) usage is by far the most common associated factor in women; 85% to 90% of patients have typically used oral contraceptives for more than 5 years (94a–97) (Table 4). There is a general feeling that the risk of OCS-related HCA may be declining in the current era of low-dose estrogen preparations (98).

HCA is also associated with sex hormone imbalance in the context of the use of anabolic/androgenic steroids (usually 17-alpha-alkylated variants used to treat hypogonadism and chronic anemia and taken by body builders) and anti-estrogens, such as danazol and clomiphene, and in Klinefelter's syndrome and other disorders that lead to increased endogenous sex steroids (3,96,99–102). Patients with apparent HCA, no history of estrogen or androgen use, and no metabolic disease should probably be investigated for abnormal secretion of sex steroids (101). Associated metabolic disorders include glycogen storage disease (most commonly type Ia), familial diabetes mellitus, and Hurler's disease (102–104). Rare associations with severe combined immunodeficiency (104) and familial adenomatous polyposis have been reported (105).

Patients with HCA often show initial signs of acute abdominal pain, which most often stems from intratumoral hemorrhage. Intraperitoneal rupture occurs in less than one-third of patients and is frequently associated with shock (3,95,96,106–108). About one-third of patients have an abdominal mass; only occasionally (less than 10% to 20%) is HCA an incidental finding. Serum AFP levels are within the normal range. Rare associations include AA amyloidosis (109) and production of adenocorticotropic hormone with elevated cortisol levels (110).

Pathologic Findings

Macroscopic Features

HCA is most commonly found as a solitary (70% to 80%), often subcapsular, sharply demarcated or encapsulated mass (3,95,96,104,107) in the right lobe of an otherwise normal liver (Fig. 6A). It is pedunculated in 10% of cases. The size is quite variable (1 to 38 cm), but the majority are larger than 10 cm in diameter. HCAs arising in association with androgen use or metabolic disease are more frequently multiple (3,96,104). The cut surface has a variegated appearance, related to the proportion of viable tan hepatocellular component, yellow necrotic foci, white infarcted areas, and red blood clot. The tumor is generally more pale than the adjacent nonneoplastic parenchyma. Now and then, excessive lipofuscin accumulation causes the tumor to have a slate-gray or black appearance, or bile production imparts a green hue. Fibrous septa (3,95,107) or a multilobated appearance (111) are uncommon macroscopic features. Rare cases of coexistent FNH are well documented (2).

Microscopic Features

HCA is a neoplasm composed of normal-sized or slightly enlarged hepatocytes in cords that are one to two cells thick. By definition, bile ducts, ductules, and portal tracts are absent within HCA, but thin-walled veins, often accompanied by arterial branches, are frequently distributed throughout the tumor (Fig. 6B). Although the hepatocellular cords are frequently closely approximated, giving a sheetlike appearance, they are actually separated by sinusoids that contain inconspicuous Kupffer cells (112). Little sinusoidal CD34 immunoreactivity was identified in one case report (113). The reticulin framework is generally intact, but it may be focally decreased (2,4). Hepatocellular rosettes (pseudoglands) may be found in association with bile production.

The hepatocytes of HCA possess acidophilic, clear or vacuolated (glycogen or fat), or hydropic cytoplasm that may contain a variable amount of lipofuscin or, less commonly, hemosiderin. PAS-positive, diastase-resistant globules or granules may be found; these are often positive by the immunoperoxidase technique for alpha$_1$-antitrypsin (A$_1$AT) but not for AFP. Megamitochondria and Mallory's hyalin in association with steatonecrosis have been reported (2,3,114). The tumor cell nuclei are round, usually single, and similar in size to those of the adjacent nonneoplastic liver. Multinucleation has been described in about 10% of cases, but the nuclei are bland and unlike the tumor giant cells of HCC (3).

TABLE 4. *Clinical and pathologic features helpful in the differential diagnosis of benign and malignant hepatocellular tumors in adults and children*

Features	Associated cirrhosis/chronic liver disease						
	Absent					Present	
	HCA	FNH	NRH	Fetal HBL[a]	MRN[b]	Usual HCC[c]
Clinical						
Peak age (decade)	3rd–4th	3rd–4th	5th–7th	1st (90% ≤ 5 yrs)	5th–6th	6th–7th (U.S.A.)
M/F	1:15	1:6–15	1:1	2:1	2–3:1	3–4:1 (U.S.A.)
Usual presentation	Acute abdominal pain	Asymptomatic	Portal hypertension	Abdominal mass	Screening for HCC	Abdominal pain, mass; screening
Associated conditions	OCS use (85–90%), androgens, metabolic disorders	OCS use (66–95%), cavernous hemangioma, multiple FNH syndrome[d]	CT disease, myelolymphoproliferative disorders, drugs/toxins, vascular disorders, other	5% congenital anomaly, FAP		
Serum AFP	Normal range	Normal range	Normal range	90% elevated	Normal range or range of chronic liver disease	60–80% elevated
Macroscopic						
Number of nodules	70–80% single	70–80% single	Numerous	70–80% single	Usually >1	Usually >1
Nodule diameter	75% ≥10 cm	75–80% ≤5 cm	0.1–4+ cm	50% 10–12 cm	90% <1.5 cm	Variable
Cut surface often	Tan-white, often hemorrhagic	Tan, nodular, rarely hemorrhagic or dilated vessels[d]	Tan-white, rarely hemorrhagic	Tan-brown, green, necrotic	Similar to adjacent liver; may be paler or bile stained	Tan-grey, green, necrotic
Fibrous septa/scar	Rare	Usually present	Absent	Absent	Absent	Absent
Microscopic						
Portal tracts	Absent	Absent	Present ± portal venopathy	Absent	Present, often distorted	Absent
Hepatocyte plate thickness	1–2 cells (sheet like)	1–2 cells	1–2 cells	2–3 cells, alternating light/dark pattern	1–2 cells	Typically >3 cells
Nuclear atypia, macronucleoli	Rare	Absent	Rare	Absent or rare	Absent	Present
Mitoses	Absent or rare	Absent	Absent	Rare or absent	Absent[d]	Common
Septa (arteries, bile ductules, inflammation; few portal veins, bile ducts)	Absent	Present	Rare (large nodules)	Absent	May be present	Absent
Nontriadal (intranodular) arteries	Common	Absent or rare	Rare (large nodules)	—	Absent or rare	Common
Hepatocytes inside and outside nodule vary in size, plate arrangement	Absent	Absent	Present	Absent	Possible[e]	Absent

AFP, alpha-fetoprotein; CT, connective tissue; FAP, familial adenomatous polyposis; FNH, focal nodular hyperplasia; HBL, hepatoblastoma; HCA, hepatocellular adenoma; HCC, hepatocellular carcinoma; MRN, macroregenerative nodule; NRH, nodular regenerative hyperplasia; OCS, oral contraceptive steroids.

[a] Clinical and macroscopic data are given for HBL in general, with histologic data solely for fetal component.
[b] Data contrasting MRN with borderline nodule and well-differentiated HCC found in Table 5.
[c] "Usual" in this table refers to moderately differentiated (grades 2–3) HCC and does not include the fibrolamellar variant. (See Table 15 for this variant.) Only 10–30% of usual HCCs arise in a normal liver.
[d] Two or more FNHs plus one or more of the following: hepatic hemangioma, systemic structural arterial defects, or brain tumors, such as meningioma or astrocytoma (see text for further details).
[e] Associated large portal vein occlusion could cause a diffuse nodular hyperplasia pattern within an MRN.

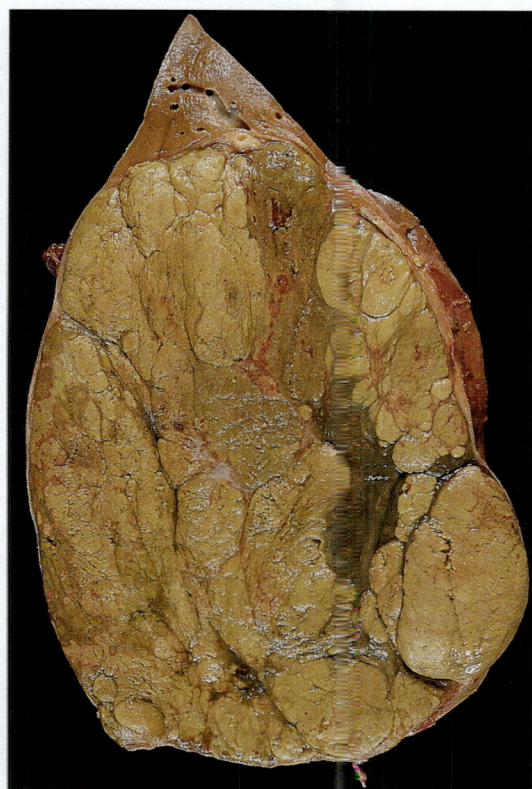
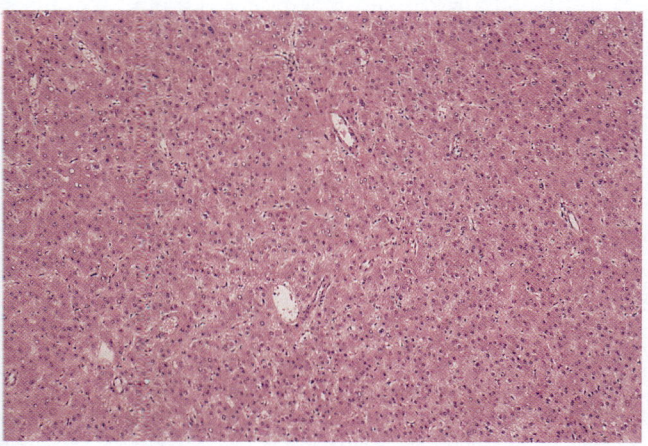

FIG. 6. Hepatocellular adenoma (HCA). **A:** Large HCA with foci of necrosis and hemorrhage that give it a lobulated appearance. (Kindly contributed by Robert E. Lee, M.D., University of Pittsburgh Medical Center, Pittsburgh, PA.) **B:** At the microscopic level, this neoplasm demonstrates cords and sheets of cytologically bland hepatocytes without portal tracts or bile ducts (for exceptions, see text). Within the mass, arterial and venous channels are unassociated with fibrous septa. A definitive diagnosis of HCA should not be made on a biopsy specimen, since histologic evaluation of the completely excised lesion is required to rule out well-differentiated hepatocellular carcinoma. The serum alpha-fetoprotein level should be within the normal reference range.

Nucleoli are generally inconspicuous and the intranuclear vacuoles frequently seen in HCC are absent. Focal cellular pleomorphism and prominent nucleoli may occasionally be noted, particularly in long-standing lesions. Mitoses are virtually never seen, and blood vessel invasion is absent. To date, p53 immunoreactivity has not been identified (115). Extramedullary hematopoiesis and noncaseating epithelioid granulomas are rarely found (2,96). The so-called oncocytic liver cell adenoma may represent an oncocytic variant of HCC (116).

Various degenerative changes have been described in HCA. Dilated sinusoids and larger blood-filled (peliotic) spaces may occasionally be noted. From time to time a myxoid stroma has been seen (117). Areas of necrosis, infarction, and hematoma may develop, particularly in the center of the tumor. Organization of these foci may lead to the accumulation of hemosiderin-laden macrophages and the formation of fibrous scars with a lamellar pattern (3). Blood vessels at the periphery of HCA often show characteristic changes. Arteries demonstrate myxoid degeneration and fibrosis of the intima with reduplication of the internal elastic lamina, while marked smooth-muscle proliferation may cause venous luminal obliteration. Occasionally, thrombosis may occur.

Androgen-related hepatocellular tumors, which are typically multiple, may appear on histologic evidence to be identical to the usual adenoma or demonstrate marked cellular pleomorphism, prominent nucleoli, and extensive pseudogland formation, thus resembling HCC (3,96,99,100,102). Peliosis hepatis and cholestasis are often present in the adjacent liver. The absence of a classic trabecular pattern, a relatively low nuclear to cytoplasmic ratio, and the absence of vascular invasion aid in making the histopathologic distinction from HCC. Since most of these tumors regress with androgen withdrawal and well-documented reports of metastasizing lesions are rare, it appears reasonable to consider most of these tumors that resemble HCC as atypical HCA unless the serum AFP level is elevated, cirrhosis is present (potentially related to transfusion-associated chronic viral hepatitis), clear-cut histologic features of malignancy are evident, or there are well-documented metastases.

While some investigators have distinguished those patients with numerous (usually more than ten) apparent adenomas as a distinct clinicopathologic group (those with multiple hepatocellular adenomatosis or liver adenomatosis) (118), it is believed that many of these cases represent other entities, such as NRH, the multiple FNH syndrome, regenerative nodules, or WD-HCC (4). Making the distinction between patients with multiple, rigidly defined adenomas and those with only one mass does not appear warranted.

Differential Diagnosis, Treatment, and Outcome

Radiographic findings, such as decreased or absent uptake on scintigraphy, centripetal hypervascularity with a central hypovascular region on angiography, and the absence of a central scar on CT or MRI aid in distinguishing HCA from FNH. In a significant number of cases, however, a precise diagnosis cannot be made, and differentiating HCA from HCC also remains a problem (9,98,106–108). The definitive diagnosis often rests with the pathologist. Discriminating HCA (Table 4) from other benign hepatocellular tumors, HCC, and possibly normal liver may be impossible with small tissue biopsies and FNA or at the time of frozen section (11,98). Foci of well-differentiated (grade 1) HCC and areas of FNH (particularly the progressive type) may be indistinguishable from HCA (2,101,119,120). It is therefore prudent not to make a definitive diagnosis of HCA on any biopsy or incompletely excised specimen with bland hepatocytes. A combination of clinical (normal serum AFP level, age more than 3 years old, presence of metabolic disease) and histologic features (larger cell size and the absence of an alternating light and dark cytoplasmic pattern) favors HCA over pure fetal HBL.

Certain situations may cause diagnostic confusion between HCA and FNH. Large HCA may be associated with conspicuous compression artifact of the adjacent liver at the interface with the mass, characterized by portal tracts with chronic inflammation, bile ductule proliferation, and the formation of short fibrous septa (96). Portal tracts may become trapped within the periphery of HCA. The location of these structures, which include portal vein branches and interlobular bile ducts (which are lacking in FNH) as well as hepatic artery branches, resolves any diagnostic problem. The presence of fibrous scars in HCA could cause diagnostic confusion. The lack of arteries and bile ductules in these scars distinguishes them from the fibrous septa of FNH. The absence of large oncocytic hepatocytes with prominent nucleoli aids in differentiating HCA from FL-HCC. Pseudoglandular spaces in HCA should not be misconstrued as interlobular bile ducts.

There have been several reports of regression of HCA after withdrawal of OCS, but this is not always the case. The possibility of rupture persists; this complication is almost always the cause of the sporadic deaths related to this tumor (96,106–108). While malignant transformation of HCA is considered rare, few unresected cases have had long-term follow-up (4,111,121–125). It has recently been estimated that about 10% of unresected HCAs will go on to develop HCC (125). This may take place many years after the original diagnosis, even after OCS withdrawal and apparent HCA resolution. The risk of HCC developing in the context of HCA related to glycogen storage disease type Ia is well known and generally affects young adult men (103).

Because it appears likely that HCA represents the precursor lesion for many HCCs arising in the normal liver (similar to the situation of macroregenerative and dysplastic nodules in the cirrhotic liver) (Fig. 14), HCAs should be completely excised if it is technically feasible. In the circumstance of very large or multiple lesions, liver transplantation can be considered (60,106–108). Close follow-up of patients with HCAs that have been incompletely excised, demonstrate cellular pleomorphism, or arise in the absence of exogenous hormones is indicated because of incomplete data regarding their natural history.

Focal Nodular Hyperplasia

Clinical Features

FNH (Table 4) is found mainly in women of reproductive age (80% to 95%; peak, third and fourth decades). Overall, 7% to 15% of cases occur in the pediatric age group, in which FNH represents 2% to 10% of all pediatric hepatic tumors (3,4,6A,94–96,98,106–108,126,127). An association with glycogen storage disease type Ia has been reported (128). FNH is most frequently detected as an incidental finding (50% to 80%) at the time of laparotomy, during radiographic investigation of another disorder, or at autopsy, where it is identified in about 1% of cases (129). An abdominal mass (10% to 15%) is the most common complaint in symptomatic patients. Oral contraceptive use, reported in 65% to 95% of cases, may promote FNH growth but does not appear to induce FNH formation. Generally these tumors remain static over time, but upon occasion they can significantly increase in size (progressive type) (119). Serum AFP levels are within the normal range.

FNH appears to represent a local hyperplastic response of hepatocytes to a vascular anomaly, particularly an arterial malformation, although associations with portal vein atresia and spontaneous intrahepatic portosystemic shunt have been reported (4,119,126,129). Although FNH overall has been found with coexisting hepatic cavernous hemangiomas (CHs) in about 20% of cases (129,130), multiple FNHs more frequently have this association. Patients with multiple FNHs who have one or more other lesions, including hepatic hemangioma, systemic arterial structural defects (arterial dysplasia, Klippel-Trenaunay-Weber syndrome, brain telangiectasia, and berry aneurysm), or brain tumors (astrocytoma and meningioma), are considered to have the multiple FNH syndrome (4,129,131). Portal hypertension may be present. Hepatic nodules in patients with Osler-Weber-Rendu disease, the Budd-Chiari syndrome, and cirrhosis (LRNs) may resemble FNH, but in light of the fact that the surrounding liver is not normal, by definition these are not considered FNH ("FNH-like" nodules) (4).

Pathologic Findings

Macroscopic Features

FNH most often appears as a solitary (70% to 80%) subcapsular, circumscribed but unencapsulated, bulging, tan, nodular mass that typically is less than 5 cm in diameter (Fig. 7A). Infrequently, FNHs may be larger than 10 to 20 cm and occupy an entire lobe. Less than 5% are pedunculated. The surrounding liver is essentially normal. The mass is characteristically dissected into multiple smaller nodules by fibrous septa that, in the majority of cases, join to form one or more central or eccentric retracted scars. Lesions smaller than 1 cm often lack a central scar, while multiple scars are more common in large tumors (4). Hemorrhage, necrosis, and infarction are unusual findings; they are typically associated with oral contraceptive use. Macroscopic

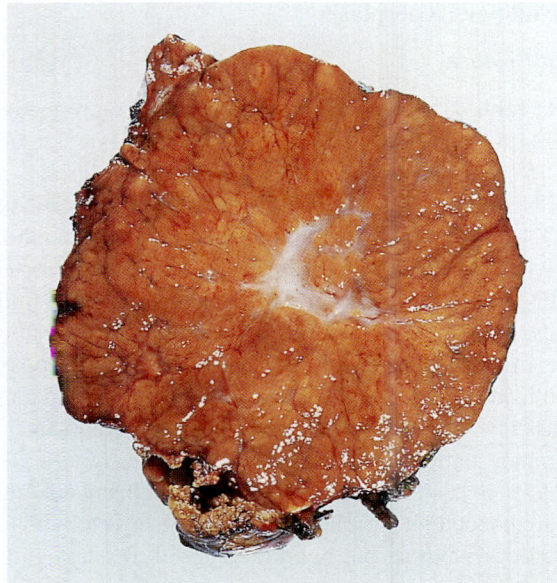

FIG. 7. Focal nodular hyperplasia (FNH), solid (usual) type. **A:** Note the central stellate scar and tan, nodular parenchyma. **B:** Low-power view shows "cirrhosis-like" architecture surrounding a central fibrous body with tortuous blood vessels (trichrome). **C:** The fibrous septa contain many bile ductules in the region of the limiting plate and a mixed acute and chronic inflammatory infiltrate simulating biliary-type cirrhosis. Note the presence of large arterial branches and the absence of an interlobular bile duct and portal vein. Hepatocyte plates are one to two cells thick. When all characteristic histologic findings are present in a needle biopsy of a mass in an otherwise normal liver in a patient with a normal serum alpha-fetoprotein level, the diagnosis "suggestive of FNH" can be made. The clinician, however, should be aware of several caveats (see text).

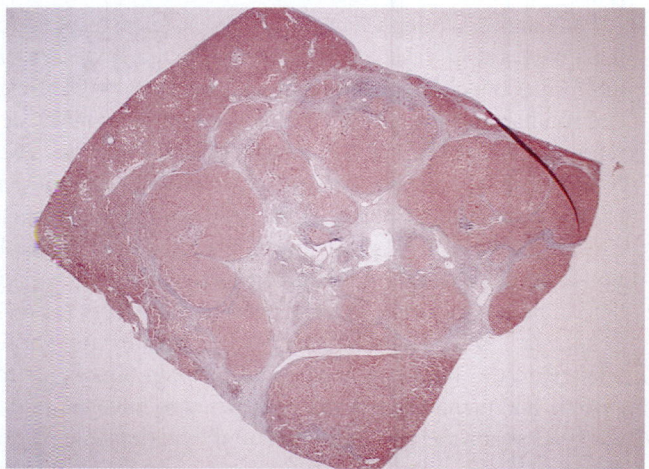
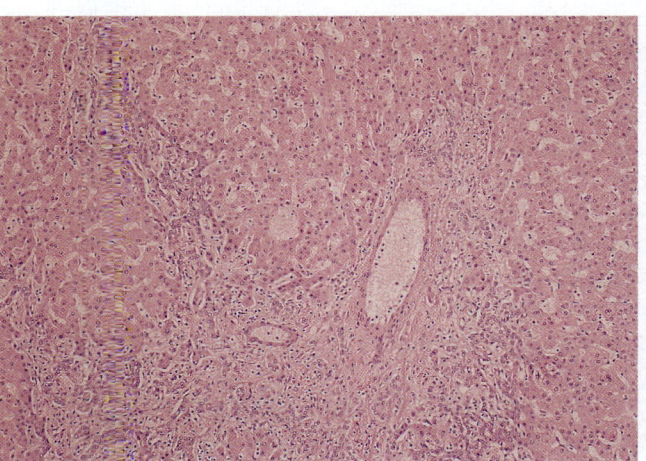

bile staining is virtually never seen unless FNH is coincidentally associated with extrahepatic biliary obstruction. This lack of bile staining is a helpful diagnostic feature that aids in making the distinction between FNH and FL-HCC, which is frequently bile-stained. Rare cases of coexistent FNH and HCA are well documented (2). The telangiectatic type of FNH is distinguished in macroscopic features from the much more common solid type described earlier by the presence of multiple dilated vascular channels in the center of the mass, which may resemble hemangioma or peliosis. This variant is more frequently found in the multiple FNH syndrome (4,129).

Microscopic Features

FNH has a uniform internal structure characterized by nodules of hepatocytes surrounded by fibrous/fibromyxoid septa that contain artery branches, bile ductules at the parenchymal interface in association with chronic and/or acute inflammation, and a distinct paucity or absence of interlobular bile ducts and portal vein branches (Fig. 7B,C). The degree of bile ductule proliferation is variable but sometimes is quite excessive and simulates a bile duct adenoma. The ductules appear to arise from the limiting plate region, possibly from undifferentiated progenitor cells or from ductular metaplasia of hepatocytes (132). The normal hepatic acinar structure is lacking; hence, portal tracts and terminal veins are absent. In the region of the scar(s), the collagen is quite dense, and numerous thick-walled arteries, which often demonstrate fibromuscular hyperplasia and myxoid degeneration, are noted (2–4,95,96). Rarely, lone arterial branches with scanty stroma are seen in the parenchyma within a few millimeters of the adjacent septa (119). In the telangiectatic variant, numerous small, dilated vessels (resembling hemangioma) are seen centrally, and the adjacent sinusoids are markedly dilated (4,129).

The hepatocellular nodule consists of a proliferation of 1- to 2-cell-thick hepatocyte plates separated by sinusoids containing inconspicuous endothelial and Kupffer cells with an intact reticulin framework. In the periseptal region the sinusoids may become capillarized. In size and overall appearance, the hepatocytes themselves are similar to those in the surrounding liver, although they may be somewhat larger and paler and may incorporate variable quantities of fat or glycogen. PAS-positive hyaline globules or granules that contain A_1AT on immunohistochemistry have been reported (95). Histologic features of chronic cholestasis (pseudoxanthomatous change, copper deposits, Mallory's hyalin, and even small foci of bile pigment) are typically noted adjacent to the septa, presumably related to the absence of interlobular bile ducts. Therefore, the histologic features overall resemble a biliary type of cirrhosis with ductopenia and arterialized nodules. Nuclear pleomorphism, prominent nucleoli, mitotic figures, and p53 immunoreactivity (115) are not found in FNH. The polyclonal versus monoclonal nature of FNH is the subject of controversy (133).

Differential Diagnosis, Treatment, and Outcome

Since there have been no documented cases of incompletely excised or unexcised FNHs that subsequently developed into HCC, even after long-term follow-up, and since FNH-related deaths are virtually unknown, a nonoperative approach is desirable in cases detected by radiography. FNH is suggested when CT or MRI shows a mass with a central scar, when angiography or Doppler ultrasound discloses centrifugal hypervascularity, or when technetium-99 sulfur colloid scan shows normal or increased uptake. One study reported a sensitivity of 70% for a preoperative diagnosis of FNH, and imaging studies were only rarely associated with false positives (98). Diagnostic confusion with HCA and HCC (especially the fibrolamellar variant, related to the presence of a central scar and, rarely, calcification in FNH), however, is well documented. If the imaging studies show conflicting results or the patient has persistent symptoms, laparotomy should be performed. In this situation, superficial lesions should be completely resected. Needle and wedge biopsies from deep lesions can be submitted for frozen section to avoid performing a technically difficult resection.

Some clinicians prefer to obtain percutaneous guided core biopsies of lesions detected on radiography, although others frown on this practice because of the risk of bleeding, problems in histologic interpretation of small biopsy fragments, and the danger of tumor tracking if the mass is subsequently found to be malignant (106–108). In resection specimens the diagnosis of FNH is usually straightforward (Table 4), but small biopsies should be interpreted with caution, using close clinicopathologic correlation. FNA biopsies are not useful to support a diagnosis of FNH (11). Clinicians should be made aware of all the diagnostic pitfalls, even when a core biopsy diagnosis is made in the optimal clinicopathologic context ("suggestive of FNH").

If the tissue specimen demonstrates only normal-appearing hepatocytes, distinguishing it from normal liver, HCA, WD-HCC, or a macroregenerative nodule may be impossible, whereas if fibrous septa and bile ductules are noted, making the distinction from cirrhosis (particularly the biliary type) becomes difficult. Arterialized fibrous septa typical of FNH are not found in HCA but may be found in chronic liver diseases, including the Budd-Chiari syndrome (4,133a). Arteries without stroma adjacent to hepatocytes (intranodular nontriadal arteries) are a rare finding in FNH (119) but are typical of HCA and borderline (dysplastic) nodules in cirrhosis. Nodular hyperplasia in a small cuff of arterialized hepatic tissue surrounding FL-HCC and potentially other hepatic masses can mimic FNH on microscopic examination; thus, sampling always becomes an issue, even when the radiologist feels that he or she is in the mass (30,31).

Treatment of patients obviously requires a flexible approach. If a nonoperative treatment is contemplated, there should be periodic follow-up, including more imaging studies, to ensure that there has been no change in mass size. Levels of serum markers, such as AFP and des-γ-carboxy-prothrombin (DCP), that might be elevated in HCC should be obtained as a baseline. All oral contraceptives should be discontinued.

Nodular Regenerative Hyperplasia (Diffuse Nodular Hyperplasia with No or Few Fibrous Septa, Nodular Transformation)

Clinical Features

NRH (Tables 4 and 5) represents a monoacinar nodular hyperplasia of hepatocytes diffusely distributed throughout the liver. It occurs in association with no or few fibrous septa, thus distinguishing it from cirrhosis (4). The rate at which NRH is found at autopsy ranges from 0.6% to 2.6% overall; the condition is present in about 5% of the elderly population. While it is usually an incidental autopsy finding (4), 38% to 57% of reported patients in two studies had associated portal hypertension (135,136), a finding that often leads to a mistaken clinical diagnosis of cirrhosis.

Patients typically show symptoms in the fifth to seventh decades of life, but NRH can develop at all ages, even in childhood (3,134–137). An ever expanding array of disorders has been associated with NRH, but occasionally none is found (Table 5). Most often there is a related connective tissue disease (particularly rheumatoid arthritis), a myeloproliferative or lymphoproliferative disorder, a vascular disorder, or previous exposure to one of several drugs/toxins typically administered after transplantation or for treatment of malignancy (134–139). There is frequently a mild to moderate elevation of the serum alkaline phosphatase level. The serum AFP level is within the normal limits, except potentially in the few reported patients with associated HCC. In one study only one-third of deaths among patients with NRH were related to liver disease (135).

TABLE 5. *Nodular regenerative hyperplasia: associated conditions[a]*

Immunologic disorders
    Connective tissue diseases
        Rheumatoid arthritis ± Felty's syndrome
        Systemic lupus erythematosis
        Progressive systemic sclerosis
        Raynaud's phenomenon
    Glomerulonephritis
    Cryoglobulinemia
    Common variable immunodeficiency
    Autoimmune hemolytic anemia
    Myasthenia gravis
    Hyper-/hypothyroidism
    Idiopathic thrombocytopenic purpura
Neoplastic disorders
    Myeloproliferative disorders
    Lymphoproliferative disorders
    Primary and secondary hepatic carcinomas
Drugs and toxins
    Azathioprine
    Chemotherapeutic agents
    Toxic oil syndrome (? adulterated rapeseed oil)
    Arsenic
    Vinyl chloride
    Corticosteroids
    Anabolic steroids
    Contraceptive steroids
Vascular disorders
    Obliterative portal venopathy
    Extrahepatic portal vein thrombosis
    Arteritis
    Hepatic venous outflow obstruction[b]
    Peliosis hepatis
    Primary pulmonary hypertension
Transplantation
    Kidney, bone marrow, liver, heart
Miscellaneous disorders
    Precirrhotic primary biliary cirrhosis and other chronic liver diseases
    Idiopathic portal hypertension and related disorders
    Generalized mastocytosis[c]
    Sarcoidosis
    Tuberculosis
    Krabbe's disease
    Down's syndrome

[a] Overlap exists among many of the indicated categories.
[b] Any cause from the hepatic venules (venoocclusive disease) all the way to the heart (congestive heart failure), either thrombotic or nonthrombotic, may result in nodular-regenerative hyperplasia. Because the nodules in these disorders may be patchy with more congestion and fibrous sepatation, some prefer to use the term nodular hyperplasia rather than nodular regenerative hyperplasia (4).
[c] Technically a myeloproliferative disorder, but not demonstrated definitively to be neoplastic.

Most cases of NRH appear to result from disturbed hepatic circulation, most commonly involving occlusion of portal vein branches, which leads to a heterogeneous blood supply. The size and distribution of the nodules is determined by the caliber of the occluded vessel. The possibility of a neoplastic process, however, has not been excluded in some cases. Although NRH has been associated with nearly 7% of cases of HCC arising in a noncirrhotic liver, it is unclear whether NRH acts as a precursor lesion or is secondary to the tumor (portal vein invasion) or results from the effects of chemotherapy (139).

Pathologic Findings

Macroscopic Features

The liver is generally of normal or low weight, although it may be heavier, particularly in patients with myeloproliferative disorders. The capsular surface is finely granular, while the parenchyma is diffusely replaced by multiple white-tan nodules separated by congested internodular parenchyma. Nodule size is typically 1 to 3 mm, but it can vary up to many centimeters in diameter (Fig. 8A). Upon occasion, hemorrhage or infarction is present in large nodules. The macroscopic appearance is often mistaken for cirrhosis or metastatic tumor. A prominence of large nodules in the perihilar region in some cases accounts for the former use of the term partial nodular transformation.

Microscopic Features

NRH has three basic histopathologic features (Fig. 8B,C): (a) nodules of hyperplastic hepatocytes (usually arising from the periportal region, each with a single, often centrally located, portal tract) distributed diffusely throughout the liver and juxtaposed with (b) regions of internodular hepatocyte atrophy (typically centrilobular), often associated with sinusoidal congestion/dilatation and compression of central veins, and (c) an absence or paucity of fibrosis, which distinguishes NRH from cirrhosis or FNH. The intranodular hepatocyte plates typically are one to two or more cells thick and show little variation in nuclear size. The hepatocytes making up small nodules appear similar to those in the surrounding parenchyma. As nodules enlarge, the hepatocytes often show an increased amount of clear or vacuolated (fat/glycogen) cytoplasm. Cholestasis, at times associated with pseudoglandular spaces (cholestatic rosettes), may be noted. Lipofuscin is absent, in contrast to the lipofuscin-laden internodular atrophic hepatocytes. Large-cell change (LCC; dysplasia) of hepatocytes is seen in less than one-half of cases (135,136). Extramedullary hematopoiesis, which may exist in the absence of a hematopoietic disorder, is a rare finding (134,135).

The different orientations of the liver cell plates in adjacent nodules and the internodular sinusoidal dilatation with hepatocyte atrophy (which may be patchy) are perhaps the best clues at scanning magnification for diagnosing NRH on hematoxylin and eosin–stained sections. A reticulin stain, which nicely highlights this pattern and the condensed reticulin fibers often seen at the periphery of the nodules, is of great utility in evaluating core biopsies. Use of this stain is

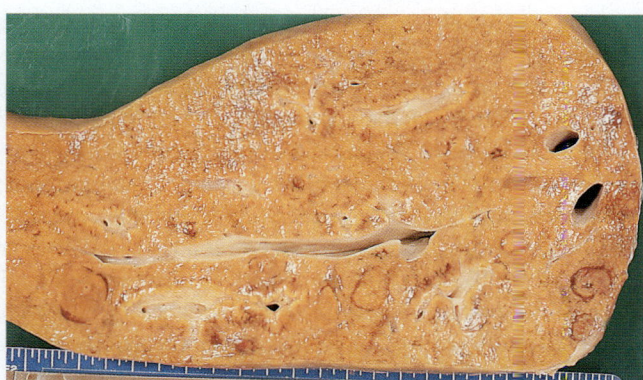
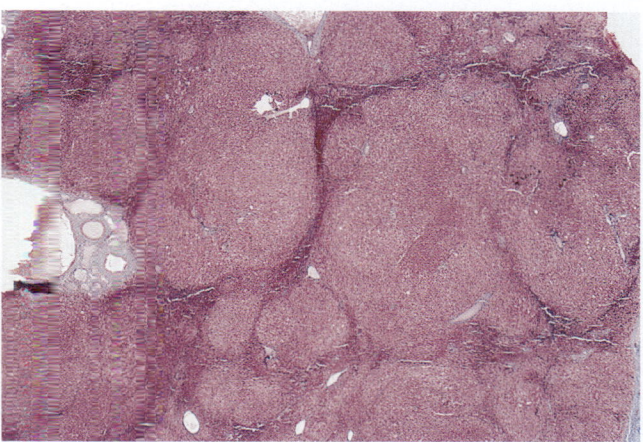
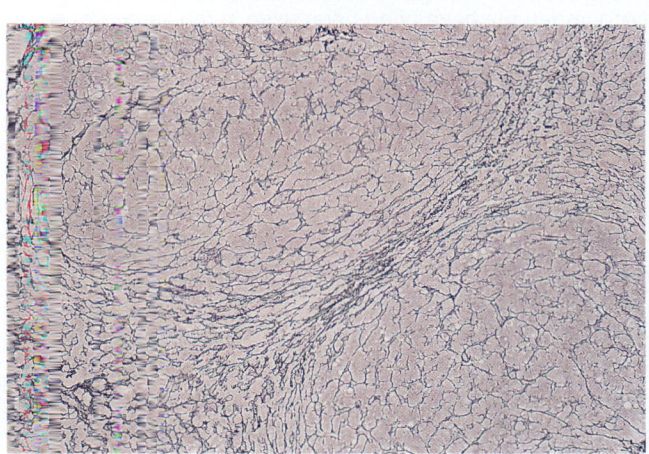

FIG. 8. Nodular regenerative hyperplasia. **A:** Liver at autopsy shows innumerable nodules varying from 1 mm to about 1 cm in diameter. Larger nodules are often surrounded by a hyperemic rim. This patient had systemic lupus erythematosis and primary pulmonary hypertension. (Kindly contributed by Kathy Saldo, M.D., Medical College of Pennsylvania, Philadelphia, PA.) **B:** Low-power view, demonstrating nodules of uniform, bland hepatocytes; a lack of fibrous septa; and the presence of perinodular congestion. The lack of fibroinflammatory septa distinguishes this lesion from cirrhosis, in terms of histologic characteristics (trichrome). **C:** Higher-power view depicts the nodular architecture, collapse of reticulin and atrophy of hepatocytes at the periphery of nodules and thickening of hepatocyte plates within the nodules, as highlighted by the reticulin stain.

advised in cases of an apparently normal biopsy in the clinical context of portal hypertension.

Although portal tracts may appear normal on histologic evaluation, morphometric studies have demonstrated a variable degree of narrowing of portal vein branches (obliterative portal venopathy) (134). Rarely, arteritis can be seen. In some cases portal vein branches show evidence of sclerosis with or without thrombosis (recent or remote) or complete obliteration. Large nodules (often perihilar) may evidence associated occlusion of large intrahepatic portal vein branches or of the extrahepatic portal vein.

Differential Diagnosis

A biopsy diagnosis of NRH must be thoroughly correlated with clinical data to avoid misdiagnosis. The major differential diagnostic considerations include nonmass lesions, such as cirrhosis; NRH superimposed upon another primary hepatic disorder, such as precirrhotic primary biliary cirrhosis; lesions of the noncirrhotic portal hypertension group (idiopathic portal hypertension, incomplete septal cirrhosis, etc.), with which NRH overlaps (see Chapter 36 by Dr. Snover); and an incidental focus of nodular hyperplasia (hyperplastic focus) (134,138). Large adenoma-like nodules appear to form by confluence of smaller monoacinar nodules; associated portal tracts may be difficult to identify, since the triadal structures may be obliterated and disappear. Arterial vessels may predominate within the portal tracts, and intranodular arteries can be found, particularly in the context of hepatic venous outflow obstruction (e.g., Budd-Chiari syndrome) (133a). These nodules may be difficult to distinguish from HCA, macroregenerative or low-grade dysplastic nodules, or even FNH (4,133a) unless the variable orientation of the liver plates in the confluent nodules of NRH can be seen, the typical features of NRH outside the nodule can be identified, or, in the context of hepatic venous outflow obstruction, marked congestion with or without fibrous septation is noted.

Macroregenerative and Borderline (Dysplastic) Nodules

The use of radiographic imaging studies to screen patients with cirrhosis for HCC, as well as the increasing use of liver transplant surgery in these patients, has led to the detection of atypical hepatocellular nodules that do not meet the histologic criteria for HCC (4,140–149). These nodules are usually similar in color and texture to the surrounding liver (from which they are well demarcated), although they may be paler or more bile stained. They are well circumscribed by a thin rim of fibrous tissue, similarly to other small nodules present in the liver; a thick fibrous capsule is not evident. The nodules demonstrate a histologic spectrum of changes

TABLE 6. *Nonmalignant hepatocellular nodules in the cirrhotic liver: preferred terminology with related terminology from the literature*[a]

Macroregenerative (or Large Regenerative) Nodule
  Macroregenerative nodule, type I
  Ordinary macroregenerative nodule
  Adenomatous hyperplasia
  Hepatocellular pseudotumor
Borderline (Dysplastic) Nodule
  Macroregenerative nodule, type II
  Atypical macroregenerative nodule
  Atypical adenomatous hyperplasia
  Normotrabecular hepatocellular carcinoma
  Hepatocellular carcinoma, grade 1 (Edmondson, Steiner)[b]

[a] Preferred term or terms in bold (ref. 4). Rarely, these nodules are found in the precirrhotic liver. Other terms are to be discouraged but have often been used in the literature. Dysplastic nodules can be subtyped as low and high grade.
[b] Some cases (ref. 120).

ranging from an appearance identical to the surrounding cirrhotic liver to features falling just short of the morphologic criteria considered diagnostic of HCC.

On histologic evaluation, there are two types of nodules, although the terms used to describe them have varied worldwide (Table 6). Laudable attempts to standardize the nomenclature have been made by international groups of pathologists (4,143), but problems in classification will continue to exist until further molecular/genetic studies are able to better define the earliest premalignant changes on the one hand and the biologic potential for metastasis on the other. Validation of the reproducibility and clinical utility of these schemas is needed. Because imaging studies and serum AFP levels (normal or within the range seen in chronic liver disease) cannot readily differentiate these nodules or distinguish them from small HCC (less than 2 cm; serum AFP level more than 200 ng/ml in only about 25% of patients) (149), pathologists are increasingly asked to solve this dilemma through the evaluation of biopsy material. This necessitates familiarity with nodule terminology, pitfalls in differential diagnosis and reporting, and the treatment of patients.

Macroregenerative Nodules

MRNs are usually multiple and measure 0.5 to 1.5 cm, but now and then they can be 5 cm or more in diameter (Fig. 9A). They are found in 15% to nearly 50% of cirrhotic livers and are three to four times more common than borderline nodules (BNs). Similar nodules are rarely encountered in precirrhotic chronic liver disease or in the context of severe acute liver injury. The hepatocytes within these multiacinar nodules are identical to those in the surrounding extranodular liver and may demonstrate any histologic abnormality (including bile pigment and pseudoglands) characteristic of the underlying disease (Fig. 9B,C). The presence of random nonspecific findings, such as steatosis, clear-cell change, hemosiderin, or Mallory bodies, by themselves do not place the nodule into the borderline category.

The hepatocellular plates are one or two cells thick. Portal tracts are scattered throughout the nodule in fragmented strands of fibrous tissue, although they are frequently diminished compared with the extranodular liver. Often they have a variable degree of structural distortion; portal veins may be obliterated, and interlobular bile ducts may sometimes be absent, leaving lone septal arteries. Bile ductules are often prominent. Few, if any, intranodular (nontriadal) arteries are discernible. The reticulin framework is intact or minimally decreased, and there is little or no evidence of sinusoidal capillarization (lack of sinusoidal immunoreactivity for factor VIII–related antigen or CD34, laminin, collagen type IV, and α-smooth-muscle actin–positive perisinusoidal cells) (146,150).

Proliferation marker studies (proliferating cell nuclear antigen, Ki-67, AgNORs) suggest a proliferative capacity that is similar or diminished compared with that of the extranodular liver. Clonality has been verified in 43% of what appear, on histologic evidence, to be otherwise typical cirrhotic nodules (151). It has been suggested by analogy that some apparent MRNs may be clonal (146); therefore, according to the definition of the International Working Party (see later section on Differential Diagnosis and Reporting), these would be considered low-grade dysplastic nodules (4). Other MRNs may arise via local disturbance of blood flow akin to the situation with large nodules in NRH.

Borderline (Dysplastic) Nodules

BNs are frequently multiple, coexist with MRNs, and are rarely larger than 2 cm. They have been reported in about 5% to 15% of cirrhotic livers and may be found in livers with only mild scarring. On macroscopic examination they cannot be distinguished from MRNs (Fig 9A). One problem with previous nodule terminology is that it was based primarily on size and therefore shed little light on the earliest findings indicative of neoplasia. The International Working Party removed the size criterion and has now defined a dysplastic nodule as being 1 mm or more in diameter and having either histologic features indicative of presumed genetic alteration (characterized by "the presence of nuclear or cytoplasmic alterations and the topographic clustering of such variations to form recognizable subpopulations of cells") or proof of genetic alteration (clonality, etc.) without definitive histologic features of malignancy (4). The subpopulation may be discerned at scanning magnification as a "nodule in nodule" configuration. If the population of cells is less than 1 mm, the term dysplastic focus is used. Dysplastic nodules have been further subdivided arbitrarily into low and high grades, depending on the degree of histologic abnormality.

In dysplastic (borderline) foci or nodules, the hepatocytes typically demonstrate the histologic features of small-cell change (small-cell dysplasia), characterized by smaller size, a greater nuclear to cytoplasmic ratio (and, hence, greater nuclear density, i.e., a larger number of nuclei per unit area),

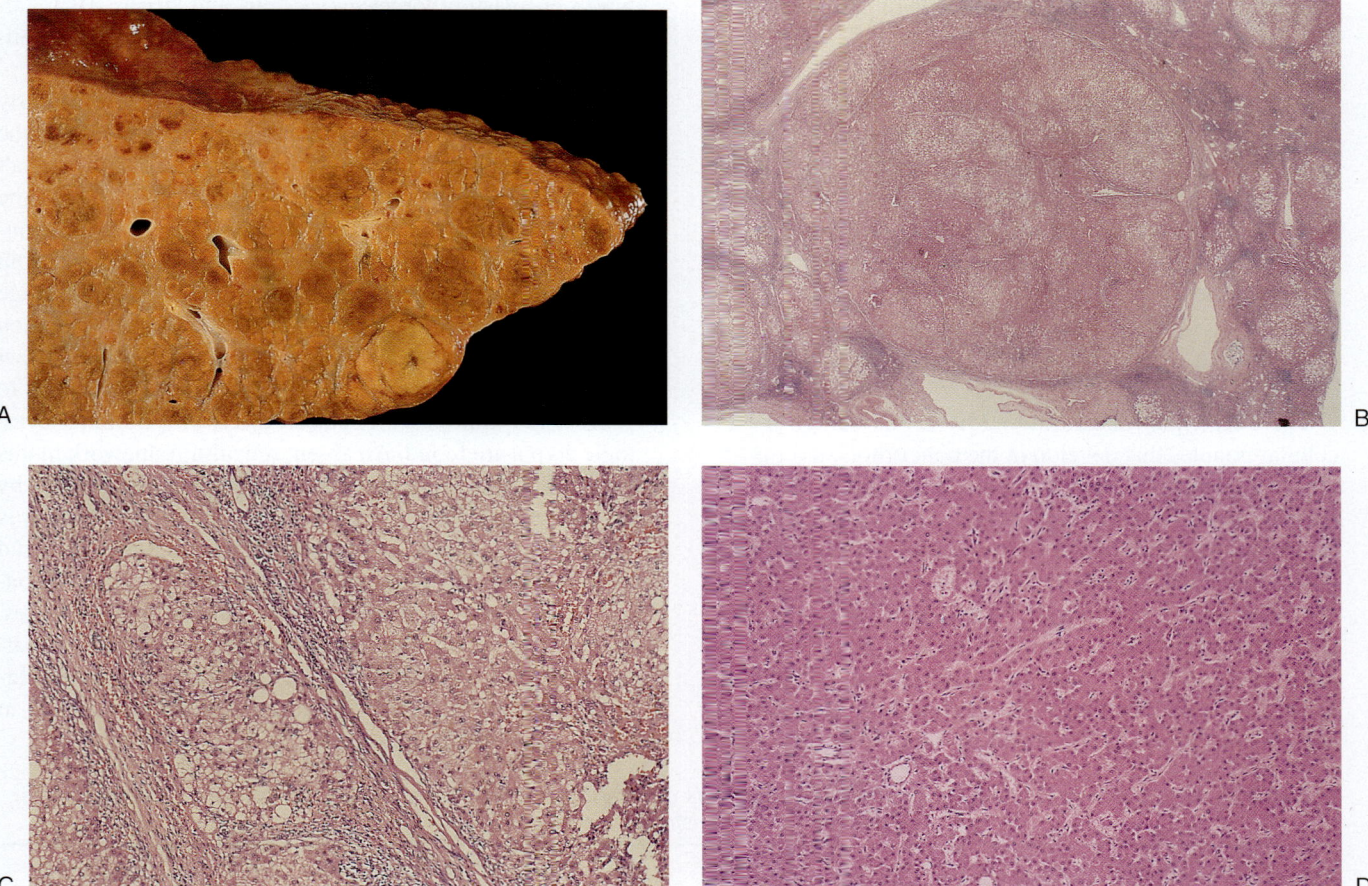

FIG. 9. Macroregenerative and borderline (dysplastic) hepatocellular nodules (MRNs and BNs). **A:** A 1-cm tan nodule distinct from other nodules in this cirrhotic liver. MRNs cannot be distinguished from BNs or small HCC based solely on the macroscopic appearance. (Kindly contributed by Randall G. Lee, M.D., University of Pittsburgh Medical Center, Pittsburgh, PA.). **B and C:** Histologic similarity of MRN to adjacent smaller cirrhotic nodules. Note the multiple portal tracts in MRN and the absence of small-cell change (MRN, right side in C). (Kindly contributed by Linda D. Ferrell, M.D., University of California at San Francisco, San Francisco, California.) **D:** BN demonstrating small-cell change (dysplasia) and non-triadal (intranodular) arteries. A definitive diagnosis of MRN or BN cannot be made on the basis of biopsy, since exclusion of HCC requires histologic evaluation of the entire nodule.

and often a more basophilic cytoplasm in comparison with the surrounding extranodular hepatocytes (Fig. 9D). A few pseudoglands, modest nuclear abnormalities, rare mitoses, and isolated liver plates that are three cells wide may be identified. Uniformly enlarged nucleoli are absent. Inclusion of LCC (large-cell change) as a diagnostic feature is the subject of controversy, but it appears to be reasonable when LCC is present in more than randomly scattered cells within the nodule (4,146). Portal tracts are usually present, but they may be structurally abnormal (see earlier section on MRN). Intranodular (nontriadal) arteries are often conspicuous and are a useful clue for diagnosis (150; Randall G. Lee, M.D., personal communication). Proliferative activity is generally similar to that of the adjacent cirrhotic liver unless subnodules are present. Capillarization of the sinusoids (see section on MRN) is more common than with MRNs. Immunoreactivity for AFP is rarely noted (149).

Association with Hepatocellular Carcinoma

Although the premalignant role of MRNs is still debated, BNs are generally considered an important precursor to HCC (146). MRNs are often static or may disappear (about 25%) after radiographic follow-up, but BNs do not regress and often increase in size (147,151,152). Patients with MRNs (without associated BNs) much less frequently have or subsequently show signs of HCC compared with BNs in the following contexts: liver explants (15–20% vs. 66%) (44,146), after clinical follow-up (0–17% vs. 50–70%) (47,151,152), or at autopsy (41% vs. 100%) (144). The HCC may be found as a distinct subpopulation ("nodule in nodule") within the preexisting nodule or within the adjacent liver. Whether the major pathway for the development of HCC is via these nodules requires further investigation, as the determination of the point at which tiny foci of HCC are capable of metastasis (see the discussion of precancerous lesions in the section on HCC and Fig. 14).

Therapeutic intervention (ablation or resection) must be seriously considered after a histologic diagnosis of BN, because it has a strong proclivity to develop into HCC and because HCC may already be present either within the nodule (sampling) or in the adjacent liver. Patients with apparent MRNs should be followed up with an appropriate imaging study at more frequent intervals than the usual patient with cirrhosis (146).

Differential Diagnosis and Reporting

The differential diagnosis of MRNs and benign hepatocellular nodules that develop in the noncirrhotic liver is usually straightforward, especially when dealing with a resection specimen for which the nature of the surrounding liver is known. Distinguishing the two may be impossible in biopsy specimens. Features useful in differential diagnosis are summarized in Table 4. Separation of low-grade dysplastic nodules from MRNs, and of high-grade dysplastic nodules from HCC, may be impossible on histologic grounds, but features useful in differential diagnosis are summarized Table 7. Criteria for making the distinction between dysplastic (borderline) lesions and "early" HCC (alternatively called "well," "very well," or "highly differentiated" HCC) are still evolving (4,141,148).

Probably the most reliable diagnostic indicator of early HCC is a nuclear density of more than 2 compared with the extranodular liver (in clinical practice performed by gestalt rather than morphometry). This parameter represents the number of nuclei per unit area and is a reflection of the nuclear to cytoplasmic ratio. It should be remembered that in liver cell atrophy, the nuclear density may fall into the range seen in HCC; therefore, it is important to pay close attention to other histologic details. Definitive stromal or portal tract invasion is diagnostic of HCC, but it may be difficult to prove when thin cords of hepatocytes with minimal cytologic atypia are found. An absent reticulin framework in this situation favors HCC, as does separation of these cords by collagen. Vascular invasion is diagnostic of HCC, but it is virtually never seen in these early lesions. Residual portal tracts can be present in small HCC (less than 2 cm), and nontriadal arteries are common. Other morphologic features, such as hepatocyte plates more than three cells thick, "floating trabecula" with adjacent dilated sinusoids, and more significant nuclear atypia and mitoses, are more often seen in higher-grade HCC.

TABLE 7. Histologic features useful in differential diagnosis of benign, borderline (dysplastic), and malignant hepatocellular nodules typically arising in the cirrhotic liver[a]

Histologic feature	MRN	Borderline nodule Low grade	Borderline nodule High grade	WD-HCC	MD-HCC
Primary diagnostic utility					
Mitoses, at least moderate (>5/10 HPF)	−	−	−	−	+
Hepatocellular plates >3 cells thick	−	−	−	−	+
Reticulin uniformly < normal	−	−	−	−	+
Positive endothelial markers (endothelium)	−	−	?	+/−	+
Uniformly prominent nucleoli	−	−	−	−	+
Nuclear density >2× normal	−	−	−	+	+
Irregular nuclear contour, ≥ moderate	−	−	−	+	+
Nuclear hyperchromasia	−	−	+	+	+
Intranodular (nontriadal) arteries	−	+	+	+	+
Subpopulations ("clonelike")	−	+	+	+	+
Secondary diagnostic utility					
Invasion of stroma or portal tracts[b]	−	−	−	+	+
Mitoses, few (1–5/10 HPF)	−[c]	+	−	+	
Nuclear density >1.3× normal	−	−	+	+	+
Irregular nuclear contour, mild	−	−	+	+	+
Pseudoglands	−[d]	+	−	+	
Cytoplasmic basophilia/clear-cell change	−	−	+	+	+
Resistance to iron accumulation in iron-loaded liver ("iron free foci")	−	?	+	+	+

MRN, macroregenerative nodule; HCC, hepatocellular carcinoma; HPF, high-power field; MD-, moderately differentiated; WD-, well differentiated.

[a] Modified from ref. 4. The presence of any one feature in the primary group is highly suggestive of one of the nodules with a "+" in that column. Features in the second group have diagnostic utility, but to a lesser degree. The absence of a feature with a "+" does not exclude the diagnosis in that column.
[b] Stromal/portal tract invasion was placed in the secondary group by the International Working Party until more published data are available evaluating the criteria for diagnosis.
[c] Mitoses can occur whenever necroinflammatory changes or cholestasis is present.
[d] Pseudoglands may be present when the extranodular liver demonstrates this finding, usually in association with cholestasis.

Since architectural features are quite important in the evaluation of this spectrum of lesions, core biopsy is favored over FNA if a biopsy is performed; cell block evaluation with reticulin staining, however, may be useful (1,24,147,153). Use of both biopsy methods has been suggested by some authors to maximize both sensitivity and specificity. An additional biopsy from the extranodular liver is desirable for comparison. Both pathologist and clinician should realize that, in the context of chronic liver disease, a core or FNA biopsy diagnosis of a hepatocellular nodule that does not reveal definitive signs of HCC should be regarded with caution, since sampling is always an issue. A diagnosis of hepatocellular nodule of uncertain malignant potential may be preferable to borderline (or dysplastic) nodule in such a biopsy specimen, because without a complete resection, it is impossible to exclude HCC (4). Close correlation with the size of the lesion and results of serum AFP testing is advised in order to institute appropriate treatment of patients.

Malignant Hepatocellular Tumors

Hepatocellular Carcinoma

Epidemiologic Factors

Malignant epithelial tumors account for about 98% of all primary hepatic malignancies, with HCC representing by far (about 85–90%) the single most common histologic type (3). In children from most parts of the world, HCC accounts for 30% to 40% of all primary hepatic malignancies (5,85,116,154), although it is the most common cause of pediatric hepatic malignancy in regions of high incidence of hepatitis B virus (HBV) and HCC (155). Although it is relatively uncommon in North America and Western Europe, HCC is one of the most prevalent malignant tumors worldwide (eighth most prevalent worldwide, 22nd most common in the U.S.A.), accounting for 500,000 to one million cases per year. It is responsible for only 0.5% to 2% of cancer deaths in regions of low incidence, while making up 20% to 40% of cancer deaths in regions of high incidence, such as sub-Saharan Africa, China, and Japan (3,156–158). The male-to-female ratio is 3:1 to 6:1; however, when HCC arises in a normal liver, there is no or little sexual preference. Patients usually show symptoms in the sixth or seventh decade of life in regions of low incidence and in the third or fourth decades in locations where HCC is common.

Pathogenesis

Factors important in the pathogenesis of HCC are summarized in Table 8 (3,103,156–158). Virtually any condition associated with chronic hepatic injury (usually cirrhosis) may predispose toward HCC; in fact, about 20% of patients who die of cirrhosis show signs of HCC at autopsy. In high-risk countries in Africa and some parts of Asia, hepatitis B–related chronic liver disease (usually perinatally acquired) is the most important risk factor, while in Japan, hepatitis

TABLE 8. *Factors implicated in the pathogenesis of hepatocellular carcinoma (HCC)*

Chronic hepatic injury (60–90%)
  Cirrhosis (most common)
  Chronic hepatitis only (far less common) (HBV ≫ HCV)
Specific etiologies
  High rate of associated HCC (>15%)
    HBV[a]
    HCV[a]
    Hereditary hemochromatosis
    Hereditary tyrosinemia
    Porphyria cutanea tarda
    Hypercitrullinemia[b]
    Membranous obstruction of the inferior vena cava
  Intermediate rate of associated HCC (~5–15%)
    Alcohol[a]
    Alpha$_1$-antitrypsin deficiency
    Glycogen storage disease (types 1 and 3)[b]
    Autoimmune hepatitis (?)
  Low rate to rare presence of associated HCC (<5%)
    Primary biliary cirrhosis
    Primary sclerosing cholangitis
    Hereditary fructose intolerance[b]
    Paucity of intrahepatic bile ducts[b]
    Progressive intrahepatic cholestasis (Byler's disease)
    Congenital hepatic fibrosis
    Biliary atresia
    Wilson's disease
    Oral contraceptive steroids[b]
    Anabolic–androgenic steroids[b,c]
    Cardiac cirrhosis
    Exposure to various chemicals/toxins, including aflatoxin B$_1$[d]

Data from refs. 3, 99, 103, 156–158.
[a]Most important specific etiologies associated with HCC worldwide. Multiple factors may act in a synergistic fashion, most frequently associated with cirrhosis.
[b]Conditions where HCC uniformly occurs in a noncirrhotic liver. Occasionally other conditions such as chronic hepatitis B or alpha$_1$-antitrypsin deficiency or, rarely, chronic hepatitis C, alcoholic liver disease, or hereditary hemochromatosis, will lead to HCC in the absence of cirrhosis.
[c]Although hepatic tumors associated with anabolic–androgenic steroid usage may have the histologic appearance of HCC, biologically malignant behavior (metastasis) is rare.
[d]While aflatoxin B$_1$ has been strongly associated with the occurrence of HCC in regions of high incidence and in experimental animals, its role as a carcinogen has not been proved in humans. The presence of a putative aflatoxin-specific G to T mutation at codon 249 of the p53 gene is of interest. Chronic exposure to vinyl chloride, pesticides/herbicides, and other organic chemicals have occasionally been reported in association with HCC. Cigarette smoking has shown inconsistent association with HCC.

C–related cirrhosis is most common. In the developed Western world, the origin of the majority of cases of cirrhosis associated with HCC is unknown, but in cases with known sources, hepatitis C and alcohol appear to be most common. Multiple etiologic factors may act in a synergistic fashion, leading to chronic liver disease with perhaps an increased risk of HCC. The annual risk of HCC developing in a cirrhotic liver is estimated at 1% to 6%, with the risk generally being highest in the context of viral sources and hereditary hemochromatosis (159). The possibility that HCC in the normal liver may arise from HCA (Fig. 4) and the association of HCC and NRH have been discussed in their respective sections (4,121–125,139).

It is believed that chronic liver injury leads to sustained hepatocyte hyperplasia, increased susceptibility to various carcinogens, and greater risk of chromosomal damage. Aberrant expression of proto-oncogenes, the expression of mutated forms of these genes, and/or mutation of suppressor genes, such as p53 (115), may lead to a selective growth advantage for a clone of cells that eventually acquires a malignant phenotype. Allelic losses of at least ten different chromosomes have been described in HCC (160). To date, neither HBV nor hepatitis C virus (HCV) has been found to be directly oncogenic. HCV does not integrate into the hepatocyte genome; conversely, HBV does integrate, but at random sites in different tumors.

Clinical Findings

Patients with symptomatic HCC typically show initial signs of abdominal pain, fullness or a mass, or features indistinguishable from cirrhosis. Only rarely (3–5%) are metastases or local spread the initial manifestation (161–166); bone, lung, gastrointestinal tract, skin, oral cavity, male breast, ovary, and testis have all been reported as metastatic sites. HCC accounts for about 70% of all malignant neoplasms found in the cirrhotic liver in regions of low incidence. While up to 30% of HCCs in North America may arise in a normal liver, it is much more likely that a malignant tumor in the normal liver represents a metastasis (2% HCC vs. 98% hepatic metastasis) (158,167). This point should be borne in mind when considering a diagnosis of HCC in the normal liver (see later discussion of FL-HCC). HCC in the noncirrhotic liver generally appears at a later stage and with a larger mass than HCC arising in patients with cirrhosis.

Periodic screening of patients with chronic liver disease for HCC, using a combination of ultrasonography and serum levels of AFP, has become accepted practice by hepatologists and has led to the diagnosis of many small (less than 2 cm), asymptomatic HCCs. Data proving a reduction in mortality and cost-effectiveness, however, are lacking (159). About 80% of cases of HCC in Japan are detected in this manner or at the time of a regular medical check-up (161).

Serum AFP levels remain the most useful marker for HCC. The level of serum des-γ-carboxy prothrombin (DCP) has been suggested as a useful marker (60–90% sensitive, 85% specific); tests may be positive in nearly 30% of AFP-seronegative patients (149,168–170). Serum AFP levels are elevated (more than 10 to 20 ng/ml) in about 70% to 80% of patients (specificity, 90%). It is frequently detectable at levels greater than 200 ng/ml in HBV- and HCV-related cases (about 75%); however, tumors arising in the context of alcohol-related cirrhosis (65%), those found in the noncirrhotic liver (33%), or those less than 2 cm in diameter (25%; additionally, the DCP level is increased in only about 5% of this group) less often show elevations of this magnitude, and serum AFP may even be undetectable.

Serum AFP levels may also be elevated, but rarely above 400 to 500 ng/ml, in several benign conditions, such as acute and chronic viral hepatitis and cirrhosis. In chronic viral liver disease, increases in serum AFP are often episodic and correlate with increased transaminases. Sustained AFP increases suggest HCC, but the time course of serum AFP is not totally reliable in predicting HCC, and, as mentioned earlier, HCC can develop in the absence of elevated serum AFP. Malignant neoplasms often associated with very high levels (more than 1,000 ng/ml) of serum AFP include HCC, HBL, and germ cell tumors containing a yolk sac component. Such elevations have been reported, though rarely, with intrahepatic cholangiocarcinoma (ICC), mesenchymal hamartoma, polycystic liver disease, nonhepatoid malignancies of the pancreas (islet cell carcinoma, pancreatoblastoma, acinar cell carcinoma), and certain carcinomas of the lung, kidney, and ovary. High AFP levels are common with hepatoid adenocarcinomas arising at various sites (particularly those of foregut origin) (56,168,171).

Pathologic Features of Small Hepatocellular Carcinoma

Macroscopic Features. By definition, small HCC is less than 2 cm in diameter (4,148,172). It may be invisible on gross inspection and may be recognized only at the microscopic level, often within a BN. Usually, a nodule with a distinct fibrous capsule and/or fibrous septa is noted (Fig. 10A). Nodules with indistinct borders are also found, particularly when the tumor's diameter is less than 1.5 cm. The nodules bulge from the cut surface, do not evidence necrosis, and often have a gray-white, green or yellow appearance, reflecting fatty change within tumor cells. Definitively making the distinction from MRNs or BNs on the basis of gross features is usually not possible. Data suggest that small, early HCC often changes its characteristics at a size of 1 to 2 cm, when it may develop some of the gross (capsule) and microscopic (higher histologic grade) characteristics of advanced HCC.

Microscopic Features. Virtually all tumors less than 1 cm consist of WD-HCC with relatively thin trabeculae (less than or equal to three cells thick) of small hepatocytes showing little cellular or structural atypia (early HCC) (Fig. 10B,C) (148). WD-HCC is principally distinguished from borderline foci/nodules, from which it may arise (nodule in a nodule), by a nuclear density greater than twice normal and by mild but definite nuclear atypia (hyperchromasia, irregular nuclear contours) (discussed in greater detail in the section on borderline nodules and in Table 7). Nucleoli are often inconspicuous. As the nodule of HCC enlarges, there is clonal dedifferentiation, often in a "nodule in a nodule" fashion. The moderate or poorly differentiated foci are always found to-

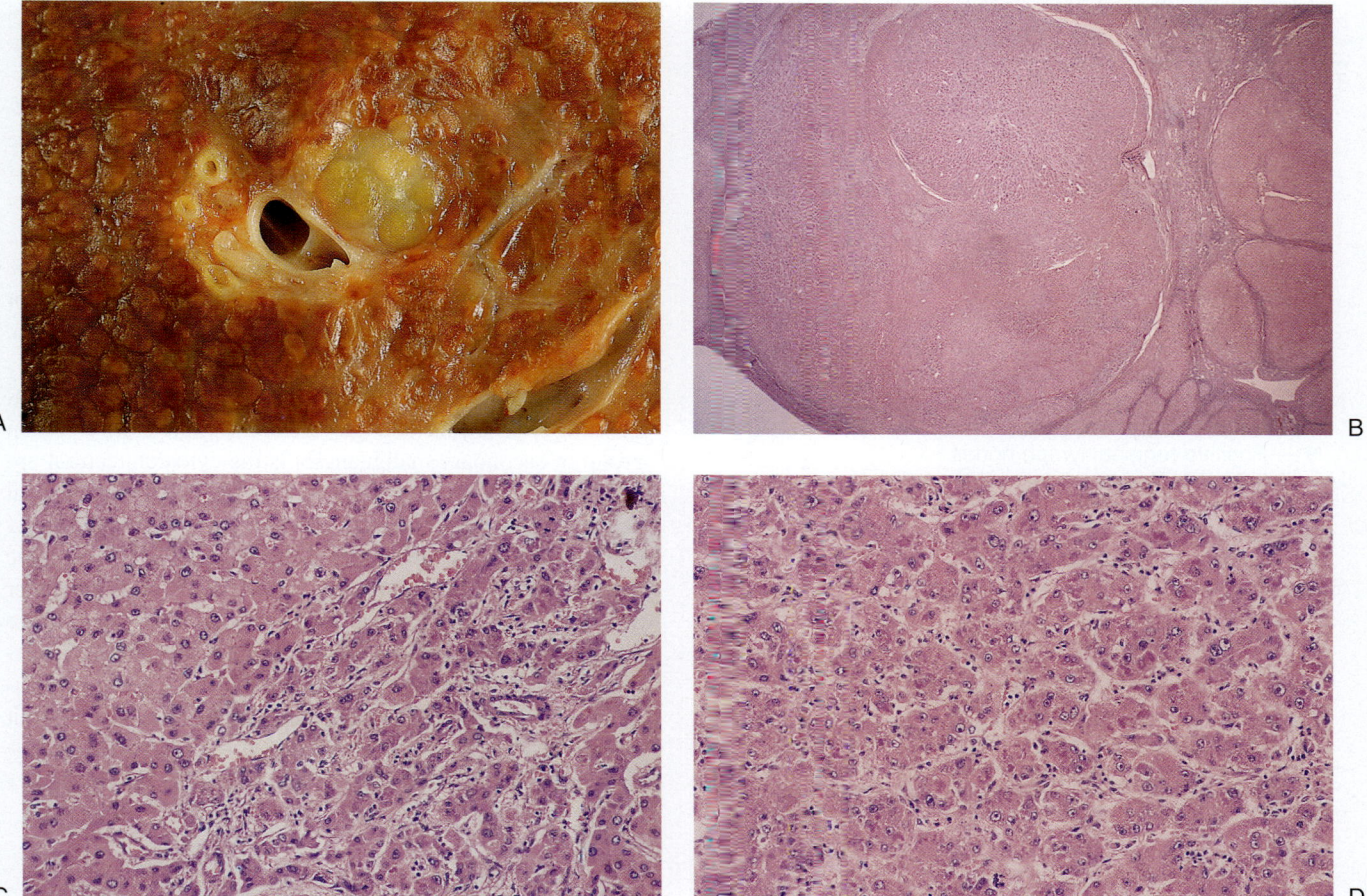

FIG. 10. Small hepatocellular carcinoma (HCC) (definition, less than 2 cm). **A:** A 1-cm HCC. Note fibrous septation and green (bile) color. Distinction from macroregenerative and borderline nodules must be made on the basis of microscopy. Proximity to large blood vessels (as seen in figure) with subsequent invasion might favor the rare occurrence of metastasis from an HCC of this size. **B:** "Nodule in nodule" appearance of small HCC (upper center) arising in a borderline nodule. **C:** Focus of very well differentiated HCC characterized by thin trabeculae of hepatocytes with high nuclear density (more than twice normal), mild nuclear atypia, and stromal reaction (right side). A few Mallory bodies are noted. Small-cell change is evident in the surrounding borderline nodule on the left side. **D:** Other portions of this small HCC display larger tumor cells with more significant nuclear atypia, more prominent nucleoli, and abundant Mallory bodies. (Kindly contributed by Randall G. Lee, M.D., University of Pittsburgh Medical Center, Pittsburgh, PA.)

ward the center of the nodule, with a peripheral component of WD-HCC that diminishes with increasing tumor size (Fig. 10D) (173). Fatty or clear-cell change, noted in 40% of cases, sometimes with Mallory bodies (i.e., steatohepatitis), can obscure the diagnostic cytoarchitectural features and make biopsy diagnosis equivocal. Stromal and portal tract invasion may occur, but vascular invasion is quite rare (148).

Advanced Hepatocellular Carcinoma

Macroscopic Features. The macroscopic appearance depends on the presence or absence of cirrhosis and portal vein thrombosis as well as the size of the tumor (3,172,174,175). Tumors arising in a normal liver usually grow as a homogeneous mass, occasionally with satellite nodules (massive or expanding type), while those associated with cirrhosis often grow as one or more relatively large nodules (nodular type) or numerous smaller nodules (diffuse type) that may themselves, in gross terms, simulate cirrhosis (cirrhotomimetic). An alternate classification emphasizes the tumor–nontumor interface, dividing HCC into expanding (discrete boundary), spreading (poorly defined tumor border), multifocal (multiple discrete nodules), and indeterminate (25%) types (174). A tumor capsule has been found in the majority of cases reported in Japan (172), while this feature has been found less frequently in North America (158). Staging criteria for primary liver carcinoma (HCC and cholangiocarcinoma) are listed in Table 9; they principally depend on the size, number, and location (one or more lobes) of the tumor nodule(s) and the presence or absence of vascular invasion (176).

TABLE 9. pTMN staging of primary hepatic epithelial malignancies[a]

T—Primary tumor
  T1—Solitary mass, ≤2 cm, without vascular invasion
  T2—Solitary mass, ≤2 cm, with vascular invasion, or multiple masses, one lobe, all ≤2 cm without vascular invasion, or solitary mass, >2 cm, without vascular invasion
  T3—Solitary mass, >2 cm, with vascular invasion, or multiple masses, one lobe, ≤2 cm, with vascular invasion, or multiple masses, one lobe, >2 cm, with or without vascular invasion
  T4—Multiple masses in more than one lobe, or invasion of major branch of portal or hepatic vein, or invasion of adjacent organs other than gallbladder
N—Regional lymph nodes
  N0—Negative regional lymph nodes
  N1—Positive regional lymph nodes
M—Distant metastases
  MX—Cannot be assessed
  M0—No distant metastases
  M1—Distant metastases present
Stage groupings
  Stage I—T1N0M0
  Stage II—T2N0M0
  Stage IIIA—T3N0M0
  Stage IIIB—T1N1M0, T2N1M0, T3N1M0
  Stage IVA—T4 any N M0
  Stage IVB—any T any N M1

Modified from ref. 176. Vascular invasion includes either macroscopic or microscopic involvement of vessels.

The liver is enlarged by one or more tumor nodules that are soft, tan-gray, or green (bile stained) and often demonstrate foci of hemorrhage and necrosis (3,172) (Fig. 11). Occasionally, HCC may be pedunculated. Separate tumor nodules may represent multicentric growth or may be monoclonal, arising via intrahepatic portal vein metastases (small, early cases vs. larger, more advanced cases, respectively) (177). Macroscopic portal vein, hepatic vein, and bile duct invasion is noted in 35% to 80%, 20% to 25%, and 1% to 7% of cases, respectively. Involvement of the inferior vena cava, sometimes with extension into the right atrium, may be found (71).

Microscopic Features. The most helpful feature in distinguishing HCC from cholangiocarcinoma or the more common group of secondary malignancies is the cytoarchitectural appearance of the tumor cells, which resembles that of normal hepatocytes typically arranged (at least focally) in a trabecular pattern outlined by sinusoids (2,3,158,172,175). Histologic grading of HCC was devised by Edmundson and Steiner nearly 50 years ago; subsequently, other, similar systems have been proposed (2,120,158,172) (Table 10). More than one histologic grade is often present within a given tumor; most tumors are moderately differentiated (grades 2 to 3). Without definite evidence of hepatocellular differentiation, a malignant epithelial tumor in the liver should be regarded as a poorly differentiated carcinoma that is most likely metastatic.

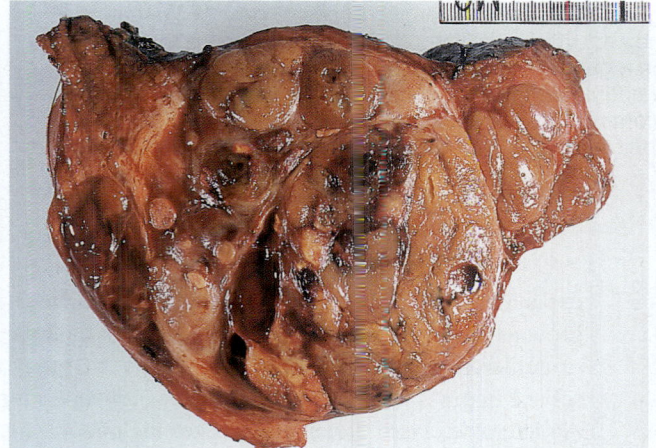
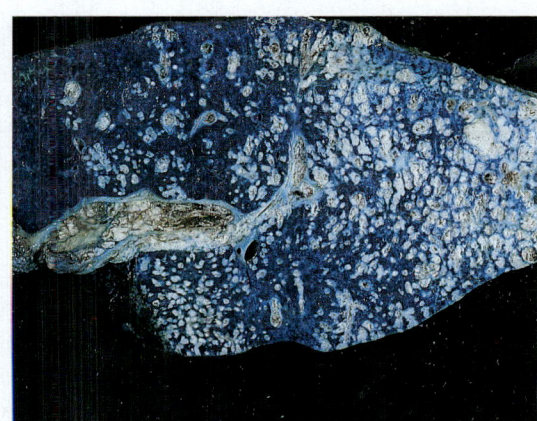
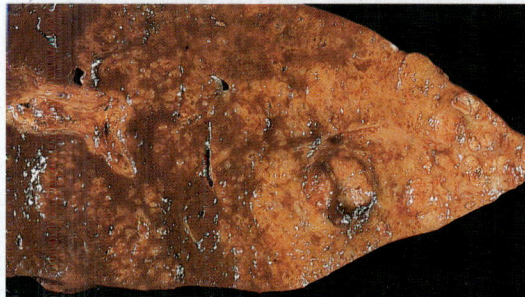

FIG. 11. Hepatocellular carcinoma (HCC), macroscopic appearance. **A:** Encapsulated type (with extracapsular extension), with multiple foci of necrosis, arising in a cirrhotic liver of an American woman. **B:** Lower panel: Diffuse pattern of hepatocellular carcinoma with extensive portal vein invasion arising in a patient with hereditary hemochromatosis. Note the ruddy appearance of the cut surface. Upper panel: The striking amount of hemosiderin (blue) present in the nonneoplastic parenchyma is evident after submersion in Gomori's iron reagent. Note unstained white areas representing foci of HCC that characteristically lack hemosiderin.

TABLE 10. *Histologic grading of hepatocellular carcinoma*[a]

<u>Well differentiated (Grades I/II of Edmondson and Steiner)</u>
  Thin plates, three or fewer hepatocytes thick, that are typically smaller than normal, demonstrate minimal nuclear atypia, and have a nuclear density greater than twice that of the nonneoplastic liver. Fatty change and pseudoglandular architecture are common. Clear-cut histologic distinction from hepatocellular adenoma may not be possible in some cases without finding other, more poorly differentiated foci and knowing the status of the nonneoplastic liver. This pattern is typical of small (<2 cm) HCC.

<u>Moderately differentiated (Grades II/III of Edmondson and Steiner)</u>
  Typically characterized by a trabecular pattern in which tumor cells are arranged in plates more than three cells thick. Tumor cells are larger and have more abundant eosinophilic cytoplasm and distinct nucleoli, compared with well-differentiated tumors. Pseudoglandular structures and bile are usually seen, and tumor giant cells may be present. This is the most common type of differentiation seen in advanced (>2 cm) HCC.

<u>Poorly differentiated (Grades III/IV of Edmondson and Steiner)</u>
  Tumor cells have larger and more hyperchromatic nuclei and are typically arranged in a compact (solid) growth pattern with rare or no trabeculae or bile. Pleomorphism may be prominent and spindle-cell or small-cell areas may be seen. May be difficult to recognize as hepatocellular in origin.

[a] Modified from refs. 2, 4, 120, 172. More than one pattern is frequently seen in tumors larger than 1.5 cm diameter.

Multiple tissue blocks may be required for appropriate tumor classification because the microscopic appearance may be quite variable, even within a given tumor. In advanced HCC, cell size may be larger or smaller than that of the adjacent nonneoplastic hepatocytes, and the nuclear to cytoplasmic ratio is increased. Growth at the tumor/nonneoplastic liver interface is usually of the replacing type (infiltrating the cell plates), although poorly differentiated variants often have a sinusoidal pattern of spread similar to that of metastatic poorly differentiated and small-cell carcinomas, lymphoma, and angiosarcoma (172,175). Occasionally, HCC may grow in an expansive fashion, compressing the adjacent nonneoplastic parenchyma.

HCC is typically associated with little tumor-induced stroma, which accounts for its soft nature. Significant fibrosis occurs in about 5% of cases (scirrhous and fibrolamellar variants of HCC), and vascular lakes are sometimes noted in the tumor, simulating peliosis hepatis (pelioid pattern) (2,3,158,172). As HCC progresses from a small to an advanced type, the extent of sinusoidal capillarization (sinusoidal immunoreactivity for factor VIII–related antigen or CD34, laminin, collagen type IV and α-smooth-muscle actin–positive perisinusoidal cells) increases, as does the number of intranodular (nontriadal) arteries (146,150, 178). The World Health Organization (WHO) (2) recognizes five histologic patterns and four cytologic variants of HCC.

Histologic Patterns. These patterns are frequently found together in the same tumor. Although they are important for the pathologist to recognize as part of the morphologic spectrum of HCC, only the fibrolamellar type appears to have prognostic significance (2,3,158,172).

1. *Trabecular (sinusoidal, platelike).* This pattern, which is nearly always found in some part of HCC, appears as a distorted caricature of the normal liver cell plates (Fig. 12A,B). The trabeculae vary in thickness and are surrounded by sinusoids lined by flattened endothelial cells and a variable number of macrophages (Kupffer cells). The reticulin framework is generally absent, although rarely it may even be accentuated.
2. *Compact (solid).* This variant of the trabecular pattern is seen in 5% to 15% of HCCs. Adjacent trabeculae merge to form sheets compressing the sinusoids, making them inconspicuous (Fig. 12C). Distinguishing this picture from regenerating hepatocytes when the HCC is well to moderately differentiated, or from large-cell carcinoma of extrahepatic origin when the HCC is obviously malignant, may be a problem in a small biopsy specimen. The cells at the periphery of the trabeculae may have a more columnar appearance.
3. *Pseudoglandular (acinar, adenoid).* This is seen as the dominant pattern in 5% to 10% of cases, but it is present at least focally in an additional third of tumors and may be mistaken for adenocarcinoma (primary or secondary) or HCC combined with cholangiocarcinoma (Fig. 12D). The spaces usually represent dilated bile canaliculi and are lined by cells with the cytologic features of malignant hepatocytes mentioned earlier. Bile and/or eosinophilic, hyaline, PAS-positive diastase-resistant material may be found in the lumen. Marked cystic dilatation of these spaces may yield a thyroid-like appearance. Complex communication of the canaliculi may produce a pseudopapillary pattern. Mucicarmine stain of the luminal contents has been inconsistently reported as negative or occasionally positive. This variation depends on whether a given author uses mucicarmine positivity as a criterion to distinguish the pseudoglandular variant from combined HCC and cholangiocarcinoma. Intracytoplasmic mucin is absent. Glandlike spaces may also be formed by palisading of tumor cells around dilated sinusoids or by central degeneration of trabeculae.
4. *Fibrolamellar.* This type comprises 1% to 5% of all HCCs in the U.S.A., but it is quite rare in regions with high rates of HCC. It is discussed in detail later.
5. *Scirrhous.* This variant accounts for less than 1% to 2% of all HCCs. It is discussed later, in the section on sclerosing hepatic carcinoma.

Cytologic Appearance and Variants. The tumor cells are usually polygonal and have (a) distinct cell membranes, (b) a higher nuclear to cytoplasmic ratio compared with normal hepatocytes, (c) abundant, finely granular eosinophilic cytoplasm, and (d) a round nucleus often containing coarse chro-

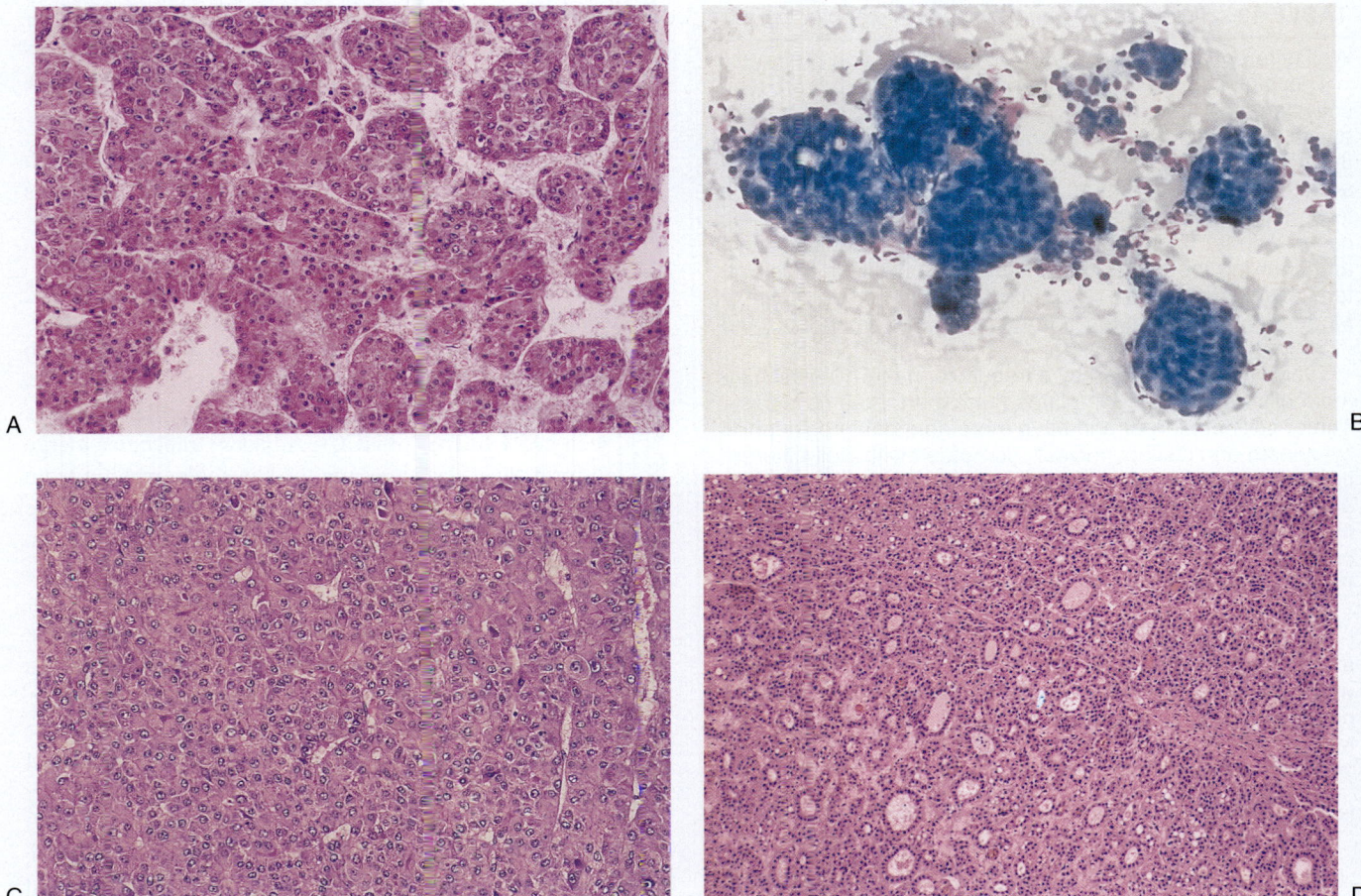

FIG. 12. Hepatocellular carcinoma (HCC), microscopic features. **A:** Classic trabecular pattern. The trabeculae shown in this photomicrograph are more than three cells thick and are covered by a layer of flattened endothelial cells. The tumor cells resemble hepatocytes, containing round nuclei, granular eosinophilic cytoplasm, and well-defined cell borders. Compared with normal hepatocytes, however, the nuclear to cytoplasmic ratio is higher, and nucleoli are variably prominent. **B:** Fine-needle aspiration (FNA) specimen demonstrating architectural and cytologic features similar to those seen in A. (Kindly contributed by Prabodh K. Gupta, M.D., Hospital of the University of Pennsylvania, Philadelphia, PA.) **C:** Compact pattern. **D:** Pseudoglandular pattern. Note proteinaceous material or bile within several lumina. Rarely, this pattern may give a "thyroid-like" appearance.

matin and a thickened or irregular nuclear membrane. Although nucleoli are often prominent, this is not a consistent finding; prominent nucleoli can certainly be seen in a wide variety of malignancies. Intranuclear cytoplasmic invaginations are a common, albeit nonspecific, finding in HCC. The following categories are recognized cytologic variants of HCC.

1. *Pleomorphic (giant cell)*. Tumor giant cells, often multinucleated and quite hyperchromatic, predominate in this variant, which comprises less than 5% of all HCCs (Fig. 12E). Marked loss of cell cohesion is typical. Tumor giant cells may be found in 15% to 30% of HCCs. Numerous bland, osteoclast-like giant cells have also been described, sometimes with focal ossification (179). The histogenesis of these bland cells is unclear. Extensive sectioning may be required to find evidence of typical HCC.

2. *Clear cell*. As the name implies, this variant is characterized by tumor cells with prominent clear cytoplasm due to loss of cytoplasmic glycogen and/or fat in the embedding process (Fig. 12F). It is the predominant appearance in 5% to 16% of cases; however, 20% to 40% of all HCCs contain a few clear cells. Nuclear features at times can be quite bland. Differentiating this type from metastatic renal, adrenal, or ovarian carcinoma may be impossible on purely histologic grounds. To aid in differential diagnosis, other portions of the tumor should be carefully examined for foci of typical HCC. Immunohistochemical (see later discussion and Table 12) evidence of bile canaliculi (polyclonal carcinoembryonic antigen; p-CEA) or use of other markers of hepatocyte differentiation may be invaluable. An elevated serum AFP and the absence of a mass in the indicated extra-

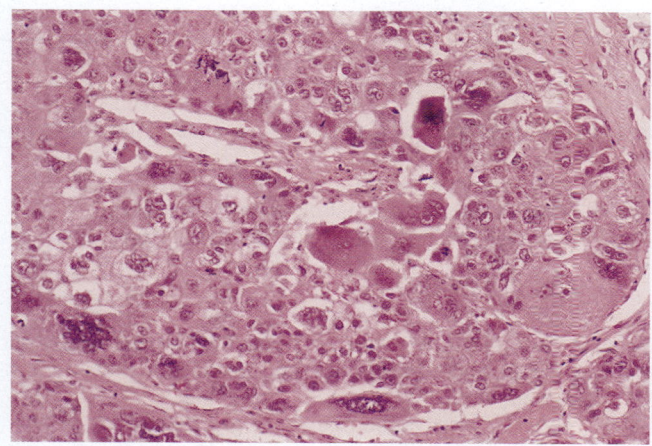
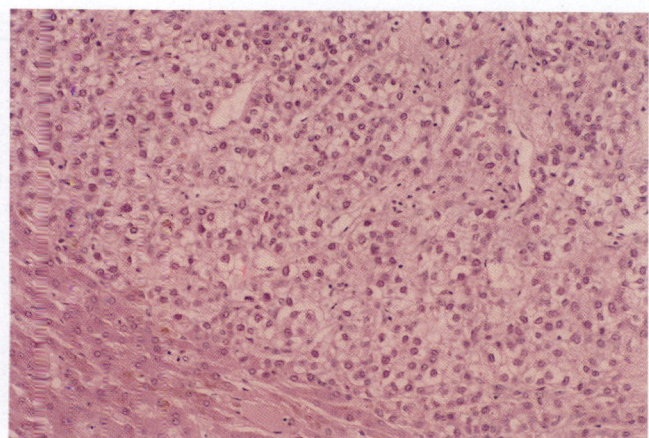
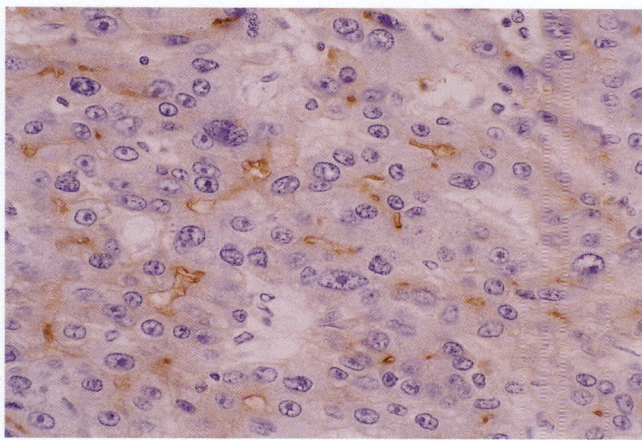

FIG. 12. (*continued*) Hepatocellular carcinoma (HCC), microscopic features. **E:** Pleomorphic (giant-cell) variant. **F:** Clear-cell variant. Differential diagnosis from other clear-cell neoplasms may be quite difficult (see text). **G:** Canalicular pattern with polyclonal carcinoembryonic antigen (cross-reacts with biliary glycoprotein 1) immunoreactivity. When the demonstrated pattern is seen in a malignant neoplasm, it is diagnostic of HCC. Tangential sections showing luminal staining of glands from adenocarcinoma or trapped nonneoplastic hepatocytes should not be misinterpreted as HCC.

hepatic organs favor a hepatic primary, but the former feature does not appear to be entirely specific (168).

3. *Oncocyte-like*. Intensely eosinophilic and coarsely granular cytoplasm due to numerous mitochondria characterize FL-HCC (see later discussion). Occasionally, a minority population of these cells is found in an usual HCC, and rarely this cell type predominates without the characteristic stroma of FL-HCC (116,180).

4. *Sarcomatoid (spindle cell, pseudosarcomatous)*. Of all HCCs, 1% to 9% exhibit a prominent sarcomatoid component characterized by spindle-shaped cells that suggest a diagnosis of fibrosarcoma or malignant fibrous histiocytoma (181). Sometimes these tumors have been reported as carcinosarcoma or malignant mixed tumors, particularly when foci of more differentiated sarcomas (osteosarcoma, chondrosarcoma, leiomyosarcoma, rhabdomyosarcoma) are noted (2,3). Separate nodules of carcinoma (HCC or cholangiocarcinoma) and differentiated sarcoma have also been described. In sarcomatoid HCC, pleomorphic and osteoclast-like giant cells, as described earlier, may be seen, thereby overlapping with the giant-cell variant. Occasionally, portions of the spindle-cell component may appear so bland as to simulate a benign process. Cytokeratin (CK) immunoreactivity, seen in about 60% of cases, supports an epithelial origin, but spindle-cell immunoreactivity for mesenchymal markers (such as HHF-35, smooth-muscle actin, desmin, KP-1, and S-100) can be detected from time to time. Diligent search in resection specimens nearly always reveals typical foci of HCC, although finding such foci can be difficult in biopsy specimens. The serum AFP level is less frequently elevated, and extrahepatic metastases are more common in this variant compared with the usual HCC.

Cytoplasmic Deposits and Immunohistochemistry. Identification of several cytoplasmic deposits and use of a panel of immunohistochemical stains that work in routinely processed tissues may assist the pathologist with diagnostically challenging cases (Tables 11 and 12). It must be recognized that reported sensitivities and specificities may vary with case mix (degree of differentiation of HCC, number and type of non-HCC cases examined, etc.) and size of specimen. Care must be used when employing immunohistochemical stains in hepatic tissue, since false positives can occur when improper dilutions of antibody are used, endogenous biotin is not blocked, tissue handling is suboptimal, or specimen size is minute. While the staining characteristics of included nonneoplastic hepatic tissue give a useful guide for the performance characteristics of the antibody, trapped immunoreactive nonneoplastic hepatocytes should not be misinterpreted as tumor cell positivity.

TABLE 11. *Hepatocellular carcinoma—cytoplasmic deposits and inclusions*

Deposit/inclusion	Sensitivity (%)	Comments
Diagnostically useful		
Absence of cytoplasmic mucin	100	May be present in combined HCC-CC, CC or metastatic adenocarcinoma
Bile	5–33	Virtually pathognomonic of HCC
Copper/copper-binding protein	7–41	To date, negative in CC and metastatic adenocarcinoma
Mallory's hyalin	2–25	In malignant neoplasm, virtually pathognomonic of HCC
Hyaline globules	10–15	Highly suggestive of HCC in malignant hepatic tumor, but metastatic adenocarcinoma and neuroendocrine carcinoma may demonstrate these deposits
PAS-positive DR		AFP, A_1AT, A_1ACT, giant lysosomes, other glycoproteins
PAS-negative		Megamitochondria, apoptotic bodies, albumin, fibrinogen, other proteins
Ground glass/pale bodies	5–10	Fibrinogen, other serum proteins; HBsAg (usually represents trapped nonneoplastic cells)
Of interest, but not diagnostically useful		
Fat, glycogen (clear cells)	20–40	Predominant in 5–16% of cases
Hemosiderin	Rare, trace amounts	True even in HCC arising in hereditary hemochromatosis
Lipofuscin-like pigment	Rare	When prominent, liver may be black (Dubin-Johnson-like)

Data primarily from refs. 158, 175, 182, 187, 188.
AFP, alpha-fetoprotein; A_1AT, alpha$_1$-antitrypsin; A_1ACT, alpha$_1$-antichymotrypsin; CC, cholangiocarcinoma; DR, diastase resistant; HBsAg, hepatitis B surface antigen; HCC, hepatocellular carcinoma; PAS, periodic acid–Schiff.

Bile located within neoplastic cells or tubular lumina is pathognomonic of HCC, but it is found in less than one-third of cases and is not evident in poorly differentiated tumors (Fig. 12D) (182). The presence of bile canaliculi is also diagnostic. Other than in HCC, bile and bile canaliculi have been identified only in hepatoid adenocarcinomas of varied primary sites (171). Routine immunohistochemical testing (Table 12) using unabsorbed polyclonal anti-CEA antiserum or certain monoclonal CEA (m-CEA) antibodies, each of which cross-reacts with canalicular biliary glycoprotein 1, demonstrates bile canaliculi (canalicular pattern) in 70% to 80% of HCCs (range, 24–90%) (183–186) (Fig. 12G).

Canalicular CEA staining remains the most useful and most thoroughly investigated immunohistochemical marker in the differential diagnosis of HCC, although one drawback is that this pattern of immunoreactivity is most frequently seen in better differentiated tumors. About 50% of poorly differentiated tumors lack immunoreactivity. A false-positive HCC interpretation of a canalicular pattern may result from inclusion of immunoreactive nonneoplastic hepatocytes within the tumor, misinterpretation of an incomplete membrane pattern as canalicular in location, or misinterpretation of periluminal immunoreactivity in adenocarcinomas as staining of dilated canaliculi. The rate of cytoplasmic p-CEA immunoreactivity in HCC is quite inconsistent and unimportant in terms of diagnosis; however, cytoplasmic immunoreactivity with m-CEA antisera is uncommon, and, for this reason, absence of immunoreactivity with this antibody may be diagnostically useful (183–186).

Several different types of eosinophilic hyaline globules, both intra- and extracellular, have been described in 10% to 15% of HCCs. They are usually PAS positive, resist predigestion with diastase, and often display immunoreactivity for AFP, A_1AT, or alpha$_1$-antichymotrypsin (A_1ACT). Granular cytoplasmic immunoreactivity is more typical of these three antigens. Immunoreactivity for A_1AT and A_1ACT is nonspecific and is not useful in differential diagnosis. The finding of a hepatic tumor with immunoreactivity for AFP is very suggestive of HCC, and its presence in poorly differentiated tumors may be of particular diagnostic utility. However, other neoplasms (such as HBL; adenocarcinomas of the pancreas, stomach, and lung; and yolk sac tumor) may demonstrate this antigen; the sensitivity in reported series varies from 15% to 70% (185,186). AFP has been found now and then in the adjacent nonneoplastic liver (149,184). Measuring serum AFP by modern techniques is more sensitive than finding immunohistochemical evidence of AFP in tumor tissue; therefore, use of the former method may be more cost-effective.

Mallory's hyalin has been found in 2% to 25% of cases, often in focal areas of the tumor or in individual tumor nodules (153,187). In a malignant hepatic tumor, it is diagnostic of HCC. In this context, it is also commonly detected in surrounding nonneoplastic hepatocytes, even in the absence of alcoholic liver disease. Mallory's hyalin has also been reported in HCA and FNH (2,114). Pale eosinophilic ("ground glass") cytoplasmic inclusions, noted from time to time in HCC, may contain fibrinogen, other serum proteins, or hep-

TABLE 12. *Hepatocellular carcinoma—immunohistochemistry*

	Sensitivity (%)	Comments
Greatest diagnostic utility		
p-CEA (canalicular staining)	50–90	Near 100% specificity; beware trapped nonneoplastic hepatocytes and mimics of canalicular pattern in non-HCC; often negative in PD-HCC
AFP	15–70	90–95% specific; lacks sensitivity; may be positive in PD-HCC
m-CEA (noncanalicular staining)	0–10	Rarely positive in HCC; 60–75% CC or met adenoca positive
HepPar-1[a]	80	90% specificity; beware trapped nonneoplastic hepatocytes; rarely CC or met adenoca positive
ERY-1[a]	90	~95% specificity (little data); may be found in renal cell Ca, yolk sac tumor, TCC; staining often focal; normal hepatocytes positive
Some diagnostic utility		
Hepatocyte CK (8, 18) vs. other CKs	94–100 vs. 30–60	Lack of specificity, but of use if only "hepatocyte CK" positive
CD34 (endothelium)	50–100	Rare positivity in cirrhotic liver, HCA, FNH; prominent in advanced HCC; 50% of small WD-HCC are negative
Least diagnostic utility and/or little data		
Alpha$_1$-microglobulin	95	Near 90% specificity; need more data
Albumin	nearly 100	Frequent false positives, prominent background staining
Inhibin	5–90	Higher rate appears to be false positive, biotin not blocked
PTHrP	0	All CC positive; met adenoca may be positive (best in frozen tissue)
A$_1$AT	55–93	Lack of specificity and/or sensitivity
EMA	40	Lack of specificity and/or sensitivity
B72.3	5–10	Lack of specificity and/or sensitivity
Ber-EP4	35	Lack of specificity and/or sensitivity
HMFG-2	20	Lack of specificity and/or sensitivity
Cu-18	10	Lack of specificity and/or sensitivity
TPA	30 (weak)	Lack of specificity and/or sensitivity
Leu-M1/CD15	5–30	Lack of specificity and/or sensitivity
Ferritin	45–70	Lack of specificity and/or sensitivity
Factor XIIIa	65–70	Lack of specificity and/or sensitivity
Synaptophysin	5–10	Focal positivity does not exclude HCC (vs. NE tumor)
Chromogranin	5	Focal positivity does not exclude HCC (vs. NE tumor)

A$_1$AT, alpha$_1$-antitrypsin; adenoca, adenocarcinoma; AFP, alpha-fetoprotein; Ca, carcinoma; CC, cholangiocarcinoma; CEA, carcinoembryonic antigen; CK, cytokeratin; Cu, copper; EMA, epithelial membrane antigen; ERY-1, erythropoiesis-associated antigen; FNH, focal nodular hyperplasia; HCA, hepatocellular adenoma; HCC, hepatocellular carcinoma; HepPar-1, hepatocyte paraffin 1; HMFG, human milk fat globulin; m, monoclonal; met, metastatic; NE, neurcendocrine tumor; p, polyclonal; PD, poorly differentiated; PTHrP, parathyroid hormone–related peptide; TPA, tissue polypeptide antigen; TCC, transitional cell carcinoma; WD, well differentiated.
[a] Promising but need further study.
Data primarily from refs. 183–186, 190–192, 234.

atitis B surface antigen (HBsAg) or may be undefined (188). Ground-glass inclusions have also been termed pale bodies, particularly in FL-HCC. Fibrinogen-containing ground-glass inclusions have been reported in 5% to 10% of cases of usual HCC. Most HBsAg-positive cells represent nonneoplastic hepatocytes trapped within the tumor.

Copper-binding protein (Shikata's orcein stain) and copper (rhodanine stain) have been detected in up to 41% of HCCs, but they have not been found to date in other primary or secondary hepatic malignancies (182,189). Hemosiderin is rarely found in HCC, even in the context of hereditary hemochromatosis. Calcification is also quite rare in untreated cases, except in the fibrolamellar variant.

HepPar-1 is a recently described monoclonal antibody that reacts with a hepatocyte-specific epitope, the exact nature of which is unknown. Its staining pattern suggests organelle localization, possibly mitochondrial (186). Studies from the University of Pittsburgh have shown performance characteristics similar to p-CEA, with 82% sensitivity and 90% specificity. Drawbacks to the use of this antibody are that it is not commercially available, that published data come from only one institution, that occasional staining of non-HCC malignancies has been described, and that there are false positives due to staining of trapped nonneoplastic hepatocytes and insensitivity of identification of poorly differentiated HCC (50%)—findings similar to those described earlier for p-CEA. Erythropoiesis-associated antigen (ERY-1; not commercially available) was found in 89% of HCCs in one study, but few additional data are available. Immunoreactivity has also been found in renal cell carcinoma, yolk sac tumor, and transitional cell carcinoma (184).

Initial reports suggested that malignant liver cells express a lineage-specific CK profile (hepatocytes express CKs 8 and 18, molecular weights 52 kd and 45 kd, respectively; bile ducts express CKs 7 and 19, molecular weights 54 kd and 40 kd, respectively). Nearly all other epithelial malignancies (except renal cell carcinoma and neuroendocrine tumors) possessed CKs in addition to those considered hepatocyte specific (183,185,186,190,191). These studies employed multiple monoclonal antibodies that were specific for a single CK or used a combination of antibodies specific for multiple CKs (for example, immunoreactivity with CAM 5.2 and CKs 8, 18, 19 but not with AE-1, which in the liver is specific for CK 19, or AE1/AE3, which contains a small amount of CK 8 but typically does not react with normal hepatocytes) that allowed for distinction between hepatocyte CK and other CKs. The initial enthusiasm has waned, because HCCs (up to 60%, particularly moderate and poorly differentiated tumors) and even nonneoplastic hepatocytes have been found to frequently modify their CK expression and express nonhepatocyte CKs (other than CKs 8 and 18), therefore limiting their diagnostic utility.

Albumin immunoreactivity is often described in the context of HCC; however, leakage of proteins normally found at high concentrations in the serum into tumor cells of various malignancies often gives false-positive results. *In situ* hybridization for albumin mRNA appears to be highly sensitive, but focal positivity was detected in one-third of peripheral cholangiocarcinomas (PCCs) (192). Whether this positivity represents trapped nonneoplastic hepatocytes is unclear; further study of this method is needed. Other antigens that have been studied lack specificity for HCC and do not appear to be diagnostically useful.

In summary, many investigators currently use a mucicarmine stain and a panel of p-CEA (canalicular pattern), m-CEA, and AFP antibodies when evaluating diagnostically challenging cases. HepPar-1 and ERY-1 may prove to complement and enhance the performance characteristics of this approach; more data on these antibodies are needed.

Fine Needle Aspiration. The pathologist must rely on both cytologic and architectural features when evaluating a hepatic FNA for the presence of HCC, adopting an approach similar to that used in making a histologic diagnosis (10–13,16,18,20–27). The aspirates are generally highly cellular, and the tumor cells are polygonal with centrally placed hyperchromatic nuclei and variably prominent nucleoli. The nuclear to cytoplasmic ratio is typically increased, varying with the degree of differentiation. Naked tumor cell nuclei are common and should not be confused with signs of lymphoma. Intranuclear cytoplasmic invaginations and the various cytoplasmic deposits (bile, hyaline globules, Mallory's hyalin), described in the section on histologic features, can be identified in cytologic preparations. Cytoplasmic vacuolation (clear-cell HCC) may simulate signet cell adenocarcinoma or pleomorphic liposarcoma.

Careful attention to the appearance of tumor cell aggregates on smear preparations will often yield findings analogous to the architectural patterns identified in cell blocks and core biopsies (Fig. 12B). A trabecular pattern is recognized on smears by finding either branching sinusoids, lined by elongated endothelial cells, that are flanked on both sides by several layers of polygonal tumor cells (central pattern) or trabeculae of malignant hepatocytes that are invested by endothelial cells (peripheral pattern). Slender trabeculae may mimic the papillary fronds of adenocarcinoma. The solid (compact) pattern is characterized by cohesive sheets of tumor cells with only a few endothelial cells. Naked tumor cell nuclei are often quite conspicuously associated with this pattern. In the pseudoglandular form, the polygonal tumor cells are arranged in rosettes or acini, sometimes surrounding a droplet of bile or proteinaceous material. Tumor giant cells and malignant spindle cells may be noted.

The sensitivity of guided FNA for diagnosing hepatic malignancy in most recent series is 90% to 96%, with a specificity of 90% to 100% (8,12,18). The preparation of cell blocks (microhistology), which can be done in 70% to 85% of cases, increases the sensitivity of a malignant diagnosis by 10% to 20% and allows the pathologist to perform routine special stains and immunohistochemistry, thus increasing the specificity of diagnosis. Moderately differentiated HCC, as in histologic material, is most easily diagnosed.

False-negative diagnoses of HCC are related either to very well differentiated tumors that are difficult to identify on the basis of cytology as being neoplastic or to poorly differentiated tumors that are difficult to distinguish as hepatocellular in origin. The presence of monotonous nuclear atypia and nuclear crowding and the absence of a reticulin framework in cell blocks may be helpful in the differential diagnosis of relatively well differentiated HCC versus benign hepatic conditions (153). On the other hand, false-positive diagnoses are usually due to the presence of reactive or dysplastic hepatocytes in a cirrhotic liver. Reactive hepatocytes generally demonstrate a continuum of morphologic changes. This variability is helpful in distinguishing reactive from malignant hepatocytes.

Two studies of cytologic smears prepared from hepatic FNAs employed stepwise logistic regression analysis to aid in distinguishing HCC from other tumors and nonneoplastic conditions. The presence of at least two of three criteria (polygonal cells with centrally placed nuclei, malignant cells separated by sinusoidal endothelial cells, and bile) was considered by Bottles et al. to be 97% sensitive and 100% specific for HCC compared with other malignancies (27). Cohen et al. (26) found that the presence of the following three features was 87% specific and 100% sensitive for the diagnosis of HCC versus nonneoplastic conditions: an increased nuclear to cytoplasmic ratio, a trabecular pattern, and atypical naked nuclei. Please consult the section on the utility of liver biopsy for tumor diagnosis at the beginning of the chapter for more general data concerning hepatic FNA biopsy.

DNA Analysis and Molecular Biology

HCC is hyperploid or aneuploid in 50% to 92% of cases (193–195). In the study of Koike et al. (194), the hepatocytes of cirrhotic patients who did not show signs of HCC after 5 years of follow-up were typically diploid, whereas nondiploid populations were frequently found in those patients in whom HCC developed within 3 years. With increasing size, tumors are more likely to be nondiploid (193). In one study, aneuploidy was found to be an independent adverse risk factor for postoperative tumor recurrence (195).

While immunohistochemical and molecular studies of HCC have detected various oncogene (bcl-2, c-erb-B-2, c-myc, c-ras, c-met) and suppressor gene (p53, nm23, RB) products as well as loss of heterozygosity involving at least ten different chromosomes, to date the role of such studies in diagnostic hepatopathology has not been defined (115,160). Proliferative activity (proliferating cell nuclear antigen, Ki-67, MIB-I, etc.) appears to increase with decreasing degrees of HCC differentiation (196).

Precancerous Lesions

Large-cell change (LCC) of hepatocytes (formerly called liver cell dysplasia or large-cell dysplasia), as first described by Anthony in 1973, is characterized on cytology by atypical hepatocytes demonstrating nuclear and cytoplasmic enlargement, nuclear pleomorphism with hyperchromasia, multinucleation, and a relatively normal nuclear to cytoplasmic ratio. These changes take place in groups of hepatocytes or entire cirrhotic nodules (Fig. 13) (4,146,197–200). The affected cells are easily seen at scanning magnification and often show a predilection for periseptal locations. They often form loose clusters with intermingled normal-appearing hepatocytes; they do not form expansile aggregates deforming the surrounding hepatic architecture. An association with prolonged cholestasis has been postulated (199). LCC is frequently found in chronic liver diseases, particularly in hepatitis B–related cirrhosis, and it has been reported in 25% to 85% of cases associated with HCC.

Although it was initially suggested that LCC is a precancerous lesion, it is now considered by many investigators not to be a direct precursor of HCC; in fact, it may represent a concurrent change in the hepatocyte's normal process of terminal differentiation, with polyploidization driven by ongoing hepatocellular injury (200). The fact that these cells typically arise in cirrhosis, are often binucleated, have increased or abnormal DNA content but little proliferative activity, a higher rate of apoptosis, and few described genetic abnormalities supports this hypothesis. While several longitudinal

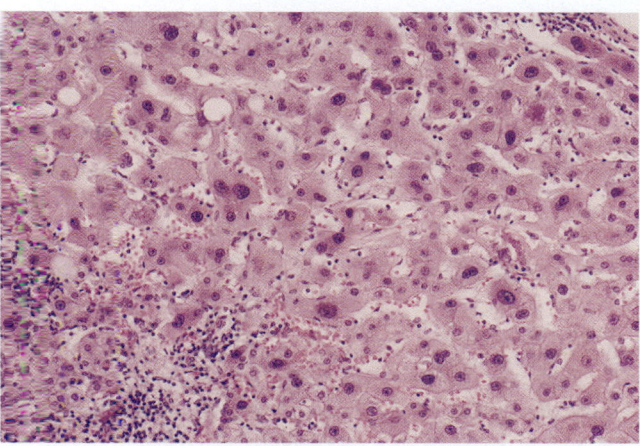

FIG. 13. Large-cell change (dysplasia). The role of this finding as a potential precursor to hepatocellular carcinoma continues to be controversial. See Fig. 9D for small-cell change (dysplasia).

studies suggest that patients with LCC have a three- to fivefold increased risk of developing HCC, its positive predictive value in biopsy specimens is quite low (about 20%) (200). Any signs of LCC noted in biopsies should probably be recorded in the surgical pathology report; however, whether patients with this finding should undergo more frequent surveillance is conjectural, since the utility of screening programs in general has not been validated (159).

While the role of LCC as a premalignant lesion has been contested, many investigators feel that small-cell change (small-cell dysplasia) may be the important link to HCC (Fig. 9D) (4,148,201). The rarity (about 5% of cirrhotic livers) (199) and focal nature of this finding make study of this process quite difficult. Nonetheless, the results of experimental data in animals, as well as its morphologic similarity to WD-HCC, suggest that it is likely a premalignant lesion. The morphologic appearance of these cells, their presence in borderline (dysplastic) nodules (which are important in the pathogenesis of HCC), and problems in their differential diagnosis have been discussed earlier in the chapter (see the section on BNs and Table 7). In the normal liver the possibility that HCC arises from HCA or an adenoma-like lesion (possible grade 1 HCC) has been hypothesized (111, 121–125). Figure 14 summarizes some of the features considered potentially important in the evolution of HCC (202).

Differential Diagnosis

The clinicopathologic features distinguishing HCC from the benign hepatocellular masses have been summarized in Table 4. One rare benign hepatic tumor that can present a diagnostic challenge is angiomyolipoma, particularly when the epithelioid component is prominent and a reticulin-sparse trabecular pattern is present (203) (Table 13). The presence of a spindle-cell component; fat, tortuous, thick-walled blood vessels; immunoreactivity of the epithelioid cells for

TABLE 13. Tumors other than usual adenocarcinomas that can be misdiagnosed as hepatocellular carcinoma: confusing pathologic features and helpful diagnostic clues[a]

Tumor type	Confusing pathologic features	Clues to correct diagnosis	
		Routine histology	Immunohistochemistry
Neuroendocrine	Similar cytoarchitectural patterns and CK pattern, hyaline globules; HCC can demonstrate focal +Cg, Syn	Stippled chromatin, nucleoli usually not prominent, sclerosis, peritumoral capillary network	Diffuse, strong + Syn, Cg; − p-CEA (canalicular), HepPar-1, AFP, etc.
Clear-cell carcinoma	Similar cytoarchitectural patterns and CK pattern as clear-cell HCC	Prominent vascular pattern may be present	− p-CEA, HepPar-1, AFP, etc.
RCC (non-clear cell)	Similar cytoarchitectural patterns and CK profile as HCC	Prominent vascular pattern may be present	− p-CEA, HepPar-1, AFP, etc.
Squamous cell ca	Solid sheets and trabeculae, eosinophilic cytoplasm	Intercellular bridges, keratin, sclerosis	− p-CEA, HepPar-1, AFP, etc.
Melanoma	Epithelioid cells and replacing growth pattern can simulate trabecular pattern; prominent nucleoli; intranuclear inclusions common; + S-100 and HMB-45 have been reported in HCC	No well-formed epithelial features, spindle cells, melanin pigment	Diffuse, strong + HMB-45; − CK, − p-CEA, HepPar-1, AFP, etc.
Angiomyolipoma	Epithelioid cells, eosinophilic or clear cytoplasm; may have trabecular pattern with little reticulin; HMB-45 has been reported in HCC	Spindle cells; fat, tortuous, thick-walled blood vessels	Diffuse, strong + HMB-45 in epithelioid cells; ± MSA and SMA; − CK, − p-CEA, HepPar-1, AFP, etc.
Prostate adenoca	Can have sheetlike growth pattern, large cells with abundant cytoplasm, round nuclei with prominent nucleoli	Cytoplasm more basophilic; glands usually noted with careful searching; cytoplasmic mucin may be present	+PSA, PSAP; − p-CEA, AFP, HepPar-1, etc.
Angiosarcoma	Thickened cords of hepatocytes; + CD34, other endothelial markers in endothelial cells lining cords; CK can be positive in these cells; CD34 etc. also + in endothelial cells lining sinusoids of HCC	Hepatocytes are cytologically bland; endothelial cells are prominent and pleomorphic; in HCC endothelial cells are inconspicuous; spindle-cell and cavernous foci may be present	+ CD34, other endothelial markers in pleomorphic endothelial cells
Other sarcoma	Bland to pleomorphic spindle cells ± differentiated sarcoma elements can be present in HCC (sarcomatoid variant, carcinosarcoma)	For diagnosis of HCC need to demonstrate differentiated foci	+ CK, AFP would favor HCC; otherwise not helpful

[a] Clinical history and results of imaging studies, including the location of dominant masses, the results of tumor marker studies (AFP, PSA, etc.), and, potentially, review of other biopsy material may prove invaluable in a given case. All of the tumors in this table typically are found in livers that lack cirrhosis or evidence of chronic liver disease (some angiosarcomas are exceptions) in comparison with HCC in which cirrhosis is typical.

Adenoca, adenocarcinoma; AFP, alpha-fetoprotein; ca, carcinoma; CEA, carcinoembryonic antigen; Cg, chromogranin; CK, cytokeratin; HCC, hepatocellular carcinoma; HepPar-1, hepatocyte paraffin 1; HMB, human melanoma black; MSA, muscle-specific actin; p, polyclonal; PSA, prostate-specific antigen; PSAP, prostate-specific acid phosphatase; RCC, renal cell carcinoma; SMA, smooth-muscle actin; Syn, synoptophysin.

HMB-45 and actin (muscle-specific and smooth-muscle types); and negativity for CK aid in making the correct diagnosis.

It is usually more difficult for the pathologist to make the distinction between HCC and the much more common group of metastatic carcinomas (particularly adenocarcinomas as well as ICC. It should be emphasized again that HCC develops much less often in the normal liver and much more frequently in the cirrhotic liver compared with metastatic tumors (167). For this reason, it behooves the pathologist to always consider the possibility of metastasis when evaluating a malignant liver tumor. Many of these differential diagnostic features have been alluded to earlier and are summarized in Table 14.

Specific mention should also be made of a few malignant tumors that can at times be quite difficult to differentiate

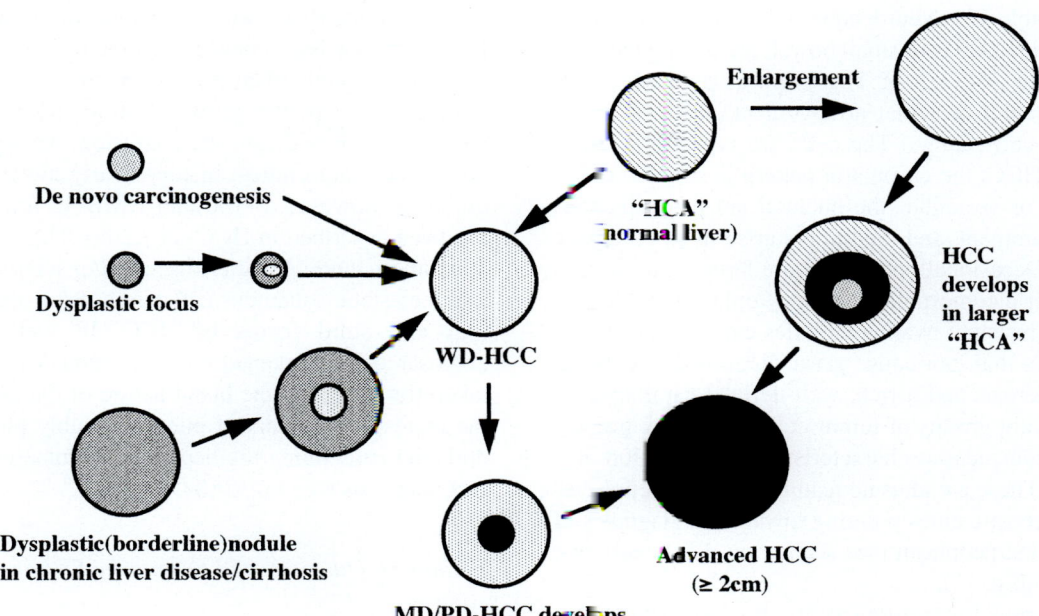

FIG. 14. Possible evolution of hepatocellular carcinoma (HCC) in chronic liver disease/cirrhosis and in the normal liver. Whether HCC developing within dysplastic nodules in the context of chronic liver disease represents the major pathway to HCC is unknown. A "nodule in nodule" pattern is common, with foci of well-differentiated HCC arising centrally in a clonelike manner, subsequently being replaced in lesions larger than 1 cm by moderately (MD) or poorly differentiated (PD) HCC. As in chronic liver disease/cirrhosis, HCC in the normal liver could arise *de novo* or from a dysplastic focus. Hepatocellular adenoma (HCA) or adenoma-like lesions (possible grade 1 HCC) could provide fertile soil for the development of some cases, as could nodular regenerative hyperplasia (not shown; modified from ref. 202).

TABLE 14. *Hepatocellular carcinoma (HCC) vs. metastatic carcinoma and cholangiocarcinoma: microscopic features useful in differential diagnosis*[a]

Characteristic	HCC	Adenocarcinoma (primary and metastatic)	Poorly differentiated carcinoma
Nonneoplastic liver	Typically cirrhotic	Cirrhosis uncommon	Cirrhosis uncommon
Growth at tumor margin	Replacement	Often sinusoidal	Often sinusoidal
Main growth pattern	Trabecular	Glands	Sheets, individual cells
Fibrous stroma	Minimal[b]	Often prominent	Variable
Intranuclear inclusions	Common	Uncommon	Uncommon
Prominent nucleolus	Typical	Often	Variable
Tumor cell cytoplasm			
General features	Often abundant; eosinophilic granular, clear	Variable	Variable
Bile	Occ. present	Absent[c]	Absent[c]
Cu, Cu-binding protein	Occ. present	Absent	Absent
Hyaline globules	Occ. present	Rare	Rare
Mallory bodies	Occ. present	Absent	Absent
Mucin	Absent	Often present	Absent
p-CEA (canalicular pattern)	Often present	Absent	Absent
m-CEA (noncanalicular)	Rarely present	Often present	?
HepPar-1	Often present	Rarely present	?
AFP	Occ. present	Rarely present	Absent
"Hepatocyte CK" only	Often present	Absent	?

AFP, alpha-fetoprotein; CEA, carcinoembryonic antigen; CK, cytokeratin; Cu, copper; HepPar-1, hepatocyte paraffin 1; m, monoclonal; Occ., occasionally; p, polyclonal.

[a] Clinical history and results of imaging studies, including location of dominant masses, the results of tumor marker studies (AFP, etc.), and, potentially, review of other biopsy material, may prove invaluable in a given case.

[b] The fibrolamellar and scirrhous variants of HCC are exceptions, since they contain a prominent fibrous stroma.

[c] Bile may very rarely be present in or around peripheral tumor cells when there is extensive cholestasis in the adjacent liver (passive uptake).

from HCC (Table 13). Neuroendocrine tumors, which usually arise in the pancreas or small bowel, are among the most challenging (Fig. 15) (3,204). These tumors can have a conspicuous trabecular or acinar arrangement and focal oncocytic or clear-cell change. The cells are typically smaller than those of HCC, the chromatin pattern is stippled rather than clumped or vesicular, the nucleoli are inconspicuous rather than prominent, and the tumors arise in an otherwise normal liver. Occasionally, the cells are larger, and there is random nuclear pleomorphism. Even cytoplasmic PAS-positive, diastase-resistant hyaline globules can be seen. These are all features that can cause great diagnostic confusion (205,206). Sclerosis and a rich, well-defined capillary network surrounding groups of tumor cells in varying proportions may be conspicuous characteristics. Calcification may also be noted. These are unusual features in HCC, representing major diagnostic clues pointing toward the diagnosis of a neuroendocrine neoplasm (see section on neuroendocrine neoplasms and Fig. 17).

Diffuse, strong immunoreactivity for neuroendocrine markers (synaptophysin, chromogranin) helps in distinguishing a neuroendocrine neoplasm from HCC, but focal immunoreactivity with these antibodies has sometimes been described in HCC (186,207,208). Evidence of hepatocellular differentiation on immunohistochemistry (canalicular pattern with p-CEA, etc.) or ultrastructural confirmation of neurosecretory granules may be helpful in individual cases.

The problem of clear-cell carcinomas of varied origin and clear-cell HCC has previously been discussed in the section on this variant. Renal cell carcinoma of the non-clear-cell type, with its trabecular and tubular architecture, granular eosinophilic cytoplasm, and identical CK profile (CKs 8 and 18), can mimic HCC, neuroendocrine tumors, and even HCA. Moreover, one has to beware that the biopsy itself may have been inadvertently obtained from a renal mass (see Fig. 1).

Melanoma can also grow within the liver in a trabecular pattern and cause diagnostic confusion. An appropriate antibody panel and clinical history nearly always resolve this dilemma; however, S-100 and HMB-45 immunoreactivity has been described in HCC (207,208). The presence of keratinization, intercellular bridges, and/or sclerosis helps separate metastatic squamous cell carcinoma from macrotrabecular and solid forms of HCC. In well-differentiated angiosarcoma, thickened cords of hepatocytes can be mistaken for HCC, but the bland nature of the hepatocytes and the increased numbers of plump, variably pleomorphic endothelial cells lining the hepatic trabeculae lead to the correct diagnosis (see Fig. 24B).

Treatment, Outcome, and Prognostic Factors

Patients with HCC usually survive only a few months after diagnosis (158,161); rarely, spontaneous tumor regression has been reported (161). The prognosis of patients with HCC is determined not only by HCC stage (Table 9) but also by the functional status of the underlying liver (209). Palliation with percutaneous ethanol injection, cryoablation, and transcatheter arterial chemo-embolization, with or without suspension in the iodized oily carrier substance Lipiodol, has been employed with some success in inoperable cases. The most common causes of death are cachexia, gastrointestinal bleeding, and hepatic failure. Spontaneous tumor rupture accounts for about 10% of deaths. At the time of autopsy 50% to 75% of patients show signs of metastases. These occur more frequently in patients without cirrhosis, presumably because they live longer. The lung and the porta hepatis lymph nodes are the most common metastatic sites. Bone, adrenal gland, gallbladder, and virtually any site in the body can be involved (3,172). While documentation of extrahepatic spread of single HCC nodules less than or equal to 3 cm in diameter is difficult to find in the literature (210), one incidental HCC, 1.5 cm in diameter, in the University of Nebraska liver transplant series was associated with an adrenal metastasis and the death of the patient (210a; C. A. Roberts, personal communication).

In selected patients, hepatic resection and transplantation provide the only possibility for cure. Because there can be tracking of tumor along sites of needle biopsy, even with FNA, some investigators feel that in the appropriate clinical context (i.e., mass in a cirrhotic liver with significant serum AFP elevation), surgical therapy should be performed without preoperative biopsy (16,17,106,108). Five-year survival after resection is often reported as 20% to 30%, but with careful selection of patients (noncirrhotic/compensated cirrhosis, tumors less than or equal to 5 cm), 5-year survival rates can exceed 50% (209). One of the major drawbacks of surgery, however, is the high recurrence rate (50% to 80%), even when patients are

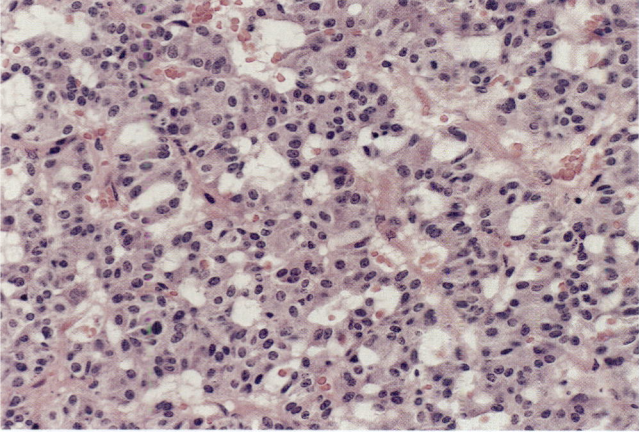

FIG. 15. Neuroendocrine neoplasm in the liver. This histologic pattern was present in a wedge biopsy obtained from a large, solitary hepatic mass arising in the otherwise normal liver of a 70-year-old woman. Features favoring a neuroendocrine tumor rather than HCC include the small cell size; the presence of bland nuclei with homogeneous, stippled chromatin; and the absence of prominent nucleoli. Immunohistochemical staining for neuroendocrine markers was diffusely positive, while canalicular polyclonal carcinoembryonic antigen immunoreactivity was absent. Electron microscopy demonstrated numerous dense-core neurosecretory granules.

carefully selected, with small tumors and negative (more than or equal to 1 cm) resection margins (211). Since only a minority of recurrences are found in the region of the resected stump, undetected micrometastases or new multicentric disease (rather than incomplete tumor removal) appear to be responsible for most recurrences.

Although various studies differ in their results, tumor size, number and location (one or both lobes) of tumor nodules, the presence of vascular invasion, and the presence or absence of cirrhosis are the most important prognostic variables for HCC that the pathologist can identify in resection specimens (209,212,213). The first three are reflected in the TMN staging system (Table 9). In addition, the distance of the tumor from the resection margin (greater or less than 1 cm or at inked margin), the presence or absence of a tumor capsule and capsular invasion, and, possibly, the degree of HCC differentiation should be clearly noted by the pathologist in the surgical pathology report, since these parameters may also have prognostic import. More data are required to evaluate whether a florid lymphocytic inflammatory infiltrate, DNA ploidy status, PCNA labeling index, detection of products of various oncogene/suppressor genes (c-myc, c-met, p-53) in tissue sections, and the presence of circulating albumin or AFP m-RNA by polymerase chain reaction are of prognostic significance (213–219).

Theoretic considerations favor hepatic transplantation over resection for curative therapy of HCC, since this procedure also eliminates the predisposing condition (i.e., cirrhosis), although reinfection with hepatitis B or C can be a long-term problem. Studies have found that if transplantation is limited to solitary HCC less than or equal to 5 cm or to multiple nodules each less than 3 cm, the recurrence rate is minimal, and the survival rate at 4 years is similar to that of non-HCC patients. Long-term studies are needed to evaluate the relative merits of transplantation versus resection (209,220).

Fibrolamellar Hepatocellular Carcinoma

Clinical Features

A distinctive variant of HCC with prolonged survival has been reported under a variety of names that emphasize the characteristic cytologic and stromal changes of this tumor. These names include eosinophilic HCC with lamellar fibrosis, HCC, polygonal cell type with fibrous stroma, fibrolamellar oncocytic hepatoma, and fibrolamellar hepatocellular carcinoma (FL-HCC), among others (2,3,121,122,158, 221–224) (Table 15). This variant most frequently arises in the noncirrhotic liver (about 90%) of young patients (peak, third decade; age range, 5 to 85 years; less than 20% over age 40). It accounts for 1% to 5% of all cases in North America and Western Europe and is quite rare in regions of high incidence of HCC (110,121,132,122,172,221,225). Men and women are equally affected. Patients usually have clinical findings similar to those of typical HCC, although initially these symptoms are vague and often overlooked. Rarely, gynecomastia and Budd-Chiari syndrome have been reported.

TABLE 15. *Fibrolamellar hepatocellular carcinoma (FL-HCC): distinguishing clinicopathologic features from the usual HCC*

	FL-HCC	Usual HCC
Clinical features		
% HCC	1–5%	95–99%
Epidemiologic factors		
Age	Peak, 3rd decade	6th–7th decade
Sex (male/female)	1:1	3–6:1
Serum markers (% elevated)		
AFP	10–15%	60–80%
DCP	100%	60–90%
NT, B_{12} $UB_{12}BC$	Often increased	Rarely increased
Imaging studies		
Calcification	40–80%	≤5% (no RX)
Central scar	50–70%	Rare
Resectability	48–75%	10–20%
Macroscopic features		
% Solitary	75%; left > right lobe	Uncommon
Fibrous septa, scar	10–63%	Absent
Necrosis, hemorrhage	Occasional (larger tumors)	Common
Associated cirrhosis	<10%	60–90%
Microscopic features		
Cell size, shape	Larger	Smaller
Cytoplasm		
Abundance	More	Less
Granularity	More	Less
Pale bodies	50%	≤10%
Hyaline globules	50%	10–15%
Stroma	Prominent lamellar bands	Scant
EM (mitochondria)	Numerous	Less common
Survival (5 yr)		
Overall	25–30%	0–7%
Resected	56–75%	20–30%

AFP, alpha-fetoprotein; DCP, des-γ-carboxy prothrombin; NT, neurotensin; $UB_{12}BC$, unsaturated B_{12} binding capacity; RX, treatment.

While serum AFP levels are elevated in only about 10% to 15% of cases (levels only rarely exceeding 1,000 ng/ml), serum DCP levels are uniformly elevated (225). Serum vitamin B_{12}, unsaturated B_{12} binding capacity, and plasma neurotensin levels are frequently elevated in these patients; in association with DCP determination, these parameters may be useful in diagnosis and monitoring the response to therapy. Differential diagnosis may be quite difficult on radiographic evidence, particularly with FNH, because FNH and FL-HCC often demonstrate a central scar. Calcification, however, is much more common in FL-HCC than FNH (40–80% vs. approximately 1%, respectively). Rarely, FL-HCC has the appearance of an abscess or multicystic mass. The pathogenesis of this tumor is unknown; there are no convincing cases suggesting malignant transformation of preexisting FNH to FL-HCC (30,31).

Pathologic Findings

Macroscopic Features. The majority of cases involve the left lobe, but it is not uncommon for both lobes to be affected. The tumors are firm, with a tan-white, gray, or brown color; they are often focally bile stained and may be necrotic or hemorrhagic (Fig. 16A). They are typically large (mean, 13 cm; range, 3 to 25 cm), solitary (75%), and well circumscribed, and they bulge from the cut surface and are dissected into multiple nodules by radiating fibrous septa (10% to 63%), which often merge to form a central stellate scar. This pattern may also be evident in metastases (222). As is apparent from the macroscopic description, distinguishing it from FNH may be difficult at surgery; however, the presence of grossly detectable bile staining and a diameter greater than 5 cm strongly suggest FL-HCC (30). The adjacent nonneoplastic liver is almost always unremarkable; however, a few cases with grossly distinctive abutting zones of arterialized nodular hepatocyte hyperplasia histologically simulating FNH, as well as distinct remote FNH lesions, have been described (30,31,221).

Microscopic Features. The tumor consists of large polygonal cells with abundant granular eosinophilic cytoplasm (oncocytes), sharply defined cell borders, and a large vesicular nucleus with a prominent nucleolus (Fig. 16B,C). These neoplastic hepatocytes are separated into nests, columns, or variably sized sheets by parallel, hyalinized

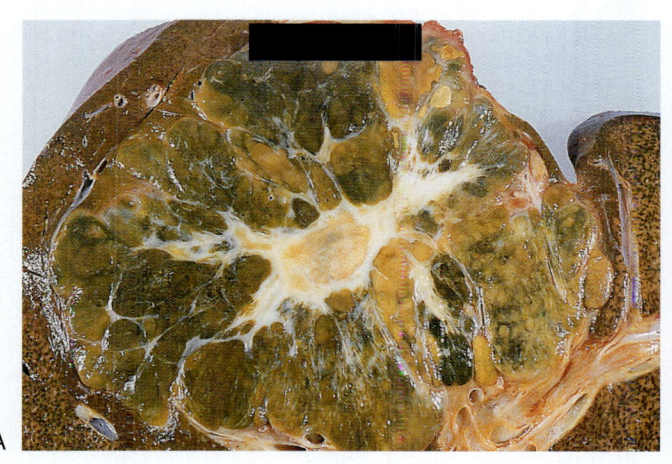
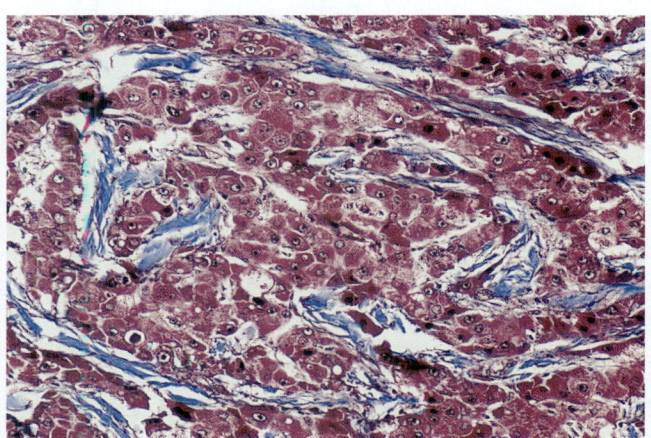
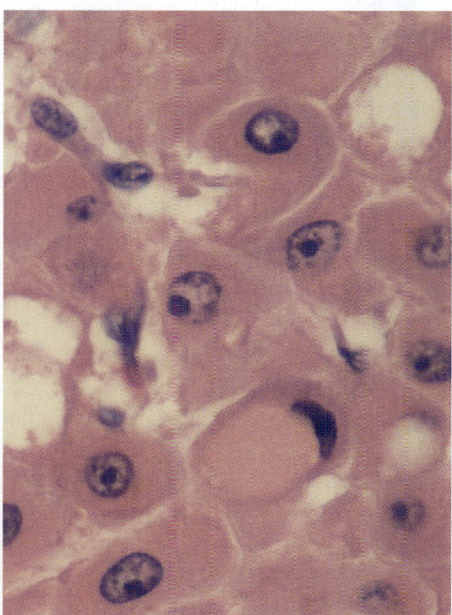
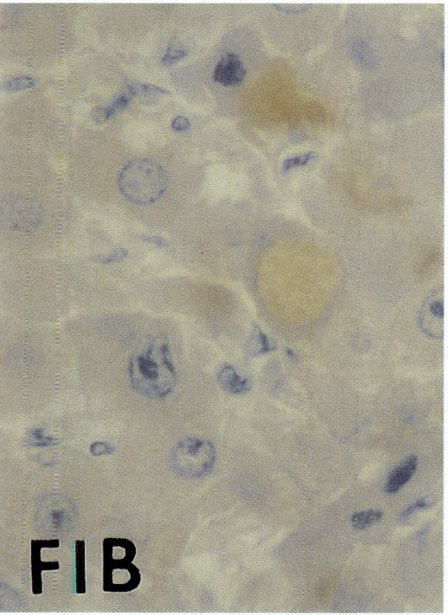

FIG. 16. Hepatocellular carcinoma, variants with prominent fibrosis. **A:** Fibrolamellar variant (FL-HCC). Note the central stellate scar. Bile, as seen in this tumor (green in photograph), aids in distinguishing FL-HCC from focal nodular hyperplasia at the time of surgery (see Fig. 7A). **B:** At the microscopic level, FL-HCC is characterized by large, polygonal, malignant hepatocytes with dense, eosinophilic, granular cytoplasm, discrete cell borders, vesicular nuclei, and prominent nucleoli. Lamellar fibrous strands separate the cords of tumor cells (trichrome). **C:** Pale bodies (ground-glass cells) are often found in hematoxylin and eosin–stained sections of FL-HCC (left panel). They are immunoreactive for fibrinogen (FIB, right panel) (immunoperoxidase, fibrinogen).

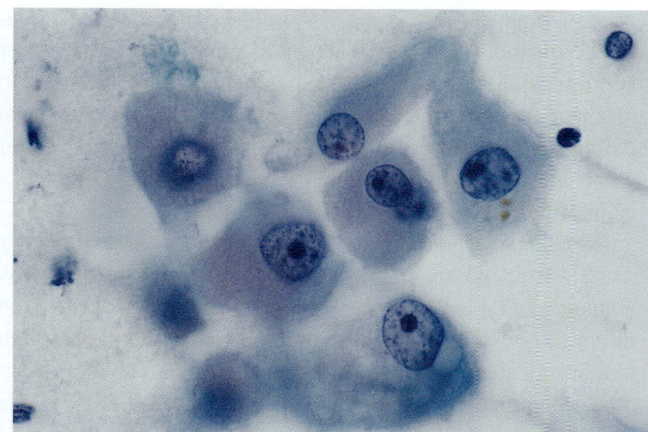
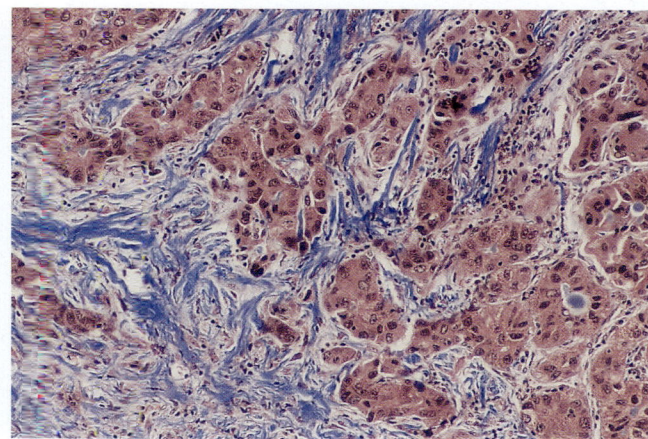
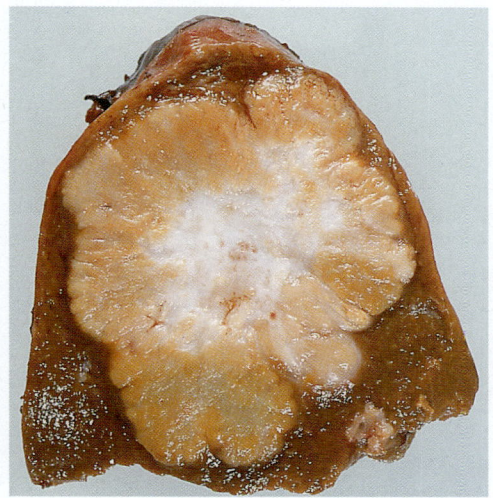

FIG. 16. (*continued*) Hepatocellular carcinoma, variants with prominent fibrosis. **D:** Fine-needle aspiration (FNA) specimen demonstrates discohesive, large, polygonal hepatocytes (note the size compared with that of lymphocytes) with the same cytologic features as described in B. Bile is present in one of the cells. Fibrous tissue is lacking, but it is sometimes seen in FNA specimens. The cytologic appearance, when evaluated in the context of the clinical and radiographic imaging studies, is suggestive of FL-HCC. **E:** Scirrhous (sclerosing) pattern of hepatocellular carcinoma (S-HCC). Although somewhat similar to FL-HCC on gross inspection, the central fibrosis in S-HCC is more diffuse and does not demonstrate radiating fibrous bands, as is often seen in FL-HCC. **F:** In S-HCC, compared with FL-HCC, the tumor cells are smaller, the nuclei usually are not vesicular, the nucleoli are not as round and prominent, and the cytoplasm is less granular and abundant. Pseudoglandular features are often present, and distinctly lamellar fibrosis is lacking. On clinical examination, hypercalcemia may be noted.

bands of relatively acellular collagen (thus the term "fibrolamellar") that may contain small, thick-walled arteries. One may see focal nuclear pleomorphism; a trabecular, adenoid, or pelioid pattern; areas of conventional HCC; or a relative lack of fibrosis. In smears prepared from FNA specimens, the tumor cells are generally noncohesive, although small cell groups and trabeculae may be evident (Fig. 16D). Strands of collagen may be noted, but they are often inconspicuous (10,11).

Mitoses are infrequent, but areas of necrosis and vascular invasion are not uncommon. Seen on electron microscopy, the cytoplasm contains numerous mitochondria, thus conforming to the definition of an oncocyte. The presence of "dense core" neuroendocrine-like granules does not indicate a neuroendocrine derivation. Eosinophilic hyaline globules, which may be PAS positive and resist diastase digestion or which may be PAS negative, are often present (50% of cases). Immunoreactivity for alpha-1-antitrypsin (AAT) is quite common, but AFP has only rarely been found. Cytoplasmic bile and copper or copper-binding protein (as manifestations of cholestasis) are seen in the majority of cases. Occasionally, intracytoplasmic fat and Mallory's hyalin are identified. Rarely, intracytoplasmic mucin is detected, in which case the tumor can be classified as a form of combined HCC-cholangiocarcinoma (226).

So-called cytoplasmic pale bodies, identical to the pale, eosinophilic, ground-glass inclusions described from time to time in the usual HCC, are noted in about 50% of cases (Fig. 16C). These contain fibrinogen and have been associated on ultrastructural examination with intracytoplasmic lumina/bile canaliculi or an accumulation of rough endoplasmic reticulum (221,227). Calcification seen on radiography corresponds to tumor necrosis with a foreign body–type giant-cell reaction. The CK profile and immunoreactivity for other tumor markers (including neurotensin and other neuroendocrine markers) do not differ significantly from those of the usual HCC (221). The rate of allelic loss appeared to be less than that of usual HCC in one small series (228).

Differential Diagnosis

Tumors in the differential diagnosis include (a) primary tumors, such as FNH, usual and scirrhous HCC, cholangiocarcinoma, and adenosquamous/squamous carcinoma with prominent sclerosis; (b) metastatic tumors, such as squamous cell carcinoma or adenocarcinoma arising in the breast or pancreas, which may be associated with a prominent sclerotic stroma, and (c) neuroendocrine (islet cell, carcinoid, paraganglioma/pheochromocytoma) tumors, which are nearly always metastatic. None of these malignant tumors have the proclivity of FL-HCC to affect young people.

The lack of hepatocellular anaplasia and the cytologic features distinguish FNH from FL-HCC, although the gross features may be similar. While HCC may have focal oncocytic features (which may, upon occasion, be extensive), the full-blown picture of FL-HCC by definition is lacking (116,180). The presence and amount of usual HCC in a tumor predominantly composed of FL-HCC should be noted. Adenosquamous/squamous cell carcinomas will often show evidence of keratinization and are easily distinguished from FL-HCC. In metastatic carcinomas and sclerosing hepatic carcinoma, the collagen is generally more dense and homogeneous, rather than forming the discrete lamellar bands characteristic of FL-HCC (2,3,229) (Fig. 16E,F). The tumor cells in scirrhous HCC are smaller and often display a glandular or pseudoglandular pattern. Nucleoli are less prominent, and the cytoplasm is less abundant and granular. Table 13 reviews features helpful in the differential diagnosis from neuroendocrine tumors. Although hyalinized fibrous bands may be found in neuroendocrine tumors, in general, they lack the lamellar pattern (Fig. 17). It is

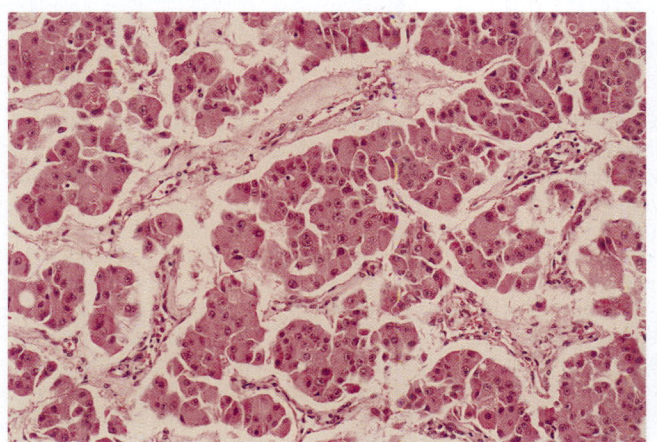

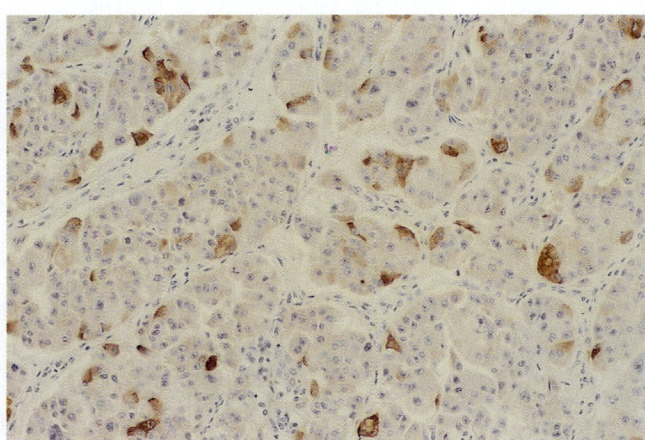

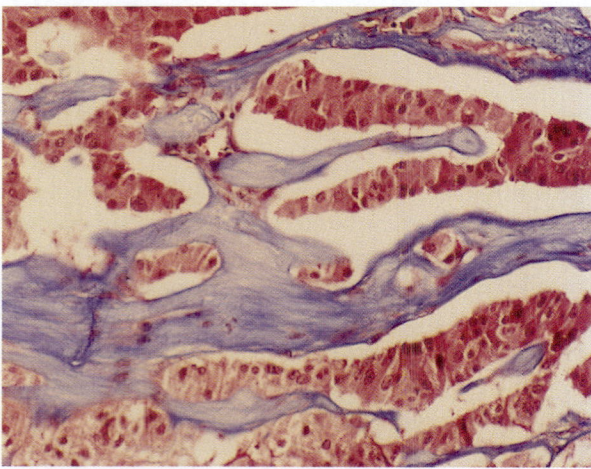

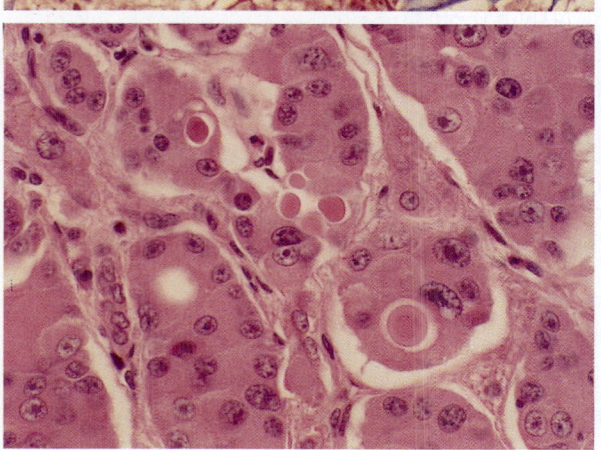

FIG. 17. Metastatic neuroendocrine neoplasm in the liver (from pancreas) simulating the fibrolamellar variant of hepatocellular carcinoma (FL-HCC). **A:** Rarely, neuroendocrine neoplasms can be confused with FL-HCC when they are composed of cords and nests of rather large cells with granular, eosinophilic cytoplasm and conspicuous nucleoli that are separated by fibrovascular septa. **B:** The presence of sclerotic fibrous bands (upper panel, trichrome) and cytoplasmic hyaline globules (lower panel) can cause further diagnostic confusion. In FL-HCC, however, neither an organoid pattern nor a prominent capillary network are seen. **C:** Immunohistochemistry for chromogranin is floridly positive in this case; a canalicular pattern with polyclonal carcinoembryonic antigen was lacking (not shown). Neuroendocrine granules were present on electron microscopy. (Kindly contributed by Ronald Jaffe, M.D., Children's Hospital of Pittsburgh, Pittsburgh, PA.)

important to note that an organoid appearance with a prominent peritumoral capillary network, which is so characteristic of endocrine lesions, is not seen in FL-HCC, and neuroendocrine tumors lack histologic or immunohistochemical evidence of hepatocellular differentiation.

Treatment and Outcome

The tumors of patients with FL-HCC are more frequently resectable, and these patients have a better outcome compared with patients with the usual HCC (even when tumor is found in a noncirrhotic liver) (Table 15) (221,225). Hepatic transplantation may be considered if the clinical situation precludes resection. Isolated metastases have been resected with long-term survival. The high incidence of nondiploid tumors and the fact that the tumor stroma resembles highgrade HCC (collagen types I, III, and VI, with a prominent tenascin meshwork and little laminin or type IV collagen) are discordant with the relatively favorable prognosis of this variant (230). Metastases most frequently involve abdominal lymph nodes, peritoneum, and lung.

Combined Hepatocellular Carcinoma–Cholangiocarcinoma

Less than 5% of primary hepatic carcinomas demonstrate an intimate admixture of both unequivocal HCC and cholangiocarcinoma (hence, combined HCC-CC), the latter characterized by cells with a cuboidal to columnar shape, less abundant and more amphophilic cytoplasm, less conspicuous nucleoli, gland formation, and mucin production (2,3,226,231). Rarely, intracytoplasmic mucin and bile have even been found in the same cell (231). A sarcomatoid component may be present (226,232). Associated cirrhosis is common. Separate HCC and CC, no matter how closely situated in the liver, are best considered "collison tumors" rather than combined HCC-CC (2). A tumor that has foci only suggestive but not diagnostic of both HCC and CC should be considered an undifferentiated carcinoma and is likely a metastasis. Metastases from combined HCC-CC may evidence HCC, CC, or combined HCC-CC.

The frequent presence of pseudoglandular spaces in HCC should not be misconstrued as a component of cholangiocarcinoma and is the most common problem in differential diagnosis. Although the presence of intracytoplasmic mucin is considered an objective marker for biliary differentiation, intraluminal mucicarmine-positive secretory material has been considered to indicate pseudoglandular HCC by some, but not all, investigators. A "biliary type" CK profile has been suggested as helpful in defining the cholangiocarcinoma component; this profile, however, seems to lack specificity (see discussion under HCC and Tables 12 and 14).

Sclerosing Hepatic Carcinoma

Sclerosing hepatic carcinoma (SHC) is not a distinct histopathologic entity, but represents a clinicopathologic entity in which a primary hepatic carcinoma (HCC, CC, or HCC-CC) is associated with a diffuse, dense, hyalinized stroma (scirrhous or sclerosing) and frequently hypercalcemia and hypophosphatemia in the absence of bone metastases (2,3,229). SHC represents about 3% of all primary hepatic neoplasms, excluding hemangiomas. Cirrhosis or hepatic fibrosis is noted in about 50% of cases.

A single, large, white-gray, firm, circumscribed mass, often with a serrated border, is typically found on macroscopic examination. There are often multiple satellite nodules. Although the sclerosis may be accentuated centrally, resulting in a retracted appearance, the stellate scar or radiating fibrous septa often seen in FNH or FL-HCC are absent (Fig. 16E). This gross appearance is easily mistaken for metastatic carcinoma, although central necrosis is unusual.

At the microscopic level, the tumor cells in scirrhous HCC are somewhat smaller than in the usual HCC, and there is a great tendency for the tumor trabeculae to undergo pseudoglandular (acinar) transformation as one proceeds from the periphery to the central fibrous core (Fig. 16F). Scirrhous CC is similar to the usual cholangiocarcinoma, except that the fibrous stroma is more diffusely distributed throughout the tumor. When the neoplastic cells are arranged as narrow tubular structures resembling bile ductules, the term cholangiolocellular carcinoma is used. Parathyroid hormone–related peptide has been verified by immunohistochemical studies in a few cases (scirrhous HCC and CC) with hypercalcemia (233,233a); however, it has also been found in the usual CC, metastatic adenocarcinoma, and reactive bile ductules in the absence of hypercalcemia (234). It has not yet been found in the usual HCC.

Differential Diagnosis

On needle biopsy, this tumor is frequently interpreted as metastatic carcinoma, particularly from the pancreas. Only rarely, however, does metastatic carcinoma feature dense sclerosis to the degree seen in SHC. Differentiation from FL-HCC has been discussed previously. As with cholangiocarcinoma in general, a definitive diagnosis of scirrhous CC cannot be made on the basis of the biopsy appearance alone. SHC can be distinguished from epithelioid hemangioendothelioma (EH), which often has a densely fibrotic stroma, by the finding of tumor cell positivity for factor VIII–related antigen, CD34, or other endothelial markers and by the absence of mucin in EH (235) (Table 21).

Hepatoblastoma

Clinical Features

HBL represents the most common primary hepatic tumor in children, accounting for about 50% of all primary pediatric hepatic malignancies and up to 0.5% of all pediatric tumors (Table 2) (3,5,6,85–87,236–238). Nearly 70% and 90% of cases occur by 2 years and 5 years of age, respectively.

Four percent of patients show signs at the time of birth, and 3% are diagnosed after the age of 15 years (oldest patient reported, 84 years). There is a male predominance (2:1) (Tables 16 and 17) (236,239). Patients generally have initial symptoms of an abdominal mass; 5.5% of patients have an associated congenital abnormality. Occasionally, one may see precocious puberty related to human chorionic gonadotropin production by the tumor (236). Patients with familial adenomatous polyposis have a risk 500 to 1,000 times that of the general population, although this neoplasm develops in less than 1% of such families (87). Calcification is often noted on radiography. The serum AFP level is elevated in up to 90% of cases, usually with very high titers. Mesenchymal hamartoma, also a consideration in this age group, may now and then be characterized by markedly elevated serum AFP (5).

While the etiologic factors of HBL are unknown, maternal occupational exposure to several environmental agents (metals, petroleum products, paints, pigments) may play an important part (240). There is no association with the usual risk factors for HCC, including cirrhosis. A variety of cytogenetic abnormalities have been identified in HBL, with trisomy 2 and trisomy 20 being the most consistent changes (236,241). Abnormalities of chromosome 11, including loss of heterozygosity at 11p15.5 (location of the insulin-like growth factor 2 gene, IGF2), and a tumor suppressor gene distinct from WT1 have been found by some investigators (242). These results are of interest because IGF2 is necessary for normal early development of the liver. Overexpression and mutation of p53 have sometimes been reported to be present in HBL (243).

Pathologic Features

Macroscopic Appearance. HBL is typically a tan-green, solitary (70% to 80%) mass that can be (a) smooth or lobulated and (b) solid and/or cystic. It develops most often in the right lobe, measures 3 to 20 cm (average, 10 to 12 cm) in diameter, and is often partially encapsulated. Tumors with a prominent mesenchymal component are often firm and may be calcified; necrosis and hemorrhage are more common than in purely epithelial HBL. Macroscopic invasion of the portal or hepatic veins is noted in less than 10% of cases (6).

TABLE 16. *Hepatoblastoma: histologic patterns, diagnostic clues and prognostic factors[a]*

Histologic pattern (rate)	Architecture	N/C ratio	Nucleolus	Pleomorphism	Mitoses (10 HPF)	Comment
Epithelial type (56%)						
Fetal (31%)	Trabeculae 2–3 cells thick; light/dark pattern; EMH	Low	Small	Minimal	<2	Best prognosis of all patterns but appears related to stage
Embryonal (19%)	Sheets, ribbons, trabeculae, acini, pseudorosettes; EMH	Higher	Often large	Frequent	>2	—
Macrotrabecular (3%)	Frequent trabeculae >10 cells thick	Variable	Variable	Variable	Variable	May be associated with poorer outcome; difficult ddx with HCC
Small-cell undifferentiated (3%)	Discohesive sheets of small, uniform cells, ± mucoid stroma	Highest	Variable	Minimal	>2	Uniformly poor outcome, few cases studied; other patterns needed for ddx with small round-cell tumors; + CK
Mixed epithelial mesenchymal type (44%)	Spindle-oval cells, frequent osteoid, rarely other differentiated sarcomatoid elements	High	Variable	Minimal	—	"Osteoblasts" + CK; mixed HBL may be favorable prognostic factor
Nonteratoid (34%)						—
Teratoid (10%)						Problem of overlap with germ cell tumors

CK, cytokeratin; ddx, differential diagnosis; EMH, extramedullary hematopoiesis; HBL, hepatoblastoma; HCC, hepatocellular carcinoma; HPF, high-power field; N/C, nuclear to cytoplasmic ratio.
[a] Rates taken from ref. 236.

TABLE 17. *Hepatoblastoma (HBL) and childhood hepatocellular carcinoma (HCC): differential diagnosis*[a]

Feature	HBL	HCC
Clinical feature		
Age	90% <5 yrs	90% >5 yrs
Sex (M:F)	1.5–2:1	1.7–11:1
Macroscopic appearance		
Single mass	70–80%	15–40%
Cirrhosis	Absent	5–25% (hepatitis B virus, metabolic disease)
Microscopic appearance		
Trabeculae	Usually 2–3 cells thick, occasionally macrotrabeculae	Often >2–3 cells thick
Cell size vs. nonneoplastic hepatocytes	Same size or smaller	Usually larger, well differentiated HCC can be smaller
Tumor giant cells	Rarely present	Common
Intranuclear inclusions	Absent	Common
Cytoplasmic hyaline globules	Absent	Common
Extramedullary hematopoiesis	Often present	Absent

[a] Data from refs. 5, 6, 85, 87, 236.

Microscopic Appearance. HBLs may be classified as either epithelial (56%) or mixed epithelial–mesenchymal (44%); they are subclassified into six patterns (Table 16) (2,236). In one study, a diagnosis of HBL was considered possible by FNA biopsy in 80% of cases, but subtyping was less reliable (14). In resection specimens, approximately one paraffin block for each centimeter of tumor should be prepared to ensure adequate sampling and, thus, appropriate classification of the histologic pattern (6a).

The epithelial component (Fig. 18) is usually divided into irregular lobules by collagenous septa and may be subclassified as described in the listing given in this section. Foci of extramedullary hematopoiesis may be found in the sinusoids of either the fetal or the embryonal patterns, but they are

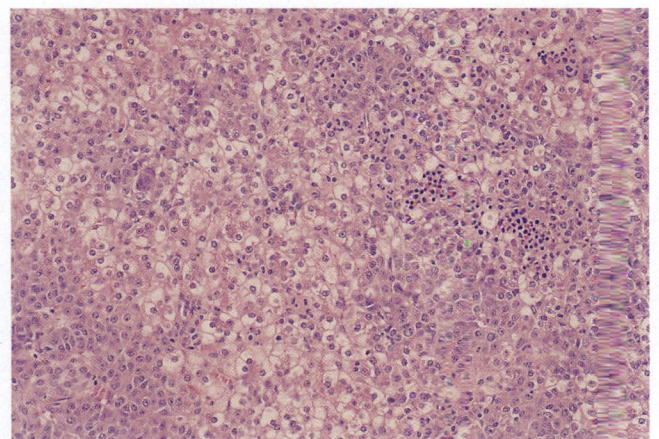

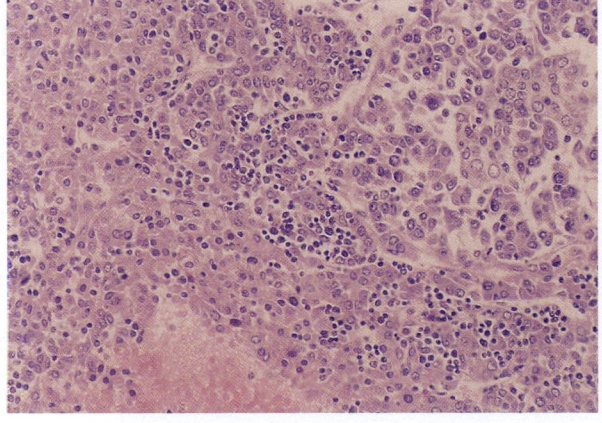

FIG. 18. Hepatoblastoma, epithelial subtypes. **A:** The fetal pattern, most resembling normal hepatocytes, often demonstrates "light" and "dark" foci related to the conspicuous presence or relative absence of glycogen and fat, respectively. Extramedullary hematopoiesis at right of photomicrograph. (Kindly contributed by Ronald Jaffe, M.D., Children's Hospital of Pittsburgh, Pittsburgh, PA.) **B:** Lower panel: The embryonal pattern is characterized by cells that have a higher nuclear to cytoplasmic ratio with greater nuclear pleomorphism (right side). The surrounding fetal component demonstrates extramedullary hematopoiesis. Upper panel: Small-cell undifferentiated pattern.

more often noted in the former. Rarely, foci of rhabdoid-type cells have been found, as have multinucleated giant cells containing human chorionic gonadotropin in the context of precocious puberty (87). Focal immunoreactivity with chromogranin has been reported in fetal and embryonal cells; it does not indicate neuroendocrine derivation. Embryonal-type cells demonstrate CKs 8, 18, and 19, but fetal-type cells are immunoreactive for CKs 8 and 18 and only weakly for 19. This finding supports the concept that embryonal-type cells can differentiate into fetal-type cells in a manner akin to normal hepatic differentiation (191,244).

1. Fetal pattern (31%). In this pattern the hepatocytes are similar in size to or smaller than those seen in the adjacent nonneoplastic liver. They have a slightly higher nuclear to cytoplasmic ratio and inconspicuous nucleoli. They are uniform and polyhedral, have distinct cell membranes, display minimal pleomorphism, occasionally contain bile, and often demonstrate an alternating light (representing the prominence of glycogen and fat) and dark pattern. Mitoses are typically rare (less than two per ten high-power fields). The tumor cells are arranged in trabeculae two to three cells thick, separated by sinusoids lined by endothelial cells that demonstrate strong immunoreactivity with CD34 (245). Portal tracts, bile ducts, and ductules are absent.
2. Embryonal pattern (19%). In addition to fetal cells, one sees less-differentiated, poorly cohesive cells that may form sheets, ribbons, acini, papillary formations (yolk sac in appearance), and/or trabeculae of variable thicknesses. Vascular lakes (pelioid foci) are often found in this subtype, as are mitoses and necrosis. Compared with the fetal pattern, the tumor cells have more poorly defined cell borders, more basophilic cytoplasm, a higher nuclear to cytoplasmic ratio, coarser chromatin, and more prominent nucleoli.
3. Macrotrabecular pattern (3%). This pattern is characterized by trabeculae that are ten or more cells (fetal, embryonal, or HCC-like with more abundant cytoplasm) thick, noted as a repetitive pattern throughout the tumor. The occasional presence of macrotrabeculae in a tumor does not warrant this designation.
4. Small-cell undifferentiated pattern (3%). The least differentiated pattern of HBL, this type is characterized by discohesive sheets of rather uniform small cells with scanty cytoplasm; indistinct cell borders; oval, hyperchromatic nuclei; and, now and then, prominent nucleoli and mitotic activity similar to those of small-cell carcinoma arising at other sites. The tumor cells are CK positive and bile negative. Irregular hyalinized septae may separate the tumor cells. Alternatively, the stroma may be quite mucoid (244,246). Other patterns of HBL must be present in order to make the diagnosis of the small-cell variant.
5. Mixed epithelial and mesenchymal pattern (44%). A varied mixture of epithelial (fetal/embryonal) and mesenchymal (primitive/differentiated) cell types characterizes this pattern. The primitive mesenchymal component has oval to spindle-shaped cells with little cytoplasm, often located within or adjacent to the neoplastic epithelial component. Mature fibrous septa, myxoid zones, and, most frequently, osteoid are noted; chondroid and rhabdomyoblastic foci are rare. Osteoid has been reported to be more common after chemotherapy (247). Both the primitive spindle cells and cells resembling osteoblasts within osteoid may demonstrate CK immunoreactivity, suggesting sarcomatoid metaplasia of the epithelial component (244).

The mixed pattern can be subdivided into those tumors with teratoid features (10%; keratinized squamous epithelium, intestinal epithelium, skeletal muscle, mature bone and cartilage, melanin pigment, and neuroectodermal structures) and those without these features (34%) (86,236,238). HBL combined with either yolk sac tumor or teratoma has rarely been described (83,248).

Differential Diagnosis

As in adults, in children the most common malignant hepatic tumors are metastases, usually neuroblastoma, lymphoma, rhabdomyosarcoma, and Wilms' tumor (236). Diagnosis of HBL on histologic evidence ordinarily is not difficult; however, in one Intergroup study of HBL, about 10% of cases were misdiagnosed, and these cases represented mainly metastases (87). Occasionally, a tumor with a predominantly or exclusively small-cell component may be difficult to distinguish from the small, round tumors mentioned earlier. The presence of more differentiated foci of HBL as well as the immunohistochemical phenotype (CK positive; leukocyte common antigen, neurofilament, and desmin negative) aid in distinguishing the small-cell variant of HBL from other neoplasms (244). Electron microscopy may also be helpful to differential diagnosis. The presence of cells resembling hepatocytes and the absence of a renal mass eliminate Wilms' tumor from the differential diagnosis. Features separating HBL from benign hepatocellular tumors and childhood HCC are summarized in Tables 4 and 17, respectively. Foci of the macrotrabecular variant of HBL may be indistinguishable from HCC in terms of histologic characteristics.

Pure sarcomas, such as undifferentiated (embryonal) sarcoma (88), are excluded from the diagnosis of HBL if an epithelial component is present, but this feature may be absent in biopsy specimens. Because HBL can demonstrate nonhepatic endodermal epithelial and mesenchymal elements, as well as embryonal foci similar to those of yolk sac tumor, the possibility of a metastatic or primary hepatic germ cell tumor must be considered (82,83,247). The focal character of the teratoid areas in HBL is an important feature in differential diagnosis (5,86). Although the histogenesis of the malignant rhabdoid tumor is unsettled, it should be separated from HBL (249). Patients with malignant rhabdoid tumor have a serum AFP level that is normal for their age.

TABLE 18. *Staging of hepatoblastoma according to the Children's Cancer Study Group[a]*

Stage I—Complete resection
Stage II—Microscopic residual disease only
Stage III—Gross residual disease or positive lymph nodes or spilled tumor
Stage IV—Metastases

[a] Modified from ref. 236.

Treatment, Outcome, and Prognostic Factors

A successful outcome is largely dependent on the ability to completely excise the tumor. The HBL staging system of the Children's Cancer Study Group (Table 18) is usually used, but the TNM system (Table 9) has also been employed; no differences in survival rates have been found between the two systems (6a,236,250,251). Previously, the tumors of only about 40% of patients were considered resectable (stages I and II), but with chemotherapy the rate of resection has dramatically increased to over 90%, and 50% to 70% of patients have survived long-term (87,236,251). Recurrences are usually detected within 36 months, but they may be delayed up to 5 years. Metastatic or recurrent disease limited to the lung is treated aggressively. Metastases, usually to regional lymph nodes and lung, have been reported at the time of death in 46% of patients (85). Liver transplantation may be the best alternative when disease appears to be limited to the liver but is unresectable by standard techniques.

Some researchers have suggested that the histologic pattern is of prognostic importance and that completely resected fetal tumors have a better prognosis (85,87,237). Other investigators have found, however, that when corrected for age, sex, and stage of disease, the histologic pattern is generally not an independent predictor of prognosis, although the uncommon small-cell undifferentiated and macrotrabecular patterns do appear to correlate with a poorer prognosis (236,250). Further study is needed, but increased mitotic activity seems to be an important unfavorable prognostic factor independent of stage, whereas the presence of osteoid or other components of mixed HBL may be associated with a favorable prognosis (236,237). The prognostic significance of vascular invasion and aneuploidy requires further investi-

TABLE 19. *Benign, solid, intrahepatic biliary tumors and tumor-like lesions: features useful in their differential diagnosis and separation from adenocarcinoma*

Feature	Bile duct hamartoma[a]	Bile duct adenoma	Reactive bile ductular proliferation in collapse[b]	Adenocarcinoma (primary and metastatic)
Clinical				
Incidental finding	Always	Always	No	Rare
Macroscopic				
Subcapsular location only	Almost always	Almost always	No	Rare
Multiple nodules	Common	Uncommon	Often	Common
Largest nodule size (cm)			Variable	
≤0.5	Almost always	Most common (60%)		Rare
>0.5, ≤2	Rare	Less common (40%)		Occasional
>2	Never	Never		Typical
Nodule border	Well circumscribed	Well circumscribed	Irregular	Infiltrative
Microscopic				
Portal tracts	Typical location	Often trapped in nodule	Incorporated	May be invaded
Ducts (glands)				
With small/absent lumina	Uncommon	Typical	Typical	Variable
With ectatic lumina	Typical	Rare	Rare	Variable
With bile	Common	Absent	Possible	Absent
With cytoplasmic mucin	Uncommon	Often present	Uncommon	Common
Pleomorphism, mitoses	Absent	Absent	Slight/rare	Common
Prominent nucleoli	Absent	Absent	Slight	Common
Vascular/lymphatic invasion	Absent	Absent	Absent	Common
Parenchymal/sinusoidal invasion	Absent	Absent	Absent	Common
Prominent lymphocytes	Absent	Common	Absent	Rare[c]
Fibrous stroma	Often sclerotic	Often sclerotic	Loose/sclerotic	Often sclerotic

[a] In congenital hepatic fibrosis, identical ducts in sclerotic stroma extensively link adjacent portal tracts.
[b] Reactive ductular proliferation in the common context of cirrhotic septa or biliary tract disease demonstrates components of the portal triad to a variable degree and is often surrounded by neutrophils (cholangiolitis). Florid ductular proliferation in FNH can mimic bile duct adenoma.
[c] Rare cases with focal or substantial lymphoepithelioma-like carcinoma pattern (Epstein-Barr virus positive) have been described.

gation (237,250,252). The surgical pathology report should disclose, where appropriate (resection vs. biopsy specimen), the status of the resection margin; the number, size, and distribution (one one or both lobes) of the tumor nodules; the histologic subtype; and the mitotic rate.

Benign Tumors and Tumor-Like Lesions of the Intrahepatic Bile Ducts

While there is some controversy as to whether bile duct hamartoma (BDH) and bile duct adenoma (BDA) are distinct lesions (2,253–255) or part of a morphologic spectrum (257), the separation of these lesions and reactive bile ductular proliferation from metastatic adenocarcinoma or cholangiocarcinoma is of the utmost importance. Surgeons occasionally suspect that these lesions represent hepatic metastases at the time of possible resection of another gastrointestinal malignancy. The pathologist's interpretation at the time of frozen section often dictates subsequent therapy (see the section on intraoperative consultation). While interpretation of the frozen section is often straightforward, it may occasionally be impossible to rule out adenocarcinoma definitively if only a small biopsy sample of these lesions is available for review. The features helpful in differential diagnosis are presented in Table 19. A rare multicystic mass with characteristics of both BDH and BDA and epithelial atypia has been reported as biliary adenofibroma (258).

Cysts and cystadenomas have been discussed previously, in the section on hepatic cysts.

Bile Duct Hamartoma (von Meyenburg Complex)

BDHs are small, incidental, clinically asymptomatic lesions currently being detected with greater frequency by more sensitive imaging studies (259). They have been reported in 0.7% to 27% of all autopsies (depending on sampling) and in 0.6% of needle biopsy specimens (256,260). Nearly 75% of livers with hepatic cysts and 10% of patients with ADPKD have BDHs; conversely, about 20% of livers with BDH have associated hepatic cysts (44). BDH may represent part of the spectrum of ductal plate malformation and may be related to ADPKD, CHF, or other genetic disorders, but the possibility that they may stem from inflammation or ischemia has not been excluded (44,45). Cholangiocarcinoma has occasionally been reported in association with BDHs (261).

When evaluated macroscopically (Table 19), BDHs appear as single or multiple (20% have four or more nodules) (44), subcapsular, gray-white or occasionally green nodules less than 0.5 cm in diameter. From time to time they are so numerous as to be mistaken by the surgeon or pathologist for metastatic carcinoma, abscesses, or granulomas. At the microscopic level, BDHs are discrete lesions found either within or directly adjacent to portal tracts (Fig. 19A). They

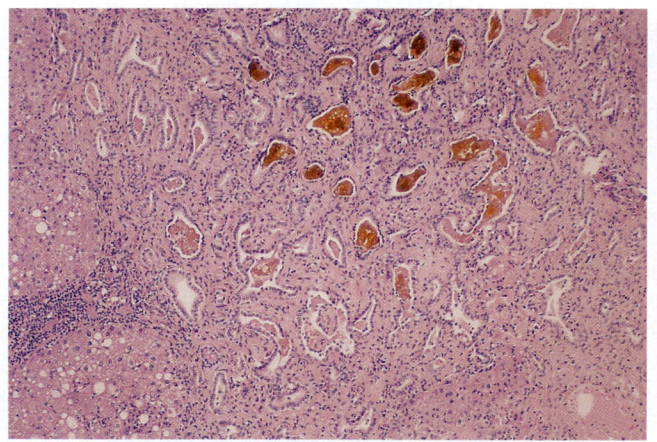
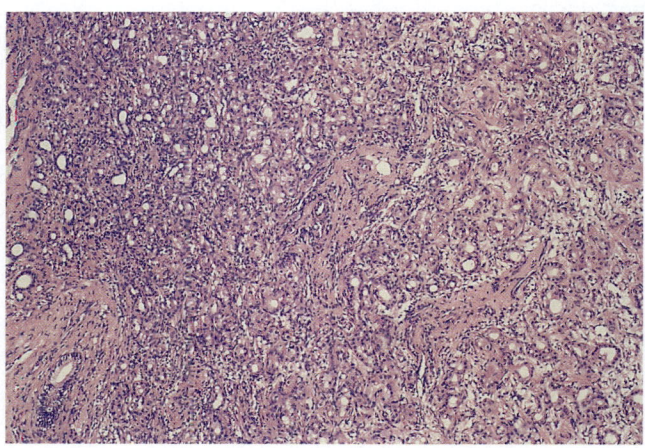
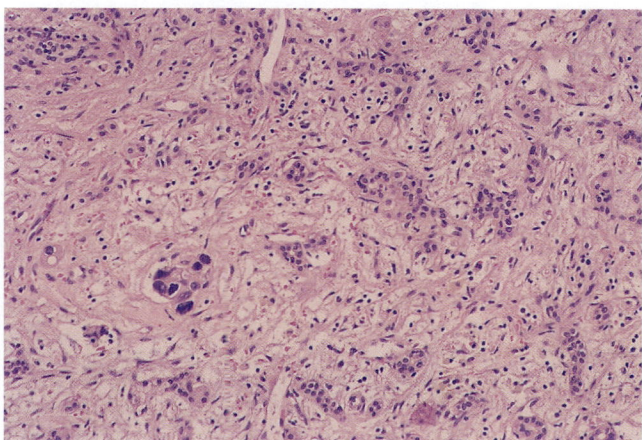

FIG. 19. Benign bile duct lesions. **A:** Rounded collection of ectatic, angulated bile ducts embedded in a fibrotic stroma, characteristic of a bile duct hamartoma. Note intraluminal bile. **B:** The bile duct adenoma contains numerous small tubules. Lumina are often inapparent. Cytoplasmic mucin may be prominent, but bile is absent. No cytologic atypia or mitoses are found. **C:** Postnecrotic collapse (after chemotherapy for metastatic carcinoma) demonstrates prominent reactive bile ductule proliferation. Note one of the very rare foci of residual carcinoma present in this case (left of center).

consist of a collection of ectatic, branched bile ducts that have a characteristic tubular or angulated appearance. The duct lining is made up of a single layer of bland, low columnar, cuboidal, or flattened epithelium. The lumina frequently contain amorphous eosinophilic material and/or bile; bile is absent in other biliary epithelial tumors. Intracytoplasmic mucin may be present. A dense, usually hyalinized, collagenous stroma separates the bile ducts and often merges imperceptibly with the normal portal tract collagen. Stromal lymphocytic or neutrophilic infiltrate is usually absent or is quite sparse, although intraluminal microabscesses associated with reactive epithelial changes may be noted (2).

Bile Duct Adenoma

While the term bile duct adenoma has often been used in the literature interchangeably with bile duct hamartoma, it appears to be a distinct entity (253,255) (Table 19). Like BDH, this much less frequently reported tumor is always an incidental finding. Nearly 40% of cases were originally considered either suggestive or diagnostic of adenocarcinoma (primary or metastatic) at the time of referral in one series (253), emphasizing the importance of familiarity with this lesion. It has been theorized that BDAs arise from foci of reactive bile ductule proliferation or are hamartomas, developmental defects, or neoplasms. One immunohistochemical study has proposed a derivation from peribiliary glands (255).

BDAs are well circumscribed (but not encapsulated), firm, gray-white or tan, subcapsular nodules, although they sometimes appear as subcapsular scars. Nearly 85% are solitary, and about 10% of cases have more than two nodules (253). Sixty percent of BDAs are 5 mm or less in diameter, and 7% are larger than 1 cm; the maximal diameter is 2 cm. At the microscopic level, one sees a compact network of ductal structures with a simple tubular appearance or a more complex tortuous arrangement embedded in a variable amount of fibrous stroma that may be sclerotic or edematous and infrequently is calcified or contains granulomas (Fig. 19B). The tubular lumina are often very small or inapparent, indistinguishable on histologic evaluation from bile ductules (cholangioles). Cystic change is uncommon.

The cuboidal/low columnar lining epithelium has more cytoplasm and paler nuclei than that of the interlobular bile ducts present within portal tracts in the adjacent liver or trapped within the lesion. Although intracytoplasmic mucin can be found, cytoplasmic or intraluminal bile is absent. Two BDAs have been described that also had intraductular and periductular nests of bland, round cells, which showed histologic and immunohistochemical signs of neuroendocrine differentiation (262). Nuclear pleomorphism and hyperchromasia, prominent nucleoli, mitoses, and vascular/lymphatic invasion are all absent in BDA, supporting its distinction from adenocarcinoma. Inflammatory cells—particularly lymphocytes, but also neutrophils—may be noted both within and at the periphery of the lesion. Lymphoid aggregates may be conspicuous at the interface with the adjacent liver (253). In rare instances, the lymphoid component is so prominent that the possibility of lymphoma may be considered. Follow-up of resected BDAs has indicated that it has a benign clinical course; however, the potential for malignant transformation has not been excluded (253).

Reactive Bile Ductule Proliferation

Prominent reactive bile ductular proliferation is typically encountered in the context of cirrhotic septa or biliary tract disorders, but it can also be quite florid in the variably sized scars or nodules seen in many forms of parenchymal collapse (atrophy) (42,94a,257,263) and in FNH (129,203). Reactive bile ductular proliferation can usually be distinguished from BDH and BDA based on the clinical context of the lesion as well as histologic features (lack of angulated duct structures, typically no dense sclerosis except with collapse, possible presence of bile, and frequent finding of periductular neutrophils) (Table 19).

When a mild degree of biliary epithelial nuclear atypia and even a rare mitosis are noted in broad scars or masslike foci of collapse, distinction from adenocarcinoma (cholangiocarcinoma or metastatic adenocarcinoma) can be challenging in needle or even wedge biopsy specimens. Both reactive bile ductule proliferation and minute residual foci of carcinoma may be present after chemotherapy, resulting in a confusing histologic picture (Fig. 19C). Such features as more severe nuclear atypia with irregular nuclear contours, prominent nucleoli, nuclear hyperchromasia, an increased nuclear to cytoplasmic ratio, and uniform dense sclerosis favor adenocarcinoma. The finding of invasive cell nests and/or glands infiltrating the adjacent parenchyma or vascular invasion clinches the diagnosis. Complete surgical excision may be necessary to resolve the issue in some cases.

Malignant Tumors of the Intrahepatic Bile Ducts

Intrahepatic Cholangiocarcinoma (ICC)

Classification

Malignant tumors can arise from any portion of the biliary tree, from the level of the bile ductule to the ampulla of Vater; more than 95% are adenocarcinomas (3,64,120, 264–266). ICCs account for 3% to 35% (usually 10–20%) of all primary malignant hepatic tumors. It is more common in regions of the world where HCC is less prevalent and is reportedly endemic in Southeast Asia. The term ICC is used variably by different authors. Some authors use it strictly for tumors arising away from the hilum (peripheral cholangiocarcinoma, PCCs), while others also include tumors developing within the porta hepatis from the region of the right or left hepatic duct, their confluence, their segmental or finer intrahepatic branches, or from adjacent peribiliary glands (hilar CC). Because the clinicopathologic features of hilar CC more closely resemble extrahepatic CC, these tumors will be discussed in the chapter "Gallbladder and Extrahepatic Bile Ducts."

Clinical, Epidemiologic, and Pathogenetic Features

Patients with PCC usually show signs of abdominal pain, general malaise, fever, and weight loss in the sixth or seventh decade of life, at a time when their tumors are quite large. The intraductal variant often is associated with right-upper-quadrant pain, fever, and jaundice because of duct obstruction by tumor or tumor-related mucus production. Men and women are similarly affected, except for a strong male predominance in cases associated with PSC. Most patients with ICC have no predisposing condition; in about 10% to 20% of cases, however, hepatolithiasis, PSC, liver fluke infestation, and, rarely, other conditions precede its development, the common thread among them being chronic bile stasis and cholangitis (Table 20) (3,264).

About 10% to 30% of patients with primary sclerosing cholangitis (PSC) and 5% to 10% of patients with hepatolithiasis are found to have CC; not unusually the tumors go undetected on clinical examination and are incidentally found at the time of resection, transplantation, or autopsy (267,268). The presence of tumors in a patient under age 40 should suggest the possibility of associated PSC and chronic idiopathic inflammatory bowel disease (particularly ulcerative colitis) (267). Nonbiliary cirrhosis is found in less than 5% of cases; when it is present, a careful search for combined HCC-CC should be made (264). Biliary cirrhosis stemming from a predisposing condition may be present; alternatively, biliary fibrosis may be induced by the tumor-related biliary obstruction.

Most investigators have found the serum AFP level to be undetectable; however, levels higher than 1,000/ng/ml have been reported from time to time. Associated paraneoplastic syndromes are much less common than with HCC, although hypercalcemia is occasionally found (see the discussion of sclerosing hepatic carcinoma) (229,233a,234). A dysplasia-carcinoma sequence appears to be operative and has been documented in the context of chronic proliferative cholangitis (264,266–269). In all, 10% to nearly 25% of cases express p53 protein on immunohistochemical studies, but there is wide variation in Ki-ras point mutations (8–82%), depending on the group of patients studied (264,270). C-met and c-erb B-2 gene products have also been identified, but expression of transforming growth factor-alpha (TGFα) is unusual compared with the findings in HCC.

Macroscopic Features. The disease can be divided into three types: massive, multinodular, and diffuse (numerous nodules less than 1 cm in diameter throughout the liver), although classification according to pattern of spread (intraductal type, periductal spreading type simulating sclerosing cholangitis, and nodular type) is useful (3,264). Multiple nodules result from varying degrees of intravascular or intraductal spread (265). Tumors can be staged similarly to HCC, as seen in Table 9. The typical tumor is a large (often 7–10 cm or more), single, gray-white, firm tumor mass with infiltrative margins and smaller satellite nodules arising in a noncirrhotic liver (Fig. 20A). Central umbilication is not unusual, particularly in those nodules located under Glisson's capsule. A peripheral hyperemic zone, frequently noted with metastatic adenocarcinoma, is not a feature of PCC. Intraductal CCs appear as variably sized, often multifocal, pink-white, papillary excrescences within dilated ducts (Fig. 20B). Portal and hepatic vein invasion occurs in cholangiocarcinoma, but at a rate somewhat lower than that of HCC (272).

Microscopic Features. Most cases of CC demonstrate a variable degree of glandular (ductal, tubular) differentiation and mucin production (well, moderately, and poorly differentiated) with a moderate amount of densely fibrotic, occasionally calcified stroma (Fig 20C,D). In well-differentiated cases, the glands are lined by cuboidal to low columnar cells that contain a moderate amount of pale, sometimes slightly granular cytoplasm. The size of the cells and nuclei is generally smaller and the nucleoli less prominent than in HCC. Although bile is not produced by cholangiocarcinomas, it may be found at the periphery of the neoplasm, in the lumina of trapped nonneoplastic bile ducts, within hepatocytes, extravasated into the stroma, or even in tumor cells (passive uptake) when there is extensive cholestasis in the adjacent liver. A trabecular pattern may be found, simulating HCC, but collagenous stroma, rather than sinusoids, surround the cords of tumor cells; bile canaliculi as well as bile are absent (2).

Special variants are found at least focally in about 10% of cases (271,272). Mucinous (copious extracellular mucin in a solid tumor), signet cell (never the sole component), adenosquamous (adenocarcinoma with unequivocal squamous differentiation), mucoepidermoid, and sarcomatoid variants are recognized by the WHO (2). In addition, cholangiolocellular (resembling nonneoplastic bile ductules), clear-cell (sometimes with papillary features), rhab-

TABLE 20. *Intrahepatic cholangiocarcinoma: predisposing and premalignant conditions*

No predisposing conditions (80–90%)
Predisposing conditions (10–20%)
    Chronic cholangitis (by far most common)
        PSC/CUC (Western countries)
        Hepatolithiasis (Far East, including Japan)
        Liver fluke infestation
            Clonorchis sinensis (Hong Kong, Canton)
            Opisthorchis viverrini (Thailand)
    Ductal plate malformation
        Hepatic cysts
        Bile duct hamartomas
        Congenital hepatic fibrosis
        Congenital dilatation of the intrahepatic bile ducts (Caroli's disease)
    Toxins/drugs
        Hereditary hemochromatosis
        Thorotrast
        Anabolic steroids
    Nonbiliary cirrhosis (<5%)
Premalignant conditions
    Dysplasia (intraluminal, flat, and papillary, including most, if not all, "biliary papillomatosis"; peribiliary glands)

PSC, primary sclerosing cholangitis; CUC, chronic ulcerative colitis (much less commonly, Crohn's disease).

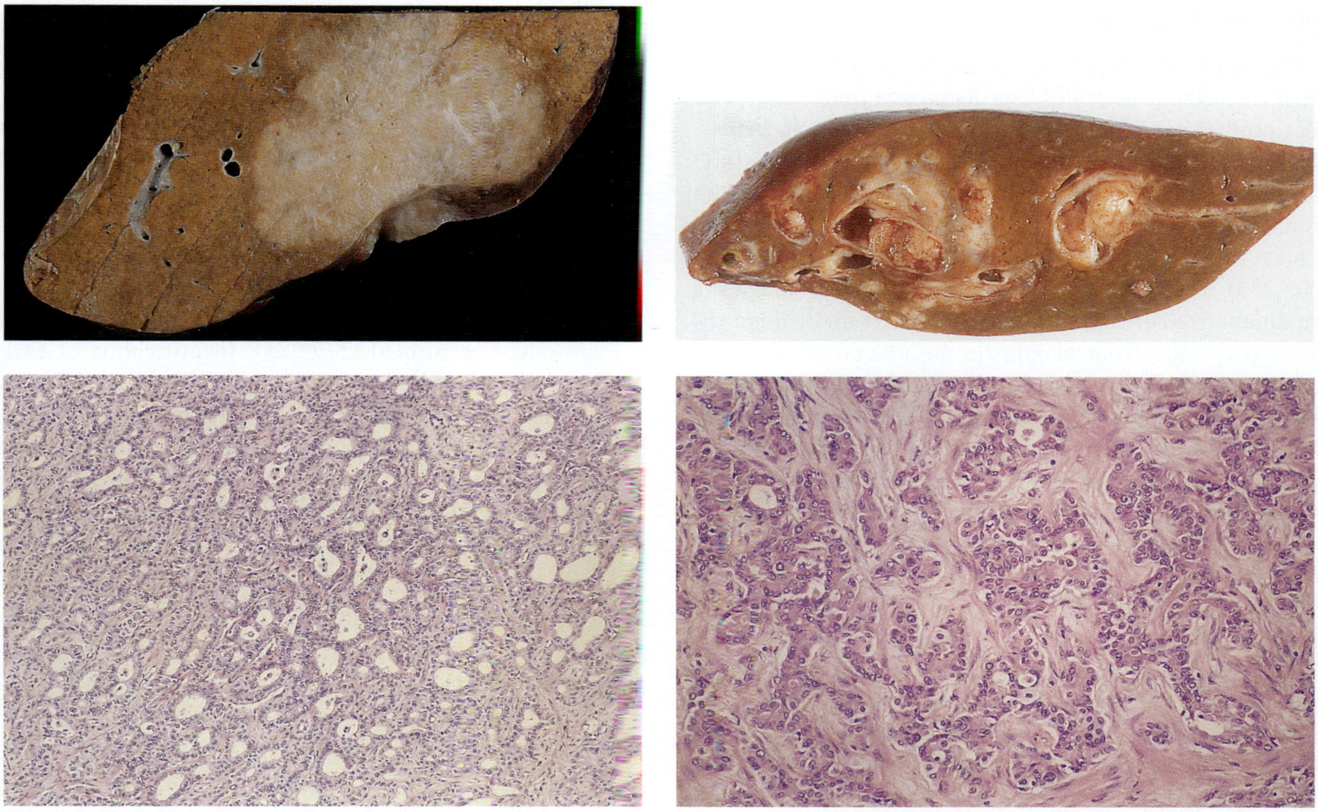

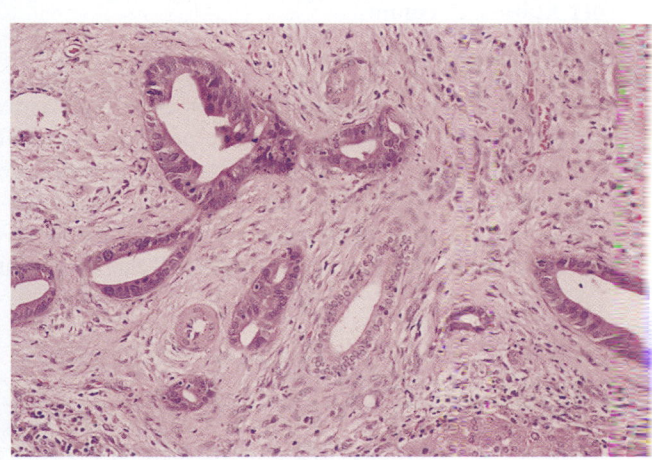

FIG. 20. Intrahepatic cholangiocarcinoma. **A:** Large, tan, homogeneous, firm mass with infiltrative borders typical of peripheral cholangiocarcinoma. **B:** Uncommon, predominately intraductal variant of cholangiocarcinoma. Note extensive intraductal growth. Only minute foci of parenchymal invasion were identified on microscopy. **C:** Microscopic appearance of well-differentiated cholangiocarcinoma with prominent glandular (ductal, tubular) pattern and scanty fibrous stroma. Although the histologic features resemble those of bile ducts, a metastatic tumor, particularly from the pancreas or extrahepatic biliary tree, cannot be ruled out. **D:** Dense sclerosis is often present in cholangiocarcinoma. Hypercalcemia may be present, particularly when fibrosis is extensive (form of sclerosing hepatic carcinoma). **E:** Metastatic adenocarcinoma from the colon invades the portal tract and simulates bile duct dysplasia/cholangiocarcinoma.

doid, and even lymphoepithelioma-like carcinoma (associated with Epstein-Barr virus) variants have been described (120,229,264,265,271–274a). Combined CC-carcinoid has also been reported (275). Squamous and adenosquamous types probably represent different degrees of squamous metaplasia in adenocarcinoma (264). They often have been reported to be at least partially cystic, thus overlapping with tumors reported as variants of cystadenocarcinoma (49,50,271).

Intraductal CCs are predominately papillary, with regions of nonpapillary flattened epithelium (264,265,269). By definition, this tumor type is noninvasive; however, as with intraductal neoplasms at extrahepatic sites, it has the potential to invade into and beyond the duct wall. In terms of the architecture, the intraductal proliferation is similar to that of villous adenomas found at extrahepatic sites and consists of fibrovascular cores lined by a single layer of columnar, mucin-containing epithelium in association with flat, similar epithelium lining the remainder of the duct. Most authors have used the term intraductal CC for cases in which high-grade dysplasia (including carcinoma *in situ*) is present; terms such as adenoma, biliary papillomatosis, adenomatosis, or even borderline tumor have been applied for cases with a lesser degree of dysplasia (2,70,256,264,266,269). Reproducibility and the practical implications of the grade of dysplasia in these lesions need further investigation. Of practical importance for the pathologist is the fact that these lesions should be submitted in their entirety to exclude the possibility of invasion. The patient should be carefully evaluated for the possibility of similar lesions elsewhere in the biliary tree.

Differential Diagnosis

The pathologist faces a major challenge in attempting to establish a diagnosis of PCC: its distinction from benign bile duct proliferations, metastatic adenocarcinoma, and HCC. Now and then there may be problems in differentiating PCC from benign solid bile duct tumors (hamartoma and adenoma) and reactive bile duct proliferation, particularly in the context of small biopsies and a lack of clinical information (203,253). The features helpful to this differential diagnosis are summarized in Table 19. The parameters for distinguishing hyperplastic from neoplastic intraductal changes are identical to those described for the extrahepatic biliary tree (see "Gallbladder and Extrahepatic Biliary Tree"). Dysplasia within peribiliary glands should not be mistaken for invasive adenocarcinoma, although the pathologist should carefully look for the latter when the former is present.

Making the distinction between PCC and metastatic adenocarcinoma, particularly from the gallbladder, pancreas, extrahepatic biliary tree, and breast, is impossible on histologic grounds. Although dysplastic foci in nearby bile ducts favor a primary tumor, metastatic foci within portal tracts or even growing along the biliary epithelium can mimic this finding, particularly in the case of metastatic colon cancer (Fig. 20E) (276). At present, there are no specific tumor markers useful in distinguishing cholangiocarcinoma from other forms of adenocarcinoma. The diagnosis of PCC is therefore one of exclusion. The histologic, histochemical, and immunohistochemical features that aid in separating HCC from PCC have been discussed in the section on HCC and are summarized in Table 14. Epithelioid hemangioendothelioma (EH) is distinguished from PCC by its vasoablative nature; the presence of cytoplasmic immunoreactivity for factor VIII–related antigen, CD34, or other endothelial cell markers; and the absence of intracellular mucin (Table 21) (235).

Treatment and Outcome

Patients with PCC generally have a dismal outcome; they die in a matter of months. The adenosquamous and sarcomatoid variants have been associated with a poorer prognosis, but multivariate analysis has not yet been performed (270,271). Even in the minority of patients treated with "curative" resection, the median survival is only 13 to 34 months, with a 5-year survival of about 30% (277). Since recurrence is nearly universal after transplantation for CC, even when the tumor is an incidental finding, this procedure is no longer performed (277,278). Identification of early hepatic recurrence in biopsy specimens may be difficult; recurrence is characterized on cytology by single or small clusters of malignant, CK-positive cells in the sinusoids (278). Patients die as a result of extensive tumor growth, hepatic failure, gastrointestinal bleeding, or infection. At autopsy, 75% of patients with PCC have metastases, usually to porta hepatis lymph nodes, peritoneal surfaces, lung, bone, and adrenal gland (3).

Biliary Cystadenocarcinoma

See section on cysts and pseudocysts.

Other Epithelial Tumors

Neuroendocrine Neoplasms

Although nearly all hepatic neuroendocrine neoplasms represent metastases, usually from the pancreas or small bowel, a few unique cases of apparent primary tumors have been described (3,204,275,279,280). Two primary pheochromocytomas have also been reported (3,281). Focal immunoreactivity for "neuroendocrine markers" can be seen in

TABLE 21. *Pathologic features aiding in the differential diagnosis of epithelioid hemangioendothelioma and carcinoma (primary and secondary) containing a densely sclerotic stroma*

Feature	Epithelioid hemangioendothelioma	Scirrhous HCC	Scirrhous CC or MET ADENOCA
Hepatic acinar structure	Zonal pattern	Destroyed	Destroyed
Infiltrative borders	Present	Absent	±
Marked venous invasion	Present	Absent	Absent
Atypical sinusoidal endothelial cells	Present	Absent	Absent
Intracytoplasmic lumina (vacuoles)			
Endothelial markers (CD34, CD31, FVIIIRAg)	Positive	Negative	Negative
Mucin	Negative	Negative	Positive
Bile	Negative	±	Negative
Other immunohistochemical markers			
p-CEA (canalicular)	Negative	Frequently present	Negative
HepPar-1	Negative	Frequently present	Negative
AFP	Negative	Occasionally present	Negative
Cytokeratin (including CK 8, 18, 19)	Occasionally positive	Positive	Positive
Electron microscopy			
Weibel-Palade bodies	Often present	Absent	Absent

AFP, alpha-fetoprotein; CC, cholangiocarcinoma; CK, cytokeratin; FVIIIRAg, factor VIII–related antigen; HCC, hepatocellular carcinoma; HepPar-1, hepatocyte paraffin 1; MET ADENOCA, metastatic adenocarcinoma; p-CEA, polyclonal antisera to carcinoembryonic antigen.

otherwise typical HCC or CC and does not alter the diagnosis (186,207,208). Features helpful in the differential diagnosis of neuroendocrine tumors and the usual HCC or FL-HCC have been delineated in their respective sections earlier in the chapter, in Table 13, and in Figs. 15 and 17.

MESENCHYMAL TUMORS

Of the benign mesenchymal tumors, those of vascular origin are by far the most common. In fact, most other tumors in this category are only rarely encountered by the practicing pathologist. Primary hepatic sarcomas are exceedingly unusual, accounting for only 1% to 2% of all malignant primary tumors arising in the liver (3,282). Among these tumors, angiosarcoma and EH in adults and undifferentiated sarcoma in children are found most frequently. The diagnosis of primary hepatic sarcoma depends on ruling out a metastatic lesion. In one report, only 60% of hepatic sarcomas initially believed to be primary were confirmed as such after a more extensive workup. The retroperitoneum was the typical site of an occult primary (283).

Benign Vascular Tumors

Cavernous Hemangioma

Clinical Features

The cavernous hemangioma (CH) is the most common primary hepatic tumor and is usually an incidental finding. It is detected in about 1% of routinely performed autopsies (3) and in 20% of autopsies entailing extensive investigation (260); it accounts for more than 50% of resected benign hepatic masses (284). These tumors are found at all ages and in both sexes, although they are most frequently seen in adults. They predominate in women in most surgical series (3–5:1), and these patients are more often symptomatic (abdominal pain). Only 10% of lesions are found to enlarge slightly (a few centimeters) on follow-up, with anecdotal reports of enlargement due to pregnancy or use of oral contraceptives (285). CHs appear more often in patients with FNH and related lesions, particularly when the lesions are multiple (multiple FNH syndrome) (126,129,130). Asymptomatic CH need not be treated (usually by resection); it need only be observed if the diagnosis is secure, because the natural history of CH is essentially complication free (285).

Giant CHs have generally been defined as larger than 4 cm in diameter, although some authors prefer a cutoff of 10 cm before using this term. Spontaneous rupture, thrombocytopenia (Kasabach-Merritt syndrome), Budd-Chiari syndrome, and hypofibrinogenemia are possible, but rare, complications (3,285). MRI can identify more than 90% of CHs; other imaging studies are somewhat less sensitive. Sclerotic lesions can defy radiographic diagnosis (1,9). FNA and core biopsies have been performed, with little morbidity, in cases found to be atypical on radiography or when a metastasis is suspected on clinical evaluation. Some researchers have found that FNA specimens are often inadequate for interpretation (8,10,11,28,286).

Pathologic Features

CHs are usually solitary (70–90%) and less than 2 to 4 cm in diameter, although in surgical series, over 75% are more than 4 cm (285). Occasionally they may be so large as to replace an entire lobe. The typical CH is soft, red-purple, and well circumscribed. They can be found beneath the capsule or deep within the parenchyma; sometimes (though rarely) they are present as pedunculated, extrahepatic (on clinical examination) masses. On sectioning, the lesion usually collapses as blood oozes from its surface, imparting a meshwork-like appearance (Fig. 21A). At the microscopic level, rather large, but somewhat variably sized, vascular spaces are lined by flattened endothelial cells that cover a wall composed of paucicellular fibrous and often myxoid tissue (Fig. 21B). Some of the septa appear to be incomplete and project into the lumen. Larger septa may contain thick-walled blood vessels and trapped bile ducts. Thrombosis, calcification, phleboliths, and even abscess formation can be found.

As the hemangioma ages, sclerosis may begin centrally and sometimes extends to involve virtually the entire lesion, masking its vascular nature both in macroscopic terms and on radiography (*sclerosed hemangioma*, estimated at less than or equal to 5% of all CHs) (198,257,284). In these lesions the cavernous vascular spaces become almost totally obliterated; the lesion assumes a gray-white-tan, sometimes umbilicated, gross appearance that can simulate metastatic carcinoma, especially when noted in patients with multiple CHs (Fig. 21C,D) (257). CHs that are virtually obliterated appear to represent one of the precursors of the "solitary necrotic nodule" of the liver (287). Elastic and trichrome stains may help expose the vascular nature of such sclerotic lesions.

The appearance on FNA is dominated by blood with scattered and often inconspicuous clusters of (as well as individual) endothelial cells with oval to elongated nuclei (sometimes demonstrating a longitudinal groove), delicate and finely dispersed chromatin, inconspicuous nucleoli, and scanty cytoplasm (10,11). A few unremarkable liver cells may be seen.

Differential Diagnosis

The diagnosis of CH is usually straightforward. Solitary capillary hemangiomas are extremely rare and are of no clinical significance. In hereditary hemorrhagic telangiectasia (Rendu-Osler-Weber disease), the liver is frequently involved but rarely symptomatic. Telangiectatic lesions, composed of dilated veins and small capillaries, are present throughout the liver. They appear to arise in relation to portal tracts and are frequently found in fibrous septa. The liver may demonstrate regenerative nodules resembling FNH (4,134). In diffuse hemangiomatosis, a rare disorder of

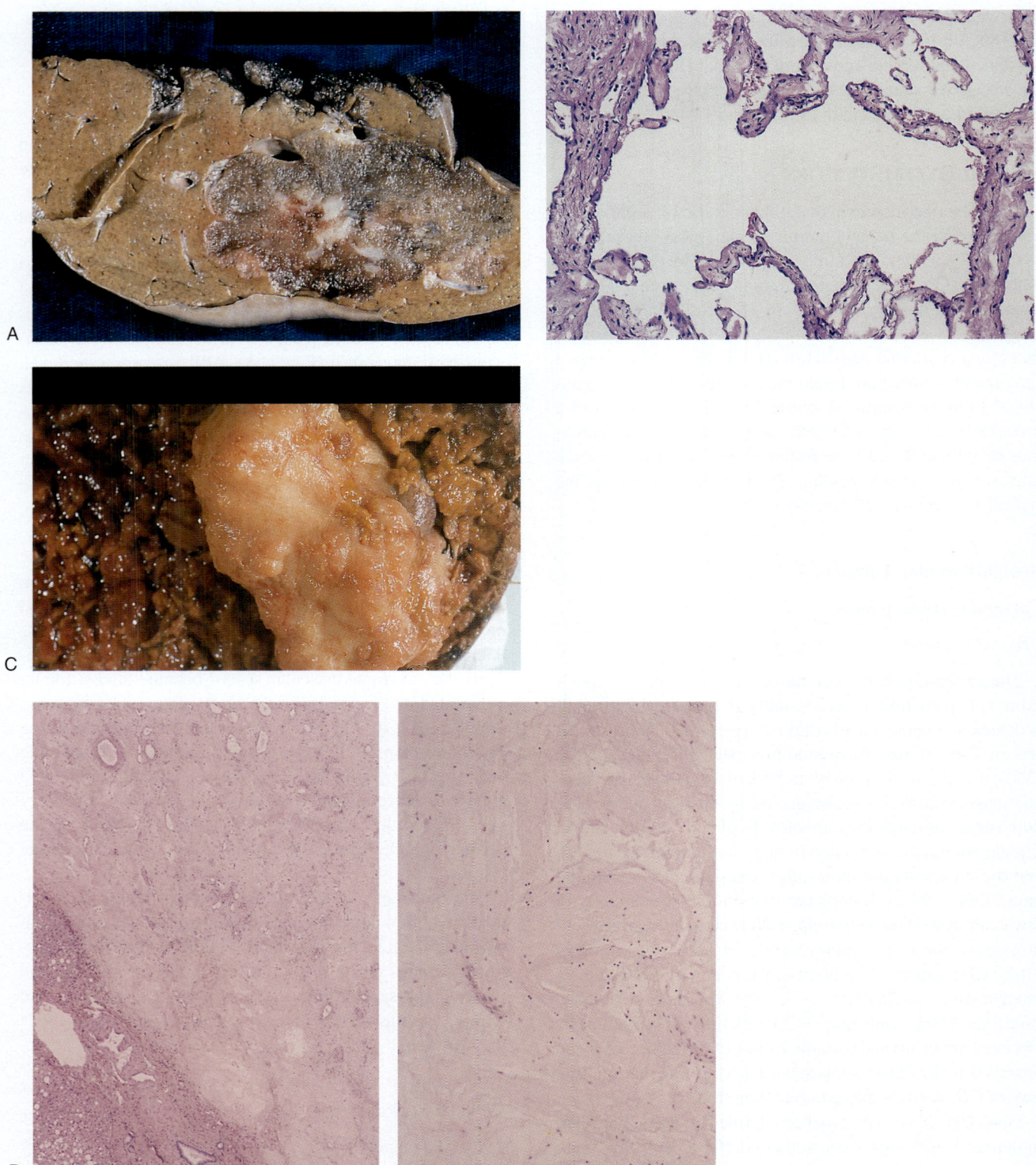

FIG. 21. Cavernous hemangioma. **A:** Resected "giant," cavernous hemangioma (after formalin fixation). The spongy nature of the tumor is evident. Central white areas represent fibrosis. **B:** Cavernous hemangioma. Large vascular spaces lined by flattened endothelial cells rest on a fibrous wall. **C:** Sclerosed hemangioma. The vascular origin of the tumor is inapparent on macroscopic examination. **D:** Left panel: Low-power view demonstrates dense sclerosis and scattered blood vessels. Right panel: Outlines of previous cavernous vascular spaces, now sclerosed, are apparent.

adults, numerous small, poorly circumscribed hemangiomatous nodules are frequently found in the portal tracts, may nearly replace the entire liver, and upon occasion become sclerosed. Other organs (bone, lung) may be involved (3,284). Peliosis hepatis is discussed later.

Hepatic lymphangiomas are extremely rare, and most of those previously reported probably represent mesenchymal hamartomas, the source of confusion being the fluid-filled alveolar spaces bounded by stroma often found in the latter lesion (88). Hepatic lymphangiomatosis is a rare disorder characterized by a large, solitary mass or multiple lesions (3,5,288). Systemic lymphangiomatosis (involvement of spleen, lung, bone, soft tissue, etc.) may or may not be present. A single case of hepatic hemangioblastoma has been reported in a patient with von Hippel–Lindau disease (289). Infantile hemangioendothelioma (IHE) (see next section) may have foci indistinguishable from CH (3,5,284). Sclerosed hemangioma should not be confused with other benign or malignant masses (benign fibrous tumor, inflammatory pseudotumor, EH, sclerosing carcinoma, etc.) that may have prominent sclerosis.

Infantile Hemangioendothelioma (IHE)

Clinical Features

Infantile hemangioendothelioma (IHE) is the most common mesenchymal tumor of the liver in childhood, and it also accounts for about 20% of all primary pediatric hepatic tumors (3,5,6,6A,284,290,291). Nearly 90% of patients are less than 6 months of age at the time of diagnosis. There is a slight female predominance. Roughly one-half of the cases are discovered incidentally at autopsy. The typical initial signs include an abdominal mass (48%) and high-output cardiac failure (15%) (291); severe thrombocytopenia and bleeding diathesis due to platelet sequestration (Kasabach–Merritt syndrome) or rupture may occur. In all, 10% to 40% of patients have cutaneous hemangiomas, usually of the cavernous type, and hemangiomas of other organs may be present (291). The serum AFP level is usually normal for age but now and then it may be elevated, leading clinicians to suggest HBL (291,292).

Macroscopic Features. IHEs may be solitary or multicentric. The tumor nodules are 0.2 to 15 cm (mean, 4 cm) in diameter and are characteristically circumscribed but not encapsulated. Smaller lesions are red to tan, soft, and spongy, while larger nodules are often variegated, with a red to brown periphery and a gray to white, scarred, sometimes umbilicated center with focal hemorrhages and flecks of calcification.

Microscopic Features. IHE most frequently is well demarcated, although in 35% of cases an infiltrative border is seen, which is best illustrated with immunohistochemical testing for CK (CK 8, 18, and 19 highlight trapped hepatocytes and bile ducts) (291). Two histologic subtypes have been recognized, those with pure type 1 change and those with at least focal type 2 change accounting for about 80%

and 20% of cases, respectively (290,291). Although the point is frequently debated, type 2 change appears now to be considered equivalent to angiosarcoma (282). The presence of pericytes in IHE is still the subject of controversy, but the endothelial nature of the lining cells is easily demonstrated by electron microscopy or immunohistochemical tests (factor VIII–related antigen, CD34, CD31).

Type 1 change is characterized by a rather orderly proliferation of small, capillary-like or slightly irregular, dilated, relatively bloodless vascular spaces (Fig. 22) lined by a continuous layer of endothelial cells with bland, plump, round to oval nuclei that may focally occlude the lumen. Variable amounts of loose to dense connective tissue separate the vascular channels. Mitoses are rare. Trapped cords of hepatocytes, which occasionally contain bile plugs, can be found, particularly at the periphery of the lesion. Small bile ducts, which may be numerous, are usually interspersed among the blood vessels and also are most prominent at the lesion's edge. Extramedullary hematopoiesis is present in about 60% of cases (291), usually within vascular lumina. Cavernous foci are often present in the center (60%) and may also be found peripherally in a few cases. Regressive changes (thrombosis, fibrosis, myxoid change, calcification) are noted in nearly 70% of cases, particularly in larger lesions. Type 2 change is characterized by poorly formed, often irregularly shaped, branching vascular structures lined by larger, more hyperchromatic and pleomorphic endothelial cells. Mitotic activity is more pronounced.

Differential Diagnosis

Differentiation of IHE from angiosarcoma may be difficult, particularly in a small biopsy specimen. If only type 1 features are noted, the distinction should not be a problem, although sampling artifact is a consideration. An infiltrative margin should not be interpreted as indicating malignancy. As noted earlier, some investigators consider type 2 IHE to represent a form of pediatric angiosarcoma (282). Hypercel-

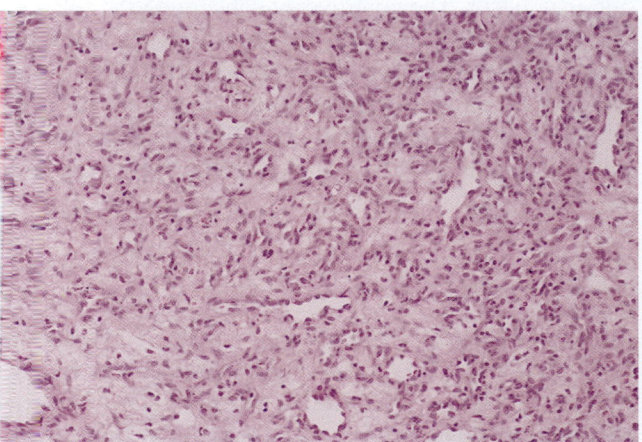

FIG. 22. Infantile hemangioendothelioma. Compressed vascular spaces are lined by plump, but rather bland endothelial cells. Bile ductules are often admixed (not shown).

lular whorls of malignant spindle cells, often with intracellular eosinophilic hyaline globules (kaposiform features), and malignant vascular channels characterize most pediatric angiosarcomas (293). Identical hyaline globules, however, have rarely been found in IHE, but the malignant spindle-cell component is absent. In addition, patients with pediatric angiosarcoma are typically older than 1.5 yrs. The presence of extrahepatic tumors in patients with IHE should not be misconstrued as metastases.

Regions of IHE with abundant myxoid stroma should not be confused with mesenchymal hamartoma; conversely, vascular proliferation in mesenchymal hamartoma should not be misinterpreted as IHE. Adequate sampling should reveal the characteristic histologic features of either lesion (88). The presence of calcification in a lesion initially regarded as mesenchymal hamartoma should suggest the possibility of IHE. The numerous small blood vessels and bile ducts found in IHE are absent in CH. Other entities in the differential diagnosis of IHE can be found in the earlier section on CH.

Treatment, Outcome, and Prognostic Factors

In one study, 70% of patients survived after a mean follow-up of 7.7 years; all deaths occurred within 1 month of diagnosis (291). Multivariate analysis demonstrated that congestive heart failure and jaundice were the factors most often associated with death, but multiple nodules and the absence of cavernous differentiation were also related to an adverse outcome (291). The percentage of cells in S+G2/M, assessed by flow cytometry, did not have a significant effect on outcome, while DNA aneuploidy appeared to be associated with a poorer prognosis, but too few cases were available for statistical analysis. The presence of type 2 change and increased mitoses did not indicate a poorer prognosis in this study. Solitary, well-situated lesions may be resected, whereas in other cases steroids have been used, and radiotherapy, arterial embolization, and even transplantation have been performed. Spontaneous regression may occur. The controversy concerning the relationship of type 2 IHE and angiosarcoma has been alluded to earlier; interpretation of previously reported cases (often based solely on biopsy material) demonstrating "dedifferentiation" or "transformation" of IHE to angiosarcoma is quite difficult and may be a matter of semantics (5,6,294–296).

Peliosis Hepatis

Peliosis hepatis is characterized by multiple blood-filled cysts in the liver. This nonneoplastic disorder was first reported in association with wasting diseases, such as tuberculosis or cancer. Today it is most commonly associated with the use of drugs such as anabolic or contraceptive steroids, danazol, or azathioprine. It is also seen in the immunocompromised host (particularly those infected with human immunodeficiency virus) in the form of *bacillary peliosis hepatis* (due to *Bartonella henselae*). Many other conditions (including liver transplantation, multicentric Castleman's disease, NRH, and hematologic malignancy) have been associated with this disorder (99,203,297–300).

Peliosis hepatis is usually an incidental autopsy finding, but severe hepatic dysfunction and even hepatic rupture have been reported. On macroscopic examination, multiple, round, red-purple, blood-filled spaces, 0.2 to 5 cm in diameter, impart a honeycomb appearance to the liver. At the microscopic level, "blood lakes" are bounded by hepatic cords that may or may not have an endothelial lining (Fig. 23). The spaces are frequently continuous, with dilated sinusoids in the adjacent hepatic parenchma. Organizing thrombus, periluminal fibrosis, and adjacent foci of hepatocellular necrosis can also be found. Proposed initiating events for the formation of the blood-filled cavities include hepatocellular necrosis, sinusoidal blockade due to veno-occlusive disease, and direct toxicity to the sinusoidal barrier.

Infection with *B. henselae*, the causative bacterium of cat scratch disease, may result in bacillary peliosis hepatis in severely immunocompromised patients (nearly always those with acquired immunodeficiency syndrome). Cystic blood-filled spaces with a fibromyxoid stroma containing a proliferation of small blood vessels (resembling granulation tissue) and a few spindle cells are noted; identical lesions may be found in the spleen. Clumps of stromal, purple to blue-gray, granular material represent the bacteria, which are best visualized with a Warthin-Starry stain. A definitive diagnosis of *B. henselae* infection can be made by PCR (203,300). Patients respond dramatically to therapy with erythromycin or doxycycline.

So-called *lipopeliosis* represents sinusoidal engorgement by extravasated lipid (not blood and hence not truly peliosis) stemming from preservation injury in allografts with steatosis (301). It is an uncommon occurrence (5% of allografts), and clinical outcome depends on the extent of hepatocellular necrosis.

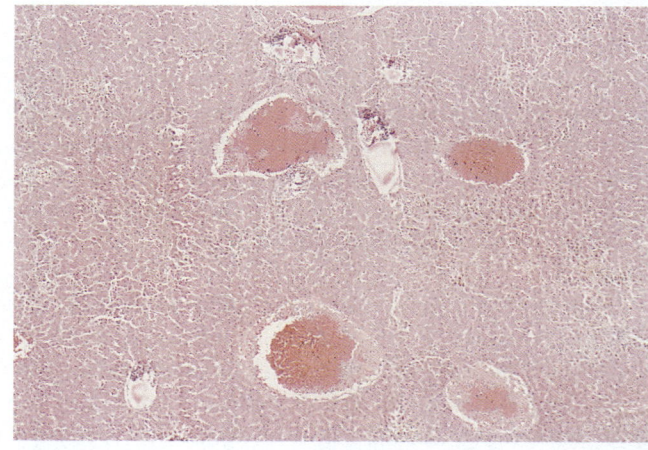

FIG. 23. Peliosis hepatis. Blood lakes with no particular zonal distribution within hepatic parenchyma.

Malignant Vascular Tumors

Angiosarcoma

Clinical, Epidemiologic, and Pathologic Features

Hepatic angiosarcoma (HAS) is the most common primary malignant mesenchymal tumor of the adult liver (3,282,302,303), but overall it is quite rare, representing only 0.4% of all primary hepatic malignancies in one large autopsy series (3). About 200 cases of HAS are diagnosed annually worldwide, with an estimated annual occurrence of ten to 20 cases in the U.S.A. (302). It is usually found in men (3–4:1) in their sixth or seventh decade of life. HAS rarely develops in childhood (282,293). Although an unknown percentage of cases may arise in the context of IHE (5,6,294–296), the more alarming type 2 variant of hemangioendothelioma, in terms of histologic features, is now considered by some researchers to be equivalent to HAS (282).

The majority of patients have initial symptoms of abdominal pain, fatigue, weight loss, or an abdominal mass. Portal hypertension is rarely evident early on. Major bleeding episodes and death have resulted from both thick-needle and FNA biopsies; therefore, nonoperative biopsy should be avoided (302–304). Synchronous cholangiocarcinoma and/or HCC may occur in Thorotrast or vinyl chloride—associated cases (282).

Overall, 25% to 42% of HAS are associated with the etiologic factors summarized in Table 22 (302,303). An uncommon p53 mutation (A:T to T:A transversion) has been found in 50% of vinyl chloride–associated cases, but not in sporadic HAS or those related to Thorotrast (305). In exposed patients, routinely stained paraffin-embedded material demonstrates thorium dioxide (Thorotrast), lying free or in macrophages, evident either as brown-gray refractile, but not birefringent, granules 0.3 to 10 m in diameter or as larger aggregates. It is an alpha emitter; the alpha tracts can be demonstrated by autoradiography. The presence of thorium can be established by gamma and x-ray spectroscopy as well as energy-dispersive x-ray microanalysis (282). The HAS induced by known environmental agents (a) are almost always associated with prolonged latent periods (often 20 to 35 years or more), (b) are accompanied by evidence of chronic liver disease with fibrosis (or cirrhosis) in the adjacent hepatic parenchyma, (c) appear to develop through a series of precursor stages with simultaneous hypertrophy of both hepatocytes and sinusoidal lining cells as well as nuclear enlargement and hyperchromasia of the latter cell type, and (d) are indistinguishable in pathologic terms from the larger group of idiopathic cases (303,282).

Macroscopic Features. Most commonly, HAS is multicentric and involves both lobes (3,282). Individual tumor foci are quite variable in size, have ill-defined borders, and often demonstrate alternating hemorrhagic and gray-white solid nodules with large blood-filled cavities (Fig. 24A). Reticular deposits of yellow chalky material, often quite noticeable just underneath the hepatic capsule, are characteristic of Thorotrast. Splenic atrophy with chalky deposits is typical of Thorotrast-related cases, whereas the spleen is usually enlarged in cases not associated with this agent.

Microscopic Features. The malignant endothelial cells that characterize HAS are plump, often elongated or pleomorphic, with hyperchromatic nuclei, variably sized nucleoli, pale eosinophilic cytoplasm, and poorly defined cell borders (Fig. 24B,C). Epithelioid cells with more conspicuous cytoplasm and generally prominent nucleoli, bizarre tumor giant cells, and nodules of spindle cells simulating fibrosarcoma may be seen. Mitotic activity is common. The tumor cells are usually seen growing in one or more layers along preformed sinusoids that maintain contact with thickened hepatic cords (sinusoidal, scaffold-like, or trabecular pattern). Cholestatic hepatocellular rosettes with bile plugs may be evident. Progressive sinusoidal obliteration by tumor cells leads to hepatocyte atrophy and variably sized cavities (cavernous or peloid pattern), which are filled with blood and lined by tumor cells that may demonstrate a papillary configuration. In 75% of cases, tumor invasion of portal or hepatic vein branches can be found on microscopy, an obvious explanation for the prevalent foci of necrosis seen in this tumor. Extramedullary hematopoiesis is often present. Tumor cells have variably been reported to demonstrate phagocytic behavior (3,282).

Immunoreactivity for endothelial markers (CD34, CD31, factor VIII–related antigen, *Ulex europaeus* lectin) is nearly always present in tumor cells in vasoformative foci, but it may be absent in non- or poorly vasoformative areas (282,306,307). CK immunoreactivity has been found in 12% of cases (306). Demonstration of Weibel-Palade bodies by electron microscopy may confirm the diagnosis, but it is rarely necessary. In one series, most cases of childhood angiosarcoma evidenced (in addition to malignant vasoformative foci) small whorls of spindle cells that often demonstrated PAS-positive intracytoplasmic globules, simulating Kaposi's sarcoma (KS) (kaposiform features) (293).

TABLE 22. *Hepatic angiosarcoma: associated etiologic agents/conditions*[a]

Idiopathic (58–75%)
Associated agents/conditions (25–42%)
Thorotrast[b]
Vinyl chloride[b]
Inorganic arsenic[b]
Androgenic steroids[b]
Copper sulfate
Estrogenic steroids
Phenelzine
Radiotherapy
Chemotherapeutic agents
Hereditary hemochromatosis (cirrhotic stage)

[a] Data from references 282, 302, 303. Cases potentially arising from preexisting benign vascular tumors, such as infantile hemangioendothelioma and a unique case of cavernous hemangioma, are excluded.
[b] By far the most commonly associated agents.

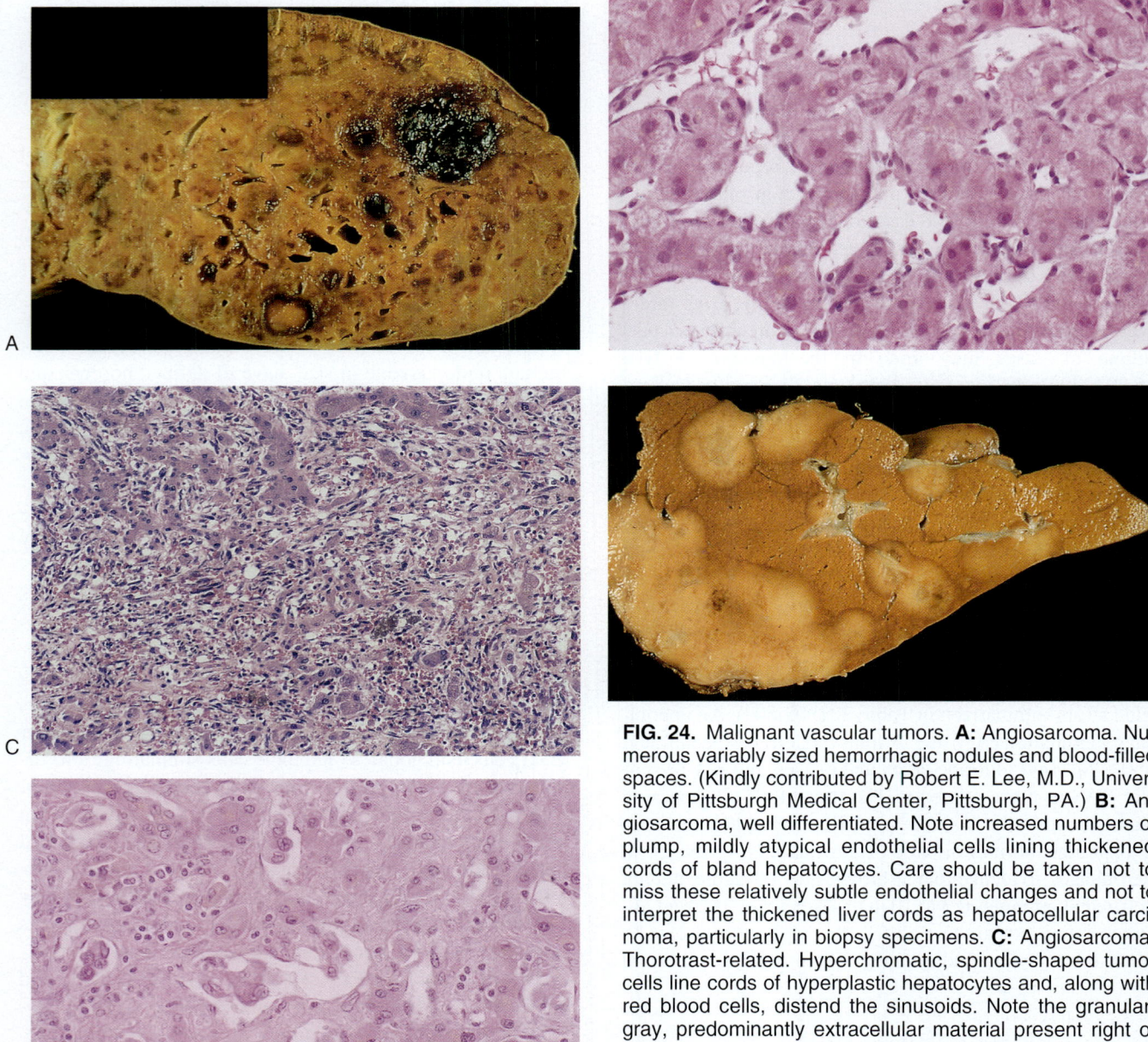

FIG. 24. Malignant vascular tumors. **A:** Angiosarcoma. Numerous variably sized hemorrhagic nodules and blood-filled spaces. (Kindly contributed by Robert E. Lee, M.D., University of Pittsburgh Medical Center, Pittsburgh, PA.) **B:** Angiosarcoma, well differentiated. Note increased numbers of plump, mildly atypical endothelial cells lining thickened cords of bland hepatocytes. Care should be taken not to miss these relatively subtle endothelial changes and not to interpret the thickened liver cords as hepatocellular carcinoma, particularly in biopsy specimens. **C:** Angiosarcoma, Thorotrast-related. Hyperchromatic, spindle-shaped tumor cells line cords of hyperplastic hepatocytes and, along with red blood cells, distend the sinusoids. Note the granular, gray, predominantly extracellular material present right of center, that represents Thorotrast. **D:** Epithelioid hemangioendothelioma. Multiple tan-gray, firm, focally confluent nodules with infiltrative borders. Several of the nodules involve venous structures. The tumor's gross appearance belies its endothelial origin. (Kindly contributed by Robert E. Lee, M.D., University of Pittsburgh Medical Center, Pittsburgh, PA.). **E:** Epithelioid hemangioendothelioma. The outer zone of the tumor at the interface with adjacent liver. Note extensive involvement of portal vein branch, growth along sinusoids with compression of hepatocytes, and mild inflammatory reaction.

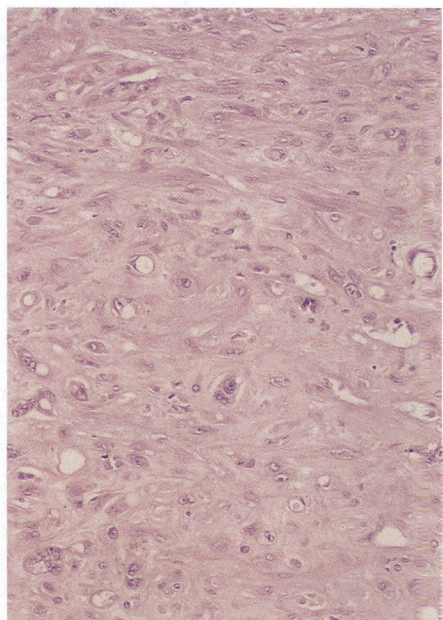 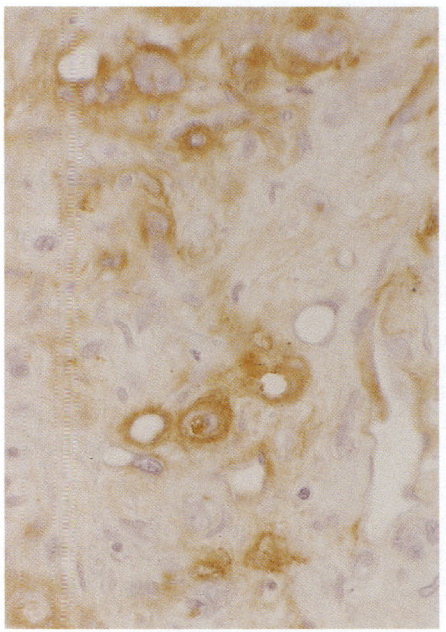

FIG. 24. (*continued*) Malignant vascular tumors. **F:** epithelioid hemangioendothelioma. Left panel: Epithelioid and dendritic tumor cells with focally vacuolated cytoplasm are embedded in a fibromyxoid matrix. This histologic picture can be confused with adenocarcinoma. Right panel: Factor VIII–related antigen immunoreactivity is present in the tumor cell cytoplasm and outlines intracytoplasmic vacuoles, indicating the vascular nature of the tumor cells (incipient vascular lumina) (immunoperoxidase, factor VIII–related antigen).

Differential Diagnosis

The diagnosis of HAS can sometimes be quite difficult. In one review, only 50% of cases of HAS were correctly diagnosed on histologic evidence (302). Subtle foci may not be readily recognized as HAS and can be mistaken for reactive, inflammatory, congestive, or fibrosing disorders. The plump, at least slightly atypical lining cells noted in HAS are not seen in reactive conditions, however. Although the histologic features may occasionally be subtle, particularly in inadvertently obtained biopsy specimens, the atypical cytologic features will be appreciated once consideration is given to this diagnosis.

The sinusoidal pattern of HAS must also be differentiated from HCC. In HCC it is the hepatocytes and not the endothelial cells that are atypical in terms of cytologic characteristics, and the sinusoidal lining cells are relatively inconspicuous. While sinusoidal endothelial cells in normal liver only rarely are immunoreactive for endothelial markers, positive endothelial staining in HCC is common but does not indicate endothelial neoplasia (146,150).

Kaposi's sarcoma (KS) may be confused with solid foci of spindle cells in HAS (see above under microscopic description); however, a clinical history indicating extrahepatic nodules, the absence of other foci typical of HAS, the distinctly portal distribution of the lesion, and, notably, the presence of acquired immunodeficiency syndrome (AIDS) facilitate the diagnosis of this tumor (203,282,308). Distinguishing HAS from EH, the other important primary malignant hepatic vascular neoplasm (235), is considered below and in Table 23. The finding of only a few atypical intrasinusoidal cells raises the possibility of leukemia, lymphoma, or a poorly differentiated carcinoma. The clinical findings as well as a panel of immunohistochemical studies (leukocyte common antigen, myeloperoxidase, CK, endothelial markers, etc.) should aid in differential diagnosis, but recall that HAS may be CK positive.

Treatment and Outcome

Hepatic failure and intraabdominal bleeding are responsible for about 75% of deaths; most patients die within six months. At autopsy, more than 60% of patients have metastases, most frequently to the lung, but making the distinction between metastases and extrahepatic multicentric growth is virtually impossible.

Epithelioid Hemangioendothelioma

Clinical and Pathologic Features

EH is a malignant endothelium-derived neoplasm with an unpredictable natural history that most frequently develops in middle-aged women (Table 23) (235,282,309–313). It is the second most common primary hepatic sarcoma seen at the Armed Forces Institute of Pathology (314). Patients most frequently show initial signs of abdominal pain or weight

TABLE 23. *Clinicopathologic features of angiosarcoma and epithelioid hemangioendothelioma*

Feature	Epithelioid hemangioendothelioma	Angiosarcoma
Clinical features		
Sex (male/female)	1:1.6	3–4:1
Mean age (range), yrs	47 (3–86)	53 (<1, >80)
Etiologic factors	None well documented	25–42%; Thorotrast, VC, arsenic, androgens, etc.
Symptoms and signs		
Abdominal pain, mass	Most common	Most common
Intraabdominal bleeding	Rare	30%
Asymptomatic	50%	Virtually never
Thrombocytopenia	No	50%
Radiographic features		
Abdominal films, calcification	20%	Virtually never; Thorotrast causes radiodensity
Angiography	Typically avascular	Typically vascular
Pathologic features		
Macroscopic		
Multiple nodules	80%	70%
Nodule size (cm)	<1–12 cm; rarely cirrhotomimetic	<1–5
Nodule appearance	White-gray, tan, firm, infiltrative borders	Blood cysts, spongy, occasionally white, firm
Microscopic		
Zonation	Present	Absent
Tumor cellularity	Scanty in fibrotic areas	Abundant
Spindle and epithelioid cells	Present	Present
Intracytoplasmic lumina	Prominent	Inconspicuous
Marked nuclear pleomorphism	Absent	Present
Sinusoidal/venous invasion	Extensive	Extensive
Stroma	Myxoid/dense sclerosis, 30% calcification	Scant, focally fibrotic, no calcification
Extramedullary hematopoiesis	Absent	Often present
Tumor cell immunohistochemistry		
Endothelial markers	Positive	Positive
Cytokeratin	Occasionally positive	Occasionally positive
Adjacent liver	Usually normal, rarely NRH or cirrhosis	Fibrosis, cirrhosis common with known etiologic factors
Outcome	Unpredictable, 19% alive at 5 yrs	Dismal, 3% alive at 2 yrs

NRH, nodular regenerative hyperplasia; VC, vinyl chloride.

loss, and, rarely, hepatic rupture or liver failure occur. Manifestations of hepatic venous outflow obstruction may result from involvement of major hepatic vein branches or terminal hepatic venules. In about 40% of cases, EH may be an incidental finding. Abdominal plain radiographs show calcification in about 20% of patients. By angiography, EH has usually been described as avascular, and CT scan typically demonstrates peripheral nodules with capsular retraction.

The etiology of EH is unknown. While OCS use has been suggested as an etiologic factor, this theory has not been supported by case-control studies (2). Vinyl chloride exposure has been reported in two cases. It has also been suggested that EH represents a neoplastic analogue of wound healing (312). Definitive diagnosis is best made by core or wedge biopsy or in cell block material, since the cytologic features are not distinctive (315).

Macroscopic Features. In nearly 80% of cases, there are multiple nodules that involve both lobes. Nodule size varies from less than 1 to 12 cm in diameter. They are typically described as white, gray-white, or tan, firm, sometimes gritty masses with ill-defined borders (Fig. 24D). When the nodules are quite small, the macroscopic picture may deceptively mimic cirrhosis (284,312). Conversely, a few cases of NRH, related to neoplastic obliterative venous changes, and cirrhosis have been reported in association with EH. The vascular nature of the tumor cannot be appreciated on gross examination.

Microscopic Features. A zonal pattern is often seen in EH, reflecting the evolutionary changes in this neoplasm. At the lesion's periphery, scanning magnification demonstrates a cellular sinusoidal proliferation in zone 1 (periportal), with residual intact hepatocytes and scanty myxoid stroma. Portal tracts may appear deceptively normal, but closer inspection often shows tufts of tumor cells within portal vein branches (Fig. 24E). Progressive neoplastic sinusoidal obliteration results in a midzone characterized by atrophic hepatocyte plates, a few bile ductules, and increasing quantities of variably inflamed myxochondroid stroma that becomes progressively sclerotic, paucicellular, and sometimes calcified (30%) as one progresses toward zone 3 (perivenular).

Recognition of the sclerotic zone alone as neoplastic may be impossible on histologic evidence. Partial or total luminal obliteration of terminal hepatic venules and larger hepatic vein branches by tufts or sessile clusters of tumor cells is typical; trichrome or elastic stains may be necessary for vessel identification.

The tumor cells, best characterized in the midzone, are embedded in the myxohyaline matrix in nests; short, single-file cords; or as single cells, simulating carcinoma. Two different cell types—dendritic and epithelioid—have been described, with isolated transitional forms (Fig. 24F). The dendritic cells are spindle-shaped or stellate, with branching processes that appear to connect adjacent cells. Their nuclei are vesicular, sometimes folded, and contain small nucleoli, while the cytoplasm is eosinophilic.

Epithelioid cells are more rounded, with a greater amount of eosinophilic cytoplasm. Nuclei are generally round, with mild to moderate atypia and often prominent eosinophilic nucleoli. Once in awhile, mitoses will be evident. The most striking and potentially misleading characteristic of these cells is the presence of one or more well-defined intracytoplasmic vacuoles of variable size ("blister cells," incipient vascular lumina), which may contain erythrocytes (a diagnostic clue). These features may lead to diagnostic confusion with signet ring adenocarcinoma, but mucin stains are always negative, and the vacuoles demonstrate immunoreactivity for CD34 or other endothelial markers but are negative for CEA (Fig. 24F) (311,313).

Care should be used in the interpretation of CK immunoreactivity, since nearly 15% of EHs are positive for this marker; trapped nonneoplastic hepatocytes or bile ductules will also be positive (311). Fusion of blister cells or the focal presence of a few well-formed neovascular channels can impart a granulation tissue-like appearance to the tumor. Anastomosing vessels are absent. Ultrastructural examination reveals Weibel-Palade bodies, characteristic of endothelial cells, and numerous intermediate filaments, which are responsible for the epithelioid histologic appearance. Detection of early EH recurrence in hepatic allografts may be quite difficult, but immunohistochemical stains for endothelial markers (particularly CD34) help by decorating rare atypical tumor cells found adjacent to areas of perivenular fibrosis (313).

Differential Diagnosis

The differential diagnosis requires consideration of conditions that are neoplastic (metastatic adenocarcinoma, particularly the signet cell type; scirrhous cholangiocarcinoma or HCC; neuroendocrine neoplasms; and chondro- and leiomyosarcoma) and nonneoplastic (sclerosed hemangioma, scar, collapsed fibrotic parenchyma, granulation tissue, cirrhosis, and veno-occlusive disease). Small biopsies can be quite misleading, as evidenced by the relatively frequent (30%) incorrect initial diagnoses in cases subsequently proved to be EH. Before the seminal report from the Armed Forces Institute of Pathology, many cases were misdiagnosed as sclerosing cholangiocarcinoma (235). The features distinguishing EH from this tumor and adenocarcinoma in general have been delineated earlier.

Neuroendocrine tumors may show signs of dense sclerosis and cords of tumor cells, but other features characteristic of these tumors are usually present and make the diagnosis straightforward. Positive immunoreactivity of EH with putative neuroendocrine markers (PGP 9.5, NSE) should not lead one astray from the correct diagnosis (207). Compact foci of spindle cells with abundant eosinophilic cytoplasm may be confused with leiomyosarcoma, and the fact that about 25% of EH evidence smooth-muscle actin may also confuse the issue (311). The myxochondroid stroma can be misinterpreted as indicating chondrosarcoma. Many spindle-cell tumors in addition to EH are CD34 positive, and for this reason immunoreactivity for this marker alone should not be considered diagnostic of EH (313). Table 21 lists features that aid in distinguishing EH from primary and metastatic carcinoma, whereas Table 23 compares the clinicopathologic features of EH and conventional angiosarcoma. There may also be lesions that are borderline between EH and epithelioid angiosarcoma (313).

Sclerosed hemangiomas do not display cytologic atypia, are well circumscribed, do not invade veins, and are less cellular than EH, but residual small capillaries can mimic blister cells (203). In postnecrotic collapse or atrophy of hepatic parenchyma, there are often bile ductules in a loose or sclerotic stroma with preserved portal tracts. These features may superficially mimic EH. Immunohistochemical testing for CK and endothelial markers may be useful in diagnostically challenging cases. The presence of neoplastic cells in the occlusive lesions of efferent veins distinguishes EH from non-neoplastic causes of venous outflow obstruction. Making the distinction between primary hepatic EH and metastatic EH, particularly from the lung, requires clinicopathologic correlation. It is unclear whether this tumor can develop in a multicentric fashion.

Treatment and Outcome

Although survival rates are much better than for conventional HAS, the clinical course of EH is unpredictable. Some patients die within months of initial diagnosis, while 26 of 137 patients (19%) in the series from the Armed Forces Institute of Pathology were known to have survived for at least 5 years, with the longest survival being 27 years (311). Tumor cellularity was found to be the only histologic feature of prognostic importance in that report. Treatment of EH is the subject of controversy; resection is usually performed if possible, and hepatic transplantation has led to improved survival even in selected unresectable cases showing signs of extrahepatic disease (282,309). Patients can live for years with metastatic disease. Extrahepatic involvement (lung, omentum/mesentery, lymph nodes) has been detected in about 50% of cases.

Kaposi's Sarcoma

Hepatic involvement by KS for all practical purposes is found only in patients with AIDS (203,282,308). While hepatic KS is not responsible for morbidity or mortality, KS lesions are seen in 12% to 25% of fatal cases in this population of patients, almost always in association with KS lesions elsewhere. The tumor, which seems to be induced by human herpesvirus 8, develops as small hemorrhagic spongy nodules that may sometimes reach a diameter of 5 to 7 cm (308). The portal tract is the site of origin for most lesions, often with preservation of the portal triad, but there may be extension for a variable distance into the adjacent parenchyma. The histologic patterns, from vasoformative channels to hyaline globule-containing spindle cells, resemble those described at extrahepatic sites. Peliotic lesions probably related to intrasinusoidal tumor extension may be seen, particularly at the lesion's periphery. Immunoreactivity for CD31 and CD34 is consistently found in the spindle cells In the context of AIDS, making the distinction from other malignancies is generally not a problem, but peliotic foci must be distinguished from bacillary peliosis hepatis.

Other Benign Mesenchymal Tumors

Fatty Tumors

Angiomyolipoma and Related Tumors

Nearly 60 cases of hepatic angiomyolipoma (AML) have been described—their number has markedly increased since the advent of CT scan and ultrasound studies (257,316). The mean age at diagnosis is 50 years (range, 9–79 years), and there is a slight female predominance. Only 6% are associated with tuberous sclerosis, and only rarely have they been reported in association with renal AMLs. Patients are often asymptomatic (40%), although rupture has been reported upon occasion. These masses are well circumscribed, solitary, and usually yellow, but they may be gray or white. Necrosis may be seen in the larger tumors. The background liver is normal. The tumor is composed of varying quantities of mature adipose tissue (rarely with hibernoma-like cells), thick-walled blood vessels, and smooth-muscle cells. Extramedullary hematopoiesis is seen in about 40% of cases (angiomyomyelolipoma or angiomyelolipoma). Extensive sampling may be required to demonstrate all components; limited sampling could explain the rare reported examples of lipoma or leiomyoma.

The smooth-muscle cells may be spindle-shaped or epithelioid; the latter cell type may have a clear or eosinophilic cytoplasm. Areas of prominent cellularity, nuclear pleomorphism with intranuclear inclusions, and tumor giant cells raise the possibility of a metastatic or primary sarcoma, while the presence of a trabecular epithelioid growth pattern can be quite alarming and can be misinterpreted as HCC (see Table 13). Typically, there are few mitoses and the nuclear to cytoplasmic ratio is relatively low. The epithelioid cells may contain PAS-positive crystals, are positive for HMB-45 and negative for CK, and may reveal premelanosome-like structures on electron microscopy. They should not be mistaken for metastatic melanoma.

Hepatic pseudolipoma (pseudolipoma of Glisson's capsule) is a rare tumor found embedded in a concavity on the surface of the liver. It represents a trapped epiploic appendage, in some cases related to previous surgery. Degenerative changes (fat necrosis, calcification, ossification) are often present (257,317). *Focal fatty change* of hepatocytes is considered in this section because it can simulate a lipomatous tumor. These foci have been detected with ultrasound or CT scan and can mimic metastatic carcinoma or an abscess on radiography or at laparotomy (257,318,319). Patients often have such conditions as obesity, diabetes mellitus, alcoholism, or other disorders that predispose to dyslipidemia. Focal fatty change is usually subcapsular, may be single or multiple, varies in size up to nearly 10 cm in diameter, and generally has a yellow-white appearance. At the microscopic level, steatosis either diffusely or focally affects the hepatic lobule; the adjacent liver is unremarkable. Foreign body–type granulomatous reactions can be seen in degenerated foci (257). Typically, the size of the lesion remains stable over time, although regression has been noted with amelioration of the underlying condition.

Inflammatory Myofibroblastic Tumor (Inflammatory Pseudotumor) and Other Fibroinflammatory Masses

Clinical Features

Inflammatory myofibroblastic tumor (IMT), also known as inflammatory pseudotumor, is a nonneoplastic solid mass that has been misdiagnosed both on radiography and on the basis of pathologic evidence as a malignant tumor (257,320,321). Patients with hepatic IMT are usually adult men (mean age 37 years; range, 10 months to 83 years; male/female ratio, 3:1) with initial symptoms of intermittent low-grade fever, vague abdominal pain, and weight loss. Involvement of hilar structures may result in portal hypertension or biliary obstruction. Surgical excision is curative, although regression without surgery has been reported. While most cases have been associated with an uneventful outcome, there have been rare fatalities; a few cases have recurred as either sarcoma (322) or follicular dendritic cell tumor (323). Anything less than total excision of the lesion should be interpreted with great caution and diagnostic restraint by the pathologist, since many hepatic masses of varied types can be associated with an fibroinflammatory reaction (324).

Pathologic Features and Differential Diagnosis

The masses are well circumscribed and solitary in more than two-thirds of cases. Nodule size varies from 1 to 25 cm. The cut surface has a variegated appearance; infarction may be present. Occasionally, the mass may extend outside the liver into the inferior vena cava (321) or contiguous retroperitoneal soft tissue (257). The number and type of inflammatory cells, as well as the extent of fibrosis, vary both within a given lesion and from case to case. Plasma cells (polyclonal) often predominate, but inconsistent proportions of lymphocytes (including lymphoid follicles), neutrophils, eosinophils, macrophages, and oval to spindle-shaped stromal cells, are found. The stroma is typically quite fibrotic, with a whorled, laminated appearance or dense sclerotic zones that may be confused with sclerosing hemangioma, EH, benign nerve sheath tumors, leiomyoma, solitary fibrous tumor, sarcomatoid carcinoma, or sarcomas (such as malignant fibrous histiocytoma). Myxoid foci may also be present, but a vascular component is minimal.

The stromal cells may simulate binucleated or mononuclear Reed-Sternberg cells, causing misdiagnosis as Hodgkin's disease, however they are CD15 and CD30 negative (323). The stromal cells typically are said to have immunohistochemical and ultrastructural features of myofibroblasts (320). A follicular dendritic cell immunophenotype (CD21 and CD35 positive) containing clonal Epstein-Barr virus, however, has been reported, indicating that some tumors initially classified as IMT actually represent follicular dendritic cell tumors (323,325). CK immunoreactivity (36%) has been reported in one large series of IMTs, but the rate in hepatic lesions was not specifically stated (326).

The inflammatory infiltrate can also be confused with non-Hodgkin's lymphoma, *Rosai-Dorfman disease*, or even the plasma cell variant of *Castleman's disease* (257,326a). Occlusive phlebitis, multinucleated giant cells, foamy histiocytes, and granulomas have all been reported in cases of IMT; these features should be distinguished from tumefactive granulomatous lesions, such as *sarcoidoma* (sarcoid pseudotumor), *tuberculoma*, *syphilitic gumma*, and *malakoplakia* (2,257,327). Zones of suppuration separate *abscesses* and *pyogenic cholangiohepatitis* from IMT, but organizing regions of these lesions are identical to IMT on histologic assessment, and making the distinction in individual cases may be a matter of semantics. Although bacteria have only rarely been isolated from IMT, both the clinical and pathologic features suggest an infectious origin in many cases.

Solitary (Fibrosing) Necrotic Nodules

Solitary necrotic nodules may be single or multiple and vary from 0.2 to 2.5 cm in diameter; they are located just beneath the anterior border of the liver (2,328). On histologic examination, a central necrotic core is surrounded by a hyalinized fibroelastic capsule. Other findings include central calcification and a prominent reticulin pattern that may either be collapsed or suggest the previous presence of hyperplastic hepatocyte plates. Although the majority appear to represent sclerosed hemangiomas, this group is most likely heterogeneous; infection (parasites, old granulomas), trauma, hyalinized bile duct hamartomas, and even degenerated benign hepatocellular nodules are other possible etiologic sources. On radiography, they can simulate metastatic disease.

Other Mesenchymal Nodules

A few hepatic tumors have been reported as *solitary fibrous tumor* (CK negative, CD34 positive), *chondroma* (history of parotid pleomorphic adenoma), *leiomyoma*, or *lipoma* (3,329,330,330a); in the latter two instances, careful search for other components of angiomyolipoma is warranted (257,316). Even with a bland appearance, metastasis (particularly from the gastrointestinal tract, female pelvic organs, and retroperitoneum) should be excluded when considering the possibility of a primary benign nonvascular mesenchymal tumor.

Other Malignant Mesenchymal Tumors

Undifferentiated (Embryonal) Sarcoma

Clinical Features

Although hepatic sarcomas are very rare in adults, they make up nearly 10% of all pediatric hepatic tumors (3,5,6,6a,282,314,331–338) (see Table 2). The undifferentiated (embryonal) sarcoma, also called mesenchymal sarcoma or malignant mesenchymoma, is by far the single most common neoplasm in this group (Table 24). More than 50% of patients are between 6 and 10 years of age, and more than 90% of such tumors occur by age 21. There is no sexual preference. Manifestations are typically those of an abdominal mass and/or abdominal pain.

Pathologic Features

Tumor size often exceeds 10 cm and can be as large as 30 cm in diameter. On macroscopic examination, there is a single, well-demarcated, soft, globular mass that frequently has cystic, gelatinous, hemorrhagic, and necrotic foci. Microscopic examination reveals a pseudocapsule surrounding a neoplasm that is composed predominately of spindle, oval, or stellate cells with ill-defined cell borders (Fig. 25). The nuclei contain stippled chromatin and usually inconspicuous nucleoli. The tumor cells are embedded in an abundant myxoid stroma that contains many thin-walled veins. Cell density may be quite variable, the cells forming fascicles in some foci and being relatively scanty in others. Multinucleated and cytologically bizarre tumor cells with prominent eosinophilic cytoplasm and numerous mitotic figures are usually present. These features have been seen in FNA biopsies (338).

Hyaline globules that are PAS positive and diastase resistant are often found both within the cytoplasm of tumor cells and in the stroma. They occasionally have alpha-1-antitrypsin (AIAT), but not AFP immunoreactivity. Trapped hepatocytes and benign cystically dilated structures resembling bile ducts

TABLE 24. *Undifferentiated (embryonal) sarcoma, embryonal rhabdomyosarcoma, and mesenchymal hamartoma: differential diagnosis*

Feature	Mesenchymal hamartoma	Undifferentiated (embryonal) sarcoma	Embryonal rhabdomyosarcoma[a]
Peak age, sex (M/F)	75% ≤ 1 yr (2–3:1)	50% 6–10 yrs (1:1)	Typically 2–6 yrs (1:1–2)
Clinical features	Abdominal mass	Abdominal mass, pain	Jaundice, abdominal mass, pain
Macroscopic features	Myxoid mass with fluid-filled cysts	Extensive necrosis, hemorrhage, and myxoid foci	Polypoid myxoid mass extending into bile duct
Microscopic features			
Tumor cells			
Spindle cells	Cytologically bland	Anaplastic	Anaplastic (cambium layer)
Giant cells	Absent	Present	Present, occasionally cross-striations
IHC: muscle markers[b]	Variable/negative	Variable/negative	Usually positive/variable
PAS-positive-DR globules	Negative	Positive	Negative
EM (thick and thin filaments)	Absent	Absent/rare	Sometimes positive (sampling)
Stroma	Quite myxoid	Variably myxoid	Myxoid under cambium layer
Bile ducts	Integral part of tumor, often cystically dilated	Usually considered "trapped"	Duct epithelium covers intraluminal tumor projections
Prognosis	Excellent—deaths related to operative complications; a few cases associated with US	Poor, but improving; a few survivors >5 yrs	Poor, but improving; a few survivors >5 yrs

EM, electron microscopy; IHC, immunohistochemistry; PAS-positive-DR, periodic acid–Schiff—positive, diastase resistant; US, undifferentiated sarcoma.

[a] Data cited are for embryonal rhabdomyosarcoma of the hepatobiliary tree in general, because purely intrahepatic tumors are so rare.

[b] Muscle markers: muscle-specific actin, desmin, Myo D1, myoglobin.

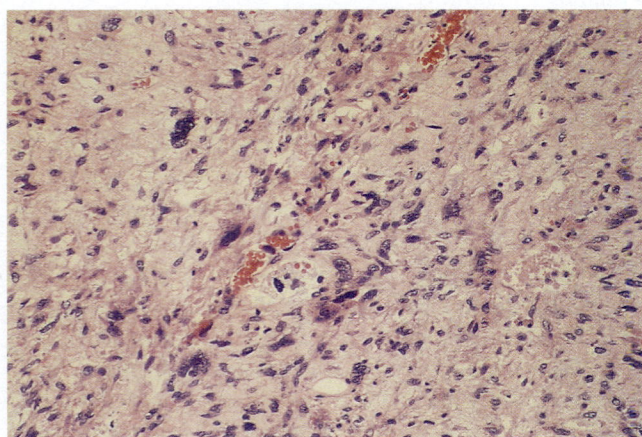

FIG. 25. Undifferentiated (embryonal) sarcoma. The pleomorphic nature of the spindle cells easily distinguishes this neoplasm from mesenchymal hamartoma, although both have abundant myxoid stroma (see Fig. 5). The lack of a cambium layer or strap cells, and absence of conspicuous immunoreactivity for muscle markers aid in making the distinction from embryonal rhabdomyosarcoma. Focal areas of differentiated sarcoma have been described in this tumor, and a relationship to rhabdomyosarcoma has been postulated.

are frequently identified at the tumor's periphery, often within the pseudocapsule but sometimes blending into the sarcoma. Atypical cytologic features in these epithelial elements have been interpreted as reactive or degenerative phenomena. Other histologic features include organizing thrombi, necrosis, and extramedullary hematopoiesis.

A few studies of flow cytometric DNA analysis have been reported; a high growth fraction was typical and aneuploidy was present in three of seven cases (332,338). It is unclear whether these features are of prognostic significance. Ultrastructural examination has generally revealed features consistent with a mesenchymal origin, now and then demonstrating foci of smooth-muscle, skeletal muscle, fat, and, rarely, cells with epithelial features (333,335,336). Immunohistochemical studies have indicated variable immunoreactivity with antibodies to desmin, muscle-specific actin, and CK, but not myoglobin (332,333,335,336). The consensus is that undifferentiated sarcoma is a primitive mesenchymal neoplasm, possibly derived from a primitive multipotential precursor cell that may have foci of differentiated sarcoma. Some cases may arise from clinically inapparent mesenchymal hamartomas (92).

Differential Diagnosis

The major features helpful in differentiating this tumor from mesenchymal hamartoma and embryonal rhabdomyosarcoma are summarized in Table 24 (5,88,282, 333,335). The sarcomatoid (spindle cell) variant of HCC as well as the mixed form of HBL should also be considered in the differential diagnosis. A normal serum AFP and the absence of typical foci of HCC or epithelial HBL are helpful discriminating features. Definitive diagnosis may be impossible in small biopsy specimens, and prominent central necrosis may obscure the diagnosis. Resection specimens should be adequately sectioned (one section per centimeter of tumor).

Treatment and Outcome

Initially, the prognosis was regarded as bleak, with a median survival of less than 1 year (331). Newer studies have emphasized better survival with complete resection, with or without associated combination chemotherapy, and long-term disease-free survival (more than 10 years) has been reported (334). Metastases to lung, pleura, and peritoneum are common; invasion of the vena cava with extension into the right atrium rarely occurs (282,331).

Fibrosarcoma and Malignant Fibrous Histiocytoma

About 40 cases have been reported as primary fibrosarcomas in the literature (282,339,340). They are typically single hepatic masses in middle-aged or elderly men. About 20% of reported cases are associated with cirrhosis, while a similar number are associated with hypoglycemia. From time to time they have appeared posttransplantation (340). Less than 20 cases of malignant fibrous histiocytoma have been reported (339). Patients with these malignant fibroblastic tumors almost always die of tumor-related disease within 1 year of diagnosis. Extensive sampling is always required to rule out sarcomatoid HCC or CC (181,272). In particular, sarcomatoid HCC should be considered when cirrhosis is present.

Leiomyosarcoma

About 60 cases of presumed primary hepatic leiomyosarcoma had been published in the literature by 1992, excluding those arising in the ligamentum teres or inferior vena cava and Epstein-Barr virus–associated cases in children or adults infected with the human immunodeficiency virus or posttransplantation in pediatric patients (282,314,340, 341). Well-defined criteria for distinguishing benign from malignant primary hepatic smooth-muscle tumors are not available, because too few cases have been studied. Most patients with leiomyosarcoma have died within 2 years of diagnosis. EH may focally simulate leiomyosarcoma (235).

Rhabdomyosarcoma

Rhabdomyosarcoma, which typically develops in children 3 to 4 years of age, rarely involves the hepatobiliary tree (342,343). The liver and hepatic ducts are the site of origin in only 4% and 10% of cases, respectively; nearly all of the remaining cases arise in the common bile duct. Secondary spread into the liver from extrahepatic foci is common. Since most patients show initial signs of obstructive jaundice, this tumor is discussed in greater detail in the chapter "Gallbladder and Extrahepatic Biliary Tree." A relationship to undifferentiated sarcoma has been suggested (333,334,343). Important features distinguishing this tumor from undifferentiated sarcoma and mesenchymal hamartoma are presented in Table 24. The presence of Myo D_1 and myoglobin immunoreactivity in rhabdomyosarcoma aid in discriminating rhabdomyosarcoma from *malignant rhabdoid tumor* (249).

Other Sarcomas

Primary hepatic liposarcoma, osteogenic sarcoma, and malignant schwannoma are extremely rare, but cases have been reported (344,345,346).

Primary Hepatic Lymphoma

Primary hepatic lymphoma is quite rare, representing less than 0.5% of all extranodal lymphomas in North America (347). Although about 100 cases have been reported as such in the literature, acceptance on the part of investigators of lymph node, bone marrow, and splenic involvement in addition to hepatic tumor foci for inclusion in this diagnosis has varied, leading to differing descriptions of clinicopathologic features (340,347–350a). A practical definition includes clinical manifestations mainly caused by liver involvement and the absence of distant lymphadenopathy or other overt clinicopathologic evidence of systemic disease. Liver involvement in disseminated disease and in the context of hepatosplenic ($\gamma\delta$) lymphoma, as well as specific histologic features, are discussed in the following section on metastatic tumors.

Cases among men outnumber those among women by 3:1, and there is a broad age spectrum (7 to 87 years; median, 55 years) (347). Patients have been reported with one of the following clinical pictures with variably abnormal liver tests, with or without the presence of "B" symptoms: (a) abdominal pain with hepatomegaly, (b) immunocompromise (chemotherapy for another disease, immunosuppresion related to transplantation, or AIDS), or (c) cirrhosis with incidental finding of lymphoma. A pathogenetic role for HBV, HCV, and autoimmune conditions has been suggested in a few cases (351).

The usual gross appearance is of a single large mass or multiple masses, often clinically considered to represent metastatic carcinoma or HCC. A diffuse pattern is much less common and clinically may mimic hepatitis. All cases have been non-Hodgkin's lymphomas (NHLs), with more than 75% representing the diffuse large-cell type. Most cases are of B-cell lineage; several reports of primary hepatic T-cell lymphomas suffer from incomplete characterization (350). Reported cases cover the gamut of lymphoma histologic subtypes, including follicular, lymphoplasmacytoid, mantle cell, small noncleaved, anaplastic large-cell, T-cell rich B-cell, MALT, and angiocentric variants (347–354). Primary hepatic follicular dendritic cell tumors have also been described (323,325).

Lymphoma may be misdiagnosed as carcinoma, chronic hepatitis, primary biliary cirrhosis, granulomatous infection, inflammatory pseudotumor, or even venous outflow obstruction (Budd-Chiari syndrome) because lymphomas may contain foci of extensive hemorrhagic necrosis. Pathologists should always consider the diagnosis of lymphoma in any liver biopsy with a lymphocytic infiltrate, paying close attention to the cytologic and architectural characteristics of the lymphoid infiltrate. The use of immunohistochemical stains for leukocyte common antigen, B- and T-cell markers, and CK aid in making the distinction from carcinoma (Table 25). In one review of 45 patients, 66% survived 2 years (347). Further follow-up data are needed. Treatment has included surgery ("curative" surgery to date has been associated with the best prognosis), chemotherapy, and radiotherapy. Immunocompromised patients and those with cirrhosis do quite poorly.

OTHER TUMORS

Heterotopias of adrenal, pancreatic, and splenic origin have been described (2,3,42). Pancreatic acini, found in the liver in 4% of autopsies within large and medium-sized portal tracts, demonstrated communication with bile duct lumina in one study (355). Islets were not found in this study. Functioning adrenal rest tumors appear to be quite rare, but they are well documented. The tumors considered in the differential diagnosis of adrenal heterotopia are metastatic adrenal and renal carcinomas, HCA and carcinoma, and other tumors with clear-cell features. *Plexiform neurofibromatosis*, *schwannoma*, and *malignant rhabdoid tumor* may now and then arise in the liver (249,346,356). The latter tumor should be distinguished from those with focal rhabdoid features, which have been described in HBL (87), cholangiocarcinoma, (273) and rhabdomyosarcoma.

METASTATIC TUMOR IN THE LIVER

Solid Tumors

Clinical Features

In the United States and many other countries, metastatic tumor accounts for about 98% of all hepatic malignancies and is found in nearly 4% of all liver biopsies (3,357). Forty percent of patients dying from cancer have hepatic metas-

TABLE 25. Conditions simulating leukemia and lymphoma in the liver[a]

Condition	Predominant distribution of infiltrate		Key diagnostic features
	Portal	Sinusoidal	
Usual acute/chronic hepatitis	+	±	Portal infiltrate often polymorphic; lack of uniformly atypical lymphocytes; lymphoid aggregates sometimes with germinal centers; rarely, ddx of low-grade lymphoma, CLL, and chronic hepatitis (usually chronic hepatitis C) is a problem; clinical features and immunophenotyping may help in these cases; sinusoidal beading may be prominent with HCV infection; lobular disarray uncommon with lymphoma/leukemia
EBV, CMV mononucleosis; toxoplasmosis	+	+	Lymphoid cells may be large and atypical; history and serologies essential for diagnosis
Hemophagocytic syndromes	±	+	Bland histiocytes with prominent erythrophagocytosis; associated conditions include infections (viral, bacterial, fungal, parasitic) in patients with primary/secondary immunodeficiency and T-cell lymphomas
Tropical splenomegaly	−	+	Sinusoidal beading of normal-appearing lymphocytes; history of malaria
Myeloid metaplasia (EMH)	±	+	Chronic myeloproliferative and myelophthisistic disorders; lack of cytologic atypia and presence of several cell lines against diagnosis of leukemia
Carcinoma	±	+	Small cell carcinoma—nuclear molding, stippled chromatin; IHC negative for LCA, often positive for NE markers, CK
			Poorly differentiated carcinoma—focal cohesive clusters; IHC negative for LCA, positive for CK

CK, cytokeratin; CLL, chronic lymphocytic leukemia; CMV, cytomegalovirus; ddx, differential diagnosis; EBV, Epstein-Barr virus; EMH, extramedullary hematopoiesis; HCV, hepatitis C virus; IHC, immunohistochemistry; LCA, leukocyte common antigen (CD45RB); NE, neuroendocrine.

tases. In the cirrhotic liver, however, primary hepatic malignancies (nearly always HCC) are more common than metastatic tumors, representing 77% and 23% of all hepatic malignancies, respectively (167). The sensitivity of ultrasonography and CT for detecting metastatic disease is about 85%, but it is considerably lower when lesions are few and smaller than 2 cm (1). Carcinomas of the lung, breast, colon, and pancreas account for the overwhelming majority of hepatic metastases in adults, whereas metastatic neuroblastoma, Wilms' tumor, and rhabdomyosarcoma are most common in the pediatric age group (3,87,314,357). In one pediatric study, 10% of cases submitted as primary hepatic tumors were misdiagnosed; these tumors frequently represented metastases (87).

Carcinomas of the pancreas, stomach, and lung are the tumors most likely to be found in adults in conjunction with hepatic metastases and an inapparent primary site. Clinical features are quite inconsistent; patients can often be asymptomatic. Infrequently, fulminant hepatic failure can take place; because of the diffuse replacement of the liver in these cases, radiographic studies may not show a space-occupying lesion (358). Obstructive jaundice, massive intraperitoneal hemorrhage, and features mimicking cirrhosis are other unusual manifestations (282). In general, patients with hepatic metastases die within 1 year, but notable exceptions include patients with metastatic neuroendocrine neoplasms and neuroblastoma and a select subgroup (approximately 5%) of patients with metastatic colon carcinoma. In the latter instance, 5-year survival rates of 25% to 39% have been reported after resection of hepatic metastases (359).

Pathologic Features

The tumor deposits are multiple in 90% to 95% of cases (3,357). They can be discrete or confluent, varying from less than 1 mm to many centimeters in diameter. Upon occasion, there may be diffuse replacement of the liver parenchyma such that nodules cannot be identified on gross inspection. The macroscopic appearance is quite variable depending on the cell type and the degree of associated hemorrhage and necrosis. Metastatic colon cancer usually forms large umbilicated nodules with extensive foci of necrosis and fibrosis; calcification is sometimes seen. Umbilication and calcification are uncommon findings in usual HCC but can be found in the fibrolamellar variant, EH, and cholangiocarcinoma. Prominent hemorrhage suggests choriocarcinoma, angiosarcoma, or thyroid carcinoma. Squamous cell carcinomas typically have a grumous necrotic center, whereas several other tumors (small-cell carcinoma, sarcoma, seminoma) often have the appearance of fish flesh. Metastatic carcinoma (generally from the breast) may result in a macroscopic aspect simulating hepar lobatum, stemming from the effects of chemotherapy-related tumor regression, parenchymal collapse, and scar contraction. Only rare residual tumor cells may be found (Fig. 19C) (263).

Metastases usually retain the histologic features found at the primary site, including the degree of stromal reaction (sparse with small-cell carcinoma; conspicuous with adenocarcinomas, particularly from the breast, pancreas, and stomach). Therefore, comparison of the histologic features of the liver tumor with those of any previous malignancy should be standard practice and helps confirm the metastatic nature of the lesion. The cells of small-cell carcinoma often appear larger than in the original transbronchial biopsy specimen, which is probably related to better cell preservation.

Intrasinusoidal growth is much more typical of poorly differentiated adenocarcinoma and small-cell carcinoma than of primary tumors; extensive vascular invasion may also be noted. Melanoma and other metastases may replace the hepatic cords and grow in a trabecular pattern complete with an endothelial lining. This replacing-type growth pattern should not be interpreted as origin from hepatocytes. In difficult cases immunohistochemistry testing is essential. In general, metastatic adenocarcinoma from the pancreas, extrahepatic biliary tree, and gastrointestinal tract cannot be distinguished from primary ICC. Invasion along portal tracts may be particularly deceptive and can even simulate high-grade bile duct dysplasia (Fig. 20E) (276,360). The problems of distinguishing metastatic neuroendocrine neoplasms (Figs. 15 and 17) and metastatic carcinomas from HCC and other primary hepatic tumors are covered earlier in this chapter (Tables 13, 14, 19, and 21).

Leukemia and Lymphoma

Clinical Features

Pathologists must always consider a diagnosis of lymphoma or leukemia in liver biopsy specimens (chance favors the prepared mind) whenever a mononuclear infiltrate is encountered. Even if a definitive diagnosis cannot be made, the clinician can be guided in the right direction, and additional material can be obtained for performance of flow cytometry, molecular analysis, or other studies. Familiarity with the varied clinical characteristics of these disorders helps us not to be caught off guard. Patients with hepatic lymphoma can be divided into four basic clinical patterns: (a) those with disseminated disease with incidental involvement found during staging procedures or at autopsy (most common) (361,362), (b) those with disseminated disease who show initial signs of fulminant hepatic failure simulating hepatitis (rare) (363), (c) those with hepatosplenic ($\gamma\delta$) T-cell lymphoma (rare) (364), and (d) those with primary hepatic lymphoma (rare; see preceding section) (347–354).

Liver involvement is present at diagnosis in about 5% to 10% and 15% to 40% of patients with Hodgkin's Lymphoma (HL) and NHL, respectively (361,362). Small lymphocytic and small cleaved B-cell lymphomas and T-cell lymphomas more frequently demonstrate hepatic infiltration compared with large B-cell lymphomas. Hepatic involvement without splenic infiltration is exceedingly rare in both HL and NHL.

Leukemias frequently involve the liver, but only rarely are they associated with hepatic dysfunction. Patients may from time to time present clinically with fulminant hepatic failure (363).

Pathologic Features

Large B-cell lymphoma typically produces one or more bulky white-tan masses, whereas small cleaved B-cell lymphoma usually demonstrates a diffuse pattern of miliary nodules. HL may be associated with either pattern. Leukemias characteristically cause organ enlargement, but only rarely, except in chronic lymphocytic leukemia (CLL), does one see discrete nodules. Diagnostic findings may be quite focal and missed on small biopsy specimens.

At the microscopic level, the pathologist must first distinguish the neoplastic hematolymphoid disorders from the much more common group of inflammatory liver diseases as well as from poorly differentiated and small-cell carcinomas (Table 25). A few small, irregular lymphocytes are often seen in the portal tracts in these disorders and should not be misconstrued as lymphoma; however, conspicuous uniform expansion of portal tracts by sheets of round or cleaved lymphocytes, typically with little interface hepatitis (piecemeal necrosis), suggests lymphoma. On the other hand, the presence of large lymphoid cells in a liver biopsy should always raise a red flag, even if they are surrounded by numerous bland-appearing lymphocytes (Fig. 26) (354).

A granulomatous component is not uncommon in both NHL and HL and should not be dismissed as infection, sarcoid or cholestatic disease. Immunohistochemical stains can be useful in distinguishing lymphoma from other malignancies and in immunophenotyping the tumor, as discussed in the chapter "Lymph Nodes." Important morphologic features of the more common leukemias, lymphomas, and related disorders, including the preferential distribution of the infiltrate, cytologic appearance, and use of ancillary techniques, are summarized in Table 26.

A definitive diagnosis of hepatic involvement by HL is made when portal-based atypical mononuclear cells with prominent nucleoli are found in the context of the usual polymorphous fibroinflammatory background in a patient in whom a diagnosis has first been established on lymph node biopsy. Diagnostic Reed-Sternberg cells are only rarely encountered (361). Nonspecific portal or lobular inflammatory infiltrates are seen in about one-third of biopsies and do not imply involvement by HL (365). A cholestatic syndrome may result from extensive hepatic replacement, intrahepatic bile duct damage and profound loss (vanishing bile duct syndrome) with ductule proliferation, even in the absence of direct hepatic involvement or extrahepatic biliary obstruction (314,366). Care should be taken not to misdiagnose HL as abscess, IMT, or follicular dendritic cell tumor (257,320,323,325,367).

B-cell lymphomas typically cause predominant portal tract expansion with relatively little sinusoidal permeation. Large-cell lymphomas, however, may occasionally cause prominent sinusoidal infiltration (361). Hepatosplenic ($\gamma\delta$) T-cell lymphoma shows striking evidence of sinusoidal involvement by medium-sized lymphocytes, with condensed nuclear chromatin, inconspicuous nucleoli, and a rim of eosinophilic cytoplasm that may mimic hairy cell leukemia (364). The immunophenotype (CD3 positive, CD4 and CD8 negative), receptor phenotype ($\gamma\delta$ T-cell), and cytogenetic profile (often isochromosome 7q, trisomy 8) aid in the differential diagnosis. Other peripheral T-cell lymphomas may also have a prominent sinusoidal component. At times, the sinusoidal component can be easily overlooked, since it may be quite focal, particularly when it is accompanied by reactive hepatocellular changes.

Lymphomatous infiltrates often appear "nodular," forming compact aggregates in patients with both diffuse and follicular disease. Only rarely, however, are true neoplastic follicles seen in the liver in patients with follicular center-cell lymphomas. Since morphologic diversity takes place in patients with NHL, the liver may display only a small cleaved cell infiltrate, whereas a diagnosis of the large-cell or mixed small- and large-cell type may have been made previously at another site. A monotonous or polymorphic lymphoid infiltrate may be found in posttransplantation lymphoproliferative disorders; it involves both portal tracts and sinusoids (340,368). An acute Epstein-Barr viral syndrome may also affect the liver, representing part of the wide clinicopathologic spectrum of Epstein-Barr virus–related disease in transplant patients (369).

The liver may be involved in *Langerhans cell histiocytosis (histiocytosis X)*, which forms portal or parenchymal

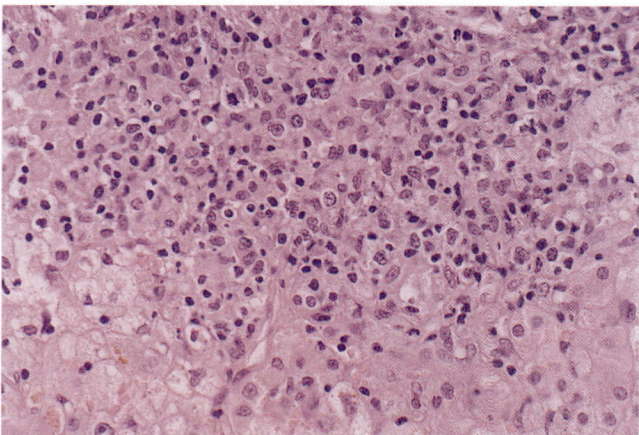

FIG. 26. Large-cell lymphoma involving the portal tract in a patient with "cholestatic hepatitis." Modest splenomegaly and a 40-pound weight loss, but no lymphadenopathy, were associated clinical features. The diagnostic malignant lymphoid cells affected only a minority of portal tracts and were often present only focally in involved areas. Adjacent hepatocytes demonstrate cholestatic features. Immunohistochemical stains may be helpful in determining the lymphoma immunophenotype (B cell in this case). Pathologists must always consider a diagnosis of malignancy when a patient shows signs of "hepatitis." Careful assessment of focal findings, with particular attention to cytologic detail, may prove lifesaving in patients with hematolymphoid malignancy.

TABLE 26. Histopathologic aspects of hepatic involvement by leukemia and lymphoma[a]

Neoplastic process	Predominant distribution of infiltrate		Key diagnostic features
	Portal	Sinusoidal	
Lymphoma			
NHL			
Most B-cell types	+	±	Most B-cell lymphomas preferentially involve portal tracts. Involvement by SL, MC and MZ lymphomas may occasionally be difficult to distinguish from chronic hepatitis, but the lymphomas are monotonous and usually demonstrate a greater degree of rounded portal tract expansion. Large-cell and high-grade lesions often form confluent masses. May appear granulomatoid or be associated with well-formed granulomas. IHC for CD20 may be useful.
Peripheral T-cell types	±	+	Typically preferential sinusoidal involvement. Variation in lymphocyte size and shape. Angiocentric lymphoma (T-cell or NK) may be found. May be granulomatoid or associated with well-formed granulomas. IHC for CD3, CD45RO (UCHL-1) may be useful.
PTLD	+	+	Polymorphous plasmacytoid infiltrate or monomorphous large-cell infiltrate; may respond to tapering of immunosuppression. Nearly always B-cell lineage.
Hodgkin's lymphoma	+	−	R-S variants in appropriate background; evidence of HL at other sites and immunoreactivity for CD15, CD30 helpful; may be granulomatoid or associated with well-formed granulomas; possible vanishing bile duct syndrome
MH/THL	±	+	Large cells with multilobed nuclei and ample eosinophilic cytoplasm; erythrophagocytosis; CD68, MAC 387 positive; exclude T- and B-cell lymphomas
Leukemia			
AML, CML	±	+	AML—blasts (IHC for myeloperoxidase, neutrophil elastase, etc. or Leder stain helpful); CML—spectrum of myeloid precursors
ALL, CLL	+	±	ALL—blasts; CLL—monomorphic small-cell lymphoid population, dense chromatin
Hairy cell	+	+	Abundant clear cytoplasm often separates round or reniform nuclei, causing "beads on a string" sinusoidal pattern. Nucleoli typically inconspicuous. Peliosis-like spaces (angiomatoids) often present; pancytopenia common.
ATL	±	+	Spectrum of neoplastic lymphocytes; pleomorphic/polylobated circulating cells.
LLGL	±	±	Small, round lymphocytes often with abundant pale cytoplasm. May morphologically resemble hairy cell leukemia or other disorders of small lymphocytes. NK and T-cell subtypes. Neutropenia and rheumatoid arthritis often present. Granular lymphocyte on peripheral blood smear.
Langerhans' cell histiocytosis (HX)	+	±	S-100 and CD1a-positive Langerhans cells may damage bile ducts, resulting in sclerosing cholangitis. Aggregates or diffuse infiltration of sinusoids may be seen. Cirrhosis may result and necessitate liver transplantation.
Generalized mastocytosis	+	+	Normal liver contains only a few (~4/mm^2) mast cells utilizing IHC for tryptase, preferentially in portal tracts. In GM the subtle presence of round or spindled, degranulated mast cells is easily overlooked. Leder stain or tryptase IHC is often essential for diagnosis. Obliterative portal venopathy, venoocclusive disease, NRH, and cirrhosis are all reported.

ALL, acute lymphoblastic leukemia; AML, acute myeloid leukemia; ATL, acute T-cell leukemia/lymphoma; CLL, chronic lymphocytic leukemia; CML. chronic myeloid leukemia; GM, generalized mastocytosis; HL, Hodgkin's lymphoma (disease); HX, histiocytosis X; IHC, immunohistochemistry; LLGL, leukemia of large granular lymphocytes; MC, mantle cell; MH/THL, malignant histiocytosis/true histiocytic lymphoma; MZ, marginal zone; NHL, non-Hodgkin's lymphoma; NK, natural killer cell; NRH, nodular regenerative hyperplasia; PTLD, posttransplant lymphoproliferative disorder; R-S, Reed-Sternberg cell; SL, small lymphocytic.

[a] Given the relatively small size of most liver biopsies, occasionally a diagnosis of "suspicious" rather than lymphoma is rendered. Additional tissue from extrahepatic sites may be necessary to confirm the diagnosis. Additionally, even when diagnostic of lymphoma/leukemia, distinguishing among the various categories may not be possible solely with routine histology and immunohistochemical stains performed in paraffin-embedded tissue. Fresh tissue may be required for flow cytometry, frozen section immunohistochemistry, or molecular studies for T- and B-cell gene rearrangements.

Data are primarily from references 361, 362, 364, 368, 370, 372, 373, 376, 377.

nodules or diffusely infiltrates the sinusoids (370). Langerhans cell histiocytosis may result in sclerosing cholangitis, leading to biliary cirrhosis. This syndrome accounts for 15% to 20% of all sclerosing cholangitis in children and preferentially, but not exclusively, affects the intrahepatic ducts. Langerhans cells are often quite difficult to identify in patients with advanced liver disease. Immunohistochemical staining for CD1a and S-100 protein may aid in their detection.

Generalized mastocytosis is associated with hepatic involvement, hepatomegaly, and portal hypertension (typically noncirrhotic) in about 40% to 60%, 25% to 75%, and 10% of cases, respectively (371,372). Portal tracts are reported to be most prominently affected, but sinusoidal spread is also common. Definitive identification of mast cells may be quite difficult in hematoxylin and eosin–stained sections; immunohistochemical staining for tryptase may be invaluable (control numbers of mast cells in normal and chronic liver diseases have been published) (Table 26) (373). Portal fibrosis is seen in the majority of cases; occasionally, bridging fibrosis or even cirrhosis can be found. Obliterative portal venopathy, veno-occlusive disease, and NRH have all been described and are likely responsible for cases of noncirrhotic portal hypertension. Extramedulary hematopoiesis is found in nearly 50% of cases. Generalized mastocytosis can simulate chronic cholestatic syndromes in clinical features (374). *Multiple myeloma* may involve portal tracts and sinusoids or form large deposits (375).

Patients with myeloid leukemia (AML,CML) or those who are in a leukemic phase of lymphoma typically have infiltrates with a principally sinusoidal component, while lymphoid leukemias (ALL,CLL) predominate in the portal tracts. In hairy cell leukemia, both portal and sinusoidal regions are involved in about 90% of cases (376). Sinusoidal "beading" is characteristic; small cavities lined by hairy cells and containing these cells and blood (angiomatoids, pseudosinuses, peliosis-like spaces) are found in 16% to 64% of cases (Fig. 27). The tumor cells usually express routine B-cell markers (CD20) in paraffin-embedded material; definitive characterization frequently requires additional studies, including flow cytometry (CD11c, CD25, CD103 positive) and cytochemistry (tartrate-resistant, acid phosphatase positive).

Epithelioid granulomas of uncertain origin have been detected in 12% to 25%, 2% to 10%, 20%, and 20% to 32% of cases of HL, NHL, cutaneous T-cell lymphoma, and hairy cell leukemia (361,377,378), respectively. The presence of granulomas alone does not imply involvement by the neoplastic process and, in the case of HL, is considered a favorable prognostic feature (361).

REFERENCES

Introduction

1. Saini S. Imaging of the hepatobiliary tract. *N Engl J Med* 1997;336:1889–1894.
2. Ishak KG, Anthony PP, Sobin LH. *Histological typing of tumors of the liver*, 2nd ed. Berlin: Springer-Verlag, 1994.
3. Craig JR, Peters RL, Edmondson HA. Tumors of the liver and intrahepatic bile ducts. In: Hartmann WH, Sobin LH, editors, *Atlas of tumor pathology*, 2nd series, fascicle 26. Washington, D.C.: Armed Forces Institute of Pathology, 1989.
4. International Working Party. Terminology of nodular hepatocellular lesions. *Hepatology* 1995;22:983–993.
5. Weinberg AG, Finegold MJ. Primary hepatic tumors in childhood. In: Finegold M, ed. *Pathology of neoplasia in children and adolescents*. Philadelphia: WB Saunders, 1986:333–372. (Bennington JL, ed. Major problems in pathology, vol. 18.)
6. Dehner LP. Hepatic tumors in the pediatric age group: a distinctive clinicopathologic spectrum. In: Rosenberg HS, Rolande RP, eds. *Perspectives in pediatric pathology*, vol. 4. Chicago: Year Book Medical Publishers, 1978:217–268.

Specimen Handling

6a. Stocker JT. An approach to handling pediatric liver tumors. *Am J Surg Pathol* 1998;109[Suppl 1]:S67–72.

Intraoperative Consultation

7. Ferrell LD, Roberts JP. Liver. In: Intraoperative consultations in surgical pathology. Ranchod M, ed. *Pathology: State of the art reviews* 1996;3:367–378.

The Utility of Liver Biopsy for Tumor Diagnosis

8. Tao L-C. Liver and pancreas. In: Bibbo M, ed. *Comprehensive cytopathology*, 2nd ed. Philadelphia: WB Saunders, 1997:827–846.
9. Bennett WF, Bova JG. Review of hepatic imaging and a problem-oriented approach to liver masses. *Hepatology* 1990;12:761–775.
10. Silverman JF, Geisinger KR. Liver. In: *Fine needle aspiration cytology of the thorax and abdomen*. New York: Churchill Livingstone, 1996;89–134.
11. Ljung BM, Ferrell LD. Fine needle aspiration biopsy of the liver: diagnostic problems. In: Ljung BM, ed. Fine-needle aspiration biopsy. *Pathology: State of the art reviews* 1994;3:161–184.

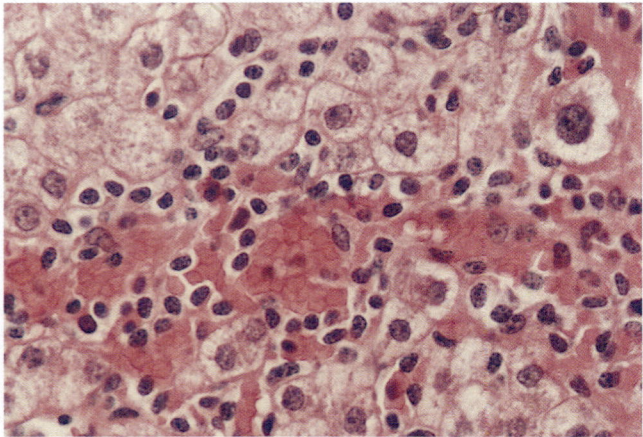

FIG. 27. Hairy cell leukemia (HCL), angiomatoid lesion. The sinusoids are congested and focally lined by round to slightly indented lymphoid cells. These foci are called angiomatoids (or pseudosinuses) and occur in 16% to 64% of liver biopsies from patients with HCL. Note the "beading" pattern and separation of the tumor cells in the adjacent sinusoids. A definitive diagnosis of HCL requires ancillary studies performed on fresh tissue (TRAP stain, flow cytometry for cell-surface markers).

12. Pisharodi LR, Lavoie R, Bedrossian CWM. Differential diagnostic dilemmas in malignant fine-needle aspirates of liver: a practical approach to final diagnosis. *Diagn Cytopathol* 1995;12:364–371.
13. Silverman JF, Gurley M, Holbrook T, Joshi VV. Pediatric fine-needle aspiration biopsy. *Am J Clin Pathol* 1991;95:653–659.
14. Us-Krasovec M, Pohar-Marinsek Z, Golough R, Jereb B, Ferlan-Marolt V, Cerar A. Hepatoblastoma in fine needle aspirates. *Acta Cytol* 1996;40:450–456.
15. Drinkovic I, Brkljacic B. Two cases of lethal complications following ultrasound-guided percutaneous fine-needle biopsy of the liver. *Cardiovasc Intervent Radiol* 1996;19:360–363.
16. Houn H-Y, Sanders MM, Walker EM, Pappas AA. Fine needle aspiration in the diagnosis of liver neoplasms: a review. *Ann Clin Lab Sci* 1991;21:2–11.
17. Isobe H, Imari Y, Sakai H, Sakamoto S, Nawata H. Subcutaneous seeding of hepatocellular carcinoma following fine-needle aspiration biopsy. *J Clin Gastroenterol* 1993;17:350–352.
18. Dusenbery D, Ferris JV, Thaete FL, Carr BI. Percutaneous ultrasound-guided needle biopsy of hepatic mass lesions using a cytohistologic approach: comparison of two needle types. *Am J Clin Pathol* 1995;104:583–587.
19. Boyce HW. Laparoscopy. In: Schiff L, Schiff ER. *Diseases of the liver*, 7th ed. Philadelphia: JB Lippincott, 1993:226–239.
20. Axe SR, Erozan YS, Ermatinger SV. Fine-needle aspiration of the liver: a comparison of smear and rinse preparations in the detection of cancer. *Am J Clin Pathol* 1986;86:281–285.
21. Sangalli G, Livraghi T, Giordano F. Fine needle biopsy of hepatocellular carcinoma: improvement in diagnosis by microhistology. *Gastroenterology* 1989;96:524–526.
22. Sole M, Calvet X, Cuberes T, et al. Value and limitations of cytologic criteria for the diagnosis of hepatocellular carcinoma by fine needle aspiration biopsy. *Acta Cytol* 1993;37:309–316.
23. Bret PM, Labadie M, Bretaqualle M, et al. Hepatocellular carcinoma: diagnosis by fine needle biopsy. *Gastrointest Radiol* 1989;13:253–255.
24. Borzio M, Borzio F, Macchi R, et al. The evaluation of fine-needle procedures for the diagnosis of focal lesions in cirrhosis. *J Hepatol* 1994;20:117–121.
25. Kung ITM, Chan S-K, Fung K-H. Fine-needle aspiration in hepatocellular carcinoma: combined cytologic and histologic approach. *Cancer* 1991;67:673–680.
26. Cohen MB, Haber MM, Holly EA, et al. Cytologic criteria to distinguish hepatocellular carcinoma from nonneoplastic liver. *Am J Clin Pathol* 1991;95:125–130.
27. Bottles K, Cohen MB, Holly EA, et al. A step-wise regression analysis of hepatocellular carcinoma: an aspiration biopsy study. *Cancer* 1988;62:558–563.
28. Terriff BA, Gibney RG, Scudamore CH. Fatality from fine-needle aspiration biopsy of a hepatic hemangioma. *AJR* 1990;154:203–204.

Histologic Findings Adjacent to Liver Tumors

29. Gerber MA, Thung SN, Bodenheimer HL, et al. Characteristic histologic triad in liver adjacent to metastatic neoplasm. *Liver* 1986;6:85–88.
30. Saul SH, Titelbaum DS, Gansler TS, et al. The fibrolamellar variant of hepatocellular carcinoma: its association with focal nodular hyperplasia. *Cancer* 1987;60:3049–3055.
31. Saxena R, Humphreys S, Williams R, Portmann B. Nodular hyperplasia surrounding fibrolamellar carcinoma: a zone of arterialized liver parenchyma. *Histopathology* 1994;25:275–278.

Cystic Masses

32. Witzleben CL. Cystic diseases of the liver. In: Zakim D, Boyer TD, eds. *Hepatology: a textbook of liver disease*, 3rd ed. Philadelphia: WB Saunders, 1996:1630–1649.
33. Frey CF, Zhu Y, Suzuki M, Isaji S. Liver abscess. *Surg Clin North Am* 1989;69:259–271.
34. Bryan RT, Michelson MK. Parasitic infections of the liver and biliary tree. In: Surawicz C, Owen RL, eds. *Gastrointestinal and hepatic infections*. Philadelphia: WB Saunders, 1995;405–454.
35. Goldman IS, Brandborg LL. Parasitic diseases of the liver. In: Zakim D, Boyer TD, eds. *Hepatology: a textbook of liver disease*, 3rd ed. Philadelphia: WB Saunders, 1996:1206–1231.
36. De Cock KM, Reynolds TB. Amebic and pyogenic liver abscess. In: Schiff L, Schiff ER, eds. *Diseases of the liver*, 7th ed. Philadelphia: JB Lippincott, 1993:1320–1337.
37. Seeto R, Rockey DC. Pyogenic liver abscess: changes in etiology, management, and outcome. *Medicine* 1996;75:99–113.
38. Canto MIF, Diel AM. Bacterial infections of the liver and biliary system. In: Surawicz C, Owen RL, eds. *Gastrointestinal and hepatic infections*. Philadelphia: WB Saunders, 1995:355–389.
38a. Vadillo M, Corbella X, Pac V, Fernandez-Viladrich P, Pujol R. Multiple liver abscesses due to *Yersinia enterocolitica* discloses primary hemochromatosis: three case reports and review. *Clin Infect Dis* 1994;18:938–941.
39. Ammann RW, Eckert J. Cestodes: Echinococcis. *Gastroenterol Clin North Am* 1996;25:655–689.
40. Spark AK, Connor DH, Neafie RC. Echinococcis. In: Binford CH, Conner DH, eds. *Pathology of tropical and extraordinary diseases*. Washington, D.C.: Armed Forces Institute of Pathology, 1976: 530–533.
41. Khuroo MS, Wani NA, Javid G, et al. Percutaneous drainage compared with surgery for hepatic hydatid cysts. *N Engl J Med* 1997; 337:881–887.
42. Ishak KG, Sharp HL. Developmental abnormality and liver disease in childhood. In: MacSween RNM, Anthony PP, Scheuer PJ, eds. *Pathology of the liver*, 3rd ed. Edinburgh: Churchill Livingstone, 1994;83–122.
43. Karhunen PJ, Penttilä A, Liesto K, et al. Benign bile duct tumors, nonparasitic liver cysts and liver damage in males. *J Hepatol* 1986; 2:89–99.
44. Redston MS, Wanless IR. The hepatic von Meyenburg complex with hepatic and renal cysts. *Mod Pathol* 1996;9:233–237.
45. Desmet VJ. Congenital diseases of intrahepatic bile ducts: variations on the theme "ductal plate malformation." *Hepatology* 1992;16: 1069–1083.
46. Brock JS, Pachter HL, Schreiber J, Hofstetter SR. Surgical diseases of the falciform ligament. *Am J Gastroenterol* 1992;67:757–758.
47. Terada T, Nakanuma Y, Kono N, Ueda K, Kadoya M, Matsui O. Ciliated hepatic foregut cyst: a mucus histochemical, immunohistochemical, and ultrastructural study in three cases in comparison with normal bronchi and intrahepatic bile ducts. *Am J Surg Pathol* 1990;14:356–363.
48. Hornstein A, Batts KP, Linz LJ, Chang CD, Galvanek EG, Bardawil RG. Fine-needle aspiration of ciliated hepatic foregut cysts: a report of three cases. *Acta Cytol* 1996;40:576–580.
49. Banbury J, Conlon KC, Ghossein R, Brennan MF. Primary squamous cell carcinoma within a solitary nonparasitic hepatic cyst. *J Surg Oncol* 1994;57:210–212.
50. Bloustein PA. Association of carcinoma with congenital cystic conditions of the liver and bile ducts. *Am J Gastroenterol* 1977;67: 40–46.
51. Azizah N, Paradinas FJ. Cholangiocarcinoma co-existing with developmental liver cysts: a distinct entity different from liver cystadenocarcinoma. *Histopathology* 1980;4:391–400.
52. D'Agata IDA, Jonas M, Perez-Atayde AR, Guay-Woodford LM. Combined cystic disease of the liver and kidney. *Semin Liver Dis* 1994;14:215–228.
53. Cobben JM, Breuning MH, Schoots C, et al. Congenital hepatic fibrosis in autosomal-dominant polycystic kidney disease. *Kidney Int* 1990;38:880–885.
54. Pirson Y, Lannoy N, Peters D, et al. Isolated polycystic liver disease as a distinct genetic disease, unlinked to polycystic kidney disease 1 and polycystic kidney disease 2. *Hepatology* 1996;23:249–252.
55. Kwok MK, Lewin KJ. Massive hepatomegaly in adult polycystic liver disease. *Am J Surg Pathol* 1988;12:321–324.
56. McCormick SE, Sjogren MH, Goodman ZD. Diagnostic problem in clinical hepatology: a 22-year-old man with a liver mass and markedly elevated serum alpha feto-protein. *Semin Liver Dis* 1994;14:395–403.
57. Gabow PA, Johnson AM, Kaehny WD, et al. Risk factors for the development of hepatic cysts in autosomal dominant polycystic kidney disease. *Hepatology* 1990;11:1033–1037.
58. Grunfeld J-P, Albouze G, Jungers P, et al. Liver changes and complications in adult polycystic kidney disease. *Adv Nephrol* 1985;14:1–20.
59. Pliskin A, Cualing H, Stenger RJ. Primary squamous cell carcinoma originating in congenital cysts of the liver. *Arch Pathol Lab Med* 1992;116:105–107.
60. Tepetes K, Selby R, Webb M, et al. Orthotopic transplantation for benign hepatic neoplasms. *Arch Surg* 1995;130:153–156.

61. Fozard JBJ, Wyatt JI, Hall RI. Epithelial dysplasia in Caroli's disease. *Gut* 1989;30:1150–1153.
62. Dayton MT, Longmire WP, Tompkins RK. Caroli's disease: a premalignant condition? *Am J Surg* 1983;145:41–48.
63. Darioca PJ, Tuthill R, Reed RJ. Cholangiocarcinoma arising in congenital hepatic fibrosis. *Arch Pathol* 1975;99:592–595.
64. Nakanuma Y, Sasaki M, Terada T, Harada K. Intrahepatic peribiliary glands of humans. II. Pathological spectrum. *J Gastroenterol Hepatol* 1994;9:80–86.
65. Okuda K, Sugita S, Tsukada E, et al. Pancreatic pseudocyst in the left hepatic lobe: a report of two cases. *Hepatology* 1991;13:359–363.
66. Seidman JD, Yale-Loehr AJ, Beaver B, Sun C-CJ. Alimentary duplication presenting as an hepatic cyst in a neonate. *Am J Surg Pathol* 1991;15:695–698.
67. Verbeke C, Harle M, Sturm J. Cystic endometriosis of the upper abdominal organs: report on three cases and review of the literature. *Pathol Res Pract* 1996;192:300–304.
68. Wheeler DA, Edmundson HA. Cystadenoma with mesenchymal stroma (CMS) in the liver and bile ducts: a clinicopathologic study of 17 cases, 4 with malignant change. *Cancer* 1985;56:1434–1445.
69. Devaney K, Goodman ZD, Ishak KG. Hepatobiliary cystadenoma and cystadenocarcinoma: a light microscopic and immunohistochemical study of 70 patients. *Am J Surg Pathol* 1994;18:1078–1091.
70. Longnecker DS, Terhune PG. The case for parallel classification of biliary tract and pancreatic neoplasms. *Mod Pathol* 1996;9:828–837.
71. Buetow PC, Buck JL, Pantongrag-Brown L, et al. Biliary cystadenoma and cystadenocarcinoma: clinical-imaging-pathologic correlation with emphasis on the importance of ovarian stroma. *Radiology* 1995;196:805–810.
72. Pinto MM, Kaye AD. Fine needle aspiration of cystic liver lesions: cytologic examination and carcinoembryonic antigen assay of cyst contents. *Acta Cytol* 1989;33:852–856.
73. Horsmans Y, Laka A, Van Beers BE, Descamps C, Gigot J-F, Geubel AP. Hepatobiliary cystadenocarcinoma without ovarian stroma and normal CA 19-9 levels: unusually prolonged evolution. *Dig Dis Sci* 1997;42:1406–1408.
74. Subramony C, Herrera GA, Turbat-Herrera EA. Hepatobiliary cystadenoma: a study of five cases with reference to histogenesis. *Arch Pathol Lab Med* 1993;117:1036–1042.
75. Kawarda Y, Taoka H, Mizumoto R. A report of cystic bile duct carcinoma of the liver and proposal of a new classification. *Gastroenterol Jpn* 1991;26:80–89.
76. Unger PD, Thung SN, Kaneko M. Pseudosarcomatous cystadenocarcinoma of the liver. *Hum Pathol* 1987;18:521–523.
77. Tomimatsu M, Okuda H, Saito A, et al. A case of biliary cystadenocarcinoma with morphologic and histochemical features of hepatocytes. *Cancer* 1989;64:1323–1328.
78. Wolf HK, Garcia JA, Bossen EH. Oncocytic differentiation in intrahepatic biliary cystadenocarcinoma. *Mod Pathol* 1992;5:665–668.
79. Lazaridis KN, Kamath PS. Image of the month. *Gastroenterology* 1997;113:366–367.
80. George DH, Murphy F, Michalski R, Ulmer BG. Serous cystadenocarcinoma of the pancreas: a new entity? *Am J Surg Pathol* 1989;13:61–66.
81. Kim YII, Kim ST, Lee GK, Choi BI. Papillary cystic tumor of the liver: a case with ultrastructural observation. *Cancer* 1990;65:2740–2746.
82. Morinaga S, Nishiya H, Inafuku T. Yolk sac tumor combined with hepatocellular carcinoma. *Arch Pathol Lab Med* 1996;120:687–690.
83. Conrad RJ, Gribbin D, Walker NI, Ong TH. Combined cystic teratoma and hepatoblastoma of the liver: probable divergent differentiation of an uncommitted hepatic precursor cell. *Cancer* 1993;72:2910–2913.
84. Kim SN, Chi JG, Kim YW, et al. Neonatal choriocarcinoma of liver. *Pediatric Pathol* 1993;13:723–730.
85. Lack EE, Neave C, Vawter GF. Hepatoblastoma: a clinical and pathologic study of 54 cases. *Am J Surg Pathol* 1982;6:693–705.
86. Manivel C, Wick MR, Abenoza P, Dehner LP. Teratoid hepatoblastoma: the nosologic dilemma of solid embryonic neoplasms of childhood. *Cancer* 1986;57:2168–2174.
87. Finegold MJ. Tumors of the liver. *Semin Liver Dis* 1994;14:270–281.
88. Stocker JT, Ishak KG. Mesenchymal hamartoma of the liver: report of 30 cases and review of the literature. *Pediatr Pathol* 1983;1:245–267.
89. Drachenberg CB, Papadimitriou JC, Rivero MA, Wood C. Adult mesenchymal hamartoma of the liver: report of a case with light microscopic, FNA cytology, immunohistochemistry, and ultrastructural studies and review of the literature. *Mod Pathol* 1991;4:392–395.
90. Otal TM, Hendricks JB, Pharis P, Donnelly WH. Mesenchymal hamartoma of the liver: DNA flow cytometric analysis of eight cases. *Cancer* 1994;74:1237–1242.
91. Lennington WJ, Page DL, Gray GF. Mesenchymal hamartoma of liver: a regional ischemic lesion of a sequestered lobe. *Am J Dis Child* 1993;147:193–196.
92. Lauwers GY, Grant LD, Donnelly WH, et al. Hepatic undifferentiated (embryonal) sarcoma arising in a mesenchymal hamartoma. *Am J Surg Pathol* 1997;21:1248–1254.
93. Manivel JC, Pettinato G, d'Amore ESG. Mesenchymal hamartoma of the liver: immunohistochemical and ultrastructural study of 8 cases. *Lab Invest* 1991;64:93A.

Benign and Borderline Hepatocellular Tumors

94. Lory J, Schweizer W, Blumgart LH, Zimmerman A. The pathology of the atrophy/hypertrophy complex of the liver: a light microscopic and immunohistochemical study. *Histol Histopathol* 1994;9:541–554.
94a. Rooks J, Ory HW, Ishak KG. Epidemiology of hepatocellular adenoma: the role of contraceptive steroids. *JAMA* 1979;242:644–648.
95. Christopherson WM, Mays ET, Barrows GH. Liver tumors in young women: a clinical pathologic study of 201 cases in the Louisville registry. In: Fenoglio C, Wolf M, eds. *Progress in surgical pathology*, vol 2. New York: Masson Publishers, 1980:187–205.
96. Ishak KG. Hepatic neoplasms associated with contraceptive and anabolic steroids. In: Lingerman CH, ed. *Carcinogenic hormones: Recent results in cancer research*. New York: Springer-Verlag, 1979:73–128.
97. Edmundson HA, Reynolds TS, Henderson B, Benton B. Liver cell adenoma associated with use of oral contraceptives. *N Engl J Med* 1976;294:470–472.
98. Cherqui D, Rahmouni A, Charlotte F, et al. Management of focal nodular hyperplasia and hepatocellular adenoma in young women: a series of 41 patients with clinical, radiological, and pathological correlations. *Hepatology* 1995;22:1674–1681.
99. Ishak KG, Zimmerman HJ. Hepatotoxic effects of the anabolic/androgenic steroids. *Semin Liver Dis* 1987;7:230–236.
100. Soe KL, Soe M, Gluud C. Liver pathology associated with the use of anabolic-androgenic steroids. *Liver* 1992;12:73–79.
101. Grange JD, Guechot J, Legendre C, et al. Liver adenoma and focal nodular hyperplasia in a man with high endogenous sex steroids. *Gastroenterology* 1987;93:1409–1413.
102. Deugnier Y, Yurlin B. Other causes of hepatocellular carcinoma. In: Okuda K, Tabor E, eds. *Liver cancer*. New York: Churchill Livingstone, 1997:97–110.
103. Bianchi L. Glycogen storage disease I and hepatocellular tumors. *Eur J Pediatr* 1993;152[Suppl]:S63–70.
104. Resnick MB, Kozakewich HPW, Perez-Atayde AR. Hepatic adenoma in the pediatric age group: clinicopathologic observations and assessment of cell proliferative activity. *Am J Surg Pathol* 1995;19:1181–1190.
105. Bala S, Wunsch PH, Ballhausen WG. Childhood hepatocellular adenoma in familial adenomatous polyposis: mutations in adenomatous polyposis gene and p53. *Gastroenterology* 1997;112:919–922.
106. Reddy KR, Schiff ER. Approach to a liver mass. *Semin Liver Dis* 1993;13:423–435.
107. Nagorney DM. Benign hepatic tumors: focal nodular hyperplasia and hepatocellular adenoma. *World J Surg* 1995;19:13–18.
108. Jenkins RL, Johnson LB, Lewis WD. Surgical approach to benign liver tumors. *Semin Liver Dis* 1994;14:178–189.
109. Cosme A, Horcajada JP, Vidaur F, Ojeda E, Torrado J, Arenas JI. Systemic AA amyloidosis induced by oral contraceptive-associated hepatocellular adenoma: a 13-year follow-up. *Liver* 1995;15:164–167.

110. Khoo US, Nicholls JM, JSK Lee, Saing H, NG IOL. Cholestatic liver cell adenoma in a child with hirsutism and elevated levels of cortisol and ACTH. *Histopathology* 1994;25:586–588.
111. Ferrell LD. Hepatocellular carcinoma arising in a focus of multilobular adenoma: a case report. *Am J Surg Pathol* 1993;17:525–529.
112. Goodman ZD, Mikel UV, Lubbers PR, et al. Kupffer cells in hepatocellular adenomas. *Am J Surg Pathol* 1987;11:191–196.
113. Scott FR, El-Refaie A, More L, Scheuer PJ, Dhillon AP. Hepatocellular carcinoma arising in an adenoma: value of QBend 10 immunostaining in diagnosis of hepatocellular carcinoma. *Histopathology* 1996;28:472–474.
114. Heffelfinger S, Irani DR, Finegold MJ. "Alcoholic hepatitis" in a hepatic adenoma. *Hum Pathol* 1987;18:751–754.
115. Ojanguren I, Ariza A, Castella EM, Fernandez-Vasalo A, Mate JL, Navas-Palacios JJ. p53 immunoreactivity in hepatocellular adenoma, focal nodular hyperplasia, cirrhosis and hepatocellular carcinoma. *Histopathology* 1995;26:63–68.
116. Salisbury JR, Portmann BC. Oncocytic liver cell adenoma. *Histopathology* 1987;11:533–539.
117. Galassi A, Pasquinelli G, Guerini A, Martinelli G, Venza E. Benign myxoid hepatocellular tumor. *Liver* 1995;15:233–235.
118. Flejou J-F, Barge J, Menu Y, et al. Liver adenomatosis: an entity distinct from liver adenoma? *Gastroenterology* 1985;89:1132–1138.
119. Sadowski DC, Lee SS, Wanless IR, Kelly JK, Heathcote EJ. Progressive type of focal nodular hyperplasia characterized by multiple tumors and recurrence. *Hepatology* 1995;21:970–975.
120. Edmondson HA, Steiner PE. Primary carcinoma of the liver: a study of 100 cases among 48,900 necropsies. *Cancer* 1954;7:462–503.
121. Goodman ZD, Ishak K. Hepatocellular carcinoma in women: probable lack of etiologic association with oral contraceptive steroids. *Hepatology* 1982;2:440–444.
122. Lack EE, Neave C, Vanter GF. Hepatocellular carcinoma: review of 32 cases in childhood and adolescence. *Cancer* 1983;52:1510–1515.
123. Gordon SC, Reddy KR, Livingstone AS, et al. Resolution of a contraceptive steroid induced hepatic adenoma with subsequent evolution into hepatocellular carcinoma. *Ann Intern Med* 1986;105:547–549.
124. Janes CH, McGill DB, Ludwig J, Krom AF. Liver cell adenoma at age of 3 years and transplantation 19 years later after development of carcinoma: a case report. *Hepatology* 1993;17:583–585.
125. Foster JH, Berman MM. The malignant transformation of liver cell adenomas. *Arch Surg* 1994;129:712–717.
126. Wanless IR, Mawdsley C, Adams R. The pathogenesis of focal nodular hyperplasia of the liver. *Hepatology* 1985;5:1194–1200.
127. Raymond D, Plaschkes J, Luthy AR, Leibundgut K, Hirt A, Wagner H-P. Focal nodular hyperplasia of the liver in children: review of follow-up and outcome. *J Pediatr Surg* 1995;30:1590–1592.
128. Takamura M, Mugishima H, Oowada M, Harada K, Uchida T. Type Ia glycogen storage disease with focal nodular hyperplasia in siblings. *Acta Pediatr Jpn* 1995;37:510–513.
129. Wanless IR, Albrecht S, Bilbao J, et al. Multiple focal nodular hyperplasia of the liver associated with vascular malformations of various organs and neoplasia of the brain: a new syndrome. *Mod Pathol* 1989;2:456–462.
130. Ndimbie OK, Goodman ZD, Chase RL, et al. Hemangiomas with localized nodular proliferation of the liver: a suggestion on the pathogenesis of focal nodular hyperplasia. *Am J Surg Pathol* 1990;14:142–150.
131. Haber M, Reuben A, Burell M, Oliverio P, Salem RR, West AB. Multiple focal nodular hyperplasia of the liver associated with hemihypertrophy and vascular malformations. *Gastroenterology* 1995;108:1256–1262.
132. Roskams T, Vos RDE, Desmet V. "Undifferentiated progenitor cells" in focal nodular hyperplasia of the liver. *Histopathology* 1996;28:291–299.
133. Paradis V, Laurent A, Flejou J-F, Vidaud M, Bedossa P. Evidence for the polyclonal nature of focal nodular hyperplasia of the liver by the study of X-chromosome inactivation. *Hepatology* 1997;26:891–895.
133a. Tanaka M, Wanless IR. Pathology of the liver in Budd-Chiari syndrome: portal vein thrombosis and the histogenesis of veno-centric cirrhosis, veno-portal cirrhosis, and large regenerative nodules. *Hepatology* 1998;27:488–496.
134. Wanless IR. Micronodular transformation (nodular regenerative hyperplasia) of the liver: a report of 64 cases among 2,500 autopsies and a new classification of hepatocellular nodules. *Hepatology* 1990 11:787–797.
135. Stromeyer FW, Ishak KG. Nodular transformation (nodular "regenerative" hyperplasia) of the liver: a clinicopathologic study of 30 cases. *Hum Pathol* 1981;12:60–71.
136. Colina F, Alberti N, Solis JA, Martinez-Tello FJ. Diffuse nodular regenerative hyperplasia of the liver (DNRH): a clinicopathologic study of 24 cases. *Liver* 1989;9:253–265.
137. Moran CA, Mullick FG, Ishak KG. Nodular regenerative hyperplasia of the liver in children. *Am J Surg Pathol* 1991;15:449–454.
138. Washington K, Lane KL, Meyers WC. Nodular regenerative hyperplasia in partial hepatectomy specimens. *Am J Surg Pathol* 1993;17:1151–1158.
139. Nzeako UC, Goodman ZD, Ishak KG. Hepatocellular carcinoma and nodular regenerative hyperplasia: possible pathogenetic relationship. *Am J Gastroenterol* 1996;91:879–884.
140. Furuya K, Nakamura M, Yamamoto Y, et al. Macroregenerative nodule of the liver: a clinicopathologic study of 345 autopsy cases of chronic liver disease. *Cancer* 1988;61:99–105.
141. Nagato Y, Kondo F, Kondo Y, et al. Histological and morphometrical indicators for a biopsy diagnosis of well-differentiated hepatocellular carcinoma. *Hepatology* 1991;14:473–478.
142. Ferrell L, Wright T, Lake J, Roberts J, Ascher N. Incidence and diagnostic features of macroregenerative nodules vs. small hepatocellular carcinoma in cirrhotic livers. *Hepatology* 1992;16:1372–1381.
143. Ferrell LD, Crawford JM, Dhillon AP, Scheuer PJ, Nakanuma Y. Proposal for standardized criteria for the diagnosis of benign, borderline, and malignant hepatocellular lesions arising in chronic advanced liver disease. *Am J Surg Pathol* 1993;17:1113–1123.
144. Terada T, Terasaki S, Nakanuma Y. A clinicopathologic study of adenomatous hyperplasia of the liver in 209 consecutive cirrhotic livers examined by autopsy. *Cancer* 1993;72:1151–1156.
145. Hytiroglou P, Theise ND, Schwartz M, Mor E, Miller C, Thung SN. Macroregenerative nodules in a series of adult cirrhotic liver explants: issues of classification and nomenclature. *Hepatology* 1995;21:703–708.
146. Theise ND. Macroregenerative (dysplastic) nodules and hepatocarcinogenesis: theoretical and clinical considerations. *Semin Liver Dis* 1995;15:360–371.
146a. Mion F, Grozel L, Boillot O, Paliard P, Berger F. Adult cirrhotic liver explants: precancerous lesions and undetected small hepatocellular carcinomas. *Gastroenterology* 1996;111:1587–1592.
147. Borzio M, Borzio F, Croce A, et al. Ultrasonography-detected macroregenerative nodules in cirrhosis: a prospective study. *Gastroenterology* 1997;112:1617–1623.
148. Kondo Y. Pathology of early hepatocellular carcinoma and preneoplastic lesions in the liver. In: Okuda K, Tabor E, eds. *Liver cancer.* New York: Churchill Livingstone, 1997:135–153.
149. Theise ND, Hytiroglou P, Ferrell L, Schwartz M, Miller C, Thung SN. Macroregenerative nodules in cirrhosis are not associated with elevated serum or stainable tissue alpha-fetoprotein. *Liver* 1995;15:30–34.
150. Terada T, Nakanuma Y. Arterial elements and perisinusoidal cells in borderline hepatocellular nodules and small hepatocellular carcinoma. *Histopathology* 1995;27:333–339.
151. Kondo F, Ebara M, Sugiura N, et al. Histological features and clinical course of large regenerative nodules: evaluation of their precancerous potentiality. *Hepatology* 1990;12:592–598.
152. Takayama T, Makuuchi M, Hirohashi S, et al. Malignant transformation of adenomatous hyperplasia to hepatocellular carcinoma. *Lancet* 1990;336:1150–1153.
153. Bergman S, Graeme-Cook F, Pitman MB. The usefulness of the reticulin stain in the differential diagnosis of liver nodules on fine-needle aspiration biopsy cell block preparations. *Mod Pathol* 1997;10:1258–1264.

Malignant Hepatocellular Tumors

154. Ishak KG, Glunz PR. Hepatoblastoma and hepatocarcinoma in infancy and childhood: report of 47 cases. *Cancer* 1967;20:396–422.
155. Ni Y-H, Chang M-H, Hsu H-Y, et al. Hepatocellular carcinoma in childhood: clinical manifestations and prognosis. *Cancer* 1991;68:1737–1741.
156. Wands JR, Blum HE. Primary hepatocellular carcinoma. *N Engl J Med* 1991;325:729–731.

157. Bosch FX. Global epidemiology of hepatocellular carcinoma. In: Okuda K, Tabor E, eds. *Liver cancer*. New York: Churchill Livingstone, 1997:13–28.
158. Nzeako UC, Goodman ZD, Ishak KG. Hepatocellular carcinoma in cirrhotic and noncirrhotic livers: a clinico-histopathologic study of 804 North American patients. *Am J Clin Pathol* 1996;105:65–75.
159. Collier J, Sherman M. Screening for hepatocellular carcinoma. *Hepatology* 1998;27:273–278.
160. Geissler M, Gesien A, Wands JR. Molecular mechanisms of hepatocarcinogenesis. In: Okuda K, Tabor E, eds. *Liver cancer*. New York: Churchill Livingstone, 1997:59–88.
161. Okuda K. Clinical presentation and natural history of hepatocellular carcinoma and other liver cancers. In: Okuda K, Tabor E, eds. *Liver cancer*. New York: Churchill Livingstone, 1997:1–12.
162. Mucitelli DR, Zuna RE, Archard HO. Hepatocellular carcinoma presenting as an oral cavity lesion. *Oral Surg Oral Med Oral Pathol* 1988;66:701–705.
163. Young RH, Patter HTV, Scully RE. Hepatocellular carcinoma metastatic to the testis. *Am J Clin Pathol* 1987;87:117–120.
164. Chen L-T, Chen C-Y, Jan C-M, et al. Gastrointestinal tract involvement in hepatocellular carcinoma: clinical, radiological and endoscopic studies. *Endoscopy* 1990;22:118–123.
165. Nappi O, Ferrara G, Ianniello G, Wick MR. Metastatic hepatocellular carcinoma of the breast, simulating gynecomastia: diagnosis by fine-needle aspiration biopsy. *Diagn Cytopathol* 1992;8:588–592.
166. Young RH, Gersell DJ, Clement PB, Scully RE. Hepatocellular carcinoma metastatic to the ovary: a report of three cases discovered during life with discussion of the differential diagnosis of hepatoid tumors of the ovary. *Hum Pathol* 1992;23:574–580.
167. Melato M, Laurino L, Mucli E, et al. Relationship between cirrhosis, liver cancer, and hepatic metastases: an autopsy study. *Cancer* 1989;64:454–459.
168. Taketa K. Alpha-fetoprotein: reevaluation in hepatology. *Hepatology* 1990;12:1420–1432.
169. Nomura F, Ohnishi K, Tanabe Y. Clinical features and prognosis of hepatocellular carcinoma with reference to serum alpha-fetoprotein levels. *Cancer* 1989;64:1700–1707.
170. Weitz IC, Lieberman HA. Des—carboxy (abnormal) prothrombin and hepatocellular carcinoma: a critical review. *Hepatology* 1993;18:990–997.
171. Roberts CC, Colby TV, Batts KP. Carcinoma of the stomach with hepatocyte differentiation (hepatoid adenocarcinoma). *Mayo Clin Proc* 1997;72:1154–1160.
172. Kojiro M. Pathology of hepatocellular carcinoma. In: Okuda K, Tabor E, eds. *Liver cancer*. New York: Churchill Livingstone, 1997:165–187.
173. Kenmochi K, Sugihara S, Kojiro M. Relationship of histologic grade of hepatocellular carcinoma (HCC) to tumor size, and demonstration of tumor cells of multiple different grades in single small HCC. *Liver* 1987;7:18–26.
174. Okuda K, Peters RL, Simson IW. Gross anatomic features of hepatocellular carcinoma from three disparate geographic areas. *Cancer* 1984;54:2165–2173.
175. Nakashima T, Kojiro M. Pathologic characteristics of hepatocellular carcinoma. *Semin Liver Dis* 1986;6:259–266.
176. American Joint Committee on Cancer. Liver (including intrahepatic bile ducts). In: *Cancer staging manual*, 5th ed. Philadelphia: Lippincott–Raven Publishers, 1997:97–101.
177. Sheu J-C, Huang G-T, Chou H-C, et al. Multiple hepatocellular carcinomas at the early stage have different clonality. *Gastroenterology* 1993;105:1471–1476.
178. Bhattacharya S, Davidson B, Dhillon A. Blood supply of early hepatocellular carcinoma. *Semin Liver Dis* 1995;15:390–401.
179. Hood DL, Bauer TW, Leibel SA, McMahon JT. Hepatic giant cell carcinoma: an ultrastructural and immunohistochemical study. *Am J Clin Pathol* 1990;93:111–116.
180. Fukunaga N, Fujioka A, Tanaka K, Toyama R. Oncocytic hepatocellular carcinoma with numerous globular hyaline bodies. *Pathol Int* 1996;46:286–291.
181. Maeda T, Adachi E, Kajiyama K, Takenaka K, Sugimachi K, Tsuneyoshi M. Spindle cell hepatocellular carcinoma: a clinicopathologic and immunohistochemical analysis of 15 cases. *Cancer* 1996;77:51–57.
182. Callea F. Natural history of hepatocellular carcinoma as viewed by the pathologist. *Appl Pathol* 1988;6:105–116.
183. Christensen W, Boitnott JB, Kuhajda FP. Immunoperoxidase staining as a diagnostic aid for hepatocellular carcinoma. *Mod Pathol* 1989;2:8–12.
184. Ganjei P, Nadji M, Albores-Saavedra J, Morales AR. Histologic markers in primary and metastatic tumors of the liver. *Cancer* 1988;62:1994–1998.
185. Ma CK, Zarbo RJ, Frierson HF, Lee MW. Comparative immunohistochemical study of primary and metastatic carcinomas of the liver. *Am J Clin Pathol* 1993;99:551–557.
186. Minervini MI, Demetris AJ, Lee RG, Carr BJ, Madariaga J, Nalesnik MA. Utilization of hepatocyte-specific antibody in the immunohistochemical evaluation of liver tumors. *Mod Pathol* 1997;10:686–692.
187. Nakanuma Y, Ohta G. Is Mallory body formation a preneoplastic change? A study of 181 cases of liver bearing hepatocellular carcinoma and 82 cases of cirrhosis. *Cancer* 1985;55:2400–2404.
188. Nakashima O, Sugihara S, Eguchi A, Taguchi J, Wantanabe J, Kojiro M. Pathomorphologic study of pale bodies in hepatocellular carcinoma. *Acta Pathol Jpn* 1992;42:414–418.
189. Guigui B, Mavier P, Lescs M-C, et al. Copper and copper-binding protein in liver tumors. *Cancer* 1988;61:1155–1158.
190. Hurlimann J, Gardiol D. Immunohistochemistry in the differential diagnosis of liver carcinomas. *Am J Surg Pathol* 1991;15:280–288.
191. Van Eyken P, Desmet VJ. Cytokeratins and the liver. *Liver* 1993;13:113–122.
192. D'Errico A, Baccarini P, Fiorentino M, et al. Histogenesis of primary liver carcinomas: strengths and weaknesses of cytokeratin profile and albumin mRNA detection. *Hum Pathol* 1996;27:599–604.
193. Wenming C, Mengchao W. The biopathologic characteristics of DNA content of hepatocellular carcinomas. *Cancer* 1990;66:498–501.
194. Koike Y, Kamijyo K, Suzuki Y, et al. DNA content of hepatocytes in various stages of liver cirrhosis. *Liver* 1985;5:156–161.
195. Okada S, Shimada K, Yamamoto J, et al. Predictive factors for postoperative recurrence of hepatocellular carcinoma. *Gastroenterology* 1994;106:1618–1624.
196. Ojanguren IO, Ariza A, Latjos M, Castella E, Mate JL, Navas-Palacios JJ. Proliferating cell nuclear antigen expression in normal, regenerative, and neoplastic liver: a fine needle aspiration cytology and biopsy study. *Hum Pathol* 1993;24:905–908.
197. Anthony PP. Primary carcinoma of the liver: a study of 282 cases in Ugandan Africans. *J Pathol* 1973;116:37–48.
198. Crawford JM. Pathologic assessment of liver cell dysplasia and benign liver tumors: differentiation from malignant tumors. *Semin Diagn Pathol* 1990;7:115–128.
199. Natarajan S, Theise ND, Thung SN, Antonio L, Paronetto F, Hytiroglou P. Large-cell change of hepatocytes in cirrhosis may represent a reaction to prolonged cholestasis. *Am J Surg Pathol* 1997;21:312–318.
200. Lee RG, Tsamandas AC, Demetris AJ. Large cell change (liver cell dysplasia) and hepatocellular carcinoma in cirrhosis: matched case-control study, pathological analysis, and pathogenetic hypothesis. *Hepatology* 1997;26:1415–1422.
201. Wantanabe S, Okita K, Harada T, et al. Morphologic studies of liver cell dysplasia. *Hum Pathol* 1983;51:2197–2205.
202. Kojiro M, Sugihara S, Nakashima O. Pathomorphologic characteristics of early hepatocellular carcinoma. *Gann Monograph on Cancer Research* 1991;38:29–37.
203. Ferrell L. Malignant liver tumors that mimic benign lesions: analysis of five distinct lesions. *Semin Diagn Pathol* 1995;12:64–76.
204. Norgaard T, Bardram L. Endocrine liver tumor differential diagnosis from hepatocellular carcinoma. *Histopathology* 1985;9:777–778.
205. Ordoñez NG, Manning JT, Hanssen G. Alpha-1-antitrypsin in islet cell tumors of the pancreas. *Am J Clin Pathol* 1983;80:277–282.
206. Lack EE. Pathology of the adrenal and extra-adrenal paraganglia. In: LiVolsi VA, ed. *Major problems in pathology*. Philadelphia: WB Saunders, 1994:244.
207. Wang J, Dhillon AP, Sankey EA, et al. Neuroendocrine differentiation in primary neoplasms of the liver. *J Pathol* 1991;163:61–67.
208. Zhao M, Laissue JA, Zimmerman A. Neuroendocrine differentiation in hepatocellular carcinomas (HCCs): immunohistochemical reactivity is related to distinct tumor cell types, but not to tumor grade. *Histol Histopathol* 1993;8:617–626.
209. Bruix J. Treatment of hepatocellular carcinoma. *Hepatology* 1997;25:259–262.

210. Ko S, Nakajima H, Kanehiro H, et al. Liver transplantation for hepatocellular carcinoma: consideration from the findings on autopsy. *Transplant Proc* 1996;28:1691–1692.
210a. Roberts CA, Markin RS, Wisecarver JL, Radio SJ. Malignant tumors in 894 consecutive explanted native livers: the University of Nebraska experience. *Lab Invest* 1998;78:156A.
211. Bathe OF, Scudamore CH, Caron NR, Buczkowski A. Resection of hepatocellular carcinoma. In: Okuda K, Tabor E, eds. *Liver cancer*. New York: Churchill Livingstone, 1997:511–535.
212. The liver cancer study group of Japan. Predictive factors for long term prognosis after partial hepatectomy for patients with hepatocellular carcinoma. *Cancer* 1994;74:2772–2780.
213. Adachi E, Maeda T, Matsumata T, et al. Risk factors for recurrence in human small hepatocellular carcinoma. *Gastroenterology* 1995;108:768–775.
213a. Wada Y, Nakashima O, Kutami R, Yamamoto O, Kojiro M. Clinicopathologic study on hepatocellular carcinoma with lymphocytic infiltration. *Hepatology* 1998;27:407–414.
214. Abou-Elella A, Gramlich T, Fritsch C, Gansler T. c-myc amplification in hepatocellular carcinoma predicts unfavorable prognosis. *Mod Pathol* 1996;9:95–98.
215. Ueki T, Fujimoto T, Yamamoto H, Okamoto E. Expression of hepatocyte growth factor and its receptor, the c-met proto-oncogene, in hepatocellular carcinoma. *Hepatology* 1997;25:619–623.
216. Hayashi H, Sugio K, Matsumata T, Adachi E, Takenaka K, Sugimachi K. The clinical significance of p53 gene mutation in hepatocellular carcinoma from Japan. *Hepatology* 1995;22:1702–1707.
217. Jwo S-C, Chiu J-H, Chau G-Y, Loong C-C, Lui W-Y. Risk factors linked to tumor recurrence of human hepatocellular carcinoma after hepatic resection. *Hepatology* 1992;16:1367–1371.
218. Funaki NO, Tanaka J, Seto S-I, Kasamatsu T, Kaido T, Imamura M. Hematogenous spreading of hepatocellular carcinoma cells: possible participation in recurrence in the liver. *Hepatology* 1997;25:564–568.
219. Barbu V, Bonnand A-M, Hillaire S, et al. Circulating albumin messenger RNA in hepatocellular carcinoma: results of a multicenter prospective study. *Hepatology* 1997;26:1171–1175.
220. Mazzaferro V, Regalia E, Doci R, et al. Liver transplantation for the treatment of small hepatocellular carcinomas in patients with cirrhosis. *N Engl J Med* 1996;334:693–699.
221. Berman MM, Libbey P, Foster JH. Hepatocellular carcinoma. Polygonal cell type with fibrous stroma: an atypical variant with favorable prognosis. *Cancer* 1980;46:1448–1455.
222. Craig JR, Peters RL, Edmondson HA, Omata M. Fibrolamellar carcinoma of the liver: a tumor of adolescents and young adults with distinctive clinicopathologic features. *Cancer* 1980;46:372–379.
223. Craig JR. Fibrolamellar carcinoma: clinical and pathologic features. In: Okuda K, Tabor E, eds. *Liver cancer*. New York: Churchill Livingstone, 1997:255–262.
224. Berman MA, Burnham JA, Sheahan DG. Fibrolamellar carcinoma of the liver: an immunohistochemical study of nineteen cases and a review of the literature. *Hum Pathol* 1988;19:784–794.
225. Pinna AD, Iwatsuki S, Lee RG, et al. Treatment of fibrolamellar hepatoma with subtotal hepatectomy or transplantation. *Hepatology* 1997;26:877–883.
226. Goodman ZD, Ishak KG, Langloss JM. Combined hepatocellular-cholangiocarcinoma: a histologic and immunohistochemical study. *Cancer* 1985;55:124–135.
227. An T, Ghatak N, Kastner R, et al. Hyaline globules and intracellular lumina in a hepatocellular carcinoma. *Am J Clin Pathol* 1983;79:392–396.
228. Ding S-F, Delhanty JDA, Bowles L, Dooley JS, Wood CB, Habib NA. Infrequent chromosome allele loss in fibrolamellar carcinoma. *Br J Cancer* 1993;67:244–246.
229. Omata M, Peters RL, Tatter D. Sclerosing hepatic carcinoma: relationship to hypercalcemia. *Liver* 1981;1:33–49.
230. Scoazec J-Y, Flejou J-F, D'Errico A, et al. Fibrolamellar carcinoma of the liver: composition of the extracellular matrix and expression of cell-matrix and cell-cell adhesion molecules. *Hepatology* 1996;24:1128–1136.
231. Haratake J, Hashimoto H. An immunohistochemical analysis of 13 cases with combined hepatocellular and cholangiocellular carcinoma. *Liver* 1995;15:9–15.
232. Nakajima T, Kubosawa H, Kondo Y, et al. Combined hepatocellular-cholangiocarcinoma with variable sarcomatous transformation. *Am J Clin Pathol* 1988;90:309–312.
233. Albar JP, De Miguel F, Esbrit P, Miranda R, Fernandez-Flores A, Sarasa JL. Immunohistochemical detection of parathyroid hormone–related protein in a rare variant of hepatic neoplasm (sclerosing hepatic carcinoma). *Hum Pathol* 1996;27:728–731.
233a. Davis JM, Sadasivan R, Dwyer T, Veldhuizen PV. Case report: cholangiocarcinoma and hypercalcemia. *Am J Med Sci* 1994;307:350–352.
234. Roskams T, Willems M, Campos RV, Drucker DJ, Yap SH, Desmet VJ. Parathyroid hormone–related peptide expression in primary and metastatic liver tumours. *Histopathology* 1993;23:519–525.
235. Ishak KG, Sesterhenn IA, Goodman ZD, et al. Epithelioid hemangioendothelioma of the liver: a clinicopathologic and follow-up study of 32 cases. *Hum Pathol* 1984;165:839–852.
236. Stocker JT, Conran RM. Hepatoblastoma. In: Okuda K, Tabor E, eds. *Liver cancer*. New York: Churchill Livingstone, 1997:263–278.
237. Haas JE, Muczynski KA, Krailo M, et al. Histopathology and prognosis in childhood hepatoblastoma and hepatocarcinoma. *Cancer* 1989;64:1082–1095.
238. Dehner LP, Manivel JC. Hepatoblastoma: an analysis of the relationship between morphologic subtypes and prognosis. *Am J Pediatr Hematol Oncol* 1988;104:301–307.
239. Harada T, Matsuo K, Kodama S, Higashihara H, Nakayama Y, Ikeda S. Adult hepatoblastoma: case report and review of the literature. *Aust N Z Surg* 1995;65:686–688.
240. Buckley JD, Sather H, Ruccione K, et al. A case-control study of risk factors for hepatoblastoma. *Cancer* 1989;64:1169–1176.
241. Ding S-F, Michail NE, Habib NA. Genetic changes in hepatoblastoma. *J Hepatol* 1994;20:672–675.
242. Akmal SN, Yun K, MacLay J, et al. Insulin-like growth factor 2 and insulin-like growth factor binding protein 2 expression in hepatoblastoma. *Hum Pathol* 1995;26:846–851.
243. Oda H, Nakatsuru Y, Imai Y, Sugimura H, Ishikawa T. A mutational hot spot in the p53 gene is associated with hepatoblastomas. *Int J Cancer* 1995;60:786–790.
244. Abenoza P, Manivel C, Wick M, et al. Hepatoblastoma: an immunohistochemical and ultrastructural study. *Hum Pathol* 1987;18:1025–1035.
245. Ruck P, Xiao J-C, Kaiserling E. Immunoreactivity of sinusoids in hepatoblastoma: an immunohistochemical study using UEA-1 and antibodies against endothelium-associated antigens, including CD34. *Histopathology* 1995;26:451–455.
246. Joshi VV, Kaur P, Ryan B, et al. Mucoid anaplastic hepatoblastoma. *Cancer* 1984;54:2035–2039.
247. Saxena R, Shafford EA, Davenport M, et al. Chemotherapy effects on hepatoblastoma. *Am J Surg Pathol* 1993;17:1266–1271.
248. Cross SS, Variend S. Combined hepatoblastoma and yolk sac tumor of the liver. *Cancer* 1992;69:1323–1326.
249. Scheimberg I, Cullinane C, Kelsey A, Malone M. Primary hepatic malignant tumor with rhabdoid features. *Am J Surg Pathol* 1996;20:1394–1400.
250. Von Schweinitz D, Wischmeyer P, Leuschner I, et al. Clinico-pathological criteria with prognostic relevance in hepatoblastoma. *Eur J Cancer* 1994;30A:1052–1058.
251. Geiger JD. Surgery for hepatoblastoma in children. *Curr Opin Pediatr* 1996;8:276–282.
252. Schmidt D, Wischmeyer P, Leuschner I, et al. DNA analysis in hepatoblastoma by flow and image cytometry. *Cancer* 1993;72:914–919.

Benign Tumors and Tumor-Like Lesions of the Intrahepatic Bile Ducts

253. Allaire GS, Rabin L, Ishak KG, Sesterhenn IA. Bile duct adenoma: a study of 152 cases. *Am J Surg Pathol* 1988;12:708–715.
254. Nakanuma Y. Non-neoplastic nodular lesions in the liver. *Pathol Int* 1995;45:703–714.
255. Bhathal PS, Hughes NR, Goodman ZD. The so-called bile duct adenoma is a peribiliary gland hamartoma. *Am J Surg Pathol* 1996;20:858–864.
256. Colombari R, Tsui W. Biliary tumors of the liver. *Semin Liver Dis* 1995;15:402–413.
257. Craig JR. Pseudoneoplastic lesions of the liver and the biliary tree. In: Wick MR, Humphrey PA, Ritter JR, eds. *Pathology of pseudoneoplastic lesions*. Philadelphia: Lippincott–Raven Publishers, 1997:157–182.

258. Tsui W, Loo KT, Chow LTC, Tse CCH. Biliary adenofibroma: a heretofore unrecognized benign biliary tumor of the liver. *Am J Surg Pathol* 1993;17:186–192.
259. Lev-Toaff AS, Bach AM, Wechsler RJ, Hilpert PL, Gatalica Z, Rubin R. The radiographic and pathologic spectrum of biliary hamartomas. *AJR* 1995;165:309–313.
260. Karhunen PJ, Penttilä A, Liesto K, et al. Occurrence of benign hepatocellular tumors in alcoholic men. *Acta Path Microbiol Immunol Scand A* 1986;94:141–147.
261. Dekker A, Ten Kate FJW, Terpstra OT. Cholangiocarcinoma associated with multiple bile-duct hamartomas of the liver. *Dig Dis Sci* 1989;34:952–958.
262. O'Hara BJ, McCue PA, Miettinen M. Bile duct adenomas with endocrine component: immunohistochemical study and comparison with conventional bile duct adenomas. *Am J Surg Pathol* 1992;16:21–25.
263. Gravel DH, Begin LR, Brisson M-L, Lamoureux E. Metastatic carcinoma resulting in hepar lobatum. *Am J Clin Pathol* 1996;105:621–627.

Malignant Tumors of the Intrahepatic Bile Ducts

264. Nakanuma Y, Hoso M, Terada T. Clinical and pathologic features of cholangiocarcinoma. In: Okuda K, Tabor E, eds. *Liver cancer*. New York: Churchill Livingstone, 1997:279–290.
265. Nakajima T, Kondo Y, Miyazaki M, Okui K. A histopathologic study of 102 cases of intrahepatic cholangiocarcinoma: histologic classification and modes of spread. *Hum Pathol* 1988;19:1228–1234.
266. Callea F, Sergi C, Fabbretti G, Brisigotti M, Cozzutto C, Medicina D. Precancerous lesions of the biliary tree. *J Surg Oncol* 1993;3[Suppl]:131–133.
267. Bergquist A, Glaumann H, Persson B, Broome U. Risk factors and clinical presentation of hepatobiliary carcinoma in patients with primary sclerosing cholangitis: a case control study. *Hepatology* 1998;27:311–316.
268. Chen M-F, Jan Y-Y, Wang C-S, et al. A reappraisal of cholangiocarcinoma in patients with hepatolithiasis. *Cancer* 1993;71:2461–2465.
269. Ohta T, Nagakawa T, Ueda N, et al. Mucosal dysplasia of the liver and the intraductal variant of peripheral cholangiocarcinoma in hepatolithiasis. *Cancer* 1991;68:2217–2223.
270. Ohashi K, Nakajima Y, Kanehiro K, et al. Ki-ras mutations and p53 protein expressions in intrahepatic cholangiocarcinomas: relation to gross tumor morphology. *Gastroenterology* 1995;109:1612–1617.
271. Maeda T, Takenaka K, Taguchi K, et al. Adenosquamous carcinoma of the liver: clinicopathologic characteristics and cytokeratin profile. *Cancer* 1997;80:364–371.
272. Nakajima T, Tajima Y, Sugano I, Nagao K, Kondo Y, Wada K. Intrahepatic cholangiocarcinoma with sarcomatous change: clinicopathologic and immunohistochemical evaluation of seven cases. *Cancer* 1993;72:1872–1877.
273. Honda M, Enjoji M, Saki H, Yamamoto I, Tsuneyoshi M, Nawata H. Case report: intrahepatic cholangiocarcinoma with rhabdoid transformation. *J Gastroenterol Hepatol* 1996;11:771–774.
274. Vortmeyer AO, Kingma DW, Fenton RG, Curti BD, Jaffe ES, Duray PH. Hepatobiliary lymphoepithelioma-like carcinoma associated with Epstein-Barr virus. *Am J Clin Pathol* 1998;109:90–95.
274a. Tihan T, Blumgart L, Klimstra DS. Clear cell carcinoma of the liver: an unusual variant of peripheral cholangiocarcinoma. *Hum Pathol* 1998;29:196–200.
275. Alpert LI, Zak FG, Werthamer S, Bochetto JF. Cholangiocarcinoma: a clinicopathologic study of five cases with ultrastructural observations. *Hum Pathol* 1974;5:709–728.
276. Riopel MA, Klimstra DS, Godellas CV, Blumgart LH, Westra WH. Intrabiliary growth of metastatic colonic carcinoma: a pattern of intrahepatic spread easily confused with primary neoplasia of the biliary tract. *Am J Surg Pathol* 1997;21:1030–1036.
277. Berdah SV, Delpero JR, Garcia S, Hardwigsen J, Le Treut YP. A western surgical experience of peripheral cholangiocarcinoma. *Br J Surg* 1996;83:1517–1521.
278. Masada CT, Markin RS. Cholangiocarcinoma following orthotopic liver transplantation: a unique pattern of recurrence diagnosed using immunohistochemical stains. *J Clin Gastroenterol* 1994;18:155–158.
279. Barsky SH. Hepatocellular carcinoma with carcinoid features. *Hum Pathol* 1984;15:892–894.
280. Andreola S, Lombardi L, Audiso RA, et al. A clinicopathologic study of primary hepatic carcinoid tumors. *Cancer* 1990;65:1211–1218.
281. Jaeck D, Paris F, Welsch M, et al. Primary hepatic pheochromocytoma: a second case. *Surgery* 1995;117:586–590.
282. Ishak KG. Malignant mesenchymal tumors and some other nonhepatocellular tumors of the liver. In: Okuda K, Tabor E, eds. *Liver cancer*. New York: Churchill Livingstone, 1997:291–314.
283. Forbes A, Portmann B, Johnson P, Williams R. Hepatic sarcomas in adults: a review of 25 cases. *Gut* 1987;28:668–674.
284. Craig JR. Mesenchymal tumors of the liver. In: Diagnostic problems for the surgical pathologist. *Pathology: State of the art reviews* 1994;3:141–160.
285. Farges O, Daradkeh S, Bismuth H. Cavernous hemangiomas of the liver: Are there any indications for resection? *World J Surg* 1995;19:19–24.
286. Tung GA, Cronan JJ. Percutaneous needle biopsy of hepatic cavernous hemangioma. *J Clin Gastroenterol* 1993;16:117–122.
287. Sundaresan M, Lyons B, Akosa AB. "Solitary" necrotic nodules of the liver: an aetiology reaffirmed. *Gut* 1991;32:1378–1380.
288. Haratake J, Koide O, Takeshita H. Hepatic lymphangiomatosis: report of two cases, with an immunohistochemical study. *Am J Gastroenterol* 1992;87:906–909.
289. Rojiani AM, Owen DA, Berry K, et al. Hepatic hemangioblastoma: an unusual presentation in a patient with von Hippel-Lindau disease. *Am J Surg Pathol* 1991;15:81–86.
290. Dehner LP, Ishak KG. Vascular tumors of the liver in infants and children: a study of 30 cases and review of the literature. *Arch Pathol* 1971;92:101–111.
291. Selby DM, Stocker JT, Waclawiw MA, Hitchcock CL, Ishak K. Infantile hemangioendothelioma of the liver. *Hepatology* 1994;20:39–45.
292. Lehrnbecher T, Frauendienst-Egger G, Schrod L, Marx A, Harms D, von Stockhausen H-B. Haemangioendothelioma in a preterm infant associated with highly elevated alpha-fetoprotein. *Eur J Pediatr* 1996;155:423–424.
293. Selby DM, Stocker JT, Ishak KG. Angiosarcoma of the liver in childhood: a clinicopathologic and follow-up study of 10 cases. *Pediatric Pathol* 1992;12:485–498.
294. Noronha R, Gonzalez-Crussi F. Hepatic angiosarcoma in childhood: a case report and review of the literature. *Am J Surg Pathol* 1984;8:863–871.
295. Falk H, Herbert JT, Edmonds L, et al. Review of four cases of childhood hepatic angiosarcoma: elevated environmental arsenic exposure in one case. *Cancer* 1981;47:382–391.
296. Strate S, Rutledge JC, Weinberg AG. Delayed development of angiosarcoma in multinodular infantile hepatic hemangioendothelioma. *Arch Pathol Lab Med* 1984;108:943–944.
297. Taxy JB. Peliosis: a morphologic curiosity becomes an iatrogenic problem. *Hum Pathol* 1978;9:331–340.
298. Scheuer PJ, Schachter LA, Mathur S. Peliosis hepatis after liver transplantation. *J Clin Pathol* 1990;43:1036–1037.
299. Molina T, Delmer A, Le Tourneau A, et al. Hepatic lesions of vascular origin in multicentric Castleman's disease, plasma cell type: report of one case with peliosis hepatis and another with perisinusoidal fibrosis and nodular regenerative hyperplasia. *Pathol Res Pract* 1995;191:1159–1164.
300. Koehler JE, Sanchez MA, Garrido CS, et al. Molecular epidemiology of *Bartonella* infections in patients with bacillary angiomatosis-peliosis. *N Engl J Med* 1997;337:1876–1883.
301. Cha I, Bass N, Ferrell LD. Lipopeliosis: an immunohistochemical and clinicopathologic study of five cases. *Am J Surg Pathol* 1994;18:789–795.
302. Falk H, Herbert J, Crowley S, et al. Epidemiology of hepatic angiosarcoma in the United States: 1964–1974. *Environ Health Perspect* 1981;41:107–113.
303. Locker GY, Doroshow JH, Zwelling LA, Chabner BA. The clinical features of hepatic angiosarcoma: a report of four cases and review of the English literature. *Medicine* 1979;58:48–64.
304. Wong JW, Bedard YC. Fine-needle aspiration biopsy of hepatic angiosarcoma: report of a case with immunocytochemical findings. *Diagn Cytopathol* 1992;8:380–383.
305. Soini Y, Welsh JA, Ishak KG, Bennett WP. p53 mutations in primary hepatic angiosarcomas not associated with vinyl chloride exposure. *Carcinogenesis* 1995;16:2879–2881.

306. Ohsawa M, Naka N, Tomita Y, Kawamori D, Kanno H, Aozasa K. Use of immunohistochemical procedures in diagnosing angiosarcoma. *Cancer* 1995;75:2867–2874.
307. Miettinen M, Lindenmayer E, Chaubal A. Endothelial cell markers CD31, CD34, BNH9 antibody in H- and Y-antigens: evaluation of their specificity and sensitivity in the diagnosis of vascular tumors and comparison with von Willebrand factor. *Mod Pathol* 1994; 7:82–90.
308. Ioachim HL, Adsay V, Giancotti FR, et al. Kaposi's sarcoma of internal organs. *Cancer* 1995;75:1376–1385.
309. Kelleher MB, Iwatsuki I, Sheahan DG. Epithelioid hemangioendothelioma of liver: clinicopathologic correlation of 10 cases treated by orthotopic liver transplantation. *Am J Surg Pathol* 1989;13:999–1008.
310. Lauffer JM, Zimmermann A, Triller J, Baer HU. Epithelioid hemangioendothelioma of the liver: a rare hepatic tumor. *Cancer* 1996;78:2318–2327.
311. Makhlouf HR, Ishak KG, Goodman ZD. Epithelioid hemangioendothelioma of the liver: a clinicopathological and follow-up study of 137 cases. *Lab Invest* 1998;78:154A.
312. Demetris AJ, Minervini M, Raikow RB, Lee RG. Hepatic epithelioid hemangioendothelioma: biological questions based on pattern of recurrence in an allograft and tumor immunophenotype. *Am J Surg Pathol* 1997;21:263–270.
313. Tsang WYW, Chan JKC. The family of epithelioid vascular tumors. *Histol Histopathol* 1993;8:187–212.
314. Goodman ZD. Nonparenchymal and metastatic malignant tumors of the liver. In: Haubrich WS, Schaffner F, Berk JE, eds. *Bochus Gastroenterology*, 5th ed. Philadelphia: WB Saunders, 1994:2488–2500.
315. Chen KTK. Cytology of epithelioid hemangioendothelioma. *Diagn Pathol* 1996;14:187–188.
316. Nonomura A, Mizukami Y, Kadoya M. Angiomyolipoma of the liver: a collective review. *J Gastroenterol* 1994;29:95–105.
317. Sasaki M, Harada K, Nakanuma Y, Wantanabe K. Pseudolipoma of Glisson's capsule: report of six cases and review of the literature. *J Clin Gastroenterol* 1994;19:75–78.
318. Brawer MK, Austin GE, Lewin KL. Focal fatty change of the liver, a hitherto poorly recognized entity. *Gastroenterology* 1980;78: 247–252.
319. Caturelli E, Costarelli L, Giordano M, et al. Hypoechoic lesions in fatty liver: quantitative study by histomorphometry. *Gastroenterology* 1991;100:1678–1682.
320. Shek TWH, Ng IOL, Chan KW. Inflammatory pseudotumor of the liver: report of four cases and review of the literature. *Am J Surg Pathol* 1993;17:231–238.
321. Broughan TA, Fischer WL, Tuthill RJ. Vascular invasion by hepatic inflammatory pseudotumor: a clinicopathologic study. *Cancer* 1993;71:2934–2940.
322. Zavaglia C, Barberis M, Gelosda F, et al. Inflammatory pseudotumor of the liver with malignant transformation: report of two cases. *Ital J Gastroenterol* 1996;28:152–159.
323. Selves J, Meggetto F, Brousset P, et al. Inflammatory pseudotumor of the liver: evidence for follicular dendritic reticulum cell proliferation associated with clonal Epstein-Barr virus. *Am J Surg Pathol* 1996;20:747–753.
324. Schwartz RE, Reynolds JC, Lotze MT. "Pseud-pseudotumor" of the liver: adenocarcinoma presenting as inflammatory pseudotumor. *Dig Dis Sci* 1994;39:2679–2684.
325. Shek TWH, Ho FCS, Ng IO, Chan AC, Ma L, Srivastava G. Follicular dendritic cell tumor of the liver: evidence for Epstein-Barr virus–related clonal proliferation of follicular dendritic cell. *Am J Surg Pathol* 1996;20:313–324.
326. Coffin CM, Watterson J, Priest JR, Dehner LP. Extrapulmonary inflammatory myofibroblastic tumor (inflammatory pseudotumor): a clinicopathologic and immunohistochemical study of 84 cases. *Am J Surg Pathol* 1995;19:859–872.
326a. Mosnier J-F, Flejou J-F, Degos F, et al. Plasma cell variant of Castleman's disease localized to the liver: a case report. *Euro J Gastroenterol* 1996;8:169–172.
327. Robertson SJ, Higgins RB, Powell C. Malakoplakia of liver: a case report. *Hum Pathol* 1991;22:1294–1295.
328. Tsui WMS, Yuen RWS, Chow LTC, Tse CCH. Solitary necrotic nodule of the liver: parasitic origin? *J Clin Pathol* 1992;45:975–978.
329. Barnoud R, Arvieux C, Pasquier D, Pasquier B, Letoublon C. Solitary fibrous tumor of the liver with CD34 expression. *Histopathology* 1996;28:551–554.
330. Reinertson TE, Fortune JB, Peters JC, Pagnotta I, Balint JA. Primary leiomyoma of the liver: a case report and review of the literature. *Dig Dis Sci* 1992;37:622–627.
330a. Fried RH, Wardzala A, Willson RA, Sinanan MN, Marchioro TL, Haggitt R. Benign cartilaginous tumor (chondroma) of the liver. *Gastroenterology* 1992;103:678–680.
331. Stocker JT, Ishak KG. Undifferentiated (embryonal) sarcoma of the liver: report of 31 cases. *Cancer* 1978;42:336–348.
332. Leuschner I, Schmidt D, Harms D. Undifferentiated sarcoma of the liver in childhood: morphology, flow cytometry, and literature review. *Hum Pathol* 1990;21:68–76.
333. Lack EE, Schloo BL, Azumi N, et al. Undifferentiated (embryonal) sarcoma of the liver: clinical and pathologic study of 16 cases with emphasis on immunohistochemical features. *Am J Surg Pathol* 1991;15:1–16.
334. Urban CE, Mache CJ, Schwinger W, et al. Undifferentiated (embryonal) sarcoma of the liver in childhood. *Cancer* 1993;72:2511–2516.
335. Aoyama C, Hachitanda Y, Sato JK, et al. Undifferentiated (embryonal) sarcoma of the liver: a tumor of uncertain histogenesis showing divergent differentiation. *Am J Surg Pathol* 1991;15:615–624.
336. Parham DM, Kelly DR, Donnelly WH, Douglass EC. Immunohistochemical and ultrastructural spectrum of hepatic sarcomas of childhood: evidence for a common histogenesis. *Mod Pathol* 1991;4: 648–653.
337. Chou P, Mangkornkanok M, Gonzalez-Crussi F. Undifferentiated (embryonal) sarcoma of the liver: ultrastructure, immunohistochemistry, and DNA ploidy analysis of two cases. *Pediatr Pathol* 1990; 10:549–562.
338. Krishnamurthy SC, Datta S, Jambhekar NA. Fine needle aspiration cytology of undifferentiated (embryonal) sarcoma of the liver: a case report. *Acta Cytol* 1996;40:567–570.
339. Pinson CW, Lopez RR, Ivancev K, Ireland K, Sawyers JL. Resection of primary hepatic malignant fibrous histiocytoma, fibrosarcoma, and leiomyosarcoma. *South Med J* 1994;87:384–391.
340. Penn I. Posttransplantation de novo tumors in liver allograft recipients. *Liver Transplant Surg* 1996;2:52–59.
341. Davidoff AM, Hebra A, Clark BJ, et al. Epstein-Barr virus–associated hepatic smooth muscle neoplasm in a cardiac transplant recipient. *Transplantation* 1996;61:515–517.
342. Ruymann FB, Raney B, Crist WM, et al. Rhabdomyosarcoma of the biliary tree in childhood. *Cancer* 1985;56:575–581.
343. Cote RJ, Urmacher C. Rhabdomyosarcoma of the liver associated with long-term oral contraceptive use: possible role of estrogens in the genesis of embryologically distinct liver tumors. *Am J Surg Pathol* 1990;14:784–790.
344. Kim YI, Yu ES, Lee KW, et al. Dedifferentiated liposarcoma of the liver. *Cancer* 1987;60:2785–2790.
345. von Hochstetter AR, Hattenschwiler J, Vogt M. Primary osteosarcoma of the liver. *Cancer* 1987;60:2312–2317.
346. Fiel MI, Schwartz M, Min AD, Sung MW, Thung SN. Malignant Schwannoma of the liver in a patient without neurofibromatosis. *Arch Pathol Lab Med* 1996;120:1145–1147.
347. Ohsawa M, Aozasa K, Horiuchi K, et al. Malignant lymphoma of the liver: report of five cases and review of the literature. *Dig Dis Sci* 1992;37:1105–1109.
348. Anthony PP, Sarsfield P, Clarke T. Primary lymphoma of the liver: clinical and pathological features of 10 patients. *J Clin Pathol* 1990;43:1007–1013.
349. Lei KI-K, Chow JH-S, Johnson PJ. Aggressive primary hepatic lymphoma in Chinese patients: presentation, pathologic features and outcome. *Cancer* 1995;76:1336–1343.
350. Isaacson PG, Banks PM, Best PV, McClure SP, Muller-Hermelink HK, Wyatt JI. Primary low grade hepatic B-cell lymphoma of mucosa-associated lymphoid tissue (MALT)-type. *Am J Surg Pathol* 1995;19:571–575.
350a. Zafrani ES, Gaulard P. Primary lymphoma of the liver. *Liver* 1993;13:57–61.
351. Mohler M, Gutzler F, Kallinowski B, Goeser T, Stremmel W. Primary hepatic high grade non-Hodgkin's lymphoma and chronic hepatitis C infection. *Dig Dis Sci* 1997;42:2241–2245.
352. Weichhold W, Labouyrie E, Merlio JPH, Masson B, de Mascarel A. Primary extramedullary plasmacytoma of the liver: a case report. *Am J Surg Pathol* 1995;19:1197–1202.
353. O'Brien CB, Pollack B, Furth E, Fox K, Schnall MD. Primary hepatic angiocentric lymphoma. *Dig Dis Sci* 1997;42:427–430.

354. Khan SM, Cottrell BJ, Millward-Sadler GH, Wright DH. T-cell rich B-cell lymphoma presenting as liver disease. *Histopathology* 1993;23:217–224.

Other Tumors

355. Terada T, Nakanuma Y, Kakita A. Pathologic observations of intrahepatic peribiliary glands in 1,000 consecutive autopsy livers: heterotopic pancreas in the liver. *Gastroenterology* 1990;98:1333–1337.
356. Ghalib R, Howard T, Lowell J, et al. Plexiform neurofibromatosis of the liver: case report and review of the literature. *Hepatology* 1995;22:1154–1157.

Metastattic Tumor in the Liver

357. Pickren JW, Tsukada Y, Lane WW. Liver metastases: analysis of autopsy data. In: Weiss L, Gilbert HA, eds. *Liver metastasis*. Boston: GK Hall Medical Publishers, 1982:2–18.
358. Myszor MF, Record CO. Primary and secondary malignant disease of the liver and fulminant hepatic failure. *J Clin Gastroenterol* 1990;12:441–446.
359. Fong Y, Blumgart LH, Cohen AM. Surgical treatment of colorectal metastases to the liver. *CA Cancer J Clin* 1995;45:50–62.
360. Ohtsuka M, Miyazaki M, Itoh H, et al. Routes of hepatic metastasis of gallbladder carcinoma. *Am J Clin Pathol* 1998;109:62–68.
361. Jaffe ES. Malignant lymphomas: pathology of hepatic involvement. *Semin Liver Dis* 1987;7:257–268.
362. Harris AC, Ben-Ezra JM, Contos MJ, Kornstein MJ. Malignant lymphoma can present as hepatobiliary disease. *Cancer* 1996;78:2011–2019.
363. Shehab TM, Kaminski MS, Lok ASF. Acute liver failure due to hepatic involvement by hematologic malignancy. *Dig Dis Sci* 1997;42:1400–1405.
364. Francois A, Lesesve J-F, Stamatoullas A, et al. Hepatosplenic gamma/delta T-cell lymphoma: a report of two cases in immunocompromised patients, associated with isochromosome 7q. *Am J Surg Pathol* 1997;21:781–790.
365. Leslie KO, Colby TV. Hepatic parenchymal lymphoid aggregates in Hodgkin's disease. *Hum Pathol* 1984;15:808–809.
366. Hubscher SG, Lumley MA, Ellas E. Vanishing bile duct syndrome: a possible mechanism for intrahepatic cholestasis in Hodgkin's disease. *Hepatology* 1993;17:70–77.
367. Zaman A, Bramely PN, Wyatt J, et al. Hodgkin's disease presenting as liver abscesses. *Gut* 1991;32:959–962.
368. Nalesnik MA, Jaffe R, Starzl T, et al. The pathology of posttransplant lymphoproliferative disorders occurring in the setting of cyclosporine A–prednisone immunosuppression. *Am J Pathol* 1988;133:173–192.
369. Randawa PS, Markin RS, Starzl TE, Demetris AJ. Epstein-Barr virus–associated syndromes in immunosuppressed liver transplant recipients: clinical profile and recognition on routine allograft biopsy. *Am J Surg Pathol* 1990;14:538–547.
370. Zandi P, Panis Y, Debray D, Bernard O, Houssin D. Pediatric liver transplantation for Langerhans' cell histiocytosis. *Hepatology* 1995;21:129–133.
371. Horny H-P, Kaiserling E, Campbell M, et al. Liver findings in generalized mastocytosis: a clinicopathologic study. *Cancer* 1989;63:532–538.
372. Mican JM, Di Bisceglie AM, Fong T-L, et al. Hepatic involvement in mastocytosis; clinicopathologic correlations in 41 cases. *Hepatology* 1995;22:1163–1170.
373. Farrell DJ, Hines JE, Walls AF, Kelly PJ, Bennet MK, Burt AD. Intrahepatic mast cells in chronic liver diseases. *Hepatology* 1995;22:1175–1181.
374. Kyriakou D, Kouroumalis E, Konsolas J, et al. Systemic mastocytosis: a rare cause of noncirrhotic portal hypertension simulating autoimmune cholangitis. Report of four cases. *Am J Gastroenterol* 1998;93:106–108.
375. Thiruvengadam R, Penetrante RB, Goolsby HJ, et al. Multiple myeloma presenting as space-occupying lesions of the liver. *Cancer* 1990;65:2784–2786.
376. Roquet ML, Zafrani ES, Farcet JP, et al. Histopathological lesions of the liver in hairy cell leukemia: a report of 14 cases. *Hepatology* 1985;5:496–500.
377. Huberman MS, Bunn PA, Matthews MJ, et al. Hepatic involvement in the cutaneous T-cell lymphomas: results of percutaneous biopsy and peritoneoscopy. *Cancer* 1980;45:1683–1685.
378. Hansen KB, Kristensen IB. Granulomas of the spleen and liver in hairy cell leukemia. *Acta Pathol Microbiol Immunol Scand A* 1984;92:157–160.

CHAPTER 38

Gallbladder and Extrahepatic Biliary Tree

Scott H. Saul

Because approximately 600,000 cholecystectomies are performed each year in the United States, and because gallstone-related disease accounts for an estimated overall cost of more than five billion dollars annually, it behooves the pathologist to be familiar with the normal anatomy, histologic characteristics, and pathologic states of this organ (1). While the advent of laparoscopic cholecystectomy has revolutionized the manner in which routine gallbladder surgery is performed, it has not altered the type of specimen that the pathologist receives for processing. With few exceptions, the diagnosis of disorders of the gallbladder is quite straightforward, with most diseases being associated with cholelithiasis. Bile duct resections represent unusual specimens for most pathologists. When they are encountered at the time of frozen section, they often present a great diagnostic challenge, even for pathologists with extensive experience.

THE GALLBLADDER

Normal Anatomy and Histology

The gallbladder is a pear-shaped saccular structure that lies in a fossa on the posterior aspect of the right hepatic lobe. Its dimensions vary with the quantity of bile it contains (up to 40–70 ml) and the degree of wall tension (relaxed vs. contracted state). It is frequently cited as being 10 cm in length and 4 cm in width in normal adults, with a mural thickness of 1 to 2 mm (2–4). It is divided into three parts: the distal fundus, which extends beyond the anterior liver margin; the large central body; and the neck, which narrows as it joins the cystic duct. A dilatation in the region of the neck, termed Hartmann's pouch, is believed to result from chronic inflammation. Proximally, the mucosa of the cystic duct is thrown into folds (spiral valve of Heister) by the presence of thin groups of smooth-muscle fibers. This valve helps regulate the degree of gallbladder distension. The normal gallbladder (without gallstones) contains sterile bile.

The gallbladder wall has several layers and differs structurally from the other hollow organs of the gastrointestinal tract (Fig. 1). The mucosal layer is thrown into branching folds that vary in number and height, being more prominent when the organ is in the contracted state. The surface epithelium consists of uniform, tall columnar cells that contain oval basally located nuclei, with absent or inconspicuous nucleoli, and pale sulfomucin-rich cytoplasm, which may have a few small, apical vacuoles. Alpha-1-antitrypsin, alpha-1-antichymotrypsin, and scant superficial carcinoembryonic antigen (p-CEA, unabsorbed only), but not lysozyme, are normally found in the surface columnar epithelial cells. Inconspicuous, narrow ("pencil"), columnar and oval basal epithelial cells, as well as a few intraepithelial T lymphocytes, may be found. Goblet cells and melanocytes are absent. Rokitansky-Aschoff sinuses, which are analogous to acquired intestinal diverticula, are discussed in the section on chronic cholecystitis. Tubuloalveolar mucus (sulfo-, sialo-, and neutral mucin)–secreting glands are normally found only in the region of the neck. Although they resemble metaplastic pyloric glands on histologic examination, they differ ultrastructurally and also lack lysozyme (5). These glands represent the only site of neuroendocrine cells in the normal gallbladder (5).

The lamina propria (sometimes erroneously referred to as the submucosa) is composed of loose connective tissue containing blood vessels, lymphatics, and small numbers of lymphocytes, plasma cells, macrophages, and mast cells. Neutrophils are absent. The muscular layer, composed of loosely arranged bundles of circular, longitudinal, and oblique smooth-muscle fibers, directly abuts the lamina propria, without an intervening submucosa. Its thickness is variable. There are no well-defined circular and longitudinal layers; thus, it resembles the muscularis mucosae rather than the muscularis externa found elsewhere in the gastrointestinal tract. The perimuscular connective tissue layer (subserosa, adventitia), composed of differing amounts of collagen, elas-

---

S. H. Saul: Department of Pathology, Chester County Hospital, West Chester, Pennsylvania 19380.

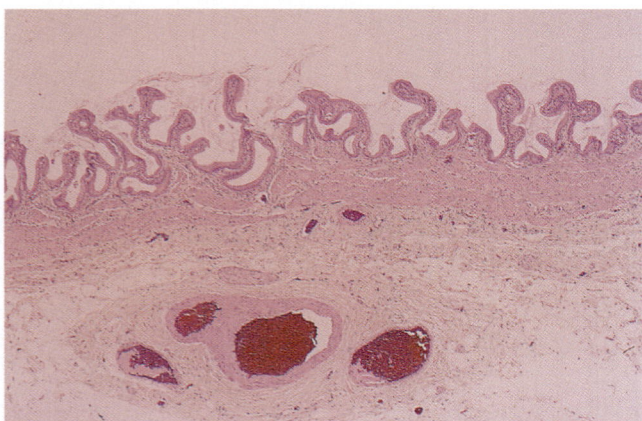

FIG. 1. Normal histologic features of the gallbladder (fundus and body). Note the mucosal, muscular, and perimuscular layers. The mucosa is thrown into branching folds, the height of which depends on the degree of distension of the organ. No pyloric or intestinal-type epithelium is evident. Rare lymphocytes are present in the lamina propria. Mucous glands similar to those seen in pyloric metaplasia are normally present only in the neck region.

tic tissue, and fat, contains blood vessels, lymphatics, nerves, and scattered paraganglia. Ganglion cells may be found in all subepithelial regions of the gallbladder wall.

Aberrant bile ducts (Lushka ducts), often possessing a collar of fibrous tissue, have been reported in the subserosa of about 10% of cholecystectomy specimens. They are believed to communicate with the intrahepatic bile ducts but have only rarely been reported to open into the gallbladder lumen (2,6). They do not communicate with Rokitansky-Aschoff sinuses. Larger accessory bile ducts, which join with the cystic or hepatic ducts, may be present within the gallbladder bed. The serosal layer (peritoneum) lines the portion of the gallbladder not directly attached to the liver.

Routine Specimen Processing

Prompt fixation is advisable, since the mucosa is quite susceptible to bile-related autolysis. A total of three full-thickness sections (one each from the fundus, body, and neck/cystic duct region) of the gallbladder are routinely taken and placed in one cassette. Pericystic duct lymph nodes should also be sampled. If gallstones are not readily apparent, the bile should be strained to assess for minute stones or "floating" cholesterol polyps, and the relative viscosity of the bile should be noted in the gross description of the specimen (see discussion under Cholesterol Stones). Small masses or polyps should be entirely submitted and additional sections taken from any suspicious areas of mural thickening. Several full-thickness sections should be taken from larger masses, to include the area of deepest mural penetration. The cystic duct resection margin should be examined in cases of carcinoma. If hepatic wedge or segmental resection for gallbladder carcinoma is performed, the extent of tumor penetration into the liver should be documented, as should the status of the hepatic margin.

Congenital Abnormalities

Congenital abnormalities of the gallbladder are uncommon. They can be divided into four groups: anomalies of shape, number, or position and heterotopias (4). The *Phyrigian cap*, representing an angulation of the distal fundus, is considered an anatomic variant by some researchers and an acquired abnormality by others. It has been detected in about 5% of cholecystograms. A small mucosal fold containing a disorganized muscle layer occasionally can be shown to account for this finding if the gallbladder is fixed in the distended state and the sections are longitudinal. *Diverticula* are usually solitary, vary in size from 0.6 to 8 cm, and can develop anywhere within the gallbladder. Only rarely are they true congenital anomalies, possessing all layers of the gallbladder wall. More commonly they are pseudodiverticula (Rokitansky-Aschoff sinuses), related to cholelithiasis/cholecystitis. Therefore, similarly to (pseudo)diverticula found in the colon, they lack a complete muscular wall. *Cysts* appear macroscopically to be separate from the gallbladder; however, they probably begin as pseudodiverticula, with progressive occlusion of their communication with the gallbladder lumen. Congenital cysts are rare.

Multiseptate gallbladders, which may be congenital or acquired, contain multiple (between three and 10) communicating compartments lined by columnar epithelium (Fig. 2). Stones may be present, but typically not in children. The congenital hourglass gallbladder, divided into proximal and distal portions by a central constriction, is a variant of the transverse septate gallbladder. The acquired form, in which the septum is composed of inflamed fibrous tissue or adenomyomatous hyperplasia, is much more common.

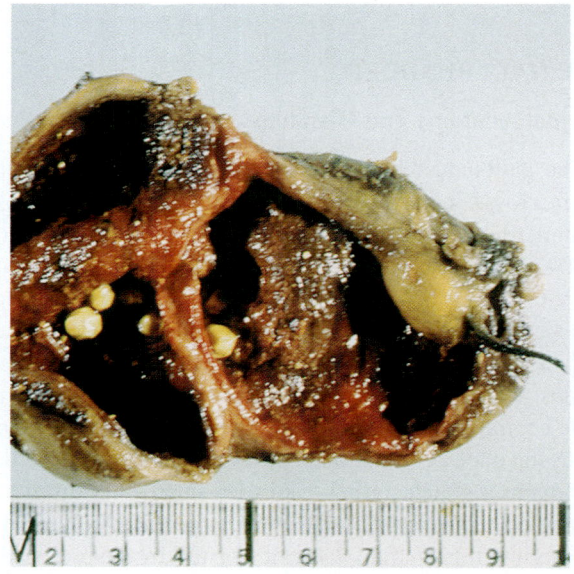

FIG. 2. Multiseptate gallbladder. Note three compartments, two of which contain gallstones. Cholecystitis/cholelithiasis appears to have been important in the pathogenesis of this example of multiseptate gallbladder, since fibroinflammatory septa were seen on microscopic examination.

Agenesis is rare; approximately 50% of cases are incidental autopsy findings. The cystic duct is usually absent as well. Choledocholithiasis is more common in these patients, and varied congenital anomalies may be encountered. Clinical symptoms may mimic those of cholecystitis or cholangitis (3). Although agenesis has little clinical importance in childhood, the hypoplastic gallbladder has several important associations. For example, in patients with extrahepatic biliary atresia, only a fibrous cord may remain in the gallbladder fossa. At the microscopic level, the site of the gallbladder consists of compressed epithelium-lined structures, fibrous tissue, strands of smooth muscle, and an inflammatory infiltrate. These findings are similar to those seen in the porta hepatis. A *small (micro-) gallbladder* (less than 2–3 cm in length, 0.5–1.5 cm in width) can be found in association with idiopathic neonatal (giant cell) hepatitis, $alpha_1$-antitrypsin deficiency, and cystic fibrosis. Differentiating congenital hypoplasia from postinflammatory scarring can be quite difficult. *Duplication* and *triplication* of the gallbladder have been reported; such cases are classified according to the arrangement of the cystic ducts.

Abnormal position of the gallbladder is quite rare. The aberrant sites have been summarized by Weedon (4) as left-sided, with or without situs inversus; intrahepatic; retroplaced (including retroperitoneal); suprahepatic (including above the diaphragm); or in a transverse position within the falciform ligament, lesser sac, or abdominal wall. The wandering (floating) gallbladder has a long mesentery or no firm attachment to the liver and is at risk of torsion.

Heterotopias now and then occur, typically as incidental findings (3,4,6). These nodules of ectopic tissue are nearly always less than 2.5 cm in diameter. Hepatic nodules are most common (7). They typically are attached to the gallbladder serosa and may be suspended by a mesenteric stalk. In this location they should be distinguished from fragments of normal liver that may detach from the region of the gallbladder bed at the time of cholecystectomy. Less commonly, hepatic nodules may be found within the gallbladder wall. Gastric (oxyntic-type mucosa) heterotopias may develop as intramural nodules, plaques, or polyps or may be an incidental microscopic finding. Peptic ulceration may be found in the adjacent mucosa, but it is uncommon (8). Heterotopic pancreatic tissue contains acinar tissue and, occasionally, islets of Langerhans; it may be responsible for acute pancreatitis limited to the gallbladder (9). Thyroid and adrenal cortical heterotopias are quite rare (4).

Cholesterolosis

Cholesterolosis, found in about 20% of cholecystectomy specimens, is characterized by the accumulation of cholesterol esters and triglyceride in aggregates of subepithelial macrophages and, to a lesser extent, in the gallbladder epithelium itself (4,10,11). Patients with this condition are typically adult women. Cholesterolosis is usually asymptomatic, but patients with acalculous biliary pain and cholesterolosis may clinically improve after cholecystectomy (12). Although the origin of cholesterolosis is unknown, most theories stress that either supersaturation of the bile with cholesterol, which is found in many but not all cases, or abnormal lipid transport across the mucosa leads to the formation of the lipid deposits. Bile cholesterol supersaturation is also seen with cholesterol gallstones. The fact that more than 50% of surgically resected gallbladders but only 10% of autopsied gallbladders with cholesterolosis have gallstones (usually cholesterol type), however, demonstrates the inconsistent relationship between these two conditions. There is no association of cholesterolosis with elevated blood cholesterol.

In most cases, the macroscopic appearance of cholesterolosis consists solely of yellow, nonpolypoid, punctate deposits in a diffuse or focal distribution (Fig. 3). When they are extensive, these deposits have been compared to the yellow-gray seeds that dot the surface of a strawberry—hence, the term strawberry gallbladder. This form is only rarely detected by sonography. Cholesterol polyps (20% of cases) may be found in the presence or absence of nonpolypoid cholesterolosis (see Nonneoplastic polyps and Table 4). Detached polyps have been implicated as the source of acute pancreatitis (4). Small, yellow particles of lipid may be found floating in the bile.

On microscopic inspection, clusters of foamy macrophages are visible in the lamina propria. Nearly always there is associated villous mucosal hyperplasia; the macrophages are initially found at the tips of the elongated villi. The overlying epithelial cells may also contain lipid droplets. Oil red O and other lipid stains show the nature of the intracytoplasmic deposits on frozen sections. Occasionally, foamy macrophages may also be found deeper within the gallbladder wall. Lipofuscin pigment has been described in both the foam cells and epithelium in this condition. Inflammation of the gallbladder wall itself is typically absent or mild.

Cholelithiasis

Clinical Features

Cholelithiasis is the most prevalent disorder of the biliary system (1,13–15). At least 10% of the adult population of the United States harbor gallstones. In the pediatric age group gallstones are quite uncommon (0.13–0.22%). Stones grow for the first 2 to 3 years, after which their growth stabilizes; 85% of all gallstones are less than 2 cm in diameter. Ultrasound surveys have shown a female to male ratio of 2–3:1 in the younger adult age groups and an increasing female prevalence with age. After age 60, the prevalence of gallstones in men and women is 10% to 15% and 20% to 40%, respectively, while the incidence of new gallstone formation becomes essentially equal.

Major risk factors include older age (peak, sixth and seventh decades), female sex, multiple pregnancies, obesity or rapid weight loss, hypertriglyceridemia and low HDL cholesterol (but not elevated serum cholesterol), ethnic pre-

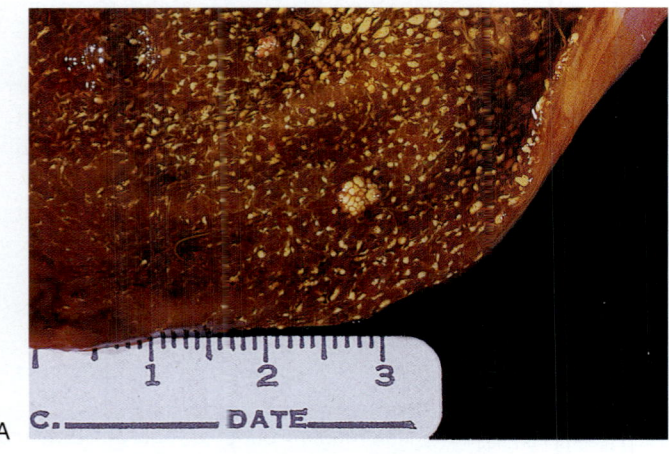
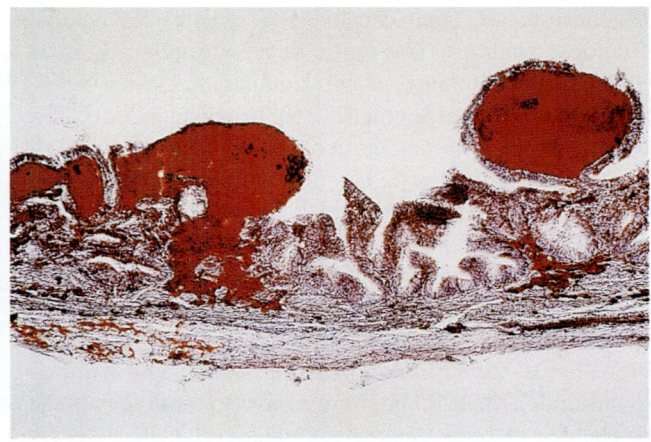
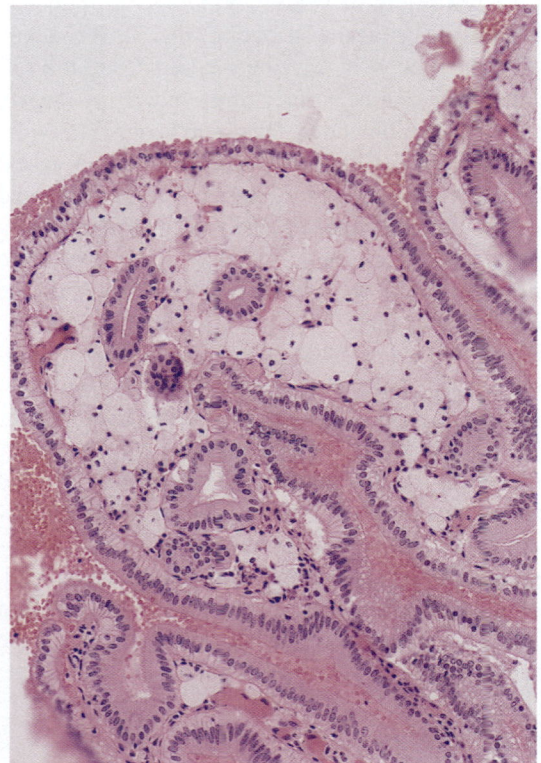

FIG. 3. Cholesterolosis. **A:** Diffuse, speckled appearance (strawberry gallbladder) with formation of minute cholesterol polyps. **B:** Numerous foamy macrophages in the lamina propria. **C:** Oil red O stain shows a high content of neutral lipid. (Kindly contributed by Virginia A. LiVolsi, M.D., Hospital of the University of Pennsylvania, Philadelphia, PA.).

disposition (high prevalence among Mexican-Americans and Native Americans in the United States, Scandinavians, and Chileans), total parenteral nutrition, diseases of the ileum (such as Crohn's disease), and the use of several drugs (estrogenic agents, clofibrate and related antihyperlipidemic agents, octreotide, and ceftriaxone). Hematologic disorders (sickle cell disease, hereditary spherocytosis, thalassemia major) account for many of the cases of gallstones among children, but other risk factors, such as those noted earlier, are playing a more prominent role. Risk factors and gender predisposition vary with gallstone type, as outlined in Table 1.

Although the majority of gallstones are clinically silent, episodes of biliary colic (severe, generally recurrent right-upper-quadrant/epigastric pain) are typically reported in symptomatic patients. Ultrasonography is the diagnostic method of choice; it has a 95% sensitivity and specificity for gallstones larger than 2 mm in diameter with an accompanying acoustic shadow. Gallbladder sludge—the usual gallstone precursor, which represents viscous, bile-containing glycoprotein; precipitated calcium bilirubinate; and tiny cholesterol crystals—can also be detected. It is associated with a natural history similar to macroscopic cholelithiasis. Ten to 25% of gallstones (including 20% of cholesterol stones and 50% of pigment stones) are radiopaque, depending on their calcium content, and, therefore, can be seen on abdominal plain films.

Treatment of gallbladder stones is recommended only for symptomatic patients, although a few groups of asymptomatic patients are exceptions (children, Native Americans, and patients with sickle cell disease, porcelain gallbladder,

TABLE 1. *Gallstones: features helpful in differential diagnosis*

	Type of gallstone			
	Cholesterol (75–85%)		Pigment (15–25%)	
Clinical features	Pure	Mixed	Black	Brown
Frequency	10%	70–80%	10–25%	Rare (U.S.A.); 15–25% (Japan)
Female/male	2–3:1	2–3:1	1.25:1	1.25:1
Increase with age	Yes	Yes	Yes	Yes
Infected bile[a]	10–100%	10–100%	Uncommon	Nearly 100%
Assoc. conditions	Obesity, rapid weight loss, diabetes mellitus, ileal disease, multiple pregnancies, ethnic predisposition, TPN, several drugs		Old age, chronic hemolysis, cirrhosis, sclerosing cholangitis	Infected bile
Radiodense	Lucent	20%	50%	Lucent
Appearance				
Usual no.	Single	Multiple	Multiple	Multiple
Usual size (cm)	Often 2–4	0.2–3.0	0.2–0.5	0.2–0.5
Color	White-yellow	Variable	Shiny, black/brown	Dull, brown
Shape	Round to oval	Faceted and round	Irregular	Irregular
Cut surface	Crystalline	Crystalline	Crystalline/amorphous	Laminated
Major components	Cholesterol (≥90%)	Cholesterol (60–89%), Ca bili, inorganic Ca salts, mucin glycoprotein	Ca bili, inorganic Ca salts, mucin glycoprotein	Ca bili, Ca salts of FFA, mucin glycoprotein
Usual GB histology	Cholesterolosis	Cholecystitis	Normal	Cholecystitis

Bili, bilirubinate; Ca, calcium; FFA, free fatty acids; TPN, total parenteral nutrition; GB, gallbladder
[a] Highest rates found in association with acute cholecystitis and choledocholithiasis with cholangitis.

or gallstones larger than 3 cm diameter) (13). Laparoscopic cholecystectomy is the procedure of choice in most instances; it is performed to avoid the 1% to 2% annual risk of complications (acute and chronic cholecystitis, choledocholithiasis, cholangitis, empyema, gallstone ileus, acute pancreatitis, possibly gallbladder cancer) that can result from untreated symptomatic cholelithiasis. *Mirizzi's* syndrome, a rare complication, results when impaction of a stone in the gallbladder neck/cystic duct results in extrinsic compression or obstruction of the common bile duct (CBD), causing jaundice. One series found a higher rate of associated gallbladder carcinoma (15a). Nonsurgical options (oral and contact dissolution therapy, extracorporeal shock-wave lithotripsy) are rarely used.

Classification

Gallstones are composed of various combinations of insoluble components of bile, including cholesterol, calcium bilirubinate, inorganic and organic calcium salts, bile salts, and mucin glycoproteins (Table 1). Although typically found within the gallbladder lumen, they may occasionally be intramural. Two broad classes of stones, cholesterol and pigment, are recognized, accounting for 75% to 85% and 15% to 25% of gallstones, respectively, in the United States (Fig. 4). Another, rare type is the calcium carbonate stone, which is gray-white and amorphous. Calcium carbonate can also be found as a thick, inspissated, cream-gray to yellow-green, putty-like, radiopaque material (milk of calcium or limey bile) filling the gallbladder lumen. Stones within the gallbladder are usually of a single type; only rarely (~1%) have black and cholesterol stones been encountered together within the same gallbladder (16). The presence of biliary sludge should be noted at the time of description of the gross features of the gallbladder, as well as the approximate number, size, and type of gallstones.

Cholesterol Stones (75–85%, U.S.A.)

Cholesterol stones by definition are composed of more than 60% to 70% cholesterol by weight. The basic units of this gallstone type are crystals of cholesterol monohydrate, which precipitate when cholesterol is no longer soluble in micelles, or vesicles, of bile (13,14). Those stones containing 90% or more cholesterol are termed pure; they account for about 10% of all gallstones. They are typically yellow-white, single, round, and smooth; have a crystalline or laminated cut surface; and measure up to 4 cm in diameter. Stones with a lower cholesterol content are designated mixed. They are usually smaller, multiple, and faceted or round, with a crystalline or laminated cut surface and a dark core.

Development of a cholesterol stone progresses through three stages, with gallbladder hypomotility playing an im-

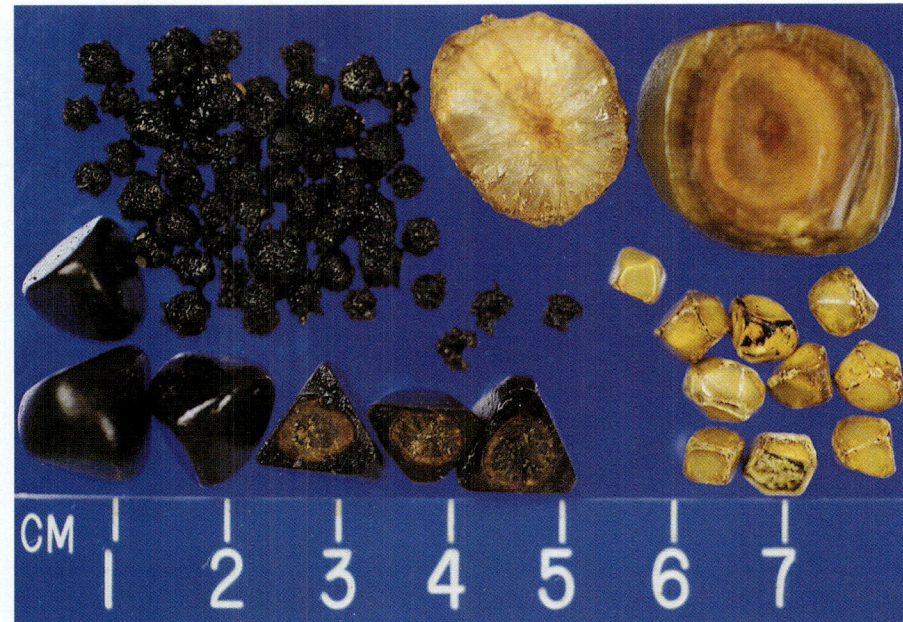

FIG. 4. Gallstones, varied macroscopic appearances. Note that clusters of gallstones from a given patient tend to be of similar size. Upper left: Black pigment stones with "jack-like" appearance. Lower left: Mixed cholesterol stones (intact and cut surface) with mixed cholesterol/pigment core and pigment shell. Upper right: Cut surface of pure cholesterol (toward midline) and mixed cholesterol stones. Lower right: Mixed cholesterol gallstones. Note the faceted appearance and dark core seen in cross section.

portant pathogenetic role: (a) Supersaturation of the bile with cholesterol (lithogenic bile), which is dependent on the ratio of cholesterol, phospholipid, and bile salts, is a necessary but not sufficient condition for stone formation. (b) Nucleation (crystallization of cholesterol monohydrate from a supersaturated solution) is viewed as an interaction between the absolute degree of cholesterol supersaturation and the outcome of a balance between the activity of mucin glycoprotein nucleation inhibitors and promotors. (c) Stone growth is a poorly understood process encouraged by bile stasis and mucin hypersecretion. Growth of multiple stones appears to occur in "generations," with those equal in size growing at the same rate and being of one generation and those of varying size probably representing different generations.

Pigment Stones (15–25%, U.S.A.; Most Common Worldwide)

Pigment stones typically contain less than 25% to 30% cholesterol. They can be divided into two different types: black and brown. Black stones arise in sterile bile and are composed of either pure calcium bilirubinate or polymer-like complexes comprising calcium, large quantities of mucin glycoproteins, and copper. They look black or deep brown, resist crushing, have an irregular shiny surface, and, on fracturing, have a glasslike, featureless appearance. Most patients with black stones have no predisposing conditions (except for advanced age). These stones, however, are the ones most commonly associated with chronic hemolytic conditions, cirrhosis, and sclerosing cholangitis. Increased unconjugated bilirubin in the bile, with or without decreased levels of bile acids, is the important factor in the pathogenesis of these stones.

Brown stones are rarely found in gallbladders in the United States (≤1%); however, they account for a greater proportion (15–70%) of gallstones in the Orient, although this high rate seems to be declining. They are much softer than black stones and have a rough, flaky appearance. Alternating brown and tan layers are found on cross section, representing noncrystalline calcium bilirubinate and calcium salts of fatty acids, respectively. Brown stones are found in the context of biliary stasis and infection (bacteria, particularly *Escherichia coli*, and parasites). In fact, rod-shaped bacteria are a consistent component of brown pigment stone nuclei, with bacterial phospholipases being responsible for the liberation of the free fatty acids that complex with calcium to form calcium salts. Hydrolysis of conjugated bilirubin to its unconjugated form by β-glucuronidases of bacterial or pancreatico-hepatobiliary origin appears to be important in the pathogenesis of this type of stone.

Choledocholithiasis and Intrahepatic Stones

Stones in the common bide duct (CBD) may arise de novo (primary) or originate from the gallbladder (secondary). They are found in the common duct in 10% to 15% of patients who undergo cholecystectomy; occasionally they are missed at the time of operation. Recent data from the United

States indicate that nearly 40% of CBD stones are brown stones, a much higher prevalence than found in the gallbladders of this population, suggesting that a large proportion of such stones arise de novo in the CBD (17). Primary common duct and intrahepatic stones (hepatolithiasis) are most prevalent in the Orient. They are typically brown stones associated with recurrent pyogenic cholangitis (also known as chronic proliferative or Oriental cholangitis) (18). Endoscopic retrograde cholangiopancreatography (ERCP) is the gold standard for detecting common duct stones (95% sensitive and specific), since ultrasound detects only 50% of cases (13). Intrahepatic black stones may be found in the context of primary sclerosing cholangitis (PSC) (19). They are most frequently encountered in the longer and more tortuous left hepatic duct and its branches. Histologic features in the gallbladder suggestive of choledocholithiasis or other causes of large duct obstruction are described later in this chapter (see the discussion of the gallbladder in extrahepatic bile duct obstruction and chronic cholestatic disorders).

From time to time, pathologists are asked to evaluate biliary drainage specimens, usually obtained from ERCP, for the presence of cholesterol crystals (Meltzer-Lyon test) (10). The bile should be examined immediately at room temperature for the presence of typical notched, birefringent platelike crystals of cholesterol, other forms of cholesterol crystals (helical, thread, arc-like, needle-shaped, etc.), and calcium bilirubinate crystals. Most patients with such crystals and acalculous biliary pain are symptom free after cholecystectomy.

Biliary Fistulas and Gallstone Ileus

Biliary-enteric fistulas, almost always a consequence of gallstone disease, are found in 0.2% to 5% of patients undergoing surgical procedures for nonmalignant conditions of the biliary tract. Calculus-induced inflammation and necrosis of the gallbladder or bile duct wall lead to intestinal adhesions with subsequent fistula formation. In only 10% of cases are non-stone-related causes implicated, such as penetrating peptic ulcers of the stomach or duodenum (4). The gallbladder is involved in nearly 90% of biliary-enteric fistulas; the cholecystoduodenal type is most common (more than 50%), followed by cholecystocolonic and choledochoduodenal fistulas. The patients typically show initial signs of biliary tract disease or, less commonly, peptic ulcer disease. The radiographic finding of air within the biliary tree is diagnostic. The mortality rate is about 15%.

Most gallstones passing into the intestine do so uneventfully, but in about 20% of cases bowel obstruction occurs ("gallstone ileus") (4). Impacted stones are usually single and 3–4.5 cm in diameter. Typically, gallstone ileus involves the distal ileum (65–80%), followed by the jejunum (20%), colon (3–5%, usually sigmoid) and, rarely, the appendix. The stones are assumed to have entered through a cholecystoenteric fistula, although this connection may have closed by the time of initial clinical examination. The gallbladder is usually small, fibrotic, and surrounded by adhesions. Stones passed from the CBD through the ampulla of Vater into the duodenum are, in general, too small to cause obstruction. Stones formed *in situ* within the bowel (enteroliths), which are usually composed of bile acids, may be mistaken for gallstones (20).

Hydrops and Mucocele

In hydrops, the gallbladder is distended, and bile is replaced by a secretion of the epithelium that is clear and watery (hydrops) or cloudy and mucoid (mucocele) (4). Together, hydrops and mucocele account for about 3% of pathologic conditions of the adult gallbladder. Stones impacted in the ampulla or cystic duct account for virtually all cases in adults; rarely, primary neoplasms or external compression by neoplastic or nonneoplastic conditions in this region may cause hydrops/mucocele. Perforation of a mucocele has been reported to cause pseudomyxoma peritonei, but mucinous cystic neoplasm of the gallbladder should be excluded.

Pediatric cases of hydrops/mucocele are typically acute and may be associated with a wide spectrum of infectious/inflammatory causes, including Kawasaki syndrome. Inflammatory narrowing of the cystic duct or compression of this structure by adjacent enlarged lymph nodes is the likely cause. Ultrasonography is a useful diagnostic tool in this context. In adult cases, which are generally of long duration, the gallbladder wall is usually thickened as the result of fibrous replacement of the muscular layer. Rarely, muciphages may be present on histologic examination and may simulate signet cell adenocarcinoma. In pediatric cases, where obstruction is often acute, the wall is generally thin. The epithelium is flattened, and inflammation is variable but usually sparse in both age groups. Varying numbers of Rokitansky-Aschoff sinuses may be present.

Cholecystitis

Acute Cholecystitis

Clinical Features and Pathogenesis

While biliary colic is considered the most common clinical manifestation of gallstone disease, acute cholecystitis is the typical complication (13). The frequency with which acute cholecystitis is found in cholecystectomy specimens differs among institutions because of variability in clinical treatment of these patients. Overall, 5% to 10% appears to be a reasonable estimate (4). About 90% to 95% of cases are associated with gallstones (acute calculous cholecystitis); in the remainder, stones are lacking (acute acalculous cholecystitis) (4,10,13). Ultrasonography and hepatobiliary scintigraphy are the diagnostic imaging methods of choice.

Patients in the gallstone-related group have a mean age of nearly 60 years, are more often female (female to male ratio, 1.5:1), and typically show initial signs of abdominal pain, right-upper-quadrant tenderness, nausea, vomiting, fever, leukocytosis, and slight jaundice. Prominent elevation of the serum bilirubin usually indicates coexistent choledocholithiasis, which is found in about 50% of jaundiced patients with acute cholecystitis (13). While intermittent obstruction of the cystic duct/gallbladder neck by a stone is responsible for biliary colic, acute cholecystitis results when the stone becomes impacted, leading to chronic obstruction. This results in increased intraluminal pressure, vascular compromise, stasis and concentration of bile within the gallbladder lumen, mucosal damage with release of cellular enzymes, and activation of a cascade of inflammatory mediators (13). Bacterial infection of gallbladder bile is found in about 50% of cases (range, 9–100%) and is believed to be a secondary phenomenon (4,13,21). Aerobes (*E. coli, Enterobacter, Enterococcus, Klebsiella*) predominate over anaerobes (*Clostridium, Peptostreptococcus, Bacteroides*), and in a minority of cases the bile show signs of infection with several microbes.

Patients with acute acalculous cholecystitis are typically male (female to male ratio, 1:2), more than 50 years of age, and quite debilitated. Many of the features found in acute calculous cholecystitis may be lacking; patients may have only fever or hyperamylasemia. One or more associated conditions or factors may be found in approximately 50% of cases: severe trauma; bacterial sepsis; shock; burns; cancer; diabetes mellitus; multiple blood transfusions; previous surgery; torsion; noncalculous obstruction of the cystic duct or CBD due to neoplasm, fibrosis, or congenital anomaly; or vasculitis. More than 50% of cholecystectomies performed on hospitalized or postoperative patients recovering from trauma or burns are for acalculous disease (13). The possibility of cocaine-induced acute cholecystitis should be considered in a young and otherwise healthy patient if vascular thrombosis is noted and other portions of the gastrointestinal tract are affected (21*a*). Cytomegalovirus (CMV), cryptosporidia, and microsporidia may be associated with acalculous cholecystitis as well as with a syndrome of sclerosing cholangitis in patients with the acquired immunodeficiency syndrome (AIDS) (see AIDS-related Cholecystitis and Fig. 8).

The definitive treatment for acute cholecystitis is cholecystectomy. Left untreated, localized perforation develops in about 10% of patients with acute cholecystitis, while free perforation and peritonitis develop in 1% (13). The overall mortality rate for acute calculous cholecystitis is about 1%, but, as expected, that for the acalculous variety is much greater (10–50%). Perforation is associated with a 20% rate of mortality (4). Findings of early, severe, acute cholecystitis in the donor gallbladder at the time of liver transplantation have been correlated with poor graft function (22).

Pathologic Findings

The pathologic features of the gallbladder wall in acute cholecystitis are the same regardless of the presence or absence of gallstones. The macroscopic appearance, which often consists of an enlarged, distended, and discolored organ with congested subserosal vessels, serosal exudate, a thickened wall (up to 2 cm) characterized by edema and hemorrhage, mucosal exudate, and ulcers with intraluminal blood clot mixed with bile and pus (termed empyema when it is marked), is typically much more dramatic for the surgeon *in vivo* compared with what is seen by the pathologist in the formalin-fixed state (4). If chronic cholecystitis has preceded the acute episode, the gallbladder may be normal in size or even small. Florid acute cholecystitis may result in focal or diffuse mural infarction (gangrenous cholecystitis) in perhaps 15% to 20% of cases, with perforation developing in 25% of this subgroup (4). Overgrowth of gas-producing organisms (most commonly *C. perfringens*) in the gallbladder wall (emphysematous cholecystitis) is associated with mural gangrene (4) and is radiographically identified by pneumobilia (4,13).

The degree and character of the histologic changes are proportional to the severity and duration of the initial insult, the interval of time until the organ is removed, and the presence/absence of previous chronic cholecystitis (Fig. 5). At the microscopic level, the earliest changes seen in the first few days after the onset of symptoms are prominent edema, vascular congestion, hemorrhage, and fibrin deposition, noted principally in the perimuscular connective tissue and adjacent muscle. This is the cause of the characteristic marked mural thickening often detected by ultrasonography. Mucosal and mural necrosis may be seen, with neutrophils peaking between the third and fifth days (4). Reactive epithelial atypia, including nuclear pleomorphism and mitotic figures, is sometimes a conspicuous histologic feature. The epithelial atypia tends to be proportional to the degree of reactive stromal atypia. A diagnosis of dysplasia should be made only with great caution in the presence of extensive ulceration or acute inflammation (Table 6) (6).

"Tissue culture–like" (myo)fibroblastic proliferation characteristic of a healing wound begins by the fifth day, is generally most pronounced in the perimuscular connective tissue, and peaks between the ninth and tenth days. Lymphocytes, plasma cells, eosinophils, and pigment-laden macrophages may be seen at about this time at any level of the gallbladder wall. The organization phase may last for several months. These more "chronic" histopathologic features (organizing/resolving acute or subacute cholecystitis) probably account for disagreement between the clinician and the pathologist regarding the "acute" or "chronic" nature of the cholecystitis. The histopathologic picture may be even more confusing, since coexistent features of classic chronic cholecystitis are quite common. The exact terminology employed by the pathologist in these contexts has no clinical relevance to subsequent treatment of the patient.

Chronic Cholecystitis

Clinical Features

The overwhelming majority of cholecystectomies are performed for symptomatic cholelithiasis (biliary colic) related

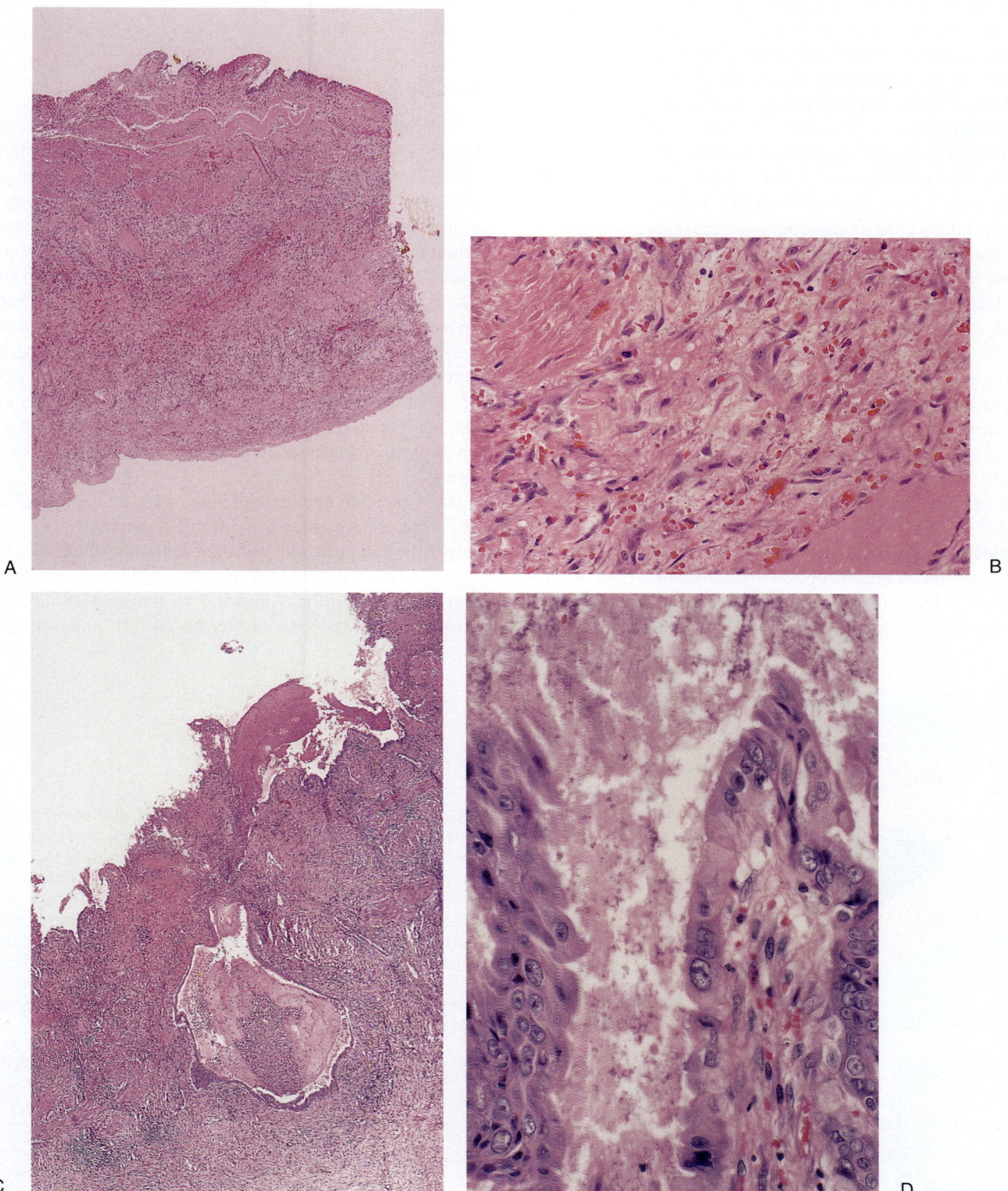

FIG. 5. Acute cholecystitis. **A:** Note the prominent thickening of perimuscular connective tissue related to edema and (myo)-fibroblastic proliferation. **B:** Higher-power view of "tissue culture–like" (myo)-fibroblastic proliferation, which may display prominent reactive changes. **C:** Mucosal ulceration with inspissated inflammatory debris in Rokitansky-Aschoff sinus. **D:** Marked reactive epithelial atypia in the region of ulcer. These changes should not be misinterpreted as dysplasia.

to intermittent obstruction of the gallbladder neck/cystic duct by one or more gallstones (13). Abnormal bile and/or gallstone-related chronic mucosal irritation are other important factors in the induction of mural damage and chronic cholecystitis. Chronic cholecystitis is virtually always associated with cholelithiasis (95%) and is the most common pathologic finding in surgically resected gallbladders. There is a female predominance (female to male ratio, 3:1), and patients typically show symptoms in the fifth and sixth decades. In addition to biliary colic, complications of gallstone disease (acute cholecystitis, choledocholithiasis, acute pancreatitis, gallstone ileus, etc.) may also lead to the diagnosis.

Bacteria are found in cultured bile in 11% to 30% of cases, with a flora similar to that discussed in the section concerning acute cholecystitis (21). The identification (mainly by polymerase chain reaction and rarely by histology) of several bile-resistant *Helicobacter* species from gallbladder bile (even though they are considered secondary invaders) in cases of chronic cholecystitis has emphasized the need for further investigation of the microecology of bile in health and disease (23,24). Very rarely, *Giardia lamblia* may be found just above the surface epithelium in cases of chronic cholecystitis, particularly in patients with IgA deficiency, achlorhydria, or malabsorption (4). *Salmonella typhi* may be present in the gallbladder in chronic carrier states. Chronic cholecystitis, often with prominent lymphoid aggregates (follicular cholecystitis; see discussion below), is frequently noted.

Pathologic Features

The pathologic correlate of biliary colic is part of the spectrum of chronic cholecystitis; however, there is little correlation between the severity of the symptoms and the histologic findings (13). The macroscopic features vary according to several factors, including the degree of outlet obstruction, inflammation, and fibrosis (4). The gallbladder is often contracted, although it may be normal or even increased in size. The wall is variably thickened, and adhesions may be noted on its external surface (Fig. 6A). A pearly white appearance is typical of the radiodense porcelain gallbladder. The importance of this unusual condition, found in less than 0.5% of cholecystectomies, is its association with gallbladder carcinoma (about 20% of cases; see discussion below) (4,25). Prophylactic cholecystectomy is recommended for this condition.

As with acute cholecystitis, the histopathologic findings of chronic cholecystitis demonstrate a spectrum of changes (Fig. 6B). The mucosal folds may be flattened, ulcerated, or normal. The amount and distribution of chronic inflammation (patchy vs. diffuse, mucosal vs. transmural), mural fibrosis, and endarteritis obliterans are all quite variable.

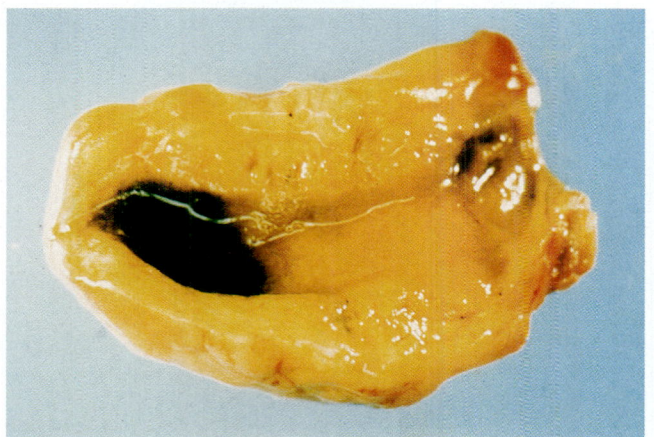

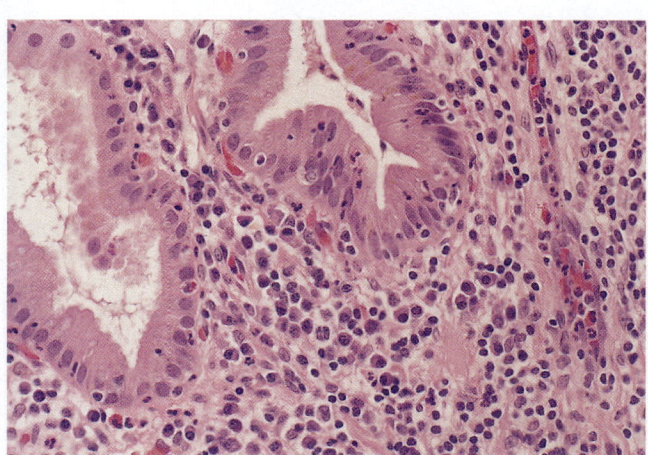

FIG. 6. Chronic cholecystitis. **A:** Marked thickening of the gallbladder wall, as seen in this photograph, may simulate carcinoma. **B:** Mild chronic inflammation, several Rokitansky-Aschoff sinuses, and modest smooth-muscle hypertrophy in a typical case of chronic cholecystitis. **C:** Chronic active (neutrophils, particularly intraepithelial) cholecystitis with prominence of lamina propria plasma cells. Particularly when these histologic features are diffuse and superficial and occur in an acalculous gallbladder, the possibility of primary sclerosing cholangitis or another cause of extrahepatic bile duct obstruction should be considered.

Mononuclear cells, particularly T lymphocytes, predominate, with lesser numbers of plasma cells and histiocytes. An inconsistent number of eosinophils may be present (26). In 20% of cholecystectomy specimens in one study, only a few scattered lymphocytes were found (26). The dividing line, on histologic examination, between minimal chronic cholecystitis and the normal gallbladder is debatable; diagnostic category used at the time of case signout varies among different observers in my experience (Fig. 1).

When intraepithelial neutrophils are noted, the term chronic active cholecystitis can be used, which is analogous to terminology used at other gastrointestinal sites (Fig. 6C). In the absence of gallbladder stones, this feature may suggest CBD obstruction of varied origin (27). A diagnosis of dysplasia should be made only with great caution, when there is extensive ulceration or acute inflammation (Fig. 5) (6). An abundance of plasma cells, particularly in an acalculous gallbladder, warrants exclusion of PSC (Fig. 6C) (see The Gallbladder in Extrahepatic Bile Duct Obstruction and Chronic Cholestatic Disorders) (27,28). In rare cases of chronic cholecystitis there may be a discontinuous band of collagen under the surface epithelium, similar to that seen in collagenous colitis (personal observation). The clinical significance of this finding, if any, is unknown.

Rokitansky-Aschoff sinuses represent diverticular herniations of the epithelium mucosa into and through the muscular layer and are found in about 90% of cases of chronic cholecystitis (Fig. 6). They often contain inspissated bile and may rupture, forming localized bile granulomas. In the normal gallbladder these sinuses are few in number and only infrequently penetrate into the smooth muscle (2). The adjacent muscular layer is often thickened. Hyperplastic and metaplastic (pyloric, gastric surface-like, intestinal) changes in the mucosa are not uncommon (discussed later on p. 17). Elastic tissue deposition may be quite pronounced in the muscular and/or perimuscular connective tissue layers. Neuromatous hyperplasia and amputation neuromas with a similar mural distribution have also been reported. Extensive mural deposition of hyalinized collagen, with foci of dystrophic calcification, characterize the porcelain gallbladder. Patients in whom the mucosa has been denuded may be at lower risk of carcinoma (29).

Chronic cholecystitis demonstrates poorly formed lymphoid aggregates in about 5% of cases. This feature is usually distinguishable from the less common (0.4%) finding of many well-formed lymphoid follicles, with germinal centers, located throughout the gallbladder wall (follicular cholecystitis) (30). On macroscopic examination, the follicles may appear as elevations of the mucosa 1 mm to several millimeters in size and are sometimes termed lymphoid polyps (see Table 4). This condition has been described more often in patients with typhoid fever, and it also has been reported in patients with PSC (30,31).

Adenomyomatous Hyperplasia (Adenomyomatosis)

Adenomyomatous hyperplasia, sometimes referred to as "diverticular disease of the gallbladder," is an acquired condition characterized by numerous extensions of the surface epithelium into, and often beyond, the thickened gallbladder muscular layer (Rokitansky-Aschoff sinuses). Inspissated bile concretions may be found within the diverticula. Varying degrees of epithelial hyperplasia are typically present; less frequently, metaplastic changes are noted (3,4,6,32). Distinguishing the condition from chronic cholecystitis can be somewhat arbitrary; however, the diagnosis of adenomyomatous hyperplasia should not be used for the finding of an isolated Rokitansky-Aschoff sinus. It has been reported with varying rates of frequency in cholecystectomy specimens (<1–33%), depending on the criteria employed for diagnosis. Symptomatic cases in the absence of gallstones have been cured by cholecystectomy; however, the majority of cases are asymptomatic.

Adenomyomatous hyperplasia can be divided into generalized (diffuse or cholecystitis glandularis proliferans), segmental, or localized (adenomyoma) types (Fig. 7). In the generalized and segmental types, the wall may be up to five times normal thickness and possess a velvety mucosal surface. Nearly all cases of the localized form are found in the fundus. In this type, the nodules vary from 0.5 to 2.5 cm in diameter and have a gray-white cut surface that often contains multiple cysts (Table 4). The nodules are unencapsulated and may be entirely subserosal (3). Inversion of the gallbladder is a possible complication (33).

At the microscopic level, glands lined by columnar to cuboidal epithelium are embedded in bundles of smooth muscle. The surface epithelium, which does not necessarily communicate with the underlying glands, frequently has a papillary configuration. The circumscribed nature of the lesion, the lack of nuclear atypia, and the intimate relationship with smooth muscle distinguish this lesion from carcinoma, although the presence of reactive epithelial atypia may make this distinction quite difficult in rare instances. Dysplasia and adenocarcinoma have now and then been reported in association with adenomyomatous hyperplasia (34,35). While perineural and intraneural invasion is generally an excellent indicator of malignancy in the biliary tree, these features have been reported in this benign condition, akin to entrapment of benign epithelial elements at other sites, such as the breast and pancreas (36).

Although chronic cholecystitis, often of mild degree, has been noted in more than 80% of cases of adenomyomatous hyperplasia, the association with cholelithiasis has been less consistent. Most investigators believe the mucosal (pseudo)diverticula are related to increased intraluminal pressure resulting from abnormal muscle contractility, but they may be primary phenomena.

Other Forms of Cholecystitis

AIDS-related Cholecystitis

In the largest reported series of cholecystectomy specimens in patients with AIDS, French et al. (37) found that 93% of resected gallbladders showed evidence of cholecys-

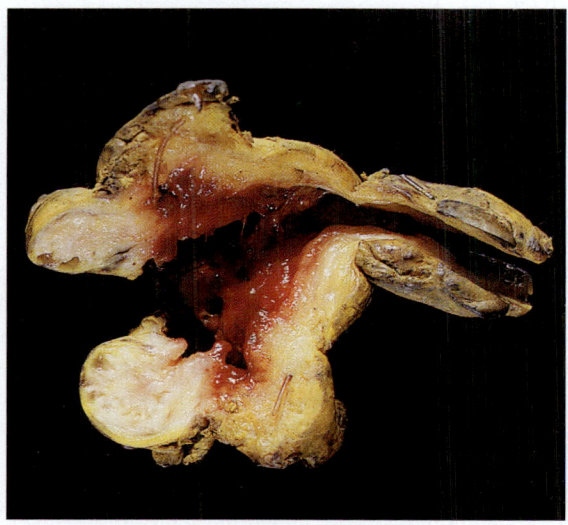 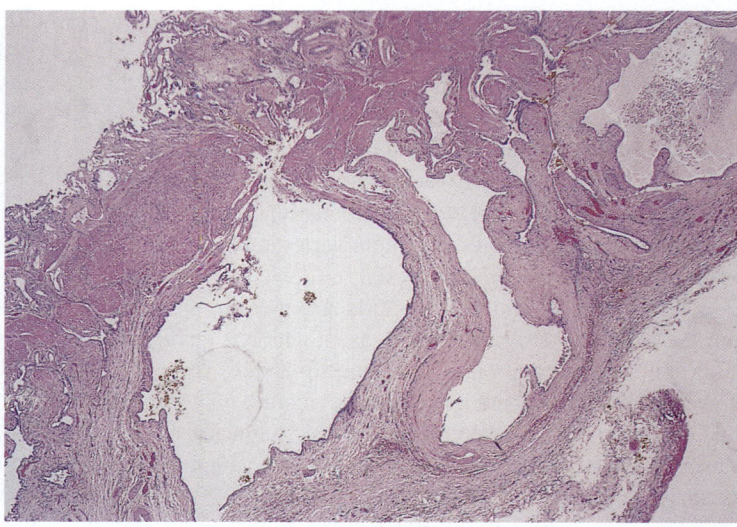

FIG. 7. Adenomyoma. **A:** Typical fundal location. Note the cystic nature and adjacent thickening (muscular) of the gallbladder wall. **B:** Proliferation of epithelium and smooth muscle with formation of irregular glandular spaces (cystically dilated Rokitansky-Aschoff sinuses).

titis; 73% of cases were acalculous, and 53% of these were idiopathic (Table 2). Opportunistic infection was found in nearly 40% of all cases, but in only 7% was the gallbladder the initial site at which the organism was detected. Opportunistic infections were absent in 29 patients infected with the human immunodeficiency virus (but who were not classified as having AIDS by Centers for Disease Control and Prevention criteria). Cryptosporidia (Fig. 8), CMV, microsporidia, and other pathogens were found, respectively, in 23%, 21%, 8%, and 2% of all AIDS cases, and the incidence of combined CMV/cryptosporidia infection was higher than that of each organism alone. Microsporidia (more commonly *Enterocytozoon bieneusi* than *Septata intestinalis*) were nearly always identified on hematoxylin and eosin–stained sections. It should be remembered that *S. intestinalis* may be found within both epithelium and lamina propria macrophages. The histologic findings can be subtle, as evidenced by the fact that 15% of cases originally diagnosed as

TABLE 2. *Results of cholecystectomy in 107 patients with AIDS*

Histologic finding	Number (%)
Normal gallbladder	7 (6%)
Cholesterolosis alone	1 (1%)
Cholecystitis	99 (93%)
Acalculous	72 (73%)
Idiopathic	38 (53%)
Opportunistic infection	34 (47%)
Calculous	27 (27%)
Gallstones only	21 (78%)
Opportunistic infection	6 (22%)
Acute; acute/chronic	16 (16%)
Chronic	83 (84%)
Minimal/mild	34 (41%)
Moderate/severe	49 (59%)
Opportunistic infection	39 (39%)
Cryptosporidium + CMV	15 (15%)
Cryptosporidium alone	8 (8%)
Microsporidia[a]	8 (8%)
CMV alone	6 (6%)
Isospora belli	1 (1%)
Pneumocystis carinii	1 (1%)
Kaposi's sarcoma	1 (1%)

AIDS, acquired immunodeficiency syndrome; CMV, cytomegalovirus.

[a] *Enterocytozoon bieneusi*, six cases; *Septata intestinalis*, two cases.

Adapted from ref. 37.

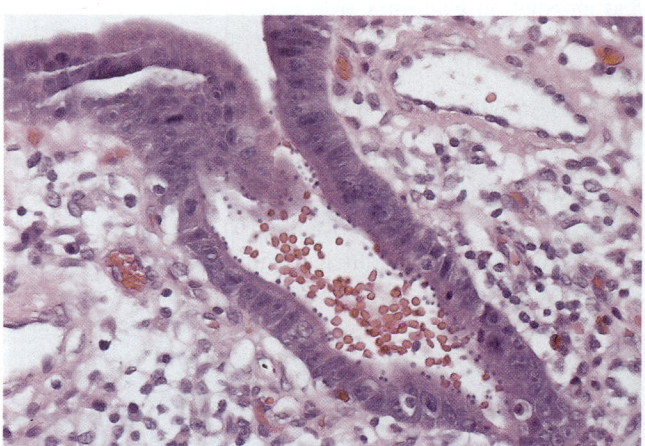

FIG. 8. Cryptosporidiosis (AIDS patient). Note the numerous small, round, basophilic organisms closely apposed to the luminal border of the gallbladder epithelium. This parasite is responsible for the single most common type of opportunistic infection, either alone or in association with CMV, seen in the gallbladder in AIDS patients. (Kindly contributed by Min Sohn, M.D., Graduate Hospital, Philadelphia.)

idiopathic acalculous cholecystitis showed evidence of microsporidia on review. Histopathologic changes were most marked in gallbladders demonstrating CMV; in these cases, erosions and deep ulcers were readily evident. In other studies, *Candida albicans* and the *Mycobacterium avium complex* have also been described.

Eosinophilic Cholecystitis

Since about 20% of resected gallbladders have eosinophils and a prominence of eosinophils in an otherwise polymorphic infiltrate is a relatively common finding in organizing (subacute) acute cholecystitis, it has been suggested that the term eosinophilic cholecystitis should be restricted to an inflammatory infiltrate composed nearly entirely of eosinophils (Fig. 9) (26). This variant is uncommon, found in less than 1% to just over 5% of surgically resected gallbladders. The figure approaches 15% if all cases in which the inflammatory infiltrate is composed of more than 50% eosinophils are included. The infiltrate often involves the muscular layer, but it may be transmural or restricted to the mucosa. There may be associated fibroblastic proliferation (4,26). The pericystic duct lymph node may also demonstrate prominent eosinophils. While most patients have gallstones, acalculous cases also occur.

A localized idiosyncratic reaction to biliary contents may be responsible for the tissue eosinophilia in most cases; however, associations with several drugs/therapies (erythromycin, ampicillin, cephalosporins, interleukin-2 plus lymphokine-activated killer cells), peripheral eosinophilia, hypereosinophilic syndrome, atopy, eosinophilic enterocolitis or appendicitis, parasitic infection, and/or biliary obstruction (eosinophilic cholangitis) have been reported (4,26,38–40). It is probably wise for pathologists to check the peripheral blood eosinophil count and correlate it with clinical data when eosinophils are conspicuous, because they may be the first clinicians to suspect the possibility of a systemic syndrome (Fig. 9). Gallbladder involvement by granulomatous angiitis with eosinophilia (Churg-Strauss syndrome) should be distinguished from eosinophilic cholecystitis where vasculitis is absent (41).

Xanthogranulomatous Cholecystitis and Related Lesions

Xanthogranulomatous cholecystitis is a variant of chronic cholecystitis (nearly always with cholelithiasis) found in 0.5% to 1.8% of all surgically excised gallbladders (6,26, 42,43). Although small intramural foci containing foamy (cholesterol) macrophages or macrophages laden with pigment (ceroid, bile, less frequently iron), bile, cholesterol clefts and multinucleated giant cells (foreign body or Touton types) can be found in the usual case of chronic cholecystitis, in up to 10% of cases these deposits can be detected macroscopically and simulate a neoplasm (Fig. 10). The lesions appear on gross examination as yellow-brown, well-demarcated foci of mural thickening, with or without ulceration, varying in size up to 3 cm in diameter. Sessile masses occasionally protrude into the lumen.

At the microscopic level, the infiltrate has been described as focal, multinodular, or diffuse. In addition to the above-mentioned histiocytes, it also contains variable numbers of lymphocytes, plasma cells, and neutrophils. The terms chole- and cholecystic granuloma have been used for these lesions; however, the more descriptive phrases xanthogranulomatous cholecystitis, foreign body granuloma, and ceroid granuloma emphasize the predominant component in a given lesion. Ulceration of the gallbladder mucosa and/or rupture of Rokitansky-Aschoff sinuses with extravasation of bile represent the inciting events. Rare cases with Michaelis-Gutman bodies have been described, justifying a diagnosis of malacoplakia (44). Some authors believe infection plays a role, because xanthogranulomatous inflammatory infiltrates have been associated with bacterial infection in the kidney and at other sites. The association between xanthogranulomatous cholecystitis and gallbladder adenocarcinoma appears to be a chance event (43).

The differential diagnosis includes carcinoma, sarcoma (particularly malignant fibrous histiocytoma), inflammatory myofibroblastic tumor (inflammatory pseudotumor), and other granulomatous processes. The cytologically bland nature of the infiltrate and awareness that this entity exists will prevent misdiagnosis as malignancy. There is overlap with inflammatory myofibroblastic tumor, and classification probably represents differences in semantics in cases with prominent (myo)fibroblastic proliferation (45). Granulomas associated with *M. tuberculosis*, fungi, Crohn's disease, primary biliary cirrhosis (PBC), and various parasites have rarely been reported in the gallbladder (4,46,47). The histologic appearance of infectious granulomas is different from xanthogranulomatous cholecystitis, and organisms can be demonstrated

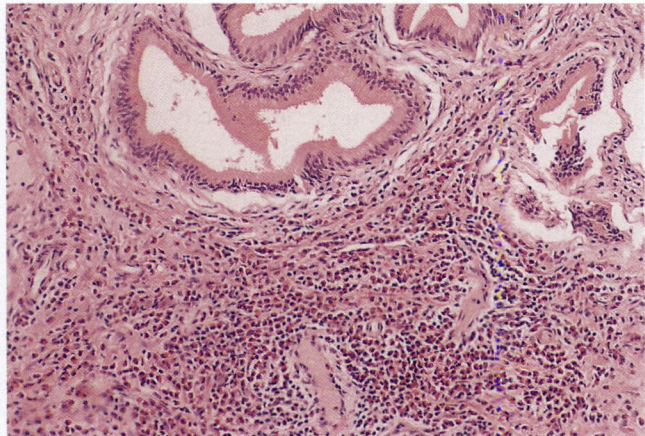

FIG. 9. Eosinophilic cholecystitis. Note the nearly "pure" infiltrate of eosinophils. The peripheral blood white blood cell count was found to be 10,000, with 19% eosinophils. Subsequent workup led to upper endoscopy and biopsy; the diagnosis was eosinophilic gastroenteritis. This is the exception, not the rule, in cases of eosinophilic cholecystitis.

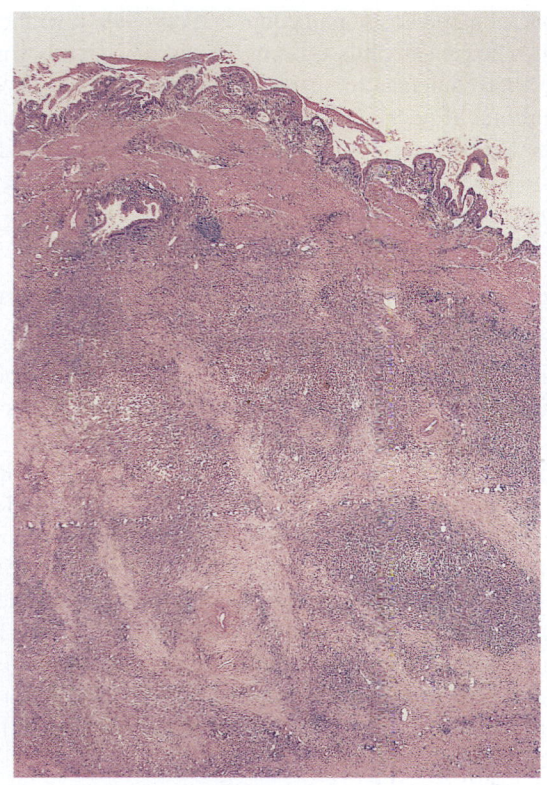
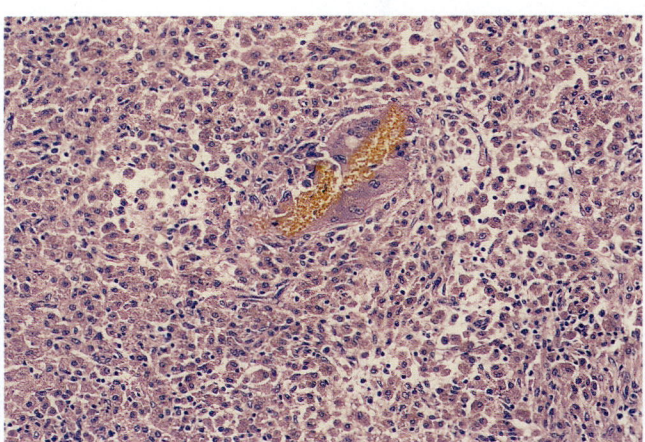

FIG. 10. Xanthogranulomatous cholecystitis. **A:** Low-power view. A pattern of usual chronic cholecystitis is evident, with Rokitansky-Aschoff sinus, muscular hypertrophy, chronic inflammation, and fibrosis. The gallbladder wall also shows signs of a dense cellular infiltrate. **B:** High-power view. The dense cellular infiltrate consists of numerous foamy macrophages. Near the center of the photomicrograph, multinucleated giant cells are seen engulfing bile.

by special stains and/or culture. Granulomatous vasculitis with eosinophilia has also been reported (41). Melanosis of the gallbladder displays a lipofuscin-like pigment within the lining epithelium and, less commonly, in macrophages in the underlying lamina propria (4). These features and the absence of a significant mural inflammatory reaction are quite distinct from xanthogranulomatous cholecystitis.

The Gallbladder in Extrahepatic Bile Duct Obstruction and Chronic Cholestatic Disorders

Patients with PSC often have abnormal gallbladders, although the prevalence of cholelithiasis is only 9% to 26% (28,48). Except for Jessurun et al. (28), investigators have not been able to readily distinguish diseased gallbladders in PSC patients from those in patients with chronic calculous cholecystitis or with PBC (28,47–50). This discrepancy may have to do with the diagnostic criteria employed or the number of gallbladders evaluated. Lymphoid aggregates have variably been found to be more common in gallbladders of PSC patients versus those with PBC or chronic calculous cholecystitis, but this is of little diagnostic value. Jeffrey et al. (47) found prominent intraepithelial lymphocytosis (T cells; "lymphocytic cholecystitis") in three of six patients with PSC, but this finding was also noted in a patient with PBC. Now and then, granulomas have been reported in gallbladders of patients with PBC (47).

Jessurun et al. have suggested that the presence of a diffuse, bandlike, superficial, chronic inflammatory infiltrate with a predominance of plasma cells is specific to PSC; however, less than 50% of PSC patients showed signs of this constellation of findings (28) (Fig. 6C). It is prudent for the pathologist to check the clinical history and laboratory data, looking for a history of ulcerative colitis and/or chronic serum alkaline phosphatase elevation in patients with these findings, particularly in an acalculous gallbladder. Moreover, the presence of chronic "active" (intraepithelial neutrophils) cholecystitis in an acalculous gallbladder should suggest the possibility of PSC as well as other nonneoplastic (choledocholithiasis) or neoplastic forms of extrahepatic bile duct obstruction (27). Benign and malignant epithelial neoplasms of the gallbladder and biliary tree are seen with increased frequency in patients with PSC; therefore, the gallbladders of these patients must be carefully evaluated (50) (see Primary Sclerosing Cholangitis).

Vasculitis

Vasculitis is a rare finding associated with cholecystitis (41, 51,52). Only 20% of patients have gallstones or sludge. The vasculitis is most often limited to the gallbladder, although it may be associated with synchronous or subsequent systemic involvement. Polyarteritis nodosa, which is seen to involve the gallbladder at autopsy in 10% to 40% of cases (51), is the most common type, representing 60% of cases in one series (41). Systemic vasculitis is most likely to develop in patients who also have connective tissue disease and/or elevated autoantibody titers; a patient with cryoglobulinemia has been reported (51).

Other reported types of gallbladder vasculitis include small-vessel vasculitis (often leukocytoclastic), Churg-Strauss angiitis (granulomatous angiitis with eosinophilia), and phlebitis (predominance of lymphocytes, occasionally a granulomatous component with giant cells) (Fig. 11) (41). Phlebitis appears to be a localized phenomenon. Chemical cholecystitis and vasculitis have been noted as complications of intrahepatic arterial chemotherapy (52). Nuclear atypia of the stromal and epithelial cells may be conspicuous findings in such cases. Secondary vascular damage, which may lead to luminal obliteration, is common in cholecystitis, as it is in other disorders where inflammation and ulceration are prominent features. Compared with primary vasculitis, it is present in proportion to the degree of mural inflammatory change and is not found in areas of the gallbladder that are normal or nearly normal.

Papillary Hyperplasia, Metaplasia, and Dysplasia

Papillary Hyperplasia

Papillary (villous) hyperplasia has been separated into the rare primary type (<1% of routine cholecystectomy specimens) and the much more frequently encountered secondary type, which has been reported in association with inflammatory disorders (chronic cholecystitis/cholelithiasis, adenomyomatous hyperplasia, PSC, ulcerative colitis) and cholesterolosis (6,53–55) (Table 3, Fig. 12A). An association with anomalous arrangement of the pancreaticobiliary duct (AAPBD) has also been described; it is unclear what percentage of these cases had been classified as primary or secondary (53a). Secondary hyperplasia has been reported in

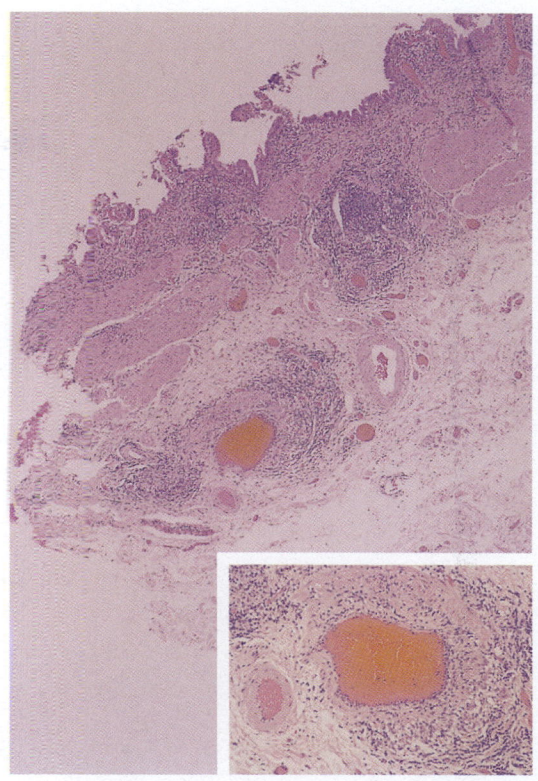

FIG. 11. Phlebitis (lymphocytic and granulomatous). Note the inflammatory infiltrate involving vein and sparing artery in the perimuscular layer. Associated chronic cholecystitis is present. Inset: Lymphocytic and granulomatous infiltrate in the vein wall. This is a rare finding within the gallbladder. To date, it appears to be a localized phenomenon; however, as with other forms of gallbladder vasculitis, the possibility of systemic disease should always be considered.

TABLE 3. *Papillary hyperplasia, metaplasia, and dysplasia: classification, diagnostic features, and frequency*

Classification	Diagnostic features	Reported prevalence
Papillary hyperplasia	Papillary mucosal folds; single layer of bland columnar (biliary-type) epithelium	<1% (primary)[a] 5–100% (secondary)[b] 38.5–87% (AAPBD)[b]
Metaplasia		
Pyloric gland	Glands lined by flattened to columnar cells with large quantities of cytoplasmic mucin	66–84%[a]
Gastric surface	Tall columnar cells with basal nuclei and conspicuous neutral cytoplasmic mucin replacing surface epithelium	25–50%[a]
Intestinal	Goblet cells, neuroendocrine cells, mucin-containing columnar cells, Paneth cells; rarely, nonmucin-containing absorptive cells with thick brush border	12–52%[a]
Squamous	Typical squamous mucosa	≤0.1%[a]
Dysplasia		
Low grade	Nuclear crowding, hyperchromatism, and elongation; nuclei confined to basal half of cell; pseudostratification; small nucleoli	<1–34% (~5–10%)[a]
High grade (includes CIS)	Nuclear/cytoplasmic ratio increased, nuclei often more rounded with prominent nucleoli, irregular nuclear membranes and chromatin clearing, often more pseudostratification	1.4–3.5%[a]

AAPBD, anomalous arrangement of the pancreaticobiliary duct; CIS, carcinoma *in situ*
[a] In consecutive cholecystectomies, without other associated conditions
[b] In particular conditions.

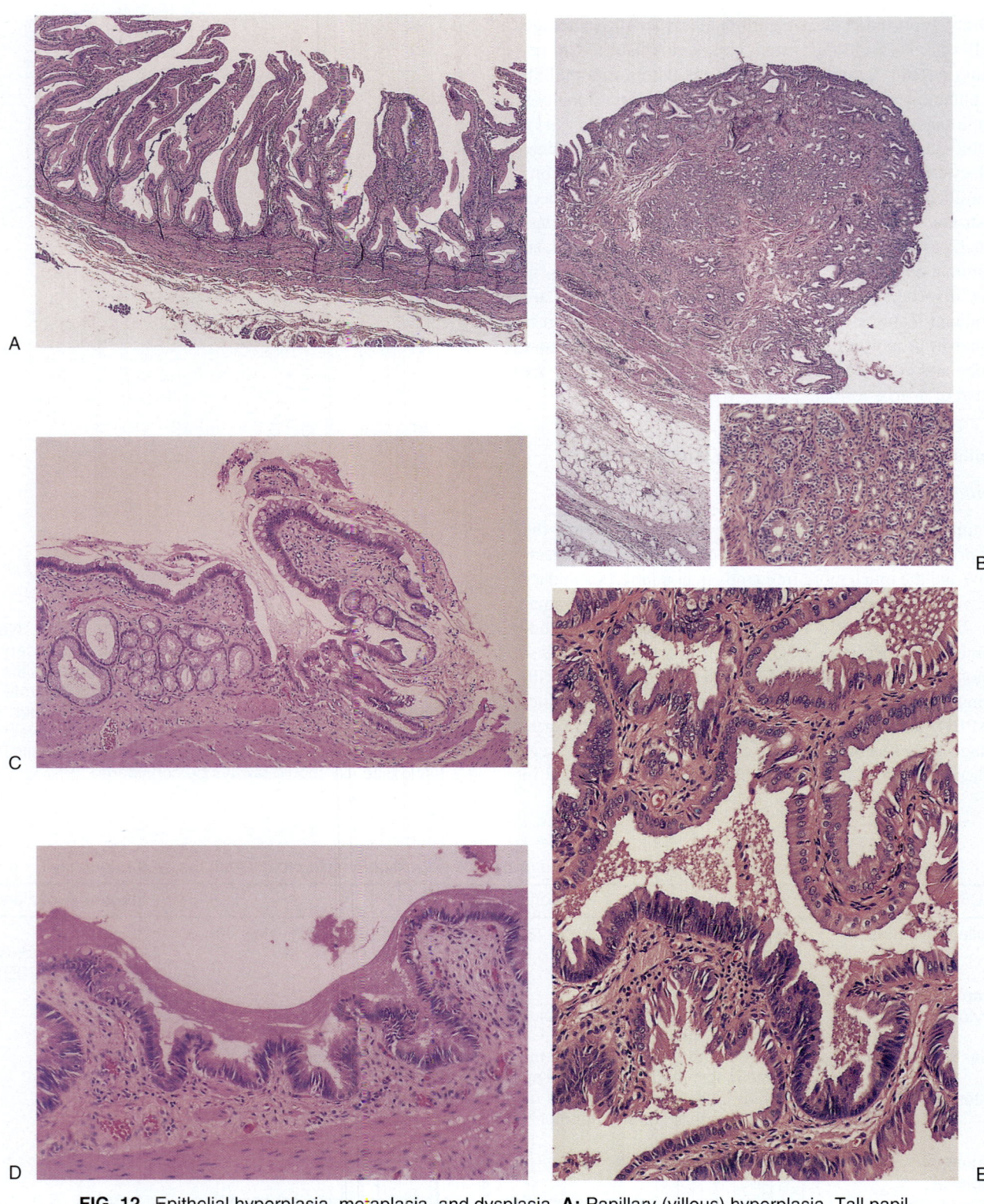

FIG. 12. Epithelial hyperplasia, metaplasia, and dysplasia. **A:** Papillary (villous) hyperplasia. Tall papillary projections of gallbladder epithelium. Note the bland cytologic features and basal orientation of nuclei. **B:** Pyloric metaplasia may be found in flat or polypoid mucosa. In this example, it is part of a hyperplastic polyp. The absence of dysplasia excludes tubular adenoma of the pyloric gland type. Inset: High-power view of pseudopyloric glands shows basal, sometimes flattened, nuclei and prominent cytoplasmic mucin content. **C:** Intestinal metaplasia. Also note the underlying metaplastic pyloric glands. **D:** Dysplasia, low grade. Crowding and hyperchromaticity of elongated nuclei are present within surface epithelium. **E:** Dysplasia, high grade. The nuclei featured just below the center of the photomicrograph are quite hyperchromatic, crowded, and stratified. Note the abrupt transition from adjacent nondysplastic epithelium.

5% to 22% of gallbladders with cholelithiasis and in up to 100% of those with cholesterolosis. AAPBD is found in 1% to 3% of patients undergoing ERCP and has been associated with papillary hyperplasia in 38.5% to 87% of patients, including children.

Papillary hyperplasia is not readily identified on casual macroscopic inspection, although with careful observation, a velvety mucosal thickening can often be detected. The secondary type has a focal or segmental distribution, while the primary type may also diffusely involve the gallbladder mucosa and even the extrahepatic bile ducts. At the microscopic level, elongated and crowded papillary mucosal folds are covered by a single layer of biliary-type columnar epithelium with basally situated nuclei. Although superimposed metaplasia and dysplasia may be found in the secondary type, they have not been described in cases of primary papillary hyperplasia. Prominent subnuclear vacuoles have been noted in primary papillary hyperplasia of the CBD, but they have not yet been reported in the gallbladder. A previously described "spongioid" or glandular pattern of mucosal hyperplasia most likely represents tangential sectioning of the papillary pattern. Hyperplasia in flat gallbladder epithelium has been reported, but it is poorly characterized. It is typified by mild crowding that can be seen adjacent to a mucosal erosion.

Metaplasia

Metaplastic epithelium in the gallbladder can be divided into two major groups, namely, gastric (pyloric gland and surface epithelial) and intestinal, although one must also consider the quite rare squamous variety (6,55–59) (Fig. 12B, C; Table 3). The changes increase in frequency with age, are more numerous in the context of gallstones, can be quite focal, and can involve any region of the organ.

Pyloric gland (pseudopyloric, antral, or mucous gland) metaplasia is most common—it is found in 66% to 84% of cholecystectomy specimens (Fig. 12B). Lobules of metaplastic pyloric glands are usually scattered in the lamina propria, although they may extend through the muscular layer. Small mucosal nodules or polyps may result, often associated with overlying papillary hyperplasia. They have often been reported in the literature as a form of hyperplastic polyp (Table 4) (60). The term adenoma should not be used in this context unless dysplasia is evident (see the section on adenoma); making the distinction may occasionally be difficult (55). The glands resemble gastric pyloric glands on microscopic, histochemical, and ultrastructural examination, but they differ in several respects from the mucous glands normally found in the gallbladder neck (see section on normal anatomy). The metaplastic glands are lined by cells with flattened to columnar, basally oriented nuclei and numerous apical mucin droplets.

Class III mucin and lysozyme, characteristic of gastric pyloric glands, have been demonstrated in all cases examined to date (58,61). While gastric pyloric glands contain only neutral mucin, histochemical analysis of pseudopyloric glands has verified neutral and, occasionally, sialo- and sulfomucins. Variations from the normal gastric antral cytoplasmic pepsinogen profile in some cases, as well as the finding of a small-intestinal mucin antigen in others, suggest that incomplete intestinal metaplasia occurs in the context of pseudopyloric metaplasia before it can be detected on morphologic grounds alone (61,62). Superimposed histologically identifiable intestinal metaplasia and/or dysplasia may also be seen.

Foci of gastric surface epithelial metaplasia are found somewhat less often than the pyloric type (59). On histologic inspection, these epithelial cells are taller and contain much more cytoplasmic mucin than those that normally line the gallbladder. Similarly to normal gastric lining cells, large quantities of neutral mucin are usually detected on histochemical study; however, the occasional finding of sialomucin again suggests the development of some degree of incomplete intestinal metaplasia (58). Normal gallbladder lining epithelium contains only sulfomucin (2).

Intestinal metaplasia represents replacement of the normal epithelium by cells with an intestinal phenotype (goblet cells, endocrine cells, Paneth cells, and absorptive cells, rarely with a distinct brush border) and has been reported in 12% to 52% of gallbladders removed for cholelithiasis or chronic cholecystitis (55,57–59) (Fig. 12C). The goblet cells typically contain sialomucin and initially appear at the tips of the mucosal folds. The intestinal cells extend laterally and downward, with glandlike structures expanding the lamina propria. Associated pyloric gland metaplasia is common. Serotonin-containing cells are the typical type of endocrine cells (59). Infrequently, intestinal metaplasia may form a polyp (55). Squamous metaplasia is rare (≤0.1% of cholecystectomy specimens) (3,4,63). It may be associated with porcelain gallbladder or squamous dysplasia or be found adjacent to invasive squamous cell carcinoma.

Dysplasia

Gallbladder dysplasia, as at other gastrointestinal sites, represents a neoplastic intraepithelial proliferation in which columnar or cuboidal cells (very rarely squamous cells) are characterized by a varying degree of nuclear pleomorphism and hyperchromatism, nucleolar enlargement, variation in nuclear/cytoplasmic ratio, cellular crowding, pseudostratification, and other architectural changes (3,6,64–72) (Fig. 12D, E; Table 3). It may be associated with or represent the superficial component of an invasive carcinoma.

Terms such as epithelial atypia, atypical hyperplasia, and atypical adenomatous hyperplasia have been employed in the past for dysplasia or related gallbladder findings, but their use should be abandoned. While the World Health Organization classification distinguishes dysplasia from carcinoma *in situ* (CIS) (6), gastrointestinal pathologists tend to separate dysplasia into two grades—low and high—with the latter including CIS (73). There are no data that indicate any

TABLE 4. Benign polyps

Type	Diagnostic features Macroscopic	Diagnostic features Microscopic	Prevalence In consecutive cholecystectomy specimens	Prevalence Of benign polyps
All benign polyps			<1–10%	—
Nonneoplastic				90%
Cholesterol	1–15 mm, yellow, soft; typically multiple, pedunculated; may detach	Mucosal projections with numerous lipid-laden macrophages		50–90%
Hyperplastic/metaplastic	<5 mm, brown-gray, sessile or pedunculated; granular or villiform; usually multiple	Nodular proliferation of pyloric-type glands most common; focal papillary hyperplasia		25%
Adenomyoma	5–25 mm; located in fundus, typically in muscular layer; gray-white cystic cut surface	Cystically dilated glands embedded in bundles of smooth muscle		15–25%
Inflammatory	3–15 mm, red-gray-brown; typically single, sessile	Chronically inflamed granulation tissue; edematous or fibrous stroma; occasionally "phyllodes-like glands"		15%
Lymphoid	<5 mm; pale, round nodules; often 20 or more	Hyperplastic lymphoid follicles (follicular cholecystitis); germinal centers often poorly developed in muscle or adventitia		0–5%
Neoplastic				10%
Adenoma	3–25 mm, red-brown; 67–90% single; sessile or short stalk; papillary or smooth surface; "papillomatosis," numerous papillary adenomas	Tubular architecture with pyloric gland features most common; occasionally squamoid (spindle cell) or squamous metaplasia; papillary architecture typically with intestinal features; higher grades of dysplasia more common in papillary/intestinal types; invasive carcinoma rare if polyp is <1 cm		10%
Miscellaneous	Variable	Heterotopias, leiomyoma, granular cell tumor, etc.		<1%

clinical utility for either stratification schema in terms of cholecystectomy specimens, although both schema distinguish noninvasive neoplastic epithelium from invasive adenocarcinoma. It should be noted, however, that epidemiologic studies have included cases reported as CIS in the category "carcinoma," and Tis (in situ tumor) is a designation in the TMN staging system of gallbladder cancer (Table 5).

Although dysplastic foci can sometimes be identified as granular mucosal patches or mucosal excrescences on macroscopic examination, they are usually found only after evaluation of routine histologic sections. The dysplastic epithelium can be found in flat mucosa, line tubules or papillae, or extend into Rokitansky-Aschoff sinuses (Table 6) or metaplastic pyloric glands, in which case it can be misinterpreted as invasive adenocarcinoma (Fig. 16B). The lack of a desmoplastic stroma is a useful differentiating feature. A rare form of *in situ* signet ring cell carcinoma has been described (73a). Dysplastic cells contain neutral and sialomucins rather than sulfomucin, which is present in normal gallbladder epithelium. Goblet cells are evident in one-third of cases; less often, additional "intestinal" components (Paneth and neuroendocrine cells) or an appearance resembling colonic dysplasia is seen (65).

Reported rates of dysplasia in series of consecutive cholecystectomy specimens vary from less than 1% (70) up to 34% (Table 3) (64,69,71,72). Reasons for the wide discrepancy include the patient populations studied, the number of sections examined, and the criteria for histologic diagnosis. Severe dysplasia or CIS was found in only 1.4% to 3.5% of cases in the two series with the highest rates of dysplasia (64,71). As with the problems often encountered in inflammatory bowel disease, the distinction of true dysplastic (neoplastic) changes from reactive epithelial atypia in the context

TABLE 5. *TNM staging of gallbladder carcinoma*

TNM staging	Definition	% in surgical series	5-year survival rate after surgical resection
Primary tumor (T)			
TX	Primary tumor cannot be assessed	—	—
Tis	Carcinoma in situ (high-grade dysplasia)	1.4–3.5%	100%
T1	Tumor invades lamina propria or muscle layer	5–10%	55–100%
	T1a tumor invades lamina propria	—	90–100%
	T1b tumor invades muscular layer	—	55–75%
T2	Tumor invades perimuscular connective tissue, no extension beyond serosa or into liver	10–15%	15–65%
T3	Tumor perforates the serosa or directly invades one adjacent organ or both findings (extension ≤2 cm into liver	15–30%	10–25%
T4	Tumor extends >2 cm into liver and/or into two adjacent organs	50–65%	2–25%
Regional lymph nodes (N)			
NX	Regional lymph nodes cannot be assessed		
N0	No regional lymph node metastases		
N1	Metastases in cystic duct, pericholedochal, and/or hilar lymph nodes		
N2	Metastases in peripancreatic (head only) periduodenal, periportal, celiac, and/or superior mesenteric lymph nodes		
Distant metastases (M)			
MX	Distant metastases cannot be assessed		
M0	No distant metastases		
M1	Distant metastases		
Stage grouping			
0	Tis, N0, M0		
I	T1, N0, M0		
II	T2, N0, M0		
III	T1, N1, M0; T2, N1, M0; T3, N0 or N1, M0		
IVA	T4, N0 or 1, M0		
IVB	Any T, N2, M0; any T, any N, M1		

Staging system adapted from ref. 103. Survival data estimated from refs. 85, 86, 95, 107, 108 and other articles in the literature. Variability in survival data depends on case selection, stage, type of surgical procedure including extent of lymph node dissection, and thoroughness of gallbladder sectioning by the pathologist.

of cholecystitis can sometimes be a problem, and it is likely that many cases previously reported as dysplasia would now be regarded as reactive in nature (Table 6) (3,6,65,70). Since the gallbladder has been removed, this is generally an academic issue unless the cystic duct margin is involved.

Reactive/regenerative changes demonstrate a heterogeneous cell population, including atypical as well as atrophic and pencil-like cells, and lack the abrupt transition from normal epithelium that is seen in dysplasia. Reactive epithelial atypia is characterized by cells with large vesicular nuclei with some degree of hyperchromasia, prominent nucleoli, and, often, basophilic cytoplasm. Mitotic figures are common. The epithelial atypia tends to be proportional to the degree of reactive stromal atypia. A diagnosis of dysplasia should be made only with great caution when there is extensive ulceration or acute inflammation (6). DNA ploidy studies performed in paraffin-embedded material do not appear to be helpful in distinguishing dysplasia from reactive atypia (65). When dysplasia is found in a routine section of a gallbladder, the gross specimen should be reevaluated and the organ extensively sectioned to exclude invasive carcinoma. Some investigators prefer the "jelly-roll technique" (3). Gallbladder aspiration may detect dysplastic cells (3,6).

(Hyperplasia) Metaplasia-Dysplasia-Carcinoma Sequence

As at other sites, such as the stomach, esophagus, and bile ducts, a metaplasia-nonpolypoid dysplasia-carcinoma sequence appears to be the major pathway to invasive gallbladder carcinoma (59,66,70,71,74,75). The importance of epithelial hyperplasia in this cascade of events is unclear, although the high rate of associated papillary hyperplasia (38–87%) in AAPBD and the increased incidence of associated gallbladder carcinoma (15–77% of patients) in this condition are of interest (53a). Recent work reporting higher proliferative activity and K-ras mutation in AAPBD-related hyperplastic epithelium requires further study (53a).

Metaplastic and high-grade dysplastic mucosa have been seen adjacent to gallbladder carcinoma in 73% to 92% and 85% of cases, respectively. The relative importance of pyloric versus intestinal metaplasia in this sequence is contro-

TABLE 6. *Microscopic staging of gallbladder carcinoma: problems and solutions*

Primary tumor (T)	Problem	Solution
Tis vs. reactive	Reactive epithelial atypia vs. carcinoma in situ (high-grade dysplasia)	A problem generally more of academic and epidemiologic interest than of clinical importance since the gallbladder has been removed. Heterogeneity of the epithelial atypia, lack of abrupt transition from normal epithelium, and presence of stromal atypia and associated acute inflammation and ulceration all favor a reactive process.
Tis/T1 vs. T2	Understaging may result from inadequate sampling	When considering a diagnosis of Tis or T1, the gallbladder should be extensively sampled and sometimes entirely submitted.
Tis vs. T1a	In situ carcinoma/high-grade dysplasia vs. lamina propria invasion	The presence of a stromal reaction and/or single infiltrating tumor cells indicates lamina propria invasion. Other features, such as a complicated glandular architecture, are subjective, as is the case with similar assessments at other gastrointestinal sites.
Tis vs. T1b/T2	Dysplasia/in situ carcinoma involving Rokitansky-Aschoff sinuses vs. invasion of muscular or perimuscular layers	Infiltrative pattern of small glands parallel, rather than perpendicular, to surface, as well as desmoplastic stroma favor invasive carcinoma.
T1b vs. T2	Mural fibrosis obliterates distinction of muscular and perimuscular layers	Look for areas of wall uninvolved by tumor, and extrapolate from these regions. Reporting depth of invasion in millimeters, as measured from the surface, may give the best estimate of depth of mural penetration in some instances.

versial; however, dysplasia can be found in both types of epithelium (56,65,66,71). Expression of p53 protein has been identified by immunohistochemistry in 0%, 0%, 0% to 33%, 46%, and 40% to 92% of cases of normal epithelium, metaplasia, dysplasia, CIS, and gallbladder carcinoma, respectively (76,76a). Loss of heterozygosity (LOH) of p53 and DCC genes, however, has been detected in normal and metaplastic epithelium, suggesting that molecular abnormalities may precede histologic/immunohistochemical changes (76a). Kozuka et al. suggested that an adenoma (polypoid dysplasia)-carcinoma sequence, similar to that in the colon, may sometimes be operative in the gallbladder (67). "Malignant change," defined variably as CIS or invasive carcinoma in the literature, has been found in 10% to 39% of adenomas, while "adenomatous residue" has been detected in 8% to 9% of cases of invasive carcinoma (60,64,67,74). In the extensive experience of Albores-Saavedra and Henson, only four examples of invasive adenocarcinoma arising in adenoma were found (65). Given that gallbladder adenomas are less common than adenocarcinomas, they are unlikely to be precursor lesions in most instances and, therefore, appear to play a minor role in the pathogenesis of gallbladder carcinoma.

Tumors

Benign Polyps

General Considerations

The prevalence of benign gallbladder polyps in cholecystectomy specimens ranges from <1% to 10% (3,10,60, 77,78) (Table 4). In many early series, authors used the terms adenoma and papilloma rather indiscriminately, not necessarily distinguishing neoplastic from nonneoplastic polyps. Better use of standardized nomenclature has helped eliminate this problem (6). Gallbladder polyps are typically incidental findings, first detected at the time of ultrasonography, computed tomography, or cholecystectomy. Symptoms may result from associated cholelithiasis/cholecystitis or, rarely, from occlusion of the cystic duct by the polyp. Individual polyp types cannot reliably be distinguished by imaging studies, nor can they be separated from small invasive carcinomas (77,78). Cholecystectomy should be performed for all radiographically detected polyps 1 cm or more in diameter, to minimize the risk of malignancy. Smaller polyps unassociated with gallstones can be followed with ultrasound exams every 3 to 6 months (10).

Nonneoplastic Polyps

About 90% of benign gallbladder polyps are nonneoplastic, making up a histologically diverse group of innocuous, small (generally <1 cm) excrescences (4,10,55,60,77,78). Adenomyoma, which may be somewhat larger, has been discussed previously (see Adenomyomatous Hyperplasia). Cholesterol polyps account for 50% to 90% of benign polyps. While they occur in about 10% of patients with diffuse or fecal cholesterolosis (see Cholesterolosis), polyps are often, and perhaps even more commonly, found in the absence of a background of nonpolypsed cholesterolosis (4,55). They are best characterized as small (4–15 mm in diameter), multiple, soft, yellow, pedunculated, and often multilobulated (Fig. 3).

Their size is frequently overestimated by ultrasound, which is perhaps related to their multiplicity (77).

Hyperplastic/metaplastic polyps account for about 25% of benign polyps. They can be pedunculated or sessile, are typically multiple, and measure no more than 5 mm in diameter. They represent focal, elevated, granular or villiform foci in an otherwise hyperplastic/metaplastic mucosa (see earlier discussion of these topics). At the microscopic level, the polyp usually shows evidence of nodular hyperplasia of pyloric glands, although focal papillary hyperplasia or some combination of the two may be seen (Fig. 12B). Other histologic changes, such as intestinal metaplasia and/or dysplasia, may be superimposed on these lesions. Distinguishing this polyp from tubular adenoma of the pyloric gland type may occasionally be difficult (see Adenoma below). The absence of parietal and chief cells aids in making the distinction from gastric heterotopia. From time to time, intestinal metaplasia may form a nodule and hence be considered a polyp (55). A polypoid hyperplastic mucosal lesion with a "sea anemone–like" configuration has been described in a 2-year-old patient with metachromatic leukodystrophy (79).

Inflammatory polyps, representing 15% of benign polyps, demonstrate a spectrum of fibroinflammatory change stemming from cholecystitis (55,60). They are sessile, single or multiple, up to 1.5 cm in diameter, and similar in color to the surrounding mucosa. The characteristic histologic picture is that of chronically inflamed granulation tissue (granulation tissue polyp) that can have a variable lining of columnar epithelium or glands deep within the polyp. More abundant fibrous tissue, which may contain scattered ductlike structures reminiscent of a phyllodes tumor (fibrous polyp), may be found.

Lymphoid polyps are uncommon, pale, round, sessile or pedunculated mucosal elevations (up to 5 mm diameter) caused by hyperplastic lymphoid follicles typically seen on a background of follicular cholecystitis (30,55,60). Often 20 or more tiny nodules can be discerned on macroscopic examination. Germinal centers are more prominent superficially and may be more poorly developed in the muscular layer and adventitia. An association with nodular lymphoid hyperplasia of the small bowel has been reported on occasion. As is seen at other gastrointestinal sites with lymphoid hyperplasia, the overlying epithelium may show focal, mild, reactive nuclear atypia. The absence of both cytologic atypia and well-developed lymphoepithelial lesions, as well as the presence of germinal centers and polyclonality, aid in differentiating it from various types of non-large-cell lymphoma.

Neoplastic Polyps (Adenoma)

Adenomas, which by definition demonstrate at least low-grade dysplasia, are rare. They are found in about 0.5% of cholecystectomy specimens and make up 10% of all benign polyps (3,6,10,55,60,77). Now and then, they have been found in children (80). Adenomas have been reported in association with Gardner's syndrome, Peutz-Jeghers syndrome, and AAPBD (55). They have a short stalk or are sessile, are typically single (66–90%) and characteristically red-brown, and measure less than 2 cm in diameter. The surface may be smooth or mulberry-like or have a granular, papillary, or cauliflower-like appearance. When there are several, they can occupy a large portion of the mucosal surface. In "papillomatosis" (adenomatosis), the entire mucosal surface of the gallbladder may be replaced by several papillary adenomas; multicentric involvement of the extra- or intrahepatic bile ducts or pancreatic duct may also be found (6,55,81). Papillomatosis demonstrates a broad histologic spectrum of dysplasia (low to high grade) analogous to intraductal neoplasia within the main pancreatic duct (pancreatic intraductal papillary mucinous neoplasms), and, as is the case with its pancreatic analogue, it may be associated with invasive adenocarcinoma (3,6,55).

Adenomas can be divided by architectural features into tubular (80%), papillary (15%), and tubulopapillary (5%) types (6,55). They can be classified in cytologic terms as either pyloric gland or intestinal types. Ninety percent of tubular adenomas are the pyloric gland type, composed of closely packed, sometimes cystically dilated, dysplastic pyloric-type glands lined by columnar to cuboidal cells with vesicular or hyperchromatic nuclei (Fig. 13A). Distinguishing them from nodular pyloric gland hyperplasia remains quite subjective in cases with minimal cytologic atypia. Focal areas of intestinal metaplasia (20%), squamoid (spindle cell) morules (10–20%), or even frank squamous metaplasia (5%) may be seen (55,81a). They may extend into the Rokitansky-Aschoff sinuses. The remainder of the tubular adenomas resemble those found in the colon; they more often demonstrate high-grade dysplasia. Papillary (villous) adenomas contain a preponderance of papillary structures with fine or coarse connective tissue cores resembling those seen in the intestine (Fig. 13B). High-grade dysplasia is more usually found in papillary than tubular adenomas. In tubulovillous adenomas, papillary and tubular architecture each account for at least 20% of the polyp.

Because of the well-differentiated nature of many gallbladder carcinomas, distinguishing adenoma from noninvasive papillary carcinoma is subjective and arbitrary; the term adenoma is used infrequently in the literature for lesions larger than 20–25 mm in diameter or for those with high-grade dysplasia (3). Since the importance for the patient resides with the risk for metastasis regardless of the designation, the entire lesion should be submitted for microscopic examination to rule out invasion, and this analysis should be documented in the surgical pathology report. The relatively small role played by adenomas in the pathogenesis of gallbladder carcinoma is discussed in the section entitled (Hyperplasia) Metaplasia-Dysplasia-Carcinoma Sequence.

Other Benign Tumors

After excluding benign mucosal polyps and adenomyoma (which is often considered a polyp), the remaining benign

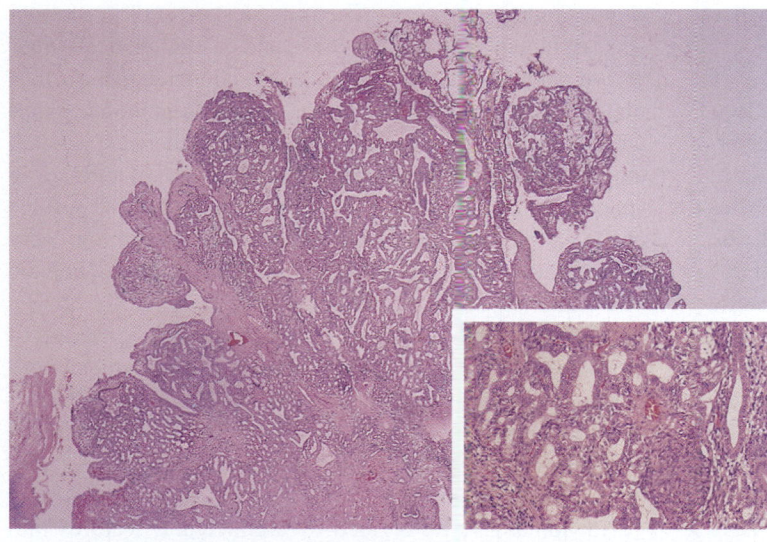
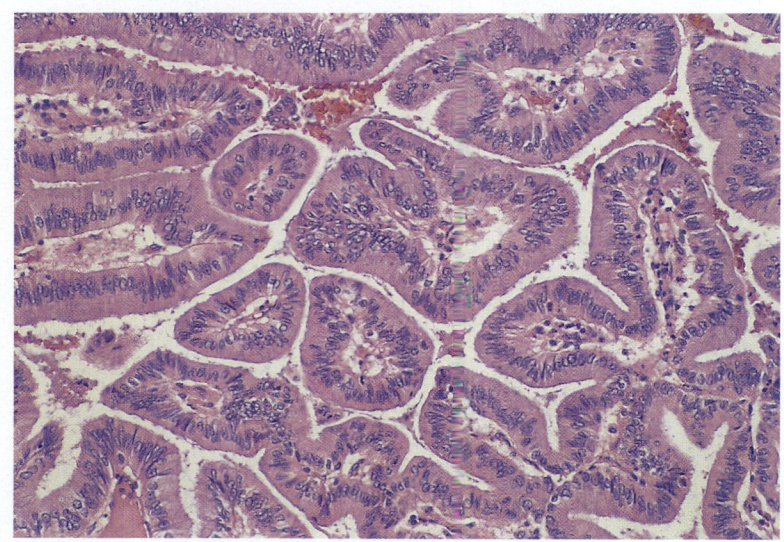

FIG. 13. A: Tubular adenoma, pyloric gland type with squamoid (spindle-cell) morule. Inset: Note the dysplastic nature of the epithelium and squamoid morule at the lower left. **B:** Papillary (villous) adenoma. Papillary proliferation of dysplastic epithelium. Adenomas must be entirely submitted to rule out invasive adenocarcinoma. The adjacent mucosa should be carefully evaluated to rule out multicentricity.

gallbladder masses are quite rare (<0.1% of cholecystectomy specimens) and do not cause diagnostic problems (10). Heterotopias, hemangioma, leiomyoma, lipoma, osteoma, granular cell tumor, paraganglioma, lymphangioma, ganglioneuromatosis (almost always in association with multiple endocrine neoplasia, type IIB), and other tumors have all been described (3,4,10,60,82). It is unclear whether some of the tumors termed neurofibromas in the literature are truly neoplasms or actually represent traumatic neuromas related to chronic cholecystitis or some other insult. Biliary cystadenomas, identical to those that more frequently arise in the liver and extrahepatic bile ducts, may now and then be found in the gallbladder (83).

Gallbladder Carcinoma

Clinical and Epidemiologic Factors

Carcinoma of the gallbladder is the most common malignancy of the biliary tract and the fifth most common malignancy of the gastrointestinal tract, with an incidence of 2.5 cases per 100,000 population per year (4,84–89). The incidence varies considerably worldwide and even within the same country among different ethnic groups. Higher rates are found in Chile, Mexico, Bolivia, and Japan, while in the U.S.A., Hispanic-Americans and southwestern Native Americans are affected more frequently. Gallbladder carcinoma is found in 1% to 2% and 0.1% of open and laparoscopic cholecystectomies, respectively, and causes 6,500 deaths annually in the United States. It is a disorder primarily of the elderly (mean age, 65 years; 90% are in their sixth decade or older). About 10% of gallbladders removed from patients more than 65 years of age harbor invasive carcinoma. This malignancy occurs more frequently in women (2–3:1), and cholelithiasis is found in 70% to 90% of patients. The risk of carcinoma developing in a patient with cholelithiasis is only 1% to 3%, but the risk appears to be higher when the stones are larger than 3 cm in diameter. Other associated conditions, which account for a minority of cases of gallbladder carcinoma, include porcelain gallbladder (4,25,84), Mirizzi syndrome (15A), AAPBD and choledochal cyst (53a,90–92), ulcerative colitis/PSC (50), familial adenomatous polyposis/Gardner's syndrome (93), and Peutz-Jeghers syndrome (94).

The clinical signs of gallbladder carcinoma mimic those of benign disease until the tumor invades surrounding structures, causing pain, jaundice, anorexia, and weight loss. By the time a correct preoperative diagnosis is made (about 50% of cases), the case is usually inoperable (95). Hypercalcemia, leukocytosis, and high serum levels of human chorionic gonadotropin and alpha-fetoprotein (73a) have all been reported, but rarely. Serum CEA and CA 19-9 levels are frequently elevated, but these markers lack specificity. Gallbladder carcinoma may even appear as an apparent primary tumor at another site, such as the ovary (96) or skin (97).

Although the collective experience with fine-needle aspiration (FNA) biopsy of the gallbladder is quite limited (98), one study of 88 patients with gallbladder masses yielded a sensitivity and specificity for carcinoma of 88.5% and 100%, respectively (99). Guided FNA of masses may play a role in confirming the diagnosis of malignancy in patients with advanced carcinoma and thus obviate the need for diagnostic laparotomy in this group. Problems with specimen adequacy and low sensitivity hinder the clinical utility of bile exfoliative cytology. An increasing number of small polypoid gallbladder carcinomas are being detected with ultrasonography; they make up 10% to 22% of all polyps in two series (see Benign Polyps for clinical management of gallbladder polyps) (10,77,78).

Pathologic Features

Macroscopic Appearance. The gross appearance of gallbladder carcinoma varies considerably. Small tumor nodules or thickened plaques may be indistinguishable from chronic cholecystitis and are first recognized by the pathologist serendipitously on examination of routine histologic sections (about 10–15% of cases). The majority of tumors grow as infiltrative gray-white masses, although papillary tumors typically form bulky intraluminal polypoid lesions (Fig. 14) (3,4,8–,100). While most tumors appear to originate in the fundus (60%), followed by the body (30%) and neck (10%), not infrequently the entire gallbladder wall may be involved (3,4). Because of local spread, it may be impossible to distinguish tumors arising in the gallbladder neck from those arising in the cystic duct. The gallbladder may appear distended (with or without hydrops) or contracted, depending on the presence or absence of cystic duct/gallbladder neck obstruction, the volume of intraluminal tumor, and the degree of desmoplastic response to mural invasion. Extension into the adjacent liver, which is present in about 80% of patients at the time of surgical evaluation, may result in encasement and even obliteration of the gallbladder (84,95).

Nearly all (98–99%) gallbladder malignancies are carcinomas, and 75–90% are pure adenocarcinomas (Fig. 15). Up to 75% of the latter are classified as well or moderately differentiated types, with variably sized glands that do not have distinctive features (73a,89). The superficial portion of gallbladder carcinoma is often well differentiated, while the

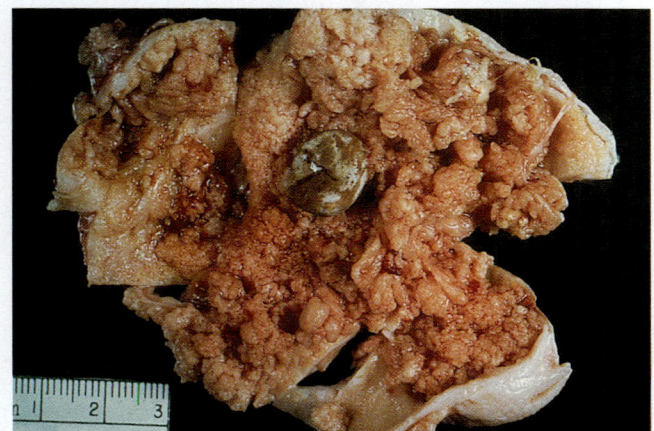

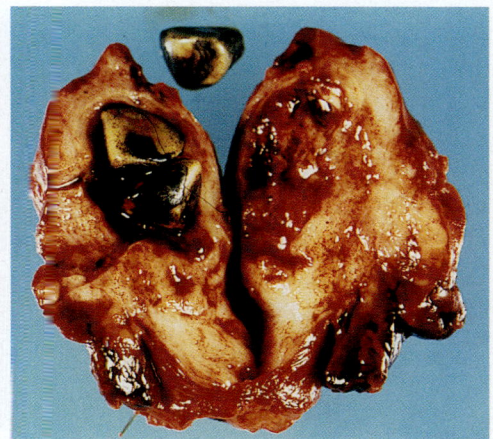

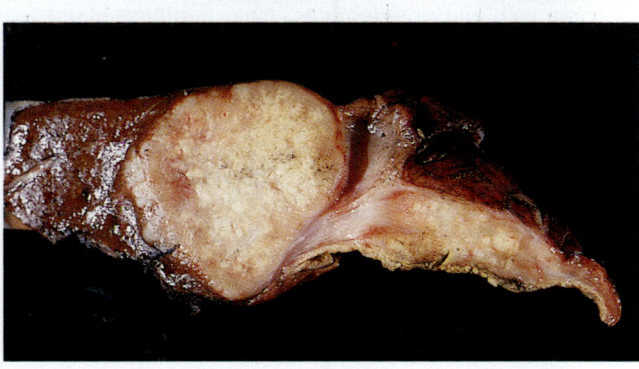

FIG. 14. Gallbladder adenocarcinoma, macroscopic appearance. **A:** Papillary type. Nearly the entire mucosal surface is involved. While papillary carcinoma has been associated with a better prognosis, this appears to be a reflection of the stage of disease. Many reported "papillary carcinomas" have been noninvasive. **B:** Diffuse thickening of the wall due to cancer may be impossible to distinguish on macroscopic evaluation from chronic cholecystitis (see Fig. 6A). Note gallstones, which are present in 70% to 90% of cases. **C:** There is extension through the gallbladder wall (right) into adjacent liver (left) (cholecystectomy with wedge liver resection, termed extended cholecystectomy).

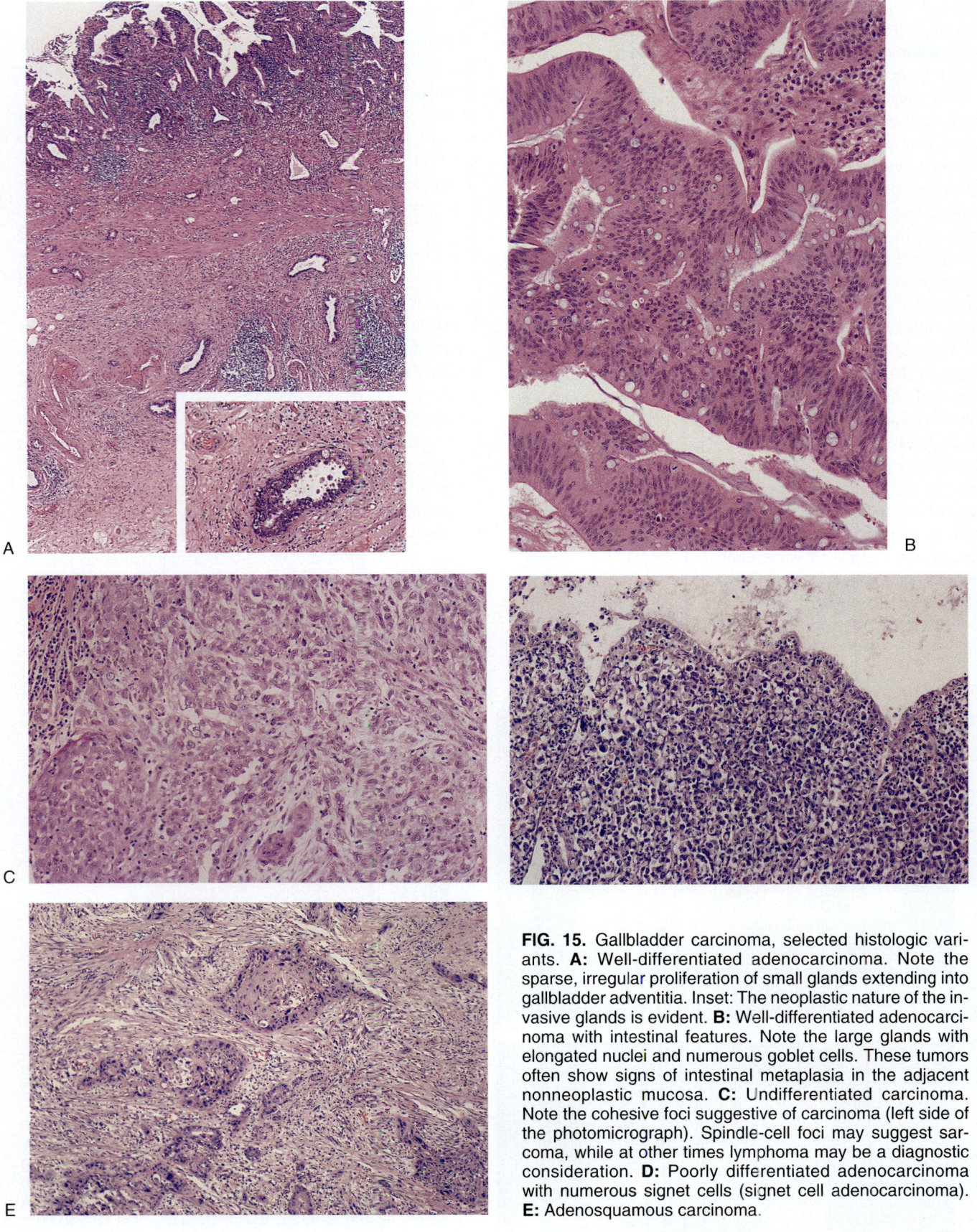

FIG. 15. Gallbladder carcinoma, selected histologic variants. A: Well-differentiated adenocarcinoma. Note the sparse, irregular proliferation of small glands extending into gallbladder adventitia. Inset: The neoplastic nature of the invasive glands is evident. B: Well-differentiated adenocarcinoma with intestinal features. Note the large glands with elongated nuclei and numerous goblet cells. These tumors often show signs of intestinal metaplasia in the adjacent nonneoplastic mucosa. C: Undifferentiated carcinoma. Note the cohesive foci suggestive of carcinoma (left side of the photomicrograph). Spindle-cell foci may suggest sarcoma, while at other times lymphoma may be a diagnostic consideration. D: Poorly differentiated adenocarcinoma with numerous signet cells (signet cell adenocarcinoma). E: Adenosquamous carcinoma.

deeper portion frequently demonstrates moderately or poorly differentiated foci (66). Rarely (1%), a well-differentiated adenocarcinoma may show a striking degree of intestinal differentiation (3,101). These tumors often have a superficial papillary architecture. The papillae and glands are sometimes lined with many goblet cells and, occasionally, Paneth and neuroendocrine cells, although a pattern with fewer goblet cells and more columnar cells with a distinct apical brush border (colonic type) has also been described. Lesser degrees of intestinal or pyloric metaplasia are frequently found in gallbladder adenocarcinomas, presumably related to the metaplasia-dysplasia-carcinoma sequence that was discussed earlier in this chapter (65,74,75).

Callea et al. documented a well-differentiated adenocarcinoma that contained globules that were periodic acid–Schiff (PAS) positive, diastase resistant and demonstrated alpha$_1$-antitrypsin immunoreactivity (102). The patient was heterozygous for the Z allele (Pi SZ). Other distinctive forms of adenocarcinoma include papillary (4–20%), colloid (mucinous) (4–7%), and signet cell (up to 3%) types (3,89). As stressed earlier in this chapter, making the distinction between noninvasive papillary carcinoma and papillary adenoma is often a moot point; regardless of what the noninvasive component is called, it is important for the pathologist to extensively section the specimen to detect invasion. This may require submitting the entire gallbladder. Foamy histiocytes of cholesterolosis (cytokeratin negative, mucin negative) and the rare presence of muciphages (cytokeratin negative, mucin positive) in a gallbladder with hydrops must be distinguished from the features of signet cell carcinoma (cytokeratin positive, mucin positive) (73a).

Very unusual cribriform, clear-cell, and pseudoangiosarcomatous variants of primary adenocarcinoma need to be distinguished, respectively, from metastatic breast carcinoma (in situ component and foci of usual gallbladder carcinoma, no clinical evidence or history of breast cancer), metastatic renal cell carcinoma (foci of usual adenocarcinoma and mucin production, CEA and cytokeratin 7 immunoreactivity, no clinical evidence or history of renal cell carcinoma) or primary clear-cell squamous carcinoma (absence of keratinizing squamous cells), and angiosarcoma (absence of immunoreactivity with endothelial markers) (73a). A pattern simulating the alveolar variant of infiltrating lobular breast cancer has also been described. The clear-cell adenocarcinoma variant is rich in glycogen. It may have focal sub- and supranuclear vacuoles reminiscent of secretory endometrium, as well as hepatoid foci. There may be a significant elevation of serum alpha-fetoprotein and immunoreactivity for this marker (73a). Choriocarcinoma-like foci have also been described.

Undifferentiated carcinoma (sarcomatoid, pleomorphic, giant-cell, or spindle cell carcinoma) accounts for 5% to 10% of cases and is characterized by varying numbers of cells that are most often quite large, pleomorphic, polygonal, or spindle-shaped. Occasionally, tumor cells have large vesicular nuclei with prominent nucleoli and may simulate lymphoma (Fig. 15C). Multinucleated tumor giant cells are prevalent. Intra- or extracellular PAS-positive hyaline globules can be found in 10% of cases; they sometimes demonstrate immunoreactivity for alpha-fetoprotein (3,73a). Rarely, osteoclast-like giant cells may be seen. They may be conspicuous and, along with mononuclear cells, give an appearance mimicking giant-cell tumor of bone. In sarcomatoid carcinoma, foci of well- to moderately differentiated adenocarcinoma or squamous cell carcinoma have been described, after extensive sectioning, in two-thirds and one-fifth of cases, respectively. Focal tumor cell cytokeratin immunoreactivity is found in 70% of cases, but osteoclast-like giant cells show negative results. Cases of sarcomatoid carcinoma with differentiated foci of sarcoma (chondro-, osteo-, rhabdomyosarcoma) are often referred to as "carcinosarcoma" or "malignant mixed tumor" (3,4,6,102a).

Squamous differentiation is reported in 5% to 10% of gallbladder carcinomas, with a variable predominance of either adenosquamous or pure squamous carcinoma (Fig. 15E) (3,4,63,84,89,100). Pure squamous cell carcinoma is probably quite rare (≤2%) if many sections are taken looking for a focal glandular component. The squamous component arises in regions of squamous metaplasia and dysplasia of the overlying columnar mucosa. Small (oat) cell carcinoma represents another rare variant of gallbladder carcinoma, the largest series reporting 29 cases (73a). The histopathologic, immunohistochemical, and ultrastructural features are identical to those found at other sites. Small foci of squamous cell carcinoma and well-differentiated adenocarcinoma may be found in 6% and 30% of cases, respectively.

Prognostic Factors and Outcome

The prognosis of gallbladder carcinoma is dismal, with less than a 5% 5-year survival rate in most major series and a median survival of less than 6 months (84,95). Surgical series, where there is a great deal of case selection bias and a variety of operations employed, report 5-year survival rates as high as 25% to 65% (95). Although macroscopic type (papillary vs. infiltrative) and histologic grade appear to correlate with outcome, by far the most significant independent predictor of outcome is the stage of disease at the time of diagnosis (Table 5) (3,84–86,95,100,103). The rare sarcomatoid and small-cell variants are associated with a uniformly poor prognosis; most patients die within a few months of diagnosis (73a). Molecular biologic studies have demonstrated K-ras codon 12 mutation, p53 protein expression, and APC gene mutation in 10% to 84%, 40% to 92% and 0% to 22% of cases, respectively, but these data are of little clinical import (53a,76,76a,104). Similarly, although 90% of cases are nondiploid by flow cytometric DNA analysis, ploidy analysis does not appear to be a useful prognostic indicator (105). The role of AgNOR parameters as prognostic factors requires further study (105).

The pathologist should document precisely the extent of mural invasion by the tumor on the pathology report; staging should be performed according to the TNM system (103). The status of the cystic duct margin (presence/absence of dysplasia or invasive carcinoma) should also be stated. Table 5 defines the staging parameters using the TNM system and estimates from the literature the percentage of cases of each type and their outcomes. Potential problems for the pathologist in the microscopic staging of gallbladder carcinoma and their potential solutions are highlighted in Table 6 (also Fig. 16). Although nearly all cases of carcinoma confined to the mucosa (T1a) have been cured by simple cholecystectomy, the outcome of patients with disease extending into, but not through, the muscular layer (T1b) does not appear to be nearly as favorable (86,106). Perhaps this result is explained by the study of Ouchi et al. (107), in which lymphatic and venous invasion was detected only when tumor extended at least into the muscular layer. Up to 15% of T1 lesions have positive lymph nodes (108).

Variations in survival rates in different studies for tumors confined to the gallbladder (T1,2) probably relate to the degree of tumor sampling by the pathologist and whether lymph node sampling has been performed by the surgeon. Usually, patients with gallbladder cancer have tumor extending into the liver or distant metastases (T3,4) (~80%). Most of these patients die within 2 years, although radical surgery may prolong their survival. Local spread to the stomach, duodenum, colon, or peritoneal surfaces may also take place. Regional lymph node metastases are present in 50% to 80% of patients at the time of presentation. This is an ominous finding, associated only rarely with long-term survival, particularly when the involved nodes are located beyond the region of the cystic duct and CBD. Hematogenous metastases to liver and lung are the form of metastasis most frequently of clinical significance. The most important pathway for the development of hepatic metastases is angiolymphatic spread along portal tracts from areas of direct hepatic invasion (109). Tumors arising in the gallbladder neck are those most inclined to spread via intraductal extension into the CBD or externally into the hepatoduodenal ligament (95); these features are poor prognostic findings.

While simple cholecystectomy appears to be adequate treatment for T1 (particularly T1a) tumors, the role of aggressive surgery (including wedge/segmental hepatic resection and regional lymphadenectomy) for more advanced lesions remains the subject of controversy in patients with potentially resectable tumors (85,95,107,108); it may be appropriate in selected cases. Recurrent tumor at the trocar sites has been reported from 1 month to 2 years in more than 20 cases after laparoscopic cholecystectomy for incidental gallbladder carcinoma. For this reason, some investigators have recommended excision of all port sites and even postoperative radiotherapy when inapparent carcinoma is detected after this procedure (87,88).

Other Primary Malignant Neoplasms

Sarcomas are quite rare; they constitute approximately 1.5% of malignant gallbladder tumors. Leiomyosarcoma, rhabdomyosarcoma, angiosarcoma, osteogenic sarcoma, chondrosarcoma, and neurofibrosarcoma have all been reported (3,4,110,111). Kaposi's sarcoma and smooth-muscle

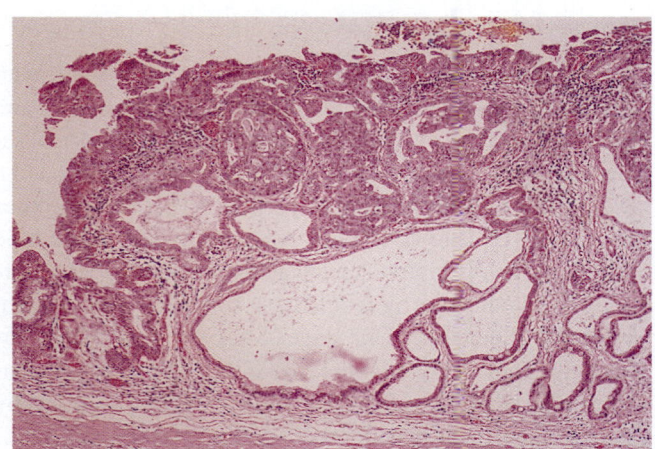
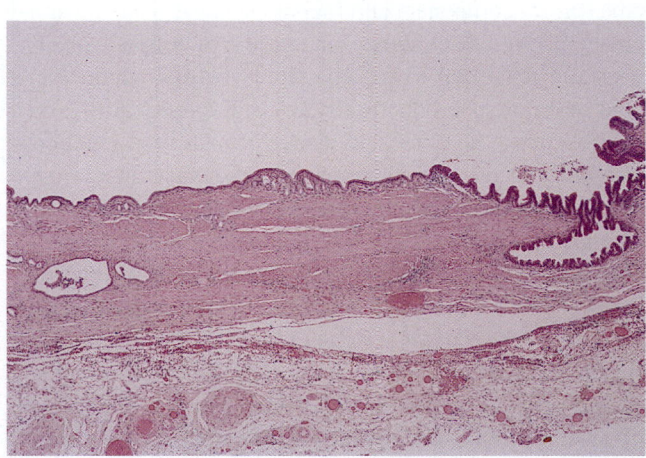

FIG. 16. Gallbladder carcinoma: Problems in staging. **A:** Tis (in situ tumor) versus T1a. While definitive lamina propria invasion is not identified (Tis), the distinction between lamina propria invasion and high-grade dysplasia (including carcinoma *in situ*), as at other gastrointestinal sites, does not appear to be particularly reproducible among pathologists in my experience. Extensive sectioning and, perhaps, submission of the entire gallbladder may be required to exclude definite invasion. Simple cholecystectomy is the treatment for both Tis and T1a. **B:** Dysplasia extending along the Rokitansky-Aschoff sinus (right). This finding should not be interpreted as invasion into the perimuscular layer (T2). Note the nondysplastic Rokitansky-Aschoff sinus (left).

nodules ("leiomyoma") have been found in AIDS patients (37,112). So-called *carcinosarcomas* (malignant mixed tumors), which demonstrate malignant epithelial (adenocarcinoma, squamous cell carcinoma) and differentiated mesenchymal (chondro-, osteo-, and rhabdomyosarcomatous foci) components, are considered variants of sarcomatoid carcinoma by many investigators. They are often polypoid, quite bulky, and necrotic (3,4,102a). Patients typically die within 6 months of diagnosis. Before a diagnosis of pure sarcoma is considered, extensive sectioning should be done to exclude the possibility of an epithelial component.

Carcinoid tumors may sometimes be associated with the carcinoid syndrome (3,4,113,114). They are usually small, single, white-yellow, mural nodules. Although metastases have been reported in about one-third of cases designated as carcinoids, some of those with more aggressive behavior are perhaps best classified as moderately or poorly differentiated *neuroendocrine carcinomas* or variants of *small-cell carcinoma*. Combined carcinoid-adenocarcinoma (invasive or in situ) has been described, sometimes with prominent goblet cells.

Although *malignant melanoma* has been reported as arising de novo within the gallbladder, some authors feel that virtually all of these cases represent metastases from regressed cutaneous lesions (3,4,115,116). The finding of junctional activity in the gallbladder mucosa adjacent to the tumor is usually regarded as indicating the primary nature of the tumor; however, its presence in one reported case of metastatic melanoma challenges the specificity of this finding (116). Primary lymphoma of the gallbladder is exceedingly rare (117).

Metastatic Tumors

Involvement of the gallbladder by metastatic tumor has been reported in 0.025% of all autopsies and in 5.8% of patients dying from carcinoma (4). If only blood-borne metastases are considered, malignant melanoma (Fig. 17) and lung carcinoma may be the most common secondary tumors to affect the gallbladder. Metastases to the gallbladder have been reported even from thin melanomas (118). In other series, in which direct extension from other abdominal sites or serosal implants as part of peritoneal carcinomatosis were not specifically excluded, carcinomas from the stomach, breast, colorectum, ovary, and pancreas were the most common neoplasms metastatic to the gallbladder. Most cases of lymphomatous involvement of the gallbladder are secondary, as is multiple myeloma, which is rarely reported (4). Secondary lymphoma is typically associated with involved adjacent lymph nodes. Angiotropic lymphoma ("malignant angioendotheliomatosis") has been described in the gallbladder (119). There is a documented case of a patient with idiopathic myelofibrosis in whom the presence of myeloid metaplasia in the gallbladder clinically mimicked acute cholecystitis (120).

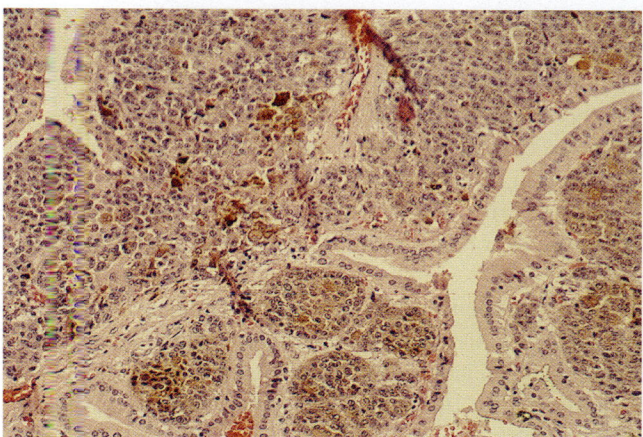

FIG. 17. Metastatic melanoma. Note the brown melanin pigment. (Kindly contributed by Virginia A. LiVolsi, M.D., Hospital of the University of Pennsylvania, Philadelphia, PA.).

THE EXTRAHEPATIC BILE DUCTS

Normal Anatomy and Histology and Routine Specimen Processing

The right and left hepatic ducts (3–4 mm in diameter) usually join to form the common hepatic duct (CHD) in the hilum (porta hepatis) within approximately 1 cm after their exit from the liver (2,121). These ducts reside between the two serous layers of the hepatoduodenal ligament. Because the hepatic duct junction is hidden within the porta hepatis, tumors arising here may escape detection at the time of laparotomy in up to 70% of cases. In 10% to 30% of people, two segmental ducts drain the right hepatic lobe and join separately with the left hepatic duct, CHD, or cystic duct.

The CHD, which has a diameter of 0.2 to 0.8 cm, descends 1 to 5 cm, where it joins with the cystic duct (usually 1–3 cm length) to form the CBD. The CBD continues 1.5 to 9 cm, passing behind the pancreas, and enters the second portion of the duodenum, where it typically joins with the pancreatic duct (common channel) before emptying into the ampulla of Vater. The diameter at its midportion varies from 0.4 to 1.3 cm, and the wall thickness is about 1 mm. The CBD thickens at about 2 mm from the duodenal wall owing to an increase in smooth muscle, resulting in a 50% narrowing in its intraduodenal portion (sphincter choledochus).

Bile duct mucosa has a reticular macroscopic appearance owing to the presence of many tiny pits (sacculi of Beale), which represent infoldings of the surface epithelium. Unevenly distributed peribiliary glands (mucous glands), which can be found in large intrahepatic ducts or within any of the extrahepatic bile ducts, empty into the sacculi. They have a lobular architecture, may be found at any level of the bile duct wall, and are surrounded by a layer of fibroconnective tissue. Preservation of the lobular architectural pattern and the fact that these benign glands have not been reported to invade nerves aid in their distinction from well-differentiated adenocarcinoma.

The surface epithelium consists of a single layer of tall columnar cells identical histologically and histochemically to those of the gallbladder, although they contain less mucin. The peribiliary glands and surface epithelium may be immunoreactive for pancreatic and salivary gland alpha-amylase, trypsin, and lipase (122). It is unclear whether scattered neuroendocrine cells identified by immunohistochemistry are a normal or metaplastic finding related to pancreaticobiliary disease.

The subepithelial region is composed of dense, hypocellular connective tissue. Lymphocytes are sparse. Beneath this subepithelial region is a loose connective tissue layer that contains elastic fibers and a varying numbers of smooth-muscle fibers (fibromuscular layer), but no well-defined, pure muscle layer. The amount of elastic tissue in the duct wall increases dramatically with age. Smooth muscle is more prominent and forms bundles in the distal CBD, as indicated earlier, and a few pancreatic acini and ducts may be found in the duct's intrapancreatic portion.

Bile duct resections should be sampled extensively—submission of the entire specimen for histologic evaluation is a reasonable approach, because distinguishing fibroinflammatory lesions from adenocarcinoma may be quite difficult at this site. Specimen orientation in terms of designation of various branch points (hepatic ducts, cystic duct, etc.) and margins requires close cooperation with the surgical team before tissue processing. Resection margins must be sampled. If wedge or segmental hepatic resection is also performed, extension of neoplasm into the liver and the hepatic margin must be assessed.

Congenital Anomalies

Extrahepatic Biliary Atresia

Extrahepatic bile duct atresia (EHBDA) is the most frequent extrahepatic cause of cholestasis in neonates; it accounts for one-third of all cases of neonatal cholestasis (121–124). The condition is found in about one in 10,000 to 15,000 live births worldwide, with girls being affected more often than boys (2–3:1). Most of these children are products of uncomplicated pregnancies. Associated congenital anomalies, including cardiovascular defects and polysplenia, have been reported in 10% to 25% of cases. Only rarely have familial cases been reported. The condition is characterized by clinical signs of persistent conjugated hyperbilirubinemia. The origin and pathogenesis of EHBDA are unknown; infectious (CMV, reovirus type III, Epstein Barr virus, rubella, rotavirus group C), ischemic, toxic (exogenous and endogenous) and structural AAPBD sources have been suggested.

EHBDA is characterized by total or focal complete fibrous obliteration of the lumen of major hepatic ducts and/or the CBD, which results in lack of bile flow into the duodenum. The most advanced stage of complete obliteration typically involves the distal CHD; more proximally the changes are often less severe. The underlying pathologic process in EHBDA is an acquired destructive sclerosing inflammatory disorder that results in replacement of the bile duct(s) by a threadlike cord embedded in fibrous tissue in the porta hepatis, often with an associated small gallbladder. Ongoing bile duct damage leads to progressive loss of intrahepatic ducts; over a variable period of time biliary cirrhosis results. Some, but not all, studies have reported that the presence of patent hilar bile ductal structures with lumina larger than 100 to 400 µm or an area of all bile duct structures larger than 50,000 µm^2 may be associated with a more favorable outcome after portoenterostomy (Kasai procedure). The differential diagnosis on liver biopsy in terms of other causes of neonatal cholestasis is beyond the scope of this discussion (see the chapter by Snover).

EHBDA is the most common cause of death from liver disease in children and the most common pediatric disorder referred for liver transplantation (about 50% of pediatric liver transplants). Portoenterostomy should be performed before the child reaches 10 to 12 weeks of age. After this time, the prevalence of cirrhosis is so high that hepatic transplantation, which is associated with up to 75% 5-year survival, is the treatment of choice. Since the 10-year survival rate after the Kasai procedure is only 16% to 30%, liver transplantation is essential in patients who have undergone portoenterostomy, when there are signs of liver failure or decreased bile flow.

Choledochal Cysts

Choledochal (bile duct) cysts are found in one in 13,000 to 15,000 and one in 1,000 live births in the United States and Japan, respectively (121,125). They are more common in girls (female to male ratio, 3:1). Although they are usually discovered in the first decade of life, choledochal cysts can be found at any age. They are not familial. Abdominal pain, a mass, and jaundice are typical clinical findings. Spontaneous rupture can occur. While ultrasonography and computed tomography are the initial imaging methods of choice, cholangiography yields a definitive diagnosis and allows for cyst classification. An AAPBD has been reported in 40% to 90% of cases (90,92,126). Reflux of pancreatic enzymes into the bile duct may lead to duct damage and dilatation, as has been shown in experimental models (126).

Todani et al. divided biliary cysts into five types (127): type 1, segmental or diffuse fusiform dilatation of the CBD, accounting for 50% to 90% of all cases; type 2, diverticulum of the CBD, typically protruding from the lateral wall and often pedunculated; type 3, dilatation of the intraduodenal portion of the CBD (choledochocele); type 4, multiple cysts of extrahepatic bile ducts with (4A) or without (4B) cysts of the intrahepatic ducts; and type 5, one or more cysts of the intrahepatic ducts (Caroli's disease). Stones are found in 1% to 30% of all cases. The cysts are either spherical or fusiform; they can contain up to 1,500 ml of bile and obtain a maximum diameter of 15 cm.

Wall thickness varies from 2 to 10 mm. The wall is composed of dense fibrous tissue with scattered elastic and smooth-muscle fibers and a variable chronic inflammatory infiltrate. The cysts may have a focal columnar epithelial lining and scattered glands in 20% to 60% of cases. A lining of duodenal mucosa is typically found in the choledochocele. Several authors have noted hyperplastic, metaplastic (intestinal type), and even dysplastic epithelial changes, suggesting a relationship to the subsequent development of carcinoma (126,128,129) (see discussion below). Liver biopsy may show features of extrahepatic obstruction, including secondary biliary cirrhosis. The treatment of choice is complete cyst removal with biliary reconstruction, usually with Roux-en-Y anastomosis. Simple decompression should be performed only when complicated anatomy precludes resection.

Biliary tract carcinoma arises in about 2% to 8% of all patients with a choledochal cyst; the risk is 20 times greater than in the general population (92,128,129). The mean age at diagnosis of cancer is 34 years; however, there are striking age-related differences. In Voyles' review of the literature, less than 1% of patients who underwent initial operation in the first decade subsequently showed signs of biliary tract carcinoma, compared with 6.8% and 14.3% operated on in the second decade or later, respectively. Seventy-six percent of all malignant cases were in patients who were initially diagnosed after 20 years of age, and 40% of the carcinomas were detected more than 2 years after initial surgery. Fifty-five percent of the carcinomas are found in the wall of the choledochal cyst itself, while 30% and 15% arise in the gallbladder and bile ducts (intra- and extrahepatic), respectively (92). The most common histologic pattern is well-differentiated adenocarcinoma; however, giant-cell and squamous cell carcinoma, as well as rhabdomyosarcoma, have been described (3,125).

Sclerosing Cholangitis

Secondary Sclerosing Cholangitis

Sclerosing cholangitis represents a fibroinflammatory process of the biliary tree, occurring as a consequence of a wide variety of insults; it may lead to chronic cholestasis, biliary cirrhosis, portal hypertension, and hepatic failure. Both the extrahepatic and intrahepatic bile ducts may be affected in different ways, as may the ampulla of Vater (papillary stenosis). Sclerosing cholangitis is divided into primary (see Primary Sclerosing Cholangitis) and secondary types (Table 7). Usually, a localized stricture develops in a region where biliary tract surgery (usually cholecystectomy) has been performed or, less frequently, as a complication of choledocholithiasis or even cholelithiasis (Mirizzi syndrome) (1,4,15a,130,131). Hepatic lobar atrophy can result (132). Many benign processes can lead to sclerosing cholangitis, and several malignancies can simulate this process on imaging studies either by invading the bile duct wall or through the effects of lymph node metastases (Table 8).

Varying degrees of fibrosis, inflammation, and ulceration can be seen in the duct wall, as can foreign body granulomas; differentiating this condition from carcinoma may be difficult (133).

Bacteria, including aerobes and anaerobes, can be cultured from the bile in nearly all cases. Mass lesions (inflammatory myofibroblastic tumor/inflammatory pseudotumor), as well as so-called eosinophilic cholangitis, have been described (40,134). *Cryptococcus* organisms (Fig. 18) and *Candida* sp may cause strictures and polypoid intraluminal defects of the CBD, respectively, in nonimmunocompromised patients (135,136). In patients with AIDS, cryptosporidia, microsporidia, CMV, and the *Mycobacterium avium complex* may be associated with significant biliary fibroinflammatory disease (AIDS cholangiopathy), and squamous metaplasia has been reported upon occasion (37,137). Compression of the CBD related to lymphadenopathic bacillary angiomatosis has also been described in this patient pop-

TABLE 7. *Sclerosing cholangitis: classification*[a]

Primary sclerosing cholangitis (PSC)
  "Rule of the 70s"[b]
    70% males
    70% <45 years of age
    ≥ 70% have chronic IIBD
Secondary sclerosing cholangitis
  Biliary obstruction
    Choledocholithiasis
    Postoperative strictures
    Chronic pancreatitis
    Choledochal cyst
    Extrahepatic biliary atresia
  Infection
    Parasites/fungus
    Immunodeficiency states
      Congenital
      AIDS
  Toxins
    Intraarterial (hepatic) FUDR
    Intraductal formalin (leakage from treatment of echinococcal cyst)
  Ischemia
    Chronic liver allograft rejection
    Trauma
  Other
    Chronic graft vs. host disease
    Sarcoidosis
    Eosinophilic cholangitis
    Langerhans cell histiocytosis (histiocytosis X)
    Systemic mastocytosis
  Malignancy
    Bile duct, pancreatic and ampullary adenocarcinoma
    Hepatocellular carcinoma
    Metastatic carcinoma
    Lymphoma

FUDR, fluorodeoxyuridine; IIBD, idiopathic inflammatory bowel disease (most commonly chronic ulcerative colitis); AIDS, acquired immunodeficiency syndrome.
[a] Some entities could be placed in more than one category. For example, intraarterial FUDR could also be listed under "ischemia."
[b] From ref. 133.

TABLE 8. *Sclerosing cholangitis and bile duct carcinoma: helpful and challenging features in microscopic differential diagnosis in the extrahepatic bile ducts*

Features	Sclerosing cholangitis	Bile duct carcinoma
Helpful features		
Papillary surface	Rare	Occasionally
Lobular pattern of peribiliary glands often preserved	Yes	No
Concentric fibrosis around peribiliary glands	Yes	No
Infiltrating glands between lobules	No	Yes
Perineural invasion	No	Often
Mucin pools in stroma	Rare	Occasionally
Marked cytologic atypia of cells lining glands	No	Often (focal)
Challenging features		
Normal surface epithelium may be present	Yes	Yes
Inflammatory component of variable intensity	Yes	Yes
Distortion of the normal lobular architecture of the peribiliary glands	Occasionally	Typical
Prominent mural fibrosis	Yes	Yes
Reactive epithelial atypia	Yes	Yes
Oncocytic metaplasia of peribiliary glands	Rarely reported	?
Dysplasia involving peribiliary glands	Occasionally[a]	Often
Coexistence of PSC and BD CA	Yes	Yes

BD CA, bile duct carcinoma; PSC, primary sclerosing cholangitis.
[a] Dysplasia has rarely been reported to affect peribiliary glands in PSC. It must be distinguished from invasive adenocarcinoma, but coexistent foci of invasion should be carefully sought.

ulation (138). Fibroinflammatory changes in the hilum, particularly in patients with cirrhosis and portal vein thrombosis, may result in the formation of multiple hilar cysts (139). These cysts have been discussed in the chapter on hepatic tumors.

Primary Sclerosing Cholangitis

Secondary forms of sclerosing cholangitis are much more common than PSC. PSC is a chronic cholestatic disorder of unknown origin that can involve the entire biliary tract, from the ampulla of Vater to the small intrahepatic bile ducts, or the gallbladder. It is frequently associated with chronic idiopathic inflammatory bowel disease (chronic IIBD), although only a minority (3–7.5%) of patients with chronic IIBD associated PSC (28,47,49,50,121,130,131,133, 140,141). Colectomy, in patients with associated chronic IIBD, has no effect on the clinical course of PSC. Cholangiocarcinoma is an important complication of PSC (see later discussion). The "rule of the 70s" applies to this disease, since approximately 70% of patients are males, have associated chronic IIBD (90–95% ulcerative colitis, 5–10% Crohn's disease), and are younger than 45 years of age (133). More than 200 cases have been reported in children. While most patients have pancolitis that predates the diagnosis of PSC, the two disorders may be detected at the same time, or PSC may even be detected first. Because colitis may be entirely asymptomatic, patients with PSC should undergo colonoscopy with biopsy to rule out quiescent disease and to search for dysplasia/carcinoma, which may occur more often in this subset of chronic IIBD patients.

PSC has been associated with many other disorders (often autoimmune or sclerosing processes), such as Riedel's disease, retroperitoneal and mediastinal fibrosis, orbital pseudotumor, Sjögren's syndrome, and "angioimmunoblastic lymphadenopathy," but these associations have mainly been case reports and may be anecdotal. Clinical features of chronic pancreatitis have been reported in 15% to 25% of patients, with nearly all patients demonstrating some degree of pancreatic fibrosis at autopsy. The pancreatitis may have a striking lymphoplasmacellular infiltrate, overlapping with so-called lymphoplasmacytic sclerosing pancreatitis with cholangitis and, perhaps, with pancreatic inflammatory myofibroblastic tumor (inflammatory pseudotumor) (134,142, 143).

Patients may show initial signs of fever, fatigue, and cholangitis; in up to 40% of cases, however, they are asymptomatic and are identified solely by an elevated serum alkaline phosphatase level on screening biochemistry tests. At the time of diagnosis, an elevated serum alkaline phosphatase level, mildly increased transaminases, and variably increased bilirubin are frequently noted. The presence of autoimmune markers (ANA, ASMA; <5% AMA) and hypergammaglobulinemia in one-third to one-half of patients may make the clinical distinction from autoimmune hepatitis ambiguous, particularly in children. Haplotype studies suggest an association with several alleles, particularly DR52a and Dw2.

Cholangiography, particularly ERCP, is the diagnostic method of choice. ERCP shows the characteristic short annular strictures separated by normal or slightly dilated duct segments in the extra- and intrahepatic bile ducts (beaded appearance). Dominant strictures (10–15%), which usually occur in the hilum, may simulate cholangiocarcinoma (Klatskin tumor). In the rare situation (~5%) in which PSC is apparently limited to the small intrahepatic ducts (small-

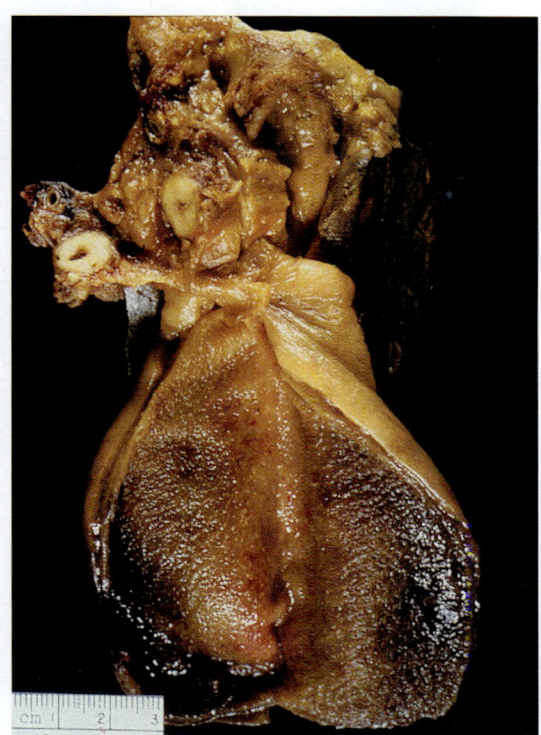
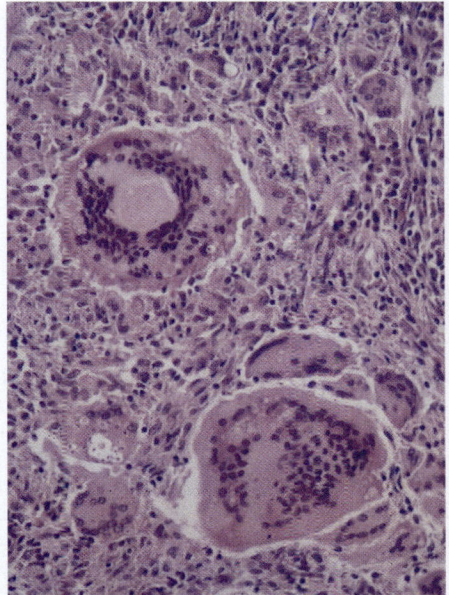
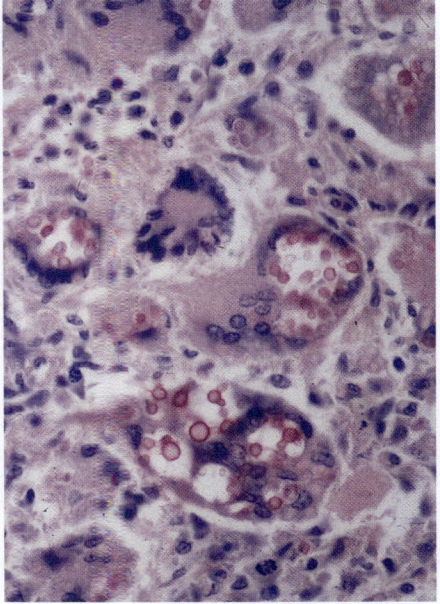

FIG. 18. Sclerosing cholangitis stemming from *Cryptococcus* infection (Contributed by Thomas Miller, M.D., Pittsburgh, PA.). **A:** Note (middle left) the marked thickening of the bile duct, which cannot be distinguished on macroscopic evaluation from primary sclerosing cholangitis or bile duct carcinoma. **B:** Granulomatous inflammation. Numerous mucicarmine-positive cryptococci are engulfed by multinucleated giant cells (right panel).

duct PSC), the cholangiogram shows normal results, but typical liver biopsy findings are present (see chapter by Snover).

The involved extrahepatic ducts are quite thickened (fibrous cords), and their appearance has been compared by the surgeon to that of a thrombosed blood vessel (Fig. 19). The walls of the extrahepatic bile ducts normally have a prominent fibroelastic component that increases with age, which often makes impossible any microscopic distinction from sclerosing cholangitis based only on the degree of fibrosis. In PSC, the inflammatory component (mixed, with predominance of lymphocytes and plasma cells) is quite variable and may be absent. The inflammation is often accentuated just under the surface epithelium and around the peribiliary glands, which may show cystic dilatation and even oncocytic change (144). Squamous metaplasia is rarely noted. A few lymphoid follicles may be visible.

The pathologist must realize, however, that the fibroinflammatory changes are quite nonspecific and do not aid in distinguishing PSC from most secondary forms. The intrahepatic bile ducts, however, may be the site of virtually pathognomonic changes (see chapter by Snover). Therefore, biopsy of the extrahepatic ducts is to be discouraged unless

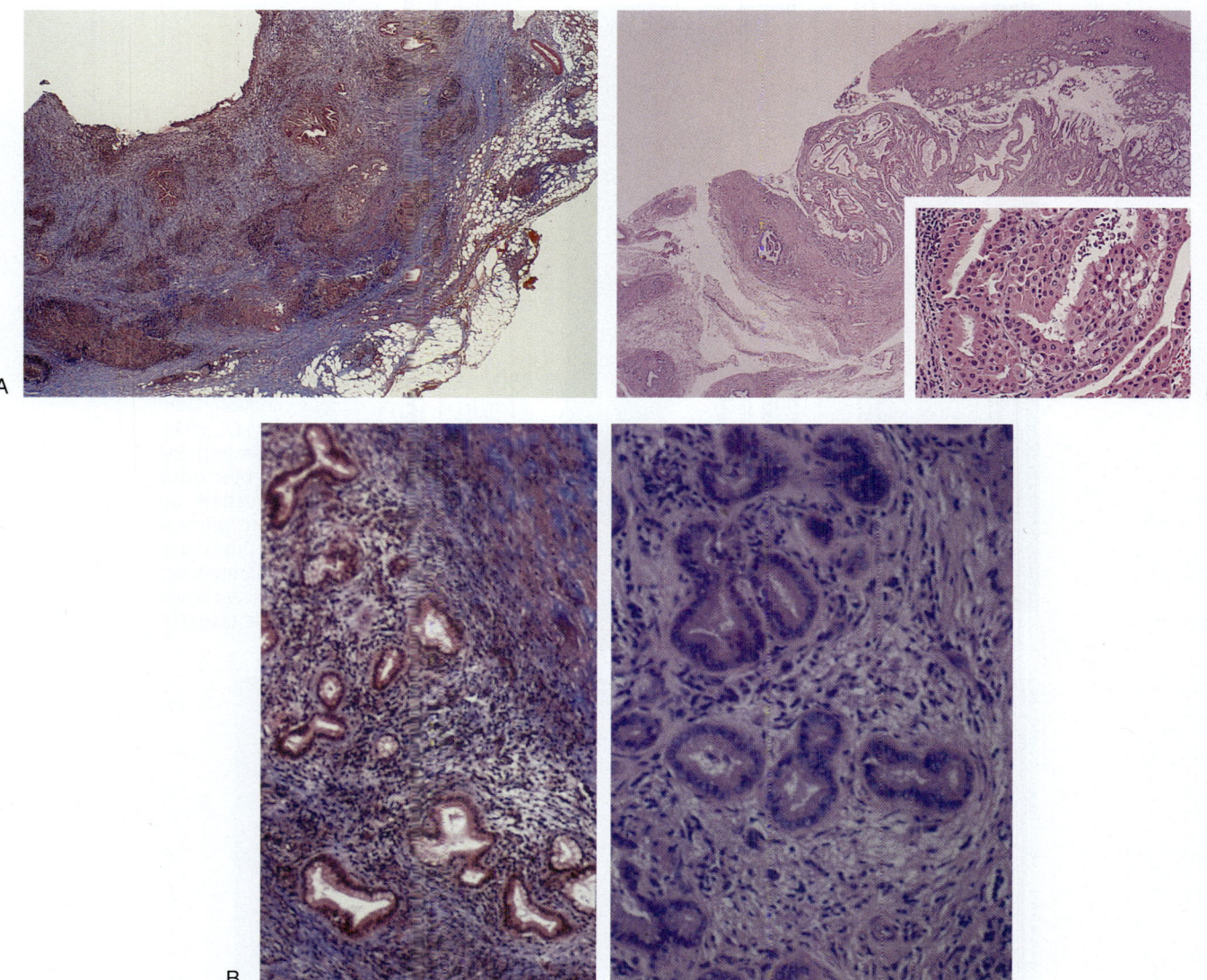

FIG. 19. Primary sclerosing cholangitis, common bile duct. **A:** The bile duct wall is thickened by fibrosis and chronic inflammation. Lobular units are demarcated by fibrosis (trichrome stain). **B:** Lobular architecture is recognizable, but somewhat distorted in both panels of this photomicrograph. The higher-power view at right demonstrates glands with hyperchromatic nuclei without prominent nucleoli. In some cases, distortion of lobular architecture and reactive epithelial changes can make distinguishing primary sclerosing cholangitis from bile duct carcinoma quite difficult in frozen as well as permanent sections (trichrome stain). (See Fig. 21 for comparison with bile duct adenocarcinoma.). **C:** Peribiliary glands with cystic dilatation and oncocytic change. Inset: High-power view shows prominent oncocytic change. The mild epithelial atypia was considered indeterminate for dysplasia, probably negative. (Kindly contributed by Randall G. Lee, M.D., Presbyterian University Hospital, Pittsburgh, PA.)

there is a clinical suspicion of bile duct carcinoma or in the unusual situation of a possible infectious process.

When specimens from the extrahepatic bile ducts in patients with suspected PSC are obtained in order to rule out malignancy, a frozen section is often requested. The absence of tumor in a few specimens certainly does not rule out malignancy. On the other hand, carcinoma and PSC may coexist (see below). Distortion of the architecture of the bile duct wall and reactive epithelial changes in sclerosing cholangitis may make the distinction from adenocarcinoma quite difficult on histologic evidence, particularly if the frozen section is not of optimal quality (Fig. 19) (145,146). Maintenance of the lobular pattern of the peribiliary glands, which are often surrounded by concentric fibrosis, is typical of PSC, while the pattern of gland infiltration in adenocarcinoma is more random. Occasionally, however, mural fibrosis will isolate individual benign glands in PSC, thus simulating malignancy. On the other hand, in adenocarcinoma, many lobular units may be intact, but deceptively bland well-differentiated tumor may percolate between them. While the presence of a papillary epithelial component is virtually found only in neoplastic disorders, the absence of surface epithelial changes epithelial changes does not exclude tumor extending in an intramural fashion. The presence of perineural invasion should be actively sought out, because it may be the only feature diagnostic of malignancy. These and other features helpful in the differential diagnosis are summarized in Table 8.

Although PSC may have a variable course, it eventually leads to biliary cirrhosis and liver failure, with a median survival of 9 to 12 years. Cholangitis and cholelithiasis/choledocholithiasis are complicating factors. PSC represents the fourth most common cause of liver transplantation in adults, resulting in more than 75% survival at 5 years. After transplantation, patients with chronic IIBD must continue to undergo colonic surveillance, since colon cancer represents the most frequent cause of death in this context.

Cholangiocarcinoma (extra- or intrahepatic) has been reported to develop in association with PSC in 10% to 43% of cases, depending on the manner in which malignancy was ascertained (clinical features, at the time of transplantation, or at autopsy) (147,148). It may be multifocal and usually occurs one to two decades earlier than in the general population. Dysplasia, which may be papillary and extend into peribiliary glands, has been documented (149). The reported histologic features span the spectrum of so-called biliary papillomatosis (see discussion of gallbladder adenoma and the chapter "Masses of the Liver"). Gallbladder carcinoma and, rarely, hepatocellular carcinoma (fibrolamellar and usual types) have also been reported (50,150).

Benign Tumors

Benign tumors at this site are unusual—they are one-tenth as common as extrahepatic bile duct carcinomas. In general, they are small, measuring 1 cm up to a few centimeters in diameter. While gallbladder polyps are often asymptomatic, those arising in the extrahepatic bile ducts often cause obstruction. Approximately 75% are adenomas (incorrectly termed papilloma or polyp) (151,152). The CBD is the usual location; however, 25% are located in the hilar region, making their surgical excision quite challenging. Because the mucosal surface area is 50 to 100 times greater in the gallbladder compared with the extrahepatic biliary tree, it is not surprising that adenomas at the latter site are much less common (3).

Adenomas may be single or multiple and pedunculated or sessile; they have tubular, tubulopapillary (tubulovillous), or papillary (villous) histologic features. They are defined on microscopy by dysplasia, which may vary from low to high grade (including CIS). Only a total excision, with complete examination of the lesion and its base, excludes the presence of invasive carcinoma. Ultrasound-guided biopsy may aid in the diagnosis of an epithelial neoplasm (153). Curettage is inadequate treatment, because nearly 25% of lesions recur (152). Papillomatosis (adenomatosis), a rare disorder characterized by several recurring papillary adenomas often associated with excess mucus secretion and involvement of other portions of the biliary tree, has been discussed in the section on adenoma of the gallbladder and in the chapter "Masses of the Liver".

As with adenomas elsewhere, when high-grade dysplasia is present, making the distinction from intraductal carcinoma (papillary carcinoma) is quite subjective. The presence of invasive foci should be carefully excluded (6,55,154). The extrahepatic bile ducts are the site of nearly 15% of all hepatobiliary cystadenomas. These may be multicentric and also involve the liver (155). Only complete excision excludes cystadenocarcinoma. The pathologic features of this lesion have been covered in the chapter "Masses of the Liver".

Granular cell tumor is the most common benign nonepithelial tumor of the extrahepatic biliary tree (Fig. 20) (6). This type constituted 9% of benign extrahepatic bile duct tumors in one series (151). As with granular cell tumors in other areas, these tumors of the biliary tree are most frequently found in young to middle-aged black women (65%); 15% are multifocal, but only rarely are they multifocal within the extrahepatic biliary tree itself (156,157). Traumatic neuromas most commonly occur in the cystic duct after cholecystectomy, but they have also been reported in the absence of previous surgery (158,159). While they are usually asymptomatic, they can grow into the common hepatic bile duct or CBD and even extend into the liver, producing obstructive jaundice. These haphazard proliferations of nerve fascicles may be difficult to distinguish from neurofibroma (160).

Other benign masses reported in this location include cholesterol polyps, inflammatory myofibroblastic tumor (inflammatory pseudotumor; see the discussion under the heading Primary Sclerosing Cholangitis), leiomyomas, fibromas, fibroadenomas, adenomyomas, and paragangliomas (3,134, 151,152,161–163). Pancreatic, gastric, and duodenal heterotopias have also been described (3,164).

Malignant Tumors

Carcinoma

Clinical and Epidemiologic Features

About 99% of extrahepatic bile duct malignancies are carcinomas. They are found in 0.012% to 0.54% of autopsy specimens and 0.3% to 1.8% of biliary trees at the time of operation (3,86,165). If one excludes carcinomas arising in the ampulla of Vater, extrahepatic bile duct carcinoma is two to three times less common than cancer of the gallbladder. Its incidence is about one per 100,000 population in the United States, but it develops more frequently in Native Americans, Mexicans, Israelis, and Japanese. Tumors are most frequently detected in the late seventh or early eighth decades and only rarely before the age of 40 years. There is a slight male predominance (male to female ratio, 1.3:1). In patients with ulcerative colitis/PSC (147–149) and choledochal cyst (92,128,129), the diagnosis is usually made two decades earlier than in the general population.

More than 90% of patients show signs of jaundice; epi-

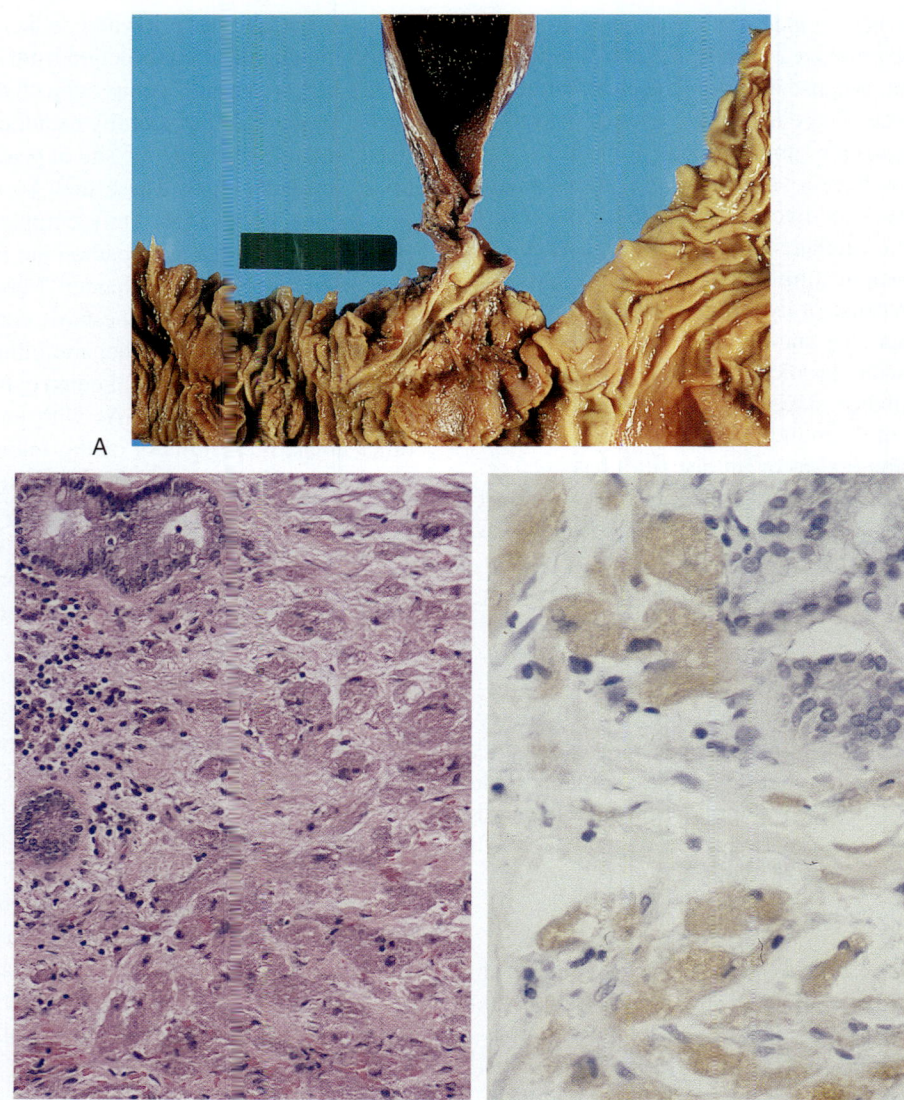

FIG. 20. Granular cell tumor, common bile duct. **A:** Note the tapered narrowing of the common bile duct below the gallbladder. **B:** The left panel shows the typical histologic appearance of a granular cell tumor. The right panel displays strong tumor cell immunoreactivity for S-100 (immunohistochemistry, S-100). (Kindly contributed by Ann Ainsworth, M.D., Bryn Mawr Hospital, Bryn Mawr, PA.)

gastric pain, weakness, and pruritus are often present. Hepatomegaly, with chronic biliary obstruction, is frequently seen; biliary cirrhosis may result. Less often, one may find compensatory lobar hypertrophy when hepatic duct or portal vein obstruction by tumor has led to lobar atrophy on the affected side (atrophy–hypertrophy complex). About 20% of patients have had prior biliary tract surgery; in these cases the tumor was either overlooked or interpreted as benign disease. In patients with tumors located above the hepatic duct bifurcation or with incomplete CBD obstruction, serum alkaline phosphatase levels may be elevated in the absence of elevated serum bilirubin. Serum CA 19-9 and CA 50 may also be elevated, but levels may fall when obstruction is relieved. Only rarely do bile duct cancers masquerade as primary tumors of other sites, such as the ovary (96).

Although many conditions characterized by biliary tract stasis and infection have been associated with extrahepatic bile duct carcinoma, they are detected in only a minority of patients. These conditions include PSC, chronic ulcerative colitis (rarely Crohn's disease), choledochal cyst, AAPBD, *Clonorchis sinensis* and *Opisthorchis viverrini* infestation, cystic fibrosis, familial polyposis coli, chronic typhoid carrier states, biliary giardiasis, and thorotrast exposure (53a,86, 90–92,128, 129,147–149,165,166). Cholelithiasis is present in about one-third of patients, but in less than 10% are stones found in the bile ducts themselves. Sonography and computed tomography often are used as screening procedures to detect duct dilatation; however, cholangiography (percutaneous for proximal lesions, endoscopic for distal lesions) is the imaging technique of choice to show the precise location and extent of the lesion (86,165).

Because it has now been recognized that the preoperative

diagnosis of bile duct carcinoma, particularly sclerosing proximal tumors, may be incorrect in 30% of cases, several investigators have stressed the importance of obtaining a tissue diagnosis, particularly if surgical resection is not performed (86,167). Material for diagnosis can be obtained from bile drainage, from brushings obtained at the time of cholangiography, from guided FNA biopsy when a mass is identified, or from endobiliary biopsy utilizing special forceps (168,169). The diagnostic sensitivity in cases of carcinoma varies greatly in different series and for different techniques but is least sensitive for bile cytology. The other methods report a sensitivity in the range of 65% to 80%. Because tumor cells exfoliate into bile, care must be taken by surgeons and interventional radiologists to avoid peritoneal spillage and the possibility of implantation metastases (170).

Pathologic Features

Macroscopic Appearance. Extrahepatic bile duct carcinoma is best divided into two groups, perihilar (70%), and distal (30%), because this classification correlates with anatomic distribution and surgical treatment (86). Perihilar tumors involve, or at least require resection of, the hepatic duct bifurcation (Klatskin tumors), and they are managed with a variety of operative or nonoperative interventions. Although some perihilar tumors have been classified as intrahepatic cholangiocarcinomas, their clinical presentation, typically with jaundice, is that of extrahepatic bile duct cancers (Fig. 21A). Distal tumors involve the distal extrahepatic or intrapancreatic portions of the bile duct and may be amenable to pancreaticoduodenectomy (Whipple procedure). Infrequently, diffuse tumors can be found in both compartments.

Extrahepatic bile duct carcinomas may be divided into sclerosing, nodular, or, less often (20%), polypoid-papillary types; however, overlap is the rule (3,145,171). Sclerosing lesions, which can resemble nonneoplastic strictures, appear as gray-white, annular, ductal thickenings (up to 1 cm). They may be discrete or extend for 4 cm or more. The exact limits of the tumor may be difficult to detect, on both gross and microscopic inspection, owing to the prominent associated desmoplastic reaction. Extension beyond the duct wall into adjacent structures is common. Circumscribed, firm, gray-white, nodular lesions, usually no more than 2 cm in diameter, often project into the duct lumen and extend through the duct wall. Papillary tumors are gray-pink and friable, may be multifocal, and occasionally are noninvasive (overlap with multiple adenomas/papillomatosis; see earlier discussion).

Microscopic Appearance. The histopathologic features of bile duct carcinomas are essentially the same as those of cancers that arise in the gallbladder (see earlier discussion). Virtually 90% to 95% of bile duct cancers are pure adenocarcinomas (3,89,172,173), the overwhelming majority of which are predominately well or moderately differentiated

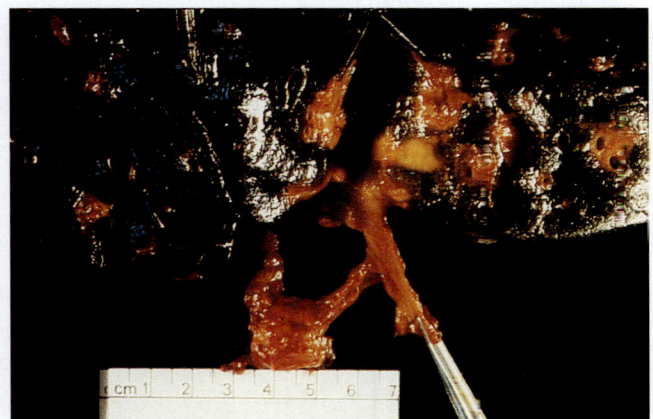

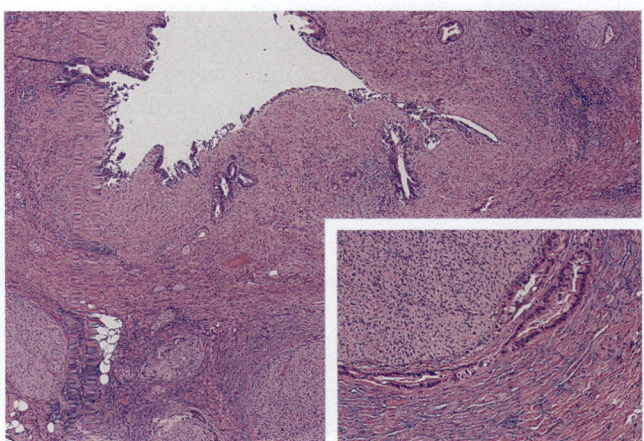

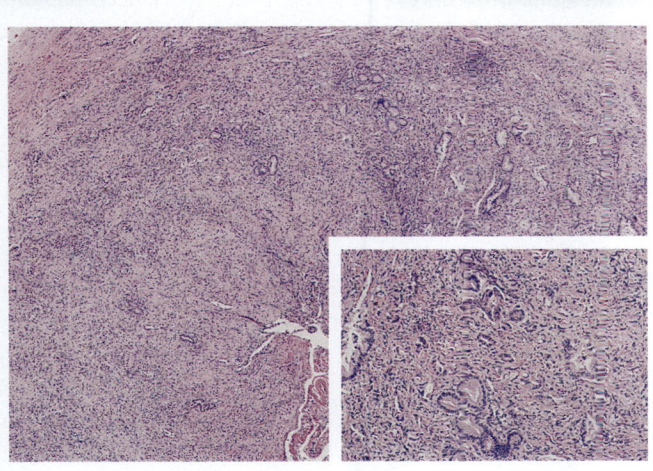

FIG. 21. Bile duct adenocarcinoma. **A:** A tumor nodule is present at the hepatic duct bifurcation (Klatskin tumor, perihilar cholangiocarcinoma). Although the adenocarcinoma appears to be relatively well circumscribed, foci of hepatic involvement are conspicuous findings, typical of this deceptive tumor (kindly contributed by Robert E. Lee, M.D., Presbyterian University Hospital, Pittsburgh, PA.) **B:** Well-differentiated adenocarcinoma with deceptive minimal mural invasion but extensive perineural invasion. Inset: High-power view shows the well-differentiated nature of the tumor in the perineural region. **C:** Moderate to poorly differentiated adenocarcinoma causes extensive mural thickening. Inset: Numerous small malignant glands are seen, as are a few residual nonneoplastic glands.

(Fig. 21B,C). Clear-cell, adenosquamous (mucoepidermoid), undifferentiated (pleomorphic, sarcomatoid, giant cell), squamous cell, and small-cell carcinomas have all been reported (3,73a,89). Well-differentiated adenocarcinomas demonstrate conspicuous gland formation although poorly differentiated foci are not uncommon deep within the wall (145,171,173). Papillary foci are occasionally present and are almost always seen in noninvasive tumors. Mucin is almost always evident within tumor cells and glandular lumina; it may form large pools in the stroma (colloid or mucinous type). The individual tumor cells are cuboidal or columnar, often containing vesicular nuclei and prominent nucleoli.

Some tumors are so well differentiated that a diagnosis of malignancy may not be possible based solely on the cytologic features of one or a few glands. The malignant glands may be widely dispersed in the fibrotic stroma, sometimes beneath a normal epithelial lining, adding to the difficulty of making the initial diagnosis and interpreting the margins of resection. The bile duct wall is characteristically thickened by a prominent desmoplastic response to the tumor. Perineural invasion, a feature diagnostic of malignancy at this site, is often present, depending on the size of the specimen and the degree of sampling. This feature can be extremely useful in well-differentiated cases. Lymphatic and venous invasion, necrosis, and a chronic inflammatory infiltrate are typical findings.

The depth of mural penetration and the status of the proximal, distal, and radial (circumferential surgical cleavage plane) margins should be indicated on the final surgical pathology report (174). Positive margins have been reported in 28% to 89% of cases; this finding is a particular problem in perihilar cases (165). High-grade dysplasia/CIS may be found a considerable distance from the primary tumor and may explain some bile duct stump recurrences (65).

(Hyperplasia) Metaplasia-Dysplasia-Carcinoma Sequence

As in the gallbladder, a metaplasia-dysplasia-carcinoma sequence can arise in the extrahepatic bile ducts. There is a similar, but fading, controversy regarding the relative importance of dysplasia versus adenoma (65,171,173,175). The importance of papillary hyperplasia is unclear. Papillary hyperplasia has been described in the extrahepatic ducts (53), and in one case it was mentioned as a potential precursor to dysplasia (149). Prominent subnuclear vacuoles similar to those seen in secretory endometrium have been described (55). In rare cases, differentiating papillary hyperplasia from dysplasia may be quite difficult (Fig. 22). Latio found metaplastic foci (intestinal, pyloric) adjacent to 80% of tumors (173). They contained a high content of nonsulfated acid mucins and neutral mucins, compared with the presence of only sulfomucins in normal bile duct epithelium. Dysplastic changes were seen in the mucosa adjacent to all tumors in that study and in 75% of cases reported in the three-dimensional mapping study of Suzuki et al. (175). In this detailed study, 42% of cases had multifocal areas of carcinoma, generally arising in zones of dysplasia. Kozuka et al. reported residual adenoma adjacent to 21% of tumors, including 75% of papillary adenocarcinomas (171). Rare foci of squamous metaplasia may provide the substrate for development of squamous cell carcinoma.

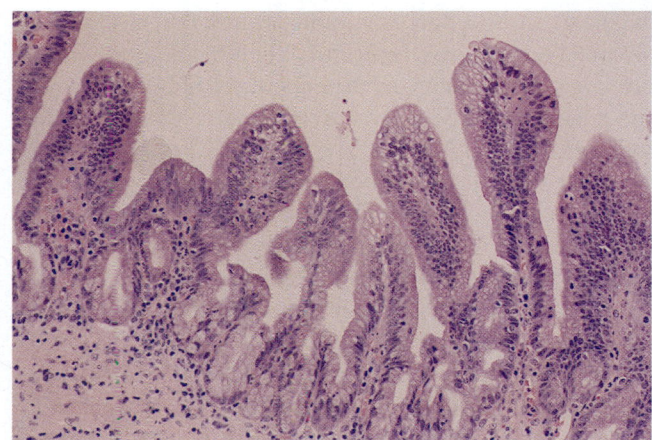

FIG. 22. Papillary hyperplasia of the common bile duct, with mild epithelial atypia and a few intraepithelial neutrophils. Indeterminate for dysplasia. Other foci (not shown) demonstrated convincing evidence of dysplasia. Differentiating hyperplasia from dysplasia can be difficult in the bile duct, particularly in small foci. A spectrum from hyperplasia to high-grade dysplasia, with foci of invasive adenocarcinoma, has been described in cases of so-called papillomatosis. This sequence is similar to that seen in pancreatic papillary intraductal mucinous neoplasms. (Kindly contributed by Mary P. Bronner, M.D., and Cyrus E. Rubin, M.D., University of Washington Medical Center, Seattle, WA.)

Differential Diagnosis

The presence of well-differentiated glands lined by cytologically bland cells in a densely fibrotic and often chronically inflamed wall can make the distinction of carcinoma from sclerosing cholangitis on frozen and permanent sections quite difficult even for the most experienced pathologists (145,146). These confusing histologic features tend to be more frequently encountered in the proximal segment of the extrahepatic bile ducts (3). Careful attention to the random pattern of gland infiltration, the presence of perineural invasion, and other features summarized in Table 8 (Figs. 19 and 21) and in the discussion of primary sclerosing cholangitis, aid in making a correct diagnosis of malignancy.

Differentiation of primary bile duct carcinomas that extend into adjacent organs (such as the pancreas, liver, ampulla, duodenum, gallbladder, stomach, and colon) from primary tumors arising at these sites may be impossible based solely on histologic grounds. The pathologist must also be aware that tumors from these local sites may directly spread into the extrahepatic biliary tree and that others (breast, colon, ovary, kidney) may metastasize there and simulate a primary tumor. Intraductal spread ("embolization") from tumors located in the hepatic parenchyma (hepatocellular carcinoma, cholangiocarcinoma, metastatic colon carcinoma) and even renal cell carcinoma may sometimes result in biliary obstruction and clinically mimic bile duct carcinoma (86,176).

Prognosis, Treatment, and Outcome

The prognosis of these tumors is dismal; the 5-year survival rate is about 5% (86,165). Most patients die within four months of diagnosis. The tumors of about 25% of patients are resectable; however, rates as high as 50% have been reported, particularly with distal tumors. Palliative therapy includes surgical biliary-intestinal bypass procedures as well as operative and nonoperative techniques for biliary intestinal drainage. Carefully selected patients with resectable perihilar tumors may have 5-year survival rates of 10% to 35%, with somewhat higher rates for distal tumors. The role of adjuvant radiotherapy or chemotherapy is unproved, and transplantation is generally not performed. Prognosis is most closely related to the stage of disease and to location (perihilar worse than distal), although resection margin status, nutritional status, and the presence of underlying sepsis are also important (86,177).

Staging based on the TNM system is similar but not identical to that used for gallbladder carcinoma (Table 5) (178). Patients with the uncommon T1 tumor (limited to subepithelial connective tissue or the fibromuscular layer) had a 60% 5-year survival rate in one study (177). Papillary adenocarcinomas are more likely to be only superficially invasive. The incidence of perineural and lymphatic invasion correlates directly with the depth of invasion (3,145,171,178). Overexpression of p53 protein has been described in 38% to 54% of cases (179,180), but this does not appear to be an independent predictor of survival. Only a small number of cases have been studied, however. Causes of death include liver failure, cholangitis, and sepsis. Metastatic disease is found at initial presentation and at autopsy in 15% to 30% and 30% to 75% of patients, respectively, with regional

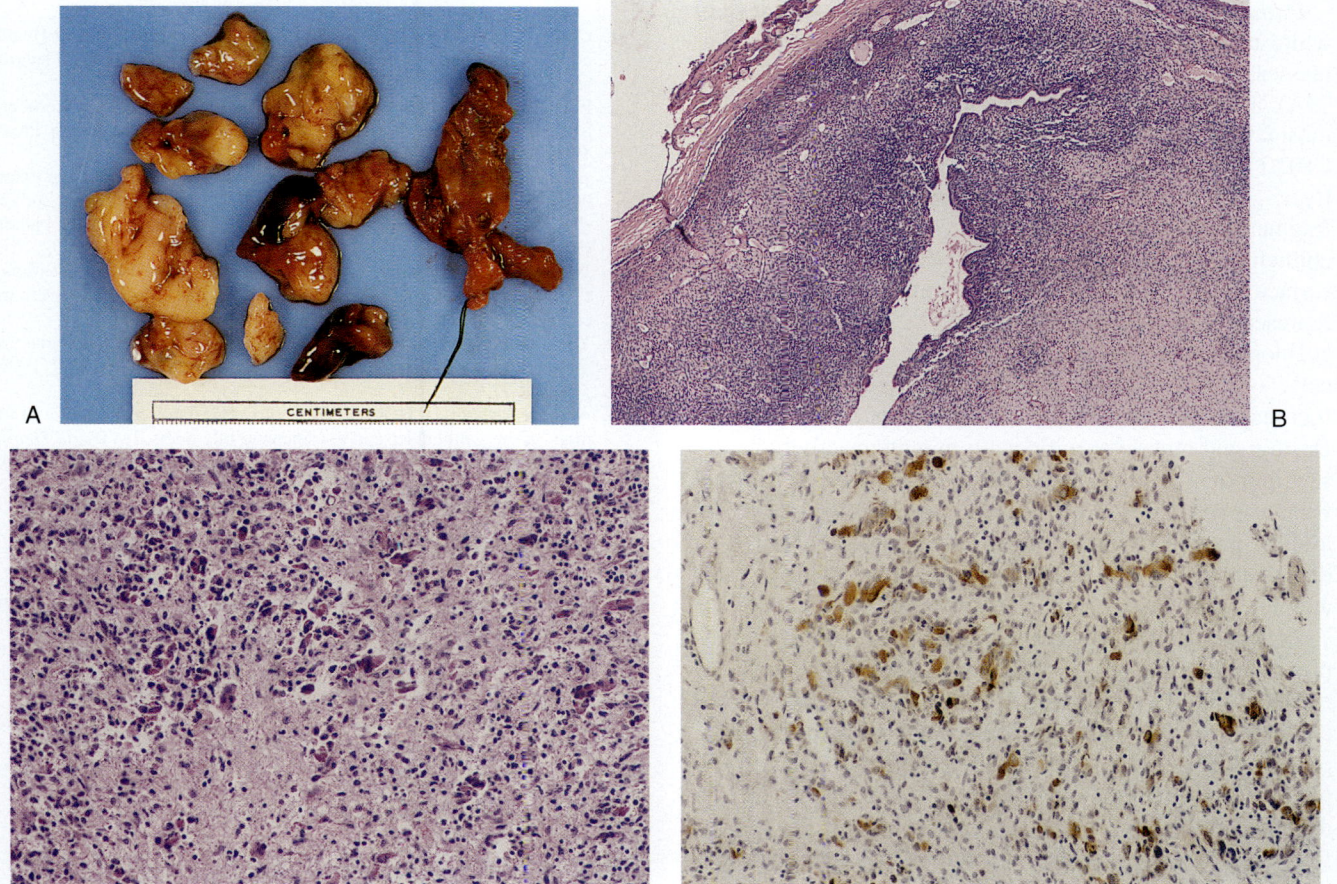

FIG. 23. Embryonal rhabdomyosarcoma (botryoid subtype). **A:** "Grapelike" (botryoid) fragments of tumor removed from the common bile duct are seen on the left. The right side of the photograph shows a portion of the duct. **B:** Condensed (cambium) layer composed primarily of primitive cells under the biliary epithelium. **C:** Focally, many rhabdomyoblasts with prominent eosinophilic cytoplasm are present. **D:** Prominent desmin immunoreactivity is evident, particularly in the more differentiated cells (immunohistochemistry, desmin). (Kindly contributed by Jane Chatten, M.D., Children's Hospital of Philadelphia, Philadelphia, PA.)

lymph nodes, liver, and peritoneum being the most common sites of disseminated disease (3,86,172).

Rare Primary Malignant Tumors

Embryonal Rhabdomyosarcoma

Clinical Features. Sarcomas account for far less than 1% of all bile duct malignancies; of these malignancies, embryonal rhabdomyosarcoma is most common (3,89). Less than 1% of rhabdomyosarcomas are found in the biliary tree. Tumors arising in the extrahepatic biliary tree are extremely rare in childhood; embryonal rhabdomyosarcoma is by far the most common of these unusual tumors (181,182). After choledochal cysts, it is probably the main cause of obstructive jaundice in children past infancy. Patients with rhabdomyosarcoma of the bile ducts are typically first seen at 3 to 4 years of age with malaise, fever, weight loss, and jaundice. A single case of rhabdomyosarcoma (alveolar subtype) has been described in an adult (183). There is no sexual preference. Ultrasonography and computed tomography aid in distinguishing this tumor from choledochal cyst by displaying the solid nature of the tumor.

Pathologic Features. The tumor consists of several white-tan, edematous, polypoid (botryoid or grapelike) masses, which cause partial or total luminal obstruction (Fig. 23A). Tumor size varies from 3 to 14 cm in diameter. The most common site within the extrahepatic biliary tree is the CBD (77%), followed by the hepatic duct (12%) and the liver, gallbladder, and ampulla (4% each). The polypoid fragments are usually covered by a layer of flattened biliary epithelium, although the lining may be denuded. Beneath the surface is a dense zone of primitive round to elongated cells representing the cambium layer (Fig. 23B,C). The deeply eosinophilic cytoplasm in some of the latter cells ("strap cells") represents rhabdomyoblastic differentiation. Some foci may be paucicellular with an abundant myxoid stroma. Desmin and muscle-specific actin immunoreactivity is present in nearly all cases, while myoglobin positivity is somewhat less sensitive (184). Recently, MyoD1 (myogenic regulatory protein) expression has been touted as being of diagnostic utility. The electron microscopic finding of thick and thin filaments also confirms the diagnosis.

Treatment and Outcome. Treatment with a multidisciplinary approach (surgery, combination chemotherapy, and radiotherapy) has occasionally resulted in long-term survival compared with the uniformly poor outcome reported previously (182). Metastases have been documented in about 40% of cases, mostly to regional lymph nodes, with only 15% to distant sites. Extension into the liver is common. For the differential diagnosis of the intrahepatic component versus undifferentiated sarcoma and mesenchymal hamartoma, see Table 24 in the chapter "Masses of the Liver" by Saul.

Other Tumors

Nearly 20 carcinoid tumors have been reported; they are typically without an associated hormonal syndrome (185). Cystadenocarcinoma, "carcinosarcoma" (sarcomatoid carcinoma), malignant fibrous histiocytoma, leiomyosarcoma, malignant melanoma, and lymphoma have all been described from time to time as primary malignancies arising in the extrahepatic bile ducts (3,89,186–188).

Metastatic Tumors

Metastatic carcinoma from various sites (including the colon, stomach, pancreas, breast, and kidney; see previous discussion of differential diagnosis), as well as lymphoma, may occasionally cause extrahepatic obstruction (86,176, 189–191). Typically the main site of involvement is the porta hepatis lymph nodes, but duct infiltration and intraductal growth may be the predominant finding. Metastatic malignant melanoma has also been described (192).

REFERENCES

The Gallbladder

General/Normal Anatomy and Histology/Specimen Processing

1. Gollan JL, Bulkley GB, Diehl AM, et al. National Institutes of Health consensus development conference statement on gallstones and laparoscopic cholecystectomy. *Am J Surg* 1993;165:390–398.
2. Frierson HF. Gallbladder and extrahepatic biliary tree. In: Sternberg SS, ed. *Histology for pathologists*, 2nd ed. New York: Raven Press, 1997:593–611.
3. Albores-Saavedra J, Henson DE. Tumors of the gallbladder and extrahepatic ducts. In: Hartman WH, ed. *Atlas of tumor pathology*, 2nd series, fascicle 22. Washington D.C.: Armed Forces Institute of Pathology, 1986.
4. Weedon D. Diseases of the gallbladder. In: MacSween RMN, Anthony PP, Scheuer PJ, Burt AD, Portmann BC, eds. *Pathology of the liver*, 3rd ed. New York: Churchill Livingstone, 1994:513–534.
5. Yamamoto M, Nagako S, Tahara E. Endocrine cells and lysozyme immunoreactivity in the gallbladder. *Arch Pathol Lab Med* 1986; 110:920–927.
6. Albores-Saavedra J, Henson DE, Sobin LH. Histological typing of tumors of the gallbladder and extrahepatic bile ducts. In: *World Health Organization international classification of tumors*, 2nd ed. New York: Springer-Verlag, 1991.

Congenital Abnormalities

7. Tejada E, Danielson C. Ectopic or heterotopic liver (choristoma) associated with the gallbladder. *Arch Pathol Lab Med* 1989;113:950–952.
8. Lamont N, Winthrop AL, Cole FM, Langer JC, Issenman RM, Finkel KC. Heterotopic gastric mucosa in the gallbladder: a cause of chronic abdominal pain in a child. *J Pediatr Surg* 1991;26:1293–1295.
9. Qizilbash A. Acute pancreatitis occurring in heterotopic pancreatic tissue in the gallbladder. *Can J Surg* 1976;19:413–414.

Cholelithiasis/Choledocholithiasis/Cholecystitis

10. Bilhartz LE. Acute acalculous cholecystitis, adenomyomatosis, cholesterolosis, and polyps of the gallbladder. In: Feldman M, Sleisenger MH, Scharschmidt BF, eds. *Sleisenger and Fordtran's gastrointestinal and liver disease: pathophysiology/diagnosis/management*, 6th ed. Philadelphia: WB Saunders, 1998:993–1005.
11. Sahlin S, Stahlberg D, Einarsson K. Cholesterol metabolism in liver and gallbladder mucosa of patients with cholesterolosis. *Hepatology* 1995;21:1269–1275.
12. Kmiot WA, Perry EP, Donovan IA, et al. Cholesterolosis in patients with chronic acalculous biliary pain. *Br J Surg* 1994;81:112–115.

13. Bilhartz LE, Horton JD. Gallstone disease and its complications. In: Feldman M, Sleisenger MH, Scharschmidt BF, eds. *Sleisenger and Fordtran's gastrointestinal and liver disease: pathophysiology/diagnosis/management*, 6th ed. Philadelphia: WB Saunders, 1998: 948–972.
14. Johnston DE, Kaplan MM. Pathogenesis and treatment of gallstones. *N Engl J Med* 1993;328:412–421.
15. Rescorla FJ. Cholelithiasis, cholecystitis, and common bile duct stones. *Curr Opin Pediatr* 1997;9:276–282.
15a.Redaelli CA, Buchler MW, Schilling MK, et al. High incidence of Mirizzi syndrome and gallbladder carcinoma. *Surgery* 1997; 121:58–63.
16. Cetta F, Lombardo F, Malet PF. Black pigment gallstones with cholesterol gallstones in the same gallbladder: 13 cases in a surgical series of 1,226 patients with gallbladder stones. *Dig Dis Sci* 1995;40:534–538.
17. Malet PF, Dabezies MA, Huang G, Long WB, Gadcz TR, Soloway RD. Quantitative infrared spectroscopy of common bile duct stones. *Gastroenterology* 1988;94:1217–1221.
18. Kim M-H, Sekijima J, Lee SP. Primary intrahepatic stones. *Am J Gastroenterol* 1995;90:540–548.
19. Crowther RS, Soloway RD. Pigment gallstone pathogenesis: from man to molecules. *Semin Liver Dis* 1990;10:171–180.
20. Singelton JM. Calcific enterolith obstruction of the intestine. *Br J Surg* 1970;57:234–236.
21. Csendes A, Burdiles P, Maluenda F, Diaz JC, Csendes P, Mitru N. Simultaneous bacteriologic assessment of bile from gallbladder and common bile duct in control subjects and patients with gallstones and common duct stones. *Arch Surg* 1996;131:389–394.
21a.Boutros HH, Pautler S, Chakrabarti S. Cocaine-induced ischemic colitis with small-vessel thrombosis of colon and gallbladder. *J Clin Gastroenterol* 1997;24:49–53.
22. Khettry U, Dwarakanath S, Pinson CW, Jenkins RL, Arkin CF. Histopathology of the donor gallbladder removed at orthotopic liver transplantation: correlation with graft function. *Hum Pathol* 1991; 22:437–441.
23. Fox JG, Dewhirst FE, Shen Z, et al. Hepatic *Helicobacter* species identified in bile and gallbladder from Chileans with chronic cholecystitis. *Gastroenterology* 1998;114:755–763.
24. Blaser MJ. Helicobacters and biliary tract disease. *Gastroenterology* 1998;114:840–845.
25. Ashur H, Siegal B, Oland Y, Adam YG. Calcified gallbladder (porcelain gallbladder). *Arch Surg* 1978;113:594–596.
26. Dabbs DJ. Eosinophilic and lymphoeosinophilic cholecystitis. *Am J Surg Pathol* 1993;17:497–501.
27. Chitkara YK. Pathology of the gallbladder in common bile duct obstruction: the concept of ascending cholecystitis. *Hum Pathol* 1993; 24:279–283.
28. Jessurun J, Bolio-Solis A, Manivel JC. Diffuse lymphoplasmacytic acalculous cholecystitis: a distinctive form of chronic cholecystitis associated with primary sclerosing cholangitis. *Hum Pathol* 1998; 28:512–517.
29. Shimizu M, Miura J, Tanaka T, Itoh H, Saitoh Y. Porcelain gallbladder: relation between its type by ultrasound and incidence of cancer. *J Clin Gastroenterol* 1989;11:471–476.
30. Estrada RL, Brown NM, James CE. Chronic follicular cholecystitis: radiological, pathological and surgical aspects. *Br J Surg* 1960; 48:205–209.
31. Thorpe MEC, Scheuer PJ, Sherlock S. Primary sclerosing cholangitis, the biliary tree and ulcerative colitis. *Gut* 1967;8:435–448.

Adenomyomatous Hyperplasia

32. Meguid MM, Aun F, Bradford ML. Adenomyomatosis of the gallbladder. *Am J Surg* 1984;147:260–262.
33. Burnett RA, McKay AJ. Inversion of the gallbladder. *Am J Clin Pathol* 1989;91:594–596.
34. Aldridge MC, Gruffaz F, Castaing D. Adenomyomatosis of the gallbladder: a premalignant lesion? *Surgery* 1991;109:107–110.
35. Katoh T, Nakai T, Hayashi S, Satake T. Noninvasive carcinoma of the gallbladder arising in localized adenomyomatosis. *Am J Gastroenterol* 1988;83:670–674.
36. Albores-Saavedra J, Henson DE. Adenomyomatous hyperplasia of the gallbladder with perineural invasion. *Arch Pathol Lab Med* 1995; 119:1173–1176.

AIDS-Related Cholecystitis

37. French AL, Beaudet LM, Benator DA, Levy CS, Kass M, Orenstein JM. Cholecystectomy in patients with AIDS: clinicopathologic correlations in 107 cases. *Clin Infect Dis* 1995;21:853–858.

Eosinophilic Cholecystitis

38. Felman RH, Sutherland DB, Conklin JL, Mitros FA. Eosinophilic cholecystitis, appendiceal inflammation, pericarditis, and a cephalosporin-associated eosinophilia. *Dig Dis Sci* 1994;39:418–422.
39. Tajima K, Katagiri T. Deposits of eosinophil granule proteins in eosinophilic cholecystitis and eosinophilic colitis associated with hypereosinophilic syndrome. *Dig Dis Sci* 1996;41:282–288.
40. Rosengart TK, Rotterdam H, Ranson JHC. Eosinophilic cholangitis: a self-limited cause of extrahepatic biliary obstruction. *Am J Gastroenterol* 1990;85:582–585.
41. Burke AP, Sobin LH, Virmani R. Localized vasculitis of the gastrointestinal tract. *Am J Surg Pathol* 1995;19:338–349.

Xanthogranulomatous Cholecystitis and Related Lesions

42. Goodman Z, Ishak KG. Xanthogranulomatous cholecystitis. *Am J Surg Pathol* 1981;5:653–659.
43. Franco V, Aragona F, Genova G, Florena AM, Stella M, Campesi G. Xanthogranulomatous cholecystitis: histopathological study and classification. *Pathol Res Pract* 1990;186:383–390.
44. Charpentier P, Prade M, Bognel C, Gadenne C, Duvillard P. Malakoplakia of the gallbladder. *Hum Pathol* 1983;14:827–828.
45. Cors A, Bosman C. Chronic cholecystitis with features of diffuse inflammatory pseudotumor: a clinico-pathological case study and review of the literature. *Ital J Gastroenterol* 1995;27:252–255.
46. Post AB, van Stolk R, Broughan TA, Tuthill RJ. Crohn's disease of the gallbladder. *J Clin Gastroenterol* 1993;16:139–142.

The Gallbladder in Extrahepatic Bile Duct Obstruction and Chronic Cholestatic Disorders

47. Jeffrey GP, Reed WD, Carrello S, Shilkin KB. Histological and immunohistochemical study of the gall bladder lesion in sclerosing cholangitis. *Gut* 1991;32:424–429.
48. Brandt DJ, MacCarty RL, Charboneau JW, LaRusso NF, Wiesner RH, Ludwig J. Gallbladder disease in patients with primary sclerosing cholangitis. *Am J Roentgenol* 1988;150:571–574.
49. Netto G, Klintmalm G, Albores-Saavedra J. Gallbladder morphology in liver explants of primary sclerosing cholangitis (PSC) and primary biliary cirrhosis (PBC). *Lab Invest* 1998;78:67A.
50. Herzog K, Goldblum JR. Gallbladder adenocarcinoma, acalculous chronic lymphoplasmacytic cholecystitis, ulcerative colitis. *Mod Pathol* 1996;9:194–198.

Vasculitis

51. Fish DE, Evans DJ, Pusey CD. Gallbladder vasculitis: a report of two cases. *Histopathology* 1993;23:584–585.
52. Marymount JV, Dakil ASR, Travers H, Houshoulder DF. Chemical cholecystitis associated with hepatic arterial chemotherapy delivered by a permanently implanted pump. *Hum Pathol* 1985;16:986–990.

Papillary Hyperplasia/Metaplasia/Dysplasia

53. Elving G, Silvonen E, Teir H. Mucosal hyperplasia of the gallbladder in cases of cholecystolithiasis. *Acta Chir Scand* 1969;135:519–521.
53a.Tanno S, Obara T, Fujii T, et al. Proliferative potential and K-ras mutation in epithelial hyperplasia of the gallbladder in patients with anomalous pancreaticobiliary ductal union. *Cancer* 1998;83: 267–275.
54. Yamamoto M, Nakajo S, Ito M, Tahara E. Primary mucosal hyperplasia of the gallbladder. *Acta Pathol Jpn* 1988;38:393–398.

55. Albores-Saavedra J, Vardaman CJ, Vuitch F. Non-neoplastic polypoid lesions and adenomas of the gallbladder. In: Rosen PP, Fechner RE, eds. *Pathology annual*, part 1. Norwalk: Appleton and Lange, 1993:145–177.
56. Yamigawa H, Tomiyama H. Intestinal metaplasia-dysplasia-carcinoma sequence of the gallbladder. *Acta Pathol Jpn* 1986;36:989–997.
57. Kozuka S, Hachisuka K. Incidence by age and sex of intestinal metaplasia in the gallbladder. *Hum Pathol* 1984;15:779–784.
58. Tsutsumi Y, Nagura H, Osamura Y, Wantanabe K, Yanaihara N. Histochemical studies of metaplastic lesion of the human gallbladder. *Arch Pathol Lab Med* 1984;108:917–921.
59. Albores-Saavedra J, Nadji M, Henson DE, Ziegels-Weissman J, Mones JM. Intestinal metaplasia of the gallbladder: a morphologic and immunohistochemical study. *Hum Pathol* 1986;17:614–620.
60. Yamaguchi K, Enjoji M. Gallbladder polyps: inflammatory, hyperplastic and neoplastic types. *Surg Pathol* 1988;1:203–213.
61. Tatematsu M, Furihata C, Miki K, et al. Complete and incomplete pyloric gland metaplasia of human gallbladder. *Acta Pathol Jpn* 1987;37:39–46.
62. De Boer WGRM, Rees JW, Nayman J. Inappropriate mucin production in gallbladder metaplasia and neoplasia: an immunohistochemical study. *Histopathology* 1981;5:295–303.
63. Hanada M, Shimizu H, Takami M. Squamous cell carcinoma of the gallbladder associated with squamous metaplasia and adenocarcinoma in situ of the mucosal columnar epithelium. *Acta Pathol Jpn* 1986;36:1879–1886.
64. Albores-Saavedra J, Alcantra-Vazquez A, Cruz-Ortiz H, Herera-Goepfert R. The precursor lesions of invasive gallbladder carcinoma: hyperplasia, atypical hyperplasia and carcinoma in situ. *Cancer* 1980;45:919–927.
65. Albores-Saavedra J, Henson DE. Gallbladder and extrahepatic bile ducts. In: Henson DE, Albores-Saavedra J, eds. *Pathology of incipient neoplasia*, 2nd ed. Philadelphia: WB Saunders, 1993:167–181.
66. Latio M. Histogenesis of epithelial neoplasms of human gallbladder. II. Classification of carcinoma on the basis of morphological features. *Pathol Res Pract* 1983;178:57–66.
67. Kozuka S, Tsubone M, Yasui A, Hachisuka K. Relation of adenoma to carcinoma in the gallbladder. *Cancer* 1982;50:2226–2234.
68. Albores-Saavedra J, Manrique JJ, Angeles Angeles A, Henson DE. Carcinoma in situ of the gallbladder. *Am J Surg Pathol* 1984;8:323–333.
69. Ojeda VJ, Shilkin KB, Walter MN-I. Premalignant epithelial lesions of the gallbladder: a prospective study of 120 cholecystectomy specimens. *Pathology* 1985;17:451–454.
70. Dowling GP, Kelly JK. The histogenesis of adenocarcinoma of the gallbladder. *Cancer* 1986;58:1702–1708.
71. Latio M. Histogenesis of epithelial neoplasms of human gallbladder. I. Dysplasia. *Pathol Res Pract* 1983;178:51–56.
72. Yamagiwa H. Mucosal dysplasia of the gallbladder: isolated and adjacent lesions to carcinoma. *Jpn J Cancer Res* 1989;80:238–243.
73. Riddell RH, Goldman H, Ransohoff DF, et al. Dysplasia in inflammatory bowel disease: standardized classification with provisional implications. *Hum Pathol* 1983;14:931–968.
73a. Albores-Saavedra J, Molberg K, Henson DE. Unusual malignant epithelial tumors of the gallbladder. *Semin Diagn Pathol* 1996;13:326–338.
74. Kijima H, Watanabe H, Iwafuchi M, Ishihara N. Histogenesis of gallbladder carcinoma from investigation of early carcinoma and microcarcinoma. *Acta Pathol Jpn* 1989;39:235–244.
75. Nakajo S, Yamamoto M, Tahara E. Morphometrical analysis of gallbladder adenoma and adenocarcinoma with reference to histogenesis and adenoma-carcinoma sequence. *Virchows Arch A Pathol Anat Histopathol* 1990;417:49–56.
76. Ajiki T, Onoyama H, Yamamoto M, et al. p53 protein expression and prognosis in gallbladder carcinoma and premalignant lesions. *Hepatogastroenterology* 1996;43:521–526.
76a. Wistuba II, Sugio K, Hung J, et al. Allele-specific mutations involved in the pathogenesis of endemic gallbladder carcinoma in Chile. *Cancer Res* 1995;55:2511–2515.

Benign Polyps and Tumors

77. Toda K, Souda S, Yoshikawa Y, Momiyama T, Ohshima M. Significance of laparoscopic excisional biopsy for polypoid lesions of the gallbladder. *Surg Laparosc Endosc* 1995;5:267–271.
78. Kubota K, Bandai Y, Noie T, Ishizaki Y, Teruya M, Makuuchi M. How should polypoid lesions of the gallbladder be treated in the era of laparoscopic cholecystectomy? *Surgery* 1995;117:481–487.
79. Warfel KA, Hull MT. Villous papilloma of the gallbladder in association with leukodystrophy. *Hum Pathol* 1984;15:1192–1194.
80. Barzilai M, Lerner A. Gallbladder polyps in children: a rare condition. *Pediatr Radiol* 1997;27:54–56.
81. Almagro VA. Diffuse papillomatosis of the gallbladder. *Am J Gastroenterol* 1985;80:274–278.
81a. Takei K, Watanabe H, Itoi T, Saito T. p53 and Ki-67 immunoreactivity and nuclear morphometry of "carcinoma-in-adenoma" and adenoma of the gall-bladder. *Pathol Int* 1996;46:908–917.
82. Chen KTK. Osteomas of the gallbladder. *Arch Pathol Lab Med* 1994;118:755–756.
83. Devaney K, Goodman ZD, Ishak KG. Hepatobiliary cystadenoma and cystadenocarcinoma: a light microscopic and immunohistochemical study of 70 patients. *Am J Surg Pathol* 1994;18:1078–1091.

Carcinoma

84. Piehler JM, Crichlow RW. Primary carcinoma of the gallbladder. *Surg Clin Obstet* 1978;147:929–942.
85. Jones RS. Carcinoma of the gallbladder. *Surg Clin North Am* 1990;70:1419–1427.
86. Pitt HA, Dooley WC, Yeo CJ, Cameron JL. Malignancies of the biliary tree. *Curr Probl Surg* 1995;32:1–90.
87. Yamaguchi K, Chijiwa K, Ichimiya H, et al. Gallbladder carcinoma in the era of laparoscopic cholecystectomy. *Arch Surg* 1996;131:981–985.
88. Sandor J, Ihasz M, Fazekas T, Regoly-Merei J, Batorfi J. Unexpected gallbladder cancer and laparoscopic surgery. *Surg Endosc* 1995;9:1207–1210.
89. Carriaga MT, Henson DE. Liver, gallbladder, extrahepatic bile ducts, and pancreas. *Cancer* 1995;75:171–190.
90. Misra SP, Dwivedi M. Pancreaticobiliary ductal union. *Gut* 1990;31:1144–1149.
91. Ohta T, Nagakawa T, Ueno K, et al. Clinical experience of biliary tract carcinoma associated with anomalous union of the pancreaticobiliary ductal system. *Jpn J Surg* 1990;20:36–43.
92. Komi N, Tamura T, Miyoshi Y, Kunitomo K, Udaka H, Takehara H. Nationwide survey of cases of choledochal cyst: analysis of coexistent anomalies, complications and surgical treatment in 645 cases. *Surg Gastroenterol* 1984;3:69–73.
93. Walsh N, Qizilbash A, Banerjee R, Waugh GA. Biliary neoplasia in Gardner's syndrome. *Arch Pathol Lab Med* 1987;111:76–77.
94. Wada K, Tanaka M, Yamaguchi K, Wada K. Carcinoma and polyps of the gallbladder associated with Peutz-Jeghers syndrome. *Dig Dis Sci* 1987;32:943–946.
95. Bartlett DL, Fong Y, Fortner JG, Brennan MF, Blumgart LH. Long-term results after resection for gallbladder cancer: implications for staging and management. *Ann Surg* 1996;224:639–646.
96. Young RH, Scully RE. Ovarian metastases from carcinoma of the gallbladder and extrahepatic bile ducts simulating primary tumors of the ovary: a report of 6 cases. *Int J Gynecol Pathol* 1990;9:60–72.
97. Krunic A, Martinovic N, Calonje E, Milinkovic M. Cutaneous metastatic adenocarcinoma of gallbladder origin presenting as carcinoma of unknown primary. *Int J Dermatol* 1995;34:360–362.
98. Dodd LG, Moffatt J, Hudson ER, Layfield LJ. Fine-needle aspiration of primary adenocarcinoma. *Diagn Cytopathol* 1996;15: 151–156.
99. Zargar SA, Khuroo MS, Mahajan R, Jan GM, Shah P. US-guided fine needle aspiration biopsy of gallbladder masses. *Radiology* 1991;179:275–278.
100. Yamaguchi K, Enjoji M. Carcinoma of the gallbladder: a clinicopathology of 103 patients and a newly proposed staging. *Cancer* 1988;62:1425–1432.
101. Albores-Saavedra J, Nadji M, Henson DE. Intestinal-type adenocarcinoma of the gallbladder: a clinicopathologic and immunohistochemical study of seven cases. *Am J Surg Pathol* 1986;10:19–25.
102. Callea F, Stuyck JM, Massi G, et al. Alpha 1 antitrypsin (AAT) deposits in gallbladder adenocarcinoma and liver in partial AAT deficiency (PiSZ phenotype). *Am J Clin Pathol* 1982;78:878–883.
102a. Lumsden AB, Mitchell WE, Vohman MD. Carcinosarcoma of the

gallbladder: a case report and review of the literature. *Am Surg* 1988;54:492–494.
103. American Joint Commission on Cancer. Gallbladder. In: *Cancer staging manual*, 5th ed. Philadelphia: Lippincott–Raven Publishers, 1997:103–108.
104. Itoi T, Wantanabe H, Ajioka Y, et al. APC, K-ras codon 12 mutations and p53 gene expression in carcinoma and adenoma of the gall-bladder suggest two genetic pathways in gall-bladder carcinogenesis. *Pathol Int* 1996;46:333–340.
105. Nishizawa-Takano J-E, Ayabe H, Hatano K, Yamaguchi H, Tagawa Y. Gallbladder cancer: a comparative study among clinicopathologic features, AgNORs, and DNA content analysis. *Dig Dis Sci* 1996; 41:840–847.
106. Kimura W, Shimada H. A case of gallbladder carcinoma with infiltration into the muscular layer that resulted in relapse and death from metastasis to the liver and lymph nodes. *Hepatogastroenterology* 1990;37:86–89.
107. Ouchi K, Owada Y, Matsuno S, Sato T. Prognostic factors in the surgical treatment of gallbladder carcinoma. *Surgery* 1987;101:731–737.
108. Wilkinson DS. Carcinoma of the gall-bladder: an experience and review of the literature. *Aust N Z J Surg* 1995;65:724–727.
109. Ohtsuka M, Miyazaki M, Itoh H, et al. Routes of hepatic metastasis of gallbladder carcinoma. *Am J Clin Pathol* 1998;109:62–68.

Other Primary Malignant Neoplasms

110. Willen R, Willen H. Primary sarcoma of the gallbladder: a light and electron microscopical study. *Virchows Arch A Pathol Anat Histopathol* 1982;396:91–102.
111. White J, Chan Y-F. Epithelioid angiosarcoma of the gallbladder. *Histopathology* 1994;24:269–271.
112. Toma P, Loy A, Pastorino C, Derchi LE. Leiomyomas of the gallbladder and splenic calcifications in an HIV-infected child. *Pediatr Radiol* 1997;27:92–94.
113. Jutte DL, Bell RH, Penn I, Powers J, Kolinjivadi J. Carcinoid tumor of the biliary tree: case report and literature review. *Dig Dis Sci* 1986;32:763–769.
114. Resnick MB, Jacobs DO, Brodsky GL. Multifocal adenocarcinoma in situ with underlying carcinoid tumor of the gallbladder. *Arch Pathol Lab Med* 1994;118:933–934.
115. Heath DI, Womack C. Malignant melanoma of the gall bladder. *J Clin Pathol* 1988;41:1073–1077.
116. Murphy MN, Lorimer SM, Glennon PE. Metastatic melanoma of the gallbladder: a case report and review of the literature. *J Surg Oncol* 1987;34:68–72.
117. Chatila R, Fiedler PN, Vender RJ. Primary lymphoma of the gallbladder: case report and review of the literature. *Am J Gastroenterol* 1996;91:2242–2244.

Metastatic Tumors

118. Langley RGB, Bailey EM, Sober AJ. Acute cholecystitis from metastatic melanoma to the gall-bladder in a patient with low-risk melanoma. *Br J Dermatol* 1997;136:279–282.
119. Laurino I, Melato M. Malignant angioendotheliomatosis (angiotropic lymphoma) of the gallbladder. *Virchows Arch A Pathol Anat Histopathol* 1990;417:243–246.
120. Payan HM, Grossman W, Pelaez M. Acute surgical abdomen and myelofibrosis. *Mod Pathol* 1989;2:70–72.

The Extrahepatic Ducts

Normal Anatomy and Histology/Routine Specimen Processing

121. Suchy FJ. Anatomy, anomalies and pediatric disorders of the biliary tract. In: Feldman M, Scharschmidt BF, Sleisenger MH, eds. *Sleisenger and Fordtran's gastrointestinal and liver disease: pathophysiology/diagnosis/management*, 6th ed. Philadelphia: WB Saunders, 1998:905–928.
122. Terada T, Kida T, Nakanuma Y. Extrahepatic peribiliary glands express alpha-amylase isozymes, trypsin and pancreatic lipase: an immunohistochemical analysis. *Hepatology* 1993;18:803–808.

Congenital Anomalies

123. Desmet VJ, Callea F. Cholestatic syndromes of infancy and childhood. In: Zakim D, Boyer TD, eds. *Hepatology: a textbook of liver disease*, vol. 2. Philadelphia: WB Saunders, 1996:1649–1698.
124. Mieli-Vergani G, Howard ER, Mowat AP. Liver disease in infancy: a 20 year perspective. *Gut* 1991;[Suppl]:S123–S128.
125. Ryckman FC, Noseworthy J. Neonatal cholestatic conditions requiring surgical reconstruction. *Semin Liver Dis* 1987;7:134–154.
126. Oguchi Y, Okada A, Nakamura T, et al. Histopathologic studies of congenital dilatation of the bile duct as related to an anomalous junction of the pancreaticobiliary ductal system: clinical and experimental studies. *Surgery* 1988;103:168–173.
127. Todani T, Wantanabe Y, Narusoe M, Tabuchi K, Okajima K. Congenital bile duct cysts: classification, operative procedures, and review of 37 cases including cancer arising from choledochal cysts. *Am J Surg* 1977;134:263–269.
128. Rossi RL, Silverman ML, Braasch JW, Munson JL, Remine SG. Carcinomas arising in cystic conditions of the bile ducts. *Ann Surg* 1987;205:377–384.
129. Voyles CR, Smadja C, Shands C, Blumgart LH. Carcinoma in choledochal cysts: age-related incidence. *Arch Surg* 1983;118:986–988.

Sclerosing Cholangitis

130. Bass NM. Sclerosing cholangitis and recurrent pyogenic cholangitis. In: Feldman M, Scharschmidt BF, Sleisenger MH, eds. *Sleisenger and Fordtran's gastrointestinal and liver disease: pathophysiology/diagnosis/management*, 6th ed. Philadelphia: WB Saunders, 1998:1006–1025.
131. Viering LM. Hepatobiliary complications of ulcerative colitis and Crohn's disease. In: Zakim D, Boyer TD. *Hepatology: a textbook of liver disease*, 3rd ed. Philadelphia: WB Saunders, 1996:1366–1405.
132. Czerniack A, Soreide O, Gibson RN, et al. Liver atrophy complicating benign bile duct strictures, surgical and interventional radiologic approaches. *Am J Surg* 1986;152:294–300.
133. Ludwig J. Surgical pathology of the syndrome of primary sclerosing cholangitis. *Am J Surg Pathol* 1989;13[Suppl]:43–49.
134. Walsh SV, Evangelista F, Khettry U. Inflammatory myofibroblastic tumor of the pancreaticobiliary region. *Am J Surg Pathol* 1998;22:412–418.
135. Bucuvalas JC, Bove KE, Kaufman RA, Gilchrist MJR, Oldham KT, Balistreri WF. Cholangitis associated with *Cryptococcus neoformans*. *Gastroenterology* 1985;88:1055–1059.
136. Gupta NM, Chaudhary A, Talwar P. Candidial obstruction of the common bile ducts. *Br J Surg* 1985;72:13.
137. Bonacini M. Hepatobiliary complications in patients with immunodeficiency virus infection. *Am J Med* 1992;92:404–411.
138. Krafcrian TD, Radner AB, Alcorn JM, Haghighi P, Fang FC. Biliary obstruction caused by epithelioid angiomatosis in a patient with AIDS. *Am J Med* 1990;89:820–822.
139. Nakanuma Y, Sasaki M, Terada T, Harada K. Intrahepatic peribiliary glands of humans. II. Pathologic spectrum. *J Gastroenterol Hepatol* 1994;9:80–86.
140. Balan V, LaRusso NF. Hepatobiliary disease in inflammatory bowel disease. *Gastroenterol Clin North Am* 1995;24:647–669.
141. Roberts SK, Ludwig J, LaRusso NF. The pathobiology of biliary epithelia. *Gastroenterology* 1997;112:269–279.
142. Kawaguchi K, Koike M, Tsuruta K, Okamoto A, Tabata I, Fujita N. Lymphoplasmacytic sclerosing pancreatitis with cholangitis: a variant of primary sclerosing cholangitis extensively involving the pancreas. *Hum Pathol* 1991;22:387–395.
143. Knisely AS, Lee RG. Pancreatic histopathology in patients with primary sclerosing cholangitis. *Mod Pathol* 1996;9:135A.
144. Terada S, Nakanuma Y, Unoura M, Kaneko S, Kobayashi K. Involvement of peribiliary glands in primary sclerosing cholangitis: a histopathologic study. *Intern Med* 1997;36:766–770.
145. Weinbren K, Mutum SS. Pathologic aspects of cholangiocarcinoma. *J Pathol* 1983;139:217–238.
146. Qualman J, Haupt HM, Bauer TW, Taxy J. Adenocarcinoma of the hepatic duct junction: a reappraisal of the histologic criteria of malignancy. *Cancer* 1984;53:1545–1551.
147. Nashan B, Schlitt HJ, Tusch G, et al. Biliary malignancies in primary

sclerosing cholangitis: timing for liver transplantation. *Hepatology* 1996;23:1105–1111.
148. Rosen CB, Nagorney DM. Cholangiocarcinoma complicating primary sclerosing cholangitis. *Semin Liver Dis* 1991;11:26–30.
149. Ludwig J, Wahlstrom E, Batts K, Wiesner RH. Papillary bile duct dysplasia in primary sclerosing cholangitis. *Gastroenterology* 1992; 102:2134–2138.
150. Ismail T, Angrisani L, Hubscher S, McMaster P. Hepatocellular carcinoma complicating primary sclerosing cholangitis. *Br J Surg* 1991;78:360–361.

Benign Tumors

151. Dowdy GS, Olin WG, Shelton EL, Waldron GW. Benign tumors of the extrahepatic ducts. *Arch Surg* 1962;85:503–513.
152. Burhans R, Myers RT. Benign neoplasms of the extrahepatic biliary ducts. *Am Surg* 1971;37:161–166.
153. Jennings PE, Rode J, Coral A, Dowsett J, Lees WR. Villous adenoma of the common hepatic duct: the role of ultrasound in management. *Gut* 1990;31:558–560.
154. Lam CM, Yuen ST, Yuen WK, Fan ST. Biliary papillomatosis. *Br J Surg* 1996;83:1712–1715.
155. Devaney K, Goodman ZD, Ishak KG. Hepatobiliary cystadenoma and cystadenocarcinoma: a light microscopic and immunohistochemical study of 70 patients. *Am J Surg Pathol* 1994;18:1078–1091.
156. Eisen RN, Kirby WM, O'Quinn JL. Granular cell tumor of the biliary tree: a report of two cases and a review of the literature. *Am J Surg Pathol* 1991;15:460–465.
157. Mulhollan TJ, Ro JY, El-Naggar AK, Sahin AA, Ayala AG. Granular cell tumor of the biliary tree. *Am J Surg Pathol* 1992;16:204–205.
158. Larson DM, Storsteen KA. Traumatic neuroma of the bile ducts with intrahepatic extension causing obstructive jaundice. *Hum Pathol* 1984;15:287–290.
159. Peison B, Benisch B. Traumatic neuroma of the cystic duct in the absence of previous surgery. *Hum Pathol* 1985;16:1168–1169.
160. Walsh MM, Drew M, Bleiweiss IJ. Neurofibroma of the common bile duct: a case report and review of the literature. *Int J Surg Pathol* 1997;4:245–248.
161. Ikoma A, Ueno T, Tanaka K, Saisho A, Yoshica A, Taira A. Cholesterol polyp of the common bile duct. *Am J Gastroenterol* 1995;90:1534–1535.
162. Ikei S, Mori K, Yamane T, Katafuchi S, Hirota M, Akagi M. Adenofibromatous hyperplasia of the extrahepatic bile duct: a report of two cases. *Jpn J Surg* 1989;19:576–582.
163. Legakis NC, Stamatiadis AP, Papadimitriou-Karapanou C, Apostolidis NS. Adenomyoma of the common bile duct. *Arch Surg* 1990;125:543.
164. Galloway PG. Heterotopic duodenum in the cystic duct. *Arch Pathol Lab Med* 1984;108:666–668.

Carcinoma and the (Hyperplasia)–Metaplasia–Dysplasia–Carcinoma Sequence

165. Vauthey J-N, Blumgart LH. Recent advances in the management of cholangiocarcinomas. *Semin Liver Dis* 1994;14:109–114.
166. Lees CD, Hermann RE. Familial polyposis coli associated with bile duct cancer. *Am J Surg* 1981;141:378–380.
167. Wetter LA, Ring EJ, Pellegrini CA, Way LW. Differential diagnosis of sclerosing cholangiocarcinomas of the common hepatic duct (Klatskin tumors). *Am J Surg* 1991;161:57–63.
168. Mansfield JC, Griffin SM, Wadehra V, Matthewson K. A prospective evaluation of cytology from biliary strictures. *Gut* 1997;40:671–677.
169. Kubota Y, Takaoka M, Tani K, et al. Endoscopic transpapillary biopsy for diagnosis of patients with pancreaticobiliary ductal strictures. *Am J Gastroenterol* 1993;88:1700–1704.
170. Verbeek PCM, van der Heyde MN, Ramsoekh T, Bosma A. Clinical significance of implantation metastases after surgical treatment of cholangiocarcinoma. *Semin Liver Dis* 1990;10:142–144.
171. Kozuka S, Tsubone M, Hachisuka K. Evolution of carcinoma in the extrahepatic bile ducts. *Cancer* 1984;54:65–72.
172. Sons HU, Borchard F. Carcinoma of the extrahepatic bile ducts: a postmortem study of 65 cases and review of the literature. *Surg Oncol* 1987;34:6–12.
173. Latio M. Carcinoma of the extrahepatic bile ducts: a histopathologic study. *Pathol Res Pract* 1983;178:67–72.
174. Bosma A. Surgical pathology of cholangiocarcinoma of the liver hilus (Klatskin tumor). *Semin Liver Dis* 1990;10:85–90.
175. Suzuki M, Takahashi T, Ouchi K, Matsuno S. The development and extension of hepatohilar bile duct carcinoma: a three-dimensional tumor mapping in the intrahepatic biliary tree visualized with the aid of a graphics computer system. *Cancer* 1989;64:658–666.
176. Miyagishima T, Ohnishi S, Chuma M, et al. Intraluminal tumor of the common bile duct as a metastasis of renal cell carcinoma. *Intern Med* 1996;35:720–723.
177. Mukhlesur MD, Bhuiya R, Nimura Y, et al. Clinicopathologic studies on perineural invasion of bile duct carcinoma. *Ann Surg* 1992;215: 344–349.
178. American Joint Commission on Cancer. Extrahepatic bile ducts (sarcomas and carcinoid tumors are not included). *Cancer staging manual*, 5th ed. Philadelphia: Lippincott–Raven Publishers, 1997: 109–112.
179. Washington K, Gottfried MR. Expression of p53 in adenocarcinoma of the gallbladder and bile ducts. *Liver* 1996;16:99–104.
180. Diamantis I, Karamitopoulou E, Perentes E, Zimmermann A. p53 protein immunoreactivity in extrahepatic bile duct and gallbladder cancer: correlation with tumor grade and survival. *Hepatology* 1995;22:774–779.

Other Primary Malignant Tumors

181. Lack E, Perez-Atayde AR, Schuster SR. Botryoid rhabdomyosarcoma of the biliary tract: report of five cases with ultrastructural observations and literature review. *Am J Surg Pathol* 1981;5:643–652.
182. Ruymann FB, Raney B, Crist WM, Lawrence W, Lindberg RD, Soule EH. Rhabdomyosarcoma of the biliary tree in childhood: a report from the intergroup rhabdomyosarcoma study. *Cancer* 1985; 56:575–581.
183. Aldabagh SM, Shibata CS, Taxy JB. Rhabdomyosarcoma of the common bile duct in an adult. *Arch Pathol Lab Med* 1986;110:547–550.
184. Eusebi V, Ceccarelli C, Gorza L, Schiaffino S, Bussolati G. Immunohistochemistry of rhabdomyosarcoma: the use of four different markers. *Am J Surg Pathol* 1986;10:293–299.
185. Hao L, Friedman AL, Navarro VJ, West B, Robert ME. Carcinoid tumor of the common bile duct producing gastrin and serotonin. *J Clin Gastroenterol* 1996;23:63–65.
186. O'Shea JS, Shah D, Cooperman AM. Biliary cystadenocarcinoma of extrahepatic duct origin arising in previously benign cystadenoma. *Am J Gastroenterol* 1987;82:1307–1310.
187. Washburn WK, Noda S, Lewis WD, Jenkins RL. Primary malignant melanoma of the biliary tract. *Liver Transplant Surg* 1995;1:103–106.
188. Brouland JP, Molimard J, Nemeth J, Valleur P, Galian A. Primary T-cell rich B-cell lymphoma of the common bile duct. *Virchows Arch A Pathol Anat Histopathol* 1993;423:513–517.

Metastatic Tumors

189. Stellato TA, Zollinger RM, Shuck JM. Metastatic malignant biliary obstruction. *Am Surg* 1987;53:385–388.
190. Franco D, Martin B, Smadja C, Szekely A-M, Rougier P. Biliary metastases of breast carcinoma: the case for resection. *Cancer* 1987;60:96–99.
191. Fidas P, Carey RW, Grossbard ML. Non-Hodgkin's lymphoma presenting with biliary obstruction. *Cancer* 1995;75:1669–1677.
192. Verbanck JJ, Rutgeerts LJ, van Aelst FJ, et al. Primary malignant melanoma of the gallbladder, metastatic to the common bile duct. *Gastroenterology* 1986;91:214–218.

CHAPTER 39

Anus and Perianal Area

Donald A. Antonioli and Henry D. Appelman

EMBRYOLOGY

The anal canal develops from the distal portion of the hindgut. Originally a cloaca, the hindgut is divided by the downgrowth of the urogenital septum into anterior urogenital and posterior alimentary compartments. Distally, the endodermally derived hindgut is separated from the perianal ectoderm by the anal membrane. The latter ruptures at approximately the seventh week of gestation, at which time the urogenital septum has also completely formed; thus, the normal anatomic relationships are established. Recent investigations have demonstrated that the anal membrane is located more distally (well below the anal valves) than originally believed; after it ruptures, squamous epithelium of ectodermal origin extends upward to line the anal canal to the level of the anal valves (1).

NORMAL ANATOMY

The anal canal is defined by the proximal and distal ends of the internal anal sphincter, which is the thickened, most distal part of the internal circular layer of the muscularis propria; it is continuous with the same layer of the rectal muscularis propria. The anal canal varies in length, but is approximately 4 cm in living patients and 3 cm in fixed specimens. On its mucosal surface is a series of vertical columns called the *anal columns* or *columns of Morgagni*. These are connected at their distal ends by a horizontal row of tissue folds referred to as the *anal valves*. These structures are most easily identified in children; they often become obscure or obliterated as patients age. The valves also may become more protruded with increasing age (1). Depressions between the columns are referred to as the *anal sinuses* or *sinuses of Morgagni* (Fig. 1A).

The circumferential dentate line is formed by the anal valves at the bases of the anal columns. If the usual landmarks are not visible, the dentate line should be defined by the location of the sinuses (1). Walls (2) has defined the upper margin of the anal canal as the level of insertion of the levator ani muscle. This area is partly lined by rectal columnar mucosa. Thus, when this definition is accepted, a small amount of distal rectal mucosa is included in the anal canal.

At flexible sigmoidoscopic or colonoscopic examination, the anal mucosa is often difficult to visualize because the endoscope quickly slips through the anal canal into the wider and longer rectum. The best views of the anus are obtained either on retroflex examinations with the flexible endoscopes or by using the rigid anoscope. However, subtle alterations in anal mucosal architecture indicative of neoplastic processes may be missed unless the endoscopic procedure is directed toward a detailed anal examination.

Histologically, the anal canal can be divided into three zones: an upper or proximal colorectal zone, a middle anal transitional zone (ATZ), and a lower or distal squamous zone (3). The colorectal zone mucosa is similar to rectal mucosa, but compared to rectal mucosa, the crypts are normally shorter and more irregular in shape and orientation than in the colon, and the lamina propria may contain more smooth muscle fibers, which extend upward from the muscularis mucosae. These normal findings should not be interpreted as evidence of chronic inactive proctitis; they may be nothing more than the consequence of chronic physiologic prolapse of the distal-most columnar mucosa.

Diseases occurring in this proximal columnar zone are indistinguishable from those occurring in the rectum. Thus, for example, adenocarcinomas arising here are identical with colorectal carcinomas, and they should be included with the colorectal neoplasms rather than making them a specific type of anal canal carcinoma. However, some studies, such as a recent national cancer data base report, include these adenocarcinomas in the category of anal neoplasms, thus confusing the data and making comparative analyses difficult (4).

The ATZ extends upward from the dentate line for vari-

D. A. Antonioli: Department of Pathology, Beth Israel Deaconess Medical Center, and Harvard Medical School, Boston, Massachusetts 02215.

H. D. Appelman: Department of Pathology, University of Michigan Medical Center, Ann Arbor, Michigan 48109-0054.

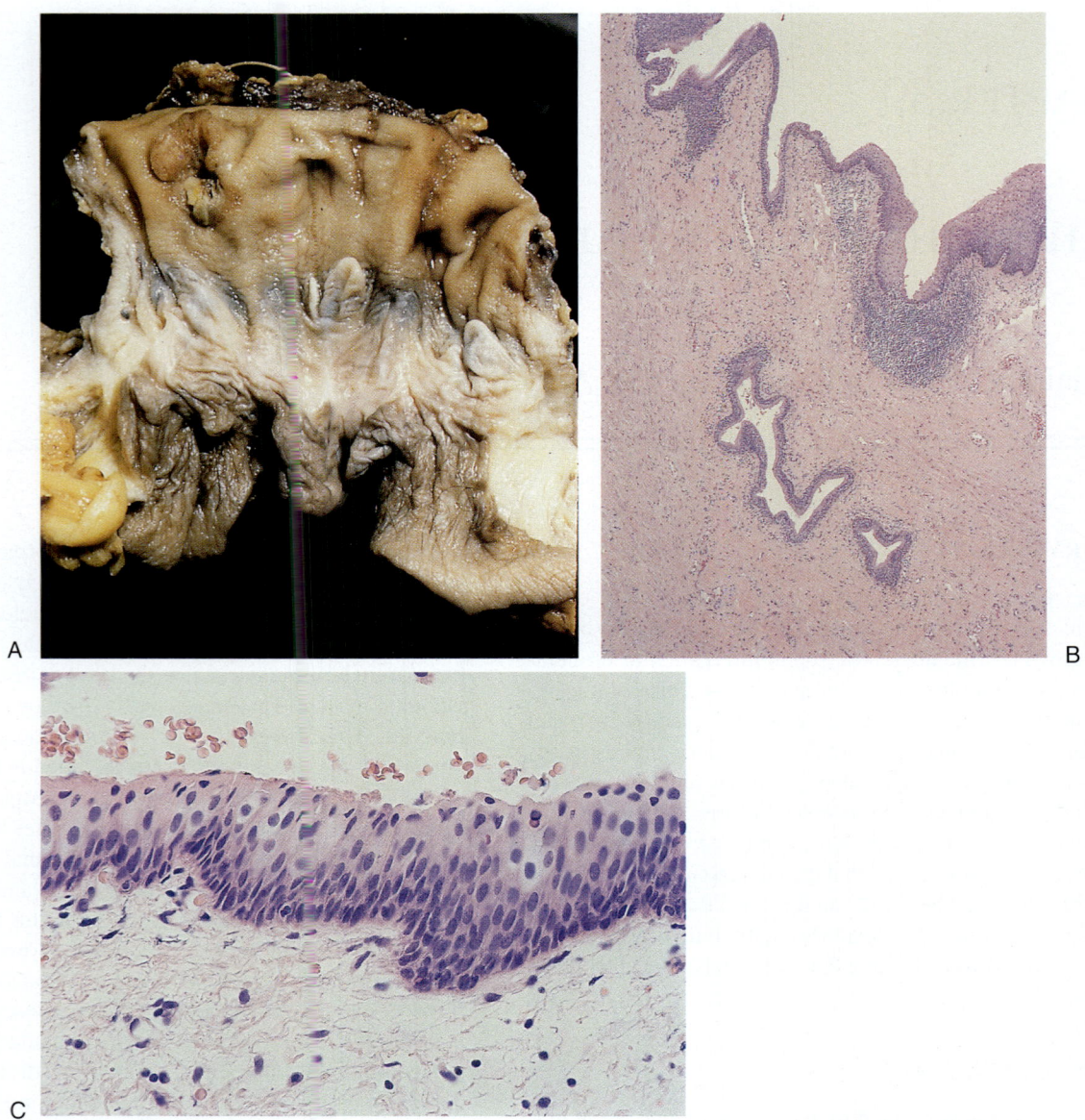

FIG. 1. A: Gross specimen of the anal canal. The vertical columns of Morgagni are evident; between them are the slightly depressed anal sinuses. The anal valves are not easily identified. A rectal cancer is also evident on the right side of the photograph. **B:** Low-power view of the anal transitional zone (ATZ), showing the surface epithelium and an anal gland. **C:** High-power view of the characteristic ATZ epithelium, which is multilayered and composed of uniform medium-sized cells.

able distances (from barely discernible to 2.0 cm in different specimens) to join the colorectal zone. It may contain a variety of epithelia. The most typical variant ("ATZ epithelium") is four to nine cells thick and is composed of relatively small cells surmounted by a layer of cuboidal, polygonal, or mucinous columnar cells. The nature of this epithelium is unclear: It has features of both metaplastic squamous mucosa and of urothelium (3,5). The ATZ may also contain colorectal crypts (especially in its upper part) and areas of mature squamous epithelium. Endocrine cells and melanocytes are also normal epithelial constituents (6).

The melanocytes are typically most numerous in the distal squamous zone, rare in the ATZ, and not present in the colorectal zone (7). However, in patients with anal melanomas, melanocytes have also been found in the colorectal zone. Six to eight anal glands, with their characteristic multilayered epithelium and intraepithelial mucinous cysts, extend from the ATZ into the submucosa (see Fig. 1B and C). Some penetrate the internal anal sphincter (3), whereas others extend distally or proximally beneath the anal epithelium.

The distal squamous zone has a flat, nonkeratinized squamous mucosa with melanocytes but without glands. It merges distally with perianal skin, the latter characterized by keratinization of the squamous epithelium and by the presence of hair follicles and apocrine glands (1).

Refer to standard textbooks for a discussion of the vasculature and innervation of the anal canal.

NONNEOPLASTIC DISEASES INTRINSIC TO THE ANUS

Congenital Abnormalities

Embryologic abnormalities involving the anal canal occur in approximately 1 in 5,000 births and include stenosis and absence of the anal canal, imperforate anus, fistulas, and anorectal duplications and cysts (1,8). Some of these conditions, as well as Hirschsprung's disease (aganglionic megacolon), are discussed in Chapter 33. In the evaluation of patients suspected of having Hirschsprung's disease, ganglion cells are normally absent or sparse in the anorectal wall for at least 1 to 2 cm above the dentate line (1,9). Therefore, biopsy specimens obtained to detect ganglion cells in the submucosal plexus should always be taken from above this zone.

Hemorrhoids

If there is deterioration of the connective tissue and smooth muscle that normally anchor the anal submucosal vascular sinusoids, the sinusoids may prolapse and form hemorrhoids. Bleeding is the major sign of hemorrhoids; pain occurs only when they are strangulated and thrombosed (10). Portal hypertension is not associated with an increased prevalence of hemorrhoids, but rather with more severe bleeding related to elevated portal venous pressure and, possibly, defects in coagulation (1,11).

Chronically prolapsed or thrombosed hemorrhoids may be resected. Microscopically, excision specimens contain dilated thick-walled submucosal vessels and sinusoidal spaces, often with thromboses and adjacent hemorrhage. The surface epithelium varies depending on the site of origin of the hemorrhoid within the anal canal; thus, it may be colorectal, ATZ type, or squamous.

All tissues excised as clinical hemorrhoids should be examined histologically. Hemorrhoids are common, but any anal neoplasm may present clinically as hemorrhoids. Furthermore, the ATZ and squamous epithelium covering the hemorrhoids may contain flat or papillary condylomas, a variety of squamous hyperplasias and the whole gamut of dysplasia, *in situ* carcinoma, and superficially invasive carcinoma (see section on Neoplastic Diseases Intrinsic to the Anus). Furthermore, the stroma may contain unexpectedly florid inflammation that may raise the possibility of infections (such as herpes or syphilis) or even Crohn's disease (CD) (1,8,10). A careful search for viral cytopathic changes should be undertaken. In particular, an inflammatory infiltrate rich in plasma cells may signify syphilitic infection.

Anal Tags, Papillae, and Fibroepithelial Polyps

Anal tags, also known as fibroepithelial polyps, are projections of submucosa and overlying mucosa, the latter usually being squamous. The submucosa contains the loose fibrous tissue with scattered blood vessels that is characteristic of anal submucosa in general. However, some anal tags contain large, multinucleated, stellate-shaped stromal cells (12). These tags often have the clinical appearance of hemorrhoids, and they are usually resected and submitted to the pathologist as hemorrhoids; however, they do not contain dilated thick-walled varices, any evidence of hemorrhage (recent or old), or organizing thrombi. They are identical to cutaneous acrochordons and may be the same as some forms of hypertrophied anal papillae (Fig. 2) (12,13)

Inflammatory Cloacogenic Polyp

Inflammatory cloacogenic polyps (ICP) occur predominantly in middle-aged patients whose most common complaint is rectal bleeding of variable (but often lengthy) duration. The polyps, which are located within the anal canal, are single or multiple, variable in size (but generally in the 1.0 to 2.0 cm range), and usually sessile. Thus, they clinically and grossly mimic hemorrhoids and are usually resected because they are diagnosed as hemorrhoids (14,15). The pathogenesis is presumably prolapse, with subsequent ischemic damage and repair of the proximal anal mucosa. ICPs resemble the polypoid variants of the solitary rectal ulcer syndrome and other colonic mucosal prolapse syndromes. They also have been described in two patients with CD (but without documented anal involvement) and distal to one rectal carcinoma. However, the ICPs may be unrelated to the other diseases. Simple excision is usually curative (14).

Histologically, the features of ICP are variable (Fig. 3). They may have a tubulovillous architecture, often with crypts extending into the submucosa, an appearance similar

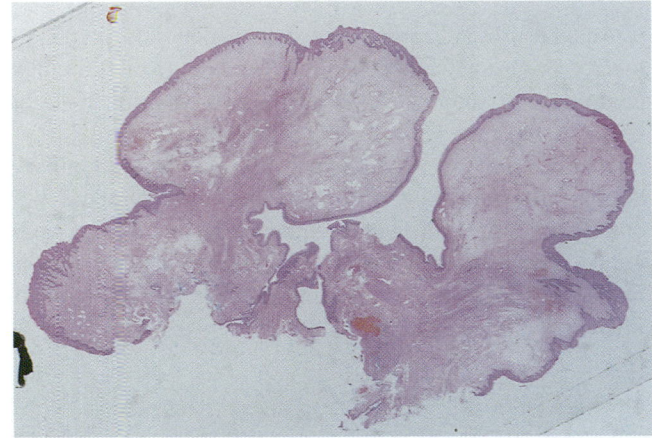

FIG. 2. Low-power view of anal fibroepithelial polyps (anal tags; hypertrophied anal papillae). The submucosa is formed of loose connective tissue containing thin-walled blood vessels.

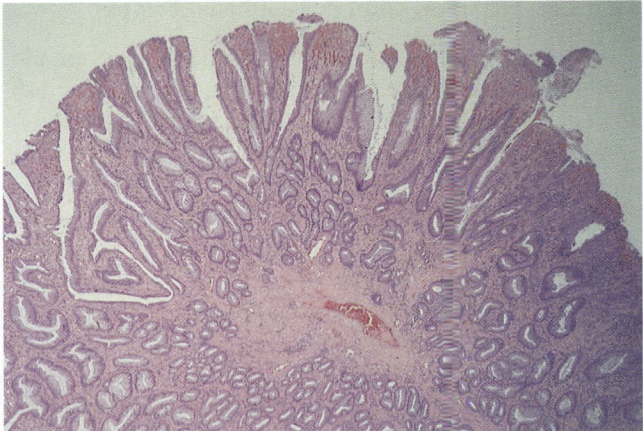

FIG. 3. Inflammatory cloacogenic polyp. Typical features include the elongated, irregular crypts, the eroded surface with exudate, and strands of smooth muscle in the lamina propria.

to colitis cystica profunda. The muscularis mucosae is thickened and irregular, frequently extending as fibromuscular strands into the lamina propria. This appearance is reminiscent of the mucosa in other colorectal mucosal prolapse syndromes. The epithelium is a mixture of squamous and colorectal, usually with patches of ATZ-type mucosa as well. The villiform surface commonly is focally eroded and covered by exudate. The adjacent epithelium may be regenerative or hyperplastic. Because of the combination of villi and hyperplastic epithelium, ICPs may superficially resemble villous adenomas (14,15). However, these lesions should not be misdiagnosed as colorectal-type adenomas, and the submucosal cystic crypts should not be misinterpreted as invasive carcinoma. Recognition of the benign epithelial nuclear cytology, the lack of desmoplasia, and the typically eroded villiform surface of ICP should eliminate diagnostic errors.

Fissures and Fistulas

Anal fissures are common posttraumatic lesions, typically located posteriorly in the midline (8). Anal fistulas are also common and usually develop secondary to chronic infection of the anal glands. Many are idiopathic, but they are also frequent occurrences in patients with CD. On microscopic examination, specimens from fistulas contain acute and chronic inflammation with granulation tissue, foreign body giant cells, and, occasionally, granulomas. ATZ or squamous epithelium may extend into the tract and partially epithelialize it.

Crohn's Disease

In CD, the anal canal is involved in about 25% of patients with small intestinal disease and 75% of those with colonic disease (16). The anal findings in CD are varied and include fissures, fistulas, ulcers, abscesses, and tags. Anal involvement, which rarely may be the first manifestation of CD, tends to pursue a benign course, but late malignant complications have been reported (see section on Adenocarcinoma) (16–20).

In CD, the most characteristic finding is granulomas, which may or may not contain multinucleated giant cells, are nonnecrotic, and are not associated with foreign material. From a practical standpoint, the diagnosis of CD cannot be made with confidence on a biopsy of an anal fissure, fistula, or inflammatory polyp unless the patient has known CD elsewhere. However, CD can be suspected if a biopsy from an anal fissure, fistula, or tag contains small, tight, nonnecrotizing granulomas close to the mucosa, especially in a young person with no other explanation for fissures or fistulas. Patients with disseminated tuberculosis may also have anal disease with granulomas. Tuberculous granulomas are generally caseating, and stains for acid-fast bacilli may be positive. Cultures, if they are positive for tubercle bacilli, may be helpful for precisely categorizing a particular specimen (8).

Lymphoid Polyps

Although they are most common in the distal rectum, benign lymphoid polyps may also develop in the colorectal-mucosa–lined upper anal canal. Grossly, they are usually small and may be superficially eroded. Microscopically, they consist of enlarged lymphoid follicles or clusters of follicles with reactive germinal centers, usually covered by columnar mucosa with occasional patches of ATZ-type epithelium (21). The pathogenesis of these benign lesions is obscure. They may be more common in children than adults, but we have noticed an unusually large number in young women. They are not associated with lymphoma.

NEOPLASTIC DISEASES INTRINSIC TO THE ANUS

Although uncommon, malignancies of the anal canal encompass a complex array of neoplasms arising in diverse locations within the canal (Table 1). The most confusing groups in terms of nomenclature have been the tumors arising from the surface epithelium of the ATZ and distal squamous mucosa, which have been variously categorized as "squamous," "basaloid," "cloacogenic," and "transitional." The World Health Organization recognizes the following anal carcinomas: squamous cell (keratinizing, nonkeratinizing, and basaloid), adenocarcinoma (rectal type, of anal glands, and within anorectal fistulas), small-cell carcinoma, and undifferentiated carcinoma (22). Refer to recent reviews for further discussion of these various categories (3,8,21,23).

Surface Epithelial Carcinomas of the Anal Transitional Zone and Squamous Zone

In this chapter, we classify all these surface epithelial carcinomas of the ATZ as variants of squamous-cell carcinoma

TABLE 1. *Types and sites of origin of anal canal malignancies*

Neoplasm	Site of origin in anal canal		
	Colorectal zone (upper)	Anal transitional zone (middle)	Squamous zone (lowest)
Adenocarcinoma of colorectal type	+		
Squamous-cell carcinoma		+	+
Basaloid carcinoma		+	
Melanoma		+	+
Carcinoid	+	+	
Small-cell carcinoma	+	+	
Mucinous adenocarcinoma[a]		−	

[a] May also be associated with chronic fistulas and congenital duplications. Site of origin uncertain.
Modified from ref. 6.

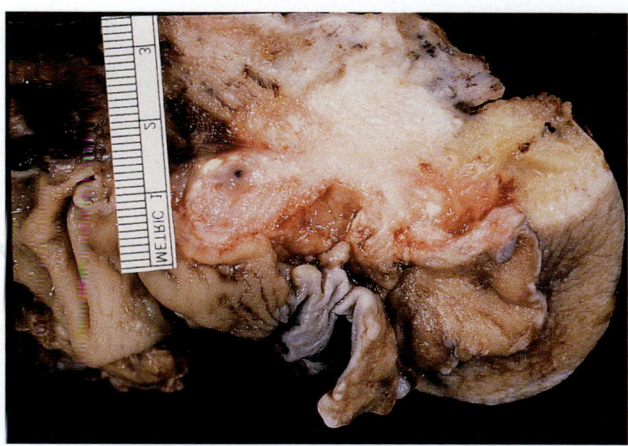

FIG. 4. Cross-section through an anal canal squamous-cell carcinoma. The central portion of the cancer is ulcerated. Note the upward, deep, and distal extension of the tumor.

for several reasons. First, the precise meaning of terms such as "cloacogenic" and "transitional" is not agreed upon by all authors. Also, recent advances in knowledge about the embryology of the anal canal have cast doubt on the validity of the term "cloacogenic" (1). Ultrastructurally, the ATZ mucosa is complex; rather than being a urothelial-type of transitional epithelium, it has both squamous and transitional characteristics (5). Furthermore, many of these neoplasms have a mixed histology; classification as to predominant cell type may be subjective and is dependent on the extent of tissue sampling (24). Finally, although earlier studies suggested differences in prognosis between patients with the basaloid-type of cloacogenic carcinoma when compared to those with squamous-cell carcinoma, recent large series have demonstrated that, in general, the histology of the tumor is not a variable of clinicopathologic significance.

Squamous-Cell Carcinomas

Squamous-cell carcinomas of the anal canal, which account for 1% to 2% of all colonic and anal malignancies (25–27), occur chiefly in middle-aged patients with a marked female predominance that varies from 5:1 to 3:2, depending on the population studied (3,23–25,28,29). Rectal bleeding is the most common presenting feature, followed by anorectal pain or a mass (17,24,25).

Pathologic Features

Grossly, the carcinomas are typically nodular and often ulcerated. Most are large (more than 3 to 4 cm in diameter) when first diagnosed (21). They invade deeply into the wall and spread distally and proximally. Some cancers that extend upward beneath the columnar mucosa of the proximal anus and distal rectum may invade that mucosa, producing an erosion, ulcer, or polypoid projection proximal to the primary site of the carcinoma, which is in the more distal ATZ (Figs. 4 and 5).

The histologic features are variable (Fig. 6). There may be well-developed squamous-cell carcinoma, which is focally keratinizing and resembles invasive carcinoma of the cervix. In some tumors, squamous areas are pleomorphic. The basaloid pattern is characterized by small, crowded, undifferentiated cells with focal, generally imperfect, palisading of peripheral nuclei in the tumor nests. The center of these nests often contains tiny foci of keratinization and variably sized geographic areas of granular necrosis. The basaloid pattern can be distinguished from upward extension of basal cell carcinoma originating in perianal skin because of the necrosis, the generally larger cells of the basaloid carcinoma, its more numerous mitoses, and its more flagrant invasive growth pattern (3). Also, the basal cell carcinomas have the

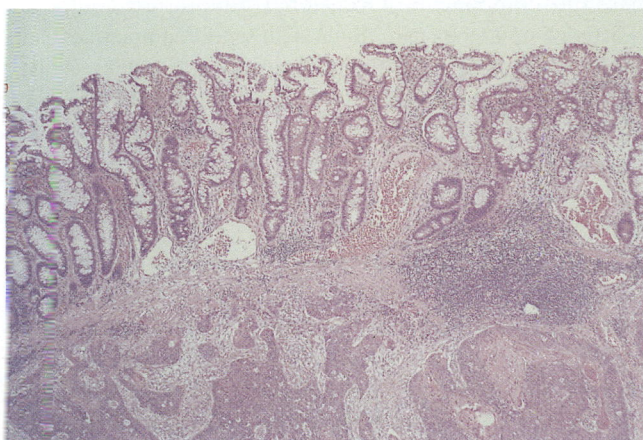

FIG. 5. Anal squamous cell carcinoma has extended upward in the submucosa into the distal rectum. Invasion by such tumors into the mucosa may be detected in rectal biopsies. The rectal mucosa itself has features of prolapse.

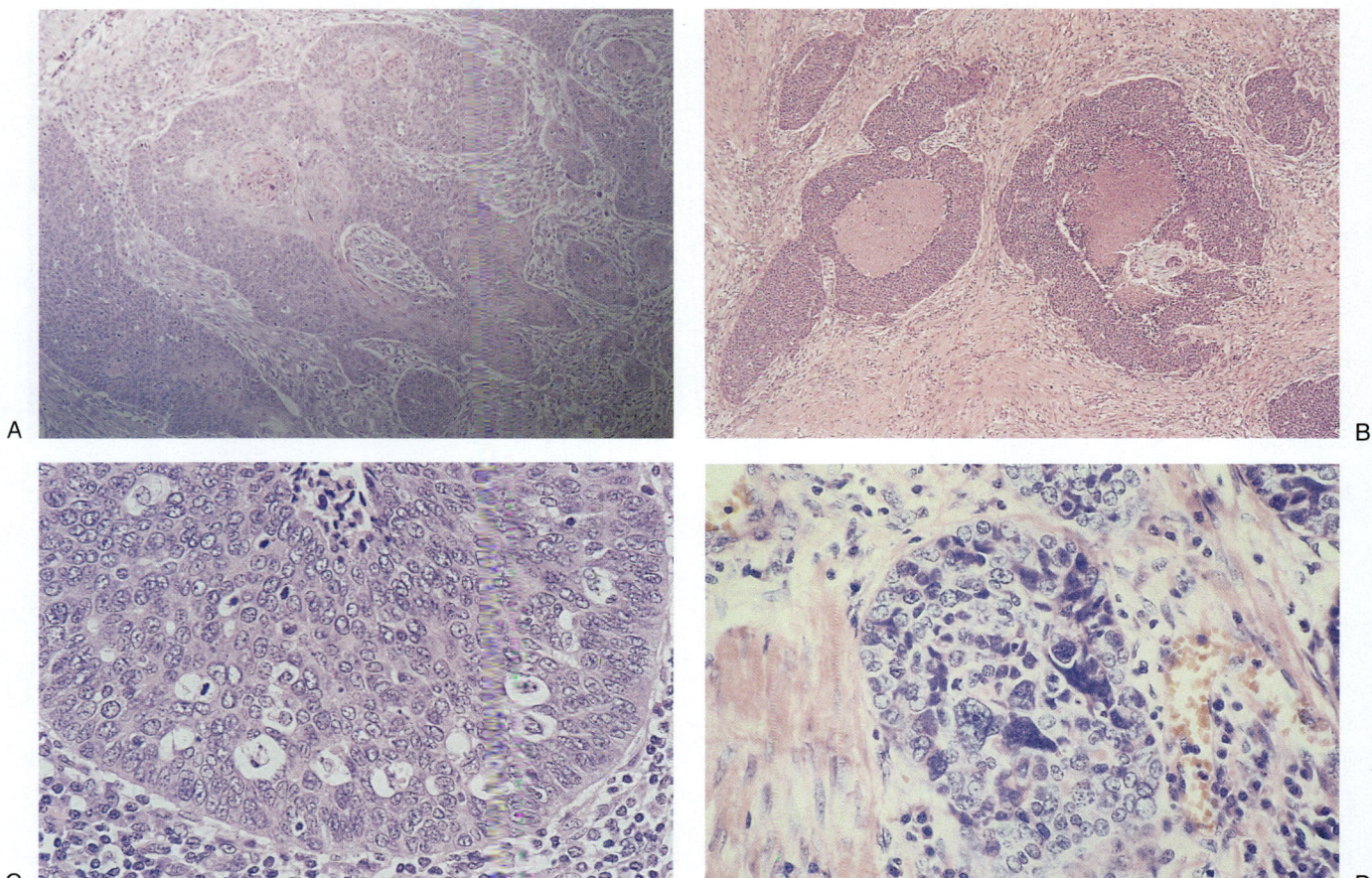

FIG. 6. Histologic aspects of anal squamous cell carcinoma. **A:** Area of invasive tumor with squamous pearl formation. **B:** Typical basaloid growth pattern, with a suggestion of peripheral palisading and central necrosis of tumor nodules. **C:** Microcyst formation in an area of basaloid carcinoma. **D:** Poorly differentiated (pleomorphic) carcinoma. Multiple different histologic patterns are often present in a single anal squamous cancer.

characteristic basophilic desmoplastic stroma that is seen in identical tumors of the skin.

In some anal carcinomas, there are equal squamous and basaloid components. Occasional tumors are composed mostly of squamous carcinoma with scattered mucin cells or mucin-containing cysts, so that, to a limited degree, they may resemble mucoepidermoid tumors of salivary gland origin (3,23,27). Finally, some tumors contain all or a large variety of patterns. Common to all types are scattered microcysts within the epithelium that do not contain mucin, but are either empty or contain debris.

Because of the tendency of these carcinomas to undermine the mucosa proximally and secondarily invade the distal rectum or proximal columnar-lined anus, and because of the difficulty in examining the anus endoscopically, rectal biopsies positive for squamous carcinomas may actually be of neoplasms that arise distally. It has been our experience that biopsies of ATZ carcinomas most commonly contain crypts on the surface, with the basaloid or squamous components located in the submucosa and extending into the base of the mucosa, sometimes appearing to replace crypts.

Prognostic Features

The most important factor determining outcome is the stage of disease; the importance of the histologic grade of the neoplasm is too widely variable among studies to be useful (3,23–26,28–30). The prognosis of anal canal squamous malignancies is related to depth of invasion, the status of regional lymph nodes, and the presence of distant metastases. The tumors are staged as follows: stage A tumors are either intraepithelial or superficially invasive; stage B tumors penetrate into the muscularis propria or adjacent pelvic tissues; stage C tumors have regional node metastases; and stage D tumors are unresectable, either because of massive local spread or distant metastases (27). The 5-year survival rate after attempts at curative therapy varies from 50% to 70% in different series (24,25,26,28,31). Small lesions (less than 2.0 cm in diameter) confined to mucosa and submucosa (stage A) and with well-differentiated histology are associated with 100% survival (26,29). Extension of tumor into or through the muscularis propria into perianal soft tissue (stage B) decreases 5-year survival to 20% to 30%, as does the presence of regional nodal metastases (stage C) (23,26,29). Recurrences are commonly confined to the pelvis, but distant metastases (chiefly to liver and lung—stage D) may occur (21,23,25,26,32). Recent data also suggest that aneuploidy may be an independent indicator of poor prognosis (30). The tumors may be treated by surgery or by radiation and/or chemotherapy (28,33). However, recent treatment programs have emphasized the nonsurgical approach, so surgical specimens of anal canal squamous carcinomas have become rarities (30,31).

Precursor Lesions

Precursor lesions and etiologic factors for anal epidermoid tumors are currently being studied. Condylomas, squamous-cell dysplasias, and carcinoma *in situ* (anal canal intraepithelial neoplasia [ACIN]), with histologic features like those of cervical intraepithelial neoplasia, have been identified adjacent to invasive cancers and as incidental findings in small resection specimens (usually hemorrhoidectomy tissue) (Fig. 7) (3,34–38). Like its cervical counterpart, ACIN can be divided into three grades: I (mild dysplasia), II (moderate dysplasia), and III (severe dysplasia and carcinoma *in situ*). Grade I lesions are considered low grade, whereas grades II and III lesions are high grade.

Epidemiologic and *in situ* hybridization studies suggest that some forms of ACIN and some forms of invasive squamous-cell carcinoma are associated with human papilloma virus (HPV) infection (especially genotypes 16 and 18 and, less commonly, 6 and 11), (38–42). In one study (43), the predominantly basaloid carcinomas were not associated with HPV infection, whereas the predominantly squamous-cell carcinomas were. However, in two subsequent studies (44,45), the predominantly basaloid carcinomas were more likely to contain HPV RNA or HPV DNA than were the predominantly squamous-cell carcinomas. It currently appears that there is no difference in HPV associations based on tumor morphology. The probability of detecting HPV sequences in anal carcinomas is related to the sensitivity of the technique used, with the polymerase chain reaction giving the highest yield of positive cases (42,45). There may also be geographic and population differences in the HPV association with anal cancer (46). Finally, there is some suggestion that tumors containing HPV DNA are more highly proliferative and more likely to be aneuploid than those that are negative (47).

Studies of genetic sequences in anal squamous carcinoma are limited. In one study, C-*myc* oncogene expression seems to have been important in some cases (48). The cases of ACIN with this oncogene expression were more likely to have adjacent invasive carcinoma than those that either

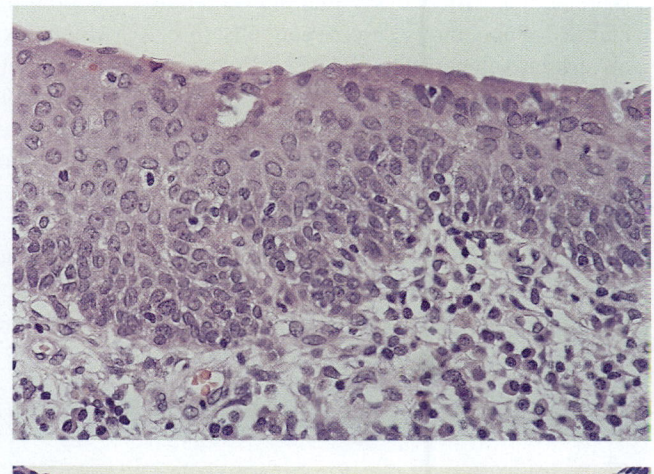

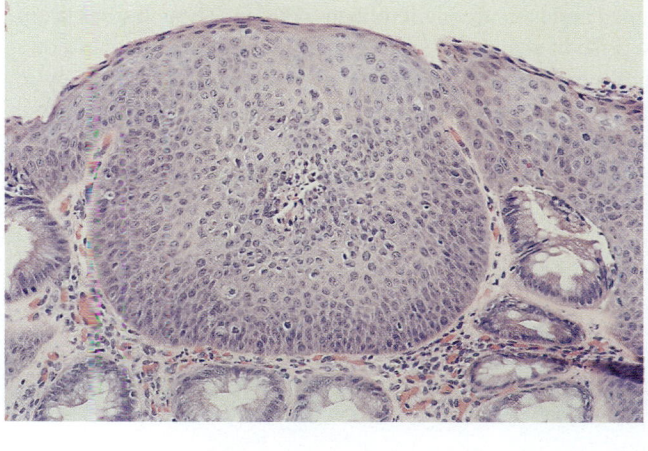

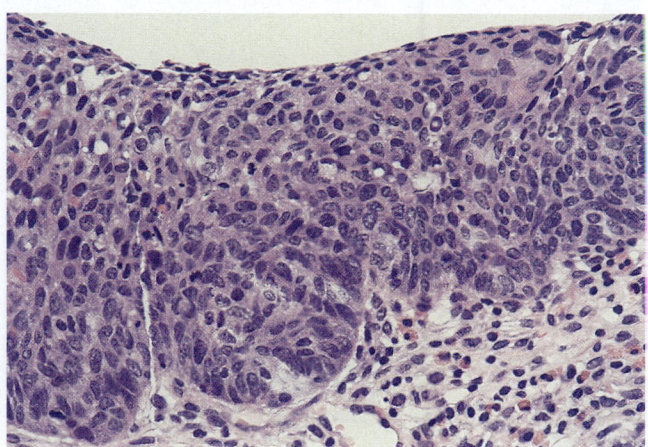

FIG. 7. Histologic spectrum of anal canal intraepithelial neoplasia (ACIN). **A:** ACIN, low grade (mild dysplasia). **B:** ACIN, high grade (moderate dysplasia). **C:** ACIN, high grade (severe dysplasia/carcinoma *in situ*). Dysplastic epithelium occupies the full thickness of the mucosa.

lacked expression or had little of it. In another study, Ki-*ras* oncogene mutations were not found to be important in the development of these tumors (49).

Risk factors for anal epidermoid tumors include receptive anal intercourse, heavy smoking, a history of sexually transmitted diseases, immunosuppression, and, in females, the presence of lower genital tract squamous neoplasia (34,38–41,50–58). Analogies to the genes of cervical and vulvar neoplasia are numerous (59). There may also be an increased risk of anal squamous neoplasms in patients with CD, especially those with chronic fistulas (60,61).

Finding ACIN as an incidental lesion in a hemorrhoid or anal tag presents a problem in management. Available data from two small series (37,38) indicate that the hemorrhoidectomy or tag resection is probably curative, but follow-up may be advisable until more data become available. However, there is no specific program for such follow-up. Cytologic examination of anal swabs may become important (62).

The Highly Differentiated Invasive or Inverted Squamous Lesion Occurring in a Background of Hyperkeratosis and Inflammation

There is a highly differentiated squamous lesion that appears to be invasive, being composed of large, relatively mature, squamous cells except at the base, where at the edges of the infiltrating nests, the cells may appear more undifferentiated and have frequent mitoses (Fig. 8). These lesions seem to arise in anal canal squamous epithelium that is acanthotic and hyperkeratotic, usually with lymphoid and plasmacytic infiltrates in the superficial submucosa. These changes have been designated as leukoplakia (63,64). The presumably invasive lesion probably is similar to some cases reported as keratoacanthoma of the anus (65). However, most of them have no central keratin-filled crater. There are few data regarding follow-up, but it appears from the few cases described that local excision is probably curative.

Adenocarcinoma

Most adenocarcinomas involving the anal canal are the result of either downward extension from a primary site in the distal rectum or, as discussed in Normal Anatomy, they are tumors that arise from the columnar epithelium in the upper anal canal (3). These are considered to be rectal, not anal, carcinomas. However, there is a group of mucinous adenocarcinomas that arise within the anal canal, usually in older patients. The site of origin is not well established, but it may be within congenital anorectal duplications. It is also possible that these carcinomas may arise from the anal glands, but that assumption can only be proven by finding intraepithelial neoplasia in those glands, and that feature has not been established. Some of these carcinomas also occur in patients with anal fissures or fistulas. A few cases have developed in patients with CD (66–70).

Often, the patients with anal canal adenocarcinomas have had a long history of perianal disease, including fistulas and abscesses, and they may even have had previous operations for these conditions. Occasionally, these tumors form large buttock masses that may become ulcerated. In all cases, the rectal mucosa is uninvolved. Histologically, these adenocarcinomas may be annoyingly well differentiated, so much so that it may be difficult to separate them from trapped, cystic anal glands. Almost all are mucinous carcinomas with glandular or tubular structures lined by relatively uniform mucus-producing columnar epithelium. The cancers often have large mucus-filled cysts that may contain free-floating clumps of mucinous carcinoma cells (Fig. 9). Mucus extravasation often results, and there may be an imperfect granulomatous reaction to this extravasated mucin that should not be confused with infection or CD-type granulomas (66–68). On occasion, the carcinoma may erode through the anal mucosa, especially in the ATZ, where it may be detected by biopsy.

The tumors often have an indolent course, with gradual progression over many years. Prognosis after definitive resection is good, but many of these tumors are extensive at the

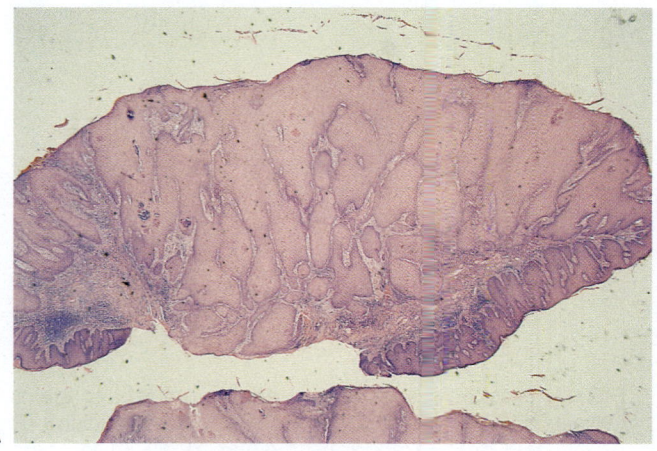 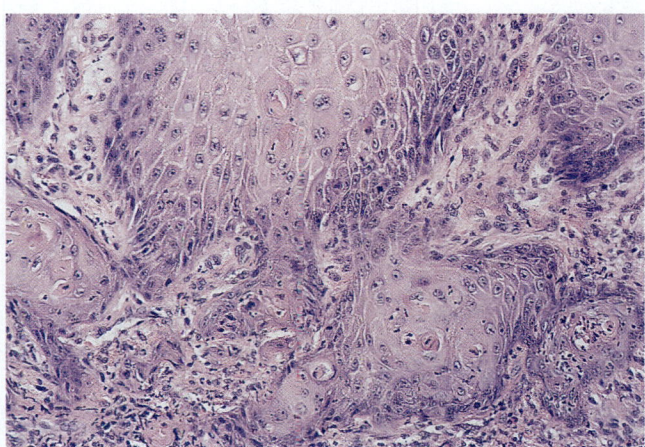

FIG. 8. A: Low-power view of a well-differentiated inverted squamous cell carcinoma of the anal canal. **B:** Base of the cancer, demonstrating invasive squamous cell carcinoma.

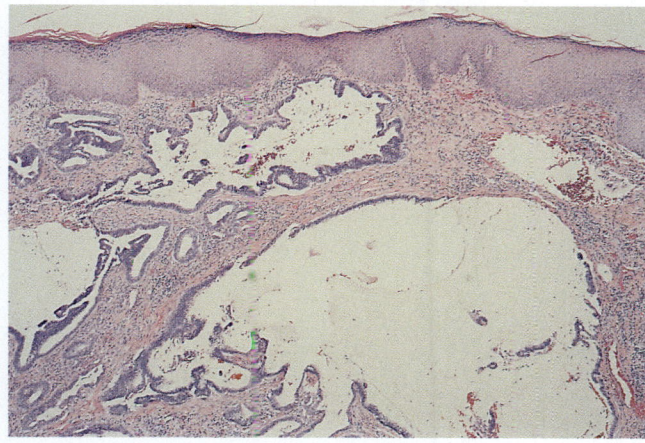

FIG. 9. Mucinous adenocarcinoma, infiltrating the submucosa of the anal canal. Note the dilated, mucin-filled cysts containing groups of neoplastic cells.

time of discovery because of the frequently long histories of fissures or fistulas. The differential features of perianal mucinous adenocarcinoma and rectal adenocarcinoma are listed in Table 2. Well-differentiated adenocarcinomas, especially those producing large quantities of mucin, can arise as primary carcinomas deep within the wall of the anal canal. Such carcinomas are not necessarily distal extensions of rectal carcinomas.

Carcinoid Tumors

Carcinoid tumors may arise in the upper glandular zone or ATZ of the anal canal, but they are generally classified as rectal carcinoid tumors (see Chapter 34). The majority are small tumors; those less than 2.0 cm in diameter and confined to the mucosa and submucosa can be locally excised and have an excellent prognosis. Anorectal carcinoids are associated with a second metachronous or synchronous neoplasm (typically a colonic adenocarcinoma) in up to 30% of cases in some series (3,71).

Small-Cell (Neuroendocrine) Carcinoma

Small-cell carcinomas are rare tumors that may involve the anorectum and have the same light-microscopic and ultrastructural features as pulmonary small-cell (oat-cell) carcinomas (see chapter 26). They present as nodular infiltrative lesions that are usually disseminated at the time of diagnosis; the 5-year survival rate is only 10% in the most optimistic series (26,72,73). Staining with antibodies to chromogranin may be negative because of the sparsity of neurosecretory granules in the tumor cells, but other immunoperoxidase studies such as the use of antibodies to synaptophysin, neuron-specific enolase, and Leu 7 may be helpful in distinguishing small-cell carcinoma from the basaloid variant of anal squamous-cell carcinoma in difficult cases (72,73). (See Table 9 concerning the immunohistochemistry of undifferentiated colorectal neoplasms in Chapter 34.)

Melanoma

Anal melanomas (AM), which account for 0.5% to 2.0% of all melanomas, usually present clinically with rectal bleeding, pain, and a mass, the same presentation as hemorrhoids or anal polyps (74–76). Partly as a result of this clinical picture, they are usually detected late in their course and are advanced tumors at the time of diagnosis (75).

Grossly, AM are most frequently polypoid, pigmented, and located at or adjacent to the dentate line. However, pigmentation is absent in about 20% of cases, or it may be obscured by hemorrhage (74–76). Microscopically, AMs exhibit the same range of features and immunohistochemical reaction patterns as melanoma of the skin (see Chapter 3), but, as with melanomas arising in other mucous membranes, AMs commonly are of the acrolentiginous type. The invasive cells are predominantly the epithelioid and spindle types; desmoplastic tumors also occur (75,77). As with melanomas elsewhere, the most useful characteristics for differentiating AM from other anal malignancies are melanin production, a nesting growth pattern, junctional changes, and appropriate immunocytochemistry, including positive staining with antibodies to S-100 protein and the melanoma marker, HMB-45 (35,76). The junctional change, however, may be obscured in ulcerated tumors, even when numerous sections are obtained. As the melanomas extend proximally, they tend to invade the columnar mucosa, separating the crypts in a pattern identical with that seen in lymphomas (Fig. 10).

The prognosis is poor, with a 5-year survival rate of about 15%. Although the histologic type of the AM does not affect survival, the thickness of the tumor (as measured from the top of the overlying intact mucosa or top of ulcerated tumor) appears to influence the outcome: AMs that are 2.0 mm or

TABLE 2. *Differential features of perianal mucinous adenocarcinoma versus rectal adenocarcinoma*

Feature	Perianal mucinous adenocarcinoma	Rectal adenocarcinoma
Origin	Anal ducts? Duplications? Fistulas?	Rectal mucosa
Histology	Mucinous	Variable; mucinous uncommon
Rectal mucosa	Not involved	Mass, possibly ulcerated; may be residual adenoma at a margin
Fistula	Common	No
Frequency	Rare	Common
Buttock mass	Possible	Rare
Invasion	Laterally into buttock	Rectal wall
Discharge	Gelatinous	Bloody
Constipation	Rare	Common

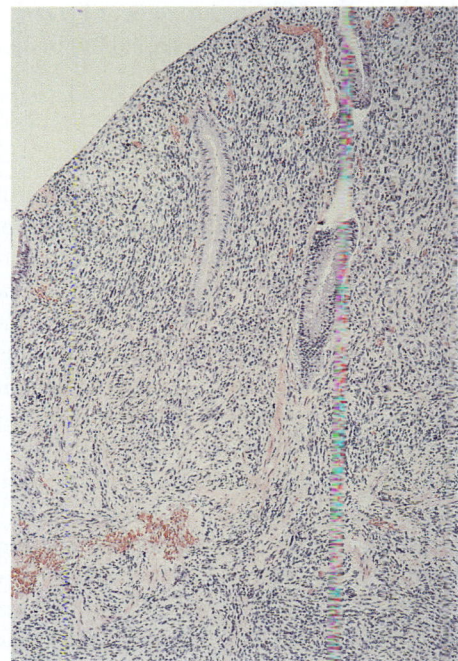
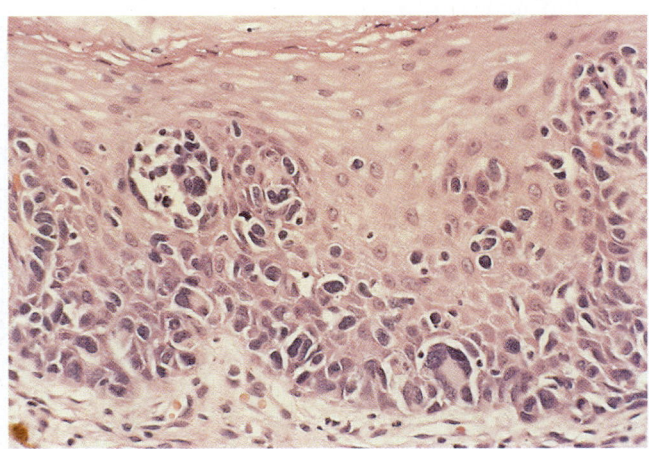

FIG. 10. A: Malignant melanoma infiltrating prolapsed mucosa of the proximal anal canal. This pattern of infiltration mimics that of lymphoma. **B:** Junctional component of an anal canal melanoma.

less in thickness have an excellent prognosis when compared to all thicker AMs (78).

Basal Cell Carcinoma

Anal basal cell carcinoma is extraordinarily rare, accounting for no more than 0.2% of anorectal tumors (79,80). It usually arises in the lowest third of the anal canal or in the perianal skin, may extend upward into the ATZ, and clinically presents with bleeding, pain, and/or a mass (79,80). The microscopic features are like those of basal cell carcinomas of the skin (see Chapter 2). The major differential diagnostic consideration, particularly in biopsy specimens, is to rule out an anal squamous-cell carcinoma with basaloid features (see Surface Epithelial Carcinoma of the Anal Transitional Zone and Squamous Zone). Wide local excision with negative margins is curative (80).

PERIANAL SKIN

In about 25% of cases, vulvar and perianal squamous-cell carcinoma *in situ* (Bowen's disease) extends into the anal canal, often into the ATZ, so that the canal must be carefully evaluated in such patients (51). Extramammary Paget's disease may likewise involve the anal canal up to the dentate line (Fig. 11) (3). Anal and perianal Paget's disease is often associated with an underlying carcinoma of the rectum, which is either concurrent with the discovery of the Paget's disease or develops later. The frequency of this association, however, varies from one study to another (81). Granular cell tumors may occur in the perianal area and mimic hemorrhoids. The appearance is identical with that of granular cell tumors elsewhere, but in the perianal area the accompanying hyperplasia of the overlying squamous epithelium may be particularly florid and mimic squamous-cell carcinoma (21,82). Soft tissue neoplasms and lymphoma may involve the anal canal and perianal skin; they have the same features as their counterparts in other organ systems (83).

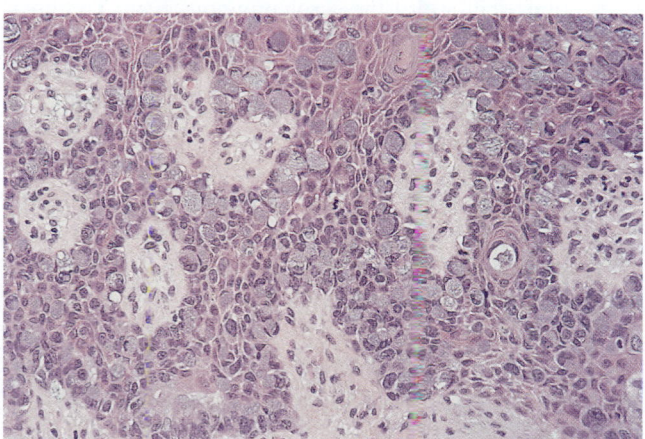

FIG. 11. Paget's disease involving anal squamous mucosa. Note the presence of intraepithelial mucin-containing cells, many with a "signet ring" configuration. This lesion was associated with an invasive adenocarcinoma higher in the anal canal.

REFERENCES

Embryology and Normal Anatomy

1. Fenger C. Anal canal. In: Sternberg SS, ed. *Histology for pathologists*, 2nd ed. Philadelphia: Lippincott-Raven, 1997:551–571.
2. Walls EW. Observations on the microscopic anatomy of the human anal canal. *Br J Surg* 1958;45:504–514.

3. Fenger C. Anal canal tumors and their precursors. In: Rosen PP, Fechner RE, eds. *Pathology annual 1988,* part I. Norwalk, CT: Appleton & Lange, 1988:45–66.
4. Myerson RJ, Karnell LH, Menck HR. The national cancer data base report on carcinoma of the anus. *Cancer* 1997;80:805–815.
5. Gillespie JJ, MacKay B. Histogenesis of cloacogenic carcinoma: fine structure of anal transitional epithelium and cloacogenic carcinoma. *Hum Pathol* 1978;9:579–587.
6. Fenger C, Lyon H. Endocrine cells and melanin-containing cells in the anal canal epithelium. *Histochem J* 1982;14:631–639.
7. Clemmensen OJ, Fenger C. Melanocytes in the anal canal epithelium. *Histopathology* 1991;18:237–241.

Congenital Anomalies

8. Morson BC, Dawson IMP. *Gastrointestinal pathology,* 3rd ed. Oxford: Blackwell Scientific Publications, 1990.
9. Blisard KS, Kleinman R. Hirschsprung's disease: a clinical and pathologic overview. *Hum Pathol* 1986;17:1189–1191.

Hemorrhoids

10. Birkett DH. Hemorrhoids—diagnostic and treatment options. *Hosp Pract* [off Ed] January 30, 1988;99–108.
11. Johansen K, Bardin J, Orloff MJ. Massive bleeding from hemorrhoidal varices in portal hypertension. *JAMA* 1980;244:2084–2085.

Anal Tags, Papillae and Fibroepithelial Polyps

12. Schinella RA. Stromal atypia in anal papillae. *Dis Colon Rectum* 1976;19:611–613.
13. Schutte AG, Tolentino MG. A second study of anal papillae. *Dis Colon Rectum* 1971;14:435–450.

Inflammatory Cloacogenic Polyp

14. Saul SH. Inflammatory cloacogenic polyp: relationship to solitary rectal ulcer syndrome/mucosal prolapse and other bowel disorders. *Hum Pathol* 1987;18:1120–1125.
15. Lobert PF, Appelman HD. Inflammatory cloacogenic polyp: a unique inflammatory lesion of the anal transitional zone. *Am J Surg Pathol* 1981;5:761–766.

Inflammatory Conditions

16. Ward CS, Dunphy EB, Jagoe WS, Sheahan DG. Crohn's disease limited to the mouth and anus. *J Clin Gastroenterol* 1985;7:516–521.
17. Williams DR, Coller JA, Corman ML, Nugent FW, Veidenhemier MC. Anal complications in Crohn's disease. *Dis Colon Rectum* 1981;24:22–24.
18. Buchmann P, Keighley MR, Allan RN, Thompson H, Alexander-Williams J. Natural history of perianal Crohn's disease. Ten year follow-up: a plea for conservatism. *Am J Surg* 1980;140:642–644.
19. Platell C, MacKay J, Collopy B, Fink R, Ryan P, Woods R. Anal pathology in patients with Crohn's disease. *Aust N Z J Surg* 1996;66:5–9.
20. Taylor BA, Williams GT, Hughes LE, Rhodes J. The histology of anal skin tags in Crohn's disease: an aid to confirmation of the diagnosis. *Int J Colorect Dis* 1989;4:197–199.
21. Helwig EB. Neoplasms of the anus. In: Norris HT, ed. *Pathology of the colon, small intestine, and anus.* New York: Churchill Livingstone, 1991:303–327.

Squamous Cell Carcinoma

22. Jass JR, Sobin LH. Histologic typing of intestinal tumors. *International histological classification of tumors,* 2nd ed. World Health Organization. New York: Springer-Verlag, 1990:41–47.
23. Dougherty BG, Evans HL. Carcinoma of the anal canal: a study of 79 cases. *Am J Clin Pathol* 1985;83:159–164.
24. Schraut WH, Wang C-H, Dawson PJ, Block GE. Depth of invasion, location, and size of cancer of the anus dictate operative treatment. *Cancer* 1983;51:1291–1296.
25. Singh R, Nime F, Mittelman A. Malignant epithelial tumors of the anal canal. *Cancer* 1981;48:411–415.
26. Boman BM, Moertel CG, O'Connell MJ, et al. Carcinoma of the anal canal: a clinical and pathologic study of 88 cases. *Cancer* 1984;54:114–125.
27. Williams GR, Talbot IC. Anal carcinoma—a histological review. *Histopathology* 1994;25:507–516.
28. Salmon RJ, Zafrani B, Labib A, Asselain B, Girodet J. Prognosis of cloacogenic and squamous cancers of the anal canal. *Dis Colon Rectum* 1986;29:336–340.
29. Frost DB, Richards PC, Montague ED, Giacco GG, Martin RG. Epidermoid cancer of the anorectum. *Cancer* 1984;53:1285–1293.
30. Shepherd NA, Scholefield JH, Love SB, England J, Northover JMA. Prognostic factors in anal squamous carcinoma: a multivariate analysis of clinical, pathological and flow cytometric parameters in 235 cases. *Histopathology* 1990;16:545–555.
31. Tanum G, Tveit K, Karlsen KO, Hauer-Jensen M. Chemotherapy and radiation therapy for anal carcinoma: survival and late morbidity. *Cancer* 1991;67:2462–2466.
32. Clark H, Petrelli N, Herrera L, Mittelman A. Epidermoid carcinoma of the anal canal. *Cancer* 1986;57:400–406.
33. Meeker WR, Sickle-Santanello BJ, Philpott G, Kenady D, Bland KI, Hill GH, Popp MB. Combined chemotherapy, radiation and surgery for epithelial cancer of the anal canal. *Cancer* 1986;57:525–529.
34. Cooper HS, Patchefsky AS, Marks G. Cloacogenic carcinoma of the anorectum in homosexual men: an observation of four cases. *Dis Colon Rectum* 1979;22:557–558.
35. Fenger C, Nielsen VT. Precancerous changes in the anal canal epithelium in resection specimens. *Acta Pathol Microbiol Immunol Scand [A]* 1986;94:63–69.
36. Fenger C, Nielsen VT. Intraepithelial neoplasia in the anal canal. *Acta Pathol Microbiol Immunol Scand [A]* 1986;94:343–349.
37. Fenger C, Nielsen VT. Dysplastic changes in the anal canal epithelium in minor surgical specimens. *Acta Pathol Microbiol Immunol Scand [A]* 1981;89:463–465.
38. Foust R, Dean P, Stoler M, Moinuddin S. Intraepithelial neoplasia of the anal canal arising in hemorrhoidal tissue: a study of 19 cases. *Hum Pathol* 1991;22:528–534.
39. Tax JB, Gupta PK, Gupta JW, Shah KV. Anal carcinoma: microscopic condyloma and tissue demonstration of human papillomaviruses capsid antigens and viral DNA. *Arch Pathol Lab Med* 1989;113:1127–1131.
40. Gall AA, Saul SH, Stoler MH. In situ hybridization analysis of human papillomavirus in anal squamous cell carcinoma. *Mod Pathol* 1989;2:439–443.
41. Bogomoletz WV, Potet F, Molas G. Condylomata acuminata, giant condyloma acuminatum (Buschke-Lowenstein tumor) and verrucous squamous carcinoma of the perianal and anorectal region: a continuous precancerous spectrum? *Histopathology* 1985;9:1155–1169.
42. Zaki SR, Judd R, Coffield LM, Greer P, Rolson H, Evatt BL. Human papillomavirus infection and anal carcinoma: retrospective analysis by in situ hybridization and the polymerase chain reaction. *Am J Pathol* 1992;140:1345–1355.
43. Wolber R, Dupuis B, Thiyagaratnam P, Owen D. Anal cloacogenic and squamous carcinomas: comparative histological analysis using in situ hybridization for human papillomavirus DNA. *Am J Surg Pathol* 1990;14:176–182.
44. Higgins GD, Uzelin DM, Phillips GE, Pieterse AS, Burrell CJ. Differing characteristics of human papillomavirus RNA-positive and RNA-negative anal carcinomas. *Cancer* 1991;68:561–567.
45. Duggan MA, Bores VF, Inoue M, McGregor SE. Human papillomavirus DNA in anal carcinomas: comparison of in situ and dot blot hybridization. *Am J Clin Pathol* 1991;96:318–325.
46. Scholefield JH, Kerr IB, Shepherd NA, Miller KJ, Bloomfield R, Northover JMA. Human papillomavirus type 16 DNA in anal cancers from six different countries. *Gut* 1991;32:674–676.
47. Noffsinger AE, Hui Y-Z, Suzuk L, et al. The relationship of human papillomavirus to proliferation and ploidy in carcinoma of the anus. *Cancer* 1995;75:958–967.
48. Ogunbiyi OA, Scholefield JH, Rogers K, Sharp F, Smith JHF, Polacarz SV. C-myc oncogene expression in anal squamous neoplasia. *J Clin Pathol* 1993;46:23–27.
49. Hiorns LR, Scholefield JH, Palmer JG, Shepherd NA, Kerr IB. Ki-*ras*

oncogene mutations in non-HPV-associated anal carcinoma. *J Pathol* 1990;161:99–103.
50. Croxson T, Chabon AB, Rorat E, Barash IM. Intraepithelial carcinoma of the anus in homosexual men. *Dis Colon Rectum* 1984;27:325–330.
51. Schlaerth JB, Morrow CP, Nalick RH, Gaddis O. Anal involvement by carcinoma *in situ* of the perineum in women. *Obstet Gynecol* 1984;64:406–411.
52. Nash G, Allen W, Nash S. Atypical lesions of the anal mucosa in homosexual men. *JAMA* 1986;256:873–876.
53. Frisch M, Glimelius B, van den Brule AJC, et al. Sexually transmitted infection as a cause of anal cancer. *N Engl J Med* 1997;337:1350–1358.
54. Daling JR, Weiss NS, Hislop TG, Maden C, Coates RJ, et al. Sexual practices, sexually transmitted diseases, and the incidence of anal cancer. *N Engl J Med* 1987;317:973–977.
55. Palefsky JM, Gonzales J, Greenblatt RM, Ahn DK, Hollander H. Anal intraepithelial neoplasia and anal papillomavirus infection among homosexual males with group IV HIV disease. *JAMA* 1990;263:2911–2916.
56. Noffsinger A, Witte D, Fenoglio-Preiser CM. The relationship of human papillomaviruses to anorectal neoplasia. *Cancer* 1992;70:1276–1287.
57. Scholefield JH, Hickson WGE, Smith JHF, Rogar K, Sharp F. Anal intraepithelial neoplasia: part of a multifocal disease process. *Lancet* 1992;340:1271–1273.
58. Surawicz CM, Kirby P, Critchlow C, Sayer J, Dunphy C, Kiviat N. Anal dysplasia in homosexual men: role of anoscopy and biopsy. *Gastroenterology* 1993;105:658–666.
59. Syrjanen KJ. Human papillomavirus (HPV) infections of the female genital tract and their associations with intraepithelial neoplasia and squamous cell carcinoma. In: Sommers C, Rosen PP, Fechner RE, eds. *Pathology annual 1986,* Part I. Norwalk, CT: Appleton-Century-Crofts, 1986:53–89.
60. Slater G, Greenstein A, Aufses AH. Anal carcinoma in patients with Crohn's disease. *Ann Surg* 1984;199:348–350.
61. Buchman AL, Ament ME, Doty J. Development of squamous cell carcinoma in chronic perineal sinus and wounds in Crohn's disease. *Am J Gastroenterol* 1991;86:1829–1832.
62. Palefsky JM, Holly EA, Hogeboom CJ, Berry JM, Jay N, Darragh TM. Anal cytology as a screening tool for anal squamous intraepithelial lesions. *J Acquir Immune Defic Syndr Hum Retrovirol* 1997;5:415–422.
63. Bender MD, Lechago J. Leukoplakia of the anal canal. *Am J Dig Dis* 1976;21:872–876.
64. Donaldson DR, Jass JR, Mann CV. Anal leukoplakia. *Gut* 1988;46:A1368.
65. Jensen SL, Sjolin K-E. Keratoacanthoma of the anus. *Dis Colon Rectum* 1985;28:743–745.

Adenocarcinoma

66. Prioleau PG, Allen MS, Roberts T. Perianal mucinous adenocarcinoma. *Cancer* 1977;39:1295–1299.
67. Lee SH, Zucker M, Sato T. Primary adenocarcinoma of an anal gland with secondary perianal fistulas. *Hum Pathol* 1981;12:1034–1037.
68. Jones EA, Morson BC. Mucinous adenocarcinoma in anorectal fistulae. *Histopathology* 1984;8:279–292.
69. Chaikhouni A, Regueyra RI, Stevens JR. Adenocarcinoma in perianal fistulas of Crohn's disease. *Dis Colon Rectum* 1981;24:639–643.
70. Nelson RL, Prasad ML, Abcarian H. Anal carcinoma presenting as a perirectal abscess or fistula. *Arch Surg* 1985;120:632–635.

Other Neoplasms

71. Nauheim KS, Zeitels J, Kaplan EL, et al. Rectal carcinoid tumors—treatment and prognosis. *Surgery* 1983;94:670–676.
72. Wick MR, Weatherby RP, Weiland LH. Small cell neuroendocrine carcinoma of the colon and rectum: clinical, histologic and ultrastructural study and immunohistochemical comparison with cloacogenic carcinoma. *Hum Pathol* 1987;18:9–21.
73. Schwartz AM, Orenstein JM. Small-cell undifferentiated carcinoma of the rectosigmoid colon. *Arch Pathol Lab Med* 1985;109:629–632.
74. Mason JK, Helwig EB. Anorectal melanoma. *Cancer* 1966;19:39–50.
75. Wanebo HJ, Woodruff JM, Farr GH, Quan SH. Anorectal melanoma. *Cancer* 1981;47:1891–1900.
76. Cooper PH, Mills SE, Allen MS Jr. Malignant melanoma of the anus. *Dis Colon Rectum* 1982;25:693–703.
77. Ackermann DM, Polk HC, Schrodt GR. Desmoplastic melanoma of the anus. *Hum Pathol* 1985;16:1277–1279.
78. Weinstock MA. Epidemiology and prognosis of anorectal melanoma. *Gastroenterology* 1993;104:174–178.
79. White WB, Schneiderman H, Sayre JT. Basal cell carcinoma of the anus-clinical and pathological distinction from cloacogenic carcinoma. *J Clin Gastroenterol* 1984;6:441–446.
80. Niehsen OV, Jensen SL. Basal cell carcinoma of the anus—a clinical study of 34 cases. *Br J Surg* 1981;68:856–857.
81. Armitage NC, Jass JR, Richman PI, Thompson JPS, Phillips RKS. Paget's disease of the anus: a clinicopathological study. *Br J Surg* 1989;76:60–63.
82. Johnston J, Helwig EB. Granular cell tumors of the gastrointestinal tract and perianal region: a study of 74 cases. *Dig Dis Sci* 1981;26:807–816.
83. Ioachim HL, Antonescu C, Giancotti F, Dorset B, Weinstein MA. EBV-associated anorectal lymphomas in patients with acquired immune deficiency syndrome. *Am J Surg Pathol* 1997;21:997–1006.

IX

Urinary Tract and Male Genital System

CHAPTER 40

Developmental Abnormalities of the Kidney

Jay Bernstein and Enid Gilbert-Barness

RENAL HYPOPLASIA

Hypoplastic kidneys are, by definition, developmentally small, although normally differentiated (1). The condition probably results from altered interaction between metanephric blastema and ureteric bud, resulting in the induction of insufficient renal parenchyma, involving either the number of lobes or the number of nephrons. Hypoplastic kidneys are rarely familial, despite a few reported exceptions to that rule. A form of oligomeganephronic renal hypoplasia in the renal developmental field defect appears to be autosomal recessive (2). The distinction between small kidneys with normally differentiated parenchyma and small kidneys with abnormally differentiated parenchyma is clinically difficult, usually depending on histopathologic evaluation, but the distinction is important to both prognosis and genetic counseling. Hypoplastic kidneys must also be differentiated from atrophic kidneys, in which segmental loss of parenchyma results from intrarenal reflux and renal scarring and in which the remnant parenchyma undergoes compensatory hypertrophy. Much of the literature regarding small kidneys has not followed these distinctions.

The evaluation of renal size requires standards of normal renal growth. Kidney size increases during childhood and decreases after middle age. The range of ±2 SD covers a span from about 50% to 150% of the mean. As a rule of thumb, an otherwise normal kidney weighing less than 50% of the expected weight, or less than 60 g in the adolescent and adult, can be regarded as hypoplastic.

The most common type of renal hypoplasia, in the intended sense of a developmentally small kidney with normally differentiated parenchyma, is oligonephronic hypoplasia, known in the French literature as *oligoméganéphronie* (3). The original French name derives from the observation that these kidneys contain a reduced number of nephrons that become enlarged, perhaps as the result of compensatory hypertrophy. There are two types of oligomeganephronia; one is a solitary sporadic type with no associated anomaly, and the other is a syndromic type that is a part of a complex anomaly of 4p deletion syndrome and possibly other related chromosomal deletion syndromes (4). Renal hypoplasia has been found in approximately 15% of Down's syndrome patients (5). The condition is usually bilateral, with exceptions accounted for by contralateral renal agenesis and contralateral renal dysplasia. Clinical characteristics include recurrent dehydration, unexplained fever, growth retardation, and a failure to thrive. Affected infants suffer an early onset of polyuria, with salt-wasting and severe polydipsia that progresses, after a relatively stable period of moderate azotemia, to chronic renal failure over a period of 10 to 12 years (3). Oligonephronic kidneys are typically very small, with mean weights of approximately 20 g each, less than one fourth of the expected normal weight in children. The kidneys may contain a reduced number of lobes, but the calyces and pelves are normally formed, with no calyceal recesses, blind calyces, or atrophic renal segments. The distinctive features become apparent on histopathologic examination, which shows a reduced number of glomeruli in the microscopic field (3). The glomeruli are clearly enlarged, with diameters more than twice normal, and it is advisable in evaluating biopsy specimens to refer to age-matched controls for determination of glomerular size (Fig. 1). The glomeruli typically have an open appearance, with patent glomerular capillaries, until the stage of declining renal function and renal failure, when segmental and global glomerular sclerosis supervene. There may be hypertrophy and hyperplasia of the juxtaglomerular complexes, even though most children are normotensive, at least until the stage of chronic renal failure. Some mesangial hypercellularity is also present. The convoluted tubules are also greatly enlarged and may be dilated to form small cysts. Immunofluorescence microscopy and electron microscopy are noncontributory. The finding of decreased metanephric blastema in the kidneys from an 18-week fetus and its ab-

---

J. Bernstein: William Beaumont Hospital, Royal Oak, Michigan 48073.

E. Gilbert-Barness: Department of Pathology, Tampa General Hospital, Tampa, Florida 33601.

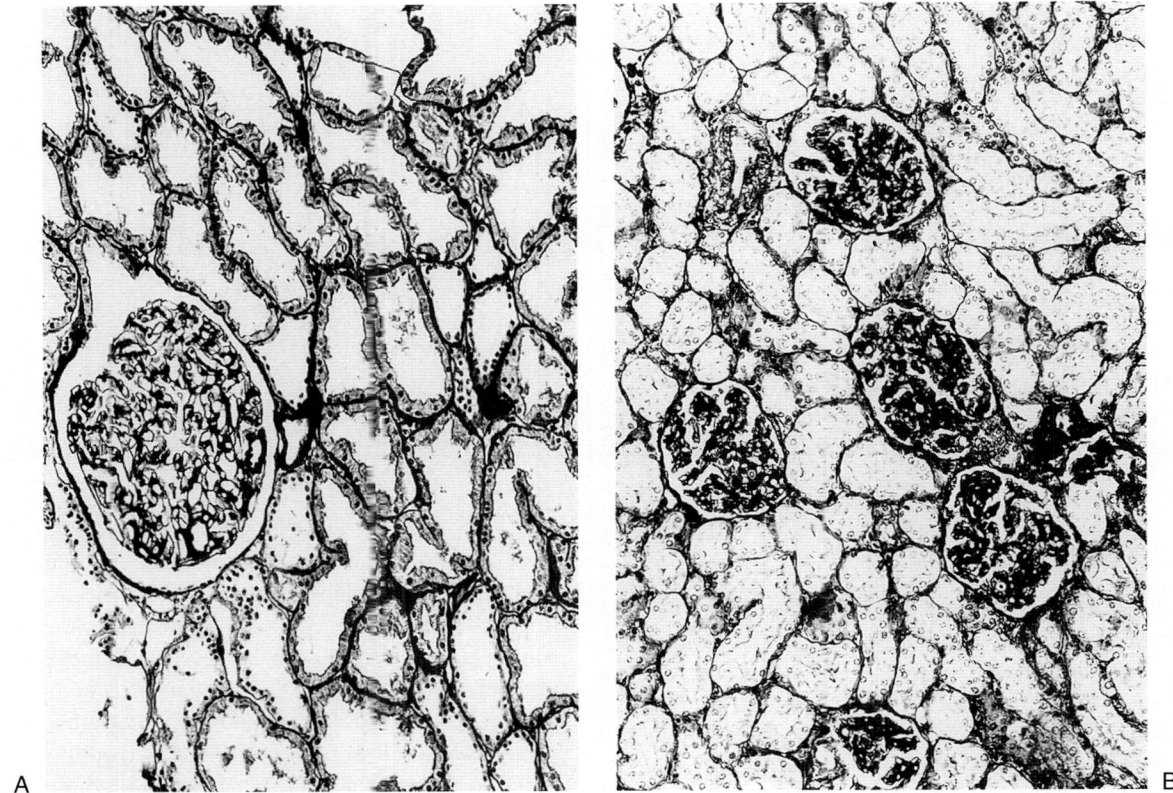

FIG. 1. Oligonephronic hypoplasia. The renal biopsy specimen **(A)** from an 11-year-old girl with bilaterally small kidneys contains large patent glomeruli and large dilated tubules. Compare with normal age-matched control kidney **(B)**. Periodic acid-Schiff stains; both ×120.

sence in the kidney of a liveborn preterm infant of 33 weeks' gestation support the hypothesis that a primary deficiency of metanephric blastema may be a pathogenetic mechanism of oligomeganephronia (6). Isolated bilateral renal hypoplasia has been well characterized in fetuses with oligohydramnios and with impaired fetal renal function (7). The association of optic nerve colobomas, renal anomalies, and vesicoureteral reflux makes up a unique autosomal dominant syndrome in which molecular investigations have determined a single nucleotide deletion in the PAX2 gene (8). Furthermore, mutations in the PAX2 gene with the renal coloboma syndrome with hypoplasia have been identified.

Another form of developmental hypoplasia is the unirenicular or unipapillary kidney, an uncommon developmental abnormality that is usually unilateral (9). Histopathologic studies show normally developed parenchyma, with focal glomerular sclerosis. Bilateral involvement results in the same clinical characteristics and the same evolution as does oligonephronic hypoplasia.

Unilateral renal hypoplasia—the unilateral small kidney, dwarf kidney, doll's kidney—is likely to be an incidental finding. In the literature, descriptions of recurrent infection and bouts of fever and pain probably relate to recurrent infection in association with vesicoureteric reflux and renal scarring. Unilateral, true hypoplasia lacks clear clinicopathologic correlations. The opposite kidney, however, may undergo compensatory hypertrophy, with complications resulting from renal enlargement and increased susceptibility to trauma, infection, and nephrolithiasis. The frequency of hypertension is not known.

RENAL DYSPLASIA

Dysplastic kidneys are, by definition, abnormally differentiated, as shown by abnormal structural organization with abnormally developed metanephric elements. The features that can be regarded as clearly dysplastic are metaplastic cartilage, primitive ducts, and lobar disorganization (Fig. 2) (1,10). Metaplastic cartilage customarily appears within the cortex as bars and nests of hyaline cartilage. Primitive ducts, which may be cystic, are altered collecting ducts lined with undifferentiated epithelium and surrounded by fibromuscular collars. Incomplete and abnormal corticomedullary relationships and rudimentary medullary development constitute lobar disorganization. The incompletely developed medullary pyramids are deficient in vasa recta and Henle's loops and are associated with incomplete calyceal and forniceal development. These renal abnormalities bear a strong relationship to other urinary tract malformations, including ureteral atresia and urethral valves, suggesting that urinary obstruction or urinary reflux during metanephric development leads to renal dysplasia (1). In the early stages of multicystic dysplasia kidney (MCDK), normal nephrogenesis occurs in what seems to be a normal metanephric blastema;

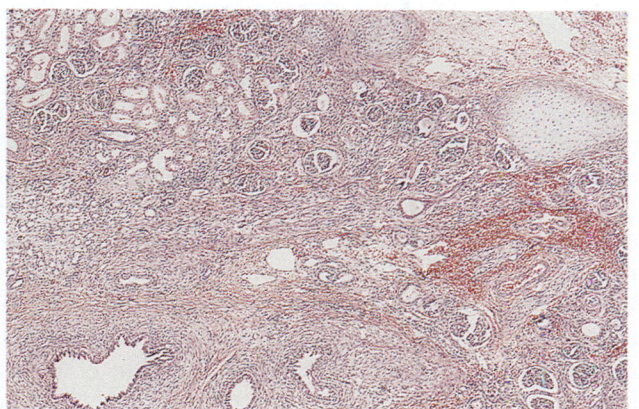

FIG. 2. Elements of renal dysplasia. The essential features of renal dysplasia are shown in hypoplastic dysplasia with patent urinary tract from a newborn boy with a nonfunctioning right kidney. The cortex contains a nest of metaplastic cartilage, and the medulla contains primitive ducts that are lined with undifferentiated epithelium and surrounded by fibromuscular collars. There is lobar disorganization, evidenced by a rudimentary medullary pyramid that lacks vasa recta and recurrent loops and is barely demarcated from the surrounding connective tissue of the renal sinus.

however, an intrinsic abnormality in the branching morphogenesis of the ureteric duct might be responsible for the development of the histopathologic changes (11). This association with urinary tract abnormalities holds in about 90% of cases; in the remaining 10%, the occurrence of hereditary and syndromal dysplasia, unaccounted for by urinary tract obstruction, implicates other pathogenetic factors.

Dysplastic kidneys are often cystic, and the most common variety perhaps is the multicystic kidney (12). Multicystic dysplasia, characterized by an enlarged, misshapen, irregularly cystic kidney (Fig. 3), is closely related to aplastic dysplasia, characterized by a small, barely recognizable, rudimentary, solid nubbin. The difference is in the degree of cyst formation, and all degrees intermediate between the two prototypes exist. The seemingly disorganized structure of the multicystic kidney is accounted for by the severity of cyst formation, and both multicystic and aplastic kidneys contain rudimentary lobes and lobules of metanephric tissue, with variable deficiencies of nephrons and ducts. Both contain relatively solid central areas, from which branching primitive ducts radiate to the periphery as incompletely differentiated branches of the ureteric bud. The septa among the cysts in multicystic kidneys contain rudimentary lobules consisting of branching collecting ducts in close relation to caps of cortical glomeruli and convoluted tubules. Cysts arise as ductal dilatations, usually in the periphery of the kidney, and they communicate (13). Metaplastic cartilage, when present, is also located peripherally, but cartilage is not always present. Some multicystic kidneys contain masses of undifferentiated cells, referred to as *nodular blastema* (12,14–16). Nodular blastema carries a risk of neoplasia, and it may be related to the rare development of Wilms' tumors in multicystic kidneys. Renal cell carcinoma has also been described as a complication of multicystic kidney (17,18).

Multicystic kidneys are almost always associated with ureteral atresia and pyelocalyceal occlusion (19), and the ureter may be partially absent (see Fig. 3) (20). The presence of patent pelvis and calyces in a cystic dysplastic kidney indicates some other type of dysplasia. Cases described in the literature as hydronephrotic multicystic kidney (21), with low ureteral atresia and dilated pelves, are probably variants of obstructive dysplasia and congenital hydronephrosis. Aplastic kidneys also have atretic ureters, but the association is not as clear because several types of small dysplastic kidneys have been grouped together under that heading. Kidneys with atretic ureters do not get infected and are not subject to reflux (22); the occurrence of chronic pyelonephritis in a predominantly dysplastic kidney indicates lower urinary tract obstruction with probable vesicoureteric reflux.

Multicystic and aplastic kidneys are nonfunctional, even though the multicystic kidney may concentrate contrast medium during high-dose excretory urography (23,24) or radionuclide during renal scans (25). Multicystic kidneys are in a dynamic state in early life, and serial ultrasound examinations have shown that the cysts change in size and assume different configurations (26) and that they may regress postnatally (27–30). Deregulation of cell survival in cystic and dysplastic renal development may be related to fulminant apoptosis that occurs in null mutations of *bcl-2*, an oncogene that suppresses apoptosis, and may contribute to the progressive destruction of functional kidney tissue in cystic kidneys and the spontaneous involution reported in cystic dysplastic kidneys (31,32).

The multicystic kidney is usually detected in the newborn as a flank mass; sonography shows large, spherical cysts with nondelineation of the renal sinus (33,34). There is a high frequency of contralateral renal and urinary tract abnor-

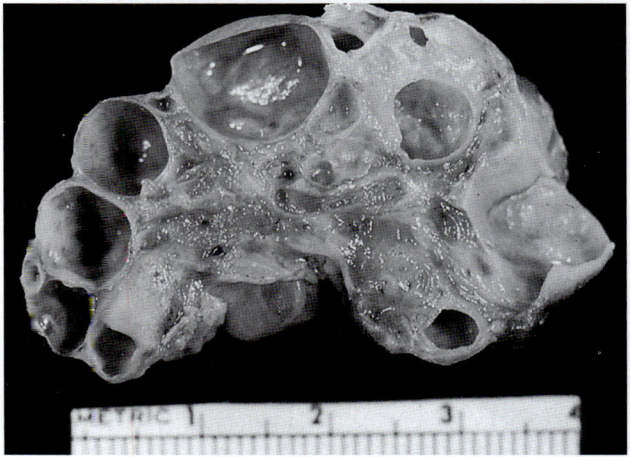

FIG. 3. Multicystic dysplasia. This kidney in a 2-day-old girl is enlarged and cystic. The cysts are predominantly peripheral around a core containing branching collecting ducts. There is pyelocalyceal occlusion; a ureter was not identifiable in the specimen.

malities (35,36), perhaps as high as 40% (37). Malformations of other systems are common, especially congenital heart disease and esophageal or intestinal atresia. Multicystic kidneys are usually unilateral, occasionally bilateral.

Routine treatment, until recently, was nephrectomy, partly because of diagnostic uncertainty and partly because of the fear of neoplasia. There is a trend toward conservative management (38,39), with careful follow-up for any suspicious change in status. That approach, however, is not without controversy (40, 41). An indication for nephrectomy is hypertension, which typically remits after surgery (42,43).

Renal dysplasia may accompany almost any type of congenital urinary tract obstruction, including urethral atresia, posterior urethral valves, anterior urethral diverticulum, and prune belly syndrome (Fig. 4). A similar pattern of subcapsular cystic renal dysplasia occurs in some patients with congenital hydronephrosis caused by ureteral obstruction. The renal abnormality takes the form of deficient medullary development and of cystic cortical dysplasia (1,44). The renal cysts in dysplasia associated with lower tract obstruction are usually smaller than are those in multicystic kidneys (45).

The cortex may contain nests of metaplastic cartilage, sometimes nodules of blastema. The cysts arise, for the most part, in peripheral primitive collecting ducts and collecting tubules, which are admixed with rudimentary glomeruli and convoluted tubules. The abnormal glomeruli and convoluted tubules result partly from arrested development, mostly from involutional and regressive changes in partially formed structures (1). The changes in both cortex and medulla appear to result from the effect of urinary obstruction on development of the outer cortex after nephrons in the inner cortex have begun to excrete urine. The cortical and medullary changes run a spectrum from very mild to extremely severe, and the abnormality is frequently asymmetrical, with more frequent involvement of the left kidney. The key to that discrepancy, even in relatively severe congenital bladder outlet obstruction, may be asymmetrical vesicoureteric reflux, typically more severe on the left than on the right (46,47). Contralateral vesicoureteric reflux is a complication of unilateral MCDK (48–50). Complete bladder outlet obstruction caused by urethral atresia is, on the other hand, almost always associated with bilateral renal dysplasia (41).

Because obstructive uropathies can be diagnosed before birth by ultrasonography (51), intrauterine surgical relief of the urinary tract obstruction has been tried but remains highly controversial (52). The clinical picture and the treatment are complicated by a high frequency of nonurinary tract malformations (53). Some boys with posterior urethral valves develop renal failure very early in life, whereas others, presumably those with less severe obstruction, have minimal symptoms into the third decade of life. Obstructed kidneys are easily infected, and therapy includes removal of obstruction and elimination of vesicoureteric reflux.

Another form of obstructive dysplasia occurs in duplex kidneys, in which one of the ureters has an abnormal bladder insertion and terminates in an ectopic ureterocele. Those circumstances, usually affecting the upper pole ureter, are associated with severe obstruction, resulting in dysplasia (54–56). The other pole may be partially obstructed as the ureterocele enlarges; this pole may then become hydronephrotic, although it is otherwise normally formed. At other times, lower pole reflux may be associated with dysplasia of the lower renal segment (56). Nodular renal blastema occurs in some multicystic kidneys and duplicated kidneys with ureteral ectopy (14,57), perhaps conferring the risk of neoplasia, including Wilms' tumor and renal cell carcinoma (58).

Renal dysplasia is encountered in about 10% of refluxing kidneys (59). The dysplastic changes in these circumstances are usually focal, consisting of clusters of primitive ducts and sometimes of cartilage bars, either in scarred and atrophic segments or adjacent to them (Fig. 5). The presence of dysplasia is interpreted as the result of intrauterine reflux during metanephric development rather than as acquired postnatal change.

Some dysplastic kidneys, like those in obstructive uropathy, retain limited functional capabilities and have unobstructed urinary systems (10). The patent ureter may be par-

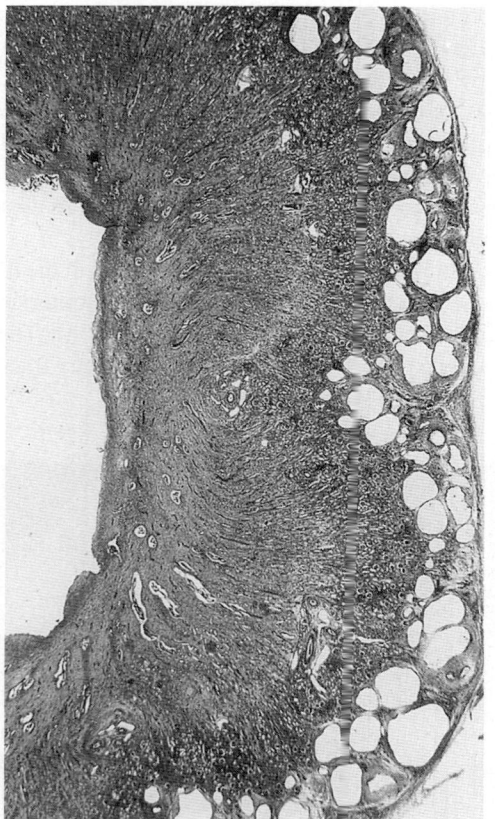

FIG. 4. Obstructive dysplasia. This kidney in a newborn boy with bilateral hydronephrosis secondary to posterior urethral valves contains a dysplastic outer cortex, whereas the inner cortex is normally differentiated. The cysts reside in dilated primitive collecting ducts and tubules. The medulla is poorly differentiated, lacking recurrent loops and vasa recta as the result of both pressure effect and altered medullary differentiation.

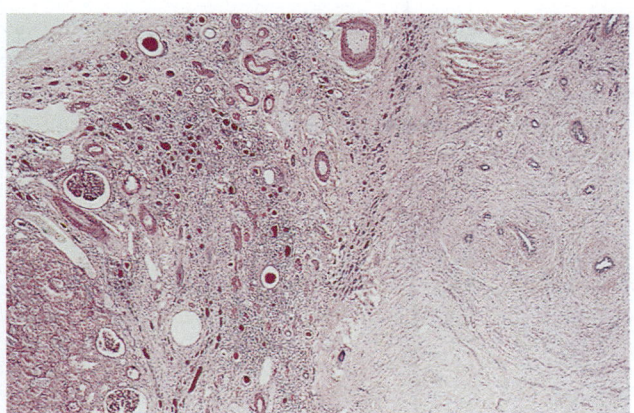

FIG. 5. Reflux nephropathy with segmental atrophy and focal renal dysplasia. A small, 37-g left kidney from a 7-year-old hypertensive girl with a history of vesicoureteric reflux contains an atrophic renal segment, sharply demarcated from relatively normal cortex to the left. The abnormal segment contains microcystic tubules with a chronic inflammatory cell infiltrate. Note the preferential loss of glomeruli and the relatively prominent, thick-walled arterioles. To the right of the atrophic segment is a collection of primitive ducts, presumably arising from abnormal metanephric differentiation secondary to intrauterine intrarenal reflux. Periodic acid-Schiff stain.

tially obstructed, or dilated or atrophic, but it has the potential for vesicoureteric reflux and ascending infection, with the complications of pyelonephritis and secondary nephrolithiasis. These dysplastic kidneys are difficult to categorize into a single morphologic pattern. Therefore, they lack a generally accepted terminology, and the term hypoplastic dysplasia has been suggested to convey the idea that they are small and partially functional. They have pelves and calyces, which are sometimes dilated, and lobar development is highly variable, with thin cortices (see Fig. 2). Evaluation of both biopsy and nephrectomy specimens leads to recognition of dysplastic elements in the form of cartilage, primitive ducts, and rudimentary medullary pyramids.

Large and diffusely cystic dysplastic kidneys with patent urinary tracts occur principally in malformation syndromes, occasionally as isolated malformations. They are not to be confused with multicystic kidneys, because the clinical and genetic implications are considerably different. The kidneys superficially resemble those of autosomal recessive "infantile" polycystic kidney disease, because they have the same reniform external configuration and a finely cystic external surface. Careful gross examination of the sectioned kidney, however, discloses a pattern of rounded rather than elongated cysts, and the medullary pyramids and calyces are severely underdeveloped. The cysts in diffuse cystic dysplasia arise principally within primitive collecting ducts, although portions of the nephron also become cystic, as in Meckel syndrome (60). In many specimens, however, there is a striking paucity of nephrons. Some clusters of glomeruli and convoluted tubules are present among the cysts, but normal cortical organization into medullary rays and cortical labyrinth is usually obscured. The association of Dandy-Walker malformation and cystic dysplastic kidneys, as well as occipital encephalocele and polydactyly, may represent pleiotropy/heterogeneity (61); however, familial renal-hepatic-pancreatic dysplasia and Dandy-Walker cyst appear to be a separate syndrome. Likewise, Dandy-Walker malformation, cystic renal dysplasia, and hepatic fibrosis may be within the phenotypic expression of Meckel syndrome or a distinct syndrome. Cartilage is seldom present. Diffuse cystic dysplasia occurs regularly in Meckel syndrome (63,64); it occurs less often in a group of disorders that includes several forms of short-limbed chondrodysplasia, Zellweger syndrome, glutaric aciduria type 2, and renal-hepatic-pancreatic dysplasia (65). In all of these syndromes, the liver contains a biliary abnormality similar to that of autosomal recessive polycystic kidney disease and congenital hepatic fibrosis. Specific diagnosis depends on recognition of the syndrome, because the renal abnormality is similar in all of them.

An important clinical question about renal dysplasia concerns the risk of recurrence. Dysplasia, unlike polycystic kidney disease, may be truly unilateral, and it does not eventually involve a previously normal opposite kidney. The risk of inheritance of nonsyndromal dysplasia is small, empirically not significantly different from zero (66). Nonetheless, there is minimal risk of recurrence of multicystic and aplastic kidneys in subsequent siblings, in that both malformations occur in the hereditary renal adysplasia syndrome, which comprises unilateral dysplasia, unilateral agenesis, and lethal bilateral agenesis, usually in a dominant pattern of inheritance (67–70). A balanced translocation in one case of bilateral multicystic dysplasia has been reported. There is also a small risk of recurrence in obstructive dysplasia secondary to posterior urethral valves, because the valves have a low familial incidence (71). The risk of recurrence is much greater in diffuse cystic dysplasia, in which the risks are those of the associated syndrome.

Multicystic kidneys, which are often diagnosed by prenatal sonography, undergo an evolution to shrinkage and even disappearance (72). The kidney occasionally enlarges, a fluctuation attributable to cyst enlargement, but the general trend toward shrinkage often leads to the ultimate equivalent of agenesis (72).

CONGENITAL HYDRONEPHROSIS

Most congenitally hydronephrotic kidneys contain normal parenchyma, apart from the compression effects of pelvic dilatation. That observation, namely, the lack of altered metanephric differentiation, suggests that the obstruction is commonly acquired late in gestation, possibly even after the cessation of nephrogenesis at 36 weeks. The hydronephrosis may also become more severe during the last month of gestation, with regression postnatally (73). The obstruction is most often at the ureteropelvic junction. Congenital hydronephrosis is usually due to an intrinsic abnormality of a short segment of the ureteral muscle. Aberrant branches of the renal artery crossing the upper ureter or renal pelvis have also been implicated, but there is usually an associated intrinsic abnormality of the ureteral musculature, so that the role of the vessels in causing obstruction is unclear (74). Patients with ureteropelvic junction obstruction with a differential function of less than 35% have a high probability of significant histologic changes on biopsy and a low probability of postoperative improvement in differential function (75,76). Urethral obstruction is considered the major etiologic factor in the development of bilateral fetal uropathy and presumably the prune-belly phenotype. Such cases are virtually always associated with pulmonary hypoplasia or immaturity, resulting in respiratory insufficiency at birth (77). Vesicoureteric reflux is emerging as the most common urologic finding in infants with prenatal hydronephrosis (78). Postnatal reconstructive surgery is usually effective in preserving and sometimes in restoring renal function (79). Some congenitally hydronephrotic kidneys, especially those that are very large ("giant hydronephrosis"), may be dysplastic (80,81). Pelvicaliceal stenosis is generally marked. They have cystic capsular surfaces, and histopathologic examination shows dysplasia in the outer cortex and hydronephrotic changes in the medulla. They should, despite certain morphologic similarities, be differentiated from multicystic kidneys.

Neonatal hydronephrosis is being detected with increasing frequency. The majority of these cases have a tendency to resolve during infancy. Hydronephrosis is an anatomical entity that is not synonymous with obstruction (82).

Hereditary hydronephrosis is a rare condition but several families are described in the literature. The inheritance pattern is autosomal dominant (McKusick number 143400) but the exact etiology of the hydronephrosis is not clear. However, linkage with the HLA region on chromosome 6 has been shown previously. One family was reported as not showing linkage to this region, giving further evidence of genetic heterogeneity in this condition (83). One of the loci for hereditary hydronephrosis has been assigned to chromosome 6p (84).

CONGENITAL NEPHROMEGALY

Compensatory growth and hypertrophy of one kidney can occur when the contralateral kidney is severely diseased, dysplastic, or congenitally absent.

Renal enlargement from an increased amount of renal parenchyma occurs in the Wiedemann-Beckwith syndrome (exomphalos, macroglossia, and gigantism) (85) and the Perlman syndrome (macrosomia, islet-cell hypertrophy, unusual facies, and renal hamartomas) (87,87). The kidneys in both syndromes are excessively lobulated and contain dysplastic medullary pyramids, sometimes with small cysts. The medullary abnormality has often been characterized clinically and radiographically as medullary sponge kidney (88), despite the clear morphologic evidence of dysplasia and the clear differences from typical medullary sponge kidney. Histopathologic examination of cortical tissue reveals persistent nephrogenesis, nodular blastema, and nephroblastomatosis. The occurrence of nephroblastomatosis imposes an increased risk of Wilms' tumor, as seen also in hemihypertrophy syndromes. The Wiedemann-Beckwith syndrome carries an increased risk of adrenal carcinoma, hepatoblastoma, and brainstem glioma (89). The Wiedemann-Beckwith syndrome is a dominant mutation, whereas Perlman syndrome is autosomal recessive. Nonetheless, some of the Wiedemann-Beckwith manifestations, for example, umbilical hernia and macroglossia, have been seen to develop postnatally (90).

RENAL TUBULAR DYSGENESIS

An unusual cause of neonatal oliguria, usually after a gestation complicated by oligohydramnios, is renal tubular dysgenesis (RTD) (91–93). Oligohydramnios may be delayed, however, becoming evident after the 20th week of gestation (94), which makes early diagnosis difficult even when the condition is suggested by family history. The renal abnormality has been associated with widely patent cranial fontanels (94,95). The kidneys are commonly, although not necessarily, enlarged, containing an increased number of nephrons (92). The cortical tubules are lined with densely packed columnar cells that histochemically bind peanut lectin and immunohistochemical reaction for epithelial

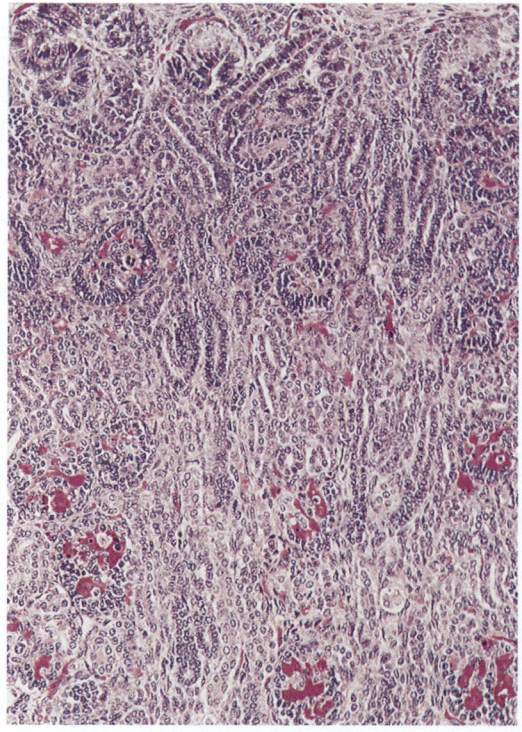

FIG. 6. Renal tubular dysgenesis. The convoluted tubules of the cortical labyrinth are lined with abnormally differentiated cells that lack the features of proximal tubular epithelium. The collecting tubules are also poorly differentiated, and the glomeruli seem crowded.

membrane antigen is positive, suggesting that the tubular segments are of collecting duct origin (Fig. 6). The glomeruli appear to be crowded together, therefore, and the medullary pyramids are smaller than normal.

Immunohistochemical demonstration of very large amounts of renin within preglomerular arteries suggests vasoconstriction and greatly reduced glomerular perfusion (96). Microdissection study has demonstrated marked shortening of all the nephron segments from the glomeruli to the collecting tubules, rather than an isolated abnormality of the proximal convoluted tubules (97).

Recognition of this condition is of great importance for family counseling, because it has been shown to have an autosomal recessive inheritance (94). The renal abnormality has also been linked to treatment of maternal hypertension with angiotensin-converting enzyme (ACE) inhibitors (98,99) and to maternal use of cocaine (93,100,101).

A renal abnormality bearing some similarities to that found in familial renal tubular dysgenesis, occurs after maternal use of nonsteroidal antiinflammatory drugs (NSAIDs). The same effect on fetal urine output and amniotic fluid volume is common to all NSAIDs and the risk of fetal renal injury may be common to all (102). Abnormal fetal renal tubular development and oligohydramnios have been attributed to treatment of pregnant women with indomethacin (103), a drug used as a tocolytic agent and inhibitor of fetal urine output. Fetuses in twin pregnancies with polyhydramnios are at increased risk of NSAID-associated renal injury.

Renal tubular dysgenesis should be obvious by the 30th week of gestation. Metzman and colleagues (104) have described partial tubular differentiation at 20 and 22 weeks, with the suggestion that regressive changes contribute to the pathogenesis of RTD.

Ischemia may play a role in RTD. Reduced renal blood flow, whether from primary renin–angiotensin abnormalities or ACE-inhibitor–mediated fetal hypotension, may contribute to poor tubular growth and differentiation, as suggested by Landing and associates (105), and lack of angiotensin II as growth factor may play a key role in both the familial and ACE-I–induced RTD (105). RTD has been reported in association with meconium ileus in neonatal hemosiderotic liver disease.

RENAL SEGMENTAL ATROPHY (SEGMENTAL "HYPOPLASIA," ASK-UPMARK KIDNEY)

Despite continuing controversy, the principal cause of small kidneys with segmental or lobar atrophy is vesicoureteric reflux with intrarenal reflux (106–109). Segmental hypoplasia is an outmoded concept, and the term *Ask-Upmark kidney* can be dropped from the lexicon. However, not all patients with this abnormality have demonstrable vesicoureteric reflux at the time of clinical evaluation, and other causes have been considered, such as localized vascular insufficiency. The possibility of localized developmental arrest was suggested in early descriptions of the abnormality (110), and that explanation still receives support. One of the arguments advanced in its favor is the occurrence of renal dysplasia in the abnormal segments (111), but the altered metanephric development is probably a consequence of intrauterine reflux. Serial radiographic studies have demonstrated that the segmental lesion initially develops in unscarred kidneys of normal size (112). The frequent paucity of inflammatory cells in the abnormal segments, as well as in the remainder of the kidney, has been taken as evidence that the lesion could not have arisen from reflux and chronic pyelonephritis; however, inflammatory infiltrates undoubtedly clear and the point needs to be evaluated also in relation to sterile intrarenal reflux and its consequences.

The characteristic abnormality is a shrunken lobe containing an attenuated cortex and an effaced medullary pyramid. The cortex typically seems to lack glomeruli and to consist of microcystic tubules plugged with colloid casts, so-called aglomerular hypoplasia (see Fig. 5). A few specimens contain easily recognizable, collapsed glomeruli, indicating that the obsolete glomeruli and eventually the tubules are resorbed to leave a fibrous scar without identifiable nephrons (108). The arcuate and interlobular arteries are, until the end-stage fibrous scar, prominent as the result of cortical shrinkage and their own medial hypertrophy. Cavernous, thin-walled vessels can be traced into the renal sinus, where, despite their resemblance to dilated lymphatics, they connect with renal vein tributaries. The medullary pyramids contain a reduced number of ducts and a paucity or absence of vasa recta and recurrent loops. The ducts sometimes have a primitive appearance, taken as evidence of renal dysplasia (see Fig. 5). These features are typically found in very small kidneys, partly accounting for the interpretation that the kidneys are hypoplastic; the kidneys have weights of 40 g or less, even in adult patients.

The presence of lobar or segmental atrophy in pyelonephritic and in dysplastic kidneys can be taken as evidence of reflux nephropathy. The abnormal segments in kidneys damaged by reflux are initially at the poles, with later involvement of middle segments. The remnant kidney undergoes compensatory hypertrophy, sometimes with a deceptively bland histopathologic appearance, overshadowing the adjacent shrunken lobes. Segmental glomerular sclerosis in hypertrophied glomeruli of the remnant kidney is associated with proteinuria, sometimes in the nephrotic range, and glomerular sclerosis is an important factor in progression to end-stage renal failure (113–115). The other important factor is frequent bilaterality of the reflux.

Many of the patients come to medical attention because of hypertension, not always with a history of recurrent urinary tract infection. The evaluation of nephrectomy specimens from patients with renal hypertension may seem to show only a small kidney with normal parenchyma, and thorough examination of the entire pyelocalyceal system is necessary in order to identify shrunken and atrophic segments.

CYSTIC KIDNEY DISEASES

Polycystic disease of the kidney in children comprises two genetically different disorders, one with autosomal recessive inheritance and an onset typically in childhood and the other with an autosomal dominant inheritance and an onset occasionally in childhood. The clinical, morphologic, and radiographic characteristics overlap, and differentiation may become apparent only on extensive investigation of the family. Nonetheless, the distinction between these disorders is important for prognostication and family counseling. Renal cystic disease also occurs in several hereditary syndromes, particularly tuberous sclerosis. Glomerulocystic disease is a morphologic term descriptive of the renal abnormality occurring in some cases of childhood autosomal dominant polycystic kidney disease, tuberous sclerosis, and certain other syndromes. Some of these cystic diseases are encountered by the surgical pathologist in renal biopsy specimens. A classification of renal cystic diseases is listed in Table 1.

Autosomal Recessive Polycystic Kidney Disease

Autosomal recessive polycystic kidney disease (AR-PKD) is a rare condition with an incidence of between 1 in 6,000 to 1 in 14,000 births. The gene has been mapped to the short arm of chromosome 6. It may consist of several clinically and morphologically overlapping syndromes (116), each with autosomal recessive inheritance, or it may be a single disorder subject to modification by gene linkages and epigenetic factors (65). In this discussion, AR-PKD is considered as one genetic disorder, with different phenotypes (117) that, in a sense, relate to differences in severity of expression. There is no confirmed evidence of genetic heterogeneity. Newborn infants typically have nonfunctioning, enlarged, diffusely cystic kidneys; the livers contain enlarged portal areas with apparent biliary proliferation. Older infants have less severely enlarged kidneys, with less functional impairment and less severe cyst formation, and the same hepatic abnormality. Some older children and adults have asymptomatic renal involvement, with very few cysts, and progressive portal fibrosis, known as *congenital hepatic fibrosis* (118), leading to portal hypertension. Although certain generalizations can be stated, sharp distinctions among these groups cannot be made. More than one pattern has occurred among affected siblings in the same family (119–122).

Newborns with the severe form of the disease die shortly after birth, usually because of respiratory insufficiency. Many of them have the Potter sequence, with its characteristic facies, secondary to oligohydramnios, and pulmonary hypoplasia leads to the postnatal complications of severe respiratory distress. The kidneys are often huge, together exceeding 300 g. They have a reniform configuration and a normal lobar structure, but they are spongy and externally finely cystic. The cysts are located in collecting ducts and tubules (123–126), which appear to be elongated sacs lined with cuboidal epithelium (Fig. 7A). Lectin markers (e.g., peanut lectin) clearly identify cysts as dilated collecting ducts (127); the lectins may also bind to distal tubular segments (60,128). The cystic ducts on the cut surface run from medulla to outer cortex, and the dilated medullary ducts tend to have a more rounded appearance than do the cortical ducts. The cortex is commonly edematous, accounting for some of the increased weight of the kidney and separating the individual nephrons so that they seem to be reduced in number. The medullary pyramids, apart from the cysts, are normally formed, and the essential architecture of the kidney appears, therefore, to be normal. The livers contain enlarged portal areas with an increased number of biliary profiles that form an array of anastomosing channels (see Fig. 7B). However, the biliary structures are flattened sacs rather than ducts (129–131), and occasional specimens contain gross cysts. Cysts in viscera other than liver and kidney are rare in homogeneous populations of AR-PKD, and their presence may be clues to other syndromes.

Older infants have more irregular renal cyst formation, and asymptomatic older children may have very few cysts. The cysts are located predominantly in the outer medulla (132). The histopathologic picture becomes complicated, however, because of tubular atrophy and interstitial fibrosis (Fig. 8). The cortical cysts often have a rounded appearance, suggesting localized obstruction. Dilated convoluted tubules become mildly cystic, perhaps as the result of secondary local obstruction. Whether the disease in those patients in whom renal insufficiency later develops progresses by additional cyst formation (133) or by tubular atrophy and interstitial fibrosis (131) is uncertain, although the former appears to be uncommon. The hepatic abnormality, although essentially the same as that in infants, becomes increasingly

TABLE 1. *Classification of renal cystic disease*

1. Polycystic disease
    A. Autosomal recessive polycystic kidney disease (AR-PKD)
        (i) Classic infantile polycystic diseases
        (ii) AR-PKD and congenital hepatic fibrosis in older individuals
    B. Autosomal dominant polycystic kidney disease (AD-PKD)
        (i) Classic adult polycystic disease
        (ii) AD-PKD in infants (glomerulocystic disease)
2. Glomerular cystic disease
3. Localized cystic disease
4. Renal cysts associated with syndromes of multiple malformations
5. Medullary cystic disease
    A. Medullary sponge kidney
    B. Familial nephronophthisis-medullary cystic disease (FN-MCD complex)
6. Multilocular renal cysts
7. Renal dysplasia with cysts
8. Simple renal cysts
9. Acquired renal cystic disease
10. Miscellaneous extrarenal cysts

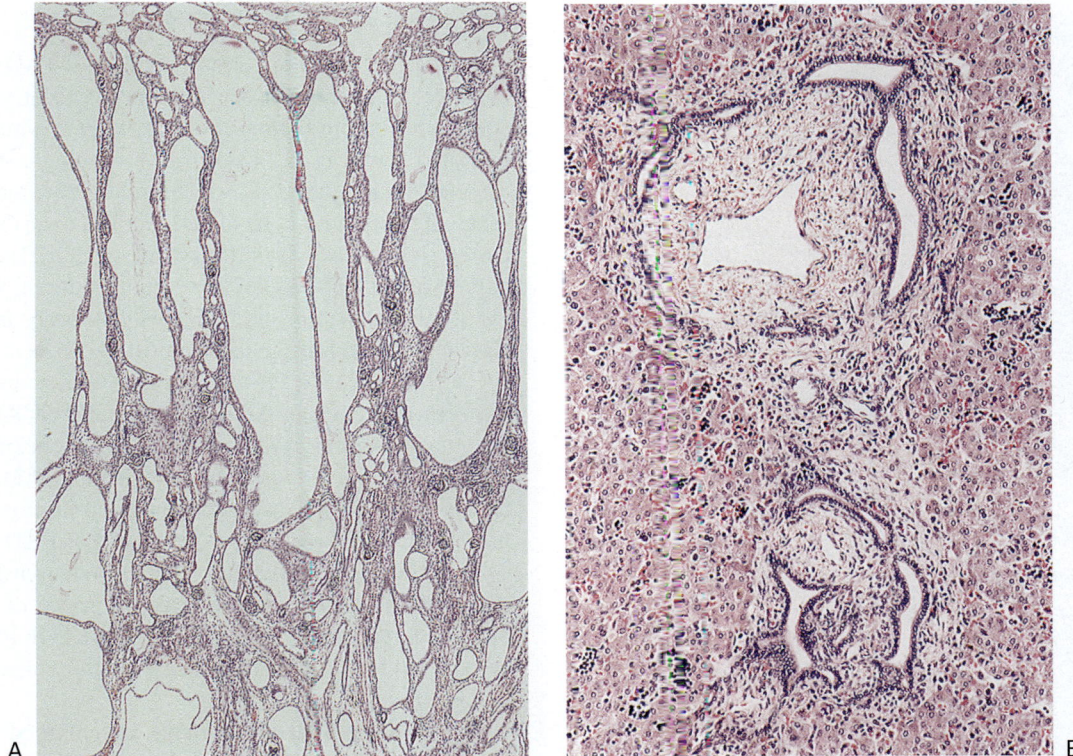

FIG. 7. Autosomal recessive, infantile polycystic disease in a newborn. The kidney **(A)** contains dilated collecting ducts that form elongated cortical cysts. Nephrogenesis is relatively normal, with mild tubular dilatation and mild interstitial fibrosis. The liver **(B)** contains enlarged portal areas with the appearance of proliferating bile ducts that are, in fact, interconnecting sacs resulting from abnormal biliary differentiation.

fibrotic with time. Perilobular fibrosis and regenerative nodules may result in a pattern resembling micronodular cirrhosis (134). It is thought that portal hypertension results from presinusoidal obstruction, but there may also be an element of postsinusoidal obstruction (135), because central perivenous fibrosis is relatively common (136). Although the abnormal portal biliary passages commonly contain plugs of inspissated bile, hepatocellular changes and intralobular cholestasis do not usually occur, except in the presence of superimposed infection. Ascending suppurative cholangitis is a relatively common complication (134,137), probably related to biliary dilatation and stasis. Nonobstructive ectasia of the intrahepatic ducts, known as Caroli disease, occurs in a small proportion (perhaps 10%) of patients with AR-PKD (134,138,139). The same or very similar intrahepatic biliary abnormalities are seen in conjunction with other hereditary syndromes with renal cystic or dysplastic changes, notably the Meckel, Jeune, and Zellweger syndromes. It has also been described in some patients with juvenile nephronopthisis. All these conditions, like AR-PKD, are inherited as autosomal recessive traits.

The histopathologic diagnosis of AR-PKD in a newborn with typical, severe renal involvement is usually straightforward. The abnormality must be differentiated, as discussed previously, from diffuse cystic dysplasia, which has different morphologic characteristics. The diagnosis often can be confirmed by a liver biopsy, but open-wedge biopsies are preferable to percutaneous needle biopsies for this purpose. The histopathologic diagnosis of the renal abnormality in older children, however, can be difficult, as attested to by some confusion in the literature and by difficulties in evaluating individual cases. The hallmark of AR-PKD in the older child is medullary ductal ectasia (140), but urography has been supplanted by sonography, which shows variably enlarged kidneys with increased echogenicity (141). The sonographic appearances are similar to those of autosomal dominant PKD in childhood and of glomerulocystic kidney disease. Liver biopsies in older children may also be helpful by showing the characteristic biliary abnormality.

Older patients have variable progression of the renal abnormality (142). In some, renal insufficiency develops in early childhood, and others remain asymptomatic into adulthood. Patients typically have a concentrating defect and impaired acidification unrelated to reduced glomerular filtration. Systemic hypertension develops in almost all patients, and cerebral arterial aneurysms, although less common than in patients with dominant PKD, do occur. Portal hypertension and its complications also develop in older children and

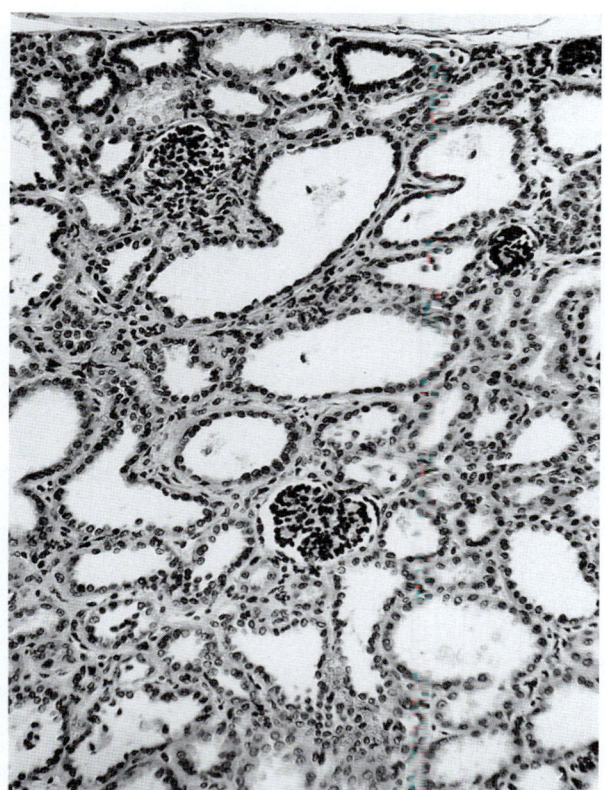

FIG. 8. Autosomal recessive, infantile polycystic disease in a 9-month-old infant with enlarged kidneys, renal insufficiency, radiographic medullary ductal ectasia, and congenital hepatic fibrosis. The biopsy specimen contains dilated cortical collecting tubules, with irregular dilatation and atrophy of convoluted tubules. There is diffuse interstitial fibrosis.

young adults. Some patients have both renal insufficiency and portal hypertension, whereas others have only mild urinary concentrating defects. Clinical evidence of hepatocellular dysfunction may develop in relation to biliary infection, but patients are ordinarily not jaundiced.

The differential diagnosis in older children includes other causes of progressive renal insufficiency with a concentrating defect, the most common of which is familial juvenile nephronophthisis, a form of hereditary interstitial nephritis. That abnormality is often accompanied by medullary cysts, and the kidneys are very small because of severe cortical atrophy. Urographic studies do not, therefore, visualize the medullary cysts, and sonographic studies may be equivocal. A small proportion of patients with nephronophthisis have had hepatic involvement in the form of portal fibrosis. More commonly associated abnormalities include pigmentary retinal degeneration (renal-retinal dysplasia) and skeletal dysplasia.

Fetal ultrasonography offers the possibility of prenatal diagnosis of AR-PKD. The fetal kidneys are enlarged bilaterally and have increased echogenicity. Ultrasonic diagnosis is straightforward when other siblings are known to be affected, but in an index case, distinction from other forms of cystic disease, such as diffuse cystic dysplasia or glomerulocystic disease, may be difficult.

Autosomal Dominant Polycystic Disease

Autosomal dominant polycystic disease (AD-PKD) occasionally has an early onset in the newborn or young infant, sometimes before the onset of clinically apparent renal disease in a parent (125,143–146). Morphologic studies of the affected infants have shown the relatively frequent occurrence of glomerular cysts (131,147,148), to an extent that so-called glomerulocystic kidney disease (GCKD) is a common expression of AD-PKD in very young children. Several studies of affected parent and fetus by DNA-probe analysis have shown the same linkage to chromosome 16 as in classic AD-PKD (149–151). In GCKD, parental ultrasound should be performed to exclude AD-PKD; neonatal GCKD may antedate the appearance of classic AD-PKD in one of the parents.

AD-PKD is genetically heterogeneous (152). Linkage to chromosome 16 has been demonstrated in most cases, perhaps 90%, who have what is designated as PKD I. Studies in some families, however, have failed to demonstrate a locus on chromosome 16, indicating the presence of at least one other genotype, tentatively designated PKD II. PKD II seems to be a milder form of the disease, with expression later in life.

The kidneys in affected infants are enlarged and hyperechoic, much like the kidneys in typical recessive disease (143,153). Young infants may have renal insufficiency and die of renal failure, but some of them seem to stabilize, with survival into the second or third decade. Very severe cortical cystic disease is accompanied by abnormal medullary development, a form of dysplasia (125,148). In older children identified by clinical screening as having more typical AD-PKD, with localized cysts, renal insufficiency does not ordinarily develop until adulthood (154). Hepatic involvement, with biliary dysgenesis resembling that of AR-PKD, occurs in approximately 10% of young children. Children also may have hypertension and cerebral berry aneurysms.

The kidneys in older children, as in adults, commonly contain irregularly clustered small cysts, and the cysts are lined with hyperplastic epithelium such as that seen in adult patients (Fig. 9). Light-, transmission-, electron-, and scanning electron-microscopic studies of AD-PKD kidneys have shown micropapillary epithelial hyperplasia with small intracystic and intraductal polyps, and the epithelial hyperplasia is believed to contribute to cyst formation by causing luminal obstruction (155–158). The cysts arise in collecting ducts and in all portions of the nephron, as shown by lectin-binding studies (127) that confirm older microdissection studies. Only a minority of nephrons, probably less than 20%, become cystic, and the disease progresses by cyst enlargement, with compression of parenchyma, rather than by recruitment of new cysts (159). Cyst enlargement, with increased renal volume, correlates also with the clinical development of hypertension (160). Cysts often become infected (161,162), and there is a very high frequency of nephrolithiasis (163). Hepatic cysts increase in frequency with age (164) and become infected (166). A few families have had a liver abnormality indistinguishable from congenital hepatic fibrosis in

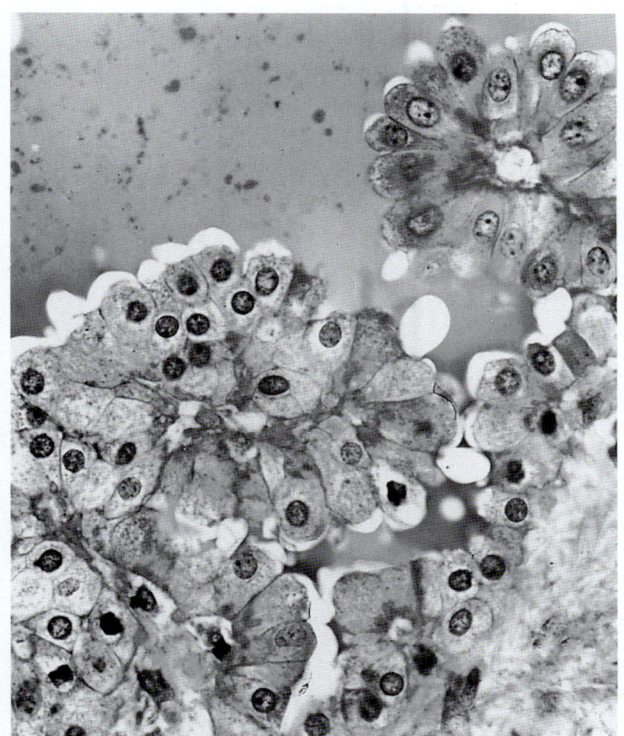

FIG. 9. Autosomal dominant adult polycystic disease. The cysts are lined with hyperplastic epithelium thrown into irregular folds and papillations. The micropapillary hyperplasia contributes to cyst formation by causing luminal obstruction, and the epithelial hyperplasia poses an increased risk of neoplasia. Azure-II-methylene blue stain.

AR-PKD (167). Cardiac valvular lesions, intracranial aneurysms, and colonic diverticula also develop (131).

In addition to AR-PKD, the differential diagnosis in early infancy includes diffuse cystic dysplasia, tuberous sclerosis, and other syndromes with diffuse renal involvement. One of the more difficult diagnostic problems in children is caused by asynchronous and asymmetrical onsets (168–170). A condition of nonprogressive, unilateral, localized cystic disease has been described (171), but long-term follow-up is necessary to exclude the possibility of eventual bilateral involvement.

Tuberous Sclerosis

Renal involvement in tuberous sclerosis, including benign and malignant angiomyolipomas, cysts, and carcinomas, affects approximately one half of patients with the syndrome (172,173). Angiomyolipomas, which in general are rarely malignant (174), increase in frequency in older patients. Severe cystic disease occurs more often in children and is a cause of chronic renal failure (175). Renal cell carcinoma, usually well differentiated, occurs with a higher-than-expected frequency and is often bilateral and multiple.

Studies have indicated locus heterogeneity in tuberous sclerosis, like that in AD-PKD, with disease-determining genes on chromosomes 9 and 16. The mutant genes occur in small regions of telomeric chromosome bands, that on chromosome 9 (designated TSC1) at 9q34.3 and that on chromosome 16 (called TSC2) at 16p13.3. In about 50% of patients, tuberous sclerosis is associated with renal cystic change, a feature that has been better appreciated since modern diagnostic imaging techniques have allowed the recognition of even quite small renal cysts. Deletion of the TSC2 and PKD 1 genes is associated with severe infantile polycystic kidney disease—a contiguous gene syndrome (176).

Three findings suggest that the tuberous sclerosis genes are tumor suppressor genes. First, loss of heterozygosity (LOH) on chromosome 16p13 and 9q34 has been demonstrated in TSC lesions, consistent with tumor suppressor functions for the TSC1 and TSC2 genes. Second, germline TSC2 gene mutations appear to inactivate TSC2. Third, specific 16p13 LOH has been found in some sporadic angiomyolipomas (177).

Severe cystic disease in infancy causes renal enlargement, moderate renal insufficiency, and severe hypertension (178). The renal manifestations sometimes precede the obvious development of other stigmata. The cystic disease may present as unilateral renal enlargement (179). The cysts are lined with a distinctive, hyperplastic epithelium seemingly unique to this syndrome (Fig. 10) (180), and cellular hyperplasia is

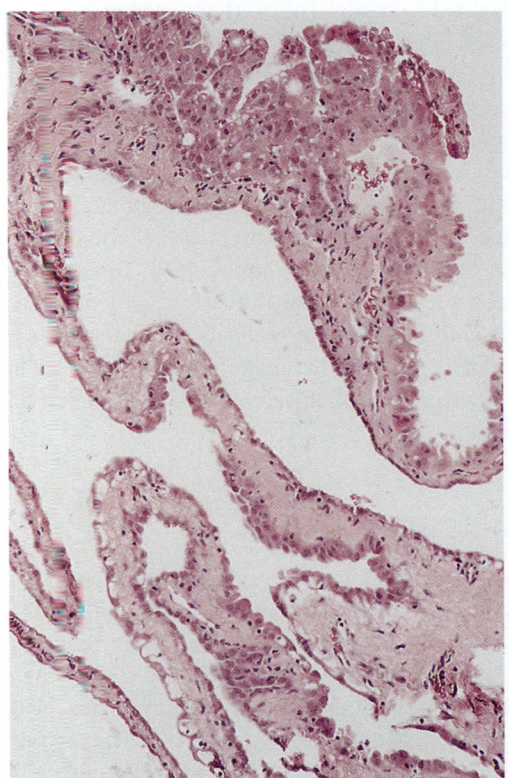

FIG. 10. Tuberous sclerosis. The cysts in a hypertensive 18-month-old infant with greatly enlarged kidneys are lined by a distinctive, possibly unique form of epithelial hyperplasia in which the cells are very large and deeply eosinophilic. The epithelium is frequently piled up in small intracystic masses. The epithelial hyperplasia contributes to the cyst formation as well as to an increased risk of neoplasia. Although the diagnosis of tuberous sclerosis had not been suspected clinically, examination after renal biopsy showed shagreen patches.

probably responsible for both cyst formation and an increased risk of neoplasia (157). The cysts occasionally predominate in glomeruli, with the histologic appearance of glomerulocystic kidney disease. Cysts and angiomyolipomas often coexist, and large angiomyolipomas are prone to rupture and cause life-threatening hemorrhage (172). Carcinomas may coexist with the other two lesions or arise independently. Although the number of reports is small, patients with carcinoma have been relatively young, and the tumors have been both bilateral and multiple, and clear-cell, high-grade spindle-cell, and granular-cell morphology have been described. Positive immunostaining for HMB-45 was present in four of six cases. There is controversy in the literature over the extent of surgical resection required for treatment (181,182). Renal oncocytoma in children is suggestive of tuberous sclerosis.

Von Hippel-Lindau Disease

Von Hippel-Lindau disease (VHL) is a condition inherited as an autosomal dominant trait characterized by a variable combination of retinal angiomatosis, cerebellar angiomas, and cysts and tumors of abdominal organs, particularly the pancreas and kidneys. The VHL disease tumor suppressor gene maps to chromosome 3p25-26. Germline mutations in the VHL tumor suppressor gene predisposes to renal cell carcinoma, hemangioblastoma of the central nervous system, and pheochromocytoma.

Renal cysts are found in two thirds of patients with VHL disease. Cysts are usually multiple and bilateral and are often lined with hyperplastic, atypical cells that form mural nodules of intracystic carcinoma (157). Renal adenocarcinoma develops in about one third of the patients, and in 15% it is bilateral. Diagnosis of renal adenocarcinoma is made an average of 15 years earlier than in sporadic cases. The carcinomas are usually well differentiated, with a relatively good prognosis.

Glomerulocystic Disease

Glomerular cysts have long been recognized in infants' kidneys, occurring in a variety of primary and secondary disorders (147,148). The abnormality occurs in both infants and adults, sometimes with a family history suggesting autosomal dominant inheritance. Glomerular cysts may be the morphologic expression of early-onset AD-PKD, as previously discussed. Clear evidence of heterogeneity comes from the recognition of glomerular cysts in tuberous sclerosis, brachymesomelia-renal syndrome, oral-facial-digital syndrome type I, trisomy 13, Zellweger syndrome, and renal dysplasia. A rare form of glomerulocystic disease in hypoplastic kidneys has an autosomal dominant inheritance (183). Many cases, however, cannot be refined further and remain as idiopathic glomerulocystic disease (Fig. 11) (184,185). A dominantly transmitted GCKD with a genetic

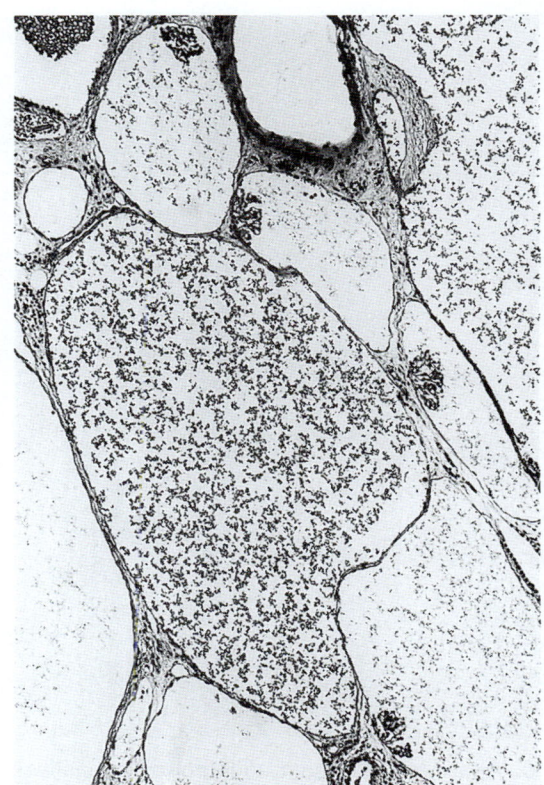

FIG. 11. Glomerulocystic kidney. The kidney contains a large number of glomerular cysts in an infant with renal insufficiency, large kidneys, negative family history, and no obvious malformations.

locus distinct from PKD1 and PKD2 loci has been described in a large three-generation African-American family (186).

REFERENCES

1. Bernstein J. Developmental abnormalities of the renal parenchyma—hypoplasia and dysplasia. *Pathol Annu* 1968;3:213–247.
2. Mitényi M, Czeizel AE, Balogh L, Detre Z. Autosomal recessive acrorenal syndrome. *Am J Med Genet* 1992;43:789–790.
3. Royer P, Habib R, Mathieu H, Courtecuisse V. L'hypoplasie rénale bilatéral congénitale avec réduction du nombre et hypertrophie des néphrons chez l'enfant. *Semin Hôp Paris* (Ann Pédiatr) 1962;38: 753–766.
4. Park SH, Chi JE G. Oligomeganephronia associated with 4p deletion type chromosomal anomaly. *Pediatr Pathol* 1993;13:731–740.
5. Ariel I, Wells TR, Singer DB. The urinary system in Down syndrome: a study of 124 autopsy cases. *Pediatr Pathol* 1991;11:879–888.
6. Foster SV, Hawkins EP. Deficient metanephric blastema—a cause of oligomeganephronia? Pediatr Pathol 1994;14:935–943.
7. Boyd T, Rosen S, Redline RW, Genest DR: Nondysplastic fetal renal hypoplasia associated with severe oligohydramnios: clinical, pathologic, and morphometric findings. *Pediatr Pathol Lab Med* 1995;15: 485–501.
8. Schimmenti LA, Pierpont ME, Carpenter BLM, et al. Autosomal dominant optic nerve colobomas, vesicoureteral reflux, and renal anomalies. *Am J Med Genet* 1995;59:204–208.
9. Smith SJ, Cass AS, Aliabadi H, et al. Unipapillary kidney: a case report and literature review. *Urol Radiol* 1984;6:43–47.
10. Bernstein J. The morphogenesis of renal parenchymal maldevelopment (renal dysplasia). *Pediatr Clin North Am* 1971;18:395–407.
11. Matsell DG, Bennett T, Goodyer P, et al. The pathogenesis of multicystic dysplastic kidney disease: insights from the study of fetal kidneys. *Lab Invest* 1996;74:883.

12. Vellios F, Garrett RA. Congenital unilateral multicystic disease of the kidney. A clinical and anatomic study of seven cases. *Am J Clin Pathol* 1961;35:244–254.
13. Saxton HM, Golding SJ, Chantler C, Haycock GD. Diagnostic puncture in renal cystic dysplasia (multicystic kidney). Evidence on the aetiology of the cysts. *Br J Radiol* 1981;54:555–561.
14. Gaddy CD, Gibbons MD, Gonzales ET Jr, Finegold MJ. Obstructive uropathy, renal dysplasia and dysplasia and nodular renal blastema: is there a relationship to Wilms tumor? *J Urol* 1985;134:330–333.
15. Dimmick JE, Johnson HW, Coleman GU, Carter M. Wilms tumorlet, nodular renal blastema and multicystic renal dysplasia, part 2. *J Urol* 1989;142:484–485.
16. Noe HN, Marshall JH, Edwards OP. Nodular renal blastema in the multicystic kidney, part 2. *J Urol* 1989;142:486–488.
17. Barrett DM, Wineland RE. Renal cell carcinoma in multicystic dysplastic kidney. *Urology* 1980;15:152–154.
18. Birken G, King D, Vane D, Lloyd T. Renal cell carcinoma arising in a multicystic dysplastic kidney. *J Pediatr Surg* 1985;20:619–621.
19. Pathak IG, Williams DI. Multicystic and cystic dysplastic kidneys. *Br J Urol* 1963;36:318–331.
20. Griscom NT, Vawter GF, Fellers FX. Pelvoinfundibular atresia: the usual form of multicystic kidney: 44 unilateral and two bilateral cases. *Semin Roentgenol* 1975;10:125–131.
21. Felson B, Cussen LJ. The hydronephrotic type of unilateral congenital multicystic disease of the kidney. *Semin Roentgenol* 1975;10:113–123.
22. Risdon RA. Renal dysplasia. I. A clinico-pathological study of 76 cases. II. A necropsy study of 41 cases. *J Clin Pathol* 1971;24:57–71.
23. Leonidas JC, Strauss L, Krasna IH. Roentgen diagnosis of multicystic renal dysplasia in infancy by high dose urography. *J Urol* 1972;108:963–965.
24. Warshawsky AB, Miller KE, Kaplan GW. Urographic visualization of multicystic kidneys. *J Urol* 1977;177:94–96.
25. Carey PO, Howards SS. Multicystic dysplastic kidneys and diagnostic confusion on renal scan. *J Urol* 1988;139:83–84.
26. Hashimoto BE, Filly RA, Callen PW. Multicystic dysplastic kidney in utero: changing appearance on US. *Radiology* 1986;159:107–109.
27. Pedicelli G, Jequier S, Bowen A, Boisvert J. Multicystic dysplastic kidneys: spontaneous regression demonstrated with US. *Radiology* 1986;160:23–26.
28. Avni EF, Thoua Y, Lalmand B, et al. Multicystic dysplastic kidney: natural history from in utero diagnosis and postnatal follow-up. *J Urol* 1987;138:1420–1424.
29. Vinocur L, Slovis TL, Perlmutter AD, et al. Follow-up studies of multicystic dysplastic kidneys. *Radiology* 1988;167:311–315.
30. Gordon AC, Thomas DFM, Arthur RJ, Irving HC. Multicystic dysplastic kidney: is nephrectomy still appropriate? Part 2. *J Urol* 1988;140:1231–1234.
31. Al-Khaldi N, Watson AR, Zuccollo J, et al. Outcome of antenatally detected cystic dysplastic kidney disease. *Arch Dis Child* 1994;70:520–522.
32. Winyard PJD, Nauta J, Lirenman DS, et al. Deregulation of cell survival in cystic and dysplastic renal development. *Kidney Int* 1996;49:135–146.
33. Bearman SB, Hine PL, Sanders RC. Multicystic kidney: a sonographic pattern. *Radiology* 1976;118:685–688.
34. Stuck KJ, Koff SA, Silver TM. Ultrasonic features of multicystic dysplastic kidney: expanded diagnostic criteria. *Radiology* 1982;143:217–221.
35. Greene LF, Feinzaig W, Dahlin DC. Multicystic dysplasia of the kidney: with special reference to the contralateral kidney. *J Urol* 1971;105:482–487.
36. Krull F, Hoyer PF, Habenicht R, et al. Die multizystische Nierendysplasie. *Monatsschr Kinderheilkd* 1990;138:202–205.
37. Kleiner B, Filly RA, Mack L, Callen PW. Multicystic dysplastic kidney: observations of contralateral disease in the fetal population. *Radiology* 1986;161:27–29.
38. Bloom DA, Brosman S. The multicystic kidney. *J Urol* 1978;120:211–215.
39. Lennert Th, Tetzner M, Er M, et al. Multicystic renal dysplasia: nephrectomy versus conservative treatment. *Contrib Nephrol* 1988;67:183–187.
40. Hartman GE, Smolik LM, Schochat SJ. The dilemma of the multicystic dysplastic kidney. *Am J Dis Child* 1986;140:925–928.
41. Webb NJA, Lewis MA, Bruce J, et al. Unilateral multicystic dysplastic kidney: the case for nephrectomy. *Arch Dis Child* 1997;76:31–34.
42. Susskind MR, Kim KS, King LR. Hypertension and multicystic kidney. *Urology* 1989;34:362–366.
43. Kullendorff CM. Surgery in unilateral multicystic kidney. *Z Kinderchir* 1990;45:235–237.
44. Cussen LJ. Cystic kidneys in children with congenital urethral obstruction. *J Urol* 1971;106:939–941.
45. Sanders RC, Nussbaum AR, Solez K. Renal dysplasia: sonographic findings. *Radiology* 1988;167:623–626.
46. Hoover DL, Duckett JW Jr. Posterior urethral valves, unilateral reflux and renal dysplasia: a syndrome. *J Urol* 1982;128:994–997.
47. Greenfield SP, Hensle TW, Berdon WE, Wigger HJ. Unilateral vesicoureteral reflux and unilateral nonfunctioning kidney associated with posterior urethral valves—a syndrome? *J Urol* 1983;130:733–738.
48. Kaneko K, Suzuki Y, Yabuta K, Miyano T. Abnormal contralateral kidney in unilateral multicystic dysplastic kidney disease. *Pediatr Radiol* 1995;25:275–277.
49. Selzman AA, Elder JS. Contralateral vesicoureteral reflux in children with a multicystic kidney. *J Urol* 1995;153:1252–1254.
50. Atiyeh B, Husmann D, Baum M. Contralateral renal abnormalities in multicystic-dysplastic kidney disease. *J Pediatr* 1992;121:65–67.
51. Barth RA, Mindell HJ. Renal masses in the fetus and neonate: ultrasonographic diagnosis. *Semin Ultrasound CT MR* 1984;5:3–18.
52. Harrison MR, Golbus MS, Filly RA, et al. Fetal surgery for congenital hydronephrosis. *N Engl J Med* 1982;306:591–593.
53. Blane CE, Barr M, DiPietro MA, et al. Renal obstructive dysplasia: ultrasound diagnosis and therapeutic implications. *Pediatr Radiol* 1991;21:274–277.
54. Newman LB, McAlister WH, Kissane J. Segmental renal dysplasia associated with ectopic ureteroceles in childhood. *Urology* 1974;3:23–26.
55. Perrin E, Persky L, Tucker A, Chrenka B. Renal duplication and dysplasia. *Urology* 1974;4:660–664.
56. Gartell PC, MacIver AG, Atwell JD. Renal dysplasia and duplex kidneys. *Eur Urol* 1983;9:65–68.
57. Cromie WJ, Engelstein MS, Duckett JW Jr. Nodular renal blastema, renal dysplasia and duplicated collecting systems. *J Urol* 1980;123:100–102.
58. Oddone M, Marino C, Sergi C, et al. Wilms' tumor arising in a multicystic kidney. *Pediatr Radiol* 1994;24:236–238.
59. Ambrose SS, Parrott TS, Woodard JR, Campbell WG Jr. Observations on the small kidney associated with vesicoureteral reflux. *J Urol* 1980;123:349–351.
60. Holthöfer H, Kumpulainen T, Rapola J. Polycystic disease of the kidney: evaluation and classification based on nephron segment and cell-type specific markers. *Lab Invest* 1990;62:363–369.
61. Gennuardi M, Dionisi-Vici C, Sabetta G, et al. Cerebro-reno-digital (Meckel-like) syndrome with Dandy-Walker malformation, cystic kidneys, hepatic fibrosis, and polydactyly. *Am J Med Genet* 1993;47:50–53.
62. Hunter ACW, Jimenez C, Tawagi FGR. Familial renal-hepatic-pancreatic dysplasia and Dandy-Walker cyst: a distinct syndrome? *Am J Med Genet* 1991;41:201–207.
63. Fraser FC, Lytwyn A. Spectrum of anomalies in the Meckel syndrome, or: "Maybe there is a malformation syndrome with at least one constant anomaly." *Am J Med Genet* 1981;9:67–73.
64. Rapola J, Salonen R. Visceral anomalies in the Meckel syndrome. *Teratology* 1985;31:193–201.
65. Bernstein J. Hepatic and renal involvement in malformation syndromes. *Mt Sinai J Med* 1986;53:421–428.
66. Al Saadi AA, Yoshimoto M, Bree R, et al. A family study of renal dysplasia. *Am J Med Genet* 1984;19:669–677.
67. Buchta RM, Viseskul C, Gilbert EF, et al. Familial bilateral renal agenesis and hereditary renal adysplasia. *Z Kinderheilkd* 1973;115:111–129.
68. McPherson E, Carey J, Kramer A, et al. Dominantly inherited renal adysplasia. *Am J Med Genet* 1987;26:863–872.
69. Squires EC, Morden RS, Bernstein J. Renal multicystic dysplasia. An occasional manifestation of the hereditary renal dysplasia syndrome. *Am J Med Genet* 1987;3[Suppl]:279–284.
70. Murugasu B, Cole BR, Hawkins EP, et al. Familial renal adysplasia. *Am J Kidney Dis* 1991;18:490–494.
71. Milliken LD, Hodgson NB. Renal dysplasia and urethral valves. *J Urol* 1972;103:960–962.
72. Bernstein J, Risdon RA. Renal system. Part I-Kidneys and urinary tract. In: Gilbert-Barness E, ed. *Potter's pathology of the fetus and infant*. St. Louis: Mosby-Year Book, 1997.

73. Kleiner B, Callen PW, Filly RA. Sonographic analysis of the fetus with ureteropelvic junction obstruction. *AJR Am J Roentgenol* 1987;148:359–363.
74. Allen TD. Congenital ureteral strictures. *J Urol* 1979;104:196.
75. Stock JA, Krous HF, Heffernan J, et al. Correlation of renal biopsy and radionuclide renal scan; differential function in patients with unilateral ureteropelvic junction obstruction. *J Urol* 1996;154:716–718.
76. Fine RN. Diagnosis and treatment of fetal urinary tract abnormalities. *J Pediatr* 1992;121:333.
77. van Velden DJJ, de Jong G, van der Walt JJ. Fetal bilateral obstructive uropathy: a series of nine cases. *Pediatr Pathol Lab Med* 1995;15:245–258.
78. Dudley JA, Hawarth JM, McGraw ME, et al. Clinical relevance and implications of antenatal hydronephrosis. *Arch Dis Child* 1997;76:F31–F34.
79. Bernstein GT, Mandell J, Lebowitz RL, et al. Ureteropelvic junction obstruction in the neonate, part 2. *J Urol* 1988;140:1216–1221.
80. Uson AC, Levitt SB, Lattimer JK. Giant hydronephrosis in children. *Pediatrics* 1969;44:209–216.
81. Allen P, Condon VR, Collins RE. Multilocular cystic hydronephrosis secondary to congenital (ureteropelvic junction) obstruction. An adjunct to diagnosis with intravenous urography. *Radiology* 1963;80:203–207.
82. Tripp BM, Homsy YL. Neonatal hydronephrosis—the controversy and the management. *Pediatr Nephrol* 1995;9:503–509.
83. McHale D, Porteous MEM, Wentzel J, Burn J. Further evidence of genetic heterogeneity in hereditary hydronephrosis. *Clin Genet* 1996;50:491–493.
84. Izquierdo L, Porteous M, Paramo PG, Connor JM. Evidence for genetic heterogeneity in hereditary hydronephrosis caused by pelviureteric junction obstruction, with one locus assigned to chromosome 6p. *Hum Genet* 1992;89:557–560.
85. Beckwith JB. Macroglossia, omphalocele, adrenal cytomegaly, gigantism and hyperplastic visceromegaly. *Birth Defects* 1969;5(2):188–196.
86. Perlman M, Goldberg GM, Bar-Ziv J, Danovitch G. Renal hamartomas and nephroblastomatosis with fetal gigantism: a familial syndrome. *Pediatrics* 1973;83:414–418.
87. Perlman M, Levin M, Wittels B. Syndrome of fetal gigantism, renal hamartomas, and nephroblastomatosis with Wilms' tumor. *Cancer* 1975;35:1212–1217.
88. Chesney RW, Kaufman R, Stapleton FB, Rivas ML. Association of medullary sponge kidney and medullary dysplasia in Beckwith-Wiedemann syndrome. *J Pediatr* 1989;155:761–764.
89. Kosseff Al, Hermann J, Gilbert EF, et al. Studies of malformation syndromes of man. XXIX. The Wiedemann–Beckwith syndrome. Clinical, genetic and pathogenetic studies of 12 cases. *Eur J Pediatr* 1976;123:139–166.
90. Chitayat D, Rothchild A, Ling E, et al. Apparent postnatal onset of some manifestations of the Wiedemann-Beckwith syndrome. *Am J Med Genet* 1990;36:434–439.
91. Allanson JE, Pantzar JT, MacLeod PM. Possible new autosomal recessive syndrome with unusual renal histopathological changes. *Am J Med Genet* 1983;16:57–60.
92. Voland JP, Hawkins EP, Wells TR, et al. Congenital hypernephronic nephromegaly with tubular dysgenesis: a distinctive inherited renal anomaly. *Pediatr Pathol* 1985;4:231–245.
93. Schwartz BR, Lage JM, Pober BR, Driscoll SG. Isolated congenital renal tubular immaturity in siblings. *Hum Pathol* 1987;17:1259–1263.
94. Swinford AE, Bernstein J, Toriello HV, Higgins JV. Renal tubular dysgenesis: delayed onset of oligohydramnios. *Am J Med Genet* 1989;32:127–132.
95. Russo R, D'Armiento M, Vecchione R. Renal tubular dysgenesis and very large cranial fontanels in a family with acrocephalosyndactyly S.C. type. *Am J Med Genet* 1991;39:482–485.
96. Bernstein J, Barajas L. Renal tubular dysgenesis: evidence of abnormality in the renin-angiotensin system. *J Am Soc Nephrol* 1994;5:224.
97. Ariel I, Wells TR, Landing BH, et al. Familial renal tubular dysgenesis: a disorder not isolated to proximal convoluted tubules. *Pediatr Path Lab Med* 1995;15:915–922.
98. Cunniff C, Jones KL, Phillipson J, et al. Oligohydramnios sequence and renal tubular malformation associated with maternal enalapril use. *Am J Obstet Gynecol* 1990;162:187–189.
99. Sedman AB, Kershaw DB, Bunchman TE. Recognition and management of angiotensin converting enzyme inhibitor fetopathy. *Pediatr Nephrol* 1995;9:382–385.
100. van der Heijden BJ, Carlus C, Narcy F, et al. Persistent anuria, neonatal death, and renal microcystic lesions after prenatal exposure to indomethacin. *Am J Obstet Gynecol* 1994;171:617–623.
101. Kaplan BS, Restaino I, Reval DS, et al. Renal failure in the neonate associated with in utero exposure to non-steroidal anti-inflammatory agents. *Pediatr Nephrol* 1994;8:700–704.
102. Voyer LE, Drut R, Méndez J. Fetal renal maldevelopment with oligohydramnios following maternal use of piroxicam. *Pediatr Nephrol* 1994;8:592–594.
103. Restaino I, Kaplan BS, Kaplan P, et al. Renal dysgenesis in a monozygotic twin: association with in utero exposure to indomethacin. *Am J Med Genet* 1991;39:252–257.
104. Metzman RA, Husson MA, Dellers EA. Renal tubular dysgenesis: a description of early renal maldevelopment in siblings. *Pediatr Pathol* 1993;13:239–248.
105. Landing BH, Ang SM, Herta N, et al. Labeled lectin studies of renal tubular dysgenesis and renal tubular atrophy of postnatal renal ischemia and end-stage kidney disease. *Pediatr Pathol* 1994;14:87–99.
106. Benz G, Willich E, Schärer K. Segmental renal hypoplasia in childhood. *Pediatr Radiol* 1976;5:86–92.
107. Johnston JH, Mix LW. The Ask-Upmark kidney: a form of ascending pyelonephritis? *Br J Urol* 1976;48:393–398.
108. Arant BS Jr, Sotelo-Avila C, Bernstein J. Segmental "hypoplasia" of the kidney (Ask-Upmark). *J Pediatr* 1979;95:931–939.
109. Risdon RA. The small scarred kidney of childhood: a congenital or an acquired lesion? *Pediatr Nephrol* 1987;1:632–637.
110. Habib R, Courtecuisse V, Ehrensperger J, Royer P. Hypoplasie segmentaire du rein avec hypertension artérielle chez l'enfant. *Ann Pediatr* (Paris) 1965;41:262–279.
111. Habib R. Pathology of renal segmental corticopapillary scarring in children with hypertension: the concept of segmental hypoplasia. In: Hodson J, Kincaid-Smith P, eds. *Reflux nephropathy*. New York: Masson, 1979:220–239.
112. Shindo S, Bernstein J, Arant BS Jr. Evolution of renal segmental atrophy (Ask-Upmark kidney) in children with vesicoureteric reflux: radiographic and morphologic studies. *J Pediatr* 1983;102:847–854.
113. Bhathena DB, Weiss JH, Holland NH, et al. Focal and segmental glomerular sclerosis in reflux nephropathy. *Am J Med* 1980;68:886–892.
114. Torres VE, Velosa JA, Holley KE, et al. The progression of vesicoureteral reflux nephropathy. *Ann Intern Med* 1980;92:776–784.
115. Morita M, Yoshiara S, White RHR, Raafat F. The glomerular changes in children with reflux nephropathy. *J Pathol* 1990;162:245–253.
116. Lieberman E, Salinas-Madrigal L, Gwinn JL, et al. Infantile polycystic disease of the kidneys and liver: clinical, pathological and radiological correlations and comparison with congenital hepatic fibrosis. *Medicine* (Baltimore) 1971;50:277–318.
117. Kaplan BS, Kaplan P, Rosenberg HK, et al. Polycystic kidney diseases in childhood. *J Pediatr* 1989;115:867–880.
118. Kerr DNS, Warrick CK, Hart-Mercer J. A lesion resembling medullary sponge kidney in patients with congenital hepatic fibrosis. *Clin Radiol* 1962;13:85–91.
119. Chilton SJ, Cremin BJ. The spectrum of polycystic disease in children. *Pediatr Radiol* 1981;11:9–15.
120. Gang DL, Herrin JT. Infantile polycystic disease of the liver and kidneys. *Clin Nephrol* 1986;25:28–36.
121. Landing BH, Wells TR, Claireaux AE. Morphometric analysis of liver lesions in cystic disease of childhood. *Hum Pathol* 1980;11[Suppl]:549–560.
122. Kaplan BS, Kaplan P, Chadarevian J-P, et al. Variable expression of autosomal recessive polycystic kidney disease and congenital hepatic fibrosis within a family. *Am J Med Genet* 1988;29:639–647.
123. Potter EL. Normal and abnormal development of the kidney. Chicago: Year Book, 1972:141–153.
124. Heggö O, Natvig JB. Cystic disease of the kidneys. Autopsy report and family study. *Acta Pathol Microbiol Immunol Scand [A]* 1965;64:459–469.
125. Rapola J, Kääriäinen H. Polycystic kidney disease: morphological diagnosis of recessive and dominant polycystic kidney disease in infancy and childhood. *APMIS* 1988;96:68–76.
126. Kissane JM. Renal cysts in pediatric patients: a classification and overview. *Pediatr Nephrol* 1990;4:69–77.

127. Faraggiana T, Bernstein J, Strauss L, Churg J. Use of lectins in the study of histogenesis of renal cysts. *Lab Invest* 1985;53:575–579.
128. Verani R, Walker P, Silva FG. Renal cystic disease of infancy: results of histochemical studies: a report of the Southwest Pediatric Nephrology Study Group. *Pediatr Nephrol* 1989;3:37–42.
129. Jørgensen M. The ductal plate malformation. *Acta Pathol Microbiol Immunol Scand [A]* 1977;257[Suppl]:1–88.
130. Landing BH, Wells TR, Reed GB, Narayan MS. Diseases of the bile ducts in children. In: Gall EA, Mostofi FK, eds. *The liver.* Baltimore: Williams & Wilkins, 1973:480–509.
131. Bernstein J. Hereditary renal disease. In: Churg J, et al, eds. *Kidney disease—present status.* Baltimore: Williams & Wilkins, 1979: 295–326.
132. Helczynski L, Wells TR, Landing BH, Lipsey AI. The renal lesion of congenital hepatic fibrosis: pathologic and morphometric analysis, with comparison to the renal lesion of infantile polycystic disease. *Pediatr Pathol* 1984;2:441–445.
133. Dupond JL, Miguet JP, Carbillet JP, et al. Polykystose rénale, principale expression de la fibrose hépatique congénitale. 3 observations. *Nouv Presse Med* 1979;8:2885–2888.
134. Bernstein J, Stickler GB, Neel IV. Congenital hepatic fibrosis: evolving morphology. *APMIS* 1988;4[Suppl]:17–26.
135. Clermont RJ, Maillard J-N, Benhamou J-P, Fauvert R. Fibrose hépatique congénitale. *Can Med Assoc J* 1967;97:1272–1278.
136. Bernstein J. Hepatic involvement in hereditary renal syndromes. *Birth Defects* 1978;23:115–130.
137. Alvarez F, Hadchouel M, Bernard O. Latent chronic cholangitis in congenital hepatic fibrosis. *Eur J Pediatr* 1982;139:203–205.
138. Williams R. Non-obstructive dilatation of the intrahepatic biliary tree with cholangitis. *Q J Med* 1972;41:477–489.
139. Alvarez F, Bernard O, Brunelle F, et al. Congenital hepatic fibrosis in children. *J Pediatr* 1981;99:370–375.
140. Gleason DC, McAlister WH, Kissane J. Cystic disease of the kidneys in children *AJR Am J Roentgenol* 1967;100:135–146.
141. Metreweli C, Garel L. The echographic diagnosis of infantile renal polycystic disease. *Ann Radiol* (Paris) 1980;23:103–107.
142. Kaplan BS, Fay J, Shah V, et al. Autosomal recessive polycystic kidney disease. *Pediatr Nephrol* 1989;3:43–49.
143. Fellows RA, Leonidas JC, Beatty EC, Jr. Radiologic features of "adult type" polycystic kidney disease in the neonate. *Pediatr Radiol* 1976;4:87–92.
144. Kaplan BS, Rabin I, Nogrady MB, Drummond KN. Autosomal dominant polycystic renal disease in children. *J Pediatr* 1977;90:782–783.
145. Kaye C, Lewy PR. Congenital appearance of adult-type (autosomal dominant) polycystic kidney disease. Report of a case. *J Pediatr* 1974;85:807–810.
146. Taitz LS, Brown CB, Blank CE, Steiner GM. Screening for polycystic kidney disease: importance of clinical presentation in the newborn. *Arch Dis Child* 1987;62:45–49.
147. Joshi VV, Kasznica J. Clinicopathologic spectrum of glomerulocystic kidneys. Report of two cases and a brief review of literature. *Pediatr Pathol* 1984;2:171–186.
148. Bernstein J, Landing BH. Glomerulocystic kidney diseases. In: Bartsocas C, ed. Genetics of kidney disorders, progress in clinical and biological research, vol 305. New York: Alan R. Liss, 1989:27–43.
149. Reeders ST, Zerres K, Gal A, et al. Prenatal diagnosis of autosomal dominant polycystic kidney disease with a DNA probe. *Lancet* 1986;ii:6–8.
150. Ceccherini I, Lituania M, Cordone MS, et al. Autosomal dominant polycystic kidney disease: prenatal diagnosis by DNA analysis and sonography at 14 weeks. *Prenat Diagn* 1989;9:751–758.
151. Novelli G, Frontali M, Baldini D, et al. Prenatal diagnosis of adult polycystic kidney disease with DNA markers on chromosome 16 and the genetic heterogeneity problem. *Prenat Diagn* 1989;9:759–767.
152. Gabow PA. Polycystic kidney disease: clues to pathogenesis. *Kidney Int* 1991;40:989–996.
153. Garel L, Sauvegrain J, Filiatrault D. Dominant polycystic disease of the kidney in a newborn child. Report of one case. *Ann Radiol* (Paris) 1983;26:183–186.
154. Sedman A, Bell P, Manco-Johnson M, et al. Autosomal dominant polycystic kidney disease in childhood: a longitudinal study. *Kidney Int* 1987;31:1000–1005.
155. Evan AP, Gardner KD Jr, Bernstein J. Polypoid and papillary epithelial hyperplasia: a potential cause of ductal obstruction in adult polycystic disease. *Kidney Int* 1979;16:743–750.
156. Gregoire JR, Torres VE, Holley KE, Farrow GM. Renal epithelial hyperplastic and neoplastic proliferation in autosomal dominant polycystic kidney disease. *Am J Kidney Dis* 1987;9:27–38.
157. Bernstein J, Evan AP, Gardner KD Jr. Epithelial hyperplasia in human polycystic kidney diseases. Its role in pathogenesis and risk of neoplasia. *Am J Pathol* 1987;129:92–101.
158. Grantham JJ, Geiser JL, Evan AP. Cyst formation and growth in autosomal dominant polycystic kidney disease. *Kidney Int* 1987;31: 1145–1152.
159. Bernstein J. Morphology of human renal cystic disease. In: Cummings NB, Klahr S, eds. *Chronic renal disease.* New York: Plenum Publishing, 1985;47–54.
160. Gabow PA, Chapman AB, Johnson AM, et al. Renal structure and hypertension in autosomal dominant polycystic kidney disease. *Kidney Int* 1990;38:1177–1180.
161. Sklar AH, Caruana RJ, Lammers JE, Strauser GD. Renal infections in autosomal dominant polycystic kidney disease. *Am J Kidney Dis* 1987;10:81–88.
162. Schwab SJ, Bander SJ, Klahr S. Renal infection in autosomal dominant polycystic kidney disease. *Am J Med* 1987;82:714–718.
163. Torres VE, Erickson SB, Smith LH, et al. The association of nephrolithiasis and autosomal dominant polycystic kidney disease. *Am J Kidney Dis* 1988;11:318–325.
164. Gabow PA, Johnson AM, Kaehny WD, et al. Risk factors for the development of hepatic cysts in autosomal dominant polycystic kidney disease. *Hepatology* 1990;11:1033–1037.
165. Telenti A, Torres VE, Gross JB Jr, et al. Hepatic cyst infection in autosomal dominant polycystic kidney disease. *Mayo Clin Proc* 1990;65:933–942.
166. Cobben JM, Breuning MH, Schoots C, et al. Congenital hepatic fibrosis in autosomal-dominant polycystic kidney disease. *Kidney Int* 1990;38:880–885.
167. Gabow PA. Autosomal dominant polycystic kidney disease—more than a renal disease. *Am J Kidney Dis* 1990;16:403–413.
168. Anton PA, Abramowsky CR. Adult polycystic renal disease presenting in infancy: a report emphasizing the bilateral involvement. *J Urol* 1982;128:1290–1291.
169. Farrell TP, Boal DK, Wood BP, et al. Unilateral abdominal mass: an unusual presentation of autosomal dominant polycystic kidney disease in children. *Pediatr Radiol* 1984;14:349–352.
170. Porch P, Noe NP, Stapleton FB. Unilateral presentation of adult-type polycystic kidney disease in children. *J Urol* 1986;135:744–746.
171. Cho KJ, Thornbury JR, Bernstein J, et al. Localized cystic disease of the kidney: angiographic-pathologic correlation. *AJR Am J Roentgenol* 1979;132:891–895.
172. Stillwell TJ, Gomez MR, Kelalis PP. Renal lesions in tuberous sclerosis. *J Urol* 1987;138:477–481.
173. Narla LD, Slovis TL, Watts FB, Nigro M. The renal lesions of tuberosclerosis (cysts and angiomyolipoma)—screening with sonography and computerized tomography. *Pediatr Radiol* 1988;18: 205–209.
174. Ferry JA, Malt RA, Young RH. Renal angiomyolipoma with sarcomatous transformation and pulmonary metastases. *Am J Surg Pathol* 1991;15:1083–1088.
175. Okada RD, Platt MA, Fleishman J. Chronic renal failure in patients with tuberous sclerosis: association with renal cysts. *Nephron* 1982; 30:85–88.
176. Brook-Carter PT, Peral B, Ward CJ, et al. Deletion of the TSC2 and PKD1 genes associated with severe infantile polycystic kidney disease—a contiguous gene syndrome. *Nat Genet* 1994;8:328.
177. Bjornsson J, Short MP, Kwiatkowski DJ, Henske EP. Tuberous sclerosis-associated renal cell carcinoma; clinical, pathological, and genetic features. *Am J Pathol* 1996;149:1201–1208.
178. Bernstein J, Robbins TO, Kissane JM. The renal lesions of tuberous sclerosis. *Semin Diagn Pathol* 1986;3:97–105.
179. Miller D, Cray ES, Lloyd DL. Unilateral cystic disease of the neonatal kidney: a rare presentation of tuberous sclerosis. *Histopathology* 1989;14:529–532.
180. Bernstein J, Brough AJ, McAdams AJ. The renal lesion in syndromes of multiple congenital malformations: cerebrohepatorenal syndrome, Jeune's asphyxiating thoracic dystrophy; tuberous sclerosis; Meckel's syndrome. In: Bergsma D, ed. Fifth conference on the clinical delineation of birth defects. *Birth Defects* 1974;10(4):35–43.

181. Shapiro RA, Skinner DG, Stanley P, Edelbrock HH. Renal tumors associated with tuberous sclerosis: the case for aggressive surgical management. *J Urol* 1984;132:1170–1174.
182. Srinivas V, Herr HW, Hajdu EO. Partial nephrectomy for a renal oncocytoma associated with tuberous sclerosis. *J Urol* 1985;133:263–265.
183. Kaplan BS, Gordon I, Pincott J, Barratt TM. Familial hypoplastic glomerulocystic kidney disease: a definite entity with dominant inheritance. *Am J Med Genet* 1989;34:569–573.
184. Taxy JB, Filmer RB. Glomerulocystic kidney. Report of a case. *Arch Pathol Lab Med* 1976;100:186–188.
185. McAlister WH, Siegel MJ, Shackelford G, et al. Glomerulocystic kidney. *AJR Am J Roentgenol* 1979;133:536–638.
186. Sharp CK, Bergman SM, Stockwin JM, et al. Dominantly transmitted glomerulocystic kidney disease: a distinct genetic entity. J Am Soc Nephrol 1977;8:77–84.

CHAPTER 41

Adult Renal Diseases

Tibor Nádasdy and Fred G. Silva

APPROACH TO CLASSIFICATION

The kidney reacts in a limited number of ways (i.e., patterns) to myriad injurious agents, and the clinical manifestations corresponding to these reactions are also circumscribed. The location and the type of injury, and the renal host response, are important in defining the histopathologic manifestations and in determining the clinical course of the patient (1–7). There are several categories by which one can classify renal disease: clinical, etiologic, immunopathologic, and morphologic.

Renal disease also can be characterized by several clinical syndromes: nephritic syndrome (red blood cells and red blood cell casts in the urine), nephrotic syndrome (3.5 g or more of proteinuria per 24 hours, with edema and hyperlipidemia), nonnephrotic proteinuria, isolated hematuria, and acute or chronic renal failure. The problem with this classification is that a variety of renal patterns of injury (each with different therapies and outcomes) may lead to the same syndrome; thus, clinical determination of the syndrome is not very precise. We often do not know the exact origin of the disease process in an individual patient. That is unfortunate, because if we knew the agent(s) leading to a given disease process, and if we were able to eliminate it (assuming the renal injury is not too far advanced), then the renal process might well resolve. The immunopathologic system of classification will be discussed later.

We will order our survey of the pathologic basis of renal disease according to a diagnostic algorithm or decision tree; in essence, this is the schema by which many renal pathologists consciously or subconsciously arrive at a diagnosis based on morphologic features. Careful, systematic study of the renal tissues by light microscopy (LM) [as well as by immunofluorescence (IF) and electron microscopy (EM)] will enable the pathologist to subclassify the pattern and type of injury. We have to emphasize that correlation of morphologic findings with clinical data is of great importance in making the diagnosis. No final or definitive renal biopsy diagnosis should be made without relevant clinical data.

The first part of this interpretive approach calls for study of each of the four renal components (glomeruli, tubules, interstitium, and vessels) to determine which is most severely affected. Each renal compartment must be assessed individually for the type and degree of change, as described by Pirani et al. (5) and Silva et al. (6). It should be decided which compartment of the kidney is the most severely involved (primary involvement). If there are less prominent changes in other compartments as well (secondary involvement), determine the light microscopic patterns, and follow an algorithmic approach.

The first diagnostic step in the interpretation of glomerular disease is to ascertain, on thin sections (2- to 3-μm paraffin or plastic), whether the glomeruli are hypercellular (Table 1). Normocellularity is defined by the World Health Organization (WHO), and others, as no more than three cells in an individual glomerular mesangial region—in thin, 2- to 3-μm sections—away from the vascular pole (2) (Fig. 1). Obviously, increased section thickness could result in apparent hypercellularity. If the tuft hypercellularity is severe and leads to closure of the glomerular capillaries [true glomerulonephritis (GN)], one has to decide whether the hypercellularity is within the glomerular tuft (intracapillary proliferative GN) or outside the glomerular tuft in Bowman's space (extracapillary proliferative GN). Some authors have used the term proliferative GN for such hypercellular lesions. There is evidence that the hypercellularity can result not only from the proliferation of native glomerular cells (i.e., mesangial and/or endothelial) but also from infiltration of blood-borne mononuclear and/or polymorphonuclear leukocytes.

T. Nádasdy: Department of Pathology, Johns Hopkins Hospital, Baltimore, Maryland 21205.

F. G. Silva: Department of Pathology, University of Oklahoma, Health Sciences Center, Oklahoma City, Oklahoma 73104.

TABLE 1. Algorithm of morphologic interpretation of glomerular patterns

	The true glomerulonephritides			The nonglomerulonephritic glomerulonephropathies		
A. Is there glomerular hypercellularity (with closure of capillary lumens):	Glomerular hypercellularity (usually nephritic)	or		Minimal glomerular hypercellularity (usually nephrotic)		
B. Is the hypercellularity:	Intracapillary	or	Extracapillary (crescents) Crescentic GN	Mesangium normal Minimal-change nephrotic syndrome or Membranous glomerulo-nephropathy (EM: Subepithelial deposits)	Diffuse mesangial prominence Diffuse mesangial hypercellularity or Diabetic nephropathy (EM: thick GBM)	Segmental Mesangial Sclerosis Focal segmental sclerosis
C. Is the hypercellularity:	Diffuse ↓ (1) Acute postinfectious GN (2) Membrano-proliferative GN	or	Focal ↓ Focal GN (SLE, collagen-vascular diseases, infective endocarditis, etc.)			

TISSUE SAMPLING AND PREPARATION

Renal biopsy samples usually are obtained by percutaneous or open renal biopsy or by nephrectomy. The biopsy is divided for LM, IF, and EM. The specimen should be handled very carefully to avoid squeezing and compression, preferably by wooden sticks instead of forceps. A needle biopsy specimen should be divided under a dissecting microscope. This microscope allows for visualization and differentiation of the renal cortex and medulla. The medulla shows parallel structures (vasa recta and collecting ducts); on the other hand, the cortex appears irregular, and its glomeruli usually are visible as small red capillary conglomerates. Even anemic glomeruli can be seen as vague shadows of small balls, if one adjusts the micrometer screw.

We recommend cutting away two small (1 mm) pieces with glomeruli for EM, a small (2 to 3 mm) piece with glomeruli for IF, and the remaining tissue for paraffin sections for LM. If no dissecting microscope is available, the best method is to cut 1-mm pieces from both ends of the biopsy specimen for EM and two 2-mm pieces for IF and submit the rest for routine paraffin processing for LM. When an excised kidney is received, it is important to bisect the kidney properly in order to make the entirety of the pyelocalyceal system and renal papillae visible. This is done by orienting the kidney longitudinally in one hand and carefully and slowly cutting into the renal cortex with a long knife. When one just enters a portion of the renal collecting system, it should be opened with scissors along the pyelocalyceal system. The accompanying renal artery, renal vein, and ureter should always be examined in terms of gross and microscopic features. After obtaining kidney tissues that are as fresh as possible, it is necessary to process the tissue quickly and appropriately for IF and EM, if it is deemed necessary (one should remember that it is better to have appropriately processed tissue and not need it than to need it and not have it).

Tissue for LM should be placed in buffered formalin. The fixed tissue can be embedded either in paraffin or plastic. The latter provides better structure; if necessary, ultrathin sections can be cut for EM. The disadvantages of plastic are that the tissue may not be suitable for certain methods that can be performed on paraffin sections (immunohistochemistry, in situ hybridization, etc.) and that preparation of plastic-embedded sections is more time-consuming and expensive. For diagnosis of medical diseases of the kidney, slides are routinely stained for LM with hematoxylin and eosin, periodic

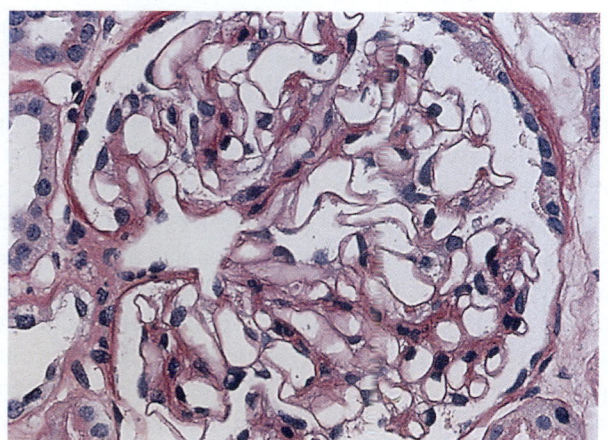

FIG. 1. Normal glomerulus. The glomerulus is normal in size and cellularity. The glomerular capillary lumens are patent, and the glomerular capillary wall appears thin and delicate [periodic acid–Schiff (PAS)]. The first decision in the analysis of glomerular lesions is to determine whether there is hypercellularity and closure of the glomerular capillary lumens. Special stains, such as PAS and methenamine silver, are especially helpful in this regard.

acid–Schiff (PAS), methenamine silver, and trichrome. Thin (2 to 3 µm) sections are extremely important. Special stains, such as Congo red for amyloid (the only exception to the need for thin sections), elastic stains, iron stains, and PTAH, or Lendrum stains for fibrin, may be useful.

Ideally, the tissue for IF should be snap-frozen, usually in isopentane or methylbutane, and cooled in liquid nitrogen, after having been surrounded by OCT frozen-section material. EM material is best diced into 1-mm cubes with a sharp razor blade (after cleaning off the oil with alcohol or xylene) and then placed in cold glutaraldehyde or Carson's formalin as soon as possible. It is imperative to transfer this tissue carefully with a small wooden stick or forceps by capillary action (do not squeeze or compress the tissue). If necessary, tissue with glomeruli for EM may be retrieved from the paraffin blocks, though the ultrastructure is usually suboptimal.

A question that is frequently asked concerns the size of an adequate biopsy specimen and how many glomeruli it should contain. In certain cases, a single glomerulus may be enough to make a diagnosis (e.g., membranous GN). In focal glomerular diseases (e.g., early-stage focal segmental glomerulosclerosis), however, a sampling error cannot be excluded even if many glomeruli are examined (8).

IMMUNOFLUORESCENCE

Tissue snap-frozen for direct IF should be cut as thin as possible (2 to 4 µm) and stained with antisera known to be relatively monospecific for IgG, IgM, IgA, kappa and lambda light chains, C3, C1q, FRA [fibrin(ogen)-related antigens], and albumin. Other antisera, such as antibodies to properdin, C4, and IgE, are applied by some laboratories. The following IF characteristics should be evaluated in every renal biopsy.

1. Is the deposition granular (probably immune complex) or linear (classic antiglomerular basement membrane [anti-GBM] antibodies [Table 2])? It should be noted, however, that linear staining is neither sufficient nor necessary for the definitive diagnosis of anti-GBM-induced GN.

2. What region of the glomerulus is staining—capillary wall or mesangium? Is this in an area of segmental sclerosis (Table 2)? If so, it would raise the possibility of nonspecific nonimmunologic trapping, especially if one found only IgM, C3, and FRA.

3. What class of immunoglobulin and fraction of complement is being deposited? Are both types of light chains positive, or just one? It is important to determine the class of immunoglobulin because the immunoglobulin classes may correlate with specific diseases. For example, IgA can be seen in systemic lupus erythematosus (SLE), often associated with a "full house" of immunoglobulins, whereas IgA alone might suggest either Berger's disease (IgA nephropathy) or anaphylactoid purpura [Henoch-Schönlein purpura (HSP)]. Finding C3 without C1q would suggest that the alternate complement pathway is involved, especially when it is accompanied by properdin.

4. Is the deposition of purported immune material associated with nonimmunologic material, such as albumin? In areas of plasmatic insudation, all plasma proteins flow into the region—not only immunoglobulins and complement but also albumin and FRA. If all are found, one is less certain of a primary immunologic phenomenon.

5. How intense is the fluorescence? Grading the image/background signal may be quite subjective, but a skilled eye can easily distinguish a mild, moderate, or strong reaction. This is important in certain diseases, such as IgA nephropathy, where, for example, IgA pre- or co-dominance in the glomerular deposits is required for the diagnosis. Examination of the extraglomerular structures (tubules, interstitium, vessels) is also important, although relevant deposits in these compartments are less common.

ELECTRON MICROSCOPY

EM is especially useful in the diagnosis of medical diseases of the kidney; indeed, one of the first uses of EM in medicine was in renal disease. The most important role of EM in the context of a diseased glomerulus is the identifi-

TABLE 2. *Algorithm of interpretation of glomerular immunofluorescence patterns*

Linear capillary wall fluorescence	Granular mesangial	Granular capillary wall (usually with mesangial deposits)	Diffuse "smudgy" mesangial and capillary wall
Anti-GBM disease (IgG, C3)	IgA nephropathy	Finely granular (membranous GN with or without SLE)	AL amyloidosis (usually lambda)
Monoclonal immunoglobulin deposition disease (mostly kappa light chain)	WHO class II lupus ("full house")	Coarsely granular (MPGN, WHO class III or IV lupus nephritis)	Fibrillary GN (IgG)
Diabetic nephropathy (IgG, albumin)	C1q nephropathy	—	Monoclonal immunoglobulin deposition disease
Dense deposit disease (ribbonlike, thick C3)	IgM in idiopathic nephrotic syndrome	—	—
Rarely fibrillary GN (IgG)	Other mesangioproliferative GN	—	—

TABLE 3. *Algorithm of interpretation of ultrastructural findings: discrete immune-type electron-dense deposits present*

Subepithelial	Intramembranous (usually combined with mesangial)	Subendothelial	Mesangial	Combined subendothelial subepithelial, and mesangial
Membranous GN	Dense deposit disease	MPGN	IgA nephropathy	Lupus (WHO classes III and IV)
Lupus (WHO class V)	GN related to endocarditis, deep-seated abscesses	Lupus (WHO class III and IV)	Henoch-Schönlein purpura	MPGN type III
Postinfectious GN		Cryoglobulinemic GN (microtubular substructure)	Lupus (WHO class II)	GN related to endocarditis, deep-seated abscesses
			C1q nephropathy Rare other forms of mesangioproliferative GN	

cation of discrete electron-dense immune-type deposits (Tables 3 and 4) (8). In immune-mediated glomerular disease, EM is useful in determining the presence and the exact site of the deposits [which is often difficult to determine by IF, especially if deposits are present along the glomerular capillary wall (subendothelial versus subepithelial)]. In certain diseases, the presence of glomerular subendothelial deposits (especially if large and in the peripheral glomerular capillary walls) indicates more active disease (as in SLE). Glomerular mesangial deposits are present in many diseases, such as SLE and IgA nephropathy (Berger's disease). A subtype of mesangial deposit is the paramesangial deposit, located immediately beneath the GBM covering the mesangium. From a practical point of view, paramesangial deposits do not differ from other mesangial deposits. Rarely, EM allows one to make a specific diagnosis (as in Alport's hereditary nephropathy with the characteristic diffuse splitting, splintering, rarefaction, and thinning of the GBM).

GENERALIZATIONS ABOUT GLOMERULAR DISEASES

The following points are important in understanding glomerular diseases.

1. A variety of renal morphologic patterns can lead to the same clinical syndrome; for example, nephritic syndrome and hematuria can be caused by hereditary nephropathy, membranoproliferative GN (MPGN), Berger's disease (mesangial IgA nephropathy), acute proliferative GN, and so on. Nephrotic syndrome can be provoked by a variety of diseases, such as minimal change nephrotic syndrome (MCNS), focal sclerosis, membranous glomerulonephropathy, diabetic nephropathy, or amyloid.

2. One disease may produce distinct patterns of renal injury. SLE is one example; in this instance, disparate patterns of injury might each have a different prognosis.

3. A distinctive type of pathologic pattern or process may be caused by or associated with many different diseases:

TABLE 4. *Algorithm of interpretation of ultrastructural findings: no discrete immune-type electron-dense deposits present*

Normal GBM	Diffusely abnormal GBM	Subendothelial fluffy electron-lucent material	Finely granular deposits	Fibrillary/microtubular deposits
Minimal change disease, FSGS	Diffuse thinning Thin GBM disease, Early Alport's syndrome	All forms of thrombotic microangiopathies, including malignant hypertension	Monoclonal immunoglobulin deposition disease	Amyloidosis, fibrillary GN, cryoglobulinemic GN, diabetic glomerulosclerosis, collagen type III glomerulopathy
	Diffuse thickening Diabetes, hypertension, long-standing ischemia (also wrinkling)			
	Diffuse lamellation/splitting Alport's syndrome			

MPGN (a pattern) can be seen in SLE, hepatitis C infection, and various other infections.

4. Renal biopsy is thought to be specific to, and diagnostic of, only a few conditions, as in Alport's hereditary nephropathy. Thus, diagnostic renal pathology is an integrated process wherein one must analyze and collate all the clinical data and results of LM, EM, and IF studies to arrive at the best diagnosis.

5. One renal syndrome may be associated with different diseases and yet have a common pathogenetic mechanism of action (e.g., crescentic GN can be seen in a variety of diseases, such as SLE, anaphylactoid purpura, acute GN; in all of these conditions, the crescents are probably related to FRAs and other proteins that reach Bowman's space through breaks or "gaps" in the GBM).

THE HYPERCELLULAR OR TRUE OR "PROLIFERATIVE" GLOMERULONEPHRITIDES (GLOMERULAR DISEASES ASSOCIATED WITH NEPHRITIC SYNDROME)

Acute Diffuse Intracapillary Proliferative Glomerulonephritis (Usually Acute Postinfectious Glomerulonephritis or Poststreptococcal Glomerulonephritis)

Epidemiology

This condition has become less prevalent after the advent of antibiotics. It is more frequently seen in warm climates. Epidemic outbreaks may occur among people living in crowded, highly populated communities in which poor hygiene and malnutrition are common. It occurs at any age, but it is primarily a disease of children.

Clinical Symptoms

This is a nephritic syndrome that develops 1 to 4 weeks after an episode of pharyngitis or skin infection caused most often by nephritogenic streptococcus types 12, 4, 1, and 49. Serum complement is at least temporarily low in about 90% of patients. The antistreptolysin O titer is high.

Light Microscopic Features

In the acute phase of postinfectious GN, all glomeruli are enlarged, and all glomerular tufts are extremely hypercellular (owing either to proliferation of native cells or to exudation of polymorphonuclear leukocytes and other inflammatory cells) (Fig. 2). Severe intracapillary hypercellularity leads to closure of the glomerular capillary lumens (9,10). There may be a slight increase in the amount of mesangial matrix, and, now and then, mesangial cell interposition between the glomerular endothelium and the GBM may be noted. In some cases, crescents may be present; occasionally they are abundant. Erythrocytes, red blood cell casts, and a few polymorphonuclear leukocytes may be seen in the tubu-

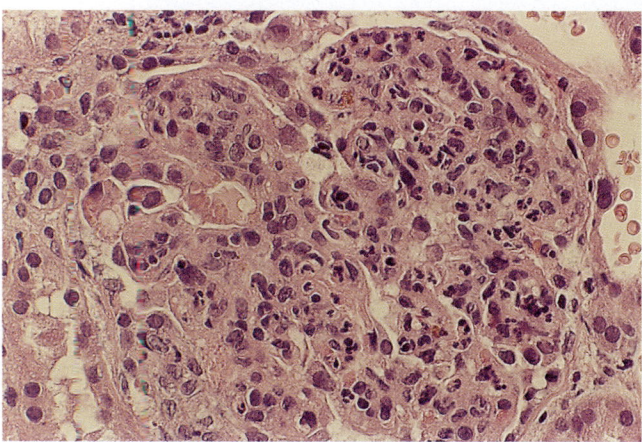

FIG. 2. Poststreptococcal glomerulonephritis. Note the prominent intracapillary hypercellularity with obliterated glomerular capillary lumina and the presence of polymorphonuclear cells.

lar lumens. Small collections of interstitial inflammatory cells can be noted. Vessels are usually normal (9,10).

Immunofluorescence Characteristics

There are granular, "lumpy-bumpy," glomerular capillary wall deposits of IgG and C3 (and sometimes IgM and other immunoreactants) in a diffuse and global distribution (Fig. 3). From time to time, C3 may be the only immunoreactant (9–11).

Electron Microscopic Features

The presence of discrete, electron-dense, large, glomerular, subepithelial deposits ("humps") is the most characteristic finding (Fig. 4). These humps are semilunar and vary in

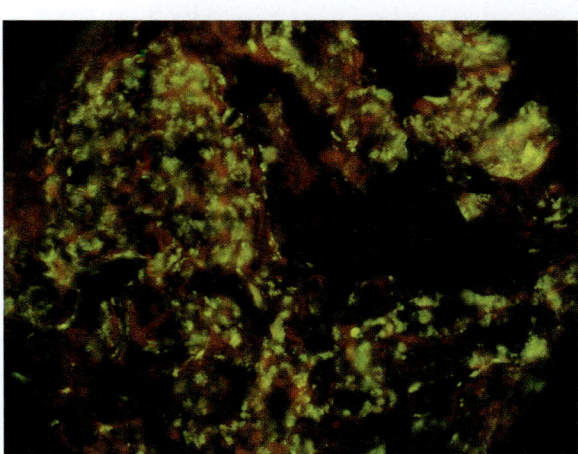

FIG. 3. Immunofluorescence picture of postinfectious (poststreptococcal) glomerulonephritis. There are generalized, lumpy-bumpy, granular glomerular capillary wall and mesangial deposits (anti-C3; ×400).

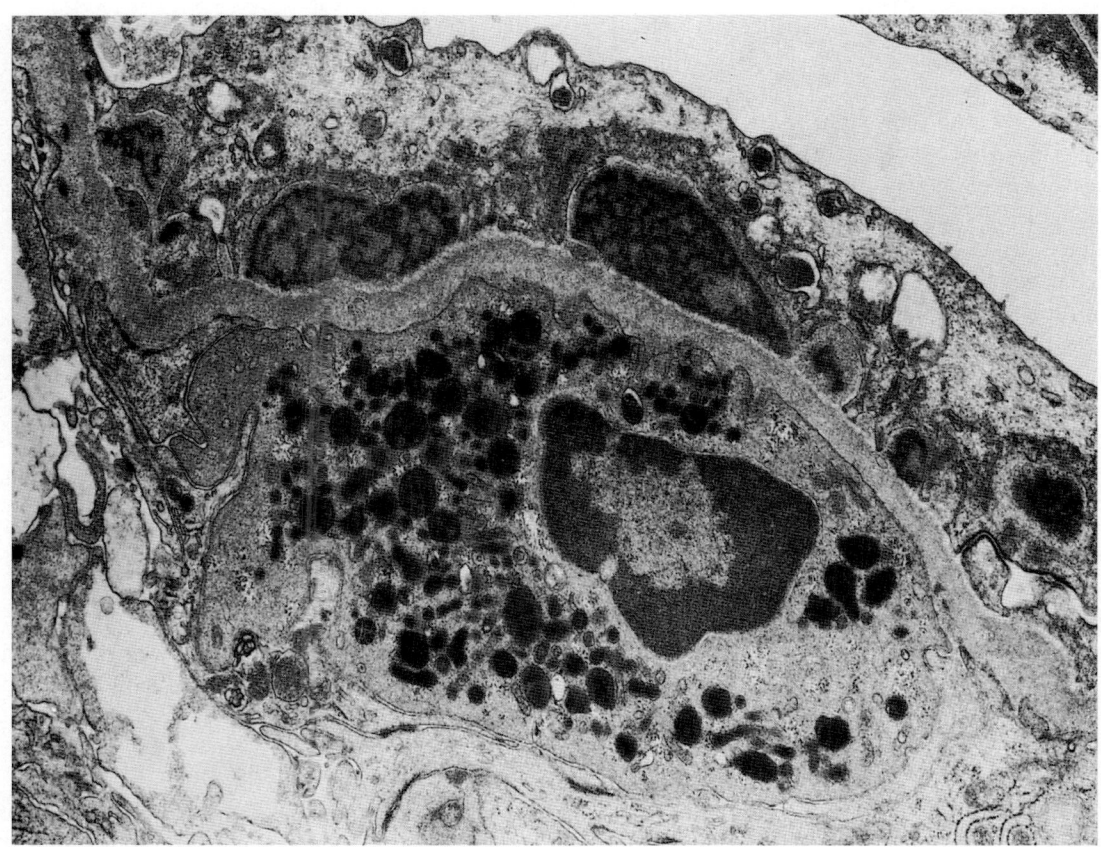

FIG. 4. Postinfectious glomerulonephritis. Note the discrete, electron-dense glomerular subepithelial deposit (hump). There is a polymorphonuclear leukocyte attached to the inner surface of the glomerular basement membrane (uranyl acetate, lead citrate; ×15,000).

shape, size, and number. Small, electron-dense deposits are sometimes noted in the glomerular mesangial and subendothelial regions as well.

Differential Diagnosis

Other diseases that may show the light microscopic pattern of intracapillary proliferative GN are MPGN; cryoglobulinemic GN; and acute GN associated with endocarditis, deep-seated visceral abscesses, or infected atrioventricular shunts ("shunt nephritis"). In these conditions, the GN may show a focal pattern by LM, but the immune deposits are present in every glomerulus (10). Diffuse proliferative lupus nephritis may also show a pattern similar to postinfectious GN.

Outcome

The prognosis (especially in children) is very good; patients usually recover from this "one-shot serum sickness" over a period of weeks to months (12). Subepithelial humps and neutrophils disappear from the glomeruli in 6 to 8 weeks. A slightly increased amount of mesangial matrix and/or more numerous glomerular cells can be detected for 1 to 2 years; proteinuria and/or hematuria may also persist for some time. Transition to a slowly progressive GN has not been well documented, and many such reported cases probably represent a chronic underlying form of GN with superimposed acute postinfectious GN. The prognosis in adults is more variable and is the subject of controversy, but it appears to be good.

Etiologic Factors and Pathogenesis

Glomerular deposition of circulating immune complexes formed by antibodies, coupled with streptococcal antigens and complement, appears to be the most important pathogenetic factor.

Membranoproliferative Glomerulonephritis

MPGN is subdivided into three types, based on the location of immune deposits on EM. The clinical behavior and outcome are very similar in all three types. For this reason, they will be discussed under MPGN type I.

Membranoproliferative Glomerulonephritis, Type I (Synonym: Mesangiocapillary Glomerulonephritis)

Epidemiology

It is a disease of all ages. MPGN types II and III are less common than type I.

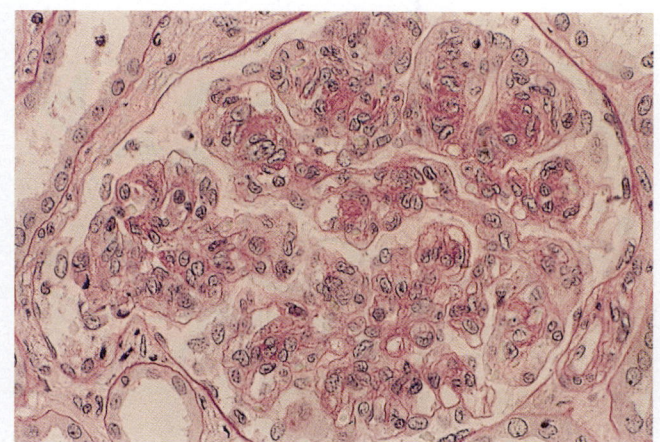 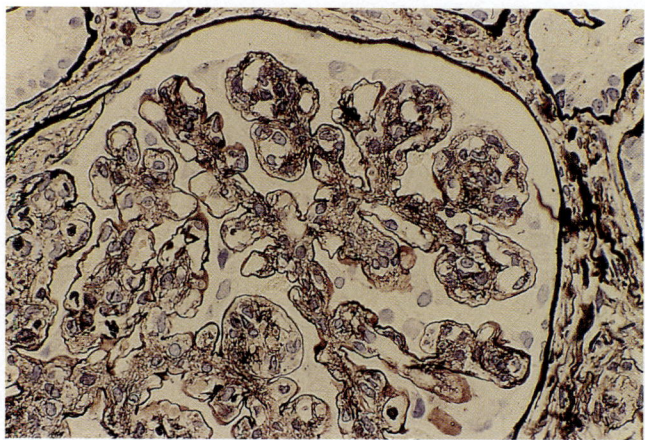

FIG. 5. Membranoproliferative glomerulonephritis. **A:** Note the hypercellular and lobulated glomerulus with many double contours of the capillary basement membrane (periodic acid–Schiff). **B:** Methenamine silver stain is best for detecting doubling (tram-tracking) of the basement membrane. Mesangial cells are frequently interposed between the silver-positive basement membrane and the endothelium (mesangial cell interposition).

Clinical Symptoms

Patients may show initial signs of the nephritic or the nephrotic syndrome or both. Low serum complement is common in all three types. C3 nephritic factor(s) (IgG autoantibodies against complement inhibitory proteins) are frequently found in patients' serum samples (13).

Light Microscopic Features

The glomeruli are diffusely enlarged, with marked intracapillary hypercellularity, lobular accentuation, and thickening of the glomerular capillary walls by large, abundant subendothelial deposits (Fig. 5). There is "tram-tracking" or "reduplication" of the glomerular capillary wall caused by circumferential mesangial cell interposition (mesangial cells spreading between the adjacent glomerular endothelium and the GBM), with creation of a new inner GBM-like material, which gives rise to the double or the reduplicated GBM (Fig. 5) (14–16). Occasionally, there may be a focal pattern, which usually becomes diffuse MPGN in subsequent biopsies (17). Crescents may be present, and tubulointerstitial disease typically correlates with the severity and duration of the GN.

Immunofluorescence Characteristics

Large, granular, confluent, glomerular capillary wall and mesangial deposits of C3 (Fig. 6) are evident. IgG deposition is noted in about two-thirds of biopsy samples. Once in awhile, other immunoreactants with less intense fluorescence are noted.

Electron Microscopic Features

There are widespread electron-dense, glomerular subendothelial deposits of varying sizes (Fig. 7); sometimes they are large and confluent, resembling the "wire loop" lesions in severe lupus nephritis. Circumferential mesangial cell interposition is frequently seen. Glomerular mesangial and subepithelial deposits (even a few humps) may be present.

Differential Diagnosis

A membranoproliferative pattern may be associated with a variety of diseases and conditions (14,18), with or without the glomerular deposition of immunoreactants. The term MPGN should be applied to conditions in which the charac-

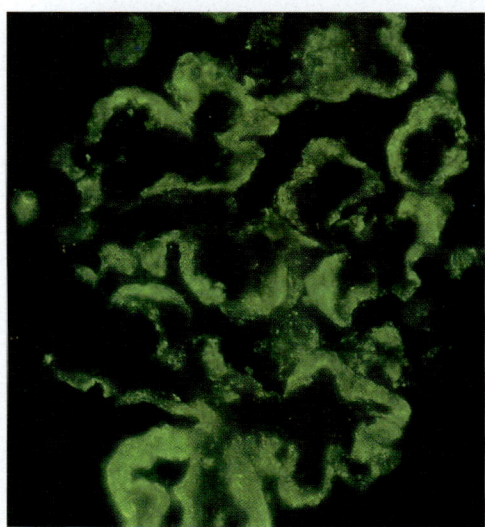

FIG. 6. Immunofluorescence of membranoproliferative glomerulonephritis type I. There is generalized glomerular capillary wall involvement, with broad deposits (anti-C3, ×450).

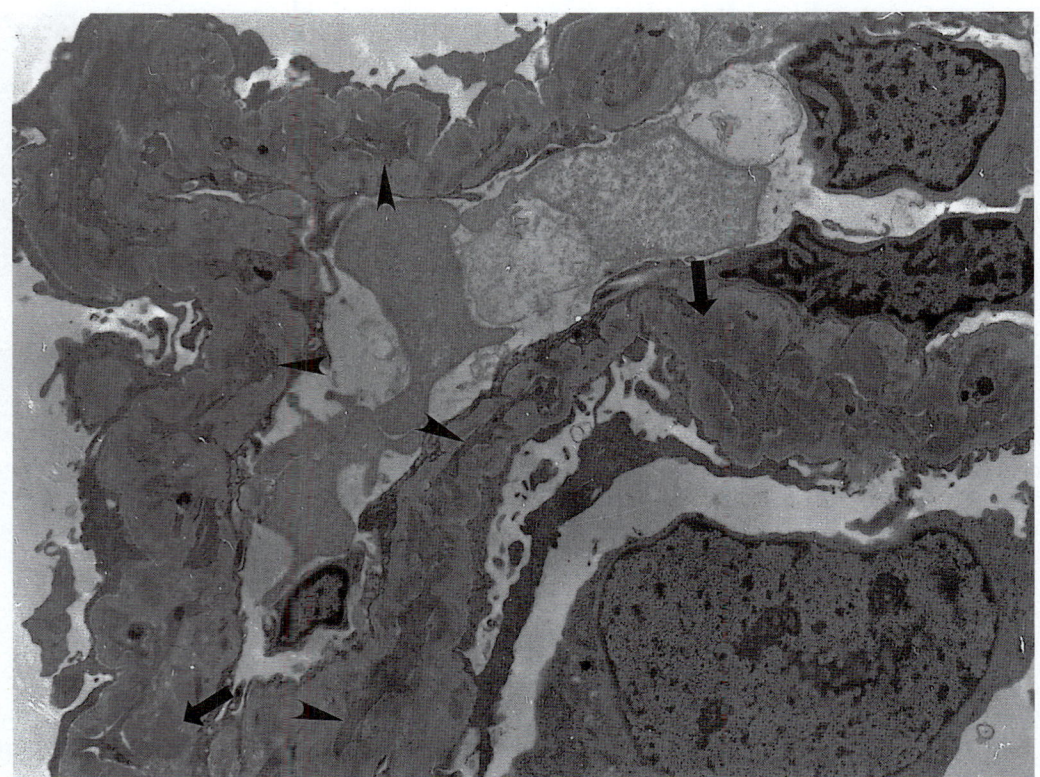

FIG. 7. Ultrastructure of membranoproliferative glomerulonephritis type I. Note that in addition to subendothelial and intramembranous electron-dense deposits (*arrows*), mesangial cell processes representing mesangial cell interposition (*arrowheads*) are also present (uranyl acetate, lead citrate, ×5,000).

teristic glomerular immune deposits can be identified. Diseases in which a membranoproliferative pattern can be noted include the following list.

1. Postinfectious (intracapillary proliferative) GN.
2. Other infective glomerulonephritides (e.g., endocarditis, deep-seated abscesses, infected shunts, schistosomiasis, and hepatitis C infection). MPGN associated with hepatitis C is usually indistinguishable from type I MPGN (19,20); in fact, many cases previously diagnosed as MPGN are probably hepatitis C–associated MPGNs. Because patients with hepatitis C virus–associated MPGN also have cryoglobulinemia, there is an overlap with cryoglobulinemic GN. Not all cases of hepatitis C–associated MPGN, however, have glomerular capillary cryoglobulin thrombi.
3. Cryoglobulinemic GN (with or without hepatitis C virus infection). The distinctive feature is the presence of glomerular, intracapillary, "hyaline"(cryoglobulin) thrombi.
4. Hepatic glomerulosclerosis is associated with chronic liver disease, usually cirrhosis. Glomeruli may resemble MPGN, but IF shows either IgA predominance or nonspecific fluorescence (21).
5. Idiopathic lobular GN without immune complex deposition may represent an advanced, "burned out" form of MPGN, but it may also be a distinct diagnostic entity (see also the differential diagnosis of diabetic glomerulosclerosis) (22).
6. Monoclonal immunoglobulin (light chain) deposition disease.
7. Diabetic glomerulosclerosis.
8. Transplant glomerulopathy.
9. LCAT (lecithin-cholesterol acyltransferase) deficiency, a rare hereditary disease of young persons. Glomerular mesangial and subendothelial lipid deposition is characteristic (23).

Outcome

MPGN type I is generally slowly progressive, and the overall long-term renal prognosis is poor. The recurrence rate after renal transplant is about 30% (24,25).

Etiologic Factors and Pathogenesis

MPGN is classically thought to be a chronic immune complex disease stemming from chronic antigenemia. The origin is most likely a combination of factors; infections, complement activation, complement deficiency, genetic predisposition, cellular and humoral immunity, and other factors have been implicated. A subset of cases has been associated with hepatitis C virus infection; these patients also have type II cryoglobulinemia (19,20).

Membranoproliferative Glomerulonephritis, Type II (Synonym: Dense Deposit Disease)

Light Microscopic Features

In general, this condition shows features similar to type I MPGN, but occasionally the glomeruli are relatively unremarkable or may show other patterns. Such patterns include focal segmental reduplication of the GBM, diffuse glomerular capillary wall thickening with less glomerular hypercellularity (resembling membranous GN), focal GN, or even crescentic GN (26–29). The characteristic GBM deposits stain with thioflavin T and frequently also with fat stains.

Immunofluorescence Characteristics

Granular, glomerular, mesangial and linear (which may be discontinuous) capillary loop deposits of C3, properdin, and, less often, immunoglobulins and C4 are evident. It is frequently apparent that C3 is present along the margins of, but not within, the dense intramembranous deposits (Fig. 8). This contributes to a double-linear appearance of the glomerular capillary wall and a ring appearance around the mesangial deposits (mesangial rings) on IF (30).

Electron Microscopic Features

The large, dense, glomerular, intramembranous deposits seen on EM, often involving long segments of the GBM, are unique and pathognomonic. The deposits may be discontinuous, occasionally even subendothelial (Fig. 9). There may be similar deposits in the nearby mesangial regions. Glomerular subepithelial deposits (humps) may also be present. Deposits similar to the GBM deposits often develop in Bowman's capsule and in tubular basement membranes (TBMs) and have even been noted in the basement membranes of other organs, such as the liver, spleen, and eye.

Differential Diagnosis

The differential diagnosis of MPGN type II is broader than that of type I MPGN at the light microscopic level because of its more variable appearance. EM is diagnostic.

Outcome

The outcome is similar to that of MPGN type I. Recurrent disease appears in almost every transplant, but it usually does not influence graft function and graft survival (24,25).

Etiologic Factors and Pathogenesis

The source of the disease is obscure. In our opinion, it most likely represents a disease unrelated to other forms of MPGN.

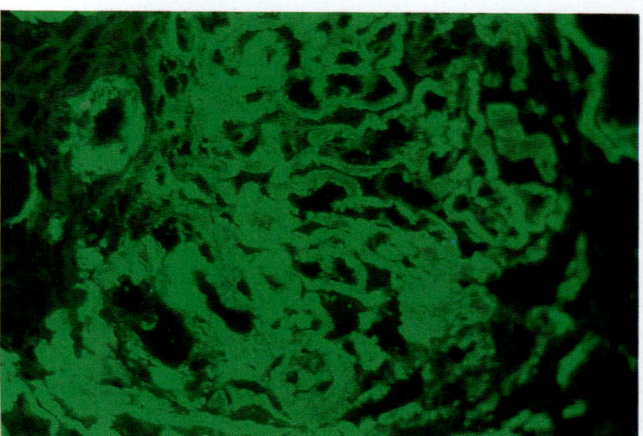

FIG. 8. Immunofluorescence of membranoproliferative glomerulonephritis type II. Note the diffuse capillary loop and mesangial deposits. In several glomerular capillary loops, the intensity of the fluorescence is stronger along the margin of the positive capillary walls (anti-C3; ×450).

Membranoproliferative Glomerulonephritis, Type III

This is a less well characterized and somewhat variably defined variant of MPGN with extensive subendothelial, subepithelial, and transmembranous deposits evident on EM and subsequent widespread disruption of the GBM (Fig. 10) (31,32). Otherwise, it is not different from MPGN type I.

Diffuse Extracapillary Proliferative Glomerulonephritis (Synonyms: Crescentic Glomerulonephritis, Rapidly Progressive Glomerulonephritis)

General Considerations

Crescentic GN is a pattern caused by, or associated with, a large number of different disease entities (Table 5). Crescents are defined by the WHO as two or more cell layers between the parietal and visceral epithelia of the glomerulus. The exact definition of diffuse crescentic GN varies; some authors require at least 50% of glomeruli to contain crescents, whereas others require 80%.

Crescents are often associated with gaps, or "focal disruptive lesions," of the GBMs through which large proteins [such as fibrin(ogen)] and cells are thought to pass (33). It is this passage of fibrin(ogen) and cells (and possibly other growth factors) that is thought to be the stimulus for crescent formation. The cellular crescents consist of large polyhedral cells most likely derived from glomerular epithelial cells and macrophages as well as other inflammatory cells (Fig. 11A). Occasionally, giant cells give the crescent a granulomatous appearance. Glomerular tuft necrosis, which is usually segmental, may occur in severe forms (Fig. 11B). The presence of fibrin is a common finding in cellular crescents.

These cellular crescents quickly transform into fibrocellular crescents with the appearance of myofibroblasts and de-

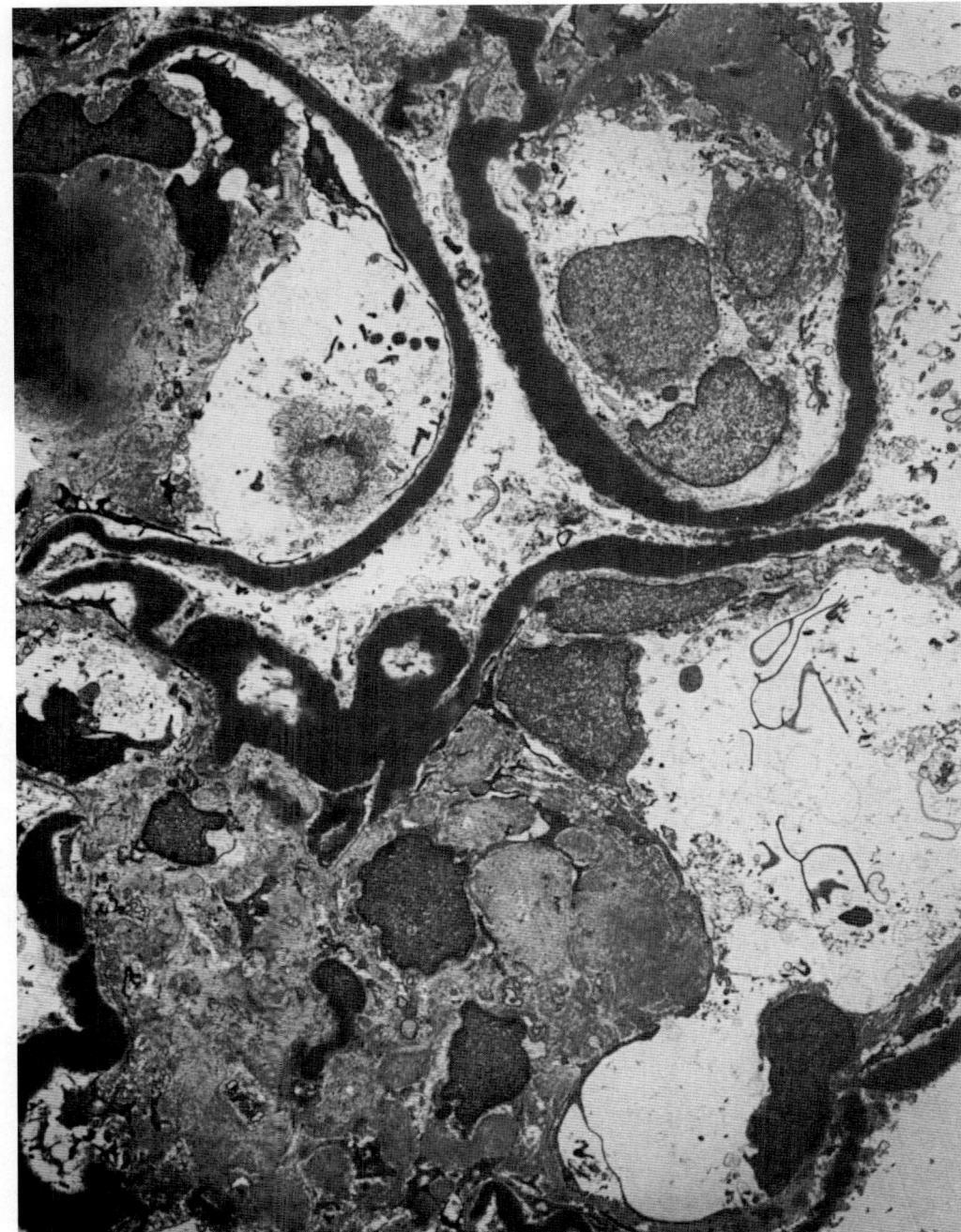

FIG. 9. Membranoproliferative glomerulonephritis type II (dense-deposit disease). Note that these three glomerular capillary walls have very electron-dense intramembranous deposits. This is pathognomonic of dense-deposit disease (uranyl acetate, lead citrate; ×4,000).

TABLE 5. *Diseases associated with crescentic glomerulonephritis*

Granular deposits by IF	Linear immunoglobulin deposits by IF	No deposits (pauci-immune)

Idiopathic immune complex–mediated crescentic GN
Secondary forms
  MPGN
  Postinfectious
  IgA nephropathy
  Lupus
  Others
	Anti-GBM disease (Goodpasture syndrome)
	Monoclonal immunoglobulin deposition disease
		Systemic vasculitides
		  Wegener's granulomatosis
		  Microscopic polyangitis
		Renal limited form

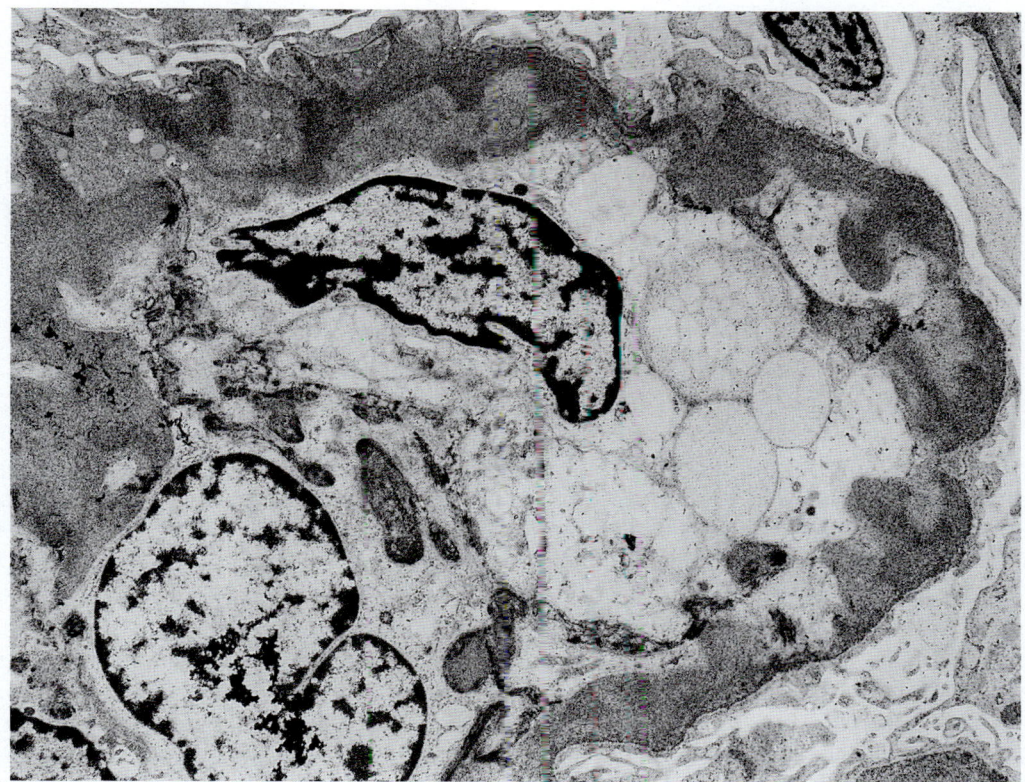

FIG. 10. Membranoproliferative glomerulonephritis type III. Note the widespread disruption of the dark (silver impregnated) glomerular basement membrane by deposits that are only slightly or not at all electron dense (silver impregnation of ultrathin section; ×9,000).

position of extracellular matrix, including interstitial collagen (Fig. 11C). Eventually, fibrous crescents develop, consisting mainly of collagen and a few fibroblasts (Fig. 11D). It is possible that myofibroblasts/fibroblasts migrate into Bowman's capsule through gaps in the Bowman's capsular basement membrane. It may be difficult to differentiate an old fibrous crescent (Fig. 11D) from Bowman's space fibro-

sis in obsolescent glomeruli (Fig. 12). A good (but not absolutely reliable) way to make the distinction is to perform a PAS reaction, which stains the basal lamina of Bowman's capsule. If the Bowman's capsular basement membrane is disrupted, the lesion probably represents an old crescent (Fig. 11D); if not, the glomerulus may simply be obsolescent (Fig. 12).

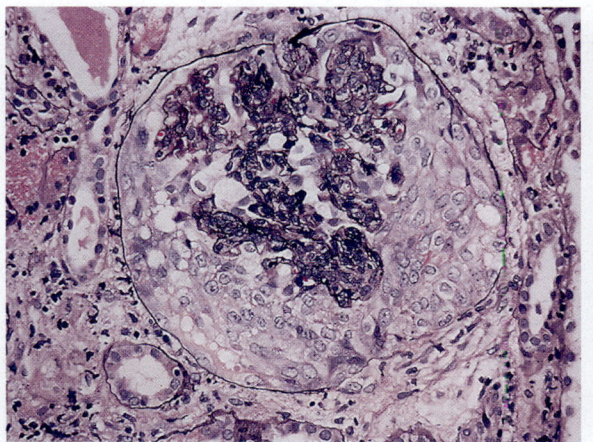
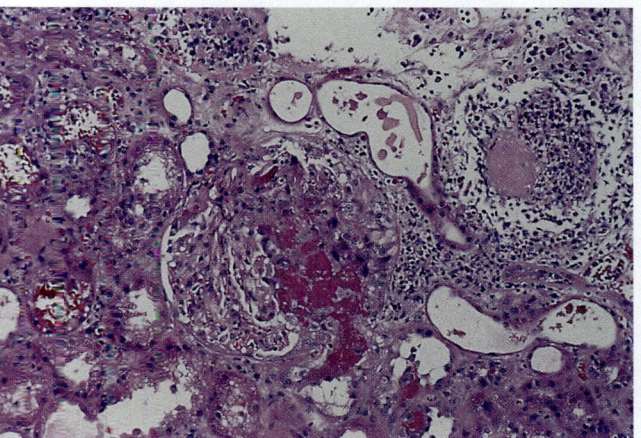

FIG. 11. Various appearances of crescents in crescentic glomerulonephritis. **A:** The glomerular tuft is compressed by this large cellular crescent. Note the rupture in the Bowman's capsular basement membrane (methenamine silver). **B:** There is segmental necrosis and crescent formation in this antineutrophil cytoplasmic autoantibody–associated crescentic and necrotizing glomerulonephritis.

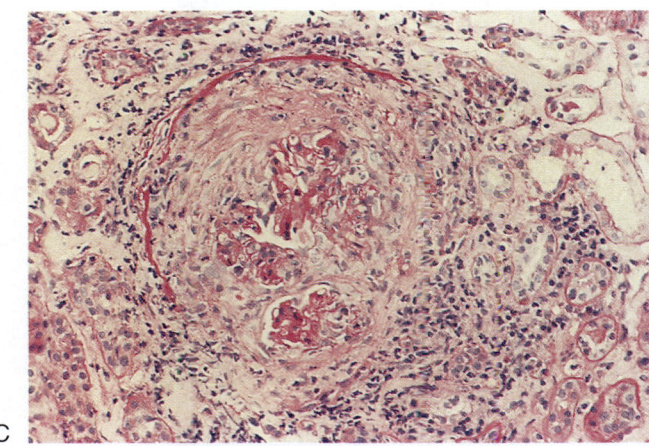 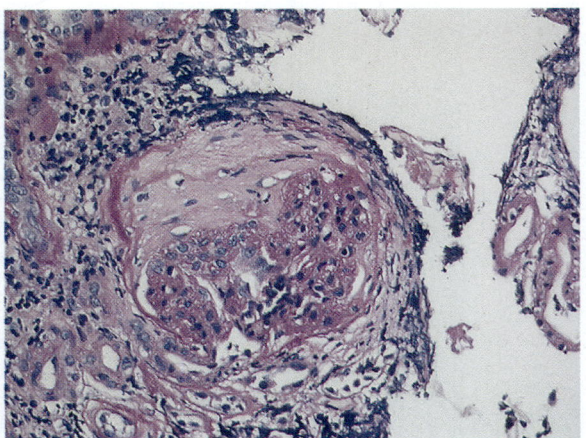

FIG. 11. (continued) **C:** Fibrocellular crescent. Note that the crescent is less cellular compared with A and has more collagen. Also note the extensive disruption of Bowman's capsule [periodic acid–Schiff (PAS)]. **D:** A fibrous crescent compresses a portion of the underlying glomerular tuft. Note the rupture in the Bowman's capsular basement membrane (PAS).

Inspecting glomeruli with the least amount of morphologic injury (i.e., those glomeruli without advanced crescents) by light IF and EM is always important, because if crescentic GN stems from a well-defined underlying glomerular disease (such as SLE, HSP, acute postinfectious GN, and others), the noncrescentic, or least involved, glomeruli may show diagnostic changes of the underlying disease.

Crescentic GN is classified by IF and EM findings into three types (Table 5): (a) pauci-immune, in which no or only insignificant deposits are noted; (b) anti-GBM disease, with intense linear deposits of IgG along the GBM (Fig. 13); and (c) immune complex crescentic GN, with diffuse granular IF and discrete immune-type, electron-dense deposits visible on EM. In idiopathic (or primary) immune complex crescentic GN, no underlying pattern of a well-defined immune complex GN (such as MPGN, SLE, postinfectious GN, etc.) is found. In the secondary forms, the pattern of an underlying well-defined immune complex GN can be recognized in better preserved or noncrescentic glomeruli.

Pauci-immune Crescentic and Necrotizing GN

Epidemiology

The incidence of this form of crescentic GN in renal biopsy material appears to be increasing. This is probably the most common form of crescentic GN seen today (particularly if we disregard immune complex glomerulonephritides with secondary crescent formation). It develops most often in the elderly population, and it rarely occurs in children.

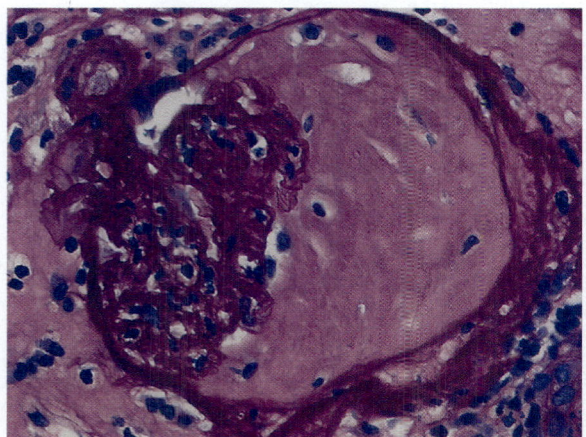

FIG. 12. Obsolescent glomerulus. Note the retracted, collapsed glomerular capillary loops that stain positive for periodic acid–Schiff (PAS) and the pale collagen filling Bowman's capsule around it. The Bowman's capsular basement membrane is wrinkled and lamellated but continuous.

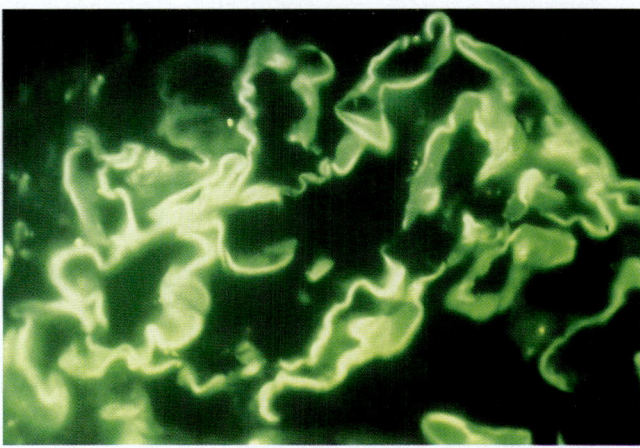

FIG. 13. Linear staining in a patient with anti-glomerular basement membrane antibody–mediated crescentic glomerulonephritis (Goodpasture's disease) (anti-IgG; ×1,000).

Clinical Symptoms

Acute renal failure, usually with nephritic syndrome, is the rule. The disease can be renal-limited or associated with systemic vasculitis, such as Wegener's granulomatosis or polyarteritis (usually with the microscopic form, also called microscopic polyangiitis, microscopic polyarteritis, or hypersensitivity vasculitis). In cases with vasculitis, symptoms of multiorgan involvement are typical. Antineutrophil cytoplasmic autoantibodies (ANCAs) are detected in about 90% of patients, irrespective of whether the disease is limited to the kidney or is systemic (34,35). ANCAs originally were detected by IF, and two subtypes, based on fluorescence pattern, were described. So-called pANCA shows perinuclear fluorescence in alcohol-fixed neutrophil granulocytes, whereas cANCA shows a diffuse cytoplasmic fluorescence. Radioimmunoassay is a more sensitive and specific method to detect ANCA. It has become clear that pANCAs are antibodies to myeloperoxidase, and cANCAs are antibodies against proteinase 3, a serine protease in the azurophilic granules of neutrophils. Patients with Wegener's granulomatosis usually have cANCA, whereas patients with polyarteritis and kidney-limited disease have predominantly pANCA (34,35). It is interesting that in a certain percentage of patients with ANCA-positive crescentic GN, anti-GBM antibodies also can be detected.

Light Microscopic Features

Pauci-immune crescentic and necrotizing GN can be diffuse or focal. In addition to crescents, segmental glomerular tuft necrosis and fibrin exudate in the crescents are typical findings (Fig. 11 A,B) (34,35). Noncrescentic glomeruli and glomeruli with small crescents usually show no or little intracapillary hypercellularity. In the glomeruli with large crescents, the compressed glomerular tuft may appear hypercellular because of nuclear crowding. Secondary interstitial nephritis, composed mainly of lymphocytes and macrophages, is almost always present. Eosinophils and plasma cells frequently are found in the interstitial infiltrate. Vascular necrosis is rarely seen in renal biopsy material, even when GN is associated with systemic vasculitis, because of the focally involved vessels and the limited tissue sample.

Immunofluorescence Characteristics

Immunofluorescence portrays negative or nonspecific findings. Some glomerular tuft C3 may be noted. Fibrinogen is frequently found in crescents or in necrotic glomerular segments.

Electron Microscopic Features

No, or only very few, small, immune-type, electron-dense deposits are visible. Electron-dense fibrin strands and wisps, with their typical periodicity, gaps, and ruptures in the GBM, and other features of severe glomerular injury are commonly seen.

Differential Diagnosis

IF and EM are necessary to exclude immune complex GN or anti-GBM disease. Certain cases with ANCAs may also have anti-GBM antibodies (see discussion of anti-GBM disease). It is worth noting that ANCAs can be detected in certain diseases that are not usually associated with crescentic GN, such as "collagen-vascular diseases," inflammatory bowel disease, and some infectious diseases (35).

Outcome

In untreated cases, there is rapid development of irreversible glomerulosclerosis and scarring. With aggressive treatment (cyclophosphamide plus steroids), however, the 2-year patient and renal survival rates are above 70% in ANCA-associated cases (34–36). The results of good long-term follow-up studies are not yet available. Whether crescents can resolve is open to question. It appears likely that small crescents, causing little glomerular tuft destruction, may heal with segmental Bowman's capsule fibrosis and disruption with or without glomerular capillary loop adhesions. If the glomerular tuft is affected as well, the healing process will result in segmental or global glomerulosclerosis and scarring (Fig. 14). The number of glomeruli involved by crescents is a good predictor of outcome. The recurrence rate of pauci-immune crescentic GN in renal transplants seems to be relatively low, probably because of the continuous immunosuppressive treatment of transplant recipients.

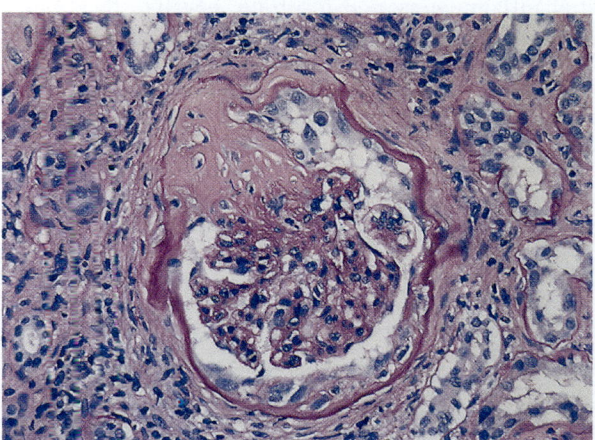

FIG. 14. Segmental scarring in a glomerulus—the consequence of healed focal necrotizing glomerulonephritis in this patient. Note that the adhesion between Bowman's capsule and the glomerular tuft is only faintly positive with periodic acid–Schiff (PAS) reaction and represents mostly collagen.

Etiologic Factors and Pathogenesis

There is some evidence that ANCAs have a pathogenetic role, but this has not yet been proved. Alternatively, the presence of ANCAs may be the result of severe tissue damage.

Anti-glomerular Basement Membrane Disease

Epidemiology

This is the least common form of the three subtypes of crescentic glomerulonephritides. In our experience, it is found in less than 0.5% of all renal biopsy specimens. It is a disease mainly affecting adults and is rare in children. It is more common in whites than in blacks.

Clinical Symptoms

The renal-limited form manifests as acute renal failure and nephritic syndrome. If GN is associated with pulmonary hemorrhage, the condition is classified as Goodpasture's syndrome. If, in addition, anti-GBM antibodies are also evident, it is properly termed Goodpasture's disease. The exact definitions for Goodpasture's syndrome (or disease) vary from investigator to investigator; it is important to be aware of a particular researcher's criteria for this diagnosis. It appears that most investigators consider only cases with anti-GBM antibodies to be Goodpasture's syndrome (or disease). Anti-GBM antibodies in the serum are best detected by radioimmunoassay (37).

Light Microscopic Features

There is no way to distinguish anti-GBM disease from other forms of crescentic GN by LM alone (Fig. 11). The crescent formation may be focal or diffuse. Glomerular necrosis is typical. The noncrescentic glomeruli usually do not show prominent intracapillary hypercellularity. An interstitial inflammatory cell infiltrate, just like that found in other forms of crescentic GN, is often present.

Immunofluorescence Characteristics

Intense linear staining for IgG and C3 along the glomerular capillary walls is characteristic (Fig. 13). C3 may be weaker than IgG, and, in certain cases, only IgG is detected. Linear staining for IgG may be found along TBMs, reflecting anti-TBM antibodies. When there is intense linear immunofluorescent staining, a search for anti-GBM antibodies in the circulation or eluted from the patient's kidneys is in order. Indirect IF, using the patient's serum placed on normal kidneys, is the easiest method, but it is neither specific nor sensitive.

Electron Microscopic Features

EM is not helpful in differentiating anti-GBM disease from pauci-immune crescentic and necrotizing GN, because no, or only very few, vague, small, electron-dense deposits can be detected in either case.

Differential Diagnosis

Linear staining for IgG by IF is neither necessary nor sufficient for the diagnosis of anti-GBM antibody-induced GN. The diagnosis must be confirmed by the presence of circulating anti-GBM antibodies in patients' serum samples. The best system today, in terms of sensitivity and specificity, is the radioimmunoassay for circulating anti-GBM antibodies (37). False-positive, mild, linear staining by IF may be noted in patients with a variety of diseases, such as diabetes mellitus, "benign or essential hematuria," SLE, acute postinfectious GN, or renal allografts—and even in 10% of supposedly normal kidneys from autopsy. There are certain other diseases in which linear glomerular capillary loop staining is present, occasionally in association with crescents.

In dense-deposit disease, the immunoreactant is C3 (characteristically there is no IgG), and under higher magnification the linear staining may have a double contour (see earlier discussion). In monoclonal immunoglobulin deposition disease (mostly light chain deposition disease), only one of the light chains is deposited (usually kappa). In fibrillary GN, linear glomerular capillary IgG fluorescence can be noted, but it is usually interrupted and segmental. In all of these conditions, mesangial staining with the same immunoreactants also is seen, and EM and laboratory data will help in establishing the correct diagnosis.

Finally, we have to reiterate that there is an overlap between ANCA-associated crescentic GN and anti-GBM disease. Approximately 30% of patients with anti-GBM antibodies also have ANCAs (37). It is possible that in these cases, anti-GBM antibodies appear following severe destruction of the GBM and subsequent release of GBM material into the circulation.

Outcome

The prognosis is poor. End-stage renal disease (ESRD) develops in most patients within a short period of time. Aggressive therapy may somewhat improve the outcome, but results are far worse than in ANCA-associated forms. Plasmapheresis may be helpful in the elimination of circulating anti-GBM antibodies. Poor prognostic indicators are oligoanuria at onset and diffuse involvement of glomeruli by crescents and necrosis (37,38). The recurrence rate in renal transplants is low, probably owing to the associated continuous immunosuppressive therapy. Delaying transplantation also lowers the chance of recurrence. In 50% of patients with transplants who have had anti-GBM disease, linear GBM staining may be noted, but this is rarely accompanied by crescent formation and nephritic syndrome (24,25).

Etiologic Factors and Pathogenesis

Binding of anti-GBM antibodies to the GBM epitopes and subsequent complement activation initiate the inflammatory response and tissue injury. The Goodpasture epitope is on the alpha 3 chain of type IV collagen. Why anti-GBM antibodies appear is unknown. Cross-reaction with environmental antigens, including infectious agents, is one possibility. The best "experimental" model has been established in humans. Classic anti-GBM disease will develop in some patients with Alport's syndrome, who lack or have an aberrant Goodpasture epitope, when they undergo transplantation with normal kidneys (which have the normal Goodpasture epitope) (39).

Idiopathic (or Primary) Immune Complex Crescentic Glomerulonephritis

Immune deposits are present in the glomeruli, but the pattern is not consistent with any of the known immune complex glomerulonephritides, such as MPGN, lupus, postinfectious GN, IgA nephropathy, and others. If one of the well-defined patterns of immune complex GN is identified, crescentic GN is considered to be secondary and is best defined as crescentic MPGN, crescentic postinfectious GN, or another form (40).

Epidemiology

Idiopathic immune complex crescentic GN is rare. The secondary forms (crescentic GN superimposed on a well-defined immune complex GN) are more common.

Clinical Symptoms

The clinical picture is not different from that of other forms of crescentic GN (see relevant earlier sections), except for negative ANCA and anti-GBM antibodies.

Light Microscopic Features

In essence, similar to other forms of crescentic GN. Glomerular intracapillary hypercellularity is more frequently evident than in other forms. In contrast, glomerular necrosis is probably less frequent.

Immunofluorescence Characteristics

There is obvious granular staining for IgG and/or C3 and sometimes IgM in the mesangium and frequently along the glomerular capillary loops as well. If strong IgA and C1q staining is noted, the possibility of IgA nephropathy, HSP, or lupus nephritis should be considered.

Electron Microscopic Features

Discrete, immune-type, electron-dense deposits are usually noted in the mesangium and scattered in or along the GBM. The distribution of these deposits in idiopathic immune complex crescentic GN does not follow a well-defined pattern (such as in membranous GN or postinfectious GN).

Differential Diagnosis

An underlying pattern of a well-known primary immune complex GN (such as SLE, HSP, IgA nephropathy, etc.) should be considered. Careful examination of the LM, IF, and EM patterns in the most well-preserved glomeruli is the best method to differentiate idiopathic (primary immune complex) crescentic GN from the secondary forms.

Outcome

The prognosis of idiopathic (primary) immune complex crescentic GN is poor, in light of the fact that it usually is resistant to therapy. The secondary forms may have somewhat better outcomes, particularly crescentic poststreptococcal GN. There is not enough information regarding the recurrence rate in renal transplants, but, in general, the recurrence rate of crescentic GN is low.

Etiologic Factors and Pathogenesis

Immune complex deposition probably plays an important role.

The Issue of Pulmonary-Renal Syndrome

Pulmonary hemorrhage and/or infiltrate associated with GN can be seen in many conditions other than anti-GBM antibody-induced GN. Such cases are frequently designated "pulmonary-renal syndrome" (41). In fact, fewer than one-third (much fewer, according to some) of patients with pulmonary hemorrhage and/or infiltrate and glomerular disease actually have demonstrable anti-GBM disease. Pulmonary hemorrhage and infiltrate in association with GN can be seen in anti-GBM antibody-induced disease; vasculitides, including Wegener's granulomatosis; cryoglobulinemia; SLE; penicillamine therapy; HSP; and in cases of GN combined with pulmonary edema or pneumonia.

Focal Glomerulonephritis

Focal GN is a pattern of reaction to renal injury in which some, but not all, of the glomeruli are seen on histologic examination to have areas of severe hypercellularity, with closure of capillary loops, necrosis, and/or sclerosis (42–44) (Figs. 14 and 15). If the term focal is to be used in a diagnostic report, the exact percentage of affected glomeruli should be stated. The remaining glomeruli appear relatively normal on LM. Frequently, glomerular involvement is segmental, affecting only a portion of a glomerulus. The pattern of focal segmental glomerular hypercellularity may be caused by, or associated with, a number of disease processes, such as SLE,

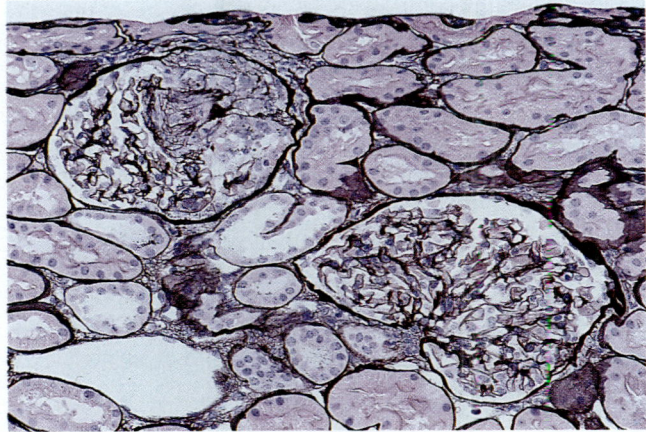

FIG. 15. Focal glomerulonephritis in a case of systemic lupus erythematosus. Note that the one glomerulus appears to be normal on light microscopy, whereas in the other glomerulus, segmental glomerular capillary loop disruption and crescent formation are present (methenamine silver).

infective endocarditis, deep-seated visceral abscess, infected atrioventricular shunts (shunt nephritis), polyarteritis nodosa (usually the microscopic form), Wegener's granulomatosis and other vasculitides, IgA nephropathy/ HSP (anaphylactoid purpura), Goodpasture's syndrome (disease), the cellular lesion in focal segmental glomerular sclerosis (FSGS), the edge of renal infarcts, malignant hypertension, scleroderma, and, from time to time, many other renal diseases.

Many glomerular processes termed focal are not truly focal; they are focal only as seen by LM. For example, in patients with focal GN in Berger's disease (IgA nephropathy), HSP, SLE, or the early stages of anti-GBM-induced GN, there are widespread, diffuse glomerular immune deposits noted on IF and/or EM. What is focal are the manifestations of diffuse deposition of immune and immune-like materials on LM. In diseases where no immune complex deposition can be detected, such as in many vasculitides and ANCA-associated glomerulonephritides, the process truly appears to be focal. Focal GN can heal with FSGS and scarring (Fig. 14). The distinction between healed focal GN (as in a treated SLE or polyarteritis) and true focal sclerosis may occasionally be difficult to make; this question is addressed by Whitworth et al. (44).

THE NONGLOMERULONEPHRITIC GLOMERULONEPHROPATHIES (GLOMERULAR CAPILLARY WALL LESIONS LEADING TO THE NEPHROTIC SYNDROME)

These diffuse, glomerular capillary wall lesions are characterized by predominant or exclusive involvement of the glomerular capillary walls (with little change, at least in the early stages, in the mesangial regions). The glomerular tufts are usually not hypercellular. The patterns described here are almost always associated with marked proteinuria and quite often with the nephrotic syndrome.

Minimal Change Nephrotic Syndrome (Synonyms: Nil Disease, Lipoid Nephrosis, Minimal Change Disease)

Epidemiology

This pattern occurs primarily and not infrequently in children, although it may also be noted in adults. It is the most common cause of nephrotic-range proteinuria in children and adolescents (45).

Clinical Symptoms

Severe proteinuria, usually in conjunction with nephrotic syndrome (edema, hypoalbuminemia, hyperlipidemia, and lipiduria) is the leading symptom. Proteinuria is selective in the majority of cases (urine protein consists mainly of albumin and low-molecular-weight proteins with little IgG), compared with the findings in other glomerular diseases that feature the nephrotic syndrome, such as FSGS, in which proteinuria is frequently nonselective (high-molecular-weight proteins, such as immunoglobulins, are also present in the urine). Microscopic hematuria may occur, but it is not characteristic. Renal function remains normal for the most part, but acute renal failure may develop in adults, particularly elderly patients. The blood pressure characteristically remains normal. Serum complement levels are also normal.

Light Microscopic Features

The renal parenchyma appears normal. In adults, and particularly in the elderly, there may be a few obsolescent glomeruli, with very mild focal interstitial fibrosis and tubular atrophy. If MCNS is associated with interstitial nephritis, a nonsteroidal antiinflammatory drug (NSAID)–induced renal disease should be suspected (see discussion of acute interstitial nephritis). Several minor LM changes have been found in what seems to be otherwise typical MCNS, such as mild mesangial prominence and hypercellularity (Fig. 16).

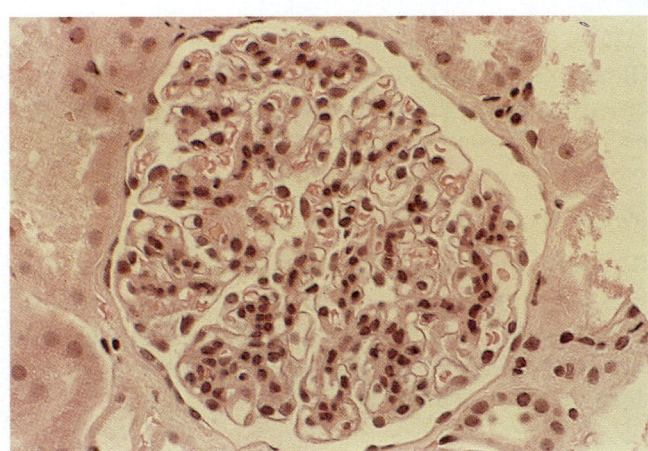

FIG. 16. Mesangial hypercellularity and prominence in a case of idiopathic nephrotic syndrome. Except for the mesangial changes, the clinical history and immunofluorescence and electron microscopy findings were suggestive of minimal change nephrotic syndrome.

The International Study of Kidney Disease in Children has shown that these minor variants do not seem to affect the patient's response to steroids and that most of these patients appear to have a good prognosis (46). The adhesion and localized sclerosis of a glomerular capillary loop to Bowman's capsule, adjacent to the origin of the proximal tubule, have been designated "glomerular tip lesion" (Fig. 17) (47). Tip lesions can develop in a variety of diseases, including MCNS, and do not influence outcome (48). Ectatic glomerular capillary lumina and slightly prominent podocytes may be seen. Tubular protein resorption droplets (also called hyaline droplets) are frequently found (Fig. 18). These are usually PAS positive and sometimes (but not always) methenamine silver positive.

Immunofluorescence Characteristics

IF results are negative in most cases. Positive glomerular IF for IgM and C3 has been noted in some patients. These are often cases with mild mesangial prominence (see glomerular wall lesions). Immunoreactants other than IgM may also be present in otherwise typical MCNS, apparently without major clinical significance (49); in such cases, MCNS should be considered only if there are no electron-dense deposits by EM.

Electron Microscopic Features

The most striking finding is the extensive loss of glomerular visceral epithelial cell foot processes (so-called fusion, which is not really fusion but rather effacement of visceral epithelial cell foot processes) (Fig. 19); no other prominent ultrastructural lesions of the glomerular capillary wall are usually noted. Immune-type, electron-dense deposits are absent. Many investigators believe that the effacement of the foot processes stems from enhanced permeability of the glomerular capillary wall. It is important to note that foot process effacement may not be obvious in biopsy specimens taken after steroid treatment. Other nonspecific glomerular visceral epithelial cell changes, such as intracytoplasmic lipid and protein droplets, hypertrophy of the visceral epithelium with microvillous transformation, and basal condensation of intracytoplasmic microfilaments, are also frequently seen.

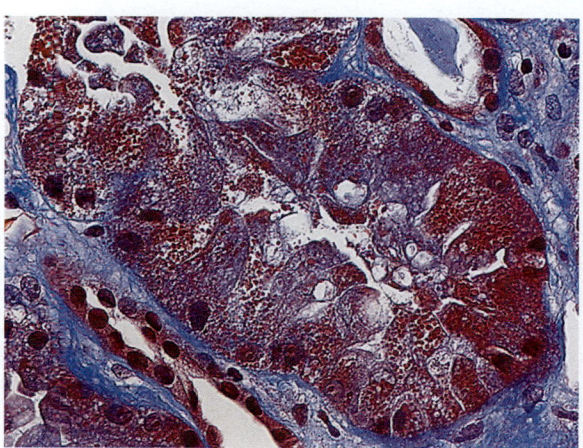

FIG. 18. Prominent protein resorption droplets in the proximal epithelium of a nephrotic patient (Masson's trichrome).

Differential Diagnosis

The main differential diagnostic problem is FSGS. A sampling error (absence of diagnostic segmentally sclerotic/hyalinized glomeruli) is difficult to exclude, particularly in biopsy specimens containing fewer than ten glomeruli and in superficial specimens not containing the corticomedullary junction and juxtamedullary glomeruli (see later section on FSGS). The paraffin block of the biopsy material should be entirely step-cut to make sure that every available glomerulus is examined. Even though FSGS cannot be established in the absence of diagnostic segmental lesions, there are certain clinical and histologic features that favor FSGS: microscopic hematuria, nonselective proteinuria, enlarged glomeruli, and focal interstitial fibrosis with tubular atrophy.

In adults, particularly in elderly patients with severe proteinuria and glomeruli that appear normal on LM, early-stage membranous GN or early-stage amyloidosis should be considered. These conditions can easily be confirmed or excluded by IF, EM, and Congo red stain. A few patients with mesangial IgA deposition (IgA nephropathy) may have nephrotic syndrome and normal-appearing glomeruli; it is interesting to note that most of them respond to steroids.

Outcome

Most patients respond to steroids with complete resolution of proteinuria. Some patients will become steroid dependent (proteinuria recurs following the tapering of steroids); others may be steroid resistant. Many of the steroid-resistant patients turn out to have FSGS on follow-up biopsy.

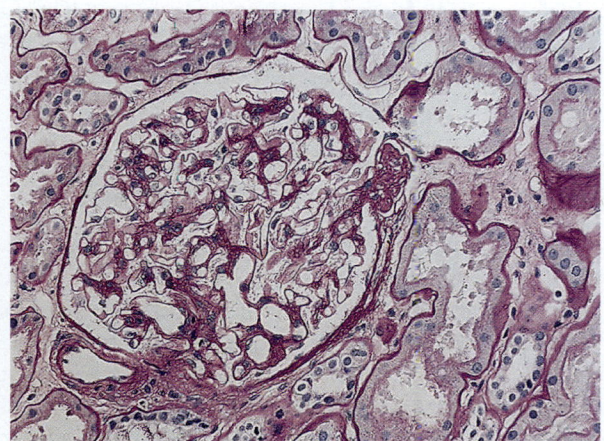

FIG. 17. Glomerular tip lesion. Note glomerulosclerosis and hyalinosis at the origin of the proximal tubule (periodic acid–Schiff).

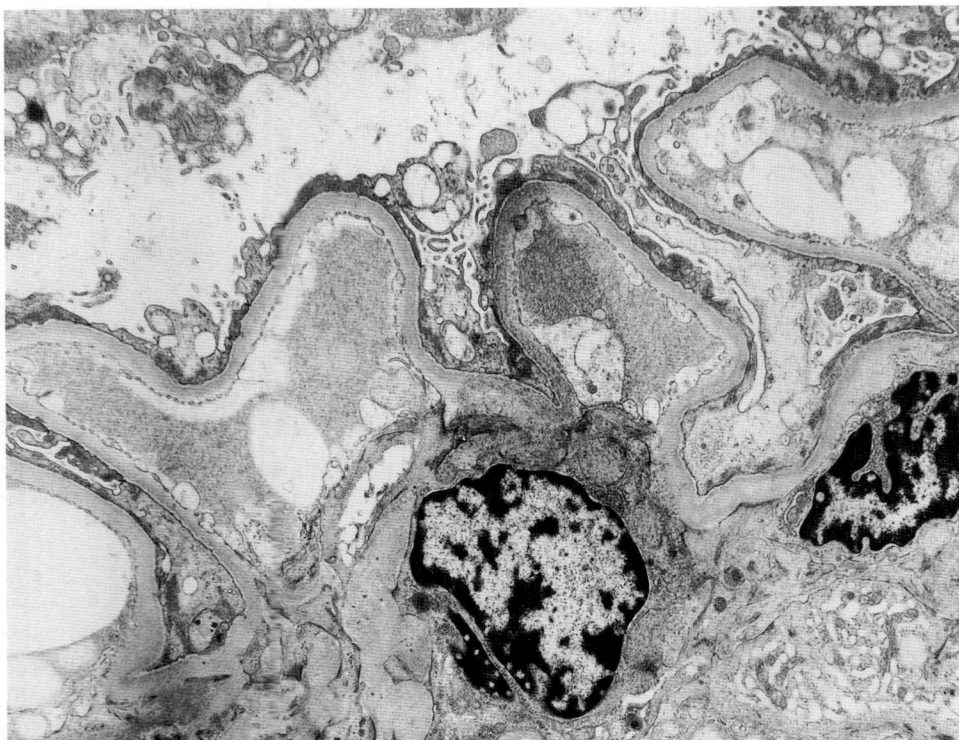

FIG. 19. Minimal change nephrotic syndrome. On ultrastructural examination, the foot processes of the visceral epithelial cells show total effacement. They form a continuous layer of cytoplasm on the outer surface of the glomerular basement membrane (uranyl acetate, lead citrate; ×3,600).

Etiologic Factors and Pathogenesis

The origin of MCNS and the mechanism of action of the marked proteinuria are unclear. On the basis of circumstantial evidence, some researchers have suggested that MCNS stems from an immune disorder. Both cellular and humoral immune responses have been implicated. The source of proteinuria is also unclear, but loss of the fixed glomerular capillary polyanionic layer(s), which normally lead to the negative charge of the glomerular capillary wall, may allow albumin and other negatively charged proteins to seep through in increasing amounts. Circulating serum factors, cytokines that amplify glomerular capillary permeability, may also be of importance (50,51). MCNS is not always idiopathic; it may be associated with a variety of NSAIDs. In such cases of MCNS, interstitial nephritis also may develop. Symptoms usually regress upon withdrawal of the drug (52).

Diffuse Mesangial Hypercellularity in Idiopathic Nephrotic Syndrome

The association of diffuse mesangial hypercellularity (DMH) and idiopathic nephrotic syndrome (INS) was first described in 1970 (Fig. 16). Various studies have verified that DMH is present in 2% to 8% of patients with INS. This histopathologic form is thought by some investigators to be a variant of MCNS, clinically associated with an increased incidence of hematuria; in some series, it has been reported to have a less favorable response to steroid therapy.

The response of children with DMH and nephrotic syndrome to treatment with steroids and/or cytotoxic agents is relatively poor compared with patients with MCNS, although the long-term renal prognosis appears to be good (at least in published short follow-up studies) (53,54). Some cases of nephrotic syndrome combined with DMH may represent undiagnosed FSGS; follow-up biopsies of these cases may show definite signs of FSGS. The majority of cases, however, probably represent a variant of MCNS with a greater than usual mesangial reaction. It has been shown that mesangial hypercellularity in MCNS may be a transient feature (49). In our opinion, DMH in INS should be considered a MCNS, particularly if the patient is steroid sensitive or dependent. If steroid resistance and, in particular, renal impairment develop, FSGS (i.e., undiagnosed FSGS) most likely lies in the background.

Glomerular Mesangial IgM Deposition in Idiopathic Nephrotic Syndrome (So-Called IgM Nephropathy)

In 1978, two groups independently described mesangial deposition of IgM in renal biopsy samples that otherwise appeared to indicate the presence of MCNS (Fig. 20) (55,56). Since that time, many reports of this so-called IgM nephropathy have been published, but the lesion continues to be the subject of controversy. In our opinion, the presence of mesangial IgM in the absence of other immunoreactants merely represents a disturbance in the mesangial transport of macromolecules and should not be considered an entity separate from MCNS (45).

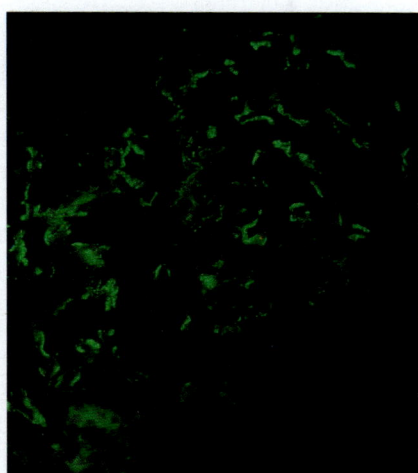

FIG. 20. Mild to moderate mesangial IgM deposits on immunofluorescence in this case of minimal change nephrotic syndrome (anti-IgM; ×400).

Several observations support our hypothesis. (a) Reports that compare cases with and without mesangial IgM within a distinct glomerular morphologic pattern did not find a difference in outcome (45). (b) In cases where IgM is the only immunoreactant, EM usually does not show electron-dense, immune-type deposits in the mesangium, except for a few vague electron densities. If discrete electron-dense deposits are present, other immunoreactants, such as IgG, IgA, C3, and C1q, are almost always evident on IF. (c) Mesangial IgM deposition may be present in normal kidneys (e.g., autopsies, donor kidney biopsies). (d) Mesangial IgM may disappear on follow-up biopsies (49). (e) We do not know the incidence of mesangial IgM in cases of steroid-sensitive MCNS because such cases are not subjected to biopsy.

In spite of these arguments, we do not think that the presence of mesangial IgM is a totally innocent finding that should be disregarded. It probably represents mesangial dysfunction, and its presence, particularly in steroid-resistant cases, is a further argument in favor of the possibility that there is underlying early-stage FSGS. Rarely, we have seen cases with mesangial IgM and C3 in which small electron-dense deposits were evident on EM. These small deposits may truly represent IgM containing mesangial immune complexes, but their significance is unknown.

C1q Nephropathy

Epidemiology

This rare condition occurs mainly in children, adolescents, and young adults (57,58).

Clinical Symptoms

Severe proteinuria, often with nephrotic syndrome, is the predominant finding. Microscopic hematuria is common.

Light Microscopic Features

Normal renal parenchyma; mesangial prominence, usually with some hypercellularity; and FSGS have been described.

Immunofluorescence Characteristics

Predominant mesangial C1q staining in the absence of SLE is a prerequisite for the diagnosis. In addition to C1q, IgG, IgA, IgM, and C3 may be seen; indeed, sometimes all are present (57,58).

Electron Microscopic Features

Electron-dense, immune-type deposits are always present in the mesangium. Glomerular subendothelial or subepithelial deposits are rarely seen.

Differential Diagnosis

SLE should be excluded before making the diagnosis. Lupus patients with histologically normal glomeruli and mesangial deposits by IF and EM (WHO class II lupus nephritis) may have prominent mesangial C1q deposits but do not have nephrotic-range proteinuria. Endothelial tubuloreticular inclusions (frequently seen in lupus) are usually absent in C1q nephropathy. Minimal change disease and FSGS are easy to exclude on IF and EM.

Outcome

These patients usually have a poor response to steroids. Adequate long-term follow-up data are not yet available. ESRD has reportedly developed in some patients, while others did not progress to this stage.

Etiology and Pathogenesis

The origins of this condition are unclear.

Focal Segmental Glomerular Sclerosis (Focal Sclerosis)

It is important to emphasize that the pattern of FSGS and hyalinosis is nonspecific and that this pattern is associated with a variety of diseases. FSGS can be primary (idiopathic) or secondary. The secondary forms are associated with an identified underlying primary disorder (59–62). The diagnosis of idiopathic FSGS should be made only after careful clinicopathologic correlation and exclusion of other possible underlying conditions (secondary forms).

Epidemiology

FSGS is one of the glomerular lesions that most frequently leads to progressive renal insufficiency in children. In major renal pathology laboratories in the United States, the proportion of biopsy samples with FSGS is on the rise; it represents the most frequently seen glomerular pattern, not only in children but also in adults, in whom it reaches or surpasses the incidence of membranous GN (62–64). This is not the case in Europe and Asia, where IgA nephropathy is the most common glomerular disease and where membranous GN is the typical cause of INS in adults. It is interesting that in the United States, African-Americans are at considerably higher risk of FSGS than whites (62–64). There is a male predominance in most studies. While the incidence of various forms of FSGS is rising, FSGS associated with intravenous drug abuse (heroin-associated nephropathy) is almost disappearing in the New York City area despite the continuing high incidence of heroin abuse (65).

Clinical Symptoms

The disease is characterized by severe proteinuria; 70% to 80% of patients have overt nephrotic syndrome. There is often associated microhematuria, hypertension, and poorly selective proteinuria (as opposed to MCNS with "highly selective" proteinuria: albuminuria but no passage of larger proteins into the urine).

Light Microscopic Features

Some, but not all, glomeruli are affected (focal involvement) (Fig. 21A). Typically, in the affected glomeruli only a portion of the glomerular tuft (segmental involvement) shows closure and collapse of glomerular capillary lumens, increase in extracellular (mesangial) matrix, lining up of prominent visceral epithelium ("visceral epithelial cell caps") along the sclerotic loops, and adhesions or synechiae (Fig. 21B,C) (61,62,66). In the early stages, the segmental lesion may appear hypercellular (cellular lesion) (Fig. 21B). There may also be regions of superimposed hyalinosis [plasma protein insudation in sclerotic regions (Fig. 21C, Table 6), between the GBM and endothelium] and intracapillary foam cell accumulation. Because of the frequent presence of hyalinosis, the disease is also called focal segmental glomerular sclerosis and hyalinosis (FSGSH), although hyalinosis is not invariably present.

The uninvolved segments of the glomerulus appear to be normal on histologic evaluation, but eventually, with disease progression, the entire glomerular tuft will undergo sclerosis with or without hyalinosis (global involvement) (Fig. 22). The segmental process is thought by many investigators to

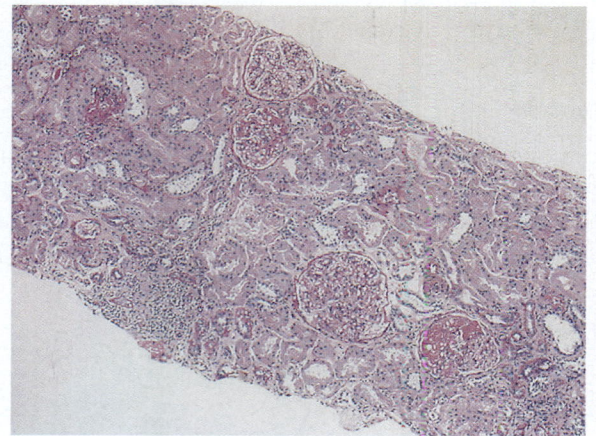
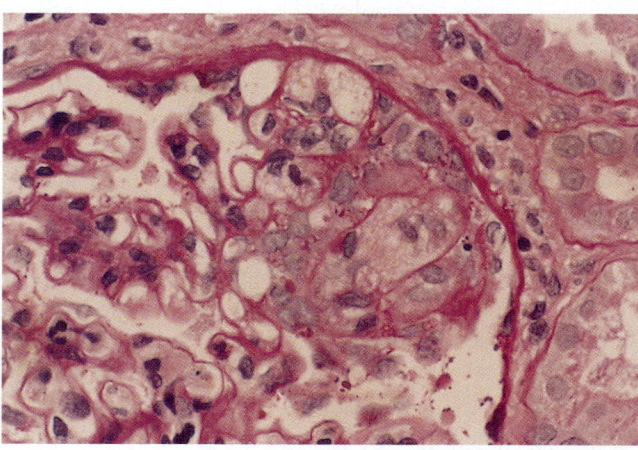

FIG. 21. Various appearances of glomeruli in focal segmental glomerular sclerosis (FSGS). **A:** Some glomeruli show segmental sclerosis and hyalinosis, while others are unremarkable or enlarged [periodic acid–Schiff (PAS)]. **B:** This picture shows a cellular (probably early) segmental lesion in FSGS. Note the segmental hypercellularity with intracapillary foam cells and prominent podocytes. The uninvolved segments of the glomerulus are unremarkable (PAS). **C:** Methenamine silver stain is the best method to show hyalinosis in areas of sclerosis; hyaline is silver negative, whereas sclerosis is silver positive.

TABLE 6. *Morphologic differential diagnosis of homogeneous acellular glomerular material*

Stain	Hyalinosis	Sclerosis	Amyloid	Fibrosis	Fibrin thrombus
H&E (eosinophilia)	+++	+++	++	++	+++
PAS	+++	+++	+	++	+
MS	−	+++	−	+	−
Trichrome (Masson's)	Red/blue	Blue	Blue	Blue	Dark red
Congo red	−	−	+++	−	−

H&E, hematoxyin and eosin; PAS, periodic acid–Schiff; MS, methenamine silver.

begin in the juxtamedullary glomeruli and usually, but not always, at the vascular pole or hilum of the involved glomerulus, especially near the afferent arteriole. The other glomeruli are normal on histologic examination or may show glomerular visceral epithelial cells. Glomerular enlargement is a common finding in FSGS. Mesangial prominence and hypercellularity away from the regions of focal and segmental sclerosis may be noted in FSGS, just as in MCNS (see earlier discussion). Tubular atrophy, interstitial fibrosis and inflammation, and arteriolar hyalin are frequently present.

Immunofluorescence Characteristics

In the regions of segmental sclerosis, IgM and C3 are frequently present. This may be related to nonimmune absorption of the large molecule IgM (900,000 d in molecular weight) in the sclerotic areas, with complement possibly secondarily activated locally. Diffuse mesangial IgM can be seen, comparable to that in cases of MCNS (see earlier discussion). Weak, patchy fluorescence for fibrinogen is occasionally visible in glomerular capillaries.

Electron Microscopic Features

All glomerular capillaries (even in glomeruli that look normal on LM) display visceral epithelial cell foot process effacement, while the sclerotic regions show evidence of increased mesangial matrix, capillary collapse, and prominence of the overlying visceral epithelial cells. Vacuolation and focal detachment of the visceral epithelial cells from the GBM are frequently noted. Discrete, immune-type, electron-dense deposits are not present; however, a few small mesangial, variably electron-dense deposits may be visible. It is important not to misinterpret glomerular hyalinosis as immune deposits. Hyaline is a bulky, amorphous, electron-dense material frequently admixed with lipid droplets (Fig. 23). It usually forms in sclerotic areas with collapsed/sclerotic capillary loops right below the GBM and frequently contains lipid droplets. A good clue to their differentiation is to look at glomerular segments with normal-appearing glomerular capillary loops and mesangium away from sclerotic areas. In cases of segmental hyalinosis, no deposits will be seen in these areas, whereas in cases of immune complex GN, deposits will generally be found throughout the glomerulus.

Differential Diagnosis

The differential diagnosis of FSGS and MCNS is discussed in the section on MCNS. Focal segmental sclerosis in glomeruli is a pattern of renal response and not a specific disease entity (59,62). Some of the diseases and conditions in

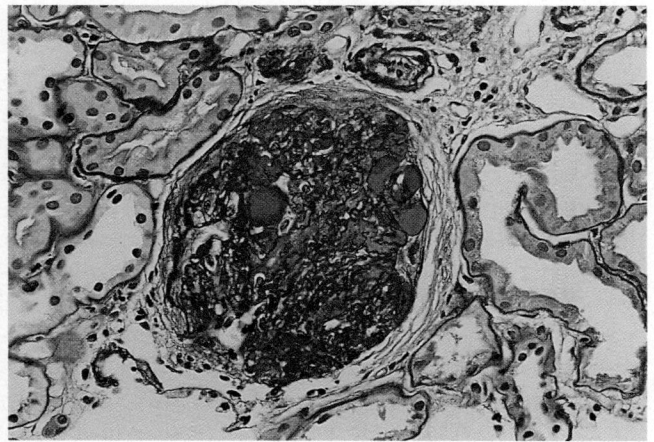

FIG. 22. Global sclerosis and hyalinosis in a glomerulus. The hyalinized areas are more homogeneous (periodic acid–Schiff).

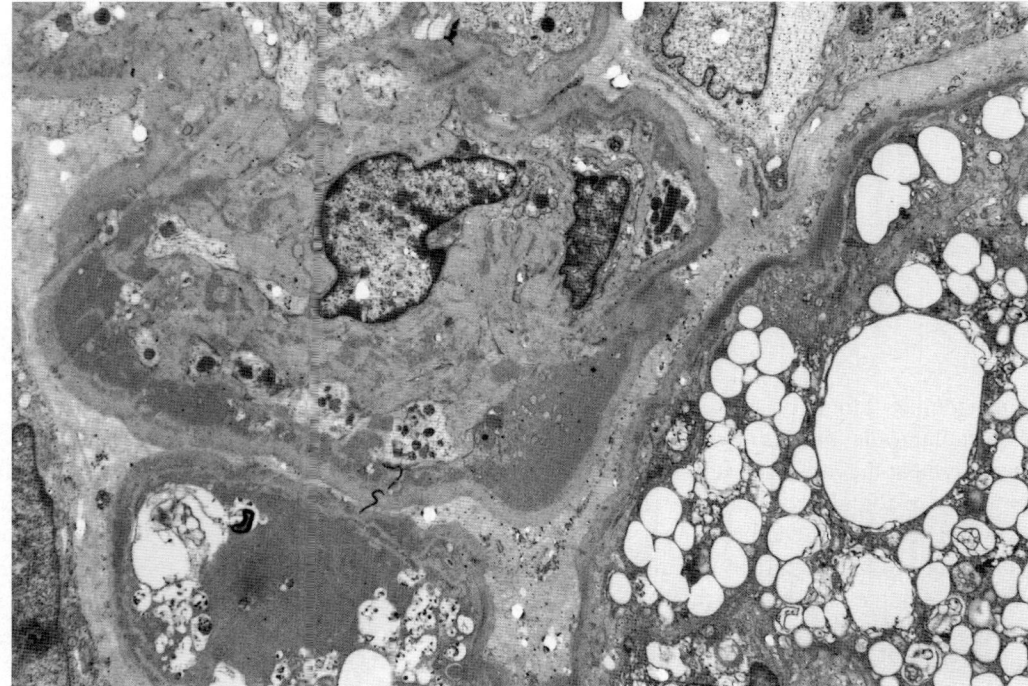

FIG. 23. Focal segmental glomerular sclerosis and hyalinosis. On ultrastructural inspection, hyaline deposits are homogeneous, electron-dense, and somewhat similar to immune deposits. One distinguishing feature is that hyaline deposits may contain lipid vacuoles. Note the intracapillary foam cell in the right-lower corner (uranyl acetate, lead citrate; ×1,600).

which segmental glomerulosclerosis may occur are IgA nephropathy, membranous GN, dense-deposit disease, "healed" focal GN, heroin-associated nephropathy, human immunodeficiency virus–associated nephropathy (HIVAN), collapsing glomerulopathy, long-standing hypertension (see benign nephrosclerosis), reduced renal mass (hyperperfusion/hyperfiltration injury, e.g., oligomeganephronic hypoplasia, other forms of renal hypoplasia/dysplasia renal ablation/nephrectomy), morbid obesity, Alport's syndrome, congenital cyanotic heart disease, sickle cell disease, and chronic pyelonephritis/reflux nephropathy

This list is far from complete, and, in fact, a segmentally sclerotic glomerulus can be an incidental finding or a late, final common pathway of severe glomerular injury. It is most important in differential diagnosis to carefully correlate the clinical history, clinical symptoms, and laboratory findings with the results of LM, IF, and EM. The diagnosis of idiopathic FSGS should be made in the appropriate clinical context only if secondary causes can be excluded.

Outcome

Idiopathic FSGS is a slowly progressive disease. Most patients fail to respond to therapy from the beginning. The more glomeruli affected by segmental or global sclerosis and hyalinosis, and the more widespread the interstitial fibrosis with tubular atrophy, the worse the prognosis. Some investigators suggest that mesangial hypercellularity is an indicator of unfavorable outcome, but this theory could not be confirmed by others. Clinical indicators of poor outcome include increased serum creatinine at the time of biopsy, high blood pressure, and severe nephrotic-range proteinuria resistant to therapy. African-Americans apparently have a more rapid progression (60,62). The recurrence rate of FSGS in renal transplants is about 30%. Young age, development of renal failure within 3 years of diagnosis, and, possibly, mesangial prominence predispose to recurrent disease (67). Once there is a recurrence, the recurrence rate in subsequent grafts is more than 80%.

Etiologic Factors and Pathogenesis

The pathogenesis of FSGS may involve immunologic, genetic, toxic, or systemic factors as well as mesangial dysfunction, coagulation, or hemodynamic factors. Whether the primary lesion is mesangial, visceral epithelial, capillary wall, or hemodynamic is not known. It has been suggested by Brenner and co-workers (68) that progressive loss of nephron mass may, through loss of normal reflex vasoconstriction of the afferent arteriole, allow (a) hyperperfusion of the remaining glomeruli, with increased capillary pressure across the glomerular capillary wall and subsequent hyperfiltration (hyperperfusion/hyperfiltration injury), and (b) functional mesangial changes and, eventually, development of FSGS irrespective of the pattern of initial glomerular damage. Thus it may be a common final pathway of progressive glomerular injury. This may be true in many conditions, but the fact that a certain percentage of cases of idiopathic FSGS recur very shortly after transplantation (with severe proteinuria), and that these cases show repeated recurrence in subsequent grafts, is very much in favor of a systemic circulating factor in at least this subpopulation of cases. There is some evidence for the existence of such factors(s) (50).

The Issue of Focal Global Glomerulosclerosis in Idiopathic Nephrotic Syndrome

Focal global glomerulosclerosis associated with INS is considered to be a separate entity in several studies. These cases appear to be responsive to steroids and have outcomes similar to those of MCNS; some of them, however, progress to ESRD (69). We have strong doubts that seeing one, or a few, sclerotic glomeruli admixed with normal glomeruli in nephrotic patients warrants a separate diagnosis. It is possible to see a few obsolescent glomeruli (up to 10% in adults under the age the age of 40) in any condition, even in normal kidneys and in MCNS (Fig. 12) (70). Thus, it is important to decide in such instances whether the glomerulus is truly sclerotic or obsolescent (for comparison see Figs. 12 and 22). A useful hint, when the glomerulus in question contains hyalinosis, is that hyalinosis is not present in obsolescent glomeruli. If true sclerotic glomeruli are seen—particularly in association with hyalinosis—a primary glomerular disease, such as FSGS (idiopathic or secondary), should be considered. One has to remember that in conditions with the pattern of FSGS, one might miss the diagnostic segmental lesions but see globally sclerotic glomeruli.

Human Immunodeficiency Virus–associated Nephropathy (Synonym: Human Immunodeficiency Virus–positive Collapsing Glomerulopathy) and Collapsing Glomerulopathy

HIVAN is discussed as a variant of FSGS in most textbooks and reviews. There are some similarities between the glomerular morphologic findings in HIVAN and idiopathic FSGS; still, we believe that the morphologic features and, in particular, the clinical behavior of HIVAN are different enough to consider this a separate disease. On the other hand, HIVAN and collapsing glomerulopathy in HIV-negative patients are so similar that they most likely represent the same, or very closely related, diseases.

Epidemiology

HIV-positive African-American male patients are most often affected, but African-American women also get the disease (71–73). HIVAN is unusual in whites. The HIV-negative form of collapsing glomerulopathy is less typical, but it also primarily affects African-Americans (74,75).

Clinical Symptoms

The disease is characterized by severe, usually nephrotic-range proteinuria with a relatively short clinical history. Renal impairment is evident at the time of diagnosis. HIVAN may be an early manifestation of HIV infection, and it is not unusual for a patient's HIV-positive status to be discovered on a renal biopsy suggestive of HIVAN. Collapsing glomerulopathy in HIV-negative patients has very similar clinical features.

Light Microscopic Features

The characteristic glomerular lesion is a predominantly collapsing type of focal glomerulosclerosis that is segmental or, more frequently, global (Fig 24) (71–77). The collapsing capillary loops are best appreciated by PAS or methenamine silver stains. The podocytes are particularly prominent; they are swollen, typically fill the entire Bowman's space, and

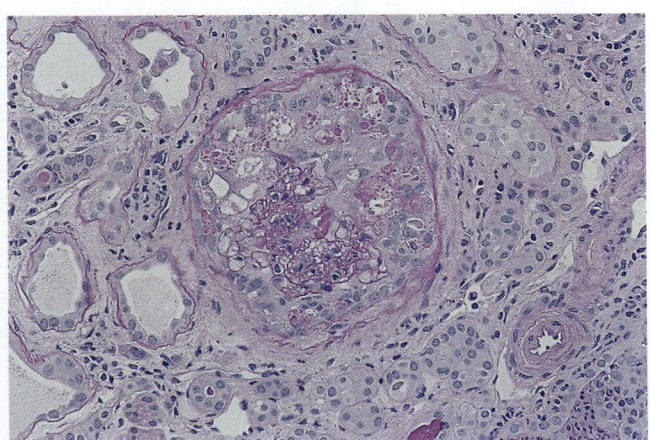
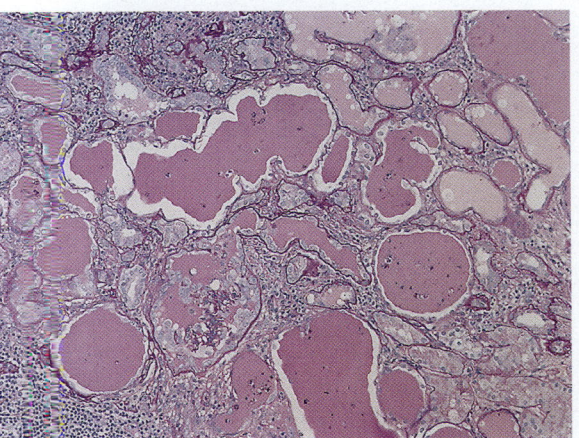

FIG. 24. Human immunodeficiency virus–associated nephropathy. **A:** The most characteristic lesion is glomerular capillary loop collapse surrounded by prominent podocytes resembling crescents. These podocytes usually contain large protein resorption droplets that are periodic acid–Schiff (PAS) positive. Also note the inflammatory cell infiltrate in the surrounding interstitium (PAS). **B:** On lower magnification, it is apparent that in addition to the collapsing glomerular lesion, prominent interstitial disease, with microcystic tubular dilatation and an inflammatory cell infiltrate, is present (PAS).

may contain large protein droplets in the cytoplasm. Unlike idiopathic FSGS, the tubulointerstitial changes are also very characteristic. There is usually quite striking interstitial fibrosis with tubular loss and atrophy at the time of diagnosis. A distinctive (but not specific) finding is microcystic dilatation of a few tubules, with a scalloping outline (Fig. 24). Large numbers of protein resorption droplets are frequently seen in hypertrophic proximal tubular epithelial cells. A prominent mononuclear interstitial infiltrate, which consists mainly of lymphocytes and macrophages, is almost invariably present.

Immunofluorescence Characteristics

As in FSGS, the findings on IF are negative or nonspecific.

Electron Microscopic Features

A distinctive, but nonspecific change is the presence of endothelial tubuloreticular inclusions (Fig. 25). These inclusions are most likely not part of the renal disease process, but rather a response to HIV infection. They reflect high interferon alpha levels and are also called interferon footprints. They are also frequently seen in lupus nephritis. Discrete, electron-dense, immune-type deposits are not part of HIVAN.

Differential Diagnosis

HIVAN must be distinguished from other forms of FSGS, including idiopathic FSGS and heroin-associated nephropathy (62,77). Heroin-associated nephropathy is more reminiscent of idiopathic FSGS than of HIVAN on histologic and clinical grounds. Changes characteristically seen in HIV-positive and HIV-negative collapsing glomerulopathy, and less frequently in other forms of FSGS, are collapsing glomerulosclerosis with prominent podocytes, prominent chronic and acute tubulointerstitial disease with microcystic dilatation of tubules, and endothelial tubuloreticular inclusions on EM. The only difference between HIVAN and the HIV-negative form of collapsing glomerulopathy is the presence of tubuloreticular inclusions in HIVAN. Of course, any kind of renal disease, such as immune complex glomerulonephritides, can develop in HIV-positive patients, just as in the general population (79); they should not be diagnosed as HIVAN.

Outcome

ESRD develops in most patients within weeks or months of clinical onset. This is true for both HIVAN and HIV-negative collapsing glomerulopathy.

Etiology and Pathogenesis

The pathogenesis of HIVAN is unclear. There is no convincing evidence that direct HIV infection of renal parenchymal cells is responsible for the changes. The preponderance in African-American men indicates a genetic predisposition.

Membranous Glomerulonephritis (Synonyms: Membranous Nephropathy, Membranous Glomerulonephropathy, Epimembranous or Extramembranous Glomerulonephritis)

Membranous GN is another morphologic pattern that can be either idiopathic (primary) or associated with a variety of disorders (see the section on pathogenesis) (80).

Epidemiology

Membranous GN is the most common cause of idiopathic nephrotic syndrome in nondiabetic adults, particularly in the elderly, in most parts of the world. It is relatively rare in children.

Clinical Symptoms

The condition usually begins with the insidious development of marked proteinuria (usually with the nephrotic syndrome). Microscopic hematuria and hypertension may be present.

Light Microscopic Features

In early-stage cases, the glomeruli may appear normal, and the diagnosis can be rendered only on the basis of IF and EM. The histologic picture is usually characteristic and identifiable in more advanced stages. There is diffuse thickening

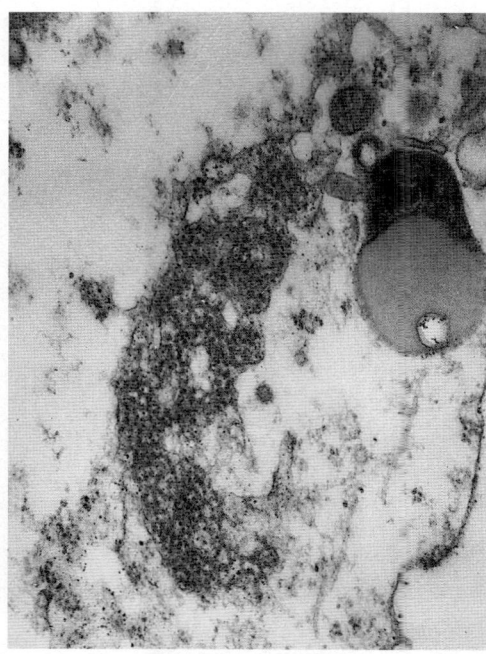

FIG. 25. Endothelial tubuloreticular inclusion in a glomerular capillary of a patient with human immunodeficiency virus–associated nephropathy (uranyl acetate, lead citrate; ×22,000).

of the glomerular capillary walls (Fig. 26A,B) as the result of electron-dense deposits on the epithelial side of the GBM, with or without the formation of methenamine silver–positive projections of GBM-like material (so-called spikes) between these deposits (81,82). Note that the spikes (basement membrane surrounding the deposits), and not the deposits, are silver positive. If the glomerular capillary wall is cut en face or if the disease is advanced and the nonargyrophilic deposits are engulfed by basement membrane material, a moth-eaten or Swiss cheese–like appearance of the thickened GBM is noted in methenamine silver–stained sections (Fig. 26B). Masson's trichrome stain sometimes reveals the fuchsinophilic subepithelial deposits if they are large enough. The glomeruli usually are not hypercellular. In some cases, however, mesangial prominence with or without hypercellularity may be noted, as will superimposed focal segmental sclerosis (the latter is especially obvious in advancing stages) (83).

FIG. 27. Immunofluorescence picture of a glomerulus in membranous glomerulonephritis. Note the diffuse, finely granular deposits outlining the glomerular capillary walls (anti-IgG; ×250).

Immunofluorescence Characteristics

Diffuse, granular, glomerular capillary wall deposits of IgG (100% of cases), C3 (75% of cases), and sometimes other immunoreactants are virtually diagnostic of this disease (Fig. 27). Mesangial deposits may be present.

Electron Microscopic Features

EM is the best method for diagnosing membranous GN. There are numerous glomerular, subepithelial, electron-dense, immune-type deposits close to each other throughout the capillary loops (Fig. 28). As the disease progresses, basement membrane–like material will protrude between the deposits. Mesangial electron-dense deposits, though not characteristic, may develop even in the absence of lupus nephritis (34).

Staging of Membranous GN

A widely used staging system was introduced by Ehrenreich and Churg (81), reflecting the morphologic stage of the disease based particularly on ultrastructural examination. In stage I, there are subepithelial deposits without spikes. Stage II has basement membrane spikes between the subepithelial deposits. By stage III, most deposits are engulfed by the

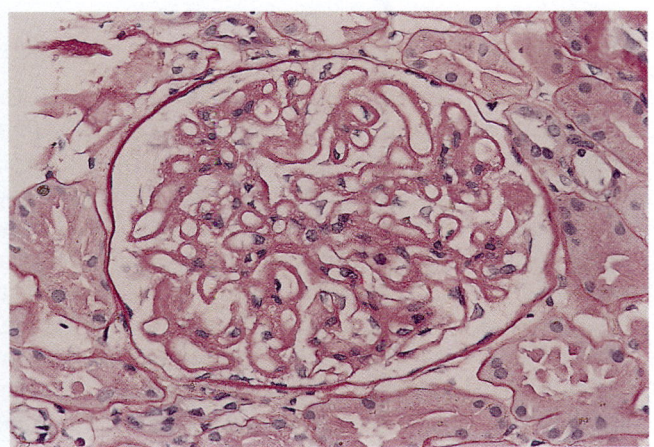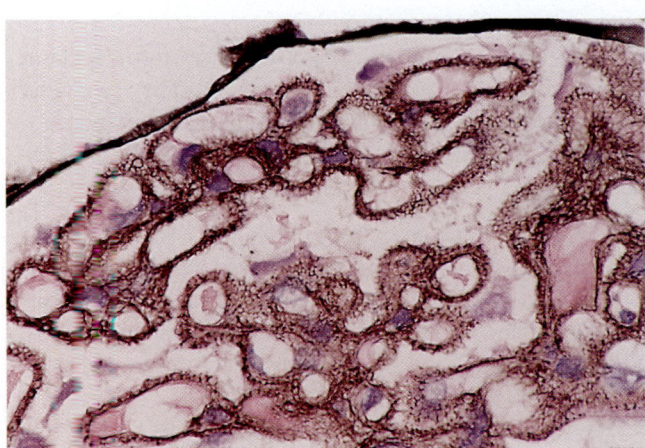

FIG. 26. Membranous glomerulonephritis. A: Note the diffusely thickened, rigid glomerular capillary walls [periodic acid–Schiff (PAS)]. B: Methenamine silver stain shows the argyrophilic spikes on the subepithelial surface of the glomerular basement membrane. These spikes represent basement membrane material protruding between the silver-negative immune deposits. En face sectioning of these spikes or deposits completely engulfed by basement membrane material will result in holes in the basement membrane (methenamine silver).

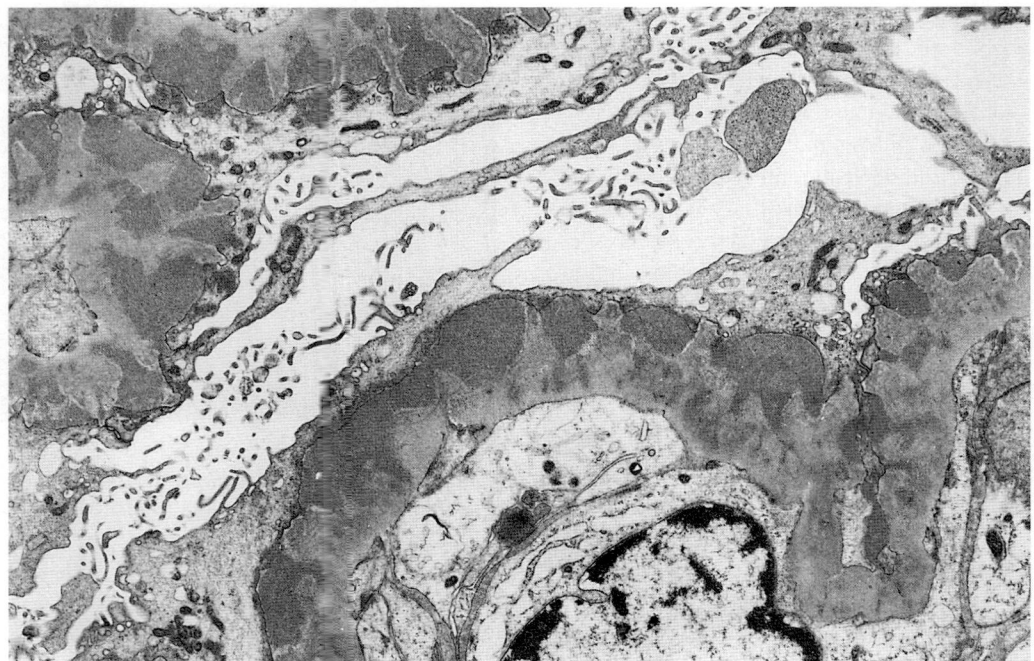

FIG. 28. Ultrastructural appearance of membranous glomerulonephritis. There are many, discrete, immune-type, electron-dense subepithelial deposits between which spikes of glomerular basement membrane–like material protrude toward Bowman's space (uranyl acetate, lead citrate; ×3,800).

thickened basement membrane; some deposits are still electron dense, while others have an electron-lucent appearance ("washed out" deposits). In stage IV, there are vague, washed-out deposits in the markedly thickened GBM. Stages III and IV may give the GBM a so-called tram-track appearance if impregnated with silver. There are many overlaps between these stages, and it is debatable whether this staging of membranous GN has any prognostic value.

Differential Diagnosis

Membranous GN is a morphologic pattern noted in association with many disorders. These secondary forms account for 20% to 25% of cases in many series (80). They cannot be differentiated from idiopathic membranous GN by morphologic features alone. There are several secondary associations.

1. SLE (class V lupus nephritis). In lupus-associated membranous GN there are always mesangial deposits. Endothelial tubuloreticular inclusions are usually present, and IF characteristically shows a "full house" pattern (in addition to IgG and C3, other immunoreactants, such as IgA, C1q, and IgM are also present) (84).
2. Infections (hepatitis B, sometimes hepatitis C, syphilis, etc.) (85,86).
3. Neoplasms. Carcinomas of the lung, gastrointestinal tract, and breast are found, particularly in patients above the age of 60 years (80,87).
4. Toxins and therapeutic agents (gold, mercury, d-penicillamine).
5. A number of diseases, such as rheumatoid arthritis, thyroiditis, inflammatory bowel disease, and others (80).

Other glomerular diseases are easy to differentiate by IF and EM. On LM only, early-stage membranous GN may be indistinguishable from MCNS or early-stage amyloidosis, which also can cause severe proteinuria. In advanced stages, LM features may resemble those of diffuse diabetic glomerulosclerosis or other advanced sclerosing glomerular diseases with glomerular capillary loop thickening and sometimes FSGS (83).

Outcome

Membranous GN is typically a very slowly progressive disease. The overall 10-year survival is between 77% and 90% (88). Segmental glomerular sclerosis, prominent interstitial fibrosis with tubular atrophy, very heavy proteinuria, and high blood pressure portend a more rapid progression. Secondary forms usually regress if the underlying cause can be eliminated. Renal vein thrombosis is a fairly typical complication of membranous GN, as well as of other glomerular diseases, leading to longstanding nephrotic syndrome (89). The recurrence rate of membranous GN in renal transplants appears to be relatively low, but this rate is difficult to assess because membranous GN is the most common de novo glomerular disease in renal allografts.

Etiologic Factors and Pathogenesis

There is good evidence, at least in experimental models, that many, if not most, examples of membranous GN represent *in situ* immune complex formation (i.e., circulating antibody binding to antigens normally present, or previously localized, along the glomerular capillary walls) rather than the deposition of circulating immune complexes along the glomerular capillary wall (90). Besides IgG and C3, the deposits also contain the terminal C5B-9 complex (the membrane attack complex), which is excreted in the urine (91). The causes of secondary forms were listed earlier.

Diabetic Nephropathy

Epidemiology

Diabetic nephropathy is the most common cause of ESRD in the United States.

Clinical Symptoms

Microalbuminuria is the first warning sign of renal disease in diabetic patients (92,93). With time, proteinuria becomes more and more severe and less selective. Eventually, most patients will experience nephrotic-range proteinuria and renal failure. Hypertension is common. Microscopic hematuria may occur, but it is not typical. Advancing renal disease usually shows good correlation with eyeground changes, but not always. In fact, most kidney biopsy samples with evidence of diabetic glomerulosclerosis are from patients with renal disease in the absence of eyeground changes, which may be an indication for renal biopsy.

Light Microscopic Features

There are no substantial histologic differences in the renal changes caused by type I and type II diabetes (93–95). These characteristic lesions are seen in the glomeruli and arterioles (Fig. 29): diffuse glomerulosclerosis (diffuse thickening of the GBM and diffuse increase in mesangial matrix) (Fig. 29A), nodular glomerulosclerosis (Kimmelstiel-Wilson mesangial nodules) (Fig. 29B), insudative changes (fibrin

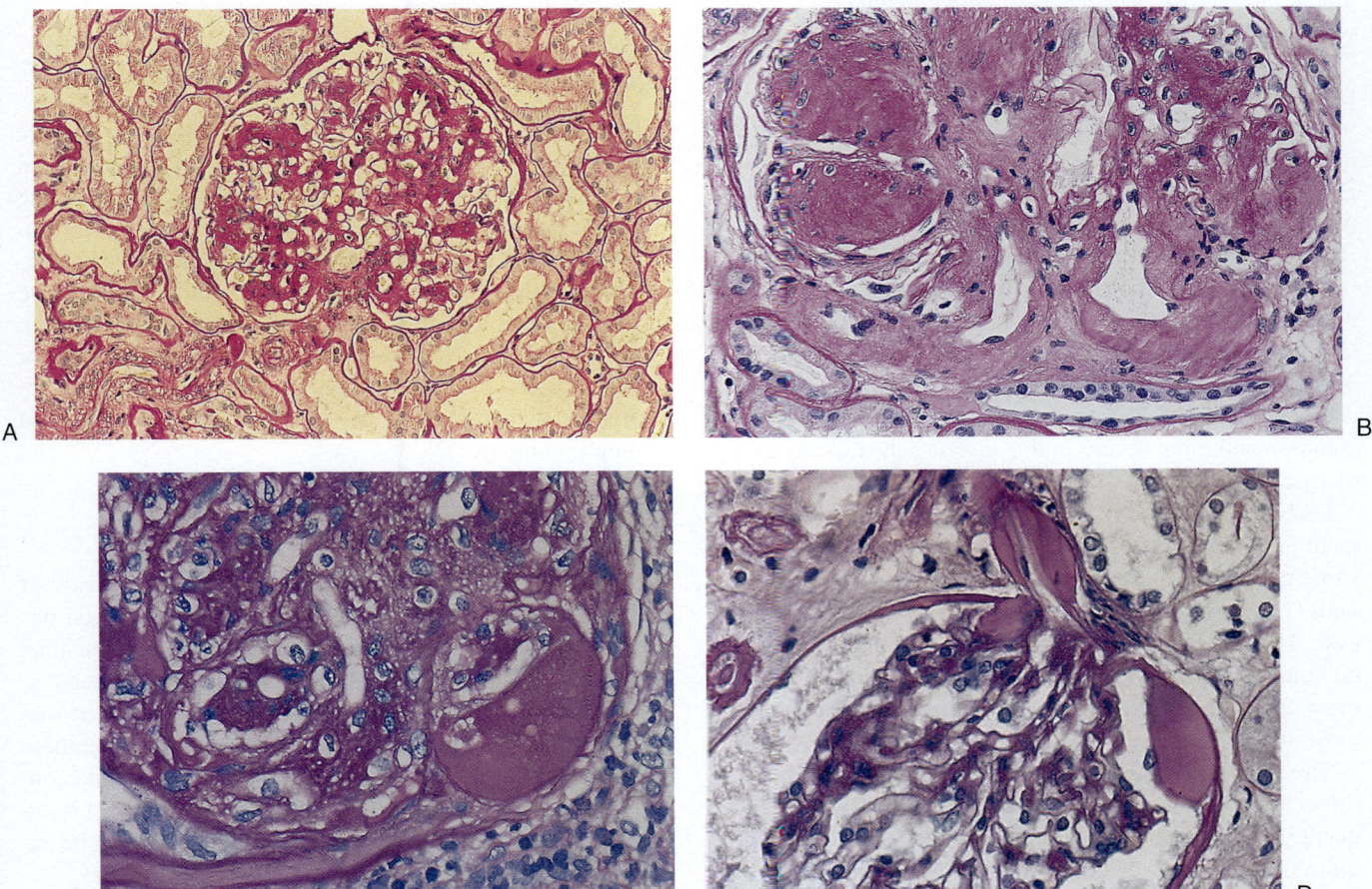

FIG. 29. Various appearances of diabetic glomerulosclerosis. **A:** In diffuse diabetic glomerulosclerosis, there is diffuse widening of the mesangium, occasionally with mild hypercellularity [periodic acid–Schiff (PAS)]. **B:** Nodular diabetic glomerulosclerosis. Note the acellular glomerular nodules occasionally surrounded by thickened glomerular capillaries. Also note the hyaline change in both the afferent and efferent arterioles (PAS). **C:** Prominent hyaline insudation (fibrin cap) in a glomerulus with diabetic glomerulosclerosis (PAS). **D:** Capsular drop is an area of circumscribed hyaline change in Bowman's capsule, protruding into Bowman's space. Also note the arteriolar hyaline change (PAS).

caps, capsular drops) (Fig. 29C,D), and prominent arteriolar hyalinosis that frequently involves both the afferent and efferent arterioles (Fig. 29B).

Diffuse diabetic glomerulosclerosis is characterized by an increase in the amount of mesangial matrix in all mesangial regions of all glomeruli, associated with diffuse thickening of the GBM. GBM thickening may not be detected by LM, because the GBM must be at least two to three times the normal thickness to be recognized as thickened by LM (Fig. 29A).

Nodular diabetic glomerulosclerosis was first described by Kimmelstiel and Wilson in 1936, hence, the name Kimmelstiel-Wilson nodule. There are sclerotic nodules in one or more intercapillary or mesangial regions of the glomerular tuft (Fig. 29B). These somewhat acellular nodules are often peripheral and laminated (with silver stain) and consist, on morphologic inspection, of material with the same staining properties as mesangial matrix and GBM. The acellular nodule may be surrounded by dilated glomerular capillary loops (microaneurysms). Nodular glomerulosclerosis is almost always superimposed upon preexisting diffuse diabetic glomerulosclerosis. The number of nodules tends to increase with the clinical duration of diabetes.

The insudative glomerular lesions consist of the so-called fibrin cap (Fig. 29C) and the capsular drop (Fig. 29D). Originally named exudation, the term insudation more correctly describes the phenomenon. Both insudative lesions are the result of accumulation of plasma proteins (hyalinosis)—between the glomerular endothelium and the GBM in the fibrin cap and between the parietal epithelial cell and Bowman's capsule in the capsular drop (another lesion that Kimmelstiel thought was pathognomonic of diabetes). These insudative lesions are more common in more severe patterns of diabetic glomerulosclerosis. Neither insudative lesion is pathognomonic of diabetic nephropathy, but both are more common and more severe in this disorder than in any other disease.

Diabetic glomerulosclerosis appears to favor the development of GN. Postinfectious GN seems to be the typical GN superimposed on diabetic glomerulosclerosis (96). Membranous GN is another frequently superimposed glomerular disease. The association of membranous GN with diabetes may be coincidental, however, because membranous GN is the most common form of GN in the elderly, the population most often affected by type II diabetes.

The renal arterioles show insudative changes similar to those found in the glomeruli (arteriolar hyalinosis). Frequently, both afferent and efferent arterioles (the efferent are quite characteristic of diabetes) show signs of prominent hyalinosis (Fig. 29B). Fibrous intimal thickening is a routine finding in arteries. These changes may be seen in the absence of hypertension and develop concomitantly with the glomerular changes.

Tubular changes include protein resorption droplets in the proximal tubules and tubular atrophy. Interstitial fibrosis and chronic interstitial inflammation may be so pronounced as to suggest underlying chronic pyelonephritis. These long-term tubulointerstitial changes can take place in the absence of infection and are probably related to the accompanying severe vascular disease and ischemia. Severe acute and chronic pyelonephritis is not an unusual complication of diabetic nephropathy, however, and papillary necrosis, with or without pyelonephritis, is most often seen in diabetic patients (see discussion of analgesic nephropathy).

Immunofluorescence Characteristics

A mild to moderate, nonspecific, linear, glomerular capillary loop staining for IgG is typical. The binding of the IgG antibody to the GBM is nonspecific and is probably due to passive imbibition of serum proteins into the thickened, glycosylated GBM. Similar linear staining is almost always seen with antibodies to albumin. No anti-GBM antibody activity can be detected in these patients. Mild, linear IgG and albumin staining may be seen along tubular and Bowman's capsular basement membranes as well. Nonspecific deposition of the macromolecule IgM and C3 is evident in areas of sclerosis and hyalinosis.

Electron Microscopic Features

Thickening of the GBM is invariably seen in diabetic glomerulosclerosis (Fig. 30), accompanied by an increase in the mesangial matrix. In nodular glomerulosclerosis, the nodules may show a fibrillary substructure (diabetic fibrillosis), which is probably a degenerative feature of the increased glomerular extracellular matrix and should not be misinterpreted as amyloidosis or fibrillary GN (Fig. 31). Hyalin deposits have a similar appearance, as described for FSGS. Discrete immune-type, electron-dense deposits are not seen; if present, they are suggestive of a superimposed immune complex GN.

Differential Diagnosis

Sclerotic mesangial nodules are highly characteristic of diabetes mellitus, although similar lesions have been observed in some other conditions, among them, monoclonal immunoglobulin (usually kappa light chain) deposition disease, advanced MPGN, and congenital cyanotic heart disease. Amyloidosis can produce mesangial nodules, but these nodules are not sclerotic (they are silver negative) and consist of amyloid (Table 6). Idiopathic nodular GN (22) is another possibility, if all the other listed conditions can be excluded.

The sclerotic nodules in light chain deposition disease, advanced MPGN, and so-called idiopathic nodular GN differ from those in nodular diabetic glomerulosclerosis. They are usually greater in number and are more uniform within each glomerulus and throughout all glomeruli than in diabetic glomerulosclerosis. Moreover, glomerular and arteriolar hyalinosis is usually less severe than in diabetic nephropa-

Eastern countries, where it represents more than 30% of the conditions found on renal biopsy. In Europe, although slightly less frequently encountered, it is still the predominant glomerular disease (101,102). For unknown reasons, this is not the case in the United States, where membranous GN and FSGS are more often seen. IgA nephropathy is less common in African-Americans than in whites. The disease typically develops in young adults, but it may be found in any age group. HSP is much less common than IgA nephropathy and is mainly a disease of children (103).

Clinical Symptoms

Hematuria is invariably present, usually only of microscopic extent, but the disease occasionally manifests with gross hematuria and the nephritic syndrome. Episodes of gross hematuria may occur during the course of disease. Proteinuria can be very mild, but significant proteinuria (more than 0.5 g/24 hour urine) is not unusual. In some cases, even nephrotic-range proteinuria is present. Renal function is usually normal at the time of diagnosis. In HSP, the renal symptoms are identical but are associated with abdominal pain, joint pain, purpura, and other symptoms.

Light Microscopic Features

IgA nephropathy does not have a truly characteristic light microscopic appearance; it shows a variety of patterns. Perhaps the most typical and classic glomerular lesion is mesangioproliferative GN with focal or diffuse mesangial hypercellularity and widening (Fig. 32). Other patterns seen on LM include essentially normal-appearing glomeruli, focal and segmental proliferative or necrotizing GN, FSGS with or without hyalinosis, and, rarely, crescentic GN and a membranoproliferative pattern (99,100,105–107).

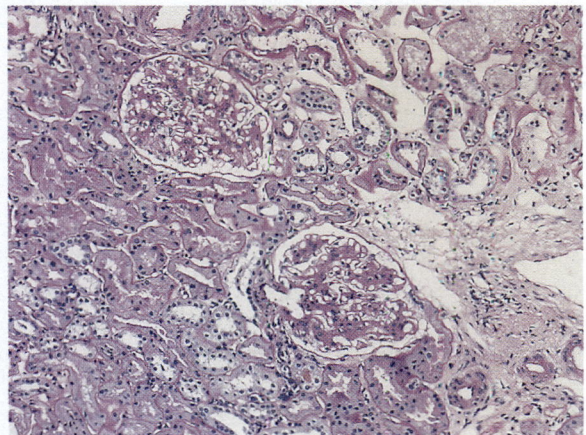

FIG. 32. IgA nephropathy (Berger's disease). Focally accentuated mesangial expansion with variable degrees of mesangial hypercellularity is a characteristic finding in the early stages. Note that in this early-stage case, no prominent tubulointerstitial changes are present (periodic acid–Schiff).

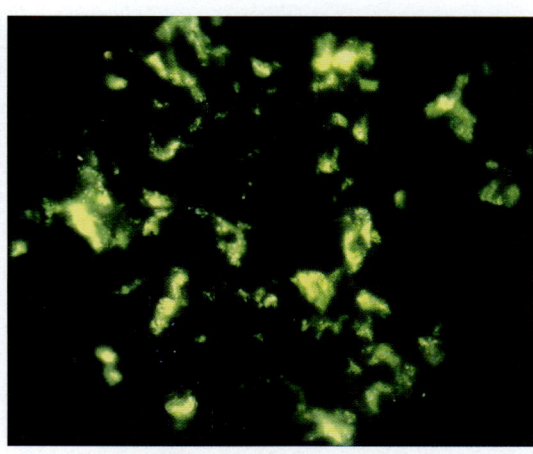

FIG. 33. IgA nephropathy. Diffuse mesangial granular immunofluorescence with an anti-IgA antibody (anti-IgA; ×500).

Immunofluorescence Characteristics

The only way to diagnose IgA nephropathy is to perform IF on a renal biopsy sample. By definition, IF studies reveal diffuse, global, and predominant, or at least co-dominant (no immunoreactant shows stronger fluorescence then IgA), mesangial IgA fluorescence in all cases (Fig. 33). IgG and IgM, sometimes of lesser intensity, are noted in about one-half to two-thirds of cases. C3 (usually of the same intensity as IgG or IgA) is found in more than three-fourths of cases. Rarely, C1q and C4 are present. FRA is also often seen, as is properdin. In addition to mesangial fluorescence, granular glomerular capillary wall staining for IgA may be found.

Electron Microscopic Features

Virtually all biopsies show electron-dense, discrete, immune-type deposits in the glomerular mesangial matrix (Fig. 34). In some (usually early-stage) cases, they are preferentially located immediately below the basement membrane covering the mesangium (these are also called paramesangial deposits). Occasionally, peripheral glomerular capillary wall deposits are noted. In a review by Navas-Palacios et al. (108) of ten series (335 patients with IgA nephropathy), only 13% of patients had glomerular subepithelial deposits, 14% had intramembranous deposits, and 17% had subendothelial deposits. These deposits are usually quite small and are virtually never as abundant and large as the peripheral glomerular capillary wall deposits seen in SLE. Other investigators have found more numerous and larger glomerular capillary wall deposits in more severe forms of IgA nephropathy.

Differential Diagnosis

Because of the variable light microscopic appearances, the differential diagnosis at the light microscopic level may include any glomerular disease. IF is essential to the differential diagnosis. Other diseases in which mesangial IgA depo-

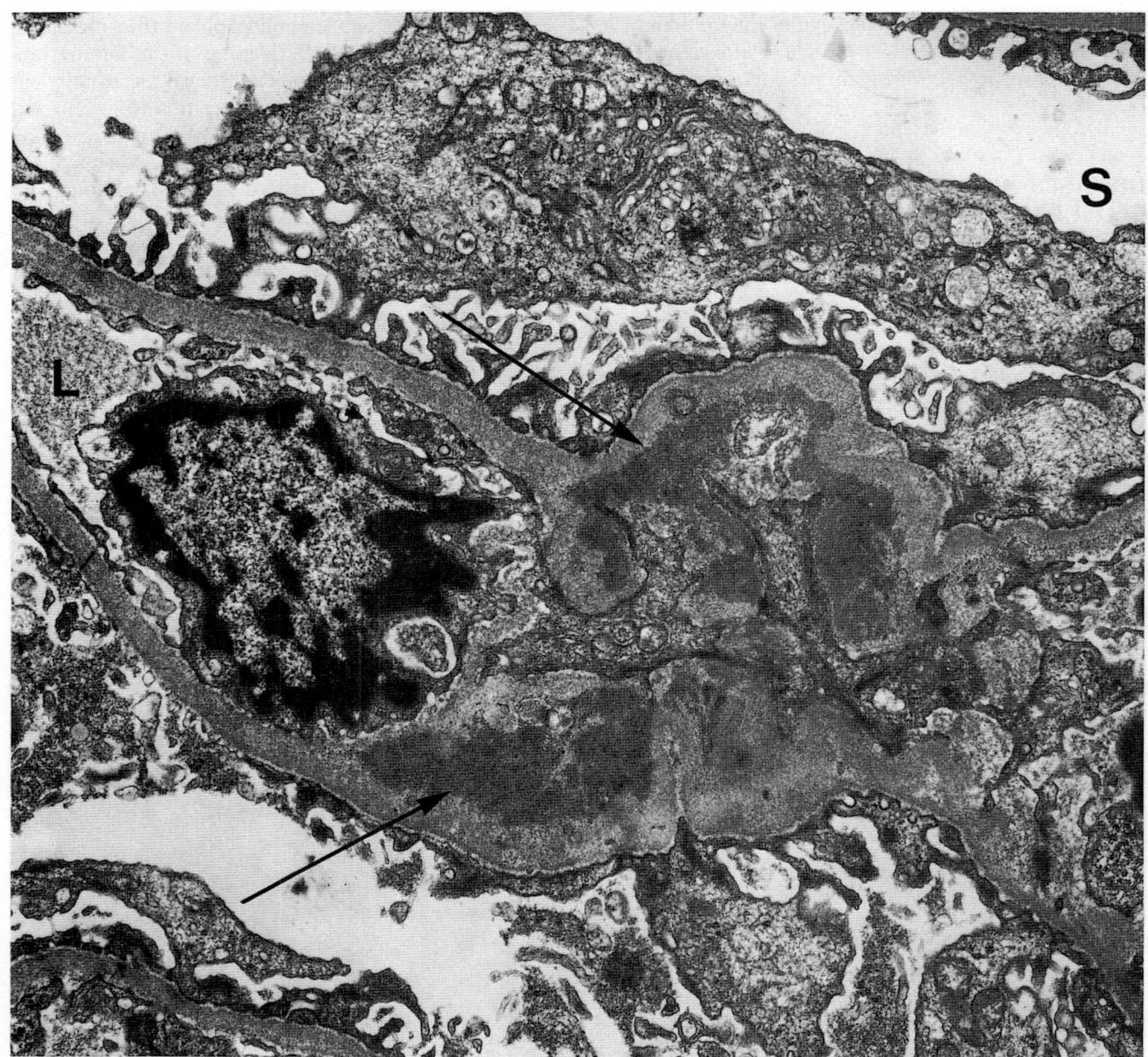

FIG. 34. IgA nephropathy. Electron micrograph shows discrete, electron-dense, immune-type deposits in the glomerular paramesangial area (*arrows*). Note that the deposits are not within the mesangial cells themselves but are just in the adjacent mesangial matrix. L, capillary lumen; S, Bowman's space (uranyl acetate, lead citrate; ×10,000).

sition can be prominent include lupus nephritis and hepatic glomerulosclerosis. In lupus nephritis IgA may be co-dominant, but it is rarely the predominant immunoreactant. In lupus nephritis, there typically is a full-house IF (most immunoreactants are positive), and EM frequently reveals endothelial tubuloreticular inclusions. Still, in some cases only clinical and laboratory data characteristic of SLE provide us with the correct diagnosis. Hepatic glomerulosclerosis may have morphologic characteristics identical to those of IgA nephropathy, including IF and EM findings. A history of chronic liver disease, usually with cirrhosis, is the only finding that distinguishes this condition. In fact, hepatic glomerulosclerosis, if accompanied by pre- or co-dominant mesangial IgA deposition, can be considered a secondary form of IgA nephropathy. As mentioned earlier, the only way HSP can be differentiated from IgA nephropathy is in terms of the presumed systemic disease in the former.

Outcome

Disease progression is usually quite slow, but a number of studies have shown that IgA nephropathy can progress to

ESRD; some series have shown that IgA nephropathy is, in fact, a major cause of ESRD. Glomerulosclerosis, widespread crescents, and interstitial fibrosis are the main morphologic signs associated with poor outcome (99–101,106,107,109–112). High blood pressure, severe proteinuria, and elevated serum creatinine levels at the time of diagnosis are clinical indicators of more rapid disease progression (101).

It appears that the prognosis of HSP in children is better than that of IgA nephropathy. Many children with HSP experience complete remission and can be considered cured. Follow-up biopsies frequently show histologic signs of improvement in renal disease, although mesangial IgA deposits rarely disappear entirely (103). The recurrence rate of mesangial IgA deposits in renal allografts is about 50% in patients with IgA nephropathy and HSP, but the recurrent disease rarely interferes with graft function (24,25). Even though glomerular IgA deposits recur in HSP patients after renal transplantation, the recurrence of systemic disease is exceptional.

Etiologic Factors and Pathogenesis

The pathogenesis of IgA nephropathy is still unclear and may be based on many factors, including immunologic abnormalities, viral/food antigens, inability to clear IgA immune deposits, and hereditary predisposition (99–102).

Thin Basement Membrane Disease (Synonyms: Thin Basement Membrane Nephropathy, Benign Recurrent Hematuria, Benign Familial Essential Hematuria, Benign Persistent Hematuria)

Epidemiology

Many patients with persistent, asymptomatic, microscopic hematuria may have thin GBMs. The disease may be familial or occur sporadically; it is found with equal frequency in adults and children.

Clinical Symptoms

The characteristic clinical picture is of symptomatic persistent or recurrent microscopic hematuria. Proteinuria is absent or mild. Renal function is normal.

Light Microscopic Features

Normal renal tissue is noted on histologic examination in most cases.

Immunofluorescence Characteristics

IF shows negative results. Sometimes mild mesangial IgM and/or C3 deposition can be seen, which is most likely nonspecific.

Electron Microscopic Features

Diffuse thinning of the GBM is required to make this diagnosis (Fig. 35) (113–115). Unfortunately, data in the literature on normal GBM thickness are somewhat variable, and the GBM thickness changes with age and differs between sexes. At birth, the GBM is about 150 nm thick, becomes thicker rapidly, and reaches a plateau by 9 to 10 years of age. Thereafter, there is only a very mild, gradual increase in thickness. Data in the literature regard normal GBM thickness in adults to be between 300 and 480 nm (115). In studies where men and women were evaluated separately, men had a GBM approximately 50 nm thicker than women. Interlaboratory variances are significant; thus, it is desirable for each laboratory to determine an age- and sex-matched normal value. Some researchers measure the lamina densa only, while others measure the entire thickness of the GBM. In our experience, the latter measurement is easier to perform and is more reliable. Dische suggests a cutoff value of normal minus 1.5 SD (115). Tiebosch et al. found a cutoff value of 264 nm useful for diagnosis (114).

Differential Diagnosis

Focal thinning of the GBM is a common nonspecific finding; diffuse prominent thinning is necessary to make the diagnosis of thin basement membrane disease. IgA nephropathy can easily be distinguished based on IF. Alport's syndrome (hereditary nephritis) may be an important differential diagnostic consideration in some cases. There is evidence that Alport's syndrome in children initially manifests as thin basement membrane disease, before the development of diagnostic GBM changes. Heterozygous women may also have thin GBM as the only morphologic manifestation. Careful evaluation of the family history and the newly available monoclonal antibodies to the alpha 3 and 5 chains of type IV collagen (see later discussion) are helpful in differential diagnosis. In some cases of benign persistent hematuria, no GBM abnormalities can be identified. In such cases, further, more detailed urologic workup is recommended.

Outcome

Thin basement membrane disease appears to be a benign condition, and most patients do not show progressive renal disease.

Etiologic Factors and Pathogenesis

The etiologic factors and pathogenesis of this disease are unknown. A diagnostic change in the composition of the GBM (unlike the situation in Alport's syndrome) has not been identified.

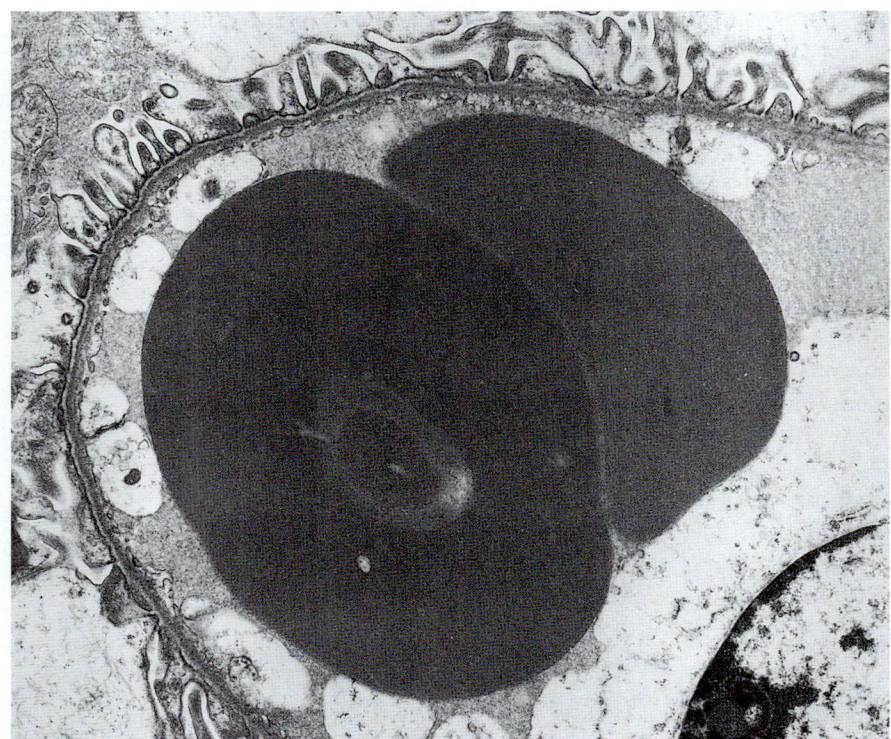

FIG. 35. Thin basement membrane disease. Note the diffusely and prominently thin glomerular basement membrane evident on electron microscopy (uranyl acetate, lead citrate; ×6,300).

Alport's Syndrome (Synonym: Hereditary Nephritis or Nephropathy)

Epidemiology

The condition is rare, and most cases show an X-linked inheritance. A few patients have been reported to have autosomal recessive inheritance (116).

Clinical Symptoms

In affected men, microscopic hematuria initially develops, which later, with disease progression, is complicated by proteinuria. Women usually have only microscopic, asymptomatic hematuria. A sensorineural hearing deficit is common. Ocular defects (anterior lenticonus), diffuse leiomyomatosis, and hematologic abnormalities (megathrombocytopenia, granulocyte abnormalities) are other, less typical associations.

Light Microscopic Features

LM can initially show normal results. In affected men, glomerulosclerosis, which can be segmental, will develop later. Interstitial fibrosis with tubular atrophy is seen in conjunction with glomerulosclerosis. The presence of interstitial foam cells in the absence of nephrotic-range proteinuria is characteristic (but not specific) of Alport's syndrome (Fig. 36). In fact, all light microscopic changes in Alport's syndrome are nonspecific.

Immunofluorescence Characteristics

Antibodies of the conventional IF panel do not show specific immunostaining. In normal (non-Alport affected) kidneys, fluorescein (or peroxidase)-labeled monoclonal antibodies to the alpha 3, alpha 4, and alpha 5 chains of type IV collagen stain the GBM, the basement membranes of distal convoluted tubules, and Bowman's capsule in a linear fashion. In X-linked Alport's syndrome, this basement membrane staining is absent (116). The staining in heterozygous women may show a mosaic pattern (interrupted or segmentally weaker staining), but

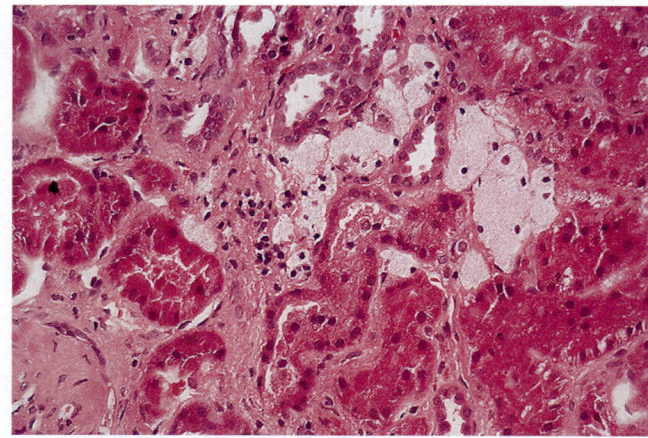

FIG. 36. Interstitial foam cells in a case of Alport's syndrome. Also note the sclerosing glomerulus in the left-lower corner.

this feature should be interpreted with caution. Appropriate controls should include, at a minimum, a renal biopsy specimen with proven Alport's syndrome and renal tissue with normal basement membranes. Rarely, alpha 5 chain staining can be seen in men with Alport's syndrome (116). Anti-GBM antibodies purified from patients with anti-GBM disease, or from those with Alport's syndrome in whom anti-GBM disease develops after transplantation, can also be used, but they are less specific. It is important to note that these immunohistochemical methods should be considered auxiliary at the present time, and the diagnosis of Alport's syndrome should not be rendered based only on these immunohistochemical findings.

Electron Microscopic Features

Diffuse splitting, splintering, and lamellation of the lamina densa and the entire GBM, with rarefactions, are the most diagnostic findings (Fig. 37) (116–119). Occasionally,

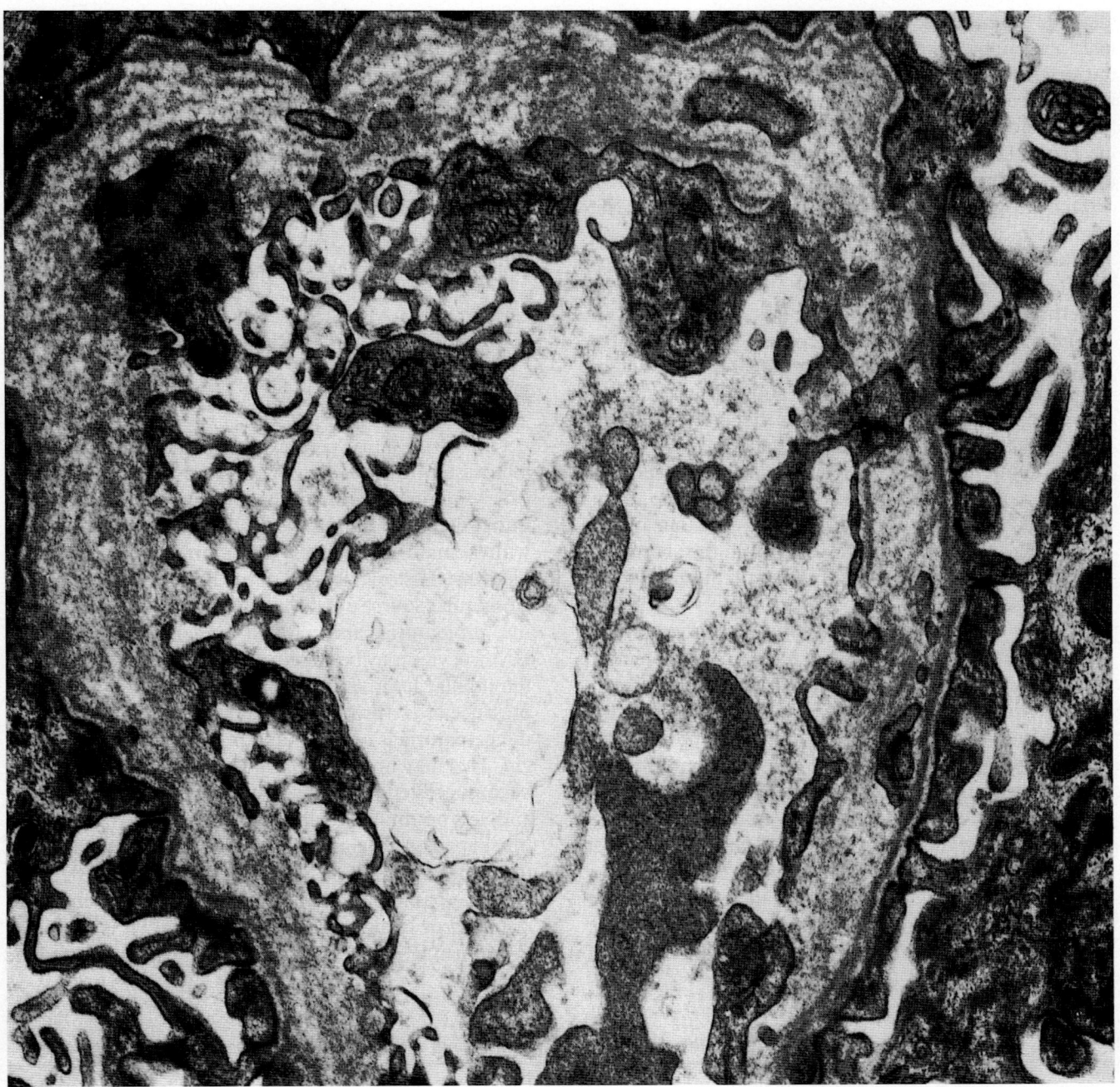

FIG. 37. Hereditary (Alport's) nephropathy. Electron micrograph shows generalized diffuse splitting, splintering, irregular thickening, and rarefaction of the glomerular capillary basement membrane. These changes can be noted in the glomerular basement membrane in a focal and segmental pattern in other nonhereditary diseases; however, if these changes are diffuse and generalized, the diagnosis of hereditary nephritis (or Alport's nephropathy) should be made (uranyl acetate, lead citrate; ×20,000).

electron-dense concretions are evident. The irregular basement membrane is usually thicker than normal. Unfortunately, these changes are not always diffuse, and, at early stages and particularly in young children, only segmental irregularities with GBM thinning are seen.

Differential Diagnosis

In a classic, fully developed case, diagnosis is straightforward. Distinguishing Alport's syndrome from thin basement membrane disease in children and in female carriers may be difficult, however. The most important differential diagnostic approach is to carefully evaluate family history. The immunohistochemical stains detailed earlier are also useful. It is important to note that focal and segmental irregularities of the GBM similar to those in Alport's syndrome can be seen in a variety of sclerosing glomerular diseases, such as FSGS; in immune complex glomerulonephritides after resorption of capillary loop deposits; and in other renal conditions (120).

Outcome

ESRD invariably develops in men in adulthood, usually at about the age of 30 years, but this can be quite variable. Women have usually an indolent course. Anti-GBM disease may develop in patients undergoing transplantation for Alport's syndrome, as a consequence of antibody formation against the alpha 5 chain of type IV collagen in patients who genetically lack normal alpha 5 chains. Fortunately, this happens only in a few patients (39).

Etiology and Pathogenesis

A single or several mutations in the COL4A5 gene on the long arm of the X chromosome are responsible for the absence of the normal alpha 5 chain in type IV collagen (116). The alpha 5 chain probably forms a network with the alpha 3 and alpha 4 chains; thus, these are not expressed in the basement membranes either. The abnormal GBM most likely will be more susceptible to injury and unable to normally regenerate, and glomerulosclerosis will result. Rare autosomal recessive and, possibly, autosomal dominant forms of Alport's syndrome also exist.

Other Findings in Patients with Asymptomatic Microscopic Hematuria

Sometimes, in the pathologic study of tissues from patients with isolated or benign essential hematuria, none of the previously cited conditions is found. Some investigators have reported mesangial IgM and/or IgG, as well as C3 deposition (in the absence of IgA), in otherwise fairly unremarkable glomeruli in these patients (121,122). It appears that the glomerulopathies with non-IgA mesangial immunoglobulin deposition have a good prognosis (123). Some patients have loin pain in association with microscopic hematuria. Usually, no glomerular abnormalities can be seen in biopsy specimens taken from patients with loin pain, and this vaguely defined condition has been called loin pain hematuria syndrome. Obliterative small arterial changes have been reported (124). There are a few patients in whom hematuria appears to be of renal origin, but no renal morphologic abnormality can be found. All these conditions appear to have a benign clinical course. As noted earlier, it is important in the renal biopsy report to note whether red blood cells are present in Bowman's space or tubules, to indicate that the hematuria is probably of glomerular origin.

DISEASES ASSOCIATED WITH ACELLULAR CLOSURE OF GLOMERULAR CAPILLARIES

The Thrombotic Microangiopathies

Thrombotic microangiopathy (TMA) is a pattern that can be seen in a variety of diseases (125–128). The classic conditions in which TMA occurs are hemolytic uremic syndrome (HUS) and thrombotic thrombocytopenic purpura (TTP). Because of the many similarities, several investigators consider them to be different clinical manifestations of the same disease and term the condition TTP/HUS (125–127). Other diseases and conditions that may be associated with TMA include postpartum renal failure, severe preeclampsia and eclampsia, malignant hypertension (malignant nephrosclerosis), acute scleroderma, drug therapy (e.g., mitomycin C, cyclosporin, FK506), primary antiphospholipid syndrome, SLE, malignancy, humoral (vascular) allograft rejection, bone marrow transplantation, radiation nephritis, and HIV infection.

Epidemiology

HUS may occur in small epidemics, particularly in children after food poisoning. This is the typical, or D+, HUS (D+ because HUS is preceded by diarrhea). The sporadic, atypical, or D−, HUS (without diarrhea) develops both in children and in adults (127,128).

Clinical Symptoms

As mentioned earlier, the epidemic (D+) form of HUS is usually associated with profuse, frequently bloody diarrhea (hemorrhagic colitis). Acute renal failure, hematuria, and variable degrees of proteinuria are the renal symptoms. Hypertension is common and may reach malignant levels. Hemolytic anemia, thrombocytopenia, fragmented red blood cells (schistocytes or fragmentocytes) in the peripheral blood, and elevated lactate dehydrogenase levels are characteristic of all forms of TMA, but these changes may be subtle.

Light Microscopic Features

The glomerular changes include thickening of the glomerular capillary walls by swollen endothelial cells and deposition of amorphous material in the capillary wall with subsequent narrowing of the glomerular capillary lumens,

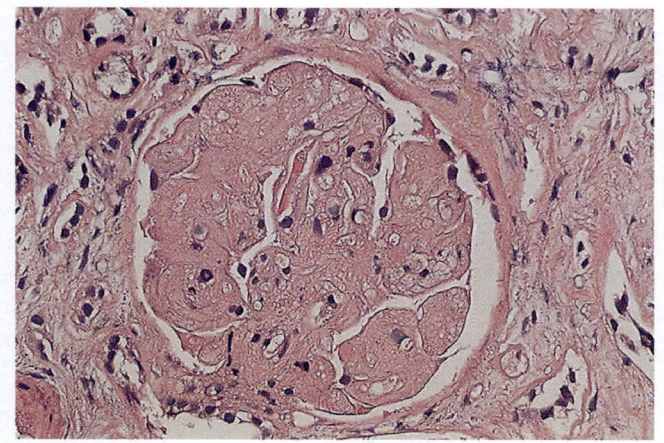
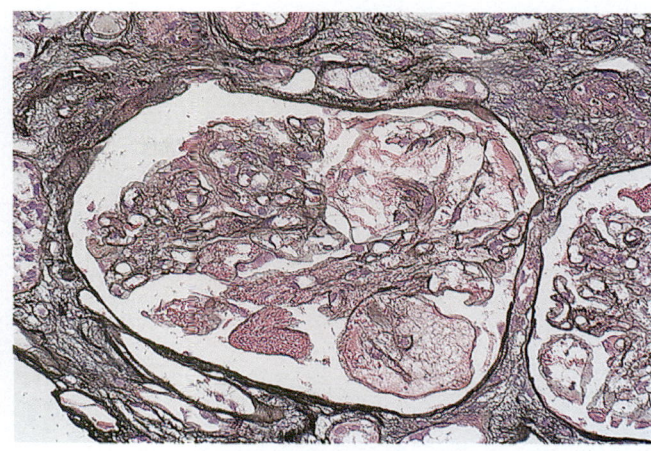
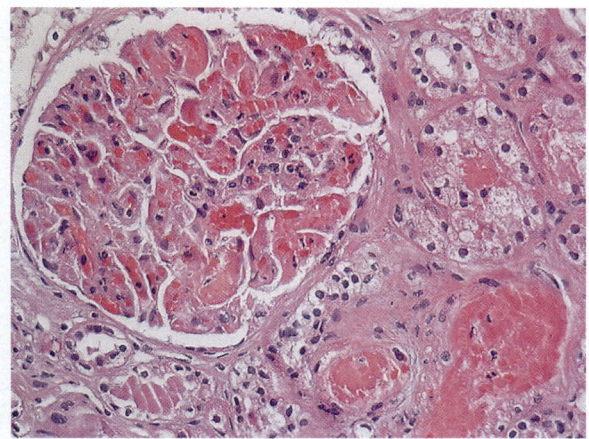

FIG. 38. Glomerular changes in thrombotic microangiopathy. **A:** A typical bloodless glomerulus. Note the obliteration of the glomerular capillary loops by slightly fibrillary, loose material. **B:** Prominent mesangiolysis and microaneurysm formation in a patient with radiation nephritis who showed initial signs of thrombotic microangiopathy. Note the fragmented red blood cells in some microaneurysms (methenamine silver). **C:** Glomerular and arteriolar thrombi are evident, but they do not have to be present to make the diagnosis of thrombotic microangiopathy.

creating "bloodless glomeruli" (Fig. 38A) (126–130). Occasionally, a membranoproliferative pattern is noted, with a double-contour appearance of the glomerular capillary wall. In some cases, particularly in TMA after bone marrow transplantation and irradiation, mesangiolysis with subsequent glomerular microaneurysm formation may be prominent (Fig. 38B). Glomerular capillary thrombi may or may not be seen (Fig. 38C). In many patients there is thickening and/or thrombosis of renal arterioles.

The preglomerular arteries and arterioles in TMA usually show two types of changes, which may overlap. (a) In intimal myxoid fibroplasia, medial smooth-muscle cells migrate into the intima, where they may show a concentric layering with severe narrowing of the lumen (so-called onion skinning) (Fig 39A). Accumulation of myxoid extracellular matrix in the thickened intima is usually seen (Fig. 39B). (b) The second type of change is "fibrinoid" necrosis with massive amounts of plasma proteins "insuding" into the vessel

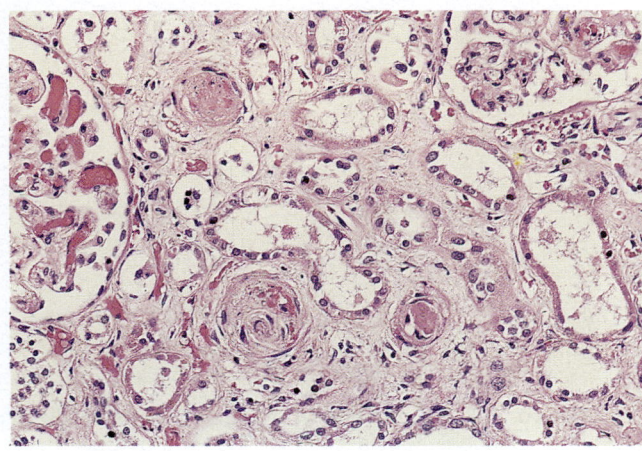
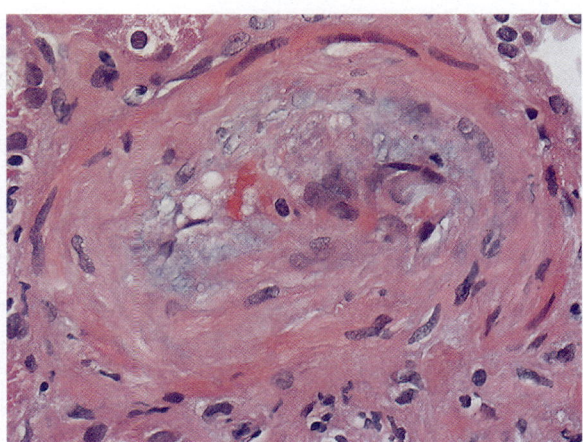

FIG. 39. Vascular changes in thrombotic microangiopathy. **A:** In this case from a patient with acquired immunodeficiency syndrome, the small arteries and arterioles show concentric thickening with insudation of fibrin and fragmented red blood cells in the wall. The glomerular capillaries are congested. **B:** Prominent mucoid intimal thickening in an interlobular artery from a case of malignant hypertension.

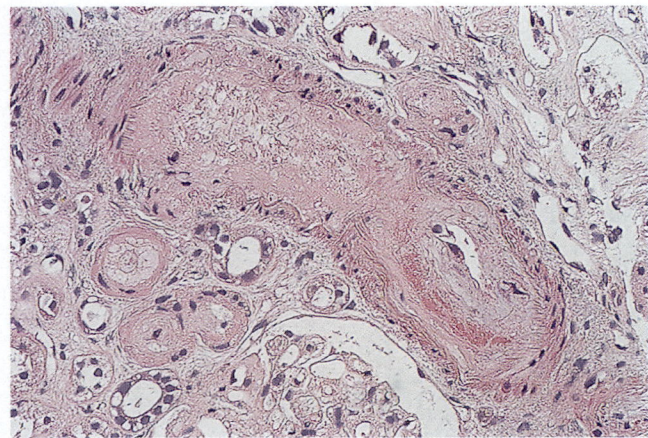

FIG. 39. (*continued*) **C:** This small artery shows very prominent, loose intimal thickening with patchy fibrinoid necrosis.

wall (Fig. 39C). In some cases of severe renal capillary thrombosis, renal cortical necrosis may develop (Fig. 40). Based on the specific compartment predominantly involved, Habib et al. (130) discriminated three patterns of TMA: the glomerular type, the vascular type, and cortical necrosis. The D+ (typical) pediatric cases tend to show mainly glomerular involvement, whereas the sporadic cases more frequently display vascular changes.

Immunofluorescence Characteristics

Glomerular and vascular fibrin/fibrinogen deposition in the lumen and/or within the vascular wall is a common finding. IgM is also frequently deposited in the mesangium, glomerular capillaries, and arteries/arterioles. C3, C1q, and IgG are seen less often. These immunoglobulin and complement deposits are thought to be nonspecific and due to activated coagulation, endothelial injury, and passive imbibition of plasma proteins.

Electron Microscopic Features

Widening of the lamina rara interna of the GBM by subendothelial electron-lucent "fluff" containing a few fibrin tactoids and cellular debris, including fragmented red blood cells, are characteristic findings (Fig. 41).

Differential Diagnosis

In our opinion, there is no reliable way to distinguish at the microscopic level between the causes of TMA. The vessels, including glomerular capillaries, react in a limited fashion to many injuries, and the morphologic and pathologic responses are somewhat nonspecific. One can differentiate between the various forms of TMA only on the basis of clinical history and findings. In some cases, even this additional information fails to clarify the sequence of events; for example, in certain cases it may be impossible to decide whether the pattern of TMA was caused by malignant hypertension or whether malignant hypertension resulted from an underlying TMA.

It may be difficult to draw a distinction between disseminated intravascular coagulation (DIC) and HUS/TTP, as well as other types of TMA. In DIC, the glomerular capillaries are occluded by intraluminal fibrin thrombi without morphologically apparent endothelial damage. Moreover, in DIC the coagulation profile is substantially more abnormal than in TMA. Still, there are many overlaps, and, in certain cases, it may be challenging to make the morphologic distinction.

Outcome

Most children with typical (D+) HUS recover fully. Atypical (D−) HUS cases and other forms of TMA have a worse outcome; ESRD frequently develops (128,129). Patients with predominantly vascular involvement are also at higher risk of ESRD. The prognosis of cortical necrosis depends primarily on the extent of necrosis. We have seen a few patients with severe cortical necrosis in the renal biopsy specimen who fully recovered on supportive therapy.

Graft survival in children who undergo transplant because of HUS does not appear to be different from overall graft survival (131). Atypical (D−) HUS may recur in renal transplants, but it is difficult to diagnose based on renal transplant biopsy alone, because vascular rejection and, now and then, cyclosporin or FK506 nephrotoxicity may cause identical morphologic changes.

Etiologic Factors and Pathogenesis

Verotoxin-producing *Escherichia coli* bacteria, particularly the O157:H7 serotype, are important in the pathogene-

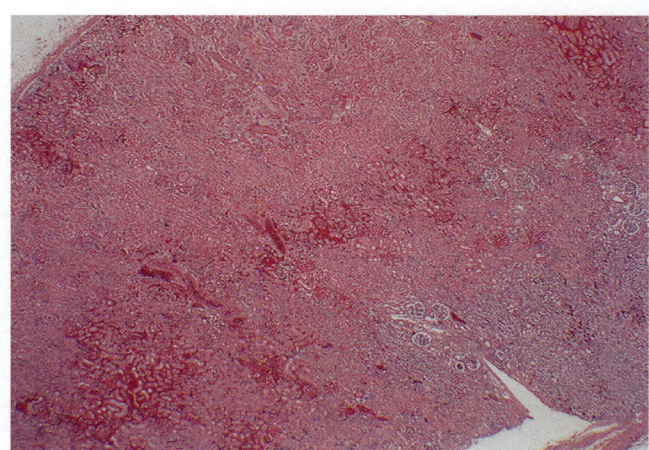

FIG. 40. Cortical necrosis in a pediatric patient with severe pneumococcal sepsis. Almost the entire renal cortex is necrotic, with hyperemic subcapsular and corticomedullary regions. The medulla and some glomeruli along the corticomedullary junction are intact.

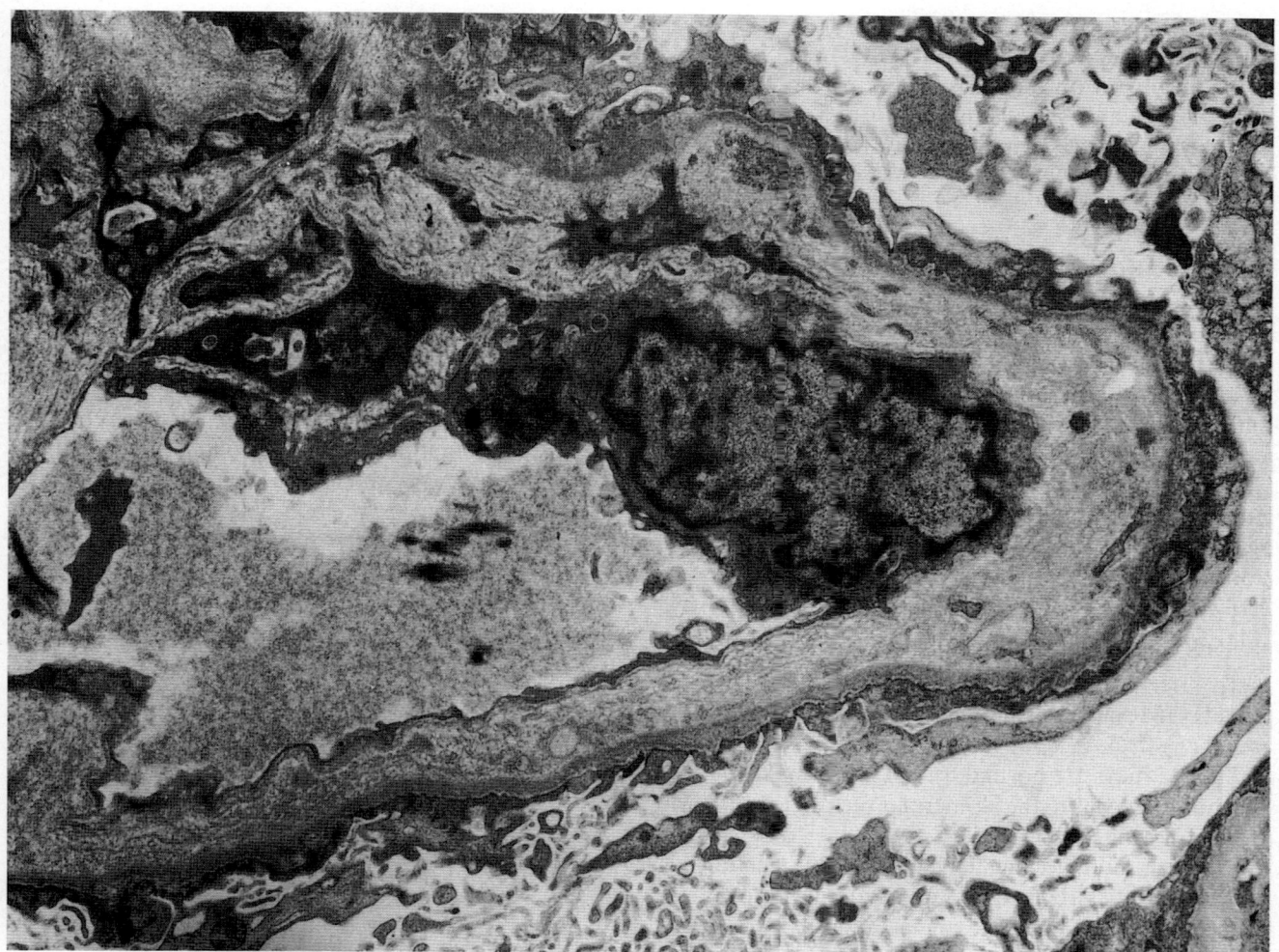

FIG. 41. Thrombotic microangiopathy. Electron micrograph of a glomerular capillary from a patient with a form of thrombotic microangiopathy (humoral rejection). Note that there is widening of the glomerular lamina rara interna by glomerular subendothelial electron-lucent, fluffy material with some migrating mesangial cells (partial mesangial interposition). These changes are not pathognomonic of humoral rejection and can be seen in any of the thrombotic microangiopathies (uranyl acetate, lead citrate; ×15,000).

sis of the epidemic (D+) forms. Other microorganisms, and a variety of other factors, play a part in the atypical forms. The common final pathway of these changes is probably endothelial damage with ongoing intramural (within the glomerular capillary wall) coagulation. The reader is referred to several articles on coagulation and the kidney and HUS (125–134).

Cryoglobulinemic Glomerulonephritis

Epidemiology

This rare disease occurs mainly in adults with type II (mixed essential) cryoglobulinemia, apparently associated with hepatitis C virus infection. Type I (monoclonal) cryoglobulinemia, for example, some cases of Waldenström's macroglobulinemia, may have similar morphologic features (20,135).

Clinical Symptoms

Patients are usually nephritic. Renal failure may develop. Cryoglobulinemia is frequently associated with systemic vasculitis; thus, a variety of symptoms due to multiorgan involvement, including purpura and arthralgia, are possible.

Light Microscopic Features

A pattern of intracapillary proliferative GN or MPGN is seen (135). The distinctive feature is the presence of glomerular, intracapillary, homogeneous "hyalin thrombi," which represent precipitated cryoglobulins (Fig. 42). A particularly large number of endocapillary monocytes can be seen in this condition (135,136). Vasculitis is rarely present in a renal biopsy specimen.

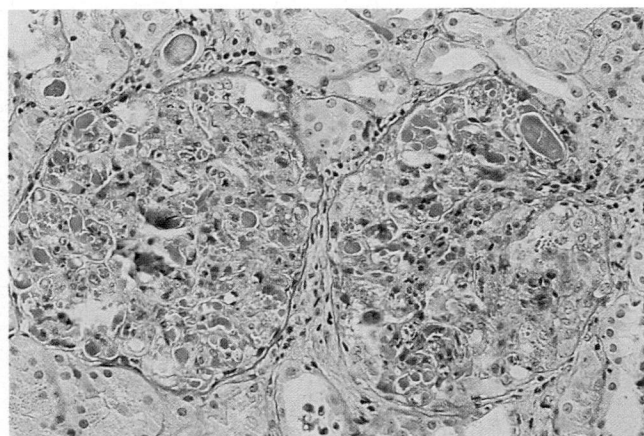

FIG. 42. Cryoglobulinemic glomerulonephritis. Note the positive cryoglobulin thrombi in many glomerular capillaries in these hypercellular glomeruli on periodic acid–Schiff stain.

Immunofluorescence Characteristics

The hyalin thrombi show positive results for IgM and IgG in cases of type II cryoglobulinemia and for IgM only in the rare type I cryoglobulinemia. Complement C3 is also frequently seen. IgG and IgM deposits may be present in the glomerular capillary walls and mesangium away from the hyalin thrombi.

Electron Microscopic Features

The cryoglobulin deposits have a distinctive microtubular/cylindrical substructure at high magnification (Fig. 43). The deposits are intracapillary or subendothelial. Occasionally, mesangial deposits are evident. There may also be deposits without this substructure.

Differential Diagnosis

Hyalin thrombus–like lesions may develop in the context of proliferative lupus nephritis, where large subendothelial deposits bulge into the glomerular capillary lumen. Fibrin thrombi are less homogeneous, and they can be differentiated by immunohistochemistry and special stains. Rarely, glomerular deposits have a microtubular substructure in the absence of cryoglobulinemia. This condition is called immunotactoid GN. Some forms of MPGN associated with hepatitis C and cryoglobulinemia can be considered cryoglobulinemic GN.

Outcome

About one-third of patients experience complete or partial remission. Others have continuous urinary abnormalities, and ESRD may develop in many of them. The disease can recur in renal allografts, but our experience is too limited to estimate a recurrence rate.

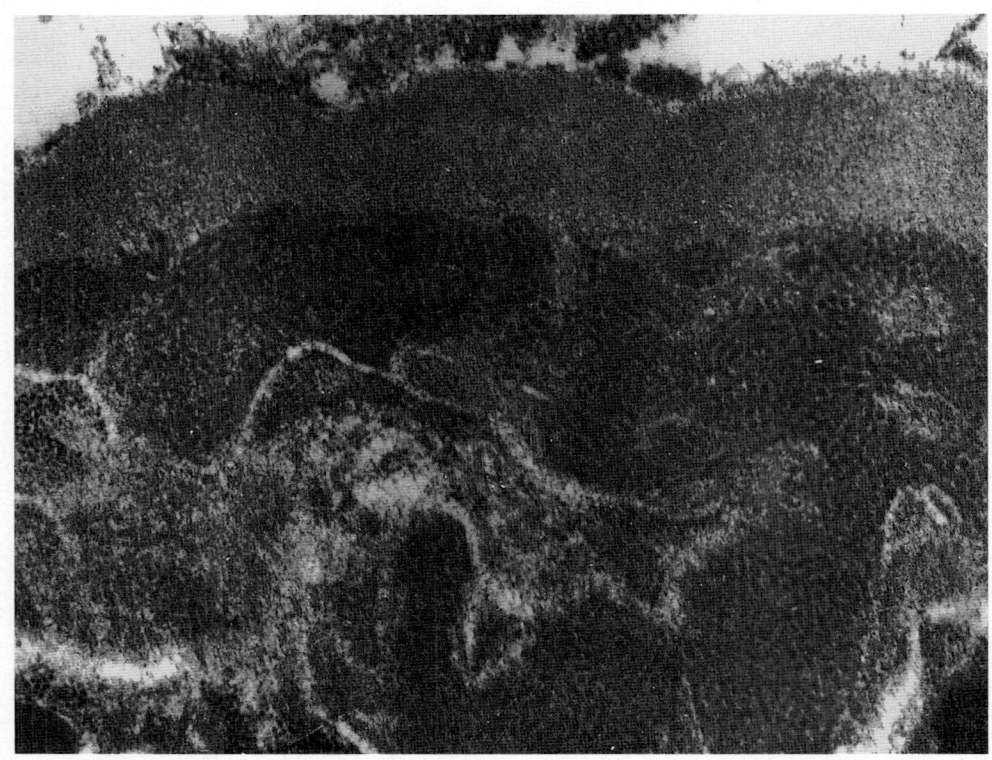

FIG. 43. Ultrastructure of cryoglobulinemic glomerulonephritis. Note the microtubular substructure of the electron-dense deposits (uranyl acetate, lead citrate; ×20,000).

Etiologic Factors and Pathogenesis

It is now clear that hepatitis C virus is the major cause of mixed essential (type II) cryoglobulinemia; it can be detected in more than 80% of cases of type II cryoglobulinemia (20). It is unclear how cryoglobulins lead to GN. The precipitated cryoglobulins may attract and activate monocytes, with a subsequent inflammatory reaction.

Amyloidosis

Epidemiology

Renal amyloidosis occurs in two groups of patients—those with plasma cell dyscrasia and those with long-standing chronic inflammatory diseases or neoplasms. In the first instance, the condition is called primary or AL amyloidosis because the amyloid is composed of monoclonal light chains (usually lambda). Only 10% to 20% of these patients have overt myeloma; the remainder have only a monoclonal spike in the serum and/or urine. In a few patients, not even that feature is detectable. The second group of patients, those with long-standing chronic inflammatory diseases (e.g., chronic osteomyelitis, rheumatoid arthritis, tuberculosis) or neoplasms (e.g., renal cell carcinoma), have a form of amyloidosis called secondary or AA amyloidosis (serum amyloid A protein-associated). Most of these patients are elderly. There are other forms of amyloid, but these are the two important types from the renal point of view (137,138).

Clinical Symptoms

Frequently, the first symptom of systemic amyloidosis is severe, often nephrotic-range proteinuria with or without renal failure. Additional symptoms depend on the involvement of other organs.

Light Microscopic Features

Renal amyloid always involves the glomeruli. It appears as homogeneous, smudgy mesangial and capillary loop deposits that are faintly PAS positive and silver negative (Table 6, Fig. 44A,B). Sometimes the silver stain reveals spiking along the glomerular capillary loops, somewhat rem-

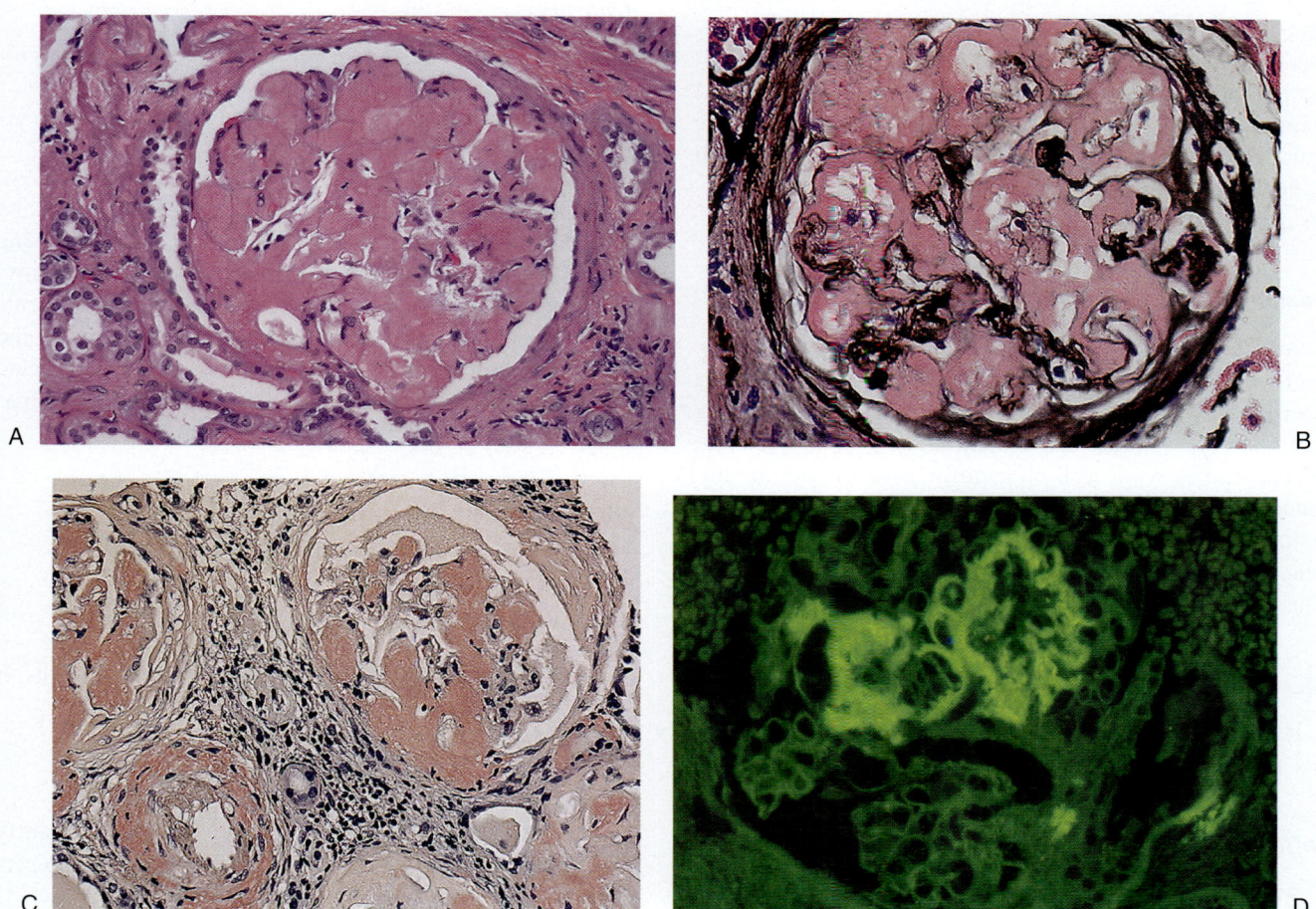

FIG. 44. Renal amyloidosis. **A:** Widespread glomerular deposition of moderately eosinophilic homogeneous material. **B:** Amyloid is silver negative (methenamine silver). **C:** Congo red stain shows positive results for amyloid deposits in the glomeruli and vessels. **D:** Positive thioflavine T stain in a glomerulus (thioflavine T fluorescence).

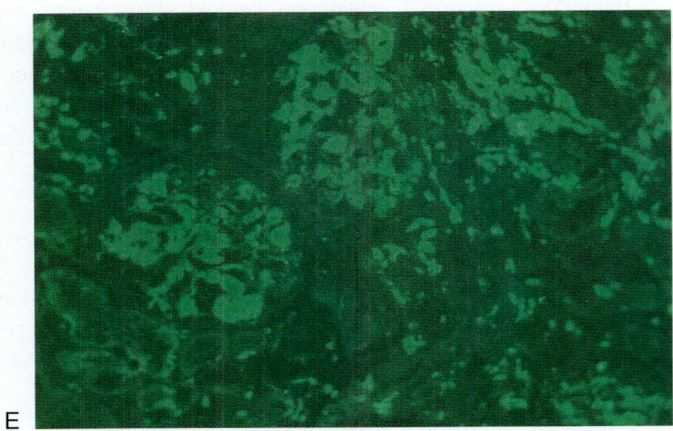
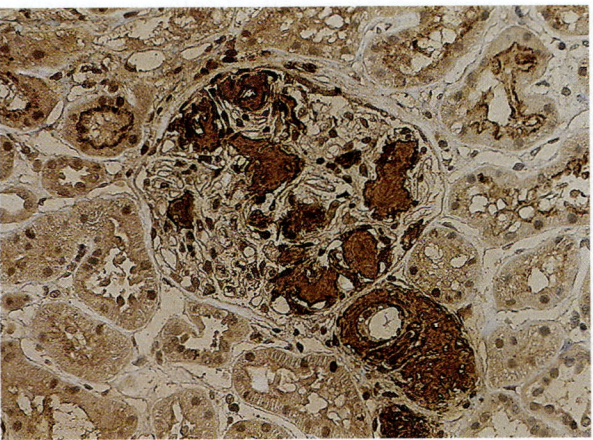

FIG. 44. (*continued*) **E:** In AL amyloidosis, immunofluorescence is characteristically positive for one of the light chains (usually lambda). Note the glomerular, vascular, and interstitial deposits (anti-lambda; ×100). **F:** In AA amyloidosis, immunoperoxidase stain is helpful in the diagnosis (anti-AA).

iniscent of membranous GN. Congo red birefringence is the most specific stain for amyloid by LM, and fluorescence of thioflavin T is the most sensitive study, in addition to EM (Fig. 44C,D). AL and AA amyloid can be differentiated by specific antibodies or by potassium permanganate pretreatment. which eliminates Congo red positivity for AA amyloid but not for AL amyloid. It is important to perform Congo red stain on at least 8-μm-thick sections. Vascular deposits are usually obvious. Amyloid deposits are also frequently seen in the interstitium and along TBMs and peritubular capillaries in more advanced cases.

Immunofluorescence Characteristics

Antibodies to light chains are sometimes, but not always, useful in the diagnosis of AL amyloid. Amyloid usually shows positive results for lambda, less frequently for kappa light chain (Fig. 44E). Good antibodies to AA amyloid are available; they work well on paraffin sections with the immunoperoxidase technique (Fig. 44F) (139). Thioflavin T stain of paraffin sections will give a bright green fluorescence (Fig. 44D), but this is not considered an IF method because thioflavin T is not an antibody.

Electron Microscopic Features

Randomly arranged, rigid, nonbranching 8- to 10-nm fibrils are virtually diagnostic of amyloidosis (Fig. 45).

Differential Diagnosis

Any lesion with advanced glomerulosclerosis and hyalinosis may raise the possibility of amyloidosis. The special stains mentioned earlier and EM make differential diagnosis straightforward in most cases (Table 6). A recently recognized entity, fibrillary GN, may simulate amyloidosis at the ultrastructural level. The fibrils in fibrillary GN are thicker (thicker than 10 nm and usually 12–24 nm), however, and stains for amyloid give negative results (see later discussion).

Outcome

The outcome is quite poor because of the relentlessly progressive systemic disease.

Etiologic Factors and Pathogenesis

As mentioned previously, monoclonal gammopathy and chronic inflammation are the most important predisposing factors for AL and AA amyloidosis, respectively, but amyloidosis develops in only a certain proportion of patients with monoclonal light chains in the serum and/or urine and elevated serum amyloid A protein levels (which is an acute phase reactant). The factors promoting amyloid fibril formation and deposition in these patients are unclear.

Fibrillary Glomerulonephritis (Synonyms: Immunotactoid Glomerulopathy, Nonamyloidotic Fibrillary Glomerulopathy)

Epidemiology

Fibrillary glomerulonephritis is a rare disease of adults. It is more common in whites than in blacks (140–144).

Clinical Symptoms

The disease is characterized by severe, frequently nephrotic-range proteinuria. Microscopic hematuria, hypertension, and renal insufficiency are also typical.

Light Microscopic Features

There are a variety of light microscopic patterns (142–144). The most frequently encountered glomerular lesion is

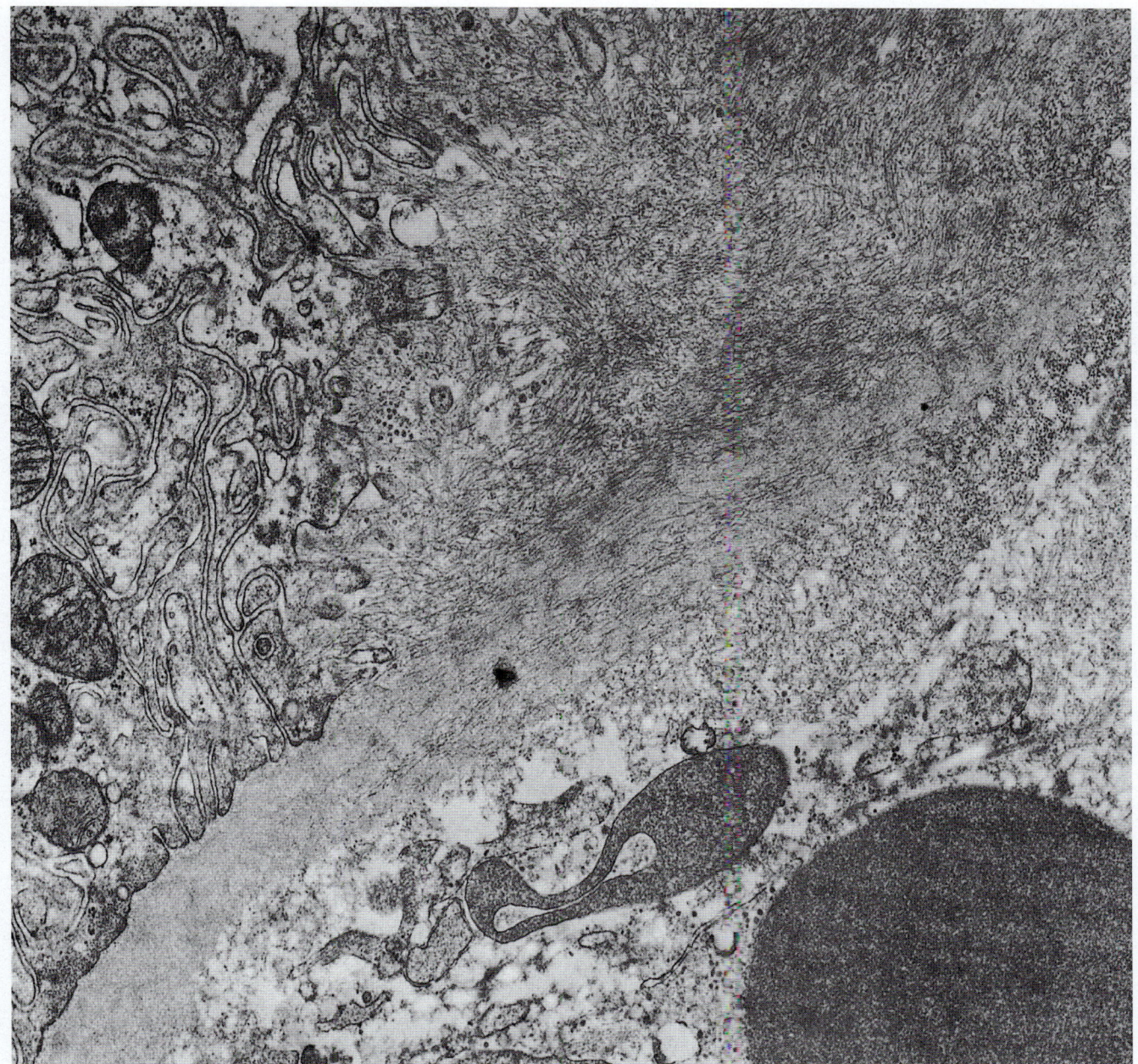

FIG. 45. Renal amyloidosis. Electron micrograph of a segment of renal tubule showing amyloidosis. Note the rigid, nonbranching fibrils (uranyl acetate, lead citrate; ×23,000).

prominent mesangial expansion with glomerular capillary wall thickening (Fig. 46). The deposited material is mostly methenamine silver negative, but it is admixed with silver-positive glomerular extracellular matrix. Crescents are present in 15% to 20% of patients.

Immunofluorescence Characteristics

Strong, diffuse, smudgy mesangial and glomerular capillary wall IgG staining is characteristic (Fig. 47). Kappa light chain fluorescence may be stronger than lambda fluorescence. C3 is frequently present. The deposited IgG is mainly of the IgG4 isotype (143).

Electron Microscopic Features

Randomly arranged, rigid fibrils, similar to amyloid fibrils but thicker than 10 nm (usually 12–24 nm) (Fig. 48), are visible. Sometimes, fibrils that are thicker than 20 to 24 nm on cross sections turn out to be microtubules (mostly 40–60 nm). Some investigators differentiate this form, calling it im-

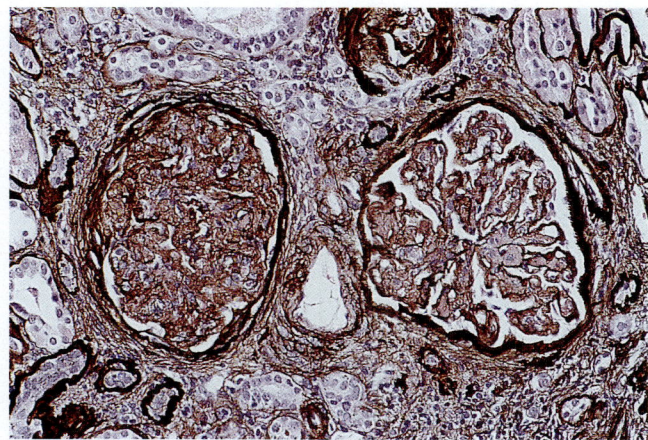

FIG. 46. Fibrillary glomerulonephritis. Note that the widened mesangium and thickened glomerular capillary loops do not stain strongly with methenamine silver stain.

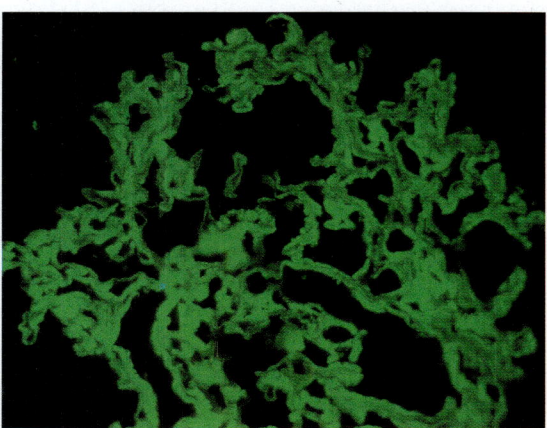

FIG. 47. Fibrillary glomerulonephritis. Prominent diffuse mesangial and capillary loop staining for IgG is characteristic (anti-IgG; ×400).

munotactoid GN as opposed to fibrillary GN. Others do not believe that this distinction is justified (140–144).

Differential Diagnosis

Amyloidosis is the most important disease to eliminate from the differential diagnosis, as discussed previously. Fibrillary GN is nonreactive with amyloid stains. Focal nonspecific fibrillary transformation of the sclerotic mesangium (such as in diabetic glomerulosclerosis) should not be diagnosed as fibrillary GN. Monoclonal gammopathy should always be considered; this condition is relatively rare in cases with microfibrils (less than 20 nm), but it is more common in cases with microtubules (usually thicker than 20 nm). If mi-

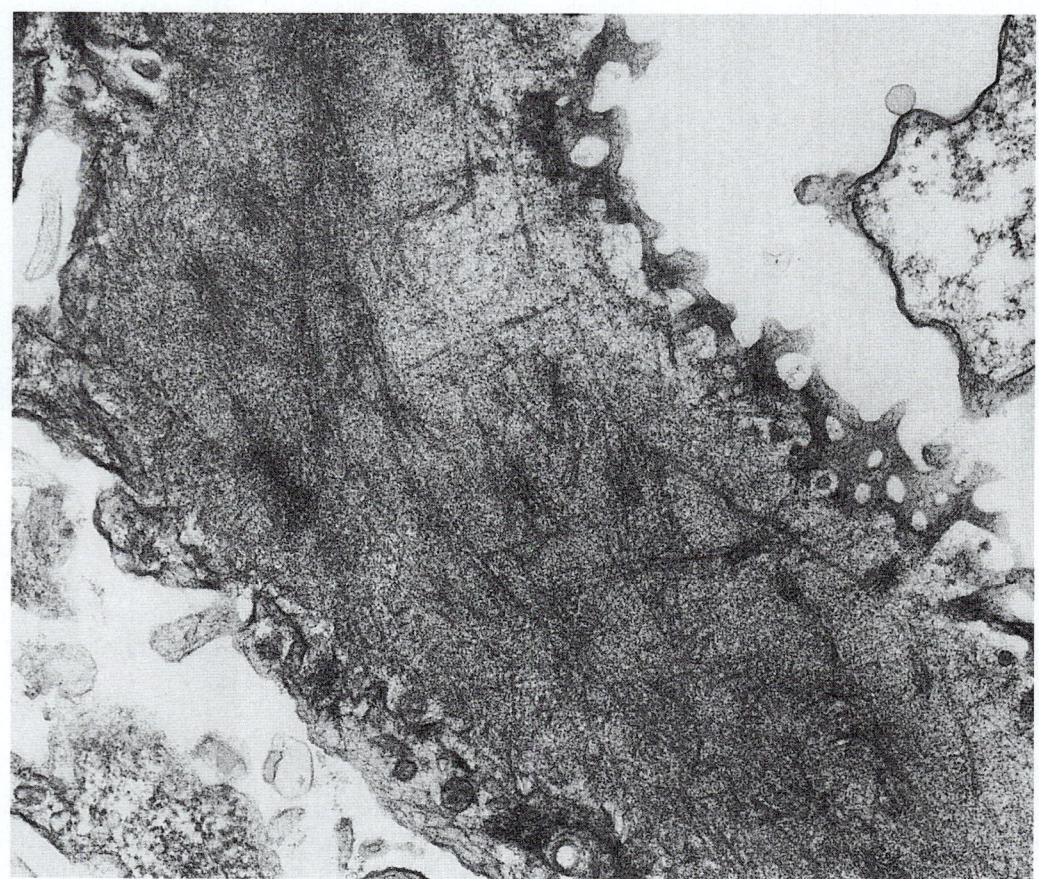

FIG. 48. Fibrillary glomerulonephritis. Note the 28-nm-thick fibrils distributed throughout the thickened glomerular capillary basement membrane (uranyl acetate, lead citrate, ×25,000).

crotubules are seen, cryoglobulinemia should also be excluded (140). In fact, if cases with cryoglobulinemia and monoclonal gammopathy are excluded, the incidence of immunotactoid GN (with microtubules) is extremely low.

Outcome

Most cases are relentlessly progressive; ESRD develops within a few months or years. Unlike the situation of amyloidosis, however, there is no compelling evidence of multiorgan involvement. It appears that fibrillary GN has a relatively high recurrence rate in renal allografts, but recurrent disease rarely interferes with graft outcome (144).

Pathogenesis

The pathogenesis is unknown. Monotypical (not monoclonal) IgG4 may have a role in the formation of fibrils.

THE NEPHROPATHIES OF SYSTEMIC LUPUS ERYTHEMATOSUS

Epidemiology

SLE is predominantly a disease of women; the female/male ratio has been reported to be between 8:1 and 13:1. In the United States, it is more common in African-Americans and in Asian women than in whites. Morphologic evidence of renal involvement in the form of glomerular immune complex deposition can be detected in almost all patients with SLE. Clinical evidence of renal disease is seen in 50% to 70% of patients (145–148).

Clinical Symptoms

The renal symptoms show good correlation with the WHO classification of lupus nephritis (see following discussion) (145–148). In class II (mesangial) lupus nephritis, microscopic hematuria is the leading symptom. Proteinuria may be present, but it is not in the nephrotic range. In classes III and IV (proliferative) lupus nephritis, nephritic syndrome, with or without nephrotic-range proteinuria, is seen. In class V (membranous) lupus nephritis, severe, usually nephrotic-range proteinuria is the most significant symptom, with microscopic evidence of hematuria. Class VI (chronic sclerosing) lupus nephritis is characterized by renal failure. Of course, other systemic signs/symptoms and the characteristic laboratory findings are evident, which are not further detailed here.

Light Microscopic Features and the Classification of Lupus Nephritis

Lupus nephritis can mimic almost any morphologic pattern, and we have to emphasize that it is not a diagnosis based primarily on morphologic features. In the absence of clinical and laboratory criteria for the diagnosis of SLE, lupus nephritis cannot be diagnosed based solely on results of renal biopsy; however, the possibility of SLE can be raised and further clinical and laboratory studies undertaken to confirm or exclude the diagnosis of lupus. The morphologic pattern of lupus nephritis has been divided by the WHO into five classes (and further subdivided within class II), to which a sixth class (chronic sclerosing GN) was later added. (2,145–148).

1. Class I: The kidney is normal by LM, EM, and IF, that is, there is no evidence of immune complex deposition or any kind of renal disease. In our opinion, this category should be omitted from this classification.
2. Class II: mesangial abnormalities.
3. Class IIa: The kidneys, including the glomeruli, are normal by LM (see Fig. 1) but have immune deposits in the glomerular mesangium on EM and IF (Fig. 51A).
4. Class IIb: Mesangial expansion and/or hypercellularity (see Fig. 16) and mesangial deposits may be evident. There are no other changes.
5. Class III: Focal proliferative GN (Fig. 15). Focal and segmental, intra- and/or extracapillary, proliferative, necrotizing and/or sclerosing lesions involve less than 50% (according to some investigators, less than 80%) of the glomeruli. Occasionally, thick, glassy glomerular capillary walls, due to large subendothelial deposits ("wire loop" lesion), are visible (Fig. 49A). If the deposits are large and bulging into the glomerular capillary lumen, they may appear as hyalin thrombi. Focal interstitial inflammation and interstitial edema are frequently found.
6. Class IV: Diffuse proliferative GN (Fig. 49). More severe lesions of the type seen in Class III involve more than 50% of glomeruli (some pathologists use a cutoff value of 80%). Usually, there is a prominent interstitial inflammatory cell infiltrate.
7. Class V: Membranous GN. The LM picture is quite similar to that of idiopathic membranous GN (see Fig. 26).
8. Class VI: Chronic sclerosing GN with advanced focal global and segmental glomerulosclerosis and interstitial fibrosis with tubular atrophy.

There may be many overlaps in this classification. The most common combinations are with class V. If a membranous pattern is combined with focal or diffuse proliferative glomerular lesions, the lupus nephritis should be classified as class III + V or class IV + V, respectively. At times, vascular changes are striking in lupus nephritis, including vascular immune complex deposition, noninflammatory necrotizing vasculopathy, TMA, and, very rarely, true vasculitis (149).

Immunofluorescence Characteristics

IF studies reveal granular immunoglobulin and complement deposition in all glomeruli (Fig. 50A–C). Typically,

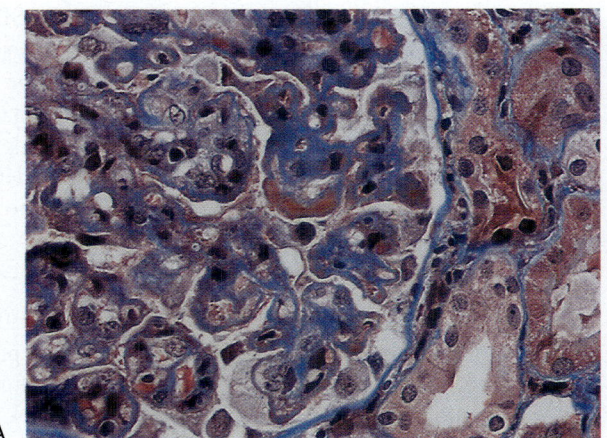
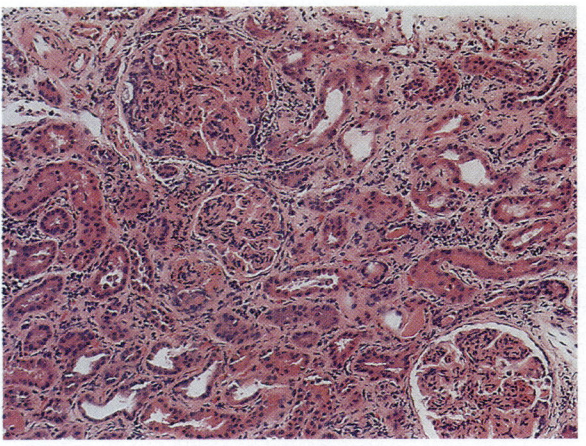

FIG. 49. Diffuse proliferative lupus nephritis (WHO class IV). **A:** Large subendothelial deposits are sometimes evident with the trichrome stain; they appear as fuchsinophilic (red), thick capillary walls, as is seen here in the center (Masson's trichrome). **B:** Note the diffusely hypercellular glomeruli and the interstitial inflammatory cell infiltrate.

there are variable combinations of IgG, IgM, C1q, C3, and IgA (full-house IF). Strong glomerular C1q staining (Fig. 50A) is rarely seen in conditions other than lupus (except, of course, C1q nephropathy). In the milder forms of renal involvement (class II), deposits are limited to the glomerular mesangium. In the more severe forms (classes III and IV), in addition to mesangial deposition, deposits extend along the glomerular capillary walls. In class V lupus nephritis, the pattern is that of membranous GN, except for consistent granular mesangial fluorescence and, frequently, full-house IF (Fig 50B). There may also be granular immunostaining along TBMs and arteries/arterioles (Fig. 50C).

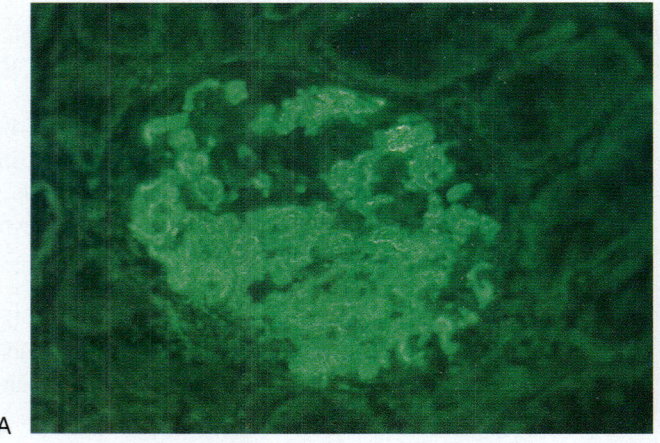
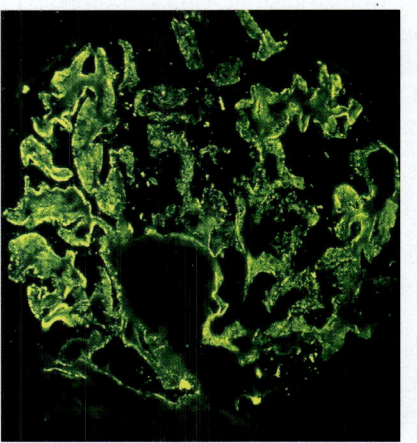
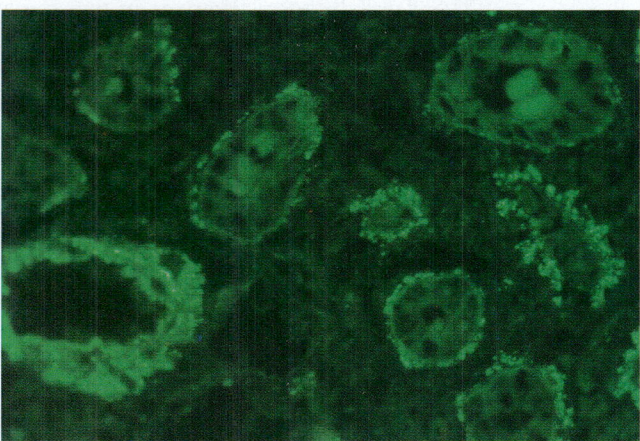

FIG. 50. Immunofluorescence of lupus nephritis. **A:** Strong granular mesangial and glomerular capillary wall staining for C1q is characteristic in diffuse proliferative lupus nephritis (anti-C1q; ×200). **B:** Membranous (WHO class V) lupus glomerulonephritis. Granular glomerular capillary and mesangial fluorescence is characteristic (anti-IgG; ×400). **C:** Granular tubular basement membrane and vascular deposits are sometimes visible. An interlobular artery is present in the lower-left corner (anti-C1q; ×200).

Electron Microscopic Features

Electron-dense deposits are always present in the glomerular mesangial areas in all of these patterns of renal involvement (150) (Fig. 51 A–C). SLE, along with Berger's disease, is one of the quintessential mesangiopathies; that is, the baseline or background upon which all patterns of SLE are superimposed is the deposition of immune reactants in the mesangial areas. When they are abundant, the mesangial deposits extend into, or are not cleared from, the adjacent glomerular subendothelial space, which is in direct continuity with the mesangium. Here, the deposits may extend peripherally along the glomerular capillary walls, leading to the thickened, glassy appearance of the glomerular capillaries (wire loops) visible on LM (Fig. 51B).

Electron-dense deposits may be seen within the basal lamina of Bowman's capsule; within the TBMs; less often in the walls of small arteries/arterioles, venules, and peritubular capillaries; and even in the interstitium. Endothelial tubuloreticular inclusions (also called myxovirus-like particles or interferon footprints) are frequently present, but they are not specific for lupus nephritis (see Fig. 25). Rarely, electron-dense deposits in lupus can have an organized substructure with curved paracrystalline structures resembling fingerprints (fingerprint deposits) (Fig. 51C).

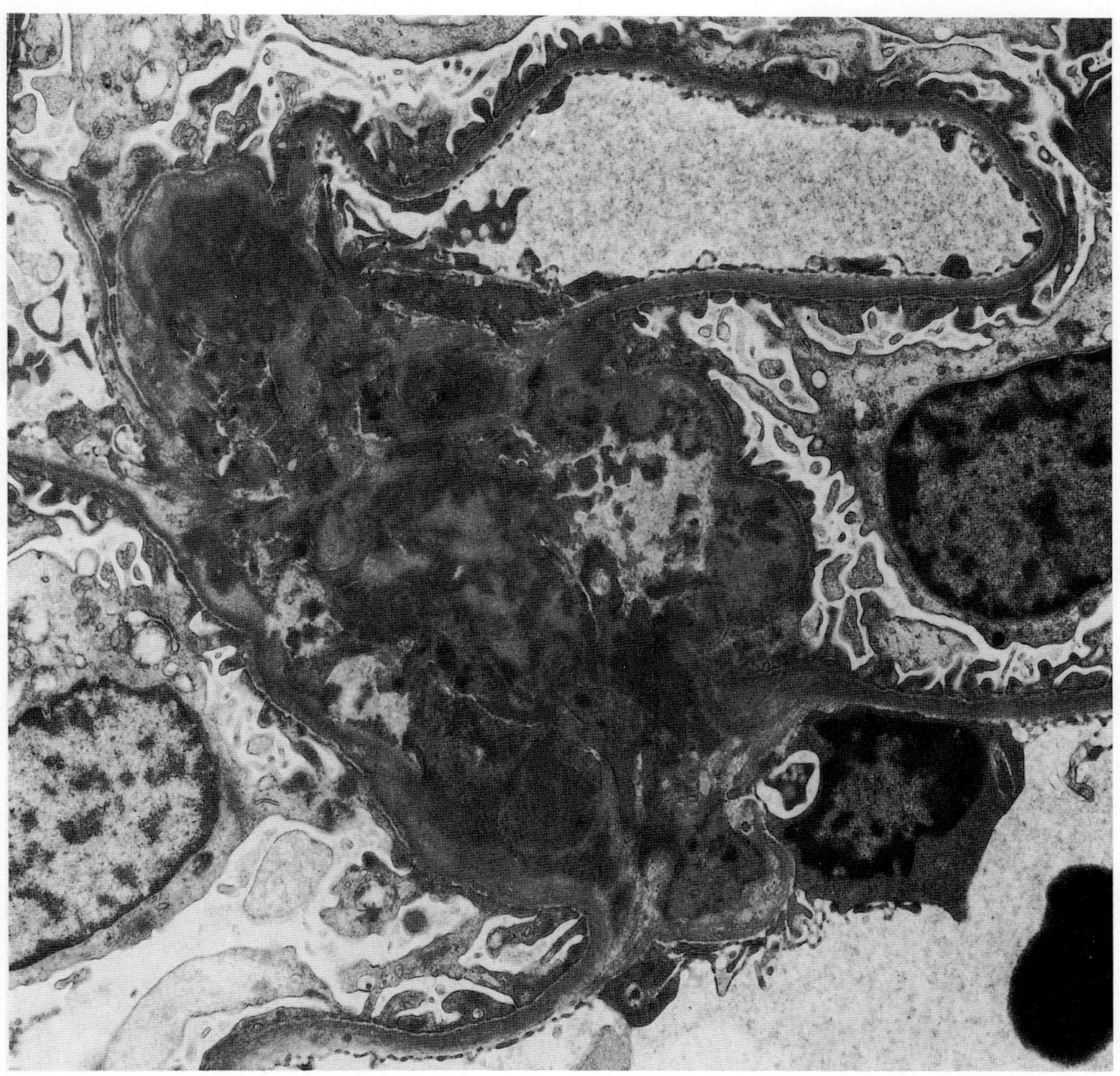

FIG. 51. Ultrastructural changes in lupus nephritis. **A:** In WHO class II (mesangial) lupus nephritis, only mesangial electron-dense deposits are seen (uranyl acetate, lead citrate; ×10,000).

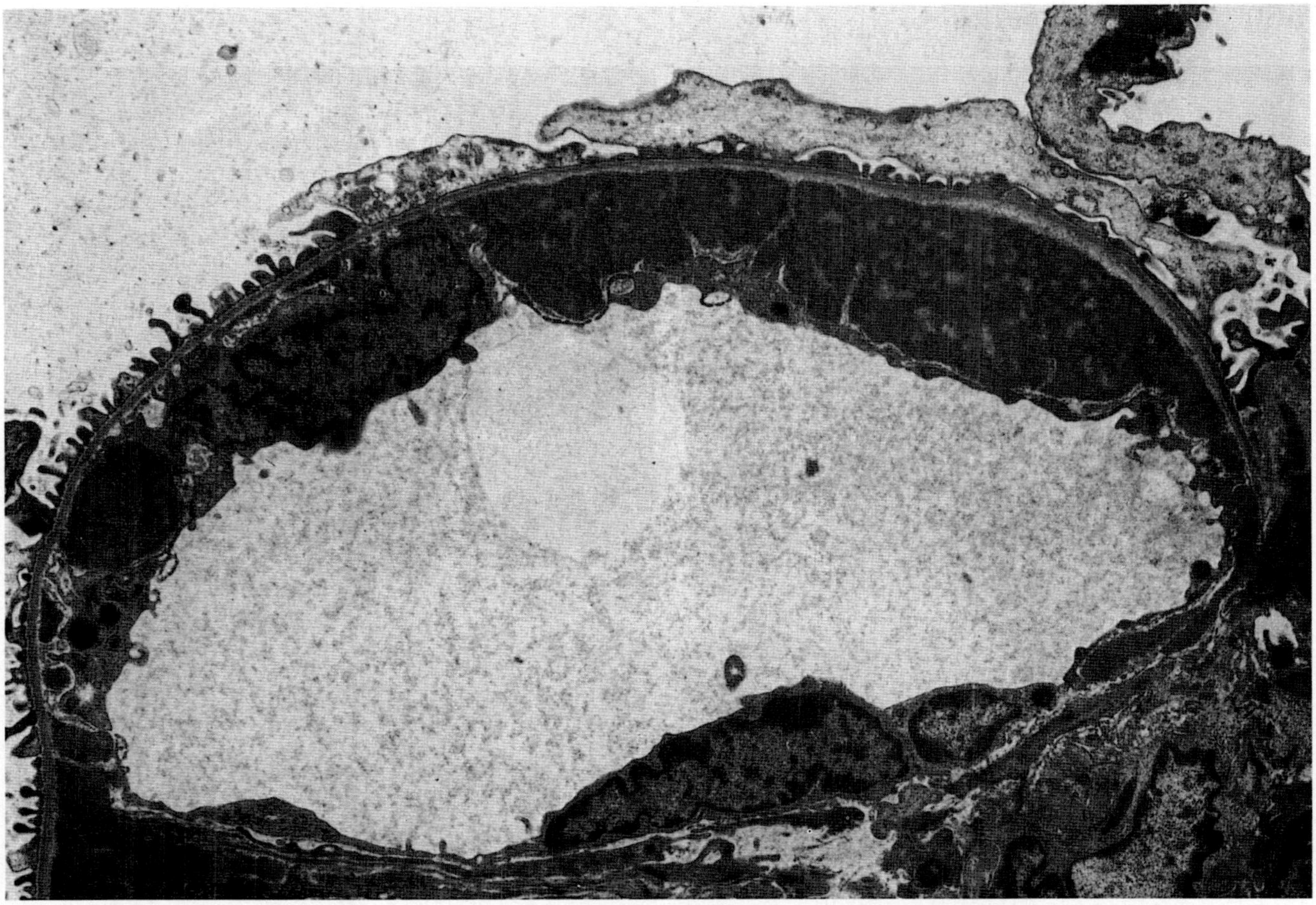

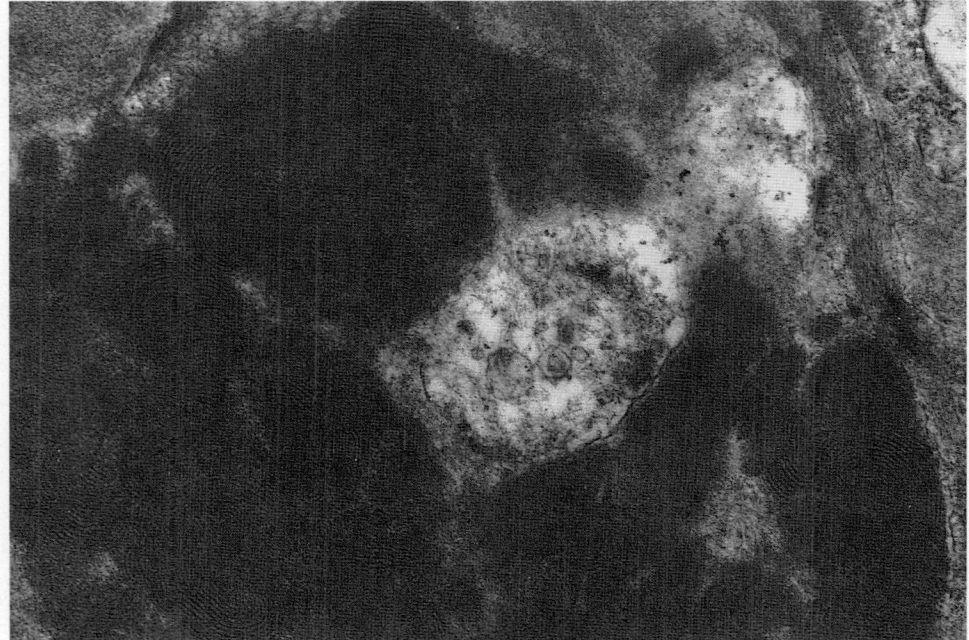

FIG. 51. (*continued*) **B:** Large, electron-dense subendothelial deposits in diffuse proliferative (WHO class IV) lupus nephritis (uranyl acetate, lead citrate; ×10,000). **C:** Occasionally, electron-dense deposits in lupus nephritis have a fingerprint-like ultrastructure (uranyl acetate, lead citrate; ×17,000).

The Issue of Activity and Chronicity

The purpose of renal biopsy in a lupus patient is not to confirm the presence of SLE but to determine the severity and type of renal involvement and provide an aid to therapeutic decisions. If lupus nephritis is florid and active, more aggressive therapy is necessary, with pulse steroids and even cyclophosphamide and possibly other immunosuppressive drugs, to prevent rapid progression to chronic renal failure. On the other hand, if the biopsy sample shows mostly severe, chronic, irreversible changes, with glomerulosclerosis and interstitial fibrosis, then aggressive therapy is not warranted because of the serious side effects of these drugs. To standardize the approach to evaluation of chronicity and activity, a widely used scoring system has been developed (151,152).

The *activity index* includes cellular crescents, (glomerular) fibrinoid necrosis/karyorrhexis, endocapillary hypercellularity, (glomerular) leukocyte infiltration, large subendothelial deposits (wire loops), and interstitial inflammation. The severity of each of these features is scored from 0 to 3, and the scores of glomerular cellular crescents and fibrinoid necrosis/karyorrhexis are multiplied by 2. Thus, the maximum score is 24. The *chronicity index* comprises glomerulosclerosis, fibrous crescents, tubular atrophy, and interstitial fibrosis. The severity of each is scored from 0 to 3, thus the maximum score is 12. The problem with this type of scoring is that it is somewhat complicated and subjective and thus not very reproducible. In addition, important signs of activity, such as TBM and vascular deposits, and other acute vascular changes should also be included.

Differential Diagnosis

Because of the variable morphologic characteristics of lupus nephritis, any immune complex GN could be listed here. Clinical and laboratory data are quite important to the diagnosis. Occasionally, IgA nephropathy and, particularly, HSP can be a problem in the context of differential diagnosis because IgA may be a co-dominant immunoreactant in lupus nephritis. C1q nephropathy is another entity that may come into the differential diagnosis because of the frequently prominent C1q staining in lupus nephritis. While the presence of many endothelial tubuloreticular inclusions favors lupus, it is not diagnostic of it.

Outcome

Class II lesions tend to remain stable or progress very slowly, whereas lesions in classes III and IV are progressive unless the activity of the acute inflammatory process can be arrested by appropriate therapy. Transformation of lupus nephritis from one pattern to another takes place in about 20% to 30% of cases that are submitted for rebiopsy (146). Very active, "hot" inflammatory lesions, including widespread glomerular necrosis and crescent formation and vascular necrosis with thrombosis, are indicators of a poor outcome (153). As in every glomerular and renal disease, the more chronic the changes (the higher the chronicity index), the poorer the outcome. The recurrence of lupus nephritis in renal transplants is very rare.

Etiologic Factors and Pathogenesis

Lupus nephritis has traditionally been thought to be the prototype of immune complex GN, owing to the deposition of circulating immune complexes. There is also evidence of possible *in situ* immune complex formation. The glomerular immune complexes have been shown to contain antibodies to a variety of nuclear constituents. It was recently postulated that increased apoptosis in lupus patients induces excessive autoantibody formation against various nuclear proteins and nucleic acid sequences (154). It is worth noting that such drugs as hydralazine, procainamide, methyldopa, and chlorpromazine (and others) can induce an SLE-like disease; renal symptoms quite similar to those of true lupus nephritis develop, but less frequently than in spontaneous SLE.

OTHER "COLLAGEN-VASCULAR" DISEASES

There can be a diverse pattern of renal injury in these conditions. Wegener's granulomatosis, microscopic polyarteritis (or hypersensitivity angiitis), and other forms of vasculitides are frequently associated with pauci-immune crescentic and necrotizing GN (see relevant section). Progressive systemic sclerosis (scleroderma), in its acute form (acute scleroderma crisis), is associated with renal histopathologic findings resembling malignant hypertension/TMA (155). In mixed connective tissue disease and other lupus-like syndromes, in which patients have some features of SLE but do not fulfill all the American Rheumatology Association criteria for the diagnosis of SLE, immune complex GN may develop, predominantly with a mesangial pattern. In primary antiphospholipid syndrome, patients may show signs of TMA (156).

Rheumatoid Arthritis

Rheumatoid arthritis, an immune-mediated systemic disorder of connective tissue, may give rise to clinical renal disease through a variety of lesions, including amyloidosis, arteritis, and chronic interstitial nephritis (related to infection or analgesic nephropathy with papillary necrosis or to use of various drugs for the treatment of rheumatoid arthritis) (157–159). Colloidal gold therapy may lead to proteinuria, and even the nephrotic syndrome, through the production of membranous GN. Gold is not present in the glomerular subepithelial deposits but can be found in tubular and interstitial cells. The exact mechanism of action leading to membranous GN following gold therapy is not known. Mesangial expansion and hypercellularity, with or without immune complex deposition, may also develop in patients with rheumatoid arthritis (160). Most patients with this disease do not experience renal involvement.

MONOCLONAL GAMMOPATHY-ASSOCIATED RENAL DISEASES

AL (Primary) Amyloidosis

This is the most common disease association with monoclonal gammopathies (161); it is discussed in the section concerning the diseases with acellular closure of glomerular capillaries.

Nonamyloidotic Monoclonal Immunoglobulin Deposition Disease (Mostly Light Chain Deposition Disease)

Epidemiology

Although it is a rare disease, it is the second most common plasma cell dyscrasia–related renal disorder (161). It is most frequently due to kappa light chain (unlike AL amyloidosis) deposition, and rarely to lambda light chain deposition. Cases of heavy chain, as well as light and heavy chain, deposition disease have been reported. The disease is found in adults and in the elderly.

Clinical Symptoms

Patients manifest heavy proteinuria with or without nephrotic syndrome. Microscopic hematuria is typical, as is renal insufficiency. Relatively few patients have overt myeloma, but a monoclonal spike in the serum and/or urine is usually (but not always) present.

Light Microscopic Features

The most characteristic lesion is nodular glomerulosclerosis. The sclerotic, acellular, mesangial nodules are quite similar to the Kimmelstiel-Wilson nodules of nodular diabetic glomerulosclerosis, but other histologic changes characteristic of diabetes (fibrin caps, capsular drops, severe arteriolar hyalinosis) are usually absent or are not prominent. Occasionally, other glomerular abnormalities, such as membranoproliferative or other intra- or extracapillary proliferative patterns, are seen (138,161–164). A characteristic tubular change is homogeneous, glassy thickening of the basement membranes of nonatrophic tubules. An interstitial mononuclear cell infiltrate may be present, but a monoclonal plasma cell population is generally not a constituent of this infiltrate.

Immunofluorescence Characteristics

Only one of the light chains (rarely, a heavy chain as well and, in exceptional cases, only a heavy chain) shows fluorescence, usually in a linear fashion along glomerular capillaries and TBMs (Fig. 52). This staining is most often only kappa chain. The mesangium is also frequently positive.

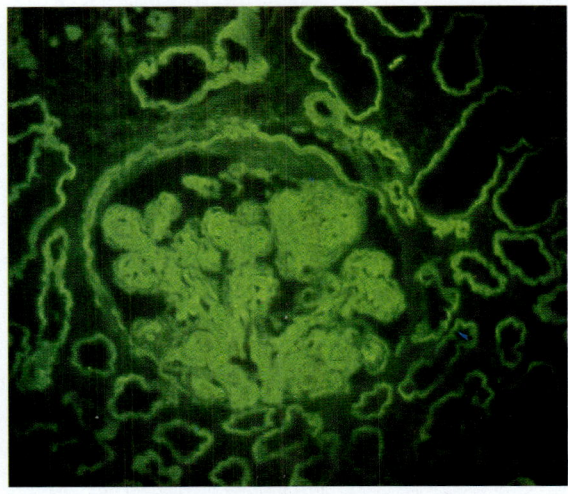

FIG. 52. In light chain deposition disease, one of the light chains (usually kappa) is deposited throughout the expanded (frequently nodular) mesangium, the glomerular capillary basement membranes, and the tubular basement membranes (anti-kappa light chain; ×140).

Electron Microscopic Features

Finely granular, electron-dense, ribbon-like, mostly continuous deposits along the subendothelial aspect of the GBM are highly characteristic (Fig. 53) (165). These finely granular deposits are also present in the mesangial matrix and, frequently, also along the interstitial (outer) aspect of the TBMs; they are rarely found in the interstitium. Occasionally, no such deposits are visible in spite of the characteristic IF. In such cases (for obscure reasons), the density of the deposits is probably not different from the basement membranes, but immunoelectron microscopy with antibodies to kappa and lambda light chains may reveal the monoclonal light chain deposits. In our experience, this study can be performed on glutaraldehyde-fixed, resin-embedded thin sections (but only with antibodies to light chains).

Differential Diagnosis

As mentioned earlier, nodular diabetic glomerulosclerosis may have a very similar light microscopic appearance. Other diseases with nodular glomerulosclerosis are discussed in the differential diagnosis section of diabetic nephropathy. If monoclonal IgG heavy chains are deposited, linear IF may raise the possibility of anti-GBM disease. In monoclonal immunoglobulin (light chain) deposition disease, the deposits now and then have a focally or more diffusely fibrillar or microtubular appearance. If only one light chain is present on IF, with a corresponding monoclonal spike in the serum and/or urine, these cases should not be diagnosed as fibrillary or immunotactoid GN. Amyloidosis should also be excluded.

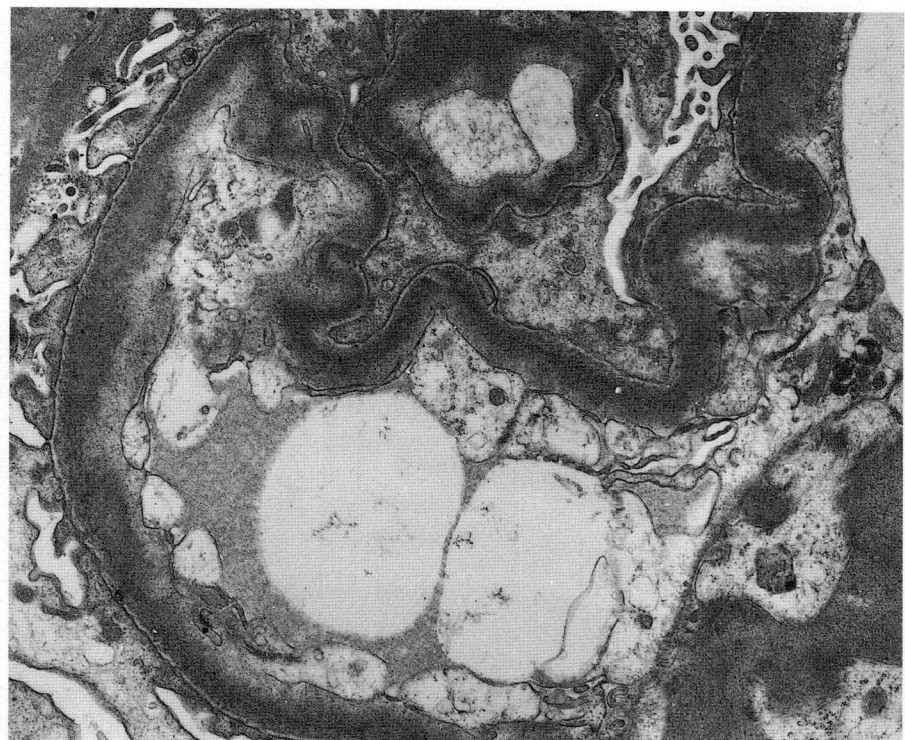

FIG. 53. Finely granular deposits along the glomerular basement membrane in a case of kappa light chain deposition disease (uranyl acetate, lead citrate; ×6,300).

Outcome

Most patients progress to ESRD within a few years following diagnosis. The disease tends to recur in renal transplants, but it appears that long-term graft survival is still possible (166).

Pathogenesis

The pathogenesis is unclear. It appears likely that local physicochemical properties of the renal extracellular matrix and the monoclonal light chain (immunoglobulin) cause excessive binding of the monoclonal light chain to certain sites. Why kappa light chains cause mainly nonamyloidotic granular deposits and lambda light chains produce fibrillary amyloid deposits is still puzzling. Circulating factors, such as amyloid P component and apolipoprotein E, may determine whether amyloid fibrils or nonamyloidotic granular deposits will form (138,164).

Myeloma Cast Nephropathy (Synonyms: Bence Jones Cast Nephropathy, Myeloma Kidney)

Epidemiology

This is the third major complication of plasma cell dyscrasia, but it is less common than amyloidosis and light chain deposition disease (161).

Clinical Symptoms

Acute renal failure and frequently severe proteinuria are the leading renal findings. Proteinuria may consist almost entirely of light chains (Bence Jones protein). Most patients have overt myeloma.

Light Microscopic Features

Numerous large, refractile, angular, usually glassy eosinophilic casts, surrounded by giant cells and macrophages, are practically diagnostic (Fig. 54) (163,167,168). The giant cells are of monocyte/macrophage, not epithelial, origin. Some casts may have faint Congo red and thioflavin T positivity. Variable numbers of interstitial inflammatory cells can be seen. The glomeruli are usually unremarkable.

Immunofluorescence Characteristics

IF is not truly helpful because the casts may contain both light chains (as a result of entrapment). Rarely, concomitant monoclonal light chain deposition is seen in glomeruli and in TBMs.

Electron Microscopic Features

EM is not helpful. The casts and the tubular epithelial cells may contain needle-shaped crystalline material (165).

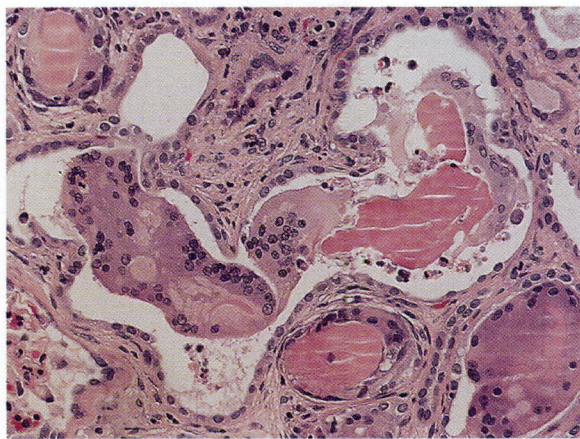

FIG. 54. Myeloma cast nephropathy. Note the glassy casts surrounded by inflammatory cells, including multinucleated giant cells.

Differential Diagnosis

Casts surrounded by inflammatory cells and macrophages can sometimes be seen in other conditions, such as some cases of acute tubular necrosis (ATN). The giant-cell reaction around the large refractile casts, however, is virtually diagnostic. Similar casts with giant cells have been reported in exceptional cases of pancreatic adenocarcinoma.

Outcome

Development of ESRD is the rule. Experience with renal transplantation is limited, but this option is not given to many patients because of the underlying multiple myeloma.

Pathogenesis

The intrinsic properties of paraproteins, facilitated by local physicochemical conditions, trigger excessive precipitation with Tamm-Horsfall protein and subsequent cast formation. The genesis of giant-cell reaction around the casts is unclear.

TUBULOINTERSTITIAL DISEASES

Often the renal tubules and interstitium are affected by the same disease process, because of the close topographical and functional association between these two renal compartments. Hence the generic encompassing term tubulointerstitial disease. One should attempt to further define a case of tubulointerstitial disease with clinical and morphologic methods whenever possible. The importance of tubulointerstitial changes in various renal diseases is stressed by several authors (169,170). It appears that renal function primarily correlates with the interstitial volume (widening due to edema, inflammation, or fibrosis) and that long-term prognosis is particularly determined by the extent of interstitial fibrosis.

Acute Tubular Necrosis

Epidemiology

ATN is the typical cause of acute renal failure in any sex and race and at any age. It is usually due to renal hypoperfusion (hypoxia), but toxic agents, hemolysis, and rhabdomyolysis can also cause ATN.

Clinical Symptoms

Acute renal failure is invariably present and is usually oligoanuric, but it can be polyuric. Typically, the urinary sediment contains granular casts, sloughed tubular epithelial cells, and, rarely, red blood cells. It is important to note that acute renal failure and ATN are not synonyms. Acute renal failure can be precipitated by a variety of conditions [e.g., ATN, acute GN (crescentic forms), acute interstitial nephritis, thrombotic microangiopathies, etc.], ATN is only one of the causes of acute renal failure, albeit the most usual. Systemic symptoms and clinical history are helpful in deciding whether ATN is due to hypoxic or toxic causes. In the more typical hypoxic form, patients frequently have cardiac insufficiency, severe peripheral circulatory disturbances, serious blood loss or hypovolemia, or compromised renal blood flow. ATN is a feared complication of shock (shock kidney).

Gross Appearance

The kidney is somewhat swollen and may have a slightly edematous, pale appearance. Frequently, the cortex is anemic and the medulla is hyperemic with a sharp demarcation of the corticomedullary junction.

Light Microscopic Features

The renal tubular epithelial abnormalities in ischemic ATN can be quite subtle, and frank necrosis of tubular epithelium is uncommon (Fig. 55A). In severe cases of toxic ATN, there is frank necrosis (coagulation necrosis) of the tubular (primarily proximal) epithelium (171,172). ATN is sometimes associated with a mild interstitial inflammatory infiltrate of lymphocytes and mononuclear cells. Occasionally, detached tubular epithelial cells leave segments of the TBM denuded (nonreplacement phenomenon). One would believe that this detachment is the consequence of tubular epithelial cell necrosis. Surprisingly, it has been shown that the majority of shed epithelial cells in voided urine from patients with ATN are still viable (173).

There is often loss of the PAS-positive brush border of proximal tubules, an abnormality that sometimes makes it difficult to distinguish proximal from distal tubules by LM. In addition, hyaline and pigmented or nonpigmented granular casts often are present in the distal tubules and collecting ducts. A variable degree of diffuse interstitial edema and accumulation of myeloid cells within the vasa recta also are common findings. Regenerative tubular epithelial changes

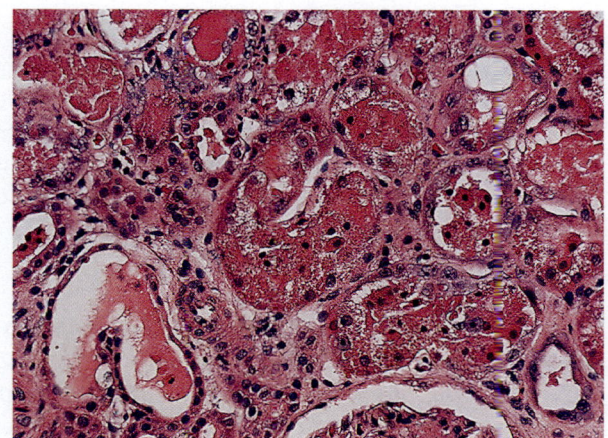 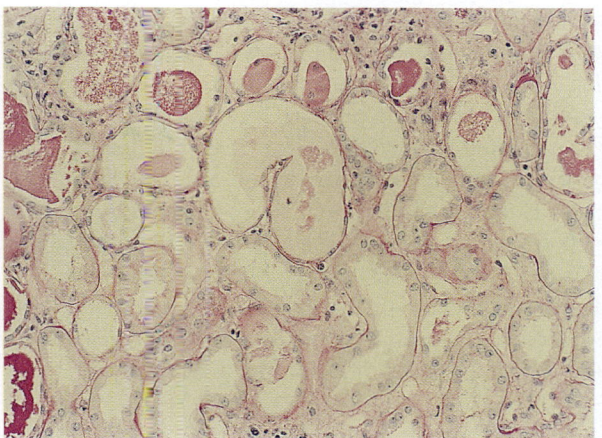

FIG. 55. Acute tubular necrosis. **A:** Note the widespread coagulative necrosis of the tubular epithelium in this severe case of acute tubular necrosis in a renal transplant. **B:** Flattening of the tubular epithelium and dilated tubular lumina as well as granular casts are characteristic findings in acute tubular necrosis, particularly in the resolving phase (periodic acid–Schiff).

almost always are evident, except in the very severe acute stage. Changes thought to represent regeneration include flattening of the epithelium, with dilatation of the tubular lumen, and variability in cell and nuclear size and configuration (large regenerative nuclei with prominent nucleoli) (Fig. 55B). Mitotic figures may be seen from time to time.

Ischemic damage involves many different portions of the nephron. Studies with nephron segment-specific tubular epithelial markers show that the regenerating tubules are both distal and proximal in origin, frequently with a slight distal predominance (174). Toxic damage usually leads to damage of that portion of the nephron most responsible for excretion of drugs and organic acids/bases, that is, the proximal tubule (171,172). In hemoglobinuric or myoglobinuric ATN, many granular casts, some of which may be pigmented, occlude the distal nephron. Immunohistochemical application of antibodies to myoglobin (or hemoglobin) is useful in the diagnosis. In severe hepatic failure with jaundice, ATN may develop, with bile pigment in the casts. This condition has been called hepatic nephrosis.

Immunofluorescence and Electron Microscopy

These techniques usually are not helpful in the diagnosis of ATN.

Differential Diagnosis

One always has to keep in mind that ATN can be seen in association with other renal diseases, such as thrombotic microangiopathies, acute pyelonephritis and acute noninfectious interstitial nephritis, crescentic and other glomerulonephritides, and MCNS. Thus, it is most important to make sure that the changes of ATN do not stem from an underlying renal disease.

At autopsy, distinguishing between true ATN and autolysis can be quite difficult. In autolysis, almost all tubular epithelial cells are diffusely sloughed off the TBM. The presence of intact nuclei in nearby cells (glomerular, vascular, tubular) suggests that the tubular injury represents true ATN. In addition, granular casts in the collecting ducts and increased numbers of myeloid cells in the vasa recta are signs favoring ATN.

Outcome

The tubular epithelium has a remarkable regenerative capacity; if there is no severe underlying and persistent disease, the outcome with supportive (dialysis) therapy is good, and patients can fully recover. Even though renal function returns to normal, we cannot be absolutely sure that histologic healing is complete, because few follow-up biopsies are now performed in these patients. It is quite possible that focal interstitial scarring will remain, particularly in cases where ATN is accompanied by TBM disruption. We have seen a few patients with protracted ATN in whom prominent interstitial fibrosis was found on follow-up biopsies. Patients who have ATN due to shock have a high mortality rate, especially if the shock is associated with multiorgan failure (175).

Etiologic Factors and Pathogenesis

The etiologic factors have been addressed. To summarize briefly, ATN can be the consequence of renal hypoperfusion/hypoxia (ischemic), systemic hypotension, renal vasoconstriction, compromise of the renal vascular bed, toxins, drugs and therapeutic agents, severe hepatic failure, rhabdomyolysis, and hemolysis. The tubular epithelium is sensitive to hypoxia and toxins and quickly undergoes widespread injury following such insults. There is evidence that renal blood flow diminishes substantially in patients with ischemic and toxic ATN, apparently as the result of arteriolar vasoconstriction (176). The renin–angiotensin system, prostaglandins, atrial natriuretic factor, and endothelin have all been implicated as mediators of this vasoconstriction. Many investigators believe that tubular obstructive casts also play an important role in the pathogenesis of acute renal failure. This obstruction would increase intratubular pressure, contributing to the back-leak of tubular fluid into the interstitium through the damaged tubular epithelium. This tubular back-leak causes increased interstitial edema (and, in fact, increased interstitial volume), which further impairs renal function.

Acute Pyelonephritis (Acute Infectious Tubulointerstitial Nephritis, Diffuse Suppurative Nephritis)

Although there is some confusion in the nomenclature, we prefer the term acute pyelonephritis as opposed to acute infectious interstitial nephritis. Acute pyelonephritis is caused by ascending bacterial infection, rarely fungal infection, and is usually preceded by infection and inflammation of the urinary tract, including the renal pelvis. In hematogenously disseminated infection, bacteria and fungi are the causative agents, but the renal pelvis is mostly not involved. Thus, the term acute pyelonephritis is nosologically incorrect; diffuse suppurative nephritis is more appropriate terminology in such cases, especially if there is abscess formation. The term acute infectious tubulointerstitial nephritis has been introduced. This, in our opinion, is rather vague wording, since it also encompasses interstitial nephritides caused by viruses. The morphologic and clinical picture of viral-induced interstitial nephritis resembles acute (noninfectious) interstitial nephritis more than acute pyelonephritis, and, in our opinion, the disease should be classed with other (nonbacterial) interstitial nephritides.

Epidemiology

Acute pyelonephritis is one of the most common acute renal diseases. It is more often found in women. In spite of the high incidence of the disease, acute pyelonephritis is rarely and incidentally seen in renal pathology practice because renal biopsies are not performed in clinically diagnosed cases.

Clinical Symptoms

Fever, lumbar tenderness and pain, dysuria, and pyuria are classic symptoms. There will be organisms in excess of 100,000 cfu/ml in the urine, a condition called significant bacteriuria. Variable degrees of renal impairment may develop in severe cases. In many patients, however, absence of some or most of the symptoms hinders diagnosis, and it is likely that many minor, subclinical episodes go unrecognized. A substantial number of patients experience urinary tract obstruction.

Gross Appearance

In ascending infection the kidney has yellow striping in the medulla and medullary rays, with scattered abscess formation throughout the renal parenchyma. In hematogenous spread, there are scattered and usually small abscesses throughout the cortex, with sparing of the medulla.

Light Microscopic Features

Large collections of polymorphonuclear leukocytes are present throughout the renal interstitium (medulla and cortex) and in tubular lumens (Fig. 56A,B) (177). Sometimes microabscesses can be seen, and tubular epithelial destruction is widespread. An associated mononuclear infiltrate of monocytes/macrophages and lymphocytes is present. There

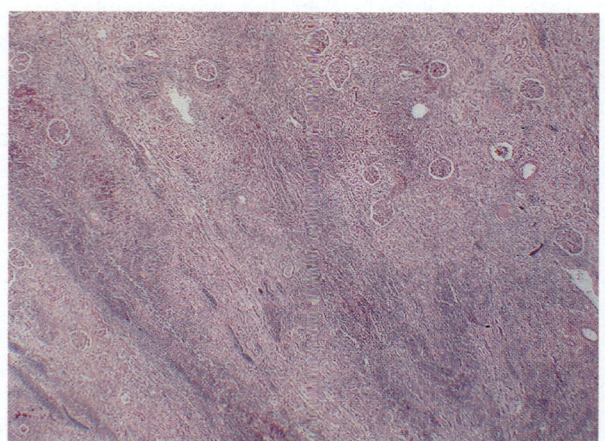
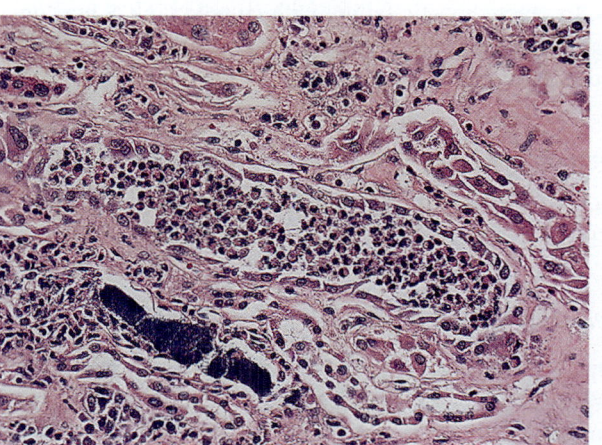

FIG. 56. Acute pyelonephritis. **A:** On low magnification, medullary and cortical stripes of inflammatory cells (mostly polymorphonuclear cells) are characteristic of an ascending infection. **B:** High magnification shows the intratubular and peritubular polymorphonuclear cells, with destruction of the tubular epithelium. There is dystrophic calcification in a tubule.

is often intense acute or chronic inflammation and even disruption of the pelvic epithelium and pyelocalyceal structures. Frequently, the pattern of inflammatory infiltrate reflects the ascending infection; stripelike involvement in the renal medulla and, in particular, severe inflammation in the medullary rays in the cortex may be noted (Fig. 56A). Bacterial or fungal stains may show the microorganism involved. In hematogenous infection (diffuse suppurative nephritis), glomerular microabscesses may be seen. The renal medulla and the pelvicocalyceal structures are usually spared in such cases.

Immunofluorescence and Electron Microscopy

These methods are not helpful to make the diagnosis.

Differential Diagnosis

In severe forms of ATN with prominent tubular epithelial necrosis, polymorphonuclears (PMNs) may be seen in tubular lumina and around damaged tubules, giving the impression of mild acute pyelonephritis. In acute (nonbacterial) interstitial nephritis, focal accumulation of PMNs may sometimes be noted around more severely affected areas with prominent tubulointerstitial injury. In such cases, most of the PMNs are around, and not in, the tubular lumina. In some cases, however, it may be difficult to make the diagnosis in a small renal biopsy specimen, and in such instances the possibility of renal infection should be raised in the renal biopsy report.

Outcome

Most cases resolve with appropriate antibiotic therapy. If the underlying predisposing condition (e.g., urinary tract obstruction) is not corrected, recurrent attacks are common, eventually leading to chronic pyelonephritis.

Etiologic Factors and Pathogenesis

Most cases develop through an ascending infection from the lower urinary tract (urinary bladder). This ascending infection is particularly common in patients with urinary obstruction and vesicoureteral reflux. Other predisposing factors include pregnancy, diabetes mellitus, and various immunosuppressive states. Rarely, the renal infection develops through a hematogenous route as a consequence of bacteremia or systemic fungal infection. Certain bacterial strains of *E. coli* cause more frequent and more severe episodes of pyelonephritis. This may be due to specific fimbriae on the bacterial surface with which they are able to adhere to urinary epithelium and tubular epithelial surfaces.

Acute Interstitial Nephritis

The terms acute and chronic interstitial nephritis refer primarily to the presence (chronic) or absence (acute) of interstitial fibrosis (178). Thus, in acute interstitial nephritis, one sees only interstitial edema, not fibrosis (179–181). Because the vast majority of cells in the interstitium are mononuclear cells (cells also seen in chronic inflammation), the terms acute and chronic do not indicate the nature of the cellular infiltrate. These mononuclear cells, if activated, can cause acute injury, which is reflected by their infiltration of tubular epithelium (tubulitis), a feature invariably present in acute interstitial nephritis. In contrast, in chronic interstitial nephritis, the mononuclear cells are mostly quiescent and localized to areas of fibrosis and scarring; tubulitis is rarely seen except in some atrophic tubules.

Epidemiology

Acute interstitial nephritis occurs in all age groups and races and in both sexes. It is primarily associated with certain drugs.

Clinical Symptoms

These patients can have a variety of clinical symptoms, but they usually do not have nephrosis, nephritis, or severe hypertension. They often experience acute renal failure with elevated serum creatinine levels, elevated BUN levels, microscopic hematuria, and/or a variety of tubular defects, such as electrolyte disturbances, inability to concentrate urine, renal tubular acidosis, and Fanconi's syndrome. There may be eosinophilia, eosinophiluria, fever, and skin rash. In NSAID-induced cases, nephrotic-range proteinuria may be associated with minimal change disease (182).

Gross Appearance

The kidney is lightly swollen and edematous.

Light Microscopic Features

The primary and most severe findings are in the interstitium (179–181). The interstitium contains a number of inflammatory cells, usually mononuclear cells (Fig. 57). Studies with monoclonal antibodies against inflammatory cell subsets indicate that the majority of infiltrating cells are T lymphocytes, with varying proportions of CD4- and CD8-positive cells. The remainder of the cells are mainly macrophages; scattered polymorphonuclear cells may also be seen. The number of B lymphocytes is relatively small (183). Eosinophils, and sometimes plasma cells, may be prominent. The presence of renal interstitial eosinophils is thought to be the result of a hypersensitivity reaction, typically due to drug allergy (usually antibiotics) (181). In our experience, however, eosinophils can be seen in any type of interstitial nephritis, and they are by no means specific to drug-induced interstitial nephritis.

The interstitial inflammatory cells frequently invade the tubular epithelium (tubulitis). The infiltrating leukocytes

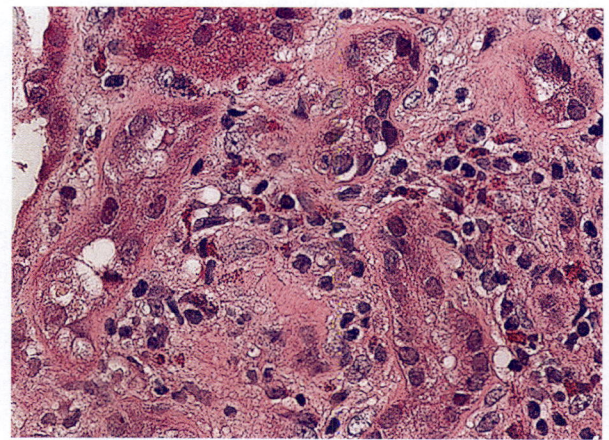 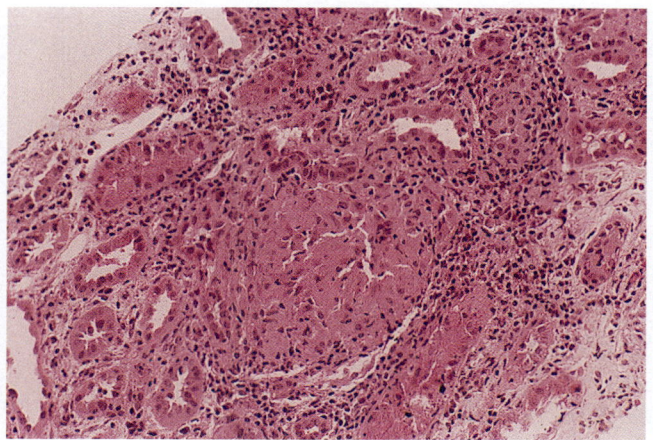

FIG. 57. Acute interstitial nephritis. **A:** Interstitial inflammation of mononuclear cells frequently admixed with eosinophils is a characteristic finding; however, eosinophils are not necessary to make this diagnosis. **B:** In this case of interstitial nephritis, granulomas with epithelial cells and giant cells are present in a case of sarcoidosis.

may cause disruption of the TBM, with subsequent spillage of tubular luminal contents (PAS-positive Tamm-Horsfall protein–containing material) into the renal interstitium. Sometimes, well-formed granulomata may be a feature of drug-induced interstitial nephritis (184). The glomeruli and vasculature are usually unremarkable.

Immunofluorescence Characteristics

IF is not informative in most cases, except for the exclusion of immune complex GN as a primary process. In exceptional cases, acute interstitial nephritis may be caused by anti-TBM antibodies or immune complex deposition along the TBM. In such cases, linear or granular TBM fluorescence is seen, respectively. In SLE, TBM deposits are not unusual, but they are primarily associated with prominent glomerular immune complex deposition (179).

Electron Microscopic Features

EM is generally not helpful. In the rare cases of TBM immune complex deposits, corresponding electron-dense deposits may be present. Sometimes viral particles can be discovered.

Differential Diagnosis

Acute pyelonephritis should be excluded (see previous discussion). It is also important to make sure that the interstitial mononuclear cell infiltrate is not the result of a primary glomerular or vascular disease. Many eosinophils are frequently seen in drug-induced interstitial nephritis (particularly that caused by antibiotics), but this is not a specific diagnostic sign because eosinophils can be found in any form of acute interstitial nephritis (185). If an infectious agent is suspected as the source (see later discussion), antibody or nucleic acid probes specific for the suspected pathogen may be useful. Typical viral inclusions are rarely seen in a renal biopsy sample. In hantavirus- or leptospira-induced interstitial nephritis, interstitial hemorrhage may be prominent. If there are epithelioid granulomas, drug-induced (NSAID) interstitial nephritis and sarcoidosis are likely; however, infectious granulomas, particularly if necrotizing granulomas are evident, should also be considered, and special stains for fungi and bacteria, including mycobacteria, should be performed.

Outcome

Prompt withdrawal of the offending drug (if it is known) and/or steroid therapy often leads to amelioration of drug-induced interstitial nephritis. Elimination of viral or other etiologic agents usually also leads to resolution. If it is not possible to identify the etiologic agent, progressive disease may develop.

Etiology and Pathogenesis

The list of agents that may directly or indirectly cause acute interstitial nephritis is very long, and the reader is referred to reviews addressing the issue (179–185). The most important pathogenetic causes and etiologic agents are secondary forms (GN, vascular disease with renal involvement, e.g., vasculitis), drugs (antibiotics, such as methicillin, other penicillin derivatives, rifampin; NSAIDs; and many others), direct infection (viruses, among them, adenovirus, polyoma virus, cytomegalovirus, other herpesviruses; rickettsia; bacteria, such as leptospira), reactivity to infection (bacteria, such as *Streptococcus beta hemolyticus, yersinia, brucella,* etc.; viruses, among them Epstein-Barr virus, HIV, etc.), systemic disease (Sjögren's syndrome, sarcoidosis), other rare associations (anti-TBM disease, toxins, metabolic and hereditary diseases, etc.), and idiopathic sources. Some agents (drugs) lead to interstitial nephritis via an immunologic pathway. They may serve as haptens or give rise to cross-reactions with tubular or interstitial antigens. Other drugs lead to a dose-dependent injury (such as amphotericin, polymyxin B, the cephalosporins, and gentamicin).

Chronic Interstitial Nephritis

In this pattern, interstitial fibrosis with tubular atrophy predominates. Glomerular and vascular changes are minor or less severe and frequently stem from the interstitial disease. A mononuclear cell infiltrate is frequently seen, but it is mostly localized to scarred, fibrotic areas, and tubulitis (except for perhaps in a few atrophic tubules) is not evident. Based on renal biopsy, only the nonspecific diagnosis of chronic interstitial nephritis can be made in most cases; it is usually not possible to render a specific diagnosis. Accurate clinical history and imaging studies on the entire shape and size of the kidney are of major importance in making an unequivocal diagnosis. Any chronic injury affecting the tubulointerstitium may cause chronic interstitial nephritis. Various forms of chronic pyelonephritis, analgesic nephropathy, and some morphologically more specific forms of the disease are discussed here.

Chronic Pyelonephritis and Reflux Nephropathy

These are related conditions, and in many publications these terms are used interchangeably. In reflux nephropathy, the primary disorder is thought to be reflux of urine into the renal parenchyma through compound renal papillae (papillae draining larger areas, usually at the upper or lower pole of the kidney, which may have a concave instead of a normal convex shape) or misshapen renal papillae. Reflux nephropathy is not initially associated with a dilated renal pelvis (nonobstructive chronic pyelonephritis). Alternatively, urinary tract obstruction may be present, with subsequent pelvic dilatation (obstructive chronic pyelonephritis) (177,186,187).

Epidemiology

The epidemiologic picture is similar to that of acute pyelonephritis. Chronic pyelonephritis is a common cause of ESRD throughout the world, particularly in women.

Clinical Symptoms

A history of recurrent urinary tract infections (usually since childhood) is most important from the point of view of clinical diagnosis. Some degree of renal insufficiency with hypertension is common. Renal imaging studies, such as intravenous or retrograde pyelography, CT scan, and voiding cystourethrogram, are important in terms of establishing pelvic and calyceal structural abnormalities and possible reflux.

Gross Appearance

In obstructive chronic pyelonephritis, there is dilation (hydronephrosis) and deformation of the renal pelvis and calyces, with atrophy and scarring of the renal parenchyma (Fig. 53) (177). In nonobstructive chronic pyelonephritis, the kidneys may not show generalized calyceal dilation, but there is dilation and deformation of a limited number of the calyces (usually upper or lower pole), with retraction and destruction of the renal papillae (usually affecting the complex concave rather than normal convex papillae). There are characteristic secondary, deep, broad-based, U-shaped scars of the overlying cortex (due to destruction of the medullary ducts of Bellini) (186). For this reason, it is important to bisect the kidney in such a manner as to see the entire pyelocalyceal system (papillae).

Light Microscopic Features

It is important to emphasize that chronic pyelonephritis is not a diagnosis that can be made on LM evidence, particularly if only a needle renal biopsy specimen is available for examination. Interstitial fibrosis, with mononuclear cell infiltrates in the fibrotic areas and tubular atrophy, is the most common finding (Fig. 59A). The chronic inflammation frequently is more severe around the renal pelvis, where large lymphoid aggregates with germinal centers may develop. So-called thyroidization of tubules (Fig. 59B) was thought to be highly characteristic, but these thyroid-type atrophic

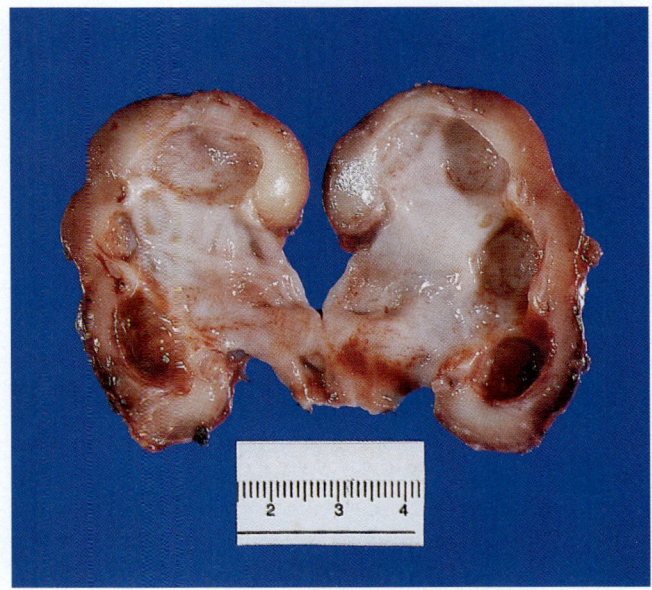

FIG. 58. Gross appearance of a kidney from a young child with advanced reflux nephropathy. Note the dilated and deformed renal pelvis and the atrophic renal parenchyma.

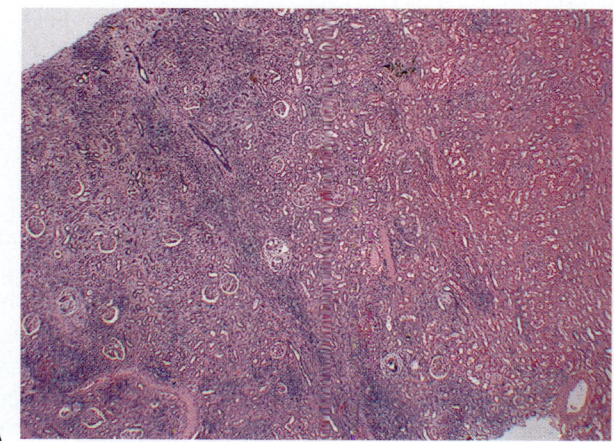
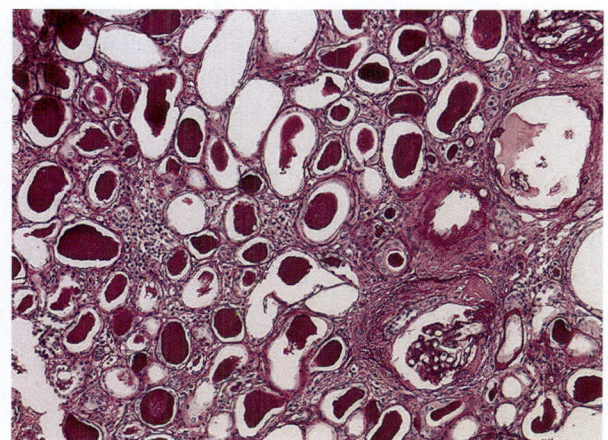

FIG. 59. Chronic pyelonephritis. **A:** Note the prominent scarring and mononuclear cell infiltrate in the renal cortex adjacent to relatively well-preserved renal parenchyma. **B:** Thyroidization of tubules in a case of advanced chronic pyelonephritis (periodic acid–Schiff).

tubules may be found in any kind of chronic renal injury. The inflammation usually does not cause tubulitis, except in atrophic tubules. An acute exacerbation, with polymorphonuclear cells in tubules and interstitium, may occur at any time.

It has been suggested that renal parenchymal destruction is most severe at the poles of the kidneys, but this frequently is not apparent, particularly in advanced cases. Interstitial deposits of Tamm-Horsfall protein in the form of large, dense, brightly PAS-positive masses represent escape of tubular contents into the interstitium either because of high intratubular pressure and subsequent rupture of tubules or because of inflammatory destruction of the tubule walls (181). There is relative sparing of the glomeruli (generally with only periglomerular fibrosis), but FSGS may develop in several forms of chronic interstitial nephritis, especially reflux nephropathy, and is often associated with variable proteinuria (usually nonnephrotic) (188,189). Changes in the arteries in the form of intimal fibrosis and "hyalinization" of arterioles may also take place.

Immunofluorescence and Electron Microscopy

These methods are not helpful to diagnosis, except to exclude superimposed glomerular diseases.

Differential Diagnosis

LM, particularly in a small renal biopsy specimen, is nonspecific. True chronic pyelonephritis is diagnosed by (a) a history of multiple urinary tract infections (presumably of the upper urinary tracts), (b) gross findings of calyceal and pelvic deformities with overlying renal parenchymal scarring, and (c) light microscopic evidence of chronic interstitial nephritis. The deep cortical scars need to be differentiated from vascular scars due to severe arterial disease. In the latter, pelvicalyceal abnormalities are generally absent, and the scar is adjacent to an occluded or severely narrowed artery. In some forms of chronic pyelonephritis, listed here, LM is important and may be the only useful diagnostic tool.

Xanthogranulomatous pyelonephritis is an uncommon inflammatory condition that can be mistaken on clinical or gross examination, and sometimes even at the microscopic level, for renal cell carcinoma (190). Because of the space-occupying nature of this lesion, a correct preoperative diagnosis may not be possible. Xanthogranulomatous pyelonephritis is usually unilateral and is characterized on gross inspection by yellow, irregular masses surrounding the renal pelvis and calyces and infiltrating and destroying adjacent renal tissue. On microscopic examination, the renal parenchyma is replaced by a granulomatous inflammatory infiltrate consisting predominantly of foamy histiocytes, a few multinucleated giant cells, and a mixture of lymphocytes, plasma cells, and neutrophils (Fig. 60). Underlying obstructive chronic pyelonephritis can be identified in most cases. *E. coli* and *Proteus mirabilis* are the most commonly identified etiologic agents.

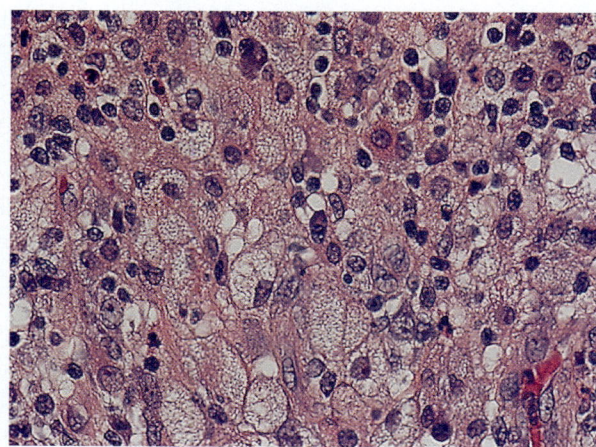

FIG. 60. Xanthogranulomatous pyelonephritis. Note the prominent foamy histiocytes admixed with mononuclear cells and a few neutrophils.

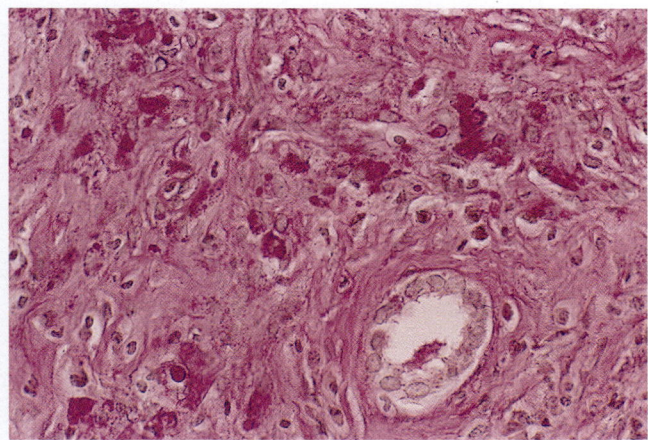

FIG. 61. Renal malacoplakia. Note the round intracytoplasmic concretions (Michaelis-Gutmann bodies) in some of the interstitial macrophages. Other macrophages contain granular cytoplasm (Hanseman cells) that is positive on periodic acid–Schiff (PAS). The diagnosis may be difficult to make without special stains (PAS).

Renal malacoplakia is characterized by large collections of PAS-positive, plump macrophages (Hanseman cells), some containing characteristic Michaelis-Gutmann bodies (iron- and calcium-laden intracytoplasmic inclusions) (Fig. 61) (191). Megalocytic interstitial nephritis is distinguished from malacoplakia by the absence of Michaelis-Gutmann bodies; however, the few published cases probably represent undiagnosed malacoplakia due to sampling error. Both of these forms of interstitial disease (and probably also xanthogranulomatous interstitial nephritis) likely are related to bacterial infections, with improper intracytoplasmic processing of the microorganisms. They may produce different appearances of the same disorder (192).

Renal tuberculosis develops in approximately 5% of patients with active tuberculosis. In addition to the kidney, other parts of the genitourinary tract are frequently affected (193). Renal tuberculosis may be part of miliary tuberculosis, with scattered, small, yellow-white tubercles, particularly in the cortex. The more traditional form represents progressive isolated organ tuberculosis. The tuberculotic granulomatous reaction gradually destroys the renal parenchyma, leaving behind cavities and large, coalescent areas of caseous material. It may be difficult to find evidence of acid-fast bacilli in advanced lesions. Renal tuberculosis often is unilateral and, thus, clinically silent. It is the classic cause of sterile pyuria. In many cases, renal tuberculosis is discovered incidentally or only at autopsy.

Outcome

Chronic pyelonephritis is a progressive disease unless the underlying course of urinary reflux (e.g., vesicoureteral reflux) or obstruction (e.g., stones) can be eradicated early.

Etiologic Factors and Pathogenesis

The typical causative agent of pyelonephritis is *E. coli*. Most cases of chronic pyelonephritis are the result of vesicoureteral and intrarenal reflux of urine, with or without obstruction and subsequent damage (177,186). This disease frequently begins in childhood in the concave compound papillae at the upper and lower poles of the kidney, in which the orifices of the Bellini ducts (in contradistinction to simple convex papillae elsewhere) are widely patent and do not close upon increased intrapelvic pressure, allowing urine contents to be refluxed into the kidney. With childhood development, the uninvolved part of the kidney continues to grow, but the affected portion of the kidney does not grow and becomes scarred. It is not known whether intrarenal reflux by itself (in the absence of infected urine) can lead to these changes.

Analgesic Nephropathy

Epidemiology

There are large geographical differences in the incidence of the disease; it varies from 0.1% to 18.1% among patients with ESRD, and the highest rate (18.1%) is in Switzerland (181,194). Other countries with a high incidence include Australia and Sweden. In the United States, the incidence has been reported to be between 1.7% and 10% among patients with ESRD in various regions. Following the withdrawal of phenacetin from the market, the incidence declined, but it remained high in many countries.

Clinical Symptoms

The most important finding is a history of analgesic abuse over several years or decades. Patients have variable degrees of renal insufficiency. Tubular damage with defects in urinary concentrating ability is a prevalent finding. Microscopic hematuria, mild proteinuria, and hypertension develop in a substantial proportion of patients. Renal imaging studies are of crucial importance in making the diagnosis: decreased renal mass, bumpy renal contours, and papillary calcifications are characteristic findings. A combination of these three features is highly specific and sensitive to the diagnosis of analgesic nephropathy (195).

Gross Appearance

The gross appearance is more characteristic than the histologic features. The kidney typically is somewhat contracted. The renal surface is bumpy, with alternating depressed and raised areas. The depressed areas represent cortical atrophy and scarring above papillary sclerosis/necrosis; the raised areas represent compensatory renal hypertrophy above the columns of Bertin (Fig. 62). The papillae are firm and shrunken, with foci of calcification and necrosis. Occasionally, the necrotic papilla is sloughed off, leaving a "raw" medullary surface behind (196).

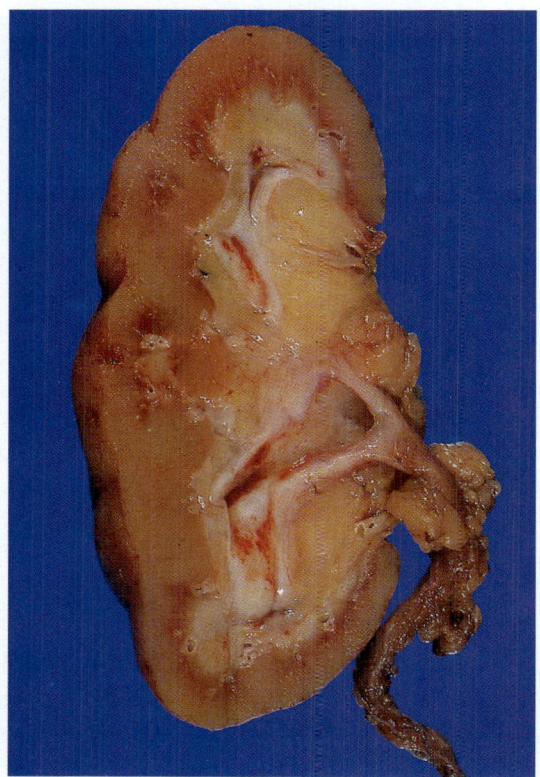

FIG. 62. Papillary necrosis. Note the atrophic cortex above the necrotic papillae.

Light Microscopic Features

The typical findings are in the medulla and renal pelvis. Early in the course of the disease, the basement membranes of the capillaries beneath the urothelial mucosa and of the thin ascending loop of Henle show substantial basement membrane thickening and calcification. At later stages, sclerosing papillary necrosis develops. This renal papillary necrosis is not associated with influx of neutrophils. The renal cortex above the necrotic papillae is atrophic, with interstitial fibrosis and tubular atrophy. The cortex in the columns of Bertin typically is spared and becomes hypertrophic. The glomeruli are spared, but, occasionally, segmental and global glomerulosclerosis is seen, as in chronic pyelonephritis (196).

Immunofluorescence and Electron Microscopy

IF and EM are not helpful to the diagnosis.

Differential Diagnosis

The pattern of scarring, papillary changes, and clinical history are distinct from those of chronic pyelonephritis. Patients with urinary tract obstruction and subsequent renal infections, however, may show signs of papillary necrosis. Diabetic nephropathy with renal papillary necrosis may give rise to somewhat similar changes, but in such cases clinical diabetes and other distinctive diabetic lesions are present. Papillary necrosis may also develop in patients with sickle cell disease (197).

Outcome

The diagnosis is usually made at a late stage, when disease progression cannot be inhibited. The incidence of transitional cell carcinoma is substantially higher among patients who have overused analgesics.

Etiology and Pathogenesis

Historically, phenacetin has been the usual cause of the disease, particularly in cases where it has been used in combination with other analgesics and caffeine. It appears that not only phenacetin but also other drugs, such as acetaminophen, in combination with salicylates and/or aspirin (which convert to salicylate during metabolism), can cause analgesic nephropathy (198,199). Analgesic drugs are highly lipophilic and easily diffuse into the medullary and papillary interstitium, where they become concentrated. Salicylates are potent depletors of glutathione. Acetaminophen metabolites are detoxified by conjugation to glutathione. If glutathione is depleted, reactive acetaminophen metabolites may produce lipid peroxides, which in turn can lead to local tissue injury, including capillary damage (198). Subsequent compromised medullary blood flow is thought to be important in the pathogenesis of papillary necrosis.

Metabolic Disorders

A variety of metabolic disorders can affect the interstitium. These are rare diseases; only the most important ones are discussed.

Nephrocalcinosis

Hypercalcemia and/or hypercalciuria (the latter usually idiopathic) may generate renal calculi (200). Renal tubular and interstitial calcification can develop (Fig. 63), and Randall's plaques (regions of papillary calcification) may serve as the nidus for renal stone development. It is quite important to perform chemical analysis on renal stones as a guide to future metabolic studies and therapy for the patient. Scattered foci of dystrophic calcification within tubular lumina may be a consequence of ATN.

Oxalosis

Oxalosis can be primary (an inborn error of oxalate metabolism) or secondary, due to increased ingestion or absorption (bowel disease) or decreased excretion (chronic renal failure) (200). Birefringent tubular and interstitial oxalate crystal deposition is widespread in the kidney (Fig. 64). In-

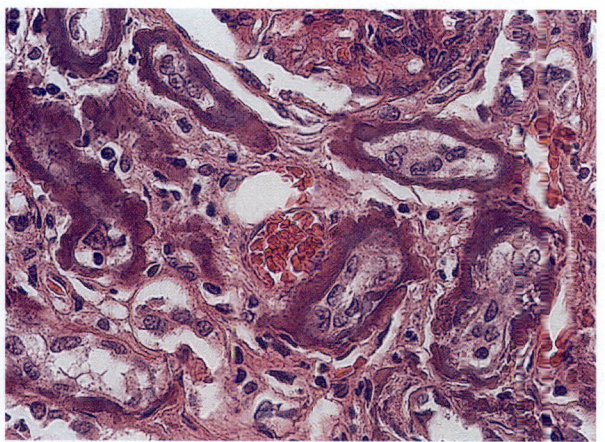

FIG. 63. Nephrocalcinosis. Basophilic calcium deposits are seen in the thickened tubular basement membranes in this kidney from a patient with hyperparathyroidism.

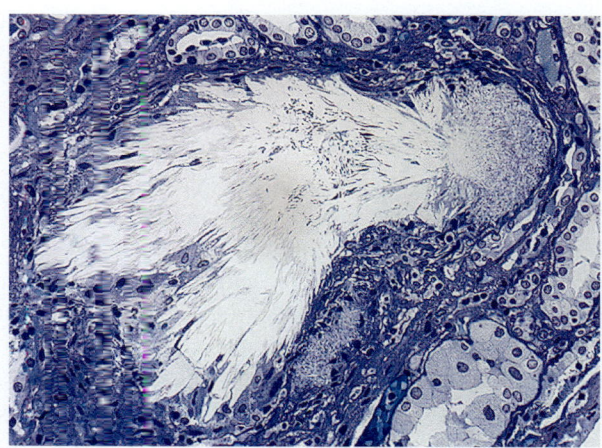

FIG. 65. Urate nephropathy. Note the interstitial accumulation of sharp-edged, elongated urate crystals surrounded by an inflammatory reaction (toluidine blue).

terstitial oxalate may induce an interstitial inflammatory reaction, occasionally with granulomas. The consequence is chronic interstitial nephritis, leading to ESRD.

Gout (Hyperuricemic Nephropathy)

Hyperuricemia also can be primary (inborn error of purine metabolism) or secondary (in which an unknown metabolic disturbance may be the predisposing factor), due to increased ingestion of purine, alcoholism, or increased breakdown of nuclear material (tumor chemotherapy). Angulated and sharp-edged urate crystals are initially deposited in the medullary tubules. Later, medullary interstitial urate accumulation with tophi develops, which induces an inflammatory response with subsequent interstitial fibrosis (Fig. 65) (201).

Cystinosis

This rare autosomal recessive metabolic disease has three forms (202). The infantile (nephropathic) form manifests early during the first 2 years of life and rapidly precipitates ESRD. The pathologic features include chronic interstitial nephritis with interstitial cystine deposits and prominent, occasionally multinucleated podocytes. The juvenile form is less aggressive, with a protracted renal course. The adult form is the least severe. Note that this disease should not be confused with cystinuria, where the proximal tubular transport of cystine is defective; the formation of cystine and mixed calculi is a usual complication.

Other Diseases

Glycogen storage disease and disturbances of lipid metabolism (e.g., Fabry's disease, lecithin-cholesterol acyl transferase deficiency) may also be associated with renal disease. In these conditions, sclerosis and deposition of lipid material may also affect the glomeruli and the vasculature.

VASCULAR LESIONS OF THE KIDNEYS

Arterial and Arteriolar Nephrosclerosis (Benign Nephrosclerosis)

Epidemiology

Hypertensive renal disease is the second most common cause of ESRD in the United States, after diabetic nephropathy; in African-Americans it is the usual cause (see the discussion of ESRD and dialysis of the kidney). Benign nephrosclerosis is probably the most common renal pathologic lesion found at autopsy. The incidence increases with age. Patients usually have a long history of benign essential hypertension, and some degree of nephrosclerosis eventually

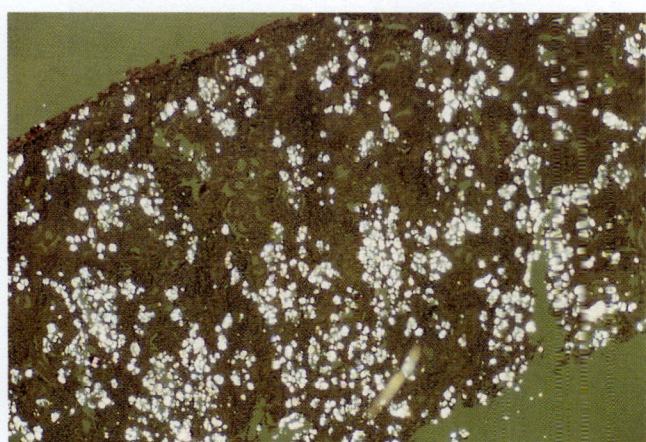

FIG. 64. Renal oxalosis. Note the large numbers of birefringent oxalate crystals in the renal cortex.

develops in the majority of patients with high blood pressure. Diabetes mellitus is a predisposing disease.

Clinical Symptoms

The WHO defines hypertension as blood pressure repeatedly more than 160/95 mm Hg. The diastolic value is of more importance. If the diastolic value does not exceed 120 mm Hg, the hypertension is conventionally designated benign. The word benign is, of course, a misnomer because this form of hypertension can have serious consequences. Most patients with mild to moderate nephrosclerosis have no urinary abnormalities and normal or close to normal renal function. A decreased glomerular filtration rate (GFR) is the first sign of renal impairment; it may be followed by an increased serum creatinine level. Proteinuria is a sign of advanced disease and may be associated with an accelerated phase of hypertension.

Gross Appearance

The kidney surface is finely granular, and the renal capsule may be adherent. The size of the kidneys is usually normal in mild to moderate cases. In advanced disease, the kidneys become shrunken, and the cortex is thinner than normal.

Light Microscopic Features

There is arterial intimal fibroplasia with migration of medial muscle cells into the intima, production of collagen and extracellular matrix, and lamination of the lamina elastica interna (also called intimal fibroelastosis) (Fig. 66A). Hyalinization of the arterioles and small interlobular arteries (hyalin arteriolosclerosis, arteriolar hyalin change) represents plasma proteins pushed or seeped into the vessel walls (Fig. 66B). These changes to some degree are virtually omnipresent in autopsied kidneys from older patients and are often found most prominently in kidneys from patients with hypertension and/or diabetes mellitus. If this vascular thickening is sufficiently severe over a period of time, "nephrosclerosis" with small subcapsular scars is found on gross examination. These scars cause small depressions of the renal surface, while the intervening normal parenchyma takes the form of small bumps. These small scars and bumps impart a granular appearance to the renal surface (203–205).

The glomeruli are unremarkable, except that there are scattered obsolescent glomeruli, particularly in the subcapsular scars (Fig. 12). True sclerotic glomeruli with hyalinosis are rarely seen (for comparison of obsolescent and sclerotic glomeruli, see Figs. 12 and 22). Glomeruli with segmental or global sclerosis and/or hyalinosis in the absence of idiopathic FSGS are suggestive of glomerular hyperperfusion/hyperfiltration injury. This condition may be seen after many years or decades of hypertension and is typically associated with an accelerated phase of hypertension and increasing (though usually not nephrotic range) proteinuria. It has been called decompensated benign nephrosclerosis by Fahr and later by Bohle (206).

Immunofluorescence and Electron Microscopy

IF and EM are not helpful.

Differential Diagnosis

If severe arteriolar hyalin change is noted, diabetes should be excluded. In decompensated benign nephrosclerosis, segmental glomerulosclerosis and hyalinosis make differentiating this condition from idiopathic FSGS impossible. A long history of hypertension, particularly if it has been poorly controlled and has signs of acceleration, and nonnephrotic-range proteinuria favor the diagnosis of benign decompen-

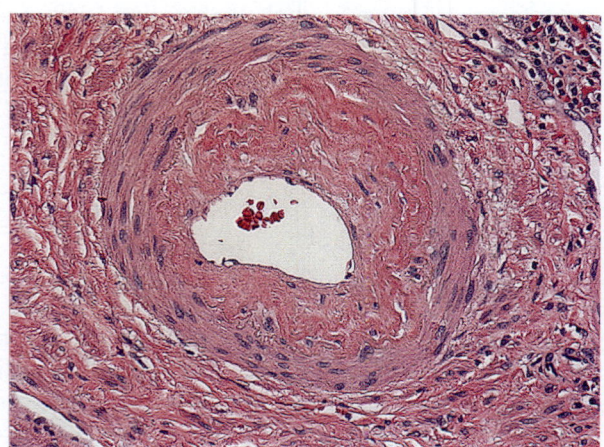
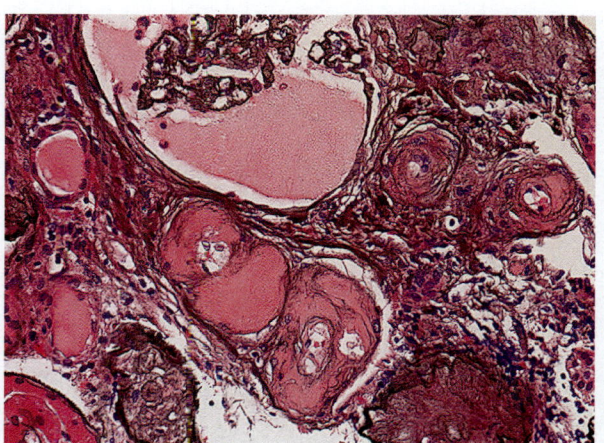

FIG. 66. Vascular changes in benign essential hypertension. **A:** This arcuate artery shows fibrous intimal thickening with lamellation of the internal elastic lamina (also called intimal fibroelastosis). **B:** Prominent arteriolar hyaline change (hyaline arteriosclerosis) is also a common finding in patients with benign essential hypertension. Note the methenamine silver–negative large arteriolar hyalin deposits.

sated nephrosclerosis. It is worth noting that idiopathic FSGS is not always associated with nephrotic-range proteinuria and that benign decompensated nephrosclerosis occasionally gives rise to nephrotic-range proteinuria. Renal biopsy changes in benign essential hypertension are nonspecific, and it may be difficult to exclude underlying diseases that cause secondary hypertension, such as chronic interstitial diseases (207). Changes of malignant nephrosclerosis may be superimposed on the other changes if the originally benign hypertension reaches a malignant phase.

Outcome

Most patients with benign arterial and arteriolar nephrosclerosis do not have clinically progressive renal disease. African-American patients, however, have a higher rate than whites of progression to ESRD due to benign essential hypertension (208). Decompensated benign nephrosclerosis is a progressive disease.

Etiologic Factors and Pathogenesis

As mentioned earlier, arterial and arteriolar nephrosclerosis develop in most patients as a result of benign essential hypertension. The intimal thickening and arteriolar hyalin change are probably the consequences of endothelial injury (perhaps mechanical). The patchy subcapsular interstitial fibrosis and tubular atrophy are most likely the results of ischemia. The scars are primarily subcapsular because the further away the tissue is from the vascular supply, the more prominent is the ischemic injury.

Malignant Nephrosclerosis

Malignant hypertension is diagnosed if the diastolic blood pressure is more than 120 mm Hg, although it is usually more than 130 mm Hg. The renal parenchymal changes associated with malignant hypertension are called malignant nephrosclerosis. These changes are quite similar to those in the various forms of TMA and are discussed in that section.

Renal Artery Stenosis

Epidemiology

The most common cause of renal artery stenosis is atherosclerosis, usually in older patients. If renal artery stenosis is seen in younger (e.g., middle-aged) patients (especially women), one should consider the possibility of a form of fibromuscular dysplasia. In Far Eastern countries, Takayasu's arteritis is also a common cause.

Clinical Symptoms

If the condition is unilateral, renovascular hypertension with high renin levels will be the result. If it is bilateral and advanced, renal failure may develop. Imaging studies, particularly renal angiography, are most important in the diagnosis.

Pathologic Features

The pathologic features of arteriosclerosis will not be detailed here. The most widely used classification of renal arterial fibromuscular dysplasia is that of Harrison and McCormack (of the combined Mayo–Cleveland Clinic study) (207). There are several rare types. Medial fibroplasia with multiple aneurysms is by far the most typical form of renal artery dysplasia and is often bilateral. The aneurysms often create a "string-of-beads" appearance on renal arteriography. There are alternating segments of disarrayed smooth muscle admixed with fibrous tissue, with very thinned muscularis: the thinned portion forms the aneurysms.

Changes affecting the kidney in the ipsilateral "protected" side with stenosis (i.e., protected from the ravages of hypertension) include diffuse renal cortical atrophy and thinning, with a smooth subcapsular surface and enlarged juxtaglomerular apparatuses (at least in the first year of stenosis). The glomeruli closely approximate each other because of diffuse tubular atrophy. The contralateral side (i.e., the nonstenosed side "exposed" to the ravages of hypertension) often shows typical, but severe arterial and arteriolar nephrosclerosis. If the hypertension is severe, fibrinoid necrosis of the renal arterioles may be present.

Differential Diagnosis

Differential diagnosis is best undertaken *in vivo* by angiography. If a segment of the renal artery is resected, histologic examination is helpful in subclassifying the lesion.

Outcome

If an early diagnosis is made, reconstructive surgery of the renal artery usually reverses hypertension. If this is not possible, unilateral nephrectomy may be necessary. Long-term prognosis also depends on the underlying disease and on how long the contralateral kidney has been exposed to the ravages of hypertension.

Etiologic Factors and Pathogenesis

As noted earlier, the usual cause of renal artery stenosis is atherosclerosis. In Far Eastern countries, Takayasu's arteritis is also a trigger. Renal artery dysplasia was detailed earlier. Other rare causes of renal artery stenosis include dissecting aortic aneurysm involving the origin of the renal arteries, thrombosis of the renal artery, and renal artery compression by tumors, such as neurofibromas in neurofibromatosis. The stenotic renal artery provokes renal hypoperfusion, which in turn induces increased renin production and activation of the renin–angiotensin system. In bilateral renal artery stenosis, in addition to initially increased renin production, diminished renal blood flow and GFR result in renal sodium and water retention, which is an important factor in maintaining and aggravating high blood pressure.

Renal Atheroembolic Disease (Cholesterol Emboli)

Epidemiology

This disease occurs mainly in elderly patients with severe atherosclerosis. An invasive procedure, such as angiography or surgical manipulation of sclerotic arteries (aorta), frequently precedes the clinical symptoms (210–211). Occasionally, renal atheroemboli may be spontaneous.

Clinical Symptoms

Acute renal failure or insidious onset of renal failure following angiography or surgery involving manipulation of the aorta is the typical clinical scenario. Livedo reticularis, acrocyanosis, low serum complement levels, and blood eosinophilia may be present. Now and then, severe proteinuria develops (211).

Light Microscopic Features

The presence of needle-shaped, sharp-edged cholesterol clefts in the lumens of arteries and arterioles or in glomeruli is diagnostic (Fig. 67). The cholesterol itself is dissolved during routine processing, but if unstained frozen sections are examined under polarized light, the birefringent cholesterol crystals are clearly visible. Examining the frozen sections in this way may be a useful ancillary method if cholesterol emboli are suspected, but the typical clefts are not seen in paraffin sections or in elderly patients with unexplained renal failure. Cholesterol crystals occluding vascular lumina are frequently surrounded by macrophages, which may form giant cells (211). Eosinophils may also be seen around the cholesterol clefts. The renal parenchyma frequently shows signs of ischemia with variable degrees of chronic changes, including interstitial fibrosis, tubular atrophy, and obsolescent glomeruli. One new report describes FSGS in several patients with renal atheroembolic disease (211).

Immunofluorescence and Electron Microscopy

IF and EM are not helpful.

Differential Diagnosis

Intravascular cholesterol clefts are diagnostic of atheroembolic disease. In patients with nephrotic syndrome, cholesterol crystals can sometimes be seen in the tubular epithelium. A PAS reaction highlights the TBM in such cases. Tubular cholesterol crystals may disrupt the tubules and cause an interstitial inflammatory reaction, which may be granulomatous. Such tubular and interstitial cholesterol deposits should not be mistaken for cholesterol emboli. It is important to note that the absence of cholesterol emboli in a renal biopsy specimen does not exclude this diagnosis, owing to possible sampling error.

Outcome

ESRD develops in most patients. Some patients have a protracted course, probably those with less severe disease. While a thromboembolus may recanalize, this is usually not the case with atheroemboli that occlude vascular lumina.

Etiologic Factors and Pathogenesis

As mentioned previously, manipulation of atherosclerotic plaques in the thoracic and abdominal aorta above the renal arteries is the most significant risk factor. Spontaneously ruptured, large, complicated, ulcerated, atherosclerotic aortic plaques may also give rise to atheroemboli; they are probably less widespread and severe.

Vasculitis

There are many somewhat confusing and usually overly complicated classifications of this condition (212). The Chapel Hill Consensus Conference classification has become widely accepted (212). Vasculitic syndromes may overlap; some (such as Churg-Strauss syndrome and Wegener's granulomatosis) are defined primarily by clinical symptoms. From the renal point of view, there are two types of vasculitis: those that are associated with crescentic GN (mostly ANCA positive) and those that are not (usually ANCA negative). This difference is also reflected in treat-

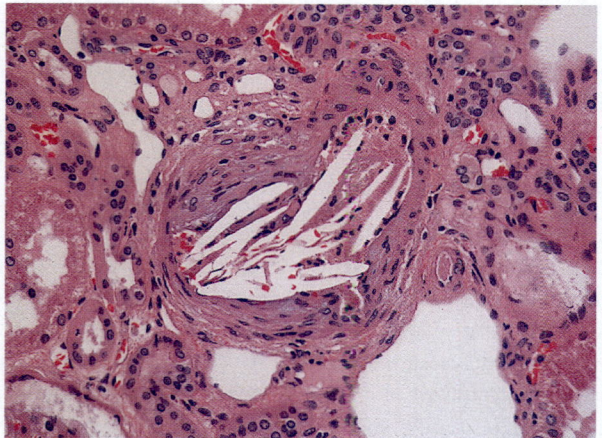

FIG. 67. Cholesterol emboli in an interlobular artery. Note the sharp-edged, needle-shaped cholesterol clefts. Cholesterol dissolves during routine processing.

ment strategies, because patients with crescentic GN require more aggressive therapy, including pulse steroids and cyclophosphamide, whereas those without crescentic GN frequently respond to steroid therapy alone.

The following vasculitides are frequently associated with crescentic GN (see also pauci-immune crescentic and necrotizing GN): Wegener's granulomatosis, microscopic polyarteritis (or polyangiitis, or hypersensitivity angiitis), cryoglobulinemic vasculitis, and HSP (IgA nephropathy but mostly not crescentic). Vasculitides usually not associated with crescentic GN include classic polyarteritis nodosa (involving medium-sized arteries), Takayasu's arteritis, giant-cell arteritis, and Kawasaki disease. Churg-Strauss syndrome (defined as vasculitis with asthma and peripheral blood eosinophilia) may or may not be associated with crescentic GN, depending on the size of vessels affected.

Vasculitis, with severe closure of the larger arteries, may lead to renal infarction. A vasculitic artery will "heal," with diffuse or segmental scarring of the vascular wall. The media may be partially or entirely replaced by fibrous tissue in these scars, and the lamina elastica is disrupted, segmentally missing, and, in some areas, severely lamellated. Where an intima still can be discerned, intimal fibroplasia is invariably present.

In our opinion, the term vasculitis should be restricted to true vasculitis with at least some necrotizing lesions showing inflammation and/or leukocytoclasia (Fig. 68). Endarteritis obliterans–like intimal fibroplasia, or a few intramural lymphocytes, do not constitute true vasculitis in our judgment, and the nosologic drift (i.e., expanding of the definition and use of the word) has added confusion to the literature. It is beyond the scope of this chapter to discuss the various vasculitides and their differential diagnoses in more detail. The interested reader is referred to monographs and reviews (212–215).

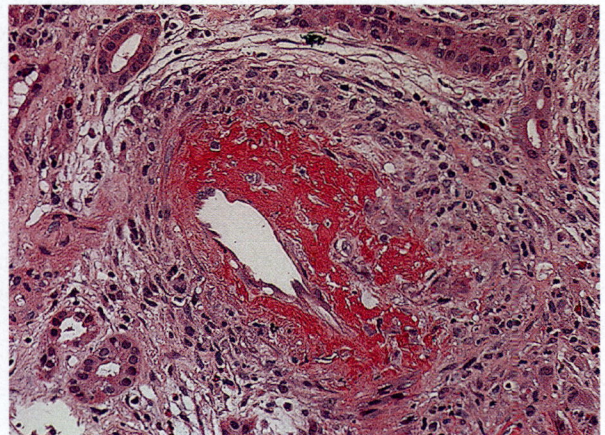

FIG. 68. A small intrarenal artery in polyarteritis nodosa. Note the fibrinoid necrosis and the inflammatory cells infiltrating the arterial wall. The process involves the entire thickness of the artery.

END-STAGE RENAL DISEASE/DIALYSIS OF THE KIDNEY

Epidemiology

In the United States, the leading cause of ESRD in white patients is diabetic nephropathy (37.1%), followed by hypertension (26.9%) and GN (13.2%). In African-Americans, the foremost cause is hypertension (39.9%), followed by diabetic nephropathy (35.8%) and GN (9.8%). Other, less typical but important causes include chronic interstitial nephritis and autosomal-dominant polycystic kidney disease (3.0% each) (215).

Clinical Symptoms

Symptoms of uremia prevail. The clinical history is important in identifying the initial cause of renal malfunction.

Gross Appearance

The kidneys typically are shrunken, but this may not be the case in diabetes and amyloidosis. The cortex is usually atrophic, and the corticomedullary junction is difficult to discern. The surface is usually granular with an adherent capsule. Large scars and a variety of other abnormalities (such as hydronephrosis in obstructive uropathy) may be visible, depending on the underlying disease.

Light Microscopic Features

Virtually any of the previously mentioned renal disorders can eventuate in advanced global glomerulosclerosis and obsolescence, tubular atrophy, and interstitial fibrosis. An interstitial mononuclear cell infiltrate is frequently seen. Tubules show four morphologic patterns. (a) Classic atrophic tubules have a thickened and wrinkled basement membrane and simplified epithelium; these mostly originate from proximal tubules (Fig. 69). (b) Endocrine-type atrophic tubules occur in clusters and have narrow lumina, pale cytoplasm, and delicate basement membranes; they resemble endocrine glands. These appear to originate primarily from distal tubules (Fig. 69). (c) Thyroid-type atrophic tubules have eosinophilic and PAS-positive homogeneous casts and a thinned epithelial lining and usually occur in clusters, resembling the follicular structure of the thyroid gland (Fig. 59B). They are of distal tubule and collecting duct origin. (d) Hypertrophic large, "super" tubules probably represent compensatory hypertrophy of remaining nephrons. They are primarily of proximal origin, but they may be of distal tubular origin (218). The presence of large numbers of endocrine-type atrophic tubules were once thought to be characteristic of ischemia (renal artery stenosis), while thyroid-type atrophic tubules were considered a hallmark of chronic pyelonephritis. This evaluation may be somewhat correct, but both endocrine-type and thyroid-type tubules are often seen admixed with many classic atrophic tubules in most

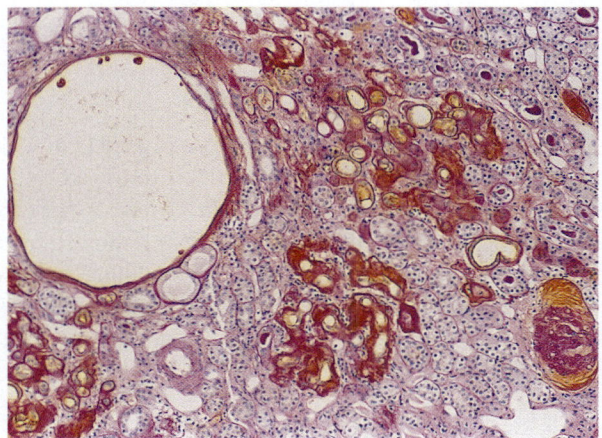

FIG. 69. End-stage renal disease. Many tubules have thick, wrinkled basement membranes (classic atrophic tubules) that stain positive on periodic acid–Schiff (PAS). Other tubules have thin basement membranes, narrow lumina, and clear cytoplasm (endocrine-type atrophic tubules). The brown apical staining in the classic atrophic tubules represents peroxidase-conjugated *Tetragonolobus purpureas* lectin staining, which is a marker of proximal tubules. Also note the cyst on the left side (PAS combined with peroxidase).

kidneys with ESRD; thus, they cannot be considered pathognomonic of any underlying renal condition.

Obliterative lesions of the arterial intima are always present in end-stage kidney disease, even if vascular disease is not an initiating factor (217). In such cases the intima is loose and less condensed, and the lamina elastica interna typically does not show the prominent lamellation seen in intimal fibroelastosis due to hypertension. This intimal thickening is also termed fibrocollagenous, and the vascular changes are called disuse arteriopathy or adoptive intimal fibrosis. It has been suggested that the intima thickens to accommodate the arterial lumen to the reduced blood flow in the atrophic kidney. Long-standing dialysis apparently aggravates this fibrocollagenous intimal thickening.

Occasionally, embryonal hyperplasia of Bowman's capsule, juxtaglomerular granular cell hyperplasia, unusual epithelial growth, interstitial smooth-muscle cell nodules associated with vessels, and other miscellaneous changes may be noted (217,219). Many of these changes develop long after dialysis treatment.

Immunofluorescence and Electron Microscopic Features

If relatively well-preserved glomeruli are available for examination, IF and EM changes may be diagnostic in cases of glomerular disease.

Differential Diagnosis

Attempts should be made, through investigation of clinical and pathologic features, to ascertain the original disease, because it may influence the outcome of renal transplantation (recurrent disease). Frequently, because of the advanced chronic changes, it is impossible to determine the underlying renal disease. Severe progressive disease of one renal compartment leads to changes in the other renal compartments. In many cases, however, changes characteristic of the disease that led to ESRD are present.

In chronic GN, most glomeruli are sclerotic, but there still may be relatively well-preserved glomeruli with diagnostic changes. In chronic tubulointerstitial nephritis, there may be many sclerotic and obsolescent glomeruli, but even in very advanced cases many normal-appearing glomeruli are present. The characteristic gross findings of pyelonephritis or analgesic nephropathy are usually recognizable. In primary vascular disease, the arterial changes of prominent fibrointimal thickening and luminal narrowing are striking. Arteriolar hyalin change is frequently noted. There is widespread parenchymal atrophy. Most of the glomeruli are obsolescent, while others are ischemic, with glomerular tuft simplification and capillary wall wrinkling and thickening. Normal glomeruli may still may be evident. There is widespread tubular atrophy with interstitial fibrosis. Large focal scars may be seen if healed infarcts are present.

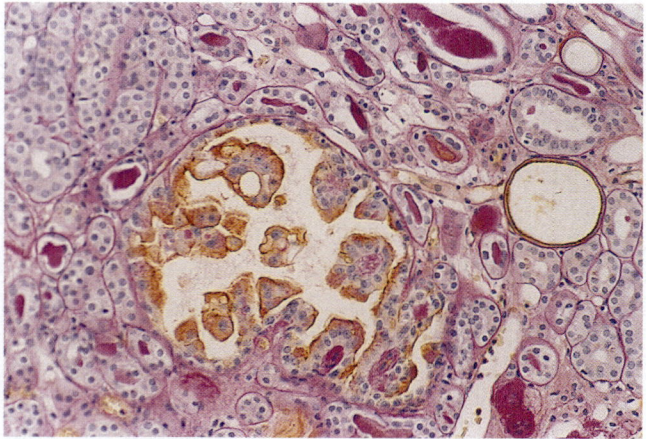

FIG. 70. Hyperplastic cyst in a case of acquired cystic kidney disease. The epithelium of this small cyst shows papillary projections. The brown color on the surface of the cyst's epithelium represents peroxidase-conjugated *Tetragonolobus purpureas* lectin stain, indicating the proximal tubular origin of this cyst. Also note the mainly endocrine-type atrophic tubules in the surrounding renal parenchyma (combination of periodic acid–Schiff and peroxidase).

Etiologic Factors and Pathogenesis

The most important causes are discussed earlier. The pathogenesis is obviously very diverse, but eventually all chronic and progressive renal diseases lead to the pattern of ESRD.

Acquired Renal Cystic Disease (ARCD)

Epidemiology

The prevalence of ARCD in dialysis populations is reported to be between 10% and 67%. This variance is due to the differences in duration of dialysis and in the criteria for diagnosis. It appears that bilateral renal cysts develop in the majority of patients who undergo dialysis for more than 5 to 10 years (217).

Clinical Symptoms

No particular symptoms are associated with ARCD. In exceptional cases, hemorrhagic cysts with perinephric hematomas develop. Another important complication is renal cell carcinoma, which is seven times more prevalent in this group than in the general population (217,220).

Gross Appearance

ARCD is diagnosed clinically if five or more cysts per kidney are found on imaging studies. We prefer the pathologic criteria set forth by Feiner et al. (221), according to which 40% of the renal parenchyma should be occupied by cysts in order to establish a diagnosis of ARCD. The weight of the kidney is frequently less than normal because it is shrunken, but sometimes, if the disease advances, substantial renal enlargement may develop. Some cysts may be hemorrhagic. Small renal cortical neoplasms are typical, and, as mentioned previously, renal cell carcinoma can be a complication.

Light Microscopic Features

The cysts lining the epithelium are quite variable; they may be flat, cuboidal, or even hyperplastic in some areas (Fig. 70) (217,219). The morphologic features of adenomas and carcinomas in ARCD are identical to those of these tumors in the general population, but papillary renal cell carcinomas appear to be more common (222).

Differential Diagnosis

The morphologic characteristics of advanced ARCD may resemble those of autosomal dominant polycystic kidney disease, but these two conditions have very different clinical histories.

Outcome

There is evidence that the cysts regress after successful renal transplantation. The possibility of renal cell carcinoma should be kept in mind, although it is a rare complication.

Etiologic Factors and Pathogenesis

The pathogenesis is unclear. Unlike other cystic diseases of the kidney, ARCD is not primarily genetically determined. The role of prolonged renal ischemia has been implicated by some investigators. The development of ARCD is clearly related to the duration of dialysis.

PATHOLOGY OF RENAL TRANSPLANTATION

With the increase in renal transplantation at almost every medical center, the pathologist is being called upon to evaluate renal transplant biopsies from patients with allografts to determine (a) whether there is evidence of allograft rejection, drug nephrotoxicity, or some other unrelated lesion and (b), if rejection is present, to predict whether the lesions are potentially reversible with therapy. The clinician usually needs an immediate diagnosis in order to undertake the necessary therapeutic measures. Many pathologists like to process the whole biopsy specimen with a fast embedding method. IF and EM are frequently not undertaken.

Except for biopsy samples examined immediately after transplant and rebiopsy specimens inspected after a short interval, we usually submit material for IF examination. If IF gives negative results, and if LM and the clinical history do not indicate glomerular disease, generally we do not perform EM. Without IF and/or EM, many recurrent or de novo glomerular diseases can be missed, and, if GN is suspected, a reliable diagnosis cannot be made. Of course, it is important to examine the thick sections taken for EM carefully under the light microscope in each case, even if ultrastructural examination is not performed. The classification of renal allograft rejection used by us is that of Dr. Kendrick A. Porter (223) and others: (a) hyperacute rejection; (b) acute rejection, either predominantly cellular (interstitial) or predominantly humoral (vascular); and (c) chronic rejection.

Hyperacute Rejection

Epidemiology

This form of rejection became very rare after the introduction of routine pretransplant cross-matching (testing the recipients for antidonor antibodies).

Clinical Symptoms

Rejection usually occurs within minutes or hours after vascular anastomosis of the allograft and is associated with primary anuria (no urine is made by the kidney from the beginning). If it is unrecognized and the kidney is not removed, graft tenderness fever may develop.

Gross Appearance

The kidney rapidly becomes mottled and turns dusky and cyanotic.

Light Microscopic Features

Sludged erythrocytes, leukocytes, and fibrin thrombi are seen in glomerular and peritubular capillaries and arterioles (Fig. 71). If the graft is not removed, renal cortical necrosis and infarction eventually develop.

Immunofluorescence Characteristics

Linear staining for complement and immunoglobulins (IgM and IgG) may be noted along the glomerular and peritubular capillary walls, but IF in the necrotic regions shows a vague, diffuse, spontaneous fluorescence, precluding interpretation of the IF study in these regions.

Electron Microscopic Features

EM studies are not helpful. Platelets, fibrin strands, and sludged red cells in capillary lumens are, of course, apparent.

Differential Diagnosis

Hyperacute rejection should not be confused with donor-derived DIC in some cadaveric donor kidneys, in which glomerular capillary thrombi are present. Inadequate preservation of cadaveric donor kidneys may cause endothelial injury, with subsequent leukocyte margination, and even fibrin deposition. Margination of leukocytes may sometimes be prominent in postperfusion biopsies, even in living related donors and in the absence of rejection. Rarely, hyperacute rejection is delayed for 1 or 2 days (delayed hyperacute rejection). In such cases, acute accelerated rejection may be a problem in terms of differential diagnosis. Acute accelerated rejection has the morphologic appearance of severe acute vascular rejection, rather than that of hyperacute rejection.

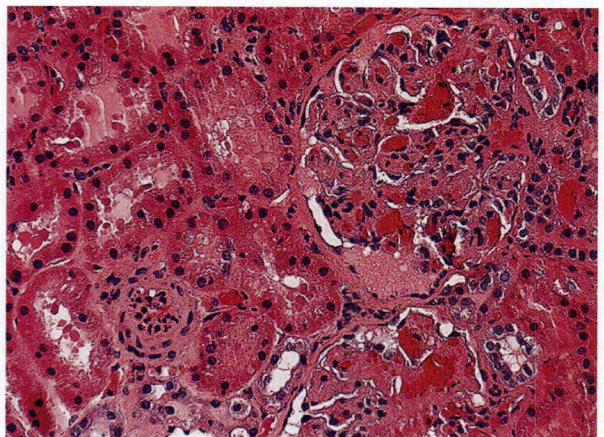

FIG. 71. Hyperacute rejection. Note the scattered glomerular capillary thrombi, capillary congestion, and prominent margination of polymorphonuclear cells in the peritubular capillaries and in an arteriole.

Outcome

Graft loss is inevitable.

Etiologic Factors and Pathogenesis

Rejection is most often due to preexisting circulating antibodies in the recipient, directed against antigens present in the grafted endothelium.

Acute Interstitial (Cellular) Rejection

Epidemiology

This is the most common type of rejection. It usually appears a few days to a few weeks after transplantation, but from time to time it develops later (late acute rejection).

Clinical Symptoms

It is important to note that there are no reliable clinical or laboratory signs of rejection. Increasing serum creatinine levels and graft tenderness are the typical features, but they are nonspecific. Lymphocytes may be seen in the urine.

Gross Appearance

The kidney is swollen and edematous.

Light Microscopic Features

There is prominent infiltration of the interstitium by lymphocytes (both CD4-positive and CD8-positive T cells, few B lymphocytes), macrophages, plasma cells, and, rarely, polymorphonuclear leukocytes and eosinophils (Fig. 72A,B) (223–226). The infiltrate is present in the peritubular interstitium (not only in the perivascular areas), which is frequently widened not only by the infiltrate but also by edema. The inflammatory cells penetrate the tubular epithelium (tubulitis) (Fig. 72C). In the absence of definite tubulitis, the diagnosis of acute interstitial rejection is questionable.

The grading of rejection is subjective. We grade acute interstitial rejection as follows (226): mild, if less than one-third of the parenchyma shows peritubular mononuclear cells with isolated tubulitis; moderate, if up to two-thirds of the parenchyma has peritubular inflammatory cells with tubulitis; and severe, if more then two-thirds of the parenchyma is affected in a similar way. In the pure form of acute interstitial rejection, no arterial changes are noted. Venulitis may be present, but its significance is uncertain. The glomeruli are unremarkable. Sometimes a moderate increase in glomerular intracapillary inflammatory cells may be seen (mild glomerulitis).

Immunofluorescence Characteristics

IF gives negative or nonspecific results. Granular or linear, patchy TBM and arteriolar staining for C3 is a typical finding, but its significance is questionable.

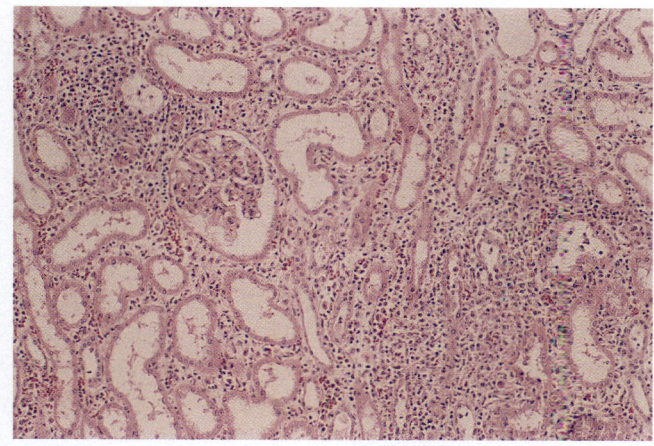
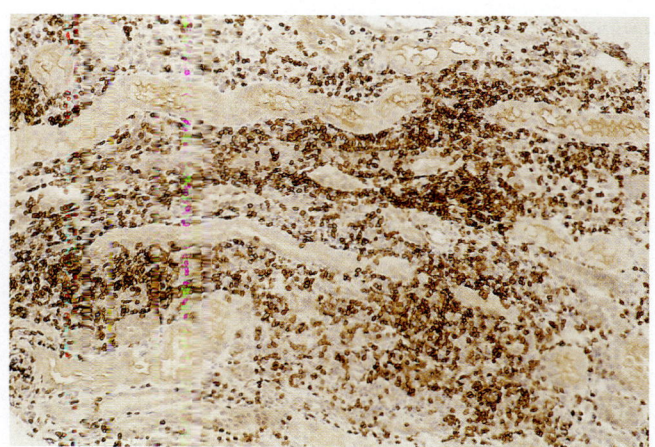
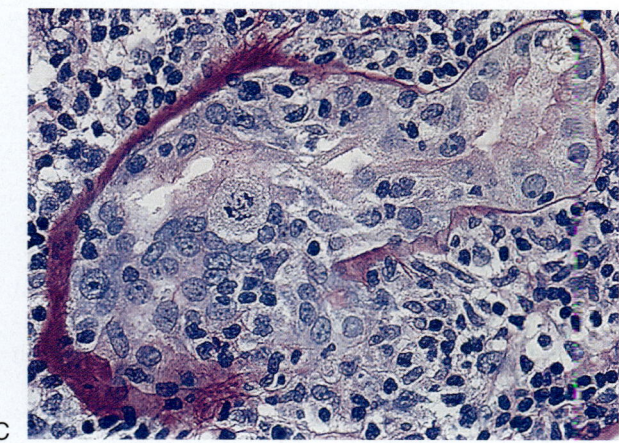

FIG. 72. Acute interstitial rejection. **A:** Note the prominent interstitial mononuclear cell infiltrate associated with interstitial edema. **B:** This immunoperoxidase stain with a CD3 antibody reveals that most of the infiltrating cells are T lymphocytes. **C:** Tubulitis. Tubulitis is the hallmark of acute interstitial rejection. Note the rupture of the tubular basement membrane (which is periodic acid–Schiff positive), with subsequent invasion of the tubular epithelium by inflammatory cells. A mitotic cell is also seen in the middle.

Electron Microscopy

EM is not helpful in diagnosing acute interstitial rejection.

Differential Diagnosis

A focal, patchy infiltrate found primarily in the perivascular and periglomerular areas (particularly if no tubulitis is noted) does not indicate true acute rejection and can be present in the context of excellent renal function. Overdiagnosing this finding as acute rejection is probably the most common mistake made in renal transplant biopsy evaluation (226). Acute vascular rejection may be missed if no diagnostic arteries are seen in the biopsy; interstitial hemorrhage, margination of inflammatory cells in the peritubular capillaries, or prominent glomerulitis are features suggestive of a vascular (humoral) component in the rejection process. It is important to exclude a posttransplant lymphoproliferative disorder (PTLD). In addition to the morphologic differences, immunohistochemistry and/or in situ hybridization for Epstein-Barr virus (EBV), as well as phenotyping of the infiltrate, are helpful in differentiating PTLD from acute rejection (see later discussion). Acute pyelonephritis should be considered if microabscesses are noted and, in particular, if there are many intratubular neutrophils. Acute interstitial nephritis unrelated to rejection is very difficult to exclude, because of the identical morphologic picture and similar phenotype of the infiltrate.

If a drug is suspected, it should be discontinued and the patient treated for rejection. If a virus is suspected, antiviral therapy is recommended, along with antirejection treatment. Careful examination of nuclei for viral inclusions and ancillary testing, such as immunohistochemistry and in situ hybridization using specific antiviral probes, are helpful in detecting viruses. It is important to note that viral inclusions (such as cytomegalovirus) can be seen in the absence of a significant inflammatory infiltrate and, alternatively, that the presence of viruses in renal parenchymal cells does not necessarily exclude the possibility of rejection. Interstitial nephritis in a renal transplant should be considered acute rejection until proved otherwise.

Outcome

Acute interstitial rejection is usually reversible with appropriate anti-rejection therapy. In our experience, late acute rejection episodes are more difficult to control and have a worse outcome. Interstitial hemorrhage is an indicator of poor outcome. Cases with large numbers of eosinophils and plasma cells appear to be also relatively poor responders to immunosuppressive therapy.

Etiologic Factors and Pathogenesis

Cellular immune response involving histocompatibility antigens is thought to be the most important factor.

Acute Vascular (Humoral) Rejection

Epidemiology

Today's immunosuppressive regimens have made this type of rejection considerably less uncommon than acute interstitial rejection. Acute vascular rejection generally develops after the second week of transplantation, usually within the first 2 months, but it may develop at any time, particularly if immunosuppression is stopped (e.g., in the context of noncompliance). Infrequently, acute vascular rejection develops within a few days, a condition called acute accelerated rejection.

Clinical Features

There are no characteristic clinical symptoms. In severe cases, deteriorating graft function may be associated with hematuria, particularly if infarcts develop. A comparable pretransplant cross-match does not exclude later acute vascular rejection; however, patients may show signs of a positive cross-match during the course of rejection, and antibodies directed against donor antigens can be detected.

Light Microscopic Features

In milder forms, there is subendothelial accumulation of inflammatory cells (intimal arteritis), occasionally with patchy necrosis of the endothelium (Fig. 73A) (223–226). In more severe cases, there is fibrinoid necrosis of the intima and media, sometimes accompanied by thrombosis (Fig. 73B). Inflammatory cells, mainly macrophages and T cells, frequently infiltrate the arterial wall. Focal interstitial hemorrhage is typical. An interstitial inflammatory cell infiltrate is usually present. Compared with acute interstitial rejection, cytotoxic T cells and macrophages are present in larger numbers (227). Inflammatory cells often accumulate in the glomerular capillaries (glomerulitis) as well as in the peritubular capillaries.

Immunofluorescence Characteristics

Occasionally, complement deposition is noted along the endothelium. Endothelial IgM and IgG deposition is rarely seen with the routine direct IF method. FRAs are frequently evident, particularly if arterial fibrinoid necrosis is present.

Electron Microscopy

EM is not helpful.

Differential Diagnosis

Sometimes it can be challenging to differentiate acute vascular rejection from TMA (usually associated with cyclosporine or FK506 treatment). In classic cases, differential diagnosis is not a problem, but there may be biopsy specimens in which acute vascular rejection is associated with thrombi and other changes of TMA (see earlier discussion), without inflammatory infiltrates of the vascular wall. Alternatively, TMA may show fibrinoid necrosis of arteries/arterioles mimicking acute vascular rejection. In such instances, we recommend omitting cyclosporine or FK506, using alternative immunosuppressants (such as mycophenolate mofetil), and initiating plasmapheresis. Vasculitis may have a histologic appearance very similar to that of acute vascular rejection, but this is rarely a differential diagnostic difficulty in everyday practice.

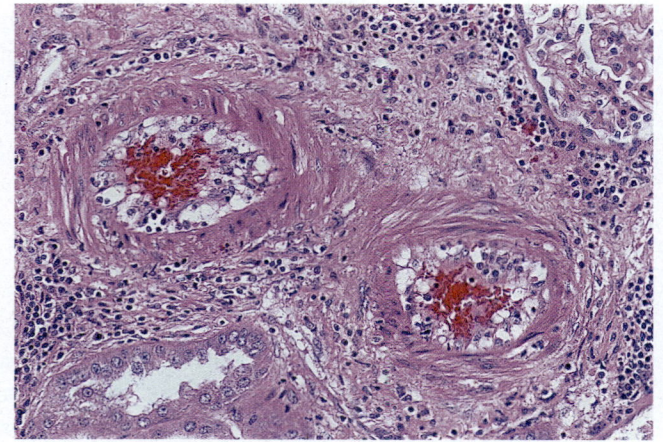 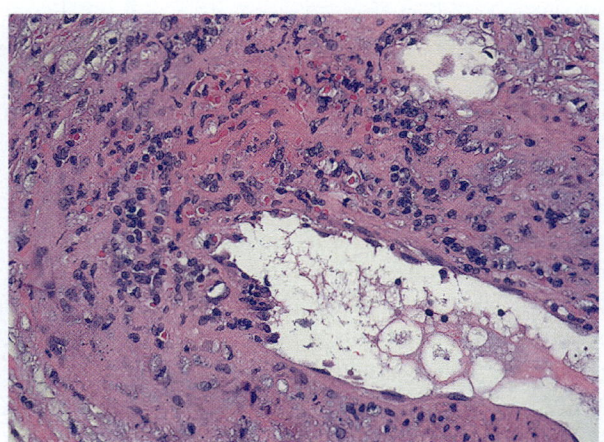

FIG. 73. Acute vascular rejection. **A:** In milder forms of acute vascular rejection, intimal arteritis (infiltration of the subendothelial space by inflammatory cells) is seen. **B:** In more severe forms, the inflammatory cell infiltrate involves the entire thickness of the vascular wall and is usually associated with fibrinoid necrosis, as is demonstrated in this arcuate artery.

Outcome

Cases of mild intimal arteritis may have an outcome comparable to acute interstitial rejection. More severe cases, particularly cases with fibrinoid necrosis of the arteries, have a poor outcome; graft failure takes place within weeks or months.

Etiologic Factors and Pathogenesis

The pathogenesis is not clear; antiendothelial antibodies (probably not just anti-major histocompatibility complex antibodies) may play an important role. There is evidence, however, that cellular immune responses are also significant to the pathogenesis of vascular lesions in the context of rejection.

Chronic Rejection

Epidemiology

With successful antirejection therapy, chronic rejection has become the most common cause of graft loss. This pattern develops several months to several years after transplantation. Sooner or later, changes suggestive of chronic rejection develop in every allograft, but in many cases it is difficult to determine whether true chronic rejection or other unrelated conditions lie in the background. In such instances, the term chronic transplant nephropathy is appropriate.

Clinical Symptoms

A gradually increasing serum creatinine level is a warning sign. Some degree of proteinuria and microscopic hematuria may be present. The proteinuria may be severe in cases of transplant glomerulopathy (and, of course, in recurrent or de novo GN).

Light Microscopic Features

The arterial lesions are probably the most important. There is narrowing of interlobar, arcuate, and interlobular arteries by intimal thickening, probably as the result of continuous or intermittent endothelial damage (Fig. 74) (223–226). The intimal thickening in chronic rejection is similar to that found in arteriosclerosis or in any form of damage to the arterial wall; however, in chronic rejection, more inflammatory cells usually are seen in the thickened intima (the vessels, just like other compartments of the kidneys, react in only a few ways to an unlimited number of injurious agents). Interstitial fibrosis with tubular atrophy is a consistent finding. The distribution of the interstitial fibrosis as well as the obliterative arteriopathy may be uneven within the graft, which occasionally leads to overdiagnosis or underdiagnosis of chronic rejection. A focal mononuclear cell infiltrate is frequently noted.

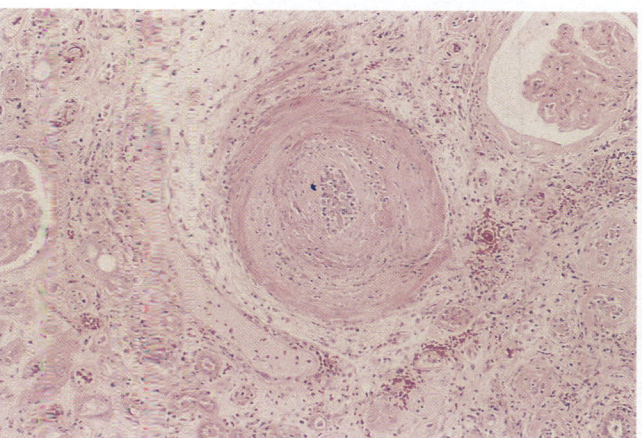

FIG. 74. Advanced obliterative transplant arteriopathy in chronic rejection. Note the prominent fibrous intimal thickening with severe narrowing of the arterial lumen. A few inflammatory cells in the intima are frequently seen, even in advanced cases. Also note the prominent atrophy of the surrounding renal parenchyma.

In inactive, quiescent chronic rejection, no tubulitis is usually noted, except in some atrophic tubules. The significance of tubulitis in atrophic tubules is unknown, but it may represent a smoldering progressive injury. In many cases of advanced chronic rejection, relatively large numbers of IgG-containing plasma cells infiltrate the graft (227). Superimposed acute rejection may appear at any time. The glomerular lesions include ischemia with focal thickening, wrinkling, distortion, or various degenerations of the GBMs. In approximately 25% of renal allografts that have functioned for more than 10 years, a peculiar glomerular lesion called transplant glomerulopathy develops. Mesangial prominence, typically with a membranoproliferative pattern, can be seen (Fig. 75). In some in-

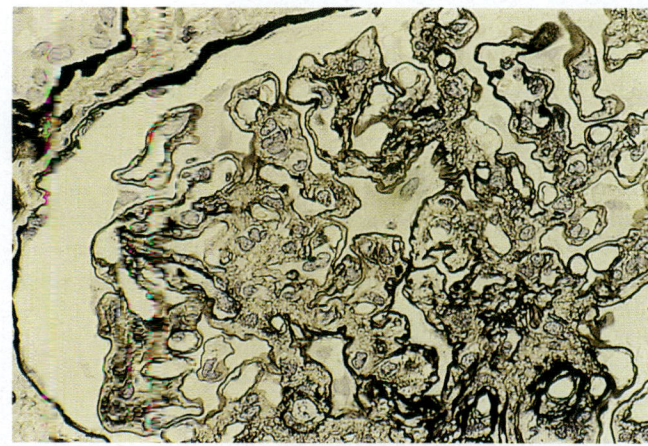

FIG. 75. Transplant glomerulopathy. In this case, the mesangial expansion is associated with capillary loop thickening and widespread doubling (tram-tracking) of the glomerular basement membrane. These changes are similar to those seen in membranoproliferative glomerulonephritis (methenamine silver).

stances, the glomerular morphologic picture resembles changes in TMA or a mixed TMA and membranoproliferative pattern (229–231). Another glomerular disease associated with chronic rejection is de novo membranous GN, which is the most common de novo GN associated with renal transplants.

Immunofluorescence Characteristics

It is important to perform IF to exclude recurrent or de novo GN. In transplant glomerulopathy, the glomerular IF findings are nonspecific; occasionally there is IgM and sometimes fibrinogen deposition.

Electron Microscopic Features

EM is important in the diagnosis of recurrent or de novo GN. In transplant glomerulopathy, glomerular subendothelial electron-lucent widening, similar to the glomerular capillary loop changes in TMA, is a characteristic finding (Fig. 41) (223,226). No discrete, well-formed electron-dense immune-type deposits are present. Otherwise, EM is not useful to the diagnosis of chronic rejection.

Differential Diagnosis

It may be difficult to differentiate chronic rejection from other chronic renal diseases that can develop in the graft but are unrelated to rejection. Among them, chronic cyclosporine toxicity has the most practical importance (Table 7). In cyclosporine toxicity, the arteriolar changes predominate (see following discussion) with relatively little obliterative intimal change in arteries. Patchy interstitial fibrosis can be seen in the context of both cyclosporine toxicity and chronic rejection. Chronic pyelonephritis/reflux nephropathy may be very difficult to diagnose in a graft (it should not be diagnosed based only on a renal biopsy specimen). The characteristic pelvic deformities or hydronephrosis with a clinical history of recurrent urinary tract infections or vesicoureteral reflux are helpful hints. Benign nephrosclerosis developing after many years is also difficult to distinguish. The history of hypertension and prominent arteriolar hyalin change may be helpful. Donor-transmitted chronic changes can be recognized only if an early posttransplant biopsy sample is available for comparison. IF and EM are important in ruling out recurrent or de novo GN, as mentioned earlier.

Outcome

The long-term outcome depends primarily on the severity of the chronic changes. Many inflammatory cells in the thickened intima of arteries indicate a progressive course, with active rejection. The presence of transplant glomerulopathy is also an indicator of an unfavorable outcome (231).

Etiologic Factors and Pathogenesis

The exact pathogenesis is unknown. Repeated or consistent low-grade endothelial injury (probably immunologically induced) is important in the development of obliterative arteriopathy. Immune injury due to repeated acute rejection episodes, which may be subclinical, and ischemia appear to be key factors in progressive tubulointerstitial injury and glomerular changes.

The Banff Classification

A new classification of rejection has begun to be used, created by a group of pathologists, nephrologists, and transplant surgeons in 1991 in Banff, Canada (235). This classification grades acute and chronic rejection. There are six diagnostic categories: normal, hyperacute rejection, borderline changes (a focal mononuclear cell infiltrate with isolated tubulitis), acute rejection, chronic rejection, and other changes not related to rejection. Acute rejection is further subdivided by grade.

1. Grade I: Moderate interstitial infiltrate with tubulitis but no vascular changes
2. Grade II: Moderate to severe interstitial infiltrate with severe tubulitis, possible mild to moderate intimal arteritis
3. Grade III: Severe intimal arteritis with fibrinoid necrosis, infarcts, interstitial hemorrhage; severity of interstitial infiltrate is irrelevant

Chronic rejection is also subdivided by grade.

1. Grade I: Mild interstitial fibrosis with tubular atrophy
2. Grade II: Moderate interstitial fibrosis with tubular atrophy
3. Grade III: Severe interstitial fibrosis and tubular atrophy and loss.

The Banff classification attempts to standardize the criteria to diagnose rejection. However, some of these criteria are not yet defined accurately. This classification can be considered a working model; minor modifications and more exact criteria are being added.

Cyclosporine Nephrotoxicity

Epidemiology

Cyclosporine is a powerful immunosuppressant widely used among transplant patients, but unfortunately it is nephrotoxic. Cyclosporine nephrotoxicity may develop not only in renal transplant patients but also in anyone taking the drug; it is a well-recognized problem, particularly in transplant patients.

Clinical Symptoms

A gradual decrease in GFR and rise in serum creatinine level are evident. In acute nephrotoxicity, renal function may not re-

Differential Diagnosis

It is very important to differentiate PTLD from acute interstitial (cellular) rejection. *In situ* detection of EBV in infiltrating cells and phenotyping of the infiltrate are helpful.

Outcome

Many cases regress following cessation of immunosuppressive therapy. Some cases will behave like true lymphomas.

Pathogenesis

EBV is most likely the causative agent.

Other Changes Seen in Transplant Specimens

ATN is common, particularly immediately after transplant. Immunosuppression may lead to infections, such as acute pyelonephritis. As discussed earlier, the incidence of recurrent GN differs in the various types of glomerulonephritides. Rarely, de novo GN develops, most commonly de novo membranous GN. Finally, donor-transmitted renal disease may sometimes be seen. It can be reliably diagnosed only in biopsy samples taken immediately after transplantation.

REVIEW OF GLOMERULAR DISEASES

Pattern Recognition in Glomerulonephropathies

I. Diffuse GN (often nephritic syndrome)
   A. Postinfectious GN
   B. MPGN (types I, II, and III)
   C. Crescentic GN
II. Focal GN
   A. Collagen vascular diseases (e.g., SLE)
   B. Crescentic GN
   C. Infective endocarditis, deep-seated abscess, etc.
III. Diffuse membranous or capillary wall lesions (no proliferation, usually nephrotic)
   A. Minimal change disease
   B. FSGS
   C. Membranous GN
   D. Diabetic glomerulosclerosis
   E. Amyloidosis
   F. Fibrillary/immunotactoid GN
IV. Glomerulonephropathies with acellular closure of capillaries (thrombi, etc.)
   A. Amyloidosis
   B. Thrombotic microangiopathies
   C. Cryoglobulinemic GN
   D. Fibrillary/immunotactoid GN
   E. Diabetes mellitus
V. Glomerulonephropathies associated with isolated ("essential") hematuria
   A. IgA nephropathy (Berger's disease)
   B. Thin-basement membrane disease
   C. Alport's syndrome (diffuse thinning, thickening, splintering, splitting of the GBM)
   D. Nonspecific changes (± IgG, ± IgM in mesangial regions)

Summary of Specific Patterns of Glomerulonephritides

I. Proliferative GN
   A. Diffuse intracapillary
      1. Diffuse postinfectious GN (poststreptococcal GN)
         a. LM: proliferative, exudative (PMNs) ± crescents
         b. IF: granular lumpy-bumpy capillary wall, IgG ± C3
         c. EM: subepithelial humps ± small subendothelial/mesangial deposits
         d. Course: resolves in vast majority of cases
         e. Dx: Anti-streptolysin O (ASO) up, serum complement down, nephritic syndrome, hypertension
      2. MPGN, type I (mesangiocapillary GN)
         a. LM: proliferative, lobulation, "tram-tracking"
         b. IF: broad capillary wall deposits; C3, IgG, ± other immunoreactants
         c. EM: subendothelial deposits ± mesangial deposits
         d. Course: progressive (many to renal failure)
         e. Dx: low serum complement, nephritic and/or nephrotic syndrome
      3. MPGN type II (dense-deposit disease)
         a. LM: many glomerular patterns (MPGN, crescentic GN, focal GN, etc.)
         b. IF: broad capillary wall deposits, C3 ± other immunoreactants, TBM and Bowman's capsule deposits
         c. EM: large, electron-dense deposits in lamina densa of GBM; ± TBM, Bowman's capsule, etc.
         d. Course: progressive (many to renal failure)
         e. Dx: low serum complement (persistent), nephritic/nephrotic syndrome
   B. Diffuse extracapillary proliferative
      1. Crescentic GN (rapidly progressive GN)
         a. LM: Over 50% of glomeruli with crescents—study the most preserved glomeruli for tuft hypercellularity
         b. IF
            (1) Granular (immune complex GN; primary [no underlying disease] or secondary [e.g., SLE, postinfectious GN, MPGN, etc])
            (2) No deposits (pauci-immune) (e.g., polyarteritis, Wegener's, vasculitis)
            (3) Linear (probably anti-GBM) (Goodpasture's disease)

c. EM: either discrete glomerular deposits anywhere (immune complex) or no obvious deposits (either anti-GBM or pauci-immune)
d. Course: rapid progression to ESRD (except postinfectious)
e. Dx: ANCA (in pauci-immune GN), anti-GBM antibodies in serum (radioimmunoassay); underlying disease

II. Glomerular capillary wall lesions (usually nephrotic syndrome)
  A. MCNS (nil disease, lipoid nephrosis, minimal change disease)
    1. LM: few if any changes
    2. IF: usually negative, possible mesangial IgM
    3. EM: only "fusion" of foot processes, ± other nonspecific changes
    4. Course: 85% responsive to steroids
  B. DMH in nephrotic syndrome
    1. LM: more than three cells in a mesangial region in a thin section away from the vascular pole
    2. IF: ± IgM in mesangial regions
    3. EM: ± mesangial deposits
    4. ? Part of MCNS or FSGS
  C. FSGS (focal sclerosis)
    1. LM: some glomeruli (especially juxtamedullary ones) with segmental sclerosis ± hyalinosis
    2. IF: usually negative except in sclerotic segments, which may have IgM ± C3
    3. EM: accumulation in sclerotic loops of matrix-like material or homogeneous, dense "hyalin"; no changes in unaffected glomeruli
    4. Course: slow progression to ESRD
  D. HIVAN (collapsing glomerulopathy)
    1. LM: collapsing glomerulosclerosis with prominent podocytes, microcystic dilatation of tubules, tubulointerstitial nephritis
    2. IF: negative or nonspecific
    3. EM: endothelial tubuloreticular inclusions
    4. Course: rapid progression to ESRD
  E. C1q nephropathy
    1. LM: normal, mesangial prominence or FSGS
    2. IF: predominant C1q (in the absence of SLE)
    3. EM: mesangial electron-dense deposits
  F. Membranous GN
    1. LM: normal to prominent, diffuse thickening of the capillary wall (± tuft hypercellularity), usually with "spikes" on silver stain
    2. IF: finely granular, diffuse capillary wall staining; IgG ± C3 and other immunoreactants
    3. EM: numerous subepithelial deposits with spikes of GBM material between
    4. Course: 1/3 progress, 1/3 remit, 1/3 proteinuria only
  G. Diabetic nephropathy
    1. LM: diffuse and/or nodular (Kimmelstiel-Wilson nodules) glomerulosclerosis
    2. IF: linear (mild to moderate and nonspecific) glomerular capillary walls for IgG and albumin
    3. EM: diffuse thickening of the GBMs and diffuse increase in mesangial matrix
    4. Course: once the BUN rises, increase in proteinuria increases; possible ESRD within a few years

III. Glomerular diseases associated with isolated hematuria
  A. IgA nephropathy (Berger's disease)
    1. LM: any glomerular pattern (mostly focal GN, mesangioproliferative GN, FSGS); can be normal
    2. IF: mesangial pre- or co-dominant granular IgA by definition (in the absence of SLE, HSP, active liver disease)
    3. EM: mesangial, discrete, dense deposits
    4. Peripheral capillary wall deposits unusual (probably a sign of severe disease)
    5. Course: 2% per year progress to ESRD
    6. ? Relationship to HSP poorly understood
  B. Thin basement membrane disease
    1. LM: normal
    2. IF: negative
    3. EM: diffuse, severely thin GBM
    4. Course: benign
  C. Alport's syndrome (familial nephritis)
    1. LM: normal, mesangial prominence or FSGS
    2. IF: negative with the routine panel
    3. EM: diffuse splintering, splitting, basket-woven appearance of GBM
    4. Course: progressive in men
  D. Minor glomerular changes
    1. LM: normal or mild mesangial prominence
    2. IF: negative or mild mesangial C3, IgM, IgG
    3. EM: normal or small electron-dense deposits
    4. Course: benign

III. Glomerular diseases with acellular closure of glomerular capillaries
  A. TMA
    1. LM: "Bloodless glomeruli," narrowing of glomerular capillaries by amorphous acellular material, endothelial swelling
    2. IF: sometimes glomerular capillary wall fibrin
    3. EM: widening of the lamina rara interna of the glomerular capillary wall by subendothelial electron-lucent fluff; seen in association with HUS/TTP, malignant hypertension, acute scleroderma, postpartum renal failure, eclampsia/preeclampsia, and other conditions.
  B. Cryoglobulinemic GN
    1. LM: usually proliferative (membranoproliferative-like), refractile, dense, thick material (hyalin thrombi) in glomerular capillary lumens
    2. IF: ± granular capillary wall staining for IgG ± IgM with glomerular capillary lumen thrombi staining for IgG and IgM

3. EM: subendothelial (± intramembranous) deposits with microtubular substructure
C. Amyloidosis
1. LM: Congo red–positive homogeneous material
2. IF: noncontributory or strong predominance of one light chain
3. EM: "rigid," nonbranching (8–10 nm) fibrils in mesangium and GBM
4. Course: poor prognosis
5. Dx: Congo red (most specific), thioflavin T fluorescence (most sensitive); antisera to AA, kappa, lambda light chains
D. Fibrillary/immunotactoid GN
1. LM: variable; most commonly mesangial expansion with glomerular capillary wall thickening
2. IF: strong mesangial and glomerular capillary wall IgG
3. EM: nonbranching fibrils or microtubules thicker than 10 nm in mesangium and glomerular capillaries
4. Course: progressive
5. Dx: Negative on Congo red and other amyloid stains

IV. Systemic lupus erythematosus
A. LM: pleomorphic
B. IF: frequently a "full house" (most immunoreactants are positive)
C. EM: deposits possibly present throughout; endothelial tubuloreticular inclusions
D. WHO classes
1. I: Normal by LM, EM, and IF (quite unusual)
2. IIA: Normal by LM, mesangial deposits by IF/EM
3. IIB: Mesangial hypercellularity only, mesangial deposits by IF/EM
4. III: Focal segmental proliferative/necrotizing/sclerosing GN (mesangial and subendothelial deposits)
5. IV: Diffuse proliferative/necrotizing/sclerosing GN (mesangial and subendothelial deposits)
6. V: Membranous GN (mesangial and subepithelial deposits)
7. VI: Advanced sclerosing GN

SHORT GLOSSARY OF IMPORTANT TERMINOLOGIES:

I. Glomeruli:

– Capsular drop: Hyalin drop sitting on Bowman's capsule and protruding into Bowman's space (Fig. 29D). Characteristic of diabetic glomerulosclerosis
– Crescent: Two or more cell layers between the visceral (podocytes) and parietal epithelium of Bowman's capsule. Cellular: Containing mainly inflammatory cells and epithelial cells. Fibrocellular: myofibroblasts with extracellular matrix are evident. Fibrous: Collagen with few fibroblasts. Bowman's capsular basement membrane is usually disrupted in all forms (Fig. 11).
– Diffuse (generalized) change: involves most (usually more than 50% [according to some more than 80%]) of glomeruli.
– Fibrin cap: See Hyalinosis
– Focal: Some, but not all, glomeruli involved
– Global: The entire glomerular tuft within a glomerulus is involved (as opposed to segmental).
– Hematuria: Can be gross (macroscopic) (coke-colored urine) or microscopic (red blood cells present by microscopic examination of urine sediment only). Caveat: Hematuria is frequently extrarenal; Red blood cell casts and dysmorphic red blood cells indicate glomerular hematuria.
– Hyalinosis (also called insudative or exudative lesion, or in diabetics, fibrin caps): Abnormal accumulation of homogenous methenamine silver negative proteinaceous material from the blood into the capillary wall (see Table 6, Figs. 21C, 22, 29C).
– Hypercellularity
  – Intracapillary (or endocapillary): Too many cells in the area bordered by the GBM (glomerular capillaries and mesangium) (Figs. 2 and 5).
– Extracapillary hypercellularity: see crescent
– Mesangial hypercellularity: more than three mesangial cells per mesangial area away from the vascular pole. In pure mesangial hypercellularity the glomerular capillaries do not contain increased number of cells and are not closed. (Figs. 16 and 32).
– Kimmelstiel-Wilson nodule: See nodular mesangial sclerosis
– Mesangial interposition: Presence of mesangial cytoplasm between the peripheral glomerular capillary basement membrane and the endothelium (Figs. 5B and 7).
– Mesangiolysis: Dissolution (necrosis?) of mesangium with subsequent coalescence of glomerular capillaries leading to glomerular microaneurysms (Fig. 38B).
– Microaneurysm: See mesangiolysis
– Nephrotic syndrome: Severe proteinuria (>3.5 g/24h) with edema, hypoalbuminemia, hypercholesterolemia, and hypercholesteroluria.
– Nephritic syndrome: Hematuria with red blood cell and granular casts, variable degree of proteinuria, and frequently, high blood pressure
– Nodular mesangial sclerosis: Methenamine-silver and PAS-positive mesangial nodules with acellular centers surrounded by frequently coalescent glomerular capillaries. Classic example is the Kimmelstiel-Wilson nodule in diabetic glomerulosclerosis. (Fig. 29B)
– Obsolescence: Retracted and collapsed glomerular capillaries around the vascular pole. Bowman's space is filled with collagen, Bowman's capsular basement membrane is usually intact. (Fig. 12)

- Segmental: Only a segment (a localized portion) of a glomerulus is involved. (Figs. 14, 15, 21)
- Sclerosis: Abnormal accumulation of methenamine silver and PAS positive glomerular extracellular matrix resembling mesangial matrix and GBM (see Table 6, Figs. 21C, 22, 29B).
- Tram-tracking: Double contour of the glomerular capillary loop best seen on silver-methenamine-stained slides. It is caused by mesangial interposition (see above), and by deposition of any glomerular subendothelial material between which and the endothelium a new layer of basement membrane is formed (e.g: membranoproliferative glomerulonephritis), or by intramembranous deposits in the GBM (e.g.: advanced membranous GN). (Figs. 5B and 75)

II. TUBULOINTERSTITIUM

- Hyalin droplets: See resorption droplets
- Isometric vacuolization: Fine diffuse vacuoles approximately of the same size in the tubular epithelial cytoplasm. Seen in osmotic nephrosis, cyclosporine toxicity, and other conditions. (Fig. 76)
- Resorption droplets: Resorbed filtered protein in tubular cytoplasm, usually PAS-positive, occasionally also methenamine-silver positive. (Fig. 18)
- Tubulitis: Infiltration of tubular epithelium by inflammatory cells. (Fig. 72C)
- Tubular atrophy: Three types: 1) "Classic": tubules with thickened, usually wrinkled, sometimes duplicated basement membranes and simplified epithelium. 2) "Endocrine": narrow tubules with thin basement membranes and in clusters, resembling endocrine glands. 3) "Thyroid": rounded tubules with simplified epithelium containing homogenous proteinaceous casts resembling thyroid follicles. (Figs. 59, 69, 70)
- Thyroidization: See tubular atrophy

III. VASCULATURE

- Hyalin change (hyalin arteriolosclerosis): Deposition of glossy, refractile, homogenous eosinophilic, PAS positive material (sometimes containing lipid droplets) in arterial walls. (Figs. 29B, 29D, 66B)
- Intimal fibrosis (intimal fibroplasia, intimal fibroelastosis): Appearance of myointimal cells with the abundant deposition of extracellular matrix between the endothelium and the media. The lamina elastica interna is frequently disrupted and lamellated. (Figs. 66A and 74)
- Intimal arteritis: Subendothelial (intimal) inflammatory cell infiltrate in transplant rejection. (Fig. 73A)
- Fibrinoid necrosis: Deposition of proteinaceous material with the staining characteristics of fibrin in the arterial/arteriolar wall. Usually associated with true necrosis of the smooth muscle cells and/or endothelium. (Fig. 73B)
- Onion skinning: Concentric layering of elongated nuclei and cells in the usually mucoid appearing intima with severely narrowed lumen. Seen in malignant hypertension, scleroderma, and sometimes in other forms of thrombotic microangiopathy. Occasionally, adventitial pericytes may show concentric layering as well. (Fig. 39A)

ACKNOWLEDGMENT

We are grateful to Gyongyi M. Nadasdy, M.D., for taking and selecting most of the color photomicrographs.

REFERENCES

General Considerations

1. Schrier RW, Gottschalk CW. *Diseases of the kidney*, 6th ed. Boston: Little, Brown and Company, 1997.
2. Churg J, Bernstein J, Glassock RJ. *Renal disease: classification and atlas of glomerular diseases*, 2nd ed. New York: Igaku-Shoin, 1995.
3. Jennette JC, Olson JL, Schwartz MM, Silva FG, eds. *Heptinstall's Pathology of the kidney*, 5th ed. Boston: Little, Brown and Company 1998.
4. Manaligod JR, Pirani CL. Renal biopsy 1985. *Semin Nephrol* 1985;5:237–239.
5. Pirani CL, Salinas-Madrigal L, Koss MN. Evaluation of percutaneous renal biopsy In: Sommers SC, ed. *Kidney pathology decennial 1966–1977*. New York: Appleton-Century-Crofts, 1975:109–163.
6. Silva FG, Nadasdy T, D'Agati V. *Renal biopsy interpretation*. New York: Churchill Livingstone, 1996.
7. Tisher CC, Brenner BM. *Renal pathology with clinical and functional correlations*, 2nd ed. Philadelphia: JB Lippincott Co, 1994.
8. Silva FG, Pirani CL. Electron microscopic study of medical diseases of the kidney: update—1988. *Mod Pathol* 1988;1:292–315.

Proliferative Glomerulonephritides

9. Spargo BH, Dodge WF, Travis LB. The relationships between the clinical course and pathologic features of poststreptococcal glomerulonephritis. *Contrib Nephrol* 1976;2:130–143.
10. Silva FG. Acute postinfectious glomerulonephritis and glomerulonephritis complicating persistent bacterial infection. In: Heptinstall RH, ed. *Pathology of the kidney*. Boston: Little, Brown and Company, 1992:297–385.
11. Sorger K, Gessler U, Hubner FK, et al. Subtypes of acute postinfectious glomerulonephritis: synopsis of clinical and pathological features. *Clin Nephrol* 1982;17:114–128.
12. Baldwin DS. Poststreptococcal glomerulonephritis: a progressive disease? *Am J Med* 1977;62:1–11.
13. Williams DG. C3 nephritic factor and mesangiocapillary glomerulonephritis. *Pediatr Nephrol* 1997;11:96–98.
14. Silva FG. Membranoproliferative glomerulonephritis. In: Heptinstall RH, ed. *Pathology of the kidney*. Boston: Little, Brown and Company, 1992:477–557.
15. Habib R, Loirat C, Gubler MC, et al. Morphology and serum complement levels in membranoproliferative glomerulonephritis. *Adv Nephrol* 1974;4:109–136.
16. Donadio JV, Holley KE. Membranoproliferative glomerulonephritis. *Semin Nephrol* 1982;2:204–216.
17. Taguchi T, Bohle A. Evaluation of change with time of glomerular morphology in membranoproliferative glomerulonephritis: a serial biopsy study of 33 cases. *Clin Nephrol* 1989;31:297–306.
18. Rennke HG. Secondary membranoproliferative glomerulonephritis. *Kidney Int* 1995;47:643–656.
19. Johnson RJ, Gretch DR, Yamabe H, et al. Membranoproliferative glomerulonephritis associated with hepatitis C virus infection. *N Engl J Med* 1993;328:465–470.
20. D'Amico G, Fornasieri A. Cryoglobulinemic glomerulonephritis: a membranoproliferative glomerulonephritis induced by hepatitis C virus. *Am J Kidney Dis* 1995;25:361–369.

21. Newell GC. Cirrhotic glomerulonephritis: incidence, morphology, clinical features, and pathogenesis. *Am J Kidney Dis* 1987;9:183–190.
22. Alpers CE, Biava CG. Idiopathic lobular glomerulonephritis (nodular mesangial sclerosis): a distinct diagnostic entity. *Clin Nephrol* 1989;32:68–74.
23. Lager DJ, Rosenberg BF, Shapiro H, Bernstein J. Lecithin cholesterol acyltransferase deficiency: ultrastructural examination of sequential renal biopsies. *Mod Pathol* 1991;4:331–335.
24. Kotanko P, Pusey CD, Levy JB. Recurrent glomerulonephritis following renal transplantation. *Transplantation* 1997;63:1045–1052.
25. Ramos EL, Tisher CC. Recurrent diseases in the kidney transplant. *Am J Kidney Dis* 1994;24:142–154.
26. Habib R, Gubler MC, Loirat C, et al. Dense deposit disease: a variant of membranoproliferative glomerulonephritis. *Kidney Int* 1975;7:204–215.
27. Sibley RK, Kim Y. Dense intramembranous deposit disease. *Kidney Int* 1984;25:660–670.
28. Southwest Pediatric Nephrology Study Group. Dense deposit disease in children: prognostic value of clinical and pathologic indicators. *Am J Kidney Dis* 1985;6:161–169.
29. Kashtan CE, Burke B, Burch G, Fisker SG, Kim Y. Dense intramembranous deposit disease: a clinical comparison of histological subtypes. *Clin Nephrol* 1990;33(1):1–6.
30. Kim Y, Vernier RL, Fish AJ, et al. Immunofluorescence studies of dense deposit disease: the presence of railroad tracks and mesangial rings. *Lab Invest* 1979;40:474–480.
31. Anders D, Agricola B, Sippel M, et al. Basement membrane changes on membranoproliferative glomerulonephritis. II. Characterization of a third type of silver impregnation of ultra thin sections. *Virchows Arch A Pathol Anat Histopathol* 1977;376:1–19.
32. Strife CF, McEnery PT. McAdams AJ, et al. Membranoproliferative glomerulonephritis with disruption of the glomerular basement membrane. *Clin Nephrol* 1977;7:65–72.
33. Southwest Pediatric Nephrology Study Group. A clinico-pathologic study of crescentic glomerulonephritis in 50 children. *Kidney Int* 1985;27:450–458.
34. Jennette JC. Antineutrophil cytoplasmic autoantibody–associated diseases: a pathologist's perspective. *Am J Kidney Dis* 1991;18:164–170.
35. Kallenberg CGM, Brouwer E, Weening JJ, Cohen Tervaert JW. Antineutrophil cytoplasmic antibodies: current diagnostic and pathophysiological potential. *Kidney Int* 1994;46:1–15.
36. Hogan SL, Nachman PH, Wilkman AS, Jennette JC, Falk RJ, and the Glomerular Disease Collaborative Network. Prognostic markers in patients with antineutrophil cytoplasmic autoantibody–associated microscopic polyangiitis and glomerulonephritis. *J Am Soc Nephrol* 1996;7:23–32.
37. Bolton WK. Goodpasture's syndrome. *Kidney Int* 1996;50:1753–1766.
38. Herody M, Bobrie G, Gouarin C, Grünfeld JP, Noel LH. Anti-GBM disease: predictive value of clinical, histological and serological data. *Clin Nephrol* 1993;40:249–255.
39. Gobel J, Olbricht J, Offner G, et al. Kidney transplantation in Alport's syndrome: long term outcome and allograft anti-GBM nephritis. *Kidney Int* 1992;38:299–304.
40. Heptinstall RH. Crescentic glomerulonephritis. In: Heptinstall RH, ed. *Pathology of the kidney*, 4th ed. Boston: Little, Brown and Company, 1992:627–675.
41. Bonsib SM, Walker WP. Pulmonary-renal syndrome: clinical similarity amidst etiologic diversity. *Mod Pathol* 1989;2:129–137.
42. Pirani CL, Silva FG. The kidney in systemic lupus erythematosus and other collagen vascular diseases. In: Churg J, Spargo BH, Mostofi FK, et al., eds. *Kidney disease: present status*. Baltimore: Williams & Wilkins, 1979:98–139 (International Academy of Pathology monograph).
43. D'Agati V, Chander P, Nash M, Mancilla-Jimenez R. Idiopathic microscopic polyarteritis nodosa: ultrastructural observations on the renal vascular and glomerular lesions. *Am J Kidney Dis* 1986;7:95–110.
44. Whitworth JA, Turner DR, Leibowitz S, et al. Focal segmental sclerosis or scarred focal proliferative glomerulonephritis? *Clin Nephrol* 1978;9:229–235.

The Glomerular Capillary Wall Lesions

45. Nadasdy T, Silva FG, Hogg RJ. Minimal change nephrotic syndrome: focal sclerosis complex (including IgM nephropathy and diffuse mesangial hypercellularity). In: Tisher CC, Brenner BM, eds. *Renal pathology with clinical and functional correlations*, 2nd ed. Philadelphia: JB Lippincott Co, 1994:330–389.
46. International Study of Kidney Disease in Children. Primary nephrotic syndrome in children: clinical significance of histopathologic variants of minimal change and of diffuse mesangial hypercellularity. *Kidney Int* 1981;20:765–771.
47. Howie AJ, Brewer DB. The glomerular tip lesion: a previously undescribed type of segmental glomerular abnormality. *J Pathol* 1984;142:205–220.
48. Howie AJ, Brewer DB. The glomerular tip lesion: a distinct entity or not? *J Pathol* 1988;154:191–192.
49. Habib R, Girardin E, Gagnadoux MR, Hinglais N, Levy M, Broyer M. Immunopathological findings in idiopathic nephrosis: clinical significance of glomerular "immune deposits." *Pediatr Nephrol* 1988;2:402–408.
50. Dantal J, Bigot E, Bogers W, et al. Effect of plasma protein adsorption on protein excretion in kidney transplant recipients with recurrent nephrotic syndrome. *N Engl J Med* 1994;330:7–14.
51. Daniel V, Trautmann Y, Konrad M, Nayir A, Schärer K. T-lymphocyte populations, cytokines and other growth factors in serum and urine of children with idiopathic nephrotic syndrome. *Clin Nephrol* 1997;47:289–297.
52. Warren GV, Korbet SM, Schwartz MM, Lewis EJ. Minimal change glomerulopathy associated with nonsteroidal antiinflammatory drugs. *Am J Kidney Dis* 1989;13:127–130.
53. Waldherr R, Bubler MC, Levy M, Broyer M, Habib R. The significance of pure diffuse mesangial proliferation in idiopathic nephrotic syndrome. *Clin Nephrol* 1978;10:171–179.
54. Southwest Pediatric Nephrology Study Group. Childhood nephrotic syndrome associated with diffuse mesangial hypercellularity. *Kidney Int* 1983;23:87–94.
55. Cohen AH, Border WA, Glassock RJ. Nephrotic syndrome with mesangial IgM deposits. *Lab Invest* 1978;38:610–619.
56. Bhasin HK, Abuelo JG, Nayak R, Esparza AR. Mesangial proliferative glomerulonephritis. *Lab Invest* 1978;39:21–29.
57. Jennette JC, Hipp CG. C1q nephropathy: a distinct pathologic entity usually causing nephrotic syndrome. *Am J Kidney Dis* 1985;6:103–110.
58. Iskandar SS, Browning MC, Lorentz WB. C1q nephropathy: a pediatric clinicopathologic study. *Am J Kidney Dis* 1991;18:459–465.
59. Rennke HG, Klein PS. Pathogenesis and significance of nonprimary focal and segmental glomerulosclerosis. *Am J Kidney Dis* 1989;13:443–456.
60. Cortes L, Tejani A. Dilemma of focal segmental glomerular sclerosis. *Kidney Int* 1996;49:S-57–S-63.
61. Schwartz MM, Korbet SM. Primary focal segmental glomerulosclerosis: pathology, histological variants, and pathogenesis. *Am J Kidney Dis* 1993;22:874–883.
62. D'Agati V. The many masks of focal segmental glomerulosclerosis. *Kidney Int* 1994;46:1223–1241.
63. Haas M, Spargo BH, Coventry S. Increasing incidence of focal-segmental glomerulosclerosis among adult nephropathies: a 20-year renal biopsy study. *Am J Kidney Dis* 1995;26:740–750.
64. Korbet SM, Genchi RM, Borok RZ, Schwartz MM. The racial prevalence of glomerular lesions in nephrotic adults. *Am J Kidney Dis* 1996;27:647–651.
65. Friedman EA, Rao TKS. Disappearance of uremia due to heroin-associated nephropathy. *Am J Kidney Dis* 1995;25:689–693.
66. Southwest Pediatric Nephrology Study Group. Focal segmental glomerulosclerosis in children with idiopathic nephrotic syndrome. *Kidney Int* 1985;27:442–449.
67. Cameron JS, Senguttuvan P, Hartley B, et al. Focal segmental glomerulosclerosis in fifty-nine renal allografts from a single centre: analysis of risk factors for recurrence. *Transplant Proc* 1989;21:2117–2118.
68. Brenner BM, Meyer TW, Hostetter TH. Dietary protein intake and the progressive nature of kidney disease: the role of hemodynamically mediated glomerular injury in the pathogenesis of progressive glomerular sclerosis in aging, renal ablation, and intrinsic renal disease. *N Engl J Med* 1982;307:652.
69. Nash MA, Griefer I, Obling H, Bernstein J, Bennett B, Spitzer A. The significance of focal sclerotic lesions of glomeruli in children. *J Pediatr* 1976;88:806–813.

70. Kaplan C, Pasternack B, Shah H, Gallo G. Age-related incidence of sclerotic glomeruli in human kidneys. *Am J Pathol* 1975;80:227–234.
71. Seney FD Jr., Burns DK, Silva FG. Acquired immunodeficiency syndrome and the kidney. *Am J Kidney Dis* 1990; 6:1–13.
72. D'Agati V, Appel GB. HIV infection and the kidney. *J Am Soc Nephrol* 1997;8:138–152.
73. Humphreys MH. Human immunodeficiency virus–associated glomerulosclerosis. *Kidney Int* 1995;48:311–320.
74. Detwiler RK, Falk RJ, Hogan SL, Jennette JC. Collapsing glomerulopathy: a clinically and pathologically distinct variant of focal segmental glomerulosclerosis. *Kidney Int* 1994;45:1416–1424.
75. Valeri A, Barisoni L, Appel GB, Seigle R, D'Agati V. Idiopathic collapsing focal segmental glomerulosclerosis: a clinicopathologic study. *Kidney Int* 1996;50:1734–1746.
76. Cohen AH, Nast CC. HIV-associated nephropathy: a unique combined glomerular, tubular, and interstitial lesion. *Mod Pathol* 1988;1:87–97.
77. D'Agati V, Suh JI, Carbone L, Cheng JT, Appel G. Pathology of HIV-associated nephropathy: a detailed morphologic and comparative study. *Kidney Int* 1989;35:1358–1370.
78. Kimmel PL, Phillips TM, Ferreira-Centeno A, Farkas-Szallasi T, Abraham AA, Garrett CT. HIV-associated immune-mediated renal disease. *Kidney Int* 1993;44:1327–1340.
79. Casanova S, Mazzucco G, di Belgiojoso GB, et al. Pattern of glomerular involvement in human immunodeficiency virus–infected patients: an Italian study. *Am J Kidney Dis* 1995;26:446–453.
80. Glassock RJ. Secondary membranous glomerulonephritis. *Nephrol Dial Transplant* 1992[Suppl 1]:64–71.
81. Ehrenreich T, Churg J. Pathology of membranous nephropathy. *Pathol Ann* 1968;3:145–186.
82. Rosen S, Tornroth T, Bernard DB. Membranous glomerulonephritis. In: Tisher CC, Brenner BM, eds. *Renal pathology*, 2nd ed. Philadelphia: JB Lippincott Co, 1994:258–293.
83. Wakai S, Magil AB. Focal glomerulosclerosis in idiopathic membranous glomerulonephritis. *Kidney Int* 1992;41:428–434.
84. Jennette JC, Iskandar SS, Dalldorf FG. Pathologic differentiation between lupus and nonlupus membranous glomerulopathy. *Kidney Int* 1983;24:377–385.
85. Venkataseshan VS, Lieberman K, Kim DU, et al. Hepatitis-B-associated glomerulonephritis: pathology, pathogenesis and clinical course. *Medicine* 1990;69:200–216.
86. Stehman-Breen C, Alpers CE, Couser WG, Willson R, Johnson RJ. Hepatitis C virus associated membranous glomerulonephritis. *Clin Nephrol* 1995;44:141–147.
87. Burstein DM, Korbet ST, Schwartz MM. Membranous glomerulonephritis and malignancy. *Am J Kidney Dis* 1993;22:5–10.
88. Cattran DC, Pei Y, Greenwood C. Predicting progression in membranous glomerulonephritis. *Nephrol Dial Transplant* 1992[Suppl1]:48–52.
89. Forero FV, Prugue NG, Morales NR. Idiopathic nephrotic syndrome of the adult with asymptomatic thrombosis of the renal vein. *Am J Nephrol* 1988;8:457–462.
90. Kerjaschki D. Molecular aspects of immune deposit formation in Heymann nephritis. *Nephrol Dial Transplant* 1992[Suppl 1]:16–20.
91. Schulze M, Donadio JV Jr., Pruchno CJ, et al. Elevated urinary excretion of the C5b-9 complex in membranous nephropathy. *Kidney Int* 1991;40:533–538.
92. Mauer SM, Steffes MW, Brown DM. The kidney in diabetes. *Am J Med* 1981;70:603–612.
93. Ritz E, Stefanski A. Diabetic nephropathy in type II diabetes. *Am J Kidney Dis* 1996;27:167–194.
94. Østerby R. Glomerular structural changes in type 1 (insulin-dependent) diabetes mellitus: causes, consequences, and prevention. *Diabetologia* 1992;35:803–812.
95. Salinas-Madrigal L, Pirani CL, Pollak VE. Glomerular and vascular insudative lesions of diabetic nephropathy: electron microscopic observations. *Am J Pathol* 1970;59:369–397.
96. Monga G, Mazzucco G, di Belgiojoso GB, Confalonieri R, Sacchi G, Bertani T. Pattern of double glomerulopathies: a clinicopathologic study of superimposed glomerulonephritis on diabetic glomerulosclerosis. *Mod Pathol* 1989;2:407–414.

Glomerular Diseases with Isolated Hematuria

97. Birch DF, Fairley KF. Haematuria: glomerular or non-glomerular? *Lancet* 1979;2:845–846.
98. Rizzoni G, Braggion F, Zacchello G. Evaluation of glomerular and nonglomerular hematuria by phase-contrast microscopy. *J Pediatr* 1983;103:370–374.
99. Emancipator SN. IgA nephropathy: morphologic expression and pathogenesis. *Am J Kidney Dis* 1994;23:451–462.
100. Silva FG, Hogg RJ. IgA nephropathy (Berger's disease). In: Tisher CC, Brenner BM, eds. *Renal pathology*. Philadelphia: JB Lippincott Co, 1989:434-493.
101. Ibels LS, Györy AZ. IgA nephropathy: analysis of the natural history, important factors in the progression of renal disease, and a review of the literature. *Medicine* 1994;73:79–102.
102. Galla JH. IgA nephropathy. *Kidney Int* 1995;47:377–387.
103. White RHR. Henoch-Schönlein nephritis: a disease with significant late sequelae. *Nephron* 1994;68:1–9.
104. Waldo FB. Is Henoch-Schönlein purpura the systemic form of IgA nephropathy? *Am J Kidney Dis* 1988;12:373–377.
105. Clive DA, Galvanek EG, Silva FG. Mesangial immunoglobulin A deposits in minimal change nephrotic syndrome: a report of an older patient and review of the literature. *Am J Nephrol* 1990;10:31–36.
106. Hogg RJ, Silva FG, Wyatt RJ, Reisch JS, Argyle JC, Savino DA. Prognostic indicators in children with IgA nephropathy: report of the Southwest Pediatric Nephrology Study Group. *Pediatr Nephrol* 1994;8:15–20.
107. Gallo GR, Katafuchi R, Neelakantappa K, Baldwin DS. Prognostic pathologic markers in IgA nephropathy. *Am J Kidney Dis* 1988;12:362–365.
108. Navas-Palacios JJ, Gutierrez-Millet LV, Usera-Sarraga G, et al. IgA nephropathy: an ultrastructural study. *Ultrastruct Pathol* 1981;2:151–161.
109. Bogenschutz O, Bohle A, Batz C, et al. IgA nephritis: on the importance of morphological and clinical parameters in the long-term prognosis of 239 patients. *Am J Nephrol* 1990;10:137–147.
110. Yoshikawa N, Ito H, Nakamura H. Prognostic indicators in childhood IgA nephropathy. *Nephron* 1992;60:60–67.
111. Packham DK, Yan HD, Hewitson TD, et al. The significance of focal and segmental hyalinosis and sclerosis (FSHS) and nephrotic range proteinuria in IgA nephropathy. *Clin Nephrol* 1996;46:225–229.
112. Haas M. IgA nephropathy histologically resembling focal-segmental glomerulosclerosis: a clinicopathologic study of 18 cases. *Am J Kidney Dis* 1996;28:365–371.
113. Rogers PW, Kurtzman NA, Bunn SM Jr, et al. Familial benign essential hematuria. *Arch Intern Med* 1973;131:257–262.
114. Tiebosch ATMG, Frederik PM, vanBreda Vriesman PJC, et al. Thin-basement-membrane nephropathy in adults with persistent hematuria. *N Engl J Med* 1989;320:14–18.
115. Dische FE. Measurement of glomerular basement membrane thickness and its application to the diagnosis of thin-membrane nephropathy. *Arch Pathol Lab Med* 1992;116:43–49.
116. Kashtan CE, Michael AF. Alport syndrome. *Kidney Int* 1996;50:1445–1463.
117. Spear GS. Alport's syndrome: a consideration of pathogenesis. *Clin Nephrol* 1973;1:336–337.
118. Churg J, Sherman RL. Pathologic characteristics of hereditary nephritis. *Arch Pathol* 1973;95:374–379.
119. Bernstein J. The glomerular basement membrane abnormality in Alport's syndrome. *Am J Kidney Dis* 1987;10:222–229.
120. Kohaut EC, Singer DB, Nevels BK, et al. The specificity of split renal membranes in hereditary nephritis. *Arch Pathol Lab Med* 1976;100:475–479.
121. van de Putte LEA, de la Riviere GB, van Breda Vriesman PJC. Recurrent or persistent hematuria: sign of mesangial immune-complex deposition. *N Engl J Med* 1974;290:1165–1170.
122. Pardo V, Berian MG, Levi DF, et al. Benign primary hematuria: clinicopathologic study of 65 patients. *Am J Med* 1979;67:817–822.
123. Copley JB. Isolated asymptomatic hematuria in the adult. *Am J Med Sci* 1986;291:101–111.
124. Weisberg LS, Bloom PB, Simmons RL, Viner ED. Loin pain hematuria syndrome. *Am J Nephrol* 1993;13:229–237.

Acellular Closure of Glomerular Capillaries

125. Remuzzi G. HUS and TTP: variable expression of a single entity. *Kidney Int* 1987;32:292–308.

126. Ruggenenti P, Remuzzi G. Malignant vascular disease of the kidney: nature of the lesions, mediators of disease progression, and the case for bilateral nephrectomy. *Am J Kidney Dis* 1996;27:459–475.
127. Laszik Z. Thrombotic microangiopathies. In: Silva FG, D'Agati VD, Nadasdy T, eds. *Renal biopsy interpretation*. New York: Churchill Livingstone, 1996:283–308.
128. Remuzzi G, Ruggenenti P. The hemolytic uremic syndrome. *Kidney Int* 1995;47:2–19.
129. Renaud C, Niaudet P, Gagnadoux MF, Broyer M, Habib R. Haemolytic uraemic syndrome: prognostic factors in children over 3 years of age. *Pediatr Nephrol* 1995;9:24–29.
130. Habib R, Levy M, Gagnadoux M, Broyer M. Prognosis of the hemolytic uremic syndrome in children. *Adv Nephrol* 1982;11:99–128.
131. Eijgenraam FJ, Donckerwolcke RA, Monnens LAH, Proesmans W, Wolff ED, vanDamme B. Renal transplantation in 20 children with hemolytic-uremic syndrome. *Clin Nephrol* 1990;33:87–93.
132. Lesesne JB, Rothschild N, Erickson B, et al. Cancer-associated hemolytic-uremic syndrome: analysis of 85 cases from a national registry. *J Clin Oncol* 1989;7:781–789.
133. Gadallah MF, El-Shahawy MA, Campese VM, Todd JR, King JW. Disparate prognosis of thrombotic microangiopathy in HIV-infected patients with and without AIDS. *Am J Nephrol* 1996;16:446–450.
134. Cohen EP, Lawton CA, Moulder JE. Bone marrow transplant nephropathy: radiation nephritis revisited. *Nephron* 1995;70:217–222.
135. D'Amico G, Colasanti G, Ferrario F, Sinico RA. Renal involvement in essential mixed cryoglobulinemia. *Kidney Int* 1989;35:1004–1014.
136. Roccatello D, Isidoro C, Mazzucco G, et al. Role of monocytes in cryoglobulinemia-associated nephritis. *Kidney Int* 1993;43:1150–1155.
137. Falk RH, Comenzo RL, Skinner M. The systemic amyloidoses. *N Engl J Med* 1997;337:898–909.
138. Gallo G, Kumar A. Hematopoietic disorders. In: Silva FG, D'Agati VD, Nadasdy T (eds), Renal Biopsy Interpretation. New York: Churchill Livingstone, 1996:259-282.
139. Noel LH, Droz D, Ganeval D. Immunohistochemical characterization of renal amyloidosis. *Am J Clin Pathol* 1987;87:756–761.
140. Korbet SM, Schwartz MM, Lewis EJ. The fibrillary glomerulopathies. *Am J Kidney Dis* 1994;23:751–765.
141. Alpers CE. Fibrillary glomerulonephritis and immunotactoid glomerulopathy: two entities, not one. *Am J Kidney Dis* 1993;22:448–451.
142. Fogo A, Qureshi N, Horn RG. Morphologic and clinical features of fibrillary glomerulonephritis versus immunotactoid glomerulopathy. *Am J Kidney Dis* 1993;22:367–377.
143. Iskandar SS, Falk RJ, Jennette JC. Clinical and pathologic features of fibrillary glomerulonephritis. *Kidney Int* 1992;42:1401–1407.
144. Pronovost PH, Brady HR, Gunning ME, Espinoza O, Rennke HG. Clinical features, predictors of disease progression and results of renal transplantation in fibrillary/immunotactoid glomerulopathy. *Nephrol Dial Transplant* 1996;11:837–842.

Systemic Lupus Erythematosus and other Collagen-Vascular Diseases

145. Berden JHM. Lupus nephritis. *Kidney Int* 1997;52:538–558.
146. Silva FG. The nephropathies of systemic lupus erythematosus. In: Rosen S, ed. *Pathology of glomerular disease*. New York: Churchill Livingstone, 1983:79–124.
147. Hill GS. Systemic lupus erythematosus and mixed connective tissue disease. In: Heptinstall RH, ed. *Pathology of the kidney*, 4th ed. Boston: Little, Brown and Company, 1992:871–951.
148. D'Agati VD. Systemic lupus erythematosus. In: Silva FG, D'Agati VD, Nadasdy T, eds. *Renal biopsy interpretation*. New York: Churchill Livingstone, 1996:181–220.
149. Appel GB, Pirani CL, D'Agati V. Renal vascular complications of systemic lupus erythematosus. *J Am Soc Nephrol* 1994;4:1499–1515.
150. Pirani CL, Olesnicky L. Role of electron microscopy in the classification of lupus nephritis. *Am J Kidney Dis* 1982;2:150–163.
151. Morel-Maroger L, Mery JP, Droz D, et al. The course of lupus nephritis: contribution of serial renal biopsies. *Adv Nephrol* 1976;6:79–118.
152. Austin HA III, Mueng LR, Joyce KM, et al. Prognostic factors in lupus nephritis: contribution of renal histologic data. *Am J Med* 1983;75:382–391.
153. Austin HA, Boumpas DT, Vaughan EM, Balow JE. High-risk features of lupus nephritis: importance of race and clinical and histological factors in 166 patients. *Nephrol Dial Transplant* 1995;10:1620–1628.
154. Tax WJM, Kramers C, vanBruggen MCJ, Berden JHM. Apoptosis, nucleosomes, and nephritis in systemic lupus erythematosus. *Kidney Int* 1995;48:666–673.
155. Donohoe JF. Scleroderma and the kidney. *Kidney Int* 1992;41:462–477.
156. D'Agati V, Kunis C, Williams G, Appel GB. Anti-cardiolipin antibody and renal disease: a report of three cases. *J Am Soc Nephrol* 1990;1:777–784.
157. Davis JA, Cohen AH, Weisbart R, Paulus HE. Glomerulonephritis in rheumatoid arthritis. *Arthritis Rheum* 1979;22:1018–1023.
158. Samuels B, Lee JA, Engleman ER, Hopper J. Membranous nephropathy in patients with rheumatoid arthritis: relationship with gold therapy. *Medicine (Baltimore)* 1978;57:319–327.
159. Sellars L, Siamopoulos K, Wilkinson R, Leohapand T, Morley AR. Renal biopsy appearance in rheumatoid disease. *Clin Nephrol* 1983 20:114–120.
160. Korpela M, Mustonen J, Pasternack A, Helin H. Mesangial glomerulopathy in rheumatoid arthritis patients. *Nephron* 1991;59:46–50.

Monoclonal Gammopathy-Associated Renal Disease

161. Sanders PW, Herrera GA, Kirk KA, Old CW, Galla JH. Spectrum of glomerular and tubulointerstitial renal lesions associated with monotypical immunoglobulin light chain deposition. *Lab Invest* 1991;64:527–537.
162. Morel-Maroger L, Verroust P. Glomerular lesions in dysproteinemias. *Kidney Int* 1974;5:249–252.
163. Silva FG, Pirani CL, Mesa-Tejada R, Williams GC. The kidney in plasma cell dyscrasias: a review and a clinicopathologic study of 50 patients. In: Fenoglio CM, Wolff M, eds. *Progress in surgical pathology*. New York: Masson, 1984:131–176.
164. Preud'Homme JL, Aucouturier P, Touchard G, et al. Monoclonal immunoglobulin deposition disease (Randall type): relationship with structural abnormalities of immunoglobulin chains. *Kidney Int* 1994;46:965–972.
165. Pirani CL, Silva F, D'Agati V, Chander P, Striker LMM. Renal lesions in plasma cell dyscrasias: ultrastructural observations. *Am J Kidney Dis* 1987;10:208–221.
166. Gerlag PGG, Loene AP, Berden JHM. Renal transplantation in light chain nephropathy: case report and review of literature. *Clin Nephrol* 1986;25:101–104.
167. Pirani CL, Silva FG, Appel GB. Tubulo-interstitial disease in multiple myeloma and other nonrenal diseases. In: *Tubulo-interstitial nephropathies*. Volume 10 of Contemporary Issues in Nephrology, Cotran R., Issue Editor; Brenner B. and Stein, J., Series Editors. Churchill Livingstone, New York, Chapter 11, 1983, pp. 287–334.
168. Start DA, Silva FG, Davis LD, D'Agati V, Pirani CL. Myeloma cast nephropathy: immunohistochemical and lectin studies. *Mod Pathol* 1988;1:336.

Tubulointerstitial Disease

169. Bohle A, Mackensen-Haen S, von Gise H. Significance of tubulointerstitial changes in the renal cortex for the excretory function and concentration ability of the kidney: a morphometric contribution. *Am J Nephrol* 1987;7:421–433.
170. Eknoyan G, McDonald MA, Appel D, Truong LD. Chronic tubulo-interstitial nephritis: correlation between structural and functional findings. *Kidney Int* 1990;38:736–743.
171. Venkatachalam MA. Pathology of acute renal failure. In: Brenner BM, Stein JH, eds. *Acute renal failure*. New York: Churchill Livingstone, 1980:79–107 (Contemporary issues in nephrology, vol. 6).
172. Solez K. Acute renal failure. In: Heptinstall RH, ed. *Pathology of the kidney*, 4th ed. Boston: Little, Brown and Company, 1992:1069–1148.
173. Racusen LC, Fivush BA, Li YL, Slatnik I, Solez K. Dissociation of tubular cell detachment and tubular cell death in clinical and experimental "acute tubular necrosis." *Lab Invest* 1991;64:546–556.
174. Nadasdy T, Laszik Z, Blick KE, et al. Human acute tubular necrosis: a lectin and immunohistochemical study. *Hum Pathol* 1995;26:230–239.
175. Bonomini V, Frascà GM, Raimondi C, Vangelista A, Scolari MP, D'Arcangelo GL. Long-term follow-up of acute renal failure. *Nephrol Dial Transplant* 1994;9:224–228.

176. Bonventre JV. Mechanisms of ischemic acute renal failure. *Kidney Int* 1993;43:1160–1178.
177. Heptinstall RH. Pyelonephritis: pathologic features. In: Heptinstall RH, ed. *Pathology of the kidney*, 4th ed. Boston: Little, Brown and Company, 1992:1489–1552.
178. Heptinstall RH. Interstitial nephritis: a brief review. *Am J Pathol* 1976;83:214–236.
179. Colvin RB, Fang LST. Interstitial nephritis. In: Tisher CC, Brenner BM, eds. *Renal pathology with clinical and functional correlations*, 2nd ed. Philadelphia: JB Lippincott Co, 1994:723–768.
180. Heptinstall RH. Interstitial nephritis. In: Heptinstall RH, ed. *Pathology of the kidney*. Boston: Little, Brown and Company, 1992:1315–1369.
181. Nadasdy T, Racusen L. Renal injury caused by therapeutic and diagnostic agents, and abuse of analgesics and narcotics. In: Jennette JC, Olson JL, Schwartz MM, Silva FG, eds. *Heptinstall's pathology of the kidney*, 5th ed. New York: Lippincott–Raven Publishers 1998;811–861.
182. Kleinknecht D. Interstitial nephritis, the nephrotic syndrome, and chronic renal failure secondary to nonsteroidal anti-inflammatory drugs. *Semin Nephrol* 1995;15:228–235.
183. D'Agati VD, Theise ND, Pirani CL, Knowles DM, Appel GB. Interstitial nephritis related to nonsteroidal anti-inflammatory agents and beta-lactam antibiotics: a comparative study of the interstitial infiltrates using monoclonal antibodies. In: Bryln GN, Giovannetti S, eds. *Contributions in nephrology*. Basel: S. Karger, 55:159–175.
184. Schwarz A, Krause PH, Keller F, Offermann G, Mihatsch MJ. Granulomatous interstitial nephritis after nonsteroidal anti-inflammatory drugs. *Am J Nephrol* 1988;8:410–416.
185. Hawkins EP, Berry PL, Silva FG. Acute tubulointerstitial nephritis in children: clinical, morphologic, and lectin studies. A report of the Southwest Pediatric Nephrology Study Group. *Am J Kidney Dis* 1989;14(6):466–471.
186. Hodson CJ. The effects of disturbance of flow on the kidney. *J Infect Dis* 1969;120:54–60.
187. International Reflux Study. Medical versus surgical treatment of primary vesicoureteral reflux: a prospective international reflux study in children. *J Urol* 1981;125:277–283.
188. Cotran RS. Glomerulosclerosis in reflux nephropathy. *Kidney Int* 1982;21:528–534.
189. Becker GJ, Kincaid-Smith P. Reflux nephropathy: the glomerular lesion and progression of renal failure. *Pediatr Nephrol* 1993;7:365–369.
190. Eble JN. Unusual renal tumors and tumor-like conditions. In: Eble JN, ed. *Tumors and tumor-like conditions of the kidneys and ureters*. New York: Churchill Livingstone, 1990:145–176.
191. Dobyan DC, Truong LD, Eknoyan G. Renal malacoplakia reappraised. *Am J Kidney Dis* 1993;22:243–252.
192. Esparza AR, McKay DB, Cronan JJ, Chazan JA. Renal parenchymal malacoplakia: histologic spectrum and its relationship to megalocytic interstitial nephritis and xanthogranulomatous pyelonephritis. *Am J Surg Pathol* 1989;13:225–236.
193. Cohen MS: Granulomatous nephritis. *Urol Clin North Am* 1986;31:647.
194. Elseviers MM, De Broe ME. The implication of analgesics in human kidney disease. In: Stuart JH, ed. *Analgesic and NSAID-induced kidney disease*. Oxford, England: Oxford University Press, 1993:32–47.
195. Elseviers MM, Waller I, Nenov D, et al. Evaluation of diagnostic criteria for analgesic nephropathy in patients with end-stage renal failure: results of the ANNE study. *Nephrol Dial Transplant* 1995;10:808–814.
196. Mihatsch MJ, Zollinger HU. The pathology of analgesic nephropathy. In: Stewart JH, ed. *Analgesic and NSAID-induced kidney disease*. Oxford, England, Oxford University Press, 1993:67–85.
197. Griffin MD, Bergstralh EJ, Larson TS. Renal papillary necrosis: a sixteen-year clinical experience. *J Am Soc Nephrol* 1995;6:248–256.
198. Duggin GG. Combination analgesic-induced kidney disease: the Australian experience. *Am J Kidney Dis* 1996;28:S39–S47.
199. Elseviers MM, De Broe ME. Combination analgesic involvement in the pathogenesis of analgesic nephropathy: the European perspective. *Am J Kidney Dis* 1996;28:S48–S55.
200. Hill GS. Calcium and the kidney, nephrolithiasis, and hydronephrosis. In: Heptinstall RH, ed. *Pathology of the kidney*, 4th ed. Boston: Little, Brown and Company, 1992:1563–1629.
201. Sommers SC, Churg J. Kidney pathology in hyperuricemia and gout. In: Yu T-F, Berger L, eds. *The kidney in gout and hyperuricemia*. New York: Futura, 1982:95.
202. Heptinstall RH. Tubular disorders and various metabolic diseases. In: Heptinstall RH, ed. *Pathology of the kidney*, 4th ed. Boston: Little, Brown and Company, 1992:1989–2043.

Vascular Lesions and the Kidney

203. Ferris TF. The kidney and hypertension. *Arch Intern Med* 1982;142:1889–1895.
204. Heptinstall RH. Hypertension. I. Essential hypertension. In: Heptinstall RH, ed. *Pathology of the kidney*, 4th ed. Boston: Little, Brown and Company, 1992:951–1028.
205. Tracy RE, Bhandaru SY, Oalmann MC, et al. Blood pressure and nephrosclerosis in black and white men and women aged 25 to 54. *Mod Pathol* 1991;4:602–609.
206. Bohle A, Ratschek M. The compensated and the decompensated form of benign nephrosclerosis. *Pathol Res Pract* 1982;174:357–367.
207. Freedman BI, Iskandar SS, Appel RG. The link between hypertension and nephrosclerosis. *Am J Kidney Dis* 1995;25:207–221.
208. Lopes AAS, Hornbuckle K, James SA, Port FK. The joint effects of race and age on the risk of end-stage renal disease attributed to hypertension. *Am J Kidney Dis* 1994;24:554–560.
209. Harrison EG, McCormack LJ. Pathologic classification of renal arterial disease in renovascular hypertension. *Mayo Clin Proc* 1971;46:161–166.
210. Mannesse CK, Blankestijn PJ, Veld AJM, Schalekamp MADH. Renal failure and cholesterol crystal embolization: a report of 4 surviving cases and a review of the literature. *Clin Nephrol* 1991;36:240–245.
211. Greenberg A, Bastacky SI, Iqbal A, Borochovitz D, Johnson JP. Focal segmental glomerulosclerosis associated with nephrotic syndrome in cholesterol atheroembolism: clinicopathological correlations. *Am J Kidney Dis* 1997;29:334–344.
212. Lie JT. Nomenclature and classification of vasculitis: plus ça change, plus c'est la même chose. *Arthritis Rheum* 1994;37:181–186.
213. Jennette JC, Falk RJ, Andrassy K, et al. Nomenclature of systemic vasculitides. *Arthritis Rheum* 1994;37:187–192.
214. Niles JL. Antineutrophil cytoplasmic antibodies in the classification of vasculitis. *Annu Rev Med* 1996;47:303–313.
215. Churg A, Churg J. *Systemic vasculitides*. New York: Igaku-Shoin, 1991.
216. The USRDS 1996 annual data report: incidence and prevalence of RSRD. *Am J Kidney Dis* 1996 28:S34–S47.
217. Hughson MD, Lajoie G. End-stage renal disease. In: Silva FG, D'Agati VD, Nadasdy T, eds. *Renal biopsy interpretation*. New York: Churchill Livingstone, 1996:357–372.
218. Nadasdy T, Laszik Z, Blick KE, Johnson DL, Silva FG. Tubular atrophy in the end-stage kidney: a lectin and immunohistochemical study. *Hum Pathol* 1994;25:22–28.
219. McManus JFA, Hughson MD. New therapies and new pathologies. *Arch Pathol Lab Med* 1979;103:53–57.
220. Hughson MD, Buchwald D, Fox M. Renal neoplasia and acquired cystic kidney disease in patients receiving long-term dialysis. *Arch Pathol Lab Med* 1986;110:592–601.
221. Feiner HD, Katz LA, Gallo GR. Acquired cystic disease of kidney in chronic dialysis patients. *Urology* 1981;12:260–264.
222. Kovacs G. High frequency of papillary renal-cell tumours in end-stage kidneys: Is there a molecular genetic explanation? *Nephrol Dial Transplant* 1995;10:593–596.

Pathology of Renal Transplantation

223. Porter KA. Renal transplantation. In: Heptinstall RH, ed. *Pathology of the kidney*, 4th ed. Boston; Little, Brown and Company, 1992:1799–1933.
224. Colvin RB. The renal allograft biopsy. *Kidney Int* 1996;50:1069–1082.
225. Solez K, Axelsen RA, Benediktsson H, et al. International standardization of criteria for the histologic diagnosis of renal allograft rejection: the Banff working classification of kidney transplant pathology. *Kidney Int* 1993;44:411–422.
226. Nadasdy T. Transplantation. In: Silva FG, D'Agati VD, Nadasdy T, eds. *Renal biopsy interpretation*. New York: Churchill Livingstone, 1996:373–401.
227. Nádasdy T, Krenács T, Kalmár KN, Csajbók E, Boda K, Ormos J. Importance of plasma cells in the infiltrate of renal allografts: an immunohistochemical study. *Pathol Res Pract* 1991;187:178–183.

228. Bia MJ. Nonimmunologic causes of late renal graft loss. *Kidney Int* 1995;47:1470–1480.
229. Maryniak RK, First MR, Weiss MA. Transplant glomerulopathy: evolution of morphologically distinct changes. *Kidney Int* 1985;27:799–806.
230. Peng-fei Z, Rao KV, Anderson WR. An ultrastructural study of the membranoproliferative variant of transplant glomerulopathy. *Ultrastruct Pathol* 1988;12:185–194.
231. Habib R, Broyer M. Clinical significance of allograft glomerulopathy. *Kidney Int* 1993;44:S95–S98.
232. Mihatsch MJ, Thiel G, Ryffel B. Morphology of cyclosporin nephropathy. *Prog Allergy* 1986;38:447–465.
233. Bergstrand A, Bohman SO, Farnsworth A, et al. Renal histopathology in kidney transplant recipients immunosuppressed with cyclosporin A: results of an international workshop. *Clin Nephrol* 1985;24:107–119.
234. Nizze H, Mihatsch MJ, Zollinger HU, et al. Cyclosporin-associated nephropathy in patients with heart and bone marrow transplants. *Clin Nephrol* 1988;30:248–260.
235. Young BA, Marsh CL, Alpers CE, Davis CL. Cyclosporine-associated thrombotic microangiopathy/hemolytic uremic syndrome following kidney and kidney-pancreas transplantation. *Am J Kidney Dis* 1996;28:561–571.
236. Zent R, Katz A, Quaggin S, et al. Thrombotic microangiopathy in renal transplant recipients treated with cyclosporin A. *Clin Nephrol* 1997;47:181–186.
237. Mihatsch MJ, Ryffel B, Gudat F. The differential diagnosis between rejection and cyclosporine toxicity. *Kidney Int* 1995;48[Suppl 52]:S63–S69.
238. Randhawa PS, Shapiro R, Jordan ML, Starzl TE, Demetris AJ. The histopathological changes associated with allograft rejection and drug toxicity in renal transplant recipients maintained on FK506: clinical significance and comparison with cyclosporine. *Am J Surg Pathol* 1993;17:60–68.
239. Randhawa PS, Tsamandas AC, Magnone M, et al. Microvascular changes in renal allografts associated with FK506 (Tacrolimus) therapy. *Am J Surg Pathol* 1996;20:306–312.
240. Nalesnik MA, Jaffe R, Starzl TE, et al. The pathology of posttransplant lymphoproliferative disorders occurring in the setting of cyclosporin A–prednisone immunosuppression. *Am J Pathol* 1988;133:173–192.
241. Randhawa P, Demetris AJ, Pietrzak B, Nalesnik M. Histopathology of renal posttransplant lymphoproliferation: comparison with rejection using the Banff schema. *Am J Kidney Dis* 1996;28:578–584.

CHAPTER 42

Adult Renal Tumors

Victor E. Reuter and Paul B. Gaudin

The majority of renal neoplasms are of epithelial origin and malignant. Renal cell carcinomas (RCCs) have been regarded as a single entity until recently. Based on the historical concept that they derive from adrenal rests in the kidney, they were called hypernephromas (1), a term that is still used occasionally. In 1959, Oberling and colleagues settled the issue by finding convincing ultrastructural evidence that these tumors arise from renal cells rather than adrenal rests (2,3).

New studies have proved conclusively that renal epithelial neoplasms are not a single tumor, but rather a group of distinguishable tumors (4,5). This understanding is based on histologic (6) as well as cytogenetic and molecular studies (7–22). This newly acquired knowledge led to a meeting of experts in the field of renal cancer, organized by Guyla Kovacs at the University of Heidelberg in Germany, which was quickly followed by a consensus conference sponsored by the Mayo Clinic, the American Cancer Society, the Union Internationale Contre le Cancer (UICC), and the American Joint Committee on Cancer (AJCC). The result was a new classification for renal neoplasms (23,24) (Table 1). It is satisfying to know that there is a close relationship between the morphologic and genetic features of the majority of these tumors (Table 2). Just as rewarding is the evidence that this new classification serves to define distinct clinical entities as well (25). Unfortunately, our newly found knowledge renders obsolete much of the old literature on renal carcinomas—especially those studies dealing with clear-cell, granular cell, or sarcomatoid tumors—since it includes a mixture of entities with diverse natural histories.

EPIDEMIOLOGY

RCC accounts for approximately 2% of all cancers (25,26). Its incidence varies among countries, with the highest rates found in North America and Scandinavia (27). This form of cancer develops twice as frequently in men as in women, and the incidence in the United States is equal among whites and blacks (26). In 1998, there will be more than 30,000 new cases of kidney cancer diagnosed and in excess of 12,000 deaths in the United States alone. More than 100,000 people per year are expected to die from this disease worldwide by the year 2000. RCC may occur at any age, but its peak incidence is in the sixth and seventh decades of life. The incidence has increased substantially over the past two decades, accompanied by an improved 5-year survival rate. Undoubtedly, both trends are due, at least in part, to improved diagnostic techniques and early detection. Over the past 15 years, we have seen a very significant decline in tumor size and pathologic stage among resected renal cancers at our institution (33).

Environmental factors play a significant role in the development of renal cancer (34–36). Cigarette smoking doubles the risk of RCC (37–38). Obesity, particularly in women, is also a risk factor (34,39). Other risk factors include hypertension, estrogen therapy, and occupational exposure to petroleum products, heavy metals, and asbestos (34,38,40,41). One case-control study based on the New Zealand cancer registry found an increased relative risk of renal cancer among firefighters and painters, both occupational groups likely to be exposed to known carcinogens (42).

The majority of renal neoplasms are sporadic. A small percentage may be hereditary, such as those conventional (clear cell) carcinomas associated with Von Hippel–Lindau disease, an autosomal dominant disorder associated with germline mutation of the VHL gene localized to chromosome 3p25.5 (43–54). In all forms of inherited renal neoplasms, tumors are more likely to be diagnosed at an early age and to be multifocal and bilateral. Von Hippel–Lindau disease is a multiple cancer syndrome; affected individuals have a predisposition to a variety of neoplasms, including RCC and renal cysts. Another mode of inheritance of conventional (clear cell) RCC is found

---

V. E. Reuter: Department of Pathology, Memorial Sloan-Kettering Cancer Center and Cornell University Medical College, New York, New York 10021.

P. B. Gaudin: Department of Pathology, Memorial Sloan-Kettering Cancer Center and Cornell University Medical College, 1275 York Avenue, New York, New York 10021.

TABLE 1. *Renal cell neoplasms: Classification*

Benign
    Oncocytoma
    Papillary (chromophil) adenoma
    Metanephric (embryonal) adenoma
    Nephrogenic adenofibroma
Malignant
    Conventional (clear cell) carcinoma
    Papillary (chromophil) carcinoma
    Chromophobe carcinoma
    Collecting duct carcinoma
    Medullary carcinoma
    Renal cell carcinoma, unclassified
Tumor of undetermined malignant potential
    Multilocular cystic renal cell carcinoma

among people with a balanced translocation between 3p and chromosome 6 or 8 (55,56). These affected patients are at higher risk of renal carcinomas but not other tumors. Hereditary forms of papillary renal cell carcinomas (PRCCs) and oncocytomas have also been described, none of which are associated with molecular abnormalities of the short arm of chromosome 3 (57,58). The former tumor is characterized by missense mutations in the MET proto-oncogene, located at chromosome 7q31-34. The genes involved in the pathogenesis of familial renal oncocytoma have yet to be defined.

GRADING AND STAGING OF RENAL TUMORS

Several systems have been proposed over the years for the grading of renal tumors, but the scheme put forth by Furhman et al. is the most widely used (60–69). This system uses nuclear grades based on nuclear size, irregularity of the nuclear membrane, and nucleolar prominence (Table 3). Although we and others have found good correlation between the Furhman nuclear grade and survival in the case of conventional (clear cell) carcinomas, application of this method may be cumbersome because it requires the pathologist to measure nuclear size. Since it is a four-tiered system, interobserver variability may be significant (69). The utility of the Furhman or any other scheme for grading papillary and chromophobe cell carcinomas remains the subject of controversy and is unproved; it should be regarded as optional until an accepted and clinically relevant classification emerges (70). There is no reason to grade oncocytomas, since they are benign tumors.

In 1969, Robson and associates published a staging scheme that has been adopted by most clinicians and pathologists and has been shown to correlate well with survival (71). During the ensuing years the AJCC, in collaboration with the UICC, published the TMN classification, in which stage I and II tumors were defined as being confined to the kidney but the former measured 2.5 cm or less (72). In 1997 this classification was modified further (73) (Table 4). Certainly, any of these classifications offers valuable prognostic

TABLE 2. *Renal cell neoplasms: Putative cell of origin, classification, and genetic correlates*

Origin	Cell type	Neoplasm
Proximal nephron	Cells of the proximal convoluted tubule	Conventional RCC • 3p− • other losses/gains
Proximal nephron	? Cells of the distal convoluted tubule	Papillary RCC • 7+, 17+, 3+, Y− • other losses/gains
Distal nephron	Intercalated cells of the renal cortex	Oncocytoma • Y−, 1− • 14−, t(11)
Distal nephron	Intercalated cells of the renal cortex	Chromophobe RCC • Y−, 1− • 2−, 6−, 10−, 13−, ...
Distal nephron	Collecting ducts of the renal medulla	Collecting duct carcinoma • 1−, 6−, 14−, 15−, 22− • 8p−, 13q−
Distal nephron	Collecting ducts of the renal medulla	Medullary carcinoma • unknown (sickle trait)

Modified from ref. 131. RCC, renal cell carcinoma.

TABLE 3. Fuhrman grading system for renal cell carcinoma[a]

Grade	Nuclear size[b]	Nuclear shape	Nucleoli	Other features
1	10 μm	Round and uniform	Inconspicuous or absent	
2	15 μm	Irregular	Present	Examined at ×400 magnification
3	20 μm	Obviously irregular	Large	Examined at ×100 magnification
4	20+ μm	Bizarre or multilobed	Large	Clumped chromatin, spindle cells

[a] We use this system for conventional (clear cell) RCC only, since its clinical utility has not been demonstrated for other tumor types.
[b] Approximate nuclear size.

information but only within specific tumor types. For example, large size and extracapsular extension do not have the same prognostic significance in cases of oncocytoma or even chromophobe carcinoma that they have for conventional (clear cell) tumors. Up to 20% of renal oncocytomas may show signs of pT3 disease, even though they are benign tumors. The mean tumor size of chromophobe carcinomas is approximately 8.0 to 9.0 cm—the largest of all renal cortical neoplasms—and yet the disease-free survival rate in virtually all published series is more than 90%. We recommend that tumors be classified using the latest TMN classification in an attempt to establish uniformity in reporting; future editions will surely correct deficiencies in the present system (74).

CONVENTIONAL (CLEAR CELL) RENAL CELL CARCINOMA

Conventional (clear cell) carcinomas comprise approximately 60% of renal tumors (Table 5). Although they are the most common of all renal cancers, their clinical and pathologic features remain poorly understood. Almost all studies published before 1995 dealing with this tumor type are flawed because of errors in classification. Perfect examples of this fact are the so-called granular and sarcomatoid carcinomas (Table 6). Rather than representing individual entities, they are morphologic variants that may arise from several tumor types. Thus, granular cell tumors may, in fact, be clear-cell RCC, chromophobe renal cell carcinoma (CRCC), or even oncocytoma. Sarcomatoid features may be seen in clear-cell RCC and in chromophobe, papillary, and collecting duct carcinomas (CDCs). To highlight the fact that clear-cell tumors may exhibit few or no cells with clear cytoplasm, the present classification regards them as conventional carcinomas, placing the term "clear cell" in parentheses to avoid confusion (23,24) (Table 1). Most important, we should never classify a tumor as a granular cell carcinoma, since this term lacks precision and could be used to describe several tumor types, ranging from fully malignant to benign.

Conventional RCCs are characterized by the loss of genetic material of the short arm of chromosome 3 (3p) 7,9,21,22,75–77). Most cases are sporadic, unilateral, and unifocal. In patients with von Hippel–Lindau disease who have clear-cell renal carcinomas, a deletion or partial deletion of chromosome 3p (52–54) with a breakpoint close to the location of the von Hippel–Lindau gene, is present in

TABLE 4. Pathologic staging of renal epithelial neoplasms[a]

Stage[b]	Robson (1969)	UICC/AJCC/TNM (1988–1992)	UICC/AJCC/TNM (1997)
1	Any size, organ-confined	2.5 cm or less, organ-confined	7 cm or less, organ-confined
2	Extension into perinephric tissue	more than 2.5 cm, organ-confined	more than 7 cm, organ-confined
3	Tumor in renal vein, vena cava, or regional lymph nodes	3a: Extension into perinephric tissue confined within Gerota's 3b: Gross tumor in renal vein(s) or vena cava	3a: Extension into perinephric tissue confined within Gerota's 3b: Gross tumor in renal vein(s) or vena cava below diaphragm 3c: Gross tumor in vena cava above diaphragm
4	Extension into adjacent organs or distant metastasis	Tumor beyond Gerota's fascia	Tumor beyond Gerota's fascia

[a] We suggest that the latest TNM classification be used, despite its failings.
[b] The numerical grade designation should be preceded by "pT" to highlight that it is pathologic rather than a clinical stage.

TABLE 5. *Epithelial tumors of the renal parenchyma: Breakdown of common histologic types in an 8-year period[a]*

Type	1989	1990	1991	1992	1993	1994	1995	1996	Total (%)
Conventional	37	38	51	47	44	51	72	56	398 (62%)
Papillary	8	7	15	14	10	12	10	9	85 (13%)
Oncocytoma	6	8	6	6	9	8	8	13	64 (10%)
Chromophobe	7	7	4	4	9	7	10	5	53 (8%)
Unclassified	4	4	6	6	7	6	7	6	46 (7%)
Total	62	64	82	77	79	84	107	91	646

[a] Primary resections performed at Memorial Sloan-Kettering Cancer Center.

practically all cases. Somatic mutations in the same region can be found in up to 60% of sporadic tumors as well. New molecular genetic studies have documented loss of heterozygosity in the distal portion of 3p (9,78–80), suggesting the presence of a tumor suppressor gene in this region (81).

Clinical Features

Men are affected more often than women in a ratio of 1.7–2.0:1. In our series of 155 patients, age at the time of diagnosis ranged from 34 to 90 years, with a mean of 61 years. There are several case reports of these tumors arising in children and young adults, although this is a rare occurrence. Hereditary conventional RCCs tend to develop at an earlier age, usually in the fourth or fifth decade of life. In sporadic disease, both kidneys are affected equally, and most tumors are solitary. Bilateral disease was documented in only 3.2% of our cases. Multifocality, defined as a collection of neoplastic clear epithelial cells with no restriction in terms of size, is present in approximately 11% of cases. Hereditary tumors are more likely to be bilateral and multifocal.

The most common symptoms at the time of diagnosis are hematuria, abdominal pain, and a palpable mass, seen in 50% to 60%, 40%, and 30% to 40% of cases, respectively (29). This classic triad occurs in less than 10% of cases. Other signs and symptoms are fairly nonspecific and include fever, night sweats, general malaise, and weight loss. At present, 50% or more of cases are diagnosed after the detection of an asymptomatic, incidental renal mass using modern imaging techniques (30–32).

Gross Features

The classic case has a golden yellow color owing to abundant intracytoplasmic lipid (Fig. 1). Higher-grade tumors contain less lipid and glycogen and may have a more varied appearance (Fig. 2). In our series the main tumor mass ranged in size from 1.8 to 21 cm, with a mean size of 8 cm. Approximately 12% showed marked cystic degenerative

TABLE 6. *Renal epithelial neoplasms: differential diagnosis*

"Granular" features	Sarcomatoid features	Papillary or tubulopapillary features
Conventional RCC	Conventional RCC	Conventional RCC
Chromophobe RCC	Papillary RCC	Chromophobe RCC
Papillary RCC	Chromophobe RCC	Papillary RCC
Oncocytoma	Collecting duct Ca. Urothelial Ca.	Collecting duct Ca. Urothelial Ca.

RCC, renal cell carcinoma; Ca., carcinoma.

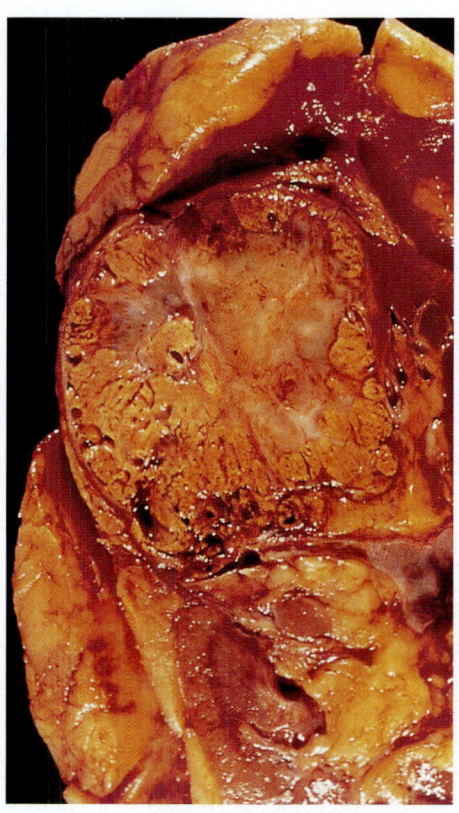

FIG. 1. The gross appearance of a conventional (clear cell) renal cell carcinoma. Lower-grade tumors are characteristically golden yellow owing to the presence of abundant cytoplasmic lipid and glycogen. This tumor also contains intratumoral hyalinization, another feature of low-grade lesions.

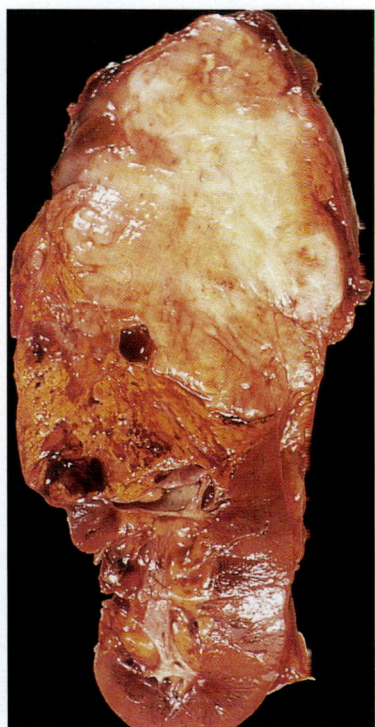

FIG. 2. The gross appearance of a conventional renal cell carcinoma with sarcomatoid features. Notice the transition between the more typical golden yellow area and the area with a tan-white color, the latter representing the high-grade spindle-cell component.

mors are more likely to have solid, pseudopapillary, or sarcomatoid areas (Fig. 4). Tumors exhibiting a pseudopapillary growth pattern, which must not be mistaken for the true papillary growth pattern typically seen in PRCCs, are characterized by peudopapillae without a true fibrovascular core. They are due to degenerative changes in areas of solid and/or acinar growth. Focal fibrosis or hyalinization due to degenerative changes is seen in more than 75% of cases, but true desmoplasia is absent or minimal. Geographic necrosis and focal hemorrhage are common histologic findings as well. These tumors may contain an inflammatory infiltrate that is predominantly lymphocytic. Calcifications and osseous metaplasia are rare findings, seen in less than 10% and 4% of cases, respectively.

In most cases the tumor cells are either polygonal or cuboidal in shape. Cell shape is more variable in higher-grade lesions. Furhman grade 4 lesions may contain bizarre, pleomorphic cells, some of which mimic the giant cells seen in some chromophobe cell tumors and angiomyolipomas (AMLs). The spindle cells seen in sarcomatoid areas should be considered as evidence of high-grade diseases. The majority of tumors show a mixture of cytoplasmic features, namely, clear or granular eosinophilic cytoplasm. Again, the cytoplasmic features can be correlated with tumor grade, since grade 1 lesions invariably contain clear cytoplasm whereas the cytoplasm of higher-grade lesions is more likely to be variably

changes, and renal vein invasion was identified on gross examination in 30%. Slightly more than half of the cases had disease extending outside the kidney (pT3 or higher). It is important to note that modern imaging techniques and early detection have brought about a significant stage migration in renal cancer. Conventional RCCs resected at our institution during the years of 1995–1997 had a mean tumor size of 5.5 cm, 2.5 cm smaller than those of the series quoted earlier herein, which included tumors resected between the years 1983 and 1985. We documented significant clinical and pathologic downstaging as well (33).

Microscopic Features

Approximately 50% of cases exhibit either a solid or an acinar growth pattern exclusively (Fig. 3). The growth pattern is characterized by solid sheets of tumors cells, compartmentalized into solid acinar structures by delicate, richly vascularized fibrous septa. In some cases the acinar pattern is less well defined, yet the prominent vascularity is retained. In the remaining cases these tumors contain a mixture of growth patterns, including cystic, papillary/pseudopapillary, tubular, and sarcomatoid. A rich capillary vascular network is prominent in all but the sarcomatoid areas. The growth pattern is loosely associated with grade, since most low-grade lesions have acinar growth, whereas higher-grade tu-

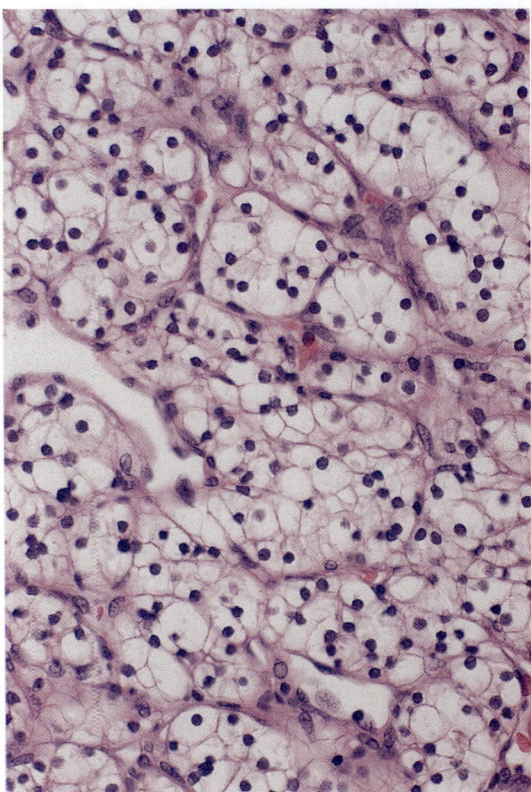

FIG. 3. Conventional (clear cell) carcinoma. Classic acinar growth pattern and clear cytoplasm in a grade 1 tumor.

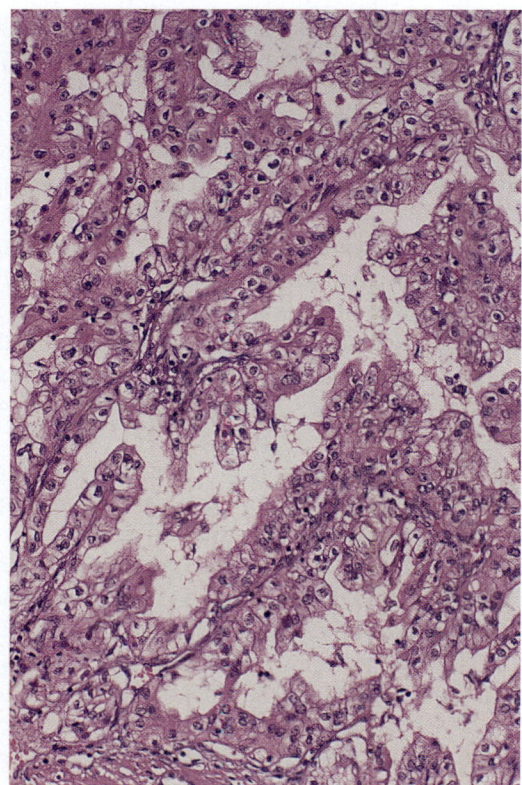

FIG. 4. Grade 2 conventional carcinoma with pseudopapillary growth.

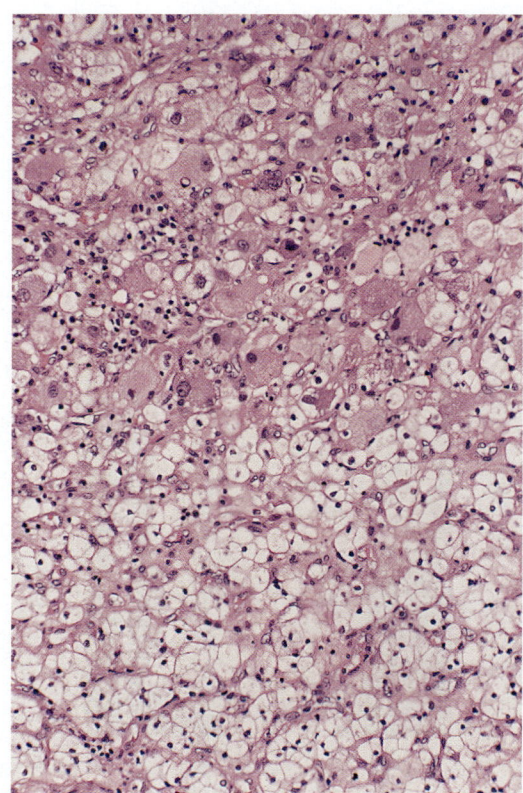

FIG. 5. Conventional (clear cell) carcinoma. Transition between grade 1 and grade 2 to 3 areas. Notice the loss of the acinar growth pattern and the cytoplasmic eosinophilia in the higher-grade areas.

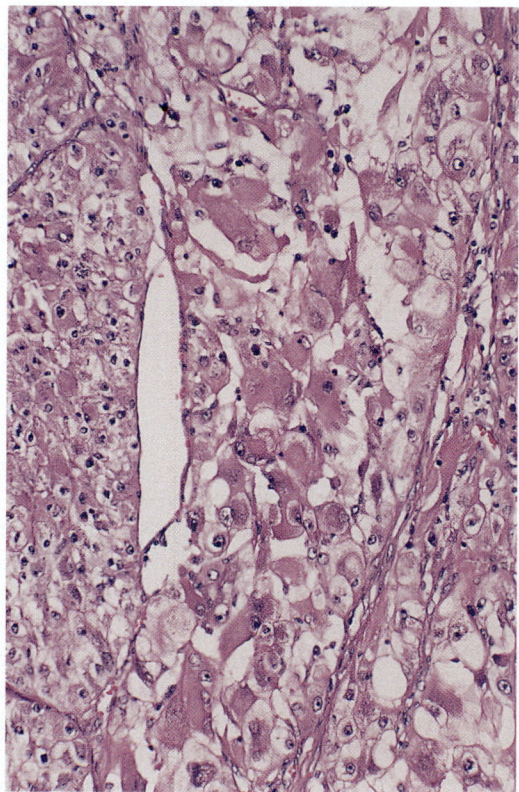

FIG. 6. Conventional (clear cell) carcinoma. Many tumor cells contain abundant eosinophilic cytoplasm.

eosinophilic and granular (Figs. 5 and 6). Some grades 3 and 4 lesions may lack clear cytoplasm altogether. These tumors should be classified as (conventional type) rather than lumping them into the category of granular cell renal carcinomas, a term that should be discarded because of its lack of specificity.

The Fuhrman nuclear grading system correlates with tumor stage and reliably stratifies patients into prognostic groups (60,62). Nevertheless, it is unfortunate that this system relies on microscopic measurements of nuclear size, since it renders it unfriendly to the user. In addition, grading schemes that group cases into four rather than two or even three categories are usually hampered by poor interobserver variability (69). In our experience, slightly less than 80% of cases are classified as grade 2 or 3 tumors, with the remainder split between grades 1 and 4. Mitotic activity is not a prominent feature of these tumors; very few cases exhibit more than five mitoses per ten high-power fields. The majority of tumors are not encapsulated, although 10% to 15% may be partially or completely surrounded by a fibrous pseudocapsule. The number of cases with renal vein invasion, extension into perinephric fat, and regional lymph node involvement has declined dramatically over the past 15 years, owing to stage migration stemming from early detection.

Differential Diagnosis

Adequate sampling and a good understanding of the morphologic diversity seen in conventional RCCs should mini-

TABLE 7. *Renal epithelial neoplasms: clinicopathologic features and survival—MSKCC*

Parameters	C-RCC[b]	Papillary[c]	Chromophobe[c]	Oncocytoma[c]
Cases studied	155	81	60	70
Male/female	1.7:1	3.8:1	1.1:1	1.3:1
Multifocality	14.2%	48.2%	12.1%	13%
Age	61	60	59	65
Size (cm)	8.0	6.4	9.0	5.2
pT1–pT2	47.8%	84%	63.8%	80%
Follow-up[a]	62.5	60.4	59.0	58.0
Outcome (DOD)	38.1%	10.5%	6.0%	0%

C-RCC, conventional (clear cell) carcinoma; DOD, dead of disease; MSKCC, Memorial Sloan-Kettering Cancer Center.
[a] Median time of follow-up.
[b] C-RCCs were consecutively resected between 1985 and 1988.
[c] Papillary, chromophobe, and oncocytic tumors were consecutively resected between 1980 and 1995.

mize errors in classification. Some tumors may be confused with PRCCs or CRCCs, but microscopic examination of all available areas should reveal areas with classic histologic features. In most cases of conventional RCC with papillary growth, this growth pattern is the result of cell drop-off, in which the tumor cells that are away from the blood supply die and those close to the vessels are preserved, thus exhibiting a pseudopapillary growth pattern. Histiocytes are unlikely to be present within the fibrovascular stalk in these pseudopapillary areas. Intracellular hemosiderin deposition is absent as well.

Papillary carcinomas are said to express cytokeratin (CK) 7, whereas conventional tumors do not. We find this approach to the differential diagnosis of limited utility, especially in challenging cases, since CK 7 expression varies with tumor grade. CRCCs have characteristic nuclear and cytoplasmic features that are only rarely seen in conventional tumors and then only focally. Diffuse cytoplasmic positivity for Hale's colloidal iron is a hallmark of chromophobe tumors, but this stain may be extremely difficult to perform and interpret. Electron microscopy is a more reliable means to resolve the differential diagnosis, but not in every case. Ultimately, cytogenetics and molecular genetics can solve problems in classification in virtually all cases, since all three lesions are associated with distinct genetic abnormalities (Table 2).

Epithelioid variants of AML can be readily misclassified as conventional RCCs and are usually assigned a high nuclear grade. The problem is compounded by the fact that some AMLs lack the morphologic diversity seen in classic cases. Close attention to morphologic features, immunohistochemical results, electron microscopic characteristics, and even cytogenetic properties can help establish the correct diagnosis. Conventional RCCs are usually immunoreactive with CK CAM 5.2 as well as epithelial membrane antigen (EMA), which is not seen in the case of AML. Alternatively, the latter stains for HMB-45 and smooth-muscle actin. Some conventional RCCs are so poorly differentiated that metastatic disease may enter into the differential diagnosis. Knowledge of the patient's medical history will help in this regard. Another tumor to be considered in the differential diagnosis is adrenocortical carcinoma, particularly in the case of upper-pole tumors. Adrenocortical tumors are not immunoreactive with EMA and rarely so with CKs, but they do express inhibin, which gives negative results in renal carcinomas.

Outcome

Disease-free and overall survival correlates with grade and stage (60,62). In our consecutive series of 155 cases accrued between 1983 and 1985 and with a median follow-up of 62.5 months, 38% of patients died of disease. Although conventional RCCs are the most virulent of all renal cortical carcinomas, survival statistics will improve as tumors are detected earlier (Tables 7 and 8). Effective systemic therapy remains elusive, making surgical resection the best chance for cure.

TABLE 8. *Renal cell carcinoma: stage versus survival for pT2 disease[a]*

Survival	C-RCC[b] (n = 61)	Papillary[b] (n = 53)	Chromophobe (n = 30)
Overall survival			
Alive	32	36	27
Dead	29	17	3
Disease-specific survival			
Not DOD	42	47	30
DOD	19	6	0
		$p = 0.02$	$p = 0.002$

C-RCC, conventional (clear cell) carcinoma; DOD, dead of disease.
[a] Median follow-up in months: C-RCC, 62.5; papillary, 60.4; chromophobe, 59.0.
[b] No follow-up in seven cases of C-RCC and three cases of papillary renal cell carcinoma.

MULTILOCULAR CYSTIC RENAL CELL CARCINOMA

Multilocular cystic renal cell carcinoma represents a rare variant of conventional (clear cell) renal carcinoma. It is estimated that these tumors constitute between 3.5% and 6% of conventional RCC (82–86), but these figures are probably too high. They have been documented in adult patients, with a mean age at diagnosis of 51 years. Few cases are included in any one publication, and follow-up information is limited. Nevertheless, none of the reported cases have progressed (82). Additional cases and better follow-up information are needed to properly assess the biologic potential of these tumors.

The gross appearance is that of a well-circumscribed, multicystic mass separated from the adjacent renal parenchyma by a fibrous pseudocapsule (Fig. 7). The size can be quite variable and has reached 13 cm in greatest dimension. The cysts are lined by thin fibrous septa, are of different sizes, and may contain serous or bloody fluid or clot. No solid masses of tumor are present.

On microscopic inspection, the thin, fibrous septa are seen to be lined by one or several layers of neoplastic epithelial cells; in many areas the epithelial lining may be absent (Fig. 8). Foamy macrophages may also line the cyst wall. Occasionally, the tumor cells exhibit papillary tufting into the cyst lumen. The tumor cells contain clear cytoplasm and Furhman grade 1 or 2 nuclei. Small collections of tumor cells may be present within the fibrous septa or in the adjacent pseudocapsule, but no expansile or solid masses of tumor are evident.

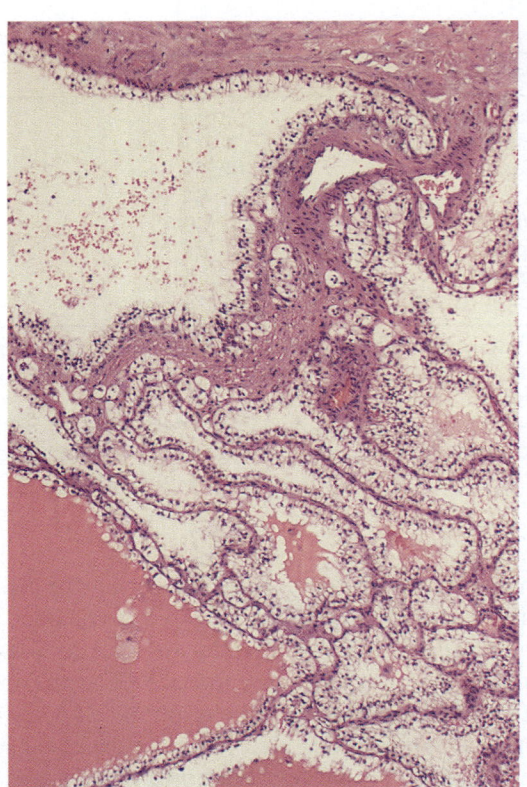

FIG. 8. Multilocular cystic renal cell carcinoma. Tumor cells line delicate fibrovascular trabeculae.

The differential diagnosis includes cystic nephroma and benign multilocular cyst of the kidney. Close attention to the epithelial lining and the fibrous cyst wall should lead to the correct diagnosis. Cystic nephromas are usually lined by a single layer of flattened or hobnail epithelium that only now and then contains clear cytoplasm. The fibrous stroma may be more cellular, resembling ovarian stroma. The septa may contain small tubules lined by bland epithelial cells, reminiscent of renal tubules. In cases where the epithelial lining is not readily apparent, immunohistochemical stains for EMA or low-molecular-weight keratins should help in identifying it.

PAPILLARY (CHROMOPHIL) RENAL CELL CARCINOMA

PRCCs comprise a minority of RCCs (6,87–90). This tumor type received little attention as a distinct morphologic entity until Mancilla-Jimenez et al. (87) published a study of 34 cases of PRCC in 1976; earlier clinical studies had suggested specific clinical characteristics for these tumors (46). The term chromophil renal carcinoma has been used to describe these tumors (6), but we have chosen to retain the designation papillary carcinoma, since it is more widely accepted and accurately describes the growth pattern of the majority of tumors.

Newer cytogenetic and molecular studies have revealed distinct findings in PRCCs that set them apart from other renal epithelial tumors (16,20). PRCCs are characterized by

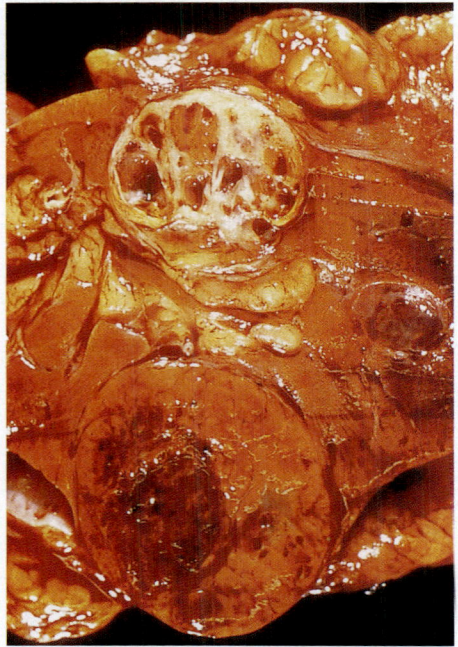

FIG. 7. Kidney containing two separate tumors that do not merge. On the bottom is a chromophobe carcinoma and on top a multilocular cystic renal cell carcinoma.

trisomy of chromosomes 7, 16, and 17 as well as loss of chromosome Y (8,12,16,17,88–95). In addition, a translocation between chromosomes X and 1 has been reported (17,94–96), and a fused novel gene has been characterized. Some investigators have suggested that tumors exhibiting only trisomy 7/17 are likely to be benign, whereas tumors exhibiting additional genetic abnormalities will behave aggressively. This hypothesis remains to be proved. Familial PRCC have mutations in the MET proto-oncogene (57,58).

While PRCCs have distinct clinical and cytogenetic features, their histomorphologic features were not well defined until recently. This fact led to difficulties in classifying renal tumors that exhibit papillary or pseudopapillary histologic characteristics. True papillae with a fibrovascular core lined by neoplastic epithelial cells is the hallmark of this tumor, but the amount of papillary component needed to classify a tumor as a PRCC is not uniformly agreed upon (5).

Clinical Features

PRCCs have been reported to represent 7% to 14% of primary epithelial renal neoplasms (12,87,88,90). In our institution they make up 13% of renal epithelial neoplasms resected in an 8-year period (Table 5). Age at diagnosis ranges from the third to eighth decade of life, with peak incidence in the sixth and seventh decades. An increasing number of cases are discovered as incidental masses during workup for unrelated causes—more than 50% of our cases were found in this fashion. The male-to-female ratio ranges from 2:1 to 3.9:1 (87–90). The majority of patients have unilateral tumors, but PRCCs are more likely to be characterized by bilateral as well as multifocal disease, the latter being reported in up to 49% of cases (97,98). Size of the dominant tumor mass can range from 1.0 cm to 18.0 cm (87–90). In a series from Memorial Hospital, the median size was 6.4 cm. Grossly visible areas of necrosis and hemorrhage, ranging from 32% to 70.5%, are typical (87,88). Of all renal epithelial tumors, PRCCs are the most likely to be surrounded by a fibrous pseudocapsule. The reported incidence of gross cystic change is quite wide ranging, varying from 9.0% to 70.5% (87,88).

Computed tomography scan and ultrasound features are nonspecific and usually reveal a solid mass that may show evidence of necrosis or calcification. Arteriography reveals either hypovascular or hypervascular tumors with equal frequency. In fact, in a case of bilateral disease seen at our institution, the tumor on one side was hypovascular, whereas the contralateral tumor was hypervascular. In approximately 25% of cases the mass is neither hypo- nor hypervascular.

Gross Features

Tumors appear as a discrete mass within the renal cortex. The size can be quite variable; in our series it ranged from 1 cm to 18 cm (median, 6.4 cm). Less than a third of cases are surrounded by a fibrous pseudocapsule. Multifocality, either macroscopic or microscopic, is present in more than 45% of cases. Most tumors exhibit a variegated appearance (Fig. 9). We have found that the color of the tumor is due in great part to the microscopic findings; tumors containing abundant foamy macrophages are tan to yellow, whereas those with intratumoral hemorrhage are dark tan to brown. Some lesions may be frankly necrotic.

Microscopic Features

The majority of PRCCs exhibit a broad morphologic spectrum, including papillary, papillary-trabecular, and papillary-solid areas (87,98–101). The classic papillary pattern is characterized by discrete papillary fronds lined by neoplastic epithelial cells and containing a central fibrovascular core, easily recognized on low magnification (Fig. 10). The papillary-trabecular areas display papillations that are delicate, elongated, and arranged in parallel fashion (Fig. 11). The fibrovascular cores, and consequently the papillary nature of the lesion, are more difficult to discern, requiring medium to high magnification. In the papillary-solid areas the papillae were closely packed, masking their true growth pattern. In cases with delicate fibrovascular cores devoid of foamy macrophages, these tumors can be mistaken for solid neoplasms (100,101).

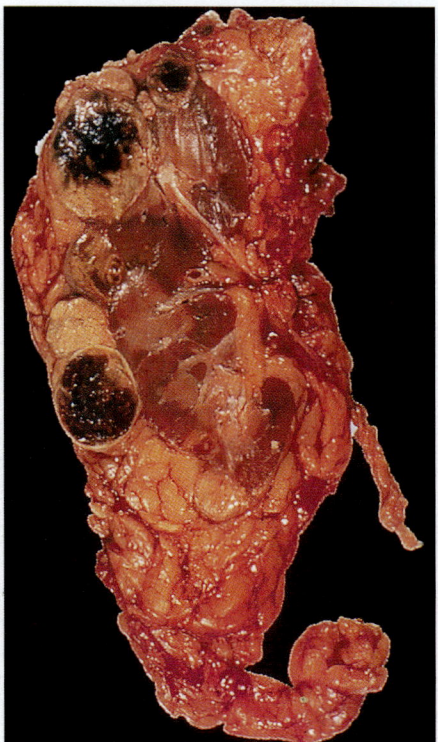

FIG. 9. Papillary renal cell carcinoma. Notice the presence of at least four grossly visible lesions. In this case, the brown-black appearance of three of the lesions is due to intratumoral hemorrhage, whereas the yellow-tan appearance of the other is due to the presence of abundant macrophages within fibrovascular cores.

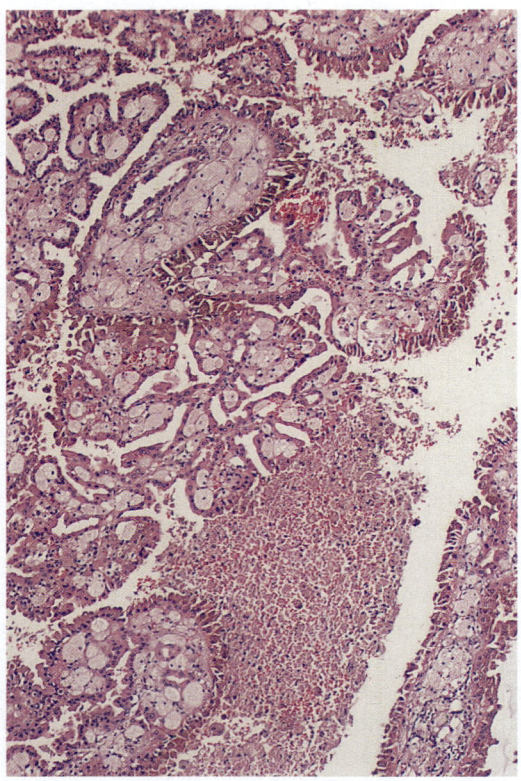

FIG. 10. Papillary renal cell carcinoma. Fibrovascular cores contain abundant histiocytes, and many tumor cells are laden with hemosiderin.

Areas containing classic papillary, papillary-trabecular, and/or papillary-solid patterns of growth are seen in almost all cases. More than half the cases exhibit other morphologic features, however, including truly solid, tubular, and/or glomeruloid growth patterns. Areas of true solid growth are made up of closely juxtaposed polygonal tumor cells, often with cytoplasmic clearing and lacking a fibrovascular core. These areas are always microscopic, never predominate, and are present adjacent to areas of more conventional PRCC. The tubular growth pattern shows evidence of small to medium-sized tubules lined by cuboidal or columnar tumor cells. The stroma between the tubular structures is usually sparse, and desmoplasia is minimal or absent.

Tumors with a glomeruloid growth pattern are composed of closely juxtaposed, small, tubule-like structures with intraluminal tufting of tumor cells (Fig. 12). In most cases, it is possible to identify two populations of tumor cells. The cells lining the tubule-like structures are cuboidal and contain scanty to moderate amounts of mostly amphophilic cytoplasm, whereas the cells tufting into the lumen are polygonal and contain more abundant, often eosinophilic cytoplasm. In rare cases the glomeruloid growth pattern predominates or comprises in virtually the entire tumor. Sarcomatoid growth may be seen infrequently and is a sign of aggressive disease (Fig. 13).

While a papillary growth pattern predominates in the majority of cases, 20% to 25% of cases show less than 50% pap-

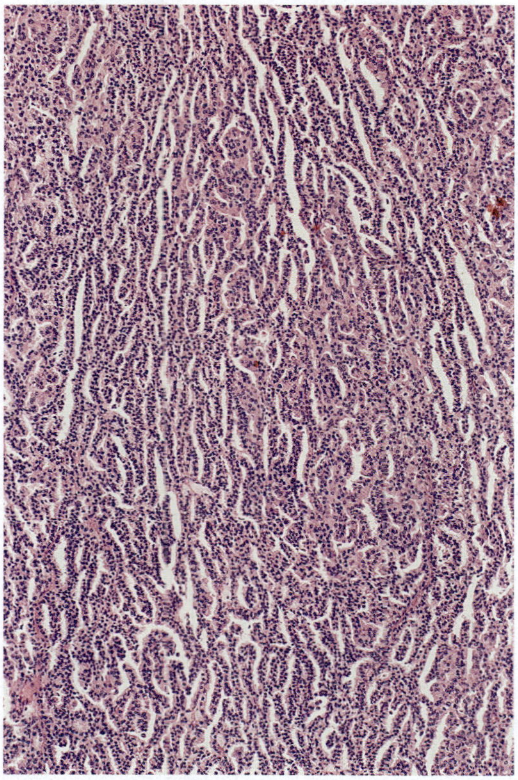

FIG. 11. Papillary renal cell carcinoma. Fibrovascular cores do not contain macrophages, and the papillae are compressed, imparting a trabecular growth pattern.

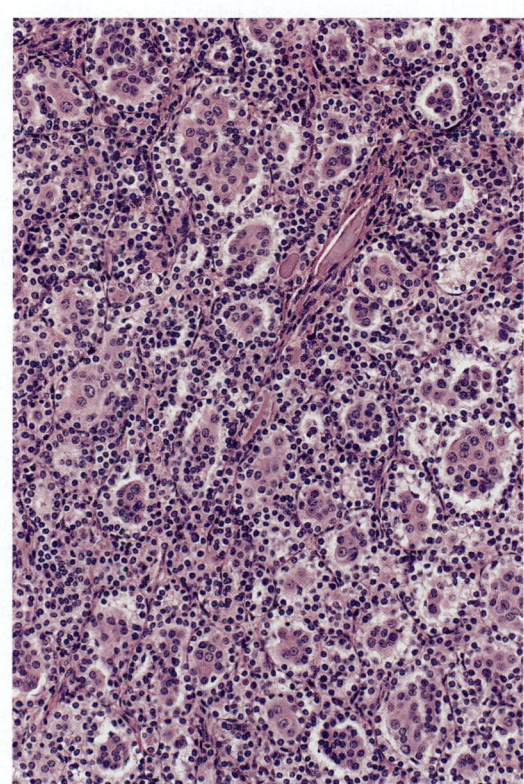

FIG. 12. Papillary renal cell carcinoma with a glomeruloid pattern of growth.

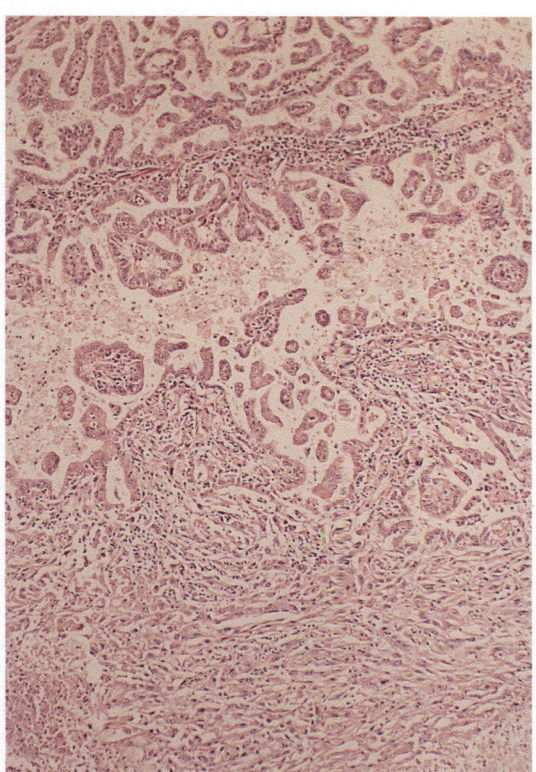

FIG. 13. Papillary renal cell carcinoma with focal sarcomatoid areas.

Outcome

The prognosis of PRCC is more favorable than that of conventional RCC and less so than that of CRCC (Tables 7 and 8). The reported 5-year disease-free survival rate varies from 79% to 92% (87,100,101). Grading remains the topic of controversy. In our series, more than 75% of cases had Furhman grade 2 nuclear features (100). Amin et al. (102) found that grade was a strong predictor of survival on univariate analysis. They also found that tumors with eosinophilic cytoplasm were likely to be high grade, whereas basophilic tumors were low grade. Delahunt and Eble divided their cases into type 1 and type 2 lesions, based on architectural and cytologic features (103) (Fig. 14). While they suggest that type 2 tumors may behave more aggressively, this fact remains to be proved on clinical grounds.

Differential Diagnosis

PRCCs may be confused principally with conventional carcinomas exhibiting papillary or pseudopapillary growth and with CDCs (Table 5). These tumors may contain tumor cells with clear cytoplasm in focal areas, especially in areas with a solid growth pattern. Conventional carcinomas may be papillary in focal areas, although this is usually due to cell drop-off in locations away from feeding vessels, which cre-

illary growth (100). In isolated cases papillary growth comprises a very minor component of the tumor. For this reason, the percentage of papillary growth should not be used to determine whether a tumor is classified as a PRCC. Renshaw et al. have shown that solid variants of PRCC contain the same genetic alterations as other classic papillary tumors (101).

The tumor cells may be cuboidal, columnar, or polygonal; the latter type are seen only in areas with a solid growth pattern. PRCCs have distinct cytologic features, the most common being cytoplasmic basophilia, amphophilia, and eosinophilia (87–89,100,102). The majority of cases contain tumor cells with different cytoplasmic features; the predominant tumor cells are either amphophilic or eosinophilic (Figs. 10–12). Tumor cells with clear cytoplasm are always a focal finding, seen predominantly in association with a solid growth pattern or in tumor cells found in close association with necrosis and degenerative changes. Nuclear features can be quite variable, ranging from small, round nuclei with inconspicuous nucleoli to large, moderately irregular nuclei containing coarse chromatin and prominent nucleoli.

Geographic necrosis is a regular finding, as is the presence of psammoma bodies and foamy macrophages within the fibrovascular stalk. At times, the fibrovascular stalk becomes hyalinized or fibrotic, masking the papillary nature of the lesion. Hemosiderin pigment may be present in the cytoplasm of the tumor cells in a patchy distribution (Fig. 10). It is common for these tumors to be surrounded by a thick fibrous pseudocapsule.

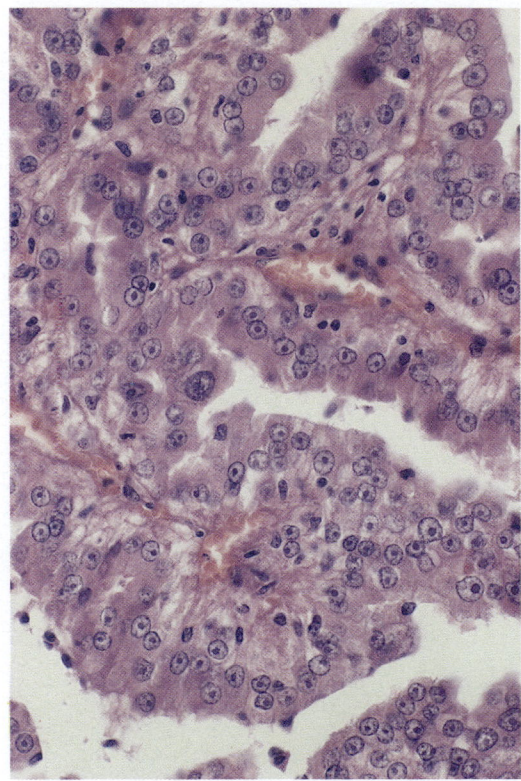

FIG. 14. Papillary renal cell carcinoma with stratification of large hyperchromatic nuclei and containing abundant eosinophilic cytoplasm. Some authors believe that these features predict more aggressive behavior.

ates a pseudopapillary appearance. Adequate sampling should clarify the issue. Psammoma bodies, hemosiderin deposition within tumor cells, and fibrovascular cores containing foamy macrophages are more likely to be seen in PRCCs. CK 7 immunoreactivity is present at least focally in many PRCCs, whereas it shows negative results in most CRCCs. This feature will not help in all cases, since CK 7 reactivity is grade-dependent; it is positive in practically all low-grade PRCCs but variably so in tumors with high-grade nuclei (103). If necessary, molecular genetics can be used to assess difficult cases.

CDCs may have a papillary growth pattern and resemble PRCCs. Nevertheless, the former tumors are centered in the medulla, are virtually always high grade, and are associated with a desmoplastic stroma. Intracytoplasmic and luminal mucin is a common feature, as is reactivity for carcinoembryonic antigen, the lectins peanut agglutinin and *Ulex europaeus*, and high-molecular-weight CK 34BE12. CK 7 may be expressed in both tumors. Again, cytogenetic studies can be used to solve difficult diagnostic problems.

Papillary (Chromophil) Adenoma

While size often correlates well with clinical outcome, characterizing a tumor as either carcinoma or adenoma based solely on size is scientifically unsound. Despite the fact that these lesions are identical to larger lesions in terms of architecture and cytologic features, it is a common practice among pathologists to use the term papillary (chromophil) adenoma to describe small papillary lesions when common sense tells us that the likelihood of metastasis is minimal. If one is to use this term at all, it should be restricted to lesions measuring 1 cm or less and containing small, regular (grade 1) nuclei (Fig. 15). Quite frankly, we hardly ever use the term, although we may describe the lesions as so-called adenomas.

CHROMOPHOBE RENAL CELL CARCINOMA

Bannasch et al. were first to report chromophobe cell tumors in the kidneys of animals exposed to nitrosomorpholine. In 1985, Thoenes et al. recognized this variant in human renal epithelial tumors and illustrated its morphologic, histochemical, and ultrastructural findings (104). During the ensuing years, our awareness of CRCC has increased dramatically, as evidenced by the increasing number of studies published on this subject (105–111). We now know that these tumors have distinct morphologic, histochemical, and ultrastructural characteristics, as well as unique molecular genetic and clinical features. Indeed, it was the discovery of the existence of human CRCCs by Thoenes, Storkel, and their collaborators that led these investigators to initiate a reassessment of the morphologic classification of renal tumors and that served as the foundation for the classification in use today (6,23,24). It is important to recognize this variant of RCC for two reasons. First, stage for stage, CRCCs have a significantly better prognosis than conventional (clear cell) RCCs (Table 7). And, second, its morphologic features may overlap somewhat with oncocytomas, a benign tumor with which it may be confused.

CRCCs are characterized genetically by loss of chromosomes 1 and Y as well as combined chromosomal losses, usually affecting chromosomes 1, 6, 10, 13, 17, and 21 (112–115). Loss of several chromosomes leads to hypodiploid tumor cells, a unique feature seen in many of these tumors (116). Abnormalities in mitochondrial DNA may be observed, but its specificity remains the subject of controversy (117). CRCCs are thought to arise from intercalated cells of the renal cortex, similarly to oncocytomas. Several investigators have drawn attention to the possible link between chromophobe and oncocytic tumors, suggesting that hybrid tumors may exist. This issue is discussed at greater length in the section on oncocytoma under the heading of oncocytosis.

Clinical Features

CRCCs comprise 6% to 11% of renal epithelial tumors. The age and sex distributions are virtually identical to those seen in the context of conventional RCCs (Table 7). In our series, the mean age at diagnosis was 59 years. Patients usually have unilateral renal masses. Of the patients who under-

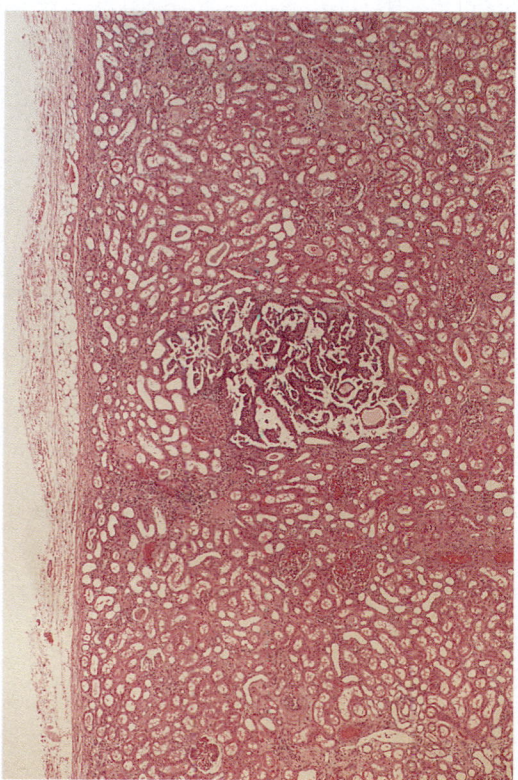

FIG. 15. Microscopic papillary neoplasm. Lesions such as this are common findings in kidneys harboring clinically evident papillary carcinomas, more than 45% of which contain multifocal disease.

went resection at our institution, 58% were asymptomatic, 30% had palpable masses, and 19% had hematuria. The tumor can involve the right and left kidneys equally; in rare instances, patients show signs of bilateral disease. Angiographic examination usually reveals a hypervascular mass, but some tumors may be hypovascular. Radiographic examination may show a central scar, similar to those seen in oncocytomas and large, low-grade conventional RCCs. The presence on radiography of a central scar in a renal neoplasm offers little diagnostic information, except to suggest the presence of a slow-growing neoplasm.

Gross Features

The gross appearance is very helpful in the diagnosis of CCRC. Characteristically, these tumors are not encapsulated and show a homogeneous beige or pale-tan cut surface (Figs. 7 and 16). Nonetheless, we and others have seen rare tumors that are dark brown and mahogany in color. A central scar is present in approximately 15% of our cases. Tumors may be quite large, ranging in size from 2.0 cm to 23.0 cm. In our series the mean size was 9.0 cm, the largest of all epithelial renal tumors. Tumors usually have a lobulated appearance and roughly one-fourth to one-third exhibit gross areas of hemorrhage or necrosis. Cystic areas are rare. Tumors are centered in the renal cortex, but this feature may be impossible to evaluate in larger neoplasms. Evidence of multifocality, either macroscopic or microscopic, is rare and was seen in only 12% of our cases. Gross involvement of the renal vein may be evident in a small number of cases, while up to a third of patients may exhibit disease that invades perirenal adipose tissue.

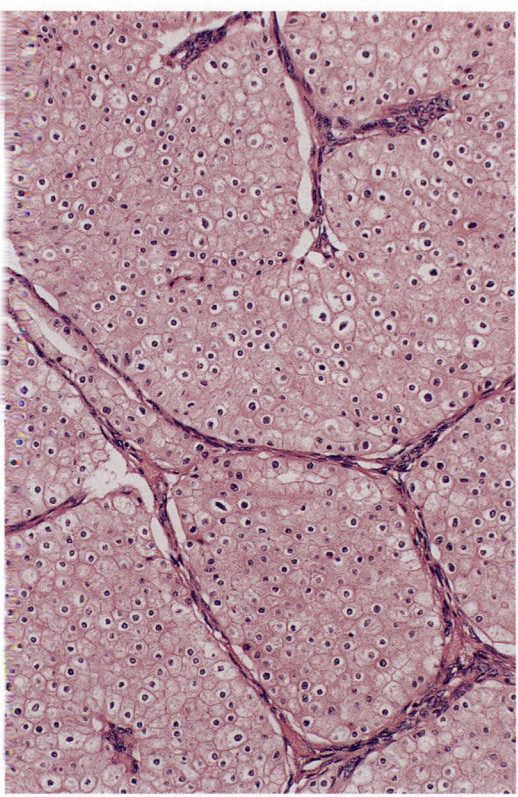

FIG. 17. Chromophobe renal cell carcinoma. The typical histologic features seen here are a solid growth pattern and perinuclear cytoplasmic clearing.

Microscopic Features

Almost all tumors are not encapsulated. The pattern of growth is predominantly solid (Fig. 17), but it may be focally admixed with tubular, trabecular, and cystic patterns (Fig. 18). A small percentage of cases may exhibit a sarcomatoid pattern of growth (Fig. 19). In fact, Akhtar et al. (118) state that CRCC may be the most common renal epithelial tumor associated with a sarcomatoid growth pattern. In most cases, islands of typical CRCC are embedded within expansive areas of spindle-cell growth. Geographic necrosis and calcification are present in 33% and 40% of cases, respectively. In our series, areas of hyalinized stroma interspersed with tumor nests were present in 41% of cases and were associated with smooth-muscle metaplasia in 26%.

The typical histologic features of CCRC consist of large, round to polygonal cells with well-defined cell borders and amphophilic to pale basophilic cytoplasm admixed with a

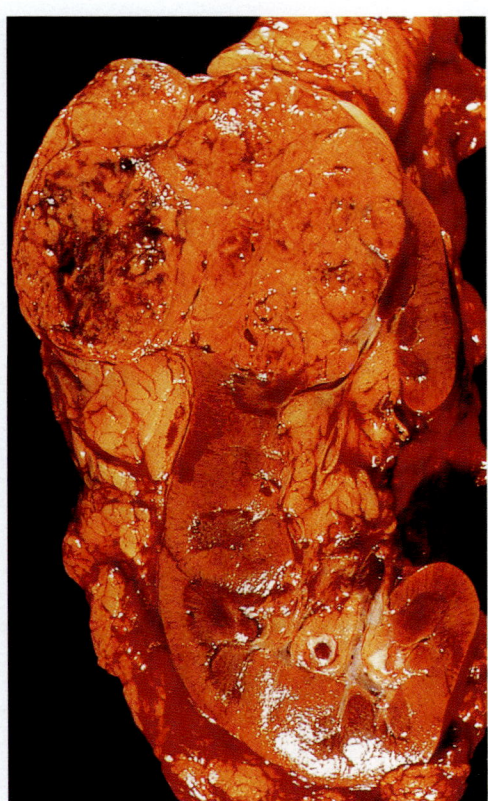

FIG. 16. Chromophobe renal carcinoma. The tumors are usually tan to light brown, never golden yellow. Areas of hemorrhage and necrosis are common, and many large lesions contain a central scar, although this one does not.

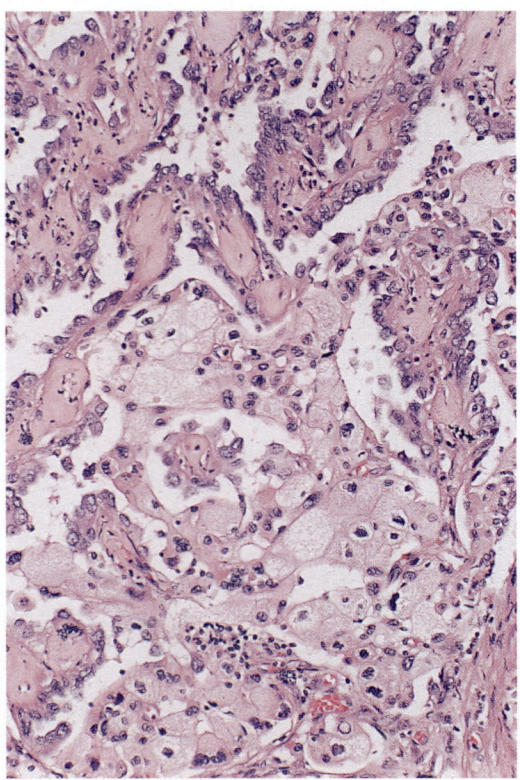

FIG. 18. Chromophobe renal carcinoma with papillary/tubular growth.

smaller population of polygonal cells with eosinophilic cytoplasm (Figs. 17 and 20). The cytoplasm is never totally clear but rather translucent and finely reticulated. Up to 25% of cases contain larger cells with abundant clear to foamy ("hydropic") cytoplasm (Fig. 20). A predominance of tumor cells with more dense eosinophilic oncocytic cytoplasm is seen in 30% of cases. The latter group of tumors constitute what has been called the eosinophilic variant of CRRC.

Although making the distinction between the typical and eosinophilic variants of CCRC is clinically unimportant, it is necessary in terms of alerting pathologists to the wide spectrum of morphologic changes seen in CCRC and avoiding misinterpretation of the tumor as oncocytoma. Perinuclear halos are invariably evident, but they are more pronounced in the typical variant. Because of the perinuclear clearing, the cytoplasmic organelles are pushed toward the periphery of the cytoplasm, thus accentuating the cell membrane. At low- to medium-power magnification, this feature gives the tumor a cobblestone appearance, also reminiscent of the membrane of plant cells as seen through the microscope (Fig. 17). The nuclei are typically hyperchromatic, elongated, and grooved, with an irregular nuclear membrane.

This nuclear cytologic picture predominates in the great majority of cases, but round nuclei with focally wrinkled contours are prominent in approximately half the cases. Round

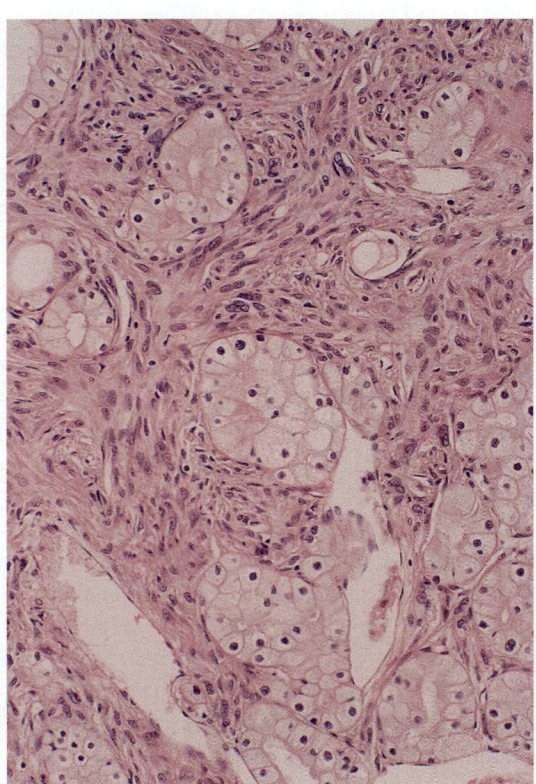

FIG. 19. Chromophobe renal cell carcinoma with a sarcomatoid pattern of growth.

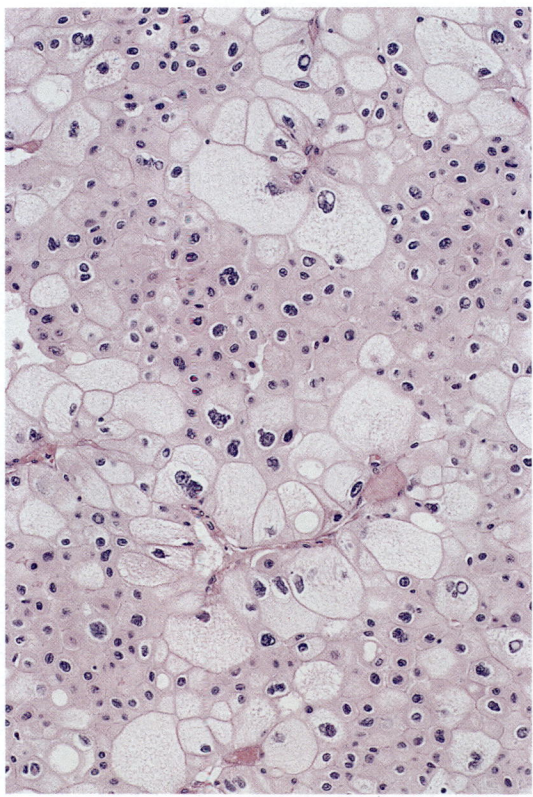

FIG. 20. Chromophobe renal cell carcinoma in which some of the tumor cells contain deeply eosinophilic cytoplasm, while others have abundant foamy cytoplasm. Notice the pronounced irregularity of the nuclear membrane.

nuclei are more likely to be seen within cells containing more eosinophilic cytoplasm. Binucleated cells are present in all cases. Focal cytologic atypia with bizarre nuclei is seen in half the cases, but this is a prominent feature in only a small minority of tumors. Mitotic activity is very low, except in sarcomatoid areas. We do not grade CRCC unless a sarcomatoid pattern is a sign of potentially aggressive (high grade) disease.

Variably granular and diffuse cytoplasmic staining with Hale's colloidal iron is reported in the majority of cases, while focal, weak, and even absent staining is seen in cases with a predominance of eosinophilic cells (105,119,120). A few cases exhibit staining of the luminal borders of acini. Hale's colloidal iron stain detects polyanionic compounds, including acid mucopolysaccharides. A unique ultrastructural feature of CRCC is the presence of cytoplasmic microvesicles (121–123) (Fig. 21). Their origin is unknown, but they are believed to represent altered mitochondria or rough endoplasmic reticulum. Bonsib et al. have shown that tissue processing for paraffin embedding results in solubilization of these vesicles and cannot be employed for the ultrastructural confirmation of a histologic diagnosis of CCRC (122). Recent work by the same author confirms the relationship between the cytoplasmic vesicles and Hale's colloidal stain in tissue that has been osmicated, a process that preserves the integrity of these vesicles (120).

Ultrastructural studies have shown that small eosinophilic cells have abundant mitochondria and a few microvesicles,

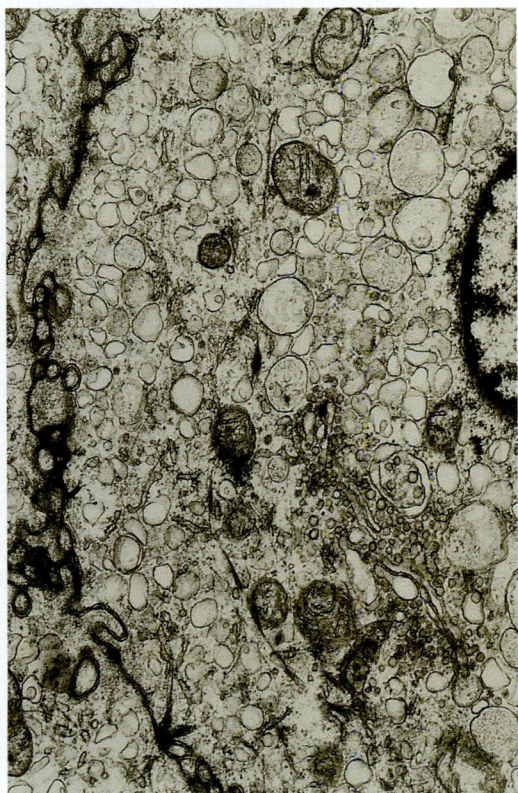

FIG. 21. Ultrastructural features of chromophobe renal carcinoma are dominated by the presence of cytoplasmic microvesicles. Scattered mitochondria are also evident.

explaining why these tumor cells show a different pattern of expression of Hale's colloidal iron (124). The vesicles and their content lack affinity for hematoxylin and eosin dyes, imparting to these cells a clear cytoplasmic appearance. Weak Hale's colloidal iron positivity has been demonstrated in other renal tumors; there is, for example, a focally diffuse distribution in oncocytoma and a droplet-like distribution in conventional RCCs and PRCCs (109). Luminal staining can be seen in the neoplastic tubules of oncocytomas. For the reasons stated here, we do not rely on Hale's colloidal iron to make a diagnosis of CRCC.

Tumor cells show immunoreactivity for EMA as well as low-molecular-weight CKs, such as CAM 5.2 and AE1. Vimentin gives positive results only in the sarcomatoid areas. High-molecular-weight CK 34BE12 tested negative in all cases we studied. While these tumors have been reported to show a characteristic staining pattern with anti-mitochondrial antibody 113-1, the staining patterns of oncocytomas and the eosinophilic variant of CRCC may overlap significantly (125).

Outcome

The prognosis of CCRC is much better than that of other types of RCC (105–107) (Tables 7 and 8). In our study, 94% of patients either were alive with no evidence of disease or died without evidence of tumor recurrence in the course of a mean follow-up period of 59 months. Only one patient succumbed to extensive CCRC disease. This patient was first seen with advanced-stage (stage IV) disease—tumor extended directly into the liver and had sarcomatoid differentiation. While classic CRCC can metastasize and kill the patient, those tumors with a sarcomatoid component are the most likely to behave in an aggressive fashion. In our series, the majority of tumors were large (with an average diameter of 9 cm), yet two-thirds of them were confined to the kidney at the time of diagnosis. Previous studies have shown similar or even a slightly higher patient survival rate (105–107). These findings further support the indolent nature of these tumors.

Differential Diagnosis

Many tumors that have been called granular RCCs in the past are actually CRCCs, while others are either conventional RCCs or oncocytomas (Table 6). Given the differing clinical behavior of these tumors, distinguishing between them is mandatory and can be performed easily in most cases by adequate sampling and by paying close attention to the growth pattern and cytologic characteristics of the tumor. Electron microscopy as well as cytogenetics may be useful in difficult cases.

ONCOCYTOMA

Oncocytoma is a benign renal epithelial neoplasm first described by Zippel in 1942 (126) and then largely ignored until the publication of 13 additional cases by Klein and Valensi (127). It is estimated that oncocytomas comprise 3.2% to 7% of all primary renal neoplasms (128–131). Over an 8-year period, oncocytomas constituted 10% of 646 renal epithelial neoplasms resected at the Memorial Sloan-Kettering Cancer Center (Table 5). Most series show a wide age distribution at diagnosis, with a peak incidence in the seventh decade of life. Men are affected nearly twice as often as women (131,132). The majority are asymptomatic at diagnosis; in these patients the disease is uncovered during examination for other unrelated, nonurologic conditions. A minority of patients show initial signs of hematuria, flank pain, or a palpable mass.

No consistent unique genetic abnormality characterizes oncocytoma, such as are found in other renal epithelial neoplasms. The most common genetic change, however, is loss of chromosomes 1 and Y (133). Less typical are translocations of chromosomes 9 and 11 [t(9;11)(p23;q13)] (134–136) and chromosomes 5 and 11 [t(5;11)(q35;q13)] (137). It is of interest that genes encoding mitochondrial DNA are found in the translocation region of chromosome 11. Familial cases have been described, but they are uncommon (58).

Gross Features

Oncocytomas are well-circumscribed, nonencapsulated neoplasms that are classically mahogany brown and less often tan to pale yellow (Fig. 22). A central, stellate, radiating scar, related to tumor size, is seen in roughly 33% of cases. For example, in one series, the mean size of tumors with a central scar was 6.5 cm, while that of tumors lacking a scar was 4.6 cm (131). One should bear in mind that low-grade conventional RCCs and CRCCs may also contain a central scar. Gross hemorrhage is present in 20% of cases, but necrosis is rare (131). Cysts and extension into perinephric adipose tissue may be encountered, but these features are unusual. Multifocal tumors are seen in up to 13% of cases and bilateral tumors in 4% (131,132).

Microscopic Features

The architectural appearance varies and consists of solid, compact nests, acini, tubules, or microcysts embedded within a hypocellular, hyalinized stroma (Figs. 23 and 24). The predominant cell type (so-called oncocyte) is round to polygonal, with granular eosinophilic cytoplasm, round and regular nuclei with evenly dispersed chromatin, and a centrally placed nucleolus (Fig. 25). A smaller population of cells with scanty granular cytoplasm, a high nuclear/cytoplasmic ratio, and dark hyperchromatic nuclei (so-called oncoblasts) may also be evident (Fig. 26). If there are microcysts, they may be filled with red blood cells (Fig. 24). The

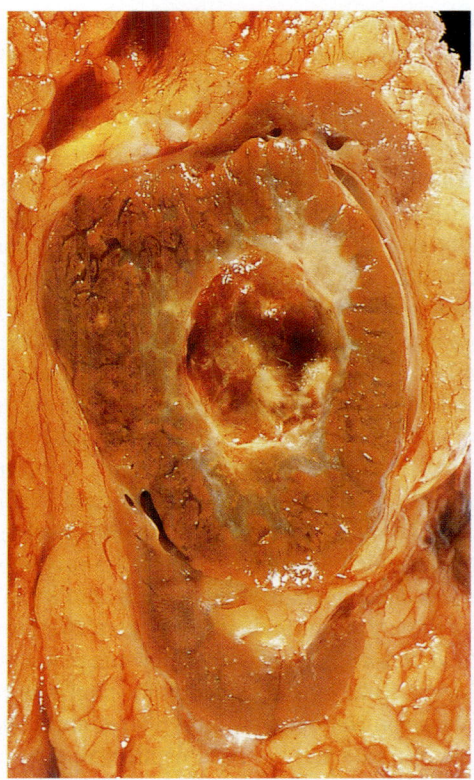

FIG. 22. Oncocytoma. The tumor is dark tan to brown and exhibits a central area of cystic degeneration and scarring, a characteristic that can be found in all types of slow-growing renal epithelial neoplasms, irrespective of the tumor type. The gross appearance of oncocytomas can overlap substantially with that seen in chromophobe tumors, especially the eosinophilic variant.

presence of a few clusters of cells with pleomorphic and hyperchromatic nuclei is typical (Fig. 27).

Mitotic activity is rare, but necrosis and atypical mitotic figures are not seen. Focal clear-cell change may be present in areas of stromal hyalinization, and these foci may superficially resemble conventional (clear cell) RCC. While small papillae or intratubular epithelial tufts may be seen in focal areas in up to 27% cases, pure or extensive papillary architecture is not a feature of renal oncocytoma. Extension into perinephric adipose tissue is found in up to 20% of cases (131,138) and vascular invasion in as many as 5% (130,131,138). Since oncocytomas are benign neoplasms, nuclear grading using the criteria of Fuhrman et al. (60) is not useful in terms of prognosis and should not be performed.

Oncocytosis

A very small subset of oncocytic tumors may show a spectrum of morphologic features besides the dominant mass. These features include extreme multifocality, oncocytic change in benign tubules, microcysts lined by oncocytic

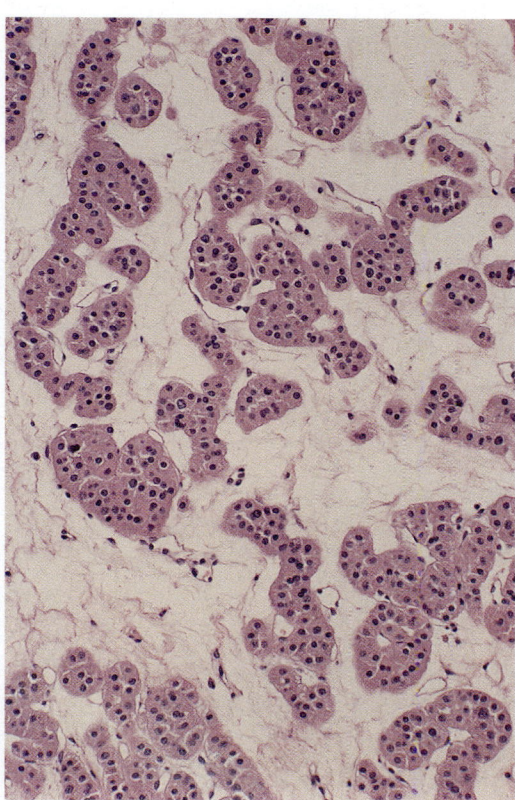

FIG. 23. Renal oncocytoma. Discrete tubules and acini are visible within a pausicellular hyalinized stroma.

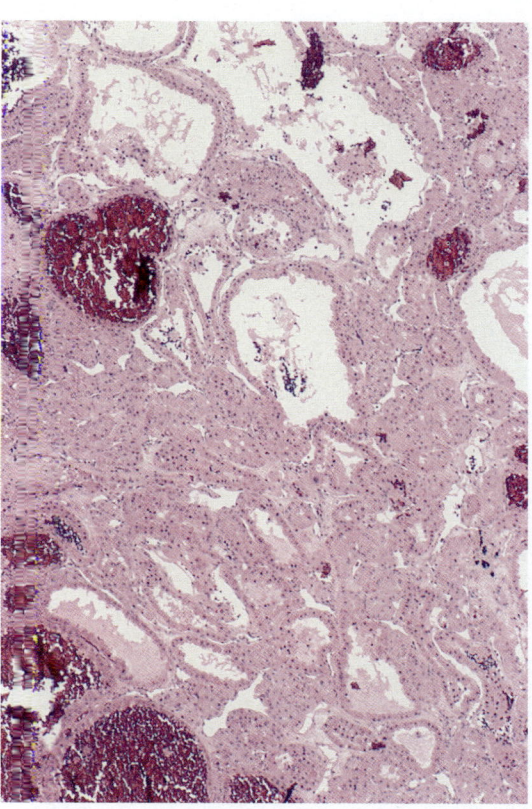

FIG. 24. Renal oncocytoma. Some of the dilated tubular structures are filled with red blood cells.

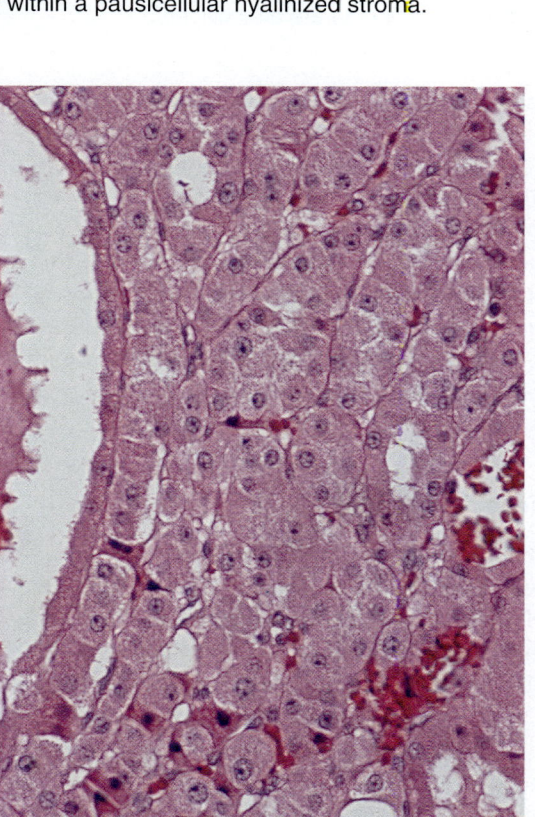

FIG. 25. High-power magnification of renal oncocytoma. Notice the densely eosinophilic cytoplasm and regular round nuclei with small but prominent nucleoli.

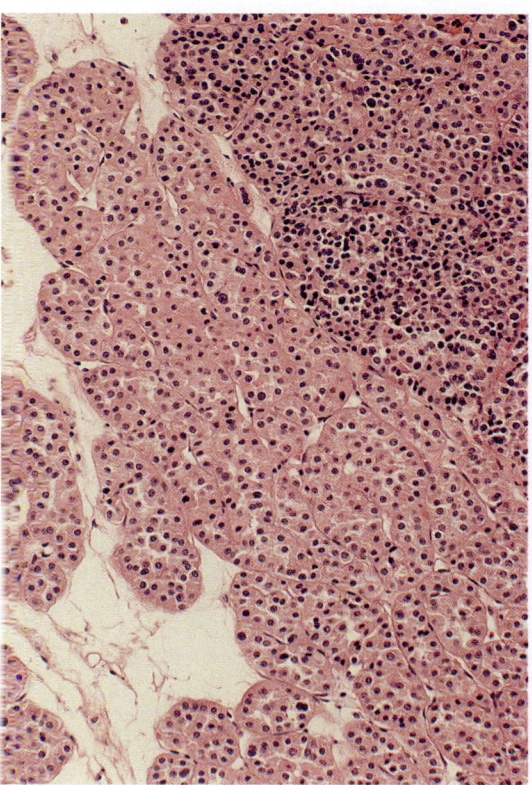

FIG. 26. Oncocytoma containing a population of cells with scanty cytoplasm, a high nuclear to cytoplasmic ratio, and small hyperchromatic nuclei (so-called oncoblasts).

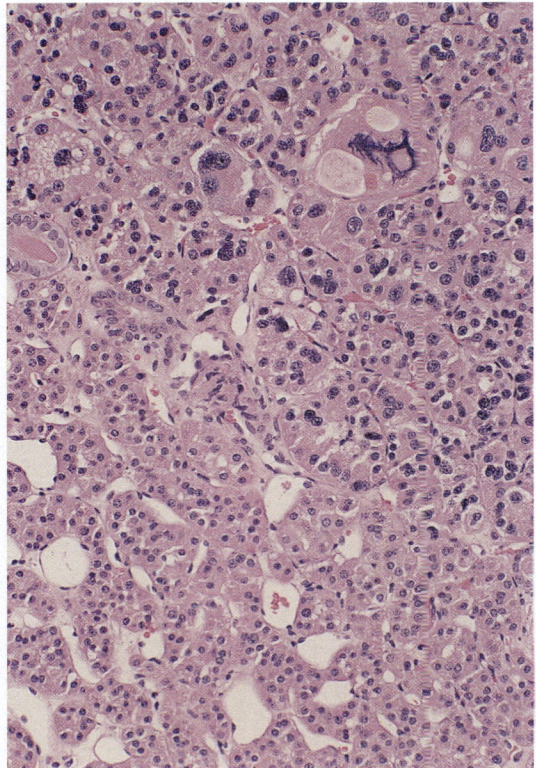

FIG. 27. Cytologic atypia can be seen in up to 30% of oncocytomas. It is believed to be a degenerative phenomenon and is virtually never associated with mitotic activity.

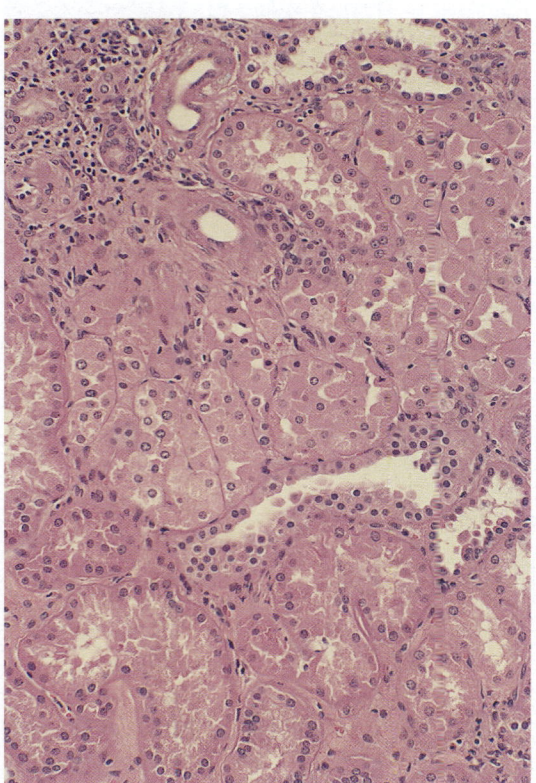

FIG. 28. Oncocytosis. Oncocytic tumor cells infiltrate between benign renal tubules.

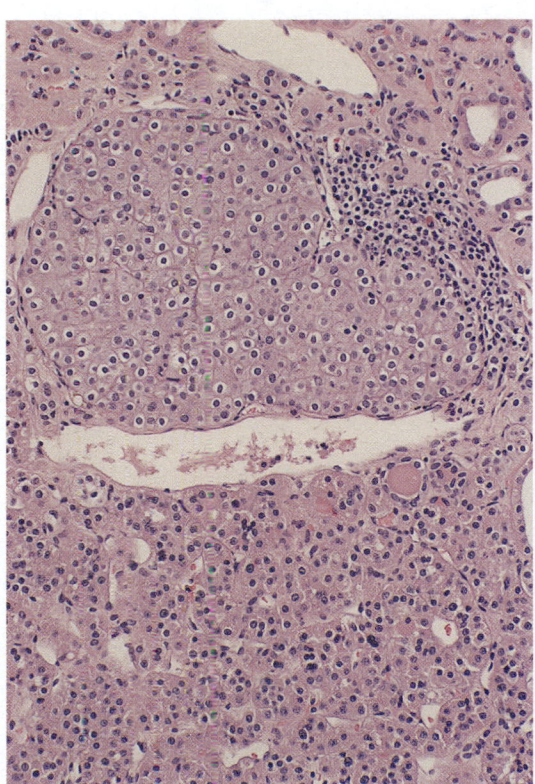

FIG. 29. Hybrid tumor. The majority of this tumor is a typical oncocytoma, but microscopic areas with features of chromophobe renal carcinoma are also evident.

cells, and neoplastic oncocytes infiltrating between benign tubules (Fig. 28). The macroscopic and microscopic oncocytic nodules usually have the morphologic and ultrastructural features of oncocytoma, but some may have either chromophobe or hybrid features (Fig. 29). We have chosen the term oncocytosis to describe the entire spectrum of morphologic changes (139). Until the clinical behavior of such hybrid tumors has been better defined, we regard them as low-grade malignant neoplasms much like pure CRCC. These rare lesions are further evidence of the possible relationship between oncocytoma and CRCC.

Differential Diagnosis

While the differential diagnosis includes any renal neoplasm with granular eosinophilic cytoplasm, tumors most likely to be confused with oncocytoma are the so-called eosinophilic variant of CRCC and epithelioid AML. The distinguishing features of oncocytoma and CRCC are outlined in Table 9. Careful attention to the distinctive architectural and cytologic characteristics of each tumor type allows for correct classification on routine hematoxylin and eosin–stained sections in the vast majority of cases. A subset of cases, however, may require ancillary studies in order to confirm the diagnosis. In this regard, electron microscopy is clearly the gold standard in distinguishing oncocytoma from CRCC.

TABLE 9. *Distinguishing features of renal oncocytoma and chromophobe RCC*

Features	Oncocytoma	Chromophobe RCC
Gross		
Color	Brown-red	Yellow-tan
Central scar	Common	Less common
Cellular		
Architecture	Nested and tubular	Solid sheets
Necrosis	Absent	Common
Cytoplasm	Densely granular	Reticular
Perinuclear halo	Absent	Present
Nuclear		
Shape	Round	Irregular, cleaved
Hyperchromatic atypical	Common	Less common
Nucleoli	Common	Small or absent
Binucleated	Common	Always
Ultrastructural	Mitochondria	Microvesicles and mitochondria
Hale's colloidal iron	Negative or luminal	Diffuse, granular

RCC, renal cell carcinoma.
Modified from ref. 131.

On ultrastructural examination, renal oncocytoma is characterized by cells containing numerous mitochondria, the majority of which are of normal size and shape, though pleomorphic forms may be seen from time to time (124). Other cytoplasmic organelles are sparse and unremarkable. Notably absent are the microvesicles typical of chromophobe tumors. Hale's colloidal iron is a less reliable means of distinguishing oncocytoma from CRCC. In the classic examples of oncocytoma, Hale's gives negative results or shows focal staining in a luminal distribution, in contrast to the diffuse cytoplasmic staining found in the classic examples of CRCC. In contrast to renal oncocytoma, the vast majority of AMLs are immunoreactive to HMB-45.

Outcome

Renal oncocytomas are benign neoplasms. This conclusion is based largely on the results of several studies that have included rigorous pathologic review and adequate clinical follow-up (131,132,138) (Table 7). Indeed, only one well-documented and acceptable case of renal oncocytoma in these series has produced a distant metastasis to the liver, which, notably, has remained stable in size for more than 5 years (131). Early reports of metastatic or malignant oncocytomas undoubtedly include tumors that today would be classified as CRCC. The Furhman nuclear grade is irrelevant in renal oncocytoma, given their uniformly indolent behavior.

COLLECTING DUCT CARCINOMA

CDC, also known as Bellini duct carcinoma, is rare, comprising less than 1% of renal epithelial tumors. Although cases had been reported earlier, it was not recognized as a clinicopathologic entity until 1986, when Lewi and Fleming described the clinical and morphologic features of six cases (140). These tumors are thought to arise within the collecting ducts of the renal medulla, and the rarity of the disease is evidenced by the fact that the largest series in the literature includes a mere 12 cases (140–145). While most authors suggest that these aggressive tumors have very distinctive morphologic features, we feel that the true spectrum of the disease remains to be defined. Many high-grade renal epithelial tumors with a papillary or papillary/tubular pattern of growth are placed in this category by default. Until this entity is better defined in terms of its morphologic, clinical, and genetic characteristics, we have chosen to place all but the classic cases into the unclassified category.

The genetic and molecular genetic findings of fewer than 25 cases of CDC have been reported (146–150). Fuzesi et al. (150) studied three cases and found consistent monosomy of chromosomes 1, 6, 14, 15, and 22. Polascik et al. (146) found loss of heterozygosity of chromosomal arm 1q in ten of 18 cases. This group subsequently reported that the minimal area of deletion is located at 1q32.1-32.2 (148). It is important to note that of all the tumors studied, none has shown trisomy 7/17 or losses of chromosome 3, features seen in PRCC and conventional RCC, respectively.

Clinical Features

CDCs may occur at any age; the mean age at diagnosis is approximately 53 years, with a range of 13 to 83 years. Nevertheless, the overall impression of most experts is that these tumors tend to develop in younger patients. In the series of six cases reported by Kennedy and collaborators, the mean age was 34 years (141). Hematuria is the most common initial symptom, followed by pain, weight loss, and the presence of a palpable mass. The aggressive nature of most of these tumors is evidenced by the fact that more than 50% of patients have metastatic disease, at the time of initial diagnosis.

Gross and Microscopic Features

CDCs are centered in the medulla; large tumors may occupy the cortex as well (Fig. 30). They are unifocal, solid, tan-white, and firm, and they may contain cysts as well as gross evidence of hemorrhage and necrosis. Most lesions are poorly circumscribed and often extend into the renal sinus and hilar fat. The histologic features of classic tumors are neoplastic ducts, tubules, and papillae in a fibrotic or desmoplastic stroma (141–143). The complex tubules and papillae are lined by tumor cells with eosinophilic, basophilic, or amphophilic cytoplasm; high-grade nuclei; and prominent nucleoli (Fig. 31). Focal spindle-cell differentiation is not unusual, and rare cases may be frankly sarcomatoid. The papillae rarely, if ever, contain foamy macrophages, but polymorphonuclear cells and lymphocytes may be abundant within the surrounding stroma. Psammoma bodies are uncommon. Dysplastic or frankly neoplastic cells may be present within adjacent renal tubules (Fig. 32).

Cytoplasmic and luminal mucin may be present and is a helpful distinguishing feature. Several reports have ver-

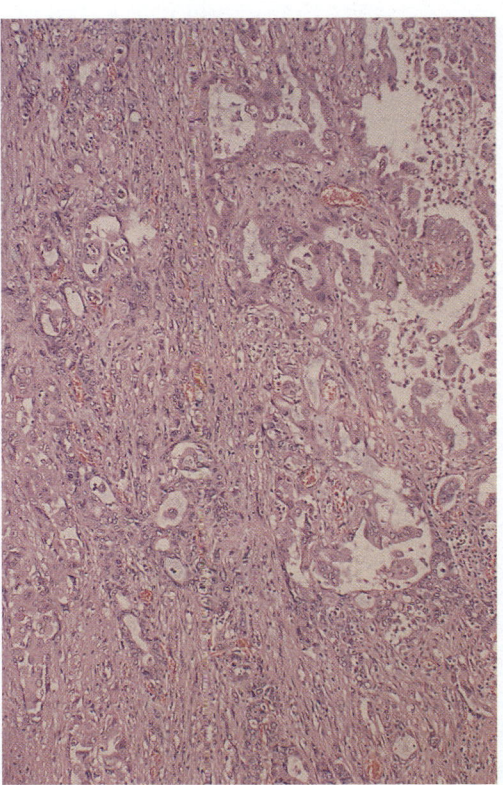

FIG. 31. Collecting duct carcinoma. Tubular and papillary structures are lined by tumor cells with high-grade nuclei. The tumor is frequently associated with marked stromal desmoplasia.

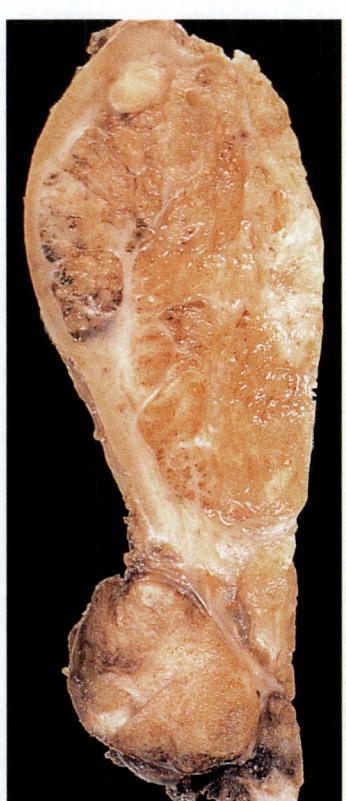

FIG. 30. Collecting duct carcinoma. The tumor is located in the medullary portion of the kidney and spares the cortex. A regional lymph node is enlarged and replaced by tumor.

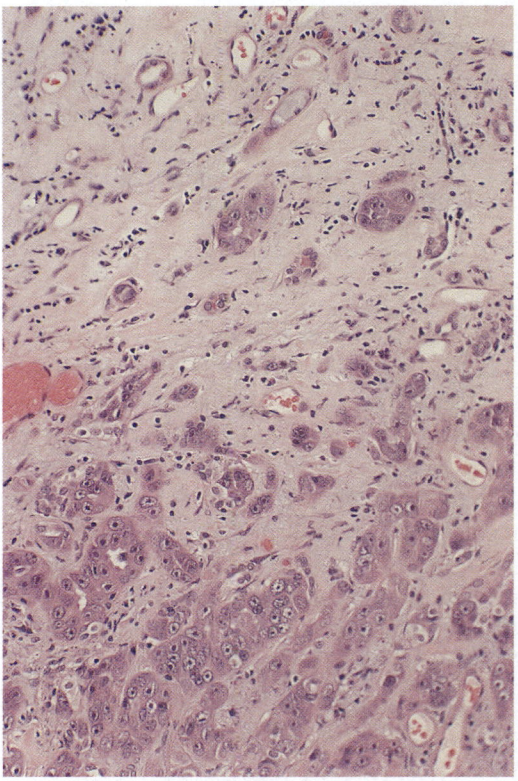

FIG. 32. Collecting duct carcinoma. Neoplastic cells within adjacent medullary tubules. This feature can be seen in association with high-grade urothelial tumors of the renal pelvis as well.

ified a characteristic immunohistochemical profile, which includes immunoreactivity for carcinoembryonic antigen, peanut lectin agglutinin, and *Ulex europaeus* agglutinin (141–143). CK 34BE12 and CK 7 may give positive results as well. While this immunophenotype may help distinguish CDC from PRCC, it is not specific. In fact, this exact staining profile may be seen in medullary carcinomas as well as urothelial tumors, including those arising in the renal pelvis.

The morphologic spectrum of CDC has been expanded to include not only sarcomatoid lesions but also low-grade tumors characterized by a tubulocystic pattern of growth, tumor cells with low-grade nuclei, and mucin production (151,152). While these tumors may represent the low-grade spectrum of CDC, we await further evidence that they are indeed of collecting duct origin. To our knowledge, none of these low-grade lesions has been studied at the molecular level.

Outcome

Classic cases are characterized by aggressive behavior. More than 50% of patients have signs of metastatic disease when they are first seen, and most die within 24 months of diagnosis. Nodal, osseous, and visceral metastases are common, and the metastases to bone are usually osteoblastic.

Differential Diagnosis

Classic tumors do not present much of a diagnostic dilemma. In other cases, the differential diagnosis may include PRCC, medullary carcinoma, and, more often, urothelial carcinoma (Table 10). PRCCs are rarely associated with desmoplastic stroma, and the papillae are more likely to contain foamy macrophages. Histochemical, immunohistochemical, and genetic features can also aid in classifying these tumors. Distinguishing between high-grade urothelial carcinoma and CDC may present a more formidable challenge, since both may be associated with inflamed, fibrotic, or desmoplastic stroma and may contain neoplastic cells within renal tubules. In addition, both may have a tubular or tubulopapillary pattern of growth and a similar immunophenotype. Intracytoplasmic mucin may be seen in urothelial tumors as well. In our experience, the best way to resolve this differential diagnosis is by sampling the renal pelvis well, looking for *in situ* urothelial carcinoma. Molecular studies may also be of diagnostic utility.

MEDULLARY CARCINOMA

In 1995, Davis et al., from the Armed Forces Institute of Pathology (153), reported a unique group of tumors affecting predominantly young patients of African-American descent. These tumors appeared to be centered in the medulla of the kidney, had distinctive morphologic features, and followed a very aggressive clinical course. They are believed to arise from the distal portions of the collecting ducts. Patients ranged in age from 11 to 39 years, with a mean of 22 years. The disease predominately affected males, especially patients under the age of 25. The mean tumor size was 7.0 cm; sizes ranged from 4.0 to 12.0 cm. All patients were believed to have a sickle cell trait, except for one, who had hemoglobin SC disease. The association of this disease with young patients with the sickle cell trait, whether of African-American, Mediterranean, or other ancestry, has been confirmed in other reports (154–158). Other characteristic genetic abnormalities have yet to be defined.

These tumors share many morphologic features with collecting duct carcinoma and, in fact, are believed to be a particularly virulent variant of that entity (142–143). Tumors are composed of cells with high-grade nuclei and prominent nucleoli arranged in solid nests or irregular tubules (Fig. 33). Microcystic or reticular growth reminiscent of that seen in yolk sac tumors is also common (Fig. 34). Areas resembling adenoid cystic carcinoma have also been described. The surrounding stroma is usually fibrotic or desmoplastic and infiltrated by abundant inflammatory cells, mostly polymorphonuclear cells.

As previously mentioned, medullary carcinomas are very aggressive tumors. Most cases reported showed signs of metastatic disease at the time of diagnosis. We have seen

TABLE 10. *Distinguishing features between papillary renal cell, collecting duct, and urothelial carcinoma*

	Papillary RCC	Collecting duct Ca	Urothelial Ca
Papillary/tubular pattern	Yes	Yes	Yes
Nuclear grade	Any	Usually high	Usually high
Stromal desmoplasia	Uncommon	Common	Common
Macrophages in papilla	Common	No	No
"Dysplastic" tubules	No	Occasionally	Occasionally
Intracytoplasmic mucin	No	Common	Occasionally
Multifocality	Common	Uncommon	Uncommon
Immunohistochemistry			
CEA	Negative	+/−[a]	+/−[a]
PNA	Negative	+/−[a]	+/−[a]
UEA	Negative	+/−[a]	+/−[a]
CK 7	+/−[a]	+/−[a]	+/−[a]

RCC, renal cell carcinoma; Ca., Carcinoma; CEA, Carcinoembryonic antigen; PNA, peanut lectin; UEA, *Ulex* lectin; CK 7, cytokeratin 7.
[a] May be positive or negative.

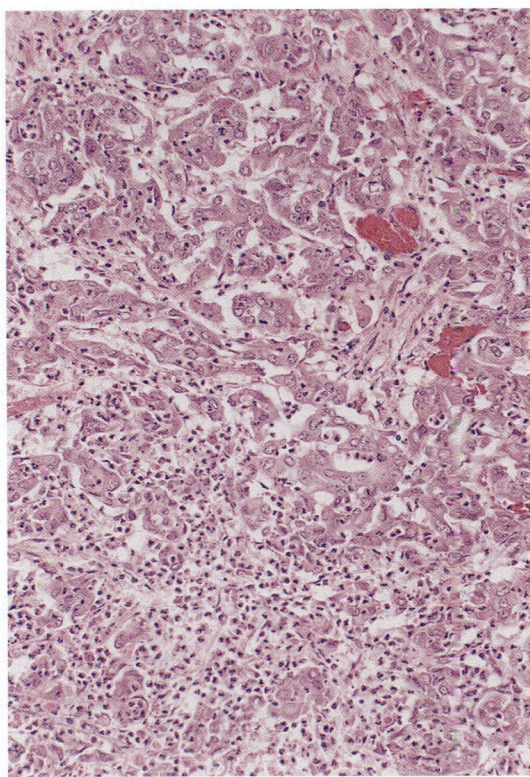

FIG. 33. Medullary carcinoma. Tumor cells are arranged in nests and cords and exhibit high-grade nuclei and varying amounts of eosinophilic or amphophilic cytoplasm. The surrounding stroma contains many inflammatory cells, predominantly polymorphonuclear cells.

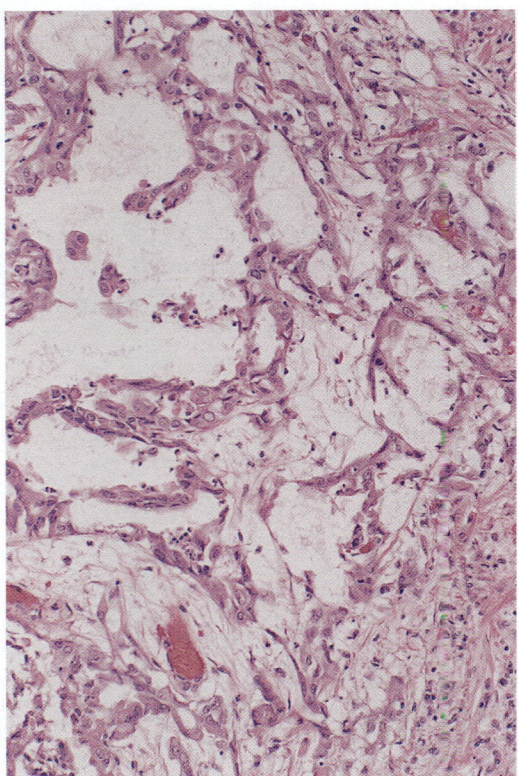

FIG. 34. Medullary carcinoma with an endodermal sinus-like growth pattern.

several cases in our institution; all but one have shown initial signs of metastatic disease as well. In the series reported by Davis et al., the mean survival was 15 weeks (153). The differential diagnosis includes collecting duct and high-grade urothelial carcinoma. Careful sampling and attention to the clinical features of the case may be needed to accurately classify the tumor. In our experience, the immunohistochemical features of all three tumor types overlap significantly, nullifying its diagnostic utility (156).

ADULT MESOBLASTIC NEPHROMA

Adult mesoblastic nephroma (cystic hamartoma, leiomyomatous renal hamartoma, solid and cystic biphasic tumor) is rare and has generally been the subject of isolated case reports or small series of cases (159–167). Patients have ranged from 19 to 78 years of age, and women have outnumbered men by a margin of 10 to 1. Initial signs and symptoms usually include a palpable abdominal or flank mass, flank pain, or hematuria. In one study, most were incidental findings (159). Imaging studies are not diagnostic but do reveal a solid or solid and cystic mass in most cases. Although adult mesoblastic nephroma is similar in many respects to the congenital form of mesoblastic nephroma, a number of differences have been described. Indeed, some authors believe that the lesion referred to herein as adult mesoblastic nephroma bears no relationship to childhood mesoblastic nephroma.

Gross Features

Tumors are solid or solid and cystic, tan to yellow, and well circumscribed and encapsulated; they have ranged in size from 2 cm to 24 cm. In some cases, a cystic component predominates and is associated with solid mural nodules (163). In others, the appearance may mimic multilocular cystic RCC (159). Like the congenital form, involvement of the renal hilus and compression of the pelvocalyceal system is common; however, gross infiltration into adjacent renal parenchyma is not seen. Necrosis may be present but is not typical (161).

Microscopic Features

In adults, the classic pattern of mesoblastic nephroma predominates over the cellular pattern. Like the congenital form, the adult form is a biphasic tumor composed of mesenchymal (stromal) and epithelial components (Fig. 35). The nature of the latter components is uncertain; some authors consider them to be entrapped renal tubules, while others view them as neoplastic elements. The mesenchymal component is characterized by fascicles and sheets of spindle cells showing variable degrees of smooth-muscle, fibroblastic, or myofibroblastic differentiation with interspersed collagen. In some cases, the mesenchymal component resembles ovarian stroma (159).

Stromal cellularity is less pronounced than that of the con-

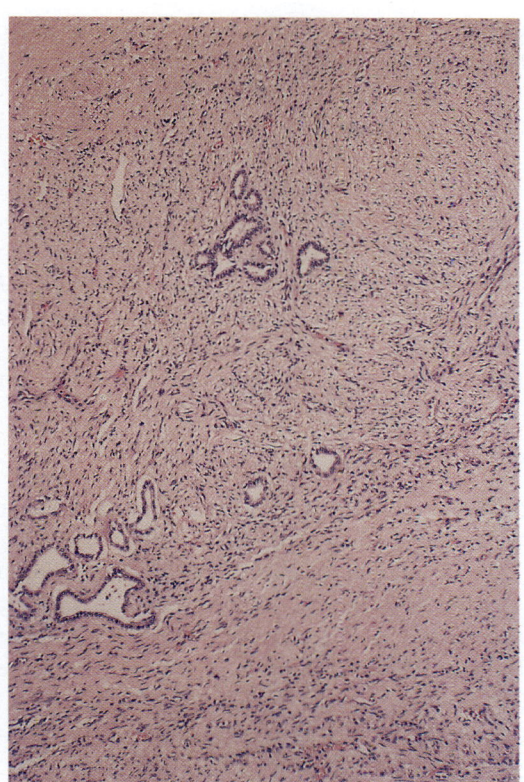

FIG. 35. Mesoblastic nephroma. A biphasic appearance with mesenchymal and epithelial components is evident.

genital form, and mitotic figures, hemorrhage, and necrosis are uncommon. Mature adipose tissue has rarely been described as a constituent of adult mesoblastic nephroma (164,166); it is unclear whether it represents entrapped or heterologous stromal elements. The epithelial components vary from round and regular tubules to more complex structures that show papillations and cystic dilatation. They are lined by cuboidal to flattened epithelium that may display clear-cell change or have a hobnail appearance. Unlike what is seen in the congenital form, the epithelial components may be found interspersed throughout the mesenchymal components and not merely restricted to the periphery of the tumor nodules.

The immunohistochemical profile of the mesenchymal component reflects the degree of smooth-muscle differentiation seen on routine hematoxylin and eosin–stained sections. The epithelial components show positive results for both low- and high-molecular-weight CKs and *Ulex europaeus* (161,166). Positive reactions with antibodies to estrogen receptors have been described in at least a subset of cases.

Outcome

All reported cases of adult mesoblastic nephroma have behaved in a benign manner after surgical excision, though one recurred locally 21 years after resection (162). The recurrent tumor invaded the liver and was composed exclusively of spindle cells.

CYSTIC NEPHROMA

Cystic nephroma is mentioned earlier, in the discussion on the differential diagnosis of multilocular cystic RCC. The majority of affected adults are female, and most tumors are asymptomatic or take the form of a palpable abdominal mass. On gross inspection, cystic nephroma is well circumscribed and composed of several noncommunicating cysts that vary in size and contain clear fluid (Fig. 36). Solid, expansile, mural nodules; hemorrhage; and necrosis are not found in the disease. At the microscopic level, the cysts are lined by flattened, cuboidal, or hobnail cells, and the septa are composed of fibrous tissue of varying cellularity, at times having the appearance of ovarian-type stroma (Fig. 37). The fibrous septa may contain microscopic cysts lined by bland cuboidal cells reminiscent of renal tubules. Sarcomas have been known to arise from cystic nephromas, although this is a rare occurrence (Fig. 38). Most are undifferentiated embryonal-type tumors (82,168).

JUXTAGLOMERULAR CELL TUMOR

The first example of juxtaglomerular cell tumor was reported in 1967 by Robertson et al. (169), who described a young male patient with hypertension and a small renal neoplasm. The following year, Kihara and colleagues (170) reported a similar neoplasm in a young female patient and proposed the term juxtaglomerular cell tumor. Since then, well over thirty cases have been reported in the English-language literature (171–174). Most patients are diagnosed in the second and third decades of life and now and then in the sixth

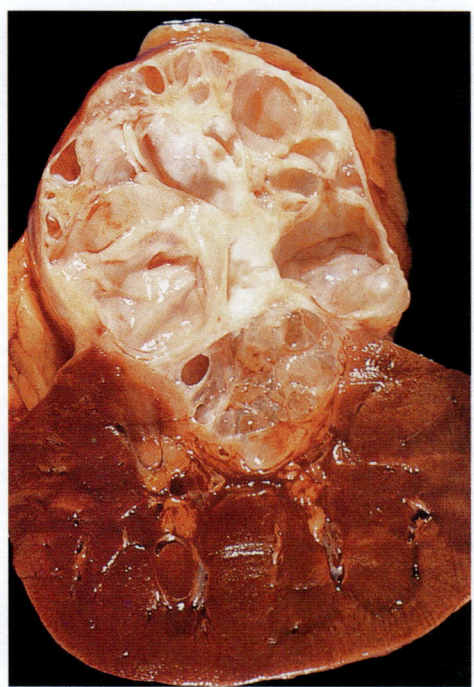

FIG. 36. Cystic nephroma. Photo shows gross features of a well-circumscribed multilocular cystic neoplasm.

and seventh decades (172,175). Signs and symptoms of hyperreninism are the hallmark of this tumor; they include hypertension, hyperaldosteronism, and hypokalemia. Women have outnumbered men by a margin of roughly 1.5:1.

In hypertensive patients suspected of having juxtaglomerular cell tumor, radiologic studies are often helpful in ruling out other causes of hypertension. Renal arteriography shows the majority of juxtaglomerular cell tumors to be hypovascular and helps rule out renal artery stenosis. Computed tomography shows a hypovascular and solid mass in most cases. Renal vein catheterization and selective measurement of renin values may help lateralize small tumors.

Gross Features

Juxtaglomerular cell tumors are well encapsulated, unilateral, and solitary and typically based in the cortex (Fig. 39). They range from light tan to yellow. Most are solid, though small cysts may be present. The majority of juxtaglomerular cell tumors are 2 cm to 3 cm in diameter, but tumors smaller than 1 cm and larger than 6 cm in diameter have been reported (176,177).

Microscopic Features

The histologic appearance of juxtaglomerular cell tumor is highly variable. The classic examples have a glomoid appearance and are composed of sheets of homogeneous, round to polygonal cells with clear to slightly eosinophilic cytoplasm and distinct cell borders. Others consist of sheets

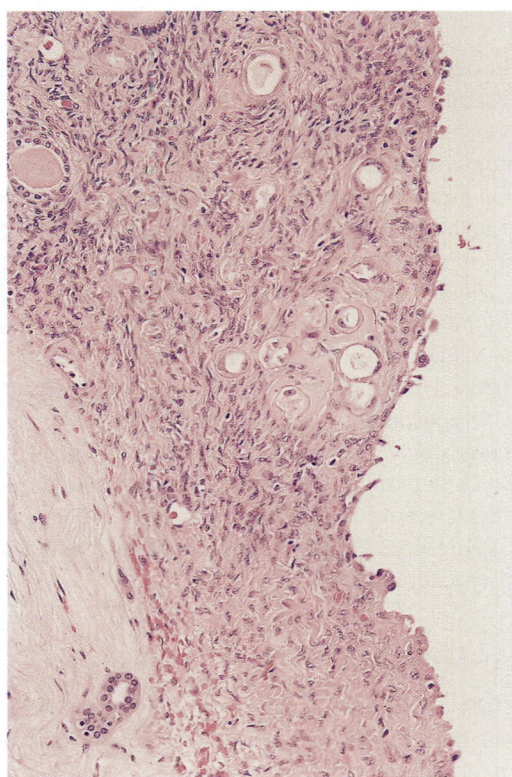

FIG. 37. Cystic nephroma. Hematoxylin and eosin stain shows a cyst wall lined by a single layer of hobnail cells. Notice the primitive, ovarian-like stroma within the cyst wall.

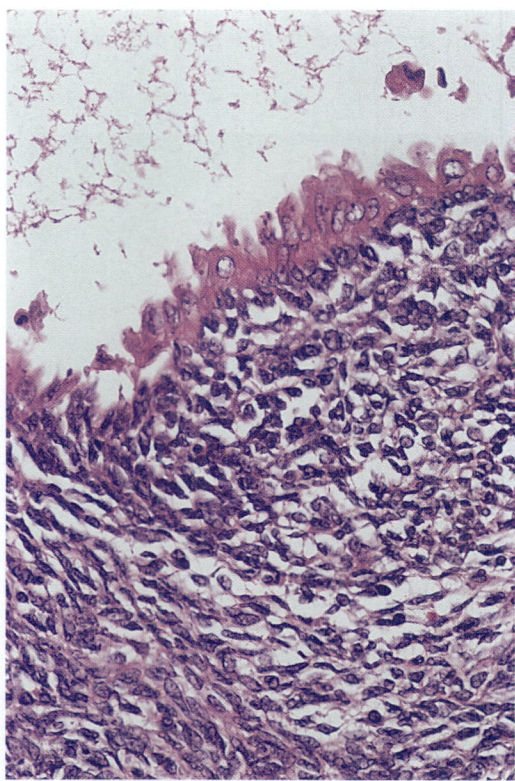

FIG. 38. Cystic nephroma with sarcomatous transformation. In this case, the mesenchymal component is primitive and undifferentiated.

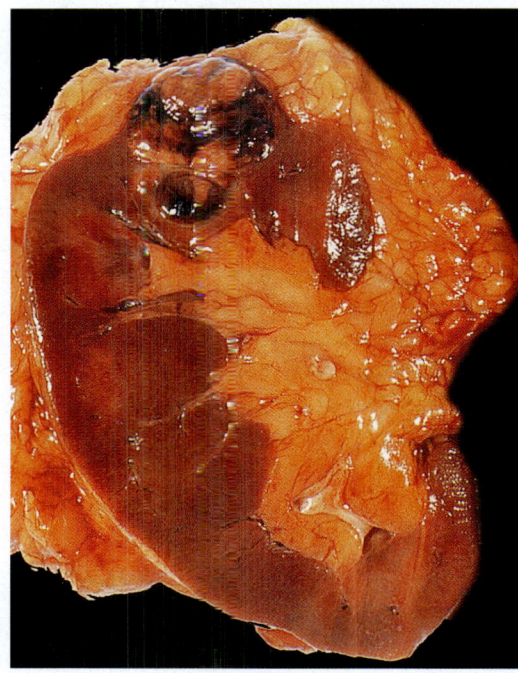

FIG. 39. Juxtaglomerular cell tumor with the gross appearance of a discrete hemorrhagis and a fleshy mass within the upper pole.

or irregular cords of polygonal to spindle-shaped cells with indistinct cell borders. Numerous capillaries and branching blood vessels and sinusoids similar to those of hemangiopericytoma are typically found. The stroma may be scanty or consist of large areas of hyalinized or myxoid fibrous tissue; it often contains a scattered lymphoplasmacytic infiltrate. Some tumors have well-developed tubules lined by a population of cuboidal cells similar to collecting duct epithelium. A papillary pattern has been described in which the neoplastic cells form papillary fronds lined by cuboidal cells (174). Pleomorphism and mitotic activity are uncommon.

Periodic acid–Schiff and Bowie stains reveal cytoplasmic granules in a subset of cells. Immunohistochemistry shows diffuse positive staining with antibodies to renin and vimentin (171,173). Variable numbers of common muscle actin (HHF-35)– and smooth-muscle actin–positive cells may be found; neuroendocrine markers give negative results. CK stains label the cuboidal epithelium of the tubules but not the polygonal or spindle cells. Electron microscopy shows distinctive membrane-bound rhomboid and polygonal granules that are immunoreactive with antibodies to renin (Fig. 40).

Outcome

Juxtaglomerular cell tumors are benign neoplasms. Surgical resection of the affected kidney cures systemic hypertension in the majority of patients.

CARCINOID TUMOR

Well over 20 cases of renal carcinoid have been reported in the English-language literature (178–185). Most patients have been diagnosed in the fifth through seventh decades of life, but the case of one patient as young as 13 years has been reported (186). Men and women are affected equally. Initial signs and symptoms are typically nonspecific and include flank pain, vague abdominal discomfort, or hematuria. Whereas many cases are discovered incidentally after radiologic staging of other malignancies, overt endocrine disturbances, including the carcinoid syndrome, are uncommon (31,186–189).

Gross Features

Renal carcinoids are well circumscribed and often encapsulated, tan to yellow, solid, and fleshy tumors that frequently show areas of hemorrhage and necrosis or cystic degeneration (Fig. 41). Reported tumors have ranged in size from 2 to 30 cm in greatest dimension (mean, 9 cm). Diffuse infiltration of renal parenchyma is not a feature of renal carcinoid, but invasion of perinephric adipose tissue and renal veins has been documented (190). Two examples have been described in horseshoe kidneys (185,191).

Microscopic Features

Renal carcinoids are similar to carcinoids found at other sites. The neoplastic cells are arranged in nests or trabeculae

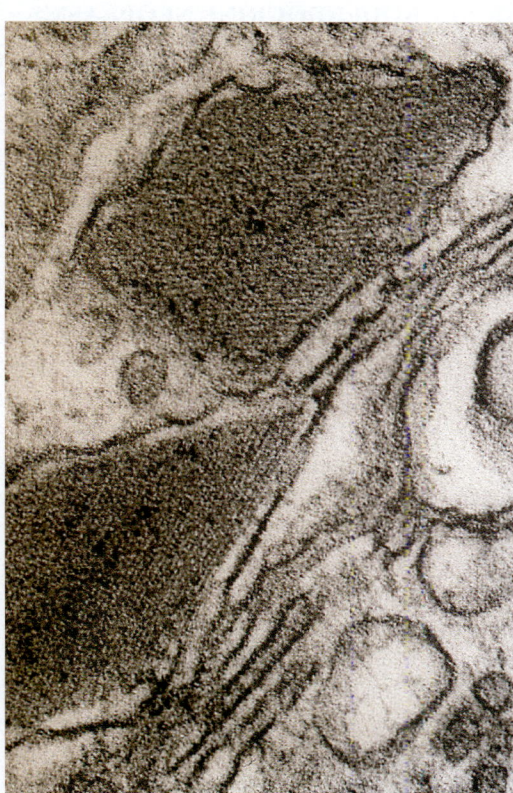

FIG. 40. Juxtaglomerular cell tumor. Ultrastructure reveals typical membrane-bound rhomboid crystals.

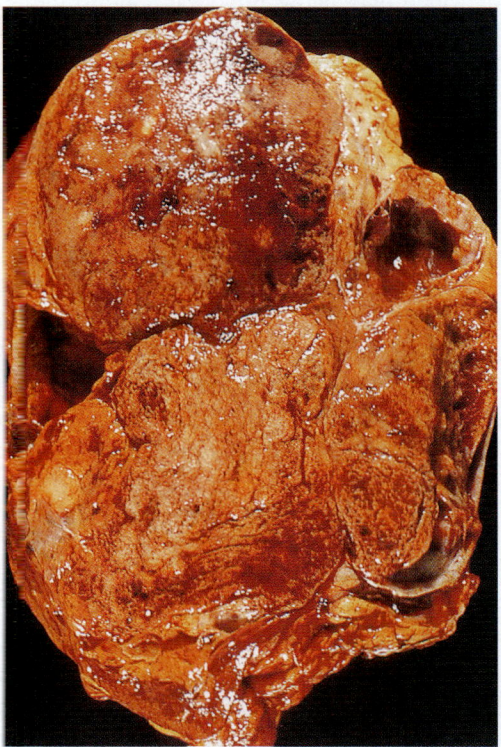

FIG. 41. Renal carcinoid. A large, hemorrhagic, and fleshy mass occupies the majority of the renal parenchyma.

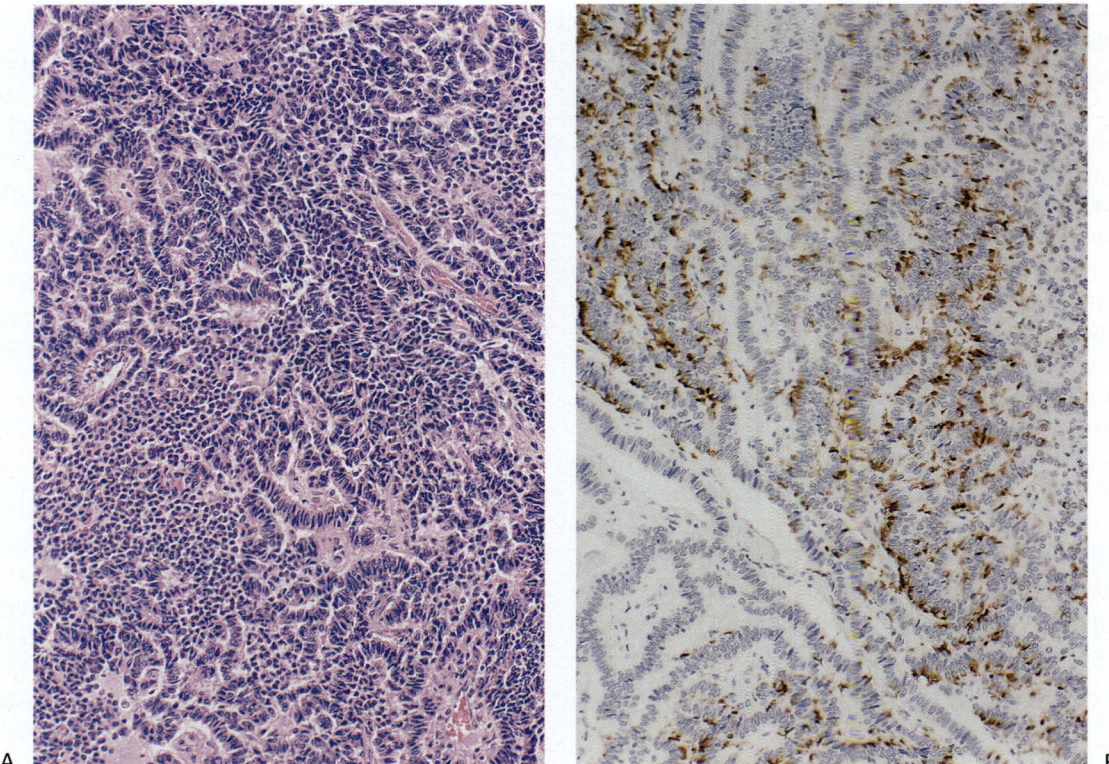

FIG. 42. Renal carcinoid. **A:** Hematoxylin and eosin stain reveals obvious neuroendocrine differentiation. **B:** Tumor cells are immunoreactive with chromogranin.

and are supported by a well-vascularized stroma, the presence of which may be an important clue to the diagnosis (192,193) (Fig. 42a). Nuclei are round and regular, though focal pleomorphism may be seen (181); mitotic figures and vascular invasion are uncommon (184). Two cases have been described as components of cystic teratoma (194) or teratoid malformation (195) of the kidney. In most cases, argyrophilic stains show positive results, while argentaffin stains negative (184). By immunohistochemistry, renal carcinoids show positive reactions to a variety of neuroendocrine markers and polypeptides, including neuron-specific enolase, chromogranin, synaptophysin, serotonin, somatostatin, pancreatic polypeptide, and glucagon (179–181,195) (Fig. 42b). As with hindgut carcinoids, positive reactions to prostate-specific acid phosphatase have been reported (179,196). Electron microscopy confirms the presence of dense-core granules.

Outcome

In roughly one-third of patients, metastases to such sites as regional lymph nodes, liver, lung, and bone have developed (179,190,197,198); several patients have died of disease (181,199). As with carcinoids found elsewhere in the body, the histologic features do not predict outcome. In one study, however, mitotic activity and pleomorphism were greatest in tumors that metastasized and ultimately led to death (181).

OTHER NEURODENDOCRINE NEOPLASMS

Primary renal small-cell carcinoma (200–203), pheochromocytoma (204–207), and neuroblastoma (208–210) have been documented. Small-cell carcinomas are large, locally invasive neoplasms that often show signs of regional or distant metastases.

PRIMITIVE NEUROECTODERMAL TUMOR

Seventeen cases of primary renal primitive neuroectodermal tumor (PNET) have been described, all within the past decade (211–221). The recognition of PNET at this site has undoubtedly been greatly enhanced by advances in molecular genetic techniques, including reverse transcription polymerase chain reaction and fluorescence *in situ* hybridization (FISH), which allow confirmation of the PNET/Ewing sarcoma specific t(11;22) and t(21;22). Patients have ranged in age from 4 to 61 years; the majority are in the second and third decades of life. Initial signs and symptoms are nonspecific and similar to those of other renal mass lesions.

Renal PNETs tend to be large at diagnosis and may entirely replace the underlying renal parenchyma. The reported sizes have ranged from 4 cm to 24 cm (mean, 16 cm). Invasion into adjacent tissues, including perinephric adipose tissue, renal vein, or inferior vena cava, may be seen. On gross examination, PNETs are tan-white to gray and contain areas

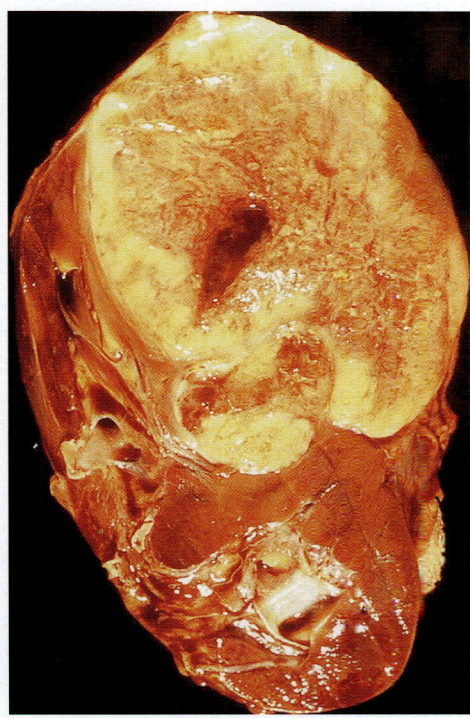

FIG. 43. Primitive neuroectodermal tumor. The gross and morphologic features are similar to those appearing at other sites.

broma are benign renal cortical neoplasms (225,226). Affected patients have ranged in age from the first through the ninth decades of life, and females have outnumbered males by a 2:1 margin. While the initial signs and symptoms are nonspecific and similar to those associated with other renal mass lesions, polycythemia has been reported in as many as 12% of patients (225,227).

Cytogenetic studies have failed to show consistent genetic abnormalities in metanephric adenoma. Some authors have found normal or variants of normal karyotypes (226, 229–231). Others have found trisomies of chromosomes 7 and 17 and loss of sex chromosomes by classic cytogenetics (232) or FISH (233), suggesting a close relationship of metanephric adenoma to PRCC. None have shown abnormalities of 11p in metanephric adenoma, which argues against a relationship to Wilms' tumor.

GROSS FEATURES

Metanephric adenoma and nephrogenic adenofibroma are well circumscribed, cortex-based neoplasms that most often are not encapsulated but may be surrounded by a thin or grossly visible capsule (Fig. 44). They are solid, range from tan to yellow, and often exhibit areas of necrosis, hemorrhage, and cystic degeneration. Calcifications may be apparent on gross examination.

of hemorrhage, necrosis, and cystic degeneration (Fig. 43). At the microscopic level, they resemble PNETs found elsewhere and consist of sheets of monotonous cells with scanty cytoplasm traversed by thin, fibrous bands. Perivascular pseudorosettes may be evident, but true rosettes are unusual. Expression of the MIC2 gene product (p30/32), as determined by immunohistochemistry using the O13 or HBA71 antibody, is a characteristic feature of PNET/Ewing sarcoma and a useful part of a diagnostic immunohistochemical panel (212,215,220,222,223).

One must bear in mind that lymphoblastic lymphoma and, occasionally, other neoplasms react with HBA71 and O13 (224). The majority of PNETs show positive results with antibodies to vimentin and neuron-specific enolase, while a minority are positive with S-100 protein and CK. Electron microscopy demonstrates primitive cells with interdigitating cell processes containing a few dense-core granules and microtubules. As previously mentioned, the finding of the characteristic t(11;22) and t(21;22) using a variety of techniques, including classic cytogenetics, reverse transcription polymerase chain reaction, and FISH, may help confirm the diagnosis of renal PNET.

METANEPHRIC ADENOMA AND NEPHROGENIC ADENOFIBROMA

Metanephric adenoma (embryonal adenoma, nephrogenic nephroma) and the closely related nephrogenic adenofi-

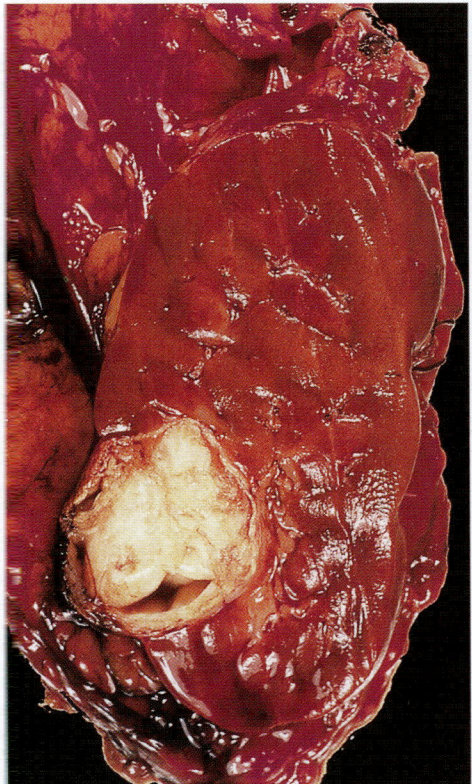

FIG. 44. Metanephric adenoma. Well-circumscribed light tan mass located within the cortex. These lesions can be heavily calcified.

MICROSCOPIC FEATURES

Metanephric adenoma is characterized by tightly packed small tubules separated by a modest amount of stroma (Fig. 45). While a solid or sheet-like growth pattern may be seen and may superficially mimic blastema, careful inspection usually reveals the presence of collapsed, compact tubules. Cytoplasm is scanty; nuclei are small and round to ovoid and often overlap. Nucleoli are typically inconspicuous, and mitotic figures are rare. Papillary or glomeruloid components are seen in roughly half of cases, often associated with microcalcifications, including psammoma bodies (Fig. 45). Multifocal tumors are rare, and bilateral tumors have not been reported. In one series of 50 patients with metanephric adenoma (225), four had concurrent conventional (clear cell) RCC either in the same kidney (three patients) or the contralateral kidney (one patient). Secondary changes, including hyalinization, hemorrhage, and necrosis, are common. Nephrogenic adenofibroma is a biphasic neoplasm composed of an epithelial component identical to that of metanephric adenoma and a mesenchymal component consisting of bland fibroblast-like cells arranged in interlacing fascicles with focal hyalinization and myxoid change (227). The latter tumor resembles mesoblastic nephroma.

Ancillary Studies

Less than half of the reported cases have been evaluated by immunohistochemistry or electron microscopy. Antibodies to pan-CK and vimentin are positive in the large majority of cases (225–231). Positive reactions with EMA are uncommon and confined to areas showing papillary cystic tubular configurations (226,227,230). Electron microscopy shows varying numbers of microvilli and a few cytoplasmic organelles consisting mainly of free ribosomes and mitochondria (226,228–230).

Differential Diagnosis

Wilms' tumor and papillary renal carcinoma are important considerations in the differential diagnosis. In contrast to Wilms' tumor, metanephric adenoma manifests, at most, rare mitotic activity, is composed of bland cells with small nuclei, and neither contains blastemal elements nor is associated with nephrogenic rests. Distinguishing some cases of PRCC from metanephric adenoma may pose a more difficult diagnostic challenge. Unlike metanephric adenoma, however, PRCC frequently contains numerous foamy histiocytes, is multifocal in up to half of cases, and is often associated with foci of tubulopapillary hyperplasia/adenoma in the adjacent renal parenchyma.

WILMS' TUMOR (NEPHROBLASTOMA)

While Wilms' tumor is the most common genitourinary malignancy in children, it is only rarely seen in patients older than 16 years of age (234–238). The gross and microscopic appearance of the adult form is similar to that of the childhood form. Genetic abnormalities found in tumors from children, such as loss of material from 11p and isochromosome 7q, have also been described in adults (239,240). Compared with children, adults are diagnosed with higher-stage disease and have a poorer prognosis.

ANGIOMYOLIPOMA

AMLs are distinctive neoplasms composed of diverse combinations of smooth muscle, adipose tissue, and vasculature. Although they are usually found within the kidneys, they may develop at extrarenal sites, including liver (241,242), lungs (243), lymph nodes (244–246), and retroperitoneal soft tissues (247–249). While less than half of all cases occur in patients with tuberous sclerosis, it is estimated that AML will develop in 80% of patients with tuberous sclerosis (250–252). AMLs appear to be related to a family of mesenchymal tumors that include lymphangioleiomyomatosis; clear-cell sugar tumors of the lung, pancreas, and uterus; and cardiac rhabdomyomas (253). Indeed, all are composed of varying proportions of smooth muscle, epithelioid cells, adipose tissue, and vasculature and are immunoreactive with the antibody HMB-45 (253–258).

Gross Features

AMLs are not encapsulated and well circumscribed and have pushing rather than infiltrative borders. In one pub-

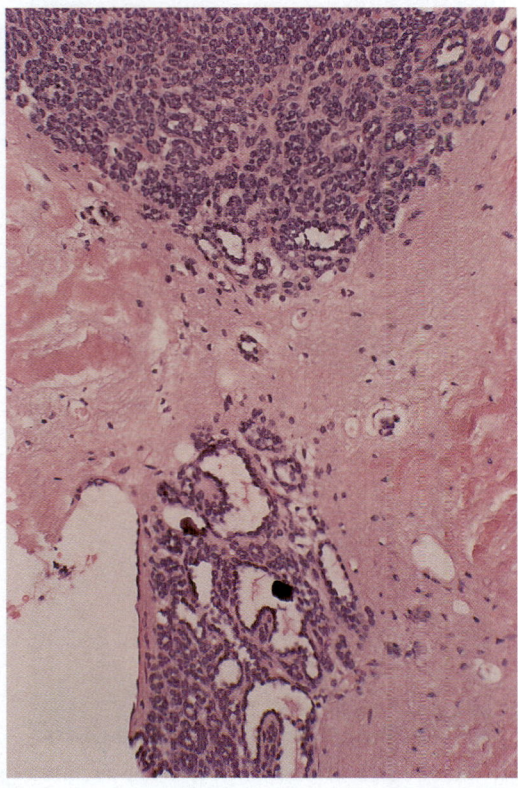

FIG. 45. Metanephric adenoma. Papillary and tubular structures lined by a monotonous population of tumor cells with small, regular nuclei and minimal amounts of cytoplasm.

lished series of 45 AMLs from Memorial Sloan-Kettering Cancer Center (259), the mean size was 6 cm (range, 0.5 cm to 25 cm). The color and consistency vary and reflect the relative proportion of adipose tissue and smooth muscle unique to each neoplasm. The classic examples are distinctive and contain soft, yellow regions admixed with more firm, tan regions (Fig. 46). Tumors composed predominantly of adipose tissue may be confused with well-differentiated liposarcoma (248), while others constituted predominantly of smooth muscle may be confused with leiomyosarcoma of sarcomatoid RCC. Small foci of hemorrhage are common, but extensive intratumoral hemorrhage is rare (259). The majority of tumors are unilateral and unifocal. The presence of bilateral or multifocal tumors strongly suggests the diagnosis of tuberous sclerosis.

Microscopic Features

AMLs are composed of differing amounts of adipose tissue, smooth muscle, and vasculature (Fig. 47). More than 90% of tumors contain at least focal areas of mature adipose tissue (259). Fat cells resembling lipoblasts are rarely seen. The smooth-muscle component ranges from fascicles of elongated spindle cells with cigar-shaped nuclei to sheets of epithelioid cells with abundant eosinophilic granular cytoplasm. The smooth-muscle cells often appear to originate and radiate from vessel walls. The morphologic features of the vascular component are inconsistent. Thickened and hyalinized vessels with eccentric lumens are seen in most cases (Fig. 48). Tumors composed predominantly of spin-

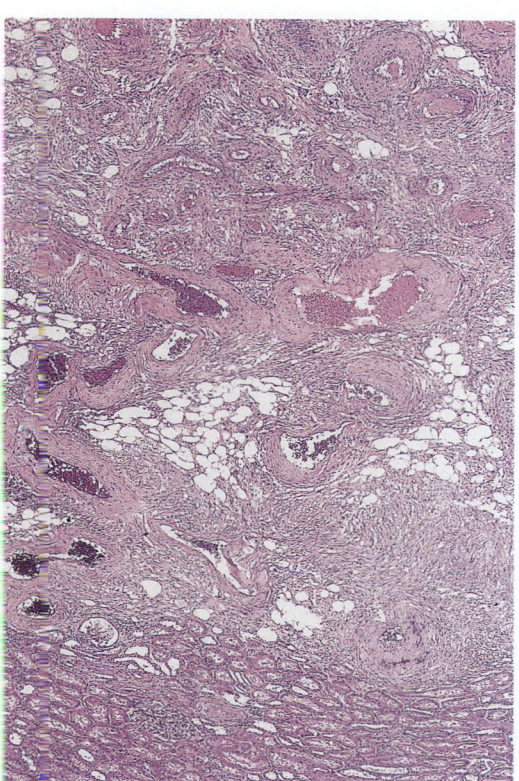

FIG. 47. Angiomyolipoma. The classic appearance is of malformed vessels, spindled myoid cells, and mature fat.

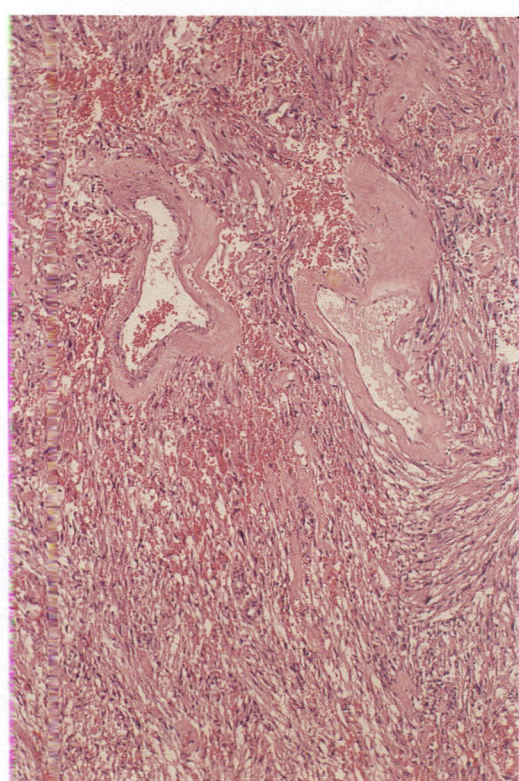

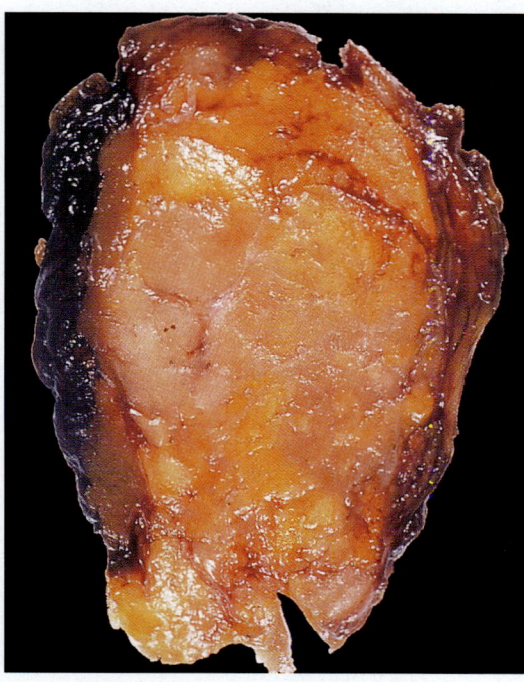

FIG. 46. Partial nephrectomy of an angiomyolipoma. The typical gross appearance shows a mixture of yellow (fatty) and tan (smooth muscle) areas.

FIG. 48. Angiomyolipoma composed of malformed vessels and spindled myoid cells. In some cases, the abnormal vessels are less apparent, which may lead to an erroneous diagnosis of leiomyosarcoma. Despite the hypercellularity and nuclear atypia, mitoses are very rare.

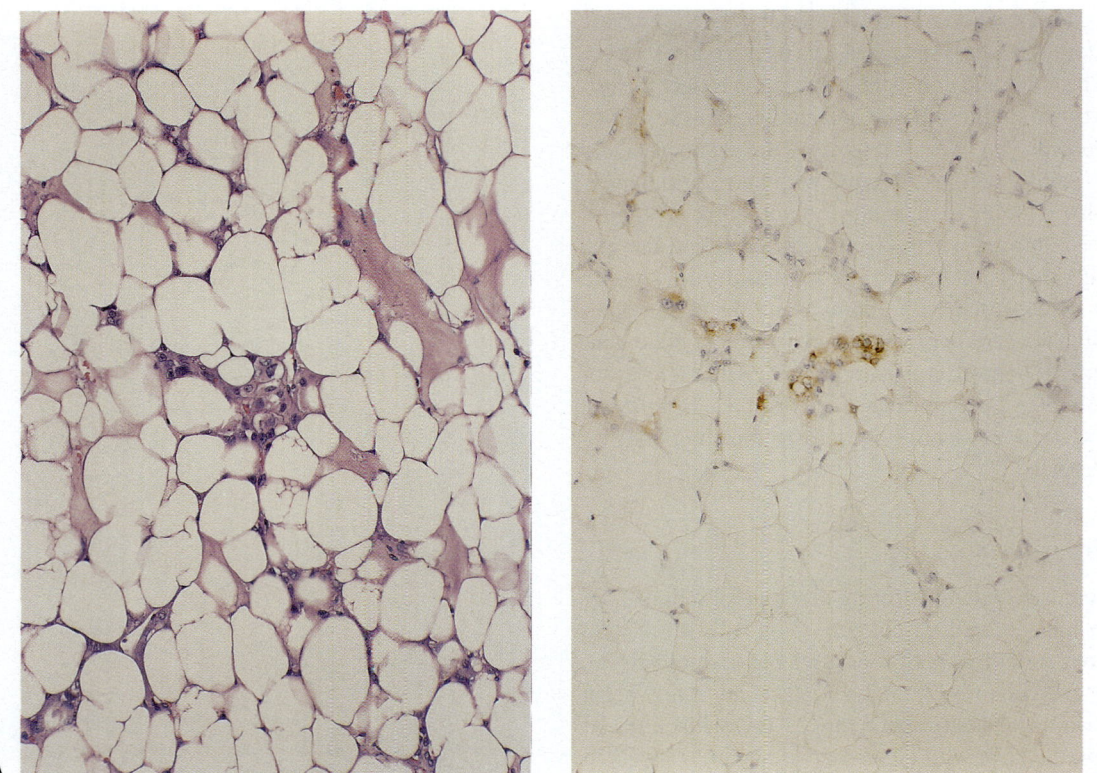

FIG. 49. Angiomyolipoma composed predominantly of mature adipose tissue, often confused with well-differentiated liposarcoma. **A:** Notice the plump epithelioid cells lining small-caliber vessels (hematoxylin and eosin stain). **B:** Immunoreactivity for HMB-45 is evident in perivascular epithelioid cells.

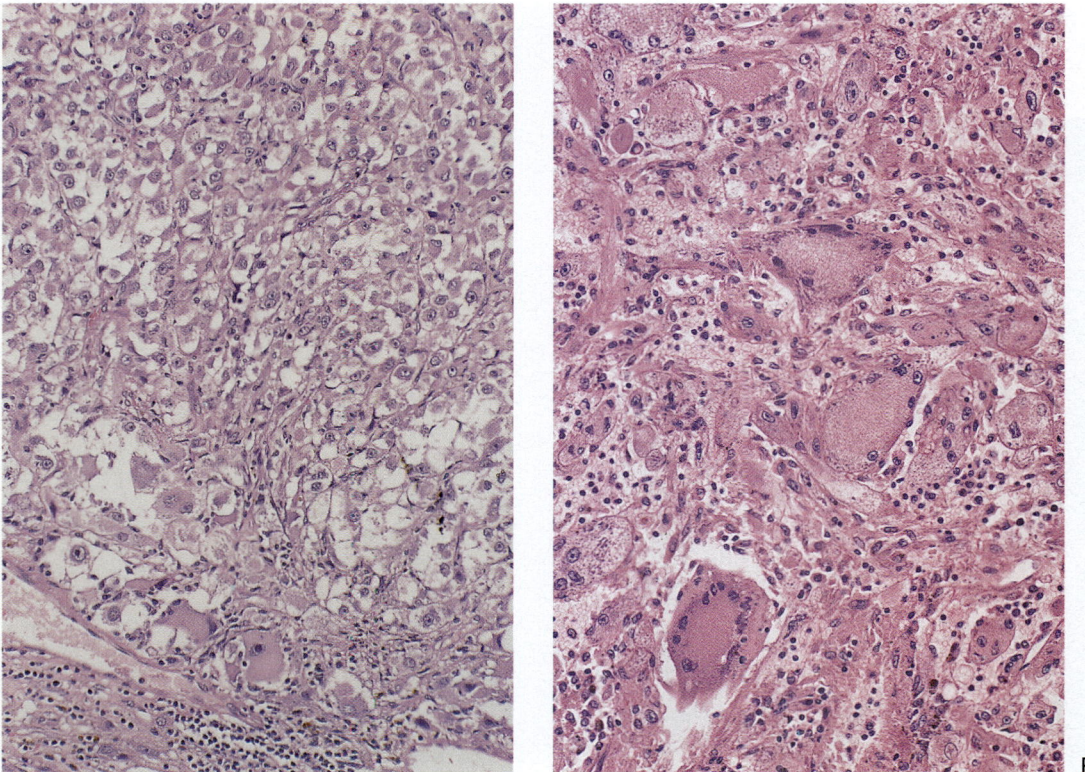

FIG. 50. Epithelioid angiomyolipoma. **A:** Epithelioid cells exhibit variably clear and granular cytoplasm, easily confused with high-grade renal cell carcinoma. **B:** Admixture of epithelioid and multinucleated giant cells.

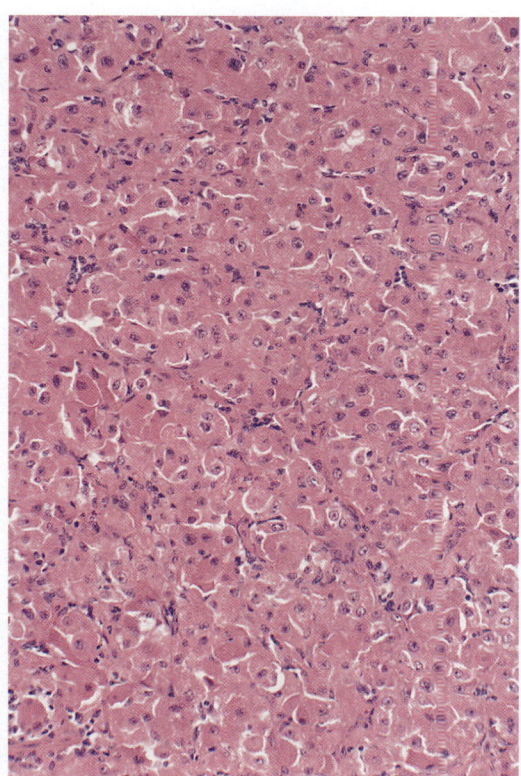

FIG. 51. Epithelioid angiomyolipoma composed exclusively of tumor cells with oncocytic cytoplasm, so-called renal epithelioid oxiphilic neoplasm.

dled smooth muscle frequently contain thin-walled vessels with a hemangiopericytoma-like architecture. Plump epithelioid cells often surround vasculature structures and may provide an important clue to the diagnosis, particularly in tumors constituted mainly of adipose tissue (Fig. 49a,b). Mitotic activity is rare.

The epithelioid variant of AML is made up either exclusively or predominantly of polygonal cells with densely eosinophilic cytoplasm (Fig. 50a,b). Varying degrees of nuclear atypia are seen, including cells with multilobulated nuclei and multinucleated forms. Focal cytoplasmic clearing, similar to that seen in so-called spider cells of cardiac rhabdomyomas, may be present. Extensive intratumoral hemorrhage and necrosis are more common in the epithelioid variant than in the classic histologic types. Rare examples of AML composed predominantly of epithelioid cells with densely eosinophilic cytoplasm reminiscent of oncocytoma have been described under the rubric renal epithelioid oxiphilic neoplasm (REON) (Fig. 51).

Ancillary Studies

In a subset of cases, periodic acid–Schiff stains reveal the presence of diastase-resistant cytoplasmic granules and rod-shaped crystals, primarily within perivascular epithelioid cells. While these crystals have an ultrastructural appearance similar to renin granules, they do not stain with either Bowie's or antibodies to renin (260). Antibodies to several melanoma-related antigens, including HMB-45 and A-103 (Melan-A/MART-1), are at least focally positive in the majority of cases (261–265) (Fig. 52). In general, 5% to 10% of cells are immunoreactive with these antibodies (259). The epithelioid smooth-muscle-cell components are most consistently positive with these antibodies, though the spindled smooth-muscle and adipose tissue components also may be positive. This observation is of particular importance in the subset of AMLs with a predominance of adipose tissue or spindled smooth muscle. In a subset of cases, ultrastructural examination reveals spherical structures with internal lamellations, suggestive of aberrant melanosomes. Rare type 2 premelanosomes and rhomboid crystals may also be seen (266,267).

Outcome

The overwhelming majority of AMLs behave in a benign fashion. The primary complication is retroperitoneal hemorrhage, which can be fatal (268–271). In this regard, size has been shown by many researchers to be an important factor for hemorrhage, prompting the recommendation that tumors larger than 4 cm be resected to avoid this complication. Renal failure may complicate massive bilateral disease, particularly in patients with tuberous sclerosis (272,273). Invasion of contiguous organs occurs rarely and has resulted in death (274).

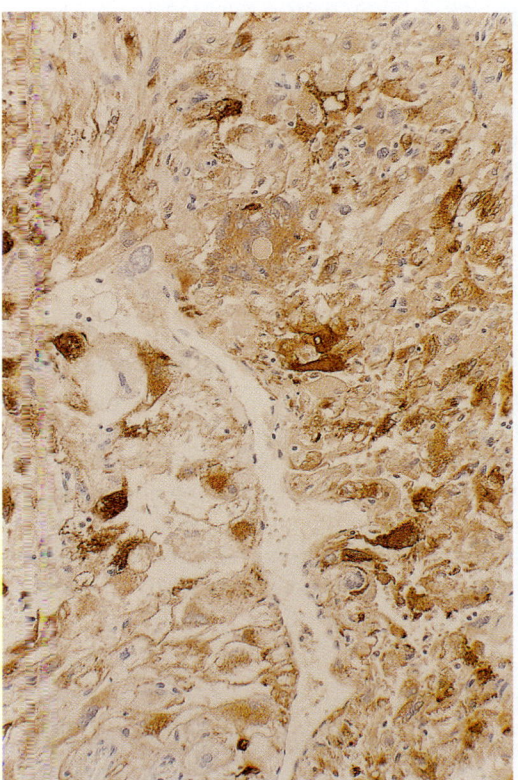

FIG. 52. Angiomyolipoma. HMB-45 immunoreactivity within epithelioid cells.

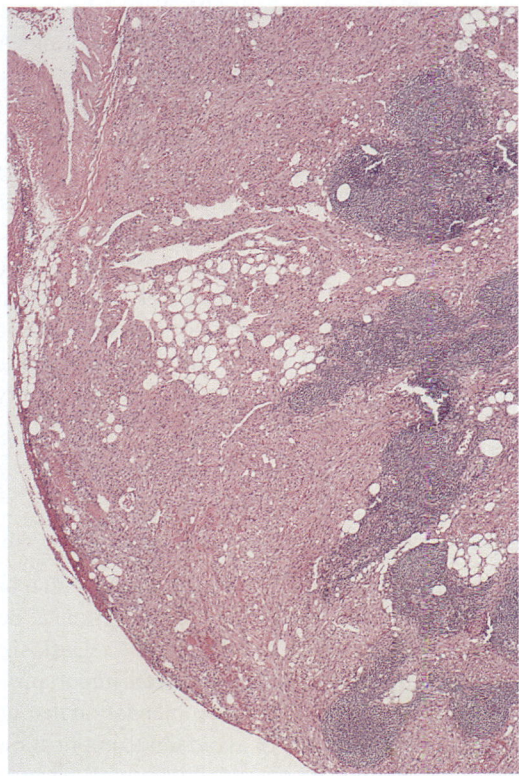

FIG. 53. Angiomyolipoma within a renal hilar lymph node, which is probably a sign of multifocality rather than metastasis.

Some patients with AML of the kidney also have AMLs involving noncontiguous sites, particularly regional lymph nodes (244–246) (Fig. 53). Most investigators consider these cases to represent multifocal rather than metastatic disease, since no patient has died from disease progression. Rare examples of sarcomatous transformation to high-grade leiomyosarcoma with subsequent distant metastases have been reported (275,276).

LIPOMA

Intrarenal lipoma is a rare neoplasm predominantly found among middle-aged women (277). Symptomatic lesions are most often associated with flank or abdominal pain and less often with hematuria. None have been reported in patients with tuberous sclerosis. The gross and microscopic features are similar to those of lipomas found at other sites. Careful examination of several tissue sections and immunohistochemical testing with antibodies to HMB-45 may be necessary to rule out the diagnosis of AML.

LIPOSARCOMA

Primary liposarcoma of the kidney is rare (278,279). More often, primary liposarcomas in the retroperitoneum secondarily involve the kidneys or perirenal tissues. In this regard, careful examination of the gross specimen is helpful in distinguishing primary versus secondary renal liposarcoma, though in some cases definitive differentiation may be impossible. For practical purposes, however, this distinction is most likely of little clinical significance, since therapy is surgical resection regardless of the primary site and because even intrarenal tumors may recur and show dedifferentiation after primary resection (279). It is of far more importance to distinguish between predominantly lipomatous AMLs and well-differentiated liposarcomas. Adequate sampling of the tumor for histologic examination and immunohistochemical testing using antibodies to HMB-45 are helpful to the differential diagnosis. All reported renal liposarcomas have been of the well-differentiated or myxoid types.

LEIOMYOMA

Acceptable examples of renal leiomyoma are rare (280,281). Tumors range from incidental, microscopic lesions found at autopsy to symptomatic masses as large as 37 kg (280). The gross and microscopic features are similar to those of leiomyoma at other sites. As is the case with smooth-muscle neoplasms arising in the retroperitoneum, mitotic activity, nuclear atypia, necrosis, and large size favor the diagnosis of leiomyosarcoma. The differential diagnosis includes mesoblastic nephroma and AML.

LEIOMYOSARCOMA

Primary renal sarcomas are estimated to comprise roughly 1% of all renal neoplasms; the majority are leiomyosarcomas (278,282). Patients most often experience symptoms of flank or abdominal pain or a palpable mass. Many tumors appear to arise from the renal capsule, while others arise from within the kidney or hilar blood vessels (278,282,283) (Fig. 54). Extension into perirenal adipose tissue and adjacent organs is common. Tumors tend to be large at diagnosis, and the majority of reported cases have been at least 10 cm in greatest dimension. On gross inspection, they are firm, white to tan, and multinodular or lobulated. Hemorrhage and necrosis are unusual. At the microscopic level, most are composed of fascicles of tapered spindle cells with blunt, ovoid nuclei. Like smooth-muscle tumors found elsewhere, mitotic activity, nuclear atypia, necrosis, and large size are indicative of malignancy. The prognosis is poor, though rare long-term survivors have been reported (278,282). The differential diagnosis includes sarcomatoid RCC and AML. In this regard, we recommend reserving tissue for possible electron microscopic studies in the case of any renal neoplasm with a gross appearance suggestive of sarcoma.

MEDULLARY FIBROMA (RENOMEDULLARY INTERSTITIAL CELL TUMOR)

Medullary fibroma (renomedullary interstitial cell tumor) is most often an unsuspected finding uncovered at the time of autopsy (284,285). An association between multiple medullary fibromas and systemic hypertension has been re-

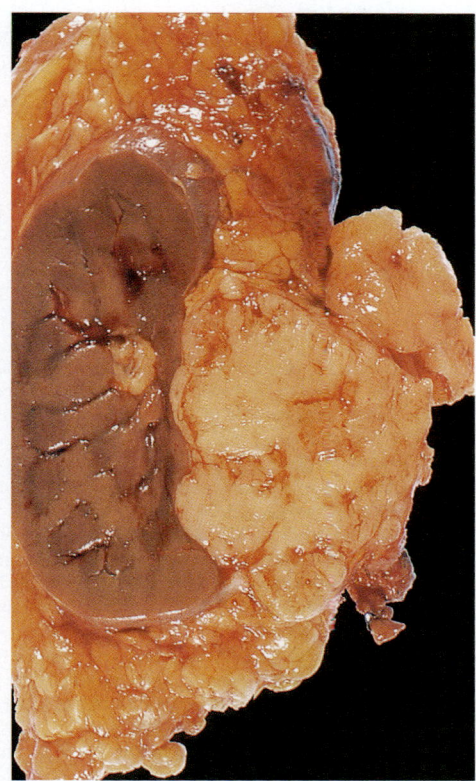

FIG. 54. Leiomyosarcoma occupying the renal hilum. It may be impossible to determine whether the tumor arises in the renal capsule or within adjacent soft tissue.

ported (285). On gross examination, these tumors, found within the renal medulla, are well circumscribed and tan to white. Most measure less than 5 mm in greatest dimension. On microscopic inspection, they consist of bland stellate cells set within a loose to densely sclerotic collagenous background (Fig. 55). Entrapped tubules may be seen at the periphery of the nodules.

OTHER MESENCHYMAL NEOPLASMS

A wide variety of other mesenchymal neoplasms now and then develop in the adult kidney and have generally been the subject of case reports or small case series. Benign tumors include solitary (localized) fibrous tumor (286,287), schwannoma (288–290), neurofibroma (291), myxoma (292), hemangioma (293,294) (Fig. 56), and lymphangioma (295,296). The four reported examples of solitary fibrous tumors were well circumscribed and apparently arose from the renal capsule. Peripheral nerve sheath tumors may arise from the renal hilum (290) and compress the adjacent kidney, or they may arise from within the renal parenchyma (289).

Primary renal hemangiopericytoma (Fig. 57) is rare and should be distinguished in its gross features from retroperitoneal hemangiopericytoma with secondary renal involvement (278,297,298) and in microscopic characteristics from juxtaglomerular cell tumor. Renal rhabdomyosarcomas in

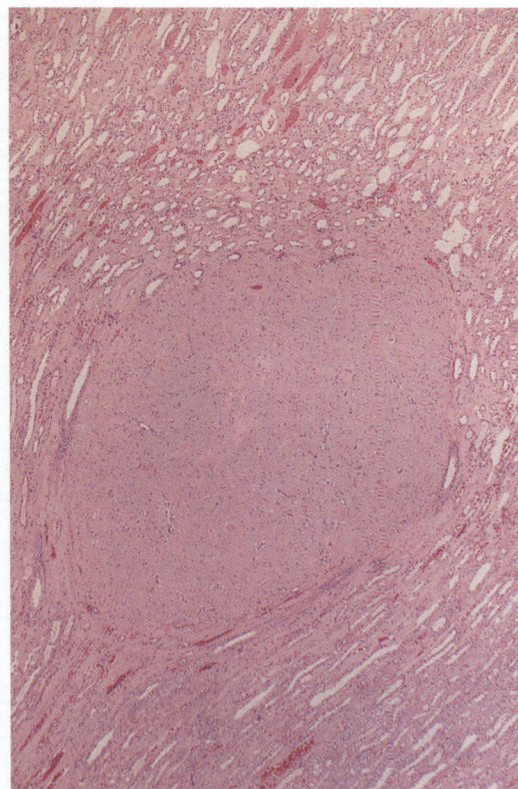

FIG. 55. Medullary fibroma (renomedullary interstitial cell tumor).

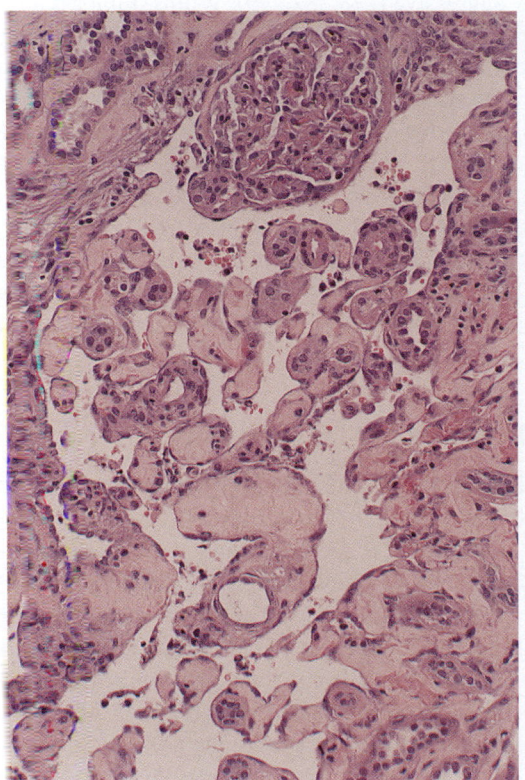

FIG. 56. Renal hemangioma. Tortuous endothelial-lined vessels infiltrate between normal renal tubules and glomeruli.

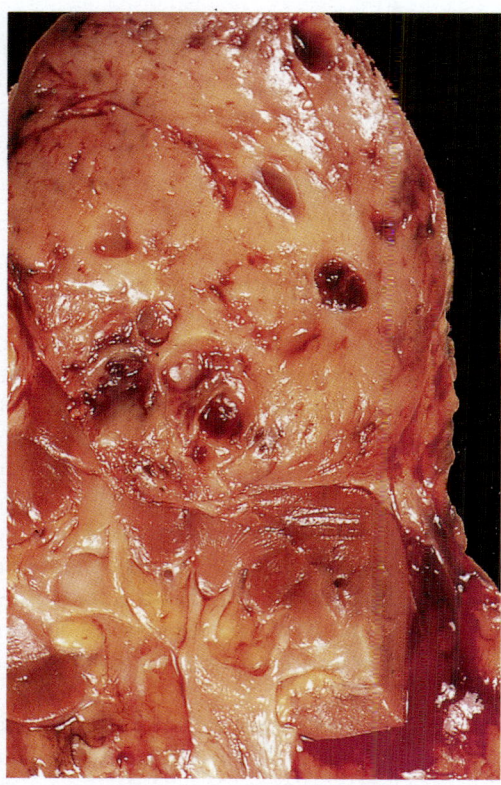

FIG. 57. Hemangiopericytoma. A tan, fleshy mass contains multiple hemorrhagic and cystic areas.

the adult are most often of the pleomorphic type and are highly aggressive (278,282,299). Wilms' tumor is an important consideration in the differential diagnosis. Acceptable cases of renal rhabdomyosarcoma should have clear-cut evidence of skeletal muscle differentiation by immunohistochemical testing or electron microscopic examination. Malignant fibrous histiocytoma (282,300–302), fibrosarcoma (282), osteogenic sarcoma (303,304), mesenchymal chondrosarcoma (305), chondrosarcoma (306), malignant mesenchymoma (307), and angiosarcoma (308,309) have also been described. Here, too, consideration should be given to sarcomatoid RCC before making the diagnosis of primary renal sarcoma.

HEMATOLOGIC MALIGNANCIES

Malignant lymphoma only rarely appears in the form of a primary, extranodal renal neoplasm (310–316). More often, renal involvement is secondary and is seen as a component of late-stage, generalized malignant lymphoma (316). Even in the context of generalized disease, however, clinical manifestations attributable to renal involvement are exceptional. This is remarkable, given that autopsy confirmation of renal parenchymal extension is seen in as many as 50% of patients with non-Hodgkin's lymphomas. On gross examination, primary renal lymphoma most often consists of a solitary, large, well-circumscribed intrarenal or hilar mass and less often consists of diffuse parenchymal infiltration. In histologic features, large-cell and noncleaved small cell lymphomas are more often low-grade lymphomas. Examples of renal plasmacytoma have also been described (317,318). Renal involvement by leukemia is most often bilateral and diffuse (316) and infrequently results in renal failure (319) or is the initial site of disease (320).

REFERENCES

1. Grawitz PA. Die Entstehung von Nierentumoren aus Nebennierengewebe. *Arch Klin Chir* 1984;30:824–834.
2. Oberling C, Rivière M, Haguenan F. Ultrastructure of clear cell epitheliomas of the kidney (hypernephroma or Grawitz tumor) and its implications for the histogenesis of the tumors. *Bull Cancer Assoc Franc* 1959;46:356–358.
3. Oberling C, Rivière M, Haguenan F. Ultrastructure of clear cells in renal carcinomas and its importance in the determination of their renal origin. *Nature* 1960;186:402–403.
4. van den Berg E, Van der Hout AH, Oosterhuis JW, et al. Cytogenetic analysis of epithelial renal-cell tumors: relationship with a new histopathological classification. *Int J Cancer* 1993;55:223–227.
5. Weiss LM, Gelb AB, Medeiros LJ. Adult renal epithelial neoplasms. *Am J Clin Pathol* 1995;103:624–635.
6. Thoenes W, Storkel S, Rumpelt JH. Histopathology and classification of renal cell tumors (adenomas, oncocytomas and carcinomas): the basic cytological and histopathological elements and their use for diagnostics. *Pathol Res Pract* 1986;181:125–143.
7. Kovacs G, Szucs S, deRiese W, Baumgartel H. Specific chromosome aberrations in human renal cell carcinoma. *Int J Cancer* 1987;40:171–180.
8. DalCin P, Gaeta J, Huben R, Li FP, Prout GR, Sandberg AA. Renal cortical tumors: cytogenetic characterization. *Am J Clin Pathol* 1989;134:27–34.
9. Kovacs G, Erlandson R, Boldog F, et al. Consistent chromosome 3p deletion and loss of heterozygosity in renal cell carcinoma. *Proc Natl Acad Sci U S A* 1988;85:1571–1575.
10. Kovacs G, Frisch S. Clonal chromosome abnormalities in tumor cells from patients with sporadic renal cell carcinomas. *Cancer Res* 1989;49:651–659.
11. Fleming S. The impact of genetics on the classification of renal carcinoma. *Histopathology* 1993;22:89–92.
12. Kovacs G, Wilkens L, Papp T, de Riese W. Differentiation between papillary and nonpapillary renal cell carcinomas by DNA analysis. *J Natl Cancer Inst* 1989;81:527–530.
13. Kovacs G, Fuzesi L, Emanual A, Kung HF. Cytogenetics of papillary renal cell tumors. *Genes Chromosom Cancer* 1991;3:249–255.
14. Kovacs G, Kung H. Non-homologous chromatid exchange in hereditary and sporadic renal cell carcinomas. *Proc Natl Acad Sci U S A* 1991;88:194–198.
15. Kovacs G. Molecular differential pathology of renal tumours. *Histopathology* 1993;22:1–8.
16. Presti JC Jr, Rao PH, Chen Q, et al. Histopathological, cytogenetic, and molecular characterization of renal cortical tumors. *Cancer Res* 1991;51:1544–1552.
17. Meloni AM, Bridge J, Sandberg AA. Reviews on chromosome studies in urological tumors. I. Renal tumors. *J Urol* 1992;148:253–265.
18. Fleming S. The impact of genetics on the classification of renal carcinoma. *Histopathology* 1993;22:89–92.
19. Hughson MD, Johnson LD, Silva FG, Kovacs G. Nonpapillary and papillary renal cell carcinoma: a cytogenetic and phenotypic study. *Mod Pathol* 1993;6:449–456.
20. Presti JC Jr, Reuter VE, Cordon-Cardo C, et al. Allelic deletions in renal tumors: histopathological correlations. *Cancer Res* 1993;53:80–83.
21. Yoshida MA, Ohyashiki K, Ochi H, et al. Cytogenetic studies of tumor tissue from patients with nonfamilial renal cell carcinoma. *Cancer Res* 1986;46:2139–2147.
22. Carrol PR, Murty VVS, Reuter VE, et al. Abnormalities at chromosome region 3q11.2-14 characterize clear cell carcinoma. *Cancer Genet Cytogenet* 1987;26:253–259.
23. Kovacs G, Akhtar M, Beckwith BJ, et al. The Heidelberg classification of renal cell tumours. *J Pathol* 1997;183:131–133.

24. Storkel S, Eble JN, Adlakha K, et al. Classification of renal cell carcinoma. *Cancer* 1997;80:987–989.
25. Motzer RJ, Bander NH, Nanus DM. Renal-cell carcinoma. *N Engl J Med* 1996;335:865–875.
26. Kosary CL, McLaughlin JK. Kidney and renal pelvis. In: Miller BA, Ries LAG, Hankey BF, et al., eds. *SEER cancer statistics review, 1970–1990*. Bethesda: National Cancer Institute, 1993. (NIH publication no. 93–2789, XI.1-XI.22.)
27. Parkin DM, Pisani P, Ferlay J. Estimates of the worldwide incidence of eighteen major cancers in 1985. *Int J Cancer* 1993;54:594–606.
28. Pisani P, Parkin DM, Ferlay J. Estimates of the worldwide mortality from eighteen major cancers in 1985: implications for prevention and projection of future burden. *Int J Cancer* 1993;54:891–903.
29. Richie AWS, Chisholm GD. The natural history of renal carcinoma. *Semin Oncol* 1983;10:390–400.
30. Porena M, Vespasiani G, Rosi P, et al. Incidentally detected renal cell carcinoma: role of ultrasonography. *J Clin Ultrasound* 1992;20:395–400.
31. Konnack JW, Grossman HB. Renal cell carcinoma as an incidental finding. *J Urol* 1985;134:1094–1096.
32. Thompson IM, Peck JM. Improvement in survival of patients with renal cell carcinoma: the role of the serendipitously detected tumor. *J Urol* 1988;140:487–490.
33. Bryant DA, Scheinfeld AG, Russo P, et al. Conventional renal cell carcinoma: a clinicopathologic study of 183 cases from 1991 to 1994. *Mod Pathol* 1998;11:77a(abst).
34. Mellemgaard A, Lindblad P, Schlehofer B, et al. International renal-cell cancer study. III. Role of weight, height, physical activity and use of amphetamines. *Int J Cancer* 1995;60:350–354.
35. Mandel JS, McLaughlin JK, Schlehofer B, et al. International renal-cell cancer study. IV. Occupation. *Int J Cancer* 1995;61:601–605.
36. Wolk A, Gridley G, Niwa S, et al. International renal-cell cancer study. VII. Role of diet. *Int J Cancer* 1996;65:67–73.
37. McLaughlin JK, Mandel JS, Blot WJ, et al. A population-based case-control study of renal cell carcinoma. *J Natl Cancer Inst* 1984;72:275–284.
38. Yu MC, Mack TM, Hanisch R, et al. Cigarette smoking, obesity, diuretic use, and coffee consumption as risk factors for renal cell carcinoma. *J Natl Cancer Inst* 1986;77:351–356.
39. Wolk A, Lindblad P, Adami H-O. Nutrition and renal cell cancer. *Cancer Causes Control* 1996;7:5–18.
40. Lindblad P, Mellemgaard A, Schlehofer B, et al. International renal-cell cancer study. V. Reproductive factors, gynecologic operations and exogenous hormones. *Int J Cancer* 1995;61:192–198.
41. Mellemgaard A, Engholm G, McLaughlin JK, et al. Risk factors for renal cell carcinoma in Denmark. I. Role of socioeconomic status, tobacco use, beverages and family history. *Cancer Causes Control* 1994;5:105–113.
42. Delahunt B, Bethwaite PB, Nacey JN. Occupational risk of renal cell carcinoma: a case-control study based on the New Zealand cancer registry. *Br J Urol* 1995;75:578–582.
43. Bugert P, Kovacs G. Molecular differential diagnosis of renal cell carcinoma. *Am J Pathol* 1996;149:2081–2088.
44. Steiner G, Sidransky D. Molecular differential diagnosis of renal carcinoma: from microscopes to microsatellites. *Am J Pathol* 1996;149:1791–1795.
45. Wagner JR, Linehan WM. Molecular genetics of renal cancer. *Semin Urol Oncol* 1996;14:244–249.
46. Richards FM, Payne SJ, Zbar B, et al. Molecular analysis of de novo germline mutations in the von Hippel–Lindau disease gene. *Hum Mol Genet* 1995;4:2139–2143.
47. Poston CD, Jaffe GS, Lubensky IA, et al. Characterization of the renal pathology of a familial form of renal cell carcinoma associated with von Hippel–Lindau disease: clinical and molecular genetic implications. *J Urol* 1995;153:22–26.
48. Linehan WM, Lerman MI, Zbar B. Identification of the von Hippel–Lindau (VHL) gene: its role in renal cancer. *JAMA* 1995;273:564–570.
49. Suzuki H, Ueda T, Komiya A, et al. Mutational state of von Hippel–Lindau and adenomatous polyposis coli genes in renal tumors. *Oncology* 1997;54:252–257.
50. Zbar B, Tory K, Merino M, et al. Hereditary papillary renal cell carcinoma. *J Urol* 1994;151:561–566.
51. Zbar B, Glenn G, Lubensky I, et al. Hereditary papillary renal cell carcinoma: clinical studies in 10 families. *J Urol* 1995;153:907–912.
52. King CR, Schminke RN, Arthur T, et al. Proximal 3p deletion in renal cell carcinoma cells from a patient with von Hippel–Lindau disease. *Cancer Genet Cytogenet* 1987;27:345–348.
53. Jordan DK, Patil SR, Divelbiss JE, et al. Cytogenetic abnormalities in tumors of patients with von Hippel–Lindau disease. *Cancer Genet Cytogenet* 1989;42:227–241.
54. Cohen MD, Goodman BK, Lubin MB, et al. Cytogenetic characterization of renal cell carcinoma in von Hippel–Lindau syndrome. *Cancer* 1990;65:1150–1154.
55. Cohen AJ, Li FP, Berg S, et al. Hereditary renal-cell carcinoma associated with a chromosomal translocation. *N Engl J Med* 1979;301:592–595.
56. Pathak S, Strong LC, Ferrell RE, et al. Familial renal cell carcinoma with a 3;11 chromosome translocation limited to tumor cells. *Science* 1982;217:939–941.
57. Schmidt L, Duh F-M, Chen F, et al. Germline and somatic mutations in the tyrosine kinase domain of the MET proto-oncogene in papillary renal carcinomas. *Nature Genet* 1997;16:68–73.
58. Duh F-M, Scherer SW, Tsui L-C, et al. Gene structure of the Met proto-oncogene. *Oncogene* 1997;15:1583–1586.
59. Weirich G, Glenn G, Junker K, et al. Familial renal oncocytoma: clinicopathologic study of 5 families. *J Urol* 1998;160:335–340.
60. Fuhrman SA, Lasky LC, Limas C. Prognostic significance of morphologic parameters in renal cell carcinoma. *Am J Surg Pathol* 1982;6:655–663.
61. Schoumann M, Warter A, Ross M, Bollock C. Renal cell carcinoma: statistical study of survival based on pathological criteria. *World J Urol* 1984;2:109–113.
62. Medeiros LJ, Gelb AB, Weiss LM. Renal cell carcinoma: prognostic significance of morphologic parameters in 121 cases. *Cancer* 1988;61:1639–1651.
63. Goldstein NS. The current state of renal cell carcinoma grading. *Cancer* 1997;80:977–980.
64. Medeiros LJ, Jones EC, Aizawa S, et al. Grading of renal cell carcinoma. *Cancer* 1997;80:990–991.
65. Hermanek P, Schrott KM. Evaluation of the new tumor, nodes and metastases classification of renal cell carcinomas. *J Urol* 1990;144:238–242.
66. Hermanek P, Sigel A, Chlepas S. Histological grading of renal cell carcinoma. *Eur Urol* 1976;2:189–191.
67. Syrjanen K, Hjelt L. Grading of human renal adenocarcinoma. *Scand J Urol Nephrol* 1978;12:49–55.
68. Skinner DG, Colvin RB, Vermillion CD, et al. Diagnosis and management of renal cell carcinoma. *Cancer* 1971;28:1165–1177.
69. Langan D, Conroy R, Barry-Walsh C, et al. A comparative analysis of grading systems in renal carcinoma. *Histopathology* 1994;24:473–476.
70. Amin MB, Corless CL, Renshaw AA, Tickoo SK, Kubus J, Schultz DS. Papillary (chromophil) renal cell carcinoma: histomorphologic characteristics and evaluation of conventional pathologic prognostic parameters in 62 cases. *Am J Surg Pathol* 1997;21:621–635.
71. Robson CJ, Churchill BM, Anderson W. The results of radical nephrectomy for renal cell carcinoma. *J Urol* 1969;101:297–301.
72. Beahrs OH, Henson DE, Hutter RVP, Kennedy BJ, eds. *Handbook for staging of cancer*. American Joint Committee on Cancer, 4th ed. Philadelphia: JB Lippincott Co, 1993.
73. Fleming ID, Cooper JS, Henson DE, eds. *AJCC cancer staging manual*. American Joint Committee on Cancer, 5th ed. Philadelphia: JB Lippincott Co, 1997.
74. Guinan P, Sobin LH, Algaba F, et al. TMN staging in renal cell carcinoma. *Cancer* 1997;80:992–993.
75. Nordenson I, Ljungberg B, Roos G. Chromosomes in renal carcinoma with reference to intratumor heterogeneity. *Cancer Genet Cytogenet* 1988;32:35–41.
76. Walter TA, Berger CS, Sandberg AA. The cytogenetics of renal tumors. Where do we stand, where do we go? *Cancer Genet Cytogenet* 1989;43:15–34.
77. Teyssier JR, Ferre D. Chromosomal changes in renal cell carcinoma: no evidence for correlation with clinical stage. *Cancer Genet Cytogenet* 1990;45:197–205.
78. Zbar B, Brauch H, Talmadge C, Linehan M. Loss of alleles of loci on the short arm of chromosome 3 in renal cell carcinoma. *Nature* 1987;327:721–724.
79. van der Hout AH, Kok K, van den Berg E, et al. Direct molecular analysis of a deletion of 3p in tumors from patients with sporadic renal cell carcinoma. *Cancer Genet Cytogenet* 1988;32:281–285.

80. Anglard P, Tory K, Brauch H, et al. Molecular analysis of genetic changes in the origin and development of renal cell carcinoma. Cancer Res 1991;51:1071–1077.
81. Ogawa O, Kakehi Y, Ogawa O, et al. Allelic loss at chromosome 3p characterizes clear cell phenotype of renal cell carcinoma. Cancer Res 1991;51:949–953.
82. Eble JN, Bonsib SM. Extensively cystic renal neoplasms: cystic nephroma, cystic partially differentiated nephroblastoma, multilocular cystic renal cell carcinoma, and cystic hamartoma of renal pelvis. Semin Diagn Pathol 1998;15:2–20.
83. Murad T, Komaiko W, Oyasu R, et al. Multilocular cystic renal cell carcinoma. Am J Clin Pathol 1991;95:633–637.
84. Taxy JB, Marshall FF. Multilocular renal cysts in adults: possible relationship to renal adenocarcinoma. Arch Pathol Lab Med 1983;107:633–637.
85. Tamura Y, Okamura K, Ogura H, et al. Multilocular cystic renal cell carcinoma: report of 2 cases. Acta Urol Jpn 1990;36:437–441.
86. Sakurai M, Sugimura Y, Satani H, et al. Multilocular cystic renal cell carcinoma: a report of two cases. Acta Urol Jpn 1993;39:45–49.
87. Mancilla-Jimenez R, Stanley RJ, Blath RA. Papillary renal cell carcinoma: a clinical, radiologic, and pathologic study of 34 cases. Cancer 1976;38:2469–2480.
88. El Naggar AK, Ro JY, Ensign LG. Papillary renal cell carcinoma: clinical implication of DNA content analysis. Hum Pathol 1993;24:316–321.
89. Kovacs G. Papillary renal cell carcinoma: a morphologic and cytogenetic study of 11 cases. Am J Pathol 1989;134(1):27–34.
90. Kovacs G. Molecular differential pathology of renal cell tumours. Histopathology 1993;22:1–8.
91. Henn W, Zwergel T, Wullich B, Thonnes M, Zang KD, Seitz G. Bilateral multicentric papillary renal tumors with heteroclonal origin based on tissue-specific karyotype instability. Cancer 1993;72(4):1315–1318.
92. Ishikawa I, Shikura N, Ozaki M. Papillary renal cell carcinoma with numeric changes of chromosomes in a long-term hemodialysis patient: a karyotype analysis. Am J Kidney Dis 1993;21(5):553–556.
93. van den Berg E, van der Hout AH, Oosterhuis JW, et al. Cytogenetic analysis of epithelial renal-cell tumors: relationship with a new histopathological classification. Int J Cancer 1993;55(2):223–227.
94. deJong B, Molenaar IM, Leeuw JA, Idenberg VJS, Oosterhuis JW. Cytogenetics of a renal adenocarcinoma in a 2 year-old child. Cancer Genet Cytogenet 1986;21:165–169.
95. Shipley JM, Birdsall S, Clark J, et al. Mapping the X chromosome breakpoint in two papillary renal cell carcinoma cell lines with a t(X;1)(p11.2;q21.2) and the first report of a female case. Cytogenet Cell Genet 1995;71(3):280–284.
96. Sidhar SK, Clark J, Gill S, et al. The t(X;1)(p11.2;q21.2) translocation in papillary renal cell carcinoma fuses a novel gene to the TFE3 transcription factor gene. Hum Mol Genet 1996;5(9):1333–1338.
97. Renshaw AA, Corless CL. Papillary renal cell carcinoma: histology and immunohistochemistry. Am J Surg Pathol 1995;19(7):842–849.
98. Lager DJ, Huston BJ, Timmerman TG, Bonsib SM. Papillary renal tumors: morphologic, cytochemical, and genotypic features. Cancer 1995;76:669–673.
99. Renshaw AA, Corless CL. Papillary renal cell carcinoma: histology and immunohistochemistry. Am J Surg Pathol 1995;19:842–849.
100. Reuter VE, Scheinfeld AG, Hamed G, et al. Papillary renal cell carcinoma: clinicopathologic study of 81 tumors. Am J Surg Pathol 1998 (in press).
101. Renshaw AA, Zhang H, Corless CL, et al. Solid variants of papillary (chromophil) renal cell carcinoma: clinicopathologic and genetic features. Am J Surg Pathol 1997;21:1203–1209.
102. Amin MB, Corless CL, Renshaw AA, et al. Papillary (chromophil) renal cell carcinoma: histologic characteristics and evaluation of conventional pathologic parameters in 62 cases. Am J Surg Pathol 1997;21:621–635.
103. Delahunt B, Eble JN. Papillary renal cell carcinoma: a clinicopathologic and immunohistochemical study of 105 tumors. Mod Pathol 1997;10:537–544.
104. Thoenes W, Storkel S, Rumpelt H-J. Human chromophobe cell renal carcinoma. Virchows Arch B Cell Pathol 1995;48:207–217.
105. Thoenes W, Storkel S, Rumpelt H-J, et al. Chromophobe cell renal carcinoma and its variants: a report on 32 cases. J Pathol 1988;155:277–287.
106. Akhtar M, Kardar H, Linjawi T, et al. Chromophobe cell carcinoma of the kidney: a clinicopathologic study of 21 cases. Am J Surg Pathol 1995;19:1245–1256.
107. Crotty TB, Farrow GM, Lieber MM. Chromophobe cell renal carcinoma: clinicopathologic features of 50 cases. J Urol 1995;154:964–967.
108. Cochand-Priollet B, Molinie V, Bougaran J, et al. Renal chromophobe cell carcinoma and oncocytoma: a comparative morphologic, histochemical, and immunohistochemical study of 124 cases. Arch Pathol Lab Med 1997;121:1081–1086.
109. DeLong WH, Sakr W, Grignon D. Chromophobe renal cell carcinoma: a comparative histochemical and immunohistochemical study. J Urol Pathol 1996;4:1–8.
110. Renshaw AA, Henske EP, Loughlin KR, et al. Aggressive variants of chromophobe renal cell carcinoma. Cancer 1996;78:56–61.
111. Bonsib SM, Lager DJ. Chromophobe cell carcinoma: analysis of five cases. Am J Surg Pathol 1990;14:260–267.
112. Bugert P, Gaul C, Weber K, et al. Specific genetic changes of diagnostic importance in chromophobe renal cell carcinomas. Lab Invest 1997;76:203–208.
113. Schwerdtle RF, Storkel S, Neuhaus C, et al. Allelic losses at chromosomes 1p, 2p, 6p, 10p, 13q, 17p, and 21q significantly correlate with the chromophobe subtype of renal carcinoma. Cancer Res 1996;56:2927–2930.
114. Kovacs A, Kovacs G. Low chromosome number in chromophobe renal cell carcinomas. Genes Chromosom Cancer 1992;4:267–268.
115. van den Berg E, van der Hout AH, Oosterhuis JW, et al. Cytogenetic analysis of epithelial renal-cell tumors: relationship with a new histopathological classification. Int J Cancer 1993;55:223–227.
116. Akhtar M, Al-Sohaibani MO, Haleem A, et al. Flow cytometric DNA analysis of chromophobe cell carcinoma of the kidney. J Urol Pathol 1996;4:15–23.
117. Kovacs A, Storkel S, Thoenes W, Kovacs G. Mitochondrial and chromosomal DNA alterations in human chromophobe renal cell carcinomas. J Pathol 1992;167:273–277.
118. Akhtar M, Tulbah A, Kardar AH, et al. Sarcomatoid renal cell carcinoma: the chromophobe connection. Am J Surg Pathol 1997;21:1188–1195.
119. Storkel S, Steart PV, Drenckhahn D, Thoenes W. The human chromophobe cell renal carcinoma: its probable relation to intercalated cells of the collecting duct. Virchows Arch B Cell Pathol 1989;56:237–245.
120. Bonsib SM. Renal chromophobe cell carcinoma: the relationship between cytoplasmic vesicles and colloidal iron stain. J Urol Pathol 1996;4:9–14.
121. Thoenes W, Baum H-P, Storkel S, Muller M. Cytoplasmic microvesicles in chromophobe cell renal carcinoma demonstrated by freeze fracture. Virchows Arch B Cell Pathol 1987;54:127–130.
122. Bonsib SM, Bray C, Timmerman TG. Renal chromophobe cell carcinoma: limitations of paraffin-embedded tissue. Ultrastruct Pathol 1993;17:529–536.
123. Gerharz C-D, Moll R, Storkel S, et al. Ultrastructural appearance and cytoskeletal architecture of the clear, chromophilic, and chromophobe types of human renal cell carcinoma in vitro. Am J Pathol 1993;142:851–859.
124. Erlandson RA, Shek TW, Reuter VE. Diagnostic significance of mitochondria in four types of renal epithelial neoplasms: an ultrastructural study of 60 tumors. Ultrastruct Pathol 1997;21:409–417.
125. Tickoo SK, Amin MB, Linden MD, et al. Antimitochondrial antibody (113-1) in the differential diagnosis of granular renal cell tumors. Am J Surg Pathol 1997;21:922–930.
126. Zippel L. Zur Kenntnis der Onkocytonen. Virchows Arch A Pathol Anat Histopathol 1942;308:360–382.
127. Klein MJ, Valensi QJ. Proximal tubular adenomas of kidney with so-called oncocytic features: a clinicopathologic study of 13 cases of a rarely reported neoplasm. Cancer 1976;38:906–914.
128. Choi H, Almagro UA, McManus JT, Norback DH, Jacobs SC. Renal oncocytoma: a clinicopathologic study. Cancer 1983;51:1887–1896.
129. Frydenberg M, Eckstein RP, Saalfield JA, Breslin FH, Alexander JH, Roche J. Renal oncocytomas: an Australian experience. Br J Urol 1991;67:352–357.
130. Lieber MM, Tomera KM, Farrow GM. Renal oncocytoma. J Urol 1981;125:481–485.
131. Perez-Ordonez B, Hamed G, Campbell S, et al. Renal oncocytoma: a clinicopathologic study of 70 cases. Am J Surg Pathol 1997;21:871–883.

132. Amin MB, Crotty TB, Tickoo SK, Farrow GM. Renal oncocytoma: a reappraisal of morphologic features with clinicopathologic findings in 80 cases. *Am J Surg Pathol* 1997;21:1–12.
133. Crotty TB, Lawrence KM, Moertel CA, et al. Cytogenetic analysis of six renal oncocytomas and a chromophobe cell renal carcinoma: evidence that -Y, -1 may be a characteristic anomaly in renal oncocytomas [Comments]. *Cancer Genet Cytogenet* 1992;61:61–66.
134. Fuzesi L, Gunawan B, Braun S, Boeckmann W. Renal oncocytoma with a translocation t(9;11)(p23;q13). *J Urol* 1994;152:471–472.
135. Neuhaus C, Dijkhuizen T, van den Berg E, et al. Involvement of the chromosomal region 11q13 in renal oncocytoma: case report and literature review. *Cancer Genet Cytogenet* 1997;94:95–98.
136. Walter TA, Pennington RD, Decker HJ, Sandberg AA. Translocation t(9;11)(p23;q12): a primary chromosomal change in renal oncocytoma. *J Urol* 1989;142:117–119.
137. van den Berg E, Dijkhuizen T, Storkel S, et al. Chromosomal changes in renal oncocytomas: evidence that t(5;11)(q35;q13) may characterize a second subgroup of oncocytomas. *Cancer Genet Cytogenet* 1995;79:164–168.
138. Davis CJJ, Mostofi FK, Sesterhenn IA, Ho CK. Renal oncocytoma: clinicopathological study of 166 patients. *J Urogen Pathol* 1991;1:41–52.
139. Tickoo SK, Reuter VE, Amin MB, et al. Renal oncocytosis; morphologic spectrum and morphogenetic considerations: a study of 10 cases. *Mod Pathol* 1998;11:97a(abst).
140. Fleming S, Lewi HJE. Collecting duct carcinoma of the kidney. *Histopathology* 1986;10:1131–1141.
141. Kennedy SM, Merino MJ, Linehan WM, et al. Collecting duct carcinoma of the kidney. *Hum Pathol* 1990;21:449–456.
142. Amin MB, Varma MD, Tickoo SK, et al. Collecting duct carcinoma of the kidney. *Adv Anat Pathol* 1997;4:85–94.
143. Srigley JR, Eble JN. Collecting duct carcinoma of the kidney. *Semin Diagn Pathol* 1998;15:54–67.
144. Rumpelt HJ, Storkel S, Moll R, et al. Bellini duct carcinoma: further evidence for this rare variant of renal cell carcinoma. *Histopathology* 1991;18:115–122.
145. Dimopoulos MA, Logothesis CJ, Markowitz A, et al. Collecting duct carcinoma of the kidney. *Br J Urol* 1993;71:388–391.
146. Polascik TJ, Cairns P, Epstein JI, et al. Distal nephron tumors: microsatellite allelotype. *Cancer Res* 1996;56:1892–1895.
147. Schoenberg M, Cairns P, Brooks JD, et al. Frequent loss of chromosome arms 8p and 13q in collecting duct carcinoma (CDC) of the kidney. *Genes Chromosom Cancer* 1995;12:75–80.
148. Steiner G, Cairns P, Polascik TJ, et al. High-density mapping of chromosomal arm 1q in renal collecting duct carcinoma: region of minimal deletion at 1q32.1-32.2. *Cancer Res* 1996;56:5044–5046.
149. Gregori-Romero MA, Morell-Quadreny L, Llombart-Bosch. Cytogenetic analysis of three primary Bellini duct carcinomas. *Genes Chromosom Cancer* 1996;15:170–172.
150. Fuzesi L, Cober M, Mittermayer C. Collecting duct carcinoma: cytogenetic characterization. *Histopathology* 1992;21:155–160.
151. MacLennan GT, Farrow GM, Bostwick DG. Low-grade collecting duct carcinoma of the kidney: report of 13 cases of low-grade mucinous tubulocystic renal carcinoma of possible collecting duct origin. *Urology* 1997;50:679–684.
152. Baer SC, Ro JY, Ordonez NG, et al. Sarcomatoid collecting duct carcinoma: a clinicopathologic and immunohistochemical study of five cases. *Hum Pathol* 1993;24:1017–1022.
153. Davis CJ, Mostofi FK, Sesterhenn IA. Renal medullary carcinoma: the seventh sickle cell nephropathy. *Am J Surg Pathol* 1995;19:1–11.
154. Figenshau RS, Basler JW, Ritter JH, et al. Renal medullary carcinoma. *J Urol* 1998;159:711–713.
155. Avery RE, Harris JE, Davis CJ, et al. Renal medullary carcinoma: clinical and therapeutics aspects of a newly described tumor. *Cancer* 1996;78:128–132.
156. Rodriguez-Jurado R, Gonzalez-Crussi F. Renal medullary carcinoma: immunohistochemical and ultrastructural observations. *J Urol Pathol* 1996;4:191–203.
157. Friedrichs P, Larsen P, Canby E, et al. Renal medullary carcinoma and sickle cell trait. *J Urol* 1997;157:1349–1351.
158. Herring JC, Schmetz MA, Digan AB, et al. Renal medullary carcinoma: a recently described highly aggressive renal tumor in young black patients. *J Urol* 1997;157:2246–2247.
159. Adsay V, Grignon D, Eble J, Jones E, Srigley J. Solid and cystic biphasic tumor of the adult kidney. *Mod Pathol* 1998;11:74a(abst).
160. Block NL, Grabstald HG, Melamed MR. Congenital mesoblastic nephroma (leiomyomatous hamartoma): first adult case. *J Urol* 1973;110:380–383.
161. Durham JR, Bostwick DG, Farrow GM, Ohorodnik JM. Mesoblastic nephroma of adulthood: report of three cases. *Am J Surg Pathol* 1993;17:1029–1038.
162. Levin NP, Damjanov I, Depillis VJ. Mesoblastic nephroma in an adult patient: recurrence 21 years after removal of the primary lesion. *Cancer* 1982;49:573–577.
163. Pawade J, Soosay GN, Delprado W, Parkinson MC, Rode J. Cystic hamartoma of the renal pelvis. *Am J Surg Pathol* 1993;17:1169–1175.
164. Prats Lopez J, Palou Redorta J, Morote Robles J, Martinez Perez E, Luiz Marcellan C. Leiomyomatous renal hamartoma in an adult. *Eur Urol* 1988;14:80–82.
165. Trillo AA. Adult variant of congenital mesoblastic nephroma. *Arch Pathol Lab Med* 1990;114:533–535.
166. Truong LD, Williams R, Ngo T, et al. Adult mesoblastic nephroma: expansion of the morphologic spectrum and review of literature. *Am J Surg Pathol* 1998;22:827–839.
167. Tuban A, Kardar AH, Akhtar M. Mesoblastic nephroma in an adult. *J Urol Pathol* 1997;6:67–73.
168. Antonescu C, Bisceglia M, Reuter VE, et al. Sarcomatous transformation of cystic nephroma in adults. *Mod Pathol* 1997;10:69a(abst).
169. Robertson PW, Klidjian A, Harding LK, Walters G, Lee MR, Robb-Smith AH. Hypertension due to a renin-secreting renal tumour. *Am J Med* 1967;43:963–976.
170. Kihara I, Kitamura S, Hoshino T, Seida H, Watanabe T. A hitherto unreported vascular tumor of the kidney: a proposal of "juxtaglomerular cell tumor." *Acta Pathol Jpn* 1968;18:197–206.
171. Bocet R, Taylor M, Vachalova H, Pycha K. Juxtaglomerular cell tumor: an immunohistochemical, electron-microscopic, and in situ hybridization study. *Am J Surg Pathol* 1994;18:837–842.
172. Squires JP, Ulbright TM, De Schryver-Kecskemeti K, Engleman W. Juxtaglomerular cell tumor of the kidney. *Cancer* 1984;53:516–523.
173. Tanaka T, Okumura A, Mori H. Juxtaglomerular cell tumor. *Arch Pathol Lab Med* 1993;117:1161–1164.
174. Tetu B, Vaillancourt L, Camilleri JP, Bruneval P, Bernier L, Tourigny R. Juxtaglomerular cell tumor of the kidney: report of two cases with a papillary pattern. *Hum Pathol* 1993;24:1168–1174.
175. Baruch D, Corvol P, Alhenc-Gelas F, et al. Diagnosis and treatment of renin-secreting tumors: report of three cases. *Hypertension* 1984;6:760–766.
176. Dunnick NR, Hartman DS, Ford KK, Davis CJ Jr, Amis ES Jr. The radiology of juxtaglomerular tumors. *Radiology* 1983;147:321–326.
177. More IA, Jackson AM, MacSween RN. Renin-secreting tumor associated with hypertension. *Cancer* 1974;34:2093–2102.
178. el-Naggar AK, Troncoso P, Ordonez NG. Primary renal carcinoid tumor with molecular abnormality characteristic of conventional renal cell neoplasms. *Diagn Mol Pathol* 1995;4:48–53.
179. Gonzalum JR, Lloyd RV. Primary renal carcinoid: case report and literature review. *Arch Pathol Lab Med* 1993;117:855–858.
180. Huettner PC, Bird DJ, Chang YC, Seiler MW. Carcinoid tumor of the kidney with morphologic and immunohistochemical profile of a hindgut endocrine tumor: report of a case. *Ultrastruct Pathol* 1991;15:655–661.
181. Raslan WF, Ro JY, Ordonez NG, et al. Primary carcinoid of the kidney: immunohistochemical and ultrastructural studies of five patients. *Cancer* 1993;72:2660–2666.
182. Rudrick E, Nguyen GK, Lakey WH. Carcinoid tumor of the renal pelvis: report of a case with positive urine cytology. *Diagn Cytopathol* 1995;12:360–363.
183. Takesima Y, Inai K, Yoneda K. Primary carcinoid tumor of the kidney with special reference to its histogenesis. *Pathol Int* 1996;46:89–90.
184. Unger PD, Russell A, Thung SN, Gordon RE. Primary renal carcinoid. *Arch Pathol Lab Med* 1990;114:68–71.
185. van den Berg E, Gown AS, Oosterhuis JW, et al. Carcinoid in a horseshoe kidney: morphology, immunohistochemistry, and cytogenetics. *Cancer Genet Cytogenet* 1995;84:95–98.
186. Hannah J, Lippe B, Lai-Goldman M, Bhuta S. Oncocytic carcinoid of the kidney associated with periodic Cushing's syndrome. *Cancer* 1988;61:2136–2140.
187. Gleeson MH, Bloom SR, Polak JM, Henry K, Dowling RH. Endocrine tumour in kidney affecting small bowel structure, motility, and absorptive function. *Gut* 1971;12:773–782.

188. Hamilton I, Reis L, Bilimoria S, Long RG. A renal vipoma. *Br Med J* 1980;281:1323–1324.
189. Resnick ME, Unterberger H, McLoughlin PT. Renal carcinoid producing the carcinoid syndrome. *Med Times* 1966;94:895–896.
190. McDonald EC, Mukai K, Burke BA, Sibley RK. Primary carcinoid tumor of the kidney: a light and electron microscopic and immunohistochemical study. *J Urol* 1983;130:333–335.
191. Acconcia A, Miracco C, Mattei FM, de Santi MM, Del Vecchio MT, Luzi P. Primary carcinoid tumor of kidney: light and electron microscopy and immunohistochemical study. *Urology* 1988;31: 517–520.
192. Gaudin PB, Rosai J. Florid vascular proliferation associated with neural and neuroendocrine neoplasms: a diagnostic clue and potential pitfall. *Am J Surg Pathol* 1995;19:642–652.
193. Gaudin PB, Rosai J. Vascular proliferation: authors' reply [Letter]. *Am J Surg Pathol* 1996;20:386–387.
194. Kojiro M, Ohishi H, Isobe H. Carcinoid tumor occurring in cystic teratoma of the kidney: a case report. *Cancer* 1976;38:1636–1640.
195. Fetissof F, Benatre A, Dubois MP, Lanson Y, Arbeille-Brassart B, Jobard P. Carcinoid tumor occurring in a teratoid malformation of the kidney: an immunohistochemical study. *Cancer* 1984;54:2305–2308.
196. Azumi N, Traweek ST, Battifora H. Prostatic acid phosphatase in carcinoid tumors: immunohistochemical and immunoblot studies [Comments]. *Am J Surg Pathol* 1991;15:785–790.
197. Ghazi MR, Brown JS, Warner RS. Carcinoid tumor of kidney. *Urology* 1979;14:610–612.
198. Stahl RE, Sidhu GS. Primary carcinoid of the kidney: light and electron microscopic study. *Cancer* 1979;44:1345–1349.
199. Cauley JE, Almagro UA, Jacobs SC. Primary renal carcinoid tumor. *Urology* 1988;32:564–566.
200. Capella C, Eusebi V, Rosai J. Primary oat cell carcinoma of the kidney. *Am J Surg Pathol* 1984;8:855–861.
201. Essenfeld H, Manivel JC, Benedetto P, Albores-Saavedra J. Small cell carcinoma of the renal pelvis: a clinicopathological, morphological and immunohistochemical study of 2 cases. *J Urol* 1990;144: 344–347.
202. Morgan KG, Banerjee SS, Eyden BP, Barnard RJ. Primary small cell neuroendocrine carcinoma of the kidney. *Ultrastruct Pathol* 1996;20:141–144.
203. Tetu B, Ro JY, Ayala AG, Ordonez NG, Johnson DE. Small cell carcinoma of the kidney: a clinicopathologic, immunohistochemical, and ultrastructural study. *Cancer* 1987;60:1809–1814.
204. Bezirdjian DR, Tegtmeyer CJ, Leef JL. Intrarenal pheochromocytoma and renal artery stenosis. *Urol Radiol* 1981;3:121–122.
205. Preger L, Gardner RE, Kawala BO, Steinbach HL. Intrarenal pheochromocytoma: preoperative angiographic diagnosis. *Urology* 1976;8:194–196.
206. Rothwell DL, Vorstman B, Patton I, Allan JS. Intrarenal pheochromocytoma. *Urology* 1983;21:175–177.
207. Simon H, Carlson DH, Hanelin J, Kleeman F, Feen D. Intrarenal pheochromocytoma: report of a case. *J Urol* 1979;121:805–807.
208. Baumgartner GC, Gaeta J, Wajsman Z, Merrin C. Neuroblastoma presenting as renal cell carcinoma in an adult. *Urology* 1975;6:376–378.
209. Gohji K, Nakanishi T, Hara I, Hamami G, Kamidono S. Two cases of primary neuroblastoma of the kidney in adults. *J Urol* 1987;137:966–968.
210. Shende A, Wind ES, Lanzkowsky P. Intrarenal neuroblastoma mimicking Wilms' tumor. *N Y State J Med* 1979;79:93.
211. Chan YF, Llewellyn H. Intrarenal primitive neuroectodermal tumour. *Br J Urol* 1994;73:326–327.
212. Furman J, Murphy WM, Jelsma PF, Garzotto MG, Marsh RD. Primary primitive neuroectodermal tumor of the kidney: case report and review of the literature. *Am J Clin Pathol* 1996;106:339–344.
213. Grouls V. [Primary, primitive (peripheral) neuroectodermal tumor (PNET) of the kidney] [Letter]. *Pathologe* 1994;15:246–246.
214. Gupta NP, Singh BP, Raina V, Gupta SD. Primitive neuroectodermal kidney tumor: 2 case reports and review of the literature. *J Urol* 1995;153:1890–1892.
215. Marley EF, Liapis H, Humphrey PA, et al. Primitive neuroectodermal tumor of the kidney: another enigma. A pathologic, immunohistochemical, and molecular diagnostic study. *Am J Surg Pathol* 1997; 21:354–359.
216. Mentzel T, Bultitude MI, Fletcher CD. [Primary primitive neuroectodermal tumor of the kidney in an adult: clinico-pathologic and immunohistochemical case report]. *Pathologe* 1994;15:124–128.
217. Mor Y, Nass D, Raviv G, Neumann Y, Nativ O, Goldwasser B. Malignant peripheral primitive neuroectodermal tumor (PNET) of the kidney. *Med Pediatr Oncol* 1994;23:437–440.
218. Quezado M, Benjamin DR, Tsokos M. EWS/FLI-1 fusion transcripts in three peripheral primitive neuroectodermal tumors of the kidney. *Hum Pathol* 1997;28:767–771.
219. Rodriguez-Galindo C, Marina NM, Fletcher BD, Parham DM, Bodner SM, Meyer WH. Is primitive neuroectodermal tumor of the kidney a distinct entity? *Cancer* 1997;79:2243–2250.
220. Sheaff M, McManus A, Scheimberg I, Paris A, Shipley J, Baithun S. Primitive neuroectodermal tumor of the kidney confirmed by fluorescence in situ hybridization. *Am J Surg Pathol* 1997;21:461–468.
221. Takeuchi T, Iwasaki H, Ohjimi Y, et al. Renal primitive neuroectodermal tumor: an immunohistochemical and cytogenetic analysis. *Pathol Int* 1996;46:292–297.
222. Fellinger EJ, Garin-Chesa P, Glasser DB, Huvos AG, Rettig WJ. Comparison of cell surface antigen HBA71 (p30/32MIC2), neuron-specific enolase, and vimentin in the immunohistochemical analysis of Ewing's sarcoma of bone. *Am J Surg Pathol* 1992;16:746–755.
223. Perlman EJ, Dickman PS, Askin FB, Grier HE, Miser JS, Link MP. Ewing's sarcoma: routine diagnostic utilization of MIC2 analysis. A Pediatric Oncology Group/Children's Cancer Group Intergroup study. *Hum Pathol* 1994;25:304–307.
224. Riopel M, Dickman PS, Link MP, Perlman EJ. MIC2 analysis in pediatric lymphomas and leukemias. *Hum Pathol* 1994;25:396–399.
225. Davis CJ Jr, Barton JH, Sesterhenn IA, Mostofi FK. Metanephric adenoma: clinicopathological study of fifty patients. *Am J Surg Pathol* 1995;19:1101–1114.
226. Jones EC, Pins M, Dickersin GR, Young RH. Metanephric adenoma of the kidney: a clinicopathological, immunohistochemical, flow cytometric, cytogenetic, and electron microscopic study of seven cases. *Am J Surg Pathol* 1995;19:615–626.
227. Hennigar RA, Beckwith JB. Nephrogenic adenofibroma: a novel kidney tumor of young people. *Am J Surg Pathol* 1992;16:325–334.
228. Bouzourene H, Blaser A, Francke ML, Chaubert P, Bouzourene N. Metanephric adenoma of the kidney: a rare benign tumour of the kidney [Letter]. *Histopathology* 1997;31:485–486.
229. Gatalica Z, Grujic S, Kovatich A, Petersen RO. Metanephric adenoma: histology, immunophenotype, cytogenetics, ultrastructure. *Mod Pathol* 1996;9:329–333.
230. Nonomura A, Mizukami Y, Hasegawa T, Ohkawa M. Metanephric adenoma of the kidney: an electron microscopic and immunohistochemical study with quantitative DNA measurement by image analysis. *Ultrastruct Pathol* 1995;19:481–488.
231. Granter SR, Fletcher JA, Renshaw AA. Cytologic and cytogenetic analysis of metanephric adenoma of the kidney: a report of two cases. *Am J Clin Pathol* 1997;108:544–549.
232. Brown JA, Sebo TJ, Segura JW. Metaphase analysis of metanephric adenoma reveals chromosome Y loss with chromosome 7 and 17 gain. *Urology* 1996;43:473–475.
233. Brown JA, Anderl KL, Borell TJ, Qian J, Bostwick DG, Jenkins RB. Simultaneous chromosome 7 and 17 gain and sex chromosome loss provide evidence that renal metanephric adenoma is related to papillary renal cell carcinoma. *J Urol* 1997;158:370–374.
234. Abratt RP, du Freez HM, Kaschula R. Adult Wilms' tumor: cisplatin and etoposide for relapse after adjuvant chemotherapy. *Cancer* 1990;65:890–892.
235. Arrigo S, Beckwith JB, Sharples K, D'Angio G, Haase G. Better survival after combined modality care for adults with Wilms' tumor: a report from the National Wilms' Tumor Study. *Cancer* 1990;66: 827–830.
236. Hentrich MU, Meister P, Brack NG, Lutz LL, Hartenstein RC. Adult Wilms' tumor: report of two cases and review of the literature. *Cancer* 1995;75:545–551.
237. Williams G, Colbeck RA, Gowing NF. Adult Wilms' tumour: review of 14 patients. *Br J Urol* 1992;70:230–235.
238. Winter P, Vahlensieck W Jr, Miersch WD, Vogel J, Gokel JM, Hellerich U. Wilms' tumor in adults: review of 10 cases. *Urol Int* 1996;57:67–71.
239. Fletcher JA, Renshaw AA. Isochromosome 7q in adult Wilms' tumor. *Cancer Genet Cytogenet* 1996;86:168–169.
240. Kozman HM, Clarke JM, Little MH, Smith PJ. Molecular genetic evidence for common pathogenesis of childhood and adult Wilms' tumor. *Cancer Genet Cytogenet* 1989;38:121–125.
241. Goodman ZD, Ishak KG. Angiomyolipomas of the liver. *Am J Surg Pathol* 1984;8:745–750.

242. Terris B, Flejou JF, Picot R, Belghiti J, Henin D. Hepatic angiomyolipoma: a report of four cases with immunohistochemical and DNA-flow cytometric studies. *Arch Pathol Lab Med* 1996;120:68–72.
243. Guinee DGJ, Thornberry DS, Azumi N, Przygodzki RM, Koss MN, Travis WD. Unique pulmonary presentation of an angiomyolipoma: analysis of clinical, radiographic, and histopathologic features. *Am J Surg Pathol* 1995;19:476–480.
244. Abdulla M, Bui HX, Del Rosario AD, Wolf BC, Ross JS. Renal angiomyolipoma: DNA content and immunohistochemical study of classic and multicentric variants. *Arch Pathol Lab Med* 1994;118:735–739.
245. Ansari SJ, Stephenson RA, Mackay B. Angiomyolipoma of the kidney with lymph node involvement. *Ultrastruct Pathol* 1991;15:531–538.
246. Ro JY, Ayala AG, el-Naggar A, Grignon DJ, Hogan SF, Howard DR. Angiomyolipoma of kidney with lymph node involvement: DNA flow cytometric analysis. *Arch Pathol Lab Med* 1990;114:65–67.
247. Fegan JE, Shah HR, Mukunyadzi P, Schutz MJ. Extrarenal retroperitoneal angiomyolipoma. *South Med J* 1997;90:59–62.
248. Hruban RH, Bhagavan BS, Epstein JI. Massive retroperitoneal angiomyolipoma: a lesion that may be confused with well-differentiated liposarcoma [Comments]. *Am J Clin Pathol* 1989;92:805–808.
249. Wang LJ, Lim KE, Wong YC, Chen CJ. Giant retroperitoneal angiomyolipoma mimicking liposarcoma. *Br J Urol* 1997;79:1001–1002.
250. Bernstein J, Robbins TO. Renal involvement in tuberous sclerosis. *Ann N Y Acad Sci* 1991;615:36–49.
251. Stillwell TJ, Gomez MR, Kelalis PP. Renal lesions in tuberous sclerosis. *J Urol* 1987;138:477–481.
252. van Baal JG, Fleury P, Brummelkamp WH. Tuberous sclerosis and the relation with renal angiomyolipoma: a genetic study on the clinical aspects. *Clin Genet* 1989;35:167–173.
253. Bonetti F, Pea M, Martignoni G, et al. Clear cell ("sugar") tumor of the lung is a lesion strictly related to angiomyolipoma: the concept of a family of lesions characterized by the presence of the perivascular epithelioid cells (PEC). *Pathology* 1994;26:230–236.
254. Bonetti F, Chiodera PL, Pea M, et al. Transbronchial biopsy in lymphangiomyomatosis of the lung: HMB45 for diagnosis [Comments]. *Am J Surg Pathol* 1993;17:1092–1102.
255. Chan JK, Tsang WY, Pau MY, Tang MC, Pang SW, Fletcher CD. Lymphangiomyomatosis and angiomyolipoma: closely related entities characterized by hamartomatous proliferation of HMB-45-positive smooth muscle [Comments]. *Histopathology* 1993;22:445–455.
256. Flieder DB, Travis WD. Clear cell "sugar" tumor of the lung: association with lymphangioleiomyomatosis and multifocal micronodular pneumocyte hyperplasia in a patient with tuberous sclerosis. *Am J Surg Pathol* 1997;21:1242–1247.
257. Gaffey MJ, Mills SE, Zarbo RJ, Weiss LM, Gown AM. Clear cell tumor of the lung: immunohistochemical and ultrastructural evidence of melanogenesis [Comments]. *Am J Surg Pathol* 1991;15:644–653.
258. Hoon V, Thung SN, Kaneko M, Unger PD. HMB-45 reactivity in renal angiomyolipoma and lymphangioleiomyomatosis. *Arch Pathol Lab Med* 1994;118:732–734.
259. Bryant DA, Gaudin PB, Hutchinson B, Erlandson RA, Reuter VE. Angiomyolipoma of the kidney: a histologic and immunohistochemical study of 39 cases. *Mod Pathol* 1998;11:77a(abst).
260. Mukai M, Torikata C, Iri H, et al. Crystalloids in angiomyolipoma: I. A previously unnoticed phenomenon of renal angiomyolipoma occurring at a high frequency. *Am J Surg Pathol* 1992;16:1–10.
261. Ashfaq R, Weinberg AG, Albores-Saavedra J. Renal angiomyolipomas and HMB-45 reactivity. *Cancer* 1993;71:3091–3097.
262. Hoon V, Thung SN, Kaneko M, Unger PD. HMB-45 reactivity in renal angiomyolipoma and lymphangioleiomyomatosis. *Arch Pathol Lab Med* 1994;118:732–734.
263. Jungbluth AA, Busam KJ, Gerald WL, et al. A103: an anti-melan-a monoclonal antibody for the detection of malignant melanoma in paraffin-embedded tissues. *Am J Surg Pathol* 1998;22:595–602.
264. Kaiserling E, Krober S, Xiao JC, Schaumburg-Lever G. Angiomyolipoma of the kidney. Immunoreactivity with HMB-45: light- and electron-microscopic findings. *Histopathology* 1994;25:41–48.
265. Pea M, Bonetti F, Zamboni G, et al. Melanocyte-marker-HMB-45 is regularly expressed in angiomyolipoma of the kidney. *Pathology* 1991;23:185–188.
266. Yum M, Ganguly A, Donohue JP. Juxtaglomerular cells in angiomyolipoma. *Urol* 1984;24:283–286
267. Weeks DA, Malott RL, Arnesen M, Zuppan C, Aitken D, Mierau G. Hepatic angiomyolipoma with striated granules and positivity with melanoma-specific antibody (HMB-45): a report of two cases. *Ultrastruct Pathol* 1991;15:563–571.
268. Azmy AF, Stephenson J, Ziervogel M. Angiomyolipoma causing life-threatening hematuria in a child with tuberous sclerosis. *J Pediatr Surg* 1989;24:1308–1309.
269. Beh WP, Barnhouse DH, Johnson SH, Marshall MJ, Price SEJ. A renal cause for massive retroperitoneal hemorrhage: renal angiomyolipoma. *J Urol* 1976;116:372–374.
270. O'Donnell M, Fleming S. Angiomyolipoma of kidney: a cause of recurrent retroperitoneal haemorrhage. *Br J Urol* 1995;76:521–522.
271. Vasko JS, Brockman SK, Bomar RL. Renal angiomyolipoma: a rare cause of spontaneous massive retroperitoneal hemorrhage. *Ann Surg* 1965;161:577–581.
272. Kalra OP, Verma PP, Kochhar S, Jha V, Sakhuja V. Bilateral renal angiomyolipomatosis in tuberous sclerosis presenting with chronic renal failure: case report and review of the literature. *Nephron* 1994;68:256–258.
273. Neumann HP, Bruggen V, Berger DP, et al. Tuberous sclerosis complex with end-stage renal failure. *Nephrol Dial Transplant* 1995;10:349–353.
274. Farrow GM, Harrison EGJ, Utz DC, Jones DR. Renal angiomyolipoma: a clinicopathologic study of 32 cases. *Cancer* 1968;22:564–570.
275. Ferry JA, Malt RA, Young RH. Renal angiomyolipoma with sarcomatous transformation and pulmonary metastases. *Am J Surg Pathol* 1991;15:1083–1088.
276. Lowe BA, Brewer J, Houghton DC, Jacobson E, Pitre T. Malignant transformation of angiomyolipoma. *J Urol* 1992;147:1356–1358.
277. Dineen MK, Venable DD, Misra RP. Pure intrarenal lipoma: report of a case and review of the literature. *J Urol* 1984;132:104–107.
278. Farrow GM, Harrison EG Jr, Utz DC, Re Mine WH. Sarcomas and sarcomatoid and mixed malignant tumors of the kidney in adults. I. *Cancer* 1968;22:545–550.
279. Mayes DC, Fechner RE, Gillenwater JY. Renal liposarcoma. *Am J Surg Pathol* 1990;14:268–273.
280. Clinton-Thomas CL. A giant leiomyoma of the kidney. *Br J Urol* 1955;43:497–501.
281. Fisher KF, van Blerk PJ. Childhood leiomyoma of kidney. *Urology* 1983;21:74–75.
282. Srinivas V, Sogani PC, Hajdu SI, Whitmore WF Jr. Sarcomas of the kidney. *J Urol* 1984;132:13–16.
283. Ng WF, Chan KW, Chan YT. Primary leiomyosarcoma of renal capsule. *J Urol* 1985;133:834–835.
284. Lerman RJ, Pitcock JA, Stephenson P, Muirhead EE. Renomedullary interstitial cell tumor (formerly fibroma of renal medulla). *Hum Pathol* 1972;3:559–568.
285. Mullick T, Hutchins GM. Multiple medullary fibromas of the kidney are associated with systemic hypertension. *Mod Pathol* 1998;8:80a(abst).
286. Fain JS, Eble J, Nascimento AG, Farrow GM, Bostwick DG. Solitary fibrous tumor of the kidney: report of four cases. *J Urol Pathol* 1996;4:227–238.
287. Gelb AB, Simmons ML, Weidner N. Solitary fibrous tumor involving the renal capsule. *Am J Surg Pathol* 1996;20:1288–1295.
288. Ma KF, Tse CH, Tsui MS. Neurilemoma of kidney: a rare occurrence. *Histopathology* 1990;17:378–380.
289. Somers WJ, Terpenning B, Lowe FC, Romas NA. Renal parenchymal neurilemoma: a rare and unusual kidney tumor. *J Urol* 1988;139:109–110.
290. Steers WL, Hodge GB, Johnson DE, Chaitin BA, Charnsangavej C. Benign retroperitoneal neurilemoma without von Recklinghausen's disease: a rare occurrence. *J Urol* 1985;133:846–848.
291. Freund ME, Crocker DW, Harrison JH. Neurofibroma arising in a solitary kidney. *J Urol* 1967;98:318–321.
292. Melamed J, Reuter VE, Erlandson RA, Rosai J. Renal myxoma: a report of two cases and review of the literature. *Am J Surg Pathol* 1994;18:187–194.
293. Schofield D, Zaatari GS, Gay BB. Klippel-Trenaunay and Sturge-Weber syndromes with renal hemangioma and double inferior vena cava. *J Urol* 1986;136:442–445.
294. Wang T, Palazzo JP, Mitchell D, Petersen RO. Renal capsular hemangioma. *J Urol* 1993;149:1122–1123.
295. Anderson E, Knibbs DR, Ludwig ME, Ely MG. Lymphangioma of the kidney: a pathologic entity distinct from solitary multilocular cyst. *Hum Pathol* 1992;23:465–468.

296. Joost J, Schafer R, Altwein JE. Renal lymphangioma. *J Urol* 1977;118:22–24.
297. Asa SL, Bedard YC, Buckspan MB, Klotz PG, Bain J, Steinhardt MI. Spontaneous hypoglycemia associated with hemangiopericytoma of the kidney. *J Urol* 1981;125:864–867.
298. Ordonez NG, Bracken RB, Stroehlein KB. Hemangiopericytoma of kidney. *Urology* 1982;20:191–195.
299. Grignon DJ, McIsaac GP, Armstrong RF, Wyatt JK. Primary rhabdomyosarcoma of the kidney: a light microscopic, immunohistochemical, and electron microscopic study. *Cancer* 1988;62:2027–2032.
300. Joseph TJ, Becker DI, Turton AF. Renal malignant fibrous histiocytoma. *Urology* 1991;37:483–489.
301. Osamura RY, Watanabe K, Yoneyama K, Hayashi T. Malignant fibrous histiocytoma of the renal capsule: light and electron microscopic study of a rare tumor. *Virchows Arch A Pathol Anat Histopathol* 1978;380:327–334.
302. Takashi M, Murase T, Kato K, Koshikawa T, Mitsuya H. Malignant fibrous histiocytoma arising from the renal capsule: report of a case. *Urol Int* 1987;42:227–230.
303. Mortensen PH. Primary osteogenic sarcoma of the kidney. *Br J Urol* 1989;63:101–102.
304. O'Malley FP, Grignon DJ, Shepherd RR, Harker LA. Primary osteosarcoma of the kidney: report of a case studied by immunohistochemistry, electron microscopy, and DNA flow cytometry. *Arch Pathol Lab Med* 1991;115:1262–1265.
305. Malhotra CM, Doolittle CH, Rodil JV, Vezeridis MP. Mesenchymal chondrosarcoma of the kidney. *Cancer* 1984 54:2495–2499.
306. Nativ O, Horowitz A, Lindner A, Many M. Primary chondrosarcoma of the kidney. *J Urol* 1985;134:120–121.
307. Mead JH, Herrera GA, Kaufman MF, Herz JH. Case report of a primary cystic sarcoma of the kidney, demonstrating fibrohistiocytic, osteoid, and cartilaginous components (malignant mesenchymoma). *Cancer* 1982;50:2211–2214.
308. Kern SB, Gott L, Faulkner J. Occurrence of primary renal angiosarcoma in brothers. *Arch Pathol Lab Med* 1995;119:75–78
309. Tsuda N, Chowdhury PR, Hayashi T, et al. Primary renal angiosarcoma: a case report and review of the literature. *Pathol Int* 1997;47:778–783.
310. Farrow GM, Harrison EG Jr, Utz DC. Sarcomas and sarcomatoid and mixed malignant tumors of the kidney in adults. II. *Cancer* 1968;22:551–555.
311. Ferry JA, Harris NL, Papanicolaou N, Young RH. Lymphoma of the kidney: a report of 11 cases [Comments]. *Am J Surg Pathol* 1995;19:134–144.
312. Osborne BM, Brenner M, Weitzner S, Butler JJ. Malignant lymphoma presenting as a renal mass: four cases. *Am J Surg Pathol* 1987;11:375–382.
313. Parveen T, Navarro-Roman L, Medeiros LJ, Raffeld M, Jaffe ES. Low-grade B-cell lymphoma of mucosa-associated lymphoid tissue arising in the kidney [Comments]. *Arch Pathol Lab Med* 1993;117:780–783.
314. Salem Y, Pagliaro LC, Manyak MJ. Primary small noncleaved cell lymphoma of kidney. *Urology* 1993;42:331–335.
315. Tsang K, Kneafsey P, Gill MJ. Primary lymphoma of the kidney in the acquired immunodeficiency syndrome [Comments]. *Arch Pathol Lab Med* 1993;117:541–543.
316. Xiao JC, Walz-Mattmuller R, Ruck P, Horny HP, Kaiserling E. Renal involvement in myeloproliferative and lymphoproliferative disorders: a study of autopsy cases. *Gen Diagn Pathol* 1997;142:147–153.
317. Igel TC, Engen DE, Banks PM, Keeney GL. Renal plasmacytoma: Mayo Clinic experience and review of the literature. *Urology* 1991;37:385–389.
318. Kandel LB, Harrison LH, Woodruff RD, Williams CD, Ahl ETJ. Renal plasmacytoma: a case report and summary of reported cases. *J Urol* 1984;132:1167–1169.
319. Phillips JK, Bass PS, Majumdar G, Davies DR, Jones NF, Pearson TC. Renal failure caused by leukaemic infiltration in chronic lymphocytic leukaemia. *J Clin Pathol* 1993;46:1131–1133.
320. Bagg MD, Wettlaufer JN, Willadsen DS, Ho V, Lane D, Thrasher JB. Granulocytic sarcoma presenting as a diffuse renal mass before hematological manifestations of acute myelogenous leukemia. *J Urol* 1994;152:2092–2093.

CHAPTER 43

Renal Neoplasms of Childhood

J. Bruce Beckwith

Pediatric renal neoplasms present special challenges for surgical pathologists. Like other embryonal neoplasms, they are often undifferentiated. Their histologic diversity includes mimicry of other renal and extrarenal neoplasms, with a potential for clinically significant diagnostic errors. Advances in therapy and clinicopathologic correlation have resulted in tumor-specific treatment approaches that depend entirely on accurate diagnosis and staging. Because fewer than 500 pediatric renal neoplasms are diagnosed annually in the United States, most pathologists have no chance to become familiar with this topic through daily experience. This is especially true for the less common entities and unusual variants, many of which have important clinical implications, yet occur only a few times annually in the entire nation.

The focus of this chapter is on the evaluation of these specimens in the diagnostic laboratory, emphasizing differential diagnosis and staging. General reviews of clinical, biologic, and molecular aspects of these neoplasms are available elsewhere (1–4). This presentation is distilled primarily from the experience of the National Wilms Tumor Study (NWTS) Pathology Center. This Center has carried out centralized pathologic review of the majority of pediatric renal tumor specimens in North America since 1969, providing an unprecedented opportunity for clinicopathologic correlations related to these uncommon tumors.

RECOMMENDATIONS FOR HANDLING PEDIATRIC TUMOR NEPHRECTOMY SPECIMENS

Pediatric renal tumors are usually large and friable, with a capsule that is under considerable tension because of rapid tumor growth. Displacement artifact, capsular retraction during sectioning, and distortion of renal anatomy often interfere with accurate staging of these specimens. The following suggestions can help to minimize diagnostic and staging errors:

1. Avoid intraoperative frozen sections whenever possible. Pediatric renal tumors present significant potential for diagnostic error, even with a complete set of optimally prepared permanent sections. Intraoperative frozen sections obviously amplify that potential and should be reserved for those instances in which the nature of the operative procedure will be determined by the result. Biopsies obtained before nephrectomy will also result in upstaging of a tumor that might otherwise have been stage I.
2. Nephrectomy specimens should be submitted intact. Bivalving the specimen in the operating room usually results in uncontrolled retraction of the tense tumor capsule, extravasation of tumor over the specimen surfaces, and other artifacts that compromise accurate staging. It is essential that the surgeon orient the intact specimen for the pathologist, pointing out sites of special concern, such as capsular defects. It should then be transported to the laboratory for photography and careful planning of the initial incision.
3. Be sure to record the specimen weight. The current NWTS trial (NWTS-5) includes nephrectomy specimen weight as an eligibility variable for one arm of the study. Failure to weigh the specimen may invalidate the case for this study.
4. The capsules of pediatric nephrectomy specimens should not be stripped. This procedure can destroy evidence of infiltration by tumor cells and often distorts the periphery of the renal cortex, where nephrogenic rests are most likely to be found.
5. Inking the surface is strongly recommended. Inking before bivalving the specimen will help identify misleading appearances produced by capsular retraction. It also facilitates recognition of artifacts due to smearing of tumor cells over the specimen surface during sectioning.
6. Placement of the initial bivalving incision requires careful consideration. The primary objectives of the initial

---

J. B. Beckwith: Department of Pathology and Laboratory Medicine, Division of Pediatric Pathology, Loma Linda University, Loma Linda, California 92350.

cut are to establish the relation of tumor to kidney and to obtain fresh tissue for special studies. Because tumors often arise eccentrically within the kidney, neither the center of the specimen nor its largest diameter is a reliable indicator of the optimal plane of section. The ureteral stump and hilar vessels are clues to the orientation of the kidney within bulky, distorted specimens. The primary incision should, whenever possible, avoid sites of suspected capsular disruption.

7. The surfaces of the bivalved specimen are ideal for initial pilot sections and for specimens requiring special processing. Tumor usually bulges above the freshly sectioned surface, providing optimal samples for electron microscopy, cytologic and ploidy studies, cytogenetic and molecular studies, frozen specimens, and so on. Be sure to include normal kidney tissue in the specimens for biologic studies, to facilitate recognition of tumor-specific abnormalities. Foci of parenchymal abnormality suggesting precursor lesions (nephrogenic rests) also should be sampled for histologic and biologic studies. After we have obtained these initial samples, the specimen remains sufficiently intact for demonstration to interested clinicians.

8. After initial sampling, fix the specimen for a few hours or overnight before completion of sampling. Before fixing, a series of slices should be made with a large-bladed knife, parallel to the initial incision, at intervals of about 2 cm, avoiding sites of capsular concern. The specimen can then be opened like a book and submerged in a large container of formalin or other routine fixative. The container should be capped to prevent environmental contamination and placed in a refrigerator. Refrigeration retards autolysis during fixative penetration, and hardens fat, minimizing retraction artifact and enhancing the firmness of tissue blocks. For these reasons, sections obtained after refrigerated fixation are optimal for staging purposes. In most cases, the advantages of this step justify the minor delay in final reporting. Microwave fixation is a rapid alternative to refrigerated formalin for laboratories experienced in its use.

9. Obtain most random tumor sections from the periphery of the tumor. One section taken from the periphery of the tumor usually yields more information than several from its interior, although any grossly distinctive internal foci should be sampled. Peripheral sections, in addition to tumor structure, reveal the invasive pattern, which is useful in evaluating differential diagnosis. Most important, they provide information critical to accurate staging.

10. The presence or absence of multicentric tumor origin should be documented, and apparently normal renal parenchyma must be generously sampled. Nephrogenic rests have important implications concerning the risk of contralateral Wilms tumor (WT) development, and other significant renal changes are often encountered.

11. Document the exact site from which each block is obtained. A diagram, polaroid photograph, photocopy of the opened specimen, or other graphic record will help identify the site of each block. This step is often critical for recognition of staging problems, and for evaluation of focal versus diffuse anaplasia in WT, as discussed later in this chapter.

STAGING

Stage is the major determinant of therapy and prognosis for most pediatric renal tumors. Table 1 presents the staging scheme currently used by the NWTS. This includes a significant recent change with respect to the staging of tumor in the renal sinus. Although this scheme may seem straightforward, it contains several pitfalls and weaknesses. Accurate staging is dependent on precise documentation of all parameters involved, as well as effective communication between clinicians and pathologists.

Significance of the Renal Sinus

The renal sinus, illustrated in Fig. 1, is the concave region on the medial aspect of the kidney, which contains the major renal vessels and portions of the pelvicalyceal system. The renal sinus is the principal route by which tumor cells pass from the renal parenchyma to metastatic sites. It is therefore essential that this region be examined carefully in all neoplastic nephrectomy specimens. Tumor in sinus vessels can

TABLE 1. *Staging of pediatric renal tumors (NWTS-5)*

Stage I	Tumor is limited to kidney and is completely resected
	Renal capsule intact, not penetrated by tumor
	No tumor invasion of veins or lymphatics of renal sinus
	No nodal or hematogenous spread
Stage II	Tumor extends beyond kidney but completely resected
	Tumor penetrates renal capsule with margins clear
	Tumor in lymphatics or veins of renal sinus
	Tumor in renal vein with margin not involved
	Biopsy (except FNA) or local intraoperative spillage confined to flank
	No residual tumor, no nodal or hematogenous metastases
Stage III	Residual tumor or nonhematogenous metastases confined to abdomen
	Involved abdominal nodes
	Peritoneal contamination or tumor implant
	Gross residual tumor in abdomen
	Resection margins involved by tumor
Stage IV	Hematogenous metastases or spread beyond abdomen
Stage V	Bilateral renal tumors
	When possible, a substage designation should be provided, according to stage of the most advanced individual tumor (e.g., stage V, substage I)

FNA, fine-needle aspiration.

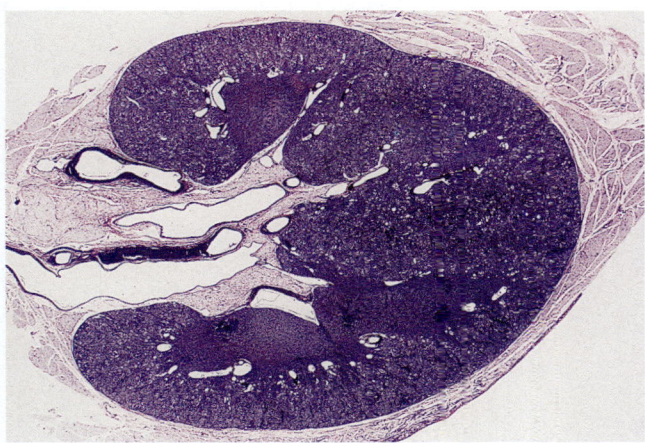

FIG. 1. Transverse section of kidney. The renal sinus is the concave region on the medial side of the organ, containing numerous large vessels.

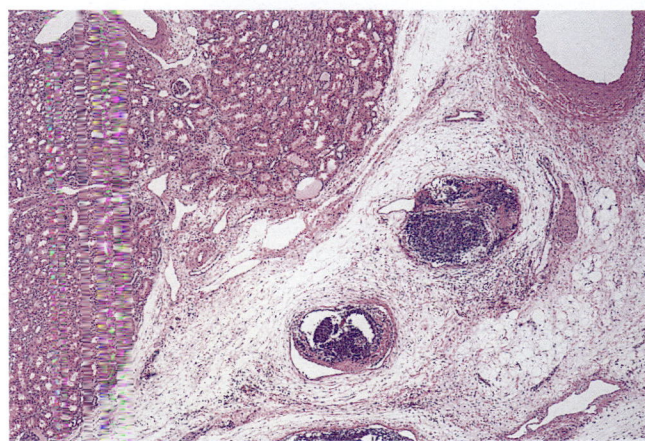

FIG. 3. Renal sinus, showing tumor invading vascular structures. Absence of capsule over adjacent cortex facilitates recognition of the renal sinus in sections.

often be identified in the gross specimen (Fig. 2). In microscopic sections, the sinus is easily recognized when pelvicalyceal structures or medullary pyramids are present on the section. Less well known is the fact that renal cortex lining the sinus is unencapsulated, facilitating recognition of sections from the renal sinus that do not include pelvicalyceal structures (Fig. 3). Dense capsules surround the pelvis and calyces and extend along the adjacent medullary pyramids, but usually disappear at the junction with cortex within the sinus (4).

On previous NWTS trials, the hilar plane was the major basis for distinguishing stage I from II in the renal sinus. This plane is an arbitrary one that connects the medial borders of the upper and lower poles and has no intrinsic anatomic significance. Not surprisingly, the hilar plane proved unsatisfactory as a staging criterion. It is usually distorted or obscured by tumor growth, is evaluable only during initial gross evaluation, and cannot be confirmed by secondary reviewers.

Beginning with NWTS 5 (August 1995), the hilar plane was abandoned as a criterion for staging. Staging of tumor within the sinus is primarily determined by the presence or absence of tumor in venous or lymphatic vessels (5). Any tumor involving these vascular structures is upstaged, regardless of relations to the hilar plane. Figure 3 illustrates tumor in vessels of the renal sinus. Vascular involvement is considered unequivocal when tumor fills venous or lymphatic lumens, is attached to the intima, or invades the vessel wall. Less certain is the presence of tumor cells lying free in the lumen, raising the question of displacement artifact. The presence of prominent artifactual tumor spread elsewhere on the slide may favor artifact over true vascular involvement. Admixture of intraluminal tumor cells with blood favors true vascular invasion. Tumor in arterial lumens is assumed to represent artifactual displacement unless the arterial wall is invaded.

Soft-tissue infiltration in the sinus, including the wall or lumen of the pelvicalyceal system, is acceptable for stage I, unless it potentially involves the medial sinus margin or invades vessels of the pelvic wall. Beware of bulky masses of apparent soft-tissue invasion in the sinus, as intravascular tumor can eventually efface vascular walls, mimicking soft-tissue invasion.

Whereas recognition of tumor in the renal sinus is usually not difficult, it is often challenging to evaluate the medial sinus margin. Involvement of resection margins is a criterion for stage III in the NWTS staging scheme. The medial margin is not demarcated by a fascia or other anatomic structure, and this region of the specimen consists of the ragged connective tissues surrounding the resected renal vessels. Sometimes it is possible to obtain an adequate transverse section through this region, especially after using the refrigerated fixation technique recommended earlier (Fig. 4).

A potential source of staging error is the renal vein margin. Veins usually retract when severed, and tumor protruding from the vein margin in the nephrectomy can produce a false impression of margin involvement. In this situation, the

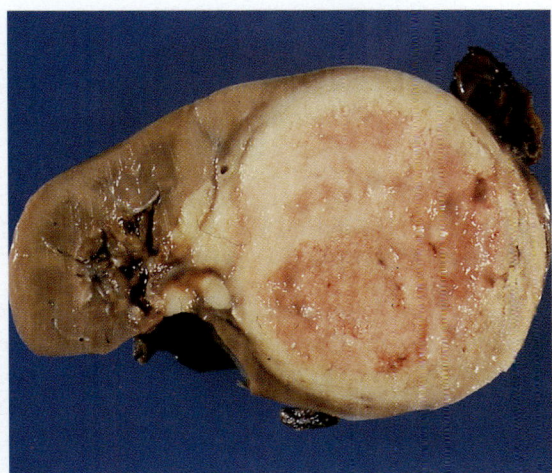

FIG. 2. Wilms tumor with small rounded extensions within renal sinus.

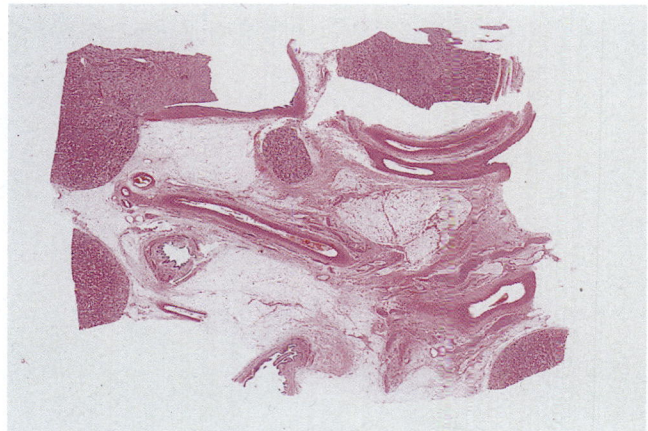

FIG. 4. Medial sinus margin. This transverse section documents that the margin is free of tumor.

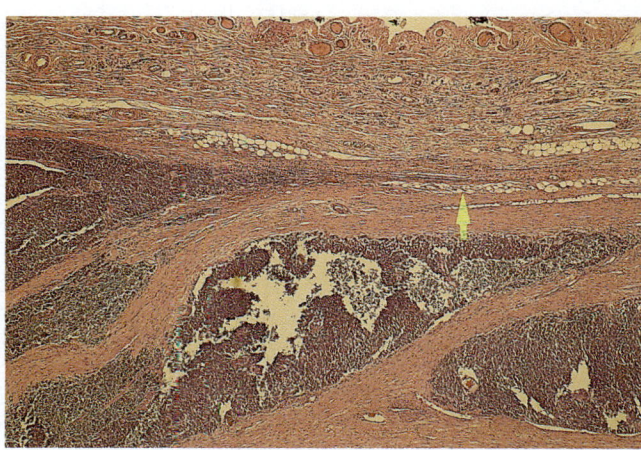

FIG. 5. Blastemal cells of Wilms tumor are in the same layer as nearby perirenal fat cells (arrow). This tumor is stage II despite the presence of an overlying capsule.

surgeon usually has a more accurate perception of whether tumor was entered during venous transection. The vein margin should be designated as positive when tumor invades the wall at that site, and when the surgeon reports that tumor was entered during venous transection. Effective communication between surgeon and pathologist can often prevent staging errors.

Evaluation of the Capsule

In the NWTS staging schema, the renal capsule, not the "tumor capsule," is the defining criterion for invasion beyond the external surface of the kidney. The tumor capsule is often a composite of several layers that become fused as the tumor enlarges. A tumor growing within the kidney may sequentially acquire some or all of the following capsular investments: (a) an intrarenal pseudocapsule, composed of compressed or reactive connective tissue within the renal parenchyma; (b) the renal capsule; (c) a perirenal pseudocapsule, composed of compressed or reactive connective tissues in the perirenal adipose layers; and finally (d) the perirenal (Gerota's) fascia. These layers tend to form a composite capsule that can defy precise analysis or lead to erroneous downstaging.

Stage I lesions may invade, but must not have penetrated, the renal capsule. Formation of a pseudocapsule in perirenal fat can obscure the fact that tumor cells have penetrated beyond the renal capsule. Sections taken from the edge, where protruding tumor abuts on the cortical surface, are often helpful in recognizing this situation, as the position of the renal capsule can often be identified with precision. By tracking laterally from the outermost tumor cells, it is often possible to recognize that these cells are within the same tissue layer as perirenal fat (Fig. 5).

Some tumors are associated with a peritumoral granulation tissue response. This "inflammatory pseudocapsule" may cause adhesions to adjacent structures, mimicking tumor invasion. Inflammatory pseudocapsules can result from perirenal hemorrhage, tumor necrosis, pyelonephritis, or preoperative tumor rupture. Viable tumor cells are not commonly found within inflammatory pseudocapsules. An inflammatory pseudocapsule is not a basis for upstaging an otherwise stage I tumor on the NWTS, although its presence was associated with somewhat higher relapse rates for stage I WT in one study (6).

Evaluation of Lymph Nodes

Tumor involvement of abdominal lymph nodes is a basis for a stage III designation by the NWTS group. Nodal involvement by undifferentiated blastemal cells may be subtle, as tumor cells may not appear much larger than lymphocytes. Even a single definite tumor cell in the marginal sinus of a regional node will mandate upstaging to stage III status on the NWTS. Sometimes an immunostain for leukocytes can be useful in determining whether a small cluster of cells in a nodal sinus represents tumor or lymphocytes (7).

Several nodal changes may falsely suggest the presence of metastases. The most frequent of these "pseudometastatic" phenomena is the presence of aggregates of Tamm–Horsfall protein containing extravasated renal tubular epithelium. The epithelium of nephrons obstructed by tumor is often dislodged and transported to marginal sinuses of hilar nodes. Swollen venular endothelium and mesothelial inclusions can also be mistaken for metastatic tumor (7).

PEDIATRIC RENAL NEOPLASMS: DIFFERENTIAL DIAGNOSTIC CONSIDERATIONS

The major renal neoplasms of childhood are listed in Table 2, including their relative prevalence, and the estimated annual incidence in the United States. With the exception of nonanaplastic WT, each entity is so rare that many pathologists will not encounter one in a lifetime, although they may enter into the differential diagnosis on multiple occasions.

TABLE 2. *Primary renal tumors of childhood*

Diagnosis	Relative percentage	Estimated no./yr (U.S.)
Wilms tumor		
Nonanaplastic	80	400
Anaplastic	5	25
Mesoblastic nephroma	5	25
Clear cell sarcoma of kidney	4	20
Rhabdoid tumor	2	10
Miscellaneous	4	20
Conventional ("clear cell") carcinoma		
Papillary carcinoma		
Medullary carcinoma		
PNET, renal neuroblastoma		
Angiomyolipoma		
Lymphoma		
Other rare or ill-defined tumors		

PNET, peripheral neuroectodermal tumor.

WILMS TUMOR (NEPHROBLASTOMA)

Wilms tumor (WT) is the most likely consideration for any pediatric renal neoplasm, except during the first 3 months of life. WT and most other eponymous designations should be spelled without the possessive apostrophe (8). The erroneous designation "Wilm's," which appears in a majority of pathology narrative reports submitted to the NWTS Pathology Center, can be avoided by following this rule.

Clinical Features

WT has a peak incidence between 2 and 5 years, with 90% being diagnosed by age 6 years (9,10). Rare cases are encountered in adults, but many tumors referred to our center as adult WT prove to be other neoplastic entities, including peripheral neuroectodermal tumors, renal carcinoids, sarcomatoid renal cell carcinoma, papillary renal carcinoma, renal sarcomas, and metanephric adenomas. The concept that WT of adults has a worse prognosis than its pediatric counterpart is probably due in part to diagnostic errors in cases reported in the literature.

For general information concerning clinical and molecular aspects of WT, references 2 and 3 are recommended.

Several dysmorphic syndromes are associated with a high risk of developing this neoplasm (3). No single cytogenetic or molecular abnormality has been consistently abnormal either in WT specimens or in patients predisposed to WT. The WT1 gene, located on chromosome 11p13, is consistently involved in the pathogenesis of the WT associated with aniridia and genital anomalies, and with the Denys–Drash syndrome (pseudohermaphroditism, severe glomerulopathy, and WT). Patients with aniridia usually have interstitial deletions of most or all of the 11p13 band, whereas patients with Denys–Drash syndrome are characterized by point mutations in the WT1 gene. However, this gene is probably normal in at least 50% of sporadic WT specimens (3). WT occasionally shows a familial distribution, with a distribution usually suggesting autosomal dominant transmission, possibly by several distinct mutations (11).

Many abnormal substances have been identified in the blood or urine of patients with WT, including acquired von Willebrand factor, active and inactive renin, erythropoietin, and neuron-specific enolase (12). These may contribute to unusual presenting symptoms in some patients, such as coagulopathy, hypertension, and polycythemia. Although some of these are occasionally useful in monitoring an individual patient for relapse, none occurs with a frequency that would justify use as a screening test (12). Abnormal circulating mucin has been described with some WT as well as several other malignant neoplasms. This appears as finely granular material on routinely stained blood smears and can cause anomalous results from automated hematology analyzers (12,13).

The most common sites of metastasis are regional nodes, lungs, and liver. Spread to other organs is rare, even in advanced cases.

Gross Features

WT typically is seen as a unicentric, spherical mass that is sharply demarcated from renal parenchyma (Figs. 2 and 6). Approximately 10% of cases are seen with multifocal primary tumors (Fig. 7). Multicentricity is associated with an increased likelihood of tumor formation in the remaining kidney. Bilateral renal tumors are initially present in 5% to 6% of cases.

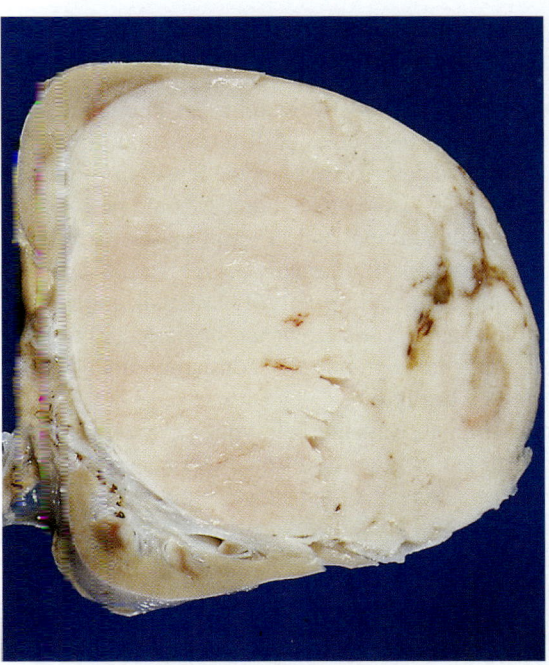

FIG. 6. Wilms tumor.

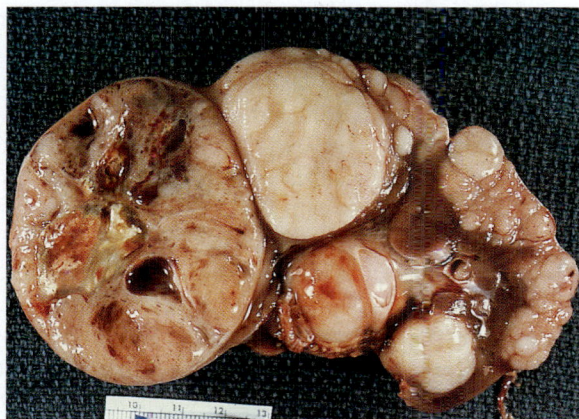

FIG. 7. Multicentric Wilms tumor.

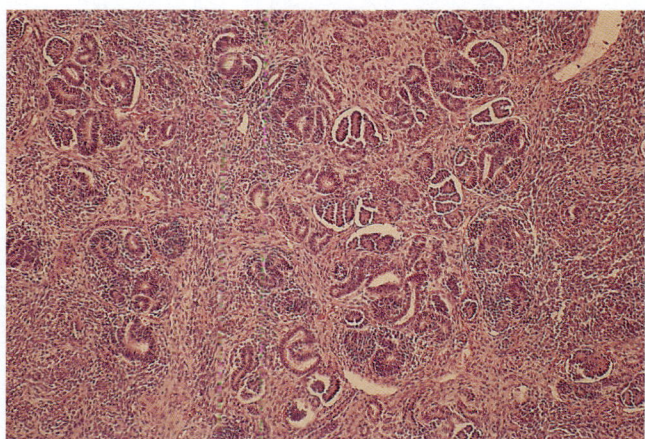

FIG. 8. Triphasic Wilms tumor.

The sectioned surface of WT is usually pale gray and uniform, but focal hemorrhage, necrosis, and cyst formation are commonly encountered. The texture is usually soft and friable, contributing to displacement artifacts during specimen manipulation, but tumors with abundant stroma may have a dense, myomatous consistency. Calcification is relatively uncommon. Prominent septa often impart a nodular appearance.

WT can arise anywhere in the cortex or medulla, usually compressing and distorting renal parenchyma around its margin. Rarely exophytic tumors connected to the renal surface by a narrow pedicle may mimic extrarenal WT. Polypoid masses in the pelvicalyceal lumen may occur either as extensions from the intrarenal mass or as separate tumors arising within the pelvic wall. The renal vein and its branches are often filled by tumor thrombus that can extend via the inferior vena cava into the right atrium.

Microscopic Features

WTs are rivaled only by teratomas in their diversity of cell and tissue types and stages of differentiation. Space permits illustration and description of only a few of the histologic appearances of WT, and other sources should be consulted for additional illustrations and descriptive details (1,4). Most specimens exhibit, to a variable degree, the so-called triphasic appearance, including cells of blastemal, stromal, and epithelial lineage (Fig. 8). However, biphasic and monophasic lesions are relatively common, consisting of any one or two of these cell lineages.

Each of the three major cell types can present a spectrum of patterns and degrees of differentiation, accounting for the remarkable diversity of appearances characterizing various WTs. Generally, however, there is relatively little variation in histologic appearance from region to region within the same tumor.

Blastemal Patterns

The blastemal cells of WT are small, closely packed cells with a high nuclear-to-cytoplasmic ratio, revealing little or no evidence of differentiation toward epithelial or stromal cell types at the light-microscopic level. Their nuclei are usually round or oval, with moderately coarse chromatin. Nucleoli are usually small, multiple, and relatively inconspicuous. Blastemal cells form several distinctive aggregation patterns, which can be divided into two broad categories, based on their structure and degree of invasiveness:

Diffuse Blastemal Pattern

Monomorphous, relatively noncohesive sheets of blastemal cells with aggressively invasive margins characterize this pattern (Fig. 9). It is the most consistently aggressive pattern of WT (14). As shown in Table 3, this pattern rarely is seen with stage I disease, and a majority are seen with stage III or IV tumor. Fortunately, most tumors with the diffuse blastemal pattern prove responsive to modern therapeutic protocols (14), so this pattern remains in the "favorable histology" category of the NWTS. In metastatic sites, the diffuse blastemal pattern can be readily confused with other small blue cell tumors of childhood, and ultrastructural or other special studies may be required to establish the correct diagnosis.

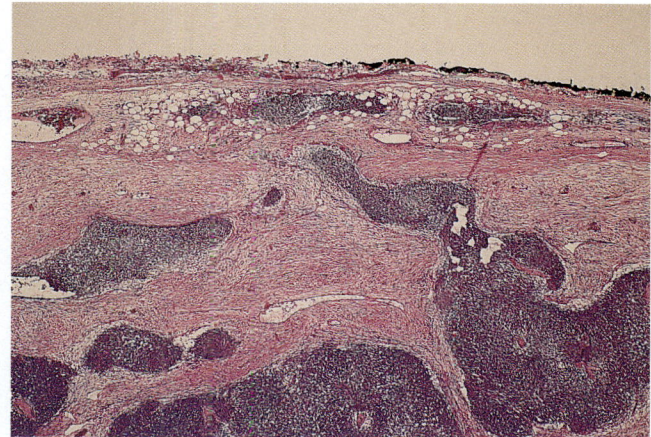

FIG. 9. Wilms tumor: diffuse blastemal pattern, showing aggressive invasiveness.

TABLE 3. *Selected histologic patterns versus stage distribution in Wilms tumor*[a]

Histologic pattern	Stage distribution (%)				Number
	I	II	III	IV	
Tubular	81	13	2	4	123
Diffuse blastemal	4	19	47	30	249
Organoid blastemal	32	28	24	16	429
Mixed	37	31	21	--	1,178

[a] NWTS-4, extracted and modified from ref. 14, with permission.

TABLE 4. *Epithelial patterns in Wilms tumor*

Patterns of cells resembling nephrogenesis
  Tubular
  Glomeruloid
  Papillary
  Transitional
Heterologous cell types
  Mucinous cells
  Squamous cells
  Neural cells
  Neuroendocrine cells

Organoid Blastemal Patterns

These patterns are characterized by sharply outlined nests of blastemal cells in a myxoid mesenchymal background. They usually lack the invasive behavior seen with the diffuse blastemal pattern and have sharply defined margins at the advancing edge of the tumor (Fig. 10). Several organoid patterns may be seen, of which the following three are the most common:

Serpentine Blastema. This pattern features serpiginous, anastomosing cords of blastemal cells in a loose, stellate, or spindled stroma (see Fig. 10). It is among the most distinctive patterns in WT and can help to distinguish WT from other blue cell neoplasms of childhood.

Nodular Blastema. This resembles the serpentine pattern, but has rounded blastemal nests instead of cell cords.

Basaloid Blastema. The basaloid form resembles the serpentine or nodular patterns, except that the blastemal cell clusters are outlined by a layer of cuboidal or columnar cells.

Epithelial Patterns

Epithelial differentiation in WT produces a variety of cell types and degrees of differentiation, as listed in Table 4. Most of these recapitulate events in normal nephrogenesis. Others are foreign to the normal kidney.

Tubular differentiation is the most frequent epithelial pattern. This ranges from vague hints at tubular formation in blastemal foci to highly differentiated tubules resembling nephronic elements in mature kidneys. True tubular lumens are present in most specimens (Fig. 11), and their presence strongly favors WT over neuroblastoma or other primitive neural tumors. As shown in Table 3, specimens in which tubular differentiation is predominant tend to be less aggressive, and most are seen as stage I tumors (14). Although not usually invasive, tubular-predominant WT often shows rapid growth, and it is not uncommon to find huge tumors that remain encapsulated within the kidney.

Glomerular differentiation, present in many WTs, ranges from simple papillary formations barely suggesting glomerulogenesis to mature tumor glomeruli closely resembling those of normal kidneys. Large, complex papillary structures sometimes lead to diagnostic confusion with papillary renal carcinomas. Heterologous epithelial cell types include mucinous differentiation (Fig. 12) and squamous cells.

Stromal Patterns

Table 5 lists the principal stromal cell types seen in WTs. Immature myxoid and spindled mesenchymal cells are present in most specimens. Skeletal muscle is the most common heterologous cell type, and usually attains a high degree of differentiation (Fig. 13). The presence of skeletal muscle in WT must not be confused with renal rhabdoid tumor, which is discussed later in this chapter. Although the term fetal rhabdomyomatous nephroblastoma is sometimes used to describe

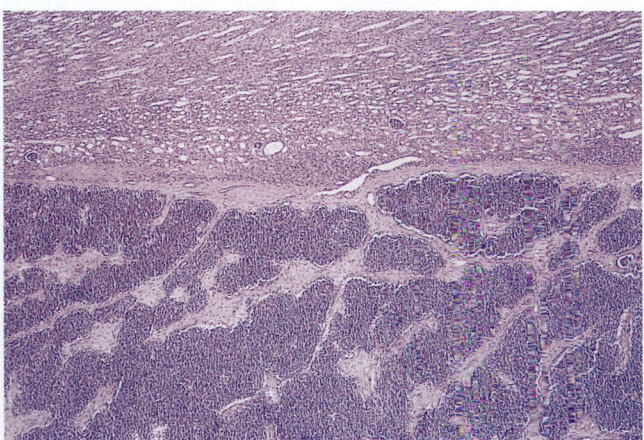

FIG. 10. Wilms tumor: serpentine blastemal pattern.

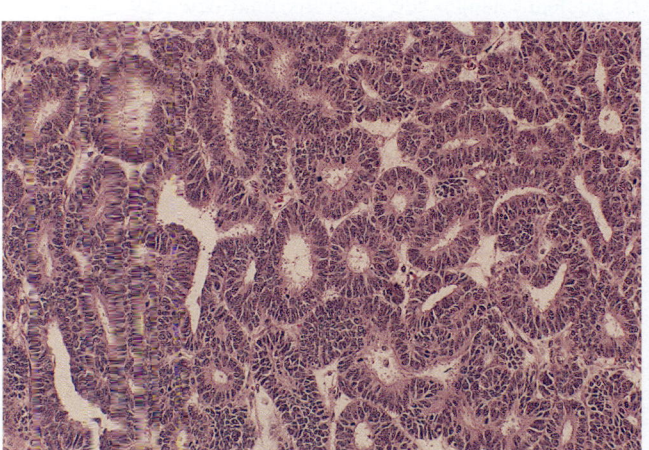

FIG. 11. Wilms tumor: tubular predominant pattern.

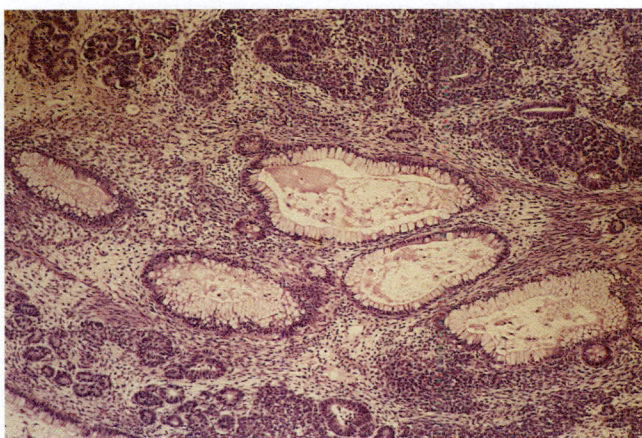

FIG. 12. Teratoid Wilms tumor containing mucinous epithelial cells.

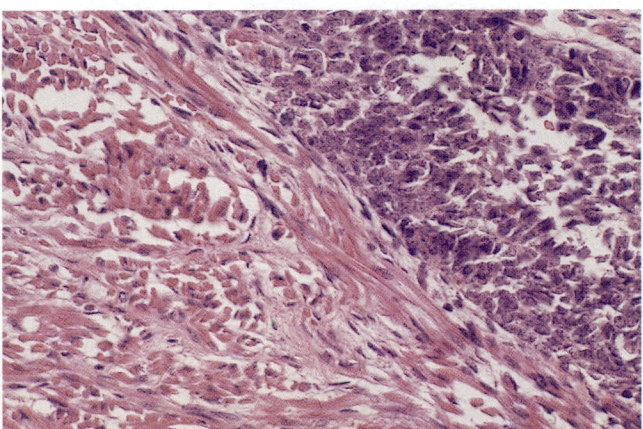

FIG. 13. Wilms tumor with skeletal muscle and blastemal cells.

WTs with abundant skeletal muscle (15,16), we have not been enthusiastic about the use of subdesignations for WT patterns. The structural diversity of WT could ultimately engender an endless number of separate designations for various morphologic patterns. Only subtypes with fundamental clinical or biologic implications deserve separate designations.

Effects of Therapy on Wilms Tumor Histology

Modern chemotherapy has been extremely effective in the management of most WT cases, and chemotherapy before nephrectomy is now used for many cases of bilateral, metastatic, or unresectable lesions. Chemotherapy usually results in massive necrosis of immature and actively proliferating cell types in WT, whereas slowly replicating and differentiated cell types are commonly unaffected. For example, tumors composed mostly of mature skeletal muscle show little clinical regression with chemotherapy, despite ablation of all malignant cells (16). The presence of mature or slowly replicating cells with few mitotic figures does not necessarily imply treatment failure, and treated WT cases can be staged according to the distribution of viable, mitotically active foci of persistent tumor (17). Cells with anaplastic nuclear changes are generally unaffected by chemotherapy and have the same significance as in untreated WT (17).

Ultrastructural and Immunohistochemical Studies

Ultrastructural study is rarely necessary to establish a diagnosis of WT but can occasionally be very helpful in distinguishing this lesion from other undifferentiated neoplasms. The ultrastructural features of WT and other childhood renal tumors were detailed elsewhere (18,19).

Immunohistochemistry has been used productively in studies of WT biology and differentiation but to date has limited usefulness in diagnosis. The diversity of cell lines and degrees of differentiation imparts a correspondingly varied profile of immunohistochemical results (20). Blastemal cells may yield either positive or negative results for vimentin and cytokeratin (21), whereas various differentiating cell lines will give results according to their patterns of differentiation. Positive results for desmin with negative stains for other muscle markers has been suggested as a characteristic feature of WT blastemal cells and might prove helpful in distinguishing this entity from other undifferentiated tumors of childhood (22).

Anaplastic Nuclear Changes: The Marker of Unfavorable Histology in Wilms Tumor

Approximately 4.5% of WTs entered in the NWTS contain cells with huge hyperchromatic nuclei, associated with multipolar mitotic figures (4,23,24). Anaplastic nuclear changes are the only criteria of "unfavorable histology" in WTs, and all WTs lacking these changes are designated by the NWTS as having "favorable histology." Clear cell sarcomas of kidney and rhabdoid tumors also are included in the unfavorable histology category but are considered separate neoplastic entities and not variants of WT. Anaplasia is almost never seen in WT diagnosed during the first year and is rare in the second year of life. Its relative frequency increases after that age, and it is found in approximately 10% of WTs diagnosed after age 5 years.

Anaplastic nuclear changes reflect extreme polyploidy and are usually apparent under low magnification (Fig. 14). The features of anaplasia as defined by the NWTS include (a) markedly enlarged tumor cell nuclei with increased chromatin content, and (b) multipolar or obviously polyploid mi-

TABLE 5. Stromal cells in Wilms tumor

Undifferentiated	Adipose cells
Myxoid	Cartilage
Fibroblasts, myofibroblasts	Osteoid, bone
Smooth muscle	Neuroglial
Skeletal muscle	

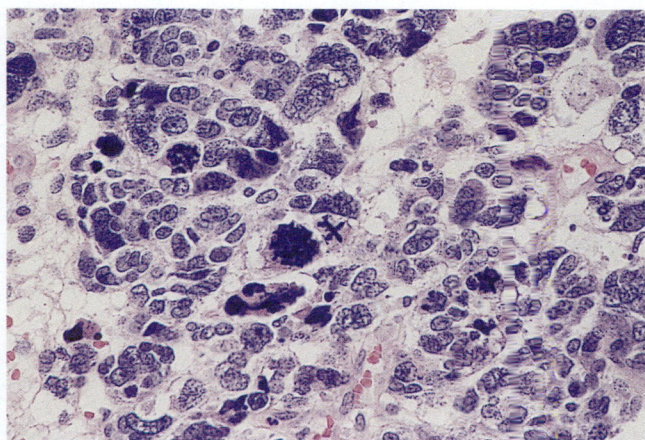

FIG. 14. Anaplastic Wilms tumor, with nuclear pleomorphism and multipolar mitotic figures.

totic figures. Multipolar mitotic figures are the most unequivocal criterion for polyploidy. We designated as anaplastic a few WT specimens in which polyploid mitotic figures were found in the absence of severe nuclear gigantism. It is important to distinguish multipolar mitotic figures from minor mitotic anomalies resulting from uneven separation of metaphase plates. This error will be avoided if we require that each limb of a mitotic figure be as large as or larger than diploid mitotic plates, as shown in Fig. 15.

New Definitions for Focal and Diffuse Anaplasia

Until recently, the presence of anaplastic nuclear changes in any region of a WT was considered prognostically significant. However, it has subsequently become apparent that anaplastic nuclear changes are an indicator of increased resistance to adjuvant therapy and not a marker of increased tumor aggressiveness (23). This concept implies that the prognosis for a patient with anaplastic WT is determined by the completeness of surgical removal of anaplastic cells. If the resistant cells are confined within the resected primary tumor, and not represented in extrarenal extensions or metastases, the outcome should be similar to that for patients with nonanaplastic WT. Based on this consideration, we revised our original definitions for "focal" anaplasia (FA) and "diffuse" anaplasia (DA) (24). The original definition of FA required that anaplasia be present in fewer than 10% of microscopic fields examined (25), regardless of the sites where anaplasia was demonstrated. Cases with FA, according to the original definition, fared somewhat better than those with DA on the first four NWTS trials, but the difference did not attain statistical significance and did not justify treating them less intensively.

We devised more restrictive criteria for FA that emphasized the distribution and location of anaplasia, rather than its relative amount. This definition proved to be successful in distinguishing a subset of anaplastic WT with good prognosis (24), and is the one being used to determine intensity of therapy on NWTS-5. The new definition of FA includes only those WTs meeting all of the following criteria:

1. Anaplasia is confined to one or more discrete sites within the primary tumor and is not present in tumor extensions or extrarenal sites.
2. Tumor cells outside anaplastic foci show no "nuclear unrest" (nuclear or mitotic abnormalities that approach, but do not quite attain, that degree of severity required for a designation of anaplasia).

In some specimens, the criteria of anaplasia are unequivocally met on only one or two slides, but other sections reveal widespread nuclear unrest. These appearances suggest that the cells are in transition toward anaplastic morphology. For this reason, nuclear unrest that is widespread, or present in extrarenal sites, excludes a case from the FA category.

Any WT not meeting this revised definition of FA is designated as DA. Any one of the following situations will justify assignment to the DA category:

1. Nonlocalized anaplastic changes.
2. Anaplastic changes or nuclear unrest in invasive sites, or any extrarenal deposits.
3. Localized anaplastic changes in a tumor showing severe nuclear unrest more diffusely.
4. Anaplasia in a random biopsy specimen.
5. Anaplasia involving the edge of one or more sections, and the site(s) from which the sections were taken cannot be determined.

Anaplastic foci are clearly demarcated from adjacent nonanaplastic tumor (Fig. 16). Whereas most cases in the FA category have a single focus, we have accepted tumors with as many as four small foci as FA, when each anaplastic focus was clearly demarcated and entirely surrounded by nonanaplastic tumor (24). Anaplastic foci are usually a few millimeters in diameter but can be larger if their localized nature is clearly documented. When anaplastic changes extend

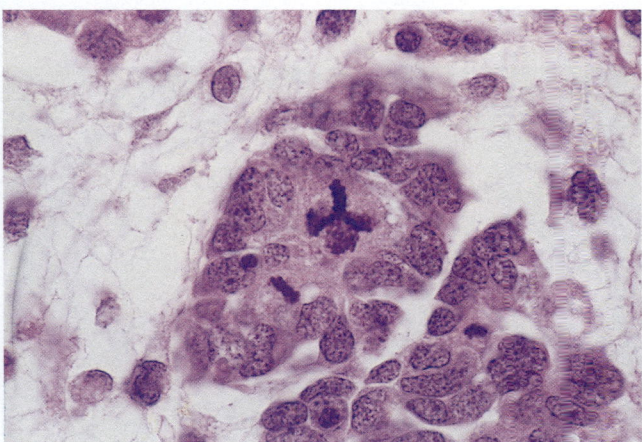

FIG. 15. Anaplastic Wilms tumor, showing multipolar mitotic figure. Each arm of the abnormal figure is as large as the adjacent normal-sized metaphase plate.

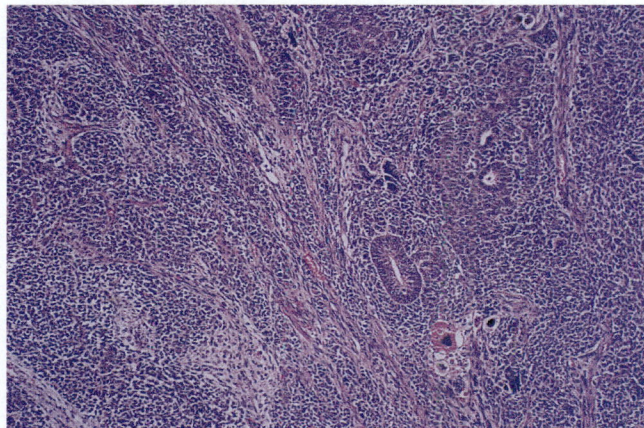

FIG. 16. Focal anaplasia. The right half shows a portion of the anaplastic focus, sharply demarcated from the nonanaplastic remainder of the tumor.

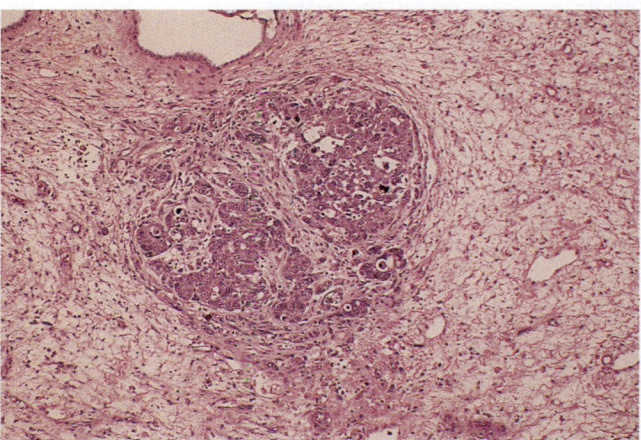

FIG. 17. Focal anaplasia after chemotherapy. This minute anaplastic nodule persists in an otherwise necrotic background.

to the edge of several sections, it is important to determine whether the sections showing anaplasia were all from the same focus. This determination depends on careful documentation of the site from which each tumor section was obtained and is one reason this point was emphasized in the first part of this chapter.

For children with stage II to IV WT, the distinction of FA from DA as currently defined has major prognostic and therapeutic significance (24). Patients with WTs with advanced-stage disease, whose primary nephrectomy specimen contains FA, have a prognosis similar to that of patients with similar stage nonanaplastic WT. The adverse prognostic significance of anaplasia in WT is limited to tumors with DA. On the current NWTS trial, patients with FA WT are treated similar to those with nonanaplastic WT of comparable stage, whereas those with stage II to IV DA WT are treated more aggressively than on previous NWTS studies.

The following caveats concerning anaplastic WT deserve emphasis:

1. Diffuse anaplasia in stage I WT is not associated with worse outcome, even with conventional therapy. These patients can be spared the intensive therapeutic approaches and poor prognosis associated with advanced-stage WT with DA. It is therefore essential that pathologists take extreme care fully to document the stage I status of a seemingly localized WTs manifesting DA.
2. Diffuse anaplasia is usually apparent in the majority of tumor sections. Anaplastic cells were found in more than half the tumor sections in 77% of specimens with DA, and in more than one fourth of slides in 98% of cases (24).
3. Once anaplasia has been identified in a case of WT, the threshold for designating its presence elsewhere can be lowered. A single gigantic nucleus or polyploid mitosis is sufficient evidence that anaplasia also is present in another site (23,24).
4. Enlarged nuclei in differentiated skeletal muscle cells of a WT do not signify anaplasia unless accompanied by multipolar mitotic figures. Anaplastic nuclear changes in embryonal muscle fibers are considered significant.
5. The cytologic criteria for anaplasia are the same in specimens removed after chemotherapy. The recognition of focal anaplasia is usually easier in specimens from treated patients. These foci, being generally resistant, continue to enlarge during the period of therapy. Even minute anaplastic foci stand out in sharp contrast in the necrotic or atrophic background (Fig. 17).

Cystic Variants of Wilms Tumor

Scattered cysts are commonly encountered in conventional WT, but rarely the tumor is composed entirely of cystic spaces and delicate septa, without an expansile solid component. These lesions are encapsulated and clearly demarcated from adjacent renal parenchyma (Fig. 18). For tumors that are entirely composed of mature cells, as shown in Fig. 19, the term cystic nephroma (CN) is recommended

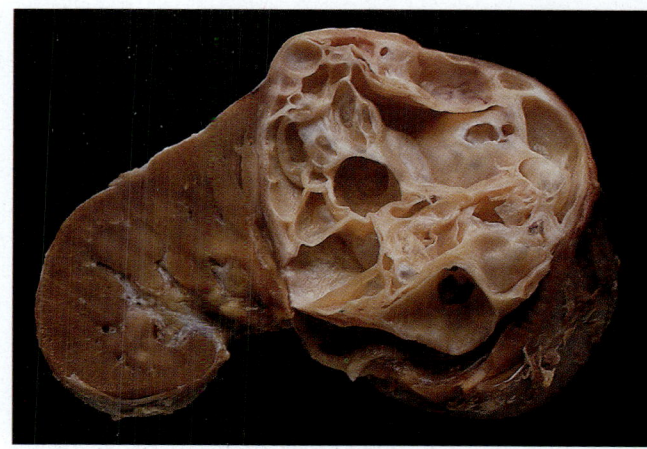

FIG. 18. Cystic nephroma.

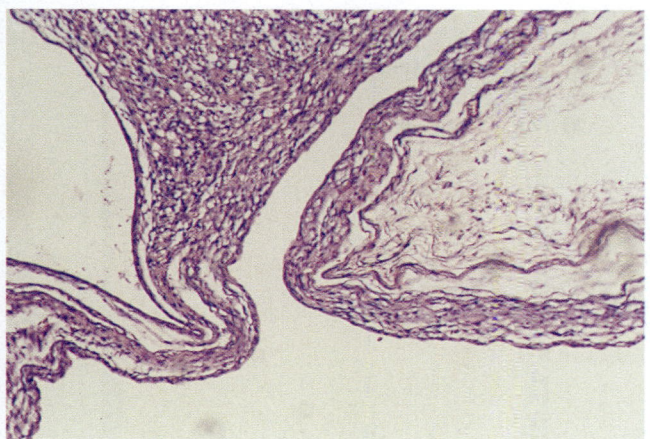

FIG. 19. Cystic nephroma: septa contain only mature cells.

(26). This term conveys the concept of a benign cystic neoplasm more clearly than the alternative designation "multilocular cyst." If the septa contain embryonal cell types, the designation cystic, partially differentiated nephroblastoma (CPDN) is appropriate (Fig. 20). CPDN appears to be a transitional stage in the development of pediatric CN, and these lesions seem to represent a "hyperfavorable" end of the WT spectrum. The epithelial cells lining the cysts of CN and CPDN range from flattened to columnar, and often are of the "hobnail" type, with prominent acidophilic cytoplasm that is more abundant at the apex than the base. The cysts often have distinct walls composed of maturing spindle cells.

The distinction of CN from CPDN has little or no clinical importance when the lesion has been cleanly and completely resected, because both lesions are curable by resection alone. If resection is incomplete or associated with tumor spill, a slight potential for recurrence may exist (26).

The differential diagnosis of CN and CPDN includes localized variants of polycystic renal disease (27), which can produce grossly cystic masses localized to a portion of one kidney. These differ from CN and CPDN in that cysts are mingled with renal cortical and medullary elements, and the abnormal region is not demarcated by a distinct pseudocapsule. CN and CPDN are sharply encapsulated lesions, with no normal renal elements inside the capsule. Localized cystic renal dysplasia can be distinguished by the presence of typical features or renal dysplasia, including primitive ducts, maldeveloped nephrons, and the frequent presence of cartilage. Localized lymphatic lesions of the kidney, including cystic lymphangiectasis and lymphangioma, can mimic the gross appearances of these tumors, as can an occasional multicystic clear cell sarcoma of kidney or mesoblastic nephroma. Multilocular cystic renal cell carcinoma, characterized by cells with clear cytoplasm lining the cysts (28), is rarely encountered in pediatric patients. Cystic WT is distinguished by the presence of solid, expansile regions that replace or distort the cystic spaces, rather than being passively molded by the cysts.

Nephrogenic Rests and Nephroblastomatosis

In more than 30% of kidneys resected for WT, the renal parenchyma contains one or more regions of persistent embryonal tissue, representing precursor lesions of WT. These lesions have been given many names in the past, for which we have suggested the generic term nephrogenic rests (NRs). This term applies to all putative precursor lesions of WT or their nonneoplastic derivatives (29,30). The presence of multiple or diffusely distributed NRs is termed nephroblastomatosis. This term is most commonly applied when the rests are in an active state of cellular proliferation and are large enough to be grossly visible or apparent on imaging studies.

NRs have a dynamic life history that can produce a variety of appearances. This feature led to complex schemes of classification, with varying terminology. Our classification is based on the assumption that the structure of NRs reflects both the dynamic state and the history of an individual rest. This scheme was presented in more detail elsewhere (4,29,30), and only a brief summary can be provided here.

Two fundamental categories of NRs are recognized, based on their topographic relation to the renal lobe. These are designated perilobar nephrogenic rests (PLNRs; Figs. 21 and 22) and intralobar nephrogenic rests (ILNRs; Figs. 23 and 24). ILNRs may occur anywhere in the renal lobe, including the peripheral cortex. They often also occur within the renal sinus, including in the walls of the pelvicalyceal system. They have a more varied structure than do PLNRs and are characterized by their interstitial location between nephrons, whereas PLNRs usually are discrete structures that are clearly demarcated from adjacent nephrons. The major features distinguishing ILNRs from PLNRs are summarized in Table 6.

Rests of either major category may be further classified based on their developmental fates. An individual NR may

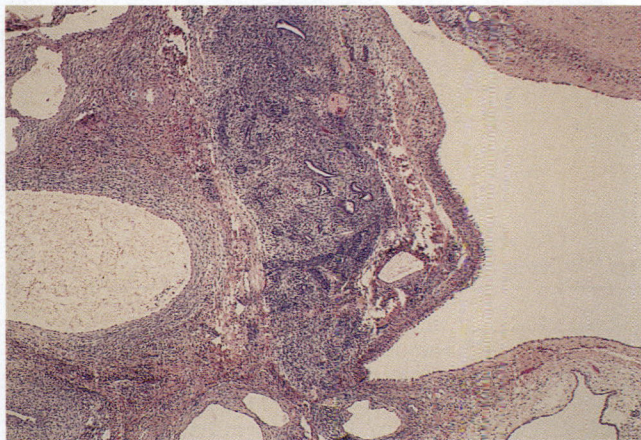

FIG. 20. Cystic, partially differentiated nephroblastoma (CPDN). This lesion resembled cystic nephroma grossly, but embryonal elements are present in the septa.

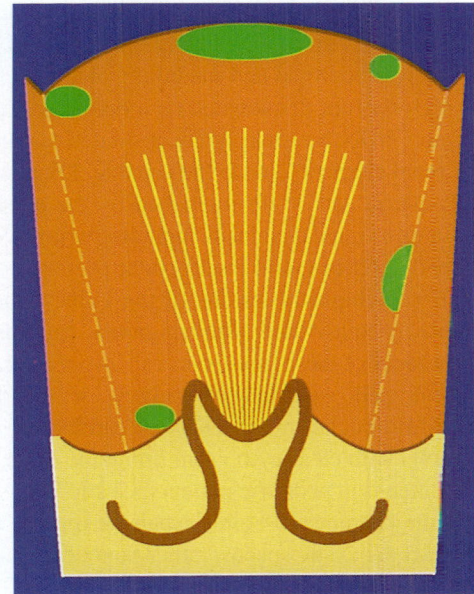

FIG. 21. Perilobar nephrogenic rests. Characteristic locations are shown in green.

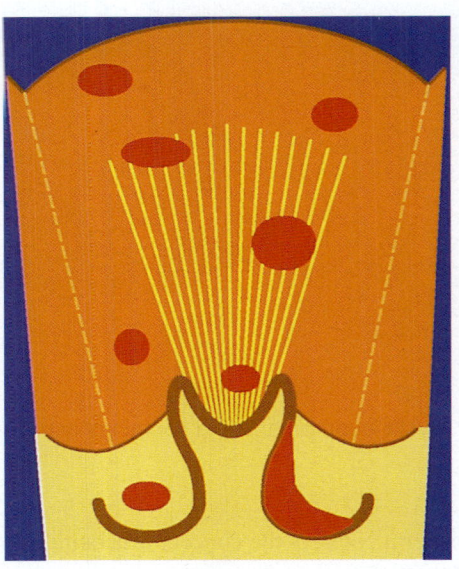

FIG. 23. Intralobar nephrogenic rests. Characteristic locations are shown in red.

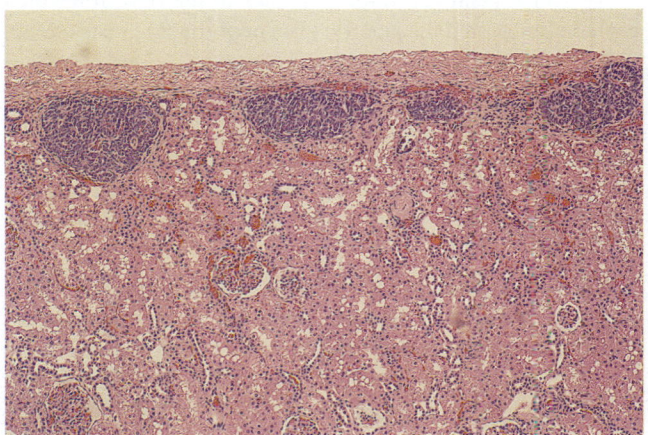

FIG. 22. Perilobar nephrogenic rests. Small, incipient blastemal rests at the lobar surface. Note sharply defined border and lack of intermixed nephrons within the rests.

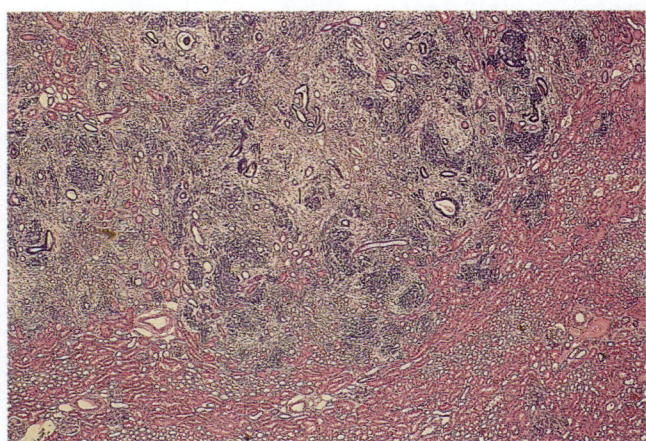

FIG. 24. Intralobar nephrogenic rest. Note the intermixed normal nephrons and indistinct borders.

TABLE 6. *Perilobar versus intralobar rests*

Feature	Perilobar rests	Intralobar rests
Site in renal lobe	Periphery	Random; cortex, medulla, sinus
Margins	Clearly demarcated	Poorly demarcated
Relation to nephrons	No nephrons within rest	Dispersed between nephrons
Composition	Blastemal or tubular; stroma scanty or sclerotic	Tubules, blastema, cysts; stroma usually predominates
Number	Usually numerous	Often single

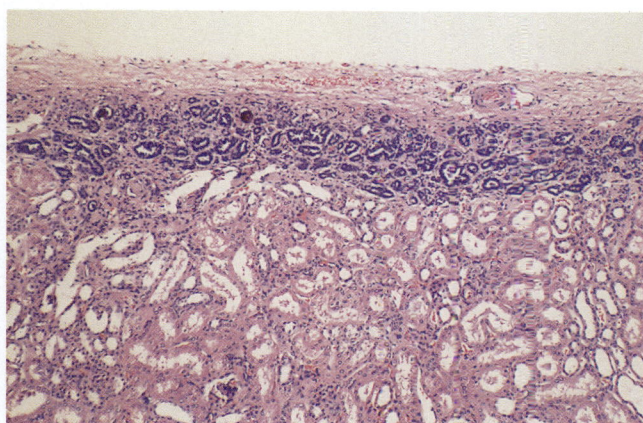

FIG. 25. Sclerosing perilobar nephrogenic rests. Tubular structures are lined by single layers of basophilic cells in a sclerotic, hypocellular background.

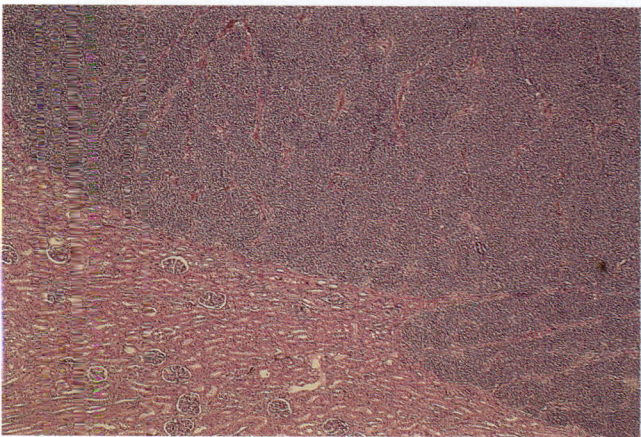

FIG. 27. Hyperplastic perilobar nephroblastomatosis, showing lack of compression or pseudocapsule formation at edge of lesion.

undergo any of the following fates, several of which often occur sequentially over time:

1. It may remain unchanged in size or composition, even for many years, as a tiny, microscopic blastemal focus similar to that in Fig. 21 (dormant NR).
2. The most common fate of NRs is maturation, sclerosis, and eventual disappearance (sclerosing NRs and obsolescent NRs). A typical sclerosing PLNR is shown in Fig. 25.
3. Hyperplastic NRs represent coordinated proliferation of all susceptible cells of the rest, as distinguished from a clonal neoplastic process originating in a single cell of the rest. Hyperplasia may produce large masses that can exhibit active growth and numerous mitotic figures, and a section from the interior of a hyperplastic NR may be indistinguishable from WT. Diffuse hyperplastic growth, involving all or most cells of a rest, tends to preserve the original shape of the rest. When PLNRs form a continuous layer of embryonal cells at the lobar surface, hyperplastic proliferation will produce a thick "rind" of abnormal tissue at the renal surface, as seen in Fig. 26. Ovoid and lenticular masses result from hyperplasia of NRs that originally had these shapes. An irregular-shaped, multinodular appearance will result if only some of the cells are capable of proliferation (30). An important feature distinguishing actively hyperplastic NRs from WT is the usual absence of a pseudocapsule at the interface between hyperplastic NRs and renal parenchyma (Fig. 27).
4. Neoplastic induction is assumed to represent a clonal event originating in single cells of a rest, resulting in WT or benign adenomas. Rapidly growing tumors originat-

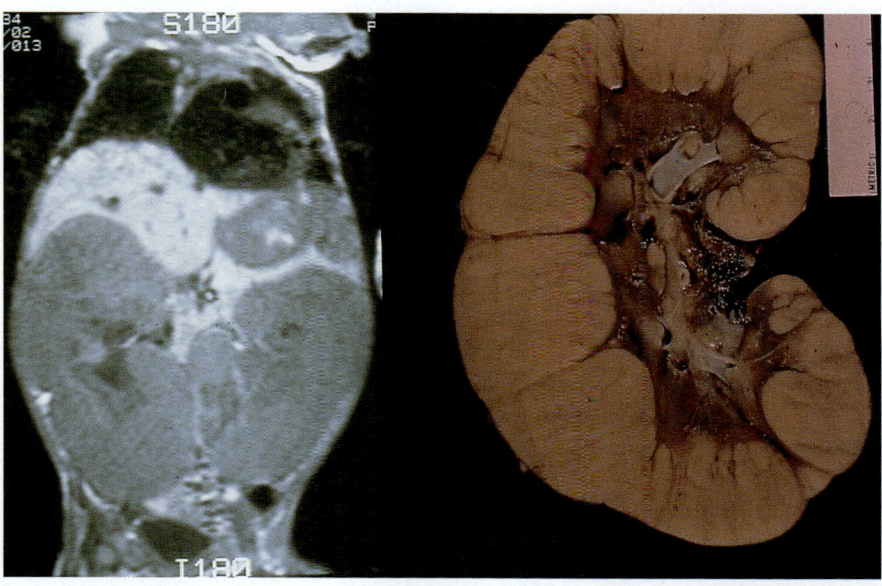

FIG. 26. Diffusely hyperplastic perilobar nephroblastomatosis, with computed tomography image showing similar changes in both kidneys.

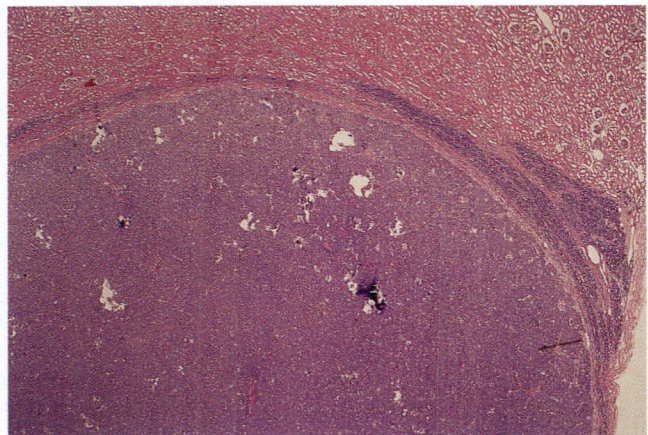

FIG. 28. Early Wilms tumor. Spherical blastemal mass compressing adjacent remnants of perilobar rest.

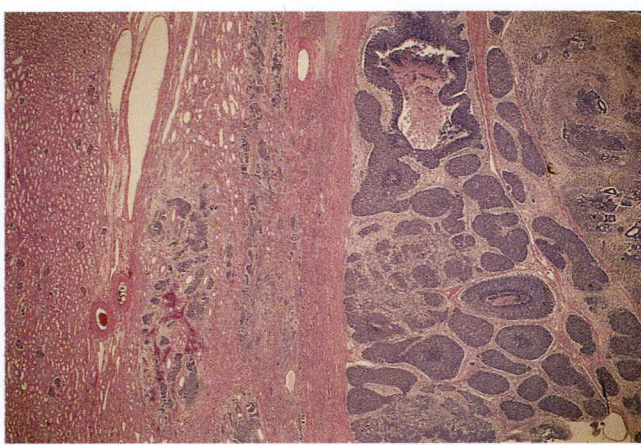

FIG. 30. Intralobar nephrogenic rest adjacent to Wilms tumor.

ing at a single point (or cell) will tend to grow equally in all directions, forming spherical, expansile nodules with compressed rest remnants often present at the periphery (Fig. 28).

Relations between the various developmental fates of NRs are shown diagrammatically in Fig. 29. An individual rest commonly progresses through several of these stages sequentially. For example, an incipient or dormant rest may undergo hyperplastic proliferation, followed by a phase of growth arrest, maturation, and regression. This will result in a large but inactive-appearing lesion. Ultimately, one or more cells within the regressing rest may be induced to form WT. The arrows in Fig. 29 show the possible pathways a rest might follow in its journey toward obsolescence or neoplasia.

ILNRs are most often found at the tumor–kidney interface, where they can be misinterpreted as infiltrating tumor cells or effaced by tumor compression. A helpful feature distinguishing ILNRs at the edge of a WT is the poorly defined, irregular outer border of the ILNR, which contrasts with the sharp, pushing border between the tumor and the rest (Fig. 30).

The presence of NRs in a kidney removed for WT is correlated with an increased risk for subsequent tumor formation in the remaining kidney (29). When a carefully sampled kidney is free of rests, the risk of this unfortunate event is extremely low. The possibility of subsequent WT developing in the remaining kidney should be considered in planning the follow-up of patients whose nephrectomy specimen reveals the presence of NRs in addition to WT.

Differential Diagnosis of Wilms Tumor

Triphasic Wilms Tumor

This pattern rarely presents a problem in diagnosis, except when small biopsies are obtained from large retroperitoneal masses of uncertain origin. In this setting, other mixed neoplasms might deserve consideration, including teratoma, hepatoblastoma, pancreatoblastoma, teratoma, mesothe-

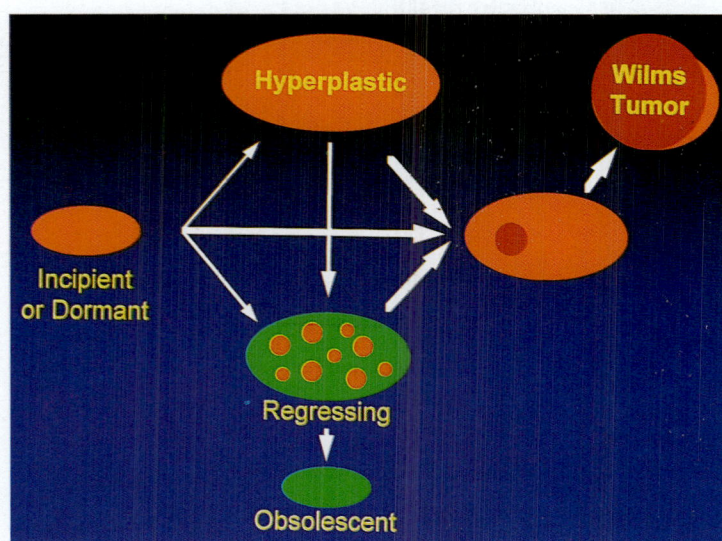

FIG. 29. Diagram showing relations of various fates of nephrogenic rests.

lioma, synovial sarcoma, and desmoplastic small-cell tumor with divergent differentiation (31). In the absence of nephrogenic differentiation or the distinctive blastemal aggregation patterns cited earlier, ancillary studies such as immunohistochemistry or electron microscopy may be required to distinguish some of these lesions from WT. Molecular studies such as the distinctive EWS-WT1 gene fusion in desmoplastic small-cell tumor (32) are increasingly important in the diagnosis of some entities that might be confused with WT. Epithelioid differentiation in clear cell sarcoma of the kidney presents another consideration in the differential diagnosis, as discussed later in this chapter.

WT with extensive heterologous differentiation ("teratoid WT") is easily confused with immature teratoma. Renal teratomas are extremely rare, and some of the reported cases represent teratoid WT. Teratomas are characterized by heterologous organoid differentiation (recognizable differentiation into organs or body parts other than the one in which the tumor arises, such as gut wall or trachea). WT, like other mixed tumors, may contain one or more cell types found in another organ, but these have histioid differentiation, characterized by random juxtaposition of various cell types, without the consistent structural organization characteristic of developing or mature organs.

Blastemal Wilms Tumor Versus Other Small Blue Cell Tumors of Childhood

This problem is most likely to arise when dealing with biopsies from metastatic sites or from large abdominal tumors of uncertain origin. The distinctive aggregation patterns of blastemal WT, or the focal presence of differentiating cells, often will reveal the diagnosis. Early tubular differentiation in WT can sometimes be confused with rosettes of neuroblastoma or neuroepithelioma. However, early tubular structures usually have cells neatly aligned to form a single layer around the future lumen, whereas neuroblastic rosettes are aggregated more randomly around the central zone and are less consistently aligned. The presence of lumens confirms tubular differentiation, and neurofibrils are diagnostic of a neuroblastic pseudorosette. Neuroblastic rosettes do rarely occur in WT, but usually only in teratoid WTs, which are not likely to be confused with neuroblastomas or primitive neuroectodermal tumors (PNETs). Immunostains, electron microscopy, molecular diagnostic techniques, circulating tumor markers, tissue culture, and other special studies may sometimes be required to confirm the nature of a small blue cell tumor.

Epithelial Predominant Wilms Tumor Versus Papillary Renal Cell Carcinoma

This dilemma is most often encountered in tumors from adolescents or adults, and is sometimes difficult to resolve with certainty. The adenomatous precursor lesions of papillary renal cell carcinoma (PRCC) may resemble epithelial-predominant nephrogenic rests (33), and epithelial-predominant WTs can have a predominantly papillary architecture. It is conceivable that a developmental relation exists between these seemingly discrete entities. Sometimes PRCCs have a prominent tubular or solid component (34). Molecular or cytogenetic studies may be helpful, because PRCC characteristically contains increased copies of chromosomes 7 and 17, and, in tumors from male patients, deletion of Y (35,36). Unequivocal glomerular differentiation, characteristic blastemal aggregation patterns, or the presence of heterologous cell types can confirm the diagnosis of WT. Positive staining for cytokeratin 7 has been advocated as a useful marker for PRCC (37–39), but we encountered focal positive staining for this epitope in many WTs. This stain is likely to be helpful only when diffusely positive or entirely negative.

Epithelial Wilms Tumor Versus Conventional (Clear Cell) Renal Carcinoma

Composite tumors with regions of both WT and clear cell renal carcinoma (CCRC) have been reported (40). Our experience with these composite neoplasms suggests that the nuclear grade of the carcinomatous component has the same significance as in conventional CCRCs. Those WTs containing grade I or II CCRCs will generally behave as WT, whereas higher grade carcinomatous elements are more likely to have carcinomatous metastases and resistant tumor biology. A limited biopsy from one of these composite tumors may reveal only one component, leading to an apparent diagnostic discrepancy when subsequent specimens reveal the other component.

Stromal-Predominant Wilms Tumor Versus Mesoblastic Nephroma and Sarcomatous Renal Tumors

This topic is discussed in the sections on these entities.

MESOBLASTIC NEPHROMA

Mesoblastic nephroma (MN) is a distinctive infantile renal neoplasm composed of monomorphous spindle cells (41,42). Although it comprises only 2% to 3% of pediatric renal tumors, MN is the most common renal neoplasm in the first 3 months of life. Sixty-two percent of cases in our files were diagnosed in the first 3 months of life, and the median age was 2 months. Ninety percent were diagnosed in the first year. Cases reported as MNs of adults and adolescents are, in our opinion, unconvincing examples of this neoplasm, and this diagnosis should be considered suspect in any patient beyond the second year of life. MN is generally associated with good outcome, and most cases are treated by nephrectomy alone. However, recurrences and metastases do occur in about 5% of cases.

In recent years, a substantial proportion of the MNs in our files were detected during fetal sonography. Hydramnios is common during gestation, and nonimmunologic fetal hydrops was reported. Hyperreninism, hypercalcemia, and coagulopathy or shock from tumor rupture during delivery also were reported in some cases.

Gross Appearance

MN arises unicentrically, and usually appears to have arisen deep within the parenchyma near the renal sinus. The renal sinus and adjacent structures on the medial side of the kidney are major sites of extrarenal spread of MN. Surgeons and pathologists must pay particular attention to the medial margin of the resection specimen in dealing with potential MN specimens. This is no simple matter. The medial specimen margin is notoriously difficult to evaluate, and it is rarely possible to be certain that it is free of involvement by MN.

The appearance of the sectioned surface is variable. Some specimens have a tough, whorled appearance resembling leiomyoma, but soft, friable tumors are more frequently encountered (Fig. 31). Hemorrhage, necrosis, and cyst formation are present to some degree in a majority of specimens. These findings are too often present in cases with good outcome to serve as useful markers of adverse prognosis.

Microscopic Appearance

MN is generally categorized into a "classic," fibromatosis-like subtype and a "cellular" pattern resembling fibrosarcomas. Variable combinations of these patterns are often seen, as the cellular pattern commonly arises with a background of the classic pattern.

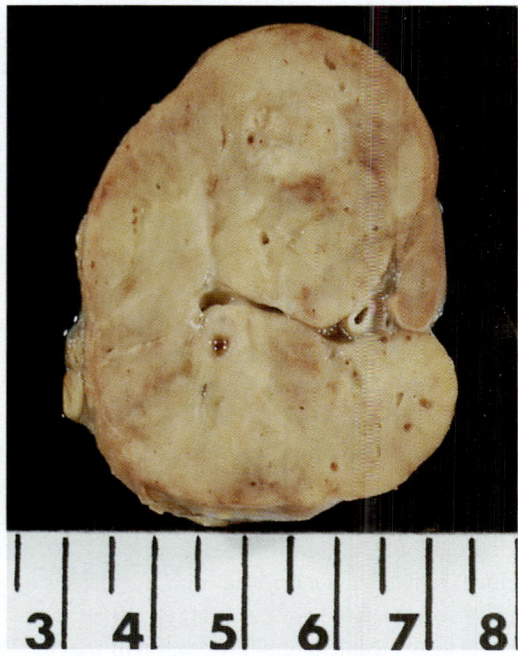

FIG. 31. Mesoblastic nephroma.

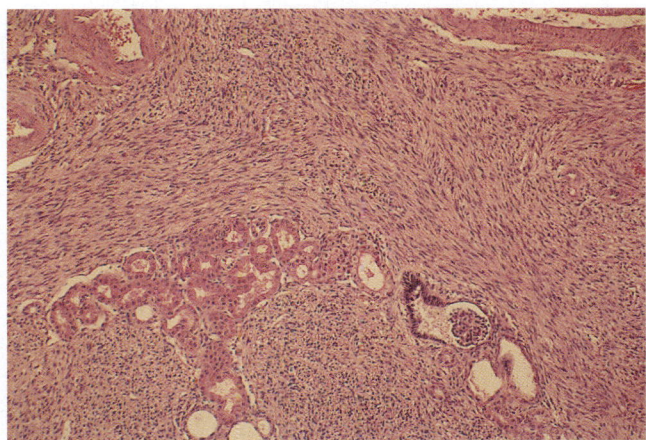

FIG. 32. Mesoblastic nephroma, classic pattern. Embryonal metaplasia involving parietal layer of a Bowman's capsule is seen near lower right corner.

Classic Mesoblastic Nephroma

The original descriptions of MN emphasized this pattern, which is characterized by relatively low cell density, low to moderate numbers of mitotic figures, and long tongues of tumor extending radially into adjacent kidney and soft tissue (Figs. 32–34). The term classic is appropriate in the historical sense, but this is not the most common subtype of MN. Among the first 350 cases recently reviewed in our files, only 24% were of the pure classic pattern. In addition to involving the renal sinus and adjacent soft tissues (see Fig. 33), classic MN also extends into perirenal fat, where its advancing edge often shows angiomatous vascular proliferation (see Fig. 34). Cartilage or other dysplastic changes may be found in the renal parenchyma adjacent to tumor, sometimes becoming surrounded by tumor. The interdigitating borders of the lesion entrap renal tubules and glomeruli, and the entrapped epithe-

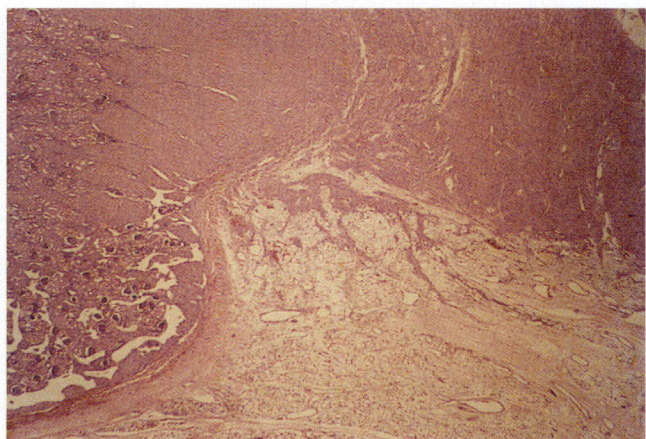

FIG. 33. Mesoblastic nephroma, classic pattern, with massive invasion of fat on medial border of kidney. Note irregular invasive borders.

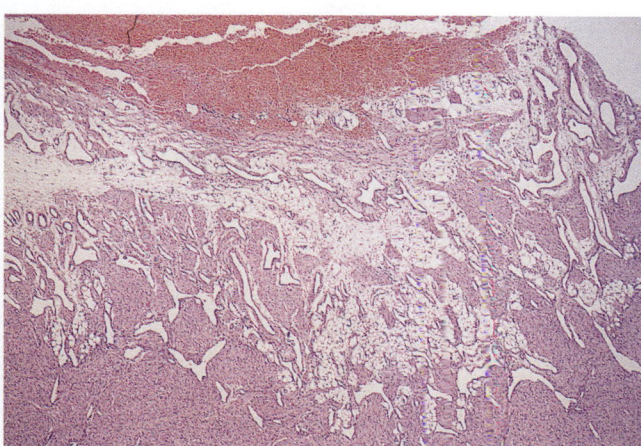

FIG. 34. Mesoblastic nephroma, classic pattern. Invasion into perirenal fat, with angiomatous appearance of advancing edge.

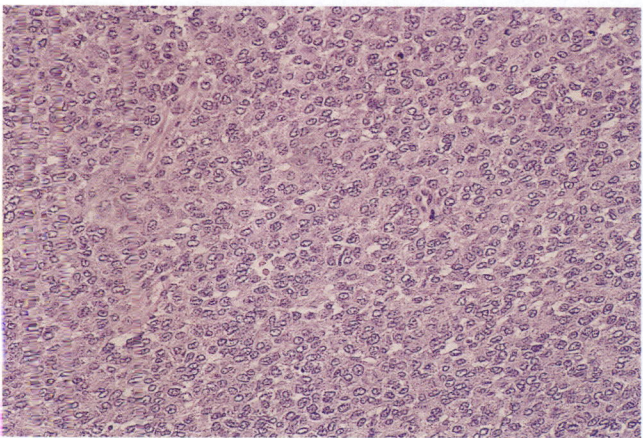

FIG. 36. Mesoblastic nephroma, cellular type, "plump cell" pattern.

lial cells abutting on tumor often undergo "embryonal metaplasia," producing tall cuboidal to columnar cells that must not be misinterpreted as evidence for WT (see Fig. 32). Tumors of the pure classic pattern are usually small, with nephrectomy specimens rarely exceeding 100 grams.

Cellular Mesoblastic Nephroma

Cellular MN is characterized by densely packed spindle cells with a high mitotic rate. This is the predominant or exclusive pattern in 66% of MN specimens in our files. Composite specimens, composed of both cellular and classic patterns, are not uncommon (Fig. 35). Because cellular foci grow faster than those of the classic pattern, they will eventually become the dominant component. Remnants of the classic pattern at the periphery of cellular MNs may be interpreted as a reactive pseudocapsule. MN of the cellular type can have an interdigitating border similar to that of classic MN, but as they enlarge, most will develop a pushing border. Cellular MN may attain very large size, with nephrectomy specimens sometimes exceeding 1 kg.

Two major histologic subtypes of cellular MN can be identified. The most common of these is a "plump cell" pattern characterized by large spindled or polygonal cells with abundant cytoplasm and variably enlarged, vesicular nuclei that may contain large nucleoli (Fig. 36). These cells may form diffuse sheets or interlacing bundles. The prominent nucleoli and cytoplasm of this subtype and the infantile age at diagnosis can lead to confusion with rhabdoid tumor. The features favoring plump cell MN over rhabdoid tumor are (a) less-invasive tumor margins, with a tendency toward encapsulation; (b) predominantly spindled cells; and (c) usual absence of cytoplasmic inclusions.

The other, less commonly encountered histologic subtype of cellular MN is one that can be described as a blue cell variant (Fig. 37). This closely resembles infantile fibrosarcoma. Both subtypes of cellular MN have numerous mitotic figures. Like infantile fibrosarcoma, both subtypes often show evidence of increased ploidy, with increased numbers of sev-

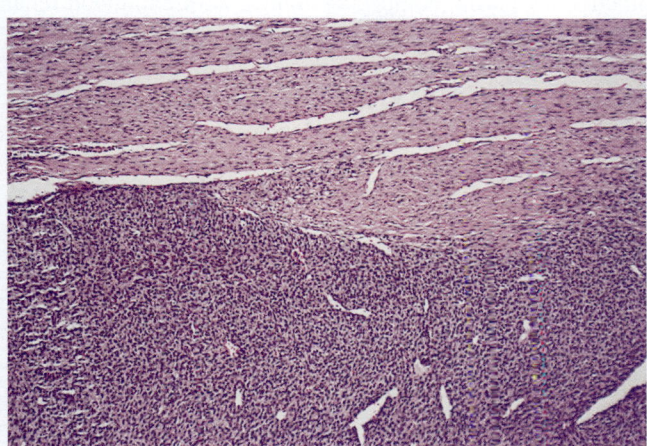

FIG. 35. Mixed classic and cellular mesoblastic nephroma.

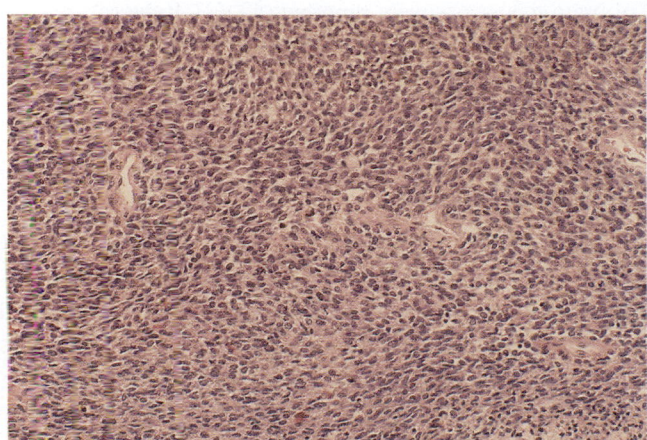

FIG. 37. Mesoblastic nephroma, cellular type, "blue cell" pattern.

eral chromosomes, most commonly including chromosome 11 (43,44).

Immunohistochemistry and Ultrastructure

Immunostains are of limited value in the diagnosis of MN, except where the differential diagnosis includes entities with a different staining spectrum. The cells of MN stain in a fashion consistent with myofibroblasts or smooth-muscle cells (42,45). Ultrastructural studies reveal features consistent with fibroblasts or myofibroblasts. Abundant rough endoplasmic reticulum (RER) with branching and anastomosing profiles are a prominent feature in most specimens, and primitive cell junctions are often found (46).

Clinical Behavior

The sarcomatous appearances of cellular MNs do not by themselves imply a high likelihood of recurrence or metastasis if the lesion is completely resected, and the vast majority of cellular MNs are cured by nephrectomy alone. The critical issue in evaluating nephrectomy specimens containing MN is to establish whether the lesion was completely resected. This is usually impossible to establish with certainty, especially on the medial aspect of the specimen. For this reason, in the majority of cases, we recommend close follow-up by imaging studies. Because only about 5% of MNs are associated with subsequent metastasis or relapse, the initial use of adjuvant therapy is not usually recommended unless there is known residual tumor. The duration of intensive follow-up can be relatively brief, because 29 of 31 relapsed cases in our files recurred within 1 year of nephrectomy. MNs of older infants and children are somewhat more likely to behave aggressively than those in neonates, but 20% of our relapsed cases were diagnosed in the first week of life.

Recurrent MN is usually limited to the retroperitoneum or peritoneum and tends to remain in the site of first relapse. The lung is the most common metastatic site, and a few cases of brain metastasis were reported (47,48). Relapses may respond to adjuvant therapy, but some are highly resistant, and complete surgical removal of recurrent disease is advisable whenever possible.

Differential Diagnosis

The three neoplasms most likely to be confused with MN in the infantile kidney are WT, clear cell sarcoma of the kidney, and rhabdoid tumor. Because most MNs are managed by resection alone, and the latter two entities are treated with aggressive and potentially dangerous regimens, the establishment of a correct diagnosis has exceptional clinical implications. Only WT is considered here, because the differential approach to clear cell sarcoma and rhabdoid tumor is discussed in their respective sections.

Mesoblastic Nephroma Versus Wilms Tumor

It is uncommon for untreated WT to be composed predominantly of stromal cells, but rare examples do occur. In most of these, the presence of immature or mature skeletal muscle readily excludes the diagnosis of MN. Embryonal metaplastic changes in nephrons surrounded by MN cells are sometimes misinterpreted as tubular or papillary elements in a WT.

The most common errors in interpretation involve specimens removed after chemotherapy. Treatment often ablates the embryonal, proliferating elements of a WT but tends to spare stromal cells. The resultant appearances can readily be confused with MN in some specimens. The following features are helpful in the differential diagnosis:

1. A diagnosis of MN should be considered suspect in a patient who has received prior therapy, unless the clinical and other features are characteristic.
2. Most MN are diagnosed in the first 3 months, whereas WT is relatively uncommon at this age. Only 10% of MNs are diagnosed after 1 year, and almost none after 2 years.
3. The cellular composition of the lesion is usually the most helpful feature. Most WTs express a diversity of cell types and tissue patterns. Blastemal foci do not occur in a MN, and skeletal muscle is never seen. Nodules of entrapped cartilage and squamous pearls may occur in MN and should not be taken as evidence for WT.
4. The growth pattern is helpful when the interdigitating, irregular border of MN is present. However, cellular MN often has a sharp, pushing border, similar to that of most WTs.
5. Bilaterality or the presence of nephrogenic rests or both strongly favor WT, although MN rarely can coexist with nephrogenic rests in the adjacent kidney (49).

CLEAR CELL SARCOMA OF THE KIDNEY

Clear cell sarcoma of the kidney (CCSK) is a rare and distinctive neoplasm, composing about 5% of childhood renal tumors. Despite its rarity, this entity is responsible for a significant proportion of the diagnostic discrepancies in cases submitted to the NWTS. CCSK is capable of mimicking, or being mimicked by, every other major pediatric renal tumor (4). Because this neoplasm has a propensity for widespread metastases and for recurrence after therapy, it is included in the "unfavorable histology" category of the NWTS (4,50–53). The designation "bone metastasizing renal tumor of childhood" also was used for this neoplasm. CCSK metastases occur in a variety of sites, including some that are unusual for WT metastases, such as bone, brain, and soft tissues. The prognosis has been improved substantially by the addition of doxorubicin to the therapeutic regimen (54), so the establishment of a correct diagnosis for CCSK has great clinical significance.

Epidemiology and Clinical Aspects

CCSK is rarely diagnosed in the first 6 months of life, but increases rapidly thereafter, peaking in the second and third years. Its incidence decreases rapidly thereafter, but occasional cases are observed in adolescents and young adults. The male-to-female ratio among cases in our files is 1.3:1. No case of confirmed bilateral primary CCSK is known to us, nor are we aware of a case that had a syndrome associated with WT or NRs in the resected kidney.

The clinical biology of CCSK is quite distinctive. It often has a relatively slow growth rate, and most cases are first seen with apparently low-stage disease. In a recent NWTSG report of 120 cases, 71% had stage I or II disease, and only 5% had hematogenous metastases (54). Survival was only 25% for patients treated with dactinomycin and vincristine as the only chemotherapeutic agents, compared with 72% for patients who also received doxorubicin. Several points concerning relapse and metastasis of CCSK deserve emphasis:

1. The distribution of metastatic sites is far wider than for WT.
2. First recurrences may be seen many years after diagnosis (55). Children with this diagnosis must be followed up closely for a longer period than required for most WTs.
3. Recurrences after therapy may have a deceptively bland appearance, suggesting low-grade fibromatosis or myxoma. A lump appearing anywhere in a child with a history of CCSK should be viewed as a potential metastasis until proven otherwise.
4. Relapses are not uncommon in patients whose original tumor was stage I or II, especially those who do not receive doxorubicin (54). This implies that occult metastases had already occurred by the time of diagnosis, and appearances suggesting localization to kidney can be deceptive. Patients with stage I CCSK should be treated more aggressively than those with stage I WT.

Gross Appearance

The tumor is always unicentric, and we know of no bilateral examples. The shape of the lesion is often irregular (Fig. 38), with a distinct tumor–kidney junction. Tumors are usually relatively small, with nephrectomy specimens usually weighing in the 300- to 600-gram range. The color is variable, but a glistening, gelatinous surface is often seen. Cysts are common and may be so prominent as to suggest cystic nephroma on gross or imaging studies (56). Smaller examples of CCSK usually suggest an origin deep within the renal parenchyma, possibly in a medullary pyramid. Multicentric origin is not a feature, and precursor lesions have not been identified.

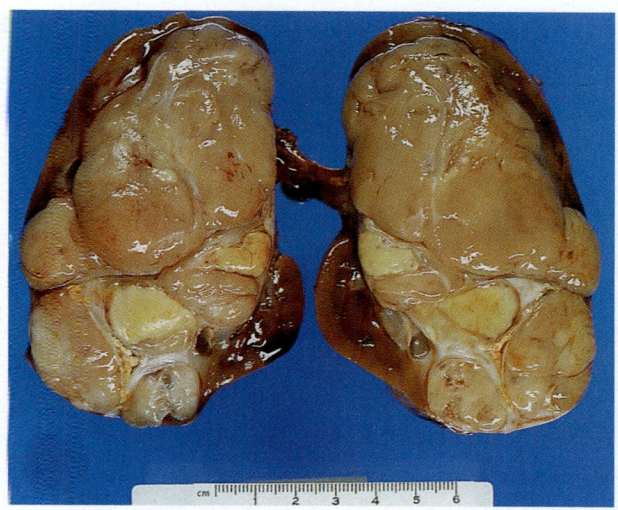

FIG. 38. Clear cell sarcoma of kidney.

Microscopic Appearance

Most CCSKs have typical appearances that can readily be distinguished from WT and other renal tumors of childhood, but variations on the classic patterns can produce the most difficult problems in differential diagnosis of any lesion discussed in this chapter. For an extended discussion of CCSK variant appearances, and more illustrations than are possible here, see reference 4.

The diagnosis can often be suspected before putting the slide on the microscopic stage, when we observe a uniform, pale gray–blue appearance to the H&E slide. This differs from most WTs, which tend to have either a uniform dark blue color or to have blue regions sharply demarcated from pink-staining regions, depending on the relative proportions of blastema, primitive tubules, and stroma in the lesion. Under low magnification, most CCSKs appear monomorphous, without the prominent lobulation usually seen with WT.

The appearance of the tumor–kidney junction is quite characteristic (see Fig. 38). CCSK usually has a scalloped border that appears fairly sharp under low power, with a thick pseudocapsule. Under higher magnification, the border tends to appear less sharply defined because of the percolation of single cells a short distance into the surrounding tissues or the tumor capsule. This growth pattern tends to surround and isolate individual nephrons (Fig. 39), which is rarely if ever seen with WT. The diffuse blastemal pattern of WT is more aggressive, usually producing a broader zone of invasiveness that surrounds islands of renal parenchyma rather than isolating single nephrons. The entrapped tubules are usually confined to the peripheral 2 to 3 cm of a CCSK. Their epithelium commonly shows embryonal metaplastic changes similar to those in MN, and the resultant basophilic epithelium invites confusion with WT (Fig. 40).

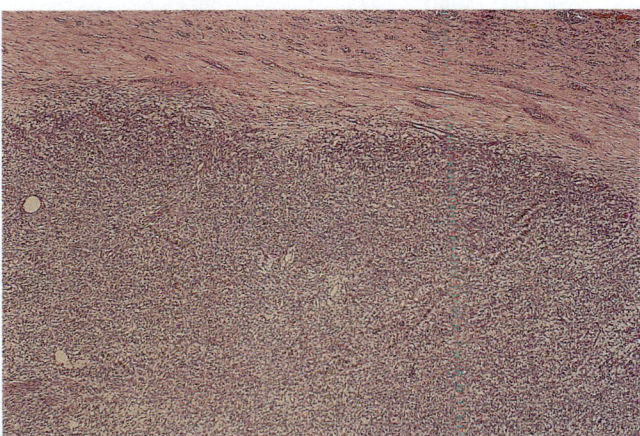

FIG. 39. Clear cell sarcoma of kidney, with characteristic scalloped, slightly indistinct margin and adjacent pseudocapsule formation.

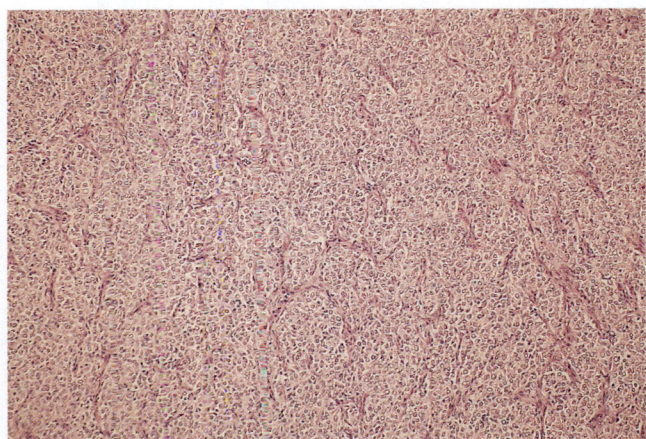

FIG. 41. Clear cell sarcoma of kidney, classic pattern.

Classic Pattern

The hallmark of this pattern is an evenly distributed network of vascular septa, connected at frequent intervals by transverse arcades (Fig. 41). These fibrovascular septa subdivide the tumor into a conspicuous pattern of cords and nests, averaging six to ten cells in width, composed of polygonal cells that usually lack distinct cytoplasmic borders (Fig. 42). Cells within the cords are less densely packed than those of blastemal WT, and overlapping nuclei are less frequent. Nuclear chromatin is usually finely granular, with inconspicuous nucleoli. In well-fixed specimens, the nuclear chromatin pattern is a helpful clue to the diagnosis, but we must beware of using this criterion alone, because it is influenced markedly by the timing and type of fixation. Delayed or imperfect fixation may cause clumping of chromatin in CCSK, and some fixatives may make the chromatin of WT appear finely granular. Mitotic figures are variable in number but are usually less numerous than those in WT.

The cytoplasm usually lacks distinct borders and encloses vacuoles of extracellular mucopolysaccharides, which are a distinctive and prominent feature of most CCSKs, and contribute to their usually pale appearance on stained slides. These vacuoles may appear empty or contain blue-stained granular material, depending on the fixative and staining technique used. The name currently used for this entity can sometimes be misleading, because some CCSKs contain cells that are neither palely stained nor vesicular. Some CCSKs contain cells with tingible, usually eosinophilic, sharply demarcated cytoplasm. These tingible cells can be present either focally or diffusely.

Variant Patterns

CCSK is easily confused with other neoplasms because the classic pattern is often modified, presenting alterations that mimic other neoplasms to a sometimes striking degree (4). Fortunately, the classic pattern of CCSK predominates in most specimens and is present focally in most tumors with variant patterns. However, the pathologist unaware of these variant patterns is likely to diagnose CCSK as another neo-

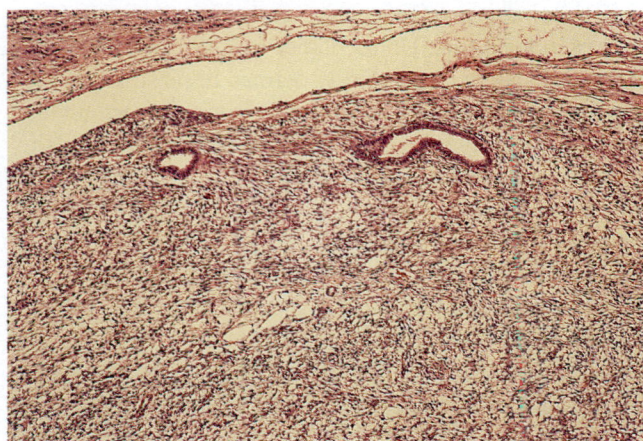

FIG. 40. Clear cell sarcoma of kidney, entrapped, isolated collecting ducts showing embryonal metaplasia.

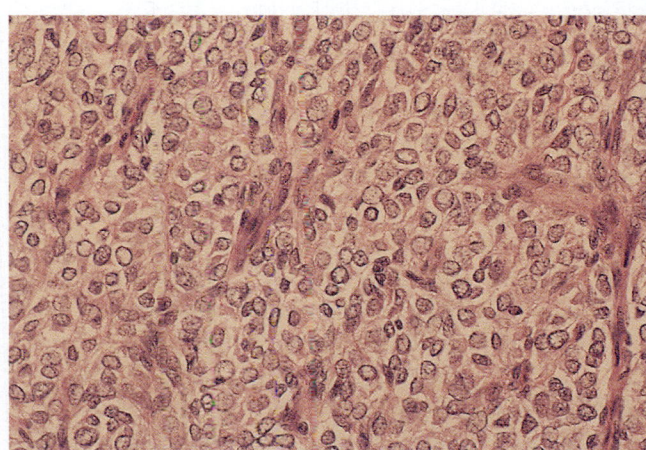

FIG. 42. Clear cell sarcoma of kidney, classic pattern, showing characteristic nuclear features.

plasm with different therapeutic and prognostic implications.

In the descriptions that follow, we refer to the "cord cells" and "septal cells" of the classic pattern, as most of the pattern alterations can be conceptualized as alterations in one or both of these components.

Epithelioid Patterns

Condensation of cord cells of the classic CCSK pattern can produce striking epithelioid arrangements, as shown in Fig. 43. These condensations usually form ribbons, but sometimes they form true tubules (57). These epithelioid formations conform to the pattern of the original cell cords and can be either straight or undulating in configuration. The epithelioid pattern is often associated with an increased mitotic rate, and epithelioid foci may form expansile nodules within the tumor. It is the epithelioid variants of CCSK that are most easily mistaken for WT. In several examples we have studied with immunohistochemistry, these epithelioid structures have been negative for epithelial markers, in contrast to the epithelial cells in WT.

Spindle Cell Patterns

Spindle cell variants seem to result from two mechanisms. Proliferation of septal cells, as shown in Fig. 44, can produce wide spindle cell septa that compress or obliterate the cell cords. Intersections of these hyperplastic septal cells often resemble the storiform arrangements seen with fibrohistiocytic tumors. Spindled transformation of cord cells imparts a spindled pattern with preservation of thin fibrovascular septa (Fig. 45).

Myxoid and Sclerosing Patterns

Most CCSKs contain abundant mucopolysaccharide, apparently produced by the cord cells (Fig. 46). This material

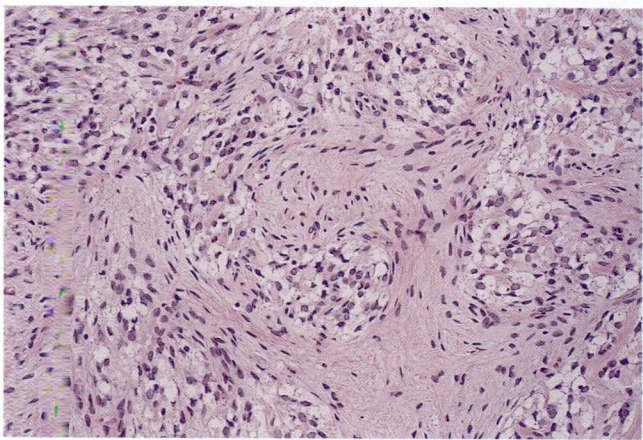

FIG. 44. Clear cell sarcoma of kidney. Spindled pattern due to hyperplasia of septal cells.

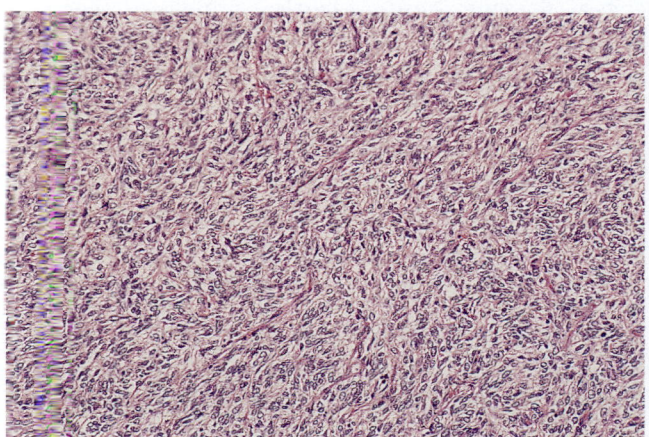

FIG. 45. Clear cell sarcoma of kidney. Spindled transformation of cord cells.

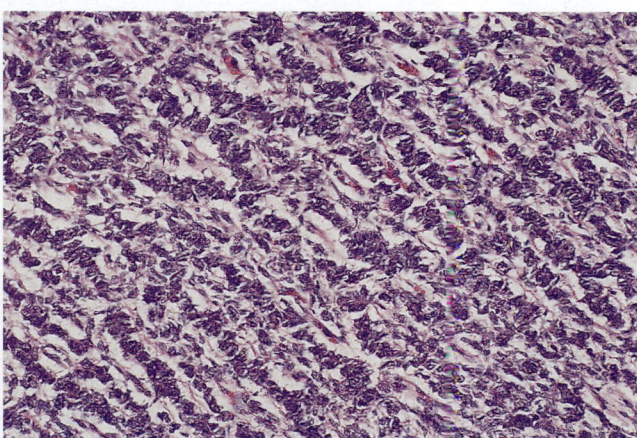

FIG. 43. Clear cell sarcoma of kidney. Epithelioid pattern.

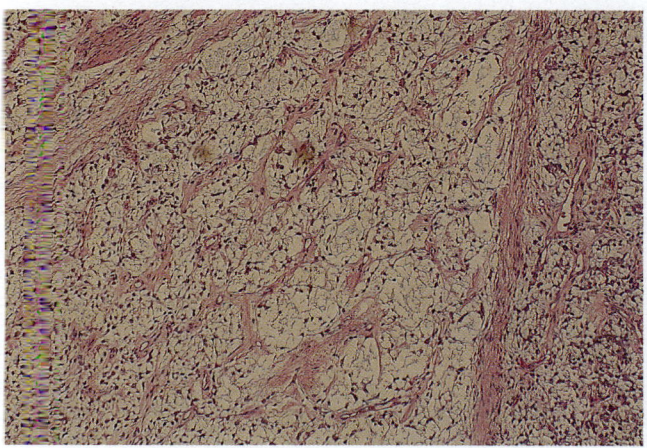

FIG. 46. Clear cell sarcoma of kidney. Myxoid pattern.

separates cord cells and is primarily responsible for the pale appearance of CCSK that suggested its name. It often occupies more volume than the tumor cells themselves and forms large pools or cystic spaces. As it accumulates, the tumor cells become progressively more isolated and eventually degenerate. As the cells producing this mucoid material disappear, mucus production ceases, and the mucoid material becomes denser, eosinophilic, and hyaline in appearance. Hyaline sclerosis is extremely common in CCSK. Complete replacement of cell cords by hyaline sclerosis often preserves the original cord pattern with retention of the vascular septa, imparting a "chicken-wire" appearance (Fig. 47). It may also form more diffuse zones of dense stromal sclerosis, surrounding individual tumor cells and sometimes imparting an osteosarcoma-like appearance. Dense stromal sclerosis is relatively uncommon in untreated WT, and this finding can be a clue to the diagnosis of CCSK or rhabdoid tumor.

Cystic Patterns

Cysts in CCSK usually result from coalescence of mucoid material, producing unlined spaces of varying size. Cysts lined by epithelium reflect dilatation of entrapped tubules.

Palisading Pattern

Nuclear palisading resembling neurilemoma is focally prominent in about 15% of CCSK specimens. In our experience, this feature has not been associated with positive staining for S-100 protein.

Monstrocellular Pattern

Rarely CCSK contains foci with gigantic, pleomorphic nuclei and bizarre mitotic figures, resembling the appearance of anaplastic sarcomas. This appearance, especially in metastatic sites, can be very misleading.

Ultrastructure and Immunohistochemistry

Ultrastructural studies yielded few clues to the cell of origin of CCSK (1,4,18,19,51,52). The tumor cells are characterized by a high nuclear-to-cytoplasmic ratio, with nuclear shapes that are more irregular and variable than would be expected from light microscopy. The cytoplasm is usually tenuous, with elongated irregular processes surrounding abundant intercellular matrix. This latter feature is responsible for the vacuoles often seen with the light microscope. Although true desmosomes are not seen, primitive cell junctions may be numerous. Cytoplasmic filaments are sometimes present, but rarely if ever do they form the conspicuous arrays seen in rhabdoid tumors. The cytoplasm tends to be poor in organelles. Immunohistochemistry has afforded little new insight into the histogenesis of CCSK, except to exclude various potential cells of origin for this enigmatic neoplasm, but only a small number of observations have been reported (20,58). Vimentin is readily demonstrable in nearly all specimens, but other intermediate filament stains are consistently negative, as are epithelial markers, which decorate only entrapped tubules. Stains for neural and muscle markers are also negative, in our experience.

Differential Diagnosis

The distinction of CCSK from other renal tumors can be extremely difficult, even for those with extensive experience in pediatric pathology. The following clues are often helpful.

Clear Cell Sarcoma of the Kidney Versus Wilms Tumor

Some blastemal WT are richly vascular, and the vessel pattern may mimic that of CCSK. Examination under low magnification often reveals the distinctive organoid blastemal patterns of WT. The following clues also are helpful:

1. Blastemal WTs are more densely cellular than are CCSKs. When cells are closely packed and most nuclei are overlapping, WT is more likely than CCSK.
2. Heterologous tissues such as skeletal muscle are never seen in CCSK. The presence of a focus resembling CCSK in an otherwise unequivocal WT can safely be ignored.
3. Multicentric and bilateral CCSKs have not been reported.
4. Sclerotic, hyalinized stroma in an untreated tumor favors CCSK over WT.
5. Fine nuclear chromatin pattern favors a diagnosis of CCSK, although this feature is susceptible to fixation and processing artifacts. Chromatin patterns must always be evaluated in the context of other histologic features.

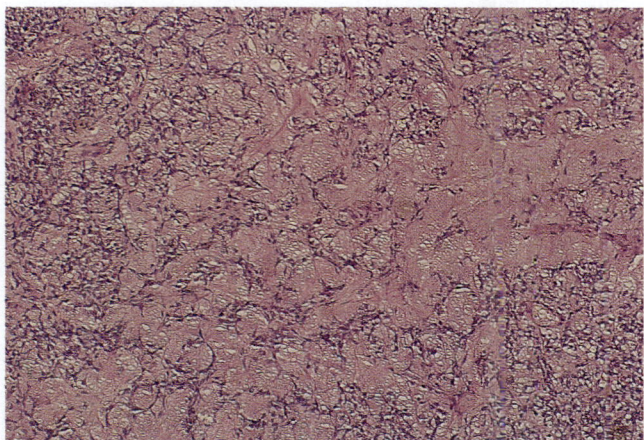

FIG. 47. Clear cell sarcoma of kidney. Sclerosing pattern with hyalinized cell cords and persisting "chicken-wire" pattern of septa.

Clear Cell Sarcoma of the Kidney Versus Mesoblastic Nephroma

Cellular MN sometimes has considerable resemblance to spindled variants of CCSK, and the age ranges of these two entities overlap. Small foci resembling CCSK may occur in MN, suggesting that these entities might be pathogenetically related. We know of no such case that has had an untoward outcome, so we advise treating a tumor as MN when the predominant pattern suggests that diagnosis.

RHABDOID TUMOR OF THE KIDNEY

Rhabdoid tumor of the kidney (RTK) is a rare but important neoplasm, first recognized in a review of the first NWTS as a histologically distinctive and clinically aggressive renal neoplasm of young infants (25). RTK composes approximately 2% of renal tumors entered on the NWTS.

After the recognition and acceptance of this infantile renal tumor as a neoplastic entity with distinctive cytologic and clinical features (59), it was soon recognized that tumors with similar cytologic features occurred in many other sites, in patients of all ages. Initially these were considered extrarenal or adult rhabdoid tumors (RTs). However, that concept was clouded by increasing awareness that many neoplasms of defined nature could contain cells resembling those of RTK. Thus arose a lively and sometimes contentious debate concerning the existence, nature, and significance of "extrarenal RT" and "adult RT," and of "true RT" versus "pseudo RT" (60–63). This debate still rages, occupying vast numbers of pages in pathology journals, and is likely to continue until the nature of the cell constituting RTK is defined and accepted. Until that time, we contend that most but not all cases of extrarenal RT are probably other entities with focal or diffuse expression of cells resembling those of RT. A small number of cases with aggressive infantile tumors arising outside the kidney seem to be convincing examples of extrarenal RT. For the present, we follow the approach suggested by Gaffney and Breathnach (60) of designating those tumors of uncertain nature that resemble RTK, but do not fulfill the full clinical and pathologic profile of RTK, as "malignant undifferentiated neoplasms of undetermined nature, with rhabdoid features." This approach avoids the necessity for drawing a line in the sand before knowing where it should be drawn.

Clinical Features

RTK has a distinctive predilection for infants (64), with a median age of 13 months. Our earlier review included three children aged 5 to 8.5 years. However, the two children older than 5 years recently were reclassified as having medullary renal carcinoma with sickle cell trait, discussed later. The oldest case that we now accept as having RTK in our files was diagnosed at age 60 months. This diagnosis should be considered unlikely in any patient older than 3 years and extremely suspect beyond 5 years.

Approximately 15% of RTK cases in our files were associated with PNET of the posterior fossa midline (65) (Fig. 48). These central nervous system (CNS) tumors generally resembled medulloblastomas. Most occurred synchronously with the renal tumor, but others preceded or followed the renal tumor by as much as 3 years, suggesting that they are separate primary tumors. RTK metastases to the brain retain the typical cytologic features of the renal tumor and lack a consistent midline posterior fossa location.

Hypercalcemia is a commonly observed first finding in young infants with RTK, which is also encountered in some infants with MN, but not with other pediatric renal tumors. Secretion of parathormone or prostaglandin E_2 is the apparent mechanism in most cases (66). We have seen a few cases with symmetrical RT in both kidneys, suggesting bilateral primary RTK, although metastasis from one kidney to the other could not be excluded. Familial recurrence was reported in infant female siblings with paravertebral RT (67), and our files contain slides from a boy who developed RTK at 7 months, whose male twin developed the same tumor at the age of 2 years. A distinctive cutaneous lesion, designated "neurovascular hamartoma," was associated with RTK in a few cases (68) and may represent another clue that RTK is part of a systemic diathesis.

Rhabdoid tumor is among the most malignant neoplasms of childhood, and despite the intensified therapeutic regimens of recent NWTS trials, the prognosis for this neoplasm remains poor. Patients develop widespread hematogenous and lymphatic metastases to bone, brain, and other sites not often involved with WT metastases, and death, usually within 1 year of diagnosis, occurs in more than 75% of patients (64).

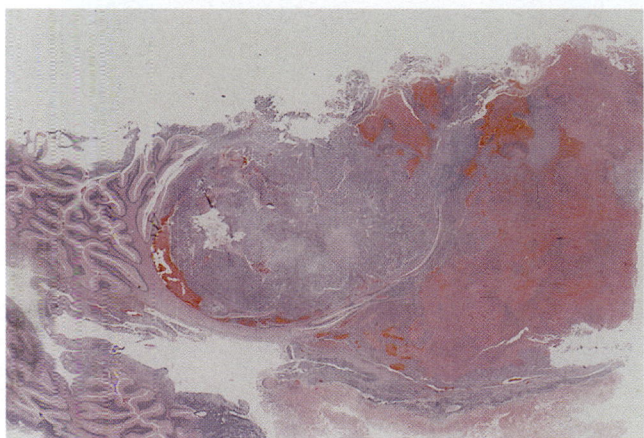

FIG. 48. Primitive neuroepithelioma of cerebellar vermis producing hydrocephalus, with simultaneous rhabdoid tumor of kidney.

Gross and Microscopic Appearance

Most RTKs are relatively small, because dissemination usually occurs early in the course of this tumor (64). Hemorrhage and necrosis are commonly seen, whereas satellite nodules in the renal parenchyma or capsular invasion or both often betray the aggressiveness of this neoplasm (Fig. 49). Most cases are at an advanced stage when diagnosed, even in the newborn period.

Microscopic appearances are monomorphous, and the tumor–kidney junction is usually poorly defined, because of aggressive invasion by relatively noncohesive tumor cells into adjacent vessels and soft tissues. This aggressive appearance is an important clue to the diagnosis, and, in specimens lacking this feature, other diagnoses must be seriously considered. The cytologic features are distinctive, but tumor cells are highly susceptible to fixation artifact, and we must take care to ensure prompt and complete fixation of thin tissue slices. In our experience, fixatives such as B5 yield more consistently good results than does formalin. In optimally fixed sections, the cells of RTK are relatively large and usually rounded or polygonal, with abundant cytoplasm that is usually eosinophilic or amphophilic (Fig. 50). With suboptimal fixation, RTK often has smudged, somewhat basophilic cytoplasm, somewhat resembling the appearances of large cell lymphomas (Fig. 51).

The nuclear features of RTK are distinctive. Nuclei are relatively large and vesicular, with exceptionally prominent nucleoli (see Fig. 50). Nuclei may be lobulated, and sometimes mimic the nuclei of Reed–Sternberg cells. Cytoplasmic inclusions are a characteristic feature (see Fig. 50). These inclusions are eosinophilic and usually appear homogeneous, but with optimally fixed specimens, we can sometimes perceive a whorled, somewhat fibrillary texture under

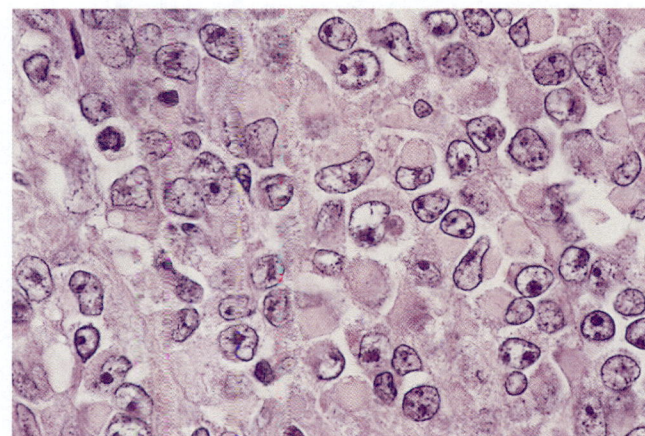

FIG. 50. Rhabdoid tumor of kidney. Appearance in optimally fixed and stained specimen.

high magnification. Cytoplasmic inclusions are variably prominent, and sometimes are sparsely distributed, requiring extensive search. They are often found most readily near foci of necrosis.

Ultrastructural Features

Detailed reviews of this topic are available (1,18,58, 59,64). The most distinctive ultrastructural feature of RTK consists of whorled arrays of intermediate filaments that are responsible for the cytoplasmic "inclusions" seen with the light microscope. However, it is important to recognize that whorled filamentous masses are not specific for RTK. The most important role of the ultrastructural study of RT is in evaluating or establishing alternative diagnoses, such as rhabdomyosarcoma or neuroendocrine neoplasms (62).

Immunohistochemistry

Polyphenotypic immunohistochemical results are commonly observed in RTK, which limits the value of im-

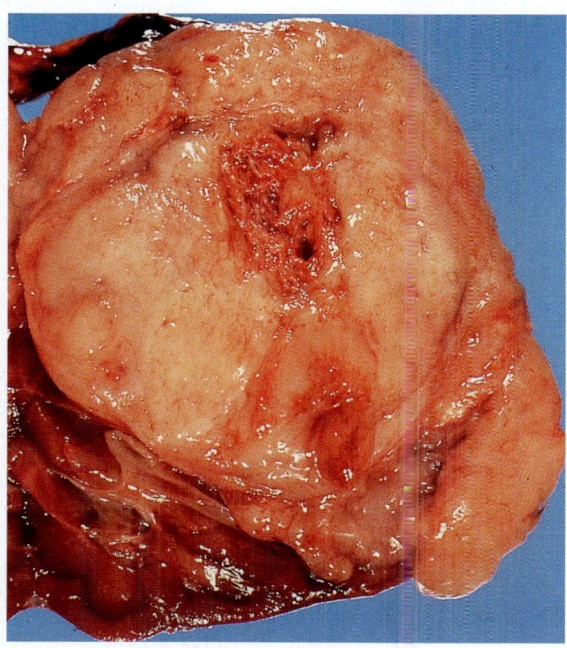

FIG. 49. Rhabdoid tumor of kidney.

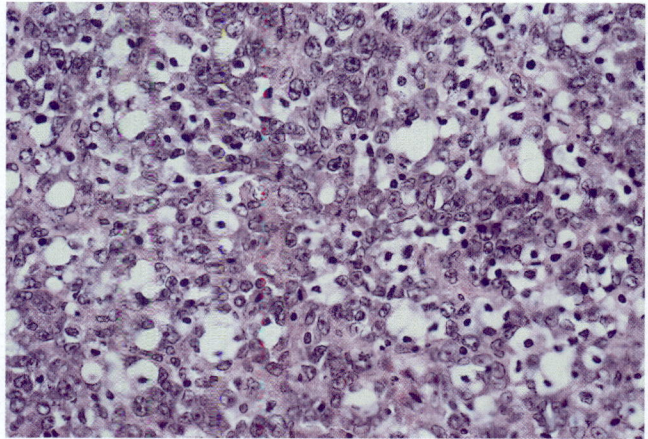

FIG. 51. Rhabdoid tumor of kidney. Appearance in suboptimally fixed specimen.

munostains in establishing this diagnosis. Vimentin is almost always expressed in RTK, and coexpression of cytokeratin and epithelial membrane antigen is frequently observed (63,64). We observed nonspecific positivity for many epitopes when the positive results are limited to the cytoplasmic inclusions (64), possibly reflecting nonspecific entrapment or binding of antibody in the dense filamentous masses. Some cases of RT express positive results for a number of epitopes more diffusely in the cytoplasm (63).

Molecular and Cytogenetic Studies

Although a variety of cytogenetic and molecular results were reported for RTK (63), the most frequently encountered finding reported is loss of heterozygosity involving chromosome 22q11-12, and less commonly also for 11p15.5 (69). Monosomy for chromosome 22 was reported in some cases of RT of the CNS (70). In an infant with synchronous PNET of the pineal region and RTK, the brain tumor showed monosomy 22, whereas the renal tumor had disomy for this chromosome, supporting the concept that these tumors are related but separate primary neoplasms (71).

Differential Diagnosis

A variety of renal tumors of both children and adults can adopt appearances that mimic RTK to a considerable degree.

Medullary Renal Carcinoma

This recently delineated neoplastic entity occurs predominantly, if not exclusively, in patients with sickle cell trait (72). It is thought to arise from distal cells of the collecting duct, is highly invasive, uniformly lethal, and has a predilection for children and young adults. In our experience, MRC is by far the most important renal neoplasm mimicking RTK (73). Most of the cases of MRC in our files were referred to as possible RTK. The oldest cases in our earlier review of RTK (64) were black children who subsequently were found to have evidence of sickle cell trait and are now considered as having had MRC. These tumors have many features in common, including similar nuclear features, abundant eosinophilic cytoplasm, and marked clinical aggressiveness. Structures resembling the inclusions of RTK are present in some cases, although more commonly, we encountered vacuoles lined by microvilli. Features distinguishing MRC from RTK include age older than 5 years and the presence of sickled erythrocytes, which are usually found without difficulty in routinely processed sections.

Rhabdoid Tumor of the Kidney Versus Wilms Tumor

Both blastemal and myogenic elements of WT contain cytoplasmic inclusions resembling those of RTK (61). The former can often be recognized by the presence under low power of a distinctive serpentine blastemal pattern. Other distinctly nephrogenic features, or heterologous cells such as skeletal muscle, will facilitate the correct diagnosis in most instances. The huge nucleoli characteristic of RTK are not seen in WT, with the exception of some anaplastic specimens.

Rhabdoid Tumor of the Kidney Versus Mesoblastic Nephroma

The plump cell variant of MN often has vesicular nuclei with prominent nucleoli, and a rare MN contains foci with hyaline cytoplasmic inclusions. The predominance of spindled patterns and the far less invasive tumor periphery will reveal that a tumor with these features is more likely an MN than a rhabdoid tumor.

Rhabdoid Tumor of the Kidney Versus Clear Cell Sarcoma of the Kidney

The rare occurrence of prominent nucleoli focally in CCSK rarely can lead to difficulty in distinguishing these entities. The presence of classic histologic and cytologic features of CCSK is the major clue to the correct diagnosis in such instances. CCSKs lack the extreme invasiveness of RTKs and are generally more indolent-appearing neoplasms.

RENAL CARCINOMAS IN CHILDREN

Renal cell carcinoma (RCC) is discussed in detail in the preceding chapter, and only those aspects of the topic relevant to childhood are noted here.

Conventional (Clear Cell) Renal Carcinoma

Conventional RCC during childhood is distinctly uncommon, but when it does occur, it seems not to differ clinically or biologically from comparable RCC of adults (74). The youngest case in our files was diagnosed at age 5 days. RCC in adolescents is an occasional sequela of radiotherapy for other lesions during infancy or early childhood. Tuberous sclerosis or von Hippel–Lindau disease is rarely associated with renal carcinoma in childhood.

Xp1.2 Renal Carcinoma

Whereas most conventional RCCs are associated with an abnormality on chromosome 3p, a distinctive variant was recently recognized to be associated with translocations that consistently involve the p11.2 region of the X chromosome (75,76). This subtype has a particular predilection for children and young adults and may account for a substantial proportion of cases of childhood RCC. Histologically, most reported cases showed a combination of clear or granular cells with significant regions of papillary architecture (Fig. 52).

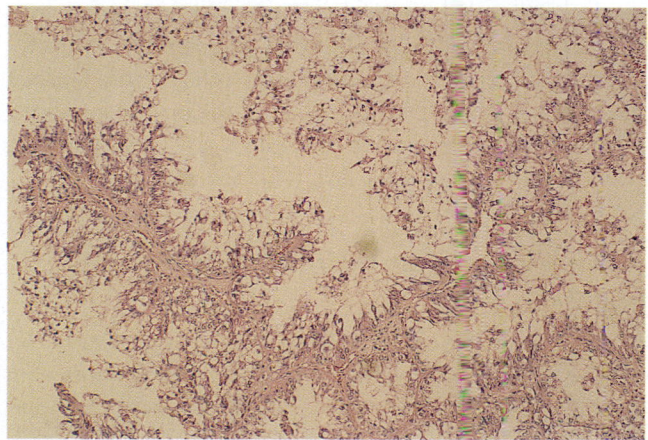

FIG. 52. Renal cell carcinoma associated with Xp11.2 breakpoint translocation. Papillary architecture is prominent, with clear cell cytologic features.

Papillary Renal Carcinoma

This entity was discussed earlier in the section on differential diagnosis of epithelial predominant WT. It remains to be determined whether a significant biologic relation exists between some cases of papillary renal carcinoma, nephrogenic rests, and WT.

Medullary Renal Carcinoma

MRC recently emerged as an important entity, usually occurring only in patients with sickle cell trait (72). This neoplasm was discussed in the section on RTK, as in our experience, it is the renal tumor most likely to be confused morphologically with RTK. We encountered MRC in patients as young as 6 years, and the median age of 29 patients in our files was 13 years (73).

MISCELLANEOUS RENAL NEOPLASMS

Primitive Neuroepithelial Tumor of Kidney

Primary renal PNET is another entity to be considered in the differential diagnosis of undifferentiated blue cell tumors of the kidney. This lesion is encountered mainly in adolescent and young adult patients (77–79). These account for a substantial proportion of tumors submitted to us as blastemal WT of adolescent or adult patients and might account for some of the adverse prognosis assigned to "adult WT." The characteristic 11;22 translocation usually found in Ewing sarcoma and other peripheral PNETs was identified in some specimens and is a useful way to confirm the diagnosis in suspected cases. Also helpful in the diagnosis is immunohistochemical staining for CD99. Although this was reported to be positive in some blastemal WT (80), our experience suggests that the characteristic cytoplasmic surface-staining pattern observed in other peripheral PNETs is rarely if ever observed in WT blastemal cells.

Metanephric ("Nephrogenic") Adenofibroma and Metanephric Adenoma

A distinctive neoplasm of the kidney in pediatric and young adult patients was first reported in 1992 and designated "nephrogenic adenofibroma" (81). This neoplasm is a composite of a somewhat undifferentiated spindle cell component and an adenomatous component identical to the lesion now termed metanephric adenoma (82) (Fig. 53). Some specimens also contain a higher grade epithelial component that we originally viewed as possible collecting duct carcinoma, but which may be more closely related to papillary renal carcinoma. Because the adenomatous component of nephrogenic adenofibroma is so nearly identical to metanephric adenoma, the designation metanephric adenofibroma was suggested as a potentially better designation than the term originally used (81), a suggestion we accept. We therefore suggest using the designation metanephric adenofibroma (MAF) in future references to this lesion.

MAF may be a link between several diverse entities, including WT, MN, metanephric adenoma, and papillary renal carcinoma, but much more work remains before these potential relations are elucidated.

Ossifying Renal Tumor of Infancy

This rare infantile neoplasm usually is seen clinically as a calcified mass located predominantly within the pelvicalyceal system (4,83). It is often thought to represent a staghorn calculus on imaging studies, but surgical exploration reveals dense adherence to the renal parenchyma, usually in the region of a medullary papilla. Microscopically, the lesion consists of a spindle cell stroma similar to that of mesoblastic nephroma, with variably large regions of osteoid material. This lesion is apparently benign.

Renal Lymphoma

The kidney is a frequent site of involvement in leukemia and disseminated lymphoma. Less commonly, it is the pre-

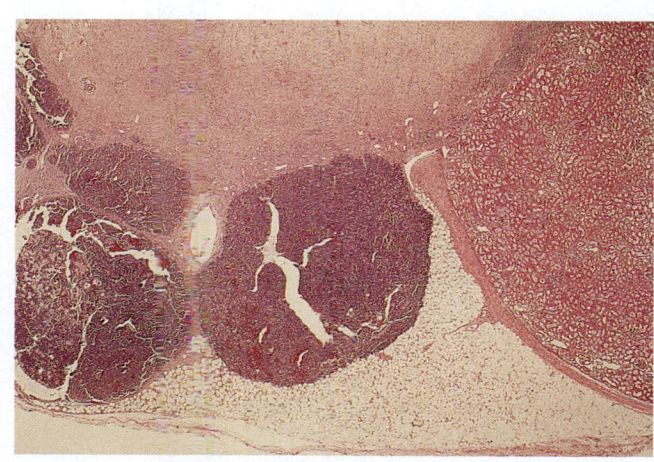

FIG. 53. Metanephric adenofibroma.

senting site for non-Hodgkin's lymphomas, so this entity must be considered in the differential diagnosis of bilateral and multicentric renal tumors of children and adolescents. The majority of reported cases in children are of B-cell lineage, but T-cell lymphoma in the kidneys also has been reported (84).

Miscellaneous Renal Neoplasms Usually Diagnosed in Adults

Most neoplasms of the adult kidney rarely involve the kidneys of children, but those that have no distinctive features in the pediatric patient are not discussed in this chapter.

ACKNOWLEDGMENTS

The innumerable pathologists and clinicians who have contributed materials and information to the NWTS Pathology Center and to the consultation files of the author have provided the indispensable foundation for all my work. The NWTS committee members, NWTS Pathology Fellows, and the staff of the NWTS Data and Statistical Center, directed by Norman Breslow, PhD, have all made major contributions. This work was supported in part by USPHS grant CA 42326.

REFERENCES

1. Parham DM. Renal neoplasms. In: Parham DM, ed. *Pediatric neoplasia: morphology and biology.* Philadelphia: Lippincott-Raven, 1996: 33–64.
2. Green DM, Coppes MJ, Breslow NE, et al. Wilms tumor. In: Pizzo PA, Poplack DG, eds. *Principles and practice of pediatric oncology.* 3rd ed. Philadelphia: Lippincott-Raven, 1997:733–759.
3. Coppes MJ, Campbell CE, Williams BRG. *Wilms tumor: clinical and molecular characterization.* Austin, TX: RG Landes, 1995.
4. Beckwith JB. Tumors of infancy and childhood. In: Murphy WM, Beckwith JB, Farrow GM, eds. *Tumors of the kidney, bladder, and related urinary structures: atlas of tumor pathology,* 3rd series, Fascicle 11. Washington DC: Armed Forces Institute of Pathology, 1994:12–91
5. Beckwith JB. National Wilms tumor study: an update for pathologists *Pediatr Dev Pathol* 1998;1:79–84.
6. Weeks DA, Beckwith JB. Relapse-associated variables in stage I, favorable histology Wilms' tumor. *Cancer* 1987;60:1204–1212.
7. Weeks DA, Beckwith JB, Mierau GW. Benign nodal lesions mimicking metastases from pediatric renal neoplasms: a report of the National Wilms' Tumor Study pathology center. *Hum Pathol* 1990;21: 1239–1244.
8. Coppes MJ, Beckwith JB. Eponyms in medicine: possessive or nonpossessive? *J Pediatr* 1993;122:165.
9. Breslow NG, Beckwith JB, Ciol M, Sharples K. Age distribution of Wilms' tumor: report from the National Wilms' Tumor Study. *Cancer Res* 1988;48:1653–1657.
10. Breslow N, Olshan A, Beckwith JB, Green DM. Epidemiology of Wilms tumor. *Med Pediatr Oncol* 1993;21:172–181
11. Breslow NE, Olson J, Moksness J, Beckwith JB, Grundy P. Familial Wilms tumor: a descriptive study. *Med Pediatr Oncol* 1996;27: 398–403.
12. Coppes M. Serum biological markers and paraneoplastic syndromes in Wilms tumor. *Med Pediatr Oncol* 1993;12:213–221.
13. Schaub CR, Farhi DC. Circulating mucin in Wilms tumor and nephroblastomatosis: effect on leukocyte counts. *Arch Pathol Lab Med* 1988;112:656–657.
14. Beckwith JB, Zuppan CE, Browning NG, et al. Histological analysis of aggressiveness versus responsiveness in Wilms tumor. *Med Pediatr Oncol* 1996;27:422–428.
15. Wigger HJ. Fetal rhabdomyomatous nephroblastoma: a variant of Wilms tumor. *Hum Pathol* 1976;7:613–623.
16. Saba LMB, de Camargo B, Gabriel-Arana M. Experience with six children with fetal rhabdomyomatous nephroblastoma: review of the clinical, biologic, and pathologic features. *Med Pediatr Oncol* 1998;30: 152–155.
17. Zuppan CW, Beckwith JB, Weeks DA, et al. Effect of preoperative therapy on Wilms' tumor histology: analysis of cases from the third National Wilms' Tumor Study. *Cancer* 1991;68:385–394.
18. Mierau GW, Beckwith JB, Weeks DA. Ultrastructure and histogenesis of the renal tumors of childhood: an overview. *Ultrastruct Pathol* 1987;11:313–333.
19. Weeks DA, Mierau GW, Malott RL, Beckwith JB. Practical electron microscopy of pediatric renal tumors. *Ultrastruct Pathol* 1996;20: 31–33.
20. Wick MR, Cherwitz DL, Manivel C, Sibley R. Immunohistochemical findings in tumors of the kidney. In: Eble JN, ed. *Tumors and tumor-like conditions of the kidneys and ureters.* New York: Churchill Livingstone, 1990:207–247.
21. Abeda FW, Molenaar WM, de Leij L, Thijs-Ipema AH. Heterogeneity of Wilms tumour blastema: an immunohistological study. *Virchows Arch A Pathol Anat* 1989;414:263–271.
22. Folpe AL, Patterson K, Gown AM. Antibodies to desmin identify the blastemal component of nephroblastoma. *Mod Pathol* 1997;10: 895–900.
23. Zuppan CW, Beckwith JB, Luckey DW. Anaplasia in unilateral Wilms' tumor: a report from the National Wilms' Tumor Study pathology center. *Hum Pathol* 1988;19:1199–1209.
24. Faria P, Beckwith JB, Mishra K, et al. Focal versus diffuse anaplasia in Wilms tumor: new definitions with prognostic significance: a report from the National Wilms Tumor Study Group. *Am J Surg Pathol* 1996;20:909–920.
25. Beckwith JB, Palmer NF. Histopathology and prognosis of Wilms tumor: results from the first national Wilms tumor study. *Cancer* 1978;41:1937–1948.
26. Joshi VV, Beckwith JB. Multilocular cyst of the kidney (cystic nephroma) and cystic, partially differentiated nephroblastoma: terminology and criteria for diagnosis. *Cancer* 1989;64:466–479.
27. Cho KJ, Thornbury JR, Bernstein J, Heidelberger KP, Walter JF. Localized cystic disease of the kidney: angiographic-pathologic correlations. *AJR Am J Roentgenol* 1979;132:891–895.
28. Murad T, Komaiko W, Oyasu R, Bauer K. Multilocular cystic renal cell carcinoma. *Am J Clin Pathol* 1991;95:633–637.
29. Beckwith JB, Kiviat NB, Bonadio JF. Nephrogenic rests, nephroblastomatosis, and the pathogenesis of Wilms' tumor. *Pediatr Pathol* 1990; 10:1–36.
30. Beckwith JB. Precursor lesions of Wilms tumor: clinical and biological implications. *Med Pediatr Oncol* 1993;21:158–168.
31. Gerald WL, Miller HK, Battifora H, et al. Intra-abdominal desmoplastic small round-cell tumor: report of 19 cases of a distinctive type of high-grade polyphenotypic malignancy affecting young individuals. *Am J Surg Pathol* 1991;15:499–513.
32. Gerald WL, Ladanyi M, de Alava E, Rosai J. Desmoplastic small round cell tumor: a recently recognized tumor type associated with a unique gene fusion. *Adv Anat Pathol* 1995;2:341–345.
33. Kovacs G, Kovacs A. Parenchymal abnormalities associated with papillary renal cell tumors: a morphologic study. *J Urol Pathol* 1993;1: 301–12.
34. Renshaw AA, Zhang H, Corless CL, Fletcher JA, Pins MA. Solid variants of papillary (chromophil) renal cell carcinoma: clinicopathological and genetic features. *Am J Surg Pathol* 1997;21:1203–1209.
35. Palmedo G, Fischer J, Kovacs G. Fluorescent microsatellite analysis reveals duplication of specific chromosomal regions in papillary renal cell tumors. *Lab Invest* 1997;77:633–8.
36. Kattar MM, Grignon DJ, Wallis T, et al. Clinicopathologic and interphase cytogenetic analysis of papillary (chromophilic) renal cell carcinoma. *Mod Pathol* 1997;10:1143–50.
37. Gatalica Z, Kovatovich A, Miettinen M. Consistent expression of cytokeratin 7 in papillary renal-cell carcinoma: an immunohistochemical study in formalin-fixed, paraffin-embedded tissues. *J Urol Pathol* 1995;3:205–12.
38. Amin MB, Corless CL, Renshaw AA, et al. Papillary (chromophil) renal cell carcinoma: histomorphologic characteristics and evaluation of conventional pathologic prognostic parameters in 62 cases. *Am J Surg Pathol* 1997;21:621–35.
39. Delahunt B, Eble JN. Papillary renal cell carcinoma: a clinicopathologic and immunohistochemical study of 105 tumors. *Mod Pathol* 1997;10:537–44.

40. Allsbrook WC, Boswell WC, Takahashi H, et al. Recurrent renal cell carcinoma arising in Wilms' tumor. *Cancer* 1991;57:690–695.
41. Bolande RP. Congenital mesoblastic nephroma of infancy. *Perspect Pediatr Pathol* 1973;1:227–250.
42. Pettinato G, Manivel JC, Wick MR, Dehner LP. Classical and cellular (atypical) congenital mesoblastic nephroma: a clinicopathologic, ultrastructural, immunohistochemical, and flow cytometric study. *Hum Pathol* 1989;20:682–690.
43. Schofield DE, Yunis EJ, Fletcher JA. Chromosome aberrations in mesoblastic nephroma. *Am J Pathol* 1993;143:714–724.
44. Mascarello JT, Cajulis TR, Krous HF, Carpenter PM. Presence or absence of trisomy 11 is correlated with histologic subtype in congenital mesoblastic nephroma. *Cancer Genet Cytogenet* 1994;77:50–54.
45. Nadasdy T, Roth J, Johnson DL, et al. Congenital mesoblastic nephroma: an immunohistochemical and lectin study. *Hum Pathol* 1993;24:413–419.
46. O'Malley DP, Mierau GW, Beckwith JB, Weeks DA. Ultrastructure of congenital mesoblastic nephroma. *Ultrastruct Pathol* 1996;20:417–427.
47. Heidelberger KP, Ritchey ML, Dauser RC, McKeever PE, Beckwith JB. Congenital mesoblastic nephroma metastatic to the brain. *Cancer* 1993;72:2499–2502.
48. Schlesinger AE, Rosenfield NS, Castle VP, Lasty R. Congenital mesoblastic nephroma metastatic to the brain: a report of two cases. *Pediatr Radiol* 1995;25:S73–S75.
49. Vujanic GM, Sandstedt B, Dijoud F, Harms D, Delemarre JFM. Nephrogenic rest associated with a mesoblastic nephroma: what does it tell us? *Pediatr Pathol Lab Med* 1995;15:469–475.
50. Sandstedt BE, Delemarre JFM, Harms D, Tournade MF. Sarcomatous Wilms' tumour with clear cells and hyalinization: a study of 38 tumours from the SIOP nephroblastoma file. *Histopathology* 1987;11:273–285.
51. Sotelo-Avila C, Gonzalez-Crussi F, Sadowinski S, Gooch WM, Pena R. Clear cell sarcoma of the kidney: a clinicopathologic study of 21 patients with long-term follow-up study. *Hum Pathol* 1986;16:1219–1230.
52. Haas JE, Bonadio JF, Beckwith JB. Clear cell sarcoma of the kidney with emphasis on ultrastructural studies. *Cancer* 1984;54:2978–2987.
53. Marsden HB, Lawler W. Bone metastasizing renal tumor of childhood: histopathological and clinical review of 38 cases. *Virchows Arch A Pathol Anat Histopathol* 1980;387:341–351.
54. Green DM, Breslow ME, Beckwith JB, Moksness J, Finklestein JZ, D'Angio GJ. Treatment of children with clear-cell sarcoma of the kidney: a report from the National Wilms Tumor Study Group. *J Clin Oncol* 1994;12:2132–2137.
55. Kusumakumary P, Chellam VG, Rojymon J, Hariharan S, Krishnan NM. Late recurrence of clear cell sarcoma of the kidney. *Med Pediatr Oncol* 1997;28:355–357.
56. Beckwith JB. The John Lattimer Lecture: Wilms tumor and other renal tumors of childhood: an update. *J Urol* 1986;136:320–324.
57. Schmidt D, Harms D, Evers KG, Bliesner JA, Beckwith JB. Bone metastasizing renal tumor (clear cell sarcoma) of childhood with epithelioid elements. *Cancer* 1985;56:609–613.
58. Mierau GW, Weeks DA, Beckwith JB. Anaplastic Wilms tumor and other clinically aggressive childhood renal neoplasms: ultrastructural and immunocytochemical features. *Ultrastruct Pathol* 1989;13:225–248.
59. Haas JE, Palmer NF, Weinberg AG, Beckwith JB. Ultrastructure of malignant rhabdoid tumor of the kidney: a distinctive renal tumor of children. *Hum Pathol* 1981;12:646–657.
60. Gaffney EF, Breathnach F. Diverse immunoreactivity and metachronous ultrastructural variability in fatal primitive childhood tumor with rhabdoid features. *Arch Pathol Lab Med* 1989;113:1322–1324.
61. Weeks DA, Beckwith JB, Mierau GW, Zuppan CW. Renal neoplasms mimicking rhabdoid tumor of kidney: a report from the national Wilms' Tumor Study pathology center. *Am J Surg Pathol* 1991;15:1042–1054.
62. Parham DM, Weeks DA, Beckwith JB. The clinicopathologic spectrum of putative extrarenal rhabdoid tumors. *Am J Surg Pathol* 1994;18:1010–1029.
63. Wick MR, Ritter JH, Dehner LP. Malignant rhabdoid tumors: a clinicopathologic review and conceptual discussion. *Semin Diagn Pathol* 1995;12:233–248.
64. Weeks DA, Beckwith JB, Mierau GW, Luckey DW. Rhabdoid tumor of kidney: a report of 111 cases from the National Wilms' Tumor Study pathology center. *Am J Surg Pathol* 1989;13:439–458.
65. Bonnin JM, Rubinstein LJ, Palmer NF, Beckwith JB. The association of embryonal tumors originating in the kidney and in the brain: a report of seven cases. *Cancer* 1984;54:2137–2146.
66. Jayabose S, Iqbal K, Newman L, et al. Hypercalcemia in childhood renal tumors. *Cancer* 1988;61:788–791.
67. Lynch HT, Shurin SM, Dahms BB, Izant RJ, Lynch J, Danes BS. Paravertebral malignant rhabdoid tumor in infancy: in vitro studies of a familial tumor. *Cancer* 1983;52:290–296.
68. Perez-Atayde AR, Newbury R, Fletcher JA, Barnhill R, Gellis S. Congenital "neurovascular hamartoma" of the skin: a possible marker of malignant rhabdoid tumor. *Am J Surg Pathol* 1994;18:1030–1038.
69. Schofield DA, Beckwith JB, Sklar J. Loss of heterozygosity at chromosomes 22q11-12 and 11p15.5 in renal rhabdoid tumors. *Genes Chromosomes Cancer* 1996;15:10–17.
70. Biegel J, Rorke LB, Packer R, Emanuel BS. Monosomy 22 in rhabdoid or atypical tumors of the brain. *J Neurosurg* 1990;73:710–714.
71. Fort DW, Tonk VS, Tomlinson GE, Timmons CF, Schneider NR. Rhabdoid tumor of the kidney with primitive neuroectodermal tumor of the central nervous system: associated tumors with different histologic, cytogenetic, and molecular findings. *Genes Chromosomes Cancer* 1994;11:146–152.
72. Davis CJ, Mostofi FK, Sesterhenn IA. Renal medullary carcinoma: the seventh sickle cell nephropathy. *Am J Surg Pathol* 1995;19:1–11.
73. Abrahams J, Drachenberg M, Beckwith JB. Medullary renal carcinoma (MRC): a report of 28 new cases [Abstract]. *Mod Pathol* 1998;11:74A.
74. Leuschner I, Harms D, Schmidt D. Renal cell carcinoma in children: histology, immunohistochemistry, and follow-up of 10 cases. *Med Pediatr Oncol* 1991;19:33–41.
75. Tomlinson GE, Nisen PD, Timmons CF, Schneider NR. Cytogenetics of a renal cell carcinoma in a 17 month-old child: evidence for Xp11.2 as a recurring breakpoint. *Cancer Genet Cytogenet* 1991;57:11–17.
76. Tonk V, Wilson KS, Timmons CN, Schneider NR, Tomlinson GE. Renal cell carcinoma with translocation (X;1): further evidence for a cytogenetically defined subtype. *Cancer Genet Cytogenet* 1995;81:72–75.
77. Takeuchi T, Iwasaki H, Ohjimi Y, et al. Renal primitive neuroectodermal tumor: an immunohistochemical and cytogenetic analysis. *Pathol Int* 1996;46:292–297.
78. Sheaff M, McManus A, Scheimberg I, Paris A, Shipley J, Baithun S. Primitive neuroectodermal tumor of the kidney confirmed by fluorescence in situ hybridization. *Am J Surg Pathol* 1997;21:461–468.
79. Marley EF, Liapis H, Humphrey PA, et al. Primitive neuroectodermal tumor of the kidney: another enigma: a pathologic, immunohistochemical, and molecular diagnostic study. *Am J Surg Pathol* 1997;21:354–359.
80. Weidner N, Tjoe J. Immunohistochemical profile of monoclonal antibody O13: antibody that recognizes glycoprotein p30/32 MIC2 and is useful in diagnosing Ewings sarcoma and peripheral neuroepithelioma. *Am J Surg Pathol* 1994;18:486–494.
81. Hennigar RA, Beckwith JB. Nephrogenic adenofibroma: a novel kidney tumor of young people. *Am J Surg Pathol* 1992;16:325–334.
82. Strong JW, Ro JY. Metanephric adenoma of the kidney: a newly characterized entity. *Adv Anat Pathol* 1996;3:172–178.
83. Sotelo-Avila C, Beckwith JB, Johnson JE. Ossifying renal tumor of infancy: a clinicopathologic study of nine cases. *Pediatr Pathol Lab Med* 1995;15:745–762.
84. Camitta BM, Casper JT, Kun LE, Lauer SJ, Starshak RJ, Oechler HW. Isolated bilateral T-cell renal lymphoblastic lymphoma. *Am J Pediatr Hematol/Oncol* 1986;8:8–12.

CHAPTER 44

The Urothelial Tract: Renal Pelvis, Ureter, Urinary Bladder, and Urethra

Victor E. Reuter and Myron R. Melamed

GENERAL CONSIDERATIONS

The epithelium of the urinary bladder and urethra is entirely derived from endoderm of the urogenital sinus, whereas the lamina propria, muscularis propria and adventitia develop from the surrounding splanchnic mesenchyme. During early embryologic development, the caudal portions of the mesonephric ducts contribute to the formation of the mucosa of the bladder trigone but are eventually replaced by endoderm (1). The renal pelvis and ureters are mesodermally derived. Despite their different histogenesis, all of the urinary excretory passages are lined by so-called transitional epithelium, which is perhaps better referred to as urothelium.

The wall of the urinary bladder is formed of four layers: (a) epithelium (urothelium), (b) lamina propria, (c) muscularis propria, and (d) adventitia or serosa (2,3). The thickness of the urothelium varies, as does the shape of the epithelial cells, depending on the degree to which the bladder is distended. In the empty bladder, the epithelium can be five to eight cells thick. The deepest (basal) cells have a cuboidal or columnar shape, above which are several layers of irregularly polyhedral cells. The most superficial or luminal layer consists of large, sometimes binucleated eosinophilic cells with abundant cytoplasm and a rounded free surface. They are descriptively called umbrella cells (2). In the distended bladder, the epithelial lining can be as few as two cells thick, with a basal layer of cuboidal cells and a superficial layer of elongated and flattened cells; umbrella cells are inconspicuous.

A thin basement membrane separates the urothelium from the underlying lamina propria. The latter is formed of abundant connective tissue containing a rich vascular network, lymphatic channels, sensory nerve endings, and a few elastic fibers. The lamina propria varies in thickness in the empty versus the distended bladder, but is generally thinner in the areas of the trigone and bladder neck. It is important to note that wisps of smooth muscle may be found within the superficial lamina propria, either isolated or forming a complete or incomplete muscularis mucosae (3,4). These superficial muscle fascicles must not be confused with the smooth-muscle bundles of the muscularis propria, because this might result in errors of tumor staging and treatment (Fig. 1). The muscularis propria has loosely anastomosing, ill-defined internal and external longitudinal layers and a more prominent middle circular layer of muscle. In the bladder neck of the male subject, the fascicles of the muscularis propria are continuous with the fibromuscular tissue of the prostate, whereas in the female subject, they are continuous with the muscle fibers in the wall of the urethra (2). The outermost layer of the viscus is an adventitia of connective tissue; only the superior surface is covered by serosa of the pelvic peritoneum. The renal pelvis and ureters have a similar structure of urothelium, lamina propria, and in the ureter, a relatively thick muscularis that increases gradually from proximal to distal ureter.

The main blood supply to the bladder comes from branches of the internal iliac arteries; the superior vesical arteries supply the anterior and superior aspects of the bladder, and the inferior vesical arteries supply the bladder base (5). The veins of the urinary bladder form the vesical venous plexuses and drain mainly into the internal iliac veins. The lymphatic channels of the superior regions of the bladder drain into the external iliac lymph nodes. The lymphatic drainage of the ureters is complex. The upper portion drains into lateral aortic lymph nodes similar to the renal pelvis. The middle portion drains into the common iliac lymph nodes, whereas the inferior portion drains into either the common, external, or internal iliac lymph nodes (5). The urethral lymphatics drain into sacral and internal iliac lymph nodes.

V. E. Reuter: Department of Pathology, Memorial Sloan-Kettering Cancer Center and Cornell University Medical College, New York, New York 10021.

M. R. Melamed: Department of Pathology, New York Medical College, Valhalla, New York 10595.

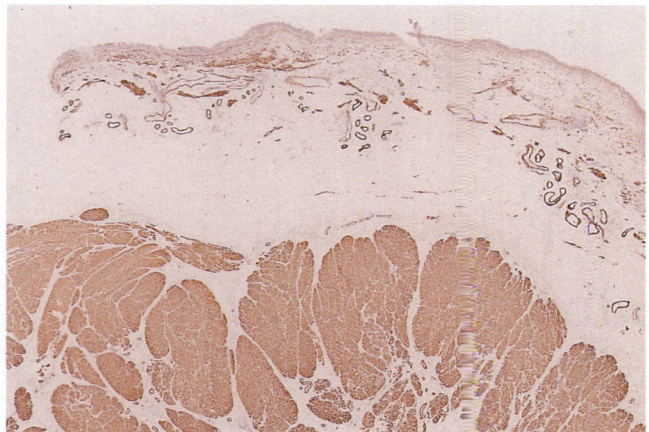

FIG. 1. Wall of urinary bladder, immunohistochemical stain for smooth-muscle actin. Notice the small fascicles of smooth muscle (muscularis mucosae) within the lamina propria, adjacent to medium-sized blood vessels.

The adult empty bladder has the shape of a four-sided inverted pyramid and is enveloped by the vesical fascia (5). The superior surface faces superiorly and is covered by the pelvic parietal peritoneum. The posterior surface, also known as the base of the bladder, faces posteriorly and inferiorly. It is separated from the rectum by the uterine cervix and the proximal portions of the vagina in female subjects and by the seminal vesicles and the ampulla of the vasa deferentia in male subjects (Fig. 2A and B). These posterior anatomic relations are very important clinically. Because most vesicle neoplasms arise in the posterior wall adjacent to the ureteral orifices, invasive tumor may extend into adjacent soft tissue and organs. The intimate relations to the previously mentioned organs explain why hysterectomy and partial vaginectomy are indicated at the time of radial cystectomy in women. Conversely, we know that seminal vesicle involvement is a bad prognostic sign in bladder carcinoma in men, a reflection of high pathologic stage.

The bladder bed (structures on which the bladder neck rests) is formed posteriorly by the rectum in male and vagina in female subjects. Anteriorly and laterally, it is formed by the internal obturator and levator ani muscles as well as the pubic bones. These structures may be involved in advanced tumors occupying the anterior, lateral, or bladder neck regions and render the patient inoperable.

The most anterosuperior point of the bladder is known as the apex and is located at the point of contact of the superior surfaces and the two inferolateral surfaces. The apex marks the point of insertion of the median umbilical ligament and consequently is the area where urachal carcinomas occur.

INFLAMMATORY DISORDERS

The many organisms that may cause cystitis include bacteria, viruses, fungi, and protozoa. Cystitis also may be result from calculus or other local trauma, radiation, or chemotherapy (6). The majority of cases of both acute and chronic cystitis show nonspecific histologic features of inflammation and do not require description here, but several inflammatory processes can be distinguished by their clinical or pathologic features.

Tuberculous cystitis tends to involve the bladder adjacent to the ureteral orifices, consistent with the observation that the majority of cases are associated with and presumably caused by renal tuberculosis. It is now a rare disease in most

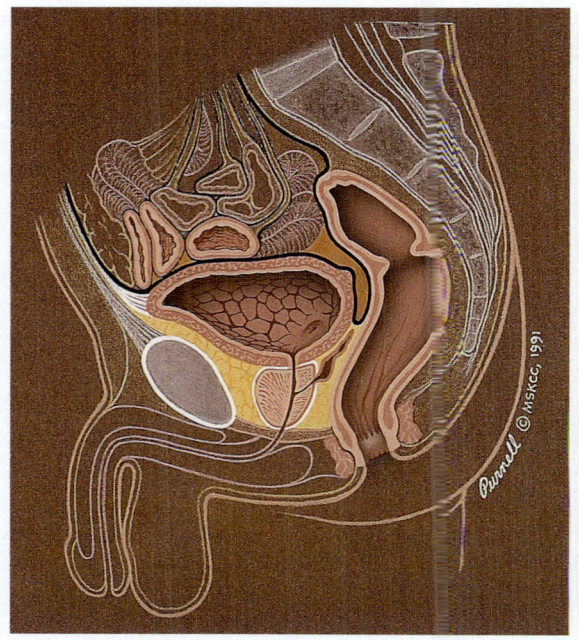
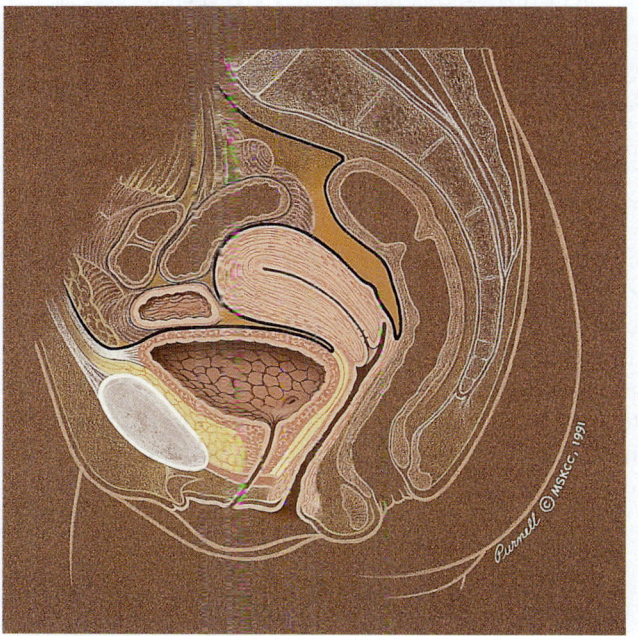

FIG. 2. Anatomic relations between the urinary bladder and the urethra. **A:** Male subject. **B:** Female subject.

countries. Histologically, we see caseating granulomas with Langerhans giant cells mostly in the lamina propria and often with mucosal ulceration. Appropriate stains should reveal the presence of acid-fast bacilli (7,8) (Fig. 3). Noncaseating granulomas are commonly seen after intravesical therapy with bacillus Calmette-Guérin (BCG) but rarely will special stains reveal the presence of acid-fast organisms. A nonspecific granulomatous inflammation with foreign-body giant cells also can be seen after transurethral biopsies.

Schistosomal cystitis is common in the Nile Valley and sub-Saharan Africa but rarely seen in the United States. It is usually due to infestation with *Schistosoma haematobium* and rarely with *S. mansoni*. The ova are deposited in veins of the muscularis propria of the bladder where they degenerate and become permeable. Eosinophilic material (antigen–antibody complex) surrounds the ovum and incites a marked inflammatory response, characterized initially by necrosis and a pleocellular inflammatory reaction rich in eosinophils (9). The overlying epithelium may become ulcerated. As the process becomes chronic, it is characterized by perioval fibrosis with surrounding lymphocytes, histiocytes, and giant cells forming a foreign-body granulomatous reaction. Dystrophic calcifications are frequent. The overlying epithelium may become hyperplastic or undergo proliferative changes of cystitis cystica, cystitis glandularis, or squamous metaplasia (10). Patients with chronic schistosomal cystitis have a high incidence of carcinoma of the bladder (9–11) (see section on squamous carcinoma).

Polypoid cystitis refers to an exophytic, inflammatory lesion for the most part causally related to the presence of indwelling catheters (12). It is seen mostly on the dome and posterior wall of the bladder, and is characterized histologically by normal or mildly hyperplastic urothelium overlying a congested, chronically inflamed, and markedly edematous stroma (13,14). Although these exophytic lesions may mimic papillary carcinoma or papilloma grossly, they can be easily distinguished histologically as an inflammatory pseudopolyp.

Eosinophilic cystitis is a rare process seen clinically with episodes of marked urinary frequency, dysuria, and not infrequently with gross hematuria (15–18). The cystoscopic appearance in adults is often suggestive of carcinoma because of nodular or masslike lesions that may be hyperemic, ulcerated, or frankly necrotic (19). Histologically, the inflammatory changes are acute, chronic, or both. The acute stage is characterized by edema, congestion, and an inflammatory infiltrate containing eosinophils and lymphocytes. The eosinophilic infiltrate is more prominent in the cases that have muscle necrosis. The chronic stage is characterized by fewer or absent eosinophils and by fibrosis in the lamina propria and interspersed among the superficial muscle layers. The overlying epithelium may undergo proliferative changes (Von Brunn's nests, cystitis cystica) or squamous metaplasia (19).

Eosinophilic cystitis is most commonly encountered in children and women and is often associated with allergic disorders and peripheral blood eosinophilia (17–19). It also may affect elderly men, and in these cases, is often associated with the trauma of transurethral resection of the prostate or bladder, concomitant bladder cancer, and so on.

Interstitial cystitis (Hunner's ulcer) is also a rare and poorly understood inflammatory process that is of possible autoimmune origin. It usually affects middle-aged women (20). The clinical symptoms are frequently severe and disabling and include urinary frequency, urgency, dysuria, and hematuria, as well as perineal or suprapubic pain (21). Cystoscopy is required to establish the diagnosis. It may reveal a distensible bladder with characteristic pinpoint petechial hemorrhages and one or several ulcerations that may be present anywhere in the bladder but are not a prerequisite for the diagnosis. In other cases, there may be a contracted, nondistensible bladder and a Hunner's ulcer (22). Histologically, there is edema and congestion of the lamina propria and, in a few cases, either ulcerated or denuded mucosa. Along with a nonspecific inflammatory infiltrate, we should observe numerous mast cells, not only in the lamina propria but also throughout the muscularis propria (23,24). Patchy fibrosis of the lamina propria or superficial muscularis propria may be encountered. The diagnosis of interstitial cystitis can be made only after other causes have been ruled out and repeated urine cultures for bacteria, fungi and viruses are negative.

Follicular cystitis is a term that has been used to describe the presence of lymphoid follicles with germinal centers in the wall of the urinary bladder (25). The term is a misnomer

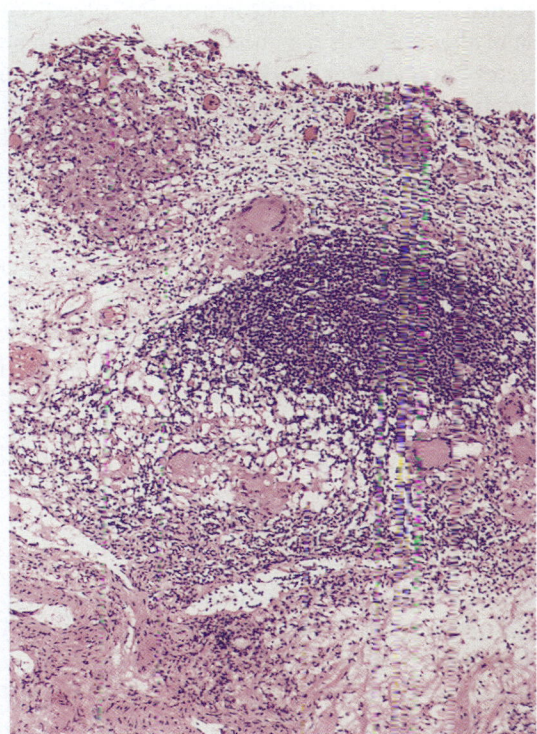

FIG. 3. Granulomatous cystitis after intravesical bacille Calmette-Guérin (BCG), characterized by a marked chronic inflammatory infiltrate and granulomas within the lamina propria.

because it does not necessarily indicate inflammation. On the other hand, it does sometimes follow infection, repeated transurethral biopsies, or the instillation of intravesical chemotherapeutic agents or BCG.

Plasma cell granuloma (inflammatory pseudotumor) has been described involving the urinary bladder (26). Histologically, it is identical to the inflammatory pseudotumors more commonly seen in the lung and other sites, exhibiting a mixed lymphocytic/histocytic cell infiltrate containing abundant mature polyclonal plasma cells. The lesion is discrete, often surrounded by a fibrous pseudocapsule, and can be quite large. The differential diagnosis will include lymphoma and, if the histiocytic proliferation is exuberant, anaplastic carcinoma or sarcoma. A more detailed description is given later in the section on inflammatory pseudosarcomatous lesions of the bladder.

Pyelitis and ureteritis are usually nonspecific and may occur as a consequence of renal lithiasis or lower urinary tract obstruction.

Urethritis is more commonly encountered in men than women and usually as a result of *Neisseria gonorrhea* or other sexually transmitted organisms including *Chlamydia* and *Mycoplasma*. *Gonococcus, Chlamydia,* and *Trichomonas* are common causes of urethritis in women (27).

Urethral caruncles are small, highly vascular, usually polypoid inflammatory lesions commonly seen in elderly women. They may be painful and associated with hematuria. Histologically, caruncles usually resemble small hemangiomas, often with intense acute and chronic inflammatory cellular infiltrate. The overlying urothelium may be hyperplastic, ulcerated, or exhibit squamous or glandular metaplasia (Fig. 4) (28).

Urethral valves occur more frequently in male than in female subjects. They may be asymptomatic but generally cause some degree of obstruction, inflammation, and hematuria. Posterior urethral valves are usually associated with bladder neck hypertrophy (29).

IATROGENIC CYSTITIS/RADIATION CYSTITIS

Radiation cystitis may be acute or chronic and can occur any time the bladder is included in the treatment field. The clinical severity and histologic features of radiation cystitis are both time and dose dependent; 5% of patients receiving 6,000 rads to the bladder will develop late clinical symptoms of radiation cystitis, whereas 50% of patients will have the same fate if the dose is 7,000 rads (30). Clinically, the acute symptoms of radiation cystitis may appear as early as 4 to 6 weeks after initiation of therapy, whereas late symptoms appear as much as 10 years later (31). The toxic effects of irradiation are enhanced if administered in conjunction with cyclophosphamide (32).

Microscopically, the early changes are characterized by marked edema and hyperemia. The edema produces thickened mucosal folds, resulting in a characteristic gross appearance, which was termed cystitis by Koss (33). These changes may be accompanied by desquamation and, rarely, superficial ulceration of the bladder epithelium (34). At this stage, the urothelium can take on very atypical cytologic features mimicking and sometimes indistinguishable from carcinoma *in situ*. The cells may become enlarged with prominent, hyperchromatic nuclei. However, the altered epithelial cells are typically more bizarre than cells of carcinoma *in situ*, with giant cells and multinucleated cells that lack the crisp nuclear detail of nonirradiated cells. These changes are temporary and should disappear within 3 months of cessation of radiation therapy (33).

The late radiation-induced changes include collagenization of the lamina propria and muscular fibers, myointimal proliferation or hyalinization of the media of arterioles, and often ulceration with abundant fibrinous exudate. Atypical fibroblasts are invariably present in the scarred lamina propria. The urothelium may be atrophic or hyperplastic and still exhibit focal radiation-induced atypia (31).

HEMORRHAGIC CYSTITIS

In the late 1950s, systemic administration of cyclophosphamide was found to cause hemorrhagic cystitis (Fig. 5). At times hematuria could be massive and uncontrollable, sometimes requiring cystectomy. Phillips et al. (35) showed that the tissue damage that led to hemorrhagic cystitis was caused by a topical effect of the metabolic byproducts of cyclophosphamide, which were excreted through the kidney. The occurrence of hemorrhagic cystitis appears to be unre-

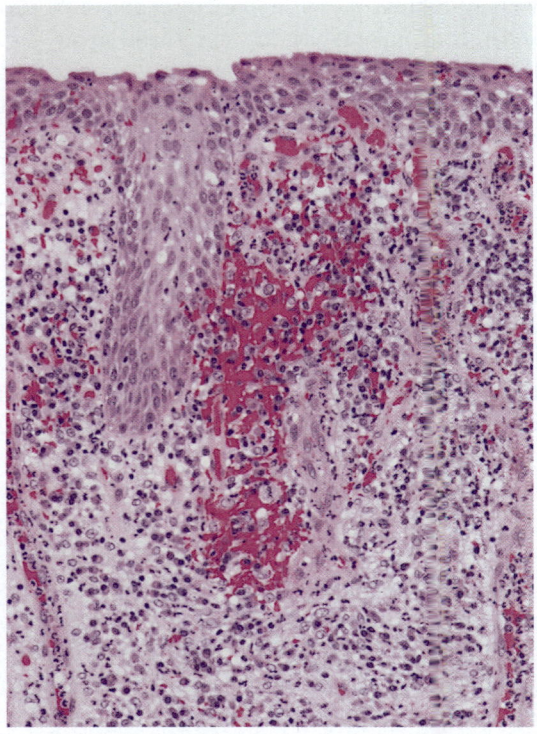

FIG. 4. Urethral caruncle. Congested and hemorrhagic lamina propria with a marked inflammatory infiltrate and overlying squamous metaplasia.

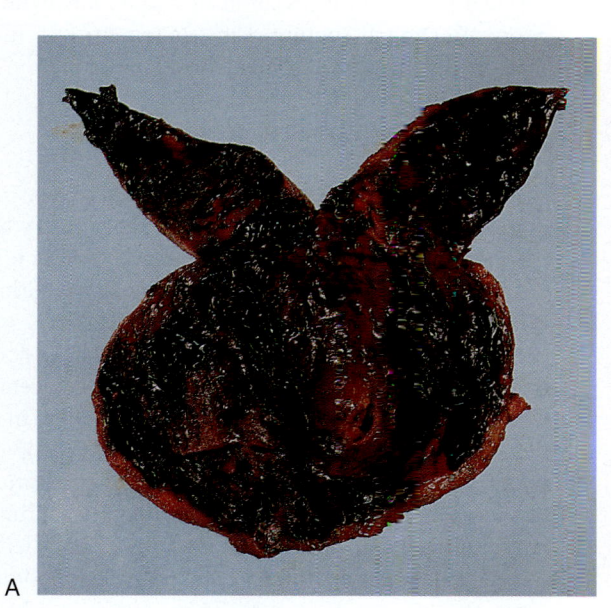
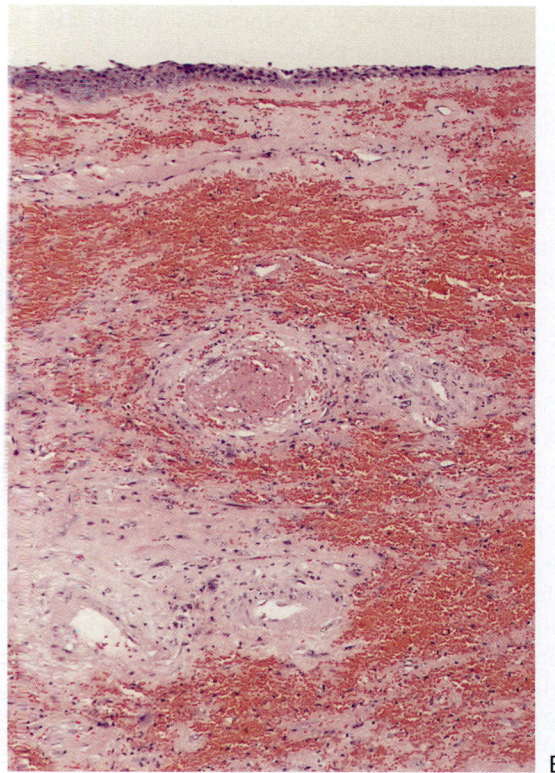
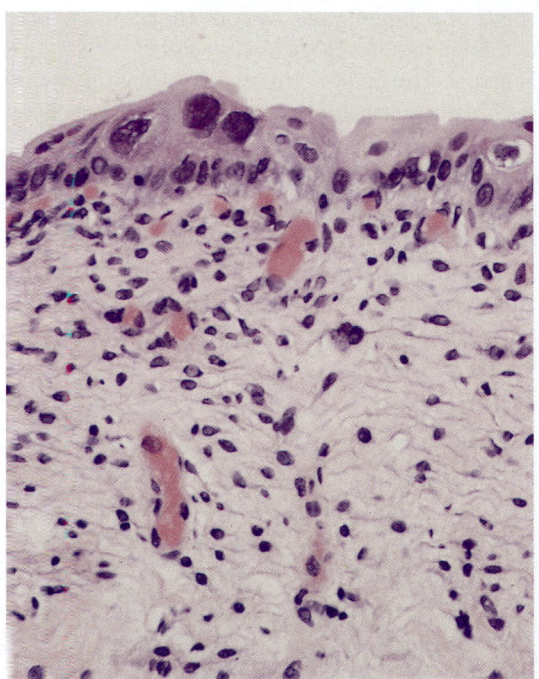

FIG. 5. A: Hemorrhagic cystitis resulting from cyclophosphamide therapy. Cystectomy was necessary because of intractable bleeding. **B:** Hemorrhagic cystitis after cyclophosphamide therapy. Characteristically the surface urothelium is ulcerated or thinned, and there is extensive hemorrhage in the bladder wall. **C:** Urothelial atypia after cyclophosphamide therapy. Several superficial and suprabasal cells are enlarged, markedly hyperchromatic, and pleomorphic.

lated to dose and was reported in roughly 3% of patients receiving the drug (36,37). Currently patients are treated with forced fluids, and the incidence of hemorrhagic cystitis has been sharply reduced. More recently, another alkylating agent, busulfan, has been implicated as a rare cause of hemorrhagic cystitis (38).

Microscopically, the bladder is characterized by marked edema and hemorrhage throughout the lamina propria, with extensive ulceration and an associated fibrinopurulent exudate. Where not ulcerated, the epithelium may be thinned and atypical. During the regenerative stage, macrophages and fibroblasts populate the lamina propria, whereas the overlying epithelium exhibits an increased mitotic rate, increased thickness, and marked atypia (35,37).

ENDOMETRIOSIS

Approximately 200 cases of vesical endometriosis have been described, making the urinary bladder the most common site of involvement within the urinary tract (39–41). Classically, it affects women between the second and fifth decades of life but may rarely be seen in postmenopausal women receiving exogenous estrogen (42). Vesical endometriosis was described in men with prostate carcinoma who were receiving exogenous estrogen therapy (43,44).

Clinically, patients are first seen with pelvic pain and possibly hematuria. A mass is frequently apparent either by palpation or cystoscopic examination. The lesion may reside in the superficial or deep layers of the vesical wall or in the adjacent perivesical soft tissue, so that a simple transurethral biopsy may not always provide a diagnostic sample. Microscopically, the lesion resembles endometriosis elsewhere; endometriumlike glandular epithelium is present in association with endometrial stromal cells and recent or old hemorrhage. Rarely we find only glands or stroma. In the former case, the differential diagnosis must include infiltrating adenocarcinoma, which is distinguished from the uniform and orderly glands of endometriosis by sometimes subtle differences in cytologic and histologic architecture.

The occurrence of endometriosis in men is intriguing. Most likely it represents activation of müllerian nests by exogenous estrogens (43,44).

Endometriosis may involve the ureter. The involvement is usually unilateral and most common in the lower third (45,46). Implantation is extrinsic to the ureter in most cases, although it also may be intramural. It may produce obstructive or irritative symptoms and endoscopically can be confused with carcinoma. Endometriosis involving the urethra is extremely rare.

Recently Clement and Young (47) described endocervicosis of the urinary bladder in women of childbearing age. Patients had a mass in the posterior wall or posterior dome. Microscopically, the lesion is characterized by extensive involvement of the wall by benign or mildly atypical endocervical glands. Extravasation of mucin was evident in all cases after gland rupture. Like endometriosis, this lesion must be distinguished from adenocarcinoma.

MALAKOPLAKIA

Malakoplakia is an unusual but distinctive type of inflammatory reaction of unknown etiology. The urinary bladder is the most common site of involvement, although it has been described in other genitourinary and nongenitourinary sites (48–50). On gross examination, malakoplakia is solitary or confluent yellow nodules or plaques. The larger nodules are centrally umbilicated or ulcerated, and the adjacent mucosa is hyperemic. The lesions may be seen anywhere in the bladder and vary greatly in size and number. Cystoscopically, the nodules or plaques of malakoplakia may be confused with carcinoma. Histologically, the lesion involves primarily the lamina propria and is characterized by a well-demarcated, mixed inflammatory infiltrate in which epithelioid histiocytes predominate (Fig. 6A). These histiocytes have abundant eosinophilic or amphophilic cytoplasm within, which are round or oval inclusions called Michaelis–Guttman bodies (Fig. 6B). These inclusions may stain with hematoxylin or eosin and are concentrically laminated calcopherites that stain for iron as well as calcium. The bodies are found within the interstitium as well as within histiocytes. The typical nodule of epithelioid histiocytes is often surrounded by lymphoid aggregates with germinal centers. The overlying urothelium may be ulcerated, hyperplastic, or metaplastic. In long-standing lesions, the characteristic infiltrate is replaced by fibrosis and scarring.

As previously mentioned, the etiology of malakoplakia re-

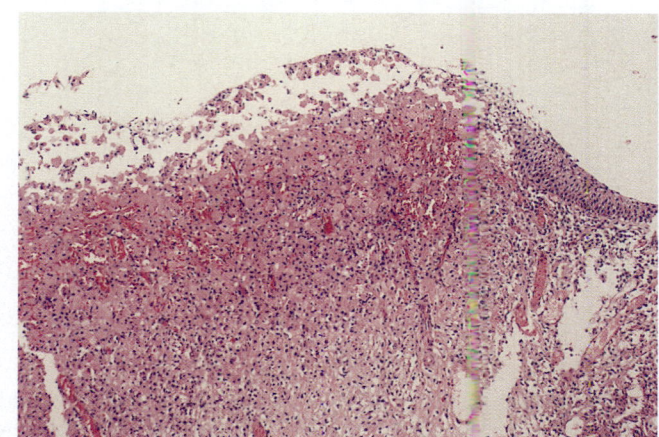 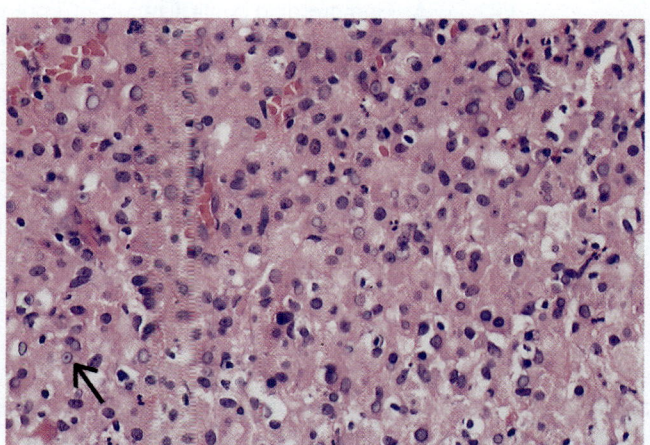

FIG. 6. A: Malakoplakia of the urinary bladder. The surface urothelium is thinned or denuded, and the lamina propria is densely infiltrated by histiocytes. At low power, we can discern the overall nodular appearance, which can be easily confused for carcinoma at cystoscopy. **B:** Malakoplakia. High-power view reveals densely packed epithelioid histiocytes, some of which contain Michaelis–Guttman bodies (arrow).

mains unknown, although it is generally believed to be a peculiar response to infection, perhaps the result of a disturbed immune response or abnormal macrophage or lysosomal activity in the host (51–54).

Malakoplakia has also been described in the renal pelvis, ureter, and urethra, the latter being the least frequent. Multifocal involvement along the entire urothelial tract also has been reported. In the ureter, it is often associated with obstruction (55,56).

AMYLOIDOSIS

The bladder can be involved in cases of systemic amyloidosis but rarely is the primary site of this disease (57). The usual clinical presentation is that of hematuria. On cystoscopy, a localized amyloid tumor will be seen as an elevated mass that can be confused with an invasive neoplasm. Less frequently, the disease may diffusely involve the bladder wall. Microscopically, the amyloid protein is an eosinophilic, afibrillar material deposited preferentially in the lamina propria and extending into the connective tissue surrounding muscle fascicles (Fig. 7) (58). Less frequently, and usually in systemic amyloidosis, there are perivascular amyloid deposits. Congestion and hemorrhage are common, but inflammatory cells are scanty unless the overlying epithelium is ulcerated. A few fibroblastlike cells are usually interspersed within the eosinophilic material. Special stains such as Congo red, crystal violet, or van Gieson will help to establish the diagnosis. Patients with localized lesions are usually successfully managed by transurethral resection, but patients with more diffuse involvement may require more radical surgery to control the bleeding (59).

In descending order of frequency, amyloid deposits also were described in the ureter, renal pelvis, and urethra (60–63). At all sites, it is associated with hematuria, and in ureter and renal pelvis may also cause obstruction.

DIVERTICULA

Bladder diverticula are relatively common, yet their etiology remains controversial. Most investigators agree that they occur from increased intravesical pressure as a result of obstruction distal to the diverticulum (64–66). The obstruction brings about compensatory muscle hypertrophy and eventual mucosal herniation in areas of weakness (Fig. 8). Others believe that at least some diverticula are a consequence of congenital defects in the bladder musculature, and they cite as evidence cases of diverticula in young patients without evidence of obstruction (67,68). The most common sites of diverticula are adjacent to the ureteral orifices, the bladder dome (probably related to a urachal remnant), and the region of the internal urethral orifice. Grossly we see distortion of the external surface of the bladder. The diverticula may be widely patent but are usually narrow in symptomatic patients. The mucosa adjoining the diverticulum is usually hyperemic or ulcerated. There may be epithelial hyperplasia, and the muscularis propria is hypertrophic. Very commonly there is inflammation involving the lamina propria and muscularis. The wall of the diverticulum itself consists of urothelium and underlying connective tissue, similar to the bladder mucosa with lamina propria. Few if any muscle fascicles will be identified in the majority of cases of acquired diverticula. The true "congenital" diverticula contain a thinned outer muscle layer. Infrequently the epithelium lining the sac will undergo squamous or glandular metaplasia due to local irri-

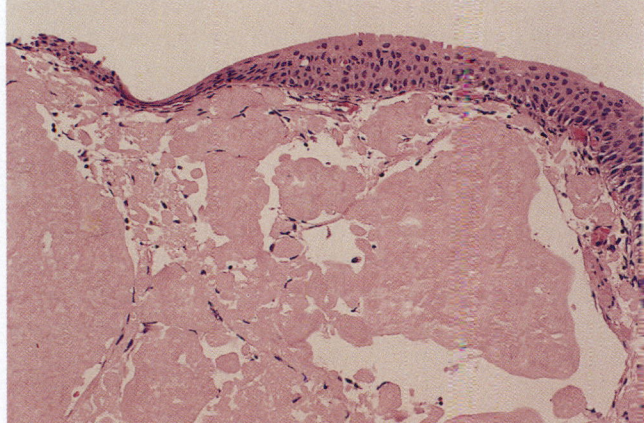

FIG. 7. Amyloidosis. There is an eosinophilic, afibrillar material deposited within the lamina propria. An inflammatory infiltrate is usually minimal or absent.

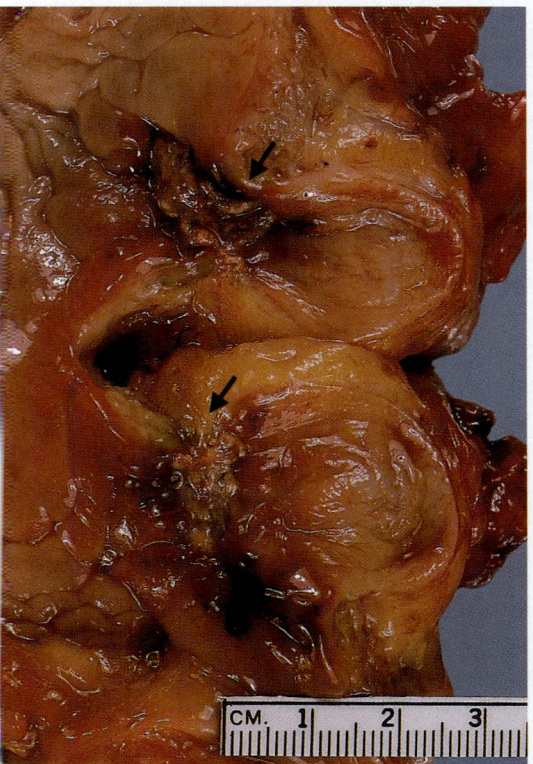

FIG. 8. Bladder diverticulum. Notice the diverticular orifice (arrows), which is hyperemic and ulcerated.

tation associated with urine stasis, infection, or stone. In these cases, it is not unusual for the diverticular wall to become extensively fibrotic.

Major complications of bladder diverticula include infection, lithiasis with subsequent obstruction, and carcinoma (69–71). It is believed that 2% to 7% of patients with bladder diverticula will develop an associated neoplasm, presumed to result from the chronic inflammatory stimuli mentioned. The neoplasms may develop at the os or may occur within the diverticula, making endoscopic evaluation difficult. Although transitional cell carcinomas (TCCs) predominate, there is a relative increase in the incidence of squamous carcinoma and adenocarcinoma associated with squamous or glandular metaplasia in the lining urothelium. Sarcomas and at least one carcinosarcoma also were reported in association with vesical diverticula, but we believe that most of these cases represent sarcomatoid metaplasia of high-grade carcinomas (71).

Diverticula also may occur in the ureter (72) and urethra. The overwhelming majority of urethral diverticula occur in women (73,74). They may be asymptomatic but usually are seen with irritative symptoms or dribbling. Complications of urethral diverticula are similar to those of the bladder (73). It is not uncommon to see the diverticular sac lined by metaplastic glandular or squamous epithelium and, if neoplasms occur, these tend to be either glandular or squamous (75,76).

REACTIVE PROLIFERATIVE CHANGES OF THE UROTHELIUM: BRUNN'S NESTS, CYSTITIS CYSTICA, AND CYSTITIS GLANDULARIS

The most common reactive proliferative change within the urothelium is the formation of Brunn's nests, which represent invaginations of the surface urothelium into the underlying lamina propria. In some cases these solid nests of benign-appearing urothelium may lose continuity with the surface and are isolated within the lamina propria, where they become cystic because of an accumulation of cellular debris or mucin. The term cystitis cystica was coined to de-

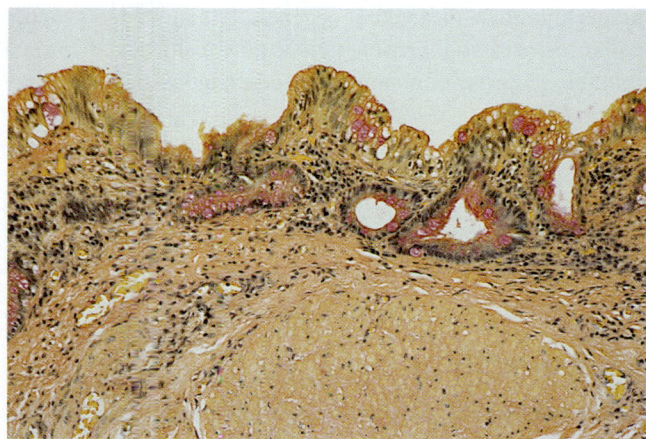

FIG. 10. Glandular (intestinal) metaplasia of the urothelium. Notice mucin-producing goblet cells in surface urothelium as well as in cystitis glandularis.

scribe this lesion (Fig. 9). The lining epithelium of these small cysts is composed of one or several layers of flattened transitional or cuboidal epithelium. In some cases, the epithelial lining undergoes glandular metaplasia, giving rise to what is called cystis glandularis. The cells become cuboidal or columnar and mucin secreting; some are transformed into goblet cells (Fig. 10). These processes also occur in the renal pelvis and ureter, where they are called pyelitis or ureteritis cystica, or glandularis, respectively.

Brunn's nests, cystitis cystica, and cystitis glandularis form a continuum of proliferative or reactive changes seen along the entire urothelial tract, and it is common to see all three in the same specimen. Most investigators believe that they occur as a result of local inflammatory insult (77,78). Nevertheless, these proliferative changes are seen in the urothelium of patients with no evidence of local inflammation so that it is possible that they also represent either normal histologic variants or the residual effects of old inflammatory processes (79,80).

Much has been written about the association of Brunn's nests, cystitis cystica, and especially cystitis glandularis and urothelial carcinoma (80–83). The high incidence of these proliferative changes in normal bladder suggests that they are not likely premalignant changes and that there is no cause–effect relation between their presence and the appearance of bladder cancer. It is true that one or all of these changes are commonly present in biopsy specimens containing bladder cancer, but the coexistence may be coincidental, or the cancer itself may produce the local inflammatory insult that causes them and not vice versa. The fact that exceptional cases may occur in which carcinoma clearly arises within the epithelium of these reactive lesions does not alter this argument (82,83).

METAPLASIA OF THE UROTHELIUM

Metaplasia refers to a change in morphology of one cell type into another type, which is considered aberrant for that

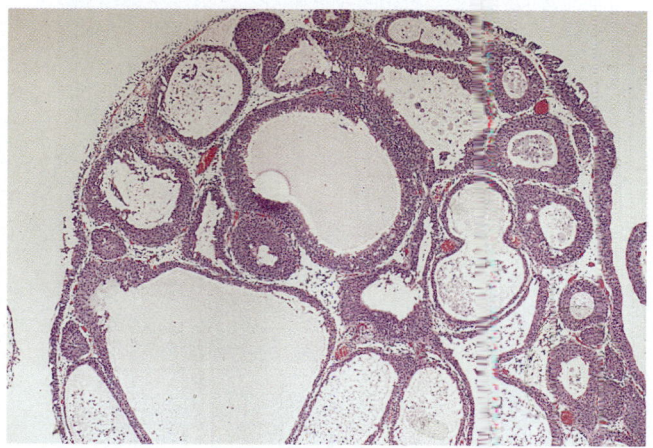

FIG. 9. Cystitis cystica. Cystic nests of benign-appearing urothelium located within the lamina propria.

location. Transitional epithelium frequently undergoes either squamous or glandular metaplasia, presumably as a response to chronic inflammatory stimuli such as urinary tract infection, calculi, diverticuli, or frequent catherization (78,80).

Squamous metaplasia, particularly in the area of the trigone, is a common finding in women and is responsive to estrogen production. This type of squamous metaplasia is characterized by abundant intracytoplasmic glycogen and lack of keratinization, making it histologically similar to vaginal or cervical squamous epithelium (Fig. 11). Under other conditions, the metaplastic squamous epithelium undergoes keratinization and may exhibit parakeratosis and even a granular layer. This metaplastic epithelium is not preneoplastic *per se*, but under some circumstances may lead to squamous carcinoma (84). This is the sequence of events, for example, in patients with long-stading schistosomiasis of the urinary bladder or in the case of squamous carcinoma arising in bladder diverticula (11,65). In these cases it may be possible to observe keratinizing squamous metaplasia adjacent to *in situ* and invasive squamous carcinoma.

The most common site of glandular metaplasia of the urothelium is the bladder, in the form of cystitis glandularis. Nevertheless, it may also occur within surface urothelium, usually as a response to chronic inflammation or irritation, and also in cases of bladder extrophy (85,86). The epithelium is composed of tall columnar cells with mucin-secreting goblet cells (Fig. 11), frequently strikingly similar to colonic or small intestinal epithelium in which we might identify even Paneth's cells. Several cases of villous intestinal-type metaplasia of the entire bladder were described, and these may be associated with mucosuria (Fig. 12) (87–89).

As with squamous metaplasia, glandular metaplasia is not of itself a precancerous lesion but may eventually undergo neoplastic transformation in some cases (86).

So-called nephrogenic adenoma is a distinct metaplastic lesion characterized by aggregates of cuboidal or hobnail cells with clear or eosinophilic cytoplasm and small discrete

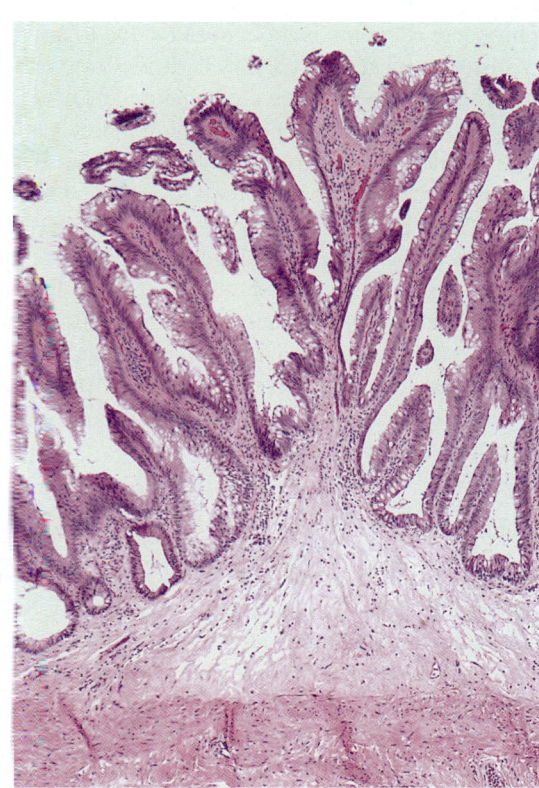

FIG. 12. Villous adenoma of the urinary bladder. This lesion occupied the entire surface of the bladder, and the patient had mucosuria. Notice the discontinuous superficial muscle layer (muscularis mucosae) within the lamina propria.

nuclei without prominent nucleoli (90). These cells line thin papillary fronds on the surface or form tubular structures within the lamina propria of the bladder (Fig. 13). The tubules are often surrounded by a thickened and hyalinized basement membrane and do not incite a stromal response. Variable numbers of acute and chronic inflammatory cells are commonplace within the bladder wall.

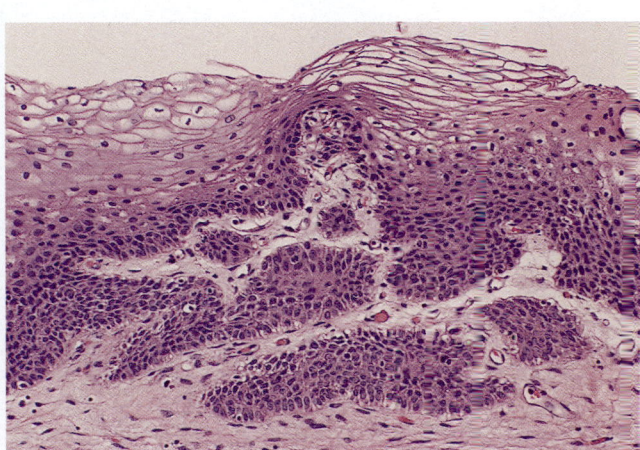

FIG. 11. Squamous metaplasia. This is commonly seen in biopsy material from the trigone in women. Notice the glycogen-containing squamous cells.

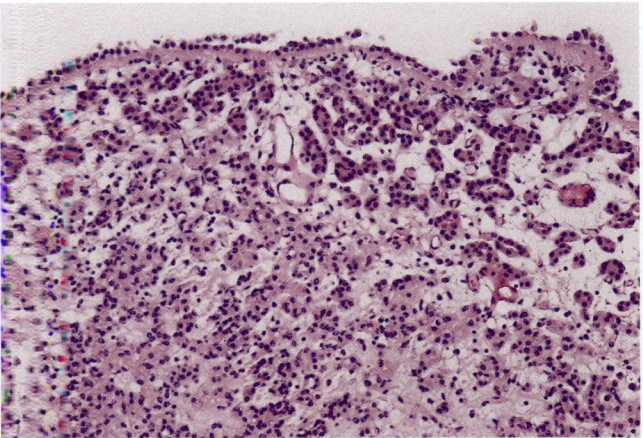

FIG. 13. Nephrogenic adenoma. This proliferative urothelial lesion is characterized by aggregates of cuboidal cells with scant eosinophilic cytoplasm forming small tubules within the lamina propria. Occasionally, these cells line discrete papillary structures.

Nephrogenic adenoma is thought to be due to an inflammatory insult or local injury (91–93). It was originally described in the trigone and given its name because it was thought to arise from mesonephric rests. We now know that nephrogenic adenoma may occur anywhere in the urothelial tract, being described even in urethral diverticula (94–97). It is important in that it may be seen as an exophitic mass mimicking carcinoma grossly and suggesting adenocarcinoma, microscopically. The benign or mildly atypical histologic appearance of the cells, arranged in characteristic tubules surrounded by a prominent basement membrane, should ensure the correct diagnosis. Given the fact that this lesion is metaplastic rather than neoplastic, we prefer the term nephrogenic metaplasia.

INVERTED PAPILLOMA

Inverted papillomas are relatively rare lesions that may occur anywhere along the urothelial tract and may be confused clinically and pathologically with TCC (98,99). In order of decreasing frequency, they occur in the bladder, renal pelvis, ureter, or urethra (100–106). Patients usually have hematuria. Cytoscopically, the lesions are polypoid and either sessile or pedunculated. The mucosal surface is smooth or nodular, without villous or papillary fronds. Microscopically, the surface transitional epithelium is compressed but otherwise unremarkable. It is undermined by invaginated cords and nests of transitional epithelium, which occupy the lamina propria (Fig. 14). The accumulation of these endophytic growths gives the lesion its characteristic polypoid gross appearance. The urothelial cells forming the cords are benign, exhibiting normal maturation and few mitoses. They are similar to the cells of bladder papillomas, differing only in that the epithelial cords are endophytic and consequently more closely packed. Frequently the cells are oval or spindle shaped. Epithelial nests may become centrally cystic, dilated, and even lined by cuboidal epithelium. Some cases of urothelial carcinoma exhibit an endophytic pattern of growth and mimic inverted papilloma (107–108). The cytologic features of the tumor cells, irregularity of the epithelial nests, and the presence of a stromal reaction offer us clues as to the correct diagnosis.

The cords of transitional epithelium in the lamina propria represent invagination, not invasion. As such, there are no fibrous reactive changes within the stroma. Although mitotic figures can be seen, they are rare, regular, and located at or near the basal layer of the epithelium. Inverted papillomas are discrete lesions and do not exhibit an infiltrative border (100,101).

The etiology of these rare lesions is unclear. Most investigators believe that, similar to other proliferative lesions such as Brunn's nests and cystitis cystica, they are a reactive, proliferative process resulting from a noxious insult. They are not premalignant, although in exceptional cases, they have been associated with carcinoma (102–104,109). Given the rarity of this association, we consider it incidental.

CONDYLOMA

Condylomata acuminata are common, sexually transmitted benign tumors caused by a human papillomavirus. They

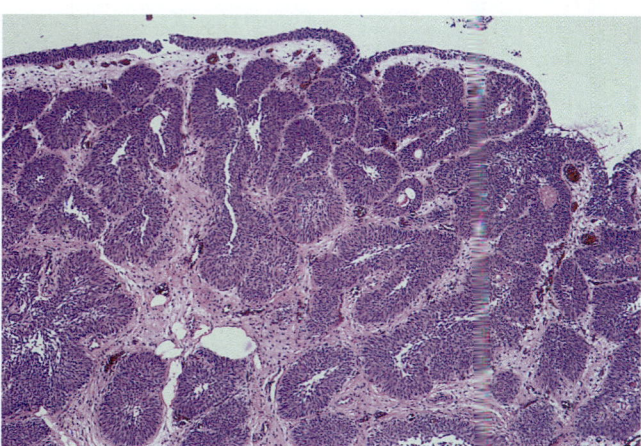

FIG. 14. Inverted papilloma. Invaginated fronds of histologically benign urothelium occupy the lamina propria and give the overlying mucosa a polypoid or nodular appearance.

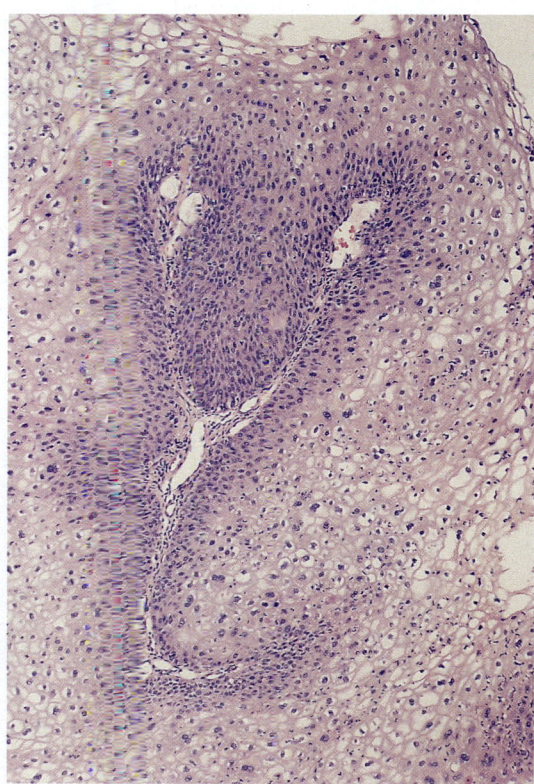

FIG. 15. Condyloma acuminatum. The urothelium has undergone squamous metaplasia, and the epithelial cells exhibit perinuclear cytoplasmic clearing and hyperchromatic pleomorphic nuclei (koilocytosis).

occur most frequently on mucocutaneous surfaces of the external genitalia, perineum, and anus, but extension into the urethra is not uncommon, occurring in up to 20% of cases. On rare occasions they may involve the bladder or even exceptionally the ureters (110–112). Condyloma affecting the bladder only is rare. The lesions may be discrete but there is a tendency towards diffuse involvement. Macroscopically the lesions are smooth, pink–tan, and papillary. If there is diffuse involvement, the urothelial surface takes on a velvety appearance. Microscopically the lesions are characterized by papillary fronds lined by hyperplastic, metaplastic squamous epithelium, which sometimes is hyperkeratotic. Typically, many of the epithelial cells have a perinuclear halo, an empty or clear area of the cytoplasm surrounding an eccentrically placed, hyperchromatic, and irregular nucleus; these cells have been given the descriptive name of koilocytes (Fig. 15). Immunohistochemical stains using anti-papillomavirus antibodies or a hybridizing nucleic acid probe will identify the cells containing the virus. They also may be cultured for positive identification.

Condylomata of the urinary tract may cause irritative symptoms and hematuria. Discrete lesions are managed by transurethral resection, but diffuse disease usually necessitates more radical surgery. We also must be aware of the risk of carcinomatous transformation in condylomata and the development of verrucous or infiltrating squamous carcinoma (113,114).

INFLAMMATORY PSEUDOSARCOMATOUS LESIONS OF THE BLADDER

Several lesions involve the urinary bladder and mimic sarcomas. They have been described under a variety of names but share many histologic and clinical features. In 1984 Proppe et al. (115) reported on nine cases of spindle cell tumors, two of which involved the bladder and three the prostatic urethra, all appearing within months of a transurethral (TUR) resection. They named the lesions "postoperative spindle cell nodules of the genitourinary tract." These apparently benign proliferative lesions are characterized histologically by plump or elongated spindle cells, which infiltrate the bladder wall and focally can destroy muscle. The lesion can be quite cellular (Fig. 16A). A prominent feature of these tumors is a delicate network of small blood vessels in an edematous or myxoid stroma with little to moderate collagen deposition. Mitotic figures may be present and even frequent, but they are not atypical. The surface urothelium is usually ulcerated with an acute inflammatory cell infiltrate superficially and chronic inflammatory infiltrate scattered throughout the remainder of the lesion.

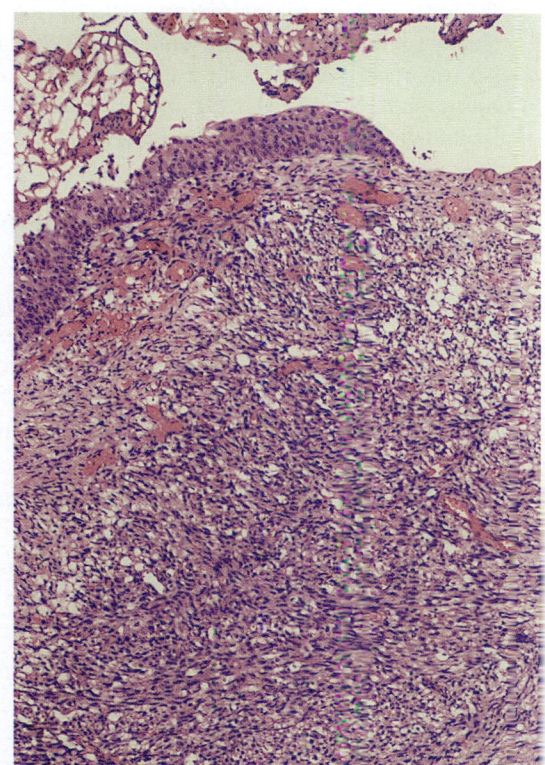 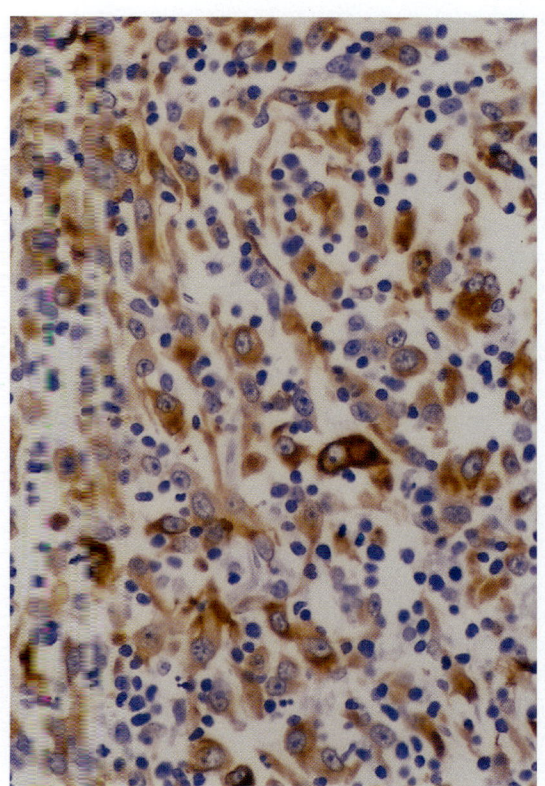

FIG. 16. Postoperative spindle cell nodule. The morphologic features may overlap with other reactive as well as neoplastic conditions. **A:** A densely cellular infiltrate contains spindle cells, inflammatory cells, and a rich vascular network. **B:** Cytokeratin stain showing strong immunostaining in myofibroblasts exhibiting epithelioid features.

Histologically similar lesions were described by other authors and called "inflammatory pseudotumor" (116,117), "pseudosarcomatous fibromyxoid tumor" (118), and "pseudosarcomatous myofibroblastic proliferation" (119). The lesions were either pedunculated or polypoid, with a low mitotic rate. They appeared either spontaneously or in a background of chronic cystitis and differed from the cases reported by Proppe in that they were not necessarily related to a recent operative procedure. A similar pseudosarcomatous lesion was reported by Roth (120). Invasive or metastatic TCC may incite a pseudosarcomatous stromal reaction that may be confused with a pseudotumor or with sarcoma (121).

The differential diagnosis usually is with leiomyosarcoma and spindle cell carcinoma (122–124). A reactive pseudosarcomatous lesion should always be suspected of postoperative spindle cell nodules involving the bladder. The best clues to their benign nature are a delicate but abundant vascular network, absence of atypical mitotic figures, edematous or myxoid stroma, and a sprinkling of chronic inflammatory cells deep within the lesion. Tumor cells will usually have the features of reactive myofibroblasts with large, epithelioid nuclei and abundant eosinophilic cytoplasm. Immunohistochemical studies or electron microscopy may be of help to prove the fibroblastic or myofibroblastic nature of the cells. Nevertheless, extreme caution is warranted in the interpretation of the immunohistochemical stains, because the atypical spindle cells may be positive for cytokeratins (Fig. 16B), vimentin, and actin (122).

UROTHELIAL CARCINOMA

Epidemiology

More than 51,000 new cases of bladder cancer occur in the United States each year, with more than 10,500 people dying of the disease. Seventy-five percent of patients are first seen with "superficial" disease, whereas 20% and 5% are seen with invasive and metastatic disease, respectively. Carcinoma of the bladder affects men more than women at a ratio of 3 to 4:1. This difference is probably accounted for by differences in smoking habits and occupational exposure in the two sexes. The incidence of bladder cancer differs between counties, between different states and counties in this country, and between adjacent urban and rural areas, also suggesting that social, occupational, environmental, or dietary factors might promote the development of bladder cancer (125).

In 1895 Rehn demonstrated an increased risk of bladder cancer in dye industry employees. Since then, a substantial number of industrially used aromatic amines such as naphthylamines, benzidine, and biphenyls have been identified as human bladder carcinogens (125–127). Occupational exposure to these organic amines has been associated with a relatively high incidence of bladder cancer. These occupations include chemical, dyestuff, rubber, paint, and textile manufacturing, as well as laboratory work, leather work, and printing (127–129).

Although it is still somewhat controversial, it is generally accepted that cigarette smokers have an increased relative risk of developing bladder cancer: up to 4 times the risk of the general population (125). It also has become clear that the relative risk of developing cancer increases with cigarette smoking, but not with cigar or pipe smoking, suggesting that inhalation is an important factor. Although it is uncertain which components in cigarette smoke are carcinogenic, prime suspects include 2-naphthylamine, nitrosamines, and tryptophan metabolites (130,131).

An increased risk in coffee drinkers also has been reported, but this association remains much more controversial (132). No direct or causal relation between coffee comsumption and human bladder cancer has been established, nor has there been convincing evidence for a carcinogenic effect of other foodstuffs such as artificial sweeteners (133–135). Despite the established importance of occupational and environmental factors in the development of bladder cancer, a great proportion of bladder tumors occur among nonsmokers and persons without occupational exposure to bladder carcinogens. This suggests that other factors, perhaps related to diet, could promote the development of bladder cancer. Armstrong and Doll (136) showed a higher incidence of bladder cancer in association with a high-fat diet, and the low incidence of bladder cancer in the Japanese population may be related to a low dietary fat intake.

Another factor that must be considered among the causes of bladder cancer is prolonged local irritation of the mucosa, which may play a role in patients with bladder diverticula, calculi, extrophy, and schistosomiasis. Urothelial carcinoma also was reported after long use of certain phenacetin-containing analgesics (137,138) and after treatment with the alkylating drug cyclophosphamide (139), as have rare cases of sarcoma (140).

Classification of Malignant Urothelial Tumors

Approximately 90% of malignant bladder tumors are TCCs. The remaining 10% comprise all other types of carcinoma, a small number of sarcomas, and miscellaneous tumors. The types of carcinoma arising in the urothelium are listed in Table 1.

It is not uncommon to see focal areas of squamous or glan-

TABLE 1. *Classification of urothelial carcinomas*

Urothelial (transitional cell) carcinoma
Urothelial carcinoma with mixed epithelial features
Squamous cell carcinoma
   Verrucous carcinoma
Adenocarcinoma
   Enteric type
   Clear cell ("mesonephric") type
   Signet-ring cell type
Small cell/neuroendocrine carcinoma
Sarcomatoid (spindle cell) carcinoma
Carcinosarcoma
Lymphoepitheliomalike carcinoma
Nested variant of urothelial carcinoma
Micropapillary carcinoma
Microcystic carcinoma

dular differentiation in transitional cell (urothelial) carcinomas, especially in intermediate- and high-grade tumors. We believe these still should be classified as TCCs. The term carcinoma with mixed epithelial features should be reserved for tumors that exhibit prominent areas of two or more histologic types, in which case the histologic tumor types present should be reported. The diagnosis of adenocarcinoma, squamous cell carcinoma or small-cell carcinoma should be reserved for tumors in which those are essentially pure patterns or at most there are only very focal areas of concomitant conventional TCC. Sarcomatoid carcinoma refers to those tumors exhibiting tumor cells with spindle cell features, whereas carcinosarcoma describes a high-grade carcinoma with areas of mesenchymal differentiation, be it leiomyosarcoma, rhabdomyosarcoma, chondrosarcoma, or osteosarcoma. Admittedly, distinction between the latter types is arbitrary because sarcomatoid carcinoma and carcinosarcoma are a morphologic continuum representing different degrees of differentiation within an epithelial tumor.

Staging of Bladder Cancer

The usefulness of any staging scheme is directly related to its ability to discriminate between prognostic groups. In 1946, Jewett and Strong (141,142) first demonstrated the importance of the depth of infiltration as a prognostic variable in bladder cancer and proposed a staging scheme that was later modified by Marshall (143). A similar classification was later adopted by the American Joint Committee on Cancer (AJCC) (144). As evidenced in Table 2, it is quite simple to convert from one staging classification to the other. The ability of these staging schemes to discriminate between clinically distinct prognostic groups is evidenced in Table 3. Many investigators showed a statistically significant survival difference between patients with noninvasive tumors, tumors confined to lamina propria, and those with muscle infiltration (145–148). The former are treated with transurethral resection and possibly intravesical chemotherapy, whereas patients with "muscle-infiltrating tumors" (at least T2 lesions) are offered radical cystectomy. For this reason, the pathologist must be very careful in assessing depth of invasion in a biopsy specimen. The few wisps of smooth muscle that are commonly seen within the lamina propria (see section describing the

TABLE 2. *Pathologic staging of bladder carcinoma*

Jewett–Marshall	Depth of invasion	AJCC (144)
O	Noninvasive	Pa, Pis
A	Lamina propria	P1
B$_1$	Superficial; ½ muscularis propria	P2a
B$_2$	Deep; ½ muscularis propria	P2b
C	Perivesical fat	P3a,b
D$_1$	Prostate, vagina, uterus	P4a
	Pelvic and/or abdominal wall	P4b

Pa, papillary *in situ*; Pis, flat *in situ*.

TABLE 3. *Five-year survival according to stage at the time of cystectomy*

Stage	Smith et al.[a] (%)	Pagano et al.[b] (%)
Pis[c]	71	70
P$_1$	67	75
P$_2$	60	63
P$_3$	50	31
P$_4$	16	21

[a] From ref. 145, with permission.
[b] From ref. 146, with permission.
[c] The patient may have had invasive tumor removed by prior transurethral resection.

anatomy of the bladder) must not be mistaken for fascicles of the muscularis propria in coming to a decision about the depth of invasion (Fig. 17) (4). To be certain the tumor is infiltrating muscularis propria, we must see tumor cells among broad bundles of smooth muscle (Fig. 18). The presence of muscle infiltration should be reported only when it is certain that the tumor has penetrated into the muscularis propria.

In invasive disease, the most powerful prognostic factor is stage. Pathologic staging takes on greater importance because we know that clinical over- or understaging may occur in up to 40% of cases. Unfortunately, pathologic staging also has its problems, specifically as it pertains to invasion of the lamina propria (pT1) (148–152). Identification of lamina propria invasion is usually straightforward but certainly not in all cases. Some may be "difficult to classify," and a decision as to the presence of invasion depends on the criteria used by the pathologist. This fact has resulted in wide variability in the reported incidence of T1 in individual series, accompanied by equally disparate rates in progression.

Interobserver variability in pathology is well known. Aside from the inherent subjectivity of our field, the major cause of this variability is the lack of widely accepted, reproducible criteria for identifying lamina propria invasion in biopsy material. Compounding the problem are technical issues, including our inability to orient biopsy specimens properly, resulting in tangential sectioning, "crush," and cautery artefact brought about by the biopsy procedure itself, as well as distortion of anatomic landmarks caused by prior biopsy or intravesical therapy. During the past few years, we have developed better morphologic criteria to identify T1 disease. It is apparent that noninvasive disease [Ta and carcinoma *in situ* (CIS)] behaves quite differently from superficially invasive (T1) tumors, and as such, probably should not be classified together for prognostic and treatment purposes.

Several morphologic criteria are useful in the determination of lamina propria invasion (Table 4). Growth-pattern characteristics of the epithelium are very important. One of the common difficulties in determining superficial invasion is the fact that several benign, proliferative urothelial lesions, such as Brunn's nests, inverted papilloma, nephrogenic metaplasia manifest as pseudoinvasive nests of urothelium within the lamina propria. The problem is often compounded by the

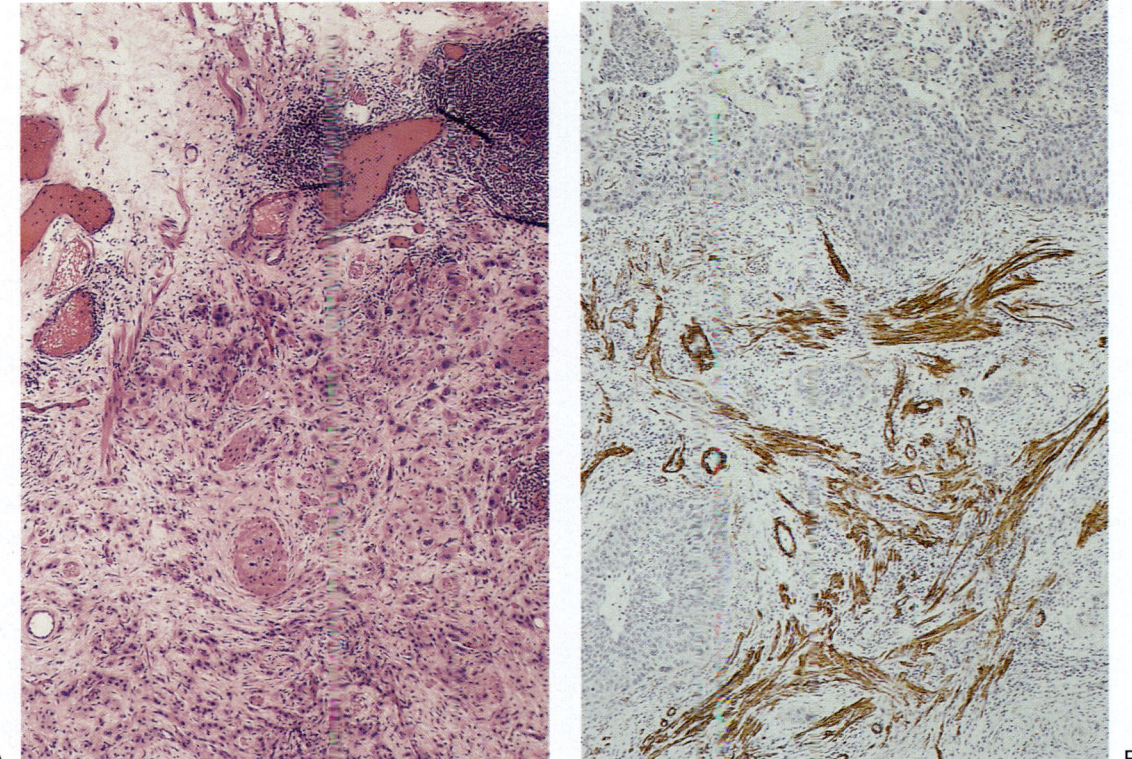

FIG. 17. Transitional cell carcinoma infiltrating lamina propria (pT1). **A:** Tumor cell surrounding small smooth-muscle fascicles commonly seen at this site (muscularis mucosae). **B:** Immunostain against actin (HHF-35) highlights disrupted muscularis mucosae infiltrated by tumor.

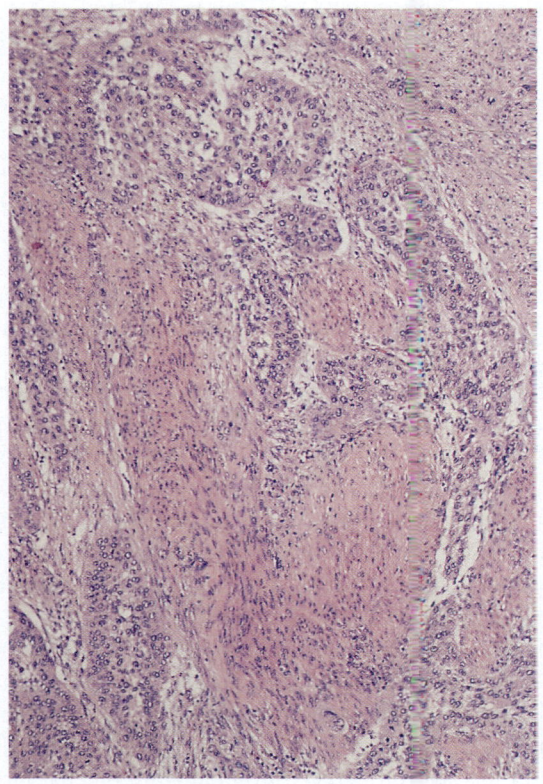

FIG. 18. Transitional cell carcinoma infiltrating muscularis propria (pT2). Tumor nests surround large fascicles of smooth muscle.

unoriented nature of the specimen. Tangentially sectioned, densely packed noninvasive papillary tumors exhibit a stroma–epithelium interface that is smooth and regular. In cases of true invasion, we are likely to see variably sized and irregularly shaped nests or individual tumor cells percolating through the stroma. The morphologic appearance of the basement membrane also may supply useful information. When dealing with tangential sections through noninvasive disease or when urothelial carcinoma involves Brunn's nests, the basement membrane preserves a regular contour, whereas it is frequently absent in the cases of true invasion. This feature may be assessed on H&E, although in many cases, additional clues are needed, including the presence of a parallel array of thin-walled vessels that evenly line the basement membrane of noninvasive nests but that are lacking in cases of invasive tumors. Another useful parameter is the assessment of stromal reaction. The stroma of the lamina propria adjacent to an invasive tumor is commonly altered when compared with uninvolved bladder wall. This stromal reaction usually consists

TABLE 4. Morphologic criteria to determine lamina propria invasion

- Growth-pattern characteristics
- Morphologic appearance of the basement membrane
- Assessment of stromal/host reaction
- Presence of retraction artifact
- Presence of paradoxical differentiation

of a fibroblastic stromal proliferation, sometimes with myxoid change. The stromal reaction may be quite cellular, adopting a pseudosarcomatous appearance, or it may consist of a minimal increase in fibroblasts. The invasive nests may be accompanied by a peritumoral inflammatory response. If this inflammatory response is brisk, it may obscure the stromal hypercellularity. On occasion, invasive nests may be surrounded by a collagenous stroma, which is not seen in the uninvolved lamina propria. Whereas the majority of bladder tumors with unquestionable lamina propria invasion exhibit some sort of stromal reaction, microinvasive disease usually does not, making its identification even more difficult. Another important feature of invasion is the presence of retraction artifact around individual tumor cells or nests of cells. This feature may be of great utility in identifying microinvasive disease and is often confused with lymphatic invasion. Nevertheless it is important to remember that this feature may be very difficult to assess in areas exhibiting cautery or crush artifact. The final clue to identifying lamina propria invasion is the presence of paradoxical differentiation. This feature is particularly helpful in microinvasive disease in which the invasive tumor cells may acquire abundant, eosinophilic cytoplasm, similar to that seen in microinvasive uterine cervical cancer. At low and medium magnification, these microinvasive cells appear to be more differentiated than the overlying noninvasive disease.

With few exceptions, such as the nested variant of TCC, the criteria enumerated allow us consistently and reproducibly to separate superficial bladder tumors into noninvasive (Ta and CIS) tumors and those that have invaded the lamina propria (T1), the latter having a significantly worse prognosis. In a cohort of 180 patients with superficial bladder cancer seen at Memorial Hospital and treated with transurethral resection alone, the progression rate of noninvasive tumors was 2.85 per 100 person/year whereas for T1 lesions, it was more than double, 6.86 per 100 person/year. Other investigators have reached similar findings, and urologists are now debating whether T1 tumors should be treated more aggressively. If this is the case, pathologists will experience additional pressure to stage these tumors accurately.

Several investigators attempted to subclassify T1 tumors based on their depth of invasion. Younes et al. (153) subclassified T1 tumors into three groups, based on whether invasion was limited to above the muscularis mucosa (T1a), reached the level of the muscularis mucosa (T1b), or extended beyond the muscularis mucosa (T1c). In their series of 50 cases, T1a and T1b tumors had a 5-year survival rate of 75% compared with 11% in the T1c group. Hasui et al. (154) used a slightly different subclassification scheme but arrived at similar results, that T1 tumors that infiltrate to or near the muscularis mucosa had a higher progression rate that those that did not (53.5% vs. 6.7%, $p < 0.01$). In a larger study, Angulo et al. (155) confirmed these findings but also reached the important conclusion that, by using the presence of muscularis mucosa or large blood vessels as determining factors, subdividing the superficial bladder wall into lamina propria (T1a) and submucosa (T1b) could be done in only 58% of TUR specimens. If we are to subdivide these tumors, it is clear that we need additional criteria to apply to all specimens. Much work remains to be done before we can incorporate this information into the pathology report.

Urothelial (Transitional Cell) Carcinoma

Approximately 98% of malignant tumors arising in the urinary bladder are of epithelial origin, and of these, 90% are TCC. The highest incidence is in the sixth and seventh decades of life, and men are affected more often than women at a ratio of 3 to 4:1. Most TCCs at initial diagnosis are papillary and superficial, and as many as 70% are characterized by a prolonged clinical course over which the patient experiences multiple recurrences after local resection without tumor progression (156,157). In contrast, a smaller but significant percentage of patients are first seen with tumors that have an aggressive clinical course over a short period of time. A number of pathologic features are accurate predictors of the clinical course of bladder cancer. The most important are depth of invasion, if any, at presentation, multiplicity (multifocality), a history of prior urothelial tumors, tumor size, and grade. Tumor size and grade are not so important an influence on the recurrence rate as tumor multiplicity (multifocality), a history of tumors, and depth of invasion at diagnosis (156–161). As a rule, only high-grade tumors will develop regional lymph node metastasis. Cytologically benign papillary tumors may and do "recur," but do not invade. Tumors are as likely to recur at a different site in the bladder, indicating multifocal occurrence rather than recurrence of the original tumor.

Pathologic stage is the most potent predictor of survival in TCC. Although a 5-year survival rate of approximately 75% is to be expected in patients with no more than lamina propria invasion at the time of cystectomy, 5-year survival rates for tumors infiltrating muscularis propria or perivesical fat are 40% and 20%, respectively (Table 3) (162). Similarly, regional lymph node metastasis at the time of cystectomy is more frequent in tumors infiltrating muscularis propria or perivesical fat. Some urothelial tumors exhibit an endophytic pattern of growth, at times mimicking inverted papilloma (107,108). In such cases, it may be quite difficult to determine the presence of stomal invasion, especially in biopsy material.

Tumor configuration is another important prognostic variable. Papillary tumors tend to be of lower grade, of earlier stage, and of less aggressive behavior than do nonpapillary tumors (158,160,163,164). Kakizoe et al. (165) studied 186 cystectomies and found that tumors with a nodular (sessile) configuration were seen at a higher stage when compared with exclusively papillary tumors. Survival was adversely ($p < 0.01$) affected in the former group. Small-vessel infiltration also affects prognosis. Fossa et al. (161) found that in a group of patients with superficial bladder carcinoma, those who had lamina propria small-vessel invasion had a significantly higher risk of subsequent tumor progression. Larsen et al. (166) disagreed that lymphatic invasion is of clinical significance in pT1 disease, but they raised the valid issue that the presence of lymphatic invasion may be very difficult to evaluate by light microscopy alone (Fig. 19). Only five of 36 biopsies originally diagnosed with vascular invasion were confirmed when immunohistochemistry studies were used to identify endothelial cells. Heney et al. (160) reported on 86 patients who underwent radical cystectomy for invasive carcinoma infiltrating at least into muscularis propria. Those who exhibited small-vessel invasion had regional lymph node metastasis in 38% of cases and a 5-year survival rate of 30%, whereas those patients who did not have small-vessel invasion had a regional lymph node metastatic rate and survival rate of 16% and 52%, respectively.

These data clearly illustrate that a number of histologic features are useful predictors of the clinical course of bladder cancer. Pathologists should make it a point to comment on these features at the time of evaluation and reporting of bladder biopsy and cystectomy specimens (see Table 5). In evaluating biopsy specimens, the pathologist should state what components of the bladder wall are represented (i.e., mucosa, lamina propria, muscularis propria). If the epithelial surface is ulcerated or denuded, it should be so stated; and if a tumor is present, we should establish the histologic type (transitional), pattern of growth (papillary, nodular), tumor grade, and depth of invasion. The presence or absence of small-vessel involvement should be noted. The status of the adjacent mucosa should be evaluated, especially with reference to CIS. In cystectomy specimens, we should comment as well on the location and size of the lesion(s), status of mucosal and soft-tissue margins, status of adjacent organs (urethra, ureters, prostate), as well as location, number, and status of regional lymph nodes. This information will allow the clinician to offer a more exact opinion as to the prognosis of the patients and the better to choose between available therapeutic options.

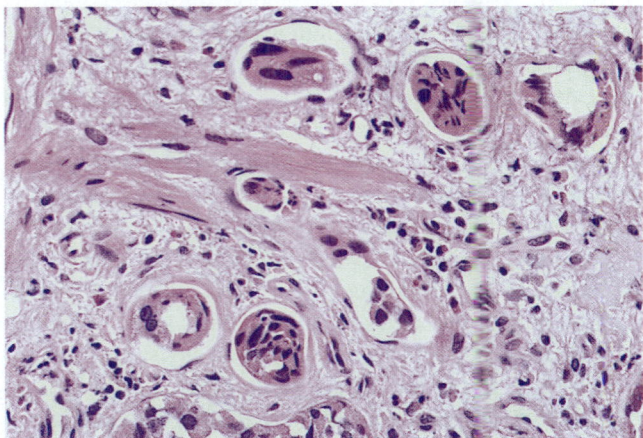

FIG. 19. Tissue retraction may mimic vascular invasion. This problem is most commonly seen in the lamina propria and in transurethral resection specimens.

TABLE 5. *Pathologic evaluation of bladder tumors*

I. Biopsy
  A. Gross description (unnecessary if embedded *in toto*)
    1. Number of pieces and dimensions
    2. Proportion of tissue embedded
  B. Microscopic description
    1. Evaluation of epithelial surface (intact, ulcerated, denuded)
    2. Depth of bladder wall included in biopsy
    3. Histology (TCC, adeno, etc.)
    4. Pattern of growth (papillary, nodular, etc.)
    5. Grade
    6. Extent (depth) of invasion
    7. Lymphatic/vascular invasion
    8. Pattern of infiltration (tentacular, broad front, mixed)
    9. Status of adjacent mucosa
II. Cystectomy
  A. Gross description
    1. Overall dimensions
    2. Location and size of lesions
    3. Depth of infiltration
    4. Urethra, ureters, prostate, seminal vesicles
    5. Margins (mucosal and soft tissue)
    6. Lymph nodes
  B. Microscopic description
    1. Evaluation of distant mucosa
    2. Evaluation of adjacent structures
      a. Ureters, urethra, prostate, seminal vesicles, cervix
    3. Margins
    4. Lymph nodes
      a. Location and number identified
      b. Number with tumor
        i. Tumor type
        ii. Extent of involvement
        iii. Extranodal extension
    5. Pathologic stage

TCC, transitional cell carcinoma.

Grading of Papillary Urothelial Lesions

The most common tumors of the urinary tract (excluding prostate) are papillary tumors of urothelial origin (Fig. 20). They frequently are multiple and often recur after being removed, yet most of these tumors are easily managed by local resection. Patients who have had papillary tumors of the bladder are at risk of developing invasive carcinoma, and some very experienced pathologists regard nearly all papillary tumors as carcinoma (167,168). We consider papillary tumors that are composed of orderly, cytologically benign, or minimally atypical epithelium to be biologically benign (Fig. 21), thus avoiding the term carcinoma. Up to this time we classified them as papillomas but, following the results of a consensus meeting among members of the classification committee of the World Health Organization and the International Society of Urological Pathologists, now call them papillary urothelial neoplasms of low malignant potential (LMP). Papillary tumors containing cytologically malignant cells are classified as papillary carcinomas of low or high grade, depending on the cytologic appearance of the cells and their growth-pattern characteristics (Figs. 22 and 23). The evidence to support this latter classification is very strong.

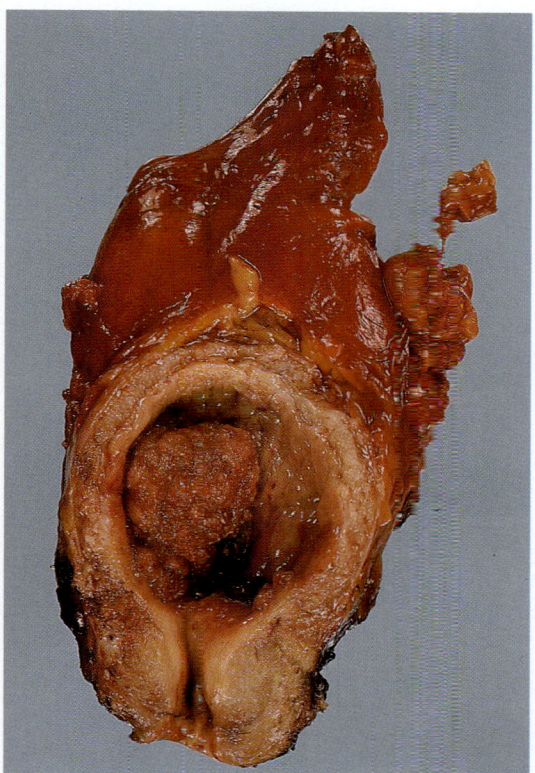

FIG. 20. Cystectomy specimen revealing a single polypoid tumor occupying the right posterior and lateral surface of the bladder. Whereas most transitional cell carcinomas are multiple, approximately one-third are solitary.

First, it is worth noting that papillary tumors of the bladder left untreated may grow profusely within the bladder without invading through the wall or metastasizing, a fact noted by pathologists in the 19th century who did not regard these growths as malignant tumors. More than 30 years ago, Nichols and Marshall reported that the 5-year survival of patients with papilloma (low-grade papillary tumors) was exactly that of the age-matched general population. However, this was not true of cytologically high-grade tumors. Ash (159) recognized this as early as 1940 in his adaption of Broder's cytologic grading system for the classification of papillary transitional cell tumors, grades I to IV. Mostofi et al. (167) later modified Ash's classification for the World Health Organization, distinguishing a class of papillomas from TCC, grades I, II, and III. Their definition of papilloma was very conservative, restricted to the approximately 1% of patients who had a usually solitary, delicate papillary tumor with no more than eight cell layers of normal-appearing transitional epithelium on a fibrovascular core. Koss (168) later accepted this definition in his influential monograph on tumors of the urinary bladder, published for the Armed Forces Institute of Pathology (AFIP), although he permitted no more than seven cell layers.

The accumulating data from an increasing number of clinicopathologic studies indicated that these definitions are too narrowly drawn, that many of the grade I papillary "carcinomas" so defined are in fact biologically benign and should be classified as papillomas. Detailed histologic studies, includ-

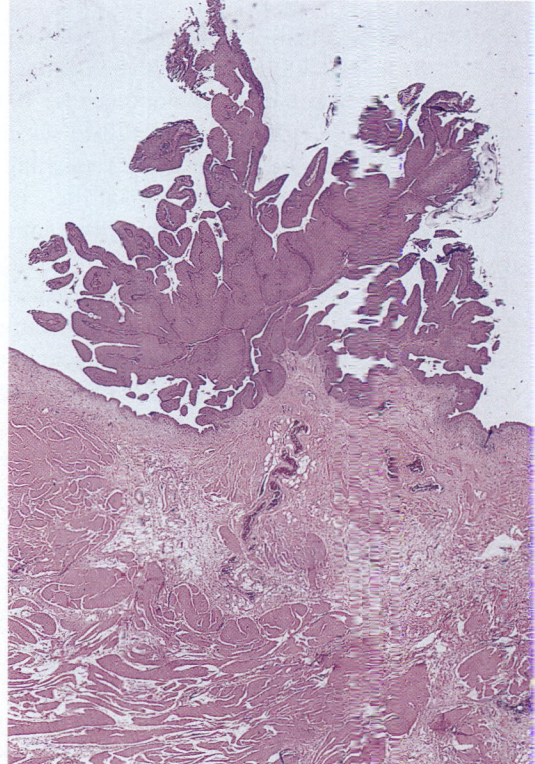
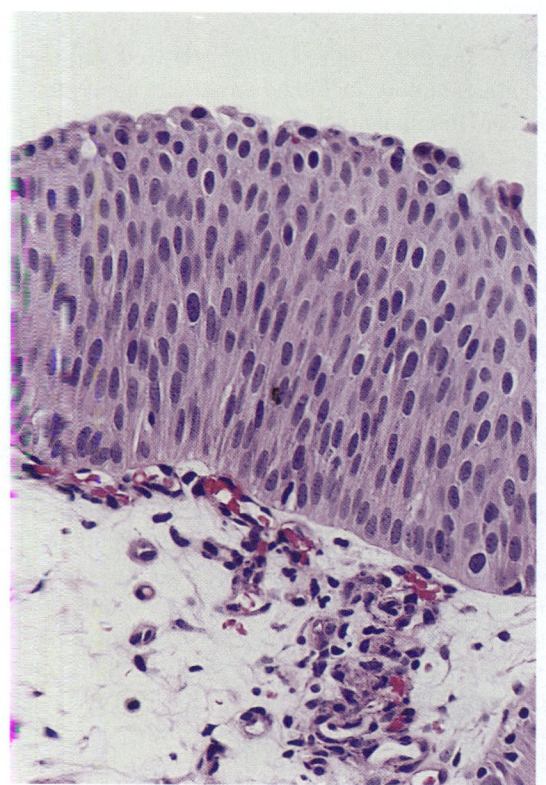

FIG. 21. Papillary urothelial neoplasm of low malignant potential (LMP). **A:** Papillary fronds lined by variably thickened epithelium surrounding a fibrovascular core. **B:** Cell layers are increased as compared with normal urothelium, but cytologically, the cells are oriented in an orderly fashion and lack pleomorphism. The chromatin pattern is homogeneous.

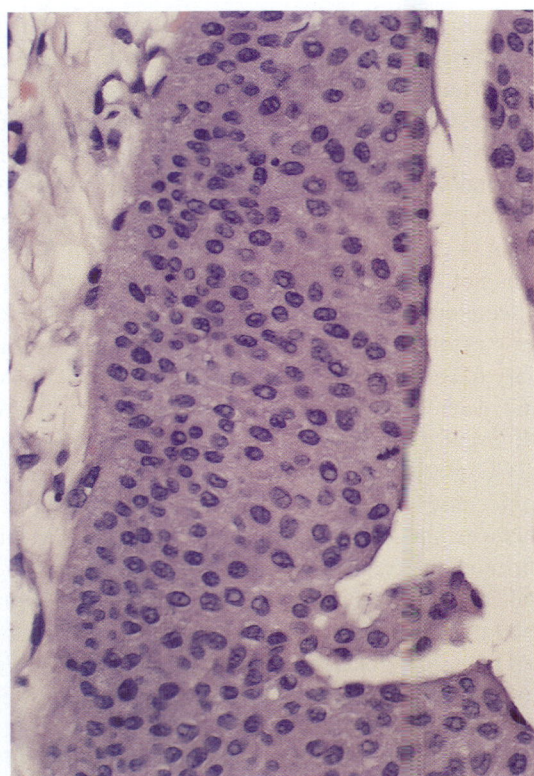

FIG. 22. Papillary urothelial (transitional cell) carcinoma, low grade. Individual cells lack orientation relative to the basement membrane (disorder). The chromatin pattern is somewhat variable, and there is mild to moderate pleomorphism.

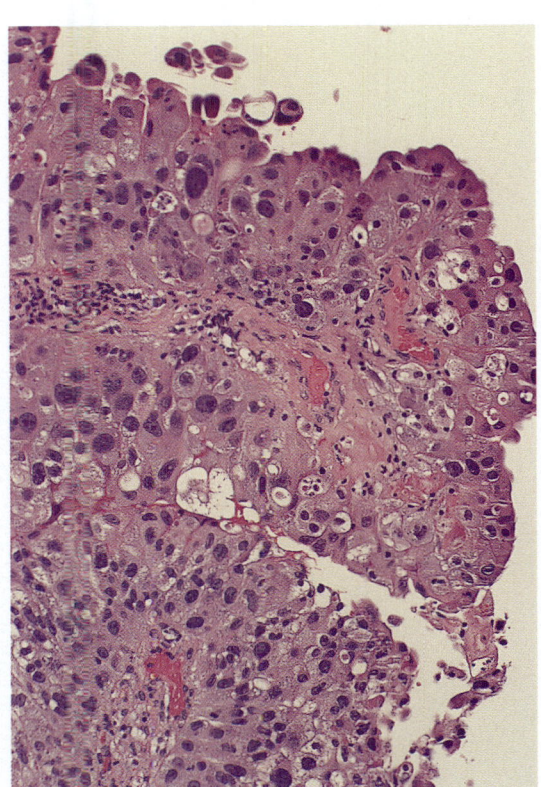

FIG. 23. Papillary urothelial (transitional cell) carcinoma, high grade. The neoplastic cells are pleomorphic and hyperchromatic and exhibit no orientation relative to the basement membrane.

ing some that mapped the entire bladder showed that the low-grade papillary tumors, including those with hyperplastic epithelium and minimal atypia, are noninvasive. It is the flat, nodular, or papillary tumors with cytologically malignant epithelium that give rise to the great majority of invasive carcinomas (170–174). Long-term clinical follow-up studies also confirmed the benign nature of the low-grade papillary tumors. Bergkvist et al. (175) followed up 300 patients with bladder tumors for 8 years, and of 64 (21%) who had low-grade tumors, only one died of bladder cancer, and that one was believed to have died of a new carcinoma that developed 5 years later. One hundred seventy-two of the 236 patients with higher-grade tumors died of their bladder cancer. Lerman et al. (176), in a study from Memorial Sloan–Kettering, reported on 125 patients with papilloma (now called papillary urothelial neoplasm of LMP), defined by the broader cytologic criteria we favor, and followed up for 10 to 20 years. Whereas nearly half recurred, only 5% later developed CIS, and another 5% developed invasive carcinoma; in no case was there invasion at the site of histologically benign papilloma, suggesting both by location and late occurrence that these were new tumors. In other studies, Heney et al. (159) reported only 2% of 92 patients with grade I TCC developed a more anaplastic tumor over a period of 36 months; Gilbert et al. (177) reported that nine (5%) of 155 patients with grade I TCC developed high-grade and muscle-invading tumors, whereas 41% did not have a single recurrence after no less than 5 years' follow-up. Recently Jordan et al. (178) studied 400 patients with transitional cell tumors classified by WHO criteria and monitored for 10 to 20 years; of 91 with grade I TCC, only seven (8%) subsequently developed more advanced tumors; the remaining 84 had no progression of disease and had normal life expectancy, although some had recurrent tumors of the same type. Fifty-five (60%) patients had no recurrences.

Some of the most interesting and informative data came from the National Bladder Cancer Collaborative Group A Program (NBCCG) (156). In that multiinstitutional study, it was found that when recurrences did occur in patients with low-grade TCC, they were as likely as not to be at sites different from the original. This, of course, suggests that the clinical recurrences were actually new tumors, and that their formation was due to the neoplastic diathesis of an unstable urothelium. They are manifestations of the multifocal origin of tumor in these patients. Althausen et al. (174) studied the normal-appearing mucosa adjoining low-grade papillary tumors and found that most of the invasive carcinomas developing later were in patients who had CIS or atypia in the adjacent flat mucosa. Presumably most invasive carcinomas develop from mucosa that has CIS or develops it over a period after resection of the papillary tumor. That CIS frequently is present elsewhere in the bladder mucosa of patients with low-grade papillary tumors is strongly suggested by other data from the NBCCG. Positive exfoliative cytology was found in 43% of the patients with grade 1 tumors (papillomas) (179). Because benign papillary lesions (WHO grade I tumors) do not shed cytologically malignant cells, they must be coming from other areas of occult carcinoma or CIS.

This information as well as the experience of many experienced pathologists led to changes in the classification of bladder tumors. This is evidenced in the grading scheme proposed by Murphy in the latest Atlas of Tumor Pathology (182), as well as the similar classification agreed on by many uropathologists from throughout the world at a recent meeting sponsored by the International Society of Urological Pathologists (Table 6). In addition, it is quite likely that the upcoming revision of the WHO classification will adopt many of the changes as well. Tumors previously called papillary carcinoma, grade 1, in the present WHO classification are now called papillary neoplasms of LMP. Carcinomas, whether papillary or invasive, are devided into low grade and high grade based on the degree of cytologic and growth-pattern abnormalities. The morphologic criteria on which this novel classification is based has its roots in the work of Bergkvist et al. (175) in the 1960s and later modified and expanded on by Busch et al. (180). Tumors classified as grade 1 by Busch et al. are now LMP, grade 2A are low grade, and grade 2B and 3 are high grade.

In summary, probably 20% or more of papillary bladder tumors are cytologically benign or exhibit low-grade cytologic atypia with or without epithelial hyperplasia. They are biologically benign, do not invade, and should be classified as papillary neoplasms of LMP rather than papillary carcinomas grade I. These tumors often recur but usually do so at the same histologic grade (LMP). The fewer than 10% that do progress will do so only after increasing in grade or developing flat CIS.

Carcinoma may develop within an existing LMP lesion as it does within flat epithelium. This transformation may be focal or multifocal. Alternatively, carcinomatous transformation may be diffuse within the papillary tumor. The distinction between low-grade and high-grade carcinoma is based on the cytology and growth-pattern characteristics of the tumor. Higher-grade tumors are more anaplastic, with cells having larger, more hyperchromatic, irregular, and coarsely textured nuclei, a more disorderly arrangement (see Fig. 23). Mitoses may be numerous and atypical. As a tumor increases in grade, mitoses tend to occur away from the basal layer. In general, the higher the grade, the more discohesive the tumor cells become.

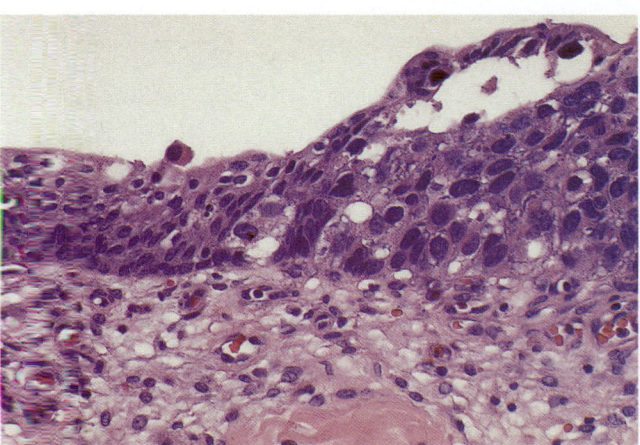

FIG. 24. Carcinoma *in situ*. Markedly hyperchromatic and pleomorphic cells occupy portions of the urothelium. They lack polarity in relation to the basement membrane.

Carcinoma *In Situ*

Unless it is specifically described within a papillary tumor, CIS usually refers to a nonpapillary (flat) mucosa in which the normal urothelium has been transformed into or replaced by cancer cells that have not invaded through the basement membrane (Figs. 24–26). CIS is a high-grade lesion and easily recognized because the cytologic abnormalities are obvious, similar to those seen in high-grade papillary tumors. We cannot and do not make the diagnosis of low-grade CIS. To cover the spectrum of minimal cytologic atypias, some pathologists have adopted the term dysplasia (179,182–186). It is a term that suggests specificity where none exists and that suggests clinical significance where none has been demonstrated, especially in cells with mild to moderate cytologic abnormalities in which these changes overlap significantly

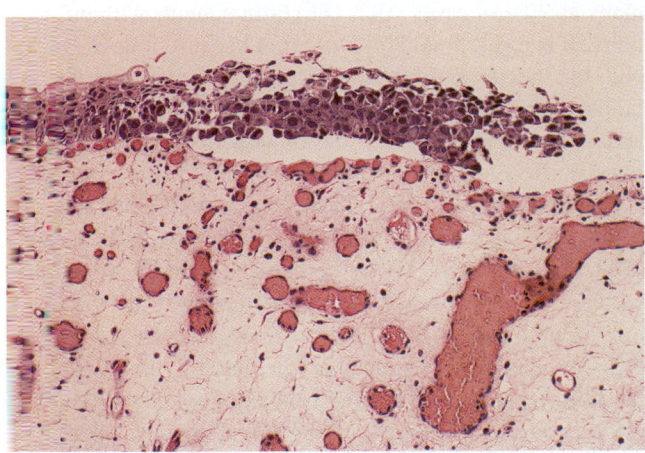

FIG. 25. Carcinoma *in situ*. Notice the propensity of the neoplastic cells to become detached from the basement membrane, a feature that explains the value of urine cytology in the diagnosis and surveillance of this disease.

TABLE 6. *Classification of papillary urothelial neoplasms*

Murphy (182)	WHO/Koss (167/168)	WHO/ISUP[a]
Papilloma	Papilloma ↔	Papilloma
	Grade 1 ↔	LMP[b]
Low grade ←	Grade 2	→ Low grade
High grade ←	Grade 3	→ High grade

From refs. 167, 168, and 182, with permission.
[a] Classification agreed on at a meeting of the International Society of Urological Pathology and the World Health Organization.
[b] Papillary urothelial neoplasm of low malignant potential

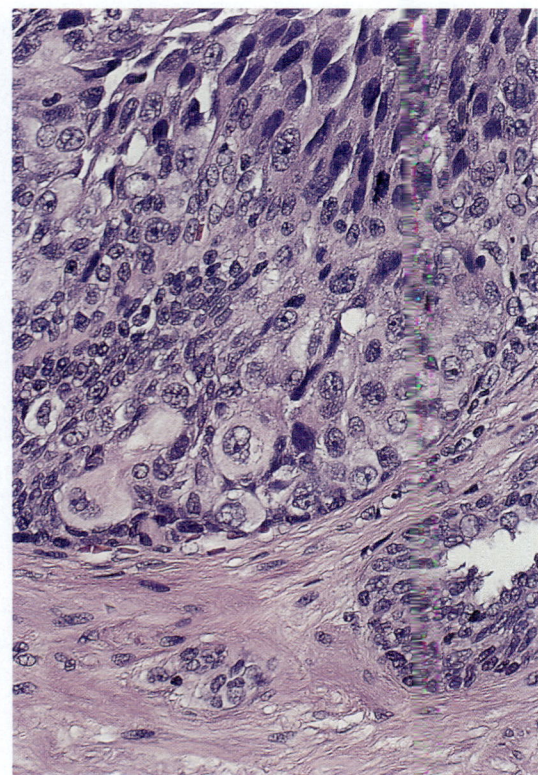

FIG. 26. Carcinoma *in situ* of a periurethral prostatic duct.

with those seen in reactive conditions. Nondiagnostic atypias or atypias of unknown significance are best reported as such. Carcinomatous transformation, even minute areas of carcinomatous transformation, if so recognized, should be classified as CIS. If we are to use the term dysplasia at all, it should be limited to those cases in which we are certain that the cytologic abnormalities seen are neoplastic yet short of CIS. Distinction from what has been called severe dysplasia and CIS suffers from great interobserver variability (187). As such, these should be called CIS.

Flat CIS is most often found in association with papillary or invasive carcinoma, in which it has been reported in as many as 90% of cases (182–186) or in patients with prior tumors. It is rarely found *ab initio,* not because it does not occur, but because the cytologic studies, cystoscopy, and biopsy necessary to detect this disease and establish the diagnosis are seldom carried out on patients with minimal or nonspecific symptoms. A substantial proportion of patients with CIS alone are asymptomatic. Symptoms, when they appear, suggest cystitis: dysuria, frequency and nocturia (185,186,188–193). Gross hematuria, usually associated with tumor, is rare; however, most patients with CIS do have microscopic hematuria. Cystoscopically also the mucosa appears to be inflamed, with an erythematous, velvety, or cobblestone appearance differing from banal cystitis only by the often discrete boundaries of the gross changes compared with the diffuseness of cystitis. The epithelium in areas of CIS is only loosely cohesive; cells readily desquamate, and the epithelium has a rapid turnover rate. Thus there is extensive exfoliation from even limited areas of CIS, making urine cytology a very sensitive means of detection and diagnosis. It is common for biopsies of areas of CIS to exhibit a predominantly denuded bladder wall (so-called erosive cystitis), making cytology that much more important in establishing a correct diagnosis. Whereas some patients may have only a limited focus of CIS, most in whom the diagnosis is made have multifocal or diffuse involvement.

The clinical presentation and natural history of CIS were first described by Melamed (194), and later by Farrow et al. (195). They agreed that, if left untreated, most cases of CIS will progress to invasive cancer. Zincke et al. (193) studied 70 patients who had had cystectomy for CIS, and of these, 34% exhibited microinvasion. All invasive foci were adjacent to CIS. Melamed (194) reported on 25 patients, of whom nine (36%) developed invasive cancer in less than 5 years; the remaining 16 patients all had had cystectomy because of the high risk of invasion. Nevertheless, not all patients with CIS will develop subsequent invasive disease (196).

There is good clinical evidence that CIS spreads within the mucosa from its focus or foci of origin before and after invasion occurs. For the most part, this simply reflects a gradual enlargement of the area of involvement, which, in patients who have had cystectomy for carcinoma, will involve the distal ureter in at least 15% of cases and the proximal urethra in a similar number. Thus frozen-section examination of the ureter should be carried out at the surgical-resection margin to be sure that it is proximal to any involvement of ureter by CIS. In some cases, extension of CIS is by pagetoid infiltration of the cancer cells into the adjacent normal epithelium (Figs. 26 and 27) (197–199).

The treatment of flat CIS, like that of superficial papillary tumors, is generally conservative, in an effort to retain the bladder for as long as possible. Areas of involvement are delineated by cystoscopic mapping biopsies, resected or fulgurated endoscopically, and followed by a series of intravesical

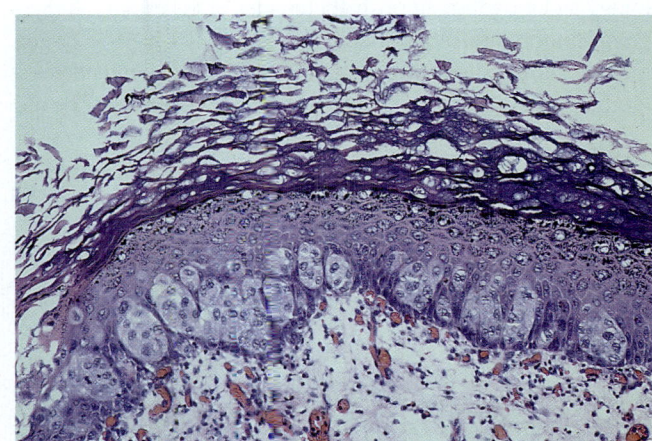

FIG. 27. Pagetoid spread of transitional cell carcinoma. Notice nests of neoplastic cells undermining urothelium, which has undergone squamous metaplasia and is hyperkeratotic. This patient had a long history of recurrent bladder tumors.

instillations of BCG. The patients are then monitored by cytologic and periodic cystoscopic examinations.

Squamous Carcinoma

The diagnosis of squamous cell carcinoma (SCC) should be reserved for those tumors that are predominantly keratin forming (Fig. 28). They constitute 2% to 7% of urothelial cancers, except in the Middle East along the Nile Valley, where, as a consequence of the endemic nature of schistosomiasis, they are the most common form of cancer (9,200,201). These tumors tend to be sessile, ulcerated, and infiltrative at the time of diagnosis. The histologic hallmarks of pearl formation, intercellular bridges, and keratotic cellular debris are those of squamous carcinoma at any site. With the exception of the verrucous variant, most of these carcinomas are moderately or poorly differentiated and more deeply invasive at the time of diagnosis than are the majority of TCCs. Their generally poor prognosis can be attributed to the typically advanced stage at diagnosis, but stage for stage, prognosis is similar for SCC and TCC (201).

Squamous carcinoma of the urothelial tract is thought to arise through a process of metaplasia of the urothelium. A large percentage of patients with SCC have squamous metaplasia of the adjacent urothelium. Many have a history of severe, long-term chronic inflammation associated with stones, chronic infection, biharziasis, and, in a few, systemic chemotherapy with cyclophosphamide (202).

Godwin and Hanash (9) reviewed a series of 160 cases of bladder carcinoma seen at King Faisal Hospital in Saudi Arabia. Of these, approximately one third were associated with schistosomiasis, 72% of which had SCC. Whereas 41% of patients in the nonschistosomiasis group had noninvasive disease or infiltration limited to the lamina propria, only 8% of *Schistosoma*-related tumors were seen at these early stages.

Verrocous carcinoma (Fig. 29) is a rare variant of squamous carcinoma more commonly seen in the oral cavity,

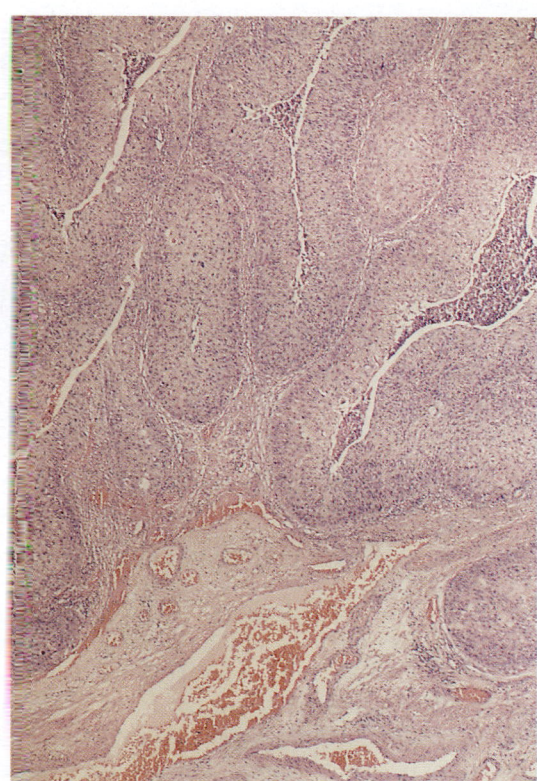

FIG. 29. Verrucous carcinoma. This rare variant of squamous carcinoma may occur rarely along the urinary tract.

anus, or genital areas. It is a very low-grade, orderly carcinoma that is clinically indolent but capable of invasion and capable of causing death. Few cases involving the bladder have been reported, usually in association with schistosomiasis or condyloma acuminatum (203–206).

Adenocarcinoma

Primary pure adenocarcinomas of the bladder are rare, representing no more than 2.5% of all malignant vesical neoplasms. As with squamous carcinoma, they arise through a process of metaplasia of the urothelium and are frequently associated with long-standing local irritation (207–213). They constitute up to 90% of carcinomas associated with bladder extrophy. They can arise anywhere on the bladder surface, although a large percentage originate from the trigone and posterior wall. A major clinical difference as compared with TCC is that two thirds of adenocarcinomas are single discrete lesions, whereas TCCs tend to be multifocal (207,208). Grossly the tumors can be papillary, nodular, or flat and ulcerated. Microscopically the tumor is most often composed of colonic-type glandular epithelium and often contains abundant extracellular mucin (Fig. 30). However, some tumors are very cellular, cytologically less well differentiated, and do not contain extracellular mucin. Regardless of histologic pattern, cystitis cystica et glandularis or surface glandular metaplasia is commonly present in the adjacent benign urothelium. Most adenocarcinomas have infiltrated

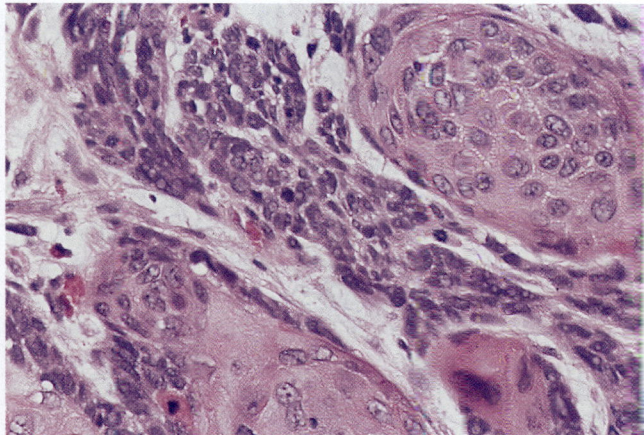

FIG. 28. Nests of squamous carcinoma within high-grade urothelial cell carcinoma. Isolated areas of squamous differentiation do not warrant classifying the tumor as a squamous cell carcinoma.

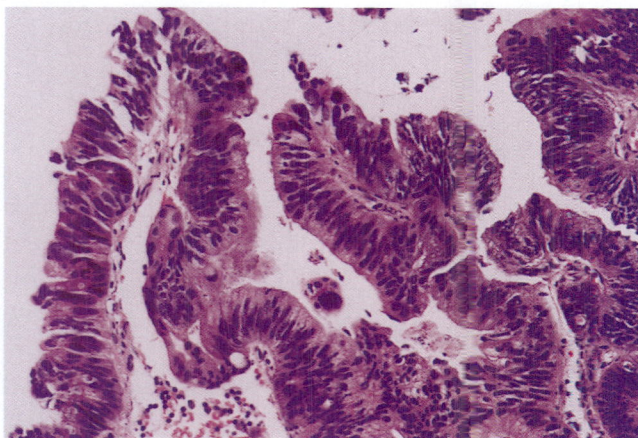

FIG. 30. Adenocarcinoma of the bladder in a transurethral resection specimen. The morphologic features of this lesion overlap with those seen in colorectal adenocarcinoma.

deeply at the time of initial diagnosis, which most likely accounts for their poor prognosis. Stage for stage, they appear to have survival similar to that of TCC (211–213).

In the differential diagnosis, we must first consider the possibility of adenocarcinoma involving the bladder either by metastasis or by direct invasion (Fig. 31). For this reason, it is important to identify CIS. This can be difficult because of extensive ulceration and may require taking many sections of adjacent mucosa. Of course, it also is necessary to rule out other possible primary sites. Tumors that directly invade the bladder and mimic primary vesical adenocarcinoma include those arising in rectum, prostate, appendix, and endometrium (214–216).

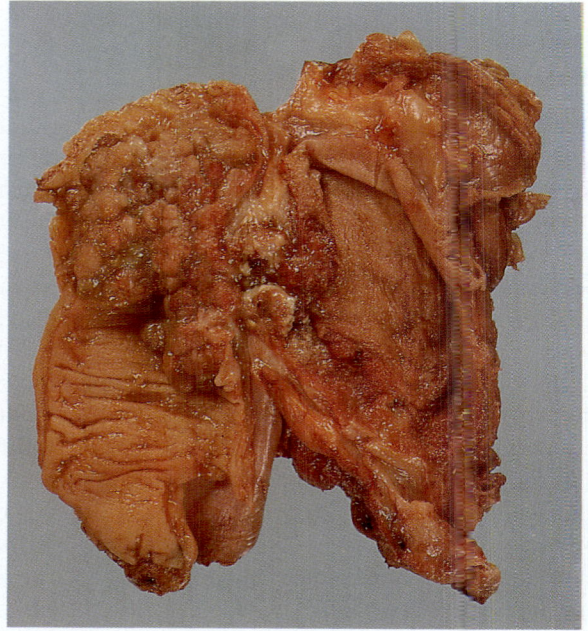

FIG. 31. Villous adenocarcinoma of the rectum with invasion of the posterior wall of the bladder. Within the bladder is a discrete villous tumor that may be mistaken for a primary vesical neoplasm on cystoscopy.

Signet-ring cell carcinoma of the bladder is a rare variant of adenocarcinoma with fewer than 50 cases reported in the English literature (217–221). It is not uncommon to see signet-ring cells within mucinous carcinomas, but we reserve the term signet-ring cell carcinoma to those tumors composed almost entirely of signet-ring or poorly differentiated round cells with intracytoplasmic mucin, and without abundant extracellular mucin. Except for their larger size, the cells are cytologically similar to those of mammary lobular carcinoma. Confirming origin in the bladder by finding CIS may be very difficult. It is not unusual to find a dense layer of signet-ring cells within the lamina propria directly below a denuded basement membrane (Fig. 32A). These tumors tend to infiltrate the bladder wall diffusely, giving it an indurated and thickened quality similar to the "linitis plastica" seen in gastric signet-ring cell carcinomas (Fig. 32B). The tumor also commonly infiltrates extensively throughout adjacent soft tissue, making primary resection for cure virtually impossible. In the differential diagnosis, we must rule out direct extension, usually from a rectal or prostatic carcinoma, or metastasis from stomach or lobular carcinoma of the breast or other organs (222).

Mesonephric or clear cell adenocarcinoma is a rare variant characterized by cuboidal tumor cells forming ductlike or tubelike structures similar to certain adenocarcinomas of the kidney (Fig. 33). These tumors initially were thought to arise from mesonephric nests in the trigone area, but we now consider that they arise through a process of metaplasia of the surface urothelium (223–225). They can begin anywhere on the bladder surface. In some cases, the tumor cells have clear cytoplasm and hobnail appearance mimicking clear cell adenocarcinomas of the female genital tract (225). It is important not to mistake these tumors for nephrogenic adenomas. Mesonephric adenocarcinomas are high-grade, infiltrating carcinomas with frequent mitoses and nuclear pleomorphism, all of which are absent in nephrogenic metaplasia.

Urachal Carcinoma

The urachus is a thick tubelike structure formed in the embryo as the allantois involutes. It extends from the bladder dome to the umbilicus. After birth it becomes a fibrous cord called the median umbilical ligament. If remnants of the allantois (endoderm) remain within the ligament, they may develop into cysts as well as epithelial neoplasms. Such remnants have been found in 25% to 35% of bladders at the time of autopsy, usually in the dome, but also along the anterior and rarely along the posterior bladder wall (226). The epithelial lining usually is transitional in type, but in 33% of cases will be glandular. Neoplasms arising from the urachal remnant are usually adenocarcinomas, and they account for as much as 22% to 35% of vesical glandular neoplasms (227,228). Most adenocarcinomas have enteric features and are mucinous; some may have a signet-ring cell component (229). Squamous cell, transitional cell, and anaplastic carcinomas also arise from the urachus (230). Rare cases of vil-

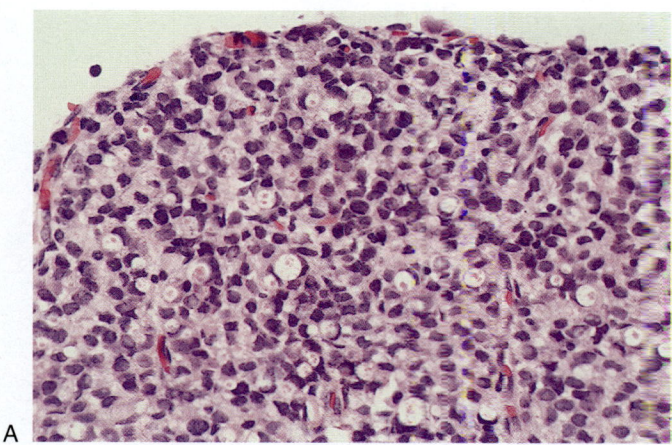
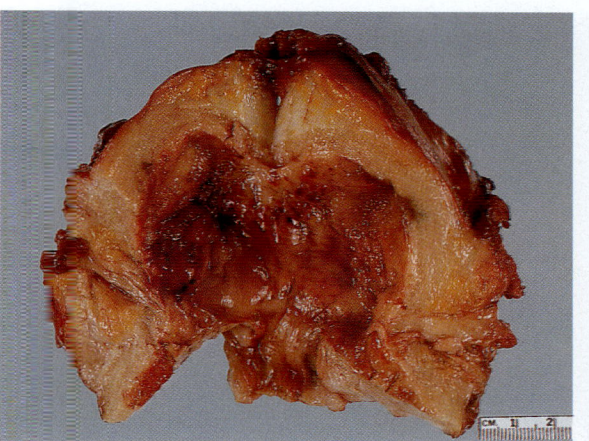

FIG. 32. Signet-ring cell carcinoma of the bladder. **A:** Notice dense layer of signet-ring cells beneath a denuded urothelial basement membrane. The vesical wall is diffusely infiltrated by undifferentiated round cells and signet-ring cells. **B:** The cystectomy specimen reveals a thickened and indurated viscus without an apparent intraluminal mass.

lous adenomas of the urachus have been reported, sometimes associated with mucosuria, suggesting communication with the bladder lumen (231).

Because the urachus is usually found along the free surface of the bladder, urachal carcinomas are frequently amenable to partial cystectomy. Because the entire length of the median umbilical ligament may harbor urachal remnants that may develop carcinoma synchronously or metachronously (232), the surgery of choice should include *en bloc* resection of the entire length of the ligament, including the umbilicus (Fig. 34).

Several criteria must be met to establish the diagnosis (208). The bladder involvement by tumor should be localized to an area usually at or near the dome, in relation to the median umbilical ligament. The overlying bladder urothelium may be ulcerated but no CIS or glandular metaplasia will be present (other than cystitis glandularis). Very often this issue is difficult to address because the overlying epithelium is ulcerated or previously sampled. Rarely will the urachal tumor communicate directly with the bladder surface (Fig. 35). On sectioning the bladder, we find that the tumors are either intramural or extramural, with involvement of the median umbilical ligament, which should be identified if at all possible (see Fig. 34B). Occasionally urachal remnants will be found. The differential diagnosis includes metastatic adenocarcinoma and adenocarcinoma arising in the bladder surface. The latter is usually associated with an intraluminal mass and the diagnosis is established by finding CIS or extensive glandular metaplasia of the adjacent urothelium.

Small Cell/Neuroendocrine Carcinoma

An increasing number of highly aggressive small cell undifferentiated carcinomas are being described arising in the bladder (233–236). Histologically they resemble oat cell or intermediate cell types of small-cell carcinoma of lung (Fig. 36A). In most cases they are associated with CIS of the urothelium and show microscopic areas of high-grade carcinoma of other histologic patterns, usually TCC but also adenocarcinoma, SCC, or spindle cell carcinoma. As a group, they are histochemically, immunohistochemically, and by electron microscopy similar to their pulmonary counterparts. Like them, many of these tumors have neuroendocrine features (Fig. 36B) (233). Some have been associated with hy-

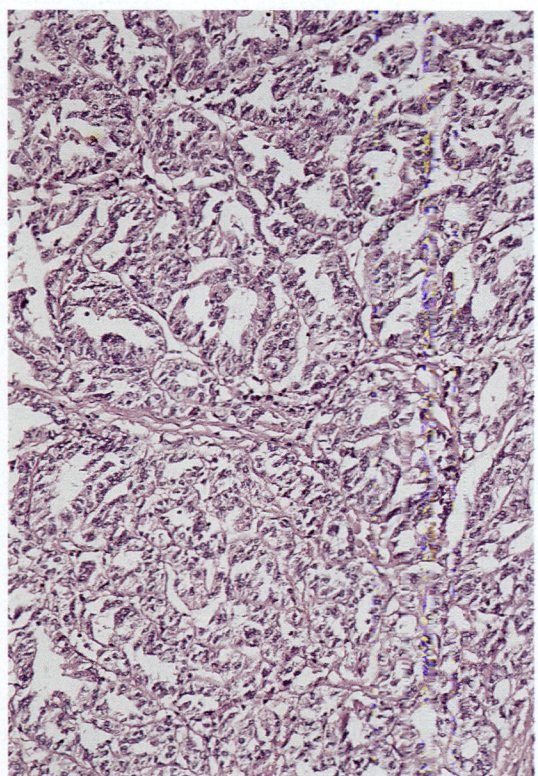

FIG. 33. So-called mesonephric adenocarcinoma is characterized by cuboidal tumor cells forming ductlike or tubulelike structures. The tumor may have clear-cell features and may mimic clear cell adenocarcinoma of the female genital tract.

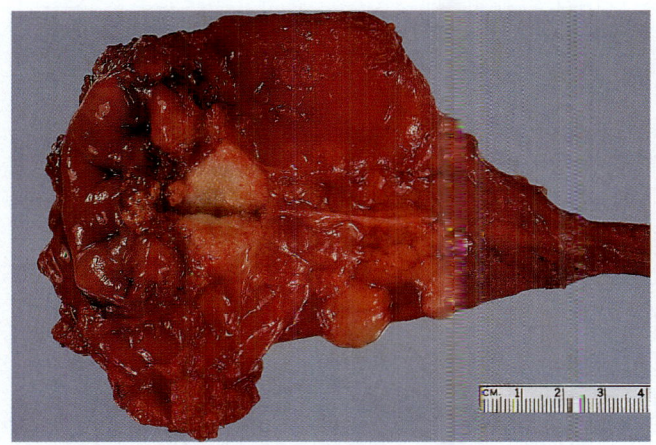
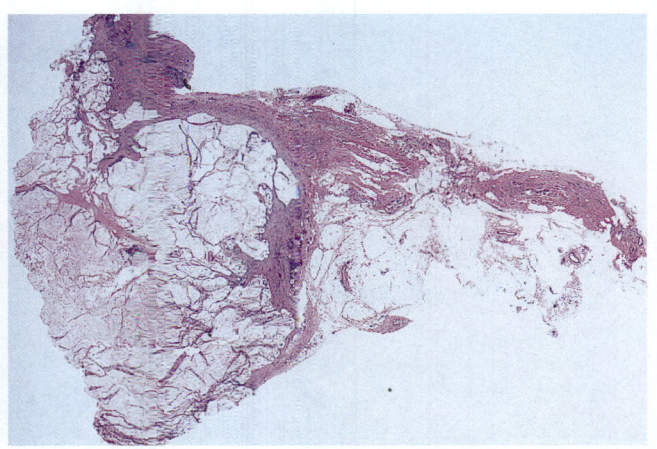

FIG. 34. Urachal carcinoma. **A:** Surgical specimen consists of the dome of the bladder, pervesical fat, medial umbilical ligament, and umbilicus (not seen). Notice tumor within thickened bladder wall. **B:** A mucinous tumor is present within the wall of the urinary bladder and infiltrates along the median umbilical ligament.

percalcemia (235). Whereas we saw one case with inappropriate secretion of antidiuretic hormone, it is interesting that Ucci et al. (237), by using immunohistochemical techniques, identified neuroendocrine cells in several cases of urothelium exhibiting squamous metaplasia, inverted papilloma, nephrogenic adenoma, and adenocarcinoma. Smith (238), in the course of an ultrastructural study of urothelial CIS, found neurosecretory granules in five of 15 cases, including three cases of "dysplasia" and two of CIS. One of eight control (normal) biopsies showed similar granules. Small-cell/neuroendocrine carcinomas should be considered high-grade tumors. They usually are seen at an advanced stage; up to one third of patients have metastases at the time of diagnosis. It is possible that these patients will benefit from therapy similar to that used in small-cell carcinoma of the lung.

Other Epithelial Tumors

A group of malignant tumors of mixed epithelial and sarcomatoid patterns have been described under different names by various authors: sarcomatoid carcinoma, metaplastic carcinoma, spindle and giant cell carcinoma, carcinosarcoma, and malignant mesodermal mixed tumor. These are tumors of mixed histology, highly variable in appearance, and not easily classified. The term mesodermal mixed tumor seems inappropriate because the bladder is endodermally derived. Metaplastic carcinoma is ambiguous and uninformative; myriad metaplastic changes can occur in urothelium, including osteoid. Stromal osteoid metaplasia also was described in association with urothelial carcinoma (239,240). Sarcomatoid carcinoma and spindle and giant cell carcinoma are descriptive terms that accurately state the histogenesis and morphologic appearance of the tumor (241–243). Perhaps they represent the best choice for a name. These are invariably high-grade tumors, and it may be difficult to establish their epithelial origin because they are often ulcerated (Fig. 37). The overlying and adjacent urothelium should be searched for CIS, and the tumor examined carefully for a transition from epithelial to spindle cell pattern. Electron microscopy as well as immunohistochemical stains for cytokeratins, carcinoembryonic antigen (CEA), or human chorionic gonadotropin (HCG) may be of help in establishing epithelial origin. It must be understood that a bladder tumor with undifferentiated spindle cell pattern is more likely to be of epithelial than of mesenchymal origin because true sarcomas of the bladder are very rare; most are readily recognized myosarcomas. As previously mentioned, sarcomatoid carcinomas are high-grade tumors whose prognosis correlates with depth of invasion. Some cases may be associated with a striking myxoid or sclerosing appearance mimicking an inflammatory pseudotumor (246).

The term carcinosarcoma should be reserved for those very rare cases in which a tumor exhibits biphasic differentiation: carcinoma and sarcoma (247–250). The sarcoma must be differentiated along one or several mesenchymal pathways such as muscle (myosarcoma), cartilage (chondrosarcoma), or bone (osteosarcoma) (Fig. 38). In this respect, the histologic criteria are similar to those of mesoder-

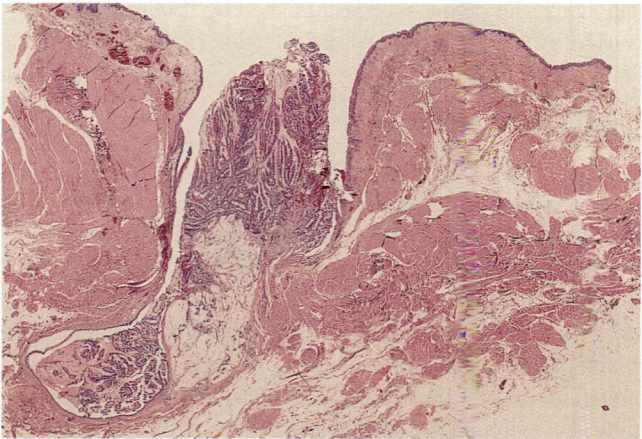

FIG. 35. Urachal carcinoma. Papillary and mucin-producing adenocarcinoma involves intramural urachal cyst and extends into the lumen of the bladder.

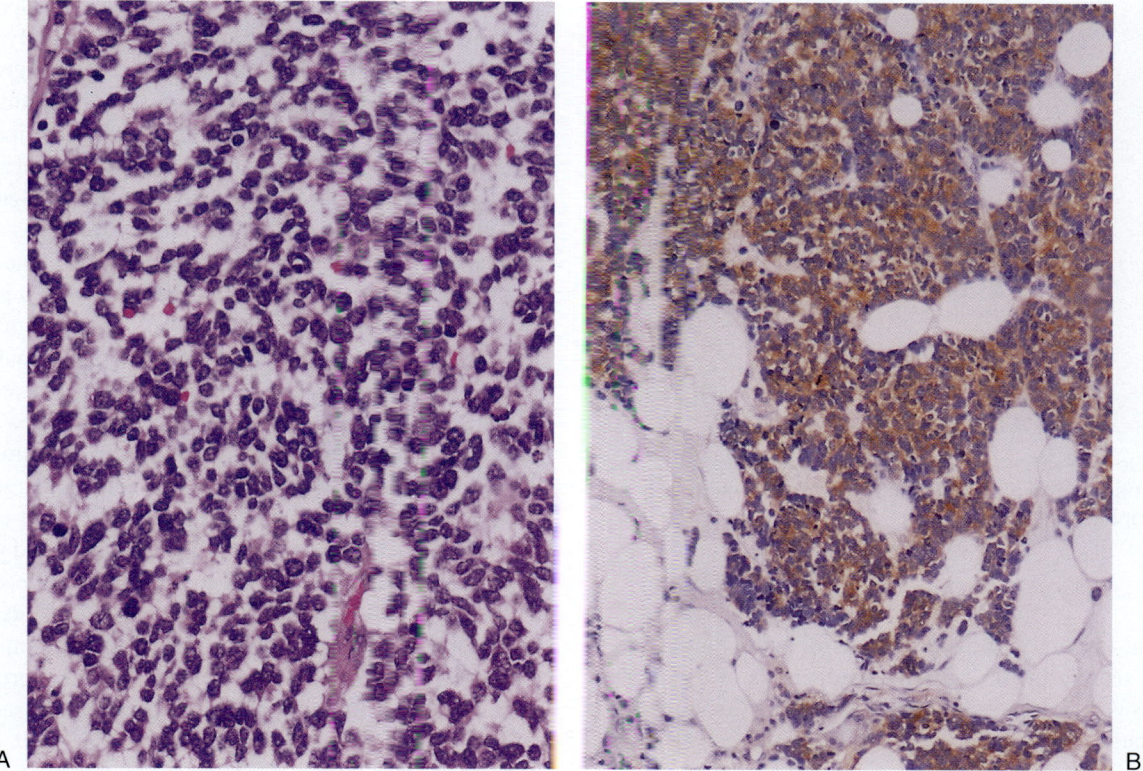

FIG. 36. Small cell carcinoma of the urinary bladder. **A:** Histologic features are similar to those of small cell carcinoma of the lung and other sites. **B:** This tumor had neuroendocrine differentiation, as evidenced by chromogranin immunostaining.

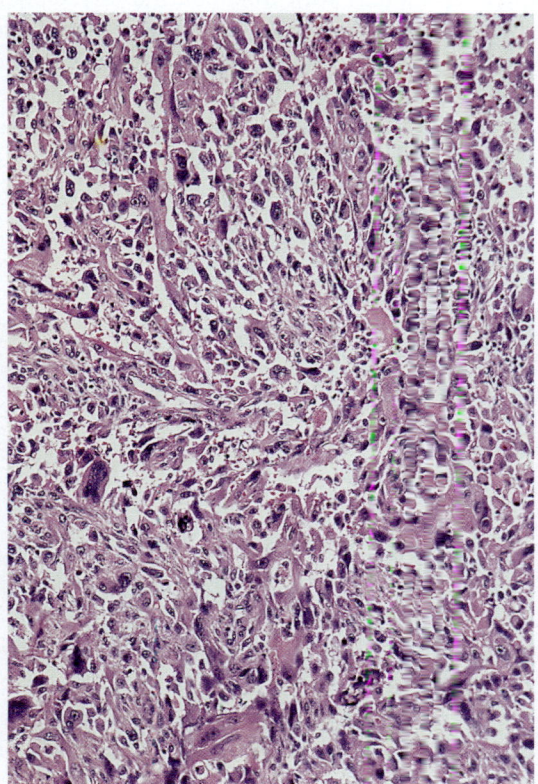

FIG. 37. Sarcomatoid (spindle cell) carcinoma of the bladder.

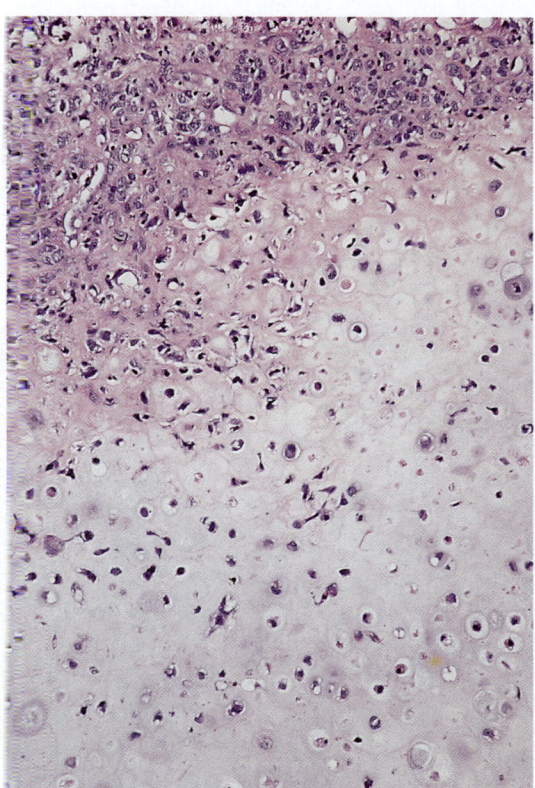

FIG. 38. Carcinosarcoma. Chondrosarcoma component within a high-grade urothelial carcinoma of the renal pelvis.

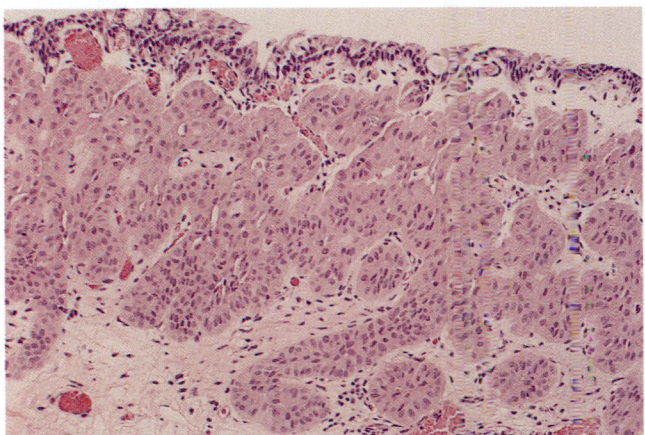

FIG. 39. Nested variant of urothelial carcinoma. Irregular and confluent nests of mildly atypical urothelial cells infiltrating the lamina propria.

mal mixed tumors with heterologous or homologous elements, as seen in the uterus. The histogenesis of these rare neoplasms is not clear, but possiblities include (a) neoplastic transformation of adjacent epithelial and mesenchymal tissues (so-called collision tumor), or (b) heterologous differentiation within either component. We regard sarcomatoid carcinomas and carcinosarcomas as a spectrum of the same disease: different degrees of differentiation within a high-grade epithelial neoplasm.

A rare but important variant of urothelial carcinoma that may violate many of these rules is the nested or deceptively bland TCC (107,108,251). These aggressive neoplasms usually have a very innocuous appearance, especially at low- and medium-power magnification (Fig. 39). They are often confused with cystitis cystica, cystitis glandularis, nephrogenic metaplasia, and inverted papilloma but can be differentiated from these by the presence of poorly defined and confluent nests, which may infiltrate deeply into the bladder wall, including muscularis propria and beyond. Rarely invasive urothelial carcinoma may exhibit a microcystic growth pattern, mimicking benign conditions such as cystitis glandularis (252). Close examination of the cytologic features of the lining cells as well as the presence of conventional carcinoma in adjacent areas, should lead us to the correct diagnosis.

Another rare variant of urothelial carcinoma has been termed lymphoepithelioma (253,254). As the name suggests, these urothelial carcinomas are associated with a prominent lymphocytic infiltrate (Fig. 40). The tumor cells have minimal cytoplasm and are of high cytologic grade, making their identification at low and intermediate magnification difficult. It is not uncommon for these tumors to be misinterpreted as lymphomas, although immunohistochemical studies will easily clarify the issue. Some authors suggested that lymphoepitheliomas of the bladder are a distinct entity that is more likely to respond to radiation therapy and platinum-based chemotherapy. Too few cases have been described for us to accept this hypothesis. Amin et al. (255) described a group of urothelial carcinomas that contained a micropapillary component resembling ovarian papillary serous carcinoma. The micropapillary growth pattern was seen in the noninvasive components of the tumor as well as in the metastasis, confirming the high-grade nature of the tumor (Fig. 41). In some cases, micropapillary growth was focal, whereas in others, it predominated.

Several cases of vesical choriocarcinoma have been described (255–260). Certainly these represent high-grade urothelial carcinomas with trophoblastic differentiation. Syncytiotrophoblasts have been described in high-grade tumors of other organs including lung and breast. Tumor cells may express HCG by immunohistochemistry, and these patients may exhibit associated increased levels of serum HCG (260). Rarely TCC may contain scattered touton-type giant cells (Fig. 42). They are of no known clinical significance.

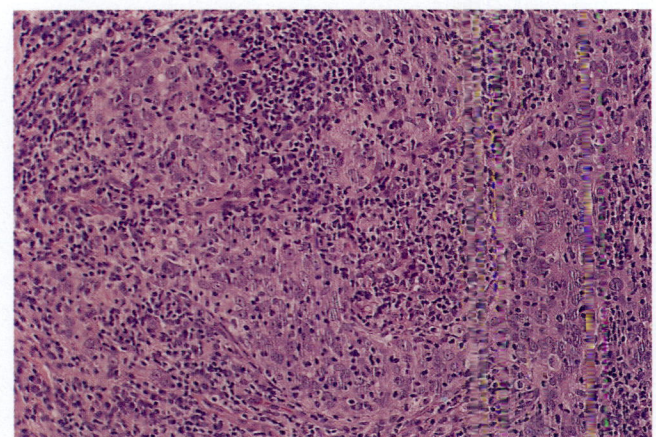
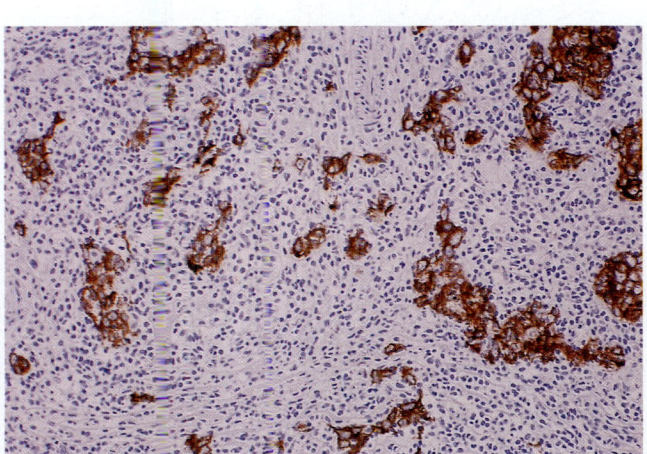

FIG. 40. Lymphoepithelioma of the bladder. **A:** Irregular nests of cytologically high-grade urothelial carcinoma surrounded by a dense lymphocytic infiltrate. **B:** Immunohistochemical stain for cytokeratin, CAM 5.2, highlights the infiltrating carcinoma cells.

CARCINOMA OF THE RENAL PELVIS AND URETER

The overwhelming majority of upper urinary tract tumors are transitional cell type, with a small number being either squamous cell type or glandular. In a review of 2,566 primary urothelial tumors at Memorial Hospital by Batata et al. (251), tumors of the renal pelvis and ureter each represented 4%. These patients usually are first seen with gross painless hematuria (Fig. 43). Accurate clinical staging before resection is difficult because of their relative inaccessibility. As with bladder tumors, stage, grade, and multicentricity are accurate predictors of future biologic behavior (262–265). Recurrences are frequent. Nocks et al. (263) reported that 41% of patients with renal pelvic tumors had urothelial tumors elsewhere either previously, concomitantly, or subsequently. Approximately 20% developed subsequent bladder tumors. Batata et al. (261) reported that 27 (65%) of 41 cases of primary ureteral carcinoma developed tumors in other parts of the urinary tract (Fig. 44). Conversely, approximately 20% of patients with bladder cancer will develop upper urinary tract disease, and at least 9% will have CIS in the resected portion of ureter (266).

URETHRA

Urethral Polyps

Benign polypoid and papillary lesions of the urethra include inflammatory polyps, caruncle, urothelial papillomas,

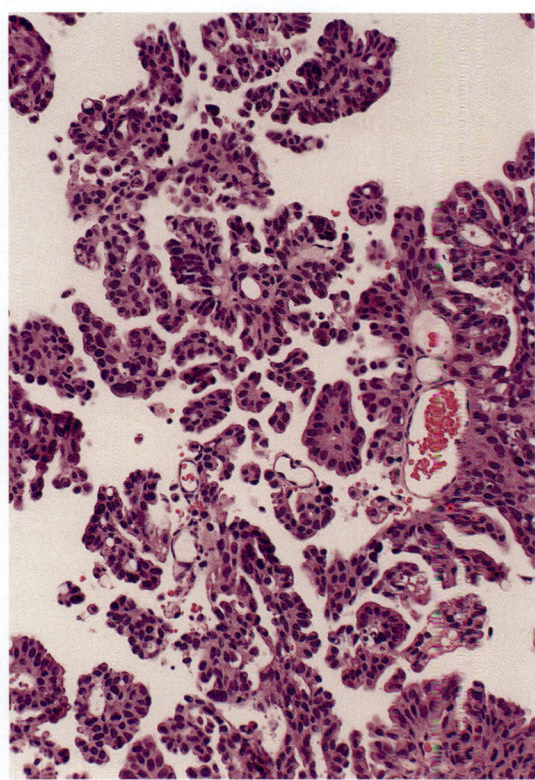

FIG. 41. Urothelial carcinoma with a micropapillary growth pattern. Micropapillary growth is seen in a small subset of high-grade disease and may be present in the noninvasive, invasive, and metastatic components.

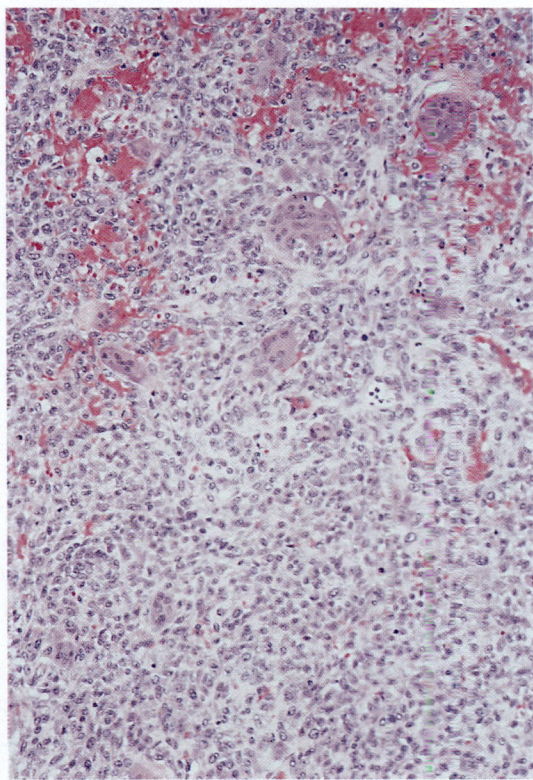

FIG. 42. Transitional cell carcinoma with osteoclastlike giant cells. These cells may be numerous and can be seen in primary and metastatic sites.

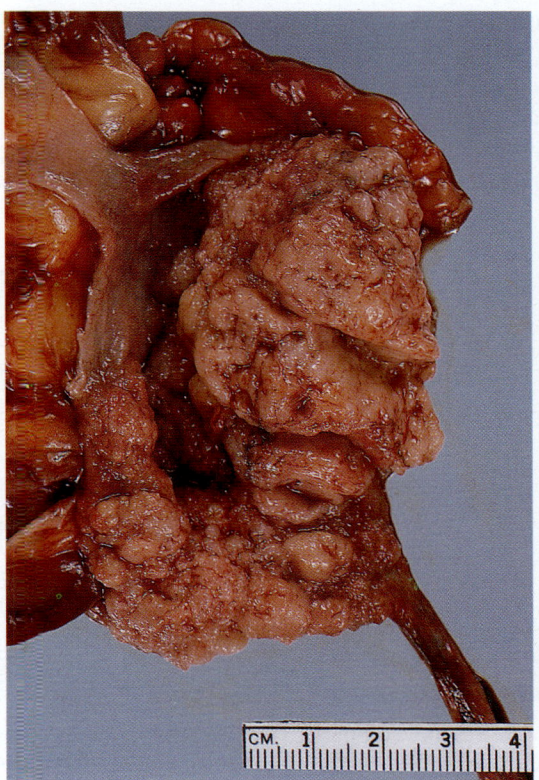

FIG. 43. Transitional cell carcinoma of the renal pelvis. Papillary tumors fill and distort the renal pelvis.

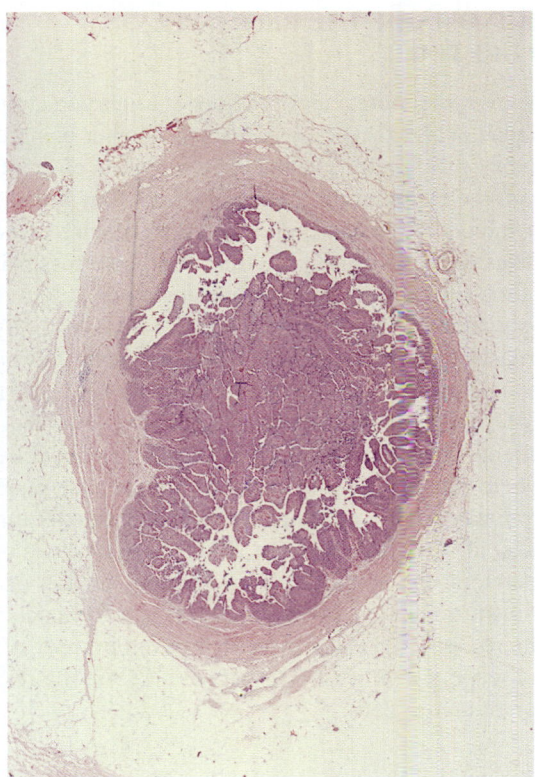

FIG. 44. Papillary transitional cell carcinoma, multifocal, filling and distending the ureteral lumen.

nephrogenic adenomas, and polyps lined by columnar, prostatic-type epithelium (267–269). They all may be seen with dysuria and hematuria. The histologic features of the first four lesions were described earlier. Polyps lined by prostatic-type epithelium (prostatic urethral polyps) may be solitary or multiple. Histologically, they are characterized by a papillary or filiform fibrovascular core covered by glandular epithelium, which is usually two cells thick (Fig. 45). The

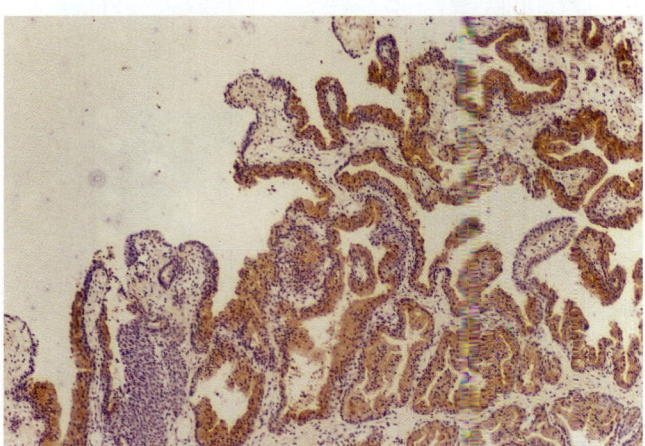

FIG. 45. Prostatic urethral polyp. Benign-appearing prostatic glandular epithelium largely replaces the urothelium (periodic acid–Schiff immunostain). These polyps are common endoscopic findings but are rarely sampled by experienced urologists.

luminal layer is columnar, whereas the basal layer is cuboidal or flat. The polyps also may contain acini, some with corpora amylacea. The histologic appearance is that of benign prostatic epithelium, and several investigators showed that the majority of these will stain strongly for prostate specific antigen (PSA) and prostate specific acid phosphatase (PSAP) by using immunohistochemical techniques (268;269). Similar lesions were described by Remick and Kumar (269) arising in the bladder, and they also expressed PSA and PSAP. Some of the polyps have urothelium lining the outer surface but contain prostatic acini within the polyp. Walker et al. (268) described one case with extensive adenomatous change exhibiting stratification of enlarged and elongated nuclei, nuclei atypia, and cytoplasmic eosinophilia. This lesion resembled an endometrial polyp yet stained for PSA and PSAP.

The histogenesis of these benign polyps with prostatic-type epithelium is unclear but possibilitites include (a) activation of embryonic nests, (b) overgrowth of the urothelium by proliferating prostatic epithelium, and (c) metaplasia. Whatever their etiology, these polyps are benign. Nevertheless, they may be seen in association with an underlying prostatic adenocarcinoma.

Young boys may develop posterior urethral polyps, with mild symptoms of bladder-outlet obstruction and sometimes hematuria. The polyps are usually located in the area of the verumontanum. Histologically they are characterized by a congested or edematous fibrovascular stroma lined by transitional epithelium. At times the stroma may be fibrotic. These lesions have been described as congenital posterior urethral polyps (270) or fibroepithelial polyps (271).

Carcinoma of the Urethra

Primary carcinoma of the urethra is rare, but major differences exist between tumors arising in this and other urothelial sites (272,273).

The male urethra may be divided into four anatomic regions; prostatic, membranous, bulbous, and penile. Tumors arising in the prostatic and membranous portions are usually transitional cell type and are most commonly associated with bladder tumors. Involvement of periurethral ducts should be distinguished from invasion into prostatic stroma because the latter indicates a much worse prognosis (274,275). Exclusive involvement of the prostatic urethra is rare. As expected, these tumors do not express PSA or PSAP antigens and are not hormone responsive. When high-grade TCC involves prostatic ducts, it can be quite difficult to differentiate from prostatic duct adenocarcinoma.

Tumors arising from the bulbous or membranous urethra are most commonly squamous cell type and rarely associated with vesical neoplasms (Fig. 46). Prognosis in these cases depends on grade and stage, although tumors arising in the fixed (proximal) portion of urethra have a worse prognosis than those arising in the pendulous (distal) portions (276,277).

Adenocarcinomas are rare and thought to arise from the

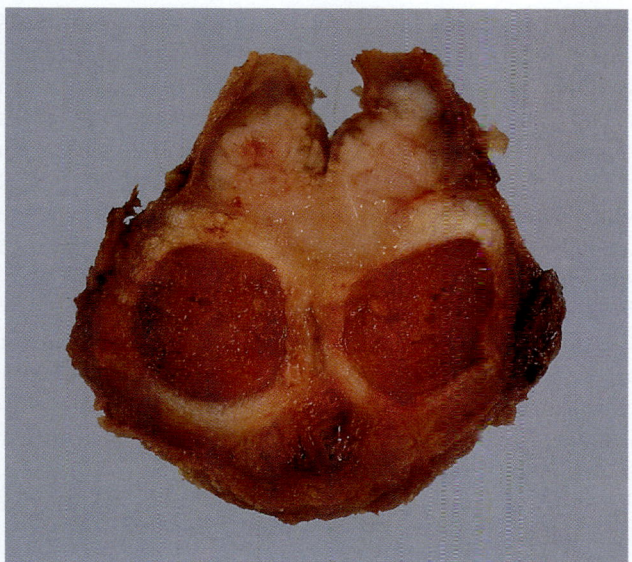

FIG. 46. Carcinoma of the penile urethra. Tumor obliterates the corpus spongiosum and infiltrates the septum but does not appear to involve the corpora cavernosa.

Sarcomas of the Urothelial Tract

Primary sarcomas of the urinary bladder are rare but more common in male than in female subjects. The majority are of muscle origin and compose fewer than 0.04% of all malignant tumors of the urinary bladder (281–283). Myosarcomas may occur in any age group, but rhabdomyosarcomas predominate in children, whereas leiomyosarcomas predominate in adults. In children, 27% of rhabdomyosarcomas arise in the genitourinary tract (284,285). Most are embryonal rhabdomyosarcoma and exophytic, with or without a "botryoid" gross appearance. Microscopically the tumor is often myxoid with a dense concentration of tumor cells, including strap cells and rhabdomyoblasts below the basement membrane, forming a so-called "cambium" layer. Rare cases of vesical rhabdomyosarcoma have been described in adults, and these may have embryonal, pleomorphic, or alveolar patterns (286). In general, rhabdomyosarcomas have a poor prognosis, although combination therapy with surgery and chemotherapy has improved survival, at least in the pediatric age group.

Leiomyosarcomas are more commonly seen in adults, although cases have been reported in children (281,283,287). The tumors are usually well circumscribed and may protrude into the lumen and ulcerate the overlying urothelium. Size is variable. Sarcomatoid carcinoma and carcinosarcoma may mimic leiomyosarcoma and must be excluded by adequate sampling of the specimen and appropriate histochemical, immunohistochemical, and electron-microscopic studies. We must also rule out reactive spindle cell nodules, which may occur after local surgery or trauma. These reactive lesions are composed of spindle cells that appear to be of smooth-muscle origin and have an increased mitotic rates. They are distinguished from sarcoma by their vascularity, a prominent inflammatory infiltrate, and well-defined margins that are not infiltrative (115,120).

Other sarcomas that have been described in the bladder include malignant fibrous histiocytoma (288,289), osteosar-

periurethral glands or through a process of metaplasia of the surface urothelium.

Urethral carcinomas are more common in women than in men (272,273) and usually are epidermoid (278–280). Anatomically the female urethra can be divided into the proximal two-thirds and the distal one-third. Tumors arising in the proximal two-thirds usually have transitional cell features and are associated with vesical neoplasms. Tumors of the distal third are usually squamous cell type. It is well to remember that carcinomas involving the urethra may not be primary in this organ but instead may be invading from a primary carcinoma of neighboring genital organs. As in men, primary adenocarcinomas are thought to arise from periurethral glands (Fig. 47) or from metaplastic urethral mucosa.

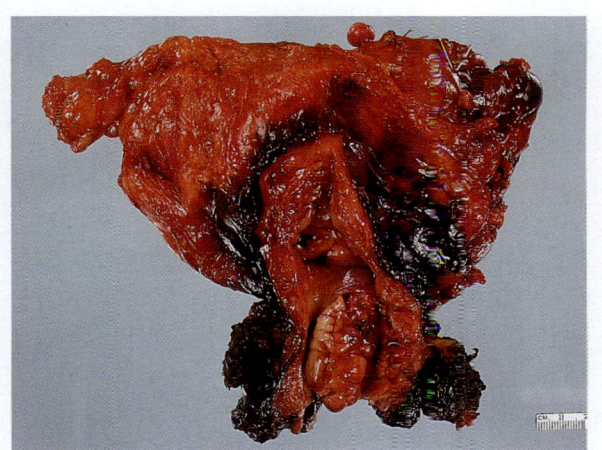
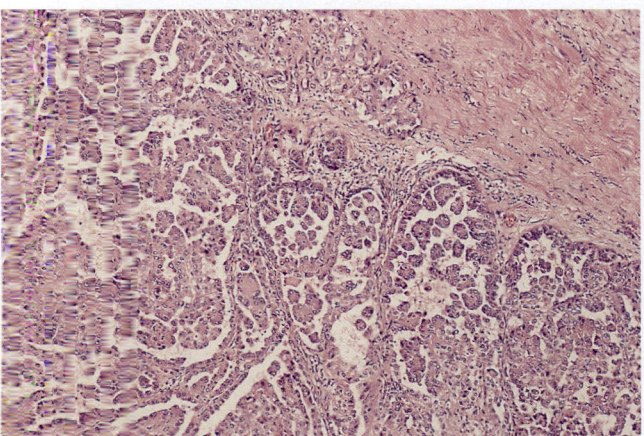

FIG. 47. A: Polypoid carcinoma of the female urethra. **B:** Papillary adenocarcinoma of the female urethra. These tumors arise from periurethral glands or from metaplasia of the surface epithelium.

coma (290), fibrosarcoma (291), and liposarcoma (292). Although it is possible for these tumors to arise in the bladder, it is more likely that they originate in other sites and involve the bladder secondarily.

MISCELLANEOUS TUMORS

Rare cases of benign mesenchymal neoplasms of the urinary tract have been described. These include leiomyoma (293), fibroma (294), neurofibroma (295), and hemagioma (296,297). Several cases of hemangiopericytoma have been described arising within the urinary bladder (298), as have granular cell tumors (myoblastomas). They usually behave in a benign fashion after complete local excision (299,300).

Malignant melanomas may arise in the urinary bladder or urethra but are more commonly metastatic to these sites (301,302). To establish the bladder as the primary site, we must identify *in situ* melanoma within or adjacent to the invasive melanoma and rule out a metastasis from another site (Fig. 48). The melanoma may be multifocal or present along the urethra as satellites of a vulvar or penile melanoma. Rare cases of melanosis also were described (302).

Hematologic neoplasms arising in the urinary tract are rare and difficult to diagnose on endoscopic biopsy (303–306). Chaitin et al. (303) reported six cases with initial manifestations in the lower urinary tract: four were lymphomas, two were plasmacytomas, and one was granulocytic sarcoma. Occasinally urothelial carcinomas may mimic malignant lymphoma (306).

A small number of carcinoid tumors are described arising in the bladder (307,308). This should not surprise us because endocrine cells have been described in normal and neoplastic urothelium (237,238). Nevertheless, we must rule out metastasis or direct invasion from the vermiform appendix or elsewhere. The differential diagnosis with paraganglioma may be difficult. Paragangliomas (extraadrenal pheochromocytoma) can arise in the bladder wall, probably from nests of paraganglionic cells that migrate along with sympathetic ganglia (309–311). These tumors affect men and women equally, and if the tumor is functional, the patient may experience sustained or paroxysmal hypertension. More than 90% of these tumors behave in a benign fashion. Special stains or electron microscopy might help in establishing the diagnosis. If paraganglioma is suspected at the time of surgery, the tumor should be placed in Zenker's fixative. Within minutes, the tumor will acquire a dark brown color.

Steeper and Rosai (312) described a mesenchymal tumor arising in renal peripelvic soft tissue of women, which they called aggressive angiomyxoma. It is characterized histologically by myxoid and vascular components and clinically by a locally infiltrative behavior and multiple recurrences. These patients may have urinary irritative or obstructive symptoms.

Cytology, Flow Cytometery, and Blood Group Antigens in Urothelial Tumors

Cytology

Cytologic examination of voided urine is the simplest and one of the most effective techniques for the detection of urothelial carcinoma and for monitoring conservative therapy. It is based on the identification of spontaneously exfoliated cancer cells stained by a modified Papanicolaou technique and examined by conventional light microscopy (313). The technique is highly specific. It is most sensitive in cases of high-grade carcinoma and CIS, and least sensitive in cases of papilloma or ulcerating, infiltrating carcinoma that is surfaced by an inflammatory exudate.

In a normal individual, voided urine is sparsely cellular, and exfoliated urothelial cells are few. These cells most probably come from the superficial, "umbrella" cell layer. They are relatively large cells, with large, round or ovoid,

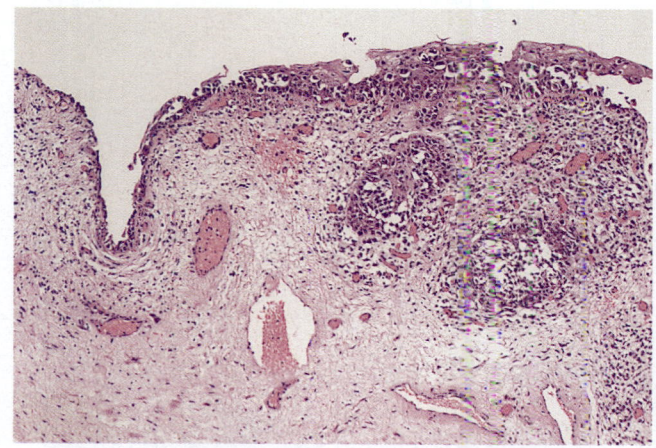 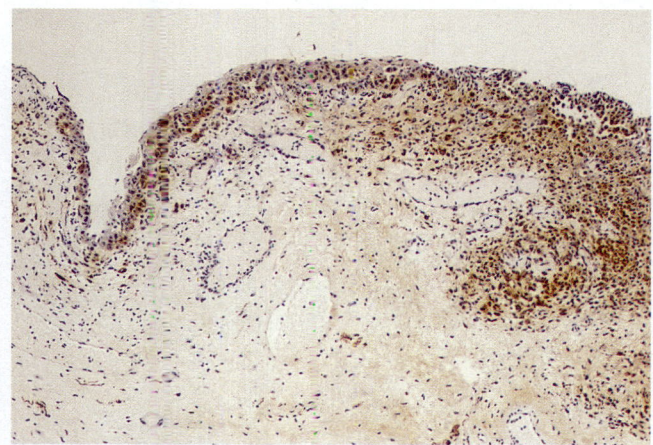

FIG. 48. Melanoma of the urinary bladder. **A:** Neoplastic melanocytes infiltrate the epithelium singly and in nests. If melanin is absent, this lesion may be difficult to distinguish from carcinoma. **B:** S-100 positivity in neoplastic cells.

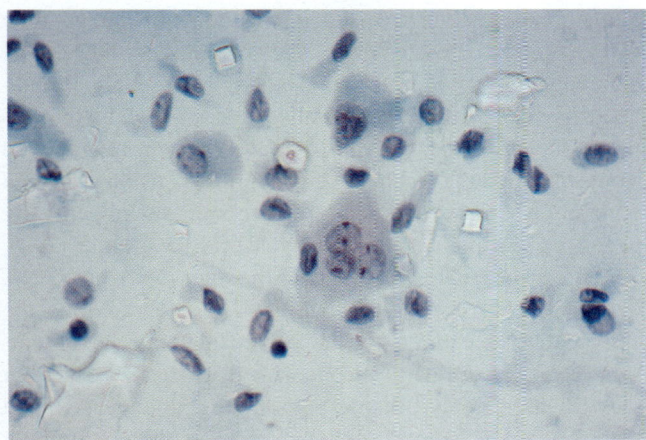

FIG. 49. Catheterized specimen showing benign urothelial cells. Multinucleated cell in the center is result of instrumentation.

smoothly contoured nuclei and delicate chromatin (Fig. 49). The cytologically malignant cells of urothelial carcinomas proliferate more rapidly than the normal urothelium and, because they have lost intercellular junctions, dissociate and exfoliate more readily. Thus cytologic specimens of voided urine contain a disproportionate number of cancer cells, even from very localized lesions. The cancer cells differ from normal in that they have increased nuclear DNA and abnormal chromatin structure. Nuclei are hyperchromatic and usually enlarged; chromatin is coarsely textured; and nuclear configuration is irregular (Fig. 50).

Cells are usually shed singly from CIS and show the nuclear changes of carcinoma without much cell-to-cell variation and without great deviation of overall cellular size and shape from normal. Occasional red blood cells are present in almost all cases, but the background is otherwise "clean" (Fig. 51) (314). Invasive carcinomas are marked by much greater variability in nuclear and cellular shape and size, by cancer cells with larger often bizarre nuclei, by more evidence of epidermoid differentiation, and by cancer cell groups that may include poorly formed "pearls" (see Fig. 50). There is evident and often marked inflammation in the background with degenerating inflammatory cellular debris as well as red blood cells (313).

Evidence is mounting that invasive carcinoma arises from CIS, which in turn may develop in the flat mucosa or in papillary tumors. Patients with a history of benign papilloma have a demonstrably "unstable" epithelium and are at risk of developing CIS, which may be in the flat mucosa. Because at least 25% of patients with CIS are asymptomatic (190,191), it is difficult to estimate the frequency of this disease in the general population. Clearly it is too infrequent to warrant screening except in selected populations known to be at risk. Screening may include industrial workers exposed to chemical carcinogens (127,315); it certainly includes any patient with a history of bladder tumor; and it probably should include any adult patient with persisting or unexplaining urologic symptoms or recurrent cystitis. Farrow et al. (195) carried out cytologic examinations of the urine on 25,000 unselected urologic patients at the Mayo Clinic and found unsuspected CIS in some middle-income populations, considered sufficient to justify screening.

All noted, the especificity of cytologic diagnoses is very high, approaching 100%; it is rare not to confirm carcinoma or CIS in patients who have clearly positive cytology, although in some cases this has required many months or even years of careful repeated examinations until an occult carcinoma is found. Sensitivity is somewhat less and depends on two factors: tumor grade and whether tumor cells break through the mucosal surface and are exfoliated. It is seldom possible to identify papillomas, for example, because the exfoliated cells (by definition) are benign (316). Low-grade bladder tumors will be identified by cytology in about half the cases, whereas high-grade tumors and CISs can be identified in 90% or more of cases (164). The probability of find-

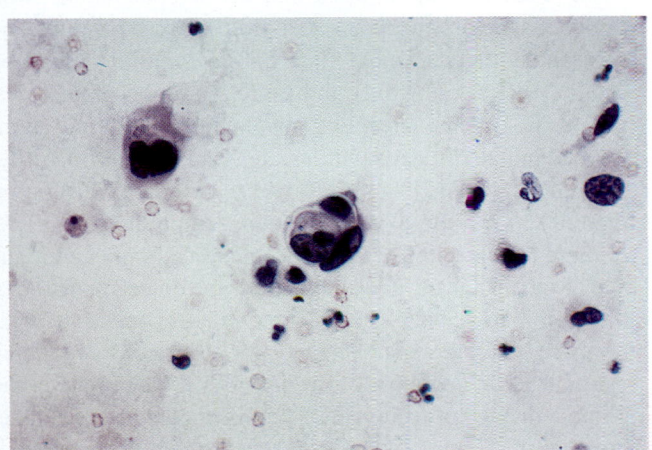
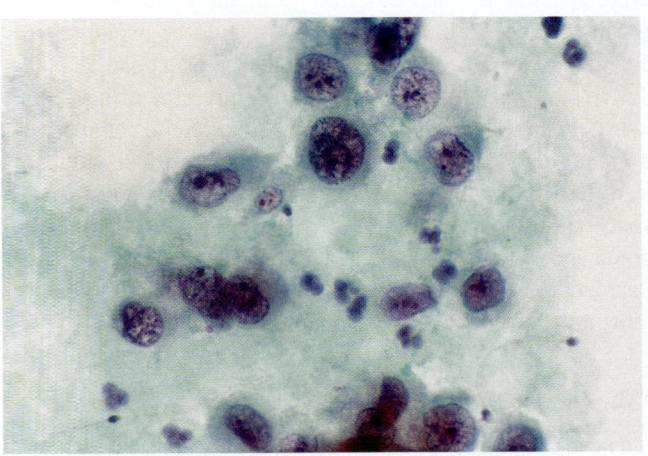

FIG. 50. A and B: Cytology of invasive bladder carcinoma showing malignant pearl and single malignant cells with varying inflammatory background.

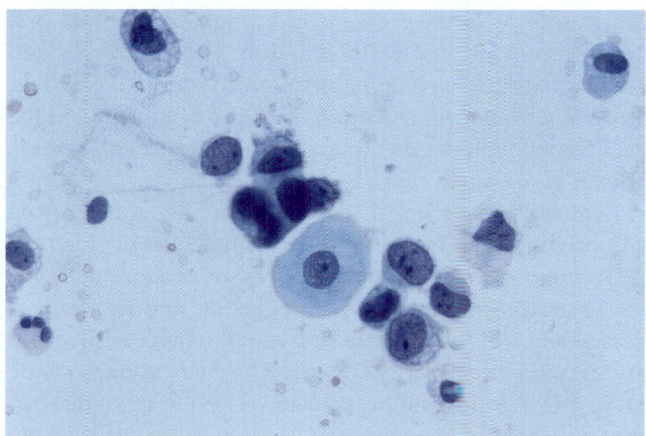

FIG. 51. Cytology of carcinoma *in situ* of bladder showing single malignant cells with obvious increase in nuclear-staining intensity, increased nuclear/cytoplasmic ratio, and irregular nuclear membrane but relatively normal overall cell size and "clean" background.

ing cancer cells and making a positive diagnosis increased with an increasing number of examinations, and at least three are recommended for good sampling. Of course, it may not be possible to identify an ulcerating, infiltrating carcinoma that is surfaced by matted, fibrinopurulent exudate and does not shed many (or any) tumor cells into the urinary stream.

The cytology of upper tract tumors is the same as that of the bladder. Thus the absence of bladder tumor in a patient with positive urinary cytology strongly suggests an upper tract tumor. However, it must be emphasized that it is quite possible to overlook an occult carcinoma or CIS of the bladder, sometimes even after multisite biopsies are taken. To resolve this dilemma, two other procedures are useful: (a) cytologic examination of a bladder irrigation specimen, which increases exfoliation of bladder epithelium and contains no upper tract cells; and (b) separately collected ureteral catheterized urines for cytology. An upper-tract tumor should shed cancer cells into the corresponding ureteral urine specimen, whereas cytology of the opposite ureteral specimen and the bladder irrigation would be negative. An occult bladder cancer would be evidenced by a positive bladder irrigation cytology and negative ureteral urines. One word of caution: specimens obtained by ureteral catheterization and bladder irrigation show cytologic artifacts that can lead the inexperienced cytologist into an erroneous diagnosis of carcinoma. Cytologic atypias that may mimic carcinoma are seen also in patients with chronic calcareous cystitis, bladder stones, after irradiation, and after chemotherapy, most notably with cyclophosphamide.

Flow Cytometry

During the last few years, there has been increasing interest in the cytologic detection and treatment monitoring of bladder cancer by flow cytometry. In this technique, bladder epithelium is dislodged by saline irrigation, either at the time of cystoscopy or by catheter. The specimen is much more cellular than a voided urine, which contains only spontaneously exfoliated epithelial cells. Clusters of cells that are not dissociated and any tissue fragments present are removed by sieving, and the resultant single-cell suspension is stained with any one of several DNA fluorochromes. We generally preferred the metachromatic dye acridine orange (AO), which can be made to differentially stain DNA and RNA (317). Others use propidium iodine (PI) after treating the cells with RNase to remove the RNA. Under special circumstances, DAPI or one of the Hoechst dyes may be used, but they are used rarely because both require an expensive and inconvenient ultraviolet light source for excitation. Staining is carried out in suspension, and the cells in suspension are forced in single file through the quartz channel of the flow cytometer, where they pass through narrowly focused excitation beam of the instrument, one cell at a time. For AO- or PI-stained cells, an argon ion laser is used that emits blue light near the excitation maximum of both dyes (488 nm). As each cell flowing through the channel interrupts the blue laser light, it emits a green (AO) or red (PI) fluorescence flash that is proportional to DNA content. The fluorescence emission is captured and measured by appropriately filtered photomultiplier tubes, and the results are recorded by a dedicated computer. In practice, 5,000 cells are measured from each specimen, usually within 10 to 20 seconds, and a histogram provided by computer shows the distribution of DNA measurements per cell (317). Most of the exfoliated urothelial cells of the normal bladder are nonproliferating (G_0G_1) and have diploid DNA content, equal to that of control peripheral blood lymphocytes (Fig. 52). Perhaps 6% to 8% of the cells are cycling and have increased DNA content to double the diploid level (S to G_2M phase), including the occasional binucleated umbrella cells. The proportion of proliferating cells may be increased to 12% (or rarely even higher) in cases of cystitis or bladder stone, in which there is marked inflammation, loss of epithelium, and regeneration. In most cases of carcinoma, there is a well-defined population of tumor cells with abnormal (aneuploid) DNA content, and sometimes there is more than one aneuploid population (multiclonal; see Fig. 52). In a smaller proportion of cases, there is no definite aneuploid population, but there is an increased number of cells with greater than diploid DNA (hyperdiploid cells). These probably include proliferating diploid and aneuploid cells. We found, empirically, that 16% or more hyperdiploid cells also is an indicator of carcinoma.

The advantage of flow cytometry is the objective nature of the examination, which does not require the considerable experience and judgment necessary for accurate conventional cytologic examination. It also provides a quantitiative and graphic display of results that simplifies comparisons of sequential studies, for example, during the course of intravesical BCG treatment (318) or after conservative resection (319). The major disadvantage is that bladder irrigation is re-

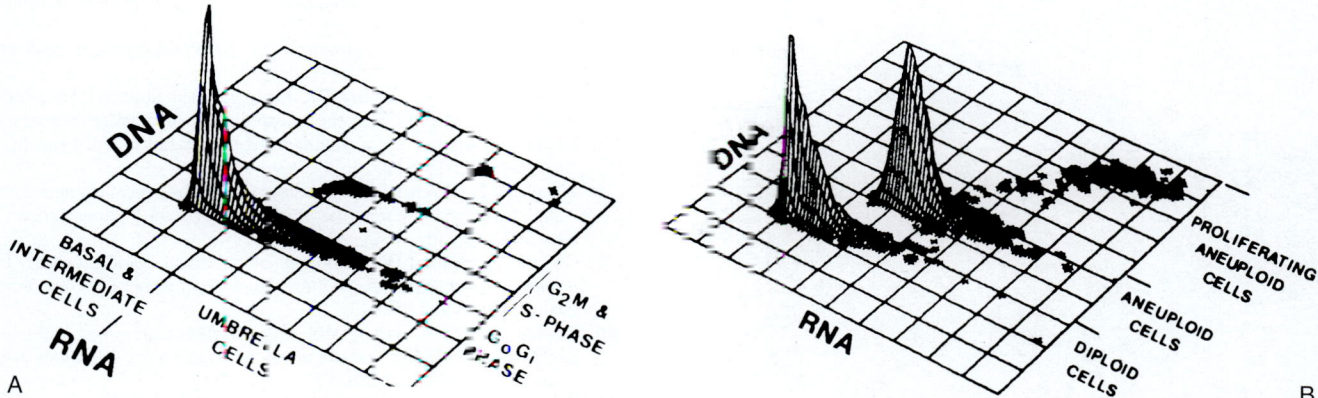

FIG. 52. Flow cytometry DNA/RNA measurements of bladder irrigation specimens. **A:** Normal bladder. **B:** Carcinoma. The number of cells at each measurement point is indicated by the height of the histogram. Note that the majority of cells in the normal bladder have a uniform (diploid) DNA content, and most have relatively low RNA content. Only 6% to 8% of the normal bladder epithelial cells have increased DNA content, mostly proliferating cells in S-G2M phase of the cycle, but also some binucleated umbrella cells. The bladder carcinoma is characterized by a population of aneuploid (tumor) cells with increased DNA content, as well as the normal diploid population. There is also an increased number of proliferating cells in the tumor population.

quired to obtain the large numbers of well-preserved cells needed for flow cytometry. Thus the technique is applicable in examination of patients suspected of tumor or at sufficient risk to require either catheterization or cystoscopy, and is useful for monitoring patients with a history of tumor; it is not suitable for screening unselected populations.

The sensitivity of flow cytometry, overall, is in the range of 85%, as good as or better than conventional cytology (320), partly because of the better sampling and partly because of the nature of the technique. The diagnosis of carcinoma is based entirely on the distribution of measurements of DNA content per urothelial cell, and small populations of tumor cells may be obscured in the presence of many leukocytes or histiocytes. Increased sensitivity probably can be obtained by using another marker: a monoclonal antibody, for example, to distinguish urothelial from other cells before

analyzing DNA distribution. There are also monoclonal antibodies that appear to distinguish low-grade from high-grade tumors (321) or to estimate percentage of DNA-synthesizing cells (322) potentially useful for subclassification according to biologic behavior or growth rate. Thus the eventual application of flow cytometry may lie not so much in detection as in characterization of bladder tumors.

Blood Group–Related Antigens

Blood group antigens (BGAs) are a family of cell-surface carbohydrate structures that were originally detected on the surface of erythrocytes. Through the years, it has become clear that these antigens are expressed in many other tissues. We now know that they undergo predictable changes during tissue differentiation and maturation, as well as during malig-

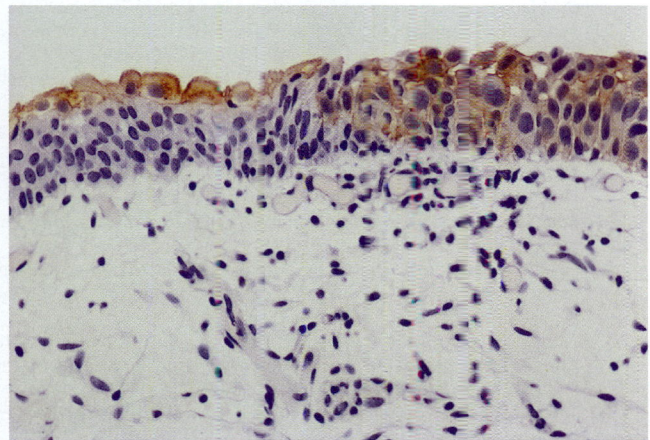
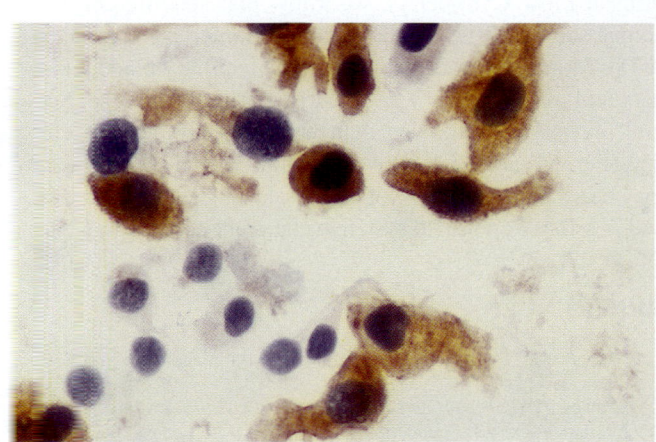

FIG. 53. A and B: Expression of Lewis-X blood group antigen in carcinoma *in situ*. Notice that in normal urothelium, expression is limited to the umbrella cells. Lewis-X–positive tumor cells in bladder irrigation specimen.

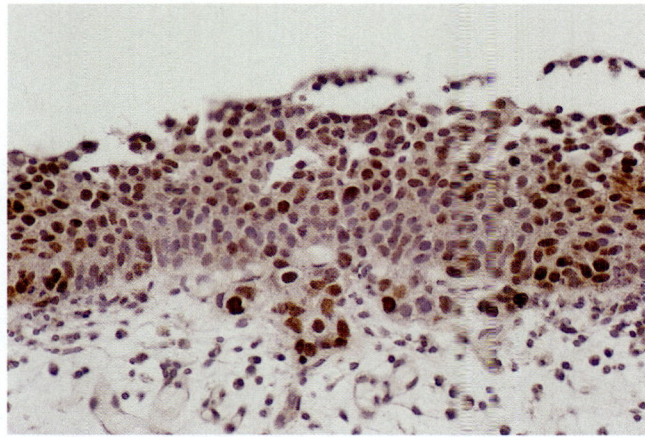

FIG. 54. Nuclear overexpression of p53 protein in carcinoma *in situ* and superficial T1 disease.

nant transformation. During transformation altered synthesis or partial degradation of oligosaccharide chains can thus result in deletion of normally expressed BGA, as well as neoexpression of precursor structures. These precursor structures may be identified on cells by using antibodies directed against the specific blood group–related antigens (Fig. 53). Whereas it is clear that blood group–related antigens undergo predictable alterations during neoplastic transformation, it is still unknown whether they can be used clinically to predict disease progression or to detect early recurrence (323–327).

Genetics and Molecular Genetics of Urothelial Carcinoma

We have made great strides in the genetic and molecular genetic characterization of solid tumors, including bladder cancer (328,329). Nevertheless, it is fair to assume that our knowledge in this area will continue to grow as we enter into the new millenium. We hope to use our new-found knowledge to to classify and treat these tumors in a more precise manner. Other than abnormalities in the DNA index (see section on Flow Cytometry), we know that specific chromosomes such as 7, 9, and 15 undergo numerical aberrations (330). Monosomy 9 is evident in most papillary bladder cancers and may serve as a good early marker of disease. Several investigators showed that the tumor-suppressor genes p53 (Fig. 54) and Rb are involved in urothelial neoplasia and may be accurate predictors of progression, metastasis, survival, and possibly response to systemic chemotherapy (331–335).

REFERENCES

1. Moore KL. *The developing human.* 3rd ed. Philadelphia: WB Saunders, 1982:267.
2. Fawcett DW. *Bloom and Fawcett: a textbook of histology.* 11th ed. Philadelphia: WB Saunders, 1986:787–790.
3. Reuter VE. Urinary bladder and ureter. In: Sternberg SS, ed. *Histology for pathologists.* 2nd ed. New York: Raven Press, 1997:835–847.
4. Ro JY, Ayala AG, El-Naggar A. Muscularis mucosa of urinary bladder: importance for staging and treatment. *Am J Surg Pathol* 1987;11:668–673.
5. Moore KL. *Clinically oriented anatomy.* 2nd ed. Baltimore: Williams & Wilkins, 1985:265.
6. Peterson RO. *Urologic pathology.* 2nd ed. Philadelphia: Lippincott, 1992:295–297.
7. Lage JM, Bauer WC, Kelley DR, Ratliff TL, Catalona WJ. Histologic parameters and pitfalls in the interpretation of bladder biopsies in bacillus Calmette-Guérin treatment of superficial bladder cancer. *J Urol* 1986;35:916–919.
8. Murphy WM, Soloway MS, Finebaum PJ. Pathological changes associated with topical chemotherapy for superficial bladder cancer. *J Urol* 1981;126:461–464.
9. Godwin JT, Hanash K. Pathology of bilharzial bladder cancer. In: *Bladder cancer part A: pathology, diagnosis and surgery.* New York: Alan R Liss, 1984:95–143.
10. Khafagy MM, El-Bolkainy MN, Mansour MA. Carcinoma of the bilharzial urinary bladder: a study of the associated mucosal lesions in 86 cases. *Cancer* 1972;30:150–159.
11. Zahran MM, Kamel M, Mooro H, Issa A. Bilharziasis of urinary bladder and ureter: comparative histopathologic study. *Urology* 1976;8:73–79.
12. Milles G. Catheter-induced hemorrhagic pseudopolyps of the urinary bladder. *JAMA* 1965;93:968–969.
13. Eklund P, Johansson S. Polypoid cystitis: a catheter associated lesion of the human bladder. *Acta Pathol Microbiol Immunol Scand (A)* 1979;87:179–184.
14. Buck EG. Polypoid cystitis mimicking transitional cell carcinoma. *J Urol* 1984;131:963.
15. Palubinskas AJ. Eosinophilic cystitis: case report of eosinophilic infiltration of the urinary bladder. *Radiology* 1960;75:589–591.
16. Brown EW. Eosinophilic granuloma of the bladder. *J Urol* 1960;83:665–668.
17. Frensilli FJ, Sacher EC, Keegan GT. Eosinophilic cystitis: observations on etiology. *J Urol* 1972;107:595–596.
18. Rubin L, Pincus MB. Eosinophilic cystitis: the relationship of allergy in the urinary tract to eosinophilic cystitis and the pathophysiology of eosinophilia. *J Urol* 1974;112 457–460.
19. Hellstrom HR, Davis BK, Shonnard JW. Eosinophilic cystitis: a study of 16 cases. *Am J Clin Pathol* 1979;72:77–84.
20. Hunner GL. A rare type of bladder ulcer in woman: a report of cases. *Boston Med Surg J* 1915;172:660–662.
21. Parivar F, Bradbrook RA. Interstitial cystitis. *Br J Urol* 1986;58:239–244.
22. Messing EM, Stamey TA. Interstitial cystitis: early diagnosis, pathology, and treatment. *Urology* 1978;12:381–392.
23. Larsen S, Thompson SA, Hald T, et al. Mast cells in interstitial cystitis. *Br J Urol* 1982;54:283–286.
24. Collan Y, Alfhan O, Kivilaakso E, Oravisto KJ. Electron microscopic and histologic findings on urinary bladder epithelium in interstitial cystitis. *Eur Urol* 1976;2:242–247.
25. Sarma KP. On the nature of cystitis follicularis. *J Urol* 1970;104:709–714.
26. Jufe R, Molinolo AA, Fefer SA, Meiss RP. Plasma cell granuloma of the bladder: a case report. *J Urol* 1984;131:1175–1176.
27. Wallin JE, Thompson SE, Zaidi A, Wong KH. Urethritis in women attending an STD clinic. *Br J Vener Dis* 1981;57:50–54.
28. Elbadawi A, Malhoski WE, Frank IN. Mucinous urethral caruncle. *Urology* 1978;12:587–590.
29. Saraf PG, Valvo JR, Frank IN. Congenital urethral posterior valves in an adult. *Urology* 1984;24:55–57.
30. Rubin R. *Radiation biology and radiation pathology syllabus.* Chicago: American College of Radiology, 1975:210.
31. Fajardo LF, Berthrong M. Radiation injury in surgical pathology. Part 1. *Am J Surg Pathol* 1978;2:159–195.
32. Jayalakshmamma B, Pinkel D. Urinary bladder toxicity following pelvic irradiation and simultaneous cyclophosphamide therapy. *Cancer* 1976;38:701–707.
33. Koss LG. Tumors of the urinary bladder fascicle 11 (2nd series). In: *Atlas of tumor pathology.* Washington, DC: Armed Forces Institute of Pathology, 1975:99–102.
34. Warren S. Effects of radiation on normal tissues, Vol 11, effects of radiation on the urinary system. *Arch Pathol* 1942;34:1079–1084.
35. Philips FS, Sternberg SS, Cronin AP, Vidal PM. Cyclophosphamide and urinary bladder toxicity. *Cancer Res* 1961;21:1577–1589.
36. Lawrence HJ, Simone J, Aur RJA. Cyclophosphamide-induced hemorrhagic cystitis in children with leukemia. *Cancer* 1975;36:1572–1576.

37. Beyer-Boon ME, De Voogt HJ, Schaberg A. The effects of cyclophosphamide treatment on the epithelium and stroma of the urinary bladder. *Eur J Cancer* 1978;14:1029–1035.
38. Pode D, Perlberg S, Steiner D. Busulfan-induced hemorrhagic cystitis. *J Urol* 1983;130:347–348.
39. Nixon WCW. Endometriosis of the bladder. *Lancet* 1940;1:405–406.
40. Fein RL, Horton BF. Vesical endometriosis: a case report and review of the literature. *J Urol* 1966;95:45–50.
41. Lichtenfeld FR, McCauley RT, Staples PP. Endometriosis involving the urinary tract: a collective review. *Obstet Gynecol* 1961;17:762–768.
42. Stewart WW, Ireland GW. Vesical endometriosis in a postmenopausla woman: a case report. *J Urol* 1977;118:480–481.
43. Pinkert TC, Catlow CE, Straus R. Endometriosis of the urinary bladder in a man with prostatic carcinoma. *Cancer* 1979;43:1562–1567.
44. Randolph Schrodt G, Alcorn MO, Ibanez J. Endometriosis of the male urinary system: a case report. *J Urol* 1980;124:722–723.
45. Rangmade CF. Pelvic endometriosis and ureteral obstruction. *Am J Obstet Gynecol* 1975;122:463–469.
46. Rosenberg SK, Jacobs H. Endometriosis of the upper ureter. *J Urol* 1979;121:512–513.
47. Clement PB, Young RH. Endocervicosis of the urinary bladder: a report of six cases of a benign müllerian lesion that may mimic adenocarcinoma. *Am J Surg Pathol* 1992;16:533–542.
48. Melicow MM. Malakoplakia: report of case, review of literature. *J Urol* 1957;78:33–40.
49. Smith BH. Malakoplakia of the urinary tract: a study of 24 cases. *Am J Clin Pathol* 1965;43:409–417.
50. Melamed MR. The urinary sediment cytology in a case of malakoplakia. *Acta Cytol* 1962;6:471–474.
51. Lou TY, Teplitz C. Malakoplakia: pathogenesis and ultrastructural morphogenesis: a problem of altered macrophage (phagolysosomal) response. *Hum Pathol* 1974;5:191–207.
52. Damjanov I, Katz SM. Malakoplakia. *Pathol Annu* 1981;16(2):103–126.
53. Stanton MJ, Maxted W. Malakoplakia: a study of the literature and current concepts of pathogenesis, diagnosis and treatment. *J Urol* 1981;125:139–146.
54. Lewin KJ, Fair WR, Steigbigel RT, Winberg CD, Droller MJ. Clinical and laboratory studies into the pathogenesis of malakoplakia. *J Clin Pathol* 1976;29:354–363.
55. Nieh PT, Althausen AF. Malakoplakia of the ureter. *J Urol* 1979;122:701–702.
56. Sharma TC, Kagan HN, Sheils JP. Malakoplakia of the male urethra. *J Urol* 1981;125:885–886.
57. Malek RS, Greene LF, Farrow GM. Amyloidosis of the urinary bladder. *Br J Urol* 1971;43:189–200.
58. Farah RN, Benson DO, Fine G, Dorman PJ. Primary localized amyloidosis of bladder. *Urology* 1979;13:200–202.
59. Akhtar M, Valencia M, Thomas AM. Solitary primary amyloidosis of urinary bladder. *Urology* 1978;12:721–724.
60. Primrose JN, McKean M, Desai S. Primary amyloidosis of ureter. *Urology* 1985;25:650–652.
61. Dias R, Ferrandes M, Patel RC, Shaderevian J, Lavengood RW. Amyloidosis of renal pelvis and urinary bladder. *Urology* 1979;24:401–404.
62. Vasudevan P, Stein AM, Pinn VW, Rao CN. Primary amyloidosis of urethra. *Urology* 1981;27:181–183.
63. Dounis A, Bourounis M, Mitropoulos D. Primary localized amyloidosis of urethra. *Eur Urol* 1985;11:344–345.
64. Miller A. The aetiology and treatment of diverticulum of the bladder. *Br J Urol* 1958;30:43–56.
65. Kertsschmer HL. Diverticula of the urinary bladder: a clinical study of 236 cases. *Surg Gynecol Obstet* 1940;71:491–503.
66. Fox M, Power RF, Bruce AW. Diverticulum of the bladder: presentation and evaluation of treatment of 115 cases. *Br J Urol* 1962;34:286–298.
67. Schiff M, Lytton B. Congenital diverticulum of the bladder. *J Urol* 1970;104:111–115.
68. Barrett DW, Malek RS, Kelalis PP. Observations on vesical diverticulum in childhood. *J Urol* 1976;116:234–236.
69. Abeshouse BS, Goldstein AE. Primary carcinoma in a diverticulum of the bladder: a report of four cases and a review of the literature. *J Urol* 1943;49:534–547.
70. Faysal MH, Freiha FS. Primary neoplasia in vesical diverticula: a report of 12 cases. *Br J Urol* 1978;53:141–143.
71. Ward MP. Sarcoma of vesical diverticula. *Br J Urol* 1958;30:57–59.
72. Cochran ST, Waisman J, Barbaric ZL. Radiographic and microscopic findings in multiple ureteral diverticula. *Diagn Radiol* 1980;137:631–636.
73. Coddington CC, Knab DR. Urethral diverticulum: a review. *Obstet Gynecol Surv* 1983;38:357–364.
74. Gesch I, Kummer M, Bettes M. Congenital urethral diverticula in boys. *Eur Urol* 1983;9:139–141.
75. Tesluk H. Primary adenocarcinoma of female urethra associated with diverticula. *Urology* 1981;27:197–199.
76. Gea PC, Ward JN, Lavengood RW, Gray GF. Mesonephoric adenocarcinomas in urethral diverticula. *Urology* 1977;10:58–61.
77. Morse HD. The etiology and pathology of pyelitis cystica, ureteritis cystica and cystitis cystica. *Am J Pathol* 1928;4:33–50.
78. Mostofi FK. Potentialities of bladder epithelium. *J Urol* 1954;71:705–714.
79. Goldstein AMB, Fauer RB, Chinn M, Kaempf MJ. New concepts on formation of Brunn's nests and cysts in the urinary tract mucosa. *Urology* 1978;11:513–517.
80. Wiener DP, Koss LG, Sablay B, Freed SZ. The prevalence and significance of Brunn's nests, cystitis cystica and squamous metaplasia in normal bladders. *J Urol* 1979;122:317–321.
81. Davies G, Castro JE. Cystitis glandularis. *Urology* 1977;10:128–129.
82. Edwards PD, Hurm RA, Jaeschke WH. Conversion of cystitis glandularis to adenocarcinoma. *J Urol* 1972;108:568–580.
83. Lin JI, Tseng CH, Choy C, Yong HS, Marsidi PS, Pilloff B. Diffuse cystitis glandularis associated with adenocarcinomatous change. *Urology* 1980;15:411–415.
84. Tanrenbaum M. Inflammartory proliferative lesion of the urinary bladder: squamous metaplasia. *Urology* 1976;7:428–429.
85. Engel RM, Wilkson HA. Bladder extrophy. *J Urol* 1970;104:699–704.
86. Nielsen K, Nielson KK. Adenocarcinoma in extrophy of the bladder: the last case in Scandinavia? A case report and review of literature. *J Urol* 1983;130:1180–1182.
87. Assor D. A villous tumor of the bladder. *J Urol* 1978;119:287–288.
88. Miller DC, Gang DL, Gauris V, Alroy J, Ucci AA, Parkhurst EC. Villous adenoma of the bladder: a morphologic or biologic entity? *Am J Clin Pathol* 1983;79:728–731.
89. Newman J, Antonakopoulos GN. Widespread mucous metaplasia of the urinary bladder with nephrogenic adenoma. *Arch Pathol Lab Med* 1985;109:560–563.
90. Bagnavan BS, Tiamson EM, Wenk RE, Berger BW, Hamamoto G, Eggleston JC. Nephrogenic adenoma of the urinary bladder and urethra. *Hum Pathol* 1981;12:907–916.
91. Stilment MM, Sivoky MB. Nephrogenic adenoma associated with intravesical bacillus Calmette-Guérin treatment: a report of two cases. *J Urol* 1986;135:359–361.
92. Navarre RJ, Loening SA, Narayana A, Culp DA. Nephrogenic adenoma: a report of nine cases and review of the literature. *J Urol* 1982;127:775–779.
93. Molland EA, Trott PA, Paris MI, Blandy JP. Nephrogenic adenoma: a form of adenomatous metaplasia of the bladder: a clinical and electron microscopical study. *Br J Urol* 1976;48:453–462.
94. Ford TF, Watson GM, Cameron KM. Adenomatous metaplasia (nephrogenic adenoma) of urothelium: an analysis of 70 cases. *Br J Urol* 1985;57:427–433.
95. Blacklock ARE, Geddes JR, Black JW. Mucinous and squamous metaplasia of the renal pelvis. *J Urol* 1983;130:544–545.
96. Satodate R, Koike H, Sasou S, Ohori T, Nagare Y. Nephrogenic adenoma of the ureter. *J Urol* 1984;131:332–334.
97. Peterson LJ, Matsumoto LM. Nephrogenic adenoma in urethral diverticulum. *Urology* 1978;11:193–195.
98. DeMeester LT, Farrow GH, Utz DS. Inverted papilloma of the urinary bladder. *Cancer* 1975;36:505–513.
99. Henderson DW, Allen PW, Bourne AJ. Inverted urinary papilloma: report of five cases and review of the literature. *Virchows Arch Pathol Anat Histol* 1975;336:177–186.
100. Caro DJ, Tesler A. Inverted papilloma of the bladder: a distinct urological lesion. *Cancer* 1978;42:708–713.
101. Anderstrom C, Johansson S, Pettersson S. Inverted papilloma of the urinary tract. *J Urol* 1982;127:1132–1134.
102. Lazarevic B, Garret R. Inverted papilloma and papillary transitional cell carcinoma of urinary bladder: report of four cases of inverted papilloma, one showing papillary malignant transformation and review of the literature. *Cancer* 1978;42:1904–1911.

103. Whitesel JA. Inverted papilloma of the urinary tract: malignant potential. *J Urol* 1982;127:539–540.
104. Stein BS, Rosen S, Kendall R. The association of inverted papilloma and transitional cell carcinoma of the urothelium. *J Urol* 1984;131:751–752.
105. Assor D. Inverted papilloma of the renal pelvis. *J Urol* 1976;116:654.
106. Lausten GS, Anagnostaki L, Thomsen OF. Inverted papilloma of the upper urinary tract. *Eur Urol* 1984;10:67–70.
107. Young RH, Oliva E. Transitional cell carcinoma of the urinary bladder that may be underdiagnosed: a report of four invasive cases exemplifying the homology between neoplastic and non-neoplastic transitional cell lesions. *Am J Surg Pathol* 1996;20:1448–1454.
108. Amin M, Gomez JA, Young RH. Urothelial transitional cell carcinoma with endophytic growth patterns: a discussion of patterns of invasion and problems associated with assessment of invasion in 18 cases. *Am J Surg Pathol* 1997;21:1057–1068.
109. Uyama T, Moriwaki S. Inverted papilloma with malignant change of renal pelvis. *Urology* 1981;17:200–201.
110. Bissada NK, Cole AT, Fried FA. Extensive condyloma acuminata of the entire male urethra and the bladder. *J Urol* 1974;112:201–203.
111. DeBenedictis TJ, Marmar JL, Praiss DE. Intraurethra condyloma acuminata: management and review of the literature. *J Urol* 1977;118:767–769.
112. Keating MA, Young RH, Carr CP, Nikrui N, Herey NM. Condyloma acuminatum of the bladder and ureter: case report and review of the literature. *J Urol* 1985;133:465–467.
113. Libby JM, Frankel JM, Scadino PT. Condyloma acuminatum of the bladder and associated urothelial malignancy. *J Urol* 1985;134:134–136.
114. Walther M, O'Brien DP, Birch HW. Condylomata acuminata and verrucous carcinoma of the bladder: case report and literature review. *J Urol* 1986;135:362–365.
115. Proppe KH, Scully RE, Rosai J. Postoperative spindle-cell nodules of the genitourinary tract resembling sarcomas: a report of eight cases. *Am J Surg Pathol* 1984;8:101–108.
116. Nochomovitz LE, Orenstein JM. Inflammatory pseudotumor of the urinary bladder: possible relationship to nodular fasciitis. *Am J Surg Pathol* 1985;9:366–373.
117. Jones EC, Clement PB, Young RH. Inflammatory pseudotumor of the urinary bladder: a clinicopathological, immunohistochemical, ultrastructural, and flow cytometric study of 13 cases. *Am J Surg Pathol* 1993;17:264–274.
118. Ro JY, Ayala AG, Ordonez NG, Swanson DA, Badaian RJ. Pseudosarcomatous fibromyxoid tumor of the urinary bladder. *Am J Clin Pathol* 1986;86:583–590.
119. Albores-Saavedra J, Manivel JC, Essenfeld H, et al. Pseudosarcomatous myofibroblastic proliferations in the urinary bladder of children. *Cancer* 1990;66:1234–1241.
120. Roth JA. Reactive pseudosarcomatous response in urinary bladder. *Urology* 1980;16:635–637.
121. Mahadevia PS, Alexander JE, Rojas-Corona R, Koss LG. Pseudosarcomatous stromal reaction in primary and metastatic urothelial carcinoma: a source of diagnostic difficulty. *Am J Surg Pathol* 1989;13:782–790.
122. Wick MR, Brown BA, Young RH, Mills SE. Spindle-cell proliferations of the urinary tract: an immunohistochemical study. *Am J Surg Pathol* 1988;12:379–389.
123. Reuter VE. Sarcomatoid lesions of the urogenital tract. *Semin Diagn Pathol* 1993;10:188–201.
124. Young RH. Spindle cell lesions of the urinary tract. *Histol Histopathol* 1990;5:505–512.
125. Wynder EL, Goldsmith R. The epidemiology of bladder cancer: a second look. *Cancer* 1977;40:1246–1268.
126. Clayson DB. Occupational bladder cancer. *Prev Med* 1976;5:228–244.
127. Ward E, Carpenter A, Markowitz S, Roberts D, Halperin W. Excess number of bladder cancers in workers exposed to ortho-toluidine and aniline. *J Natl Cancer Inst* 1991;83:501–506.
128. Anthony HM, Thomas GM. Tumors of the urinary bladder: an analysis of the occupations of 1030 patients in Leeds, England. *J Int Cancer Inst* 1970;45:879–895.
129. Cole P, Hoover R, Friedell GH. Occupation and cancer of the lower urinary tract. *Cancer* 1972;29:1250–1260.
130. Cole P. Lower urinary tract. In: Schottenfeld D, ed. *Cancer epidemiology and prevention*. Springfield: Charles C Thomas, 1975:233–262.
131. Wynder EL, Underdonk J, Mantel N. An epidemiological investigation of cancer of the bladder. *Cancer* 1963;16:1388–1407.
132. Cole P. Coffee-drinking and cancer of the lower urinary tract. *Lancet* 1971;302:1335–1337.
133. Cohen SM, Arai M, Jacobs JB, Friedell GH. Promoting effect of saccharin and dl-tryptophan in urinary bladder carcinogenesis. *Cancer Res* 1979;39:1207–1217.
134. Kessler II. Non-nutritive sweeteners and human bladder cancer: preliminary findings. *J Urol* 1976;115:143–146.
135. Morrison AS, Buing JE. Artificial sweeteners and cancer of the lower urinary tract. *N Engl J Med* 1980;302:537–541.
136. Armstrong B, Doll R. Environmental factors and cancer incidence and mortality in different countries, with special references to dietary practices. *Int J Cancer* 1975;15:617–631.
137. Gaaker HA, Ruiter HJ. Carcinoma of the renal pelvis following abuse of phenacetin-containing analgesic drugs. *Br J Urol* 1979;51:188–192.
138. Lomax-Smith JD, Seymour AE. Neoplasia in analgesic nephropathy: a urothelial field change. *Am J Surg Pathol* 1980;4:565–572.
139. Fairchild WV, Spencer CR, Soloway HD, Gangai MP. The incidence of bladder cancer after cyclophosphamide therapy. *J Urol* 1979;122:163–164.
140. Seo IS, Clark SA, McGovern FD, Clark DL, Johnson EH. Leiomyosarcoma of the urinary bladder: thirteen years after cyclophosphamide therapy for Hodgkin's disease. *Cancer* 1985;55:1597–1603.
141. Jewett HJ, Strong GH. Infiltrating carcinoma of the bladder: relation of depth of penetration of the bladder wall to incidence of local extension and metastases. *J Urol* 1946;55:366–372.
142. Jewett HJ. Carcinoma of the bladder: influence of depth infiltration on the 5-year results following complete extirpation of the primary growth. *J Urol* 1952;67:672–676.
143. Marshall VF. The relation of the preoperative estimate to the pathologic demonstration of the extent of vesical neoplasms. *J Urol* 1952;68:714–723.
144. American Joint Committee on Cancer. In Fleming ID, Cooper JS, Henson DE, et al, eds. *AJCC cancer staging manual.* 5th ed. Philadelphia: Lippincott-Raven, 1997:241–243.
145. Smith JA, Batata M, Grabstald H. Preoperative irradiation and cystectomy for bladder cancer. *Cancer* 1982;49:869–873.
146. Pagano F, Bassi P, Galetti TP. Results of contemporary radical cystectomy for invasive bladder cancer: a clinicopathologic study with an emphasis on the inadequacy of the tumor, nodes, and metastases classification. *J Urol* 1991;145:45–50.
147. Richie JP, Skinner DG, Kaufman JJ. Radical cystectomy for carcinoma of the bladder: 16 years experience. *J Urol* 1975;113:186–189.
148. Abel PD. Prognostic indices in transitional cell carcinoma of the bladder. *Br J Urol* 1988;62:235–239.
149. Herr HW, jaske G, Sheinfeld J. The T_1 bladder tumor. *Semin Urol* 1990;8:254–261.
150. Reuter VE. Pathology of bladder cancer: assessment of prognostic variables and response to therapy. *Semin Oncol* 1990;17:524–532.
151. Abel PD, Henderson D, Bennett MK, Hall RR, Williams G. Differing interpretations by pathologists of the pT category and grade of transitional cell cancer of the bladder. *Br J Urol* 1988;62:339–342.
152. Abel PD, Williams G. Should pT1 transitional cell cancers of the bladder still be classified as superficial? *Br J Urol* 1988;62:235–239.
153. Younes M, Sussman J, True LD. The usefulness of the level of the muscularis mucosae in the staging of invasive transitional cell carcinoma of the urinary bladder. *Cancer* 1990;66:543–548.
154. Hasui Y, Osada Y, Kitada S, Nishi S. Significance of invasion to the muscularis mucosae on the progression of superficial bladder cancer. *Urology* 1994;43:782–786.
155. Angulo JC, Lopez JI, Grignon DJ Sanchez-Chapado M. Muscularis mucosa differentiates two populations with different prognosis in stage T1 bladder cancer. *Urology* 1995;45:47–53.
156. National Cancer Collaborative Group A (NBCCGA). Surveillance, initial assessment and subsequent progress of patients with superficial bladder cancer in a prospective longitudinal study. *Cancer Res* 1977;37:2907–2910.
157. Loening S, Narayana A, Yoder L, et al. Factors influencing the recurence rate of bladder cancer. *J Urol* 1980;123:29–31.
158. Kern WH. The grade and pathologic stage of bladder cancer. *Cancer* 1984;53:1185–1189.
159. Heney NM, Ahmed S, Flanagan MJ, et al. Superficial bladder cancer: progression and recurrence. *J Urol* 1983;130:1083–1086.

160. Heney NM, Proppe K, Prout GR, Griffin PP, Shipley WU. Invasive bladder cancer: tumor configuration, lymphatic invasion and survival. *J Urol* 1983;130:895–897.
161. Fossa SD, Reitan JB, Ous S, Odegaard A, Loeb M. Prediction of tumor progression in superficial bladder carcinoma. *Eur Urol* 1985;11:1–5.
162. Skinner DS. Current state of classification and staging of bladder cancer. *Cancer Res* 1977;37:2838–2842.
163. Brawn PN. The origin of invasive carcinoma of the bladder. *Cancer* 1982;50:515–519.
164. Prout GR, Griffin PP, Shipley WU. Bladder carcinoma as a systemic disease. *Cancer* 1979;43:2531–2539.
165. Kakizoe T, Tobisu K, Takai K. Relationship between papillary and nodular transitional cell carcinoma in the human urinary bladder. *Cancer Res* 1988;48:2293–2303.
166. Larsen MP, Steinberg GC, Brendler CB. Use of *Ulex europaeus* agglutinin (UEA-1) to distinguish vascular and pseudovascular invasion in transitional cell carcinoma of the urinary bladder with lamina propria invasion. *Mod Pathol* 1990;3:83–88.
167. Mostofi FK, Sobin LH, Torloni H. Histological typing of urinary bladder tumors: international classification of tumors. No. 10. Geneva: WHO, 1973.
168. Koss LG. Tumors of the urinary bladder. Fascicle 11 (2nd series). In: *Atlas of tumor pathology*. Washington, DC: Armed Forces Institute of Pathology, 1975:16.
169. Ash JE. Epithelial tumors of the bladder. *J Urol* 1940;44:135–145.
170. Friedell GH, Parija GC, Nagy GK, Soto EA. The pathology of human bladder cancer. *Cancer* 1980;45:1823–1831.
171. Koss LG. Mapping of the urinary bladder: its impact on the concepts of bladder cancer. *Hum Pathol* 1979;10:533–548.
172. Soto EA, Friedell GH, Tiltman AJ. Bladder cancer as seen on giant histologic sections. *Cancer* 1977;39:447–455.
173. Kakizoe T, Matsumoto K, Nishio Y, Kishi K. Analysis of 90 step-sectioned cystectomized specimens of bladder cancer. *J Urol* 1984;131:467–472.
174. Althausen AF, Prout GR, Daly JJ. Non-invasive papillary carcinoma of the bladder associated with carcinoma in situ. *J Urol* 1976;116:575–580.
175. Bergkvist A, Lungqvist A, Moberger G. Classification of bladder tumours based on the cellular pattern. *Acta Chir Scand* 1961;130:371–378.
176. Lerman RI, Hutter RVP, Whitmore WF. Papilloma of the urinary bladder. *Cancer* 1970;25:333–342.
177. Gilbert HA, Logan JL, Kagan AR, et al. The natural history of papillomy transitional cell carcinoma of the bladder and its treatment in an unselected population on the basis of histologic grading. *J Urol* 1978;119:488–492.
178. Jordan AM, Weingarten J, Murphy WM. Transitional cell neoplasms of the bladder: can biologic potential be predicted from histologic grading? *Cancer* 1987;60:2766–2774.
179. National Bladder Cancer Cooperative Group A. Cytology and histopathology of bladder cancer cases in prospective longitudinal study. *Cancer Res* 1977;37:2911–2915.
180. Busch C, Engberg A, Norlen BJ, Stenkvist B. Malignancy grading of epithelial bladder tumours. *Scand J Urol Nephrol* 1977;11:143–148.
181. Malmstrom P-U, Busch C, Norlen BJ. Recurrence, progression and survival in bladder cancer: a retrospective analysis of 232 patients with >5-year follow-up. *Scand J Urol Nephrol* 1987;21:185–195.
182. Murphy WM, Beckwith JB, Farrow GM. Tumors of the kidney, bladder and related urinary structures. In: *Atlas of tumor pathology, fascicle 13*, 3rd series. Washington, DC: Armed Forces Institute of Pathology, 1994:198–233.
183. Murphy WM. Current topics in the pathology of bladder cancer. *Pathol Annu* 1983;25:1–25.
184. Murphy WM, Irving CC. The cellular features of developing carcinoma in murine bladder. *Cancer* 1981;47:514–522.
185. Murphy WM, Soloway MS. Developing carcinoma (dysplasia) of the urinary bladder. *Pathol Annu* 1982;17(1):197–217.
186. Nagy GK, Frable WJ, Murphy WM. The classification of premalignant urothelial abnormalitites: a delphi study of the National Bladder Clinical Collaborative Group A. *Pathol Annu* 1982;17(1):219–233.
187. Amin MB, Grignon DJ, Eble JN, et al. Intraepithelial lesions of the urothelium: an interobserver reproducibility study with proposed terminology and histologic criteria [Abstract]. *Mod Pathol* 1997;10:69A.
188. Koss LG, Nakaniski I, Freed SZ. Nonpapillary carcinoma in situ and atypical hyperplasia in cancerous bladders: further studies of surgically removed bladders by mapping. *Urology* 1977;9:442–455.
189. Murphy WM, Nagy GK, Rao MK, et al. "Normal" urothelium in patients with bladder cancer: a preliminary report from the National Bladder Cancer Collaborative Group A. *Cancer* 1979;44:1050–1058.
190. Prout GR, Griffin PP, Daly JJ, Heney NM. Carcinoma in situ of the urinary bladder with and without associated vesical neoplasms. *Cancer* 1983;52:524–532.
191. Kakizoe T, Matumoto K, Nishio Y, Ohtani M, Kishi K. Significance of carcinoma in situ and dysplasia in association with bladder cancer. *J Urol* 1985;133:395–398.
192. Utz DC, Farrow GM, Rife CC, Segura JW, Zincke H. Carcinoma in situ of the bladder. *Cancer* 1980;45:1842–1848.
193. Zincke H, Utz DC, Farrow GM. Review of Mayo Clinic experience with carcinoma in situ. *Urology* 1985;26(4 suppl):39–46.
194. Melamed MR, Vousta NG, Grabstaldt H. Natural history and clinical behavior of in situ carcinoma of the human urinary bladder. *Cancer* 1964;17:1533–1545.
195. Farrow GM, Utz DC, Rife CC, Greene LF. Clinical observations on sixty-nine cases of in situ carcinoma of the urinary bladder. *Cancer Res* 1977;37:2794–2798.
196. Weinstein RS, Miller AW, Pauli BU. Carcinoma in situ: comments on the pathobiology of a paradox. *Urol Clin North Am* 1980;7:523–531.
197. Turner AG. Pagetoid lesions associated with carcinoma of the bladder. *J Urol* 1980;123:124–126.
198. Tomaszewski JE, Koral OC, LiVolsi VA, Connor AM, Wein A. Paget's disease of the urethral meatus following transitional cell carcinoma of the bladder. *J Urol* 1986;135:368–370.
199. Powel FC, Bjornsson J, Doyle JA, Cooper AJ. Genital Paget's disease and urinary tract malignancy. *J Am Acad Dermatol* 1985;13:84–90.
200. Faysal MH. Squamous cell carcinoma of the bladder. *J Urol* 1981;126:598–599.
201. Newman DM, Brown JR, Jay AC, Pontius EE. Squamous cell carcinoma of the bladder. *J Urol* 1968;112:66–67.
202. Wall FL, Clausen KP. Carcinoma of the urinary bladder in patients receiving cyclophosphamide. *N Engl J Med* 1975;293:271–273.
203. Walther M, O'Brien D, Birch HW. Condyloma acuminata and verrucous carcinoma of the bladder: case report and literature review. *J Urol* 1986;135:362–365.
204. El Sebai I, Sherif M, El Bolkaimy MN, et al. Verrucose squamous carcinoma of the bladder. *Urology* 1974;4:407–410.
205. Wyatt JK, Craig I. Verrucous carcinoma of urinary bladder. *Urology* 1980;16:97–99.
206. Holck S, Jorgensen L. Verrucous carcinoma of urinary bladder. *Urology* 1983;21:435–437.
207. Wheeler JD, Hill WT. Adenocarcinoma involving the urinary bladder. *Cancer* 1954;7:119–135.
208. Mostofi FK, Thomson RV, Dean AL. Mucous adenocarcinoma of the urinary bladder. *Cancer* 1955;8:741–758.
209. Hicks BN, Heney NM, Daly JJ. Primary adenocarcinoma of urinary bladder. *Urology* 1983;21:26–29.
210. Anderstrom C, Johansson SL, von Schultz L. Primary adenocarcinoma of the urinary bladder: a clinicopathologic and prognostic study. *Cancer* 1983;52:1273–1282.
211. Grignon DJ, Ro JY, Ayala AG, Johnson DE, Ordoñez NG. Primary adenocarcinoma of the urinary bladder: a clinicopathologic analysis of 72 cases. *Cancer* 1991;67:2165–2172.
212. Jones WA, Gibbons RP, Correa RJ, Cummings KB, Tate J. Primary adenocarcinoma of the bladder. *Urology* 1980;15:119–122.
213. Malek RS, Rosen JS, O'Dea MJ. Adenocarcinoma of the bladder. *Urology* 1983;20:357–359.
214. Dean AL, Mostofi FK, Thompson RV. A restudy of the first fourteen hundred tumors in the bladder tumor registry. *J Urol* 1954;71:571–590.
215. Melicow MM. Tumors of the urinary bladder: a clinicopathological analysis of over 2,500 specimens and autopsies. *J Urol* 1955;74:498–521.
216. Eischoff W, Bohn N. Adenocarcinoma of the appendix penetrating the bladder. *J Urol* 1980;123:123–126.
217. Braun EV, Ali M, Fayemi O, Beaugard E. Primary signet-ring cell carcinoma of the urinary bladder: review of the literature and report of a case. *Cancer* 1981;47:1430–1435.
218. Poore TE, Egbert B, Jahnke R, Kraft K. Signet ring cell adenocarcinoma of the bladder: linitis plastica variant. *Arch Pathol Lab Med* 1981;105:203–204.

219. Choi H, Lamb S, Pintar K, Jacobs SC. Primary signet-ring cell carcinoma of the urinary bladder. *Cancer* 1984;53:1985–1990.
220. Bernstein SA, Reuter VE, Carroll PR, Whitmore WF. Primary signet ring cell carcinoma of the urinary bladder. *Urol* 1988;31:432–436.
221. Grignon DJ, Ro JY, Ayala AG, Johnson DE. Primary signet ring cell carcinoma of the urinary bladder. *Am J Clin Pathol* 1991;95:13–20.
222. Pontes JE, Oldford JR. Metastatic breast carcinoma to the bladder. *J Urol* 1970;104:839–842.
223. Skor AB, Warren MM. Mesonephric adenocarcinoma of the bladder. *Urology* 1977;10:64–65.
224. Schultz RE, Block MJ, Tomaszewski JE, Brooks JSJ, Hanno PM. Mesonephric adenocarcinoma of the bladder. *J Urol* 1984;132:263–265.
225. Young RH, Scully RE. Clear cell adenocarcinoma of the bladder and urethra: a report of three cases and review of the literature. *Am J Surg Pathol* 1985;9:816–826.
226. Schubert GE, Paukovic MB, Bethke-Bedurftig BA. Tubular urachal remnants in adult bladders. *J Urol* 1982;127:40–42.
227. Johnson DE, Hodge GB, Abdul-Karim FW, Ayala AG. Urachal carcinoma. *Urology* 1985;26:218–221.
228. Jakse G, Schneider HM, Jacobi GH. Urachal signet-ring cell carcinoma, a rare variant of vesical adenocarcinoma: incidence and pathological criteria. *J Urol* 1978;120:764–766.
229. Alonso-Gorrea M, Mompo-Sanchis JA, Jorda-Cuevas M, Froufe A, Jimenez-Cruz JF. Signet ring cell adenocarcinoma of the urachus. *Eur Urol* 1985;11:282–284.
230. Ghazizadeh M, Yamamoto S, Kurokawa K. Clinical features of urachal carcinoma in Japan: review of 157 patients. *Urol Res* 1983;11:235–238.
231. Eble JN, Hull MT, Rowland RG, Hostetter M. Villous adenoma of the urachus with mucosuria: a light and electron microscopic study. *J Urol* 1986;135:1240–1244.
232. Hayman J. Carcinoma of the urachus. *Pathology* 1984;16:167–171.
233. Mills SE, Wolfe JT, Weiss MA, et al. Small cell undifferentiated carcinoma of the urinary bladder: a light microscopic, immunohistochemical and ultrastructural study of 12 cases. *Am J Surg Pathol* 1987;11:606–617.
234. Davis BH, Ludwig ME, Cole SR, Pastuszak WT. Small neuroendocrine carcinoma of the urinary bladder: report of three cases with ultrastructural analysis. *Ultrastruct Pathol* 1983;4:197–204.
235. Reyes CV, Soneru I. Small cell carcinoma of the urinary bladder with hypercalcemia. *Cancer* 1985;56:2530–2533.
236. Grignon DJ, Ro JY, Ayala AG, et al. Small cell carcinoma of the urinary bladder: a clinicopathologic analysis of 22 cases. *Cancer* 1992;69:527–536.
237. Ucci AA, Alroy J, Tallberg K, Gauris VE, Dayal DeLellis R. Neuroendocrine cells in squamous metaplasia, inverted papillomas, and adenocarcinomas of the urinary bladder [Abstract]. *Lab Invest* 1985;52:71A.
238. Smith A. Neurosecretory cells in carcinoma in situ of the urinary bladder: an incidental finding. *Ultrastruct Pathol* 1985;8:267.
239. Toma H, Yamashita N, Nakazawa H, Yamaguchi Y. Transitional cell carcinoma with osteoid metaplasia. *Urology* 1986;27:174–176.
240. Eble JN, Young RH. Stromal osseous metaplasia in carcinoma of the bladder. *J Urol* 1991;145:823–825.
241. Komatsu H, Kinoshita K, Mikata N, Honma Y. Spindle and giant cell carcinoma of the bladder: report of three cases. *Eur Urol* 1985;11:141–144.
242. Hotlz F, Fox JE, Abell MR. Carcinoma of the urinary bladder. *Cancer* 1972;29:294–304.
243. Jao W, Soto JM, Gould VE. Squamous carcinoma of bladder with pseudosarcomatous stroma. *Arch Pathol* 1975;99:461–466.
244. Sen SE, Malek RS, Farrow GM, Lieber MM. Sarcoma and carcinosarcoma of the bladder in adults. *J Urol* 1985;133:29–30.
245. Schoborg TW, Saffos RO, Rodriguez AP, Scott C. Carcinoma of the bladder. *J Urol* 1980;124:724–727.
246. Jones EC, Young RH. Myxoid and sclerosing sarcomatoid transitional cell carcinoma of the urinary bladder: a clinicopathologic and immunohistochemical study of 25 cases. *Mod Pathol* 1997;10:908–916.
247. Kanno J, Sakamoto A, Washizuka M, Kawai T, Kasuga T. Malignant mixed mesodermal tumor of bladder occurring after radiotherapy for cervical cancer: report of a case. *J Urol* 1985;133:854–856.
248. Smith JA, Herr HA, Middleton RG. Bladder carcinosarcoma: histologic variation in metastatic lesions. *J Urol* 1983;129:829–831.
249. Kusaba Y, Yushita Y, Suzu H, et al. Carcinosarcoma of the bladder. *J Urol* 1984;131:118–119.
250. Tungekar MF, Al Adnani MS. Sarcomas of the bladder and prostate: the role of immunohistochemistry and ultrastructure in diagnosis. *Eur Urol* 1986;12:180–183.
251. Drew FA, Furman J, Civantos F, Murphy WM. The nested variant of transitional cell carcinoma: an aggressive neoplasm with innocuous histology. *Mod Pathol* 1996;9:989–994.
252. Young RH, Zukerberg LR. Microcystic transitional cell carcinomas of the urinary bladder: a report of four cases. *Am J Clin Pathol* 1991;96:635–639.
253. Amin MB, Ro JY, Lee KM, et al. Lymphoepithelioma-like carcinoma of urinary bladder. *Am J Surg Pathol* 1994;18:466–473.
254. Holmang S, Borghede G, Johansson SL. Bladder carcinoma with lymphoepithelioma-like differentiation: a report of 9 cases. *J Urol* 1998;159:779–782.
255. Amin MB, Ro JY, El-Sharkawy T, et al. Micropapillary variant of transitional cell carcinoma of the urinary bladder, histologic pattern resembling ovarian papillary serous carcinoma. *Am J Surg Pathol* 1994;18:1224–1232.
256. Dennis PM, Turner AG. Primary choriocarcinoma of the bladder evolving from a transitional cell carcinoma. *J Clin Pathol* 1984;37:503–505.
257. Gallagher L, Lind R, Oyasu R. Primary choriocarcinoma of the urinary bladder in association with undifferentiation carcinoma. *Hum Pathol* 1984;11:793–795.
258. Shah VM, Newman J, Crocker J, et al. Ectopic B-human chorionic gonadotropin production by bladder urothelial neoplasia. *Arch Pathol Lab Med* 1986;110:107–111.
259. Yamase HT, Wurzel RS, Nich PT, Gondes B. Immunohistochemical demonstration of human chorionic gonadotropin in tumors of the urinary bladder. *Ann Clin Lab Sci* 1985;15:414–417.
260. Kawamura J, Rhinsho K, Taki Y, et al. Choriocarcinoma and undifferentiated cell carcinoma of the bladder with gonadotropin secretion. *J Urol* 1979;121:684–686.
261. Batata MA, Whitmore WF, Hilaris BS, Tukita N, Grabstald H. Primary carcinoma of the ureter: a prognostic study. *Cancer* 1975;35:1626–1632.
262. Grabstald H, Whitmore WF, Melamed MR. Renal pelvic tumors. *JAMA* 1971;218:845–854.
263. Nocks BN, Perrone TA, Heney NM, Griffin PP, Daly JJ, Prout GR. Transitional cell carcinoma of the renal pelvis. *Urology* 1982;19:472–477.
264. McCarron JP, Mills C, Vaugh ED. Tumors of the renal pelvis and ureter: current concepts and manangement. *Semin Urol* 1983;1:75–81.
265. Johansson S, Angervall L, Bengtsson U, Wahlqvist L. A clinicopathologic and prognostic study of epithelial tumors of the renal pelvis. *Cancer* 1976;37:1376–1383.
266. Linker DG, Whitmore WF. Ureteral carcinoma in situ. *J Urol* 1975;113:777–780.
267. Craig JR, Hart WR. Benign polyps with prostatic-type epithelium of the urethra. *Am J Clin Pathol* 1975;63:343–347.
268. Walker AN, Fechner RE, Mills SE, Perry JM. Epithelial polyps of the prostatic urethra: a light-microscopic and immunohistochemical study. *Am J Surg Pathol* 1983;7:351–356.
269. Remick DG, Kumar NB. Benign polyps with prostatic-type epithelium of the urethra and the urinary bladder: a bladder suggestion of histogenesis based on histologic and immunohistochemical studies. *Am J Surg Pathol* 1984;8:833–839.
270. Foster RS, Garrett RA. Congenital posterior urethral polyps. *J Urol* 1986;136:670–672.
271. Gunther I, Abrams HJ, Sutton AP, Buchbinder MI. Fibroepithelial polyp of the verumontanum: a case report and review of the literature. *J Urol* 1979;121:525–526.
272. Schellhammer PF. Urethral carcinoma. *Semin Urol* 1983;1:82–89.
273. Grabstald H. Tumors of the urethra in men and women. *Cancer* 1973;32:1236–1255.
274. Schellhammer PF, Whitmore WF. Transitional cell carcinoma of the urethra in men having cystectomy for bladder cancer. *J Urol* 1976;115:56–60.
275. Bearhs IJ, Fleming TR, Zincke H. Risk of local urethral recurrence after radical cystectomy for bladder cancer. *J Urol* 1984;131:264–266.
276. Ray B, Canto AR, Whitmore WF. Experience with primary carcinoma of the male urethra. *J Urol* 1977;117:591–594.

277. Melicow MM, Roberts TW. Pathology and natural history of urethral tumors in males. *Urology* 1978;11:83–89.
278. Bracken RB, Johnson DE, Miller LS, Ayala AG, Gomez JJ, Rutledge F. Primary carcinoma of the female urethra. *J Urol* 1976;116:188–192.
279. Roberts TW, Melicow MM. Pathology and natural history of urethral tumors in females: review of 65 cases. *Urology* 1977;10:42–45.
280. Johnson DE, O'Connell JR. Primary carcinoma of the female urethra. *Urology* 1983;21:42–45.
281. Mackenzie AR, Whitmore WF, Melamed MR. Myosarcomas of the bladder and prostate. *Cancer* 1968;22:833–844.
282. Russo P, Brady MS, Conlon K, et al. Adult urological sarcoma. *J Urol* 1992;147:1032–1037.
283. Weitzner S. Leiomyosarcoma of urinary bladder in children. *Urology* 1978;12:450–452.
284. Maurer HM. The inter-group rhabdomyosarcoma study (NIH): objectives and clinical staging classification. *J Pediatr Surg* 1975;10:977–978.
285. Scholtmeijer RJ, Tromp CG, Hazebroeck FWJ. Embryonal rhabdomyosarcoma of the urogenital tract in childhood. *Eur Urol* 1983;9:69–74.
286. Hendricksen C, Zetterlund CG, Boisen P, Pattersson S. Large rhabdomyosarcoma of the urinary bladder in an adult. *Scand J Urol Nephrol* 1985;19:237–239.
287. Swartz DA, Johnson DE, Ayala AG, Watkins DL. Bladder leiomyosarcoma: a review of 10 cases with five-year followup. *J Urol* 1985;1333:200–202.
288. Henriksen OB, Mogensen P, Engelholm A. Inflammatory fibrous histiocytoma of the bladder. *Acta Pathol Microbiol Immunol Scand (A)* 1982;90:333–337.
289. Turner AG. Malignant fibrous histiocytoma involving the bladder. *Br J Urol* 1985;57:237–238.
290. Berenson RJ, Flynn S, Freiha FS, Kempson R, Torti FM. Primary osteogenic sarcoma of the bladder. *Cancer* 1986;57:350–355.
291. Foote JW, Seemayer TA, Duigan JP. Desmoid tumor involving the bladder: case report. *J Urol* 1975;114:147–149.
292. Rosi P, Selli C, Carni M, Rosi MF. Myxoid liposarcoma of the bladder. *J Urol* 1983;130:560–561.
293. Lake MH, Kossow AS, Bokinsky G. Leiomyoma of the bladder and urethra. *J Urol* 1981;125:742–743.
294. Murao T, Kamoi M, Asano K. Fibroma of the bladder: a light and ultrastructural study of a case with review of the literature in Japan. *Acta Med Okayama* 1979;33:113–120.
295. Winfield HN, Catalona WJ. An isolated plexiform neurofibroma of the bladder. *J Urol* 1985;134:542–543.
296. Fuleihan FM, Cordonnier JJ. Hemagioma of the bladder: report of a case and review of the literature. *J Urol* 1969;102:581–585.
297. Proca E. Haemangioma of the bladder. *Br J Urol* 1977;4:60.
298. Baumgartner G, Gaeta J, Wajsman Z, Merrin C. Hemangiopericytoma of the urinary bladder: a case report and review of the literature. *J Surg Oncol* 1976;8:281–286.
299. Fletcher MS, Aker M, Hill JT, Pryor JP, Whimster WF. Granular cell myoblastoma of the bladder. *Br J Urol* 1985;57:109–110.
300. Mouradian JA, Coleman JW, McGovern JH, Gray GF. Granular cell tumor (myoblastoma) of the bladder. *J Urol* 1974;112:343–345.
301. Ainsworth AM, Clark WH, Mastrangelo M, Conger KB. Primary malignant melanoma of the urinary bladder. *Cancer* 1976;37:1928–1936.
302. Alroy J, Ucci AA, Heaney JA, Mitcheson HD, Gavris VE, Woods W. Multifocal pigmentation of prostatic and bladder urothelium. *J Urol* 1986;136:96–97.
303. Chaitin BA, Manning JT, Ordonez NG. Hematologic neoplasms with initial manifestations in lower urinary tract. *Urology* 1984;23:35–42.
304. Makinen J, Alfthan O, Vuori J. Malignant lymphoma of the urinary bladder: a report of two cases. *Eur Urol* 1979;5:45–47.
305. Ferry JA, Young RH. Malignant lymphoma of the genitourinary tract. *Curr Diagn Pathol* 1997;4:145–169.
306. Zukerberg LR, Harris NL, Young RH. Carcinomas of the urinary bladder simulating malignant lymphoma: a report of five cases. *Am J Surg Pathol* 1991;15:569–576.
307. Yang CH, Krzyaniak K, Brown W, Kurtz SM. Primary carcinoid tumor of urinary bladder. *Urology* 1985;26:594–597.
308. Colby TV. Carcinoid tumor of the bladder. *Arch Pathol Lab Med* 1980;104:199–200.
309. Albores-Saavedra J, Maldonado ME, Ibarra J, Rodriguez H. Pheochromocytoma of the urinary bladder. *Cancer* 1969;23:1110–1118.
310. Leetsma JE, Price EB. Paraganglioma of the urinary bladder. *Cancer* 1971;28:1063–1073.
311. Lieberman PH. Consultation case. *Am J Surg Pathol* 1977;1:83–84.
312. Steeper TA, Rosai J. Aggressive angiomyxoma of the female pelvis and perineum: report of nine cases of a distinctive type of gynecologic soft-tissue neoplasms. *Am J Surg Pathol* 1983;7:463–475.
313. Koss LG. Tumors of the urinary tract and prostate. In: Koss LG, ed. *Diagnostic cytology*. 3rd ed. Philadelphia: JB Lippincott, 1979:767–794.
314. Boutsa NG, Melamed MR. Cytology of in situ carcinoma of the human urinary bladder. *Cancer* 1963;16:1307–1316.
315. Koss LG, Melamed MR, Ricci A, Melick WF, Kelly RE. Carcinogenesis in the human urinary bladder: observations after exposure to paraaminodiphenyl. *N Engl J Med* 1965;272:767–770.
316. Wolinska W, Melamed MR, Klein FA. Cytology of bladder papilloma. *Acta Cytol* 1985;29:817–822.
317. Melamed MR, Mullaney PF, Mendelsohn ML, eds. *Flow cytometry and testing*. New York: John Wiley, 1979.
318. Badalament RA, Gay H, Whitmore WF Jr, et al. Monitoring intravesical bacillus Calmette-Guérin treatment of superficial bladder carcinoma by serial flow cytometry. *Cancer* 1986;58:2751–2757.
319. Devonec M, Darzynkiewicz Z, Whitmore WF Jr, Melamed MR. Flow cytology for follow-up examinations of conservatively treated low stage bladder tumors. *J Urol* 1981;126:166–170.
320. Badalament RA, Hermansenn DK, Kimmel M, et al. The sensitivity of bladder wash flow cytometry, bladder wash cytology, and voided cytology in the detection of bladder carcinoma. *Cancer* 1987;60:1423–1427.
321. Fradet Y, Cordon-Cardo C, Thomson T, et al. Cell surface antigens of human bladder cancer defined by mouse monoclonal antibodies. *Proc Natl Acad Sci U S A* 1984;81:224–228.
322. Dolbeare F, Gratzner H, Pallavicini MG, Gray JW. Flow cytometric measurement of total DNA content and incorporated bromodeoxyuridine. *Proc Natl Acad Sci U S A* 1983;80:5573–5577.
323. Cordon-Cardo C, Lloyd KO, Finstad CL, et al. Immunoanatomic distribution of blood group antigens in human urinary tract: influence of secretor status. *Lab Invest* 1986;55:444–454.
324. Cordon-Cardo C, Reuter VE, Lloyd Ko, et al. Blood group antigens in human urothelium: enhanced expression of precursor, X and Y determinants in urothelial carcinoma. *Cancer Res* 1988;48:4113–4120.
325. Limas C, Lange P, Fraley EE, Vassella RL. A, B, H antigens in transitional cell tumors of the urinary bladder: correlation with clinical course. *Cancer* 1979;44:2099–2107.
326. Juhl B, Harton SH, Hainau B. A, B, H antigen expression in transitional cell carcinomas of the urinary bladder. *Cancer* 1986;57:1768–1775.
327. Sheinfeld J, Reuter VE, Melamed MR, et al. Enhanced bladder cancer detection with the Lewis-x antigen as a marker of neoplastic transformation. *J Urol* 1990;143:285–288.
328. Sidransky D, Messing E. Molecular genetics and biochemical mechanisms in bladder cancer; oncogenes, tumor suppressor genes, and growth factors. *Urol Clin North Am* 1992;19:629–639.
329. Cordon-Cardo C, Reuter VE. Alterations of tumor suppressor genes in bladder cancer. *Semin Diagn Pathol* 1997;14:123–132.
330. Waldman M, Carroll PR, Kerschmann R, et al. Centromeric copy number of chromosome seven is strongly correlated with tumor grade and labeling index in human bladder cancer. *Cancer Res* 1991;51:3807–3813.
331. Presti JC, Reuter VE, Galan T, Rair WR, Cordon-Cardo C. Molecular genetic alterations in superficial and locally advanced human bladder cancer. *Cancer Res* 1991;51:5405–5409.
332. Fujimoto K, Yamada Y, Okajima E, Kakizoe T, Sasaki H, Sugimura T. Frequent association of p53 gene mutation in invasive bladder cancer. *Cancer Res* 1992;52:1393–1398.
333. Sidransky D, Von Eschenbach A, Tsai YC, et al. Identification of p53 gene mutations in bladder cancers and urine samples. *Science* 1991;252:706–709.
334. Cordon-Cardo C, Wartinger D, Petrylak D, et al. Altered expression of retinoblastoma protein and known prognostic variables in locally advanced bladder cancer. *J Natl Cancer Inst* 1992;84:1256–1261.
335. Cairns P, Proctor AJ, Knowles MA. Loss of heterozygosity at the RB locus is frequent and correlates with muscle invasion in bladder carcinoma. *Oncogene* 1991;6:2305–2309.

CHAPTER 45

The Prostate and Seminal Vesicles

Jonathan I. Epstein and Kirk J. Wojno

ANATOMY AND HISTOLOGY

The prostate gland is a functional conduit that allows urine to pass from the urinary bladder to the urethra and adds nutritional secretions to the sperm to form semen during ejaculation. The function of the many secreted products of the prostate, including prostate-specific antigen (PSA) is incompletely understood (1,2). The normal adult prostate weighs approximately 20 g and is roughly funnel shaped. The basal portion of the prostate lies immediately beneath the bladder neck, and the apical region of the prostate rests directly above the urogenital diaphragm. The prostatic urethra runs vertically through the center of the gland and is bent anteriorly at the level of the verumontanum (3). Posteriorly, the prostate and seminal vesicles are separated from the rectum by a thin, filmy layer of connective tissue known as Denonvillier's fascia. At the most apical portion of the gland, the skeletal muscle of the urogenital diaphragm extends into the prostate. Striated muscle continues in the anterior, anterolateral, and, to a lesser extent, posterior regions of the gland to form a sleeve around the prostate (4,5). Although mostly exterior to the gland, these skeletal muscle fibers extend into the peripheral portion of the prostate gland. Consequently the finding of a few benign-appearing prostatic glands admixed with skeletal muscle fibers does not indicate that the glands are neoplastic, and the finding of adenocarcinoma of the prostate admixed with skeletal muscle fibers is likewise not diagnostic of extraprostatic extension by carcinoma. The identification of skeletal muscle fibers in surgical specimens is not associated with an increase in incontinence (6). The prostate gland consists of concentric inner and outer zones where clinically detectable carcinomas predominantly affect the outer region of the gland, and benign prostatic hyperplasia involves the central inner aspect of the gland (7).

For practical purposes, McNeal's model is often simplified such that the central inner periurethral aspect of the prostate is termed the "transition zone," and the outer peripheral aspect is referred to as the "peripheral zone" and includes the "central zone," which is located toward the base of the prostate (5,) (Fig. 1).

Microscopically the prostate is composed of glandular epithelium and fibromuscular stroma. The duct and glandular system is arranged in a complex architectural pattern. The ducts consist of elongated branching tubular structures and end blindly in rounded acini. Ducts cut in cross section are indistinguishable from acini. The luminal surfaces of benign prostate glands often have undulating contours and papillary infoldings. These glands are lined by three distinct epithelial cell populations; secretory cells, basal cells, and neuroendocrine cells. The luminally located secretory cells are terminally differentiated and stain positively with prostate-specific antigen, prostatic acid phosphatase, and other enzymes. The nonneoplastic secretory cells have been noted to contain acid and neutral mucins, lipofuscin, and melanin (8–10). Basal cells are peripherally located in the gland between the secretory cells and the basement membrane. They are football- to cigar-shaped with the long axis parallel to the basement membrane. The basal cells may either have a finely granular, uniformly distributed chromatin pattern or prominent nucleoli, often have a prominent nuclear groove, and stain with high-molecular-weight keratin (34Be12) 34BE12 (11–13). Basal cells are thought to represent the stem cell compartment within the prostate (14). Neuroendocrine cells are irregularly distributed throughout the ducts and acini and are difficult to recognize without the use of special staining techniques. Their exact function is unknown, but it is thought that they function in a paracrine fashion to regulate adjacent cells.

BENIGN PROSTATIC HYPERTROPHY

The prostate slowly enlarges from birth to puberty. Thereafter, the prostate rapidly increases in size until the ages of 21 to 30 years, at which point, the prostate weighs, on average,

---

J. I. Epstein: Department of Pathology, The Johns Hopkins Hospital, Baltimore, Maryland 21287.

K. J. Wojno: Department of Pathology, The University of Michigan, Ann Arbor, Michigan 48109-0054.

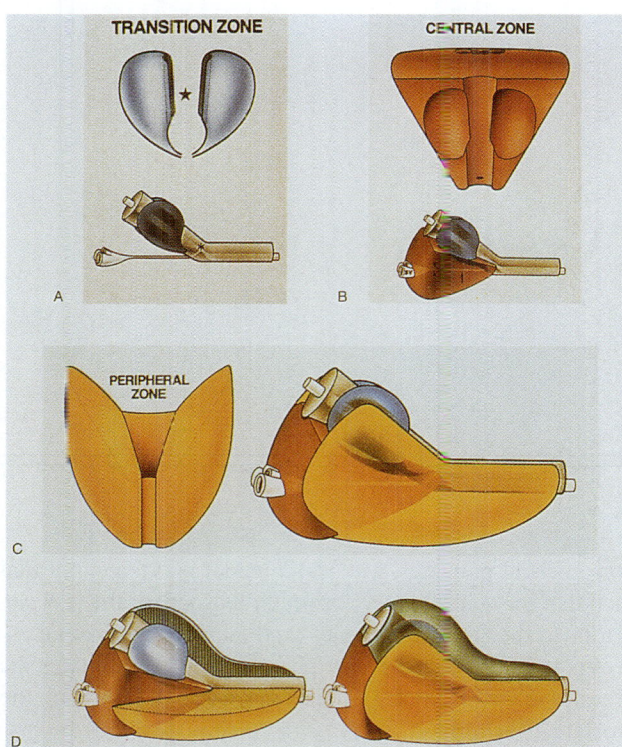

FIG. 1. McNeal's model of zonal anatomy of the prostate.

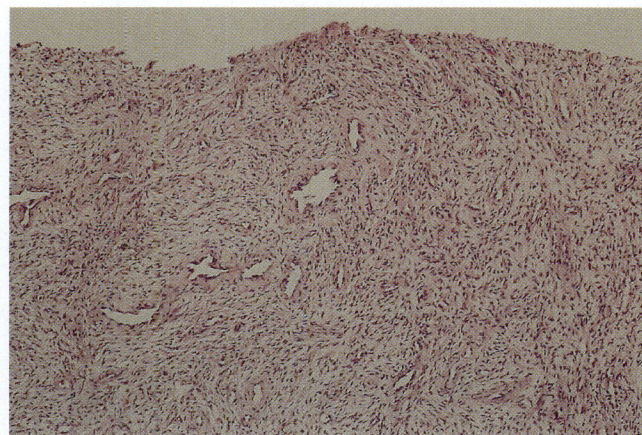

FIG. 2. Stromal nodule of hyperplasia on needle biopsy. Nodules are composed of loose mesenchyme containing prominent small round vessels.

20 g (15). The frequency of benign prostatic hypertrophy (BPH) is extremely low in men younger than 40 years, after which its development increases steadily to the point at which BPH is the most common urologic disorder in men. Symptomatic BPH increases proportionately with increasing age.

Franks (7) described a spectrum of five histologic subtypes of BPH and their differing epithelial and stromal components ranging from pure stromal to nearly pure epithelial nodules. The earliest BPH nodules are predominantly stromal and are composed mainly of fibrous tissue admixed with some smooth muscle (16). These stromal nodules are located submucosally in the periurethral region and seldom reach large size except near the bladder neck, where they may protrude as a solitary midline mass into the bladder lumen (Fig. 2).

The larger and more numerous BPH nodules are almost always more laterally situated and tend to occur in the transition zone (3) (Fig. 3). These laterally placed nodules are predominantly glandular from inception and are the cause of most clinically evident BPH. Histologically, the glandular component is made up of nodules of small and large acini, some showing papillary infoldings infoldings and projections containing central fibrovascular cores, and others that are dilated and cystic (Fig. 4). The luminal secretory epithelium comprises tall columnar cells with pale-staining granular cytoplasm and round euchromatic nuclei with inconspicuous nucleoli. Situated beneath the secretory cells is the basal cell layer, composed of cells with scant cytoplasm and oval nuclei oriented horizontally, parallel to the basement membrane. The stromal component often shows both fibrous and smooth-muscle elements. Less commonly, BPH nodules may be found within the peripheral zone (17).

The nearly pure epithelial nodules have been labeled adenosis (atypical adenomatous hyperplasia) (18) (see p. 19). Although adenosis can be a morphologic mimic of carcinoma and has been suggested as a possible precursor lesion, it has no known association with cancer (19).

Within areas of BPH, we often find nodules or a diffuse stromal infiltrate of lymphocytes and plasma cells in a periglandular distribution. However, in the majority of cases, these findings have not been identified with an infectious process or clinical symptoms of prostatitis (20,21). Whereas acute inflammation appears to correlate with serum PSA increases, there are conflicting studies as to the effect of chronic inflammation (22,23). Because the histologic finding of inflammation does not correlate with clinical prostati-

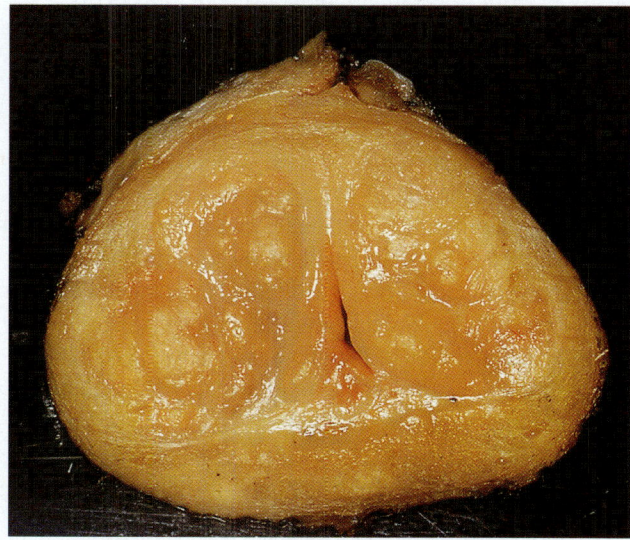

FIG. 3. Gross photograph of benign prostatic hyperplasia.

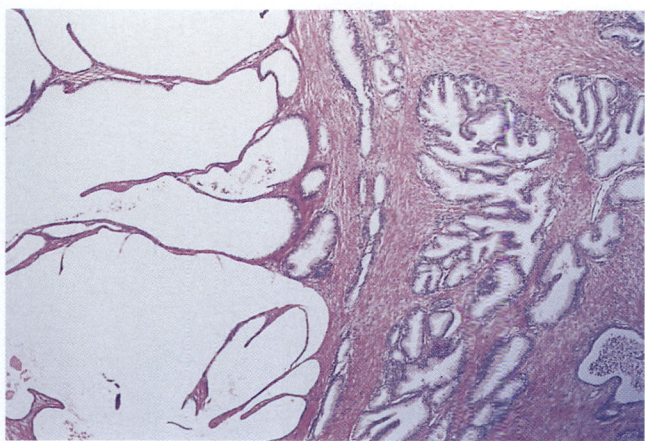

FIG. 4. Benign prostatic hyperplasia composed of nodules of cystically dilated glands and hyperplastic glands.

tis, we do not sign out surgical specimens as showing "acute prostatitis" or "chronic prostatitis," but rather as showing "acute inflammation" or "chronic inflammation."

In approximately 20% to 25% of specimens removed for BPH, prostatic infarcts can be found, ranging in size from a few millimeters to 5 cm (16,24). In the acute phase, discrete foci of coagulative necrosis involve the epithelium and connective tissue. Healed infarcts can be identified by areas of dense scar formation. Grossly, they appear yellow or mottled with a hemorrhagic margin and are somewhat firmer than the surrounding prostatic tissue. Patients with acute prostatic infarcts have glands twice as large as those in patients without infarcts and are more prone to have acute urinary retention or histories of gross hematuria. Because the infarcts are often small and not close to the urethra, the symptoms may not be due to the infarcts but, instead, may be due to the larger size of the glands containing them. Surrounding acute prostatic infarcts, we can often see islands of immature squamous metaplasia (25) (Fig. 5). These nests rarely show keratinization and can easily be distinguished from squamous carcinoma by their lack of pleomorphism and the localized nature of the process to the area immediately adjacent to the infarct.

PROSTATIC INFECTIONS

Bacterial Prostatitis

Although acute and chronic prostatitis make up a significant portion of urologic practice, they are usually diagnosed clinically and treated with antibiotics, without the need for surgical intervention. Consequently, the histologic examination of specimens removed for symptomatic prostatitis is uncommon. Whereas it is difficult to distinguish histologically chronic infectious prostatitis from nonspecific chronic inflammation seen in hyperplasia, acute bacterial prostatitis is characterized by sheets of neutrophils within and around acini, intraductal desquamated cellular debris, and stromal edema and hyperemia. Although microabscess formation is not uncommon, the advent of effective antibiotics led to a vast decline in the incidence of symptomatic prostatic abscess formation. The most common type of prostatic abscess formation is in individuals with preexisting bladder-outlet obstruction in whom a prostatic abscess develops as a result of a lower urinary tract infection (26). Much less frequently, prostatic abscesses arise by dissemination from an extraurinary source of infection, the most common being staphylococcal infections involving the skin.

Mycotic Prostatitis

Of the deep mycoses, the largest number of prostatic infections are observed with blastomycosis, coccidiomycosis, and cryptococcosis. Cases also have been reported of histoplasmosis, paracoccidiomycosis, and aspergillosis of the prostate (27). Most, if not all, cases of mycotic prostatitis occur in the setting of systemic hematogenous dissemination.

Tuberculous Prostatitis

The incidence of prostatic involvement in systemic tuberculosis ranges from 3% to 12%, with more than 90% of these cases also showing lung involvement (28,29). In cases with urogenital tuberculosis, the prostate is involved in 75% to 95% of the cases. However, in only 7% to 13% of the cases of uro-

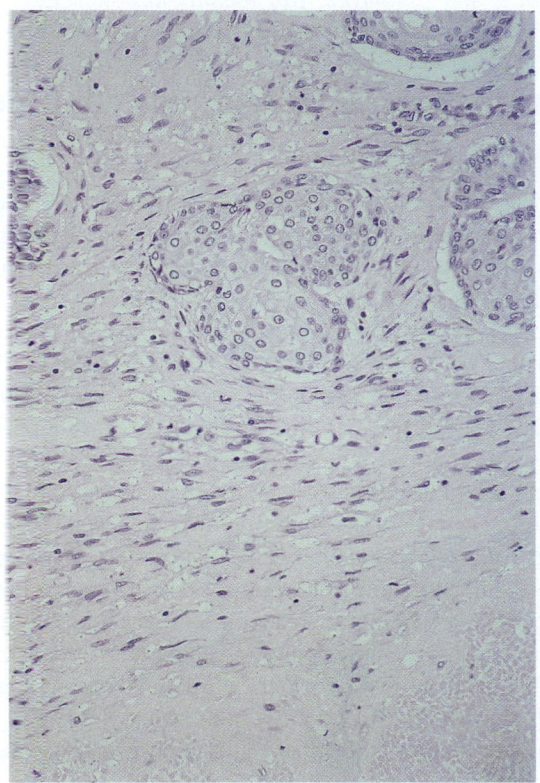

FIG. 5. Infarct (bottom) with adjacent squamous metaplasia.

genital tuberculosis is the prostate the sole organ involved. Systemic tuberculous prostatitis is rarely seen in today's surgical pathology practice as a result of (a) the declining incidence of the disease and (b) the presence of other nonprostatic signs and symptoms of infection, leading to diagnosis and treatment.

A more recent form of tuberculous involvement of the prostate is that following bacillus Calmette-Guérin (BCG) immunotherapy for superficial transitional cell cancer of the bladder. The granulomas may be small, noncaseating, and close to the urethral surface. These granulomas are expected after BCG therapy and are usually seen in follow-up biopsies done to evaluate urothelial atypia. In addition, larger noncaseating and caseating granulomas may be found throughout the prostate, resulting in an abnormal rectal examination or in increased serum PSA levels (30–31). Regardless of the histologic pattern of BCG-related granulomatous prostatitis or the presence or absence of acid-fast bacilli on special stains, patients have remained asymptomatic and require no specific therapy. Patients are monitored for systemic signs and symptoms, because on rare occasions, disseminated tuberculosis after BCG has been reported.

Miscellaneous Infections

Other infections involving the prostate, some of which are more commonly seen in developing countries, are exceedingly rare in today's practice of surgical pathology in this country. These include brucellosis, schistosomiasis, amoebic prostatitis, syphilis, actinomycosis, and infection by atypical mycobacteria (32–38). The role of *Trichomonas vaginalis* and *Chlamydia trachomatis* in nonbacterial prostatitis remains controversial (39–41).

NONINFECTIOUS INFLAMMATORY CONDITIONS

Nonspecific Granulomatous Prostatitis

The most commonly diagnosed noninfectious granulomatous process within the prostate is termed nonspecific granulomatous prostatitis (42,43). The lesion consists of a lobular dense infiltrate of lymphocytes, plasma cells, and histiocytes (Fig. 6). Many of the histiocytes have a foamy appearance, and some are multinucleated. Neutrophils and eosinophils make up a smaller component of the inflammatory infiltrate (Fig. 7). These dense nodules of inflammation tend to obscure and efface ductal and acinar elements. The earliest lesion of nonspecific granulomatous prostatitis consists of dilated ducts and acini filled with neutrophils, debris, and desquamated epithelial cells (Fig. 6). Focal rupture of these ducts and acini results in a localized granulomatous and chronic inflammatory reaction. The extension of the infiltrate into surrounding ductal and acinar units accounts for the characteristic lobular pattern of more advanced nonspecific granulomatous prostatitis. In most cases, there is little histologic similarity between nonspecific granulomatous prostatitis and infectious granulomatous inflammation of the prostate. Although discrete small granulomas can be seen

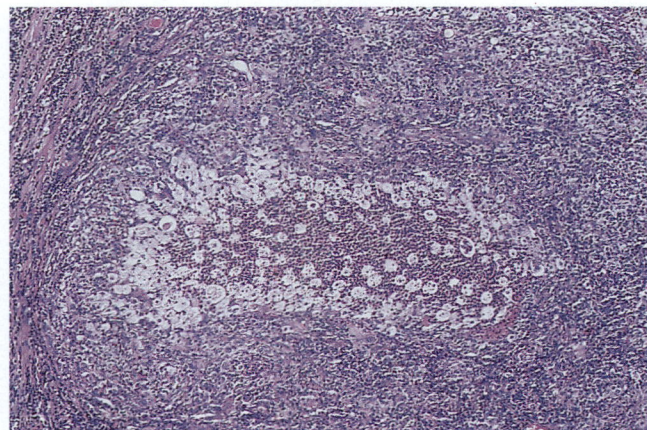

FIG. 6. Nonspecific granulomatous prostatitis with dilated prostatic ducts containing numerous neutrophils and foamy histiocytes. Note lobular configuration.

with nonspecific granulomatous prostatitis, they are always seen with the early lesion surrounding a ruptured dilated duct or acinus. Areas of necrosis within the center of small lesions of nonspecific granulomatous prostatitis contain numerous neutrophils. Older lesions of nonspecific granulomatous prostatitis show a more prominent fibrous component. Nonspecific granulomatous prostatitis is thought to result from a local foreign-body reaction to ruptured prostatic secretions and contents and tends to resolve spontaneously. Clinically, the symptoms are those of either urinary obstruction or a severe lower urinary tract infection. The average age at time of diagnosis is in the early sixties, with a wide age range from the twenties to the very elderly. The major significance of this lesion is that the rectal examination in nonspecific granulomatous prostatitis commonly reveals nodularity or induration such that carcinoma of the prostate is often suspected. Nonspecific granulomatous prostatitis, in particular cases with prominent epithelioid histiocytes, may be misdiagnosed as adenocarcinoma of the prostate on needle biopsy (44)

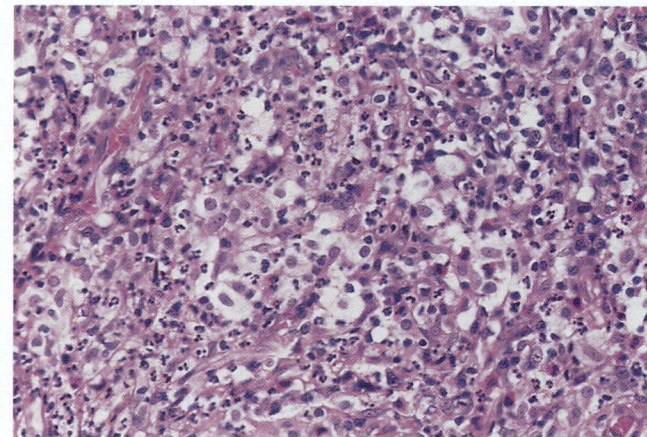

FIG. 7. Nonspecific granulomatous prostatitis consisting of foamy histiocytes, neutrophils, lymphocytes, and plasma cells. Eosinophils also may be noted.

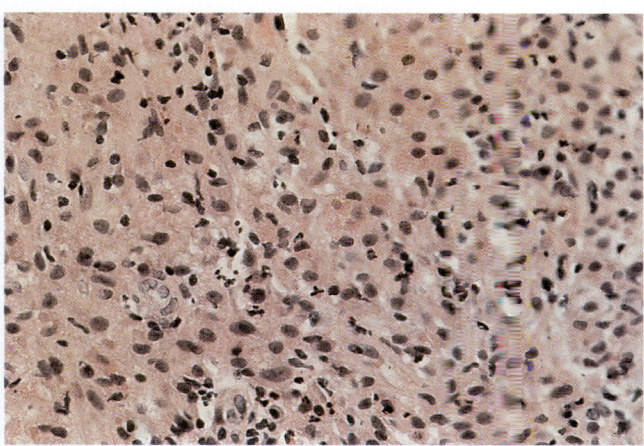

FIG. 8. Nonspecific granulomatous prostatitis with epithelioid histiocytes mimicking prostate cancer.

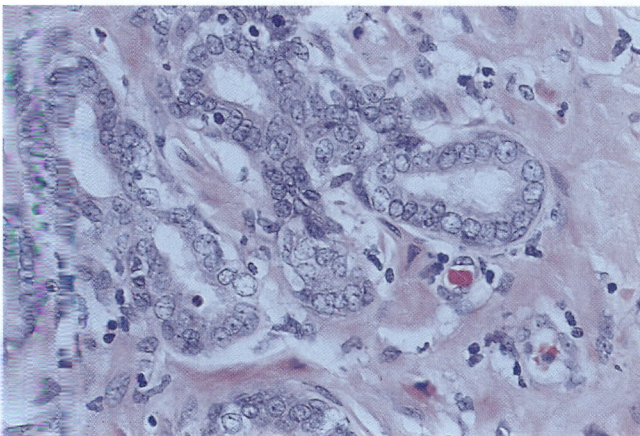

FIG. 10. Chronic inflammation resulting in reactive nuclear atypia and occasional prominent nucleoli in atrophic glands.

(Fig. 8). The finding of plasma cells, neutrophils, and eosinophils helps to identify the lesion as prostatitis. The clustering of the epithelioid histiocytes around partially ruptured acini, which may sometimes be appreciated on needle biopsy, contrasts with the diffuse nature of high-grade prostate cancer. If difficulty persists, immunohistochemical stains for histiocytic markers and epithelial markers can differentiate the two entities (45). As a result of the inflammation, reactive architectural and cytologic atypia may occur (Figs. 9 and 10).

Posttransurethral Resection Granulomas

Posttransurethral resection (post-TUR) granulomas are composed of a central region of fibrinoid necrosis surrounded by palisading epithelioid histiocytes (46) (Fig. 11). The numbers of granulomas seen in a case may range from one to ten. Although lesions can assume a multitude of round, ovoid, triangular, and rectangular shapes, a somewhat characteristic configuration is that of long, tortuous granulomas dissecting the tissue. In the tissue surrounding the necrobiotic granulomas, multinucleated giant cells and granulomas without central necrosis are common findings. Inflammation surrounding the granulomas is usually minimal consisting predominantly of lymphocytes and plasma cells with scattered eosinophils. The post-TUR intervals with which these granulomas may be identified range from 9 days to 52 months. When the interval between TUR resections is approximately 1 month or less, abundant eosinophils can be identified. Before the recognition of this disorder, post-TUR granulomas with numerous eosinophils had been reported in the literature as allergic granulomatous prostatitis. The post-TUR granuloma appears to be a reaction to altered epithelium and stroma from the trauma of previous cautery. Although within the center of most post-TUR granulomas, there is only amorphous fibrinoid material, in some cases, there may be necrotic epithelial and stromal components. The recognition of similar granulomas after cautery in

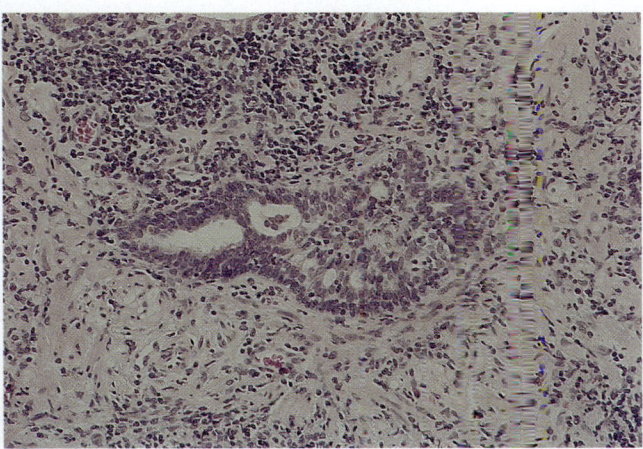

FIG. 9. Reactive benign cribriform prostatic gland due to inflammation.

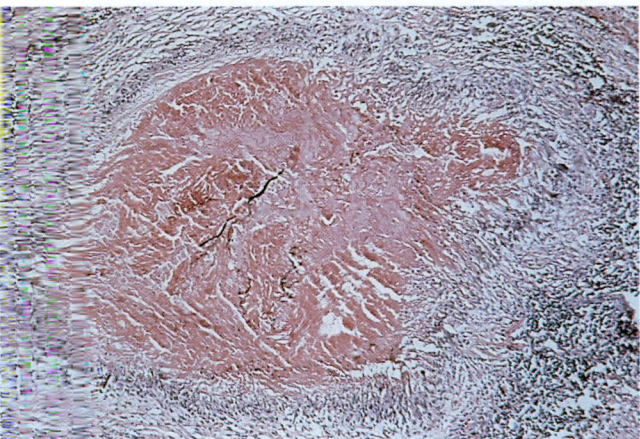

FIG. 11. Posttransurethral resection granuloma with central fibrinoid necrosis and surrounding palisading histiocytes.

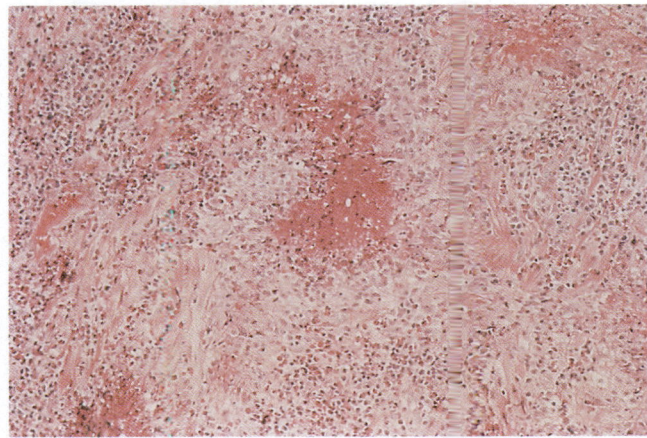

FIG. 12. Allergic granulomatous prostatitis with multiple small foci of eosinophilic necrosis surrounded by abundant eosinophils. (Courtesy of Dr. B.S. Bhagavan, Baltimore, Maryland.)

other sites argues against the process resulting solely from altered epithelium or secretions unique to the prostate. Rarely similar linear granulomas may be seen after needle biopsy. Post-TUR granulomas appear to be incidental findings and are commonly seen in radical prostatectomy specimens removed for carcinoma when a prior TUR resection was performed. The lesion is so characteristic and histologically distinct from infectious granuloma that stains for organisms are not necessary.

Allergic Granulomatous Prostatitis

Allergic granulomatous prostatitis, as a reflection of a more generalized allergic reaction, is an exceedingly uncommon condition (47). It is characterized histologically by multiple small, ovoid necrobiotic granulomas surrounded by numerous eosinophils (Fig. 12). The regularity of the size and shape of these granulomas and the extensive infiltration of eosinophils throughout the stroma, not just surrounding the granulomas, separates this entity from that of post-TUR granulomas with eosinophils. When numerous eosinophils are present in a lesion of nonspecific granulomatous prostatitis, it also should be distinguished from allergic granulomatous prostatitis. Of the 12 patients with allergic granulomatous prostatitis reported in the literature, all had either asthma or evidence of systemic allergic reactions at the time of diagnosis of the prostatic lesions, and the majority of affected individuals had increased blood eosinophil counts. Most important, in a few cases, similar granulomas were found systemically, and in one individual were a contributing factor in his death. Consequently recognition of this disease, as well as distinguishing it from other granulomatous prostatic lesions with eosinophils, is important if prompt and aggressive treatment with steroids is to be instituted.

Malakoplakia

Malakoplakia of the prostate has uncommonly been reported in the world literature; histologically they are indistinguishable from those occurring in other sites (48). The ages of the patients with prostatic malakoplakia range from 47 to 85 years. Clinically the symptoms are nonspecific, and on rectal examination, the prostate is enlarged and suggestive of carcinoma.

BENIGN NONNEOPLASTIC CONDITIONS

Amyloid

Some 2% to 10% of prostates with BPH or carcinoma contain vascular amyloid deposits (49,50). A higher incidence of prostatic amyloidosis is seen in patients with multiple myeloma, primary amyloidosis of the kidney, or chronic debilitating diseases. The location of amyloid in these cases is in vessels and subepithelial areas. Corpora amylacea also often nonspecifically stain for amyloid.

Calculi and Calcification

Prostatic calculi are those calculi that are found within the tissues or acini of the gland and should be distinguished from urinary calculi found within the prostatic urethra (51,52). Although prostatic calculi are common, they are usually asymptomatic and are discovered incidentally during diagnostic procedures performed for other conditions. Prostatic calculi are present in 70% to 100% of the glands studied at autopsy. The majority are found in men older than 50 years. Generally prostatic calculi are multiple and small, with an average diameter of less than 5 mm. Larger ones ranging in size up to 4 cm, however, have been identified. They are brownish gray, as well as round to ovoid, and they usually have a smooth surface. They are more often found within large central prostatic ducts and, when peripherally located, may sometimes be found in cystic cavities. Histologically, the calculi appear stratified in concentric layers resembling calcified corpora amylacea. Current studies suggested that prostatic calculi form by the consolidation and calcification of corpora amylacea or by calcification of precipitated prostatic secretions or both. Abscess formation caused by prostatic calculi is an uncommon complication. This situation may occur in patients who have urinary tract infections resistant to antimicrobial therapy, in which the prostatic calculi are infected and provide a continual source of prostatic urinary infection. In addition to the uncommon occurrence of infected prostatic calculi, prostatic calculi are significant in that they may be confused on clinical examination with carcinoma of the prostate.

Cysts

Prostatic cysts can be subdivided into utricle cysts and retention cysts (53,54). Most utricle cysts lie outside the prostate between the bladder and rectum, with the orifice of the cyst located at the prostatic utricle. The patients range in age from 2 months to 75 years, with a median age of 26 years. In approximately 25% of the cases, abnormalities of the external genitalia can be identified, and in about 10% of the cases, there is unilateral renal dysgenesis or agenesis. Histologically, the cyst walls may lack an epithelial lining or may be composed of columnar, cuboidal, transitional or, less frequently, squamous epithelium. In approximately 10% of the cases, calculi are formed within the cyst. Other associations include four cases of cystadenoma and isolated cases of squamous cell carcinoma and adenocarcinoma arising in the cysts. Retention cysts arise when prostatic acini become distended with clear fluid. Clusters of dilated prostatic glands may appear hypoechoic on transrectal ultrasound, mimicking carcinoma. Because small asymptomatic dilated prostatic acini may frequently be found, the term retention cyst should be reserved only for those cysts that are symptomatic. Defined accordingly, the cysts range in size from 1 to 2 cm, are usually unilocular, and are found adjacent to the urethra. Histologically, the cysts are lined with flattened prostatic glandular epithelium or transitional epithelium.

Melanocytic Lesions

In general, "blue nevus" has been used to denote melanin confined to ovoid or elongated melanocytes in the prostatic stroma, and "melanosis" used for prostatic lesions with melanin present in both the stroma and glandular epithelium (9). Prostatic blue nevi account for approximately 65% of these cases. In about 50% of cases, there is grossly evident pigment, measuring up to 2 cm. Microscopically, blue nevi show numerous melanin-filled spindle-shaped cells in a fibromuscular stroma. Ultrastructurally, the cells appear to be melanocytes with melanosomes in different stages of differentiation. In a few cases, foci of adenocarcinoma of the prostate also were noted to contain melanin. Nonneoplastic and neoplastic prostatic epithelial cells with melanin contain only mature stage 4 melanosomes, suggesting that epithelial

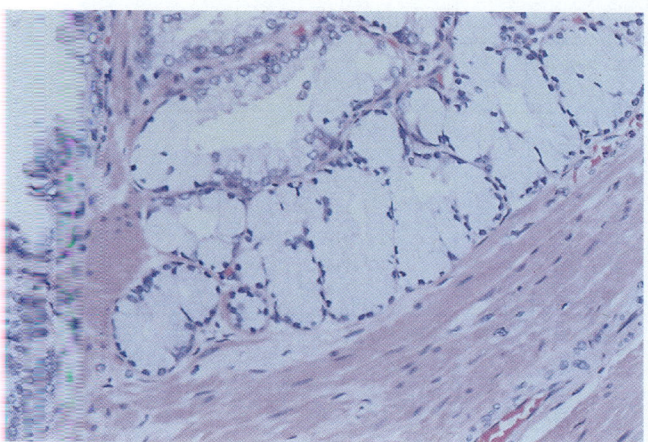

FIG. 14. Mucinous metaplasia of the prostate.

melanin results from a transfer of pigment from the stromal melanocytes. These melanotic lesions are benign. Rare reports of a malignant melanoma, apparently primary, whose first clinical manifestation was in the prostate gland were reported (55).

Miscellaneous Benign Lesions

Rare cases of prostatic endometriosis, Wegener's granulomatosis, and vasculitis were reported with prostatic symptoms (56–59). Other benign lesions reported in the prostate include ganglioneuroma, mucinous metaplasia, xanthoma, and Paneth's cell metaplasia (60–63) (Figs. 13 and 14). Prostatic cystadenomas are large tumorlike lesions with the appearance of BPH. They were reported to arise in the retrovesicle space, either attached to the prostate by a pedicle or apparently separate from the prostate (64). Occasionally these lesions are intraprostatic and are differentiated from BPH only when they are composed of a well-circumscribed nodule occupying one side of an otherwise nonhyperplastic gland.

ADENOCARCINOMA OF THE PROSTATE

Approximately one of every five American men will be diagnosed with prostate cancer in their lifetime, and about 3% will die of it. The American Cancer Society estimated 209,900 new cases of adenocarcinoma of the prostate in 1997, which well surpassed lung cancer as the most prevalently diagnosed carcinoma in men. There were projected to be 41,800 deaths attributable to prostate cancer in 1997, second only to deaths resulting from lung cancer (65).

The incidence of adenocarcinoma of the prostate found at autopsy increases with age and varies depending on the method of sampling the gland. Especially in men younger than 50 years, increased numbers of carcinomas of the prostate are identified by step-sectioning the gland rather than by examining only random sections of the prostate (66–69) (Table 1). The carefully done study of medical ex-

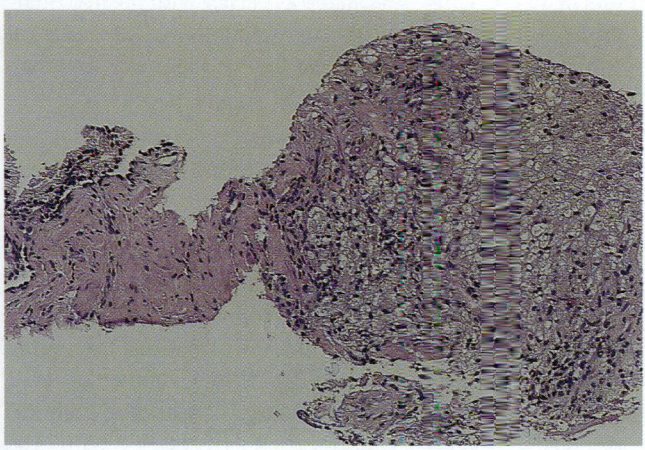

FIG. 13. Xanthoma of the prostate.

TABLE 1. Incidence of carcinoma of prostate at autopsy

Age range (yr)	Random sections (%)	Step sections (%)
<30	0	0
30–49	0–0.2	4
40–49	0–3.8	4.9–17
50–59	6.4–29	10.4–14
60–69	12.5–30.2	17.8–23
70–79	17.4–40	21–41
80–89	26–66.7	29–54

Data from refs. 66–69, with permission.

aminer cases by Sakr (70) highlighted the high incidence (34%) of histologically diagnosable but clinically inapparent prostate cancer in men younger than 50 years who die of trauma (70). This raises the question as to whether the apparent increase in prostate cancer incidence is due to PSA screening or is a true phenomenon.

Men younger than 50 years have a broad spectrum of disease, ranging from small insignificant tumors to advanced incurable cancer. Young men who are candidates for radical prostatectomy do not have a worse prognosis after surgery than do older men. These men may be diagnosed in the workup of other genitourinary symptoms unrelated to the prostate or because of a family history of prostate cancer (71,72). Older studies that claimed an almost universally dismal prognosis for this group predated the use of serum PSA tests and contained many men with large tumors obstructing the urethra (73).

Adenocarcinoma of the prostate in childhood and adolescence is rare, with approximately five cases in patients younger than 10 years and 21 cases between the ages of 10 and 21 years reported (74). Patients tend to have obstructive symptoms and at an advanced stage, showing a metastatic pattern similar to that seen in adults. The tumors are almost uniformly poorly differentiated and are not responsive to treatment, with an average survival ranging between 3 and 10 months.

Most studies demonstrated that black patients are first seen with a higher stage of disease than white patients and thus have an overall greater mortality rate from prostate cancer (75). However, stage for stage, black and white patients have equivalent survival figures, although recent studies showed an earlier time to biochemical failure (76,77).

The incidence of clinically detected adenocarcinoma of the prostate varies significantly among nations. In particular, Scandinavian countries have relatively high rates, and Asian nations have very low rates (65,75). It is of note that the incidence of incidentally discovered adenocarcinoma of the prostate at autopsy is relatively uniform among different nations. On migration of persons from low- to high-incidence countries, the rate of clinical prostate cancer increases, suggesting a role for environmental factors (78).

Staging Classification

In the United States, the most frequently used clinical staging system for prostatic adenocarcinoma is the TNM system. Stages T1a and T1b adenocarcinoma of the prostate are clinically unsuspected tumor that is discovered in either TURP or enucleation specimens removed for BPH (see p. 1923). Stage T1c disease refers to nonpalpable prostate cancer is found on needle biopsy, usually performed for an abnormal serum PSA determination (see p. 1924). Stage T2 is defined as palpable tumor localized to the prostate. Clinical stage T2 disease is further subcategorized into stages T2a and T2b, depending on whether unilateral or bilateral tumor is present. Stage T3 represents tumor that has extended out of the prostate gland (see p. 1925). Stage T3 is further subclassified into T3a and T3b, depending on whether the extraprostatic tumor is without or with seminal vesicle invasion, respectively. Stage N1 disease indicates the presence of metastases to regional lymph nodes, and M1 represents distant metastasis (see p. 1925). As with all staging systems, we must be aware of whether we are referring to the clinical or pathologic stage. For example, a patient with clinical stage T2b disease that appears, on rectal examination, to be confined to the prostate may eventually be upstaged to stage T3 disease if his prostatectomy specimen is shown to have tumor extending out of the gland.

There is no officially sanctioned pathologic staging system, but a consensus panel proposed the following modifications to the TNM system, which should be used for pathologic staging of prostate cancer until the American Joint Committee on Cancer adopts an official pathologic staging system (79). A radical prostatectomy performed for stage T1 disease is staged as T2 or T3, depending on whether tumor is organ confined. Pathologic stage T2 is left unmodified and represents organ-confined disease, as laterality has not proven to be of any prognostic value. Stage T2+ represents tumor with no identifiable tumor in extraprostatic adipose tissue but with a positive margin (capsular incision). T3a is subdivided according to focal versus established tumor in extraprostatic adipose tissue, by using one high-power field for semiquantitive estimate of the amount of extraprostatic tumor. T3a+ or T3b+ is the same as earlier with positive margins. T4 is controversial but usually refers to extensive invasion into the detrussor muscle at the bladder neck, and T4+ is the same with a positive margin.

Presentation of Disease: Means of Establishing Diagnosis

Stage T1a-b prostate cancer refers to tumor that is unsuspected clinically and that is incidentally discovered in specimens usually removed for benign prostatic hypertrophy. With the advent of numerous treatment options, including pharmacologic and thermal therapies, the number of TUR resection specimens seen in the surgical pathology laboratory has markedly decreased. Conversely, with the widespread use of serum PSA testing, the number of nonpalpable cancers diagnosed by needle biopsy (stage T1c) has markedly increased (80,81). In patients with an abnormality noted on rectal examination or an abnormal serum PSA, tissue obtained for histologic examination will usually be obtained by core biopsy. Despite the controversies as to the efficacies of prostate cancer screening, it is nonetheless being adopted within the urologic community. The controversies center around the high false-negative and false-positive rates. The sensitivity of transrectal ultrasonography (TRUS) in identifying tumors greater than 5 mm is only approximately 60% and is therefore falling out of favor (82). False-positive ultrasound examinations may result from inflammation, cystic dilatation of prostate glands, prostatic intraepithelial neoplasia (PIN; see p. 1914), atrophy, and fibrosis from prior TUR (83). Approximately 50% of organ-confined tumor and 33% with extraprostatic extension are associated with normal serum PSA levels (84). Elevated serum PSA levels also may be due to nodular hyperplasia, prostatic biopsy, and inflammation. Recently attempts to factor in the volume of BPH as a contributor to serum PSA levels resulted in a measurement called PSA density (PSAD) or, synonymously, PSA index. The serum PSA level is divided by the volume of the prostate, as calculated by TRUS, yielding PSA per gram of tissue. Because carcinoma produces more PSA per gram of tissue than does BPH, a high PSAD may be a better indication of carcinoma than the use of the uncorrected PSA value (85). Another technique to enhance screening that has been recently proposed is PSA velocity, in which the change of PSA per unit time is measured (86). More recently, age-specific PSA reference ranges and percentage free PSA have become additional tools in the prostate cancer screening armamentarium (87). Age-specific reference ranges try to increase sensitivity and specificity of the test by accounting for the increasing PSA seen with aging. Most prostate cancer allows the complex form of PSA into the serum, whereas BPH tends to release the free form of PSA into the circulation. Therefore a low percentage of free PSA is suggestive of cancer (1,88,89). Screening by some method is recommended in young (40 to 50 years) men with a strong family history of prostate cancer (90).

Core biopsy of the prostate may be performed via a transrectal or rarely a transperineal route. The core-biopsy needle varies from a 14-gauge Tru-CUT needle to the more recently introduced 18-gauge spring-driven Biopty gun (C. R. Bard, Inc., Covington, GA, U.S.A.). The Biopty gun is usually used transrectally, with or without ultrasound guidance. Because of its thin gauge, multiple biopsies may be performed either concurrently or in follow-up. In addition to performing a biopsy of the area of palpable abnormality, most authors recommend random systematic biopsies to enhance detection (91). The false-negative rate with core biopsies of the prostate is approximately 25% from 12% to 28% (92). These figures vary depending on the type of biopsy performed, the degree of palpable abnormality, and the number of biopsies performed. In general, transrectal biopsies are more accurate than transperineal. Specimens should be considered unsatisfactory when there is only minimal or no prostatic glandular or stromal tissue. Cores of prostatic tissue containing only stroma are not unsatisfactory specimens and may represent biopsy of a predominantly stromal nodule of hyperplasia. Negative biopsies of prostates that are clinically suggestive of carcinoma are not uncommon and may not represent a false-negative biopsy, because only about 50% of nodular prostates contain carcinoma (93). A rare complication after perineal needle biopsy is that of tumor seeding the perineal needle tract (94). Most of these cases have been poorly differentiated adenocarcinomas. Recently tumor seeding in soft tissue away from the biopsy site also has been noted in radical prostatectomy specimens, in which most of the carcinomas were intermediate grade and some diagnosed via transrectal needle biopsy (95).

Adenocarcinoma of the prostate also may be diagnosed in the workup for metastatic carcinoma of unknown origin. The importance of identifying these tumors as being of prostatic origin is that even widespread metastatic prostate carcinoma may be hormonally responsive, and treatment may lead to dramatic and sometimes long-term symptomatic relief of both local and distant tumor growth. Because the bones are a common site of presentation for prostate cancer, immunoperoxidase stains for prostate-specific acid phosphatase (PSAP) or PSA or both should be performed on all cases of metastatic adenocarcinoma to the bone in men without known primaries. Prostate carcinoma also shows a tendency to metastasize to left-sided cervical or other supradiaphragmatic lymph nodes, often as the first manifestation of prostate cancer (96). Before immunohistochemical staining for PSA and PSAP became readily available, most of the cases that were recognized were histologically suggestive of prostate cancer. Subsequently, it has been shown that prostate cancers metastatic to supradiaphragmatic lymph nodes are often poorly differentiated and may not be suggestive of prostate carcinoma histologically. Furthermore, patients may have normal rectal examinations and an absence of metastatic bone disease. Despite the high grade of these tumors, either PSA or PSAP staining will be present in almost all cases. By using immunoperoxidase for PSA and PSAP, metastatic prostate carcinoma should therefore be ruled out in all men older than 45 years with carcinoma of unknown primary in left-sided supradiaphragmatic lymph nodes, even in the absence of clinical or pathologic features suggesting prostate cancer.

Pathologists should also be attuned to prostate carcinoma seen as a rectal mass (97). In some cases, the prostate cannot be palpated because of the rectal tumor. In the remaining cases, the gland may be either unremarkable or suggestive of carcinoma. Cases may or may not have increased acid phosphatase levels or bone metastases at the time of presentation. The lesions have ranged in location from the anal verge to 17 cm from the anal verge. Grossly, the lesion may be indistinguishable from a colonic primary, growing as an annular stenosing or eccentric mass. Although most prostate carcinomas that invade the rectum lack mucosal involvement, approximately 20% of the cases may invade the rectal mucosa, further mimicking a colonic primary. Most of the cases have been described as poorly differentiated histologically. The finding of submucosal tumor in the colon that lacks an in situ component and is not histologically typical of colonic adenocarcinoma should suggest the possibility of an extrinsic tumor, and immunohistochemical staining with PSA and PSAP should be performed. We must be aware that rectal carcinoids react with antibodies to PSAP (98).

Grade

The most widely used grading system is the Gleason system. The Gleason system is based on the glandular pattern of the tumor as identified at relatively low magnification (99,100) (Figs. 15 through 21). In contrast to some of the other proposed systems for grading prostate carcinoma, cytologic features play no role in the grade of the tumor. Both the primary (predominant) and the secondary (second most prevalent) architectural patterns are identified and assigned a grade from 1 to 5, with 1 being the most differentiated and 5 being undifferentiated.

When Gleason compared his grading system with survival rates, it was noted that in tumors with two distinct tumor patterns, the observed number of deaths generally was between the number expected on the basis of the primary pattern and that based on the secondary pattern. Because both the primary and secondary patterns were considered influential in predicting prognosis, a combined Gleason grade resulted, obtained by the addition of the primary and secondary

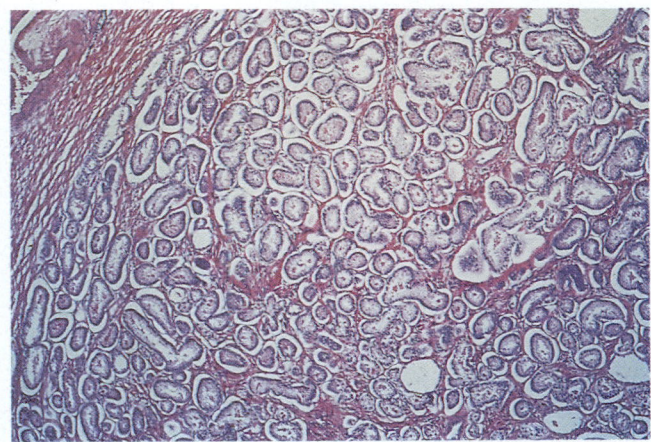

FIG. 16. Gleason pattern 1 tumor composed of a circumscribed nodule of uniform, single, separate, closely packed glands.

grades. If a tumor had only one histologic pattern, then for uniformity, the primary and secondary scores were given the same grade. The combined Gleason grades range from 2 (1 + 1 = 2), which represents tumors uniformly composed of Gleason pattern 1 tumor, to 10 (5 + 5 = 10), which represents totally undifferentiated tumors. A tumor that is predominantly Gleason pattern 3 with a lesser amount of Gleason pattern 5 has a combined Gleason grade of 8 (3 + 5 = 8), just as does a tumor that is predominantly Gleason pattern 5 with a lesser amount of Gleason pattern 3 tumor (5 + 3 = 8). Therefore stating the Gleason grade in the form of a simple mathematical equation, as noted, rather than as a single number, gives the most insight into the true nature of the neoplasm. The Gleason grading system has become the de facto standard for the grading of prostate cancer.

The advantages of the Gleason grading system are (a) it is easy to learn and apply because it is based on low-magnifi-

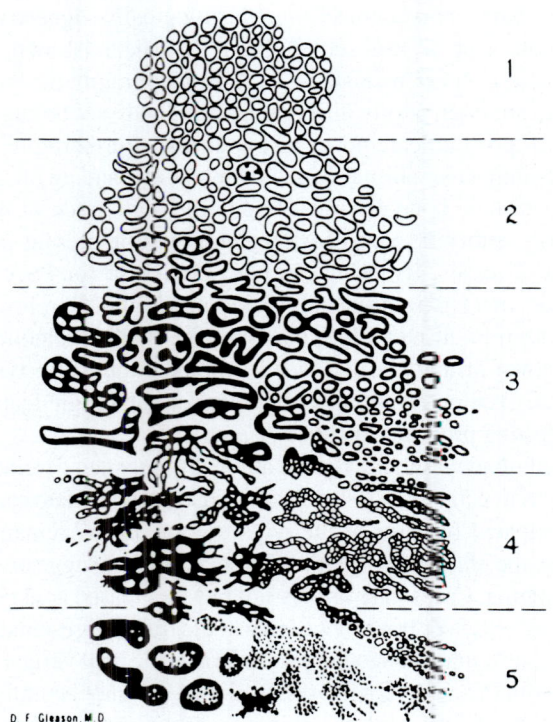

FIG. 15. Schematic diagram of the Gleason grading system (courtesy of Dr. D.F. Gleason, Minneapolis, Minnesota.)

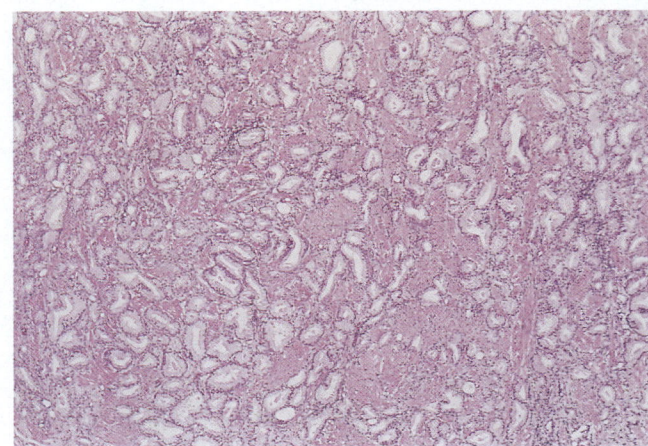

FIG. 17. In Gleason pattern 2. Although the tumor is still fairly circumscribed, at the edge of the tumor nodule, there can be minimal extension by neoplastic glands into the surrounding nonneoplastic prostate. The glands in pattern 2 are still single and separate, yet they are more loosely arranged and not quite so uniform as in pattern 1.

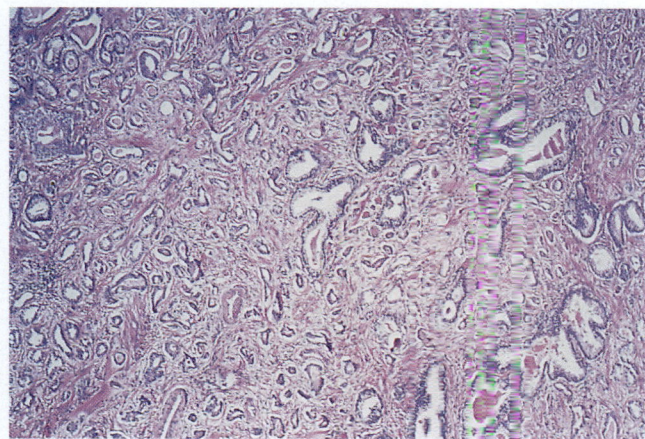

FIG. 18. Pattern 3 tumor infiltrates in and among the non-neoplastic prostate, with the glands having marked variation in size and shape. Many of the glands are smaller than those seen in pattern 1 or 2 tumors. Smoothly circumscribed cribriform nodules of tumor also are classified as pattern 3.

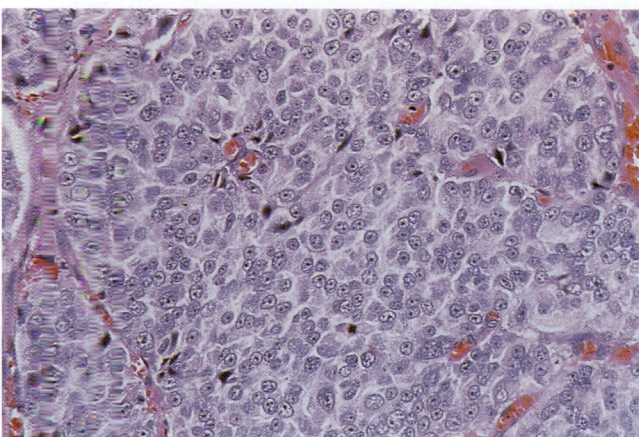

FIG. 20. The Gleason pattern 5 tumor shows no glandular differentiation with either solid masses of cells or individually infiltrating cells.

cation pattern recognition; and (b) it is less time consuming than the grading systems that examine cytologic features. Much of the Gleason grading system's ease of application results from the availability of a simplified illustration of the grading system by Gleason, which can be readily referred to when first learning the system (Fig. 15). Two older studies demonstrated good interobserver and intraobserver reproducibility with the Gleason system with agreements to within one combined Gleason grade of more than 80% and 90%, respectively (101,102). However, more recent studies showed only moderate interobserver reproducibility among academic and private pathologists (103,104). In the past, Gleason sums of 2 to 4 were considered to be low grade; Gleason sums of 5 to 7 to be intermediate grade; and Gleason sums of 8 to 10 to be high grade. However, it has been demonstrated that Gleason 7 tumor is more aggressive than Gleason 5 to 6 and should not be lumped together as intermediate-grade tumor (105,106). The strength of the Gleason system is its discriminatory capability between the various Gleason sums, which may be lost when various Gleason sums are combined together in an analysis.

One of the most frequent causes of discordant grading is the assessment of tumors that bridge two grades. As shown on Gleason's schematic diagram (Fig. 15), there is a continuum of differentiation between the various Gleason patterns such that the grade assigned at the extremes of a particular Gleason pattern may be somewhat subjective. Another reason for grading discrepancies is the presence of more than two grades. Gleason's system and most of the other grading systems were developed predominantly on needle biopsy and TUR specimens, in which it is uncommon for more than two grades to be represented. In prostatectomy specimens, however, tumors with multiple grades are not infrequent. Gleason states that only the primary and secondary patterns should be incorporated into the grade. If more than two grades exist in Gleason's system, they should be commented on in a note.

The Gleason grade on biopsy material has been shown to correlate fairly well with that of the subsequent radical

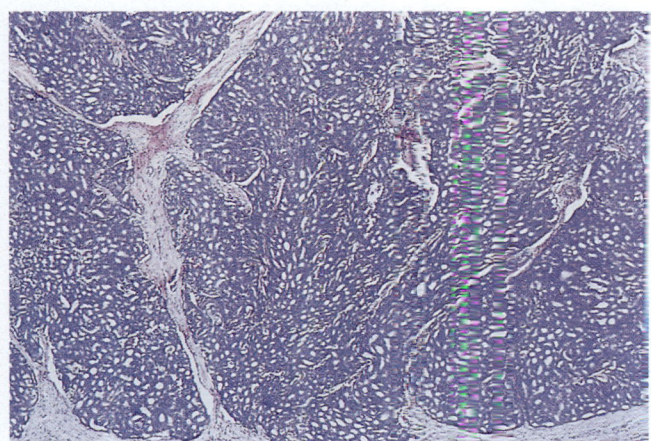

FIG. 19. In Gleason pattern 4 tumor, the glands are no longer single and separate, as seen in patterns 1 through 3, and are composed of fused glands with ragged infiltrating edges.

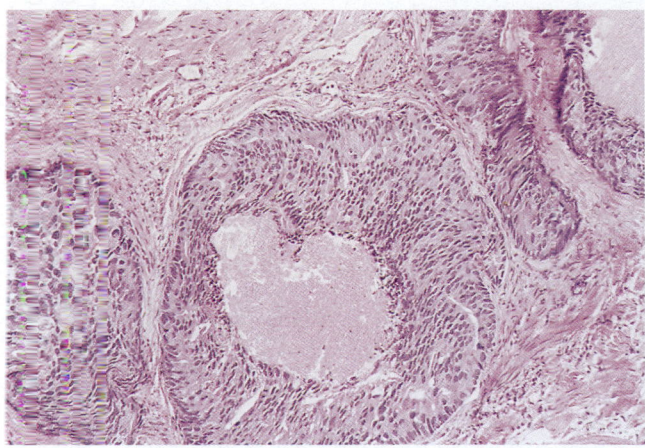

FIG. 21. Gleason pattern 5 with central comedonecrosis.

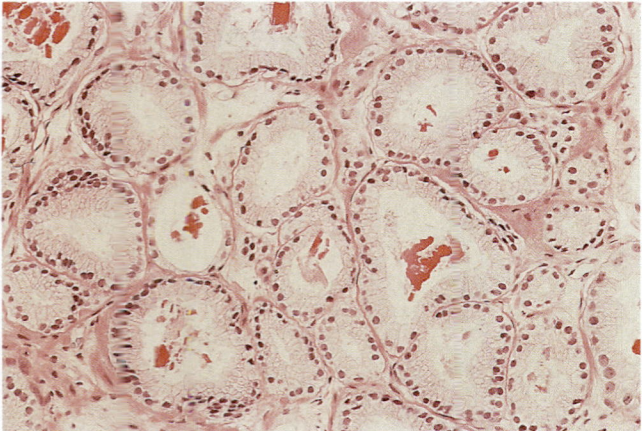

FIG. 22. Low-grade tumor on needle biopsy consisting of closely packed, fairly large, open, uniform glands with numerous crystalloids.

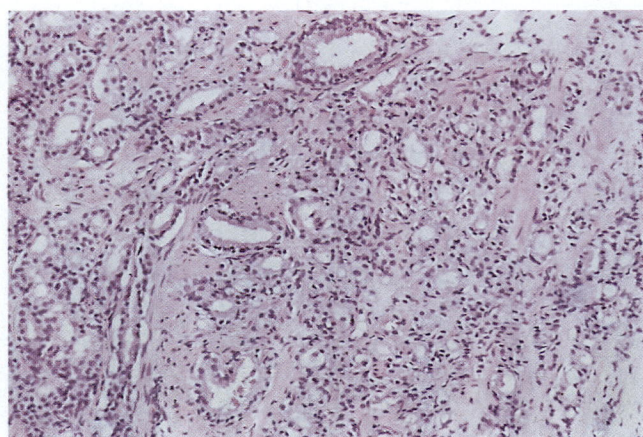

FIG. 24. Adenocarcinoma, Gleason grade 3 + 4 = 7. Note well-formed glands consistent with Gleason pattern 3 (lower left) compared with fused glands of Gleason pattern 4 (upper right).

prostatectomy (107–109). Two large series comparing radical prostatectomy specimens and their diagnostic biopsies showed a correlation to within one combined Gleason grade in approximately 73% of the cases (107,108). An equally large number of cases have been studied in our own institution, showing a correlation to within one combined Gleason grade of 85% (109). One of the most frequent errors in grading needle-biopsy material is to grade the tumor as combined Gleason grade 2 to 4, with the subsequent prostatectomy showing a primary Gleason pattern of 3, resulting in combined Gleason grades of 6 or sometimes 5. A bias when evaluating needle-biopsy specimens is that tumors with combined Gleason grades of 2 to 4 are uncommonly present on needle-biopsy material, because palpable tumors are usually of a higher grade (110). These low grades should be assigned only when the tumor is composed of closely apposed larger, open, uniform glands (Fig. 22). The tendency to undergrade needle-biopsy material results from the minimal amount of tumor in the needle biopsy and the consequent difficulty in appreciating either the infiltrative nature of the tumor or the variability in size and shape of the neoplastic glands, features that are characteristic of Gleason pattern 3. A feature of Gleason pattern 3 tumor that may be more readily identifiable on limited material is that the glands with Gleason pattern 3 are smaller than those of patterns 1 or 2. Consequently, if the tumor on needle-biopsy material is composed of small glands, or the glands are seen infiltrating between nonneoplastic prostatic glands, the tumor is graded 3 + 3 = 6, even though there may be only a few malignant glands present (Fig. 23). If the glands are somewhat more open, larger, and more uniform than a combined Gleason grade 6, yet are still infiltrative, a combined Gleason grade of 5 is assigned. If the glandular pattern is not so well defined as a combined Gleason grade 6 with some loss of discrete gland formation, a combined Gleason grade of 7 is given (Fig. 24). An unavoidable cause of discrepant grading between the biopsy and subsequent prostatectomy specimen is that due to sampling error by the needle biopsy. Because in TUR material there is greater sampling of the prostate and more tissue, the better to appreciate the overall architecture of the tumor, the grades assigned to TUR material tend to be more accurate than those given on needle-biopsy specimens.

Multifocality of prostate cancer contributed some confusion in the application of the Gleason grading system, both on needle-biopsy and on radical-prostatectomy specimens. In radical-prostatectomy specimens, it is not uncommon to have a Gleason score 5 to 7 tumor in the peripheral zone and small multifocal Gleason score 2 to 4 cancers in the transition zone. We comment on and assign a separate Gleason score to the main or index tumor. Commenting on every small multifocal low-grade tumor is optional, as these lesions do not affect prognosis. It is more controversial on needle biopsies whether to assign a separate Gleason score to each involved core or to assign a single Gleason score based on all the involved cores.

The ultimate value of any grading system is its ability to

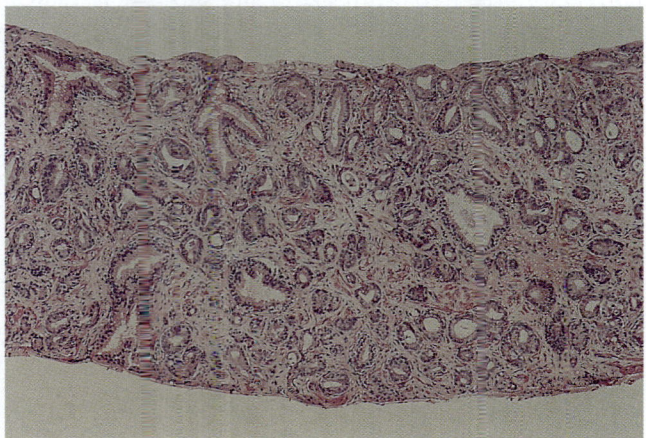

FIG. 23. Adenocarcinoma of the prostate, Gleason grade 3 + 3 = 6 on needle biopsy. Note small glands infiltrating in and among larger benign glands.

be of predictive value in terms of prognosis. Both Gleason's data with 2,911 patients and a similar study from Memorial Sloan–Kettering with long-term follow-up demonstrated a good correlation between prognosis and the combined Gleason grade (111,112). When the stage of disease was factored in with the grade, even better prognostic results were obtained.

The major weakness of the Gleason grading system is that, although at both the low and high ends of the Gleason system we have fairly accurate predictive ability, the prognosis of the remaining patients is uncertain. This preponderance of patients who are left with an indeterminate prognosis is not unique to the Gleason system and is a criticism that also may be applied to any of the other grading systems for prostate cancer.

Recently Partin et al. calculated on a large group of patients the prediction of stage based on preoperative PSA, biopsy Gleason score, and clinical stage (113). Because of the large number of patients in this study, the confidence intervals are quite narrow, which should allow translation to individual patient-care decisions. The positive lymph node rate for various Gleason scores is reported as follows: 2 to 4, less than 1%; 5 to 6, 2% to 3%; 7, 10%; and 8 to 10, 20%.

The concept of tumor dedifferentiation over time is controversial and under intense study. Although early studies suggested that grade progression may occur over time if a tumor is left in situ, this study is flawed by the use of androgen-deprivation therapy, which is now known to cause morphologic changes that can mimic dedifferentiation (114).

Extent of Cancer on Biopsy

There are few data as to how the extent of cancer on needle biopsy should be recorded. Our own results show that only the number of involved cores and bilaterality add to the prediction of pathologic stage, beyond that provided by biopsy grade and serum PSA values. Nevertheless, it is the convention to provide additional quantification when diagnosing cancer on needle biopsy. We record the number of positive cores and the percentage positivity of each core. When cores are fragmented, and this is difficult to determine, we record the percentage involvement of the entire specimen part.

Microscopic Diagnosis

The types of difficulty encountered in diagnosing adenocarcinoma of the prostate depend on whether we are evaluating needle-biopsy material or TUR resection specimens. In needle-biopsy material, there exists the risk of overdiagnosing atrophic glands and seminal vesicles as carcinoma, as well as underdiagnosing adenocarcinoma because of the limited amount of tumor present.

Atrophic glands stand out at scanning magnification because of their open lumina lined by cells with a high nuclear-to-cytoplasmic ratio, resulting in a very basophilic appearance to the glands (Fig. 25). When there is an increased number of crowded atrophic glands, the term postatrophic hyperplasia is used (115). Within the center of these small atrophic glands, there may be seen a dilated gland surrounded by fibrosis. These small glands, despite their atrophic appearance, have an increased proliferation rate (116). In contrast, gland-forming adenocarcinomas at low magnification usually appear pale/amphophilic with cells showing abundant cytoplasm and basally situated nuclei (Fig. 26). The high nuclear-to-cytoplasmic ratio seen in atrophic glands is usually present only in poorly differentiated adenocarcinomas of the prostate, which lack discrete well-formed glands. Recently atrophic adenocarcinomas have been recognized. The most useful criteria to establish a diagnosis of atrophic

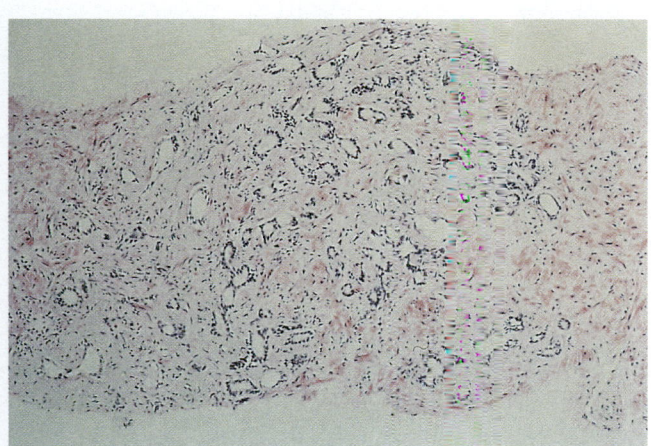

FIG. 25. Needle biopsy showing sclerotic atrophy with an infiltrative appearance.

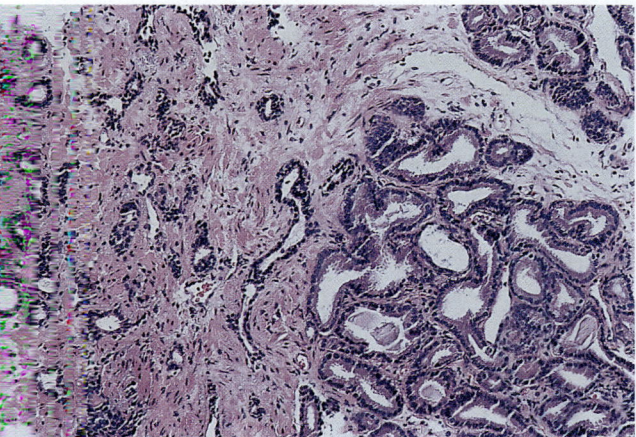

FIG. 26. Benign prostatic atrophy (left) compared with adenocarcinoma with amphophilic cytoplasm (right). Even compared with an amphophilic appearing carcinoma, atrophy appears more basophilic at low power.

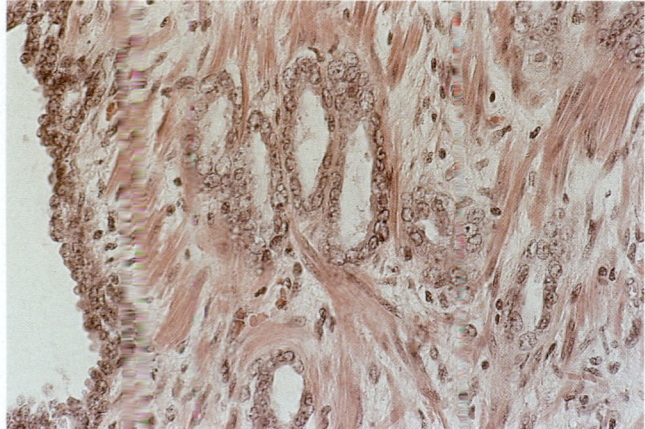

FIG. 27. Atrophic adenocarcinoma of the prostate with very prominent nucleoli.

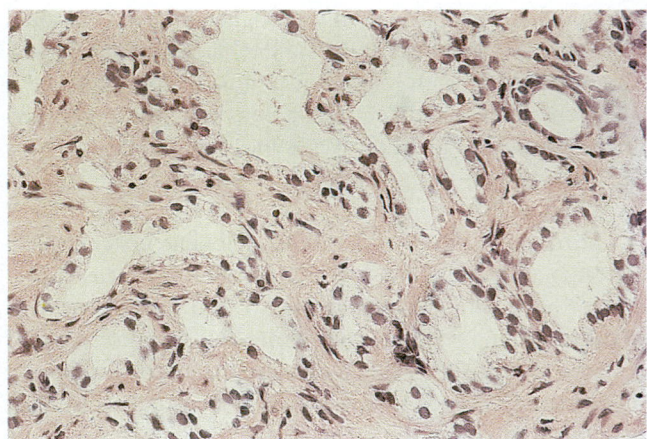

FIG. 29. Needle biopsy showing glands with partial atrophy.

adenocarcinoma are (a) an infiltrative pattern of growth, (b) the presence of macronucleoli (Fig. 27), (c) increased nuclear size, and (d) the presence of adjacent, nonatrophic cancer (Fig. 28). An important feature, which may not necessarily be readily identifiable in atrophic glands, is the presence of a basal cell layer. The use of keratin antibodies specific for prostatic basal cells is helpful in identifying basal cells in atrophic glands. Atrophic prostate cancer is rarely encountered on prostate needle biopsy (2%) but must be recognized to prevent underdiagnosis (117).

Small glands with partial atrophy may also have a disorganized infiltrative appearance and be misdiagnosed as carcinoma (118). In partial atrophy, the small glands appear similar to adjacent larger benign glands; the small glands have pale-to-clear attenuated cytoplasm with small, somewhat crinkly or irregular nuclei without nucleoli (Fig. 29). Again, basal cell–specific cytokeratin staining is useful in this situation.

Another potential source of overdiagnosing prostatic adenocarcinoma is the presence of seminal vesicles or seminal vesicle–type epithelium on needle biopsy. We must remember that the lining of the ejaculatory ducts is similar to that of the seminal vesicles and traverses the posterior prostate from the base to the level of the verumontanum and is therefore subject to biopsy. Given the limited tissue, it is difficult to recognize the architectural pattern of the seminal vesicles. A common finding on needle biopsy of the seminal vesicle is to see at the tip or at the edge of the core of tissue an irregular row of glandular epithelium that represents the lining of the central dilated seminal vesicle lumen, because the core of tissue fractures at this interface (Fig. 30). Surrounding this lumen may be numerous small glandular diverticula of the seminal vesicle, which may be confused with carcinoma. The presence of prominent lipofuscin granules within seminal vesicle epithelium is an important diagnostic aid. We should be aware that normal prostate glands also may demonstrate lipofuscin pigment with refractile red–brown granules corresponding to lysosomes (10). In addition, seminal vesicles characteristically have scattered cells showing prominent nu-

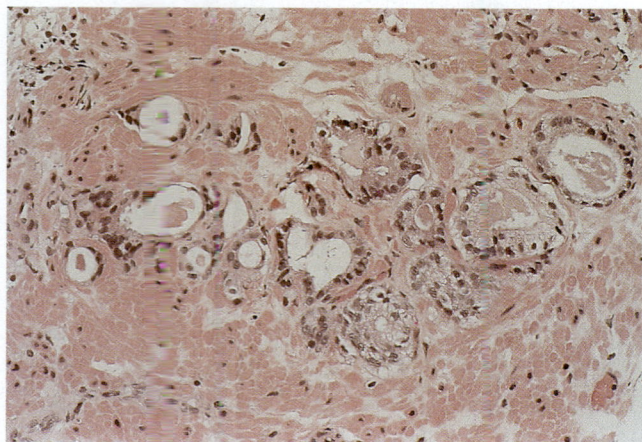

FIG. 28. Atrophic adenocarcinoma of the prostate (left) merging with more typical adenocarcinoma of the prostate (right).

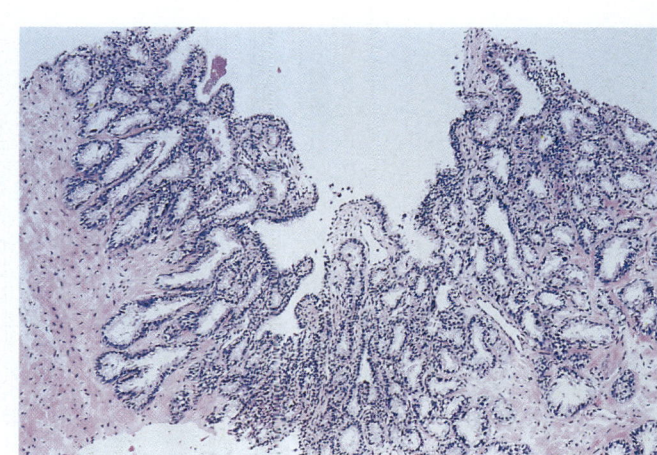

FIG. 30. Needle biopsy of seminal vesicles showing multiple small glands arranged around central lumen.

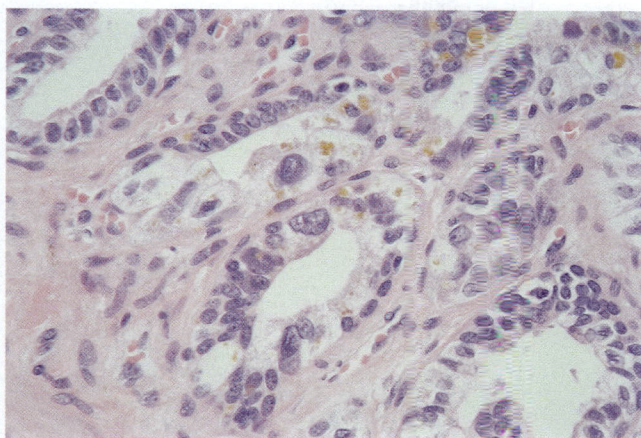

FIG. 31. Scattered markedly atypical nuclei with a degenerative appearance, characteristic of seminal vesicle epithelium. Prominent lipofuscin pigment noted.

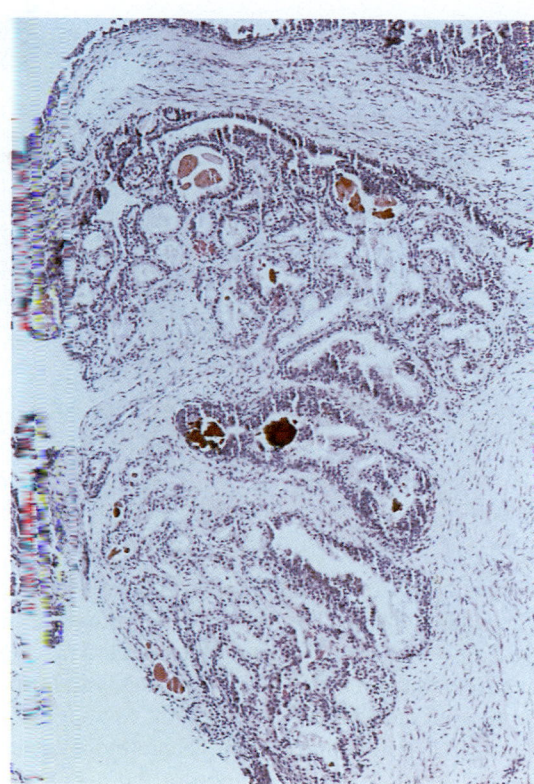

FIG. 33. Verumontanum mucosal gland hyperplasia consisting of crowded glands beneath urethra (top). Glands contain distinctive orange–red concretions and corpora amylacea.

clear atypia; these cells also exhibit hyperchromasia, which often obscures nuclear details (Fig. 31). Despite their marked enlargement and often bizarre shapes, these cells lack mitotic activity and commonly appear degenerated in nature, similar to what is seen with radiation atypia. The disparate finding within seminal vesicles of markedly atypical nuclei present within well-formed glandular structures differs from the histologic appearance of prostate cancer, in which gland-forming, well-differentiated or moderately differentiated carcinoma has only slight or moderate nuclear atypia. Even in poorly differentiated prostatic carcinoma, which lacks glandular differentiation, we rarely see the severe atypia that is present within scattered seminal vesicle epithelial cells. Seminal vesicle–type epithelium is also PSAP (not always PSA) negative and high-molecular-weight cytokeratin can distinguish between the two tissue types.

Other lesions that may be misdiagnosed as adenocarcinoma are Cowper's glands (Fig. 32), xanthomas (Fig. 13), verumontanum mucosal gland hyperplasia (Fig. 33), nephrogenic adenoma of the prostatic urethra, and mesonephric hyperplasia (61,119–122).

A more common problem with the evaluation of needle-biopsy material from the prostate is not the overdiagnosis of carcinoma, but rather the underdiagnosis of carcinoma as a result of the limited amount of tumor present (123). Not uncommonly, biopsies of adenocarcinoma of the prostate yield several cores of tissue containing benign glands and stroma,

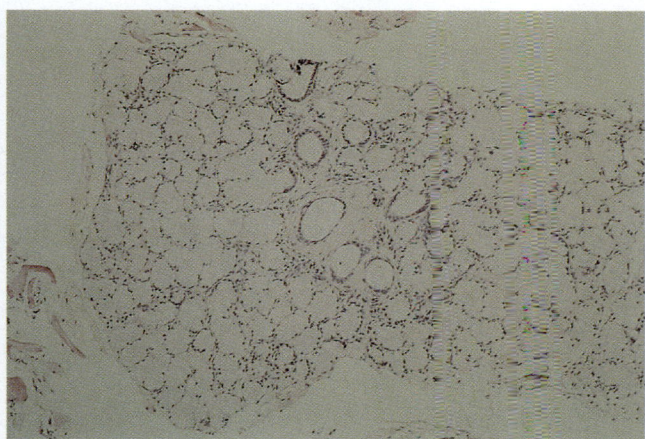

FIG. 32. Cowper's gland on needle biopsy. Note dimorphic population with duct surrounded by mucinous glands. The lesion is present in skeletal muscle.

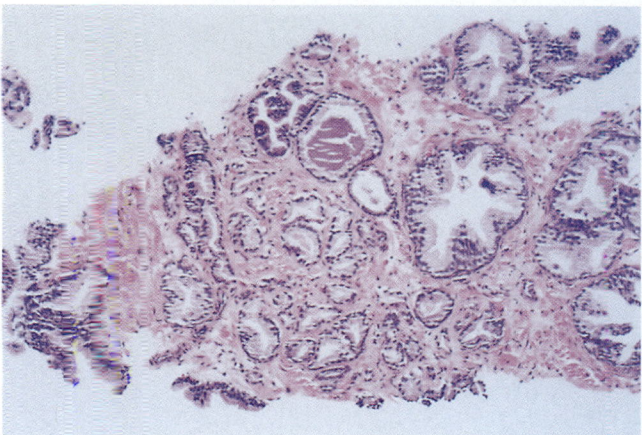

FIG. 34. Small focus of intermediate-grade prostate carcinoma infiltrating between nonneoplastic glands.

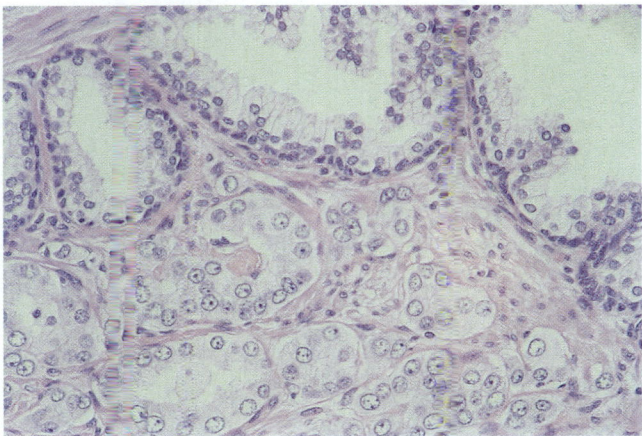

FIG. 35. Neoplastic glands composed of a single layer of cells with enlarged nuclei, some with prominent nucleoli.

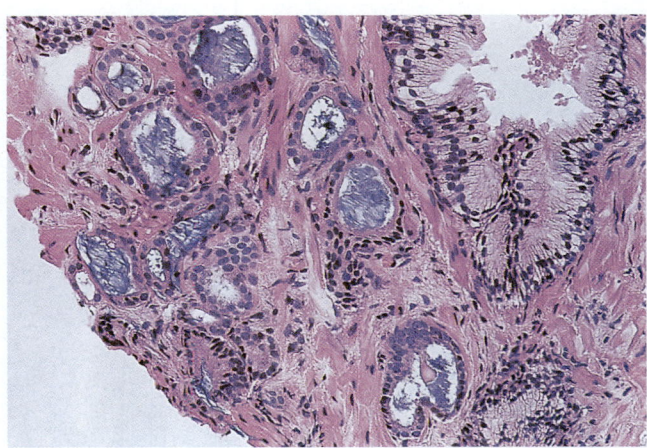

FIG. 37. Adenocarcinoma of the prostate with blue-tinged mucinous secretions seen on H&E.

with only a few neoplastic glands insinuating themselves within the benign tissue. The recognition of prostatic cancer in these cases rests on both the architectural abnormalities resulting from the infiltrating neoplastic glands and the cytologic features of the neoplastic epithelium. Although it is difficult to appreciate architecture on needle-biopsy material, we can still develop an appreciation of the evenly spaced larger benign glands with papillary infolding and two cell types separated by a moderate amount of prostatic stroma. In cases with a minimal amount of carcinoma on needle biopsy, we find small glands infiltrating the stroma between larger benign glands (Fig. 34). In most cases of limited cancer on needle biopsy, there are cytologic differences in the malignant glands when compared with surrounding benign glands (Fig. 35). Although the finding of prominent nucleoli in the small glands is reassuring, it is not necessary to diagnose carcinoma. Often, only significant nuclear enlargement discriminates cancer from the surrounding benign glands. In addition to differentiating nuclear features, neoplastic glands may have amphophilic cytoplasm contrasted with the pale-to-clear cytoplasm of adjacent benign glands (Fig. 36). Intraluminal pink acellular dense secretions or blue-tinged mucinous secretions seen in small suggestive glands may be additional features that help to differentiate malignant from benign glands, given their greater frequency in malignancy (Fig. 37). Other findings that are uncommonly seen in benign glands that may aid in the diagnosis of cancer include prostatic crystalloids (see p. 1913) and mitoses (Fig. 38). Rather than relying on any one of these features as the sole diagnostic criterion, the finding of several of these features should be used to diagnose limited cancer (Table 2). Occasionally we may see small glands infiltrating haphazardly in the stroma or crowded between normal glands, which is diagnostic of carcinoma, even if the glands lack cytologic atypia (Fig. 39). If the architectural or cytologic features or both are diagnostic of cancer, searching for a basal cell layer tends to confound rather than to help. Thin, hyperchromatic, elongated, fibroblastic nuclei commonly surround neoplastic glands, mimicking a basal cell layer, and stratification of neoplastic cells due to tangential sectioning also may be confused with a basal cell layer. An equivocal diagnosis may be rendered when there are only a few glands with slight nu-

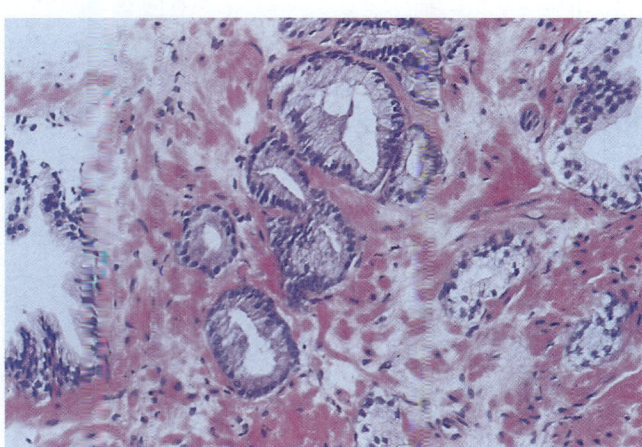

FIG. 36. Small glands of infiltrating adenocarcinoma with amphophilic cytoplasm noted between larger pale-staining benign glands.

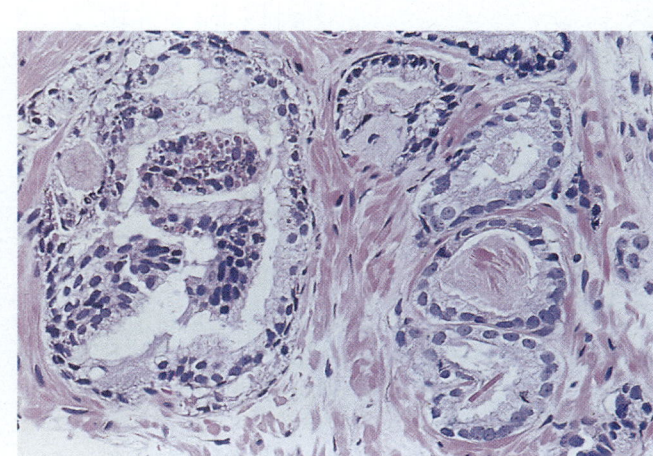

FIG. 38. Adenocarcinoma with small glands with enlarged nuclei, crystalloids, and mitotic figure. Adjacent benign prostate glands contains lipofuscin pigment.

TABLE 2. *Helpful features in the needle-biopsy diagnosis of adenocarcinoma on H&E-stained sections*

Features diagnostic of adenocarcinoma
    Perineural invasion
    Mucinous fibroplasia (collagenous micronodules)
    Glomerulations
Features favoring the diagnosis of cancer
(diagnosis based on a constellation of features)
Architecture
    Small glands in between larger benign glands
    Crowded glands that stand out from adjacent benign glands
Cytology
    Prominent nucleoli
    Nuclear enlargement
    Hyperchromatic nuclei
    Amphophilic cytoplasm
    Mitotic figures
Luminal contents
    Blue mucinous secretions
    Pink amorphous secretions
    Crystalloids in small infiltrating glands (i.e. not adenosis)
Adjacent findings
    High grade PIN either away from small atypical glands or in presence of numerous small atypical glands, such that tangential sectioning or outpouching off of PIN not possible

PIN, prostatic intraepithelial neoplasia.

TABLE 3. *Features that elicit caution in the diagnosis of adenocarcinoma on needle biopsy*

Atypical glands associated with acute or chronic inflammation (rule out reactive atypia) or both
Atrophic cytoplasm (distinguish atrophy from atrophic cancer)
Small crowded glands merging in with similar appearing more recognizable larger benign glands (rule out adenosis)
Small crowded glands with corpora amylacea (rule out adenosis)
Large cytologically atypical glands with papillary infolding or luminal undulations (rule out PIN)
Few small cytologically atypical glands immediately adjacent to PIN (rule out outpouching or tangential sectioning off of PIN)

PIN, prostatic intraepithelial neoplasia.

clear or cytoplasmic differences or both that are suggestive yet not diagnostic of cancer. The presence of atrophy or inflammation associated with suggestive glands often leads to an equivocal diagnosis, because benign glands with these features may mimic cancer (Table 3). Because benign prostate glands show some heterogeneity in their staining with basal cell antibodies (i.e., basal cell–specific cytokeratin, clone designation 34 βE12), negative staining for basal cell–specific cytokeratin in only a few glands suggestive of cancer is not proof of their malignancy. If there are numerous atypical glands that are negative for basal cell–specific cytokeratin, a diagnosis of carcinoma may be rendered (Fig. 40). In cases of atrophy or inflammation, positive basal cell–specific cytokeratin staining may definitively label a focus as benign.

An unusual pattern of adenocarcinoma seen on needle biopsy that may be underdiagnosed involves cancers with voluminous xanthomatous cytoplasm in which nuclei are small and often show no or minimal atypia, termed foamy gland carcinoma; intraluminal pink homogeneous secretions are often present (Fig. 41) (124). The identification of this type of cancer hinges on recognizing that the cytoplasm is unique to malignant glands, and the small, round nuclei are more uniformly hyperchromatic and round without a hint of a basal cell layer, as compared with normal glands. Nucleoli are often difficult to visualize because of marked hyperchromasia.

Another finding, virtually diagnostic of carcinoma, although infrequently seen in limited material, is the presence of perineural invasion (123) (Fig. 42). Although perineural indentation by benign prostatic glands has been reported, the glands in these cases appear totally benign and are present at only one edge of the nerve rather than circumferentially involving the perineural space, as can be seen in carcinoma (125) (Fig. 43). In rare cases, there is crushed cellular atypical tissue intimately associated with nerves. Similarly, in some cases, there is a crushed cellular focus in which the differential rests between poorly differentiated adenocarcinoma and crushed stroma or inflammation. The identification of this tissue as epithelial and of prostatic origin by the use of

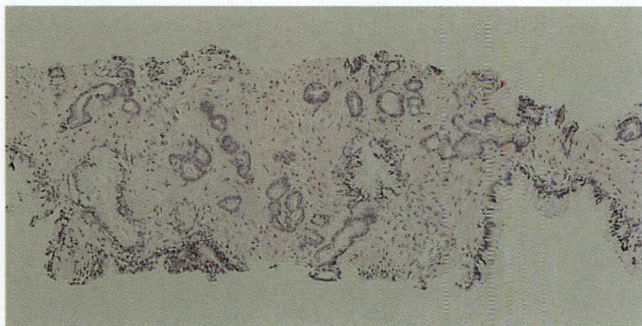

FIG. 39. Adenocarcinoma of the prostate, Gleason grade 3 + 3 = 6. Infiltrative appearance among benign glands is diagnostic of cancer.

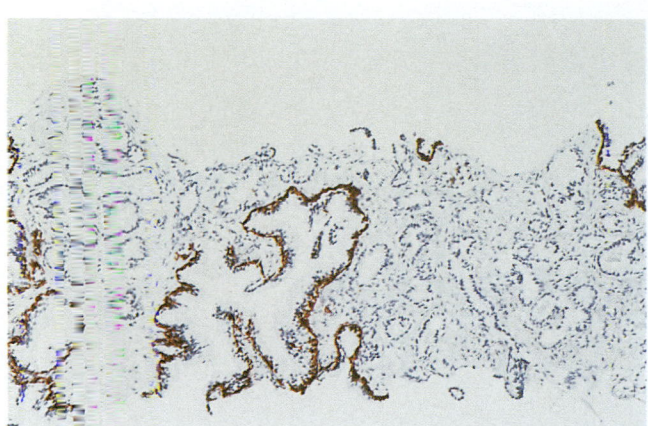

FIG. 40. High-molecular-weight cytokeratin stain of Fig. 34 showing lack of basal cells in small glands, consistent with adenocarcinoma.

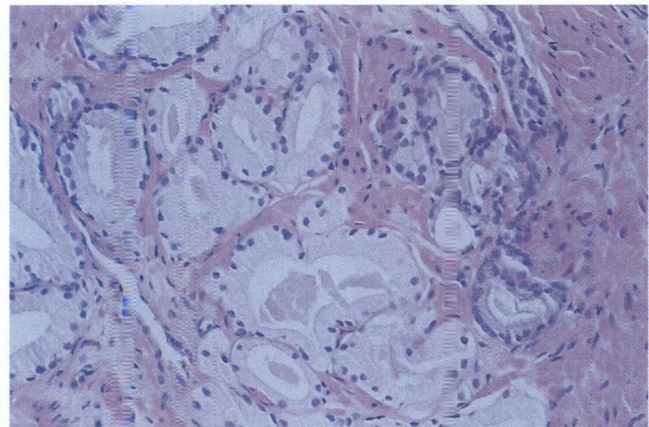

FIG. 41. Adenocarcinoma of the prostate with abundant xanthomatous cytoplasm, small nuclei, and pink homogeneous intraluminal secretions. Compare cytoplasm with more typical adenocarcinoma (right).

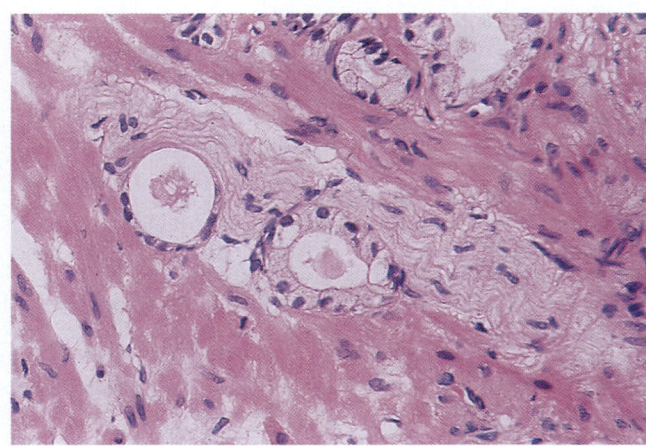

FIG. 43. Perineural indentation by benign prostate gland.

antisera to PSA and PSAP may help to establish the diagnosis of prostatic carcinoma. Other findings that have been described only in cancer are collagenous nodules (mucinous fibroplasia; Fig. 44) and glomerulations (126,127) (Fig. 45). Whereas we have seen cases in which the only carcinoma on needle biopsy showed perineural invasion, cancers composed of collagenous nodules and glomerulations are almost invariably accompanied by ordinary carcinoma.

The importance of not underdiagnosing prostatic adenocarcinoma on needle biopsy relates to the relatively high false-negative rates with needle biopsy of prostatic carcinoma. Consequently, diagnosing a small focus of adenocarcinoma of the prostate on needle-biopsy material as atypical but not diagnostic of carcinoma does not guarantee that repeated biopsy or biopsies will obtain diagnostic material. Furthermore, a limited amount of cancer on needle biopsy does not necessarily equate with a limited amount of cancer in the corresponding radical prostatectomy specimen (80). Therefore in those cases in which the histologic material is strongly suggestive of carcinoma, but the pathologist does not feel

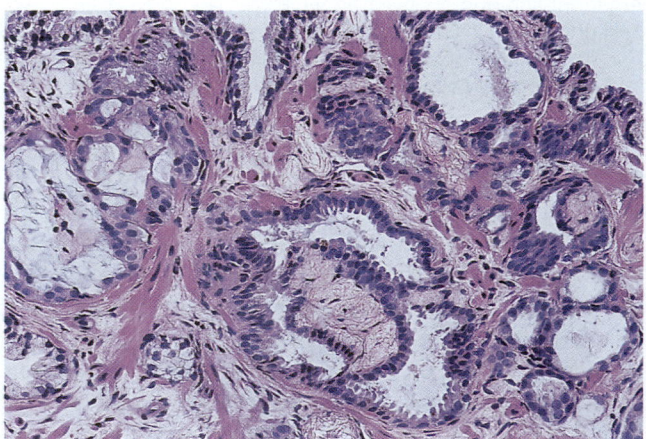

FIG. 44. Collagenous nodules with mucin undergoing organization to delicate loose fibrosis.

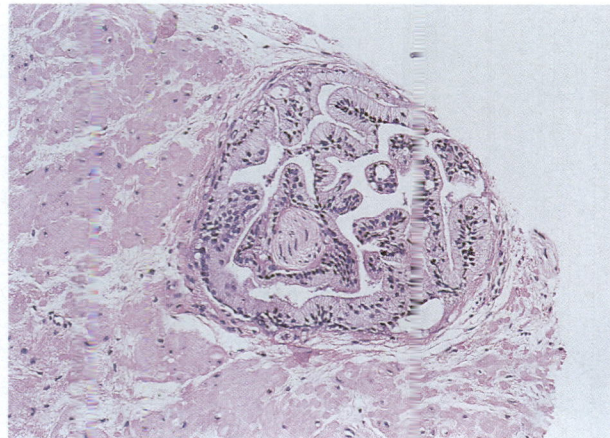

FIG. 42. Adenocarcinoma of the prostate with perineural invasion. Occasionally glands with perineural invasion will show papillary infolding, mimicking a benign gland.

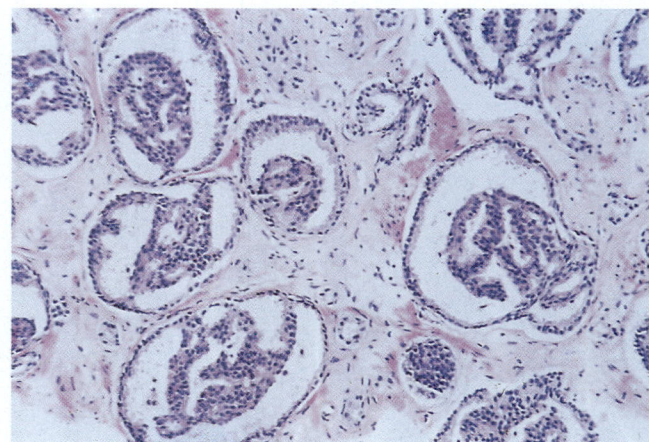

FIG. 45. Glomerulations with adenocarcinoma showing cribriform formation that is not transluminal, resembling glomeruli.

TABLE 4. *Diagnostic criteria for adenosis*

Adenosis	Low-grade carcinoma
Features seen at low magnification	
Lobular growth	Infiltrative/haphazard
Small crowded glands admixed with larger glands	May be pure population of small crowded glands
Features seen at high magnification	
Huge (≥3 μm) nucleoli absent	Occasionally huge nucleoli present
Small glands share cytoplasmic and nuclear features with admixed larger benign glands	Small glands differ from surrounding benign glands in cytoplasmic or nuclear features or both
Pale, clear cytoplasm	May have amphophilic cytoplasm
Blue-tinged mucinous secretions rare	Blue-tinged mucinous secretions common
Corpora amylacea common	Corpora amylacea rare
Occasional glands with basal cells	Basal cells absent
Basal cell–specific anti-keratin antibodies stain basal cells in some small glands	Small glands are not immunoreactive with basal cell–specific anti-keratin antibodies

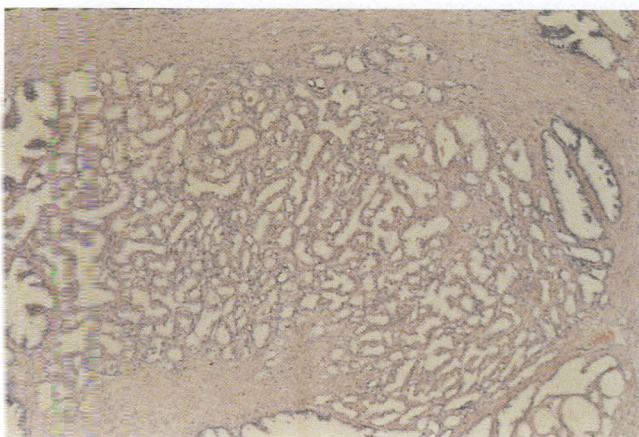

FIG. 46. Low magnification of adenosis. Lesion is very lobular with only minimal infiltration at perimeter. Small crowded glands mimicking cancer merge with more typically benign glands (left).

histology is better appreciated. Similarly, atrophic glands are more readily recognized on TUR specimens by their frequent arrangement in lobules.

The greatest difficulty with TUR material is the distinction of low-grade adenocarcinoma from adenosis. Adenosis is the most common lesion mimicking low-grade adenocarcinoma (Tables 4 and 5). Some common synonyms include small glandular hyperplasia, atypical adenomatous hyperplasia, and adenomatous hyperplasia (18,132,133). We must be cognizant that the definition of adenosis has varied according to the author. We define adenosis on the basis of a constellation of features, rather than relying on any one finding. Adenosis at low magnification is composed of numerous crowded, small, pale-staining glands that resemble a nodule of low-grade adenocarcinoma of the prostate (Fig. 46). Whereas both adenosis and low-grade adenocarcinoma consist of glands that are relatively noninfiltrative, in adenosis the glands tend to have a lobular configuration. In contrast, the glands in low-grade adenocarcinoma are arranged in a haphazard array, with glands often appearing to infiltrate into the stroma at right angles to each other (Fig. 47). In

comfortable in establishing the diagnosis, and subsequent biopsies do not show carcinoma, the material should be sent for a consulting opinion rather than assuming that the first material was not carcinoma. The incidence of atypical glands on needle biopsy is approximately 4% to 6% (128–131). The use of high-molecular-weight cytokeratin can reduce the rate of these atypical diagnoses. Approximately 40% to 50% of cases with an atypical diagnosis will have cancer on repeated biopsy. Although patients with an elevated PSA and an atypical biopsy are more likely to have cancer on repeated biopsy, even men with lower PSA values have a significant risk of cancer, and the biopsy should be repeated.

Given the recently recognized increased risk of progression in patients with small foci of low-grade adenocarcinoma, it should be noted that the diagnosis of low-grade adenocarcinoma, even if present in a small amount on transurethral resection material, is not inconsequential and may lead to prostatectomy in young men.

On TUR material, the overdiagnosis of seminal vesicles as carcinoma is less likely than on needle biopsy because its

TABLE 5. *Nondiagnostic features in differential of adenosis versus carcinoma*

Features shared in adenosis and cancer
Crowded (back-to-back) glands
Intraluminal crystalloids
Medium-sized (<3 μm) nucleoli
Scattered poorly formed glands and single cells
Minimal infiltration at periphery of nodule

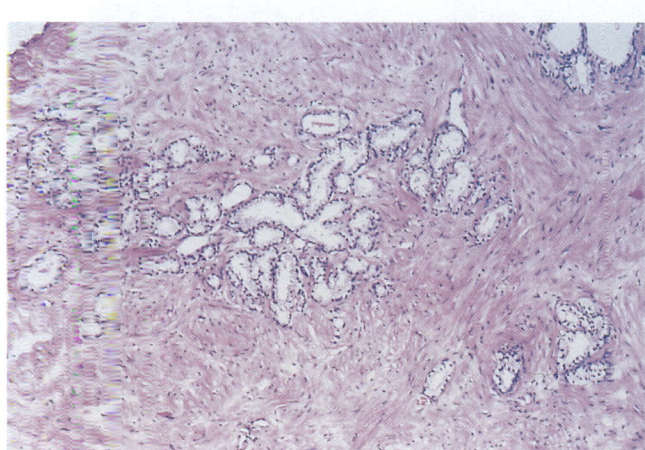

FIG. 47. Low-grade adenocarcinoma of the prostate with an infiltrative appearance. Glands infiltrate at right angles to each other.

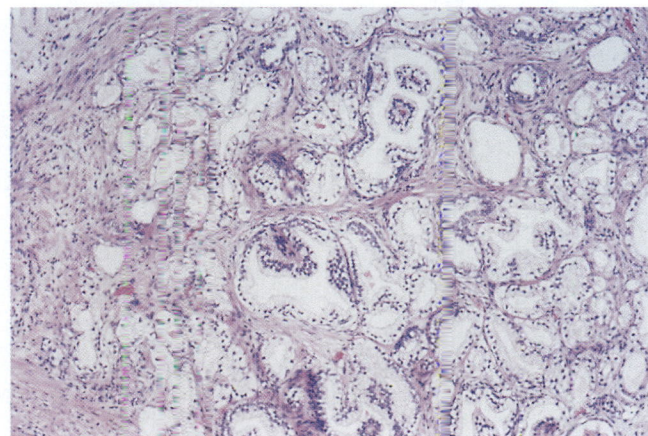

FIG. 48. Adenosis showing lobular collection of crowded glands. Note benign glands with papillary infoldings admixed with small crowded glands showing similar nuclear and cytoplasmic features.

adenosis, there is a gradual transition between the small glands suggestive of carcinoma and adjacent more recognizably benign glands; some of the features seen in the benign glands include branching, larger, more irregular shapes, and papillary infoldings (Fig. 48). On the other hand, glands of low-grade adenocarcinoma stand out in sharp contrast to surrounding benign glands. Whereas we should be able to say with confidence, when assessing a focus of adenocarcinoma of the prostate, which are the benign glands and which are malignant, in adenosis, this distinction cannot be made. At higher magnification, the cells of adenosis have pale-to-clear cytoplasm, similar to that of surrounding normal benign glands (Fig. 49). Although some adenocarcinomas have pale-clear cytoplasm, others have more amphophilic cytoplasm. In general, in adenosis, the nuclei have at most only small nucleoli.

This description is accurate for most cases of adenosis. Some atypical cases of adenosis have features that may lead to even further confusion with carcinoma, including: (a) minimal infiltration away from the edge of the nodule of adenosis, (b) a minor component of poorly formed glands and even single cells, and (c) fairly prominent nucleoli (18,133,134). Very large prominent nucleoli are, however, incompatible with adenosis. One of the key distinguishing features between carcinoma and benign glandular proliferations mimicking carcinoma is the lack of a basal cell layer in all adenocarcinomas of the prostate. However, the use of basal cells as a diagnostic criteria in adenosis is difficult for several reasons. First, basal cells visible by light microscopy are present in only a minority of the glands of adenosis within a given nodule. In addition, the distinction of a flattened basal cell layer from closely apposed fibroblasts can be extremely difficult. The use of certain keratin antibodies that selectively stain basal cells within the prostate can help to diagnose adenosis, especially when there are some atypical features. Within a nodule of adenosis, between 10% and 100% (mean, two thirds) of the glands will show some staining of basal cells with basal cell–specific cytokeratin (11). The staining may be difficult to interpret because within a given gland, it is often patchy and consists of a flattened attenuated rim of immunoreactivity located beneath the secretory cell layer (Fig. 50). This staining also tends to be sensitive to various lengths of formalin fixation and must be titrated accordingly. We have seen rare cases of cancers in which the tumor cells showed moderate staining for high-molecular-weight cytokeratin. In contrast to benign glands, there was no immunoreactivity of cells in a basal cell distribution. Positive staining of benign glands adjacent to carcinoma can be distinguished from adenosis based on the morphologic differences between the immunoreactive benign and the negative-stained malignant glands; in a nodule of adenosis, glands that lack basal cell–specific cytokeratin staining are identical to adjacent immunoreactive glands. Also, basal cells in benign glands tend to stain uniformly and intensely, in contrast to the patchy staining in adenosis. Adenosis tends to be located centrally within the gland, such

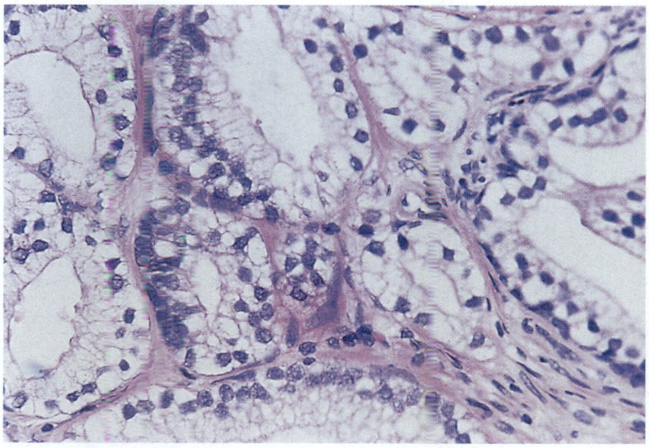

FIG. 49. Higher magnification of adenosis showing glands with pale-to-clear cytoplasm, relatively benign-appearing nuclei, and a focally identifiable basal cell layer.

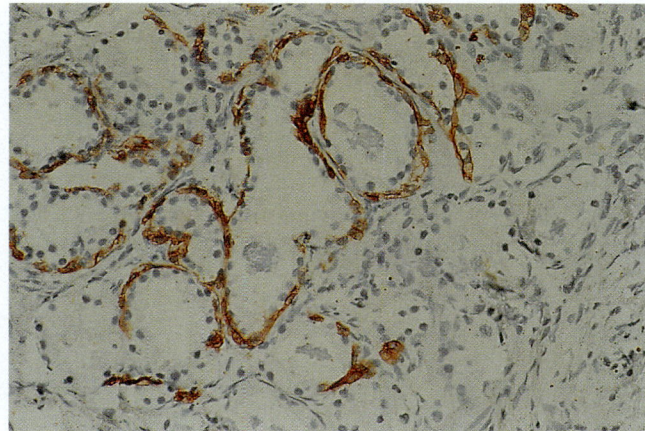

FIG. 50. Basal cell–specific cytokeratin (34BE12) immunostaining demonstrates a patchy basal cell layer surrounding some of the glands within a nodule of adenosis.

that it is most commonly seen in TUR resection specimens. In TUR resection specimens, we usually have an entire nodule of adenosis to evaluate; it would be highly unlikely for the entire focus to show no immunoreactivity with basal cell–specific cytokeratin. Consequently, the lack of basal cell–specific cytokeratin staining in a nodule of glands in which we are deciding between adenosis and low-grade adenocarcinoma is highly supportive of the diagnosis of adenocarcinoma. Another feature that is more common in low-grade adenocarcinoma than adenosis is the presence of crystalloids (Figs. 22 and 38) (135). Prostatic crystalloids are dense, eosinophilic, crystalloid structures that appear in various geometric shapes. These crystalloids can be found in approximately 60% of prostatic adenocarcinomas, preferentially in well-differentiated tumors.

Crystalloids also were identified in a few instances in benign-appearing glands adjacent to cancers and may also be seen in adenosis. If crystalloids are seen in benign glands on needle biopsy, there is no increased likelihood of cancer on repeated biopsy (136). Because crystalloids may be seen in adenosis and in even totally benign glands, the finding of crystalloids is not diagnostic of carcinoma. When we strongly favor carcinoma, the finding of prostatic crystalloids may provide the extra bit of evidence to yield a definitive diagnosis of cancer, given their greater frequency in carcinoma. If the differential diagnosis is between adenosis and low-grade adenocarcinoma (i.e., a lobular collection of crowded glands), the presence of crystalloids is not helpful. If the focus consists of small atypical glands infiltrating between larger benign glands, in which adenosis is not in the differential, then the findings of crystalloids can help to establish a malignant diagnosis.

Numerous studies claimed that acid mucin is absent in benign glands and may be seen in approximately two thirds of well- or moderately differentiated adenocarcinomas of the prostate (137). However, it was demonstrated that adenosis also frequently contains acid mucin secretions (8). This finding does not negate the usefulness of finding blue-tinged mucinous secretions on hematoxylin–eosin (H&E) sections, given its rarity in adenosis. Because adenosis can uncommonly demonstrate these features, only if there are other findings favoring a diagnosis of carcinoma should these features be used to help establish a definitive diagnosis of carcinoma. Adenosis may be seen in approximately 1% of needle-biopsy specimens (133) (Figs. 51 and 52).

Because keratin staining of adenosis is often patchy and may be present in only a minority of the glands within a nodule, the lack of basal cell staining on a needle biopsy with more limited tissue is not so definitive. The positive staining of glands suggestive of adenosis on needle biopsy, however, is diagnostic of adenosis and rules out carcinoma. The relation of adenosis to carcinoma is still controversial. Most of the studies suggesting a link between adenosis and adenocarcinoma of the prostate included cases that would currently be regarded as carcinoma or PIN. There currently does not appear to be strong evidence that patients with adenosis have an increased risk of adenocarcinoma, either at the time of diagnosis or in the future (19).

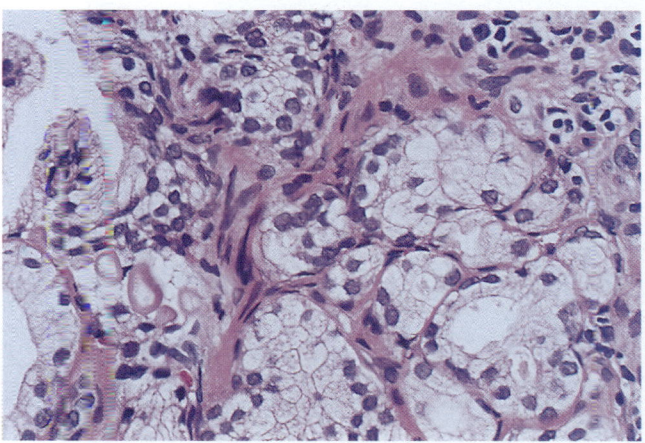

FIG. 52. Adenosis on needle biopsy showing crowded glands with pale-to-clear cytoplasm and benign-appearing nuclei, which are similar to adjacent more recognizably benign glands (left). Stains for high-molecular-weight cytokeratin were positive in this case, demonstrating basal cells.

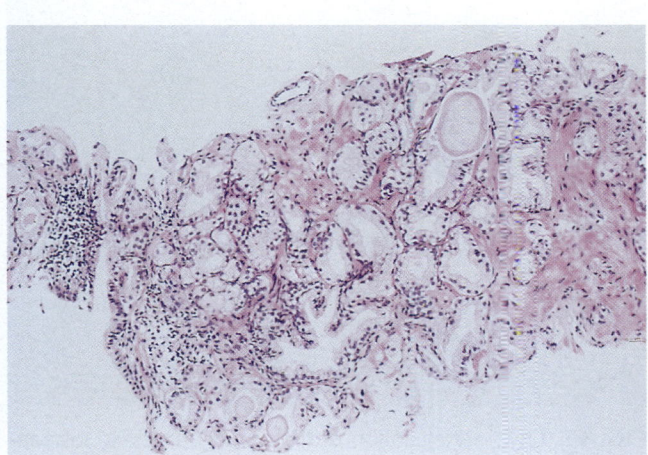

FIG. 51. Crowded glands of adenosis on needle biopsy.

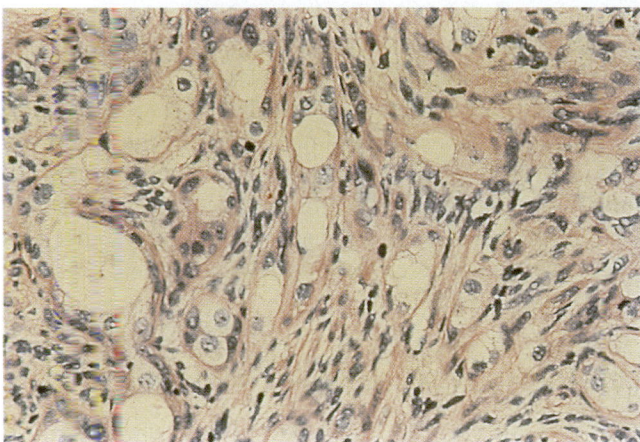

FIG. 53. Sclerosing adenosis showing glands of adenosis (left) merging with cytologically similar cords and spindle cells (right)

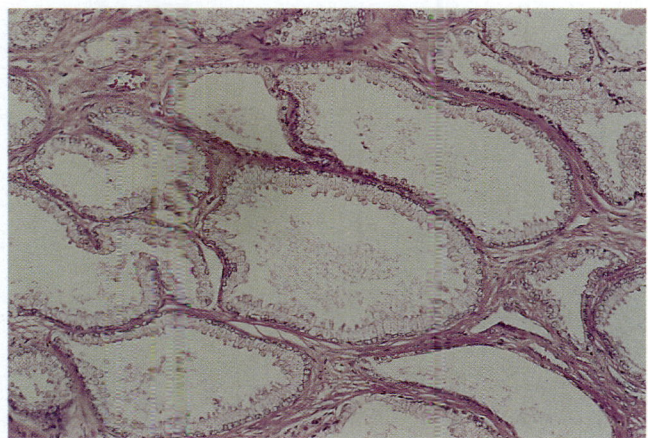

FIG. 54. Low-grade adenocarcinoma showing large back-to-back glands in which the luminal surfaces have an even straight edge without papillary infoldings, and cells have abundant cytoplasm. Stains for high-molecular-weight cytokeratin were negative in these glands.

A variant of adenosis that may be confused with intermediate- to high-grade adenocarcinoma of the prostate is sclerosing adenosis of the prostate (138). Sclerosing adenosis consists of small, relatively localized foci of well- and poorly formed glands (Fig. 53). The glands resemble ordinary adenosis yet merge with cytologically similar cords and individual cells. Nucleoli may be fairly prominent. A thick hyaline basement membrane–like sheath invests some of the glands. Between the glands and individual epithelial cells, there is a cellular spindle-cell component. In contrast to sclerosing adenosis, adenocarcinomas with this appearance are more extensive and lack both the cellular spindle-cell component and the periglandular hyaline sheath. Immunohistochemistry with actin and S-100 demonstrate that there is myoepithelial cell differentiation to the basal cells around the glands in sclerosing adenosis and in the spindle cells between the glands (139). In contrast, adenocarcinomas of the prostate lack basal cells. Sclerosing adenosis also differs from ordinary benign prostate glands, in which basal cells lack myoepithelial cell differentiation (140).

Rarely prostatic adenocarcinomas may resemble benign glands and be composed of numerous, crowded, large, open glands (127). The neoplastic glands have a crisp, even luminal surface without papillary infoldings or ruffling (Fig. 54). The glands lack a basal cell layer and have abundant tall cytoplasm with small, round, uniform, basally situated nuclei. Comparably sized benign glands would have papillary infoldings, inculations, or ruffling of their luminal border or have atrophic cytoplasm.

PROSTATIC INTRAEPITHELIAL NEOPLASIA

In 1986 McNeal and Bostwick (141) published an article on a premalignant lesion of the prostate that they termed intraductal dysplasia. Intraductal dysplasia was subcategorized into three grades. Grade 1 (mild) was characterized by increased nuclear size with increased variability of nuclear size, along with irregular focal crowding and multilayering. Grade 2 (moderate) has features similar to grade 1, with hyperchromatism and occasional small prominent nucleoli. The hallmark of grade 3 (severe) intraductal dysplasia was the finding of numerous large prominent nucleoli. Over the ensuing years, the diagnostic criteria proposed by McNeal and Bostwick have generally been adopted as the accepted method of grading cytologically atypical lesions within the prostate. The other term introduced to describe the same lesion is prostatic intraepithelial neoplasia (PIN) (142). PIN-1 is synonymous with mild dysplasia, PIN-2 with moderate dysplasia, and PIN-3 with severe dysplasia. The convention is to call PIN-1 low-grade PIN and to combine PIN-2 and PIN-3 as high-grade PIN. PIN-2 and PIN-3 are combined as high-grade PIN because the two grades cannot be reliably distinguished, and the distinction lacks clinical significance (143).

Although PIN is characterized by nuclear atypia, there are often accompanying architectural abnormalities (144). At low magnification, PIN is characterized by glands that are separated by a modest amount of stroma and have a normal overall architectural pattern (Fig. 55). These glands resemble benign glands in that they branch, are large, and have papillary and undulating luminal surfaces. However, at low magnification, glands with high-grade tend to have a basophilic appearance, caused by a combination of features, including enlarged nuclei, hyperchromatism, overlapping of the nuclei, epithelial hyperplasia, and amphophilic cytoplasm. The earliest form of high-grade PIN is characterized by an increase in nuclear size with prominent nucleoli, without significant epithelial hyperplasia (Fig. 56). Often the basal cell layer is still visible, and the demarcation between dysplastic and normal nuclei is often abrupt. With more pronounced forms of high-grade PIN nuclei become more piled up and develop micropapillary projections composed of tall epithelial buds lacking fibrovascular cores (Fig. 57). An interesting phenomenon in PIN is that, within these epithelial projec-

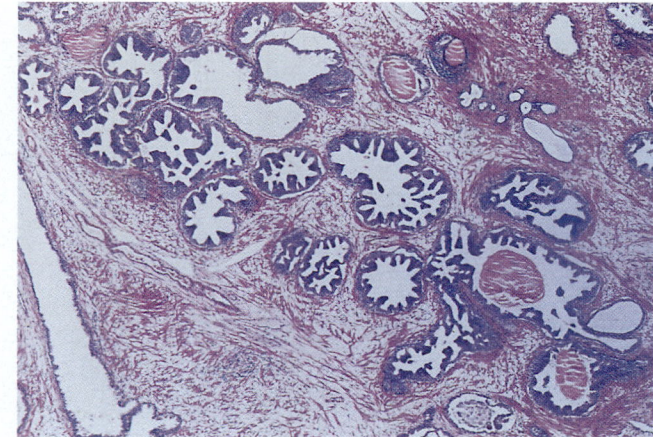

FIG. 55. Low magnification of high-grade prostatic intraepithelial neoplasia (PIN), showing glands with a normal architectural pattern yet a basophilic appearance.

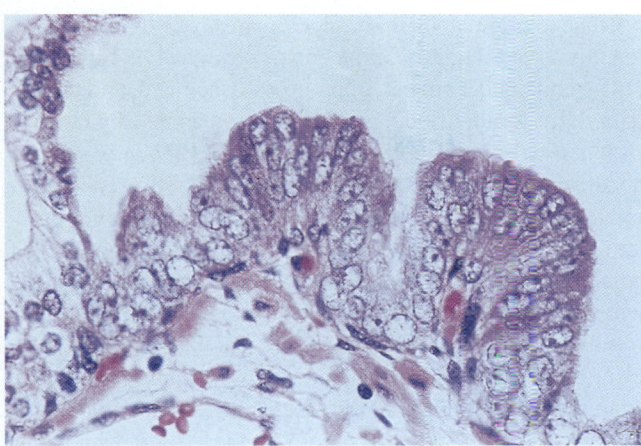

FIG. 56. Basophilia of gland with high-grade prostatic intraepithelial neoplasia (PIN) due to nuclear stratification and high nuclear-to-cytoplasmic ratio with large nuclei and prominent nucleoli. Note in left portion of field within a single gland, the abrupt transition between benign-appearing nuclei and PIN nuclei.

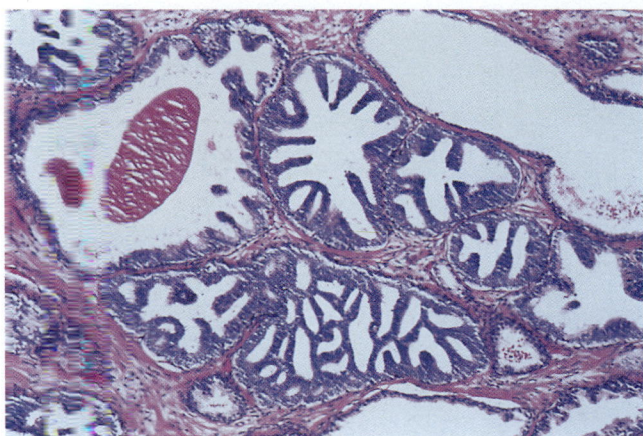

FIG. 58. High-grade prostatic intraepithelial neoplasia (PIN) with cribriform pattern.

tions, the nuclei toward the center of the gland tend to have a more bland cytologic appearance compared with the nuclei peripherally located up against the basement membrane. The grade of PIN is assigned based on assessment of the nuclei peripherally located up against the basement membrane rather than the more bland-appearing nuclei toward the center of the gland. With further epithelial hyperplasia, more complex architectural patterns appear, such as Roman bridge and cribriform formation (Fig. 58). Unusual variants of high-grade PIN, including those with signet ring, mucinous, and neuroendocrine features, were also described (145).

The major differential diagnosis of PIN is with acinar (ordinary) and ductal adenocarcinomas of the prostate. Cytologically, high-grade PIN may be indistinguishable from infiltrating acinar carcinoma. The diagnosis of infiltrating carcinoma is made when the cytologically atypical glands are too small or crowded to be benign glands replaced by cytologically atypical cells (PIN). In contrast to PIN, ductal adenocarcinomas in many cases are centrally located, have papillary formations with fibrovascular cores, show prominent cribriform patterns often with extensive comedonecrosis, and reveal more diffuse cytologic atypia. Cribriforming PIN may be indistinguishable from cribriforming acinar carcinoma (143). Carcinoma should be diagnosed only when the cribriforming glands are back to back, or when many such glands are negative for basal cell–specific cytokeratin. In some cases high-grade PIN is surrounded by a few small atypical glands. It may be difficult to distinguish between outpouchings or tangential sections of high-grade PIN and

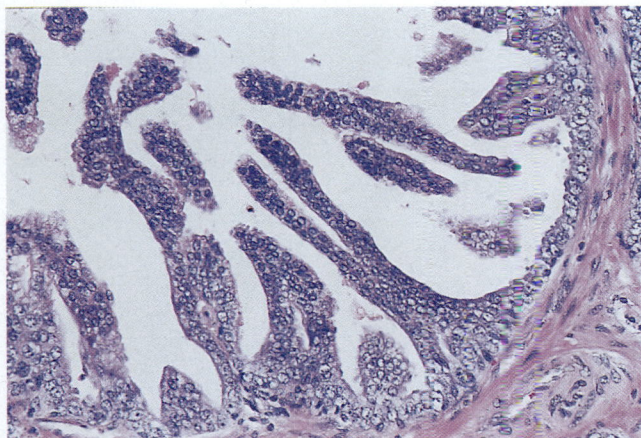

FIG. 57. Prominent tall papillary tufts within high-grade prostatic intraepithelial neoplasia (PIN). Nuclei appear more benign toward the luminal surface of the papillary projections. Note large nuclei with frequent nucleoli, diagnostic of high-grade PIN, toward the edge of the gland up against the basement membrane.

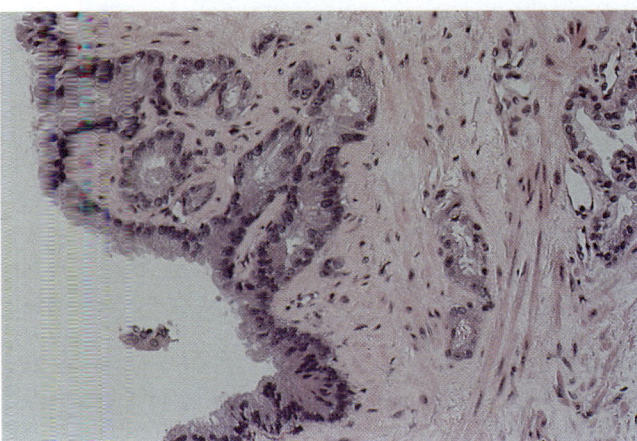

FIG. 59. High-grade prostatic intraepithelial neoplasia (PIN; left) with only a few atypical small glands. We cannot distinguish between PIN and adjacent infiltrating carcinoma versus outpouchings or tangential sections off of high-grade PIN.

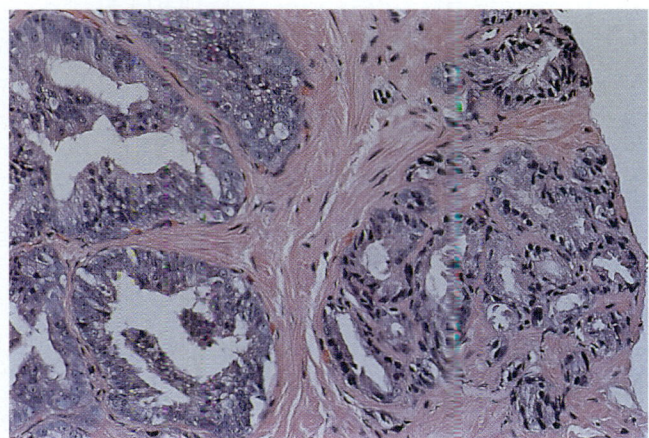

FIG. 60. High-grade prostatic intraepithelial neoplasia (PIN; left) with adjacent small atypical glands. The number of small atypical glands and their greater distance away from the high-grade PIN is diagnostic of infiltrating carcinoma with adjacent high-grade PIN.

PIN with associated infiltrating carcinoma. The greater distance of the small atypical glands away from the high-grade PIN and the greater number of small crowded atypical glands favor the diagnosis of infiltrating carcinoma associated with high-grade PIN (143) (Figs. 59 and 60). The presence of prominent nucleoli in high-grade PIN differentiates it from low-grade PIN (Fig. 61). These two lesions can usually be reproducibly distinguished, but problems arise in cases in which there is prominent cytologic atypia yet no prominent nucleoli (143). There are also cases in which the degree of nucleolar prominence is borderline; some authorities may regard these as low-grade PIN and others as high-grade PIN. These features contribute to the varying incidences of high-grade PIN reported on needle biopsy, ranging from 4% to 16%, with most studies in the 4% to 5% range (146).

Much of the indirect evidence associating PIN with carcinoma of the prostate has come from studies examining differences between prostate glands with carcinoma and prostate glands without carcinoma (147). Low-grade PIN is common in benign glands, and its distinction from normal histology is difficult and subjective (143). For this reason, we do not comment on low-grade PIN in the prostate.

It is difficult to arrive at specific numbers for the incidence of high-grade PIN in benign prostate glands as compared with prostates with cancer, as most of the pertinent studies are older, from when data for PIN-2 and PIN-3 were separately recorded.

Other evidence supporting a relation with high-grade PIN and carcinoma include an increase in the size and the number of PIN foci in glands with carcinoma as compared with glands without carcinoma; with increasing amounts of PIN, there are a greater number of multifocal carcinomas; PIN is more common in the peripheral zone of the prostate, correlating with the predilection for most adenocarcinomas of the prostate to originate in this region; in areas of PIN, there is often the appearance of adjacent microinvasive carcinoma (148); and histochemical, immunohistochemical, and genetic data show parallel findings with carcinoma and PIN (147).

When only high-grade PIN (PIN-2 or PIN-3) is seen on needle biopsy, repeated biopsy reveals infiltrating carcinoma in approximately 50% of cases (147). This sampling problem results from the ubiquitous presence of high-grade PIN adjacent to peripherally located dominant tumor nodules, where the PIN may be extensive. Whether those with benign follow-up biopsies will also eventually be shown to have carcinoma is unknown. The findings of an abnormal rectal examination, an abnormal transrectal ultrasound, or PIN-3 as opposed to PIN-2 were not helpful in identifying which men had infiltrating carcinoma on subsequent biopsy. The presence of a persistently elevated serum PSA level was the only finding seen more frequently in patients who were eventually shown to have carcinoma. We recommend that when only high-grade PIN is identified on biopsy, the biopsy be repeated to look for infiltrating carcinoma. When cancer is found on repeated biopsy, it may be anywhere in the gland, not only at the site of the initially biopsy of high-grade PIN. Consequently, when high-grade PIN is found on biopsy, a full sextant biopsy should be performed to look for cancer (149). We must be aware that high-grade PIN may appear as a hypoechoic lesion, even if there is no infiltrating carcinoma (83). PIN by itself does not give rise to increased serum PSA levels (150).

The significance of high-grade PIN on TUR is not so clear, although these men appear to be at increased risk for subsequent discovery of cancer (151). In an elderly patient with high-grade PIN on TUR, often no further workup is instituted. In a younger man, a more aggressive workup to rule out a clinically significant tumor is warranted. If high-grade PIN is found on TUR and the specimen has not been put through entirely, the remainder should be processed to look for infiltrating carcinoma.

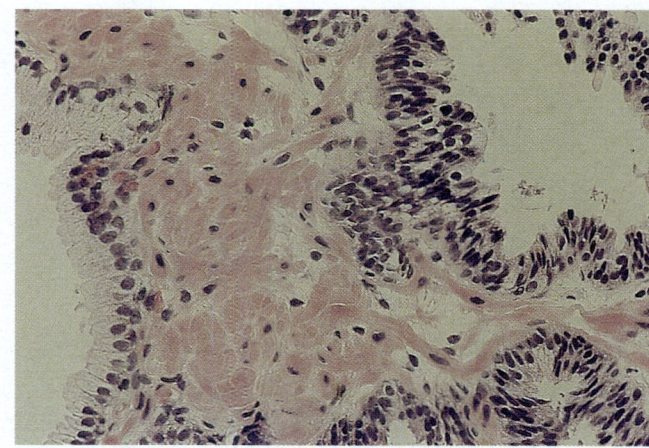

FIG. 61. Low-grade prostatic intraepithelial neoplasia (PIN) with slight enlargement of nuclei and stratification, yet no prominent nucleoli.

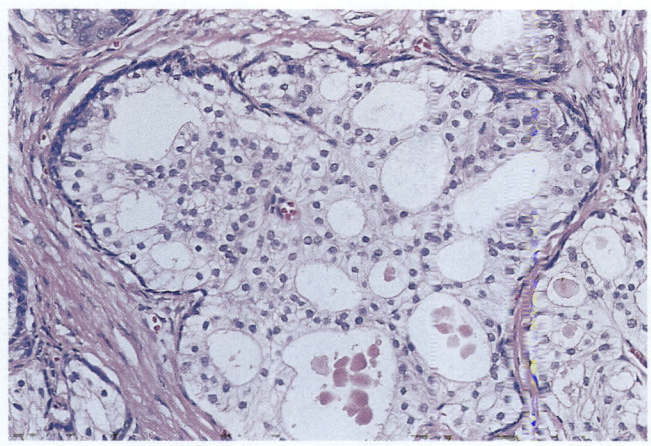

FIG. 62. Clear cell cribriforming hyperplasia showing cribriforming glands with clear cytoplasm, benign-appearing nuclei, and a well-defined basal cell layer surrounding many of the glands.

The one piece of evidence we have for premalignant lesions in other organs (i.e., cervix) that is lacking in the prostate is the natural history of high-grade PIN. When PIN is diagnosed, there is no method to determine whether (a) there is not already infiltrating carcinoma at that site, or (b) when infiltrating carcinoma evolves, has it done so in the immediate vicinity of the PIN. Because we do not yet know what percentage of patients with PIN will develop infiltrating carcinoma over a given follow-up interval, most authorities do not prefer the term carcinoma in situ (CIS). CIS has implications that these lesions will develop into infiltrating carcinoma at a sufficiently high frequency that may lead some aggressive clinicians to treat these lesions in a radical fashion. Given that there is still controversy as to whether even infiltrating adenocarcinoma of the prostate should always be treated aggressively, it is doubtful that these potential precursor lesions should be treated with aggressive therapy until their natural history is better understood. Additional questions have been raised as to whether low-grade centrally located adenocarcinomas are as closely related to PIN as are peripherally located intermediate-grade adenocarcinomas. These questions highlight the one negative aspect of the term "PIN," which by virtue of its parallel terminology to that of cervical intraepithelial neoplasia (CIN; used for the cervix) implies a greater knowledge of the biology of PIN and its relation to invasive carcinoma than is currently available.

Benign Cribriforming Lesions Mimicking PIN and Carcinoma

Clear-cell cribriforming hyperplasia consists of numerous cribriforming glands with clear cytoplasm that may grow either in a nodular pattern or as a more infiltrative lesion (152) (Fig. 62). Differentiating clear-cell cribriforming hyperplasia from PIN or carcinoma is the fact that the cells in clear-cell cribriforming hyperplasia have distinctive clear cytoplasm and benign-appearing nuclei with at most small nucleoli. The other diagnostic feature in clear-cell cribriforming hyperplasia is the presence of a strikingly prominent basal cell layer around many of the cribriforming glands.

A variation of normal histology is the finding of prominent Roman bridge and cribriform formation up at the base of the prostate in the central zone (Fig. 63). The lack of cytologic atypia in these glands again distinguishes this cribriforming pattern from that of cribriforming PIN or cribriforming carcinoma.

CLINICAL STAGE T2 (PALPABLE) CARCINOMA

Methods of Processing Radical Prostatectomy Specimens

In institutions that do not totally embed radical prostatectomy specimens, the following is the optimal method to sample the prostate (153). Routine sections include: (a) amputation of the distal (apical) 1 cm of the prostate and serial sections of this specimen parallel to the urethra (Fig. 64); (b) either a thin shave of the proximal (base) margins or amputation of the base analogous to that described for the apex; (c) base of seminal vesicles; and (d) right and left vas deferens margins. In addition, after serial sectioning of the prostate perpendicular to the urethra, sections are submitted in which gross tumor is identified. Gross tumor may be identified by examination of the posterior and posterolateral horseshoe-shaped peripheral zone of the prostate looking for asymmetry in size, color, and density of tissue between right and left halves of the prostate (Fig. 65). In more than 85% of prostates, gross tumor will be identified. Submission of the prostate in this manner will allow detection of more than 90% of positive margins, extraprostatic extension, and seminal vesicle invasion with, on average, a submission of only 12 to 3 cassettes (see later for description of lymph node examination).

Whole-mount sectioning of the prostate provides more esthetically pleasing sections for teaching and publications, yet

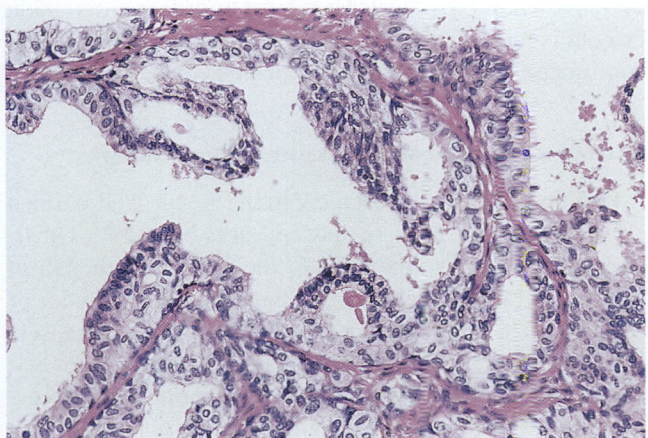

FIG. 63. Benign Roman bridge and cribriform formation seen normally in the central zone at the base of the prostate. Note lack of nuclear atypia.

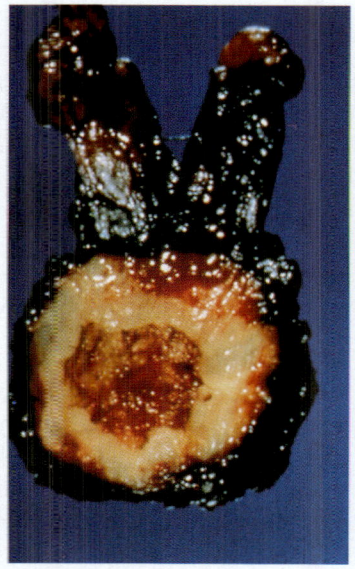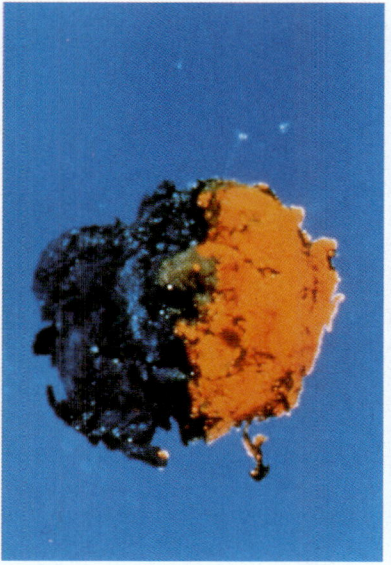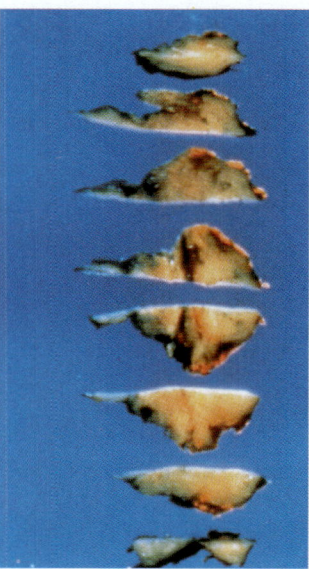

FIG. 64. Handling of the apical margin. The distal 1 cm is amputated, inked to designate left versus right, and then serially sectioned parallel to the urethra.

the information obtained by using routine sections is identical, and in a small minority of cases, routinely processed thinly sliced sections will identify positive margins not identified by using thicker slices of tissue, which is necessary for whole-mount processing.

Tumor Location

Stage T2 adenocarcinomas of the prostate in almost all cases show predominantly peripherally located carcinoma up against the edge of the prostate (154,155). In a few cases, large centrally located tumors may extend peripherally and be palpated and diagnosed on needle biopsy. Only when a peripherally located tumor becomes very large does it extend anteriorly and centrally. Tumors tend to predominate within the posterior and posterolateral aspects of the gland. Tumors that appear to be unilateral on rectal examination will have bilateral tumor in approximately 70% of cases when examined pathologically. The presence of multifocal adenocarcinoma of the prostate is more than 85% (154). However, in many of these cases of bilateral or multifocal tumor (or both), the other tumors are small, low grade, and clinically insignificant. Significant bilateral tumor may be composed of discrete right and left tumor nodules or a single, large, confluent tumor mass involving both sides.

Progression After Radical Prostatectomy

The finding of postradical prostatectomy serum PSA levels above the female range is the most sensitive means of detecting progression. However, whether these patients with elevated serum PSA levels have local or distant progression or both is unclear. Proven local recurrence requires biopsy confirmation of tumor within the prostatic bed.

Extraprostatic Extension (Capsular Penetration)

Histologically, the prostatic capsule is not well defined (156). In some areas, there may appear to be a fibrous or fibromuscular band at the edge of the prostate, although in other areas, normal prostatic glands extend out to the edge of the prostate without any appearance that there is a capsule (Fig. 66). In most areas, there appears to be no apparent histologic barrier between the prostatic and periprostatic tissue. Nevertheless, we not uncommonly see a wall of prostatic carcinoma along the edge of the gland without extension into the adjacent soft tissue, demonstrating that the edge of the prostate physiologically acts as a fairly effective barrier (Fig.

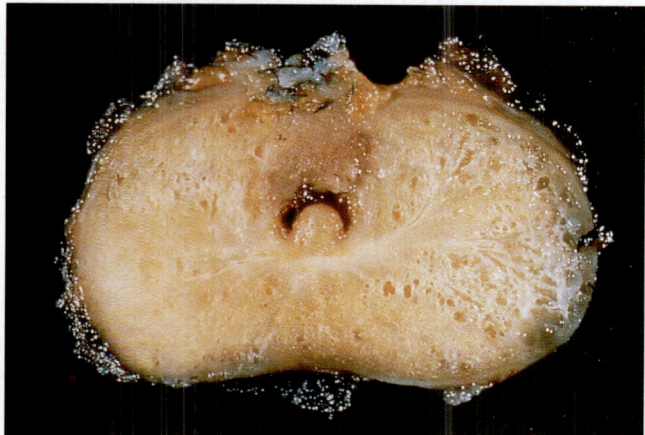

FIG. 65. Gross appearance of adenocarcinoma of the prostate. Note more solid, homogeneous, gray–white appearance to carcinoma (left) as compared with contralateral benign prostate with a more spongy appearance.

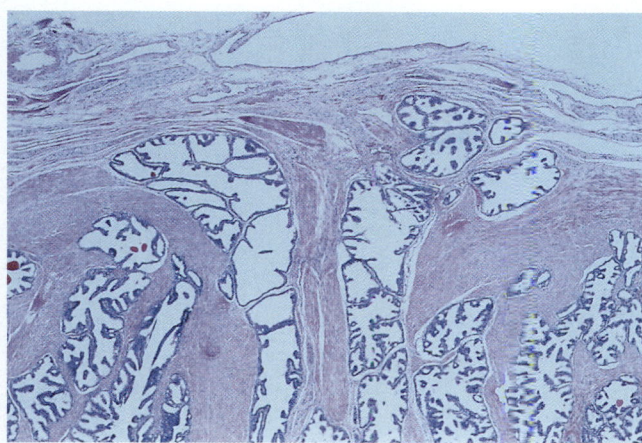

FIG. 66. Edge of the prostate toward the base of the gland. Benign glands appear to extend out of the prostate with no well-defined prostatic capsule.

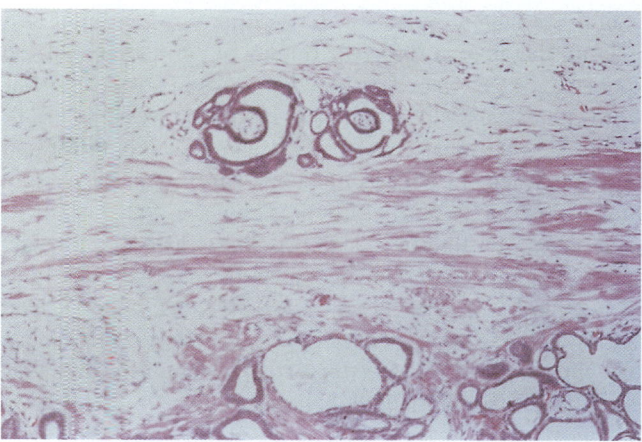

FIG. 68. Focal extraprostatic extension with only a few neoplastic glands situated exterior to the edge of the prostate.

67). Although the prostate lacks a discrete capsule, the term capsular penetration is often used to a convenient method of describing tumor that has extended out of the prostate into periprostatic soft tissue. Some authors use the term capsular invasion when they believe that the "capsule" is infiltrated by tumor, but the tumor does not extend out of the prostate. Because "capsular invasion" is almost always present and because of the ambiguity as to where the prostatic stroma stops and the capsule begins, we do not recognize capsular invasion. Difficulty in diagnosing extraprostatic extension arises when the tumor has penetrated the prostatic gland and induces a dense desmoplastic response in the periprostatic adipose tissue. Because of the desmoplastic response, it can be difficult to judge whether the tumor has extended out of the gland or is within the fibrous tissue of the prostate. The best way of assessing whether extraprostatic extension has occurred is to look at the adjacent edge of the prostate on scanning magnification where there is no tumor and follow the edge of the gland to the area in question to see whether the normal rounded contour of the gland has been altered by a protuberance corresponding to extension of tumor into the periprostatic tissue (157). Stage T2 adenocarcinomas of the prostate have a tendency to extend out of the prostate via perineural space invasion (158). Perineural invasion by itself does not worsen prognosis, because perineural invasion merely represents extension of tumor along a plane of decreased resistance and not invasion into lymphatics (159). Extraprostatic extension preferentially occurs posteriorly and posterolaterally, paralleling the location of most stage T2 adenocarcinomas. Even with clinically organ-confined tumor, there is microscopic extraprostatic extension in 50% of cases. The degree of extraprostatic extension varies from only a few glands outside the prostate, which we term focal extraprostatic extension, to cases with more extensive extraprostatic spread that we designate established extraprostatic extension (Figs. 68 and 69). The degree of extrapro-

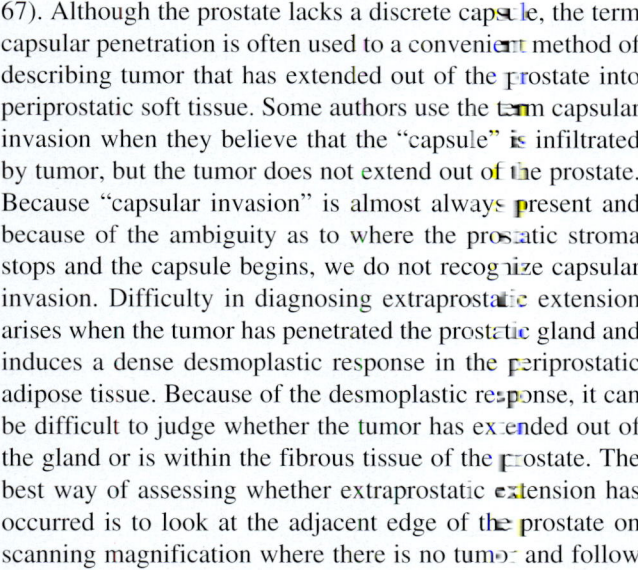

FIG. 67. Adenocarcinoma of the prostate extending to the edge of the prostate but not into periprostatic tissue.

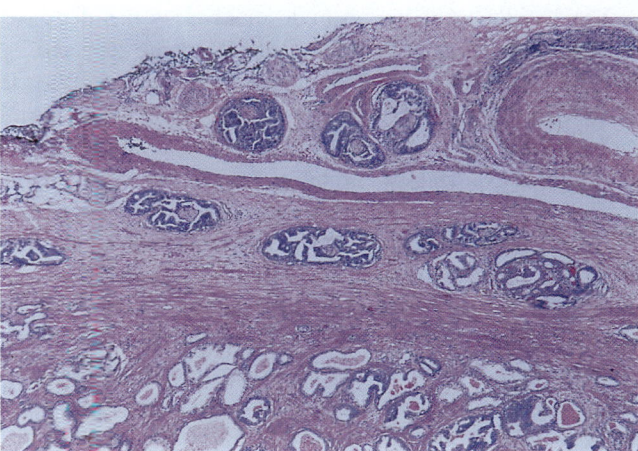

FIG. 69. Established extraprostatic extension with multiple neoplastic glands exterior to the prostate. Glands show prominent perineural invasion. Margins are still negative, as tumor does not extend to the inked edge of the gland.

static extension correlates with risk of progression after radical prostatectomy (105). The finding of perineural invasion on needle biopsy has been shown to have a strong association with extraprostatic extension in the corresponding radical prostatectomy specimen and is worth searching for and recording when diagnosing adenocarcinoma of needle biopsy (160). There are conflicting studies as to the independent prognostic significance of perineural invasion of needle biopsy (161,161a). Widely excising the neurovascular bundle on the side of perineural invasion seen on biopsy can lead to a decrease in the incidence of positive margins (162). Potency may still be preserved in patients who have had a unilateral neurovascular bundle removed.

Seminal Vesicle Invasion

Although both seminal vesicle invasion and extraprostatic extension are pathologic stage T3 disease, seminal vesicle invasion is a much more dire prognostic finding, with a 75% progression rate after surgery (163). In our material, of the 69 cases with positive seminal vesicles, only 20% were free of progression 5 years after radical prostatectomy. The most common route of seminal vesicle invasion we have noted is through spread of the tumor out of the gland at the base with growth and extension into periseminal vesicle soft tissue and eventually into the seminal vesicles. Less commonly, there may be direct extension through the ejaculatory ducts into the seminal vesicles or direct extension from the base of the prostate into the wall of the seminal vesicles. Least commonly, there may be discrete metastases to the seminal vesicle. Seminal vesicle invasion may be identified by examining the base of the seminal vesicles, because this is always the first region to be invaded by carcinoma. Seminal vesicle invasion should be diagnosed when tumor invades the muscular coat of the seminal vesicle (Fig. 70).

Lymph Node Metastases

The incidence of lymph node metastases has declined markedly in recent years as earlier tumors are detected by screening techniques. The incidence of nodal metastases is related to the clinical stage, preoperative PSA level, and biopsy grade (113). Because the presence of nodal metastases indicates a lack of curability, surgeons will often perform staging pelvic lymphadenectomies with frozen sections; if positive nodes are found, the surgery is aborted. Even when the lymph nodes are grossly uninvolved, we can identify more than two thirds of microscopic metastases with random frozen sections (164). In particular, small indurated nodes provide the highest yield. When microscopic metastases are identified at the time of frozen section, many urologists will abort the radical prostatectomy because the procedure will not be curative. Other urologists will perform radical prostatectomy in the face of microscopic metastases for local control if the patient has a relatively long life ex-

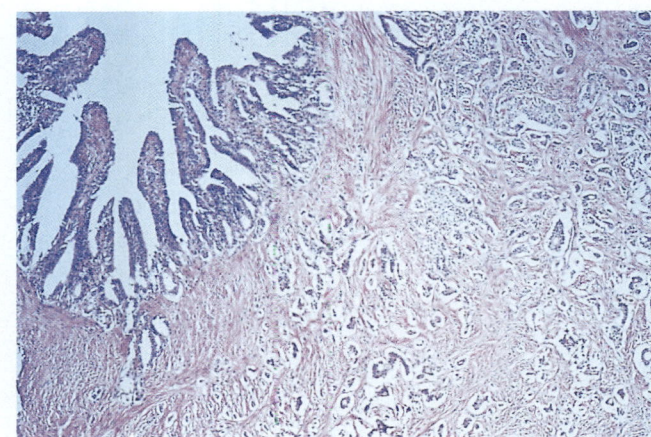

FIG. 70. Adenocarcinoma of the prostate invading the seminal vesicles.

pectancy. It has been demonstrated that patients with positive lymph nodes who undergo radical prostatectomy will all have progression indicative of distant occult metastases. Nonetheless, the overall 5- and 10-year projected actuarial survival rates for patients with positive nodes who undergo radical prostatectomy is 97% and 62%, respectively. In cases in which the preoperative biopsy score is less than 8, the time to onset of distant metastases is sufficiently long that our surgeons proceed in these instances with radical prostatectomy even if the nodes are involved (165). Consequently, we freeze pelvic nodes only when the biopsy score is 8 to 10. Another option is to freeze nodes only in cases in which the risk of metastases is sufficiently high, based on preoperative parameters (113). The extent of nodal metastases and, in some studies, the histologic appearance of the nodal metastases correlate with progression (see later for discussion on DNA) (166). We routinely submit all of the tissue removed during lymphadenectomy because the modified lymphadenectomy contains relatively scant tissue and in 5% of cases with lymph node metastases, the only metastases have been present in a small lymph node that was unidentifiable grossly.

Grade

Several studies have correlated core biopsy and radical prostatectomy grade (107–109). In general, a Gleason score of 5 to 6 on biopsy corresponds to the same grade in the radical prostatectomy in 64% of the cases. When the Gleason grade is equal or higher than 7 on biopsy, the radical prostatectomy was the same in 87.5% of the cases. It is reasonable to assign a full Gleason score even to small foci of cancer on needle biopsy, as it has been demonstrated that the grade assigned to these minimal cancers is just as accurate compared with cases with more extensive cancer on biopsy. Both the preoperative Gleason grade and the Gleason grade assigned to the radical prostatectomy specimen correlate with final pathologic stage (109,167). Gleason score 7 tumor has a significantly higher progression rate than tumors with the Gleason score of 5 or 6 (105) (Fig. 71). This finding emphasizes that tumors of Gleason scores 5 to 7 should not be considered together as intermediate-grade tumor. In radical prostatectomy specimens seen at Johns Hopkins Hospital, only 6% of cases are assigned a Gleason score of 2 to 4, and 9.7%, a Gleason score of 8 to 9. Gleason score 2 to 4 tumors tend to occur in the transition zone (periurethral region) where the tumors tend to be fairly small and of low stage and not detected on needle biopsy. In contrast, high-grade tumors less commonly come to radical prostatectomy, as many of these tumors are advanced and not as amenable to surgery.

Margins of Resection

Much of the difficulty in assessing the prostatic margins of resection is due to the close relation of the prostate to surrounding structures such as the urogenital diaphragm, pelvic sidewall, rectum, and bladder neck. At many sites, only 1 to 2 mm of soft tissue separates the prostate from the rectum and pelvic sidewall (168). Consequently, on pathologic examination of radical prostatectomy specimens, we often find only a scant amount of periprostatic tissue. The incidence of positive margins will vary according to the clinical stage of the patients. It may range from 7% for T1c (nonpalpable) tumors to 30% to 40% for larger palpable lesions (169,170).

The apex is one of the most frequent sites of a positive margin (171). There are conflicting studies as to the significance of a sole positive margin at the apex (172,173). The value of frozen sections of the distal margin at the time of radical prostatectomy is questionable because often the urologist has taken as much tissue as possible at the site. Removal of additional tissue risks injuring the urogenital diaphragm and increasing postoperative incontinence. The proximal margin in radical prostatectomy specimens consists of the bladder neck, composed of thick muscle bundles. Positive proximal margins usually correlate with extensive tumor.

In clinical stage T2 carcinomas, the anterior margin is involved infrequently (3% to 4%). Dissection of the anterior region of the gland is performed by cutting smooth muscle so that any tumor extending to the inked edge of the gland is considered to be a positive margin. We consider tumor in this region extending to the ink as showing extraprostatic extension because the surgeon transects this region as far anteriorly away from the prostate as possible.

Posterior, posterolateral, and lateral sites account for a sizable proportion of positive margins. They parallel the location of most stage T2 carcinomas. In particular, these sites are disproportionately involved toward the apex of the prostate. In assessing these margins of resection, it is critical to determine first whether the tumor has extended out of the prostate or is confined to the gland. When prostate cancer extends out of the prostate, the tumor in almost all cases induces a marked desmoplastic response, in which tumor adheres to the gland (Fig. 69). Whether the tumor is organ confined or shows extraprostatic extension, the cleavage plane that the urologist dissects is usually between the tumor and the uninvolved periprostatic adipose tissue. When the tumor is confined to the gland, the capsular surface has a smooth, rounded contour at low magnification. In these cases, the prostate is often covered only by a filmy connective tissue layer (Fig. 72) that may be inapparent or easily disrupted during intra- or postoperative handling of the prostate, leading to the picture seen in Fig. 73. In these cases, even if the tumor extends just to the inked surface of the prostate, the margins are considered negative for tumor because the tumor is confined to the prostate and has been removed in its entirety. When tumor extends out of the prostate, the contour of the prostate at scanning magni-

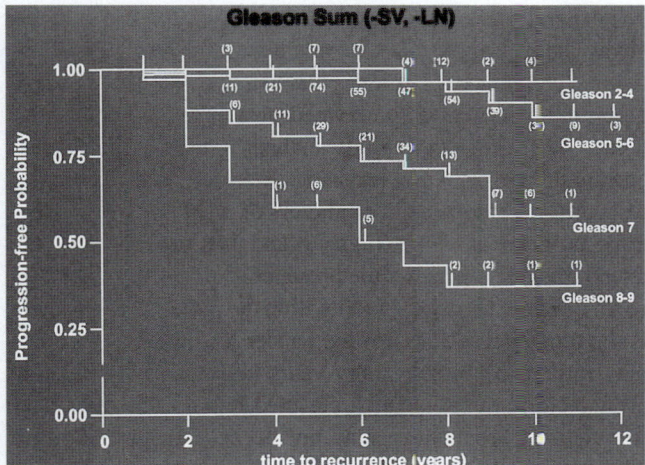

FIG. 71. Correlation of Gleason sum of cancer in radical prostatectomy specimen with progression after surgery.

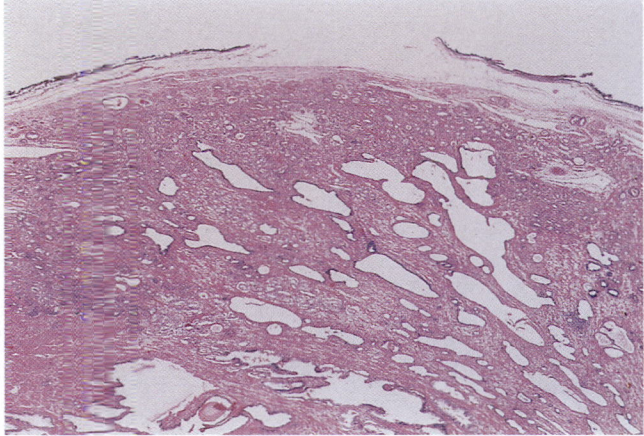

FIG. 72. Organ-confined adenocarcinoma of the prostate. Edge of the prostate has a smooth rounded border. Flimsy periprostatic soft tissue may be easily disrupted.

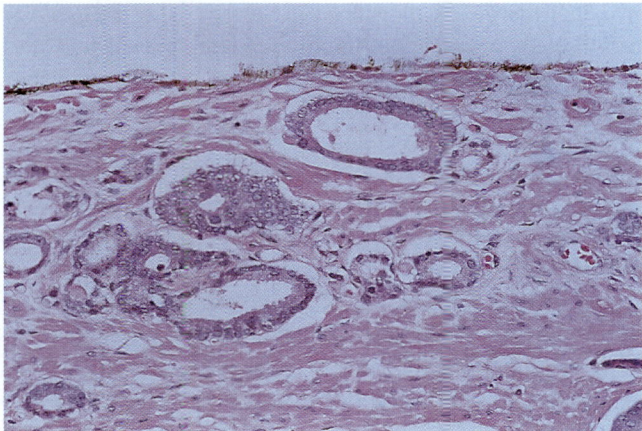

FIG. 73. Adenocarcinoma extending close to the inked edge of the gland, which has a smooth rounded surface. This margin is negative for tumor and is associated with a low risk of progression.

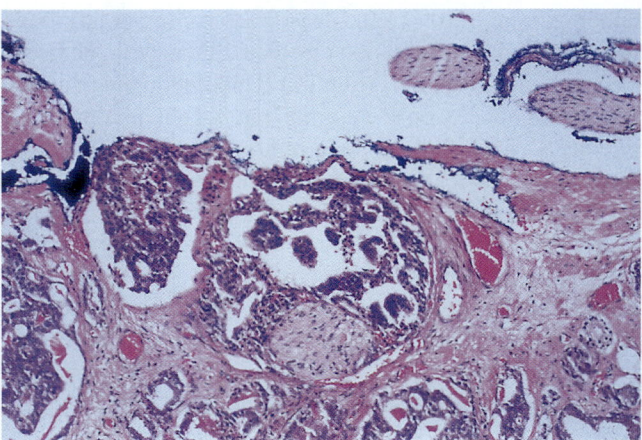

FIG. 75. Adenocarcinoma of the prostate, which has extended out of the prostate where the surgeon transected tumor, resulting in a shaggy, irregular surface of the gland. The tumor in this region extends to the inked margin and is therefore positive for tumor.

fication will have an irregular surface. In these cases with extraprostatic extension, the adequacy of resection will depend on whether the tumor extends to the inked margin (Fig. 69). However, even in these cases, if there is only a scant amount of benign soft tissue separating the tumor from the ink, the margin should be considered negative. Two studies showed that close (less than 1 mm) margins are perfectly adequate margins in radical prostatectomy specimens (174,175). The importance of distinguishing between posterior and posterolateral and lateral is that one of the few sites that the urologist may modify is in the posterolateral regions bilaterally in the regions of the neurovascular bundle (Fig. 74). The neurovascular bundles run along this aspect of the gland and have been shown to be a major contributor to potency. The surgeon, based either on preoperative or intraoperative factors, can decide whether to spare the neurovascular bundles (i.e., leave them within the patient for potency), at which point we will find only a scant amount of periprostatic soft tissue in the posterolateral regions of the gland. Alternatively, the surgeon can sacrifice (resect) the neurovascular bundle, resulting in an additional approximately 5 mm of soft tissue in this region. In contrast, laterally and posteriorly, the surgeon cannot take additional tissue because of the presence of pelvic sidewall and rectum. In general, most authorities recognize that judicious preservation of one or both of the neurovascular bundles can be performed without compromising removal of cancer. Some authorities recommended routine removal of the bundle on the side of the dominant tumor. In most cases when the posterolateral margin is positive, there are other positive margins for which sacrifice of the neurovascular bundle would not have resulted in negative margins (Fig. 75). We also must recognize that positive margins in radical prostatectomy specimens do not always necessarily mean that tumor has been left in the patient. Even when margins are thought to be positive, additional tissue removed from that site does not always show tumor (174). In only approximately 50% of patients with positive margins is there showed evidence of progression as measured by elevated postoperative serum PSA levels (172). In a multivariate analysis, Gleason grade, presence and degree of extraprostatic extension, and margins of resection are independent predictors of postradical prostatectomy progression (105) (Figs. 76 and 77). In addition to the uncertainty as to whether the presence of positive margins always translates into tumor left within the patient locally, there is the recognition that prostate cancer left in small amounts may remain occult for many years because of its indolent growth (176). Consequently, elevated PSAs as the only measurement of progression may not necessarily translate into clinical progression. Because of the uncertainty as to whether positive margins always translate into residual tumor left within the patient, as well as to the lack of definitive data showing effectiveness of adjuvant therapy, many authorities

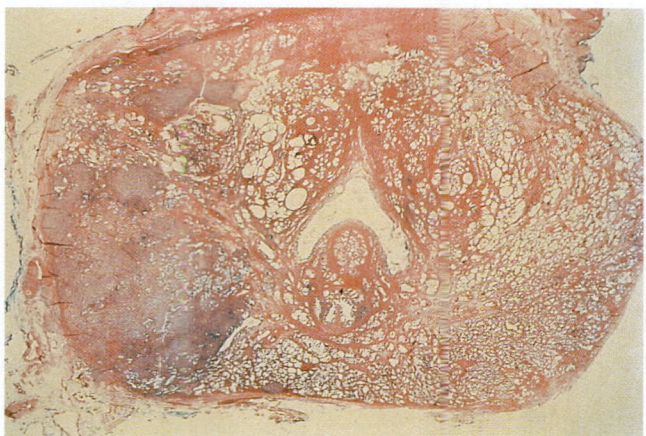

FIG. 74. Whole-mount cross section of prostate showing posterolateral unilaterally resected neurovascular bundle (lower left) and contralateral region posterolaterally where neurovascular bundle has been spared (lower right).

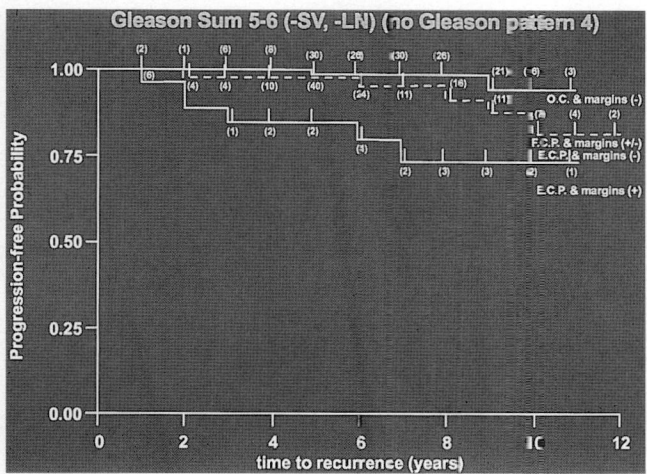

FIG. 76. Kaplan–Meier curves showing progression after radical prostatectomy for Gleason score 5 to 6 tumor. Prognosis is stratified by extent of extraprostatic extension and margin status. FCP, focal extraprostatic extension; ECP, established extraprostatic extension.

will monitor patients who have positive margins until progression is demonstrated before administering adjuvant therapy. In addition to noting the sites of positive margins, some indication as to the extent of positive margins also should be noted.

Tumor Volume

Tumor volume in the radical prostatectomy specimen correlates well with pathologic stage and Gleason grade in clinical stage T2 cancers (106,177,178). In addition to measurements of cubic centimeters, the percentage of the specimen involved by tumor also correlated well with pathologic stage (179). Lim-

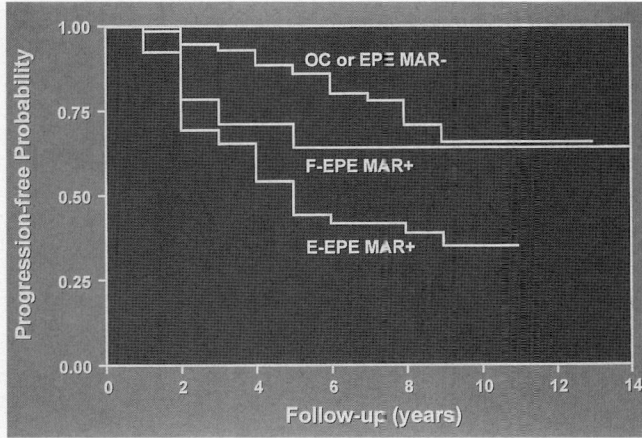

FIG. 77. Kaplan–Meier curve showing progression after radical prostatectomy for Gleason score 7 tumor. Progression is stratified by extent of extraprostatic extension and margin status. OC, organ confined; EPE, extraprostatic extension; F-EPE, focal extraprostatic extension; E-EPE, established extraprostatic extension; MAR −, margins negative; MAR +, margins positive.

ited tumor volume on the needle biopsy, by itself, does not necessarily indicate limited cancer in the corresponding radical prostatectomy specimen (80,180). Preoperatively, both rectal examination and transrectal ultrasound significantly underestimate tumor volume. Tumor volume does not independently predict postradical prostatectomy progression once grade and pathologic stage are determined (181). Consequently it is not essential that tumor volume be calculated for clinical purposes in radical prostatectomy specimens. Rather, there should be some overall subjective indication of tumor volume to identify those cases with minute amounts of tumor with an excellent prognosis and those with extensive tumor and a worse prognosis. Although in general, larger tumors are high grade and small tumors low grade, exceptions occur. There is a tendency to hypothesize that tumors begin as low-grade tumors, and on reaching a certain size, dedifferentiate into higher-grade lesions, accounting for the relation between size and grade. Alternatively, high-grade tumors may be high grade at their inception, yet because of their rapid growth are detected at an advanced size (182). Similarly, low-grade tumors may evolve so slowly that they tend to be detected at lower volumes.

Ploidy

Although most studies showed that ploidy weakly correlates with pathologic stage and tumor behavior, there are conflicting studies as to whether ploidy offers independent prognostic information beyond that of routinely measured parameters. Consequently, ploidy is not recommended for routine clinical use (183,184). One situation in which there is evidence that ploidy may be of prognostic importance in patients undergoing radical prostatectomy is in patients with nodal metastases. Some studies demonstrated that patients who have undergone radical prostatectomy with positive nodes, who have diploid tumors, do significantly better than patients with nondiploid tumors (185)). The data also suggest that early hormonal therapy in patients with diploid tumors can offer a survival advantage.

Vascular Invasion

Vascular invasion is uncommonly identified in radical prostatectomy specimens, seen in 7% of tumors smaller than 4 cc (most tumors seen today at radical prostatectomy are smaller than 2 cc) (186). Although vascular invasion correlates with other adverse findings (i.e., extraprostatic extension, grade, margins, tumor volume), studies are conflicting as to whether vascular invasion offers independent prognostic information beyond those of routinely noted findings (186–188).

CLINICAL STAGES T1A AND T1B CANCER (DETECTED ON TURP)

Stages T1a and T1b disease refers to prostatic carcinoma that is unsuspected clinically and is incidentally discovered in specimens usually removed for BPH. In approximately

16% of TUR specimens taken for presumed BPH, carcinoma is identified (189). Stages T1a and T1b carcinomas are much more heterogeneous than tumors in other stages. Tumor may be clinically unsuspected because (a) there are only small amounts of scattered tumor, (b) the tumor is predominantly centrally or anteriorly located, (c) the tumor diffusely infiltrates the prostate without resulting in induration or a clinically detectable nodule, or (d) the tumor is well defined and peripherally located but still is not palpable for reasons that remain to be clarified. As we would expect, the biologic behavior of tumor in these situations differs considerably. The system that is gaining widespread acceptance is based on the percentage of the specimen involved by tumor, with 5% being the cutoff between stages T1a and T1b (189). There is controversy as to whether intermediate-grade tumor (Gleason score 5 to 5) should be included in the stage T1a category. Data from our long-term follow-up study of untreated cancer occupying less than 5% of the TURP specimen showed that intermediate-grade tumor had the same progression rate as low-grade tumor. In addition, there was no difference in prediction of either residual tumor volume or tumor extent in radical prostatectomies performed for stage T1a disease whether the TUR tumor was of low or intermediate grade. Consequently, we believe that intermediate-grade tumor should be considered stage T1a disease as long as it is less than 5%. In the study of Cantrell et al. (189) of untreated stage A carcinomas found on TURP, when less than 5% of the specimen was involved by tumor and the tumor was not high grade (stage T1a), only 2% progressed at 4 years after diagnosis, in comparison with 32% progression in patients with specimens containing more than 5% of cancer or high-grade tumor (Gleason score 7 to 10) of any quantity (stage T1b). Although the risk of progression at 4 years with stage T1a cancer was low, recently between 16% and 25% of men with untreated stage T1a prostate cancer and longer (8 to 10 years) follow-up have had clinically evident progression (189). The significance of these studies, in general, relates only to treatment of stage T1a tumors in relatively young men, because studies demonstrated that the chance of older men dying of other causes is greater than the risk of progression with their prostate cancer. There are multiple options for the management of men with stage T1a prostate carcinoma. Because on average only 10% of stage T1a patients have been upstaged by repeated TUR, and even those patients who are not upstaged are still at risk of progression, this procedure is in general not recommended (189). Another option has been the performance of TRUS after diagnosis of carcinoma by TUR, possibly with accompanying needle biopsies of the peripheral region of the gland. This treatment option is currently unproven. Difficulty arises because post-TUR scarring mimics carcinoma on TRUS, and with ultrasound it is difficult to visualize the anterior portion of the gland. The other option for treatment of relatively young men with stage T1a prostate cancer who are at increased long-term risk of progression is radical prostatectomy (190). In the largest series of 64 totally embedded radical prostatectomy specimens performed for stage T1a prostate cancer, 6% had no residual cancer, 74% had minimal cancer, and 20% had substantial cancer. Those with substantial cancer had tumor volumes comparable to those seen in stages T1b and palpable carcinoma. The other treatment option for patients with stage T1a cancer is to monitor PSA levels (191). Patients who have increased post-TUR serum PSA levels have been shown to have a higher likelihood of having significant residual tumor within the prostate and may be good candidates for radical prostatectomy.

Patients with stage T1b prostate cancer are in general treated with either radiotherapy or radical prostatectomy (192). Stage T1b tumors are more heterogeneous in grade, location, and volume than are stage T2 carcinomas (192). Stage T1b cancers tend to be lower grade and located within the transition zone (periurethral region) as compared with palpable cancers. The relation between tumor volume and pathologic stage also differs, in that centrally located carcinomas may grow to a large volume before reaching the edge of the gland and extending out of the prostate, whereas stage T2 tumors that begin peripherally show extraprostatic extension at relatively lower volumes (192–194). This poor correlation between volume and pathologic stage is also attributable to the lower grade in many stage T1b cancers. Despite some overlap between stages T1a and T1b disease, T1b tumors have in general greater tumor volumes, worse pathologic stage, and a higher rate and more rapid interval to progression than do stage T1a. Although the subclassification of incidental tumors found on TURP to stage T1a and T1b disease is imperfect, it remains a useful system to separate patients in terms of their relative tumor aggressiveness.

Regardless of the staging systems used to separate stage T1a and T1b disease, all stage T1b tumors will be detected by processing between six and eight cassettes of a TUR specimen. By processing eight to ten cassettes, more than 90% of stage T1a lesions will be identified (189). Depending on the institution, all TUR tissues may be examined in relatively young men (younger than 65 years) in whom aggressive therapy for stage T1a disease might be pursued. When cancer is incidentally found on TURP, algorithms have been developed as to whether and how much additional sampling of the TURP specimens is needed (195).

STAGE T1C CANCER (NONPALPABLE CANCER DETECTED ON NEEDLE BIOPSY)

With widespread use of PSA tests, an increasing number of tumors are diagnosed and treated when they are nonpalpable on digital-rectal examination. Stage T1c tumors are more extensive than small cancers found on transurethral resection and less extensive than clinically palpable tumors. Although the majority of stage T1c cancers are significant tumors warranting definitive therapy, approximately 25% of these tumors detected by needle biopsy are thought to be "insignificant" tumors. A combination of relatively low PSA values and minimal findings of cancer on needle biopsy can help predict preoperatively which patients may have insignificant tumors and who might be candidates for conservative therapy (80,169). Repeated sextant biopsies in men who are considered candidates for expectant therapy are problematic, in that even when the repeated biopsy is negative, men may have significant tumors (196). Investigators are currently evaluating whether more extensive repeated sampling of the prostate in these cases will give a better indication of which tumors are truly insignificant. In a growing number of cases, these insignificant tumors may be so small that they are difficult to detect pathologically at radical prostatectomy. Exceptionally, there may be no identifiable cancer in the radical prostatectomy specimen, despite tumor seen on the preoperative needle biopsy (197,198).

CLINICAL STAGE T3 (NON–ORGAN CONFINED) DISEASE

In general, patients with clinical stage T3 prostate cancer are not candidates for radical prostatectomy and are usually treated with radiotherapy. Stage T3 disease encompasses both those with extraprostatic extension alone and those with seminal vesicle involvement, the latter associated with a much worse prognosis. Between 50% and 60% of clinical stage T3 prostate cancers have lymph node metastases at the time of diagnosis. More than 50% of patients with clinical stage T3 disease develop metastases in 5 years, and 75% of these patients die of prostate carcinoma within 10 years.

METASTATIC DISEASE (NODAL AND DISTANT)

Treatment of patients with nodal metastases disease with radical prostatectomy was discussed earlier. Distant metastases appear within 5 years in more than 85% of these patients who receive no further treatment. Pelvic lymph nodes examined at the time of radical prostatectomy may contain foamy xanthomatous histiocytes. These may be seen as a reaction to a hip prosthesis or in men with nodal metastases who have received preoperative hormonal therapy (199,200).

In patients with distant metastases, the mortality is approximately 15% at 3 years, 80% at 5 years, and 90% at 10 years. Of the patients who relapse after endocrine therapy, most die within the first year, and 90% die within 2 years.

After lymph node metastases, bone metastases are the next most frequent site of metastatic prostate carcinoma. Among bone metastases, metastases to the spine are most frequent; other common sites are the ribs, sternum, ileum, and femur (201). More than 90% of bone metastases from prostate carcinoma are either osteoblastic or mixed blastic and lytic. Lung metastases from prostate carcinoma are extremely common at autopsy, and almost all cases have bone involvement as well (202). Metastatic lesions usually take the form of multiple small nodules or diffuse lymphatic spread rather than large metastatic deposits. Clinically, prostate carcinoma metastatic to the lung is usually asymptomatic. A not uncommon site of metastatic prostate carcinoma diagnosed before death is the testes (203). Prostate carcinoma is the most common tumor to spread to the testes and is usually diagnosed as an incidental finding at orchiectomy done for widely metastatic disease. Numerous cases have been reported of men treated with estrogen for carcinoma of the prostate who then developed carcinomas within their breasts. Although some of these cases may represent a second primary tumor, most are examples of metastatic prostate carcinoma to the breast (204). Almost all of these patients have been terminal, with widespread prostate cancer metastases. In most cases, metastatic prostate carcinoma to the breast is not suspected clinically and is diagnosed only after careful examination at autopsy. In view of the relatively small number of primary male breast carcinomas and the widespread use of estrogen therapy and resultant gynecomastia, it is unlikely that a strong causal relation exists between estrogen administration or gynecomastia and breast cancer in men. The use of immunohistochemical staining for PSAP and PSA can distinguish between a primary breast carcinoma and metastatic prostate cancer, although we should recognize that some cross-reactivity in breast carcinomas has been reported with PSAP and PSA. Other rare manifestations of metastatic prostate carcinoma are those of skin and penile metastases (205). In general, there is a tendency for the metastases from a carcinoma of the prostate to be less well differentiated than the primary tumor.

EVALUATION OF PROSTATIC SPECIMENS AFTER ENDOCRINE OR RADIATION THERAPY

With antiandrogen therapy, the neoplastic acini appear small and shrunken and atrophic (206,207) (Fig. 78). Cytologically, small intracytoplasmic vacuoles may coalesce to form large, swollen, ballooned cells (Fig. 79). The eccentrically displaced nuclei become condensed, hyperchromatic, and pyknotic. Stromal vacuolization also may be apparent.

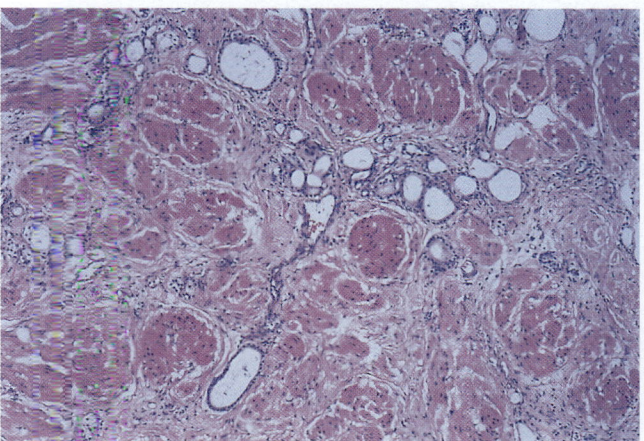

FIG. 78. Atrophic adenocarcinoma of the prostate after hormone therapy. Glands infiltrate in and among thick smooth muscles consistent with invasion of bladder neck.

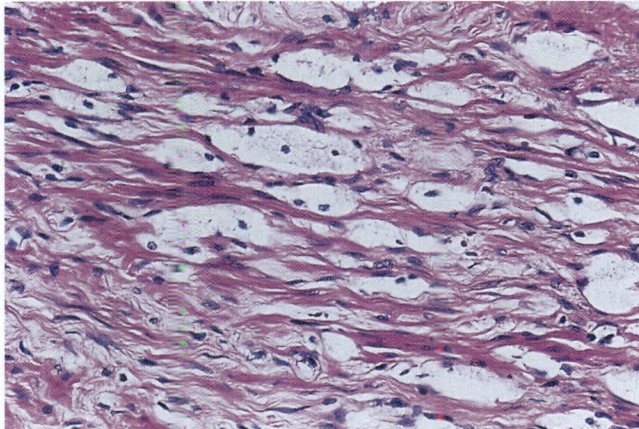

FIG. 79. Adenocarcinoma after hormone therapy, showing tumor cells with pyknotic nuclei and foamy cytoplasm resembling histiocytes.

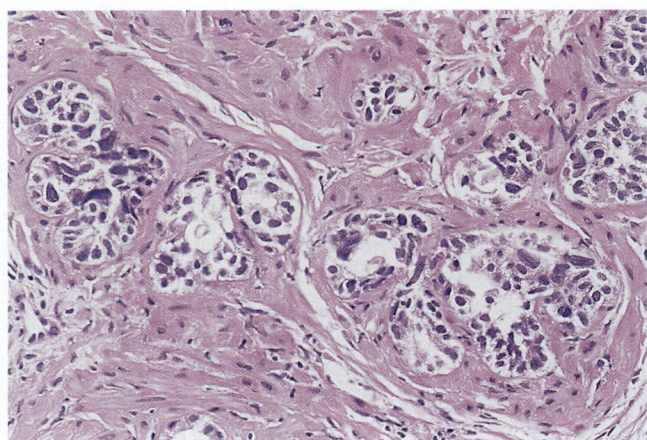

FIG. 80. Benign prostate glands showing radiation effect.

Even in tumors that have responded well to therapy, small clumps of unaltered tumor cells can usually be identified. Along with these changes, estrogen therapy results in squamous metaplasia of both benign and malignant prostatic glands (208). The diffuse nature of this squamous metaplasia is characteristic of hormone therapy, because the only other situation in which squamous metaplasia occurs within the prostate is in the immediate vicinity of healed prostatic infarcts. Other changes with antiandrogen therapy seen in the nonneoplastic tissue include atrophy of the glandular epithelium, basal cell hyperplasia, and stromal fibrosis.

Margin assessment after androgen deprivation can be difficult. There have been reports of decreased incidence of positive margins in patients treated with androgen deprivation (209). These studies are flawed in that they do not admit that margin status is much more difficult to evaluate in these specimens in which it may be hard just to find tumor. Use of ancillary studies, such as immunoperoxidase staining with cytokeratin, should provide better assessment of margin status. Studies addressing the long-term effects of preoperative androgen deprivation are still under way, although thus far, neoadjuvant hormone therapy has not led to a reduction of the progression rate after radical prostatectomy.

After radiation therapy, most tumors retain their pretreatment architectural pattern (210). The predominant finding is the decrease in the number of neoplastic glands. Usually we do not find an increase in nuclear pleomorphism within the irradiated neoplastic cells. Within the nonneoplastic prostatic glands, radiation results in an increased number of atrophic glands, squamous metaplasia of the glands, and cytologic atypia (Fig. 80). The stromal atypia characteristic of radiation elsewhere is not usually seen. Because radiation-induced cytologic atypia of nonneoplastic glands is common, the distinction between residual carcinoma and radiation change is best made by evaluating the architectural pattern of the glands rather than the cytologic features. Keratin immunohistochemistry can aid in the diagnosis of irradiated prostate by identifying basal cells (211).

Because prostatic cancer does not regress immediately after irradiation, the evaluation of a postradiation biopsy is useful only if the biopsy is obtained at least 6 months after completion of radiation therapy, with most authorities advising a 12- to 18-month interval. Some studies demonstrated that the morphologic appearance of the cancer after radiotherapy correlates with prognosis (212). Although a system has been proposed to quantify the degree of radiation effect on the cancer, currently the convention is merely to record the presence or absence of tumor, without commenting on treatment effect.

Because androgen deprivation and radiation therapy can result in morphologic changes resembling high-grade prostate cancer, it was agreed on by the consensus panel that tumors showing treatment effect should not be graded (213). In cases after radiation or hormonal therapy in which the tumor does not show treatment effect, it is reasonable to assign a Gleason grade.

IMMUNOHISTOCHEMICAL TECHNIQUES

Immunohistochemical staining for PSAP and PSA in tumor cells has provided pathologists with a reliable means of determining the prostatic origin of metastases (98). Among the low- and intermediate-grade prostatic adenocarcinomas, in either the primary or metastatic site, all but a few cases will show immunoreactivity with both antisera. In fact, there is an inverse correlation between tissue PSA immunoperoxidase staining and Gleason grade such that the highest Gleason grade has the weakest staining. Between 5% and 10% of poorly differentiated prostatic carcinomas without glandular differentiation will show no immunoreactivity with one of the two antibodies. In addition, between 25% and 59% of these poorly differentiated tumors will show only focal (1% to 25% tumor cell staining) immunoreactivity, such that in limited biopsy material, a false-negative result may occur. Although some studies claimed superiority of PSA over

PSAP in staining prostatic carcinoma, others demonstrated poorly differentiated prostatic carcinomas that lack PSA staining yet still maintain their immunoreactivity with antisera to PSAP. A similar variability as to the sensitivity of PSA and PSAP in metastatic tumors in decalcified bone marrow sections was reported. Because in some cases, antisera to PSA is more sensitive in identifying prostatic tumors, and in other cases, PSAP gives superior results, both antisera should be used when we are trying to establish whether the tumor is of prostatic origin. When both antisera are used, only a rare case will be negative with both markers, regardless of the tumor differentiation. Monoclonal antisera to PSAP have relatively low sensitivity, compared with polyclonal antisera.

With only a few exceptions, immunoperoxidase staining for PSA and PSAP is highly specific for prostatic tissue. Weak false-positive staining for PSAP has been reported in several breast and renal cell carcinomas, granulocytes, islet cells, gastric parietal cells, and hepatocytes (98) In addition, PSA immunoreactivity was reported in breast carcinoma, melanoma, and lung carcinomas (214–216). In cases with this differential diagnosis, it is prudent to require staining with both PSA and PSAP before rendering a diagnosis of metastatic prostate cancer. In addition, because some adenocarcinomas of the bladder and rectal carcinomas have been shown to be strongly reactive with antisera to PSAP and not PSA, these tumors should be ruled out on clinical and histologic grounds in PSAP-positive, PSA-negative tissue (98). For example, in a poorly differentiated tumor occurring in the bladder and prostate in which the differential diagnosis is between a high-grade prostatic adenocarcinoma and a transitional cell carcinoma, focal strong PSAP staining in the absence of PSA staining can be used reliably to make the diagnosis of prostatic adenocarcinoma, because PSAP false positivity has not been described in transitional cell carcinomas. However, in more well-differentiated glandular tumors within the bladder or prostate, focal PSAP staining without PSA reactivity would be unusual in prostatic tumors, making it necessary to rule out a bladder adenocarcinoma on the basis of either clinical or histologic features. Less problematically, PSA and PSAP may be seen in cystitis cystica and cystitis glandularis, male and female periurethral glands, and male anal glands (98). PSA positivity also was noted in urachal remnants and female paraurethral gland cancers (98).

After hormonal therapy, there may be a decrease in immunoreactivity with PSA and PSAP, but most tumors show persistent immunopositivity with both antisera (98). In tumors treated with radiation, PSAP immunoreactivity is maintained in all but a few cases.

Basal cell–specific keratin antibodies can identify basal cells in glandular patterns sometimes confused with carcinoma, such as basal cell hyperplasia, atrophic glands, adenosis, and radiated benign glands (11—13,211,217,218) (Fig. 50). It also can be used as an additional feature in diagnosing limited cancer on needle biopsy (Fig. 40). It was shown to decrease the rate of equivocal diagnosis in both academic centers and private settings (13,219). The absence of basal cells cannot be used as a sole criterion for the diagnosis of cancer because of the occasional regions of the prostate with pale, difficult-to-visualize staining of basal cells (220). The presence of basal cells, however, allows a definitive diagnosis of a benign mimic of cancer. For proper use, this antibody should be titrated on appropriate control tissue that has both cancer and benign prostate glands and has been subject to the same fixation and processing conditions as the needle-biopsy specimens on which there is anticipated use. Bench needle biopsies from radical prostatectomy specimens that are immediately fixed and processed as a diagnostic biopsy serve as an optimal control. Tissues not optimally fixed and handled (such as TURP or prostatectomy specimens) are not good positive controls for this type of analysis. Immunohistochemistry to laminin and type IV collagen cannot be used to differentiate adenocarcinoma from its mimickers, because adenocarcinomas produce basement membrane material (221).

VARIANTS OF PROSTATIC ADENOCARCINOMA

Mucinous Adenocarcinoma

Mucinous adenocarcinoma of the prostate gland is one of the least common morphologic variants of prostatic carcinoma (222,223). A lack of precision in the definition of these mucinous neoplasms resulted in reports that overstated the incidence of this lesion. Much of the confusion in the terminology for this entity arises from the lack of recognition that between 60% and 90% of prostatic adenocarcinomas secrete mucosubstances, depending on the histochemical technique used. Only when extracellular mucin is secreted in sufficient quantity to result in pools of mucin should the term "mucinous" be used (Fig. 81). If the mucinous area occupies only a small portion of the tumor, it should not be called a "mucinous prostatic carcinoma" but rather a "prostatic adenocarcinoma with focal mucinous areas." With criteria developed for mucinous carcinomas of other organs, the diagnosis of

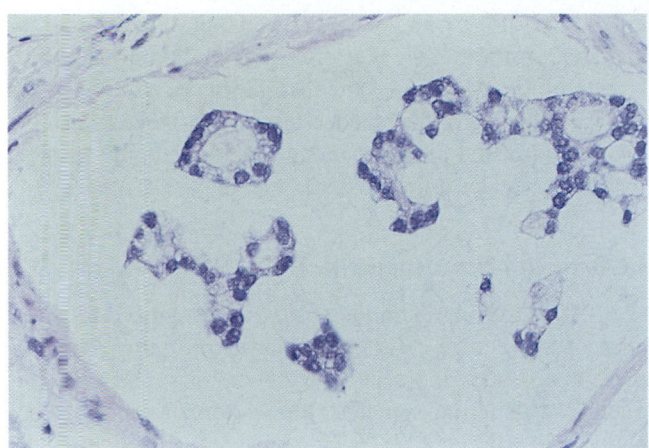

FIG. 81. Mucinous adenocarcinoma of the prostate with glands of adenocarcinoma floating within mucin.

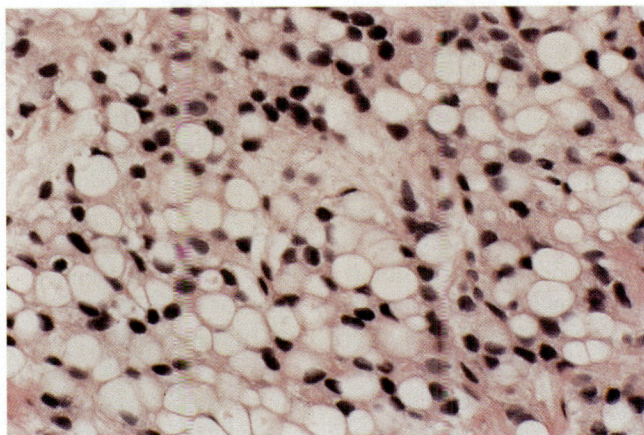

FIG. 82. Adenocarcinoma of the prostate with signet ring cell–like features.

mucinous adenocarcinoma of the prostate gland should be made when at least 25% of the tumor resected contains lakes of extracellular mucin. Histologically, mucinous adenocarcinomas of the prostate are predominantly intermediate-grade tumors in which a cribriform pattern tends to predominate in the mucinous areas. They have an aggressive biologic behavior and, like nonmucinous prostate carcinomas, have a propensity to develop bone metastases with advanced disease. In contrast to bladder adenocarcinomas, mucinous adenocarcinoma of the prostate rarely contain signet cells. Some carcinomas of the prostate will have a signet-ring cell appearance, yet the vacuoles do not contain intracytoplasmic mucin (224) (Fig. 82). Only a few cases of prostate cancer have been reported with mucin-positive signet cells (225). Another histologic growth pattern found in mucinous carcinomas of the bladder but not in those of the prostate gland is that of tall columnar epithelium, resembling both normal and neoplastic colonic epithelium lining mucinous lakes. In ruling out a mucinous adenocarcinoma of the bladder infiltrating the prostate, we must be aware that some bladder adenocarcinomas will show focal, yet intense, immunoreactivity with antisera to PSAP (98). In these cases, the use of antisera to PSA, along with the clinical and light-microscopic appearance of the tumor, is useful in excluding an extraprostatic tumor. Mucinous adenocarcinomas, analogous to those originating in the bladder, also may arise from colonic metaplasia of the prostatic urethra and invade the prostate without a bladder primary (226).

Lesions with Neuroendocrine Differentiation

In 1971, Azzopardi and Evans (227) recognized the presence of argentaffin cells within normal prostates. Most of these neuroendocrine cells contain serotonin and (less frequently) calcitonin, somatostatin, or human chorionic gonadotropin (HCG) (228). They can be recognized on H&E-stained sections by their basally located deeply eosinophilic fine cytoplasmic granules. Coarser eosinophilic clumped granules located throughout the cytoplasm represent lipofuscin or lysosomes. In histologically typical adenocarcinomas of the prostate, we also may find similar-appearing eosinophilic cells that are argyrophilic and on electron microscopy are seen to contain neurosecretory granules (Fig. 83). These cells may stain for serotonin, adrenocorticotropic hormone (ACTH), calcitonin, HCG, or neuron-specific enolase (NSE). Even in ordinary adenocarcinomas of the prostate without light-microscopic evidence of neuroendocrine differentiation, up to 47% may show neuroendocrine differentiation when evaluated with immunohistochemistry for multiple neuroendocrine markers. Most of these cases show no clinical evidence of ectopic hormonal secretion. It remains controversial whether neuroendocrine (NE) differentiation in adenocarcinoma of the prostate is independently associated with more aggressive behavior (228–232). Several cases were reported in which a "carcinoid" appearance of the tumor was present either as the sole histologic pattern or admixed with more typical adenocarcinoma of the prostate (233). In none of these cases has a carcinoid syndrome been present. All such cases have been positive with antisera for PSA and PSAP and have clinically behaved like ordinary prostate carcinomas, except for one case of a prostatic carcinoid tumor in a child with MENIIb syndrome (234). Although most of these tumors showing NE differentiation (including the presence of neurosecretory granules) have not produced clinical symptoms, several cases have produced ACTH in sufficient quantity to result in Cushing's syndrome. ACTH production also was present in several typical-appearing adenocarcinomas.

Small-cell carcinomas of the prostate have a cytologic appearance similar to that found in small-cell carcinomas of the lung (235–237). In approximately 50% of the cases, the tumors are mixed small-cell carcinoma and adenocarcinoma of the prostate (Fig. 84). Neurosecretory granules have been demonstrated within several prostatic small-cell carcinomas.

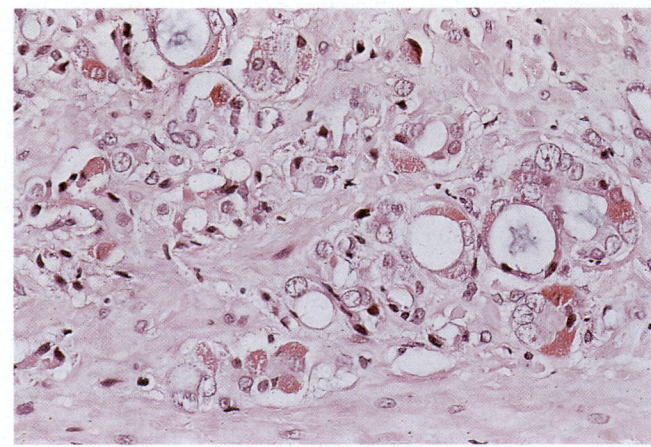

FIG. 83. Adenocarcinoma of the prostate with fine, eosinophilic cytoplasmic granules corresponding to neuroendocrine differentiation. Immunostaining revealed strong positivity with human chorionic gonadotropin.

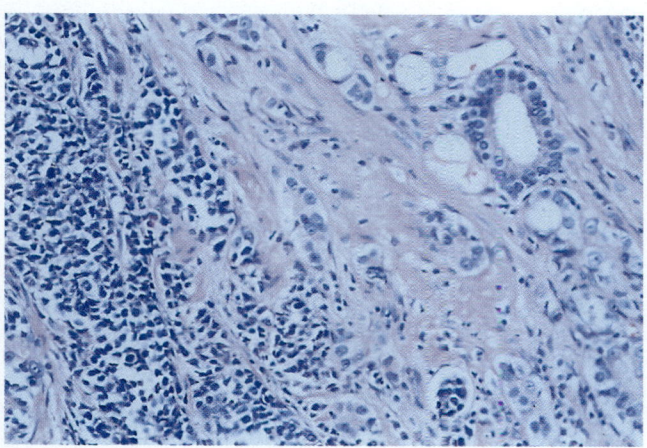

FIG. 84. Small-cell carcinoma of the prostate admixed with ordinary adenocarcinoma of the prostate (right).

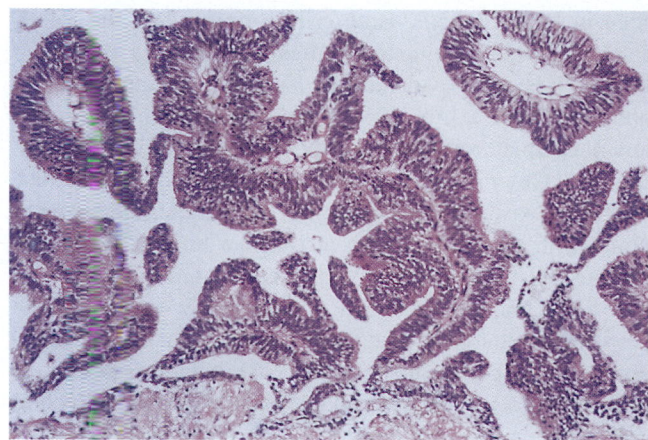

FIG. 85. Papillary prostatic duct adenocarcinoma showing tall pseudostratified columnar epithelium with dark cytoplasm.

With immunohistochemical techniques, the small-cell component may be positive for NSE and negative for PSA and PSAP, positive for PSA and PSAP with negative immunoreactivity for NSE, or negative for all three antigens. Although most small-cell tumors of the prostate lack clinically evident hormone production, they account for the majority of prostatic tumors with clinically evident ACTH or antidiuretic hormone production. The average survival of patients with small-cell carcinoma of the prostate is less than 1 year. There is no difference in prognosis between patients with pure small-cell carcinomas and those with mixed glandular and small-cell carcinomas. Similarly, the pattern of immunostaining does not affect survival. The appearance of a small-cell component in the course of adenocarcinoma of the prostate usually indicates an aggressive terminal phase of the disease, with the manifestations and patterns of tumor spread still resembling those of typical adenocarcinoma of the prostate. The heterogeneity of prostatic small-cell tumors suggests that they arise from multipotential prostatic epithelial cells that may express divergent differentiation.

Several case reports of pheochromocytomas originating in the prostate also were reported (238). Paraganglia, which are typically found just exterior to the prostate, may be sampled on biopsy or TURP and can be confused with adenocarcinoma of the prostate (239).

Prostatic Duct Adenocarcinoma

Whereas most adenocarcinomas of the prostate are of acinar origin, between 0.4% and 0.8% of prostatic carcinomas arise from prostatic ducts (240–242). In about 5% of prostatic carcinomas, tumors showing both ductal and acinar differentiation are found. When prostatic duct adenocarcinomas arise in the large primary periurethral prostatic ducts, they may grow as an exophytic lesion into the urethra, most commonly in and around the verumontanum. Tumors arising in the more peripheral prostatic ducts may or may not have a urethral component. Cytologically, prostatic duct adenocarcinomas are characterized by tall columnar pseudostratified epithelial cells with abundant, usually amphophilic, cytoplasm that may also be pale or clear. In the exophytic component of prostatic duct adenocarcinomas, the cells are usually arranged along papillae (Fig. 85). Another pattern seen with ductal tumors is that of cribriform formations, which, although it may be seen in the exophytic urethral component of the lesion, is more commonly seen in its infiltrating component. The cribriform pattern is formed by back-to-back large acini with intraglandular epithelial bridging, resulting in the formation of slitlike lumens (Fig. 86). Prostatic duct adenocarcinomas also may invade as single glands lined by tall columnar epithelial cells, unlike the cuboidal cells that characterize typical acinar prostatic carcinoma. Prostatic duct adenocarcinomas with a cribriform pattern may be difficult to distinguish from cribriforming PIN. Features favoring ductal carcinoma include back-to-back or irregular glands, extensive comedonecrosis, more prominent nuclear atypia throughout the glands, and a papillary component with fibrovascular cores, as opposed to the micropapillary tufts

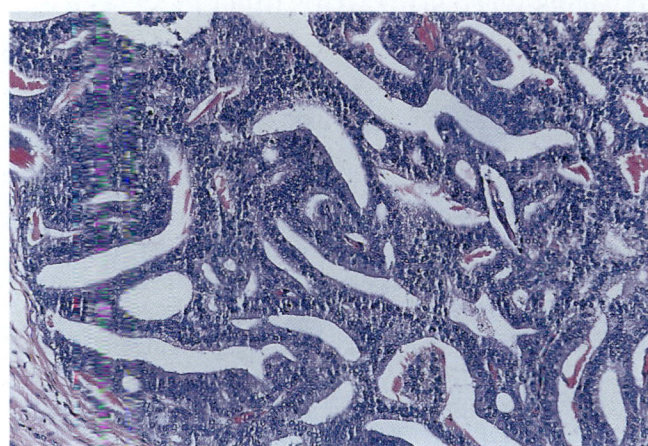

FIG. 86. Cribriform pattern of prostatic duct adenocarcinoma.

seen in PIN (Fig. 57). Both cribriforming PIN and cribriforming ductal adenocarcinomas may show a preserved basal cell layer as evidenced by basal cell–specific cytokeratin staining (243). In most of the cases with mixed acinar and ductal features, the two components are intimately commingled. Other relations seen between the two types include (a) the coexistence of a centrally located duct adenocarcinoma with a peripherally located acinar tumor, and (b) the finding of a prostatic tumor with ductal features in which acinar differentiation was seen in either prior or subsequent biopsies. Similarly, the metastases from a ductal adenocarcinoma may be purely ductal, acinar, or mixed. Because of the histologic resemblance to endometrial carcinoma, as well as their tendency to arise around the verumontanum (a müllerian remnant), prostatic duct adenocarcinomas were initially considered to be of endometrial origin and were designated endometrioid carcinomas of the prostate. Subsequent studies refuted the existence of an endometrial carcinoma of the prostate, showing them to be reactive with PSAP and PSA. When compared with men with typical acinar carcinomas, men with ductal tumors are of similar age and demonstrate a greater tendency to have either obstructive symptoms or hematuria. Although some of the exophytic ductal tumors are relatively indolent, most prostatic duct adenocarcinomas have a fairly aggressive course. In contrast to typical acinar prostate carcinoma, a smaller proportion of ductal adenocarcinomas respond well to hormone therapy. Prostatic duct adenocarcinomas, in which at least 50% of the tumor shows ductal differentiation, are large and of advanced pathologic stage, with almost all showing extraprostatic extension, 50% positive margins, 40% seminal vesicle invasion, and 27% metastases to pelvic lymph nodes (244). Almost half of the patients treated with radical prostatectomy manifest recurrent disease at intervals of only 3 to 18 months after radical prostatectomy. The prognostic significance of a minor ductal component in an acinar carcinoma is unknown. Tumors are often underestimated clinically because rectal examination and serum PSA levels may be normal.

TUMORS WITH SQUAMOUS DIFFERENTIATION

Pure primary squamous carcinoma of the prostate is rare (0.5% of prostate tumors) and is associated with a poor survival (245). These tumors develop osteolytic metastases, do not respond to hormone therapy, and do not develop increased serum PSA with metastatic disease. More commonly, squamous differentiation occurs in the primary and metastatic deposits of adenocarcinomas that have been treated with hormone therapy (246). Squamous carcinoma was reported after luteinizing hormone–releasing hormone agonist, flutamide, and radiation seed implantation for prostate cancer (247,248). After therapy, the prostate may develop squamous metaplasia only in benign glands or, in some cases, in some of the neoplastic glands as well, resulting in an adenosquamous carcinoma (Fig. 87). The metastases may be adenosquamous carcinoma or pure squamous

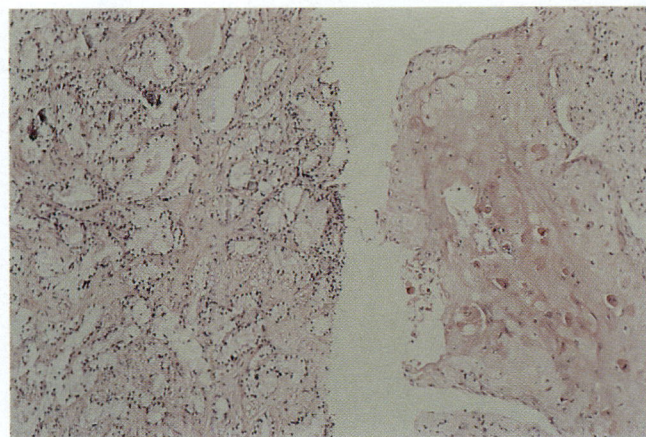

FIG. 87. Adenosquamous carcinoma.

carcinoma; in some cases, the squamous component may be PSA or PSAP positive (249). There also were rare reports of adenosquamous carcinoma of the prostate in which there was no previous therapy.

TRANSITIONAL CELL LESIONS

Transitional epithelium within the prostate is found predominantly within the periurethral (central) prostatic ducts, although more peripheral prostatic ducts and even some acini may also be lined by transitional epithelium. These changes are referred to as transitional cell metaplasia (250).

Primary transitional cell carcinoma of the prostate without bladder involvement accounts for 1% to 4% of all prostate carcinomas (251). Primary transitional cell carcinoma of the prostate should not be called periurethral prostatic duct carcinoma, as sometimes reported in the literature, because this term may be confused with prostatic duct adenocarcinomas. Microscopically, an in situ component is usually present that consists of nests of neoplastic cells, often with central necrosis filling prostatic ducts. Sometimes a continuum from transitional cell hyperplasia without atypia to atypical transitional cell hyperplasia to CIS can be seen (252). Rarely transitional cell CIS has taken a papillary form within large dilated prostatic ducts. In cases of primary transitional cell carcinoma of the prostate, stromal invasion is almost always identified (253). The invasive component of transitional cell carcinoma of the prostate is characterized by small nests of tumor cells with a greater degree of anaplasia and mitotic figures than usually is seen in even poorly differentiated prostatic adenocarcinoma (127) (Fig. 88). In a minority of primary transitional cell carcinomas of the prostate, an adenocarcinomatous component may also be identified. Although Greene et al. (253) claimed that one third of the cases of primary transitional cell carcinoma of the prostate have areas of adenocarcinoma, this number is probably overstated, in that the adenocarcinomatous component in this study and others is described as high grade and probably represents poorly differentiated transitional cell carcinoma in some of the

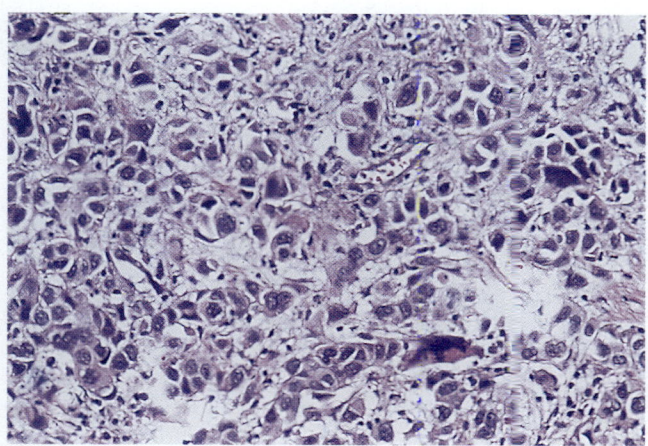

FIG. 88. Infiltrating transitional cell carcinoma in the prostate. Cells are more pleomorphic than is poorly differentiated prostate cancer. See Fig. 20 for comparison.

cases. These studies lacked the use of immunohistochemistry for PSA and PSAP to distinguish between poorly differentiated transitional cell carcinoma and poorly differentiated prostatic adenocarcinoma. Primary transitional cell carcinomas of the prostate show a propensity to infiltrate the bladder neck and surrounding soft tissue such that more than 50% of the patients are first seen with stage T3 or T4 tumors. Twenty percent of the patients have distant metastases, with bone, lung, and liver being the most common sites. In contrast to adenocarcinoma of the prostate, bone metastases tend to be osteolytic. Treatment of stage T3 disease with radiation results in a 5-year survival of approximately 34%. In the minority of cases with tumor localized to the prostate (T2), radical surgery resulted in long-term disease-free survival in several patients.

More commonly, transitional cell carcinoma involves prostatic ducts and acini in patients with a history of flat CIS of the bladder who have been treated over a period of months to years with intravesicle topical chemotherapy (254–257). Between 35% and 45% of cystoprostatectomies performed for transitional cell carcinoma contain prostatic involvement. However, this number is dependent on the amount of histologic sampling of the prostate tissue and may be much higher in completely mapped specimens (258). Whereas the intravesicle therapy may effectively rid the bladder of tumor, the chemotherapy does not treat effectively the prostatic urethra and does not reach the underlying prostatic ducts and acini. To rule out extension of tumor into the prostate, patients who are treated conservatively for CIS of the bladder undergo periodic deep transurethral biopsies of the prostatic urethra and underlying prostate. The finding of intraductal transitional cell carcinoma usually leads to radical cystoprostatectomy. If cystoprostatectomy is performed and only intraductal transitional cell carcinoma is present, the prostatic involvement does not worsen the prognosis, which is determined by the stage of the bladder tumor (259). Intraductal transitional cell carcinoma of the prostate appears to involve the prostate via direct extension from the overlying urethra, which is usually involved by CIS. Intraductal transitional cell carcinoma within the prostatic ducts may appear histologically as nests of neoplastic transitional epithelium filling prostatic ducts or as neoplastic transitional cells insinuating themselves beneath the secretory and basal cell layer (Fig. 89). The most subtle form of prostatic involvement is by pagetoid spread. When prostatic stromal invasion occurs, there are cords and single cells of infiltrating carcinoma, inducing a desmoplastic stromal response (Fig. 89). Intraductal and infiltrating transitional cell carcinoma involving the prostate tends to be seen in higher-stage bladder tumors, in which the patients have a poor prognosis, attributable to either the advanced bladder or the prostatic disease. A minority of these cases will have low-stage bladder tumor and a poor prognosis, demonstrating the adverse effect of prostatic stromal infiltration (259). It is therefore prognostically important to identify prostatic stromal invasion in cases with intraductal transitional cell carcinoma, especially in patients with low-stage bladder tumor. Extensive sampling of the periurethral area in cystoprostatectomy specimens performed for transitional cell carcinoma is necessary to identify and evaluate the prostate for transitional cell carcinoma. The finding of prostatic involvement by transitional cell carcinoma also is associated with a higher risk for urethral recurrence and usually leads to prophylactic urethrectomy (260).

In cystoprostatectomy specimens removed for bladder cancer there is an increased risk of adenocarcinomas of the prostate (~6%) (261–262). Careful sampling of the peripheral regions of the prostate in these specimens to search for adenocarcinoma of the prostate should also be performed.

Finally, we may find direct invasion from a bladder transitional cell carcinoma into the stroma of the prostate, where there is no in situ component within the prostatic ducts. This situation is associated with a dramatic decrease in the prognosis of transitional cell carcinoma of the bladder and is equivalent in survival to cases with local metastases.

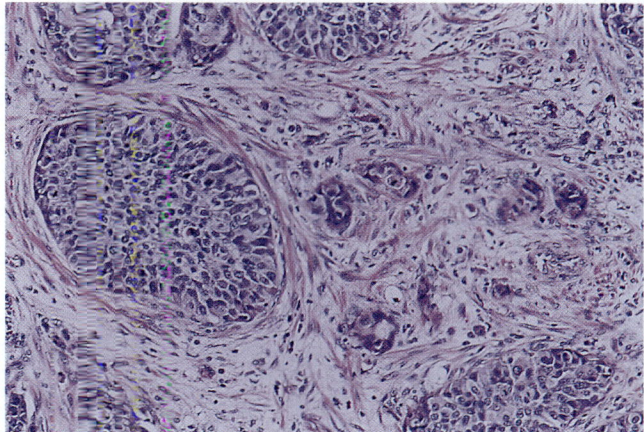

FIG. 89. Intraductal transitional cell carcinoma with rounded nests. Stromal invasion characterized by cords and single cells of infiltrating transitional cell carcinoma.

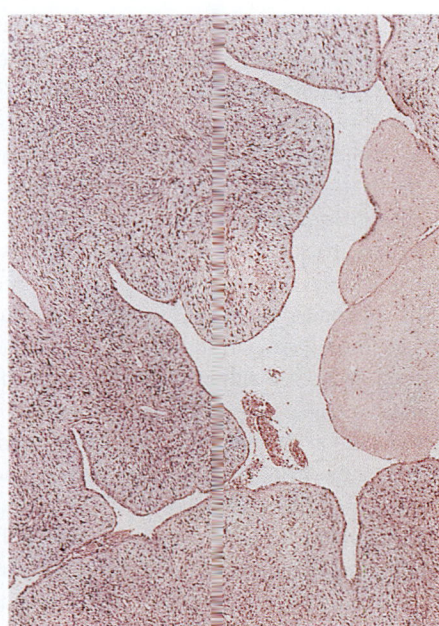 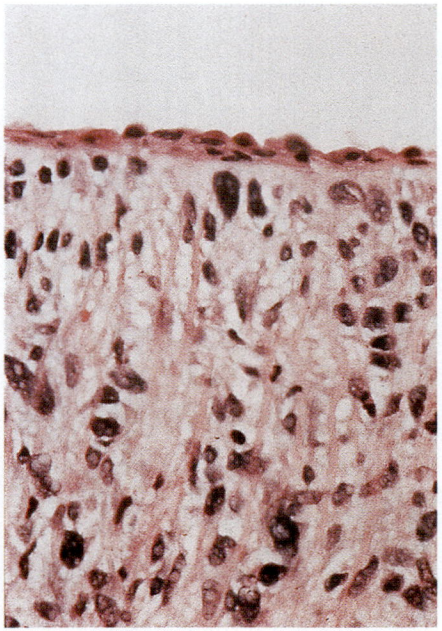

FIG. 90. Stromal sarcoma of the prostate (malignant phyllodes tumor).

MESENCHYMAL TUMORS

Benign soft-tissue tumors of the prostate are rare, the most common being leiomyomas. The difficulty in diagnosing a leiomyoma of the prostate is that we often may find small stromal nodules with the histologic appearance of leiomyomas in prostates with hyperplasia (16). These stromal nodules, although they contain abundant smooth muscle, lack the well-organized fascicles of a leiomyoma and do not have the other degenerative features commonly seen in leiomyomas, such as hyalinization, necrosis, and calcification. Large single symptomatic leiomyomas of the prostate are rare; most are seen with symptoms of BPH (263).

Sarcomas and related proliferative lesions of specialized prostatic stroma are rare. In a large series of 22 cases, lesions were classified into prostatic stromal proliferations of uncertain malignant potential and prostatic stromal sarcoma (malignant phyllodes tumor) based on the degree of stromal cellularity, presence of mitotic figures, necrosis, and stromal overgrowth (264) (Fig. 90). There were several different patterns of stromal proliferations of uncertain malignant potential, including those that resemble benign phyllodes tumor seen in the breast (Figs. 91 and 92). Although most cases of prostatic stromal proliferations of uncertain malignant potential do not behave in an aggressive fashion, occasional cases have been documented to recur rapidly after resection and progress to stromal sarcoma. Small incidentally discovered prostatic lesions with the structure of fibroadenomas also were described (265).

Sarcomas (exluding those of specialized prostatic stroma) of the prostate account for 0.1% to 0.2% of all malignant pro-

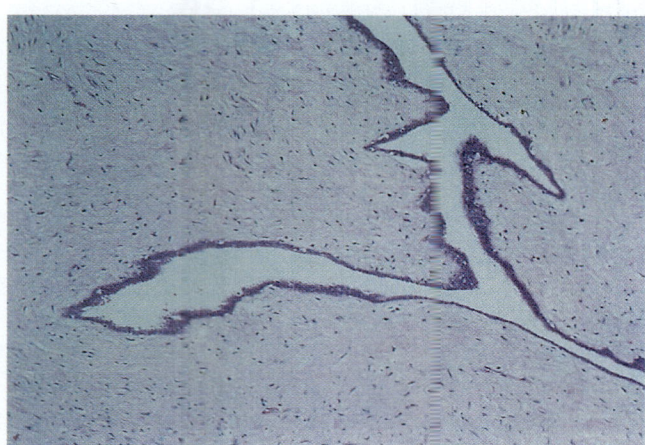

FIG. 91. Stromal proliferation of uncertain malignant potential with appearance of benign phyllodes tumor.

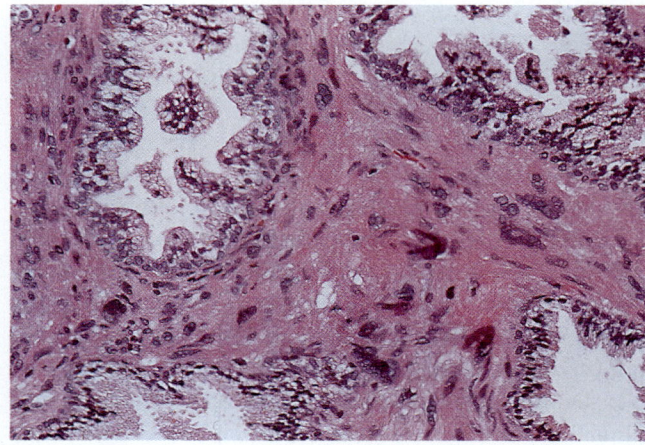

FIG. 92. Stromal proliferation of uncertain malignant potential consisting of scattered atypical yet degenerative-appearing stromal cells between benign glands.

static tumors. Rhabdomyosarcoma is the most frequent mesenchymal tumor within the prostate and is seen almost exclusively in childhood. Rhabdomyosarcomas of the prostate occur from infancy to early adulthood, with an average age at diagnosis of 5 years (266). Most patients are first seen with stage 3 disease, in which there is gross residual disease after incomplete resection or biopsy only. A smaller, but significant, proportion of patients are seen with distant metastases. Localized tumor that may be completely resected is only rarely present. Histologically, most prostate rhabdomyosarcomas are of the embryonal subtype. Because of their large size at the time of diagnosis, the distinction between rhabdomyosarcoma originating in the bladder and that arising in the prostate is often impossible. After the development of effective chemotherapy for rhabdomyosarcomas, those few patients with localized disease (stage 1) or microscopic residual regional disease (stage 2) stand an excellent chance of being cured. The majority of patients with gross residual disease (stage 3) have remained without evidence of disease for a long time, but approximately 15% to 20% die of their tumor. The prognosis for patients with metastatic tumor (stage 4) is more dismal, with most patients dying of the tumor.

Leiomyosarcomas are the most common sarcomas involving the prostate in adults (267). The majority of patients are between ages 40 and 70 years, although in some series, up to 20% of leiomyosarcomas occurred in young adults or children. Leiomyosarcomas ranged in size between 2 and 24 cm, with a mean size of 95 cm. After either local excision or resection of prostatic leiomyosarcomas, the clinical course tends to be characterized by multiple recurrences. Metastases, when present, are usually found in the lung and liver. The average survival with leiomyosarcoma of the prostate is between 3 and 4 years.

A benign reactive spindle-cell lesion, which may simulate a leiomyosarcoma, may rarely occur after recent TUR resection for BPH (268). The important features that distinguish this postoperative spindle-cell nodule from sarcoma are the lack of nuclear pleomorphism, absence of atypical mitoses, relatively small size, and history of a recent resection not showing the lesion. Another pseudosarcomatous lesion of the prostate was described in which there is no history of TUR resection, and the histology resembles the postoperative spindle-cell nodule, with areas having the appearance of granulation tissue (269). Although there are numerous synonyms, the preferred term is pseudosarcomatous fibromyxoid tumor.

Other rare mesenchymal tumors of the prostate are malignant peripheral nerve sheath tumors, angiosarcomas, hemangiopericytomas, malignant fibrous histiocytomas, and hemangiomas (270–274).

BASAL CELL HYPERPLASIA/CARCINOMA

A spectrum of basaloid lesions ranging from hyperplasia to carcinoma exists in the prostate with a proposed classification of basal cell hyperplasia, basal cell hyperplasia with

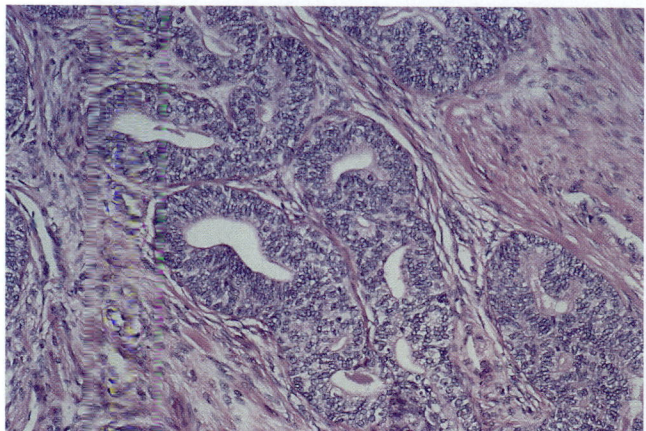

FIG. 93. Basal cell hyperplasia characterized by glandular structures with multiple cell layers.

prominent nucleoli (atypical basal cell hyperplasia), basal cell adenoma, florid adenoid basal cell tumor, and adenoid cystic/basaloid carcinoma (275–277). These lesions are relatively uncommon and occur in 6% to 8% of cases (278). Basal cell hyperplasia, also known as "fetalization of the prostate," is characterized by collections of small solid nests of uniform cells similar to those of the normal prostatic basal cells (Fig. 93). The cells are often arranged in a palisading configuration around the edge of the nests and may demonstrate acinar differentiation with central lumen formation. Basal cell hyperplasia may be admixed with ordinary BPH, be present as distinct nodules, or have a diffusely infiltrative appearance. When a well-formed distinct nodule of basaloid nests is formed, the term "basal cell adenoma" is sometimes used, although others prefer to consider these lesions more pronounced examples of basal cell hyperplasia. In these more prominent basaloid proliferations, we also may find cribriform patterns as well as solid nests. Basal cell hyperplasia with its multiple cell layers that stain with basal

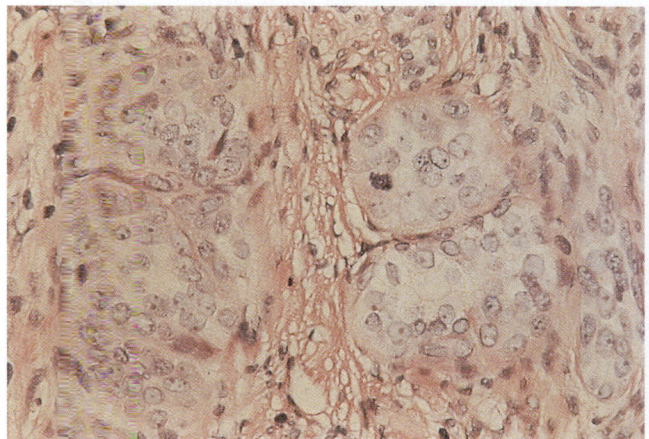

FIG. 94. Basal cell hyperplasia with prominent nucleoli and mitotic figures. In contrast to prostatic intraepithelial neoplasia (PIN), there are increased number of small rounded glands, many of which appear solid.

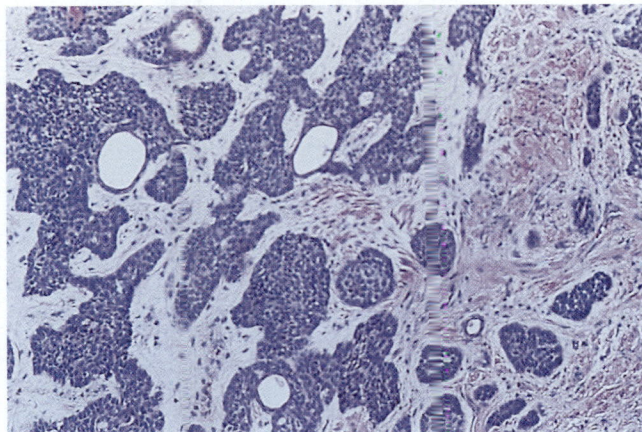

FIG. 95. Basaloid carcinoma of the prostate with desmoplastic stromal reaction. In contrast, basal cell hyperplasia usually lacks a stromal response.

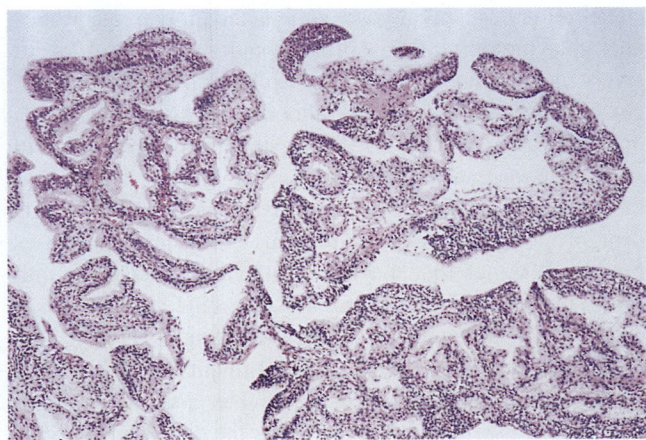

FIG. 96. Prostatic urethral polyp lined by transitional and prostatic epithelium, with its core containing benign prostatic glands.

cell–specific keratin, differs from the usual pattern of prostatic adenocarcinoma, which contains a single layer of epithelial cells with abundant cytoplasm. We should recognize that some examples of basal cell hyperplasia have prominent nucleoli that must be distinguished from both PIN and adenocarcinoma (276,277) (Fig. 94). There are some cribriforming basaloid lesions of the prostate in which their designation is controversial. Some authors believe that these should be regarded as adenoid basal cell tumors of uncertain malignant potential. Others think that some of these lesions are within the spectrum of basal cell hyperplasia. In contrast to cribriforming basal cell hyperplasia, basaloid carcinomas demonstrate either a desmoplastic stromal response, perineural invasion, necrosis, or widespread infiltration into surrounding tissue. Basaloid carcinomas also have been referred to as adenoid cystic carcinomas of the prostate (276,279,280) (Fig. 95). These basaloid carcinomas appear to have relatively low malignant potential in that metastases have not been reported from these lesions. The distinction of basal cell hyperplasia, adenoid basal cell tumor, and basaloid carcinoma of the prostate cannot be performed by using basal cell antibodies because all three of these entities show similar positive immunoreactivity.

URETHRAL POLYPS

Urethral polyps are usually single, polypoid lesions found within the prostatic urethra in and around the verumontanum (281,282). Commonly the lesions result in gross and microscopic hematuria and less frequently result in hemospermia, dysuria, and frequency. Lesions have been described from adolescence to the elderly, with conflicting reports as to the most commonly involved age group. Several of these lesions also were described within the bladder, usually around the trigone. The surface of urethral polyps often appears papillary, with the broad papillae lined by either transitional cells, prostatic epithelial cells, or a combination of both (Fig. 96). The cores of the papillary projections contain prostatic stroma and often prostatic glands. The glands may be closely packed, and in some areas they may be cystically dilated at the periphery. These broad fingerlike projections of urethral polyps differ from the delicate fibrovascular cores seen in low-grade papillary transitional cell neoplasms and from the thin villi seen in prostatic duct adenocarcinomas arising from the central urethral ducts. Urethral polyps are totally benign. Cases that have been reported as villous polyps of the urethra represent papillary prostatic duct adenocarcinomas and should not be considered variants of urethral polyps (283). In lesions reported as villous polyps, the glandular epithelium resembles the epithelium in colonic villous adenomas, in contrast to the epithelium lining urethral polyps, which is indistinguishable from normal prostatic glandular epithelium. Various proposals for the origin of urethral polyps include (a) acquired lesions after prior instrumentation, (b) postpubertal hyperplasia, (c) ectopic prostatic tissue, and (d) extrinsic hyperplasia or evagination of glandular epithelium into the urethral lumen.

Other benign polypoid lesions found in the prostatic urethra that should be distinguished from the urethral polyps include nephrogenic adenomas and papillary pseudotumors of the prostatic urethra composed of large edematous urethral mucosal folds, and papillary urothelial hyperplasia (121,284).

HEMATOLOGIC LESIONS

Extramedullary hematopoiesis is the one benign hematologic lesion that has been reported in the prostate (285).

Hematologic malignancies have been found involving the prostate or lymph nodes or both in 1.2% of prostatectomy specimens (286). The malignancies detected in one large series included Hodgkin's disease, hairy cell leukemia, chronic lymphocytic leukemia, or low-grade small lymphocytic lymphoma.

Primary prostatic lymphoma without lymph node involvement appears to be much less common than secondary infiltration of the prostate (287). Most reported lymphomas have been of the large-cell and small cleaved-cell types with a diffuse pattern. Lymphomas with a nodular pattern involving the prostate are seen infrequently. The entire spectrum of malignant lymphomas seen at other sites may become manifest in the prostate, including undifferentiated lymphomas, angiotropic lymphomas, Hodgkin's disease, myeloma, and T-cell lymphomas, as well as a case of pseudolymphoma (288). Malignant lymphoma involving the prostate appears to carry a poor prognosis regardless of patient age, stage at presentation, histologic classification, or treatment regimen. The poor prognosis of prostatic lymphoma is related to the generalized disease that eventually results rather than to prostatic involvement.

The most common form of leukemic involvement of the prostate is that of chronic lymphocytic leukemia, although monocytic, granulocytic, and lymphoblastic leukemias also were described in the prostate (289). Most patients have known leukemia or have the diagnosis established at the time of workup for urinary symptoms. It is often unclear whether the prostatic leukemic infiltrate in chronic lymphocytic leukemia is an incidental finding in patients with BPH or the cause of their obstructive symptoms.

MISCELLANEOUS MALIGNANT PROSTATIC TUMORS

Carcinosarcomas of the prostate are rare, with only a handful of cases reported (290). The glandular components of carcinosarcomas are moderately and poorly differentiated adenocarcinomas (Gleason grades from 7 to 10, mean of 9 in one series). In one large series, the sarcoma component was mostly high grade and consisted mostly of osteosarcoma and leiomyosarcoma, with rare cases of fibrosarcoma, malignant fibrous histiocytoma, chondrosarcoma, and rhabdomyosarcoma. Most of the cases have a dismal prognosis, with metastatic lesions variably showing a spectrum from purely glandular metastases to mixed carcinosarcomatous lesions to purely sarcomatous metastases. Although some lesions spread in a pattern similar to that seen in adenocarcinoma of the prostate, others behaved more like sarcomas, with prominent lung involvement. Adenocarcinoma was the dominant histologic pattern in seven cases and sarcoma in 14.

Excluding hematopoietic neoplasms, the prostate even at autopsy is rarely involved by metastatic tumor. Metastases from malignant melanoma and carcinoma of the lung predominate (291).

Other malignant tumors of the prostate include cases of malignant mixed tumor resembling that of the salivary gland, endodermal sinus tumor, rhabdoid tumor, and prostatic carcinoma with oncocytic changes (292—295).

NEW TECHNIQUES AND BIOMARKERS

There has been a tremendous proliferation of putative prostate cancer biomarkers in recent years. These can be placed into several broad categories with some degree of overlap: tumor-suppressor genes, oncogenes, proliferation markers, programmed cell death (apoptosis), DNA content (ploidy), angiogenesis, and morphometry (296–299).

Among the markers pathologists are currently called on to address are DNA ploidy (see p. 1923), NE differentiation (see p. 1923), and angiogenesis. Several studies demonstrated that quantification of the microvasculature within prostate cancers is prognostic (300–304).

Although in general, many of these markers correlate with tumor grade and show differences between hyperplasia, PIN, and carcinoma, the overlap among groups limits their use for clinical practice. Even those with better prognostic attributes are limited by technical difficulty, lack of standardization, and little overall added performance over the combination of standard available parameters (Gleason grade, PSA, clinical stage, pathologic stage, and margin status). Even though the Gleason grading system has been criticized on the basis of reproducibility, at least the issue has been addressed in the literature. With many of the newer techniques, there has been little study of reproducibility and no attempt at standardization. A complicating factor is the multifocality of prostate cancer and the question as to which cells in a sample should be analyzed for a given biomarker to give optimal prognostication. The future holds many possibilities and much responsibility for the rational use of new technology in a cost-effective manner.

SEMINAL VESICLES

Seminal vesicle cysts may be congenital, or they may be acquired as a result of obstruction resulting from inflammation (305). Both types of seminal vesicle cysts are usually unilateral and unilocular and histologically resemble dilated seminal vesicles lined by either flattened or papillary epithelium. Seminal vesicle cysts are usually found in men in their twenties, and all except one have been unilateral. Not infrequently, ipsilateral renal agenesis is identified (306); in some cases, ectopic ureters may enter the cysts (307).

Seminal vesicle cystadenomas are found incidentally in elderly men (308). The lesions are multilocular and are lined by a single layer of columnar or cuboidal epithelium. The cyst walls contain a nondescript fibromuscular stroma, which may be inflamed.

Primary carcinoma of the seminal vesicles or retrovesicle space, before the development of immunohistochemical techniques to identify PSAP and PSA, were difficult to distinguish from secondary involvement by prostatic adenocarcinoma (309,310). Histologically, a wide range of microscopic patterns was reported. Some of the tumors resemble those of Gleason pattern 3 or Gleason pattern 4 prostate carcinoma. Others resemble prostatic duct adenocarcinomas with tall columnar epithelium and a micropapillary pattern. Seminal vesicle adenocarcinomas may be mucinous with epithelial cords and poorly formed glands floating within mucin, or they may appear as mucinous lakes lined by tall columnar colonic-appearing epithelium. Other reported seminal vesicle carcinomas have been undifferentiated. Most patients die without surgery as a result of the unresectability of the tumor. Of the ten cases reported since 1956 in which the diagnosis was made before autopsy, half were dead in less than 18 months. Of those patients surviving more than 18 months, all were treated with estrogen, orchiectomy, or both. In addition to ruling out invasion from the prostate by the use of antisera to PSA and PSAP, which do not stain seminal vesicle neoplasms, extension from a rectal carcinoma or "rectal shelf" tumor also must be excluded primarily on clinical grounds. Carcinoembryonic antigen (CEA) immunoreactivity has not been observed in all seminal vesicle carcinomas and is not useful in differentiating it from a rectal primary. Although most tumors are unilateral, rare bilateral seminal vesicle adenocarcinomas have been reported (311).

Sarcomas of the seminal vesicle are even more rare than carcinomas. As with carcinomas, many of the published cases are poorly documented in terms of both the origin of tumor and the histologic subtype. Well-documented cases of angiosarcoma and leiomyosarcoma of the seminal vesicles have been reported (312,313).

Like similar tumors in the breast and prostate, phyllodes tumors of the seminal vesicle have been rarely reported (314). They should be considered of high grade and malignant when there is significant mitotic activity, stromal pleomorphism, and stromal overgrowth.

Rare primary germ-cell tumors of the seminal vesicle were reported such as seminoma and choriocarcinoma (315,316). These probably arise from germ cells entrapped there during fetal development.

ACKNOWLEDGMENT

We would like to thank Mathew J. Petzi, M.D. for taking some of the new color photomicrographs in this chapter.

REFERENCES

1. Sokoll LJ, Chan DW. Prostate-specific antigen: its discovery and biochemical characteristics. *Urol Clin North Am* 1997;24(2):253–258.
2. Partin AW, Coffey DS. The molecular biology, endocrinology, and physiology of the prostate and seminal vesicles. In: Walsh PC, Retik AB, Vaughan ED Jr, Wein AJ. eds. *Campbell's urology.* 7th ed. Philadelphia: Saunders, 1998:1381–1428.
3. McNeal JE. Normal and pathologic anatomy of prostate. *Urology* [Suppl] 1981;17:11–16.
4. Kost LV, Evans GW. Occurrence and significance of striated muscle within the prostate. *J Urol* 1964;92:703–70.
5. Manley CB, Jr. The striated muscle of the prostate. *J Urol* 1966;95:234–240.
6. Graversen PH, England DM, Madsen PO, et al. Significance of striated muscle in curettings of the prostate. *J Urol* 1988;139:751–753.
7. Franks LM. Benign nodular hyperplasia of the prostate: a review. *Ann R Coll Surg* 1954;14:92–106.
8. Epstein JI, Fynheer J. Can acid mucin histochemistry differentiate adenosis from prostate adenocarcinoma? *Hum Pathol* 1992;23:1321–1325.
9. Ro JY, Grignon DJ, Ayala AG, Hogan SF, Tetu B, Ordonez NG. Blue nevus and melanosis of the prostate: electron microscopic and immunohistochemical studies. *Am J Clin Pathol* 1988;90:530–535.
10. Brennick JB, O Connell JS, Dickersin GR, et al. Lipofuscin pigmentation (so-called melanosis) of the prostate. *Am J Surg Pathol* 1994;18:446–454.
11. Hedrick L, Epstein JI. Use of basal cell specific cytokeratin as an adjunct in the diagnosis of prostate carcinoma. *Am J Surg Pathol* 1989;13:389–396.
12. Brawer MK, Peehl DM, Stamey TA, et al. Keratin immunoreactivity in the benign and neoplastic human prostate. *Cancer Res* 1985;45:3663–3667.
13. Wojno KJ, Epstein JI, The utility of basal cell-specific anti-cytokeratin antibody (34 beta E12) in the diagnosis of prostate cancer: a review of 228 cases. *Am J Surg Pathol* 1995;19(3):251–60.
14. Bonkhoff H, Stein U, Remberger K. Multidirectional differentiation in the normal, hyperplastic, and neoplastic human prostate: simultaneous demonstration of cell-specific epithelial markers. *Hum Pathol* 1994;25:42–46.
15. Berry SJ, Coffey DS, Walsh PC, Ewing LL. The development of human benign prostatic hyperplasia with age. *J Urol* 1984;132:474–479.
16. Moore RA. Benign hypertrophy of the prostate: a morphologic study. *J Urol* 1943;50:680–710.
17. Kerley SW, Corica FA, Qian J, Myers RP, Bostwick DG. Peripheral zone involvement by prostatic hyperplasia. *J Urol Pathol* 1997;6:87–94.
18. Gaudin PB. Epstein JI. Adenosis of the prostate: histologic features in transurethral resection specimens *Am J Surg Pathol* 1994;18:863–870.
19. Renedo D, Poy E, Oesterling J, Wojno K. Clinical significance and distinction of adenosis from low grade adenocarcinoma of the prostate on TURP. *Mod Pathol* 1995;8:468A.
20. Kohnen PW, Drach GW. Patterns of inflammation in prostatic hyperplasia: a histologic and bacteriologic study. *J Urol* 1979;121:755–760.
21. Nielsen ML, Asnaes S, Hattel T. Inflammatory changes in the noninfected prostate gland: a clinical, microbiological and histological investigation. *J Urol* 1973;110:423–426.
22. Nadler RB, Humphrey PA, Smith DS. Catalona WJ, Ratliff TL. Effect of inflammation and benign prostatic hyperplasia on elevated serum prostate specific antigen levels. *J Urol* 1995;154:407–413.
23. Hasui Y, Marutsuka K, Asada Y, Ide H, Nishi S, Osada Y. Relationship between serum prostate specific antigen and histological prostatitis in patients with benign prostatic hyperplasia. *Prostate* 1994;25:91–96.
24. Baird HH, McKay HW, Kimmelstiel P. Ischemic infarction of the prostate gland. *South Med J* 1950;43:234–240.
25. Mostofi FK, Morse WH. Epithelial metaplasia in prostatic infarction. *Arch Pathol Lab Med* 1951;51:340–345.
26. Trapnell J, Roberts M. Prostatic abscess. *Br J Surg* 1970;57:565–568.
27. Wise GJ, Silver DA. Fungal infections of the genitourinary system. *J Urol* 1993;149:1377–1388.
28. Auerbach O. Tuberculosis of the genital system. *Q Bull Sea View Hosp* 1942;7:188–207.
29. Moore RA. Tuberculosis of the prostate gland. *J Urol* 1937;37:372–384.
30. Oates RD, Stilmant MM, Freedlung MC, Siroky MB. Granulomatous prostatitis following Bacillus Calmette-Guerin immunotherapy of bladder cancer. *J Urol* 1988;140:751–754.
31. Mukamel E, Konichezky M, Engelstein D, Cytron S, Abramovici A, Servadio C. Clinical and pathological findings in prostates following intravesical Bacillus Calmette-Guerin instillations. *J Urol* 1990;144:1399–1400.
32. Kelalis PP, Greene LF, Weed LA. Brucellosis of the urogenital tract: a mimic of tuberculosis. *J Urol* 1962;88:347–353.
33. DeSouza E, Katz DA, Dwarzack DL, Long G. Actinomycosis of the prostate. *J Urol* 1985;133:290–291.
34. Goff DA, Davidson RA. Amebic prostatitis. *South Med J* 1984;77:1053–1054.
35. Houston W. Primary hydatid cyst of the prostate gland. *J Urol* 1975;113:732–733.
36. Lee LW, Burgher LW, Price EB, Cassidy E. Granulomatous prostatitis: association with isolation of mycobacterium kansasii and mycobacterium fortuitum. *JAMA* 1977;237:2408–2409.
37. Thompson L. Syphilis of the prostate. *Am J Syph* 1920;4:323–341.
38. Zaher MF, El-deeb AA. Bilharziasis of the prostate: its relation to bladder neck obstruction and its management. *J Urol* 1971;106:257–261.

39. Shurbaji MS, Gupta PK, Myers J. Immunohistochemical demonstration of chlamydial antigens in association with prostatitis. *Mod Pathol* 1988;1:348–351.
40. Gardner WA, Culberson DE, Bennett BD. Trichomonas vaginalis in the prostate gland. *Arch Pathol Lab Med* 1986;110:430–432.
41. Doble A, Thomas BJ, Walker MM, Harris JRW, Witherow OR, Taylor-Robinson D. The role of chlamydia trachomatis in chronic abacterial prostatitis: a study using ultrasound guided biopsy. *J Urol* 1989;141:332–333.
42. Kelalis PP, Greene LF, Harrison EG, Jr. Granulomatous prostatitis: a mimic of carcinoma of the prostate. *JAMA* 1965;191:111–113.
43. Tanner FH, McDonald JR. Granulomatous prostatitis: a histologic study of a group of granulomatous lesions collected from prostate glands. *Arch Pathol* 1943;36:358–370.
44. Oppenheimer JR, Kahane H, Epstein JI. Granulomatous prostatitis on needle biopsy -characterization and clinical correlation of 124 cases. *Arch Pathol Lab Med* 1997;121:724–729.
45. Presti B, Weidner N. Granulomatous prostatitis and poorly differentiated prostate carcinoma: their distinction with the use of immunohistochemical methods. *Am J Clin Pathol* 1991;95:330–334.
46. Epstein JI, Hutchins GM. Granulomatous prostatitis: distinction among allergic, nonspecific and posttransurethral resection lesions. *Hum Pathol* 1984;15:818–825.
47. Kelalis PP, Harrison EG, Jr, Greene LF. Allergic granulomas of the prostate in asthmatics. *JAMA* 1964;188:963–967
48. Shimizu S, Takimoto Y, Niimura T, et al. A case of prostatic malacoplakia. *J Urol* 1981;126:277–279.
49. Lupovitch A. The prostate and amyloidosis. *J Urol* 1972;108:301–302.
50. Wilson SK, Buchanan RD, Stone WJ, Rhamy RK. Amyloid deposition in the prostate. *J Urol* 1973;110:322–323.
51. Hassler O. Calcifications in the prostate gland and adjacent tissues: a combined biophysical and histological study. *Pathol Microbial (Basel)* 1968;31:97–107.
52. Menon M, Parulkar BG, Drach GW. Urinary lithiasis: etiology, diagnosis, and medical management. In: Walsh PC, Retik AB, Vaughan ED, Wein AJ. eds. *Campbell's urology*. Philadelphia: WB Saunders, 7th ed. 1998;2716–2717.
53. Magri J. Cysts of the prostate gland. *Br J Urol* 1960;32:295–301.
54. Schuhrke TD, Kaplan GW. Prostatic utricle cysts (mullerian duct cysts). *J Urol* 1978;119:765–767.
55. Wang CJ, Chen YT, Shun CT, Lai MK. Primary malignant melanoma of the prostate. *J Urol* 1995;154:1865.
56. Lopez-Beltran A. Vasculitis involving the prostate: report of two cases. *Path Case Reviews* 1996;1:70–73.
57. Beckman EN, Leonard GL, Pintado SO, Sternberg WH. Endometriosis of the prostate. *Am J Surg Pathol* 1985;9:374–379
58. Vaught WW, Wilson TM, Raife MJ, Horne DW. Wegener granulomatosis: prostatic involvement and bladder outlet obstruction. *Urology* 1989;34:43–45.
59. Cheatam DE, Sowell DS, Dulaney RB. Hepatitis B antigen-associated periarteritis nodosa with prostatic vasculitis. *Ann Intern Med* 1981;141:107–108.
60. Nassiri M, Ghazi C, Stivers JR, Nadji M. Ganglioneuroma of the prostate: a novel finding in neurofibromatosis. *Arch Pathol Lab Med* 1994;118:938–939.
61. Sebo TJ, Bostwick DG, Farrow GM, Eble JN. Prostatic xanthoma: a mimic of prostatic adenocarcinoma. *Hum Pathol* 1994;25:386–389.
62. Grignon DJ, O Malley FP. Mucinous metaplasia in the prostate gland. *Am J Surg Pathol* 1993;17:287–290.
63. Weaver MG, Abdul-Karim FW, Srigley J. Paneth cell-like change of the prostate gland: a histological, immunohistochemical, and electron microscopic study. *Am J Surg Pathol* 1992;16:62–68.
64. Lim DJ, Hayden RT, Murad T, Nemcek AA Jr, Dalton DP. Multilocular prostatic cystadenoma presenting as a large complex pelvic cystic mass. *J Urol* 1993;149:856–859.
65. Cancer facts & figures: a cancer journal for clinicians 1994;44:4–28.
66. Franks LM. Latent carcinoma of the prostate. *J Pathol Bacteriol* 1954;68:603–616.
67. Halpert B, Schmalhorst WR. Carcinoma of the prostate in patients 70 to 79 years old. *Cancer* 1966;19:695–698.
68. Moore RA. The morphology of small prostatic carcinoma. *J Urol* 1935;33:224–234.
69. Schmalhorst WR, Halpert B. Carcinoma of the prostate gland in patients more than 80 years old. *Am J Clin Pathol* 1962;32:170–173.
70. Sakr WA, Haas GP, Cassin BF, Pontes JE, Crissman JD. The frequency of carcinoma and intraepithelial neoplasia of the prostate in young male patients. *J Urol* 1993;150:379–385.
71. Ropel MA, Polascik TJ, Partin AW, Walsh PC, Epstein JI. Pathologic findings and progression after radical prostatectomy in men less than 50 years old: a study of 140 cases. *Urolog Oncol* 1995;1:80–83.
72. Ruska KM, Walsh PC, Kahane H, Epstein JI. Prostate needle biopsy and adenocarcinoma in men <40 years of age. *Mod Pathol* 1998;11:94A.
73. Aprikian AG, Zhang ZF, Fair WR. Prostate adenocarcinoma in men younger than 50 years. *Cancer* 1994;74:1768–1777.
74. Shimada H, Misugi K, Sasaki Y, Iizuka A, Nishihira H. Carcinoma of the prostate in childhood and adolescence: report of a case and review of the literature. *Cancer* 1980;46:2534–2542.
75. American cancer society, cancer Facts and figures. Atlanta: 1997.76.
76. Levine RL, Wilchinsky M. Adenocarcinoma of the prostate: a comparison of the disease in blacks versus whites. *J Urol* 1979;121:761–762.
77. Moul JW, Douglas TH, McCarthy WF, McLeod DG. Black race is an adverse prognostic factor for prostate cancer recurrence following radical prostatectomy in an equal access health care. *J Urol* 1996;155:1667–1673.
78. Carter HB, Piantadosi S, Issacs JT. Clinical evidence for and implications of the multistep development of prostate cancer. *J Urol* 1990;143:742–746.
79. Schröder F, Denis HL, Fair WR, et al. The TNM classification of prostate cancer. *Prostate* [Suppl] 1992;4:129–138.
80. Epstein JI, Walsh PC, CarMichael M, Brendler CB. Pathological and clinical findings to predict tumor extent of non-palpable (stage T1c) prostate cancer. *JAMA* 1994;271:368–374.
81. Partin AW. Oesterling J. The clinical usefulness of prostate specific antigen update. *J Urol* 1994;152:1258–1368.
82. Rifkin MD, Zerhouni EA, Gatsonis CA, et al. Comparison of magnetic resonance imaging and ultrasonography in staging early prostate cancer: results of a multi-institutional cooperative trial. *N Engl J Med* 1990;323:621–626.
83. Hammerer UM, Sheth S, Walsh PC, Holtz PM, Epstein JI. Stage B adenocarcinoma of the prostate: transrectal US and pathologic correlation of non-malignant hypoechoic peripheral zone lesions. *Radiology* 1991;180:101–104.
84. Oesterling JE, Chan DW, Epstein JI, et al. Prostate-specific antigen in the pre- and post-operative evaluation of localized prostatic cancer treated with radical prostatectomy. *J Urol* 1988;139:766–772.
85. Benson MC, Whang IS, Pantuck A, et al. Prostate specific antigen density a means of distinguishing benign prostatic hypertrophy and prostate cancer. *J Urol* 1992;147:815–816.
86. Carter HB, Pearson JD, Metter J, et al. Longitudinal evaluation of prostate-specific antigen levels in men with and without prostate disease. *JAMA* 1992;267:2215–2220.
87. Richardson TD, Oesterling JE, Age-specific reference ranges for serum prostate-specific antigen. *Urol Clin N Am* 1997;24:339–51.
88. McCormack RT, Rittenhouse HG, Finlay JA, et al. Molecular forms of prostate-specific antigen and the human kallikrein gene family: a new era. *Urology* 1995;45:729–744.
89. Vashi AR, Wojno KJ, Henricks W, et al. Determination of the "reflex range" and appropriate cutpoints for percent free prostate-specific antigen in 413 men referred for prostatic evaluation using the AxSYM system. *Urology* 1997;49:19–27.
90. Steinberg GD, Carter BS, Beaty TH, Childs B, Walsh PC. Family history and the risk of prostate cancer. *Prostate* 1990;17:337–347.
91. Hodge KK, McNeal JE, Terris MK, Stamey TA. Random systematic versus directed ultrasound guided transrectal core biopsies of the prostate. *J Urol* 1989;142:71–75.
92. Keetch DW, Catalona WJ, Smith DS. Serial prostatic biopsies in men with persistently elevated serum prostate specific antigen values. *J Urol* 1994;151:1571–1574.
93. Hudson PB, Stout AP. Prostatic cancer: comparison of physical examination and biopsy for detection of curable lesions. *NY State J Med* 1966;66:351–355.
94. Moul JW, Miles BJ, Skoog ST, McLeon DG. Risk factors for perineal seeding of prostate cancer after needle biopsy. *J Urol* 1989;142:86–88.
95. Bastacky S, Walsh PC, Epstein JI. Needle biopsy associated tumor tracking of adenocarcinoma of the prostate. *J Urol* 1991;145:1003–1007.

96. Cho KR, Epstein JI. Metastatic prostatic carcinoma to supradiaphragmatic lymph nodes: a clinicopathologic and immunohistochemical study. Am J Surg Pathol 1987;11:457–463.
97. Fry DE, Amin M, Harbrecht PJ. Rectal obstruction secondary to carcinoma of the prostate. Ann Surg 1979;189:488–492.
98. Epstein JI. PSAP and PSA as immunohistochemical markers. Urol Clin N Am 1993;20:757–770.
99. Gleason DF, Mellinger GT, the VACURG. Prediction of prognosis for prostatic adenocarcinoma by combined histologic grading and clinical staging. J Urol 1974;111:58–64.
100. Mellinger GT, Gleason DF, Bailar J. The histology and prognosis of prostatic cancer. J Urol 1967;97:331–337.
101. Bain GO, Koch M, Hanson J. Feasibility of grading prostatic carcinomas. Arch Pathol Lab Med 1982;106:265–267.
102. Harada M, Mostofi FK, Corle DK, Byar DP, Trump BF. Preliminary studies of histologic prognosis in cancer of the prostate. Cancer Treat Rep 1977;61:223–225.
103. Allsbrook WC, Lane RB, Lane CG, Mangold KA, Johnson M, Epstein JI. Interobserver reproducibality of Gleason's grading system for prostate carcinoma. Mod Pathol 1997;10:68a.
104. Allsbrook W, Lane R, Jr., Lane C, et al. Interobserver reproducibility of Gleason s grading system 1. Urologic pathologists. Mod Pathol 1998;11:75A.
105. Epstein JI, Partin AW, Sauvageot J, Walsh PC. Prediction of following radical prostatectomy: a multivariate analysis 721 men with long-term follow-up Am J Surg Pathol 1996;20:286–292.
106. McNeal JE, Villers AA, Redwine EA, Freiha FS, Stamey TA. Histologic differentiation, cancer volume, and pelvic lymph node metastasis in adenocarcinoma of the prostate. Cancer 1990;66:1225–1233.
107. Spires SE, Cibull ML, Wood DP, Miller S, Spires SM, Banks ER. Gleason histologic grading in prostatic carcinoma: correlation of 18-guage core biopsy with prostatectomy. Arch Pathol Lab Med 1994;118:705–708.
108. Bostwick DG. Gleason grading of prostatic needle biopsies: correlation with grade in 316 matched prostatectomies. Am J Surg Pathol 1994;18:796–803.
109. Steinberg DM, Sauvageot J, Piantadosi S, Epstein JI. Correlation of prostate needle biopsy and radical prostatectomy Gleason grade in academic and community settings. Am J Surg Pathol 1997;21:566–576.
110. Epstein JI, Steinberg GD. The significance of low grade prostate cancer on needle biopsy: a radical prostatectomy study of tumor grade, volume, and stage of the biopsied and multifocal tumor. Cancer 1990;66:1927–1932.
111. Gleason DF. The veterans administrative cooperative urologic research group: Histologic grading and clinical staging of prostatic carcinoma. In: Tannenbaum M. ed. Urologic pathology: the prostate. Philadelphia: Lea & Febiger, 1977;171–198.
112. Sogani PC, Israel A, Lieberman PH, Lesser ML, Whitmore WF. Gleason grading of prostate cancer: a predictor of survival. Urology 1985;25:223–227.
113. Partin AW, Kattan MW, Subong EN, et al. Combination of prostate-specific antigen, clinical stage, and Gleason score to predict pathological stage of localized prostate cancer: a multi-institutional update. JAMA 1997;277:1445–51.
114. Brawn PN. The dedifferentiation of prostate carcinoma. Cancer 1983;52:246–251.
115. Cheville JC, Bostwick DG. Postatrophic hyperplasia of the prostate: a histologic mimic of prostatic adenocarcinoma. Am J Surg Pathol 1995;19:1068–1076.
116. Ruska KM, Sauvageot J, Epstein JI. Histology and cellular kinetics of prostatic atrophy. Am J Surg Pathol 1998;22:1073–1077.
117. Cina SJ, Epstein JI. Adenocarcinoma of the prostate with atrophic features. Am J Surg Pathol 1997;21:289–295.
118. Oppenheimer JR, Epstein JI. Partial atrophy in prostate needle cores-another diagnostic pitfall for the surgical pathologist. Am J Surg Pathol 1998;22:440–445.
119. Cina SJ, Silberman MA, Kahane H, Epstein JI. The diagnosis of Cowpers glands on prostate needle biopsy. Am J Surg Pathol 1997;21:550–555.
120. Gaudin PB, Wheeler TM, Epstein JI. Verumontanum mucosal hyperplasia (VMGH) in prostatic needle biopsy specimens: a mimic of low-grade prostatic adenocarcinoma. Am J Clin Pathol 1995; 104:620–626.
121. Malpica A, Ro JY, Troncoso P, Ordonez NG, Amin MB, Ayala AG. Nephrogenic adenoma of the prostatic urethra involving the prostate gland: a clinicopathologic immunohistochemical study of eight cases. Hum Pathol 1994;25:390–395.
122. Gikas PW, Del Buono EA, Epstein JI. Florid hyperplasia of mesonephric remnants involving prostate and periprostatic tissue: possible with adenocarcinoma. Am J Surg Pathol 1993;17:454–460.
123. Epstein JI. Diagnostic criteria of limited adenocarcinoma of the prostate on needle biopsy. Hum Pathol 1995;26:223–229.
124. Nelson RS, Epstein JI. Prostatic carcinoma with abundant cytoplasm: foamy gland carcinoma. Am J Surg Pathol 1996;20:419–426.
125. Carstens PHB. Perineural glands in normal and hyperplastic prostates. J Urol 1980;123:686–688.
126. Bostwick DG, Wollan P, Adlakha K. Collagenous micronodules in prostate cancer. a specific but infrequent diagnostic finding. Arch Pathol Lab Med 1995;119:444–447.
127. Epstein JI. Interpretation of prostate biopsies. 2nd ed. New York: Raven Press, 1996.
128. Cheville JC, Reznlicek MJ, Bostwick DG. The focus of atypical glands, suspicious for malignancy in prostatic needle biopsy specimens:incidence, histologic features, and clinical follow-up of cases diagnosed in a community practice. Am J Clin Pathol 1997;108: 633–640.
129. Iczkowski KA, MacLennan GT, Bostwick D. Atypical small acinar proliferation suspicious for malignancy in prostate needle biopsies: cliical significance in 33 cases. Am J Surg Pathol 1997;21:1489–1495.
130. Chan TY, Epstein JI. Follow-up of atypical prostate needle biopsies. Urology (In press).
131. Allen EA, Kahane H, Epstein JI. Repeat biopsy strategies for men with atypical diagnoses on initial prostate needle biopsy. Urology (in press)
132. Bostwick DG, Srigley J, Grignon D, et al. Atypical adenomatous hyperplasia of the prostate: morphologic criteria for its distinction from well-differentiated carcinoma. Hum Pathol 1993;24:819–832.
133. Gaudin PB, Epstein JI. Adenosis of the prostate: histologic features in needle biopsy specimens. Am J Surg Pathol 1995;19:737–747.
134. Kramer CE, Epstein JI. Nucleoli in low-grade prostate and adenosis. Hum Pathol 1993;24:618–623.
135. Ro JY, Grignon DJ, Troncoso P, Ayala AG. Intraluminal crystalloids in whole-organ sections of prostate. Prostate 1988;13:233–239.
136. Henneberry JM, Kahane H, Epstein JI. The significance of intraluminal crystalloids in benign prostatic glands on needle biopsy. Am J Surg Pathol 1997;21:725–728.
137. Pinder SE, McMahon RFT. Mucins in prostatic carcinoma. Histopathology 1990;16:43–46.
138. Sakamoto N, Tsuneyoshi M, Enjoji M. Sclerosing adenosis of the prostate: histopathologic and immunohistochemical analysis. Am J Surg Pathol 1991;15:660–667.
139. Jones EC, Clement PB, Young RH. Sclerosing adenosis of the prostate gland: a clinicopathologic and immunohistochemical study of 11 cases. Am J Surg Pathol 1991;15:1171–1180.
140. Srigley JR, Dardick I, Warren R, Hartwick R, Klotz L. Basal epithelial cells of human prostate gland are not myoepithelial cells. A comparative immunohistochemical and ultrastructural study with the human salivary gland. Am J Pathol 1990;136:957–966.
141. McNeal JE, Bostwick DG. Intraductal dysplasia: a pre-malignant lesion of the prostate. Hum Pathol 1986;17:64–71.
142. Bostwick DG, Brawer MK. Prostatic intra-epithelial neoplasia and early invasion in prostate cancer. Cancer 1987;59:788–794.
143. Epstein JI, Grignon DJ, Humphrey PA, et al. Interobserver reproducibility in the diagnosis of intraepithelial neoplasia. Am J Surg Pathol 1995;19:873–886.
144. Bostwick DG, Amin MB, Dundore P, Marsh W, Schultz DS. Architectural patterns of high-grade prostatic intraepithelial neoplasia. Hum Pathol 1993;24:298–310.
145. Reyes AO, Swanson PE, Carbone JM, Humphrey PA. Unusual histologic types of high-grade prostatic intraepithelial neoplasia. Am J Surg Pathol 1997;21:1215–1222.
146. Wills ML, Hamper UM, Partin AW, Epstein JI. Incidence of high-grade prostatic intraepithelial neoplasia in sextant needle biopsy specimens. Urology 1997;49:367–373.
147. Haggman MJ, Macoska JA, Wojno KJ, Oesterling JE. The relationship between PIN and prostate cancer: critical issues. Urology 1997;158:12–22.
148. McNeal JE, Villers AA, Redwine EA, Freiha FS, Stamey RA. Microcarcinoma in the prostate: its association with duct-acinar dysplasia. Hum Pathol 1991;22:644–652.
149. Shepherd D, Keetch DW, Humphrey PA, Smith DS, Stahl D. Repeat

biopsy strategy in men with isolated prostatic intraepithelial neoplasia on prostate needle biopsy. *J Urol* 1996;156:460–463.
150. Ronnette BM, CarMichael MJ, Carter HB, Epstein JI. Does intraepithelial neoplasia result in elevated serum prostate specific levels? *J Urol* 1993;150:386–389.
151. Gaudin PB, Sesterhenn IA, Wojno KJ, Mostofi FK, Epstein JI. Incidence and clinical significance of high-grade prostatic intraepithelial neoplasia in TURP specimens. *Urology* 1997;49:558–563.
152. Ayala AG, Srigley JR, Ro JY, Abdul-Karim FW, Johnson DE. Clear cell cribriform hyperplasia of prostate: report of 10 cases. *Am J Surg Pathol* 1986;10:665–671.
153. Hall GS, Kramer CE, Walsh PC, Epstein JI. Evaluation of radical prostatectomy specimens: a comparative analysis of various sampling methods. *Am J Surg Pathol* 1992;16:315–324.
154. Byar DP, Mostofi FK, the Veterans Administrative cooperative urologic research groups. Carcinoma of the prostate; prognostic evaluation of certain pathologic features in 208 radical prostatectomies. *Cancer* 1972;30:5–13.
155. McNeal JE. Origin and development of carcinoma in the prostate. *Cancer* 1969;23:24–34.
156. Ayala AG, Ro JY, Babaian R, Troncoso P, Grignon DJ. The prostatic capsule: does it exist? Its importance in the staging and treatment of prostatic carcinoma. *Am J Surg Pathol* 1989;13:21–27.
157. Epstein JI. The evaluation of radical prostatectomy specimens performed for carcinoma of the prostate: therapeutic and prognostic implications. *Pathol Ann* 1991;26:159–210.
158. Villers AA, McNeal JE, Redwine EA, Freiha FS, Stamey TA. The role of perineural space invasion in the local spread of prostatic adenocarcinoma. *J Urol* 1989;142:763–768.
159. Hassan MO, Maksem J. The prostatic perineural space and its relation to tumor spread. *Am J Surg Pathol* 1980;4:143–148.
160. Bastacky SI, Walsh PC, Epstein JI. Relationship between perineural tumor invasion on needle biopsy and radical prostatectomy capsular penetration in clinical stage B adenocarcinoma of the prostate. *Am J Surg Pathol* 1993;17:336–341.
161. Egan AJM, Bostwick DG. Prediction of extraprostatic extension of prostate cancer based on needle biopsy findings: perineural invasion lacks significance on multivariate analysis. *Am J Surg Pathol* 1997;21:1496–1500.
161a. Stone NN, Stock RG, Parikh D, Yeghiayan P, Unger P. Perineural invasion and seminal vesicle involvement predict pelvic lymph node metastasis in men with localized carcinoma of the prostate. *J Urol* 1998;160:1722–1726.
162. Holmes F, Walsh PC, Pound CR, Epstein JI. Excision of the neurovascular bundle at radical prostatectomy in cases with perineural invasion on needle biopsy. *Mod Path* 1998;11:84A.
163. Epstein JI, CarMichael M, Walsh, PC. Adenocarcinoma of the prostate invading the seminal vesicle: definition and relation of tumor, grade, and margins of resection to prognosis. *J Urol* 1993;149:1040–1045
164. Epstein JI, Oesterling JE, Eggleston JC, Walsh PC. Frozen section detection of lymph node metastases in prostatic carcinoma: accuracy in grossly uninvolved pelvic lymphadenectomy specimens. *J Urol* 1986;136:1234–1237.
165. Sgrignoli AR, Walsh PC, Steinberg GD, Steiner MS, Epstein JI. Prognostic factors in men with stage D1 prostate cancer: identification of patients less likely to benefit from radical surgery. *J Urol* 1994;152:1077–1081.
166. Brawn P, Kyhl D, Johnson C, III, Pandya P, McCord R. Stage D1 prostate carcinoma: the histologic appearance of nodal metastases and its relationship to survival. *Cancer* 1990;65:538–543.
167. Oesterling JE, Brendler CB, Epstein JI, Kimball AW, Walsh PC. Correlation of clinical stage, serum prostatic acid phosphatase, and preoperative Gleason grade with final pathologic stage in 275 patients with clinically localized adenocarcinoma of the prostate. *J Urol* 1987;138:92–98.
168. Lepor H, Gregerman M, Crosby R, Mostofi FK, Walsh PC. Precise localization of the autonomic nerves from the pelvic plexus to the corpora cavernosa; a detailed anatomic study of the adult male pelvis. *J Urol* 1985;133:207–212.
169. Carter HB, Sauvageot J, Walsh PC, Epstein, JI. Prospective evaluation of men with stage T1C adenocarcinoma of the prostate. *J Urol* 1997;157:2206–2209.
170. Epstein JI. Incidence and significance of positive margins in radical prostatectomy specimens. *Urol Clin N Am* 1996;23:651–663.

71. Stamey TA, Villers AA, McNeal JE, Link PC, Freiha FS. Positive surgical margins at radical prostatectomy: importance of the apical dissection. *J Urol* 1990;143:1166–1173.
72. Epstein JI, Pizov G, Walsh PC. Correlation of pathologic findings with progression following radical retropubic prostatectomy. *Cancer* 1993;71:3582–3593.
173. Fesseha T, Sakr W, Grignon D, Banerjee M, Wood DP Jr, Pontes JE. Prognostic implications of a positive apical margin in radical prostatectomy specimens. *J Urol* 1997;158:2176–2179.
174. Epstein JI. Evaluation of radical prostatectomy capsular margins of resection: the significance of margins designated as negative, closely approaching, and positive. *Am J Surg Pathol* 1990;14:626–632.
175. Epstein JI, Sauvageot J. Do close but negative margins in radical prostatectomy specimens increase the risk of post-operative progression? *J Urol* 1997;157:241–243.
176. Oesterling JE, Epstein JI, Walsh PC. Long-term autopsy findings following radical prostatectomy. *Urology* 1987;29:584–588.
177. Stamey TA, McNeal JE, Freiha FS, Redwine EA. Morphometric and clinical studies on 68 consecutive radical prostatectomies. *J Urol* 1988;139:1235–1241.
178. Partin AW, Epstein JI, Cho KR, Gittelsohn AM, Walsh PC. Morphometric measurement of tumor volume and per cent of gland involvement as predictors of pathological stage in clinical stage B prostate cancer. *J Urol* 1989;141:341–345.
179. Humphrey PA, Vollmer RT, Ackerman LV. Percentage carcinoma as a measure of prostatic tumor size in radical prostatectomy tissues. *Mod Pathol* 1997;10:326–333.
180. Cupp MR, Bostwick DG, Myers RP, Oesterling JE. The volume of prostate cancer in the biopsy specimen cannot reliably predict the quantity of cancer in the radical prostatectomy specimen on an individual basis. *J Urol* 1995;153:1543–1548.
181. Epstein JI, Carmichael M, Partin AW, Walsh PC. Is tumor volume an independent predictor of progression following radical prostatectomy? A multivariate analysis of 185 clinical stage B adenocarcinomas of the with five years follow-up. *J Urol* 1993;149:1478–1481.
182. Epstein JI, CarMichael MJ, Partin AW. Small high grade adenocarcinoma of the prostate in radical prostatectomy specimens for non-palpable disease: pathogenic and clinical implications. *J Urol* 1994;151:1587–1592.
183. Adolfsson J. Prognostic value of deoxyribonucleic acid content in prostate cancer: a review of current results. *Int J Cancer* 1994;58:211–216.
184. Shankey TV, Kallioniemi OP, Koslowski JM, et al. Consensus review of the clinical utility of DNA content cytometry in prostate cancer. *Cytometry* 1993;14:497–500.
185. Winkler HZ, Rainwater LM, Myers RP, et al. Stage D1 prostatic adenocarcinoma: significance of nuclear DNA patterns studied by flow cytometry. *Mayo Clin Proc* 1988;63:103–112.
186. McNeal JE, Yemoto CEM. Significance of demonstrable vascular space invasion for the progression of prostatic adenocarcinoma. *Am J Surg Pathol* 1996;20:1351–1360.
187. Bahnson RR, Dresner SM, Gooding W, Becich MJ. Incidence and prognostic significance of lymphatic and vascular invasion in radical prostatectomy specimens. *The Prostate* 1989;15:149–155.
188. Salomao DR, Graham SD, Bostwick DG. Microvascular invasion in prostate cancer correlates with pathologic stage. *Arch Pathol Lab Med* 1995;119:1050–1054.
189. Ebie JN, Epstein JI: Stage A carcinoma of the prostate. In: *Pathology of the prostate, seminal vesicles, and male urethra.* Bostwick (consultant ed.) New York: Churchill Livingstone, (Roth LM, ed.) Contemporary issues in Surgical Pathology, 1990:61–82.
190. Larsen MP, Carter HB, Epstein JI. Can stage A1 tumor extent be predicted by transurethral resection tumor volume, per cent, or grade? A study of 64 stage A1 radical prostatectomies with comparison to prostates removed for stage A2 and B disease. *J Urol* 1991;146:1059–1063.
191. Carter HB, Partin AW, Epstein JI, Chan DW, Walsh PC. The relationship of prostate specific antigen levels and residual tumor volume in stage A prostate cancer. *J Urol* 1990;144:1167–1171.
192. Christensen WN, Partin AW, Walsh PC, Epstein JI. Pathologic findings in stage A2 prostate cancer: relation of tumor volume, grade and location to pathologic stage. *Cancer* 1990;65:1021–1027.
193. Greene DR, Wheeler TM, Egawa S, Dunn JK, Scardino PT. A comparison of the morphological features of cancer arising in the transition zone and in the peripheral zone of the prostate. *J Urol* 1991;146:1069–1076.

194. McNeal JE, Price HM, Redwine EA, Freiha FS, Stamey TA. Stage A versus stage B adenocarcinoma of the prostate: morphological comparison and biological significance. *J Urol* 1988; 139:61–65.
195. McDowell PR, Fox W, Epstein JI. Is submission of remaining tissue necessary when incidental carcinoma of the prostate is found on resection? *Hum Pathol* 1994;25:493–497.
196. Epstein JI, Walsh PC, Sauvageot J, Carter HB. Utility of repeat sextant and transition zone biopsies for assessing extent of prostate cancer. *J Urol* 1997;158:1886–1890.
197. DiGiuseppe JA, Sauvageot, J Epstein JI. Increasing incidence of minimal residual cancer in radical prostatectomy specimens. *Am J Surg Pathol* 1997;21 174–178.
198. Goldstein NS, Begin LR, Grody WW, Novak JM, Qian J, Bostwick DG. Minimal or no cancer in radical prostatectomy specimens. *Am J Surg Pathol* 1995;19:1002–1009.
199. Albores-Saavedra J, Vuitch F, Delgado R, Wiley E, Hagler H. Sinus histiocytosis of pelvic lymph nodes after hip replacement: a histiocytic proliferation induced by cobalt-chromium and titanium. *Am J Surg Pathol* 1994;18:83–90.
200. Schned AR, Gormley EA. Florid xanthomatous pelvic lymph node reaction to metastatic prostatic adenocarcinoma: a sequela of preoperative androgen deprivation therapy. *Arch Pathol Lab Med* 1996;120:96–100.
201. Jacobs SC. Spread of prostatic cancer to bone. *Urology* 1983;21:337–344.
202. Varkarakis MJ, Winterberger AR, Gaeta J, Moore RH, Murphy GP. Lung metastases in prostatic carcinoma. *Urology* 1974;3: 447–452.
203. Haupt HM, Mann RB, Trump DL, Abeloff ML. Metastatic carcinoma involving the testis: clinical and pathologic distinction from primary testicular neoplasms. *Cancer* 1984;54:709–71.
204. Green LK, Klima M. The use of immunohistochemistry in metastatic prostatic adenocarcinoma to the breast. *Hum Pathol* 1991;22:242–263.
205. Venable DD, Hastings D, Mistra RP. Unusual metastatic patterns of prostate adenocarcinoma. *J Urol* 1983;130:980–985.
206. Franks LM. Estrogen-treated prostatic cancer: the variation in responsiveness of tumor cells. *Cancer* 1960;13:490–501.
207. Têtu B, Srigley JR, Boivin JC, et al. Effect of combination endocrine therapy (LHRH agonist and flutamide) on normal prostate and prostatic adenocarcinoma. *Am J Surg Pathol* 1991;15:111–120.
208. Bainborough AR. Squamous metaplasia of prostate following estrogen therapy. *J Urol* 1952;68:329–336.
209. Poppel HV, Ridder DD, Elgamal AA, et al. Neoadjuvant hormonal therapy before radical prostatectomy decreases the number of positive surgical margins in stage T2 prostate cancer: interim results of a prospective randomized trial. *J Urol* 1995;154 429–434.
210. Bostwick DG, Egbert BM, Fajardo LF. Radiation injury of the normal and neoplastic prostate. *Am J Surg Pathol* 1982;6:541–551.
211. Brawer MK, Nagle RB, Pitts W, Freiha FS, Gamble SL. Keratin immunoreactivity as an aid to the diagnosis of persistent adenocarcinoma in irradiated human prostates. *Cancer* 1989;63:454–460.
212. Crook JM, Bahadur YA, Robertson SJ, Perry GA, Esche BA. Evaluation of radiation effect, tumor differentiation, and prostate specific antigen staining in sequential prostate biopsies after external beam radiotherapy for patients with prostate carcinoma. *Cancer* 1997;79:79–81.
213. Algaba F, Epstein JI, Aldape HC, et al. International consultation on PIN and pathologic staging of prostate cancer, Workgroup 5. *Cancer* 1996;78:376–381
214. Bodey B, Bodey B Jr, Kaiser HE. Immunocytochemical detection of prostate specific antigen expression in human primary and metastatic melanomas. *Anticancer Res* 1997;17(3C):2343–6.
215. Howarth DJ, Aronson IB, Diamandis EP. Immunohistochemical localization of prostate-specific antigen in benign and malignant breast tissues. *Br J Cancer* 1997;75;1646–51.
216. Alanen KA, Kuopio T, Koskinen PJ, Nevalainen TJ. Immunohistochemical labelling for prostate specific antigen in non-prostatic tissues. *Pathol Res Prac* 1996;192:233–7.
217. O Malley EP, Grignon DJ, Shum DT. Usefulness of immunoperoxidase staining with high-molecular-weight cytokeratin in the differential diagnosis of small-acinar lesions of the prostate. *Arch A Pathol Anat* 1990;417:291–296.
218. Shah IA, Schlageter MO, Stinnett P, Lechago J. Cytokeratin immunohistochemistry as a diagnostic tool for distinguishing malignant from benign epithelial lesions of the prostate. *Mod Pathol* 1991;4:220–224.
219. Kahane H, Sharp JW, Shuman GB, Dasilva G, Epstein JI. Utilization of high molecular weight cytokeratin on prostate needle biopsies in an independent laboratory. *Urology* 1995;45:981–6,.
220. Putzi M, Wojno KJ. Characterization of apparent false negative staining for 34Be12 in BPH nodules. *Mod Pathol* 1998;12(1)93A.
221. Sinha AA, Gleason DF, Wilson MJ, et al. Immunohistochemical localization of laminin in the basement membranes of normal, hyperplastic, and neoplastic human prostate. *Prostate* 1989;15: 299–313.
222. Epstein JI, Lieberman PH. Mucinous adenocarcinoma of the prostate gland. *Am J Surg Pathol* 1985;9:299–308.
223. Ro JY, Grignon J, Ayala AG, Fernandez PL, Ordonez NG, Wishnow KI. Mucinous adenocarcinoma of the prostate: histochemical and immunohistochemical studies. *Hum Pathol* 1990;21: 593–600.
224. Ro JY, Naggar A, Ayala AG, Mady DR, Ordonez NG. Signet-ring cell carcinoma of prostate. *Am J Surg Pathol* 1988;12:453–460.
225. Uchijima Y, Ito H, Takahashi M, Yamashina M. Prostate mucinous adenocarcinoma with signet ring cell. *Urology* 1991;36:267–268.
226. Tran KP, Epstein JI. Mucinous adenocarcinoma with urinary bladder differentiation arising from the prostatic urethra: distinction from mucinous adenocarcinoma of the prostate. *Am J Surg Pathol* 1996; 20:1346–1350.
227. Azzopardi JG, Evans DJ. Argentaffin cells in prostatic carcinoma: differentiation from lipofuscin and melanin in prostatic epithelium. *J Pathol* 1971;104:247–251.
228. di Sant'Agnese PA, Cockett AT. Neuroendocrine differentiation in prostatic malignancy. *Cancer* 1996;78:357–61.
229. Aprikian AG, Cordon-Cardo C, Fair WR, et al. Neuroendocrine differentiation in metastatic prostatic adenocarcinoma. *J Urol* 1994; 151:914–919.
230. Weinstein MH, Partin AW, Veltri RW, Epstein JI. Neuroendocrine (NE) differentiation in prostate cancer: enhanced prediction of progression following radical prostatectomy. *Hum Pathol* 1996; 27:683–687.
231. Theodorescu D, Broder SR, Boyd JC, Mills SE, Frierson HF. Cathepsin D and chromogranin A as predictors of long term disease specific survival after radical prostatectomy for localized carcinoma of the prostate. *Cancer* 1997;80:2109–2119.
232. Krijnen JL, Bogdanowicz JF, Seldenrijk CA, Mulder PG, van der TH. The prognostic value of neuroendocrine differentiation in adenocarcinoma of the prostate in relation to progression of disease after therapy. *J Urol* 1997;158:171–4.
233. Egan AJM, Youngkin TP, Bostwick DG. Mixed carcinoid-adenocarcinoma of the prostate with spindle cell carcinoid: the spectrum of neuroendocrine differentiation in prostatic neoplasia. *Path Case Rev* 1996;1:65–69.
234. Whelan T, Gatfield CT, Robertson S, Carpenter B, Schillinger JF. Primary carcinoid of the prostate in conjunction with multiple endocrine neoplasia IIb in a child. *J Urol* 1995;153:1080–1082.
235. Oesterling JE, Hauzeur CG, Farrow GM. Small cell anaplastic carcinoma of the prostate: a clinical, pathological and immunohistological study of 27 patients. *J Urol* 1992;147:804–807.
236. Ro JY, Têtu B, Ayala AG, Ordonez NG. Small cell carcinoma of the prostate: immunohistochemical and electron microscopic studies of 18 cases. *Cancer* 1987;59:977–982.
237. Têtu B, Ro JY, Ayala AG, et al. Small cell carcinoma of prostate. Part 1: a clinicopathologic study of 20 cases. *Cancer* 1987;59:1803–1809.
238. Dennis PJ, Lewandowski AE, Rohner TJ, Weidner WA, Mamourian AC, Stern DR. Pheochromocytoma of the prostate: an unusual location. *J Urol* 1989;141:130–132.
239. Ostrowski ML, Wheeler TM. Paraganglia of the prostate: location, frequency, and differentiation from prostatic adenocarcinoma. *Am J Surg Pathol* 1994;18:412–420.
240. Bostwick DG, Kindrachuk RW, Rouse RV. Prostatic adenocarcinoma with endometrial features; clinical, pathologic, and ultrastructural findings. *Am J Surg Pathol* 1985;9:595–609.
241. Epstein JI, Woodruff J. Prostatic carcinomas with endometrioid features: a light microscopic and immunohistochemical study of 10 cases. *Cancer* 1986;57:111–119.
242. Greene LF, Farrow GM, Ravits JM, Tomera FM. Prostatic adenocarcinoma of ductal origin. *J Urol* 1979;121:303–305.
243. Samaratunga H, Singh M. Distribution pattern of basal cells detected by cytokeratin 34 beta E12 in primary prostatic duct adenocarcinoma. *Am J Surg Pathol* 1997;21:435–40.
244. Christensen WN, Walsh PC, Epstein JI. Prostatic duct adenocarcinoma: findings at radical prostatectomy. *Cancer* 1991;67:2118–2124.

245. Little NA, Wiener JS, Walther PJ, Paulson DF, Anderson EE. Squamous cell carcinoma of the prostate: 2 cases of a rare malignancy and review of the literature. *J Urol* 1993;149:137–9.
246. Devaney DM, Dorman A, Leader M. Adenosquamous carcinoma of the prostate: a case report. *Hum Pathol* 1991;22:1045–1050.
247. Miller VA, Reuter V, Scher HI. Primary squamous cell carcinoma of the prostate after radiation seed implantation for adenocarcinoma. *Urology* 1995;46:111–3.
248. Braslis KG, Davi RC, Nelson E, Civantos F, Soloway MS. Squamous cell carcinoma of the prostate: a transformation from adenocarcinoma after the use of a luteinizing hormone-releasing hormone agonist and flutamide. *Urology* 1995;45:329–31.
249. Acetta PA, Gardner WA. Squamous metastases from prostatic adenocarcinoma. *Prostate* 1982;3:515–521.
250. Yantiss RK, Young RH. Transitional cell metaplasia in the prostate gland: a survey of its frequency and features based on 103 consecutive prostatic biopsy specimens. *J Urol Path* 1997;7:71–80.
251. Sawczuk I, Tannenbaum M, Olsson CA, White RD. Primary transitional cell carcinoma of prostatic periurethral ducts. *Urology* 1985;25:339–343.
252. Ullman AS, Ross OA. Hyperplasia, atypism, and carcinoma in situ in prostatic periurethral glands. *Am J Clin Pathol* 1967;47:497–504.
253. Greene LF, O Dea MJ, Dockerty MB. Primary transitional cell carcinoma of the prostate. *J Urol* 1976;116:761–763.
254. Schellhammer PF, Bean MA, Whitmore WF Jr. Prostatic involvement by transitional cell carcinoma: pathogenesis, patterns, and prognosis. *J Urol* 1977;118:399–403.
255. Mahadevia PS, Koss LG, Tar IJ. Prostatic involvement in bladder cancer: prostate mapping in 20 cystoprostatectomy specimens. *Cancer* 1986;58:2096–2102.
256. Matzkin H, Soloway MS, Hardeman S. Transitional cell carcinoma of the prostate. *J Urol* 1991;146:1207–1212.
257. Wood DP, Montie JE, Pontes JE, Medendorp SV, Levin HS. Transitional cell carcinoma of the prostate in cystoprostatectomy specimens removed for bladder cancer. *J Urol* 1989;141:346–349.
258. Sakamoto N, Tsuneyoshi M, Naito S, Kumazawa J. An adequate sampling of the prostate to identify prostatic involvement by urothelial carcinoma in bladder cancer patients. *J Urol* 1993;149 318–21.
259. Esrig D, Freeman JA, Elmajian DA, et al. Transitional cell carcinoma involving the prostate with a proposed staging classification for stromal invasion. *J Urol* 1996;156:1071–6.
260. Hardeman SW, Soloway MS. Urethral recurrence following radical cystectomy. *J Urol* 1990;144:666–669.
261. Kabalin JN, McNeal JE, Price HM, Freiha FS, Stamey TA. Unsuspected adenocarcinoma of the prostate in patients undergoing cystoprostatectomy for other causes: incidence, histology and morphometric observations. *J Urol* 1989;141:1091–1094.
262. Montie JE, Wood DP, Pontes JE, Boyett JM, Levin HS. Adenocarcinoma of the prostate in cystoprostatectomy specimens removed for bladder cancer. *Cancer* 1989;63:381–385.
263. Michaels MM, Brown HE, Favino CJ. Leiomyoma of prostate. *Urology* 1974;3:617–620.
264. Gaudin PB, Rosai J, Epstein JI. Sarcomas and related proliferative lesions of specialized prostatic stroma. *Am J Surg Pathol* 1998;22:148–162.
265. Kafandaris PM, Polyzonis MB. Fibroadenoma-like foci in human prostatic nodular hyperplasia. *Prostate* 1983;4:33–35.
266. Hays DM, Raney RB, Lawrence W, Soule EH, Gehan EA, Tefft M. Bladder and prostatic tumors in the intergroup rhabdomyosarcoma study (IRSI): results of therapy. *Cancer* 1982;50:1472–1482.
267. Cheville JC, Dundore PA, Nascimento AG, et al. Leiomyosarcoma of the prostate: report of 23 cases. *Cancer* 1995;76:1422–1427.
268. Proppe KH, Scully RE, Rosai J. Postoperative spindle cell nodules of genitourinary tract resembling sarcoma. *Am J Surg Pathol* 1984;8:101–108.
269. Sahin AA, Ro JY, El-Naggar AK, Ordóñez NG, Babaian RJ, Ayala AG. Pseudosarcomatous fibromyxoid tumor of the prostate. A case report with immunohistochemical, electron microscopic, and DNA flow cytometric analysis. *Am J Clin Pathol* 1991;96:253–258.
270. Chin W, Fay R, Ortega P. Malignant fibrous histiocytoma of prostate. *Urology* 1986;27:363–365.
271. Reyes JW, Shinozuka H, Garry P, Putong PB. A light and electron microscopy study of a hemangiopericytoma of the prostate with local extension. *Cancer* 1977;40:1122–1126.
272. Schuppler J. Malignant neurolemmoma of prostate gland. *J Urol* 1971;105:903–905.
273. Smith DM, Manivel C, Kappa D, Uecker J. Angiosarcoma of the prostate report of 2 cases and review of the literature. *J Urol* 1986;135:382–384.
274. Sudaras varao D, Banerjea S, Nageswararao A, Rao NV. Hemangioma of the prostate: a case report. *J Urol* 1973;110:708–709.
275. Grignon DJ, Ro JY, Ordonez NG, Ayala AG, Cleary KR. Basal cell hyperplasia, adenoid basal cell tumor, and adenoid cystic carcinoma of the prostate gland: an immunohistochemical study. *Hum Pathol* 1988;19:1425–1433.
276. Epstein JI, Armas OA. Atypical basal cell hyperplasia of the prostate. *Am J Surg Pathol* 1992;16:1205–1214.
277. Devaraj LT Bostwick DG. Atypical basal cell hyperplasia of the prostate. Immunophenotypic profile and proposed classification of basal cell proliferations. *Am J Surg Pathol* 1993;17:645–659.
278. Mittal BV, Amin MB, Kinare SG. Spectrum of histopathologic lesions in 185 consecutive prostate specimens. *J Postgrad Med* 1989;35:157–161.
279. Frankel K, Craig JR. Adenoid cystic carcinoma of the prostate. *Am J Clin Pathol* 1974;62:639–645.
280. Denholm SW, Webb JN, Howard GCW, et al. Basaloid carcinoma of the prostate gland: histogenesis and review of the literature. *Histopathology* 1992;20:151-155.
281. Butterick JD, Schnitzer B, Abell MR. Ectopic prostatic tissue in urethra: a clinicopathological entity and a significant cause of hematuria. *J Urol* 1971;105:97–104.
282. Remick DG, Kumar NB. Benign polyps with prostatic-type epithelium of the urethra and the urinary bladder. *Am J Surg Pathol* 1984;8:833–839.
283. Walker AN, Mills SE, Fechner RE, Perry JM. Endometrial adenocarcinoma of the prostatic urethra arising in a villous polyp: a light microscopic and immunoperoxidase study. *Arch Pathol Lab Med* 1982;106:624–627.
284. Seninel a R, Thurm J, Feiner H. Papillary pseudotumor of the prostatic urethra: proliferative papillary urethritis. *J Urol* 1974;111:38–40.
285. Humphrey PA, Vollmer RT. Extramedullary hematopoiesis in the prostate. *Am J Surg Pathol* 1991;15:486–490.
286. Ferris MK, Hausdorff J. Freiha FS. Hematolymphoid malignancies diagnosed at the time of radical prostatectomy. *J Urol* 1997;158:457–1459.
287. Bostwick DG, Mann RB. Malignant lymphoma involving the prostate. A study of 13 cases. *Cancer* 1985;56:2932–2938.
288. Ferry JA, Young RH. Malignant lymphoma of the genitourinary tract. *Current Diagnostic Pathology* 1997;4:145–169.
289. Cajai YF, Burke M. Leukemic infiltration of the prostate: a case study and clinicopathologic review. *Cancer* 1976;38:2442–2446.
290. Dundore PA. Cheville JC. Nascimento AG. Farrow GM. Bostwick DG. Carcinosarcoma of the prostate. Report of 21 cases. *Cancer* 1995;76:1035–1042.
291. Zin TA. Huben R. Lane W. Pontes JE. Englander LS. Secondary tumors of the prostate. *J Urol* 1985;133:615–616.
292. Elfors TO, Aho HJ, Kekomaki M. Malignant rhabdoid tumor of the prostate region: immunohistological and ultrastructural evidence for epithelial origin. *Virchows Arch [A]* 1985;406:381–388.
293. Manrique U, Albores-Saavedra J, Orantes A, Brandt H. Malignant mixed tumor of the salivary gland type, primary in the prostate. *Am J Clin Pathol* 1978;70:932–937.
294. Tay HP, Bidair M, Shabaik A, Gilbaugh JH III, Schmidt JD. Primary yolk sac tumor of the prostate in a patient with Klinefelter s syndrome. *J Urol* 1995;153:1066–1069.
295. Pinto JA, Gonzalez JE, Granadillo MA. Primary carcinoma of the prostate with diffuse oncocytic changes. *Histopathol* 1994;25:286–288.
296. Wang YZ, Wong YC. Oncogenes and tumor suppresser genes in prostate cancer: a review. *Urol Oncol* 1997;3:41–46.
297. Isaacs JT. Molecular markers for prostate cancer metastasis. Developing diagnostic methods for predicting the aggressiveness of prostate cancer. *Am J Pathol* 1997;150:1511–1521.
298. Gao X. Porter AT, Grignon DJ, Pontes JE, Honn KV. Diagnostic and prognostic markers for human prostate cancer. *The Prostate* 1997;31:264–281.
299. Bostwick DG, Pacelli A, Lopez-Beltran A. Molecular biology of prostatic intraepithelial neoplasia. *The Prostate* 1996;29:117–134.
300. Silberman MA, Partin AW, Veltri RW, Epstein JI. Tumor angiogene-

300. sis correlates with progression after radical prostatectomy but not with pathological stage in Gleason sum 5 to 7 adenocarcinoma of the prostate. *Cancer* 1997;79:772-779.
301. Bostwick DG, Wheeler TM, Blute M, et al. Optimized microvessel density analysis improves prediction of cancer stage from prostate needle biopsies. *Urology* 1996;48:47–57.
302. Campbell SC. Advances in angiogenesis research: relevance to urological oncology. *J Urol* 1997;158:1663–1674.
303. Lissbrant IF, Stattin P, Damber JE, Bergh A. Vascular density is a predictor of cancer-specific survival in prostatic carcinoma. *The Prostate* 1997;33:38–45.
304. Hall MC, Troncoso P, Pollack A, Zhau HY, Zagars GK, Chung LWK, von Eschenbach AC. Significance of tumor angiogenesis in clinically localized prostate carcinoma treated with external beam radiotherapy. *Urology* 1994;44:869–875.
305. Ejeckam GC, Covatsos S, Lewis AS. Cyst of seminal vesicle associated with ipsilateral renal agenesis. *Urology* 1984;24:372–374.
306. Rappe BM, Meuleman EH, Debruyne FJ. Seminal vesicle cyst with ipsilateral renal agenesis. *Urol Int* 1993;50:54–56.
307. Schnitzer B. Ectopic ureteral openings into vesicle: a report of 4 cases. *J Urol* 1965;93:576–581.
308. Damjanov I, Apic R. Cystadenoma of seminal vesicles. *J Urol* 1974;111:808–809
309. Benson RC, Jr, Clark WR, Farrow GM. Carcinoma of the seminal vesicle. *J Urol* 1984;132:483–485.
310. Zenklusen HR, Weymouth G, Rist M, Mihatsch MJ. Carcinosarcoma of the prostate in combination with adenocarcinoma of the prostate and adenocarcinoma of the seminal vesicles. A case report with immunocytochemical analysis and review of the literature. *Cancer* 1990;66:998–1001
311. Ormsby AH, Haskell R, Ruthven SE, Mylne GE. Bilateral primary seminal vesicle carcinoma. *Pathology* 1996;28:196–200.
312. Lamont JS, Hesketh PJ, de las Morenas A, Babayan RK. Primary angiosarcoma of the seminal vesicle. *J Urol* 1991;146:165–167.
313. Schned AR, Ledbetter JS, Selikowitz SM. Primary leiomyosarcoma of the seminal vesicle. *Cancer* 1986;57:2202–2206.
314. Fain JS, Cosnow I, King BF, Zincke H, Bostwick DG. Cystosarcoma phyllodes of the seminal vesicle. *Cancer* 1993;71:2055–61.
315. Fairey AE, Mead GM, Murphy D, Theaker J. Primary seminal vesicle choriocarcinoma. *Br J Urol* 1993;71:756–7.
316. Adachi Y, Rokujyo M, Kojima H, et al. Primary seminoma of the seminal vesicle: report of a case. *J Urol* 1991;146:857–859.

CHAPTER 46

Nonneoplastic Diseases of the Testis

Howard S. Levin

The testis is a paired organ suspended in the scrotum by a spermatic cord. Attached to each testis is an epididymis that connects the rete testis to the vas deferens. Each testis weighs approximately 12 to 19 g and averages 4.5 × 2.5 × 3 cm (1,2). The testis is covered by a mesothelium-lined fibrous capsule, the tunica albuginea, and lies within a mesothelium-lined cavity, the tunica vaginalis. Posteriorly, the tunica albuginea extends into the testis. In this area, the mediastinum testis, blood vessels, lymphatics, and nerves extend into the testis, and the rete testis communicates with the efferent ducts. Connective tissue septa derived from the tunica vasculosa divide the testis into approximately 250 lobules of one to four seminiferous tubules each, between which are loose connective tissue, clusters of Leydig cells, blood vessels, lymphatics, and nerves (2).

Adult seminiferous tubules measure approximately 150 to 250 μm in diameter. Each tubule is lined by a multilayered epithelium in which the least mature cells lie against the basement membrane and the most mature cells define the lumen of the tubule (Fig. 1A). The seminiferous epithelium is composed of six defined cellular associations arranged in the seminiferous tubules in a mosaic pattern (3). Not all associations culminate in fully mature spermatids. Separating groups of germ cells are Sertoli cells, which are oriented perpendicular to the basement membrane. Spermatids are embedded in the apical portion of Sertoli cells. Tubules are lined by a basal lamina, peripheral to which are layers of myoid cells that stain positively for desmin, muscle-specific actin, and vimentin (Fig. 1B). Leydig cells lie in loose connective tissue between seminiferous tubules. These are variably shaped, often polyhedral, and are in proximity to blood vessels. The cells are about 20 μm in diameter and contain nucleolated round nuclei and eosinophilic, sometimes vacuolated cytoplasm. Within the cytoplasm are varying amounts of brown lipochrome pigment. Some cells contain eosinophilic crystals of Reinke, which may be seen in long or cross section and have a crystalline ultrastructural appearance (Fig. 2A).

On ultrastructural examination, adult Sertoli cells have convoluted nuclei and prominent nucleoli. The basal cytoplasm contains lipid droplets, glycogen, spherical and elongated mitochondria, thin filaments, and a Golgi complex. Charcot–Böttcher crystals, which are elongated bundles of parallel microfilaments that measure up to 25 μm in length and 1 μm in width and extend in various directions, may be present within the cytoplasm and may be seen on light microscopy (Fig. 2B). Adjacent to the junctions of Sertoli cells are bundles of parallel filaments and cisternae of endoplasmic reticulum.

The functions of the Sertoli cell have only recently become recognized, and it is obvious that the Sertoli cell is not a passive structure (4). Junctions between Sertoli cells are among the tightest in the body and divide the seminiferous tubule into an outer basal compartment containing spermatogonia and preleptotene spermatocytes and an inner adluminal compartment containing more mature forms. Junctions develop at puberty and define the blood–testis barrier, which gives the adluminal compartment a protected environment. Human Sertoli cells in cell culture secrete androgen-binding protein (ABP) and are responsive to follicle-stimulating hormone (FSH) (5). In rats, ABP is synthesized by the Sertoli cell. This protein binds testosterone (T) and is concentrated in the epididymis. Other substances synthesized by the Sertoli cell include transforming growth factor X, transferrin, ceruloplasmin, testibumin, inhibin, sulfated glycoprotein 2, creatine phosphokinase, lactic dehydrogenase, alkaline phosphatase, and γ-glutamyl transferase (5–8). In cultures of Sertoli cells from rat testes, it was shown that the Sertoli cells metabolize progesterone substrate to T and other androgens (9). Aromatization of T to estradiol occurs in the Sertoli cell under FSH control (10). Sertoli cells in rats contain androgen receptors, suggesting that androgen activity in germ cells is mediated through Sertoli cells (4). Sertoli cells produce inhibin, which suppresses FSH secre-

---

H. S. Levin: Department of Anatomic Pathology, The Cleveland Clinic Foundation, Cleveland, Ohio 44195.

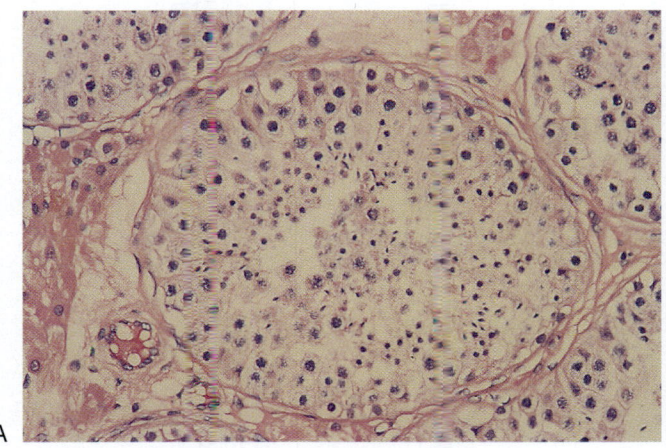 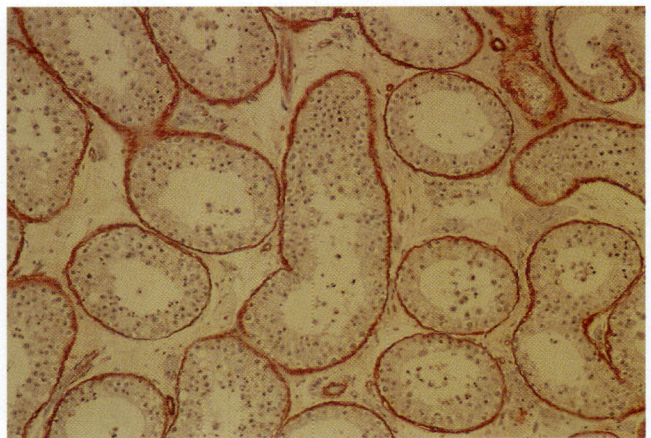

FIG. 1. A: Normal spermatogenesis in a 34-year-old. A cluster of Leydig cells is present at the left. **B:** Immunoperoxidase stain for actin stains myoid cells. The section is from testis of a 36-year-old with seminoma.

tion from rat anterior pituitary cells *in vitro* (9). Sertoli cells also have phagocytic and spermatogenesis-regulating capability. The fetal and postnatal Sertoli cell secretes antimüllerian hormone (AMH) (11). Thus the Sertoli cell has important effects on differentiation, spermatogenesis, and endocrine function.

EMBRYOLOGY

At the time of conception, fertilization of an X-bearing egg by a Y-bearing sperm determines the formation of the testis. It is believed that a genetic switch named testis-determining factor (TDF), localized on the Y chromosome, diverts the primordial gonads to form testes. A single Y-located gene named sex-determining region Y (SRY) is thought to be the TDF (12). At about week 5 of development, the coelomic epithelial cells and the underlying mesenchyme along the medial portions of the mesonephros become thickened and are designated the genital ridges (13). Primary sex cords develop in the genital ridges and extend into the mesenchyme. Primordial germ cells, visible in week 4 of gestation in the yolk sac, migrate along the dorsal mesentery of the hindgut into the genital ridges and in week 6 are within the sex cords. At 7 weeks, the sex cords separate from the surface lining. Straight tubules and rete testis form, and Leydig cells, having developed from the mesenchyme, are present in large numbers between seminiferous tubules. Sertoli cells (derived from the sex cords) and germ cells compose the seminiferous tubules. Mesonephric tubules form the efferent ducts, which connect the rete testis with the epididymal duct. Under the influence of T produced locally by Leydig cells, the ipsilateral mesonephric duct develops into epididymis, vas deferens, and seminal vesicle. Sertoli cells produce AMH, which causes ipsilateral regression of mülle-

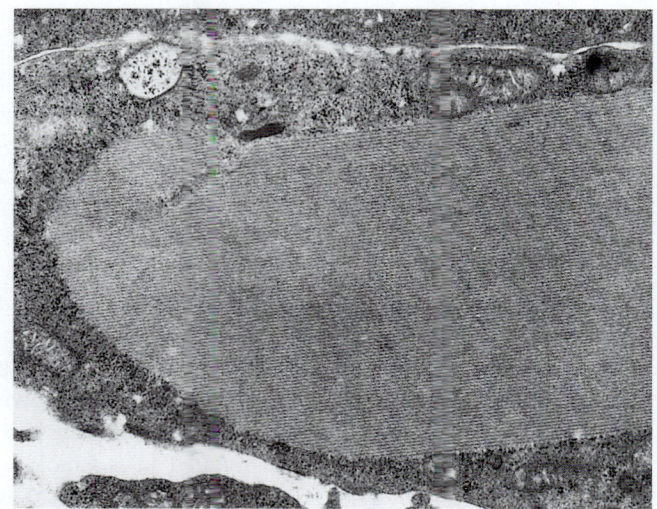 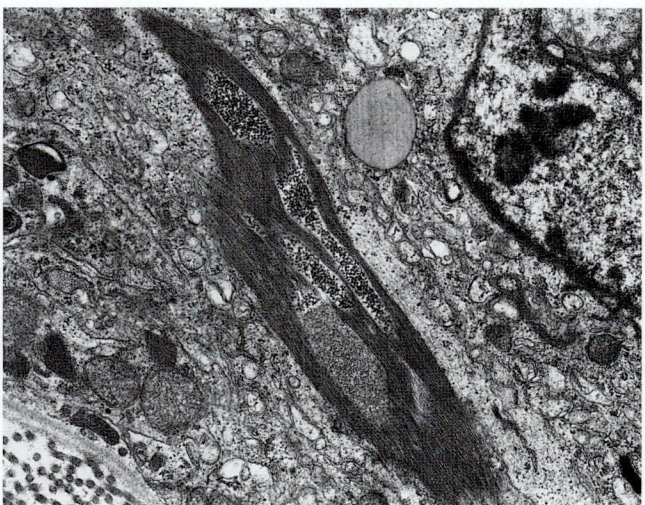

FIG. 2. A: Electron micrograph of Reinke's crystal within a Leydig cell. Longitudinal section of crystal demonstrates parallel lamellae. ×23,000. **B:** Electron micrograph of Charcot–Böttcher crystal. Parallel bundles of microfilaments in an intracytoplasmic location within a Sertoli cell. ×21,000.

rian duct structures. The schedule of development of the testes and the excurrent duct system is an intricate one, depending for its integrity on the Y chromosome, migrating germ cells, and Leydig and Sertoli cells, as well as their products. Faulty anlage or mistiming lead to defects in function and structure of gonads and excurrent ducts.

POSTNATAL DEVELOPMENT

After birth, there is rapid regression of Leydig cells, which are usually no longer visible by light microscopy after about age 4 months. During this time, seminiferous tubules are essentially aluminal and contain numerous immature Sertoli cells and rare fetal spermatogonia. Immature Sertoli cells are characterized by scant cytoplasm and round nuclei with inconspicuous nucleoli.

Although earlier studies indicated that testicular development is static during the first years of life (14), stereologic studies showed progressive increase in testicular volume from birth to adulthood (15). This increase is not sufficient during the first 5 or 6 years to produce distinctive changes by light-microscopic study (Fig. 3). In Müller and Skakkebaek's study (15), mean tubular diameter was constant through year 5, with slight enlargement through year 14, and a significant increase in diameter in the tubules of 14- to 17.9-year-olds. The numeric density of germ cell nuclei per tubule increased progressively from age 5, as did the total number of germ cells per boy. Seminiferous tubules occupied about half the testicular volume before puberty and about 67% from age 14 to 17.9 years. By 8 years, primary spermatocytes may be evident. Development becomes progressive thereafter. Sertoli cells become more mature with increased eosinophilic cytoplasm and oval, often nucleolated, nuclei. Mitotic figures are not seen in Sertoli cells. Spermatogenesis and spermiogenesis may be seen by year 11. Leydig cells, usually not evident histologically after 4 months, reappear as soon as 8 years and are more numerous at 11 through 14 years (16). They have been described ultrastructurally in boys 3 through 8 years and presumably are present earlier. Leydig cells contain steroidogenic hormones, aromatase (17), nitric oxide synthase (18), substance P, and methionine–enkephalin immunoreactivity (19). After spermatogenesis has been completed, the testis resembles the adult testis. Changes related specifically to advancing age are not readily discernible in an individual testis. No one feature characterizes the senescent testis. After age 40 years, serum luteinizing hormone (LH) and FSH increase, and serum T values slowly decrease (20). Weights of testes are similar in young and older men, but the percentage of total testicular weight represented by the tunica albuginea and the thickness of the tunica albuginea are greater in older adults. The weight of testicular parenchyma is similar or reduced in older men, but the daily sperm production per testis and per gram of testis is greater in young men (21). With increasing age, there is reduced volume of parenchyma, seminiferous tubules, and seminiferous epithelium; in addition, the number of Sertoli cells is reduced per gram, per testis, and per seminiferous tubule (21,22). Germinal cell degeneration occurs in the testes of both younger and older men during spermatogonial mitosis and meiosis, as well as during spermiogenesis. Additional degeneration occurs during meiosis of older men (23). Older men show reductions in the number of non-Leydig interstitial and myoid cells (23). Johnson (23) and Kaler and Neaves (24) described reduced numbers of Leydig cells in the testes of older men. Honoré (25), however, indicated that there is Leydig cell hyperplasia, but this was not assessed in a quantitative fashion. He also described tubular sclerosis, focal mononuclear cell infiltration, capsular smooth-muscle hyperplasia, and dilation of the rete testis. Johnson (23) described increased thickness of myoid cells and extracellular components in older men, but no difference in the volume density of myoid cells, and he interpreted the changes as secondary to reduction in tubule length.

In the human, in general, spermatogenic and hormonal function do not abruptly cease. It is difficult to determine causes of the various changes, but decrease in hormonal function is probably at least partly due to a loss of about 80 million Leydig cells per decade (24). Tubular sclerosis occurs in testes of men with arteriosclerosis, but the fact that arteriosclerosis specifically causes the changes remains to be proven (25). Reduced function and altered structure of the testis in older men have multiple etiologies, including reduced nutrition and intercurrent disease.

CONGENITAL ABNORMALITIES

Cryptorchidism

The congenital abnormality most frequently encountered by the pathologist is the cryptorchid testis. Specimens may be obtained occasionally as a result of complications such as

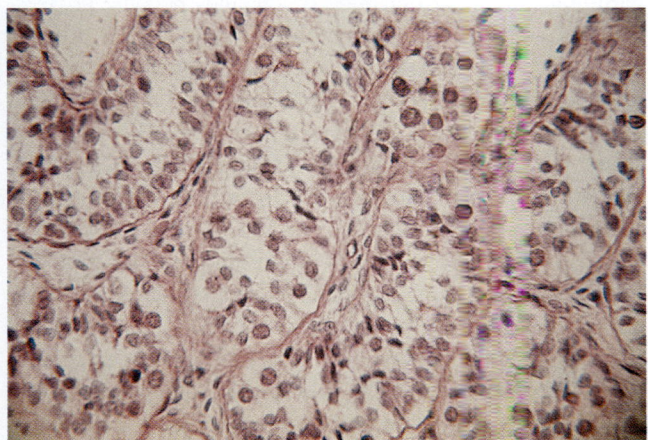

FIG. 3. Prepubertal testis from a 3-year-old. Aluminal tubules contain numerous undifferentiated Sertoli cells and spermatogonia centrally in tubules and along the basement membranes.

the development of a tumor or torsion or at the time of orchiopexy. The etiology of testicular maldescent is being increasingly understood, and its causes include abnormalities in a number of areas: the integrity of the anterior abdominal wall, T production, an intact hypothalamic–pituitary–testicular axis including a possibly reduced surge of gonadotropins at age 50 to 90 days (27), and the anatomy of the inguinal canal and the gubernaculum (28). Testes may be intraabdominal, intracanalicular, ectopic, or retractile (28). The last condition is not considered truly cryptorchid by some and appears to be more susceptible to spontaneous descent or descent after hormonal therapy (29). If the gonad spontaneously descends, the pathologist will not have an opportunity to examine it. However, if orchiopexy is performed intrapubertally or postpubertally, the surgeon may obtain a small biopsy. The histologic appearance may vary with age, testicular position, and prior hormonal therapy. Hadziselimovic et al. (27) found hypoplasia of Leydig cells, normal germ cell counts, and defective maturation of gonocytes into adult dark spermatogonia in boys aged 30 to 120 days with cryptorchidism. Huff et al. (30) found that the number of germ cells decreased when secondary degeneration of untransformed gonocytes led to a decreased total germ cell count. Hedinger (31) and Huff et al. (30) pointed out that there are fewer germinal cells per seminiferous tubule after the first year of life in the cryptorchid testis than in the normally descended testis. Nistal et al. (32) classified prepubertal undescended testes into four groups according to tubular diameter, tubular–fertility index (TFI; the number of tubules with germ cells), Sertoli cell index (SCI; the number of Sertoli cells per transverse tubular section), and the mean tubular diameter (MTD). The most severely involved testes showed reduced TFI, reduced SCI, and decreased MTD. These authors believed that orchiopexy improves the chance for fertility only in those cases with minimal alterations (i.e.,

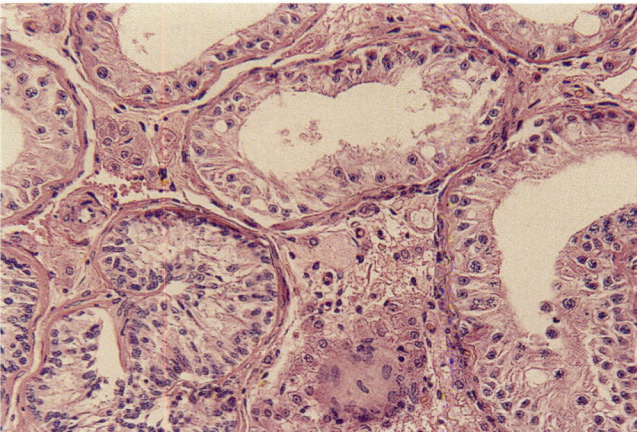

FIG. 4. Cryptorchid testis from a 17-year-old. Postpubertal seminiferous tubules are lined by Sertoli cells. The tubule at the right also has primary spermatocytes. Tubules at bottom left are lined by immature Sertoli cells and are persistent immature tubules (Pick's adenoma).

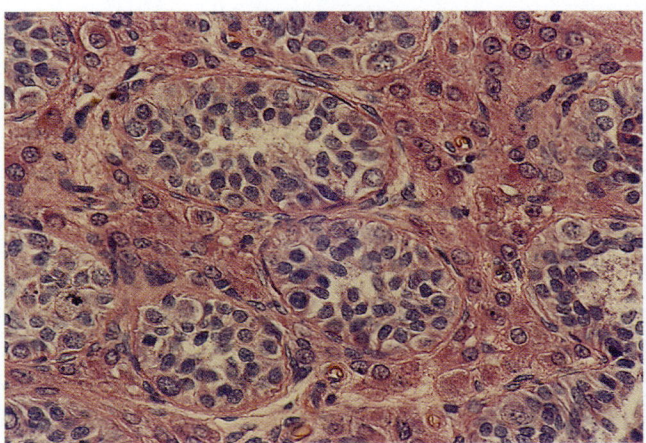

FIG. 5. Fourteen-year-old with biopsy of a cryptorchid testis after hormonal therapy. Small aluminal tubules contain numerous Sertoli cells and occasional spermatogonia placed against the basement membrane. Prominent Leydig cells have been stimulated by administered luteinizing hormone.

slight tubular hypoplasia). The more severely affected prepubertal testes will develop postpubertal hypospermatogenesis, maturation arrest, and germinal cell aplasia or hypoplasia (Fig. 4). Tunica propria thickening of the seminiferous tubules develops in the first year of life (33). Surgeons are treating cryptorchid patients earlier than previously, often after a trial of human chorionic gonadotropin or gonadotropin-releasing hormone (GnRH) (29). Biopsies after such therapy in the first years of life contain clusters of stimulated Leydig cells that ordinarily would have regressed (Fig. 5). Biopsies of cryptorchid testes at any age should be examined for the presence and numbers of germinal cells, tubular size, the presence of malignant intratubular germ cells, and other abnormalities. Other changes include ring-shaped tubules, intratubular calcifications, and an increased amount of interstitial tissue (32). Swerdlow et al. (34), however, indicated that cryptorchid patients who had testicular biopsy at the time of orchiopexy had an increased risk of developing malignant germ cell tumors. After puberty, changes become progressively more apparent and include obvious tunica propria thickening with reduced actin, increased vimentin, and the presence of low-molecular-weight keratins (8 and 18) in myoid cells, reduced tubular diameter, tubular sclerosis, interstitial fibrosis, and more prominent Leydig cells. Nistal et al. (35,36) also described oncocytic changes, vacuolation, and athrocytosis (apical granules) in Sertoli cells of retractile testes, and these were subsequently found in testes with germinal cell aplasia, macroorchidism, interstitial orchitis, acquired immunodeficiency syndrome (AIDS), male pseudohermaphroditism, and in a testis associated with varicocele.

Undescended testes are susceptible to torsion, infarction, and the development of germinal cell neoplasms. When torsion occurs in the undescended testis of an adult, the gonad is likely to harbor a malignant germinal tumor. Germ cell tumors of almost any type may develop in a disproportionately high number of cryptorchid testes, with a

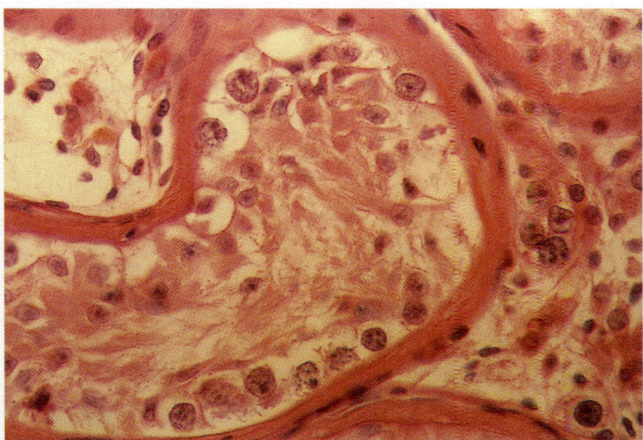

FIG. 6. Malignant intratubular and interstitial germ cells in an intraabdominal cryptorchid testis of a 26-year-old with prune-belly syndrome.

risk of up to 35 times that of a patient with descended testes. More recent studies indicate a relative risk of 5.2 to 7.5 for the development of testicular germ cell malignancy relative to the population of male subjects with descended testes (34,37). Of germ cell tumors, only spermatocytic seminoma has not been reported occurring in an undescended testis. Undescended testes of postpubertal individuals are unlikely to be capable of fertility, other than with assisted reproductive techniques. In undescended prepubertal testes, malignant intratubular germ cells occur only rarely. Of utmost importance is the finding of malignant cells within the tubules or within the interstitium or both, if they exist at any age (Fig. 6). Malignant intratubular germ cells may be very few and can be overlooked. Immunoperoxidase stains for placental alkaline phosphatase can be performed on sections of cryptorchid testes so that malignant germ cells are not overlooked. Malignant intratubular germ cells have been identified in the testes of men with prior orchiopexy in up to 8% of cases (38), a higher incidence than is found in testis biopsies from infertile patients (0.5% and 1.1%) (39,40). Such malignant cells have the potential to develop into clinically important germ-cell tumors of varying types. The postpubertal cryptorchid testis is often surgically removed. Gross examination of the organ should be carefully performed, and any scars, infarcts, or nodules should be noted. Scars or infarcts may be the site of regressed tumors, and small nodules of approximately 1 mm diameter may represent clusters of persistent immature tubules, the so-called Pick's adenomas or tubular congeries (see Fig. 4). Patients with metastatic germ-cell neoplasms may have a testis removed in an attempt to discover and treat the primary tumor. In this situation, the entire testis should be sectioned and submitted, whether the testis is undescended or normal in position. The source of metastatic tumors may be found only in scars, which sometime contain calcifications.

Anorchia

Anorchia is a rare occurrence in clinically cryptorchid individuals. In a phenotypically normal male subject, if the vas deferens is present, there had to have been a functioning ipsilateral testis during gestation. There are two reasons for failure to discover the gonad at the time of surgical exploration: either it does not exist, or the urologist failed to find it. In the former circumstance, the gonad will have disappeared sometime after induction of the wolffian duct system, regression of the müllerian duct, and formation of external genitalia (approximately week 16 of gestation) (41,42). This is an example of testicular regression syndrome (*vide infra*) and may be due to a variety of causes, including intrinsic gonadal disorder, infection, trauma, torsion, or prenatal hormone-induced atrophy resulting from overproduction of androgens (41). When regression occurs before seminiferous tubule and Leydig cell formation, there is ipsilateral absence of the wolffian duct system and failure of regression of the müllerian duct system.

The urologist may call on the pathologist in the course of surgical exploration to determine if testicular tissue is present. Fibrosis, hemosiderin deposition, calcification, or Leydig cells near the epididymis or proximal portion of the vas deferens indicate the position of the former testis. When frozen section shows only fat, connective tissue, or epididymis, a separate intraabdominal testis cannot be excluded (43). All tissue should be examined histologically. The presence of vas deferens or epididymis or both and histologic changes should be noted, and it should be indicated that this is the probable location of the former testis. The presence of venous structures next to the vas deferens or epididymis should be noted, because a testis probably cannot be present without a gonadal vein (44). The contralateral descended testis is usually enlarged in an individual with monoorchism.

Polyorchism

Polyorchism may be seen as an abnormal intrascrotal or intraabdominal structure suggestive of tumor, maldescent, or torsion (41). Testes may each have an individual epididymis and vas deferens that join distally, a single epididymis that joins both testes and leads to a single vas deferens, or discordant connection of the excurrent duct system to the testes (42). The spermatogenic function of the testes is variable. Tumors have rarely been reported in polyorchism (42).

Testicular–Splenic Fusion

Fusion of testicular and splenic tissue involves only the left testis. Fusion may be continuous, attaching to the spleen, or discontinuous with intrascrotal splenic nodules attached to the spermatic cord, epididymis, appendices of the epididymis or testis, or the testis itself; the nodules may, in some cases, lie within the testis or may be unattached in the scrotum. Putschar and Manion (45) reported four cases and summarized 26 other cases of splenic gonadal fusion. Twelve of 30 cases were discontinuous. There was a 9:1 male-to-female ratio. Five cases had peromelia (severe congenital malformations of the extremities) identical to that seen in thalidomide embryopathy (46). The etiology of testicular–splenic fusion has not been established. Coexistence of this lesion with limb-bud anomalies suggests that it is produced in week 5 to 8 of gestation. How the spleen and gonad intermingle is not clear. It is not known whether the discontinuous form was continuous at one time. Limb-bud anomalies occur in both forms. The intrascrotal lesion may enlarge and become symptomatic as a result of circumstances that produce splenomegaly, such as infection (45). A variety of changes may be present in the testis, including atrophy and fibrosis. In a case I reviewed, seminiferous tubules adjacent to splenic tissue showed focal germinal cell aplasia and hypoplasia.

Adrenal Cortical Rests

Rests of adrenal cortex occur in the testis, adjacent to the testis, or in the spermatic cord and epididymis in 4% to 15% of individuals (42). They are small, rounded, yellow structures composed of adrenal cortical tissue. No adrenal medullary tissue is present in the cortical rests. In congenital adrenal hyperplasia, multiple masses histologically similar to Leydig cell tumors occur in the testes and peritesticular areas, although the cells do not contain crystals of Reinke (*vide infra*). In cases of Nelson's syndrome that have an adrenocorticotropic hormone (ACTH)-producing pituitary tumor, similar bilateral masses occur after bilateral adrenalectomy, and because the source of ACTH production is neoplastic, ACTH is not suppressed by administered corticosteroids. In the case reported by Johnson and Scheithauer (47), nodules of eosinophilic cells of probable adrenocortical origin were present in both testes and the left spermatic cord. In the orchiectomy specimens, the testicular parenchyma adjacent to the intratesticular masses was devoid of Leydig cells because of absent LH secretion resulting from irradiation and surgical resection of the pituitary. Irradiation, however, failed to control the ACTH-producing pituitary adenoma. Regression of the native Leydig cells in this case further suggests origin of the testicular tumors to be ACTH-sensitive cells of probable adrenocortical origin. Leydig cell tumors are rarely bilateral.

ACQUIRED ABNORMALITIES

Torsion and Infarction

Torsion of the spermatic cord may occur within the tunica vaginalis or external to it, so-called intravaginal or extravaginal torsion. Most torsions occur intravaginally and result from high insertion of the tunica vaginalis on the spermatic cord. In this circumstance, the testis is not attached to the scrotal wall posteriorly and is suspended on a longer-than-normal spermatic cord, the so-called bell-clapper abnormality. Intravaginal torsion, the complete or incomplete twisting of the cord within the tunica vaginalis, generally occurs in adolescents and young adults. Torsion may be greater than 360°. Torsion that lasts less than 6 hours probably will not cause a testicular infarct. If torsion lasts longer than 24 hours, the testis almost certainly will infarct (48). Thus testicular torsion should be diagnosed and treated promptly. Torsion is a direct cause of infertility when it results in infarct or atrophy. Even if the testis is judged not to have been infarcted and is treated with orchiopexy, there is a substantial possibility that atrophy may ensue. Thomas et al. (49) studied 54 patients 4 years (mean elapsed time) after torsion and orchiopexy and found 45 to have atrophy of the affected testis. The degree of atrophy correlated with the duration of torsion. Patients who had torsion for more than 10 hours had a 50% decrease in testicular volume. Most patients with unilateral torsion and orchiopexy had an abnormal semen analysis at the time of study, which might have resulted from an immunologic event at the time of torsion, from subclinical torsion of the nonorchiopexed testis, or from an abnormality of the untorsed testis unrelated to the occurrence or therapy of torsion.

The pathologist usually is not part of the preoperative diagnostic or operative treatment of the patient. It is only when viability of the testis is in doubt that a frozen section is requested. With present techniques, frozen section can usually determine whether testicular parenchyma has been infarcted. If the frozen section is quickly fixed with alcohol and acetic acid, lysis of red cells may diminish the appearance of interstitial hemorrhage.

Pathologists have generally been cavalier with regard to completely studying testes excised after torsion. It is not usually possible grossly to determine the degree of torsion in such specimens, and sections are usually taken merely to verify the presence of infarct without carefully analyzing the spectrum and location of changes. Thus sections of testis often do not help us to determine the duration of infarction.

In cases I have studied from available biopsy and orchiectomy specimens, histologic changes have been noted that may be useful in determining the duration of the torsion. Up to six hours after torsion, the testis shows venous congestion and interstitial hemorrhage. A biopsy at 5½ hours showed no nuclear pyknosis (Fig. 7A). At 9½ hours, polymorphonuclear leukocytes (PMNs) were in the walls of capillaries, and there was severe interstitial hemorrhage but no definite infarction. At 4 days, there was hemorrhagic infarction and coagulative necrosis of testicular parenchyma with a PMN reaction. Infarct and granulation tissue were present in specimens obtained 1 and 2 months after onset of torsion (Fig. 7B). Thus infarcts of 4 days to 2 months showed complete infarction (Fig. 7C). If a section is not taken at the periphery of the infarct, granulation tissue will not be recognized. We have seen mummification of a testis that had been atrophic for 23 years. Fibrosis and calcium deposition also may occur in ancient infarcts.

Testicular pain simulating torsion may result from other causes. The small vessel vasculitis of Henoch–Schönlein

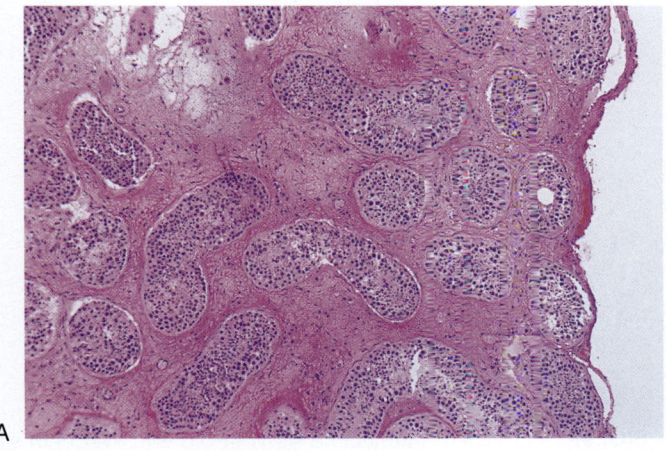
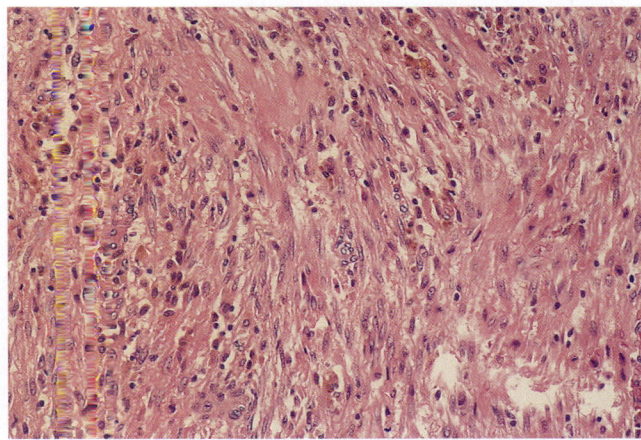
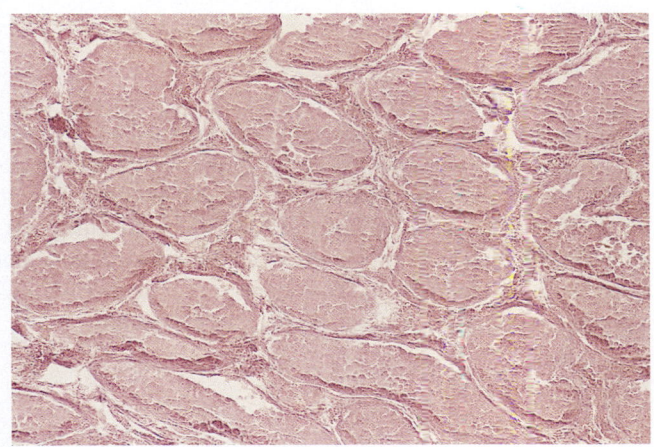

FIG. 7. A: Spermatic cord torsion for 5 1/2 hours in a 14-year-old. Testis shows marked interstitial hemorrhage but no necrosis of germinal cells. **B:** Active granulation tissue at the periphery of an infarct of approximately 3 months' duration in a 17-year-old. **C:** Infarct of 1 month's duration in a 17-year-old.

purpura may necessitate a scrotal exploration, but with the urologist's observation that the testis is grossly normal, usually no tissue is removed (50,51). Torsion of the appendix testis may mimic testicular torsion and result in a specimen of appendix testis that has undergone torsion with or without infarction.

Although bilateral torsions occur rarely, it is good surgical practice to anchor the testis that has not undergone torsion to prevent it from doing so. I saw one case in which failure to anchor the remaining testis after orchiectomy for infarct was followed by torsion, infarction, and orchiectomy of the second testis, with resultant anorchia. In general, extravaginal torsions occur in infancy and are rarer than intravaginal torsion.

Varicocele

Varicocele is an abnormal dilatation and tortuosity of veins in the pampiniform plexus of the spermatic cord. It is probably caused by insufficiency of venous valves, involves the left side in 90% of cases, and is bilateral in about 10% (52). Varicocele involving the right side exclusively is extremely rare and may be associated with situs inversus (a vascular abnormality), venous thrombosis, or venous compression resulting from a space-occupying mass (53). Although many men with varicoceles have fathered children (54), a greater percentage of infertile men have varicocele than do the normal population (55). Ligation or occlusion of the left spermatic vein may improve the fertility rate as well as the quality of semen (56,57). Numerous theories have been advanced regarding the abnormalities in spermatogenesis in patients with varicocele, including (a) hypothalamic–hypophyseal–gonadal axis insufficiency, (b) venous stasis leading to carbon dioxide pressure–oxygen pressure imbalance or build-up of testicular metabolites, (c) elevated temperature, and (d) reflux of adrenal metabolites into the gonadal vein (52).

The pathologist rarely examines a varicocele or a large portion of one. Usually a cross section of spermatic vein shows only variable thickening of the vein wall with fibrosis. Testis biopsies may be obtained at the time of high ligation or balloon occlusion of the left spermatic vein. Biopsies of either testis will show similar nonspecific morphologic changes consisting of decreased spermatogenesis with sloughing of immature germinal cells, degeneration of germ cells, and increased numbers of Leydig cells (Fig. 8). Bonanni et al. (58), by using DNA flow cytometry of cells from fine-needle aspiration (FNA) biopsy of the testis, demonstrated reduced percentage of haploid cells and increased percentage of diploid cells, indicating greater damage in the testis ipsilateral to the varicocele. Agger and Johnsen (59) used a scoring system

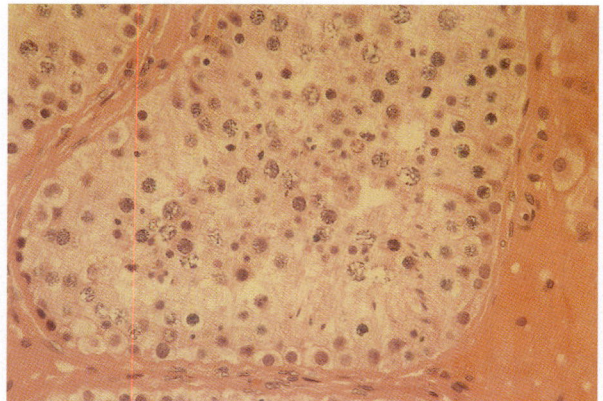

FIG. 8. Biopsy of right testis in a 30-year-old with a varicocele. Seminiferous tubule shows mild tunica proprial thickening and hypospermatogenesis.

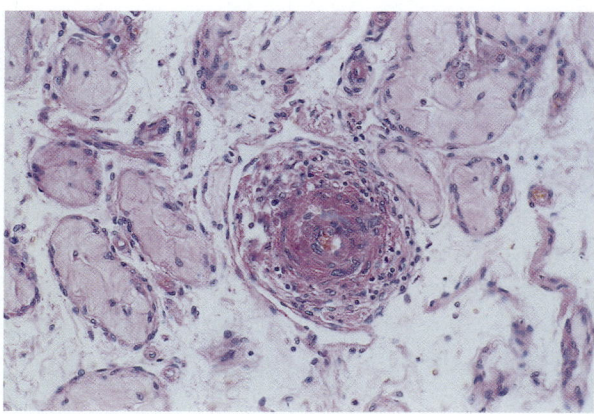

FIG. 9. Necrotizing arteritis in a 49-year-old with Wegener's granulomatosis.

and found improvement in testicular histology 1 year after venous ligation. Andres et al. (60) demonstrated fibrosis of veins with narrowing of their lumens in two of six patients in addition to changes of hypospermatogenesis. They suggested that altered venous flow may contribute to testicular dysfunction. Jones et al. (61) described changes in 13 adolescents that included peritubular sclerosis, small-vessel sclerosis, marked premature germ cell sloughing in more than 50% of tubules, and reduced numbers of germ cells. Saypol et al. (62), working with an experimental model of induced varicoceles in rats and dogs, suggested that increased blood flow led to increased temperature, which led to decreased spermatogenesis and eventually to seminiferous tubular atrophy and decreased blood flow. The prognosis for fertility in patients surgically treated for varicocele has been estimated at 40% to 55% (56,57).

TESTICULAR INVOLVEMENT IN SYSTEMIC DISEASE

Vasculitis

Systemic vasculitis frequently involves the testes. The most extensively studied cases are those of polyarteritis nodosa, but testicular involvement also was identified in cases of Wegener's granulomatosis, dermatomyositis, Henoch–Schönlein purpura, typhus, acute myelogenous leukemia, hairy cell leukemia, and Goodpasture's syndrome (63–66). Occasional patients have vasculitis of the testis without systemic vasculitis (64,65). Spermatic cord involvement has been documented in Buerger's disease (67). From a diagnostic point of view, blind biopsy of an asymptomatic testis is unlikely to yield a positive diagnosis. Dahl et al. (63) found that 38 of 44 patients with known polyarteritis nodosa had diagnostic lesions in the testis at postmortem examination. Dividing the autopsy testes into portions of biopsy size, they found lesions diagnostic of polyarteritis in 22% of the segments. Testis biopsy is most valuable in patients with testicular symptoms. The biopsy should be from a painful, enlarging, or shrinking testis and should consist of a wedge containing capsule, tunica vasculosa (the vascular zone beneath the tunica albuginea), and testicular parenchyma. In light of the focal nature of the lesions of vasculitis, the paraffin block should be serially sectioned if initial sections do not yield a diagnosis (Fig. 9). Biopsy of a testis with vasculitis might contain an infarct rather than vasculitis itself.

Amyloidosis

Systemic amyloidosis may uncommonly involve the testis (68). Amyloid deposition occurs in relation to blood vessels of the interstitium and, to a much smaller degree, in the walls of the seminiferous tubules. Seminiferous tubules with or without amyloid show reduced spermatogenesis. In examination of testicular specimens with marked hyaline thickening of the seminiferous tubules, the extent and texture of the hyaline change may suggest the differential diagnosis of amyloid. This diagnosis is unlikely unless there is extensive thickening of interstitial blood vessel walls. I know of no recorded case of amyloid deposition manifesting as a tumor of the testis.

PATHOLOGY OF MALE INFERTILITY

There are several ways to approach the pathology of the testis in the infertile male. Classifications have been oriented toward both morphologic changes and their etiology (69). I use a classification that is principally morphologic but that uses known or suspected clinical associations in the case of karyotypic abnormalities and excurrent duct obstruction (Table 1).

To obtain maximal information from the biopsy, there should be clinical input regarding medical history, semen analysis, physical findings, and the results of serum gonadotropin measurements. These should not alter the interpretation of the biopsy, but instead should offer meaningful explanation of the changes and may help with prognostic implications.

TABLE 1. *Histologic changes in testes in male infertility*

Normal spermatogenesis
Hypospermatogenesis
Maturation arrest
Germinal cell aplasia
Germinal cell aplasia with focal spermatogenesis
Testicular changes associated with karyotypic abnormalities
Tubular sclerosis and interstitial fibrosis (end-stage testis)
Active spermatogenesis compatible with excurrent duct obstruction

Normal Spermatogenesis

When the biopsy findings correspond to a fully functioning testis (i.e., insofar as we can tell from the biopsy, all tubules are actively undergoing spermatogenesis; see Fig. 1), a diagnosis of normal spermatogenesis is made. One way to determine what is normal spermatogenesis is to study a group of well-fixed testes from forensic autopsies in cases of sudden death. The landmark article by Heller and Clermont (3) contains information regarding spermatogenesis and the structure of the normal testis. They point out the mosaic appearance of the testis and demonstrate that not every tubule viewed in cross or longitudinal section has complete spermatogenesis. Sperm counts cannot be precisely correlated with testis biopsy findings, but the number of late spermatids correlates best with sperm counts. Once the diagnosis of normal spermatogenesis is made, an attempt should be made to correlate structure with clinical data. An important determination is whether the patient has excurrent duct obstruction, as discussed later. Histologically normal spermatogenesis may occur in patients with normal sperm counts and low motility. Ultrastructural evaluation of semen may point out structural abnormalities in spermatozoa of men with normal sperm counts, such as in patients with round-headed sperm or in patients with the immotile-cilia syndrome (70).

Hypospermatogenesis

Hypospermatogenesis characterizes a reduced degree of spermatogenesis, but not one that stops at a particular point in the sequence of spermatogenesis. It is characterized by appreciable reduction in the number of germinal cells (see Fig. 8). It may result in a thinning in the number of epithelial layers. Changes in occasional tubules are interpreted as mild, and significant reductions in numbers of germ cells in virtually all tubules are interpreted as severe. Almost invariably there are other changes, including tunica propria thickening with increased collagen deposition and interstitial fibrosis. Some tubules may show sclerosis, and there may be an appearance of germinal cell disorganization and sloughing into the tubular lumens. Tubular sclerosis may be only focal within the testis, and such changes should not be assumed to be generalized. Sloughing and disorganization may be, at least in part, a function of the technical aspects of obtaining or processing the biopsy. Leydig cells should be present in the angles between the tubules. In general, there is no accurate way to relate their numbers to the level of serum T. There are several methods of evaluating the numbers of Leydig cells in biopsy specimens (2,27). Only when Leydig cells are absent or virtually absent is their number likely to be associated with a low level of serum T. When Leydig cells appear numerous, particularly when there is coalescence of Leydig cell groups or if nodules are evident, there is probably an increased level of serum LH.

The finding of hypospermatogenesis does not indicate the etiology of the changes. Such changes are not etiologically specific and may occur in a variety of circumstances, including (a) exposure to toxins or excess heat, (b) varicocele, or (c) hypothyroidism.

Maturation Arrest

The diagnosis of complete maturation arrest is rendered when the germ cells in the seminiferous tubules mature only to a certain point. If spermatogenesis is perceived in a diagrammatic fashion, the appearance suggests that a line exists beyond which germ-cell maturation does not extend. Cells with irregular, dense nuclei may be present in the lumens of some tubules and may represent abortive attempts at further maturation or degenerating cells, possibly spermatids (Fig. 10). In incomplete maturation arrest, the appearance is similar, except that a few late spermatids are evident along the luminal border of a few seminiferous tubules. In both complete and incomplete maturation arrest, tubules are usually reduced in diameter, but there may be no increase in tubule wall thickening or histologic abnormality of interstitium or Leydig cells.

The specific etiology of the changes cannot be predicted from the histology. The same clinical situations that produce hypospermatogenesis may result in germinal cell arrest (69). In addition, as described later, postpubertal gonadotropin de-

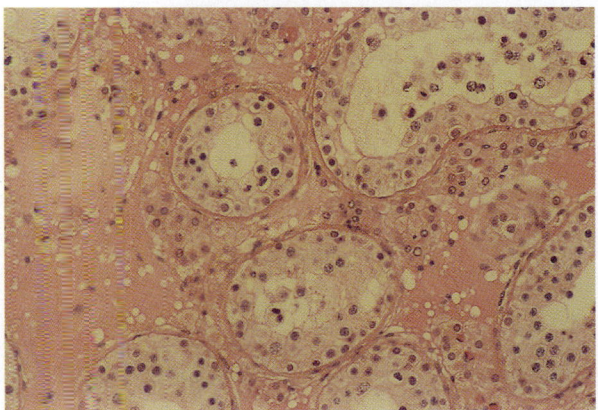

FIG. 10. Complete maturation arrest in a 49-year-old. Spermatogonia, primary spermatocytes, and degenerated intratubular cells are present in small tubules.

ficiency, alkylating agent therapy, and radiation therapy may produce similar changes at some stage of injury.

Correlation of structure and sperm count is usually quite good in cases of maturation arrest. In patients with complete maturation arrest, sperm counts are usually zero. When a few sperm are present in ejaculates, the biopsy showing complete maturation arrest may not be representative of both testes, and tubules with late spermatids must be present elsewhere in the testes. When fresh testis biopsies have been minced in patients undergoing assisted reproductive techniques, some testes with a diagnosis of complete maturation arrest have been found to contain spermatozoa. Patients with incomplete maturation arrest are usually oligospermic.

Germinal Cell Aplasia

In biopsies of germinal cell aplasia (GCA), seminiferous tubules of reduced diameter are lined exclusively by postpubertal Sertoli cells, hence the synonym Sertoli-cell-only syndrome (Fig. 11A). Sertoli cells are oriented perpendicular to the basement membrane; often cells in small groups along the length of the tubules are parallel to one another, giving an appearance of palm trees waving in a breeze. The appearance of postpubertal Sertoli cell nuclei is probably best recognized in biopsies of GCA, in which the nuclear indentations and nucleoli can be seen in some cells (Fig. 11B). Charcot–Böttcher crystals may sometimes be seen in Sertoli cells as thin, almost imperceptible, eosinophilic lines extending in various directions (see Fig. 2B). Nistal et al. (36) described variations in Sertoli cell structure in testes in prepubertal gonadotropin deficiency, cryptorchidism, estrogen treatment, chemotherapy, and del Castillo's syndrome. Leydig cells are usually normal in appearance, but they may appear numerous because of reduced tubular diameter and relative increase in their number.

Testes show GCA in del Castillo's syndrome, in which phenotypically normal men have small soft testes, normal secondary sex characteristics, normal levels of serum T, azoospermia, and increased or high-normal levels of serum FSH (71). Occasionally a biopsy has the appearance of GCA with scattered spermatogonia and is characterized as germinal cell hypoplasia. Biopsies with GCA or germinal cell hypoplasia should be carefully examined to make certain that tubules do not harbor malignant intratubular germ cells. Such cells might be overlooked if few in number and might be misinterpreted if fixation were suboptimal. It must be recognized that alkylating agents and irradiation in sufficient doses over a significant time may produce loss of germ cells and result in the appearance of GCA (see Fig. 11A). In these therapeutic situations, such changes may be reversible over a prolonged period.

Germinal Cell Aplasia and Focal Spermatogenesis

Testis biopsies demonstrating GCA with focal spermatogenesis contain two populations of tubules. The smaller tubules exhibit GCA, and tubules of increased diameter show spermatogenesis that is usually reduced (Fig. 12). Some tubules, particularly those cut longitudinally, may demonstrate contiguous stretches of only Sertoli cells next to areas with spermatogenesis, indicating that a given tubule may harbor both changes. Patients having bilateral biopsies may show GCA on one side and GCA with focal spermatogenesis or other findings contralaterally. Patients with GCA and focal spermatogenesis usually have a profoundly reduced sperm count.

The etiology of GCA with focal spermatogenesis is not apparent from the biopsy. It may be surmised that tubules in some parts of the testis were not populated by germinal cells during intrauterine development, or that postnatally, includ-

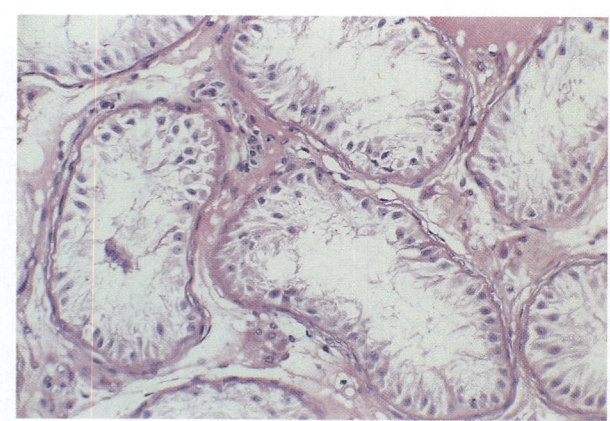
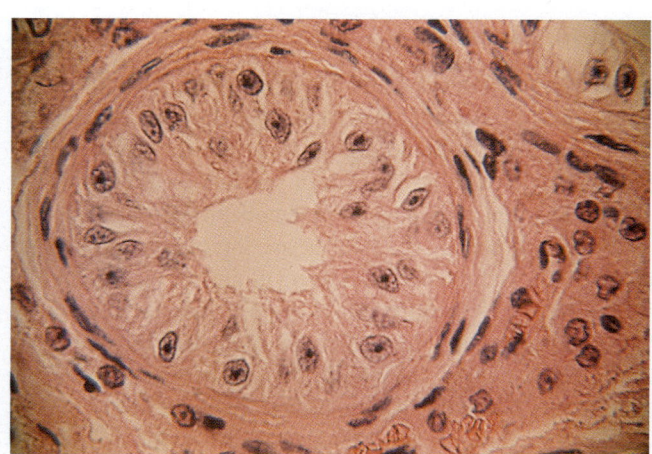

FIG. 11. **A:** Germinal cell aplasia in an adult testis after chemotherapy for acute lymphocytic leukemia. The biopsy is identical to idiopathic germinal cell aplasia. **B:** Idiopathic germinal cell aplasia in an adult demonstrating undulating nuclear borders, prominent nucleoli, and perpendicular orientation of Sertoli cells to basement membrane.

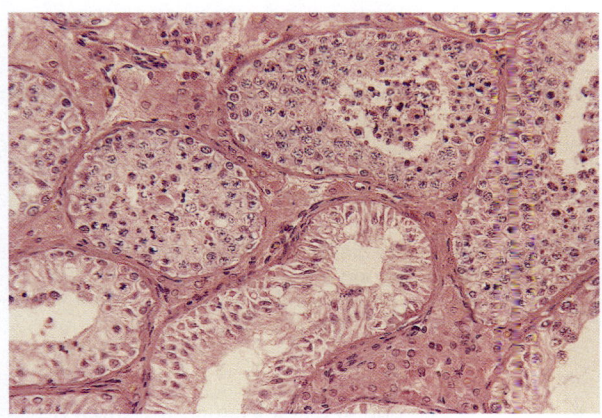

FIG. 12. Germinal cell aplasia and focal spermatogenesis in an adult. One tubule (below) is lined by Sertoli cells. The others are undergoing spermatogenesis.

ing childhood and adulthood, there was a loss of germ cells, resulting in the picture of tubules with and without germinal cells. If the latter were the case, there might be further loss of germ cells, resulting eventually in the appearance of GCA.

Karyotypic Abnormalities

The best-known karyotypic abnormality associated with a characteristic appearance of the testis is Klinefelter's (KF) syndrome (72), which is characterized by a karyotype of 47XXY, sometimes a eunuchoid habitus, reduced body and pubic hair, gynecomastia in 40% to 80% of cases, extremely small testes, and an increase of serum FSH and sometimes LH. It should be pointed out that the structure of the testes may be normal after birth but that the number of intratubular germ cells in biopsies of children is reduced (73). Some prepubertal testes may contain only Sertoli cells lining tubules. After puberty, the testes usually have a severely altered structure, with reduced spermatogenesis, tubular sclerosis, and Leydig cell nodules (Fig. 13). Although some biopsies show absolutely no spermatogenesis, others may show a degree of spermatogenesis. The presence of sperm in the ejac-

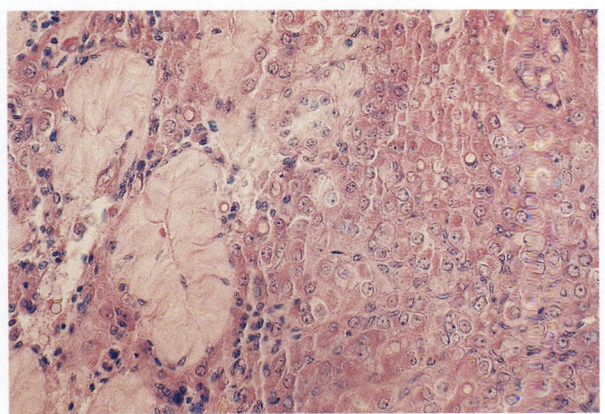

FIG. 13. Biopsy of an adult with Klinefelter's syndrome. A nodule of Leydig cells is at the periphery of sclerotic tubules.

ulate does not absolutely militate against the diagnosis of KF. Indeed Tournaye et al. (74) found spermatozoa in four of nine apparently nonmosaic 47XXY patients in wet preparations from testicular biopsies. The classic histologic appearance of KF may occur in the absence of karyotypic abnormalities. Other disease processes may occur in patients with KF, but only breast carcinoma occurs with increased frequency. It has been stated, but not proved, that breast cancer occurs in these patients with the same frequency as in adult females (75). Rare germ cell tumors were reported in testes of patients with KF (76). One case of epidermoid cyst was reported in a patient with KF, and we studied another (77). At least six intracranial germ cell tumors, mostly seminoma, were reported in association with KF (78).

Changes identical to KF may occur in patients with a 46XX karyotype. These patients are designated as having de la Chapelle's syndrome and are generally shorter than KF patients, with sparse pubic and facial hair, occasional gynecomastia, and possibly reduced size of penis, testes, and prostate (79). These patients may have had an XXY karyotype and may have lost or translocated the Y chromosome early in development. Serum gonadotropin levels are usually increased; serum T level is usually reduced. The fragile X mutation has rarely been found in KF patients with bilateral micro-orchidism (80).

Tubular Sclerosis and Interstitial Fibrosis

Although sclerotic seminiferous tubules may be found in biopsies with hypospermatogenesis and frequently are found in cryptorchid testes or those with karyotypic abnormalities, it is rare that biopsies are composed exclusively of sclerotic tubules. This appearance may follow acquired gonadotropin deficiency or remote chronic orchitis or ischemia, or it may occur without a known etiology. Such changes may be accompanied by interstitial fibrosis and loss of Leydig cells and, if present bilaterally and involving the entire testicular parenchyma, can functionally be characterized as end-stage testis.

Excurrent Duct Obstruction

Obstruction of the excurrent duct system distal to the rete testis occurs in about 10% of biopsies of infertile patients (69). The cause of obstruction may be congenital or acquired. Obstruction may result from agenesis or atresia of part of the excurrent duct system (e.g., the epididymis or vas deferens) or from atrophy resulting from inspissated secretions in cystic fibrosis. Acquired obstruction may result from infection or voluntary sterilization. Occasional inadvertent ligation of the vas deferens may occur during herniorrhaphy or varicocele ligation.

The clinicopathologic triad in patients with excurrent duct obstruction consists of azoospermia, normal-sized testes, and active, although not necessarily normal, spermatogenesis (Fig. 14). In a series of nine patients with previous vol-

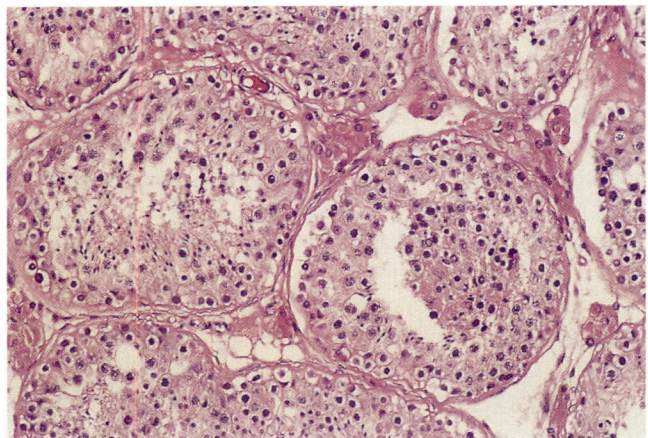

FIG. 14. Active spermatogenesis in a 28-year-old with agenesis of the vas deferens.

TABLE 2. *Histologic findings in testes after biopsy at vasovasotomy*

All testes showed active spermatogenesis, germinal cell disorganization, and sloughing
No testes revealed tubular basement membrane thickening, Leydig cell, or vascular abnormalities
Twelve of 18 testes showed some degree of tunica proprial thickening
Four of 18 testes showed some degree of interstitial fibrosis
Two of 18 testes contained sperm granulomas

untary sterilization 1 to 8 years earlier, we found a variety of changes in biopsies of nine pairs of testes at the time of vasovasotomy (Table 2).

Varying degrees of vasitis nodosum characterized the removed segments of vas deferens. This entity was composed of proliferated ductal structures within and through the wall of the vas deferens (81) (Fig. 15A). Associated changes were fibrosis, sperm granulomas (Fig. 15B), varying degrees of chronic inflammation, elastic tissue proliferation in blood vessel walls, and neural proliferation resembling traumatic neuroma. The ductal structures were lined by cuboidal or columnar epithelium, and some cells were ciliated. Invasion of blood vessels and nerves was described in vasitis nodosum (82,83). Spermatozoa were present within some ductal lumens (Fig. 15A). Similar lesions were reported rarely without history of prior surgery or trauma (84). The infiltrative pattern may resemble adenocarcinoma, but the history and intraluminal sperm, if present, militate against the diagnosis of malignancy.

Jarow et al. (85) reported that testicular interstitial fibrosis was the histologic factor that adversely affected prognosis for fertility in patients who underwent vasovasostomy after vasectomy. Other changes in their patients were increased thickness of the tubular wall, increased cross-sectional tubular area, and decreased numbers of Sertoli cells and spermatids. Spermatogenesis occurs in the face of obstruction for many years. It is surprising to note that patients with agenesis of the vas deferens biopsied in their twenties have significant spermatogenesis and scant interstitial fibrosis (see Fig. 14).

Men may have partial obstruction of the excurrent duct system. This is identified when there is a significant disparity between the sperm count and the degree of spermatogenesis identified in testicular biopsy specimens. Silber and Rodriguez-Rigau (86) found that a correlation can be made between the number of late elongate spermatids found in round cross sections of seminiferous tubules and the number of sperm per milliliter in the semen analysis of unobstructed men. Useful figures obtained from the curve in their article indicated that if the number of late spermatids per round cross section counts are 45, 40, 20, and 6 to 10, the sperm counts should be approximately 85, 45, 10, and 3 million/ml, respectively. If the sperm count corresponds to the number of late spermatids in the biopsy specimen, there is no evi-

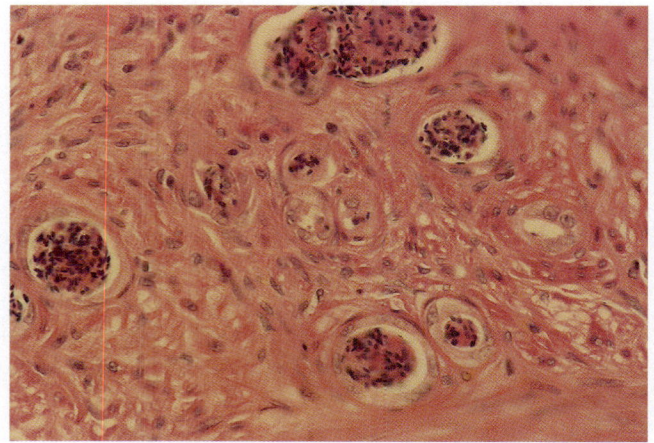
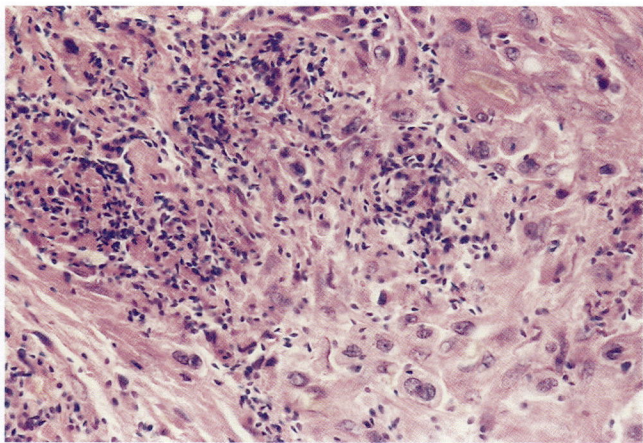

FIG. 15. A: Vasitis nodosum. Proliferated ductal structures within smooth-muscle wall of vas deferens. Spermatozoa stuff duct lumens. **B:** Sperm granuloma. Aggregates of histiocytes, many of which contain spermatozoa.

dence of obstruction. A sperm count that is appreciably lower than expected from biopsy findings is evidence of partial excurrent duct obstruction. The authors indicated that at least 20 tubules should be counted. However, 20 properly oriented tubules may not be present in a biopsy (86).

GONADOTROPIN DEFICIENCY

Prepubertal Gonadotropin Deficiency

The date of onset of puberty differs in different individuals and is dependent on genetic and environmental influences. Bhasin and Swerdloff (87) indicated that the mean age of entry into puberty is 11.6 years, with a range of 9 to 13 years. Federman (88) indicated that delayed puberty is the failure of adolescent development to occur by age 16. Testicular development and function depend on the integrity of the hypothalamic–pituitary–testicular axis. There must be timely and adequate release of GnRH, which stimulates release of FSH and LH. Anything that interferes with this sequence leads to prepubertal gonadotropin deficiency. A patient is considered to have prepubertal gonadotropin deficiency if gonadotropins have never been secreted in a normal fashion.

Depending on the cause and site of the lesion, a patient may have selective gonadotropin deficiency, deficiency of both LH and FSH, or GnRH deficiency resulting in LH or FSH deficiency or both. A variety of syndromes are associated with prepubertal gonadotropin deficiency, including the Laurence–Moon–Biedl, Carpenter, Lowe, multiple lentigines, Prader–Willi, Rud, and Kallmann syndromes (89). Almost all patients have other major congenital anomalies and are unlikely to have biopsies performed. Although patients with Kallmann's syndrome are usually adolescents or young adults, their testes have a prepubertal structure. The major clinical finding in this syndrome is anosmia or hyposmia. Other findings include cleft palate or lip, color blindness, and short fourth metacarpals. This syndrome is related to GnRH deficiency (89). Weiss et al. (90) reported a 17-year-old boy with an XY karyotype and pubertal delay in whom serum immunoreactive LH concentration was twice as high as normal, serum FSH was normal, and serum T was low. A single amino acid substitution of arginine for glutamine in amino acid 54 of the LH β subunit eliminated the ability of LH to bind to its receptors. The biopsy was reported as showing an arrest of spermatogenesis, although no illustration or description was provided. No Leydig cells were identified. The medical history, response to therapy, and demonstration that the absence of biologic activity in LH was due to its inability to bind to its receptors suggest that this is a definable form of prepubertal gonadotropin deficiency (90).

In general, testicular biopsies are rarely indicated in prepubertal gonadotropin deficiency, and measurements of serum gonadotropins and serum T, along with the results of GnRH and clomiphene administration, are usually sufficient to render a diagnosis. However, it is important that pathologists recognize prepubertal gonadotropin deficiency so that the lesion can be properly classified and treated in the rare clinical situation in which a biopsy occurs and so that the relation to pathologic changes in the hypothalamus and pituitary gland can be ascertained in autopsied cases.

The structure of the testes in prepubertal gonadotropin deficiency is that of a prepubertal child and is abnormal only in that it is inappropriate for the patient's age. Tubules are small, generally aluminal, and populated by prepubertal-type Sertoli cells and scattered spermatogonia. There is no further maturation of germ cells. Interstitial connective tissue is loose without recognizable Leydig cells. When fertility is desired, patients are usually treated with combinations of human gonadotropins. When fertility is not a consideration, androgen therapy will produce masculinization (89). In the former situation, gonadotropin treatment with FSH and LH will produce maturation of testes characterized by development of normal-appearing Leydig cells and complete spermatogenesis. The testis may achieve a histologically normal appearance if gonadotropin replacement is maintained, and fertility may result from therapy (91,92).

Postpubertal Gonadotropin Deficiency

In addition to combined LH and FSH deficiency, patients may rarely experience selective LH or FSH deficiency. The former patients have been called fertile eunuchs (93). These patients have active spermatogenesis and low semen volume. Testicular tubules have a postpubertal appearance with active spermatogenesis, but Leydig cells are absent or reduced in number. Serum levels of FSH are normal, and serum levels of T and LH are diminished (94). Isolated FSH deficiency has been described in rare infertile men with normal-sized testes, normal basal LH and T, low serum FSH, and normal sperm counts, oligospermia, or azoospermia. Testis biopsies in three cases revealed hypospermatogenesis, spermatogenesis with germ-cell aplasia, and incomplete maturation arrest (95,96).

Testicular changes may be produced by hypothalamic or pituitary dysfunctions caused by trauma, surgery, neoplasms, irradiation, or exogenous or endogenous estrogens or androgens. The histologic changes tend to be progressive. With a continuing or untreated insult, there is regression of spermatogenesis progressing through incomplete maturation arrest, complete maturation arrest, germ-cell hypoplasia, germ-cell aplasia, and possibly totally sclerotic tubules without cells. The walls of the seminiferous tubules become progressively thickened and fibrotic (Fig. 16). If there is a complete loss of gonadotropin production, Leydig cells disappear, and the interstitium is fibrotic. High-dose prolonged estrogen therapy given to adult transsexual patients before orchiectomy produces immature-appearing Sertoli cells, germ-cell hypoplasia with tunica proprial thickening, and atrophy of Leydig cells (Fig. 17) (97). Low-dose estrogen therapy for adenocarcinoma of the prostate in older men usually produces arrested maturation of germ cells and subtotal atrophy of Leydig cells. Morphologic and functional

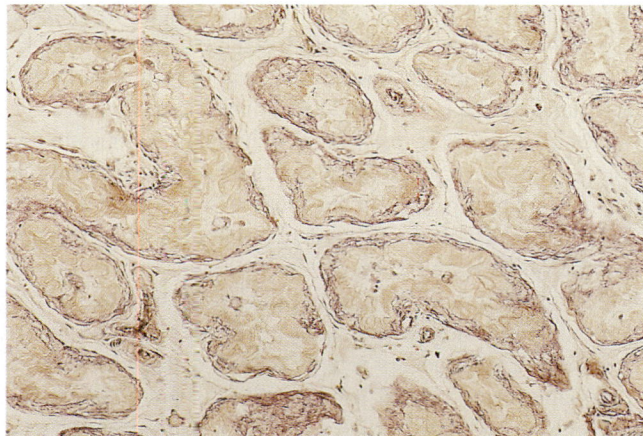

FIG. 16. Postpubertal gonadotropin deficiency characterized by tubular sclerosis and absence of Leydig cells in a 48-year-old who had a pituitary adenoma excised 9 years earlier and who received no gonadotropin therapy. Purple line at periphery of tubule demonstrates elastic tissue.

alterations of the testes may be reversed by gonadotropin administration if it is given soon after the onset of gonadotropin deficiency (98,99). That long-term androgen replacement does not preclude gonadotropin-induced improvement was demonstrated in a man who had 11 years of androgen replacement and who fathered a child after 5 weeks of HCG/HMG treatment (100).

Macroorchidism

Testicular enlargement was described in cases of fragile X syndrome, sexual precocity, testotoxicosis, and in patients with microadenomas of the pituitary secreting FSH (101). In patients with macroorchidism and fragile X syndrome, seminiferous tubules may be combinations of normal, dilated,

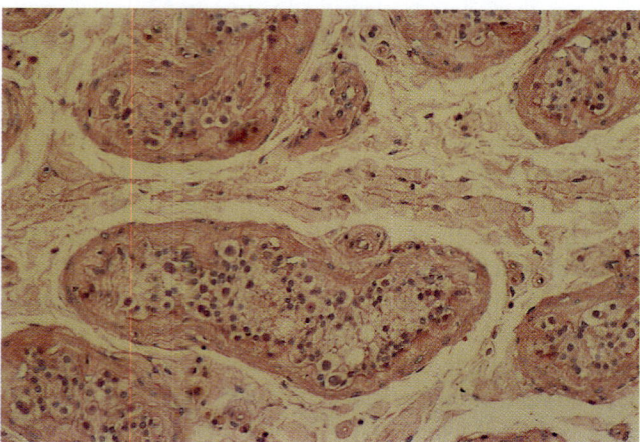

FIG. 17. Orchiectomy specimen from 27-year-old transsexual previously treated with estrogen. Tubules have thickened tunica propria and contain Sertoli cells and spermatogonia. Leydig cells are atrophic.

and atrophic tubules with mature or immature-appearing Sertoli cells (102).

TESTICULAR BIOPSY

The pathologist receives, processes, and interprets the testis biopsy and should advise urologists in obtaining a proper biopsy. Testis biopsies are obtained for a variety of reasons, and with changing patterns of medical practice, criteria for biopsy will vary. Traditionally biopsies have been obtained to evaluate infertility, diagnose vasculitis, determine viability in cases of torsion, discover malignant germinal cells in patients with increased risk of malignancy, or identify the presence of lymphoma cells after chemotherapy. More recently, because of the availability of assisted reproductive techniques, biopsies have been used to identify the presence of spermatozoa or even spermatids. Spermatozoa or spermatids were identified in all ten testis biopsies of patients with obstructive azoospermia and biopsies of 21 of 41 patients with nonobstructive azoospermia (103). Biopsies are presently used as a source from which to obtain spermatozoa or spermatids to use therapeutically in assisted reproductive techniques. Sperm has been obtained from testicular sperm extraction (TESE) and microsurgical epididymal sperm aspiration (MESA) and is used for intracytoplasmic sperm injection (ICSI), wherein a single sperm is injected into an egg, producing a fertilized egg. Tournaye et al. (104) published a series of 124 infertile men who underwent TESE for ICSI. No spermatozoa were removed in 10 (8%). Motile sperm were found in 59% of patients. The fertilization rate in the remaining 114 couples was 58%, (i.e., two pronuclei in 18 hours). The fertilization rate was lower in patients with germ-cell aplasia and maturation arrest than in patients with normal spermatogenesis and hypospermatogenesis. The cleavage rate was 55% (cleaving embryos showed 50% or fewer anucleate fragments). At the time of publication, seven patients had delivered, and 14 pregnancies were ongoing. It is difficult to sift through data to find a take-home-baby rate, but in this study, it appears to be 21 (18%) in 114 ICSI couples, not an astronomic rate, but better than 0. Even if the rate of a normal delivered child were higher, cost precludes this being a universal treatment now. The cost of a live birth for ICSI has been estimated at $87,000, counting the cost of failed attempts (105).

It was found that sperm may be present in the testes of patients who have biopsies diagnosed as GCA or complete maturation arrest (CMA) (104). Tournaye (104) found spermatozoa in biopsies and wet preparations in four of six patients with GCA and nine of 11 patients with CMA. This would indicate that either the pathologist did not recognize late spermatids in the biopsies, or the biopsies were not representative of the testis. Perhaps both are true in some cases. It is probably not important if a pathologist does not see a rare sperm in the biopsy of an oligospermic patient, as long as the clinician recognizes that there is a significant possibility that sperm may be present. I reviewed several cases that

I diagnosed as GCA in the past, subserially sectioned them, and still did not find late spermatids. It is possible to stain a fresh ejaculate with nuclear-fast red picroindigocarmine and identify rare spermatozoa with heads that stain red and tails that stain blue (106). This will indicate to the urologist that the patient produces spermatozoa, although it will not be possible to determine whether spermatozoa were produced in one or both testes.

The ability to produce pregnancy and live births with ICSI raises many ethical questions. It may be that in addition to studying testicular biopsies in infertile men, pathologists will eventually do molecular diagnostic tests on sperm or single blastomeres to help to assure that the sperm and ovum do not harbor deleterious genes. This has already been done in a fetus whose parents had the cystic fibrosis F508 mutation (107).

Biopsy of all cases of infertility is no longer necessary unless assisted reproductive techniques will be used. Prognosis for fertility in men with oligospermia or azoospermia, small testes, and markedly increased serum FSH is virtually nil with therapy other than assisted reproductive techniques. The diagnosis of KF can be made with analysis of karyotypes of peripheral lymphocytes, obviating the need for invasive procedures. In recent years the discrimination of primary testicular abnormality from excurrent duct obstruction has been a frequent reason for testicular biopsy.

Some patients have an increased risk of developing testicular germ-cell malignancies. These include patients with cryptorchid testes (including testes with previous orchiopexy), those with a contralateral germ-cell testicular tumor or a history of one, and patients with infertility (38–40,108). In such patients, the presence of neoplastic intratubular or interstitial germ cells may be difficult to recognize. The plasma membranes of malignant intratubular and interstitial germ cells stain positively for placental alkaline phosphatase with immunoperoxidase stains, in contrast to nonmalignant germinal cells in male subjects older than 1 year, which do not stain for this enzyme. Seminoma and malignant intratubular germ cells were discovered in testis biopsies of rare patients undergoing TESE for ISCI (109).

A caveat should be issued whenever a testis biopsy is reviewed, always look for malignant intratubular germ-cell neoplasia. I diagnosed carcinoma *in situ* (MITGCN) on several infertility biopsies. In the large study of ICSI described earlier, two of 124 patients had MITGCN (104). This is about the same incidence as Nüesch-Bachmann and Hedinger (40) and Skakkabaek (39) reported in their original studies of testis biopsies of infertile men. I recommend a second look in every testis biopsy.

Because patients with acute lymphoblastic leukemia may relapse initially in the testes, bilateral testicular biopsies may be performed on completion of the chemotherapy regimen. Usually, malignant lymphoid cells produce enlargement of the testis or a palpable mass; however, in a small percentage of cases, leukemic infiltrates are clinically imperceptible (110,111). If neoplastic infiltrates are sparse, it may be important to perform immunohistochemical studies on frozen, formalin and B5-fixed tissue, preparation for which should be made before the biopsy.

Method

Open testis biopsies are generally obtained under local anesthesia. An incision is made in the tunica albuginea, pressure is exerted on the testis, and a small amount of testis (up to 5 mm) herniates through the incision (112). This is removed and atraumatically dropped into a suitable fixative. This method is optimal for most uses but will not obtain tunica vasculosa in cases of possible vasculitis, for which a wedge biopsy containing tunica albuginea and underlying parenchyma is more satisfactory. It is possible to prepare touch preparations with the biopsy specimen followed by immediate spraying with hair spray and subsequent processing as a cytologic smear, but care should be taken not to crush the tissue. Patients were studied with reported success by using material from FNA. FNA was found to be more sensitive and equally specific as testis biopsy for sperm detection and equally sensitive and specific as the biopsy touch imprint. FNA also was used to map the testis to identify foci of sperm (113) and to aspirate sperm for ICSI. Touch preparation at the time of testis biopsy and H&E staining allows all cell types to be rapidly identified. The distinction can be made between maturation arrest at the late spermatid level and excurrent duct obstruction (114). Percutaneous testis biopsy with a spring-loaded biopsy gun presently used for prostatic needle-biopsy diagnosis was successfully used for the diagnosis of male infertility (115).

Fixation

One of the major problems in evaluating testis biopsies in infertility is the quality of the preparation. Unfortunately, 10% formalin introduces significant artifact in testicular specimens. Nuclei tend to shrink and appear denser, tubular margins have a somewhat undulating appearance, and tubules shrink slightly, creating a larger interstitial space. Nevertheless, diagnoses can be made on formalinized, albeit suboptimal, tissue. Optimal fixation is rendered with Bouin's and Hollande's solutions, which eliminate artifacts introduced by formalin (116). Nuclear detail is superior, aiding in identification of cell types and in ascertaining whether enlarged germinal cells along the basement membrane are giant spermatogonia or malignant germ cells (117). Urologists should have Bouin's or Hollande's solutions available before the biopsy. I had difficulty staining malignant intratubular germ cells for placental alkaline phosphatase by using Bouin's fixed material.

Special Stains

In general, a 4-μm section stained with H&E is sufficient for diagnosis. Certain special stains may be helpful. Masson's trichrome stain is useful in demonstrating the presence of increased tubular and interstitial collagen and will stain Reinke's crystals red. Periodic acid–Schiff (PAS) stain identifies cytoplasmic glycogen and will stain the eosinophilic granules rarely seen in the cytoplasm of Sertoli cells in some cryptorchid and other testes (35,36). Elastic tissue stains demonstrate elastic fibers in the walls of postpubertal tubules and are helpful in evaluating blood vessels in cases of suspected vasculitis.

Electron Microscopy

In cases of infertility, ultrastructural analysis is generally of no diagnostic help. If it is deemed desirable to obtain tissue for electron-microscopic study, a small portion of the biopsy can be immediately sectioned with a razor blade and placed into glutaraldehyde for processing.

EFFECTS OF DRUGS ON THE TESTIS

A variety of drugs and chemicals influence the function of the testis. In general, pathologists do not see biopsy material from patients who are exposed to these drugs, and evaluations of drug-exposed patients are usually based on analysis of semen and serum in conjunction with clinical history and physical examination.

The three circumstances in which pathologists have seen testicular specimens after drug therapy were (a) after estrogen therapy for prostatic cancer, (b) after chemotherapy for acute lymphocytic leukemia (ALL), and (c) rarely after orchiectomy in patients with metastatic testicular germ-cell tumors who had received chemotherapy before orchiectomy. In the latter patients, dense fibrous scars are almost always also identified. Although biopsies in cases of ALL are taken for the purpose of identifying leukemia, the effect of chemotherapy can be identified in germinal epithelium. Because multiple drugs are used, it is not possible to be certain which have produced changes in germinal epithelium. Single drugs have produced testicular changes, and it is assumed that these drugs have the same effects when used in multiple drug regimens.

The alkylating agent is the major class of anticancer drug that produces testicular changes. These are primarily in the seminiferous tubules, are dose related, and may result in GCA. Some patients treated with cyclophosphamide, an alkylating agent, will recover spermatogenic function and fertility. Buchanan et al. (118) treated 26 adult males with cyclophosphamide. All became azoospermic after 6 months and remained so while taking the drug. The mean period between cessation of treatment and the reappearance of spermatozoa was 31 months and ranged from 15 to 49 months. In two of four patients with GCA, spermatogenesis returned. Pregnancies occurred in the wives of three of 12 patients in whom spermatogenesis returned. We have seen active spermatogenesis in a 19-year-old patient treated for ALL, but with limited exposure to cyclophosphamide. That patient had a minor degree of interstitial fibrosis in the posttreatment biopsy, which showed no tumor. It may be that the production of interstitial fibrosis is important in the pathogenesis of infertility after chemotherapy. Neither azoospermia nor GCA absolutely militates against future fertility after chemotherapy (119,120). As in patients treated with ionizing radiation, recovery of spermatogenesis may take many months after completion of therapy. Estrogens are no longer used to treat prostate cancer, but pathologists may see the effects of other androgen-deprivation therapies in the future. Some men who have been treated with cisplatin-based chemotherapy regimens for metastatic germ-cell tumors before orchiectomy demonstrated persistence of invasive germ-cell tumors and malignant intratubular germ cells in the orchiectomy specimens. In addition, seminiferous tubules without malignant cells demonstrated marked atrophy with spermatogonial arrest or GCA. In four patients with biopsy of the contralateral testis, similar changes were present (121).

Drugs other than alkylating agents produced damage in seminiferous tubules. Methotrexate in a patient with psoriasis (122) and cytosine arabinoside in patients with ALL (123) produced damage in seminiferous tubular epithelium. 1,2-Dibromo-3 chloropropane (DBCP) caused testicular damage in petrochemical workers. Biopsies showed reduction in all types of germ cells. Semen quality was improved within 18 to 21 months after last contact with the drug (124). Patients exposed to DBCP also showed GCA in biopsy specimens. The testicular target cell in rats treated with DBCP was not established (125). Strauss (126) summarized the effects of sex steroids, anticancer drugs, halogenated organic compounds, and heavy metals on the testes of humans and experimental animals. Histologic material in human men subjected to chemical substances is extremely limited and often of poor quality. Because of this, the complex interaction between cells in the testis and the variability of the time–dose relation, it is extremely difficult to determine cell-specific toxicity for an individual substance (125).

EFFECTS OF IRRADIATION ON THE TESTIS

Ionizing irradiation produces changes in the germ-cell population, tunica propria of seminiferous tubules, and blood vessels. Except for the possibility of a nuclear accident, pathologists are unlikely to observe acute testicular injury after exposure to a large dose of irradiation. Such changes were reported by Liebow et al. (127) in 1949 and were summarized by Jordan in 1971 (128). The latter report also summarized the late changes of those exposed to irradiation at Hiroshima and Nagasaki and found that increased tubular sclerosis and vascular hyalinization were found in Hiroshima survivors within 1,400 meters from the hypocenter with more than 300-rad exposure. Tubular sclerosis and tubule wall thickening increased with age, but the proportion of men with Leydig cell hyperplasia decreased with age in all exposure categories (128).

Patients receiving radiation exposure incident to therapy for a malignant tumor elsewhere such as Hodgkin's disease, seminoma of the opposite testis, or ALL receive fractionated doses whose effect on the testis depends on the total dose and duration of therapy. Germ cells are not uniformly sensitive to irradiation. Type B spermatogonia are the most radiosensitive, with damage at dosage levels greater than 0.08 Gy (129). Spermatocytes are damaged at 2 to 3 Gy, whereas spermatids appear undamaged at 4 to 6 Gy. Many patients exposed to irradiation may have only temporary infertility. Azoospermia was reported in patients receiving 0.35 Gy of fractionated radiation and may be permanent in fractionated doses greater than 2 Gy (130). Spermatogenesis recovers after radiation exposure, with histologic recovery occurring earlier after lower doses. Hahn et al. (131) studied 26 men after unilateral orchiectomy and radiotherapy for seminoma. The patients received an average of 0.78 Gy to the contralateral testis. Oligospermia occurred in 4 to 16 weeks, and azoospermia occurred in 10 to 30 weeks. Recovery of sperm in semen first occurred within 30 to 80 weeks. With doses less than 0.6 Gy, recovery of sperm in semen or improvement from profound oligospermia occurred in 21 to 41 weeks. With doses between 0.6 and 1.48 Gy, recovery or improvement occurred in 47 to 88 weeks. Smithers et al. (132) reported that of 74 men treated with radiation for a testis tumor, 34 fathered 52 children after irradiation therapy. In patients receiving radiation alone or with chemotherapy for testicular germ-cell tumors, recovery of the contralateral testis depended on radiation dose. Adjuvant chemotherapy delayed recovery, and recovery was decreased in patients with low pretreatment total sperm counts and in patients older than 25 years (133).

There are no pathognomonic histologic changes in patients exposed to therapeutic levels of irradiation. The changes will mimic those described in infertility patients and will resemble hypospermatogenesis, maturation arrest, germ-cell hypoplasia, or GCA.

In 20 patients with malignant intratubular germ cells, irradiation of 20 Gy obliterated malignant cells. After therapy the structure of the testis was that of GCA. Leydig cell function was partially impaired (134). Irradiation caused changes in Leydig cell function with increased basal LH levels and a reduced testosterone/LH ratio (135). Morphologic changes to the Leydig cells were not described. Patients treated for thyroid carcinoma with ^{131}I have increased serum FSH, but morphologic changes in the testes were not described (136).

TESTICULAR CYSTS

Cysts of the testis have been increasingly recognized since the use of ultrasonography (US). Gooding et al. found 10% of 307 men who underwent US had cysts (137). These are in all segments of the testis and the tunica albuginea. In 233 inguinal explorations for cancer, 16 cysts of the testis, including five epidermoid cysts and six tunica albuginea cysts, were described (138). Epithelial cysts of the rete testis, efferent ducts, and testicular parenchyma were described. Albugineal cysts were lined by cuboidal to columnar, ciliated, and nonciliated cells. The parenchymal cysts were lined by flattened cuboidal nonciliated cells (139). These cysts do not have malignant potential. With increased sophistication of radiologic techniques, urologists are more likely locally to excise cysts and subject them to frozen section.

EPIDIDYMIS

The rete testis extends from the end of the seminiferous tubules as straight ducts that enter the mediastinal rete and through the extratesticular bullae retis. The rete is lined by flattened to columnar epithelium with numerous microvilli (2). The rete may undergo cystic transformation as a result of obstruction or in patients with renal disease in hemodialysis. The latter changes resemble, to some extent, those in renal cysts in acquired renal cystic disease (140).

Eight to 15 efferent ducts extend from the rete testis to the head of the epididymis. Efferent duct lumens are narrower than those of the epididymis and are lined by columnar cells with cilia and microvilli, basal cells, and also contain occasional lymphocytes (2). The epithelium of the epididymal duct is pseudostratified and contains basal cells, clear cells, and much taller chief cells with microvilli, lipid, and lipofuscin. Striking diastase-resistant, PAS-positive intranuclear inclusions are present within epididymal epithelial cells as well as within the vas deferens and less commonly in the seminal vesicles (141). The epididymis is composed of a head, body, and tail and is a single, long, coiled duct with a smaller diameter as it approaches the vas deferens. The epithelium of the epididymis rests on a basement membrane, beneath which are contractile cells, which stain positively for actin, and fibroblasts. In the midepididymis, the contractile cells become well defined, forming an inner and outer longitudinal and an intermediate circular smooth-muscle layer. Around the coils of the duct are collagen, elastic fibers, and blood vessels (142).

Congenital lesions that cause obstruction of the excurrent ducts include complete or partial absence of the epididymis and dissociation of the epididymis from the testis (42). These lesions may be associated with absence or atresia of the vas deferens. The predominant cause of epididymal obstruction is epicidymitis. *Chlamydia trachomatis* and *Neisseria gonorrheae* are the most frequent causes in sexually active men younger than 35 years. In men older than 35 years, epididymitis is associated with acquired obstruction, urinary tract disease, and bacterial organisms that cause infection (143). The organisms usually reach the epididymis in an ascending manner via the duct or lymphatics. Many other bacteria have produced blood-borne infections of the epididymis and the testis (144). Acute epididymitis may rarely be followed by a suppurative process resulting in abscess. In acute epididymitis, the epididymis is enlarged and covered with fibrin. The epididymal duct may contain pus and may rupture, producing sperm granulomas. After acute inflam-

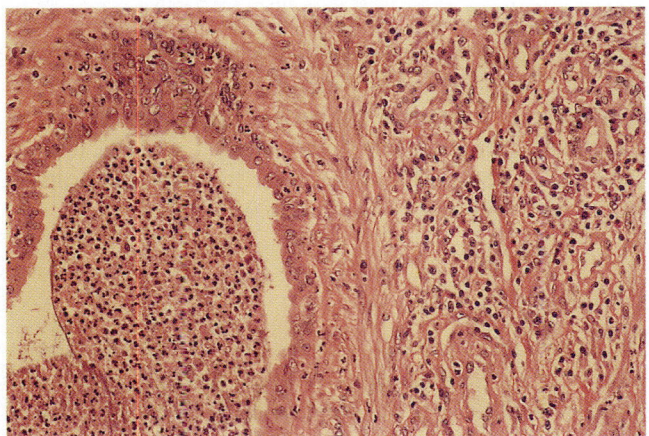

FIG. 18. Acute and chronic epididymitis in a 65-year-old. Duct contains numerous polymorphonuclear leukocytes (PMNs) and a few histiocytes. PMNs are present within and adjacent to duct epithelium. The interstitium contains principally lymphocytes and plasmacytes.

mation, a healing process will result in a fibrotic epididymis with a narrowed epididymal duct (144). The number of chronic inflammatory cells is extremely variable in cases of chronic and healed epididymitis (Fig. 18). Cytomegalovirus infection of the epididymis may occur in patients with AIDS or renal transplantation (145,146).

Epididymal cysts usually present as masses that transilluminate and may be associated with infertility. Cysts up to several centimeters in diameter are usually gray–white and translucent, unilocular or multilocular, and involve the rete testis, efferent duct, or the head of the epididymis. They are in continuity with the excurrent duct system and, therefore, contain motile or nonmotile sperm in cyst fluid. Epithelial cysts are termed spermatoceles (Fig. 19A). Their epithelium varies from flat to pseudostratified (Fig. 19B). Sections may demonstrate only denuded epithelium lying on fibromuscular tissue, and the diagnosis may be made only by finding spermatozoa. Rarely the epithelium may be tall columnar. Mural papillomas lined by ciliated and nonciliated columnar epithelium occurred rarely (147). Sperm from a ruptured spermatocele may be present in a fibrotic hydrocele sac and may look histologically similar to a spermatocele with denuded epithelium.

In cases of distal excurrent duct obstruction, the epididymis may be dilated (148). Spermatozoa may fill and distend the epididymal duct, and there may be macrophages containing multiple sperm in the epididymal lumen. Spermatic granulomas result from rupture of the epididymal duct with spillage of sperm into the interstitial tissues, causing an inflammatory reaction consisting initially of PMNs and later of mononuclear cells, histiocytes that may contain spermatozoa, and brown pigment (148,149). Fibrosis and calcification may be present in older lesions, and duct epithelium may show squamous metaplasia. Glassy and Mostofi (149) described spermatic granulomas ranging from 3 mm to 3 cm in diameter, usually in the upper pole in patients with a history of acute or chronic epididymitis, vasectomy, or trauma. The lesions varied from yellow to yellow–brown to white, depending on the relative amounts of lipid in macrophages, pigment from epididymal epithelial cells, inflammatory cells, and fibrosis.

INFECTIOUS DISEASE

The surgical pathologist does not deal frequently with infectious diseases of the testis. However, when they occur, such cases may not be recognized as infectious problems, and suboptimal treatment may result.

Bacterial Disease

Bacterial infections usually extend to the testis directly from the epididymis and are manifest as epididymoorchitis,

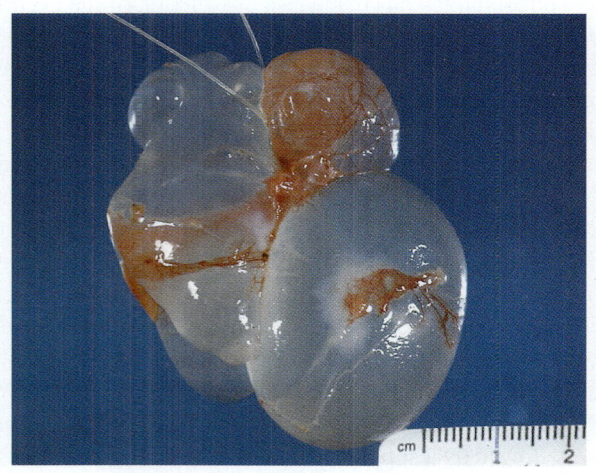
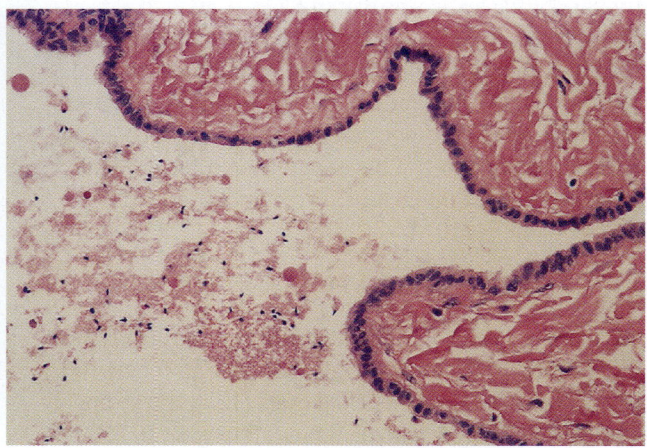

FIG. 19. A: Translucent multilocular spermatocele in 48-year-old. Touch preparation demonstrated motile spermatozoa. **B:** Cuboidal epithelial lining with underlying fibrous tissue in spermatocele. Lumen contains numerous spermatozoa.

but they may also reach the testis via lymphatics and blood vessels. Various types of bacteria have caused orchitis, including *Escherichia coli,* brucella, staphylococci, streptococci, members of the Klebsiella and Salmonella groups, and actinomyces (150). Abscesses may follow acute orchitis and may result in marked destruction of testicular parenchyma. Brucellosis may involve the testis and epididymis in up to 20% of cases (151). In this infection, the tubule-oriented inflammatory process, accompanied by the massive interstitial mononuclear inflammatory process, has a somewhat granulomatous appearance and resembles nonspecific granulomatous orchitis. Morgan (150) described tuberculoid granulomata in the tunica albuginea and spermatic cord in brucellosis.

Mycobacterial Disease

Testicular involvement by *Mycobacterium tuberculosis* is always the result of infection elsewhere and is a relatively frequent cause of granulomatous orchitis. Infection generally spreads directly from the epididymis or via the bloodstream. In the older medical literature, involvement was usually bilateral and associated with an enlarged, dilated epididymis. In early disseminated tuberculosis, 1- to 3-mm nodules are distributed in testicular parenchyma. Fistulae may involve the scrotum. The histologic changes resemble those in tuberculosis in other organs. Necrotic granulomas are usually present, but not all granulomas are necrotic. Much of the inflammatory process away from granulomatous areas is mononuclear and nonspecific. Caseous lesions with necrotic foci tend to be located near the epididymis. In five of eight cases studied by Kahn and McAninch (152), acid-fast bacilli were identified. Culture should be performed to identify the microorganism specifically, because *M. kansasii* and *M. avium-intracellulare* also produced necrotizing granulomas of the testis (153).

Although rarely seen in the United States, leprosy is common elsewhere in the world. Testicular involvement is divided into three phases: a vascular phase with lepra cells stuffed with acid-fast bacilli in blood vessel walls and interstitium; an interstitial phase with obliterative endarteritis, clusters of Leydig cells, interstitial fibrosis, variable numbers of histiocytes containing acid-fast bacilli and reduced spermatogenesis; and an obliterative phase with complete fibrosis, no demonstrable seminiferous tubules, diminished vascularity, and very rare acid-fast bacilli (154). The last two phases tend to merge. Gynecomastia is not infrequent in patients with testicular leprosy. In Egypt, substantial series of infertile patients were reported with leprosy. In the United States, because of our unfamiliarity with leprosy, the diagnosis may not be considered either clinically or pathologically in a patient with a unilateral testicular mass resected as a possible tumor. In early-phase lesions, Fite–Faroco stain should demonstrate the numerous acid-fast organisms.

Fungal Infections

Various fungal organisms produce clinically important infections in the testis and may be seen as part of a systemic illness or as a surgical lesion of the testis. Organisms that have been identified in testicular infections include blastomyces, actinomyces, *Histoplasma capsulatum, Trichophyton mentagraphytes,* and *Coccidioides immitis* (155,156). In fungal orchitis the histologic appearance of the inflammation usually resembles that of similar infections elsewhere. The need to identify the specific infectious agent is illustrated by Monroe's case of *H. capsulatum* infection of the testis interpreted as a sperm granuloma and not further treated, resulting in fungal involvement of the adrenal glands and death 2 years after orchiectomy (155).

Rickettsial Infections

Orchitis was described in patients with typhus and Q fever (157). In typhus the vasculitis manifests by large numbers of organisms in swollen capillary endothelial cells with accompanying vascular thrombi.

Viral Infections

Numerous viral infections have involved the testis, including mumps, variola, varicella, ECHO, lymphocytic choriomeningitis, group B arbor virus, influenza, Dengue fever, sandfly fever, and coxsackie B virus (158,159). Epstein–Barr virus also affects the testis when that organ is involved in infectious mononucleosis.

Mumps

As a result of childhood immunization, clinical mumps is now a rarity. It has been well studied, however, and helps to understand the evolution of other orchitides (160). Acutely, there is edema of the tunica albuginea and interstitium, congestion of the tunica vasculosa, and interstitial lymphocytic aggregation and hemorrhage. This progresses to a mixed lymphocyte–PMN interstitial infiltration with patchy irregular hemorrhage and focal inflammation of the seminiferous tubules. Intratubular inflammation is composed of numerous PMNs and a few histiocytes. Eventually, spermatogenic cells become necrotic, leaving only Sertoli cells, some of which will disappear from tubules. The process becomes more intense with interstitial lymphocytic and histiocytic inflammation, tubules filled with inflammatory debris, and tubule walls infiltrated by lymphocytes and plasma cells. When infertility occurs as a result of mumps, it is due to the extensiveness and bilaterality of the process. Orchitis rarely occurs prepubertally. Conversely, 20% of postpubertal males who develop mumps have an associated orchitis. Of that group, atrophy develops in about one third, but infertility is infrequent. Werner (161) estimated that fewer than 2% of all patients with mumps had infertility as a result of orchitis. In cases of healed orchitis, there may be virtually no inflammation, with only foci of tubular sclerosis and tubules with reduced numbers of germ cells and residual Sertoli cells marking the site of the orchitis.

Spirochetal Infections

The fibrotic type of acquired syphilis generally occurs in a painless, enlarged testis with a peritubular interstitial mononuclear cell infiltration, small seminiferous tubules containing reduced numbers of germinal epithelial cells, and peritubular fibrosis. In the gummatous form, the testis is enlarged and irregular or nodular. Discrete gummas are seen grossly. Microscopically, these show coagulative necrosis with a peripheral zone of lymphocytes, plasma cells, and occasional histiocytic giant cells. Obliterative endarteritis may be present. Fibromatous and gummatous changes may be present in the same testis. Spirochetes are usually not identifiable in the fibromatous stage, but are present in the gummatous stage (162).

Acquired Immunodeficiency Syndrome

The testis is usually not a site of clinical disease in patients with AIDS. However, at autopsy, testes show markedly decreased spermatogenesis, arrested maturation, and GCA with tunica proprial thickening, tubular hyalinization, interstitial inflammation, reduced numbers of Leydig cells, and interstitial fibrosis (163,164). Toxoplasmosis, tuberculosis, histoplasmosis, candidiasis, *M. avium-intracellulare,* and cytomegalovirus infection were described in testes of AIDS patients (146,163–167). DePaepe et al. (166) demonstrated a 39% incidence of cytomegalovirus, *M. avium-intracellulare,* and toxoplasma infection in the testes of a series of 56 autopsies.

Anti-HIV P17 monoclonal antibody was identified in eight of 14 autopsy testis specimens from AIDS patients. These were present in one or several degenerating germ cells and surrounding Sertoli cells (167). Polymerase chain reaction (PCR)-amplified HIV-1 DNA localized to many spermatogonia, spermatocytes, and rare spermatids of AIDs patients. The germ cells may serve as the primary source of spread of the virus (168). Kaposi's sarcoma was rarely identified in the testis and epididymis of AIDS patients (146). Testicular germ cell tumors of various types are being identified in AIDS patients (169). The overall mortality rate due to testicular germ-cell tumors is similar to that of nonimmunosuppressed patients with germ-cell tumors (170).

Nonspecific Granulomatous Orchitis and Malakoplakia

Nonspecific granulomatous orchitis (NSGO), despite its unknown but probably infectious etiology, is a definable clinical–pathologic entity. The disease usually is seen as a unilateral, firm, enlarged tender mass in the testis of a middle-aged man and may be preceded by a flulike illness (171). Rare cases have been bilateral. Epidydimal sperm granulomas may be present. The testis is enlarged by a homogeneous tan infiltrate that obscures testicular architecture and may involve the epididymis. The gross appearance resembles that of lymphoma, leukemia, and malakoplakia (Fig. 20A). Microscopically, large numbers of lymphocytes and plasma cells infiltrate the interstitium, surround seminiferous tubules, widen tubular walls, and may be in tubule lumens (Fig. 20B). Although there are no true granulomas in NSGO, the tubular orientation of the inflammation, sometimes with histiocytes and occasional multinucleated giant cells, gives the lesion a somewhat granulomatous micro-

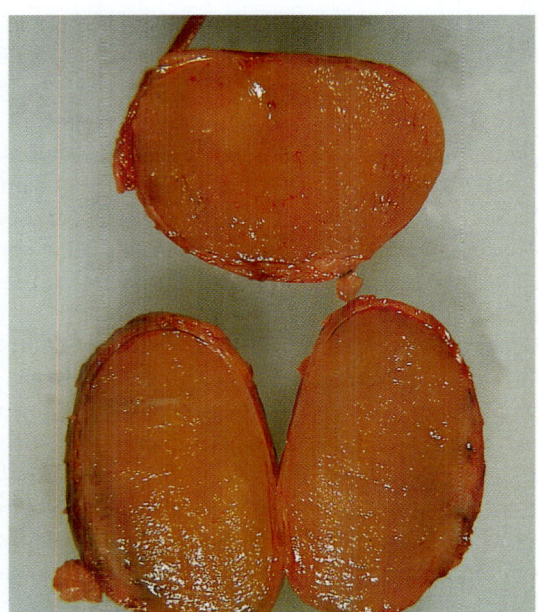
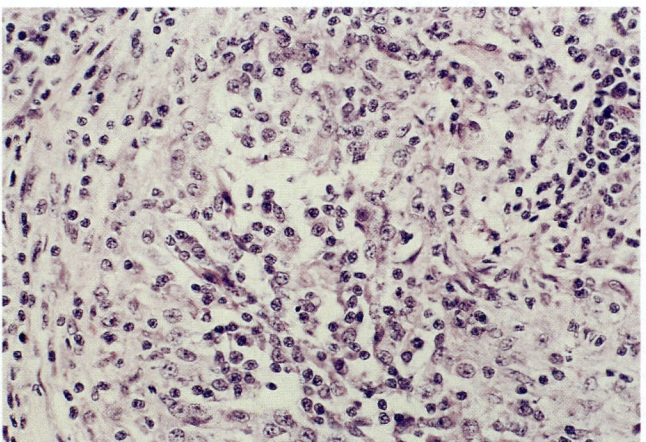

FIG. 20. Nonspecific granulomatous orchitis in 45-year-old man with a 6-month history of unilateral testicular enlargement and fever. **A:** Testis (34 gm) with uniform, tan parenchyma. **B:** Mixed inflammatory cell infiltrate contains lymphocytes, plasmacytes, and histiocytes and involves tubules and interstitium. Case contributed by Dr. Gurdev Garewal of Maple Heights, Ohio.

scopic appearance. Various etiologies that have been suggested include trauma, reaction to extravasated sperm, autoimmune disease, urinary tract infection with retrograde spread via the vas deferens, and venous thrombosis involving the spermatic cord. The prodromal symptoms similarity to the clinical, gross, and microscopic findings of bacterial orchitis, and the occasional response to antibiotics suggest that NSGO is of bacterial origin. The two important distinctions that must be made are between NSGO and infections caused by specific organisms and between NSGO and malignant lymphoma. I suggest that when an infection of the testis is suspected, fresh tissue should be taken from the excised testis. A frozen section should be prepared and tissue should be cultured for bacterial, acid-fast, and fungal organisms, stained for spirochetes, and placed in glutaraldehyde for ultrastructural study. In this way, a specific cause can be identified if present. If malignant lymphoma is a diagnostic consideration on frozen section, tissue can be processed for a complete lymphoma workup. In general, the distinction between NSGO and malignant lymphoma is not difficult. NSGO tends to retain a tubule-oriented granulomatous appearance and has a mixed cell population, whereas malignant lymphoma tends to have a more diffuse monomorphic infiltrate that compresses and obliterates tubules.

Testicular malakoplakia is an orchitis of bacterial origin that closely resembles NSGO clinically, grossly and sometimes microscopically. The testes are usually large, yellow, tan, or brown, and sometimes contain abscesses (172). The process sometimes involves the epididymis. The distinctive histologic change is the same as that seen in malakoplakia in other parts of the body, with sheets of eosinophilic histiocytes in the interstitium and sometimes in the tubules. The pathognomonic change is the presence of laminated calcific Michaelis–Gutmann bodies microscopically, or bacteria within phagolysosomes in the histiocytes demonstrated by ultrastructural study. If the gross specimen is handled as described, optimally fixed tissue will be available for ultrastructural study.

INTERSEX SYNDROMES

Intersex refers to syndromes in which there is a discordance among at least two of the following: genetic sex, gonadal sex, genital tract sex, and phenotypic sex. The pathologist may anticipate that an individual has an intersex problem based on the pathologic findings. However, in many instances, the cytogenetic, anatomic, biochemical, and clinical facts of the case must be known before the most accurate diagnosis is possible. In most instances, the surgical pathologist's role begins with a pathologic specimen. This may be a biopsy of a gonad, potential gonad, tumor, segment of indeterminate tissue, or major resection of a specimen that could include gonads and the entire wolffian or müllerian duct systems or both. If other than a biopsy, the pathologist and the surgeon should review the gross specimen together, determine the laterality of structures, and photograph the specimen for future reference. All parts of the specimen should be labeled so that the presence of ductal structures can be related to gonadal tissue.

To understand the pathology of intersex syndromes, we must understand the development of the gonads and the male and the female reproductive tracts not only in the three dimensions of space, but also in the dimension of time (173). If the timetable of gonadal and reproductive tract development is understood, the findings in intersex cases make more sense, and diagnostic possibilities become reduced.

In human development, the presence of the Y chromosome determines the formation of a testis. Germ cells migrate into the genital ridge, and tubule formation is recognizable by day 45. Wolffian duct development commences on day 25 and continues thereafter. Müllerian duct formation commences on day 43. If no Y chromosome is present, the gonad develops into an ovary. In the presence of a Y chromosome, a testis develops. Sertoli cells, which derive from the genital ridge, secrete AMH approximately 62 days after fertilization. This protein causes regression of the müllerian duct, which is normally completed by days 75 to 80. This effect is ipsilateral and depends on the proximity of a gonad with competent Sertoli cells. If Sertoli cells are not present in one gonad, the müllerian duct will not regress ipsilaterally, and in such a situation, the uterus and upper vagina will be present in some form. Shortly after the beginning of müllerian regression, Leydig cells appear at about day 64 and begin production of T, which continues throughout intrauterine development. T also acts ipsilaterally and causes development of the wolffian duct (i.e., the epididymis, vas deferens and seminal vesicles if androgen receptors are present and qualitatively sufficient). If no T is produced, wolffian duct degeneration begins at about day 75 and is completed about day 84. Systemic production of androgens, administration of androgens to the mother, or production of androgens by a maternal tumor or by fetal congenital adrenal hyperplasia may cause the development of the wolffian duct system. Masculinization of external genitalia commences after T production on about day 70. T itself will not cause complete development. The external genitalia and urogenital sinus anlage must have androgen receptors and must contain 5 α-reductase, which converts T to dihydrotestosterone (DHT). The latter causes development of external genitalia, which is completed between days 120 and 140. DHT causes elongation of the phallus. If ovaries or no gonads are present, the internal ducts are female. If DHT is not present, external genitalia will have a female phenotype (173).

Classification of intersex has been done in a variety of ways based on sex chromosomes; on types of pseudohermaphroditism; on androgen-receptor defects; on sources of primary gonadal defect including testicular regression syndrome, Leydig cell agenesis, defects in T and DHT synthesis; and on external phenotypes (11,173–175). Major types of intersex involving the testis are described later.

Male Pseudohermaphroditism

Male pseudohermaphroditism exists when the karyotype is XY, the gonads are testes, and the phenotype is ambiguous or female.

Persistent Müllerian Duct Syndrome

Persistent müllerian duct syndrome (PMDS) is a recessive autosomal disorder. The phenotypic male with PMDS has normal external genitalia, unilateral or bilateral cryptorchidism, sometimes an empty hemiscrotum, normal wolffian duct derivatives, and a uterus, usually with two fallopian tubes within an inguinal hernia (174) (Fig. 21A–E). This entity has been termed hernia uteri inguinale. Cases are most frequently identified in infants and children, but have been first diagnosed in adults as well. PMDS may be associated with testicular degeneration before or after birth (176). Similar hernial contents can occur in mixed gonadal dysgenesis

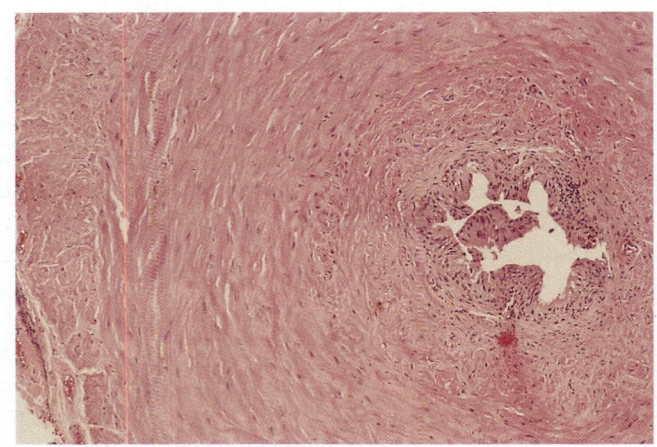
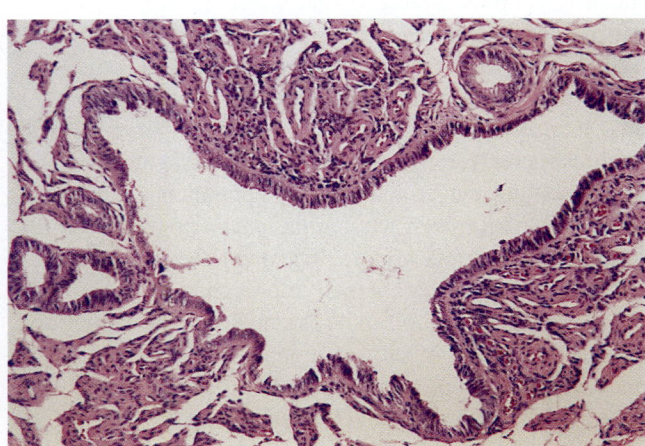
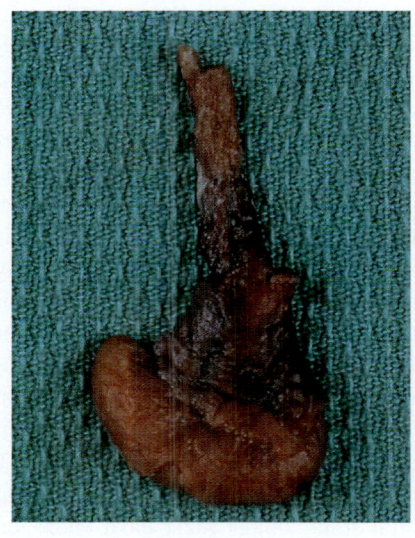
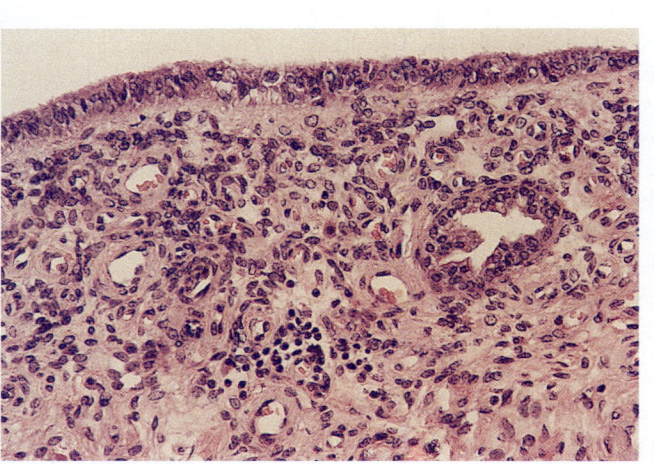
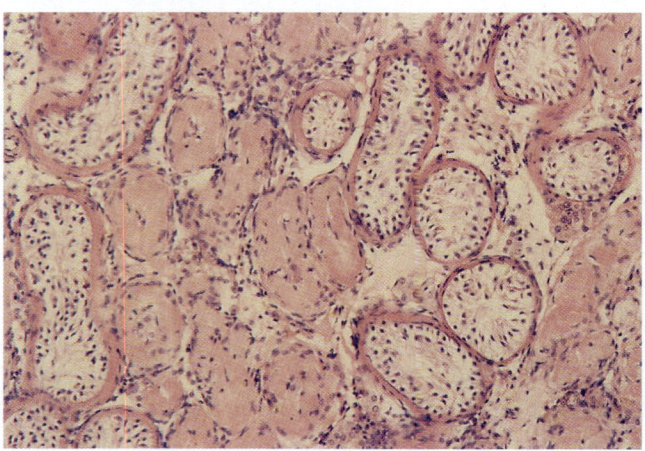

FIG. 21. Persistent müllerian duct syndrome in a 42-year-old man with three children. **A:** Normal vas deferens was identified in left vasectomy specimen. **B:** Müllerian duct remnant was identified in right "vasectomy" specimen. **C:** Persistent müllerian duct structures were subsequently identified in an intrascrotal hernia. **D:** Rudimentary uterus with surface epithelium, endometrial-type stroma, and gland. **E:** Testis biopsy demonstrates tubules lined only by Sertoli cells and sclerotic tubules. Elsewhere, tubules were undergoing spermatogenesis. (Case contributed by Dr. Arlington Kuklinca of Youngstown, Ohio, and Dr. Linda Olmstead of Warren, Ohio.)

(MGD). It is important to examine gonadal tissue to distinguish PMDS from MGD, because bilateral gonadectomies are usually performed because of an increased risk of germ-cell neoplasms in MGD. Germ-cell tumors of all types including malignant intratubular germ-cell neoplasia may occur in PMDS, with an incidence of approximately 15%. PMDS is due to a lack of AMH activity caused by a mutation in the AMH gene on the short arm of chromosome 19 or an abnormality of the end-organ receptor gene on chromosome 12. Testicular structure may not be diagnostic because of the age of the patient and the presence of cryptorchidism, and should be interpreted in the context of the gross findings.

Testicular Regression Syndrome

Testicular regression syndrome (TRS) consists of a range of findings that occur in paucigonadal or agonadal individuals of male, female, or ambiguous phenotype who have had no gonadal or testicular formation or who have had damage and regression of testicular tissue. The findings consist of a constellation of developmental defects of the wolffian duct, variable müllerian duct development, and external genitalia phenotype that results from gonadal absence and depends on the chronology of a gonadal injury (174). Anorchia is an example of TRS and is usually discovered in the workup of a cryptorchid male subject. Fibrosis, hemosiderin deposition, and dystrophic calcification in relation to vas deferens identifies the site of the former testis.

Defects in Adrenal Cortical Hormone Synthesis Associated with Congenital Adrenal Hyperplasia

Five enzymatic defects involving 20,22-desmolase, 3-β-hydroxysteroid dehydrogenase, 17-α hydroxylase, 17,20-desmolase, and 17β-hydroxysteroid dehydrogenase may cause male pseudohermaphroditism (174). The location and severity of the enzyme defect will determine the pattern of glucosteroid, mineral corticoid, and sex-steroid synthesis. Genetic males have cryptorchidism, variably developed wolffian duct systems, absent müllerian duct derivatives, and female or ambiguous external genitalia (174). 20,22-Desmolase deficiency is incompatible with survival, and 3-β-hydroxysteroid dehydrogenase deficiency may also cause death in infancy. This form and the other enzyme defects have been identified in adults. The morphologic changes in the testes are those found in cryptorchid testes. Cases of 17β-hydroxysteroid dehydrogenase have been mistaken for cases of incomplete androgen insensitivity syndrome (174). In those defects involving mineral corticoid and glucocorticoid synthesis, the early clinical diagnosis of congenital adrenal hyperplasia (CAH) is extremely important so that therapy can be initiated as early as possible.

21-Hydroxylase and 11-hydroxylase deficiencies do not cause male pseudohermaphroditism. However, 21- and 11-hydroxylase and 17β-hydroxysteroid dehydrogenase deficiencies may be associated with the development of masses that resemble Leydig cell tumors in and adjacent to the testes (Fig. 22). These masses occur bilaterally in response to ACTH stimulation of ectopic adrenocortical cells or ACTH-sensitive Leydig cells. The clinical recognition that these masses are part of the adrenogenital syndrome will obviate orchiectomy because corticosteroid therapy usually will cause regression of the masses. Surgery may be necessary for masses that will not regress. Isosexual precocity may be associated with this form of CAH. However, testicular and peritesticular masses may develop later in life in unrecognized, untreated cases, presumably with a less severe enzyme defect.

Androgen Insensitivity Syndrome

Complete androgen insensitivity syndrome (AIS), also known as testicular feminization, is the most frequent cause of male pseudohermaphroditism. The etiologic defect is the lack of androgen receptor, because of which T and DHT are unable to affect the developing wolffian duct system and external genitalia. Lack of androgen receptor is due to a variety of mutations in the androgen-receptor gene on the X chromosome (177). The prototypic patient is a tall phenotypic female with well-formed breasts, absent or scanty pubic and axillary hair, and a shallow vagina because of the absent contribution by the müllerian duct. The patient also has bilateral cryptorchidism with intraabdominal, inguinal, or labial testes and usually has absent wolffian and müllerian duct derivatives (174). The testes often have a characteristic, if not diagnostic gross appearance with a tan to brown parenchyma and multiple white nodules from millimeter size up to 24 cm in diameter (Fig. 23). A smooth-muscle mass may be present medial to the testis, and cysts of wolffian or müllerian duct origin may be present at the lateral pole of the testis (174). The microscopic appearance of the testis also is characteristic (see Fig. 23). Seminiferous tubules are small and are composed mostly of immature

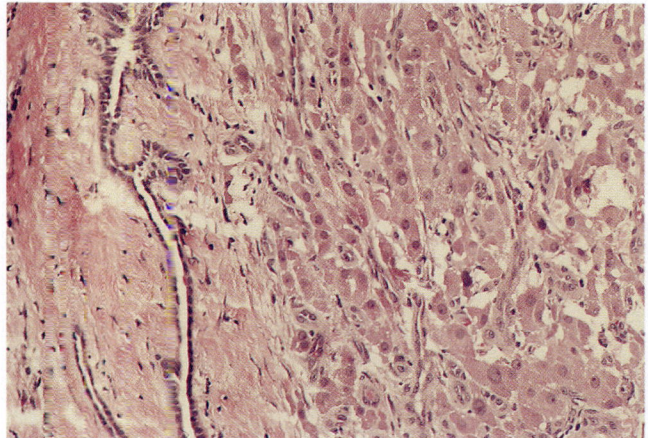

FIG. 22. Five-year-old with 21-hydroxylase deficiency with a nodule of adrenocorticotropic hormone (ACTH)-sensitive cells compressing the rete testis.

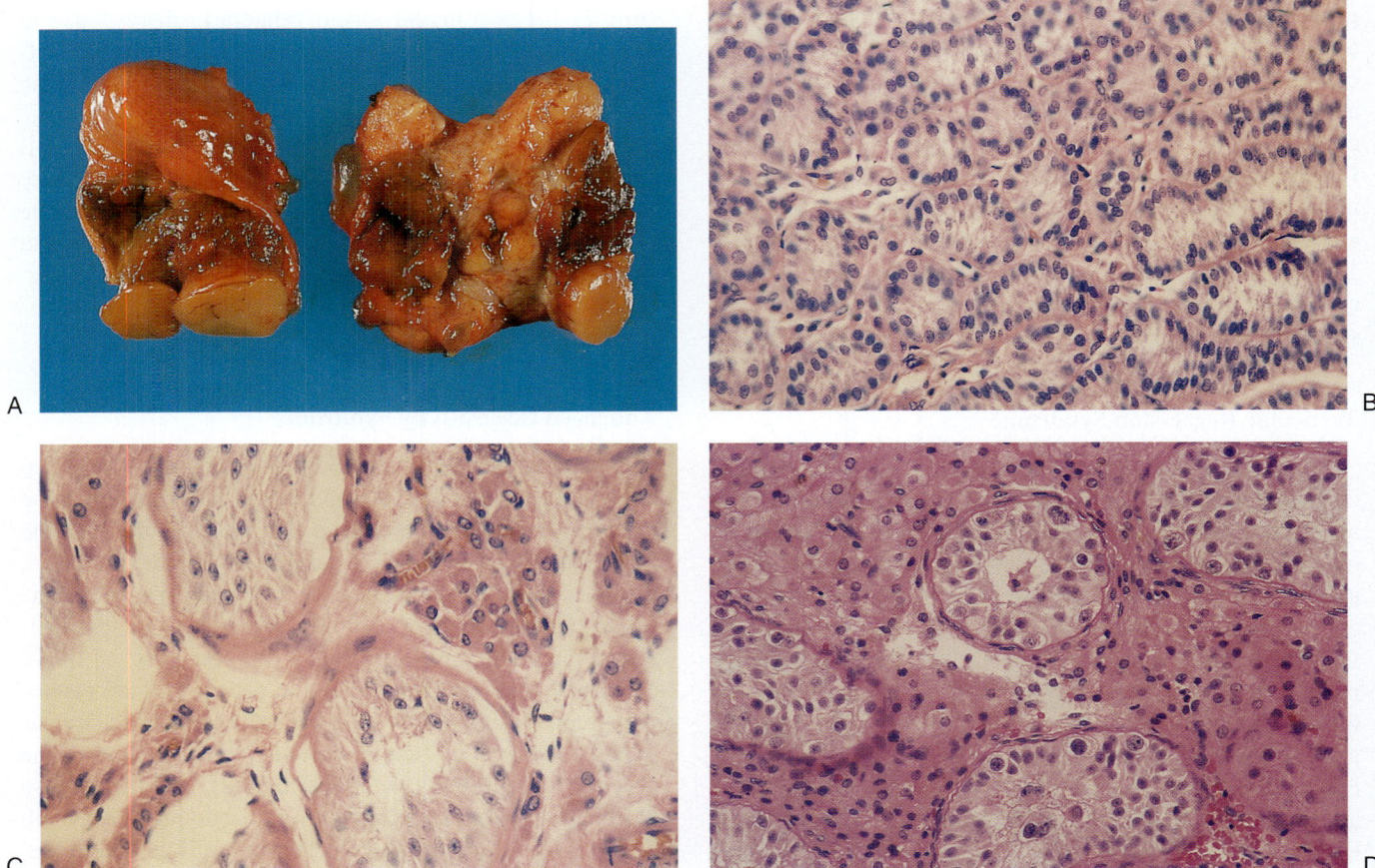

FIG. 23. Complete androgen insensitivity syndrome. **A–C:** In a 17-year-old. **A:** Bilateral testes demonstrating dark brown parenchyma and pale Sertoli cell adenomas. **B:** Sertoli cell adenoma composed of small tubules lined by immature-appearing Sertoli cells. Rare Leydig cells are present between the tubules. **C:** Testis adjacent to Sertoli cell adenoma demonstrates Leydig cells and adult seminiferous tubules with germinal cell aplasia. **D:** Malignant intratubular germ cells in cryptorchid testis of 18-year-old with complete androgen insensitivity syndrome. Marked hyperplasia of Leydig cells.

Sertoli cells. Mature Sertoli cells may be present. Spermatogonia are usually sparse, and spermatocytes have been reported. There is marked Leydig cell hyperplasia, and Rutgers and Scully (174) indicated that most cases have an ovarian-type stroma. The nodules are composed of small tubules populated almost exclusively by immature Sertoli cells with few germ cells. In cases I have seen, the nodules are demarcated from surrounding tissue. Because of their increased tubular density, Sertoli cell immaturity, and reduced numbers of Leydig cells relative to the surrounding parenchyma, the nodules have been called Sertoli cell adenomas based on the predominant Sertoli cell composition and on their often impressive size (see Fig. 23). However, they have not evolved into malignant tumors, and because they share all of the elements of the surrounding testis, they are probably of hamartomatous origin.

Complete AIS may be seen as inguinal hernias or labial masses at birth, primary amenorrhea, infertility, or a tumor mass. If testes are sampled incident to hernial repair, the diagnosis can be made early in life. At puberty, the absence of menarche may instigate investigation and enable the diagnosis to be made. Rarely when amenorrhea has been ignored, the diagnosis is made after an infertility workup. The presence of a pelvic mass caused by a germ-cell tumor or so-called Sertoli cell adenoma may be the presenting feature. Some cases have been discovered in the evaluation of familial cases of AIS.

Neoplasms may occur in complete AIS. The most important of these are of germ-cell origin. MITGCN has been identified in infancy, adolescence, and adulthood, so that the tubules should be carefully studied in biopsies obtained at any age (see Fig. 23). Germ-cell tumors have an increased incidence with increasing age in AIS, and all types have been reported. The frequency of malignant tumors was estimated at more than 30% by age 50 years (174). Because of the risk of malignancy, gonadectomy should occur after or before completion of puberty. One case of bilateral Leydig cell tumors has been reported in a case of partial AIS (178).

A variety of syndromes with ambiguous external genitalia, quantitatively or qualitatively abnormal androgen receptors, and variable wolffian duct development have been given a variety of names and eponyms. Such patients are now characterized as partial or incomplete AIS or Reifenstein's syndrome. Testes in these cases may be cryptorchid and show typical changes. There are rare cases in which a phenotypically normal male has infertility associated with a mild defect in androgen receptors (174).

Gonadal Dysgenesis

Gonadal dysgenesis consists of a spectrum of disorders with ambiguous genitalia, persistent müllerian duct structures, wolffian duct derivatives, karyotypes having a Y chromosome, and the potential for neoplastic transformation of gonads. The entities in this spectrum include MGD (Fig. 24), pure gonadal dysgenesis (PGD), and dysgenetic male pseudohermaphroditism (DMPH). MGD was the term used by Sohval (179) in 1963 for a group of intersex patients with asymmetric gonadal development including (a) a testis on one side and a contralateral streak gonad, (b) a testis and contralateral gonadal agenesis, (c) hypoplastic gonads with rudimentary tubules in one, or (d) a streak gonad with a contralateral tumor. Davidoff and Federman (180) considered a testis or gonadal tumor on one side and a rudimentary streak gonad or no gonad on the other side as MGD. Because of insufficient or delayed production of AMH by the dysgenetic gonad, müllerian structures are invariably present. Some patients may have hernia uteri inguinale. The majority of cases have bilateral fallopian tubes. Inadequate or delayed production of T by the dysgenetic gonad causes incomplete masculinization of the external genitalia and poor development of the ipsilateral wolffian duct structures. External genitalia may be normal male, ambiguous, or normal female. Most patients at birth have ambiguous genitalia, and approximately two thirds are raised as females. At puberty, phenotypic females often develop signs of virilization. Patients may have stigmata of Turner's syndrome. The 45 XO/46 XY mosaic karyotype is most common, followed by 46 XY, and less frequently by other mosaic karyotypes with a Y chromosome–containing cell line (144). In postpubertal patients reported by Wallace and Levin (181), the seminiferous tubules ranged from totally sclerotic to having mild hypospermatogenesis. Oxyphilic granular Sertoli cells were focally present in two patients, one with a scrotal testis and the other with a cryptorchid testis. Testes in prepubertal patients have a prepubertal appearance. A streak gonad consists of ovarian-type stroma with no primordial ovarian follicles (Fig. 25). Streak ovaries are streak gonads with primordial follicles or germ cells.

PGD is characterized by bilateral streak gonads, internal müllerian structures, a 46 XY karyotype, and a female phenotype without signs of Turner's syndrome (174). DMPH is characterized by bilateral dysgenetic testes, persistent müllerian structures, cryptorchidism, and inadequate virilization. XC/XY mosaicism may be present. In adults, spermatogenesis and fertility are absent. Because of the overlap in syndromes, similar karyotypes, similar phenotypes, susceptibility of gonads for neoplastic transformation, and the inability to distinguish the type of gonad in those harboring tumors, we and others consider PGD and DMPH as part of the syndrome of MGD (181).

Rutgers and Scully (174) indicated that tumors develop in 9% to 30% of patients with MGD. The most common tumor is gonadoblastoma, a neoplasm composed of intimately admixed germ cells and sex-cord cells in circumscribed nests with focal or diffuse calcification. In about 50% of cases, malignant germ cells invade stroma and form a germinoma (seminoma). Other types of germ-cell tumors also may occur. Approximately one sixth of germinomas arising in gonadoblastomas are bilateral. Gonadoblastomas do not metastasize but have been shown to express malignant intratubular germ-cell markers (182). Germ-cell tumors occurring in association with gonadoblastoma may metastasize. Gonadoblastomas may not be evident in association with germ-cell tumors arising in dysgenetic gonads. This may be due to overgrowth of the gonadoblastoma or origin of the germ-cell

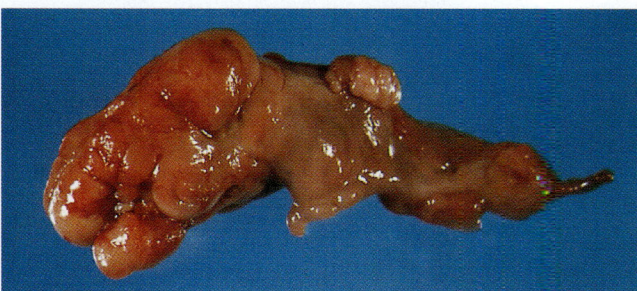

FIG. 24. Mixed gonadal dysgenesis in an 8 1/4-year-old phenotypic female patient with bilateral gonadoblastoma and germinoma. Left streak gonad containing gonadoblastoma and germinoma 7 cm in maximum dimension with a cerebriform configuration and a flat streak at the base.

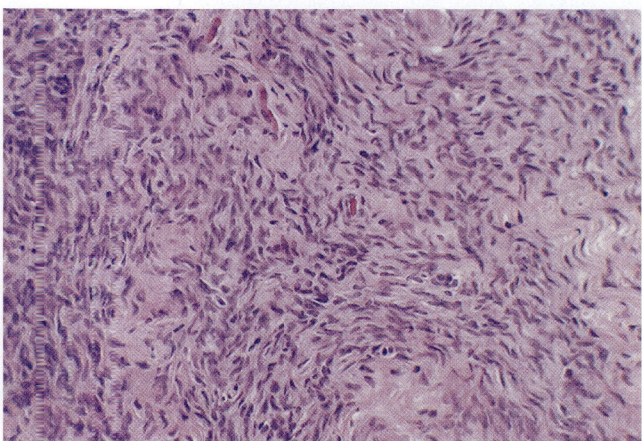

FIG. 25. Right streak gonad with ovarian-type stroma and no ovarian follicles in a 20-year-old phenotypic female patient with mixed gonadal dysgenesis, bilateral gonadoblastomas, and a left-sided germinoma.

tumor in MITGCN. Of 15 cases of MGD studied, Wallace and Levin (181) found seven, all phenotypic females, with gonadal tumors. These patients had five gonadoblastomas, four germinomas, and one MITGCN. One patient had a gonadal stromal tumor (181). Juvenile granulosa cell tumor also was reported in patients with an abnormal karyotype containing a Y chromosome (183). Because of the risk of development of malignant germ-cell tumors, it is recommended that gonads be removed at the time of diagnosis of MGD.

True Hermaphroditism

Ovarian and testicular tissue is found in the same patient either as bilateral ovotestes, as an ovotestis on one side and contralateral ovary or testis, or as an ovary and contralateral testis. The ovotestis is the most frequent gonad. Generally, the testicular and ovarian segments of the ovotestis are end-to-end. The ovarian part is generally normal, but the testicular component is abnormal and only rarely contains spermatogonia. Streak gonads are never found. Malignant germ-cell tumors including gonadoblastoma rarely occur in testicular tissue. Brenner tumor, mucinous cystadenoma, and endometriotic cysts were reported in ovarian tissue.

REFERENCES

1. Dym M. The male reproductive system. In: Weiss L, Greep RO, eds. *Histology*. 4th ed. New York: McGraw-Hill, 1977:979–1021.
2. Trainer TD. Testis and excretory duct system. In: Sternberg SS, ed. *Histology for pathologists*. New York: Raven Press, 1992:731–747.
3. Heller CG, Clermont Y. Kinetics of the germinal epithelium in man. In: Pincus G, ed. *Recent progress in hormone research*. Vol 20. New York: Academic Press, 1964:545–575.
4. Smith RG, Lipshultz LI. Infertility. In: Rajfer J, ed. *Urologic endocrinology*. Philadelphia: WB Saunders, 1986:325–345.
5. Lipshultz LI, Murthy L, Tindall DJ. Characterization of human Sertoli cells in vitro. *J Clin Endocrinol Metab* 1982;55:228.
6. Nakazumi H, Sasano H, Maehara I, et al. Transforming growth factor-α, epidermal growth factor, and epidermal growth factor receptor in human testis obtained from biopsy and castration: immunohistochemical study. *Tohoku J Exp Med* 1996;178:381–388.
7. Steger K, Rey R, Kliesch S, et al. Immunohistochemical detection of immature Sertoli cell markers in testicular tissue of infertile adult men: a preliminary study. *Int J Androl* 1996;19:122–128.
8. Carreau S. Human Sertoli cells produce inhibin in vitro: an additional marker to assess the seminiferous epithelium development. *Hum Reprod* 1995;10:1947–1949.
9. Steinberger A. The Sertoli cell and its role in spermatogenesis. In: Frajese G, ed. *Oligozoospermia: recent progress in andrology*. New York: Raven Press, 1981:35–43.
10. Vigersky RA. Testis: normal testicular physiology. In: Rajfer J, ed. *Urologic endocrinology*. Philadelphia: WB Saunders, 1986:196–215.
11. Rajfer J. Disorders of sexual differentiation. In: Rajfer J, ed. *Urologic endocrinology*. Philadelphia: WB Saunders, 1986:17–40.
12. Poulat F, Girard F, Chevron M-P, et al. Nuclear localization of the testis determining gene product SRY. *J Cell Biol* 1995;128:737–748.
13. Moore KL. *The developing human: clinically oriented embryology*. 3rd ed. Philadelphia: WB Saunders, 1982:271–280.
14. Sniffen RC. The testis. 1. The normal testis. *Arch Pathol* 1950;50:259.
15. Müller J, Skakkebaek NE. Quantification of germ cells and seminiferous tubules by stereological examinations of testicles from boys who suffered from sudden death. *Int J Androl* 1983;6:143.
16. Prince FP. Ultrastructure of immature Leydig cells in the human prepubertal testis. *Anat Rec* 1984;209:165.
17. Brodie A, Inkster S. Aromatase in the human testis. *J Steroid Biochem Mol Biol* 1993;44:549–555.
18. Davidoff MS, Middendorff R, Mayer B, et al. Nitric oxide/cGMP pathway components in the Leydig cells of the human testis. *Cell Tissue Res* 1997;287:161–170.
19. Schulze W, Davidoff MS, Holstein A-F. Are Leydig cells of neural origin? Substance P-like immunoreactivity in human testicular tissue. *Acta Endocrinologica (Copenh)* 1987;115:373–377.
20. Baker HWG, Burger HG, de Kretser DM, et al. Changes in the pituitary-testicular system with age. *Clin Endocrinol* 1976;5:349.
21. Johnson L, Petty CS, Neaves WB. Influence of age on sperm production and testicular weights in men. *J Reprod Fertil* 1984;70:211.
22. Johns ML, Zane RS, Petty CS, Neaves WB. Quantification of the human Sertoli cell population: its distribution, relation to germ cell numbers, and age related decline. *Biol Reprod* 1984;31:785–795.
23. Johnson L. Spermatogenesis and aging in the human. *J Androl* 1986;7:331.
24. Kaler LW, Neaves WB. Attrition of the human Leydig cell population with advancing age. *Anat Rec* 1978;192:513–518.
25. Honoré LH. Ageing changes in the human testis: a light microscopic study. *Gerontology* 1978;24:58.
26. Regadera J, Nistal M, Paniagua R. Testis, epididymis and spermatic cord in elderly men: correlation of angiographic and histologic studies with systemic arteriosclerosis. *Arch Pathol Lab Med* 1985;109:663.
27. Hadziselimovic F, Herzog B, Huff DS, Menardi G. The morphometric histopathology of undescended testes and testes associated with incarcerated inguinal hernia: a comparative study. *J Urol* 1991;146:627–629.
28. Rajfer J, Walsh PC. *Testicular descent: original article series*. Vol XIII, no. 2. New York: The National Foundation, 1977:107–122.
29. Rajfer J, Handelsman DJ, Swerdloff RS, et al. Hormonal therapy of cryptorchidism. *N Engl J Med* 1986;314:466.
30. Huff DS, Hadziselimovic F, Snyder HM, et al. Post-natal testicular maldevelopment in unilateral cryptorchidism. *J Urol* 1989;142:546–548.
31. Hedinger C. Histopathology of the cryptorchid testes. In: Bierich JR, Giarola A, eds. *Proceedings of the Serona Symposia*. Vol 25. New York: Academic Press, 1979:29–38.
32. Nistal M, Paniagua R, Diez-Pardo JA. Histologic classification of undescended testes. *Hum Pathol* 1980;11:666.
33. Mininberg DT, Rodger JC, Bedford JM. Ultrastructural evidence of the onset of testicular pathologic conditions within the first year of life. *J Urol* 1982;128:782.
34. Swerdlow AJ, Higgins CD, Pike MC. Risk of testicular cancer in cohort of boys with cryptorchidism. *BMJ* 1997;314:1507–1511.
35. Nistal M, Paniagua R. Infertility in males with retractile testes. *Fertil Steril* 1984;41:395.
36. Nistal M, Garcia-Rodeja E, Paniagua R. Granular transformation of Sertoli cells in testicular disorders. *Hum Pathol* 1991;22:131–137.
37. Prener A, Engholm G, Jensen OM. Genital anomalies and risk for testicular cancer in Danish men. *Epidemiology* 1996;7:14–19.
38. Krabbe S, Berthelsen JG, Volsted P, et al. High incidence of undetected neoplasia in maldescended testes. *Lancet* 1979;1:999.
39. Skakkebaek NE. Carcinoma in situ of the testis: frequency and relationship to invasive germ cell tumours in infertile men. *Histopathology* 1978;2:157.
40. Nüesch-Bachmann IH, Hedinger C. Atypische spermatogonien als prakenzerose. *Schweiz Med Wochenschr* 1977;107:795.
41. Federman DD. Disorders of gonadal development: mixed gonadal dysgenesis: dysgenetic male pseudohermaphroditism: agonadism. In: *Abnormal sexual development*. Philadelphia: WB Saunders, 1968:84–88.
42. Nistal M, Paniagua R. Congenital anomalies of the testis and the epididymis. In: *Testicular and epididymal pathology*. New York: Thieme-Stratton, 1984:72–93.
43. Smith NM, Byard RW, Bourne AJ. Testicular regression syndrome: a pathological study of 77 cases. *Histopathology* 1991;19:269–272.
44. Weiss RM, Glickman MG. Localization and management of nonpalpable undescended testes. *Surg Clin North Am* 1980;60:1253.
45. Putschar WGJ, Manion WC. Splenic-gonadal fusion. *Am J Pathol* 1956;32:15.
46. Mellin GW, Katzenstein M. The saga of thalidomide (concluded): neuropathy to embryopathy, with case reports of congenital anomalies. *N Engl J Med* 1962;267:1238.
47. Johnson RE, Scheithauer B. Massive hyperplasia of testicular adrenal rests in a patient with Nelson's syndrome. *Am J Clin Pathol* 1982;77:501–507.

48. Williamson RCN. Torsion of the testis and allied conditions. *Br J Surg* 1976;63:465.
49. Thomas WEG, Cooper MJ, Crane GA, Williamson RCN. Testicular exocrine function after torsion. *Lancet* 1984;2:1357.
50. O'Regan S, Robitaille P. Orchitis mimicking testicular torsion in Henoch-Schönlein's purpura. *J Urol* 1981;126:834.
51. Mikuz G, Hofstadter F, Hager J. Testis involvement in Schönlein-Henoch purpura. *Pathol Res Pract* 1979;165:323.
52. Turner T. Varicocele: still an enigma. *J Urol* 1983;129:695.
53. Sayfan J, Adam YG. Right sided varicocele associated with situs inversus. *Fertil Steril* 1978;30:716.
54. Kursh E. What is the incidence of varicocele in a fertile population? *Fertil Steril* 1987;48:510.
55. Greenberg SH. Varicocele and male fertility. *Fertil Steril* 1977;28:699.
56. Dubin L, Amelar RD. Varicocelectomy: 986 cases in a 12 year study. *Urology* 1977;10:446.
57. Cockett ATK, Takihara H, Consentino MJ. The varicocele. *Fertil Steril* 1984;41:5.
58. Bonanni G, Calcagno A, Mammana G, et al. DNA flow cytometry of left and right testes in normospermic patients affected by left varicocele. *Hum Reprod* 1997;12:64–67.
59. Agger P, Johnsen SG. Quantitative evaluation of testicular biopsies in varicocele. *Fertil Steril* 1978;29:52.
60. Andres TL, Trainer TD, Lapenas DJ. Small vessel alterations in the testes of infertile men with varicocele. *Am J Clin Pathol* 1981;76:378.
61. Jones MA, Sharp GH, Trainer TD. The adolescent varicocele: a histopathologic study of 13 testicular biopsies. *Am J Clin Pathol* 1988;89:321–328.
62. Saypol DC, Howards SS, Turner TT. Influence of surgically induced varicocele on testicular blood flow, temperature, and histology in adult rats and dogs. *J Clin Invest* 1981;68:39.
63. Dahl EV, Baggenstoss AH, DeWeerd JH. Testicular lesions of periarteritis nodosa with special reference to diagnosis. *Am J Med* 1960;218:222.
64. Lie JT. Isolated polyarteritis of testis in hairy-cell leukemia. *Arch Pathol Lab Med* 1988;112:646–647.
65. Shurbaji MS, Epstein JI. Testicular vasculitis: implications for systemic disease. *Hum Pathol* 1988;19:186–189.
66. Huisman TK, Collins WJ Jr, Voulgarakis GR. Polyarteritis nodosa masquerading as a primary testicular neoplasm: a case report and review of the literature. *J Urol* 1990;144:1236–1238.
67. Tartakoff J, Hazard JB. Thromboangitis obliterans of the spermatic cord. *N Engl J Med* 1938;218:173.
68. Montie JE, Stewart BH. Massive bladder hemorrhage after cystoscopy in a patient with secondary systemic amyloidosis. *J Urol* 1973;109:49.
69. Wong W, Strauss FH, Warner NE. Testicular biopsy in the study of male infertility. I. Testicular causes of infertility. II. Post-testicular causes of infertility. III. Pretesticular causes of infertility. *Arch Pathol* 1973;95:151, 160. 1974;98:1.
70. Zamboni L. The ultrastructural pathology of the spermatozoon as a cause of infertility: the role of electron microscopy in the evaluation of semen quality. *Fertil Steril* 1987;48:711–734.
71. Del Castillo EB, Trabucco A, De la Balze FA. Syndrome produced by absence of the germinal epithelium without impairment of the Sertoli or Leydig cells. *J Clin Endocrinol* 1947;7:493.
72. Klinefelter HF Jr, Reifenstein EC, Albright F. Syndrome characterized by gynecomastia, aspermatogenesis without a-Leydigism, and increased excretion of follicle stimulating hormone. *J Clin Endocrinol* 1942;8:615.
73. Ferguson-Smith, MA. Chromatin-positive Klinefelter's syndrome (primary microrchidism) in a mental-deficiency hospital. *Lancet* 1958;1:928.
74. Tournaye H, Staessen C, Liebaers, et al. Testicular sperm recovery in nine 47,XXY Klinefelter patients. *Hum Reprod* 1996 11:1644–1649.
75. Evans DB, Crichlow RW. Carcinoma of the male breast and Klinefelter's syndrome: is there an association? *CA Cancer J Clin* 1987;37:246.
76. Carroll PR, Morse MJ, Koduru PPK, Chaganti RSK. Testicular germ cell tumor in patient with Klinefelter syndrome. *Urology* 1988;31:72–74.
77. Baniel J, Perez JM, Foster RS. Benign testicular tumor associated with Klinefelter's syndrome. *J Urol* 1994;151:157–158.
78. Prall JA, McGavran L, Greffe BS, Partington MD. Intracranial malignant germ cell tumor and the Klinefelter syndrome: case report and review of the literature. *Pediatr Neurosurg* 1995;23:219–224.
79. De la Chapelle A. Analytic review: nature and origin of males with XX sex chromosomes. *Am J Hum Genet* 1972;24:71.
80. Pecile V, Filippi G. Screening for fra (X) mutation and Klinefelter syndrome in mental institutions. *Clin Genet* 1991;39:189–193.
81. Civantos F, Lubin J, Rywlin AM. Vasitis nodosa. *Arch Pathol* 1972;94:355.
82. Balogh K, Travis WD. Benign vascular invasion in vasitis nodosa. *Am J Clin Pathol* 1985;83:426.
83. Balogh K, Travis WD. The frequency of perineurial ductules in vasitis nodosa. *Am J Clin Pathol* 1984;82:710.
84. Taxy JB. Vasitis nodosa: two cases. *Arch Pathol Lab Med* 1973;102:643.
85. Jarow JP, Budin RE, Dym M, Zirkin BR, Noren S, Marshall FF. Quantitative pathologic changes in the human testis after vasectomy: a controlled study. *N Engl J Med* 1985;313:1252.
86. Silber SJ, Rodriguez-Rigau LJ. Quantitative analysis of testicular biopsy: determination of partial obstruction and prediction of sperm count after surgery for obstruction. *Fertil Steril* 1981;36:480–485.
87. Bhasin S, Swerdloff RS. Puberty. In: Rajfer J, ed. *Urologic endocrinology*. Philadelphia: WB Saunders, 1986:299–315.
88. Federman DD. Disorders of puberty in phenotypic males. In: *Abnormal sexual development*. Philadelphia: WB Saunders, 1968:162–178.
89. Glass AR, Vigersky RA. Hypogonadism. In: Rajfer J, ed. *Urologic endocrinology*. Philadelphia: WB Saunders, 1986:216–237.
90. Weiss J, Axelrod L, Whitcomb RW, Harris PE, Crowley WF, Jameson JL. Hypogonadism caused by a single amino acid substitution in the B subunit of luteinizing hormone. *N Engl J Med* 1992;326:179–183.
91. Burris AS, Rodbard HW, Winters SJ, Sherins RJ. Gonadotropin therapy in men with isolated hypogonadotropic hypogonadism: the response to human chorionic gonadotropin is predicted by initial testicular size. *J Clin Endocrinol Metab* 1988;66:1144–1151.
92. Liu L, Banks SM, Barnes KM, Sherins RJ. Two year comparison of testicular responses to pulsatile gonadotropin-releasing hormone and exogenous gonadotropins from the inception of therapy in men with isolated hypogonadotropic hypogonadism. *J Clin Endocrinol Metab* 1988;67:1140–1145.
93. McCullagh EP, Beck JC, Schaffenburg CA. A syndrome of eunuchoidism with spermatogenesis, normal urinary FSH and low or normal ICSH ("fertile eunuchs"). *J Clin Endocrinol Metab* 1953;13:489.
94. Faiman C, Hoffman DL, Ryan RJ, Albert A. The fertile eunuch syndrome: demonstration of isolated luteinizing hormone deficiency by radioimmunoassay technique. *Mayo Clin Proc* 1968;43:661.
95. Maroulis GB, Parlow AF, Marshall JR. Isolated follicle-stimulating hormone deficiency in man. *Fertil Steril* 1977;28:818.
96. Al-Ansari A-K, Khalil TH, Kelani Y, Mortimer CH. Isolated follicle-stimulating hormone deficiency in men: successful long term gonadotropin therapy. *Fertil Steril* 1984;42:618.
97. Schulze C. Response of the human testis to long term estrogen treatment: morphology of Sertoli cells, Leydig cells and spermatogonial cells. *Cell Tissue Res* 1988;251:31–43.
98. Gemzell C, Kjessler B. Treatment of infertility after partial hypophysectomy with human pituitary gonadotropins. *Lancet* 1964;1:644.
99. MacLeod J, Pazianos A, Ray BS. Restoration of human spermatogenesis by menopausal gonadotropins. *Lancet* 1964;1:1196.
100. Hammar M, Berg AA. Long term androgen replacement therapy does not preclude gonadotropin induced improvement of spermatogenesis. *Scand J Urol Nephrol* 1990;24:17–19.
101. Heseltine D, White MC, Kendall-Taylor P, DeKretser DM, Kelly W. Testicular enlargement and elevated serum inhibin concentrations occurring in patients with pituitary microadenomas secreting follicle stimulating hormone. *J Endocrinol* 1989;31:411–423.
102. Nistal M, Martinez-Garcia F, Regadera J, et al. Macro-orchidism: a clinicopathologic approach. *J Urol* 1994;151:1155–1161.
103. Chen CS, Chu SH, Laiym, et al. Reconsideration of testicular biopsy and follicle-stimulating hormone measurement in the era of intracytoplasmic sperm injection for non-obstructive azoospermia? *Hum Reprod* 1996;11:2176–2179.
104. Tournaye H, Liu J, Nagy PZ, et al. Correlation between testicular histology and outcome after intracytoplasmic sperm injection using testicular spermatozoa. *Hum Reprod* 1996;11:127–132.

105. Kolettis PN, Thomas AJ. Vasoepididymostomy for vasectomy reversal: A critical assessment in the era of intracytoplasmic sperm injection. *J Urol* 1997;158:467–470.
106. Hendin BN, Patel B, Levin HS, Thomas AJ, Agarwal A. Presence of spermatozoa and spermatids in the semen of men with germinal cell aplasia. *J Urol* 1997;157:448 (abstract).
107. Liu J, Lissens W, Silber S, et al. Birth after preimplantation diagnosis of the cystic fibrosis F508 mutation by polymerase chain reaction in human embryos resulting from intracytoplasmic sperm injection with epididymal sperm. *JAMA* 1994;272:1858–1860.
108. Berthelsen JG, Skakkebaek NE, von der Maase H, Sorensen BL. Screening for carcinoma in situ of the contralateral testis in patients with germinal testicular cancer. *Br Med J* 1982;285:1683.
109. Novero V Jr., Silber S, Goossens A, et al. Seminoma discovered in two males undergoing successful testicular sperm extraction for intracytoplasmic sperm injection. *Fertil Steril* 1996;65:1051–1054.
110. Nachman J, Palmer NF, Sather HN, et al. Open-wedge testicular biopsy in childhood acute lymphoblastic leukemia after two years of maintained therapy: diagnostic accuracy and influence on outcome: a report from Children's Cancer Study Group. *Blood* 1990;75:1051–1055.
111. Miller DR, Leikin SL, Albo VC, Sather H, Hammond GD. Three versus five years of maintenance therapy are equivalent in childhood acute lymphoblastic leukemia: a report from the Children's Cancer Study Group. *J Clin Oncol* 1989;7:316–325.
112. Levin HS, Thomas, AJ, Jr. Testicular biopsy. *AUA Update Series* 1985;4:2.
113. Turek PJ, Cha I, Ljung B-M. Systematic fine-needle aspiration of the testis: correlation to biopsy and results of organ mapping for mature sperm in azoospermic men. *Urology* 1997;49:743–748.
114. Kim ED, Greer JA, Abrams, et al. Testicular touch preparation cytology. *J Urol* 1996;156:1412–1414.
115. Harrington TG, Schauer D, Gilbert BR. Percutaneous testis biopsy: an alternative to open testicular biopsy in the evaluation of the subfertile man. *J Urol* 1996;156:1647–1651.
116. Rowley MJ, Heller CG. The testicular biopsy: surgical procedure, fixation, and staining techniques. *Fertil Steril* 1966;27:177.
117. Sigg C, Hedinger C. The frequency and morphology of giant spermatogonia in the human testis. *Virchows Arch Cell Pathol* 1983;44:115.
118. Buchanan JD, Fairley KF, Barrie JU. Return of spermatogenesis after stopping cyclophosphamide therapy. *Lancet* 1975;2:156.
119. Stricker S, Crosby K, Carey RW. Paternity after chemotherapy-induced sterility in Hodgkin's disease. *N Engl J Med* 1981;304:1175.
120. Dieckmann K-P, Loy V. Intratesticular effects of cisplatin-based chemotherapy. *Eur Urol* 1995;28:25–30.
121. Simmonds PD, Mead GM, Lee AHS, et al. Orchiectomy after chemotherapy in patients with metastatic testicular cancer. *Cancer* 1995;75:1018–1024.
122. Sussman A, Leonard JM. Psoriasis, methotrexate and oligospermia. *Arch Dermatol* 1980;116:215.
123. Shalet SM, Hann IM, Lendon M, Morris-Jones PH, Beardwell CG. Testicular function after combination chemotherapy in childhood for acute lymphocytic leukemia. *Arch Dis Child* 1981;56:275.
124. Lipshultz LI, Ross CE, Whorton D, Milby T, Smith R, Joyner RE. Dibromochloropropane and its effect on testicular function in man. *J Urol* 1980;124:464.
125. Nolte T, Harleman HJ, Jahn W. Histopathology of chemically induced testicular atrophy in rats. *Exp Toxic Pathol* 1995;47:267–286.
126. Strauss FH, II. The testis. In: Riddell RH, ed. *Pathology of drug induced and toxic diseases.* New York: Churchill Livingstone, 1982;279–295.
127. Liebow AA, Warren S, DeCoursey E. Pathology of atomic bomb casualties. *Am J Pathol* 1949;25:853.
128. Jordan SW. Late gonadal radiation effects. *Hum Pathol* 1971;2:551.
129. Rowley MJ, Leach DR, Warner GA, Heller CG. Effect of graded doses of ionizing radiation on the human testis. *Radiat Res* 1974;59:665.
130. Ash P. The influence of radiation on fertility in man. *Br J Radiol* 1980;53:271.
131. Hahn EW, Feingold SM, Simpson L, et al. Recovery from aspermia induced by low-dose radiation in seminoma patients. *Cancer* 1982;50:337.
132. Smithers DW, Wallace DM, Austin DE. Fertility after unilateral orchidectomy and radiotherapy for patients with malignant tumors of the testis. *Br J Med* 1973;4:77.
133. Hansen PV, Trykker H, Svennekjaer IL, Huolby J. Long term recovery of spermatogenesis after radiotherapy in patients with testicular cancer. *Radiother Oncol* 1990;18:117–125.
134. Giwercman A, von der Maase H, Berthelsen JG, et al. Localized irradiation of testes with carcinoma in situ: effects on Leydig cell function and eradication of malignant germ cells in 20 patients. *J Clin Endocrinol Metab* 1991;73:596–603.
135. Ogilvy-Stuart AL, Shalet SM. Effect of radiation on human reproductive system. *Environ Health Perspect Suppl* 1993;101 (suppl 2):109–116.
136. Pacini F, Gasperi M, Fugazzola L, et al. Testicular function in patients with differentiated thyroid carcinoma treated with radioiodine. *J Nucl Med* 1994;35:1418–1422.
137. Gooding GAW, Leonhardt W, Stein R. Testicular cysts: US findings. *Radiology* 1987;163:537–538.
138. Haas GP, Shumaker BP, Cerny JC. The high incidence of benign testicular tumors. *J Urol* 1986;136:1219–1220.
139. Nistal M, Iñiguez L, Paniagua R. Cysts of the testicular parenchyma and tunica albuginea. *Arch Pathol Lab Med* 1989;113:902–906.
140. Nistal M, Santamaria L, Paniagua R. Acquired cystic transformation of the rete testis secondary to renal failure. *Hum Pathol* 1989;20:1065–1070.
141. Madara JL, Haggitt RC, Federman M. Intranuclear inclusions of the human vas deferens. *Arch Pathol Lab Med* 1978;102:648–650.
142. Vendrely E. Histology of the epididymis in the human adult. *Prog Reprod Biol* 1981;8:21.
143. Berger RE. Sexually transmitted diseases. In: Walsh PC, Gittes RF, Perlmutter AD, Stamey TA, eds. *Campbell's urology.* 5th ed. Philadelphia: WB Saunders, 1986:900–946.
144. Mikuz G, Damjanov I. Inflammation of the testis, epididymis, peritesticular membranes and scrotum. In: Sommers SC, Rosen PP, eds. *Pathology annual.* Norwalk: Appleton-Century Crofts, 1982:101–128.
145. McCarthy JM, McLoughlin MG, Shackleton CR, et al. Cytomegalovirus epididymitis following renal transplantation. *J Urol* 1991;146:417–419.
146. Dalton ADA, Harcourt-Webster JN. The histopathology of the testis and epididymis in AIDS a post-mortem study. *J Urol* 191;163:47–52.
147. Mostofi FK, Price EP Jr. Tumors of the testis: tumors of the male genital system. In: Firminger H, *Atlas of tumor pathology,* second series, fascicle 8. Washington, DC: Armed Forces Institute of Pathology, 1973: 165.
148. Nistal M, Paniagua R. Disorders secondary to obstruction of the epididymis and vas deferens. In: Nistal M, Paniagua R, eds. *Testicular and epididymal pathology.* New York: Thieme Stratton, 1984:278–287.
149. Glassy FJ, Mostofi FK. Spermatic granulomas of the epididymis. *Am J Clin Pathol* 1956;26:1303.
150. Morgan AD. Inflammation and infestation of the testis and paratesticular structures. In: Pugh RC, ed. *Pathology of the testis.* Oxford: Blackwell Scientific, 1976:79–138.
151. Hunt AC, Bothwell PW. Histological findings in human brucellosis. *J Clin Pathol* 1967;20:267.
152. Kahn RI, McAninch JW. Granulomatous disease of the testis. *J Urol* 1980;23:868.
153. Hepper NGG, Karlson AG, Leary FJ, Soule EH. Genitourinary infection due to *Mycobacterium kansasii*. *Mayo Clin Proc* 1971;46:387.
154. Grabstald H, Swan LL. Genitourinary lesions in leprosy with special reference to the problem of atrophy of the testis. *JAMA* 1952;149:1287.
155. Monroe M. Granulomatous orchitis due to *Histoplasma capsulatum* masquerading as sperm granuloma. *J Clin Pathol* 1974;27:929.
156. Hironaga M, Okazaki N, Saito K, Watanabe S. *Trichophyton mentagrophytes* granulomas: unique systemic dissemination to lymph nodes, testes, vertebrae and brain. *Arch Dermatol* 1983;119:482.
157. Wolbach SB, Todd JC, Palfrey FW. *The etiology and pathology of typhus.* Cambridge: Harvard University Press, 1922:173, 216, 222.
158. Riggs S, Sanford JP. Viral orchitis. *N Engl J Med* 1962;266:990.
159. Craighead JE, Mahoney EM, Carver DH, Naficy K, Fremont-Smith P. Orchitis due to coxsackievirus group B, type 5. *N Engl J Med* 1962;267:498.
160. Gall EA. The histopathology of acute mumps orchitis. *Am J Pathol* 1947;23:637.
161. Werner CA. Mumps orchitis and testicular atrophy. *Ann Intern Med* 1950;32:1075.

162. Pessin SB. The lower urinary tract and male genitalia. In: Anderson WAD, ed. *Pathology.* 2nd ed. St Louis: CV Mosby, 1953:605–645.
163. Reichert CM, O'Leary TJ, Levens DL, Simrell CR, Macher AM. Autopsy pathology in acquired immunodeficiency syndrome. *Am J Pathol* 1983;112:357.
164. Welsh K, Finkbeiner W, Alpers CE, et al. Autopsy findings in the acquired immune deficiency syndrome. *JAMA* 1984;252:1152.
165. Nistal M, Santana A, Paniagua R, Palacios J. Testicular toxoplasmosis in two men with the acquired immunodeficiency syndrome (AIDS). *Arch Pathol Lab Med* 1986;110:744.
166. DePaepe ME, Guerrieri C, Waxman M. Opportunistic infections of the testis in the acquired immunodeficiency syndrome. *Mt Sinai J Med* 1990;57:25–29.
167. DaSilva M, Shevchuk MM, Cronin WJ, et al. Detection of HIV-related protein in testes and prostates of patients with AIDS. *Am J Clin Pathol* 1990;93:196–201.
168. Nuovo GJ, Becker J, Simsir A, et al. HIV-1 nucleic acids localize to the spermatogonia and their progeny: a study by polymerase chain reaction in situ hybridization. *Am J Pathol* 1994;144:1142–1148.
169. Wilkerson M, Carroll PR. Testicular carcinoma in patients positive and at risk for human immunodeficiency virus. *J Urol* 1990;144:1157.
170. Leibovitch I, Baniel J, Rowland RG, et al. Malignant testicular neoplasms in immunosuppressed patients. *J Urol* 1996;155:1938–1942.
171. Wegner HEH, Loy V, Dieckmann K-P. Granulomatous orchitis—analysis of clinical presentation, pathological anatomic features and possible etiologic factors. *Eur Urol* 1994;26:56–60.
172. Brown RC, Smith BH. Malacoplakia of the testis. *Am J Clin Pathol* 1965;43:409.
173. Robboy SJ, Welsh WR. Classification of intersex. In: *Weekly pathology update,* vol 1, 1980:1–8.
174. Rutgers JL, Scully RE. Pathology of the testis in intersex syndromes. *Semin Diagn Pathol* 1987;4:275–291.
175. Coulam CB. Testicular regression syndrome. *Obstet Gynecol* 1979;55:44–49.
176. Imbeaud S, Rey R, Berta P, et al. Testicular degeneration in three patients with the persistent müllerian duct syndrome. *Eur J Pediatr* 1995;154:187–190.
177. Patterson MN, McPhaul MJ, Hughes IA. Androgen insensitivity syndrome. *Baillieres Clin Endocrinol Metab* 1994;8:379–404.
178. Jockenhövel F, Rutgers JKL, Mason JS, et al. Leydig cell neoplasia in a patient with Reifenstein syndrome. *Exp Clin Endocrinol* 1993;101:365–370.
179. Schwal AR. Mixed gonadal dysgenesis: a variety of hermaphroditism. *Am J Hum Genet* 1963;15:155–158.
180. Davidoff F, Federman DD. Mixed gonadal dysgenesis. *Pediatrics* 1973;52:725–742.
181. Wallace TM, Levin HS. Mixed gonadal dysgenesis: a review of 15 patients reporting single cases of malignant intratubular germ cell neoplasia of the testis, endometrial adenocarcinoma, and a complex vascular anomaly. *Arch Pathol Lab Med* 1990;114:679–688.
182. Jorgensen N, Müller J, Jaubert, et al. Heterogeneity of gonadoblastoma germ cells: similarities with immature germ cells, spermatogonia and testicular carcinoma in situ cells. *Histopathology* 1997;30:177–186.
183. Young RH, Lawrence WD, Scully RE. Juvenile granulosa cell tumor: another neoplasm associated with abnormal chromosomes and ambiguous genitalia. *Am J Surg Pathol* 1985;9:737–743.

CHAPTER 47

Testicular and Paratesticular Tumors

Thomas M. Ulbright and Lawrence M. Roth

The testis measures about 4.5 × 2.5 × 3 cm and weighs 20 g (1). It is largely surrounded by a small extension of peritoneal cavity, the tunica vaginalis, with the visceral layer of this peritoneal sac lying on the tough fibrous capsule of the testis, the tunica albuginea. A small amount of fluid separates the visceral from the parietal layers of the tunica vaginalis, both of which are lined by mesothelium. The testicular parenchyma is mostly occupied by the seminiferous tubules with their components of various germ cells and Sertoli cells. The interstitium contains Leydig cells, blood and lymphatic vessels, fibroblasts, myofibroblasts, and occasional lymphocytes, plasma cells, and macrophages. The seminiferous tubules converge to empty into the rete testis at the testicular hilum, and these in turn anastomose with the efferent tubules that penetrate the tunica albuginea and coil to form the head of the epididymis. The epididymis is applied to much of the posterior surface of the testis and gives rise to the ductus (vas) deferens, which empties into the seminal vesicle.

Not unexpectedly, given the rapid proliferative rate of the self-renewing spermatogonia, the vast majority of testicular tumors are of germ cell origin and, like the totipotent germ cells from which they arise, may differentiate along several pathways. The distinction of seminoma from the nonseminomatous germ cell tumors remains of critical clinical importance. Tumors of nongerminal origin, while relatively uncommon, are frequent diagnostic problems, from the standpoint of both classification and prognosis. These include Leydig cell tumors, Sertoli cell tumors, granulosa cell tumors, and less specific forms of sex cord-stromal tumor. The non-Leydig cell elements of the testicular interstitium may also be sources for neoplasms, as may the ductal system

T. M. Ulbright: Department of Pathology, Indiana University School of Medicine, Indianapolis, Indiana, and Director of Anatomic Pathology, Indiana University Hospital, Indianapolis, Indiana 46202-5280.

L. M. Roth: Department of Pathology, Indiana University School of Medicine, Indianapolis, Indiana, and Director of Surgical Pathology, Indiana University Hospital, Indianapolis, Indiana 46202-5280.

of the testis. The mesothelium that lines the tunica vaginalis testis may give rise to mesotheliomas, as well as provide the basis, through müllerian metaplasia, for the formation of epithelial tumors more typically identified in the ovary. A distinctive form of mesothelioma with a benign natural history, the adenomatoid tumor, also derives from paratesticular mesothelium but is categorized separately. Mesothelium may also be the source for the recently described desmoplastic small round cell tumor of the paratestis (2). The paratesticular area has a rich component of supporting mesenchymal cells as well as embryonic remnants that allow for a truly diverse number of paratesticular tumors. A general classification of testicular and paratesticular neoplasms is shown in Table 1.

GROSS EXAMINATION

Ideally, orchiectomy specimens should be examined fresh as soon as possible following surgical excision. Far too often the excised testis with tumor is placed intact into a container with fixative, and the dissection delayed until a convenient time. The tunica albuginea is a formidable barrier to the penetration of fixative, and this approach leads to autolytic changes that can result in diagnostic confusion.

A radical orchiectomy typically consists of the testis and the surrounding tunica vaginalis with a variable length of spermatic cord. The specimen should be weighed, measured in three dimensions, and the length of the cord specified. We recommend submission of spermatic cord sections, including the margin of the cord, prior to incision of the testis in order to minimize artifactual contamination (3). The tunica vaginalis (parietal layer) should be inspected for irregularities and possible tumor penetration, and subsequently incised. Fluid present between the two layers of the tunica vaginalis should be noted. Any abnormalities of the tunica should be blocked for microscopic examination. With the opening of the tunica vaginalis, the external aspect of the testis (the tunica albuginea) becomes apparent, and it should be inspected for possible tumor transgression. Next, a sharp

TABLE 1. *Classification of testicular tumors*

I. Germ cell neoplasms (90–95%)[a]
II. Sex cord–stromal neoplasms (4%)
   A. Leydig cell tumor (3%)
   B. Sertoli cell tumor (1%)
      Variant: sclerosing Sertoli cell tumor
      Variant: large cell calcifying Sertoli cell tumor
   C. Sertoli-Leydig cell tumor (rare)
   D. Granulosa cell tumors (<1%)
      Variant: adult type (rare)
      Variant: juvenile type
   E. Tumors in the fibroma/thecoma group (rare)
   F. Mixed and indeterminant (unclassified) sex cord–stromal tumors (<1%)
III. Mixed germ cell–sex cord–stromal neoplasms (<1%)
   A. Gonadoblastoma (0.5%)
   B. Other mixed germ cell–sex cord–stromal tumors (rare)
IV. Tumors of "passenger" and non-Leydig, interstitial cells
   A. Lymphoma (? 1% as true primary neoplasm)
   B. Plasmacytoma (rare) and multiple myeloma
   C. Granulocytic sarcoma and leukemic infiltrates (rare as primary manifestation)
   D. Miscellaneous others, including epidermoid cysts, mesenchymal tumors, and metastatic tumors (1–2%)
V. Neoplastic and nonneoplastic "tumors" of the rete testis
   A. Cystic dysplasia
   B. Adenomatous hyperplasia
   C. Adenoma
   D. Adenocarcinoma
VI. Neoplastic and nonneoplastic "tumors" of the tunica albuginea and mesothelium
   A. Hydrocele
   B. Splenic-gonadal fusion
   C. Meconium periorchitis
   D. Nodular and diffuse fibrous proliferation
   E. Fibroma
   F. Fibrous tumor of pleural-type
   G. Mesothelioma
   H. Ovarian-type epithelial tumors
   I. Desmoplastic small round cell tumor
   J. Miscellaneous others
VII. Epididymal tumors
   A. Adenomatoid tumor
   B. Papillary cystadenoma
   C. Adenocarcinoma
   D. Melanotic neuroectodermal tumor of infancy
VIII. Spermatic cord tumors
   A. Lipoma
   B. Liposarcoma
   C. Rhabdomyosarcoma
   D. Aggressive angiomyxoma
   E. Angiomyofibroblastoma
   F. Miscellaneous (predominantly mesenchymal) tumors

[a] Estimated percentage of testicular tumors with primary manifestation in the testis; see Table 3 for germ cell tumor classification.

knife should be used to bisect the testis along its long axis in a plane that extends into the testicular hilum (i.e., toward the head of the epididymis). If desired, photographs and samples for electron microscopy and special studies (flow cytometry and cytogenetics) may be obtained at this point, although these are primarily for investigative rather than diagnostic purposes. Additional parallel cuts at 2- to 3-mm intervals should be made, followed by thorough fixation in a generous volume of fixative (10% neutral buffered formalin is adequate). After fixation, any tumor should be described and measured, and its relationship to the tunica albuginea and the hilar structures noted. Blocks of the different-appearing areas should be submitted, with a minimum number being one block per centimeter of maximum tumor dimension. Foci of hemorrhage and necrosis should be noted and included in the blocks for microscopic examination. We recommend at least ten blocks of cases that have the gross appearance of seminoma (or submission of all of the tumor, if it can be accomplished in ten blocks or less) because nonseminomatous elements can be identified focally in such cases and often determine an entirely different therapy. A block that includes the testicular hilum should be submitted. The epididymis should be incised by serial, parallel cuts from head to tail, any abnormalities noted, and an appropriate block submitted. Finally, a block of nonneoplastic testicular parenchyma should be submitted. Care must be taken during the entire dissection since testicular tumors are often cellular and friable, leading to artifactual implantation of tumor on surfaces and tissue spaces, including vascular lumina (3).

STAGING

Much of the clinicopathologic significance of testicular tumors hinges upon an understanding of the staging of testicular cancer. Unfortunately, no single system of staging has proved entirely satisfactory, and a variety of staging systems remain in use. Several of the more commonly used ones are summarized in Table 2. These systems recognize an early stage tumor (designated I or A) that is clinically confined to the testis; a stage of early dissemination (II or B) in which metastases are confined to the retroperitoneum; and a more advanced metastatic status (III or C) in which metastatic deposits are present above the diaphragm. Refinements of these basic categories may then take into account such factors as the number of metastases and overall size of the metastatic deposits (Table 2).

GERM CELL TUMORS

Classification

As seen in Table 1, the overwhelming majority of primary testicular tumors are of germ cell origin. A further subclassification of this group of testicular tumors is provided in Table 3. The classification in Table 3 represents a modification of the classification of the World Health Organization (WHO) (4) and is based on work originally performed by a number of contributors (5–9). Unfortunately, there remains a lack of uniform acceptance of the WHO classification, with a second major system stemming from the work of Collins and Pugh (10) in Great Britain. The classification of the British Testicular Tumour Panel (BTTP) recognizes two major categories

TABLE 2. Staging systems for testicular cancer

TNM system (AJCC and UICC)[a]		Stage grouping for AJCC/UICC system	
Tx	Unknown status of testis	Stage 0	Tis, N0, M0, S0
T0	No apparent primary (includes scars)	Stage IA	T1, N0, M0, S0
Tis	Intratubular tumor, no invasion	Stage IB	T2–T4, N0, M0, S0
T1	Testis and epididymis only; no vascular invasion or penetration of tunica albuginea	Stage IS	Any T, N0, M0, S1–S3
		Stage IIA	Any T, N1, M0, S0–S1
T2	Testis and epididymis with vascular invasion or through tunica albuginea to involve tunica vaginalis	Stage IIB	Any T, N2, M0, S0–S1
		Stage IIC	Any T, N3, M0, S0–S1
T3	Spermatic cord	Stage IIIA	Any T, any N, M1a, S0–S1
T4	Scrotum	Stage IIIB	Any T, any N, M0–M1a, S2
Nx	Unknown nodal status	Stage IIIC	Any T, any N, M0–M1a, S3; any T, any N, M1b, any S
N0	No regional node involvement		
N1	Node mass or single nodes ≤2 cm; ≤5 nodes involved		
N2	Single node 2–5 cm or multiple nodes ≤5 cm; >5 nodes positive		
N3	Node mass >5		
Mx	Unknown status of distant metastases		
M0	No distant metastases		
M1a	Nonregional nodal or lung metastases		
M1b	Distant metastasis other than nonregional nodal or lung metastases		
Sx	No marker studies available		
S0	All marker levels normal		

	LDH*	hCG (mIU/ml)	AFP (ng/ml)
S1	<1.5 × N +	<5,000 +	<1,000
S2	1.5–10 × N or	5,000–50,000 or	1,000–10,000
S3	>10 × N or	>50,000 or	>10,000

Boden/Gibb[b]	Memorial Sloan Kettering	Royal Marsden[c,d]	M.D. Anderson[e]	Skinner[f]	Mass. Gen.[g]
A Testis only	A Testis and adnexa only	I Testis only IM cont. positive serologic evidence of tumor after orchiectomy	I Testis only	A Testis only	I Testis only
B Regional nodal involvement	B Infradiaphragmatic nodal metastases		IIA Negative lymphangiogram but pathology positive reoperationed nodes	B Infradiaphragmatic involvement	II Retroperitoneal involvement
C Spread beyond retroperitoneal nodes	B1 <5 cm		IIB Positive lymphangiogram	B1 <6 nodes, no extranodal	IIA <2 cm
	B2 5 to 10 cm	II Infradiaphragmatic nodal involvement	IIIA Supraclavic. nodes	B2 >6 nodes or any node >2 cm	IIB ≥2 cm
	B3 >10 cm	IIA <2 cm	IIIB1 Gynecomastia lacking gross tumor	B3 Bulky disease (>5 cm)	III Supraclavicular and mediastinal involvement
	C Spread beyond retroperitoneal nodes	IIB 2 to 5 cm	IIIB2 Lung metastasis (no more than 5 nodules per lung and not >2 cm)	C Supradiaphragmatic involvement	
		IIC >5 cm	IIIB3 Advanced lung		
		III supraclavicular or mediastinal involvement	IIIB4 Advanced abdominal or obstructive uropathy		
		IV Extranodal metastases	IIIB5 Visceral disease, excluding lung		
		IVL Lung metastases			
		IVH Liver metastases			

AFP, alpha-fetoprotein; AJCC, American Joint Committee on Cancer; hCG, human chorionic gonadotropin; LDH, lactate dehydrogenase; Mass. Gen., Massachusetts General Hospital; TNM, tumor, nodes, metastases; UICC, Union Internationale Contra Cancre.

*LDH levels expressed as elevations above upper limit of normal (N).
[a]Reproduced from ref. 632, with permission.
[b]Adapted from ref. 633.
[c]Adapted from ref. 191.
[d]Adapted from ref. 634.
[e]Adapted from ref. 635.
[f]Adapted from ref. 636.
[g]Adapted from ref. 637.

TABLE 3. *Classification of testicular germ cell tumors*

Precursor lesion
    Intratubular germ cell neoplasia (unclassified type equivalent to carcinoma *in situ*)
Tumors of one histologic type
    Seminoma
        Variant: seminoma with syncytiotrophoblast cells
    Spermatocytic seminoma
        Variant: spermatocytic seminoma with a sarcomatous component
    Embryonal carcinoma
    Yolk sac tumor (Endodermal sinus tumor)
    Trophoblastic tumors
        Choriocarcinoma
            Variant: "monophasic" choriocarcinoma
        Placental site trophoblastic tumor
    Teratoma
        Mature teratoma
        Immature teratoma
        Teratoma with a secondary malignant component
        Monodermal variants
            Carcinoid (pure and with teratomatous elements)
            Primitive neuroectodermal tumor
            Others
Tumors of more than one histologic type
    Mixed germ cell tumors (specify individual components)
    Variants: polyembryoma and diffuse embryoma

TABLE 4. *Comparison of nomenclatures of the WHO-based system and the British Testicular Tumour Panel (BTTP) classification*

Modified WHO classification	BTTP classification
Tumors of one histologic type	
Seminoma	Seminoma
Spermatocytic seminoma	Spermatocytic seminoma
Embryonal carcinoma	Malignant teratoma, undifferentiated (MTU)
Yolk sac tumor	Yolk sac tumor (pure neoplasms only)
Teratoma	
Mature	Teratoma, differentiated (TD)
Immature	TD
With a sarcomatous or carcinomatous component	Malignant teratoma, intermediate (MTI)
Choriocarcinoma (pure)	Malignant teratoma, trophoblastic (MTT)
Mixed germ cell tumors	
Embryonal carcinoma & mature and/or immature teratoma	MTI
Yolk sac tumor & mature and/or immature teratoma	MTI
Seminoma and teratoma	Combined tumor (seminoma & TD)
Seminoma & embryonal carcinoma	Combined tumor (seminoma & MTU)
Choriocarcinoma & embryonal carcinoma	MTT
Choriocarcinoma & teratoma	MTT
Choriocarcinoma & seminoma	Combined tumor (MTT & seminoma)

Adapted from refs. 13 and 638.

of testicular germ cell tumors—seminoma and teratoma—with the further subdivision of the teratoma category into differentiated, intermediate, undifferentiated, and trophoblastic types (11). The basis for the BTTP classification appears to be the incorrect concept that seminomas are of germ cell origin but that other tumors (i.e., those in the teratoma category) are derived from embryonically displaced blastomeres (12). A comparison of the two classifications is shown in Table 4. We continue to urge the use of the modified WHO system, since it not only is based on histogenetically correct concepts but also permits comparison of therapies for similar entities, unlike the BTTP classification that "lumps" dissimilar entities under a common nomenclature (13).

Histogenesis

The histogenetic relationships among the various morphologic types of germ cell tumors has been a matter of continued interest and controversy. Recent evidence from ultrastructural (14), cytogenetic (15), and ploidy analyses (15–18) suggests that the traditional scheme (Fig. 1) of two divergent pathways leading to seminoma and embryonal carcinoma is incorrect. Instead there are numerous observations to support that seminoma may act as a common precursor lesion, having developed from intratubular germ cell neoplasia (IGCN), that may then transform into embryonal carcinoma or, more rarely, directly into other forms of germ cell tumor such as yolk sac tumor (19) and choriocarcinoma. Embryonal carcinoma may also (apparently more commonly) transform to these other forms of germ cell tumor. The basis for considering seminoma the common precursor includes

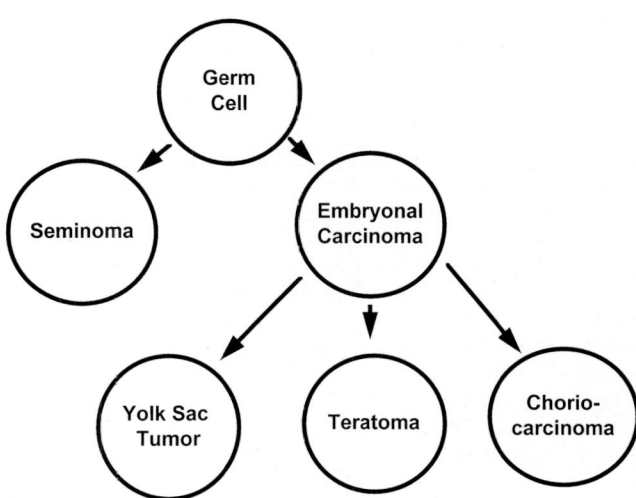

FIG. 1. Traditional model of testicular germ cell tumor histogenesis hypothesizes that seminoma and embryonal carcinoma form by two divergent pathways, and that other types of germ cell tumor are derived from embryonal carcinoma. (Adapted from ref. 14, with permission.)

the ultrastructural identification of epithelial differentiation in some seminomas (14) and the higher ploidy values of seminoma compared to the nonseminomatous tumors (15–18)—an observation consistent with the loss of cancer suppressor genes as a mechanism for evolution to the nonseminomatous tumors. Morphologic observations support apparent direct transformation of seminoma to yolk sac tumor (19) and embryonal carcinoma (5). Furthermore, the common presence of a distinctive karyotypic abnormality—isochromosome (12p)—in IGCN, seminoma, and the nonseminomatous tumors (15) implies a common sequence of origin stemming from IGCN. It is furthermore logical to consider seminoma the invasive derivative of IGCN (unclassified type[IGCNU], see below) given the strikingly similar morphology, immunohistochemistry, ultrastructure, DNA content, content of nucleolar organizer regions, and lectin binding patterns of these two lesions (15,18,20–25). It therefore seems most reasonable to believe that germ cell tumors begin as IGCNU that may then pursue several courses: (a) extratubular invasion (which we recognize as seminoma) that may either remain stable or transform to nonseminomatous tumors; (b) simultaneous extratubular invasion and transformation to nonseminomatous tumors (i.e. an extremely transient seminoma phase); and (c) intratubular transformation into nonseminomatous neoplasms that subsequently invade the interstitium. Srigley and co-workers (14) proposed a new model of histogenesis for testicular germ cell tumors that appears to accommodate most of these considerations. We have further modified it to account for certain aberrant observations involving childhood germ cell tumors, to incorporate the key role of IGCNU in this process, and to allow for specific forms of intratubular differentiation (Fig. 2).

Epidemiology

Germ cell tumors of the testis have an interesting, although poorly understood, epidemiology. First of all, they occur predominantly (with the exception of spermatocytic seminoma) in young men—most commonly from 15 to 45 years of age—although a smaller peak occurs in childhood, and there are rare cases that occur in the elderly. For unclear reasons, the incidence of testicular germ cell tumors has increased progressively in the 20th century, as verified by independent studies in several different countries (26–29), with the exception of cohorts born during World War II in Nazi-occupied countries (30), thought, perhaps, to be related to poor nutrition. Some authorities consider this increase to be of epidemic proportions. The most recent annual incidences are on the order of 9 per 100,000 male population in

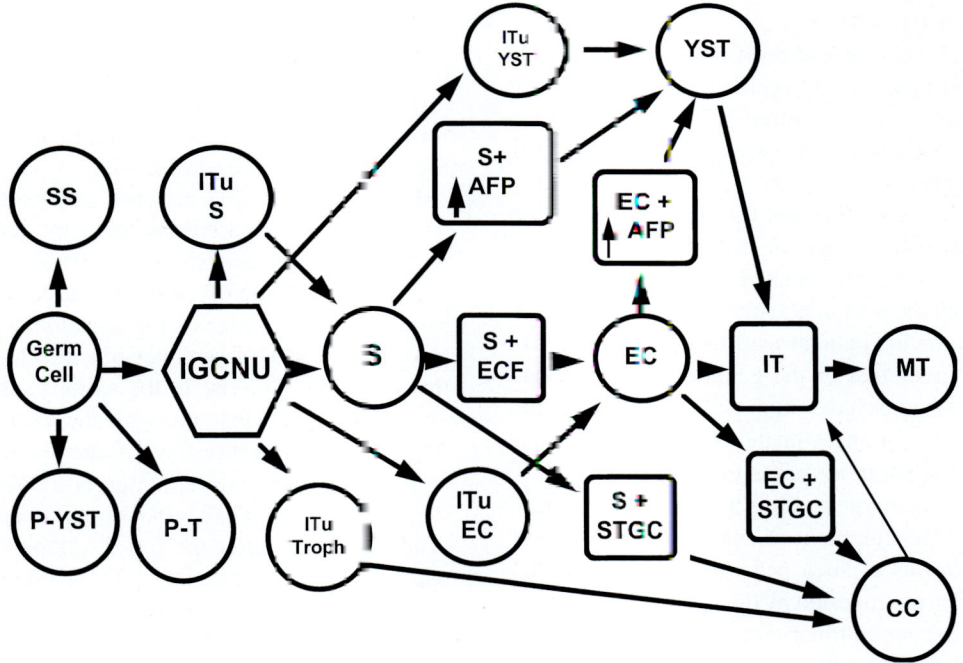

FIG. 2. New model of testicular germ cell tumor histogenesis. IGCNU represents the common precursor lesion to the vast majority of germ cell tumors (excluding, however, spermatocytic seminoma and perhaps the pediatric forms of yolk sac tumor and teratoma). Invasion of IGCNU results in seminoma that may then transform into a variety of other germ cell tumor types, with intermediate phases being recognized. In some instances, there is intratubular transformation of IGCNU into nonseminomatous forms, which may then also invade the interstitium. (Modified from ref. 631.) AFP, alpha-fetoprotein; CC, choriocarcinoma; EC, embryonal carcinoma; ECF, early carcinomatous features; IGCNU, intratubular germ cell neoplasia, unclassified; IT, immature teratoma; ITu, intratubular; P-T, pediatric teratoma; P-YST, pediatric yolk sac tumor; S, seminoma; SS, spermatocytic seminoma; STGC, syncytiotrophoblast giant cells; T, teratoma; Troph, trophoblast cells; YST, yolk sac tumor; *thin arrow,* more speculative step; smaller print indicates rare lesions.

Denmark and Switzerland, the countries with the highest rates of testicular germ cell tumors, but the annual incidence in the United States white population is not far behind, on the order of 5 to 6 per 100,000 male population. Racial variations in the incidence of testicular cancer are quite apparent—the nonwhite populations in the United States have a substantially lower incidence than does the white population. In fact, the only nonwhite population with a comparably high incidence is the Maoris of New Zealand (31,32). Testicular germ cells tumors furthermore occur more commonly among professional workers and those of higher socioeconomic class than among laborers and those of lower socioeconomic class (29,33–37). Isolated reports have implicated exposures to certain agents or association with particular occupations as being of potential etiologic importance (29,33,34,38–41), but no consistent pattern has emerged from a variety of studies (31,37). Exposure to estrogenic compounds *in utero* is implicated in some studies (42), as is a familial history of breast cancer (43), early birth order (44), certain human leukocyte antigen (HLA) haplotypes (45–47), Marfan syndrome (48), Down syndrome (48,49), and the dysplastic nevus syndrome (50). Klinefelter's syndrome does not appear to be associated with testicular germ cell tumors but is positively associated with mediastinal germ cell tumors (48,51). No linkage of testicular cancer with smoking, alcohol consumption, radiation exposure, or prior vasectomy is established (31,52).

There are several well-defined positive associations with testicular germ cell tumors: (a) cryptorchidism, (b) a prior testicular germ tumor, (c) a familial history of testicular germ cell tumors, (d) certain intersex syndromes, and (e) oligospermic infertility.

Cryptorchidism remains the best established risk factor for testicular germ cell tumors. In many series, approximately 10% of the cases are associated with past (corrected) or present cryptorchidism (53–59). Increased risk for testis cancer among cryptorchid patients is most commonly calculated at 10 to 14 times that of the general population, although more recent studies have suggested that a fourfold elevated risk is a more accurate estimate (60). The mechanism by which cryptorchidism predisposes to germ cell tumor is unclear, but it has been suggested it is a marker for generalized embryonic maldevelopment of the genitourinary system, and that the testes of such patients are "dysgenetic" (61). This conclusion is supported by the association of cryptorchidism with other genitourinary tract anomalies (62–64), and the finding of a bilaterally elevated risk for testicular germ cell tumors in patients with unilateral cryptorchidism (65–68). The failure of orchidopexy, at least in most studies, to reduce the elevated risk is supportive of this hypothesis (59,65,69).

Because of the elevated risk of cryptorchid patients for testicular germ cells tumors, it has been suggested that they have diagnostic testicular biopsies to evaluate for the presence of the precursor lesion, IGCNU (see below). Such biopsies appear to be a worthwhile procedure in cryptorchid patients; IGCNU is detected in from 2% to 8% of such patients (70–74). Follow-up studies of patients with IGCNU have verified a high rate of development of invasive testicular germ cell tumors—(50% at 5 years (75))—but an essential absence of invasive germ cell tumors in cryptorchid patients with negative biopsies (72). Such biopsies should be bilateral, and the suggested time is between ages 18 and 20 years, since the reliability of identifying IGCNU at an earlier age is in doubt (73).

Patients with a prior history of testicular germ cell tumor are at increased risk for the development of another germ cell tumor in the residual testis—from 2% to 5% of such patients developed bilateral tumors (76–79). There is an especially increased risk if the residual testis is atrophic or cryptorchid (80,81) or there is a family history of testicular cancer (82,83). Intervals of more than a decade may occur between such metachronous testicular cancers (84), although some may present synchronously, and 50% of second tumors occur within 3 to 5 years (76,81). Again, biopsy of the remaining testis appears to be an effective method of identifying patients at risk for a second primary testicular germ cell tumor (85). Some advocate biopsy of the opposite testis at the initial orchiectomy (86).

There is growing evidence of a familial basis to some testicular germ cell tumors (87–89), with an approximate 2% frequency of testicular cancer in the first-degree male relatives of patients with testicular germ cell tumors compared to 0.4% in a control population (90). Patients with testicular cancer and a familial history are at apparent increased risk for bilateral tumors, with bilateral involvement occurring in 8% to 14% of such cases (82,87).

It is also clear that patients with certain intersex syndromes are at increased risk for germ cell tumors. Patients with gonadal dysgenesis who carry a Y chromosome develop germ cell tumors at an increased rate—most often in association with a preexisting gonadoblastoma (91,92). Approximately 30% of such patients develop gonadoblastoma that may then give rise to the various subtypes of invasive germ cell tumor. Patients with the androgen insensitivity (testicular feminization) syndrome should also be considered at increased risk, although at a somewhat lesser rate (93,94). Most germ cell tumors in the androgen insensitivity syndrome occur after the full development of female secondary sexual characteristics (93,95), but occasional cases are reported in younger patients (96), making the timing of prophylactic gonadectomy somewhat controversial. Gonadal biopsy may successfully identify IGCNU in at-risk patients with gonadal dysgenesis and the androgen insensitivity syndrome (97,98), even during childhood (99).

The independent linkage of testicular germ cell tumors with oligospermic infertility remains less well established than with the other four factors. There is no question that male infertility patients have an elevated risk of testis cancer, with IGCNU being identified in about 1% of such patients (74,100–102). The association of cryptorchidism and gonadal dysgenesis with infertility, however, complicates this analysis, thus casting doubt that infertility is an independent risk factor (103).

Intratubular Germ Cell Neoplasia

The term *intratubular germ cell neoplasia* (IGCN) refers both to a lesion that was originally described by Skakkebaek as "carcinoma *in situ*" of the testis, as well as to differentiated forms of intratubular germ cell tumor. The more commonly occurring lesion described by Skakkebaek is now subcategorized as intratubular germ cell neoplasia unclassified (IGCNU) because it is associated with the entire spectrum of germ cell tumors, with the exception of spermatocytic seminoma. The term *carcinoma in situ* is no preferred because IGCNU is not an epithelial lesion. When patients with IGCNU were prospectively followed, invasive germ cell tumors developed in 50% by 5 years of follow-up (104). In additional support of its precursor role, IGCNU is identified at increased frequency in patients known to be at increased risk for testicular germ cell tumors. Thus, IGCNU is identified in 2% to 8% of cryptorchid patients (70–74); in 5% of the contralateral testes of patients with a prior testicular germ cell tumor (85,105); in 0.4% to 1% of patients with infertility (100–102); and at high rates in selected cases of gonadal dysgenesis and the androgen insensitivity syndrome (97,106). IGCNU is also observed in virtually all cases of invasive germ cell tumors of the testis in adults if residual seminiferous tubules are present (107–109), although it is not seen with spermatocytic seminoma (75). Furthermore, its association with the childhood forms of testicular germ cell tumor (yolk sac tumor and teratoma) is controversial, with some studies claiming an absence of associated IGCNU in these cases (110,111), but others disputing this absence (112,113). (One can at least say the association of IGCNU with childhood testicular germ cell tumors is much less conspicuous than in postpubertal patients.)

In postpubertal patients, IGCNU most commonly appears as germ cells with enlarged, hyperchromatic nuclei and clear cytoplasm (often having retraction artifact in formalin-fixed material) aligned along the basal portion of the seminiferous tubules (Fig. 3). Nucleoli are conspicuous, and mitoses are frequent. The Sertoli cells are often displaced toward the lumen, and spermatogenesis in the affected segment of tubule is almost always absent (Fig. 3), although it may appear normal in adjacent tubules. The affected tubules usually have thickened peritubular basement membranes. As IGCNU progresses, the Sertoli cells may be replaced and a pattern resembling so-called intratubular seminoma may develop. Pagetoid spread of IGCNU into the rete testis is common (114). Although there is little experience with IGCNU in children, rare cases suggest that the neoplastic cells are not basally located in the prepubertal testis but are dispersed at various levels, with the more typical pattern evolving as the patient ages (75,115).

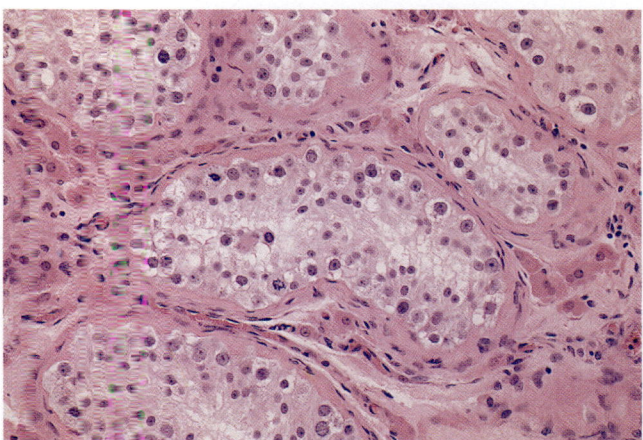

FIG. 3. IGCNU consisting of cells with enlarged nuclei, prominent nucleoli, and clear cytoplasm along the basal aspect of seminiferous tubules lacking spermatogenesis. Sertoli cells are displaced toward the lumen.

The great majority of cases of IGCNU are periodic acid-Schiff (PAS)-positive (Fig. 4), diastase-sensitive (109), but similar positivity may also be identified in nonneoplastic spermatogonia and Sertoli cells (116). A more specific method is immunostaining with antibodies directed against placental alkaline phosphatase; placental-like alkaline phosphatase (PLAP) was detected in 231 of 237 (97%) cases of IGCNU in several series (116–119). Unlike PAS stains, PLAP-positivity did not occur in nonneoplastic spermatogonia, although very rare cases showed very focal PLAP-positivity in spermatocytes (119). PLAP staining is usually membrane accentuated (Fig. 5). Antibodies M2A and 43-9F and those with specificities against glutathione S-transferase and the *c-kit* proto-oncogene have also successfully identified IGCNU with very high sensitivities (21,120–123). Several ultrastructural studies of IGCNU have identified features similar to those of seminoma (74,124–127); another study noted a similar distribution of nucleolar organizing regions in IGCNU and seminoma (23).

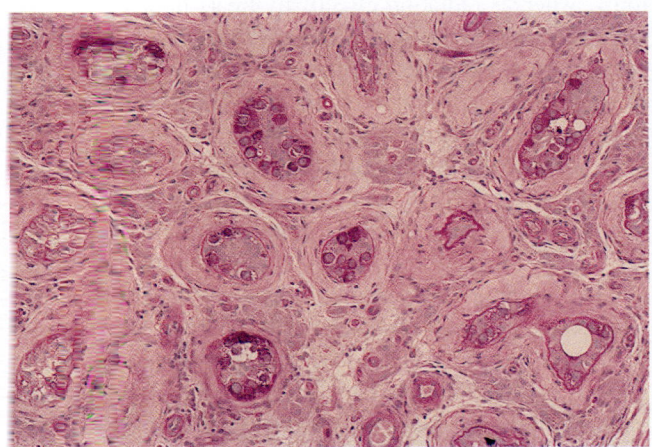

FIG. 4. Strong PAS-positivity in IGCNU.

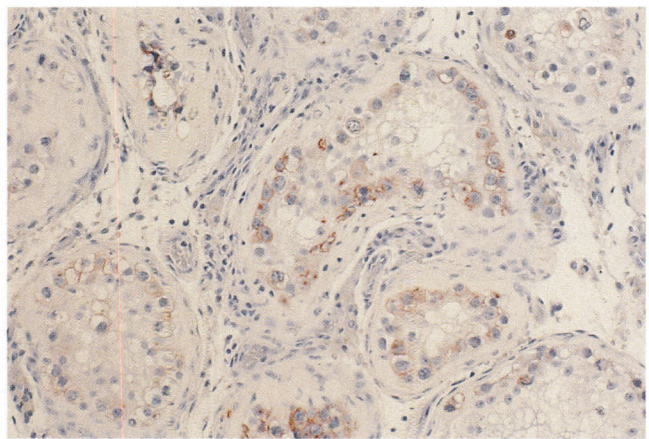

FIG. 5. PLAP-positivity in IGCNU with the characteristic membranous pattern.

Testicular biopsies detect IGCNU in at-risk patients with a high sensitivity, and the recommended approach is to take one or two 3-mm biopsies per testis (128). A negative result on adequate biopsies is excellent reassurance of no increased risk of testicular cancer since only one patient among more than 1,500 with negative biopsies for IGCNU developed a germ cell tumor in follow-up studies extending to 8 years (86). It remains controversial as to whom should be screened; many authorities suggest screening biopsies in patients with a history of cryptorchidism, prior testicular cancer, and somatosexual ambiguity in the presence of a Y chromosome. The need to biopsy patients with oligospermic infertility is not clear (86). Such bilateral screening biopsies in cryptorchidism should generally be performed in late adolescence (86). There is a much greater probability of a positive biopsy for IGCNU in the presence of testicular atrophy (86).

The treatment of IGCNU is controversial. Because of the high rate of progression to an invasive tumor, there is a growing tendency to recommend intervention rather than close follow-up. Unilateral IGCNU is treated by orchiectomy, whereas radiation effectively treats bilateral IGCNU but also causes permanent sterility. In patients with IGCNU opposite a testis with an invasive germ cell tumor, the chemotherapy administered for the invasive tumor has sometimes eradicated the contralateral IGCNU, but this is not a consistently effective form of treatment (86,129–131).

Seminoma

Pure seminoma (including cases with scattered trophoblastic elements) represents about 50% of all testicular germ cell tumors (132,133) and occurs at an average age of 40 years (132), which is 5 to 10 years older than patients with nonseminomatous germ cell tumors (5,132). Seminoma is very rare in children (134). Between 80% and 90% of patients with seminoma have initial symptoms of testicular swelling or other palpable abnormalities (11,135), and testicular pain occurs in about 10% to 20% of cases (11,135). Presenting symptoms secondary to metastases, most commonly lumbar back pain due to retroperitoneal spread, are relatively unusual, occurring in about 1% to 3% of cases (11,135). Only rare patients may develop gynecomastia due to elevations of human chorionic gonadotropin (hCG) secondary to intermixed trophoblastic elements. Paraneoplastic exophthalmos is rarely described (136,137). There may be a higher proportion of seminomas among cryptorchid patients with germ cell tumors than in the general population with testicular germ cell tumors (53).

Serum hCG levels are mildly to moderately elevated in about 10% of patients with clinical stage I seminoma and in about 25% of patients with metastatic involvement (138), although testicular vein hCG is elevated in a much higher proportion of cases (139). Elevated serum hCG correlates with trophoblast cells in the tumor. Alpha-fetoprotein (AFP) is not produced by seminoma cells, and an elevated serum AFP in a patient with an apparently pure seminoma is generally indicative of nonsampled nonseminomatous elements, although mild AFP elevation may reflect liver disease, including metastatic hepatic involvement (140) and, in one study, were not associated with a different behavior (141). Serum PLAP levels are also elevated in about 50% of patients with seminoma (142).

The cut surface of the tumor is cream-colored to tan to pink and lobulated to multinodular (Fig. 6), with a fleshy quality and a tendency to bulge above the surrounding parenchyma. Punctate foci of hemorrhage may correspond to foci of syncytiotrophoblast cells (143). Well-defined foci of yellow necrosis may be present, but extensive hemorrhage and necrosis are unusual. Extension through the tunica albuginea or into the epididymis occurs in less than 10% of cases (9).

On microscopic examination seminomas may show a diffuse, sheet-like pattern (Fig. 7) or a confluent multinodular

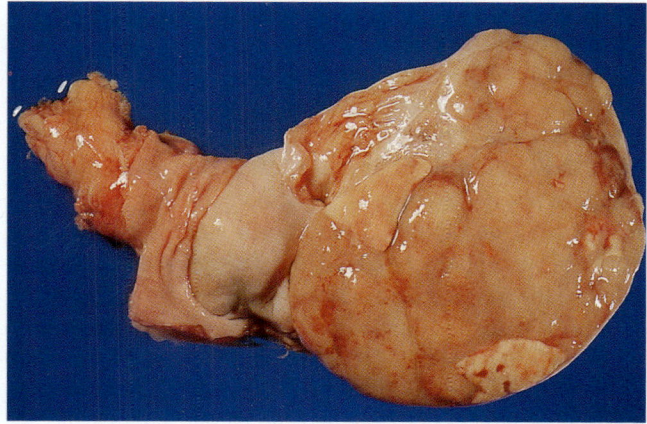

FIG. 6. Seminoma with a light tan, lobulated cut surface. Punctate foci of hemorrhage may indicate intermixed syncytiotrophoblast elements. Note small focus of necrosis at bottom. (Photograph courtesy of S.F. Cramer, M.D., Rochester General Hospital, Rochester, New York.)

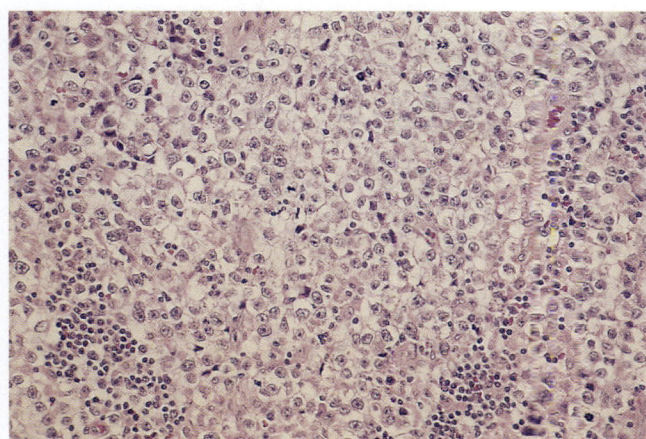

FIG. 7. Seminoma with sheet-like arrangement of cells with clear cytoplasm, well-defined cell membranes, and nuclei with prominent, central nucleoli. Note lymphoid infiltrate.

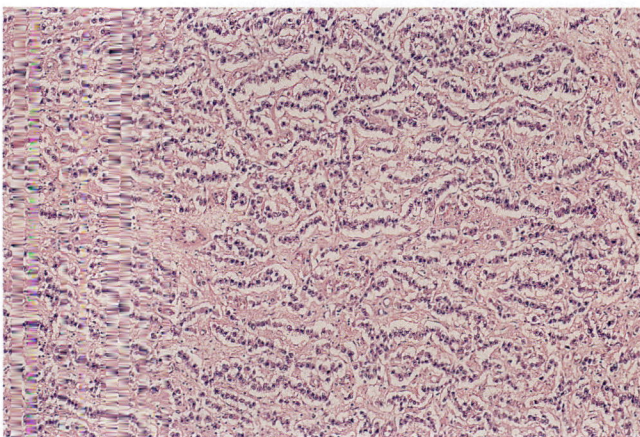

FIG. 9. Seminoma with cords of tumor cells.

pattern (Fig. 8). There often is an interstitial pattern at the periphery of the tumor as neoplastic cells surround but do not destroy seminiferous tubules. In some cases tubular preservation persists in the center of the neoplasm. A peripheral, cord-like pattern reflects the tendency for interstitial growth (Fig. 9) that is occasionally predominant. Branching, fibrous septa often course through seminomas (Fig. 8). Extensive zones of scarring may occur, with obliteration of major portions of the tumor. Rarely a tubular (or pseudotubular) pattern may occur, usually as a focal finding (144,145) (Fig. 10).

Seminoma cells characteristically have clear to lightly eosinophilic cytoplasm and central nuclei, often with slightly squared edges, and one or two large central nucleoli (Fig. 7). The cells are closely apposed, with well-defined cytoplasmic borders. An abundant amount of cytoplasm causes the nuclei to be well spaced and nonoverlapping (Fig. 7). In poorly fixed specimens, however, cytoplasmic autolysis occurs, obscuring the cell borders and causing apparent nuclear overlapping, thus creating confusion with solid patterns of embryonal carcinoma (see below).

Lymphocytic infiltrates occur in virtually all seminomas. They are often most intense in and around the fibrous trabeculae but also intermingle with the tumor cells (Figs. 7 and 8). Germinal center formation can develop in some cases, but most of the lymphoid elements mark as T cells (146–150), have gamma/delta receptors (151), and appear to produce a cytotoxic effect on the tumor (152) and promote granuloma formation (151). A granulomatous reaction occurs in up to 50% of the cases (9) and varies from scattered clusters of epithelioid histiocytes to well-defined granulomas with characteristic Langhans giant cells. An extensive granulomatous reaction can, in rare cases, obliterate almost all evidence of the underlying seminoma, thus causing a misdiagnosis of granulomatous orchitis (see chapter by Levin). It is therefore crucial to examine closely any testis with an extensive granulomatous reaction for residual seminoma cells before accepting such a case as granulomatous orchitis. PLAP immunostains can prove useful (see below) in identifying residual seminoma cells in this circumstance.

Edema may occur in seminomas, with the separation of tumor cells by small, cystic spaces (Fig. 11). This pattern may therefore mimic the microcystic pattern of yolk sac tumor;

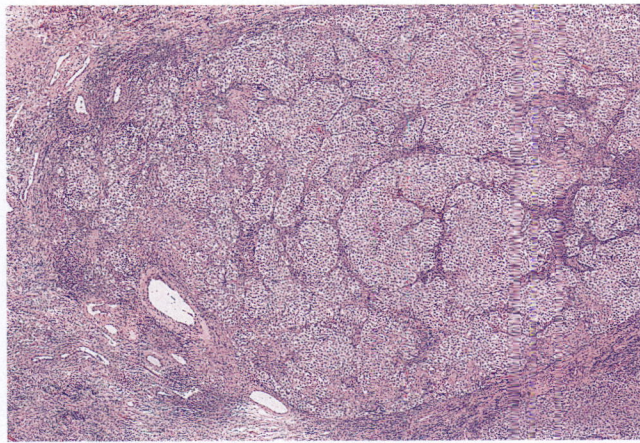

FIG. 8. Multinodular seminoma with subdivision of nodules by branching, fibrous septa containing lymphocytes.

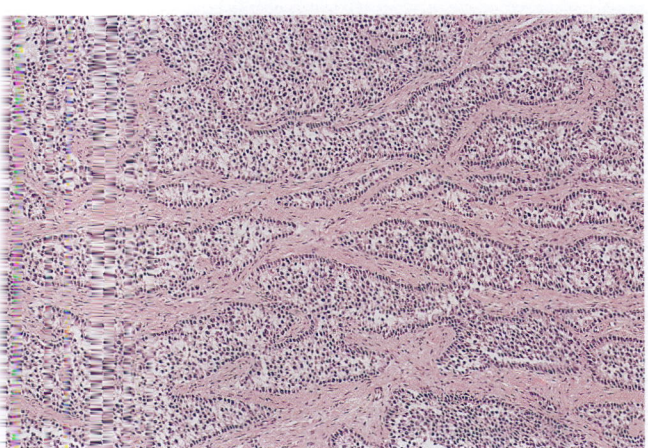

FIG. 10. "Tubular" pattern in seminoma that must be distinguished from Sertoli cell tumor.

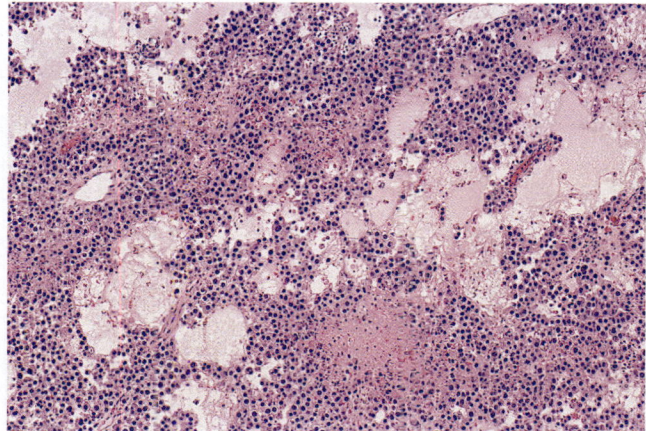

FIG. 11. Edema in seminoma causing a microcystic pattern. Note the irregular shapes of the cysts and the exfoliated cells within some of them.

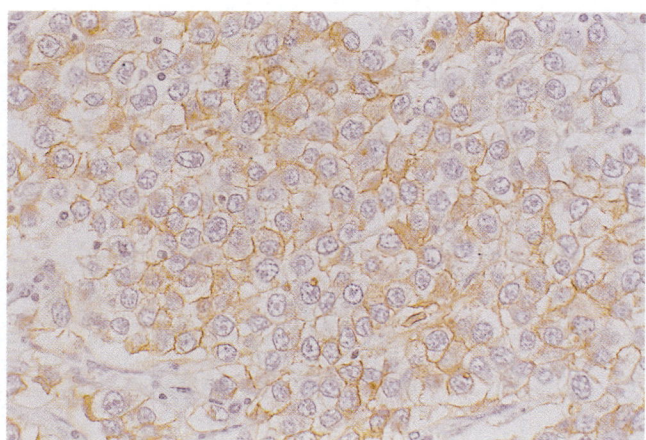

FIG. 13. PLAP-positivity in a seminoma showing the typical membrane-accentuated pattern.

distinction can usually be made based on the typical seminomatous appearance of the surrounding tumor and the more irregular nature of the cystic spaces, with the frequent presence of intracystic, exfoliated seminomatous cells and edema fluid.

In up to 20% of seminomas, larger trophoblast cells are identified in a scattered pattern (153,154). Sometimes these cells have a distinctly syncytiotrophoblastic appearance with multinucleation and/or intracytoplasmic lacunae (Fig. 12). In other cases they appear as large mononucleated cells. They are often located adjacent to capillaries and may be associated with microfoci of hemorrhage. A nodular growth of trophoblast cells is lacking, which, in conjunction with the absence of a cytotrophoblast component, permits distinction from choriocarcinoma.

Most seminomas contain glycogen, and PAS stains are usually positive. PLAP immunostains are positive, usually with a membrane-accentuated pattern, in up to 98% of cases (116,155–157) (Fig. 13). Seminomas may also contain cytokeratins 8 and 18 (158) and less commonly cytokeratins 4, 17, and 19 (159–161). Intermingled trophoblast cells are positive for cytokeratins 8, 18, and 19 (159). Positivity of seminomas with antibodies directed against cytokeratins 8 and 18 (e.g., CAM 5.2) may therefore be seen [usually in isolated cells but rarely more diffusely (156,160,162)] in up to 73% of cases (159). Most routinely processed seminomas, however, are negative with broad-spectrum cytokeratin antibodies lacking these specificities, although such antibodies generally produce strong and diffuse staining in nonseminomatous germ cell tumors. The combination of PLAP-positivity and AE1/AE3 negativity (in paraffin sections) can assist in the diagnosis of seminoma (163). Immunostains for hCG highlight the intermingled trophoblast cells seen in some seminomas (153,154,156,164,165).

On electron microscopic study, seminomas are primitive cells, often having large aggregates of glycogen and simple cellular organelles that are polarized in the cytoplasm (14,166,167). Cell membranes are closely apposed, but junctions are usually primitive and few. The nuclei have intricate nucleoli but an evenly dispersed euchromatin. Srigley and co-workers (14) described seminomas with epithelial differentiation, including well-defined desmosomes and surface microvilli.

Seminomas have a DNA index of 1.66 (16), which is significantly higher than in nonseminomatous tumors (16,18). In addition, isochromosome (12p) or other chromosome 12 anomalies are identified on karyotypic analysis (168–170).

Differential Diagnosis

Solid patterns of embryonal carcinoma may be confused with seminoma. Poorly defined cell borders, nuclear overlapping, and nuclear irregularity and pleomorphism are features of embryonal carcinoma that differ from well-fixed seminomas. Furthermore, embryonal carcinomas lack the regular fibrous septa of seminoma. Cytokeratin stains may also prove useful in this differential diagnosis (see above). It is clear that some seminomas have more pleomorphic foci

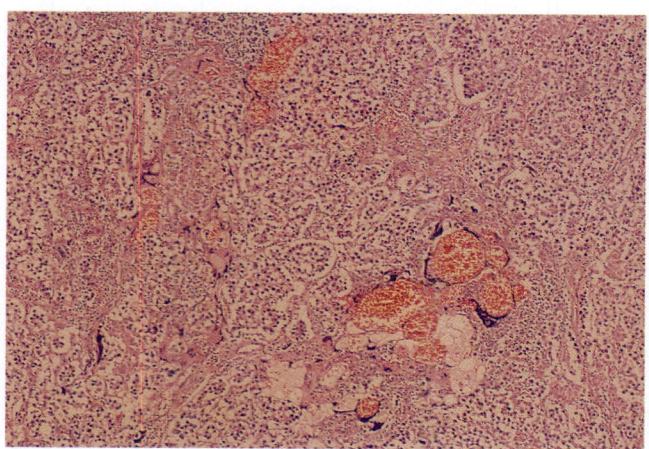

FIG. 12. Seminoma with syncytiotrophoblast cells having lacunae with red blood cells.

than others; we require, however, definite evidence of epithelial differentiation in the form of papillae or glands or disproportionate cytokeratin reactivity in the pleomorphic zones before recognizing nonseminomatous differentiation.

Solid patterns of yolk sac tumor may also resemble seminoma, but these are usually associated with more characteristic yolk sac tumor patterns. If only a small biopsy is available, solid pattern yolk sac tumor often shows suggestions of true microcyst formation, unlike seminoma. (The edematous seminoma with cystic areas has already been discussed.) Cytokeratin stains may also prove useful in difficult cases, with yolk sac tumor being positive for AE1/AE3 and seminoma often being negative or only focally and weakly positive in routinely processed sections. AFP stains are also frequently positive in yolk sac tumor and are negative in seminoma. Hyaline globules and intercellular basement membrane are commonly identified in yolk sac tumor and are almost never seen in seminomas (171). Lymphomas involving the testis may be confused with seminoma. Although primary testicular lymphomas do occur, most cases of testicular involvement represent spread from an extratesticular site. Bilateral involvement in an older patient is a clinical feature in favor of lymphoma over seminoma (172–176). Paratesticular involvement on gross examination is more common in lymphoma (176). Lymphomas often have an extensive interstitial pattern with relative tubular preservation (173,174,177) and usually lack the clear cytoplasm and well-defined cell borders of seminoma. The nuclei of lymphomas are frequently irregular and less uniform than those of seminoma. The great majority of seminomas are associated with IGCNU, but lymphomas are not. PLAP immunostains are positive in most seminomas but are negative in lymphomas (163), whereas lymphoid markers show the opposite pattern (156). The distinction of seminoma with a tubular pattern from Sertoli cell tumor is discussed below.

Seminomas are extremely sensitive to radiation and chemotherapy, and these modalities represent the primary forms of treatment following orchiectomy. Most patients with clinical stage I seminoma receive radiation directed at the ipsilateral inguinal and iliac lymph nodes as well as to the abdominal paraaortic and paracaval nodes. Recent studies suggest that early stage patients may not need pelvic radiation in the absence of prior inguinal surgery or scrotal involvement (178,179). Cure rates exceeding 95% can be expected for these patients (180–184). Some interest has developed in managing clinical stage I patients with seminoma by close follow-up after orchiectomy, with further treatment reserved for those who relapse—a surveillance-only approach. This approach has received more support in the management of nonseminomatous tumors since relapse in seminomas is more difficult to detect due to its relative marker negativity and greater tendency for late recurrences (185,186). The identification of vascular invasion (187), as well as large size (>6 cm) (188), may be a contraindication for a surveillance-only approach. In patients with metastatic seminoma to the retroperitoneum, those with less bulky disease are treated with radiation with cure rates of 90% to 96% (134,189,190). With bulky retroperitoneal seminoma or supradiaphragmatic involvement, cisplatin-based chemotherapy is now the preferred treatment. Survival for these patients when so treated is approximately 80% (191,192).

The most important prognostic factor in seminoma is tumor stage (which includes tumor bulk). There is controversy concerning the significance of elevated hCG levels in patients with seminoma; there is growing evidence that patients with more than a moderate hCG elevation have a poorer overall survival (193–195). The presence of a lymphoid infiltrate and prominent granulomatous reaction may confer a somewhat improved prognosis (6), but this may be of borderline significance (196,197). The recognition of a histologically defined "anaplastic seminoma" with a worse prognosis remains controversial. It is clear that the original criterion (198), based on the mitotic rate of seminomas, is not effective in recognizing an aggressively behaving subset of seminomas (199,200). Often tumors classified as anaplastic seminomas are either poorly fixed seminomas, with obscuring of the diagnostic features, or solid-pattern embryonal carcinomas.

Spermatocytic Seminoma

Spermatocytic seminoma is an unusual but generally distinctive germ cell tumor first recognized by Masson (201). It constitutes about 1% to 2% of all testicular germ cell tumors (132,202) and therefore is 25 to 40 times less common than classic seminoma. It is particularly important to recognize spermatocytic seminoma and distinguish it from classic seminoma because the implications for treatment differ significantly.

Patients with spermatocytic seminoma are older than most testicular germ cell tumor patients, with an average age of 50 to 60 years (132,202,203) and rare occurrence in patients younger than 30 (203). Most present with painless testicular enlargement (202,203), which can be of several years' duration. Bilateral involvement, usually asynchronous, occurs in 9% of cases (202). Unlike classic seminoma, which can occur in extragonadal sites as a primary tumor (where it is designated germinoma), spermatocytic seminoma has never been described as originating in any site other than the testis. It does not appear to be linked to cryptorchidism (202,204), as are other testicular germ cell tumors, and probably does not share other epidemiologic features with the usual forms of testicular germ cell tumors. The usual serum markers are negative (202,203).

Grossly, spermatocytic seminomas are usually multinodular with a cut surface that varies from gray-white and fleshy to tan and gelatinous (Fig. 14). Hemorrhage and necrosis may occur, as well as extratesticular extension (203,205).

At low power, nodules of diffuse sheets of cells may be interrupted by edema-filled spaces (Fig. 15). If edema is extensive, a nested, pseudoglandular, or even trabecular pattern can develop. The stroma is typically not conspicuous, and

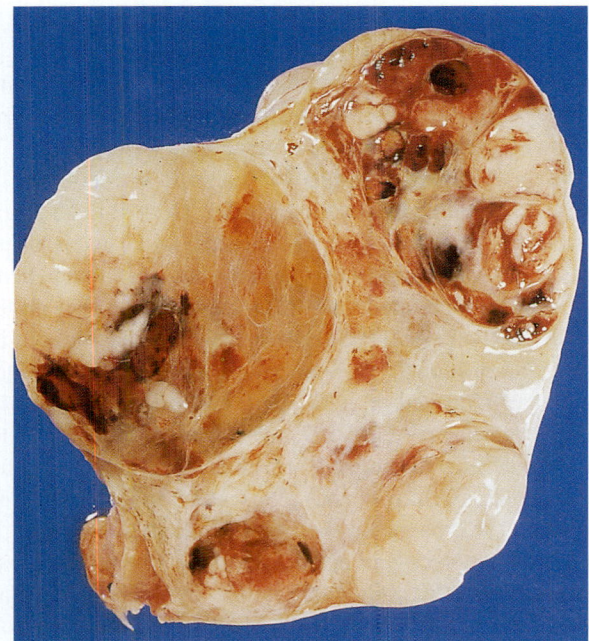

FIG. 14. Spermatocytic seminoma with fleshy, gelatinous, and hemorrhagic nodules. (Photograph courtesy of S.F. Cramer, M.D., Rochester General Hospital, Rochester, New York.)

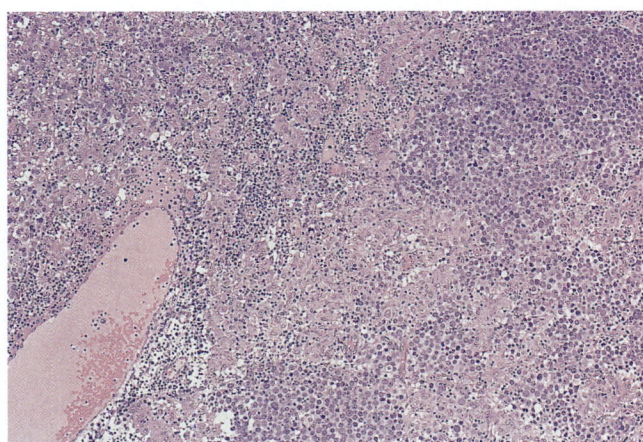

FIG. 16. Extremely unusual spermatocytic seminoma with granulomatous and lymphocytic reactions. (Case courtesy of R.H. Young, M.D., Harvard Medical School, Boston, Massachusetts.)

the regular fibrous septation of classic seminoma is absent. Also there is usually no, or only a scant, predominantly perivascular lymphoid infiltrate, although a rare case may show a more extensive lymphoid component. Granulomas are virtually always absent, although we have seen a unique case with prominent granulomas (Fig. 16). Vascular invasion can occasionally be identified (203).

The most distinctive feature of spermatocytic seminoma is its cellular polymorphism. The cells generally have uniformly round nuclei but they vary in diameter from 6 to 100 μm. Three cellular populations are described—small lymphocyte-like cells averaging 6 to 8 μm in diameter; intermediate-sized cells averaging 15 to 20 μm in diameter; and giant cells, averaging 50 to 100 μm in diameter (Fig. 17). The lymphocyte-like cells actually have smudged chromatin and more cytoplasm than a true lymphocyte; the character of the chromatin supports the viewpoint that it is degenerate. The intermediate cells are most common and have round nuclei with granular chromatin, variably prominent nucleoli, and pale to eosinophilic cytoplasm. Some have distinctive filamentous chromatin reminiscent of the "spireme" chromatin identified in meiosis of primary spermatocytes (Fig. 18). The giant cells may be uninucleate or multinucleated with prominent nucleoli; some may also have a spireme chromatin (Fig. 18). The mitotic rate is often high. Recently, an anaplastic variant of spermatocytic seminoma was described (206); it consists of a relatively monomorphic population of intermediate cells with prominent nucleoli, with foci of typical spermatocytic seminoma elsewhere (Fig. 19). The immunohistochemistry, ultrastructure, and clinical course of these cases, however, was typical for spermatocytic seminoma (206).

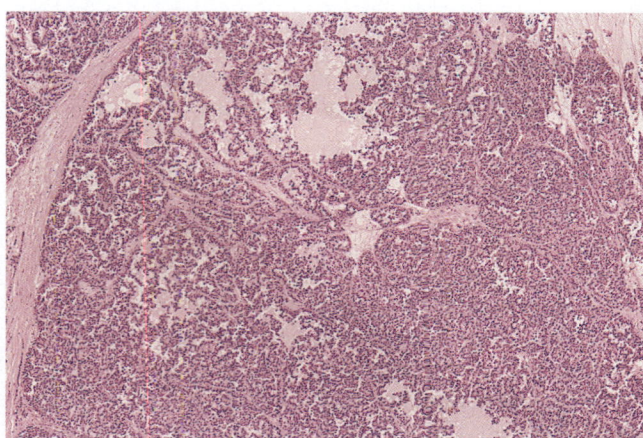

FIG. 15. Nodule of spermatocytic seminoma with edema-filled spaces.

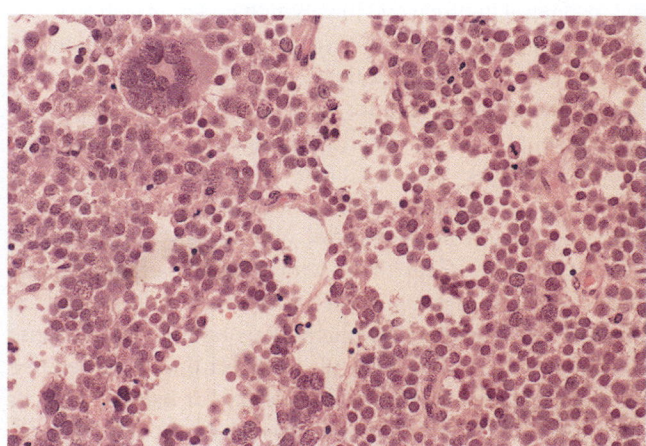

FIG. 17. Polymorphic appearance of spermatocytic seminoma, with small, lymphocyte-like, intermediate, and giant cells.

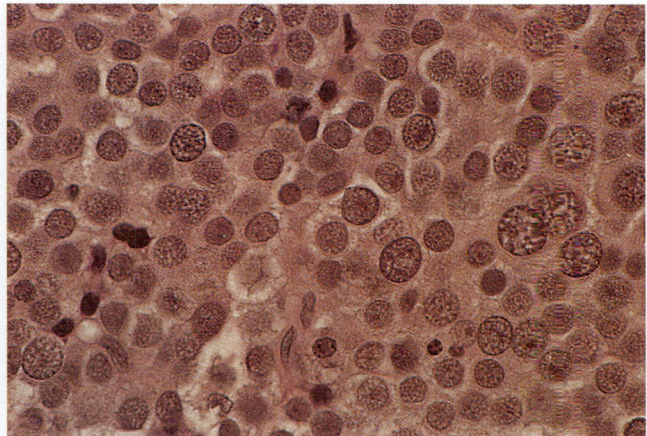

FIG. 18. High magnification of spermatocytic seminoma showing filamentous (spireme) chromatin in some of the larger cells and the typical round nuclei.

Intratubular growth of spermatocytic seminoma occurs commonly, and probably such foci are the basis for the development of separate nodules of tumor. Unlike most other forms of testicular germ cell tumor, with the possible exception of childhood cases (110,111), spermatocytic seminomas are not associated with IGCNU (207).

Immunostains are negative for vimentin, actin, desmin, AFP, hCG, carcinoembryonic antigen (CEA), and leukocyte common antigen (LCA) (203,208,209). Staining for PLAP is generally reported as negative (203,208,210), although some investigators have reported rare PLAP-positive tumors cells in a minority of cases (203,209). Cytokeratins are usually negative, although a rare case may show cytoplasmic positivity for cytokeratin 18 (159).

On ultrastructural examination one study described meiotic-like chromosomal structures in spermatocytic seminomas (211), but another failed to find these (212). Primitive junctions can be identified as well as a Golgi apparatus, ribosomes, mitochondria, and a peripheral layer of basement membrane (211,212). Intercytoplasmic bridges may form between adjacent cells (213). Glycogen is usually absent or sparse.

Because of the distinctive meiotic-type chromatin in some cells of spermatocytic seminomas, it has been proposed that the tumor develops from meiotic cells. However, haploid DNA values have not been identified (207,209,212,214), and lectin-binding studies do not support advanced spermatogenic differentiation (215).

Spermatocytic seminoma is most likely to be confused with classic seminoma. Table 5 lists the clinical and pathologic features that distinguish these two neoplasms.

Despite its alarming microscopic appearance, spermatocytic seminoma metastasizes only exceedingly rarely. There is only one well-documented case of metastasis (204,216); adequate treatment therefore consists of orchiectomy alone.

In recent years, several cases of spermatocytic seminoma combined with sarcoma have been described (203,217,218). These tumors occurred in older men, just like uncomplicated spermatocytic seminomas, but there was often a history of recent, accelerated growth. Grossly, they tended to have a more hemorrhagic, necrotic appearance with a whorled appearance on cut surface (217,218). The sarcomatous component was intimately intermingled with the typical appearing spermatocytic seminoma and usually had an undifferentiated, spindle cell appearance, with two cases showing rhabdomyoblastic differentiation (203,217,218) (Fig. 20). Unlike uncomplicated spermatocytic seminoma, these tumors behaved aggressively, with about 50% of the patients developing metastatic disease and dying of the tumor (203,217,218). The disseminated tumor in all cases consisted only of the sarcomatous component and tended to have a hematogenous metastatic pattern, involving the lung most frequently.

Embryonal Carcinoma

Embryonal carcinoma is a germ cell neoplasm composed of primitive epithelial cells arranged in solid, papillary, and glandular configurations. As a pure neoplasm, embryonal carcinomas are relatively uncommon, representing only about 2% of germ cell tumors in a referral series (219); however, an embryonal carcinoma component is found in most (87%) of the nonseminomatous neoplasms (132). Therefore, most of the studies that have examined the clinical and pathologic correlates of embryonal carcinoma are based on series of mixed germ cell tumors with a predominant embryonal carcinoma component. The declining frequency of pure embryonal carcinomas over the years—from about 20% (5,9) to 2% (219)—reflects the recognition of teratomatous and yolk sac tumor elements in neoplasms previously considered embryonal carcinomas and that are now classified as mixed germ cell tumors.

Embryonal carcinomas tend to occur in patients about 10 years younger [average age—31 years (132)] than those with seminomas. Most patients present with a testicular mass, which may be associated with pain. Unlike seminoma, which is limited to the testis at presentation in 70% of the cases,

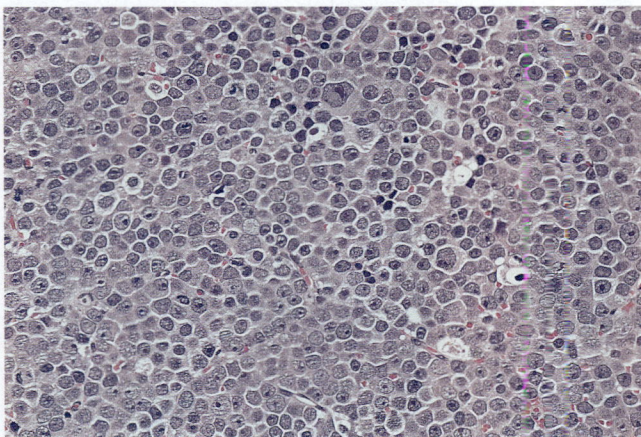

FIG. 19. Anaplastic spermatocytic seminoma with a predominance of intermediate cells with prominent nucleoli

TABLE 5. *Comparison of the clinical and pathologic features of spermatocytic seminoma with classic seminoma*

	Spermatocytic seminoma	Classic seminoma
Proportion of germ cell tumors	2%	40% to 50%
Sites	Testis only	Testis, ovary (dysgerminoma), mediastinum, pineal, RP
Cryptorchidism association	No	Yes
Bilaterality	9%	2%
Association with other forms of germ cell tumor	No	Yes
Association with IGCNU	No	Yes
Composition	3 cell types, with denser cytoplasm, round nuclei	1 cell type, often clear cytoplasm, less regular nuclei
Intercellular edema	Common	Uncommon
Stroma	Scanty	Prominent
Lymphoid reaction	Rare	Prominent
Granulomas	Very rare	Often prominent
Growth pattern	Often intratubular	Often interstitial
Glycogen	Absent to scant	Abundant
PLAP staining	Absent	Prominent
hCG staining	Absent	Present in 10%
Metastases	Very rare	Common

hCG, human chorionic gonadotropin; IGCNU, intratubular germ cell neoplasia, unclassified; PLAP, placental-like alkaline phosphatase; RP, retroperitoneum.
Adapted from refs. 326 and 205.

66% of patients with a tumor composed predominantly of embryonal carcinoma have metastases at diagnosis (220), and presenting symptoms may therefore be related to metastatic disease, including back pain, dyspnea, cough, hemoptysis, hematemesis, and neurologic symptoms. Gynecomastia may occur in a minority of patients and generally is a reflection of hCG production by an intermixed trophoblastic component (strictly speaking, not a pure embryonal carcinoma). Sometimes widespread metastases are present in the face of a clinically occult primary tumor (221) (see below).

Patients with pure embryonal carcinomas usually do not have serum AFP elevation (219), although rare embryonal carcinoma cells may stain positively for AFP on immunohistochemistry (156,222). The high rate of positivity for AFP reported by some (223) reflects the frequent association of embryonal carcinoma with a yolk sac tumor component. Similarly, hCG elevations reflect trophoblastic differentiation and imply that the tumor is not a pure embryonal carcinoma. Elevated serum levels of lactate dehydrogenase (LDH) occur in about 60% of patients with advanced stage disease (224), and elevation of PLAP may also be seen (142).

On gross examination, embryonal carcinomas are usually pale-gray, poorly demarcated tumors associated with hemorrhage and necrosis (Fig. 21) with an average diameter of 2 to 3 cm (6). Extratesticular spread is present in about 20% of cases (9).

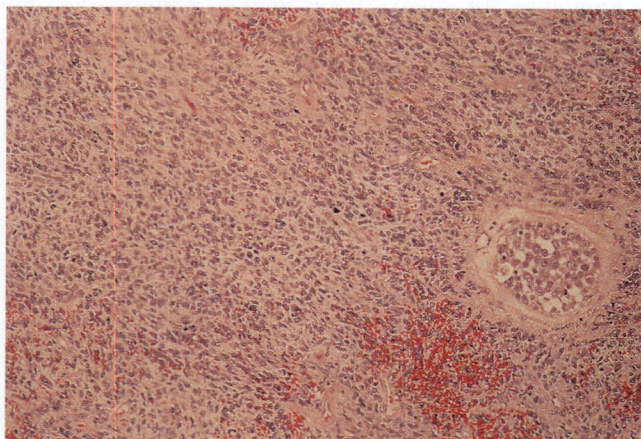

FIG. 20. Rhabdomyosarcoma associated with spermatocytic seminoma. Residual intratubular spermatocytic seminoma is apparent *(right center)*. (Case courtesy of R.H. Young, M.D., Harvard Medical School, Boston, Massachusetts.)

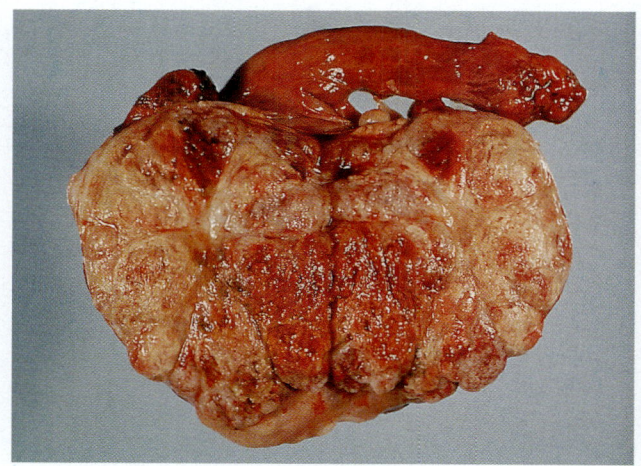

FIG. 21. Hemorrhagic and necrotic appearance of a tumor consisting predominantly of embryonal carcinoma.

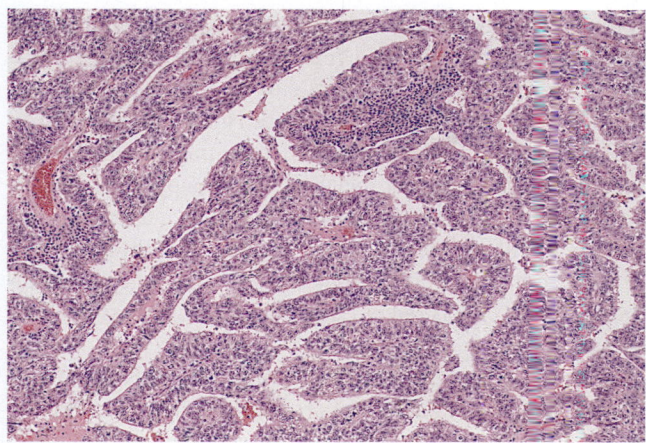

FIG. 22. Papillary pattern of embryonal carcinoma with fibrous cores.

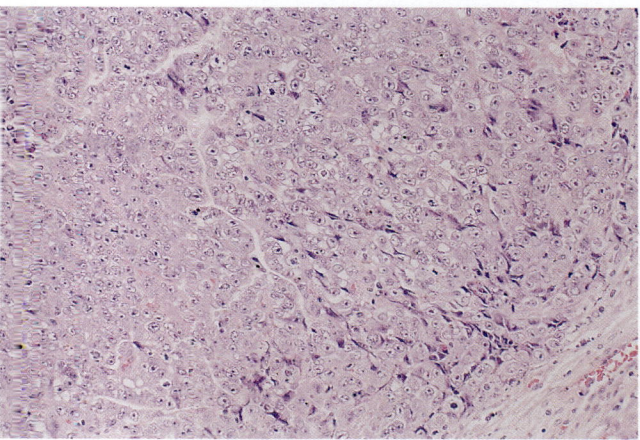

FIG. 24. Solid pattern of embryonal carcinoma. Note numerous intermixed cells with "smudged" nuclei.

On microscopic examination, there are typically nodules of large cells with prominent zones of eosinophilic coagulative necrosis. Within these nodules several patterns may occur. The tumor may be arranged in papillae that may have stromal cores (Fig. 22) or consist purely of epithelium, with intervening slit-like spaces. When the papillae have prominent vessels, a "pseudoendodermal sinus" pattern occurs (225). Glandular patterns are common, with cuboidal to columnar tumor cells arranged around luminal spaces (Fig. 23). Solid patterns have a sheet-like proliferation of tumor cells (Fig. 24). Intermingled cells with a dark, smudged appearance are common and characteristic (Fig. 24) but are nonspecific. Occasionally, such cells can be difficult to distinguish from trophoblastic elements, causing concern about choriocarcinoma. Immunostaining for hCG is useful in resolving this problem. Usually, however, such cells appear to represent a degenerative population.

On high-power examination embryonal carcinoma cells, in routine paraffin sections, are generally polygonal with amphophilic to lightly basophilic cytoplasm and ill-defined cytoplasmic borders (Fig. 25). The nuclei are large, often irregularly shaped, with vesicular chromatin interspersed with clumps of heterochromatin, and having one or more, centrally located, large nucleoli. Often the routine histologic appearance is that of nuclear crowding such that nuclei appear to overlap, although in plastic sections this finding is seen to be an effect of the section thickness. The mitotic rate is generally very brisk.

A doubled-layered pattern of embryonal carcinoma has been described in which ribbons of columnar embryonal carcinoma cells are accompanied by a parallel layer of smaller, flattened cells (225) (Fig. 26). The AFP-positivity of the smaller cell component as well as its appearance indicate that this pattern represents a mixed germ cell tumor with a yolk sac tumor component.

It is common to identify intratubular embryonal carcinoma adjacent to an invasive lesion. Such intratubular foci often show extensive necrosis and may ultimately undergo total necrosis and calcify. If there is similar regression of the primary neoplasm (see below), the presence of such

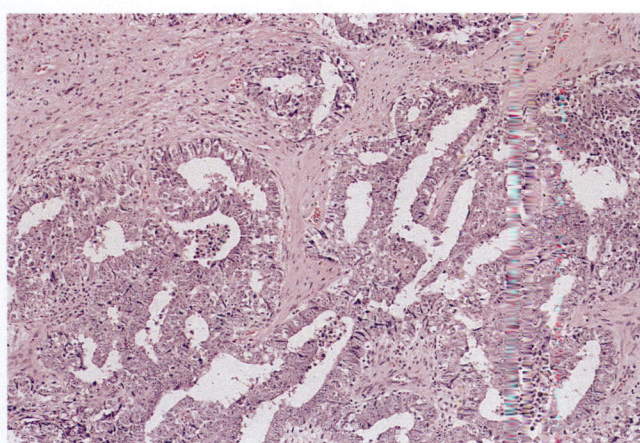

FIG. 23. Glandular pattern of embryonal carcinoma with columnar cells.

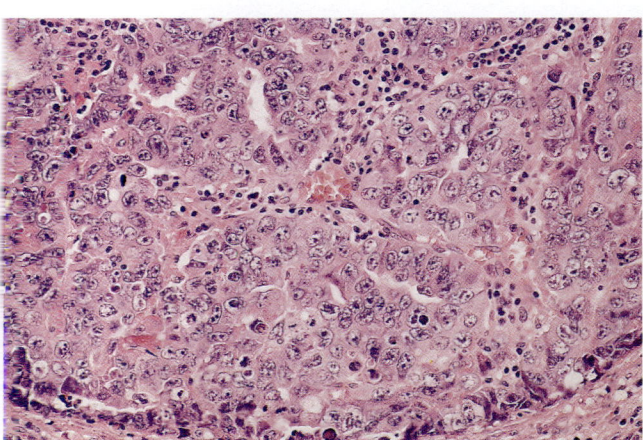

FIG. 25. Embryonal carcinoma with crowded, vesicular nuclei, prominent nucleoli, and poorly defined cell borders.

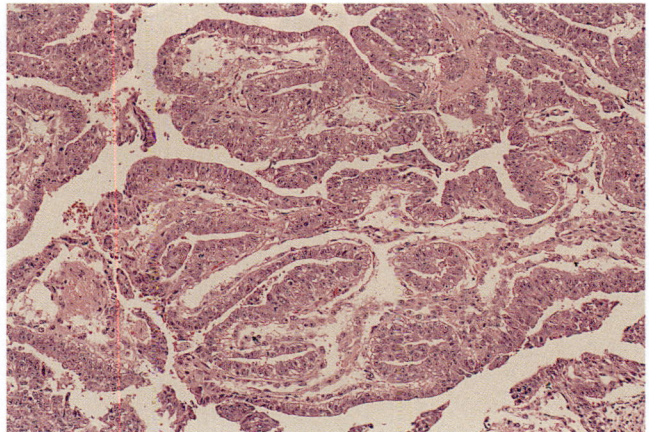

FIG. 26. A so-called double-layered pattern of embryonal carcinoma with processes having an outer layer of embryonal carcinoma cells and an inner layer of flat to cuboidal cells. We regard such cases as mixed germ cell tumor (embryonal carcinoma and yolk sac tumor).

intratubular calcified concretions (hematoxylin-staining bodies) may provide good evidence of the former presence of an embryonal carcinoma (or other germ cell tumor type) in the testis (226).

A source of controversy is the extent that an embryonal carcinoma may have a stromal component. There is a tradition of permitting a primitive neoplastic mesenchymal component to be associated with the typical epithelial cells of embryonal carcinoma (Fig. 27) and yet retain classification of such tumors as pure embryonal carcinoma (4,9), rather than embryonal carcinoma with a teratomatous component. The rationale for this approach is that such a finding represents a reiteration of primitive embryonic development. There is also some evidence that embryonal carcinomas with and without a primitive mesenchymal component have a similar biology based on the experience of the BTTP (11), although these data antedate current treatments. We nonetheless feel that such a stromal component should compose only a minority of the embryonal carcinoma and retain an undifferentiated appearance, consisting of oval to spindle cells lacking light microscopic features of recognizable mesenchymal tissue such as cartilage or muscle. Von Hochstetter and Hedinger (133) have discussed the problem of a stromal component in embryonal carcinoma and noted inconsistencies between the WHO-based approach and the British approach on this question. More than a minor stromal component or light microscopic evidence of differentiation of the stroma places such tumors into a mixed germ cell tumor category consisting of embryonal carcinoma and immature teratoma.

With the advent of surveillance-only protocols in patients with nonseminomatous tumors (see below), it is important to assess an embryonal carcinoma for vascular invasion and extratesticular extension. Artifactual implants of embryonal carcinoma occur easily during tissue cutting because of its extremely cellular and friable nature (3). Intravascular implants consist of loosely cohesive cells that do not conform to the shape of the vessel but lie randomly in the luminal space. They are often associated with implants that are "buttered" on the surface of the testis and spermatic cord (3). True vascular invasion consists of cohesive groups of cells that conform to the shape of the vessel (Fig. 28) or are adherent to its wall by thrombotic material. Vascular invasion is usually easiest to appreciate at the periphery of the main tumor. Intratubular neoplasm may mimic vascular invasion; the identification of residual Sertoli cells in such cases as well as staining for endothelial markers can be of assistance.

Immunohistochemical stains may assist in the diagnosis of embryonal carcinoma. From 0% to 33% of morphologically typical embryonal carcinomas stain positively for AFP (156,165,222,227,228), with a higher frequency of positivity in the embryonal carcinoma component of a mixed germ cell tumor (222,227), probably indicating its capacity for transformation to yolk sac tumor. PLAP is positive in 86% to 97% of embryonal carcinomas (116,156,229), and cytokeratin is positive in 95% to 100% of cases (156,230), although epithelial membrane antigen (EMA) positivity occurs in only 2% (156). The presence of cytokeratins other than 8 and 18

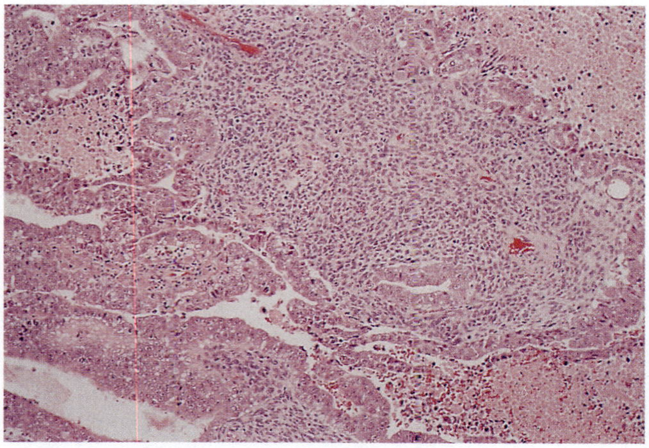

FIG. 27. Undifferentiated, neoplastic stroma associated with the typical-appearing epithelium of embryonal carcinoma.

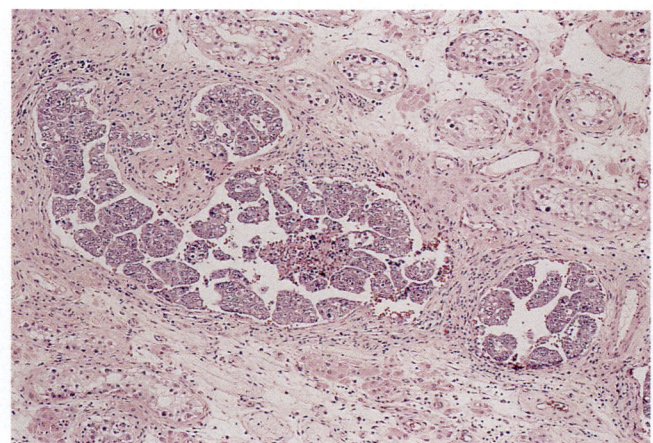

FIG. 28. Vascular invasion by an embryonal carcinoma, with conformation of the tumor to the vessel lumen.

in embryonal carcinomas contrasts with the limited reactivity (mainly confined to cytokeratins 8 and 18 in scattered cells) of most seminomas (159–161). Ki-1 (CD30) may be identified in most embryonal carcinomas (Fig. 29) and therefore cannot be relied on for differentiation of embryonal carcinoma from anaplastic, large cell lymphoma; it is uncommonly seen in other types of germ cell tumor (231–233). Although embryonal carcinomas are not difficult to recognize in the testis, an embryonal carcinoma presenting in a metastatic site may be extremely difficult to distinguish from an undifferentiated carcinoma of nongerminal type. The presence of PLAP-positivity and EMA-negativity in such cases can be of significant diagnostic assistance. Other stains that may be positive in some embryonal carcinomas include alpha$_1$-antitrypsin, Leu 7, vimentin, LDH, ferritin, and human placental lactogen (156,222,234,235).

On ultrastructural examination, embryonal carcinomas appear as poorly differentiated adenocarcinomas, forming small glandular spaces with tight junctional complexes and a peripheral basal lamina (14,236). The Golgi complex is usually prominent, and the nucleus quite irregular in shape with a large, complex nucleolus and cytoplasmic inclusions.

Cytogenetic analysis of embryonal carcinomas has identified the i (12p) marker chromosome in many cases (169), with a general correlation between the aggressiveness of the tumor and the number of copies of i (12p) (159). Other chromosome 12 anomalies occur in some cases (237). Expression of several proto-oncogenes by embryonal carcinomas has been reported (238–240).

Differential Diagnosis

Embryonal carcinomas must be distinguished from several other types of tumor. It is most important to distinguish embryonal carcinoma from seminoma because seminomas, at least in lower stage disease, are treated with radiation therapy whereas metastatic embryonal carcinomas are generally treated with polyagent chemotherapy and surgery. This important differential diagnosis has been discussed above. Solid-pattern yolk sac tumors may be confused with embryonal carcinomas; however, usually other patterns of yolk sac tumor permit this distinction. In small specimens, solid-pattern yolk sac tumor can usually be distinguished from embryonal carcinoma by virtue of the smaller size of its cells and nuclei and its less pleomorphic nature. The presence of hyaline globules or basement membrane deposits favors yolk sac tumor (171), as does AFP-positivity and CD30-negativity. Often tumors composed predominantly of embryonal carcinoma have foci of contiguous yolk sac tumor composed of smaller, vacuolated tumor cells, often in a myxoid background. Large cell lymphomas may be confused with embryonal carcinomas but usually occur in older patients with extratesticular disease. Lymphomas often have an interstitial pattern, always lack IGCNU, are negative for PLAP and cytokeratin (163), and are usually positive for LCA and other lymphoid markers (156,176). The most difficult diagnosis is the distinction of embryonal carcinoma in an extragonadal site from a metastatic undifferentiated carcinoma. The helpful immunostaining patterns for this problem have been discussed above; mucin stains may be helpful as well since embryonal carcinomas lack cytoplasmic mucin, which may be identified in poorly differentiated carcinomas of somatic origin. The electron microscopic demonstration of the long tight junctions of embryonal carcinoma may also be helpful in this context (236).

There has been a revolution in the treatment of patients with nonseminomatous germ cell tumors, including embryonal carcinoma, that has resulted in a much improved prognosis. Forty years ago the survival of such patients was about 30% (6) but currently it is in excess of 90% (241). The form of treatment following radical orchiectomy is stage dependent. For clinical stage I disease there is controversy regarding the best approach; one school of thought advocates retroperitoneal lymph node dissection (RPLND) (especially of the nerve-sparing type to avoid the complication of postoperative ejaculatory failure) in all such patients (242). If pathologic evaluation confirms a lack of nodal metastases, these patients may be followed without receiving chemotherapy (unless relapse develops later). Patients with pathologically confirmed metastases may receive polyagent, cisplatin-based chemotherapy or be followed depending on the extent of nodal involvement and the reliability of the patient. A 98% to 100% survival can be anticipated for this group of clinical stage I patients as a whole (241).

Another approach to clinical stage I patients is to follow them closely after orchiectomy without doing RPLND. Several studies have suggested that the relapse rate is too high in some patients with certain pathologic findings in the orchiectomy specimen to place them on a surveillance-only protocol. It is therefore crucial for the pathologist to provide all of the clinically relevant pathologic observations for these cases. The features in the orchiectomy specimen that have been associated with excess relapse in clinical stage I patients include vascular/lymphatic invasion (243–259); advanced local stage (i.e., spread into extratesticular structures or possibly into the rete testis) (244,249,250,260); a tumor

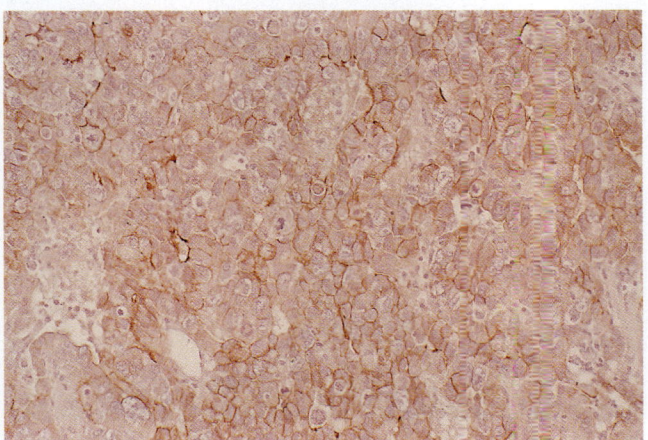

FIG. 29. Positivity for Ki-1 antigen in embryonal carcinoma.

composition of predominantly embryonal carcinoma (248,257,261), pure embryonal carcinoma (247,262), any embryonal carcinoma (246,249,252,259,263), embryonal carcinoma unassociated with teratoma (245), embryonal carcinoma in excess of 2 ml (264,265), the absence of yolk sac tumor (252) or mature teratoma (259), a teratomatous component of <50% (244,248), the presence of choriocarcinoma (250), and high S-phase or proliferation indices (262, 264,266). In a summary of the results of several surveillance-only trials, 544 of 560 patients (97%) were disease-free on last follow-up, with 72% of the patients needing no treatment after orchiectomy (245). There is ongoing interest in identifying features in the orchiectomy specimens that would permit accurate prediction of high or low probabilities of relapse.

For patients with nonbulky retroperitoneal metastases, treatment is RPLND and either close follow-up or limited-course adjuvant chemotherapy. Survivals exceeding 95% are expected (241). In more advanced stage disease, the usual treatment is initial cisplatin-based chemotherapy followed by resection of residual masses, if any exist. This group of patients has an overall survival of 70% to 80% (191,267). Pathologic findings in the resected residual tissue often determine the need for additional therapy (268).

For patients with disseminated disease, the prognosis appears to depend on factors including tumor bulk (192, 267,269–271), levels of serum markers (192,269–273), and proliferative index (272).

Yolk Sac Tumor

Teilum's (274–276) studies provided the evidence that the neoplasm we now recognize as yolk sac tumor is of germ cell origin with differentiation toward the yolk sac and allantoic membranes. Yolk sac tumor is the most common form of testicular tumor in prepubertal children in whom it occurs as a pure neoplasm at a mean age of 17 to 18 months (277,278), with an age range from the newborn period to 9 years (279). In postpubertal patients it is much more commonly a component of a mixed germ cell tumor. In Talerman's (280) study there was a 44% frequency of a yolk sac tumor component in prospectively examined, nonseminomatous germ cell tumors. Childhood yolk sac tumor is not associated with cryptorchidism and occurs with roughly equivalent frequencies in black and white populations (281). Both childhood and adult cases most commonly present with a testicular mass, but a small proportion of adult cases have symptoms of metastatic disease or gynecomastia. Yolk sac tumor remains the most commonly overlooked component of nonseminomatous germ cell tumors (219,255).

Eighty-five percent of children presenting with yolk sac tumor have clinical stage I disease (282); there is some evidence that a yolk sac tumor component in a mixed germ cell tumor of an adult is associated with early stage disease as well (252), but this observation needs additional corroboration.

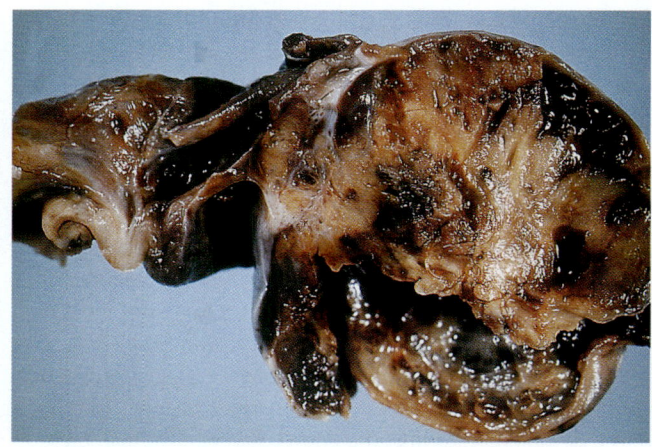

FIG. 30. Adult yolk sac tumor with areas of hemorrhage and cystic change.

From 95% to 100% of patients with tumors containing yolk sac tumor elements have elevated levels of serum AFP (283,284). This provides both an important diagnostic aid, as well as a means of monitoring therapy and detecting recurrences. It is important, however, not to overinterpret high AFP levels in young children since physiologic AFP elevations may occur (285).

On gross examination, yolk sac tumor may appear as a nonencapsulated, gray to tan to yellow nodule, often with cystic change or a myxoid quality (Fig. 30). Hemorrhagic and necrotic areas are common, more so in adult cases. Pediatric cases are usually more homogeneous, often appearing as a solid, yellow/tan myxoid nodule (Fig. 31).

There are numerous patterns associated with yolk sac tumor, making it a truly polymorphous neoplasm. Fortunately, most of the time these patterns are intermixed, thus facilitating their recognition. The following classification of yolk sac tumor patterns represents a modification of Talerman's

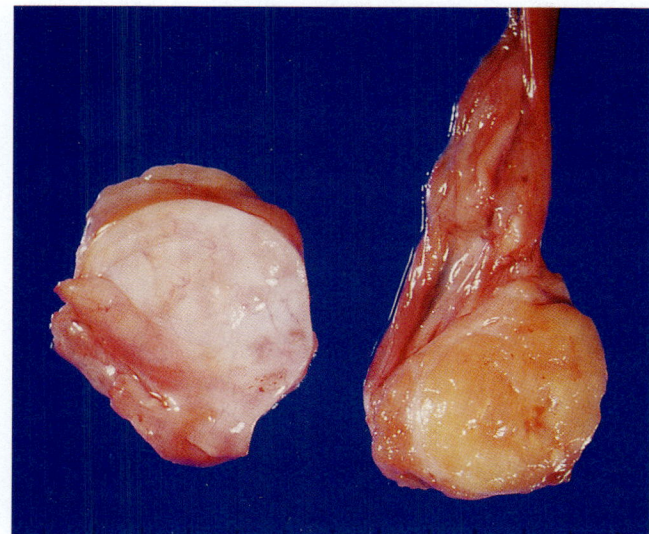

FIG. 31. Pediatric yolk sac tumor, with solid, yellow, myxoid nodule.

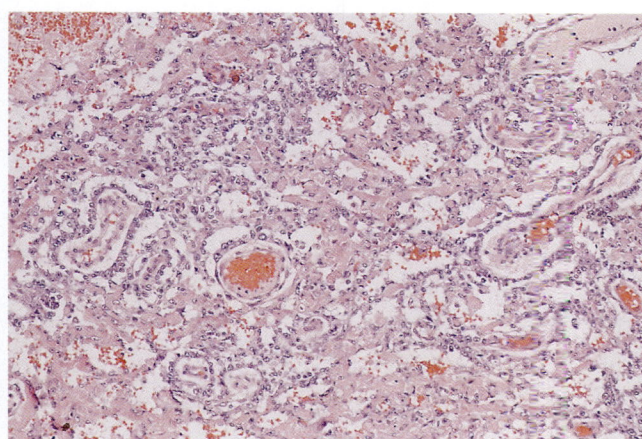

FIG. 32. Endodermal sinus pattern of yolk sac tumor. Note also extensive basement membrane deposits indicative of parietal differentiation.

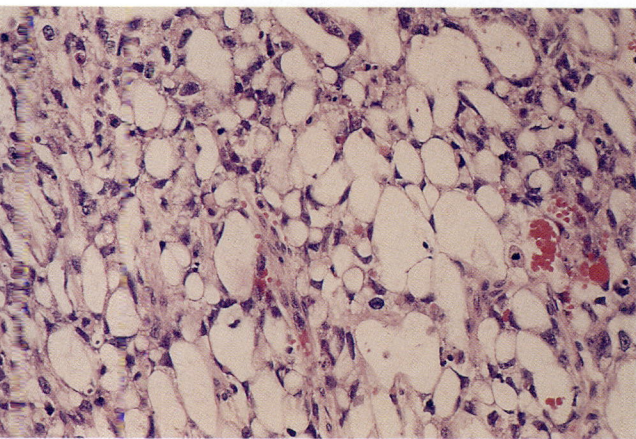

FIG. 34. Microcystic or reticular pattern of yolk sac tumor. Many cells resemble lipoblasts.

(286) work; the 11 patterns are (a) endodermal sinus (also designated perivascular or festoon); (b) reticular (microcystic, honeycomb); (c) macrocystic; (d) papillary; (e) solid; (f) glandular-alveolar; (g) myxomatous; (h) sarcomatoid; (i) polyvesicular vitelline; (j) hepatoid; and (k) parietal.

The endodermal sinus pattern is characterized by a central vessel in a core of mesenchyme that is mantled by a cuboidal to columnar layer of malignant cells and that is recessed into a cystic space (Fig. 32). These structures are referred to as "glomeruloid" or Schiller-Duval bodies. In addition, this pattern has fibrous cores of tissue draped (or "festooned") by tumor cells that alternate with "labyrinthine" spaces (Fig. 33).

The reticular pattern is most common and consists of a network of tumor cells with prominent cytoplasmic vacuolation, thus creating a microcystic or honeycomb appearance (Fig. 34). Sometimes the cells, because of the extensive vacuolation, have a morphology similar to lipoblasts or signet-ring cells. A cord-like arrangement may be identified, associated with a myxoid background, that blends gradually into a myxomatous pattern (see below). Larger cysts may develop in some yolk sac tumors, usually in association with a reticular (microcystic) pattern, to produce a macrocystic pattern. It is likely they derive from coalescence of microcysts.

Some yolk sac tumors form cystic spaces into which papillary processes project (Fig. 35). These papillae may contain fibrous cores or simply be composed of papillary processes of epithelium. Typically the cells have relatively scant cytoplasm, with high nuclear to cytoplasmic ratios and some "hobnail" configurations. Intracystic, detached clusters of cells are frequent.

The solid pattern has a sheet-like configuration of cells that may resemble seminoma, although there is often a focal microcystic tendency, and the fibrous septation and prominent lymphoid component of seminoma are lacking (Fig. 36). Often the cells have clear cytoplasm and well-defined borders, similar to seminoma, but there is an association with other yolk sac tumor patterns. Occasionally the cells are small and primitive, resembling blastema (Fig. 37). In our opinion, some tumors classified as solid pattern yolk sac

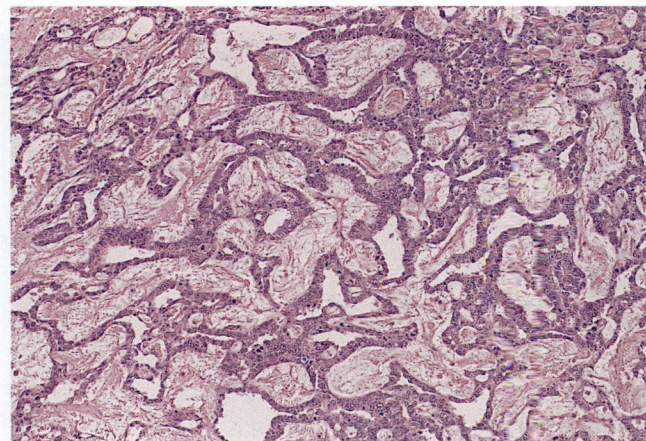

FIG. 33. Festoons of epithelium on fibrovascular cores and anastomosing, "labyrinthine" spaces characteristic of the endodermal sinus pattern.

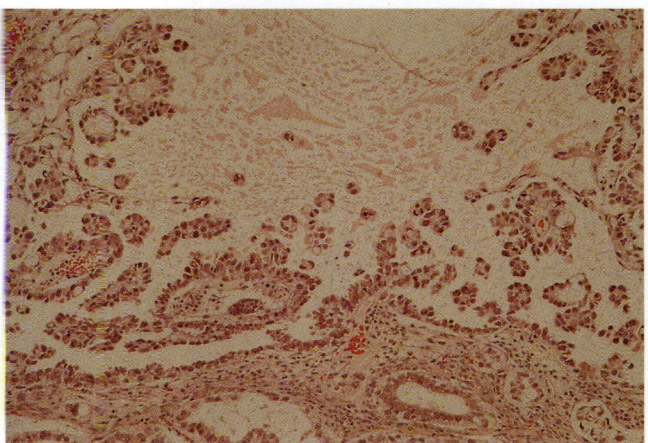

FIG. 35. Papillary pattern of yolk sac tumor, with "hobnail" cells.

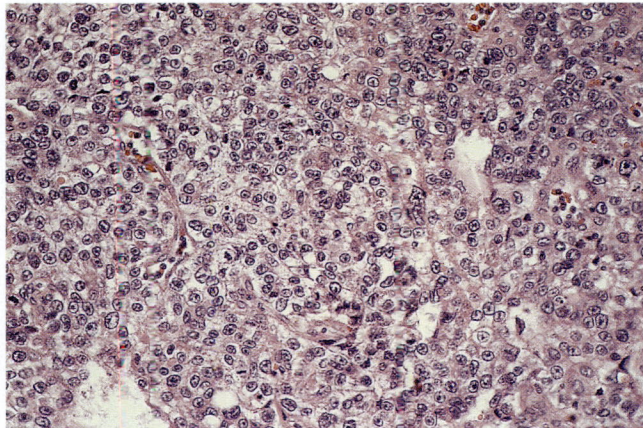

FIG. 36. Solid pattern of yolk sac tumor. Note microcystic tendency and absence of lymphoid infiltrate and fibrous septa.

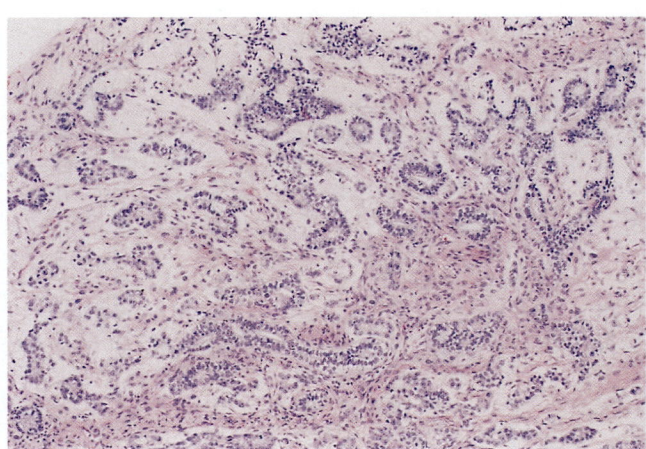

FIG. 38. Glandular pattern of yolk sac tumor.

tumor represent seminoma with transformation to yolk sac tumor (19); other examples, however, are true yolk sac tumors with a diffuse, sheet-like pattern. Cytokeratin stains (see below) are useful in separating these two possibilities.

Distinct glands may occur in yolk sac tumor, often developing from cystic, alveolar-like spaces lined by flattened epithelium. Thirty-four percent of yolk sac tumors had such glandular differentiation in one study (171). The glands have a primitive appearance, often with enteric features including an apical brush border (Fig. 38). They may have extensive subnuclear vacuolation, similar to early secretory phase endometrial glands. An anastomosing or branching arrangement is common, and, rarely, a predominant or pure glandular pattern occurs, although this appears to be more common in ovarian (287) rather than testicular yolk sac tumors (288). Differentiation of purely glandular yolk sac tumors from teratomas can be problematic; staining for AFP may assist but is not specific. The branching, anastomosing pattern is typical of yolk sac tumor, and these glands lack a circumferential smooth muscle component, unlike many teratomatous glands (289).

Some yolk sac tumors are extensively myxoid, with trabeculae, thin cords, and individual cells in a mucoid stroma having a high content of hyaluronic acid (Fig. 39). Individual stellate to spindle cells trail into the myxoid and vascular stroma in apparent transition from the epithelium, but retain cytokeratin reactivity (290). Teilum (291) considered this pattern a reiteration of the extraembryonic mesenchyme of the developing embryo. Occasionally the spindle cells may undergo stromal differentiation, forming skeletal muscle (Fig. 40) and cartilage (290), and blurring the distinction between yolk sac tumor and teratoma. We believe that when such elements are intimately associated with yolk sac tumor, they should be classified as yolk sac tumor with, for instance, rhabdomyoblastic differentiation. Some of the sarcomatous tumors observed in resections following chemotherapy for metastatic testicular germ cell tumors may derive from this mesenchymal component of yolk sac tumor (290,292).

It also appears likely that the cellular, sarcomatoid foci that can be identified in occasional yolk sac tumors derive from the proliferation of the spindle and stellate cells originally associated with the myxomatous pattern. Such sarcomatoid areas generally retain cytokeratin reactivity.

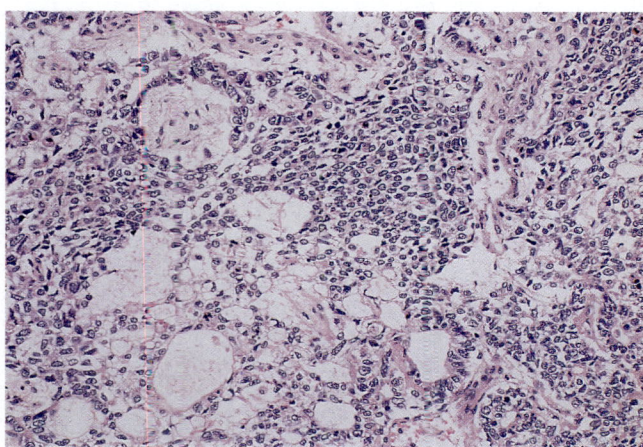

FIG. 37. Solid foci in yolk sac tumor with a blastema-like quality; microcystic foci are also present.

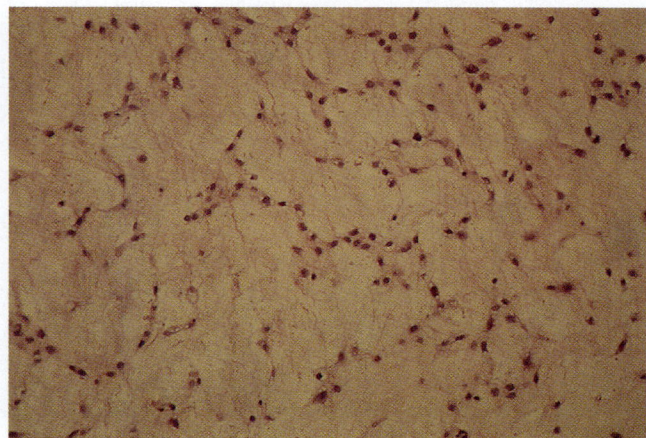

FIG. 39. Myxomatous pattern of yolk sac tumor, with thin cords of cells in an extensively mucoid stroma.

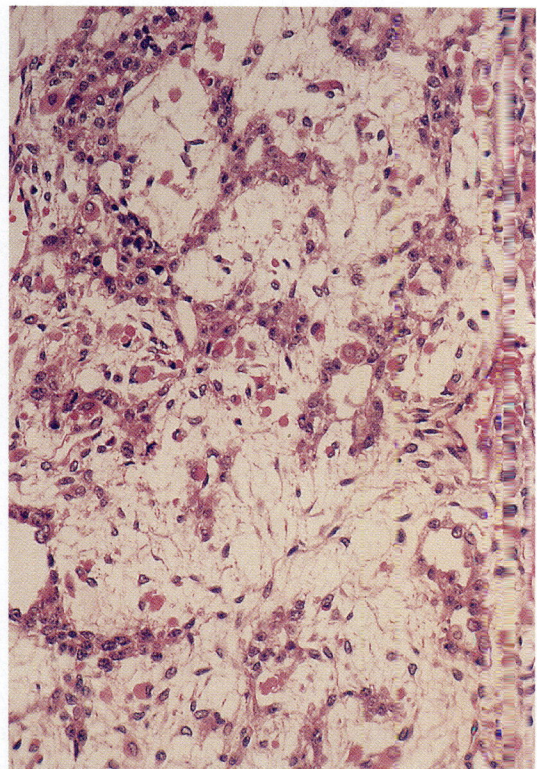

FIG. 40. Rhabdomyoblastic differentiation in a myxomatous pattern of yolk sac tumor.

The polyvesicular vitelline pattern of yolk sac tumor is relatively unusual, occurring in 8% of cases in one series (171). It consists of vesicles, often with central constrictions, lined by flattened to cuboidal to columnar cells (Fig. 41). A transition in epithelial height may occur at the point of the constriction. The columnar cells resemble primitive enteric epithelium similar to that lining the embryonic allantois. Apical and basal vacuoles may occur. Teilum (293) felt that this pattern was analogous to the embryonic subdivision of the primary yolk sac into the secondary yolk sac.

Some yolk sac tumors show definite hepatic differentiation, with clusters of polygonal cells with eosinophilic cytoplasm, round, vesicular nuclei, and prominent nucleoli (Fig. 42). These hepatoid cells may be arranged in sheet-like, trabecular, or nested patterns. Hepatoid differentiation is generally focal in about 20% of yolk sac tumors (171,294), but in rare cases may be predominant, although this would appear to be more common in ovarian tumors (295). Hepatoid foci are intensely positive for AFP and may contain hyaline globules.

A parietal pattern in yolk sac tumor refers to a predominance of extracellular basement membrane between neoplastic cells. The term takes origin from the parietal layer of the embryonic yolk sac that synthesizes a thick basement membrane known as Reichert's membrane. It is actually quite common to find foci of such parietal differentiation in yolk sac tumors—92% of cases (171)—where it can aid in their recognition and proper classification. It is seen in association with several patterns, including reticular, endodermal sinus, and solid patterns, and usually consists of focal, wispy to band-like deposits of eosinophilic matrix (Fig. 32). It is quite rare, however, to have a predominance of extracellular basement membrane such that the associated pattern is obliterated; when this occurs it is designated a parietal pattern (Fig. 43). We have seen occasional cases of metastatic yolk sac tumor following chemotherapy in which a parietal pattern occurred, and Damjanov and co-workers (296) reported a pure parietal yolk sac tumor under similar circumstances.

The reticular pattern of yolk sac tumor is the most common one (171,297); solid and macrocystic patterns are also relatively frequent (171,225), whereas hepatoid, polyvesicular vitelline, and endodermal sinus structures are relatively infrequent (171,225).

Hyaline globules commonly occur in yolk sac tumor and can aid in its recognition. These are round, eosinophilic, PAS-positive, diastase-resistant globules of variable size from 1 to 50 μm or more in diameter (Fig. 44). They also occur in other neoplasms but are uncommon in seminoma and

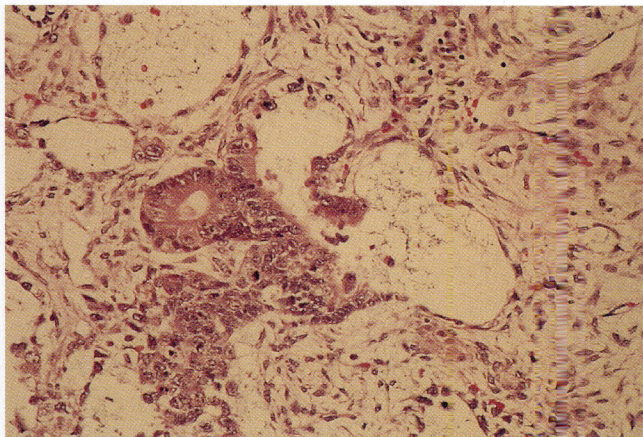

FIG. 41. Polyvesicular vitelline pattern of yolk sac tumor. Irregularly shaped and constricted vesicles lined by flattened and intestinal-type columnar epithelium.

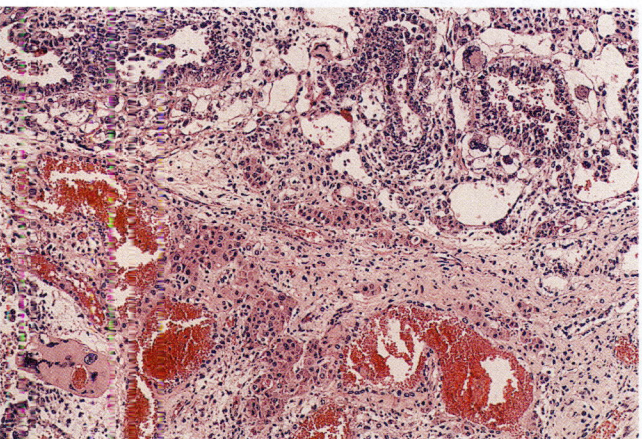

FIG. 42. Nests of polygonal hepatoid cells with abundant eosinophilic cytoplasm in a yolk sac tumor. Syncytiotrophoblast cell is also present.

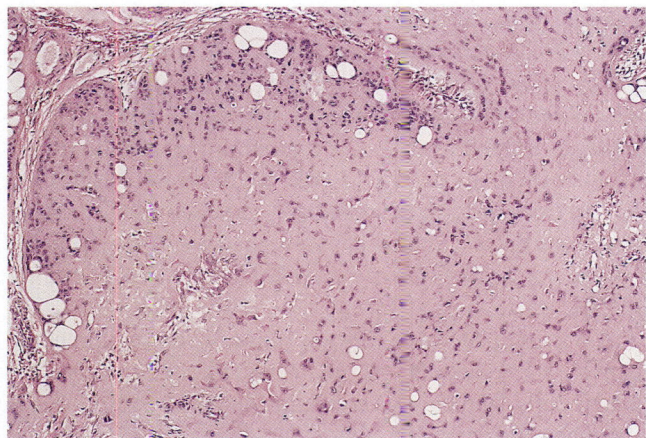

FIG. 43. Parietal pattern of yolk sac tumor. Extensive deposits of basement membrane efface most of the underlying microcystic pattern.

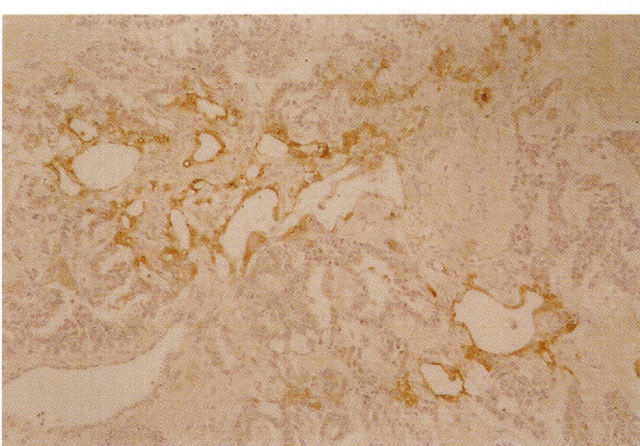

FIG. 45. AFP-positivity in a yolk sac tumor, with the characteristic patchy distribution.

embryonal carcinoma (171). They generally do not stain for AFP. Such globules should not be confused with the more irregularly shaped, band-like deposits of basement membrane that are the hallmark of parietal differentiation.

Hematopoietic foci, usually consisting of erythroblasts, are rarely identified in yolk sac tumors. IGCNU is commonly identified in the seminiferous tubules of postpubertal patients with yolk sac tumor, but perhaps not in the pediatric form of yolk sac tumor (110,298).

Alpha-fetoprotein can be identified intracellularly in most

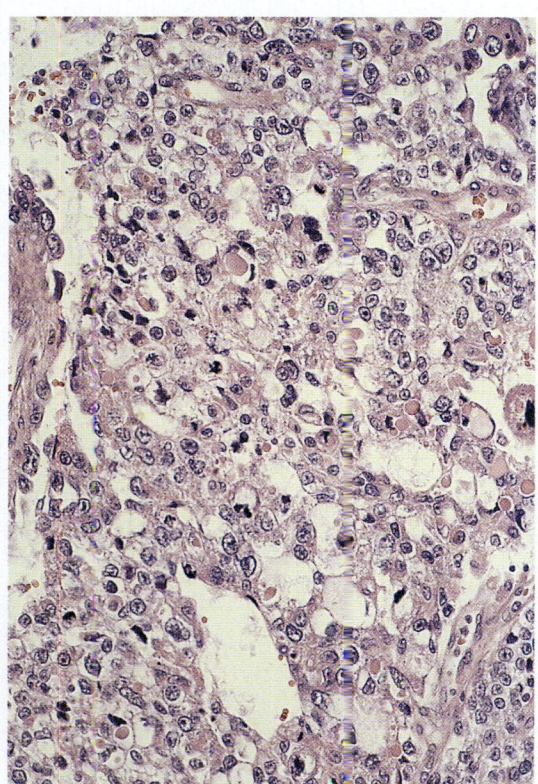

FIG. 44. Scattered, round, eosinophilic hyaline globules in a yolk sac tumor.

yolk sac tumors, with frequencies ranging from 55% to 100% (156,162,164,222); the staining is often patchy (Fig. 45). Pediatric yolk sac tumors are more likely to be AFP-negative (222). Hepatoid foci are generally intensely AFP-positive. The enteric glandular structures of yolk sac tumor may stain positively for CEA (156,171,235). Alpha$_1$-antitrypsin can be identified in roughly 50% of cases (156,164). Cytokeratin is diffusely positive in virtually all yolk sac tumors (156,299), and vimentin can be demonstrated in the stromal component (299). PLAP-staining is not as likely to be positive in yolk sac tumor as in most other types of germ cell tumor, with 39% to 85% positive (116,156,229). EMA is usually negative (156).

By electron microscopy, yolk sac tumors show epithelial cells with tight junctional complexes and apical microvilli. Extracellular basal laminar deposits may be prominent, with similar-appearing material, often with a central lucent zone, within dilated cisternae of endoplasmic reticulum (14). Glycogen is commonly seen, and the nuclei are irregular in shape with a "wandering" nucleolonema.

Differential Diagnosis

It is important to distinguish solid patterns of yolk sac tumor from seminoma, a differential diagnosis discussed above. Embryonal carcinomas lack the distinctive patterns of yolk sac tumor and have cells with larger, more pleomorphic nuclei. Hyaline globules and deposits of basement membrane are rarely seen in embryonal carcinoma (171). There are rare cases that appear to be transitional morphologies between embryonal carcinoma and yolk sac tumor, and examination of other sections usually shows both tumor types. Pediatric yolk sac tumors may be confused with juvenile granulosa cell tumors (300,301) (see below), since both share a solid and cystic pattern, show cytologic atypia, and have a high mitotic rate. Yolk sac tumor typically occurs in older children than the neonates and very young infants who characteristically develop juvenile granulosa cell tumor.

Usually the presence of other yolk sac tumor patterns resolves this differential diagnosis, as does the immunohistochemical demonstration of AFP, which is absent in juvenile granulosa cell tumor. [Serum AFP, however, may be physiologically elevated in neonatal patients (285).] Strong vimentin and weak or absent cytokeratin staining would also appear to favor juvenile granulosa cell tumor over yolk sac tumor, based on the experience with ovarian juvenile granulosa cell tumors (302,303). Glandular patterns of yolk sac tumor lack the circumferential muscle seen in the glandular components of many teratomas (289). Invasion of the rete testis by germ cell tumor elements can cause a hyperplastic epithelial reaction with intracytoplasmic hyaline globules that may be misinterpreted as a yolk sac tumor component (304) (Fig. 46). This intra-rete hyperplasia is differentiated from yolk sac tumor on the basis of the characteristic branching pattern, as seen at low magnification, and the bland cytologic features of the cells (304).

The treatment of adult patients with yolk sac tumor is similar to that of other nonseminomatous germ cell tumors (see above). The presence of a yolk sac tumor component in a testicular primary may be associated with a higher frequency of low-stage disease (252,305). The proper treatment of children with yolk sac tumors is somewhat controversial, but the current trend is toward conservative management by careful follow-up after radical orchiectomy in patients lacking clinical evidence of metastases, including postorchiectomy AFP values. This approach reflects the facts that 80% to more than 90% of children with yolk sac tumors have stage I disease (277,282,306), and there is a low rate of retroperitoneal metastases compared to pulmonary metastases (278,282, 307,308). It used to be said that children younger than 2 years old with testicular yolk sac tumor had a significantly better prognosis than those older than 2 (278), but a more recent study from the Pediatric Oncology Group reported a 91% 5-year survival and failed to identify a survival difference with respect to age (309).

It may be that adults who have a yolk sac tumor component in a metastatic lesion have a worse prognosis than those lacking a yolk sac tumor component (310), despite the opposite impact when in the testis (252). This finding probably reflects a greater chemoresistance of yolk sac tumor elements than other germ cell tumor elements. This conclusion is supported by autopsy studies that documented a much greater frequency of residual yolk sac tumor in patients dying in the chemotherapeutic era compared to those dying before effective chemotherapy (311). Chemoresistant spindle cell tumors of variable morphology probably are derived from yolk sac tumor elements and may be the source of ultimately fatal sarcomatous tumors (292).

Trophoblastic Tumors

Choriocarcinoma

Pure testicular choriocarcinomas are rare—0.3% of testicular tumors (9)—but a component of choriocarcinoma is identified in 16% of mixed germ cell tumors upon careful examination (312) typically as microfoci. Patients with pure testicular choriocarcinoma are usually in the second or third decade and often present with metastatic symptoms rather than a testicular mass; some may have no palpable testicular abnormalities on clinical examination. No cases are described in prepubertal children. Frequent presenting symptoms are hemoptysis, lumbar back pain, gastrointestinal bleeding, and neurologic abnormalities. There is often marked elevation of hCG levels and secondary endocrine abnormalities, including gynecomastia (which may also be a presenting complaint) and thyrotoxicosis (because of the thyroid stimulating hormone-like activity of hCG) (313).

On gross examination, choriocarcinomas are often small, and the testis may appear normal or atrophic from its external aspect. On cut surface a hemorrhagic and centrally necrotic nodule is generally identified, often with gray tissue at its periphery (Fig. 47).

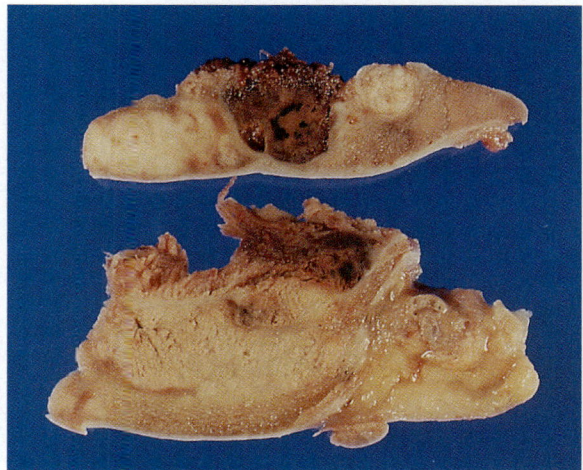

FIG. 47. Cut surface of a mixed germ cell tumor composed of choriocarcinoma and seminoma. The central hemorrhagic nodule represents the choriocarcinomatous component. (Photograph courtesy of S.F. Cramer, M.D., Rochester General Hospital, Rochester, New York.)

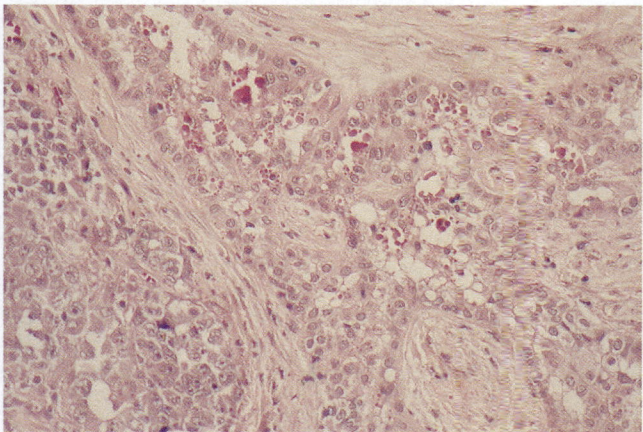

FIG. 46. Hyperplasia of the rete testis with hyaline globule formation, a lesion mimicking yolk sac tumor. Embryonal carcinoma is adjacent.

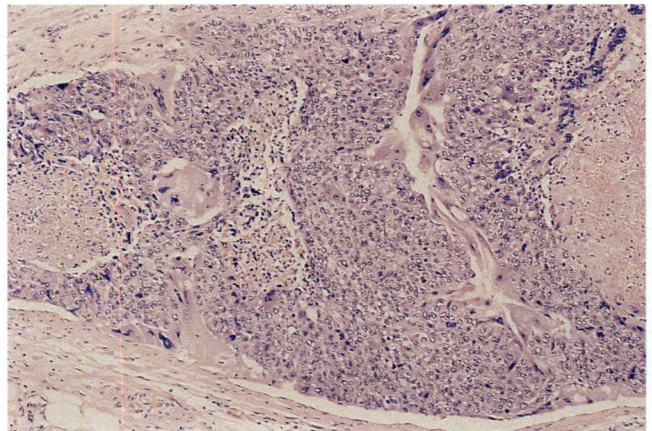

FIG. 48. Classic choriocarcinoma with clusters of lightly staining cytotrophoblast cells capped by multinucleated syncytiotrophoblast cells with dense, eosinophilic cytoplasm.

Choriocarcinomas consist of a proliferation of malignant trophoblastic cells. In its classic form, a central area of hemorrhage and necrosis is surrounded by an admixture of two distinct populations of cells—mononuclear cells with generally clear cytoplasm and mild to moderate nuclear pleomorphism (cytotrophoblast cells); and multinucleated cells, often with intracytoplasmic lacunae containing erythrocytes, that have abundant amphophilic cytoplasm (syncytiotrophoblast cells). Smudged nuclear chromatin is common in the syncytiotrophoblasts. In the better differentiated cases, the syncytiotrophoblast cells "cap" the cytotrophoblast population (Fig. 48), similar to the normal arrangement on placental villi. In other instances, the intermingling is more random. In some cases, the syncytiotrophoblast cells are a minor and relatively inconspicuous component and mainly recognizable by their more deeply staining cytoplasm and smudged nuclei. It can be difficult to distinguish such cases from embryonal carcinomas with cellular degeneration (see above). In other cases the syncytiotrophoblasts may be easily recognized but uncommon, occurring as scattered cells among sheets of cytotrophoblast cells (Fig. 49) (314). This "monophasic" pattern is one that we have more commonly seen following chemotherapy. There are rare cases in which the separation of the trophoblast elements into two populations becomes indistinct, but there is a proliferation of a spectrum of malignant trophoblasts, from small to large; this pattern, in our experience, is also more common in postchemotherapy specimens. The mitotic rate is generally high in the cytotrophoblast population, but mitoses do not occur in the syncytiotrophoblast cells.

Because of the extensive hemorrhagic necrosis of most choriocarcinomas, diagnostic foci of viable cells may require many sections. Such foci are usually peripheral, and an additional clue to the diagnosis is IGCNU in the adjacent seminiferous tubules. Pyknotic syncytiotrophoblast cells may be identified within the necrotic zone to encourage continued searching for diagnostic foci. Choriocarcinomas, like physiologic trophoblastic tissue, have a marked tendency for angioinvasion that correlates with their clinical aggressiveness.

Stains for hCG are quite valuable in helping to establish a diagnosis of choriocarcinoma and are positive in essentially all cases, mainly in the syncytiotrophoblast cells but also in scattered large mononuclear cells that may be transitional forms between cytotrophoblasts and syncytiotrophoblasts (156,164,315). Cytotrophoblasts are usually but not always hCG negative. Pregnancy-specific β_1-glycoprotein and human placental lactogen are also positive in syncytiotrophoblast and intermediate-type trophoblast cells but are negative in cytotrophoblasts (315). PLAP is positive in about 50% of choriocarcinomas (156), and CEA is positive in 25% of choriocarcinomas (156,316). Choriocarcinomas contain cytokeratins 7, 8, 18, and 19 (317). Unlike several forms of germ cell tumor, EMA is positive in a significant number of

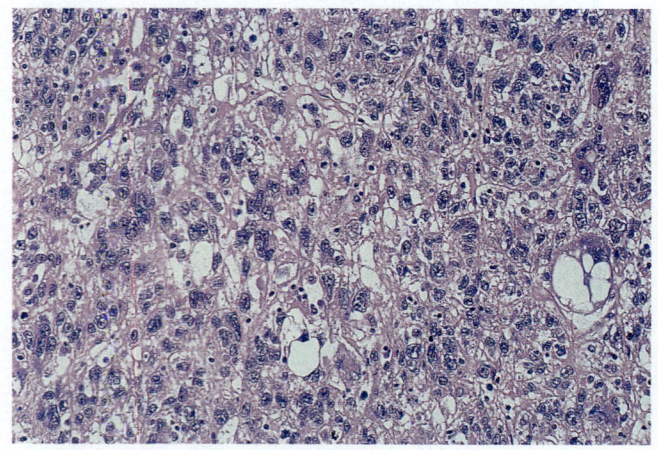
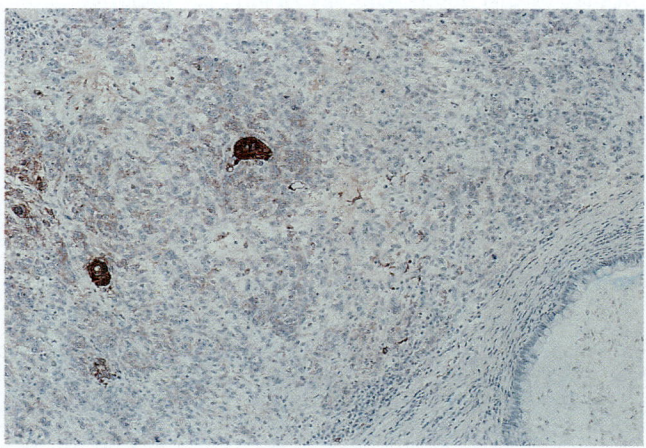

FIG. 49. A: "Monophasic" choriocarcinoma composed of pleomorphic, mononucleated cytotrophoblast cells with vacuolated cytoplasm and rare syncytiotrophoblast cells. **B:** Weak staining of the predominant cytotrophoblast cells for hCG, with strong staining of the syncytiotrophoblast cells. A teratomatous gland is negative.

choriocarcinomas (46%), mainly in the syncytiotrophoblasts (156).

Differential Diagnosis

It is important to distinguish choriocarcinoma from hemorrhagic testicular necrosis due to torsion, trauma, or clotting abnormalities. Clinically, testicular infarction usually produces painful testicular enlargement, whereas patients with choriocarcinomas often have small, nonpainful testes. On cross section infarction usually has a diffuse hemorrhagic picture, whereas a nodular area of hemorrhagic necrosis is typical of choriocarcinoma. Coagulative necrosis characterizes infarction, but residual tissue structures cannot be identified in the central hemorrhagic and necrotic areas of choriocarcinomas. The presence of IGCNU and hCG immunostains may be of additional help. It is also important to distinguish choriocarcinomas from other types of germ cell tumors that contain intermingled trophoblast cells. This distinction is based on the scattered nature of the trophoblastic elements, lack of a cytotrophoblast component, minor amounts, and absence of hemorrhagic necrosis in the latter. Embryonal carcinoma with cellular degeneration may be distinguished from choriocarcinoma by hCG stains. (It may not be possible to draw a firm distinction between embryonal carcinoma cells and a cytotrophoblast component, although a tendency for clear cytoplasm and more distinct cellular borders favors cytotrophoblasts over embryonal carcinoma cells.)

Choriocarcinomas disseminate rapidly, often via hematogenous routes. Brain involvement occurs with disproportionate frequency (318). It is treated similarly to other nonseminomatous tumors, but a significant choriocarcinomatous component in a testicular germ cell tumor probably worsens the prognosis, based on several studies in which multivariate analysis correlated a poor outcome with high hCG titers (319–321). In some studies direct identification of choriocarcinoma or "trophoblastic" elements correlated with a poorer prognosis (319,320,322,323). A choriocarcinoma syndrome has been identified in which patients have hemorrhagic visceral metastases and a high mortality despite aggressive therapy (319). Despite these findings, cures of metastatic choriocarcinoma do occur (319,324) Choriocarcinomas as a component of mixed germ cell tumors may behave less aggressively than do pure choriocarcinomas (6,325–327).

Placental-Site Trophoblastic Tumor

We have seen a single case of a trophoblastic tumor of the testis that resembled the placental-site trophoblastic tumor of the uterus. This tumor occurred in a 16-month-old infant and consisted of an interstitial proliferation of intermediate trophoblast cells (Fig. 50). The patient was well on follow-up, 8 years after orchiectomy (314). Small foci of similar appearance may be seen in some typical choriocarcinomas.

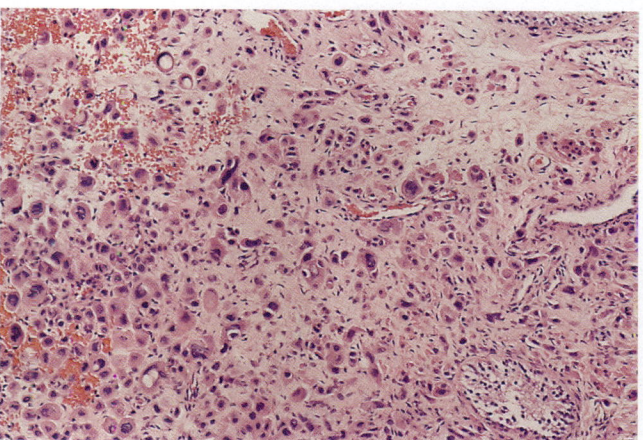

FIG. 50. Placental-site trophoblastic tumor, with an interstitial growth of intermediate trophoblasts, admixed with Leydig cells.

Teratoma

Testicular teratomas occur both in pediatric and adult patients, and their biology appears to be significantly different for these two groups. In prepubertal patients, they almost always are pure neoplasms and represent 14% of testicular germ cell tumors (the others being yolk sac tumors) (278). The mean age at diagnosis is 20 months, and occurrence beyond 4 years is unusual (278). Most patients present with a testicular mass identified by a parent. There are reported associations with congenital anomalies or diseases, including Down syndrome, Klinefelter's syndrome, hernia, hemihypertrophy, xeroderma pigmentosa, spina bifida (328), and retrocaval ureter (328,329). In adult patients, on the other hand, teratoma usually occurs as one component of a mixed germ cell tumor, with over 50% of all mixed germ cell tumors having a teratomatous component (133,330); pure cases in adults are uncommon. The adult patients have the typical features of a testicular germ cell tumor, i.e., they are generally young, present with a testicular mass, but may have symptoms secondary to metastatic involvement and may have serum marker elevations depending on the nature of the associated components.

One puzzling aspect about the biology of testicular teratomas in adults is the occasional development of nonteratomatous metastases in patients with apparently pure teratomas (327). The most likely explanation for this phenomenon, in our opinion, is the common development of the adult form of teratoma from a nonteratomatous precursor element (e.g., embryonal carcinoma) that can metastasize as such but also transform to teratoma in the testis. Transformation to teratoma in the metastatic site as well may explain cases reported as "mature teratoma metastasizing as mature teratoma" (331–334), although direct vascular/lymphatic invasion in the testis with metastasis remains another possibility (154). In support of this concept, adult patients with teratoma have the common precursor lesion of germ cell

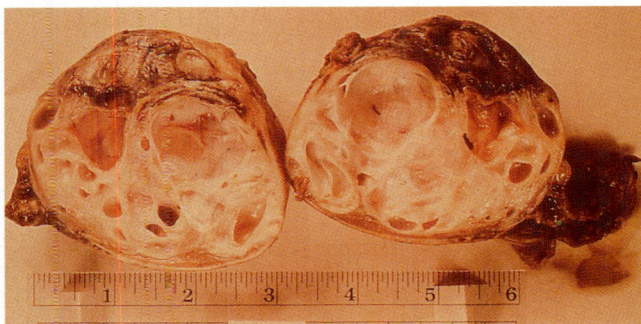

FIG. 51. Mature teratoma, with multiple cysts. (Photograph courtesy of D.J. Gersell, M.D., Washington University School of Medicine, St. Louis, Missouri.)

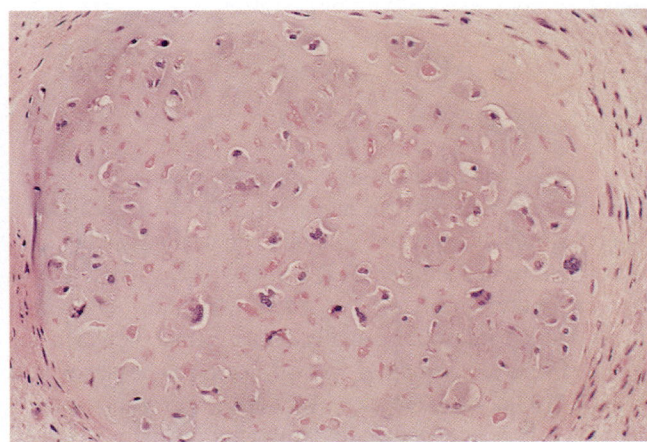

FIG. 53. Cytologic atypia of cartilage in a testicular teratoma from an adult patient.

tumors in their seminiferous tubules—IGCNU (111)—making it likely that pure teratomas in adults evolve from an initially undifferentiated tumor with an inherent capacity to transform to somatic tissues. This may not be the case for children with testicular teratomas, with reports of IGCNU lacking in such cases (111), despite the rare description of PLAP-negative atypical germ cells (335); perhaps this observation is linked with the absence of metastases in childhood testicular teratomas. It should be emphasized that although we subcategorize teratomas into mature and immature types based on their histology, a mature teratoma in an adult does *not* equate with a benign tumor.

Serum marker studies of patients with pure testicular teratomas are generally negative, although the immunohistochemical detection of AFP in teratomatous glands indicates a potential for abnormal AFP values (154,164,235). One should also be aware that in very young children there is a physiologically high AFP value (285).

On gross examination, teratomas are often multinodular, and their cut surface varies from multicystic (Fig. 51) to solid. Nodules of translucent white cartilage may be seen. The cysts may be filled with clear or mucoid fluid or keratinous material. Hair, except in the rare dermoid cyst (a specialized form of pure teratoma discussed more fully below), is unusual. Areas of immature tissue may have a fleshy, encephaloid character.

On microscopic examination, pure mature teratomas, by definition, are composed of tissues resembling adult somatic tissues (Fig. 52). Most teratomas in children, somewhat paradoxically, consist solely of mature tissues. In postpubertal patients, there is frequent cytologic atypia of such tissues that reflects their malignant potential and development from IGCNU. This is supported by the demonstration of aneuploidy (336,337). Such cytologic atypia, in our opinion, should not qualify for classification as immature, which, by definition, should be reserved for tissues resembling embryonic or fetal structures. Thus, one may find nodules of atypical cartilage (Fig. 53), gastrointestinal and respiratory epithelium with muscular cuffs, squamous islands, transitional epithelium, neuroglia, pigmented retinal epithelium, fibrous stroma, bone with active marrow, and others. Sometimes the glands are architecturally complex (Fig. 54). A granulomatous reaction to extravasated keratin is common. We are in the habit of qualitatively grading the cytologic atypia of the

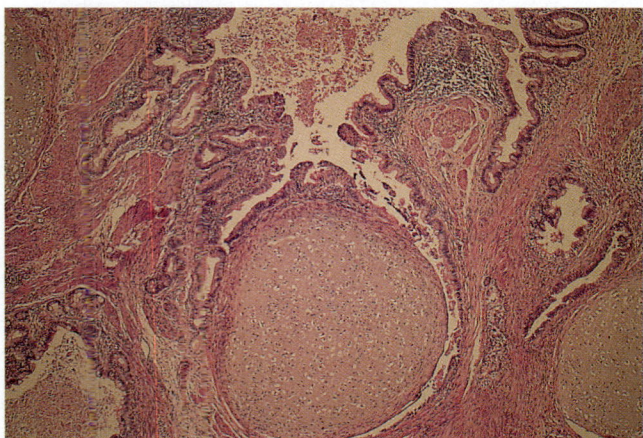

FIG. 52. Mature teratoma consisting of intestinal-type glands closely associated with smooth muscle and nodules of hyaline cartilage.

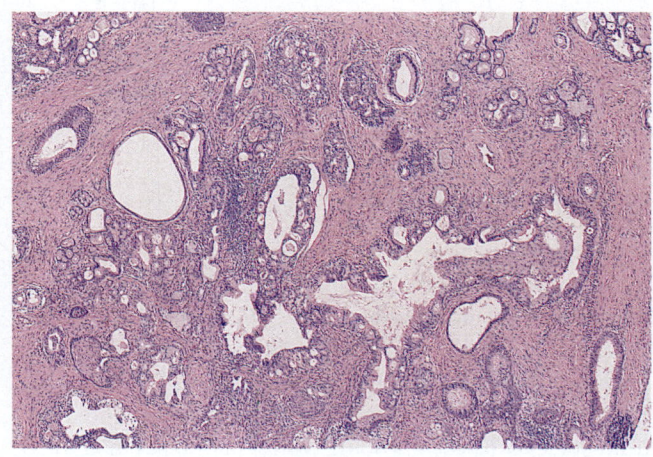

FIG. 54. Architecturally complex glands in mature teratoma.

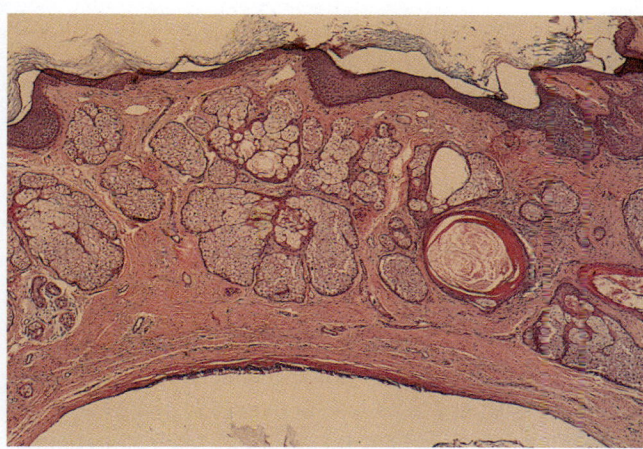

FIG. 55. Dermoid cyst lined by keratinizing, squamous epithelium with numerous sebaceous glands in its wall.

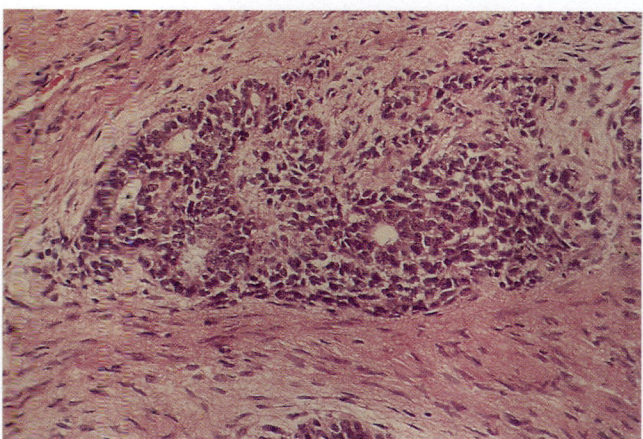

FIG. 57. Collections of primitive-appearing tubules and blastema-like cells in an immature teratoma.

elements as either low or high grade, although there is no evidence that this has any prognostic significance. On occasion, frank somatic-type malignancies can develop in mature teratomas ("mature teratoma with a secondary malignant component"), in which case a diagnosis of mature teratoma with sarcoma or carcinoma is justified (see below).

Dermoid cysts should be recognized as a distinct subcategory of mature teratoma. They are quite rare and analogous to the more commonly occurring ovarian counterpart, consisting of a cystic structure filled with keratin and hair with one or more protruding nodules on its wall. The cyst wall is lined by keratinizing squamous epithelium with sebaceous glands and hair follicles (Fig. 55), and the nodules may contain cartilage, neuroglia, or fibrous tissue (9). Metastasis is not reported in association with dermoid cysts, unlike other varieties of mature teratoma, and these lesions should, therefore, be classified separately and not lumped with mature teratoma, not otherwise specified. In the two cases we have seen, there was no IGCNU, a feature we regard as incompatible with dermoid cyst.

Immature teratoma, by definition, has tissues resembling those of embryonic or fetal development. Usually these are admixed with mature tissues. Most teratomas in postpubertal patients have some degree of immaturity. Some of the more commonly occurring immature tissue are neuroepithelium (Fig. 56) and neuroblastic-type tissues, blastomatous tissues resembling Wilms' tumor (Fig. 57), immature skeletal muscle with primitive cells admixed with differentiated muscle cells, and cuffs of immature stromal tissues, probably representing smooth muscle precursors, around islands of epithelium (Fig. 58). The recognition of such tissues justifies subcategorization as immature teratoma. We also grade the immaturity based, qualitatively, on the cellularity and mitotic activity of the immature elements and give an estimate of their extent. Thus, a small focus of highly cellular and mitotically active neuroepithelium would justify a diagnosis of teratoma with focal high-grade immature elements. A more widespread presence of modestly cellular but immature mesenchymal cuffs around glandular structures would result in a diagnosis of teratoma with moderately diffuse, low-grade immature elements. This practice, however, remains an aca-

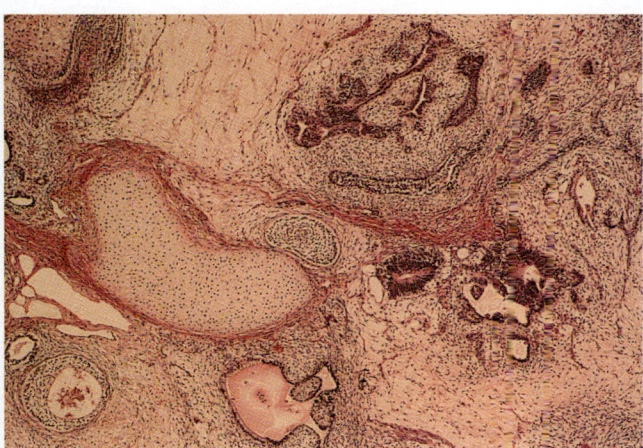

FIG. 56. Focal immature tissues in a teratoma, with small collections of embryonic-appearing neuroepithelium.

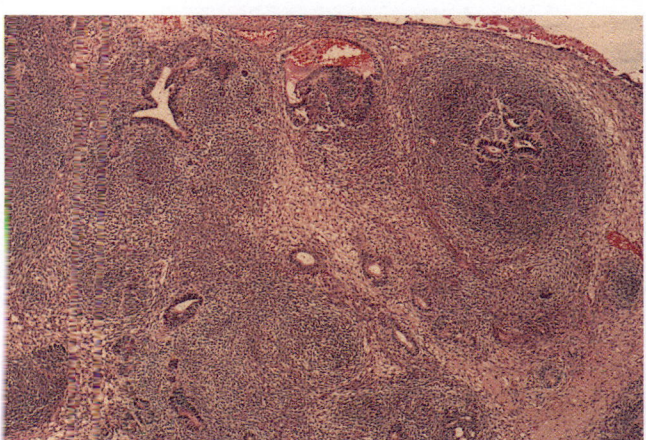

FIG. 58. Cuffs of undifferentiated, cellular mesenchyme surround islands of primitive-appearing epithelium in this immature teratoma.

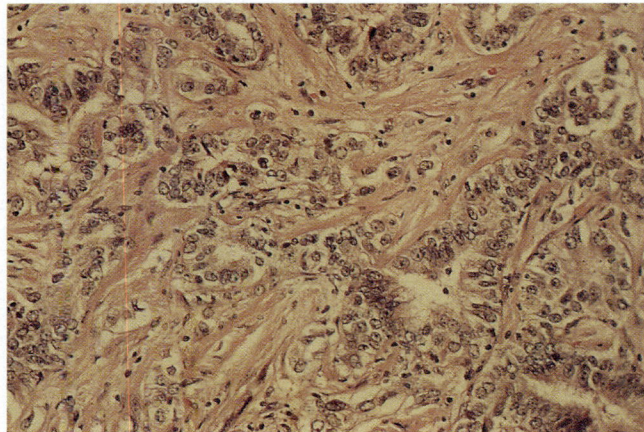

FIG. 59. Malignant glandular elements of teratoma invade the stroma, permitting a diagnosis of teratoma with adenocarcinoma.

demic exercise since no study has shown it has any prognostic significance; this is likely because of the usual association of immature teratoma with other forms of germ cell tumor that determine the prognosis.

When should a diagnosis of a secondary malignancy in a teratoma (teratoma with a secondary malignant component) be made? There are no meaningful studies to answer this question. We believe that malignancies of somatic type should be diagnosed in mature teratomas when there is evidence of stromal invasion by malignant-appearing epithelium (Fig. 59) or a sizable nodule of highly atypical stromal elements occurs. This latter criterion also applies to immature elements in teratoma, resulting in diagnoses such as primitive neuroectodermal tumor (338,339), embryonal rhabdomyosarcoma, and primitive nephroblastoma-like neoplasm (Fig. 60) only when a pure and relatively large nodule of such elements is produced and not when they remained scattered in small nests in a multifocal fashion. Our empiric guideline for a "sizable nodule" is the majority of the field area viewed with a ×4 objective. Whether such an approach is clinically significant is unknown. It should be noted that in two studies no adverse prognostic significance was associated with secondary teratomatous malignancies when identified in the testis (340), although their presence in metastatic sites was ominous (339,340), as demonstrated previously (341). Mostofi (342), however, believes that virtually all patients with postchemotherapy failure secondary to non–germ cell malignancies have similar tumors in the testicular primary.

Immunohistochemical staining of teratomas yields the expected results for the specific elements examined. Thus, neural markers are identified in neural tissues (343), cytokeratins in epithelia, vimentin in stromal tissues, and desmin in muscle (299). AFP may be seen in enteric or respiratory type glandular structures as well as in liver (154,164,235). CEA, alpha$_1$-antitrypsin, and ferritin occur in teratomatous epithelium in about 50% of cases (235), and PLAP is also positive in glandular teratomatous structures in a minority of cases (116,155,229). p53 protein may be identified in teratomatous epithelium (344).

Differential Diagnosis

It is important to distinguish mature teratoma in adults from epidermoid cysts and dermoid cysts. These latter two entities behave in a benign fashion, whereas mature teratoma has metastatic potential. An epidermoid cyst is an intratesticular, squamous epithelial-lined cyst filled with keratinous debris. No adnexal structures or other elements are present (345,346). There is no association with IGCNU (111), and the pathogenesis of the lesion is not clear. Dermoid cysts have been described above. They lack the solid component of most adult teratomas, show no immaturity or significant atypia of tissues, and are not, to our knowledge, associated with IGCNU.

Pure teratomas in prepubertal children behave as benign lesions, and orchiectomy is curative (327,347). Pure teratomas in adults are rare; they are usually associated with other germ cell elements, which determine the prognosis. At Indiana University, 63% of adults with pure teratomas had metastases, but this high proportion reflects referral bias (348). Johnson and co-workers (349) reported 18 adult patients with teratomas (some of which were associated with seminoma) who were treated by orchiectomy and RPLND, achieving a 5-year survival of 100%. It is important, however, always to be aware of the possibility of nonteratomatous elements occurring in metastatic sites in adults with pure testicular teratomas (327). Dixon and Moore (7) reported a 30% 5-year mortality of testicular teratomas. A reasonable approach in patients with pure teratomas is nerve-sparing RPLND followed by either chemotherapy or close follow-up, depending on the pathologic findings in the retroperitoneal nodes.

Carcinoid Tumor

Testicular carcinoid tumors are considered to be monodermal teratomas since, although most are pure neoplasms,

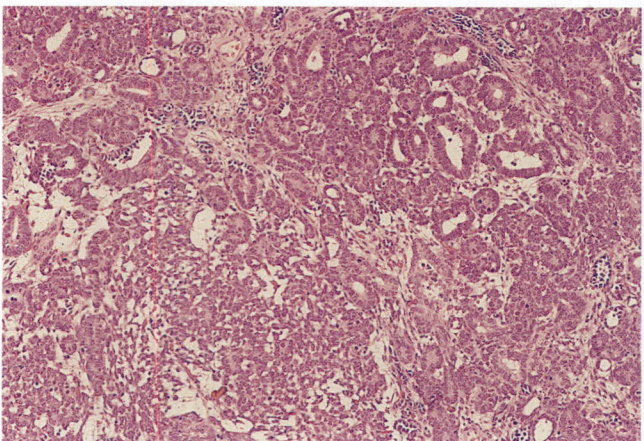

FIG. 60. A blastomatous-type tumor in a teratoma with a large collection of primitive-appearing tubules.

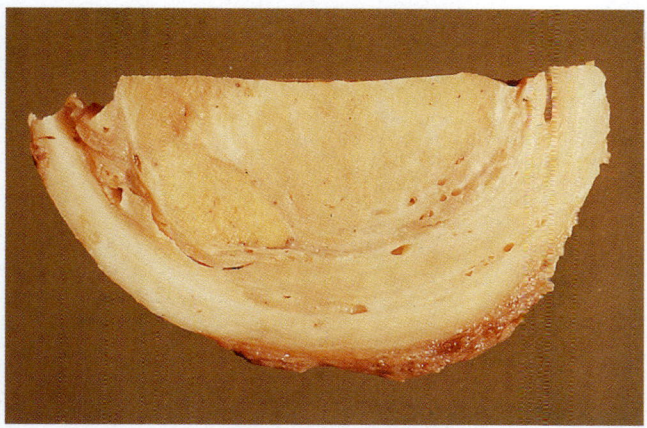

FIG. 61. Yellow cut surface and well-circumscribed margins are typical gross features of a testicular carcinoid. (Photograph courtesy of D.J. Gersell, M.D., Washington University School of Medicine, St. Louis, Missouri.)

about 20% are associated with teratomatous elements (350–352). They are rare and occur over an age range from the second to the ninth decades, with a mean age of 46 years (350–353). Most patients present with a mass, sometimes of several years' duration (352). A clinical carcinoid syndrome is infrequent, occurring in about 10% of cases, but serotonin metabolites are detected in a higher proportion (352). On gross examination, they are solid, yellow to tan, well-circumscribed nodules (Fig. 61); cysts may be identified if other teratomatous structures are present. Microscopically they generally appear similar to mid-gut carcinoid tumors, composed of islands of cells forming small acini (Fig. 62). The nuclei are round with granular chromatin, and there is granular, eosinophilic cytoplasm. Other teratomatous elements may be identified, most frequently mucinous and glandular epithelium. We have not identified IGCNU in the few pure carcinoids that we have seen. Argyrophil and argentaffin stains are positive, and serotonin, neuron-specific enolase, chromogranin, and cytokeratin may be identified immunohistochemically (352,354,355); it is also likely that other markers of mid-gut type carcinoid tumors (356) would

prove positive. Polymorphous neurosecretory granules are seen by electron microscopy (350,352,354). It is important to distinguish primary testicular carcinoids from metastatic carcinoid tumors. The presence of teratomatous elements supports a primary lesion; metastatic carcinoids are frequently bilateral, multifocal, and show lymphatic/vascular invasion, and the patients have evidence of extratesticular tumor. The general prognosis of primary testicular carcinoids is good, however, 2 of 12 patients in the series of Berdjis and Mostofi (351) developed metastatic disease, which may occur many years following orchiectomy (357). A clinical carcinoid syndrome correlates with malignant behavior, as does large tumor size (mean = 7.3 cm for malignant cases) (352). Orchiectomy with follow-up is the usual therapy.

Primitive Neuroectodermal Tumor

Primitive neuroectodermal tumors (PNET) of the testis are also considered monodermal teratomas composed of small cells arranged in diffuse sheets, tubules, rosettes, and pseudorosettes (Fig. 63) (338). They usually represent overgrowth of primitive neural elements of immature teratoma, and hence are components of germ cell tumors with teratomatous and other elements (339,358). Rarely they represent a pure testicular tumor (338,359,360). When admixed with other germ cell tumor components, distinction from immature teratoma is based on the size of the primitive neuroepithelial component, as discussed below. On gross examination, the pure cases are gray-white and partially necrotic. Microscopically, small cells with hyperchromatic nuclei are arranged in sheets, neural-type tubules, and rosettes. Neuron specific enolase (NSE), synaptophysin, chromogranin, and HBA-71 are positive in varying proportions of cases (339). Neurosecretory granules may be present on ultrastructural examination (360). In the series of Michael et al. (339), metastatic cases had a very poor outcome.

Mixed Germ Cell Tumors

Although the various types of germ cell tumors discussed in the previous sections may occur as pure tumors, it is much

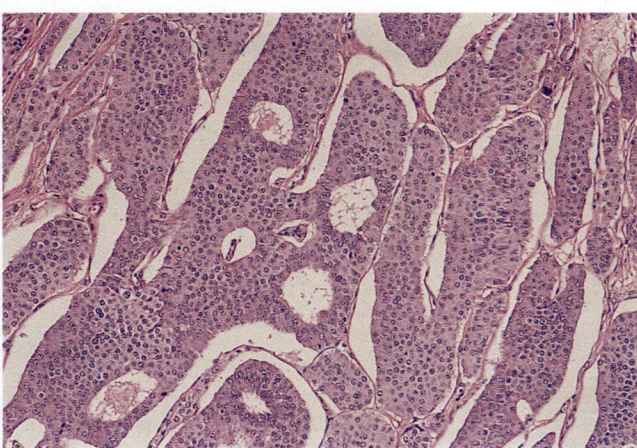

FIG. 62. Solid islands of cells with small acini are characteristic of testicular carcinoid tumor.

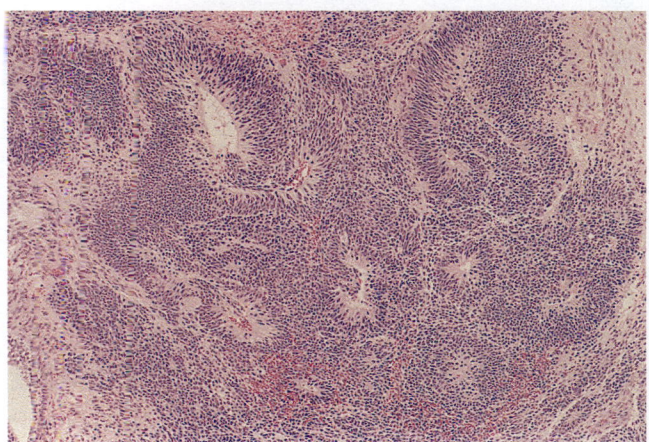

FIG. 63. Primitive neuroectodermal tumor in teratoma.

more common, except for seminoma, to see intermixtures of different neoplastic type. From 69% to 91% of the nonseminomatous testicular germ cell tumors are of mixed types (132,330). In diagnosing such cases, our recommendation is to use the term *mixed germ cell tumor,* followed by a parenthetical listing of the components with an estimate of their relative proportions in percentages. On gross examination, mixed germ cell tumors are characteristically variegated, reflecting their different components, with foci of hemorrhage and necrosis (Fig. 64). Microscopically, the appearance is identical to the various pure neoplasms. We and others (219) have noted a tendency of many pathologists to overlook foci of yolk sac tumor that characteristically develop in close association with an embryonal carcinoma component. We also regard the double-layered pattern of embryonal carcinoma described by Jacobsen (225) as an example of a mixed germ cell tumor composed of embryonal carcinoma and yolk sac tumor. There is evidence that tumors composed of embryonal carcinoma and teratoma behave in a less aggressive fashion than those consisting of pure embryonal carcinoma (361), and yolk sac tumor elements may also favorably alter the behavior of mixed germ cell tumors (252).

Polyembryoma and Diffuse Embryoma

Both polyembryoma and diffuse embryoma are distinctive forms of mixed germ cell tumors. Polyembryoma consists of small, scattered, embryo-like bodies having a central core of embryonal carcinoma cells (resembling the embryonic plate), an associated amnion-like cavity, and a yolk sac tumor component resembling the embryonic yolk sac (362,363) (Fig. 55). Syncytiotrophoblasts are often associated with the amnion-like and yolk sac–like components, and intestinal, hepatic, and squamous differentiation may occur (362). Thus, these tumors are considered to have compo-

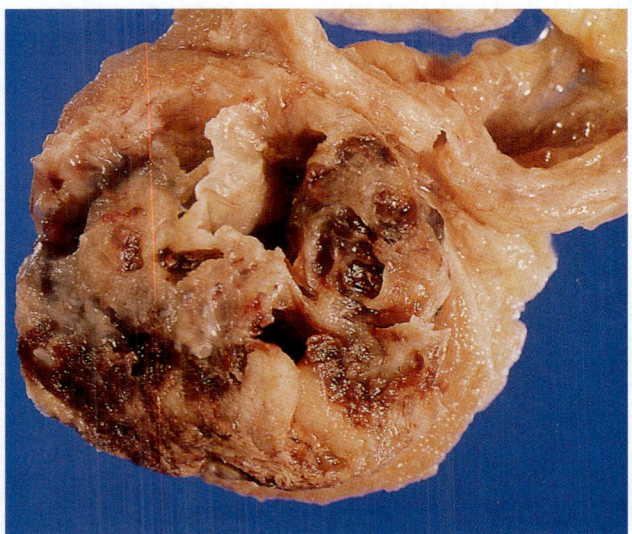

FIG. 64. Typical variegated appearance of a mixed germ cell tumor with areas of hemorrhage, necrosis, and cystic change.

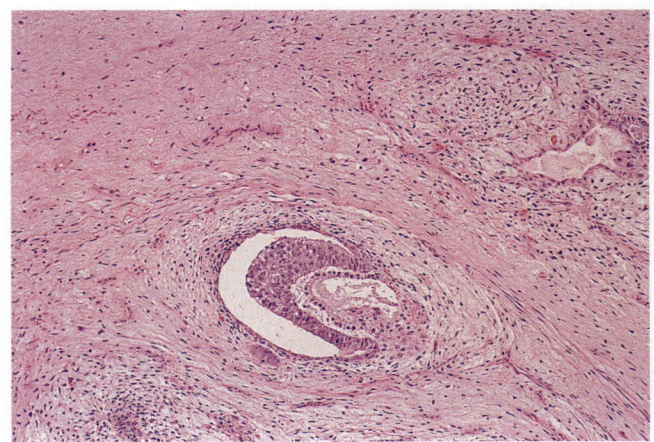

FIG. 65. Embryoid body of polyembryoma. Note amnion-like cavity, core of embryonal carcinoma, and yolk sac tumor, resembling the embryonic yolk sac.

nents of embryonal carcinoma and yolk sac tumor, and sometimes teratomatous and syncytiotrophoblastic components. Their behavior is typical of nonseminomatous germ cell tumors. In diffuse embryoma, there is a diffuse intermingling of approximately equal amounts of embryonal carcinoma and yolk sac tumor elements (Fig. 66) (364,365).

Regression of Germ Cell Tumors

Some patients with metastatic germ cell tumors are noted, either at autopsy or orchiectomy, to have testicular scars that may be associated with IGCNU, intratubular hematoxylin-staining bodies (consisting of nuclear debris and calcifications) (226), or teratomatous elements. These patients are thought to have had regression of most or all of their primary neoplasm (226). Approximately 10% of male patients dying of metastatic germ cell tumors have such "burnt-out" primary tumors (366), and it is especially likely to occur in patients with metastatic choriocarcinoma (367), but may be as-

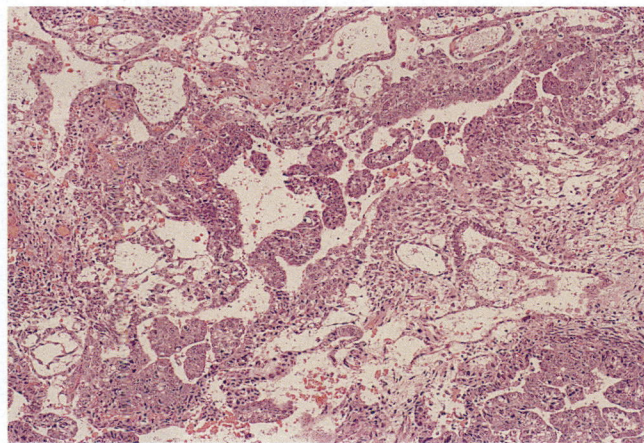

FIG. 66. Diffuse embryoma, with admixed embryonal carcinoma and yolk sac tumor in approximately equal amounts.

sociated with other germ cell tumor types as well. It is likely that most patients with isolated retroperitoneal germ cell tumors have metastatic retroperitoneal disease with tumor regression in the testis (368). On microscopic examination of the testis, there are fibrotic areas, hemosiderin-laden macrophages, chronic inflammatory cells, and often, intratubular calcifications (Fig. 67). The latter probably correspond to a complete comedo-type of intratubular tumor necrosis with dystrophic calcification. IGCNU may be identified in residual seminiferous tubules (368), and some teratomatous elements may also persist.

Postchemotherapy Resections

Patients with metastatic testicular germ cell tumors commonly undergo postchemotherapy resection of residual masses, and the interpretation of these specimens can pose problems, even to experienced pathologists (265). The diagnosis of residual, nonteratomatous germ cell tumor in these cases is often considered an indication for additional chemotherapy, whereas teratoma, necrosis, and fibrotic or reparative reactions are not (369).

Necrotic foci are often surrounded by a prominent infiltrate of foamy macrophages, sometimes containing hemosiderin, and an active fibroblastic proliferation (Fig. 68). The cytoplasmic clarity of the macrophages may cause a misinterpretation as seminoma, but the nuclei, although sometimes active-appearing with small to moderate-sized nucleoli, lack malignant features. In the central portion of the necrosis, pyknotic nuclei in the "ghost-like" outlines of tumor cells should not be considered evidence of persistent germ cell tumor.

Fibrotic foci often contain widely scattered, spindle-shaped to epithelioid-appearing cells with nuclear atypia (Fig. 69). Cytokeratin stains may highlight these cells, confirming they have an epithelial phenotype and supporting our belief they often derive from the "mesenchymal" component of yolk sac tumor (290,292). Others may represent persistent trophoblastic cells. As long as the atypical cells are widely scattered as individual or small clusters and show no or only rare mitotic figures, we do not qualify our diagnosis of fibrosis. A greater degree of cellularity or proliferative activity may merit comment, but it is unlikely to alter the future therapy—i.e., close follow-up rather than additional chemotherapy.

Persistent teratoma often shows significant cytologic atypia in both mesenchymal and epithelial components. In the absence of stromal invasion or overgrowth, this atypia has no significant impact on prognosis and is not considered an indication for additional chemotherapy (370). The development of carcinoma or sarcoma, manifest by invasion or overgrowth, is associated with an aggressive course, but the treatment primarily remains surgical excision (370).

Although most forms of germ cell tumor in postchemotherapy resections have a similar morphology as in untreated cases, we have noted a tendency for some choriocarcinomas to lack a well-defined biphasic pattern and mainly consist of

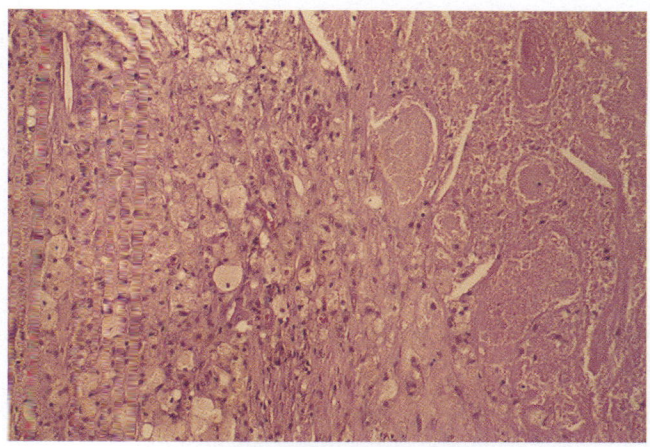

FIG. 68. Postchemotherapy specimen showing the typical coagulative necrosis surrounded by a prominent foamy macrophage reaction with cholesterol clefts.

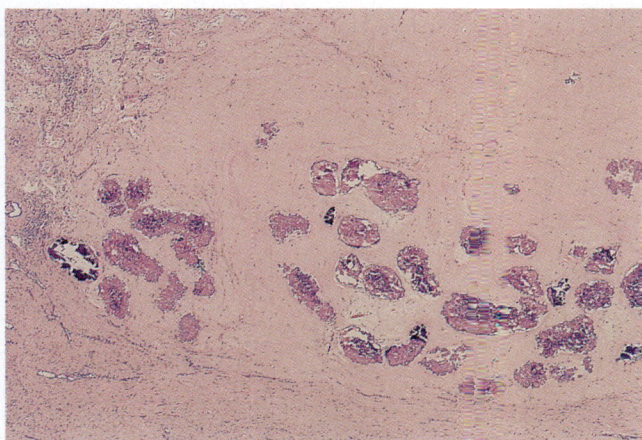

FIG. 67. "Burnt-out" germ cell tumor, with an area of scar and intratubular calcifications.

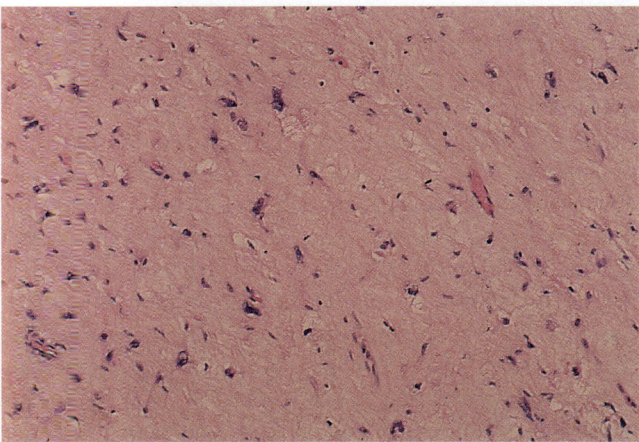

FIG. 69. Postchemotherapy specimen showing fibrous tissue containing widely scattered spindle to oval cells with degenerate-type atypia.

cytotrophoblast cells, as was noted in treated gestational choriocarcinoma (371). Marked cystic transformation of choriocarcinoma, with a lining epithelium resembling atypical, squamoid cells, may also occur and probably should not be considered a reason for additional chemotherapy, although this has not been rigorously examined. Persistent yolk sac tumor may have more prominent parietal and glandular features than in untreated patients.

SEX CORD–STROMAL TUMORS

The sex cord–stromal tumors of the testis represent a distinct minority of testicular neoplasms but a disproportionate number of diagnostic difficulties. Only about 4% of testicular tumors fall into this category (198,372), which consists of those neoplasms whose constitutive cells resemble Leydig cells, Sertoli cells, theca cells, granulosa cells, and/or fibroblasts. There are six major categories of neoplasms in this group: Leydig cell tumors, Sertoli cell tumors, Sertoli-Leydig cell tumors, granulosa cell tumors, fibromas of gonadal stromal origin, and sex cord–stromal tumors of mixed type or indeterminate origin. Ovarian tumors in the sex cord–stromal category, with the exception of fibromas, myxomas, and sclerosing stromal tumors, stain for inhibin, a glycoprotein hormone produced by normal ovarian granulosa cells and testicular Sertoli cells (373–375).

Leydig Cell Tumor

Leydig cell tumors constitute the single most common type of testicular sex cord–stromal tumor and represent about 2% to 3% of all testicular neoplasms (376). They occur over a wide age range, 2 to 90 years old (377), but are most common in the third to sixth decades (376), with a smaller peak in children 5 to 10 years old (378). The presentation depends on the age of the patient, with children, representing about 20% of cases, commonly presenting with isosexual pseudoprecocity due to androgenic hormone production by the neoplasm (379). These patients may have small, nonpalpable tumors requiring specialized methods for clinical detection. Adults, in whom additional androgenic production is more difficult to detect, more commonly present with a testicular mass (376). About 30% of adults develop gynecomastia (376), which also occurs in about 10% of children (378), in whom it is invariably superimposed on virilization. Bilateral Leydig cell tumors occur in roughly 3% of the cases (376). The familial occurrence of Leydig cell tumors in a father and his adult son has been reported (380).

On gross examination Leydig cell tumors are characteristically solid, well-circumscribed, round to lobulated nodules that vary from yellow to tan to brown to gray, with some cases having coarse fibrous bands (Fig. 70). They range from 0.5 to 10 cm in diameter, but are most commonly 2 to 5 cm (376). Foci of hemorrhage and necrosis may be identified in a minority of the cases. From 10% to 15% of the cases have extratesticular extension (376). On microscopic examina-

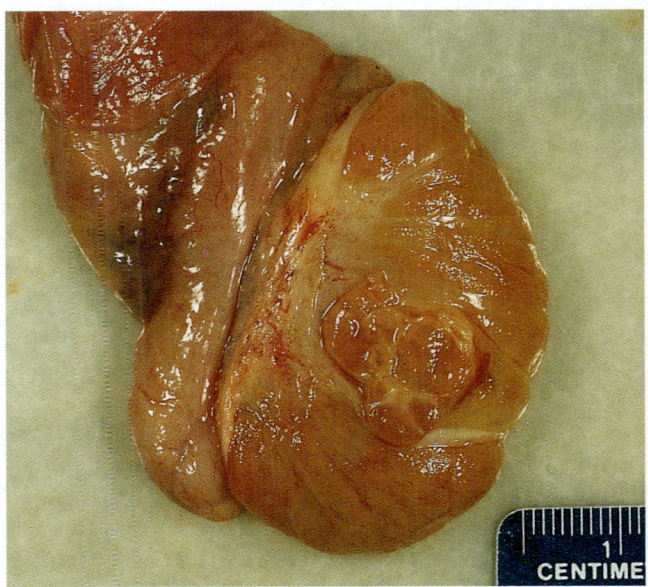

FIG. 70. Leydig cell tumor, consisting of a circumscribed, bulging, tan nodule containing fibrous bands.

tion, a diffuse, sheet-like pattern of cells is most common (Fig. 71), although small nests, ribbons, and cords (Fig. 72) may also be present in fibrous stroma. We have seen several cases with a prominent microcystic arrangement in areas. The individual cells are polygonal and usually have eosinophilic cytoplasm, although abundant lipids may cause the cells to have clear, finely vacuolated cytoplasm in some cases (Fig. 73). The nuclei are round, often with a moderate-sized central nucleolus, and can show moderate variation in diameter (Fig. 74). Mitoses are generally infrequent. Lipofuscin can be identified in the cytoplasm in a minority of the cases (Fig. 74) (generally those with a tan to brown gross appearance) and rod-shaped intracytoplasmic crystals of Reinke may be identified in up to 40% of the cases (372) (Fig. 75). A more spindled cell population can be identified in some cases; classification of those cases with a predomi-

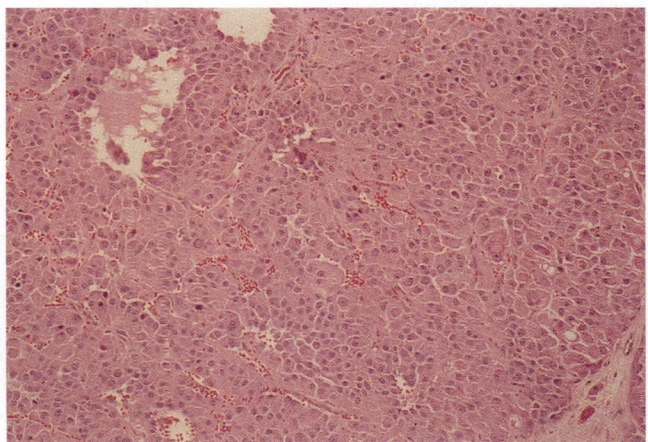

FIG. 71. Sheet-like pattern of Leydig cell tumor, with occasional small cysts.

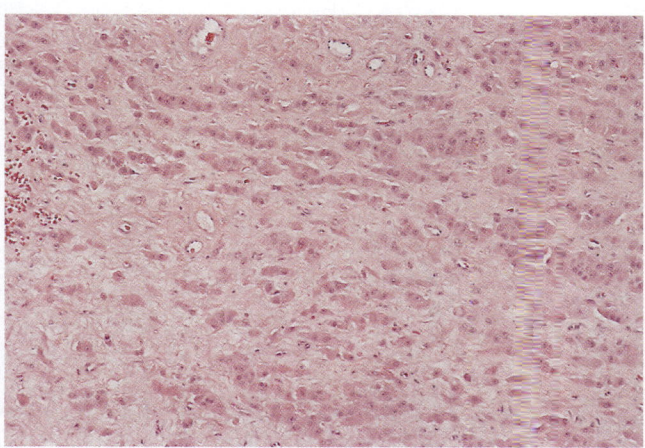

FIG. 72. Cord-like pattern of Leydig cell tumor.

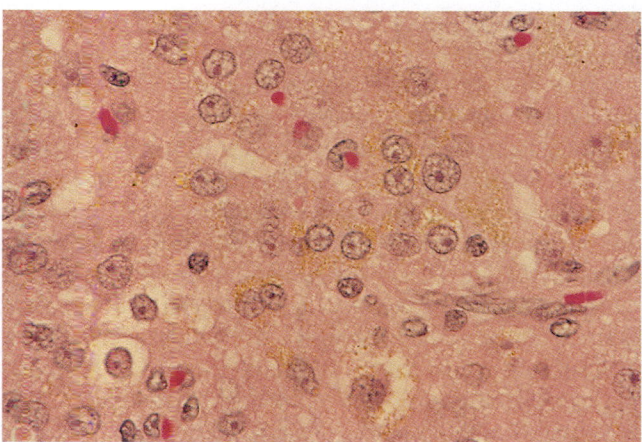

FIG. 74. Central, round nucleoli, moderate variation in nuclear size, and cytoplasmic lipofuscin in Leydig cell tumor.

nant spindle cell component as unclassified stromal tumors would appear to be preferable (377).

On ultrastructural examination, the distinctive features are those of a steroid hormone producing cell—i.e., abundant smooth endoplasmic reticulum, mitochondria with tubular cristae, and intracytoplasmic lipid droplets (381,382); in some cases, the distinctive crystals of Reinke are identified as well as membranous whorls (383). Immunostaining for vimentin is characteristically positive in Leydig cell tumors (384), and we have noted strongly positive staining for inhibin and patchy low molecular weight cytokeratin reactivity in several cases. Androgenic hormones may be demonstrated by immunohistochemistry. Enkephalin-like reactivity was described in one Leydig cell tumor (385). Variants include rare cases with ossification and psammoma bodies (386,387) (which should be distinguished from large cell calcifying Sertoli cell tumors—see below) and adipose metaplasia (388).

Differential Diagnosis

The differential diagnosis of Leydig cell tumors has been well discussed by Young and Talerman (372). In contrast to Leydig cell tumor, Leydig cell hyperplasia, as seen in Klinefelter's syndrome and other disorders, may mimic a neoplasm but produces an interstitial growth pattern that does not destroy the surrounding tubules. Ultrastructural differences between Leydig cell tumor and Leydig cell hyperplasia have been described (389). Large cell calcifying Sertoli cell tumor (LCCSCT) (see below) (390–397), is distinguished from Leydig cell tumor on the basis of its frequent multifocality, high incidence of bilaterality, more abundant stroma, calcifications, intratubular growth, and absence of Reinke crystals (372,391). Malakoplakia may resemble Leydig cell tumor but has foci of intratubular Leydig-like cells and the characteristic Michaelis-Gutmann bodies. The testicular nodules of the adrenogenital syndrome (398,399) or as seen in Nelson's syndrome (400) strongly resemble Leydig cell tumors, but are multifocal and bilateral, lack Reinke crystals, and usually contain more prominent lipofuscin (372,398). The clinical history in such cases is obviously important. Lymphomas and plasmacytomas often have an interstitial pattern, and lymphoma is more frequently bilateral; appropriate immunostains can confirm their nature. Rarely metastatic prostate cancer may mimic a Leydig cell tumor

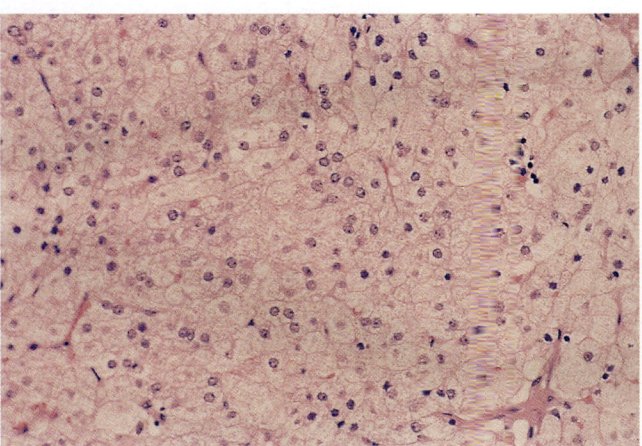

FIG. 73. Clear, vacuolated cytoplasm caused by abundant intracytoplasmic lipid in a Leydig cell tumor.

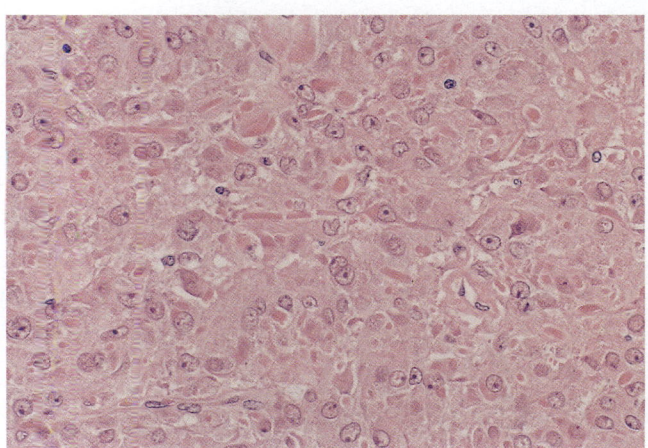

FIG. 75. Numerous Reinke crystals in Leydig cell tumor.

(372); immunostains for cytokeratins, prostate-specific antigen, and prostatic acid phosphatase should resolve the issue.

About 10% of Leydig cell tumors behave in a malignant fashion, but it is difficult, short of the presence of metastases, to predict malignancy. There is a greater likelihood of malignancy in larger tumors (>5 cm); those with infiltrative margins; in the presence of necrosis, nuclear atypia, and a mitotic rate of more than 3 per 10 high power fields; and with vascular invasion (376). Older patients are more likely to have a malignant tumor (401), but those with gynecomastia are more likely to pursue a benign course (376). Malignant behavior in a prepubertal patient has not been reported (376,379). An ossifying malignant Leydig cell tumor has been described (387). For patients with clinically malignant Leydig cell tumors, retroperitoneal lymph node dissection is often performed. Radiation and chemotherapy are usually not effective. Recurrences may develop after several years, although the mean survival for malignant Leydig cell tumors is 4 years (401).

Sertoli Cell Tumor

Sertoli cell tumor represents only about 1% of testicular tumors. Three histologic types are described: Sertoli cell tumor, not otherwise specified (NOS); sclerosing Sertoli cell tumor; and LCCSCT. Multicentric Sertoli cell tumors or variants of them (perhaps LCCSCTs—see below) or sex cord tumors with annular tubules (see chapter by Young et al., "The Ovary") are associated with the Peutz-Jeghers syndrome and gynecomastia in young boys (402,403).

Sertoli Cell Tumor, NOS

The age range is 15 to 80 years with a mean of 45 years; most patients present with a testicular mass (378,404), although occasional tumors may produce clinical estrogenic manifestations such as gynecomastia and impotency, which may therefore be presenting features (377,404). Gynecomastia in a child in the absence of virilism is an important diagnostic clue to a possible Sertoli cell tumor and contrasts with the situation in childhood Leydig cell tumor where gynecomastia does not occur in the absence of virilism (378). On gross examination, Sertoli cell tumor NOS is usually firm, yellow to gray to white, well circumscribed and solid, most commonly under 4 cm in diameter, although occasionally quite large (Fig. 76). On microscopic examination, Sertoli cell tumors NOS typically forms solid (Fig. 77) or hollow tubules and cords in a nested or diffuse arrangement with a prominent, sometimes hyalinized, intervening fibrous stroma. Cytoplasmic vacuolation may occur in some cases, causing a microcystic-type of arrangement in a tubular pattern (Fig. 78). The cytoplasm is often clear, reflecting a high lipid content, and the nuclei are oval and may have a moderate-sized nucleolus, notches, or grooves (404). Intermixture of the Sertoli cell population with a significant component of granulosa cells or sex cord–stromal elements of indetermi-

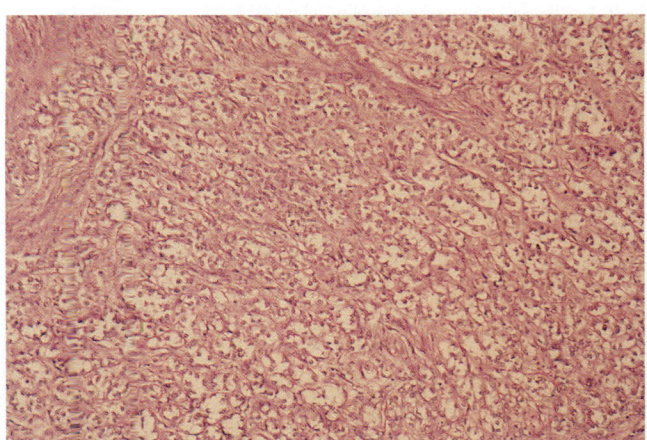

FIG. 77. Sertoli cell tumor with solid and vacuolated tubules.

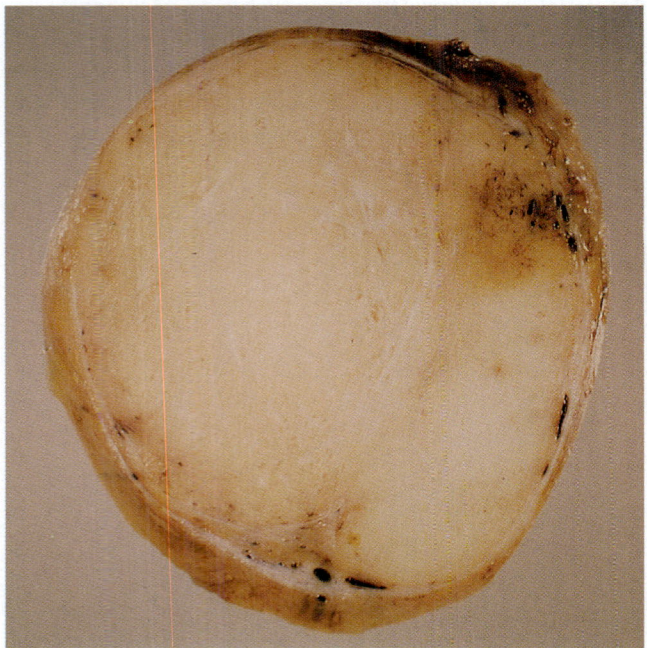

FIG. 76. Well-circumscribed, solid, gray-white Sertoli cell tumor.

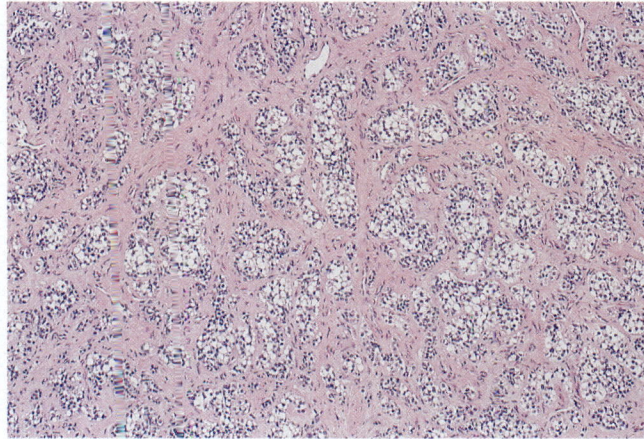

FIG. 78. Prominently vacuolated cells, causing a microcystic pattern, in a Sertoli cell tumor with well-defined tubules.

nate type places the neoplasm into a mixed sex cord–stromal or incompletely differentiated sex cord–stromal category (372). Cytokeratin, inhibin, and vimentin may be identified by immunohistochemistry (299,384,405–407). By ultrastructure, the cells are interconnected by desmosomes, and have abundant smooth endoplasmic reticulum and lipid droplets (408). By analogy with ovarian Sertoli cell tumors (409), it may be possible to demonstrate cytoplasmic Charcot-Böttcher filaments, which are considered pathognomonic of Sertoli cell differentiation. These structures, however, have more commonly been identified in LCCSCTs rather than in the NOS category (393,394).

Perhaps 10% of cases manifest malignant behavior (377,404,410,411). These are more likely to be large tumors (tumor diameter >5 cm), have a mitotic rate of >5 mitotic figures per 10 high power fields, show necrosis, have moderate to severe nuclear atypia, and/or demonstrate lymphatic/vascular invasion (411) (Fig. 79). Only one of nine benign tumors with follow-up of 5 or more years had more than one of these features, whereas five of seven malignant cases had at least three (404). In contrast to Leydig cell tumors, malignant behavior in children with Sertoli cell tumors is reported (378).

Differential Diagnosis

It is important to distinguish Sertoli cell tumor NOS from the rare seminomas with a tubular pattern (144) (Fig. 10). This distinction depends on the greater cytologic atypia in seminoma, the differences in the nature of the clear cytoplasms of the two tumors (being predominantly due to glycogen in seminoma and lipid in Sertoli cell tumor), and the association of seminoma with adjacent IGCNU, which is not seen in Sertoli cell tumor. Inhibin and PLAP immunostains may be helpful in problematic cases, as well as electron microscopy. Hyperplastic Sertoli cell nodules occur commonly in cryptorchid testes and are not infrequent in noncryptorchid testes (413,414). These are usually small, or even microscopic, lesions that consist of small tubules lined by im-

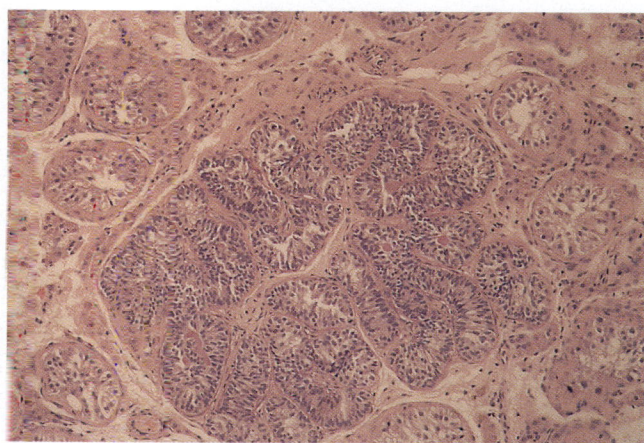

FIG. 80. Sertoli cell nodule in a cryptorchid testis consisting of small tubules lined by immature-appearing Sertoli cells and containing focal round aggregates of basement membrane.

mature Sertoli cells that occasionally have spermatogonia, unlike Sertoli cell tumor. Central, hyalinized basement membrane material is commonly identified in the tubules (Fig. 80). The testes of patients with androgen insensitivity syndrome (AIS) may contain multiple hamartomatous nodules composed of small tubules lined by Sertoli cells with intervening Leydig cells (Fig. 81); in addition, Sertoli cell adenomas, consisting of a pure proliferation of Sertoli cells arranged in small tubules, may occur in about 25% of AIS cases (95). These are categorized separately from Sertoli cell tumor NOS because they have never metastasized.

Sclerosing Sertoli Cell Tumor

Zukerberg and co-workers (415) described a variant of Sertoli cell tumor associated with prominent stromal sclerosis. These neoplasms occurred in patients from 18 to 80 years old, with a mean age of 35 years. They presented as painless testicular masses unassociated with hormonal fea-

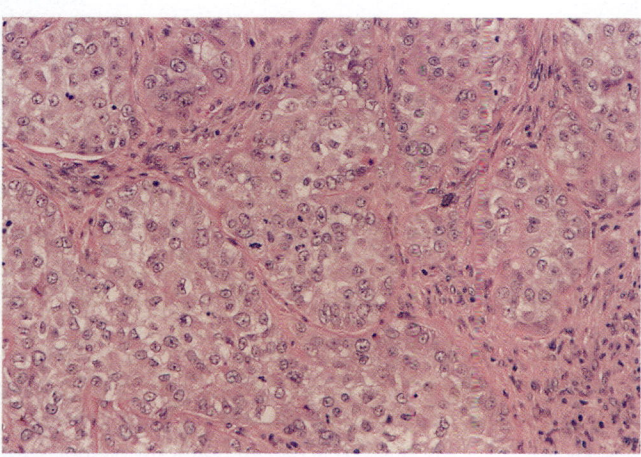

FIG. 79. Nests of cells showing significant atypia and occasional mitotic figures in a malignant Sertoli cell tumor.

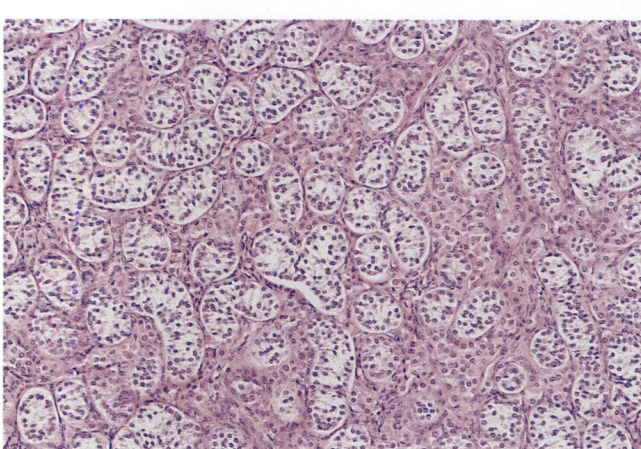

FIG. 81. A hamartomatous nodule in a patient with androgen insensitivity syndrome consists of Sertoli cell-lined tubules and intervening Leydig cells.

tures. On gross examination they were usually under 1.5 cm (although two cases were 4 cm in diameter), well-circumscribed, firm, white to tan to yellow nodules. On microscopic examination these sclerosing Sertoli cell tumors were composed of tubules, both solid and hollow, and cords of cells in a hypocellular, fibrous stroma (Fig. 82). The cells had pale cytoplasm; some had lipid vacuoles. The nuclei varied from small and hyperchromatic to large and vesicular. One of ten tumors had significant cytologic atypia and mitotic activity. Immunostains were negative except for vimentin, and follow-up did not indicate any instances of aggressive behavior. A recent report emphasizes that these tumors represent a distinct subtype of Sertoli cell tumor (416). Considerations in the differential diagnosis include carcinoid tumor (which, however, usually has a mid-gut type of pattern rather than the cord-like pattern of sclerosing Sertoli cell tumor), adenomatoid tumor (which is usually centered in paratesticular structures rather than the testis), and metastatic prostatic carcinoma (which does not form tubules and may be distinguished as well based on immunostains for prostate specific antigen and prostatic acid phosphatase) (415).

Large Cell Calcifying Sertoli Cell Tumor

About 30% of large cell calcifying Sertoli cell tumors (LCCSCT) occur in patients with the Carney syndrome or, rarely, the Peutz-Jeghers syndrome (397,402,403,417). Presenting features may therefore include the stigmata of the syndrome, which, for the Carney syndrome, include myxomas of skin, soft tissue, and heart, and myxoid lesions of the breast (418,419); lentigines of the face and lips; cutaneous blue nevi; Cushing's syndrome secondary to pigmented adrenocortical nodular hyperplasia; pituitary somatotroph adenomas (418); and psammomatous melanotic schwannomas (420). LCCSCT usually occurs in young patients (391), with a mean age of 17 years for benign cases and a mean age of 39 years for the rare malignant tumors (397). Despite the associated syndromes, most patients present with a mass; gy-

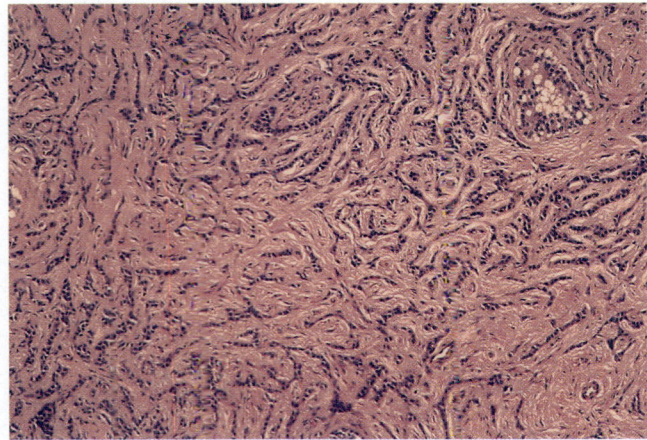

FIG. 82. Sclerosing Sertoli cell tumor, with prominent cords of tumor cells in an abundant fibrous stroma.

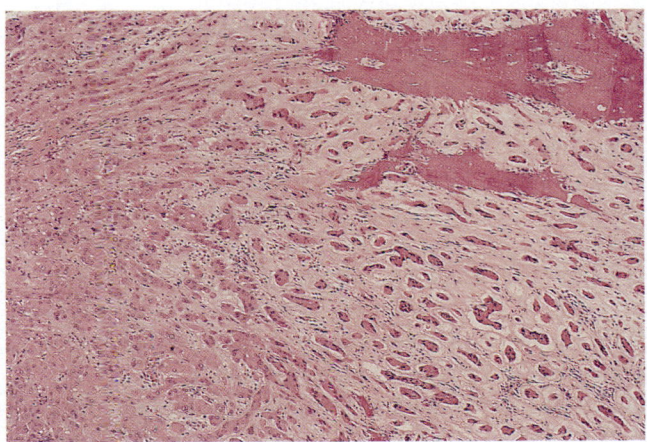

FIG. 83. Large cell calcifying Sertoli cell tumor composed of cords and nests of cells with abundant eosinophilic cytoplasm in a variably prominent stroma with focal ossification.

necomastia and isosexual pseudoprecocity may also be presenting features due to hormone production by the tumor or due to associated Leydig cell nodules (391). The tumors are usually small, most commonly under 2 cm, often bilateral [up to 25% (391,397)], and frequently multifocal (396). Bilateral and multifocal tumors are almost always syndrome associated, but solitary tumors may also be. They are typically yellow to tan with a gritty cut surface due to calcifications. On microscopic examination, nodules, nests, and cords of large, polygonal cells with abundant eosinophilic cytoplasm are identified in a myxoid to fibrous stroma, often with scattered neutrophils (Fig. 83). Intratubular tumor growth is common. Calcifications are present in about one-half of the cases; they occur both within foci of intratubular as well as extratubular tumor. The tumor cells have round to oval nuclei and may occasionally have prominent nucleoli. Mitoses are rare except in the uncommon malignant cases (391,397). Most cases are benign, but malignancy correlates with size greater than 4 cm, extratesticular growth, gross or microscopic necrosis, high-grade cytologic atypia, vascular space invasion, and a mitotic rate greater than 3 mitoses/10 high power fields. All malignant cases showed at least two of these features, whereas none of the benign cases had any of them (397). Malignant cases furthermore occurred in patients older than 25 years of age, and only one of eight was syndrome associated (397). Several ultrastructural studies of these tumors support their Sertoli cell derivation (390,394,395), including the presence of Charcot-Böttcher filaments (393). The problem of differentiating these tumors from Leydig cell tumors has been discussed above.

Sertoli-Leydig Cell Tumor

Testicular tumors with the same appearance as ovarian Sertoli-Leydig cell tumors are rare; only six acceptable cases have been identified (421). One-third of the patients had gynecomastia. The age range is wide, and only one tumor with an unusual morphology was clinically malignant (422).

These tumors are typically yellow, entirely or predominantly solid, and often are lobulated. Required for the diagnosis is an unequivocal tubular component of Sertoli cell type and/or sex cord patterns typical of ovarian Sertoli-Leydig cell tumor, as well as a neoplastic stromal component that usually contains at least focal Leydig cells. Although most of the reported cases have been of intermediate differentiation, both well (423) and poorly differentiated tumors occur. As in ovarian cases, retiform patterns (421) and heterologous elements have been described (422).

Granulosa Cell Tumor

Adult Type

Granulosa cell tumors similar to the typical granulosa cell tumors of the ovary (see chapter by Young et al.) are quite rare in the testis (424–428). They have occurred over an age range of 16 to 76 years (428) and have sometimes been associated with gynecomastia (372). They are typically circumscribed, yellow to gray, with a solid to partially cystic appearance. Microscopically they have the typical patterns of ovarian granulosa cell tumors (Fig. 84), and the usual pale nuclei with occasional or frequent nuclear grooves. They are typically strongly reactive for vimentin, with focal, weak, or absent keratin reactivity (428). Malignant behavior is rare (378,429) but should be suspected if the tumor is large (>7 cm), necrotic, hemorrhagic, or shows vascular/lymphatic invasion (428).

Juvenile Type

Juvenile granulosa cell tumors are similar in appearance to their ovarian counterpart. These tumors, however, are most commonly found in infants under 5 months of age, with a rare case occurring in a child of 21 months (300,430). Association with X/XY mosaicism has been described (431). A testicular mass is found by either a parent or physician in most cases. On gross examination there is a variable inter-

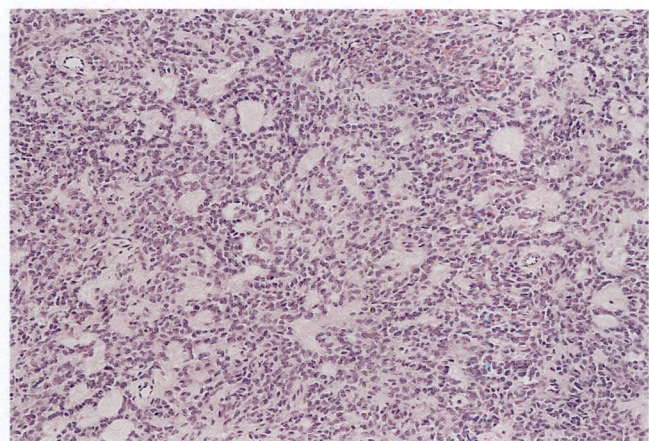

FIG. 84. Adult-type granulosa cell tumor forming Call-Exner bodies.

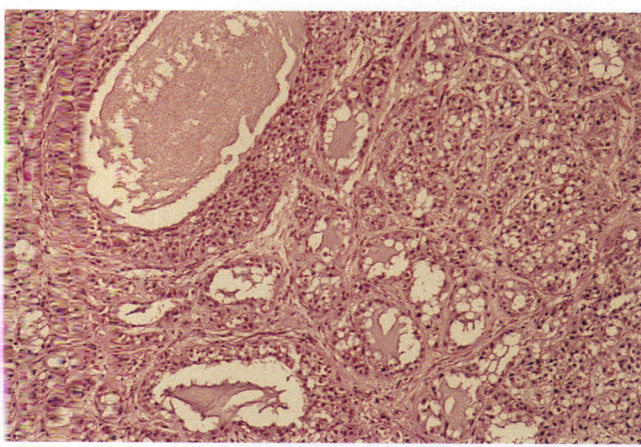

FIG. 85. Juvenile granulosa cell tumor with follicle-like spaces filled with fluid and nests of cells with pale cytoplasm.

mixture of gray to yellow solid areas and cystic foci filled with viscid fluid. On microscopic examination, there are round, follicle-like structures filled with watery-appearing, often mucicarminophilic, fluid (300) (Fig. 85). The intervening solid areas consist of nodules and sheets of cells, with frequently conspicuous stromal hyalinization. The cells have an abundant amount of pale to eosinophilic cytoplasm and hyperchromatic, round nuclei with nucleoli. Mitoses may be numerous. Despite these worrisome histologic features, this tumor behaves in a benign fashion (300,372). The major differential diagnosis is the distinction of juvenile granulosa cell tumor from yolk sac tumor, an issue that has been addressed above.

Fibromas of Gonadal Stromal Origin

Three intratesticular fibromas of gonadal stromal origin have been reported recently (432). The patients were between 28 to 35 years of age and had painless masses. On gross examination the tumors were circumscribed, yellow-white to white lesions that were up to 4 cm in diameter. On histologic examination they resembled ovarian fibromas, being composed of short, interlacing fascicles of spindle-shaped cells. In two cases small, acellular plaques of hyalinized collagen were present. Immunohistochemically, the tumor cells were strongly positive for vimentin, and were sometimes focally positive for actin and desmin.

Mixed and Unclassified Sex Cord-Stromal Tumors

This group of neoplasms consists of those cases that show either a mixture of sex cord–stromal elements (as, for instance, granulosa and Sertoli cell elements) or nonspecific forms of differentiation. They occur over a wide age range and present as testicular masses, with 15% having associated gynecomastia (372). Almost 50% have occurred in children (430). They range in size from small nodules to large masses and typically are lobulated and gray to yellow. A variable intermixture of sex cord and stromal differentiation is the usual

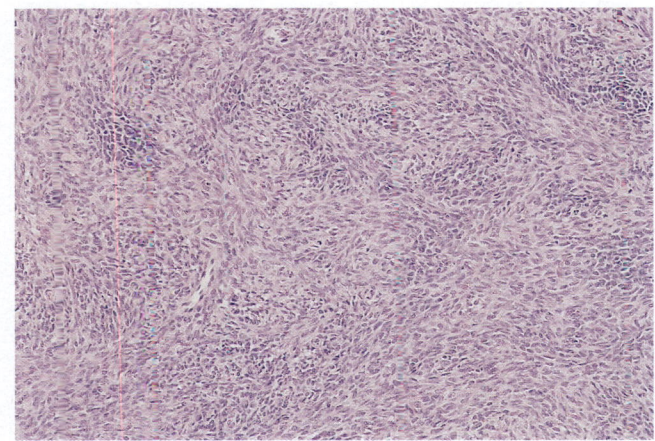
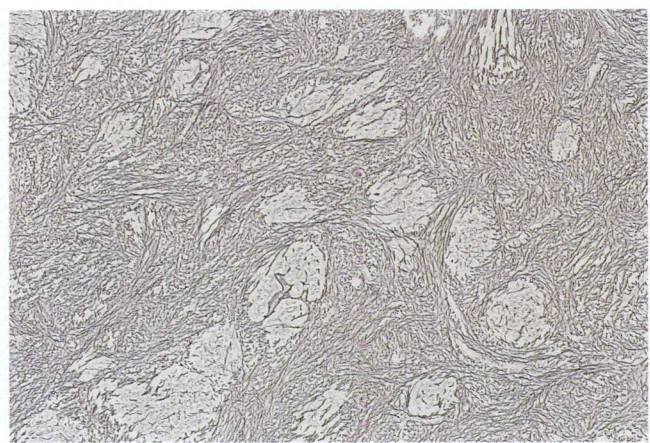

FIG. 86. A: Unclassified sex cord–stromal tumor consisting predominantly of a spindle cell, stromal-type proliferation with focal sex cord differentiation. **B:** Reticulin stain outlines the relatively inconspicuous sex cord component.

microscopic picture (Fig. 86). Pleomorphism and mitotic activity can be prominent in sarcomatoid areas. In better differentiated cases, tubules lined by Sertoli-like cells may be formed. Some of the neoplasms with a stromal pattern may be derived from peritubular, myofibroblastic cells. One study supported granulosa cell differentiation in those cases with a predominance of spindle cells (433). The behavior of this group of tumors has been benign when occurring in children under 10 years of age (430); the prognosis, however, is more guarded in older patients, with malignant behavior occurring in 20% of the cases (430). They are typically managed by orchiectomy, with retroperitoneal lymph node dissection being reserved for those patients with clinical manifestations of malignant behavior or whose pathologic findings suggest a high probability of malignant behavior. Such findings include large size, invasive growth pattern, evidence of lymphatic or vascular invasion, nuclear atypicality, high mitotic rate, and necrosis (430).

MIXED GERM CELL–SEX CORD–STROMAL TUMORS

Gonadoblastoma

Gonadoblastomas are tumors composed of an intermixture of seminoma-like germ cells and sex cord cells, probably showing Sertoli-like differentiation based on the electron microscopic demonstration of Charcot-Böttcher filaments (434,435). They almost invariably occur in patients with dysgenetic gonads and an intersex syndrome, with 80% being phenotypic females and 20% being phenotypic males (436). Bilaterality of gonadoblastomas occurs in about one-third of cases (436). Phenotypic males usually present in childhood or early adolescence with feminizing symptoms, including gynecomastia, hypospadias, and cryptorchidism. At surgical exploration, they are usually also found to have persistence of internal müllerian duct-derived structures. On karyotypic analysis, a Y-chromosome can be identified in almost all of the patients, with 46,XY and 45,X/46,XY being the most common findings (437). Grossly, gonadoblastomas are tan to yellow with diffusely gritty calcifications on the cut surface. Microscopically, the most common pattern is well-defined, rounded nests of seminoma-like cells intermingled with round to angulated sex cord cells that may form a peripheral palisade surrounded by basement membrane (Fig. 87). A cord-like growth of these two cells may also occur. Within the usual nests, aggregates of eosinophilic, hyalinized basement membrane commonly occur, and these appear to act as a nidus for the associated, often dense calcifications. Coalescence of calcifications results in irregular, mulberry-shaped foci lacking tumor cells. Outside of the nests, aggregates of Leydig-like cells (however, lacking crystals of Reinke) are seen in the stroma of about two-thirds of the cases (436,437).

Gonadoblastoma should be considered as an *in situ* form of malignant germ cell tumor. In approximately 50% of the cases, an invasive germ cell tumor develops, usually a semi-

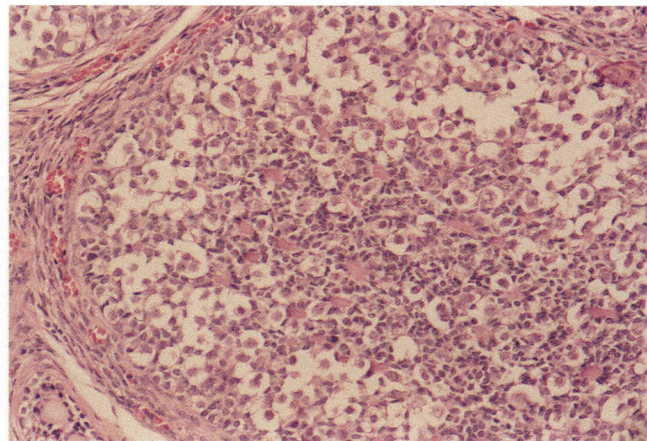

FIG. 87. Gonadoblastoma with typical circumscribed nests composed of germ cells, sex cord cells, and round islands of hyalinized basement membrane.

noma. In 8% of the cases, however, a more highly malignant germ cell tumor may occur such as embryonal carcinoma or yolk sac tumor (436). Because of the dysgenetic nature of the gonads in these patients and the frequent bilaterality of gonadoblastomas, bilateral gonadectomy is indicated in patients found to have a gonadoblastoma. A benign outcome can be expected in patients lacking an invasive germ cell component.

Mixed Germ Cell and Sex Cord–Stromal Tumors Other Than Gonadoblastoma

There are rare tumors other than gonadoblastoma that are composed of a mixture of germ cells and sex cord–stromal cells (438). We have seen several cases of sex cord–stromal tumor with entrapped germ cells that have simulated mixed germ cell–sex cord–stromal tumor (Fig. 88) (unpublished observation, 1996), so it is important that the germ cells resemble seminoma cells and not spermatogonia. The reported cases occurred in adults, with an age range of 30 to 69 years (438). They presented as a testicular mass, sometimes of long duration. Features of gonadal dysgenesis or an intersex syndrome were not identified. They were typically gray-white and solid to partly cystic (438). On microscopic examination, an admixture of large, seminoma-like cells and darkly staining sex cord–like cells were typically seen. The sex cord component resembled either adult-type granulosa cell tumor or Sertoli cell tumor. In one case, Charcot-Böttcher filaments were identified, supporting Sertoli cell differentiation (439). The degenerative changes and small nested pattern of gonadoblastoma were absent, and these features, along with the different clinical situation served to aid in the differential diagnosis. Neither overgrowth of the germ cell component to form a typical germ cell tumor nor the development of metastases has been reported (438). Orchiectomy alone, therefore, appears to be adequate treatment, with close follow-up. The experience with these neoplasms, though, is quite limited.

TUMORS OF "PASSENGER" AND NON-LEYDIG INTERSTITIAL CELLS

Lymphoma

Lymphomas may occur in the testes, most commonly representing dissemination from extratesticular sites (175), although occasionally representing a primary neoplasm of testicular origin (177). Testicular lymphoma is predominantly a disease of older men, with the mean age in several series being approximately 60 years (172–176,440,441). Although lymphomas represent only about 5% of testicular neoplasms, they compose 50% of cases in patients over age 60 years (372). Bilateral testicular involvement, usually metachronous, is common (172–175,442), occurring in about 20% of patients (443). Systemic symptoms such as fever and weight loss may be present (173). On gross examination, a fleshy white to tan to pink neoplasm that resembles seminoma is identified; however, there is a much greater likelihood of extratesticular involvement than in seminoma (176,177). The most important clue to diagnosis occurs at scanning magnification where an interstitial pattern, with relative tubular preservation, is identified (Fig. 89). Although effacement of tubules, particularly in the central portion of the tumor, may occur, they are preserved to a greater extent than in germ cell tumors. Significant sclerosis occurs in about 30% of cases, and vascular invasion is seen in about 60% (175). The great majority are of the large cell type (148,173,174,176,440,441,444), usually of B-cell immunophenotype (148,176,440), and not uncommonly having an immunoblastic appearance (176,440,444). Rare examples of Burkitt's-type lymphoma have been reported in adults (445), but it remains the most common lymphoma of childhood with testicular involvement (176,443). Hodgkin's disease uncommonly affects the testis (443,446). Ki-1–positive, anaplastic large cell lymphoma is also reported (447,448).

At high magnification, there is usually a noncohesive growth of cells with large, often irregularly shaped nuclei; large central nucleoli may be identified in immunoblastic

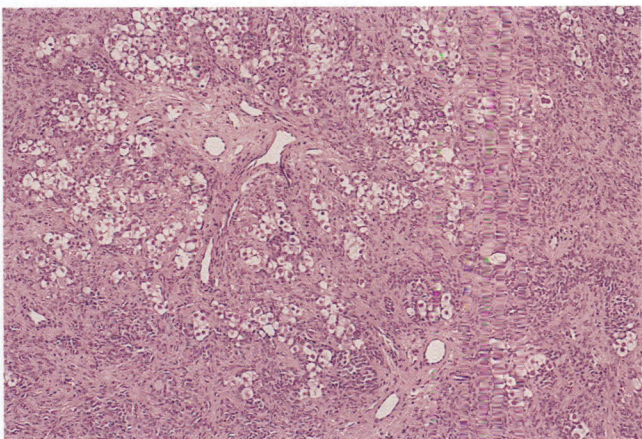

FIG. 88. Sex cord–stromal tumor with germ cells. This case, in our opinion, represents entrapped, nonneoplastic germ cells.

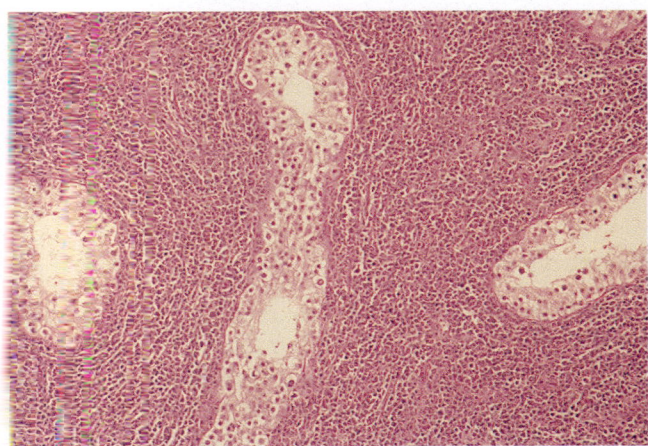

FIG. 89. Testicular lymphoma with characteristic interstitial pattern resulting in preservation of some tubules.

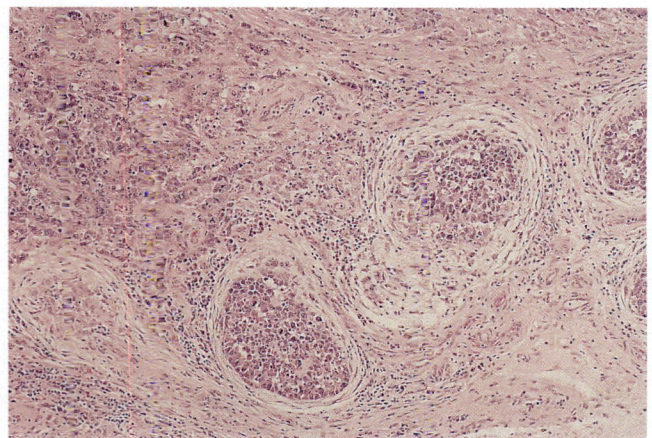

FIG. 90. Ki-1–positive, anaplastic large cell lymphoma with prominent intratubular growth, mimicking embryonal carcinoma.

types; other large cell types often have nucleoli adjacent to the nuclear membrane. Significant variation in cell size is common, as is migration into the seminiferous tubules. One of the reported Ki-1–positive anaplastic large cell lymphomas had prominent intratubular growth that simulated embryonal carcinoma (Fig. 90) (447). There is no association with IGCNU. The differential diagnosis with seminoma is discussed above. In difficult cases, PLAP and LCA immunostains can be employed to distinguish between a germ cell tumor (usually seminoma) and lymphoma; these markers are positive and negative, respectively, in germ cell tumors with an opposite pattern in lymphomas (156,163). It is also important to distinguish lymphomas from cases of chronic orchitis; these may be recognized by the more patchy nature of the infiltrate and the heterogenous character of the cells—consisting of lymphocytes, plasma cells, neutrophils, etc. Exuberant examples of such cases produce the picture of reactive lymphoid hyperplasia, reported as testicular "pseudolymphoma" (449).

Stage remains of paramount prognostic importance in patients with testicular lymphoma; those patients with true testicular primaries limited to the testis (stage IE) have a 5-year survival of 60% compared to 17% for all other stages (176). Sclerosis and unilateral involvement are favorable features, whereas all patients with bilateral involvement eventually died of tumor (176). Subclassification also has prognostic value (174,176). Progression in Waldeyer's ring has been noted in patients with testicular lymphoma (176,442,443).

Plasmacytoma

Plasmacytomas of the testis are rare. They are most commonly a manifestation of multiple myeloma, occurring in patients with a previous or concurrent diagnosis of multiple myeloma (450,451). Involvement of the testis in cases of multiple myeloma actually occurs in about 2% of cases, but this is usually clinically occult and identified only at autopsy (372). In rare cases, testicular plasmacytomas are apparently isolated findings, although such patients must be closely followed for the development of systemic involvement (450). Rarely patients may survive for decades without other manifestations (452). The mean age is about 55 years (452). Grossly, plasmacytomas are usually soft and fleshy, tan to gray/white, often with foci of hemorrhage. The microscopic findings are similar to those of plasmacytomas at other sites. Typically the tubules are effaced centrally but preserved at the periphery of the tumor. The demonstration of monoclonality by immunostains showing immunoglobulin light chain restriction assures the diagnosis (450,451).

Leukemic Infiltration and Granulocytic Sarcoma

Neoplastic infiltrates in the testis are not uncommon in the course of leukemia. About 40% to 65% of patients with acute leukemia and 20% to 35% of patients with chronic leukemia have leukemic infiltration of the testis at autopsy (446,453). Boys with acute lymphoblastic leukemia appear especially prone to develop testicular involvement, even during what appears to be an otherwise complete clinical remission, with a positive biopsy frequency of 5% to 10% in such patients (454–456). Most of the time such involvement is detectable only on biopsy, but in some cases a palpable induration or testicular enlargement may be identified on clinical examination (456). Rarely, leukemia presents as a mass prior to the establishment of the diagnosis (372). Bilateral involvement is usual. A handful of cases of granulocytic sarcoma (tumorous myeloid leukemic infiltrates) are reported (457). These resemble lymphoma on gross examination and may have prominent extratesticular involvement. On microscopic examination leukemia produces a monomorphic interstitial infiltrate, typical of the morphology of the particular leukemia. The major differential diagnoses include orchitis, lymphoma, and seminoma with an interstitial pattern. Orchitis is polymorphic, with a variety of mature inflammatory cells; the distinction of leukemia from lymphoma may be problematic and largely dependent on the clinical history, including knowledge of the peripheral blood and bone marrow. The cells of granulocytic sarcoma have somewhat smaller nuclei and less prominent nucleoli than those of centroblasts or immunoblasts, with an evenly distributed chromatin (457). Intermixed eosinophilic myelocytes are helpful but not always present. Eccentric nuclei may also cause confusion with plasmacytoma (457). Seminoma should have associated IGCNU and be PLAP-positive; good fixation should permit its recognition by light microscopy.

Epidermoid Cysts

Squamous epithelial-lined cysts (epidermoid cysts) filled with keratin are not uncommon in the testis, representing about 1% of testicular masses (345,346). Their pathogenesis is unknown, with possibilities including displacement of scrotal epithelium, metaplasia of mesothelial inclusions, and

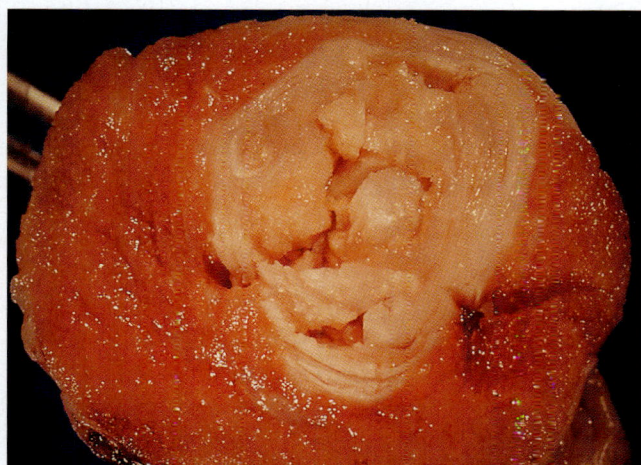

FIG. 91. Epidermoid cyst containing lamellated, white keratinous material. (Photograph courtesy of S.F. Cramer, M.D., Rochester General Hospital, Rochester, New York.)

monodermal teratomas. If they are teratomatous, they differ significantly from other forms of mature teratoma by their totally benign course (345) and lack of association with IGCNU (111,458).

They are most common from the second to fourth decades and present as a palpable mass (345). They are usually about 2 cm in diameter (372), and contain the characteristic white, grumous debris typical of keratin (Fig. 91). On microscopic examination, a fibrous wall is lined by keratinizing squamous epithelium with a granular cell layer but no skin appendages (Fig. 92). Areas of rupture may allow keratin to escape and result in a granulomatous and fibrous reaction. They are benign lesions (345,346) but must be distinguished from teratomas and dermoid cysts. The distinction from teratoma is important because of the malignant potential of teratomas and depends on the demonstration of other teratomatous elements; the presence of associated IGCNU in adult patients with teratomas is also helpful. The distinction from dermoid cysts is less important from the clinical standpoint but depends on the presence of adnexal structures associated with the squamous epithelial lining. Epidermoid cyst may be managed by conservative local excision if the diagnosis can be assured, typically by biopsies of the surrounding tubules to exclude IGCNU (458).

Mesenchymal Tumors

There are rare mesenchymal tumors of the testis that are either not obvious members of the sex cord–stromal group of neoplasms or that show evident differentiation along lines similar to those normally seen in soft tissue neoplasms. These tumors may be derived from supporting stromal cells of the testicular interstitium such as the peritubular myoid cells (459,460), endothelial cells, smooth muscle of vascular origin, or from primitive mesenchymal cells capable of various forms of differentiation (378). Rare testicular leiomyomas (461), neurofibromas (462), hemangiomas (463–465), and hemangioendotheliomas (466) are reported. Sarcomas that have been identified include osteosarcoma (467,468), fibrosarcoma (467), leiomyosarcoma (469), Kaposi's sarcoma (470), and, most commonly, rhabdomyosarcoma (471–474). It is possible that some of these cases, particularly those occurring in young patients, represent overgrowth of a sarcomatous component of a teratoma. This viewpoint is supported by one case of testicular and paratesticular rhabdomyosarcoma in a 12-year-old boy that was associated with IGCNU (475).

Metastatic Tumors

Metastases to the testis most commonly occur in patients with a known malignant tumor and therefore are usually recognizable as such. In a review of metastatic lesions to the testis, Haupt and co-workers (476) found that prostate (35%) and lung (19%) cancer accounted for over one-half of the cases with other primary tumors including malignant melanoma (9%), and carcinomas of the colon (9%) and kidney (7%). A variety of other sites gave rise to the remaining testicular metastases. [The large number of identified metastases of prostate cancer is, in part, a reflection of the greater opportunity to examine the testes in these patients because of therapeutic orchiectomies (477)]. The pathologic recognition of a testicular metastasis, however, may be difficult in those rare instances in which the testicular mass is the presenting feature of an occult neoplasm. Four of nine cases with testicular metastases masquerading as clinical primary tumors were misdiagnosed on pathologic examination as either embryonal carcinoma or Leydig cell tumor (476). Metastatic tumors presenting as testicular primaries included three cases of prostate cancer, two of lung cancer, and one each of melanoma, pancreas, stomach, colon, and liver cancer, with one carcinoid tumor (372,478). In one case, the primary site remained occult (476).

Most of the patients are older (mean age, 57 years) than patients with germ cell tumors, which may be a clue to the

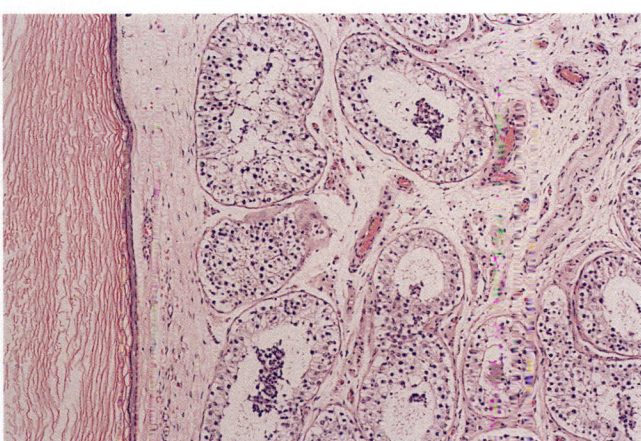

FIG. 92. Epidermoid cyst lined by keratinizing squamous epithelium and containing central masses of keratin; the adjacent seminiferous tubules lack IGCNU.

diagnosis. There is, however, overlap, and patients with metastatic stomach and small bowel cancers to the testis fall within the usual age range for germ cell tumors (479). Elevations of serum markers are less likely in cases of metastatic lesions, although some nongerminal neoplasms are associated with AFP and hCG elevations. The gross examination of a metastatic tumor is more likely to show a multinodular pattern of involvement, but diffuse involvement or a single nodule may also occur (479), and some germ cell tumors may demonstrate a multinodular pattern as well. Bilateral testicular involvement favors a metastatic process and occurs in about 20% of cases. On microscopic examination, an interstitial pattern, often with extensive lymphatic/vascular invasion, should be a clue to the possibility of metastasis (476,477). Specific forms of differentiation not typically seen in germ cell tumors may also occur. Positive mucin stains are helpful in recognizing metastatic adenocarcinomas, although teratomatous elements and yolk sac tumor elements may also show mucin positivity. The absence of associated IGCNU in testicular metastases makes the possibility of a primary germ cell tumor much less likely. Immunostaining for PLAP and EMA may prove quite helpful, given that germ cell tumors are usually PLAP-positive and EMA-negative while somatic carcinomas are often (but not always) PLAP-negative and EMA-positive (163). Immunostains specific for certain types of tumor, such as prostate specific antigen and prostatic acid phosphatase, may prove useful.

TUMORS OF THE RETE TESTIS

Pathologic processes that cause tumorous masses of the rete testis are rare. These include simple cysts of the rete testis (480), hamartomas (481), cystic dysplasia (482–485), adenomatous hyperplasia (486,487), adenofibromas (488), adenomas (489–491), cystadenomas with Sertoliform patterns (492), and adenocarcinomas (493–500). Cystic dysplasia, adenomatous hyperplasia, and adenocarcinoma will be considered in greater detail.

Cystic Dysplasia

Cystic dysplasia of the rete testis tends to present in infants and children as a testicular mass. There is cystic dilatation of the rete testis and the tubuli recti, with compression and atrophy of the seminiferous tubules. The lesion appears to be a developmental anomaly and is associated with ipsilateral renal agenesis (483–485) and renal dysplasia (482).

Adenomatous Hyperplasia

Hartwick et al. (486) described nine cases of adenomatous hyperplasia of the rete testis in men from 30 to 74 years old, with a mean age of 59 years. In three instances grossly apparent testicular hilar masses were identified that had solid and cystic appearances. These lesions consisted of tubu-lopapillary proliferations of cytologically bland cuboidal to columnar cells that projected into dilated channels of the rete testis (486). Follow-up was uneventful.

Reactive hyperplasia of the rete testis epithelium represents an incidental finding in orchiectomy specimens that may be misinterpreted as yolk sac tumor (304). This lesion is discussed above.

Adenocarcinoma

Adenocarcinoma of the rete testis has been thoroughly reviewed by Nochomovitz and Orenstein (493,501). They believe that many reported cases of cystic adenocarcinoma of the rete testis actually represent tumors of müllerian differentiation, often having the histology of serous cystadenomatous tumors of low malignant potential. These cases stand in contrast to well-established examples of rete testis adenocarcinoma that have a combination of solid, tubular, and papillary growth patterns with clear-cut stromal invasion. Well-established cases of rete testis adenocarcinoma occur over a wide age range from 31 to 91 years and have only been described in white patients (493). Most patients present with testicular pain and swelling, features of epididymitis, or, not uncommonly, an associated hydrocele (493). Nodules involving the scrotal skin are seen occasionally (498). On gross examination a typically white—but sometimes yellow, brown, gray, or tan—tumor is identified, centered in the testicular hilum, sometimes with separate nodules on the tunica vaginalis or grossly extending into the spermatic cord. Microscopically a transition between nonneoplastic and neoplastic rete epithelium may be identified. Slit-like spaces are common in the otherwise solid nests of tumor. Papillae with fibrous cores may resemble the chordae retis of the nonneoplastic rete testis. Intra-rete growth is common (Fig. 93). Tubular patterns may focally mimic Sertoli cell tumors (496), and transition from epithelial patterns to a spindle cell morphology has been described (494). Distinction

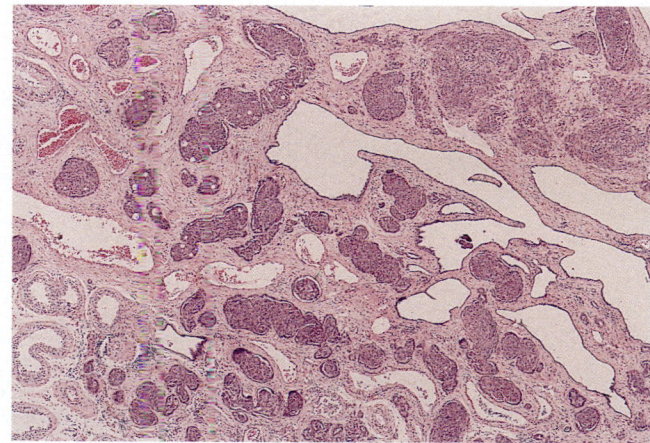

FIG. 93. Rete testis carcinoma showing solid nodules in the rete tubules and infiltrating the stroma. (Reproduced from ref. 639, with permission.)

from müllerian-type tumors is based on the hilar location, intra-rete growth, with transition from benign to malignant epithelium in some cases, and the mainly solid rather than cystic appearance.

Distinction from malignant mesothelioma may be difficult but relies on the hilar location and features, including immunohistochemistry and electron microscopy, which are employed with respect to pleural tumors (see chapter by Battifora) to assist in the distinction of adenocarcinoma from mesothelioma (493). Metastatic carcinomas are also a differential diagnostic consideration; prostate carcinoma usually stains for PSA. An appropriate history is important. The prognosis is generally poor, with only 36% of those with available follow-up disease-free after treatment (493). Lymphatic metastases to the retroperitoneum are the most common mode of spread (493), and patients who have retroperitoneal lymph node dissections have a somewhat improved outcome (502).

Miscellaneous

Two other pathologic entities of the rete testis warrant mention in passing, although they do not present with clinical masses. These are so-called nodular proliferation of calcifying connective tissue (503), which consists of intra-rete projections of hypocellular fronds of fibrous tissue, and acquired cystic transformation of the rete testis, a lesion that may be produced by obstruction or in conjunction with renal failure (504).

TUMORS OF THE TUNICA ALBUGINEA AND MESOTHELIUM

Hydrocele

There are several nonneoplastic conditions closely related to the tunica albuginea that may present as scrotal "tumors." Hydroceles result from failure of complete obliteration of the processus vaginalis; fluid may therefore accumulate between the visceral and parietal layers of the tunica vaginalis testis, either from local production or leakage from the peritoneal cavity. An accurate clinical diagnosis can usually be made by transillumination. On microscopic examination, a hydrocele sac consists of loose connective tissue with a mesothelial lining. Long-standing hydroceles may become chronically inflamed, fibrotic, and rarely develop squamous metaplasia.

Splenic-Gonadal Fusion

Splenic-gonadal fusion, with accessory splenic tissue adherent to the testis, epididymis, or spermatic cord, may present as a left testicular mass (505,506). Localization within the tunica albuginea is possible (507). A cord composed of fibrous and splenic tissue may connect the intrascrotal, accessory spleen to the normally located spleen (continuous type) (Fig. 94), or no such connection may exist (discontin-

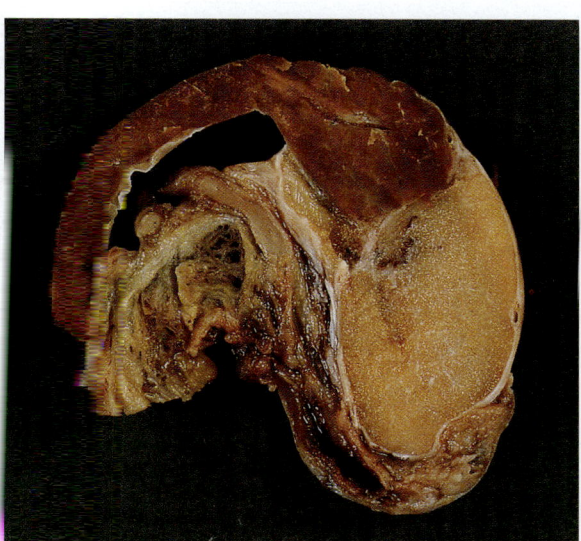

FIG. 94 Splenic-testicular fusion, continuous type. The cord-like extension of splenic tissue connected to the normally located spleen.

uous type). Limb defects and micrognathia are associated with the continuous type (507). Enlargement may occur following splenectomy or with other conditions associated with splenomegaly.

Meconium Periorchitis

Meconium periorchitis results from meconium peritonitis during fetal life; some patients may have cystic fibrosis, but probably only a minority of the cases (508). There is leakage of meconium from a perforated viscus into the peritoneum and through a patent processus vaginalis to localize in the scrotum, adherent to the tunica albuginea of the testis. Most patients present with a testicular mass in early infancy (508). A yellow-green mass is identified adherent to the testis, and microscopically a combination of pigmented macrophages, myxoid stroma, squames, and lanugo hairs is seen. Calcification may occur as well as mesothelial hyperplasia (508).

Nodular and Diffuse Fibrous Proliferation

Nodular and diffuse fibrous proliferation (NDFP) is a term proposed by Srigley and Hartwick (481) to describe the fibrous "tumors" that occur in and between the testicular tunics and less commonly involve the epididymis and spermatic cord. A variety of similar terms have been applied to these lesions, including *nodular fibrous proliferation* (509), *fibrous pseudotumor* (509–511), *chronic proliferative periorchitis* (512), and *inflammatory pseudotumor*. This lesion occurs over a wide age range, 7 to 95 years old, with a peak incidence in the third decade (481). A history of trauma or infection in some patients supports a reactive pathogenesis (509). One case was associated with retroperitoneal fibrosis (513). Most patients present with a scrotal mass (507,514), which on gross examination consists of either a diffuse, multinodular thickening of the peritesticular tissue, or a discrete nodule of firm, white tissue (481) that may reach 15 cm (507). There may be an associated hydrocele or hematocele. Microscopically there is an admixture of fibrous tissue, fibroblastic type cells, inflammatory cells, and dystrophic calcification (Fig. 95). The earlier lesions have a greater cellularity, and the later ones are more densely collagenized. Some lesions with features of myofibroblastomas are likely derived from NDFP (422). A spindle cell mesothelioma may mimic NDFP (515,516); differentiation may be achieved by immunohistochemistry and electron microscopy. Simple excision of NDFP is curative.

Additional nonneoplastic mass lesions that affect this area include mesothelial cysts (517,518), hematoceles, epidermoid cysts (9,481), and endometriosis (in rare patients taking exogenous estrogens) (519).

Fibroma

Fibromas of the testis are rare and are actually slightly more common in the testicular tunics. There appears to be two forms of fibroma. One type is analogous to the intratesticular tumor (see above), resembling the common ovarian fibroma and presumed to be derived from gonadal stromal-type cells. A second type is similar to the fibrous tumor of the pleura and may occur in relation to the tunica albuginea or in the paratestis (432). Six cases of these two types occurred in patients from 22 to 74 years old, typically as circumscribed, whorled, white nodules arising from the tunica albuginea and sometimes extending into the testis, with some cases in the paratestis (432). These lesions are typically moderately cellular, with bland spindle cells in a vascular, myxoid to collagenous stroma. The ovarian type fibromas may have the storiform patterns and hyaline fibrous plaques expected for the ovarian tumor. The pleural-type lesion typically shows the random growth of spindle cells, often with thick bands of collagen, and having CD34 reactivity (432). In contrast to NDFP, the fibromas are more cellular than the older, mature cases of NDFP and lack the inflammatory component of the early cases.

Mesothelioma

Both benign and malignant mesotheliomas of the tunica vaginalis have been described (481), with the distinction based on atypia, mitotic activity, and invasion (481,520). Malignant cases occur over an age range from childhood (521,522) to old age, with a mean age in the mid-50s (481,523). Some cases are associated with asbestos exposure (521,523–525). Most patients present with a clinical hydrocele, but at operation a multifocal, friable, papillary tumor is identified within the hydrocele sac. Cytologic examination of aspirated hydrocele fluid may permit a preoperative diagnosis (524). Grossly, tumor coats the tunica vaginalis either diffusely or in a multinodular fashion, with invasion into the surrounding structures in some cases. On microscopic examination, the pattern is usually a purely epithelial mesothelioma, with a papillary or tubulopapillary pattern having a single layer of atypical mesothelium resting on fibrovascular cores (Fig. 96). They are usually mainly exophytic, although focal stromal invasion can be identified in most cases and is good evidence of malignancy. Psammoma bodies may be identified and are therefore not necessarily indicative of a serous tumor of müllerian type. Atypical mesothelial lining cells in other portions of the hydrocele sac may be seen. Occasional cases have a spindle cell component, and a biphasic pattern is produced (520,523); rarely a pure spindle cell pattern may occur, which must be differentiated from a sarcoma. The histochemical, immunohistochemical, and ultrastructural approaches employed for the diagnosis of mesotheliomas at other sites can be employed to resolve differential diagnostic problems between serous tumors of müllerian type in purely epithelial cases and sarcomas in purely spindle cell cases. Radical orchiectomy is the usual treatment, with some patients possibly benefiting from retroperitoneal lymph node dissection (481). After a median follow-up of 22 months, 50% of 30 patients were disease-free following treatment (481). Division of malignant mesotheliomas into high-grade and low-grade categories based on pathologic and clinical evaluation may aid in prognostication (526). Distinction from mesothelial hyperplasia depends on the identification of a gross mass, complex arborizing papillae with fibrovascular cores, invasive growth, and a less frequent inflammatory background.

Ovarian-Type Epithelial Tumors

Ovarian-type epithelial tumors may occur in the testicular tunics, most likely resulting from müllerian metaplasia of mesothelium. They may also occur in the testicular parenchyma in some instances, perhaps from embryonic mesothelial inclusions (519,527,528). Most of the cases have the features of papillary serous tumor of low malignant po-

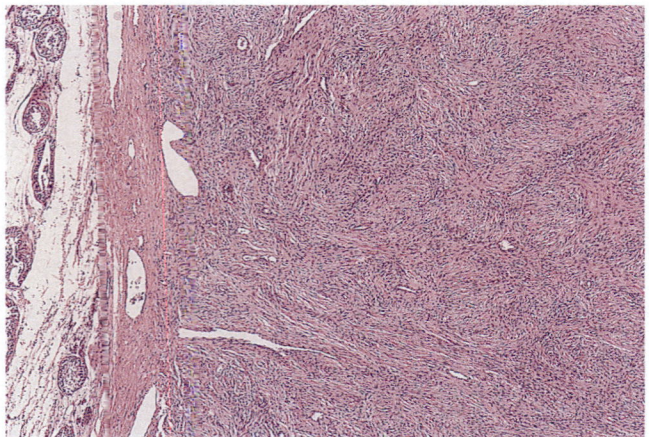

FIG. 95. Nodular fibrous proliferation of the tunica. A haphazard arrangement of fibroblastic-type cells projects from the tunica albuginea, away from the testis.

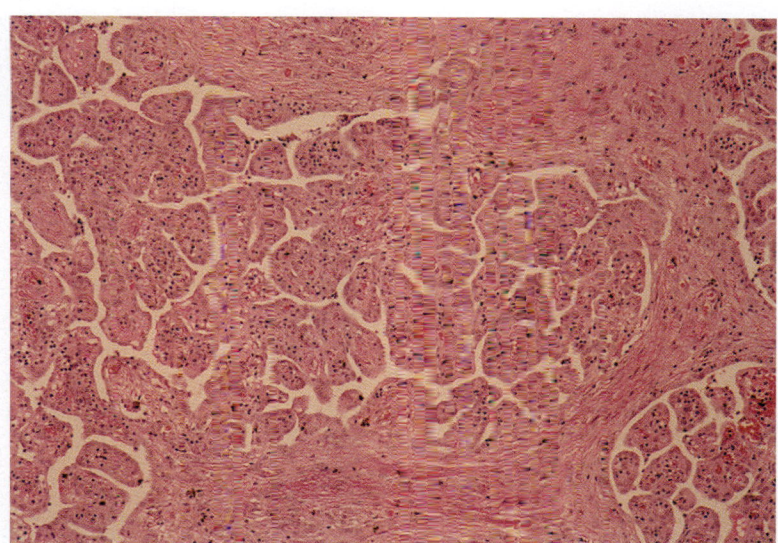

FIG. 96. Papillary mesothelioma showing fibrovascular cores covered by a single layer of cuboidal mesothelial cells. (Case courtesy of Thomas Mason, M.D., Piedmont Hospital, Atlanta, Georgia.)

tential (serous borderline tumor) (481,507,527,529–531), although serous carcinoma (532,533), endometrioid adenocarcinoma (529), benign (529,534) and malignant (529,535) mucinous tumors, benign (529,536–539) and malignant (540) Brenner tumors, and clear cell carcinoma (529) also occur. One tumor had a combination of Brenner and adenomatoid tumor morphologies (541). Most cases occur in adults who are often young; six cases of serous carcinoma occurred at a mean age of 31 years (533). Patients with paratesticular tumors have lesions involving the surfaces of the tunica vaginalis and often present with hydroceles. On gross examination, there are single or multifocal, exophytic, papillary lesions on the surfaces of the tunica vaginalis (519,542). On microscopic examination a papillary serous tumor of low malignant potential has the characteristic arborizing pattern and detached buds of epithelium, as seen in the ovary (Fig. 97), whereas serous carcinoma demonstrates destructive stromal invasion (Fig. 98). Distinction of papillary serous tumor of low malignant potential from mesothelioma is based on the broader papillae, greater degree of cellular budding and stratification, and more prominent psammoma bodies in the former. Immunohistochemistry may also assist, with papillary serous tumors typically being positive with B72.3, PLAP, Leu-M1, CA125, and sometimes CEA (528,543). Estrogen and progesterone receptors have been identified in an intratesticular case (528). The usual treatment is radical orchiectomy; patients with serous tumors of low malignant potential have had a benign clinical course (519,542), while patients with serous carcinoma have a guarded prognosis (532,533).

Desmoplastic Small Round Cell Tumor

Desmoplastic small round cell tumor (see chapter by Clement et al.) may also occur as a paratesticular mass, often

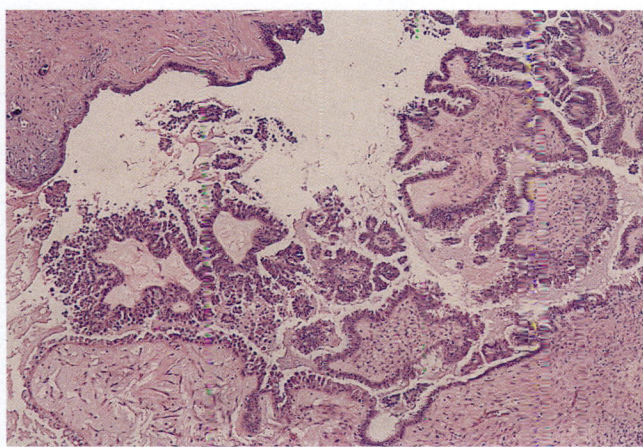

FIG. 97. Papillary serous tumor of low malignant potential, showing multiple fibrovascular cores lined by stratified cells, with prominent cellular buds.

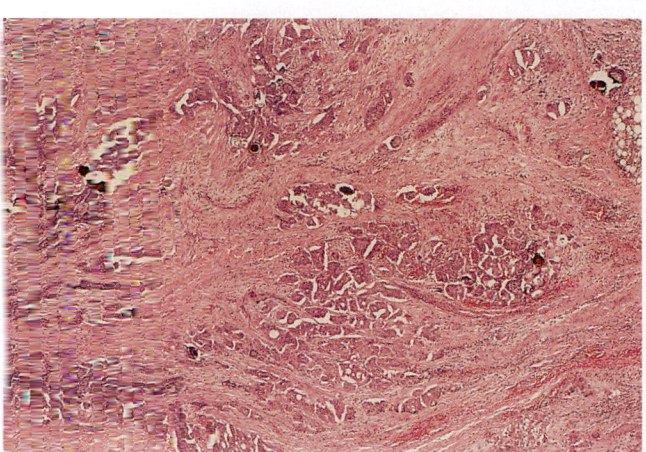

FIG. 98. Invasive, papillary serous adenocarcinoma. Note prominent desmoplasia and scattered psammoma bodies.

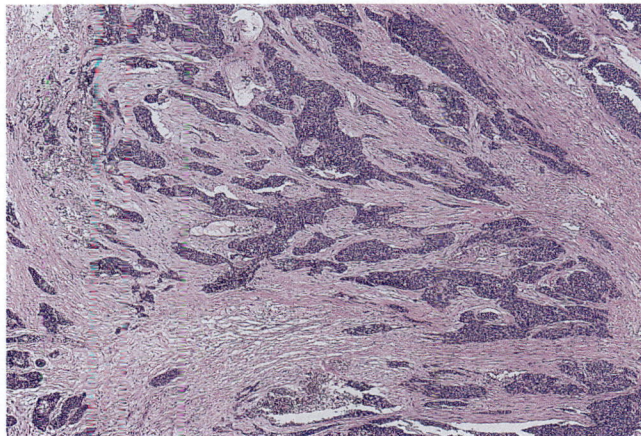

FIG. 99. Desmoplastic small round cell tumor of the paratestis, with nests and cords of cell in a desmoplastic stroma. The tumor had the characteristic polyimmunophenotypic profile.

near the epididymis, in young men (2,544). The patients present with a mass, with an average tumor diameter of 3 to 4 cm and a firm, gray-white to tan cut surface. They show the typical light microscopic features as in the abdominal cases (545,546), with nests and cords of small cells in a prominently fibrous stroma, sometimes with tubules or pseudorosettes (Fig. 99). The cells have the characteristic polyimmunophenotype, and the tumor behaves aggressively (2).

Miscellaneous Tumors

Rare leiomyomas (547,548), hemangiomas (549), malignant fibrous histiocytomas (550), neurofibromas (551), and dermoid cysts (534) of the testicular tunics are reported. Adenomatoid tumors, discussed in detail in the section on the epididymis, may also be identified separate from the epididymis, arising from the tunica vaginalis.

OTHER PARATESTICULAR TUMORS INCLUDING THOSE OF THE EPIDIDYMIS AND SPERMATIC CORD

Epididymal Tumors

Nonneoplastic lesions of the epididymis that may clinically mimic a neoplasm includes rare cysts of the epididymal appendix (481), the common spermatocele, which represents a dilated efferent ductule filled with proteinaceous fluid and degenerating spermatozoa, and rare epidermoid cysts (cholesteatomas) (346,552).

Adenomatoid Tumor

Adenomatoid tumor is the second most common paratesticular tumor (9). (Spermatic cord lipomas are the most common.) It often involves the epididymis but may also occur in the spermatic cord and testicular tunics. Growth into the testicular parenchyma is not unusual. It occurs over a wide age

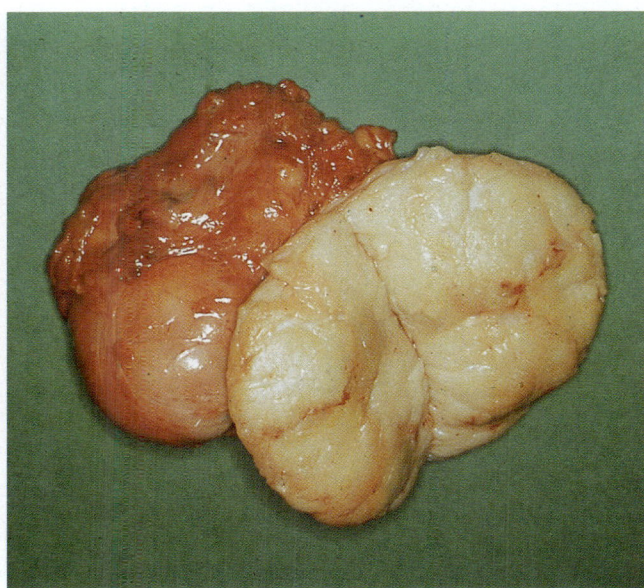

FIG. 100. Adenomatoid tumor consisting of a white, circumscribed nodule (bisected), attached to the epididymis.

range from adolescence to the elderly, with a median age in one series of 23 cases of 35 years (481). Most patients present with a painless, firm, intrascrotal mass (507). On gross examination, there is usually a well-circumscribed, firm, white to tan nodule, typically under 5 cm in diameter (Fig. 100) (372). Most commonly the head of the epididymis is affected. In some cases, ill-defined margins are present (372). On microscopic examination, solid to cystic tubules and cords of vacuolated cells are characteristic. Scattered individual cells and, occasionally, sheet-like clusters also occur. The cells lining the tubules vary from flattened to cuboidal, usually with a prominent intervening fibrous, sometimes hyalinized, stroma (Fig. 101). The cellular vacuoles may yield a signet ring-like appearance, but epithelial-type mucin is not present. The cytoplasm is typically abundant and eosinophilic, and the nuclei vesicular with small nucleoli. In

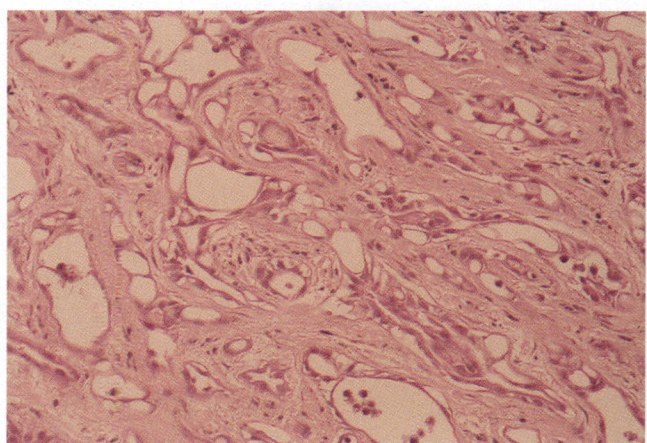

FIG. 101. Typical adenomatoid tumor consisting of tubules of cells that often have large cytoplasmic vacuoles.

some cases, there is a more cellular proliferation of cells in cords, with less distinct cytoplasmic vacuolation (Fig. 102). A prominent smooth muscle stroma may occur, leading to a designation of "adenomatoid leiomyoma" (553). Immunohistochemical studies show positivity for cytokeratin and EMA and negativity for factor VIII–related antigen and *Ulex europeus* agglutinin I, supporting a mesothelial derivation (481,525,554–558). Ultrastructural studies also support a mesothelial origin (559–565). A tumor that may mimic cellular adenomatoid tumor is epithelioid (histiocytoid) hemangioma (566), and the inclusion of such cases under the rubric of adenomatoid tumor has led to the conclusion that there are two types of adenomatoid tumor, the common mesothelial form and one of endothelial origin (556,560). We agree, however, with Banks and Mills (566) that such cases should not be diagnosed as adenomatoid tumors but designated epithelioid hemangiomas. Lack of intervening tumor cells between the tubular structures favors a vascular tumor (556), as does greater nuclear irregularity and blood in abortive luminal spaces. Distinction may be accomplished by immunohistochemistry (566). We have also seen cases of large cell calcifying Sertoli cell tumor with cord-like patterns that resembled cellular adenomatoid tumor. The testicular epicenter, frequent calcifications, intratubular growth, and weak to absent cytokeratin reactivity of such cases serve to distinguish them from adenomatoid tumor. Adenomatoid tumors behave in a benign fashion, with complete surgical excision curative.

Papillary Cystadenoma

Papillary cystadenomas are partially to completely cystic masses of the epididymal head that occur bilaterally in 40% of the cases (481). The mean age is 36 years (481,567), and most patients present with a scrotal mass. On gross examination, papillary fronds of gray-brown to yellow tissue project into a cystic, fluid-filled space. Microscopically, cores of fibrous tissue projecting into cystic spaces are covered by a single or double layer of cuboidal to columnar cells, sometimes with surface cilia or eosinophilic cytoplasmic droplets (Fig. 103). Tubules are also common, as is colloid-like proteinaceous material in the cysts (567). The cytoplasm of the tumor cells is lightly eosinophilic to clear, and the nuclear features are bland. Sixty-five percent of bilateral papillary cystadenomas occur in patients with von Hippel–Lindau syndrome, and 18% of unilateral lesions have this association (567). Conversely, 17% of males with von Hippel–Lindau disease have papillary cystadenoma of the epididymis (568). Because of the relationship to von Hippel–Lindau syndrome and the common occurrence of renal cell carcinoma in that disorder, it has been suggested that the differential diagnosis includes metastatic papillary clear cell carcinoma of the kidney and that lectin-binding patterns can discriminate these entities (569). Recently, a somatic mutation in the von Hippel–Lindau gene was reported in a sporadic case of papillary cystadenoma (570). The distinction from papillary serous tumors of low malignant potential depends on the lack of atypia, stratification, mitotic activity, and detached cell clusters in papillary cystadenomas. These are benign lesions, although a rare malignant variant has been reported (571).

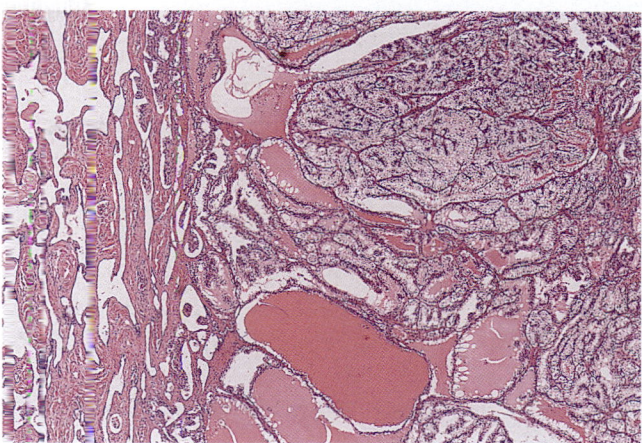

FIG. 103. Papillary cystadenoma of the epididymis showing tubules and papillae lined by clear cells and projecting into cystic spaces. Note colloid-like secretion in some spaces.

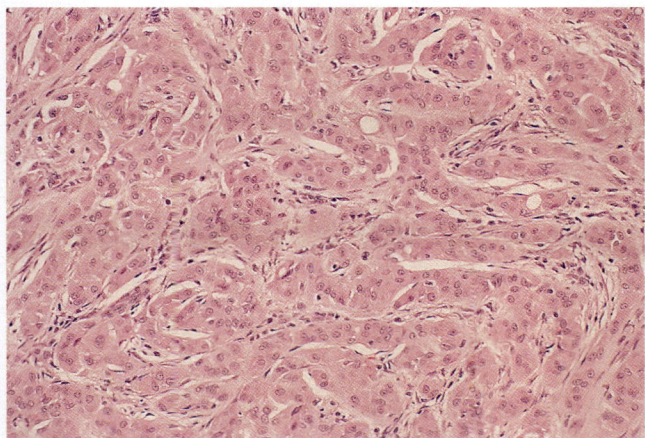

FIG. 102. More cellular adenomatoid tumor consisting of closely packed cords of cells with only focal cytoplasmic vacuoles.

Melanotic Neuroectodermal Tumor

Melanotic neuroectodermal tumor, similar in appearance to the more commonly occurring lesion of the jaw (so-called melanotic progonoma) rarely occurs in the epididymis (572–575) [and even more rarely in the testis (576)]. The patients are typically young infants, with a mean age of about 7 months and a range of 3 months to 8 years (481,575). One case was associated with elevated serum AFP (573). A well-circumscribed, brown to black nodule in the epididymal head is the usual gross appearance, although some cases are lightly colored, and the microscopic pattern is similar to that which is seen in the jaws. The prognosis is good following complete surgical excision, although these tumors should be regarded as potentially malignant since a rare epididymal case has metastasized (577). It has been suggested that the finding of an aneuploid pattern on flow cytometry may help identify the clinically malignant cases, although the experience is limited (575).

Miscellaneous Epididymal Tumors

Other tumors reported in the epididymis include leiomyoma (481,578), angiofibroma (579), palisaded myofibroblastoma (580), lymphoma (581–583), rare primary adenocarcinomas (481,517,584), often with a clear cell appearance, leiomyosarcoma (481,491,585,586), and metastatic carcinoma (587).

Spermatic Cord/Paratesticular Tumors

Nonneoplastic mesothelial cysts may cause a spermatic cord mass (481), and dermoid cysts of the spermatic cord are also reported (588).

A variety of benign and malignant tumors of soft tissue type may involve the spermatic cord/paratesticular area. The most common lesion is lipoma, including variants such as fibrolipoma and angiolipoma (481). Adults are most commonly affected, and many cases may not represent true neoplasms but lipomatous hyperplasia (481). Additional benign tumors and tumor-like lesions of this region include leiomyoma (589,590), rhabdomyoma (481,591), lymphangioma (592,593), hemangioma (481), ganglioneuroma (594), desmoid tumor (595), granular cell tumor (596), and inflammatory pseudotumor (597).

Rhabdomyosarcoma

Rhabdomyosarcoma is the most common malignant tumor of the spermatic cord, and the spermatic cord/paratesticular region is one of the more common sites of its occurrence. Most patients present with a palpable mass (598), with a peak incidence at 9 years (599); occurrence in older patients, however, is possible (600–602). A fleshy white-gray to tan-pink mass, 4 to 6 cm in diameter, is typical (Fig. 104); a mucoid consistency may be identified (598). On microscopic examination, the tumors are generally conventional embryonal rhabdomyosarcomas composed of relatively small cells with hyperchromatic nuclei and little cytoplasm admixed with other cells with rims of eosinophilic cytoplasm and sometimes more spindle-shaped cells with cytoplasmic tails (Fig. 105). Such "strap cells" may demonstrate cytoplasmic cross striations. The stroma varies from myxoid to collagenous. (See chapter by Brooks for a more comprehensive description of embryonal rhabdomyosarcoma.) A disproportionate number of paratesticular rhabdomyosarcomas have a spindle cell morphology (603,604); these, on gross examination, may have a firmer character and microscopically have a fascicular arrangement of spindle cells (Fig. 106). A minor component of conventional embryonal rhab-

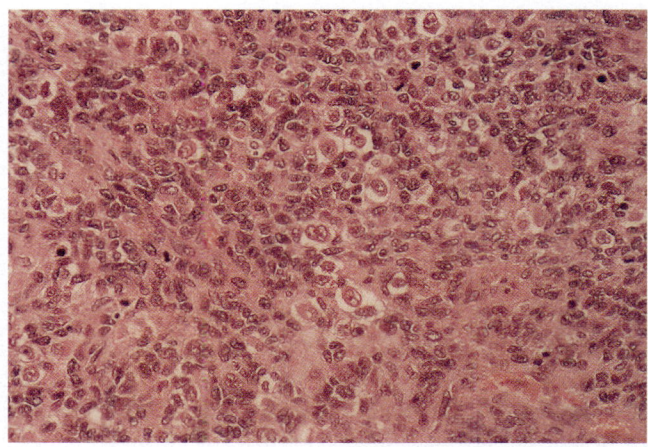

FIG. 105. Paratesticular embryonal rhabdomyosarcoma showing a predominance of poorly differentiated, small cells with hyperchromatic nuclei intermingled with rhabdomyoblasts having rims of eosinophilic cytoplasm.

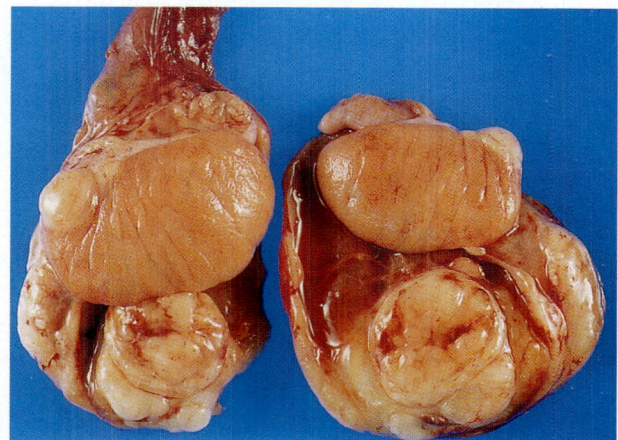

FIG. 104. Paratesticular rhabdomyosarcoma showing typical fleshy, tan neoplasm with foci of hemorrhage occurring in a dilated tunica vaginalis testis. The spermatic cord in this particular case does not appear to be the site of origin. Note nodular extension into the testicular parenchyma.

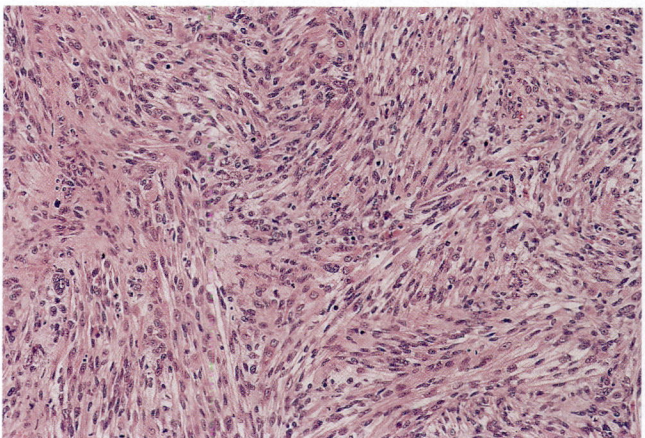

FIG. 106. Spindle cell variant of embryonal rhabdomyosarcoma, with a fascicular arrangement.

domyosarcoma is usually present. A small percentage of cases are of the alveolar type (604). The most useful immunostains appear to be desmin and muscle specific actin; however, other malignant tumors may show positivity for these markers as well. Myoglobin stains, though less sensitive, are specific. Continued use of electron microscopy is encouraged (605). Radical orchiectomy with retroperitoneal lymph node dissection is the usual form of treatment, with combination chemotherapy and radiation therapy also given to most patients (599,606). In one study, 6 of 15 patients (40%) had histologic confirmation of retroperitoneal metastases (599). [Nodal metastases have been reported in 29% of paratesticular sarcomas in general (607).] An overall survival, after proper treatment, of about 80% can be expected (481). Complete local resectability and an absence of parenchymal metastases are important favorable prognostic features (606).

Aggressive Angiomyxoma

Aggressive angiomyxoma, more commonly seen in the vulva (see chapter by Frierson and Mills), may also involve the paratesticular soft tissue in the region of the spermatic cord (412,608–610). Several patients were thought to have inguinal hernias. On gross exam, they are nonencapsulated, myxoid masses. Microscopically, bland-appearing spindle and stellate cells are widely dispersed in a myxoid stroma with prominent thick-walled, sometimes hyalinized vessels. Local recurrence is common, but metastases do not occur.

Angiomyofibroblastoma

This benign soft tissue tumor may rarely occur in the paratesticular/spermatic cord region (608) and should be distinguished from aggressive angiomyxoma based on its circumscription, alternating hypocellular and hypercellular zones, and capillary-sized vessels (see chapter by Frierson and Mills).

Miscellaneous Spermatic Cord Tumors

Other malignant or potentially malignant tumors that occur in the spermatic cord include leiomyosarcoma (601,611–616), malignant fibrous histiocytoma (617–620), fibrosarcoma (601,614,615), liposarcoma (especially the well-differentiated, sclerosing type) (481,615,621–624), plasmacytoma (481), neurogenic sarcoma (594), malignant mesenchymoma (625,626), several other poorly differentiated sarcomatous tumors (481), extrarenal Wilms' tumor (627–629), and pheochromocytoma (paraganglioma) (630).

REFERENCES

1. Giwercman A, Müller J, Skakkebaek NE. Prevalence of carcinoma in situ and other histopathological abnormalities in testes from 399 men who died suddenly and unexpectedly. *J Urol* 1991;145:77–80.
2. Cummings OW, Ulbright TM, Young RH, Dei Tos AP, Fletcher CDM, Hull MT. Desmoplastic small round cell tumors of the para-testicular region: a report of six cases. *Am J Surg Pathol* 1997;21:219–225.
3. Nazeer T, Ro JY, Kee KH, Ayala AG. Spermatic cord contamination in testicular cancer. *Mod Pathol* 1996;9:762–766.
4. Mostofi FK, Sobin LH. *Histological typing of testicular tumors* (International histological classification of tumors, No. 16). Geneva: World Health Organization, 1977.
5. Friedman NB, Moore RA. Tumors of the testis: a report on 922 cases. *Milit Surg* 1946;99:573–593.
6. Dixon FJ, Moore RA. *Tumors of the male sex organs. Atlas of tumor pathology,* 1st series, fascicles 31b and 32. Washington, DC: Armed Forces Institute of Pathology, 1952.
7. Dixon FJ, Moore RA. Testicular tumors: a clinicopathologic study. *Cancer* 1953;6:427–454.
8. Melicow MM. Classification of tumors of the testis: a clinical and pathological study based on 105 primary and 13 secondary cases in adults, and 3 primary and 4 secondary cases in children. *J Urol* 1955;73:547–574.
9. Mostofi FK, Price EB Jr. *Tumors of the male genital system. Atlas of tumor pathology,* 2nd series, fascicle 8. Washington, DC: Armed Forces Institute of Pathology, 1973.
10. Collins DH, Pugh RCB. Classification and frequency of testicular tumours. *Br J Urol* 1964;36(suppl):1–11.
11. Pugh RCB. Testicular tumours—introduction. In: Pugh RCB, ed. *Pathology of the testis.* Oxford: Blackwell Scientific, 1976:139–159.
12. Willis RA. *Pathology of tumours,* 4th ed. London: Butterworths, 1967:959–1003.
13. Mostofi FK. Comparison of various clinical and pathological classifications of tumors of testes. *Semin Oncol* 1979;6:26–30.
14. Srigley JR, Mackay B, Toth P, Ayala A. The ultrastructure and histogenesis of male germ neoplasia with emphasis on seminoma with early carcinomatous features. *Ultrastruct Pathol* 1988;12:67–86.
15. de Jong B, Oosterhuis JW, Castedo SM, Vos A, te Meerman GJ. Pathogenesis of adult testicular germ cell tumors. A cytogenetic model. *Cancer Genet Cytogenet* 1990;48:143–167.
16. Oosterhuis JW, Castedo SM, de Jong B, et al. Ploidy of primary germ cell tumors of the testis. Pathogenetic and clinical relevance. *Lab Invest* 1989;60:14–21.
17. Fossa SD, Nesland JM, Pettersen EO, Amellen O, Waehre H, Heimdal K. DNA ploidy in primary testicular cancer. *Br J Cancer* 1991;64:948–952.
18. El-Naggar AK, Ro JY, McLemore D, Ayala AG, Batsakis JG. DNA ploidy in testicular germ cell neoplasms: histogenetic and clinical implications. *Am J Surg Pathol* 1992;16:611–618.
19. Czaja JT, Ulbright TM. Evidence for the transformation of seminoma to yolk sac tumor, with histogenetic considerations. *Am J Clin Pathol* 1992;97:468–477.
20. Bailey D, Baumal R, Law J, et al. Production of monoclonal antibody specific for seminomas and dysgerminomas. *Proc Nat Acad Sci USA* 1986;83:5291–5295.
21. Giwercman A, Marks A, Bailey D, Baumal R, Skakkebaek NE. M2A—a monoclonal antibody as a marker for carcinoma-in-situ germ cells of the human adult testis. *Acta Pathol Microbiol Immunol Scand (A)* 1988;96:667–670.
22. Schulze C, Holstein AF. On the histology of human seminoma: development of the solid tumor from intratubular seminoma cells. *Cancer* 1977;39:1090–1100.
23. Delahunt B, Mostofi FK, Sesterhenn IA, Ribas JL, Avallone FA. Nucleolar organizer regions in seminoma and intratubular malignant germ cells. *Mod Pathol* 1990;3:141–145.
24. Malmi R, Söderström KO. Lectin histochemistry of embryonal carcinoma. *APMIS* 1991;99:233–243.
25. de Graaff WE, Oosterhuis JW, de Jong B, et al. Ploidy of testicular carcinoma in situ. *Lab Invest* 1992;66:166–168.
26. Osterlind A. Diverging trends in incidence and mortality of testicular cancer in Denmark, 1943–1982. *Br J Cancer* 1986;53:501–505.
27. Pike MC, Chilvers CE, Bobrow LG. Classification of testicular cancer in incidence and mortality statistics. *Br J Cancer* 1987;56:83–85.
28. Boyle P, Kaye SB, Robertson AG. Changes in testicular cancer in Scotland. *Eur J Cancer Clin Oncol* 1987;23:827–830.
29. Pearce N, Sheppard RA, Howard JK, Fraser J, Lilley BM. Time trends and occupational differences in cancer of the testis in New Zealand. *Cancer* 1987;59:1677–1682.
30. Bergstrom R, Adami HO, Mohner M, et al. Increase in testicular can-

cer incidence in six European countries: a birth cohort phenomenon. *J Natl Cancer Inst* 1996;88:727–733.
31. Forman D, Gallagher R, Moller H, Swerdlow TJ. Aetiology and epidemiology of testicular cancer: report of consensus group. *Prog Clin Biol Res* 1990;357:245–253.
32. Wilkinson TJ, Colls BM, Schluter PJ. Increased incidence of germ cell testicular cancer in New Zealand Maoris. *Br J Cancer* 1992;65:769–771.
33. Swerdlow AJ, Skeet RG. Occupational associations of testicular cancer in south east England. *Br J Indust Med* 1988;45:225–230.
34. McDowall ME, Balarajan R. Testicular cancer mortality in England and Wales 1971–80: variations by occupation. *J Epidemiol Community Health* 1986;40:26–29.
35. Ross RK, McCurtis JW, Henderson BE, Menck HR, Mack TM, Martin SP. Descriptive epidemiology of testicular and prostatic cancer in Los Angeles. *Br J Cancer* 1979;39:284–292.
36. Graham S, Gibson R, West D, Swanson M, Burnett W, Dayal H. Epidemiology of cancer of the testis in Upstate New York. *J Natl Cancer Inst* 1977;58:1255–1261.
37. Davies JM. Testicular cancer in England and Wales: some epidemiological aspects. *Lancet* 1981;1:928–932.
38. Haughey BP, Graham S, Brasure J, Zielezny M, Sufrin G, Burnett WS. The epidemiology of testicular cancer in upstate New York. *Am J Epidemiol* 1989;130:25–36.
39. Marshall EG, Melius JM, London MA, Nasca PC, Burnett WS. Investigation of a testicular cancer cluster using a case-control approach. *Int J Epidemiol* 1990;19:269–273.
40. Anonymous. Testicular cancer in leather workers—Fulton County, New York. MMWR 1989;38:105–106.
41. Ducatman AM, Conwill DE, Crawl J. Germ cell tumors of the testicle among aircraft repairmen. *J Urol* 1986;136:834–836.
42. Swerdlow AJ, Huttly SR, Smith PG. Prenatal and familial associations of testicular cancer. *Br J Cancer* 1987;55:571–577.
43. Moss AR, Osmond D, Bacchetti P, Torti FM, Gurgin V. Hormonal risk factors in testicular cancer: a case control study. *Am J Epidemiol* 1986;124:39–52.
44. Prener A, Hsieh CC, Engholm G, Trichopoulos D, Jensen OM. Birth order and risk of testicular cancer. *Cancer Causes Control* 1992;3:265–272.
45. Dieckmann KP, von Keyserlingk HJ. HLA association of testicular seminoma. *Klin Wochenschr* 1988;66:337–339.
46. Kratzik C, Aiginger P, Kuzmits R, et al. HLA-antigen distribution in seminoma, HCG-positive seminoma and non-seminomatous tumours of the testis. *Urol Res* 1989;17:377–380.
47. Oliver RT. HLA phenotype and clinicopathological behaviour of germ cell tumours: possible evidence for clonal evolution from seminomas to nonseminomas. *Int J Androl* 1987;10:85–93.
48. Dexeus FH, Logothetis CJ, Chong C, Sella A, Ogden S. Genetic abnormalities in men with germ cell tumors. *J Urol* 1988;140:80–84.
49. Braun DL, Green MD, Rausen AR, et al. Down's syndrome and testicular cancer: a possible association. *Am J Pediatr Hematol Oncol* 1985;7:208–211.
50. Sigg C, Pelloni F. Dysplastic nevi and germ cell tumors of the testis—a possible further tumor in the spectrum of associated malignancies in dysplastic nevus syndrome. *Dermatologica* 1988;176:109–110.
51. Nichols CR, Heerema NA, Palmer C, Loehrer PJ Sr, Williams SD, Einhorn LH. Klinefelter's syndrome associated with mediastinal germ cell neoplasms. *J Clin Oncol* 1987;5:1290–1294.
52. Nienhuis H, Goldacre M, Seagroatt V, Gill L, Vessey M. Incidence of disease after vasectomy: a record linkage retrospective cohort study. *BMJ* 1992;304:743–746.
53. Halme A, Kellokumpu-Lehtinen P, Lehtonen T, Teppo L. Morphology of testicular germ cell tumours in treated and untreated cryptorchidism. *Br J Urol* 1989;64:78–83.
54. Lanson Y. Epidemiology of testicular cancers. *Prog Clin Biol Res* 1985;203:155–159.
55. Javadpour N, Bergman S. Recent advances in testicular cancer. *Curr Prob Surg* 1978;15 (Feb):1–64.
56. Schottenfeld D, Warshauer ME, Sherlock S, Zauber AG, Leder M, Payne R. The epidemiology of testicular cancer in young adults. *Am J Epidemiol* 1980;112:232–246.
57. DePue RH, Pike MC, Henderson BE. Estrogen exposure during gestation and risk of testicular cancer. *J Natl Cancer Inst* 1983;71:1151–1155.
58. Henderson BE, Benton B, Jing J, Yu MC, Pike MC. Risk factors for cancer of the testis in young men. *Int J Cancer* 1979;23:598–602.
59. Pike MC, Chilvers C, Peckham MJ. Effects of age at orchidopexy on risk of testicular cancer. *Lancet* 1986;1:1246–1248.
60. Giwercman A, Grindsted J, Hansen B, Jensen OM, Skakkebaek NE. Testicular cancer risk in boys with maldescended testis: a cohort study. *J Urol* 1987;138:1214–1216.
61. Fram RJ, Garnick MB, Retik A. The spectrum of genitourinary abnormalities in patients with cryptorchidism, with emphasis on testicular carcinoma. *Cancer* 1982;50:2243–2245.
62. Sakashita S, Koyanagi T, Tsuji I, Arikado K, Matsuno T. Congenital anomalies in children with testicular germ cell tumor. *J Urol* 1980;124:889–891.
63. Li FP, Fraumeni JF Jr. Testicular cancers in children: epidemiologic characteristics. *J Natl Cancer Inst* 1972;48:1575–1582.
64. Swerdlow AJ, Stiller CA, Wilson LMK. Prenatal factors in the aetiology of testicular cancer: an epidemiological study of childhood testicular cancer deaths in Great Britain, 1953–73. *J Epidemiol Comm Health* 1982;36:96–101.
65. Senturia YD. The epidemiology of testicular cancer. *Br J Urol* 1987;60:285–291.
66. Swerdlow AJ, Huttly SRA, Smith PG. Testicular cancer and antecedent disease. *Br J Cancer* 1987;55:97–103.
67. Johnson DE, Woodhead DM, Pohl DR, Robison JR. Cryptorchidism and testicular tumorigenesis. *Surgery* 1968;63:919–922.
68. Gilbert JB, Hamilton JB. Studies in malignant testis tumors: III—incidence and nature of tumors in ectopic testes. *Surg Gynecol Obstet* 1940;71:731–743.
69. Batata MA, Chu FCH, Hilaris BS, Whitmore WF, Golbey RB. Testicular cancer in cryptorchids. *Cancer* 1982;49:1023–1030.
70. Krabbe S, Skakkebaek NE, Berthelsen JG, et al. High incidence of undetected neoplasia in maldescended testes. *Lancet* 1979;1:999–1000.
71. Pedersen KV, Bolesen P, Zetter-Lund CG. Experience of screening for carcinoma-in-situ of the testis among young men with surgically corrected maldescended testes. *Int J Androl* 1987;10:181–185.
72. Giwercman A, Muller J, Skakkebaek NE. Carcinoma in situ of the undescended testis. *Semin Urol* 1988;6:110–119.
73. Giwercman A, Bruun E, Frimodt-Moller C, Skakkebaek NE. Prevalence of carcinoma-in-situ and other histopathologic abnormalities in testes of men with a history of cryptorchidism. *J Urol* 1989;142:998–1002.
74. Gondos B, Migliozzi JA. Intratubular germ cell neoplasia. *Semin Diagn Pathol* 1987;4:292–303.
75. Skakkebaek NE, Berthelsen JG, Giwercman A, Müller J. Carcinoma-in-situ of the testis: possible origin from gonocytes and precursor of all types of germ cell tumours except spermatocytoma. *Int J Androl* 1987;10:19–28.
76. Kristianslund S, Fosså SD, Kjellevold K. Bilateral malignant testicular germ cell cancer. *Br J Urol* 1986;58:60–63.
77. Osterlind A, Berthelsen JG, Abildgaard N, et al. Incidence of bilateral testicular germ cell cancer in Denmark, 1960–84: preliminary findings. *Int J Androl* 1987;10:203–208.
78. Scheiber K, Ackermann D, Studer UE. Bilateral testicular germ cell tumors: a report of 20 cases. *J Urol* 1987;138:73–76.
79. Dieckmann KP, Boeckmann W, Brosig W, Jonas D, Bauer HW. Bilateral testicular germ cell tumors. Report of nine cases and review of the literature. *Cancer* 1986;57:1254–1258.
80. Giwercman A, Berthelsen JG, Muller J, von der Maase H, Skakkebaek NE. Screening for carcinoma-in-situ of the testis. *Int J Androl* 1987;10:173–180.
81. Zingg EJ, Zehntner C. Bilateral testicular germ cell tumors. *Prog Clin Biol Res* 1985;203:673–680.
82. Dieckmann KP, Becker T, Jonas D, Bauer HW. Inheritance and testicular cancer. Arguments based on a report of 3 cases and a review of the literature. *Oncology* 1987;44:367–377.
83. Hayakawa M, Mukai K, Nagakura K, Hata M. A case of simultaneous bilateral germ cell tumors arising from cryptorchid testes. *J Urol* 1986;136:470–472.
84. Ware SM, Heyman J, Al-Askari S, Morales P. Bilateral testicular germ cell malignancy. *Urology* 1982;19:366–372.
85. von der Maase H, Rorth M, Walbom-Jorgensen S, et al. Carcinoma in situ of contralateral testis in patients with testicular germ cell cancer: study of 27 cases in 500 patients. *BMJ* 1986;293:1398–1401.
86. Giwercman A, Skakkebaek NE. Carcinoma-in-situ (gonocytoma-in-

situ) of the testis. In: Burger H, de Kretser D, eds. *The testis*, 2nd ed. New York: Raven Press, 1989:475–491.
87. Fuller DB, Plenk HP. Malignant testicular germ cell tumors in a father and two sons. Case report and literature review. *Cancer* 1986;58:955–958.
88. Patel SR, Kvols LK, Richardson RL. Familial testicular cancer: report of six cases and review of the literature. *Mayo Clin Proc* 1990;65:804–808.
89. Forman D, Oliver RT, Brett AR, et al. Familial testicular cancer: a report of the UK family register, estimation of risk and an HLA class 1 sib-pair analysis. *Br J Cancer* 1992;65:255–262.
90. Tollerud DJ, Blattner WA, Fraser MC, et al. Familial testicular cancer and urogenital developmental anomalies. *Cancer* 1985;55:1849–1854.
91. Rutgers JL, Scully RE. Pathology of the testis in intersex syndromes. *Semin Diagn Pathol* 1987;4:275–291
92. Hughesdon PE, Kumarasamy T. Mixed germ cell tumours (gonadoblastomas) in normal and dysgenetic gonads: case reports and review. *Virchows Arch [A]* 1970;349:258–280.
93. Manuel M, Katayama KP, Jones HW. The age of occurrence of gonadal tumors in intersex patients. *Am J Obstet Gynecol* 1976;124:293–306.
94. Morris JM. The syndrome of testicular feminization in male pseudohermaphrodites. *Am J Obstet Gynecol* 1953;65:1192–1211.
95. Rutgers JL, Scully RE. The androgen insensitivity syndrome (testicular feminization): a clinicopathologic study of 43 cases. *Int J Gynecol Pathol* 1991;10:126–145.
96. Hurt WG, Bodurtha JN, McCall JB, Ali MM. Seminoma in pubertal patient with androgen insensitivity syndrome. *Am J Obstet Gynecol* 1989;161:530–531.
97. Muller J, Skakkebaek NE, Ritzèn M, Plöen L, Petersen KE. Carcinoma in situ of the testis in children with 45,X/46,XY gonadal dysgenesis. *J Pediatr* 1985;106:431–436.
98. Nogales FF Jr, Toro M, Ortega I, Fulwood HR. Bilateral incipient germ cell tumours of the testis in the incomplete testicular feminization syndrome. *Histopathology* 1981;5:511–515.
99. MacMahon RA, Cussen LJ. Detection of gonadal carcinoma in situ in childhood and implications for management. *Aust N Z J Surg* 1991;61:667–669.
100. Pryor JP, Cameron KM, Chilton CP, et al. Carcinoma in situ in testicular biopsies in men presenting with infertility. *Br J Urol* 1983;55:780–784.
101. West AB, Butler MR, Fitzpatrick J, O'Brien A. Testicular tumors in subfertile men: report of 4 cases with implications for management of patients presenting with infertility. *J Urol* 1985;133:107–109.
102. Skakkebaek NE. Carcinoma in situ of the testis: frequency and relationship to invasive germ cell tumours in infertile men. *Histopathology* 1978;2:157–170.
103. Swerdlow AJ, Huttly SR, Smith PG. Testis cancer: post-natal hormonal factors, sexual behaviour and fertility. *Int J Cancer* 1989;43:549–553.
104. Skakkebaek NE, Berthelsen JG, Muller J. Carcinoma-in-situ of the undescended testis. *Urol Clin North Am* 1982;9:377–385.
105. Berthelsen JG, Skakkebaek NE, von der Maase H, Sorensen BL, Mogensen P. Screening for carcinoma in situ of the contralateral testis in patients with germinal testicular cancer. *BMJ* 1982;285:683–1686.
106. Muller J, Skakkebaek NE. Testicular carcinoma in situ in children with the androgen insensitivity (testicular feminisation) syndrome. *BMJ* 1984;288:1419–1420.
107. Jacobsen GK, Henriksen OB, von der Maase H. Carcinoma in situ of testicular tissue adjacent to malignant germ-cell tumors: a study of 105 cases. *Cancer* 1981;47:2660–2662.
108. Skakkebaek NE. Atypical germ cells in the adjacent "normal" tissue of testicular tumours. *Acta Pathol Microbiol Scand [A]* 1975;83:127–130.
109. Coffin CM, Ewing S, Dehner LP. Frequency of intratubular germ cell neoplasia with invasive testicular germ cell tumors. Histologic and immunocytochemical features. *Arch Pathol Lab Med* 1985;109:555–559.
110. Manivel JC, Simonton S, Wold SE, Dehner LP. Absence of intratubular germ cell neoplasia in testicular yolk sac tumors in children. *Arch Pathol Lab Med* 1988;112:641–645
111. Manivel JC, Reinberg Y, Niehans GA, Fraley EE. Intratubular germ cell neoplasia in testicular teratomas and epidermoid cysts. Correlation with prognosis and possible biologic significance. *Cancer* 1989;64:715–720.
112. Jorgensen N, Muller J, Visfeldt J, Giwercman A, Skakkebaek NE. Infantile germ cell tumors associated with carcinoma-in-situ of the testis. *Onkologie* 1991;14(suppl 4):8(abst).
113. Hu LM, Phillipson J, Barsky SH. Intratubular germ cell neoplasia in infantile yolk sac tumor: verification by tandem repeat sequence in situ hybridization. *Diagn Mol Pathol* 1992;1:118–128.
114. Perry A, Wiley EL, Albores-Saavedra J. Pagetoid spread of intratubular germ cell neoplasia into rete testis: a morphologic and immunohistochemical study of 100 orchiectomy specimens with invasive germ cell tumors. *Hum Pathol* 1994;25:235–239.
115. Muller J, Skakkebaek NE, Nielsen OH, Graem N. Cryptorchidism and testis cancer. Atypical infantile germ cells followed by carcinoma in situ and invasive carcinoma in adulthood. *Cancer* 1984;54:629–634.
116. Manivel JC, Jessurun J, Wick MR, Dehner LP. Placental alkaline phosphatase immunoreactivity in testicular germ cell tumors. *Am J Surg Pathol* 1987;11:21–29.
117. Jacobsen GK, Norgaard-Pedersen B. Placental alkaline phosphatase in testicular germ cell tumours and carcinoma-in-situ of the testis: an immunohistochemical study. *Acta Pathol Microbiol Immunol Scand [A]* 1984;92:323–329.
118. Beckstead JH. Alkaline phosphatase histochemistry in human germ cell neoplasms. *Am J Surg Pathol* 1983;7:341–349.
119. Burke AP, Mostofi FK. Intratubular malignant germ cells in testicular biopsies: clinical course and identification by staining for placental alkaline phosphatase. *Mod Pathol* 1988;1:475–479.
120. Giwercman A, Lindenberg S, Kimber SJ, Andersson T, Müller J, Skakkebaek NE. Monoclonal antibody 43–9F as a sensitive immunohistochemical marker of carcinoma in situ of human testis. *Cancer* 1990;65:1135–1142.
121. Bailey D, Marks A, Stratis M, Baumal R. Immunohistochemical staining of germ cell tumors and intratubular malignant germ cells of the testis using antibody to placental alkaline phosphatase and a monoclonal anti-seminoma antibody. *Mod Pathol* 1991;4:167–171.
122. Klys HS, Whillis D, Howard G, Harrison DJ. Glutathione S-transferase expression in the human testis and testicular germ cell neoplasia. *Br J Cancer* 1992;66:589–593.
123. Hawkins E, Heifetz SA, Giller R, Cushing B. The prepubertal testis (prenatal and postnatal): its relationship to intratubular germ cell neoplasia: a combined Pediatric Oncology Group and Children's Cancer Study Group. *Hum Pathol* 1997;28:404–410.
124. Sigg C, Hedinger C. Atypical germ cells of the testis. Comparative ultrastructural and immunohistochemical investigations. *Virchows Arch [A]* 1984;402:439–450.
125. Nielsen H, Nielsen M, Skakkebaek NE. The fine structure of possible carcinoma-in-situ in the seminiferous tubules in the testis of four infertile men. *Acta Pathol Microbiol Scand [A]* 1974;82:235–248.
126. Gondos B, Berthelsen JG, Skakkebaek NE. Intratubular germ cell neoplasia (carcinoma in situ): a preinvasive lesion of the testis. *Ann Clin Lab Sci* 1983;13:185–192.
127. Albrechtsen R, Nielsen MH, Skakkebaek NE, Wewer U. Carcinoma in situ of the testis. Some ultrastructural characteristics of germ cells. *Acta Pathol Microbiol Immunol Scand [A]* 1982;90:301–303.
128. Berthelsen JG, Skakkebaek NE. Value of testicular biopsy in diagnosing carcinoma in situ testis. *Scand J Urol Nephrol* 1981;15:165–168.
129. von der Maase H, Giwercman A, Muller J, Skakkebaek NE. Management of carcinoma-in-situ of the testis. *Int J Androl* 1987;10:209–220.
130. Bottomley D, Fisher C, Hendry WF, Horwich A. Persistent carcinoma in situ of the testis after chemotherapy for advanced testicular germ cell tumours. *Br J Urol* 1990;66:420–424.
131. von der Maase H, Meinecke B, Skakkebaek NE. Residual carcinoma-in-situ of contralateral testis after chemotherapy. *Lancet* 1988;1:477–478.
132. Jacobsen GK, Barlebo H, Olsen J, et al. Testicular germ cell tumours in Denmark 1976–1980: pathology of 1058 consecutive cases. *Acta Radiol Oncol* 1984;23:239–247.
133. von Hochstetter AR, Hedinger CE. The differential diagnosis of testicular germ cell tumors in theory and practice: a critical analysis of two major systems of classification and review of 389 cases. *Virchows Arch [A]* 1982;396:247–277.
134. Perry C, Servadio C. Seminoma in childhood. *J Urol* 1980;124:932–933.
135. Nilsson S, Anderstrom C, Hedelin H, Unsgaard B. Signs and symptoms of adult testicular tumours. *Int J Androl* 1981;4(suppl):146–152.

136. Taylor JB, Solomon DH, Levine RE, Ehrlich RM. Exophthalmos in seminoma: regression with steroids and orchiectomy. *JAMA* 1978;240:860–861.
137. Mann AS. Bilateral exophthalmos in seminoma. *J Clin Endocrinol Metab* 1967;27:1500–1502.
138. Mann K, Siddle K. Evidence for free beta-subunit secretion in so-called human chorionic gonadotropin-positive seminoma. *Cancer* 1988;62:2378–2382.
139. Mumperow E, Hartmann M. Spermatic cord beta-human chorionic gonadotropin levels in seminoma and their clinical implications. *J Urol* 1992;147:1041–1043.
140. Javadpour N. Management of seminoma based on tumor markers. *Urol Clin North Am* 1980;7:773–781.
141. Nazeer T, Ro JY, Amato B, Ordonez NG, Ayala AG. Histologically pure seminoma (HPS) with elevated alpha-fetoprotein (AFP): a clinicopathologic and immunohistochemical study of ten cases. *Mod Pathol* 1996;9:79A(abst).
142. Rustin GJ, Vogelzang NJ, Sleijfer DT, Nisselbaum JN. Consensus statement on circulating tumour markers and staging patients with germ cell tumours. *Prog Clin Biol Res* 1990;357:277–284.
143. Jacobsen GK, Talerman A. *Atlas of germ cell tumours.* Copenhagen: Munksgaard, 1989.
144. Young RH, Finlayson N, Scully RE. Tubular seminoma. Report of a case. *Arch Pathol Lab Med* 1989;113:414–416.
145. Zavala-Pompa A, Ro JY, El-Naggar AK, et al. Tubular seminoma: an immunohistochemical and DNA flow cytometric study of four cases. *Am J Clin Pathol* 1994;102:397–401.
146. Bell DA, Flotte TJ, Bhan AK. Immunohistochemical characterization of seminoma and its inflammatory cell infiltrate. *Hum Pathol* 1987;18:511–520.
147. Strutton GM, Gemmell E, Seymour GJ, Walsh MD, Lavin MF, Gardiner RA. An immunohistological examination of inflammatory cell infiltration in primary testicular seminomas. *Aust N Z J Surg* 1989;59:169–172.
148. Wilkins BS, Williamson JM, O'Brien CJ. Morphological and immunohistological study of testicular lymphomas. *Histopathology* 1989;15:147–156.
149. Bentley AJ, Parkinson MC, Harding BN, Bains RM, Lantos PL. A comparative morphological and immunohistochemical study of testicular seminomas and intracranial germinomas. *Histopathology* 1990;17:443–449.
150. Akaza H, Kobayashi K, Umeda T, Niijima T. Surface markers of lymphocytes infiltrating seminoma tissue. *J Urol* 1980;124:827–828.
151. Zhao X, Wei YQ, Kariya Y, Teshigawara K, Uchida A. Accumulation of gamma/delta T cells in human dysgerminoma and seminoma: roles in autologous tumor killing and granuloma formation. *Immunol Invest* 1995;24:607–618.
152. Wei YQ, Hang ZB, Liu KF. In situ observation of inflammatory cell-tumor cell interaction in human seminomas (germinomas): light, electron microscopic, and immunohistochemical study. *Hum Pathol* 1992;23:421–428.
153. von Hochstetter AR, Sigg C, Saremaslani P, Hedinger C. The significance of giant cells in human testicular seminomas. A clinicopathological study. *Virchows Arch [A]* 1985;407:309–322.
154. Mostofi FK, Sesterhenn IA. Pathology of germ cell tumors of testes. *Prog Clin Biol Res* 1985;203:1–34.
155. Uchida T, Shimoda T, Miyata H, et al. Immunoperoxidase study of alkaline phosphatase in testicular tumor. *Cancer* 1981;48:1455–1462.
156. Niehans GA, Manivel JC, Copland GT, Scheithauer BW, Wick MR. Immunohistochemistry of germ cell and trophoblastic neoplasms. *Cancer* 1988;62:1113–1123.
157. Hustin J, Collettee J, Franchimont P. Immunohistochemical demonstration of placental alkaline phosphatase in various states of testicular development and in germ cell tumours. *Int J Androl* 1987;10:29–35.
158. Moll R, Franke WW, Schiller DL, Geiger B, Krepler R. The catalog of human cytokeratins: patterns of expression in normal epithelia, tumors, and cultured cells. *Cell* 1982;31:11–14.
159. Fogel M, Lifschitz-Mercer B, Moll R, et al. Heterogeneity of intermediate filament expression in human testicular seminomas. *Differentiation* 1990;45:242–249.
160. Denk H, Moll R, Weybora W, et al. Intermediate filaments and desmosomal plaque proteins in testicular seminomas and non-seminomatous germ cell tumours as revealed by immunohistochemistry. *Virchows Arch [A]* 1987;410:295–307.
161. Bartkova J, Rejthar A, Bartek J, Kovarik J. Differentiation patterns in testicular germ-cell tumours as revealed by a panel of monoclonal antibodies. *Tumor Biol* 1987;8:45–56.
162. Eglen DE, Ulbright TM. The differential diagnosis of yolk sac tumor and seminoma: usefulness of cytokeratin, alpha-fetoprotein, and alpha-1-antitrypsin immunoperoxidase reactions. *Am J Clin Pathol* 1987;88 328–332.
163. Wick MR, Swanson PE, Manivel JC. Placental-like alkaline phosphatase reactivity in human tumors: an immunohistochemical study of 520 cases. *Hum Pathol* 1987;18:946–954.
164. Jacobsen GK, Jacobsen M. Alpha-fetoprotein (AFP) and human chorionic gonadotropin in testicular germ cell tumours: a prospective immunohistochemical study. *Acta Pathol Microbiol Scand [A]* 1983;91:165–176.
165. Boseman FT, Giard RWM, Kruseman ACN, Knijenenburg G, Spaander PJ. Human chorionic gonadothropin and alpha-fetoprotein in testicular germ cell tumors: a retrospective immunohistochemical study. *Histopathology* 1980;4:673–684.
166. Koide O, Iwai S. An ultrastructural study on germinoma cells. *Acta Pathol Jpn* 1981;31:755–766.
167. Pierce CB Jr. Ultrastructure of human testicular tumors. *Cancer* 1966;19:1963–1983.
168. Castedo SM, de Jong B, Oosterhuis JW, et al. Cytogenetic analysis of ten human seminomas. *Cancer Res* 1989;49:439–443.
169. Delozier-Blanchet CD, Walt H, Engel E, Vuagnat P. Cytogenetic studies of human testicular germ cell tumours. *Int J Androl* 1987;10:59–77.
170. Castedo SM, de Jong B, Oosterhuis JW, et al. i (12p)-negative testicular germ cell tumors. A different group? *Cancer Genet Cytogenet* 1988;35:171–178.
171. Ulbright TM, Roth LM, Brodhecker CA. Yolk sac differentiation in germ cell tumors: a morphologic study of 50 cases with emphasis on hepatic, enteric and parietal yolk sac features. *Am J Surg Pathol* 1986;10:151–164.
172. Hamlin JA, Kagan AR, Friedman NB. Lymphomas of the testicle. *Cancer* 1972;29:1352–1356.
173. Paladugu RR, Bearman RM, Rappaport H. Malignant lymphoma with primary manifestation in the gonad: a clinicopathologic study of 38 patients. *Cancer* 1980;45:561–571.
174. Turner RR, Colby TV, MacKintosh FR. Testicular lymphomas: a clinicopathologic study of 35 cases. *Cancer* 1981;48:2095–2102.
175. Sussman EB, Hajdu SI, Lieberman PH, Whitmore WF. Malignant lymphoma of the testis: a clinicopathologic study of 37 cases. *J Urol* 1977;118:1004–1007.
176. Ferry JA, Harris NL, Young RH, Coen J, Zietman A, Scully RE. Malignant lymphoma of the testis, epididymis, and spermatic cord. A clinicopathologic study of 69 cases with immunophenotypic analysis. *Am J Surg Pathol* 1994;18:376–390.
177. Talerman A. Primary malignant lymphoma of the testis. *J Urol* 1977;118 783–786.
178. Brunt AM, Scoble JE. Para-aortic nodal irradiation for early stage testicular seminoma. *Clin Oncol* 1992;4:165–170.
179. Horwich A, Dearnaley DP. Treatment of seminoma. *Semin Oncol* 1992;19:171–180.
180. Hunter M, Peschel RE. Testicular seminoma. Results of the Yale University experience, 1964–1984. *Cancer* 1989;64:1608–1611.
181. Babaian RJ, Zagars GK. Testicular seminoma: the M.D. Anderson experience: an analysis of pathological and patient characteristics, and treatment recommendations. *J Urol* 1988;139:311–314.
182. Fossa SD, Aass N, Kaalhus O. Radiotherapy for testicular seminoma Stage I: treatment results and long-term post irradiation morbidity in 365 patients. *Int J Radiat Oncol Biol Phys* 1989;16:383–388.
183. Amichetti M, Fellin G, Bolner A, et al. Stage I seminoma of the testis: long term results and toxicity with adjuvant radiotherapy. *Tumori* 1994;80:141–145.
184. Vallis KA, Howard GC, Duncan W, Cornbleet MA, Kerr GR. Radiotherapy for stages I and II testicular seminoma: results and morbidity in 238 patients. *Br J Radiol* 1995;68:400–405.
185. Oliver RT. Limitations to the use of surveillance as an option in the management of stage I seminoma. *Int J Androl* 1987;10:263–268.
186. Kageyama S, Ueda T, Yamauchi T, et al. Mediastinal lymph node metastasis 38 months after surveillance for stage I seminoma: a case report. *Hinyokika Kiyo* 1994;40:1021–1025.
187. Marks LB, Rutgers JL, Shipley WU, et al. Testicular seminoma: clinical and pathological features that may predict para-aortic lymph node metastases. *J Urol* 1990;143:524–527.

188. Banerjee D, Warde PR, Gospodarowicz MK, et al. Stage I testicular seminoma managed by surveillance alone: is flow cytometric DNA analysis of predictive value for relapse. *Mod Pathol* 1996;9:70A(abst).
189. Doornbos JF, Hussey DH, Johnson E. Radiotherapy for pure seminoma of the testis. *Radiology* 1975;116:401–404.
190. Thomas GM, Rider WD, Dembo AJ, et al. Seminoma of the testis: results of treatment and patterns of failure after radiation therapy. *Int J Radiat Oncol Biol Phys* 1982;8:165–174.
191. Morse MJ, Whitmore WF. Neoplasms of the testis. In: Walsh PC, Gittes RF, Perlmutter AD, Stamey TA, eds. *Campbell's urology*. Philadelphia: WB Saunders, 1986:1535–1582.
192. Peckham M. Testicular cancer. *Acta Oncol* 1988;27:439–453.
193. Motzer RJ, Bosl GJ, Geller NL, et al. Advanced seminoma: the role of chemotherapy and adjuvant surgery. *Ann Intern Med* 1988;108:513–518.
194. Fossa A, Fossa SD. Serum lactate dehydrogenase and human chorionic gonadotropin in seminoma. *Br J Urol* 1989;63:408–415.
195. Dieckmann K-P, Due W, Bauer HW. Seminoma testis with elevated serum beta-HCG—a category of germ cell cancer between seminoma and nonseminoma. *Int Urol Nephrol* 1989;21:175–184.
196. Evensen JF, Fosså SD, Kjellevold K, Lien HH. Testicular seminoma: histological findings and their prognostic significance for stage II disease. *J Surg Oncol* 1987;36:166–169.
197. Johnson DE, Gomez JJ, Ayala AG. Histologic factors affecting prognosis of pure seminoma of the testis. *South Med J* 1976;69:1173–1174.
198. Mostofi FK. Testicular tumors: epidemiologic, etiologic, and pathologic features. *Cancer* 1973;32:1186–1201.
199. Zuckman MH, Williams G, Levin HS. Mitosis counting in seminoma: an exercise of questionable significance. *Hum Pathol* 1988;19:329–335.
200. von Hochstetter AR. Mitotic count in seminomas—an unreliable criterion for distinguishing between classical and anaplastic types. *Virchows Arch [A]* 1981;390:63–69.
201. Masson P. Etude sur le seminome. *Rev Canad Biol* 1946;5:361–387.
202. Talerman A. Spermatocytic seminoma: clinicopathological study of 22 cases. *Cancer* 1980;45:2169–2176.
203. Burke AP, Mostofi FK. Spermatocytic seminoma: a clinicopathologic study of 79 cases. *J Urol Pathol* 1993;1:21–32.
204. Eble JN. Spermatocytic seminoma. *Hum Pathol* 1994;25:1035–1042.
205. Scully RE. Spermatocytic seminoma of the testis: a report of 3 cases and review of the literature. *Cancer* 1961;14:788–794.
206. Albores-Saavedra J, Huffman H, Alvarado-Cabrero I, Ayala AG. Anaplastic variant of spermatocytic seminoma. *Hum Pathol* 1996;27:650–655.
207. Muller J, Skakkebaek NE, Parkinson MC. The spermatocytic seminoma: views on pathogenesis. *Int J Androl* 1987;10:147–156.
208. Cummings OW, Ulbright TM, Eble JN, Roth LM. Spermatocytic seminoma: an immunohistochemical study. *Hum Pathol* 1994;25:54–59.
209. Dekker I, Rozeboom T, Delemarre J, Dam A, Oosterhuis JW. Placental-like alkaline phosphatase and DNA flow cytometry in spermatocytic seminoma. *Cancer* 1992;69:993–996.
210. Aguirre P, Scully RE, Dayal Y, DeLellis R. Placental-like alkaline phosphatase reactivity in germ cell tumors of the ovary and testis. *Lab Invest* 1985;52:2A(abst).
211. Rosai J, Khodadoust K, Silber I. Spermatocytic seminoma. II. Ultrastructural study. *Cancer* 1969;24:103–116.
212. Talerman A, Fu YS, Okagaki T. Spermatocytic seminoma. Ultrastructural and microspectrophotometric observations. *Lab Invest* 1984;51:343–349.
213. Romanenko AM, Persidsky YV, Mostofi FK. Ultrastructure and histogenesis of spermatocytic seminoma. *J Urol Pathol* 1993;1:387–395.
214. Frasik W, Okon K, Sokolowski A. Polymorphism of spermatocytic seminoma. A morphometric study. *Anal Cell Pathol* 1994;7:195–203.
215. Lee M-C, Talerman A, Oosterhuis JW, Damjanov I. Lectin histochemistry of classic and spermatocytic seminoma. *Arch Pathol Lab Med* 1985;109:938–942.
216. Matoska J, Ondrus D, Hornák M. Metastatic spermatocytic seminoma. A case report with light microscopic, ultrastructural, and immunohistochemical findings. *Cancer* 1988;62:1197–1201.
217. True LD, Otis CN, Delprado W, Scully RE, Rosai J. Spermatocytic seminoma of testis with sarcomatous transformation. A report of five cases. *Am J Surg Pathol* 1988;12:75–82.
218. Floyd C, Ayala AG, Logothetis CJ, Silva EG. Spermatocytic seminoma with associated sarcoma of the testis. *Cancer* 1988;61:409–414.
219. Mostofi FK, Sesterhenn IA, Davis CJ Jr. Developments in histopathology of testicular germ cell tumors. *Semin Urol* 1988;6:171–188.
220. Rodriguez PN, Hafez GR, Messing EM. Nonseminomatous germ cell tumor of the testicle: does extensive staging of the primary tumor predict the likelihood of metastatic disease. *J Urol* 1986;136:604–608.
221. Böhle A, Studer UE, Sonntag RW, Scheidegger JR. Primary or secondary extragonadal germ cell tumors. *J Urol* 1986;135:939–943.
222. Mostofi FK, Sesterhenn IA, Davis CJ Jr. Immunopathology of germ cell tumors of the testis. *Semin Diagn Pathol* 1987;4:320–341.
223. Javadpour N. The role of biologic tumor markers in testicular cancer. *Cancer* 1980;45:1755–1761.
224. Bosl GJ, Lange PH, Nochomovitz LE, et al. Tumor markers in advanced non-seminomatous testicular cancer. *Cancer* 1981;47:572–576.
225. Jacobsen GK. Histogenetic considerations concerning germ cell tumours. Morphological and immunohistochemical comparative investigation of the human embryo and testicular germ cell tumours. *Virchows Arch [A]* 1986;408:509–525.
226. Azzopardi JG, Mostofi FK, Theiss EA. Lesions of testes observed in certain patients with widespread choriocarcinoma and related tumors. *Am J Pathol* 1961;38:207–225.
227. Wittekind C, Wichmann T, Von Kleist S. Immunohistological localization of AFP and HCG in uniformly classified testis tumors. *Anticancer Res* 1983;3:327–330.
228. Saller D, Bahn H, Pressler H. Immunohistochemical demonstration of alpha-fetoprotein in testicular germ cell tumors. *Acta Histochem Suppl* 1986;33:225–231.
229. Burke AP, Mostofi FK. Placental alkaline phosphatase immunohistochemistry of intratubular malignant germ cells and associated testicular germ cell tumors. *Hum Pathol* 1988;19:663–670.
230. Battifora H, Sheibani K, Tubbs RR, Kopinski MI, Sun T-T. Antikeratin antibodies in tumor diagnosis: distinction between seminoma and embryonal carcinoma. *Cancer* 1984;54:843–848.
231. Pallesen G, Hamilton-Dutoit SJ. Ki-1 (CD30) antigen is regularly expressed in tumor cells of embryonal carcinoma. *Am J Pathol* 1988;133:446–450.
232. Hittmair A, Rogatsch H, Hobisch A, Mikuz G, Feichtinger H. CD30 expression in seminoma. *Hum Pathol* 1996;27:1166–1171.
233. Ferreiro JA. Ber-H2 expression in testicular germ cell tumors. *Hum Pathol* 1994;25:522–524.
234. Murakami SS, Said JW. Immunohistochemical localization of lactate dehydrogenase isoenzyme 1 in germ cell tumors of the testis. *Am J Clin Pathol* 1984;81:293–296.
235. Jacobsen GK, Jacobsen M, Clausen PP. Distribution of tumor-associated antigens in the various histologic components of germ cell tumors of the testis. *Am J Surg Pathol* 1981;5:257–266.
236. Ulbright TM, Goheen MP, Roth LM, Gillespie JJ. The differentiation of carcinomas of teratomatous origin from embryonal carcinoma. A light and electron microscopic study. *Cancer* 1986;57:257–263.
237. Samaniego F, Rodriguez E, Houldsworth J. Cytogenetic and molecular analysis of human male germ cell tumors: chromosome 12 abnormalities and gene amplification. *Genes Chrom Cancer* 1990;1:289–300.
238. Misaki H, Shuin T, Yao M, Kubota Y, Hosaka M. Expression of myc family oncogenes in primary human testicular cancer. *Nippon Hinyokika Gakkai Zasshi* 1989;80:1509–1513.
239. Tesch H, Fürbass R, Casper J, et al. Cellular oncogenes in human teratocarcinoma cell lines. *Int J Androl* 1990;13:377–388.
240. Shuin T, Misaki H, Kubota Y, Yao M, Hosaka M. Differential expression of protooncogenes in human germ cell tumors of the testis. *Cancer* 1994;73:1721–1727.
241. Leyland RG, Donohue JP. Scrotum and testis. In: Gillenwater JY, Grayhack JT, Howards SS, Duckett JW, eds. *Adult and pediatric urology*, 2nd ed. St. Louis: Mosby Year Book, 1991:1565–1598.
242. Pizzocaro G, Zanoni F, Salvioni R, Milani A, Piva L, Pilotti S. Difficulties of a surveillance study omitting retroperitoneal lymphadenectomy in clinical stage I nonseminomatous germ cell tumors of the testis. *J Urol* 1987;138:1393–1396.
243. Moriyama N, Daly JJ, Keating MA, Lin CW, Prout GR Jr. Vascular invasion as a prognosticator of metastatic disease in nonseminomatous germ cell tumors of the testis. Importance in "surveillance only" protocols. *Cancer* 1985;56:2492–2498.

244. Fung CY, Kalish LA, Brodsky GL, Richie JP, Garnick MB. Stage I nonseminomatous germ cell testicular tumor: prediction of metastatic potential by primary histopathology. *J Clin Oncol* 1988;6:1467–1473.
245. Sogani PC, Fair WR. Surveillance alone in the treatment of clinical Stage I nonseminomatous germ cell tumor of the testis (NSGCT). *Semin Urol* 1988;6:53–56.
246. Dunphy CH, Ayala AG, Swanson DA, Ro JY, Logothetis C. Clinical stage I nonseminomatous and mixed germ cell tumors of the testis. A clinicopathologic study of 93 patients on a surveillance protocol after orchiectomy alone. *Cancer* 1988;62:1202–1206.
247. Jacobsen GK, Rorth M, Osterlind K, et al. Histopathological features in stage I non-seminomatous testicular germ cell tumours correlated to relapse. Danish Testicular Cancer Study Group. *APMIS* 1990;98:377–382.
248. Wishnow KI, Johnson DE, Swanson DA, et al. Identifying patients with low-risk clinical stage I nonseminomatous testicular tumors who should be treated by surveillance. *Urology* 1989;34:339–343.
249. Javadpour N, Canning DA, O'Connell KJ, Young JD. Predictors of recurrent clinical stage I nonseminomatous testicular cancer. A prospective clinicopathologic study. *Urology* 1986;27:508–511.
250. Costello AJ, Mortensen PH, Stillwell RG. Prognostic indicators for failure of surveillance management of stage I non-seminomatous germ cell tumours. *Aust N Z J Surg* 1989;59:119–122.
251. Fosså SD, Aass N, Kaalhus O. Testicular cancer in young Norwegians. J Surg Oncol 1988;39:43–63.
252. Freedman LS, Parkinson MC, Jones WG, et al. Histopathology in the prediction of relapse of patients with stage I testicular teratoma treated by orchidectomy alone. *Lancet* 1987;2:294–298.
253. Rodriguez PN, Hafez GR, Messing EM. Nonseminomatous germ cell tumor of the testicle: does extensive staging of the primary tumor predict the likelihood of metastatic disease? *J Urol* 1986;136:604–608.
254. Hoeltl W, Pont J, Kosak D, Honetz N, Marberger M. Treatment decision for stage I non-seminomatous germ cell tumours based on the risk factor "vascular invasion." *Br J Urol* 1992;69:83–87.
255. Sesterhenn IA, Weiss RB, Mostofi FK, et al. Prognosis and other clinical correlates of pathologic review in stage I and II testicular carcinoma: a report from the Testicular Cancer Intergroup Study. *J Clin Oncol* 1992;10:69–78.
256. Sturgeon JF, Jewett MA, Alison RE, et al. Surveillance after orchidectomy for patients with clinical stage I nonseminomatous testis tumors. *J Clin Oncol* 1992;10:564–568.
257. Moul JW, McCarthy WF, Fernandez EB, Sesterhenn IA. Percentage of embryonal carcinoma and of vascular invasion predicts pathological stage in clinical stage I nonseminomatous testicular cancer. *Cancer Res* 1994;54:362–364.
258. Fernandez EB, Sesterhenn IA, McCarthy WF, Mostofi FK, Moul JW. Proliferating cell nuclear antigen expression to predict occult disease in clinical stage I nonseminomatous testicular germ cell tumors. *J Urol* 1994;152:1133–1138.
259. Gels ME, Hoekstra HJ, Sleijfer DT, et al. Detection of recurrence in patients with clinical stage I nonseminomatous testicular germ cell tumors and consequences for further follow-up: a single-center 10-year experience. *J Clin Oncol* 1995;13:1188–1194.
260. Raghavan D, Vogelzang NJ, Bosl GJ, et al. Tumor classification and size in germ-cell testicular cancer: influence on the occurrence of metastases. *Cancer* 1982;50:1591–1595.
261. Moul JW, Foley JP, Hitchcock CL, et al. Flow cytometric and quantitative histological parameters to predict occult disease in clinical stage I nonseminomatous testicular germ cell tumors. *J Urol* 1993;150:879–883.
262. de Riese WT, Albers P, Walker EB, et al. Predictive parameters of biologic behavior of early stage nonseminomatous testicular germ cell tumors. *Cancer* 1994;74:1335–1341.
263. Nicolai N, Pizzocaro G. A surveillance study of clinical stage I nonseminomatous germ cell tumors of the testis: 10-year followup. *J Urol* 1995;154:1045–1049.
264. Albers P, Miller GA, Orazi A, et al. Immunohistochemical assessment of tumor proliferation and volume of embryonal carcinoma identify patients with clinical stage A nonseminomatous testicular germ cell tumor at low risk for occult metastasis. *Cancer* 1995;75:844–850.
265. Albers P, Ulbright TM, Albers J, et al. Tumor proliferative activity is predictive of pathological stage in clinical stage A nonseminomatous testicular germ cell tumors. *J Urol* 1996;155:579–586.
266. de Riese WT, de Riese C, Ulbright TM, et al. Flow-cytometric and quantitative histologic parameters as prognostic indicators for occult retroperitoneal disease in clinical-stage-I non-seminomatous testicular germ-cell tumors. *Int J Cancer* 1994;57:628–633.
267. Einhorn LH. Chemotherapy of disseminated testicular cancer. In: Skinner DG, Lieskovsky G, eds. *Diagnosis and management of genitourinary cancer.* Philadelphia: WB Saunders, 1988:526–531.
268. Ulbright TM, Roth LM. A pathologic analysis of lesions following modern chemotherapy for metastatic germ cell tumors. *Pathol Annu* 1990;25(Pt 1):313–340.
269. Vogelzang NJ. Prognostic factors in metastatic testicular cancer. *Int J Androl* 1987;10:225–237.
270. Stoter G, Sylvester R, Sleijfer DT, et al. Multivariate analysis of prognostic variables in patients with disseminated non-seminomatous testicular cancer: results from an EORTC multi-institutional phase III study. *Int J Androl* 1987;10:239–246.
271. Mead GM, Stenning SP, Parkinson MC, et al. The Second Medical Research Council study of prognostic factors in nonseminomatous germ cell tumors. Medical Research Council Testicular Tumour Working Party. *J Clin Oncol* 1992;10:85–94.
272. Sledge GW Jr, Eble JN, Roth BJ, Wuhrman BP, Fineberg N, Einhorn LH. Relation of proliferative activity to survival in patients with advanced germ cell cancer. *Cancer Res* 1988;48:3864–3868.
273. International Germ Cell Cancer Collaborative Group. International germ cell consensus classification: a prognostic factor-based staging system for metastatic germ cell cancer. *J Clin Oncol* 1997;15:594–603.
274. Teilum G. Gonocytoma: homologous ovarian and testicular tumors I: with discussion of "mesonephroma ovarii" (Schiller: Am J Cancer 1939). *Acta Pathol Microbiol Scand* 1946;23:242–251.
275. Teilum G. "Mesonephroma ovarii" (Schiller)—an extra-embryonic mesoblastoma of germ cell origin in the ovary and the testis. *Acta Pathol Microbiol Scand* 1950;27:249–261.
276. Teilum G. Endodermal sinus tumors of the ovary and testis: comparative morphogenesis of the so-called mesonephroma ovarii (Schiller) and extraembryonic (yolk sac-allantoic) structures of the rat's placenta. *Cancer* 1959;12:1092–1105.
277. Kaplan GW, Cromie WC, Kelalis PP, Silber I, Tank ES Jr. Prepubertal yolk sac testicular tumors—report of the testicular tumor registry. *J Urol* 1988;140:1109–1112.
278. Brosman SA. Testicular tumors in prepubertal children. *Urology* 1979;13:581–588.
279. Harms D, Janig U. Germ cell tumours of childhood: report of 170 cases including 59 pure and partial yolk-sac tumours. *Virchows Arch [A]* 1986;409:223–229.
280. Talerman A. Endodermal sinus (yolk sac) tumor elements in testicular germ-cell tumors in adults: comparison of prospective and retrospective studies. *Cancer* 1980;46:1213–1217.
281. Brown LM, Pottern LM, Hoover RN, Devesa SS, Aselton P, Flannery JT. Testicular cancer in the United States: trends in incidence and mortality. *Int J Epidemiol* 1986;15:164–170.
282. Grady RW, Ross JH, Kay R. Patterns of metastatic spread in prepubertal yolk sac tumor of the testis. *J Urol* 1995;153:1259–1261.
283. Talerman A, Haije WG, Baggerman L. Serum alphafetoprotein (AFP) in patients with germ cell tumors of the gonads and extragonadal sites: correlation between endodermal sinus (yolk sac) tumor and raised serum AFP. *Cancer* 1980;46:380–385.
284. Jacobsen GK. Alpha-fetoprotein (AFP) and human chorionic gonadotropin (HCG) in testicular germ cell tumours. *Acta Pathol Microbiol Immunol Scand [A]* 1983;91:183–190.
285. Wu JT, Book L, Sudar K. Serum alpha fetoprotein (AFP) levels in normal infants. *Pediatr Res* 1981;15:50–52.
286. Talerman A. Germ cell tumors. In: Talerman A, Roth LM, eds. *Pathology of the testis and its adnexa.* New York: Churchill Livingstone, 1986:29–65.
287. Clement PB, Young RH, Scully RE. Endometrioid-like variant of ovarian yolk sac tumor. A clinicopathological analysis of eight cases. *Am J Surg Pathol* 1987;11:767–778.
288. Cohen MB, Friend DS, Molnar JJ, Talerman A. Gonadal endodermal sinus (yolk sac) tumor with pure intestinal differentiation: a new histologic type. *Pathol Res Pract* 1987;182:609–616.
289. Martinazzi M, Crivelli F, Zampatti C. Immunohistochemical study of hepatic and enteric structures in testicular endodermal sinus tumors. *Basic Appl Histochem* 1988;32:239–245.
290. Michael H, Ulbright TM, Brodhecker CA. The pluripotential nature of the mesenchyme-like component of yolk sac tumor. *Arch Pathol Lab Med* 1989;113:1115–1119.

291. Teilum G. *Special tumors of ovary and testis and related extragonadal lesions.* Philadelphia: JB Lippincott, 1976.
292. Ulbright TM, Michael H, Loehrer PJ, Donohue JP. Spindle cell tumors resected from male patients with germ cell tumors: a clinicopathologic study of 14 cases. *Cancer* 1990;65:148–152.
293. Teilum G. Classification of endodermal sinus tumor (mesoblastoma vitellinum) and so-called "embryonal carcinoma" of the ovary. *Acta Pathol Microbiol Scand* 1965;64:407–429.
294. Jacobsen GK, Jacobsen M. Possible liver cell differentiation in testicular germ cell tumours. *Histopathology* 1983;7:537–545.
295. Prat J, Bhan AK, Dickersin GR, Robboy S, Scully RE. Hepatoid yolk sac tumor of the ovary (endodermal sinus tumor with hepatoid differentiation): a light microscopic, ultrastructural, and immunohistochemical study of seven cases. *Cancer* 1982;50:2355–2368.
296. Damjanov I, Amenta PS, Zarghami F. Transformation of an AFP-positive yolk sac carcinoma into an AFP-negative neoplasm: evidence for *in vivo* cloning of the human parietal yolk sac carcinoma. *Cancer* 1984;53:1902–1907.
297. Kurman RJ, Norris HJ. Endodermal sinus tumor of the ovary: clinical and pathologic analysis of 71 cases. *Cancer* 1976;38:2402–2419.
298. Koide O, Iwai S, Baba K, Iri H. Identification of testicular atypical germ cells by an immunohistochemical technique for placental alkaline phosphatase. *Cancer* 1987;60:1325–1330.
299. Miettinen M, Virtanen I, Talerman A. Intermediate filament proteins in human testis and testicular germ-cell tumors. *Am J Pathol* 1985;120:402–410.
300. Lawrence WD, Young RH, Scully RE. Juvenile granulosa cell tumor of the infantile testis. A report of 14 cases. *Am J Surg Pathol* 1985;9:87–94.
301. Chan JK, Chan VS, Mak KL. Congenital juvenile granulosa cell tumour of the testis: report of a case showing extensive degenerative changes. *Histopathology* 1990;17:75–80.
302. Chadha S, van der Kwast TH. Immunohistochemistry of ovarian granulosa cell tumours: the value of tissue specific proteins and tumour markers. *Virchows Arch [A]* 1989;414:439–445.
303. Biscotti CV, Hart WR. Juvenile granulosa cell tumors of the ovary. *Arch Pathol Lab Med* 1989;113:40–46.
304. Ulbright TM, Gersell DJ. Rete testis hyperplasia with hyaline globule formation. A lesion simulating yolk sac tumor. *Am J Surg Pathol* 1991;15:66–74.
305. Loehrer PJ Sr, Williams SD, Einhorn LH. Testicular cancer: the quest continues. *J Natl Cancer Inst* 1988;80:1373–1382.
306. Sabio H, Burgert EO Jr, Farrow GM, Kelalis PP. Embryonal carcinoma of the testis in childhood. *Cancer* 1974;34:2118–2121.
307. Kramer SA. Pediatric urologic oncology. *Urol Clin North Am* 1985;12:31–42.
308. Drago JR, Nelson RP, Palmer JM. Childhood embryonal carcinoma of testes. *Urology* 1978;12:499–504.
309. Hawkins EP, Finegold MJ, Hawkins HK, Krischer JP, Starling KA, Weinberg A. Nongerminomatous malignant germ cell tumors in children: a review of 89 cases from the Pediatric Oncology Group, 1971–1984. *Cancer* 1986;58:2579–2584.
310. Logothetis CJ, Samuels ML, Trindade A, Grant C, Gomez L, Ayala A. The prognostic significance of endodermal sinus tumor histology among patients treated for stage III nonseminomatous germ cell tumors of the testes. *Cancer* 1984;53:122–128.
311. Nseyo UO, Englander LS, Wajsman Z, Huben RP, Pontes JE. Histological patterns of treatment failures in testicular germ cell neoplasms. *J Urol* 1985;133:219–220.
312. Jacobsen GK, Barlebo H, Olsen J, et al. Testicular germ cell tumours in Denmark 1976–1980. Pathology of 1058 consecutive cases. *Acta Radiol Oncol* 1984;23:239–247.
313. Giralt S, Dexeus F, Amato R, Sella A, Logothetis C. Hyperthyroidism in men with germ cell tumors and high levels of beta-human chorionic gonadotropin. *Cancer* 1992;69:1286–1290.
314. Ulbright TM, Young RH, Scully RE. Trophoblastic tumors of the testis other than classic choriocarcinoma: "monophasic" choriocarcinoma and placental site trophoblastic tumor: a report of two cases. *Am J Surg Pathol* 1997;21:282–288.
315. Manivel JC, Niehans G, Wick MR, Dehner LP. Intermediate trophoblast in germ cell neoplasms. *Am J Surg Pathol* 1987;11:693–701.
316. Lind HM, Haghighi P. Carcinoembryonic antigen staining in choriocarcinoma. *Am J Clin Pathol* 1986;86:538–540.
317. Clark RK, Damjanov I. Intermediate filaments of human trophoblast and choriocarcinoma cell lines. *Virchows Arch [A]* 1985;407:203–208.
318. Bedael JJ, Vugrin D, Whitmore WF Jr. Autopsy findings in 154 patients with germ cell tumors of the testis. *Cancer* 1982;50:548–551.
319. Logothetis CJ, Samuels ML, Selig DE, et al. Cyclic chemotherapy with cyclophosphamide, doxorubicin, and cisplatin plus vinblastine and bleomycin in advanced germ cell tumors: results with 100 patients. *Am J Med* 1986;81:219–228.
320. Raeth M, Schultz HP, von der Maase H, et al. Prognostic factors in testicular germ cell tumours: experiences with 1058 consecutive cases. *Acta Radiol Oncol* 1984;23:271–285.
321. Bosl GJ, Geller NL, Cirrincione C, et al. Multivariate analysis of prognostic variables in patients with metastatic testicular cancer. *Cancer Res* 1983;43:3403–3407.
322. Stoter G, Sylvester R, Sleijfer DT, et al. A multivariate analysis of prognostic factors in disseminated non-seminomatous testicular cancer. *Prog Clin Biol Res* 1988;269:381–393.
323. Taguchi T, Iwasaki A, Sugao H, Nakano E, Matsuda M, Sonoda T. Clinical statistics of germinal testicular cancer. *Nippon Hinyokika Gakkai Zasshi* 1990;81:889–894.
324. Brigden ML, Sullivan LD, Comisarow RH. Stage C pure choriocarcinoma of the testis: a potentially curable lesion. *CA* 1982;32:82–84.
325. Mostofi FK, Spaander P, Grigor K, Parkinson CM, Shakkebaek NE, Oliver RT. Consensus on pathological classifications of testicular tumours. *Prog Clin Biol Res* 1990;357:267–276.
326. Damjanov I. Tumors of the testis and epididymis. In: Murphy WM, ed. *Urological pathology.* Philadelphia: WB Saunders, 1989:324–379.
327. Pugh RCB, Cameron KM. Teratoma. In: Pugh RCB, ed. *Pathology of the testis.* Oxford: Blackwell Scientific, 1976:199–244.
328. Agostini S, Magrini SM, Simoncini R, Biti G, Villari N, Giannardi G. Association between testicular cancer and spina bifida occulta. *Acta Oncol* 1991;30:579–581.
329. Gilman PA. The epidemiology of human teratomas. In: Damjanov I, Knowles BB, Solter D, eds. *The human teratomas: experimental and clinical biology.* Clinton, NJ: Humana Press, 1983:81–104.
330. Barsky SH. Germ cell tumors of the testis. In: Javadpour N, Barsky SH, eds. *Surgical pathology of urologic diseases.* Baltimore: Williams and Wilkins, 1987:224–246.
331. Hasuda L, Leidich RB, Das S. Mature teratoma of the testis metastasizing as mature teratoma. *J Urol* 1986;135:1020–1022.
332. Kedia K, Fraley EE. Adult teratoma of the testis metastasizing as adult teratoma: case report and review of literature. *J Urol* 1975;114:535–539.
333. Cameron-Strange A, Horner J. Differentiated teratoma of testis metastasizing as differentiated teratoma in adult. *Urology* 1989;33:481–482.
334. Fogalter H, Scofield GF. Adult teratoma of the testicle metastasizing as adult teratoma. *J Urol* 1962;87:573–576.
335. Renedo DE, Trainer TD. Intratubular germ cell neoplasia (ITGCN) with p53 and PCNA expression and adjacent mature teratoma in an intact testis. An immunohistochemical and morphologic study with a review of the literature. *Am J Surg Pathol* 1994;18:947–952.
336. Oosterhuis JW, de Jong B, Cornelisse CJ, et al. Karyotyping and DNA flow cytometry of mature residual teratoma after intensive chemotherapy of disseminated nonseminomatous germ cell tumor of the testis: a report of two cases. *Cancer Genet Cytogenet* 1986;22:149–157.
337. Molenaar WM, Oosterhuis JW, Meiring A, Sleyfer DT, Koops HS, Cornelisse CJ. Histology and DNA contents of a secondary malignancy arising in a mature residual lesion six years after chemotherapy for a disseminated nonseminomatous testicular tumor. *Cancer* 1986;58:264–268.
338. Aguirre P, Scully RE. Primitive neuroectodermal tumor of the testis. Report of a case. *Arch Pathol Lab Med* 1983;107:643–645.
339. Michael H, Hull MT, Ulbright TM, Foster RS, Miller KD. Primitive neuroectodermal tumors arising in testicular germ cell neoplasms. *Am J Surg Pathol* 1997;21:896–904.
340. Ahmed T, Bosl GJ, Hajdu SI. Teratoma with malignant transformation in germ cell tumors in men. *Cancer* 1985;56:860–863.
341. Ulbright TM, Loehrer PJ, Roth LM, Einhorn LH, Williams SD, Clark SA. The development of non-germ cell malignancies within germ cell tumors. A clinicopathologic study of 11 cases. *Cancer* 1984;54:1824–1833.
342. Mostofi FK. Histological change ostensibly induced by therapy in the metastasis of germ cell tumors of testis. *Prog Clin Biol Res* 1985;203:47–60.
343. Trojanowski JQ, Hickey WF. Human teratomas express differentiated

neural antigens: an immunohistochemical study with anti-neurofilament, anti-glial filament, and anti-myelin basic protein monoclonal antibodies. *Am J Pathol* 1984;115:383–389.
344. Bartkova J, Bartek J, Lukas J, et al. p53 protein alterations in human testicular cancer including pre-invasive intratubular germ-cell neoplasia. *Int J Cancer* 1991;49:196–202.
345. Shah KH, Maxted WC, Chun B. Epidermoid cysts of the testis: a report of three cases and an analysis of 141 cases from the world literature. *Cancer* 1981;47:577–582.
346. Price EB Jr. Epidermoid cysts of the testis: a clinical and pathologic analysis of 69 cases from the testicular tumor registry. *J Urol* 1969;102:708–713.
347. Kooijman CD. Immature teratomas in children. *Histopathology* 1988;12:491–502.
348. Leibovitch I, Foster RS, Ulbright TM, Donohue JP. Adult primary pure teratoma of the testis. The Indiana experience. *Cancer* 1995;75:2244–2250.
349. Johnson DE, Bracken RB, Blight EM. Prognosis for pathologic Stage I non-seminomatous germ cell tumors of the testis managed by retroperitoneal lymphadenectomy. *J Urol* 1976;116:63–68.
350. Talerman A, Gratama S, Miranda S, Okagaki T. Primary carcinoid tumor of the testis: case report, ultrastructure and review of the literature. *Cancer* 1978;42:2696–2706.
351. Berdjis CC, Mostofi FK. Carcinoid tumors of the testis. *J Urol* 1977;118:777–782.
352. Zavala-Pompa A, Ro JY, El-Naggar A, et al. Primary carcinoid tumor of testis. Immunohistochemical, ultrastructural, and DNA flow cytometric study of three cases with a review of the literature. *Cancer* 1993;72:1726–1732.
353. Sullivan JL, Packer JT, Bryant M. Primary malignant carcinoid of the testis. *Arch Pathol Lab Med* 1981;105:515–517.
354. Ordonez NG, Ayala AG, Sneige N, Mackay B. Immunohistochemical demonstration of multiple neurohormonal polypeptides in a case of pure testicular carcinoid. *Am J Clin Pathol* 1982;78:860–864.
355. Ogawa A, Sugihara S, Nakazawa Y. A case of primary carcinoid tumor of the testis. *Gan No Rinsho* 1988;34:1629–1634.
356. Lewin KJ, Ulich T, Yang K, Layfield L. The endocrine cells of the gastrointestinal tract: tumors, part II. *Pathol Annu* 1986;21(Pt 2):181–215.
357. Hosking DH, Bowman DM, McMorris SL, Ramsey EW. Primary carcinoid of the testis with metastases. *J Urol* 1981;125:255–256.
358. Young RH, Scully RE. *Testicular tumors.* Chicago: ASCP Press, 1990.
359. Nocks BN, Dann JA. Primitive neuroectodermal tumor (immature teratoma) of testis. *Urology* 1983;22:543–544.
360. Nistal M, Paniagua R. Primary neuroectodermal tumour of the testis. *Histopathology* 1985;9:1351–1359.
361. Brawn PN. The characteristics of embryonal carcinoma cells in teratocarcinomas. *Cancer* 1987;59:2042–2046.
362. Nakashima N, Murakami S, Fukatsu T, et al. Characteristics of "embryoid body" in human gonadal germ cell tumors. *Hum Pathol* 1988;19:1144–1154.
363. Evans RW. Developmental stages of embryo-like bodies in teratoma testis. *J Clin Pathol* 1957;10:31–39.
364. Cardoso de Almeida PC, Scully RE. Diffuse embryoma of the testis. A distinctive form of mixed germ cell tumor. *Am J Surg Pathol* 1983;7:633–642.
365. de Peralta-Venturina MN, Ro JY, Ordonez NG, Ayala AG. Diffuse embryoma of the testis: an immunohistochemical study of two cases. *Am J Clin Pathol* 1994;101:402–405.
366. Bär W, Hedinger C. Comparison of histologic types of primary testicular germ cell tumors with their metastases: consequences for the WHO and the British Nomenclatures? *Virchows Arch [A]* 1976;370:41–54.
367. Lopez JI, Angulo JC. Burned-out tumour of the testis presenting as retroperitoneal choriocarcinoma. *Int Urol Nephrol* 1994;26:549–553.
368. Daugaard G, von der Maase H, Olsen J, Rorth M, Skakkebaek NE. Carcinoma-in-situ testis in patients with assumed extragonadal germ-cell tumours. *Lancet* 1987;2:528–530.
369. Donohue JP, Roth LM, Zachary JM, Rowland RG, Einhorn LH, Williams SD. Cytoreductive surgery for metastatic testis cancer: tissue analysis of retroperitoneal masses after chemotherapy. *J Urol* 1982;127:1111–1114.
370. Davey DD, Ulbright TM, Loehrer PJ, Einhorn LH, Donohue JP, Williams SD. The significance of atypia within teratomatous metastases after chemotherapy for malignant germ cell tumors. *Cancer* 1987;59:533–539.
371. Mazur MT, Lurain JR, Brewer JI. Fatal gestational choriocarcinoma: clinicopathologic study of patients treated at a trophoblastic disease center. *Cancer* 1982;50:1833–1846.
372. Young RH, Talerman A. Testicular tumors other than germ cell tumors. *Semin Diagn Pathol* 1987;4:342–360.
373. Costa MJ, Ames PF, Walls J, Roth LM. Inhibin immunohistochemistry applied to ovarian neoplasms, a novel, effective diagnostic tool. *Hum Pathol* 1997;28:1247–1254.
374. Rishi M, Howard LN, Bratthauer GL, Tavassoli FA. Use of monoclonal antibody against inhibin as a marker for sex cord-stromal tumors of the ovary. *Am J Surg Pathol* 1997;21:583–589.
375. Zheng W, Sung CJ, Hanna I, et al. Alpha and beta subunits of inhibin/activin as sex cord-stromal differentiation markers. *Int J Gynecol Pathol* 1997;16:263–271.
376. Kim I, Young RH, Scully RE. Leydig cell tumors of the testis. A clinicopathological analysis of 40 cases and review of the literature. *Am J Surg Pathol* 1985;9:177–192.
377. Wheeler JE. Testicular tumors. In: Hill GS, ed. *Uropathology.* New York: Churchill Livingstone, 1989:1047–1100.
378. Dilworth JP, Farrow GM, Oesterling JE. Non-germ cell tumors of testis. *Urology* 1991;37:399–417.
379. Kaplan GW, Cromie WJ, Kelalis PP, Silber I, Tank ES Jr. Gonadal stromal tumors: a report of the Prepubertal Testicular Tumor Registry. *J Urol* 1986;136:300–302.
380. Bokemeyer C, Kuczyk M, Schoffski P, Schmoll HJ. Familial occurrence of Leydig cell tumors: a report of a case in a father and his adult son. *J Urol* 1993;150:1509–1510.
381. Sohval AR, Churg J, Gabrilove JL. Ultrastructure of feminizing testicular Leydig cell tumors. *Ultrastruct Pathol* 1982;3:335–345.
382. Kay S, Fu Y-S, Koontz WW, Chen ATL. Interstitial-cell tumor of the testis: tissue culture and ultrastructural studies. *Am J Clin Pathol* 1975;63:366–376.
383. Sohval AR, Churg J, Gabrilove JL, Freiberg EK, Katz N. Ultrastructure of feminizing testicular Leydig cell tumors. *Ultrastruct Pathol* 1982;3:335–345.
384. Miettinen M, Wahlstrom T, Virtanen I, Talerman A, Astengo-Osuna C. Cellular differentiation in ovarian sex-cord-stromal and germ-cell tumors studied with antibodies to intermediate filament proteins. *Am J Surg Pathol* 1985;9:640–651.
385. Descheemaeker T, Fontaine P, Racadot A, et al. Enkephalin-like immunoreactivity in Leydig cell tumor. *Ann Endocrinol* 1989;50:513–516.
386. Minkowitz S, Soloway H, Soscia J. Ossifying interstitial cell tumor of the testes. *J Urol* 1965;94:592–595.
387. Balsitis M, Sokal M. Ossifying malignant Leydig (interstitial) cell tumour of the testis. *Histopathology* 1990;16:599–601.
388. Santonja C, Varona C, Burgos FJ, Nistal M. Leydig cell tumor of testis with adipose metaplasia. *Appl Pathol* 1989;7:201–204.
389. Söderström KO. Leydig cell hyperplasia. *Arch Androl* 1986;17:57–65.
390. Proppe KH, Dickersin GR. Large-cell calcifying Sertoli cell tumor of the testis: light microscopic and ultrastructural study. *Hum Pathol* 1982;13:1109–1114.
391. Proppe KH, Scully RE. Large-cell calcifying Sertoli cell tumor of the testis. *Am J Clin Pathol* 1980;74:607–619.
392. Buchino JJ, Uhlenhuth ER. Large-cell calcifying Sertoli cell tumor. *J Urol* 1989;141:953–954.
393. Waxman M, Damjanov I, Khapra A, Landau SJ. Large cell calcifying Sertoli tumor of the testis. Light microscopic and ultrastructural study. *Cancer* 1984;54:1574–1581.
394. Horn T, Jao W, Keh PC. Large-cell calcifying Sertoli cell tumor of the testis: a case report with ultrastructural study. *Ultrastruct Pathol* 1983;4:359–364.
395. Perez-Atayde AR, Nunez AE, Carroll WL, et al. Large-cell calcifying Sertoli cell tumor of the testis. An ultrastructural, immunocytochemical, and biochemical study. *Cancer* 1983;51:2287–2292.
396. Blix GW, Levine LA, Goldberg R, Talerman A. Large cell calcifying Sertoli cell tumor of the testis. *Scand J Urol Nephrol* 1992;26:73–75.
397. Kratzer SS, Ulbright TM, Talerman A, et al. Large cell calcifying Sertoli cell tumor of the testis: contrasting features of six malignant and six benign tumors and a review of the literature. *Am J Surg Pathol* 1997;21:1271–1280.
398. Rutgers JL, Young RH, Scully RE. The testicular "tumor" of the

399. adrenogenital syndrome. A report of six cases and review of the literature on testicular masses in patients with adrenocortical disorders. *Am J Surg Pathol* 1988;12:503–513.
399. Srikanth MS, West BR, Ishitani M, Isaacs H Jr, Applebaum H, Costin G. Benign testicular tumors in children with congenital adrenal hyperplasia. *J Pediatr Surg* 1992;27:639–641.
400. Johnson RE, Scheithauer B. Massive hyperplasia of testicular adrenal rests in a patient with Nelson's syndrome. *Am J Clin Pathol* 1982;77:501–507.
401. Grem JL, Robins HI, Wilson KS, Gilchrist K, Trump DL. Metastatic Leydig cell tumor of the testis: report of three cases and review of the literature. *Cancer* 1986;58:2116–2119.
402. Wilson DM, Pitts WC, Hintz RL, Rosenfeld RG. Testicular tumors with Peutz-Jeghers syndrome. *Cancer* 1986;57:2238–2240.
403. Young S, Gooneratne S, Straus FH, Zeller WP, Bulun SE, Rosenthal IM. Feminizing Sertoli cell tumors in boys with Peutz-Jeghers syndrome. *Am J Surg Pathol* 1995;19:50–58.
404. Young RH, Koelliker DD, Scully RE. Sertoli cell tumors of the testis, not otherwise specified: a clinicopathologic analysis of 60 cases. *Am J Surg Pathol* 1998;22:709–721.
405. Aguirre P, Thor AD, Scully RE. Ovarian small cell carcinoma. Histogenetic considerations based on immunohistochemical and other findings. *Am J Clin Pathol* 1989;92:140–149.
406. Aguirre P, Thor AD, Scully RE. Ovarian endometrioid carcinomas resembling sex cord-stromal tumors. An immunohistochemical study. *Int J Gynecol Pathol* 1989;8:364–373.
407. Nielsen K, Jacobsen GK. Malignant Sertoli cell tumour of the testis: an immunohistochemical study and a review of the literature. *APMIS* 1988;96:755–760.
408. Able ME, Lee JC. Ultrastructure of a Sertoli-cell adenoma of the testis. *Cancer* 1969;23:481–486.
409. Tavassoli FA, Norris HJ. Sertoli cell tumors of the ovary: a clinicopathologic study of 28 cases with ultrastructural observations. *Cancer* 1980;46:2281–2297.
410. Littleton R, Farah R, Cerny J, Ohorodnik J. Sertoli cell testicular tumors. *Urology* 1981;17:557–559.
411. Jacobsen GK. Malignant Sertoli cell tumors of the testis. *J Urol Pathol* 1993;1:233–255.
412. Iezzoni JC, Fechner RE, Wong LS, Rosai J. Aggressive angiomyxoma in males: a report of four cases. *Am J Clin Pathol* 1995;104:391–396.
413. Stalker AL, Hendry WT. Hyperplasia and neoplasia of the Sertoli cell. *J Pathol Bacteriol* 1952;64:161–168.
414. Hedinger CE, Huber R, Weber E. Frequency of so-called hypoplastic or dysgenetic zones in scrotal and otherwise normal human testes. *Virchows Arch [A]* 1967;342:165–168.
415. Zukerberg LR, Young RH, Scully RE. Sclerosing Sertoli cell tumor of the testis: a report of 10 cases. *Am J Surg Pathol* 1991;15:829–834.
416. Anderson GA. Sclerosing Sertoli cell tumor of the testis: a distinct histological subtype. *J Urol* 1995;154:1756–1758.
417. Dreyer L, Jacyk WK, du Plessis DJ. Bilateral large-cell calcifying Sertoli cell tumor of the testes with Peutz-Jeghers syndrome: a case report. *Pediatr Dermatol* 1994;11:335–337.
418. Carney JA, Gordon H, Carpenter PC, Shenoy BV, Go VLW. The complex of myxomas, spotty pigmentation, and endocrine overactivity. *Medicine* 1985;64:270–283.
419. Carney JA, Toorkey BC. Myxoid fibroadenoma and allied conditions (myxomatosis) of the breast: a heritable disorder with special associations including cardiac and cutaneous myxomas. *Am J Surg Pathol* 1991;15:713–721.
420. Carney JA. Psammomatous melanotic schwannoma: a distinctive, heritable tumor with special associations, including cardiac myxoma and the Cushing syndrome. *Am J Surg Pathol* 1990;14:206–222.
421. Ulbright TM, Young RH, Amin MB. *Tumors of the testis and scrotum.* Atlas of Tumor Pathology, 3rd series. Washington, DC: Armed Forces Institute of Pathology (in press).
422. Oosterhuis JW, Castedo SM, de Jong B, et al. A malignant mixed gonadal stromal tumor of the testis with heterologous components and i (12p) in one of its metastases. *Cancer Genet Cytogenet* 1989;41:105–114.
423. Perito PE, Ciancio G, Civantos F, Politano VA. Sertoli-Leydig cell testicular tumor: case report and review of sex cord/gonadal stromal tumor histogenesis. *J Urol* 1992;148:883–885.
424. Talerman A. Pure granulosa cell tumour of the testis. Report of a case and review of the literature. *Appl Pathol* 1985;3:117–122.
425. Düe W, Dieckmann KP, Niedobitek G, Bornhöft G, Loy V, Stein H. Testicular sex cord stromal tumour with granulosa cell differentiation: detection of steroid hormone receptors as a possible basis for tumour development and therapeutic management. *J Clin Pathol* 1990;43: 732–737.
426. Gaylis FD, August C, Yeldandi A, Nemcek A, Garnett J. Granulosa cell tumor of the adult testis: ultrastructural and ultrasonographic characteristics. *J Urol* 1989;141:126–127.
427. Nistal M, Lazaro R, Garcia J, Paniagua R. Testicular granulosa cell tumor of the adult type. *Arch Pathol Lab Med* 1992;116:284–287.
428. Jimenez-Quintero LP, Ro JY, Zavala-Pompa A, et al. Granulosa cell tumor of the adult testis: a clinicopathologic study of seven cases and a review of the literature. *Hum Pathol* 1993;24:1120–1126.
429. Matoska J, Ondrus D, Talerman A. Malignant granulosa cell tumor of the testis associated with gynecomastia and long survival. *Cancer* 1992;69: 1769–1772.
430. Lawrence WD, Young RH, Scully RE. Sex cord—stromal tumors. In: Talerman A, Roth LM, eds. *Pathology of the testis and its adnexa.* New York: Churchill Livingstone, 1986:67–92.
431. Raju U, Fine G, Warrier R, Kini R, Weiss L. Congenital testicular juvenile granulosa cell tumor in a neonate with X/XY mosaicism. *Am J Surg Pathol* 1986;10:577–583.
432. Jones MA, Young RH, Scully RE. Benign fibromatous tumors of the testis and paratesticular region: a report of 9 cases with a proposed classification of fibromatous tumors and tumor-like lesions. *Am J Surg Pathol* 1997;21:296–305.
433. Renshaw AA, Gordon M, Corless CL. Immunohistochemistry of unclassified sex cord-stromal tumors of the testis with a predominance of spindle cells. *Mod Pathol* 1997;10:693–700.
434. Ishida T, Tagatz GE, Okagaki T. Gonadoblastoma: ultrastructural evidence for testicular origin. *Cancer* 1976;37:1770–1781.
435. Roth LM, Eglen DE. Gonadoblastoma: immunohistochemical and ultrastructural observations. *Int J Gynecol Pathol* 1989;8:72–81.
436. Scully RE. Gonadoblastoma. A review of 74 cases. *Cancer* 1970;25:1340–1356.
437. Rutgers JL. Advances in the pathology of intersex syndromes. *Hum Pathol* 1991;22:884–891.
438. Matoska J, Talerman A. Mixed germ cell-sex cord stroma tumor of the testis. A report with ultrastructural findings. *Cancer* 1989;64: 2146–2153.
439. Bolen JW. Mixed germ cell-sex cord stromal tumor. A gonadal tumor distinct from gonadoblastoma. *Am J Clin Pathol* 1981;75:565–573.
440. Nonomura N, Aozasa K, Ueda T, et al. Malignant lymphoma of the testis: histological and immunohistological study of 28 cases. *J Urol* 1989;141:1368–1371.
441. Hayes MM, Sacks MI, King HS. Testicular lymphoma. A retrospective review of 17 cases. *S Afr Med J* 1983;64:1014–1016.
442. Duncan PR, Checa F, Gowing NF, McElwain TJ, Peckham MJ. Extranodal non-Hodgkin's lymphoma presenting in the testicle: a clinical and pathologic study of 24 cases. *Cancer* 1980;45:1578–1584.
443. Doll DC, Weiss RB. Malignant lymphoma of the testis. *Am J Med* 1986;81:515–524.
444. Buskirk LA, Brunkvall J, Cavallin-Ståhl E, et al. Malignant lymphoma of the testis. *Br J Urol* 1984;56:525–530.
445. Read M, Wang TY, Hescock H, Parker M, Hudson P, Balducci L. Burkitt's lymphoma of the testicle: report of 2 cases occurring in elderly patients. *J Urol* 1990;144:1239–1241.
446. Givler RL. Testicular involvement in leukemia and lymphoma. *Cancer* 1969;23:1290–1295.
447. Ferry JA, Ulbright TM, Young RH. Anaplastic large cell lymphoma presenting in the testis. *J Urol Pathol* 1997;5:139–147.
448. Akhtar M, Al-Dayel F, Siegrist K, Ezzat A. Neutrophil-rich Ki-1-positive anaplastic large cell lymphoma presenting as a testicular mass. *Mod Pathol* 1996;9:812–815.
449. Algaba F, Santaularia JM, Garat JM, Cubells J. Testicular pseudolymphoma. *Eur Urol* 1986;12:362–363.
450. Oppenheim PI, Cohen S, Anders KH. Testicular plasmacytoma. A case report with immunohistochemical studies and literature review. *Arch Pathol Lab Med* 1991;115:629–632.
451. Avitable AM, Gansler TS, Tomaszewski JE, Hanno P, Goldwein MI. Testicular plasmacytoma. *Urology* 1989;34:51–54.
452. Ferry JA, Young RH, Scully RE. Testicular and epididymal plasmacytoma: a report of 7 cases, including 3 that were the initial manifestation of plasma cell myeloma. *Am J Surg Pathol* 1997;21:590–598.
453. Kahajda FP, Haupt HM, Moore GW, Hutchins GM. Gonadal morphology in patients receiving chemotherapy for leukemia: evidence

453. for reproductive potential and against a testicular tumor sanctuary. *Am J Med* 1982;72:759–767.
454. Askin FB, Land VJ, Sullivan MP, et al. Occult testicular leukemia: testicular biopsy at three years continuous complete remission of childhood leukemia: a Southwest Oncology Group study. *Cancer* 1981;47:470–475.
455. Nesbit ME Jr, Robison LL, Ortega JA, Sather HN, Donaldson M, Hammond D. Testicular relapse in childhood acute lymphoblastic leukemia: association with pretreatment patient characteristics and treatment: a report for Children's Cancer Study Group. *Cancer* 1980;45:2009–2016.
456. Tiedemannn K, Chessells JM, Sandland RM. Isolated testicular relapse in boys with acute lymphoblastic leukaemia: treatment and outcome. *BMJ* 1982;285:1614–1616.
457. Ferry JA, Srigley JR, Young RH. Granulocytic sarcoma of the testis: a report of two cases of a neoplasm prone to misinterpretation. *Mod Pathol* 1997;10:320–325.
458. Dieckmann KP, Loy V. Epidermoid cyst of the testis: a review of clinical and histogenetic considerations. *Br J Urol* 1994;73:436–441.
459. Greco MA, Feiner HD, Theil KS, Mufarrij AA. Testicular stromal tumor with myofilaments: ultrastructural comparison with normal gonadal stroma. *Hum Pathol* 1984;15:238–243.
460. Evans HL. Unusual gonadal stromal tumor of the testis. Case report with ultrastructural observations. *Arch Pathol Lab Med* 1977;101:317–320.
461. Honore LH, Sullivan LD. Intratesticular leiomyoma: a case report with discussion of differential diagnosis and histogenesis. *J Urol* 1975;114:631–635.
462. LiVolsi VA, Schiff M. Myxoid neurofibroma of the testis. *J Urol* 1977;118:341–342.
463. Nistal M, Paniagua R, Regadera J, Abaurrea MA. Testicular capillary haemangioma. *Br J Urol* 1982;54:433.
464. D'Esposito RF, Ferraro LR, Wogalter H. Hemangioma of the testis in an infant. *J Urol* 1976;116:677–678.
465. Tada M, Takemura S, Takimoto Y, Kishimoto T. A case of cavernous hemangioma of the testis. *Hinyokika Kiyo* 1989;35:1969–1971.
466. Cricco CF Jr, Buck AS. Hemangioendothelioma of the testis: second reported case. *J Urol* 1980;123:131–132.
467. Zukerberg LR, Young RH. Primary testicular sarcoma: a report of two cases. *Hum Pathol* 1990;21:932–935.
468. Mathew T, Prabhakaran K. Osteosarcoma of the testis. *Arch Pathol Lab Med* 1981;105:38–39.
469. Yachia D, Auslaender L. Primary leiomyosarcoma of the testis. *J Urol* 1989;141:955–956.
470. Kneale BJ, Bishop NL, Britton JP. Kaposi's sarcoma of the testis. *Br J Urol* 1993;72:116–117.
471. Davis AE Jr. Rhabdomyosarcoma of the testicle. *J Urol* 1962;87:148–154.
472. Ravich L, Lerman PH, Drabkin JW, Foltin E. Pure testicular rhabdomyosarcoma. *J Urol* 1965;94:596–599.
473. Alexander F. Pure testicular rhabdomyosarcoma. *Br J Cancer* 1968;22:498–501.
474. Kumar PV, Khezri AA. Pure testicular rhabdomyosarcoma. *Br J Urol* 1987;59:282.
475. Nistal M, Fachal C, Paniagua R. Testicular carcinoma in situ associated with rhabdomyosarcoma of the spermatic cord. *J Urol* 1989;142:358–360.
476. Haupt HM, Mann RB, Trump DL, Abeloff MD. Metastatic carcinoma involving the testis: clinical and pathologic distinction from primary testicular neoplasms. *Cancer* 1984;54:709–714.
477. Bhasin SD, Shrikhande SS. Secondary carcinoma of testis—a clinicopathologic study of 10 cases. *Ind J Cancer* 1990;27:83–90.
478. Richardson PG, Millward MJ, Shrimankar JJ, Cantwell BM. Metastatic melanoma to the testis simulating primary seminoma. *Br J Urol* 1992;69:663–665.
479. Pienkos EJ, Jablokow VR. Secondary testicular tumors. *Cancer* 1972;30:481–485.
480. Tejada E, Eble JN. Simple cyst of the rete testis. *J Urol* 1988;139:376–377.
481. Srigley JR, Hartwick RWJ. Tumors and cysts of the paratesticular region. *Pathol Annu* 1990;25(Pt 2):51–108.
482. Nistal M, Regadera J, Paniagua R. Cystic dysplasia of the testis: light and electron microscopic study of three cases. *Arch Pathol Lab Med* 1984;108:579–583.
483. Tesluk H, Blankenberg TA. Cystic dysplasia of testis. *Urology* 1987;290:472–493.
484. Leissring JC, Oppenheimer ROF. Cystic dysplasia of the testis: a unique congenital anomaly studied by microdissection. *J Urol* 1973;110:362–363.
485. Fisher JE, Jewett TC Jr, Nelson SJ, Jockin H. Ectasia of the rete testis with ipsilateral renal agenesis. *J Urol* 1982;128:1040–1043.
486. Hartwick RW, Ro JY, Srigley JR, Ordoñez NG, Ayala AG. Adenomatous hyperplasia of the rete testis. A clinicopathologic study of nine cases. *Am J Surg Pathol* 1991;15:350–357.
487. Nistal M, Paniagua R. Adenomatous hyperplasia of the rete testis. *J Pathol* 1988;154:343–346.
488. Murao T, Tanahashi T. Adenofibroma of the rete testis. A case report with electron microscopy findings. *Acta Pathol Jpn* 1988;38:105–112.
489. Altaffer LF,III, Dufour DR, Castleberry GM, Steele SM Jr. Coexisting rete testis adenoma and gonadoblastoma. *J Urol* 1982;127:332–335.
490. Gupta RK. Benign papillary tumor of the rete testis. *Ind J Cancer* 1974;11:480–481.
491. Yadav SB, Patil PN, Karkhanis RB. Primary tumors of the spermatic cord, epididymis, and rete testis. *J Postgrad Med* 1969;15:49–52.
492. Jones MA, Young RH. Sertoliform rete cystadenoma: a report of two cases. *J Urol Pathol* 1997;7:47–53.
493. Nochomovitz LE, Orenstein JM. Adenocarcinoma of the rete testis: review and regrouping of reported cases and a consideration of miscellaneous entities. *J Urogenit Pathol* 1991;1:11–40.
494. Visscher DW, Talerman A, Rivera LR, Mazur MT. Adenocarcinoma of the rete testis with a spindle cell component. A possible metaplastic carcinoma. *Cancer* 1989;64:770–775.
495. Mrak RE, Husain MM, Schaefer RF. Ultrastructure of metastatic rete testis adenocarcinoma. *Arch Pathol Lab Med* 1990;114:84–88.
496. Watson PH, Jacob VC. Adenocarcinoma of the rete testis with sertoliform differentiation. *Arch Pathol Lab Med* 1989;113:1169–1171.
497. Haas GP, Ohorodnik JM, Farah RN. Cystadenocarcinoma of the rete testis. *J Urol* 1987;137:1232–1233.
498. Nochomovitz LE, Orenstein JM. Adenocarcinoma of the rete testis. Case report, ultrastructural observations, and clinicopathologic correlates. *Am J Surg Pathol* 1984;8:625–634.
499. Jacobellis U, Ricco R, Ruotolo G. Adenocarcinoma of the rete testis 21 years after orchiopexy: case report and review of the literature. *J Urol* 1981;125:429–431.
500. Burns MW, Chandler WL, Krieger JN. Adenocarcinoma of rete testis. Role of inguinal orchiectomy plus retroperitoneal lymph node dissection. *Urology* 1991;37:571–573.
501. Nochomovitz LE, Orenstein JM. Adenocarcinoma of the rete testis: consolidation and analysis of 31 reported cases with a review of miscellaneous entities. *J Urol Pathol* 1994;2:1–37.
502. Sanchez-Chapado M, Angulo JC, Haas GP. Adenocarcinoma of the rete testis. *Urology* 1995;46:468–475.
503. Nistal M, Paniagua R. Nodular proliferation of calcifying connective tissue in the rete testis: a study of three cases. *Hum Pathol* 1989;20:58–61.
504. Nistal M, Santamaria L, Paniagua R. Acquired cystic transformation of the rete testis secondary to renal failure. *Hum Pathol* 1989;20:1065–1070.
505. Putschar WG, Manion WC. Splenic-gonadal fusion. *Am J Pathol* 1956;32:15–33.
506. Walter MM, Trulock TS, Finnerty DP, Woodard J. Splenic gonadal fusion. *Urology* 1988;32:521–524.
507. Walker AN, Mills SE. Surgical pathology of the tunica vaginalis testis and embryologically related mesothelium. *Pathol Annu* 1988;25(Pt 2):125–152.
508. Dehner LP, Scott D, Stocker JT. Meconium periorchitis: a clinicopathologic study of four cases with a review of the literature. *Hum Pathol* 1986;17:807–812.
509. Thompson JE, van der Walt JD. Nodular fibrous proliferation (fibrous pseudotumour) of the tunica vaginalis testis. A light, electron microscopic and immunocytochemical study of a case and review of the literature. *Histopathology* 1986;10:741–748.
510. Corcione N, Mancini P, Cecchi M, Pingitore R. Fibrous pseudotumor of tunica vaginalis. Report of a case. *Pathologica* 1988;80:723–727.
511. Gilchrist KW, Benson RC Jr. Multifocal fibrous pseudotumor of testicular tunics. Possible clinical dilemma. *Urology* 1979;14:285–287.

512. Polsky MS, Ball TP Jr, Smith RB, Weber CH Jr. Benign fibrous paratesticular tumors. *Urology* 1976;8:174–176.
513. Nistal M, Paniagua R, Torres A, Hidalgo L, Regadera J. Idiopathic peritesticular fibrosis associated with retroperitoneal fibrosis. *Eur Urol* 1986;12:64–68.
514. Parveen T, Fleischmann J, Petrelli M. Benign fibrous tumor of the tunica vaginalis testis. Report of a case with light, electron microscopic, and immunocytochemical study, and review of the literature. *Arch Pathol Lab Med* 1992;116:277–280.
515. Benisch B, Peison B, Sobel HJ, Marquet E. Fibrous mesotheliomas (pseudofibroma) of the scrotal sac: a light and ultrastructural study. *Cancer* 1981;47:731–735.
516. Eimoto T, Inoue I. Malignant fibrous mesothelioma of the tunica vaginalis: a histologic and ultrastructural study. *Cancer* 1977;39:2059–2066.
517. Warner KE, Noyes DT, Ross JS. Cysts of the tunica albuginea testis: a report of 3 cases with review of the literature. *J Urol* 1984;132:131–132.
518. Mancilla-Jimenez R, Matsuda GT. Cysts of the tunica albuginea: report of 4 cases and review of the literature. *J Urol* 1975;114:730–733.
519. Young RH, Scully RE. Testicular and paratesticular tumors and tumor-like lesions of ovarian common epithelial and mullerian types: a report of four cases and review of the literature. *Am J Clin Pathol* 1986;86:146–152.
520. Chen KT, Arhelger RB, Flam MS, Hanson JH. Malignant mesothelioma of tunica vaginalis testis. *Urology* 1982;20:316–319.
521. Antman K, Cohen S, Dimitrov NV, Green M, Muggia F. Malignant mesothelioma of the tunica vaginalis testis. *J Clin Oncol* 1984;2:447–451.
522. Stein N, Henkes D. Mesothelioma of the testicle in a child. *J Urol* 1986;135:794.
523. Jones MA, Young RH, Scully RE. Malignant mesothelioma of the tunica vaginalis: a clinicopathologic analysis of 11 cases with review of the literature. *Am J Surg Pathol* 1995;19:815–825.
524. Japko L, Horta AA, Schreiber K, et al. Malignant mesothelioma of the tunica vaginalis testis: report of first case with preoperative diagnosis. *Cancer* 1982;49:119–127.
525. Fligiel Z, Kaneko M. Malignant mesothelioma of the tunica vaginalis propria testis in a patient with asbestos exposure: a case report. *Cancer* 1976;37:1478–1484.
526. Grove A, Jensen ML, Donna A. Mesotheliomas of the tunica vaginalis testis and hernial sacs. *Virchows Arch [A]* 1989;415:283–292.
527. Axiotis CA. Intratesticular serous papillary cystadenoma of low malignant potential: an ultrastructural and immunohistochemical study suggesting mullerian differentiation. *Am J Surg Pathol* 1988;12:56–63.
528. Carano KS, Soslow RA. Immunophenotypic analysis of ovarian and testicular mullerian papillary serous tumors. *Mod Pathol* 1997;10:414–420.
529. Young RH, Scully RE. Testicular and paratesticular tumors and tumor-like lesions of ovarian common epithelial and mullerian types. A report of four cases and review of the literature. *Am J Clin Pathol* 1986;86:146–152.
530. Remmele W, Kaiserling E, Zerban U, et al. Serous papillary cystic tumor of borderline malignancy with focal carcinoma arising in testis: case report with immunohistochemical and ultrastructural observations. *Hum Pathol* 1992;23:75–79.
531. De Nictolis M, Tommasoni S, Fabris G, Prat J. Intratesticular serous cystadenoma of borderline malignancy. A pathological, histochemical and DNA content study of a case with long-term follow-up. *Virchows Arch [A]* 1993;423:221–225.
532. Blumberg HM, Hendrix LE. Serous papillary adenocarcinoma of the tunica vaginalis of the testis with metastasis. *Cancer* 1991;67:1450–1453.
533. Jones MA, Young RH, Srigley JR, Scully RE. Paratesticular serous papillary carcinoma. A report of six cases. *Am J Surg Pathol* 1995;19:1359–1365.
534. Kellert E. An ovarian type pseudomucinous cystadenoma in the scrotum. *Cancer* 1959;12:187–190.
535. Elbadawi A, Batchvarov MM, Linke CA. Intratesticular papillary mucinous cystadenocarcinoma. *Urology* 1979;14:280–284.
536. Nogales FF Jr, Matilla A, Ortega I, Alvarez T. Mixed Brenner and adenomatoid tumor of the testis: an ultrastructural study and histogenetic considerations. *Cancer* 1979;43:539–543.
537. Ross L. Paratesticular Brenner-like tumor. *Cancer* 1968;21:722–726.
538. Goldman RL. A Brenner tumor of the testis. *Cancer* 1970;26:853–856.
539. Ross L. Paratesticular Brenner-like tumor. *Cancer* 1968;21:722–726.
540. Caccamo D, Socias M, Truchet C. Malignant Brenner tumor of the testis and epididymis. *Arch Pathol Lab Med* 1991;115:524–527.
541. Nogales FF Jr, Matilla A, Ortega I, Alvarez T. Mixed Brenner and adenomatoid tumor of the testis: an ultrastructural study and histogenetic considerations. *Cancer* 1979;43:539–543.
542. Currie JS, Ngaei G. A papilloma of epididymis of mullerian vestigial origin. *Br J Urol* 1977;49:331–334.
543. Bollinger DJ, Wick MR, Dehner LP, Mills SE, Swanson PE, Clarke RE. Peritoneal malignant mesothelioma versus serous papillary adenocarcinoma: a histochemical and immunohistochemical comparison. *Am J Surg Pathol* 1989;13:659–670.
544. Prat J, Matias-Guiu X, Algaba F. Desmoplastic small round-cell tumor. *Am J Surg Pathol* 1992;16:306–307.
545. Gerald WL, Miller HK, Battifora H, Miettinen M, Silva EG, Rosai J. Intra-abdominal desmoplastic small round-cell tumor: report of 19 cases of a distinctive type of high-grade polyphenotypic malignancy affecting young individuals. *Am J Surg Pathol* 1991;15:499–513.
546. Gonzalez-Crussi F, Crawford SE, Sun C-CJ. Intraabdominal desmoplastic small-cell tumors with divergent differentiation: observations on three cases of childhood. *Am J Surg Pathol* 1990;14:633–642.
547. Chiaramonte RM. Leiomyoma of tunica albuginea of testis. *Urology* 1983;31:344–345.
548. Aus G, Boiesen PT. Bilateral leiomyoma of the tunica albuginea. Case report. *Scand J Urol Nephrol* 1991;25:79–80.
549. Pfannenmaier NW, Wurster K, Kjelle-Schweigler M. Hemangioma of the tunica albuginea testis. *Urol Int* 1975;30:237–241.
550. Miyagi T, Ohtaki M, Rin S, Matsubara F. Intrascrotal malignant fibrous histiocytoma: a case report and review of the literature. *Fukuoka Kiyo* 1985;31:527–532.
551. Levant B, Chetlin MA. Neurofibroma of the tunica albuginea testis. *J Urol* 1948;59:1187–1189.
552. Firgree LJ, Brown DE. Cholesteatoma of the epididymis. *J Urol* 1951;65:126–127.
553. Fornanelli R, Sanna A. Adenomatoid leiomyoma and papillary cystadenoma of the epididymis. *Pathologica* 1985;77:445–448.
554. Detassis C, Pusiol T, Piscioli F, Luciani L. Adenomatoid tumor of the epididymis: immunohistochemical study of 8 cases. *Urol Int* 1986;41:232–234.
555. Earwick KW, Madri JA. An immunohistochemical study of adenomatoid tumors utilizing keratin and factor VIII antibodies: evidence for a mesothelial origin. *Lab Invest* 1982;47:276–280.
556. Eel DA, Flotte TJ. Factor VIII related antigen in adenomatoid tumors: implications for histogenesis. *Cancer* 1982;50:932–938.
557. Said JW, Nash G, Lee M. Immunoperoxidase localization of keratin proteins, carcinoembryonic antigen, and factor VIII in adenomatoid tumors: evidence for a mesothelial derivation. *Hum Pathol* 1982;13:1106–1108.
558. Urrales-Viedma M, Martos-Padilla S, Caballero-Morales T. Adenomatoid tumors. Immunohistochemical study and histogenesis. *Arch Pathol Lab Med* 1985;109:636–638.
559. Mucientes F. Adenomatoid tumor of the epididymis. Ultrastructural study of three cases. *Pathol Res Pract* 1983;176:258–268.
560. Davy CL, Tang CK. Are all adenomatoid tumors adenomatoid mesotheliomas? *Hum Pathol* 1981;12:360–369.
561. Stephenson TJ, Mills PM. Adenomatoid tumours: an immunohistochemical and ultrastructural appraisal of their histogenesis. *J Pathol* 1986;148:327–335.
562. Sidhu GS, Fresko O. Adenomatoid tumor of the epididymis: ultrastructural evidence of its biphasic nature. *Ultrastruct Pathol* 1980;1:39–47.
563. Ferenczy A, Fenoglio J, Richart RM. Observations on benign mesothelioma of the genital tract (adenomatoid tumor): a comparative ultrastructural study. *Cancer* 1972;30:244–260.
564. Taxy JB, Battifora H, Oyasu R. Adenomatoid tumors: a light microscopic, histochemical, and ultrastructural study. *Cancer* 1974;34:306–316.
565. Mackay B, Bennington JL, Skoglund RW. The adenomatoid tumor: fine structural evidence for a mesothelial origin. *Cancer* 1971;27:109–115.
566. Banks ER, Mills SE. Histiocytoid (epithelioid) hemangioma of the

566. testis. The so-called vascular variant of "adenomatoid tumor." *Am J Surg Pathol* 1990;14:584–589.
567. Wernert N, Goebbels R, Prediger L. Papillary cystadenoma of the epididymis. Case report and review of the literature. *Pathol Res Pract* 1986;181:260–264.
568. Lamiell JM, Salazar FG, Hsia YE. von Hippel-Lindau disease affecting 43 members of a single kindred. *Medicine* 1989;68:1–29.
569. Kragel PJ, Pestaner J, Travis WD, Linehan WM, Filling-Katz MR. Papillary cystadenoma of the epididymis. A report of three cases with lectin histochemistry. *Arch Pathol Lab Med* 1990;114:672–675.
570. Gilcrease MZ, Schmidt L, Zbar B, Truong L, Rutledge M, Wheeler TM. Somatic von Hippel-Lindau mutation in clear cell papillary cystadenoma of the epididymis. *Hum Pathol* 1995;26:1341–1346.
571. Wang TY, Chiang H, Huang JK, Liu HC. Papillary cystadenocarcinoma of the epididymis—report of a case. *Chung Hua i Hsueh Tsa Chih* 1990;45:139–142.
572. Murayama T, Fujita K, Ohashi T, Matsushita T. Melanotic neuroectodermal tumor of the epididymis in infancy: a case report. *J Urol* 1989;141:105–106.
573. Ricketts RR, Majmudarr B. Epididymal melanotic neuroectodermal tumor of infancy. *Hum Pathol* 1985;16:416–420.
574. Frank GL, Koten JW. Melanotic hamartoma ("retinal anlage tumour") of the epididymis. *J Pathol Bacteriol* 1967;93:549–554.
575. Pettinato G, Manivel JC, d'Amore ES, Jaszcz W, Gorlin RJ. Melanotic neuroectodermal tumor of infancy. A reexamination of a histogenetic problem based on immunohistochemical, flow cytometric, and ultrastructural study of 10 cases. *Am J Surg Pathol* 1991;15:233–245.
576. Denadai ER, Zerati Filho M, Verona CB, Martucci RC, Zerati S, Suzigan S. Tumor of the testicle: a case of melanotic neuroectodermal tumor of infancy. *J Urol* 1986;136:117–118.
577. Johnson RE, Scheithauer BW, Dahlin DC. Melanotic neuroectodermal tumor of infancy: a review of seven cases. *Cancer* 1983;52:661–666.
578. Hata R, Iizumi T, Yazaki T, Waku M. A case of primary bilateral epididymal leiomyoma. *Hinyokika Kiyo* 1989;35:1247–1249.
579. Mathew T. Angiofibroma of the epididymis. *Pathology* 1981;13:625–630.
580. Busmanis I. Paratesticular plexiform tumour of myofibroblastic origin. *Histopathology* 1991;18:178–180.
581. Schned AR, Variakojis D, Straus FH,II, Sweet DL Jr. Primary histiocytic lymphoma of the epididymis. *Cancer* 1979;43:1156–1163.
582. Heaton JPW, Morales A. Epididymal lymphoma: an unusual scrotal mass. *J Urol* 1984;131:353–354.
583. Schned AR, Variakojis D, Straus FH, Sweet DL Jr. Primary histiocytic lymphoma of the epididymis. *Cancer* 1979;43:1156–1163.
584. Salm R. Papillary carcinoma of the epididymis. *J Pathol* 1969;97:253–259.
585. Farrell MA, Donnelly BJ. Malignant smooth muscle tumors of the epididymis. *J Urol* 1980;124:151–153.
586. Helm RH, Al-Tikriti S. Primary leiomyosarcoma of the epididymis. *Br J Urol* 1986;58:99.
587. Burger R, Guthrie TH. Metastatic colonic carcinoma to epididymis. *Urology* 1973;2:566–567.
588. Ford J Jr, Singh S. Paratesticular dermoid cyst in a 6-month-old infant. *J Urol* 1988;139:89–90.
589. Sarma DP, Weilbaecher TG. Leiomyoma of the spermatic cord. *J Surg Oncol* 1985;28:318–320.
590. Belis JA, Post GJ, Rochman SC, Milam DF. Genitourinary leiomyomas. *Urology* 1979;13:424–429.
591. Tanda F, Rocca PC, Bosincu L, Massarelli G, Cossu A, Manca A. Rhabdomyoma of the tunica vaginalis of the testis: a histologic, immunohistochemical, and ultrastructural study. *Mod Pathol* 1997;10:608–611.
592. El-Badawi AA, Al-Ghorab MM. Tumors of the spermatic cord: a review of the literature and a report of a case of lymphangioma. *J Urol* 1965;94:445–450.
593. Arda S, Senocak ME, Buyukpamukèu N, Hièonmez A, Gogus S. Lymphangioma of the spermatic cord and tunica vaginalis in children. *Eur Urol* 1992;21:253–255.
594. Banks E, Yum M, Brodhecker C, Goheen M. A malignant peripheral nerve sheath tumor in association with a paratesticular ganglioneuroma. *Cancer* 1989;64:1738–1742.
595. Gluck RW, Bloiso G, Glasser J. Paratesticular desmoid tumor. *Urology* 1987;29:648–649.
596. Chung H. Granular cell tumor of the spermatic cord: a case report with light and electron microscopic study. *J Urol* 1978;120:379–382.
597. Hollowood K, Fletcher CDM. Pseudosarcomatous myofibroblastic proliferations of the spermatic cord ("proliferative funiculitis"): histologic and immunohistochemical analysis of a distinctive entity. *Am J Surg Pathol* 1992;16:448–454.
598. Rosas-Uribe A, Luna MA, Guinn GA. Paratesticular rhabdomyosarcoma. A clinicopathologic study of seven cases. *Am J Surg* 1970;120:737–791.
599. Raney RB Jr, Hays DM, Lawrence W Jr, Soule EH, Tefft M, Donaldson MH. Paratesticular rhabdomyosarcoma in children. *Cancer* 1978;42:729–736.
600. Kage M, Kojiro M, Arakawa M, Nakamura Y, Kawada H. Paratesticular rhabdomyosarcoma. *Acta Pathol Jpn* 1983;33:817–821.
601. Abell MR, Holtz F. Testicular and paratesticular neoplasms in patients 60 years of age and older. *Cancer* 1968;21:852–870.
602. Knight B, Tiltman AJ. Paratesticular rhabdomyosarcoma. Case reports. *S Afr Med J* 1986;69:702–704.
603. Cavazzana AO, Schmidt D, Ninfo V, et al. Spindle cell rhabdomyosarcoma: a prognostically favorable variant of rhabdomyosarcoma. *Am J Surg Pathol* 1992;16:229–235.
604. Leuschner L, Newton WA Jr, Schmidt D, et al. Spindle cell variants of embryonal rhabdomyosarcoma in the paratesticular region. A report of the Intergroup Rhabdomyosarcoma Study. *Am J Surg Pathol* 1993;17:221–230.
605. Parham DM, Webber B, Holt H, Williams WK, Maurer H. Immunohistochemical results of an Intergroup Rhabdomyosarcoma Study Project. *Cancer* 1991;67:3072–3080.
606. LaQuaglia MP, Ghavimi F, Heller G, et al. Mortality in pediatric paratesticular rhabdomyosarcoma: a multivariate analysis. *J Urol* 1989;142:473–478.
607. Banowsky LH, Schultz GN. Sarcoma of the spermatic cord and tunics: review of the literature, case report and discussion of the role of retroperitoneal lymph node dissection. *J Urol* 1970;103:628–631.
608. Ockner DM, Sayadi H, Swanson PE, Ritter JH, Wick MR. Genital angiomyofibroblastoma: comparison with aggressive angiomyxoma and other myxoid neoplasms of skin and soft tissue. *Am J Clin Pathol* 1997;107:36–44.
609. Clatch RJ, Drake WK, Gonzalez JG. Aggressive angiomyxoma in men: a report of two cases associated with inguinal hernias. *Arch Pathol Lab Med* 1993;117:911–913.
610. Tsang WYW, Chan JKC, Lee KC, Fisher C, Fletcher CDM. Aggressive angiomyxoma: a report of four cases occurring in men. *Am J Surg Pathol* 1992;16:1059–1065.
611. Gaffney EF, Harte PJ, Browne HJ. Paratesticular leiomyosarcoma: an ultrastructural study. *J Urol* 1984;132:133–134.
612. Donovan MG, Fitzpatrick JM, Gaffney EF, West AB. Paratesticular leiomyosarcoma. *Br J Urol* 1987;60:590.
613. Kyle VN. Leiomyosarcoma of the spermatic cord: a review of the literature and report of an additional case. *J Urol* 1966;96:795–800.
614. Gowing NFC. Paratesticular tumours of connective tissue and muscle. In: Pugh RCB, ed. *Pathology of the testis*. Oxford: Blackwell Scientific, 1976:317–333.
615. Malek RS, Utz DC, Farrow GM. Malignant tumors of the spermatic cord. *Cancer* 1972;29:1108–1113.
616. Banik S, Guha PK. Paratesticular rhabdomyosarcomas and leiomyosarcomas: a clinicopathologic review. *J Urol* 1979;121:823–826.
617. Algaba F, Trias I, Castro C. Inflammatory malignant fibrous histiocytoma of the spermatic cord with eosinophilia. *Histopathology* 1989;14:319–321.
618. Sclama AO, Berger BW, Cherry JM, Young JD Jr. Malignant fibrous histiocytoma of the spermatic cord: the role of retroperitoneal lymphadenectomy in management. *J Urol* 1983;130:577–579.
619. Smailowitz Z, Kaneti J, Sober I, Krugliak L, Sacks M. Malignant fibrous histiocytoma of the spermatic cord. *J Urol* 1983;130:150–151.
620. Williamson JC, Johnson JD, Lamm DL, Tio F. Malignant fibrous histiocytoma of the spermatic cord. *J Urol* 1980;123:785–788.
621. Pozza D, Masci P, D'Ottavio G, Zappavigna D. Spermatic cord liposarcoma in a young boy. *J Urol* 1987;137:306–308.
622. Chan Y-F, Yuen MYP, Ma LT, Li MK. Recurrent dedifferentiated liposarcoma of the spermatic cord simulating malignant fibrous histiocytoma: an immunohistochemical and ultrastructural study. *Pathology* 1987;19:99–102.

623. Vorstman B, Block NL, Politano VA. The management of spermatic cord liposarcoma. *J Urol* 1311;1984:66–69.
624. Johnson DE, Harris JD, Ayala AG. Liposarcoma of spermatic cord. *Urology* 1978;11:190–195.
625. Mhiri MN, Sellami F, Sellami M, Ben Hamed Y, Snide ML. Malignant para-testicular tumors. Apropos of 3 unusual cases. *Ann Urol (Paris)* 1989;23:23–26.
626. Stein BS, Petersen RO, Conger KB. Malignant mesenchymoma of the spermatic cord. *J Urol* 1984;131:551–552.
627. Heyns CF, Van Niekerk JT, Roussouw DJ, Burger EC, De Klerk DP. Nephroblastoma in an ovotestis of a true hermaphrodite a case report. *J Urol* 1987;137:1003–1005.
628. Orlowski JP, Levin HS, Dyment PG. Intrascrotal Wilms' tumor developing in a heterotopic renal analge of probable mesonephric origin. *J Pediatr Surg* 1980;15:679–682.
629. Taylor WF, Myers M, Taylor WR. Extrarenal Wilms' tumour in an infant exposed to intauterine phenytoin. *Lancet* 1980;2:481–482.
630. Eusebi V, Massarelli G. Phaeochromocytoma of the spermatic cord: report of a case. *J Pathol* 1971;105:283–284.
631. Srigley JR, Toth P, Edwards V. Diagnostic electron microscopy of male genital tract tumors. *Clin Lab Med* 1987;7:93–115.
632. Bosl GJ, Sheinfeld J, Bajorin DF, et al. Cancer of the testis. In: DeVita VT Jr, Hellman S, Rosenberg SA, eds. *Cancer: principles and practice of oncology*, 5th ed. Philadelphia: Lippincott-Raven, 1997:1397–1425.
633. Boden G, Gibb R. Radiotherapy and testicular neoplasms. *Lancet* 1951;2:1195–1197.
634. Hendry WF, Barrett A, McElwain TJ, Wallace DM, Peckham MJ. The role of surgery in the combined management of metastases from malignant teratomas of testis. *Br J Urol* 1980;52:38–49.
635. Johnson DE. Clinical staging. In: Donohue JP, ed. *Testis tumors*. Baltimore: Williams and Wilkins, 1983:131–144.
636. Skinner DG. Non-seminomatous testis tumors: a plan of management based on 96 patients to improve survival in all stages by combined therapeutic modalities. *J Urol* 1969;115:65–69.
637. Shipley WU. The role of radiation in the management of adult germinal testis tumors. In: Einhorn LH, ed. *Testicular tumors*. New York: Masson, 1980;47–67.
638. Pugh RCB, Parkinson C. The origin and classification of testicular germ cell tumours. *Int J Androl* 1981;4(suppl):15–25.
639. Kramer SS, Ulbright TM. Papillary serous tumor of low malignant potential of the testis: a problem in differential diagnosis. American Society of Clinical Pathologists: Check-Sample—Tumor Diagnosis and Treatment No. TD 95–2 (TD-130) 1995;22:15–29.

CHAPTER 48

The Penis

Antonio L. Cubilla, José E. Barreto, and Gustavo Ayala

There is a wide spectrum of pathologic conditions of the penis with which pathologists should be familiar, from venereal lesions such as syphilitic chancre, to bizarre conditions such as Zoon's balanitis or Tancho's nodules, to the still not clearly defined human papillomavirus (HPV)-related lesions. Systemic neoplastic and nonneoplastic diseases can secondarily involve the penis and mimic primary lesions. The methodology for the clinical and functional evaluation of the penis has greatly improved in recent years. Physicians of various specialties deal with penile organic as well as functional disorders, such as radiologists [using computed tomography (CT), nuclear magnetic resonance (NMR), and angiographic studies], internists, pediatricians, general surgeons, oncologists, urologists, and plastic surgeons. Pathologists should exchange ideas with all of them and be aware of a wide variety of diseases affecting the penis.

However, the vast majority of penile specimens submitted to surgical pathologists for evaluation are from neoplasms or from lesions that simulate tumors; this is especially true in geographic areas where cancer of the penis is epidemic. Hence, the emphasis in this chapter is on the pathologic description of the various types of penile tumors or pseudotumors.

ANATOMY

From the point of view of surgical pathology, the penis should be anatomically divided into the head, the body or shaft, and the urethra (1–3).

A. L. Cubilla: Instituto de Patología e Investigación Martín Brizuela 323 c/o Ayala Velazquez Asunción, Paraguay.

J. E. Barreto: Department of Pathology, Facultad de Medicina de la Universidad Católica, Villarica, Paraguay

G. Ayala: Department of Pathology, Baylor College of Medicine Houston, Texas.

The Glans

The glans is the site of the majority of neoplastic lesions. Grossly it is a conical cup covering the distal end of the penile shaft. The meatus urethralis is a vertical cleft located in the central portion of the glans and it is closely related to the frenulum, which is a fibrous band of tissue attaching the foreskin to the glans. The base of the glans is the glans corona, composed of an slightly elevated circumferential rim. If a resected specimen is longitudinally sectioned along its longer axis, the cut surface will show the following anatomical structures (or anatomical levels): epithelium, lamina propria (LP), corpus spongiosum (CS), albuginea (AB), corpora cavernosa (CC) (Fig. 1) (4). The epithelium is a thin, nonkeratinized stratified squamous epithelium. After circumcision, the epithelium becomes keratinized. The lamina propria is a 2- to 3-mm layer of loose connective tissue situated beneath the epithelium (Fig. 2). It contains small blood and lymphatic vessels as well as nerve branches (Fig. 3). Occasionally Vater-Pacini corpuscles can be identified. The transition between LP and CS is not always sharp. The corpus spongiosum is the principal anatomical compartment of the penis, and it is made of specialized, erectile tissue or specialized venous sinuses, which are of variable caliber and widely interconnected. The albuginea encases the adjacent corpora cavernosa and separates CS from the former. It is a triangular-shaped, thick, 2- to 4-mm band of fibrous tissue, terminating in an acute angle usually at the level of the coronal sulcus. We find, however, that in some patients the albuginea is closer to the epithelium than in others. The coronal sulcus is a narrow and circumferential cul de sac located behind the glans corona; it shows two histologic layers: the squamous epithelium, which is a continuation of and identical to the glans epithelium; and the lamina propria and the area of insertion of both the dartos and the Buck's fascia. The foreskin (5) is a delicate dependence of the shaft penis covering the glans (Fig. 4). It has four histologic layers: (a) squamous epithelium, (b) lamina propria, (c) dartos, and (d) skin (Figs. 5 and 6).

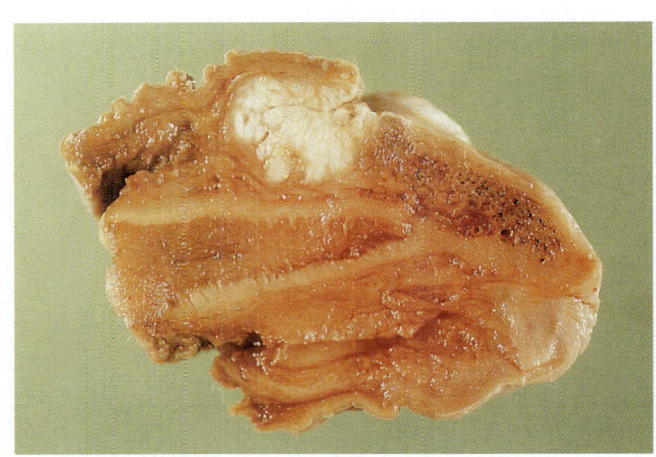
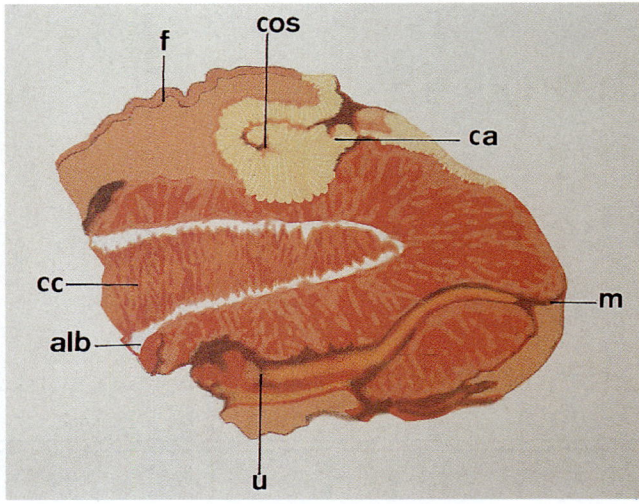

FIG. 1. A: Cut surface of partial penectomy specimen from a circumcised patient with an infiltrating squamous cell carcinoma located in the coronal sulcus. The section is longitudinal and central, including the urethra. **B:** The various penile anatomical structures and the neoplasm. f, foreskin; COS, coronal sulcus; Ca, carcinoma; CS, corpus spongiosum; M, meatus; CC, corpus cavernosum; Alb, albuginea; and U, urethra.

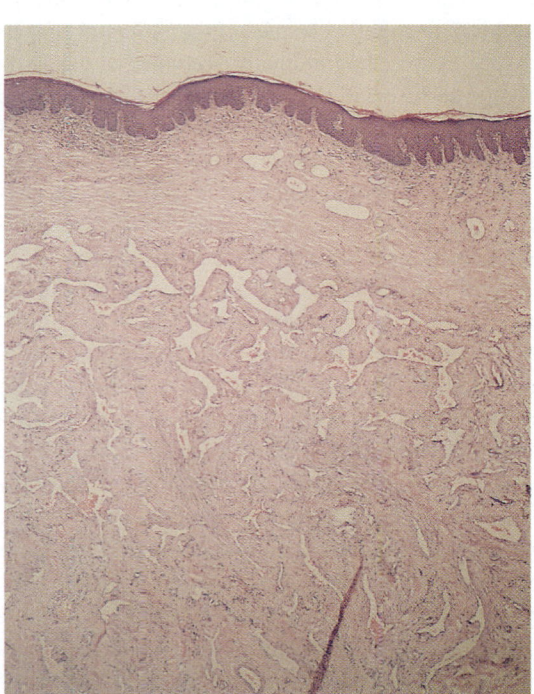

FIG. 2. Anatomy of the glans. Microscopic section showing the three anatomical layers of the glans—squamous epithelium, lamina propia, and corpus spongiosum, composed of highly vascular erectile tissue.

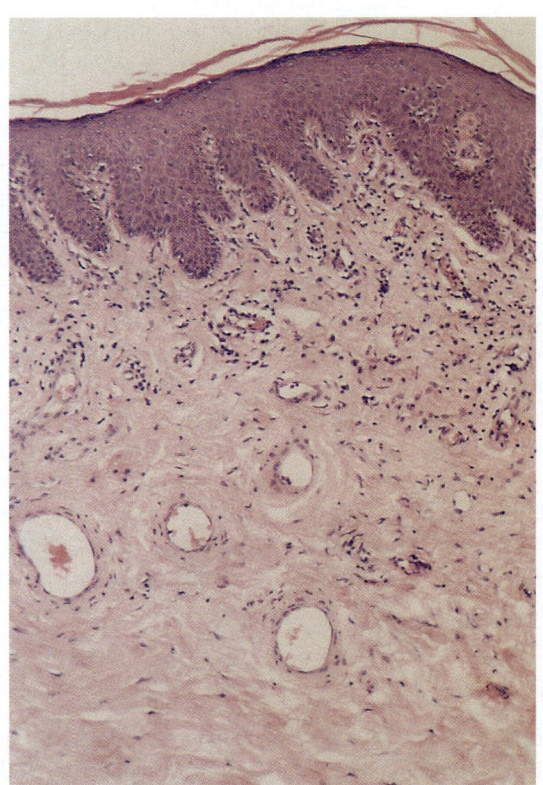

FIG. 3. Anatomy of the glans. Higher power of glans epithelium and lamina propria. The squamous epithelium is keratinized. The lamina propria shows a loose connective tissue and vascular spaces.

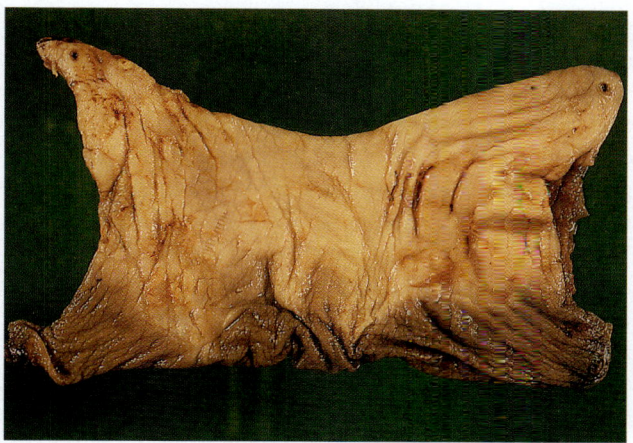

FIG. 4. Anatomy of the foreskin. Gross appearance of the foreskins of an adult male, resected because of chronic inflammation. The mucosal surface is pale beige and slightly wrinkled. The skin (bottom) is dark and hyperpigmented.

Body or Shaft

The penile body or shaft is mostly composed of two parallel, firm, rubbery cylinders—the corpora cavernosa (CC), just behind the corpus spongiosum. Like the latter, CC principal tissues are vascular erectile (Fig. 7). The numerous vascular channels are surrounded by criss-crossing of interconnected smooth muscle fibers and spaces that become tense as the cylinder expands during erection. Buck's fascia is a fibroelastic and vascular membrane that encases the CC and part of the CS. The shaft penis is covered by a thin epidermis, rugged and hyperpigmented.

Urethra

The penile urethra (Fig. 8) is in close relationship with the corpus spongiosum, which forms a protective cylindrical sheath around it. The urethral epithelium is stratified, columnar, or ciliated. Under pathologic conditions and even in the normal urethra it is common to note squamous metaplasia of urethral epithelium. Mucin-producing carcinomas can arise in urethral Littre's glans.

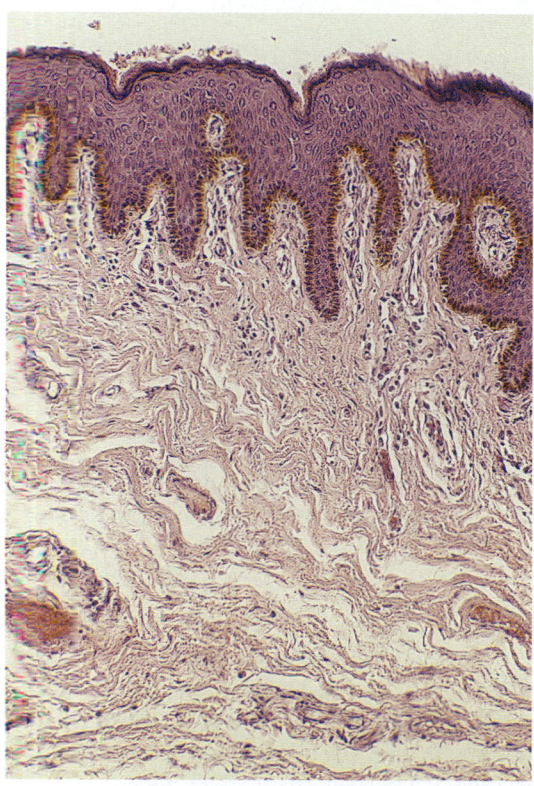

FIG. 6. Anatomy of the foreskin. Closer view of foreskin histologic layers. **A:** squamous epithelium. **B:** lamina propia.

Lymph Nodes

The inguinal lymph nodes may be classified as superficial or deep. The separation of the two types is made anatomically by a horizontal line passing through the point where the

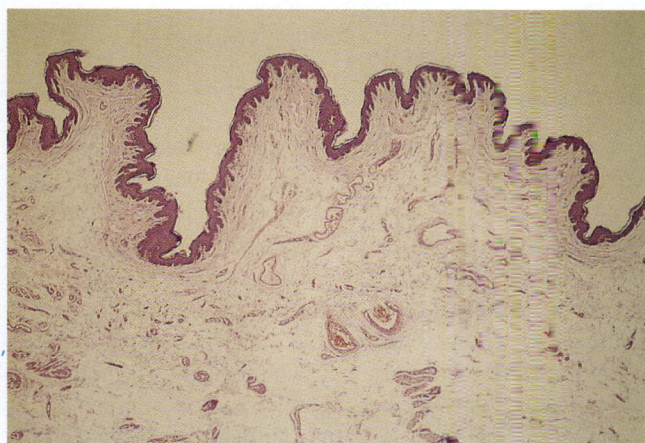

FIG. 5. Anatomy of the foreskin. Microscopic features of a normal foreskin, showing the wrinkled squamous epithelium, underlying the lamina propria and preputial dartos (bottom).

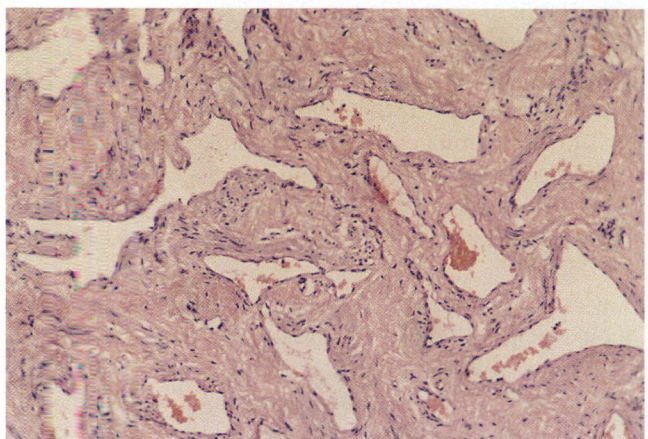

FIG 7. Anatomy of the corpus cavernosum: multiple irregular thick-walled vessels, widely interconnected, are noted conforming the erectile tissues.

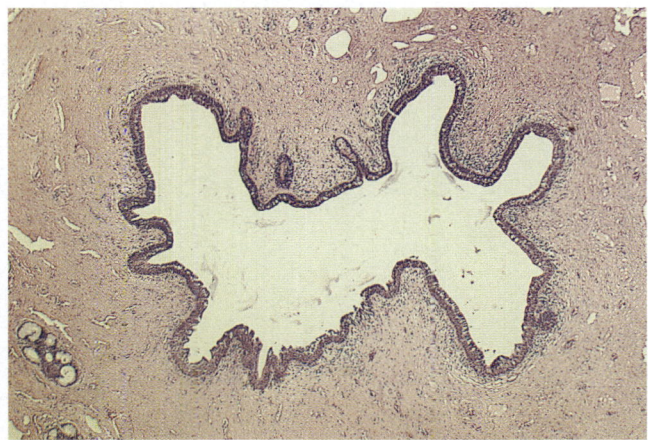

FIG. 8. Anatomy of urethra. Microscopic appearance of the urethra at the level of the penile shaft. The epithelium is transitional. There are periurethral mucous glands deep in the lamina propria.

saphenous vein enters the femoral vein. The superficial nodes (about 10–13) are located above the cribriform fascia. The group of nodes located at the superior inner quadrant are designated as "sentinel" lymph nodes, based on the belief that they are the first site of metastasis in squamous cell carcinoma (SCC) of the penis (6,7). Deep nodes are scanty (3,4) and their lymphatic vessels drain into the pelvic (iliac) lymph nodes, located externally or medially along the major iliac vessels.

ANOMALIES

Congenital anomalies of the penis are rare and a wide variety have been described (8). They range from the absolute lack of this organ to segmentary structural anomalies. Penile agenesis or aphalalia is a rare condition in which the genital tubercle fails to develop. About 70 cases have been reported. Other malformations of the genitourinary tract are associated with it. Immediate assessment is required to successfully reassign gender (9,10). Conditions in which the penis appears to be absent are concealed penis and webbed penis. In the first anomalie the penis is normally developed but it is camouflaged under fat in the suprapubic area, scrotum, perineum, or thigh (10,11). In webbed penis the scrotal skin extends to the ventrum of the penis and hides it.

Hypoplasia and hyperplasia of the penis are usually associated with endocrine abnormalities. Hypoplasias are more common than hyperplasias. The ratio of the length of the penile shaft to its circumference is normal in the cases of micropenis (10). Duplication of the penis or diphalalia is usually associated with other genitourinary anomalies such as hypospadias, bifid scrotum, duplication of the bladder, and renal agenesis. The spectrum ranges from a small accessory penis to complete duplication (10). Lateral curvature of the penis is caused by overgrowth or hypoplasia of one corporeal body. In penile torsion, a rotational defect of the penile shaft is present, caused by fibrous tissue surrounding the corpus spongiosum or by a short urethra. Chordae are usually associated with hypospadias or epispadias. Epispadias occur when the urethra opens on the dorsum of the penis. If the opening of the urethra is in the dorsal aspect of the glans it is called glandular epispadias; if it is between the pubic symphysis and the coronal sulcus, it is a penile epispadias; if it is in the penopubic junction, it is a penopubic hypospadias. This last type is the most common and is associated with urinary incontinence (11). Hypospadias occur when the urethra opens into the ventral aspect of the penis, anywhere from the glans to the perineum. The classification depends on the anatomic location of the defect. It can be glandular, coronal, penile, penoscrotal, or perineal, the most frequent being the glandular and coronal. They are the most common types of penile congenital defect. The incidence is calculated as 3.2 per 1,000 live male births. Associated anomalies include absence of the foreskin chordee, undescended testis, and inguinal hernias (11).

Cysts of the penis are rare. Median raphe cysts result from anomalies in the development of the urethral groove: from epithelial residues that are trapped in an incomplete closure of the genital folds or migration of cell groups after the closure of these folds (12,13). They occur in the midline and appear as asymptomatic, translucent subcutaneous masses in the ventral aspect of the shaft (14). Histologically, they are lined by different types of epithelium according to their embryologic origin: nonkeratinized squamous, pseudostratified columnar, mucus-producing cylindric and apocrine-like epithelium (Fig. 5). Os penis is the presence of heterotopic bone in the penis; it is usually found in the elderly and is associated with Peyronie's disease; it can also be seen in children (15). In the evolutionary scale the human species is one of the mammals whose male genital organ does not normally have an intrapenile bone or bacula (Kurt Benirschke).

INFLAMMATION

Multiple pathogenic organisms can affect the penis. These organisms can be sexually transmitted or transmitted through other means.

Bacterial Infections

Bacterial infections of the genitourinary tract are more frequent in females. The only circumstance when this situation is altered is in male newborns, especially if uncircumcised (16). Pathogenic bacteria have a greater propensity to adhere to the mucosal surface of the prepuce and therefore colonize it. The adhesion to the surface of the foreskin may be due to fimbriae as well as hydrophobic and electrostatic charges. These factors may explain why balanoposthitis is more common in uncircumcised men. Histologically a nonspecific inflammatory infiltrate is found. Uncommon cases of balanoposthitis due to *Gardnerella vaginalis* (17) and *Trichomonas* (18) have been reported. These infections are usually sexually transmitted. Gonococcal infections are also usually sexually transmitted, but they more frequently produce urethritis. They have also been reported to infect penile median raphe cysts (13).

Localized infections of the penis, if not properly controlled, can spread and produce cellulitis. This situation is more common in newborns and in immunodepressed patients. Cellulitis usually involves the scrotum and is caused by group A streptococcus, although group B streptococcus has also been reported as a causative organism (19). Deep infections of the penis are rare and usually caused by *Neisseria gonorrhoeae* (20). Mixed infections can also occur. They are usually seen as a complication of gonorrhea in patients with an underlying debilitating condition (21).

Fournier's gangrene is a necrotizing fasciitis of the genitalia (Fig. 7). Predisposing factors such as local or perineal trauma, burns, or anorectal disease added to debilitating conditions such as diabetes, leukemia, and alcoholic cirrhosis make the appropriate setting for this widespread infection (22,23). Streptococci and staphylococci are the most common causative agents in children as gram-negative bacilli and anaerobic bacteria are in the adults (22).

Mycobacterial Infections

Tuberculosis of the penis is now a rare condition. In the past it has been associated with circumcision rituals (23). It can present as a primary focus, as a direct spread from nearby areas, or by hematogenous spread in generalized tuberculosis. Histologic features do not differ from tuberculous granulomas of other sites. Papulonecrotic tuberculids, an intense necrotizing reaction owing to an hyperimmune reaction, can be found in the glans (24).

Fungal Infections

Mycotic infections of the penis can be superficial or deep. Superficial infections are caused by dermatophytes and should be suspected when nonspecific inflammation associated with hyper- and parakeratosis is seen histologically. In some instances the mycotic spores can be found in the keratinized layers of the penis. They infect the penis through local spread from more commonly affected areas such as the groin. Another pathogenic organism is *Candida albicans*. It is usually sexually transmitted and is carried asymptomatically by 15% to 20% of men. It is believed that this is a factor in recurrent candidal vaginosis. Deep mycotic infections of the penis are rare and should be considered hematogenous spread from other primary sites. *Cryptococcus neoformans* can also affect the penis (25).

Parasitic Infections

Scabies is the most common parasitic infection. When affecting the penis it is part of a generalized infection. It is caused by the mite *Sarcoptes scabiei*, hominis variety, an obligate human parasite.

Sexually Transmitted Infection

Syphilis

This sexually transmitted disease has three clinical stages. In primary syphilis a papulae enlarges and forms an ulcer with an indurated base, the hard chancre. The characteristic lesion of secondary syphilis is condyloma lata, a flat, rose to gray maculopapule. Gummas are characteristic of tertiary syphilis. Histologically an obliterative endarteritis surrounded by a predominantly plasmocytic infiltrate is the typical lesion. In primary syphilis the endarteritis can be found at the base of the ulcer. In secondary syphilis the endarteritis can be superficial or deep and is usually associated with epidermal hyperplasias such as lichen planus, psoriasiform, or spongiform pustular lesions. The infiltrate composed of plasma cells and lymphocytes obscures the dermoepidermal junction. Gummas of tertiary syphilis are granulomas with epithelioid and giant cells, obliterative endarteritis, and areas of necrosis. Reactivation of syphilis in patients infected with human immunodeficiency virus (HIV) is becoming more frequent. *Treponema pallidum*, the causative agent, can be identified with the Wharthin-Starry stain (26).

Granuloma Inguinale

Calymmatobacterium granulomatis, a gram-negative bacteria is the causative agent of this sexually transmitted disease (27). A small nonpainful nodule at the site of infection is the first clinical manifestation. The nodule ulcerates and leaves an ulcer with abundant granulation tissue in its base. Satellite lesions can be found as pseudobuboes. Histologically the most important features are (a) massive plasma cell infiltrate in the granulation tissue, (b) diffuse infiltration of leukocytes that form local collections, (c) absence or paucity of lymphocytes, and (d) large mononuclear cells with Donovan bodies. These are large intracytoplasmatic, encapsulated bipolar bodies that are better seen in crushed preparations. Wharthin-Starry stains are also used to detect them. Electron microscopy shows a capsular structure surrounding the bacteria and dense peripheral cytoplasmic inclusions in the organisms (27).

Lymphogranuloma Venereum

An obligate intracellular parasite, *Chlamydia trachomatis*, is the agent associated with this sexually transmitted disease. Clinically a painless papule or ulcer appears at the site of inoculation and then rapidly disappears. Histologically the primary penile lesion shows a flat base of granulation tissue with border zone necrosis and neutrophil reaction. The adjacent skin shows pseudoepitheliomatous hyperplasia. The inflammatory infiltrate consists of plasma cells and lymphocytes. Nonnecrotizing granulomas composed of epithelioid and a few giant cells surrounded by plasma cells can also be seen (28). The lymph nodes show focal accumulations of neutrophils in necrotic foci in the early stages. Thereafter, lymphocytic hyperplasia and massive plasma cell infiltration follow. The lymphocytic hyperplasia can be so pronounced that it can alter the architecture of the lymph node diffusely or create follicular center hyperplasia. The small suppurative foci coalesce and form the classical although not pathognomonic stellate abscess of this disease. As the lesion progresses, a marginal zone of epithelioid and giant cells and fibroblasts surround it and form the suppurative granuloma. Sinuses and tracts can develop and ultimately fibrosis can be the predominating element in the lymph node (28).

Chancroid

Chancroid or soft chancre, a disease caused by a gram-negative organism, *Haemophilus ducreyi,* can have several clinical presentations (29). All of them have as a hallmark a soft-based painful ulcer. If the ulcer is small, it is called dwarf chancroid; if the ulcer extends rapidly and is associated with a ruptured inguinal abscess, it is a giant chancroid; if there is widespread necrosis and destruction of the external genitalia, it is called a phagedenic chancroid and is caused by a superimposed infection of *Fusobacterium* organisms (29). Histologically it can be distinguished by its zonation. The uppermost layer is the ulcer base and shows necrosis, fibrin, and polymorphonuclear leukocytes. The middle layer shows abundant granulation tissue and palisading of blood vessels and thrombosis. The deepest layer shows an intense plasma and lymphoid cell infiltrate (30).

Herpes

Herpes is a sexually transmitted disease caused by a DNA virus, the type 2 herpes simplex virus. It clinically presents with multiple millimeter-sized vesicles that rupture and form painful ulcers. Histologically the skin may show intraepidermal vesicles or ulceration. The virus located inside the nuclei creates a ground-glass appearance and nuclear molding. Multinucleated giant cells with well-defined acidophilic inclusions can be seen in tissue sections, but are better seen in Tzanck preparations. Herpetic infections without vesicles have been reported in immunodepressed patients (31).

Molluscum Contagiosum

This is an infection that can be sexually transmitted and is caused by a DNA pox virus. The lesion is a 3- to 6-mm dome-shaped pearly papule with central umbilication (32). Histologically it shows lobular acanthosis of the epidermis, which causes an inverted pattern of epidermal hyperplasia. Intracytoplasmatic eosinophilic inclusions called Henderson-Paterson bodies can be identified in the stratum spinosum and granulosum.

Human Papillomavirus—Condylomas

The human papillomavirus (HPV) (33–36) has been associated with genital lesions, including the penis. They occur

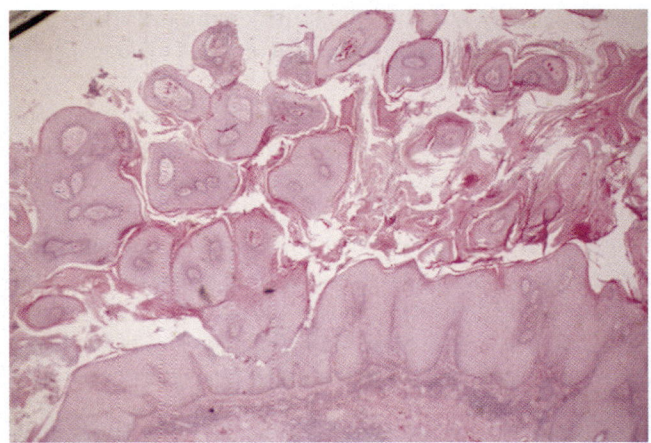

FIG. 9. Condyloma acuminatum. There is an arborizing papillomatous benign growth. The papillae are hyperkeratotic and show a central fibrovascular core. The squamous epithelium is acanthotic.

sporadically in patients with AIDS (37) or in partners of women harboring squamous intraepithelial lesions with histologic changes of HPV (38–42). The most common HPV types found in penile conditions are 6 and 11, and 16 and 18 for benign and malignant lesions, respectively (43). There are clinical and subclinical HPV-related diseases (44,45). Clinical methods of detection are visual examination, application of acetic acid, peniscopy, and brush cytology (46–48). Pathologic methods of virus identification are immunohistochemistry, *in situ* hybridization, and polymerase chain reac-

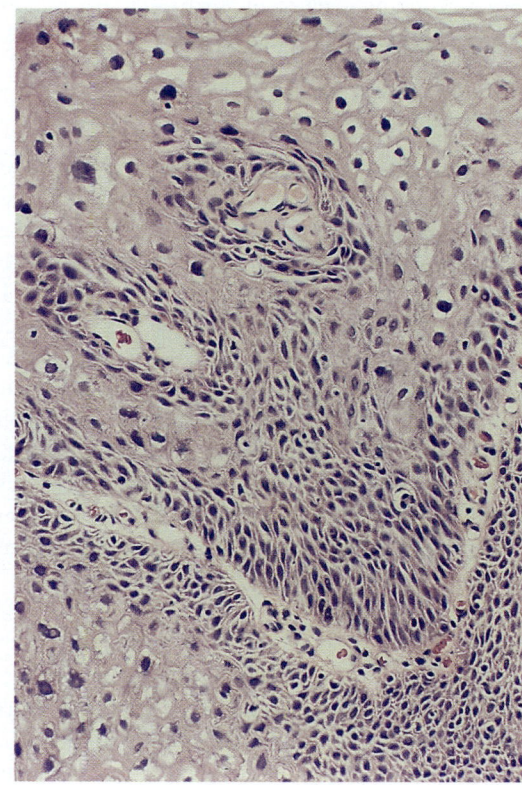

FIG. 10. Condyloma acuminatum. Acanthosis, papillomatosis, and koilocytosis are prominent.

tion (49–51). Mostly HPV is related in the penis to benign or precancerous conditions such as warts, condylomas, bowenoid papulosis, and squamous intraepithelial lesions. The frequency of the virus in malignant tumors was reported initially to be high (52–54), but recent studies demonstrated the opposite (see below). A variety of morphologic types of genital warts related to HPV has been described: condyloma acuminatum, sessile condylomas, and flat or inverted condylomas. They affect the shaft, foreskin coronal sulcus, glans, meatus, and urethra of young individuals and are often multicentric (55–57). Classical condyloma acuminatum is an elevated squamous papilloma. Grossly, they are soft, flesh-colored, cauliflower-like growths, or flat, patchy, simulating balanoposthitis (58). Microscopically, an arborescent pattern is noted, with the papillae showing a central fibrovascular cores (Fig. 9). Hyperkeratosis, acanthosis, and koilocytosis are noted (Fig. 10). The koilocytes are located near the surface of the papillae. Penile condylomas may reach large sizes (8–12 cm), and after a long history of several years of neglect may become atypical and locally destructive (giant or atypical condyloma) or may harbor carcinoma (59).

MISCELLANEOUS CONDITIONS

Phimosis

This is a condition in which the prepuce cannot be retracted, usually as a consequence of nonspecific chronic bacterial infections or congenital abnormally long foreskin. The accumulation of smegma induces a diffuse inflammation of all mucosal epithelial compartments of the glans and the foreskin. The treatment of choice is the surgical removal of the foreskin. Histologically, nonspecific lymphocytic and plasma cell infiltrates are present in the lamina propria of glans and foreskin. Vascular congestion and edema can be noted. It is important for the surgical pathologist to sample liberally the foreskin specimens from adults to rule out dysplasia, carcinoma *in situ*, or occult early invasive carcinoma. In paraphimosis the prepuce cannot be advanced over the glans and becomes trapped in the space located between the coronal sulcus and the glans corona. Unusual cases of penile infarct secondary to arterial obstruction resulting from edema have been described.

Balanitis Xerotica Obliterans (BXO)

This lesion is similar to the lichen sclerosus et atrophicus of the vulva, consisting of a diffuse atrophy of epithelium subepithelial glans and condensation of connective tissues; it can lead to the narrowing of the urethral meatus (60). It is not an unusual finding in specimens removed for phimosis or in association with carcinomas (61). In a review of 40 patients with carcinoma of the foreskin we found BXO in 37% of the specimens associated with the carcinomas. Grossly there are white gray, flat, irregular geographic atrophic areas compromising the foreskin or glans, specially the perimeatal region. In advanced cases the preputial mucosa folds disappear owing to a diminution of elastic properties of the foreskin.

These changes can result in acquired phimosis. Histologically, there is atrophy of squamous epithelium with hyperkeratosis, the rete ridges are punctate or flat. A dense eosinophilic fibrosis and edema are present, as well as a delimited band, in lamina propria. There is a nonspecific, mainly lymphocytic, inflammatory infiltrate in the deep submucosa (Fig. 11). This lesion is usually superficial, measuring no more than 3 to 4 mm in depth, and usually spares the preputial dartos and the corpus spongiosum of the glans. The relationship between the lesion and carcinoma is not well understood. It may coexist or arise subsequent to a diagnosis of carcinoma (61). An analogous lesion, lichen planus, also has been associated with squamous carcinoma (62).

Gangrenous Balanitis (Corbus's Disease)

Like scrotal Fournier's gangrene (63) this is a rapidly progressing necrotizing inflammatory process. It is due to anaerobic organisms affecting the glans penis. A total necrosis of the glans can be present (64,65). Necrotizing gangrene has also been noted in association with reaction to penile prosthesis.

Balanitis Circumscripta Plasmacellularis (Zoon's Balanitis)

This is an inflammatory condition of unknown etiology occurring in uncircumcised men (66,67); grossly, they are

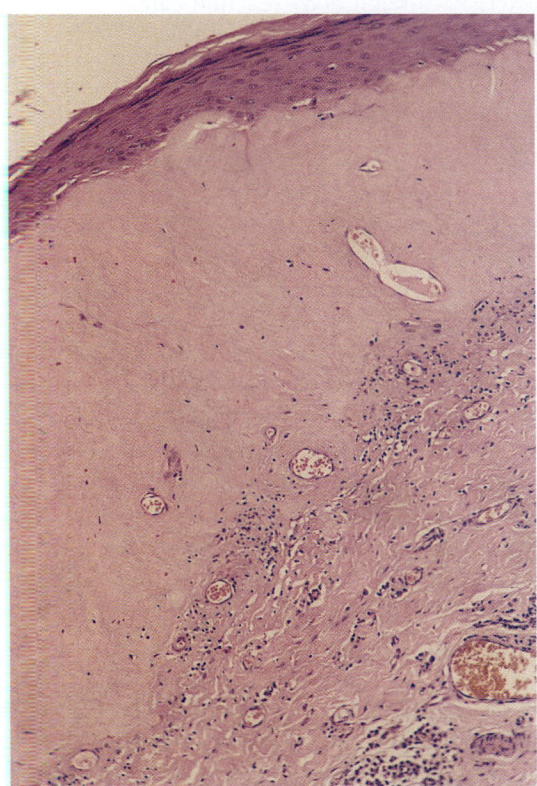

FIG. 11. Balanitis xerotica obliterans. Dense condensation and hyalinization of lamina propria connective tissue with an underlying chronic inflammatory cell infiltrate. The epithelium is atrophic and hyperkeratotic.

solitary or multiple well-defined brown to reddish plaques. The clinical appearance can simulate erythroplasia of Queyrat. Histologically, there is edema and a dense plasma cell infiltrate with the presence of histiocytes with cytoplasmic hemosiderin pigment.

Peyronie's Disease

This unusual condition of unknown etiology is characterized by dense focal fibrosis of dermis and Buck's fascia of the penile corpus. The fibrosis produces an abnormal curvature of the penis, which is painful during erection and sexual intercourse. In some cases there are several firm nodules over the mid-dorsal line. Calcification and ossification can be present (68). The nodules frequently are adherent to the albuguinea. Histologically there are dense fibrous nodules similar to the tissue found in fibromatosis, Dupuytren's contracture, and other desmoplastic conditions involving myofibroblasts. It may be the presenting complaint of the carcinoid syndrome (69). Spontaneous regression has been described.

Tancho's Nodules and Paraffinomas

It is an unusual custom among some Asiatic populations to implant foreign material under the skin of the penis to purportedly improve sexual pleasure (70). Histologically, this material causes a foreign body reaction that may need surgical resection. Such foreign substances that are injected or inserted into the penis include paraffin, silicone, or wax. A characteristic foreign body reaction called paraffinoma is produced.

Papillomatosis of Glans Corona

This is an asymptomatic benign condition showing multiple pearly gray white fibroepithelial papillomas located in the dorsal aspect of glans corona (71,72). They are characteristically arranged in two to three rows. It can be confused with condyloma acuminatum, although the diagnosis can be easily made because of the specific location of the lesions as well as the uniformity of the small papules or nodules. It may be related to excessive sexual activity. It can be seen in 20% to 30% of normal males. This lesion has been more frequently noted in male sexual partners of women carrying an HPV cervical lesion. It is likely that papillomas are not related to HPV infections; but owing to the fact that more penises are scrutinized under peniscopy, more diagnoses are being made.

Lentiginous Melanosis

This is a relatively frequent benign lesion of the glans and the foreskin (73,74). These are flat pigment macules with irregular borders. Histologically, melanotic hyperplasia with hyperpigmentation of the basal layers and elongation of the rete ridges can be noted. Melanomas of the glans can be associated with melanosis. However, a precursor role for this lesion is not well established. Biopsies of all pigmented lesion should be performed.

Mondor's Phlebitis

In this condition, very firm subcutaneous cord-like structures are located along the dorsal shaft of the penis or around the corona sulcus. They are secondary to trauma or associated with herpes simplex infections. Histologically, massive thrombosis of the superficial venous plexus of the penis is present. This condition was formerly considered to be caused by inflammation of lymphatic vessels (nonvenereal sclerosing lymphangitis) (75,76).

Other Rare Conditions

There are other rare diseases that may present grossly as tumor-like conditions in the penis. Verruciform xanthoma shows a warty like lesion characterized by acanthosis and hyper- and parakeratosis. A distinctive feature is the presence of foamy histiocytes between the elongated rete ridges (77–79). The lipogranulomas are due to injections of paraffin, silicone, or wax, and may affect the penis (80). Rare cases of Wegener's granulomatosis involving the penis has been grossly interpreted as carcinoma (81). Other rare conditions affecting the penis are inflammatory pseudotumor secondary to chronic condom catheterization (82), penile horns, ectopic sebaceous glands in the foreskin mimicking molluscum contagiosum (83), and pyogenic granulomas (84).

DERMATOLOGIC CONDITIONS THAT INCIDENTALLY AFFECT THE PENIS

There are a variety of dermatoses that can incidentally involve the penis (11). They are usually diagnosed and biopsied by dermatologists, not by the urologists. Hence, the specimens are submitted to dermatopathologists for histologic evaluation and are rarely seen by the surgical pathologist. Some of these lesions are lichen planus, lichen nitidus, lichen simplex chronicus, erythema multiforme, and psoriasis. As part of the Reiter syndrome (urethritis, conjunctivitis, arthritis, and keratodermia blennorrhagica) a balanitis circinata can be noted. These are irregular plaques located in the corona of the penis.

NEOPLASMS

Squamous Hyperplasia

A benign, not atypical acanthotic thickening of the squamous epithelium is designated as squamous hyperplasia (SH) (85). It is frequently associated with squamous cell carcinomas, particularly with the verrucous and low-grade papillary variants. SH may involve the glans, sulcus, and foreskin. Grossly, the mucosa is flat, smooth, and pearly white with occasional slightly papillary configuration, merging with an adjacent low-grade carcinoma. Microscopically, SH may present as a flat, papillary, mixed flat papillary or pseudoepitheliomatous lesion. Most of the cases are flat, showing hyperkeratosis and acanthosis, with normal maturation of squamous cells (Fig. 12). Parakeratosis, atypias or koilocytosis are not present. Papillary hyperplasia has a serrated appearance at low power; nuclear atypia is not present (Fig. 13). Pseudoepitheliomatous hyperplasia (PEH) may be confused with squamous cell carcinoma; it is most commonly associated with papillary hyperplasia and consists of a downward florid proliferation of squamous cell nests often detached from the epithelium. The nests are composed of benign, mature, nonkeratinizing squamous cells with smooth contours (Fig. 14); basal cell palisading may be noted. The most important feature differentiating PEH from carcinoma is the absence of keratinization and of stromal reaction or desmoplasia (Fig. 15). Occasionally, benign hyperplasia of basal cells may be noted especially in association with the basaloid variant of squamous cell carcinoma.

Precancerous Lesions

Penile intraepithelial precancerous lesions show a wide spectrum of degrees of cellular atypia and morphologic patterns. The designation of such lesions varies: mild, moderate, severe dysplasia; penile intraepithelial neoplasia (PIN) I, II, and III; squamous intraepithelial lesions (SIL), low and high grade, with or without HPV changes. We prefer this last terminology. Erythroplasia of Queyrat and Bowen's disease are synonymous with carcinoma *in situ* (86–91). The former term has been used for a glans location of the lesion and the latter when the lesion is situated in the skin of the shaft. Squamous intraepithelial lesions are solitary, multifocal, or more commonly, in our experience in Paraguay associated with infiltrating squamous cell carcinoma, in about two-thirds of cases. Atypical intraepithelial squamous lesions are rarely present in tissues adjacent to highly differentiated carcinomas such as the verrucous and the papillary. The gross

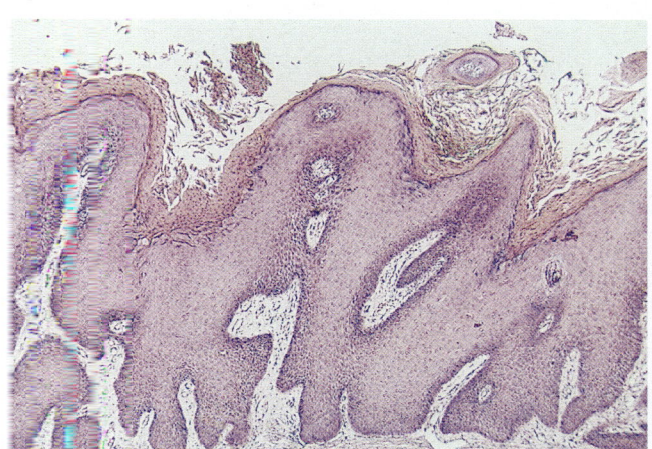

FIG. 13. Squamous hyperplasia, papillary: hyperkeratosis, acanthosis, and papillomatosis. There is a normal cell maturation without atypias. Fibrovascular cores are seen.

appearance of SIL is heterogeneous: a flat or slightly elevated pearly white or moist erythematous, or a dark brown or black macule, papula, or plaque. The contours of the lesion may be sharp or subtle, or focal or diffuse, involving most mucosal compartments. Occasionally, a granular or low papillary appearance may be noted. Microscopically, low-grade squamous intraepithelial lesion reveals atypical cells in the lower third of the epithelium (Figs. 16–18) and high-grade lesions in most of the thickness of the epithelium (Figs. 19–22). Koilocytosis may be present, especially in lesions associated with the warty (condylomatous) carcinoma.

Similar to its gross appearance, the morphologic pattern of the squamous intraepithelial lesion at the microscopic level is heterogeneous. The principal types are squamous cell, basaloid, and warty. Other morphologic features such as pleomorphic, pagetoid, small cell, and unclassified can be identified. In general, the microscopic appearance of the *in situ* process usually corresponds to the pattern of the associated invasive carcinoma, but there are exceptions. High-grade basaloid intraepithelial lesions (BSILs) are distinctive.

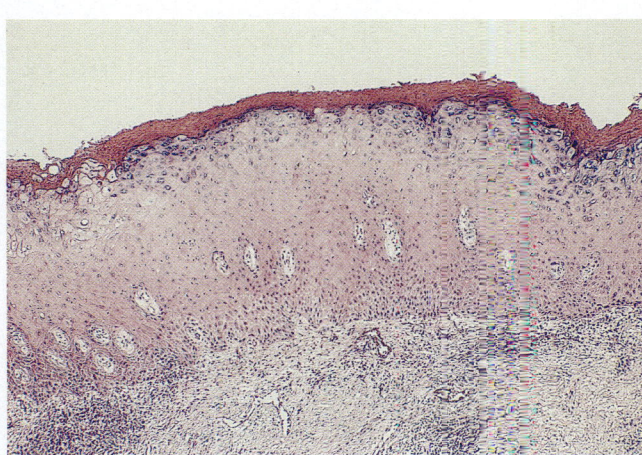

FIG. 12. Squamous hyperplasia, flat. Hyperkeratosis (orthokeratosis) and acanthosis. The limits of the epithelium and stroma is flat. Atypias are not present.

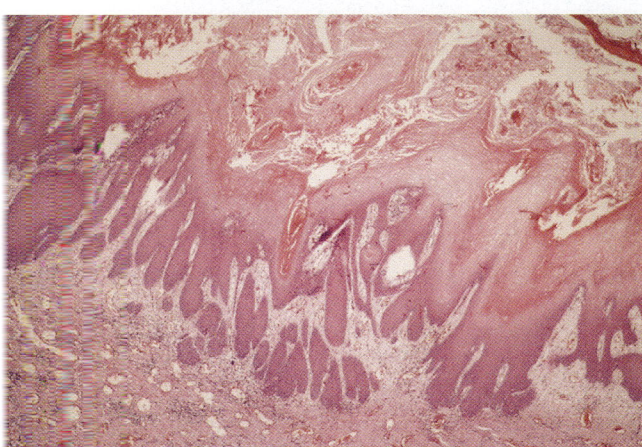

FIG. 14. Squamous hyperplasia, pseudoepitheliomatous. Downward proliferation of rete pegs, with a detachment of squamous nests into the underlying stroma.

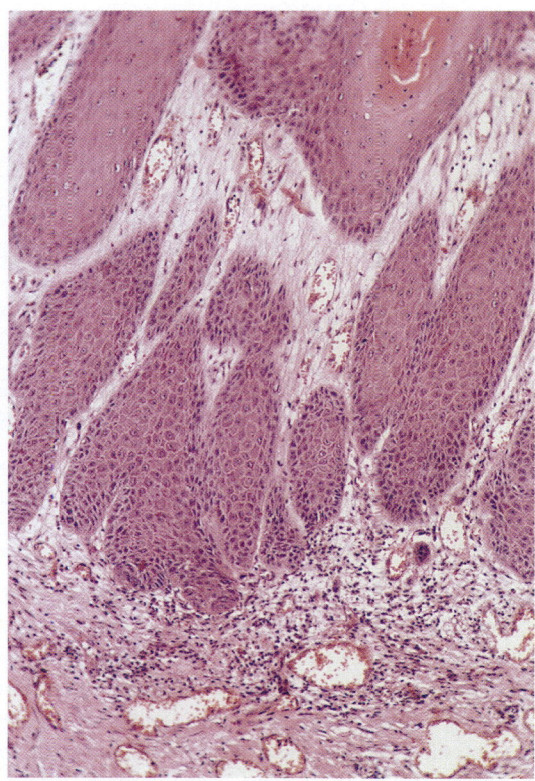

FIG. 15. Squamous hyperplasia, pseudoepitheliomatous. The nests detached from the overlying squamous epithelium are composed of orderly, nonatypical cells and peripheral palisading. No stromal desmoplastic reaction around the nests is present.

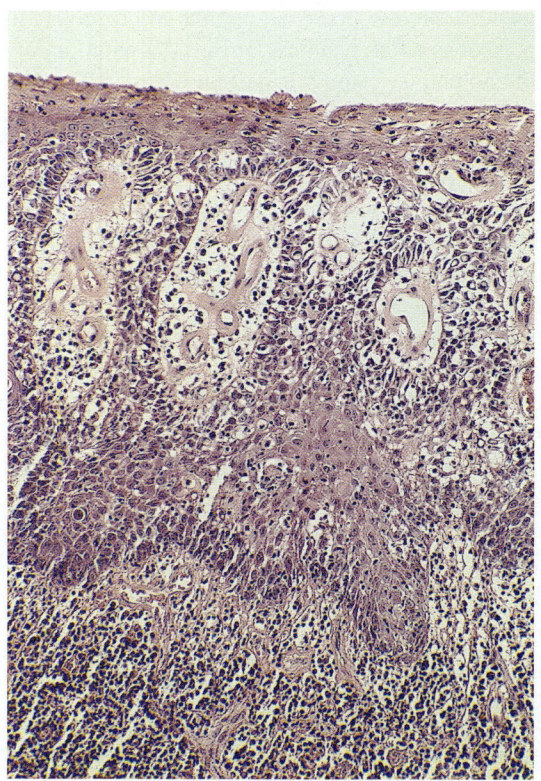

FIG. 17. Low-grade squamous intraepithelial lesions. Elongation of rete ridges, mild atypia, and a dense stromal chronic inflammatory cell infiltrate are prominent. This lesion was grossly reddish and erythroplastic.

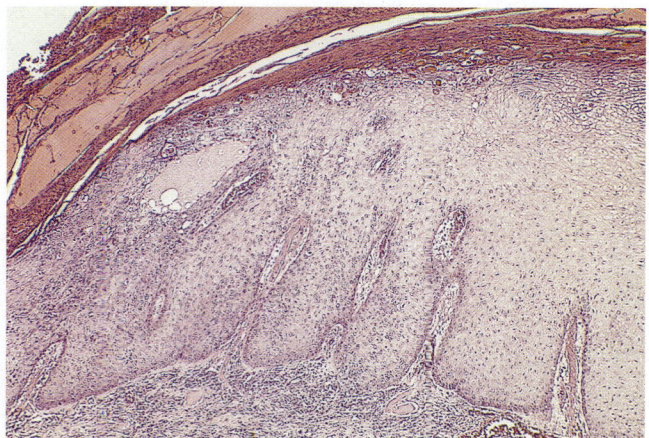

FIG. 16. Low-grade squamous intraepithelial lesion. There are hyper- and parakeratosis, acanthotic thickening, and slight cellular atypia at the lower third of the epithelium. The gross appearance of this lesion was white and leukoplakia-like.

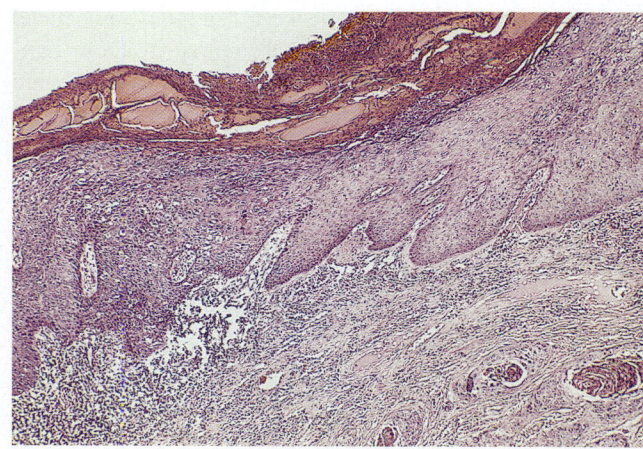

FIG. 18. Low- and high-grade squamous intraepithelial lesion.

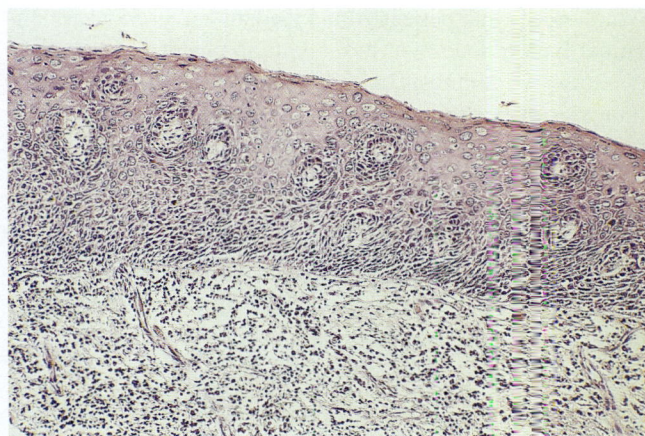

FIG. 19. Carcinoma *in situ*, usual squamous cell type. Most of the thickness of the epithelium is replaced by malignant cells with atypical nuclei and some keratinization. The underlying stroma is densely inflamed.

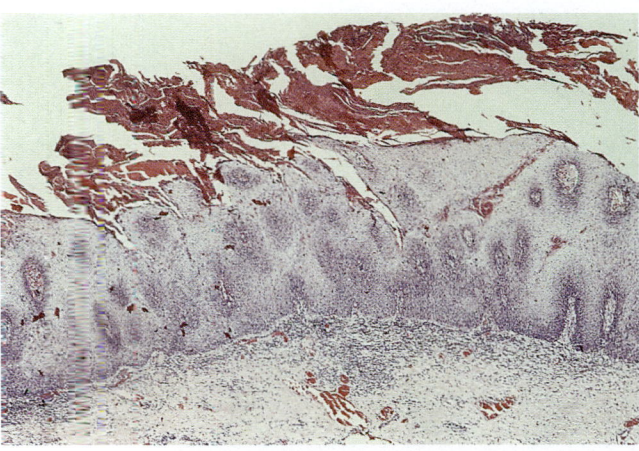

FIG. 21. Carcinoma *in situ*, warty type. Hyperkeratotic, papillary pattern of the lesion, which shows atypical koilocytosis throughout the full thickness of the epithelium.

They are entirely composed of small basophilic immature basal cells (Fig. 20); apoptotic cells may be noted. The base is usually flat, but the rete pegs may show a downward proliferation. These lesions are similar to their counterparts in the cervix and vulva (92). BSILs are present in association with more than half of invasive basaloid carcinomas of the penis, and less frequently in other subtypes of penile cancer. High-grade warty intraepithelial lesion (WSIL) is also a distinctive precancerous penile condition showing hyper- and atypical parakeratosis, marked nuclear pleomorphism, abnormal mitosis, and koilocytotic changes throughout the epithelium. A flat or slightly ulcerated papillary or spiky condylomatous growth is characteristic (Figs. 21 and 22). It is not unusual to identify mixtures of warty and basaloid patterns in the same specimen, an expected finding, since both lesions are probably related to HPV. The high-grade squamous intraepithelial lesion not otherwise specified, the most common type, is similar to carcinoma *in situ* of other sites (Fig. 19). It should be distinguished from transitional cell urethral carcinoma *in situ*, which may secondarily involve the penile meatal region (93).

Bowenoid Papulosis

In bowenoid papulosis there are multiple soft papules or macules mostly affecting the skin of the shaft, and less frequently the epithelium of the glans, sulcus, or foreskin. The lesions are present in young men, with a mean age of 30 years (94,95). The lesions may regress spontaneously (96). Histologically, an acanthotic thickening of the epithelium is noted. A spiky or flat appearance is common (Fig. 23). There

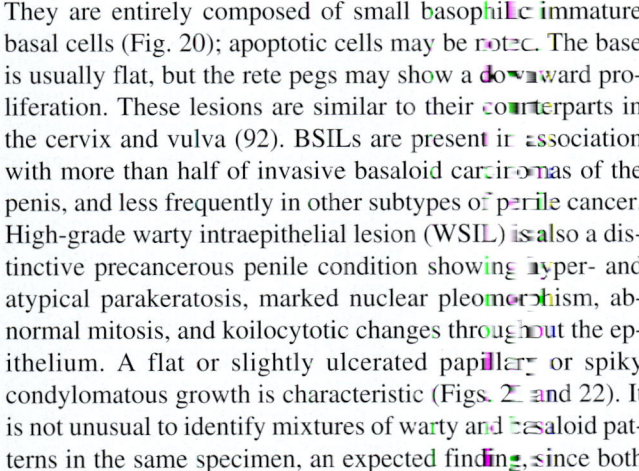

FIG. 20. Carcinoma *in situ*, basaloid type. The epithelium is replaced by small anaplastic cells. Mitotic figures are prominent.

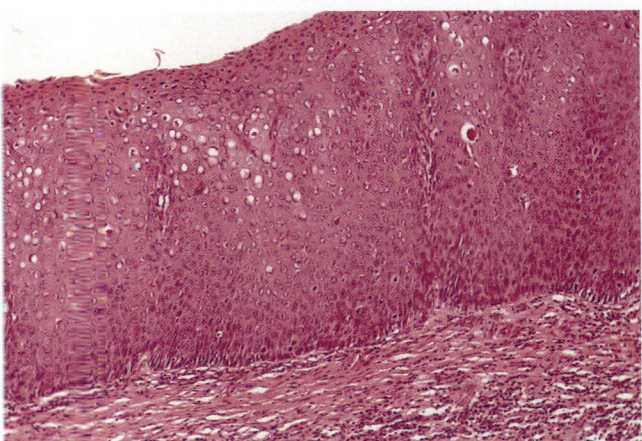

FIG. 22. Carcinoma *in situ*, warty type. Atypical parakeratosis and koilocytosis. The full thickness of the epithelium shows atypical cells.

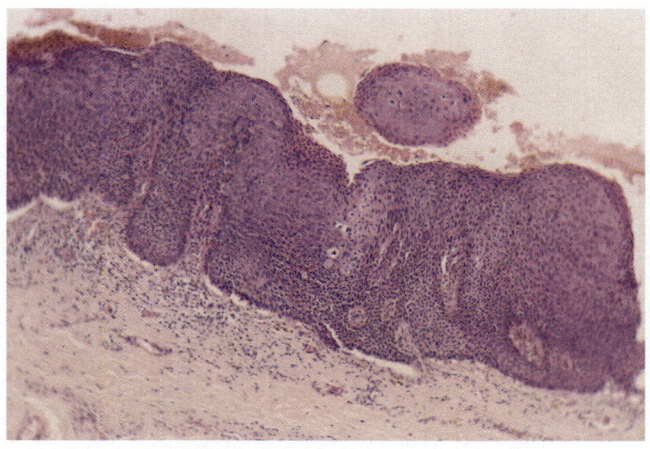

FIG. 23. Bowenoid papulosis. Acanthotic thickening of preputial mucosa in a young male with multiple lesions in the foreskin. There is a focal spiky appearance. The atypical cells are spotty. Occasional koilocytotic changes on the surface are present.

is a proliferation of small basophilic cells with a more spotty disposition of atypical cells than in carcinoma *in situ*. Mild to heavy melanin pigmentations within the lesions my be present as well as hyper- and parakeratosis (97). HPV types 16 and 18 have been associated with bowenoid papulosis (98,99). Hence a sexual transmission is suspected (100,101).

Squamous Cell Carcinoma

There is a wide geographical distribution with low frequency in the United States and Europe, where it accounts for less than 1% of all malignant male neoplasms, to higher frequencies in Africa, Latin America, and Asia (excepting Japan), where up to 20% frequency among male malignant tumors has been reported (102–107). Epidemiologic studies relate cancer of the penis to environmental factors, such as poor hygiene, and sexual habits (108,109). It is known that early circumcision prevents penile cancer, but there is greater risk for cancer in patients who underwent late circumcision. It does appear that all conditions, congenital or acquired, that restrict the motility of the foreskin, such as paraphimosis or phimosis, greatly increase the risk for the development of penile cancer (108–111). The geographic clustering of both uterine and penile cancer has led to studies suggesting a relationship between these cancers (112,113). Prior veneral infections, herpes human papillomavirus, and smoking have been implicated (113,114). A link between immunosuppression and penile cancer has been reported in transplant patients as well as in those with psoriasis treated with psoralens and ultraviolet A (PUVA) (115). More than a third of patients with squamous cell carcinoma, especially the non-HPV–related, differentiated types, are associated with BXO; it is not clear whether this association is coincidental or causally related.

The most frequent clinical presentation is of an irregular mass in the glans penis with or without palpable inguinal lymph nodes in a patient with a median age of 58 years. Inguinal lymph node metastasis with an occult penile cancer due to severe phimosis or very small size of the primary tumor are other presenting features. Hypercalcemia occurs rarely.

Classification

The vast majority of the malignant neoplasms of the penis are squamous cell carcinomas. They may be classified according to patterns of growth and histologic structure.

Patterns of Growth

The classification of SCC of the penis according to growth patterns is justified because there is a correlation with prognosis (116). More than a third of penile tumors show a mixed pattern of growth, principally those of clinically advanced stages. There are four main growth patterns:

Superficial Spreading (SS)

This pattern consists of slowly growing neoplasms widely involving mucosa and superficial anatomical layers of glans, sulcus, or foreskin (116) (Fig. 24). It is the most common pattern of growth. It does appear that, like in malignant melanomas, there are two phases of growth: initially horizontal, and in more advanced stages vertical with deep invasion of CS and CC. Rarely, tumors with this pattern of growth affect only one anatomical compartment, such as the glans or the foreskin. Grossly, there is a slightly raised white-gray granular firm neoplasm involving epithelial surfaces. Microscopically, the lesion is mostly horizontal, with three features of presentation: (a) all *in situ* carcinoma, with or without superficial infiltration in lamina propia; (b) part of the tumor is nodular and deeply or superficially invasive in this area, and the rest is *in situ*; and (c) the carcinoma is horizontal and bandlike in growth, entirely composed of a mixture of *in situ* and invasive carcinomas (Fig. 24). The most common histologic type associated with this pattern is the usual squamous cell.

Special attention should be given to the microscopic evaluation of surgical margins of resection in this type of tumor. It can extend, due to its characteristic centrifugal growth, to the urethral or skin surgical margin of resection. If a foreskin specimen is evaluated, the entire circumferential margin near the coronal sulcus should be submitted for histologic evaluation. Recurrent carcinoma in the glans, years after an incomplete removal of an SS carcinoma of the foreskin, is not uncommon.

Vertical Growth (VG)

This variant is associated with a high risk of regional metastasis and death (116). A large ulcerated or fungating mass is typical of this tumor type. The cut surface shows a

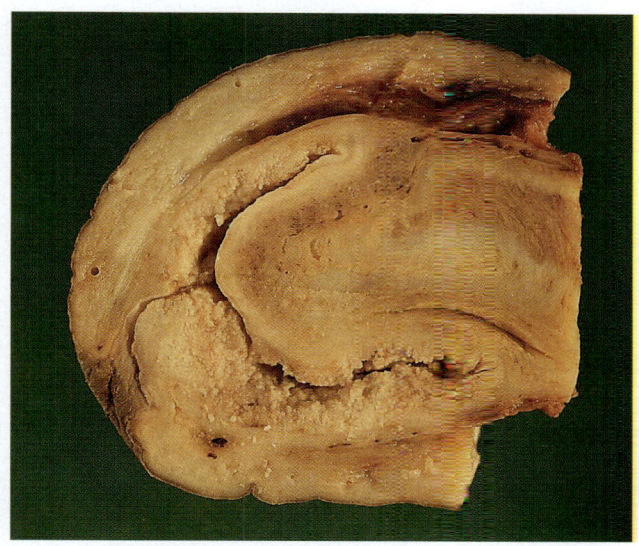 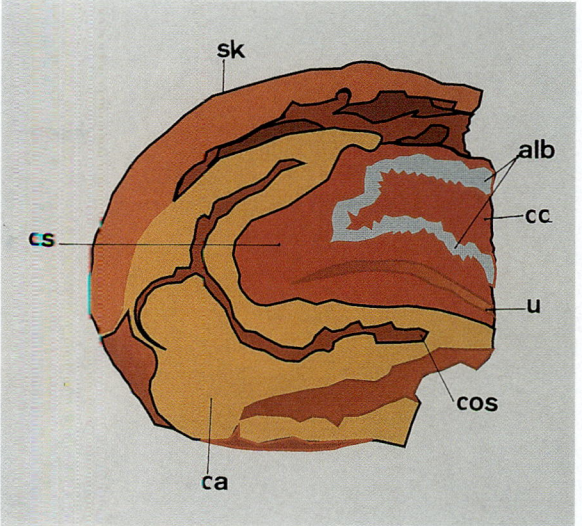

FIG. 24. Growth patterns of SCC: superficial spreading. **A:** Partial penectomy specimen of an uncircumcised man with a phimosis and a large neoplasm growing along the surfaces of all penile anatomical compartments. **B:** In the diagram in color, the tumor (ca) is shown to involve superficially the glans corpus spongiosum (cs), coronal sulcus (cos), and the foreskin. The skin of the penis (sk), the urethra (u), albuginea (alb), and corpus cavernosum (cc) are spared.

solid uniform appearance (Fig. 25). Focal necrosis is characteristic. Microscopically, the carcinoma is of high grade, with prominent vascular invasion. In some cases, rounded satellite nodules separated from the main tumor mass are noted deeply located in the CS or CC. Histologic types associated with these patterns are the basaloid, sarcomatoid, anaplastic, solid, and usual SCC.

Verruciform (Vm)

Slow-growing exophytic tumors with a well-differentiated keratotic papillary configuration are typical features (Fig. 26). These tumors are usually superficial but rarely may invade deeper structures. Approximately 25% of penile tumors are verruciform. There is an heterogeneous group of histologic types associated with this growth pattern. They are the verrucous, condylomatous (warty), papillary, and SCC (see below). Not unusually, mixed forms are noted. Benign pseudotumors (verruciform xanthomas) or benign tumors (giant condylomas) may grossly or microscopically simulate malignant verruciform lesions.

Multicentric (MC)

Two or more independent foci of carcinoma separated by benign tissues are the features of multicentric carcinomas (115) (Fig. 27). They may be clinically evident or may be a microscopic finding. The whole organ section technique facilitates the identification of neoplastic foci. MC may be synchronous or metachronous and appear in multiple compart-

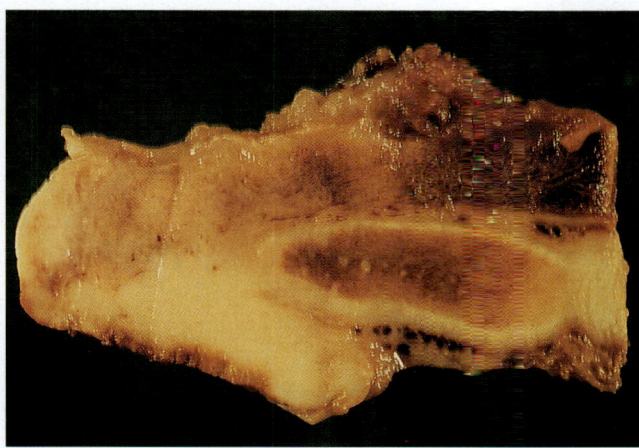 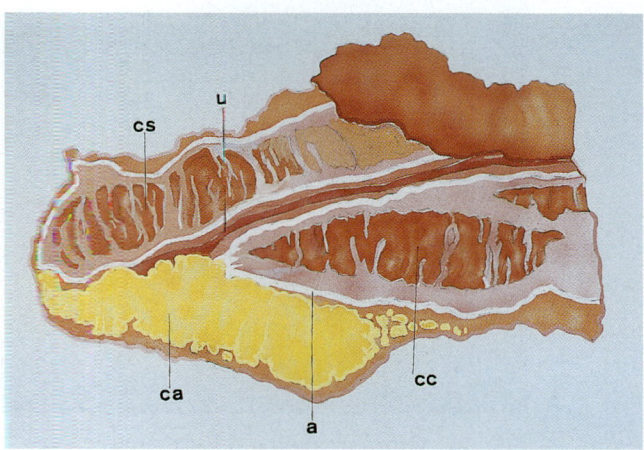

FIG. 25. Growth patterns of SCC: vertical growth. **A:** Cut surface of a partial penectomy specimen with a solid, tan neoplastic tissue located at the ventral region of the glans. **B:** A parallel section of the same specimen shows the relationship of the tumor (ca) to the urethra (u), albuginea (a), corpus spongiosum (cs), and corpus cavernosum (cc).

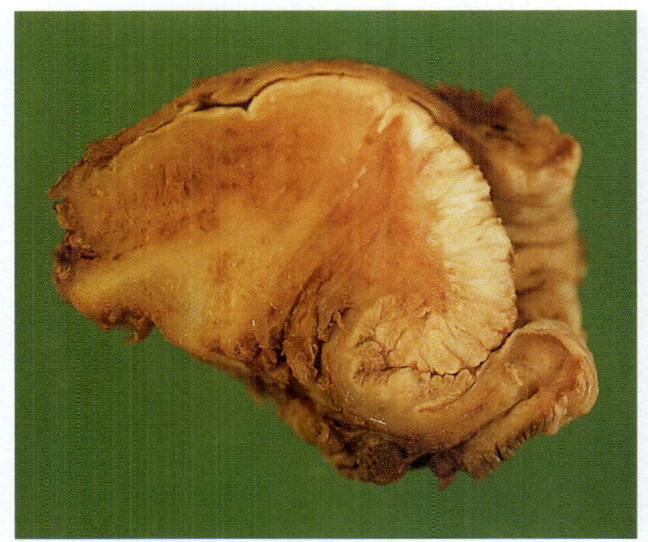 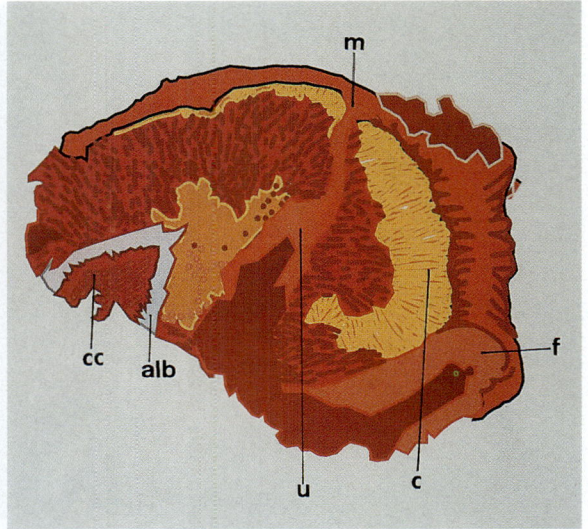

FIG. 26. Growth patterns of SCC: verruciform. **A:** Partial penectomy specimen showing a white tan papillomatous tumor on the ventral surface of the glans. **B:** The gross picture shows the cancer (c) in yellow color, with a well-demarcated border. The albuginea (alb), corpus cavernosum (cc), urethra (u), meatus (m), and foreskin are free of tumor.

ments. They are of similar or different histologic types. Their behavior is similar to that of the SS carcinomas, and patients are prone to recurrences unless all anatomical compartments are removed at surgery.

Mixed Patterns

It is not unusual to find a mixture of growths, composed of SS, VG, and MC patterns. On histologic examination, a combination of low-grade and high-grade histologic differentiation may be found.

Histologic Subtypes

Squamous cell carcinomas of the penis are similar to squamous cell neoplasms of other organs, especially vulvar, buccal, and anal carcinomas. There is a heterogeneous spectrum of morphologic patterns, most showing a conventional nonverruciform keratinizing squamous cell appearance; however, about 30% of penile tumors are made of special structures, among them the verruciform group (warty-condylomatous, verrucous, and papillary), and other patterns such as basaloid, sarcomatoid, adenosquamous, anaplastic, and mixed (117–120).

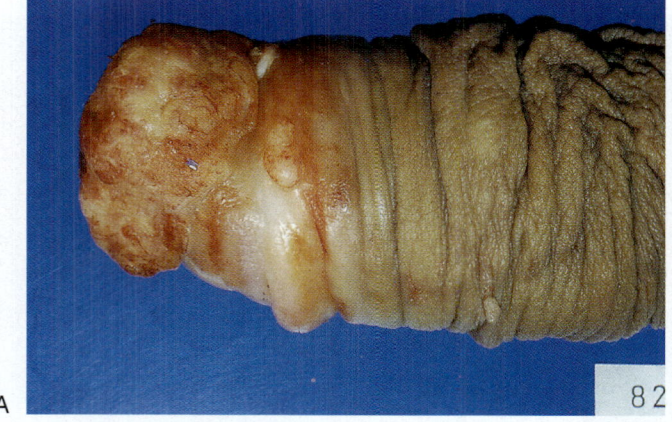 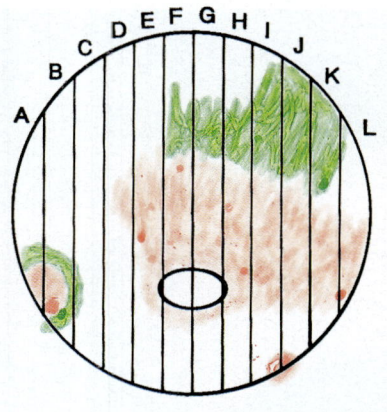

FIG. 27. Growth patterns of SCC: multicentric. **A:** Penectomy specimen showing a large, fungating mass in the distal end of the glans and a separate white smaller nodule in the rim of the glans corona. **B:** A total section organ technique (116) of the same specimen identifies three separate and independent carcinomas in the glans: carcinomas *in situ (green)*, invasive carcinoma *(orange)*.

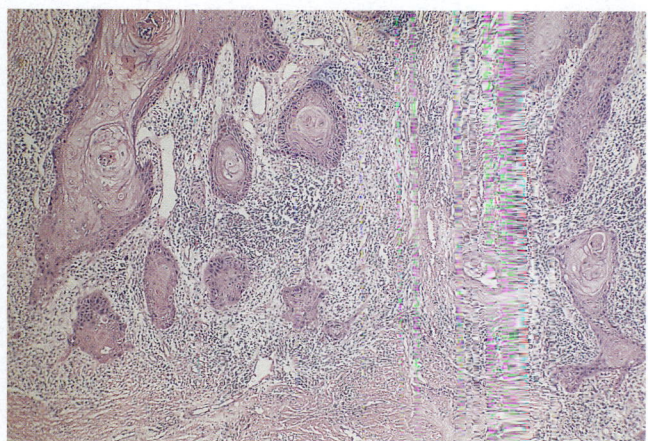

FIG. 28. Infiltrating squamous cell carcinoma, well differentiated. Mature nests of squamous carcinoma are detached from the surface invading lamina propria. The nests are irregular, with minimal atypia and show focal keratinization. There is stromal reaction around the nests. Compare with Fig. 15 to note the differences with the benign pseudoepitheliomatous hyperplasia.

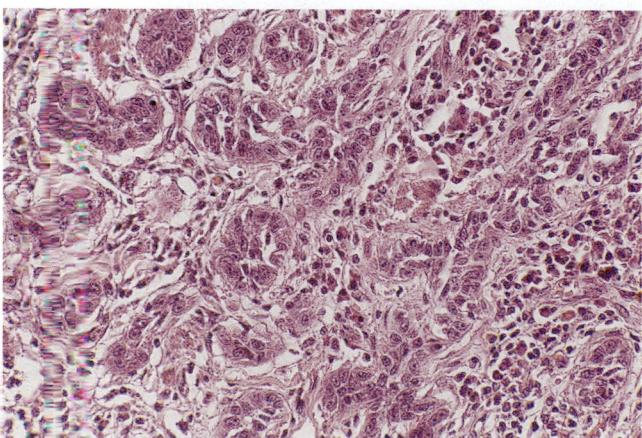

FIG. 30. Infiltrating squamous cell carcinoma, poorly differentiated, with pseudoglandular features. Nests of high-grade, nonkeratinizing carcinoma show central clear spaces due to acantholysis, simulating glandular structures.

Squamous Cell Carcinoma, Usual Type

This is the most common type of penile cancer, accounting for 70% of all cases. Clinical, treatment, and survival features are discussed elsewhere (121–131). The median age is about 58 years. Grossly, an irregular granular mass, a flat ulcerated surface, or a mixed exophytic, ulcerated appearance is seen. The cut surface shows a white to tan solid irregular tumor with either superficial or deep penetration into the various penile anatomical layers. Microscopically, an infiltrating keratinized squamous carcinoma of moderate differentiation is noted (Figs. 28 and 29). Focally, areas of poorly differentiated carcinoma can be seen; predominantly undifferentiated carcinomas of the penis are rare. Unusual patterns such as acantholytic (pseudoglandular), spindle cell, lymphoepithelioma-like, trabecular, endocrine, giant cell pleomorphic or clear cell may be seen (Figs. 30–33). The stroma shows a mild to severe chronic inflammatory infiltrate usually lymphoplasmocytic, although eosinophils may be occasionally prominent. Foreign body–type giant cell reaction to the keratin may be noted, especially in highly keratinized tumors. Desmoplasia is unusual. Associated low- or high-grade squamous intraepithelial lesions are present in two-thirds of the cases as well as squamous hyperplasia, most commonly of the flat type. BXO can be noted in the lamina propia, especially in association with low-grade carcinomas of the foreskin.

The differential diagnosis is with well-differentiated and anaplastic neoplasms. In the former category, PEH should be

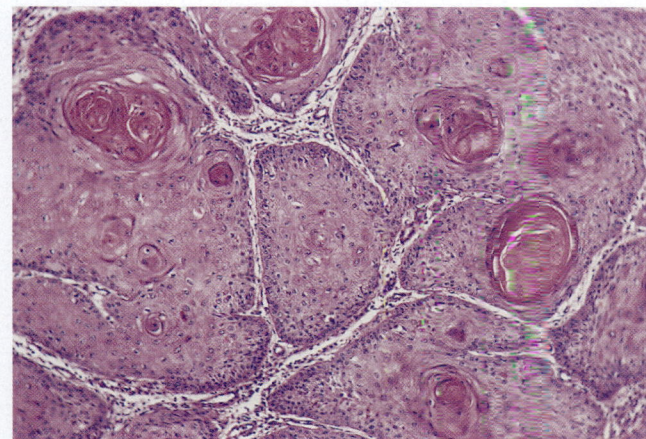

FIG. 29. Infiltrating squamous cell carcinoma, moderately differentiated. Deeply invasive keratinizing carcinoma with an interanastomosing syncytial pattern.

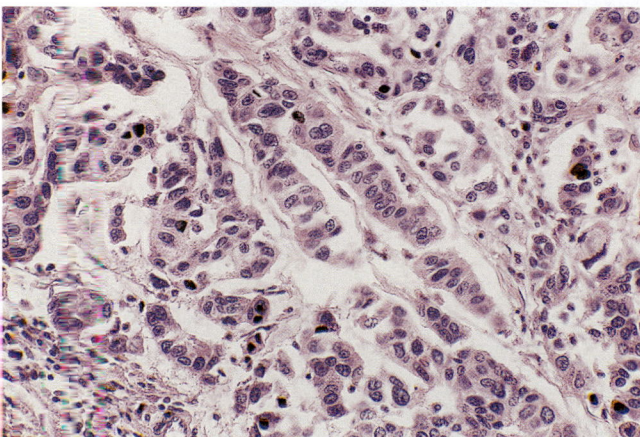

FIG. 31. Infiltrating squamous cell carcinoma, poorly differentiated, with trabecular features. Tumor cells are arranged in cords separated by loose connective tissue stroma.

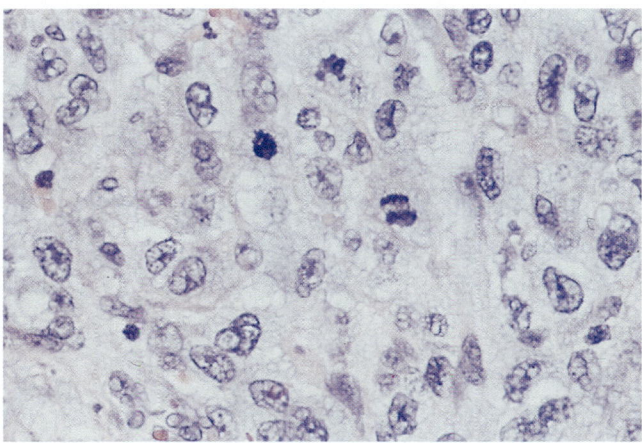

FIG. 32. Infiltrating squamous cell carcinoma, poorly differentiated, with solid pattern. High-grade carcinoma with pleomorphism and numerous mitoses.

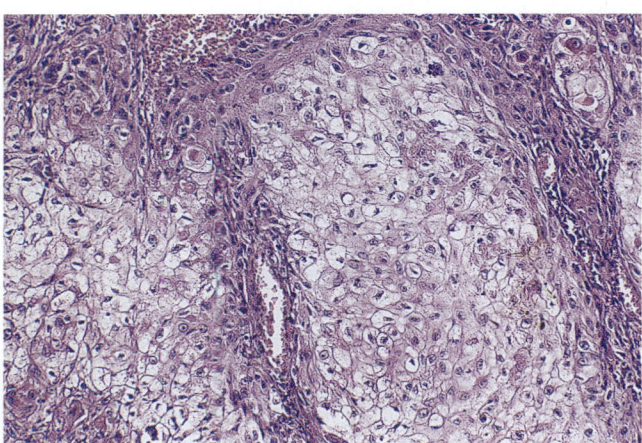

FIG. 33. Infiltrating squamous cell carcinoma, poorly differentiated, with clear cell features. Large, solid nests of invasive carcinoma without keratinization and clear cell features.

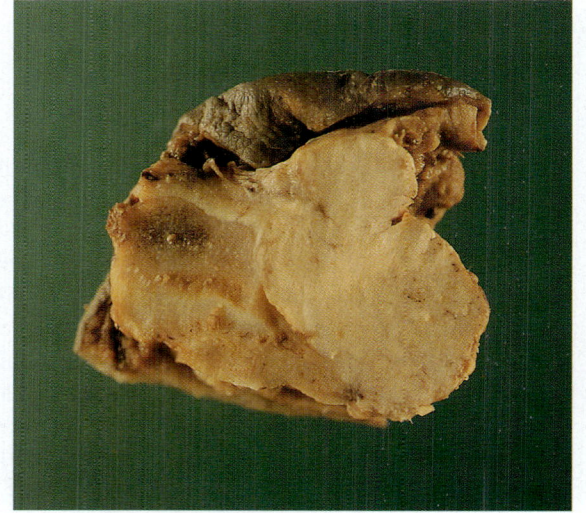
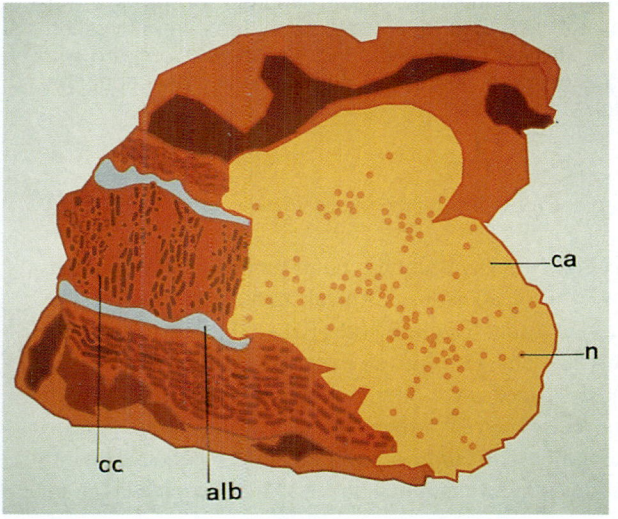

FIG. 34. Basaloid carcinoma. **A:** Gross picture of a partial penectomy specimen with a solid beige neoplasm totally replacing the glans. **B:** The tumor is depicted in yellow (ca); it infiltrates the albuginea (alb) and corpus cavernosum (cc). Note the multifocal necrotic foci within the lesion (n).

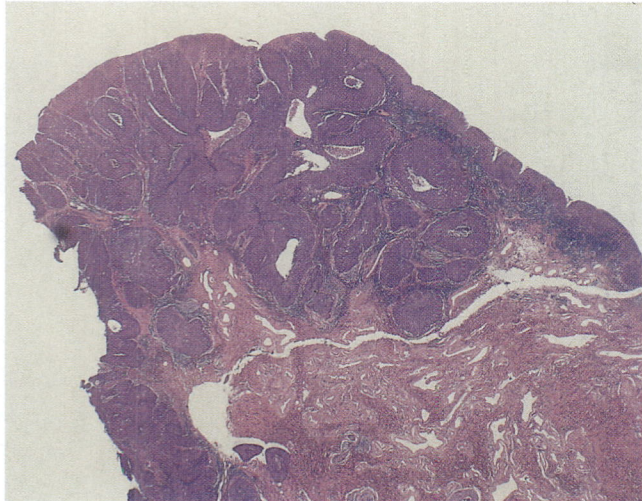

FIG. 35. Basaloid carcinoma. Solid neoplasm, composed of confluent neoplastic nests with a microcystic pattern focally invading the lamina propria and corpus spongiosum. Adjacent epithelium is thickened due to carcinoma *in situ*.

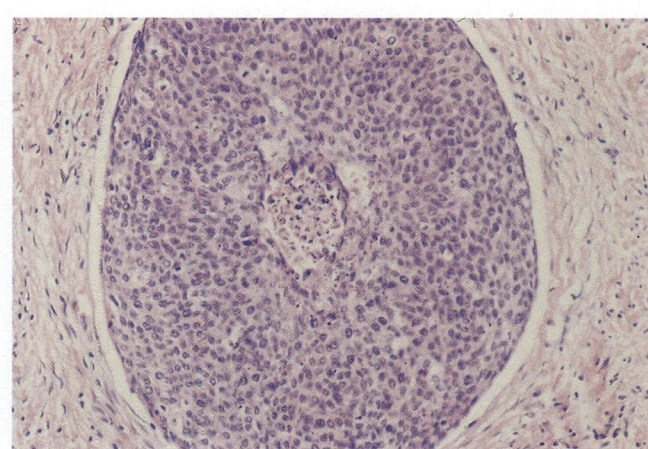

FIG. 36. Basaloid carcinoma. A neoplastic nest composed of small, uniform anaplastic, basal cells, with a central focus of necrosis. Note the peripheral clear separation shrinkage artifact.

ruled out. In PEH there are elongated rete ridges, with foci of epithelium appearing as separated from the surface by a tangential cut. These nests, however, are orderly, showing no atypias or keratinization; typically, stromal reaction or desmoplasia around the nest is not present; the contrary is seen in SCC, where atypia, keratinization, and stromal reaction are present. High-grade SCC may be confused with malignant melanoma or epithelioid angiosarcoma. Immunohistochemical stains may be of help in distinguishing them. Transitional cell urethral carcinomas should be distinguished from solid, poorly differentiated SCC. Urethral neoplasms usually affect the ventral portion of the penis and show no evidence of squamous intraepithelial atypias; the identification of transitional cell carcinoma *in situ* in urethral epithelium or the history of a previous bladder cancer would facilitate the diagnosis.

Basaloid Carcinoma

This is an aggressive, high-grade, and deeply invasive penile neoplasm, usually associated with the human papillomavirus (117,118). It accounts for 5% to 10% of all penile cancers; the median age is 52. More than half the patients show enlarged inguinal nodes due to metastasis at the time of diagnosis. The glans is the main location, and its purported site of origin is the squamous transitional junction in the meatal region. Grossly, there is a rather flat, ulcerated irregular mass; the cut surface shows a solid, tan tissue usually replacing CS, with involvement of albuginea and CC. Necrotic foci within the tumor are noted using a magnifying lens (Fig. 34). Microscopically, characteristic closely attached nests of solid tumor cells (Fig. 35) often with central comedonecrosis are noted. These islands of tissue may show a peripheral clear cleft due to retraction artifact (Fig. 36). The cells are small, similar to basal cells, showing inconspicuous nucleoli and numerous mitosis (Fig. 37). Focal keratinization in the central portion of the nest and palisading at the periphery can be seen in some cases. A peculiar, starry-sky appearance may be noted, due to apoptosis. Atypical basal cell hyperplasia and basaloid carcinoma *in situ* are frequently associated lesions. Warty carcinoma *in situ* can also be noted. The stroma may show chronic inflammatory cells or hyalinization. Perineural, lymphatic, and venous invasion are prominent. The mortality rate of patients with BC is of 59% (118).

Verruciform Carcinomas

Penile exophytic tumors with a verruciform gross appearance and low- to intermediate-grade papillary microscopic features are similar but heterogeneous. Most of these lesions may be classified according to the strict morphologic characteristics depicted in Fig. 38. After the gross and histologic evaluation of more than 50 cases of these unusual neoplasms, we think there are two principal groups of verruciform tumors: condylomatous, composed of the giant condyloma and the condylomatous (warty) carcinoma; and noncondylomatous, composed of the verrucous carcinoma and the closely related, low-grade papillary squamous cell carcinoma.

Warty (Condylomatous Carcinoma)

Warty carcinomas (WCs) are unusual, low- to intermediate-grade, slow-growing malignant tumors with a verruciform pattern and a morphologic similarity with condylomas due to its prominent HPV-related changes (85,132). They are identical to vulvar WC (92). Grossly, an exoendophytic, white-tan, cauliflower-like large tumor measuring 5 cm in average diameter is noted. The surface of the tumor may show a cobblestone appearance. The cut surface reveals a papillomatous growth, with frequent deep penetration into CS and CC, with irregular or broad contours of the neoplasm (Fig. 39). Microscopically, an arborescent papillary pattern is noted (Fig. 40). The papillae are long, undulating, rounded or spiky, with prominent fibrovascular cores and cellular pleomorphism with clear cytoplasm, similar to HPV-related changes or koilocytosis (Figs. 41 and 42). These changes are not restricted to the surface but involve the entire tumor. Intraepithelial abscesses may be prominent, especially in the basal areas. The boundary between the neoplasm and the stroma is jagged in the majority of the cases (Fig. 43). Hyperkeratosis and atypical parakeratosis are prominent. WC should be differentiated from the giant condylomas, which are benign tumors with HPV changes restricted to the superficial layers and with no pleomorphic cells. Verrucous and papillary carcinomas show no HPV-related changes. Deeply invading high-grade WC may show regional nodal metastasis. WC, from the point of view of biologic behavior, is intermediate between other types of low-grade verruciform tumors (verrucous, papillary) and the usual SCC of the penis.

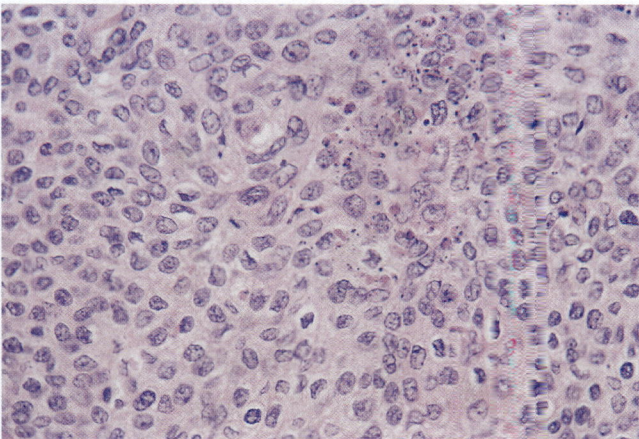

FIG. 37. Basaloid carcinoma. High power shows small ovoid to round anaplastic cells with numerous mitosis.

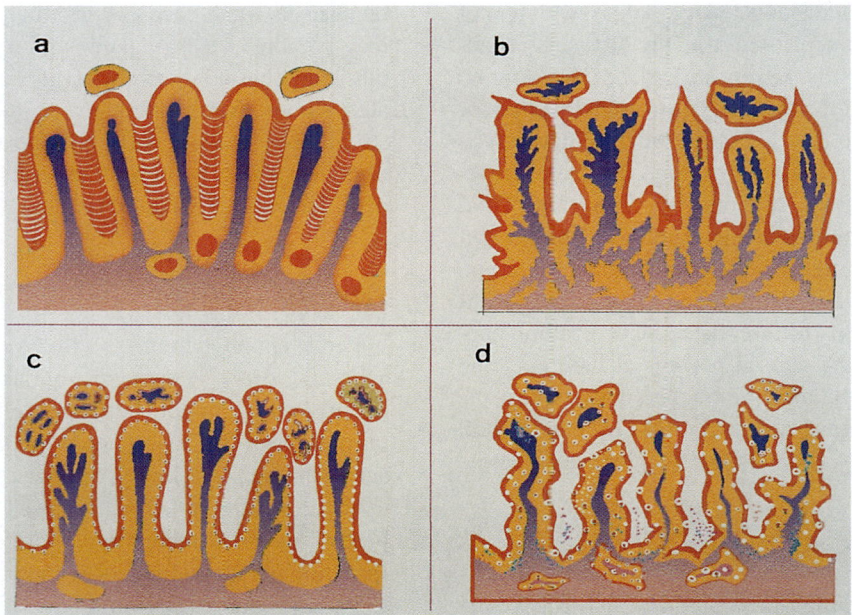

FIG. 38. Verruciform tumors. Differential features. **A:** Verrucous carcinoma: hyperkeratotic and acanthotic papillae *(yellow)* with keratin cysts. The base is broad. **B:** Papillary carcinoma: hyperkeratosis, papillomatosis, and acanthosis. Fibrovascular cores *(blue)* present. Base of lesion is irregular, infiltrative. **C:** Giant condyloma: arborescent papillae with prominent fibrovascular cores, koilocytosis *(white dots)* at the surface only and the base is broad; the cells are benign. **D:** Warty (condylomatous) carcinoma: complex arborescent papillae with fibrovascular cores and koilocytosis throughout the lesion. Microabscesses *(small dots)* are prominent and the base is jagged. Most cells show malignant features.

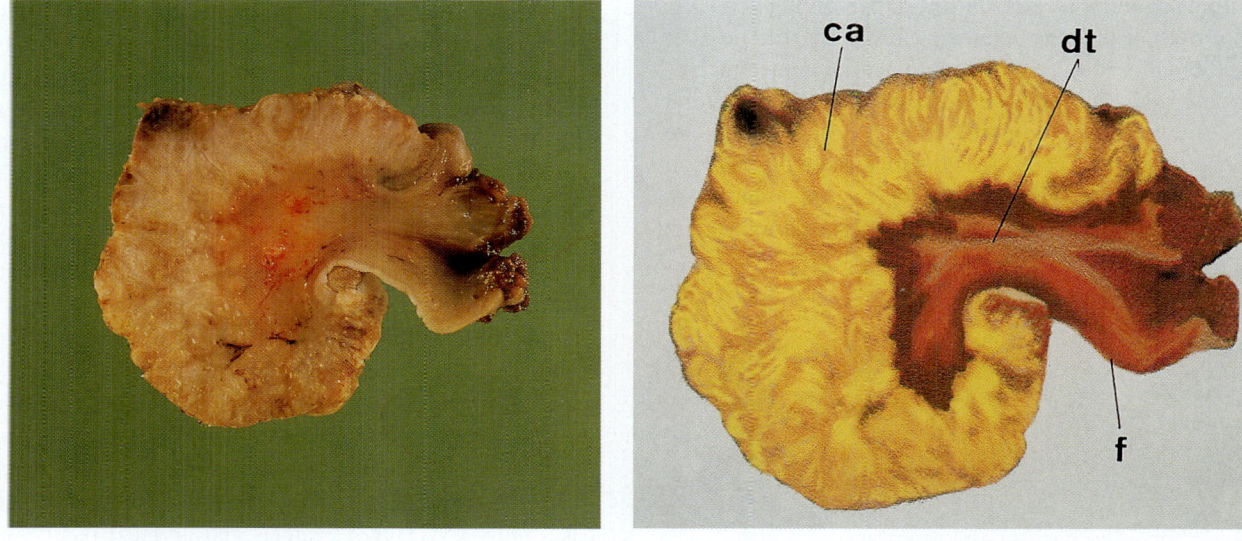

FIG. 39. Warty (condylomatous) carcinoma. **A:** Exophytic tumor located in the foreskin. The cut surface is shown with an arboriform neoplasm deeply penetrating into the preputial dartos. **B:** The papillomatous pattern of the lesion (ca) and the deep penetration into preputial dartos (dt).

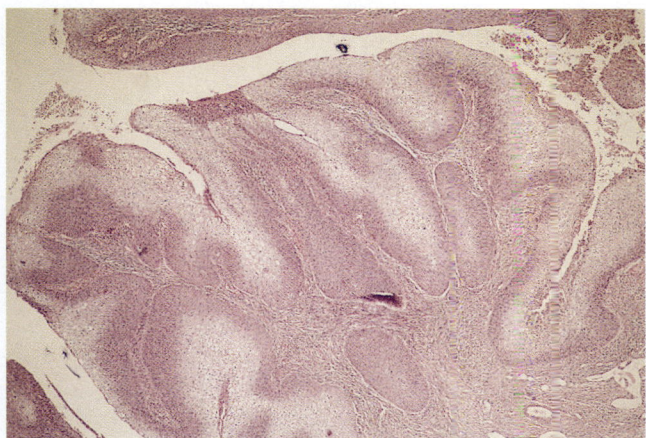

FIG. 40. Warty (condylomatous) carcinoma. An arborescent papillomatous growth is noted. The papillae are complex and show a central fibrovascular core. The similarity with the condylomas is striking except that most cells are malignant and the base of infiltration is irregular in this neoplasm.

Verrucous Carcinoma

Verrucous carcinomas (VCs) are slowly growing, extremely well differentiated variants of SCC, with an exophytic papillary appearance and characteristic broadly based boundary between tumor and underlying stroma

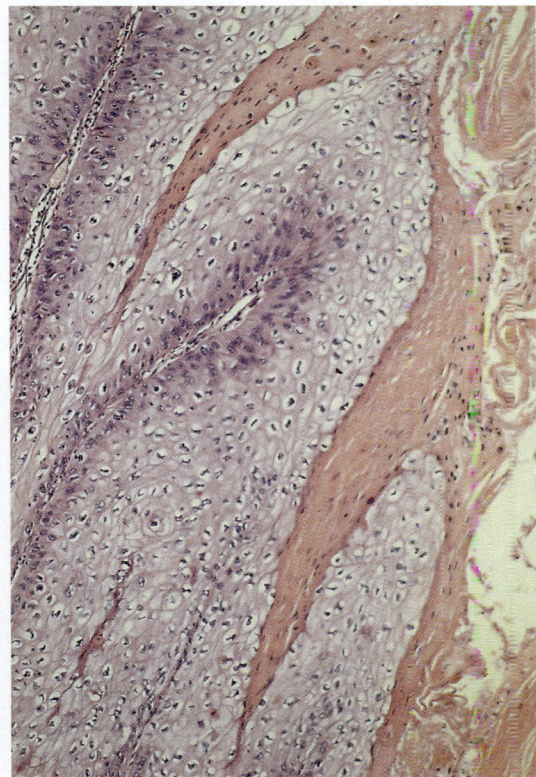

FIG. 41. Warty (condylomatous) carcinoma. Atypical parakeratosis, papillomatosis, and koilocytosis are present. Each papilla has a central fibrovascular core.

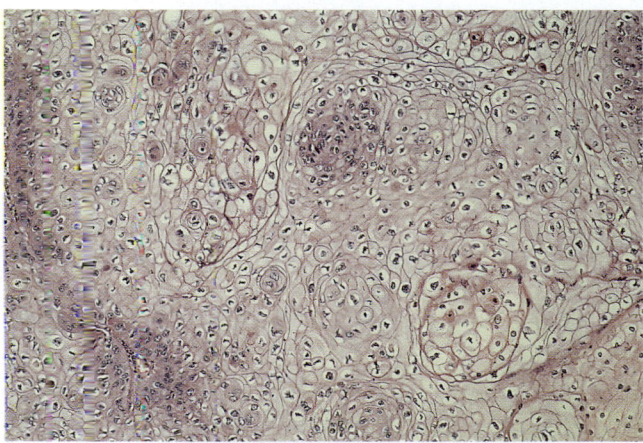

FIG. 42. Warty (condylomatous) carcinoma. The clear cell appearance of the cells is due to atypical koilocytosis.

(133,134) (Fig. 44). They are unusual neoplasms. Under the designation of verrucous carcinomas, cases of condylomas, papillary, and warty carcinomas have been published. Grossly, an exophytic white-gray neoplasm measuring about 3 cm in diameter is usual, although large destructive lesions may be identified. All penile compartments are involved, the glans being the most common site. The median age is 57 and the average duration of the disease of 56 months, the longest among all penile malignant tumors. Microscopically, hyperkeratosis, papillomatosis, and acanthosis are noted (Fig. 45). Central fibrovascular cores of the papillae may occur, but are unusual and not prominent. The cross section of the tip of the papillae shows a central keratin plug, with peripherally located tumor cells. Orthokeratosis, with presence of keratohyaline granules, is more prominent than parakeratosis. Koilocytosis is not present. Occasional vacuolated clear cells (nonkoilocytotic) may be seen at the surface. The cells are extremely well differentiated, with prominent intercellular

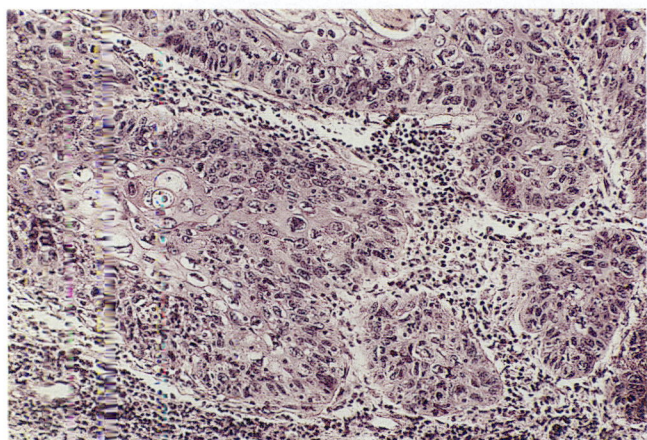

FIG. 43. Warty (condylomatous) carcinoma. A deeply invasive rests of carcinoma with a characteristic pleomorphic pattern.

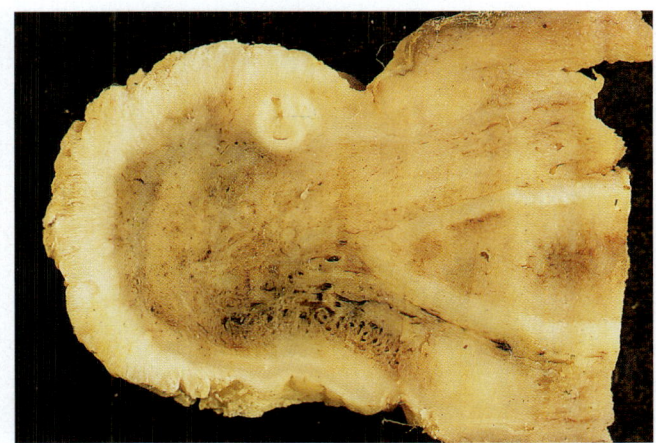
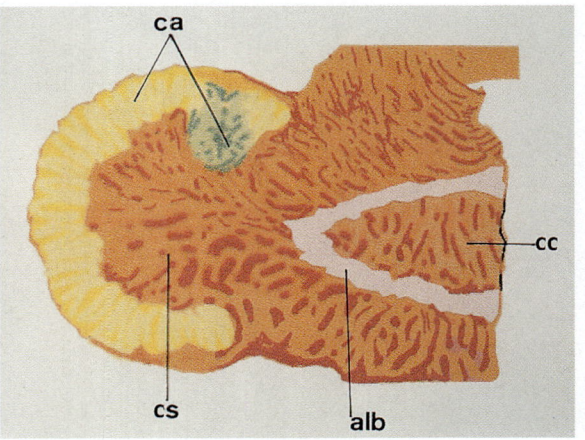

FIG. 44. Verrucous carcinoma. **A:** Exophytic lesion covering the entire glans surface. The demarcation between tumor and penile stroma is sharp. There is a nodular penetration of the neoplasm into corpus spongiosum. **B:** In the diagram the neoplasm is shown in color. Note the tumor (ca) replacement of lamina propria of the glans, and the impinging on the corpus spongiosum (cs). Coronal sulcus, albuginea (alb), and corpus cavernosum (cc) are free of lesion.

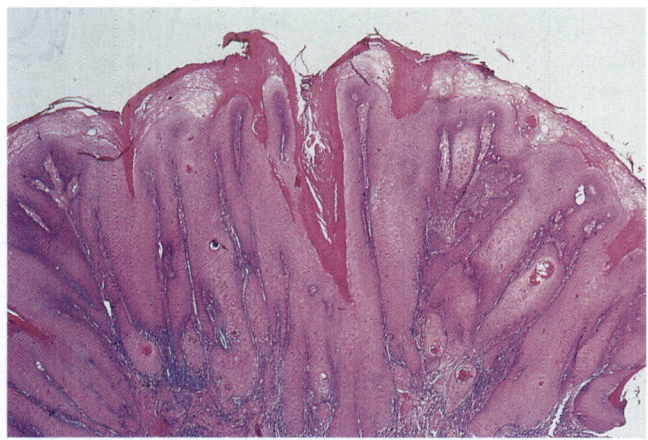

FIG. 45. Verrucous carcinoma. Hyperkeratosis, acanthosis, and papillomatosis. The papillae are composed of extremely well-differentiated cells. There are multiple keratin cysts. The fibrovascular cores are thin and not prominent.

bridges. There is minimal atypia at the base of the nests as well as rare mitosis. The base of the tumor is broad or slightly serrated (Fig. 46 and Fig. 47), deeper invasion is unusual, but in some cases it is striking. Many verrucous tumors in our experience show areas of focal invasion similar to typical squamous cell carcinoma. A dense inflammatory cell infiltrate may obscure the boundaries between tumor and stroma. Metastasis in pure verrucous carcinomas is not present. Recurrence is noted in a third of the cases due to insufficient surgery or multicentric carcinoma not identified at the time of original diagnosis. Verrucous carcinoma can be distinguished from the giant condyloma and warty carcinoma because in the VC koilocytotic changes are not present. Papillary carcinomas can be very similar to VC, but they show an invasive, jagged border and slightly more atypia as well as a definite potential for inguinal node metastasis.

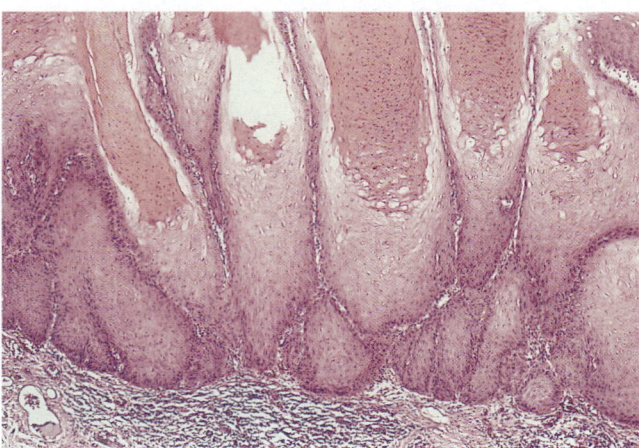

FIG. 46. Verrucous carcinoma. Papillomatous and hyperkeratotic growth with a well-demarcated boundary between tumor and stroma. There is slight atypia of basal cells.

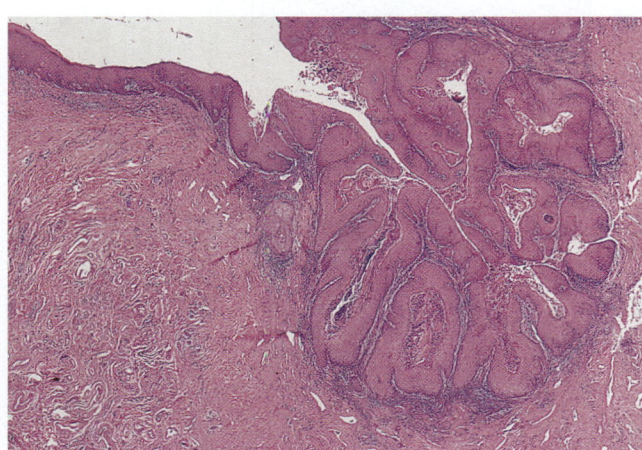

FIG. 47. Verrucous carcinoma. A keratin-filled cystic structure detached from the surface is deeply invasive into the glans corpus spongiosum.

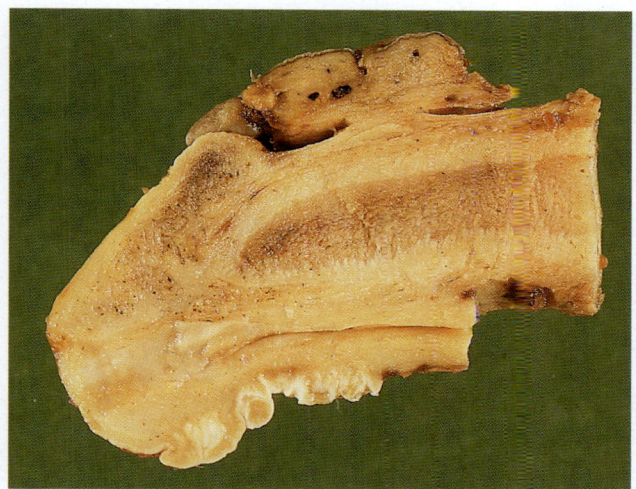 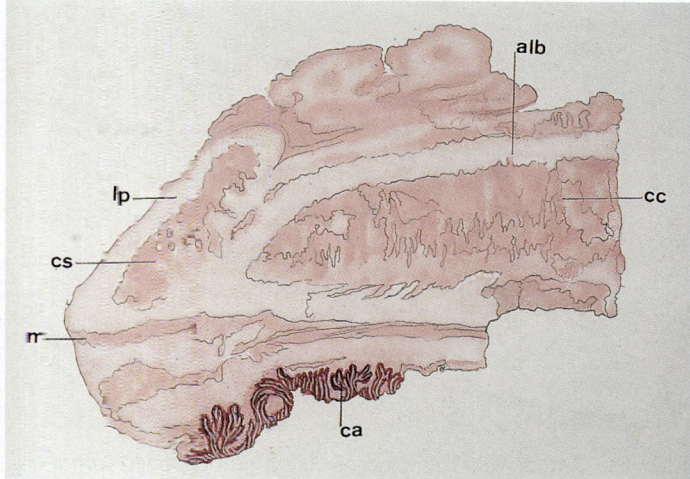

FIG. 48. Papillary carcinoma. **A:** Longitudinal hemisection of a partial penectomy specimen showing a white-beige papillary lesion in the ventral portion of the glans. **B:** The same specimen—the tumor (ca) *(purple)* shows superficial invasion of lamina propria (lp) and corpus spongiosum (cs). Urethra (u), albuginea (alb), corpus cavernosum (cc), meatus (m), and urethra (u) are free of tumor.

Papillary Carcinoma

This is an exophytic, slowly growing, low-grade squamous cell carcinoma without condylomatous features and with an irregular infiltrating margin. The diagnosis is made by exclusion of the other more specific types of verruciform tumors. It is most commonly located in the glans, although other compartments may also be involved. Inguinal lymph node metastasis is unusual. Grossly, they are large white-gray exophytic destructive lesions measuring 6 cm in average diameter, and occasionally reaching 14 cm in largest diameter. The cut surface shows a pearly white tissue with a serrated papillomatous appearance and a poor delineation of the limits between tumor and stroma (Fig. 48). Microscopically, the appearance is that of a well-differentiated papillary squamous neoplasm. Hyperkeratosis and acanthosis are prominent. The papillae are variable, short or long, with or without fibrovascular cores (Fig. 49). Keratin cysts or intraepithelial abscesses can be noted. Koilocytotic-like changes may be focally present but are never prominent. The base of the lesion is irregular and infiltrative (Fig. 50). PC should be distinguished from typical squamous cell carcinoma in which papillary features and a high degree of differentiation are not prominent. Verrucous carcinomas may be cytologically similar to PC, but the boundaries of tumor and stroma are broad and bulbous in VC and jagged in PC. Warty carcinomas are distinctively pleomorphic and koilocytotic, both features lacking in PC. Nests of infiltrating papillary carcinoma should be distinguished from those of PEH. In PC, the nests show slight atypia, keratinization, and desmoplastic stromal reaction, features not seen in PEH.

Sarcomatoid Carcinoma

These are rare, aggressive, large neoplasms characterized by a predominance of anaplastic spindle cells, occa-

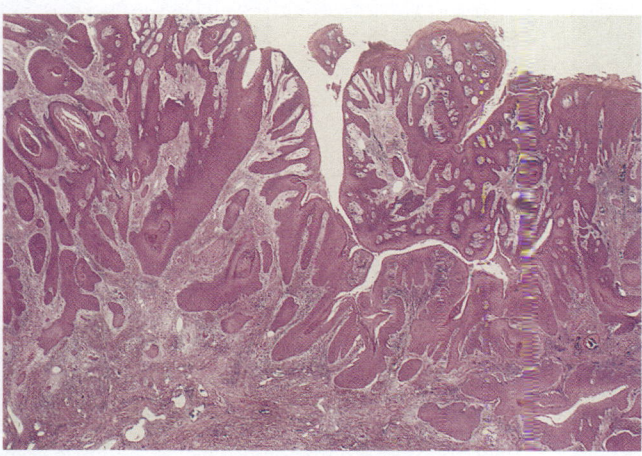

FIG. 49. Papillary carcinoma. Low-power view showing a low-grade papillomatous growth.

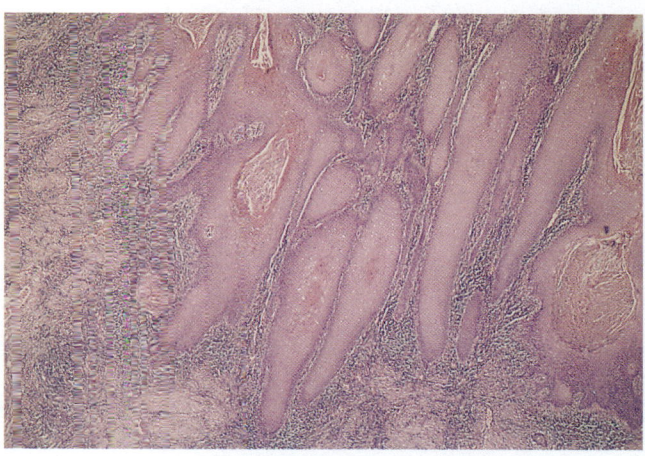

FIG. 50. Papillary carcinoma. The interphase between neoplastic islands of low-grade carcinoma and stroma are irregular; there is desmoplasia surrounding tumor nests.

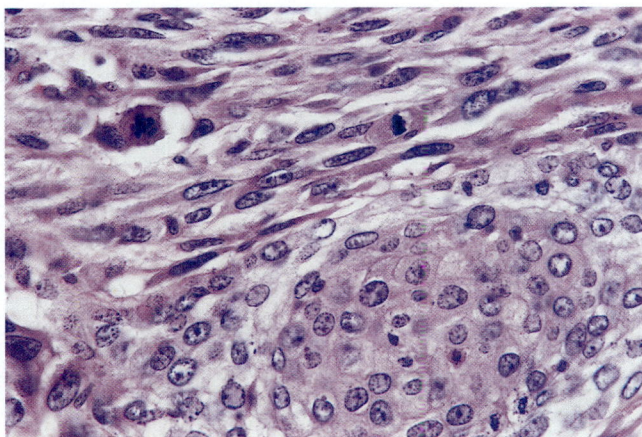

FIG. 51. Sarcomatoid carcinoma. High-grade penile tumor with a biphasic pattern: squamous and spindle cells. Both components are malignant.

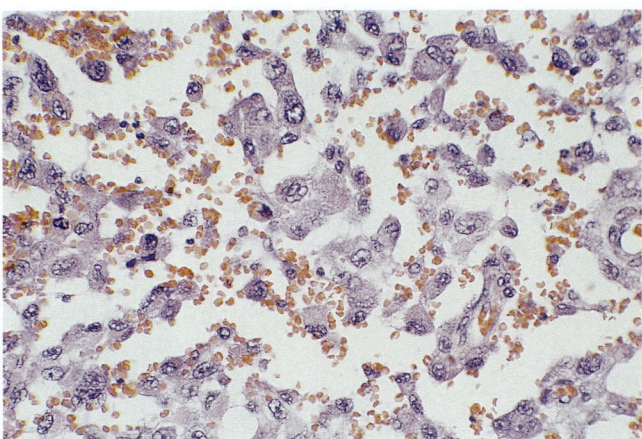

FIG. 53. Sarcomatoid carcinoma, pleomorphic. Anaplastic angiosarcomatous features of a penile carcinoma. Note the hemorrhagic and pleomorphic appearance.

sionally intermingled with giant cells, and a focal or absent conventional squamous cell carcinoma component (135,136). The median age is 60 and the most common location is the glans. Recurrences due to insufficient surgery are frequent. Grossly, a large white-gray or reddish fungating mass measuring 5 to 7 cm is noted. The cut surface shows deep invasion of CS and CC; satellite nodules, separated from the main tumor mass, can be seen in the skin of the penis or deep in the CC. Microscopically, spindle cell, pleomorphic, giant cell, or mixed squamous-spindle features are present. The sarcomatoid aspect is predominant (Figs. 51–53). Necrosis and mitosis are prominent; the presence of SCC, *in situ* or invasive, helps to determine the basic epithelial nature of this highly lethal neoplasm. Immunohistochemical stains may be necessary to rule out a sarcoma.

Adenosquamous Carcinoma

This exceedingly rare carcinoma consists of penile neoplasms, purportedly originating in misplaced glandular cells in the perimeatal region of the penis (119). Grossly, a firm granular, large neoplasm is present. In all cases deep invasion of CS is present. Microscopically a biphasic squamous cell and glandular pattern in the tumor is noted (Fig. 54). The squamous component predominates. The glands are mucin producing and stain with carcinoembryonic antigen (CEA) (Fig. 55). Low- and high-grade intraepithelial squamous lesion is present in glans mucosa. Adenosquamous carcinomas of the penis should be distinguished from the adenoid (pseudoglandular) SCC, where prominent acantholysis simulates glandular spaces but the lining is made of acantholytic squamous cells and the spaces contain keratin and necrotic debris. Adenosquamous (mucoepidermoid) carcinomas of the urethra (120) and Littre gland adenocarcinoma are located ventrally in the penis, with the usual restriction to periurethral tissue and corpora cavernosa.

Pathologic Factors Related to Prognosis

There are few studies relating pathologic factors to prognosis (137–140). The two most important pathologic factors

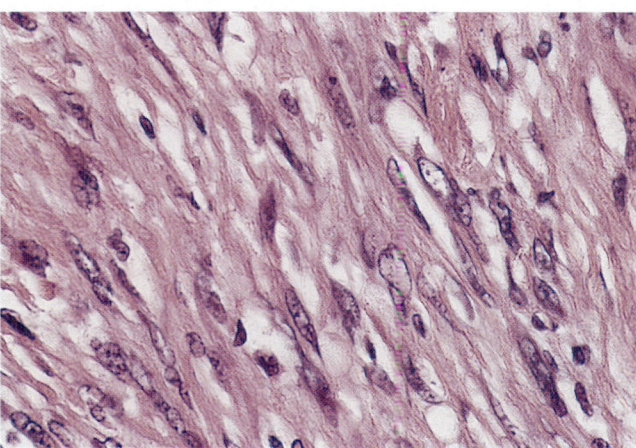

FIG. 52. Sarcomatoid carcinoma, spindle cell. Spindle cell malignant tumor simulating a sarcoma. In other areas foci of SCC are present.

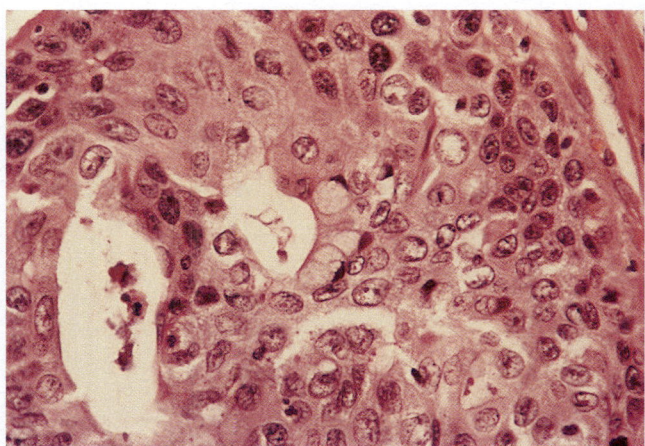

FIG. 54. Adenosquamous carcinoma. This neoplasm is composed of solid squamous carcinoma and mucin-secreting glandular features.

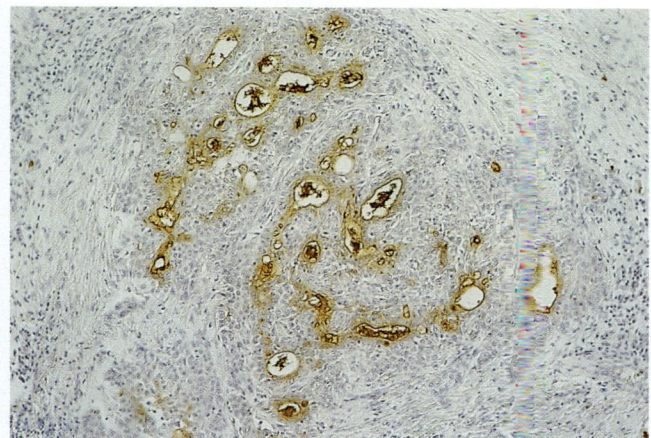

FIG. 55. Adenosquamous carcinoma. Carcinoembryonic antigen (CEA) immunostaining reveals strong positivity in the glandular areas.

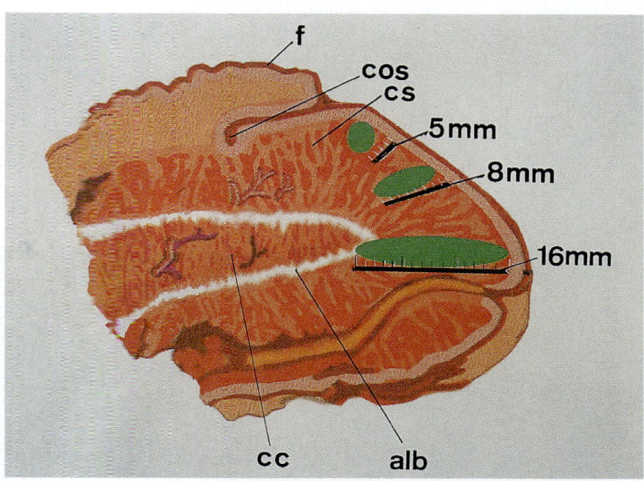

FIG. 56. Depth of invasion and prognosis. Anatomical diagram of a longitudinal section of a penectomy specimen showing an ideal representation of three moderately differentiated squamous cell carcinomas (green) with superficial (5 mm), intermediate (8 mm), and deep infiltration (16 mm) of superficial CS, deep CS, and corpus cavernosum (cc). They correspond, respectively, to null, low, and high risk of regional metastasis. Other anatomical features shown are the foreskin (f), the coronal sulcus (cos), and the albuginea (alb).

that help to predict regional and systemic metastasis in our experience are histologic grade and depth of penetration of the tumor into the various penile anatomical layers (137). Low-grade neoplasms superficially invading anatomical layers to a depth less than 6 mm usually are not associated with regional metastasis. In contrast, neoplasms of high-grade histology and deep invasion into the CS, dartos, or CC (more than 8–10 mm) are associated with a high rate of metastasis (more than 80% of the cases). It is more difficult to predict the outcome of tumors of intermediate- or high-grade histology with invasion of the CS or dartos to a depth of 5 to 10 mm (Fig. 56). In an unpublished series we found a 15% risk of metastasis in such a group of patients. Other pathologic factors predictive of poor outcome are vascular or lymphatic invasion, more than 20 mitoses, a vertical pattern of growth, and special histologic subtypes such as the basaloid, sarcomatoid, solid, anaplastic, and pseudoglandular. Carcinoma with exclusive location in the foreskin (Fig. 57) appears to carry a better prognosis than those located in the glans (141). This may be due to the higher frequency of low-grade verruciform or more superficial lesions in the prepuce.

Squamous Cell Carcinoma and HPV

A possible role of HPV in the causation of some forms of penile cancer is supported by the finding of the virus in preneoplastic and neoplastic penile lesions (142) as well as in sexual partners of women with HPV-related lesions, and the coexistence of high frequency of cervical (a well-known HPV-related neoplasm) and penile cancer in the same geographical areas (112,143–145). Some studies reported a high incidence of HPV in penile cancer (18,59,146). It does appear, however, that according to more recent reports only a subset of penile cancers are related to HPV and most are not. This was substantiated in a study of 117 specimens with SCC and its variants, using polymerase chain reaction (PCR). It demonstrated the presence of the virus in only 22% of the cases (132). This low figure is similar to that reported in other recent studies (147,148) and similar to published findings in vulvar cancer. Of interest was the finding of a correlation of HPV 16 and special subtypes of penile cancer such as the basaloid, condylomatous, and mixed condylomatous-basaloid. Other pathologic factors correlated with the presence of HPV were anatomical site (the glans), the vertical growth pattern, and poor differentiation of the tumor (132). Benign condyloma acuminatum, usually associated with HPV, may coexist with SCC of the penis (Fig. 58).

Rare and Metastatic Neoplasms

Malignant melanomas (Fig. 59) are the most commonly reported penile neoplasms (149–152) after SSC. They are rare, and mainly localized in the glans; 43% of patients with melanoma show inguinal lymph node metastasis at the time of diagnosis. The prognosis is dismal. Basal cell carcinomas arise in the skin of the shaft (Fig. 60) and show no metastatic

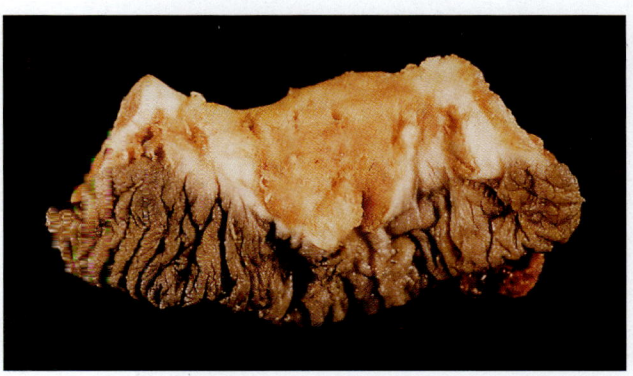

FIG. 57. Carcinoma exclusive of the foreskin. A flat beige granular tumor is present on the mucosal aspect of the foreskin, with minimal extension to the pigmented skin.

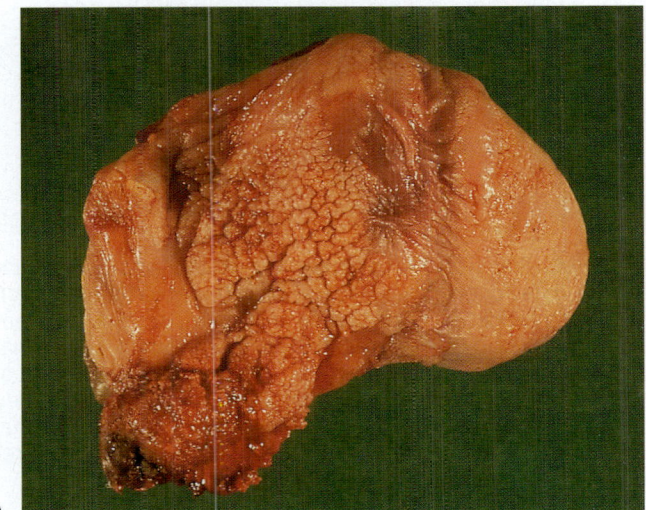
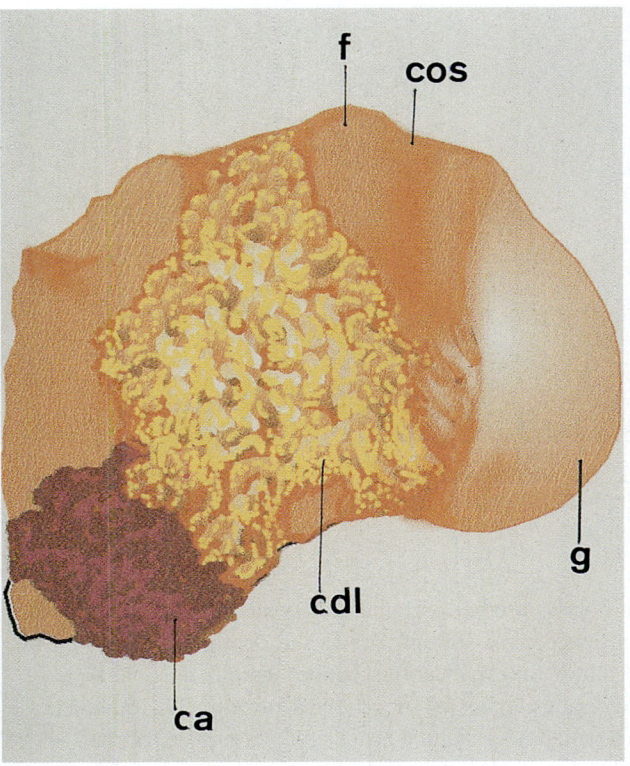

FIG. 58. Coexistence of benign condyloma acuminatum with an infiltrating squamous cell carcinoma. **A:** Partial penectomy specimen of on uncircumcised male. The foreskin has been totally retracted to show the lesion. **B:** The same specimen—the condyloma (cdl) *(yellow)*, and the malignant tumor (ca) *(purple)*. Note the cerebriform or cobblestone appearance of the condyloma and the solid granular pattern of the carcinoma. Both lesions involve the foreskin (f). The coronal sulcus (cos) and glans (g) are free of tumor.

potential (153–155). They can be multicentric (156). Sweat gland adenomas (syringomas) (Fig. 61) (157) and carcinoma with pagetoid features have also been reported. There is a great variety of benign and malignant penile soft tissue tumors, although they are rare (158). Most commonly reported are hemangiomas (159–162) lymphangiomas (163), neurofibromas (164,165), glomus tumors (166), fibrohistiocytomas (167), and granular cell myoblastomas (168,169). One of the frequent soft tissue sarcomas arising in the penis is leiomyosarcoma (170–174). Other malignant soft tissue neoplasms reported are angiosarcoma (175,176), Kaposi's sarcoma with (177,178) or without (179,180) AIDS (Fig. 62), embryonal rhabdomyosarcoma (181), malignant fibrohistiocytoma (182), epithelioid sarcoma (183), clear cell sarcoma (184), and fibrosarcoma (185). Primary lymphomas of the penis are extremely rare (186,187), as is histiocytosis (188).

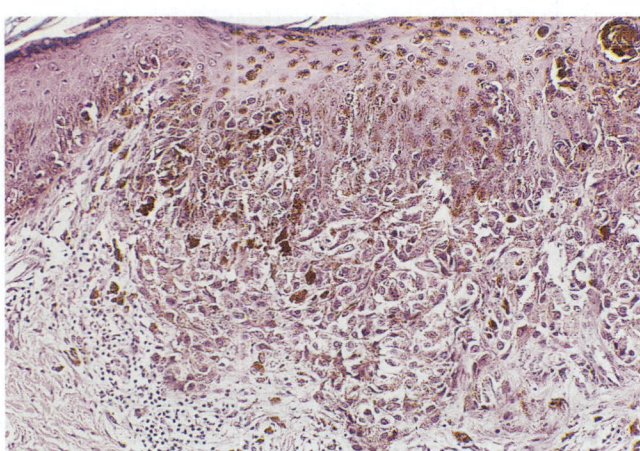

FIG. 59. Malignant melanoma. Pigmented malignant melanoma of the glans penis.

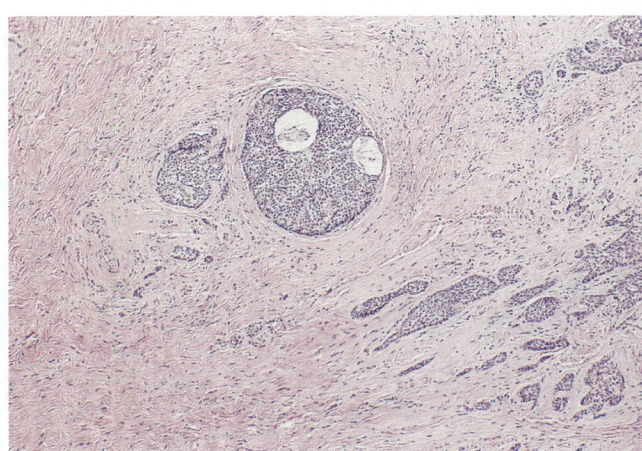

FIG. 60. Basal cell carcinoma, skin of the shaft. Nests of basal cell with peripheral palisading, with diffuse infiltration and desmoplasia.

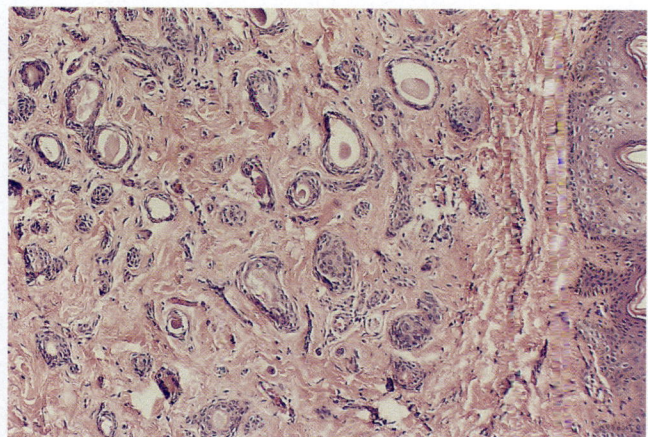

FIG. 61. Syringoma of the foreskin. Lamina propria is replaced by a sweat gland adenoma with syringomatous features. (Courtesy of Dr. Ernest Lack, Georgetown University.)

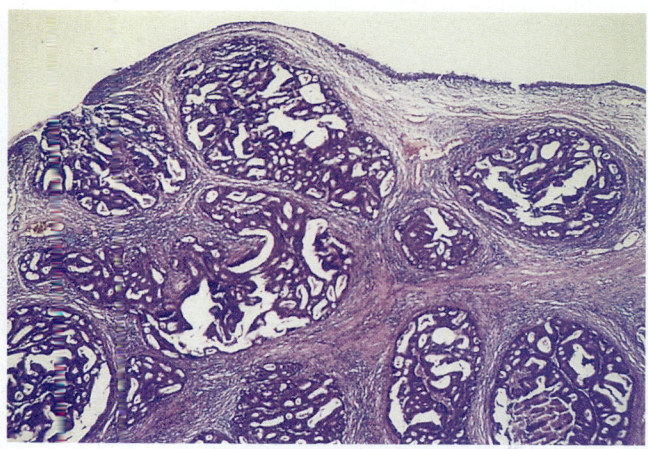

FIG. 64. Metastatic colonic carcinoma to the penis. An adenocarcinoma of colonic type involves periurethral corpus spongiosum. Additional nodules of carcinoma were found in the corpus cavernosum and fascia. (Courtesy of Dr. Carmelo Caballero, Paraguay)

Although the penis is a highly vascularized organ, metastases are unusual (189). Metastatic tumors from the urogenital area and from neighboring organs are most commonly reported (189). Urogenital, renal, urinary bladder (Fig. 63), and prostatic carcinomas have been described (190–192). Metastatic tumors from distant organs (Fig. 64) have also been described as primary sites (193,194). A prominent clinical feature of metastatic carcinoma is the so-called malignant priapism, due to massive replacement of corpora cavernosa by the neoplasm (Fig. 65).

Giant Condyloma Acuminatum (GC)

The giant condyloma (GC) is a benign, exceedingly rare exophytic arborescent papillomatous growth of the penis, sometimes referred to as Buschke-Lowenstein tumor (195). It occurs in patients slightly older than those with common

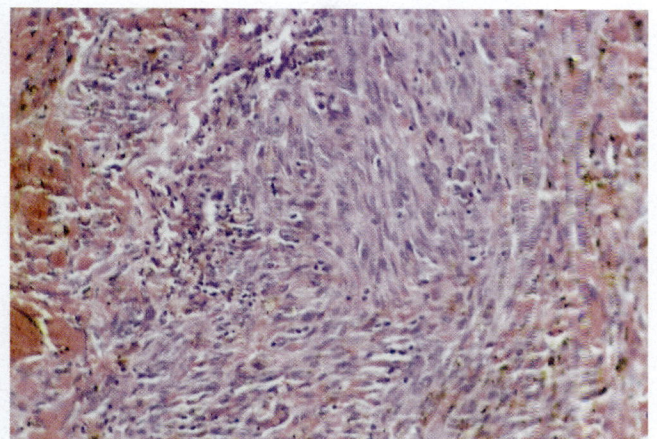

FIG. 62. Kaposi's sarcoma. This biopsy was taken from a dark-blue 3-mm lesion in the glans penis of a 42-year-old man without AIDS. The lesion shows a spindle cell growth with hemorrhagic features.

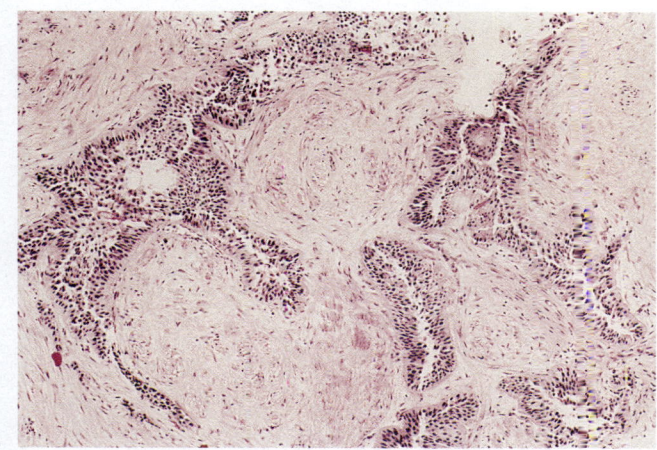 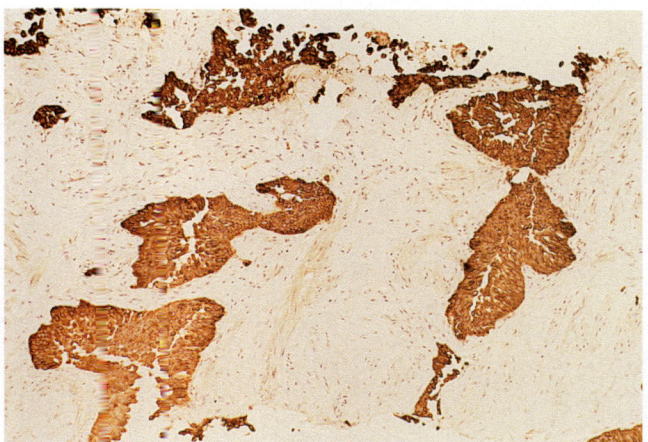

A **B**

FIG. 63. Metastatic bladder transitional cell carcinoma (TCC) of bladder to the penis. **A:** Nest of papillary TCC invading fibromuscular tissue. **B:** Immunostain for keratin shows the intramuscular metastatic carcinoma.

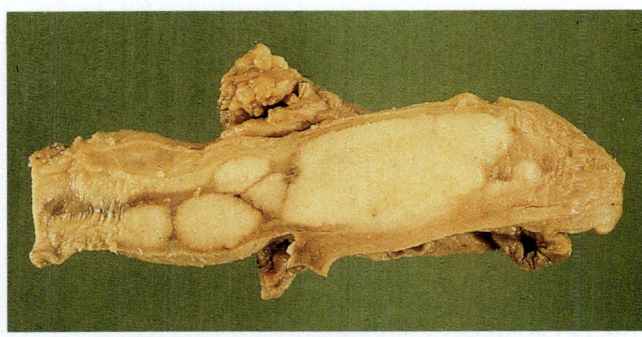
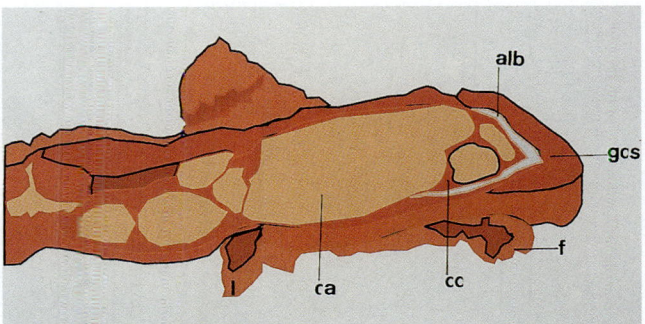

FIG. 65. Metastatic adeno-squamous cell carcinoma to the penis, primary in the prostate, with priapism. **A:** Longitudinal section of a total penectomy specimen showing multiple tan nodules of tumor filling most of the corpora cavernosa. **B:** The epithelial anatomical structures from which penile cancer usually originates (glans, sulcus, and foreskin epithelia) are not involved by the tumor. BCS, glans corpus spongiosum; f, foreskin; alb, albuginea; cc, corpus cavernosum; ca, carcinoma.

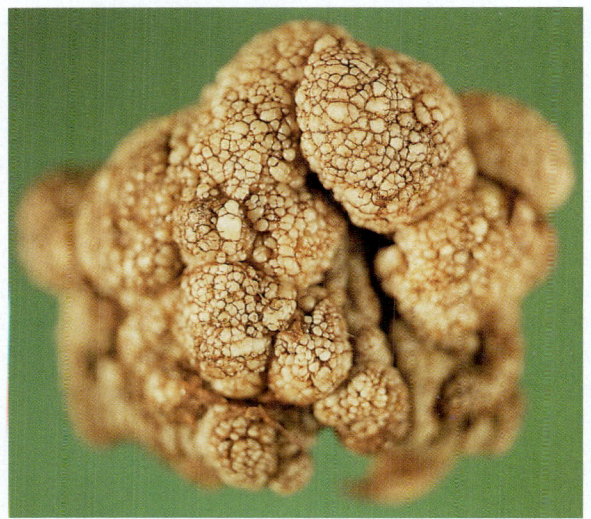

FIG. 66. Giant condyloma acuminatum. Large exophytic tumor located in the foreskin measuring 5 cm. The surface shows a typical cobblestone appearance.

condylomata and younger than those with condylomatous (warty) carcinoma, the other two HPV-related lesions of the penis. There is a long duration of the disease prior to pathologic diagnosis. Most commonly, GC affects the coronal sulcus and the foreskin, but the glans can also be involved. Grossly they are large (5–10 cm) cauliflower-like verruciform tumors, usually unicentric, with a surface showing a cobblestone or gyriform appearance (Fig. 66). The cut surface shows a papillomatous growth, with a sharp separation of the lesion from the underlying stroma. By the burrowing

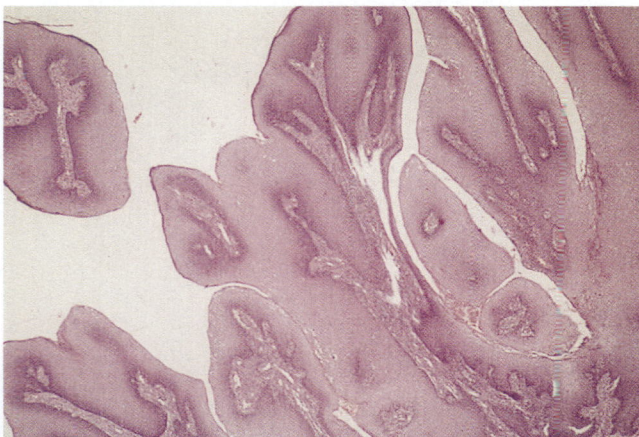

FIG. 67. Giant condyloma acuminatum. Benign papillomatosis with an arborescent pattern. Fibrovascular cores are prominent.

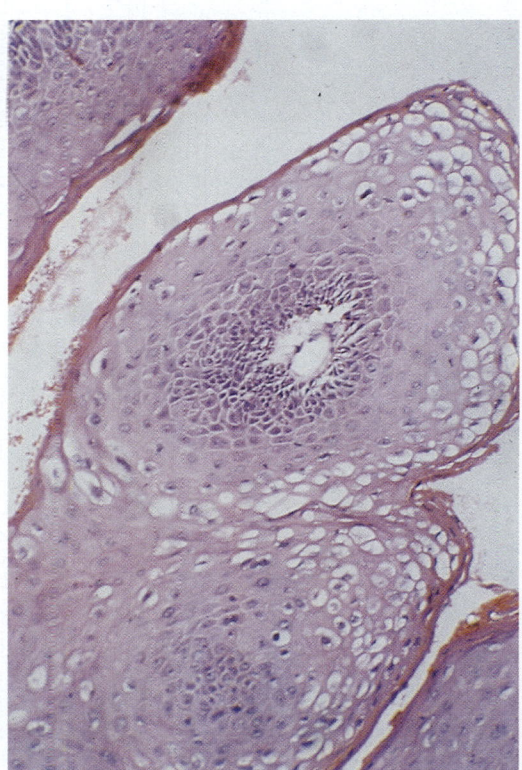

FIG. 68. Giant condyloma acuminatum. The tip of the papilla shows superficial koilocytosis. There are no significant atypical changes in the cells.

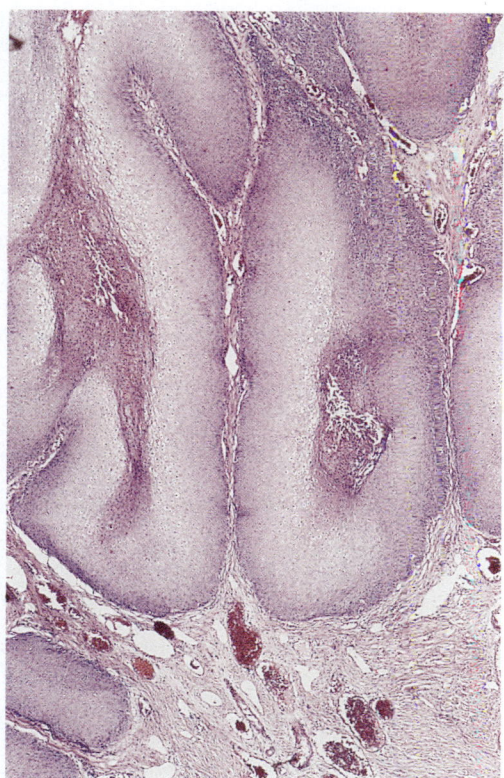

FIG. 69. Giant condyloma acuminatum. The base of the lesion invades the corpus spongiosum of the glans, with broad pushing borders.

mechanism, deep penetration of broad bands of tumor may be noted, with occasional skin fistulae. Microscopic features are identical to the common type of condyloma, with papillae showing prominent fibromuscular cores (Fig. 67), surface koilocytosis (Fig. 68), and a benign but more cellular histology, with slight atypia. The growth is more exuberant in the GC, and the base of the lesion shows a bulbous expansion into underlying tissues (Fig. 69). The differential diagnosis is with the condylomatous (warty carcinoma), a probably related tumor, which is clearly malignant histologically, with the borders between tumor and stroma being preferentially jagged. Although in the literature, GC and verrucous carcinomas have been considered the same tumor (118,133), we now think that they represent separate lesions (196). In verrucous carcinomas no evidence of koilocytosis is present and the prominence of papillae with fibrovascular cores noted in both GC and WC are not seen.

REFERENCES

1. Hricak H, Marotti M, Gilbert TJ, et al. Normal penile anatomy and abnormal penile conditions: evaluation with MR imaging. *Radiology* 1988;169:683–690.
2. Rouviere H. *Anatomy of the human lymphatic system.* Ann Arbor, MI: Edwards Broders, 1938.
3. Testut L-Latarjet A. *Tratado de anatomia humana.* Barcelona: Salvat, 1979.
4. Barreto J, Caballero C, Cubilla AL. Penis. In: Sternberg SS, eds. *Histology for pathologists.* New York: Raven Press, 1991:721–730.
5. Bloom W, Fawcett DW. *A textbook of histology,* 11th ed. Philadelphia: WD Saunders, 1991:802.
6. Cabañas RM. Anatomy and biopsy of sentinel lymph nodes. *Urol Clin North Am* 1992;19:267–276.
7. Crawford DE, Daneshgari F. Management of regional lymph drainage in carcinoma of the penis. *Urol Clin North Am* 1992;19:305–317.
8. Herbut PA. *Urological pathology.* Philadelphia: Lea & Febiger, 1952:1196–1222.
9. Oesch Y, Pinter A, Rasley P. Penile agenesis: a report of six cases. *J Pediatr Surg* 1987;22:172–174.
10. Elder J. Congenital anomalies of the genitalia. In: *Campbell's urology* 5th ed. Philadelphia: WB Saunders, 1982:1920–1937.
11. Chesney T, Murphey W. Diseases of the penis and scrotum. In: *Urologic pathology.* Philadelphia: WB Saunders, 1989:380–408.
12. Duckett JW. Advances in hypospadia repair. *Postgrad Med J* 1990;66(1):62–71.
13. Quiles DR, Betllcoh Mas I, Jimenez A, Verdeguer J, Botella R, Castells A. Gonococcal infection of the penile median raphe cyst. *Int J Dermatol* 1987;26(4):242–243.
14. Claudy A, Dutoit M, Boucheron S. Epidermal and urethral penile cyst. *Acta Dermatol Venereol (Stockh)* 1991;71:61–62.
15. Sarma D, Weilbaecher T. Human os penis. *Urology* 1990;35:349–350.
16. Fussell E, Kaach M, Cherry R, Roberts J. Adherence of bacteria to human foreskins. *J Urol* 1988;140:997–1001.
17. Burdge DR, Bowei W, Chow A. *Gardnerelia vaginalis*-associated balanoposthitis. *Sex Transm Dis* 1986;13:159–162.
18. Coldiron CB, Jacobson C. Common penile lesions. *Urol Clin North Am* 1988;15(4):671–685.
19. Brady M. Cellulitis of the penis and scrotum due to group B streptococcus. *J Urol* 1987;137:736–737.
20. Niedrach WL, Lerner R, Linke C. Penile abscess involving the corpus cavernosum. A case report. *J Urol* 1989;141:374–375.
21. Sater A, Vanderdris M. Abscess of corpus cavernosum. *J Urol* 1989;141:949.
22. Adams J, Mata J, Venable D, Culkin D, Bochini J. Fournier's gangrene in children. *Urology* 1990;35:439–441.
23. Annobil SD, Al-Hilfi A, Kazi T. Primary tuberculosis of the penis in an infant. *Tubercle* 1990;71:229–230.
24. Jeyakumar W, Ganesh R, Mohanram MS, Shanmugasundararaj A. Papulonecrotic tuberculids of the penis. *Genitourin Med* 1988;64:130–132.
25. Perfect JR, Seaworth BA. Penile cryptococcosis with review of mycotic infections of the penis. *Urology* 1985;2505:528–531.
26. Hay PE, Lam FWK, Kitchen VS, Horner S, Bridger J, Weber J. Gummatous lesions in men infected with human immunodeficiency virus and syphilis. *Genitourin Med* 1990;60:374–379.
27. Davis CM. Granuloma inguinale: a clinical, histological and ultrastructural study. *JAMA* 1970;211:632–636.
28. Smith EB, Custer RP. The histopathology of lymphogranuloma venereum. *J Urol* 1950;63(3):546–563.
29. McCarley ME, Cruz PD, Sontheimer RD. Chancroid: clinical variants from an epidemic in Dallas County. *J Am Acad Dermatol* 1988;19:330–337.
30. Sheldon WH, Heyman A. Studies on chancroid: observations of the histology with an evaluation of biopsy as a diagnostic procedure. *Am J Pathol* 1946;22:415–425.
31. Schniederman H, Robert NJ, Walker S, Memoll VA. Herpes without vesicles: limited recurrent genital lesions in an immunodebilitated host. *South Med J* 1986;79:368–370.
32. Oriel JD. Natural history of genital warts. *Br J Venereol Dis* 1971;47:1–13.
33. Couturier J, Sastre-Garaux, Schneider-Mauncury S, Labib A, Orth G. Integration of papillomavirus DNA near myc genes in genital carcinomas and its consequences for proto-oncogene expression. *J Virol* 1991;65:4534–4538.
34. Monsonego J, Magdelena H, Catalan F, Coscas Y, Serat L, Sastre X. Estrogen and progesterone receptors in cervical human papillomavirus related lesions. *Int J Cancer* 1991;48:533–539.
35. Schlegel R. Papillomavirus and human cancer. *Virology* 1990;1:297–306.
36. Woodworth CE, Waggoner S, Barnes W, Stoler MH, Dipaolo JA. Human cervical and foreskin epithelial cells immortalized by human papillomavirus DNAs exhibit dysplastic differentiation in vivo. *Cancer Res* 1990;50:3709–3715.

37. Milburn PB, Brandsma JL, Goldsman CI, Tepliztz DE, Heilman EL. Disseminated warts and evolving squamous cell carcinoma in a patient with acquired immunodeficiency syndrome. *J Am Acad Dermatol* 1988;1:401–405.
38. Barrasso R, De Brux J, Croissant O, Orth G. High prevalence of papillomavirus-associated penile intraepithelial neoplasia in sexual partners of women with cervical intraepithelial neoplasia. *N Engl J Med* 1987;317:916–923.
39. Boon ME, Schneider A, Hogenwoning CGA, Van Der Kwast TH, Bolhuis P, Kok LP. Penile studies in heterosexual partners: peniscopy, cytology, histology and immunohistochemistry. *Cancer* 1988;61:2652–1659.
40. Campion MJ, McCance DJ, Mitchell HS, Jenkins D, Singer A. Subclinical penile human papillomavirus infection and dysplasia in consorts of women with cervical neoplasia. *Genitourin Med* 1988,64:90–99.
41. Hippellainen M, Ylykoski M, Saarikiske S, Syrjanen S, Syrjanen K. Genital human papillomavirus lesions of the male sexual partners; the diagnostic accuracy of peniscopy. *Genitourin Med* 1991;67:291–296.
42. Selvey L. Bunitne DW, Kennedy L, Frazer IH. Male partners of women with human papillomavirus infection: an assessment of colposcopic abnormalities by histologic examination and human papillomavirus hybridization. *Med J Aust* 1989;150:479–481.
43. O'Brien WM, Jenson AB, Lancaster WD, Masted WC. Human papillomavirus typing of penile condylomas. *J Urol* 1989;141:863–865.
44. Rosemberg SM. Subclinical papillomaviral infection of male genitalia. *Urology* 1985;26:554–557.
45. Koronel R, Stefanon B, Pilotti S, Bandieramonte G, Rilke F, De Palo G. Genital papillomavirus infection in males: a clinicopathologic study. *Tumori* 1991;77:76–82.
46. Comite SL, Castadot MJ. Colposcopic evaluation of men with genital warts. *J Am Acad Dermatol* 1988;18:1274–1278.
47. Krebs HS, Schneider V. Human papillomavirus-associated lesions of the penis: colposcopy, cytology and histology. *Obstet Gynecol* 1987;70:299–304.
48. Von Krogh G, Syrjanen SM, Syrjanem KJ. Advantage of human papillomavirus typing in the clinical evaluation of genitoanal warts. *J Am Acad Dermatol* 1988;18:495–453.
49. Nuovo GJ, Hochman HA, Ellezri YD, Lastarria D, Comite SL, Silvers DN. Detection of human papillomavirus DNA in penile lesions histologically negative from condylomata. *Am J Surg Pathol* 1990;14:829–836.
50. Syrjanem SM, Von Krogh G, Syrjanem K. Detection of human papillomavirus DNA in anogenital condyloma using in situ hybridization applied to paraffin sections. *Genitourin Med* 1987;63:32–39.
51. Zderic SA, Carpiniello VL, Mallcy TR, Rando RF. Urologic applications of human papillomavirus typing using deoxyribonucleic acid probes for the diagnosis and treatment of genital condyloma. *J Urol* 1989;141:163–165.
52. McCance DJ, Kalache A, Ashdown K, et al. Human papillomavirus types 16 and 18 in carcinomas of the penis from Brazil. *Int J Cancer* 1986;37:55–59.
53. Varma VA, Sanchez-Lanier M, Unger ER, et al. Association of human papillomavirus with penile cancer: a study using polymerase chain reaction and in situ hybridization. *Hum Pathol* 1991;22:908–913.
54. Villa LL, Lopes A. Human papillomavirus sequences in penile carcinomas in Brazil. *Int J Cancer* 1986;37:853–855.
55. Bissada NK, Cole AT, Fried FA. Extensive condylomata acuminata of the entire male urethra and the bladder. *J Urol* 1974;112:201–203.
56. Green J, Monterio E, Gibson P. Detection of human papillomavirus DNA in semen from patients with intrameatal penile warts. *Genitourin Med* 1989;65:357–360.
57. Kateraris PM, Cossart YE, Rose BR, et al. Human papillomavirus: the untreated male reservoir. *J Urol* 1988;140:300–305.
58. Arumainayagam JT, Sumathilpa AHT, Smallman LA, Shahmanesh M. Flat condyloma of the penis presenting as patchy balanoposthitis. *Genitourin Med* 1990;66:251–253.
59. Loning T, Riviere A, Henke RP, Von Preyss S, Dorner A. Penile-anal condylomas and squamous cell cancer. *Virchows Arch [A]* 1988;413:491–498.
60. Chalmers RJG, Burton PA, Bennett R, et al. Lichen sclerosus et atrophicus: a common distinctive cause of phimosis in boys. *Arch Dermatol* 1984;120:1025–1027.
61. Bart RS, Kopft AW. Squamous cell carcinoma arising in balanitis xerotica obliterans. *J Dermatol Surg Oncol* 1978;4.556–558.
62. Bain L, Geronemus R. The association of lichen planus of the penis with squamous carcinoma in situ with verrucous squamous carcinoma. *J Dermatol Surg Oncol* 1989;15:413–417.
63. Thambi Dorai CR, Kandasami P. Fournier's gangrene: its aetiology and management. *Aust NZ J Surg* 1991;61:370–372.
64. Corbus BC, Harris FG. Erosive and gangrenous balanitis. The fourth venereal disease. *JAMA* 1909,52:1474.
65. Barile MF, et al. Penile lesions among U.S. Armed Forces personnel in Japan. *Arch Dermatol* 1962;86.273–276.
66. Zoon JI. Balanopostithe chronique circonscrite benigne a plasmocytes. *Dermatologica* 1952;105:1–7.
67. Sauteyrand P, Wong E, Mcdonald DM. Zoons balanitis (balanitis circumscripta plasmacellularis). *Br J Dermatol* 1981;105:195–199.
68. Gelbrad MK. Dystrophic penile calcification in Peyronie's disease. *J Urol* 1988;139:738–740.
69. Bivens CH, Marecek RL, Feldman JM. Peyronie's disease: a presenting complaint of the carcinoid syndrome. *N Engl J Med* 1973;289:844–845.
70. Gilmore JAI, Weingad DA, Burgdorf WHC. Penile nodules in Southeast Asian men. *Arch Dermatol* 1983;119:446–447.
71. Tannembaum MH, Becker SW. Papillae of the corona of the glans penis. *J Urol* 1965;93:391–395.
72. Winer JH, Winer LH. Hirsutoid papillomas of the coronal margin of the glans penis. *J Urol* 1955;74:375–378.
73. Revuz J, Clerice T. Penile melanosis. *J Am Acad Dermatol* 1939;20:567–570.
74. Barnhill RL, Albert LS, Shama SK, Bolgenhersh MH, Rhodes A, Sober AJ. Genital lentiginosis: a clinical and histopathologic study. *J Am Acad Dermatol* 1990;22:453–460.
75. Gharpuray MB, Tolat SN. Nonvenereal sclerosing lymphangitis of the penis. *Cutis* 1991;47:421–422.
76. Ball TP, Pickett JD, Traumatic lymphangitis of the penis. *Urology* 1975;6:594–597.
77. Crozzo DW, Vachher p, Sau P, Frishberg DP, James WD. Verruciform xanthoma: a benign penile growth. *J Urol* 1995;153:1625–1627.
78. George WM. Azadeh B. Verruciform xanthoma of the penis. *Cutis* 1989;44:167–170.
79. Kraemer BB, Schmidt WA, Foucar E, Rosen T. Verruciform xanthoma of the penis. *Arch Dermatol* 1981;117:516–518.
80. Oertel YC, Johnson FB. Sclerosing lipogranuloma of male genitalia. Review of 23 cases. *Arch Pathol Lab Med* 1977;101:321–326.
81. Nielsen GP, Pilch BZ, Black-Schaffer WS, Young RH. Wegener's granulomatosis of the penis clinically simulating carcinoma. Report of a case. *J Urol Pathol* 1996;4:265–272.
82. Nielsen GP, Rosenberg AE, Dretler SP, Young RH. An unusual pseudotumor of the penis. Report of case associated with chronic catheterzation. *J Urol Pathol* 1996;4:79–84.
83. Hassan AA. Orteza AM, Milam DF. Penile horn: review of the literature with 3 case reports. *J Urol* 1967;97:315–317.
84. Piccinno R, Carrel CF, Menni S, Brancaleon W. Preputial ectopic sebaceous glands mimicking molluscoum contagiosum. *Acta Derm Venereol (Stockh)* 1990;70:344–345.
85. Cubilla AL. Carcinoma of the penis. In consultation. *Mod Pathol* 1995;8:116–118.
86. Andersson L, Johnsson G, Brehmer-Andersson E. Erythroplasia of Queyrat—carcinoma in situ. *Scand J Urol Neurophol* 1967;1:303–306.
87. Graham JH, Helwig EB. Erythroplasia of Queyrat: a clinico-pathologic and histochemical study. *Cancer* 1973;32:1396.
88. Grossman B. Premalignant and early carcinomas of the penis and scrotum. *Urol Clin North Am* 1992;19:221–226.
89. Kaye V, Zhang G, Dehner LP, Fraley EE. Carcinoma in situ of penis. Is distinction between erythroplasia of Queyrat and Bowen's disease relevant? *Urology* 1990;36:479–482.
90. Lucia MS, Miller GJ. Histopathology of malignant lesions of the penis. *Urol Clin North Am* 1992;19:227–246.
91. Queyrat L. Erythroplasie du gland. *Bull Soc Franc Dermatol Syph* 1911;22:378–382.
92. Kurman RJ, Norris HJ, Wilkinson E. *Tumors of the cervix, vagina and vulva.* Atlas of tumor pathology, 3rd series, fascicle 4. Washington, DC: Armed Forces Institute of Pathology, 1992:202–203.
93. Metcalf JS, Lee RE, Maize JC. Epidermotropic urothelial carcinoma involving the glans penis. *Arch Dermatol* 1985;121:532–534.
94. Wade TR, Kopf AW, Ackerman AB. Bowenoid papulosis of the genitalia. *Arch Dermatol* 1979;115:306–308.

95. Wade TR, Kopf AW, Ackerman AB. Bowenoid papulosis of the penis. *Cancer* 1978;42:2078–2085.
96. Eisen RF, Bawan J, Cahn TH. Spontaneous regression of bowenoid papulosis of the penis. *Cutis* 1983;32:269–272.
97. Patterson JW, Kao GF, Graham JH, et al. Bowenoid papulosis: a clinicopathologic study with ultrastructural observations. *Cancer* 1986;57:823–836.
98. Hauser B, Gross G, Shneider A, Michele De Villiers E, Gissmann L, Wagner D. HPV-16-related bowenoid papulosis [letter]. *Lancet* 1985;106.
99. Ikenberg H, Gissmann K, Gross G, Grussendorf-Conen EI, Zur-Hausen H. Human papillomavirus type-16 related DNA in genital Bowen's disease and in bowenoid papulosis. *Int J Cancer* 1983;32:563–565.
100. Hurwitz RM, Egan WT, Murphy SH, Pontius EE, Forster ML. Bowenoid papulosis and squamous cell carcinoma of the genitalia: suspected sexual transmission. *Cutis* 1987;39:193–196.
101. Obalek S, Jablonaska S, Beadenon S, Walczak L, Orth G. Bowenoid papulosis of the male and female genitalia: risk of cervical neoplasia. *J Am Dermatol* 1986;14:433–444.
102. Dodge OG, Linsell CA. Carcinoma of the penis in Ugandan and Kenyan Africans. *Cancer* 1963;16:1255–1263.
103. Malik MO, Belail OM. Pattern of tumors of the male genitalia in the Sudan. *East Afr Med J* 1979;56:229–234.
104. Oota K. Cancer of the penis in Japan. *Rev Inst Natl Cancer* 1964;15:289–292.
105. Persky L. Epidemiology of cancer of the penis. *Recent results. Cancer Res* 1977;60:97–109.
106. Lebron RF, Riveros M. Geographical pathology of cancer of the penis. *Cancer* 1963;16:798–810.
107. Muir CS. Male and female genital tract cancer in Singapore. *Cancer* 1962;15:354–382.
108. Brinton LA, Yao LJ, Shou-de R, et al. Risk factors for penile cancer: results from a case control study in China. *Int J Cancer* 1991;47:504–509.
109. Maden C, Sherman KJ, Beckman AM, et al. History of circumcision, medical conditions and sexual activity and risk of penile cancer. *J Natl Cancer Inst* 1993;85:19–24.
110. Wolbarst AL. Circumcision and penile cancer. *Lancet* 1932;1:150–153.
111. Bissada N, Marcos R, El-Senoussi M. Post-circumcision carcinoma of the penis. *J Urol* 1986;135:283–285.
112. Martinez Y. Relationship of squamous cell carcinoma of the cervix uteri to squamous cell carcinoma of the penis among Puerto Rican women married to men with penile carcinoma. *Cancer* 1969;24:777–780.
113. Boon ME, Susanti Y, Torsche MJA, Kok LP. Human papilomavirus (HPV) associated male and female genital carcinomas in a Hindu population. The male as vector and victim. *Cancer* 1989;64:559–565.
114. Daling JR. Sherman KJ, Hislop TG, et al. Cigarette smoking and the risk of anogenital cancer. *Am J Epidemiol* 1992;135:180–189.
115. Stern RS. Genital tumors among men with psoriasis exposed to psoralens and ultraviolet A radiation (PUVA) and ultraviolet B radiation. The photochemotherapy follow up study. *N Engl J Med* 1990;322:1149–1151.
116. Cubilla AL, Barreto J, Caballero C, Ayala G, Riveros M. Pathologic features of epidermoid carcinomas of the penis. A prospective study of 66 cases. *Am J Surg Pathol* 1993;17:753–763.
117. Cubilla AL, Reuter V, Ayala G, Ocampos S, Fair W. Basaloid carcinoma of the penis: a distinct clinico-pathologic entity. *Mod Pathol* 1995;(abst).
118. Cubilla AL, Reuter VE, Gregoire L, et al. Basaloid squamous cell carcinoma: an aggressive HPV-related penile neoplasm. A report of 20 cases. *Am J Surg Pathol* (in press).
119. Cubilla AL, Ayala MT, Barreto JE, Bellasai JG, Noel JC. Surface adenosquamous carcinoma of the penis. A report of three cases. *Am J Surg Pathol* 1996;20:156–160.
120. Cubilla AL, Barreto JE, Ayala G. The penis. In: Sternberg SS, ed. *Diagnostic surgical pathology*, 2nd ed. New York: Raven Press, 1994;1949–1973.
121. Merrin CE. Cancer of the penis. *Cancer* 1980;45:1973–1979.
122. Derrick FC Jr, Lynch KM, Kretkowski C, Yarbrough WJ. Epidermoid carcinoma of the penis: computer analysis of 87 cases. *J Urol* 1973;110:303–305.
123. Hanash KA, Furlow WL, Utz DC, Harrison EG Jr. Carcinoma of the penis. A clinico-pathologic study. *J Urol* 1970;104:291–297.
124. Hardner GJ, Bhanalaph CT, Murphy GP, Albert DJ, Moore RH. Carcinoma of the penis. Analysis of therapy in 100 consecutive cases. *J Urol* 1972;108:428–430.
125. Hoppman HJ, Fraley EE. Squamous cell carcinoma of the penis. *J Urol* 1978;120:393–398.
126. Jones WG, Fossa SD. Hamers H, VanDen Bogaert W. Penis cancer: a review by the joint radiotherapy committee of the European Organization for Research and Treatment of Cancer (EORTC) Genitourinary and Radiotherapy groups. *J Surg Oncol* 1989;40:227–231.
127. Kamat MR, Kulkarni JN, Tongaonkar HB. Carcinoma of the penis: the Indian experience. *J Surg Oncol* 1993;52:50–55.
128. Narayana AS, Olney LE, Loening SA, Weirmar GW, Culp DA. Carcinoma of the penis. Analysis of 219 cases. *Cancer* 1982;49:2185–2191.
129. Ornellas AA, Seixas AL, de Moraes JR. Analyses of 200 lymphadenectomies in patients with penile carcinoma. *J Urol* 1991;146:330–332.
130. Ornellas AA, Seixas ALC, Marota A, Wisnescky A, Campos F, de Moraes JR. Surgical treatment of invasive squamous cell carcinoma of the penis: retrospective analysis of 350 cases. *J Urol* 1994;151:1244.
131. Srinivas V, Morse MJ, Herr JW, Sogani PC, Whitmore WF Jr. Penile cancer: relation of extent of nodal metastasis to survival. *J Urol* 1987;137:880–882.
132. Gregoire L, Cubilla AL, Reuter VE, Haas G, Lancaster WD. Analysis of HPV DNA in 117 penile invasive carcinomas: preferential association of virus with high grade histologic variants. *J Natl Cancer Inst* 1995;87:1705–1709.
133. Johnson DE, Lo RK, Srigley J, Ayala AG. Verrucous carcinoma of the penis. *J Urol* 1985;133:216–218.
134. Mckee PH, Lowe D, Haigh J. Penile verrucous carcinoma. *Histopathology* 1983;7:897–906.
135. Wood EW, Gardner WA, Brown FM. Spindle cell squamous carcinoma of the penis. *J Urol* 1972;107:590–591.
136. Manceni KS. Manaligod JR, Ray B. Spindle cell squamous carcinoma of the glans penis: a light and electron microscopic study. *Cancer* 1980;46:2266–2272.
137. Caballero C, Cubilla AL, Barreto J, Riveros M. Factores patológicos relacionados con metastasis inguinal en carcinoma epidermoide del glande penal. *Patología (Spain)* 1991;24:1137–1141.
138. Horenblas S, Van Tinteren HV, Delemarre JFM, Moonen LMF, Lustig V, Kroger R. Squamous cell carcinoma of the penis: accuracy of tumor, nodes and metastasis classification system, and role of lymphangiography, computerized tomography scan and fine needle aspiration cytology. *J Urol* 1991;146:1279–1283.
139. Horenblas S, Van Tinteren HV, Delmarre JFM, Moonen LMF, Lustig V, Van Waardenberg EW. Squamous cell carcinoma of the penis. III Treatment of regional nodes. *J Urol* 1993;149:492.
140. Maiche AG, Pyrhonen S, Karkinen M. Histological grading of squamous cell carcinoma of the penis: a new scoring system. *Br J Urol* 1991;67:522–526.
141. Cuella AL, Bray C, Barreto J, Caballero C. Carcinoma epidermoide del prepucio. Estudio clinico-patológico de 40 casos. *Anales de la Facultad de Ciencias Médicas. Asunción* 1992;24(1,2):187–208.
142. Iwasawa A, Kumamoto Y, Fujinaga K. Detection of human papillomavirus deoxyribonucleic acid in penile carcinoma by polymerase chain reaction and in situ hybridization. *J Urol* 1993;149:59–63.
143. Graham S. Priore R, Graham M, Browne R, Burnett W, West D. Genital cancer in wives of penile cancer patients. *Cancer* 1979;44:1870–1874.
144. Hellberg D, Nilsson S. Genital cancer among wives of men with penile cancer. A study between 1958–1982. *Br J Obstet Gynaecol* 1989;96:221–225.
145. Maiche AG, Pyrhonen S. Risk of cervical cancer among wives of men with carcinoma of the penis. *Acta Oncol* 1990;29:569–571.
146. Sarkar FH, Miles BJ, Plieth DH, Crissman JD. Detection of human papillomavirus in squamous neoplasms of the penis. *J Urol* 1992;147:389–392.
147. Weaver MG, Abdul Karin FW, Dale G, Sorensen K, Huang YT. Detection and localization of human papillomavirus in penile condylomas and squamous cell carcinomas using in situ hybridization with biotinylated DNA viral probes. *Mod Pathol* 1989;2:94–100.
148. Wiener JS, Effert PJ, Humphrey PA, Yo L, Liu ET, Walther PJ. Prevalence of HPV types 16 and 18 in squamous cell carcinoma of the penis: a retrospective analysis of primary and metastatic lesions by differential PCR. *Int J Cancer* 1992;50:694–701.

149. Das Gupta T, Grabstald H. Melanoma of the genitourinary tract. *J Urol* 1965;93:607–614.
150. Khezri AA, Dounis A, Robert JBM. Primary malignant melanoma of the penis. Two cases and a review of the literature. *Br J Urol* 1979;51:147.
151. Stilwell TJ, Zincke H, Gaffey TA, Woods JE. Malignant melanoma of the penis. *J Urol* 1988;140:72–75.
152. Begun FP, Grossman HB, Diokno AC, Sogani PC. Malignant melanoma of the penis and male urethra. *J Urol* 1984;132:123–125.
153. Goldwing D, Scott G, Klaus S. Penile basal cell carcinoma. *J Am Acad Dermatol* 1989;20:1094–1097.
154. Fegen JP, Beebe D, Persky L. Basal cell carcinoma of the penis. *Urol* 1970;104:864–866.
155. McGregor DH, Tanimura A, Weigel JW. Basal cell carcinoma of the penis. *Urology* 1982;20:320–323.
156. Peison B, Benisch B, Nicora B. Multicentric basal cell carcinoma of penile skin. *Urology* 1985;25:322–323.
157. Lo JS, Dijkstra JW, Bergfeld WF. Syringomas of the penis. *Int J Dermatol* 1990;29:309–310.
158. Dehner LP, Smith BH. Soft tissue tumors of the penis. A clinicopathologic study of 46 cases. *Cancer* 1970;25:1431–1447.
159. Senoh K, Miyazaki T, Kikuchi J, Sumiyoshe A, Kohga A. Angiomatous lesions of the glans penis. *Urology* 1981;17:194–196.
160. Mortesenn H, Murphy L. Angiomatous malformations of the glans penis. *J Urol* 1950;64:396–399.
161. Hamal HK, Goswani AK, Sharma SK, Radotre BA, Malik N. Penile venous hemangioma. *Aust NZ J Surg* 1989;59:814–816.
162. Solsona E, Ricos J, Monros J, Ibarra I, Mazcunan F. Linfangioma cavernoso de pene. *Acta Urol Esp* 1986;10:73–76.
163. Ogawa A, Watanabe K. Genitourinary neurofibromatosis in a child presenting with an enlarged penis and scrotum. *J Urol* 1986;135:755–757.
164. Dwosh J, Mininberg DT, Schlossberg J, Peterson P. Neurofibroma involving the penis in a child. *J Urol* 1984;132:988–989.
165. Maher JD, Thompson GM, Loening J, Platz CE. Penile plexiform neurofibroma: case report and review of the literature. *J Urol* 1988;139:1310–1312.
166. Macaluso JN, Sullivan JW, Tomberlin S. Glomus tumor of the glans penis. *Urology* 1985;25:409–410.
167. Kinoshita H, Okada K, Nagata Y, Kawamura N. Fibrous histiocytoma of penis. *Urology* 1985;25:544–546.
168. Stone NN, Sun CCJ, Brutscher S, Zein T. Granular cell tumor of penis. *J Urol* 1983;130:575.
169. Suarez GM, Lewis RW. Granular cell tumor of the glans penis. *J Urol* 1980;135:1252.
170. Isa SS, Almaraz R, Macgovern J. Leiomyosarcoma of the penis case report and review of the literature. *Cancer* 1984;54:939–942.
171. Greenwoon N, Fox H, Edwards EC. Leiomyosarcoma of the penis. *Cancer* 1972;29:481–483.
172. Pack GT, Trinidad SS, Humphreys GA. Primary leiomyosarcoma of the penis: report of a case. *J Urol* 1963;89:839–841.
173. McDonald MW, O'Connell JR, Monring JT, Benjamin RS. Leiomyosarcoma of the penis. *J Urol* 1983;130:788–789.
174. Smart RK. Leiomyosarcoma of the penis. *J Urol* 1984;132:356–357.
175. Hudgins TE, Hancock RA. Hemangio-endothelial sarcoma of the penis Report of a case and review of the literature. *J Urol* 1970;104:867–870.
176. Williams JJ, Mouradian JA, Hagopian BA, Gray GF. Hemangioendothelial sarcoma of penis. *Cancer* 1979;44:1146–1149.
177. Hulnes KB, Greene JB, Marcus A, et al. Kaposi's sarcoma in homosexual men. A report of eight cases. *Lancet* 1981;1:598–600.
178. Lowe FC, Lattimer DG, Metroka CE. Kaposi sarcoma of the penis in patients with acquired immunodeficiency syndrome. *J Urol* 1989;142:1475–1477.
179. Zambolin T, Simeone C, Baronchelli C, Cunico SC. Kaposi's sarcoma of the penis. *Br J Urol* 1989;63(6):645–646.
180. Conger K, Sporer A. Kaposi's sarcoma limited to glans penis. *Urology* 1985;26:173–175.
181. Ramos JZ, Pack GT. Primary embryonal rhabdomyosarcoma of the penis in a 2 year-old child. *J Urol* 1966;96:928–932.
182. Fletcher CDM, Lowe D. Inflammatory fibrous histiocytoma of the penis. *Histopathology* 1984;8:1079–1084.
183. Moore SW, Wheeler JE, Hefter LG. Epithelioid sarcoma masquerading as Peyronie's disease. *Cancer* 1975;35:1706–1710.
184. Saw D, Tse CH, Chan J, Watt CY, Ng CS, Poon YF. Clear cell sarcoma of the penis. *Hum Pathol* 1986;17:423–425.
185. Ashley DJB, Edwards EC. Sarcoma of the penis. Report of a case and review of the literature. *Br J Surg* 1957;45:170–179.
186. Gough J. Primary reticulum cell sarcoma of the penis. *Br J Urol* 1970;42:336–339.
187. Gonzalez-Campora R, Nogales FF, Lerma E, Navarro A, Matilla A. Lymphoma of the penis. *J Urol* 1981;126:270–271.
188. Myers DA, Strandjord SE, Marcus RB, Pierson KK, Walker RD. Histiocytosis X presenting as a primary penile lesion. *J Urol* 1981;126:268–269.
189. Bosch PC, Forbes KA, Kollin J, Golji H, Miller JB. Secondary carcinoma of the penis. *J Urol* 984;132:990–991.
190. Mugharbil ZH, Childs C, Tannenbaum M, Schapiro H. Carcinoma of prostate metastatic to penis. *Urology* 1985;25:314–315.
191. Perez-Meza C, Oxenhandler R. Metastatic tumors of the penis. *J Surg Oncol* 1989;42(1):11–15.
192. Hernaez Manrique I, Aurteneche JJ. Metastasis peneana de un carcinoma transicional renal. *Acta Urol Esp* 1985;9:435–436.
193. Karanjie ND, King H, Schweitzer FAW. Metastasis to the penis from carcinoma of the stomach. *Br J Urol* 1987;60:368–375.
194. Perez LM, Shumway RA, Carson CC, Fischer SR, Hudson WR. Penile metastases secondary to supraglotic squamous cell carcinoma: review of the literature. *J Urol* 1992;147:157–160.
195. Lowenstein LW. Carcinoma-like condylomata acuminata of the penis. *Med Clin North Am* 1939;23:789–795.
196. Masih AS, Stoler MH, Farrow GM, Wooldridge TN, Johansson SL. Penile verrucous carcinoma: a clinico-pathologic human papillomavirus typing and flow cytometric analysis. *Mod Pathol* 1992;5:48–55.

X

Female Reproductive System and Peritoneum

CHAPTER 49

Gestational Trophoblastic Disease

Ie-Ming Shih, Michael T. Mazur, and Robert J. Kurman

Gestational trophoblastic disease constitutes a diverse group of lesions that include placental villous abnormalities characterized by hydropic change with abnormal proliferation and maturation of trophoblast, as well as nonneoplastic and neoplastic proliferations of trophoblast unaccompanied by chorionic villi (Table 1). The diversity of lesions seen in gestational trophoblastic disease has been underscored by recent morphologic, epidemiologic, immunohistochemical and cytogenetic studies. The various forms of gestational trophoblastic disease can be defined and related to discrete pathologic aberrations occurring at different trophoblastic subpopulations and stages of trophoblastic differentiation during placentation. The recognition and separation of the individual categories of gestational trophoblastic disease is important, as each disease entity has distinctive clinical manifestations and each requires different therapeutic approaches. Furthermore, these disorders mimic growth patterns encountered in normal placental development and nonmolar abortions. Therefore, an appreciation of the morphologic manifestations of gestational trophoblastic disease is important to avoid confusing these lesions with normal physiologic changes of pregnancy.

OVERVIEW OF MORPHOLOGY AND DIFFERENTIATION OF TROPHOBLAST DURING NORMAL GESTATION

Trophoblast plays a crucial role in implantation and placentation, exhibiting a number of unique properties in accordance with its wide range of metabolic, endocrinologic, and invasive functions (1). Prior to the development of villi, the primitive trophoblast is termed *previllous trophoblast*. Our knowledge of the previllous trophoblast is limited because few specimens are available for study. After formation of villi at approximately 2 weeks of gestational age, trophoblasts on chorionic villi are termed *villous trophoblast*, whereas trophoblastic cells in all other locations are designated *extravillous trophoblastic cells*. The trophoblast in villous and extravillous locations can be broadly divided into three distinct populations based on morphologic, immunophenotypic, and functional studies (2,3) (Table 2). The cytotrophoblast is a relatively small, mononucleate cell with a distinct cell border that contains a small amount of eosinophilic cytoplasm (Fig. 1). In early gestation, the cytotrophoblast on the villous surface differentiates along two main pathways, developing into either a villous or extravillous trophoblast (1–4). On the villous surface cytotrophoblastic cells fuse to form syncytiotrophoblastic cells. Syncytiotrophoblastic cells are terminally differentiated cells that synthesize and secrete a variety of pregnancy-associated hormones including human chorionic gonadotropin (hCG). The syncytiotrophoblast is multinucleated and often the nuclei appear dark and pyknotic. The cytoplasm of syncytiotrophoblastic cells is dense and stains deeply eosinophilic to basophilic. Often, there are multiple intracytoplasmic vacuoles that result from dilatation of the endoplasmic reticulum and lacunae formed by complex infoldings of the plasma membrane. In contrast, cytotrophoblastic cells at the margin of what are destined to become anchoring villi display a morphologic spectrum of differentiation resulting in the development of intermediate trophoblastic cells within the trophoblastic columns (Fig. 1). This differentiation from cytotrophoblast to intermediate trophoblast is accompanied by gradual enlargement of the cells and their nuclei, accompanied by cytoplasmic clearing. From the trophoblastic columns, intermediate trophoblastic cells infiltrate the decidua and myometrium, and invade and replace the spiral arteries of the basal plate to establish the maternal/fetal circulation. The differentiation of intermediate trophoblast toward the distal ends of the anchoring villi and in the endomyometrium is accompanied by a decrease in cellular proliferation (5).

I-M. Shih: Department of Pathology, Johns Hopkins Hospital, Baltimore, Maryland 21287.

M. T. Mazur: Department of Pathology, Crouse Hospital, Syracuse, New York 13210.

R. J. Kurman: Departments of Pathology and Gynecology, Johns Hopkins Hospital, Baltimore, Maryland 21287

TABLE 1. Modified World Health Organization classification of gestational trophoblastic disease

Hydatidiform mole
  Complete
  Partial
Invasive mole
Choriocarcinoma
Placental site trophoblastic tumor
Epithelioid trophoblastic tumor
Miscellaneous trophoblastic lesions
  Exaggerated placental site
  Placental site nodule

The morphologic features of intermediate trophoblastic cells are quite variable depending on location (Table 2). In the trophoblastic columns we refer to the intermediate trophoblastic cells as villous intermediate trophoblastic cells. In this location they are mononucleate, larger than cytotrophoblastic cells, and polygonal with clear cytoplasm. We have termed the intermediate trophoblastic cells that infiltrate the endomyometrium of the placental site as implantation-site intermediate trophoblastic cells. In the endometrium these cells are polygonal and contain abundant amphophilic cytoplasm closely resembling the decidual cells with which they are admixed. These cells have hyperchromatic nuclei with irregular outlines and frequent deep folds or clefts. In the myometrium, implantation-site intermediate trophoblastic cells are frequently spindle-shaped and resemble the surrounding smooth muscle cells. Occasionally, mononucleate intermediate trophoblastic cells in the implantation site fuse to form multinucleated intermediate trophoblastic cells (so-called syncytiotrophoblastic giant cells) (5). Lastly, in the chorion laeve there are two distinct populations of cells, one containing eosinophilic and the other containing clear cytoplasm (6). In the past, we proposed the term *vacuolated cytotrophoblastic cells* for the cells with clear cytoplasm (6). Based on our most recent immunostaining studies (Table 2), we believe these cells represent a subpopulation of intermediate trophoblastic cells rather than a subtype of cytotrophoblastic cells and prefer the designation chorionic-type intermediate trophoblastic cells for both the cells with clear and eosinophilic cytoplasm. The functional role of chorionic-type intermediate trophoblast is not known. Thus, at present we subdivide intermediate trophoblast into three types based on its anatomical location: villous intermediate trophoblast, implantation-site intermediate trophoblast, and chorionic-type intermediate trophoblast.

TABLE 2. Morphologic and immunohistochemical features of trophoblastic cells throughout gestation

	Cytotrophoblast	Intermediate trophoblast (IT)			Syncytiotrophoblast
		Villous IT	Implantation site IT	Chorionic-type IT	
Nucleus	Single	Single	One to several	Single	Multiple
Shape	Round	Polyhedral	Variable; polyhedral to spindle	Round to polyhedral	Irregular; highly variable
Cytoplasm	Scant; clear to granular; prominent cell borders	Abundant; eosinophilic to clear prominent cell borders	Abundant; amphophilic; occasional vacuoles	Abundant; eosinophilic and clear[f]	Abundant; dense; multiple vacuoles; lacunae
Immunostaining					
Cytokeratin (AE1/AE3)	++++[a]	++++	++++	++++	++++
hCG	−	−	+(multinucleated IT)	−	++/++++[c]
hPL	−	−/+	++++	++	++/++++[c]
Mel-CAM	−	−/++++[b]	++++	++	−
PLAP	−	−	+	+++	++++
HNK-1	−	++++	−	−	−
EMA	−	−	−[d]	+++	−
Ki-67 index[e]	30%	>90%	0	3–6%	0

hCG, human chorionic gonadotropin; hPL, human placental lactogen; Mel-CAM, melanoma cell adhesion molecule (CD146); EMA, epithelial membrane antigen; PLAP, placental alkaline phosphatase; HNK-1 also known as Leu-7 and CD57.
[a]Semiquantitative scoring of proportion of cells showing a positive reaction: +, <25%; ++, 25–50%; +++, >50–75%; ++++, >75%.
[b]Mel-CAM immunointensity increases from the base to the tip of the trophoblastic column.
[c]The immunodistribution of hPL and hCG in syncytiotrophoblast is variable depending on gestational age; hCG decreases and hPL increases in intensity toward term.
[d]Some of the implantation site intermediate trophoblastic cells in the term placenta are positive for EMA.
[e]The percentage of Ki-67 positive trophoblastic cells is calculated in 300 randomly selected trophoblastic cells.
[f]The chorionic-type IT with clear cytoplasm is more often positive for PlAP. In contrast, the cells with eosinophilic cytoplasm are more often positive for hPL and Mel-CAM.

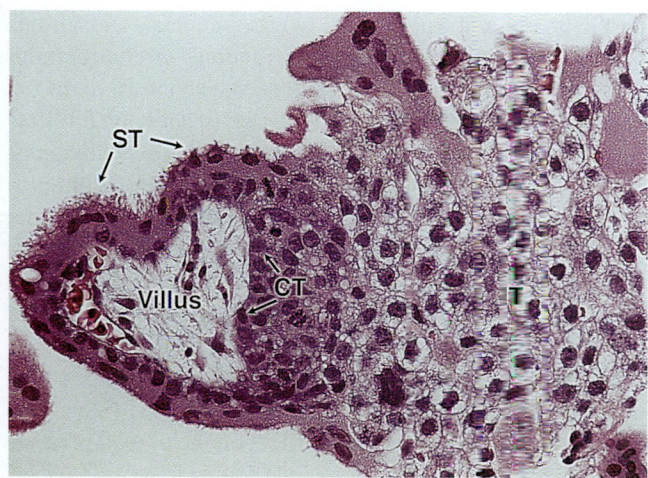

FIG. 1. Villus surface *(left)* with trophoblastic column *(right)*. Three distinct trophoblastic populations can be identified. The cytotrophoblast (CT) is a small mononucleate stem cell on the villous surface that fuses directly into the syncytiotrophoblast (ST). In contrast, cytotrophoblast cells at the margin of what is destined to become an anchoring villus, display a morphologic spectrum of differentiation merging imperceptibly into villous intermediate trophoblastic cells (IT) within the trophoblastic column. In contrast to CT, villous IT are larger and more polyhedral with abundant clear or amphophilic cytoplasm. From the trophoblastic columns, villous IT infiltrate the decidua and myometrium to become implantation-site IT or differentiate into chorionic-type IT, which are found in the chorion laeve.

The various trophoblastic subpopulations have different immunophenotypes depending on various factors including anatomical location and gestational age (5–8) (Table 2).

CLINICAL AND PATHOLOGIC FEATURES OF GESTATIONAL TROPHOBLASTIC DISEASE

Hydatidiform Mole

Hydatidiform mole, complete or partial, represents an abnormal placenta characterized by marked enlargement of chorionic villi caused by central edema of the stroma. Variable hyperplasia of the villous trophoblastic cells also is present, and this hyperplasia may be marked. A complete mole is distinguished from a partial mole by the amount of villous involvement. The edema is generalized in a complete mole, while in a partial mole the edematous change affects some of the villi. Most molar pregnancies are complete, and 25% to 43% are partial (9–11). Clinical, pathologic, and cytogenetic differences separate the two forms of hydatidiform mole, yet all molar pregnancies have the potential for persistent gestational trophoblastic disease.

Cytogenetic analysis of moles shows different mechanisms of origin for complete and partial mole. The complete mole is diploid. Usually, it is 46,XX and is androgenetic, formed from duplication of a haploid paternal genome (23X), and lacking functional maternal DNA. Over 90% of complete moles contain this paternal chromosome composition (12). The remaining group of complete moles also are androgenetic but are largely 46,XY and formed by dispermy, i.e., fertilization of an ovum lacking functional maternal chromosomes by two spermatozoa (12,13).

Partial moles are cytogenetically different (13), being triploid with two sets of chromosomes of paternal origin and a haploid maternal set (14,15). This triploid chromosomal composition is known as diandric. Usually the triploid set is XXY (58%). Less commonly it is XXX (40%) or XYY (2%) (13). Thus, a predominance of paternal chromosomes characterizes the cytogenetics of molar pregnancy. The ratio of paternal to maternal chromosomes is 2:0 in a complete mole and 2:1 in a partial mole.

Further chromosomal analyses and flow cytometric studies of ploidy in molar gestations indicate that cytogenetic distinctions between complete and partial moles are not always clear-cut (16–23). A few partial moles can be diploid (16,17,23) and occasional complete moles are triploid (17,22). Furthermore, both complete and partial moles can show marked heterogeneity in their ploidy patterns. Haploid, aneuploid and tetraploid moles, both partial and complete, rarely occur (22–24). There is no consistent association between the DNA ploidy of either a partial or a complete mole and subsequent clinical course (22).

Complete Mole

Morphologic Features

A complete mole often is voluminous, consisting of up to 500 cc or more of bloody tissue. Prior spontaneous passage of a portion of the tissue may decrease this volume substantially, however. In addition, many moles are now diagnosed earlier in pregnancy when the placenta is smaller, resulting in decreased tissue. The hallmark of the complete mole is gross, generalized villous edema (Fig. 2). Enlarged villi form grape-like, transparent vesicles measuring 1 to 2 cm across. When a complete mole is encountered in a hysterectomy specimen, the uterus is enlarged and molar vesicles protrude on opening. Only rarely is an embryo or fetus associated with a complete mole (25). In most of these cases, this represents a twin gestation, i.e., a fetus with a normal placenta and the second placenta a complete mole.

The primary histologic feature of a complete mole is generalized hydropic villous change. Most villi are edematous (Fig. 3), and many have cisterns. The latter are central, acellular, fluid-filled spaces. A small rim of mesenchyme separates the cistern from the surface layer of trophoblastic cells. Often the border of the mesenchyme with the acellular cistern is abrupt and well defined. Necrosis and patchy calcification of villous stroma may be seen.

The other hallmark of a complete mole is proliferation of villous trophoblastic cells (Fig. 3). This proliferation is irregular, affecting villi unevenly; some, including smaller villi, may show marked overgrowth of trophoblast, whereas others, including larger villi, may show little trophoblastic hyperplasia. The proliferating trophoblastic elements, com-

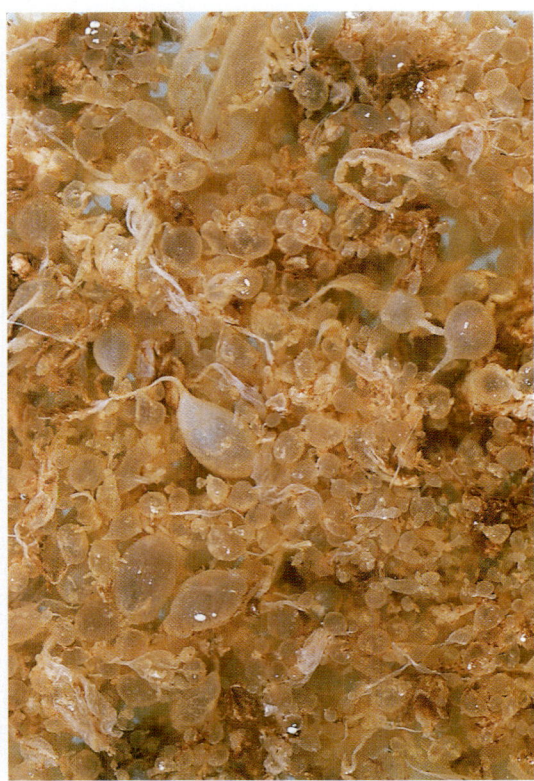

FIG. 2. Gross illustration of a complete mole, demonstrating the marked, generalized villous hydrops.

posed of syncytiotrophoblast, cytotrophoblast, and villous intermediate trophoblast, show a random, circumferential growth from the villous surface in marked contrast to the orderly growth of normal trophoblastic cells, showing proliferation from only the end of anchoring villi in early nonmolar placentas. The trophoblastic cells of a mole, in addition to being hyperplastic, often show considerable cytologic atypia (Fig. 4) with nuclear and cytoplasmic enlargement, irregularity of nuclear outlines, and hyperchromasia. The amount of trophoblastic growth is highly variable in moles; it may be exuberant, or focal and minimal. Consequently, this feature does not have to be prominent to establish the diagnosis. Furthermore, the histologic grade of the trophoblastic cells in a complete mole has no apparent effect on the overall prognosis (26).

In addition to the marked villous swelling and trophoblastic hyperplasia, a complete mole is typically characterized by an absence of development of an embryo/fetus. Neither fetal parts nor amnion is found.

Besides the proliferation of trophoblast on the villous surface, hydatidiform moles are invariably associated with hyperplasia of implantation-site intermediate trophoblastic cells, resembling an exaggerated placental site (see below) (27). The infiltrating implantation-site intermediate trophoblastic cells are generally more numerous and more atyp-

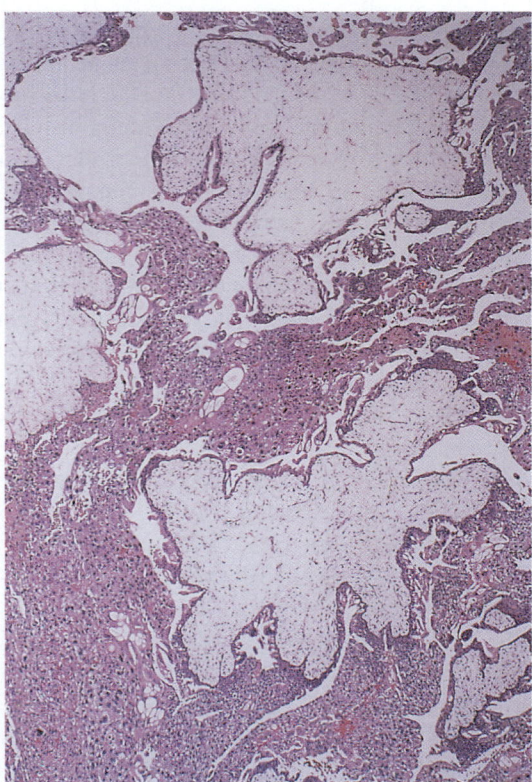

FIG. 3. Low-magnification view of complete mole, demonstrating generalized villous swelling with circumferential hyperplasia of trophoblastic cells.

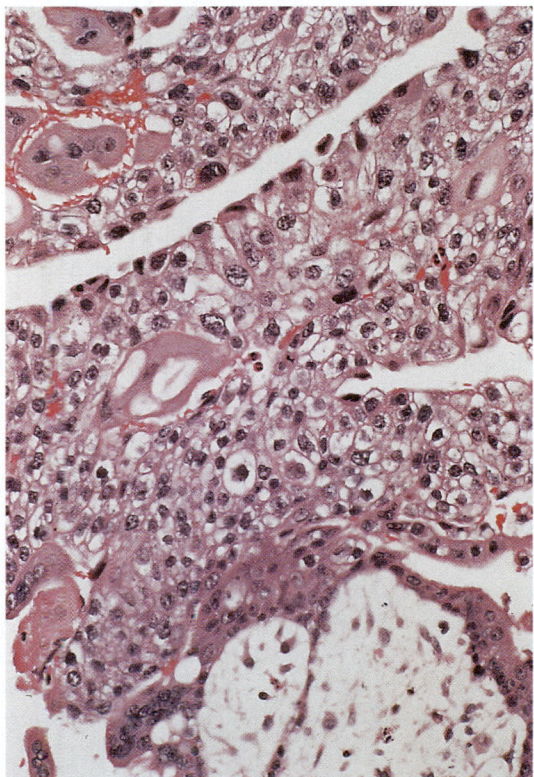

FIG. 4. High magnification of trophoblastic cells growing from the surface of a villus in a complete hydatidiform mole. A mixture of syncytiotrophoblast, cytotrophoblast, and villous intermediate trophoblast is present. Cytologic atypia accompanies the trophoblastic proliferation.

ical than those in an exaggerated placental site not associated with a hydatidiform mole. Nonetheless the immunophenotype of intermediate trophoblast in the molar implantation site is typical of implantation-site intermediate trophoblastic cells found in normal gestation. The implantation site of a hydatidiform mole has an increased Ki-67 labeling index in contrast to a labeling index of 0 in the exaggerated placental site of nonmolar gestation, suggesting that these two lesions are different despite their similar immunohistochemical features (27,28).

Partial Mole

Several features distinguish a partial mole from a complete mole. First, the amount of tissue in a partial mole is generally less than in complete mole; the total volume is often no greater than 200 cc. The gross specimen shows large, hydropic villi like those seen in a complete mole mixed with nonmolar placental tissue (29), an important distinguishing feature. In some cases of partial mole, a fetus is found and, when present, may show gross developmental abnormalities (29).

Morphologic Features

Microscopically, the hallmark of a partial mole is a mixture of large, edematous villi and small, normal-sized villi without edema (9,29) (Fig. 5). At least some of the hydropic villi show a central, acellular cistern like those seen in a complete mole. The small villi often show fibrosis. Trophoblastic hyperplasia is limited and focal, and is often confined to the syncytiotrophoblast. As in a complete mole, the trophoblastic overgrowth, where present, is haphazard and circumferential over the surface of the villi.

There are other common histologic features of a partial mole. The villi often have irregular, scalloped outlines (29). These irregular outlines produce infoldings of trophoblastic cells into the villous stroma, which, when prominent and sectioned tangentially, appear to be inclusions of trophoblast within the stroma (Fig. 6). Evidence of a fetus with fetal parts or an amnion is seen in many cases. With fetal development, villous stromal vasculature often persists, and these vessels may contain nucleated erythrocytes.

Differential Diagnosis

The differential diagnosis of a hydatidiform mole, complete or partial, usually includes early, nonmolar pregnancy. The nonmolar abortus may possess several morphologic features that mimic changes found in molar pregnancy. First, early nonmolar gestations typically are accompanied by trophoblastic proliferation that must be distinguished from the trophoblastic hyperplasia of a mole. Second, immature villi

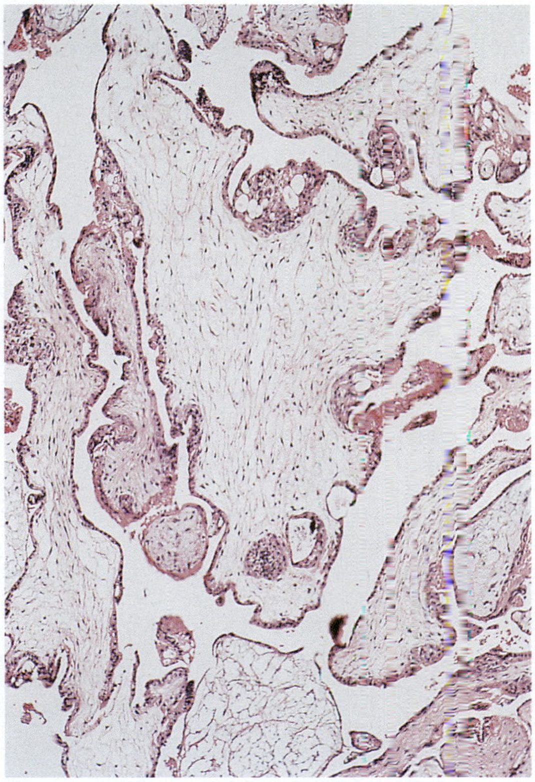

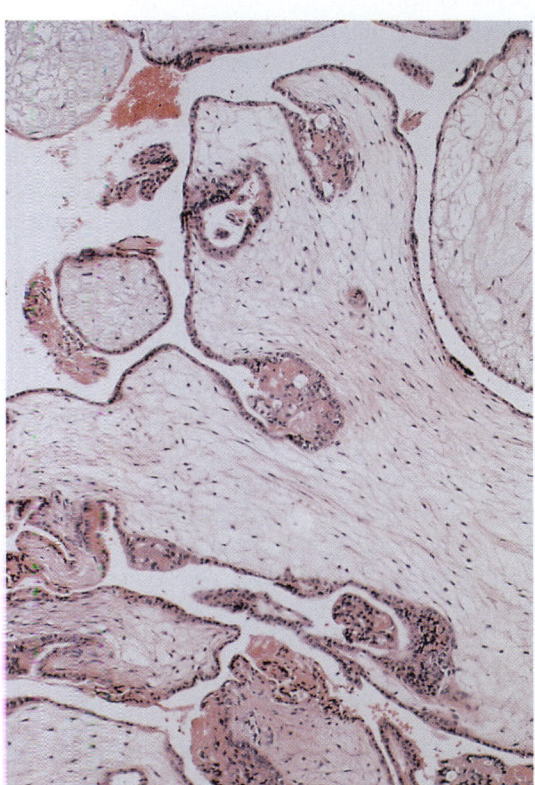

FIG. 5. A partial hydatidiform mole demonstrating a mixture of small villi and large hydropic villi with an irregular, scalloped outline.

FIG. 6. A partial mole demonstrating mild, irregular trophoblastic proliferation from the villous surface. A trophoblastic inclusion is present.

have loose, edematous stroma. Finally, the hydropic villi of the so-called blighted ovum in which there was no development of an embryo demonstrate moderate edema.

In routine abortion specimens trophoblastic proliferations from chorionic villi show polarity characterized by column-like growth of the cells from only one pole of a villus. In addition, the trophoblast in the nonmolar gestation does not show cytologic atypia like that seen in many moles, especially complete moles. The edema of the nonmolar abortus, including the blighted ovum, is separated from the molar pregnancy by degree. Most importantly, in nonmolar gestations central cistern formation is not a significant component. Edema may be present but is usually only a microscopic finding in the routine abortion. The differential diagnosis of an abortion versus a partial mole may be especially difficult, because hydropic change is less extensive in the latter condition.

Placental tissue associated with chromosomal abnormalities that are not triploid, for example trisomy, may display hydropic change and abnormal villus morphology that mimic a partial mole. These abnormal placentas are not associated with an increased risk of gestational trophoblastic disease and therefore this is an important differential diagnosis. The most useful histologic feature is the distribution of the trophoblast. In contrast to the circumferential distribution in partial mole, the trophoblast retains a polar orientation (trophoblastic column or island on one end of a villus) in these other cytogenetically abnormal placentas.

Although molar pregnancies usually present with a moderate volume of tissue, occasionally the amount of tissue is scant, and gross features helpful for anticipating the diagnosis of molar pregnancy are absent. This problem may be encountered when suction curettage causes collapse of villi onto gauze used to collect the specimen. Only histologic examination of the tissue attached to the gauze establishes the diagnosis. Repeat curettage after initial evacuation of a hydatidiform mole may contain proliferating trophoblastic cells, raising the possibility of choriocarcinoma following mole. If villi are present, however, choriocarcinoma cannot be diagnosed, and the lesion represents a persistent mole. Conversely, neither invasive mole nor choriocarcinoma are excluded, and meticulous follow-up with serum hCG titers is needed. Importantly, nonvillous trophoblastic elements after evacuation of a mole do not necessarily indicate the presence of choriocarcinoma (30). The diagnosis of choriocarcinoma requires the absence of villi, along with evidence of destructive and infiltrative growth.

Clinicopathologic Correlation

A complete mole typically presents between the 11th and 25th week of pregnancy with an average gestational age of about 16 weeks (31–33). With the routine use of ultrasound during pregnancy complete moles are being increasingly diagnosed earlier in pregnancy and therefore many of the classic presenting signs and symptoms are absent. Excessive uterine enlargement is common, and is often accompanied by other symptoms such as severe vomiting (hyperemesis gravidarum) and toxemia of pregnancy (31). Toxemia associated with molar pregnancy may be a clinical clue to the diagnosis, because this disorder generally occurs later in gestation (third trimester) with nonmolar pregnancies. Often, patients with complete mole spontaneously abort, presenting with vaginal bleeding or passage of molar vesicles. Ovarian enlargement due to multiple theca-lutein cysts (hyperreactio luteinalis) occurs in some patients with a complete mole. The hCG level is markedly elevated, especially in the tetraploid complete mole (34). Ultrasonography often discloses a classic "snowstorm" appearance.

In patients with a partial mole, the duration of pregnancy tends to be greater than in patients with a complete mole, with an average gestational age of about 19 weeks (9,35) (Table 3). Often the gestational age is greater than 20 weeks. Usually the patient presents with abnormal uterine bleeding and clinically appears to have a spontaneous or missed abortion (9,35). As with complete moles, patients with a partial mole are now diagnosed earlier because of the routine use of ultrasound in pregnancy. As a result some of the clinical differences between complete and partial moles are less clearly defined. In patients with a partial mole, the uterus is typically normal or small in size for the gestational age, and serum hCG levels generally do not show the marked elevation seen in a complete mole (36). Toxemia of pregnancy also may occur in association with a partial mole.

TABLE 3. *Comparison of complete and partial mole*

	Complete mole	Partial mole
Preoperative diagnosis		
Hydatidiform mole	+++	+/−
Spontaneous abortion	++	++
Missed abortion	+/−	+++
Heavy bleeding	+++	+
Toxemia	++	+/−
Uterus large for dates	++	+/−
Uterus small for dates	+/−	++
Fetus present	−	+
Serum hCG level	+++	+/++
Cytogenetics	XX or XY (all paternal)	XXY or XXX (2:1, paternal:maternal)
Behavior	10–30% persistent GTD	4–11% persistent GTD

hCG, human chorionic gonadotropin; GTD, gestational trophoblastic disease.

Behavior and Treatment

Many of the long-term follow-up studies of hydatidiform moles were reported before partial moles were recognized as a distinctive variant, so comprehensive comparison of the clinicopathologic features for these two forms of mole is not always feasible. Nonetheless, available data indicate that 10% to 30% of complete moles result in persistent gestational trophoblastic disease, as evidenced by a plateau or rise in hCG titers or the presence of extrauterine diseases (12,31,37,38). Reliable prognostic features have not been found. Specifically, histologic grading and expression of proliferating cell nuclear antigen (PCNA) and Ki-67 do not show correlation with the clinical outcome (39,40). Choriocarcinoma is the most serious form of persistent gestational trophoblastic disease, and occurs in about 2% to 3% of patients with complete moles (38,41). Other sequelae are persistent uterine cavity disease and an invasive mole that penetrates the myometrium or embolizes to the vagina, vulva, or lungs.

A partial mole has less risk for persistent gestational trophoblastic disease, and the percentage of patients requiring therapy following evacuation of a partial mole has ranged from 4% to 11% (9–12,35,42) with most studies showing a rate of about 5%. Importantly, there are few well-documented reports of choriocarcinoma following a partial mole; the sequelae have been persistent intrauterine disease or, rarely, an invasive mole (43,44).

Because of the risk of continued gestational trophoblastic disease, close monitoring of serum hCG levels is necessary following the diagnosis of any form of hydatidiform mole until levels fall to and remain in the normal range (12,38,45). A chest radiograph after diagnosis also is useful for detecting early pulmonary lesions, as well as providing a baseline should pulmonary disease ensue.

Invasive Mole

An invasive hydatidiform mole is almost invariably a sequela of a complete hydatidiform mole or a partial mole (33–37,46,47). The pathologic diagnosis is based on the presence of molar villi with associated trophoblastic cells in the myometrium and broad ligament or at distant sites, almost always the vagina, vulva, or lung. There are rare examples of an invasive mole showing deportation of the villi to other sites (such as paraspinal soft tissues) (48). A clinical diagnosis of invasive mole can be suspected when hCG titers plateau or rise following evacuation of a mole, but since choriocarcinoma can also supervene in this setting the clinical diagnosis should be persistent trophoblastic disease. The exact frequency of invasive mole is difficult to determine because of the lack of pathologic confirmation in most cases. Best estimates are that invasive mole is a clinically significant sequela in about 15% to 20% of patients with complete moles.

Pathologic Features

Grossly invasive mole in the uterus results in an irregular, often hemorrhagic lesion that penetrates into the myometrium. The lesion can grow through the myometrium, perforating the serosa or extending into the broad ligament and adnexa. Extracavitary hydropic villi are grossly visible in some cases, but often they are difficult to detect.

Microscopically, invasive mole has molar villi with associated trophoblastic cells, either within the myometrium, within myometrial blood vessels, or at distant sites. The villi are enlarged, but often are not as large as those of a typical complete intrauterine mole. The amount of trophoblastic proliferation around the villi of invasive mole is highly variable; there may be marked proliferation that obscures the villi. In such cases, careful sectioning and scrutiny for villi is necessary to avoid misclassification of the lesion as choriocarcinoma.

Differential Diagnosis

The differential diagnosis of invasive mole includes intracavitary noninvasive hydatidiform mole, choriocarcinoma, and placenta increta/percreta. The pathologic diagnosis of invasive mole requires clear-cut evidence of extension of molar tissue into the myometrium and its vessels, or deportation to distant sites. Marked trophoblastic proliferation associated with intracavitary hydatidiform mole does not necessarily indicate the presence of an invasive mole. An invasive mole may be difficult to distinguish from choriocarcinoma, as both entities feature a proliferation of trophoblastic cells in the myometrium, vagina, or lungs. These two disorders are distinguished by the presence or absence of chorionic villi.

Placenta increta and percreta represent growth of nonmolar placental tissue into the myometrium. These abnormal placentas lack the villous hydrops and abnormal trophoblastic proliferation found in invasive mole, and they almost always present during parturition when the placenta fails to separate from the myometrium. This presentation contrasts with an invasive mole, which usually is a sequela of an intracavitary hydatidiform mole.

Behavior and Treatment

Invasive hydatidiform mole may cause severe, life-threatening hemorrhage if it perforates the uterus or involves the parametrial tissues (49). Currently, this is an unusual event. Persistently elevated or rising serum hCG titers following evacuation of a mole may represent either an invasive mole or choriocarcinoma. Since tissue is generally not available to make the distinction, elevated serum hCG titers are usually attributed to persistent gestational trophoblastic disease without further classification. The risk of invasive mole progressing to choriocarcinoma appears to be no greater than that of progression from an intracavitary hydatidiform mole, and presumably many lesions of invasive mole would regress spontaneously if given appropriate opportunity. Nonetheless, persistent or elevated hCG titers are treated with chemotherapy often in the absence of a histologic diagnosis, and the lesions nearly always respond.

Exaggerated Placental Site

Exaggerated placental site is a benign, nonneoplastic lesion characterized by an increased number of implantation-site intermediate trophoblastic cells that extensively infiltrate the endometrium and underlying myometrium. An exaggerated placental site may occur in association with normal pregnancy or an abortion. In the past, this lesion was designated syncytial endometritis, but recently the term *exaggerated placental site* was introduced by the World Health Organization because the lesion is not inflammatory or confined to the endometrium and most of the constituent cells are not syncytial (50). An exaggerated placental site is composed of implantation-site intermediate trophoblastic cells, which display an identical immunophenotypic profile to the intermediate trophoblastic cells found in the normal implantation site, supporting the view that this lesion is an exaggeration of a normal physiologic process.

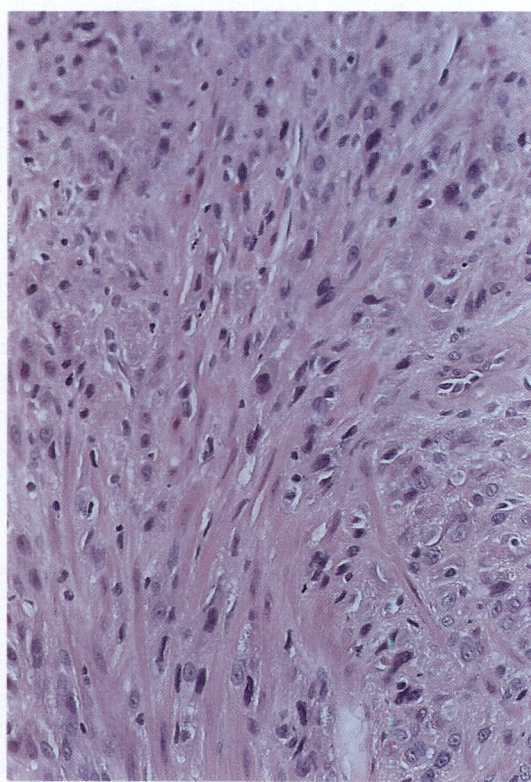

FIG. 7. An exaggerated placental site showing nests of implantation-site intermediate trophoblastic cells infiltrating the superficial myometrium. The pattern of invasion closely simulates placental-site trophoblastic tumors but is focal and not confluent.

Morphologic Features

The exaggerated placental site is defined as an increased number of implantation-site intermediate trophoblastic cells exceeding those normally present in the implantation site. Based on a review of the surgical pathology files at the Johns Hopkins Hospital, it occurs in approximately 1.6% of spontaneous and elective abortions from the early first trimester (unpublished data). The lesion is composed predominantly of mononucleate implantation-site intermediate trophoblastic cells and variable numbers of multinucleated intermediate trophoblastic cells that extensively infiltrate the endomyometrium (Fig. 7). Despite the extensive infiltration by intermediate trophoblastic cells, the overall architecture of the implantation site is not disturbed. Endometrial glands may be completely surrounded by trophoblastic cells but are not destroyed, and similarly the smooth muscle cells of the myometrium are separated by cords, nests, and individual implantation-site intermediate trophoblastic cells that diffusely infiltrate the myometrium without producing necrosis (2,51). The surrounding decidua, however, may show degeneration and necrosis typical of spontaneous abortion. Other features associated with gestation are usually present including hyalinized spiral arteries, hypersecretory glands, and chorionic villi. Despite the profuse infiltration of trophoblastic cells, the Ki-67 index of these cells is near zero, suggesting that the increased number of trophoblastic cells is not the result of de novo proliferation in the implantation site (27).

Differential Diagnosis

At times, an exaggerated placental site may be difficult to distinguish from a placental-site trophoblastic tumor (PSTT), particularly in curettings, as the diagnostic criteria for an exaggerated placental site are imprecise. There are no reliable data quantifying the amount and extent of infiltration of implantation-site intermediate trophoblast at different stages of normal gestation. Besides the overlap in the morphologic features of exaggerated placental site and PSTT, trophoblastic cells in early gestation have a primitive appearance and invade the uterine wall and spiral arteries extensively, thus invalidating the conventional histologic features used to distinguish a benign from a malignant process. The exaggerated placental site is microscopic, lacks mitotic activity, is composed of intermediate trophoblastic cells separated by masses of hyaline, and usually is admixed with decidua and chorionic villi. In contrast, a lesion unaccompanied by villi and composed of confluent masses of implantation-site intermediate trophoblastic cells that display unequivocal mitotic figures is classified as a PSTT. In addition, multinucleated trophoblastic cells are more often present in an exaggerated placental site than in a PSTT.

Recent studies show that the Ki-67 nuclear labeling index using a Ki-67–specific (MIB-1) antibody is superior to the mitotic index as a diagnostic aid in the differential diagnosis of

TABLE 4. *Immunohistochemistry in the differential diagnosis of gestational trophoblastic disease*

	Exaggerated placental site	Placental site nodule	Placental site trophoblastic tumor	Epithelioid trophoblastic tumor	Choriocarcinoma	Squamous carcinoma of cervix
CK18	++++	-+++	+++-	++++	+++	-
Inhibin-α	+	+++	+++	+++	+/++	-
Ki-67 index[a]	0	4.2 ± 3.1%	14 ± 7%	20 ± 7%	69 ± 20%	71 ± 10%
hPL	++++	+/-	+++	-/-	+/++	-
Mel-CAM	++++	+/-	+++-	-/-	+/+++	-

Semiquantitative scoring system based on the percentage of immunopositive cells:, 0%; +/-, <0-2%; +, <2-25% ++, <25-50%; +++, <50-75%; ++++, <75-100%.
[a] Mean ± standard deviation.
hPL, human placental lactogen; Mel-CAM, melanoma cell adhesion molecule.

exaggerated placental site versus PSTT (27). Specifically, the Ki-67 index (mean ± standard deviation) of the trophoblastic cells in an exaggerated placental site is near zero in contrast to 14% ± 6.9% in a PSTT (Table 4). Because Ki-67 labeling may occur in the lymphoid cells normally present at the placental site, it is important to be certain that Ki-67 labeling is assessed only in an intermediate trophoblast using strict cytologic criteria. In difficult cases, double immunostaining utilizing an antibody against Mel-CAM, which specifically defines implantation-site intermediate trophoblastic cells, can assist in this distinction. Mel-CAM, which is also designated as CD146, is a membrane glycoprotein of the immunoglobulin gene superfamily involved in cell-cell interaction that specifically identifies intermediate trophoblastic cells among the various trophoblastic populations (5,52,53). For further inquiry about the Mel-CAM antibody, please contact Dr. Shih (E-mail address: ishih@welchlink.welch.jhu.edu).

Behavior and Treatment

An exaggerated placental site is a benign trophoblastic lesion that involutes following curettage. It does not include the exaggerated placental site-like implantation site associated with moles (see above), and it is not associated with increased risk of persistent gestational trophoblastic disease. No specific treatment or follow-up is necessary. When an exaggerated placental site cannot be confidently distinguished from PSTT by morphology and immunohistochemistry, close follow-up with serial hCG titers is advisable.

Placental-Site Nodule

A placental-site nodule is a well-circumscribed hyalinized lesion composed of chorionic-type intermediate trophoblastic cells. Typically, it is incidentally found in an endometrial biopsy or endocervical curetting from a woman in the reproductive age group. It has also been found in the fallopian tube (54). A placental-site nodule may be diagnosed several years after tubal ligation, suggesting either that it can be retained in the endometrium for extended periods of time or that the lesion develops as an unrecognized pregnancy. In this latter scenario one must postulate that the tubes were incompletely transected or that they recanalized after surgery. It is generally thought that placental-site nodule represents a retained noninvoluted placental site (55-58). However, morphologic and immunohistochemical studies have shown that placental-site nodules are more closely related to chorion laeve of fetal membrane than the placental site (59). It is also conceivable that the placental-site nodule is an abnormal, i.e. blighted gestation, that never fully developed (59). This latter view is consistent with reports of these lesions as incidental findings in patients who never realized that they were pregnant. Although these patients may have had irregular bleeding, an extended period of amenorrhea was not documented.

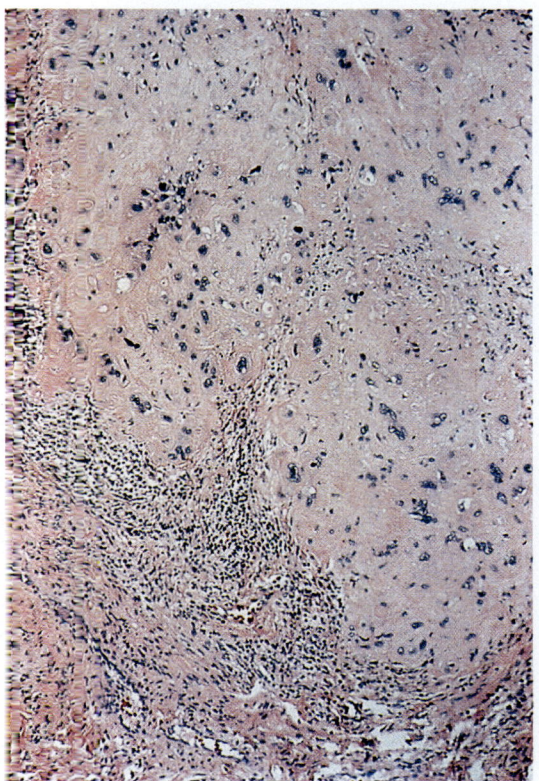

FIG. 8. A placental-site nodule in endometrial curettings showing the typical circumscribed and hyalinized appearance of the lesion at low magnification.

Pathologic Features

The placental-site nodule is a small, often microscopic finding (Fig. 8). When grossly visible, it presents as a yellow, tan, or hemorrhagic nodule measuring up to 1 cm in diameter and located in the endometrium or superficial myometrium. Microscopically, the placental-site nodule has a discrete, well-circumscribed, lobulated border sometimes showing small irregular nests of cells projecting into the surrounding tissue (pseudopods). A thin layer of chronic inflammatory cells and decidual cells often encompasses the lesion. The chorionic-type intermediate trophoblastic cells within the placental site nodule are arranged singly, in nests and cords. They are embedded in abundant eosinophilic fibrillar extracellular matrix protein, which contains type IV collagen and fibronectin of adult and oncofetal types (59). The latter finding is a prominent feature of placental-site nodules. The cells vary in size; many have relatively small uniform nuclei but others are large with mononucleate, irregular, and hyperchromatic nuclei (Fig. 9). Occasionally, scattered multinucleated cells are present. The cytoplasm of chorionic-type intermediate trophoblastic cells is abundant and eosinophilic to amphophilic, sometimes with conspicuous vacuolation. Morphologically and immunohistochemically these cells resemble those in the chorion laeve and therefore they have been designated as chorionic-type intermediate trophoblastic cells. Like all trophoblastic cells, intermediate trophoblastic cells in placental-site nodules are strongly and diffusely positive for cytokeratin. Chorionic-type intermediate trophoblastic cells in the placental-site nodule are only focally positive for human placental lactogen (hPL) and Mel-CAM, in contrast to the normal implantation site, where these antigens are highly expressed (59). Reactivity for hCG is usually absent. In contrast to implantation-site intermediate trophoblastic cell in the first trimester, the chorionic-type intermediate trophoblastic cells in placental-site nodules are positive for epithelial membrane antigen and placental alkaline phosphatase. Similar to the chorionic-type intermediate trophoblastic cells found in the fetal membranes of normal pregnancy, there is a low level of proliferation in the cells of placental-site nodules as indicated by a few scattered Ki-67 labeled nuclei (59). In contrast, in the normal implantation site and even in exaggerated placental sites the Ki-67 index of implantation-site intermediate trophoblastic cells is zero (27).

Differential Diagnosis

Placental-site nodules may be microscopically confused with PSTTs, epithelioid trophoblastic tumors, and some non-trophoblastic lesions, notably invasive keratinizing squamous carcinoma of the cervix (3,55). The small size, circumscription, extensive eosinophilic extracellular matrix, and paucity of mitotic figures distinguish this lesion from PSTT. Immunohistochemically, the placental-site nodule is diffusely and strongly positive for placental alkaline phosphatase but only focally and weakly for Mel-CAM and hPL (Table 4). In contrast, PSTT demonstrates diffuse and strong staining for Mel-CAM and hPL but shows only scattered and faint staining for placental alkaline phosphatase. The differential diagnosis of the placental-site nodule versus epithelioid trophoblastic tumor is considered in the discussion of the latter, below. The placental-site nodule can also be confused with squamous carcinoma of the cervix, especially when the placental-site nodule involves the lower uterine segment or cervix. Lack of mitotic activity or necrosis favors a placental-site nodule. In addition, cytokeratin 18 and inhibin-α are useful markers in such cases, as the placental-site nodule exhibits strong immunoreactivity for these markers, whereas squamous carcinoma of the cervix does not (Table 4) (60, 61).

Behavior and Treatment

Placental-site nodules behave in a benign fashion. Neither local recurrence nor metastasis has been reported in patients treated by either hysterectomy or curettage alone (55,56,59).

Choriocarcinoma

Gestational choriocarcinoma is a highly aggressive, malignant tumor derived from placental trophoblast. It has a high propensity for hematogenous dissemination. Furthermore, gestational choriocarcinoma, being derived from fetal cells, is a tumor allograft in the host, making it unique among human malignancies. Choriocarcinoma can arise from the

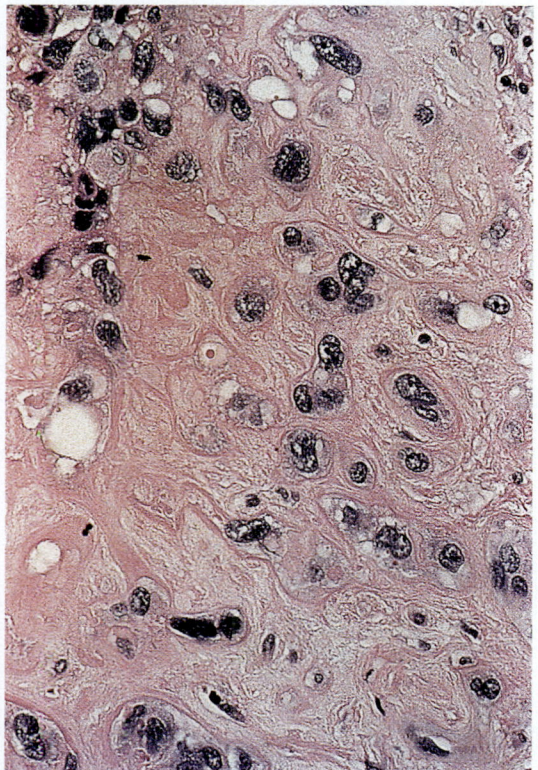

FIG. 9. A placental-site nodule with a cluster of hyperchromatic and vacuolated chorionic-type intermediate trophoblastic cells in a hyaline matrix.

previllous trophoblast of an early implantation or from the villous surface of a placenta. The more abnormal the pregnancy, the more likely that it will be followed by choriocarcinoma. Hydatidiform mole is the most common preceding gestation, with about 50% of all choriocarcinomas developing from a complete hydatidiform mole (41). About one-quarter of gestational choriocarcinomas follow abortions, and the remainder occur after or during normal pregnancies, or, rarely, within an ectopic gestation. Although patients with gestational choriocarcinoma most frequently present with abnormal uterine bleeding, choriocarcinoma not associated with a hydatidiform mole is often not suspected clinically (12,62). Choriocarcinoma may regress in the uterus without causing symptoms, and metastases can be the first sign of the tumor (62–66). There also are rare examples of long latent periods of more than 30 years between the preceding gestation and the diagnosis of choriocarcinoma (66).

Pathologic Features

On gross examination, choriocarcinoma is characterized by one or multiple circumscribed, hemorrhagic masses (49,50,67,68). This appearance is due to rapid proliferation, combined with a marked propensity to invade blood vessels. The tumors vary from small, pinpoint-sized lesions to large destructive masses. The central portion of the lesion is typically hemorrhagic and necrotic, with only a thin rim of recognizable trophoblastic cells at the periphery of the nodule (Fig. 10).

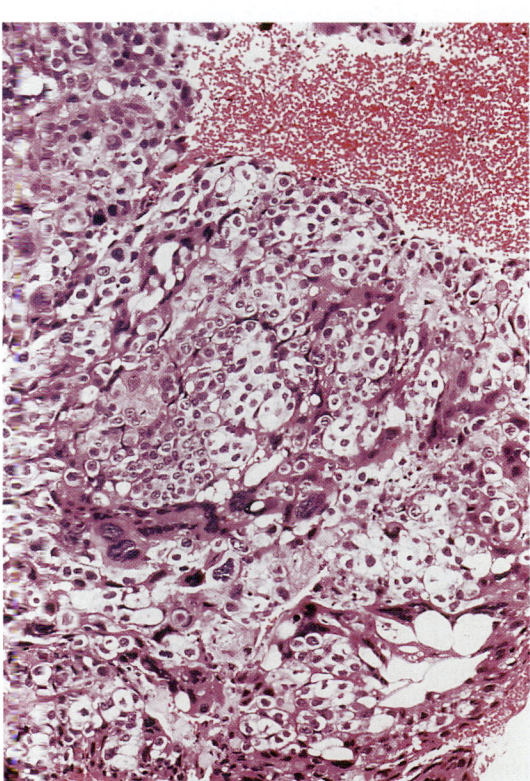

FIG. 11. Choriocarcinoma within the uterus. There is a prominent biphasic mixture of syncytiotrophoblastic and cytotrophoblastic cells with scattered intermediate trophoblastic cells intermixed.

Microscopically, the classic pattern of choriocarcinoma has been described as bilaminar, dimorphic, or biphasic. These terms refer to the distinctive alternating arrangement of mononucleate trophoblastic cells and syncytiotrophoblastic cells that characterize choriocarcinoma (63). The mononucleate trophoblastic cells can be cytotrophoblast, intermediate trophoblast, or both (Figs. 11–13). The intermediate trophoblast in choriocarcinoma resembles the primitive intermediate trophoblast in the previllous stage of placental development but may show marked variation in the degree of cytologic atypia from case to case and from field to field within a given neoplasm. Nuclear pleomorphism and hyperchromasia often is striking, and nucleoli can be prominent. The percentage of intermediate trophoblast in choriocarcinomas is highly variable, ranging from 1% to 90% of the mononucleate trophoblastic cell population (5). Multinucleated intermediate trophoblastic cells can occasionally be seen adjacent to mononucleate intermediate trophoblastic cells (5).

Because of the extensive necrosis associated with the rapid proliferation of choriocarcinoma, trophoblastic tissue may be scant, and extensive sectioning may be necessary to find the diagnostic biphasic pattern. Sometimes, following chemotherapy, syncytiotrophoblastic cells are inconspicuous throughout the tumor (63). Vascular invasion often is prominent. Chorionic villi are not a component of choriocarcinoma except for the rare cases of choriocarcinoma arising

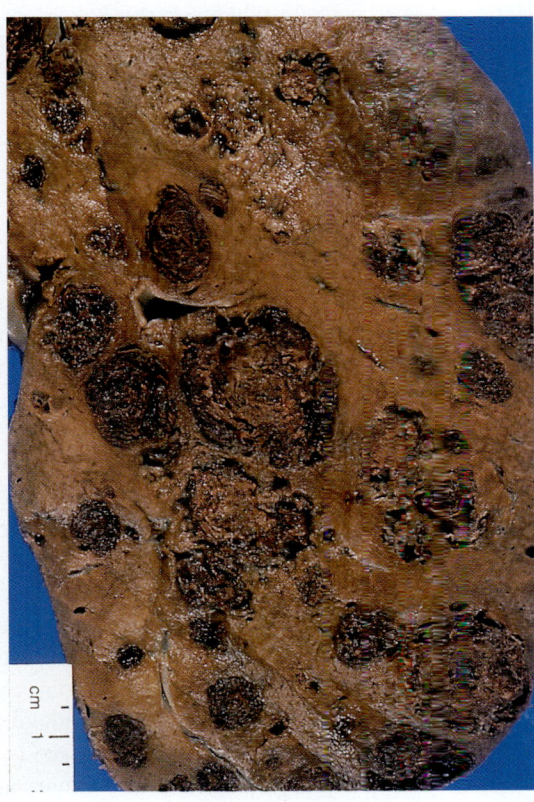

FIG. 10. Hemorrhagic nodules of choriocarcinoma metastatic to liver.

in the normally developing placenta. In the few reported cases of placental choriocarcinoma, the tumor clearly arises from the surface of normal-appearing chorionic villi that do not show hydropic change (69).

Rarely, choriocarcinoma can be seen in association with PSTT and epithelioid trophoblastic tumor. In our opinion, this mixed pattern reflects the fact that the primitive cytotrophoblast in choriocarcinoma can differentiate into implantation-site intermediate trophoblast or chorionic-type intermediate trophoblast, forming PSTT and epithelioid trophoblastic tumor, respectively.

Syncytiotrophoblast and intermediate trophoblast are hormonally active cells, so immunohistochemical studies using antibodies to beta-hCG or hPL are very helpful in evaluating cases of suspected choriocarcinoma (7). In typical choriocarcinoma, the syncytiotrophoblastic cells react intensely with beta-hCG and to a variable but lesser extent with hPL. Furthermore, the staining pattern helps to define the regular alternating network of syncytiotrophoblast that stains intensely with hCG and cytotrophoblast that is nonreactive for hCG. Intermediate trophoblastic cells also stain to some extent with hCG and hPL.

Ultrastructurally, trophoblastic cells, especially syncytiotrophoblastic cells, show marked epithelial differentiation characterized by the presence of desmosomes and tonofilaments (70). Consequently, choriocarcinoma is broadly reactive with antibodies to cytokeratin. All trophoblastic cell

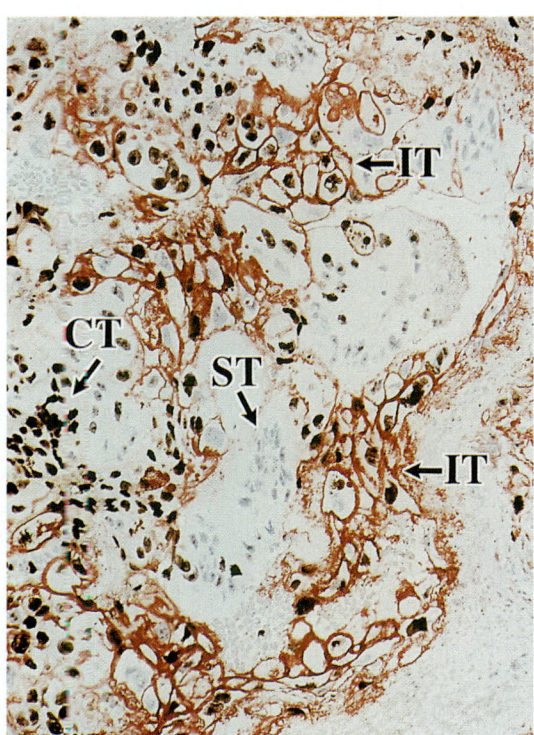

FIG. 13. Double immunostaining demonstrates the expression of Mel-CAM (red membrane staining) and Ki-67 (brown nuclear staining) in choriocarcinoma. Almost all the nuclei in the Mel-CAM negative cytotrophoblastic cells (CT) are Ki-67 positive. A large number of Mel-CAM positive intermediate trophoblastic cells (IT) are also immunoreactive for Ki-67. In contrast, the Mel-CAM negative syncytiotrophoblast (ST) is largely nonreactive for Ki-67.

types, including cytotrophoblast and intermediate trophoblast, are positive for cytokeratin (60,71).

Differential Diagnosis

In the uterus, the differential diagnosis of choriocarcinoma includes normal trophoblastic tissue from early gestation and the trophoblastic proliferation associated with hydatidiform mole, as rapidly growing trophoblast in any of these conditions results in a somewhat similar histologic picture (Fig. 14) (30). Identifying chorionic villi is important in making the correct diagnosis. Chorionic villi associated with trophoblastic proliferation represent hydatidiform mole or a nonmolar abortion specimen, except for the rare cases of choriocarcinoma arising in an otherwise normally developing placenta.

Trophoblast without villi in curettings may be suspicious for choriocarcinoma but difficult to categorize with certainty (30). The distinction between the trophoblast of an early abortus and that of choriocarcinoma is based to some extent on the quantity of the cells. In a normal abortus without villi, usually only a small amount of trophoblastic tissue is present. In choriocarcinoma, the tissue tends to be more abundant, and the trophoblastic cells predominate in the sections.

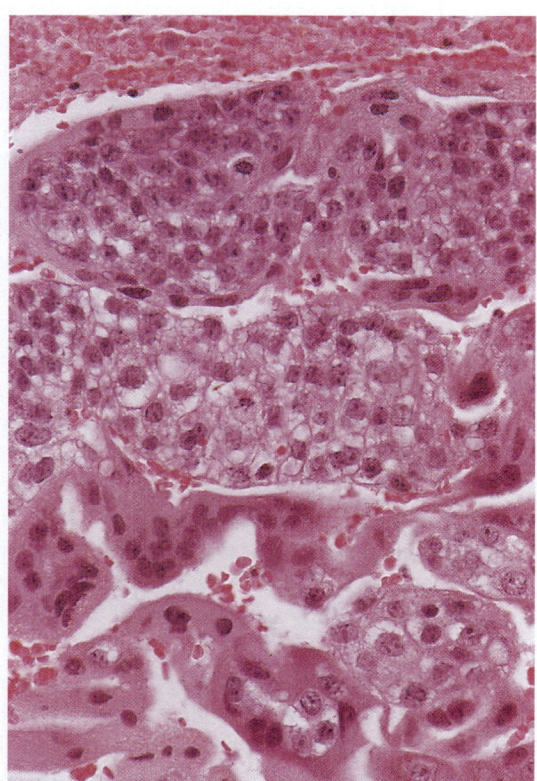

FIG. 12. High magnification of choriocarcinoma, demonstrating the alternating arrangement of syncytiotrophoblast and mononucleate trophoblast.

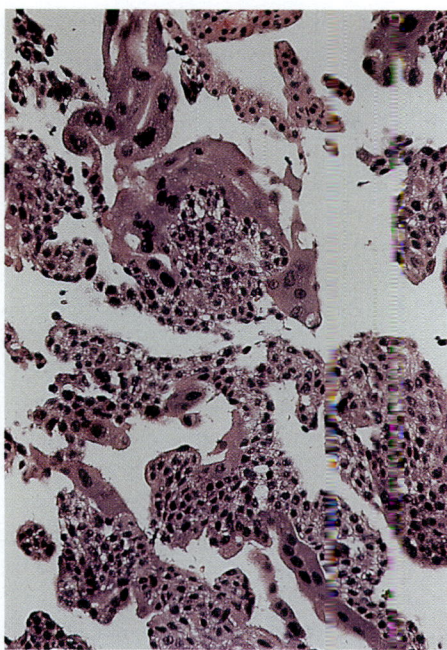

FIG. 14. An early placenta demonstrating a dimorphic pattern composed of mononucleate trophoblastic cells and syncytiotrophoblastic cells that resembles a choriocarcinoma. In contrast to choriocarcinoma, the mononucleate trophoblastic cells are smaller with less nuclear atypia and more uniform. Most importantly, villi are identified elsewhere in this specimen.

Most importantly, unlike trophoblast of an early gestation the trophoblast of choriocarcinoma is associated with necrosis as it invades adjacent tissue in a destructive manner. A careful obstetric history in such cases is extremely helpful. Atypical trophoblast without villi is more likely to represent choriocarcinoma if the preceding pregnancy was nonmolar, whereas similar trophoblastic cells after evacuation of mole may only represent persistent intrauterine mole (30). In questionable cases, careful monitoring of serum beta-hCG levels and chest radiographs help to establish the diagnosis. The differential diagnosis of PSTT versus choriocarcinoma is considered in the discussion of PSTT, below.

At extrauterine sites, the differential diagnosis includes deported invasive moles, gonadal germ cell tumors, ordinary epithelial malignancies with areas of choriocarcinomatous differentiation, and pleomorphic epithelial malignancies with tumor giant cells. Choriocarcinoma is distinguished from invasive mole by the absence of chorionic villi, especially when evaluating lesions of the lung, vagina, or vulva following molar gestation. Choriocarcinoma can be a predominant feature of some germ cell tumors, but ovarian germ cell tumors often are associated with a large adnexal mass, a helpful differential feature. In addition, germ cell tumors containing choriocarcinoma nearly always contain a mixture of other germ cell neoplasms such as dysgerminoma, teratoma, or yolk sac tumor. Pure choriocarcinoma of germ cell origin is exceedingly rare. Alpha-fetoprotein (AFP) is produced by yolk sac tumors and, less commonly, by teratomas but not by trophoblastic tumors, so immunostaining and serum AFP levels can be useful in differential diagnosis (72).

In nongestational tumors with choriocarcinomatous differentiation or with areas that mimic choriocarcinoma, the differential diagnosis may be difficult, especially in younger women in whom gestational trophoblastic disease would be highly suspect. Occasionally, primary visceral neoplasms such as carcinomas of the gastrointestinal tract, endometrium, breast, or bladder have areas of clear-cut choriocarcinomatous differentiation with syncytiotrophoblast and cytotrophoblast (73–76). In such cases, the sections usually reveal areas of typical adenocarcinoma or transitional cell carcinoma that clarify the diagnosis. When the differential diagnosis includes epithelial malignancy with giant cell change, immunohistochemistry is useful for establishing the correct diagnosis. In choriocarcinoma, the syncytiotrophoblast stains with hCG and the multinucleated intermediate trophoblast stains with hPL and Mel-CAM, whereas nontrophoblastic giant cells do not. Occasionally, an epithelial malignancy arising at an extrauterine site may focally produce hCG, hPL or Mel-CAM (77,78), and immunostaining must be correlated with the histologic pattern to arrive at the diagnosis. In questionable cases, serum beta-hCG levels are helpful as they usually are markedly elevated with choriocarcinoma but generally are only minimally elevated with other neoplasms.

Behavior and Treatment

Choriocarcinoma disseminates hematogenously. The lungs are most frequently involved (33,49,50,63,68). Other common metastatic sites include the brain, liver, and gastrointestinal tract (49,63). Metastasis to the vagina also occurs, and these may bleed profusely when biopsied. Kidney, skin, and other unusual locations may also be involved.

Prior to the development of effective cytotoxic chemotherapy, hysterectomy was the only therapy. With this treatment there was a survival rate of about 40% if no metastases were present and about 20% with metastases (79). Chemotherapy dramatically improved the prognosis. Now, the survival rate is 81% for all patients with gestational choriocarcinoma, although it is only 71% for those with metastatic disease. In comparison, the overall survival rate for all cases of persistent and metastatic gestational trophoblastic disease, which includes postmolar disease as well as diagnosed choriocarcinoma, is now over 90% (32,80).

Several prognostic factors help to predict the response to treatment. Poor prognostic factors include advanced stage disease at diagnosis, cerebral or hepatic metastases, symptoms for longer than 4 months, failure of prior chemotherapy, and a pretreatment serum beta-hCG level of greater than 40,000 mIU/ml (80–82). Metastases limited to the lung or vagina are not, by themselves, poor prognostic signs. Choriocarcinoma following a term gestation has a somewhat worse prognosis. This is attributed to delay in treatment and the presence of metastases beyond the lungs and vagina (64,83). No histologic features alone have prognostic importance. Chemotherapy may alter the histologic appearance in isolated cases (63), but the influence of such changes on the clinical outcome is not established. Some investigators suggest that all forms of gestational trophoblastic disease showing only minimal differentiation toward syncytiotrophoblast have a somewhat worse prognosis (84). Further study is needed to determine whether or not such histologic patterns do, in fact, have clinical significance.

Placental-Site Trophoblastic Tumor

The PSTT is a distinctive but rare form of trophoblastic neoplasia that develops as a result of neoplastic transformation of the implantation-site intermediate trophoblast. This tumor was described intermittently for many years by the terms *atypical chorioepithelioma*, *atypical choriocarcinoma*, *syncytioma*, *chorioepitheliosis*, and *trophoblastic pseudotumor*, but none of these terms is now appropriate (3,33). In addition, this tumor has been mistakenly classified as a sarcoma. PSTT occurs during the reproductive years, although several patients have been over 50 years of age when their tumors were diagnosed (85,86). Most patients have been parous; only a few had a preceding hydatidiform mole (86–88). Both term pregnancies and spontaneous abortions have preceded the diagnosis of PSTT. Usually, the relationship to the previous gestations is uncertain, because the PSTT is diagnosed long after the last known pregnancy. Patients with PSTT can present either with amenorrhea or with abnormal bleeding (3,86–88). Often the uterus is enlarged, and the patient is thought to be pregnant. Pregnancy tests are almost always positive when a sensitive immunologic assay is used. When progressive uterine enlargement ceases, a diagnosis of missed abortion is often made. Rarely, PSTT is associated with virilization (89,90). A few cases of PSTT have been associated with an apparently unique form of renal disease in which the nephrotic syndrome is a major component (91).

Pathologic Features

Placental-site trophoblastic tumor has a highly varied gross appearance. The tumors range from diffuse microscopic findings to tumors that enlarge and distort the fundus. Usually PSTT is circumscribed, but some are poorly demarcated. PSTT may project into the uterine cavity or grow predominantly into the myometrium. The neoplasm is soft and tan and may have areas of hemorrhage or necrosis. Many PSTT have invaded through the entire thickness of the myometrium, extending to the serosa. Perforation or extension into the broad ligament or adnexa also occurs.

Microscopically, implantation-site intermediate trophoblastic cells predominate in PSTT (2,3,5,7). The typical growth pattern is characterized by infiltration of the myometrium by large, polygonal, implantation-site intermediate trophoblastic cells that insinuate themselves between the smooth muscle fibers (Fig. 15). The cells may be present singly or in large nests or masses. Although most of the implantation-site intermediate trophoblastic cells are polyhedral, they can also be spindle cell shaped. PSTT has a secondary component of multinucleated intermediate trophoblastic cells that can have vacuolated cytoplasm. Cytotrophoblastic cells are not a conspicuous component of PSTT. PSTT is generally not associated with the presence of chorionic villi.

In addition to its cytologic features, there are several other microscopic characteristics of PSTT. One consistent finding is the extensive deposition of fibrinoid material. The intermediate trophoblastic cells of PSTT also characteristically invade blood vessels in a manner that results in replacement of the muscle wall by intermediate trophoblastic cells, and then fibrinoid material is deposited in the vessel wall, which typically maintains a central lumen (Fig. 16).

It is not possible to accurately predict the prognosis of PSTTs but some tumors display histologic features associated with a poor outcome. These tumors are composed of larger masses and sheets of cells with clear or amphophilic cytoplasm and highly atypical nuclei (Fig. 17). Necrosis is more extensive than in the benign tumors, and the mitotic count is generally higher. In benign PSTT the mean mitotic

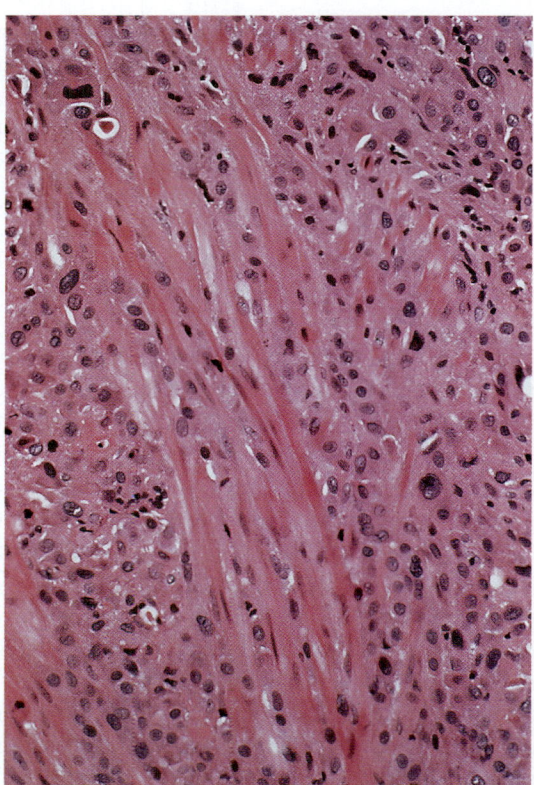

FIG. 15. A placental-site trophoblastic tumor (PSTT) with sheets of implantation-site intermediate trophoblastic cells separating smooth muscle cells of the myometrium.

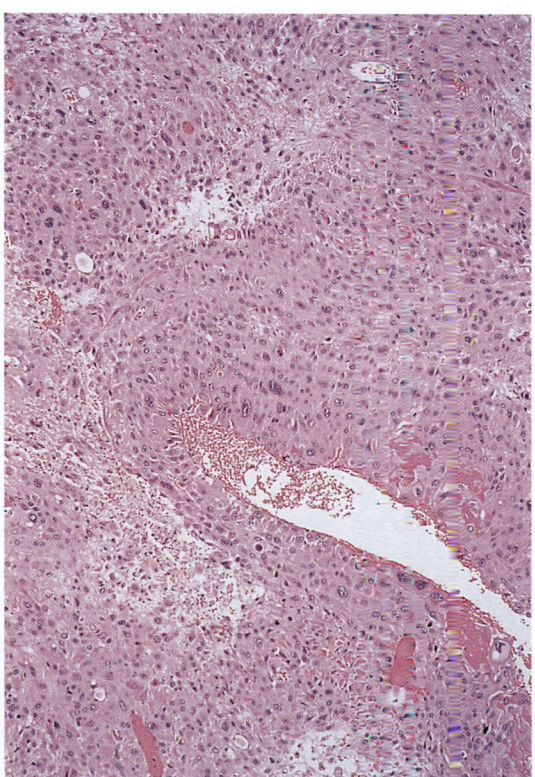

FIG. 16. A PSTT demonstrating replacement of a vascular wall by implantation-site intermediate trophoblastic cells. Note fibrinoid material in vessel wall. Characteristically, the lumen of the blood vessel is preserved.

count is 2 mitotic figures per 10 high-power fields (HPFs), with the highest reported counts being 5 mitotic figures per 10 HPFs. In contrast, malignant lesions generally have more than 5 mitotic figures per 10 HPFs. In a few fatal cases, however, the mean mitotic count was only 2 per 10 HPFs. Preliminary data suggest that Ki-67 nuclear labeling index may be a reliable indicator of prognosis, as the index is usually higher than 50% in malignant tumors, in contrast to 14% in benign ones (27). Abnormal mitotic figures can occur in either benign or malignant PSTTs.

Differential Diagnosis

Placental-site trophoblastic tumor must be differentiated from choriocarcinoma, epithelioid trophoblastic tumor, other forms of neoplasia, an exaggerated implantation site, and the placental-site nodule (3). Usually, the distinction of PSTT from choriocarcinoma is not difficult. PSTT is composed predominantly of implantation-site intermediate trophoblastic cells with occasional multinucleated intermediate trophoblastic cells. The multinucleated intermediate trophoblastic cells resemble syncytiotrophoblastic cells in choriocarcinoma but multinucleated intermediate trophoblastic cells are Mel-CAM positive and widely scattered in PSTT. This is in contrast to the syncytiotrophoblastic cells, which are Mel-CAM negative and are abundantly present in the biphasic pattern of choriocarcinoma. We have seen choriocarcinomas in which there are more intermediate trophoblast than cytotrophoblast alternating with the syncytiotrophoblast, but the biphasic pattern persisted, in contrast to the monomorphic growth of PSTT.

The PSTT has a different immunohistochemical staining pattern than choriocarcinoma. Because the tumor is composed primarily of implantation-site intermediate trophoblast, staining for hPL and Mel-CAM is diffuse throughout the neoplasm (5,7). In contrast, hCG staining is usually focal because of the lack of syncytiotrophoblastic cells and only scattered multinucleated intermediate trophoblastic cells (7) (Table 4). The tumor immunoreactivity correlates with the serum hCG titers. Typically, in choriocarcinoma the beta-hCG levels are high, ranging from 1,000 mIU/mL to over 1,000,000 mIU/mL, whereas in PSTT the levels are lower, often less than 1,000 mIU/mL.

A wide variety of other malignancies, especially epithelioid leiomyosarcoma, can mimic PSTT. The differential diagnosis from leiomyosarcoma can be difficult, as PSTT often has a highly infiltrative pattern within the myometrium, dissecting among the smooth muscle fibers and simulating origin from these cells. Helpful clues in the differential diagnosis include the distinctive pattern of vascular invasion and the deposition of fibrinoid material in PSTT, features not found in leiomyosarcomas or most other malignancies. Immunostaining for hPL and inhibin-alpha can also help to dis-

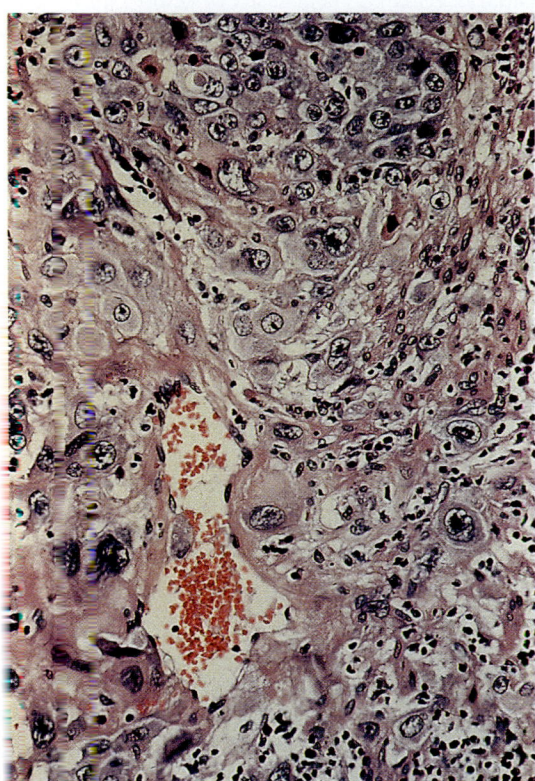

FIG. 17. Malignant PSTT composed of implantation-site intermediate trophoblastic cells with pale to clear cytoplasm.

tinguish PSTT from other malignancies (Table 4). In addition, PSTT shows diffuse immunoreactivity for cytokeratin, whereas most sarcomas do not. Other tumors may, on occasion, stain focally for inhibin-alpha and/or hPL, but the combination of the histologic features and the more diffuse and intense immunostaining for hPL and inhibin-alpha in PSTT should resolve difficult cases. Leiomyosarcoma also stains for desmin and actin while PSTT does not.

The differential diagnosis of the PSTT from exaggerated placental site, placental site nodule, and epithelioid trophoblastic tumor is considered in the specific sections describing these lesions.

Behavior and Treatment

The PSTT tends to have an indolent behavior. In most cases, the tumor remains confined to the uterus. Because of the deep myometrial penetration, perforation may occur during curettage. With PSTT, mildly elevated serum hCG levels often persist following curettage. In view of the low propensity for spread beyond the uterus, careful clinical follow-up with monitoring of serum hCG levels is a safe procedure in PSTT. A plateau or rise in hCG titers, however, signals the need for hysterectomy, in view of the apparent lack of response to chemotherapy of these neoplasms. Approximately 10% to 15% of the cases have resulted in the death of the patient (3,92–94). In the few overt malignancies, metastases involve the lungs, liver, abdominal cavity, and brain, where they have a histologic appearance similar to that of the uterine primary. Usually, metastases develop rapidly after the initial diagnosis, but one reported PSTT recurred 5 years after hysterectomy (93). Most malignant PSTTs have not responded as well to the multiagent chemotherapy that has been successfully used to treat choriocarcinoma.

Epithelioid Trophoblastic Tumor

The term *epithelioid trophoblastic tumor* was initially proposed to describe an unusual type of trophoblastic neoplasm distinct from PSTT and choriocarcinoma with features resembling a poorly differentiated carcinoma (33). A lesion with similar features termed *atypical choriocarcinoma* was first described in the lung of patients with choriocarcinoma following intensive chemotherapy (95,96). Similar tumors were subsequently identified in the uteri of patients without a history of prior gestational trophoblastic disease. Lesions that we believe are examples of epithelioid trophoblastic tumor have been also reported as multiple nodules of intermediate trophoblast following hydatidiform moles (97). Uterine epithelioid trophoblastic tumor can be seen in association with choriocarcinoma (97,98) and we have seen some tumors with features of PSTT that appear to be hybrids of the exaggerated placental-site nodule and PSTT. Epithelioid trophoblastic tumor is a rare form of gestational trophoblastic disease that occurs in women of reproductive age (15 to 48 years) (98). Like placental-site nodule and PSTT, epithelioid trophoblastic tumor can be diagnosed more than 10 years after the last known pregnancy. This is in contrast to choriocarcinoma, which is usually more closely linked to an identifiable gestational event. Epithelioid trophoblastic tumor can occur following a term pregnancy, an elective abortion, or a hydatidiform mole. Abnormal vaginal bleeding is the most common clinical presentation, and serum hCG levels are always elevated at the time of diagnosis. At times, epithelioid trophoblastic tumor is diagnosed in the lungs with or without evidence of prior gestational trophoblastic disease in the uterus (95,96,98). Based on morphologic, ultrastructural, and immunohistochemical studies, epithelioid trophoblastic tumor is a distinct trophoblastic tumor that appears to develop from neoplastic transformation of chorionic-type intermediate trophoblastic cells (95,98).

Pathologic Features

Experience with this tumor has been limited to 28 cases (95–98). On gross examination, the tumor measures 0.9 to 4.0 cm. It nearly always presents as a discrete, expansile nodule in the endomyometrium or in the lower uterine segment (Fig. 18). The cut surface of the tumor is solid, often with cystic areas and is brown-tan with areas of hemorrhage and necrosis. Microscopically, epithelioid trophoblastic tumor is composed of atypical mononucleate trophoblastic cells arranged in discrete nests and cords that in areas merge to form large sheets or masses (Fig. 19). The tumor invades in an expansile fashion. Similar to placental-site nodules, a thin rim of lympho-

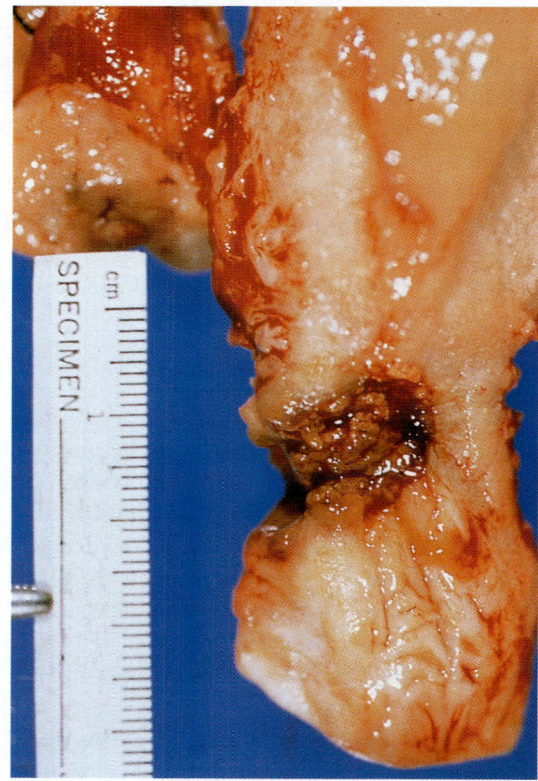

FIG. 18. Epithelioid trophoblastic tumor presenting a well-circumscribed tumor.

cytic infiltrate is occasionally found at the periphery of the expansile masses. Almost invariably, the cords and nests of cells are surrounded by fibrillar, eosinophilic, and hyaline-like material that probably represents a combination of necrotic debris from tumor cells and the extracellular matrix protein invested by the tumor cells (98). This is the same material that is found in placental-site nodules. The eosinophilic hyaline-like material is generally focal but in areas coalesces to form large aggregates. In the center of some of the nests, the dense eosinophilic material resembles keratin (Fig. 20). In areas in which cell necrosis is extensive, islands of viable tumor cells surround small blood vessels (Fig. 21). In epithelioid trophoblastic tumor, the lumina of blood vessels are preserved with occasional deposition of amorphous fibrinoid material in the wall and interstitium. Unlike the trophoblast at the early implantation site and in PSTT, the tumor cells in epithelioid trophoblastic tumors do not infiltrate and replace the vascular wall. A unique feature of epithelioid trophoblastic tumor, compared with PSTT and choriocarcinoma, is its ability to replace and reepithelialize the endocervical and/or endometrial surface epithelium. This heightens its similarity to a keratinizing squamous carcinoma, when it involves the lower uterine segment and endocervix (Fig. 22).

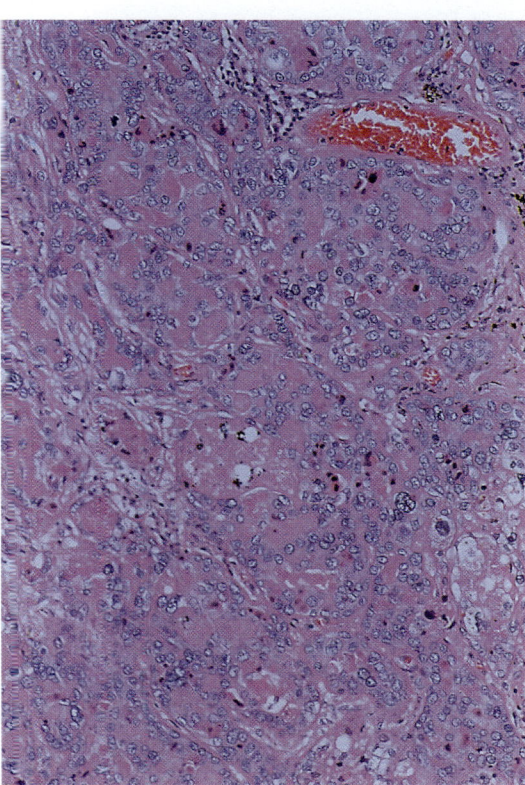

FIG. 20. Epithelioid trophoblastic tumor. Prominent cellular necrosis in the nests of trophoblastic cells is characteristic of this tumor.

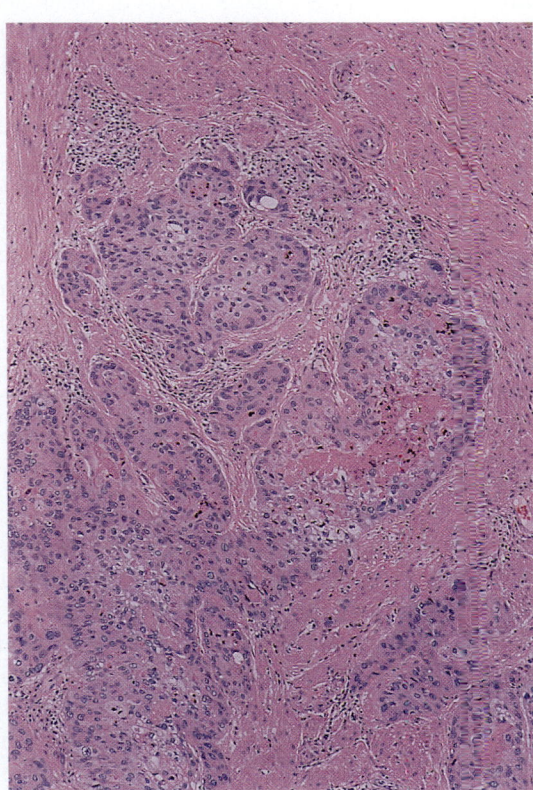

FIG. 19. Epithelioid trophoblastic tumor. The lesion is characterized by mononucleate chorionic-type intermediate trophoblastic cells forming discrete nests and cords infiltrating the myometrium. Necrosis and fibrillar eosinophilic material resembling keratin is present in the center of some of the nests and cords.

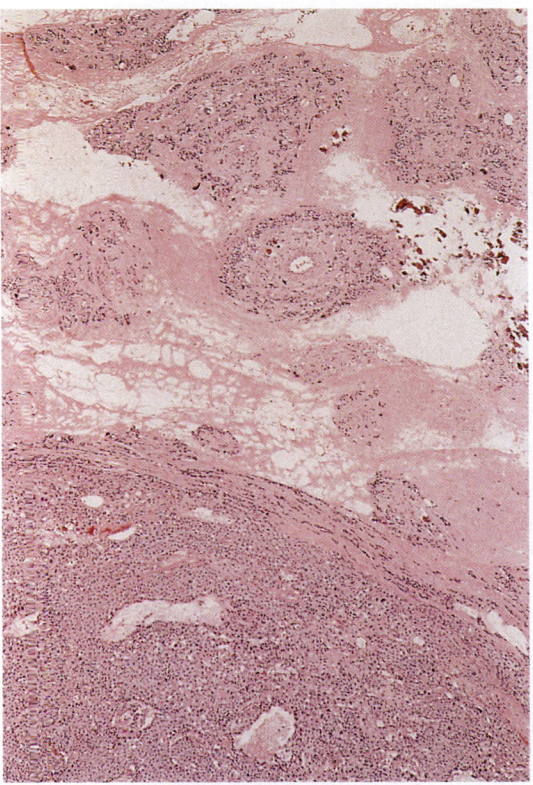

FIG. 21. Epithelioid trophoblastic tumor. Low-magnification view shows extensive areas of necrosis with several irregular islands of tumor cells surrounding small blood vessels.

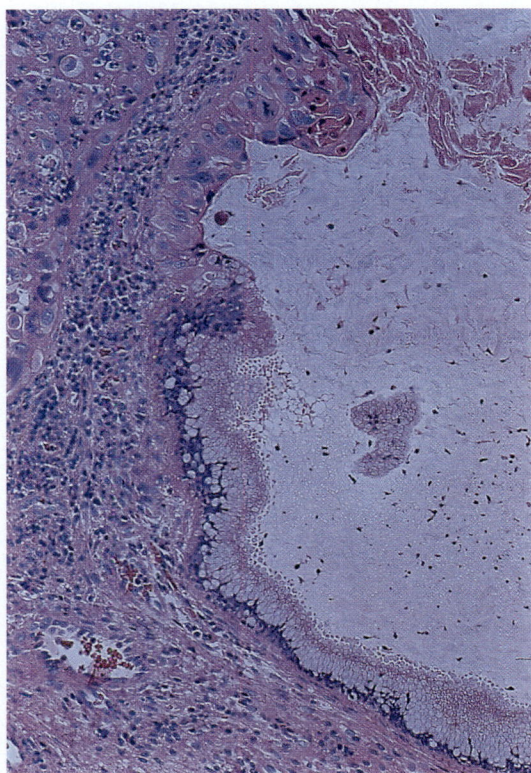

FIG. 22. Epithelioid trophoblastic tumor replacing and reepithelializing the endocervical glandular epithelium.

The predominant cells of epithelioid trophoblastic tumor are uniform in size and mononucleate with well-defined cell membranes. Generally, they are larger than cytotrophoblastic cells but smaller than implantation-site intermediate trophoblastic cells. Most of the tumor cells are rounded with uniform nuclei and eosinophilic or vacuolated cytoplasm. Prominent nucleoli are present in some cells and the mitotic count varies from 0 to 9 mitoses per 10 HPFs (40×) with an average of 2 mitoses per 10 HPFs (40×). In most cases, apoptotic cells are diffusely distributed throughout the tumor. Occasionally, larger cells resembling implantation-site intermediate trophoblastic cells are present with convoluted, irregular, and slightly vesicular nuclei and a moderate amount of eosinophilic cytoplasm. These cells are usually found singly or in small clusters. Immunohistochemically, all the cells are strongly positive for cytokeratin 18 and inhibin-alpha. However, most epithelioid trophoblastic tumors demonstrate only focal immunoreactivity with hPL, hCG, and Mel-CAM. The average Ki-67 nuclear labeling index in epithelioid trophoblastic tumor is 20% ± 7%, a range falling between that of PSTT and choriocarcinoma (Table 4) (98). Based on our recent studies (59), the cells in epithelioid trophoblastic tumors have a similar morphologic appearance and immunohistochemical profile to the cells that compose the placental-site nodule, suggesting that the epithelioid trophoblastic tumor represents the neoplastic counterpart of the placental-site nodule.

Differential Diagnosis

Although epithelioid trophoblastic tumor has distinct morphologic features, it may be confused with PSTT, placental-site nodule, and keratinizing squamous carcinoma of the cervix, especially in a biopsy or curettage specimen (98,99). At times, the growth of the tumor cells on the surface of the endocervix with replacement of the epithelium of the endocervix can make distinction from a primary cervical carcinoma very difficult. The arrangement of tumor cells in nests and cords and the eosinophilic extracellular matrix that accompanies the tumor resembles keratin and heightens its similarity to keratinizing squamous carcinoma of cervix. While epithelioid trophoblastic tumor can replace the surface epithelium and resemble a squamous intraepithelial neoplasm, epithelioid trophoblastic tumor has fewer stratified epithelial layers. In addition, the cells of epithelioid trophoblastic tumor that replace the surface epithelium tend to be more pleomorphic and are arranged parallel to the basement membrane in contrast to high-grade squamous intraepithelial lesions, which are composed of more uniform-sized cells that are aligned perpendicular to the basement membrane. Immunohistochemical reactions for cytokeratin 18 and inhibin-alpha are very helpful in the differential diagnosis of epithelioid trophoblastic tumor versus cervical carcinoma since cytokeratin 18 and inhibin-alpha are expressed in all epithelioid trophoblastic tumors but not in squamous carcinoma of the cervix (60,61) (Table 4). The focal immunoreactivity for Mel-CAM and hPL in epithelioid trophoblastic tumors is useful in the differential diagnosis of epithelioid trophoblastic tumor from PSTT, as the latter shows diffuse Mel-CAM and hPL expression (5) (Table 4). At times, epithelioid trophoblastic tumor may be difficult to distinguish from a placental-site nodule. In contrast to the former, the placental-site nodule is a microscopic and paucicellular lesion without necrosis. In addition, the Ki-67 index in epithelioid trophoblastic tumors is significantly higher than in placental-site nodules (Table 4).

Behavior and Treatment

The behavior of epithelioid trophoblastic tumor is still unclear, as the entity has only recently been recognized as a form of trophoblastic disease, and long-term follow-up is not available (33,97,98). Available data indicate that the epithelioid trophoblastic tumor, like PSTT, is less aggressive than choriocarcinoma. Among 28 reported patients, three have died and seven are living with metastasis. The remaining 18 patients are alive without evidence of disease (95–98). Three patients in these studies presented with extrauterine epithelioid trophoblastic tumor in the lungs without evidence of a primary tumor in the uterus. Unlike choriocarcinoma, epithelioid trophoblastic tumor appears to demonstrate only partial response to chemotherapy; tumors may recur or metastasize despite intensive chemotherapy (95,97,98). Hysterectomy and pulmonary resections have been used successfully in the treatment of these tumors, but there is insufficient data to evaluate the use of curettage and chemotherapy for the treatment of early lesions (95,97,98). Although the serum hCG level is only mildly elevated in most epithelioid trophoblastic tumors, as with PSTTs it appears to be useful in monitoring response to treatment. In summary, although epithelioid trophoblastic tumor and PSTT have different morphologic features, the approximate 25% metastatic rate and 10% mortality rate of epithelioid trophoblastic tumor, the low serum hCG titers, and the failure to respond to conventional chemotherapy used in the treatment of choriocarcinoma are reminiscent of the behavior of PSTT.

REFERENCES

1. Cross JC, Werb Z, Fisher SJ. Implantation and the placenta: key pieces of the development puzzle. *Science* 1994;266:1508–1518.
2. Kurman RJ, Main CS, Chen HC. Intermediate trophoblast: a distinctive form of trophoblast with specific morphological, biochemical and functional features. *Placenta* 1984;5:349–370.
3. Kurman RJ. The morphology, biology, and pathology of intermediate trophoblast—a look back to the present. *Hum Pathol* 1991;22:847–855.
4. Loke YW, King A. Human trophoblast development. In: *Human implantation-cell biology and immunology*, 1st ed. Cambridge: Cambridge University Press, 1995:32–62.
5. Shih IM, Kurman RJ. Expression of melanoma cell adhesion molecule in intermediate trophoblast. *Lab Invest* 1996;75:377–388.
6. Yeh I-T, O'Connor DM, Kurman JK. Vacuolated cytotrophoblast: a subpopulation of trophoblast in the chorion laeve. *Placenta* 1989;10:429–438.
7. Kurman RJ, Young RH, Norris HJ, Main CS, Lawrence WD, Scully RE. Immunocytochemical localization of hPL and hCG in the normal placenta and trophoblastic tumors, with emphasis on intermediate trophoblast and the placental site trophoblastic tumor. *Int J Gynecol Pathol* 1984;3:101–121.
8. Shih IM, Schnarr RL, Gearhart JD, Kurman RJ. Distribution of cells bearing the HNK-1 epitope in the human placenta. *Placenta* 1997;18:667–674.
9. Czernobilsky B, Barash A, Lancet M. Partial moles: a clinicopathologic study of 25 cases. *Obstet Gynecol* 1982;59:75–77.
10. Szulman AE, Surti U. The clinicopathologic profile of the partial hydatidiform mole. *Obstet Gynecol* 1982;59:597–602.
11. Wong LC, Ma HK. The syndrome of partial mole. *Arch Gynecol Obstet* 1984;234:161–166.
12. Berkowitz RS, Goldstein DP. Chorionic tumors. *N Engl J Med* 1996;335:1740–1748.
13. Surti U. Genetic concepts and techniques. In: Szulman AE, Buchsbaum HJ, eds. *Gestational trophoblastic disease*. New York: Springer-Verlag, 1987:111–121.
14. Szulman AE, Surti U. The syndromes of hydatidiform mole. I. Cytogenetic and morphologic correlations. *Am J Obstet Gynecol* 1978;131:665–671.
15. Jacobs PA, Szulman AE, Funkhouser J, Matsuura JS, Wilson CC. Human triploidy: relationship between parental origin of the additional haploid complement and development of partial hydatidiform mole. *Ann Hum Genet* 1982;46:223–231.
16. Sumithran E, Cheah PL, Susil BJ, Looi LM. Problems in the histological assessment of hydatidiform moles: a study on consensus diagnosis and ploidy status by fluorescent in situ hybridization. *Pathology* 1996;28:311–315.
17. Hemming JD, Quirke P, Womack C, Wells M, Elston CW, Bird CC. Diagnosis of molar pregnancy and persistent trophoblastic disease by flow cytometry. *J Clin Pathol* 1987;40:615–620.
18. Ohama K, Ueda K, Oka B, Moto E, Takenaka M, Fujiwara A. Cytogenetic and clinicopathologic studies of partial moles. *Obstet Gynecol* 1986;68:259–262.
19. Vejerslev LO, Fisher RA, Surti U, Walka N. Hydatidiform mole: cytogenetically unusual cases and their implications for the present classification. *Am J Obstet Gynecol* 1987;157:180–184.
20. Lawler SD, Fisher RA, Dent J. A prospective genetic study of complete and partial hydatidiform moles. *Am J Obstet Gynecol* 1991;164:1270–1277.
21. Vejerslev LO, Sunde L, Hansen BF, Larsen JK, Christensen IJ, Larsen G. Hydatidiform mole and fetus with normal karyotype: support of a separate entity. *Obstet Gynecol* 1991;77:868–874.
22. Lage JM, Mark SD, Roberts DJ, Goldstein DP, Bernstein MR, Berkowitz RS. A flow cytometric study of 137 fresh hydropic placentas: correlation between types of hydatidiform moles and nuclear DNA ploidy. *Obstet Gynecol* 1992;79:403–410.
23. Lage JM, Berkowitz RS, Rice LW, Goldstein DP, Bernstein MR, Weinberg DS. Flow cytometric analysis of DNA content in partial hydatidiform moles with persistent gestational trophoblastic tumor. *Obstet Gynecol* 1991;77:111–115.
24. Lage JM, Weinberg DS, Yavner DL, Bieber FR. The biology of tetraploid hydatidiform moles: histopathology, cytogenetics, and flow cytometry. *Hum Pathol* 1989;20:419–425.
25. Baergen RN, Kelly T, McGinniss J, Jones OW, Benirschke K. Complete hydatidiform mole with a coexistent embryo. *Hum Pathol* 1996;27:731–734.
26. Genest DR, Laborde O, Berkowitz RS, Goldstein DP, Bernstein MR, Lage J. A clinicopathologic study of 153 cases of complete hydatidiform mole (1980–1990)—histologic grade lacks prognostic significance. *Obstet Gynecol* 1991;78:402–409.
27. Shih IM, Kurman RJ. Assessment of proliferation activity in the differential diagnosis of placental site trophoblastic lesions and choriocarcinoma—a double immunohistochemical staining technique using Ki-67 and Mel-CAM antibodies. *Hum Pathol* 1998;28:27–33.
28. Montes M, Roberts D, Berkowitz RS, Genest DR. Prevalence and significance of implantation site trophoblastic atypia in hydatidiform moles and spontaneous abortions. *Am J Clin Pathol* 1996;105:411–416.
29. Szulman AE, Surti U. The syndromes of hydatidiform mole. II. Morphologic evolution of the complete and partial mole. *Am J Obstet Gynecol* 1978;132:20–27.
30. Elston CW, Bagshawe KD. The diagnosis of trophoblastic tumours from uterine curettings. *J Clin Pathol* 1972;25:111–118.
31. Curry SL, Hammond CB, Tyrey L, Creasman WT, Parker RT. Hydatidiform mole: diagnosis, management, and long-term follow-up of 347 patients. *Obstet Gynecol* 1975;45:1–8.
32. Hertig AT, Sheldon WH. Hydatidiform mole. A pathologico-clinical correlation of 200 cases. *Am J Obstet Gynecol* 1947;53:1–36.
33. Mazur MT, Kurman RJ. Gestational trophoblastic disease and related lesions. In: Kurman RJ, ed. *Blaustein's pathology of the female genital tract*. New York: Springer-Verlag, 1994:1049–1093.
34. Newra C, Frankforter S, Narcus JN. Clinicopathologic differences between diploid and tetraploid complete hydatidiform moles. *Int J Gynecol Pathol* 1997;16:239–244.
35. Berkowitz RS, Goldstein DP, Bernstein MR. Natural history of partial molar pregnancy. *Obstet Gynecol* 1985;66:677–681.
36. Smith EB, Szulman AE, Hinsaw W, Tyrey L, Surti U, Hammond CB. Human chorionic gonadotropin levels in complete and partial hydatidiform moles and in nonmolar abortuses. *Am J Obstet Gynecol* 1984;149:129–132.
37. Szulman AE. Complete hydatidiform mole: clinico-pathologic features. In: Szulman AE, Buchsbaum HJ, eds. *Gestational trophoblastic disease*. New York: Springer-Verlag, 1987:27–36.
38. Lurain JR, Brewer JI, Torok EE, Halpern B. Natural history of hydatidiform mole after primary evacuation. *Am J Obstet Gynecol* 1983;145:591–595.
39. Jeffers MD, Richmond JA, Smith R. Trophoblast proliferation rate does not predict progression to persistent gestational trophoblastic disease in complete hydatidiform mole. *Int J Gynecol Pathol* 1996;15:34–38.
40. Cheung ANY, Ngan HYS, Chen WZ. The significance of proliferating cell nuclear antigen in human trophoblastic disease: an immunohistochemical study. *Histopathology* 1993;22:566–571.
41. Hertig AT, Mansell H. *Tumors of the female sex organs. Part 1. Hydatidiform mole and choriocarcinoma*. Atlas of tumor pathology, section 9 fascicle 33. Washington, DC: Armed Forces Institute of Pathology, 1956.
42. Rice LW, Berkowitz RS, Lage JM, Goldstein DP, Bernstein MR. Persistent gestational trophoblastic tumor after partial hydatidiform mole. *Gynecol Oncol* 1990;36:358–362.
43. Gaber LW, Redline RW, Mostoufi-Zadeh M, Driscoll SG. Invasive partial mole. *Am J Clin Pathol* 1986;85:722–724.
44. Szulman AE, Ma HK, Wong LC, Hsu C. Residual trophoblastic disease in association with partial hydatidiform moles. *Obstet Gynecol* 1981;57:392–394.
45. Berkowitz RS, Goldstein DP. Diagnosis and management of primary hydatidiform mole. *Obstet Gynecol Clin North Am* 1988;15:491–503.
46. Takeuchi S. Nature of invasive mole and its rational treatment. *Semin Oncol* 1982;9:181–186.

47. Dehner LP. Gestational and nongestational trophoblastic neoplasia. A historic and pathobiologic survey. *Am J Surg Pathol* 1980;4:43–58.
48. Delfs E. Quantitative chorionic gonadotrophin: prognostic value in hydatidiform mole and chorionepithelioma. *Obstet Gynecol* 1957;9:1–24.
49. Elston CW. Development and structure of trophoblastic neoplasms. In: Luke YW, Whyte A, eds. *Biology of trophoblast*. New York: Elsevier, 1983:188–232.
50. Scully RE, Bonfiglio TA, Kurman RJ, Silverberg SG, Wilkinson EJ. *Gestational trophoblastic diseases. World Health Organization International Histological Classification of Tumors,* 2nd ed. Berlin: Springer-Verlag, 1994.
51. Kurman RJ. Pathology of trophoblast. In: Kaufman ed. *Pathology of reproductive failure*. New York: International Academy of Pathology, 1991;33 195–227.
52. Shih I-M, Nesbit M, Herlyn M, Kurman RJ. A new Mel-CAM (CD146)-specific monoclonal antibody, MN-4, on paraffin-embedded tissue. *Mod Pathol* 1998;11:1098–1106.
53. Shih IM, Speicher D, Hsu MY, Levine E, Herlyn M. Melanoma cell-cell interactions are mediated through heterophilic Mel-CAM/ligand adhesion. *Cancer Res* 1997;57:3835–3840.
54. Jacques SM, Qureshi F, Ramirez NC, Lawrence WD. Retained trophoblastic tissue in fallopian tubes: a consequence of unsuspected ectopic pregnancies. *Int J Gynecol Pathol* 1997;16:219–224.
55. Young RH, Kurman RJ, Scully RE. Placental site nodules and plaques—clinicopathologic analysis of 20 cases. *Am J Surg Pathol* 1990;14:1001–1009.
56. Huettner PC, Gersell DJ. Placental site nodule: a clinicopathologic study of 38 cases. *Int J Gynecol Pathol* 1994;13:191–198.
57. Shitabata PK, Rutgers JL. The placental site nodule: an immunohistochemical study. *Hum Pathol* 1994;25:1295–1301.
58. Nayar R, Snell J, Siverberg SG, Lage JM. Placental site nodule occurring in a fallopian tube. *Hum Pathol* 1996;27:1243–1245.
59. Shih I-M, Seidman JD, Kurman RJ. Characterization of distinct types of intermediate trophoblast with specific references to placental site nodules. *Hum Pathol,* 1999 (in press).
60. Shih I-M, Kurman RJ. Distribution of cytokeratin subtypes in trophoblast. Unpublished.
61. Shih I-M, Kurman RJ. Immunohistochemical localization of inhibin-alpha in the human placenta and gestational trophoblastic lesions. *Int J Gynecol Pathol,* 1999 in Press.
62. Hammond CB, Hertz R, Ross GT, Lipsett MB. Odell WD. Diagnostic problems of choriocarcinoma and related trophoblastic neoplasms. *Obstet Gynecol* 1967;29:224–229.
63. Mazur MT, Lurain JR, Brewer JI. Fatal gestational choriocarcinoma. Clinicopathologic study of patients treated at a trophoblastic disease center. *Cancer* 1982;50:1833–1846.
64. Olive DL, Lurain JR, Brewer JI. Choriocarcinoma associated with term gestation. *Am J Obstet Gynecol* 1984;148:711–716.
65. Hou PC, Pang SC. Chorionepithelioma: an analytical study of 28 necropsied cases with special reference to the possibility of spontaneous retrogression. *J Pathol Bacteriol* 1956;72:95–104.
66. Dougherty CM, Cunningham C, Mickal A. Choriocarcinoma with metastasis in a postmenopausal woman. *Am J Obstet Gynecol* 1978:132:700–701.
67. Novak E, Seah CS. Choriocarcinoma of the uterus. A study of 74 cases from the Mathieu Memorial Chorionepithelioma Registry. *Am J Obstet Gynecol* 1954;67:933–961.
68. Ober WB. Edgcomb JH, Price EB. The pathology of choriocarcinoma. *Ann NY Acad Sci* 1971;179:299–321.
69. Brewer JI, Mazur MT. Gestational choriocarcinoma: its origin in the placenta during seemingly normal pregnancy. *Am J Surg Pathol* 1981;5:267–277.
70. Duncan DA, Mazur MT. Trophoblastic tumors. Ultrastructural comparison of choriocarcinoma and placental-site trophoblastic tumor. *Hum Pathol* 1989;20:370–381.
71. Daya D, Sabet L. The use of cytokeratin as a sensitive and reliable marker for trophoblastic tissue. *Am J Clin Pathol* 1991;95:137–141.
72. Niehans GA, Manivel JC, Copland GT, Scheithauer BW, Wick MR. Immunohistochemistry of germ cell and trophoblastic neoplasms. *Cancer* 1988;62:1113–1123.
73. Kubosawa H, Nagoa K, Kondo Y. Coexistence of adenocarcinoma and choriocarcinoma in the sigmoid colon. *Cancer* 1984;54:866–868.
74. Obe JA, Rosen N, Koss LG. Primary choriocarcinoma of the urinary bladder. Report of a case with probable epithelial origin. *Cancer* 1983;52:1405–1409.
75. Savage J, Subby W, Okagaki T. Adenocarcinoma of the endometrium with trophoblastic differentiation and metastases as choriocarcinoma: a case report. *Gynecol Oncol* 1987;26:257–262.
76. Campo E, Algaba R, Palacin A, Germa R, Sole-Balcells FJ, Cardesa A. Placental proteins in high-grade urothelial neoplasms. An immunohistochemical study of human chorionic gonadotropin, human placental lactogen, and pregnancy-specific beta-1-glycoprotein. *Cancer* 1989;63:2497–2504.
77. Heyderman E, Chapman DV, Richardson TC, Calvert I, Rosen SW. Human chorionic gonadotropin and human placental lactogen in extragonadal tumors: an immunoperoxidase study of ten non-germ cell neoplasm. *Cancer* 1985;56:2674–2682.
78. Heitz PU, von Herbay G, Kloppel G, et al. The expression of subunits of human chorionic gonadotropin (hCG) by nontrophoblastic, nonendocrine, and endocrine tumors. *Am J Clin Pathol* 1987;88: 467–472.
79. Brewer JI, Smith RT, Pratt GB. Choriocarcinoma. Absolute 5 year survival rates of 122 patients treated by hysterectomy. *Am J Obstet Gynecol* 1963;85:841–843.
80. Lurain JR, Casanova LA, Miller DS, Rademaker AW. Prognostic factors in gestational trophoblastic tumors: a proposed new scoring system based on multivariate analysis. *Am J Obstet Gynecol* 1991;164:611–616.
81. Bagshawe KD. Risk and prognostic factors in trophoblastic neoplasia. *Cancer* 1976;38:1373–1385.
82. Surwit EA, Alberts DS, Christian CD, Graham VE. Poor-prognosis gestational trophoblastic disease: an update. *Obstet Gynecol* 1984;6421–26.
83. Berkowitz RS, Goldstein DP, Bernstein MR. Choriocarcinoma following term gestation. *Gynecol Oncol* 1984;17:52–57.
84. Deligdisch L, Driscoll SG, Goldstein DP. Gestational trophoblastic neoplasms: morphologic correlates of therapeutic response. *Am J Obstet Gynecol* 1978;130:801–806.
85. Nickels J, Risberg B, Melander S. Trophoblastic pseudotumor of the uterus. *Acta Pathol Microbiol Immunol Scand [A]* 1978;86:14–16.
86. Eckstein RP, Paradinas FJ, Bagshawe KD. Placental site trophoblastic tumour (trophoblastic pseudotumor): a study of four cases requiring hysterectomy including one fatal case. *Histopathology* 1982;6: 211–226.
87. Kurman RJ, Scully RE, Norris HJ. Trophoblastic pseudotumor of the uterus. *Cancer* 1976;38:1214–1226.
88. Gloor E, Hurlimann J. Trophoblastic pseudotumor of the uterus. Clinicopathologic report with immunohistochemical and ultrastructural studies. *Am J Surg Pathol* 1981;5:5–13.
89. Nagelberg SB, Rosen SW. Clinical and laboratory investigation of a virilized woman with placental site trophoblastic tumor. *Obstet Gynecol* 1985;65:527–534.
90. Nagamani M, Kaspar HG, Dinh TV, Hannigan EV, Smith E. Hyperthecosis of the ovaries in a woman with a placental site trophoblastic tumor. *Obstet Gynecol* 1990;76:931–935.
91. Young RE, Scully RE, McCluskey RT. A distinctive glomerular lesion complicating placental site trophoblastic tumor: report of two cases. *Hum Pathol* 1985;16:35–42.
92. Eckstein RP, Russell P, Friedlander ML, Tattersall MHN, Bradfield A. Metastasizing placental site trophoblastic tumor: a case study. *Hum Pathol* 1983;16:632–636.
93. Gloor E, Dialdas J, Hurlimann J, Ribolzi J, Barrelet L. Placental site trophoblastic tumor (trophoblastic pseudotumor) of the uterus with metastases and fatal outcome. *Am J Surg Pathol* 1983;7:483–486.
94. Hopkins M, Nunez C, Murphy JR, Wentz WB. Malignant placental site trophoblastic tumor. *Obstet Gynecol* 1985;66:95S–100S.
95. Mazur MT. Metastatic gestational choriocarcinoma. Unusual pathologic variant following therapy. *Cancer* 1989;63:1370–1377.
96. Jones WB, Romain K, Erlandson RA, Burt ME. Thoracotomy in the management of gestational choriocarcinoma: a clinicopathologic study. *Cancer* 1993;72:2175–2181.
97. Silva EG, Tornos C, Lage J, Ordonez NG, Morris M, Kavanagh J. Multiple nodules of intermediate trophoblast following hydatidiform moles. *Int J Gynecol Pathol* 1993;12:324–332.
98. Shih I-M, Kurman RJ. Epithelioid trophoblastic tumor—a distinctive neoplasm simulating carcinoma but differing from choriocarcinoma and placental site trophoblastic tumor. *Am J Surg Pathol* 1998;22:1393–1403.
99. Mazur MT, Kurman RJ. Gestational trophoblastic disease. In: Mazur Mt, Kurman, RJ, eds. *Diagnosis of endometrial biopsies and curettings—a practical approach*. New York: Springer-Verlag, 1995:63–88.

CHAPTER 50

The Placenta

Geoffrey Altshuler

The placenta is like a diary of gestational life. Conventional diaries often contain provocative items that ultimately are unimportant, and conversely they often contain obscure information that is the ignored harbinger of detrimental outcomes. Newborns whose placentas are abnormal often develop normally. Other newborns seemingly have little clinical aberration but they develop cerebral palsy; the placentas of those infants usually have meaningful histopathology. Surgical pathologists are thus increasingly requested to perform placental examinations. This chapter discusses the need for clinicopathologic correlation between placental pathology and the outcome of the associated neonate.

INDICATIONS FOR PLACENTAL EXAMINATION

The American College of Obstetricians and Gynecologists has suggested that routine study of the placenta is not warranted (1). Benirschke and Kaufmann (2) strongly disagree. Combined gross and light microscopic placental examinations should not be performed when normal newborns are forthcoming from normal pregnancies and deliveries. This statement should not discourage a nurse practitioner, pathologist's assistant, or pathologist from completing a gross placental checklist for all delivered specimens. An example of such an examination and report is illustrated in Table 1. In 1989 I recommended an "embed and hold" placental program (3). Complementary to the gross report, segments of umbilical cord, extraplacental membranes, and placenta can be stored in three paraffin blocks. When later needed for medical or medicolegal purposes, light microscopic slides can readily be prepared from stored paraffin blocks (3).

Any concern by a clinician should be sufficient indication for a pathologist to perform gross and light microscopic placental examination. Table 2, from Conference XIX of the College of American Pathologists (CAP) (4), summarizes indications for placental examination, recommended by a working group of pathologists, obstetricians, and neonatologists. Although the college has recently issued another list of recommendations for placental examination (5), the two statements are essentially the same.

PLACENTAL ACCESSION, STORAGE, PROCESSING AND ARTIFACTS

Because detailed methods of placental examination are available elsewhere (5–7), this chapter is not comprehensive. Placentas should never be frozen. Freezing distorts the villi, obscures meconium, and thereby compromises diagnoses. Placentas of all pregnancies and deliveries should be freshly refrigerated. Placentas not examined on the day of delivery or soon thereafter, should be stored at 4°C for 1 week. If a clinician subsequently requests a placental examination, the specimen, which otherwise would have been incinerated, is available. If a specimen needs to be sent to another medical center, it should be fixed in a volume of formalin that is at least ten times its own volume. The partially fixed item can be transported in a very small amount of the same fluid. In my opinion, Bouin's solution is an undesirable fixative. It obscures bacteria (particularly fusobacteria), compromises some immunocytochemical processing, because of its poor preservation of antigen (8), and stains laboratory equipment. The Brown and Hopps method of staining bacteria is convenient and reliable (9). Other stains may fail to show organisms. Also note the following:

1. Artifacts occur when placentas are fixed prior to examination. Depending on the specimen's size and the volume of fixative used, fixation in buffered formalin increases a placenta's weight by 7% to 12%.
2. Fixation produces distention of fetal blood vessels and, with congestion, this simulates effects of cord obstruction and fetal cardiac failure.
3. Umbilical cord vascular anastomoses are present near the placenta. To avoid an incorrect diagnosis of single

---

G. Altshuler: Department of Pathology, University of Oklahoma Health Sciences Center; Department of Pathology, Children's Hospital of Oklahoma, Oklahoma City, Oklahoma 73104.

TABLE 1. *Gross placental findings*

General
Trimmed weight: _____ g   Complete (Y/N): ___   Fixed (Y/N): ___ or Fresh (Y/N): ___
Size _ _._ × _ _._ × _._ cm   Accessory lobe (Y/N): ___ (Size _ _._ × _ _._ × _ _._ cm)

Membranes
Placental sac rupture: _____ cm from margin   Membranes edema: (Y/N) ___
Membranes insertion site: _____ % marginal; _____ % circummarginate; _____ % circumvallate
Color: Normal ___   green (G) ___   brown (B) ___   yellow (Y) ___   gray (G) ___   Combined colors _____

Cord
Knots (Number and type): True ___, Variceal or false ___; Length: ___ cm; Vessels: (3) ___ or (2) ___
Site of cord insertion: Central ___   Marginal ___   Eccentric ___   Velamentous ___
Color: Normal ___   green (G) ___   brown (B) ___   yellow (Y) ___   gray (G) ___   Combined colors _____

Placenta
Color: Normal ___   green (G) ___   brown (B) ___   yellow (Y) ___   gray (G) ___   Combined colors _____
Superficial (e.g., tan-gray) fibrinoid material: none (Y/N) ___, <25% ___, 25–50% ___, >50% ___
Amnion nodosum or any other unusual superficial lesions (Y/N): ___
Appearance of placental tissue: congested (Y/N) ___   Very pale (Y/N) ___   Unremarkable ___
Infarcts or infarction (including the distribution and the approximate amount of the placenta involved):
Focal ___   Multifocal ___   or   Diffuse ___   <25% ___, 25–50% ___, >50% ___
Abruption: (Y/N) ___   (Approximate % of placental floor involved): ___%
                         Approximate volume of blood clots: ___ ml)
Maternal floor calcification, degeneration or infarction: (Approximate % of floor involved) ___%
Other information

Comments:

TABLE 2. *Indications that require a comprehensive gross and microscopic examination by a pathologist*

Maternal conditions
  Diabetes mellitus (or glucose intolerance)
  Hypertension (pregnancy-induced)
  Prematurity (less than 32 weeks)
  Postmaturity (pregnancy longer than 42 weeks)
  Maternal history of reproductive failure (defined as one or more previous stillbirths, spontaneous abortions, or premature births)
  Oligohydramnios
  Fever
  Infection
  Maternal history of substance abuse
  Repetitive bleeding (other than minor spotting of the first trimester)
  Abruptio placentae
Fetal and neonatal conditions
  Stillbirth or perinatal death
  Multiple birth
  Congenital abnormalities
  Fetal growth retardation
  Prematurity (32 weeks or less gestation)
  Hydrops
  Viscid/thick meconium
  Admission to a neonatal intensive care unit
  Severe central nervous system depression (Apgar score of 3 or less at 5 minutes)
  Neurologic problems, including seizures
  Suspected infection
Placental conditions
  Any gross abnormality of the placenta, its membranes, or the umbilical cord

From ref. 4.

---

umbilical artery, the cord should be sampled 4 cm or more from its insertion into the placenta.

4. Fresh samples of tissue for initial fixation, prior to trimming and placement of the samples into cassettes, should be no more than 2 cm thick. This facilitates proper fixation.

5. In the Comments section of the placental report, considerations of gross findings are very pertinent. For example:

   a. A wrinkled and narrow umbilical cord typically accompanies oligohydramnios.

   b. At the decidual aspect of the extraplacental membranes, adherent fresh blood or fibrinous material, may indicate acute abruptio placentae or a remote episode of placental separation. The substantial majority of premature placental separations are followed by delivery of the fetus within 3 hours. When delivery does not occur, retroplacental blood clot compresses the adjacent placenta and produces a cupola or cup-like placental indentation.

6. Many pathologists process a total of only three slides consisting of placental tissue, extraplacental membranes, and umbilical cord. When those slides have equivocal pathology they return to the gross specimen and process additional samples. I usually obtain six slides. Those samples originate from a block with a segment of umbilical cord and membrane roll, a block with a segment of superficial placenta near the umbilical cord insertion site, two blocks of nonmarginal superficial pla-

cental tissue, and two blocks of nonmarginal placenta with maternal floor. Gross lesions should therein be included; for a small percentage of cases, more sections are needed.

7. Because dull knife blades disrupt the placental amniotic epithelium away from the underlying tissue, new blades are repeatedly needed to enable inclusion of the entire placental amnion with the underlying fetal chorionic plate and villous tissue.

NORMAL PLACENTAL DEVELOPMENT

Gross Features

The placenta should consist of a single disk, without any kind of accessory lobe. At midtrimester the umbilical cord insertion is central and, as gestation proceeds, the cord insertion becomes eccentric. The umbilical cord should have two arteries and one vein. Severe eccentricity of the cord's insertion is abnormal, as is irregular insertion of the extraplacental membranes (Fig. 1). Gross placental abnormalities are often not associated with symptomatic disease or malformation. Pathologists who only occasionally examine placentas are well advised to use photographic documentation of any seemingly major abnormality. This allows a consultant to evaluate the extent to which an apparently rare anomaly might be clinically significant.

Light Microscopic Features

To facilitate illustration of reduction in the size of villi throughout gestation, Figs. 2 to 5 are made at the same magnification. The villi of first trimester placentas are relatively large and, at their surface, they have an outer layer of syncytiotrophoblast and an inner cytotrophoblast (Fig. 2). By midtrimester, the villi are appreciably smaller; the cytotrophoblast is less appreciable and the syncytiotrophoblast includes a small population of clusters or so-called knots (Fig. 3). Often, between 20 and 30 weeks' gestation, intermediate villi have large spaces (Fig. 4). This is normal and should not be diagnosed as villous edema. That diagnosis requires the additional presence of numerous water-laden Hofbauer cells. At term, the placental villi are obviously smaller than villi of mid-trimester. The trophoblast should have readily appreciable foci of agglutinated syncytial trophoblast cells (knots) and the villi should not be enlarged by stromal cell hypercellularity, edema, or blood vessels (Fig. 5). Knowledge of these general features is sufficient to enable surgical pathologists to recognize severe dysmaturity such as chorangiosis, discussed later in this chapter.

MAJOR GROSS ABNORMALITIES

Placental Weight and Size

Although storage of fresh placentas leads to some drainage of blood from each specimen, this does not eradi-

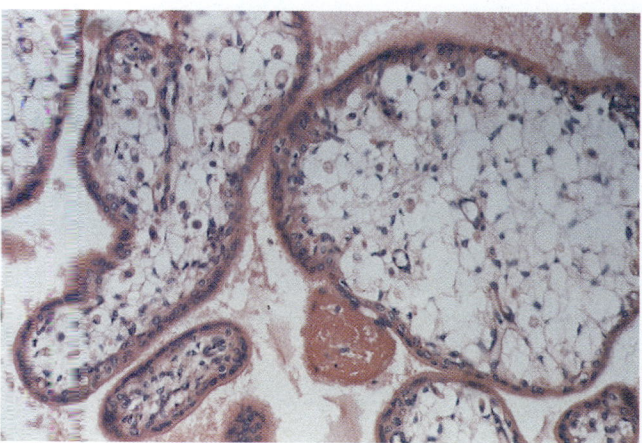

FIG. 2. Normal first trimester placental villi (12 weeks' gestation).

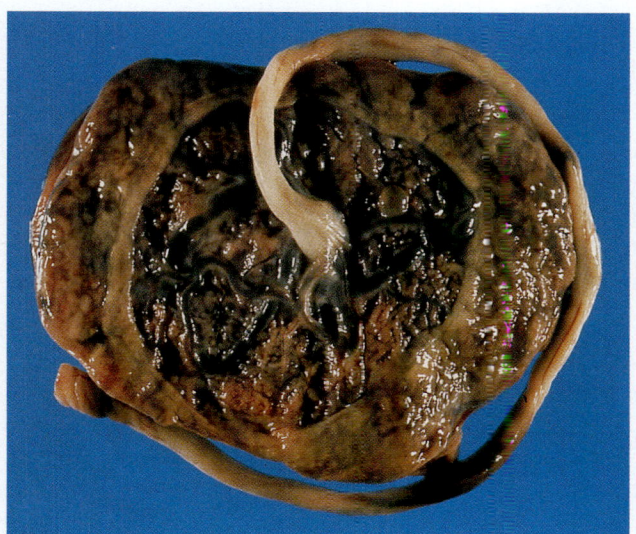

FIG. 1. Circumvallate placenta. There is a peripheral cup-like insertion of the membranes at the placental surface. When the extrachorial insertion has a flattened configuration, it is called circummarginate.

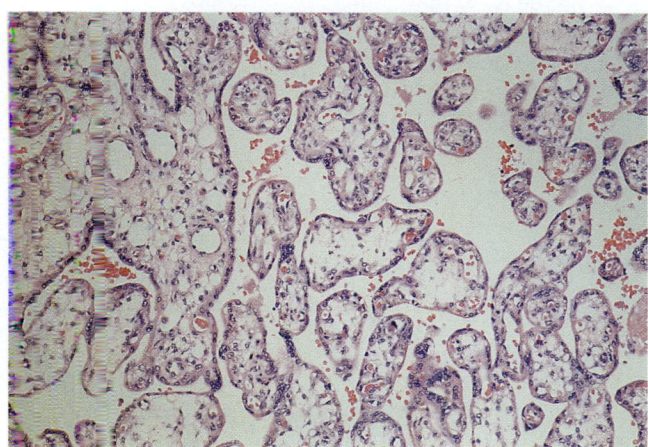

FIG. 3. Early third trimester villi (30 weeks' gestation).

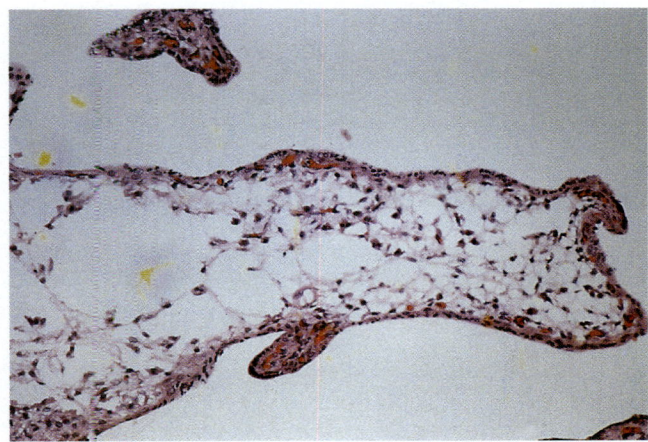

FIG. 4. Normal intermediate villus at 24 weeks' gestation. Note the prominent vascular spaces.

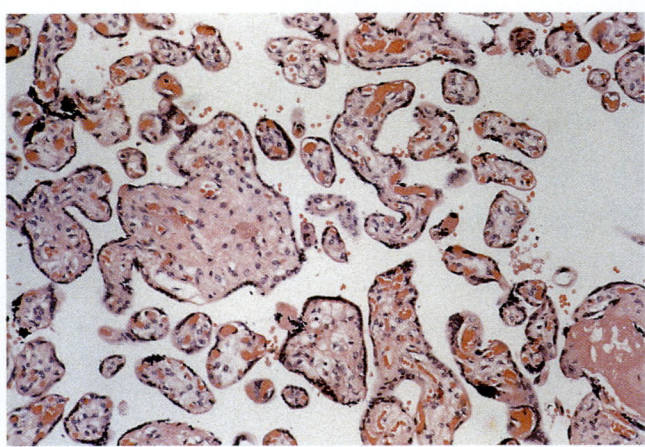

FIG. 5. Normal villi at 40 weeks' gestation. Note that the term gestation villi have dark-colored superficial focal syncytiotrophoblast knots and that these villi are appreciably smaller than those from immature placentas.

cate meaningful information of a placenta's mass and size. In my opinion, socioeconomic factors produce a significantly greater variation in placental weights than triage and storage. From various published standards, 10th percentile birth weights at each gestational age differ substantially and the differences occasionally exceed 500 g (10). Caution is thus needed in any applied consideration of fetal-placental weight ratios. This is true even when one uses the data of Benirschke and Kaufmann (2).

Table 3 lists weights obtained from my examination of 977 singleton placentas. At 20 weeks' gestation, the trimmed unfixed and fresh placenta should not exceed 150 g; at 30 weeks' gestation, 375 g; and at term, 600 g.

Clinicians know that an edematous infant at birth frequently has an edematous placenta, but that an infant with no bodily signs of edema may be born with placental edema. Maternal diabetes mellitus may then have caused reduced colloid osmotic pressure and passage of maternal fluid into the fetal placental villous tissue (11). Additionally, with maternal diabetes, uteroplacental vasculopathy may cause a thin and small placenta resultant from chronically reduced uteroplacental blood flow. The fetus then sustains abnormal growth. Relative to these considerations, Table 4 has helpful information on placental size and thickness. At and beyond 37 weeks' gestation, placentas thicker than 3.5 cm are usually abnormal. Even if they are not overtly large, they are usually heavy and are thus diagnosable as placentomegaly. The cause is usually diabetes, chronic intrauterine infection, immunohemolytic anemia, fetal-maternal hemorrhage, hydrops, or maternal anemia.

Placental Shape

Abnormal placental shapes usually are not associated with clinical problems. Accessory placental lobes or bidiscoid placentas with anastomoses between the disks can predispose a newborn to fulminant blood loss from lacerated intramembranous vessels. The same risk occurs with vascular rupture, which accompanies velamentously inserted umbili-

TABLE 3. *Placental weight by gestational age category (n = 977)*

Gestational age (weeks)	Placental weight (g): mean (SD)
<28 (n = 73)	237.0 (122.2)
28–32 (n = 132)	292.5 (96.0)
33–36 (n = 189)	384.6 (101.5)
37–40 (n = 399)	455.9 (110.1)
>40 (n = 184)	501.9 (104.1)

TABLE 4. *Placental dimensions by gestational age category (n = 225)**

Gestional age (weeks)	Placental weight (g): mean (SD)	Biggest dimension (cm): mean (SD)	Thickness (cm): mean (SD)
<28 (n = 22)	252.5 (136.6)	15.1 (3.1)	2.0 (0.50)
28–32 (n = 33)	314.3 (101.5)	17.0 (3.2)	2.5 (0.64)
33–36 (n = 37)	390.8 (119.2)	18.5 (2.6)	2.4 (0.58)
37–40 (n = 97)	456.2 (112.9)	19.4 (2.8)	2.5 (0.54)
>40 (n = 36)	496.1 (110.4)	19.7 (2.4)	2.7 (0.65)

* Reliability subsample.

cal cords (Fig. 6). When segments of placenta are retained in the uterus, postpartum bleeding and fever indicate a clinical diagnosis of placenta accreta. Gross examination of the maternal floor often then reveals ragged tissue or incomplete cotyledons. Light microscopic findings may include muscle fibers in the basal decidua. My experience has been that the histologic findings of placenta accreta can occur without accompanying postpartum maternal complications. Alternatively, particularly with mothers who have had vaginal birth after previous cesarean section, clinical signs of placenta accreta may not be accompanied by obvious gross or light microscopic placental lesions. In such cases, the basal decidua of the placenta is grossly smooth and intact, not ragged or incomplete.

Fetal Placental Surface Color

A normal fetal placental surface has a glistening light blue or blue-pink color. When acute meconium staining occurs and the meconium has been on the placenta for only a few minutes or for less than 2 hours, the placenta surface and membranes have a slimy and green appearance (Fig. 7). When the pathologist receives a specimen that has been partially covered with meconium shortly before delivery, the placenta may grossly appear normal. The longer a placenta has been exposed to meconium, the more that its appearance changes from slimy green to muddy-brown (Fig. 8). Chronic exposure of the extraplacental membranes to meconium typically causes the tissue to be slippery and edematous. Whereas placentas with slight chorioamnionitis usually are not discolored, severe or chronic chorioamnionitis has a yellow-gray or gray-blue color. Fusobacteria can cause the fetal placental surface to appear light green. When we have seen that color, we have taken a chorionic specimen for culture and have isolated fusobacteria. Acute abruptio placentae is

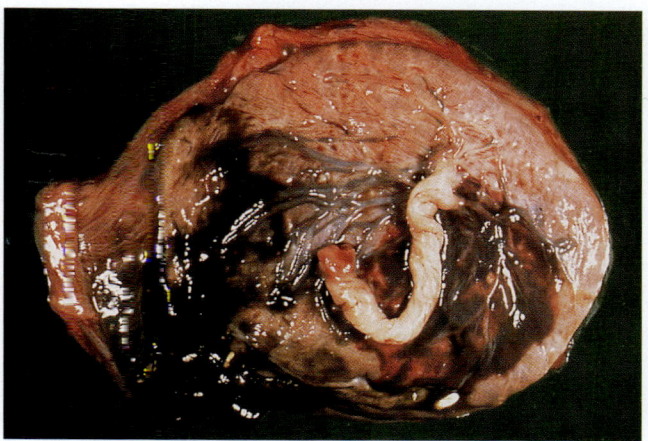

FIG. 7. Placenta with acute meconium staining and superficial meconium.

typically accompanied by loose blood clots or by blood clots that are tenuously adherent to the placental floor. A remote episode of placental abruption causes brown-tan, old fibrin and necrotic tissue to be present across the abruption site and often across adjacent retromembranous tissue of the extraplacental membranes. Light microscopic examination then reveals hemosiderin and other blood pigment. Entirely unrelated to that, and for no definitely known reason, the fetal placental surface sometimes has multifocal plaques of pink-tan or pink-orange chorionic fibrin. The size and extent of these changes should be noted in the gross description.

Insertion of the Extraplacental Membranes

Normal placentas have membranes that insert directly into their edge, with a lack of chorionic villous tissue being present lateral to the insertion of the membranes. Extrachorial

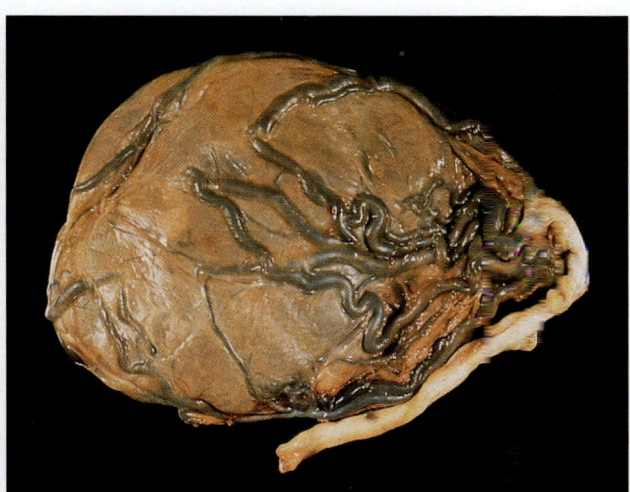

FIG. 6. Velamentous insertion of the umbilical cord. The umbilical cord is seen to insert into the placental membranes (right).

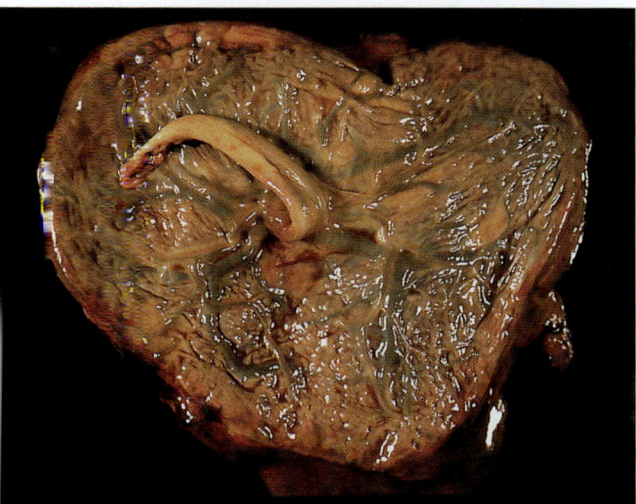

FIG. 8. Placenta with very chronic meconium staining. Note the compressed appearance of the umbilical cord near its insertion into the placenta.

placentas are either circummarginate or circumvallate. Whereas the margin of circummarginate placentas is thin and flat, circumvallate placentas have a peripheral protuberance (Fig. 1). The latter placentas result from marginal hemorrhage. In large population studies, circumvallate placentas with cysts and other gross aberrations are associated with maternal and fetal abnormalities. The mother may have an abnormal uterus and the newborn may have an overt or clinically inapparent malformation. Circummarginate placentas usually do not have an accompanying clinical problem. Severe circumvallate placentation results from repeated marginal hemorrhages. Associated manifestations include a maternal history of uterine bleeding, cramping, and hydrorrhea (12).

Fetal Placental Surface Lesions

Apart from having absent or ragged placental floor tissue, placenta accreta may manifest superficial acute hemorrhagic extravasation near the insertion of the umbilical cord. That fine film of hemorrhage results from excessive traction on the cord during the third stage of labor. Multiple 0.2 to 0.4 cm superficial amniotic lesions are either amnion nodosum or stratified squamous metaplasia. When present, they are probably most easily seen near the insertion of the umbilical cord. Amnion nodosum signifies oligohydramnios, either because of amniotic fluid leakage or because of absent or dysplastic kidneys. Amnion nodosum light microscopically

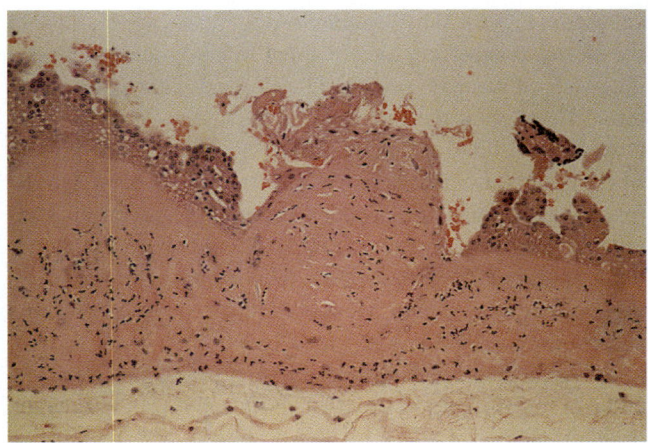

FIG. 10. Amnion nodosum and stratified squamous metaplasia.

features small nodules of protuberant proteinaceous material with entrapped squames (Fig. 9); stratified squamous metaplastic lesions have finely umbilicated gross appearances; the light microscopic appearances are similar to metaplastic stratified squamous epithelium in other organs (Fig. 10).

Cysts

Whether or not they contain blood, cysts can be present at the surface of a placenta (Fig. 11) or anywhere throughout its cotyledons. The cysts are lined by X cells (Fig. 12). This cellular tissue has a fetal origin. The cells are diffusely abundant in degenerate and ischemic placentas of growth-retarded fetuses (13,14). Their function is poorly understood but is perhaps significantly involved with prostaglandins and suppression of labor (14,15). X-cell cysts usually measure less than 3 cm in diameter. Focal or multifocal cysts of smaller size, which are not bordered by X cells or other remarkable lining, occur in partial moles and result from vil-

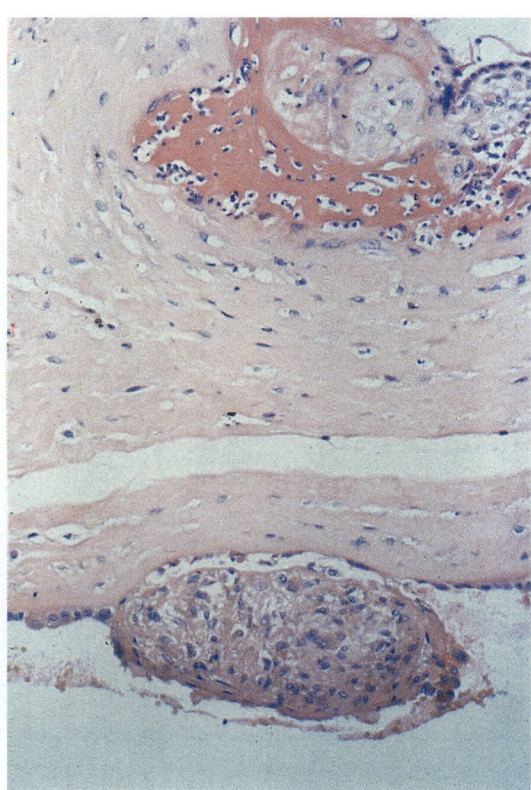

FIG. 9. Amnion nodosum.

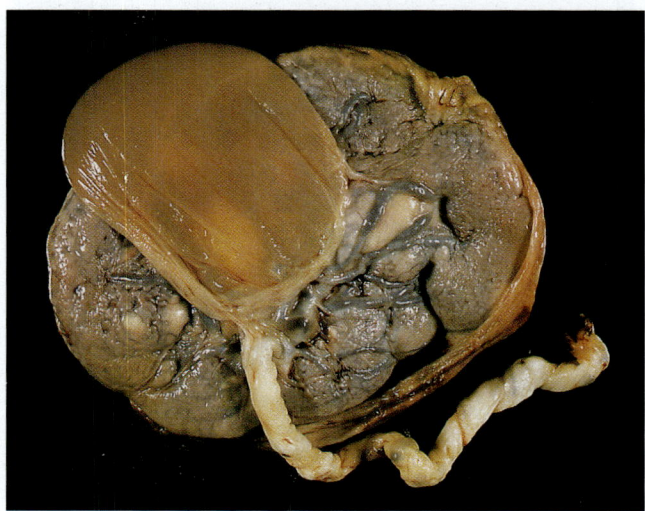

FIG. 11. Placenta with a superficial X-cell cyst.

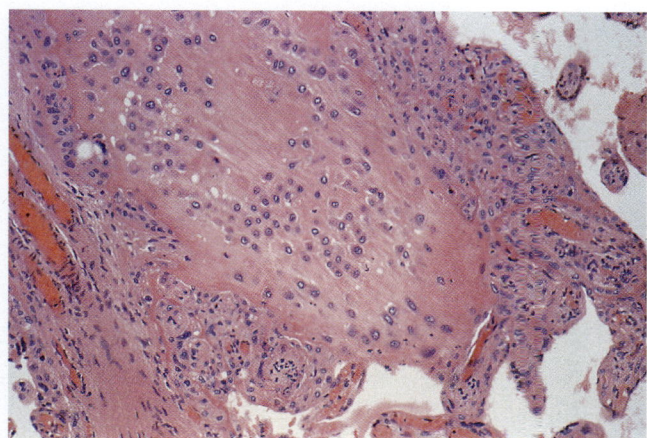

FIG. 12. A developing cyst: numerous basophilic X cells are present around proteinaceous eosinophilic material.

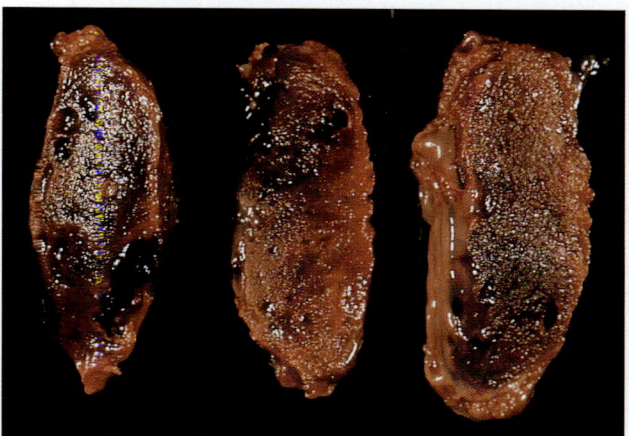

FIG. 13. Acute placental infarction.

lous stromal degeneration. This kind of cyst is rare. The accompanying fetus or newborn typically has triploidy and the fetal placental vessels have numerous nucleated red blood cells.

Infarcts and Intervillous Thrombi

Acute infarcts have a dark red-brown color in fresh tissue and their consistency is abnormal as compared to the adjacent placenta. This facilitates their recognition when one slices through a fresh specimen (Fig. 13). Reduced blood flow is present at the edge of a placenta, and focal infarction often occurs in this region. These lesions usually do not have clinically significant complications. When nonlateral infarcts are grossly seen, the pathologist should closely examine the light microscopic appearance of the tissue elsewhere. Diffuse acute and chronic ischemic change indicate reduced uteroplacental blood flow with attendant risk of perinatal morbidity and mortality (Figs. 14–16). Intervillous thrombi resemble infarcts but, in fresh tissue, they have more of an orange-tan color than the darker color of acute infarcts. By use of Sternberger's technique of peroxidase-labeling, Kaplan and her colleagues (16) demonstrated fetal hemoglobin in erythrocytes within intervillous thrombi.

Maternal Floor Infarction

A strong epidemiologic association between maternal floor infarction and recurrent reproductive failure accounts for the importance of this rare entity. From data of the Col-

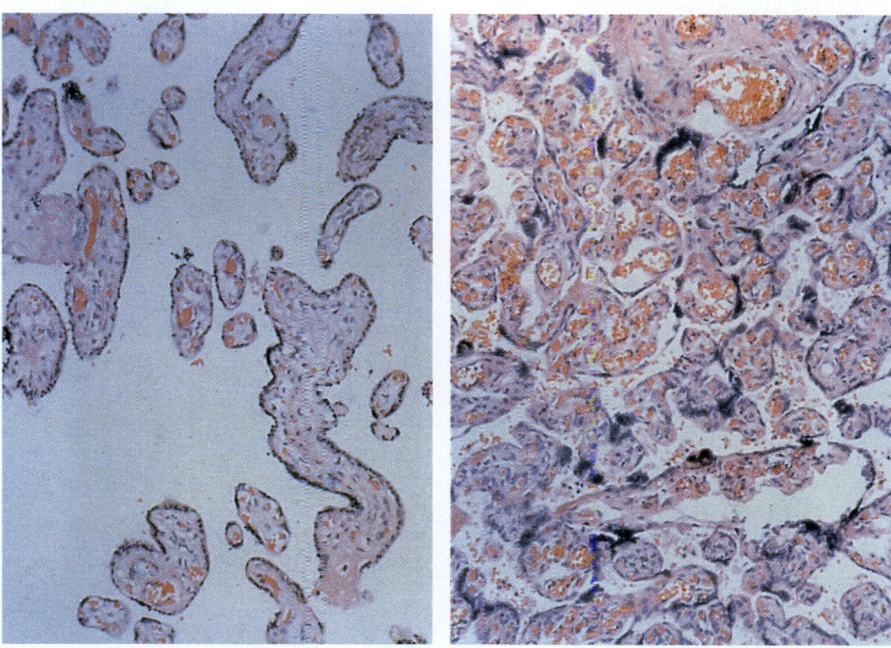

FIG. 14. Acute placental ischemic change: compare the agglutination of villi and the increased syncytial knots *(right)* with the normal tissue *(left)*.

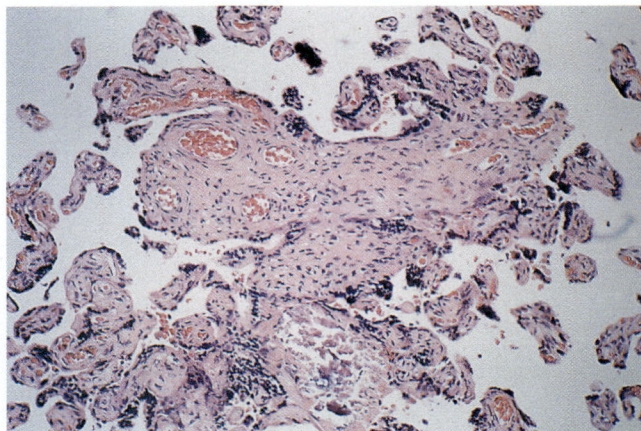

FIG. 15. Placenta with chronic ischemic change. The villi are moderately sclerotic and they have increased syncytial knots.

laborative Perinatal Study, Naeye (18) has found that 50% of gravidas with maternal floor infarction have had prior abortions and stillbirths. Because the placental villous tissue typically has severe ischemic change, freshly made cut sections are palpably firm (Fig. 17). The light microscopic diagnosis (Fig. 18) is characterized by an approximately 0.4-cm band of degenerate placental basal tissue, composed of fibrinoid material and X cells. The cause is unknown. Major basic protein (a protein first identified in eosinophilic granules) is greatly elevated in the serum of mothers whose placentas have maternal floor infarction (19).

Umbilical Cord Abnormalities

The mean length of an umbilical cord at term is between 50 and 60 cm (20). Obstruction and thrombi may occur when an umbilical cord is very long (Fig. 19). Short cords have been associated with conditions of impaired fetal mobility. Examples include oligohydramnios, maternal uterine mal-

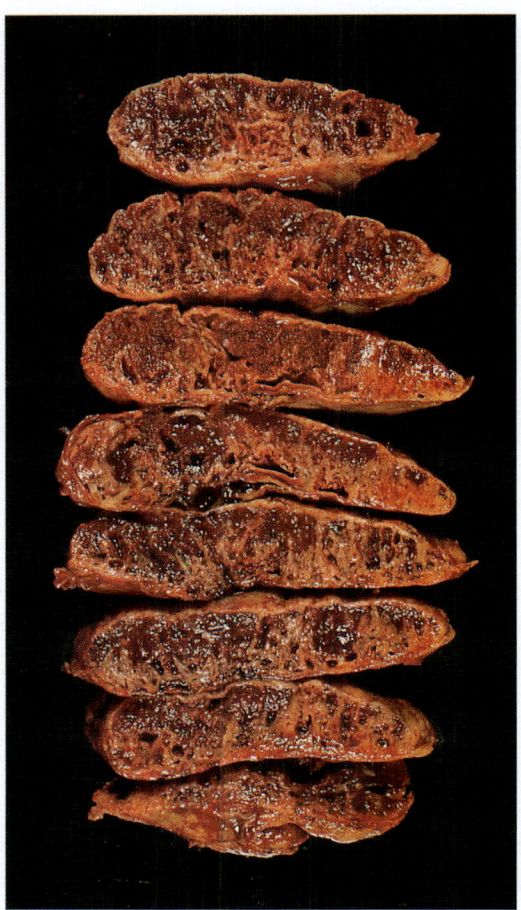

FIG. 17. Gross features of chronic placental ischemic change.

formation, the amniotic band syndrome, and congenital neuromuscular diseases. Rupture of a vessel with a cord that inserts into the placental membranes may occur during labor and cause anemia of fetal blood loss (Fig. 6). A higher incidence of deformational defects has been suggested to result

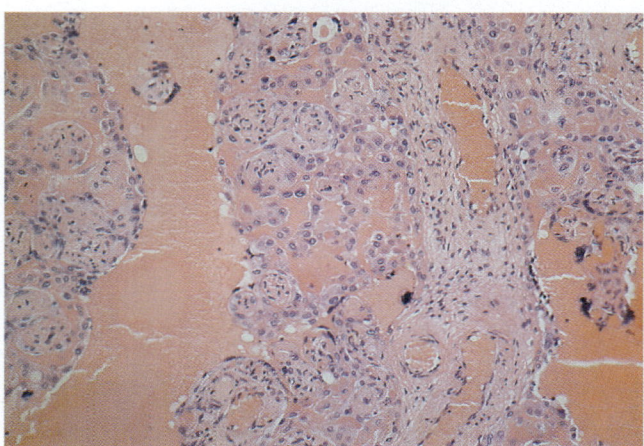

FIG. 16. Placenta with chronic ischemic change. Note the numerous X cells with the abundant fibrinoid material.

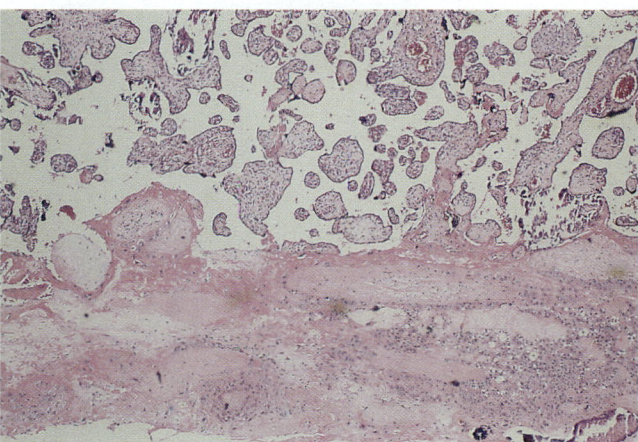

FIG. 18. Maternal floor infarction: the basal tissue features numerous basophilic X cells with diffuse eosinophilic fibrinoid material.

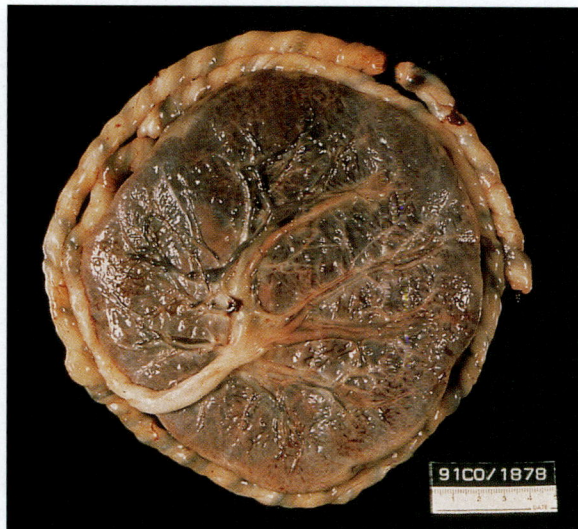

FIG. 19. Placenta with long umbilical cord. Note the superficial placental vascular thrombi ("intimal cushions") that extend across the placenta from the insertion of the cord.

from intrauterine mechanical factors that cause the fetus and placenta to compete for space at the implantation site (21).

Single umbilical artery (SUA) occurs in approximately 1% of term deliveries. Heifetz (22) has provided a major review. There is a sevenfold incidence of associated anomalies but no particular organ system is therein affected. Twins have an increased incidence of SUA and acardiac twins invariably have the anomaly. When newborns with SUA survive the neonatal period, they are at no greater risk of mortality than non-SUA neonates.

Rare omphalomesenteric duct cysts and tumors of the umbilical cord have been reviewed (23,24).

Miscellaneous Gross Abnormalities

Gross examination should include documentation of blood clots and the rupture site of the extraplacental membranes. In the absence of cesarean section, marginally ruptured membranes indicate placenta previa, resultant from implantation near the cervix. Placenta previa is a major cause of critical vaginal bleeding in the third trimester; it often requires an emergency cesarean section. Of the macroscopic placental abnormalities in Table 1, particularly note should be made of any instance of edematous and slimy membranes. This change is much more commonly seen as a consequence of chronic fetal exposure to meconium than as a manifestation of fetal hydrops. The pathologist will then probably find that the tissue has a tan color, rather than greenish discoloration. At term gestation, normal umbilical cords have a diameter of approximately 1 cm and a pearl-white color. Not uncommonly, and particularly when the gestational age exceeds 42 weeks, a 0.7-cm-diameter, wrinkled and discolored umbilical cord indicates deficient placental function and oligohydramnios. Prolonged placental exposure to meconium often grossly features a muddy or tan-brown discoloration and an accompanying flattened segment in the umbilical cord (Fig. 8). These findings warrant consideration of cord compression resulting from oligohydramnios.

DOCUMENTATION OF MICROSCOPIC PLACENTAL PATHOLOGY

Relative to light microscopic placental findings, data entry scores of zero to 3+ indicate absent, slight, moderate, or severe. They do not equate with the duration of the inflammation or with the degree of risk. For example, there are many cases of 3+ chorioamnionitis complicated by much less perinatal morbidity or mortality than that which happens with 1+ chorioamnionitis caused by group B streptococcus. The same is true for conditions other than those of infection; 1+ chorangiosis combined

TABLE 5. *A format for a light microscopic placental report*

1. Chorioamnionitis	2. Extraplacental membranitis
3. Umbilical cord vasculitis	4. Funisitis
5. Inter- or perivillositis	6. Basal villitis
7. Villitis	8. Acute intravillous hemorrhage
9. Ischemic change Acute ___ Chronic ___	10. Infarction Acute ___ Chronic ___
11. Calcification	12. Intervillous hemorrhage
13. Intervillous fibrin strands	14. Abruptio placentae
15. Fibrinoid material	16. Thrombi in villi
17. Avascular villi	18. Intravillous hemosiderin
19. Hemorrhagic endovasculopathy	20. Amnion nodosum
21. Chorangiosis	22. Dysmaturity
23. Fetal nucleated red blood cells	24. Meconium staining
25. Sickle cells	26. Hydrops

Comment: Documentation for the substantial majority of lesions is reasonably tabulated according to grades of 0, 1, 2, or 3 (slight, moderate, or severe). The following modifications are additionally useful:

Focal or multifocal villitis: (1) relatively rare and small foci of villitis within the total area of all the tissue sections (e.g., less than 5% area); (2) multifocal lesions occupying 5% to 25% of the total area of the tissue sections; (3) multifocal villitis exceeding 25% of the total tissue sections.

Fetal nucleated red blood cells: (1) presence of any immature fetal red blood cells, easily seen in placentas of premature newborns and seen with difficulty in term placentas; (2) readily recognizable such cells, at any gestational age; (3) a huge number of obvious immature erythrocytes, at any gestational age

Meconium: (1) superficial necrotic or sloughed (absent necrotic) amniotic epithelium, with meconium-laden macrophages confined to the surface; (2) ballooning of vacuolated amniotic epithelium with obvious meconium-laden macrophages adjacent to the chorionic tissue; (3) ballooning of vacuolated amniotic epithelium with a huge number of meconium-laden macrophages adjacent to the chorionic tissue and/or meconium-induced necrosis in any of the umbilical vessels.

with 1+ hydrops may be much more hazardous than 2+ chorangiosis unaccompanied by villous edema. The explanation is that the hydrops probably results from fetal heart failure or from low maternal colloid osmotic pressure caused by maternal diabetes. Alternatively, the 2+ chorangiosis may have no significant accompanying pathology.

Table 5 lists 26 items of diverse light microscopic placental histopathology (only some of which are discussed here and later in the chapter). The first four items (chorioamnionitis, extraplacental membranitis, umbilical cord vasculitis, and funisitis) result from infection that ascends from the maternal genital tract, with or without rupture of the extraplacental membranes. Table 6 gives information of a scoring system for chorioamnionitis and accompanying inflammation. This system conveys the extent of the observed pathology but does not imply the age or clinical significance of the pathologic process. Consequent to intraamniotic infection, leukoattractants in the amniotic fluid induce inflammatory cells to migrate from the placenta and umbilical cord to the fetal sac. Initially these cells were considered to originate from the mother (25), but findings from fluorescence *in situ* hybridization studies indicate that the inflammatory cells are dominantly fetal (26). Group B streptococcus, which typically produces little inflammation, is now a much more common cause of chorioamnionitis than is *Escherichia coli*. Partly for this reason, the extent of exudative inflammation with chorioamnionitis is not as severe as in previous decades (Fig. 20). Obstetricians and pathologists should thus not expect that the diagnosis is achievable from clinical and gross findings. Diagnosis of chorioamnionitis depends on light microscopic findings (Fig. 21). Similar considerations apply to umbilical vasculitis and funisitis (Fig. 22). Table 7 lists causes of chorioamnionitis, from which a precise diagnosis may be ascertainable by culture. Absence of an isolate, however, does not invalidate current opinion that chorioamnionitis is caused by infection.

Not uncommonly, newborns have pneumonia, meningitis, or sepsis, without obvious histologic chorioamnionitis. The causative microbe is then usually group B streptococcus but group A streptococcus, pneumococcus and herpes simplex virus can also be incriminated. Fetal meconium discharge is a common occurrence. In my experience, several hours of placental exposure to meconium increases the inflammation that is primarily caused by coincidental infection. This is an additional reason for caution in assignment of clinical significance to the grade or stage of histologic chorioamnionitis.

TABLE 6. *Grades of chorioamnionitis and its accompanying inflammation*

Extraplacental inflammation ("membranitis")
1. Polymorphs confined to the decidua
2. Polymorphs in the chorion and the subamniotic connective tissue
3. Necrotizing inflammation at either of the above locations

Chorioamnionitis (inflammation at the placental surface)
1. Polymorphs confined to the placental chorionic plate
2. Polymorphs throughout the chorionic plate and the subamniotic connective tissue
3. Necrotizing chorioamnionitis and/or multifocal chorionic abscesses

Umbilical cord vasculitis
(0.5) for each involved vessel plus an extra (0.5) for each severely involved vessel

Umbilical cord funisitis
(1) or focal inflammation; (2) or diffuse inflammation (3) for necrotizing inflammation (with or without calcification and/or neovascular proliferation of capillaries in umbilical vessels and/or the Wharton's jelly)

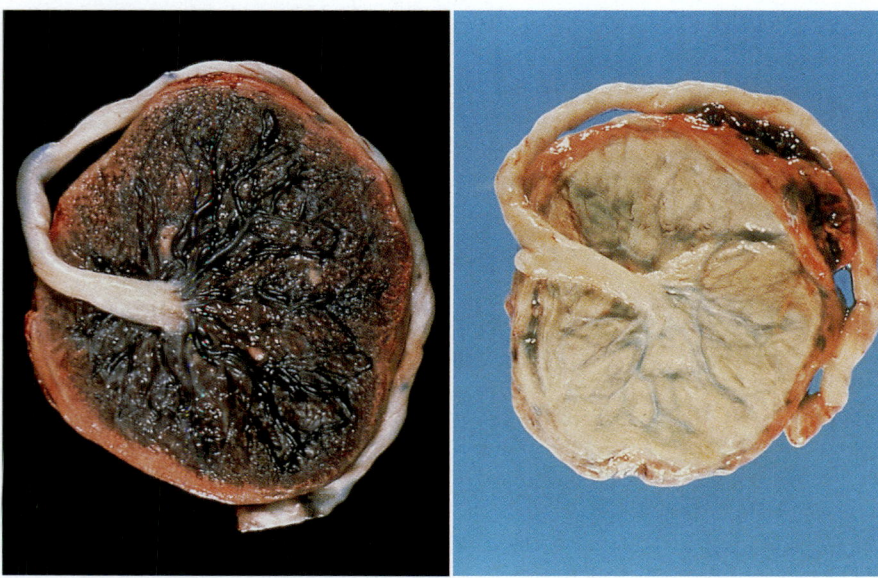

FIG. 20. Gross appearance of severe chorioamnionitis *(right)* compared with normal placenta *(left)*.

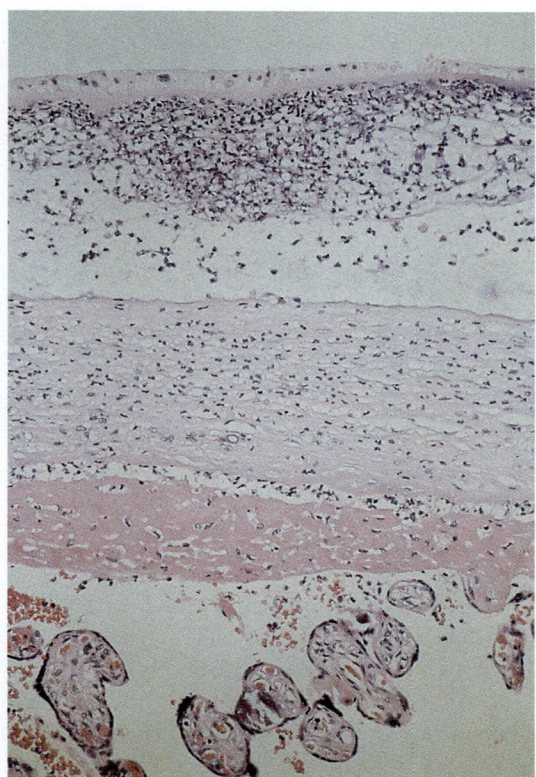

FIG. 21. Light microscopic features of stage 2 chorioamnionitis (also see Table 7).

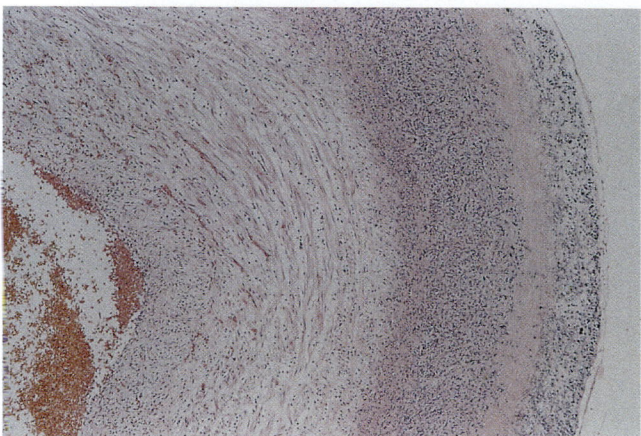

FIG. 22. Necrotizing funisitis. There are a band of necrotic inflammatory cells and another band of necrobiotic cells near the surface of the umbilical cord. Neovascularization of small capillaries is present in the vascular media.

The terms *inter-* and *perivillositis* denote inflammation between and about the villi (Fig. 23). In descending order of occurrence, placental infection by *E. coli*, *Listeria monocytogenes*, *Campylobacter*, and *Chlamydia psittaci* is uncommon or rare (27,28). With the last-mentioned infection, the inflammation is typically confined to the maternal sinusoids.

Basal villitis manifests as multifocal lymphohistiocytic infiltrates that frequently accompany villitis. In our Health Sciences Center, approximately 5% of placentas have villitis and, with all of those cases, only very rarely do we see infiltrates of lymphoctyes and plasma cells diffusely across the maternal floor.

Acute intravillous hemorrhage rarely occurs other than with abruptio placentae and it probably then happens in less than 15% of cases.

Ischemic change and infarction are very difficult to subclassify into categories that correlate with the chronology or age of causative low uteroplacental blood flow. This is un-

TABLE 7. *Patterns of chorioaminionitis*

Generic pattern	Distinctive component	Organism
Suppurative	Slight to severe	Aerobes
		Anaerobes
		Ureaplasma
Suppurative	Very slight or slight, but with fulminant early onset of pneumonia or sepsis	Group B streptococcus
		Herpes simplex virus
		Group A streptococcus
		Pneumococcus
Suppurative and/or histiocytic	Accompanying acute villitis, inter- or perivillositis	*Escherichia coli*
		Listeria monocytogenes
		Staphylococcus
		Campylobacter fetus
		Nonsyphilitic spirochetosis
Suppurative	Fetal eosinophils	Gram-positive bacteria
Suppurative	Filamentous bacteria	*Fusobacterium*
Necrotizing	Superficial umbilical cord microabscesses	*Candida* and other fungi
Variably necrotizing, with microscopic superficial vesicles and lymphoplasmacytic cells	Plasma cell funisitis and bland necrosis in the placental villi	Herpes simplex virus
Lymphoplasmacytic	Accompanying triad of plasmacytic villitis, villous endovasculitis or obliterative vasculopathy, and villous dysmaturity	Syphilis

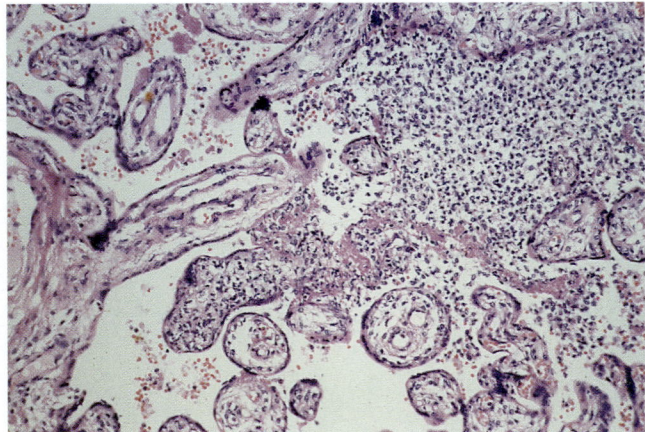

FIG. 23. Acute intervillositis, perivillositis, and villitis.

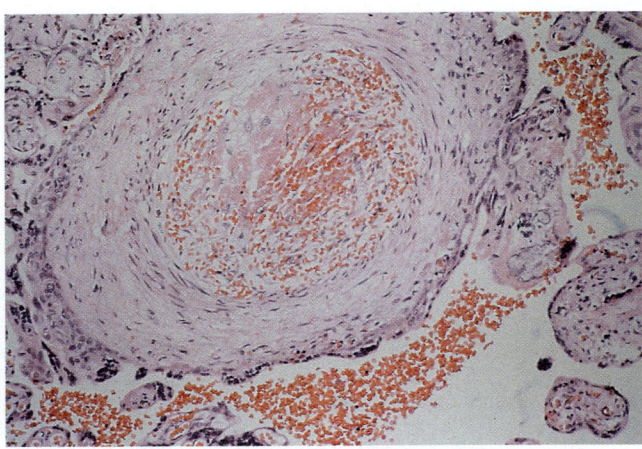

FIG. 24. Hemorrhagic endovasculopathy. Within the obliterated lumen there are fragmented red blood cells.

fortunate because, in my experience, at least 40% of light microscopically examined placentas have ischemic change and or infarction. The probable age of the histopathology is best adduced from additional consideration as to the numerical extent of accompanying fetal placental nucleated red blood cells. Using these considerations and information of the mass and size of a placenta, pathologists may be able to identify placentas that correlate with abnormally grown fetuses or newborns. Acute placental ischemic change is represented by agglutination of villi and syncytial knots in more than 30% of the villi (Fig. 14). Acute infarcts are readily identifiable by ghost-like appearance of the villi; and chronic infarcts are characterized by focal or multifocal abundance of fibrinoid material, which obliterates villous architecture and includes a multitude of X cells. With diffuse degeneration or infarction across the maternal floor, these particular chronic ischemic lesions (Fig. 16) become confluent; diagnosis of chronic infarction is then made. Often, chronic placental ischemia is manifested by shrunken, sclerotic villi with numerous condensed syncytial knots (Fig. 15).

The aforementioned changes are not the only consequences of clinically significant fetal placental hypoxia. In pregnant mothers who live in high mountainous countries, hypobaric hypoxia is the reported cause of chorangioma (29). That entity and chorangiosis probably result from capillary growth, stimulated by protracted placental tissue hypoxia (30). Clinicopathologic considerations of chorangiosis are discussed below (see Miscellaneous Pathology of Noninfectious Cause).

Calcification develops in many placentas that have fibrin or fibrinoid material. Hematoxylin and eosin staining produces a multifocal blue color. Although similar-appearing material is present along the villous basement membrane of placentas from stillbirths, the chemical is probably iron rather than calcium. When placentas with severe and diffuse calcification accompany hypoxic newborns, low uteroplacental blood flow is the probable cause. Mothers who smoke excessively have had increased placental calcification, but this is not as frequent a finding as is the calcification that is seen in the placentas of primigravidas.

Intervillous hemorrhage is a relatively frequent sign of acute abruptio placentae. With remote episode of retroplacental hemorrhage, a cupola develops when the blood clot presses against the adjacent placenta. Diagnosis of acute abruptio placentae depends on the clinical facts, but within half an hour of an acute separation the placental sinusoids typically have focal or multifocal maternal leukostasis and intervillous fibrin strands. The combination of old basal placental fibrin and hemosiderin deposits with similar material attached to adjacent extraplacental membranes indicates that placental abruption had probably occurred a day or more prior to delivery.

Intravillous hemosiderin is very uncommon, if not rare. When it does occur, one should suspect remote infection with cytomegalovirus infection or syphilis. Those infections and rubella virus attack endothelium, but rubella virus infection is now very rare.

Hemorrhagic endovasculopathy, in my opinion, is a preferable term to Sander's (31) *hemorrhagic endovasculitis.* A coterie of placental pathologists has long been aware of this important entity. It is a noninflammatory microangiopathy characterized by slight hemorrhage with fragmented red blood cells in obliterated fetal vessels (Fig. 24). The lesions commonly occur in placentas of stillborns and with diverse maternal and fetal conditions. From experimental studies, Silver and her colleagues (32) have shown that tissue hypoxia is involved in the pathogenesis of these lesions.

MULTIPLE PREGNANCY

Benirschke has provided detailed methods for the placental examination of specimens from multiple births (33) and a concise account of the placenta in twin gestation (34). In his textbook (2) and in that of Baldwin (35), there are lengthy reviews of developmental, clinicopathologic, and many

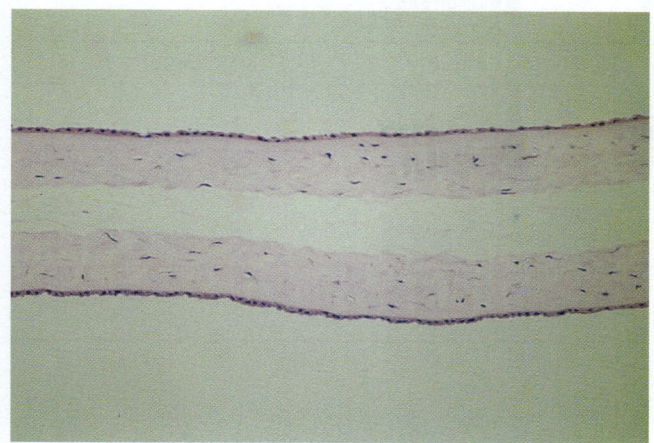

FIG. 25. Monochorionic interplacental partition.

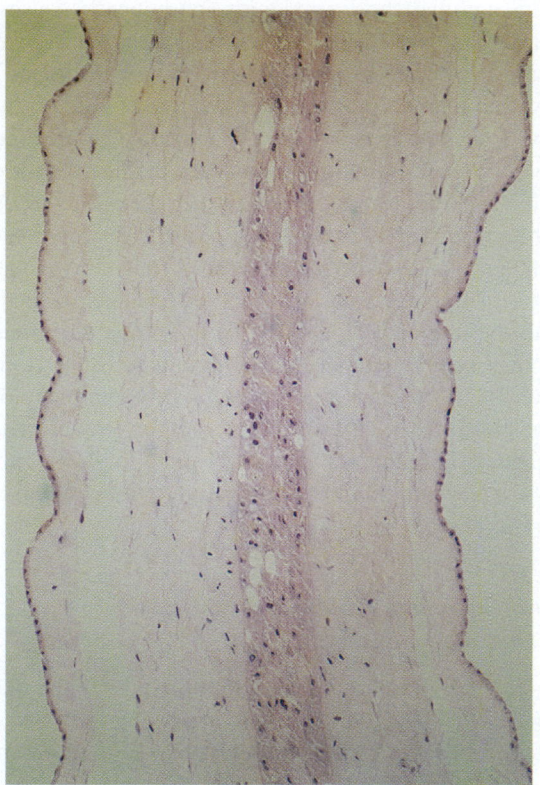

FIG. 26. Dichorionic interplacental partition.

other aspects of twins and multiple births. The examination of placentas from twins and higher multiple births is similar to that for a singleton. Tissue pieces are trimmed into five blocks from each placenta, plus blocks of each umbilical cord, placental sac, and interplacental partition. Because monochorionic twin placentas have only one disk, their interplacental partition does not include chorionic or decidual tissue (Fig. 25); it is transparent and has only two layers of amnion. Diamnionic, dichorionic placental partitions include two separate or or fused (originally bilayered) chorions (Fig. 26). They tend to be opaque and often have grossly discernible blood vessels. Whereas there are only very rare reports of human dichorionic placentas with interplacental anastomoses, monochorionic placentas always have them. These vascular connections explain the greater morbidity and mortality with monochorionic twins than with dichorionic twins and singletons (including increased chorioamnionitis).

Twin Transfusion Syndrome

Monochorionic twin placentas share artery-to-artery, vein-to-vein, and artery-to-vein anastomoses. Arterial and venous identification cannot be made by light microscopic examination. It is made from gross observation that arteries course superficially to veins. Injection of milk or colored liquid demonstrates anastomoses much more conveniently than can be done with radiographic dye. Artery-to-artery anastomoses are the most common. From an investigation of 69 monochorionic twin placentas, Machin and his colleagues (36) provided correlations of placental vascular anatomy with clinical outcomes of the associated twins. They found that the worst outcomes occurred with specimens that each had arteriovenous anastomoses and an absence of arterioarterial and venovenous anastomoses. The investigators additionally examined clinical consequences relative to equal or unequal sizes of venous fields returning blood to each twin cord (36). They affirmed the historic speculation of Schatz (37) and of later investigators (38) that large superficial placental anastomoses compensate for hemodynamic imbalance caused by transfer of blood via deep arteriovenous anastomoses. With clinically obvious chronic twin transfusion syndrome, the donor twin is small and pale and the recipient twin is large and plethoric. The donor twin suffers anemia and the recipient twin suffers high-output cardiac failure. Autopsy findings of fatal cases reveals that the donor has small organs and that the recipient has large organs. This syndrome is the major cause of midtrimester, twin-pregnancy mortality. Even prior to 20 weeks' gestation, there is a grossly obvious difference in the size of the hearts. Benirschke (39) initially proposed that thromboplastin from a dead co-twin *in utero* infuses into the survivor and causes disseminated intravascular coagulation; he later emphasized that acute exsanguination of the surviving fetus into the dead co-twin may be a more probable cause of neurologic damage (40).

Baldwin and her colleagues (35,41) have clarified many of these various complex considerations. Most such cases have occurred in the third trimester as a consequence of fetal death, invasive interventions, and fetomaternal hemorrhage (35). When the twin transfusion syndrome results from many weeks of imbalanced interplacental blood flow, the placental part of the donor twin is smaller and paler than that of the recipient twin. Thus, when fetal death complicates this syndrome and there is an apparent smaller and congested component at delivery, an acute reverse transfusion has probably followed death of the donor twin (Fig. 27). Definitive diagnosis of twin transfusion syndrome can be very elusive. One

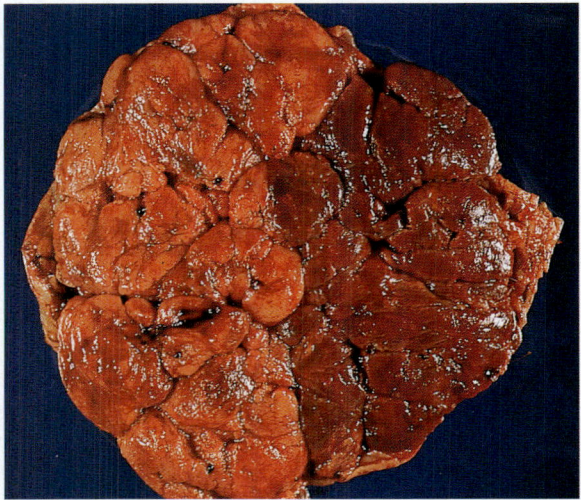

FIG. 27. Twin transfusion syndrome placentas, status post-demise of the donor twin.

cannot depend on a hemoglobin difference of greater than 5 g/dL and birth weight difference of greater than 20% (42). The clinical management of chronic transfusion syndrome has included serial amniocentesis, selective feticide, and removal of a fetus (35). In my opinion, surgical interruption of the common vasculature is preferable treatment (43,44). It has much support from the fact that the anatomical patterns of anastomoses are simple and they are readily amenable to laser occlusion (36). Also, after laser ablation of anastomoses, if one fetus dies it is impossible for acute transfusion to occur from the surviving fetus to the dead fetus. For an in-depth account of intrauterine death in multiple gestation, see Liu and colleagues (45).

PLACENTAL DIAGNOSES IN SURGICAL PATHOLOGY

Surgical pathologists who are new to placental examination should learn the range of clinically important entities that they are likely to encounter. A recent epidemiologic investigation provides such information (46). In a study of 1,252 placentas, examined because of clinical reasons (4), the most frequent pathologic findings were ischemic change (40%), meconium staining (27%), and chorioamnionitis (21%) (Table 8). Abruptio placentae, infarction, chorangiosis, and villitis of unknown etiology each accounted for less than 10% of all the reported diagnoses (Table 8). Only in 8% was the diagnosis essentially normal. For the 1,252 placentas, there were 1,636 diagnosed pathologic features. In other studies, I have found a moderately higher incidence of villitis of unknown etiology; the present 4% finding was low, probably because specimens with rare foci of villitis would not have been coded in the surgical pathology file. Of the 1,636 diagnoses coded, miscellaneous diagnoses included placentomegaly ($n = 76$), extrachorial placenta ($n = 30$), fetal thrombi ($n = 25$), intravillous hemorrhage ($n = 18$), villous edema ($n = 8$), placenta accreta ($n = 6$), and grossly abnormal appearance of no immediately apparent clinical significance ($n = 38$).

TABLE 8. *Placental features in 1252 examined placentas*

Diagnostic category	Occurrence (%)
Ischemic change	40
Meconium	27
Chorioamnionitis	21
Abruptio placentae	9
Infarction	8
Villitis of unknown etiology	4
Chorangiosis	3
Other feature	11
Normal	8

HISTOPATHOLOGY OF INFECTIOUS CAUSE

Chorioamnionitis

Historical Considerations

More than 40 years ago, Knox and Hoerner (47) postulated the pathogenesis of chorioamnionitis: "It seemed logical that an infectious process in the cervical canal might extend itself to the membranes overlying the internal os." In the ensuing 10 years, Benirschke (48) and Blanc (49) separately described pathways by which a fetus can become infected. They developed a concept that infection causes chorioamnionitis and that chorioamnionitis subsequently causes prematurity and morbid or fatal complications. Benirschke and Blanc described histologic chorioamnionitis to be the hallmark of ascending intrauterine infection, and inflammation in and between placental villi to be indicative of maternal-fetal blood-borne infection. Clinicians diagnose chorioamnionitis according to the presence of maternal fever during labor ($>37.8°C$) plus two or more of the following: maternal or fetal tachycardia, uterine tenderness, foul odor, and leukocytosis (50). Because obstetricians were frequently unable to obtain the microbiologic cause of the placental inflammation, they concluded that chorioamnionitis results from hypoxia (51). More than 30 years elapsed before many obstetricians corrected that error. For example, Romero and his colleagues (52) reported that only 1 of 11 mothers with histologic chorioamnionitis and positive amnionic fluid cultures had clinical chorioamnionitis.

Chorioamnionitis, Prostaglandins, Cytokines, and Their Complications

A recent review has included 14 references to the work of Romero's investigative team (53). Many of these studies elucidate mechanisms by which bacterial agents and inflammation cause premature onset of labor. Complex biochemical activities therein include mobilization of arachidonic acid from cell membrane phospholipids of the placenta, decidua, and extraplacental chorionic membranes, by catalytic action of phospholipase A_2. Bacteria, which are often present in those tissues, secrete high levels of phospholipase A_2 (e.g., *Fusobacterium, Bacteroides,* and *Ureaplasma*). It is particularly noteworthy that bacteria can invade the amniotic cavity by penetration through intact placental membranes. Even more important than the bacterial production of phospholipases, however, is the fact that the host's inflammatory response to infection stimulates cytokines to produce prostaglandin from the amnion and decidua (53–55). Cytokines are small proteins of 5 to 20 kd. Inflammation causes their mobilization in a way that impacts on cells in other tissues. These interleukins are thus comparable to hormones. Particular agents, such as interleukin-1 (IL-1) and tumor necrosis factor, activate phospholipases that are endogenous in lipid cell membranes. Separate from these activities that cause prematurity, cytokines directly injure the unmyelinated periventricular regions of the fetal brain, ultimately to produce periventricular leukomalacia (56,57). From the recently reviewed literature, one learns that mothers who delivered preterm are more likely to have histologic chorioamnionitis and increased amniotic fluid levels of tumor necrosis factor, IL-6, and prostaglandin E_2, than are mothers delivered at term (57).

Baergen and her colleagues (58) examined IL-1 and IL-1 receptor antagonist (Il-1ra) expression in chorioamnionitis and parturition. They postulated that a balance between proinflammatory and antiinflammatory mediators may play a role in parturition. Their concept is that chorioamnionitis may precipitate preterm labor by causing an increase or imbalance in the expression of IL-1 and IL-1ra. A major and possibly unexpected finding of the investigations was that meconium-stained necrotic umbilical vessels were immunocytochemically positive for IL-1 and IL-1ra (58).

Polymicrobial Causes of Chorioamnionitis

Recent reviews have detailed polymicrobial causes of chorioamnionitis (2,27,59). In my experience, other than for very slight inflammation caused by group B streptococcus, chorioamnionitis usually results from infection by two and more microbes. Bacterial vaginosis is diagnosed when the pH of vaginal secretions is greater than 4.5 and when *Lactobacillus* is replaced by *Bacteroides, Gardnerella vaginalis, Mycoplasma hominis, Ureaplasma urealyticum,* and *Mobiluncus* (60,61). When *G. vaginalis* is singly present in amniotic fluid, it is not a substantial pathogen; when it is present with the other aforementioned organisms, it is a significant cause of prematurity.

Fusobacteria Infection

Although fusobacteria in neonates and infants was reported in papers of 30 to 40 years ago (62,63), relatively few other papers have been written. Altshuler and Hyde

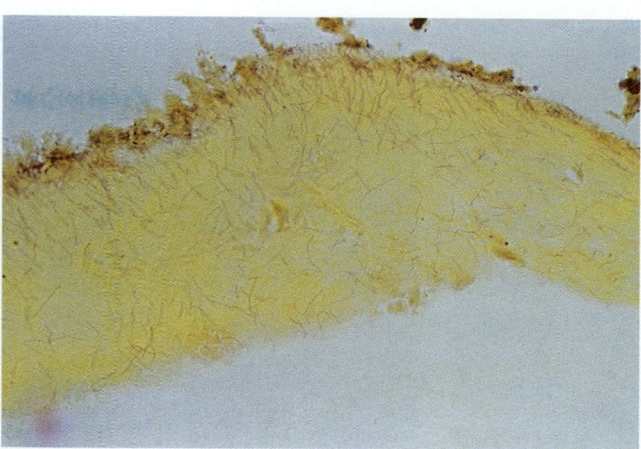

FIG. 28. Fusobacteria in amniotic tissue. The Brown and Hopps staining method shows the filamentous appearance of these anaerobic, gram-negative organisms.

(64,65) prepared antisera in rabbits and thereby validated our documentation that this infection occurs in as many as 18% placentas with histologic chorioamnionitis. Fusobacteria are very difficult to see with hematoxylin and eosin stains, and Bouin's fixation severely masks them. The organisms are pleomorphic and filamentous (Figs. 28 and 29). We initially found them with Warthin-Starry stain. Giemsa and Brown and Hopps stains (9) are much simpler to perform and are therefore preferable. Reports of fusobacterium amnionitis have been reported in the clinical literature (66). Our experience has been that, if fusobacteria are unaccompanied by other organisms, they rarely cause neonatal pneumonia, meningitis, or sepsis. Fusobacteria produce phospholipase A_2; for this reason and because of the cytokines and other mediators of accompanying inflammation, they are particularly prone to cause prematurity (67).

Mycoplasma Infection

Kundsin and colleagues (68) emphasized the role of *Mycoplasma* as a cause of chorioamnionitis and reproductive failure. In a later study of 572 placentas, these investigators found that perinatal morbidity and mortality are associated with colonization of the chorionic surface by *Ureaplasma urealyticum* or *Mycoplasma hominis* or both (69). Although the investigation included 125 perinatal deaths and 293 placentas from neonatal intensive care patients, *Chlamydia trachomatis* was not isolated from any placenta (69). This raises questions as to the investigators' methods. There have been many investigations of genital mycoplasmas (68–73). They substantiate a causal relationship between *U. urealyticum* (T-mycoplasmas), chorioamnionitis, and perinatal morbidity and mortality (70–73). *M. hominis* is a common inhabitant of the female genital tract but is less prone to produce chorioamnionitis and reproductive failure (70,73).

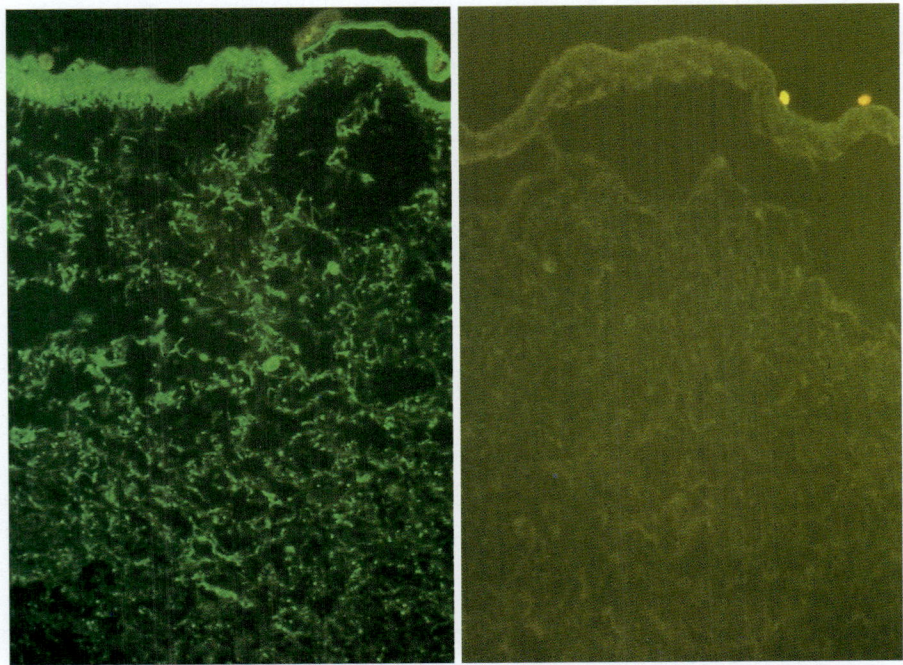

FIG. 29. Fusobacteria on immunofluorescent microscopic examination *(left)* compared with negative control *(right).*

Bacteroides Fragilis Infection

In the European literature, there are reports of infection with *Bacteroides fragilis* (74,75). The role of diagnosis by immunofluorescent light microscopic examination is emphasized (75). *B. fragilis* are very small organisms with a safety-pin configuration. On the uncommon occasion that they cause chorioamnionitis, they may thus be recognizable.

Nontypable Haemophilus Influenzae Infection

Since 1965, there have been numerous reports of neonatal infection with nontypable *Haemophilus influenzae*. Recent publications include review of 107 cases (76,77). Affected newborns have suffered pneumonia, meningitis, and sepsis, similar to that which occurs with early-onset group B, β-hemolytic streptococcus sepsis (76–79). There has been a strong association with prematurity; more than 80% of the cases have been born at less than 37 weeks' gestation (76). The associated chorioamnionitis has varied in severity (67) and has occurred with intact amniotic membranes (80). The organisms are fastidious in culture but are conveniently demonstrable by the Brown and Hopps stain (9). They are short gram-negative bacilli.

Chlamydia Trachomatis Infection

In Schachter's (81) review of chlamydia infections, he has provided extensive details of microbiology, pathogenesis, and resultant diseases. In 1981, Heggie and colleagues (82) reported chlamydia infection in 28% of 95 infants born vaginally to infected mothers; conjunctivitis occurred in 20 of 21 infants with chlamydia infection of the conjunctivae, but the chlamydia pneumonia syndrome occurred in only 3 of 18 infants with nasopharyngeal infection. Several investigators have shown associations between *Chlamydia trachomatis* (CT) infection and perinatal morbidity and mortality in humans (83–85). Their findings indicate that this infection can produce chorioamnionitis or ascending intrauterine infection. At the International Academy of Pathology Congress in 1982, Rettig and I described a rat model of CT amniotic infection syndrome. Chorioamnionitis was found in all placentas of CT fetal sac inoculations, and, by immunofluorescent light microscopic study, CT was demonstrable within the amniotic and yolk sac tissue. Inflammation was rarely present in controls. By immunohistochemical methods, chlamydia antigens have been demonstrated in 4 of 19 cases with severe endometritis (86). Given that chlamydia antibodies have been commercially available for several years, it is interesting that histologic reports of chlamydia chorioamnionitis remain conspicuously lacking.

Necrotizing Funisitis

Authors have variably used the terms *necrotizing funisitis* and *subacute necrotizing funisitis* to designate this pathology. The latter term was introduced by Navarro and Blanc (87), who described a "barber-pole" pattern of yellow-white bands between umbilical vessel(s) and the umbilical cord surface. Two phenomena cause this pathology. Amniotic fluid leukoattractants stimulate leukocytes to migrate from the umbilical vessels to the amniotic fluid, and during this emigration the fetal leukocytes are destroyed by amniotic fluid leukotoxins that diffuse through the Wharton's jelly. Light microscopic features include inflammatory cells, necrotic cell debris, and calcific material (Fig. 22). There has been an incorrect claim that necrotizing funisitis is probably a specific feature of syphilis (88). With 25 placentas from syphilitic mothers, nine of the umbilical cords had necrotizing funisitis and eight of those affected cords were spirochete positive (89,90). Almost half of the cases, however, were histologically normal (90). Findings of other investigations indicate that a range of microbes is present with these lesions (91,92). In most instances the specific cause of necrotizing funisitis is not known. Necrotizing funisitis is rare, but, because of high associated fetal and neonatal morbidity and mortality, it is important (92). Two specific kinds of necrotizing funisitis are particularly noteworthy (93–95). Herpes simplex funisitis light microscopically features necrotizing lesions with accompanying slight plasma cell infiltrates and *Candida albicans* funisitis has grossly appreciable small focal necrotizing lesions at the surface of the cord (Fig. 30).

Villitis, and Villitis of Unknown Etiology

Throughout several decades authors have described numerous and diverse kinds of villitis of polymicrobial cause. By the mid-1970s, it became apparent that the dominant majority of these lesions are villitis of unknown etiology (VUE) (96,97). Depending on demographic and sociocultural factors of populations investigated, villitis probably occurs in 6% to 14% of all newborns in Western countries (59). Fox (59) has persistently agreed with me that a viral (or fastidious microbe) is the primary cause of VUE. Others have favored an immunologic process (98–103). Findings of *in situ* hybridization investigation, with X and Y chromosome-specific probes, showed that VUE is associated with major infiltration of fetal tissue by maternal inflammatory cells (103). The number of specimens tested was small. Other in-

TABLE 9. *The etiology of villitis of unknown etiology (VUE): infection, not immunologic aberration, is probably the primary cause*

There is no histologic difference between VUE and diverse specific villitides (for example: cytomegalovirus infection, rubella virus infection, enteroviruses, mycoplasma and syphilis)

Diseases that involve antibody-mediated immunologic assault of the fetus by the mother do not manifest VUE; these include ABO and Rh blood group incompatibilities, isoimmune thrombocytopenia, maternal autoimmune diseases, and fetal-maternal transfusion; it is particularly noteworthy that VUE does not accompany chronic fetal-maternal blood transfusion because, in that condition, class I and class II major histocompatibility complex antigens are released into the maternal circulation

In the early phase of VUE, inflammatory cells migrate from the fetal villous capillaries to the trophoblast about the villus; this indicates that the primary inflammatory response is fetal; probably, as the inflammation proceeds, activated stromal macrophages produce cytokines that attract maternal leukocytes into the villus

Table developed with Scott Hyde, Ph.D.

vestigators thus need to confirm that the findings did not result from the use of an insufficiently sensitive Y probe. As shown on Table 9, nonculturable virus or some fastidious other microbe is probably the primary cause of VUE (Fig. 31). The findings of Khong (104) accord well with this opinion. He did not find any correlation of VUE and expression of major histocompatibility complex class II antigens; immunoreactivity was absent in villi that had chronic inflammation but present in villi that did not have inflammation.

Villitis of unknown etiology has been present in approximately 25% small for gestational age newborns (14). Others have also found association of villitis with intrauterine growth retardation (105–112), and there have been reports of rare fetal growth retardation occurring with mothers who have experienced recurrent VUE (101,109–111). The last such report is most remarkable because silver stains revealed medium-sized straight to slightly curved rods, that were

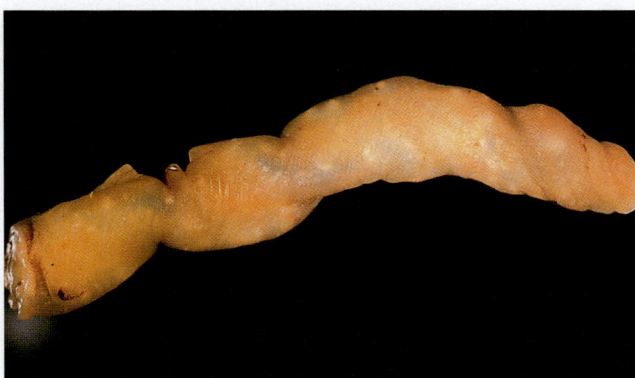

FIG. 30. Umbilical cord with multifocal, superficial yellow-gray lesions, characteristic of *Candida* infection.

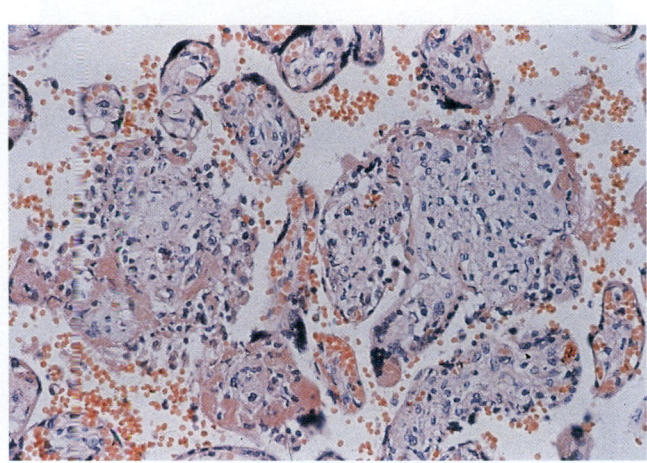

FIG. 31. Villitis of unknown etiology.

unidentifiable (111). Salafia and her colleagues (112–115) have extensively investigated and confirmed associations between villitis, histologic signs of low uteroplacental blood flow, and fetal growth retardation.

Whereas VUE is common in all populations, specific villitides are very uncommon or rare. In our Health Sciences Center, the prevalence of specific villitides is little more than 0.1%. Partly for this reason and also because extensive information of specific villitides is conveniently available in three recent reviews (2,27,59), no further discussion of villitis is herein provided.

MISCELLANEOUS PATHOLOGY OF NONINFECTIOUS CAUSE

Meconium Staining

It is important to define what one means by fetal exposure to meconium. There is a huge difference between fetal defecation at or shortly before delivery and fetal passage of meconium many hours before delivery (Fig. 32). Fox (59) states, "The reality of the situation is that, in our present state of knowledge, no inference as to the well-being or otherwise of the fetus can be drawn from the mere presence of meconium in the placental tissues" (p. 479). I disagree. Clinicians and pathologists have insufficiently recognized temporal aspects of fetal meconium discharge and the related consequences. Titles of relatively recent publications are relevant: "Meconium Aspiration Syndrome: Reflections on a Murky Subject" (116) and "Meconium Aspiration Syndrome Made Murkier" (117). The topic is so important that Benirschke (118) chose it to be one of three entities warranting obstetricians' prioritized attention. For a recent review of clinical and pathologic information, see Wiswell (119).

Meconium staining is completely different from deposition of slimy green meconium across the placental surface.

Many normal fetuses pass meconium shortly before delivery. Gentle hosing of the placenta with water washes the meconium from the tissue surface (Fig. 7). Those newborns do not have detrimental outcomes. The perspective is entirely different when a fetus has been exposed to meconium for several hours. Meconium aspiration syndrome results from fetal defecation, usually within a very few hours or minutes of delivery. Associated risks to the fetus increase with prolonged duration of fetal exposure to noxious meconium components. These temporal considerations are optimally discernible by examination of unfixed specimens, followed by light microscopic examination. After a very few hours, the extraplacental membranes become slimy and edematous and the color of the placenta and the membranes changes from dark green to tan-green, to tan-brown (Fig. 8), and to yellow-brown. During this time, soluble components of meconium diffuse into the placenta and umbilical cord, ultimately to reach and enter the placental and umbilical blood vessels. These agents stimulate vasoactivity and, as a consequence of intermittent vasocontraction, there is hypoperfusion of fetal organs (120,121). Caution is needed in considerations of the chronology of the aforementioned events. The approximation is very difficult or impossible if moderate or severe chorioamnionitis is additionally present.

In my experience, the *in vivo* presence of meconium-laden macrophages adjacent to the fetal placental chorionic plate indicates passage of fetal meconium discharge at least 2 to 3 hours prior to delivery. This time frame is similar to that ascertained from laboratory experiments (122). Numerous meconium-laden macrophages, situated extensively and deeply in the extraplacental membranes, indicate fetal meconium discharge from 6 to 12 hours before delivery (depending on one's concept of the words *numerous* and *extensively*). From clinicopathologic observations, I have found that 16 hours of intraamniotic presence of meconium has not caused any semblance of necrosis of placental and umbilical vessels. The earliest necrotic change is seen in arterial tissue (Figs. 33 and 34). Obvious necrosis in all three vessels prob-

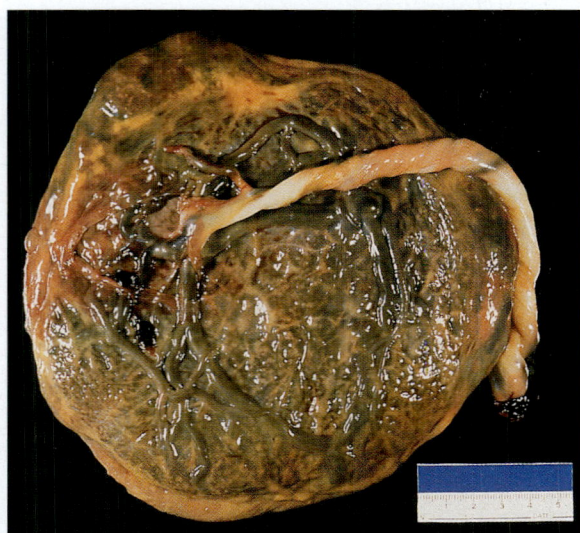

FIG. 32. Placenta with chronic meconium staining.

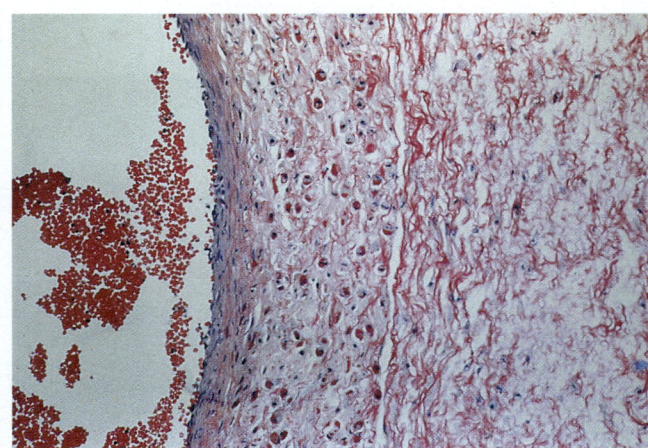

FIG. 33. Low-magnification photomicrograph of meconium-induced umbilical artery necrosis.

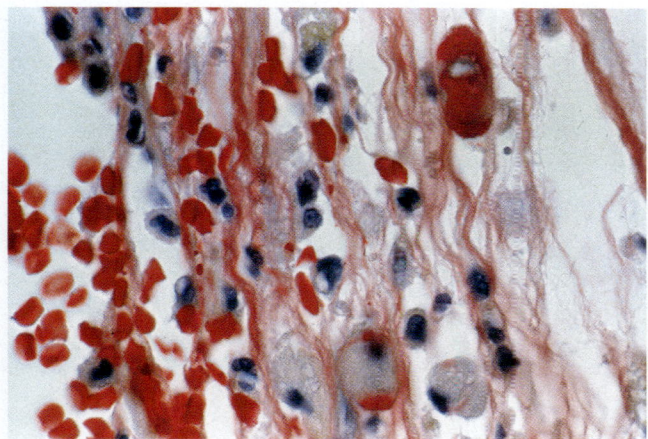

FIG. 34. High-magnification photomicrograph of meconium-induced umbilical artery necrosis. Note the gold green meconium-laden cells and the purple necrotic myocytes.

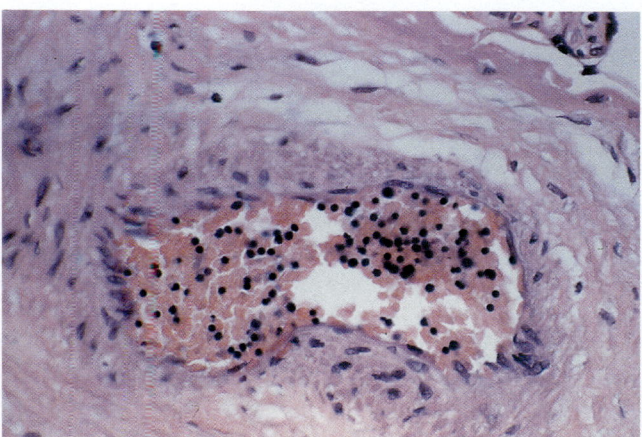

FIG. 36. Nucleated red blood cells.

ably does not occur in less than 48 hours, and the duration may be longer when grossly evident umbilical cord ulceration is additionally present (Fig. 35). Coexistent meconium-induced epithelial erosion and reparative epithelial changes, with multilayered nuclei and ballooned and vacuolated amniotic epithelial cytoplasm, are evidence of recurrent fetal meconium discharge.

Fetal Nucleated Red Blood Cells

Although this topic is comprehensively reviewed elsewhere (53,123,124), it warrants a brief discussion here. Reports more than 70 years ago documented that nucleated red blood cells are not present in the blood of normal term newborns and that these cells are a compensatory response to fetal hypoxia (125). Although Fox (126) drew attention to this in 1967, clinicians and pathologists remain insufficiently aware of relationships between nucleated red blood cells, perinatal asphyxia, fetal growth retardation, cerebral palsy, mental retardation, and other disorders. Nucleated red blood cells have a dark color. Their nuclear surface is crisply smooth and they are conspicuously smaller than mature red blood cells and lymphocytes (Fig. 36). If pathologists use the scoring system for nucleated red blood cells shown in Table 5, they will probably find that postnatal hematology laboratory counts of these cells, within the first 6 hours of delivery, will validate the histologically evident degree of elevation. Causes of histologically evident increased nucleated red blood cells include chronic or long-standing fetal hypoxia resulting from reduced uteroplacental blood flow, abruptio placentae, maternal diabetes, chronic fetal-maternal transfusion, hemolytic diseases (e.g., ABO blood group incompatibility, Rh-disease and anti-c immunohemolytic disease), acute fetal blood loss, and chromosomal disorders (e.g., trisomy 13 and trisomy 21). The first three causes and ABO blood group incompatibility are not at all uncommon; the others are rare. Rare causes of fetal blood loss include sepsis-induced fetal hemolysis, vasa previa, and laceration of intramembranous fetal vessels by intrauterine pressure catheters.

Villous Dysmaturity

Generalized villous dysmaturity, formerly called relative immaturity, implies abnormal villous maturation. The cause is usually unknown. The villi are enlarged and the trophoblast usually has deficient syncytiotrophoblast with a numerical lack of syncytial knots. When the stromal cells are increased, the term *diffuse villitis* may be reasonable (Fig. 37). The associated newborn in Fig. 37 soon developed biopsy-proven postnatal hepatitis. This diagnosis may reasonably be anticipated when, as Khudr and Benirschke (127) reported, the placenta has pigment-laden Hofbauer cells in addition to diffuse villous dysmaturity (Fig. 38).

Chorangiosis

When villous dysmaturity features villous capillary hypervascularity rather than stromal cell hypercellularity, the preferable diagnosis is chorangiosis. Placentas with choran-

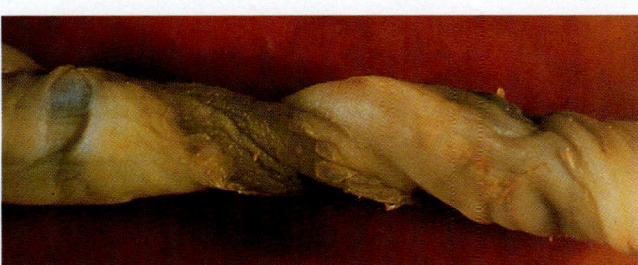

FIG. 35. Gross photograph of an umbilical cord segment with meconium-induced ulceration. The lesions have exposed underlying vessels toward each side of the cord segment.

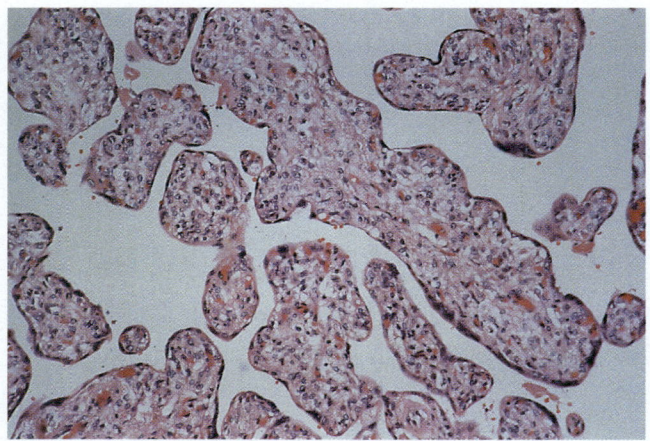

FIG. 37. Diffuse placental villous dysmaturity.

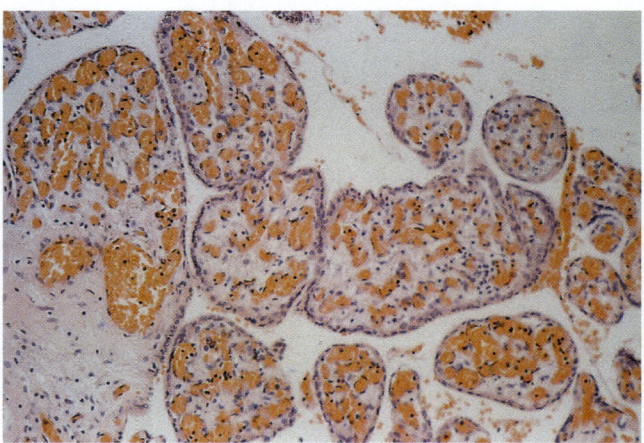

FIG. 39. Severe chorangiosis.

giosis have at least ten different microscopic fields in ten different placental areas, with ten villi that have ten capillary lumina in each villus (128). Irrespective of the fact that a vessel may be represented in more than one plane of section, normal villi rarely have more than five capillary lumina. Chorangiosis features diffuse villous hypervascularity; it is different from congestion in which there are a normal number of blood vessels. The abnormality may be obscured by slight edema or obvious hydrops and, on those occasions, pathogenetic causes have included maternal diabetes and high-output fetal cardiac failure. Severe chorangiosis is very obvious (Fig. 39).

Subacute low uteroplacental blood flow may cause additional presence of increased syncytial knots (Fig. 40). Chorangiosis never occurs in normal placentas of normal pregnancies and deliveries. It occurs in 5% of placentas from newborns hospitalized in intensive care units (128). The incidences of mortality and major congenital anomalies in the population studied were 39% and 27%, respectively. Chorangiosis has an increased incidence with diabetes and preeclampsia. In the latter disease, this results from villous capillary endothelial proliferation (129). Pregnant mothers in high mountainous countries experience hypobaric hypoxia throughout their pregnancies. They have a remarkably high number of chorangiomas in their placentas, documented from study of resin-embedded placentas (130). Because the samples did not represent large areas of various cotyledons, the extent of chorangiosis was not ascertainable.

VASCULAR RELATED ABNORMALITIES

Maternal Vessels

The literature has extensive information on uteroplacental blood vessels relative to preeclampsia and to other common diseases (2,59). Fox (59) states, "Examination of basal plate vessels, rather than placental bed biopsies, is a sub-optimal method of assessing the adequacy of the maternal uteroplacental circulation" (p. 249). Without the availability of placental bed biopsies for all cases, Khong and his colleagues (131) studied maternal intrauterine vessels from 39 patients with preeclampsia. They found a 46% incidence of acute

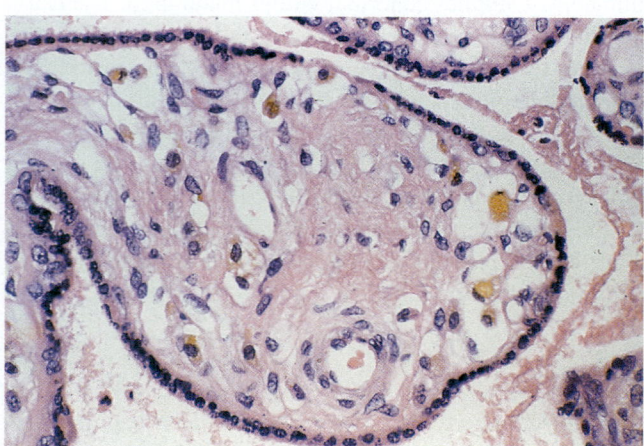

FIG. 38. Pigmented Hofbauer cells.

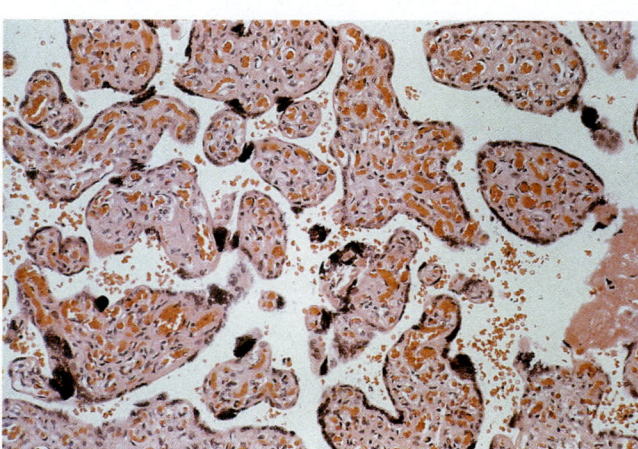

FIG. 40. Moderate chorangiosis with numerically increased syncytial knots.

atherosis; there was no statistically significant relation between acute atherosis and parity, degree of proteinuria, severity and duration of hypertension, and antihypertensive therapy. When Khong and Chambers (132) examined tissue blocks en face to the basal plate, they found significantly more vessels than the number seen in full-thickness blocks. Perhaps application of this method will contribute information relative to the etiology of early-onset preeclampsia and other conditions.

Fetal Vessels

Thrombi in the villi or at the placental surface (Fig. 19) have the potential to embolize to the fetus (133,134). They also are a risk factor for clinically diagnosed perinatal asphyxia (3) and for development of avascular villi. These latter lesions are associated with increased rates of intrauterine growth retardation, oligohydramnios, and maternal coagulation disorders (134).

CONCLUSION

This chapter began with a concept that the author coined many years ago—an opinion that the placenta is like a diary of gestational life and that, like other surgical pathology specimens, it valuably assists the clinician in the pursuit of a firm diagnosis. In considerations of the outcome of the newborn, the surgical pathologist needs clinical information that is usually not available when the initial placental examination and report are made. Because that information is often fundamentally important, I conclude that surgical pathologists should make little or no comment as to the potential effect of placental abnormalities on the prognosis of the associated newborn.

REFERENCES

1. American College of Obstetricians and Gynecologists. Placental pathology. *Committee Opinion* 1991;102:1–2.
2. Benirschke K, Kaufmann P. *The pathology of the human placenta*, 3rd ed. New York: Springer-Verlag, 1995.
3. Altshuler G. *The relationship of placental pathology to causation of detrimental pregnancy outcome in fetal and neonatal brain injury, mechanisms, management, and the risks of practice*, 2nd ed. In: Stevenson DK, Sunshine P. New York: Oxford University Press, 1997, pp. 585–601.
4. Altshuler G, Deppisch L. College of American Pathologists Conference XIX on the examination of the placenta: report of the Working Group on Indications for Placental Examination, C.A.P. Placenta Consensus Conference. *Arch Pathol Lab Med* 1991;115:701–703.
5. Langston C, Kaplan C, Macpherson T, et al. Practice guideline for examination of the placenta: developed by the Placental Pathology Practice Guideline Development Task Force of the College of American Pathologists. *Arch Pathol Lab Med* 1997;121:449–472.
6. Benirschke K. Examination of the placenta. *Obstet Gynecol* 1961;18:309–333.
7. Driscoll SG, Langston C. College of American Pathologists Conference XIX on the examination of the placenta: report of the Working Group on Indications for Placental Examination, C.A.P. Placenta Consensus Conference. *Arch Pathol Lab Med* 1991;115:704–708, 1991.
8. Williams JH, Mepham BL, Wright DH. Tissue preparation for immunocytochemistry. *J Clin Pathol* 1997;50:422–428.
9. Brown and Hopps method for gram-positive and gram-negative bacteria. In: Luna L, ed. *Manual of histologic staining methods of the Armed Forces Institute of Pathology*, 3rd ed. New York: McGraw-Hill, 1967:224–225.
10. Goldenberg RL, Cutter GR, Hoffman HJ, et al. Intrauterine growth retardation standards for diagnosis. *Am J Obstet Gynecol* 1989;161:271–277.
11. Wu PYK. Colloid osmotic pressure in the pregnant woman and the fetus. In: Polin RA, Fox WW, eds. *Fetal and neonatal physiology*. Philadelphia: WB Saunders, 1992:1316.
12. Naftolin F, Khudr G, Benirschke K, Hutchinson DL. The syndrome of chronic abruptio placentae, hydrorrhea, and circumvallate placenta. *Am J Obstet Gynecol* 1973;116:347–350.
13. Ermocilla R, Altshuler G. An enigma: the origin of "X-cells" of the human placenta and their possible relationship to intra-uterine growth retardation. *Am J Obstet Gynecol* 1973;117:1137–1140.
14. Altshuler G, Ermocilla R, Russell P. The placental pathology of the small for gestational age infant. *Am J Obstet Gynecol* 1975;121:351–359.
15. Benirschke K, Kaufmann P. *The pathology of the human placenta*, 3rd ed. New York: Springer-Verlag, 1995:193.
16. Kaplan C, Blanc WA, Elias J. Identification of erythrocytes in intervillous thrombi: A study using immunoperoxidase identification of hemoglobins. *Hum Pathol* 1982;13:554–556.
17. Benirschke K, Kaufmann P. *The pathology of the human placenta*, 3rd ed. New York: Springer-Verlag, 1995:245–250.
18. Naeye RL. Maternal floor infarction. *Hum Pathol* 1985;16:823–828.
19. Maddox DE, Butterfield JH, Ackerman SJ, Coulam CB, Gleich GJ. Elevated serum levels in human pregnancy of a molecule immunochemically similar to eosinophil granule major basic protein. *J Exp Med* 1983;158:1211–1226.
20. Moessinger AC, Blanc WA, Marone PA, Polsen DC. Umbilical cord length as an index of fetal activity: Experimental study and clinical implications. *Pediatr Res* 1982;16:109–112.
21. Robinson LK, Jones KL, Benirschke K. The nature of structural defects associated with velamentous and marginal insertion of the umbilical cord. *Am J Obstet Gynecol* 1983;146:191–193.
22. Heifetz SA. Single umbilical artery. A statistical analysis of 237 autopsy cases and review of the literature. *Perspect Pediatr Pathol* 1984;8:345–378.
23. Heifetz SA, Rueda-Pedraza ME. Omphalomesenteric duct cysts of the umbilical cord. *Pediatr Pathol* 1983;1:325–335.
24. Heifetz SA, Rueda-Pedraza ME. Hemangiomas of the umbilical cord. *Pediatr Pathol* 1983;1:385–398.
25. Kaplan C, Lowell DM, Salafia C. College of American Pathologists Conference XIX on the examination of the placenta: report of the working group on the definition of structural changes associated with abnormal function in the maternal/fetal placental unit in the second and third trimesters. *Arch Pathol Lab Med* 1991;115:709–716.
26. Sampson JE, Theve RP, Blatman RN, et al. Fetal origin of amniotic fluid polymorphonuclear leukocytes. *Am J Obstet Gynecol* 1997;76:77–81.
27. Hyde SR, Altshuler G. Placentitis. In: Connor DH, Chandler FW, Schwartz DA, Manz HJ, Lack EE, eds. *Pathology of infectious diseases*. Stamford: Appleton and Lange, 1997:1675–1693.
28. Hyde SR, Benirschke K. Gestational psittacosis: case report and literature review. *Mod Pathol* 1997;10:602–607.
29. Reshetnikova OR, Burton GJ, Milovanov AP, Fokin EI. Increased incidence of placental chorioangioma in high-altitude pregnancies: Hypobaric hypoxia as a possible etiologic factor. *Am J Obstet Gynecol* 1996;174:557–561.
30. Jackson MR, Mayhew TM, Haas JD. Morphometric studies on villi in human term placentae and the effects of altitude, ethnic grouping and sex of newborn. *Placenta* 1987;8:487–495.
31. Sander CH. Hemorrhagic endovasculitis and hemorrhagic villitis of the placenta. *Arch Pathol Lab Med* 1980;104:371–373.
32. Silver MM, Yeger H, Lines LD. Hemorrhagic endovasculitis-like lesion induced in placental organ culture. *Hum Pathol* 1988;19:251–256.
33. Benirschke K. Accurate recording of twin placentation. A plea to the obstetrician. *Obstet Gynecol* 1961;18:334–347.
34. Benirschke K. The placenta in twin gestation. *Clin Obstet Gynecol* 1990;33:18–31.
35. Baldwin VJ. *Pathology of multiple pregnancy*, 1st ed. New York: Springer-Verlag, 1994.

36. Machin G, Still K, Lalani T. Correlations of placental vascular anatomy and clinical outcomes in 69 monochorionic twin pregnancies. *Am J Med Genet* 1996;61:229–236.
37. Schatz F. Systematisches und alphabetisches Inhaltsverzeichniss von Friedrich Schatz: Placentakreisläufe eineiiger Zwillinge, ihre Entwicklung und ihre Folgen, in Band 19, 24, 27, 29, 30, 53, 55, 58, 60. *Arch Gynäkol* 1990;60:559–584.
38. Aherne W, Strong SJ, Corney G. The structure of the placenta in the twin transfusion syndrome. *Biol Neonat* 1968;12:121–135.
39. Benirschke K. Twin placenta in perinatal mortality. *NY State J Med* 1961;61:1499–1508.
40. Benirschke K. The contribution of placental anastomoses to prenatal twin damage [editorial]. *Hum Pathol* 1992;23:1319–1320.
41. Dimmick JE, Hardwick DF, Ho-Yuen B. A case of renal necrosis and fibrosis in the immediate newborn period. Association with the twin-to-twin transfusion syndrome. *Am J Dis Child* 1971;122:345–347.
42. Danskin FH, Neilson JP. Twin-to-twin transfusion syndrome: What are appropriate diagnostic criteria? *Am J Obstet Gynecol* 1989;161:365–369.
43. De Lia JE, Rogers JG, Dixon JA. Treatment of placental vasculature with a neodymium-yttrium-aluminum-garnet laser via fetoscopy. *Am J Obstet Gynecol* 1985;151:1126–1127.
44. De Lia JE, Kuhlmann RS, Harstad TW, Cruikshank DP. Fetoscopic laser ablation of placental vessels in severe previable twin-twin transfusion syndrome. *Am J Obstet Gynecol* 1995;172:1202–1211.
45. Liu S, Benirschke K, Scioscia AL, Mannino FL. Intrauterine death in multiple gestation. *Acta Genet Med Gemellol* 1992;41:5–26.
46. Beebe LA, Cowan LD, Altshuler G. The epidemiology of placental features: association with gestational age and neonatal outcome. *Obstet Gynecol* 1996;87:771–778.
47. Knox IC, Hoerner JK. The role of infection in premature rupture of the membranes. *Am J Obstet Gynecol* 1950;59:190–194.
48. Benirschke K. Routes and types of infection in the fetus and the newborn. *Am J Dis Child* 1960;99:714–721.
49. Blanc WA. Amniotic infection syndrome. *Clin Obstet Gynecol* 1959;2:715–734.
50. Gibbs RS, Blanco JD, St Clair PJ, et al. Quantitative bacteriology of amniotic fluid from women with clinical intraamniotic infection at term. *J Infect Dis* 1982;145:1–8.
51. Dominguez R, Segal AJ, O'Sullivan JA. Leukocytic infiltration of the umbilical cord Manifestation of fetal hypoxia due to reduction of blood flow in the cord. *JAMA* 1960;173:346–349.
52. Romero R, Mazor M, Morrotti R, et al. Infection and labor. VII. Microbial invasion of the amniotic cavity in spontaneous rupture of membranes at term. *Am J Obstet Gynecol* 1992;166:129.
53. Altshuler G. The role of the placenta in perinatal pathology (revisited). *Pediatr Pathol* 1996;16:207–233.
54. Mitchell MD, Trautman MS, Dudly DJ. Cytokine networking in the placenta. *Placenta* 1993;14:249–275.
55. Stallmach T, Hebisch G, Joller-Jemelka HI, Orban P, Schwaller J, Engelmann M. Cytokine production and visualized effects in the fetomaternal unit. Quantitative and topographic data on cytokines during intrauterine disease. *Lab Invest* 1995;73:384–392.
56. Dammann O, Leviton A. Intrauterine infection, cytokines, and brain damage in the preterm newborn. *Pediatr Res* 1997;42:1–8.
57. Yoon BH, Romero R, Yang SH, et al. Interleukin-6 concentrations in umbilical cord plasma are elevated in neonates with white matter lesions associated with periventricular leukomalacia. *Am J Obstet Gynecol* 1996;174:1433–1440.
58. Baergen R, Benirschke K, Ulich TR. Cytokine expression in the placenta. The role of interleukin 1 and interleukin 1 receptor antagonist expression in chorioamnionitis and parturition. *Arch Pathol Lab Med* 1994;118:52–55.
59. Fox H. *Pathology of the placenta. Major problems in pathology,* vol. 7, 2nd ed. Philadelphia: WB Saunders, 1997.
60. Spiegel CA, Amsel R, Eschenbach DA, et al. Anaerobic bacteria in nonspecific vaginitis. *N Engl J Med* 1980;303:601.
61. Westrom L, Evaldson G, Holmes KK, et al. Taxonomy of vaginosis: bacterial vaginosis, a definition. In: Mardh PA, Taylor-Robinson D, eds. *Bacterial vaginosis.* Stockholm: Almqvist & Wiksell, 1985:259–260.
62. Robinow M, Simonelli FA. Fusobacterium bacteremia in the newborn. *Am J Dis Child* 1965;110:92–94.
63. Hurst V. Fusiforms in the infant mouth. *J D Res* 1957;36:513–515.
64. Altshuler G, Hyde S. Fusobacteria: An important cause of chorioamnionitis. *Arch Pathol Lab Med* 1985;109:739–743.
65. Altshuler G, Hyde S. Clinicopathologic Considerations of Fusobacteria Chorioamnionitis. *Acta Obstet Gynecol Scand* 1988;67:513–517.
66. Easterling TR, Garite TJ. Fusobacterium: Anaerobic occult amnionitis and premature labor. *Obstet Gynecol* 1985;66:825–828.
67. Bejar R, Curbelo V, Davis C, Gluck L. Premature labor. II. Bacterial sources of phospholipase. *Obstet Gynecol* 1981;57:479–482.
68. Kundsin RB, Driscoll SG, Ming PL. Strain of mycoplasma associated with human reproductive failure. *Science* 1967;157:1573–1574.
69. Kundsin RB, Driscoll SG, Pelletier PA. Ureaplasma urealyticum incriminated in perinatal morbidity and mortality. *Science* 1981;213:474–476.
70. Shurin PA, Alpert S, Rosner B, et al. Chorioamnionitis and colonization of the newborn infant with genital mycoplasmas. *N Engl J Med* 1975;293:5–8.
71. Tafari N, Ross S, Naeye RL, et al. Mycoplasma T strains and perinatal death. *Lancet* 1976;108–109.
72. Dische MR, Quinn PA, Czegledy-Nagy E, et al. Genital mycoplasma infection. *Am J Clin Pathol* 1979;72:167–174.
73. Embree JE, Krause VW, Embil JA, et al. Placental infection with mycoplasma hominis and ureaplasma urealyticum: Clinical Correlation. *Obstet Gynecol* 1980;56:475–481.
74. Larroche CL Jr, Paul G, Helffer L, Beaudoin M. Bacteroides fragilis. Contamination materno-placento-foetale. *Arch Fr Pediatr* 1981;38:41–45.
75. Evaldson GR, Malmborg AS, Nord CE. Premature rupture of the membranes and ascending infection. *Br J Obstet Gynaecol* 1982;89:793–801.
76. Friesen CA, Cho CT. Characteristic features of neonatal sepsis due to Haemophilus influenzae. *Rev Infect Dis* 1986;8:777–780.
77. Campognone P, Singer DB. Neonatal sepsis due to nontypable Haemophilus influenzae. *Am J Dis Child* 1986;140:117–121.
78. Lilien LD, Yeh TF, Novak GM, Jacobs NM. Early-onset Haemophilus sepsis in newborn infants: Clinical, roentgenographic, and pathologic features. *Pediatrics* 1978;62:299–303.
79. Wallace RJ, Baker CJ, Quinones FJ, et al. Nontypable Haemophilus influenzae (biotype 4) as a neonatal, maternal, and genital pathogen. *Rev Infect Dis* 1983;5:123–136.
80. Winn HN, Egley CC. Acute Haemophilus influenzae chorioamnionitis associated with intact amniotic membranes. *Am J Obstet Gynecol* 1987;156:458–459.
81. Schachter J. Chlamydial infections, Part 1. *N Engl J Med* 1978;298:428–435. Part II. *N Engl J Med* 1978;298:490–495. Part III. *N Engl J Med* 1978;298:540–549.
82. Heggie AD, Lumicao GG, Stuart LA, et al. Chlamydia trachomatis infection in mothers and infants. *Am J Dis Child* 1981;135:507–511.
83. Martin DH, Koutsky L, Eschenbach DA, et al. Prematurity and perinatal mortality in pregnancies complicated by maternal chlamydia trachomatis infections. *JAMA* 1982;247:1585–1607.
84. Thompson SE, Dretler RH. Epidemiology and treatment of chlamydial infections in pregnant women and infants. *Rev Infect Dis Suppl* 1982;4:S747–S757.
85. Alexander ER, Harrison HR. Role of chlamydia trachomatis in perinatal infection. *Rev Infect Dis* 1983;5:713–719.
86. Winkler B, Reumann W, Mitao M, et al. Chlamydial endometritis. *Am J Surg Pathol* 1984;8:771–778.
87. Navarro CN, Blanc WA. Subacute necrotizing funisitis: A variant of cord inflammation with a high rate of perinatal infection. *J Pediatr* 1973;85:689–697.
88. Fojaco RM, Hensley GT, Moskowitz L. Congenital syphilis and necrotizing funisitis. *JAMA* 1989;261:1788–1790.
89. Schwartz DA, Larsen SA, Beck-Sague C, Fears M, Rice RJ. Pathology of the umbilical cord in congenital syphilis: analysis of 25 specimens using histochemistry and immunofluorescent antibody to Treponema pallidum. *Hum Pathol* 1995;26:784–791.
90. Schwartz DA, Zhang W, Larsen S, Rice RJ. Placental pathology of congenital syphilis. *Trophoblast Res* 1994;8:223–229.
91. Jacques SM, Qureshi F. Necrotizing funisitis: a study of 45 cases. *Hum Pathol* 1992;23:1278–1283.
92. Craver RD, Baldwin VJ. Necrotizing funisitis. *Obstet Gynecol* 1992;79:64–70.
93. Heifetz SA, Bauman M. Necrotizing funisitis and herpes simplex infection of placental and decidual tissues: study of four cases. *Hum Pathol* 1994;25:715–722.
94. Hyde SR, Giacoia GP. Congenital herpes infection: placental and umbilical cord findings. *Obstet Gynecol* 1993;81:852–855.

95. Benirschke K, Raphael SI. *Candida albicans* infection of the amniotic sac. *Am J Obstet Gynecol* 1958;75:200–202.
96. Altshuler G. Placental villitis of unknown etiology: Harbinger of serious disease? A four months' experience of nine cases. *J Reprod Med* 1973;11:215–222.
97. Altshuler G, Russell P. The human placental villitides. A review of chronic intrauterine infection. In: Grundmann E, Kirsten W, eds. *Current topics in pathology*. Heidelberg: Springer-Verlag, 1975;60:63–112.
98. Labarrere C, Althabe O, Telenta M. Chronic villitis of unknown aetiology in placentae of idiopathic small for gestational age infants. *Placenta* 1982;3:309–318.
99. Althabe O, Labarrere CA. Chronic villitis of unknown etiology and intrauterine growth retarded infants of normal and low ponderal index. *Placenta* 1985;6:369–373.
100. Labarrere CA, McIntyre JA, Faulk WP. Immunohistological evidence that villitis in normal human term placentas is an immunologic lesion. *Am J Obstet Gynecol* 1990;162:515–522.
101. Redline RW, Abramowsky CR. Clinical and pathologic aspects of recurrent placental villitis, *Hum Pathol* 1985;16:727–731.
102. Redline RW, Patterson P. Villitis of unknown etiology is associated with major infiltration of fetal tissue by maternal inflammatory cells. *Am J Pathol* 1993;143:473–479.
103. Redline RW. Placental pathology: a neglected link between basic disease mechanisms and untoward pregnancy outcomes. *Curr Opin Obstet Gynecol* 1995;7:10–15.
104. Khong TY. Expression of MHC class II antigens by placental villi: no relationship with villitis of unknown origin. *J Clin Pathol* 1995;48:494–495.
105. Knox WF, Fox H. Villitis of unknown aetiology: Its incidence and significance in placentae from a British population. *Placenta* 1984;5:395–402.
106. Nordenvall M, Sandstedt B. Placental villitis and intrauterine growth retardation in a Swedish population. *APMIS* 1990;98:19–24.
107. Mortimer G, MacDonald DJ, Smeeth A. A pilot study of the frequency and significance of placental villitis. *Br J Obstet Gynaecol* 1985;92:629–633.
108. Russell P. Inflammatory lesions of the human placenta. III: The histopathology of villitis of unknown aetiology. *Placenta* 1980;1:227–244.
109. Russell P, Atkinson K, Krishnan, L. Recurrent reproductive failure due to severe placental villitis of unknown etiology. *J Reprod Med* 1980;24:93–98.
110. Labarrere CA, Althabe O. Chronic villitis of unknown etiology in recurrent intrauterine fetal growth retardation. *Placenta* 1987;8:167–173.
111. Redline RW. Recurrent villitis of bacterial etiology. *Pediatr Pathol* 1996;16:995–1001.
112. Salafia CM, Vintzileos AM, Silberman L, Bantham KF, Vogel CA. Placental pathology of idiopathic intrauterine growth retardation at term. *Am J Perinatol* 1992;9:179–184.
113. Salafia CM, Vogel CA, Bantham KF, Vintzileos AM. Preterm delivery: correlations of fetal growth and placental pathology. *Am J Perinatol* 1992;9:190–193.
114. Salafia CM, Ernst LM, Pezzullo JC, Wolf EJ, Rosenkrantz TS, Vintzileos AM. The very low birthweight infant: Maternal complications leading to preterm birth, placental lesions, and intrauterine growth retardation. *Am J Perinatol* 1995;12:106–110.
115. Salafia CM, Minior VK, Pezzullo JC, Popek EJ, Rosenkrantz TS, Vintzileos AM. Intrauterine growth restriction in infants of less than thirty-two weeks' gestation: associated placental pathologic features. *Am J Obstet Gynecol* 1995;173:1049–1057.
116. Katz VL, Bowes WA Jr. Meconium aspiration syndrome: Reflections on a murky subject. *Am J Obstet Gynecol* 1992;166:171–183.
117. Wiswell TE. Meconium aspiration syndrome made murkier. *Am J Obstet Gynecol* 1992;167:1914.
118. Benirschke K. Placental pathology questions to the perinatologist. *J Perinatol* 1994;14:371–375.
119. Wiswell TE. Meconium staining and the meconium aspiration syndrome. In: Stevenson DK, Sunshine P, eds. *Fetal and neonatal brain injury mechanisms, management, and the risks of practice*, 2nd ed. New York: Oxford University Press, 1997:539–563.
120. Altshuler G, Hyde S. Meconium-induced vasocontraction: a potential cause of cerebral and other fetal hypoperfusion and of poor pregnancy outcome. *J Child Neurol* 1989;4:137–142.
121. Sepulveda WF, Gonzalez C, Cruz MA, Rudolph MI. Vasoconstrictive effect of bile acid on isolated human placental chorionic veins. *Eur J Obstet Gynecol Reprod Biol* 1991;42:211–215.
122. Miller PW, Coen RW, Benirschke K. Dating the time interval from meconium passage to birth. *Obstet Gynecol* 1985;66:459–462.
123. Altshuler G. A conceptual approach to placental pathology and pregnancy outcome. *Semin Diag Pathol* 1993;10:204–221.
124. Altshuler G, Hyde S. Clinicopathologic implications of placental pathology. *Clin Obstet Gynecol* 1996;39:549–570.
125. Lippman HS. A morphologic and quantitative study of the blood corpuscles in the new-born period. *Am J Dis Child* 1924;27:473–526.
126. Fox H. The incidence and significance of nucleated erythrocytes in the foetal vessels of the mature human placenta. *Br J Obstet Gynaecol* 1967;74:40–43.
127. Khudr G, Benirschke K. Placental lesion in viral hepatitis. *Am J Obstet Gynecol* 1972;40:381–384.
128. Altshuler G, with the assistance of a computer program written by Randy Stafford. Chorangiosis: An important placental sign of neonatal morbidity and mortality. *Arch Pathol Lab Med* 1984;108:71–74.
129. Hustin J, Foidart JM, Lambotte R. Cellular proliferation in villi of normal and pathological pregnancies. *Gynecol Obstet Invest* 1984;17:1–9.
130. Reshetnikova OS, Burton GJ, Milovanov AP, Fokin EI. Increased incidence of chorangioma in high altitude pregnancies: Hypobaric hypoxia as a possible etiologic factor. *Am J Obstet Gynecol* 1996;174:557–561.
131. Khong TY, Pearce JM, Robertson WB. Acute atherosis in preeclampsia: Maternal determinants and fetal outcome in the presence of the lesion. *Am J Obstet Gynecol* 1987;157:360–363.
132. Khong TY, Chambers HM. Alternative method of sampling placentas for the assessment of uteroplacental vasculature. *J Clin Pathol* 1992;45:925–927.
133. Wolf PL, Jones KL, Longway SR, Benirschke K, Bloor C. Prenatal death from acute myocardial infarction and cardiac tamponade due to embolus from the placenta. *Am Heart J* 1985;109:603–605.
134. Redline RW, Pappin A. Fetal thrombotic vasculopathy: The clinical significance of extensive avascular villi. *Hum Pathol* 1995;26:80–85.

CHAPTER 51

The Vulva and Vagina

Henry F. Frierson, Jr. and Stacey E. Mills

VULVA

Normal Anatomy and Histology

The vulva is covered by skin and skin-like mucous membrane. It consists of the mons pubis, labia majora and minora, clitoris (with prepuce and frenulum), vulvovaginal glands, Skene's (paraurethral) glands, vestibule, vestibular bulbs, urethral meatus, and hymen. Keratinized squamous epithelium covers most of the vulvar surface, but it becomes nonkeratinized at the introitus. The labia majora have sebaceous, eccrine, and apocrine glands, and much of their thickness is due to abundant adipose tissue. Distinctive anogenital, mammary-like glands are lined by simple columnar epithelium with apical cytoplasmic snouts; they are typically surrounded by a myoepithelial layer, a thickened basement membrane, and a cuff of loose or dense stroma (Fig. 1) (1,2). These long, coiled glands may have acini, diverticula, or short branches. They have their highest concentration in the interlabial sulcus, where they open directly onto the surface. It is believed that they are not derived from rudiments of the mammary ridges (2). The labia minora are rich in blood vessels, elastic fibers, and sebaceous glands, and have few, if any, sweat glands and little or no adipose tissue. Bartholin's glands, which are homologous to Cowper's glands in the male, are composed of lobules of mucus-secreting acini located bilaterally in the stroma of the vestibule, inferior to the hymen. They are palpable sometimes in thin women and are more easily detected when enlarged by inflammation or neoplasm (3). The major excretory duct of each Bartholin's gland empties posterolaterally at the junction of the hymenal ring and labium minus. Each major duct, as well as each of the ductules, is lined by stratified transitional-type epithelium that changes to stratified squamous epithelium at its orifice. The lesser vestibular glands (Littre's glands in the male) are lined by a single layer of tall columnar mucinous cells.

Robboy et al. (4) found from one to several hundred (usually two to ten) of these glands in 9 of 19 autopsied fetuses and young women whose vulvae were serially blocked for microscopic examination. Skene's paraurethral glands, homologues to the prostatic glands, form a network that surrounds the urethra, primarily posteriorly and laterally (5). Most of the ducts open into the distal one-third of the urethral canal. Skene's glands are lined by low columnar to tall cylindrical cells with occasional mucus-secreting cells. The paraurethral ducts are lined by columnar epithelium that changes to stratified squamous epithelium or transitional epithelium near their urethral openings.

The local environment has very important effects on vulvar skin. The various factors producing this environment have been emphasized by Lawrence (6).

The lymphatic channels of the anterior portion of the labia majora and minora and the prepuce of the clitoris drain into the superficial and deep femoral lymph nodes via the dense lymphatic network at the symphysis pubis (the presymphyseal plexus), or into the superficial inguinal lymph nodes (7). The superficial inguinal nodes form a horizontal chain between the skin and deep fascia, just inferior to the inguinal ligament. Lymph drainage ultimately proceeds to the external iliac system. Unilateral vulvar injection studies show lymph flow to contralateral pelvic nodes due to anastomotic channels between both sides of the vulva or the pelvis (8). The obturator lymph node, located in the obturator fossa of the pelvis near the obturator nerve, is often large and is found inferior and lateral to the other external iliac nodes. Cloquet's (or Rosenmuller's) lymph node is either the most superior lymph node of the deep femoral chain or the most inferior external iliac node that projects below the inguinal ligament. Way (9) noted that only about 8% of individuals have nodal tissue at this location. Iversen and Aas (8), however, using radioactive injections, found that the medial lacunar node of the external iliac chain (which perhaps is Cloquet's node) had nearly half of the total activity detected in removed pelvic nodes. In his vital dye studies, Eichner (10) noted that Cloquet's node was always involved initially and,

---

H. F. Frierson, Jr. and S. E. Mills: Department of Pathology, University of Virginia Health Sciences Center, Charlottesville, Virginia 22908.

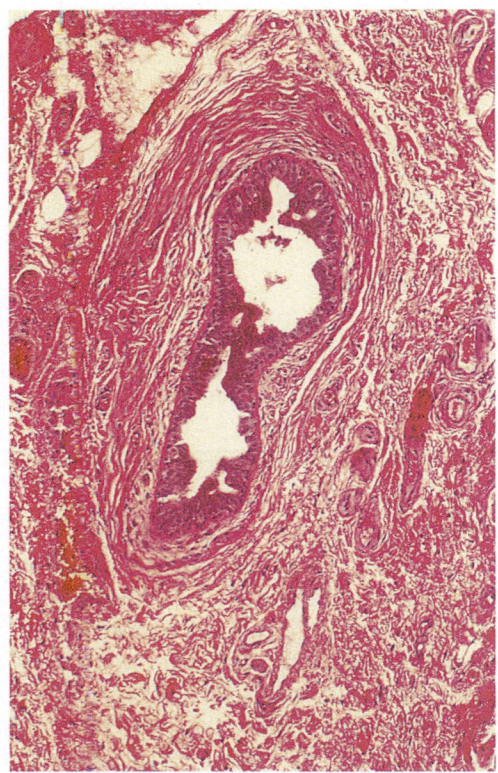

FIG. 1. Anogenital "sweat" gland. Mammary-like ducts, typically concentrated in the interlabial sulcus, usually have a prominent basement membrane and a dense or loose stromal cuff.

if it was not stained, then dye was absent in the superficial and deep femoral nodes and in the iliac nodes. The lymphatic channels of the posterior vulva reach the femoral lymph nodes, bypassing the presymphyseal plexus.

Most of the lymphatic drainage of the clitoris is into the superficial femoral lymph nodes via the presymphyseal plexus. Plentl and Friedman (7) emphasized direct lymphatic communications from the clitoris to pelvic nodes. Way (9), however, has stated that there is no evidence for spread of cancer from the clitoris to the pelvic lymph nodes without initial involvement of the inguinal lymph nodes. Moreover, Iversen and Aas (8) failed to find a direct lymphatic pathway from the clitoris to the pelvic lymph nodes.

Lymph drainage from midline vulvar structures, such as the clitoris and perineum, is often bilateral. Most unilateral vulvar squamous cell carcinomas that metastasize do so to the ipsilateral groin lymph nodes. Approximately 5% of all carcinomas located on one side of the vulva metastasize to the contralateral lymph nodes only, and 15% of unilateral cancers metastasize bilaterally (9).

Approach to Specimens

Several types of vulvar biopsy and excision specimens may be submitted to the surgical pathology laboratory. For excisions of carcinoma, it is important to identify the primary tumor, search for multifocal lesions, document the depth (thickness) of tumor penetration, check the margins of resection, and examine all lymph nodes. A labeled picture protocol is often useful to indicate the sites selected for microscopic study. Alternatively, the specimen may be placed upside down on clear plastic and photocopied. Wide excision vulvar specimens contain underlying adipose tissue and fascia. A partial vulvectomy specimen retains as much normal vulva as possible. The tissue from the "skinning" vulvectomy consists of only epidermis and dermis. The total (simple) vulvectomy specimen contains the entire vulva, including subcutaneous tissue down to the deep fascia. The traditional radical vulvectomy with lymphadenectomy is an en bloc resection of the entire vulva, inguinal skin and subcutaneous tissue, femoral and inguinal lymph nodes, and portions of the saphenous vein. At present, some surgeons have abandoned the en bloc resection, utilizing separate incisions for the inguinal node dissections. The radical hemivulvectomy is a unilateral radical vulvectomy with separate incisions for the groin dissections.

Congenital Anomalies

There are a variety of congenital abnormalities of the vulva. Most are rare. They may be categorized as genital manifestations of specific genetic anomalies, developmental defects affecting the external genitalia only, and congenital abnormalities associated with anomalies of other anatomical regions, especially the urinary and gastrointestinal tracts. A newborn with ambiguous genitalia may be a virilized female, an imperfectly masculinized male, or a true hermaphrodite. The external genitalia of a true hermaphrodite also may have primarily male or female features. Female pseudohermaphroditism results from prenatal virilization and manifests as clitoral hypertrophy and, often, labial fusion. There may be a persistent urogenital sinus or penis with a penile urethra. Most frequently, female pseudohermaphroditism is caused by congenital adrenal hyperplasia. Virilization results from excess adrenal androgens due to deficiencies in converting enzymes (11). Masculinization also develops from exposure to exogenous or maternal androgens. Although virilization is sometimes induced by exogenous testosterone or the synthetic androgen danazol (12,13), most instances have resulted from exposure to progestational compounds that were used for the treatment of threatened abortion (14,15). Female pseudohermaphroditism has resulted from maternal androgen-producing neoplasms such as luteoma of pregnancy (16–18) and Krukenberg's tumor with stromal luteinization (19–22). A purported maternal Sertoli-Leydig cell tumor causing congenital virilization more likely represents a luteoma (23). Congenital virilization also may be secondary to maternal adrenal adenoma (24–26), adrenal hyperplasia (27), or undetermined causes.

Malformations of the external genitalia are sometimes an isolated finding, but often are associated with gastrointestinal or urinary tract defects (28–30). Complete absence or duplication of the external genitalia occurs virtually always in association with multiple anomalies, many of which are not compatible with life. Severe cases of labial fusion (chiefly due to the exposure to androgens *in utero*) result in the covering of the vaginal and urethral orifices and the formation of a urogenital sinus. Labial adhesions (agglutination), which are more often an acquired condition, sometimes obstruct the urethral or vaginal orifices. Unilateral or bilateral hypertrophy of the labium minus is a common finding that, in actuality, may be a normal variant (31). An ectopic labium majus has been described (32). The clitoris may be absent, hypoplastic, hypertrophic, or bifid. Clitoral hypertrophy is most often associated with exposure to androgens *in utero,* but is also found in rare conditions such as the Beckwith-Wiedemann syndrome (11). A bifid clitoris may be a solitary abnormality, or may be found with episadias or exstrophy of the bladder (28). The hymen may be imperforate, microperforate, or rigid. An imperforate hymen is often not recognized until after puberty. A microperforate hymen is usually detected before menarche, as it results in recurring vulvovaginitis and urinary tract infections (33). A persistent urogenital membrane sinus develops from fusion of the membrane with the inner labia minora, obliterating the introitus (34). The shallow sinus is covered by a thick membrane that contains a small aperture; the vagina and urethra open separately into the sinus.

Anomalies of the urinary tract that occur with malformations of the female external genitalia include episadias, exstrophy of the bladder, and ectopic ureteral orifices. Ectopic ureters, which usually are accessory, open into the vagina or the vestibule. An ectopic ureterocele sometimes is seen as a cystic mass at the introitus (35). An ectopic anus opens more anteriorly in the perineum than normal or is found in the inferior portion of the vagina. In the persistence of the cloaca, the fused labial folds cover only a single narrow channel that empties onto the perineum via a small orifice; the bladder, genital tract, and bowel each open into this common cavity (28). In other cloacal malformations, the external appearance of the perineum is quite variable (30). A case of intestinal heterotopia resulting in a small vulvar ulcer in an adult has been described (36).

Cysts

The most common vulvar cyst, epidermoid cyst (37), occurs as a round or oval, painless nodule primarily on the anterior half of the labia majora. Frequently multiple cysts are present. The cyst is found chiefly in adults, but one report described an epidermoid cyst of the labium majus in a newborn, who also had a bifid clitoris and skeletal anomalies (38). So-called traumatic inclusion cysts, also lined by squamous epithelium and filled with keratinous debris, are found at sites of previous surgery, especially episiotomy. Some have occurred in Nigerian women and children who have undergone ritual circumcision (39).

A vulvar pilonidal cyst (or sinus) typically involves the clitoral area (40). It consists of an abscess cavity filled with hair shafts that elicit a foreign body granulomatous reaction. A squamous lining may cover the superficial portion of the sinus tract, but most of the sinus tract is surrounded by granulation tissue.

Skene's duct cyst (paraurethral cyst) is usually less than 2 cm in diameter, but may cause urethral obstruction (37). The cyst is lined by transitional epithelium, sometimes with squamous or ciliated cells (4,41–43). Although inflammation has been considered causal, most women lack a history of infection. When found in the newborn, Skene's duct cyst must be distinguished clinically from ectopic ureterocele, urethrocele, and urethral diverticulum (41). Spontaneous drainage of the cyst in the newborn occurs within a few weeks or months (43).

Hymenal cyst is the most common vulvar cyst of the female newborn (43). It is ½ to 1 cm in diameter and is lined by squamous epithelium. Spontaneous drainage of a milky fluid is characteristic.

The cyst of the canal of Nuck, similar to the hydrocele of the spermatic cord, results from incomplete obliteration of the processus vaginalis (44). This hydrocele is located along the course of the round ligament and is bordered by its occluded ends at the inguinal ring and labium majus. The nontender, elongated cyst varies in size, is occasionally multiple, and transilluminates. Unlike a hernia, it is typically irreducible. An inguinal hernia is present in one-third of the cases, however (44,45). The cyst contains clear fluid and is lined by a single layer of cuboid or flattened mesothelial cells. The cyst must be excised, as recurrence follows aspiration (45).

The mucous or mucinous cyst of the vestibule (4,46–48), virtually never seen before puberty, may be related to hormonal stimulation. Twenty percent of the cysts are multiple, and the mean size is approximately 1 cm (47). The cyst is usually unilocular and contains abundant mucoid material. It is lined by a single layer of tall columnar, mucus-secreting cells that have basal nuclei (Fig. 2). Papillary groups of cells,

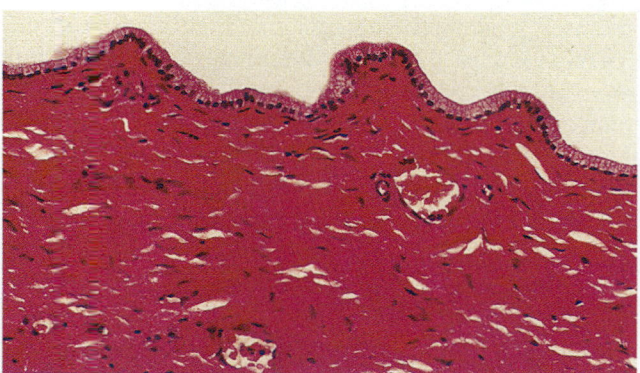

FIG. 2. Mucous cyst. The cyst is lined by a single layer of columnar, mucus-producing cells surrounded by a fibrovascular stroma.

reserve cell hyperplasia, ciliated cells, and squamous metaplasia may also be present. The lining is surrounded by a fibrovascular stroma without smooth muscle cells. A müllerian origin was postulated formerly (46), but the mucous cyst is now considered to derive from urogenital sinus (minor vestibular gland) epithelium (4,47).

Bartholin's duct cyst results from occlusion of the major duct, with persistent secretion of the glands. The cyst occurs chiefly during the reproductive years and is usually unilocular, unilateral, and nontender (37). Large cysts may block the entrance to the vestibule. Unless infected, the cyst fluid is mucoid and clear. Transitional-type epithelium is the most common lining, but cuboid, columnar, ciliated, and squamous cells may be observed in varying proportions (Fig. 3) (3). The cyst wall contains a variable number of chronic inflammatory cells and normal or atrophic acini. A papilloma of Bartholin's gland duct cyst has been described (49). Mucocele-like changes of Bartholin's gland are observed after rupture of obstructed, dilated ducts with leakage of mucin (50). Vacuolated histiocytes are conspicuous in the stroma.

Gartner's duct cyst (mesonephric or wolffian cyst) occurs less often in the vulva than in the vagina. A lining of nonmucinous, cuboid, or low columnar cells is sometimes accompanied by focal squamous metaplasia (Fig. 4). Smooth muscle fibers may be found in the cyst wall.

Fox-Fordyce disease is a chronic pruritic eruption of multiple, 1- to 3-mm papules or microcysts (51). The condition manifests in anatomical sites that have apocrine glands. It predilects the axilla and vulva, is very rare before puberty, and is uncommon after menopause. Microscopically, the superior portion of the hair follicle is obstructed by a keratin plug that also occludes the ostium of the apocrine duct. A vesicle then forms in the wall of the follicle after ductal rupture. Acanthosis and spongiosis of the follicle, dilatation of apocrine gland acini, and chronic inflammation of the dermis are also present. Multiple histologic sections are often necessary to identify the diagnostic microcysts (retention vesicles) (51).

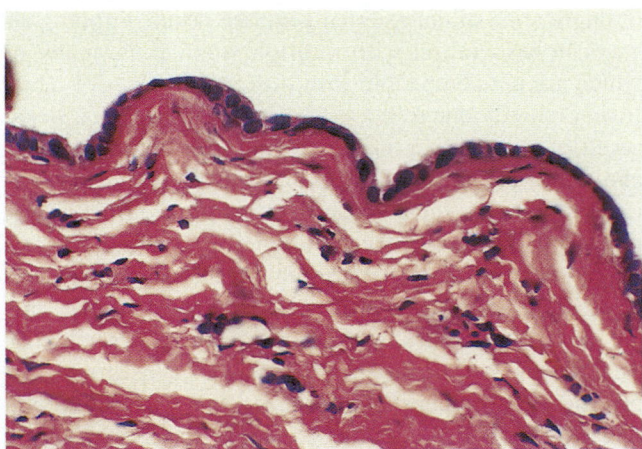

FIG. 4. Gartner's duct cyst. A single layer of cuboid, non–mucus-producing cells lines the cyst.

Endometriosis manifests as blue or red, firm, cystic nodules that enlarge cyclically with menses. Endometriotic foci are found at sites of previous surgery, especially episiotomy. Typically, postpartum endometrial curettage had been performed as a routine measure to prevent bleeding and uterine subinvolution (52).

Mammary-like vulvar glands may rarely give rise to involution cysts and hidrocystoma (53).

Infectious Diseases

Bacteria

The chancre of primary syphilis *(Treponema pallidum)* occurs as a painless, eroded papule or indurated ulcer with raised edges and a smooth, erythematous base. Microscopically, the central surface epithelium is attenuated or ulcerated. There is an intense infiltrate of lymphocytes and plasma cells in the edematous ulcer bed and prominent proliferation of capillaries with swollen endothelial cells. The characteristic spiral organisms in smears of the exudate may be visualized using darkfield examination or immunofluorescence with antitreponemal antibodies (54). In paraffin sections, the organisms may be seen with the Warthin-Starry or Levaditi stains, or with antisera using the immunoperoxidase technique (55). Secondary syphilis of the vulva, condyloma latum, manifests as moist, gray-white patches or flat-topped papules that usually appear from 3 to 6 weeks after the chancre. They are highly contagious, containing many spirochetes. Pseudoepitheliomatous hyperplasia is conspicuous and neutrophils may migrate into the epithelium. The chronic inflammatory and endothelial cell changes are similar to those of the chancre. Tertiary syphilis is rarely observed in the vulva.

Vulvar infection by *Neisseria gonorrhoeae* usually involves Skene's glands or Bartholin's glands, and is often accompanied by gonococcal cervicitis, urethritis, or proctitis. The vulvar glands are swollen and painful, with abscess for-

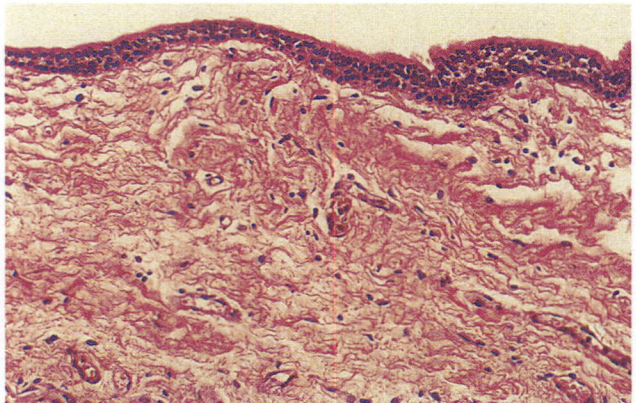

FIG. 3. Bartholin's duct cyst. The cyst is lined most often by transitional-type epithelium.

mation. Culture of the organism is essential for diagnosis. Although gonococci were believed responsible for most abscesses of Bartholin's gland, in one study they were cultured from only 17% of the abscesses that contained bacteria (56).

Granuloma inguinale *(Calymmatobacterium granulomatis)* is rare in the United States, and is largely confined to the southern states (57). It manifests as solitary or multiple, painless papules that ulcerate and have serpiginous, rolled borders. Marked tissue destruction may ensue with extensive scarring and elephantiasis (54,57). Inguinal lymphadenopathy is generally not marked. Microscopically, there is exuberant pseudoepitheliomatous hyperplasia (58), granulation tissue, and an inflammatory infiltrate with plasma cells, scattered polymorphonuclear leukocytes, and characteristic vacuolated histiocytes. The histiocytes contain 0.6- to 2-μm encapsulated rods with bipolar granules (Donovan bodies). The gram-negative bacteria are difficult to identify in hematoxylin and eosin–stained paraffin sections, but are better visualized with Wright, Giemsa, toluidine blue, or Warthin-Starry stains. They are readily apparent in Papanicolaou-stained smears (59) and in appropriately stained, thin plastic sections. The florid pseudoepitheliomatous hyperplasia must not be confused with squamous cell carcinoma. There are, however, well-documented reports of vulvar squamous cell carcinoma arising in areas of chronic granuloma inguinale infection (60,61).

Chancroid *(Haemophilus ducreyi)* is an unusual venereal disease in the United States. It begins as a small papule or pustule, usually on the vestibule. Later, painful, soft, single or multiple ulcers have ragged edges with erythematous borders. Enlarged inguinal lymph nodes with suppuration (buboes) are present in approximately one-quarter of cases (62). Beneath the surface ulceration and necrotic debris, endothelial proliferation is prominent, and there may be lumenal compromise and thrombosis. Lymphocytes and plasma cells densely populate the deep dermis. Culture isolation of the gram-negative organism is necessary for diagnosis (63).

The vulva is the least common site for tuberculosis of the female genital tract (64). Vulvar tuberculosis results from hematogenous dissemination or spread from the upper genital tract. It also may be transmitted sexually from a male partner harboring tuberculous epididymitis. Grossly, the infected vulva is ulcerated or hypertrophic, and may mimic squamous cell carcinoma. Culture is usually necessary for diagnosis, given the low sensitivity of acid-fast stains (65). Women with leprosy sometimes have vulvar involvement.

Erythrasma *(Corynebacterium minutissimum)* forms symmetrical, erythematous inguinal macules that may simulate infection with tinea or candida. The condition is asymptomatic and is almost never biopsied. The organisms are located in the horny layer of the epidermis. Diagnosis is confirmed by orange-red fluorescence with a Wood's lamp (66).

Impetigo and ecthyma may spread to the vulvar area in children. Folliculitis and erysipelas of the vulva are typically due to staphylococci and streptococci, respectively. These microorganisms, as well as a variety of other aerobic and anaerobic bacteria, may also be involved in deep abscesses, cellulitis, and necrotizing fasciitis (67). Necrotizing fasciitis is a toxic, systemic illness that follows surgery or minor trauma. The disease usually occurs in diabetics and is rapidly progressive and frequently fatal (68). Grossly, the vulva is erythematous and swollen. The superficial fascia and subcutaneous tissue are necrotic, but the underlying muscular layer is spared. Microscopically, the subcutaneous tissue shows necrosis, acute inflammation, and thrombosis and necrosis of small vessels. Bacteria can be seen in the necrotic tissue. Aggressive surgical resection is the most important therapeutic modality.

Hidradenitis suppurativa is a chronic inflammation of sites replete with apocrine glands. The disease is virtually never seen prior to puberty and has a peak incidence in the third decade of life (69). Follicular and intraepidermal apocrine duct occlusion by keratin with perifolliculitis and apocrine adenitis leads to the formation of abscesses. Chronic inflammatory cells, foreign body giant cells, granulation tissue, fibrosis, and deep sinus tracts follow destruction of cutaneous appendages. Cultures usually reveal a spectrum of bacterial pathogens (69). Surgery is the mainstay of therapy for severe cases (70).

Bacillary angiomatosis of the vulva has been reported in a patient with AIDS (71).

Chlamydia

Chlamydia trachomatis serotypes L1–L3 cause lymphogranuloma venereum and serotypes D-K are associated with sexually transmitted oculogenital disease (72).

The initial manifestation of lymphogranuloma venereum is a small, asymptomatic vesicle, papule, or ulcer, frequently on the posterior vulva (54). Swollen inguinal lymph nodes with suppuration occur after a few weeks. The histopathologic features of the ulcer include marked chronic inflammation, a few giant cells, necrosis, granulation tissue, fibrosis, and pseudoepitheliomatous hyperplasia. The lymph nodes show follicular hyperplasia and characteristic, but nonspecific, stellate microabscesses. In long-standing infection, there is extensive scarring, with strictures and fistulas of the vulva, urethra, vagina, and rectum. Chronic lymphedema and obstruction may result in elephantiasis. Squamous cell carcinoma of the vulva has been reported in women with previous infection (61). The most important technique for the identification of oculogenital chlamydia has been culture isolation. The characteristic intravacuolar organisms in vacuolated macrophages have been observed in suppurative inguinal lymphadenitis of lymphogranuloma venereum (73). They are gram-negative, stain faintly blue with H&E, and are black with the Warthin-Starry silver impregnation stain. Electron microscopy, immunohistochemistry, and polymerase chain reaction using primers for chlamydial 16S ribosomal DNA can be used to detect the organisms in tissues. *C. trachomatis* has also been isolated from duct exudate of Bartholin's gland (74).

Viruses

Herpes simplex is the most common cause of vulvar ulcers. Genital tract infection is due more often to type 2 than type 1 virus (75). An intraepithelial herpetic vesicle forms from acantholysis of the squamous epithelium due to ballooning and reticular degeneration. Subsequent rupture forms a painful superficial ulcer. The inflammatory infiltrate in the dermis varies; polymorphonuclear leukocytes and vasculitis may be present. At the periphery of the ulcers, mononucleate or multinucleated epithelial cells contain "ground-glass" nuclei or eosinophilic intranuclear inclusions. The inclusions are seen in both H&E-stained histologic sections and in Papanicolaou- or Giemsa-stained cytologic preparations.

Herpes zoster (76,77), vaccinia (78), Epstein-Barr virus (79,80), and cytomegalovirus (81) have resulted in vulvar infection. In some women with genital ulcer disease and human immunodeficiency virus (HIV) infection, no specific cause of the ulcer is found, and, hence, HIV is presumed to play a role (81).

Human papillomaviruses make up a heterogeneous group that causes squamous proliferations of the skin and mucous membranes. New genotypes continue to be reported and are defined as such when the DNA sequence has less than 50% homology with other established genomes. Infections with multiple venereal genotypes are not unusual. Only uncommonly do nonvenereal types of papillomavirus involve the vulva. Papillomavirus infection occurs anywhere on the external genitalia and is most commonly observed in women of childbearing age. Vulvar warts (condylomata acuminata) appear as pink or gray-white, soft, sessile or verrucous growths that may become confluent (Fig. 5). Vulvar vestibular squamous papillomatosis, small, sometimes pruritic growths on the vestibule, have been considered to be due to papillomavirus only in some women (82,83). Multiple papillae that lack evidence for papillomavirus represent normal anatomical variants of the vulvar vestibule, however (84,85). These uniform and symmetrical micropapillations lack the classic cytologic features of condylomata (86,87).

Recurrence of genital warts is due to reinfection or latent viral activation (88). Microscopically, condyloma acuminatum is characterized by delicate, branching fibrovascular cores (papillomatosis) lined by squamous epithelium showing acanthosis, hyperkeratosis, and parakeratosis (Fig. 6). The parabasal layer is thickened, and there is minimal nuclear enlargement and pleomorphism of parabasal cells. Orderly maturation and normal cellular polarity are retained. Mitotic figures are identifiable, but atypical mitoses are absent. Koilocytosis is the characteristic cytopathic effect of papillomavirus infection. Koilocytes are superficial or intermediate squamous cells with single or occasionally multiple, enlarged, hyperchromatic, and wrinkled nuclei. Surrounding the nucleus is a prominent clear space or "halo," which abuts a thickened zone of peripheral cytoplasm. Binucleate forms are typically present. Electron microscopic, immunohistochemical, and *in situ* hybridization studies have shown that the viral particles are concentrated in the nuclei of koilocytes and parakeratotic cells (89).

Lesions caused by human papillomaviruses should not be confused with multinucleated atypia of the vulva in which multinucleated cells are confined to the lower or middle epithelial layers (90). Unlike condyloma and intraepithelial neoplasia, surface atypia is absent and hyperchromasia, irregularity, and variation are not seen in the multinucleated cells. This focal histologic change usually occurs in young women, but it is unclear that it results in a clinically visible vulvar lesion.

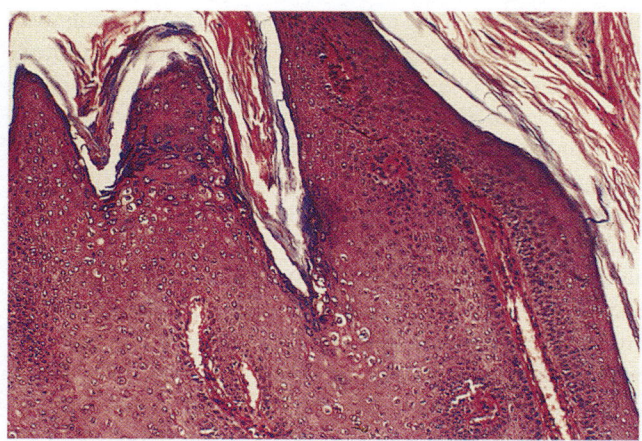

FIG. 6. Condyloma acuminatum. Acanthotic squamous epithelium is supported by fibrovascular cores. Hyperkeratosis, orderly maturation of cells, and koilocytes are characteristic.

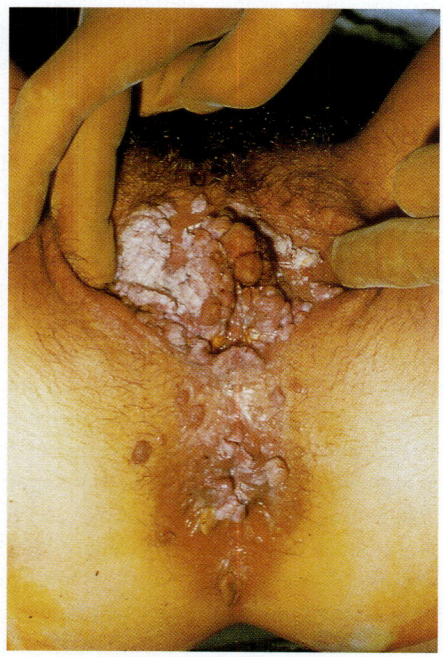

FIG. 5. Condyloma acuminatum. Genital warts may be discrete or confluent. Perianal involvement is common.

Podophyllin therapy for condyloma acuminatum may produce cytologic changes mimicking intraepithelial neoplasia. Microscopically, the effects are most pronounced within 48 hours after treatment, and are absent after 1 week (91). Typically, there is intercellular edema, necrosis of the basal one-half of the epidermis, and an edematous, inflamed papillary dermis. Mitotic figures (with a few bizarre forms) are markedly increased. Unlike intraepithelial neoplasia, orderly squamous cell maturation is present; marked nuclear atypia and dyskeratotic cells are absent.

Occasionally, papillary vulvar lesions have some features suggestive of condyloma acuminatum, but lack koilocytotic atypia. In such cases, molecular studies can be used to assess the possibility of a viral etiology; 20% to 70% of these condyloma-like lesions have detectable papillomavirus DNA (92,93). Condyloma acuminatum usually is easy to distinguish from high-grade vulvar intraepithelial neoplasia. For the latter, pleomorphic, enlarged, and hyperchromatic parabasal nuclei, disorderly maturation, and abnormal mitotic figures are conspicuous (94). The nuclei of condyloma acuminatum are diploid or polyploid, whereas those of intraepithelial neoplasia are typically aneuploid (89,95). Focal koilocytotic atypia and cellular maturation may be observed in or adjacent to intraepithelial neoplasia. In addition, some squamous proliferations of the vulva have microscopic features intermediate between condyloma and intraepithelial neoplasia. Indeed, some examples of vulvar intraepithelial neoplasia grade I represent flat condyloma acuminatum. There is abundant evidence at clinical, light microscopic, ultrastructural, immunocytochemical, and molecular levels that human papillomavirus infection is linked to premalignant and malignant squamous proliferations of the vulva (89,96–108). Human papillomavirus DNA has been noted in 80% to 100% of genital intraepithelial neoplasia and bowenoid papulosis (98,104–107). Viral DNA has also been demonstrated in verrucous carcinoma (100,101) and some types of squamous cell carcinoma of the vulva (98,102,108,109). Viral types 6 and 11 are frequently observed in vulvar condylomata acuminata (88,98,100,103,106), whereas types 16, 18, and 31 have been found more often in intraepithelial neoplasia and cancer (98,102,106–109).

Molluscum contagiosum is a DNA poxvirus that has a predilection for the vulva of postpubertal women. This mildly contagious infection appears as multiple, 1- to 4-mm papules with central umbilication. The papules often disappear spontaneously after approximately 6 months, but others may remain for several years (110). Microscopically, the follicular epithelium expands to produce rounded lobules of cells and keratinized debris (111). Eosinophilic intracytoplasmic inclusion bodies enlarge and become basophilic as they migrate from the deeper layers of the epidermis. The diagnostic viral inclusions may also be observed in cytologic material obtained by squeezing the papules.

Fungi and Parasites

Tinea cruris causes erythematous, scaly patches in the perineal, inguinal, and vulvar areas. The diagnosis is determined by culture or identification of hyphae in potassium hydroxide-treated skin scrapings.

Vulvar cutaneous candidiasis commonly accompanies vaginal infection, but should be distinguished from the more common vulvovaginal disease (112). The erythematous, pruritic lesions may involve large areas of the vulva and perineum. Small pustules are sometimes also present. Severe infection is associated with obesity and diabetes mellitus. Microscopically, the epidermis is mildly thickened and spongiotic; a chronic inflammatory infiltrate is present in the dermis. The surface contains degenerated squamous cells, polymorphonuclear leukocytes, yeast, and pseudohyphae.

Deep fungal infections of the vulva are very rare. Clinically, they may simulate necrotizing fasciitis. Phycomycosis of the vulva has been reported in a diabetic woman (113).

While superficial genital parasites are common (lice and scabies), invasive parasitic infestation of the vulva is rare in North America. Vulvar elephantiasis sometimes results from lymphatic obstruction by filariform worms. Schistosomiasis may cause ulcers or papillary nodules that simulate condylomata acuminata (114).

Miscellaneous Benign Lesions

Seborrheic keratosis and fibroepithelial polyp occur on the labia majora of middle-aged or elderly women. The latter may contain scattered pleomorphic stromal cells and appear identical to the vaginal stromal polyp (115). Identical pleomorphic stromal cells have been found in nearly 80% of adults whose vulvae were biopsied or resected for intraepithelial neoplasia or squamous carcinoma (116). Two cases of verruciform xanthoma of the vulva have been described (117). This warty lesion is characterized by acanthosis, hyperkeratosis, and parakeratosis with deep extension of the rete pegs and an associated neutrophilic infiltrate. There is also hyalinization of dermal collagen, a few lymphocytes and plasma cells, and conspicuous xanthoma cells in the papillary dermis between the rete pegs. Sebaceous gland hyperplasia forms smooth, soft dermal nodules up to 1.5 cm in diameter on the labia minora or majora (118). Minor vestibular gland adenoma occurs as a firm nodule less than 2 cm in size (119). The nodules of mucus-secreting glands have been associated with previous surgery or chronic inflammation. Some authors believe the lesion has more features of nodular hyperplasia of minor vestibular glands rather than an adenoma (120). Pilar tumor, usually found on the scalp, has been reported to occur on the vulva (121). In epidermolytic acanthoma, multiple small nodules show acanthosis, hyperkeratosis, and a prominent granular layer (122). Keratoacanthoma only rarely has been described as occurring in the vulva (123). Benign vulvar melanocytic lesions include lentigo (124,125) and nevi (congenital or acquired). The former uncommonly are multiple and large and have irregular borders. Multiple genital lentigines have been associated with cardiac abnormalities (124). Rare junctional or compound vulvar nevi in premenopausal women may be atypical and have some architectural features of melanoma, including wide lateral extent, confluence and variation in size and shape of junctional nests, and involvement of adnexal structures (126,127). Unlike melanoma, atypical vulvar nevi have a well-demarcated epidermal melanocytic component, lack melanocytes at all levels of the epidermis, and show maturation of melanocytes from the epidermis to the dermis (126). In vulvar hyperpigmentation (melanosis), there is dermal deposition of melanin but no melanocytic hyperplasia.

Vulvar vestibulitis syndrome, an idiopathic chronic condition in which there is tenderness after touching the vestibule and dyspareunia in young women, has also been termed focal vulvitis, hyperesthesia of the vulva, and infection of the minor vestibular gland (128). Grossly, there is focal erythema at the openings of the minor vestibular glands. Microscopically, there is a mild to severe chronic inflammatory infiltrate in the lamina propria and superficial stroma around the glands (Fig. 7). Usually the intensity of the infiltrate is mild or moderate. There is a predominance of T lymphocytes and plasma cells with fewer B cells (120). The surface squamous epithelium is often infiltrated by lymphocytes, and shows spongiosis, parakeratosis, or hyperkeratosis. Ductal epithelium may be infiltrated by lymphocytes but the glandular acini are typi-

TABLE 1. *Dermatologic conditions that may occur on the vulva*

Lichen simplex chronicus	Familial benign pemphigus
Allergic contact dermatitis	Bullous pemphigoid
Irritant dermatitis	Benign mucosal pemphigoid
Seborrheic dermatitis	Darier's disease
Acne	Acantholytic dermatosis
Psoriasis	Herpes gestationis
Lichen planus	Subcorneal pustular dermatosis
Vitiligo	
Erythema multiforme	Linear immunoglobulin A disease
Acanthosis nigricans	
Sweet syndrome	Epidermolysis bullosa acquisita
Pemphigus vulgaris	
Dermatitis herpetiformis	

cally not affected. Squamous metaplasia involves the duct or acinus or both. At low power, a vestibular cleft at the opening of the duct is created by extensive squamous metaplasia that may entirely replace the minor vestibular gland. Human papillomavirus may be found in only rare cases, and, hence, is not the chief etiologic factor (120,129). Vulvar vestibulitis syndrome is most successfully treated with both resection and psychological intervention (120).

A variety of dermatologic conditions may involve the vulva, either as a localized process, or as part of generalized disease (Table 1) (see Fox-Fordyce disease in the section

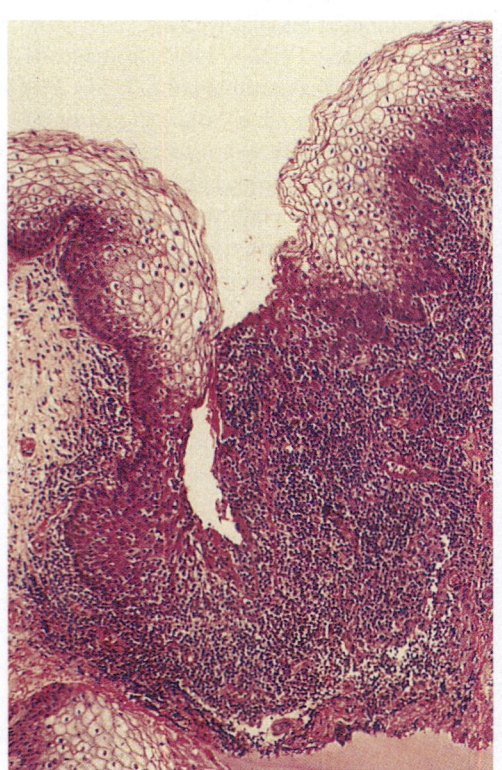 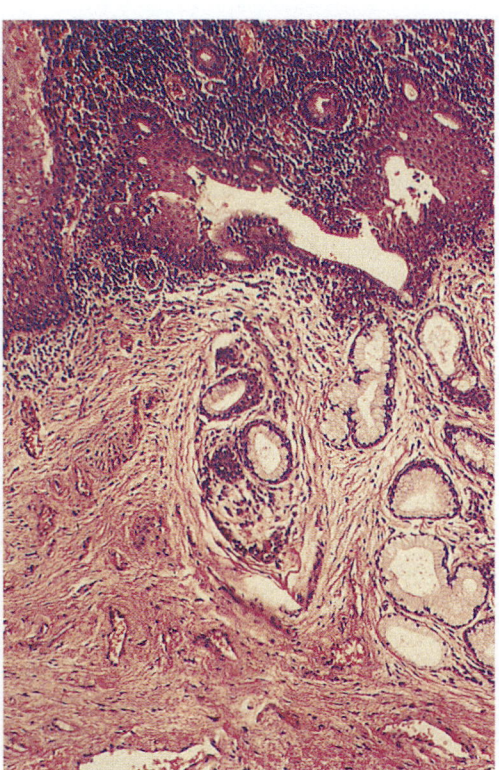

FIG. 7. Vulvar vestibulitis syndrome. A well-formed vestibular cleft is characteristic *(left)*. Also, minor vestibular glands undergo squamous metaplasia and are surrounded by chronic inflammation of variable degree *(right)*.

Cysts, above). Specific dermatoses affecting the vulva are sometimes not identified by either the gynecologist or the surgical pathologist (130). The special anatomical features of the vulva and its local environment may modify the clinical appearance of a specific dermatosis and render the clinical diagnosis more difficult.

Radiation damage to the vulva, although uncommon, results in loss of pubic hair and sclerosis of the connective tissue and blood vessels. As Reiter's syndrome is exceedingly rare in the vulva, the histopathologic features are not well categorized (131). Behçet's syndrome, a chronic, relapsing disease, manifests as small vesicles or pustules that may develop into deep ulcers. Microscopically, there is a necrotizing vasculitis with swollen endothelial cells, fibrinoid necrosis of vascular walls, and a lymphocytic perivascular infiltrate (132). Persistent red-brown or orange, glistening papules or macules and erosions are characteristic of vulvitis circumscripta plasmacellularis (133–135). The microscopic features of this idiopathic condition include an inflamed epidermis, parakeratosis, telangiectasia, and a dense dermal infiltrate of plasma cells and hemosiderin-laden macrophages.

Lipoma and fibrolipoma occur on the labium majus as solitary subcutaneous nodules and pedunculated masses (136). Sclerosing lipogranuloma, due to trauma or injection of foreign oils, is characterized by vacuolated cysts lined by adipocytes or giant cells with adjacent bands of hyalinized tissue. The lesion may be locally infiltrative and should be distinguished from liposarcoma (137). Approximately three times more vulvar leiomyomas than leiomyosarcomas have been reported (138). Criteria have been developed to predict the behavior of vulval smooth muscle tumors (138,139). Neoplasms that have at least three of the following features are considered sarcomas: 5 cm or more in diameter, infiltrating margins, 5 or more mitotic figures/10 high-power fields (HPFs), and moderate to severe cytologic atypia. Tumors with only one of these features should be considered leiomyomas, while those with two of the characteristics should be considered atypical leiomyomas. Rare leiomyomas have evolved into leiomyosarcomas (138). Epithelioid leiomyoma (139,140) appears to have a greater proclivity to recur than the usual spindle-cell type. Leiomyomas excised during pregnancy may have extensive myxoid change, hemorrhage, or foci of necrosis (139). An unusual syndrome of diffuse vulvar and gastroesophageal leiomyomatosis has been described in at least 20 patients most of whom also have Alport's syndrome (141,142). Vulvar neurofibroma occurs as an isolated lesion or as part of von Recklinghausen's disease (143,144). Rarely, there is extensive involvement of the genitourinary tract (145). Other neural tumors including schwannoma (146,147), plexiform schwannoma (148), traumatic neuroma, and paraganglioma (149) may arise in the vulva. Granular cell tumor occurs as a single (or multiple) superficial nodule on the labium majus or clitoris and strongly predilects black women (also see Malignant Neoplasms, below) (150,151). The overlying pseudoepitheliomatous hyperplasia may mimic well-differentiated squamous cell carcinoma (150). Solitary fibrous tumor (152), nodular fasciitis (153), postoperative spindle cell nodule (154), desmoid tumor (155), and genital rhabdomyoma (156) only rarely involve the vulva.

Benign vascular lesions of the vulva include capillary (strawberry) hemangioma, senile hemangioma, cavernous hemangioma, congenital dysplastic angiopathy, angiokeratoma, lobular capillary hemangioma (pyogenic granuloma) (136), and varicosities. Lobular capillary hemangioma and varicosities are seen most often during pregnancy. Cavernous hemangioma may involve the clitoris, simulating pseudohermaphroditism (157). Angiokeratomas are often multiple, 2 to 10 mm in diameter, papillary, warty, or globular lesions of the labia majora (158). They are associated with pregnancy and increased venous pressure. Microscopically, dilated, often thrombosed, capillaries are found in the upper dermis, surrounded by acanthosis and hyperkeratosis of the overlying squamous epithelium (Fig. 8). Glomus tumor, arising on the labium minus or clitoris, causes persistent pain and dyspareunia (159,160). Lymphangiomas are rarely observed on the vulva (161). Lymphangiectasis (acquired lymphangioma) arises as multiple vesicles or warty papules on the labia majora, and develops in chronic lymphedematous states after radiation therapy or surgery (162,163). Microscopically, thin-walled, ectatic lymphatic channels are located superiorly in the papillary dermis (Fig. 9).

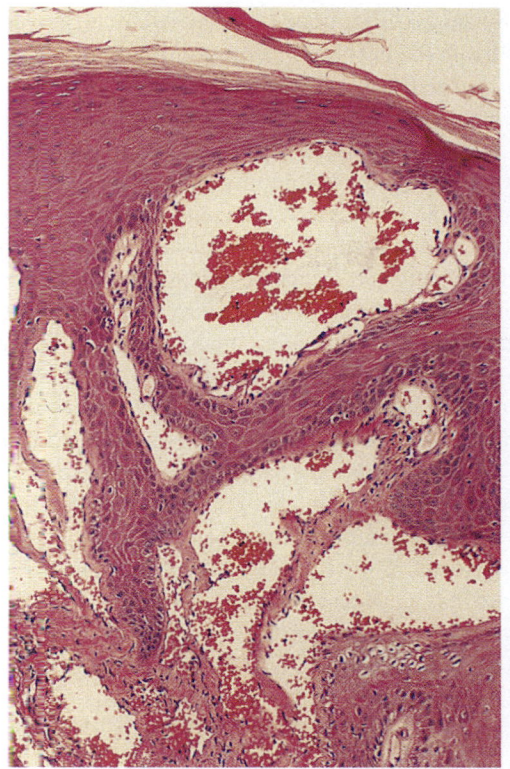

FIG. 8. Angiokeratoma. Acanthotic and hyperkeratotic squamous epithelium surrounds dilated capillaries.

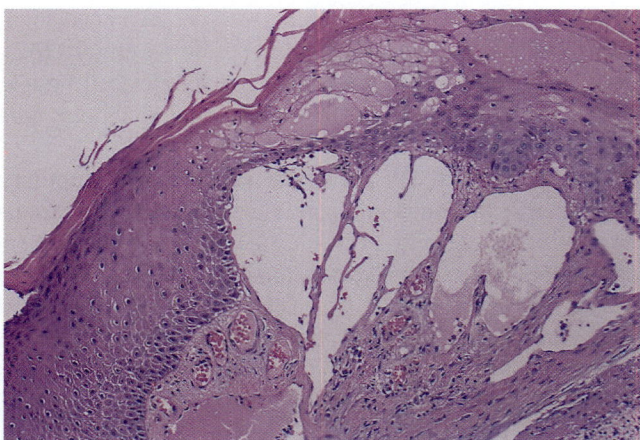

FIG. 9. Lymphangiectasis. Dilated superficial lymphatics may impart a vesicular or warty appearance.

The concept of "milk lines" and vulvar lesions derived from these rudiments has recently been challenged (2). It has been proposed that a variety of lesions that commonly occur in the breast as well as hidradenoma papilliferum and extramammary Paget's disease arise from mammary-like glands. These anogenital "sweat" glands resembling mammary ducts are found incidentally, chiefly in the interlabial sulcus (Fig. 1) (1). It is possible that most examples of accessory breast tissue develop from these anogenital sweat glands and not from caudal remnants of the milk line (1). Clinically apparent mammary-like tissue is sometimes found in the labial area and may be bilateral (164). Very rarely, a nipple is present. Because of hormone-induced swelling, vulvar mammary-like tissue becomes manifest during pregnancy or lactation. Fibrocystic changes, lactating adenoma (165), fibroadenoma (166), intraductal papilloma (167), and phyllodes tumor (168) have all developed in mammary-like breast tissue. Adenocarcinoma may also arise in vulval mammary-like tissue (169–171), and must be distinguished from conventional cutaneous adenocarcinomas of apocrine or eccrine origin and metastatic mammary carcinoma.

Crohn's disease involves the vulva by direct extension from the anus or as a discontinuous, "metastatic" ulcer. The latter shows granulomatous inflammation, acute and chronic inflammation, fibrosis, and sometimes extensive pseudoepitheliomatous hyperplasia (172). Most, but not all, patients with Crohn's vulvitis have had a history of intestinal Crohn's disease (173). A chronic granulomatous hypertrophy of the labia, vulvitis granulomatosa, resembles Crohn's disease as there is edema, fibrosis, lymphangiectasia, chronic inflammatory cells, and nonnecrotizing granulomas (173). There appears to be a relationship between vulvitis granulomatosa, cheilitis granulomatosa, and Crohn's disease. Sarcoidosis (174), malakoplakia (175,176), amyloidosis (localized or systemic) (177), calcinosis (178,179), mucinous metaplasia (180), lymphoid hamartoma (181), and ectopic salivary gland (182) of the vulva also have been described. A case of rheumatoid nodule with ulceration and lymphadenopathy clinically mimicked carcinoma (183). A lymphoma-like lesion has been reported in a patient with infectious mononucleosis (80).

Aggressive Angiomyxoma, Angiomyofibroblastoma, and Angiofibroma

Aggressive angiomyxoma occurs in the vulva, vagina, perineum, inguinal area, or pelvic soft tissues (184–187). It presents as a large, slowly growing, polypoid mass or swelling in women who are most often in their third or fourth decade of life. Grossly, the tumor is rubbery and white or soft and gelatinous. Most are at least 10 cm in greatest dimension (186). Microscopically, stellate and spindle-shaped mesenchymal cells are embedded in a loose myxoid stroma with a few collagen fibers (Fig. 10). The cells are small and bland, and lack nuclear atypia. Small or medium-sized veins and arteries within the tumor often are grouped together and may show medial hypertrophy. Blood vessels of various caliber are typically widely dilated, and extravasation of red blood cells is usual. Aggressive angiomyxoma is characteristically hypocellular and lacks necrosis and mitotic figures. Invasion of skeletal muscle and fat is usual. Small nerves are often trapped within the neoplasm. The tumor cells have fibroblastic or myofibroblastic properties ultrastructurally. Immunohistochemically, they are at least focally positive for desmin, smooth muscle actin, muscle specific actin, and vi-

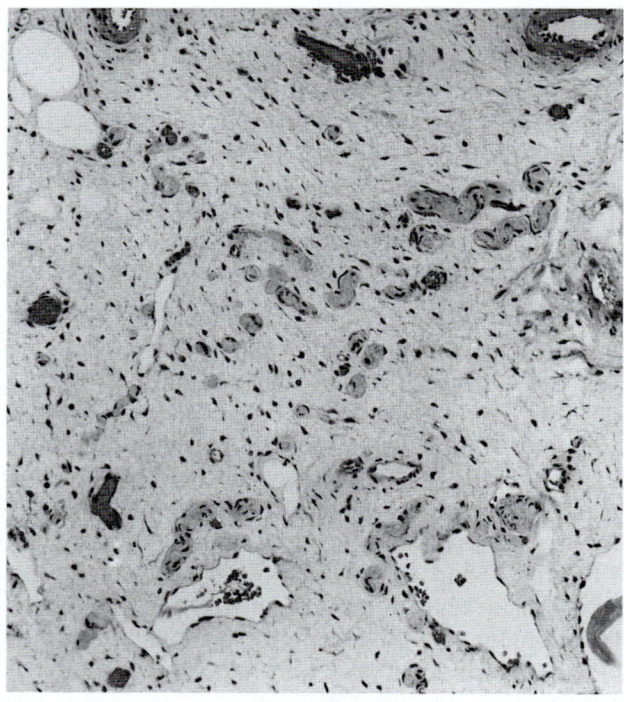

FIG. 10. Aggressive angiomyxoma. Spindle-shaped and stellate cells without nuclear atypia are loosely arranged in a myxoid stroma. Dilated blood vessels and vessels with thickened walls are frequently observed. Entrapped nerves and adipocytes are also present.

mentin (186). CD34, estrogen receptor, and progesterone receptor are also commonly present. The microscopic differential diagnosis includes neurofibroma, intramuscular myxoma, angiomyofibroblastoma, myxoid smooth muscle tumors, spindle cell lipoma, myxoid malignant fibrous histiocytoma, myxoid liposarcoma, and embryonal rhabdomyosarcoma. A few tumors have shown histologic features resembling those of angiomyofibroblastoma (187). The therapy for aggressive angiomyxoma is complete excision. Local recurrence, often many years following initial resection, is common (between 36% and 72%), but metastases have not been described. In one series of 29 patients, there were no tumor-related deaths (186).

The vulva and, to a lesser extent, the vagina are also sites of predilection for a distinctive, recently described benign soft tissue lesion that is often confused with aggressive angiomyxoma, the angiomyofibroblastoma (152,188–191). Over 50 examples of angiomyofibroblastoma have been reported. This tumor presents as a polypoid submucosal mass ranging from 0.5 to 12 cm in size. Affected women are in their third to ninth decade of life. Grossly, the tumors are sharply demarcated, tan, pink or yellow in color, with a spongy, soft to firm consistency. This appearance is not dissimilar from that of aggressive angiomyxoma. Microscopically, angiomyofibroblastomas retain their sharp circumscription and are characterized by alternating areas of hypercellularity and stromal edema with hypocellularity. There are abundant but irregularly distributed capillary-sized blood vessels or small veins, often surrounded by loose aggregates of spindled stromal cells (Fig. 11). Some stromal cells may be larger and more epithelioid or plasmacytoid in appearance. Binucleated and multinucleated stromal cells, often with linearly arranged nuclei may also be present (189). Entrapped mucosal glands or nerves are rarely present within the mass (152,188). Intralesional fat may be focal and entrapped or, less often, massive and an intrinsic component of the tumor (152). Nuclear pleomorphism is typically mild, though rare hyperchromatic, probably degenerative cells have been described. Mitotic activity is sparse with fewer than 1 mitotic figure per 10 HPFs (188,189).

Light microscopic features of angiomyofibroblastoma that distinguish it from aggressive angiomyxoma include marginal circumscription, higher cellularity, larger numbers of blood vessels lacking hyalinization or hypertrophy, often plump stromal cells with perivascular accentuation, a paucity of stromal mucin, and only rare extravasated erythrocytes (188). Immunohistochemical studies have not been of value in making this distinction as both lesions display myofibroblastic features with vimentin, desmin, and actin reactivity (188–190). Both tumors have also been shown to have stromal cells that are reactive for estrogen receptor protein (152,190). The distinction of these two lesions is important because of their different clinical behaviors. Unlike aggressive angiomyxomas, angiomyofibroblastomas do not recur following local excision. One case of angiomyofibroblastoma with sarcomatous transformation has been described, however (192).

Nucci et al. (193) have described four examples of a benign spindle cell tumor of the vulva, which is distinct from both aggressive angiofibroma and angiomyofibroblastoma. The tumor somewhat resembles spindle cell lipoma but was considered a distinct entity and was labeled cellular angiofibroma. The tumors occurred in middle-aged women and measured 1.2 to 2.5 cm in size. Follow-up was only available for two patients and both were free of disease after 12 and 19 months. Microscopically, these were monotonous, spindle cell proliferations, often admixed with small foci of mature fat. Focally prominent myxoid matrix was also noted. Small to medium-sized blood vessels with prominent mural hyalinization were common. Entrapped small nerves were encountered at the periphery of the lesion. The lesions were noted to be nonreactive for CD34, a marker often positive in spindle cell lipomas.

Dystrophy and Squamous Intraepithelial Neoplasia

Standardized terminology for vulvar dystrophy and squamous intraepithelial neoplasia has evolved over the last several decades (Table 2) (194). Biopsy of one or more vulval lesions in a particular patient is essential, because of the variable and overlapping clinical appearances for dystrophic and dysplastic conditions.

Lichen sclerosus, a persistent and recurring condition found at all ages, is seen predominantly in postmenopausal women. Two-thirds of affected children have spontaneous involution before or at puberty (195). All or any part of the vulva may be involved, with occasional extension to the perianal region and inner thighs. Lesions are often multiple, bilateral, and symmetrical (6). Initial pale pink or white maculopapules coalesce to form dry, rough, scaly plaques (Fig. 12). Advanced lesions appear wrinkled and parchment-like, with telangiectasia and ecchymoses frequently observed (196). Extensive vulvar contracture may lead to agglutina-

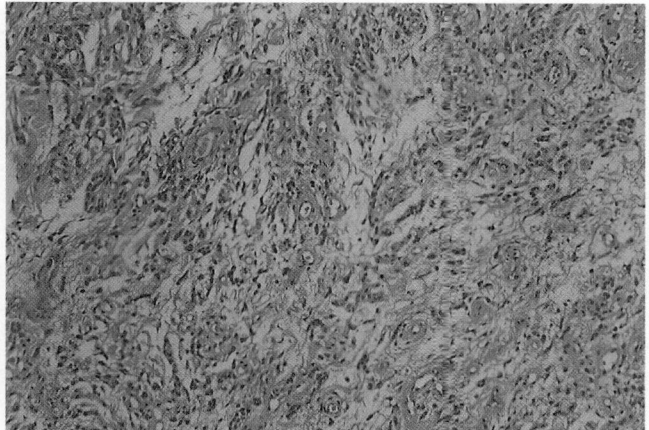

FIG. 11. Angiomyofibroblastoma. Spindled and epithelioid stromal cells are present in a loose or more dense matrix that contains capillary-sized blood vessels.

TABLE 2. *Classification of vulvar dystrophy and squamous vulvar intraepithelial neoplasia (VIN)*

Dystrophic conditions
    Lichen sclerosus
    Squamous cell hyperplasia (hyperplastic dystrophy)
    Mixed lichen sclerosus and squamous hyperplasia
Squamous intraepithelial neoplasia[a]
    VIN I (mild dysplasia)
    VIN II (moderate dysplasia)
    VIN III (severe dysplasia/carcinoma *in situ*)
Dystrophy with squamous intraepithelial neoplasia[a]
    Squamous cell hyperplasia with VIN
    Lichen sclerosus with VIN
    Mixed dystrophy (squamous hyperplasia and lichen sclerosus) with VIN

[a]The presence of changes suggestive of human papillomavirus infection should be noted.

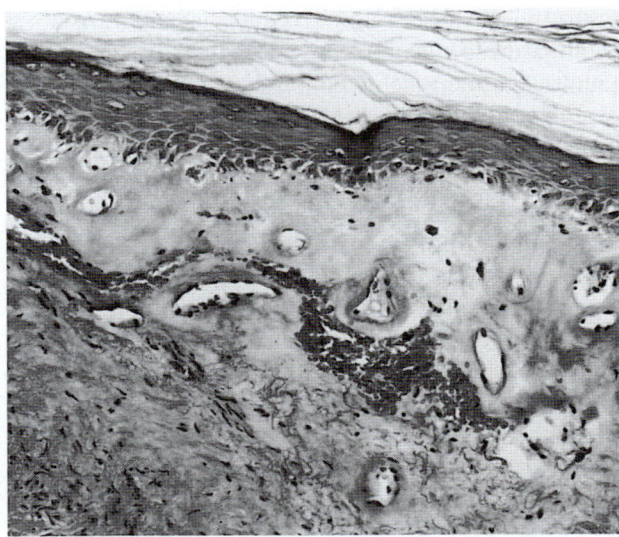

FIG. 13. Lichen sclerosus. The thin, hyperkeratotic epidermis shows basal layer vacuolization and overlies a hyalinized dermis.

tion of the labia minora and stenosis of the introitus. Microscopically, there is epithelial thinning, loss of rete pegs, hyperkeratosis, and plugging of follicles (Fig. 13). The epithelial thickness is variable, however, and may even be normal or show reactive hyperplasia. The basal cells are vacuolated and, occasionally, subepidermal bullae are present. Melanin pigment and melanocytes are lost from the epithelium. The atrophic dermis is edematous, hyalinized, and sparsely cellular. Sweat glands and pilosebaceous apparati are absent. Dermal vessels are telangiectatic or obliterated, and there is loss of elastic fibers. A variable number of lymphocytes and plasma cells lie just below the atrophic dermis. Lichen sclerosus is commonly observed in association with intraepithelial neoplasia and invasive squamous cell carcinoma (197). Hart et al. (198), however, followed 92 patients with lichen sclerosus for a median follow-up interval of 9 years. The single patient who subsequently developed an invasive squamous cell carcinoma initially had coexistent mild intraepithelial neoplasia. In the same series, each of five pa-

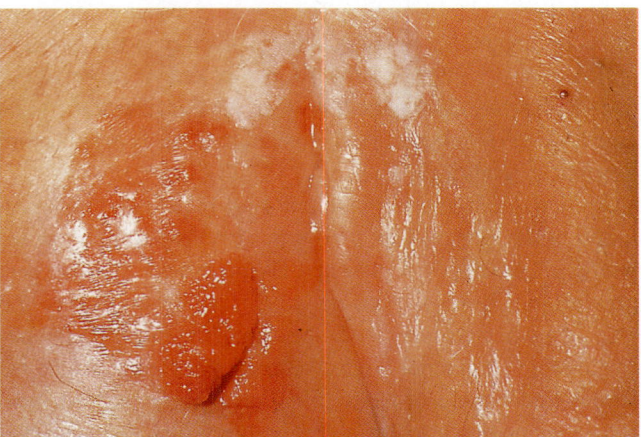

FIG. 12. Lichen sclerosus and squamous cell carcinoma. In this atrophic vulva there are white plaques, telangiectasia, and contracture. Squamous cell carcinoma is present on the left.

tients with simultaneous lichen sclerosus and invasive carcinoma had neoplasms that tended to arise in areas of minimal dystrophy or in areas of normal vulvar skin. Melanoma (199) and basal cell carcinoma (200) have occurred coincidentally with lichen sclerosus.

Squamous cell hyperplasia (hyperplastic dystrophy) in most cases is likely due to chronic irritation (chronic rubbing and the itch-scratch cycle). Although many cases likely represent lichen simplex chronicus (196), lichen simplex chronicus may be classified as a specific dermatosis. Most diagnoses of squamous hyperplasia are rendered by surgical pathologists, while dermatopathologists prefer the designation *lichen simplex chronicus* (130). It is important to classify an inflammatory lesion of the vulva as a specific dermatosis, if possible, and reserve the poorly descriptive term *squamous cell hyperplasia* for when a more specific diagnosis cannot be rendered. Two-thirds of patients with squamous cell hyperplasia are premenopausal (201). The lesions occur on the labia majora or mons and have a highly variable appearance, but are usually discrete, red or white plaques that may be multiple and lichenified (196). Scales and excoriations are often present. Microscopically, the acanthotic epidermis contains cells with orderly maturation and uniform nuclei. Hyperkeratosis is frequent, sometimes with parakeratosis and hypergranulosis. Thickened rete pegs are club-shaped or pointed and may become confluent. The dermis contains a variable number of chronic inflammatory cells and minimal edema. Thick collagen bundles lying parallel to the rete ridges are typically present in lichen simplex chronicus (6,130). Squamous cell hyperplasia may be superimposed on other dermatoses and is sometimes observed adjacent to invasive squamous cell carcinoma. The risk of development of invasive carcinoma for women treated for squamous cell hyperplasia without intraepithelial neoplasia is minimal (201).

Approximately 45% to 50% of patients with vulvar dystrophy have squamous cell hyperplasia and 40% have lichen sclerosus (201,202); 10% to 15% of the patients have mixed dystrophies. Squamous cell hyperplasia may be present adjacent to or remote from lichen sclerosus. Sometimes squamous cell hyperplasia overlies an atrophic dermis (Fig. 14). No more than 10% of biopsies of squamous cell hyperplasia have foci of intraepithelial neoplasia (6,201,202). Although studies of untreated women with long follow-up intervals are not available, there is probably only a small risk of invasive squamous cell carcinoma for women with squamous cell hyperplasia and mild intraepithelial neoplasia.

Vulvar intraepithelial neoplasia (VIN) is a designation promulgated to replace other terms for *in situ* squamous proliferations of the vulva including atypia, dysplasia, Bowen's disease, bowenoid atypia, bowenoid papulosis, erythroplasia of Queyrat, and carcinoma *in situ*, simplex type. Prior to 1970, VIN was found most often in women in the fifth or sixth decade of life (203), but currently about one-half of the patients are less than 40 years old. VIN in young women is frequently multiple and is associated with human papillomavirus infection (see human papillomavirus in the section Viruses, above). Progression to carcinoma appears to be uncommon in this age group (204). Older women with VIN more often have solitary lesions with a higher risk for progression to cancer (204). The clinical appearance of VIN is variable. The lesions may be single or multiple, and involve any portion of the vulva. Discrete or coalescent papules or macules are gray, white, red, or darkly pigmented. They may be scaly or eczematoid. Some lesions mimic condyloma grossly. Among the three grades of VIN, VIN III occurs most often; in one study about 70% of the lesions were VIN III (205). Microscopically, VIN consists of crowded cells with high nuclear-to-cytoplasmic ratios, hyperchromatic, pleomorphic nuclei, and increased numbers of mitotic figures (with abnormal forms) (94, 97). Hyperkeratosis, parakeratosis, and dyskeratotic cells are often observed (206). The dysplastic cells of VIN I (mild dysplasia) are confined to the lower one-third of the epithelium. Mitotic figures (with occasional abnormal forms) are also confined to the basal layers. Orderly, mature squamous epithelium is found overlying the dysplastic cells. Some examples of VIN I correspond to flat condyloma acuminatum. VIN I is often difficult to distinguish from reactive changes in inflammatory conditions. VIN II (moderate dysplasia) contains cells with enlarged, crowded nuclei limited to the lower two-thirds of the epithelium. Cellular maturation is present at the uppermost one-third of the epithelial surface. Mitotic figures (including abnormal forms) and dyskeratotic cells are found in the dysplastic cell layers. VIN III (severe dysplasia/carcinoma *in situ*) contains dysplastic cells that extend up more than two-thirds of the thickness of the epithelium (Fig. 15). The dysplastic cells often extend into the outer portions of hair follicles. Some examples of VIN III have cells with copious mature cytoplasm that retain dysplastic nuclei. The dysplastic cells are usually located in the basilar layers with maturation in the superficial layers. The rete pegs may be thickened and branched, and intraepithelial squamous pearls may be located at their tips (95) (Fig. 16). This differentiated or simplex type of VIN III is usually found in or adjacent to invasive squamous cell carcinoma occurring in postmenopausal women. Multinucleated, giant dysplastic cells (bowenoid cells) are frequently seen in VIN III. Koilocytotic atypia and evidence of human papillomavirus are often associated with intraepithelial neoplasia (94,99). Condyloma may be seen adjacent to VIN or there may be a gradual transition from condyloma to VIN. Some lesions have features of both VIN and condyloma (94). Human papillomavirus type 16 has emerged as the predominant type in VIN III, although other viral types have been found (106,107). In a study of 67 lesions of VIN III including both warty (bowenoid) and basaloid (nonbowenoid) types (vide infra), 90% contained type 16 or 33 by polymerase chain reaction (207).

Bowenoid papulosis (105,208), or bowenoid dysplasia (209), represents a clinical subset of VIN, in which multiple, small, red-brown papules occur chiefly in young women from 20 to 40 years of age. The lesions are sometimes found during pregnancy. Some untreated cases of bowenoid papulosis have regressed spontaneously (208,209). Human papillomavirus type 16 DNA has been documented in bowenoid papulosis (105). Some authors have reported that the cells of bowenoid papulosis show a lesser degree of dysplasia and more maturation than VIN III (208,209). It has also been noted that bowenoid papulosis tends to involve the acrosyringium and spare the acrotrichium (208,209). Although the natural history of bowenoid papulosis is not completely known, the risk of progression to invasive carcinoma appears to be low. *Bowenoid papulosis* should not be used as a specific histopathologic term.

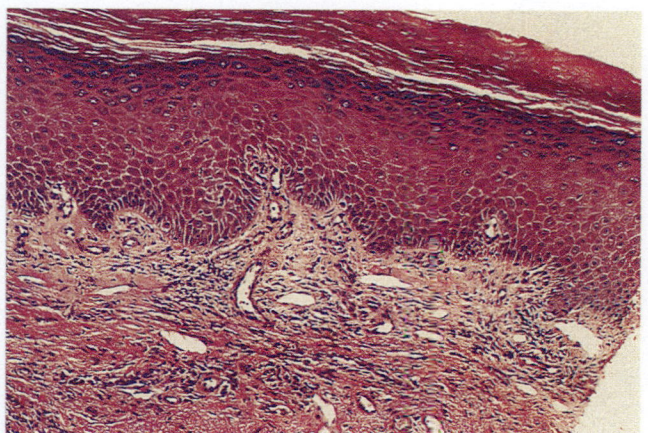

FIG. 14. Squamous cell hyperplasia and lichen sclerosus. The thickened epidermis shows hyperkeratosis, hypergranulosis, and orderly maturation of cells without nuclear atypia. The dermis contains chronic inflammatory cells and shows areas of hyalinization superficially.

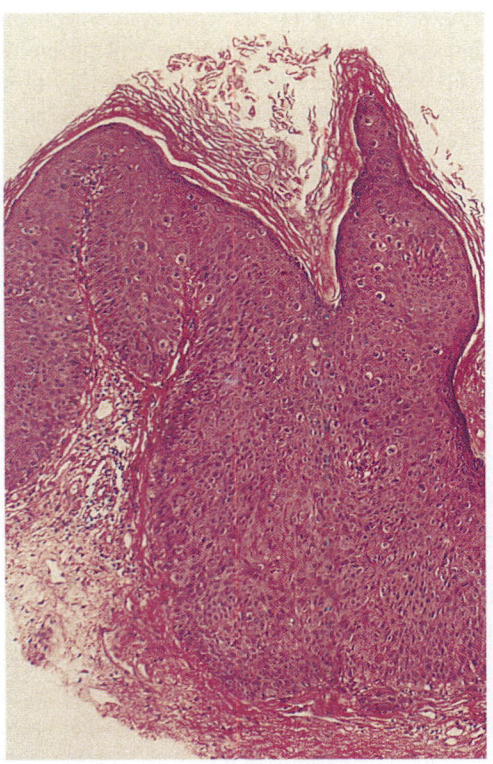
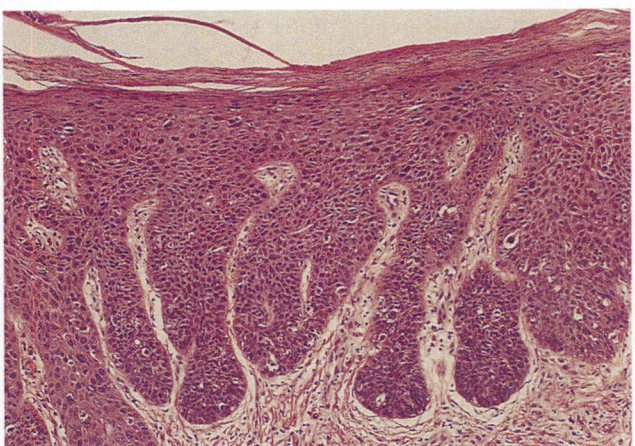

FIG. 15. Vulvar intraepithelial neoplasia (VIN), grade III. The epidermis is filled with crowded cells having high nuclear-to-cytoplasmic ratios and hyperchromatic, pleomorphic nuclei. Mitotic figures and dyskeratotic cells are numerous. VIN III often has either a warty (bowenoid) *(left)* or a basaloid *(right)* appearance.

Finally, there is emerging clinical, pathologic, and virologic evidence that VIN III can be separated into distinctive types (107). Warty (bowenoid) VIN tends to occur in younger women, has a condylomatous appearance, and often contains human papillomavirus type 16 DNA (Fig. 15). Basaloid (undifferentiated) VIN III more often occurs in older women, has a smooth surface, consists of small cells with little maturation, shows koilocytotic atypia less frequently, and less often contains human papillomavirus DNA (Fig. 15). VIN III with both warty and basaloid microscopic features has been found in about 20% to 35% of cases (107,210). Hence, there are overlapping morphologic features among warty and basaloid VIN III lesions. Simplex or differentiated VIN III typically lacks evidence for human papillomavirus and contains dysplastic cells with mature cytoplasm in the basilar layers, occasional pearl formation, and surface maturation. It occurs usually in older women in or around invasive squamous cell carcinoma. In the absence of invasive cancer, it is the least common form of VIN III. At the present time there is no clear clinical need to subtype VIN III. Treatment is usually local excision or laser vaporization. Recurrence is more common following the latter procedure (205). Approximately one-quarter of women with VIN III have persistent or recurrent disease after local excision (99,204,211,212); 2% to 10% of women treated for VIN III develop invasive squamous cell carcinoma (95,203,204, 205,211,212). In one study of incompletely excised VIN III, seven of eight patients progressed to invasive cancer within 8 years (212). The presence of invasive cancer is due to progression of intraepithelial neoplasia or to the development of carcinoma away from the area of VIN. One-fifth to one-third

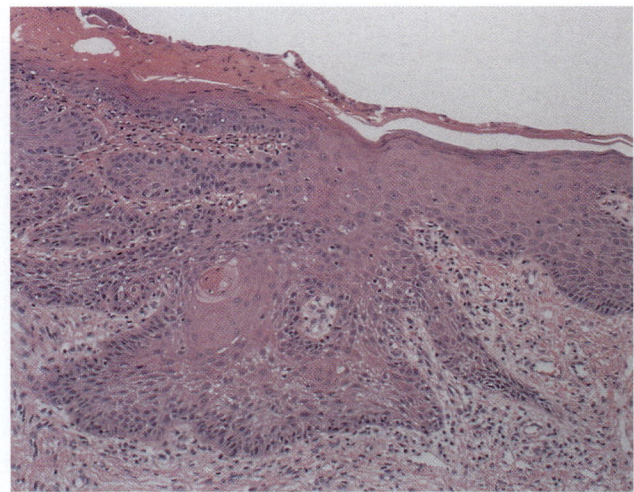

FIG. 16. Vulvar intraepithelial neoplasia (VIN), grade III. This simplex type of VIN III is usually found adjacent to invasive squamous cell carcinoma, and consists of thickened rete pegs with squamous pearl formation.

of invasive squamous cell carcinomas have adjacent foci of VIN III (197,213). Patients with VIN are at high risk for the development of dysplasia or invasive squamous cell carcinoma of the vagina and cervix; 20% to 40% of patients with VIN III have vaginal or cervical dysplasia or carcinoma (95,203,207,211).

Malignant Neoplasms

Squamous cell carcinoma accounts for approximately 90% of all primary invasive vulvar neoplasms. Three-fourths arise on the labia (usually the labia majora), and most of the remainder are located on the clitoris or fourchette (214–217). The age range is broad, but most neoplasms develop in women in the seventh or eighth decade of life (214,217,218). Very rarely are patients less than 20 years of age. Prior conditions associated with vulvar squamous cell carcinoma include human papillomavirus infection (95,97,99,106,108,109), lymphogranuloma venereum (61), granuloma inguinale (60,61), immunosuppression (219), and Fanconi's anemia (220). Overall, human papillomavirus has been detected in about 50% of vulvar squamous cell carcinomas (221). Type 16 has been the predominantly identified papillomavirus (106,108,109). There is evidence that the presence of the virus correlates with specific histologic subsets of invasive cancer (basaloid and warty), the presence of VIN, and young patient age (109,207,222). In a study of 100 squamous

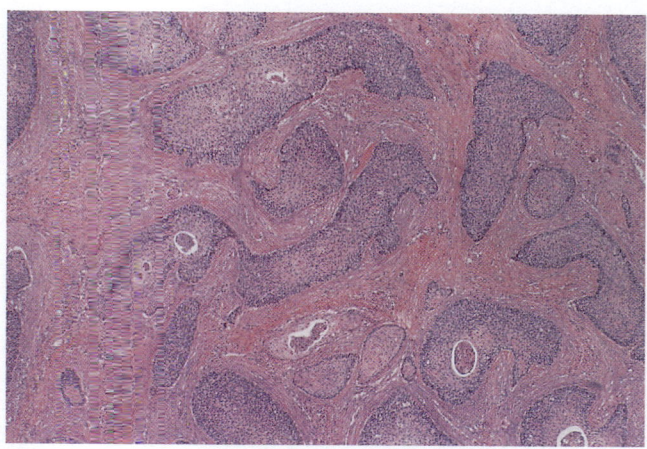

FIG. 18. Squamous cell carcinoma, basaloid type. Nests or bands of cancer contain basaloid cells and occasional central keratinization.

cell carcinomas, 7% were warty, 28% were basaloid, and 65% were keratinizing (223). Warty carcinomas have a condylomatous appearance, as the papillary surface overlies irregular jagged nests of squamous epithelium at the tumor base (Fig. 17). Cells with marked nuclear pleomorphism and features resembling koilocysts are present as well as squamous pearls found in ordinary squamous cell carcinoma. Basaloid carcinomas have sheets or bands of small, immature squamous cells with nuclear hyperchromasia and high nuclear/cytoplasmic (N:C) ratios (Fig. 18). Little or no squamous maturation is seen, but occasional abrupt keratin pearl formation may be present. Conventional squamous cell carcinomas, not otherwise specified (NOS), show overt keratinization and squamous pearls (Fig. 19). Squamous hyperplasia has been found adjacent to 83% of keratinizing carcinomas while basaloid or warty VIN was observed adjacent to 72% of the invasive warty or basaloid cancers

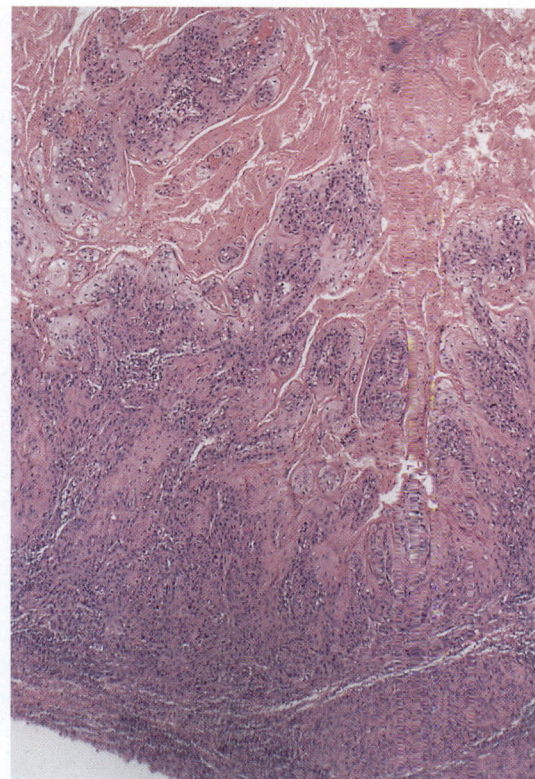

FIG. 17. Squamous cell carcinoma, warty type. The neoplasm has a papillary surface but contains cells with marked nuclear pleomorphism. Some cells resemble koilocytes.

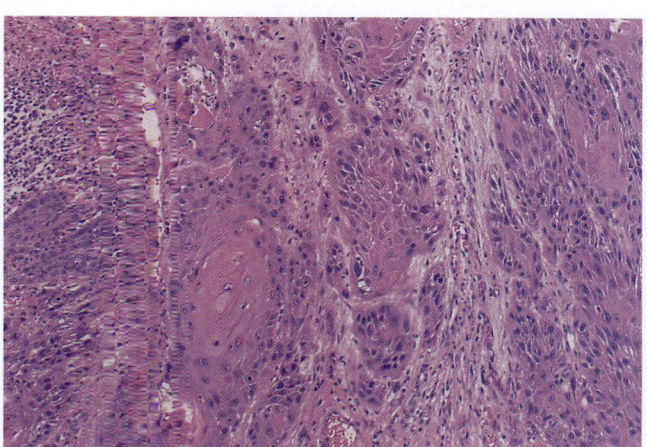

FIG. 19. Squamous cell carcinoma, keratinizing type. Most vulvar squamous cancers are keratinizing but with varying degrees of nuclear pleomorphism and cytoplasmic maturation.

(223). Keratinizing cancers occur more often in older white women, while basaloid and warty types occur chiefly in younger black women. Conventional squamous cell carcinomas in older women are less often virus related (109,222). In one study 84% of basaloid or warty carcinomas had type 16 or 33 human papillomavirus by polymerase chain reaction, while only 4% of the keratinizing squamous cell carcinomas had evidence of the virus (207). There is some evidence that the absence of human papillomavirus DNA in vulvar cancers is predictive of an adverse outcome (224). Loss of wild-type p53 function occurs either by interaction with human papillomaviral oncoproteins or by somatic mutation in those vulvar carcinomas that lack papillomavirus (225). Some women with vulvar cancer and human papillomavirus are at high risk for dysplasia and invasive carcinoma of the cervix and vagina. Hor017ding and colleagues (207) found that only 2% of women with keratinizing squamous cell carcinoma of the vulva developed cervical neoplasia, while 40% of those with basaloid or warty types of vulvar carcinoma had cervical dysplasia or carcinoma.

Grossly, squamous cell carcinomas appear as erythematous or white plaques, ulcers, nodules, or fungating, papillomatous growths (218). The important factors in surgical staging include tumor size, extension, status of the groin and pelvic lymph nodes, and distant metastasis (Table 3) (226).

TABLE 3a. *TNM surgical staging system for squamous cell carcinoma of the vulva[a]*

Primary tumor (T)	
TX	Primary tumor cannot be assessed
T0	No evidence of primary tumor
Tis	VIN III
T1	Tumor confined to the vulva/perineum, ≤2 cm in greatest dimension
T1a	As for T1 and with ≤1 mm of stromal invasion[b]
T1b	As for T1 and with >1 mm of stromal invasion[b]
T2	Tumor confined to vulva/perineum, >2 cm in greatest dimension
T3	Tumor of any size with adjacent spread to lower urethra or vagina or anus
T4	Tumor invades upper urethral mucosa, bladder mucosa, rectal mucosa, or is fixed to public bone
Regional lymph node(s) (N)	
NX	Regional lymph nodes cannot be assessed
N0	No regional lymph node metastasis
N1	Unilateral regional lymph node metastasis
N2	Bilateral regional lymph node metastasis
Distant metastasis (M)	
MX	Distant metastasis cannot be assessed
M0	No distant metastasis
M1	Distant metastasis (including pelvic lymph node metastasis)

[a]Also applies to verrucous carcinoma, Paget's disease of the vulva, adenocarcinoma not otherwise specified, basal cell carcinoma, and Bartholin's gland carcinoma, but not to malignant melanoma.
[b]The depth of invasion defined as the measurement of the tumor from the epithelial stromal junction of the adjacent most superficial dermal papilla to the deepest point of invasion.

TABLE 3b. *TNM surgical stage grouping for vulvar cancer*

Stage	T	N	M
Stage 0	Tis	N0	M0
Stage IA	T1a	N0	M0
Stage IB	T1b	N0	M0
Stage II	T2	N0	M0
Stage III	T1	N1	M0
	T2	N1	M0
	T3	N0	M0
	T3	N1	M0
Stage IVA	T1	N2	M0
	T2	N2	M0
	T3	N2	M0
	T4	Any N	M0
Stage IVB	Any T	Any N	M1

The clinical evaluation of groin lymph nodes is often unreliable. Up to 43% of clinically negative groin lymph nodes contain carcinoma microscopically (227). Conversely, up to 45% of clinically positive inguinal-femoral lymph nodes lack tumor upon microscopic examination (218).

Important pathologic factors for vulvar squamous cell carcinoma include tumor size, thickness or depth of stromal invasion, grade, pattern of infiltration, vascular invasion, perineural invasion, multifocality, margins of excision, and status of lymph nodes. Although strict criteria for grading have not been well delineated in most studies, the criteria set forth by Broders (228), originally for lip cancer, and Jakobsson (229), for carcinoma of the larynx, generally have been applied. Although the data are conflicting concerning the relationship of tumor grade to groin lymph node status and overall prognosis (217,218,230–243), many studies have shown that high-grade tumors more often metastasize to inguinal and femoral nodes, resulting in a poorer outlook (217,218,232–235,240,241,243,244). Vulvar squamous cancers have either a broad, pushing, and circumscribed front or an irregular, infiltrating margin. Tumors with an infiltrating margin may contain dissociated cells or cells forming small, angulated nests or cords that incite a prominent desmoplastic response (diffuse, stellate, or spray pattern) (Fig. 20) (232,236,239,245,246). Such neoplasms, even those that are small and superficially invasive, have a proclivity for lymph node metastasis. *Confluent growth* is a poorly defined term that often refers to an amount of tumor filling at least 1 mm of a microscopic field (233,236,237). It primarily correlates with tumor thickness and depth of stromal invasion. The use of the term *confluent* should be discouraged. Patients with squamous cancers having a marked lymphocytic stromal response may have a better prognosis than those whose tumors incite a minimal lymphoplasmacytic reaction (218,231,239). On the other hand, patients with tumors exhibiting a prominent fibromyxoid stromal response have been reported to have a poorer survival rate and more extensive lymph node metastasis than those with neoplasms lacking this stromal feature (247). Such neoplasms with a conspicuous fibromyxoid stromal reaction are most often clitoral, flat or elevated, ulcerated, and occur in older women.

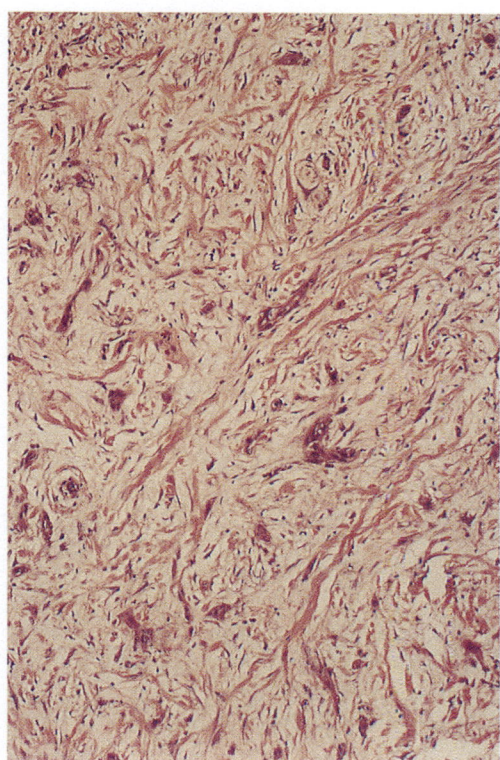

FIG. 20. Squamous cell carcinoma. Small nests and strands of cells embedded in a loose fibrous stroma characterize the "spray" pattern of invasion.

The presence of vascular permeation clearly increases the risk for nodal metastasis (233,234,236,239,240,244, 248,249). Using multiple step sections, Donaldson et al. (249) found capillary permeation in 34% of tumors that had less than 5 mm of stromal invasion and in 71% of neoplasms that had more than 5 mm of stromal infiltration; 79% of their patients with vascular invasion had inguinal lymph node metastases, as compared with only 6% of patients whose tumors lacked invasion. For stage I carcinomas, Iverson et al. (248) found that 6 of 15 tumors with vascular invasion metastasized to lymph nodes, whereas only 2 of 61 that lacked vascular permeation metastasized. The 5-year survival rate for their patients whose tumors lacked vascular invasion was 85%, compared with 52% survival for patients having neoplasms with vessel invasion (248). Some data indicate that perineural invasion, perhaps even more strongly than other histologic features of the primary lesion, is strongly predictive of lymph node metastasis (250).

Microinvasive, superficially invasive, and early invasive are descriptions for squamous cell carcinomas that are thin and have small amounts of stromal penetration (Fig. 21). Historically, these terms have not been applied uniformly. Franklin and Rutledge (241) initially defined microinvasive squamous cell carcinoma as a tumor 2 cm or less in diameter with 5 mm or less of stromal invasion; 3 mm (231,233,238) and 1 mm (251) have been used more recently as upper limits for stromal invasion. Currently, superficially invasive tumors are defined as confined to the vulva/perineum, ≤2 cm in greatest dimension, and having ≤1 mm of stromal invasion. In a literature review, Wilkinson (252) found that 15% of tumors with stromal invasion of 5 mm or less metastasized to groin lymph nodes, whereas 12% of tumors that invaded to a depth of 3 mm or less resulted in nodal metastases. In a large study of 272 women with superficial squamous cell carcinoma, 3% of tumors (one of 32) that were <1 mm thick (as measured with a ruler on the microscopic sections), 19% of those that were 3 mm thick, and 33% of neoplasms that were 5 mm thick metastasized to groin lymph nodes (253). Nodal metastases also occurred more frequently in squamous cell carcinomas that were poorly differentiated (grade 4), had capillary-like space involvement, or had a clitoral or perineal location. Each of the above factors showed a statistically significant correlation with groin lymph node metastasis in a multivariate analysis.

A variety of measuring points have been used to determine the depth of stromal invasion. The most frequently used methods for assessing tumor depth (or thickness) include (a) from the surface of the tumor (excluding the hyperkeratotic layer) to the deepest point of invasion (thickness) (232,238,239,248), (b) from the epithelial-stromal junction of the adjacent most superficial dermal papilla to the deepest point of infiltration (232,233), and (c) from the tip of the adjacent nonneoplastic rete ridge to the deepest point of invasion (238). Currently, there is controversy as to which is the optimal technique of measurement. Clearly, methods b and c cannot be used for exophytic cancers. Method b is used for the TNM staging system. We believe, however, that tumor thickness may be the simplest and most reproducible measurement. The form of measurement, whichever is preferred, should be mentioned in the pathology report. A calibrated ocular micrometer is most useful for accuracy.

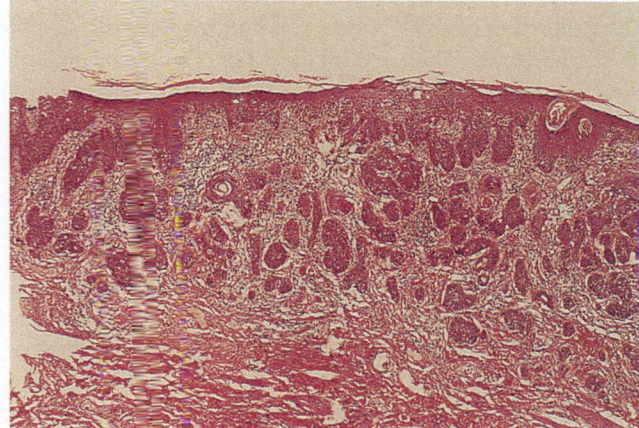

FIG. 21. Superficial squamous cell carcinoma. All superficially invasive squamous cell carcinomas of the vulva should be measured microscopically and the method of measurement should be stated in the pathology report. The maximal thickness of this lesion was 1.1 mm, as measured with an ocular micrometer.

At times, the separation of minimally invasive squamous cell carcinoma from intraepithelial neoplasia is difficult. Sections that are completely perpendicular to the tumor surface are essential for evaluation. The diagnosis of invasion is readily made when small nests or buds of cells are separate from the overlying surface. Clearly, difficulties arise in individual cases, especially for lesions that have complex, branching rete pegs.

Historically, the standard treatment for vulvar squamous cell carcinoma has been radical vulvectomy with en bloc bilateral inguinal-femoral lymph node dissection. Modern therapeutic approaches are individualized (254). More conservative operative procedures are used for small, unilateral tumors. A 1-cm tumor-free margin has been found to result in local control; in one study, there was a recurrence rate of 50% when margins were <8 mm (255). The 5-year survival rate for patients without groin node metastasis is 81% to 96% and for those with positive groin lymph nodes 43% to 66% (214–216,226,235,239,242). The mortality increases with the number of nodes involved by tumor (216,235,242), bilateral involvement of groin nodes (235,239,256), and metastasis to pelvic lymph nodes (216,235,239,240). In an analysis of 588 patients, independent predictors of positive groin nodes were high grade, suspicious or fixed/ulcerated nodes, lymphovascular invasion, older age, and greater tumor thickness (244). In that study, groin node status (number of positive nodes and laterality) and tumor diameter were important independent prognostic parameters for survival (257). More recently, other studies have shown that extracapsular growth of lymph node metastases also predicts an adverse outcome (258,259).

Adenoid squamous cell carcinoma consists of a single layer of squamous cells lining pseudoacini that contain dyskeratotic, acantholytic cells. Adenoid changes in squamous cell carcinoma may be focal or predominant (260,261). Neoplasms with a predominantly adenoid pattern are poorly differentiated and have a poor prognosis. Underwood et al. (261) noted only a 6% 5-year survival for such patients, as compared with a 77% survival for patients with conventional squamous cell carcinoma. Ultrastructurally, some adenoid squamous cancers have features suggesting glandular differentiation (261). For these cases, adenosquamous carcinoma (of possible skin appendage origin) seems a better designation (261). Spindle cell carcinoma is a rare, aggressive variant of squamous cell carcinoma of the vulva (262,263). Grossly, the tumor is often polypoid. It is composed of spindle-shaped cells (Fig. 22) and, sometimes, highly pleomorphic, sarcomatoid cells. Ulceration, hemorrhage, necrosis, and numerous mitotic figures are typical. Spindle cell carcinoma must be distinguished from melanoma and sarcoma. The diagnosis of spindle cell carcinoma is secure when foci of conventional squamous cell carcinoma or overlying intraepithelial neoplasia are observed. In histologically difficult cases, the identification of tonofilaments and desmosomes ultrastructurally finalizes the diagnosis of squamous cancer. Immunohistochemical positivity for keratin is also

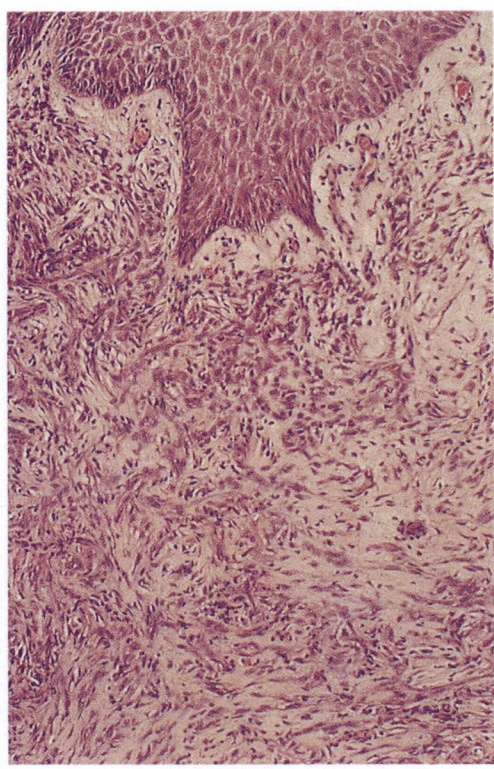

FIG. 22. Spindle cell carcinoma. This unusual variant of squamous cell carcinoma consists of dispersed, spindle-shaped cells that sometimes mimic the cells of sarcoma and melanoma.

helpful, but does not exclude certain sarcomas, such as epithelioid and synovial types. Rare cases of squamous cell carcinoma with osteosarcomatous differentiation (264) and lymphoepithelioma-like carcinoma of the vulva have been reported (265).

Verrucous carcinoma, a distinctive clinicopathologic subtype of squamous cell carcinoma, was initially documented on the vulva by Kraus and Perez-Mesa (266). This exquisitely well-differentiated tumor occurs in a broad age range, but most patients are in the sixth or seventh decade of life (267). Grossly, it is bulky, exophytic, and cauliflower-like. Ulceration is present in one-third of the cases. Microscopically, there is prominent acanthosis, hyperkeratosis, and parakeratosis (Fig. 23). The broad and elongated papillary processes generally lack well-formed fibrovascular cores. The bulbous rete pegs are well circumscribed and push deeply into the underlying tissue. Keratin microcysts are sometimes present centrally in the acanthotic pegs. Minimally pleomorphic cells are confined to the lower layers, and the overlying stratified squamous epithelium is mature. Mitotic figures are few and confined primarily to the basal layer.

The microscopic diagnosis of verrucous carcinoma is usually difficult, and appropriate clinical information is imperative. Indeed, diagnosis may be impossible with small, superficial specimens. Deep biopsies that include underlying stroma are usually necessary. The distinction from condy-

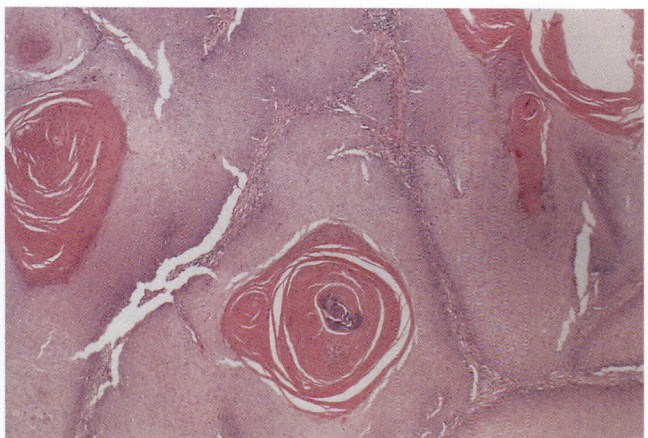

FIG. 23. Verrucous carcinoma. The acanthotic epithelium contains mature cells with minimal pleomorphism. Keratin microcysts may be very prominent.

loma and squamous cell carcinoma is often a challenge. The latter, however, typically contains cells with more nuclear pleomorphism, more mitotic figures, and has a more irregular invasive front. Although verrucous carcinoma may have vacuolated cells at the surface, the papillae lack the characteristic central fibrovascular cores seen in condyloma. The papillary fronds of verrucous carcinoma also penetrate deeper into the subepithelial tissues than the papillae of condyloma. Controversy still exists regarding the so-called giant condyloma of Buschke-Löwenstein. Whether it represents atypical condyloma, verrucous carcinoma, or warty carcinoma has been debated. Many believe that the Buschke-Löwenstein tumor represents verrucous carcinoma.

Verrucous carcinoma has been associated with human papillomavirus infection. In one study, half of the patients with verrucous carcinoma had had vulvar condylomas from 3 to 10 years previously (267). Human papillomavirus DNA (typically type 6 or 11) also has been identified in verrucous carcinoma (100,101). Warty squamous cell carcinoma with a well-differentiated upper component and small nests and cords of cells irregularly penetrating the underlying stroma should be distinguished from verrucous carcinoma because the former is a more aggressive, metastasizing lesion. Unlike verrucous carcinoma, warty squamous cell carcinoma has squamous pearls at the invasive front and more nuclear pleomorphism. Verrucous carcinoma, especially if it is massive, tends to recur and may prove fatal due to direct extension into vital structures. Inguinal-femoral lymph nodes may be enlarged, but metastases are typically absent (267). The 5-year survival rate for patients treated with complete excision alone was 94% in one study (267).

Basal cell carcinoma of the vulva occurs chiefly on the labia majora of middle-aged or elderly white women (268,269). Histologically and biologically, the tumor is identical to basal cell carcinoma elsewhere on the skin. Basal cell carcinoma with an adenoid pattern (270) must be distinguished from adenoid cystic carcinoma. The former neoplasm originates from the basal layer of the epidermis, grows in a serpiginous fashion, focally shows cribriform and gland-like patterns, and has a palisading arrangement of cells at the periphery of nests. Squamous differentiation and solid foci are also observed in adenoid basal cell carcinoma. Basal cell carcinoma of the vulva may recur following excision or new tumors may arise, but metastases are infrequent (271).

Primary adenocarcinoma of the vulva may have its origin in the epidermal appendages, mammary-like tissue, minor vestibular glands, periurethral glands (272), misplaced cloacal tissue (273), or Bartholin's gland. Approximately 40% of Bartholin's gland carcinomas are adenocarcinomas, and a similar number are squamous cell carcinomas (274,275). Most of the remaining cases include adenoid cystic carcinomas, undifferentiated carcinomas, or carcinomas having both squamous and glandular features. Tumors reported as transitional cell carcinomas are poorly described microscopically; it is likely that most, if not all, represent nonkeratinizing squamous cell carcinomas. A case of small cell undifferentiated carcinoma of Bartholin's gland has been described (276).

To be considered as a primary tumor of Bartholin's gland, a neoplasm must be located in the correct anatomical location, and the patient must not have a histologically similar neoplasm elsewhere (275). The presence of intact overlying squamous epithelium and residual normal acini adjacent to the tumor is helpful for determining origin in Bartholin's gland. In situ squamous carcinoma or adenocarcinoma in ducts or acini is also helpful, but is not essential for the diagnosis (275). A large, ulcerated tumor in the proper anatomical position might represent a Bartholin's gland carcinoma, especially if intraepithelial neoplastic changes of the adjacent skin and anus are absent. It may be impossible, however, to determine the exact origin of extensive, deeply invasive lesions.

Carcinoma of Bartholin's gland is often unsuspected, but should be considered in a woman 40 years of age or older who has any clinical abnormality of the gland. Microscopically, most of the adenocarcinomas produce mucus and are well or moderately differentiated. Approximately 10% are adenoid cystic carcinomas (277); the tumors are histologically identical to their counterparts in salivary glands and elsewhere (278). They have a propensity for perineural invasion, recurrence, and distant metastasis, but metastases to groin lymph nodes have occurred in only one instance (279).

Formerly, the standard treatment for a carcinoma of Bartholin's gland was radical vulvectomy with bilateral inguinal lymphadenectomy (274). Some authors have advocated wide local excision, ipsilateral inguinal lymphadenectomy, and radiation therapy (275). Leuchter et al. (274) noted a 52% survival for patients with negative inguinal nodes and a 36% survival for those with positive inguinal-femoral lymph nodes. Copeland et al. (275) found an overall 5-year survival rate of 84%. For 32 patients with adenoid cystic carcinoma the survival rate at 5 years was 71%, but recurrences developed in over 85% by 12 years (280).

Endodermal sinus tumor of the vulva has been described

in four patients ranging in age from 22 months to 26 years; three of the four died of disease within 2 years (281). Less than a dozen patients with vulvar Merkel cell carcinoma have been described; death within 2½ years is usual (282–287). One tumor was associated with intraepithelial neoplasia (283), and another had an invasive squamous cell carcinoma component (282).

Approximately 60% of vulvar melanomas arise on the labium minus or clitoris, and 40% occur on the labium majus (Fig. 24) (288–291). Melanoma is found primarily in white women, 70% of whom are postmenopausal (288). The lesions can be classified as superficial spreading, nodular, or acral lentiginous types (289). A case of neurotropic melanoma has been documented (291). Some authors have not applied levels of invasion, as specifically defined by Clark, stating that the papillary dermis is poorly defined or absent in certain parts of the vulva (288). A modification of Clark's system has been devised, however (288). Most vulvar melanomas are pigmented and thick. About 80% are greater than 1.5 mm thick (290). Tumor thickness ranged from 0.6 to 28.0 mm, with a median thickness of 9.0 mm in another study (289). The minimum thickness for nonsurvivors was 2.6 mm (289). In an additional study, 1 melanoma was <0.75 mm thick, 20 were between 0.76 and 3.00 mm, and 22 were >3.00 mm (292). The overall survival is approximately 30% to 40% (288–290) and correlates with the status of groin lymph nodes (290,293). In a study of 45 patients with lymphadenectomy, the 5-year survival rate was 9% for those with positive nodes and 57% for patients lacking nodal metastasis (293).

A variety of sarcomas have arisen on the vulva (138,294–313) (Table 4); leiomyosarcoma is the most common (138,294,295). Criteria for the distinction of benign and malignant smooth muscle tumors have been described in the discussion concerning leiomyoma. Two-thirds of vulvar sarcomas develop in the labium majus; most of the remainder

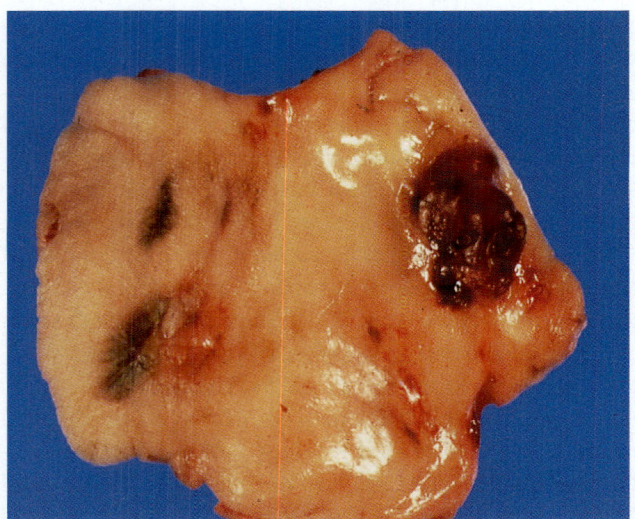

FIG. 24. A 1.5-cm nodular melanoma and two foci of precancerous melanosis are present in this excision specimen of the vulva.

TABLE 4. *Primary sarcomas of the vulva*

Sarcoma	Reference
Leiomyosarcoma	138,294,295
Malignant fibrous histiocytoma	295–297
Rhabdomyosarcoma (embryonal, alveolar)	294,298,299
Malignant schwannoma	294,295
Epithelioid sarcoma	301
Fibrosarcoma	294,295,302
Dermatofibrosarcoma protuberans	295,303
Angiosarcoma	295
Kaposi's sarcoma	304
Hemangiopericytoma	295,302
Alveolar soft part sarcoma	307
Malignant granular cell tumor	308
Liposarcoma	309
Synovial sarcoma	310
Mesenchymal chondrosarcoma	311
Epithelioid hemangioendothelioma	312
Peripheral neuroectodermal tumor	313

are found in the fourchette and the deep tissues near Bartholin's gland (295). Many of the reported epithelioid sarcomas of the vulva have features of extrarenal malignant rhabdoid tumor (300). Despite the fact that the diagnostic label for these vulvar neoplasms is controversial, the tumors often exhibit aggressive behavior (300,301).

Non-Hodgkin's lymphoma (80,314) and Hodgkin's disease (315) of the vulva are primarily manifestations of systemic disease. There are rare reports of primary plasmacytoma (316) and diffuse large cell lymphoma (immunoblastic) (317) of the labium majus.

The vulva is the most common site of Langerhans cell histiocytosis of the female genital tract (318). Except for a few examples that were localized, most were manifestations of systemic disease. Vulvar eosinophilic granuloma must be distinguished microscopically from venereal and other inflammatory diseases.

In one series of 22 metastatic carcinomas to the vulva, 10 originated from the cervix, and 8 arose in the endometrium, urethra, vagina, or ovary (319). Metastasis to the vulva may be the initial manifestation of recurrent disease. Squamous cell carcinoma metastatic to the vulva usually appears as a circumscribed, subepithelial mass, whereas metastatic adenocarcinoma tends to invade the surface epithelium. Most patients with vulvar metastases have disseminated disease and a very poor prognosis (319). There have been a few reported patients with cervical carcinoma metastatic (or implanted) to episiotomy scars (320).

Extramammary Paget's Disease, Hidradenoma Papilliferum, and Skin Appendage Neoplasms

Vulvar Paget's disease, often controversial and misunderstood, occurs in three forms: (a) most commonly, by far, it is an intraepithelial adenocarcinoma that is derived from a multipotential cell in the epidermis, adnexa, or anogenital mammary-like glands (2,171); (b) it may become an invasive adenocarcinoma, arising from intraepithelial adenocarcinoma; and (c) it may represent pagetoid extension or metastasis to the skin by a carcinoma nearby such as a primary adenocarcinoma of the cervix (321,322) or Bartholin's gland (323), or a transitional cell carcinoma of the bladder or urethra (324). Approximately 29% of patients with Paget's disease have an additional, unrelated synchronous or metachronous carcinoma, most commonly arising from the genitourinary tract, gastrointestinal tract, or breast (325).

Paget's disease is a slowly growing neoplasm of long duration that is sometimes mistaken clinically for a chronic, intractable dermatitis. Most cases occur in postmenopausal white women, chiefly in the seventh decade of life (321,326). Vulvar Paget's disease is extremely rare in black women. Grossly, Paget's disease appears as a flat or slightly raised, granular, moist, erythematous patch (Fig. 25). It primarily occurs on the labia majora, but is often extensive, involving the labia minora, perineum, perianal skin, thighs, mons, and lower abdomen. Occasionally, there is extension along the mucosa of the vagina, cervix, urethra, bladder, or ureter (324,326,327). Extension into the ducts of the periurethral glands, the mucus-secreting glands of the vestibule, and the endocervical mucous glands also occurs (321,324). Clinically, Paget's disease is sharply demarcated and may be multifocal (328). Typically, however, there is microscopic extension into grossly normal skin.

Microscopically, Paget's disease consists of large pale

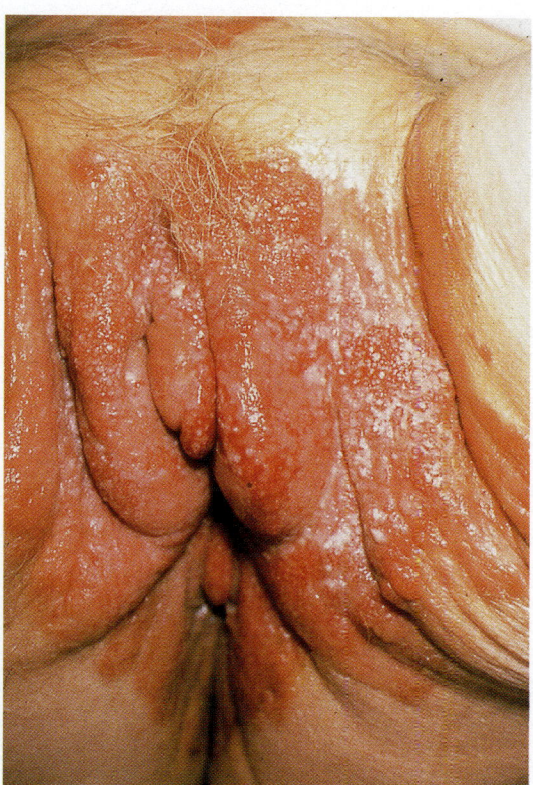

FIG. 25. Vulvar Paget's disease. Granular, erythematous patches may be localized or cover the entire vulva and perineum.

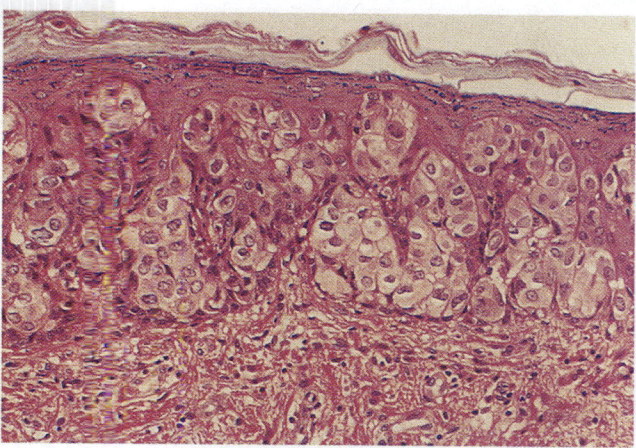

FIG. 26. Paget's disease. The epidermis contains nests of cells with abundant clear cytoplasm and large, pleomorphic nuclei with vesicular chromatin and conspicuous nucleoli.

cells, predominantly in the basal layer of the epidermis (Fig. 26). Single cells, nests, and well-formed glands are present and sometimes extend into the upper layers of the epithelium. The squamous epithelium is acanthotic, often with hyperkeratosis and parakeratosis. Paget's cells frequently involve the basal layers of pilosebaceous structures, and the ducts and acini of sweat glands (321,329,330). Paget's cells have abundant clear or eosinophilic, granular cytoplasm. Their large nuclei have vesicular chromatin and, often, prominent nucleoli. Mitotic figures are easily identified. Signet ring cells may be observed (321). Some Paget's cells are invariably positive with mucicarmine, periodic acid-Schiff (PAS) after diastase pretreatment, colloidal iron after hyaluronidase pretreatment, aldehyde fuchsin, or alcian blue stains (321,330). The dermis contains a variable number of inflammatory cells, and dermal vessels may be increased in number and size. Infrequently, patients with Paget's disease have areas of dermal invasion. It is important not to mistake intraepithelial involvement of sweat glands or ducts for invasive tumor. The cells of invasive disease infiltrate the dermis from the intraepidermal or adnexal component. They invade as cords, nests, and sheets of cells (Fig. 27). The cells may also form trabeculae, tubules, and glands with intraluminal secretions.

Immunocytochemically, Paget's cells are reactive for carcinoembryonic antigen (331,332), cytokeratin (332), and epithelial membrane antigen (332). In addition, they are immunoreactive for gross cystic disease fluid protein, which is also found in normal eccrine and apocrine cells (332). Ultrastructurally, Paget's cells have some features of apocrine or eccrine cells (333,334).

The microscopic differential diagnosis for Paget's disease includes melanoma and squamous intraepithelial neoplasia. The presence of intracytoplasmic melanin does not exclude a diagnosis of Paget's disease, as 60% of cases contain cells with a few, coarse melanin granules (330). Unlike Paget's disease, melanoma contains theques of cells at the dermal-

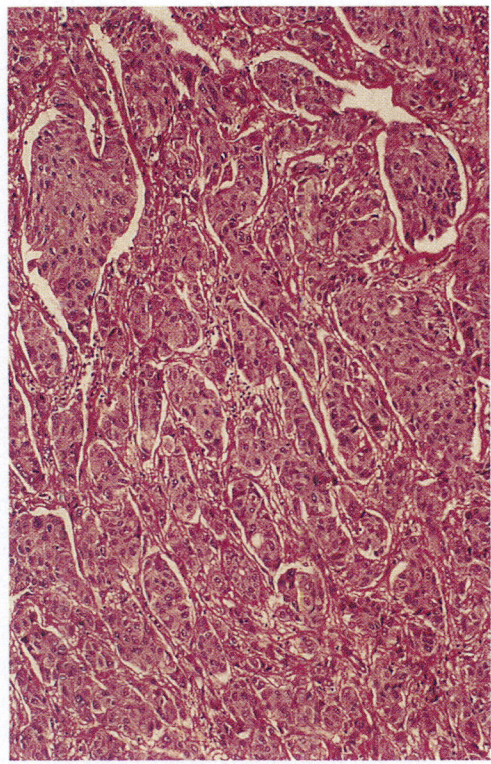

FIG. 27. Paget's disease with invasion. The dermis is infiltrated by nests of adenocarcinoma. The intraepithelial component from this case is illustrated in Fig. 26.

epidermal junction; fine, diffuse granules of melanin; and immunoreactivity with S-100 protein and HMB45 antibodies. Melanoma also lacks mucin and immunoreactivity for carcinoembryonic antigen.

Patients with Paget's disease are treated usually with wide excision or simple vulvectomy (326,329). Because the sharply demarcated clinical lesion belies microscopic extension into grossly normal epithelium, adequate margins can be obtained by frozen sections or by numerous perilesional biopsies prior to resection. Local recurrence of intraepithelial tumor develops in approximately one-third of the cases after surgical excision (321). The therapy for invasive tumor developing from Paget's disease is radical vulvectomy and bilateral inguinal-femoral lymph node dissection (326,329,335). Lymph node metastases occur in about 85% of patients with invasive anogenital disease (330). Long-term survival for patients with groin lymph node metastasis is unusual (321,329,330). The prognosis appears to be better for patients whose invasive tumors have not metastasized to inguinal-femoral lymph nodes (321,330). No large studies have correlated the thickness of invasive tumors with the status of groin lymph nodes and survival. Thin (1 mm depth of invasion) invasive tumors may metastasize to inguinofemoral lymph nodes, however (336).

Hidradenoma papilliferum (papillary hidradenoma) is virtually nonexistent in prepubertal females. In two series totaling 120 patients, no cases were found in black women (337,338). It is usually single and less than 1 cm in diameter. Eighty percent are on the labia majora or labia minora, often in or near the interlabial sulcus (337,338) (Fig. 28). Grossly, the lesion appears as a round or oval, firm nodule that sometimes ulcerates and bleeds. On cut section, the tumor is a well-circumscribed, soft, gray-white to red, solid or cystic nodule. Microscopically, hidradenoma papilliferum has papillary and complex glandular patterns (Fig. 29). Glands sometimes contain eosinophilic material and are lined by a single or double layer of cuboid cells. Papillary foci usually contain two layers of cells supported by fibrovascular stroma. The superficial cells are columnar and have basal nuclei. The smaller cells adjacent to the basement membrane are cuboid with clear cytoplasm. Mild, focal nuclear atypia and occasional mitotic figures may be observed. Some cells have overt apocrine features, which are also evident histochemically and ultrastructurally (339). Hidradenoma papilliferum often resembles intraductal papilloma or nipple adenoma of the breast. It likely derives from anogenital mammary-like glands, which are often found in or around the hidradenoma (1,2). Rare cases of *in situ* or invasive carcinoma (adenosquamous) arising in hidradenoma papilliferum have been reported (340,341).

A few mixed tumors and syringomas of the vulva have been described. The former occur on the labia majora and most are of long duration (342). Microscopically, they are identical to salivary gland mixed tumors, and probably arise from labial sweat glands. There are no convincing cases of

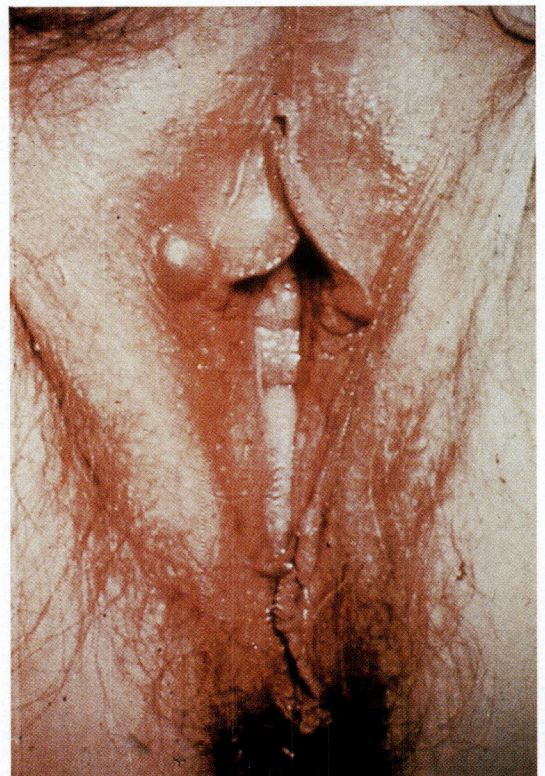

FIG. 28. Hidradenoma papilliferum. A small discrete nodule is usually seen in the interlabial sulcus.

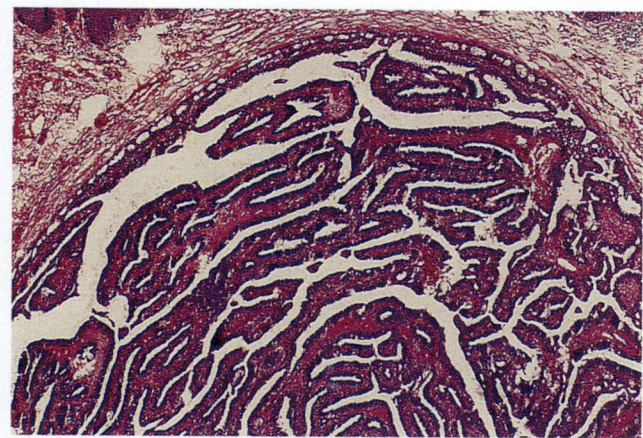

FIG. 29. Hidradenoma papilliferum. A well-circumscribed subepithelial nodule is composed of papillae having prominent fibrovascular cores.

mixed tumor arising in Bartholin's gland or malignant mixed tumor of the vulva. Vulvar syringoma, histologically identical to syringoma of the face, manifests as small papules less than 5 mm in diameter. They are found in children and young adults (343). Syringomas usually occur on both labia majora, but may be unilateral or arise on the labium minus. Vulvar lesions may be accompanied by extragenital syringomas.

Cutaneous appendage neoplasms reported as rare examples on the vulva include trichoepithelioma (344), proliferating trichilemmal tumor (345), trichoblastic fibroma (346), clear cell hidradenoma (eccrine acrospiroma) (347), ductal eccrine adenocarcinoma (348), eccrine porocarcinoma (348), clear cell hidradenocarcinoma (348), apocrine carcinoma (349), sebaceous carcinoma (350), and mucinous eccrine carcinoma (351).

VAGINA

The vagina is that segment of the female genital tract between the hymenal ring and the uterine cervix. It is lined by stratified squamous epithelium overlying a lamina propria, a muscular coat, and an adventitial layer. Keratinized epithelium, normally absent, may be found after mucosal prolapse. The squamous mucosa undergoes cyclic hormonal changes. Cytoplasmic glycogen is most abundant at the time of ovulation. Atrophy of the epithelium occurs at menopause. The lamina propria contains collagen, elastic fibers, fibroblasts, blood vessels, and lymphatic channels. A few lymphocytes are typically present. A band of loose connective tissue in the lamina propria may contain large, often stellate stromal cells whose nuclei are hyperchromatic and multiple or multilobed. The muscular coat has an inner layer of circular smooth muscle fibers and an outer longitudinal layer. The adventitia contains connective tissue with a well-developed venous plexus, lymphatics, and a few nerve branches.

The vaginal lymphatic drainage is complex, and pathways from specific regions are not always predictable (7). In general, the channels that flow from the superior, posterior vagina drain into the rectal lymph nodes and those from the superior anterior vagina lead to the interiliac nodes. Lymphatics from the middle region of the posterior wall terminate in the deep pelvic nodes. From the middle portion of the anterior wall, lymphatics lead to the lymph nodes of the lateral pelvic wall, especially the interiliac lymph nodes, or to the vesical nodes. Lymphatic channels from the distal vagina communicate with pelvic lymph nodes or with anastomoses from the vestibule that drain into lymph nodes of the femoral triangle. All portions of the vagina have lymphatic channels that drain into lateral collecting vessels around the vaginal artery, and lead to superior gluteal and, sometimes, to the common iliac nodes.

Congenital Anomalies Including Those Due to Intrauterine Exposure to Diethylstilbestrol

The vaginal anatomy is variable in patients with cloacal malformations (30). Vaginal agenesis results from defective formation of the distal portions of the müllerian ducts. Agenesis is typically associated with abnormal development of the uterus and, often, renal and skeletal anomalies (Mayer-Rokitansky-Küster-Hauser syndrome) (352–354). Vaginal biopsies from split-thickness skin grafts (neovaginas) for congenital absence reveal various changes that range from near-normal mucous membrane to skin-like (355). The microscopic appearance may depend on the amount of corium included in the transplant. Neovaginas that are not lined or are grafted with amniotic membrane or peritoneum develop a vaginal-like squamous epithelium (356,357). Mild diversion colitis sometimes occurs in isolated segments of sigmoid colon used as neovaginas (358). Longitudinal or transverse vaginal septa are either complete or partial. Transverse septa are most often observed at the junction of the middle and upper one-third of the vagina and have central or eccentric openings. Microscopically, a core of fibrovascular tissue and smooth muscle is lined on both sides by squamous epithelium (359). Mucinous glandular epithelium is generally absent. Vaginal duplication is commonly associated with duplication of the uterus. Other congenital vaginal malformations include oblique septa and distal vaginal atresia (354).

Congenital abnormalities of the vagina that result from *in utero* exposure to diethylstilbestrol (DES) include mucosal membrane, corolla-like mucosal elevation, fibrous band, apical narrowing, forniceal obliteration, transverse or longitudinal vaginal septa, and adenosis (360) (Fig. 30). Excluding adenosis, structural malformations of the vagina or cervix occur in about one-fourth of DES-exposed women (361). Adenosis is the presence of müllerian glands in the vagina after birth. This condition was documented in 1971 in women exposed *in utero* to DES, when clear cell adenocarcinoma of the vagina also was linked to this drug (362). DES had been used for over 20 years for women with high-risk pregnancies. Robboy et al. (363), using intact reproductive tracts from human embryos and fetuses grown in athymic (nude) mice, showed that *in vivo* exposure to DES resulted in

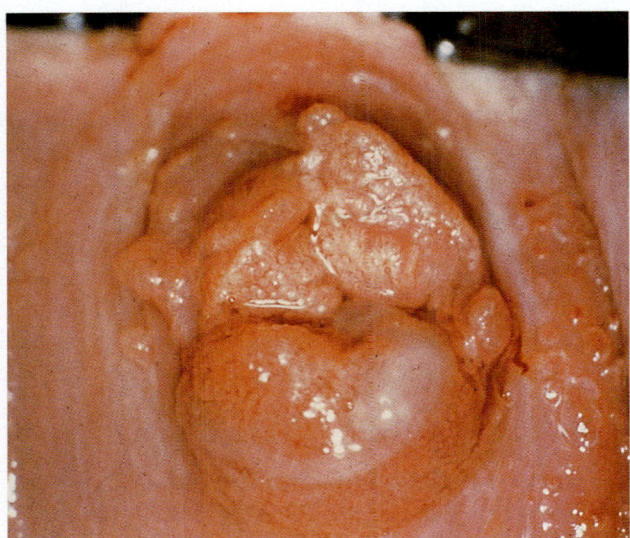

FIG. 30. DES-induced changes. In this patient with *in utero* exposure to DES, the cervix has a distorted appearance and is accompanied by vaginal adenosis.

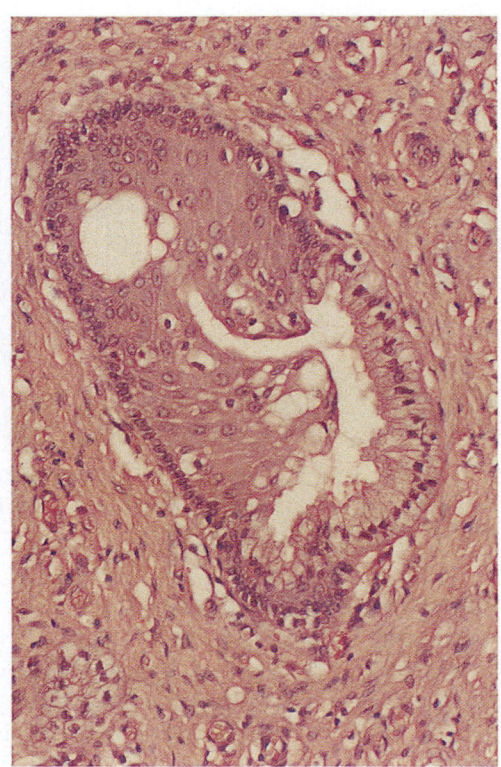

FIG. 31. Vaginal adenosis. Columnar, mucus-producing epithelium (endocervical type) is most often observed in adenosis. The glands are eventually replaced by squamous metaplasia.

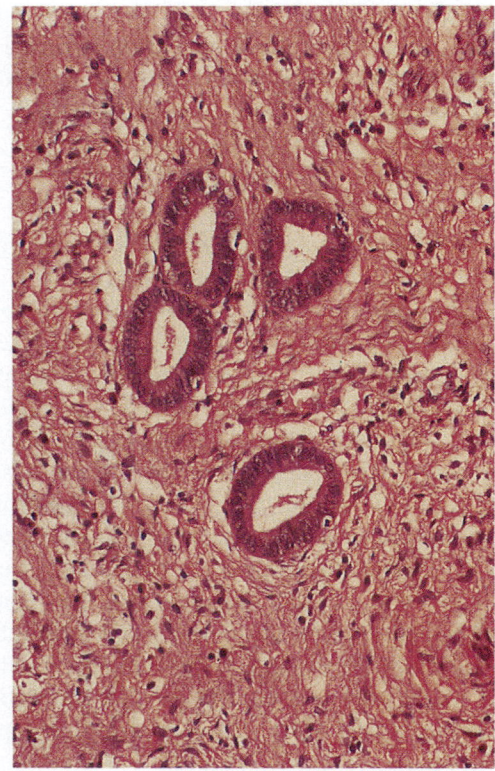

FIG. 32. Vaginal adenosis. Endometrial-type glands are sometimes present in adenosis. Unlike endometriosis, endometrial stroma is absent.

developmental anomalies of the female reproductive tract, including vaginal adenosis. The drug prevents the urogenital squamous epithelium from replacing the müllerian columnar epithelium. Adenosis, however, is not limited to women with *in utero* exposure to DES, having been identified in 2.3% of unexposed women (364). Adenosis in unexposed women may be congenital or acquired. Acquired adenosis appears to represent columnar cell metaplasia, and has been reported after topical 5-fluorouracil therapy and CO_2 laser vaporization for condyloma acuminata or intraepithelial neoplasia (365,366). Additional examples of acquired adenosis have followed other causes of vaginal epithelial trauma (366). When caused by DES, the frequency of adenosis is related to the total drug dose, the duration of pregnancy at the onset of its administration, and the duration of exposure (364,367). Almost all women exposed to DES *in utero* at or before the eighth week of pregnancy have developed adenosis, compared with only 6% exposed at or after the 15th week of gestation (364). Thirty-four percent of women with DES exposure, examined after review of their prenatal records, had vaginal epithelial changes in the form of adenosis or squamous metaplasia (367).

Adenosis occurs chiefly in the upper one-third of the vagina, but may extend to the lower two-thirds. There may be only a few glands or extensive involvement. The epithelial changes are characteristically located at the mucosal surface or in the superficial lamina propria or both. Grossly, adenosis appears as cysts or a granular red surface. Microscopically, endocervical-type mucous glands predominate, but endometrial and tubal-type glands are frequently present (Figs. 31 and 32). The glands may be simple, complex, cystic, or papillary (368). Cysts, resembling cervical nabothian cysts, are lined either by a single layer of columnar mucinous cells or occasionally by papillary fronds. Tuboendometrial glands, when present, are found in the upper vagina in approximately 20% of cases and in the lower vagina in almost 100% (369). Occasionally, small embryonic-type glands composed of low columnar or cuboid cells are found in patients exposed to DES (370). They are also found in women without a history of exposure to the drug. Rarely, intestinal metaplasia may arise in DES-induced adenosis; in the described case, the vaginal discharge was so profuse that a vaginal resection was required (371).

The microscopic appearance of adenosis in women without exposure to DES is similar to that for women with *in utero* exposure (370). With age, vaginal adenosis is replaced by squamous metaplasia. Sparse intraluminal or intracytoplasmic droplets of mucus that may be present can be detected with the mucicarmine stain (372). Squamous metaplasia is ultimately replaced by fully glycogenated squamous epithelium (373). The incidence of squamous intraepithelial neoplasia of the vagina or cervix is twice as high for women exposed to DES as for a nonexposed cohort (374).

Adenosis must be distinguished from endometriosis, clear cell adenocarcinoma, and mesonephric remnants. Mesonephric (wolffian) tubules are located deep in the lateral vaginal wall, are lined by nonciliated, nonmucinous cuboid cells, and have dense, eosinophilic luminal secretions (Fig. 33) (375). The remnants are surrounded by a loose fibrovascular stroma that may contain smooth muscle fibers. Clear cell adenocarcinoma might be confused with the glands of adenosis that undergo microglandular hyperplasia (376).

Unlike clear cell adenocarcinoma, microglandular hyperplasia consists of small, uniform, crowded glands without prominent intervening stroma. The cells contain mucin but lack glycogen. Nuclear pleomorphism and prominent nucleoli are absent.

Although adenosis composed of a variety of cell types may be found adjacent to clear cell adenocarcinoma, tuboendometrial glands are most common, being found in up to 94% of cases (377). It is hypothesized that carcinoma develops from adenosis through an intermediate form of atypical adenosis (atypical tuboendometrial glands) (377). The latter glands are seen adjacent to about 75% of vaginal clear cell adenocarcinomas (377). The glands of atypical adenosis have smooth borders, are lined by a single layer of cells, and occasionally show intraglandular bridging. Their enlarged, hyperchromatic, and pleomorphic nuclei have prominent nucleoli. Glands with severely atypical nuclei may represent *in situ* clear cell adenocarcinoma.

Infectious Diseases

Cases of infectious vaginitis are typically due to *Candida* species, *Gardnerella vaginalis* (or other agents in bacterial vaginosis), or *Trichomonas vaginalis*. Diagnostic methods include the examination of an isotonic saline wet mount preparation, a Papanicolaou-stained cervicovaginal smear, and culture isolation.

Bacteria

The replacement of the predominant lactobacilli by an assortment of other bacteria in the vaginal ecosystem has been termed *bacterial vaginosis,* which is the most common cause of abnormal vaginal discharge (378). *G. vaginalis* is responsible for many of the cases of nonspecific vaginitis (bacterial vaginosis), due to synergism with anaerobic bacteria (379). Other organisms are sometimes involved. The *G. vaginalis* coccobacillus does not invade the vaginal epithelium and does not stimulate a local inflammatory response, but often results in a gray, offensive vaginal discharge in affected women. The vaginal epithelium has a normal microscopic appearance. In a vaginal smear, the coccobacilli often reside on the surface of the superficial squamous cells (clue cells), causing the disappearance of distinct cytoplasmic borders.

N. gonorrhoeae rarely causes vaginitis in adults, but may infect children who have less resistant vaginal squamous epithelium. The chancre of primary and, later, mucous patches of secondary syphilis occasionally occur in the vagina. Granuloma inguinale and chancroid infection may involve the vagina, most often in instances of long-standing, destructive vulvar disease. Other organisms that are unusual agents in bacterial vaginitis include staphylococci, streptococci, and *Mycobacterium tuberculosis.* Some strains of *Staphylococcus aureus* produce an exoprotein (toxic shock syndrome toxin 1) that has an important role in toxic shock syndrome (380). The association of menstruation and tampon use with

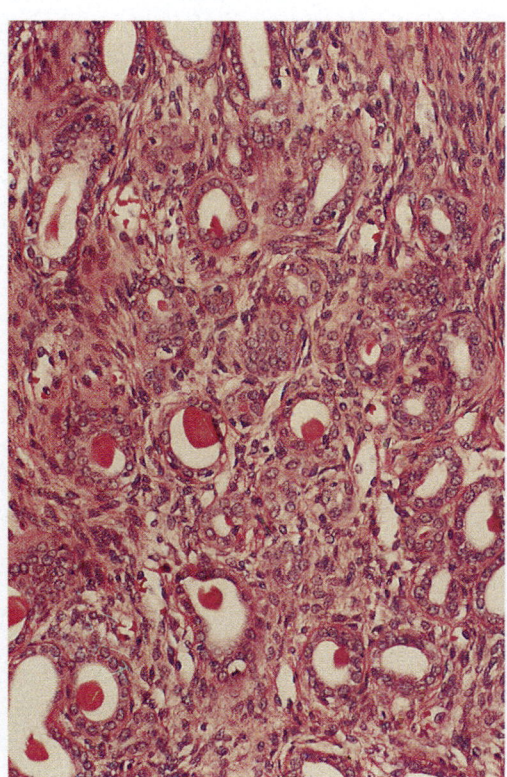

FIG. 33. Mesonephric remnants. Cuboid cells are not ciliated and do not produce mucus. Dense, eosinophilic secretions are present in the lumens.

toxic shock syndrome results from a complex interaction that includes exposure to a strain of toxin-producing *S. aureus*, lack of immunity, optimal growth conditions in the vagina for the production of toxin, and other primary and secondary mediators (381). Microscopic changes of the vagina in women who die of toxic shock syndrome include mucosal ulceration, separation of the epithelium beneath the basal layer, vascular congestion, thrombosis, acute inflammation, bacteria within the epithelium, and surface fibrin (382).

A polypoid xanthogranulomatous pseudotumor of the vagina was composed of sheets of large histiocytes with abundant eosinophilic, granular cytoplasm that mimicked granular cell tumor (383). Infection by a mucoid form of *Escherichia coli* was causative (383). Although similar to malakoplakia, the lesion lacked Michaelis-Gutmann bodies. The vagina is the most frequent site of malakoplakia when it occurs in the female genital tract (384). *E. coli* is often cultured from the urine or the specific lesion of genital malakoplakia (384).

Viruses, Chlamydia, and Mycoplasma

Herpesvirus and human papillomavirus usually involve the vagina as a part of multicentric infection. Vaginal condylomata may be flat, inverted, or warty. Using DNA hybridization techniques, human papillomavirus DNA has been identified in vaginal condylomata, (98,385), vaginal intraepithelial neoplasia (386), and verrucous carcinoma (387). Human papillomavirus types 6 and 11 have been found in vaginal condyloma (98), and types 6 and 16 have been described in vaginal intraepithelial neoplasia (98,386).

The vagina may be affected by lymphogranuloma venereum *(C. trachomatis)* as a part of severe local infection. *Mycoplasma* species and *Ureaplasma urealyticum* normally inhabit the vagina, but, rarely, each may be the predominant isolate in cases of vaginitis (388).

Fungi and Parasites

Candida (usually *C. albicans*) is a common agent in vaginitis. It is chiefly observed in women during the childbearing years, and manifests as mucosal erythema or a thick, white exudate. Histologically, there is mild acanthosis and spongiosis, with congestion and edema of the lamina propria. Lymphocytes, plasma cells, and a few neutrophils are observed in the stroma (112). The organism resides on the epithelial surface and does not penetrate the mucosa. Necrotic debris, neutrophils, and yeast form a surface exudate. About 10% of fungal vaginitis is caused by *Candida glabrata* (389).

T. vaginalis is a 15- to 20-μm, unicellular, flagellate protozoan that is sexually transmitted, primarily during the reproductive years. Some infections are asymptomatic, but in most instances the protozoan causes acute or chronic vaginitis. Histologic changes of acute infection include surface exudate, mild acute inflammation, mild acanthosis, spongiosis, congestion, edematous papillae, and small stromal hemorrhages (390). Ulceration is usually not present. Lymphocytes, plasma cells, and a few neutrophils are observed in the lamina propria. Necrotic debris and neutrophils sometimes lie on the mucosal surface. The changes are less severe in chronic infection, and no microscopic abnormalities of the epithelium are usually observed in the asymptomatic patient.

Pinworms, schistosomiasis, and *Entamoeba histolytica* (391) are unusual causes of parasitic vaginal infection.

Miscellaneous Benign Conditions

Atrophic vaginitis results from withdrawal of estrogen. The vaginal mucosa appears pale and lacks prominent rugae. Microscopically, the attenuated epithelium is reduced to the basal layer and a few overlying parabasal and intermediate-type squamous cells. The prominent basal and parabasal cells should not be mistaken for dysplastic epithelium. There may be focal ulceration. Lymphocytes, plasma cells, and a few neutrophils are present in the lamina propria. Desquamative inflammatory vaginitis, histologically similar to atrophic vaginitis, occurs characteristically in the vaginal vault of women with normal estrogen levels (Fig. 34) (392). The mucosa may be ulcerated superficially with acute and chronic inflammation, as well as stromal hemorrhage. The cause is unknown, but is believed by some to be a form of lichen planus (393). Oral cavity involvement may also be present. The condition is sometimes persistent, but it may respond to oral or intravaginal corticosteroids (392). Emphysematous vaginitis, also known as vaginitis emphysematosa, occurs usually incidentally in postpubertal women as gas-filled cysts in the superficial lamina propria (394,395). The cysts are typically multiple and measure up to 2 cm in diameter. They are surrounded by multinucleate giant cells, histiocytes, fibroblasts, or collagen (Fig. 35). Occasionally, there is a partial lining of squamous epithelium. Scattered inflammatory cells, including multinucleate giant cells and

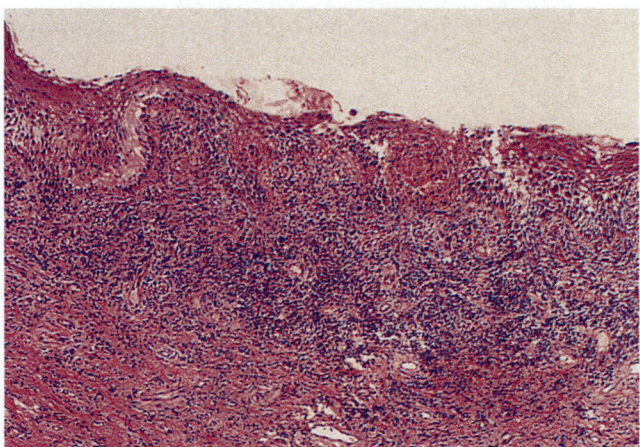

FIG. 34. Desquamative inflammatory vaginitis. Occurring in women who have normal estrogen levels, this condition microscopically shows thinning or ulceration of the epithelium and chronic inflammation.

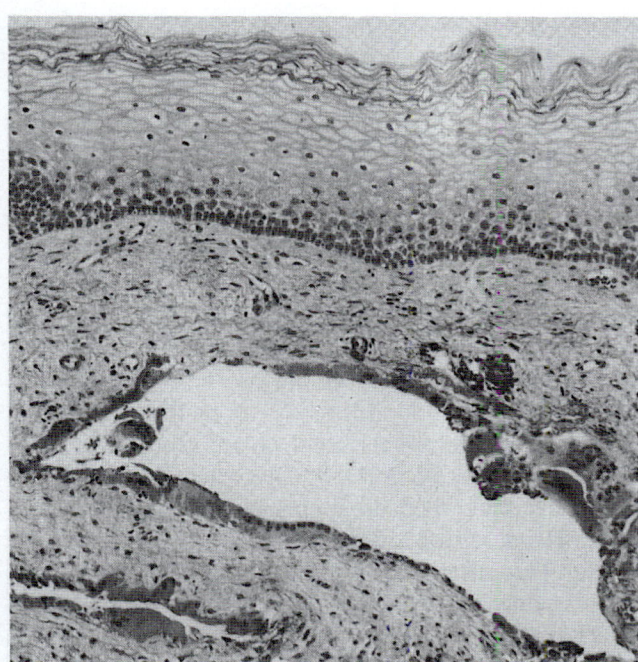

FIG. 35. Emphysematous vaginitis. The lamina propria contains cysts surrounded by multinucleate giant cells, histiocytes, fibroblasts, and collagen.

mononuclear histiocytes, are found in the surrounding fibrotic stroma. The condition has been associated with *Trichomonas* or *Gardnerella* infection and usually disappears after eradication of these organisms (394).

Noninfectious causes of vaginitis include irradiation and a variety of physical and chemical agents. Tampons, especially those of the superabsorbent variety, sometimes cause epithelial drying, layering, and ulceration (396). Granulation tissue, acute and chronic inflammation, and monofilament foreign body material (synthetic cellulose acetate) have been observed in tampon-related ulcers (397). Crohn's disease rarely involves the vagina, manifesting as enterovaginal fistulas, (398), sinuses, and abscesses. One case of ulcerative colitis that arose in colonic tissue used as a neovagina has been described (399).

Epidermal inclusion cyst occurs as a small, asymptomatic cyst in the anterior or posterior vaginal wall. In most instances it is related to previous trauma (400,401). Mucous cyst, variously located in the vagina (400,401), is unilocular and typically measures from 0.5 to 7 cm in diameter. It is lined by a single layer of columnar mucous cells, but ciliated cells and squamous metaplasia may be observed focally (400). In contrast, vaginal adenosis occurs as multiple small cysts. Gartner's duct (mesonephric) cyst is a rare vaginal cyst. It is small, single, and characteristically found along the lateral or anterolateral wall. The cyst is lined by a single layer of cuboid, nonmucinous cells. A basement membrane and smooth muscle fibers in the surrounding stroma are not always present (400). An ectopic ureter may drain into Gartner's duct cyst (402). Vaginal endometriosis arises from implantation of shed endometrial fragments into areas of trauma or, more commonly, from pelvic implants along the posterior vaginal fornix (403). The hymenal cyst (42) of the newborn is discussed in the section on vulvar cysts. Rare cases of vaginal dermoid cyst (mature cystic teratoma) have been reviewed (404).

The stromal cells of the lamina propria may undergo decidual metaplasia, giving rise to a polypoid mass or indurated ulcer that clinically suggests vaginal cancer (405). Spontaneous resolution occurs in the postpartum interval. Trophoblastic tissue in the vaginal wall, found rarely in association with normal pregnancy but in up to 10% of patients with hydatidiform mole (406,407), appears as one or more red or purple nodules that readily bleed on palpation. Trophoblastic cells and villi present in the nodules presumably result from hematogenous dissemination and should not be mistaken for choriocarcinoma. A case of vaginal ectopic pregnancy has been reported (408).

Granulation tissue, commonly found in the vaginal vault after hysterectomy, occurs chiefly within a few weeks or months after surgery, but has appeared after 14 years (409). Granulation tissue is biopsied because it simulates carcinoma clinically, and is of utmost concern in women who have had a prior hysterectomy for neoplasia. This clinical appearance also may be recapitulated by a prolapsed fallopian tube (407,410). Tubal prolapse develops most often after vaginal hysterectomy. The symptoms (abdominal pain, vaginal bleeding, discharge, or dyspareunia) usually occur within 6 months postoperatively, but may develop as late as 28 years after surgery (410). Grossly, the prolapsed tube appears as an erythematous, granular, and polypoid mass. It can be diagnosed clinically, when a probe is passed through its lumen or when its traction causes pain (410,411). Microscopically, it is easily overdiagnosed as adenocarcinoma. Marked inflammation, distortion, atypia, and a pseudoinvasive pattern are common (Fig. 36) (410,411). The diagnosis is made upon recognition of hyperplastic tubal epithelium surrounded by smooth muscle bundles. The therapy is complete excision through the vaginal cuff. Cautery, usually therapeutic for granulation tissue, is not effective (411). The finding of asymptomatic vaginal telangiectasias on routine pelvic examination has been noted as a manifestation of Osler-Weber-Rendu syndrome (412).

Ectopic thyroid and parathyroid glands in the wall of the vagina have been described (404).

Benign melanocytic lesions of the vagina include melanotic macule (lentigo) (413), atypical melanocytic hyperplasia (414), blue nevus (415), and cellular blue nevus (416). Three percent of vaginas at necropsy have melanocytes in the epithelium (417).

Vaginal stromal (fibroepithelial) polyps are generally found in adults, but may occur in newborns (418). The designation "pseudosarcoma botryoides" as a synonym for stromal polyp is confusing, and its use should be abandoned (419). The polypoid or pedunculated stromal polyp is found along the lateral walls of the lower one-third of the vagina. It is usually less than 4 cm in size and is soft or rubbery, gray-

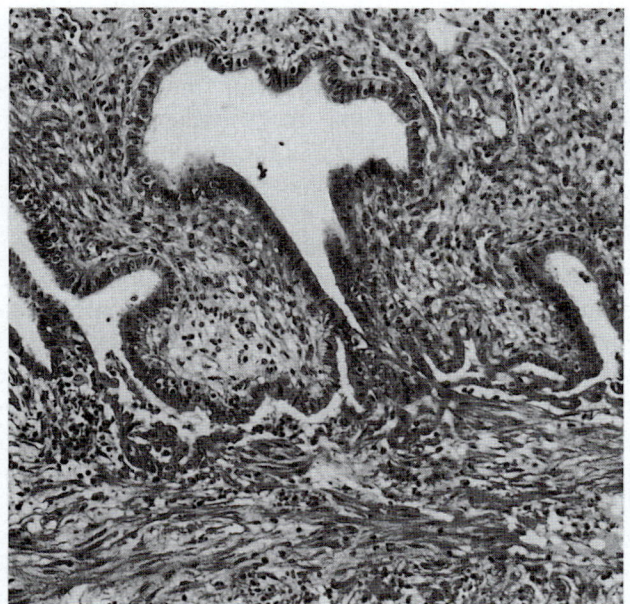

FIG. 36. Fallopian tube prolapsed into vaginal vault. Inflamed tubal glands are associated with smooth muscle bundles.

white, and covered by an intact squamous epithelium. The underlying fibrovascular stroma is loose or dense and contains abundant blood vessels (Fig. 37). Approximately one-half of the cases have atypical stromal cells with large nuclei and abundant cytoplasm. Pleomorphic, hyperchromatic, and

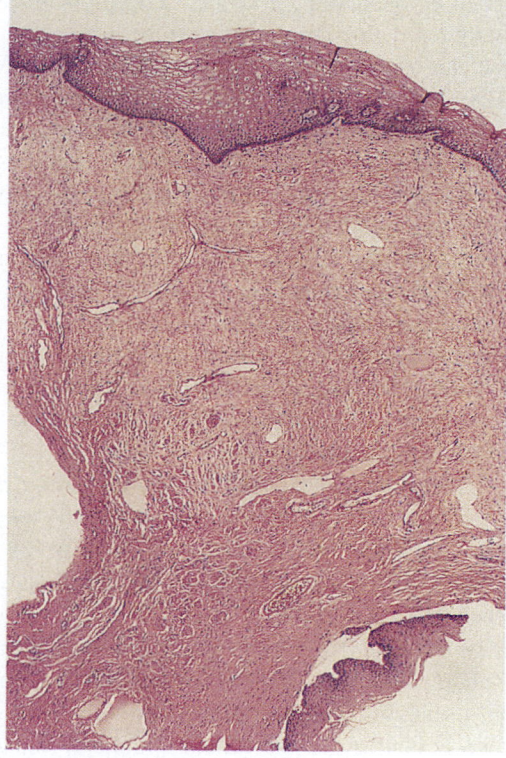

FIG. 37. Vaginal stromal polyp. In this example, dense fibrovascular stroma lies beneath an intact squamous epithelium.

occasionally multiple nuclei sometimes have prominent nucleoli. Mitotic figures are rare, but abnormal mitotic forms have been described (420). Stromal polyp may arise from expansion of the subepithelial stromal zone (116,421). About 12% of women at autopsy have stromal cells with bizarre nuclear features within the vaginal subepithelial stroma (116). Unlike rhabdomyosarcoma (which usually occurs in young children), it lacks rapid growth, invasion of adjacent tissues, hypercellularity, a cambium layer, and cells with cytoplasmic cross-striations. In addition, stromal polyps lack immunoreactivity for myoglobin. In two studies, vimentin was found in 12 of 16 and desmin in 9 of 16 polyps (422,423). Stromal polyp is cured by simple local excision.

Mesonephric papilloma is a very rare polypoid or papillary growth in the vagina or cervix of young girls generally less than 6 years of age (424–426). Loose or dense fibrovascular stroma is lined by nonmucinous cuboid cells. Tall columnar cells and squamous epithelium may be present focally. The papillae vary in size and shape, and the fibrovascular stroma may be infiltrated by neutrophils and lymphocytes. Despite its designation, there is no evidence of mesonephric derivation (426). The reported example of intramural papilloma (427) has some features of mesonephric papilloma, but also has similarities to vaginal mixed tumor.

The vaginal mixed tumor (also known as spindle cell epithelioma) is situated most often just above the hymenal ring in adults (428,429). It presents as a nonencapsulated, well-circumscribed subepithelial nodule that in most instances is not connected to the surface epithelium. Microscopically, the tumor is dissimilar to the usual mixed tumor of salivary gland, skin, or vulva, and lacks myoepithelial differentiation. Vaginal mixed tumor is composed of small spindle cells that surround nests of mature squamous cells and glands lined by mucinous epithelium (Fig. 38). A pseudopapillary arrangement, spindle-shaped cells arranged in fascicles, and hyaline stromal cores may be present. Ultrastructurally and immunohistochemically, the spindle cells have epithelial features (429). The tumor may arise from urogenital sinus-derived epithelium. A reported case of Brenner tumor (430) of the vagina has microscopic features quite similar to vaginal mixed tumor and might be an example of this neoplasm. Recurrence after local excision for vaginal mixed tumor has been reported (431), but complete excision is considered appropriate treatment for this benign neoplasm.

Rare cases of vaginal papillary müllerian cystadenofibroma (432), glomus tumor (433), and paraganglioma (434) have been documented. Benign soft tissue tumors that may arise in the vagina include leiomyoma (136,435), rhabdomyoma (156,436,437), nodular fasciitis (438), hemangioma (136), angiomyolipoma (439), angiomyofibroblastoma (189), granular cell tumor (440), neurofibroma (441), and neurofibroma with rhabdomyomatous differentiation (benign "Triton" tumor) (442). Leiomyoma is the most common vaginal mesodermal neoplasm. The authors of one study of 60 vaginal smooth muscle tumors developed criteria for malignancy that included moderate to marked cytologic atypia

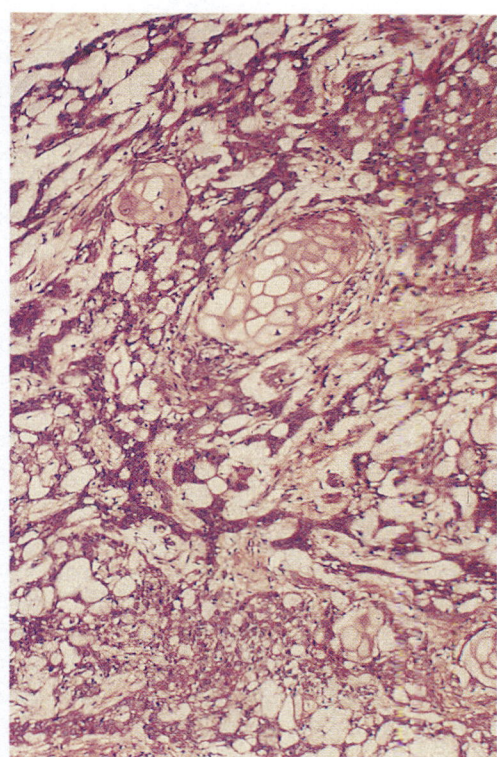

FIG. 38. Mixed tumor of vagina. This neoplasm consists of cords of hematoxylinophilic cells, gland-like spaces, and nests of mature squamous cells.

and at least 5 mitotic figures/10 HPFs (435). Leiomyomas with epithelioid features are very uncommon in the vagina.

Vaginal rhabdomyoma occurs as an asymptomatic polypoid mass in middle-aged women (436,437). The nonencapsulated, poorly circumscribed lesion generally measures less than 3 cm in diameter. Microscopically, it is distinct from both adult and fetal types of rhabdomyoma. Vaginal rhabdomyoma is composed of interlacing oval or spindle-shaped cells having large vesicular nuclei with nucleoli, but lacking overt atypia (Fig. 39). The cells lie in a collagenous or myxoid stroma that contains thin-walled blood vessels. Cells with cytoplasmic cross-striations may be abundant focally, but form only a small proportion of the total population. Large striated muscle cells may be conspicuous. Mitotic figures are generally absent. Skeletal muscle differentiation is evident ultrastructurally (436). The differential diagnosis of rhabdomyoma includes stromal polyp and sarcoma botryoides.

Reactive, postoperative sarcoma-like lesions of the vagina include spindle cell nodule (443) and fibrohistiocytic proliferation (444). Postoperative spindle cell nodule, also found in the urinary tract and elsewhere, measures up to 4 cm in diameter and is usually located at a surgical incision site. Resembling spindle cell sarcoma light microscopically, it is composed of interlacing fascicles of plump spindle cells replacing collagenous stroma and smooth muscle. Nuclei have vesicular chromatin and prominent nucleoli. Mitotic figures are numerous. Unlike in sarcoma, marked nuclear pleomorphism, hyperchromatism, and bizarre mitotic figures are absent. There is a single report of a reactive fibrohistiocytic proliferation that developed postoperatively at the vaginal apex in a woman 5 months after hysterectomy. Microscopically, it consisted of foamy histiocytes, foreign body–type giant cells, polarizable material, and bundles of spindle-shaped cells in a storiform pattern, simulating fibrous histiocytoma.

An incidental finding considered to represent transitional cell metaplasia has been seen in peri- and postmenopausal women, and should not be confused microscopically with intraepithelial neoplasia (445).

Premalignant Conditions and Malignant Neoplasms

Vaginal intraepithelial neoplasia (VAIN) and squamous cell carcinoma are often associated with intraepithelial and invasive squamous neoplasms of the cervix and vulva (446,447) and, also, human papillomavirus. This multicentricity of neoplastic disease represents a "field effect" involving the epithelium of the lower female genital tract. Squamous neoplasms that involve both the cervix and vagina are arbitrarily classified as cervical in origin, and those that involve the vagina and vulva are categorized as vulvar tumors. Criteria for the classification of *in situ* and invasive squamous lesions of the vagina that manifest following cervical *in situ* or invasive squamous tumors, as new, primary vaginal neoplasms are not standardized. Some authors have required more than a 5-year disease-free interval after treatment for cervical squamous cell carcinoma and greater than

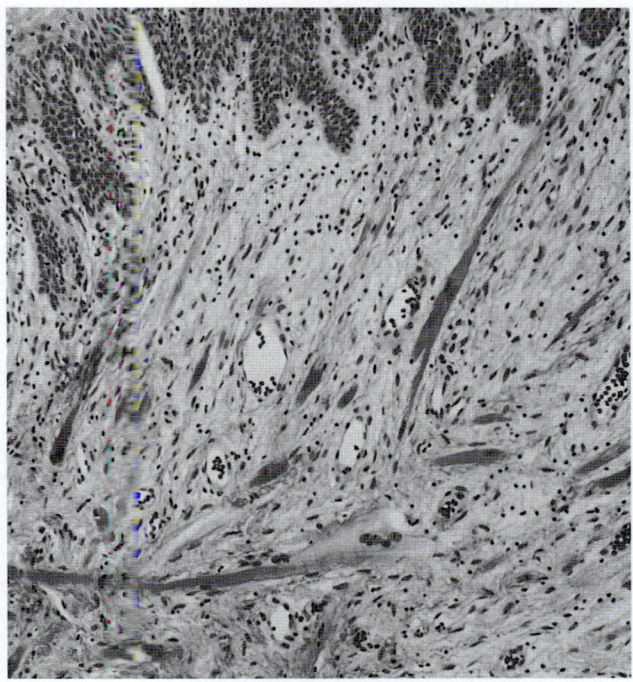

FIG. 39. Vaginal rhabdomyoma. The subepithelial tissue contains abundant long, spindle-shaped cells with dense, eosinophilic cytoplasm. Nuclei have vesicular chromatin, small nucleoli, and lack pleomorphism.

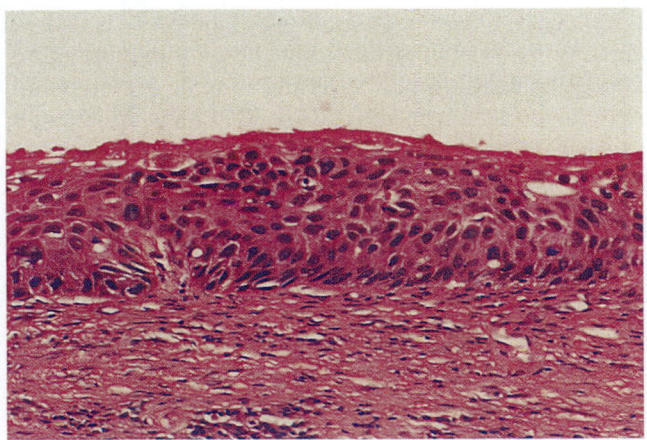

FIG. 40. Vaginal intraepithelial neoplasia, grade III. The criteria for grading squamous intraepithelial neoplasms of the vagina are the same as those for lesions of the cervix.

a 2-year disease-free interval after therapy for cervical intraepithelial neoplasia for a subsequent lesion confined to the vagina to be classified as a new, separate vaginal neoplasm (447). Hence, in situ and invasive squamous cell carcinomas involving the vagina are undoubtedly underclassified as primary vaginal lesions.

VAIN typically occurs in the upper one-third of the vagina. Although the age range is broad, most patients are postmenopausal. Approximately one-third have had prior hysterectomy for benign conditions (446). VAIN is multifocal or diffuse in about one-half of the cases (446,448). The criteria for grading VAIN [I: mild dysplasia; II: moderate dysplasia; III: severe dysplasia/carcinoma in situ (CIS)] are identical to those for grading intraepithelial neoplasia of the cervix (Fig. 40) (449). Morphologic changes of human papillomavirus infection may also be identified in or adjacent to VAIN. In one study of VAIN III, subsequent disease was noted in 12% of patients who had complete excision and 34% who had equivocal or incomplete surgical margins (446). Three of 136 women treated for VAIN III developed invasive squamous cell carcinoma after 10 to 48 months (446). In addition to excision, VAIN has been treated with laser vaporization or topical 5-fluorouracil. Differential diagnostic considerations for VAIN include atrophic squamous epithelium, reactive changes, transitional cell metaplasia, and squamous metaplasia occurring in adenosis.

Squamous cell carcinoma accounts for over 90% of all primary invasive neoplasms of the vagina (450–452). It typically arises in the upper posterior vagina of postmenopausal women. Using the polymerase chain reaction, human papillomavirus DNA (usually type 16) has been found in 8 of 14 invasive neoplasms (108). Occasionally, squamous cell carcinoma develops in young adult women. Rarely, it arises in split-thickness skin grafts created as neovaginas for women with vaginal agenesis (453,454). The TNM staging system for squamous cell carcinoma of the vagina is shown in Table 5 (455). Size of the tumor is not considered in clinical staging. Grossly, squamous cell carcinoma is nodular, ulcerative, indurative, or exophytic. Approximately one-third are keratinizing tumors (450). Adequate current data that compare grade with prognosis are incomplete. The concept of microinvasive squamous cell carcinoma of the vagina recently has been formulated as a means of identifying patients who appear to have a good prognosis and might be treated more conservatively (456). Peters et al. (456) found that six patients who had partial or complete vaginectomy for squamous cancers less than 2.5 mm thick and lacking vascular invasion were all alive without disease (follow-up, 51 to 172 months). In another study, however, one patient with a 0.4-mm-thick squamous cell carcinoma without vascular invasion died of tumor at 35 months (457). A large study is necessary to determine the relationship between thickness and prognosis for women with vaginal carcinoma. Treatment of squamous cell carcinoma is individualized; external beam or implant radiation is often preferred, with surgery reserved

TABLE 5a. *TNM staging system for squamous cell carcinoma of the vagina[a]*

Primary tumor (T)	
TX	Primary tumor cannot be assessed
T0	No evidence of primary tumor
Tis	VAIN III
T1	Tumor confined to vagina
T2	Tumor invades paravaginal tissues, but not to pelvic wall
T3	Tumor extends to pelvic wall
T4	Tumor invades mucosa of bladder or rectum or extends beyond true pelvis
Regional lymph nodes (N)	
NX	Regional lymph nodes cannot be assessed
N0	No regional lymph node metastasis
N1	Pelvic or inguinal lymph node metastasis
Distant metastasis (M)	
MX	Distant metastasis cannot be assessed
M0	No distant metastasis
M1	Distant metastasis

[a]Also includes primary adenocarcinoma of vagina.

TABLE 5b. *TNM stage grouping for vaginal cancer*

Stage 0	Tis	N0	M0
Stage I	T1	N0	M0
Stage II	T2	N0	M0
Stage III	T1	N1	M0
	T2	N1	M0
	T3	N0	M0
	T3	N1	M0
Stage IVA	T4	Any N	M0
Stage IVB	Any T	Any N	M1

for selected cases (449–452). The 5-year survival is largely determined by the clinical stage; typically it is 70% to 75% for stage I tumors and 45% to 50% overall (451,452,458).

Verrucous carcinoma invades on a broad front with a pushing border. There may be extensive local spread, with invasion of the rectum and coccyx (459). Human papillomavirus DNA has been identified in vaginal verrucous cancer (387). Spindle cell carcinoma (squamous cell carcinoma with sarcoma-like stroma) of the vagina has gross and light microscopic features similar to those neoplasms that arise in the upper aerodigestive tract (263). A case of vaginal lymphoepithelioma-like carcinoma has been documented (460).

The association of vaginal and cervical clear cell adenocarcinoma with *in utero* exposure to DES is well known (362,461,462), but up to one-third of patients lack exposure (462). Over 500 cases of vaginal and cervical clear cell adenocarcinoma have been accessioned in the Registry for Research on Hormonal Transplacental Carcinogenesis (461,462). The patients range in age from 7 to 37 years, and the median age is 19 years (461,462). The tumor is distinctly uncommon before age 12 and after age 30. Genetic instability, identified by somatic mutation of microsatellite repeats, has been found in these neoplasms, while mutations in p53, K-*ras,* the Wilms' tumor (WT1) tumor suppressor gene, and the estrogen receptor gene have been absent (453). Grossly,

the neoplasm appears as a polypoid, nodular, flat, or ulcerated mass, usually in the anterior or lateral wall of the upper vagina (464). Rarely, it is confined to the lamina propria with overlying normal squamous epithelium. Clear cell adenocarcinoma varies in size from microscopic to more than 10 cm in diameter (464). Microscopically, about 60% of cervical and vaginal tumors show a predominantly tubulocystic growth pattern (462); 20% have a predominantly solid pattern of growth, and 12% are papillary (462). A mixture of growth patterns is usual (Fig. 41). Solid sheets of tumor are composed of cells with abundant clear cytoplasm. Tubules, cysts, and papillae are lined chiefly by cells that are cuboid, hobnail, or flat. Cords of cells having eosinophilic cytoplasm may also be observed. Nuclear pleomorphism is variable. Flat cells that line dilated cysts often have a bland cytologic appearance (454). Approximately three-fourths of all neoplasms have no more than 1 mitotic figure/10 HPFs (462). Foci of atypical adenosis are usually observed adjacent to the tumor (377). Clear cell adenocarcinoma must not be confused with microglandular hyperplasia (arising in adenosis) and the Arias-Stella phenomenon (377,464). The neoplasm must also be distinguished from endodermal sinus tumor and metastatic renal cell carcinoma. Cells of clear cell adenocarcinoma contain abundant glycogen, but mucin, which may be present in the lumina of tubules, is absent in the cytoplasm. Ultrastructurally, vaginal and cervical clear cell adenocarcinomas are identical to clear cell adenocarcinomas that arise in the ovary or endometrium (465). Intracytoplasmic glycogen and short, blunt surface microvilli are conspicuous features.

The prognosis for cervical or vaginal clear cell adenocarcinoma is related primarily to the tumor stage. The overall actuarial 10-year survival rate is 79% (462). In one study, recurrences developed in almost one-fourth of the patients overall, most of whom died (464). Patients with stage I vaginal tumors have a 90% 10-year actuarial survival rate after therapy (466). When it metastasizes, clear cell adenocarci-

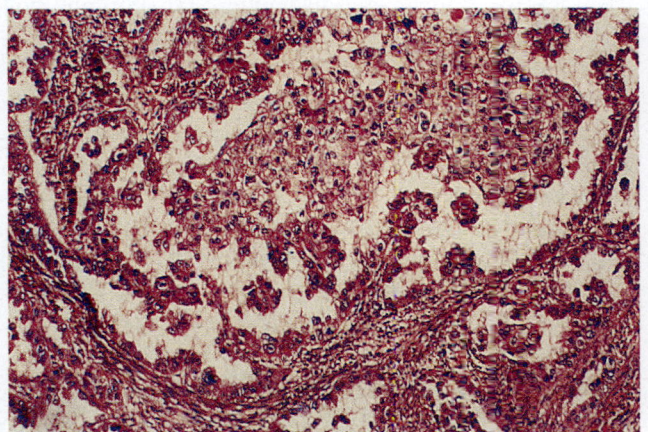 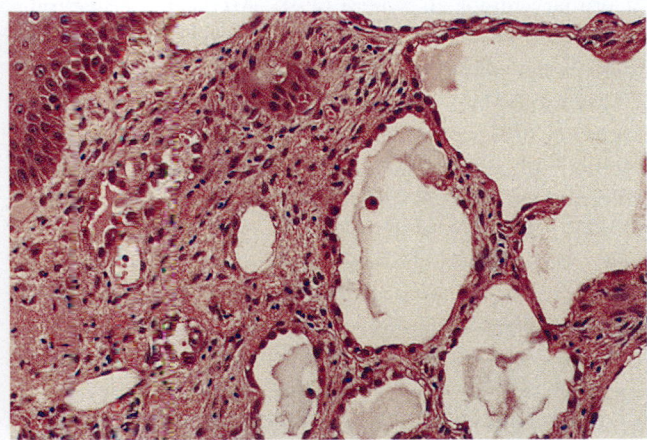

FIG. 41. Clear cell adenocarcinoma. The neoplasm consists of sheets of cells with pleomorphic nuclei and clear cytoplasm and papillae with cells having dense, eosinophilic cytoplasm *(left).* Other lesions are composed of cysts lined by cuboid or flat cells whose nuclei show only mild or moderate pleomorphism *(right).*

noma has a propensity for the pelvis, lungs, and supraclavicular lymph nodes.

Some adenocarcinomas of the vagina are papillary or mucinous, and a few have a squamous component (adenosquamous) (447). Non–clear cell adenocarcinoma (mucin-producing, intestinal-type) originating in vaginal adenosis has been documented in women with and without prior *in utero* exposure to DES (467–469). Intestinal-type adenocarcinoma rarely develops in grafts used to create neovaginas (454). Other enteric type neoplasms (adenocarcinomas and tubulovillous adenomas) may have arisen from cloacal remnants (470). Paravaginal wolffian duct (mesonephric) adenocarcinoma rarely has been described (471). Small cell undifferentiated carcinoma of the vagina usually occurs in postmenopausal women and portends a very poor prognosis (447,472,473); 85% of patients died within 1 year. One of the reported tumors also contained areas of intestinal-type adenocarcinoma (474), while another apparently arose from atypical adenosis (475). Two cases of so-called malignant mixed tumor were composed of epithelial cells arranged in tubules and acini, as well as spindle-shaped cells (476,477). Whether these tumors represent stromal sarcoma with epithelial-like elements (uterine–sex-cord–like tumor), wolffian duct (mesonephric) adenocarcinoma, spindle cell carcinoma, or benign mixed tumor is uncertain. Several examples of sarcomatoid carcinoma (malignant mixed müllerian tumor) have developed following pelvic radiation for cervical carcinoma (478).

Vaginal or paravaginal carcinoma or sarcoma sometimes arises in endometriosis. The rectovaginal septum is the most common extraovarian site for a malignant tumor occurring in endometriosis (479). Neoplasms that have originated in endometriosis of the vagina or rectovaginal septum include endometrioid adenocarcinoma, clear cell adenocarcinoma, and stromal sarcoma (478–482). Criteria promulgated for endometriosis as a source of malignancy include the presence of endometriosis near the neoplasm, histology consistent with origin from endometrial glands or stroma, and absence of a primary tumor elsewhere (479). Atypical endometrial glands, when present, provide further support for origin of carcinoma in endometriosis.

Endodermal sinus tumor of the vagina occurs in girls 3 years of age or less (483). Grossly, the neoplasm is sessile or polypoid, with areas of ulceration. On cut section, it is soft, friable, and tan-white, with areas of hemorrhage and necrosis (484). Clinically, it may simulate sarcoma botryoides. Vaginal endodermal sinus tumor is microscopically identical to pure yolk sac tumors of the ovary and testis (Fig. 42) (484). The prognosis has improved greatly since the addition of chemotherapy (483–485). Local excision plus chemotherapy appears to be the optimal treatment. Since 1970, 26 of 38 patients have survived (median follow-up, 46 months) (485).

Vaginal melanoma presents as an ulcerated, blue or black polypoid nodule most frequently in the lower one-third of the vagina of postmenopausal white women (486). The neoplasm tends to be large, as the median diameter in one series

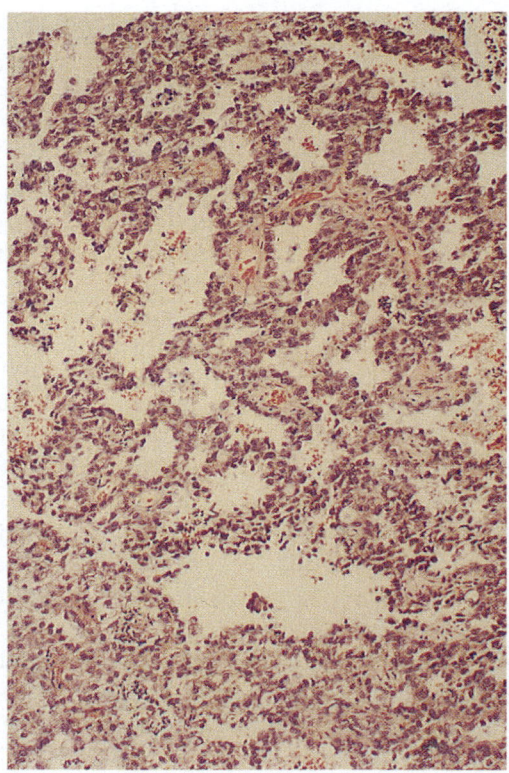

FIG. 42. Endodermal sinus tumor. Schiller-Duval bodies are not always well formed. This neoplasm occurred in a 13-month-old girl.

was 3 cm (413). Junctional activity may be extensive. Sometimes the neoplasm consists of pleomorphic cells, spindle-shaped cells, or small cells (413,486). In such instances, the differential diagnosis includes a variety of other highly malignant neoplasms. The 5-year survival rate for women with vaginal melanoma, based on a literature summary, is a dismal 7% (487).

Non-Hodgkin's lymphoma and granulocytic sarcoma (80,488) may involve the vagina as a part of widespread disease. Rarely, primary plasmacytoma (316,489) and non-Hodgkin's lymphoma (490,491) arise in the vagina. Diffuse, large-cell lymphoma appears to be the predominant subtype of vaginal lymphoma, although nodular lymphoma has also been described. Langerhans cell histiocytosis is usually found in conjunction with other genital tract or extragenital involvement (318).

A variety of sarcomas have arisen in the vagina or paravaginally (Table 6) (435,478,492–502). Leiomyosarcoma is by far the most frequent in adults; criteria for its distinction from leiomyoma are discussed under miscellaneous benign conditions of the vagina (Fig. 43) (435).

Vaginal embryonal rhabdomyosarcoma is found chiefly in infants or children up to 6 years of age (median age, 1.8 years) (492). The neoplasm often arises from the anterior vaginal wall and presents as soft botryoid nodules that fill and often protrude out of the vagina. On cut section, the smooth-surfaced nodules appear gray-white or hemorrhagic.

TABLE 6. *Primary sarcomas of the vagina*

Sarcoma	Reference
Rhabdomyosarcoma	492,494
Leiomyosarcoma	435,473,493,494
Malignant fibrous histiocytoma	496
Hemangiopericytoma	497,498
Malignant schwannoma	478,494
Endometrial stromal sarcoma	478,494,499
Fibrosarcoma	495
Alveolar soft part sarcoma	500,501
Angiosarcoma	502

Microscopically, small, round, or spindle-shaped cells with scanty cytoplasm are embedded in a myxoid stroma. A subepithelial condensation of malignant cells (cambium layer) and rhabdomyoblasts are observed. Cross-striations may be identified, sometimes after prolonged examination. Electron microscopy or immunohistochemical stains for muscle proteins in general (muscle actins, desmin) or skeletal muscle (myoglobin) may be a valuable diagnostic adjunct. The prognosis for patients with vaginal rhabdomyosarcoma has improved due to a multimodal therapeutic approach. Because of the effectiveness of chemotherapeutic agents, primary pelvic exenteration can be avoided. Only one tumor-related death was found among 24 evaluable children who were admitted to the Intergroup Rhabdomyosarcoma Study (492).

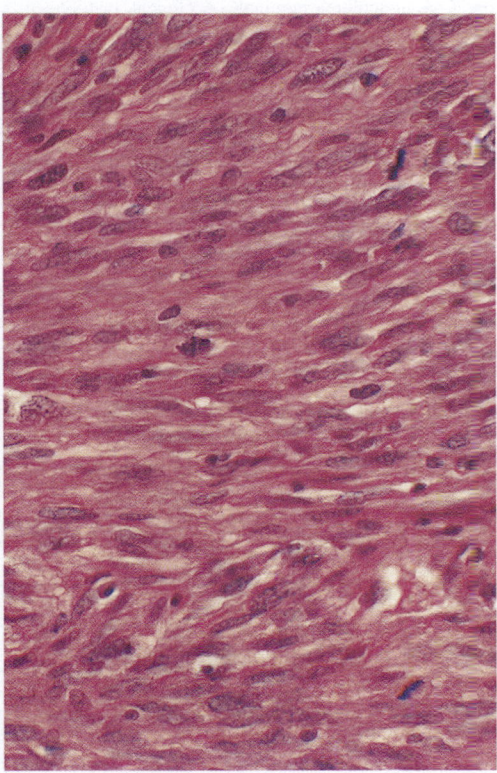

FIG. 43. Leiomyosarcoma. Malignant smooth muscle tumors of the vagina have at least moderate cytologic atypia and 5 or more mitotic figures per 10 high-power fields.

Malignant neoplasms that involve the vagina by local extension or recurrence include carcinomas of the cervix, vulva, bladder, urethra, and rectum. Very rarely, patients with a history of treatment for noninvasive papillary transitional cell carcinoma of the urinary tract develop multiple identical papillary tumors of the vagina (503). Tumors that sometimes metastasize to the vagina include carcinomas of the endometrium (504), ovary (505), kidney (506), and breast (507). Following primary therapy, approximately 9% of patients with endometrial adenocarcinoma develop vaginal recurrences, two-thirds of which are solitary (504). The recurrences may be small and resemble granulation tissue clinically. In an autopsy study of 86 women with advanced ovarian cancer, 12% had vaginal involvement (505). Gestational choriocarcinoma metastasizes to the vagina in about one-fourth of cases (407,508,509). Over 90% of choriocarcinomas metastatic to the vagina are found in the lower portion, most often in the anterior wall beneath the urethra or at the urethral orifice (508). The majority of renal cell carcinomas metastatic to the vagina arise from the left kidney, suggesting a retrograde venous route via the ovarian vein and vaginal venous plexuses. The initial presentation may be as a nodule in the vagina (506). Renal cell carcinoma is distinguishable from primary vaginal clear cell adenocarcinoma light microscopically and ultrastructurally.

REFERENCES

Vulva

1. van der Putte SCJ. Anogenital "sweat" glands. Histology and pathology of a gland that may mimic mammary glands. *Am J Dermatopathol* 1991;13:557–567.
2. van der Putte SCJ. Mammary-like glands of the vulva and their disorders. *Int J Gynecol Pathol* 1994;13:150–160.
3. Rorat E, Ferenczy A, Richart RM. Human Bartholin gland, duct, and duct cyst. Histochemical and ultrastructural study. *Arch Pathol Lab Med* 1975;99:367–374.
4. Robboy SJ, Ross JS, Prat J, Keh PC, Welch WR. Urogenital sinus origin of mucinous and ciliated cysts of the vulva. *Obstet Gynecol* 1978;51:347–351.
5. Huffman JW. The detailed anatomy of the paraurethral ducts in the adult human female. *Am J Obstet Gynecol* 1948;55:86–101.
6. Lawrence WD. Non-neoplastic epithelial disorders of the vulva (vulvar dystrophies) historical and current perspectives. *Pathol Annu* 1993;28(part 2):23–51.
7. Plentl AA, Friedman EA. *Lymphatic system of the female genitalia. The morphologic basis of oncologic diagnosis and therapy.* Philadelphia: WB Saunders, 1971:15–26, 51–56.
8. Iversen T, Aas M. Lymph drainage from the vulva. *Gynecol Oncol* 1983;16:179–189.
9. Way S. *Malignant disease of the vulva.* Edinburgh: Churchill Livingstone, 1982:13–19.
10. Eichner E. Vulvar carcinoma. *Am J Obstet Gynecol* 1961;81:1280.
11. Simpson JL. Genetic aspects of gynecologic disorders occurring in 46,XX individuals. *Clin Obstet Gynecol* 1972;15:157–182.
12. Shaw RW, Farquhar JW. Female pseudohermaphroditism associated with danazol exposure in utero. Case report. *Br J Obstet Gynaecol* 1984;91:336–389.
13. Kingsbury AC. Danazol and fetal masculinization: a warning. *Med J Aust* 1985;143:410–411.
14. Wilkins L, Jones HW Jr, Holman GH, Stempfel RS Jr. Masculinization of the female fetus associated with administration of oral and intramuscular progestins during gestation: non-adrenal female pseudohermaphrodism. *J Clin Endocrinol Metab* 1958;18:559–585.

15. Wilkins L. Masculinization of female fetus due to use of orally given progestins. *JAMA* 1960;172:1028–1032.
16. Malinak LR, Miller GV. Bilateral multicentric ovarian luteomas of pregnancy associated with masculinization of a female infant. *Am J Obstet Gynecol* 1965;91:251–259.
17. Jenkins ME, Surana RB, Russell-Cutts CM. Ambiguous genitals in a female infant associated with luteoma of pregnancy. Report of a case. *Am J Obstet Gynecol* 1968;101:923–928.
18. Verkauf BS, Reiter EO, Hernandez L, Burns SA. Virilization of mother and fetus associated with luteoma of pregnancy: a case report with endocrinologic studies. *Am J Obstet Gynecol* 1977;129:274–280.
19. Fox LP, Stamm WJ. Krukenberg tumor complicating pregnancy. Report of a case with androgenic activity. *Am J Obstet Gynecol* 1965;92:702–710.
20. Spadoni LR, Lindberg MC, Mottet NK, Herrmann WL. Virilization coexisting with Krukenberg tumor during pregnancy. *Am J Obstet Gynecol* 1965;92:981–991.
21. Connor TB, Ganis FM, Levin HS, Migeon CJ, Martin LG. Gonadotropin-dependent Krukenberg tumor causing virilization during pregnancy. *J Clin Endocrinol Metab* 1968;28:198–214.
22. Bell RJM. Fetal virilisation due to maternal Krukenberg tumour. *Lancet* 1977;1:1162–1163.
23. Brentnall CP. A case of arrhenoblastoma complicating pregnancy. *Br J Obstet Gynaecol* 1945;52:235–240.
24. Murset G, Zachmann M, Prader A, Fischer J, Labhart A. Male external genitalia of a girl caused by a virilizing adrenal tumour in the mother. Case report and steroid studies. *Acta Endocrinol* 1970;65:627–638.
25. Fuller PJ, Pettigrew IG, Pike JW, Stockigt JR. An adrenal adenoma causing virilization of mother and infant. *Clin Endocrinol* 1983;18:143–153.
26. van de Kamp JJP, van Seters AP, Moolenaar AJ, van Gelderen HH. Female pseudo-hermaphroditism due to an adrenal tumour in the mother. *Eur J Pediatr* 1984;142:140–142.
27. Kai H, Nose O, Iida Y, Ono J, Harada T, Yabuuchi H. Female pseudohermaphroditism caused by maternal congenital adrenal hyperplasia. *J Pediatr* 1979;95:418–420.
28. Dewhurst CJ. Congenital malformations of the genital tract in childhood. *Br J Obstet Gynaecol* 1968;75:377–391.
29. Lubinsky MS. Female pseudohermaphroditism and associated anomalies. *Am J Med Genet* 1980;6:123–136.
30. Hendren WH. Cloacal malformations: experience with 105 cases. *J Pediatr Surg* 1992;27:890–901.
31. Radman HM. Hypertrophy of the labia minora. *Obstet Gynecol* 1976;48:78s–80s.
32. So EP, Brock W, Kaplan GW. Ectopic labium and VATER association in a newborn. *J Urol* 1980;124:156–157.
33. Capraro VJ, Dillon WP, Gallego MB. Microperforate hymen. A distinct clinical entity. *Obstet Gynecol* 1974;44:903–905.
34. Nesbitt REL Jr, Abdul-Karim RW. Persistent urogenital membrane sinus as a clinical entity. *JAMA* 1968;205:91–94.
35. Roceretto TF, Campbell WA III. Ureterocele presenting as a perineal cyst. *Obstet Gynecol* 1980;55:54s–56s.
36. Yeoh G, Bannatyne P, Kossard S, Russell P. Intestinal heterotopia: an unusual cause of vulval ulceration. Case report. *Br J Obstet Gynaecol* 1987;94:600–602.

Cysts

37. Kaufman RH, Friedrich EG Jr, Gardner HL. Cystic tumors. In: Kaufman RH, Friedrich EG Jr, Gardner HL, eds. *Benign diseases of the vulva and vagina*, 3rd ed. Chicago: Year Book Medical, 1989:237–285.
38. Zivkovic SM. Epidermoid cyst of anterior commissure of labia majora and separated pubic bones. *Urology* 1981;17:467–468.
39. Onuigbo WIB. Vulval epidermoid cysts in the Igbos of Nigeria. *Arch Dermatol* 1976;112:1405–1406.
40. Betson JR Jr, Chiffelle TL, George RP. Pilonidal sinus involving the clitoris. A case report. *Am J Obstet Gynecol* 1962;84:543–545.
41. Kimbrough HM Jr, Vaughan ED Jr. Skene's duct cyst in a newborn: case report and review of the literature. *J Urol* 1977;117:387–388.
42. Blaivas JG, Pais VM, Retik AB. Paraurethral cysts in female neonate. *Urology* 1976;7:504–507.
43. Merlob P, Bahari C, Liban E, Reisner SH. Cysts of the female external genitalia in the newborn infant. *Am J Obstet Gynecol* 1978;132:607–610.
44. Kucera PR, Glazer J. Hydrocele of the canal of Nuck. A report of four cases. *J Reprod Med* 1985;30:439–442.
45. Block RE. Hydrocele of the canal of Nuck. A report of five cases. *Obstet Gynecol* 1975;45:464–466.
46. Hart WR. Paramesonephric mucinous cysts of the vulva. *Am J Obstet Gynecol* 1970;107:1079–1084.
47. Friedrich EG Jr, Wilkinson EJ. Mucous cysts of the vulvar vestibule. *Obstet Gynecol* 1973;42:407–414.
48. Oi RH, Munn R. Mucous cysts of the vulvar vestibule. *Hum Pathol* 1982;13:584–586.
49. Enghardt MH, Valente PT, Day DH. Papilloma of Bartholin's gland duct cyst: first report of a case. *Int J Gynecol Pathol* 1993;12:86–92.
50. Freedman SR, Goldman RL. Mucocele-like changes in Bartholin's glands. *Hum Pathol* 1978;9:111–114.
51. Shelley WB, Levy EJ. Apocrine sweat retention in man. II. Fox-Fordyce disease (apocrine miliaria). *Arch Dermatol* 1956;73:38–49.
52. Paull T, Tedeschi LG. Perineal endometriosis at the site of episiotomy scar. *Obstet Gynecol* 1972;40:28–34.
53. van der Putte SCJ, van Gorp LHM. Cysts of mammarylike glands in the vulva. *Int J Gynecol Pathol* 1995;14:184–188.

Infectious Diseases

Bacteria

54. Lynch PJ. Sexually transmitted diseases: granuloma inguinale, lymphogranuloma venereum, chancroid, and infectious syphilis. *Clin Obstet Gynecol* 1978;21:1041–1052.
55. Beckett JH, Bigbee JW. Immunoperoxidase localization of Treponema pallidum. *Arch Pathol Lab Med* 1979;103:135–138.
56. Lee YH, Rankin JS, Alpert S, Daly AK, McCormack WM. Microbiological investigation of Bartholin's gland abscesses and cysts. *Am J Obstet Gynecol* 1977;129:150–153.
57. Kuberski T. Granuloma inguinale (Donovanosis). *Sex Transm Dis* 1980;7:29–36.
58. Davis CM. Granuloma inguinale. A clinical, histological, and ultrastructural study. *JAMA* 1970;211:632–636.
59. de Boer Al, de Boer F, Van der Merwe JV. Cytologic identification of Donovan bodies in granuloma inguinale. *Acta Cytol* 1984;28:126–128.
60. Alexander LJ, Shields TL. Squamous cell carcinoma of the vulva secondary to granuloma inguinale. *Arch Dermatol* 1953;67:395–402.
61. Saltzstein SL, Woodruff JD, Novak, ER. Postgranulomatous carcinoma of the vulva. *Obstet Gynecol* 1956;7:80–90.
62. Margolis RJ, Hood AF. Chancroid: diagnosis and treatment. *J Am Acad Dermatol* 1982;6:493–499.
63. Werman BS, Herskowitz LJ, Olansky S, Kleris G, Sottnek FO. A clinical variant of chancroid resembling granuloma inguinale. *Arch Dermatol* 1983;119:890–894.
64. Brenner BN. Tuberculosis of the vulva. Case reports. *S Afr Med J* 1976;50:1798–1800.
65. Millar JW, Holt S, Gilmour HM, Robertson DHH. Vulval tuberculosis. *Tubercle* 1979;60:173–176.
66. Friedrich EG Jr. *Vulvar disease*, 2nd ed. Philadelphia: WB Saunders, 1983:126.
67. Addison WA, Livengood CH III, Hill GB, Sutton GP, Fortier KJ. Necrotizing fasciitis of vulvar origin in diabetic patients. *Obstet Gynecol* 1984;63:473–479.
68. Roberts DB. Necrotizing fasciitis of the vulva. *Am J Obstet Gynecol* 1987;157:568–571.
69. Thomas R, Barnhill D, Bibro M, Hoskins W. Hidradenitis suppurativa: a case presentation and review of the literature. *Obstet Gynecol* 1985;66:592–595.
70. Bhatia NN, Bergman A, Broen EM. Advanced hidradenitis suppurativa of the vulva. A report of three cases. *J Reprod Med* 1984;29:436–440.
71. Long SR, Whitfeld MJ, Eades C, Koehler JE, Korn AP, Zaloudek CJ. Bacillary angiomatosis of the cervix and vulva in a patient with AIDS. *Obstet Gynecol* 1996;88:709–711.

Chlamydia

72. Winkler B, Crum CP. Chlamydia trachomatis infection of the female genital tract. Pathogenetic and clinicopathologic correlations. *Pathol Annu* 1987;22:193–223.
73. Hadfield TL, Lamy Y, Wear DJ. Demonstration of chlamydia trachomatis in inguinal lymphadenitis of lymphogranuloma venereum: a light microscopy, electron microscopy and polymerase chain reaction study. *Mod Pathol* 1995;8:924–929.
74. Davies JA, Rees E, Hobson D, Karayiannis P. Isolation of Chlamydia trachomatis from Bartholin's ducts. *Br J Vener Dis* 1978;54:409–413.

Viruses

75. Kawana T, Kawagoe K, Takizawa K, Chen T, Kawaguchi T, Sakamoto S. Clinical and virologic studies of female genital herpes. *Obstet Gynecol* 1982;60:456–461.
76. Brown D. Herpes zoster of the vulva. *Clin Obstet Gynecol* 1972;15:1010–1014.
77. Sites CK, Sherer DM, Gandell DL, Woods JR Jr. Extensive vulvar and vaginal varicella necessitating abdominal delivery. *Am J Obstet Gynecol* 1990;163:1630–1631.
78. Humphrey DC. Localized accidental vaccinia of the vulva. Report of three cases and a review of the world literature. *Am J Obstet Gynecol* 1963;86:460–469.
79. Portnoy J, Ahronheim GA, Ghibu F, Clecner B, Joncas JH. Recovery of Epstein-Barr virus from genital ulcers. *N Engl J Med* 1984;311:966–968.
80. Ferry JA, Young RH. Malignant lymphoma, pseudolymphoma, and hematopoietic disorders of the female genital tract. *Pathol Annu* 1991;26:227–263.
81. LaGuardia KD, White MH, Saigo PE, Hoda S, McGuinness K, Ledger WJ. Genital ulcer disease in women infected with human immunodeficiency virus. *Am J Obstet Gynecol* 1995;172:553–562.
82. Growdon WA, Fu YS, Lebherz TB, Rapkin A, Mason GD, Parks G. Pruritic vulvar squamous papillomatosis: evidence for human papillomavirus etiology. *Obstet Gynecol* 1985;66:564–568.
83. Costa S, Rotola A, Terzano P, et al. Is vestibular papillomatosis associated with human papillomavirus? *J Med Virol* 1991;35:7–13.
84. Moyal-Barracco M, Leibowitch M, Orth G. Vestibular papillae of the vulva. Lack of evidence for human papillomavirus etiology. *Arch Dermatol* 1990;126:1594–1598.
85. de Deus JM, Focchi J, Stavale JN, de Lima GR. Histologic and biomolecular aspects of papillomatosis of the vulvar vestibule in relation to human papillomavirus. *Obstet Gynecol* 1995;86:758–763.
86. Bergeron C, Ferenczy A, Richart RM, Guralnick M. Micropapillomatosis labialis appears unrelated to human papillomavirus. *Obstet Gynecol* 1990;76:281–286.
87. Potkul RK, Lancaster WD, Kurman RJ, Lewandowski G, Weck PK, Delgado G. Vulvar condylomas and squamous vestibular micropapilloma. Differences in appearance and response to treatment. *J Reprod Med* 1990;35:1019–1022.
88. Ferenczy A, Mitao M, Nagai N, Silverstein SJ, Crum CP. Latent papillomavirus and recurring genital warts. *N Engl J Med* 1985;313:784–788.
89. Crum CP, Braun LA, Shah KV, et al. Vulvar intraepithelial neoplasia: correlation of nuclear DNA content and the presence of a human papilloma virus (HPV) structural antigen. *Cancer* 1982;49:468–471.
90. McLachlin CM, Mutter GL, Crum CP. Multinucleated atypia of the vulva. Report of a distinct entity not associated with human papillomavirus. *Am J Surg Pathol* 1994;18:1233–1239.
91. Wade TR, Ackerman AB. The effects of resin of podophyllin on condyloma acuminatum. *Am J Dermatopathol* 1984;6:109–122.
92. Nuovo GJ, O'Connell M, Blanco JS, Levine RU, Silverstein SJ. Correlation of histology and human papillomavirus DNA detection in condyloma acuminatum and condyloma-like vulvar lesions. *Am J Surg Pathol* 1989;13:700–706.
93. McLachlin CM, Kozakewich H, Craighill M, O'Connell B, Crum CP. Histologic correlates of vulvar human papillomavirus infection in children and young adults. *Am J Surg Pathol* 1994;18:728–735.
94. Crum CP, Fu YS, Levine RU, Richart RM, Townsend DE, Fenoglio CM. Intraepithelial squamous lesions of the vulva: biologic and histologic criteria for the distinction of condylomas from vulvar intraepithelial neoplasia. *Am J Obstet Gynecol* 1982;144:77–83.
95. Friedrich EG Jr, Wilkinson EJ, Fu YS. Carcinoma in situ of the vulva: a continuing challenge. *Am J Obstet Gynecol* 1980;136:830–843.
96. Ehrmann RM, Saffos RO. Condyloma acuminatum and squamous carcinoma of the vulva. *South Med J* 1977;70:591–594.
97. Shafeek MA, Osman MI, Hussein MA. Carcinoma of the vulva arising in condylomata acuminata. *Obstet Gynecol* 1979;54:120–123.
98. Gupta J, Pilotti S, Rilke F, Shah K. Association of human papillomavirus type 16 with neoplastic lesions of the vulva and other genital sites by in situ hybridization. *Am J Pathol* 1987;127:206–215.
99. Pilotti S, Rilke F, Shah KV, Delle Torre G, De Palo G. Immunohistochemical and ultrastructural evidence of papilloma virus infection associated with in situ and microinvasive squamous cell carcinoma of the vulva. *Am J Surg Pathol* 1984;8:751–761.
100. Gissmann L, de Villiers EM, zur Hausen H. Analysis of human genital warts (condylomata acuminata) and other genital tumors for human papillomavirus type 6 DNA. *Int J Cancer* 1982;29:143–146.
101. Rando RF, Sedlacek TV, Hunt J, Jenson AB, Kurman RJ, Lancaster WD. Verrucous carcinoma of the vulva associated with an unusual type of human papillomavirus. *Obstet Gynecol* 1986;67:70s–75s.
102. Durst M, Gissmann L, Ikenberg H, zur Hausen H. A papillomavirus DNA from a cervical carcinoma and its prevalence in cancer biopsy samples from different geographic regions. *Proc Natl Acad Sci USA* 1983;80:3812–3815.
103. Gissmann L, Wolnik L, Ikenberg H, Koldovsky U, Schnurch HG, zur Hausen H. Human papillomavirus types 6 and 11 DNA sequences in genital and laryngeal papillomas and in some cervical cancers. *Proc Natl Acad Sci USA* 1983;80:560–563.
104. Ikenberg H, Gissmann L, Gross G, Grussendorf-Conen EI, zur Hausen H. Human papillomavirus type-16-related DNA in genital Bowen's disease and in bowenoid papulosis. *Int J Cancer* 1983;32:563–565.
105. Gross G, Hagedorn M, Ikenberg H, et al. Bowenoid papulosis. Presence of human papillomavirus (HPV) structural antigens and of HPV 6-related DNA sequences. *Arch Dermatol* 1985;121:858–863.
106. Buscema J, Naghashfar Z, Sawada E, Daniel R, Woodruff JD, Shah K. The predominance of human papillomavirus type 16 in vulvar neoplasia. *Obstet Gynecol* 1988;71:601–606.
107. Park JS, Jones RW, McLean MR, et al. Possible etiologic heterogeneity of vulvar intraepithelial neoplasia. A correlation of pathologic characteristics with human papillomavirus detection by in situ hybridization and polymerase chain reaction. *Cancer* 1991;67:1599–1607.
108. Kiyabu MT, Shibata D, Arnheim N, Martin WJ, Fitzgibbons PL. Detection of human papillomavirus in formalin-fixed, invasive squamous carcinomas using the polymerase chain reaction. *Am J Surg Pathol* 1989;13:221–224.
109. Bloss JD, Liao S-Y, Wilczynski SP, et al. Clinical and histologic features of vulvar carcinomas analyzed for human papillomavirus status: evidence that squamous cell carcinoma of the vulva has more than one etiology. *Hum Pathol* 1991;22:711–718.
110. Lynch PJ. Molluscum contagiosum venereum. *Clin Obstet Gynecol* 1972;15:966–975.
111. Reed RJ, Parkinson RP. The histogenesis of molluscum contagiosum. *Am J Surg Pathol* 1977;1:161–166.

Fungi and Parasites

112. Kaufman RH, Friedrich EG Jr, Gardner HL, eds. Candida. In: *Benign diseases of the vulva and vagina*, 3rd ed. Chicago: Year Book Medical 1989:361–381.
113. Scott RA, Gallis HA, Livengood CH. Phycomycosis of the vulva. *Am J Obstet Gynecol* 1985;153:675–676.
114. McKee PH, Wright E, Hutt MSR. Vulval schistosomiasis. *Clin Exp Dermatol* 1983;8:189–194.

Miscellaneous Benign Lesions

115. Ostor AG, Fortune DW, Riley CB. Fibroepithelial polyps with atypical stromal cells (pseudosarcoma botryoides) of vulva and vagina. A report of 13 cases. *Int J Gynecol Pathol* 1988;7:351–360.
116. Abdul-Karim FW, Cohen RE. Atypical stromal cells of lower female genital tract. *Histopathology* 1990;17:249–253.
117. Santa Cruz DJ, Martin SA. Verruciform xanthoma of the vulva. Report of two cases. *Am J Clin Pathol* 1979;71:224–228.

118. Rocamora A, Santonja C, Vives R, Varona C. Sebaceous gland hyperplasia of the vulva: a case report. *Obstet Gynecol* 1986;68:63s–65s.
119. Axe S, Parmley T, Woodruff JD, Hlopak B. Adenomas in minor vestibular glands. *Obstet Gynecol* 1986;68:16–18.
120. Prayson RA, Stoler MH, Hart WR. Vulvar vestibulitis. A histopathologic study of 36 cases, including human papillomavirus in situ hybridization analysis. *Am J Surg Pathol* 1995;19:154–160.
121. Buchler DA, Sun F, Chuprevich T. Case report. A pilar tumor of the vulva. *Gynecol Oncol* 1978;6:479–486.
122. De Coninck A, Willemsen M, de Dobbeleer G, Roseeuw D. Vulvar localization of epidermolytic acanthoma. A light- and electron-microscopic study. *Dermatologica* 1986;172:276–278.
123. Rhatigen RM, Nuss RC. Keratoacanthoma of the vulva. *Gynecol Oncol* 1985;21:118–123.
124. Barnhill RL, Albert LS, Shama SK, Goldenhersh MA, Rhodes AR, Sober AJ. Genital lentiginosis: a clinical and histopathologic study. *J Am Acad Dermatol* 1990;22:453–460.
125. Rock B, Hood AF, Rock JA. Prospective study of vulvar nevi. *J Am Acad Dermatol* 1990;22:104–106.
126. Friedman RJ, Ackerman AB. Difficulties in the histologic diagnosis of melanocytic nevi in the vulvae of premenopausal women. In: Ackerman AB, ed. *Pathology of malignant melanoma*. New York: Masson, 1981:119–127.
127. Christensen WN, Friedman KJ, Woodruff JD, Hood AF. Histologic characteristics of vulvar nevocellular nevi. *J Cutan Pathol* 1987;14:87–91.
128. Pyka RE, Wilkinson EJ, Friedrich EG Jr, Croker BP. The histopathology of vulvar vestibulitis syndrome. *Int J Gynecol Pathol* 1988;7:249–257.
129. Wilkinson EJ, Guerrero E, Daniel R, et al. Vulvar vestibulitis is rarely associated with human papillomavirus infection types 6, 11, 16, or 18. *Int J Gynecol Pathol* 1993;12:344–349.
130. Ambros RA, Malfetano JH, Carlson JA, Mihm MC Jr. Non-neoplastic epithelial alterations of the vulva: recognition assessment and comparisons of terminologies used among the various specialties. *Mod Pathol* 1997;10:401–408.
131. Edwards L, Hansen RC. Reiter's syndrome of the vulva. The psoriasis spectrum. *Arch Dermatol* 1992;128:811–814.
132. Dodson MG, Klegerman ME, Kerman RH, Lange CF, Tressler HH, O'Leary JA. Behcet syndrome. With immunologic evaluation. *Obstet Gynecol* 1978;51:621–625.
133. Davis J, Shapiro L, Baral J. Vulvitis circumscripta plasmacellularis. *J Am Acad Dermatol* 1983;8:413–416.
134. Scurry J, Dennerstein G, Brenan J, Ostor A, Mason G, Dorevitch A. Vulvitis circumscripta plasmacellularis. A clinicopathologic entity? *J Reprod Med* 1993;38:14–18.
135. Yoganathan S, Bohl TG, Mason G. Plasma cell balanitis and vulvitis (of Zoon). A study of 10 cases. *J Reprod Med* 1994;39:939–944.
136. Kaufman RH, Gardner HL. Benign mesodermal tumors. *Clin Obstet Gynecol* 1965;8:953–981.
137. Kempson RL, Sherman AI. Sclerosing lipogranuloma of the vulva. *Am J Obstet Gynecol* 1968;101:854–856.
138. Nielsen GP, Rosenberg AE, Koerner FC, Young RH, Scully RE. Smooth-muscle tumors of the vulva. A clinicopathological study of 25 cases and review of the literature. *Am J Surg Pathol* 1996;20:779–793.
139. Tavassoli F, Norris HJ. Smooth muscle tumors of the vulva. *Obstet Gynecol* 1979;53:213–217.
140. Aneiros J, Beltran E, Garcia del Moral R, Nogales FF Jr. Epithelioid leiomyoma of the vulva. *Diagn Gynecol Obstet* 1982;4:351–355.
141. Faber K, Jones MA, Spratt D, Tarraza HM, Jr. Vulvar leiomyomatosis in a patient with esophagogastric leiomyomatosis: review of the syndrome. *Gynecol Oncol* 1991;41:92–94.
142. Siegler RW, Rothstein RI, Beecham JB, Dunn JL. Gastroesophageal-vulvar leiomyomatosis presenting over the course of 20 years. *Arch Pathol Lab Med* 1996;120:1141–1144.
143. Messina AM, Strauss RG. Pelvic neurofibromatosis. *Obstet Gynecol* 1976;47:63s–66s.
144. Schreiber MM. Vulvar von Recklinghausen's disease. *Arch Dermatol* 1963;88:320–321.
145. Gersell DJ, Fulling KH. Localized neurofibromatosis of the female genitourinary tract. *Am J Surg Pathol* 1989;13:873–878.
146. Huang HJ, Yamabe T, Tagawa H. A solitary neurilemmoma of the clitoris. *Gynecol Oncol* 1983;15:103–110.
147. White W, Shiu MH, Rosenblum MK, Erlandson RA, Woodruff JM. Cellular schwannoma. A clinicopathologic study of 57 patients and 58 tumors. *Cancer* 1990;66:1266–1275.
148. Woodruff JM, Marshall ML, Godwin TA, Funkhouser JW, Thompson NJ, Erlandson RA. Plexiform (multinodular) schwannoma. A tumor simulating the plexiform neurofibroma. *Am J Surg Pathol* 1983;7:691–697.
149. Colgan TJ, Dardick I, O'Connell G. Paraganglioma of the vulva. *Int J Gynecol Pathol* 1991;10:203–208.
150. Wolber RA, Talerman A, Wilkinson EJ, Clement PB. Vulvar granular cell tumors with pseudocarcinomatous hyperplasia: a comparative analysis with well-differentiated squamous carcinoma. *Int J Gynecol Pathol* 1991;10:59–66.
151. Slavin RE, Christie JD, Swedo J, Powell LC Jr. Locally aggressive granular cell tumor causing priapism of the crus of the clitoris. A light and ultrastructural study, with observations concerning the pathogenesis of fibrosis of the corpus cavernosum in priapism. *Am J Surg Pathol* 1986;10:497–507.
152. Laskin WB, Fetsch JF, Tavassoli FA. Angiomyofibroblastoma of the female genital tract: analysis of 17 cases including a lipomatous variant. *Hum Pathol* 1997;28:1046–1055.
153. LiVolsi VA, Brooks JJ. Nodular fasciitis of the vulva: a report of two cases. *Obstet Gynecol* 1987;69:513–516.
154. Manson CM, Hirsch PJ, Coyne JD. Post-operative spindle cell nodule of the vulva. *Histopathology* 1995;26:571–574.
155. Allen MV, Novotny DB. Desmoid tumor of the vulva associated with pregnancy. *Arch Pathol Lab Med* 1997;121:512–514.
156. di Sant'Agnese PA, Knowles DM, II. Extracardiac rhabdomyoma: a clinicopathologic study and review of the literature. *Cancer* 1980;46:780–789.
157. Kaufman-Friedman K. Hemangioma of clitoris, confused with adrenogenital syndrome. Case report. *Plast Reconstr Surg* 1978;62:452–454.
158. Imperial R, Helwig EB. Angiokeratoma of the vulva. *Obstet Gynecol* 1967;29:307–312.
159. Jagadha V, Srinivasan K, Panchacharam P. Glomus tumor of the clitoris. *NY State J Med* 1985;85:611.
160. Kohorn EI, Merino MJ, Goldenhersh M. Vulvar pain and dyspareunia due to glomus tumor. *Obstet Gynecol* 1986;67:41s–42s.
161. Brown JV, Stenchever MA. Cavernous lymphangioma of the vulva. *Obstet Gynecol* 1989;73:877–879.
162. Young AW Jr, Wind RM, Tovell HMM. Lymphangioma of vulva. Acquired following treatment for cervical cancer. *NY State J Med* 1980;80:987–989.
163. La Polla J, Foucar E, Leshin B, Whitaker D, Anderson B. Vulvar lymphangioma circumscriptum: a rare complication of therapy for squamous cell carcinoma of the cervix. *Gynecol Oncol* 1985;22:363–366.
164. Garcia JJ, Verkauf BS, Hochberg CJ, Ingram JM. Aberrant breast tissue of the vulva. Case report and review of the literature. *Obstet Gynecol* 1978;52:225–228.
165. O'Hara MF, Page DL. Adenomas of the breast and ectopic breast under lactational influences. *Hum Pathol* 1985;16:707–712.
166. Foushee JHS, Pruitt AB, Jr. Vulvar fibroadenoma from aberrant breast tissue. Report of two cases. *Obstet Gynecol* 1967;29:819–823.
167. Rickert RR. Intraductal papilloma arising in supernumerary vulvar breast tissue. *Obstet Gynecol* 1980;55:84s–87s.
168. Tbakhi A, Cowan DF, Kumar D, Kyle D. Recurring phyllodes tumor in aberrant breast tissue of the vulva. *Am J Surg Pathol* 1993;17:946–950.
169. Hendrix RC, Behrman SJ. Adenocarcinoma arising in a supernumerary mammary gland in the vulva. *Obstet Gynecol* 1956;8:238–241.
170. Guerry RL, Pratt-Thomas HR. Carcinoma of supernumerary breast of vulva with bilateral mammary cancer. *Cancer* 1976;38:2570–2574.
171. van der Putte SCJ, van Gorp LHM. Adenocarcinoma of the mammary-like glands of the vulva: a concept unifying sweat gland carcinoma of the vulva, carcinoma of supernumerary mammary glands and extramammary Paget's disease. *J Cutan Pathol* 1994;21:157–163.
172. Reyman L, Milano A, Demopoulos R, Mayron J, Schuster S. Metastatic vulvar ulceration in Crohn's disease. *Am J Gastroenterol* 1986;81:46–49.
173. Guerrieri C, Ohlsson E, Ryden G, Westermar P. Vulvitis granulomatosa: a cryptogenic chronic inflammatory hypertrophy of vulvar labia related to cheilitis granulomatosa and Crohn's disease. *Int J Gynecol Pathol* 1995;14:352–359.
174. Tatnall FM, Barnes HM, Sarkany I. Sarcoidosis of the vulva. *Clin Exp Dermatol* 1985;10:384–385.
175. Arul KJ, Emmerson RW. Malacoplakia of the skin. *Clin Exp Dermatol* 1977;2:131–135.
176. Paquin ML, Davis JR, Weiner S. Malacoplakia of Bartholin's gland. *Arch Pathol Lab Med* 1986;110:757–758.

177. Northcutt AD, Vanover MJ. Nodular cutaneous amyloidosis involving the vulva. Case report and literature review. *Arch Dermatol* 1985;121:518–521.
178. St. Clair JT, Majmudar B. Tumoral calcinosis masquerading as metastatic carcinoma. *Gynecol Oncol* 1980;10:69–74.
179. Balfour PJT, Vincenti AC. Idiopathic vulvar calcinosis. *Histopathology* 1991;18:183–184.
180. Coghill SB, Tyler X, Shaxted EJ. Benign mucinous metaplasia of the vulva. *Histopathology* 1990;17:373–375.
181. Kernen JA, Morgan ML. Benign lymphoid hamartoma of the vulva. Report of a case. *Obstet Gynecol* 1970;35:290–292.
182. Marwah S, Berman ML. Ectopic salivary gland in the vulva (choristoma): report of a case and review of the literature. *Obstet Gynecol* 1980;56:389–391.
183. Appleton MAC, Ismail SM. Ulcerating rheumatoid nodule of the vulva. *J Clin Pathol* 1996;49:85–87.

Aggressive Angiomyxoma, Angiomyofibroblastoma, and Angiofibroma

184. Steeper TA, Rosai J. Aggressive angiomyxoma of the female pelvis and perineum. Report of nine cases of a distinctive type of gynecologic soft-tissue neoplasm. *Am J Surg Pathol* 1983;7:463–475.
185. Begin LR, Clement PB, Kirk ME, Jothy S, McCaughey WTE, Ferenczy A. Aggressive angiomyxoma of pelvic soft parts. A clinicopathologic study of nine cases. *Hum Pathol* 1985;16:621–628.
186. Fetsch JF, Laskin WB, Lefkowitz M, Kindblom L-G, Meis-Kindblom JM. Aggressive angiomyxoma. A clinicopathologic study of 29 female patients. *Cancer* 1996;78:79–90.
187. Granter SR, Nucci MR, Fletcher CDM. Aggressive angiomyxoma: reappraisal of its relationship to angiomyofibroblastoma in a series of 16 cases. *Histopathology* 1997;30:3–10.
188. Fletcher CDM, Tsang WYW, Fisher C, Lee KC, Chan JKC. Angiomyofibroblastoma of the vulva. A benign neoplasm distinct from aggressive angiomyxoma. *Am J Surg Pathol* 1992;16:373–82.
189. Nielsen GP, Rosenberg AE, Young RH, Dickersin GR, Clement PB, Scully RE. Angiomyofibroblastoma of the vulva and vagina. *Mod Pathol* 1996;9:284–91.
190. Fukunaga M, Nomura K, Matsumoto K, Doi K, Endo Y, Ushigome S. Vulval angiomyofibroblastoma. Clinicopathologic analysis of six cases. *Am J Clin Pathol* 1997;107:45–51.
191. Ockner DM, Sayadi H, Swanson PE, Ritter JH, Wick MR. Genital angiomyofibroblastoma. Comparison with aggressive angiomyxoma and other myxoid neoplasms of skin and soft tissue. *Am J Clin Pathol* 1997;107:36–44.
192. Nielsen GP, Young RH, Dickersin GR, Rosenberg AE. Angiomyofibroblastoma of the vulva with sarcomatous transformation ("angiomyofibrosarcoma"). *Am J Surg Pathol* 1997;21:1104–1108.
193. Nucci MR, Granter SR, Fletcher CDM. Cellular angiofibroma: A benign neoplasm distinct from angiomyofibroblastoma and spindle cell lipoma. *Am J Surg Pathol* 1997;21:636–44.

Dystrophy and Squamous Intraepithelial Neoplasia

194. Ridley CM, Frankman O, Jones ISC, Pincus SH, Wilkinson EJ. New nomenclature for vulvar disease: International Society for the Study of Vulvar Disease. *Hum Pathol* 1989;20:495–496.
195. Wallace HJ. Lichen sclerosus et atrophicus. *Trans St Johns Hosp Dermatol Soc* 1971;57:9–30.
196. Kaufman RH, Gardner HL. Vulvar dystrophies. *Clin Obstet Gynecol* 1978;21:1081–1106.
197. Buscema J, Stern J, Woodruff JD. The significance of the histologic alterations adjacent to invasive vulvar carcinoma. *Am J Obstet Gynecol* 1980;137:902–909.
198. Hart WR, Norris HJ, Helwig EB. Relation of lichen sclerosus et atrophicus of the vulva to development of carcinoma. *Obstet Gynecol* 1975;45:369–377.
199. Friedman RJ, Kopf AW, Jones WB. Malignant melanoma in association with lichen sclerosus on the vulva of a 14-year-old. *Am J Dermatopathol* 1984;6:253–256.
200. Meyrick Thomas RH, McGibbon DH, Munro DD. Basal cell carcinoma of the vulva in association with vulval lichen sclerosus et atrophicus. *J R Soc Med Suppl* 1985;78:16–18.
201. Kaufman RH, Gardner HL, Brown D Jr, Beyth Y. Vulvar dystrophies: an evaluation. *Am J Obstet Gynecol* 1974;120:363–367.
202. Friedrich EG Jr, Burch K, Bahr JP. The vulvar clinic: an eight-year appraisal. *Am J Obstet Gynecol* 1979;135:1036–1040.
203. Buscema J, Woodruff JD, Parmley TH, Genadry R. Carcinoma in situ of the vulva. *Obstet Gynecol* 1980;55:225–230.
204. Crum CP, Liskow A, Petras P, Keng WC, Frick HC II. Vulvar intraepithelial neoplasia (severe atypia and carcinoma in situ). A clinicopathologic analysis of 41 cases. *Cancer* 1984;54:1429–1434.
205. Herod JO, Shafi MI, Rollason TP, Jordan JA, Luesley DM. Vulvar intraepithelial neoplasia: long term follow up of treated and untreated women. *Br J Obstet Gynecol* 1996;103:446–452.
206. Abell MR. Intraepithelial carcinomas of epidermis and squamous mucosa of vulva and perineum. *Surg Clin North Am* 1965;45:1179–1198.
207. Hording U, Daugaard S, Junge J, Lundvall F. Human papillomaviruses and multifocal genital neoplasia. *Int J Gynecol Pathol* 1996;15:230–234.
208. Patterson JW, Kao GF, Graham JH, Helwig EB. Bowenoid papulosis. A clinicopathologic study with ultrastructural observations. *Cancer* 1986;57:823–836.
209. Ulbright TM, Stehman FB, Roth LM, Ehrlich CE, Ransburg RC. Bowenoid dysplasia of the vulva. *Cancer* 1982;50:2910–2919.
210. van Beurden M, ten Kate FJW, Smits HL, et al. Multifocal vulvar intraepithelial neoplasia grade III and multicentric lower genital tract neoplasia is associated with transcriptionally active human papillomavirus. *Cancer* 1995;75:2879–2884.
211. Andreasson B, Bock JE. Intraepithelial neoplasia in the vulvar region. *Gynecol Oncol* 1985;21:300–305.
212. Jones RW, Rowan DM. Vulvar intraepithelial neoplasia III: a clinical study of the outcome in 113 cases with relation to the later development of invasive vulvar carcinoma. *Obstet Gynecol* 1994;84:741–745.
213. Zaino RJ, Husseinzadeh N, Nahhas W, Mortel R. Epithelial alterations in proximity to invasive squamous carcinoma of the vulva. *Int J Gynecol Pathol* 1982;1:173–184.

Malignant Neoplasms

214. Benedet JL, Turko M, Fairey RN, Boyes DA. Squamous carcinoma of the vulva: results of treatment, 1938 to 1976. *Am J Obstet Gynecol* 1979;134:201–207.
215. Barthcldson L, Eldh J, Eriksson E, Peterson LE. Surgical treatment of carcinoma of the vulva. *Surg Gynecol Obstet* 1982;155:655–661.
216. Hacker NF, Berek JS, Lagasse LD, Leuchter RS, Moore JG. Management of regional lymph nodes and their prognostic influence in vulvar cancer. *Obstet Gynecol* 1983;61:408–412.
217. Figge DC, Tamimi HK, Greer BE. Lymphatic spread in carcinoma of the vulva. *Am J Obstet Gynecol* 1985;152:387–394.
218. Gosling JRG, Abell MR, Drolette BM, Loughrin TD. Infiltrative squamous cell (epidermoid) carcinoma of vulva. *Cancer* 1961;14:330–343.
219. Choo YC. Invasive squamous carcinoma of the vulva in young patients. *Gynecol Oncol* 1982;13:158–164.
220. Kennedy AW, Hart WR. Multiple squamous-cell carcinomas in Fanconi's anemia. *Cancer* 1982;50:811–814.
221. Ansink AC, Krul MRL, de Weger RA, et al. Human papillomavirus, lichen sclerosus, and squamous cell carcinoma of the vulva: detection and prognostic significance. *Gynecol Oncol* 1994;52:180–184.
222. Toki T, Kurman RJ, Park JS, Kessis T, Daniel RW, Shah KV. Probable nonpapillomavirus etiology of squamous cell carcinoma of the vulva in older women: a clinicopathologic study using in situ hybridization and polymerase chain reaction. *Int J Gynecol Pathol* 1991;10:107–125.
223. Kurman RJ, Toki T, Schiffman MH. Basaloid and warty carcinomas of the vulva. Distinctive types of squamous cell carcinoma frequently associated with human papillomaviruses. *Am J Surg Pathol* 1993;17:133–145.
224. Monk BJ, Burger RA, Lin F, Parham G, Vasilev SA, Wilczynski SP. Prognostic significance of human papillomavirus DNA in vulvar carcinoma. *Obstet Gynecol* 1995;85:709–715.
225. Pilotti S, D'Amato L, della Torre G, et al. Papillomavirus, p53 alteration, and primary carcinoma of the vulva. *Diagn Mol Pathol* 1995;4:239–248.
226. American Joint Committee on Cancer. *AJCC cancer staging manual*, 5th ed. Philadelphia: Lippincott-Raven, 1997:181–184.

227. Way S. Carcinoma of the vulva. *Am J Obstet Gynecol* 1960;79: 692–697.
228. Broders AC. Squamous-cell epithelioma of the lip. A study of five hundred and thirty-seven cases. *JAMA* 1920;74:656–664.
229. Jakobsson PA, Eneroth CM, Killander D, Moberger G, Martensson B. Histologic classification and grading of malignancy in carcinoma of the larynx. *Acta Radiol Oncol* 1973;12:1–7.
230. Magrina JF, Webb MJ, Gaffey TA, Symmonds RE. Stage I squamous cell cancer of the vulva. *Am J Obstet Gynecol* 1979;134:453–459.
231. Andreasson B, Bock JE, Visfeldt J. Prognostic role of histology in squamous cell carcinoma in the vulvar region. *Gynecol Oncol* 1982;14:373–381.
232. Wilkinson EJ, Rico MJ, Pierson KK. Microinvasive carcinoma of the vulva. *Int J Gynecol Pathol* 1982;1:29–39.
233. Hoffman JS, Kumar NB, Morley GW. Microinvasive squamous carcinoma of the vulva: search for a definition. *Obstet Gynecol* 1983;61:615–618.
234. Husseinzadeh N, Zaino R, Nahhas WA, Mortel R. The significance of histologic findings in predicting nodal metastases in invasive squamous cell carcinoma of the vulva. *Gynecol Oncol* 1983;16:105–111.
235. Podratz KC, Symmonds RE, Taylor WF, Williams TJ. Carcinoma of the vulva: analysis of treatment and survival. *Obstet Gynecol* 1983;61:63–74.
236. Hacker NF, Berek JS, Lagasse LD, Nieberg RK, Leuchter RS. Individualization of treatment for stage I squamous cell vulvar carcinoma. *Obstet Gynecol* 1984;63:155–162.
237. Boice CR, Seraj IM, Thrasher T, King A. Microinvasive squamous carcinoma of the vulva: present status and reassessment. *Gynecol Oncol* 1984;18:71–76.
238. Dvoretsky PM, Bonfiglio TA, Helmkamp FB, Ramsey G, Chuang C, Beecham JB. The pathology of superficially invasive, thin vulvar squamous cell carcinoma. *Int J Gynecol Pathol* 1984;3:331–342.
239. Boyce J, Fruchter RG, Kasambilides E, Nicastri AD, Sedlis A, Remy JC. Prognostic factors in carcinoma of the vulva. *Gynecol Oncol* 1985;20:364–377.
240. Shimm DS, Fuller AF, Orlow EL, Dosoretz DE, Aristizabal SA. Prognostic variables in the treatment of squamous cell carcinoma of the vulva. *Gynecol Oncol* 1986;24:343–358.
241. Franklin EW III, Rutledge FD. Prognostic factors in epidermoid carcinoma of the vulva. *Obstet Gynecol* 1971;37:892–901.
242. Creasman WT, Phillips JL, Menck HR. The national cancer data base report on early stage invasive vulvar carcinoma. *Cancer* 1997;80:505–513.
243. Frankman O, Kabulski Z, Nilsson B, Silfversward C. Prognostic factors in invasive squamous cell carcinoma of the vulva. *Int J Gynecol Obstet* 1991;36:219–228.
244. Homesley HD, Bundy BN, Sedlis A, et al. Prognostic factors for groin node metastasis in squamous cell carcinoma of the vulva (a Gynecologic Oncology Group study). *Gynecol Oncol* 1993;49:279–283.
245. Crissman JD, Azoury RS. Microinvasive carcinoma of the vulva. A report of two cases with regional lymph node metastasis. *Diagn Gynecol Obstet* 1981;3:75–80.
246. Drew PA, al-Abbadi MA, Orlando CA, Hendricks JB, Kubilis PS, Wilkinson EJ. Prognostic factors in carcinoma of the vulva: a clinicopathologic and DNA flow cytometric study. *Int J Gynecol Pathol* 1996;15:235–241.
247. Ambros RA, Malfetano JH, Mihm MC Jr. Clinicopathologic features of vulvar squamous cell carcinomas exhibiting prominent fibromyxoid stromal response. *Int J Gynecol Pathol* 1996;15:137–145.
248. Iversen T, Abeler V, Aalders J. Individualized treatment of stage I carcinoma of the vulva. *Obstet Gynecol* 1981;57:85–89.
249. Donaldson ES, Powell DE, Hanson MB, van Nagell JR Jr. Prognostic parameters in invasive vulvar cancer. *Gynecol Oncol* 1981;11:184–190.
250. Rowley KC, Gallion HH, Donaldson ES, van Nagell JR, Higgins RV, Powell DE, Kryscio RJ, Pavlik EJ. Prognostic factors in early vulvar cancer. *Gynecol Oncol* 1988;31:43–49.
251. Kneale BL. Microinvasive cancer of the vulva. Report of the ISSVD Task Force. *J Reprod Med* 1984;29:454–456.
252. Wilkinson EJ. Superficially invasive carcinoma of the vulva. In: Wilkinson EJ, ed. *Pathology of the vulva and vagina*. New York: Churchill Livingstone, 1987:103–117.
253. Sedlis A, Homesley H, Bundy BN, et al. Positive groin lymph nodes in superficial squamous cell vulvar cancer. A Gynecologic Oncology Group study. *Am J Obstet Gynecol* 1987;156:1159–1164.
254. Homesley HD. Management of vulvar cancer. *Cancer* 1995;76: 2159–2170.
255. Heaps JM, Fu YS, Montz FJ, Hacker NF, Berek JS. Surgical-pathologic variables predictive of local recurrence in squamous cell carcinoma of the vulva. *Gynecol Oncol* 1990;38:309–314.
256. Rutledge FN, Mitchell MF, Munsell MF, et al. Prognostic indicators for invasive carcinoma of the vulva. *Gynecol Oncol* 1991;42:239–244.
257. Homesley HD, Bundy BN, Sedlis A, et al. Assessment of current International Federation of Gynecology and Obstetrics staging of vulvar carcinoma relative to prognostic factors for survival (a Gynecologic Oncology Group Study). *Am J Obstet Gynecol* 1991;164:997–1004.
258. van der Velden J, van Lindert ACM, Lammes FB, et al. Extracapsular growth of lymph node metastases in squamous cell carcinoma of the vulva. The impact on recurrence and survival. *Cancer* 1995;75:2885–2890.
259. Paladini D, Cross P, Lopes A, Monaghan JM. Prognostic significance of lymph node variables in squamous cell carcinoma of the vulva. *Cancer* 1994;74:2491–2496.
260. Lasser A, Cornog JL, Morris JM. Adenoid squamous cell carcinoma of the vulva. *Cancer* 1974;33:224–227.
261. Underwood JW, Adcock LL, Okagaki T. Adenosquamous carcinoma of skin appendages (adenoid squamous cell carcinoma, pseudoglandular squamous cell carcinoma, adenoacanthoma of sweat gland of Lever) of the vulva. A clinical and ultrastructural study. *Cancer* 1978;42:1851–1858.
262. Copas P, Dyer M, Comas FV, Hall DJ. Spindle cell carcinoma of the vulva. *Diagn Gynecol Obstet* 1982;4:235–241.
263. Steeper TA, Piscioli F, Rosai J. Squamous cell carcinoma with sarcomalike stroma of the female genital tract. Clinicopathologic study of four cases. *Cancer* 1983;52:890–898.
264. Parham DM, Morton K, Robertson AJ, Philip WDP. The changing phenotypic appearance of a malignant vulval neoplasm containing both carcinomatous and sarcomatous elements. *Histopathology* 1991;19:263–268.
265. Axelsen SM, Stamp IM. Lymphoepithelioma-like carcinoma of the vulvar region. *Histopathology* 1995;27:281–283.
266. Kraus FT, Perez-Mesa C. Verrucous carcinoma. Clinical and pathologic study of 105 cases involving oral cavity, larynx, and genitalia. *Cancer* 1966;19:26–38.
267. Japaze H, Dinh TV, Woodruff JD. Verrucous carcinoma of the vulva: study of 24 cases. *Obstet Gynecol* 1982;60:462–466.
268. Palladino VS, Duffy JL, Bures GJ. Basal cell carcinoma of the vulva. *Cancer* 1969;24:460–470.
269. Cruz-Jimenez PR, Abell MR. Cutaneous basal cell carcinoma of vulva. *Cancer* 1975;36:1860–1868.
270. Merino MJ, LiVolsi VA, Schwartz PE, Rudnicki J. Adenoid basal cell carcinoma of the vulva. *Int J Gynecol Pathol* 1982; 1:299–306.
271. Perrone T, Twiggs LB, Adcock LL, Dehner LP. Vulvar basal cell carcinoma: an infrequently metastasizing neoplasm. *Int J Gynecol Pathol* 1987;6:152–165.
272. Taylor RN, Lacey CG, Shuman MA. Adenocarcinoma of Skene's duct associated with a systemic coagulopathy. *Gynecol Oncol* 1985;22:250–256.
273. Tiltman AJ, Knutzen VK. Primary adenocarcinoma of the vulva originating in misplaced cloacal tissue. *Obstet Gynecol* 1978;51:330–335.
274. Leuchter RS, Hacker NF, Voet RL, Berek JS, Townsend DE, Lagasse LD. Primary carcinoma of the Bartholin gland: a report of 14 cases and review of the literature. *Obstet Gynecol* 1982;60:361–368.
275. Copeland LJ, Sneige N, Gershenson DM, McGuffee VB, Abdul-Karim F, Rutledge FN. Bartholin gland carcinoma. *Obstet Gynecol* 1986;67:794–801.
276. Jones MA, Mann EW, Caldwell CL, Tarraza HM, Dickersin GR, Young RH. Small cell neuroendocrine carcinoma of Bartholin's gland. *Am J Clin Pathol* 1990;94:439–442.
277. Abrao FS, Marques AF, Marziona F, Abrao MS, Uchoajunqueira LC, Torloni H. Adenoid cystic carcinoma of Bartholin's gland: review of the literature and report of two cases. *J Surg Oncol* 1985;30:132–137.
278. Abell MR. Adenocystic (pseudoadenomatous) basal cell carcinoma of vestibular glands of vulva. *Am J Obstet Gynecol* 1963;86:470–482.
279. Dodson MG, O'Leary JA, Orfei E. Adenoid cystic carcinoma of the vulva. Malignant cylindroma. *Obstet Gynecol* 1978; 51:26s–29s.
280. Copeland LJ, Sneige N, Gershenson DM, Saul PB, Stringer CA, Seski JC. Adenoid cystic carcinoma of Bartholin gland. *Obstet Gynecol* 1986;67:115–120.

281. Dudley AG, Young RH, Lawrence WD, Scully RE. Endodermal sinus tumor of the vulva in an infant. *Obstet Gynecol* 1983;61:76s–79s.
282. Tang CK, Toker C, Nedwich A, Zaman ANF. Unusual cutaneous carcinoma with features of small cell (oat cell-like) and squamous cell carcinomas. A variant of malignant Merkel cell neoplasm. *Am J Dermatopathol* 1982;4:537–548.
283. Bottles K, Lacey CG, Goldberg J, Lanner-Cusin K, Hom J, Miller TR. Merkel cell carcinoma of the vulva. *Obstet Gynecol* 1984;63:61s–65s.
284. Copeland LJ, Cleary K, Sneige N, Edwards CL. Neuroendocrine (Merkel cell) carcinoma of the vulva: a case report and review of the literature. *Gynecol Oncol* 1985;22:367–378.
285. Husseinzadeh N, Wesseler T, Newman N, Shbaro I, Ho P. Neuroendocrine (Merkel cell) carcinoma of the vulva. *Gynecol Oncol* 1988;29:105–112.
286. Gil-Moreno A, Garcia-Jimenez A, Gonzalez-Bosquet J, et al. Merkel cell carcinoma of the vulva. *Gynecol Oncol* 1997;64:526–532.
287. Chen KTK. Merkel's cell (neuroendocrine) carcinoma of the vulva. *Cancer* 1994;73:2186–2191.
288. Chung AF, Woodruff JM, Lewis JL Jr. Malignant melanoma of the vulva. A report of 44 cases. *Obstet Gynecol* 1975;45:638–646.
289. Johnson TL, Kumar NB, White CD, Morley GW. Prognostic features of vulvar melanoma: a clinicopathologic analysis. *Int J Gynecol Pathol* 1986;5:110–118.
290. Podratz KC, Gaffey TA, Symmonds RE, Johansen KL, O'Brien PC. Melanoma of the vulva: an update. *Gynecol Oncol* 1983;16:153–168.
291. Warner TFCS, Hafez GR, Buchler DA. Neurotropic melanoma of the vulva. *Cancer* 1982;49:999–1004.
292. Woolcott RJ, Henry RJW, Houghton CRS. Malignant melanoma of the vulva. Australian experience. *J Reprod Med* 1988;33:699–702.
293. Raber G, Mempel V, Jackisch C, et al. Malignant melanoma of the vulva. Report of 89 patients. *Cancer* 1996;78:2353–2358.
294. DiSaia PJ, Rutledge F, Smith JP. Sarcoma of the vulva. Report of 12 patients. *Obstet Gynecol* 1971;38:180–184.
295. Davos I, Abell MR. Soft tissue sarcomas of vulva. *Gynecol Oncol* 1976;4:70–86.
296. Santala M, Suonio S, Syrjanen K, Uronen MT, Saarikoski S. Malignant fibrous histiocytoma of the vulva. *Gynecol Oncol* 1987;27:121–126.
297. Taylor RN, Bottles K, Miller TR, Braga CA. Malignant fibrous histiocytoma of the vulva. *Obstet Gynecol* 1985;66:145–148.
298. Talerman A. Sarcoma botryoides presenting as a polyp on the labium majus. *Cancer* 1973;32:994–999.
299. Copeland LJ, Sneige N, Stringer CA, Gershenson DM, Saul PB, Kavanagh JJ. Alveolar rhabdomyosarcoma of the female genitalia. *Cancer* 1985;56:849–855.
300. Perrone T, Swanson PE, Twiggs L, Ulbright TM, Dehner LP. Malignant rhabdoid tumor of the vulva: is distinction from epithelioid sarcoma possible? A pathologic and immunohistochemical study. *Am J Surg Pathol* 1989;13:848–858.
301. Ulbright TM, Brokaw SA, Stehman FB, Roth LM. Epithelioid sarcoma of the vulva. Evidence suggesting a more aggressive behavior than extra-genital epithelioid sarcoma. *Cancer* 1983;52:1462–1469.
302. Hall JS, Amin UF. Fibrosarcoma of the vulva: case reports and discussion. *Int Surg* 1981;66:185–187.
303. Leake JF, Buscema J, Cho KR, Currie JL. Dermatofibrosarcoma protuberans of the vulva. *Gynecol Oncol* 1991;41:245–249.
304. Hall DJ, Burns JC, Goplerud DR. Kaposi's sarcoma of the vulva: a case report and brief review. *Obstet Gynecol* 1979;54:478–483.
305. Reymond RD, Hazra TA, Edlow DW, Bawab MS. Haemangiopericytoma of the vulva with metastasis to bone 14 years later. *Br J Radiol* 1972;45:765–768.
306. Zakut H, Lotan M, Lipnitzky M. Vulvar hemangiopericytoma. A case report and review of previous cases. *Acta Obstet Gynecol Scand* 1985;64:619–621.
307. Shen JT, D'ablaing G, Morrow CP. Alveolar soft part sarcoma of the vulva: report of first case and review of literature. *Gynecol Oncol* 1982;13:120–128.
308. Robertson AJ, McIntosh W, Lamont P, Guthrie W. Malignant granular cell tumour (myoblastoma) of the vulva: report of a case and review of the literature. *Histopathology* 1981;5:69–79.
309. Brooks JJ, LiVolsi VA. Liposarcoma presenting on the vulva. *Am J Obstet Gynecol* 1987;156:73–75.
310. Nielsen GP, Shaw PA, Rosenberg AE, Dickersin GR, Young RH, Scully RE. Synovial sarcoma of the vulva: a report of two cases. *Mod Pathol* 1996;9:970–974.
311. Lin J, Yip KMH, Maffulli N, Chow LTC. Extraskeletal mesenchymal chondrosarcoma of the labium majus. *Gynecol Oncol* 1996;60:492–493.
312. Strayer SA, Yum MN, Sutton GP. Epithelioid hemangioendothelioma of the clitoris: a case report with immunohistochemical and ultrastructural findings. *Int J Gynecol Pathol* 1992;11:234–239.
313. Scherr GR, D'Ablaing G III, Ouzounian JG. Peripheral primitive neuroectodermal tumor of the vulva. *Gynecol Oncol* 1994;54:254–258.
314. Plouffe L Jr, Tulandi T, Rosenberg A, Ferenczy A. Non-Hodgkin's lymphoma in Bartholin's gland: case report and review of literature. *Am J Obstet Gynecol* 1984;148:608–609.
315. Labes J, Ring A. Ulcerating cutaneous Hodgkin's disease of the vulva. *Am J Obstet Gynecol* 1964;89:272–273.
316. Doss LL. Simultaneous extramedullary plasmacytomas of the vagina and vulva. A case report and review of the literature. *Cancer* 1978;41:2468–2474.
317. Swanson S, Innes DJ Jr, Frierson HF Jr, Hess CE. T-immunoblastic lymphoma mimicking B-immunoblastic lymphoma. *Arch Pathol Lab Med* 1987;111:1077–1080.
318. Axiotis CA, Merino MJ, Duray PH. Langerhans cell histiocytosis of the female genital tract. *Cancer* 1991;67:1650–1660.
319. Dehner LP. Metastatic and secondary tumors of the vulva. *Obstet Gynecol* 1973;42:47–57.
320. van Dam PA, Irvine L, Lowe DG, Fisher C, Barton DPJ, Shepherd JH. Carcinoma in episiotomy scars. *Gynecol Oncol* 1992;44:96–100.

Extramammary Paget's Disease, Hidradenoma Papilliferum, and Skin Appendage Neoplasms

321. Jones RE Jr, Austin C, Ackerman AB. Extramammary Paget's disease. A critical reexamination. *Am J Dermatopathol* 1979;1:101–132.
322. McKee PH, Hertogs KT. Endocervical adenocarcinoma and vulval Paget's disease: a significant association. *Br J Dermatol* 1980;103:443–448.
323. Tcharg F, Okagaki T, Richart RM. Adenocarcinoma of Bartholin's gland associated with Paget's disease of vulvar area. *Cancer* 1973;31:221–225.
324. Powell FC, Bjornsson J, Doyle JA, Cooper AJ. Genital Paget's disease and urinary tract malignancy. *J Am Acad Dermatol* 1985;13:84–90.
325. Hart WR, Millman JB. Progression of intraepithelial Paget's disease of the vulva to invasive carcinoma. *Cancer* 1977;40:2333–2337.
326. Creasman WT, Gallager HS, Rutledge F. Paget's disease of the vulva. *Gynecol Oncol* 1975;3:133–148.
327. Lee EA, Dahlin DC. Paget's disease of the vulva with extension into the urethra, bladder and ureters. A case report. *Am J Obstet Gynecol* 1981;140:834–836.
328. Gunn RA, Gallager HS. Vulvar Paget's disease. A topographic study. *Cancer* 1980;46:590–594.
329. Lee SC, Roth LM, Ehrlich C, Hall JA. Extramammary Paget's disease of the vulva. A clinicopathologic study of 13 cases. *Cancer* 1977;39:2540–2549.
330. Helwig EB, Graham JH. Anogenital (extramammary) Paget's disease. A clinicopathological study. *Cancer* 1963;16:387–403.
331. Nadji M, Morales AR, Girtanner RE, Ziegels-Weissman J, Penneys NS. Paget's disease of the skin. A unifying concept of histogenesis. *Cancer* 1982;50:2203–2206.
332. Ordonez NG, Awalt H, Mackay B. Mammary and extramammary Paget's disease. An immunocytochemical and ultrastructural study. *Cancer* 1987;59:1173–1183.
333. Koss LG, Brockunier A Jr. Ultrastructural aspects of Paget's disease of the vulva. *Arch Pathol Lab Med* 1969;87:592–600.
334. Demopoulos RI. Fine structure of the extramammary Paget's cell. *Cancer* 1971;27:1202–1210.
335. Parmley TH, Woodruff JD, Julian CG. Invasive vulvar Paget's disease. *Obstet Gynecol* 1975;46:341–346.
336. Fine BA, Fowler LJ, Valente PT, Gaudet T. Minimally invasive Paget's disease of the vulva with extensive lymph node metastases. *Gynecol Oncol* 1995;57:262–265.
337. Meeker JH, Neubecker RD, Helwig EB. Hidradenoma papilliferum. *Am J Clin Pathol* 1962;37:182–195.
338. Woodworth H Jr, Dockerty MB, Wilson RB, Pratt JH. Papillary hidradenoma of the vulva: a clinicopathologic study of 69 cases. *Am J Obstet Gynecol* 1971;110:501–508.
339. Hashimoto K. Hidradenoma papilliferum. An electron microscopic study. *Acta Derm Venereol (Stockh)* 1973;53:22–30.

340. Pelosi G, Martignoni G, Bonetti F. Intraductal carcinoma of mammary-type apocrine epithelium arising within a papillary hydradenoma of the vulva. Report of a case and review of the literature. *Arch Pathol Lab Med* 1991;115:1249–1254.
341. Bannatyne P, Elliott P, Russell P. Vulvar adenosquamous carcinoma arising in a hidradenoma papilliferum, with rapidly fatal outcome: case report. *Gynecol Oncol* 1989;35:395–398.
342. Rorat E, Wallach RC. Mixed tumors of the vulva: clinical outcome and pathology. *Int J Gynecol Pathol* 1984;3:323–328.
343. Young AW Jr, Herman EW, Tovell HMM. Syringoma of the vulva: incidence, diagnosis, and cause of pruritus. *Obstet Gynecol* 1980;55:515–518.
344. Cho D, Woodruff JD. Trichoepithelioma of the vulva. A report of two cases. *J Reprod Med* 1988;33:317–319.
345. Avinoach I, Zirkin HJ, Glezerman M. Proliferating trichilemmal tumor of the vulva. Case report and review of the literature. *Int J Gynecol Pathol* 1989;8:163–168.
346. Gilks CB, Clement PB, Wood WS. Trichoblastic fibroma. A clinicopathologic study of three cases. *Am J Dermatopathol* 1989;11:397–402.
347. Nielsen NC. Hidroadenoma of the vulva. *Acta Obstet Gynecol Scand* 1973;52:387–389.
348. Wick MR, Goellner JR, Wolfe JT III, Su WPD. Vulvar sweat gland carcinomas. *Arch Pathol Lab Med* 1985;109:43–47.
349. Bondi R, Di Lollo S, Pagnini P. Il carcinoma delle ghiandole apocrine. *Arch Vecchi Anat Patol* 1974;59:429–446.
350. Jacobs DM, Sandles LG, Leboit PE. Sebaceous carcinoma arising from Bowen's disease of the vulva. *Arch Dermatol* 1986;122:1191–1193.
351. Rahilly MA, Beattie GJ, Lessells AM. Mucinous eccrine carcinoma of the vulva with neuroendocrine differentiation. *Histopathology* 1995;27:82–86.

Vagina

Congenital Anomalies Including Those Due to Intratuterine Exposure to Diethylstilbesterol

352. Griffin JE, Edwards C, Madden JD, Harrod MJ, Wilson JD. Congenital absence of the vagina. The Mayer-Rokitansky-Kuster-Hauser syndrome. *Ann Intern Med* 1976;85:224–236.
353. Varner RE, Younger JB, Blackwell RE. Mullerian dysgenesis. *J Reprod Med* 1985;30:443–450.
354. Evans TN, Poland ML, Boving RL. Vaginal malformations. *Am J Obstet Gynecol* 1981;141:910–920.
355. Nielsen AL, Lassen M, Nielsen IM, Medgyesi S. The fate of the split thickness skin graft in neovaginas. A pathologic study of 21 cases and a review of the literature. *Int J Gynecol Pathol* 1988;7:173–181.
356. Tozum R. Homtransplantation of the amniotic membrane for the treatment of congenital absence of the vagina. *Int J Gynaecol Obstet* 1976;14:553–556.
357. Herman CJ, v Erp A, Willemsen WNP, Mastboom JL, Vooijs GP. Artificial vaginas. *Hum Pathol* 1982;13:1100–1105.
358. Toolenaar TAM, Freundt I, Huikeshoven FJM, Drogendijk AC, Jeekel H, Chadha-Ajwani S. The occurrence of diversion colitis in patients with a sigmoid neovagina. *Hum Pathol* 1993;24:846–849.
359. Sueldo CE, Rotman CA, Cooperman NR, Rana N. Transverse vaginal septum. A report of four cases. *J Reprod Med* 1985;30:127–131.
360. Sandberg EC. Benign cervical and vaginal changes associated with exposure to stilbestrol in utero. *Am J Obstet Gynecol* 1976;125:777–789.
361. Jefferies JA, Robboy SJ, O'Brien PC, et al. Structural anomalies of the cervix and vagina in women enrolled in the Diethylstilbestrol Adenosis (DESAD) Project. *Am J Obstet Gynecol* 1984;148:59–66.
362. Herbst AL, Ulfelder H, Poskanzer DC. Adenocarcinoma of the vagina. Association of maternal stilbestrol therapy with tumor appearance in young women. *N Engl J Med* 1971;284:878–881.
363. Robboy SJ, Taguchi O, Cunha GR. Normal development of the human female reproductive tract and alterations resulting from experimental exposure to diethylstilbestrol. *Hum Pathol* 1982;13:190–198.
364. Sonek M, Bibbo M, Wied GL. Colposcopic findings in offspring of DES-treated mothers as related to onset of therapy. *J Reprod Med* 1976;16:65–71.
365. Dungar CF, Wilkinson EJ. Vaginal columnar cell metaplasia. An acquired adenosis associated with topical 5-fluorouracil therapy. *J Reprod Med* 1995;40:361–366.
366. Sedlacek TV, Riva JM, Magen AB, Mangan CE, Cunnane MF. Vaginal and vulvar adenosis. An unsuspected side effect of CO_2 laser vaporization. *J Reprod Med* 1990;35:995–1001.
367. O'Brien PC, Noller KL, Robboy SJ, et al. Vaginal epithelial changes in young women enrolled in the National Cooperative Diethylstilbestrol Adenosis (DESAD) project. *Obstet Gynecol* 1979;53:300–308.
368. Antonioli DA, Burke L. Vaginal adenosis. Analysis of 325 biopsy specimens from 100 patients. *Am J Clin Pathol* 1975;64:625–638.
369. Robboy SJ, Kaufman RH, Prat J, et al. Pathologic findings in young women enrolled in the National Cooperative Diethylstilbestrol Adenosis (DESAD) project. *Obstet Gynecol* 1979;53:309–317.
370. Robboy SJ, Hill EC, Sandberg EC, Czernobilsky B. Vaginal adenosis in women born prior to the diethylstilbestrol era. *Hum Pathol* 1986;17:488–492.
371. Merchant WJ, Gale J. Intestinal metaplasia in stilboestrol-induced vaginal adenosis. *Histopathology* 1993;23:373–376.
372. Hart WR, Townsend DE, Aldrich JO, Henderson BE, Roy M, Benton B. Histopathologic spectrum of vaginal adenosis and related changes in stilbestrol-exposed females. *Cancer* 1976;37:763–775.
373. Burke L, Antonioli D, Friedman EA. Evolution of diethylstilbestrol-associated genital tract lesions. *Obstet Gynecol* 1981;57:79–84.
374. Robboy SJ, Noller KL, O'Brien P, et al. Increased incidence of cervical and vaginal dysplasia in 3,980 diethylstilbestrol-exposed young women. Experience of the National Collaborative Diethylstilbestrol Adenosis Project. *JAMA* 1984;252:2979–2983.
375. Kurman RJ, Scully RE. The incidence and histogenesis of vaginal adenosis. An autopsy study. *Hum Pathol* 1974;5:265–276.
376. Robboy SJ, Welch WR. Microglandular hyperplasia in vaginal adenosis associated with oral contraceptives and prenatal diethylstilbestrol exposure. *Obstet Gynecol* 1977;49:430–434.
377. Robboy SJ, Young RH, Welch WR, et al. Atypical vaginal adenosis and cervical ectropion. Association with clear cell adenocarcinoma in diethylstilbestrol-exposed offspring. *Cancer* 1984;54:869–875.

Infectious Diseases

Bacteria

378. Priestley CJF, Kinghorn GR. Bacterial vaginosis. *Br J Clin Pract* 1996;50:331–334.
379. Spiegel CA, Amsel R, Eschenbach D, Schoenknecht F, Holmes KK. Anaerobic bacteria in nonspecific vaginitis. *N Engl J Med* 1980;303:601–607.
380. Bergdoll MS, Schlievert PM. Toxic shock syndrome toxin. *Lancet* 1984;2:691.
381. Todd JK, Todd BH, Franco-Buff A, Smith CM, Lawellin DW. Influence of focal growth conditions on the pathogenesis of toxic shock syndrome. *J Infect Dis* 1987;155:673–681.
382. Larkin SM, Williams DN, Osterholm MT, Tofte RW, Posalaky Z. Toxic shock syndrome: clinical, laboratory, and pathologic findings in nine fatal cases. *Ann Intern Med* 1982;96:858–864.
383. Strate SM, Taylor WE, Forney JP, Silver FG. Xanthogranulomatous pseudotumor of the vagina: evidence of a local response to an unusual bacterium (mucoid Escherichia coli). *Am J Clin Pathol* 1983;79:637–643.
384. Chen KTK, Hendricks EJ. Malacoplakia of the female genital tract. *Obstet Gynecol* 1985;65:84s–87s.

Viruses, Chlamydia, and Mycoplasma

385. Nuovo GJ, Blanco JS, Silverstein SJ, Crum CP. Histologic correlates of papillomavirus infection of the vagina. *Obstet Gynecol* 1988;72:770–774.
386. Okagaki T, Twiggs LB, Zachow KR, Clark BA, Ostrow RS, Faras AJ. Identification of human papillomavirus DNA in cervical and vaginal intraepithelial neoplasia with molecularly cloned type (group) specific DNA probes. *Int J Gynecol Pathol* 1983;2:153–159.
387. Okagaki T, Clark BA, Zachow KR, et al. Presence of human papillomavirus in verrucous carcinoma (Ackerman) of the vagina. Immunocytochemical, ultrastructural, and DNA hybridization studies. *Arch Pathol Lab Med* 1984;108:567–570.

388. Shafer MA, Sweet RL, Ohm-Smith MJ, Shalwitz J, Beck A, Schachter J. Microbiology of the lower genital tract in postmenarchal adolescent girls: differences by sexual activity, contraception, and presence of nonspecific vaginitis. *J Pediatr* 1985;107:974–981.

Fungi and Parasites

389. Friedrich EG Jr. Vaginitis. *Am J Obstet Gynecol* 1985;152:247–251.
390. Kaufman RH, Friedrich EG Jr, Gardner HL. Trichomoniasis. In: Kaufman RH, Friedrich EG Jr, Gardner HL, eds. *Benign diseases of the vulva and vagina,* 3rd ed. Chicago: Year Book Medical, 1989:382–400.
391. Munguia H, Franco E, Valenzuela P. Diagnosis of genital amebiasis in women by the standard Papanicolaou technique. *Am J Obstet Gynecol* 1966;94:181–188.

Miscellaneous Benign Conditions

392. Gardner HL. Desquamative inflammatory vaginitis: a newly defined entity. *Am J Obstet Gynecol* 1968;102:1102–1105.
393. Edwards L, Friedrich EG Jr. Desquamative vaginitis: lichen planus in disguise. *Obstet Gynecol* 1988;71:832–836.
394. Gardner HL, Fernet P. Etiology of vaginitis emphysematosa. Report of ten cases and review of literature. *Am J Obstet Gynecol* 1964;88:680–694.
395. Kramer K, Tobon H. Vaginitis emphysematosa. *Arch Pathol Lab Med* 1987;111:746–749.
396. Friedrich EG Jr, Siegesmund KA. Tampon-associated vaginal ulcerations. *Obstet Gynecol* 1980;55:149–156.
397. Danielson RW. Vaginal ulcers caused by tampons. *Am J Obstet Gynecol* 1983;146:547–549.
398. Givel JC, Hawker P, Allan RN, Alexander-Williams J. Enterovaginal fistulas associated with Crohn's disease. *Surg Gynecol Obstet* 1982;155:494–496.
399. Froese DP, Haggitt RC, Friend WG. Ulcerative colitis in the auto-transplanted neovagina. *Gastroenterology* 1991;100:1749–1752.
400. Deppisch LM. Cysts of the vagina. Classification and clinical correlations. *Obstet Gynecol* 1975;45:632–637.
401. Pradhan S, Tobon H. Vaginal cysts: a clinicopathological study of 41 cases. *Int J Gynecol Pathol* 1986;5:35–46.
402. Kjaeldgaard A, Fianu S. Classification and embryological aspects of ectopic ureters communicating with Gartner's cysts. *Diagn Gynecol Obstet* 1982;4:269–273.
403. Gardner HL. Cervical and vaginal endometriosis. *Clin Obstet Gynecol* 1966;9:358–372.
404. Kurman RJ, Prabha AC. Thyroid and parathyroid glands in the vaginal wall: report of a case. *Am J Clin Pathol* 1973;59:503–507.
405. Mathie JG. Vaginal deciduosis simulating carcinoma. *Br J Obstet Gynecol* 1957;34:720–721.
406. Haines M. Hydatidiform mole and vaginal nodules. *Br J Obstet Gynecol* 1955;62:6–11.
407. Elston CW. The histopathology of trophoblastic tumours. *J Clin Pathol Suppl* 1971;10:111–131.
408. Duckman S, Suarez J, Spitaleri J. Vaginal pregnancy presenting as a suburethral cyst. *Am J Obstet Gynecol* 1984;149:572–573.
409. Wood P. Persistence of vaginal vault granulation. *Lancet* 1986;2:918.
410. Wheelock JB, Schneider V, Goplerud DR. Prolapsed fallopian tube masquerading as adenocarcinoma of the vagina in a postmenopausal woman. *Gynecol Oncol* 1985;21:369–375.
411. Silverberg SG, Frable WJ. Prolapse of fallopian tube into vaginal vault after hysterectomy. Histopathology, cytopathology, and differential diagnosis. *Arch Pathol Lab Med* 1974;97:100–103.
412. Humphries JE, Frierson HF Jr, Underwood PB Jr. Vaginal telangiectasias: unusual presentation of the Osler-Weber-Rendu syndrome. *Obstet Gynecol* 1993;81:865–866.
413. Norris HJ, Taylor HB. Melanomas of the vagina. *Am J Clin Pathol* 1966;46:420–426.
414. Bottles K, Lacey CG, Miller TR. Atypical melanocytic hyperplasia of the vagina. *Gynecol Oncol* 1984;19:226–230.
415. Tobon H, Murphy AI. Benign blue nevus of the vagina. *Cancer* 1977;40:3174–3176.
416. Rodriguez HA, Ackerman LV. Cellular blue nevus. Clinicopathologic study of forty-five cases. *Cancer* 1968;21:393–405.
417. Nigogosyan G, de la Pava S, Pickren JW. Melanoblasts in vaginal mucosa. Origin for primary malignant melanoma. *Cancer* 1964;17:912–913.
418. Norris HJ, Taylor HB. Polyps of the vagina. A benign lesion resembling sarcoma botryoides. *Cancer* 1966;19:227–232.
419. Tobon H, McIntyre-Seltman K, Rubino M. 'Polyposis vaginalis' of pregnancy. *Arch Pathol Lab Med* 1989;113:1391–1393.
420. Chirayil SJ, Tobon H. Polyps of the vagina: a clinicopathologic study of 18 cases. *Cancer* 1981;47:2904–2907.
421. Elliott GB, Elliott JDA. Superficial stromal reactions of lower genital tract. *Arch Pathol Lab Med* 1973;95:100–101.
422. Hartmann C-A, Sperling M, Stein H. So-called fibroepithelial polyps of the vagina exhibiting an unusual but uniform antigen profile characterized by expression of desmin and steroid hormone receptors but no muscle-specific actin or macrophage markers. *Am J Clin Pathol* 1990;93:604–608.
423. Mucitelli DR, Charles EZ, Kraus FT. Vulvovaginal polyps. Histologic appearance, ultrastructure, immunocytochemical characteristics, and clinicopathologic correlations. *Int J Gynecol Pathol* 1990;9:20–40.
424. Novak E, Woodruff JD, Novak ER. Probable mesonephric origin of certain female genital tumors. *Am J Obstet Gynecol* 1954;68:1222–1242.
425. Janovski NA, Kasdon EJ. Benign mesonephric papillary and polypoid tumors of the cervix in childhood. *J Pediatr* 1963;63:211–216.
426. Norris HJ, Bagley GP, Taylor HB. Carcinoma of the infant vagina. A distinctive tumor. *Arch Pathol Lab Med* 1970;90:473–479.
427. Ulbright TM, Alexander RW, Kraus FT. Intramural papilloma of the vagina: evidence of mullerian histogenesis. *Cancer* 1981;48:2260–2266.
428. Sirota RL, Dickersin GR, Scully RE. Mixed tumors of the vagina. A clinicopathological analysis of eight cases. *Am J Surg Pathol* 1981;5:413–422.
429. Branton PA, Tavassoli FA. Spindle cell epithelioma, the so-called mixed tumor of the vagina. A clinicopathologic, immunohistochemical, and ultrastructural analysis of 28 cases. *Am J Surg Pathol* 1993;17:509–515.
430. Chen KTK. Brenner tumor of the vagina. *Diagn Gynecol Obstet* 1981;3:255–258.
431. Wright RG, Buntine DW, Forbes KL. Recurrent benign mixed tumor of the vagina. *Gynecol Oncol* 1991;40:84–86.
432. Kerner H, Munichor M. Papillary mullerian cystadenofibroma of the vagina. *Histopathology* 1997;30:84–86.
433. Spitzer M, Molho L, Seltzer VL, Lipper S. Vaginal glomus tumor: case presentation and ultrastructural findings. *Obstet Gynecol* 1985;66:86s–88s.
434. Pezeshkpour G. Solitary paraganglioma of the vagina—report of a case. *Am J Obstet Gynecol* 1981;139:219–221.
435. Tavassoli FA, Norris HJ. Smooth muscle tumors of the vagina. *Obstet Gynecol* 1979;53:689–693.
436. Gold JH, Bossen EH. Benign vaginal rhabdomyoma. A light and electron microscopic study. *Cancer* 1976;37:2283–2294.
437. Autio-Harmainen H, Apaja-Sarkkinen M, Martikainen J, Taipale A, Rapola J. Production of basement membrane laminin and type IV collagen by tumors of striated muscle: an immunohistochemical study of rhabdomyosarcomas of different histologic types and a benign vaginal rhabdomyoma. *Hum Pathol* 1986;17:1218–1224.
438. Allen PW. Nodular fasciitis. *Pathology* 1972;4:9–26.
439. Chen KTK. Angiomyolipoma of the vagina. *Gynecol Oncol* 1990;37:302–304.
440. Hertig AT, Gore H. Tumors of the female sex organs. In: *Atlas of tumor pathology,* part 2, sec. IX, fasc. 33. Washington, DC: Armed Forces Institute of Pathology, 1960:66–67.
441. Gold BM. Neurofibromatosis of the bladder and vagina. *Am J Obstet Gynecol* 1972;113:1055–1056.
442. Azzopardi JG, Eusebi V, Tison V, Betts CM. Neurofibroma with rhabdomyomatous differentiation: benign 'Triton' tumour of the vagina. *Histopathology* 1983;7:561–572.
443. Proppe KH, Scully RE, Rosai J. Postoperative spindle cell nodules of genitourinary tract resembling sarcomas. A report of eight cases. *Am J Surg Pathol* 1984;8:101–108.
444. Snover DC, Phillips G, Dehner LP. Reactive fibrohistiocytic proliferation simulating fibrous histiocytoma. *Am J Clin Pathol* 1981;76:232–235.
445. Weir MM, Bell DA, Young RH. Transitional cell metaphysis of the uterine cervix and vagina: an underrecognized lesion that may be con-

fused with high-grade dysplasia. A report of 59 cases. *Am J Surg Pathol* 1997;21:510–517.

Premalignant Conditions and Malignant Neoplasms

446. Benedet JL, Sanders BH. Carcinoma in situ of the vagina. *Am J Obstet Gynecol* 1984;148:695–700.
447. Peters WA III, Kumar NB, Morley W. Carcinoma of the vagina. Factors influencing treatment outcome. *Cancer* 1985;55: 892–897.
448. Lenehan PM, Meffe F, Lickrish GM. Vaginal intraepithelial neoplasia: biologic aspects and management. *Obstet Gynecol* 1986;68:333–337.
449. Petrilli ES, Townsend DE, Morrow CP, Nakao CY. Vaginal intraepithelial neoplasia: biologic aspects and treatment with topical 5-fluorouracil and the carbon dioxide laser. *Am J Obstet Gynecol* 1980;138:321–328.
450. Perez CA, Arneson AN, Dehner LP, Galakatos A. Radiation therapy in carcinoma of the vagina. *Obstet Gynecol* 1974;44:862–872.
451. Benedet JL, Murphy KJ, Fairey RN, Boyes DA. Primary invasive carcinoma of the vagina. *Obstet Gynecol* 1983;62:715–719.
452. Rubin SC, Young J, Mikuta JJ. Squamous carcinoma of the vagina: treatment, complications, and long-term follow-up. *Gynecol Oncol* 1985;20:346–353.
453. Hopkins MP, Morley GW. Squamous cell carcinoma of the neovagina. *Obstet Gynecol* 1987;69:525–527.
454. Munkarah A, Malone JM Jr, Budev HD, Evans TN. Mucinous adenocarcinoma arising in a neovagina. *Gynecol Oncol* 1994;52:272–275.
455. American Joint Committee on Cancer. *AJCC cancer staging manual*, 5th ed. Philadelphia: Lippincott-Raven, 1997:185–188.
456. Peters WA III, Kumar NB, Morley GW. Microinvasive carcinoma of the vagina: a distinct clinical entity? *Am J Obstet Gynecol* 1985;153:505–507.
457. Eddy GL, Singh KP, Gansler TS. Superficially invasive carcinoma of the vagina following treatment for cervical cancer: a report of six cases. *Gynecol Oncol* 1990;36:376–379.
458. Stock RG, Chen ASJ, Seski J. A 30-year experience in the management of primary carcinoma of the vagina: analysis of prognostic factors and treatment modalities. *Gynecol Oncol* 1995;56:45–52.
459. Ramzy I, Smout MS, Collins JA. Verrucous carcinoma of the vagina. *Am J Clin Pathol* 1976;65:644–653.
460. Dietl J, Horny H-P, Kaiserling E. Lymphoepithelioma-like carcinoma of the vagina: a case report with special reference to the immunophenotype of the tumor cells and tumor-infiltrating lymphoreticular cells. *Int J Gynecol Pathol* 1994;13:186–189.
461. Melnick S, Cole P, Anderson D, Herbst A. Rates and risks of diethylstilbestrol-related clear-cell adenocarcinoma of the vagina and cervix. An update. *N Engl J Med* 1987;316:514–516.
462. Senekjian EK, Hubby M, Bell DA, Anderson D, Herbst AL. Clear cell adenocarcinoma (CCA) of the vagina and cervix in association with pregnancy. *Gynecol Oncol* 1986;24:207–219.
463. Boyd J, Takahashi H, Waggoner SE, et al. Molecular genetic analysis of clear cell adenocarcinomas of the vagina and cervix associated and unassociated with diethylstilbestrol exposure in utero. *Cancer* 1996;77:507–513.
464. Robboy SJ, Scully RE, Welch WR, Herbst AL. Intrauterine diethylstilbestrol exposure and its consequences. Pathologic characteristics of vaginal adenosis, clear cell adenocarcinoma, and related lesions. *Arch Pathol Lab Med* 1977;101:1–5.
465. Dickersin GR, Welch WR, Erlandson R, Robboy SJ. Ultrastructure of 16 cases of clear cell adenocarcinoma of the vagina and cervix in young women. *Cancer* 1980;45:1615–1624.
466. Senekjian EK, Frey KW, Anderson D, Herbst AL. Local therapy in stage I clear cell adenocarcinoma of the vagina. *Cancer* 1987;60:1319–1324.
467. Ray J, Ireland K. Non-clear-cell adenocarcinoma arising in vaginal adenosis. *Arch Pathol Lab Med* 1985;109:781–783.
468. Yaghsezian H, Palazzo JP, Finkel GC, Carlson JA Jr, Talerman A. Primary vaginal adenocarcinoma of the intestinal type associated with adenosis. *Gynecol Oncol* 1992;45:62–65.
469. DeMars LR, van Le L, Huang I, Fowler WC. Primary non-clear-cell adenocarcinomas of the vagina in older DES-exposed women. *Gynecol Oncol* 1995;58:389–392.
470. Fox H, Wells M, Harris M, McWilliam LJ, Anderson GS. Enteric tumours of the lower female genital tract: a report of three cases. *Histopathology* 1988;12:167–176.
471. Hinchey WW, Silva EG, Guarda LA, Ordonez NG, Wharton JT. Paravaginal Wolffian duct (mesonephros) adenocarcinoma: a light and electron microscopic study. *Am J Clin Pathol* 1983;80:539–544.
472. Hopkins MP, Kumar NB, Lichter AS, Peters WA III, Morley GW. Small cell carcinoma of the vagina with neuroendocrine features. A report of three cases. *J Reprod Med* 1989;34:486–491.
473. Miliauskas JR, Leong AS-Y. Small cell (neuroendocrine) carcinoma of the vagina. *Histopathology* 1992;21:371–374.
474. Fukushima M, Twiggs LB, Okagaki T. Mixed intestinal adenocarcinoma-argentaffin carcinoma of the vagina. *Gynecol Oncol* 1986;23:387–394.
475. Prasad CJ, Ray JA, Kessler S. Primary small cell carcinoma of the vagina arising in a background of atypical adenosis. *Cancer* 1992;70:2484–2487.
476. Okagaki T, Ishida T, Hilgers RD. A malignant tumor of the vagina resembling synovial sarcoma. A light and electron microscopic study. *Cancer* 1976;37:2306–2320.
477. Shevchuk MM, Fenoglio CM, Lattes R, Frick HC II, Richart RM. Malignant mixed tumor of the vagina probably arising in mesonephric rests. *Cancer* 1978;42:214–223.
478. Peters WA III, Kumar NB, Andersen WA, Morley GW. Primary sarcoma of the adult vagina: a clinicopathologic study. *Obstet Gynecol* 1985;65:699–704.
479. Brooks JJ, Wheeler JE. Malignancy arising in extragonadal endometriosis. A case report and summary of the world literature. *Cancer* 1977;40:3065–3073.
480. Goldberg MI, Ng ABP, Belinson JL, Hutson ED, Nordqvist SRB. Clear cell adenocarcinoma arising in endometriosis of the rectovaginal septum. *Obstet Gynecol* 1978;51:38s–40s.
481. Kapp DS, Merino M, LiVolsi V. Adenocarcinoma of the vagina arising in endometriosis: long-term survival following radiation therapy. *Gynecol Oncol* 1982;14:271–278.
482. Berkowitz RS, Ehrmann RL, Knapp RC. Endometrial stromal sarcoma arising from vaginal endometriosis. *Obstet Gynecol* 1978;51:34s–37s.
483. Copeland LJ, Sneige N, Ordonez NG, et al. Endodermal sinus tumor of the vagina and cervix. *Cancer* 1985;55:2558–2565.
484. Young RH, Scully RE. Endodermal sinus tumor of the vagina: a report of nine cases and review of the literature. *Gynecol Oncol* 1984;18:380–392.
485. Andersen WA, Sabio H, Durso N, Mills SE, Levien M, Underwood PB Jr. Endodermal sinus tumor of the vagina. The role of primary chemotherapy. *Cancer* 1985;56:1025–1027.
486. Chung AF, Casey MJ, Flannery JT, Woodruff JM, Lewis JL Jr. Malignant melanoma of the vagina. Report of 19 cases. *Obstet Gynecol* 1980;55:720–727.
487. Lee RB, Buttoni L Jr, Dhru K, Tamimi H. Malignant melanoma of the vagina: a case report of progression from preexisting melanosis. *Gynecol Oncol* 1984;19:238–245.
488. Socinski MA, Ershler WB, Belinson JL. Coexistent breast and vaginal granulocytic sarcoma. *Gynecol Oncol* 1983;16:299–304.
489. Osanto S, Valk P, Meijer CJLM, van Amstel WJ, Willemze R. Solitary plasmocytoma of the vagina. *Acta Haematol* 1981; 66:140–144.
490. Prevot S, Hugol D, Audouin J, et al. Primary nonHodgkin's malignant lymphoma of the vagina. Report of 3 cases with review of the literature. *Pathol Res Pract* 1992;188:78–85.
491. Harris NL, Scully RE. Malignant lymphoma and granulocytic sarcoma of the uterus and vagina. A clinicopathologic analysis of 27 cases. *Cancer* 1984;53:2530–2545.
492. Hays DM, Shimada H, Rarey RB Jr, et al. Sarcomas of the vagina and uterus: the Intergroup Rhabdomyosarcoma Study. *J Pediatr Surg* 1985;20:718–724.
493. Malkasian GD Jr, Welch JS, Soule EH. Primary leiomyosarcoma of the vagina. Report of 8 cases. *Am J Obstet Gynecol* 1963;86:730–736.
494. Davos I, Abell MR. Sarcomas of the vagina. *Obstet Gynecol* 1976;47:342–350.
495. Palmer JP, Bibark SM. Primary cancer of the vagina. *Am J Obstet Gynecol* 1954;67:377–397.
496. Webb MJ, Symmonds RE, Weiland LH. Malignant fibrous histiocytoma of the vagina. *Am J Obstet Gynecol* 1974;119:190–192.
497. Hiura M, Nogawa T, Nagai N, Yorishima M, Fujiwara A. Vaginal hemangiopericytoma: a light microscopic and ultrastructural study. *Gynecol Oncol* 1985;21:376–384.
498. Buscema J, Rosenshein NB, Taqi F, Woodruff JD. Vaginal hemangiopericytoma: a histopathologic and ultrastructural evaluation. *Obstet Gynecol* 1985;66:82s–85s.

499. Ulbright TM, Kraus FT. Endometrial stromal tumors of extra-uterine tissue. *Am J Clin Pathol* 1981;76:371–377.
500. Zaleski S, Setum C, Benda J. Cytologic presentation of alveolar soft part sarcoma of the vagina. A case report. *Acta Cytol* 1986;30:665–670.
501. O'Toole RV, Tuttle SE, Lucas JG, Sharma HM. Alveolar soft part sarcoma of the vagina: an immunohistochemical and electron microscopic study. *Int J Gynecol Pathol* 1985;4:258–265.
502. Chan WWY, SenGupta SK. Postirradiation angiosarcoma of the vaginal vault. *Arch Pathol Lab Med* 1991;115:527–528.
503. Bass PS, Birch B, Smart C, Theaker JM, Wells M. Low-grade transitional cell carcinoma of the vagina —an unusual case of vaginal bleeding. *Histopathology* 1994;24:581–583.
504. Phillips GL, Prem KA, Adcock LL, Twiggs LB. Vaginal recurrence of adenocarcinoma of the endometrium. *Gynecol Oncol* 1982;13:323–328.
505. Bergman F. Carcinoma of the ovary: a clinicopathological study of 86 autopsied cases with special reference to mode of spread. *Acta Obstet Gynecol Scand* 1966;45:211–231.
506. O'Reilly AP, McLeod F, Craft I. Hypernephroma presenting as a vaginal metastasis. Case report. *Br J Obstet Gynaecol* 1984;91:812–815.
507. Jacobs AJ, Deppe G, Kessinger MA, Newland JR. Case report. Breast carcinoma metastatic to the vagina. *Acta Obstet Gynecol Scand* 1983;62:83–85.
508. Xiu-yu Y, Hong-zhao S, Yuan-e W, Min-yi T, Yan-ning Z. Vaginal metastasis of choriocarcinoma and invasive mole. Clinical and pathological characteristics, diagnosis and treatment. *Chin Med J* 1985;98:463–470.
509. Goldberg GL, Yon DA, Block B, Levin W. Gestational trophoblastic disease: the significance of vaginal metastases. *Gynecol Oncol* 1986;24:155–161.

CHAPTER 52

The Cervix

Christopher P. Crum, Gerard J. Nuovo, and Kenneth R. Lee

INFLAMMATIONS

Acute and Chronic Cervicitis

At the onset of menarche, the production of estrogens by the ovary stimulates maturation (glycogen uptake) of cervical and vaginal squamous mucosa. The glycogen provides a substrate for endogenous vaginal aerobes and anaerobes, streptococci, enterococci, *Escherichia coli,* and staphylococci. The bacterial growth produces a drop in vaginal pH, and the exposed endocervix is sensitive to these changes in chemical environment. The response is a transformation from columnar to squamous epithelium. The process and transformation is also hastened by trauma and other infections occurring in the reproductive years. As the squamous epithelium overgrows and obliterates the surface columnar papillae, it covers and obstructs crypt openings, with the accumulation of mucus in deeper crypts (glands) to form mucous (nabothian) cysts. This process is invariably associated with an inflammatory infiltrate composed of a mixture of polymorphonuclear leukocytes and mononuclear cells, erosion or ulceration, and epithelial repair (reparative atypia or dysplasia of repair). All of these components characterize what is known as chronic cervicitis.

Some degree of cervical inflammation may be found in virtually all multiparous and in many nulliparous adult women, and is usually of little clinical consequence. Principal concerns include the potential presence of organisms, which may be clinically important. Specific infections by gonococci, chlamydia, mycoplasma, and herpes (mostly type II) may produce significant acute or chronic cervicitis and should be identified for their relevance to upper genital tract disease, pregnancy complications, or sexual transmission.

Specific Infections

Clinically significant infections that can be identified or suspected by histologic examination of the cervix include herpes simplex viruses (HSV), cytomegalovirus, *Chlamydia trachomatis* and, rarely, adenovirus (1–5). HSV should be suspected and excluded in any ulcer, particularly if it is accompanied by epithelial cell necrosis and acute inflammatory exudate. The diagnostic cells contain one or multiple nuclei with either discrete inclusions or smudged (ground glass) chromatin. They are typically found at the periphery of the ulcer, in the spongiotic epithelium or as single desegregated cells. Special stains may be helpful if the diagnosis is uncertain on morphologic grounds alone. *C. trachomatis* infection does not elicit specific epithelial changes, but is closely associated with severe acute and chronic inflammatory infiltrates, repair, and follicular cervicitis (1,6,7). The latter is not a very sensitive marker for chlamydia infection, but has been shown to be more commonly associated with positive cultures than not. Thus, if follicular cervicitis is identified in a biopsy, a comment should be made in the report that this finding may be associated with chlamydia, but is not diagnostic. Chlamydia is typically identified in small inclusion vacuoles in the endocervical or reparative epithelial cells. It is uncommonly identified in more mature squamous cells. Whether these inclusion vacuoles can be identified and distinguished from noninfectious vacuoles, by histology or cytology, is controversial (8,9). Raising the suspicion of chlamydia based on these changes alone is not recommended.

INTRAEPITHELIAL AND INVASIVE SQUAMOUS NEOPLASIA

Fifty years ago, carcinoma of the cervix was the leading cause of cancer deaths in women in the United States, but the

---

C. P. Crum: Department of Pathology, Harvard Medical School; Women's and Perinatal Pathology Division, Brigham and Women's Hospital, Boston, Massachusetts 02115.

G. J. Nuovo: Director, MGN Medical Research Laboratories, Setauket, New York 11733.

K. R. Lee: Department of Pathology, Harvard Medical School; Department of Pathology, Divisions of Cytology and Women's and Perinatal Pathology, Brigham and Women's Hospital, Boston, Massachusetts 02115.

death rate has declined by two-thirds to its present rank as the eighth source of cancer mortality (after lung, breast, colon, pancreas, ovary, lymph nodes, and blood), causing about 4,500 deaths annually (10). In sharp contrast to this reduced mortality, the detection frequency of early cancers and precancerous conditions is very high. Much credit goes to the Papanicolaou smear test in detecting cervical precancers and to the accessibility of the cervix to colposcopy and biopsy. Annually there are an estimated 13,000 cases of new invasive cancer and nearly one million precancerous conditions (squamous intraepithelial lesions) of varying grade. Thus, it is evident that Pap smear screening has increased the detection of potentially curable cancers as well as the detection and eradication of preinvasive lesions, some of which would progress to cancer without intervention.

Pathogenesis

Epidemiologic data have long implicated a sexually transmitted agent, based specifically on the risk factors for cervical cancer, which include early age at first intercourse, multiple sexual partners, and a male partner with multiple previous sexual partners. All other risk factors are subordinate to these three, primarily multiple sexual partners. Potential risk factors that remain poorly understood include oral contraceptive use, cigarette smoking, parity, family history, associated genital infections, and lack of circumcision in the male sexual partner (11).

Concerning sexually transmitted agents, human papillomavirus (HPV) is currently considered an important factor in cervical oncogenesis. This virus is the known cause of the sexually transmitted vulvar condyloma acuminatum and has been isolated from vulvar and vaginal squamous cell carcinomas; it is also suspected to be an oncogenic agent in a variety of other squamous tumors or proliferative lesions of skin and mucous membranes (12).

There is mounting evidence linking human papillomavirus to cancer in general and cervical cancer in particular: (a) Human papillomavirus DNA is detected by hybridization techniques in approximately 85% of cervical cancers and in approximately 90% of cervical condylomata and precancerous lesions (12). (b) Specific human papillomavirus types are associated with cervical cancer (high risk) versus condylomata (low risk); low-risk types include types 6, 11, 42, and 44 and high-risk types 16, 18, 31, and 33 (12). (c) *In vitro* studies indicate that the high-risk human papillomavirus types have the capability to transform cells in culture, and this ability is linked to specific viral oncogenes (E6 and E7 genes), which differ in sequence between the high-risk and low-risk human papillomavirus types. Introduction of these nucleic acids into cultured keratinocytes produces morphologic changes nearly identical to precancerous changes, and under certain circumstances, these cells may form squamous tumors when injected into mice. (d) The physical state of the virus differs in cancers, being covalently linked (integrated) with the host genomic DNA. This is in contrast to free (episomal) viral DNA in condylomata and most precancerous lesions (12) (Fig. 1). (e) The E6 oncoprotein of human papillomavirus type 16 and

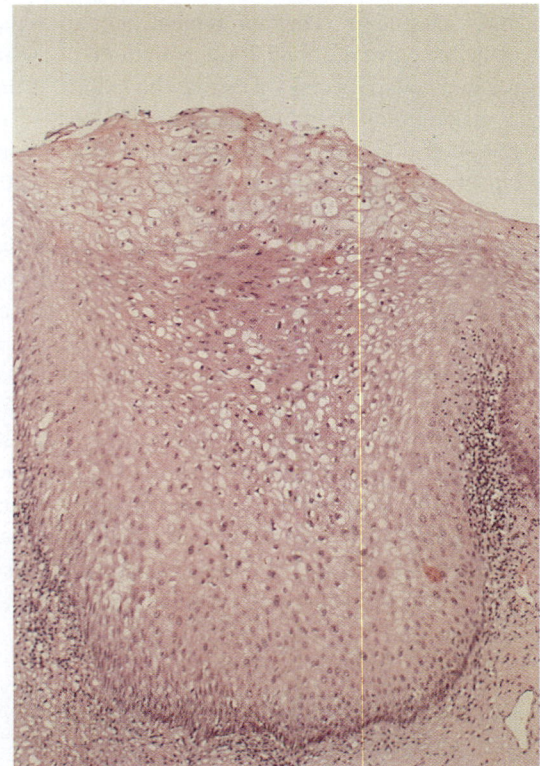 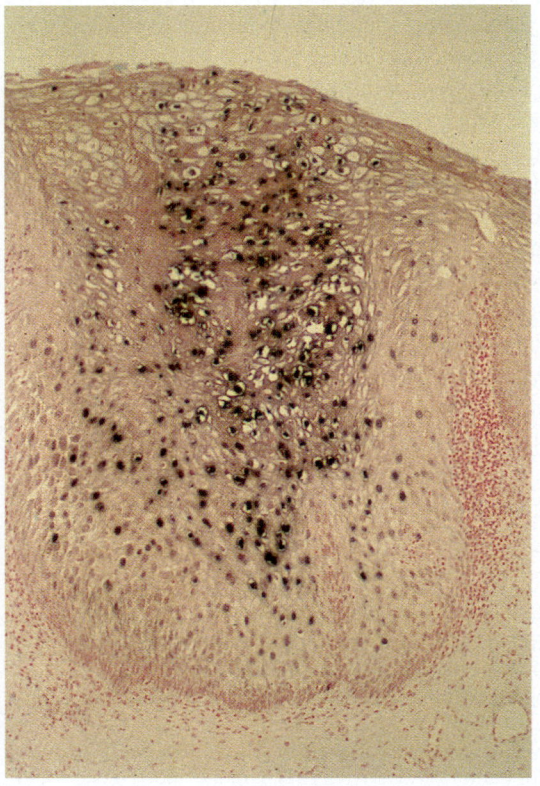

FIG. 1. Expression of papillomavirus nucleic acid in a condyloma. **A:** Hematoxylin and eosin-stained section. **B:** Distribution of DNA in the epithelium following DNA-DNA *in situ* hybridization.

TABLE 1. *Criteria for cervical diagnosis*

Findings	Diagnosis	Management
Negative, no transformation zone seen	Descriptive	Depends on cytologic and colposcopic findings
Acanthosis, parakeratosis, reactive changes	Descriptive	Depends on cytologic and colposcopic findings
Severe inflammation or follicular cervicitis, reparative changes	Descriptive	Consider treatment of inflammation, exclude chlamydia in follicular cervicitis
Flat or exophytic lesions with koilocytotic atypia, maturation, minimal parabasal atypia	Low-grade SIL (CIN I/condyloma)	Remove or follow
Filiform papillae with immature metaplasia and minimal atypia	Low-grade SIL (papillary immature metaplasia or immature condyloma)	Remove or follow
Koilocytosis, maturation, increased atypia, including parabasal distribution	High-grade SIL (CIN II)	Remove
Minimal maturation, diffuse atypia	High-grade SIL (CIN III)	Remove
Neoplastic epithelium in the ECC with preserved polarity characteristic of intraepithelial disease	Strips of neoplastic squamous epithelium consistent with (low- or high-grade) SIL	Remove
Neoplastic squamous epithelium in the ECC with loss of polarity or marked atypia	Strips of neoplastic squamous epithelium, exclude invasive carcinoma	Diagnostic cone biopsy

CIN, cervical intraepithelial neoplasia; ECC, endocervical curetting; SIL, squamous intraepithelial lesion.

18 (but not low-risk type 11) binds to the tumor suppressor gene p53 and accelerates its proteolytic degradation; the E7 protein binds to the retinoblastina gene (Rb) and displaces transcription factors normally sequestered by Rb. Both of these properties affect cell-cycle regulation. (f) Certain chromosomal abnormalities, including amplification of 3q, have been associated with cancers containing specific (HPV-16) papillomaviruses (13).

The evidence does not implicate human papillomavirus as the only factor. A high percentage of young women are infected with one or more human papillomavirus types during their reproductive years, and only a few develop cancer. Other co-carcinogens, the immune status of the individual, nutrition, and many other factors influence whether the human papillomavirus infection remains subclinical (latent), turns into a precancer, or eventually progresses to cancer. In addition, about 15% of cervical cancers are not associated with human papillomavirus, leaving open to question other pathways of cancer development, including host gene mutations (14).

The reason that Papanicolaou smear screening is so effective in preventing cervical cancer is that the majority of cancers are preceded by a precancerous lesion. This lesion may exist in the noninvasive stage for as long as 20 years and shed abnormal cells that can be detected on cytologic examination. These precancerous changes should be viewed with the following in mind: (a) they represent a continuum of morphologic change with relatively indistinct boundaries; (b) they will not invariably progress to cancer and may spontaneously regress, with the risk of persisting or progressing to cancer increasing with the severity of the precancerous change; (c) they are associated with papillomaviruses, and high-risk human papillomavirus types are found in increasing frequency in the higher grade precursors (15,16); (d) they virtually always occur at the squamocolumnar junction in the cervical transformation zone (Fig. 2).

Squamous Intraepithelial Lesions (SILs)

Cervical precancers have been classified in a variety of ways. The oldest system is the dysplasia–carcinoma *in situ* system with mild dysplasia on one end and severe dysplasia/carcinoma *in situ* on the other. Another is the cervical intraepithelial neoplasia (CIN) classification, with mild dysplasias termed CIN grade I and carcinoma *in situ* lesions termed CIN III. Still another reduces these entities to two: low-grade and high-grade intraepithelial lesions (15).

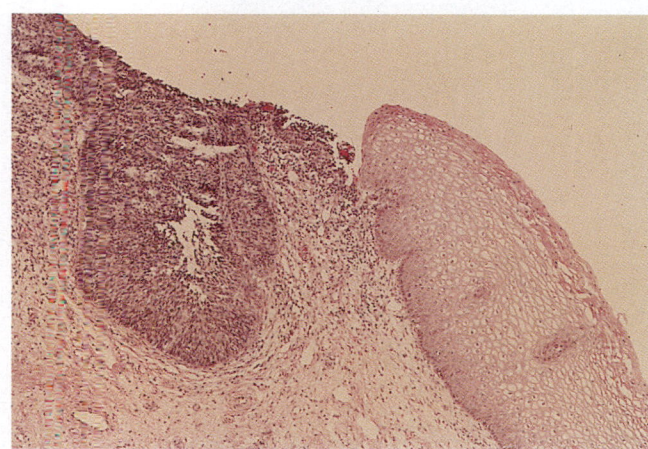

FIG. 2. Squamocolumnar junction with high-grade squamous intraepithelial lesion (HSIL).

Although the latter terminology is relatively new, the general criteria for distinguishing these entities have been published in many articles and books in the past 40 years. Recent changes in classification have depended heavily on these prior publications. One difference in the current approaches is the redefinition of CIN I, the low-grade squamous intraepithelial lesion (LSIL) as a lesion closely resembling a flat or exophytic condyloma and the use of criteria for distinguishing CIN I from CIN II or CIN III (17). The diagnostic approach to these lesions is summarized in Table 1.

Low-Grade Squamous Intraepithelial Lesions (CIN I)

Histologically, these lesions have cytologic atypia in a distribution characteristic of flat or exophytic condylomas (Fig. 3). Cervical condylomas vary in appearance from flat to slightly raised exophytic lesions that resemble condylomata of the vulva. The distinguishing features are a thickening of the epithelium (acanthosis) with koilocytotic atypia in the middle and upper portions of the epithelium. Koilocytotic atypia is a constellation of cellular changes that include variation in nuclear size and shape, wrinkled nuclei, hyperchromasia, binucleation or multinucleation, and perinuclear halos (18). The perinuclear halos vary in shape, and in koilocytes there is often a distinct zone of clearing around the nucleus with a condensation of more dense-appearing cytoplasm peripheral to the halo. Importantly, nuclear atypia is minimal in the lower half of the epithelium, there is a low mitotic index, and bizarre or abnormal mitoses are absent. Flat condylomata have a similar appearance but lack

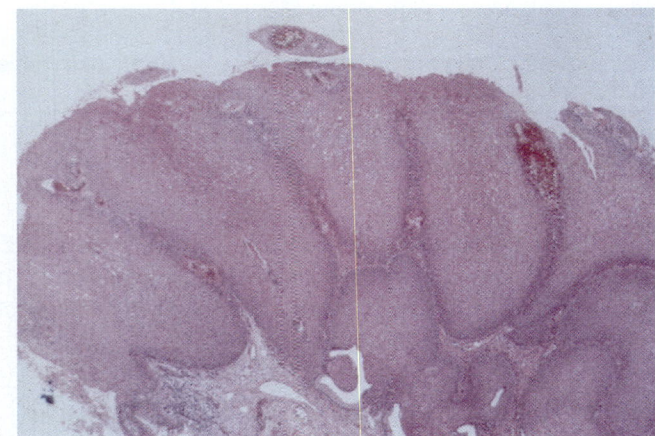
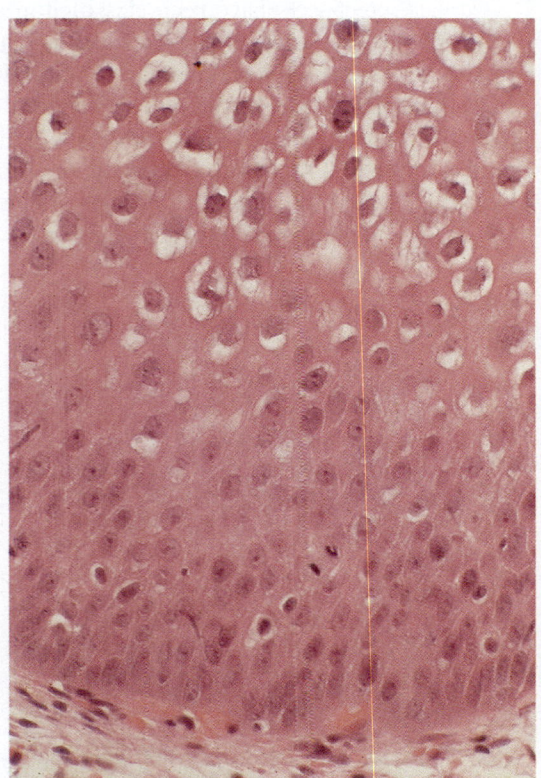
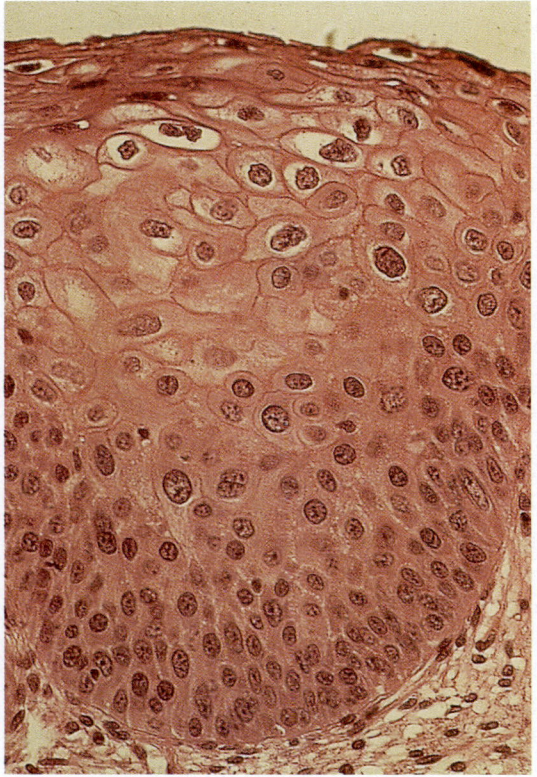

FIG. 3. Histologic features of low-grade squamous intraepithelial lesion (LSIL). **A:** Exophytic condyloma. **B:** LSIL with mild parabasal hyperplasia and koilocytosis. **C:** LSIL with expanded parabasal cell layers but minimal atypia.

the papillary architecture of an exophytic lesion. The absence of nuclear enlargement and atypia throughout the full thickness of the epithelium distinguishes LSIL from high-grade lesions (HSILs), although not necessarily a high-risk HPV (19–21).

In addition to the distribution of the nuclear atypia, the low-grade lesions exhibit the following, which parallel the findings seen on the Papanicolaou smear: (a) the nuclei retain a certain consistency in degree of irregularity, with wrinkled or round nuclear contours; (b) although the nuclei are hyperchromatic, the hyperchromasia tends to be more uniform in intensity than in HSIL.

High-Grade Squamous Intraepithelial Lesions (CIN II, CIN III)

These lesions share several morphologic features, specifically nuclear atypia in all layers of the epithelium at least in a portion of the lesion (20,21) (Fig. 4). Lesions with koilo-

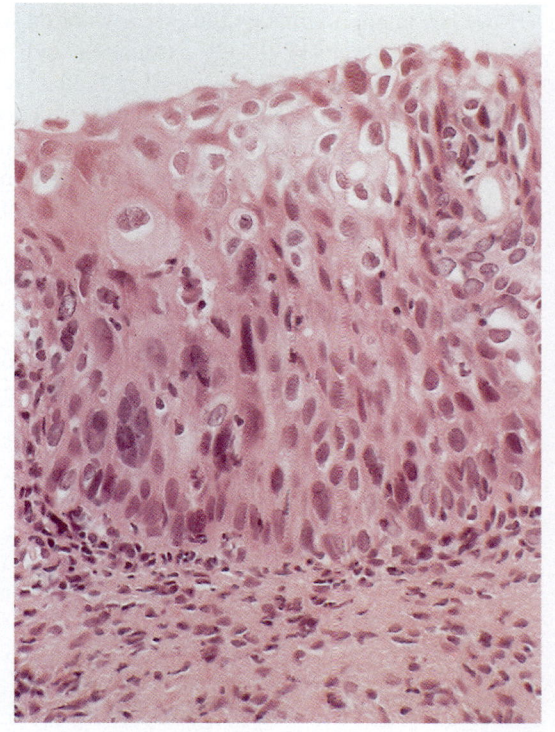
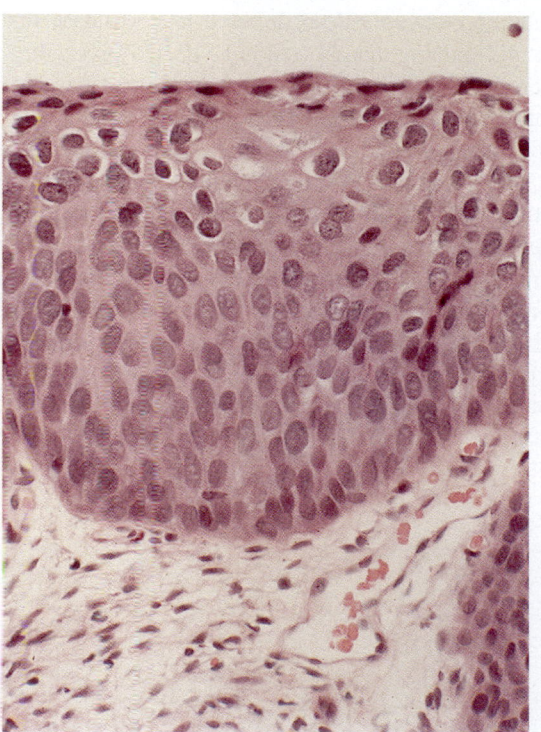
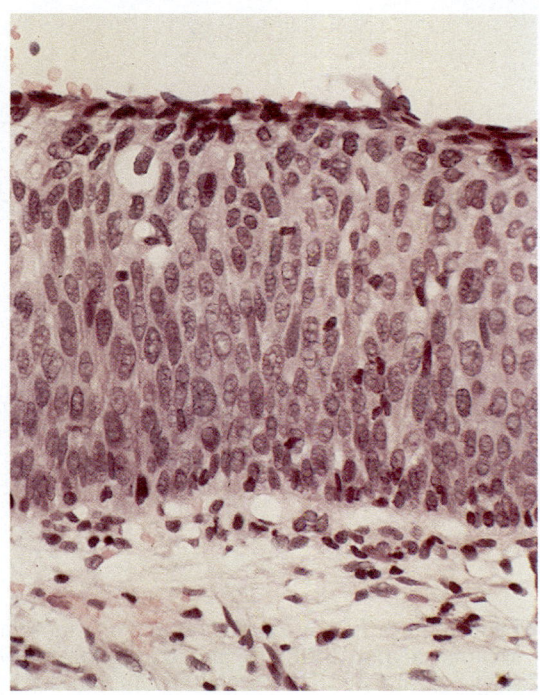

FIG. 4. Histologic features of HSIL. **A:** Cervical intraepithelial neoplasia grade II (CIN II) with focal marked atypia and loss of cell polarity. **B:** CIN II with focal maturation and diffuse nuclear atypia. **C:** CIN III.

cytotic atypia or maturation conform to the image of CIN II, whereas those without discernible maturation fall into the category of CIN III. The koilocytes may be identical to those in flat condyloma, but commonly differ by the presence of smaller, more concentric halos, and more dense nuclear hyperchromasia and/or pleomorphism. The epithelial surface of CIN II and CIN III lesions occasionally contains horizontally arranged parakeratotic cells with abnormal nuclei. In addition, nuclear atypia is present in the lower half of the epithelium in at least a portion of the lesion (Fig. 5). Paradoxically, some high-grade CIN lesions exhibit a more homogeneous population of neoplastic cells, with less variation in nuclear size and staining than is seen in LSIL. However, the nuclei are crowded, enlarged, hyperchromatic, and have a higher mitotic index than normal basal cells.

In addition to the distribution of nuclear atypia, mitotic abnormalities, and alterations in cell differentiation, HSIL differs qualitatively from LSIL in two cytologic parameters that are better appreciated on Papanicolaou smears: (a) the nuclei often vary markedly in contour; (b) the nuclei are not only hyperchromatic but contain irregularly or coarsely distributed chromatin. These nuclear abnormalities associated with high-grade precursors can be appreciated in not only the basal/parabasal cells but also frequently in intermediate and superficial cells.

Coexistence of Low- and High-Grade SIL

It should be emphasized that a portion of high-grade SILs are associated with low-grade SIL (Fig. 6). As many as three-fourths of SIL lesions of all grades have been reported to coexist with cervical condyloma (22). From 10% to 20% of LSILs on Papanicolaou smear are confirmed as HSIL on biopsy (23,24). Moreover, high-risk HPV types have been identified in low-grade SIL (25). However, the association between LSIL and HSIL varies depending on the criteria used to define LSIL. Moreover, at least one-half of high-grade SILs contain some areas of koilocytotic atypia (26). However, in approximately three-fourths of these cases, the koilocytotic atypia is closely associated with features of HSIL, including nuclear atypia in all epithelial layers. Therefore, the proportion of HSIL cases in which a classic condyloma (LSIL) merges with an HSIL is relatively small. In our experience, a significant minority of such cases reflects two separate HPV infections (Park J, Crum CP, unpublished observations).

Histologic Variations in Presentation of SIL

There are several general categories of squamous intraepithelial lesions that may prove difficult on either cytologic or biopsy interpretation:

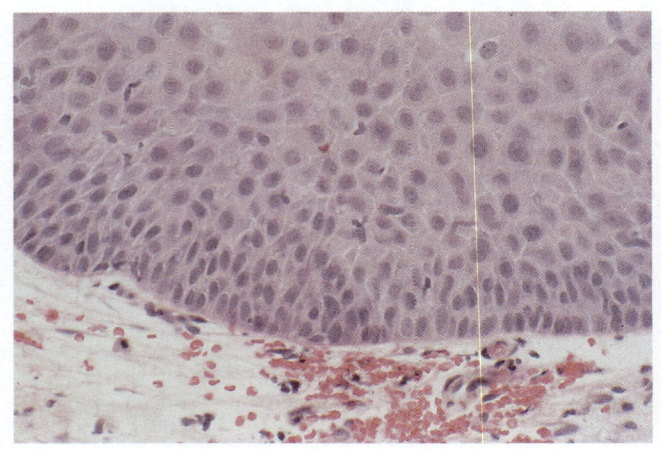
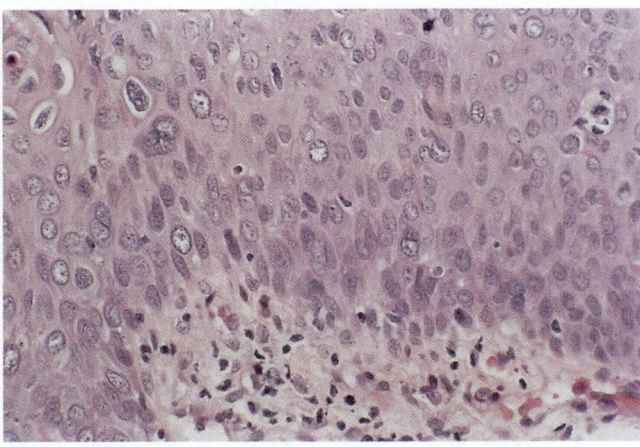

FIG. 5. Spectrum of parabasal cell changes in SILs. **A:** Minimal atypia (LSIL). **B** and **C:** Moderate and severe atypia (HSIL).

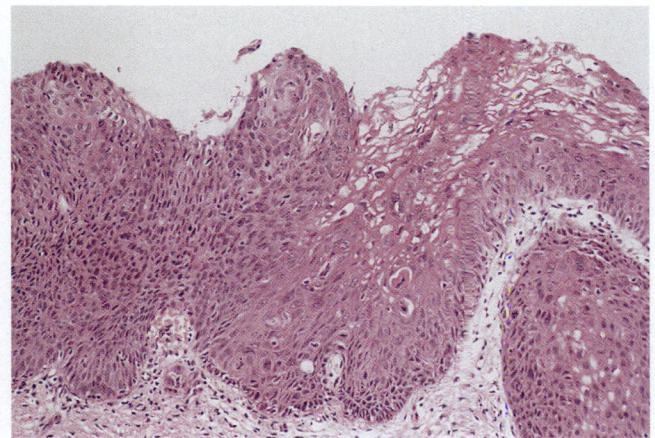

FIG. 6. Merging of LSIL *(left)* and HSIL *(right)* in an HPV-16 positive lesion.

Keratinizing SIL (Fig. 7)

This lesion is characterized by prominent superficial keratinization in addition to atypia. Practically speaking, keratinized abnormal cells on cytologic smears confer some degree of uncertainty with respect to the nature of the lesion. Keratinized cells may be seen in smears in some benign cellular reactions such as hyper- or parakeratosis, atypias of undetermined significance, some low- and high-grade SILs, and invasive squamous cell carcinomas. The diagnosis of a keratinizing SIL is based on the presence of keratinizing cells with nuclear atypia such as variation in nuclear size and staining, usually accompanied by some binucleation. Very mild atypia usually signifies a low-grade SIL. In contrast to condylomata, the nuclei in a keratinizing HSIL exhibit much greater variation in contour, dense or coarse appearing chromatin, and variable often intensely eosinophilic cytoplasm. It is important to emphasize that keratinizing high-grade lesions cannot always be distinguished cytologically from condylomata and that a report of any Papanicolaou smear with prominent atypical parakeratosis should include the possibility of a high-grade lesion (see below). Histologically, keratinizing HSIL exhibits conspicuous nuclear atypia in the lower and intermediate cell layers, similar to nonkeratinizing high-grade SIL.

Keratinizing HSIL must be distinguished not only from condylomata but also from invasive squamous cell carcinoma. In condylomata, the principal feature is nuclear hyperchromasia and binucleation within relatively small, parakeratotic cells. Irregular shapes may be present, but the nuclear-cytoplasmic ratio is usually high with uniformly distributed cytoplasm. Squamous cell carcinoma is the more likely diagnosis if one encounters tumor diathesis, very numerous atypical cells, many with bizarre shapes (tadpole cells, etc.), and prominent nucleoli.

Papillary Immature Metaplasia (PIM) (Fig. 8A,B)

This lesion is one exception to the concept that all immature lesions warrant classification as HSIL. We have previ-

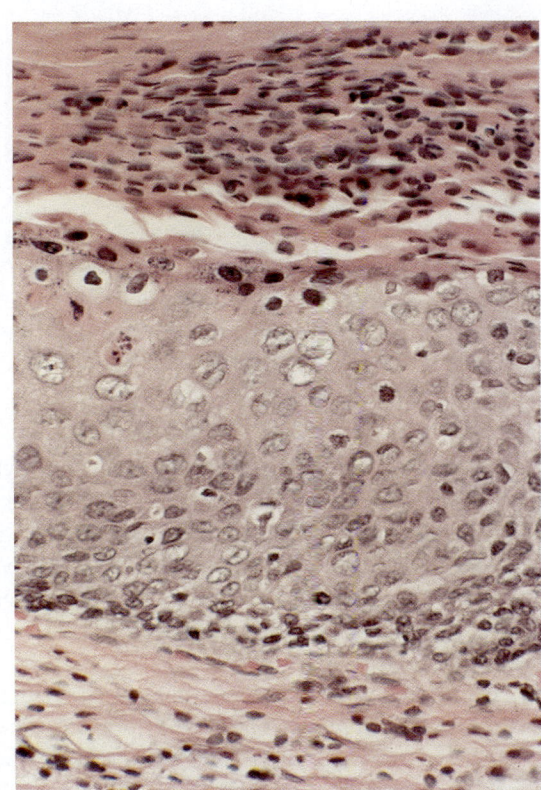
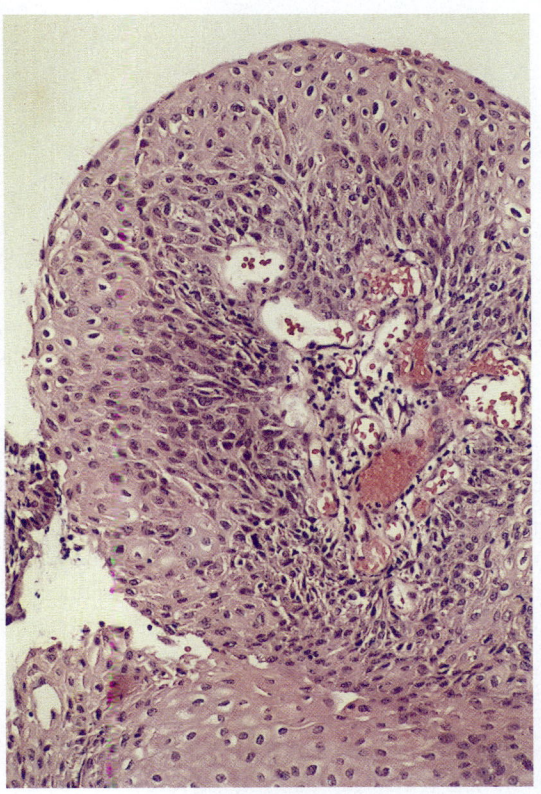

FIG. 7. Keratinizing HSIL with a dense keratinizing surface **(A)**. Papillary immature metaplasia (LSIL) **(B)**.

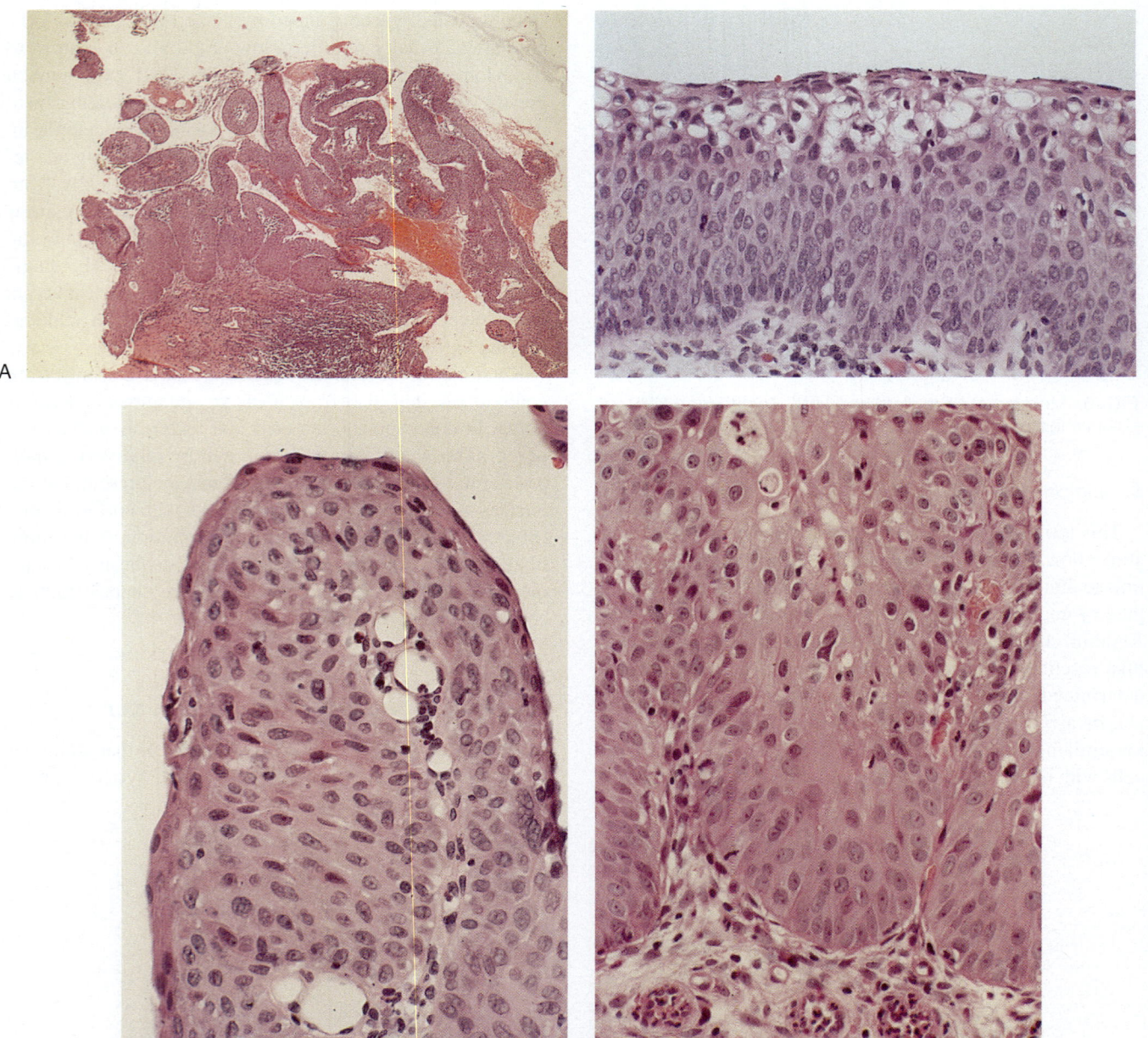

FIG. 8. SILs with metaplastic growth patterns. **A:** Papillary immature metaplasia (immature LSIL). Low-power architecture is characterized by filiform papillae, which at higher magnification **(B)** demonstrate mild atypia. **C:** HSIL with an immature metaplastic growth pattern. **D:** Reactive metaplasia for contrast.

ously identified a distinct subset of lesions (atypical immature metaplasia [AIM] or PIM) that is characterized by a proliferation of immature squamous cells with mild cytologic atypia, frequently associated with more mature areas of typical condyloma, and a tendency to extend into the endocervical canal (27–29). Koilocytotic atypia is identified in mature areas, whereas the immature areas exhibit slightly increased cellularity, with cells that have an increased nuclear/cytoplasmic ratio, smooth nuclear contours, and uniformly distributed chromatin with prominent chromocenters. Free-standing (filiform) papillae covered by these immature cells, with preservation of the surface endocervical epithelium, are a frequent feature. *In situ* hybridization studies have shown that HPV types 6/11 are present, not only in the areas that show koilocytotic atypia but also in those areas of immature metaplasia. High-risk HPV types, by contrast, are almost never seen, but we have encountered several cases in which a PIM coexisted with a separate high-grade lesion of separate HPV type (29).

Papillary immature metaplasia must be distinguished not only from reactive metaplasia, but from HSIL and papillary squamous cell carcinoma. The cytologic correlate of the immature metaplastic component is squamous cells of metaplastic appearance with nuclear enlargement, occasional binucleation, relatively uniform nuclear contours, and minimal hyperchromasia (30). It is important to emphasize that the histologic distinction of PIM from HSIL may be very difficult, depending on fixation and thickness of section. In the authors' experience, it is not uncommon to encounter immature proliferations that initially suggest papillary AIM and are eventually concluded to be HSIL. The reader should be aware of this pitfall, both in cytology and histology.

SIL with Immature Metaplastic-Type Differentiation (Fig. 8C)

Immature metaplastic lesions are discussed later in the chapter. However, worthy of mention here are those immature "metaplasias" that are in fact squamous intraepithelial lesions. This category pertains to immature flat lesions that exhibit a relatively uniform population of small metaplastic-type cells, some preservation in polarity, and, not infrequently, mucin droplets. Such lesions are distinguished as SIL by the presence of mitoses in the upper epithelial layers with anisokaryosis and nuclear pleomorphism, in contrast to conventional reactive changes (Fig. 8D). They are classified as HSIL and are distinguished from papillary immature metaplasia by the presence of greater anisonucleosis, absence of regular chromocenters, and absence of papillary morphology.

Differential Diagnosis of Squamous Intraepithelial Lesions

Typically, the diagnosis of a LSIL requires the presence of superficial nuclear atypia. The strong association between atypia and the presence of papillomavirus nucleic acids supports establishing a morphologic threshold for the diagnosis of LSIL (31). However, how this is to be distinguished from nonspecific cellular changes can be problematic. A useful approach to the diagnosis of LSIL is to apply several criteria in sequence (Fig. 8):

1. *Low power epithelial organization:* In many cases, the diagnosis of a LSIL will be suspected at low magnification (40–100×) based on the presence of epithelial alterations that are conspicuously different from surrounding epithelium. These alterations may take the form of changes in epithelial thickness, absence of metaplastic changes with columnar cells or mucin droplets, conspicuous hyperchromasia in the upper cell layers, or more subtle changes in nuclear density, cell arrangement, or halo contour in the upper epithelium.
2. *Major histologic criteria:* The next step is to assess the epithelium at higher magnification, and quantify the nuclear atypia. The distinction of a squamous intraepithelial lesion from a nonspecific process is based primarily on differences in size and staining of the intermediate and superficial cells. Technically, there should be threefold differences in size with variable staining. Hence the pathologist is searching for large, hyperchromatic nuclei (32,33). Size differences may not be as striking, however, and a combination of nuclear, cytoplasmic, and growth pattern alterations may prompt the diagnosis. In some instances the diagnosis may be made on instinct alone, although the reader is warned that instinctive diagnoses (particularly if rendered frequently) may not be reproducible.
3. *Minor histologic criteria:* In more subtle lesions certain criteria may be useful in confirming the diagnosis: (a) Binucleation is present in approximately 90% of low grade SIL. In our experience, two or more binucleate cells in a high-power (400×) field strongly supports the diagnosis of an LSIL, particularly if these nuclei are enlarged or hyperchromatic. Small, densely hyperkeratotic binucleate cells also support a diagnosis of a squamous intraepithelial lesion, resembling the atypical parakeratotic cells seen in Papanicolaou smears (34). It should be emphasized that sporadic binucleation frequently occurs in the setting of reactive epithelial changes; for this reason, binucleation is used to aid in the diagnosis rather than to make the diagnosis of LSIL per se (32,33). (b) Irregularly shaped cytoplasmic halos are another useful, if less specific feature. The halos are often punctuated by a rim of dense cytoplasm, forming an interlacing meshwork, or basket weave, in the superficial epithelial layers (32,33).

A variety of epithelial alterations may mimic koilocytosis and are illustrated in and the succeeding cases (Fig. 9). They include the following:

1. *Vaginal papillomatosis* (Fig. 9C): The increased (and at times misplaced) concern over papillomaviruses in the past 10 years has resulted in a higher index of suspicion for lesions in the vaginal mucosa. Because the vagina characteristically contains epithelial folds, excrescences or "papillae," these may be suspected clinically and sampled. The histologic appearance of such biopsies includes papillomatosis, parakeratosis, and cytoplasmic halos. However, prominent acanthosis, nuclear atypia, and atypical parakeratosis are not present. The appropriate diagnosis for biopsies of this type is "acanthosis, papillomatosis, etc., nonspecific." The term *nonspecific* properly designates these alterations as not associated with HPV nucleic acids. Molecular studies have confirmed that such changes are no more likely to harbor HPV nucleic acids than normal squamous epithelium (35,36).
2. *Reactive epithelial changes (nonspecific)* (Fig. 9A): Prominent cytoplasmic halos may be present in association with any glycogenated epithelium, and mild nuclear atypia will result if the epithelium is either directly inflamed or associated with underlying inflammation. Occasionally, reparative or reactive epithelial changes undergo incomplete maturation, in which case nuclear hyperchromasia will be present in association with the

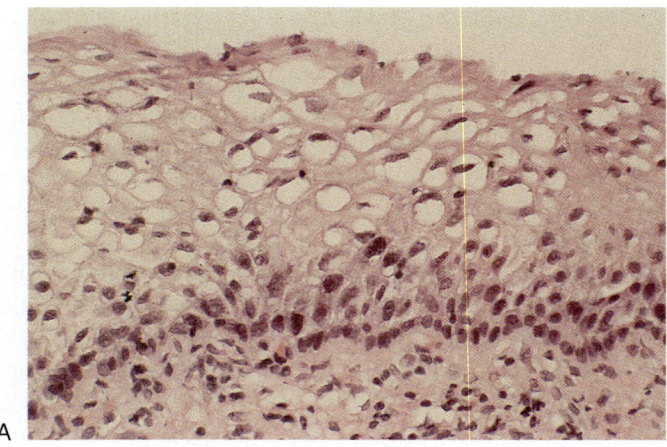
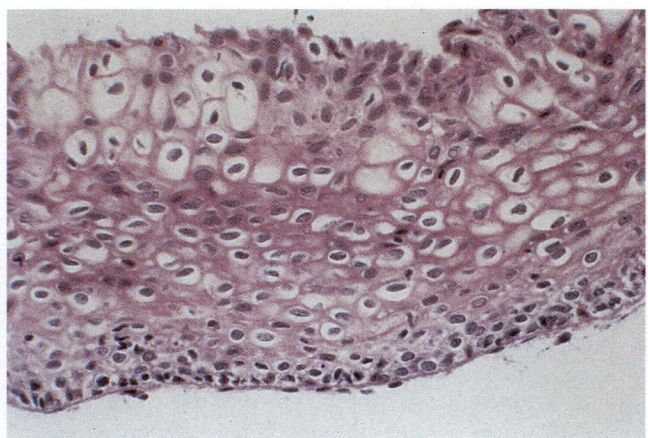
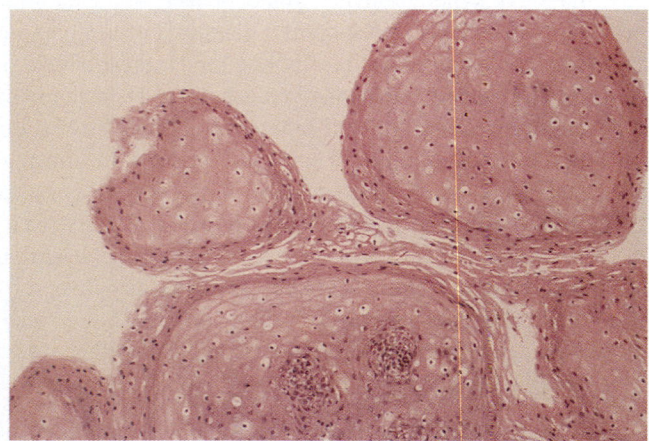

FIG. 9. Differential diagnosis of LSIL. **A:** Reactive epithelial changes with prominent cytoplasmic halos. **B:** Postmenopausal squamous atypia with pseudokoilocytosis. **C:** Vaginal papillomatosis.

cytoplasmic halos. In such cases, the most important discriminating feature is absence of variation, in either cell size or staining intensity, in the cell population. Binucleated cells may or may not be present, but are usually inconspicuous.

A second type of reactive epithelial change may exhibit semimature metaplasia with prominent binucleation. Such cases should not be confused with condyloma; the binucleated cells are usually not enlarged, and are bland in appearance, occurring in a background pattern of metaplasia (33).

3. *Postmenopausal squamous atypia* (Fig. 9B): Prior reports have identified cells resembling koilocytes in postmenopausal women (37,38). Although LSIL may occur in this age group, a spectrum of epithelial and cellular alterations may exist in menopausal or postmenopausal women, ranging from partial to complete atrophy. This spectrum includes maturation disturbances with pseudokoilocytosis, transitional metaplasia, and classic atrophic changes. In some instances, all three may be present in the same biopsy. Pseudokoilocytosis is characterized by epithelial maturation, cytoplasmic halos, and variable (usually mild) nuclear size or staining. The halos are usually round and uniform in appearance, with centrally placed nuclei. The latter are usually slightly hyperchromatic, at times elongated, and occasionally grooved. Occasionally, binucleation is present, and the process may closely mimic koilocytosis. In some cases, peripheral condensation of pale cytoplasm around the uniform halos gives a target-like or "fried egg" appearance to the cells. This pattern is similar to that produced by navicular cells in pregnancy and postpartum. It is uncommonly associated with papillomavirus nucleic acids (39–41).

Efforts to distinguish low-grade squamous intraepithelial lesions from nonspecific reactive epithelial processes have usually centered on the use of papillomavirus DNA analysis (42). More recently, preliminary studies suggest that other markers may aid in identifying HPV infected epithelium, including cell cycle proteins (Quade B, Crum CP, Dutta A, unpublished observations).

High-Grade Squamous Intraepithelial Lesions

The diagnosis of HSIL (CIN II or III) is considered when the abnormality in question either does not resemble a condyloma or, if it does, the atypia under study is not confined strictly to the superficial cell layers. Because epithelial immaturity, nuclear atypia, and inflammatory cellular changes may be present in both benign and neoplastic squamous proliferations, the distinction of reactive processes from SIL requires careful attention to the growth pattern of the epithelium, the distribution of atypia, and degree of nuclear abnormality. Nonneoplastic reactive changes include regularity of nuclear spacing, preservation of nucleoli, absence of marked variation in nuclear size, contour and staining (specifically coarse appearing hyperchromatic nuclei), and, with minor exceptions, lack of nuclear atypia in the upper epithelial layers. This latter parameter is referred to as normalization of the epithelium with maturation (Fig. 10). Nuclear atypia in the upper epithelial cell layers is present in most squamous intraepithelial lesions, irrespective of grade, but the interpretation of this parameter in the context of inflammatory change is subjective. Most reactive/reparative processes, however severe, will mature with spacing of nuclei due to cytoplasmic maturation, accompanied by either a reduction in nuclear size or regularity in nuclear morphology. Immature metaplasias and atrophy usually undergo maturation but in some instances (due to extreme immaturity or partial epithelial denudation) there may be no decrease in the nuclear-cytoplasmic ratio in the surface of the epithelium. In such cases the distinction of benign from neoplastic changes must be made on cytologic grounds, and a diagnosis of uncertainty on cytology (ASCUS) or biopsy (atypical squamous epithelium with a comment) may be necessary if there is atypia present. Occasionally nuclear enlargement and hyperchromasia may be seen near the surface of inflamed immature metaplasia, in which case the distinction of metaplasia from a SIL is based on evaluation of the entire epithelium (see below).

Reactive squamous epithelial changes that may mimic high-grade squamous intraepithelial lesions include the following (Fig. 10):

Reactive/Reparative Epithelial Changes

Epithelial alterations in this category demonstrate: (a) intercellular edema (spongiosis), (b) evenly spaced nuclei with mild to moderate enlargement but minimal anisokaryosis, (c) prominent nucleoli, (d) intraepithelial neutrophils, and (e) a tendency for superficial maturation. Nuclear enlargement may be present, but it is not accompanied by hyperchromasia or changes in nuclear spacing. Incomplete maturation may be present, but the nuclei should display regular spacing, distinct cell borders, and mild variation in staining or size. Irregularities in the parabasal cell population may accompany inflammation, but normal maturation excludes an SIL. Mild reactive/inflammatory cell changes may produce general nuclear enlargement with binucleation, and SIL is excluded by the absence of variation in nuclear staining or contour.

More marked inflammatory/reparative changes may coexist with striking hyperchromasia of the lower epithelial layers, with variably degrees of spongiosis. The higher nuclear-

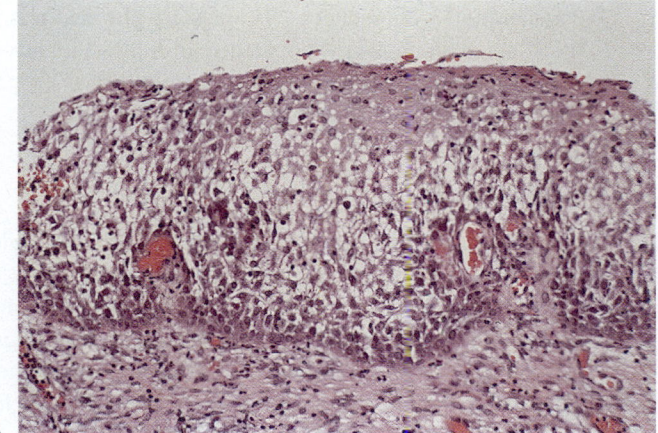
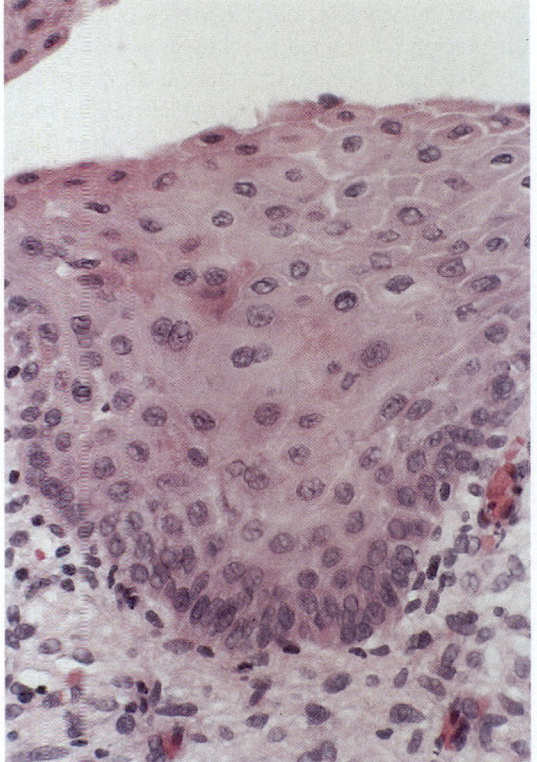
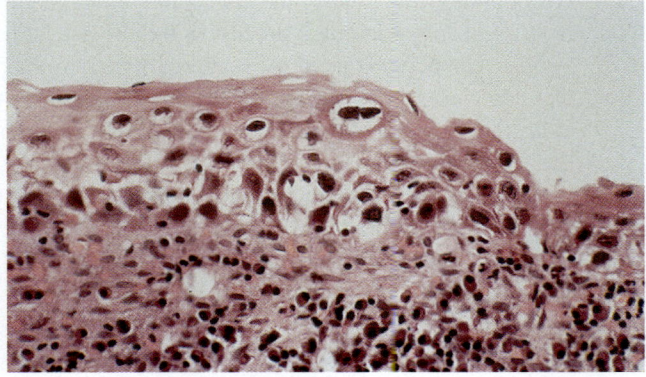

FIG. 10. Reactive epithelial changes with and without SIL. **A:** Reactive changes with spongiosis. **B:** Reactive changes with binuclated forms. **C:** Inflamed SIL, with focal marked atypia in basal superficial cells.

cytoplasmic ratio of basal/parabasal cells combined with inflammation contributes to the increased nuclear density and hyperchromasia in the lower third of the epithelium. However, in these epithelia, SIL can be excluded if there is a normalization of the epithelium near the surface (Fig. 10A,B).

The diagnosis of a SIL, either low or high grade, should be considered when features of repair—spongiosis, prominent nucleoli—are accompanied by greater than usual degrees of nuclear enlargement and hyperchromasia and when the abnormalities are present in some superficial epithelial cells (Fig. 10C). Features that should raise the question of SIL include irregular nuclear spacing or loss of polarity, discrete enlarged hyperchromatic nuclei or binucleated forms, anisokaryosis, and the presence of enlarged hyperchromatic nuclei on the surface. The evaluation of surface atypia is subjective, inasmuch as the number of abnormal cells and the characteristics of the epithelium influence interpretation. In some cases a diagnosis of uncertainty (atypical squamous epithelium) may be necessary, with a qualifying comment.

Immature Squamous Metaplasia

It is important to distinguish metaplasia from a metaplastic growth pattern. By definition, epithelial alterations associated with typical squamous metaplasia are usually nonneoplastic, particularly if characterized by mucin droplets or endocervical cells, either within the epithelium or on the surface. Surface columnar cells and mucin droplets are uncommonly (but sometimes are!) associated with high-grade precursors; surface columnar cells may be found in association with atypical immature metaplasia (immature condyloma. Immature squamous cell alterations exhibiting a metaplastic growth pattern include the following: (a) Mild reactive alterations in immature metaplasia are characterized by some variation in nuclear staining and size. (b) Acutely inflamed metaplastic epithelia with polynucleation can usually be distinguished from SIL if the nuclei are not densely hyperchromatic and the background cell population displays a uniform nuclear morphology with nucleoli. (c) Occasional surface atypia may be present in association with inflammation, but the general growth pattern of the metaplastic process should not be altered; the lower epithelial cells should exhibit a minimum of nuclear crowding or pleomorphism and display chromocenters or nucleoli. (d) If extreme degrees of nuclear enlargement and hyperchromasia are present, a squamous intraepithelial lesion should be strongly considered. (e) When nuclear enlargement and/or hyperchromasia is present in the parabasal cells of a "metaplastic" epithelium and is accompanied by nuclear crowding, surface atypia, and an absence of normal maturation, the diagnosis of an HSIL should be made.

Atrophy

The spectrum of squamous epithelial changes associated with older age includes the following: (a) maturation disturbances with pseudokoilocytosis (Fig. 9B), (b) conventional atrophy with immature but cytologically bland epithelium, (c) transitional metaplasia, (d) profound atrophy (Fig. 11A), (e) atrophy with partial maturation and focal nuclear enlargement or conspicuous nuclear hyperchromasia (Fig. 11B), and, rarely, (f) atypical atrophy in which the distinction from a SIL is virtually impossible. Features common to atrophic processes include (a) hyperchromatic but generally uniform nuclei, (b) frequent elongated and sometimes grooved nuclei, (c) absence of conspicuous atypia in the upper epithelial layers, and, importantly, (d) absence of mitotic figures. Atrophic epithelia with partial maturation and enlarged atypical nuclei make up one of the more difficult categories, and distinction from SIL is based on even spacing of nuclei with conspicuous intercellular bridges and an absence of mitotic activity.

One lesion that may mimic both atrophy and HSIL is adenoid basal cell carcinoma. These tumors exhibit sharply demarcated epithelial nests resembling crypt involvement, and if the atypia is minimal, may mimic atrophy (Fig. 11C).

Radiation Effect

Radiation effect can involve both the endocervical and squamous epithelial cells. The prominent changes include nuclear enlargement and hyperchromasia associated with abundant cytoplasm, uniform nuclear spacing with minimal crowding, a low mitotic index, and evidence of cytoplasmic degeneration with vacuoles. The nuclear chromatin is often indistinct or smudged in appearance, in contrast to the coarse chromasia associated with neoplasia. Important is the preservation of a low nuclear-cytoplasmic ratio.

Nonepithelial Alterations

These alterations include implantation site and endometrial macrophages. The placental implantation site is commonly recognized in the endometrium (43). It may mimic a neoplasm in cervical biopsies or endocervical curettings, but it is sufficiently distinctive that misdiagnosis is uncommon once the pathologist has some experience with this lesion (see below). Implantation site usually presents as an eosinophilic (by virtue of the abundant keratin positive matrix) irregularly contoured process in the superficial cervical stroma that is punctuated by scattered hyperchromatic nuclei. On closer examination, the irregular margins of the lesion are composed of a series of small, rounded borders, and the atypical nuclei are separated by abundant pale to eosinophilic matrix. Occasionally, these may present as plaque-like proliferations resembling intraepithelial lesions. Special stains for human chorionic gonadotropin or human placental lactogen are usually not helpful, as these cells often do not react for these markers. Moreover, they are strongly keratin positive. However, reactivity for placental alkaline phosphatase (PLAP) discriminates these changes from squamous epithelium (44). Endometrial macrophages

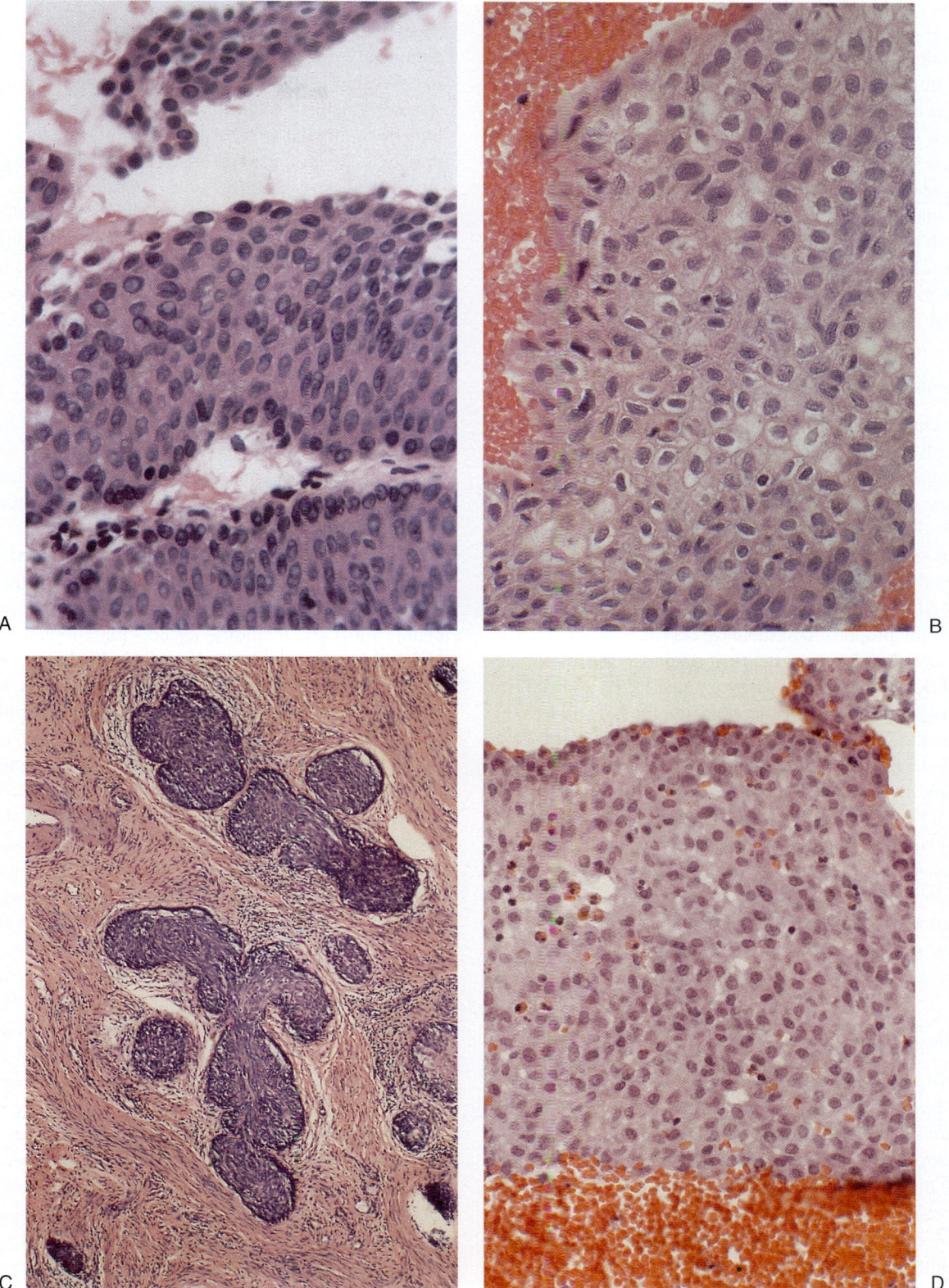

FIG. 11. Differential diagnosis of HSIL. **A:** Marked atrophy. **B:** Atrophy with reactive epithelial changes. **C:** Adenoid basal carcinoma, which may mimic either atrophy or HSIL. **D:** Epithelioid sheets of endometrial histiocytes from a curetting.

are another phenomenon that may mimic squamous lesions (Fig. 11D). We have seen occasional endometrial curettings that contained sheets of endometrial macrophages. The distinction from an epithelial neoplasm is based on the small size of the cells, the small slightly vesicular nuclei, granular cytoplasm without distinct boundaries, and a feathering of the peripheral line of demarcation without a sharp basal lamina. Mitoses may be present and eosinophils are common. In general, macrophages are commonly encountered in association with inflammatory changes or in smears from postmenopausal women and in this context are not related to neoplasia. Keratin (negative) and macrophage (positive) stains may assist in confirming the diagnosis.

Microinvasive Carcinoma

Approximately 4% to 7% of CIN lesions have been associated with superficial invasion (45,46), and a subset of invasive squamous cell carcinoma of the cervix is termed microinvasive carcinoma on the assumption that a portion of early invasive cancers can be treated conservatively by cone biopsy or simple hysterectomy. Tumor exceeding the criteria for microinvasion are managed with radical hysterectomy and pelvic lymph node dissection or radiation therapy. In recent years the proportion of invasive cervical carcinoma that invaded less than 5 mm in depth at diagnosis has increased over tenfold and currently is approximately 21% (47,48).

For the pathologist, specific concerns must be addressed when determining if a cervical squamous cell carcinoma warrants designation as microinvasive. They include (a) identifying invasion, (b) distinguishing it from noninvasive mimics, (c) applying correctly the criteria for microinvasion, and (d) advising the gynecologist regarding management. It should be emphasized that the diagnosis of microinvasion can only be made on a specimen containing the entire lesion. The specimen must have uninvolved margins and the pathologist must examine a sufficient number of sections, usually one for every 2 mm of cone thickness (49).

Diagnosis of Invasion (Fig. 12)

The criteria for microinvasive squamous cell carcinoma include the following: (a) a desmoplastic response in the adjacent stroma (Fig. 12A), (b) focal conspicuous maturation of the neoplastic epithelium with prominent nucleoli (Fig. 12B), (c) blurring of the epithelial stromal interface, and (d) loss of polarity of the nuclei at the epithelial stromal border with absence of the palisaded pattern characteristic of CIN. Three additional features include scalloping of the margins at the epithelial-stromal interface, the apparent "folding or duplication" of the neoplastic epithelium, and less commonly, the appearance of "pseudoglands" (Fig. 12C,D). Scalloping refers to fine irregularities, which are not typically seen with gland (crypt) involvement or tangential sectioning through gland involvement. Duplication of epithelium refers to the presence of vascular structures within a sheet of neoplastic epithelial cells, producing an image of incompletely formed papillae. These features aid in recognizing invasion in the presence of an intense inflammatory response, which may obscure desmoplasia on the one hand and blur the epithelial-stromal interface on the other (6). Pseudoglands are defined as discrete circumscribed nests of invasive carcinoma, usually with central necrosis, that may mimic crypt involvement. In contrast to crypts, this form of invasive carcinoma does not exhibit glandular epithelium, is often composed of multiple circumscribed nests, often contains central necrosis, and may display a loss of polarity.

Differential Diagnosis of Invasion (Fig. 13)

A previous review of 265 cases of presumed microinvasion sent to the Gynecologic Oncology Group determined that approximately one-third were overdiagnosed intraepithelial lesions (50), underscoring the potential problems in lesion interpretation. The most important mimics of microinvasion include: (a) crypt (gland) involvement that is tangentially sectioned; (b) cautery or crush artifact, including prior biopsy sites; (c) inflammatory or reparative changes in CIN, including pseudoepitheliomatous changes (Fig. 13A); and (d) blurring of the epithelial stromal interface by inflammation or other artifact (Fig. 13B). Crypt involvement is characterized by preservation of epithelial polarity, a smooth epithelial stromal interface, and, in contrast to the parameter of duplication, each nest of epithelium is discrete and separate from the adjacent one. Artifacts are usually produced by prior biopsy, in which a stromal response may be present. They should not be associated with the other parameters of invasion. Cautery or crush artifact should be recognized and reported if it hinders diagnosis. Inflammatory changes are responsible for the greatest diagnostic difficulty, inasmuch as these alterations may blur the epithelial stromal interface or, in combination with prior trauma, be associated with small nests of epithelium in the inflammatory cell infiltrates. The laboratory management of these findings is to obtain levels to determine if additional features of invasive carcinoma are present and obtain consultation if there is a question of invasion in a cone specimen. Factors influencing management include whether the areas in question are in continuity with, or within 1 mm of, the surface epithelium, are limited to one or two foci, are not associated with other parameters of invasion, including capillary-lymphatic space invasion, and are associated with clear margins. Intraepithelial lesions associated with underlying inflammation, either from secondary infection or previous biopsy, must be evaluated carefully to avoid the overdiagnosis of invasion when the epithelial stromal interface is disrupted by the inflammatory process.

Another mimic of invasion is placental implantation site (Fig. 13C,D), which was discussed above.

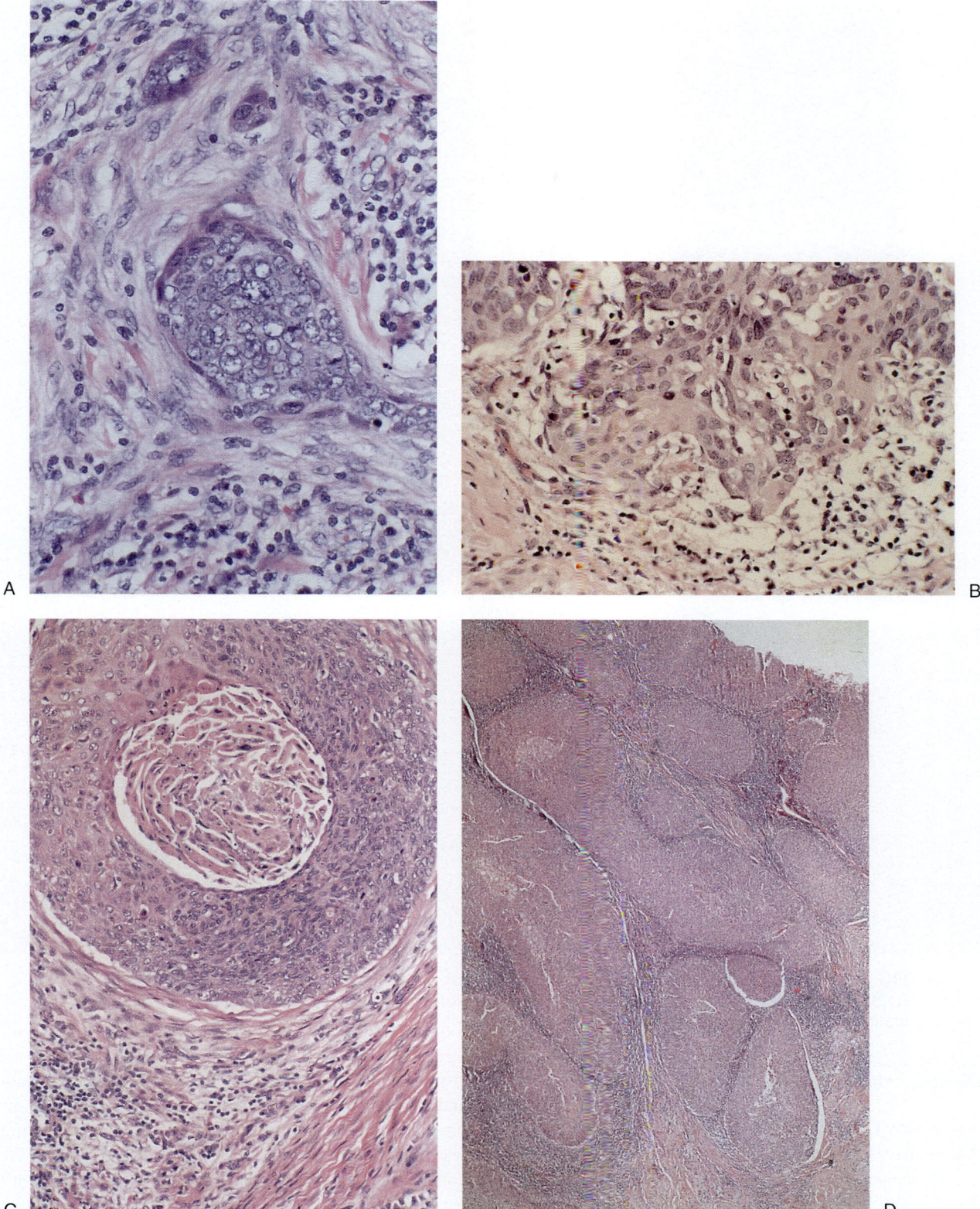

FIG. 12. Diagnosis of invasive squamous cell carcinoma. **A:** Desmoplasia. **B:** Scalloped irregular borders with absence of polarity and focal cell maturation. **C:** Pseudoglands with preservation of cell polarity combined with peripheral desmoplasia. **D:** Confluent, "reduplicating" epithelium without intervening stroma, characterizing a "pushing" invasive border.

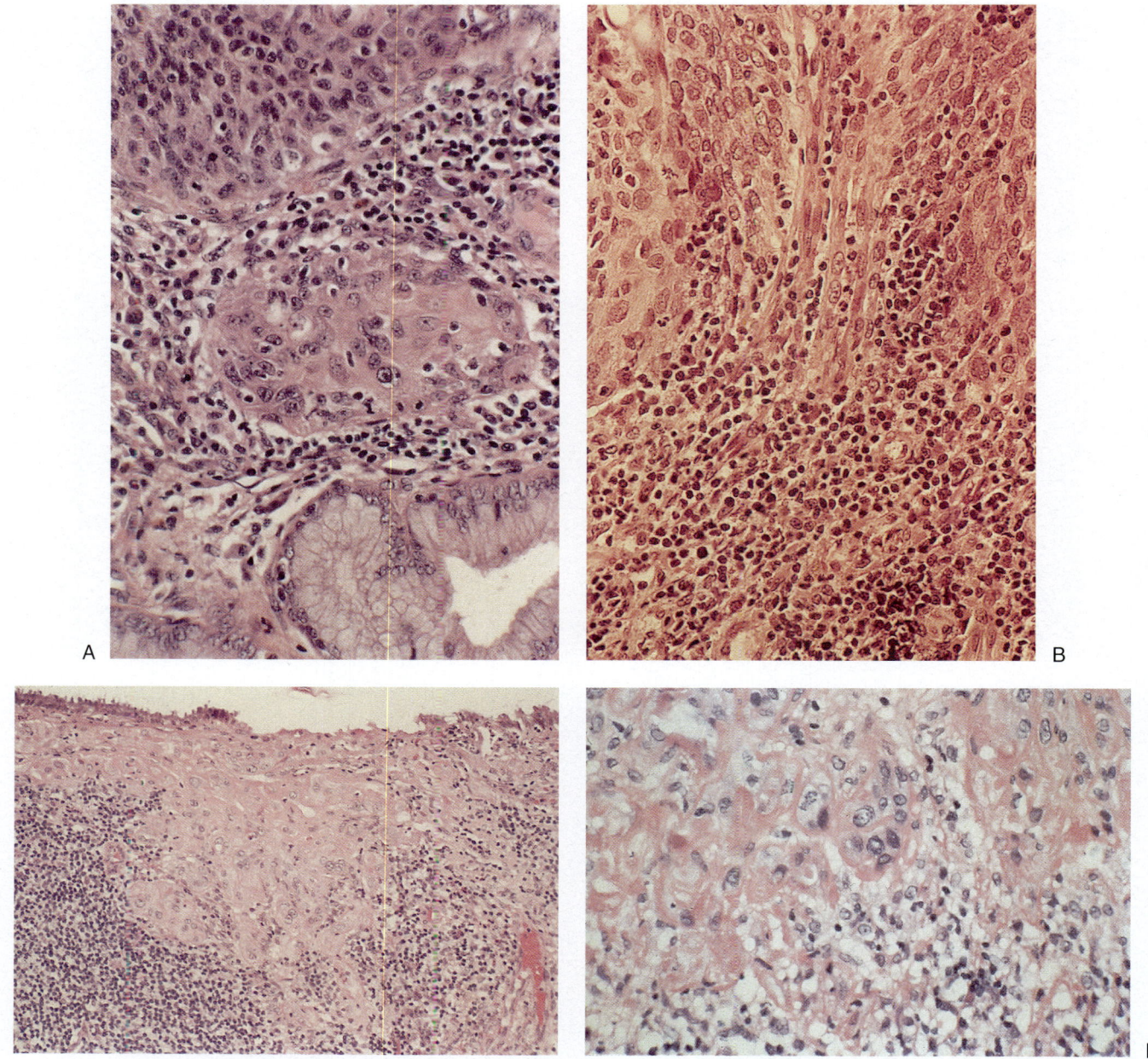

FIG. 13. Features that are not sufficient for a diagnosis of, or may be confused with, invasive carcinoma. **A:** Small discrete nests in inflamed stroma. **B:** Disruption of the epithelial-stromal interface by inflammation. **C** and **D:** Placental implantation site.

Confirming "Microinvasion"

Cone biopsy is necessary if (a) the lesion does not appear grossly invasive clinically or colposcopically and (b) if it is not clearly deeper than 3 mm in the original biopsy or does not exhibit capillary-lymphatic space invasion. Once the cone biopsy is performed, the measurement of depth of invasion should be made from the most superficial epithelial-stromal interface of the adjacent intraepithelial process. This is best accomplished using an ocular micrometer or a method of measurement that makes it possible to identify with certainty if the lesion has invaded to a depth of over 3 mm.

Three issues of potential concern when considering microinvasion are tumor depth, confluence of growth pattern, and capillary-lymphatic space invasion. Microinvasion has been defined variably depending on whether the definition was recommended by the International Federation of Gynecology and Obstetrics (FIGO) (5 mm) or the Society of Gynecologic Oncology (3 mm) (51,52). Depth of invasion and capillary lymphatic space invasion remain the most intensively studied parameters. The risk of pelvic lymph note metastases increases between 1 and 5 mm of invasion. It is estimated as high as 4.3% for lesions invading between 3.1 and 5.0 mm (53–58). In a recent review by Ostor (59), the risk of lymph node metastases increased only slightly (from <1% to 2%) as tumor depth increased from 1 to 5 mm.

Based on this estimate, Ostor questioned the premise that microinvasive carcinoma be defined by a 3 mm cutoff. However, a diagnosis of microinvasion (as defined by the therapeutic alternative of simple hysterectomy) in the United States requires that the carcinoma invade less than 3.0 mm into the stroma, based on recommendations of the Society of Gynecologic Oncology (51).

Both confluent growth patterns and capillary lymphatic space invasion correlate with depth of invasion (51,58), but their independent value is less clear. Confluence has been defined as anastomosing tongues of epithelium with pushing borders, or a lesion front of greater than 1 mm (46). Despite a report emphasizing the prognostic importance of confluent patterns of invasion, others have not found that confluence is an independent factor, once depth of invasion is controlled for (54,56,57). In his review, Ostor (59) noted an adverse outcome in less than 3% of cases with this feature. The importance of width is less certain. Burghardt and Holzer (53) proposed that tumor volume be taken into account as a more precise predictor of recurrence and metastases. They reported that lesions less than 420 mm^2 rarely recur (53). A more simplified approach places the cutoff at 10 mm in width (53).

The frequency of capillary-lymphatic space invasion (CLSI) has varied widely. Van Nagel et al. (55) reported it in 33 of 177 cases (19%) (55). In a detailed study of 91 cases of microinvasive carcinoma, Ostor (60) reported CLSI in 22 (24%) based on *Ulex uropeaus* agglutinin I (UEAI) stains (60). These figures contrast with a high of 57% reported by Roche and Norris (57). Its significance remains controversial (57). CLSI increases in frequency as a function of lesion depth, which increases the risk of lymph node metastases (50,51,54–59). Whether CLSI is a critical prognostic factor in lesions of 3.0 mm depth or less is unclear (55–57). There are three components to this issue. The first is that the interpretation of CLSI is subjective. Inflammation and retraction artifact may produce confusion in the interpretation of CLSI and special stains for vascular endothelium may or may not be helpful (Fig. 14A,B). Displacement of neoplastic epithelium into vascular spaces during injection of anesthetic or biopsy may also mimic invasion (61) (Fig. 14C). Roche and Norris recommended that CLSI not be a parameter for determining therapy due to problems in its interpretation and significance. In fact, they recommended referring to this change as *capillary-like* space involvement. This may more accurately convey the uncertainty of the diagnosis; however, in our experience the clinical response to this diagnosis is the same regardless of qualifiers. Hence, we either use the term *capillary-lymphatic space invasion* or issue a descriptive report if the diagnosis cannot be made with certainty. The second point is that the frequency of lymph node metastases associated with lesions less than 3 mm thick and having CLSI

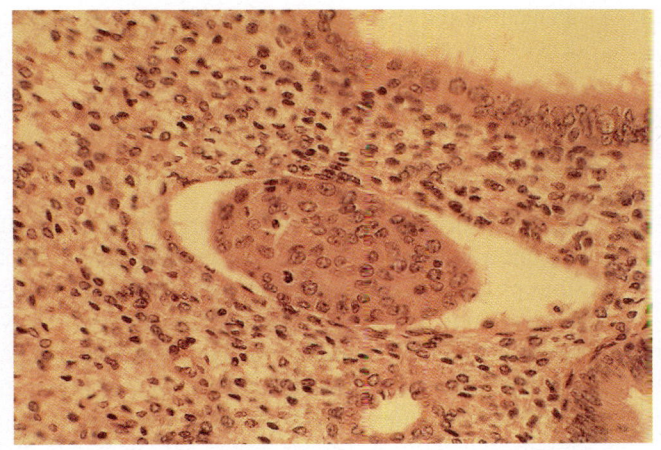
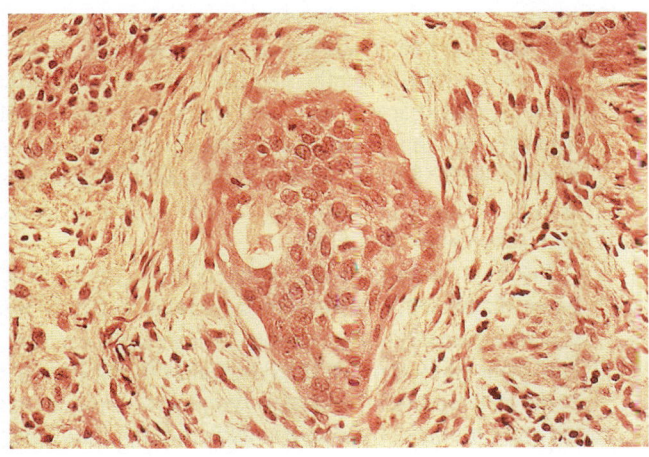
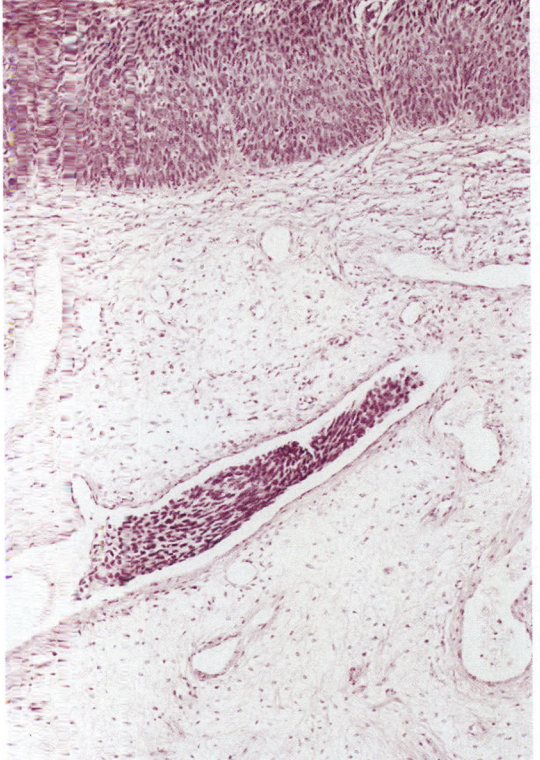

FIG. 14. Capillary-lymphatic space invasion (CLSI) and its mimics. **A:** CLSI. **B:** Retraction artifact with desmoplasia. **C:** Neoplastic epithelium (CIN III) introduced into a vascular space via injection of anesthesia.

has generally not been shown to be significantly greater than for similar depth lesions without CLSI. Van Nagell et al. found that none of 17 patients with CLSI and lesions invading less than 3.0 mm had metastases in their lymph node specimens. In a review of cases with less than 5 mm of invasion, Roche and Norris also noted no relationship between CLSI and lymph node metastases.

In his recent review, Ostor (59) noted that 6 of 12 (50%) tumors with lymph node metastases were associated with CLSI. Nevertheless, 192 of 1,036 (19%) cases with negative lymph nodes had CLSI. Similarly 18 of 36 (50%) invasive recurrences were associated with CLSI in the original tumor in contrast to 496 of 3,597 (14%) patients with no recurrence (59). CLSI has been associated with an adverse prognosis in carcinomas exceeding 3 mm in depth in most (55,58,62,63) if not all (64) reports. The implication from these multiple studies is that although CLSI is associated with cases having an adverse outcome, the vast majority of cases with CLSI do not present with histologically positive lymph nodes.

Many assumptions about managing CLSI are based on its relationship to histologically proven lymph node metastases. However, the third and infrequently discussed issue is that there are no large studies following a series of microinvasive (<3 mm) carcinomas with CLSI without lymphadenectomy. This is not trivial, because it is conceivable that the removal of lymph nodes, even reputedly negative ones, may influence prognosis. The 5-year survival of cases with pelvic lymph node involvement is approximately 50% regardless of the mode of management once metastases are diagnosed (65). This suggests that lymph node dissection may be therapeutic not only by removing microscopically visible metastases but, in some cases, by removing micrometastases missed on pathologic examination. The degree to which such micrometastases are detected may depend heavily on the exactness with which the lymph nodes are processed (66). If removal of even negative-appearing lymph nodes were to improve survival, the actual risk of metastatic disease in microinvasive lesions exhibiting CLSI could not be determined without placing the patient at risk by deferring lymphadenectomy. Kolstad (67) reported a frequency of CLSI at 13% for lesions less than 3 mm in depth. In that study, none of 50 cases of microinvasive (<5 mm) carcinoma with CLSI treated by radical hysterectomy and lymph node dissection recurred. However, four of eight patients treated by simple hysterectomy died of their disease, including lesions originally 2, 4, and 5 mm in depth). These figures imply an increased risk of recurrence in patients who do not undergo lymphadenectomy, but are not sufficient for determining the risk in women with lesions under 3 mm in depth. Moreover, it is not clear whether the increased risk conferred by CLSI can be reduced by lymphadenectomy. For example, one study found a relationship between CLSI and extrapelvic recurrences, while another found that a worse prognosis associated with CLSI was not influenced by lymph node dissection (58,62).

Presently, the nomenclature committee of the Society of Gynecologic Oncology has not accepted the diagnosis of microinvasion if CLSI is present (51). In standard practice, most oncologists request that the presence of CLSI be reported, and they usually opt for radical hysterectomy and pelvic lymphadenectomy if it is seen in a lesion less than 3.0 mm in depth. For these reasons, over- and underinterpretation of CLSI must be avoided, as has been discussed above (56).

Reporting Microinvasion

In our practice, we do not use the term *microinvasive carcinoma*, opting to report such tumors as "superficially invasive squamous cell carcinomas." As summarized above, the criteria for microinvasion may vary slightly and management may depend on multiple factors. When reviewing the biopsy, we report the largest dimensions of the lesion to aid the clinician in deciding the next step in management (i.e., cone biopsy vs. radical hysterectomy), particularly if there is no visible mass on clinical examination. In cone biopsies the following should be reported: (a) depth; (b) length of the entire lesion; (c) if length constitutes continuous tumor or is composed of multiple small foci; (d) the presence or absence of CLSI; (e) status of endocervical, ectocervical, and deep margins and, if negative, distance (in millimeters) from invasive tumor to these margins; (f) intraepithelial disease and its relationship to the margins; and (g) clear-cut glandular differentiation if present. The latter generally precludes management of the lesion as microinvasive if there is clear evidence of invasive adenocarcinoma.

Squamous Cell Carcinoma and Its Variants

Conventional Squamous Cell Carcinoma

The majority of squamous cell carcinomas evolve from a precancerous lesion (68-71). Up to two-thirds of CIN III lesions progress to cancer if untreated, and the time course for this evolution has been estimated to range from 3 to over 20 years (84,85). Squamous cell carcinoma that develops rapidly, without a defined precursor, has also been reported rarely (86). The mean age for patients with carcinoma is approximately 51 years, in contrast to approximately 28 years for those with CIN III. A subset of invasive cancers is termed occult carcinoma. These are clinically inapparent stage Ib lesions >3.1 mm in depth. The mean age for this group has been estimated at 43 years, and the 5-year survival of 96% distinguishes this group from clinical stage Ib invasive carcinoma (86% 5-year survival). Accordingly, patients with occult disease can be managed with radical hysterectomy and lymph node dissection.

Survival is most closely related to the stage of disease when diagnosed, which in turn correlates closely with the risk of regional lymph node metastases (Table 2). Spread occurs principally through the lymphatics of the cervix, which consist of superficial and deep lymphatics draining to the iliac and obturator, hypogastric and common iliac, and sacral

TABLE 2. *Clinical staging of cervical cancer (International Federation of Gynecology and Obstetrics)*

Stage	Features
0	Carcinoma *in situ* (intraepithelial neoplasia)
1	Carcinoma confined to the cervix
1a	Microinvasive carcinoma
1b	Other stage I disease, including occult
2	Extension of the carcinoma beyond the cervix without extension to the lower third of the vagina or pelvic wall
2a	No parametrial involvement
2b	Parametrial involvement
3	Extension of the carcinoma to the pelvic wall and/or lower third of the vagina; cases with hydronephrosis or nonfunctioning kidney are included unless proved to be of other cause
3a	No extension to the pelvic wall
3b	Extension to the pelvic wall and/or hydronephrosis or nonfunctioning kidney
4	Carcinoma extends beyond the true pelvis or involves the urinary bladder or rectum
4a	Spread to adjacent organs
4b	Spread to distant organs

lymph nodes, as well as lymph nodes in the posterior bladder wall (1). Approximately two-thirds of invasive squamous carcinomas are stages I or II when diagnosed. The actuarial 5-year survival drops abruptly from over 70% for stage II to 30% to 35% for stage III neoplasms.

Diagnosis

Squamous cell carcinomas have been classified according to degree of squamous differentiation (grades I–III) or according to cell type. Reagan et al. (71) subdivided squamous cancer of the cervix into (a) large cell keratinizing carcinoma, (b) large cell nonkeratinizing carcinoma, and (c) small cell carcinoma. The basis for this distinction has been the observation that large cell keratinizing carcinomas are radioresistant relative to nonkeratinizing carcinomas and that small cell carcinomas have the worst overall prognosis. In a review of five large series by Reagan and Fu (72), the average 5-year survival for stage I tumors treated by radiation therapy was 54%, 84%, and 42% for keratinizing, nonkeratinizing, and small cell carcinomas, respectively. The distinction between large cell keratinizing and nonkeratinizing squamous cell carcinoma is based primarily on the presence of intercellular bridges and keratin pearls in the former, although focal individual-cell keratinization may be present in the latter (72) (Fig. 15A). The small cell group has been more precisely defined and now consists of neoplasms that are small cell squamous cell carcinomas (Fig. 15B) and tumors that are morphologically and functionally identical to (but etiologically distinct from) small cell undifferentiated carcinoma (oat cell carcinoma, argyrophilic carcinoma, neuroendocrine carcinoma arising at other anatomic sites.

Excepting small cell undifferentiated carcinoma, classification according to cell type is not universally accepted. Not all authors have observed differences in survival between

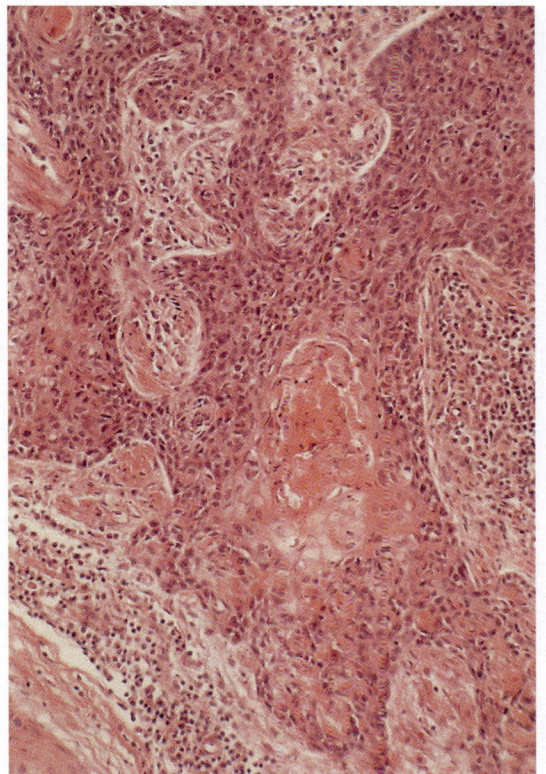
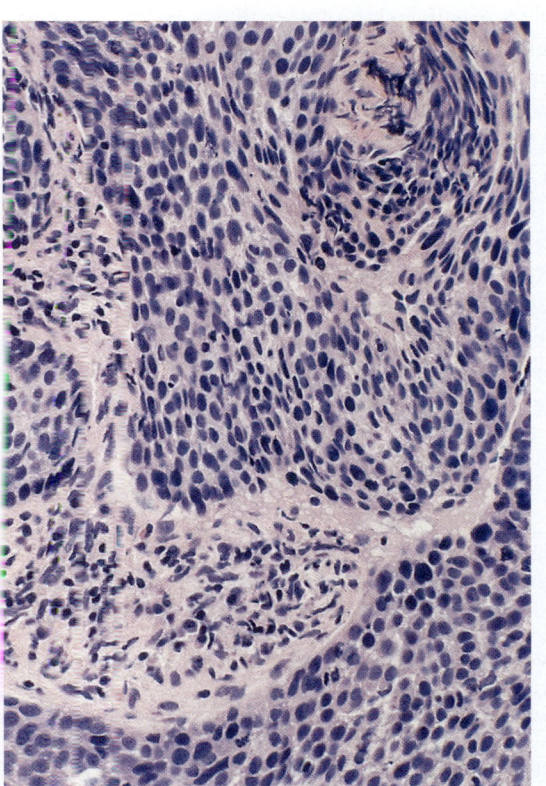

FIG. 15. Squamous cell carcinoma. **A:** Moderately differentiated (large cell squamous) carcinoma. **B:** Poorly differentiated (small cell squamous) carcinoma.

keratinizing and nonkeratinizing tumors. Randall et al. (73) found that keratinizing tumors had a greater tendency to recur locally after radiotherapy but that the frequency of distant metastases was the same for both cell types. An alternative, but accepted, approach to grading is to classify squamous cell carcinomas into the categories of well, moderately, and poorly differentiated. A summary of histologic patterns encountered is in Table 3. It should be emphasized that excepting extremely well-differentiated variants (verrucous carcinoma), management is not significantly influenced by histologic pattern per se.

Verrucous Carcinoma

Pure verrucous carcinoma of the cervix is a very rare lesion (74). The criteria for diagnosis are the same as in the vulva, and the diagnosis is one of exclusion. Verrucous carcinoma usually presents as a large sessile lesion resembling a condyloma. Histologically, it consists of a lesion with both exophytic and endophytic growth patterns, lacking the more delicate architecture of condylomata and demonstrating columns of well-differentiated epithelium expanding the underlying stroma in lieu of crypt involvement (Fig. 16A). The pattern of invasion is blunt, with minimal nuclear atypia at the epithelial-stromal interface (Fig. 16B). An intense inflammatory infiltrate has been associated with verrucous carcinoma of the cervix but is nonspecific. The differential diagnosis includes large exophytic condylomata with crypt involvement and well-differentiated squamous cell carcinomas. The latter usually exhibit finger-like or angulated invasive tongues. The presence of filiform papillary projections or marked nuclear atypia at the epithelial-stromal interface rules out verrucous carcinoma. Given the extreme rarity of this lesion, the diagnosis of verrucous carcinoma must be made with caution. Because verrucous carcinomas present grossly as large, sessile, wart-like growths, the diagnosis may be difficult without multiple biopsies or hysterectomy. Local excision is not usually possible, and extension into the adjacent pelvic tissues may occur. Very few cases are available to determine metastatic potential. None of 18 reported metastasized to lymph nodes, although the recurrence rates have been as high as 50% (74).

TABLE 3. *Histologic patterns of squamous cell carcinomas of the cervix*

Conventional squamous cell carcinoma
Well differentiated (large cell keratinizing carcinoma)
Moderately differentiated (large cell nonkeratinizing carcinoma)
Poorly differentiated (includes small cell squamous cell carcinoma)
Papillary squamous cell carcinoma
Transitional cell carcinoma
Lymphoepithelioma-like carcinoma
Verrucous carcinoma
Condylomatous carcinoma
Spindle cell (sarcomatoid) squamous cell carcinoma

Papillary Neoplasms

Papillary neoplasia of the cervix encompasses a broad spectrum of benign, potentially malignant, and clearly malignant lesions. In the benign category are conventional condylomata, and immature variants thereof. The potentially malignant category includes any filiform papillary lesion with a transitional appearance to the epithelium, a high mitotic index, a flat component, or any morphologic features resembling a high-grade intraepithelial lesion (Fig. 16C). Papillary lesions have been described in the cervix, ranging from those resembling transitional-cell papillomas to those diagnosed as papillary carcinoma *in situ* (75–78). Although the former are not invariably associated with invasive cancer, a number of filiform cervical papillomas have been observed in which deeper sampling disclosed invasive cancer (77,78). For this reason, any diagnosis of papillary high-grade SIL should be made carefully and should be based on local excision of the lesion, to rule out invasion. The differential diagnosis, as with verrucous carcinoma, includes condyloma, although the latter usually does not exhibit delicate finger-like proliferations. An occasional diagnostic problem is the presence of papillary immature metaplasia (immature condyloma), either overlying endocervical papillae or in association with condylomata (27–29). In this case, the diagnosis of papillary neoplasia can be excluded by the bland nuclear appearance, very low mitotic index, and presence of endocervical columnar cells in the lesion—features more closely associated with metaplastic epithelium than a papillary neoplasm. Nevertheless, papillary lesions resembling condylomata must be examined carefully, with particular attention to any areas that suggest a high-grade SIL or worse. If such areas exist in any large lesion, additional biopsies should be requested.

Another variant that can be distinguished from both papillary and verrucous carcinoma is condylomatous carcinoma. Such tumors exhibit prominent cytoplasmic halos around tumor cells (Fig. 16D).

Variants of Condyloma with Squamous Cell Carcinoma

Rare reports have described classic- (or almost classic)-appearing condylomata extending deeply into the endocervical canal or endometrium, some of which have been associated with invasive cancer (79,80). Lesions of this type are usually detected in endocervical or endometrial curettings. For this reason, if endocervical curettings contain abundant fragments of condyloma, or any papillary neoplasm, a cone biopsy or hysterectomy should be strongly considered to confirm or exclude invasive cancer.

Another rare variant is CIN extending into the endometrial cavity or rarely, throughout the upper genital tract (81,82). This is a particularly mysterious form of intraepithelial neoplasia displaying aggressive growth with obliteration of the upper genital tract mucosa and total replacement by the neoplastic squamous epithelium. Involvement of the ovary may

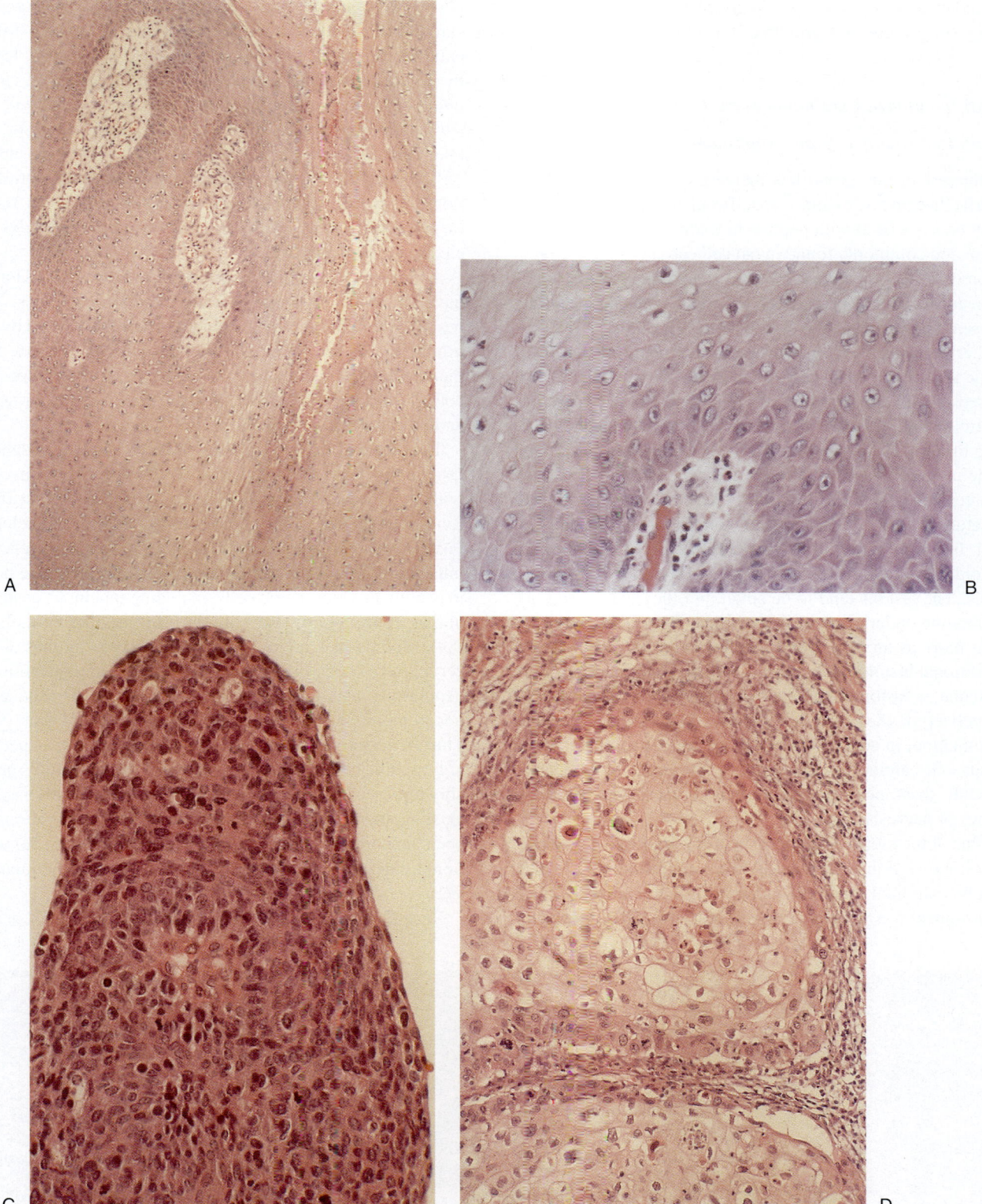

FIG. 16. Variants of squamous cell carcinoma. **A** and **B:** Verrucous carcinoma. **C:** Papillary squamous carcinoma. **D:** "Condylomatous" carcinoma, with cells resembling koilocytes.

include numerous cysts lined by neoplastic epithelium, again suggesting aggressive growth of the epithelial process.

Undifferentiated Carcinoma of the Cervix

Small Cell Undifferentiated Carcinoma

Interest in this group has increased in recent years, primarily because it exhibits specific histologic features and may be associated with peptide hormone production, a phenomenon commonly found in oat cell carcinoma of the lung. Moreover, this carcinoma, like its counterpart in the lungs, appears to have a propensity for rapid metastasis and radiosensitivity, and carries a high mortality (83).

Cervical small cell carcinoma shares many of the histologic features of small cell carcinoma of the lung. It is composed of a small, uniform cell population with hyperchromatic nuclei and a very high nuclear-to-cytoplasmic ratio. The tumor cells form irregular, loose aggregates, often with little cohesion (Fig. 17A). At times, the cells may display greater cohesion and form sheets with small acini, akin to rosettes (Fig. 17B). The nuclei contain coarse chromatin, and, because there is little cytoplasm, they often appear to "mold," as they are artifactually compressed in tissue sections. The lesions tend to be small, but they extensively infiltrate the underlying cervical stroma. Hence, they may appear more as an indurated mass than as a fungating lesion. Additional histologic features that distinguish this entity are vascular invasion, observed in up to 9% of cases by Van Nagell et al. (83), and conspicuous lack of coexisting inflammation, in contrast to most cases of conventional squamous cell carcinoma. Furthermore, by virtue of their rapid growth, these neoplasms are often characterized by broad zones of necrosis.

One of the more intriguing aspects of small cell carcinoma is its association with peptide hormone production, which can be exhibited by ultrastructural or immunohistochemical techniques in a portion of the neoplasms (84). Such neoplasms have been termed "argyrophilic carcinoma," "oat cell carcinoma," "neuroendocrine carcinoma," or "poorly differentiated carcinoid" (85–88). These observations have led to the assumption that both small cell undifferentiated carcinoma of the cervix and carcinoid tumors of the cervix are similar to other neoplasms capable of amine precursor uptake and decarboxylation (APUD) (89). These so-called APUDomas are characterized by peptide hormone production, the propensity to take up silver salts in special stains (argyrophilia), and, in a portion, dense-core granules on electron microscopy (87).

As a result of peptide hormone production, APUDomas have the ability to induce certain clinical syndromes. The best known of these is the carcinoid syndrome, caused by the production of serotonin, but neoplasms of the cervix, like their counterparts elsewhere, may also produce adrenocorticotropic hormone (ACTH), insulin, parathyroid hormone, and other substances (85,89).

The origin of these neoplasms has been a matter of debate. Originally, it was thought that all APUDomas rise from cells with a common embryonic source—the neural crest (89). Evidence that this process could occur in the cervix included Fox et al.'s (90) observation of such cells as normal cervical inhabitants. However, certain neoplasms occurring de novo may contain argyrophilic cells, including mucinous cystadenomas of the ovary that contain intestine-like epithelium (89). Moreover, carcinoids and small cell carcinomas of the cervix have been observed in association with conventional neoplasms, including adenocarcinoma *in situ,* invasive adenocarcinoma, and cervical intraepithelial neoplasms (91). Thus, it appears that, rather than originating from a specific argyrophilic cell, small cell carcinomas and carcinoids probably represent "selective differentiation," often within a preexisting, more conventional carcinoma. This observation has been supported by findings in other organs, where conventional carcinomas blend with the argyrophilic neoplasms (92).

Recently, studies of archival tissue with RNA-RNA *in situ*

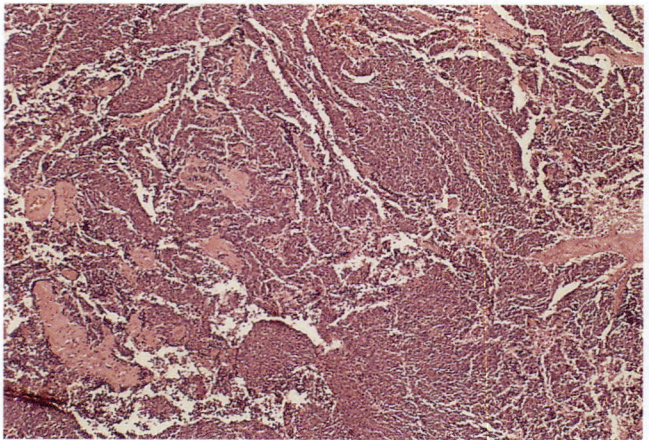 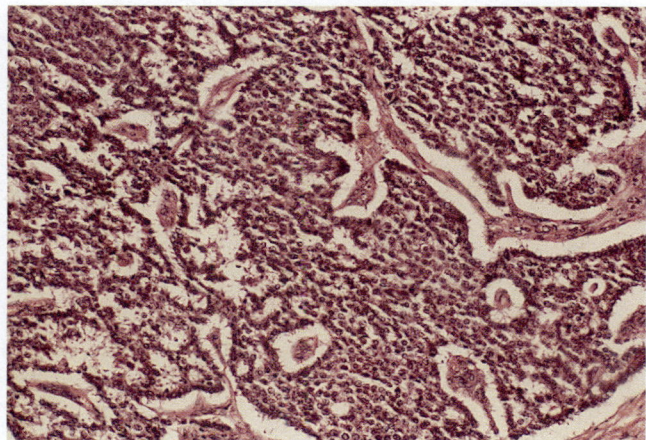

FIG. 17. Small cell undifferentiated carcinoma. **A:** At low power, irregular sheets of tumor cells haphazardly subdivided with randomly arranged fracture lines and absence of sharply demarcated nests with uniform borders (compare to Fig. 16B). **B:** Focal neuroendocrine differentiation with rosettes.

hybridization have revealed small cell undifferentiated carcinomas to be strongly associated with HPV-18 nucleic acids (93). Combined with the relatively higher association of HPV-18 with adenocarcinomas of the cervix, this information suggests that this type of HPV may have a propensity to produce neoplasms arising in endocervix reserve cells, which have a more aggressive biologic behavior.

Although certain small cell neoplasms of the cervix may exhibit functional characteristics, the major criterion for distinguishing them from conventional squamous cell carcinomas is histologic. Small cell morphology is not itself the most important consideration in making the diagnosis of small cell carcinoma. Many squamous cell carcinomas are composed of relatively small cells, but these maintain the infiltrating pattern of a conventional squamous cell carcinoma (Fig. 15). In contrast, small cell undifferentiated carcinoma not only is composed of small cells but also has the cellular characteristics and pattern of infiltration described above (94). HPV type (type 18), immunohistochemical positivity for neuroendocrine markers, and the absence of a conventional precursor lesion are more characteristic of small cell carcinoma but may be identified in conventional small cell squamous carcinomas (95). Another undifferentiated variant is *lymphoepithelioma-like carcinoma,* which resembles its nasopharyngeal counterpart and is composed of uniform undifferentiated cells with eosinophilic cytoplasm, oval vesicular nuclei, and an intense stromal inflammatory-cell infiltrate (96). Too few cases have been reported to determine if this neoplasm has a prognosis distinguishing it from squamous cell carcinoma of the cervix. Another rare variant of squamous cell carcinoma is the *spindle cell or sarcomatoid variant* (97,98). These tumors present as poorly differentiated squamous cell carcinomas with a distinct component of spindle-shaped cells. The latter are strongly keratin positive (Fig. 16).

GLANDULAR LESIONS

Benign Glandular Lesions

Benign glandular lesions of the cervix are common. Most are easily recognized. However, on occasion, florid or unusual varieties may be mistaken for malignancy. Thus, it is essential for diagnostic pathologists to be aware of the spectrum of benign glandular processes.

Endocervical Polyps

Endocervical polyps are common lesions, most often occurring in multigravidas during their fourth to sixth decades of life (98a). When symptomatic, they usually cause profuse mucoid discharge or abnormal bleeding. They are usually small (up to 1 cm in size) and single, although cases of large polyps protruding into the canal and thus mimicking a malignant tumor have been reported (99). Histologically, many different patterns may be observed. Variations include polyps containing nabothian cysts. The distinction between these and simple nabothian cysts may be arbitrary. Carcinomas arising in an endocervical polyp are very rare and, if confined to the polyp, carry a very good prognosis.

Nabothian Cysts/Tunnel Clusters

Nabothian cysts of the cervix are ubiquitous. These dilated, mucin-filled cysts may be single or multiple and may be easily visible grossly. They are lined by normal-appearing columnar cells or compressed and atrophic endocervical cells. They result from occlusion of gland ostia secondary to inflammation with entrapment of secreted mucus. Rupture and extravasation of mucin into the stroma may cause reactive changes in adjacent glands and stroma, which have sometimes been confused with neoplasia (100). Nabothian cysts may penetrate deep into the wall of the cervix and may therefore be mistaken for cystically dilated glands of invasive cervical adenocarcinoma (101). The diagnosis is established by finding benign nuclear features in the cells lining the glands, as well as a uniform, well-demarcated architectural pattern. Tunnel clusters were first described by Fluhmann (102). These blind-ended, complex, branching glandular tunnels occur in two forms that may be mixed. In one, the spaces are dilated and filled with mucin, similar to nabothian cysts (103). However, the outline of the dilated glands are scalloped, appearing as fused glands rather than a single cyst (Fig. 18A). In the other type, the glands appear as multiple, small acini or tubules and may cause more difficulty in the distinction from adenocarcinoma (104). In both types of tunnel clusters, there is a well-demarcated, lobulated architecture. This low-power appearance and the benign features of the nuclei distinguish this fairly common process from carcinoma (Fig. 18B). However, occasionally cytologic atypia and mitotic figures are seen in tunnel clusters (104). The atypia is usually focal and not as severe as that of adenocarcinoma.

Diffuse Laminar Endocervical Glandular Hyperplasia/Nonspecific Hyperplasia

A peculiar type of glandular hyperplasia in which hyperplastic glands involve the cervical stroma to a similar depth circumferentially, often accompanied by an inflammatory reaction, has been designated "diffuse laminar endocervical glandular hyperplasia" [DLEGH] (105) (Fig. 19A).

In this condition, the glands are closely packed, evenly spaced, and lined by well-differentiated mucinous epithelium with basally located nuclei that may be slightly enlarged (Fig. 19B). DLEGH has been confused with minimal deviation adenocarcinoma [adenoma malignum] (see Fig. 35); however, unlike adenoma malignum, DLEGH is always an incidental finding, lacks the deeply invasive, irregularly infiltrative appearance of an adenocarcinoma, and cytologic atypia in DLEGH does not reach the degree seen at least focally in most cases of adenoma malignum.

Some glandular hyperplasias do not fit into the categories

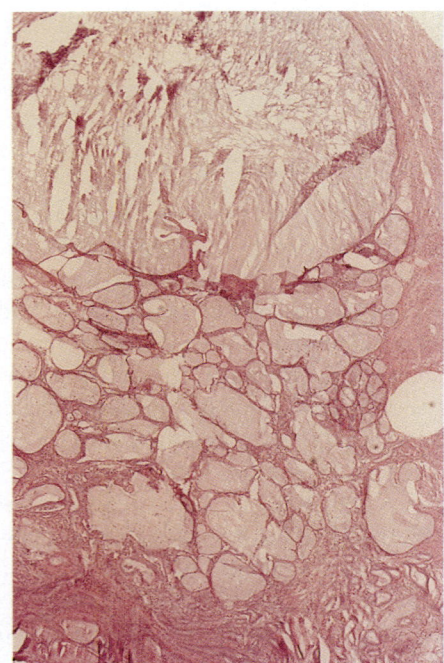
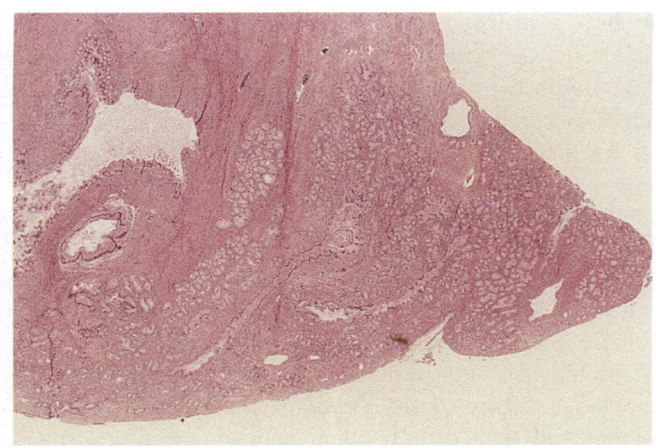

FIG. 18. A: Compact cluster of mucin-filled spaces. Small tubules in compact, well-demarcated arrangement. **B:** Tunnel clusters.

defined above and are nonspecific (100). As with tunnel clusters and DLEGH, they are usually incidental findings. In spite of a rather exuberant proliferative pattern in some cases (106,107) (Fig. 20), these hyperplastic lesions are usually well demarcated and exhibit no stromal reaction. Nuclear atypia, although sometimes present focally, is not of a sufficient degree to diagnose carcinoma. In a small biopsy specimen, these lesions may be very difficult to distinguish from well-differentiated adenocarcinoma, and a larger biopsy may be necessary.

Microglandular Hyperplasia

Microglandular hyperplasia (MGH) is a common cervical lesion, first recognized because of its having been mistaken for carcinoma (108). Typically, MGH is found in young adults and has been related to the use of oral contraceptives. However, it may occur without such a history, as well as in postmenopausal women (109,110). Although MGH is usually an incidental finding, it may cause cervical friability or grow as a polypoid mass. Microscopically, MGH is characterized by a proliferation of small back-to-back glands that may extend above the adjacent noninvolved surface. The glands are lined with cuboidal or columnar cells with prominent subnuclear and/or supranuclear vacuoles that may stain positively for mucin, but are negative for carcinoembryonic antigen (CEA) (111). Sometimes, however, the cytoplasm is eosinophilic or blends with areas of underlying immature metaplastic squamous epithelium. Within the lumina of the glands, there is mucin containing acute inflammatory cells

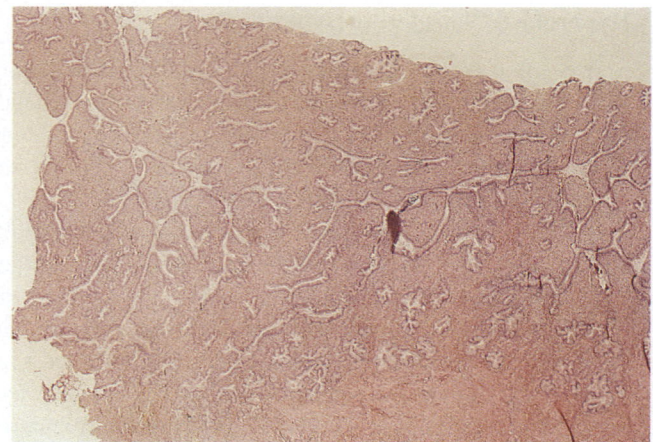
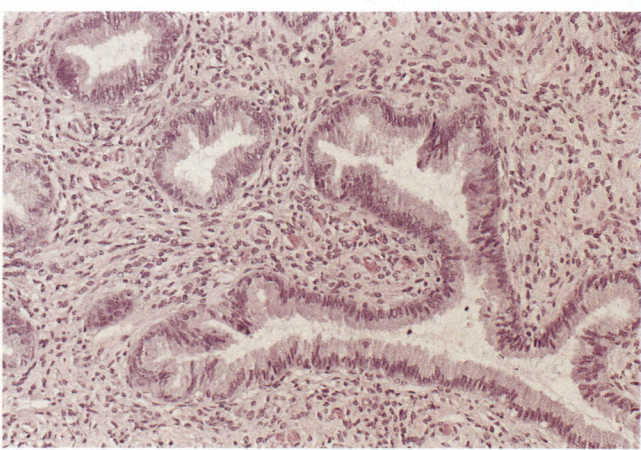

FIG. 19. Diffuse laminar endocervical gland hyperplasia. **A:** Low-power view of ramifying, evenly spaced glands with sharply delimited lower border. (With permission, Ref. 15 [part A].) **B:** High-power view of branching and tubular glands similar to those seen in minimal deviation adenocarcinoma (adenoma malignum).

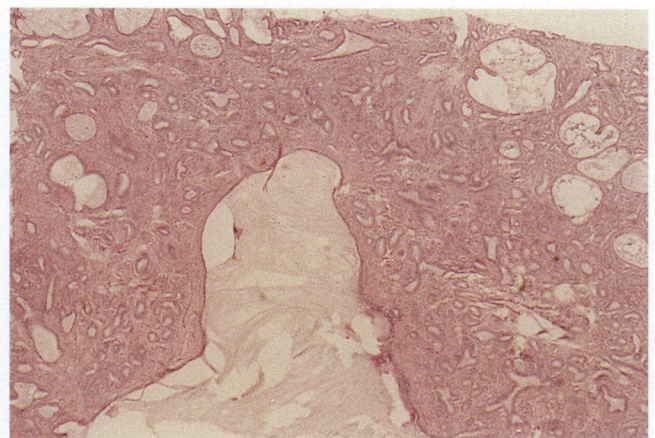

FIG. 20. Cervical gland hyperplasia. Pattern of large and small glands, consistent with mixed pattern of tunnel clusters.

(Fig. 21A, B). In the adjacent stroma there are mixed acute chronic inflammatory cells. Solid foci, signet-ring cells, extravasated mucin, a hyalinized stroma, nuclear atypia (Fig. 21C), a hobnail nuclear appearance, and epithelial mitoses may occur in MGH, causing confusion with carcinoma, particularly clear cell carcinoma (112). However, unlike clear cell carcinoma, nuclear atypia is focal. Subnuclear vacuoles and inflammatory cells are not a prominent feature of clear cell carcinoma. A microglandular hyperplasia-like mucinous endometrial adenocarcinoma has been described (113,114). This lesion may be seen in endocervical or endometrial curettings and be mistaken for cervical microglandular hyperplasia. The absence of a spectrum of cytologic changes, more uniform nuclear atypia, and the lack of immature squamous metaplastic cells peripheral to the glands help to distinguish this carcinoma from MGH. In addition, the age and clinical presentation of women with endometrial carcinoma differ from those of most women with MGH.

Mesonephric Hyperplasia

Although mesonephric remnants in the lateral wall of the cervix are not uncommon (115), mesonephric hyperplasia, which is florid enough to evoke the possibility of malignancy, is rare (116–118). Ferry and Scully (118) describe three varieties: lobular, diffuse, and ductal. In the diffuse variety, a lobulated pattern is absent, but the bland appearance of the glands, an occasional accompanying duct, and the absence of stromal reaction distinguish this lesion from malignancy (Fig. 22A). The ductal pattern, composed of larger, sometimes dilated and irregular ducts, may not be recognized as mesonephric in origin except by its location in the wall of the cervix and the characteristic micropapillary intraluminal budding of pseudostratified epithelial cells with a

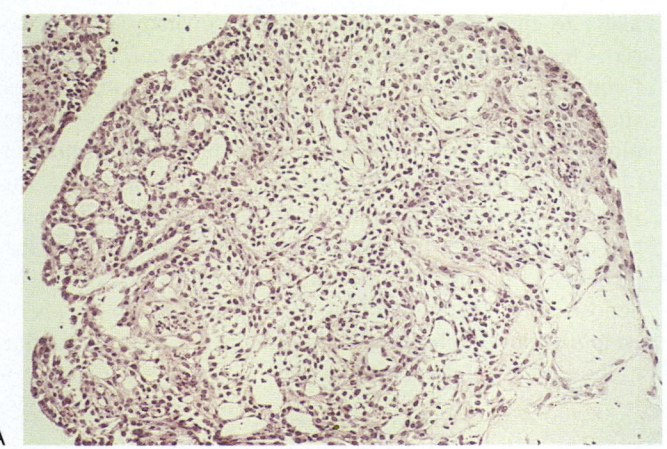

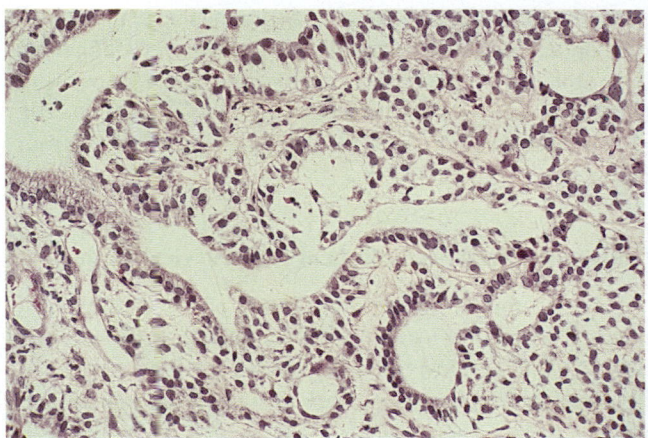

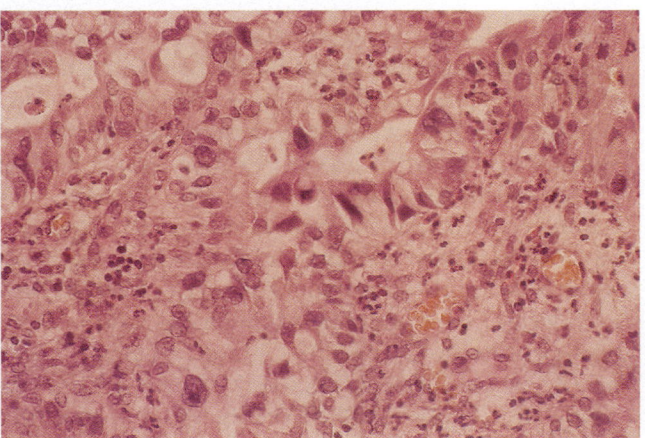

FIG. 21. Microglandular hyperplasia. **A:** Polypoid lesions with characteristic closely packed small and large glands. **B:** Cytoplasmic vacuoles, inflammatory cells, and spectrum of nuclear changes confirm the diagnosis. **C:** Nuclear enlargement and pleomorphism may cause concern for adenocarcinoma. (With permission, Ref. 15 [part C].)

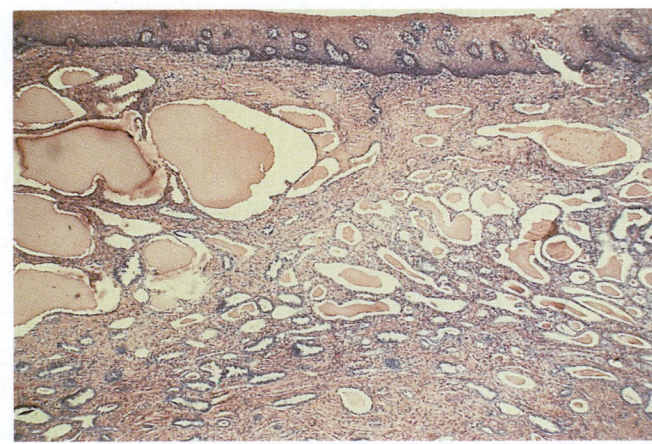 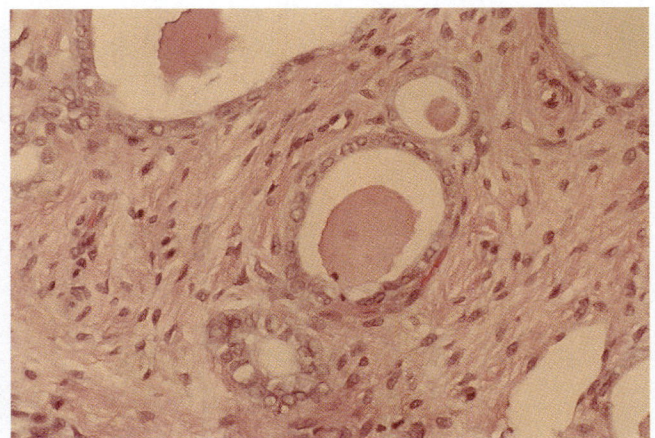

FIG. 22. Mesonephric hyperplasia. **A:** Large and small glands in a vaguely lobulated pattern contain eosinophilic material. **B:** Glands are lined by bland cuboidal cells.

benign cytologic appearance. Except in this instance, hyperplastic mesonephric glands are usually lined by small cuboidal epithelial cells that have uniform round-to-oval nuclei with rare, if any, mitotic figures (Fig. 22B). A characteristic intraglandular eosinophilic material resembling thyroid colloid is a useful clue.

Mesonephric hyperplasia must be distinguished from the very rare mesonephric adenocarcinoma, well-differentiated endocervical adenocarcinoma, and clear cell carcinoma. The number of hyperplastic glands in mesonephric hyperplasia is sometimes striking and alarming. The benign cytologic appearance, intraluminal eosinophilic material, an orderly architectural pattern, a lack of a stromal response, and a lack of involvement of the overlying endocervical mucosa all help to distinguish these hyperplastic proliferations from cancer.

Tuboendometrial Metaplasia of Endocervical Glands

Tuboendometrial metaplasia (TEM) of the endocervical glands is seen in 30% to 100% of completely examined cervices (119–123). TEM is usually seen in the upper portion of the canal and involves the deep, as well as the superficial, portions of the glands. TEM is not usually associated with gland irregularity or intraglandular cellular proliferation. However, nuclear enlargement and crowding may cause confusion with adenocarcinoma *in situ* (AIS). In contrast to those of AIS, the cells of TEM resemble fallopian tube or endometrium, often containing intercalated, serous, and ciliated cells. Nuclei are not as coarse as those of AIS, and there is a paucity or absence of mitotic figures (Fig. 23A). The location of TEM in the upper canal and in the deeper parts of the glands also distinguishes this condition from AIS, which primarily involves the squamocolumnar junction and the superficial portion of the glands. Glands with TEM may sometimes be encountered deep in the stroma and surrounded by a slightly edematous reaction, causing confusion with invasive very well differentiated endometrioid adenocarcinoma (124) (Fig. 23B). Bland nuclear chromatin and the absence of an invasive pattern distinguish TEM from carcinoma. Use of antibodies Ki67 and MIB-1 has been reported to be helpful in the distinction of TEM from AIS and adenocarcinoma (125). CEA has been less useful in this distinction, showing positivity in TEM as well as AIS (126).

Cervical Endometriosis

Endometriosis that involves the cervix is similar histologically to endometriosis encountered elsewhere (127). Two types have been described: deep and superficial. The superficial variety has been seen most often following procedures such as dilatation and curettage of the endometrium or cone biopsy (122) and is probably due to mechanical implantation of endometrial tissue. Endometriosis may be mistaken for AIS when it is superficial or for invasive endometrioid carcinoma when deep. In contrast to those lesions, however, the presence of endometrial stroma alerts one to the correct diagnosis (Fig. 24). In addition, the cells lining the glands of endometriosis are benign in appearance, with nuclei similar to those of the endometrium itself.

Endocervicitis

Reactive cytologic atypia in endocervical glands secondary to inflammatory processes is sometimes mistaken for glandular neoplasia, most often in small biopsy specimens or curettage fragments with poorly preserved nuclei. An occasionally disconcerting aspect of cervicitis is a papillary growth pattern (papillary endocervicitis) (128) (Fig. 25A). An absence of infiltrative features distinguishes inflammatory reactions from invasive adenocarcinoma, and nuclear features distinguish them from AIS. Well-preserved nuclei in cervicitis have finely stippled chromatin, sometimes with prominent nucleoli (Fig. 25B). Mitotic figures, however, may be present. The high frequency of reactive, rather than neoplastic, changes in the cervix argues for caution when

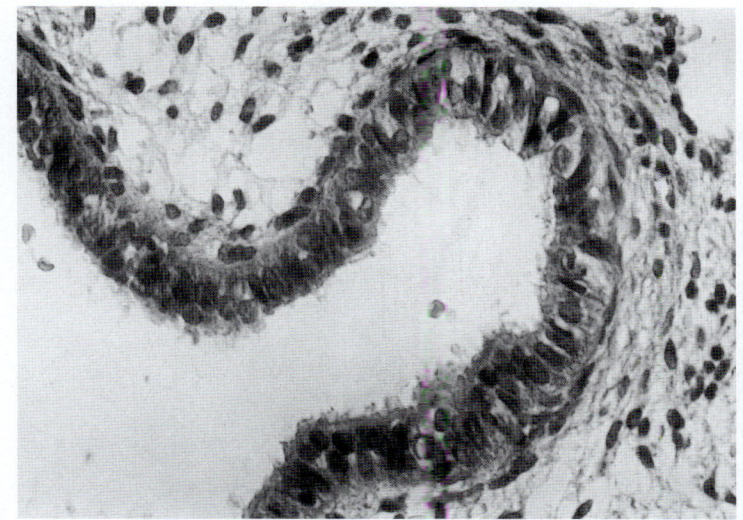
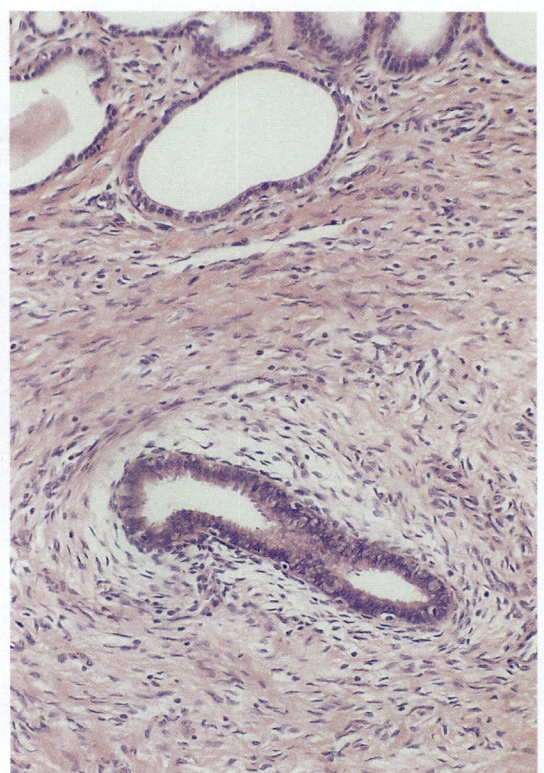

FIG. 23. Tubal metaplasia. **A:** Endocervical gland lined by crowded columnar cells with ciliated cytoplasm. **B:** Deep gland with periglandular edema, which might cause concern for invasive well-differentiated adenocarcinoma.

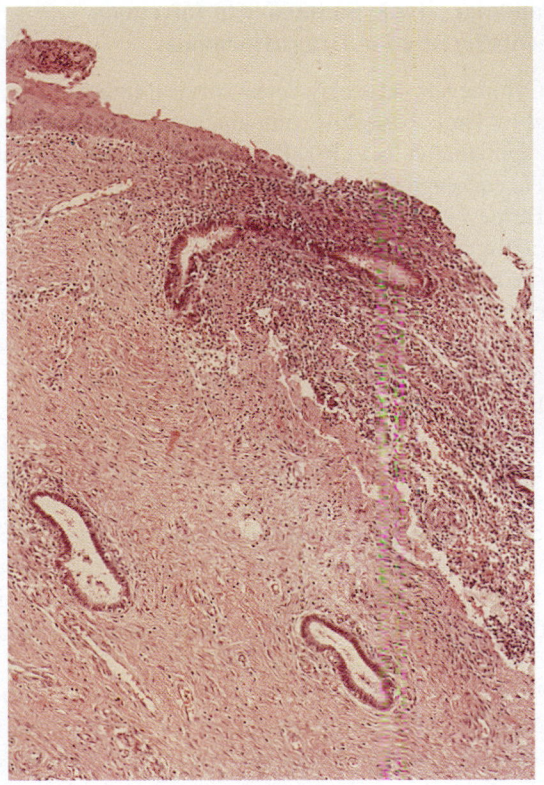
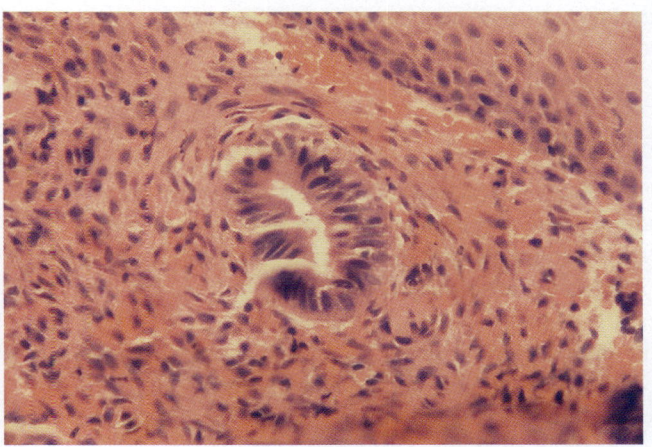

FIG. 24. Endometriosis. **A:** Darkened superficial glands might cause concern for adenocarcinoma *in situ* (AIS). **B:** Spindled stromal cells are a clue to superficial endometriosis.

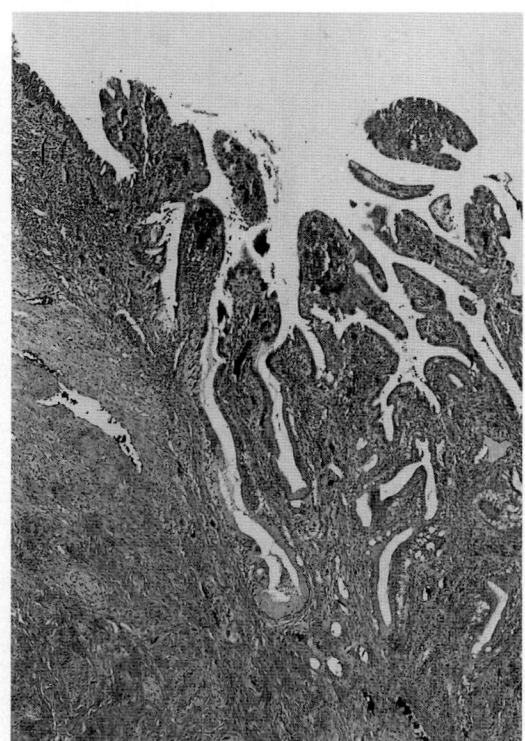
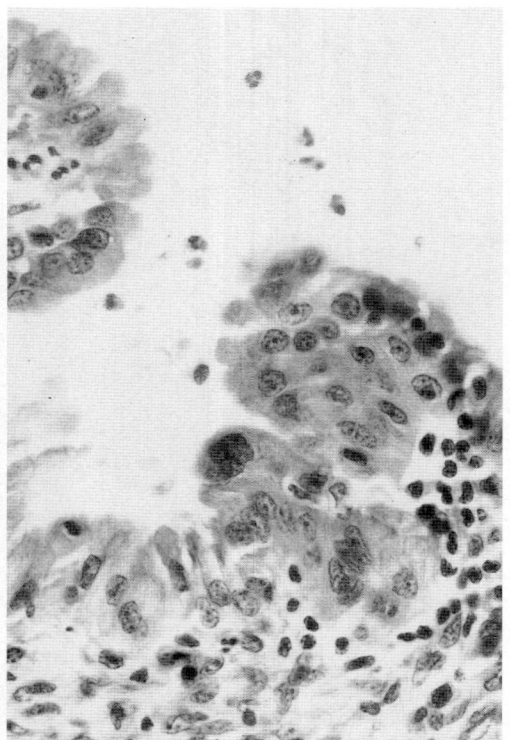

FIG. 25. Papillary endocervicitis. **A:** Papillary pattern might cause concern for adenocarcinoma. **B:** Nuclear chromatin is bland, nucleoli are prominent. (With permission, Ref. 15 [parts A and B].)

considering glandular neoplasia in an inflammatory background.

Arias-Stella Reaction

The Arias-Stella reaction (AS), more commonly seen in the endometrium, may be an incidental finding in a cervical biopsy from a pregnant or postpartum patient (129–131). With AS, glands are somewhat dilated and lined by cells with enlarged and hyperchromatic nuclei (Fig. 26A). A hobnail-like luminal protrusion of nuclei may cause confusion with clear cell carcinoma, but the changes in AS are focal, the architecture of the glands is not invasive, and the nuclei show a spectrum of atypia. Smudging of the chromatin and finely vacuolated cytoplasm are seen with AS (Fig. 26B). Of course, a history of a current or recent pregnancy is crucial to the correct diagnosis.

Müllerian Papilloma

This rare lesion, seen almost exclusively in children, presents as a papillary excrescence on the ectocervix or vagina (132) (Fig. 27A). Microscopically, it contains small papillae lined by a single layer of cuboidal epithelium without nuclear atypia or significant mitotic activity (Fig. 27B). Benign papillary adenomas may also rarely be seen in adults (133). Villous adenomas of the cervix have been reported (134, 135).

Glandular Atypia Secondary to Infectious Agents/Irradiation/Drugs/Hormones

Cytomegalovirus may cause cervical infection characterized by large, basophilic, intranuclear inclusions in glandular epithelial cells (136) (Fig. 28). Inclusions may also involve endothelial or stromal cells.

Herpesvirus may also infect endocervical glandular epithelium, although it more commonly involves the squamous epithelium (137). Multinucleated cells with ground-glass nuclear chromatin or intranuclear inclusions are characteristic and should not be confused with a neoplasm or nonspecific multinucleation of glandular epithelium.

Irradiation may cause substantial nuclear atypia of endocervical glandular epithelium (138,139). Nuclei are enlarged, pleomorphic, sometimes smudged, and may have prominent nucleoli (Fig. 29A). The chromatin, however, is fine or degenerated and the cytoplasm is abundant and sometimes vacuolated. Mitoses are uncommon. The stroma may be hyalinized or demonstrate a reactive fibroblastic change with ectatic vessels (Fig. 29B). Knowledge of the history is of course essential.

Nonspecific glandular cytologic atypia with either cytomegaly, nuclear enlargement, or multinucleation, sometimes with foamy or vacuolated cytoplasm, may be associated with use of oral contraceptives or tamoxifen therapy, or may occur without a drug history (140). A variation of this type of change with prominent eosinophilic cytoplasm has been called "atypical oxyphilic metaplasia" (141). In contrast to AIS, the cells in these types of atypia have a normal

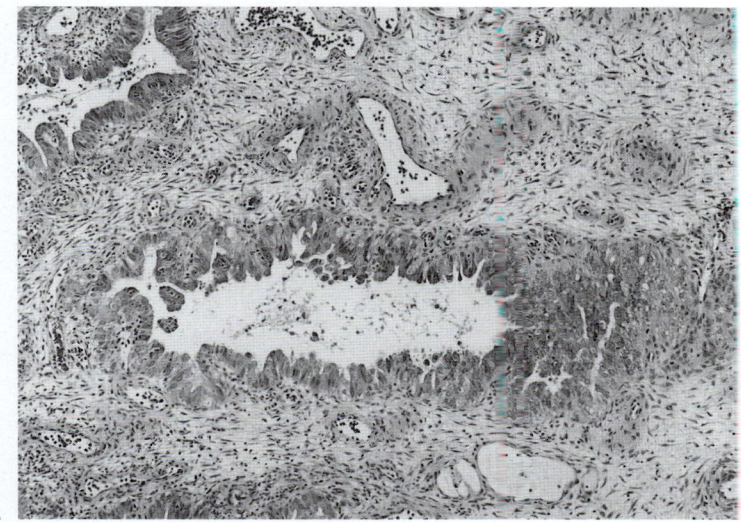

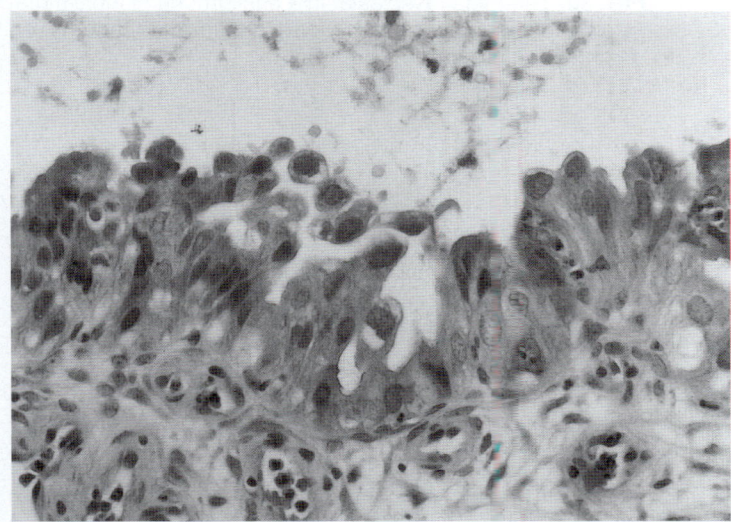

FIG. 26. Arias-Stella reaction. **A:** Dilated gland in a cervical polyp removed from a pregnant woman. **B:** 2 Hobnail nuclei with smudged chromatin, cytoplasmic vacuoles. (With permission, Ref. 15 [A and B].)

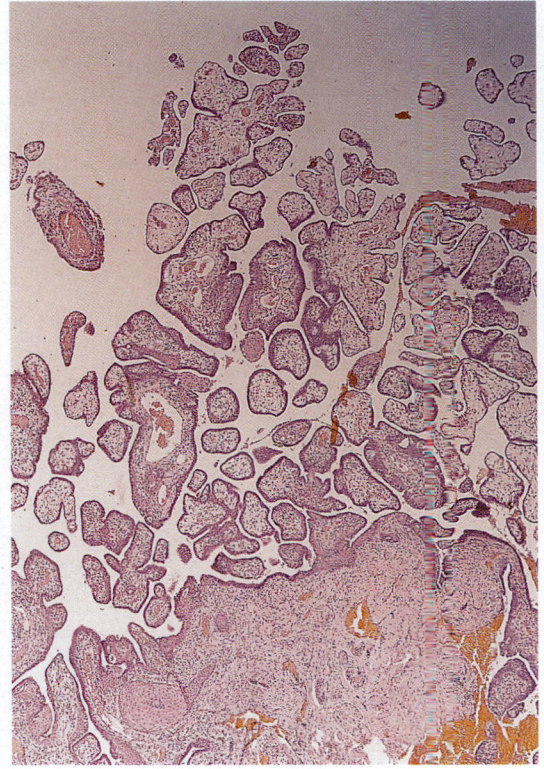

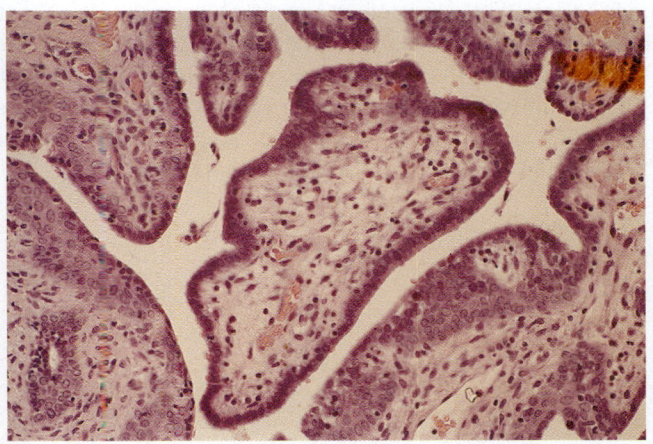

FIG. 27. Müllerian papilloma. **A:** Exophytic papillary lesion from the ectocervix in a 3-year-old girl. **B:** Fibrous cores, benign epithelial lining.

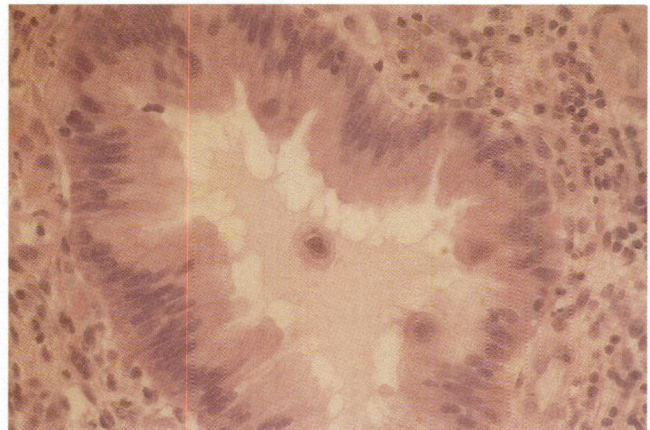

FIG. 28. Cytomegalovirus infection. Endocervical gland containing cells with characteristic intranuclear inclusions.

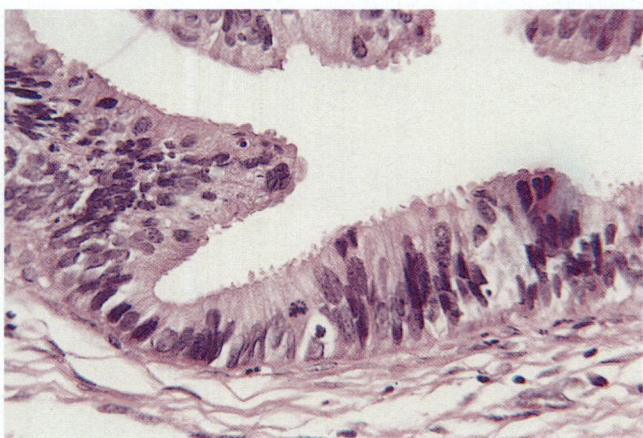

FIG. 30. Glandular dysplasia. In a background of tubal metaplasia there is increased crowding, stratification, and hyperchromasia. Note single mitotic figure.

nucleus-to-cytoplasm ratio, lack significant crowding, have bland to smudged nuclear chromatin, and lack mitotic figures.

Glandular Dysplasia

The term *endocervical glandular dysplasia* has been used for endocervical glands with cellular crowding and cytologic atypia that exhibit some but not all of the features of AIS (142–144). Dysplasia has been stratified into low-grade and high-grade categories (144). In reality, there is a continuum of nuclear atypia, crowding, loss of mucin, stratification, and tufting, sometimes superimposed on tubal metaplasia (Fig. 30). Thus, the diagnosis itself and the stratification into subcategories is difficult to reliably reproduce. Glandular dysplasia may be seen with concomitant squamous lesions, AIS, or as an isolated finding (144,145). High-grade dysplasia is likely to be a form of AIS and most cases should be so diagnosed. Incidental lesions in the low-grade category are probably nonspecific and should be designated "atypical hyperplasia" rather than "dysplasia" (146). Most cases of AIS do not have concomitant dysplasia (147), and thus many AIS cases may not be derived from a recognizable precursor lesion. Studies of HPV in glandular dysplasia have been contradictory (148–151). Considering these difficulties, the morphologic appearance of true precursors to AIS, if they exist, remains to be elucidated.

Adenocarcinoma In Situ

Adenocarcinoma *in situ* (AIS) was first described in 1953, much later than cervical squamous precursors (152). The frequency of this diagnosis has been increasing steadily since then. Perhaps some of this increase is due to increased awareness, but there also appears to have been an absolute increase in incidence. AIS is the precursor to most, but perhaps not all, forms of cervical adenocarcinoma. Evidence of this includes the following: The average age at presentation is 35 to 40 years, approximately 10 years earlier than invasive adenocarcinoma (147,153–158); 30% to 60% of cases have a concomitant squamous intraepithelial lesion; 50% to

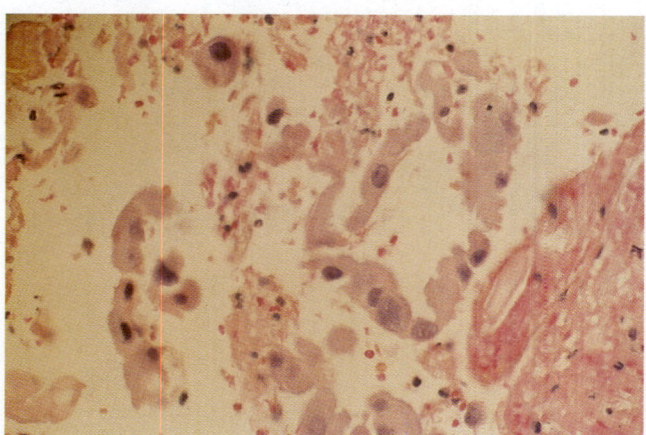
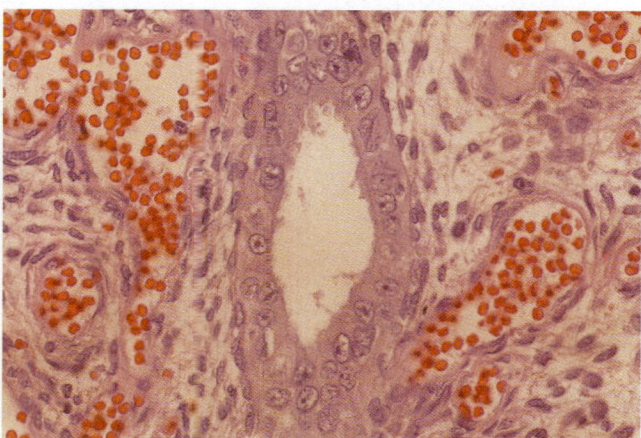

FIG. 29. Irradiation effect. **A:** Endocervical curettage specimen. Nuclei are enlarged and pleomorphic with smudged chromatin. Cytoplasm is voluminous. **B:** Endocervical gland with nucleomegaly, prominent nucleoli. Note ectatic vessels, reactive stromal cells. (With permission, Ref. 15 [B].)

90% of cases have detectable HPV in AIS cells, almost equally divided between HPV 16 and HPV 18 (148, 159–166). Individual cases of AIS have been observed to progress to invasive adenocarcinoma (167), and AIS is present adjacent to most very early invasive adenocarcinomas (157,167,168). AIS can be suspected at low power. AIS involves the glandular epithelium at the squamocolumnar junction beginning on the surface with extension into the superficial portions of the glands, sometimes with an abrupt change at a deeper level to normal endocervical cells (169–171) (Fig. 31A). Skip areas are sometimes seen with separate foci of AIS higher up in the canal, but this is uncommon (147,170). Endocervical glands are lined with slightly enlarged, crowded, and hyperchromatic nuclei. There may be expansion of the glands with an intraglandular papillary or cribriform pattern of growth. A periglandular inflammatory reaction may be present. The cells lining the glands in AIS are markedly crowded and nuclei are slightly to moderately enlarged and irregularly shaped with somewhat coarse chromatin (Fig. 31B,C). Mitotic figures are eas-

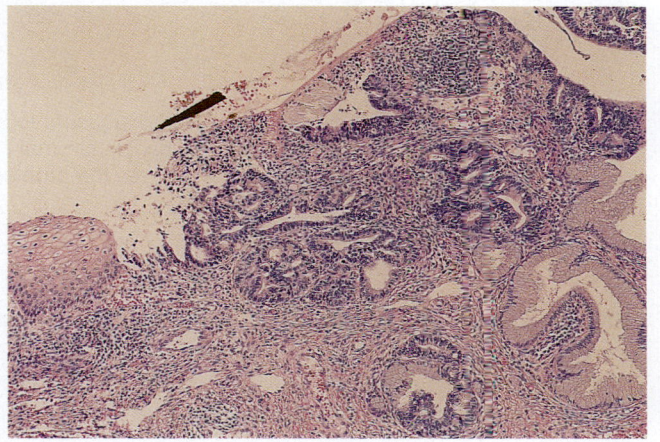
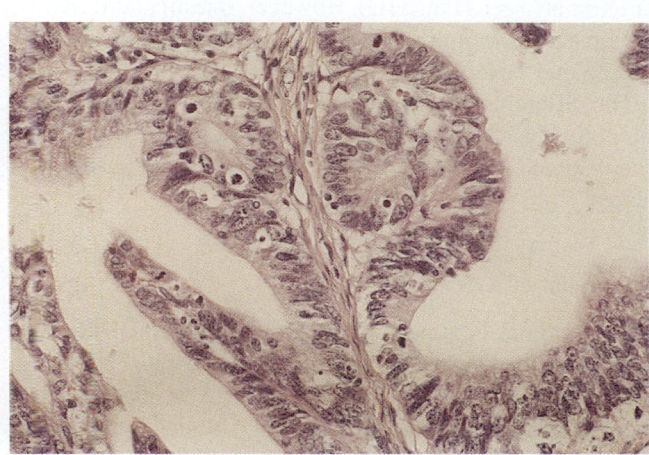
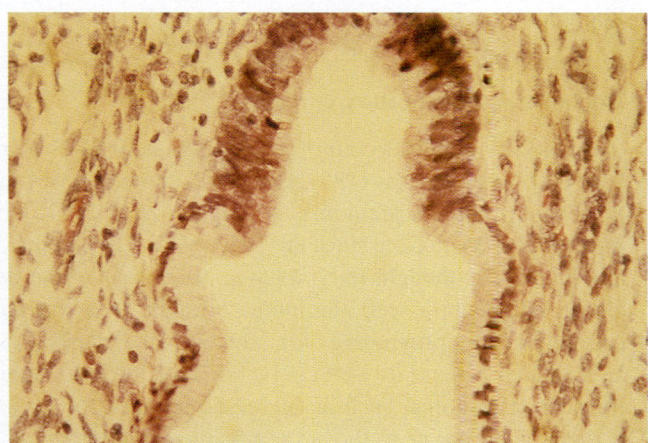
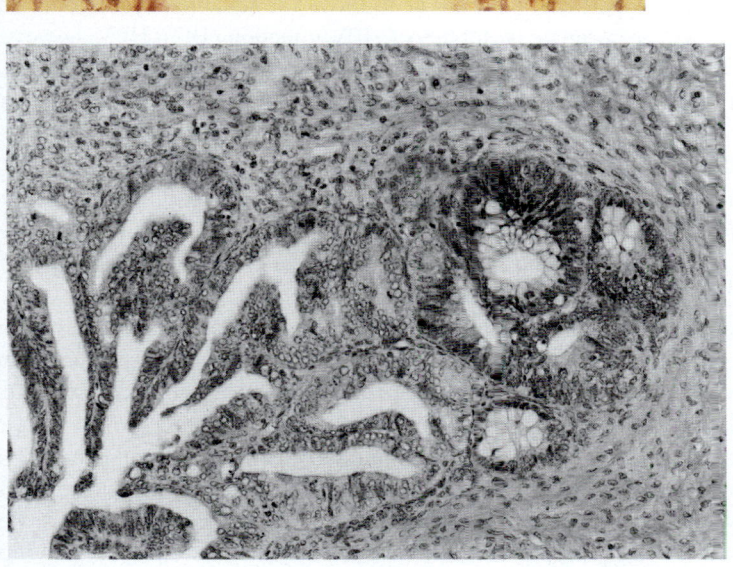

FIG. 31. Adenocarcinoma in situ (AIS). **A:** Low-power demonstrating darkened glands at squamocolumnar junction contrasting with normal glands deeper and higher in the canal. **B:** Nuclei are crowded, stratified, enlarged, and hyperchromatic. Mitotic figures and apoptotic bodies are seen. **C:** Endocervical (mucinous) type. Abrupt transition to normal epithelium in lower portion of gland. **D:** Mixed endometrioid type *(left)* and intestinal type *(right)*. (With permission, Ref. 15.)

ily found and are essential for the diagnosis. Nucleoli are usually small and inconspicuous, but in some cases may be prominent (147,171). Apoptotic bodies are frequently seen. AIS has been subclassified into endocervical, endometrioid, and intestinal types (147). The endocervical type is the most common and retains some mucinous cytoplasm (Fig. 31C), the endometrioid type mimics hyperplastic or well-differentiated malignant endometrial glands, and the intestinal type contains tall columnar cells and prominent goblet cells. These distinctions have no clinical significance and mixed varieties are seen (Fig. 31D). However, intestinal differentiation is rarely seen in nonneoplastic cervical glands, so this finding may be a clue to the presence of AIS.

The differential diagnosis of AIS includes TEM, cervicitis, nonspecific glandular atypia, and glandular dysplasia. The distinction from these lesions has been previously discussed.

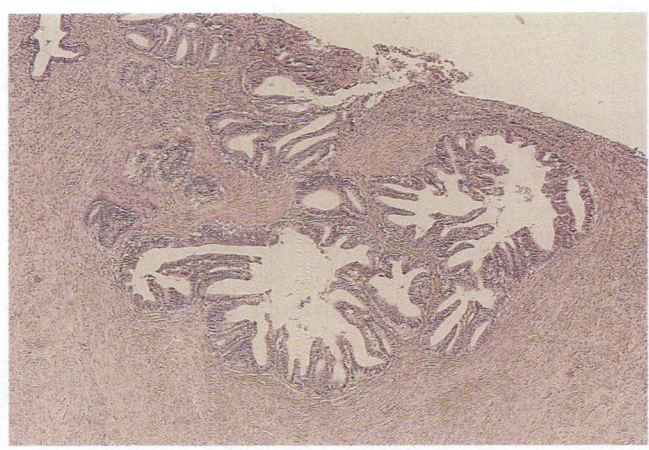

FIG. 32. AIS vs early invasion. AIS at surface adjacent to dilated irregular glands with papillary infoldings. No stromal reaction. Case was considered AIS, but illustrates the problem in ruling out invasion.

Treatment of AIS

The optimal treatment for AIS is controversial. Recent studies indicate that a cold knife cone biopsy with clear margins is not protective against recurrent AIS or invasive adenocarcinoma in all cases (172–176). This fact, combined with the difficulty in detecting recurrence by Pap smear after cone biopsy (177) is an argument for hysterectomy in selected cases.

Detection of Early Invasion

In some cases of AIS it is difficult to rule out early invasion (178). In the earliest form of invasion there is a contiguous budding of cells from the AIS gland (179). The cytoplasm in this bud is expanded, and the nuclei are vesicular with prominent nucleoli, similar to changes in early invasive squamous carcinoma. This early form of invasion by itself carries no increased clinical risk. A clinically important problem, however, occurs when AIS glands are expanded by a complex intraglandular epithelial proliferation or when AIS-like glands are separated by stroma beneath more superficial AIS (Fig. 32). In general, either a desmoplastic stromal reaction, irregularity of glandular size and shape, or the presence of AIS-like glands below the level of adjacent normal endocervical glands indicates early invasion (171) (Fig. 33). These features may be impossible to assess in a small biopsy specimen. Even in a cone biopsy, inclusion or exclusion of invasion may sometimes be very difficult.

Once invasion is recognized, there is no universally accepted definition for the upper limit of microinvasive adenocarcinoma of the cervix (180–184). However, in the largest series of such cases, in which microinvasion was defined as invasion no greater than 5 mm as measured from the surface, none of 48 women who had a pelvic node dissection had metastases in the nodes (184). However, recurrent adenocarcinoma has developed after hysterectomy in cases with lesser depths of invasion (180,182,183). Currently, the standard is to report the presence of invasion, its depth as measured from the surface, and the presence or absence of vascular space invasion. In most cases, the treatment is radical hysterectomy and pelvic node dissection for invasion of any depth; however, this practice may change as more data are accrued.

Adenocarcinoma of the Cervix

Adenocarcinomas account for approximately 15% of invasive cervical cancers (135). However, in some series the percentage of adenocarcinomas is a high as 25% (186). This rate has been increasing since the 1980s (187–189). Some of this increase is thought to be relative, secondary to the decrease in squamous cell carcinoma brought about by Pap smear screening programs (190). However, there appears to an absolute increase as well (191). Some of the risk factors for adenocarcinoma, such as increased numbers of sexual partners, are similar to those for squamous carcinoma and correlate with rates of HPV infection (192). HPV, however, is less frequently found in adenocarcinoma than in squamous carcinoma (148,193,194). Cigarette smoking has been implicated as a risk factor for squamous carcinoma but not for adenocarcinoma (192). Prolonged use of birth control pills may be related to the development of cervical adenocarcinoma (192,195–197), although this point is disputed (198). It may be that different subtypes of adenocarcinoma have different etiologies (199).

On gross examination, advanced cervical adenocarcinoma may present as an exophytic mass, an ulcerated plaque, or diffuse cervical enlargement (barrel-shaped cervix) (200). Most symptomatic patients have vaginal bleeding, pelvic pain, or pressure (186). Less commonly, patients present with a pelvic or ovarian mass (201). Most adenocarcinomas of the cervix spread in similar fashion to squamous cell carcinomas, first involving contiguous pelvic structures and pelvic lymph

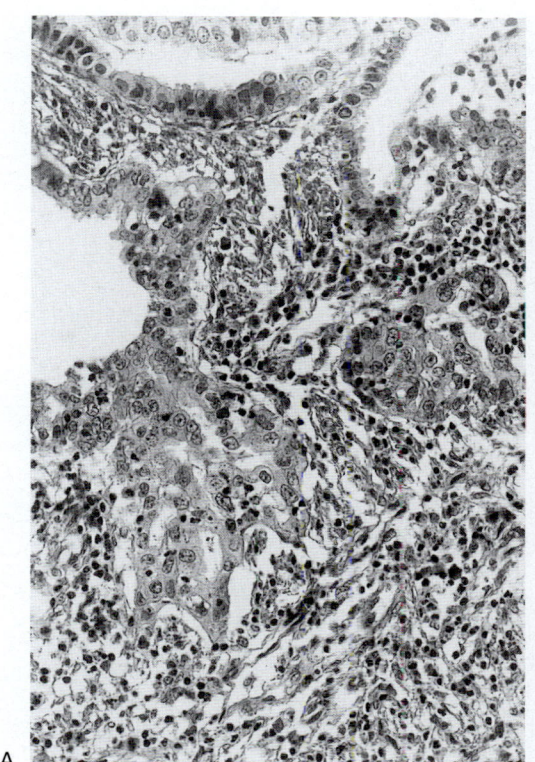 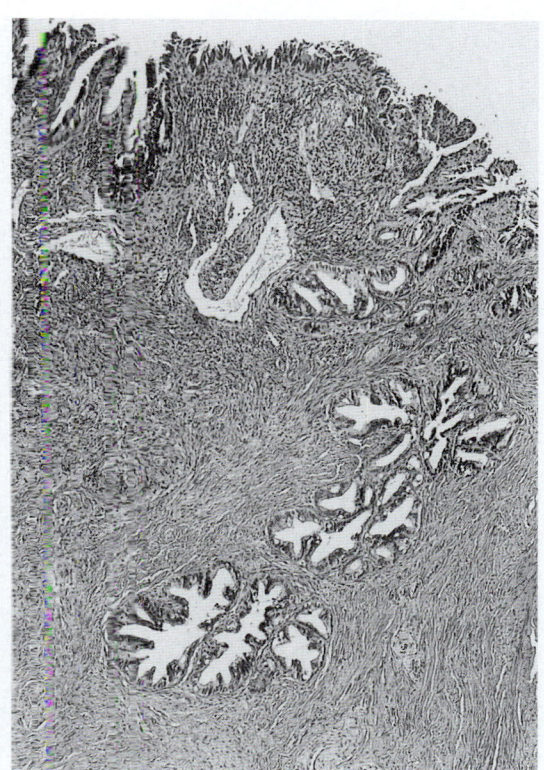

FIG. 33. Adenocarcinoma with early invasion. **A:** Jagged bud of cells protrudes into stroma from AIS gland. **B:** AIS *(top* and *left).* Glands *(lower right)* are considered invasive because of depth although gland profiles are similar to those seen in some AIS cases.

nodes. However, adenocarcinomas of the cervix more frequently metastasize to the ovaries, upper abdomen, or distant organs than do squamous carcinomas (202).

The microscopic classification of cervical adenocarcinoma is given in Table 4.

Endocervical-Type Adenocarcinoma

Approximately 70% of cervical adenocarcinomas are of the endocervical (mucinous) type (200). In this variety, the tumor cells recapitulate the mucinous columnar cell morphology of the normal endocervix to a greater or lesser degree. The tumor may contain simple, complex, or dilated glands, solid sheets, cords, or single cells (Fig. 34A–C). Mucinous differentiation may be obvious or subtle. The extent of stromal reaction may vary from none to a prominent desmoplastic or inflammatory response. In some cases, there is extravasated stromal mucin. In small lesions, AIS may be evident.

Rare variants include the intestinal subtype, with goblet, argentaffin, and sometimes Paneth cells (203,204), carcinomas with extensive extracellular mucin (colloid carcinoma) (205), and signet-ring cell carcinomas (206). Signet-ring cells in abundance are uncommon in primary cervical adenocarcinomas and, if encountered, raise the possibility of a primary malignancy elsewhere.

Adenoma Malignum (Minimal Deviation Adenocarcinoma)

This well-differentiated subtype accounts for approximately 10% of endocervical adenocarcinomas (207–212). It has been associated with Peutz-Jeghers syndrome (213), but most cases are sporadic. Adenoma malignum usually results in a diffusely enlarged, barrel-shaped cervix and may cause a vaginal discharge. Notorious for being missed by small cervical biopsies, adenoma malignum reportedly has a worse

TABLE 4. *Classification of cervical adenocarcinoma*

1. Adenocarcinoma
   a. Endocervical type
      Variants
         i. Adenoma malignum (minimal deviation adenocarcinoma)
         ii. Villoglandular
   b. Endometrioid
   c. Clear cell
   d. Serous
   e. Mesonephric
2. Adenosquamous carcinoma
      Variant: glassy cell carcinoma
3. Adenoid basal carcinoma
4. Adenoid cystic carcinoma
5. Adenocarcinoma, mixed (specify subtypes)
6. Adenocarcinoma and small cell carcinoma
7. Metastatic adenocarcinoma

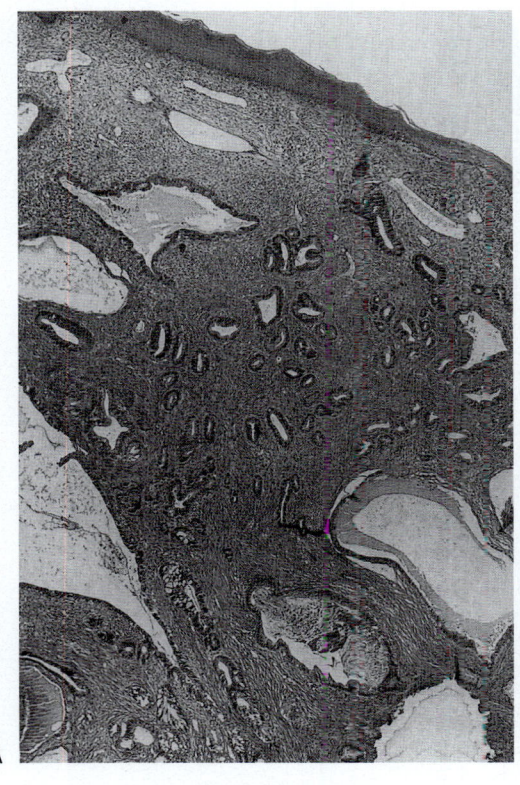
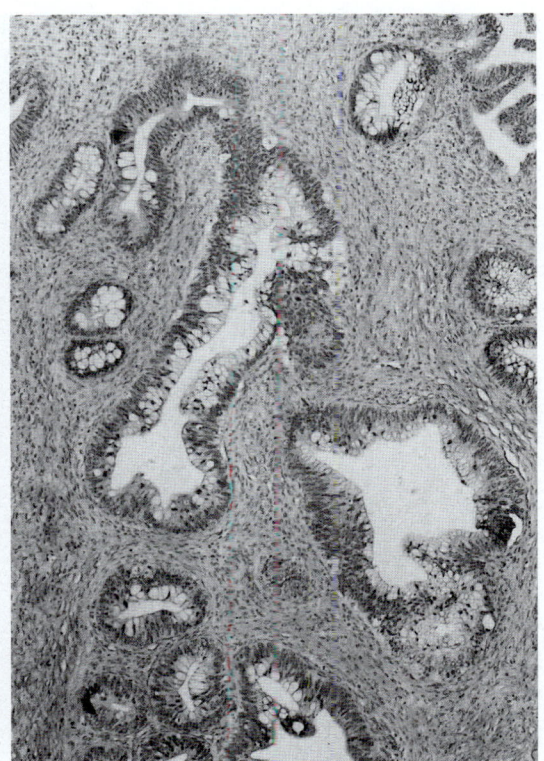
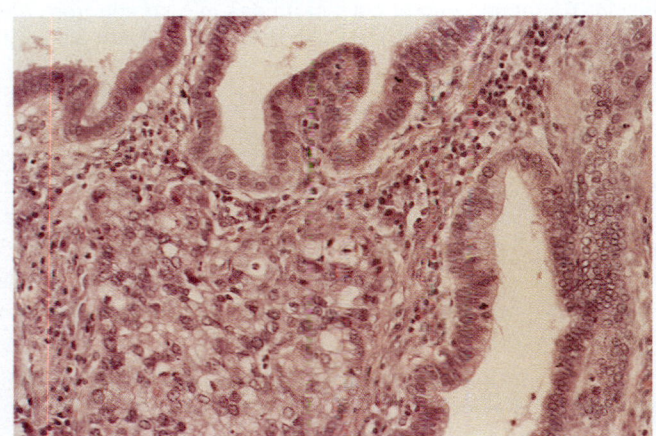

FIG. 34. Adenocarcinoma-endocervical type. **A:** Small glands and cystic glands infiltrate the stroma. Low-power pattern might be mistaken for nabothian cysts or nonspecific hyperplasia. **B:** Focal intestinal differentiation with goblet cells. **C:** Well-differentiated glands adjacent to more poorly differentiated focus. (With permission, Ref. 15 [A].)

prognosis than other forms of cervical adenocarcinoma. This may be related to the tumor's discovery at a later stage because of a lack of symptoms and the difficulty of diagnosis by Pap smear (214) or biopsy. In adequate specimens, adenoma malignum is suspected on the basis of the infiltrative appearance of either cystically dilated, irregular, or "claw-shaped" glands that permeate the endocervical stroma (Fig. 35A). These may elicit an inflammatory or desmoplastic reaction, but often no stromal reaction is seen. Perineural space invasion may be noted. The cells lining the glands are extremely well differentiated, with basally located nuclei and abundant, tall columnar cytoplasm (Fig. 35B). The nuclei are slightly larger than those of normal endocervical cells and may have a small eosinophilic nucleolus. A range of nuclear atypia, with slightly more enlargement and hyperchromasia in some foci and the presence of occasional mitotic figures, is helpful for diagnosis if present (Fig. 35C). CEA staining is reported to be positive in the cytoplasm of many of these tumors, but a negative reaction does not rule out malignancy (211,212). The differential diagnosis includes tunnel clusters, deep nabothian cysts, diffuse laminar endocervical gland hyperplasia, nonspecific gland hyperplasia, and mesonephric lesions. The most useful differential feature is the haphazard, infiltrative nature of the glands.

Villoglandular Papillary Adenocarcinoma

This variant of endocervical-type adenocarcinoma with a prominent papillary growth pattern characterized by narrow or broad papillary cores with a spindled or inflamed stroma has been recognized because of its good prognosis (215,216) (Fig. 36A) Cells lining the papillae are not significantly strat-

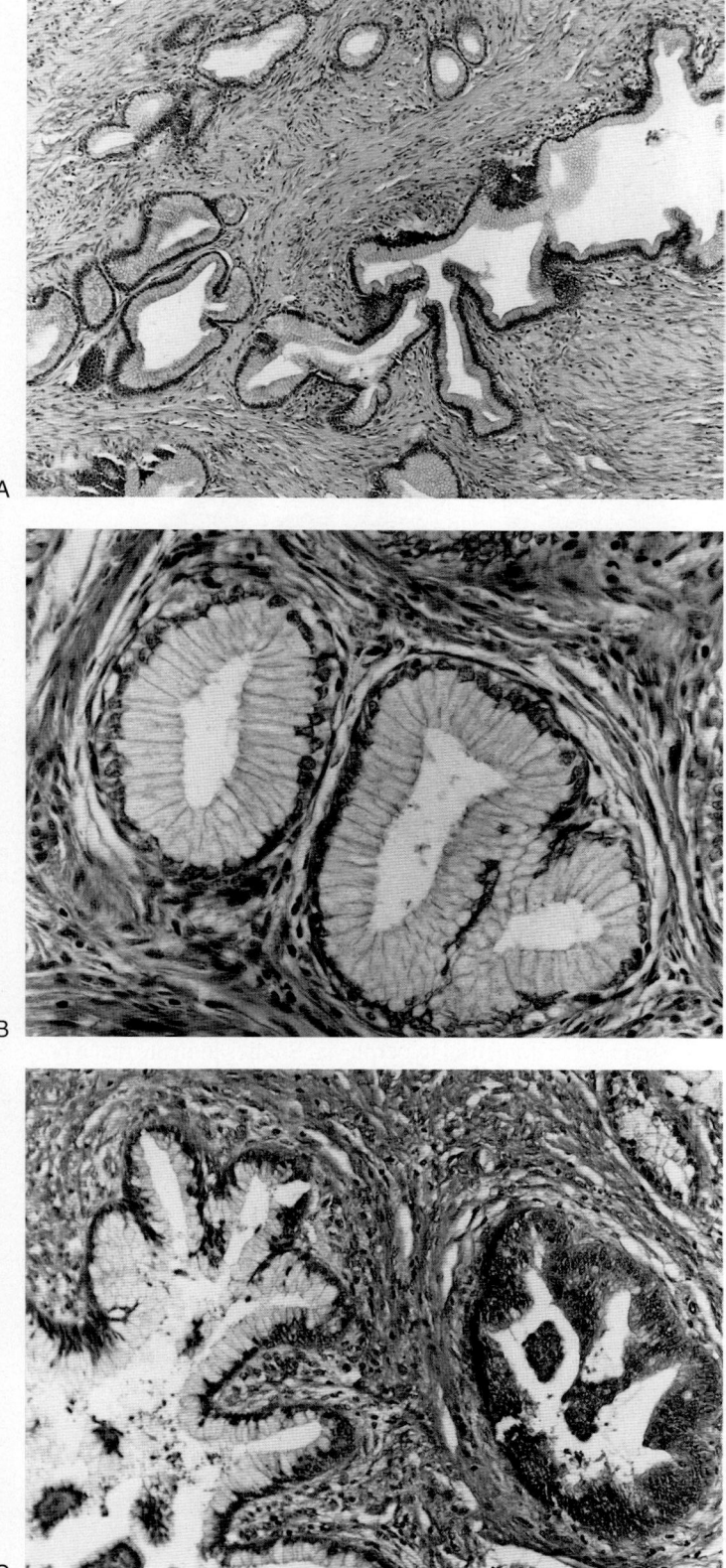

FIG. 35. A: Adenoma malignum. Large irregular gland and several smaller glands in cervical stroma. Note absence of stromal reaction. **B:** Adenoma malignum. Invasive extemely well-differentiated glands with colunar shapes. **C:** Gland with higher grade atypia, loss of mucin. Occasional more poorly differentiated glands may be seen in adenoma malignum. (With permission, Ref. 214.)

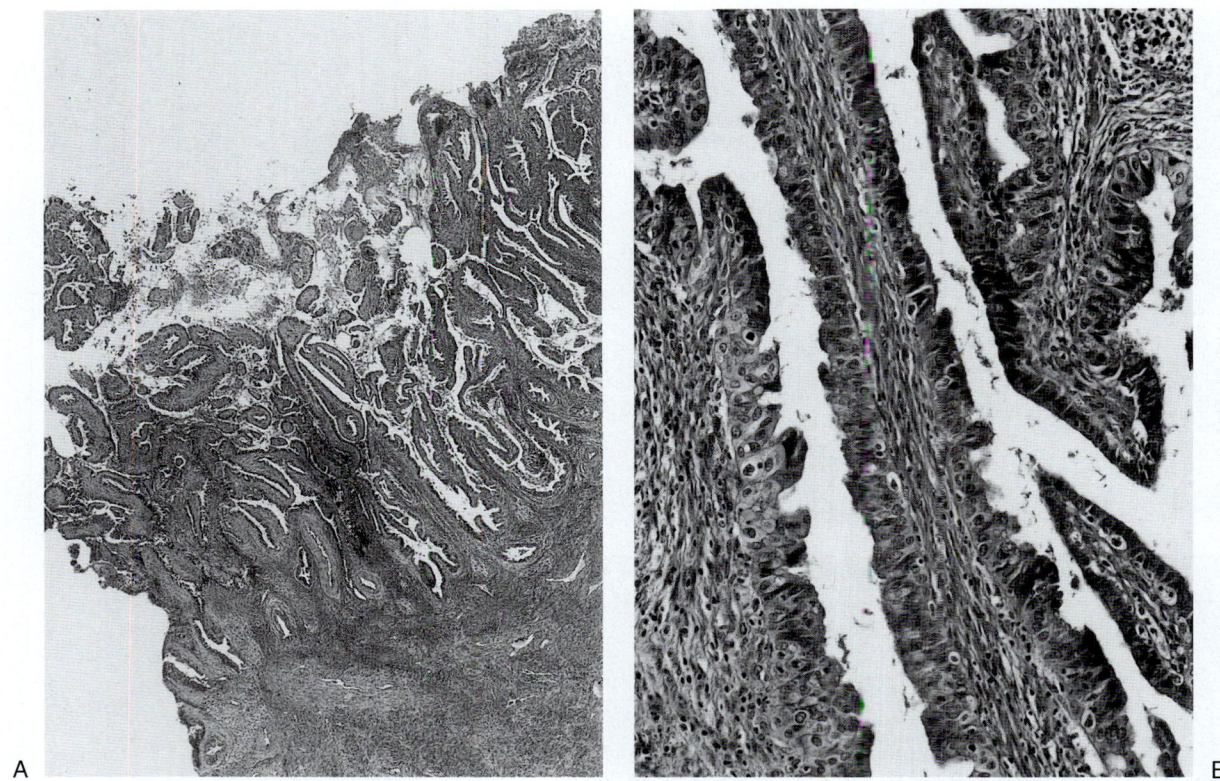

FIG. 36. Villoglandular papillary adenocarcinoma. **A:** Papillary pattern, well-demarcated lower border, AIS *(lower left)*. **B:** Well-differentiated cytologic features. (With permission Ref. 15)

ified and are well differentiated, but of a slightly higher grade of malignancy than is seen in adenoma malignum (Fig. 36B). Adjacent AIS is often present. The underlying invasive component may lose its papillary architecture but usually infiltrates as glands or tubules in a broad, confluent fashion rather than as single invasive glands. To date, no lesions that are purely of this type have metastasized (168,215,216). However, caution must be used in diagnosing villoglandular papillary adenocarcinoma if there is even a moderate degree of cytologic atypia or if there are small foci of a different type of carcinoma (217). In small biopsies or curettings, a papillary appearance does not necessarily connote invasion, as some variants of AIS may have a papillary surface (156).

Endometrioid Adenocarcinoma

The second most frequent category of pure cervical adenocarcinoma is the endometrioid type. As the name suggests, the infiltrating glands mimic those of a well to moderately differentiated carcinoma of the endometrium. Cytoplasm is scant and nuclei are more crowded and stratified than in the endocervical type (Fig. 37). It is likely that many of these cases are endocervical-type adenocarcinomas in which the mucinous epithelium is inconspicuous. In smaller lesions, AIS may be present, indicating a pathogenesis similar to the endocervical type. An occasional problem in curettage specimens is in the distinction of endometrioid cervical carcinoma from primary endometrial carcinoma that has metasta-

sized to the cervix or has exfoliated into the cervical canal. The most helpful findings in diagnosing primary endocervical carcinoma include the presence of AIS, the involvement of endocervical stroma rather than free-floating malignant glands, and, if an endometrial sample is procured, the absence of endometrial hyperplasia. Studies indicate that a positive CEA stain favors an endocervical origin (218). While this is true, the usefulness of this technique is marginal (219,220), and in most cases the diagnosis can be made on the basis of a differential curettage and clinical findings. Radiographic techniques such as magnetic resonance imaging

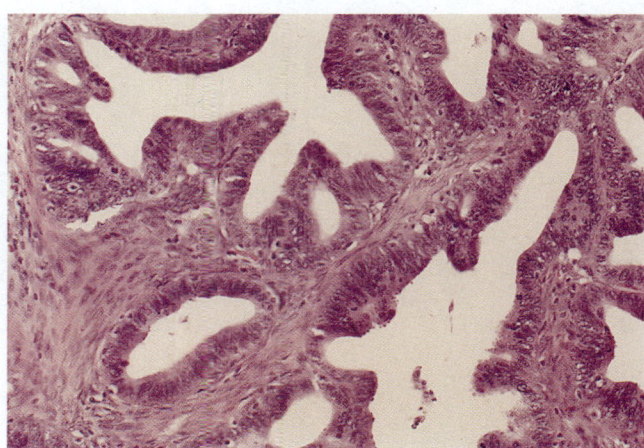

FIG. 37. Endometrioid adenocarcinoma. Glands similar to those of well-differentiated carcinoma of the endometrium.

(MRI) and ultrasound are sometimes useful in locating the center of the mass.

Excluding a primary endometrial carcinoma, the differential diagnosis includes AIS, cervical endometriosis, and TEM. These are only problematic in small biopsies, as the architectural features of carcinoma distinguish it from these lesions.

Rarely, an extremely well differentiated (minimal deviation) adenocarcinoma of the cervix is of the endometrioid rather than the endocervical type (210,221). The glands in such cases resemble endometrial glands, and nuclear atypia is slight and focal (Fig. 38). There may even be ciliated cells and apical cytoplasmic "snouts" mimicking tubal metaplasia. The lesion is distinguished from endometriosis or TEM of the cervix by its infiltrative pattern, deep extension, and focal cytologic atypia beyond that seen in these benign lesions. CEA staining was only focally positive in the two cases in which it was studied and therefore may not be of much help (222). Twelve cases have been reported with follow-up, and one patient died of her tumor (211).

Clear Cell Carcinoma

Clear cell carcinoma of the cervix is much less common than histologically similar tumors in the ovary and endometrium. It develops in young women who have been exposed in utero to diethylstilbestrol (DES) (223,224) and at a later age in those with no such exposure (225,226). In the former group, the tumor is usually centered on the ectocervix. In the latter, it may be in this location or may involve the endocervical canal. Cells contain clear or eosinophilic cytoplasm with enlarged, irregular nuclei (Fig. 39A,B). As in clear cell carcinomas arising in other organs, cells are arranged in a tubulocystic, solid, or papillary pattern. In the tubulocystic variant, the nuclei protrude into the lumina of the tubules or cysts in a hobnail pattern. Hyaline intertubular stroma or papillary cores distinguish some clear cell carcinomas.

The differential diagnosis includes microglandular hyperplasia, mesonephric hyperplasia, Arias-Stella reaction, squamous cell carcinoma, metastatic renal cell carcinoma, the very rare primary cervical yolk sac tumor in young children, and the uncommon alveolar soft part sarcoma of the cervix. Recognition of the typical patterns of clear cell carcinoma (as described above) and diffuse nuclear atypia as opposed to focal atypia distinguishes clear cell carcinoma from microglandular hyperplasia. Clear cell carcinoma may have eosinophilic material within tubules and cysts, mimicking similar material seen in mesonephric glands (Fig. 39C). However, significant and diffuse cytologic atypia is not seen in mesonephric hyperplasia. A history of pregnancy is obviously important when the Arias-Stella phenomenon is being considered. Arias-Stella nuclei may have a hobnail appearance, but glands lack the infiltrative pattern of a carcinoma, nuclear atypia is only focal, and mitotic figures are few or nonexistent. The solid variant of clear cell carcinoma can appear somewhat squamoid and must be distinguished from a squamous carcinoma, which may have clear cytoplasm due to glycogen (Fig. 39D). A search for more characteristic foci of either squamous carcinoma or clear cell carcinoma usually allows distinction. Renal cell carcinoma is rarely seen as a cervical metastasis, but may be difficult to distinguish from a primary clear cell carcinoma without knowing the history. Descriptions of yolk sac tumor and alveolar soft part sarcoma, which are only rarely seen in the cervix, are presented elsewhere in this book.

Serous Papillary Adenocarcinoma

This subtype, histologically similar to serous papillary carcinoma of the ovary and endometrium, is very rare as a primary adenocarcinoma of the cervix (227). It grows as a papillary proliferation with broad or thin fibrovascular cores, lined by pleomorphic epithelial cells with large nuclei, prominent nucleoli, and many mitotic figures. There is strat-

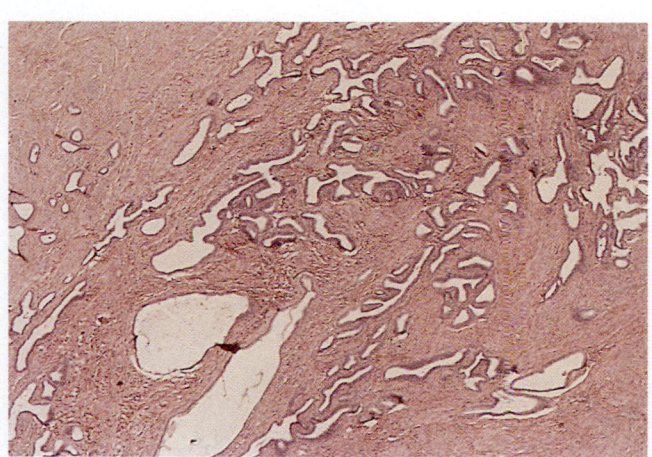
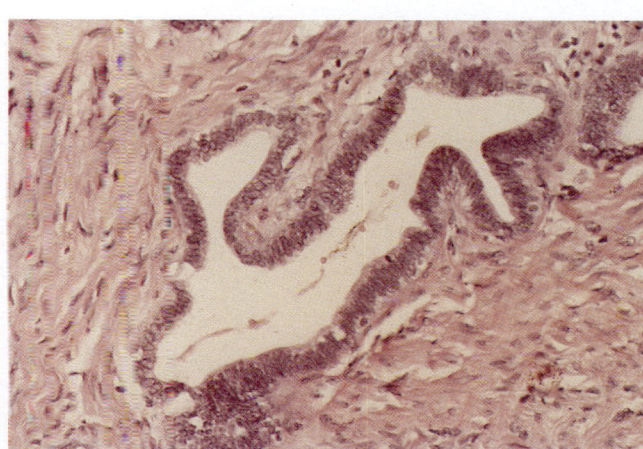

FIG. 38. Endometrioid adenocarcinoma. Minimal deviation type. **A** and **B:** Very well-differentiated infiltrating glands, no stromal reaction.

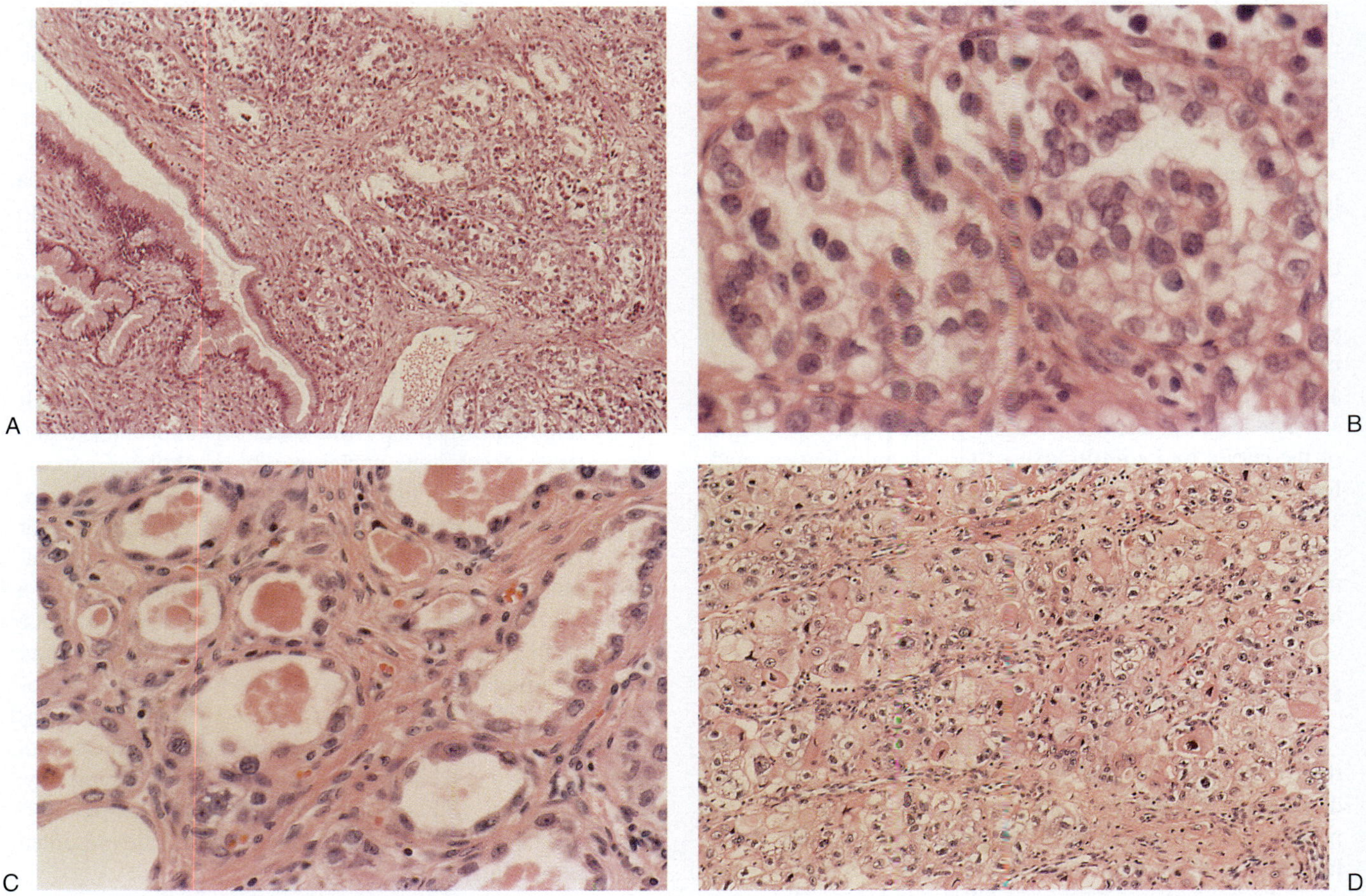

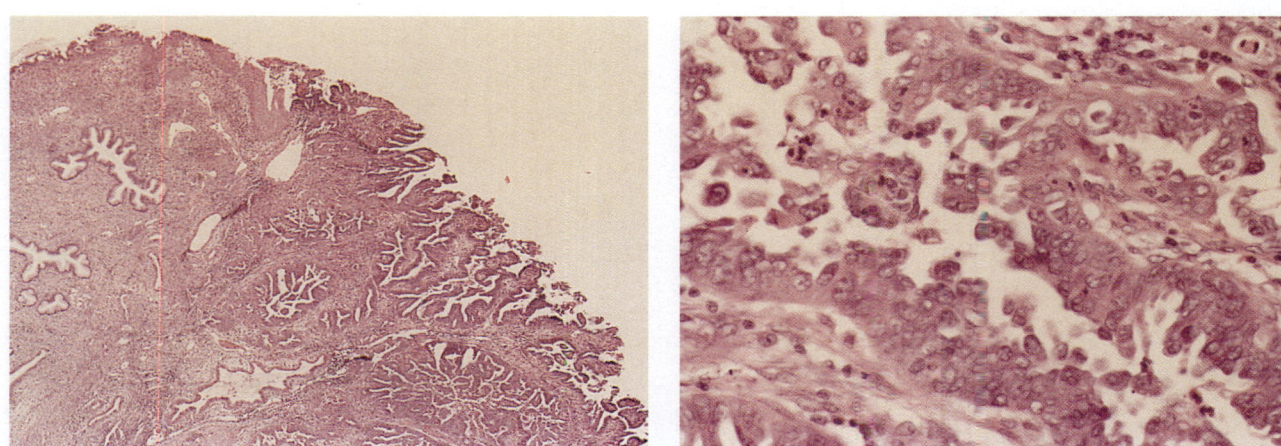

FIG. 39. Clear cell carcinoma. **A** and **B:** Tubular pattern, clear cytoplasm, moderate grade nuclei. **C:** Eosinophilic material may lead to confusion with mesonephric hyperplasia. Note atypia of nuclei, hobnail effect. **D:** Solid pattern; resembles squamous carcinoma.

ification with secondary and tertiary budding of the epithelial cells into the spaces between papillae (Fig. 40). Serous papillary carcinoma spread from the endometrium or ovary must be excluded. Papillary adenocarcinomas of the ordinary type or of the villoglandular type contain well-differentiated nuclei without cellular stratification or secondary or tertiary budding of cells. There have been too few cases of cervical serous adenocarcinoma reported to generalize about the prognosis, although in one report serous morphology was an unfavorable feature (168).

FIG. 40. Serous papillary carcinoma. **A:** Complex papillary pattern. **B:** Budding of cells, large vesicular nuclei with prominent nucleoli.

Mesonephric Adenocarcinoma

Adenocarcinomas derived from mesonephric remnants are rare. The histologic patterns are quite variable and include the ductal, retiform, tubular, solid, and sex-cord–like types (118,228). The glandular component often appears somewhat endometrioid (Fig. 41A,B). The nuclei of mesonephric carcinomas are usually of low to moderate grade. Some malignant glands contain eosinophilic secretion similar to that in mesonephric rests. A spindle cell component, resembling endometrial stromal sarcoma or other sarcoma, may merge imperceptibly with the glandular component (228) (Fig. 41C). Foci of mesonephric hyperplasia sometimes persist adjacent to the carcinoma. This finding and the lack of involvement of the surface epithelium help to suggest the correct diagnosis. Immunohistochemistry also may be helpful. Most cases are reactive for keratin, epithelial membrane antigen (EMA), and vimentin (228). The differential diagnosis of mesonephric adenocarcinoma includes mesonephric hyperplasia, endometrioid adenocarcinoma, and mixed müllerian tumor in cases with a spindle cell component. Distinction from florid examples of mesonephric hyperplasia may be difficult. However, in hyperplasia the maintenance of a lobular, noninfiltrative pattern and a lack of significant atypia are important findings. Endometrioid carcinomas are often of higher grade than mesonephric carcinoma and involve the surface as well as the deep cervical stroma without associated mesonephric hyperplasia. Mixed müllerian tumors are rare as primary cervical lesions and usually have higher grade atypia and more distinct demarcation between the epithelial and stromal component than mesonephric carcinomas with a spindle cell component. The prognosis for mesonephric carcinoma is uncertain because of the few cases reported. However, there is a suggestion that they have a more indolent course than the usual cervical carcinoma with a propensity to recur after many years (228).

Adenosquamous Carcinoma

Adenosquamous carcinomas have been said to account for between 15% and 35% of all cervical carcinomas with a glandular component. This wide variation in frequency may relate to different definitions. Many squamous cell carcinomas without an obvious glandular component stain positively for mucin (229). It is best, therefore, to limit the designation "adenosquamous" to tumors with a biphasic squamous and glandular pattern that is clearly recognizable without the use of special stains (200) (Fig. 42). The glandular component in adenosquamous carcinoma is almost always of the endocervical type. Cases with an endometrioid glandular component are classified as endometrioid adenocarcinomas with squamous differentiation, rather than adenosquamous carcinomas, in keeping with the terminol-

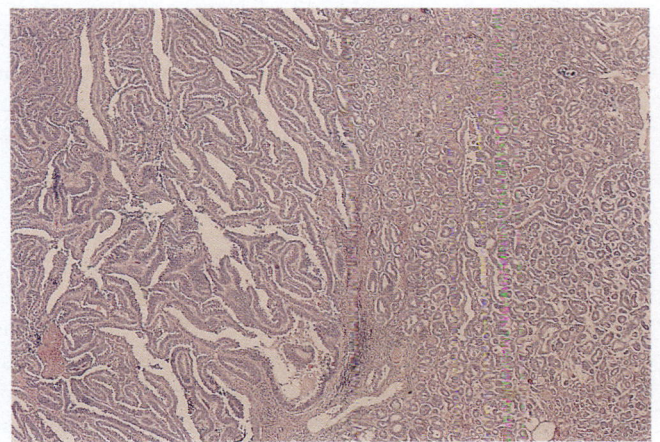
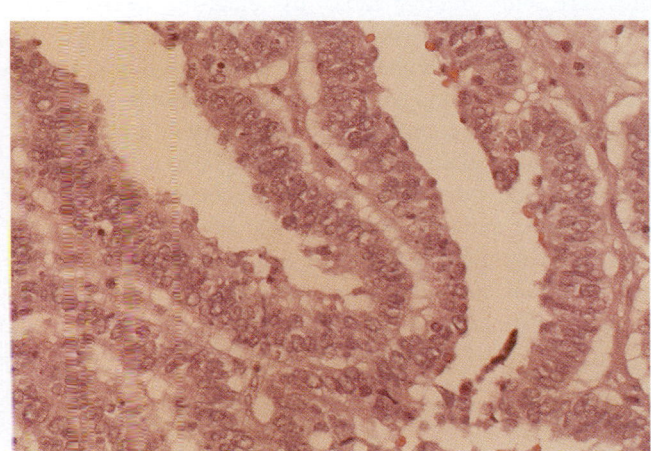
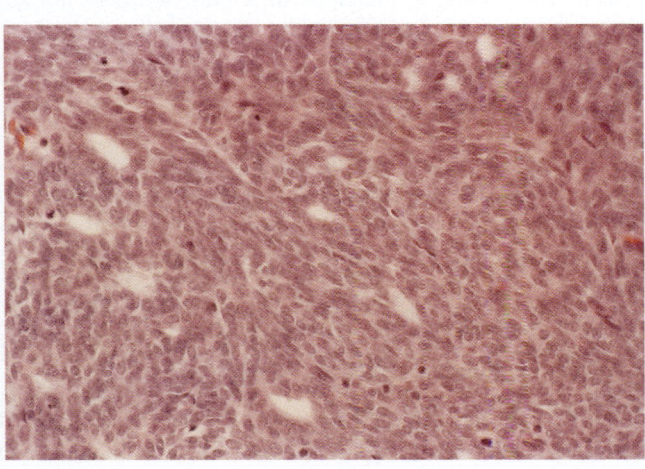

FIG. 41. Mesonephric carcinoma. **A:** Biphasic appearance with retiform appearance on *left,* tubular on *right.* **B:** Glands appear endometrioid at high power. **C:** Biphasic pattern with spindle cell component.

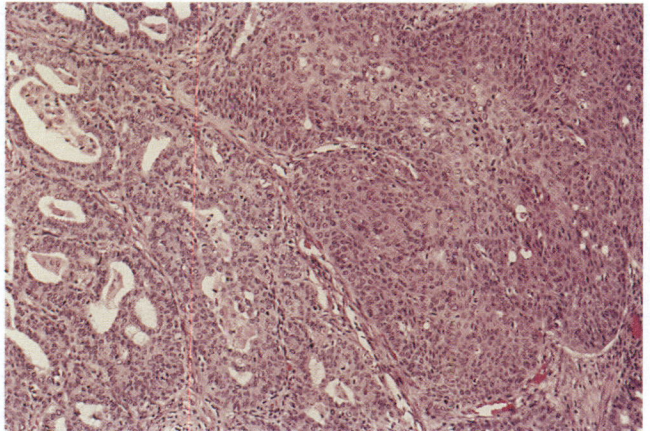

FIG. 42. Adenosquamous carcinoma. Solid squamous component merges with gland-forming area.

ogy used in primary endometrial carcinomas. Adenosquamous carcinomas have been reported to have a worse prognosis than other adenocarcinomas (168,230,231). However, some studies have not shown this to be the case (232,233).

Glassy Cell Carcinoma

Glassy cell carcinoma is considered a variant of adenosquamous carcinoma in which the differentiating features are only recognizable by electron microscopy (234–237). This tumor is characterized by a solid growth of large tumor cells with abundant eosinophilic (glassy) cytoplasm. Nuclei are large with prominent eosinophilic nucleoli, and the stroma contains an inflammatory infiltrate, often with many eosinophils (Fig. 43). The prognosis is worse than that of ordinary adenosquamous or adenocarcinoma of the cervix. Some authors emphasize that the morphology of glassy cell carcinoma merges with that seen in some cases of large cell, nonkeratinizing squamous carcinoma, from which it must be distinguished (238).

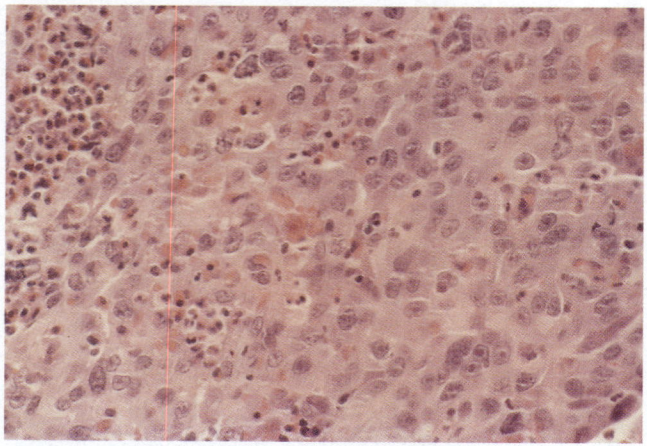

FIG. 43. Glassy cell carcinoma. Sheets of malignant cells with abundant eosinophilic cytoplasm, large nuclei with prominent nucleoli. Eosinophils in background.

Adenoid Basal Carcinoma

This uncommon form of cervical carcinoma is sometimes classified with squamous carcinomas. It occurs in elderly women, does not grow as a visible mass, and is associated with a high-grade squamous intraepithelial lesion of the surface epithelium (239–242). It appears as an infiltrate of small basaloid islands containing small cells with peripheral nuclear palisading and sometimes central squamoid or glandular differentiation, but no stromal reaction (Fig. 44). In some cases, adenoid basal carcinoma merges focally with a more typical squamous cell carcinoma. Adenoid basal carcinoma has a favorable prognosis; only 1 of 13 patients reported with follow-up data died of this cervical tumor (242).

Adenoid Cystic Carcinoma

As with adenoid basal carcinoma, this rare tumor occurs in older women but, unlike adenoid basal carcinoma, presents with a cervical mass. It grows predominantly as nests of cells in a cribriform pattern with intervening hyaline cores, resembling adenoid cystic carcinoma of the salivary glands (241,242) (Fig. 45). Because of a focal basaloid appearance, adenoid cystic carcinoma may mimic adenoid basal carcinoma to some degree, but has a higher grade of nuclear atypia, an expansile pattern of growth, and a stromal response not seen in the adenoid basal type. In some foci, tumor growth may be solid (243), and squamous differentiation may also be seen (242,243). For these reasons and because adenoid cystic carcinomas do not stain with S-100 for myoepithelial differentiation as does their salivary gland counterpart, the term *adenoid cystic* refers to the morphologic similarity with true adenoid cystic carcinoma, rather than to a similar derivation (242). The prognosis is poor.

Adenocarcinoma with Small Cell Undifferentiated Carcinoma

Small cell undifferentiated (neuroendocrine) carcinomas were described earlier in this chapter. In some cases, these tumors have focal glandular differentiation (Fig. 46). In a small biopsy specimen, the glandular cells may be the only ones seen. The finding of glandular differentiation does not alter the prognosis of this tumor, which was described earlier.

Mixed Adenocarcinomas

Besides the mixed varieties already discussed, other cervical adenocarcinomas may be composed of more than one histologic type. If a secondary component accounts for more than 10% of the entire tumor, it is designated as mixed, with each subtype identified.

Adenocarcinoma Metastatic to the Cervix

Although direct cervical extension from an endometrial carcinoma is not unusual, metastatic adenocarcinoma to the

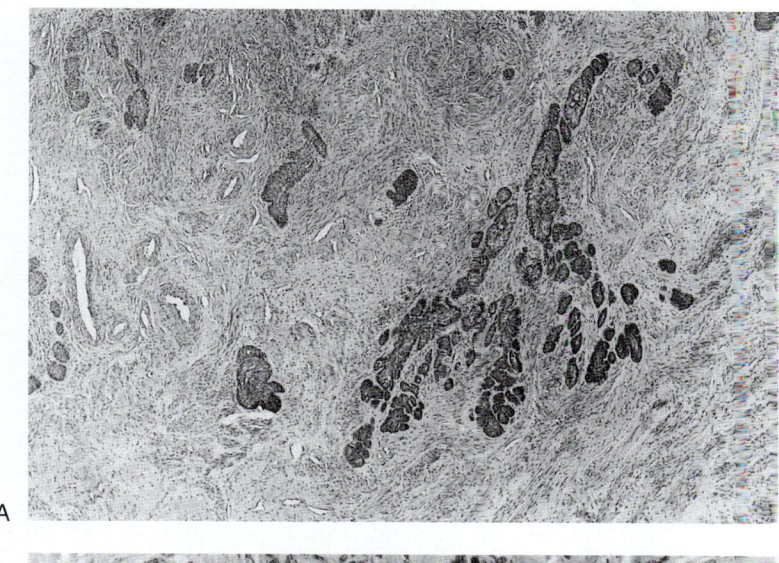
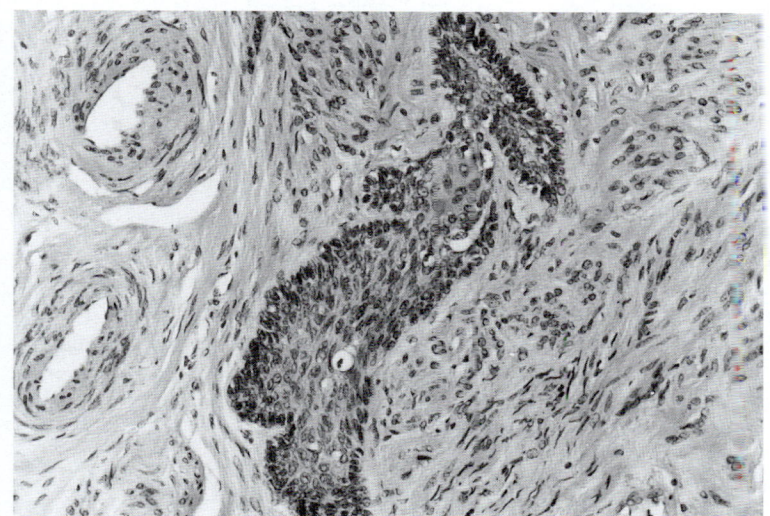

FIG. 44. Adenoid basal carcinoma. **A:** Islands of basaloid cells in cervical stroma. No stromal reaction. **B:** Centrally cells become more squamoid.

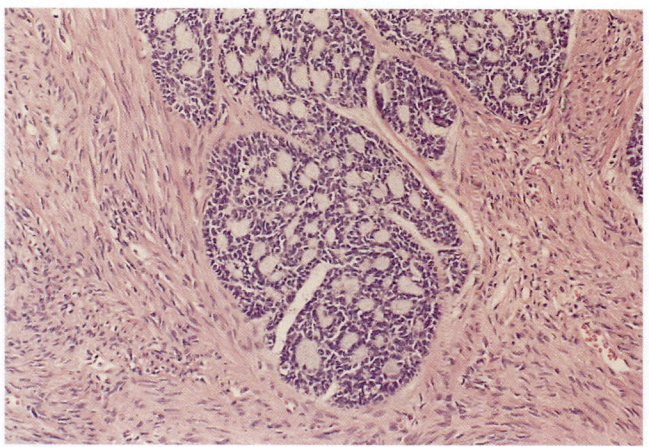

FIG. 45. Adenoid cystic carcinoma. Cribriform pattern of basaloid nuclei and eosinophilic intercellular material.

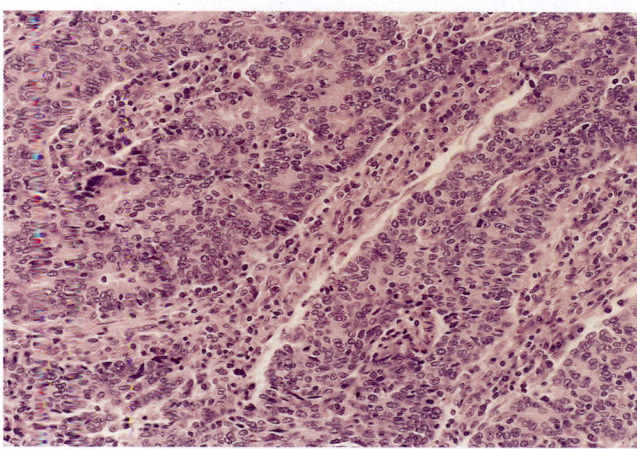

FIG. 46. Mixed adenocarcinoma and small cell undifferentiated (neuroendocrine) carcinoma.

cervix from other sites is uncommon. In most cases the primary tumor is in the ovary, colon, stomach, breast, or kidney (244). The metastasis involves the wall of the cervix, often spares the overlying epithelium and endocervical glands, and may invade lymphovascular spaces. The morphology is that of the primary tumor and differs in most cases from the usual varieties of primary cervical adenocarcinoma (Fig. 47). The clinical history is essential.

SOFT TISSUE AND OTHER NEOPLASMS OF THE CERVIX

Fibroepithelial Polyps

Occasionally, fibroepithelial polyps occur on the cervical portio and consist of a prominent connective tissue base with normal to acanthotic overlying epithelium. The differential diagnosis includes condyloma, which is distinguished by the characteristic epithelial changes, and vaginal polyps, which contain atypical stromal cells (245).

Polyps of Endometrial Origin

Polyps of endometrial origin include (a) endometrial polyps that extend through the endocervical canal; and (b) decidual polyps, which occur in pregnancy. Mixed polyps containing both endocervix and endometrium may also be seen, in which case the diagnosis of polyps of mixed type is appropriate.

Submucosal Leiomyomas

The most common benign neoplasm of the cervix is a leiomyoma, accounting for about 8% of all uterine leiomyomas. They may protrude from the endocervical canal and thus mimic an endocervical polyp, although they are typically firmer and have a whorled appearance on cut section. As would be expected, their histologic features are similar to those of uterine corpus leiomyomas, with mitotic activity being the most useful predictive factor for malignant potential. As is true of leiomyomas in general, cervical leiomyomas are frequently associated with the thick walls of blood vessels, suggesting a site of origin for these lesions.

Other Rare Variants

Other variants include (a) mesonephric papilloma, which has been reported in children; and (b) papillary adenofibroma (246,247). The latter is similar in appearance to adenofibroma of the endometrium and typically occurs in postmenopausal women. Histologically, it is characterized by blunt and branching stromal papillae covered with benign endocervical epithelium. The differential diagnosis includes (a) endocervical polyps, which lack the characteristic stromal papillary change and stromal proliferation; and (b) adenosarcoma, which contains a higher stromal mitotic index (248).

Other Benign Soft Tissue Neoplasms

Benign vascular tumors are rarely identified in the cervix and include capillary or cavernous hemangiomas. It is often difficult to differentiate such lesions from arteriovenous malformations with microvascular proliferation (249,250). Other rare benign tumors that have been reported in the cervix include lipoma, blue nevus, glioma, and lymphangioma (251–255). These lesions are usually encountered as incidental findings at the time of hysterectomy.

MALIGNANT SOFT-TISSUE NEOPLASMS

Sarcomas of the uterine cervix are very rare. They usually present in the fourth to sixth decades of life as a protruding cervical mass and/or postmenopausal or postcoital bleeding. The most frequent types reported include stromal sarcoma, leiomyosarcoma, and malignant mixed mesodermal tumors, hence paralleling sarcomas of the uterine corpus (256,257). The most common variant is stromal sarcoma, which predominates in postmenopausal women and may present as a cervical polyp. The histologic features include sheets of round to spindle-shaped cells with a high nuclear-to-cytoplasmic ratio and mitotic figures. With the exception of low-grade stromal sarcoma, these tumors appear to have a poor prognosis. Stromal sarcoma can usually be differentiated from small cell carcinoma and lymphoma by growth pattern alone, although stains for reticulin should exclude these entities. Other types of cervical sarcoma include embryonal rhabdomyosarcoma of childhood (sarcoma botryoides), Wilms' tumor, and adenosarcoma (258–260). Cervical embryonal rhabdomyosarcoma usually occurs in the first two decades and generally is associated with a better prognosis than sarcomas (including rhabdomyosarcomas) occurring in older women. Cervical adenosarcoma may also occur in adolescents and has a favorable prognosis. These tumors contain

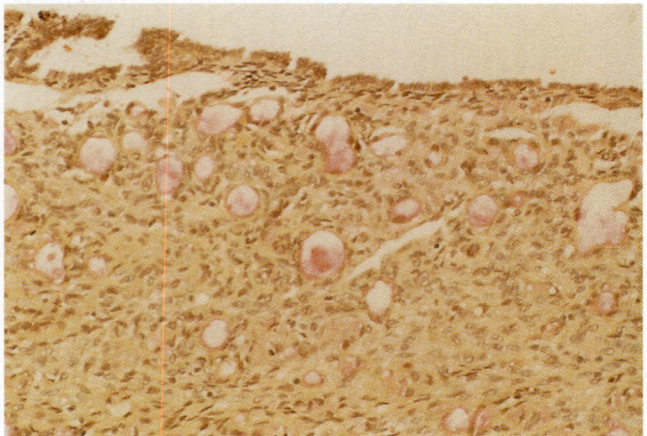

FIG. 47. Metastatic carcinoma to the cervix. Mucin stain shows cytoplasmic mucin in single cells infiltrating stroma. Note intact surface epithelium. Patient had gastric adenocarcinoma.

benign-appearing glands and a stroma that may resemble stromal sarcoma, or that may contain rhabdomyoblasts or cartilage. Chen (260) emphasized the importance of distinguishing adenosarcomas with rhabdomyoblastic elements from embryonal rhabdomyosarcomas and mixed müllerian tumors because adenosarcomas have a better prognosis (261). Most of the different subtypes of lymphoma have been identified in the cervix, usually as a manifestation of systemic disease, although primary lymphoma of the cervix also has been reported (262–264). Lymphomas usually present as a polypoid mass with typical soft, gray-white "fish flesh" appearance on cut section. Microscopically, they infiltrate stroma without destroying the native glandular architecture, a feature that, in part, distinguishes them from carcinoma. Lymphoid-specific immunohistochemical markers such as leukocyte common antigen facilitate recognition of diagnostically problematic cases. The prognosis is usually a function of the histologic subtype for the non-Hodgkin's lymphomas. When documented, lymphoma limited to the cervix is associated with a favorable prognosis (262,263).

REFERENCES

1. Kiviat NB, et al. Histopathology of endocervical infection by *Chlamydia trachomatis*, herpes simplex virus, *Trichomonas vaginalis*, and *Neisseria gonorrhea*. Hum Pathol 1990;21:831–837.
2. Stern E, Longo LD. Identification of herpes simplex virus in a case showing cytological features of viral vaginitis. Acta Cytol 1963;7:295–299.
3. Goldman RL, Bank RW, Warren NE. Cytomegalovirus infection of the cervix: an "incidental" finding of possible clinical significance. Report of a case. Obstet Gynecol 1969;34:326–329.
4. Laverty CR, Russell P, Black J, Kappagoda N, Benn RAV, Booth MA. Adenovirus infection of the cervix: Acta Cytol 1977;21:114–117.
5. Winkler BW, Crum CP. Chlamydia trachomatis infection of the female genital tract: pathogenetic and clinico-pathologic correlations. In: Rosen PP, Fechner RE, ed. *Pathology annual*. New York: Appleton-Century-Crofts, 1987:193–223.
6. Westrom L, Mardh PA. Genital chlamydial infections in the female. In: Mardh PA, Holmes KK, Oriel JD, Piot P, Schachter J, eds. *Chlamydial infections*. Amsterdam: Elsevier Biomedical Press, 1982:121–139.
7. Crum CP, Mitao M, Winkler B, Reumann W, Boon M, Richart RM. Localizing chlamydial infection in cervical biopsies with the immunoperoxidase technique. Int J Gynecol Pathol 1984;2:191–197.
8. Giampaolo C, Murphy J, Benes S, et al. How sensitive is the Papanicolaou smear in the diagnosis of infections with *Chlamydia trachomatis?* Am J Clin Pathol 1983;80:844–849.
9. Gupta PK, Lee EF, Erozan YS, Frost JK, Geddes ST, Donovan PA. Cytologic investigations of *Chlamydia* infection. Acta Cytol 1979;23:315–320.
10. *Cancer manual*, 9th ed. Boston: American Cancer Society, Massachusetts Division, 1996.
11. Herrero R, et al. Sexual behavior, venereal diseases, hygiene practices and invasive cervical cancer in a high-risk population. Cancer 1990;65:380–386.
12. Howley PM. Role of the human papillomaviruses in human cancer. Cancer Res 1991;51(suppl 18):5019s–5022s.
13. Heselmeyer K, Schrock E, du Manoir S, et al. Gain in chromosome 3q defines the transition from severe dysplasia to invasive carcinoma of the uterine cervix. Proc Natl Acad Sci USA 1996;93:479
14. Crook T, Vousden KH. Properties of p53 mutations detected in primary and secondary cervical cancers suggest mechanisms of metastasis and involvement of environmental carcinogens. Embo J 1992;11:3935–3940.
15. Crum CP, Cibas ES, Lee KR. *Pathology of early cervical neoplasia*. New York: Churchill Livingstone, 1996.
16. Crum CP, Cibas ES, Lee KR. Cervical papillomaviruses segregate within morphologically distinct precancerous lesions. J Virol 1985;54:675–681.
17. Crum CP. Redefining cervical intraepithelial neoplasia. J Surg Pathol 1995;1:159–164.
18. Meisels A, Fortin R. Condylomatous lesoins of the cervix and vagina I. Cytologic patterns. Acta Cytol 1976;20:505–509.
19. Richart RM. Cervical intraepithelial neoplasia. In: Sommers SC, ed. *Pathology annual*. New York: Appleton-Century-Crofts, 1973; 301–328.
20. Crum CP, Mitao M, Levine RU, Silverstein S. Cervical papillomaviruses segregate within morphologically distinct precancerous lesions. J Virol 1985;54:675–681.
21. Genest D, Stein L, Cibas E, Sheets E, Zitz J, Crum CP. A binary (Bethesda) system for classifying cervical cancer precursors: criteria, reproducibility and viral correlates. Hum Pathol 1993;24:730–736.
22. Saito K, Saito A, Fu YS, Smotkin D, Gupta J, Shah K. Topographic study of cervical condyloma and intraepithelial neoplasia. Cancer 1987;59:2064–2070.
23. Lee KR, Minter LJ, Crum CP. Koilocytotic atypia in Papanicolaou smears: reproducibility and biopsy correlates. Cancer Cytopathol 1997;81:10–15.
24. Hall S, Wu TC, Soudi N, Sherman ME. Low grade squamous intraepithelial lesions: cytologic predictors of biopsy confirmation. Diagn Cytopathol 1994;10:3–9.
25. Willet GD, Kurman RJ, Reid R, Greenberg M, Jenson AB, Lorincz AT. Correlation of the histologic appearance of intraepithelial neoplasia of the cervix with human papillomavirus types. Int J Gynecol Pathol 1989;8:18–25.
26. McLachlin CM, Shen L, Crum CP. High grade cervical intraepithelial neoplasia: frequency and significance of co-existing condyloma. J Surg Pathol 1995;1:165–172.
27. Crum CP, Egawa K, Fu YS, et al. Atypical immature metaplasia (AIM): a subset of human papillomavirus infection of the cervix. Cancer 1983;51:2214–2219.
28. Ward BE, Saleh AM, Williams JV, Crum CP. Papillary immature metaplasia of the cervix: A distinct subset of exophytic cervical condyloma associated with HPV-6/11 nucleic acids. Mod Pathol 1992;5:391–395.
29. Trivijitsilp P, Mosher RE, Crum CP. Papillary immature metaplasia (immature condyloma) of the cervix: a clinicopathologic analysis and comparison with papillary carcinoma. Hum Pathol, 1998;29:641–648.
30. Mosher RE. Lee KR, Trivijitsilp P, Crum CP. Cytologic correlates of papillary immature metaplasia of the cervix. Diagn Cytopathol, 1998;18:416–421.
31. Nuovo GJ, Nuovo MA, Cottral S, Gordon S, Silverstein SJ, Crum CP. Histological correlates of clinically occult papillomavirus infection of the uterine cervix. Am J Surg Pathol 1988;12:198–204.
32. Mittal KR, Chan W, Demopoulos RI. Sensitivity and specificity of various morphological features of cervical condylomas. Arch Pathol Lab Med 1990;114:1038–1041.
33. Prasad CJ, Sheets E, Selig AM, McArthur MC, Crum CP. The binucleate squamous cell: histologic spectrum and relationship to low grade squamous intraepithelial lesions. Mod Pathol 1993;6:313–317.
34. Meisels A, Morin C. Human papillomavirus induced changes. In: Meisels A, Morin C, eds. *Cytopathology of the uterine cervix*. Chicago: ASCP Press, American Society of Clinical Pathology, 1990:73–117.
35. Moya-Barracco M, Leibowitch M, Orth G. Vestibular papillae of the vulva. Lack of evidence for human papillomavirus etiology. Arch Dermatol 1990;126:1594–1598.
36. Nuovo G, Blanco J, Richart RM, Levine R, Silverstein S, Crum CP. Histological correlates of papillomavirus infection of the vagina. Obstet Gynecol 1988;72:770–774.
37. Laverty CR, Booth N, Hills E, Cossart Y, Will EJ. Noncondylomatous wart virus infection of the postmenopausal cervix. Pathology 1978;10:373–378.
38. Nuovo GJ, Cottral S, Richart RM. Occult human papillomavirus infection of the uterine cervix in postmenopausal women. Obstet Gynecol 1989;160:340–344.
39. Symmars F, Mechani L, MacConnell P, DaSilva K, Stricker B, Nuovo G. Correlation of cervical cytology and human papillomavirus DNA detection in postmenopausal women. Int J Gynecol Pathol 1992;11:204–209.
40. Jovanovic A, McLachlin M, Shen L, Welch WR, Crum CP. Post-

menopausal squamous atypia: a morphologic spectrum including "pseudokoilocytosis." *Mod Pathol* 1995;8:408–412.
41. Koss LG. Histology and cytology of pregnancy and abortion. In: Koss LG, ed. *Diagnostic cytology and its histologic basis.* Philadelphia: JB Lippincott, 1992:284.
42. McLachlin CM, Kosakevitch H, Craighill M, Crum CP. Morphologic correlates of vulvo-vaginal HPV infection in children and young adults. *Am J Surg Pathol* 1994;18:728–735.
43. Young RH, Kurman RJ, Scully RE. Placental site nodules and plaques. A clinicopathologic analysis of 20 cases. *Am J Surg Pathol* 1990;14:1001.
44. Huettner PC, Gersell DJ. Placental site nodule: a clinicopathologic study of 38 cases. *Int J Gynecol Pathol* 1994;13:191–198.
45. Boyes DA, Worth AJ, Fidler HK. The results of treatment of 4389 cases of preclinical squamous cell carcinoma. *Br J Obstet Gynaecol* 1973;77:769.
46. Savage EW. Microinvasive carcinoma of the cervix. *Am J Obstet Gynecol* 1972;113:708.
47. Ng ABP, Reagan JW: Microinvasive carcinoma of the uterine cervix. *Am J Clin Pathol* 1969;52:511.
48. Robert ME, Fu YS. Squamous cell carcinoma of the uterine cervix—a review with emphasis on prognostic factors and unusual variants. *Semin Diag Pathol* 1990;7:173.
49. Wilkinson EJ, Komorowski RA. Borderline microinvasive carcinoma of the cervix. *Obstet Gynecol* 1977;51:472.
50. Sedlis A, Sall S, Tsukada Y, et al. Microinvasive carcinoma of the uterine cervix: a clinicopathologic study. *Am J Obstet Gynecol* 1979;133:64.
51. Creasman WT, Fetter BF, Clarke-Pearson DL, et al. Management of stage IA carcinoma of the cervix. *Am J Obstet Gynecol* 1985;153:164.
52. International Federation of Gynecology and Obstetrics. *Annual report on the results of treatment on gynecologic cancer,* vol 20. Stockholm: FIGO, 1988.
53. Burghardt E, Holzer E. Diagnosis and treatment of microinvasive carcinoma of the uterine cervix. *Obstet Gynecol* 1977;49:641.
54. Hasumi K, Sakamoto A, Sugano H. Microinvasive carcinoma of the uterine cervix. *Cancer* 1980;45:928.
55. Van Nagell JR, Greenwell N, Powell DF. Microinvasive carcinoma of the cervix. *Am J Obstet Gynecol* 1983;145:981.
56. Benson WL, Norris HJ. A critical review of the frequency of lymph node metastasis and death from microinvasive carcinoma of the cervix. *Obstet Gynecol* 1977;49:632.
57. Roche WD, Norris HJ. Microinvasive carcinoma of the cervix; 30:103–136. The significance of lymphatic invasion and confluent patterns of growth. *Cancer* 1975;36:180.
58. van Nagell JR Jr, Donaldson ES, Wood EG, Parker JC Jr. The significance of vascular invasion and lymphocytic infiltration in invasive cervical cancer. *Cancer* 1978;41:228–234.
59. Ostor AG. Pandora's box or Ariadne's thread? Definition and prognostic significance of microinvasion in the uterine cervix. Squamous lesions. *Pathol Annu* 1996.
60. Ostor AG. Studies on 200 cases of early squamous cell carcinoma of the cervix. *Int J Gynecol Pathol* 1993;12:193–207.
61. McLachlin CM, Devine P, Muto M, Genest DR. Pseudoinvasion of vascular spaces: report of an artifact caused by cervical lidocaine injection prior to loop diathermy. *Hum Pathol* 1994;25:208–211.
62. Delgado G, Bundy BN, Fowler WC, et al. A prospective surgical pathological study of Stage I squamous carcinoma of the cervix: a Gynecologic Oncology Group study. *Gynecol Oncol* 1989;35:314–320.
63. Barber HRK, Sommers SC, Rotterdam H, Kwon T. Vascular invasion as a prognostic factor in stage IB cancer of the cervix. *Obstet Gynecol* 1977;52:343.
64. White CD, Morley GW, Kuman NB. The prognostic significance of tumor emboli in lymphatic and vascular spaces of the cervical stroma in Stage IB squamous cell carcinoma of the cervix. *Am J Obstet Gynecol* 1984;149:342–349.
65. van Nagell JR, Higgins RV, Powell DE. Invasive cervical cancer. In: Knapp RC, Berkowitz RS, eds. *Gynecologic oncology,* 2nd ed. New York: McGraw-Hill, 1993:192–222.
66. Girardi F, Pickel H, Winter R. Pelvic and parametrial lymph nodes in the quality control of the surgical treatment of cervical cancer. *Gynecol Oncol* 1993;50:330–333.
67. Kolstad P. Follow-up study of 232 patients with stage IA1 and 411 patients with stage IA2, squamous cell carcinoma of the cervix (microinvasive carcinoma). *Gynecol Oncol* 1989;33:265–272.
68. Fidler HK, Boyes DA, Worth AJ. Cervical cancer detection in British Columbia. *Br J Obstet Gynaecol* 1968;75:392–404.
69. Barron BA, Cahill MC, Richart RM. A statistical model of the natural history of cervical neoplastic disease: the duration of carcinoma in situ. *Gynecol Oncol* 1973;6:196–205.
70. Schiller W, Daro AF, Gollin HA, et al. Small pre-ulcerative invasive carcinoma of the cervix—the spray carcinoma. *Am J Obstet Gynecol* 1953;65:1088–1098.
71. Reagan KW, Mamanic MS, Wentz WB. Analytical study of the cells in cervical squamous cell cancer. *Lab Invest* 1957;6:241–250.
72. Reagan KW, Fu YS. Histologic types and prognosis of cancers of the uterine cervix. *Int J Radiol Oncol Biol Phys* 1979;5:1015–1020.
73. Randall ME, Constable WC, Hahn SS, et al. Results of the radiotherapeutic management of carcinomas of the cervix with emphasis on the influence of histologic classification. *Cancer* 1988;62:48–53.
74. Spratt DW, Lee SC. Verrucous carcinoma of the cervix. *Am J Gynecol* 1977;129:699.
75. Kister RW, Hertig AT. Papillomas of the uterine cervix-the malignant potentiality. *Obstet Gynecol* 1955;6:147.
76. Qizilbash A. Papillary squamous tumors of the uterine cervix. A clinical and pathological study of 21 cases. *Am J Clin Pathol* 1974;61:508.
77. Randall ME, Andersen WA, Mills SE, et al. Papillary squamous cell carcinoma of the uterine cervix. A clinicopathologic study of nine cases. *Int J Gynecol Pathol* 1986;5:1.
78. Walker AN, Mills SE. Unusual variants of uterine cervical carcinoma. *Pathol Ann* 1987;277:1987.
79. Venkateseshan VS, Woo TH. Diffuse viral papillomatosis (condyloma) of the uterine cavity. *Int J Gynecol Pathol* 1985;4:370.
80. Tiltman AJ, Atad J. Verrucous carcinoma of the cervix with endometrial involvement. *Int J Gynecol Pathol* 1982;1:221.
81. Ferenczy A, Richart RM, Okagaki T. Endometrial involvement by cervical carcinoma in situ. *Am J Obstet Gynecol* 1971;110:590.
82. Pins MR, Young RH, Crum CP, Leach IH, Scully RE. Cervical squamous carcinoma in situ with superficial extension to corpus and tubes and invasion of tubes and ovaries: Report of a case with HPV analysis. *Int J Gynecol Pathol* 1997;16:272–278.
83. Van Nagell JR, Donaldson ES, Wood EG, et al. Small cell cancer of the uterine cervix. *Cancer* 1977;40:2243–2249.
84. Barrett RJ, Davos I, Leuchter RS, Lagasse LD. Neuroendocrine features in poorly differentiated and undifferentiated carcinomas of the cervix. *Cancer* 1987;60:2325.
85. Albores-Saavedra J, Larraza P, Poucell S, et al. Carcinoids of the uterine cervix: additional observations in a new tumor entity. *Cancer* 1976;38:2328–2342.
86. Groben P, Reddick R, Askin F. The pathologic spectrum of small cell carcinoma of the cervix. *Int J Gynecol Pathol* 1985;4:42–47.
87. Mullins JD, Hilliard GD. Cervical carcinoid ("argyrophil cell carcinoma") associated with an endocervical adenocarcinoma: a light and ultra-structural study. *Cancer* 1981;47:785–790.
88. MacKay B, Osborne BM, Wharton JT. Small cell tumor of the cervix with neuroepithelial features: ultrastructural observations in two cases. *Cancer* 1979;43:1138–1145.
89. Pearce AGE. The APUD cell concept and its implications in pathology. *Pathol Annu* 1974;9 27–41.
90. Fox H, Kazzaz B, Langley FA. Argyrophil and argentaffin cells in the female genital tract and in ovarian mucinous cysts. *J Pathol Bacteriol* 1964;88:479–488.
91. Stassart J, Crum CP, Yorda EL, et al. Argyrophilic carcinoma of the cervix: a report of a case with coexisting cervical intraepithelial neoplasia. *Gynecol Oncol* 1982;13:247–251.
92. Taxi JB, Tischler AS, Insalaco SJ, et al. "Carcinoid" tumor of the breast. A variant of breast cancer? *Hum Pathol* 1981;12:170–179.
93. Stoler M, Mills SE, Gersell DJ, Walker AN. Small-cell neuroendocrine carcinoma of the cervix. A human papillomavirus type 18-associated cancer. *Am J Surg Pathol* 1991;15:28–32.
94. Gersell DJ, Mazoujian G, Mutch DG, Rudloff MA. Small-cell undifferentiated carcinoma of the cervix. A clinicopathologic, ultrastructural, and immunocytochemical study of 15 cases. *Am J Surg Pathol* 1988;12:684–698.
95. Ambros RA, Park TS, Shah KV, Kurman RJ. Evaluation of histologic, morphometric, and immunohistochemical criteria in the differential diagnosis of small cell carcinomas of the cervix with particular reference to human papillomavirus types 16 and 18 (published erratum appears in *Mod Pathol* 1992;5:40). *Mod Pathol* 1991;4:586–593.

96. Mills SE, Austin MB, Randall ME. Lymphoepithelioma-like carcinoma of the uterine cervix. A distinctive, undifferentiated carcinoma with inflammatory stroma. *Am J Surg Pathol* 1985;9:883–889.
97. Raptis S, Haber G, Ferenczy A. Vaginal squamous cell carcinoma with sarcomatoid spindle cell features. *Gynecol Oncol* 1993;49:100.
98. Ogawa K, Kim YC, Nakashima Y, Yamabe H, Takeda T, Hamashima Y. Expression of epithelial markers in sarcomatoid carcinoma: an immunohistochemical study. *Histopathology* 1987;11:511–522.
98a. Aaro LA, Jacobsen LG, Soule E. Endocervical polyps. *Obstet Gynecol* 1963;21:659–665.
99. Lippert LJ, Richart RM, Ferenczy A. Giant benign endocervical polyp: report of a case. *Am J Obstet Gynecol* 1974;118:1140–1141.
100. Young RH, Clement PB. Pseudoneoplastic glandular lesions of the uterine cervix. *Semin Diagn Pathol* 1990;8:234–249.
101. Clement PB, Young RH. Deep nabothian cysts of the uterine cervix. *Int J Gynecol Pathol* 1989;8:340–348.
102. Fluhmann CF. Focal hyperplasia (tunnel clusters) of the cervix uteri. *Obstet Gynecol* 1961;17:206–214.
103. Segal GH, Hart WR. Cystic endocervical tunnel clusters. *Am J Surg Pathol* 1990;14:895–903.
104. Jones M, Young RH. Endocervical type A (noncystic) tunnel clusters with cytologic atypia. *Am J Surg Pathol* 1996;20(11):1312–1318.
105. Jones MA, Young RH, Scully RE. Diffuse laminar endocervical glandular hyperplasia. *Am J Surg Pathol* 1991;15:1123–1129.
106. Daya D, Young RH. Florid deep glands of the uterine cervix: another mimic of adenoma malignum. *Am J Clin Pathol* 1995;103:614–617.
107. Sherrer CW, Parmley T, Woodruff JD. Adenomatous hyperplasia of the endocervix. *Obstet Gynecol* 1977;49:65.
108. Taylor HB, Irey NS, Norris HJ. Atypical endocervical hyperplasia in women taking oral contraceptives. *JAMA* 1967;202:185–187.
109. Greeley C, Schroeder S, Silverberg SG. Microglandular hyperplasia of the cervix: a true "pill" lesion? *Int J Gynecol Pathol* 1995;14:50–54.
110. Chumas JC, Nelson B, Mann WJ, Chalas E, Kaplan CG. Microglandular hyperplasia of the uterine cervix. *Obstet Gynecol* 1985;66:406–409.
111. Speers WC, Picaso LG, Silverberg SG. Immunohistochemical localization of carcinoembryonic antigen in microglandular hyperplasia and adenocarcinoma of the endocervix. *Am J Clin Pathol* 1983;79:105–107.
112. Young RH, Scully RE. Atypical forms of microglandular hyperplasia of the cervix simulating carcinoma. *Am J Surg Pathol* 1989;13:50–56.
113. Young RH, Scully RE. Uterine carcinomas simulating microglandular hyperplasia. *Am J Surg Pathol* 1992;16(11):1092–1097.
114. Zaloudek C, Hayashi G, Ryan I, Bethan Powell C, Miller T. Microglandular adenocarcinoma of the endometrium: a form of mucinous adenocarcinoma that may be confused with microglandular hyperplasia of the cervix. *Int J Gynecol Pathol* 1997;16:52–59.
115. Sherrick JC, Vega JG Congenital intramural cysts of the uterus. *Obstet Gynecol* 1962;19(4):486–493.
116. Lang G, Dallenbach-Hellweg G. The histogenetic origin of cervical mesonephric hyperplasia and mesonephric adenocarcinoma studied with immunohistochemical methods. *Int J Gynecol Pathol* 1990;9:145–157.
117. Seidman JD, Tavassoli FA. Mesonephric hyperplasia of the uterine cervix: a clinicopathologic study of 51 cases. *Int J Gynecol Pathol* 1995;14:293–299.
118. Ferry JA, Scully RE. Mesonephric remnants, hyperplasia and neoplasia in the uterine cervix: a study of 49 cases. *Am J Surg Pathol* 1990;14:1100–1111.
119. Jonasson JG, Wang HH, Antonioli Da, Ducatman BS. Tubal metaplasia of the uterine cervix: a prevalence study in patients with gynecologic pathologic findings. *Int J Gynecol Pathol* 1992;11:89–95.
120. Suh KS, Silverberg SG. Tubal metaplasia of the uterine cervix. *Int J Gynecol Pathol* 1990;9:122–128.
121. Yeh IT, Bronner M, LiVolsi VA. Endometrial metaplasia of the uterine cervix. *Arch Pathol Lab Med* 1993;117:734–735.
122. Ismail SM. Cone biopsy causes cervical endometriosis and tubo-endometrioid metaplasia. *Histopathology* 1991;18:107–114.
123. Babkowski R, Wilbur D, Rutkowski M, Facik M, Bonfiglio T. The effects of endocervical canal topography, tubal metaplasia, and high canal sampling on the cytologic presentation of nonneoplastic endocervical cells. *Am J Clin Pathol* 1996;105(4):403–410.
124. Oliva E, Clement PB, Young RH. Tubal and tubo-endometrioid metaplasia of the uterine cervix: unemphasized features which may cause problems in differential diagnosis. A report of 25 cases. *Am J Clin Pathol* 1995;103:618–623.
125. McCluggage WG, Maxwell P, McBride HA, Hamilton PW, Bharucha H. Monoclonal antibodies Ki67 and MIB1 in the distinction of tuboendometrial metaplasia from endocervical adenocarcinoma and adenocarcinoma in situ in formalin fixed material. *Int J Gynecol Pathol* 1995;14:209–216.
126. Marques T, De Angelo Andrade LAL, Vassallo J. Endocervical tubal metaplasia and adenocarcinoma in situ: role of immunohistochemistry for carcinoembryonic antigen and vimentin in differential diagnosis. *Histopathology* 1996;28:549–550.
127. Clement PB. Pathology of endometriosis. *Pathol Annu* 1990;25(1):245–295.
128. Young RH, Clement PB. Pseudoneoplastic lesions of the lower female genital tract. *Pathol Annu* 1989;24(2):189–226.
129. Cariani DJ, Guderian AM. Gestational atypia in endocervical polyps—the Arias-Stella reaction. *Am J Obstet Gynecol* 1996;95:589–590.
130. Rhatgan RM. Endocervical atypia associated with Arias-Stella change. *Arch Pathol Lab Med* 1992;116:943–946.
131. Schneider V. Arias-Stella reaction of the endocervix: frequency and location. *Acta Cytol* 1981;25:224–228.
132. Andrews CF, Jourdain L, Damjanov I. Benign cervical mesonephric papilloma of childhood. Report of a case studied by light and electron microscopy. *Diagn Gynecol Obstet* 1981;3(1):39–43.
133. Young RH, Scully RE. Invasive adenocarcinoma and related tumors of the uterine cervix. *Semin Diagn Pathol* 1990;7(3):205–227.
134. Michael H, Sutton G, Hull MT, Roth LM. Villous adenoma of the uterine cervix associated with invasive adenocarcinoma: a histologic, ultrastructural, and immunohistochemical study. *Int J Gynecol Pathol* 1986;5(2):163–169.
135. Alvaro T, Nogales F. Villous adenoma and invasive adenocarcinoma of the cervix (letter). *Int J Gynecol Pathol* 1988;7(1):96–97.
136. Brown S, Senekjian EK, Montag AG. Cytomegalovirus infection of the uterine cervix in a patient with acquired immunodeficiency syndrome. *Obstet Gynecol* 1988;71(3 Pt 2):489–491.
137. Josey WE, Nahmias AJ, Naib ZM. Viral and virus-like infections of the female genital tract. *Clin Obstet Gynecol* 1969;12(1):161–178.
138. Lesack D, Ibrahim W, Gilks CB. Radiation-induced atypia of endocervical epithelium: a histological, immunohistochemical and cytometric study. *Int J Gynecol Pathol* 1996;15:242–247.
139. Shield PW. Chronic radiation effects: a correlative study of smears and biopsies from the cervix and vagina. *Diagn Cytopathol* 1995;13:107–119.
140. Koss LG. The effects of therapeutic procedures and drugs on the epithelium of the female genital tract. In: *Diagnostic cytology and its histologic bases* Philadelphia: JB Lippincott; 1992:682–683.
141. Jones M, Young RH. Atypical oxyphilic metaplasia of the endocervical epithelium: a report of six cases. *Int J Gynecol Pathol* 1997;16:99–102.
142. Gloor E, Hurlimann J. Cervical intraepithelial glandular neoplasia (adenocarcinoma in situ and glandular dysplasia): a correlative study of 23 cases with histologic grading, histochemical analysis of mucins, and immunohistochemical determination of the affinity for four lectins. *Cancer* 1986;58:1272–1280.
143. Alva J, Lauchlins S. The histogenesis of mixed cervical carcinoma: the concept of endocervical columnar cell dysplasia. *Am J Clin Pathol* 1975;64:20–25.
144. Brown LR, Wells M. Cervical glandular atypia associated with squamous intraepithelial neoplasia: a premalignant lesion? *J Clin Pathol* 1986;39:22–28.
145. Casper G, Östör A, Quinn M. A clinicopathologic study of glandular dysplasia of the cervix. *Gynecol Oncol* 1997;64:166–170.
146. Kurman RJ, Norris HJ, Wilkinson E. Tumors of the cervix, vagina and vulva. In: *Atlas of tumor pathology*. Washington, DC: Armed Forces Institute of Pathology; 1992:78–79.
147. Jaworski RC, Pacey NF, Greenberg ML, Osborn RA. The histologic diagnosis of adenocarcinoma in situ and related lesions of the cervix uteri: adenocarcinoma in situ. *Cancer* 1988;61:1171–1181.
148. Lee KR, Howard P, Heintz NH, Collins CC. Low prevalence of human papillomavirus types 16 and 18 in cervical adenocarcinoma in situ, invasive adenocarcinoma and glandular dysplasia by polymerase chain reaction. *Mod Pathol* 1993;6:433–437.
149. Higgins CD, Phillips GE, Smith LA, Uzelin DM, Burrell CJ. High prevalence of human papillomavirus transcripts in all grades of cervical intraepithelial glandular neoplasia. *Cancer* 1992;70:136–146.

150. Tase T, Okagaki T, Clark BA, Twiggs LB, Ostrow RS, Faras AJ. Human papillomavirus DNA in glandular dysplasia and microglandular hyperplasia: presumed precursors of adenocarcinoma of the uterine cervix. *Obstet Gynecol* 1989;73:1005–1008.
151. Anciaux D, Lawrence WD, Gregoire L. Glandular lesions of the uterine cervix: prognostic implications of human papillomavirus status. *Int J Gynecol Pathol* 1997;16(2):103–110.
152. Freidell GH, McKay DG. Adenocarcinoma in situ of the endocervix. *Cancer* 1953;6:887–897.
153. Christopherson WM, Nealon N, Gray LA. Noninvasive precursor lesions of adenocarcinoma and mixed adenosquamous carcinoma of the cervix uteri. *Cancer* 1979;44:975–983.
154. Andersen ES, Arffmann E. Adenocarcinoma in situ of the uterine cervix: a clinicopathologic study of 36 cases. *Gynecol Oncol* 1989;35:1–7.
155. Ayer B, Pacey F, Greenberg M, Bousfield L. The cytologic diagnosis of adenocarcinoma in situ of the cervix uteri and related lesions: I. Adenocarcinoma in situ. *Acta Cytol* 1987;31:391–411.
156. Betsill WL, Clark AH. Early endocervical glandular neoplasia: I. Histomorphology and cytomorphology. *Acta Cytol* 1986;30:115–126.
157. Lee KR, Manna EA, Jones MA. Comparative cytologic features of adenocarcinoma in situ of the uterine cervix. *Acta Cytol* 1991;35:117–126.
158. Quizilbash AH. In situ and microinvasive adenocarcinoma of the uterine cervix: a clinical, cytologic and histologic study of 14 cases. *Am J Clin Pathol* 1975;64:155–170.
159. Bjersing L, Rogo K, Evander M, Gerdes U, Stendahl U, Wadell G. HPV 18 and cervical adenocarcinomas. *Anticancer Res* 1991;11:123–127.
160. Duggan MA, Benoit JL, McGregor ES, Masafumi I, Nation JG, Stuart GCE. Adenocarcinoma in situ of the endocervix: human papillomavirus determination by dot blot hybridization and polymerase chain reaction amplification. *Int J Gynecol Pathol* 1994;13:143–149.
161. Griffin NR, Dockey D, Lewis FA, Wells N. Demonstration of low frequency of human papillomavirus DNA in cervical adenocarcinoma in situ by polymerase chain reaction and in situ hybridization. *Int J Gynecol Pathol* 1991;10:36–40.
162. Hording U, Teglbjaerg CS, Visfeldt J, Bock JE. Human papillomavirus type 16 and 18 in adenocarcinoma of the uterine cervix. *Gynecol Oncol* 1991;46:313–316.
163. Johnson TL, Kim W, Plieth DA, Sarkar FH. Detection of HPV 16/18 DNA in cervical adenocarcinoma using polymerase chain reaction (PCR) methodology. *Mod Pathol* 1992;5:35–40.
164. Leminen A, Paavonen J, Vesterinen E, Wahlstrom T, Rantala I, Lehtinen N. Human papillomavirus type 16 and 18 in adenocarcinoma of the uterine cervix. *Am J Clin Pathol* 1991;95:647–652.
165. Milde-Langosch K, Schreiber C, Becker G, Loning T, Stegner H. Human papillomavirus detection in cervical adenocarcinoma by polymerase chain reaction. *Hum Pathol* 1993;24:590–594.
166. Stoler MH, Rhodes CR, Whitbeck A, Wolinsky SM. Human papillomavirus types 16 and 18 gene expression in cervical neoplasia. *Hum Pathol* 1992;23:117–128.
167. Boon ME, Baak JPA, Kurver PJH, Overdiep SH, Verdonk GW. Adenocarcinoma in situ of the cervix: and underdiagnosed lesion. *Cancer* 1981;48:768–733.
168. Costa MJ, McIlnay KR, Trelford J. Cervical carcinoma with glandular differentiation: histologic evaluation predicts recurrence in clinical stage I or II patients. *Hum Pathol* 1995;26:829–837.
169. Bertrand M, Lickrish GM, Colgan TJ. The anatomic distribution of cervical adenocarcinoma in situ: implications for treatment. *Am J Obstet Gynecol* 1987;157:21–25.
170. Colgan TJ, Lickrish GM. The topography and invasive potential of cervical adenocarcinoma in situ, with and without associated squamous dysplasia. *Gynecol Oncol* 1990;36:246–249.
171. Crum CP, Cibas ES, Lee KR. *Pathology of early cervical neoplasia.* New York: Churchill-Livingstone 1997:177–181.
172. Widrich T, Kennedy AW, Myers TM, Hart WR, Wirth S. Adenocarcinoma in situ of the uterine cervix: management and outcome. *Gynecol Oncol* 1996;61(3):304–308.
173. Im DD, Duska LR, Rosenshein NB. Adequacy of conization margins in adenocarcinoma in situ of the cervix as a predictor of residual disease. *Gynecol Oncol* 1995;9:179–182.
174. Paynor EA, Barakat RR, Hoskins WJ. Management and follow-up of patients with adenocarcinoma in situ of the uterine cervix. *Gynecol Oncol* 1995;57:158–164.
175. Wolf J, Levenback C, Malpica A, Morris M, Burke T, Follen Mitchell M. Adenocarcinoma in situ of the cervix: significance of cone biopsy margins. *Obstet Gynecol* 1996;88(1):82–86.
176. Denehy T, Gregori C, Breen J. Endocervical curettage, cone margins, and residual adenocarcinoma in situ of the cervix. *Obstet Gynecol* 1997;90(1):1–6.
177. Lee KR. Atypical glandular cells in cervical smears from women who have undergone cone biopsy: a potential diagnostic pitfall. *Acta Cytol* 1993;37:705–709.
178. Fu YS, Berek JS, Hillborne LH. Diagnostic problems of in situ and invasive adenocarcinomas of the uterine cervix. *Appl Pathol* 1987;5:47–56.
179. Rollason TP, Cullimore J, Bradgate MG. A suggested columnar cell morphological equivalent of squamous carcinoma in situ with early stromal invasion. *Int J Gynecol Pathol* 1989;8:230–236.
180. Teshima S, Shimosato Y, Kishi K. Early stage adenocarcinoma of the uterine cervix: histopathologic analysis with consideration of histogenesis. *Cancer* 1985;56:167–172.
181. Burghardt E. Microinvasive carcinoma in gynecologic pathology. *Clin Obstet Gynaecol* 1984;11:239–257.
182. Kaspar HG, Dinh T, Doherty MG, Hannigan EV, Kumar D. Clinical implications of tumor volume measurement in stage I adenocarcinoma of the cervix. *Obstet Gynecol* 1993;81:296–300.
183. Tsunehisa K, Toshiharu K, Kunihiro S, Satoshi A, Hiroaki K, Toshiyuki S, Toshiaki S, Hitoo N. Early adenocarcinoma of the uterine cervix. *Gynecol Oncol* 1997;65(2):281–285.
184. Östör A, Rome R, Quinn M. Microinvasive adenocarcinoma of the cervix: a clinicopathologic study of 77 women. *Obstet Gynecol* 1997;89(1):88–93.
185. Greer BE, Figge DC, Tamimi HK, Cain JM. Stage IB adenocarcinoma of the cervix treated by radical hysterectomy and pelvic lymph node dissection. *Am J Obstet Gynecol* 1989;160(6):1509–1513.
186. Miller BE, Flax SD, Arheart K, Photopulos G. The presentation of adenocarcinoma of the uterine cervix. *Cancer* 1993;72:1281–1285.
187. Vesterinen E, Forss M, Nieminen U. Increase of cervical adenocarcinoma: a report of 520 cases of cervical carcinoma including 112 tumors with glandular elements. *Gynecol Oncol* 1989;33(1):49–53.
188. Davis JR, Moon LB. Increased incidence of adenocarcinoma of uterine cervix. *Obstet Gynecol* 1975;45(1):79–83.
189. Hopkins MP, Morley GW. A comparison of adenocarcinoma and squamous carcinoma of the cervix. *Obstet Gynecol* 1991;77:912–917.
190. Nieminen P, Kallio M, Hakama M. The effect of mass screening on incidence and mortality of squamous and adenocarcinoma of the cervix uteri. *Obstet Gynecol* 1995;85:1017–1021.
191. Peters RK, Chow A, Mack TM, Bernstein TD, Henderson BE. Increased frequency of adenocarcinoma of the uterine cervix in young women in Los Angeles county. *J Natl Cancer Inst* 1986;76:423–428.
192. Ursin G, Pike MC, Preston-Martin S, d'Ablaing G 3rd, Peters RK. Sexual, reproductive, and other risk factors for adenocarcinoma of the cervix: results from a population-based case-control study. *Cancer Causes Control* 1996;7(3):391–401.
193. Duggan MA, McGregor SE, Benoit JL, Inoue M, Nation JG, Stuart GC. The human papillomavirus status of invasive cervical adenocarcinoma: a clinicopathologic and outcome analysis. *Hum Pathol* 1995;26(3):319–325.
194. Uchiyama M, Tsuyoshi I, Norihito M, Toru H, Mori M, Sugimori H. Correlation between human papillomavirus positivity and p53 gene overexpression in adenocarcinoma of the uterine cervix. *Gynecol Oncol* 1997;65:23–29.
195. Thomas DB, Ray RM. Oral contraceptives and invasive adenocarcinomas and adenosquamous carcinomas of the uterine cervix (the world health organization collaborative study of neoplasia and steroid contraceptives). *Am J Epidemiol* 1996;144(3):281–289.
196. Dallenbach-Hellweg G. On the origin and histological structure of adenocarcinoma of the endocervix in women under 50 years of age. *Pathol Res Pract* 1984;179(1):38–50.
197. Brinton LA, Tashima KT, Lehman HG, et al. Epidemiology of cervical cancer by cell type. *Cancer Res* 1987;47(6):1706–1711.
198. Jones MW, Silverberg SG. Cervical adenocarcinoma in young women: possible relationship to microglandular hyperplasia and use of oral contraceptives. *Obstet Gynecol* 1989;73(6):984–989.
199. Tenti P, Romagnoli S, Silini E, et al. Human papillomavirus types 16 and 18 infection in infiltrating adenocarcinoma of the cervix. *Am J Clin Pathol* 1996;106(1):52–56.
200. Young RH, Clement PB, Scully RE. Premalignant and malignant

glandular lesions of the uterine cervix. In: Clement PB, Young RH, eds. *Tumors and tumor-like lesions of the uterine corpus and cervix.* New York: Churchill-Livingstone, 1993.

201. Young RH, Scully RE. Mucinous tumors of the ovary associated with mucinous adenocarcinomas of the cervix: a clinicopathologic analysis of 16 cases. *Int J Gynecol Pathol* 1988;7(2):99–111.
202. Eifel PJ, Burke TW, Morris M, Smith TL. Adenocarcinoma as an independent risk factor for disease recurrence in patients with stage IB cervical carcinoma. *Gynecol Oncol* 1995;59(1):38–44.
203. Azzopardi JG, Hou LT. Intestinal metaplasia with argentaffin cells in cervical adenocarcinoma. *J Pathol Bacteriol* 1965;90:686–690.
204. Lee KR, Trainer TD. Adenocarcinoma of the uterine cervix of intestinal type containing numerous Paneth cells *Arch Pathol Lab Med* 1990;114(7):731–733.
205. Lewis TLT. Colloid (mucus secreting) carcinoma of the cervix. *Br J Obstet Gynaecol* 1971;78(2):1128–1132.
206. Moll UM, Chumas JC, Mann WJ, Patsner B. Primary signet-ring cell carcinoma of the uterine cervix. *NY State J Med* 1990;90(11):559–560.
207. McKelvey JL, Goodlin RR. Adenoma malignum of the cervix. *Cancer* 1963;16(5):549–557.
208. Silverberg SG, Hurt WG. Minimal deviation adenocarcinoma ("adenoma malignum") of the cervix. *Am J Obstet Gynecol* 1975;121(7):971–975.
209. Kaku T, Enjoji M. Extremely well-differentiated adenocarcinoma ("adenoma malignum") of the cervix. *Int J Gynecol Pathol* 1983;2(1):28–41.
210. Kaminski PF, Norris HJ. Minimal deviation carcinoma (adenoma malignum) of the cervix. *Int J Gynecol Pathol* 1983;2(2):141–152.
211. Michael H, Grawe L, Kraus FT. Minimal deviation endocervical adenocarcinoma: clinical and histologic features, immunohistochemical staining for carcinoembryonic antigen, and differentiation from confusing benign lesions. *Int J Gynecol Pathol* 1984;3(3):261–276.
212. Gilks CB, Young RH, Aguirre P, DeLellis RA, Scully RE. Adenoma malignum (minimal deviation adenocarcinoma) of the uterine cervix. A clinicopathologic and immunohistochemical analysis of 26 cases. *Am J Surg Pathol* 1989;13(9):717–729.
213. McGowan L, Young RH, Scully RE. Peutz-Jeghers syndrome with "adenoma malignum" of the cervix. A report of two cases. *Gynecol Oncol* 1980;10(2):125–133.
214. Granter SR, Lee KR. Cytologic findings in minimal deviation adenocarcinoma (adenoma malignum) of the cervix: a report of seven cases. *Am J Clin Pathol* 1996;105:327–333.
215. Jones MW, Silverberg SG, Kurman RJ. Well-differentiated villoglandular adenocarcinoma of the uterine cervix: a clinicopathologic study of 24 cases. *Int J Gynecol Pathol* 1993;12:1–7.
216. Young RH, Scully RE. Villoglandular papillary adenocarcinoma of the uterine cervix: a clinicopathologic analysis of 13 cases. *Cancer* 1989;63:1773–1779.
217. Kaku T, Kamura T, Shigematsu T, et al. Adenocarcinoma of the uterine cervix with predominantly villoglandular papillary growth pattern. *Gynecol Oncol* 1997;64(1):147–152.
218. Wahlstrom T, Korhonen M, Lindgren J, Seppala M. Distinction between endocervical and endometrial adenocarcinoma with immunoperoxidase staining of carcinoembryonic antigen in routine histologic tissue specimens. *Lancet* 1979;2(8153):1159–1160.
219. van Nagell JR Jr, Goldenberg JR Jr. Carcinoembryonic antigen staining of endometrial and endocervical carcinomas. *Lancet* 1980;1(8161):213.
220. Cohen C, Shulman G, Budgeon LR. Endocervical and endometrial adenocarcinoma. An immunoperoxidase and histochemical study. *Am J Surg Pathol* 1982;6(2):151–157.
221. Young RH, Scully RE. Minimal deviation endometrioid adenocarcinoma of the uterine cervix: a report of five cases of a distinctive neoplasm that may be misinterpreted as benign. *Am J Surg Pathol* 1993;17:660–665.
222. Rahilly MA, Williams ARW, Al-Nafussi A. Minimal deviation endometrioid adenocarcinoma of the cervix: a clinicopathologic and immunohistochemical study of two cases. *Histopathology* 1992;20:351–354.
223. Scully RE, Welch WR. Pathology of the female genital tract after prenatal exposure to diethylstilbestrol. In: Herbst Al, Bern HA, eds. *Developmental effects of diethylstilbestrol (DES) in pregnancy.* New York: Thieme-Stratton, 1981:26.
224. Nordqvist SRB, Fidler W Jr, Woodruff J, Lewis J Jr. Clear cell adenocarcinoma of the cervix and vagina: a clinicopathologic study of 21 cases with and without a history of maternal ingestion of estrogens. *Cancer* 1976;37:858–871.
225. Hart WR, Norris HJ. Mesonephric adenocarcinomas of the cervix. *Cancer* 1972;29(1):106–113.
226. Kaminski PF, Maier RC. Clear cell adenocarcinoma of the cervix unrelated to diethylstilbestrol exposure. *Obstet Gynecol* 1983;62(6):720–727.
227. Gilks CB, Clement PB. Papillary serous adenocarcinoma of the uterine cervix. A report of three cases. *Mod Pathol* 1992;5(4):426–431.
228. Clement PB, Young RG, Keh P, Östör A, Scully RE. Malignant mesonephric neoplasms of the uterine cervix. A report of eight cases, including four with a malignant spindle-cell component. *Am J Surg Pathol* 1995;19(10):1158–1171.
229. Benda J, Platz C, Buchsbaum H, Lifshitz S. Mucin production in defining mixed carcinoma of the uterine cervix: a clinicopathologic study. *Int J Gynecol Pathol* 1985;4:314–327.
230. Hopkins MP, Schmidt RW, Roberts JA, Morley GW. The prognosis and treatment of stage I adenocarcinoma of the cervix. *Obstet Gynecol* 1988;72(6):915–921.
231. Look KY, Brunetto VL, Clarke-Pearson DL, et al. An analysis of cell type in patients with surgically staged stage IB carcinoma of the cervix: a gynecologic oncology group study. *Gynecol Oncol* 1996;63(3):304–311.
232. Yazigi R, Sandstad J, Munoz AK, Choi DJ, Nguyen PD, Risser R. Adenosquamous carcinoma of the cervix: prognosis in stage IB. *Obstet Gynecol* 1990;75(6):1012–1015.
233. Shingleton HM, Bell MC, Fremgen A, et al. Is there really a difference in survival of women with squamous cell carcinoma, adenocarcinoma, and adenosquamous cell carcinoma of the cervix? *Cancer* 1995;76(suppl 10):1948–1955.
234. Glucksmann A, Cherry CP. Incidence, histology and response to radiation of mixed carcinomas (adenoacanthomas) of the uterine cervix. *Cancer* 1956;9(5):971–979.
235. Cherry CP, Glücksmann A. Histology of carcinomas of the uterine cervix and survival rates in pregnant and nonpregnant patients. *Surg Gynecol Obstet* 1961;113(6):763–776.
236. Littman P, Clement PB, Henriksen B, et al. Glassy cell carcinoma of the cervix. *Cancer* 1976;37(5):2238–2246.
237. Lotocki RJ, Krepart GV, Paraskevas M, Vadas G, Heywood M, Fung FK. Glassy cell carcinoma of the cervix: a bimodal treatment strategy. *Gynecol Oncol* 1992;44(3):254–259.
238. Costa MJ, Kenny MB, Hewan-Lowe K, Judd R. Glassy cell features in adenosquamous carcinoma of the uterine cervix. Histologic, ultrastructural, immunohistochemical, and clinical findings. *Am J Clin Pathol* 1991;96(4):520–528.
239. Baggish MS, Woodruff JD. Adenoid basal lesions of the cervix. *Obstet Gynecol* 1971;37:807–819.
240. Daroca PJ, Dhurandhar HN. Basaloid carcinoma of the uterine cervix. *Am J Surg Pathol* 1980;4:235.
241. van Dinh T, Woodruff JD. Adenoid cystic and adenoid basal carcinomas of the cervix. *Obstet Gynecol* 1985;65(5):705–709.
242. Ferry JA, Scully RE. "Adenoid cystic" carcinoma and adenoid basal carcinoma of the uterine cervix. A study of 28 cases. *Am J Surg Pathol* 1988;12(2):134–144.
243. Albores-Saavedra J, Manivel C, Mora A, Vuitch F, Milchgrub S. The solid variant of adenoid cystic carcinoma of the cervix. *Int J Gynecol Pathol* 1992;11(1):2–10.
244. Mazur MT, Hsueh S, Gersell DJ. Metastases to the female genital tract. Analysis of 325 cases. *Cancer* 1984;53:1978–1983.
245. Chirayil SJ, Tobon H. Polyps of the vagina: a clinicopathologic analysis of 18 cases. *Cancer* 1981;47:2904–2907.
246. Selzer I, Nelson H. Benign papilloma (polypoid tumor) of the cervix uteri in children. *Am J Obstet Gynecol* 1962;84:165–169.
247. Abell MR. Papillary adenocarcinoma of the uterine cervix. *Am J Obstet Gynecol* 1971;110:990–993.
248. Zaloudek CJ, Norris HJ. Adenofibroma and adenosarcoma. A clinical and pathological study of 35 benign and low grade variants of mixed mesodermal tumor of the uterus. *Cancer* 1981;48:354–366.
249. Cusmano JT. Hemangioma of the cervix. *Am J Obstet Gynecol* 1965;91:204–209.
250. Nuovo GJ, Nagler HM, Fenoglio JJ. Arteriovenous malformation of the bladder presenting as gross hematuria. *Hum Patho*l 1986;17:94–97.
251. Rilke F, Cantaboni A. Lipomas of the uterus. Presentation of 2 cases and a review of the recent literature. *Ann Obstet Gynecol* 1964;86:645.

252. Patel DS, Bhagavan BS. Blue nevus of the uterine cervix. *Hum Pathol* 1985;16:79–86.
253. Dundore W, Lamas C. Benign nevus (ephelis) of the uterine cervix. *Am J Obstet Gynecol* 1985;152:881–882.
254. Luevano-Flores E, Sotelo J, Tena-Suck M. Glial polyp (glioma) of the uterine cervix, report of a case with demonstration of glial fibrillary acidic protein. *Gynecol Oncol* 85;21:385–390.
255. Stout AP. Hemangioendothelioma: a tumor of blood vessels featuring vascular endothelial cells. *Ann Surg* 1943;118:445–464.
256. Jaffe R, Altaras M, Bernheim J, Aderet NB. Endocervical stromal sarcoma-case report. *Gynecol Oncol* 1985;22:105–108.
257. Abell MR, Ramirez JA. Sarcomas and carcinosarcomas of the uterine cervix. *Cancer* 1973;31:176–192.
258. Williamson HO, McIver FA. Sarcoma botryoides of the cervix treated by vaginal hysterectomy and subtotal vaginectomy. *Obstet Gynecol* 1968;31:689–694.
259. Bell DA, Shimm DS, Gang DL. Wilms' tumor of the endocervix. *Arch Pathol Lab Med* 1985;109:371–373.
260. Chen KTK. Rhabdomyosarcomatous uterine sarcoma. *Int J Gynecol Pathol* 1985;4:146–152.
261. Hart WR, Craig JR. Rhabdomyosarcomas of the uterus. *Am J Clin Pathol* 1978;70:217–223.
262. Lathrop JC. Views and reviews. Malignant pelvic lymphomas. *Obstet Gynecol* 1967;30:137–145.
263. Volpe R, Tirelli U, Tumolo S, et al. Stage IIe diffuse small cleaved cell lymphoma of the cervix. *Pathologica* 1983;75:887–892.
264. Freeman C, Berg JW, Cutler SJ. Occurrence and prognosis of extranodal lymphomas. *Cancer* 1972;29:252–260.

CHAPTER 53

The Uterine Corpus

Michael R. Hendrickson, Teri A. Longacre, and Richard L. Kempson

EVALUATION OF ENDOMETRIAL AND MYOMETRIAL SPECIMENS

Endometrial Samples

Among the most common specimens in day-to-day surgical pathology practice are those produced by sampling the endometrium. The typical indications for endometrial sampling are: (a) the workup of abnormal uterine bleeding, (b) the evaluation of the endometrium of women who are infertile, and (c) the monitoring of the endometrium of women being treated with hormone replacement therapy. The purpose of the sampling determines the kind of sampling technique that is most appropriate and the timing of sample acquisition.

The most commonly employed endometrial sampling techniques are dilatation and curettage (D&C) and endometrial biopsy (EMB). Curettage is, in essence, an excisional biopsy of the endometrium. If performed correctly, this is, in principle, the most complete sampling technique, even though mechanically distorting lesions, such as leiomyomas and polyps, may occasionally shield some portion of the uterine lining from the curette. D&C requires anesthesia, and there is a small but definite risk of uterine perforation or secondary amenorrhea due to postcurettage adhesions (Asherman's syndrome) (1–5). EMB, in contrast is a relatively inexpensive office procedure, and modifications in sampling instrument design since the technique's inception have reduced the discomfort of the procedure without sacrificing sampling adequacy (6–12). Claimed disadvantages of EMB is the limited sample that is obtained and its unsuitability for the diagnosis and removal of such focal lesions as endometrial polyps. In recent years, however, the status of D&C as the gold standard sampling technique has been challenged (13–15). Moreover, the diagnostic suitability of samples obtained by biopsy compare favorably with those obtained by D&C (10,16–18).

For these reasons, outpatient endometrial assessment has largely replaced in-hospital D&C (11,19). Office biopsy appears to be as effective as D&C in detecting malignancy (20). Hysteroscopy and directed biopsy, in contrast to both EMB and D&C, are particularly suited to identifying focal lesions, such as polyps and submucous leiomyomata (21,22). Transvaginal ultrasound has been extensively investigated as a screening technique for high-risk endometrial proliferations in postmenopausal women with uterine bleeding (18,23–26). In this context, a thin endometrial strip (<5.0 mm) is only rarely associated with malignancy and thus is effective in ruling out malignancy (23,27). On the other hand, it appears that as a screening test in asymptomatic women taking hormone replacement medication, EMB alone is more cost-effective than a combination of transvaginal ultrasound and EMB in those patients with a thick endometrium (28).

At a threshold value of 5.0 mm for endometrial thickness, transvaginal ultrasonography has a positive predictive value of 9% for detecting any abnormality, with 90% sensitivity and 48% specificity, and a negative predictive value of 99%. With this threshold, a biopsy would be indicated in more than half the women, only 4% of whom would have serious disease. In a patient suspected of having a malignant neoplasm, negative results on EMB do not exclude the possibility of malignancy, and it is mandatory to obtain additional tissue from such patients, whether by way of a second biopsy or formal curettage (29–32).

Patients who are being evaluated for infertility should undergo sampling well into their presumed luteal phase (2 or 3 days before their next menstrual period), as predicted by the shift in basal body temperature (BBT) or by one of several available assays designed to detect the luteinizing hormone (LH) peak (which is followed shortly by ovulation) (33–35). Some investigators have advocated conducting biopsy at the onset of uterine bleeding (36), although we and others find morphologic features in menstrual endometrium difficult to interpret. It has been proposed that midluteal biopsy sampling is more effective in evaluating luteal phase defects

---

M. R. Hendrickson, T. A. Longacre, and R. L. Kempson: Department of Pathology, Stanford University Medical Center, Stanford, California 94305.

(LPDs) (see later discussion under Other Secretory Patterns) (37). When tuberculous endometritis is a serious possibility, biopsy at the time of menstrual bleeding is recommended; in principle, this allows the maximum amount of time for diagnostic granulomata to develop and provides the best material for culture. The optimal site for endometrial sampling for infertility evaluation is the uterine fundus. This is the region of the endometrium whose morphologic characteristics reflect the maximum effect of reproductive hormones. The precise location (anterior or posterior fundus) makes little difference (38–40).

The endometrial sampling for abnormal bleeding should be undertaken during the bleeding episode itself (11,41). The indications for tissue sampling in various age groups are beyond the scope of this chapter; suffice it to say that many patients with abnormal bleeding who are not at particular risk of endometrial carcinoma (e.g., women younger than 40) are treated medically without benefit of tissue examination (42). In general, progestational agents should not be administered before diagnostic sampling, particularly in a postmenopausal patient. These agents can mask important features necessary to identify abnormal endometrial proliferative states, including adenocarcinoma. These interpretive problems are, of course, inevitable in patients taking hormone replacement medication that contains a progestogen.

The importance of correlating the morphologic features of EMB with the clinical findings—whatever the indication for sampling—cannot be overemphasized. Normal endometrial morphologic characteristics can be associated with a variety of abnormal clinical states. For example, normal morphologic features of late proliferative endometrium are obviously abnormal during what should be a patient's late luteal phase. The minimal clinical information required for interpretation in most cases includes the patient's age, the date and characteristics of the last menstrual period, the date and characteristics of the previous menstrual period, a statement about past or current administration of steroids, and an account of the current chief complaint and physical findings.

Hysterectomy Specimens

An outline containing suggestions for the handling of hysterectomy specimens removed for various reasons is supplied in Tables 1 and 2. The histologic sections taken depend very much upon the clinical questions being asked (explicitly or implicitly) and the gross abnormalities encountered during the examination of the specimen.

Myomectomy Specimens

Most myomectomies are performed in premenopausal women who wish to retain their uterus; the procedure is done either to relieve symptoms produced by the neoplasm or in an effort to enhance the woman's fertility; it may be conducted in a variety of ways—in the course of laparotomy, laparoscopically, or hysteroscopically (43–48). The gross appearance of these specimens is particularly important with regard to the question of possible leiomyosarcoma. Almost

TABLE 1. *Gross sectioning of the hysterectomy specimen for uterine corpus disease*

Uterus removed for nonneoplastic disease
  No gross pathology present
    One section each of the anterior or posterior fundal endometrium and subadjacent myometrium
    Standard cervix sections (see Cervix chapter)
  Gross pathology discovered
    See Table 2 for gross differential diagnosis.
Uterus removed for neoplastic disease
  Endometrial carcinoma
    Questions that motivate the examination
      What is the histologic type and (if appropriate) grade of the carcinoma?
      What is the surgical stage?
    Assessment of the endometrium
      Ink the serosa and the cervical or vaginal margins. Take at least three sections of the tumor to include the entire thickness of the myometrium.
    Assessment of the depth of myometrial invasion (myoinvasion)
      Record gross impression. Sections should include what appears on gross inspection to be the serosa, so they can be reoriented as histologic sections.
    Assessment of the cervix (if involvement is documented—i.e., surgical Stage II—)
      Sections should include the high endocervical canal and the lower uterine segment to include the deep lymphatics
      With extensive involvement of the cervix, give some thought to a cervical primary secondarily involving the uterine corpus
      Simultaneous primary neoplasms in both endometrium and cervix is also a possibility
      Take sections to determine if the vaginal and cervical margins of the specimen are free of carcinoma
    Assessment of the adnexa
      The ovarian hilar lymphatics of grossly normal ovaries should be sampled, particularly if the endometrial carcinoma is a high-risk type (e.g., UPSC, grade 3 endometrioid carcinoma)
      If low-grade endometrioid carcinoma is present in the ovary and if the carcinoma)
      If no tumor is seen on gross examination, take at least one section of ovarian cortex and of fallopian tube; include the ovarian hilar region
  Uterine sarcoma and mixed müllerian tumor
    Questions that motivate the examination
      What is the histologic type of the mesenchymal neoplasm and the epithelial elements, if they are present?
      What is the surgical stage?
    Protocol is much the same as for endometrial adenocarcinoma.
    If the histologic type is in doubt, more sections of tumor may be required than for adenocarcinoma.
    Check margins of resection, which requires inking.

all leiomyosarcomas deviate from the characteristic gross features of leiomyomas by being soft, hemorrhagic, and/or necrotic, and almost all leiomyosarcomas infiltrate the myometrium such that they are difficult to remove. Conversely, however, most grossly peculiar myomectomy specimens will ultimately prove to be benign when their histologic appearance has been evaluated. The preoperative administra-

TABLE 2. *Differential diagnosis of gross findings in the uterus*

Focally polypoid endometrium
  Endometrial polyp
    Multicystic cut surface
    May be sessile or pedunculated
  Submucous leiomyoma
    Firm, whorled cut surface
    Thin, focally hemorrhagic lining mucosa
  Atypical polypoid adenomyoma
    Usually located in lower uterine segment
    Circumscribed margin
  Adenofibroma
    Firm, knobby or papillary multicystic
    Not necrotic
    N.B.: Multiple sections to distinguish from adenosarcoma
  Polypoid malignancy
    Firm, friable
    Focal necrosis
    Sections taken so that myoinfiltration can be evaluated
    Neoplasms to consider
      Adenocarcinoma (unusual presentation)
      Carcinosarcoma (common presentation)
      Adenosarcoma (common presentation)
Thickened endometrium
  Secretory endometrium
    Lush, polypoid
    No necrosis
    May be hemorrhagic if close to menstruation
  Gestational endometrium
    Lush decidual reaction
    Look for evidence of pregnancy
      Placental fragments
      Gestational sac
  Hyperplastic-carcinomatous endometrium
    Lush, polypoid endometrium, particularly if there are yellow necrotic areas, should raise the possibility of adenocarcinoma, particularly if the patient is older than 40. Ink the serosa and, if patient is not known to have carcinoma, take initial sections in such a way that subsequent sections can be taken to determine depth of invasion. If carcinoma is known to be present, ink the serosa and take sections so that depth of invasion can be determined, as outlined in Table 1.

Space-occupying intramural lesions
  Leiomyoma (with/without "degeneration")
    Shells out bulging, trabeculated
    Often multiple. When multiple, we sample all up to three. If more than three, we sample at least three, being sure that unsampled tumors have the *classic* gross appearance of leiomyomas
    Wide variety of appearances
    N.B. Sample all apparent smooth-muscle neoplasms with a deviant gross appearance. Take at least one section per centimeter of diameter of any tumor that has less than diagnostic microscopic features, to rule out leiomyosarcoma or non-smooth-muscle neoplasms.
  Leiomyosarcoma
    Fish flesh consistency, hemorrhage and necrosis common
    Infiltrative margins
    Usually solitary mass with extension, rather than one of multiple masses
  Adenomyosis
    Trabeculated smooth muscle, myometrium often thickened
    If focal it merges with surrounding myometrium
    Resists shelling out (unlike leiomyoma)
  Adenomatoid tumor
    Subserosal cornual region most common site
    This neoplasm is sometimes yellow
  Low-grade endometrial stromal sarcoma
    White and fleshy
    Infiltration of myometrium may be visible on gross inspection as tongues extending from the tumor.
    Take sections from margins of the tumor in order to evaluate the presence or absence of infiltration.
Grossly visible tumor within vessels
  Low-grade endometrial stromal sarcoma
  Intravenous leiomyomatosis
  Leiomyosarcoma (rare)

NB, nota bene.

tion of gonadotropin-releasing hormone (GnRH) has been shown to reduce the size of myomata, and these agents can modify the appearance of benign smooth-muscle tumors; however, the gross and histologic correlates of this clinical shrinkage have been difficult to identify (49–54). Leiomyosarcoma in the reproductive years is very unusual. The tissue samples taken should be well fixed and, when possible, include the interface between normal myometrium and the gross lesion. Histologic sections prepared from these samples must be suitable for obtaining an accurate mitotic index (MI), that is, they must be thinly cut and well stained (Table 3).

APPROACH TO UTERINE CORPUS DIAGNOSIS: PATTERN DIAGNOSIS

Even in the absence of any previous information, the range of differential diagnostic possibilities is narrowed initially by the overall low-power microscopic appearance of the endometrium and myometrium. Most specimens fall into one of six "scanning-power groups." In our view, it is very helpful in formulating differential diagnoses to examine the endometrium and myometrium at low-power magnification and to attempt to place it into one of the following six categories. The location in the text of the differential diagnosis of each of these patterns is presented in Table 4.

Pattern 1: Proliferations Composed of Glands and Supportive Nonneoplastic Endometrial Stroma

This is the most common pattern encountered in daily practice. Diagnosis is facilitated by a systematic examination of the glands-to-stroma ratio, glandular features, stromal features, the appearance of the vessels, and pattern uniformity.

TABLE 3. *Caveats concerning mitotic activity (559–560)*

Sections thin, well stained
Strict criteria for accepting mitotic figures
  Hairy extensions of chromatin (condensed chromosomes) must be unequivocally present, extending from a central clot-like, dense mass of chromosomes. The clots may be single (metaphase) or separate (telophase). Hairy extensions from an empty center favor a nonmitosis.
  The nuclear membrane must be absent, but the cytoplasm is often discernible.
  Differential diagnosis: lymphocytes, mast cells, stripped nuclei, degenerated cells, precipitated Hematoxylin. If in doubt, do not accept it as a mitotic figure.
Begin counts in the area of highest mitotic activity.
Four sets of ten fields; use the highest count.
Counts should be performed with a binocular microscope using ×10 or ×15 wide-field eyepieces and ×40 high dry objectives. Minor variations in eyepieces and objectives do not significantly affect diagnostic interpretation.
Use mitotic counts in conjunction with the degree of cytologic atypia and the presence or absence of coagulative tumor cell necrosis (see Table 14 and smooth-muscle tumor section).

Glands-to-Stroma Ratio

The low-power evaluation of the ratio of glands to stroma leads to a further sorting into three categories. The first group shows a roughly 1:1 ratio of glands to stroma, a pattern exhibited by most normally cycling endometria and also encountered in the majority of endometria associated with dysfunctional uterine bleeding (DUB) and infertility. Second, there are endometria marked by a shift in the glands-to-stroma ratio in favor of glands. This group includes some fully developed late secretory endometria, menstrual endometria, endometrial hyperplasias, and carcinomas. Finally, we find endometria featuring a predominance of stroma, a group that includes normal decidua, some examples of atrophy, and all of the pattern 3 monophasic stromal proliferations listed later herein.

Glandular Features

The next step in narrowing the differential diagnosis of proliferations composed of glands and supportive stroma involves an examination of the cytologic features and architecture of the endometrial glands.

Cytologic Features

Atrophic and weakly proliferative glands are lined by low cuboidal to columnar cells with sparse or absent mitotic figures. Proliferating glands are lined by columnar epithelium exhibiting nuclear pseudostratification, mitotic figures, high nucleus-to-cytoplasm ratios, and elongated, ovoid nuclei with dense basophilic chromatin. Cytologic atypia in such glands is manifest by an increase in nuclear (and cell) size, increasing prominence of nucleoli, rounding of nuclei, nuclear pleomorphism, and a tendency of the cells to become stratified. These nuclear features are most pronounced in carcinoma. Parenthetically, in many carcinomas the epithelium tends to grow in a complex stratified, sheetlike pattern punctuated by sharply rounded spaces (cribriform pattern).

Secretory epithelia can be broadly divided into those manifesting early secretory, midsecretory, and late secretory changes. Early secretory epithelia feature large cytoplasmic vacuoles either in a subnuclear or in a supranuclear position; the nuclear features are those of late proliferative phase cells. Midsecretory glands are coiled, the epithelium is low columnar to cuboidal, and the cells possess an oval to round, vesicular, usually basilar nucleus with a small but discernible nucleolus. The cytoplasm is eosinophilic to clear. A dominant secretory vacuole is typically absent. Late secretory glands are fully coiled and dilated and frequently show luminal secretion and luminal border fraying. Marked cytoplasmic vacuolation associated with nuclear hyperchromasia and pleomorphism in the absence of mitotic figures is characteristic of the Arias-Stella reaction. The epithelial cells of disintegrating glands often contain karyorrhectic fragments (apoptosis).

Architecture

The normal endometrial gland is a nonbranched, coiled structure. Branching and budding of varying degrees of complexity are the hallmarks of endometrial hyperplasia and carcinoma. Occasionally, epithelial secretory changes are superimposed on the budding pattern of hyperplasia or even of carcinoma.

Stromal Features

Characteristically, endometrial stromal cells have either oblong or spindled nuclei with scanty cytoplasm that is difficult to discern (proliferative phase); alternatively, they show varying degrees of deciduation (secretory phase and pregnancy). The term deciduation refers to the transformation of a proliferative-phase stromal cell, with its dense nucleus and sparse, ill-defined cytoplasm, to one with a large, ovoid to round vesicular nucleus and abundant well-defined eosinophilic to clear cytoplasm. Lesser degrees of this transformation are known as predecidua and are representative of the normal late secretory phase of the menstrual cycle. Fibrotic spindled stroma is a property of endometrial polyps.

The Appearance of the Vessels

The distinctive feature of the normal developing endometrium is a synchronous proliferation of blood vessels, glands, and stroma. The endometrial vasculature begins as a delicate arborizing network of vessels ramifying through the developing proliferative endometrial stroma. It is this early vascular pattern that is so characteristic of endometrial stromal neoplasms. As the vasculature continues its develop-

TABLE 4. Location of Differential Diagnosis Sections in Uterine Corpus Chapter

Pattern	Page number
Pattern 1: Proliferations composed of glands and supportive nonneoplastic endometrial stroma	2205
Differential diagnosis of normal secretory endometrium	2216–2217
Atypical hyperplasia with secretory change vs. secretory carcinoma	2218
Differential diagnosis of gestationaerns	
Arias-Stella reaction vs. clear-cell carcinoma	2221
Infiltrating normal trophoblastic cells vs. mimics	2221
Differential diagnosis of nonsecretory patterns	
Atrophic vs. insufficient for diagnosis	2241
Atrophic vs. weakly proliferative	2241
Atrophic vs. endometrial hyperplasia	2242
Disordered proliferative vs. normal proliferative	2242
Disordered proliferative vs. hyperplasia	2242
Hyperplasia: nonatypical vs. atypical	2242
Atypical hyperplasia vs. grade 1 adenocarcinoma	2242–2244
Disintegrating endometria vs. adenocarcinoma	2244
Polypoid fragments of endometrium vs. endometrial polyp	2244
Endometrial polyp vs. adenofibroma vs. adenomyoma vs. atypical polypoid adenomyoma	2245
Grading adenocarcinoma: Grade 1 vs. Grade 2	2245
Grade 3 adenocarcinoma vs. other neoplasms featuring sheet-like proliferation of malignant cells	2245
Differential diagnosis of endometrium featuring squamous differentiation	
Sheetlike growth of poorly differentiated carcinoma vs. sheetlike growth of morules	2248
Differential diagnosis of endometrium featuring mucinous differentiation	
Atypical mucinous metaplasia vs. mucinous carcinoma	2250
Primary mucinous carcinoma of the endometrium vs. endocervical mucinous carcinoma	2250
Primary mucinous carcinoma vs. metastatic mucinous carcinoma	2250
Mucinous carcinoma vs. cervical microglandular hyperplasia	2250
Differential diagnosis of endometrium featuring papillary architecture	
Syncytial papillary metaplasia and villoglandular hyperplasia vs. endometrioid adenocarcinoma with villoglandular architecture	2254
Villoglandular endometrioid carcinoma vs. uterine papillary serous carcinoma	2254
Carcinosarcoma vs. uterine papillary serous carcinoma	2254
Ovarian or fallopian tube primary with secondary involvement of the endometrium	2254
Uterine papillary serous carcinoma vs. clear-cell carcinoma	2254
Differential diagnosis featuring ciliated cells	
Ciliated cell prominence in complex atypical hyperplasia vs. well-differentiated adenocarcinoma	2256
Patterns featuring a prominence of cleared cells or cells with prominent eosinophilic cytoplasm, but without visible cilia	2256
Differential diagnosis of clear cells and related differentiated types	
Clear cell carcinoma vs. other proliferations featuring cleared cells	2258
Clear cell carcinoma vs. uterine papillary serous carcinoma (see section on UPSC)	2258
Clear cell carcinoma: primary cervix vs. primary endometrium	2258
Pattern 2: Biphasic proliferations composed of glands and abundant (possibly neoplastic) stroma	2258
Differential diagnosis of mixed müllerian neoplasms	
Endometrial polyp vs. adenofibroma vs. polypoid adenomyoma vs. atypical polypoid adenomyoma	2264
Atypical polypoid adenomyoma vs. adenocarcinoma with bland squamous elements	2264
Adenofibroma vs. adenosarcoma	2264
Adenosarcoma vs. carcinosarcoma	2264
Adenosarcoma vs. pure sarcoma invading nonneoplastic endometrium and entrapping glands	2264
Adenosarcoma vs. endometrial stromal neoplasm with glandular elements	2265
Carcinosarcoma vs. sheet-like proliferations of malignant undifferentiated cells	2265
Adenomatoid mesothelioma	2290
Pattern 3: Predominately monophasic spindle-cell proliferations	2208
Differential diagnosis of endometrial stromal proliferations	
Low-grade endometrial stromal sarcoma vs. stromal nodule	2269
Low-grade endometrial stromal sarcoma vs. adenomyosis with sparse glands or glands or menstrual endometrium within vessels	2269
Low-grade endometrial stromal sarcoma vs. lymphoma/leukemia vs. carcinoma	2269
Low-grade endometrial stromal sarcoma vs. inflammation, fragmented lymphoid nodules, and immunoblasts	2270
Low-grade endometrial stromal sarcoma vs. smooth-muscle tumor, particularly intravascular smooth-muscle tumors	2270
Low-grade endometrial stromal sarcoma vs. high-grade uterine sarcoma	2270
Stromal nodule and low-grade endometrial stromal sarcoma vs. sex-cord-like tumor	2270

(Continued)

TABLE 4. *Continued*

Pattern	Page number
Adenofibroma and adenosarcoma vs. sex-cord-like tumor	2270
Endometrial stromal neoplasm vs. adenosarcoma (see differential diagnosis section of mixed müllerian neoplasms).	
Differential diagnosis of nonneoplastic smooth-muscle processes	
Differential diagnosis of smooth-muscle proliferations	
Differential diagnosis of usual leiomyoma	2282
Differential diagnosis of disseminated peritoneal leiomyomatosis	2285
Differential diagnosis of benign metastasizing leiomyoma	2286
Intravascular leiomyomatosis vs. low-grade endometrial stromal sarcoma	2287
Intravascular leiomyomatosis vs. leiomyosarcoma with vascular invasion	2287
Differential diagnosis of leiomyosarcoma	2287
Other types of sarcoma vs. high-grade leiomyosarcoma with difficult to discern smooth-muscle differentiation	2287
Well-differentiated leiomyosarcoma vs. low-grade endometrial stromal sarcoma	2287
Differential diagnosis of pure undifferentiated sarcoma other than leiomyosarcoma and low-grade endometrial stromal sarcoma	
Carcinosarcoma vs. pure sarcoma	2288
Adenosarcoma vs. pure differentiated sarcoma	2288
Mesenchymal metaplasia vs. pure heterologous sarcoma	2288
Anaplastic carcinoma vs. lymphoma/leukemia vs. pure sarcoma	2288
Pattern 4: Sheet-like proliferations composed of large, round, undifferentiated cells	2210
Lymphoma/leukemia	
Grade 3 carcinoma vs. other neoplasms forming sheetlike proliferations of malignant cells	2245
Pattern 5: Samples that feature extensive necrosis, inflammation, or disintegration	2210
Pattern 6: Scanty samples that raise the question of sampling adequacy	2210

ment during the normal secretory phase of the menstrual cycle, the vessels acquire thicker walls and become coiled; this appearance led to the designation spiral arteries. This coiling is particularly evident in the middle and superficial regions of the stratum functionalis. Poorly developed, thin-walled vessels are typically seen in the endometria in anovulatory cycles and in those reflecting the effect of progestational agents. Larger, thick-walled vessels embedded in fibrotic stroma are features of endometrial polyps.

Endometrial Pattern Uniformity

The hallmark of the normal endometrium is a uniformity of development from one portion of the stratum functionalis to another. In curettage or biopsy specimens, this implies uniformity from one fragment of endometrium to another. There are two important exceptions: fragments that derive from the region around the internal cervical os (lower uterine segment or isthmus) and fragments of the stratum basalis in the deepest (lower) part of the endometrium. The lower uterine segment is typically less responsive to hormonal stimulation than the fundal stratum functionalis, and the appearance of this region does not reflect the full impact of prevailing steroid hormone levels.

Fragments from the lower uterine segment are very often present in endometrial samples and can be identified by their spindled stromal cells separated by collagen fibers and by the presence of hybrid endometrial-endocervical glands. The stratum basalis maintains an essentially constant appearance throughout the menstrual cycle and does not exhibit the striking glandular and stromal changes of the overlying cycling stratum functionalis. The basalis is composed of small-caliber, minimally tortuous, weakly proliferative glands embedded in a cellular stroma. This stroma frequently intermingles with wisps of superficial myometrium. As a result, evaluation of the functional state of the endometrium should be carried out only on fragments of stratum functionalis that are lined by surface epithelium.

Pattern 2: Biphasic Proliferations Composed of Glands and Abundant (Possibly Neoplastic) Stroma

Entities that figure in the differential diagnosis of this pattern include endometrial polyps, atypical polypoid adenomyomas (APAs), mixed müllerian proliferations, and some of the patterns with prominent stroma discussed under the heading of pattern 1.

Pattern 3: Predominantly Monophasic Spindle-cell Proliferations

This pattern figures most prominently in the evaluation of hysterectomy or myomectomy specimens, although, from time to time, an endometrial sample will contain fragments of spindled stroma devoid or largely devoid of glands. The major differential diagnostic considerations raised by this low-power pattern are smooth-muscle neoplasms, endometrial stromal neoplasms, spindled epithelial neoplasms, pure heterologous uterine sarcomas, and undifferentiated sarcoma.

Epithelial Versus Mesenchymal Differentiation

Strategies useful in separating spindled epithelial neoplasms from spindled mesenchymal neoplasms include immunohistochemical staining and preparation of additional hematoxylin and eosin (H&E)–stained sections to search for areas of less equivocal epithelial differentiation. Normal endometrial epithelial cells express keratins, epithelial membrane antigen (EMA), and vimentin; this same pattern is found in most epithelial neoplasms, including carcinoma. Smooth-muscle cells can also express keratins, usually AE1, and less often, EMA. Smooth-muscle cells usually show positive results for muscle actin and very often for desmin. Some investigators maintain that neoplastic endometrial stromal cells have staining patterns similar to smooth muscle, but others insist that strong, diffuse desmin staining supports smooth-muscle differentiation. At present, the issue is the subject of controversy. Distinguishing uterine epithelial proliferations from mesenchymal processes should not be based on immunohistochemical staining patterns alone, but antigen expression may provide support for interpretation reached on the basis of H&E sections (55, 56). Nonneoplastic endometrial stromal cells do not express cytokeratin or EMA, and desmin staining, if positive, is usually focal.

Smooth-muscle Versus Stromal Versus Heterologous Differentiation

Under the assumption that a proliferation is mesenchymal, a number of techniques may be useful in distinguishing the possibilities. They are set out in Table 5. This topic is further discussed in the introductory section of the text devoted to smooth-muscle neoplasms.

TABLE 5. *Comparison of differentiating features for endometrial stromal cells and smooth-muscle cells (55, 518, 648, 649)*

Technique	Endometrial stromal cells	Usual smooth-muscle cells	Epithelioid smooth-muscle cells
Light microscopy			
Architecture	Haphazardly arranged cells resembling normal proliferative phase endometrial stromal cells	Cells arranged in looping, intersecting fascicles	Rounded or polygonal cells with moderate amount of cytoplasm
	Complex plexiform vascular pattern	Vascular component not complex	Foci of neoplasm often exhibiting standard smooth-muscle features
	Hyalin often abundant	—	—
Cytologic features			
Nucleus	Blunt, fusiform, uniform, bland	Elongated cigar-shaped	Round, crumpled
Cytoplasm	Scanty (on H&E and trichrome)	Moderate amount (on H&E and trichrome); typically fibrillar	Cytoplasm may be clear around the nucleus, clear at the periphery of the cell, or entirely clear; glycogen positive in slightly more than half of cases; PAS with diastase negative; mucin negative in all cases; lipid negative except for slight positivity in some
Ultrastructure	Endometrial stromal cells are undifferentiated mesenchymal cells; no myofilaments or dense bodies	Abundant, 60–80 nm, longitudinally arranged myofilaments parallel to long axis of cell; some filaments at oblique angles to these filaments	Some cases lack ultrastructural features of smooth muscle
	Intercellular collagen	Marginal spindle-shaped to oval dense bodies adjacent to plasmalemma (plaques) or along the trajectory of the filaments	
	No micropinocytotic vesicles	Micropinocytotic vesicles adjacent to plasma membrane	Rare pinocytotic vesicles
	Complex cytoplasmic processes	A few cilia	Vacuoles probably derived from swollen mitochondria
	No basal lamina	Interrupted basal lamina around individual cells (these features variably present in tumors)	No basal lamina around individual cells
Immunohistochemistry (55)	Normal endometrial stromal cells are reported to express vimentin, desmin, and muscle actin. They are negative for cytokeratin and EMA. Endometrial stromal sarcoma cells are reported to express desmin, vimentin, muscle actin, and less often cytokeratin. EMA has shown negative results to date. Sex-cord areas and glands in ESS can express cytokeratin and inhibin. Such areas show positive results for desmin and muscle actin in some reports and stain negative in others.	Essentially the same immunohistochemical profile as normal endometrial stromal cells, except that normal smooth-muscle cells may express cytokeratin.	Largely unknown for uterine tumors

H&E, hematoxylin and eosin; PAS, periodic acid–Schiff; EMA, epithelial membrane antigen; ESS, endometrial stromal sarcoma

Pattern 4: Sheet-like Proliferations Composed of Large, Round, Undifferentiated Cells

The major consideration that falls under this heading is the uterine version of the problem of the undifferentiated malignancy. In whatever organ system this diagnostic dilemma arises, it is important to cast one's net widely in terms of differential diagnosis; the undifferentiated uterine neoplasm is no exception. In addition to poorly differentiated uterine corpus primaries—grade 3 adenocarcinoma, carcinosarcoma, and high-grade undifferentiated uterine sarcomas—one must consider extension of a primary uterine cervix malignancy to the uterine corpus, metastatic carcinoma (particularly from an extragenital primary), metastatic melanoma, leukemia (including granulocytic sarcoma), and lymphoma (the usual problem being the large-cell diffuse type).

The most useful maneuvers in sorting out this differential diagnosis in our experience are submitting more tissue if it is available and performing a standard immunohistochemical panel for undifferentiated malignant neoplasms: common leukocyte antigen, S-100, and keratin stains. If these are not informative, chloroacetate esterase stains for myelogenous leukemia cells, more lymphoid markers, desmin, muscle actin, EMA, and other immunohistochemical stains can be used, depending on the H&E appearance of the tumor (see earlier discussion of epithelial vs. mesenchymal differentiation). When tissue is limited, rebiopsy may be necessary. When a proliferation's histologic appearance raises the possibility of a metastatic neoplasm, clinical history and additional clinical studies are often indicated. We have encountered several cases of cytologically bland, undifferentiated tumors infiltrating the endometrial stroma and causing abnormal endometrial bleeding; a history of lobular carcinoma of the breast was found in each of these cases.

Usually, these studies serve to narrow the possibilities to one or two processes, and examination of the hysterectomy specimen most often establishes the diagnosis. It is obviously important not to misidentify leukemia, lymphoma, melanoma, and metastatic carcinomas as primary uterine carcinomas or sarcomas, and it is rare for the procedures listed here not to prevent such an error. There are occasions, however, when even complete sampling of a malignant uterine primary neoplasm fails to reveal the direction of differentiation of the tumor. It is of some comfort that failure to distinguish primary high-grade uterine sarcoma from carcinosarcoma or poorly differentiated high-grade carcinoma is usually of little clinical consequence.

Pattern 5: Samples That Feature Extensive Necrosis, Inflammation, or Disintegration

Extensive necrosis in endometrial samples should always raise the possibility of malignancy, especially in a menopausal woman. A careful search should be made for isolated malignant cells in such a sample. Inflammatory cells are most often a normal finding in the postpartum endometrium, but sheets of polymorphonuclear leukocytes (pus) should suggest the possibility of a postpartum bacterial infection. Necrotic endometrial samples are obtained when cervical stenosis and pyometra are present; xanthomatous endometritis occurs in this context. A variety of infectious diseases may cause inflammation and necrosis when they affect the endometrium and are outlined at the end of this chapter in Table 16.

Disintegrating endometria may be encountered in a variety of situations, most often at the time of menstruation. The features of menstrual endometrium are familiar. Glands exhibiting secretory exhaustion are surrounded by a halo of disintegrating, swollen predecidual cells; often both are suspended in fibrin and blood and typically are infiltrated by varying numbers of neutrophils (57). Karyorrhectic fragments are often present in epithelial cells (apoptosis). Nonsecretory endometria, including hyperplastic endometria, may also disintegrate, and this disintegration is often marked by fibrin thrombi in vessels and stroma. On occasion, the degenerative changes in the epithelial and stromal cells of these endometria cause the stroma to collapse, which results in glandular approximation mimicking hyperplasia or carcinoma. For the same reason that a diagnosis of malignancy should be avoided in cytologic specimens composed of degenerated cells, so, too, such a diagnosis should be made only when cytologic features are well preserved in tissue sections. If the specimen exhibits degeneration and disintegration, and if carcinoma is a possibility, a second tissue sampling is warranted.

Pattern 6: Scanty Samples That Raise the Question of Sampling Adequacy

Scanty endometrial samples are commonly encountered. In this context, there are a number of diagnostic possibilities. Occasionally, an obstructing lesion shields the endometrium from the sampling instrument; more often there is little or no endometrium in the specimen either because the endometrium is atrophic (and what is present is all there is) or because of previous endometrial shedding or removal. When neoplasm is suspected, inquiries about the operative particulars—the thoroughness of the procedure and its extent—should be made and consideration given to resampling the endometrium.

THE NORMAL MENSTRUAL CYCLE ENDOMETRIUM (33,36,58–65)

Introduction

The particulars of the normal menstrual cycle are chiefly important for setting a morphologic baseline for discussion of endometrial abnormalities and for the interpretation of EMB performed for infertility. Today, biopsies are infrequently undertaken for the latter purpose in many academic institutions for reasons set out later herein (see Endometrial

Dating), but they are still relatively common in community practice. In women being evaluated for infertility there are three clinical questions of major interest.

Clinical question 1: Is there an intrinsic abnormality of the endometrium that might explain the couple's infertility (e.g., endometrial polyps, submucous leiomyomata, endometritis, hyperplasia, carcinoma)? Much of this information is provided by hysterosalpingogram, hysteroscopy, and laparoscopy—increasingly routine procedures for the workup of the infertility patient (66–69).

Clinical question 2: If the endometrium is normal, do its morphologic features provide evidence that the patient ovulated in the biopsy cycle? This amounts to deciding whether or not the endometrium is secretory. The answer to this question is also relevant for the patient undergoing EMB for abnormal bleeding in the reproductive years; the approach to the therapy of DUB depends upon whether such bleeding is ovulatory (secretory pattern of some sort) or anovulatory (nonsecretory pattern of some sort).

Clinical question 3: If the endometrium *is* secretory, is it appropriately developed for the patient's chronological dates (see Endometrial Dating)? The only importance of this observation is that under certain circumstances, the establishment of endometrial maturational delay warrants the diagnosis of LPD, a relatively uncommon condition that is thought by some researchers to be responsible for infertility and is correctable using a variety of therapies. As discussed later, LPD is defined in terms of a >3-day disparity between the woman's date of ovulation and her endometrial morphologic date, when this disparity occurs more than sporadically (see Clinicopathologic Correlation under Other Secretory Patterns). Thus, after determining that the endometrium is normal, an essential part of the evaluation of EMB from the infertility patient is to assign the endometrium a morphologic date (33,58,70–72). The following discussion provides a brief review of normal endometrial histologic characteristics.

Endometrial Dating

The first day of the menstrual cycle has conventionally been identified as the first day of menstrual flow. Menses usually lasts for fewer than 5 days and is followed by the endometrial proliferative phase, the length of which exhibits great variation (9–20 days); on average, it lasts 10 days. After ovulation, the coordinated and highly predictable series of stromal and glandular changes characteristic of the secretory (luteal) phase takes place. The traditional view is that the length of this phase is constant (14 days), and it is this alleged constancy that provides the basis for endometrial dating.

In evaluating the endometrium, it is important to carefully distinguish between the morphologic postovulatory date assigned to a morphologically normal endometrium and the chronological postovulatory date. The morphologic date is a summary characterization of the histologic development of the endometrium based upon an assessment of glandular and stromal features. Endometrial development is characterized either in terms of conventional light microscopic features or, in recent years (and in research settings), in terms of more sophisticated and reproducible morphometric semiquantitated features. The morphologic findings may be summarized in terms of postovulatory days (PODs), cycle days (CDs), or phases. For example, the morphologic pattern associated with a particular "standard" POD is assigned the number of that day: POD 12 refers to the pattern seen on the 12 h PCD of the standard cycle. Equivalently, this morphologic information can be conveyed using CD (e.g., CD 26) or phase (e.g., late secretory). The precise details of the morphologic patterns corresponding to standard cycle dates are presented in Table 6 and Fig. 1.

The chronological date is an estimate of when the patient actually ovulated and does not use any information about the morphologic appearance of the endometrium (73,74). Chronological dates are established in a variety of more or less indirect ways. Before the availability of hormonal assays, the two methods employed for assessing chronological dates were the analysis of the BBT chart (the nadir marks the time of ovulation) and back dating from the first day of the menstrual period after EMB, that is, the next menstrual period (NMP). The NMP technique makes no assumption about the length of the follicular phase but does assume that the luteal phase is 14 days in length. When this method is employed, the biopsy sample cannot be interpreted in relation to the patient's cycle until the date of her NMP is known.

Both of these methods for determining chronological dates have come under attack in recent years, and a number of replacements have been suggested. The gold standard for the estimate of the time of ovulation is ultrasonic visualization of the disappearance of the dominant follicle. This method is not employed in the routine workup of infertility patients; it is reserved for either research studies or for egg harvesting for *in vitro* fertilization therapy. Measurement of the time of the pre-ovulatory LH peak, the "LH surge," is now possible with home kits (35). Over the past 15 years, work in a number of laboratories has drawn into question the conventional wisdom about the normal menstrual cycle. Much of that wisdom was accumulated before assays were available to chart the cyclic changes of serum gonadotropins and steroids and before techniques were available to establish the woman's chronological date (75).

Several observations relevant to the evaluation of EMB for infertility have been made. The first is that the luteal phase of normally fertile and normally cycling woman is of variable length. (60,61,76–79). Landgren et al. (76) studied 68 normally menstruating women of proven fertility and confirmed that the follicular phase was highly variable (9–23 days). Surprisingly, the luteal phase, which was long thought to have a relatively fixed length of 14 days, in fact, varied from 8 to 17 days. Slightly less than half of the women studied had a luteal phase length of 14 to 15 days. The importance of this observation is that many women who have nor-

TABLE 6. *Decision tree for endometrial dating*

What type of gland is present?
- Proliferative gland (early proliferative, midproliferative, late proliferative, interval)
  - Is the gland straight or coiled?
    - Straight: early proliferative
    - Coiled: midproliferative, late proliferative, interval
  - Is there stromal edema?
    - Yes: midproliferative
    - No: late proliferative, interval
  - Are there scattered subnuclear vacuoles present, but with less than 50% of the glands exhibiting uniform subnuclear vacuolation?
    - No: late proliferative
    - Yes: interval—suggestive but not diagnostic of POD 1
- Secretory gland—vacuolated (early secretory)
  - POD 2: subnuclear vacuolation uniformly present, leading to exaggerated nuclear pseudostratification; many mitotic figures (>50% of the glands exhibit uniform subnuclear vacuolation)
  - POD 3: subnuclear vacuoles and nuclei uniformly aligned, scattered mitotic figures
  - POD 4: vacuoles assume luminal position, mitotic figures rare
  - POD 5: vacuoles uncommon, secretion in lumen of gland, nonvacuolated cells have nonvacuolated secretory appearance
- Secretory gland—nonvacuolated (midsecretory, late secretory, menstrual)
  - Is there normal stromal predeciduation?
    - No: midsecretory
      - POD 6: secretion prominent
      - POD 7: beginning stromal edema
      - POD 8: maximal stromal edema
    - Yes: late secretory, menstrual
  - Is there crumbling of the stroma?
    - No: late secretory
      - POD 9: spiral arteries first prominent
      - POD 10: thick periarterial cuffs of predecidua
      - POD 11: islands of predecidua in superficial compactum
      - POD 12: beginning coalescence of islands of predecidua
      - POD 13: confluence of surface islands; stromal granulocytes prominent
      - POD 14: extravasation of red cells in stroma; prominence of stromal granulocytes
    - Yes: menstrual
      - Crumbling stroma, hemorrhage
      - Intravascular fibrin thrombi
      - Stromal granulocytes prominent
      - Polymorphs present
      - Late menstrual: regenerative changes prominent

POD, postovulatory day.

mal fertility will have sporadic or even sequential luteal phases that are more than 2 days shorter (≥2 days) than the ideal 14 days. The term short luteal phase has been suggested for patients whose luteal phase is ≤11 days, which is regarded by many investigators as a type of LPD (see Underdeveloped Secretory Endometrium). These observations have been confirmed by many workers.

The second observation is that conventional Noyes' dating has low reproducibility (63,80,81). The poor interobserver agreement for conventional histologic dating of the endometrium using the criteria of Noyes and co-workers has been recognized for some time. Noyes and Haman report that two observers agreed on the same morphologic date 29% of the time, were within 1 day of each other in 63% of cases, and were within 2 days of each other in 82% of cases (82). These poor results have been duplicated in newer studies (40,63,80,83). As a consequence, the results of endometrial dating should be reported as a range of 2 days, to reflect this variability. Morphometric dating is more reproducible than Noyes' dating and provides insight into the development of the normal endometrium and those deviations from normal that would warrant the label LPD, but it has little practical clinical value at this time (60,61,63,80,81).

Third is the observation that endometrial morphologic features are more highly correlated with LH surge than with the NMP (78,80,84,85). As a consequence, there is a growing tendency to use as the point of reference the midcycle surge of LH (which sets ovulation into motion 24 hours after the LH peak) rather than the first day of menstrual flow (86).

Fourth is the finding that the correlation of endometrial pattern (whether assessed morphometrically or using Noyes' criteria) with the LH surge is the highest during that portion of the follicular phase and the luteal phase that straddles the day of the LH surge. Johannisson and co-workers (60,61) undertook a morphometric analysis of the EMBs of 90 apparently reproductively normal women and noted that the morphologic characteristics of the endometrium were remarkably uniform among women 3 days before the LH surge until 8 days afterward. Thus, substantial variability is present in normal women during the late luteal phase of the cycle, the usual time recommended for obtaining an EMB sample. Similar results have been reported by the Sheffield group (63,87). It seems that the timing of EMB in an infertility patient involves a trade-off between precision (first half of luteal phase better than second half) and relevance (second half provides a view of the cumulative progesterone effect over the duration of the cycle). Most workers opt for relevance.

All of these observations expose the considerable problems involved in deciding whether a secretory endometrium is appropriately developed for a woman's chronological date. It is important to note that these problems tend to call the definition of LPD into question. For these and other reasons, some clinicians involved in the treatment of infertility have raised doubts about the wisdom of incorporating EMB in the initial workup of the infertile couple. There are better ways of ruling out structural disease of the uterus (hysterosalpingogram, hysteroscopy, laparoscopy) and establishing that cycles are ovulatory (e.g., noting that cycles are regular and obtaining a midluteal progesterone level). Finally, the diagnosis of LPD may not be worth the effort and expense of EMB except in a select subset of patients (see Clinical Significance of Luteal Phase Defect) (29,73,88–90,91).

These skeptical observations notwithstanding, pathologists are still expected to assign morphologic dates to cycling en-

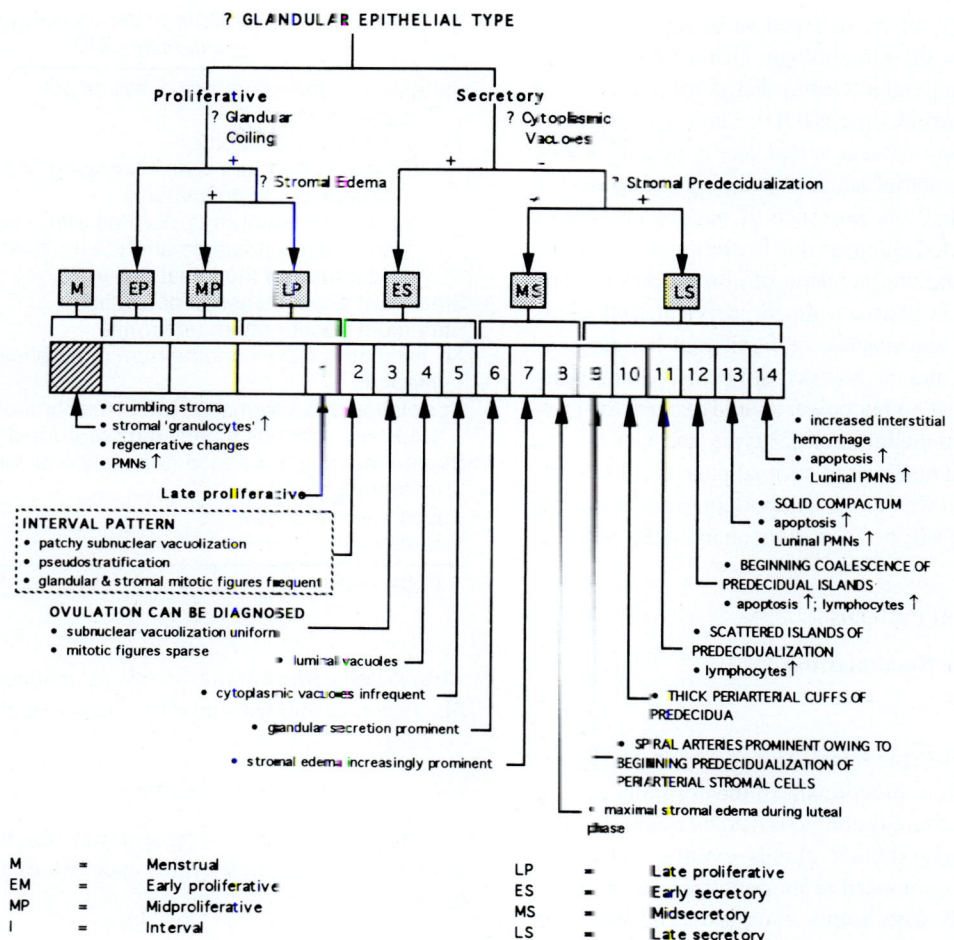

FIG. 1. Decision tree for endometrial dating (see Table 6).

dometria, and, for the biopsies of infertility patients, they may be asked to correlate that date with some estimate of the patient's chronological date. When information about ovulation in the current cycle is not available, the chronological date can be estimated by back dating. It must be said as a cautionary note, however, that back dating (using the NMP method) has been found by most workers to be inadequate for assessing the presence of corpus luteum defects (84). It is important to emphasize that the morphologic changes taking place from day to day are continuous, resulting in overlapping morphologic patterns that in most observers' views preclude reliably assigning postovulatory morphologic dates more closely than within a 48-hour interval pinpointed, on one's best guess, to the true morphologic date (e.g., the endometrium looks most like the POD 10 pattern, but the next choice of pattern would be POD 11; diagnosis: POD 10–11) (34,86).

Deciding whether a woman has ovulated by examining an EMB sample taken in what is presumed to be her late luteal phase is usually a trivial matter; the presence of a late secretory endometrium means that ovulation has taken place. Deciding whether or not ovulation has occurred in the early luteal phase is more challenging. The characteristic light microscopic postovulatory secretory changes in the en-

dometrium lag behind actual ovulation by at least 1 day. A biopsy on POD 2 will show spotty, nonuniform subnuclear vacuolation (interval pattern). Such vacuolation may be seen in late proliferative endometria as well as in other types of nonsecretory endometria and is, for this reason, not diagnostic of ovulation. Because of the ambiguous morphologic picture in the early postovulatory period, EMBs are usually conducted well into the presumed luteal phase of the cycle, preferably PODs 11 to 13. We require uniform subnuclear vacuolation in 50% of the glands before diagnosing the earliest morphologic evidence of ovulation; this evidence usually is present by POD 3.

Accurate endometrial dating requires attention to a number of details (33). Dating features should be sought only in fragments of endometrial functionalis, which are lined by surface epithelium; fragments of basalis and the lower uterine segment should be ignored. The assigned date should be of the most developed area and should be based on features near the surface epithelium (the "egg's eye view" of Noyes) (33).

There are several preconditions for assigning a morphologic date to an endometrium. Assigning a date to an EMB is obviously not possible in the absence of an adequate specimen in a noncycling endometrium (e.g., a nonsecretory pattern other than proliferative), in a patient being treated with medication that alters the morphologic characteristics of the endometrium, or in an endometrium that is inflamed or one that houses an intrauterine device (IUD). Thus, a precondition for applying the dating criteria is that one is dealing with a roughly normal endometrial pattern. Scanning-power examination should establish the presence of pattern uniformity (apart from the expected variation due to sectioning randomly oriented fragments and the inclusion of normal out-of-phase fragments of the lower uterine segment, cervical epithelium, and stratum basalis), the absence of significant budding and branching of glands, and the absence of necrosis and inflammation. Examination at higher power should exclude the presence of significant epithelial nuclear atypia and confirm the absence of significant numbers of stromal plasma cells. Table 7 lists the features that we think are important to address in the pathology report for EMB performed for an infertility workup.

Normal Endometrial Patterns

Normal Proliferative Endometrium

Description

Refer to Fig. 1 and Table 6 in conjunction with the text in this section. The stratum functionalis of the normally cycling proliferative endometrium is characterized by nonbranching, nonbudding, similarly shaped glands evenly distributed throughout a stroma composed of monomorphous, undifferentiated stromal cells with scanty cytoplasm and indistinct cell margins supplied by a uniformly developed, arborizing vasculature with thin walls (Fig. 2). Early in proliferation, the glands are tubular and of narrow caliber; as proliferation continues, they become increasingly coiled, and their caliber increases. Normal proliferative endometria are further marked by pseudostratified, mitotically active, elongated epithelial cells with dense chromatin and mitotically active stromal cells. Most of the vessels are inconspicuous and capillary-like, particularly near the endometrial surface.

TABLE 7. *The contents of the pathology report for an infertility EMB*

Statement of the adequacy of the biopsy
Suggest rebiopsy if
Sample is inadequate
If the endometrium is disintegrating and not clearly menstrual (i.e., postovulatory)
If the endometrium is disintegrating, postovulatory, but otherwise undatable and the main concern is with the adequacy of the luteal phase
Statement about evidence of ovulation
Statement about pattern uniformity
An estimate of the endometrium's morphologic date (2-day interval)
Correlation with information about the chronological date (time of LH surge or basal body temperature shift)
Statement about presence or absence of "organic disease"
Inflammation
Endometrial polyps
Submucous leiomyomas

EMB, endometrial biopsy; LH, luteinizing hormone.

Clinicopathologic Correlation

A normal proliferative pattern may also be seen in association with anovulatory cycles and with exogenous estrogen therapy.

Interval Endometrium

Description

In essence, an interval endometrium is a late proliferative endometrium in which the glands are coiled and in which less than half the epithelial cells feature spotty, nonuniform sub-

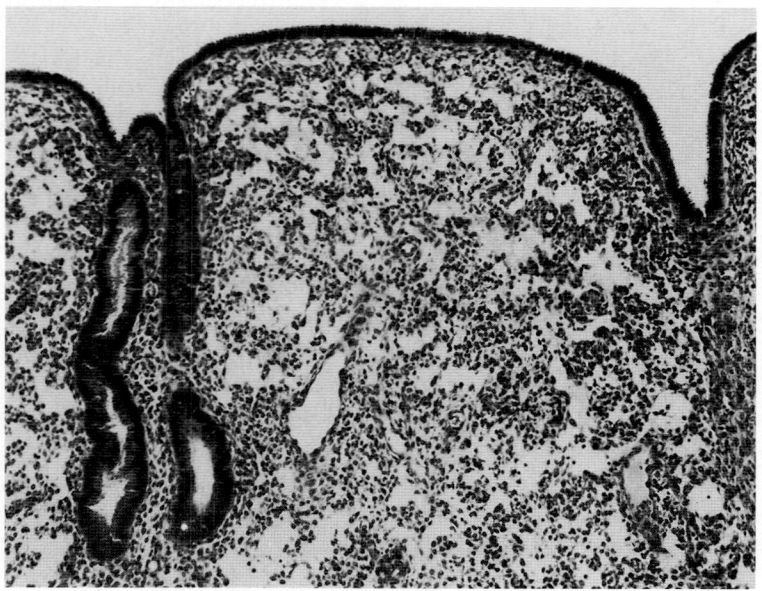

FIG. 2. Normal midproliferative endometrium. This endometrium can be identified as proliferative because elongated, dense, pseudostratified nuclei line the glands. The stroma is edematous, causing the stromal cell nuclei to be spaced apart. This appearance can be confused with a predecidual pattern, in which the nuclei are widely spaced by virtue of their cytoplasm. Confusion can be avoided by attending to the nuclear features of the glandular cells, specifically the elongated, dense nuclei characteristic of proliferative phase endometrium, and by remembering that predecidual cells have a distinct cytoplasm, often with easily discernible cytoplasmic margins.

nuclear vacuolation. Two points about the ultrastructural appearance of the endometrium during this period should be made parenthetically. First, there is ultrastructural evidence of secretion throughout the menstrual cycle; it is the relative increase in secretory activity (visible on H&E preparations) after ovulation that motivates the designation secretory phase (62). Second, the first unambiguous evidence of ovulation seen in the endometrium on ultrastructural examination is the appearance of the distinctive nucleolar channel system (62).

Clinicopathologic Correlation

The presence of this pattern is no guarantee that ovulation has occurred, even though the normal endometrium from PODs 1 to 2 has this appearance.

Normal Early Secretory Endometrium Postovulatory Days 2 to 5

Description

The endometrium during this time features coiled glands composed of cells resembling those found in the proliferative phase, but more than half the glandular cells contain relatively large cytoplasmic vacuoles. These vacuoles serve as the marker of early secretory endometria. The glands are set within a non-predeciduated stroma. The precise date assigned to such patterns depends upon the location of the cytoplasmic vacuole (subnuclear or supranuclear) and the number of mitotic figures present (Table 6, Figs. 1 and 3).

Clinicopathologic Correlation

This pattern may be accompanied by a clinical history of midcycle spotting and Mittelschmerz.

Normal Midsecretory Endometrium Postovulatory Days 6 to 8

Description

The midsecretory endometrium is characterized by fully coiled secretory glands lined by cells with round, often vesicular nuclei. The cytoplasm of such cells does not contain large cytoplasmic vacuoles, but luminal secretions may well be present. The stroma has not begun to undergo predeciduation. The fine-tuning of the postovulatory date within 48 hours in this segment of the secretory phase depends upon an evaluation of the extent of stromal edema and the prominence of the glandular luminal secretion, as summarized in Fig. 1 and Table 6. The absence of extensive vacuolation and of predecidua is the most useful marker of midsecretory endometria (Fig. 1).

Clinicopathologic Correlation

Implantation occurs during this part of the cycle. This morphologically normal pattern may be clinicopathologically (functionally) abnormal, depending upon the time of ovulation.

Normal Late Secretory Endometrium Postovulatory Days 9 to 14

Description

At the beginning of this phase in the cycle, low-power examination reveals that the spiral arteries are prominent, owing in part to the thickness of their walls but also largely to the cuffs of predeciduated stromal cells around them. Predeciduation begins initially around spiral arteries (POD 10) and then extends to form islands in the superficial reaches of the endometrial stroma. It marks the beginning of the last third of the secretory phase (Fig. 4). At the end of the late secretory phase, these decidual islands become confluent and then, as menstruation becomes imminent, are dissected by interstitial hemorrhage. Associated with the progressive predeciduation of the endometrial stroma is the increase in the number of "stromal granulocytes" (Fig. 5). These cells have bean-shaped, dense nuclei; inconspicuous cytoplasm; and cytoplasmic granules visible with special stains and occasionally on H&E preparations. These enigmatic cells, once thought to derive from the endometrial stroma, have been shown by immunoperoxidase techniques to be derived from bone marrow. Whether they are macrophages or represent subpopulations of T cells is still unresolved (92–95).

Menstrual Endometrium (59)

Description

The menstrual pattern features disintegrating fragments of fully developed secretory endometrium. The glands are di-

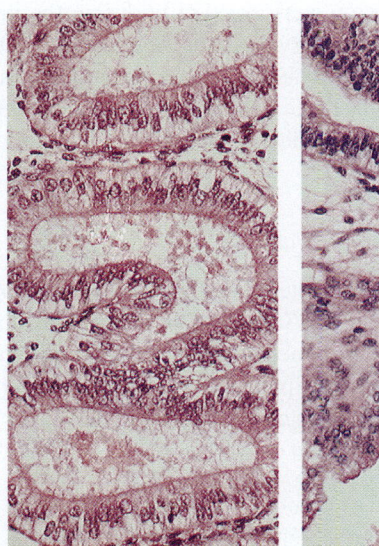
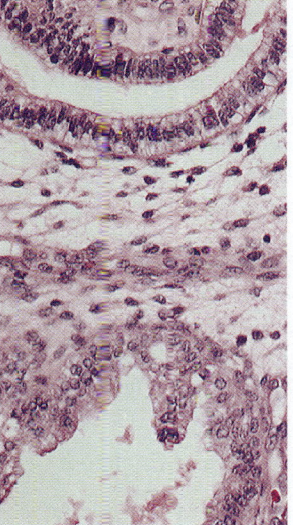

FIG. 3. Types of normal secretory epithelium. *Left*: Uniform subnuclear vacuolation is present in coiled secretory glands. *Right*: Uniform subnuclear vacuolation above and nonvacuolated secretory epithelium below.

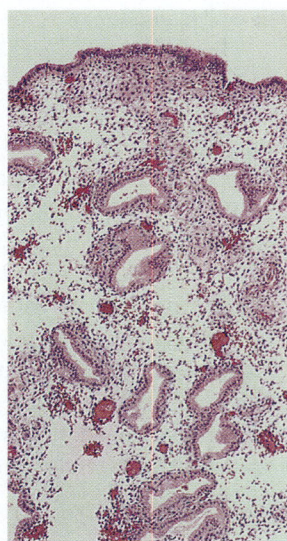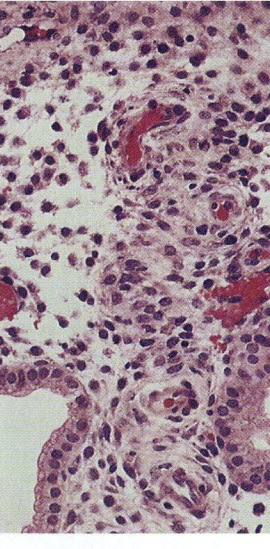

FIG. 4. Normal late secretory endometrium (postovulatory days 9 to 10). Coiled, uniform secretory glands lined by nonvacuolated secretory epithelium are set within an edematous stroma. The distinctive feature of postovulatory days 9 to 10 is the beginning of prediciduation around developed spiral arteries.

lated and lined by flattened cells, often with frayed borders (secretory exhaustion), and the stroma is fully prediciduated. Karyorrhectic fragments are present in the subnuclear area of some glands (apoptosis), the cell margins are frayed, the epithelial nuclei are pyknotic, and fibrin thrombi are present in vessels and sometimes within the stroma. Fibrin thrombi are a very useful feature in the identification of endometrial disintegration. As menstruation proceeds, the glands break up into strips, the stroma crumbles, and the epithelial cells lose cohesion.

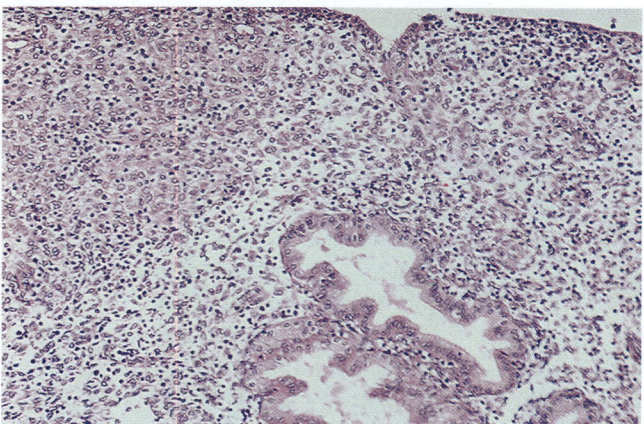

FIG. 5. Normal late secretory endometrium (postovulatory days 12 to 13). This endometrium features tightly coiled glands lined by nonvacuolated secretory epithelium set within extensively prediciduated stroma. Stromal prediciduation involves the surface endometrial stroma in a patchy fashion, and large numbers of "stromal granulocytes" are scattered throughout prediciduated cells.

Clinicopathologic Correlation

Menstrual shedding should be distinguished from shedding of abnormal endometrial tissue, for example, premature shedding of proliferative endometria, shedding of hyperplastic endometria, and sloughing of disintegrating fragments of carcinoma.

Differential Diagnosis

Compact Late Proliferative Stroma Versus Prediciduated Stroma

Prediciduation begins around spiral arteries and only later becomes confluent (Fig. 4). It is invariably accompanied by prominent spiral arteries with thicker walls than the thin-walled, capillary-like vessels of the late proliferative endometrium. Proliferative-phase stromal cells have indistinct cell margins and scanty cytoplasm, whereas decidual cells have abundant cytoplasm and more distinct cell margins. When edema is prominent, proliferative stromal cell nuclei may be spread apart and appear to have abundant cytoplasm, which can cause them to resemble decidual cells. Attention to stromal cell margins, the vascular pattern, and the nuclear features of the glandular cells will help avoid misclassifying such proliferative stromal changes as secretory.

Interval Versus Early Secretory Pattern

The importance of this distinction is that an early secretory pattern (PODs 2–3) is required before ovulation can be confidently diagnosed. We require that at least 50% of the glandular cells show uniform subnuclear vacuolation before asserting that ovulation has occurred. The reason for this prerequisite is that scattered subnuclear vacuoles can be seen in a wide variety of nonsecretory conditions, including endometrial hyperplasia and well-differentiated "secretory" carcinoma. If the biopsy is performed only during the presumed last third of the secretory phase of the cycle, this 50% rule need only rarely be invoked; if the biopsy is, in fact, taken in the presumed late luteal phase, the endometrium's maturation is substantially delayed, and it would be abnormal on that account.

Secretions in Nonsecretory Glands

The finding of secretory material in glands is entirely nonspecific and may be seen in a variety of contexts other than the midsecretory phase endometrium. In particular, luminal glandular secretions may be found in disordered proliferative endometria, hyperplasia, and carcinoma.

Nonsecretory Epithelial Cell Vacuolation

The presence of a large secretory vacuole in the cytoplasm of endometrial epithelial cells is only one cause of epithelial cell clearing. In some stages of their evolution, ciliated cells (normally present in proliferative endometria) are cleared, and lymphocytes migrating through epithelium may produce cytoplasmic clearing. Cleared cells can be seen in some patterns of squamous or morular differentiation and also in mucinous metaplasia.

Nonmenstrual Hemorrhage in Endometrial Biopsies

Hemorrhage in an endometrial sampling may be produced by a number of processes other than menstruation. Hemorrhage is a feature of any disintegrating endometrium, including those produced by estrogen-withdrawal bleeding in an anovulatory patient. It is, of course, common to see blood in any endometrial sampling, simply as a result of the operative procedure.

Isolated, Out-of-step, Cystically Dilated Glands

Isolated, cystically dilated or budded glands are commonly encountered in otherwise normal endometria, and, as isolated findings, they do not provide an adequate explanation for a patient's infertility.

Midsecretory Versus Late Secretory Endometria

In late secretory endometria, the predecidua first forms cuffs around vessels and then coalesces to form islands in the superficial endometrium. Later, these islands become confluent. Predecidua is absent in midsecretory endometria.

OTHER SECRETORY PATTERNS (70,96–102)

Deviations from the patterns expected in endometria during the normal secretory phase may sometimes be encountered, particularly in infertile women (103). The pathogenesis and significance of these changes are the subject of debate. Some researchers believe these endometria are the result of inadequate corpus luteum function, while others implicate a defect in the endometrium itself. Indeed, some of these patterns, particularly underdeveloped (out of phase) endometria, may be normal variations of no particular significance in explaining a couple's infertility. Patients with unusual secretory patterns may experience oligomenorrhea or hypomenorrhea as well as infertility.

Underdeveloped Secretory Endometria

Description

This term is used to denote two classes of deviant endometria. Into the first class fall endometria with abnormal morphologic features, in which the glands are inadequately developed. This abnormal development may take the form of inadequate coiling (suggesting deficiencies in the proliferative phase) or a deficiency in the quantity of secretion and the extent of stromal predecidual reaction (suggesting deficiencies in the luteal phase). Into the second group fall endometria with normal morphologic characteristics (i.e., they fit comfortably into one of the 14 POD morphologic pigeonholes) but are seen to be inappropriately delayed when correlated with the patient's chronological time of ovulation (as determined by an assessment of the true time of ovulation—back dating, BBT, LH surge, hormone levels, etc.).

Clinicopathologic Correlation

These underdeveloped secretory endometria are the morphologic correlates of the controversial clinical entity LPD (34,64,75 78,104,105–115). LPD is an ovulatory dysfunction that manifests at the ovarian level in the form of an insufficient production of progesterone over the lifetime of the corpus luteum and at the endometrial level through an inadequately developed secretory endometrium. Just as "polycystic ovary disease" has been recognized as a syndrome with several different etiologies featuring chronic anovulation, so, too, LPD is now recognized as a syndrome that may be caused by many different factors—hypothalamic (e.g., disturbances of prolactin secretion, exercise, and weight-loss-related endocrinopathies), ovarian (e.g., extremes of age), and endometrial (e.g., steroid receptor deficiency, mucosa overlying uterine septum, leiomyoma) (13,116) In addition, the administration of ovulation-inducing agents (e.g., clomiphene) may produce this pattern in the endometrium (117).

The gold standards for the diagnosis of LPD are one or more of the following endometrial abnormalities. The first is morphologically normal but incompletely developed secretory endometria (sampled within 2 days of menstruation) associated with a luteal phase of normal length. This is the out-of-phase (OOP) endometrium. It is traditional to judge the adequacy of endometrial maturation using the NMP method for approximating the true time of ovulation, but objections to this method were presented earlier herein. Investigators disagree on the required magnitude of the discrepancy before labeling an endometrium as OOP: some argue for ≥2 days, while others favor ≥3 days. The finding, on serial EMBs, by Davis et al. (78) of a high rate of OOP cycles in normal, fertile, cycling women suggests that the figure of ≥3 days is the threshold with the greater specificity. The use of hormonal or a combination of hormonal and strict morphologic criteria has been urged by some investigators (37,118–120).

The second abnormality is morphologically abnormal endometria featuring dysynchronous development of glands and stroma. This is particularly evident in the endometria of patients treated with ovulation-inducing medication (117). Third, there may be morphologically normal (77,100) secretory endometria associated with a luteal phase of ≤11 days' duration. As noted previously, the importance of this last pattern has been blunted by the observation that normally fertile women may, on occasion, have cycles of this length. Moreover, Smith and colleagues (100) found no statistical difference in the occurrence of luteal phases lasting ≤11 days between 35 women with unexplained infertility (9%) and 92 controls (8%).

These morphologic abnormalities must be more than sporadic to warrant a diagnosis of LPD, but the definition of what constitutes a more than sporadic abnormality varies from investigator to investigator. Some argue that LPD may be diagnosed on a single OOP biopsy sample for women considered to be at high risk (history of recurrent abortions, clomiphene treatment, patient's age ≥35 years) (34,121). In the absence of a suggestive clinical history (the usual situation), the majority of researchers require that at least two successive cycles be OOP. Balasch and Vanrell (105) suggest that a third biopsy be obtained if the first two biopsies are at variance.

Clinical Significance of Luteal Phase Defect

LPD has been confirmed in the context of nonhuman primate research, but the clinical importance of LPD is much more questionable. LPD is undoubtedly responsible for a substantial percentage of repeated early pregnancy wastage (habitual abortion) (25–60%) and is a relatively common finding in patients treated with clomiphene (20–50%). LPD may be responsible for the infertility of a small minority of patients; estimates of LPD among infertile couples range from 3% to 20%, depending upon the stringency of the criteria used to define the condition (73,90).

What is the role of LPD in infertility? Clement reviews a number of observations that cast doubt on the role of LPD in infertility (109). (a) The ability of the blastocyst to implant at ectopic sites, such as the fallopian tubes or peritoneum, suggests that the blastocyst is not particularly discriminating about the milieu in which it implants. (b) The incidence of LPD in infertile women (Noyes' dating compared with NMP ovulatory date) may not be significantly different from that of normally fertile women (122). On the other hand, more sophisticated methodology (morphometric dating compared with LH surge ovulatory dating) has shown significant differences between these two populations (123,124). (c) There are no double-blind, controlled studies in which infertile women with biopsy-diagnosed LPD have been randomized into treatment and placebo groups, with comparison of term pregnancy rates after appropriate follow-up intervals (125). Several retrospective studies have failed to show that therapy for LPD increases pregnancy rates over the spontaneous pregnancy rates in untreated patients (122). Wentz and associates conclude that "in a routine infertile population, among whom hyperprolactinemia and low body weight and other conditions were rare, the diagnosis and treatment of luteal phase inadequacy did not benefit the population in terms of pregnancy and its outcome."

Mixed Secretory Patterns

Description

This term is used when there is more than 2 days' disparity in the development of the secretory endometrium from region to region of the stratum functionalis (126).

Clinicopathologic Correlation

The clinical significance of this pattern is unknown.

Secretory Change Superimposed on Abnormal Nonsecretory Patterns (127)

Description

Secretory change may be superimposed on a disordered proliferative endometrium, endometrial hyperplasia, or carcinoma. This condition can usually be recognized, because the glands in these processes are frequently branched, whereas the glands of the normal secretory endometrium are coiled. The diagnostic importance of this phenomenon is that the features used to distinguish atypical hyperplasia (AH) from well-differentiated carcinoma may be lost or substantially altered in these circumstances. Extensive secretory change in well-differentiated endometrial adenocarcinoma is referred to as "secretory carcinoma." We require that the architectural and cytologic features of carcinoma be present before making this diagnosis (see later section that discusses carcinoma).

Clinicopathologic Correlation

Secretory changes of this sort may be produced by spontaneous ovulation or prebiopsy administration of progestational agents.

Differential Diagnosis

Atypical Hyperplasia with Secretory Change Versus Secretory Carcinoma

Although secretory carcinomas are very low grade, the architectural and cytologic features of well-differentiated carcinoma must be present before making that diagnosis. These characteristics include a rather extensive cribriform pattern,

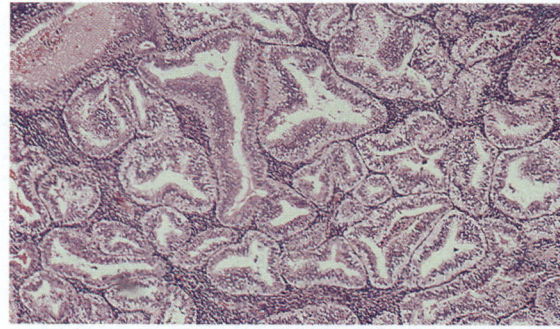

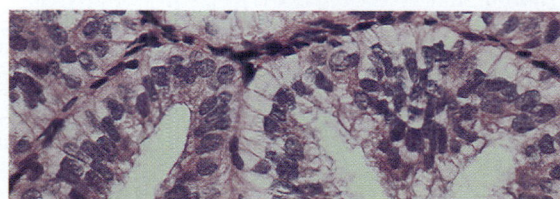

FIG. 6. Complex hyperplasia with superimposed secretory changes. *Top*: The budding and branching diagnostic of complex hyperplasia. *Bottom*: Uniform subnuclear vacuolation produced by the progesterone this patient received. This pattern must be distinguished from secretory carcinoma (see text). In secretory carcinoma, the cytologic features are those of carcinoma.

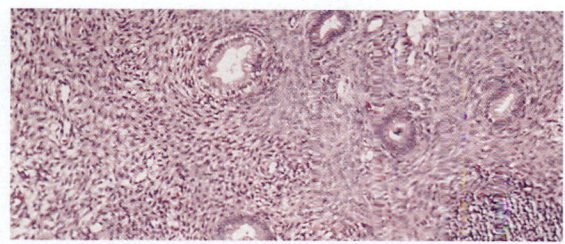
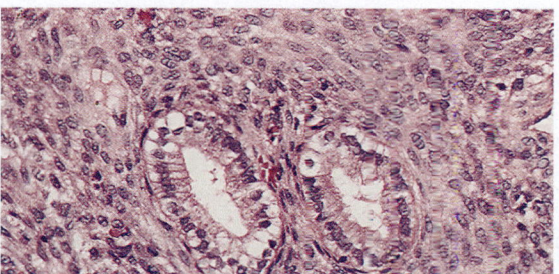

FIG. 7. The progestogen effect features underdeveloped noncoiled glands lined by patchy, vacuolated secretory epithelium set within a predeciduated stroma.

some degree of nucleomegaly, nuclear rounding, chromatin abnormalities, and mitotic figures. If most of these features are not present but the architecture is complex, we designate the process as atypical complex hyperplasia with a superimposed secretory effect and specify the degree of cytologic atypia (Fig. 6; see also Fig. 67).

Secretory Patterns Stemming from Administration of Progestational or Combined Estrogenic-progestational Agents (128–132)

It is difficult to determine the effects of progestins on an endometrium unprimed by estrogen. The morphologic patterns will depend on the initial state of the endometrium, the dose employed and the duration of treatment, and the type of drug used. Combined estrogenic-progestational agents typically produce a weakly secretory pattern characterized by underdeveloped, noncoiled glands set within a spindled, vaguely predeciduated stroma containing thin-walled vascular channels (Fig. 7) (71,129,133,134). A fully developed decidual response is sometimes seen, and the stromal cells may be atypical (128). With continued use, there is a tendency for the endometrium to become progressively thinned. At this stage it is not unusual for it to consist of only a single layer of surface epithelium covering a weakly predeciduated or spindled stroma that is only several cells thick and populated with few or no tubular glands.

GESTATIONAL ENDOMETRIUM

Following implantation, the secretory changes in the endometrium become more pronounced, and the fully developed gestational endometrium can usually be recognized on the basis of the features discussed here. Such changes in the endometrium, however, also can be seen in patients harboring an ectopic pregnancy as well as in patients receiving progestogen therapy (135,136).

Early Gestational Endometrium

Description

Hertig described changes that he considered to be indicative, but not diagnostic of early gestation (135,137): the coincidence of prominent glandular luminal secretion, prominent predeciduation, and prominent stromal edema. In the cycling endometrium, these changes assume their maxima in a sequential fashion. In early gestational endometria, their maximal development is simultaneous. In biopsy material, these secretory changes may not be particularly conspicuous (137).

Clinicopathologic Correlation

When these changes are encountered in an EMB, they are highly suggestive of early gestation, but because there is considerable overlap with late secretory changes in the cycling endometrium, they are not diagnostic. Obviously, extrauterine as well as intrauterine pregnancy can cause such endometrial changes.

Biopsing During the Cycle of Conception

The recommendation that EMBs for evaluation of the luteal phase be taken within 2 days of the onset of menses carries with it the risk that a pregnancy may be interrupted. The incidence of cycle-of-conception biopsies ranges from 1% to 4%. Several authors have examined the rate of spontaneous abortions subsequent to an EMB performed during a cycle of conception and have *not* found an increase in miscarriage rates (121,138,139). Herbert et al. (140) demonstrated the value of rapid urinary pregnancy test before luteal phase EMB, to avoid ever this potential risk. Barrier contraception during the biopsy cycle has also been recommended. Much less frequently (0.6%), the implantation site itself is recovered in a biopsy sample and is inevitably followed by abortion (141).

Fully Developed Gestational Endometrium

Description

The fully developed gestational endometrium is characterized by sheets of decidua surrounding glands lined by relatively low cuboidal or flattened cells. Some of the glands may be tubular or gaping rather than coiled. Glandular cells with inclusion-like cleared chromatin can be seen in the presence of trophoblasts. Although they resemble nuclei infected with herpesvirus, there is no evidence that virus is present in such cells (142,143). Associated findings in curettage specimens containing fully developed gestational endometria depend, of course, on the age of the gestation, and they range from primary villi and anchoring cytotrophoblastic tissue to fetal parts and placental fragments in more advanced gestations. Intermediate trophoblasts infiltrate the endometrium and the underlying myometrium in normal gestation, and these often large, bizarre-appearing cells must not be misconstrued as evidence of a gestational trophoblastic neoplasm or sarcoma.

Clinicopathologic Correlation

The unequivocal diagnosis of intrauterine pregnancy requires, in our opinion, the presence of chorionic villi, fetal parts, or unambiguous trophoblastic cells within the uterus. Immunohistochemical techniques may help identify trophoblastic cells (144,145).

Arias-Stella Reaction (146–151)

Description

This change is marked (Fig. 8) by hypersecretory glands lined by large cells with abundant clear to eosinophilic cytoplasm and irregularly shaped, hyperchromatic, smudged, enlarged nuclei exhibiting striking pleomorphism. Mitotic figures are very rare, if they are present at all. The stroma is often deciduated. The Arias-Stella reaction may be focal, and the remainder of the endometrium may or may not exhibit a secretory reaction.

Clinicopathologic Correlation

The Arias-Stella phenomenon may be found in the endometrium in a variety of contexts, including normal pregnancy, gestational trophoblastic disease, ectopic gestation, and in association with the administration of exogenous hormones. This glandular reaction may also develop in extra-endometrial sites, such as the cervix or fallopian tubes, and in foci of endometriosis (152,153).

Gestational Pattern Without Placental Tissue or Fetal Parts

Description

Endometrial samples composed entirely of decidua and secretory glands with or without Arias-Stella reaction but *unassociated* with fetal or placental tissues are *not* diagnostic of intrauterine pregnancy. On occasion, such endometria may be shed intact ("decidual cast"). Typically, the secretory development is florid and characterized by dilated glands and inspissated secretions.

Clinicopathologic Correlation

These changes are not infrequently found in the endometria of patients who have spontaneously aborted an intrauterine gestation. They may also be seen in endometria associated with ectopic gestations (154) or with a corpus luteum cyst or persistent corpus luteum or in endometria that have responded to the administration of progestational agents (151). Endometrial vascular changes similar to atherosclerosis are commonly present in the decidual vessels of intrauterine gestations, but not in those associated with ectopic pregnancy (155). It is imperative to alert the clinician to the possibility of an ectopic gestation when the patient is suspected of being pregnant and the tissue recovered from the uterus does not show unequivocal features of intrauterine gestation.

Implantation Site Reaction, Placental Site Nodules, and Subinvolution of the Placental Site (156–159)

The endometrium and myometrium beneath an implantation site is invaded by trophoblasts shortly after implantation occurs. This phenomenon has been labeled syncytial metritis (erroneously, since the reaction is not inflammatory) but is better termed implantation site reaction. Trophoblasts have enlarged, often atypical nuclei that may be arranged in a syncytium; contain mitotic figures, including abnormal forms; and may invade blood vessels. Intermediate trophoblasts, cytotrophoblasts, and syncytial trophoblasts are all present in varying numbers. The resemblance to a malig-

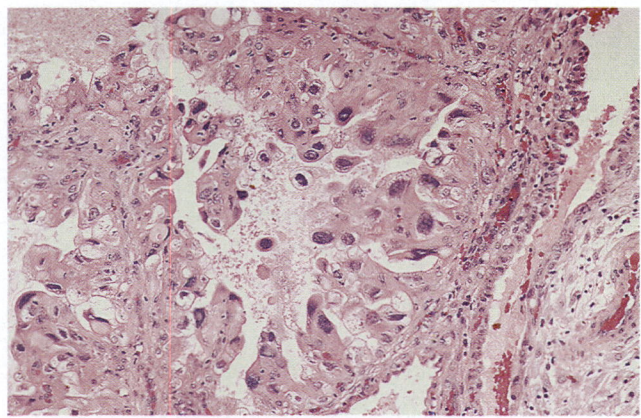
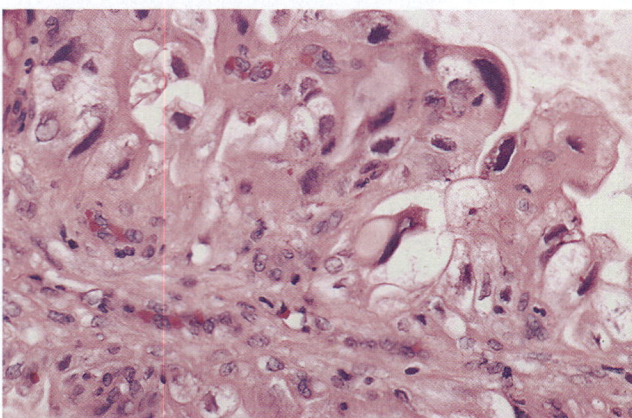

FIG. 8. Arias-Stella reaction. The endometrial glands are lined by enlarged cells with markedly hyperchromatic pleomorphic nuclei. The chromatin is smudged rather than coarse, as is the case in many carcinomas, and mitotic figures are not present. Knowledge of the age of the patient and a finding of accompanying decidua almost always allow this morphologic change to be distinguished from clear-cell carcinoma.

nant neoplasm can be striking, particularly if the infiltration is composed predominantly of intermediate trophoblasts. The latter often resemble smooth-muscle cells, and their nuclear atypia often raises the question of leiomyosarcoma. When the implantation site reaction does not promptly regress following abortion or delivery, it is designated subinvolution. Nodular aggregates of intermediate trophoblasts embedded in a hyaline matrix have been designated placental site nodules. The constituent cells are amphophilic, vacuolated, and mitotically inactive. There typically is no histologic or clinical evidence of a recent pregnancy (158,159).

Distinguishing choriocarcinoma from an implantation site is based on the bilaminar pattern of large numbers of cytotrophoblasts and syncytial trophoblasts in choriocarcinoma and the extensive hemorrhagic necrosis that is a feature of choriocarcinoma but not usually of an implantation site. Moreover, chorionic villi may be associated with an implantation site but are essentially absent in choriocarcinoma. Placental site trophoblastic tumor (PSTT) is composed of intermediate trophoblasts and shares many features with an implantation site. It is distinguished by the presence of confluent masses of intermediate trophoblasts and the absence of villi.

Syncytial trophoblasts and cytotrophoblasts predominantly produce human chorionic gonadotropin (HCG), while intermediate trophoblasts express large amounts of placental lactogen. HCG is absent in the latter cells, or expressed only in small quantities. Antibodies against these hormones are available, and they can be detected in cells in paraffin-embedded tissue sections. In addition to trophoblasts, subinvolution of the placental site is marked by patchy chronic inflammation and distended spiral arteries whose walls are composed, in part, of hyalinized decidua. These vessels (rather than retained placental fragments) are usually the culprits in postpartum hemorrhage. The chronic inflammation routinely encountered in this situation does not indicate clinically significant infection.

Differential Diagnosis

Arias-Stella Reaction Versus Clear-cell Carcinoma

Patients with the Arias-Stella reaction are in the childbearing years; they will have experienced a recent pregnancy or be pregnant, will have an HCG-producing tumor, or will have undergone hormonal therapy. The patient may be unaware of a pregnancy, however, especially if it is ectopic or has aborted. Tumors producing HCG and resulting in the Arias-Stella reaction may also be silent. Patients with clear-cell carcinoma of the endometrium are almost always postmenopausal, and their tumors are mitotically active. The cells in the Arias-Stella reaction are not mitotically active, and the chromatin is smudged rather than coarsely granular.

A stromal decidual reaction is often associated with the glands demonstrating the Arias-Stella reaction but not with the tumor glands of clear-cell carcinoma, unless the patient has received progestogen therapy. A distinctive localized endometrial proliferation associated with pregnancy has been described. It consists of a focal, microscopic epithelial proliferation featuring smoothly contoured cribriform endometrial glands lined by stratified, cytologically bland cells. The appearance is quite distinct from the Arias-Stella reaction (Fig. 3; see also Fig. 68). Despite its alarming appearance, this proliferation is unassociated with any clinical consequences (160).

Infiltrating Normal Trophoblastic Cells Versus Mimics

Normal trophoblasts invading beneath an implantation site can mimic malignant neoplasms, particularly leiomyosarcoma and choriocarcinoma. The clinical history will usually allow accurate interpretation; occasionally, immunohistochemical stains for HCG, placental lactogen, and muscle filaments will be indicated. An implantation site must be distinguished from choriocarcinoma (characterized by a lamellar pattern of syncytial trophoblasts and cytotrophoblasts as well as by extensive hemorrhage and necrosis), invasive hydatidiform mole (presence of villi), and PSTT (a mass composed mainly of intermediate trophoblasts). These neoplasms are further discussed in the chapter by Altshuler.

INFLAMMATION, NECROSIS, AND INFECTIONS (TABLE 16)

Endometritis

General Comments

The endometrium is normally populated by a variety of "inflammatory" cells, including lymphocytes (occasionally organized into follicles and germinal centers) and neutrophils or eosinophils. The latter infiltrate the stroma of late secretory, menstrual, and gestational endometria. These observations imply that specific morphologic criteria must be present before diagnosing clinically significant endometrial inflammation. These criteria are discussed in the following sections.

Acute Endometritis (161)

Description

This diagnosis requires the presence of confluent aggregates of polymorphonuclear cells (microabscesses) as well as infiltration and destruction of glandular epithelium. The diffuse infiltration of the endometrium by stromal neutrophils during menstruation should not be construed as evidence of acute endometritis (57). Chlamydial endometritis may be an acute or a mixed inflammatory process (162,163).

Nonspecific Chronic Endometritis (109,164–169)

Of the usual inflammatory cells, only plasma cells and probably eosinophils are normally absent from the endometrium. For this reason, most researchers in this field have regarded the presence of plasma cells as the sine qua non for establishing the diagnosis of chronic endometritis (71,166). Immunophenotypic techniques have largely confirmed the rarity of cells of B-lymphoid lineage (including plasma cells) in the endometrium of normal women (92–95).

Undoubtedly, large numbers of lymphocytes, lymphoid follicles, and germinal centers should be considered abnormal, but when they are present in significant numbers, there is almost always an associated plasma cell infiltrate, which should be documented before a diagnosis of chronic endometritis is made.

Description

A diagnosis of chronic endometritis requires the presence of more than rare plasma cells. In convincing examples, lymphocytes, lymphoid follicles, and histiocytes are also usually evident; the inflammatory infiltrate is often mixed. The stroma may be fibrous, and there may be glandular destruction. Xanthomatous endometritis is a form of chronic endometritis characterized by sheets of xanthoma cells.

Clinicopathologic Correlation

Chronic endometritis (as defined earlier) is usually encountered in the context of pelvic inflammatory disease, in association with the use of an IUD, or in connection with retained products of conception. Kiviat et al. found that the combination of acute inflammation (more than or equal to five PMNs per ×400 field in endometrial surface epithelium) and stromal plasma cells (more than or equal to one plasma cell per ×120 field in endometrial stroma) was a highly sensitive and specific rule for predicting the presence of culture-positive and laparoscopically visible salpingitis (170). One polymerase chain reaction study suggests that *Chlamydia trachomatis* is not implicated in mild to moderate chronic endometritis (171). This pattern has been associated with symptomatic bacterial vaginosis, a condition connected to high concentrations of potentially pathogenic aerobic and anaerobic organisms that replace the normal flora of the lower genital tract (172).

Chronic endometritis is also present in the endometrium immediately postpartum, but in this circumstance it is considered a normal finding (173). Most patients with chronic endometritis have menstrual abnormalities, and one-half of them experience pelvic pain. While florid endometritis may be a cause of infertility, the relevance of the occasional plasma cell to a couple's infertility is much less clear. Xanthomatous endometritis is seen most often in the elderly and is almost exclusively associated with cervical stenosis and pyometra (174–176).

Granulomatous Endometritis and Specific Infections

Tuberculous endometritis, characterized by a granulomatous inflammatory response, is rare in the United States but is a relatively common cause of infertility in other countries (177–179). Other causes of granulomatous endometritis as well as specific infections are listed in Table 16.

NONSECRETORY ENDOMETRIAL PATTERNS OTHER THAN NORMAL PROLIFERATIVE, INCLUDING ENDOMETRIOID ADENOCARCINOMA

Introduction

In addition to the normal proliferative endometrium of the menstrual cycle (discussed earlier), a spectrum of other nonsecretory patterns in which stroma plays a supportive role are often encountered in day-to-day practice (Fig. 9). We use the terms atrophic, weakly proliferative, disordered proliferative, hyperplastic, and carcinomatous to label the various morphologic patterns along this spectrum. With the exception of AHs and carcinomas, these patterns are normal in certain clinical conditions. For example, an atrophic endometrium is normal for the prepubertal girl and the elderly postmenopausal woman; however, it is distinctly abnormal during the reproductive years, unless the patient has been treated with hormones or suffers from ovarian failure. As a result, the clinical significance of many of these histopathologic patterns emerges only after clinicopathologic correlation. Patients with nonsecretory-type endometria may be asymptomatic; when they have symptoms they most often have experienced abnormal uterine bleeding.

If abnormal uterine bleeding occurs during the reproductive years and is not associated with a detectable uterine abnormality other than these nonsecretory patterns—again excluding AH and carcinoma—it is termed dysfunctional uterine bleeding (12). Uterine bleeding is designated abnormal if it is excessive or scanty or if it occurs at the wrong time. The clinical diagnosis of DUB should be made only after excluding other causes of uterine bleeding, including focal abnormalities (such as submucous leiomyomas and polyps), AH, carcinoma and other malignant neoplasms, gestational side effects, endometritis, and systemic coagulation abnormalities. The treatment of patients with abnormal bleeding is beyond the scope of this chapter and is discussed in several reviews (11,12,41,180–192).

Several generalizations can be derived from these sources.

1. Tissue sampling is mandatory in any patient who in clinical terms is at high risk of harboring a malignant or premalignant proliferation of the endometrium. The clinical criteria defining high risk vary from authority to authority.
2. Tissue sampling is rarely indicated in the adolescent, since abnormal bleeding is almost invariably due to anovulatory cycles and the risk of malignancy in this age group is extremely low (191,193).
3. The decision to obtain a tissue sample in patients taking hormone replacement therapy who bleed during their artificial cycle is complicated, and there are circumstances when it may not be necessary.

The endometrial patterns discussed later herein—with the exception of endometrial carcinoma and probably some forms of AH—are the morphologic reflections of alterations in prevailing serum steroid levels, whether derived from endoge-

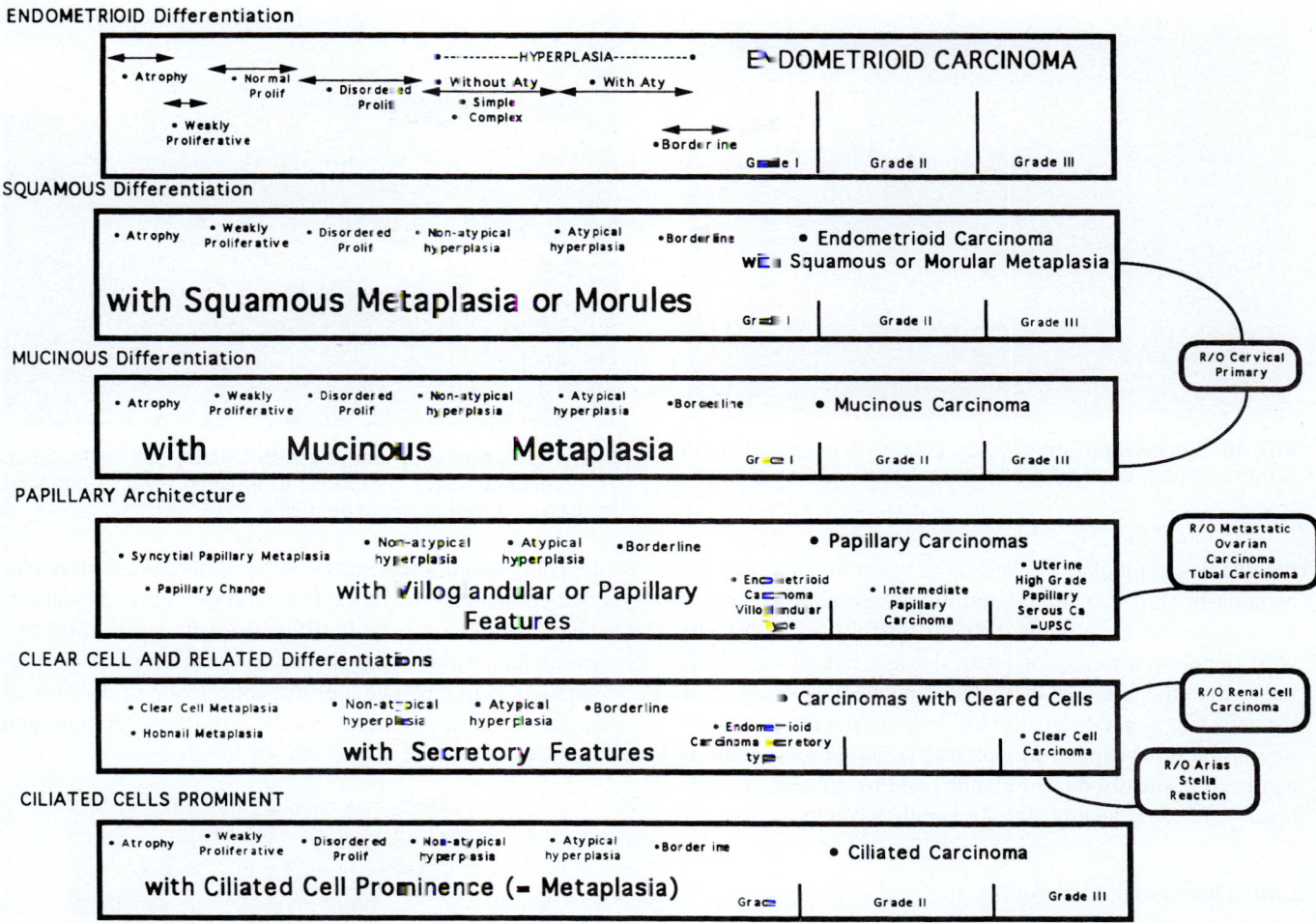

FIG. 9. The differential diagnosis of nonsecretory endometrial patterns. The epithelium of nonsecretory endometrial proliferations may have a variety of appearances. Best known is a differentiated appearance reminiscent of normal proliferative endometrium ("endometrioid"). Alternative differentiated epithelial and architectural patterns are frequently encountered; they include morular, squamous, mucinous, papillary, clear cell, and epithelial with a prominence of ciliated cells. These patterns are often mixed in a single proliferation. They can be further stratified in accordance with their architectural complexity and/or cytologic atypia. These designations are indicated in the top endometrioid strip and are bracketed by atrophy (left) and grade III carcinoma (right). The corresponding designations are indicated in the other strips; they include metaplasia for the benign proliferations and special variant carcinomas for the malignant ones. In short, this diagram can be thought of as a map of endometrial nonsecretory patterns. The histologic pattern is indicated in the vertical direction (y-axis), and the composite degree of architectural complexity and cytologic atypia is indicated in the horizontal direction (x-axis).

nous or exogenous sources. Atrophic and weakly proliferative endometria represent the appropriate response of a physiologically competent endometrium to depressed estrogen levels. Disordered proliferative endometria and hyperplastic endometria represent the physiologic normal endometrial response to elevated estrogen levels or prolonged estrogen stimulation. The reversibility of some well-differentiated endometrial adenocarcinomas using progestational agents or ovulation induction suggests that at least a subset of these proliferations may represent extreme responses of a physiologically normal endometrium to prolonged estrogen stimulation. In short, the endometrium in these circumstances can be thought of as functioning as a bioassay, reflecting in its changing morphologic features shifting serum estrogen levels.

Atrophic and Weakly Proliferative (Inactive) Endometria (194–197)

Description

Both of these terms refer to the appearance (and inferred activity) of the epithelium lining the glands of the endometria. The epithelium tends to be mitotically inactive and bland in terms of cytologic appearance. The glands are embedded in a similarly "inactive" spindled stroma that exhibits varying degrees of collagenation and practically no mitotic activity (Fig. 10). The ratio of glands to stroma is near unity, although pattern uniformity is variable. The glandular architecture may be cystic or budded, and the buds may even be closely packed, as in hyperplastic endometria; typically, however,

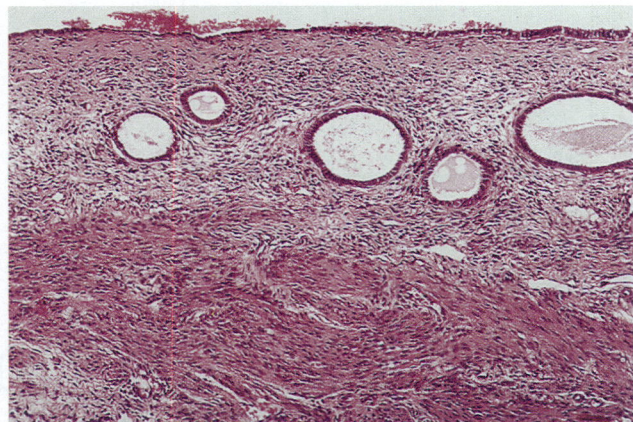

FIG. 10. Endometrial atrophy (low power). The endometrium is thin and populated by scattered, cystically dilated glands.

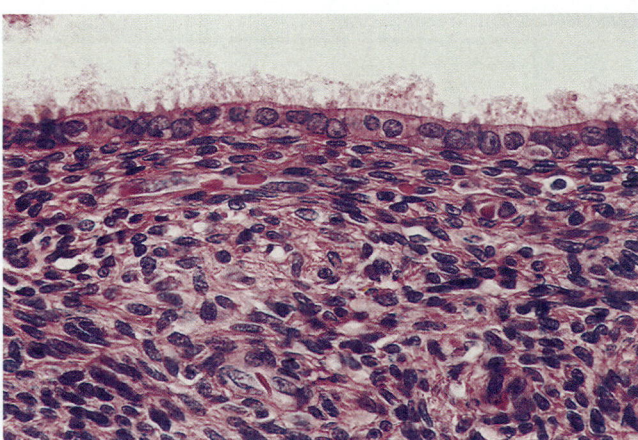

FIG. 11. Endometrial atrophy with ciliated cell metaplasia. The glandular lining is reduced to a single layer of cuboidal epithelium featuring prominent cilia.

the glands are tubular. Occasionally, the epithelium may be metaplastic (Fig. 11). Weakly proliferative endometria differ from those that are atrophic (Figs. 12–15) by virtue of cells with pseudostratified, elongated, densely basophilic nuclei rather than the cuboidal or flattened nuclei characteristic of the cells that populate an atrophic endometrium. Cystic atrophy is the term applied to endometria composed predominantly of cystically dilated glands lined by cuboidal to flattened (and consequently atrophic) epithelial cells.

Clinicopathologic Correlation

Atrophy and weakly proliferative patterns are normal in menopausal and perimenopausal women as well as prepubertal girls (197). Atrophic endometria are most commonly recovered in the endometrial biopsy sample from patients with postmenopausal bleeding (194,196). Such patterns are distinctly abnormal during the reproductive years, unless there is a history of hormonal medication. When seemingly atrophic endometrium is recovered, it is important to consider these alternatives: (a) scanty endometrial samples that consist only of basalis (make sure there is surface endometrium to evaluate), (b) samples that consist of only the lower uterine segment (look for hybrid endocervical-endometrial glands characteristic of the lower uterine segment), (c) the endometrial lining of a submucous myoma (look for rounded aggregates of smooth muscle underneath the endometrium), (d) fragments of endometrial polyp (look for other fragments in the sampling showing normal features and thick-walled vessels in the atrophic fragment), and (e) a progestogen effect (look for predecidual changes associated with underdeveloped, noncoiled glands).

Disordered Proliferative Endometrium (29,198,199)

Description

The disordered proliferative endometrium resembles the normal proliferative one in consisting of glands lined by cytologically bland, pseudostratified, proliferative, mitotically active epithelium and in having a roughly normal (unitary) ratio of glands to stroma. It differs from the normal proliferative endometrium in the absence of uniform glandular development (Fig. 16) The uniform appearance of the normal proliferative endometrium results from synchronous and

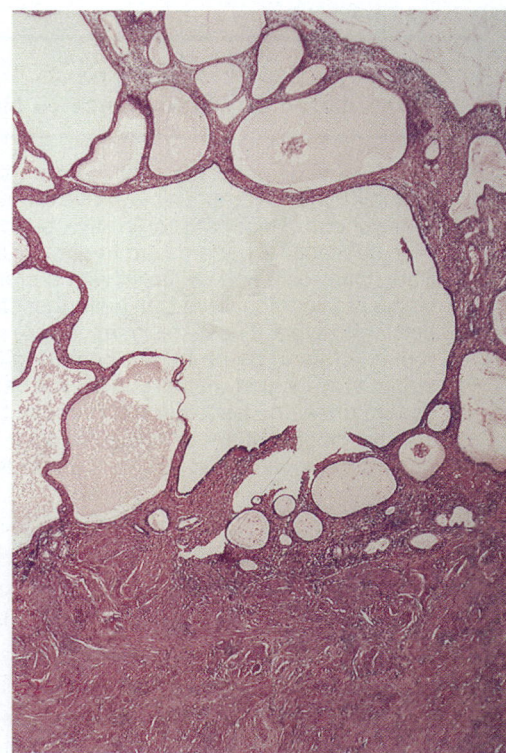

FIG. 12. Cystic atrophy (low power). The apparent shift in the glands-to-stroma ratio has come about because the glands are cystically dilated. There is no evidence of budding growth, however, and the epithelium lining the spaces is flattened. Cystic atrophy is probably the result of inspissated secretions, and it should not be confused with hyperplasia with cystically dilated glands. In the latter case, the epithelium is at least proliferative, if not atypical.

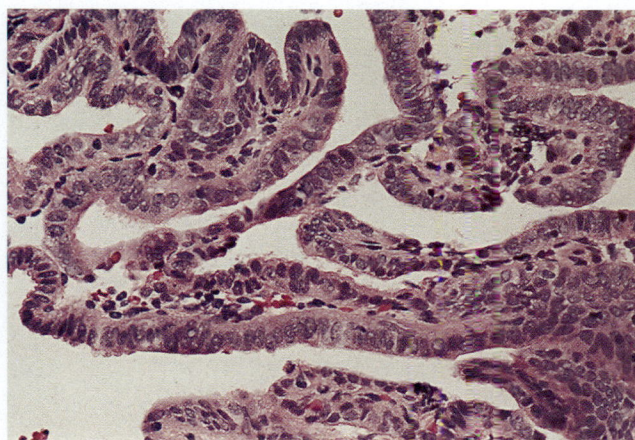

FIG. 13. Endometrial atrophy as seen in an endometrial sampling. On occasion, atrophic surface epithelium may be removed in coiled masses and may simulate hyperplasia because the glands are closely approximated.

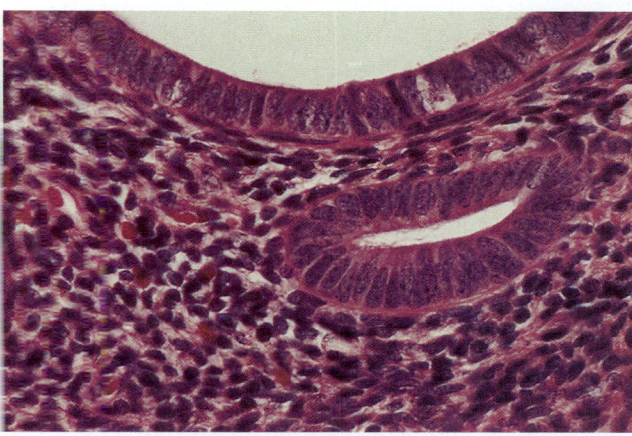

FIG. 15. Weakly proliferative endometrium (high power). Weakly proliferative endometrium features tubular glands lined by cells with pseudostratified nuclei. Mitotic figures are very sparse or absent. Such endometria differ from those with normal proliferation by virtue of the absence of mitotic figures and glandular development. They differ from atrophic endometria because the cells are pseudostratified rather than cuboidal or flattened. This is a common and normal pattern in the peri- and postmenopausal years.

coordinated growth of the fundal functionalis under the influence of estradiol. In contrast, the absence of pattern uniformity—a principal defining feature of disordered proliferative endometrium—is a result of dysynchronous growth of the functionalis (Fig. 17).

In some areas, the glands may be cystically dilated or may demonstrate varying degrees of shallow budding, while in other regions the glands are tubular, of narrow caliber, and set within abundant stroma. Metaplastic epithelium—particularly ciliated epithelium—is commonly encountered (Fig. 18). No significant cytologic atypia is present. Evidence of endometrial breakdown and hemorrhage (the morphologic correlate of abnormal bleeding) may be present and is characterized by thrombosed, thin-walled vessels and interstitial fibrin and hemorrhage (Fig. 19). Disordered proliferation differs from hyperplasia without cytologic atypia by virtue of its relatively normal ratio of glands to stroma, that is, the significant shift in the glands-to-stroma ratio in favor of glands that we require for a diagnosis of hyperplasia is absent. Thus, disordered proliferation serves as a morphologic "bridge" between normal proliferation and hyperplasia.

Clinicopathologic Correlation

This is a common and normal pattern in the perimenarchal and postmenopausal years. The functional correlates are anovulatory cycles and exogenous estrogen therapy (200).

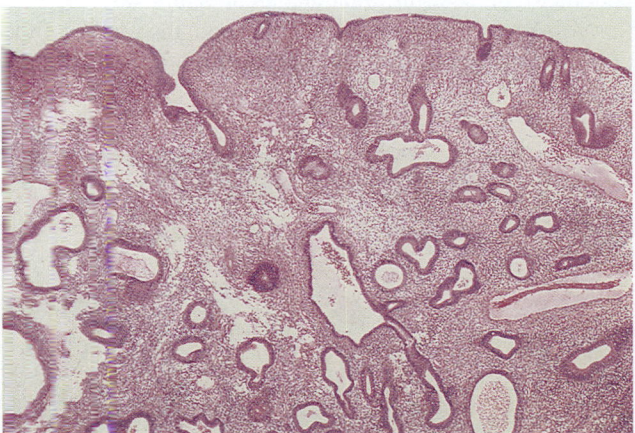

FIG. 16. Disordered proliferative endometrium (low power). This pattern features widely spaced glands that vary in size and shape. Some glands are cystically dilated, and others exhibit shallow budding. The hallmark of disordered proliferation is dysynchronous development of glands set within easily discernible stroma (see text). Disordered proliferation is common during anovulatory cycles, particularly in the perimenopausal years. We do not include this pattern in the category of hyperplasia.

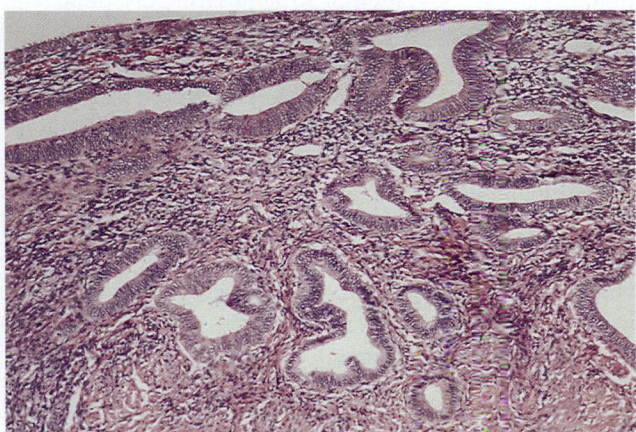

FIG. 14. Weakly proliferative (inactive) endometrium. This endometrium is thinned, but the budded and branched, widely spaced glands are lined by slightly pseudostratified epithelium.

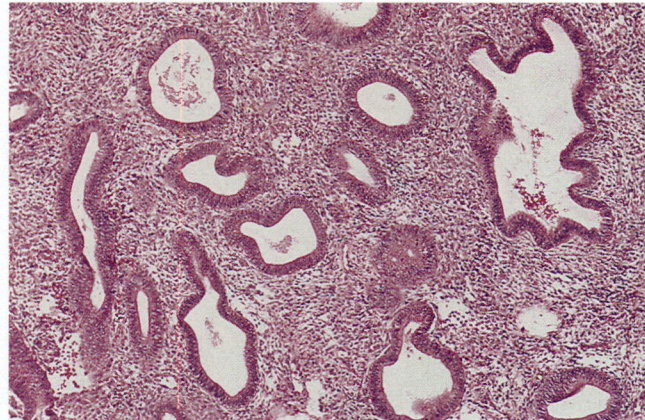

FIG. 17. Disordered proliferative endometrium (medium power). The endometrial glands have irregular shapes but are widely separated by mitotically active, proliferative-type stroma.

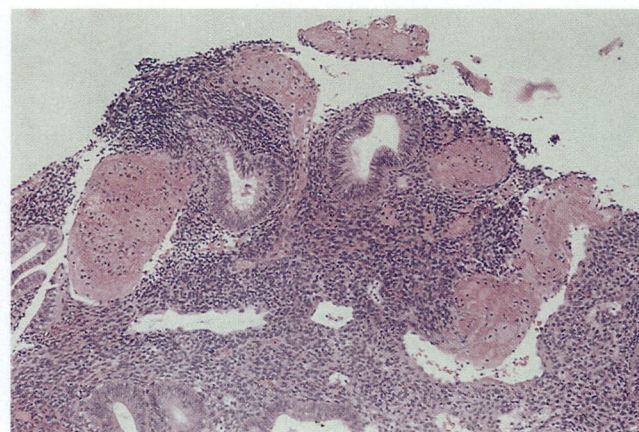

FIG. 19. Disordered proliferative endometrium. Patients with disordered proliferative endometrium typically have abnormal uterine bleeding. The morphologic correlate in the endometrial sampling is the presence of fibrin thrombi, seen here within thin-walled, distended vascular channels.

This pattern is considered by some researchers to represent hyperplasia, but hyperplasia also connotes to many clinicians a proliferation that puts the patient at increased risk of endometrial carcinoma. Because there is no evidence that patients with disordered proliferative endometria are at any greater risk of endometrial carcinoma than those without this pattern, we do not think the label hyperplasia is appropriate. Nevertheless, the International Society of Gynecologic Pathology recommends that disordered proliferation be included in the category of simple hyperplasia.

Hyperplasia (201–214)

Description

The term endometrial hyperplasia denotes a proliferating endometrium featuring glandular architectural abnormalities that result in glandular crowding and take the form of either cystic dilatation of glands (simple hyperplasia) or glandular budding (complex hyperplasia). Current taxonomy further stratifies hyperplastic endometria on the basis of their cytologic features into atypical endometrial hyperplasia and nonatypical endometrial hyperplasia, the latter term implying that significant cytologic atypia is absent (Table 8).

The characteristic architectural features of hyperplasia are glandular enlargement and budding. When it is excessive, budding leads to complex epithelial structures with numerous branching channels and papillary infoldings. Sectioning of these channels produces a pattern of closely approximated, narrow-caliber glands that, in extreme cases, can mimic the cribriform pattern characteristic of carcinoma. When growth is predominantly exophytic, "villoglandular" architecture reminiscent of villous adenoma of the gastrointestinal tract may be produced, with the formation of attenuated, thin-stalked (foliate) structures.

As emphasized earlier, nonsecretory endometria constitute a morphologic spectrum, and the lines separating neighboring entities along this spectrum are ultimately conventional, that is, they attempt to approximately demarcate morphologic categories associated with different levels of risk of subsequent invasive endometrial carcinoma. The groupings are probably more or less right; the precise lines are underspecified by currently available data. Before invoking the term hyperplasia (rather than "disordered proliferative"), we require that the glandular overgrowth be sufficiently pronounced to shift the glands-to-stroma ratio to 3:1 (i.e., such that the stroma comprises less than one-third of the volume—or cross-sectional area—of the proliferation). We incorporate in the glandular fraction both glands (including their lumens) and villoglandular structures (Figs. 20 and 21).

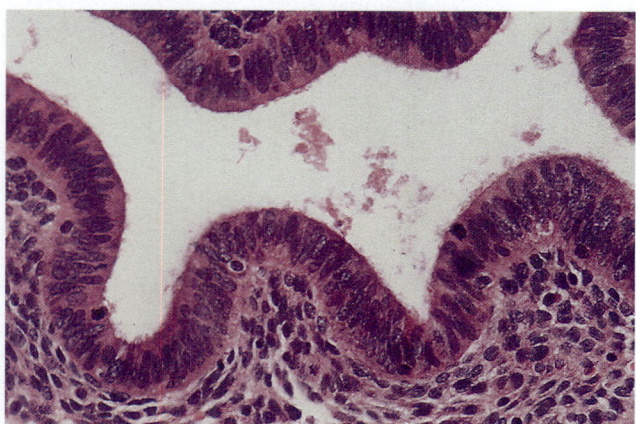

FIG. 18. Disordered proliferative endometrium (high power). This epithelium is identical in histologic features to that seen in normal late proliferative endometrium. Metaplastic epithelium is commonly encountered in this context.

TABLE 8. *Classification of endometrial hyperplasis*

Simple
Complex
Atypical (specify architecture: simple or complex)

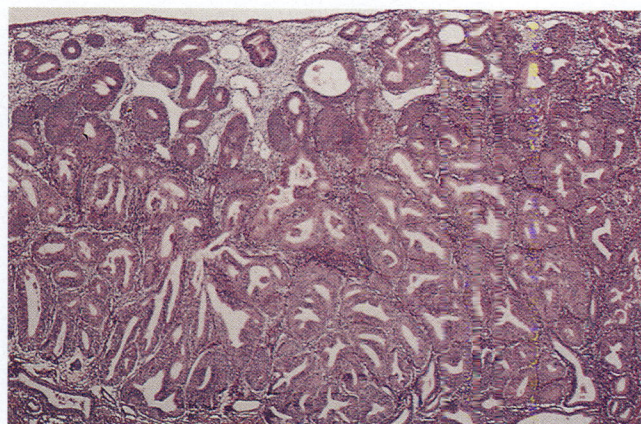

FIG. 20. Endometrial hyperplasia (low power). The term endometrial hyperplasia denotes a predominantly epithelial proliferation of nonsecretory endometrium, to the extent that stroma is a minor component of the process. This low-power photomicrograph illustrates glandular complexity. The presence or absence of atypia is based on an examination of cytologic features (which cannot be evaluated in this photomicrograph).

To qualify as hyperplastic, the epithelium must also be proliferative in its morphologic features. As a result, it should exhibit, at the very least, prominent pseudostratification; the cells may, in some cases, be stratified. The constituent cells in a hyperplastic endometrium vary from those that resemble the cells of the normal proliferative endometrium (Figs. 21 and 22) to those that show varying degrees of nuclear atypia, characterized by nuclear enlargement and irregularity, chromatin abnormalities, and prominent nucleoli. Again, these nuclear features grouped as atypia, not architectural complexity, are the defining feature

of AH. These epithelial requirements immediately eliminate from the category of hyperplasia architecturally complex endometria with atrophic or weakly proliferative epithelium.

Our criteria for minimal cytologic atypia include nuclear enlargement and very often nuclear rounding, some degree of pleomorphism, and a shift in the nuclear/cytoplasmic ratio in favor of the nuclei. The relative size of the nuclei can be estimated by comparing them to the surrounding stromal cell nuclei or those of residual normal epithelial elements. Features frequently present in severe cytologic atypia include large, prominent nucleoli; irregularity of nuclear size and shape; dispersed and clumped chromatin; and larger nuclei than are found in minimal atypia (Fig. 23). There may be disarray and jumbling of the epithelium. Intraluminal tufting and focal stratification may be found, but when it is extensive, stratification is a criterion of malignancy (see section concerning Well-Differentiated Carcinoma). Mitotic figures are almost always present in AH and may be numerous in severely atypical cases, but abnormal division figures are sparse or absent.

The glandular architectural changes encountered in hyperplasia range from endometria that contain glands with shapes similar to those found in disordered proliferation to endometria that approach the architectural complexity and cytologic atypia of well-differentiated adenocarcinoma (215–217). Many taxonomic schemes have been proposed to subdivide this continuum, resulting in a profusion of terms denoting roughly the same patterns. Moreover, some, but not all, forms of hyperplasia have been shown to be associated with an increased risk of endometrial adenocarcinoma. We think that any classification (and associated terminology) for hyperplasia should as clearly as possible (given the paucity of available data) distinguish between proliferations that are associated with an increased risk of endometrial carcinoma and

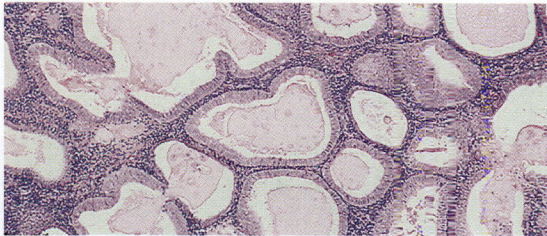

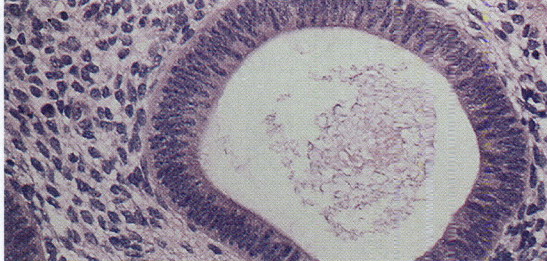

FIG. 21. Simple hyperplasia without atypia. *Top:* Cystically dilated and minimally budded glands that are separated by wisps of compressed stroma. *Bottom:* The lining epithelium is proliferative and comparable to normal late proliferative endometrium. Cytologic atypia is absent.

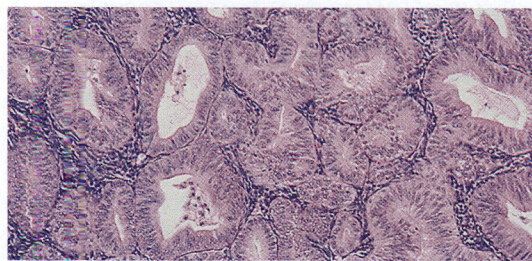

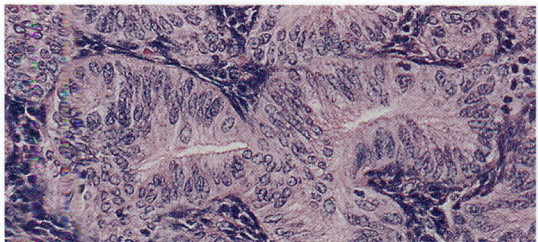

FIG. 22. Complex hyperplasia without atypia. *Top:* When hyperplastic endometria exhibit the degree of budding seen here, the term complex hyperplasia is used. *Bottom:* The epithelium lining these budded glands is not atypical.

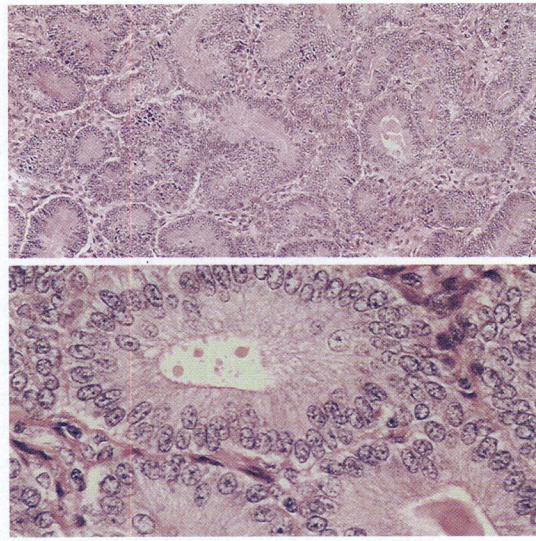

FIG. 23. Complex hyperplasia with atypia. *Top:* The budding required for a diagnosis of complex hyperplasia. *Bottom:* Cytologic atypia sufficient to warrant a diagnosis of atypical complex hyperplasia.

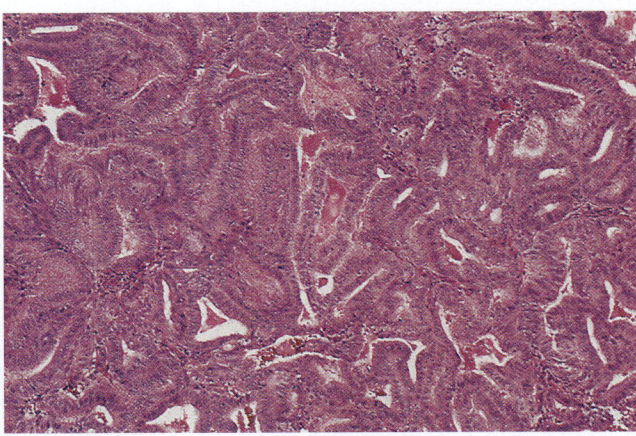

FIG. 24. Complex hyperplasia (low power). The degree of budding and channeling is more extensive than that seen in Fig. 23.

those that are not. New studies provide evidence that the presence of cytologic atypia is the best predictor of an increased risk of subsequent carcinoma (210,218).

Thus, for purposes of clinical decision-making, we think that any taxonomic scheme that is used should reflect what is known about cancer risk and hyperplasia. To do this, hyperplastic endometria are separated into two categories: hyperplasia without cytologic atypia (little or no known risk) and hyperplasia with cytologic atypia (implies significantly increased risk). The degree of cytologic atypia can be specified as minimal, moderate, and severe, although the information to date is insufficient to support this more elaborate classification scheme, that is, there is little evidence that further division of AH accurately sorts patients into low-, medium-, and high-risk groups.

The International Society of Gynecologic Pathologists has proposed a three-tiered classification as follows: (a) simple hyperplasia (which roughly corresponds to "cystic" hyperplasia and includes some of the patterns we label as disordered proliferation), (b) complex hyperplasia (hyperplasia without cytologic atypia but with architectural complexity), and (c) atypical hyperplasia (constituent cells with cytologic atypia and simple or complex architecture; rare occurrence of simple hyperplasias with atypical cells) (Figs. 24–25; Table 8). Apart from our unwillingness to trade the label disordered proliferation for simple hyperplasia, we endorse this classification for those endometria without a significant shift in the glands-to-stroma ratio and employ it in our diagnostic practice.

It has been the custom in some laboratories to grade the degree of cytologic atypia in hyperplasia, even though the evidence is not conclusive that this grading is associated with risk (203,204,210,218). The claimed advantages are several. First, the terms serve a descriptive purpose by indicating how closely the cytologic atypia of hyperplasia approaches that of well-differentiated adenocarcinoma. Second, distinguishing between benign proliferations (AH) and potentially myoinvasive proliferations (grade 1 adenocarcinoma) at the atypical end of the spectrum of hyperplasia is difficult, and many pathologists (ourselves included) like to employ a term that can be followed by such a caveat as "well-differentiated carcinoma cannot be excluded." Third, the terms are used by some clinicians (rightly or wrongly) as a guide to clinical treatment; in some institutions, patients with milder forms of AH are followed with repeated samplings, while patients with moderate and severely atypical hyperplasia often are treated with hysterectomy. We continue to grade AH for these reasons, even though we remain skeptical on the issue of whether grading provides insight into relative risk.

In most instances, hyperplastic endometria have an increased volume. On occasion, however, the architectural and cytologic criteria for hyperplasia are fulfilled, but the proliferation represents a small focus in an otherwise nonhyper-

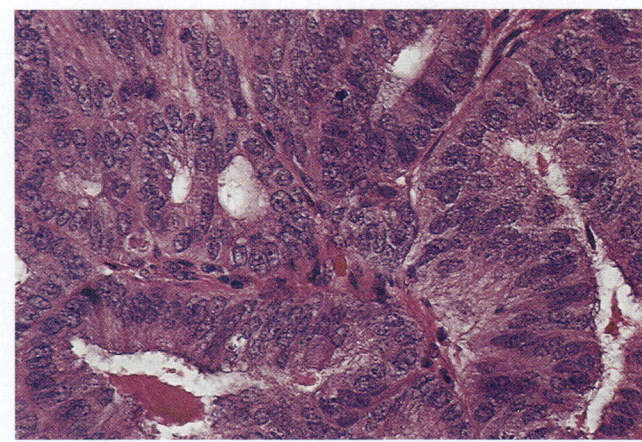

FIG. 25. Complex hyperplasia with atypia. This higher-power view of Fig. 24 shows rounding of nuclei and grainy chromatin. The cytologic features warrant a diagnosis of atypical hyperplasia.

plastic endometrium. The term focal hyperplasia seems reasonable for this finding. In other instances, the features of hyperplasia are present throughout a thin endometrium (or scanty curetting). The prognostic and therapeutic implications of these variations of hyperplasia are probably those that would attach to a more voluminous proliferation with these features.

The term epithelial metaplasia denotes the presence of epithelial cells expressing differentiated features not usually encountered to any noticeable degree in endometrial cells. This phenomenon is most often encountered in hyperplastic endometria; the details of specific metaplastic cell types and their relationship to hyperplasia are discussed in the section concerning the endometrial metaplasias.

Clinicopathologic Correlation

Most patients with either endometrial hyperplasia or atypical epithelial hyperplasia experience abnormal uterine bleeding. Endometrial hyperplasia usually occurs in the perimenopausal or postmenopausal years; in rare instances, adolescents show signs of AH (219). Most hyperplastic endometria represent the normal endometrium's response to sustained estrogen levels unrelieved by progesterone. The estrogen responsible for this process may be either endogenous (e.g., chronic anovulation) or exogenous (e.g., estrogen hormone replacement therapy) (220,221). Adjuvant tamoxifen (a nonsteroidal anti-estrogen with some estrogenic effects) has recently been reported to be associated with endometrial hyperplasia and to increase the relative risk of endometrial carcinoma (see later discussion of carcinoma) (222–225). Hyperplastic endometria without atypia and those with minimal atypia can usually be successfully treated by curettage and hormonal manipulation.

Although there is little doubt that AH is a marker for an increased risk of adenocarcinoma, the magnitude of that risk is the subject of some controversy (203,205,210,226,227) because our knowledge of the relative risk of endometrial carcinoma that attaches to various patterns found in hyperplastic endometria is meager and acquisition of new knowledge is beset by formidable methodologic problems. The morphologic definition of the target event (invasive, usually well-differentiated, endometrial adenocarcinoma) is ill-defined and a matter of ongoing debate. Moreover, the willingness of the surgeon and patient to retain the organ involved by the putative precancerous lesion in order to wait out its natural history is extremely low in the usual age group in which these hyperplasias develop. In addition, the precursor lesions are anatomically unstable; they can be shed spontaneously or they can be reversed by a change in the patient's hormonal milieu, whether through alterations in physiology or alterations produced iatrogenically. It is as though one were attempting to develop a classification of intraepithelial breast lesions in a world where researchers had no universally shared morphologic definition of invasive breast cancer (e.g., the separation of ductal carcinoma *in situ* and invasive ductal cancer was typically challenging), where the intraductal lesion changed its appearance with depressing frequency, and where any atypical lesion was treated by bilateral mastectomies.

Despite these logistical problems, most reports provide evidence that approximately 20% to 30% of women with endometrial hyperplasia characterized by glands with marked architectural complexity and crowding, in addition to some degree of cytologic atypia, will progress to adenocarcinoma (218). In the study published by Kurman and associates (210), once a patient had AH, no further insight into risk was provided by grading the degree of atypia, that is, varying degrees of cytologic atypia were not reflected in a greater or lesser risk of adenocarcinoma once it was determined that the endometrium was architecturally complex and the glands were lined by cytologically atypical cells.

To ascertain whether a patient with endometrial hyperplasia should be treated by hysterectomy, two classes of hysterectomies need to be distinguished: one performed on the climacteric or menopausal patient who is a low-risk surgical candidate ("low penalty" hysterectomy) and one performed on the patient interested in preserving her fertility or on the climacteric or menopausal patient who is a high-risk surgical candidate ("high penalty" hysterectomy). Patients in the first group usually undergo hysterectomy for benign disease (uterine prolapse, leiomyomas, dysfunctional bleeding, etc.) simply to deal with troublesome symptoms. Since fertility is no longer a relevant consideration, the risk that a life-threatening disease will develop, typically offsets whatever advantage (body image, perceived change in sexual function, etc.) there might be to retaining the uterus. In this situation, a diagnosis of AH with any degree of atypia beyond a minimal amount is sufficient to warrant hysterectomy.

Again, a diagnosis of nonatypical hyperplasia does not, in itself, warrant hysterectomy, but the severity of the patient's symptoms (e.g., dysfunctional bleeding) and the need for continued endometrial samplings may tip the balance enough to make hysterectomy the most attractive option. Patients in the high-penalty group are in a very different situation, since substantial risks attach to hysterectomy: infertility in the first subset and an increased risk of dying at the time of surgery or in the postoperative period in the second. In this high-penalty group there is literature to support treating even well-differentiated carcinoma in a nonsurgical fashion.

Is there utility in grading the degree of cytologic atypia in this circumstance? Certainly, a diagnosis of nonatypical hyperplasia is not sufficient ground to remove the uterus; however, the same may be true of a diagnosis of AH for patients in the high-risk group. For these patients, it seems that there are (or should be) no substantial changes in clinical treatment anywhere along the spectrum from disordered proliferation to markedly atypical hyperplasia. The critical end of the classification for high-risk patients is at the boundary between AH and grade 1 carcinoma or even at the interface of grades 1 and 2 carcinoma, not across any boundary within the hyperplasia group.

In summary, climacteric and menopausal women with severe or even moderate cytologic atypia are usually treated by hysterectomy if they are suitable surgical candidates. Thus, the pathologist need not label borderline, worrisome lesions as adenocarcinoma in order to remove the uterus. Occasionally, curettings contain only AH, while well-differentiated adenocarcinoma is found in the hysterectomy specimen. No harm has been done in this circumstance by the misinterpretation, since a diagnosis of carcinoma would have resulted in the identical treatment. Premenopausal women with AH who desire uterine preservation may be treated by hormonal eradication of the lesion, recurettage, and induction of ovulation (228–230).

Endometrial Polyp

Description (231)

The usual endometrial polyp is a grossly pedunculated lesion whose bulk is composed predominantly of collagenated fibrous stroma populated by cystically dilated and occasionally crowded glands lined by inactive, atrophic to weakly proliferative endometrium (Fig. 26). Sometimes endometrial stromal cells are admixed with the fibrous tissue, and on rare occasions the stromal cells may exhibit striking nuclear atypia (232). All types of endometria, however—including those showing signs of hyperplasia—can be found in polyps; now and then, adenocarcinoma, including papillary serous carcinoma or even carcinosarcoma, will be found in focal areas or diffusely throughout an otherwise characteristic polyp (233,234). The central portion of a polyp contains large, thick-walled, coiled blood vessels, and metaplastic epithelium may also be present (Fig. 27). Thus, the definition of an endometrial polyp requires a polypoid structure with a fibrous core containing large, thick-walled vessels. Rarely, polyps may be sessile. Polyps containing cycling endometrium are called functional polyps. If the stroma is made up predominantly of smooth muscle but the glands are not atypical, the term adenomyoma is used. If atypical endometrial glands are set in a predominantly smooth-muscle stroma, the polyp is called APA (see separate section on this condition).

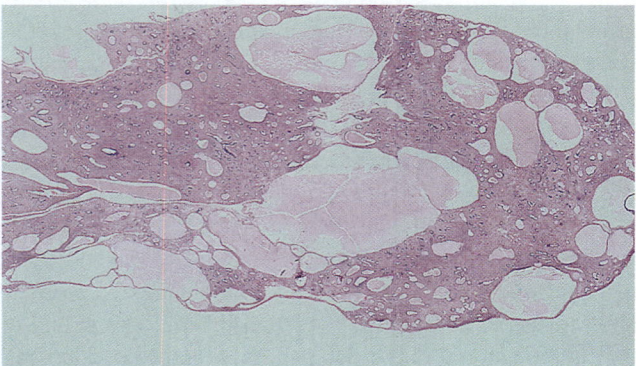

FIG. 26. Endometrial polyp (low power). This endometrial polyp features cystically dilated glands of varying sizes and shapes.

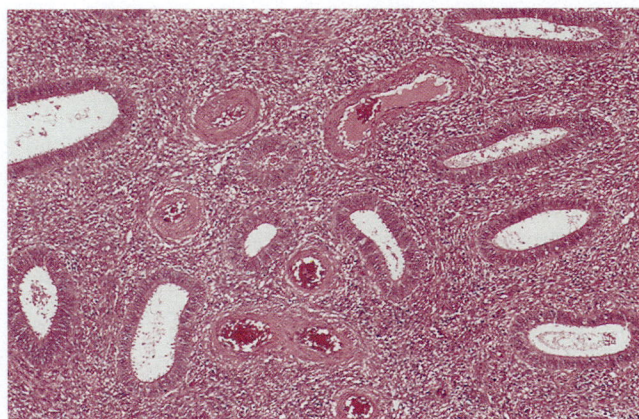

FIG. 27. Endometrial polyp (high power). The characteristic feature of an endometrial polyp is the presence of thick-walled blood vessels within the fibrous core of the polyp.

Clinicopathologic Correlation

Endometrial polyps are characteristically asymptomatic, incidental findings in perimenopausal women, but they may cause clinically significant bleeding or spotting. They are thought to be foci of retained endometrium that have become pedunculated and fibrotic over several cycles. The relationship of endometrial polyps to the subsequent development of endometrial carcinoma is uncertain. A recent case-control study showed a somewhat increased risk of carcinoma in this context (235). endometrial polyps with severe focal epithelial atypia have been associated with the administration of tamoxifen (236,237). Carcinomas developing in patients using tamoxifen are more often associated with endometrial polyps than carcinomas in other patients (238). Polypoid adenomyomas (PAs) produce similar symptoms but are distinctly less common than polyps with predominantly fibrous stroma.

Usual Endometrial Adenocarcinoma

General Description (20,214,239–241)

Endometrial adenocarcinomas, far and away the most common malignancies of the uterine corpus, are divided into endometrioid ("usual") and special variant types. In terms of their architectural and cytologic features, better-differentiated examples of endometrioid adenocarcinoma are composed of glands or villoglandular structures that resemble those found in endometrial hyperplasia; by convention the endometrioid group includes neoplasms that have a squamous component (Figs. 28). The remaining minority of endometrial adenocarcinomas are termed special variant carcinomas and are composed of cells demonstrating a type of differentiation usually encountered elsewhere in the female genital tract (Table 9). In excess of 80% of endometrial adenocarcinomas in most large series are of the endometrioid type (242–246). Because endometrioid adenocarcinomas represent the terminus along the morphologic spectrum of nonsecretory endometrium that we have been studying, it is

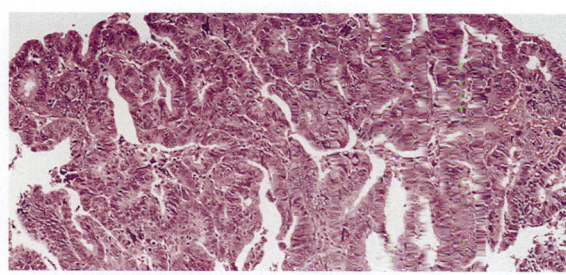
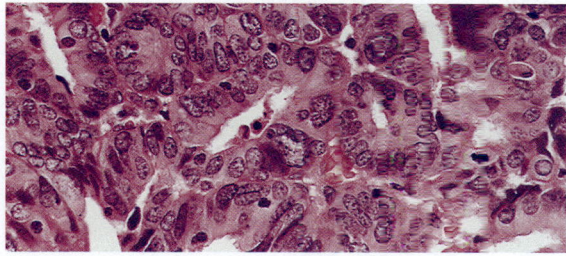

FIG. 28. Well-differentiated endometrioid carcinoma. *Top:* Closely approximated, irregularly shaped glands with very little intervening stroma. *Bottom:* Focal severe cytologic atypia. The presence of these cells warrants a diagnosis of carcinoma.

natural to discuss them in this section, accompanied by an overview of endometrial carcinoma; the specifics concerning the special variant carcinomas are discussed in the section entitled Endometria with Alternative Differentiated Epithelia.

Endometrioid adenocarcinomas exhibit a continuous spectrum of appearances. This continuum is bracketed at one end by proliferations difficult to distinguish from atypical endometrial hyperplasia and at the other end by sheet-like proliferations of malignant cells difficult to distinguish from uterine sarcomas. The typical carcinoma in the endometrioid group is easy to recognize as an adenocarcinoma because gland formation is prominent; these neoplasms are sometimes associated with squamous elements that may be malignant in cytologic features but more often are bland.

The low-power appearance of the nonsquamous elements typically conforms to one or more of three broad architectural patterns (Figs. 29 and 30). The first pattern consists of large, back-to-back, architecturally complex, compressive

TABLE 9. *Classification of endometrial carcinoma*

Endometrioid (usual) carcinoma (includes glandular and villoglandular patterns)
   Secretory (449,450,650)
   Ciliated cell (447)
   With squamous differentiation (includes adenoacanthoma and adenosquamous carcinomas—see text) (365–368)
Special variant carcinomas
   Uterine papillary serous (high-grade papillary) (416,417,420,422–430,651,652)
   Clear cell (429,449,451–457,650)
   Mucinous (387–389)
   Pure squamous cell (377–379,653)
   Mixed
   Undifferentiated (456)

"macroglands" (Figs. 31 and 32); these macroglands may, in turn, be composed of closely approximated back-to-back buds set within a delicate stromal supportive framework whose presence may be suggested only by the radial polarization of the epithelial cells. The second pattern is represented by extensively budding and branching glands with little intervening stroma, forming a complex labyrinth (Fig. 30). Third, there might be a branching, exophytic thin-stalked papillary (villoglandular) pattern, visible at low power, that is reminiscent of villous adenoma of the gastrointestinal tract. Less often, the malignant glands are composed of extensively stratified epithelium forming a gland-within-gland (cribriform) pattern uninterrupted by stromal scaffolding (Fig. 33). While most endometrioid carcinomas form easily found glands or complex, branching villoglandular structures, in high-grade carcinomas these features may be focal and, in some cases, require extensive sampling to pinpoint. A detailed morphologic description of endometrial adenocarcinoma is provided later herein.

Many clinicopathologic studies of patients with endometrioid adenocarcinoma have shown that increasing loss of glandular and villoglandular architecture (and their displacement by more and more areas of sheet-like growth) is positively correlated with progressive cytologic atypia; both of these features, in turn, are correlated with higher stages (as determined at surgery) and diminished survival rates. These clinicopathologic correlations can be charted by a numerical grading system. Similarly, some types of special variant carcinoma are associated with high-grade clinical behavior. Thus, the histologic appearance of endometrial carcinomas (whether endometrioid or a special variant subtype) provides important insight into prognosis and plays a role in determining therapy (see Clinicopathologic Correlation). The histologic assessment of an endometrial carcinoma should proceed in a stepwise fashion.

First, a histologic subtyping of endometrial carcinomas selects out two clinically aggressive special variant carcinomas—uterine papillary serous carcinoma (UPSC) and clear-cell carcinoma—that do not need to be graded because the subtype dictates outcome and one clinically low-grade carcinoma—secretory carcinoma—that does not need to be graded because it is definitionally grade 1. The remainder of the carcinomas are graded using the current modified FIGO (International Federation of Gynecology Obstetrics) system, a three-tiered classification based on an evaluation of *both* the low-power architectural appearance and the cytologic features of a neoplasm (Fig. 34). This scheme is set out in Table 10 (Figs. 30, 32, 33, 35, and 36) (247,248). We employ an essentially similar system in assigning a grade to an endometrial carcinoma.

The cytologic features we principally rely upon are nuclear pleomorphism and the prominence of nucleoli (Figs. 34 and 37). Additional features evaluated in assigning a cytologic grade include nuclear size, nuclear irregularity, and the degree of chromatin clumping. When there is discordance between the cytologic and architectural grade, we supply

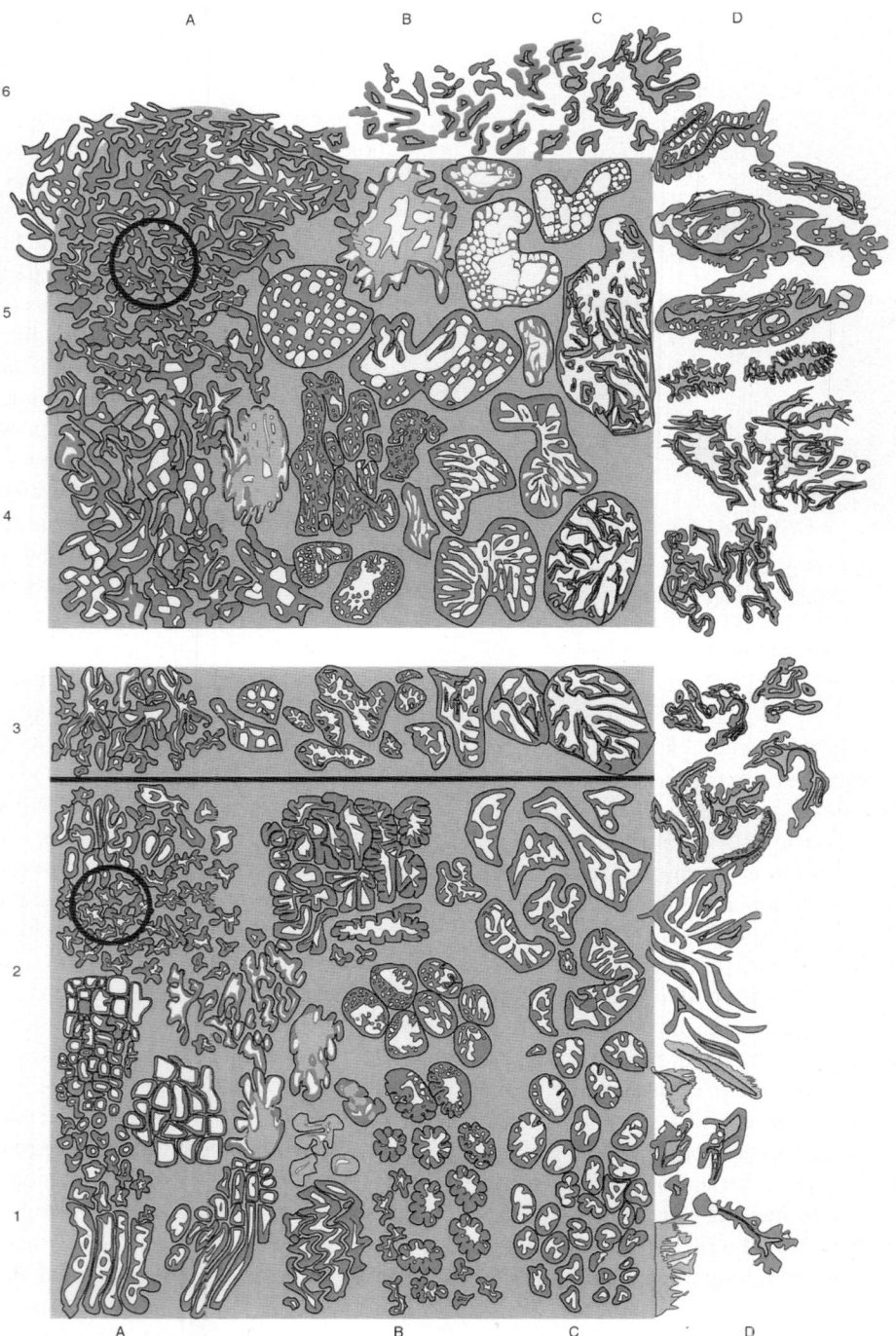

FIG. 29. A: Architectural index for well-differentiated endometrial carcinoma. Endometrial proliferations with gland patterns that map to the lower half of the chart are associated with a negligible risk of myometrial invasion and are regarded as benign. These proliferations fall within the range of endometrial hyperplasia/metaplasia and are further designated as atypical when they are associated with cytologic atypia, as depicted in Figs. 23 and 25. Occasionally, endometrial proliferations with a low architectural index contain foci with cytologic atypia sufficiently severe to warrant a diagnosis of carcinoma on the basis of cytologic features alone (usually manifest by prominent nucleoli and marked nuclear pleomorphism). In contrast, endometrial proliferations with gland patterns that map to the top half of the chart are associated with myoinvasion with sufficient frequency to warrant a diagnosis of carcinoma regardless of the cytologic features. In unusual cases, endometrial proliferations may feature architectural patterns that are ambiguous in morphologic characteristics, and these patterns are positioned along the borderline zone above the solid line in the lower half of the chart; in these cases, the diagnosis "borderline" is warranted.

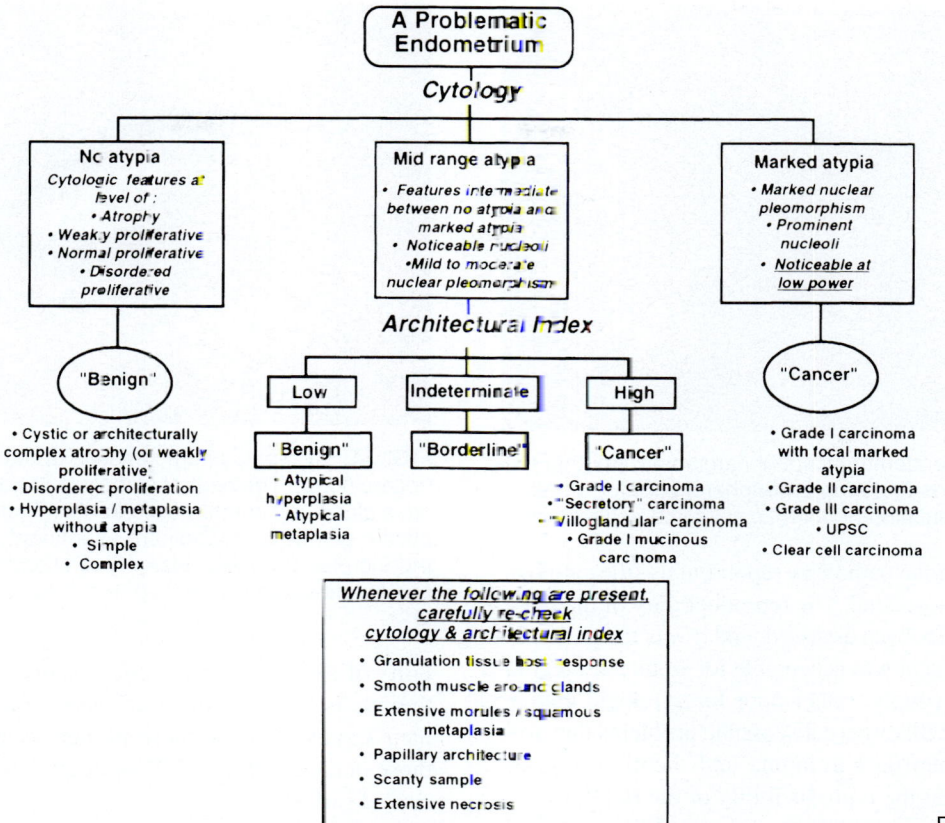

FIG. 29. *(continued)* **B:** An algorithmic approach to the diagnosis of challenging endometrial proliferations. The use of this flow chart requires an adequate sample, an evaluation of the cytologic index (prominence of nucleoli and degree of nuclear pleomorphism), and an evaluation of the architectural index, as indicated in A.

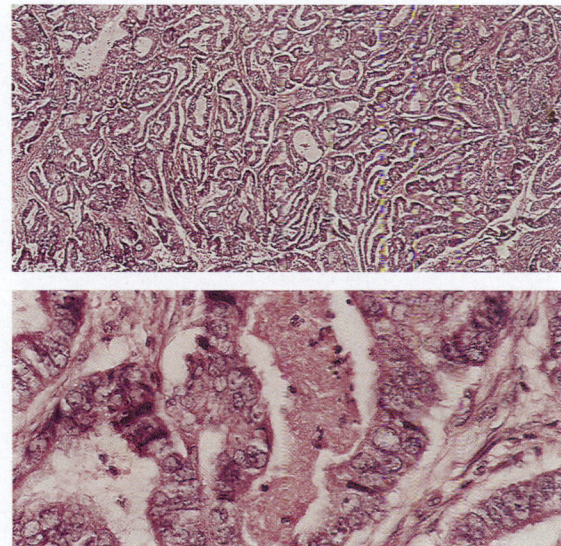

FIG. 30. Well-differentiated endometrioid carcinoma. *Top:* The complex labyrinthine growth pattern diagnostic of carcinoma. *Bottom:* Enlarged hyperchromatic cells with grainy, irregular nuclear chromatin.

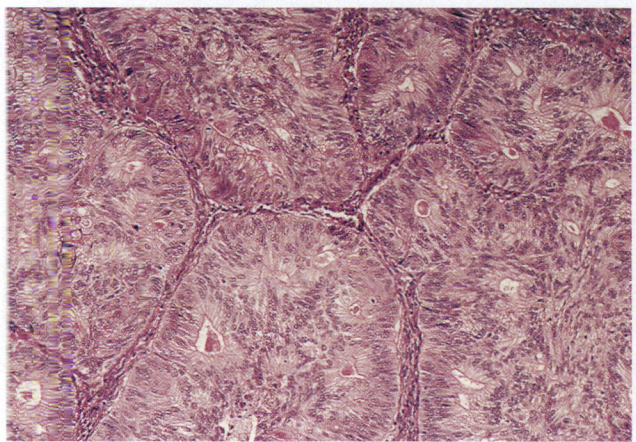

FIG. 31. Well-differentiated adenocarcinoma. In this example, the typical macroglands of carcinoma are seen. Large glands with a complex secondary structure featuring budding and branching are present.

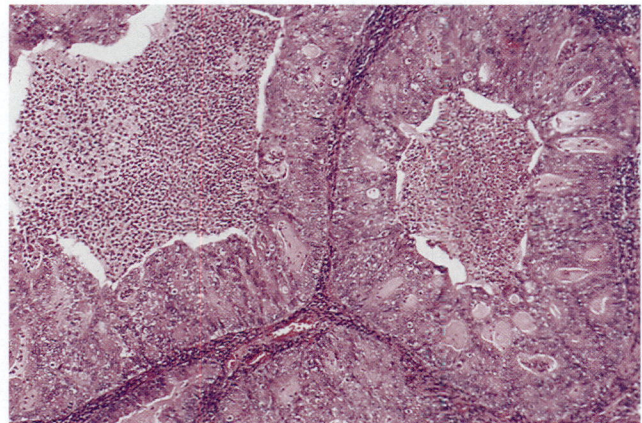

FIG. 32. Grade 1 endometrial adenocarcinoma. Another pattern of macroglands featuring a peripheral cribriform pattern and central accumulation of necrotic cells and polymorphs.

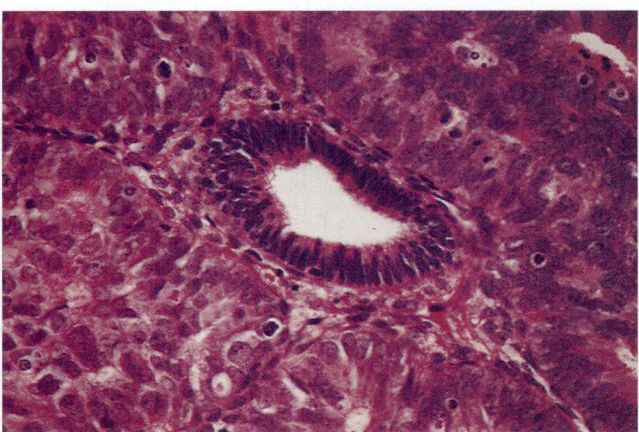

FIG. 34. Cytologic characteristics of malignant cells in adenocarcinoma. The central gland is a residual, weakly proliferative gland and contrasts markedly with the surrounding neoplastic glandular epithelium. Prominent differences include the increased nuclear size, hyperchromatism, and a higher nucleus-to-cytoplasm ratio of the carcinomatous epithelium.

both in the body of the pathology report but use the cytologic grade on the diagnosis line. The reproducibility of the FIGO modified system has been assessed, and it was found that interobserver agreement was acceptable for architectural grading but, not surprisingly, rather poor for cytologic grading (249). Sidawy and Silverberg discuss the problems that arise in grading endometrial carcinoma and mention a newer study reporting that the reproducibility of the (GOG) gynecologic oncology group/FIGO modified architectural grading scheme by three independent observers was good but that it could be improved by a two-tiered assessment of nuclear grade (250–252).

Clinicopathologic Correlation (244,245,253–257)

Most patients with endometrial carcinoma show initial signs of uterine bleeding. Given uterine bleeding, the probability of carcinoma is a strong function of the patient's age: the rate is 9% for women in their fifties, 16% for those in their sixties, 28% for those in their seventies, and 60% for those in their eighties (258). Sampling issues have been discussed earlier.

It is now apparent that many patients with endometrial adenocarcinoma fall into two loose clinicopathologic clusters or syndromes (259–262). Patients in the first group (type I) tend to be between 40 and 60 years of age (although carcinoma can develop in younger women, including, in rare instances, those in their twenties). They may have a history of

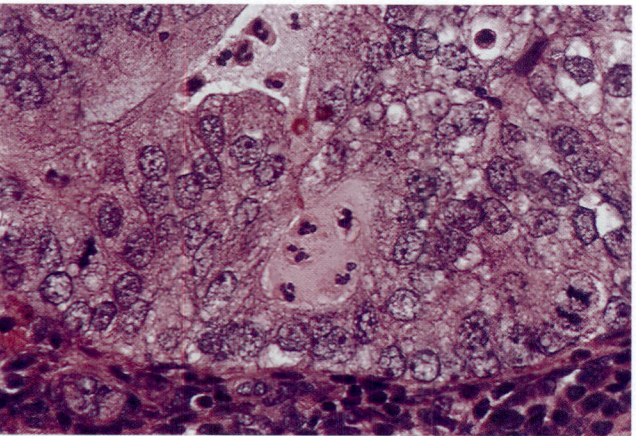

FIG. 33. Well-differentiated endometrioid adenocarcinoma (grade 1). The complex budding and branching of the periphery of the macroglands seen in the previous slide are illustrated here. The cells of the epithelial lining of these neoplastic glands are large (compare with the stromal cells) and have prominent nucleoli, rounding, and easily identified mitotic figures. The latter feature does not serve to distinguish between hyperplasia and carcinoma.

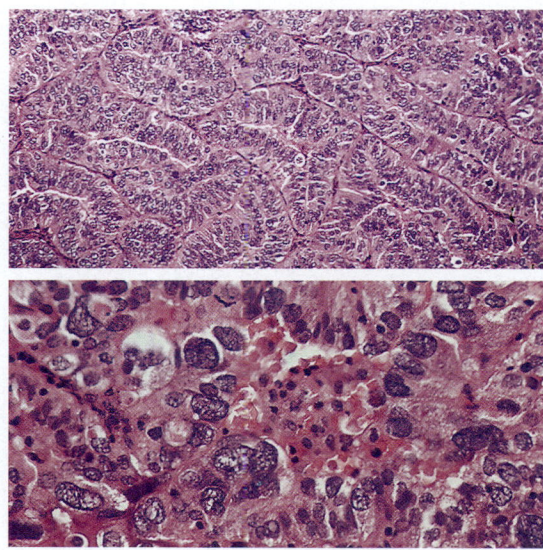

FIG. 35. Grade 2 endometrioid adenocarcinoma. *Top:* Complex budding and branching of glands separated only by thin wisps of stroma. *Bottom:* Focal severe nuclear pleomorphism, hyperchromatism, and prominent nucleoli. The architecture is that of grade 1 adenocarcinoma (extreme end of the spectrum), but the degree of cytologic atypia warrants an overall grade of moderately differentiated (grade 2).

TABLE 10. *Modified FIGO surgical staging and grading system for uterine corpus carcinoma (247,248)*

Stage I:	confined to the uterine corpus
IA:	Tumor limited to endometrium
IB:	Invasion of less than half of the myometrium
IC:	Invasion of more than half of the myometrium
Stage II:	uterine cervix involved
IIA:	Endocervical glandular involvement only
IIB:	Cervical stromal invasion
Stage III:	pelvic extension
IIIA:	Tumor invades serosa and/or adnexae and/or positive peritoneal cytology features
IIIB:	Vaginal metastasis
IIIC:	Metastases to pelvic and/or paraaortic lymph nodes
Stage IV:	extrapelvic extension
IVA:	Tumor invasion of bladder and/or bowel mucosa
IVB:	Distant metastases, including intrabdominal and/or inguinal lymph nodes

FIGO rules related to staging (with our modifications)
  Since corpus cancer is now surgically staged, procedures previously used for determination of stages are no longer applicable, such as using the findings in a fractional D&C to distinguish between stage I and stage II carcinomas.
  It is understood that there may be a small number of patients with corpus cancer who will be treated primarily with radiation therapy. If that is the case, the clinical staging adopted by FIGO in 1971 would still apply, but designation of the staging system would be noted.
  "Ideally, the width of the myometrium should be measured along with the width of tumor invasion." (We take this to be a request for the raw measurements that go into calculating the percentage involvement of the uterine wall.)
Histologic grading system
  Degree of architectural differentiation
    Grade 1 = ≤5% of a nonsquamous or nonmorular solid growth pattern
    Grade 2 = 6–50% of a nonsquamous or nonmorular solid growth pattern
    Grade 3 = >50% of a nonsquamous or nonmorular solid growth pattern
  Cytological features to be used in formulating final grade
    Notable nuclear atypia, inappropriate for the architectural grade, raises the grade of a grade 1 or grade 2 tumor by one level.
    In serous adenocarcinomas, clear-cell adenocarcinomas, and areas of squamous differentiation, nuclear grade takes precedence over architecture.

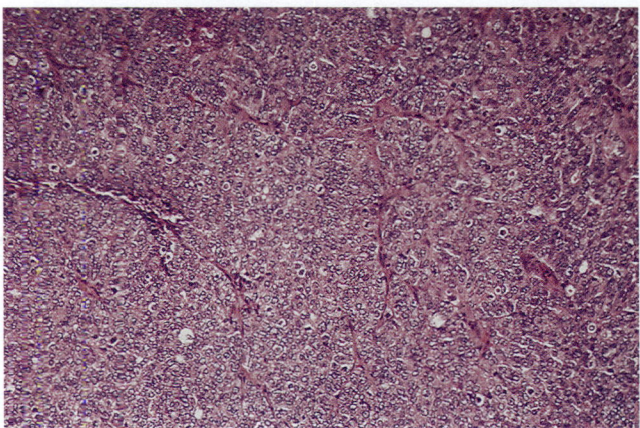

FIG. 36. Poorly differentiated (grade 3) endometrioid adenocarcinoma. This epithelial neoplasm features sheets uninterrupted by glandular lumina. At low power, a number of differential diagnostic possibilities must be considered, including malignant mixed müllerian tumor, poorly differentiated endometrioid adenocarcinoma, and primary endometrial sarcomas. Gland formation was evident elsewhere in this neoplasm.

(neither endogenous nor exogenous). In these cases, the surrounding nonneoplastic endometrium is atrophic, and there is often an *in situ* component with high-grade cytologic features. The carcinomas that develop in this group of patients are usually of the special variant type with a poor prognosis or high-grade endometrioid neoplasms that, with depressing frequency, are first found at surgery at a high stage with deep myoinvasion. They tend to be ER/PR negative, strongly express p53, and show high Ki-67 labeling (261). Needless to say, these patients are often not cured by hysterectomy. Lax and Kurman have summarized these clinical differences as well as a body of molecular genetic differences; they propose that type 1 carcinomas conform closely to the adenoma–carcinoma sequence of colonic cancer, while type II carcinomas arise rapidly from an *in situ* lesion in the context of endometrial atrophy (261,263).

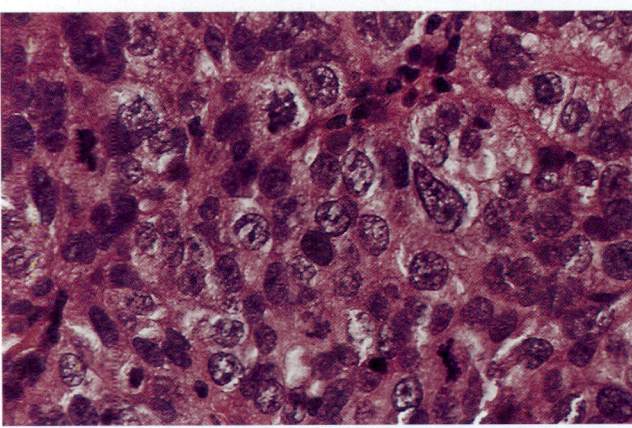

FIG. 37. In gland-forming areas of the neoplasm illustrated in Fig. 36, the cytologic features of the cells are those of grade 3 adenocarcinoma.

chronic anovulation or estrogen hormone replacement therapy, and the carcinomas are usually well-differentiated stage I, nonmyoinvasive tumors associated with endometrial hyperplasia (found either concurrently or in previous endometrial samplings) (219). Most of the tumors are estrogen and progesterone receptor (ER/PR) positive and p53 negative and express low levels of the proliferation antigen Ki-67 (261). Patients in this first group have a very favorable prognosis after hysterectomy.

In contrast, patients in the second group (type II) tend to be elderly and typically have no history of hyperestrogenism

As noted earlier, almost all patients with adenocarcinomas of the endometrium are older than age 40 at the time of diagnosis. Those few patients younger than 45 almost without exception fall into the first clinicopathologic group, that is, their neoplasms are most often well differentiated and confined to the endometrium (264–268), and they frequently have a history of anovulatory cycles or exogenous estrogen therapy; rarely, they may have a functioning ovarian tumor (269–273). Given the clinical indolence of the usual well-differentiated carcinoma in women younger than 45, we think a nonsurgical approach is acceptable for selected young women with well-differentiated (grade 1) adenocarcinoma who desire uterine preservation (274,275). Those very rare women in the reproductive years with grades 2 or 3 carcinomas should be treated like older patients with carcinomas of comparable grade.

Estrogen therapy has also been linked to an increased risk of adenocarcinoma of the endometrium among peri- and postmenopausal women. Almost all of these carcinomas are well differentiated (243,276–288). Tamoxifen is a synthetic anti-estrogen used in the treatment of breast cancer, but it has a paradoxically agonist effect on the endometrium and has been associated with the development of a number of estrogen-driven proliferations, including endometrial carcinoma. The association with endometrial carcinoma was noted in 1985; since then, several studies have shown that patients taking tamoxifen have a higher relative risk of endometrial carcinoma. The reported relative risk ranges from 2.2 to 7.5 (222,289–292). Developing cost-effective screening studies and identifying clinical features that pinpoint high-risk patients, either before the initiation of tamoxifen therapy or during its administration, are matters of debate (225,238, 293–297). Whether the carcinomas that arise in the context of tamoxifen therapy are high or low risk is also disputed (238,298–302).

Endometrial carcinoma is the most common extracolonic cancer in women with the hereditary nonpolyposis colorectal cancer syndrome (Lynch syndrome II) (303,304).

The outlook for patients with endometrial adenocarcinoma depends primarily upon three factors (in order of importance): the stage of the neoplasm, the depth of myometrial invasion, and the histologic subtype of the tumor and its grade (the third factor has been discussed earlier) (Table 10) (241,243–245,256,305–307). Accurate assignment of histologic subtype and grade (when appropriate) requires adequate sampling. Other features reported to worsen the prognosis in endometrial carcinoma include the presence of vascular invasion and uterine serosal involvement; these features should be noted in the body of the pathology report (308–311).

The presence of malignant cells in peritoneal fluids in women with endometrial adenocarcinoma is an adverse prognostic finding; however, the *independent* prognostic significance of carcinoma cells in peritoneal washings is unclear (312–315). In the most recent proportional hazards analysis of the GOG stage I and II endometrial cancer group of 895 patients, positive peritoneal cytologic features conferred a relative risk of recurrence of 1.7 for patients with metastases and 2.4 for patients without metastases (256).

Surgical Staging of Endometrial Carcinoma

Before the 1980s, endometrial carcinoma was most often staged clinically by means of preoperative clinical studies combined with a careful scrutiny of the differential curettings. The preoperative clinical stage was used to formulate therapy, which, in the past, might well include preoperative radiotherapy. Since that time, preoperative radiation has largely been abandoned (except for bulky extrauterine or cervical disease), and now the initial procedure is almost always abdominal hysterectomy. Staging and subsequent therapy are based upon the histopathologic analysis of tissue removed at the time of hysterectomy. In addition to the uterus and adnexa, peritoneal biopsies, cytologic preparations, and lymph node samplings are frequently obtained.

In many institutions, the pathologist bears some responsibility for determining which patients will undergo surgical staging. Patients with grade 3 and high-risk special variant carcinomas, as determined by preoperative biopsies, are often considered candidates for a staging procedure regardless of the presence or absence of myometrial invasion or its depth. For patients with grade 1 or 2 endometrial carcinoma, gross examination of the myometrium at the time of operation and selected frozen-section examination of apparent areas of invasion are often used to determine which patients will undergo staging (316–319). The final surgical pathologic stage assigned to a patient with endometrial carcinoma is based on complete examination of the hysterectomy specimen using permanent sections as well as intraoperative biopsies. Thus, the pathologist bears the chief responsibility for assigning the stage. The current FIGO staging and grading systems are set out in Table 10.

Assessing Myoinvasion (250,320–322)

To obtain accurate staging information, it is essential to carefully examine and intelligently section the hysterectomy specimen in a way that unambiguously reveals whether myoinvasion is present (Table 1). If it is, sections must be cut so that the maximum depth of invasion can be determined. Invasive adenocarcinomas typically infiltrate the myometrium in the form of jagged, irregular branching glands, and inflamed granulation tissue often forms around these invasive foci (Figs. 38–40). In a distressingly large number of cases, however, establishing the presence of myoinvasion is not straightforward because the normal endometrial–myometrial junction is irregular and the normal endometrium often interdigitates deeply with the myometrium. As a result, the basalis can lie deep in the myometrium.

If deeply lying basalis is involved by carcinoma, it may be difficult (sometimes impossible) to distinguish this carcinomatous involvement from superficial myoinvasion. Unless a granulation tissue host inflammatory reaction is identified, we withhold a diagnosis of myoinvasion in challenging cases involving the superficial myometrium. One is unlikely to be proved wrong by this maneuver because the behavior of endometrial carcinomas with superficial myoinvasion is essen-

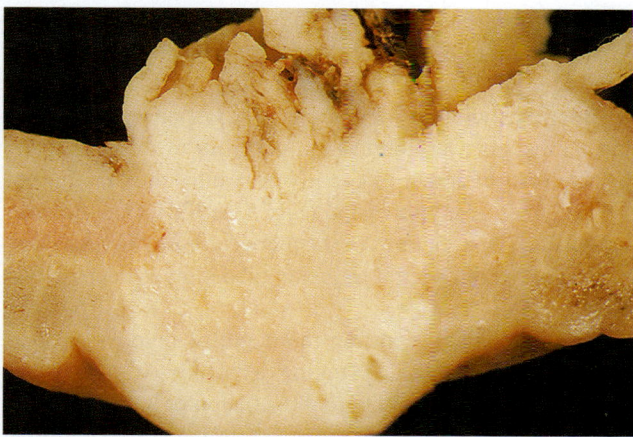

FIG. 38. Myoinvasive endometrioid adenocarcinoma (gross features). In this bivalved hysterectomy specimen, an exophytic papillary necrotic neoplasm occupies the fundal mucosa and overlies whitish, irregularly infiltrative, myoinvasive carcinoma. Assessment of the depth of myoinvasion is an important staging criterion. An accurate assessment of depth requires a careful correlation of gross and microscopic features.

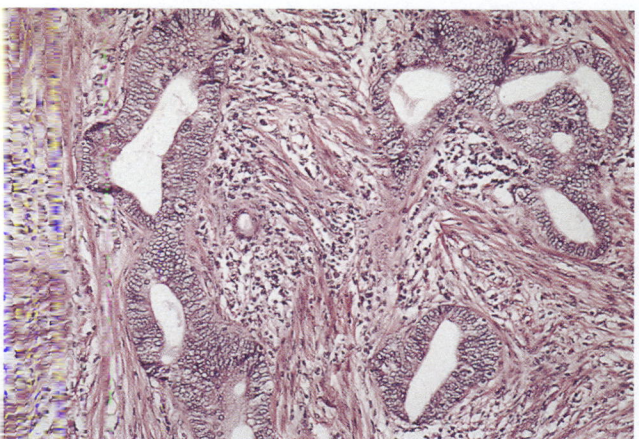

FIG. 40. A higher-power view of well-differentiated myoinvasive carcinoma. Neoplastic glands associated with the host response infiltrate the myometrium.

tially that of nonmyoinvasive carcinomas of identical grade and type. Likewise, involvement of adenomyosis by carcinoma should be distinguished from myoinvasion, since the former case does not imply a worse prognosis than carcinoma strictly limited to the endometrium (323,324).

Through sectioning to identify residual benign endometrial glands and/or endometrial stroma in suspected foci of myoinvasion is a useful way of establishing that carcinoma is confined to the endometrium or to an area of adenomyosis (Figs. 41 and 42). Moreover, neoplastic glands within deep invaginations of the endometrium or within adenomyosis usually have a blunted advancing front, a growth pattern dif-

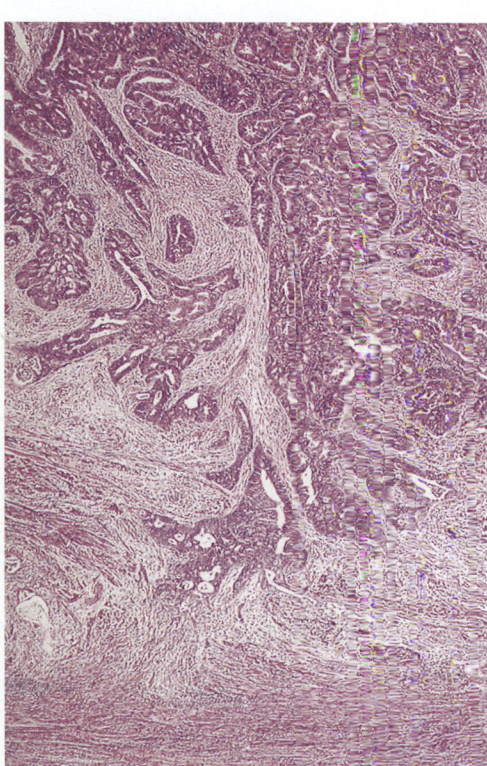

FIG. 39. Myoinvasive well-differentiated carcinoma. Myoinvasive foci feature irregularly shaped, jagged glands infiltrating the myometrium. In most cases, there is a zone of edematous and inflamed fibroblastic tissue between the normal myometrium and the infiltrating neoplastic glands.

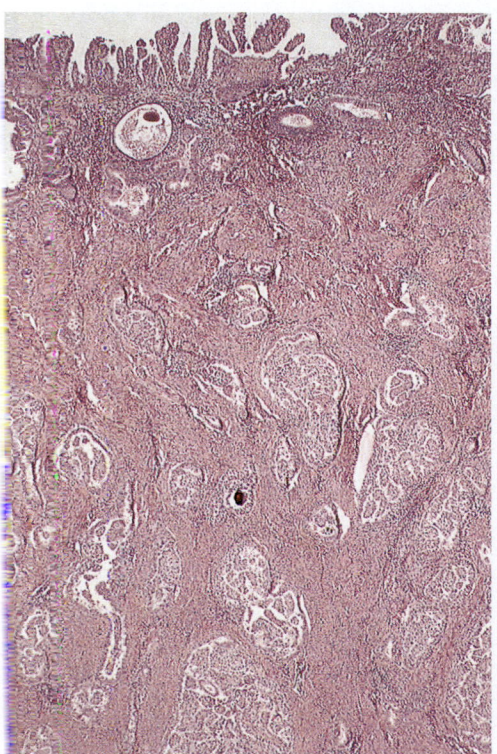

FIG. 41. Adenomyosis expanded by well-differentiated adenocarcinoma and atypical hyperplasia. The most difficult task in the staging of endometrial carcinoma is assessing the presence or absence of myoinvasion. An important mimic of myoinvasive carcinoma is the replacement of irregular extensions of basalis and adenomyosis with carcinoma.

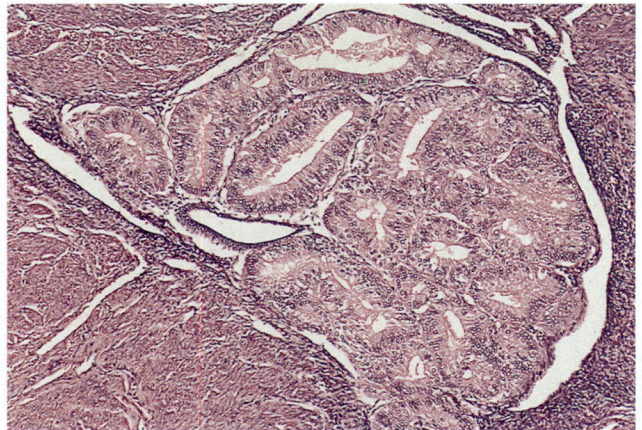

FIG. 42. A focus of adenomyosis with borderline endometrial proliferation. Features that serve to differentiate this focus from myoinvasion include the presence of residual normal endometrial glands and stroma, mixed with an atypical endometrioid proliferation. In addition, the absence of a host response is evidence against myoinvasion.

ferent from the ragged infiltration found in many carcinomas, particularly of grades 2 and 3. Foci of adenomyosis are often surrounded by hyperplastic struts of myometrium, a feature not present around myoinvasive foci of carcinoma. Despite these maneuvers, in some cases determining whether carcinoma in the myometrium represents invasion or involvement of basalis or adenomyosis may be particularly problematic. If the tumor in an ambiguous case is grade 1, we tend to consider that it represents adenomyosis or basalis involvement; if it is grade 2 or 3, we are more inclined toward the myoinvasion interpretation. In either event, when uncertainty exists after culling many sections, we state the problem, provide our best determination of whether invasion is present, and append the equivocation "invasion cannot be excluded." Occasionally, the glands forming well-differentiated carcinomas "melt" through the myometrium without inducing a host response; this condition almost always manifests in the form of massive tumor involvement of much of the myometrium, thus facilitating the diagnosis of myoinvasion (Fig. 43) (322). Occasionally, in poorly chosen sections of the uterus, nonmyoinvasive carcinoma of the intramural fallopian tube mimics deep myoinvasion.

Conventions for reporting the depth of myoinvasion are surprisingly varied. FIGO staging determines whether carcinoma has invaded the inner half or the outer half of the myometrium with measurements taken from the endometrial–myometrial junction (247,248) (Table 10), and GOG studies employ measurement in thirds, as calculated from the junction (245,256,325); other researchers have advocated measuring the distance from the deepest myoinvasive focus to the serosa (320). The compulsive pathologist reports the raw measurements (uterine wall thickness and maximum depth of myoinvasion) and the manner in which they were obtained (e.g., measuring from the endomyometrial junction to both the deepest myoinvasive point and the serosa versus measuring from the surface of the carcinoma to those two points), so that a ratio can be derived. More important, the pathologist's reporting practices should conform to those of the treating physician. We report myoinvasion in accordance with the FIGO scheme and take our measurements from the endometrial–myometrial junction.

Assessing the Status of the Cervix

Sampling of the cervix and lower uterine segment should be sufficient to determine whether the cervix is involved by carcinoma. Although the staging of endometrial carcinoma

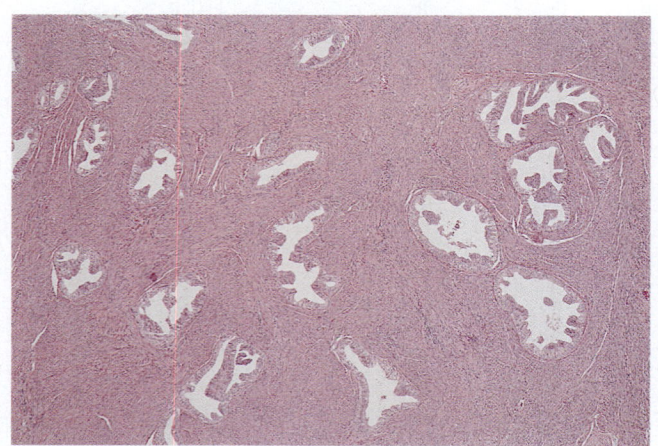
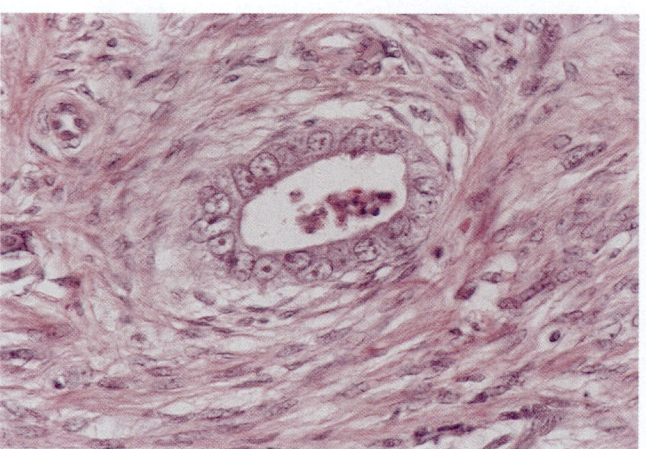

FIG. 43. "Melter" or "adenoma malignum" pattern of myoinvasion. **A:** Minimally branching, well-formed neoplastic glands diffusely infiltrate the myometrium with little or no desmoplastic or inflammatory cell response. **B:** The infiltrating glands may show only minimal cytologic atypia in areas; elsewhere, the cytologic features of carcinoma are present. Although endometrial carcinomas with diffuse myometrial infiltration are fully capable of aggressive clinical behavior, they do not appear to behave any more aggressively than those with conventional myometrial invasion.

is now done on surgical rather than clinical grounds, and the involvement of the cervix is definitively determined on the hysterectomy specimen, endocervical curettage is sometimes still performed on patients with endometrial carcinoma before hysterectomy, in an attempt to determine the status of the cervix (326). Contamination of such specimens by carcinoma actually originating from the endometrium is a common phenomenon. Consequently, it is widely held that cervical involvement should not be diagnosed unless the carcinoma actually invades cervical tissue either as a growth along the surface or as foci of cervical stromal invasion (327–329). If fragments of endometrial adenocarcinoma and fragments of normal cervix are present but separate from each other in the endocervical specimen, and the adenocarcinoma is primary in the endometrium, the prognostic implications seem to be the same as if the endocervical curettage material did not contain adenocarcinoma.

Evaluating Extrauterine Specimens Produced by the Staging Procedure

Occasionally, endometrioid adenocarcinoma is present in both the uterus and the ovary, but only at these two sites. Whether these tumors are considered to represent a primary carcinoma and a metastasis to one site from the other (and hence high-stage neoplasms arising from one of the sites) or are interpreted as simultaneous primaries (hence both stage I) has significant implications for therapy and prognosis. When both neoplasms are grade 1 and the endometrial neoplasm is not myoinvasive, we think the available published evidence supports the theory that they are simultaneous primaries; under this interpretation, adjuvant therapy is not required (330–333). Foci of AH can sometimes be seen in the uterus in association with endometrioid tumors of the ovary (see chapter by Young et al.).

Lymph nodes are often sampled in staging procedures, and foci of endosalpingiosis may be present; these foci should not be misinterpreted as adenocarcinoma (see chapter by Clement et al.). Peritoneal metastasis from an endometrial carcinoma may be mimicked by a peritoneal foreign body reaction to keratin, produced by endometrial carcinomas with prominent squamous elements and regurgitated through the fallopian tubes (334,335). An erroneous diagnosis of carcinoma in this circumstance can be avoided by not interpreting bland squamous cells on the peritoneum as carcinoma.

Nearly three-fourths of patients with adenocarcinoma of the endometrium are found to have tumors limited to the corpus at the time of hysterectomy (stage I). Another 10% have cervical involvement (stage II), while the remainder are fairly evenly divided between stages III and IV (Table 10) (245,336–338). Cervical and/or occult lymph node metastasis is detected at the time of hysterectomy in approximately 10% of patients thought to have stage I clinical symptoms of disease. These are almost exclusively patients with grade 2 or 3 carcinomas. While patients with high-stage (stages III and IV) neoplasms have a poor prognosis, those with stage I or II endometrial adenocarcinoma of the endometrioid type have excellent outcomes (stage I survival is better than 90%, while stage II is approximately 80%) (326,339,340). These survival figures are higher if the carcinoma is grade 1 and myoinvasion is minimal or absent. Stage, grade, and depth of myometrial invasion are not simply the parameters used to gauge prognosis, they also determine the need for adjuvant therapy (253,254,256,339,341,342). Surgical staging is of undoubted importance in clarifying the natural history of endometrial carcinoma; it remains an open question whether outcome is improved by this procedure (343).

There has been interest concerning the correlation between the level of ER/PR in endometrial adenocarcinoma cells and the clinical outcome using current therapies. The results of numerous studies indicate that, in general, the increasing levels of receptor protein are positively correlated with low histologic grade. Thus, it is not clear that ER/PR status provides prognostic insight over and above that furnished by the more easily determined and less costly system of grading (344–348).

Well-differentiated (Grade 1) Endometrioid Adenocarcinoma (215)

Description

The morphologic boundaries (diagnostic criteria) of well-differentiated (grade 1) endometrioid adenocarcinoma (WDCA) have been variously drawn over the years. Controversy has surrounded both the AH/WDCA morphologic threshold and the WDCA/grades 2 to 3 carcinoma morphologic threshold. Different choices of boundaries, not surprisingly, result in different statistical (or average) properties of the WDCA group: disparate percentages of myoinvasive cases, varying relapse-free survival rates, and diverse descriptions of the typical case of WDCA. What follows is a description of the typical WDCA case using our diagnostic criteria; commonly employed criteria, while differing on the assignment of cases near a boundary, would yield roughly the same description of the typical WDCA case (217,226, 349–351). In terms of its definition, WDCA must meet specific architectural and cytologic requirements (Figs. 28–34).

Architectural Abnormalities

WDCA must consist almost entirely of epithelium with very little intervening stroma; in fact, an extensive, complex epithelial growth pattern is prerequisite to the definition of WDCA. Usually the tumor has a complex glandular pattern featuring budding and branching of enlarged neoplastic macroglands, which result in the formation of side channels and papillary infoldings (Figs. 28 and 30–33). In many cases, the constituent glands form long, complex and intertwining channels that cannot be easily traced and are best detected by the microscopist's ability to view large extents of luminal spaces and epithelial bridges without crossing intervening stroma (complex budding or labyrinthine glands). It is not uncommon, however, for the tumor to have a low-power villoglandular pattern reminiscent of villous adenoma of the gastrointestinal tract, featuring either pseudostratified epithelial cells on thin, delicate stromal stalks (really sheets or folia) or a uniform layer of budded glands growing out over stalks. Both glandular and villoglandular patterns may be found in the same tumor.

Less often seen is a pattern featuring true papillae formed by collagenated stromal stalks lined by relatively bland epithelial cells; this architectural pattern is much more characteristic of clear-cell and serous carcinomas that are composed of cells with marked cytologic atypia (see Uterine Papillary Serous Carcinoma). For reasons outlined later, we require that at least 30% of the proliferation in an endometrial sampling that is considered to be carcinoma exhibit these architectural abnormalities, which we label a high architerual index, as defined in Fig. 29. Epithelial stratification uninterrupted by stroma so pronounced as to produce a cribriform pattern is relatively unusual in WDCA, but it is more common in higher-grade carcinomas. On the other hand, back-to-back buds with thin, delicate intervening stroma (confusingly also referred to as cribriform) is characteristic of WDCA.

Cytologic Abnormalities

A spectrum of cytologic atypia may be encountered in WDCA: in brief, atypia falls short of that required for grade 2 carcinoma but is at least as severe as that of AH (Figs. 33 and 34). This means that the degree of cytologic atypia for AH and WDCA may be identical; in this circumstance, WDCA is recognized on the basis of the architectural changes described in the last paragraph. The typical cytologic features of WDCA include cytomegaly, nucleomegaly, identifiable nucleoli, high nucleus-to-cytoplasm ratios, mild hyperchromasia, and easily found mitotic figures. Atypical mitotic figures may be present, but they are usually sparse. Although they are relatively unusual features, significant nuclear pleomorphism and large eosinophilic nucleoli may be seen in endometrial proliferations that otherwise do not meet the complex architectural criteria delineated in Fig. 29.

In these exceptional cases, cytologic abnormalities are often only focal and are of a degree that, if they were present to a greater extent, would confer a grade 2 diagnosis under the recently revised FIGO grading system. Our data indicate that some of these lesions invade the myometrium; hence, endometrial proliferations with this degree of cytologic abnormality should be considered carcinomas, even though the architectural complexity found in the usual carcinoma is absent. The degree of cytologic atypia overrides the architectural requirements for grade 1 adenocarcinoma. On the other hand, a few endometrial proliferations associated with myoinvasion have the glandular complexity of carcinoma but have cytologic abnormalities less severe than those usually seen in AH.

The aggressive potential of these few cases cannot be recognized in biopsy and curetting specimens. The extreme architectural complexity, however, should lead the pathologist to interpret these as borderline lesions, which will result in appropriate treatment. Extensive, marked nuclear pleomorphism with prominent, variably sized and shaped nucleoli are features of grades 2 to 3 adenocarcinoma, not of grade 1 endometrioid carcinomas. Squamous differentiation is often present; in WDCA the squamous elements characteristically are cytologically bland (adenoacanthoma) (Table 11). An approach to the evaluation of a challenging endometrial curetting is presented in Fig. 29.

While the pattern of irregular, atypical glands surrounded by a granulation tissue–like host fibrous stromal response in an endometrial curettage specimen is highly associated with the presence of myoinvasion in the subsequent hysterectomy specimen, care must be taken to exclude mimics of this infrequently encountered pattern. These mimics include foreign body reaction to keratin, nonspecific associated endometritis, and the eosinophilic, cellular fibrous stroma that is relatively nonspecifically associated with a variety of endometrial lesions but is most notably seen in benign endometrial polyps and some cases of well-differentiated adenocarcinoma. The latter type of fibrous tissue has very low predictive value for myoinvasion.

We find distinctions among types of stroma to be most challenging, and consequently we place less reliance on the finding of fibroblastic stroma than other researchers. Foam cells may be present in either hyperplastic endometria or those harboring adenocarcinoma; thus, their presence provides no additional information as to the aggressive potential of a proliferation. Extensive areas of squamous epithelium are more common in myoinvasive endometrial proliferations than in nonmyoinvasive proliferations, but the differences are insufficient for this to be a reliable discriminating feature. The problem of distinguishing AH from well-differentiated endometrial adenocarcinoma is discussed later, in the differential diagnosis section.

Not infrequently, well-differentiated adenocarcinoma cells demonstrate variation in cytoplasmic differentiation. In addition to the expected endometrioid cells, scattered ciliated cells, cells with eosinophilic cytoplasm without cilia,

TABLE 11. *International Society of Gynecologic Pathologists criteria for squamous differentiation (232)*

A solid focus of tumor in an endometrioid-type carcinoma should be considered glandular unless at least one of the following criteria suggesting squamous differentiation is present:
  Keratinization, demonstrated, with standard staining techniques
  Intercellular bridges
  Three or more of the following four criteria
    Sheet-like growth without gland formation or palisading
    Sharp cell margins
    Eosinophilic and thick or glassy cytoplasm
    Cells with significantly more abundant cytoplasm than nonsquamous tumor cells

squamous cells and morules, cells with intracytoplasmic mucin, and cells with secretory-like features may be found. Most often these different types of cells are mixed with the endometrioid cells, but well-differentiated adenocarcinomas may feature populations of mixed cells alternating with areas of monotypic differentiation. When the alternatively differentiated cells come to predominate, a diagnosis of special variant carcinoma should be considered (see later discussion of Special Variant Carcinomas).

Clinicopathologic Correlation

Grade 1 adenocarcinomas of the endometrium are almost always stage I, and the vast majority are not myoinvasive. In the Stanford series, the overall relapse-free survival rate for grade 1, stage I patients was nearly 95% (244). The figure is essentially 100% for patients with grade 1, stage I tumors confined to the endometrium. Hysterectomy is the treatment of choice for patients with WDCA for whom fertility is not a consideration. Young women with WDCA interested in preserving their childbearing capacity may be treated nonsurgically under some circumstances (see earlier discussion). Postoperative radiation therapy is often used for those patients in whom grade 1 adenocarcinoma has invaded more than a 50% thickness of the uterine wall.

Grade 2 Endometrioid Adenocarcinoma

Description

The usual grade 2 adenocarcinoma (Fig. 35) has all the architectural features of a grade 1 adenocarcinoma, except that 6% to 50% of the tumor is composed of a sheet-like proliferation of malignant cells in which glandular differentiation is either absent or barely discernible (Table 10). The constituent cells almost always have cytologic features characterized by pleomorphism and large, prominent nucleoli, which are easily recognized as malignant. Care must be taken to distinguish between a sheet-like proliferation of cytologically malignant cells and sheet-like formations produced by cytologically bland squamous cells or morules in what is otherwise grade 1 carcinoma; the latter should be ignored in assigning a grade to the carcinoma (see later section on squamous and morular differentiation and Table 11).

Clinicopathologic Correlation

The initial treatment for patients with Grade 2 carcinomas is hysterectomy and, in some patients, surgical staging. Postoperative radiation therapy is administered to patients whose carcinomas are myoinvasive. Because the clinical behavior of grades 2 and 3 adenocarcinomas of the endometrium is similar and both are distinctly more aggressive than grade 1 carcinomas, it has been suggested that grades 2 and 3 be collapsed into a single high-grade group; this would result in a simplified (and perhaps more clinically relevant) stratification of endometrial carcinoma into low- and high-grade groups. These considerations notwithstanding, we prefer to retain the three-tiered grading scheme because it allows more flexibility in the grading process.

Grade 3 Endometrioid Adenocarcinoma

Description

The definition of grade 3 adenocarcinoma (Figs. 36 and 37) requires that more than 50% of the tumor be solid or sheet-like, with cytologically high-grade undifferentiated cells (Table 10). Even if better-differentiated areas are present, the glands tend to be poorly formed. The constituent cells are easily recognized as malignant and feature marked nuclear pleomorphism and prominent nucleoli of varying sizes. Grade 3 endometrioid carcinomas sometimes contain areas of cytologically malignant squamous elements; not infrequently, grade 3 endometrioid adenocarcinomas are mixed with poor-prognosis special variant carcinomas (see the later section on squamous and morular metaplasia and Table 11). Vascular invasion is not unusual; it should be searched for and reported if present.

Clinicopathologic Correlation

Most grade 3 carcinomas have invaded the myometrium by the time of hysterectomy. We think any degree of myometrial invasion by grade 3 carcinoma warrants adjuvant therapy.

Differential Diagnosis: Nonsecretory Patterns

Atrophic Versus "Insufficient for Diagnosis"

At times, the endometrial sample may contain only fragments of the lower uterine segment. The glands in such a specimen are similar to those found in endometrial atrophy. Misinterpretation of such fragments as atrophy would mislead the clinician into believing that the endometrium had been adequately sampled when in fact it had not. This error can be avoided by paying attention to the prominent fibrotic stroma characteristic of the lower uterine segment. Even if the specimen consists entirely of atrophic endometrium, a scanty specimen may not be representative of the entire endometrium. In each instance, the diagnosis should be "insufficient for evaluation of the endometrium." In the interest of maintaining clinicopathologic harmony, it should be remembered that "insufficient for diagnosis" is not to be equated with "inadequate gynecologist"; there may be nothing more in the uterus for the sampling to obtain.

Atrophic Versus Weakly Proliferative

In the usual case, weakly proliferative glands are tubular and lined by small (relative to cells in normal proliferative glands), pseudostratified, elongated, bland cells with densely basophilic nuclei (Fig. 15). Mitoses are distinctly rare or absent. Atrophic glands are lined by flattened to cuboidal cells and may be tubular or cystically dilated (Figs. 11 and 12). Both of these patterns are normal in the perimenopausal and postmenopausal years and may be seen in endometria from patients experiencing abnormal uterine bleeding. It is of no importance to distinguish between atrophic and weakly proliferative endometria. It is important, however, to ensure that the sample is representative and that nothing else is present in curettings with this pattern. In this regard, it should be remembered that many cases of high-grade carcinoma in postmenopausal women are unaccompanied by hyperplastic endometria. In some cases of UPSC, for example, the only evidence of the malignant neoplasm in curettings will be individual malignant cells scattered among otherwise atrophic endometrial fragments.

Atrophic Endometrium Versus Endometrial Hyperplasia

Occasionally, the atrophic surface epithelium and underlying thin endometrium may be rolled up like a carpet by the sampling curette. Sectioning of this low-volume sample may yield a low-power pattern that resembles complex hyperplasia in its predominance of epithelium over stroma (Fig. 13). The addition of a few atypical-looking ciliated cells may further prompt a diagnosis of AH (Fig. 11). An awareness of this possibility and attention to the overall inactive appearance of the epithelium should lead to the correct diagnosis. Atrophic endometria may be abundant and contain cystically dilated glands (Fig. 12), which may be crowded. Distinguishing this condition from hyperplasia is based on the flattened to cuboidal cells lining the atrophic glands rather than the mitotically active, elongated to round and often enlarged cells characteristic of hyperplasia (Figs. 10-12 and 20-21).

Disordered Proliferative Versus Normal Proliferative

Both of these patterns are encountered in patients who are experiencing sporadic anovulation at the beginning and the end of the reproductive years—the perimenarche and the climacteric. The normal proliferative pattern is, of course, the usual follicular phase pattern found during the reproductive years. In addition, both of these patterns are typically seen in patients receiving exogenous estrogens. Distinguishing disordered proliferative endometria (Figs. 16–18) from proliferative endometria is of no particular importance. The essential information conveyed by a diagnosis of disordered proliferation is that the patient has not ovulated, that neither AH nor carcinoma is present, and that the specimen is judged to be representative of the uterine lining. Curettage is usually sufficient to control acute bleeding and, at least for the time being, eradicate the responsible proliferation.

Attention can then turn to tracking down the source of what is, in essence, estrogen-withdrawal bleeding and instituting appropriate hormonal manipulations. Indeed, there is a growing tendency to manage DUB without tissue sampling in patients not suspected of harboring a malignancy (72). Morphologic features that distinguish normal and disordered proliferation have been presented earlier. Weakly proliferative endometria lack the mitotic activity found in both disordered proliferative and normal proliferative endometria, and the constituent nuclei are smaller and thinner.

Disordered Proliferative Versus Hyperplasia

For a diagnosis of hyperplasia, rather than disordered proliferative endometrium (Figs. 16–22), we require that glandular overgrowth be sufficiently pronounced to shift the glands-to-stroma ratio to 3:1, that is, the stroma comprises less than one-third the volume of the proliferation. The glandular fraction includes both glands (and their lumens) and villoglandular structures.

Hyperplasia: Nonatypical Versus Atypical

The term atypical hyperplasia refers to hyperplastic endometria composed of cells with cytologic atypia (Figs. 23–25). Patients with AH have a higher risk of endometrial adenocarcinoma; those patients harboring hyperplastic endometria featuring architectural complexity *without* cytologic atypia (complex hyperplasia) apparently are not at a significant risk of endometrial carcinoma, and their endometria should not be labeled atypical (Figs. 21 and 22). The phrase "without atypia" (though redundant) may be appended, to emphasize that the risk is not that of AH. Thus, when evaluating hyperplastic endometria, the important observation is cytologic atypia in an architecturally simple or complex endometrium; only endometria with cytologic atypia should be labeled AH.

Cytologic atypia implies that most of the following features are present: enlargement and rounding of nuclei, prominence of nucleoli, chromatin clearing, hyperchromatism, and a tendency for the cells to appear piled up, with a loss of polarity. Cells with minimal atypia deviate only very slightly from those in proliferative endometria; they are larger, but still elongated, and have increased chromatin. Cells demonstrating severe atypia have the features found in grade 1 carcinoma cells, but their architectural arrangement is not as complex as is required for carcinoma (see earlier discussion). Our moderate and severe categories of atypia correspond more or less to the complex AH of Kurman et al. (210).

Atypical Hyperplasia Versus Grade 1 Adenocarcinoma

The diagnostic decision-making dilemmas in the range of AH/WDCA are notoriously challenging and were fully discussed earlier (Figs. 23–25 and 28–34). Our approach is also presented in Table 12 and Fig. 29 (214,215,217,349–351). It is important to remember that there are no known abrupt biochemical, cellular, kinetic, chromosomal, ultrastructural, or light microscopic discontinuities as one travels along the morphologic continuum from significantly atypical hyper-

TABLE 12. *An approach to the diagnosis of endometrial carcinoma in an endometrial sampling*

Endometrial feature to be explained	Malignant process that might explain the finding	Benign process that might explain the finding	Suggested solutions
Papillary architecture	Some very well differentiated carcinomas have papillary syncytial-like areas that are noninformative on the issue of benign/malignant as in the case of morules/squamous metaplasia. Endometrioid carcinoma of the villoglandular type is composed of relatively bland cells. UPSC is papillary but possesses marked cytological atypia.	Papillary syncytial metaplasia Papillary change	Careful attention to the cytological features of the proliferation Repeated sampling if indicated
Granulation tissue host response	Host response to carcinoma	Postcurettage change Reparative reaction in endometrial polyp tip or other exophytic endometrial lesion Cervical or endometrial inflammatory process	Careful search for preserved epithelial elements to evaluate; use the cytology and growth index features of the algorithm. Repeated sampling if indicated
Fibrous stroma of nongranulation tissue type	Some grade 1 carcinomas may have this type of stroma. In our experience, as many noncarcinomas as carcinomas possess this type of stroma.	Lower uterine segment Endometrial polyps Hyperplasia/metaplasia often has this type of stroma.	Careful attention to the cytologic features of the proliferation and other features of the proliferation that would identify it as one of the possibilities in the "benign" column
Smooth muscle mixed with glands	Fragments of myometrium invaded by carcinoma (possibly architecturally noncomplex and cytologically bland) Carcinoma involving the basalis or fragments of superficial myometrium	Atypical polypoid adenomyoma Atypical hyperplasia involving deep basalis or superficial adenomyosis Adenomyoma	Careful attention to cytologic features Imaging studies to identify myoinvasion Repeated sampling if indicated
Scanty sample	Truly inadequate sample; the carcinoma has not been sampled. The exophytic part of the carcinoma may have been shed. The carcinoma may not have a prominent exophytic component (e.g. some UPSCs).	Truly inadequate sample, and the endometrium is benign. Atrophy	Hysteroscopy and/or imaging studies may be helpful. Repeated sampling if indicated
Extensive necrosis	Necrotic carcinoma with no residual diagnostic cells	Any disintegrating endometrium, including menstrual endometrium, may feature necrosis.	Careful search for preserved epithelial elements to evaluate, using the cytology and growth index features of the algorithm Some high-grade carcinomas (e.g., UPSC) may shed only single diagnosable malignant cells. Repeated sampling if indicated
Extensive morules/ squamous metaplasia	The bland squamous component of a grade 1 or 2 carcinoma	Atrophy, weakly proliferative and disordered proliferative endometrium with morular/squamous elements Hyperplasia with morular/squamous metaplasia	Careful search for glandular elements to evaluate, using criteria in text In general, the squamous elements of well-differentiated carcinoma are noninformative in morphologic features on the issue of benign/malignant Repeated sampling if indicated

UPSC, uterine papillary serous carcinoma.

plasias to proliferations whose light microscopic features would compel a diagnosis of malignancy by all responsible observers (216,352–354). In short, special technology provides us with no gold standard for distinguishing the biologically benign from the biologically malignant at a fundamental level in the AH/WDCA range.

This leaves us with the admittedly unsatisfactory situation of drawing subjective lines using standard H&E cytologic and architectural features. Furthermore, this line-drawing is as much dependent on patients' values, risks of current therapies, medical–legal considerations, and professional self-interest as it is on the "objectively evaluated" morphologic features of these proliferations. It follows that even given agreement on the clinicopathologic facts of the matter (e.g., given that a pattern is correlated with some probability of finding occult distant disease at the time of diagnosis or myoinvasion in the hysterectomy specimen), a large number of plausible morphologic definitions of WDCA are still possible—one for every combination of choices about the nonhistopathologic issues listed earlier. All of these problems also arise in the separation of atypical metaplasia and the corresponding well-differentiated special variant carcinomas that feature cellular differentiation other than endometrioid. Elsewhere, we have outlined an argument for using the probability of myoinvasion in the hysterectomy specimen to motivate distinguishing between AH and WDCA (217).

Kurman and Norris have suggested one set of morphologic criteria for the diagnosis of well-differentiated endometrial adenocarcinoma (349). These workers require that one of four patterns be present before making a diagnosis of carcinoma: irregularly shaped glands embedded in fibrous tumor stroma, confluent glandular growth, an extensive papillary growth, and/or extensive squamous epithelium. The latter three patterns must be present in a contiguous area of at least 2.1 mm. Using these criteria, Kurman and Norris achieved a 90% sensitivity for picking out myoinvasion in the hysterectomy specimen (false-negative rate of 10%) and a 70% specificity for identifying myoinvasion (false-positive rate of 30%). In their series, the false-negative cases (diagnosis of AH on the sampling when myoinvasive carcinoma was present in the hysterectomy specimen) were all ones in which the tumors were only superficially myoinvasive. In our hands, these criteria have a sensitivity of 80% and a specificity of 70%.

We have explored alternative sets of criteria and, using myoinvasion in the hysterectomy specimen as the outcome variable, we find that essentially all of the predictive power of H&E criteria for distinguishing myoinvasion in these well-differentiated proliferations resides in the complex glandular and villoglandular patterns enumerated in the section devoted to well-differentiated carcinoma, as long as the required minimal cytologic features are also present (Fig. 17). For these well-differentiated borderline lesions, more elaborate rules incorporating the degree of cytologic abnormalities (nuclear pleomorphism, prominence of nucleoli), stromal features (presence of granulation tissue-like stroma, fibrous stroma, adenofibromatous or smooth muscle), and the differentiated features of the epithelium (squamous, mucinous, ciliated) could be constructed that marginally improved upon the sensitivity and specificity figures cited, but none of them stood up under cross-validation.

This impression was confirmed when various rules were tested on an entirely different set of endometria from those used to construct the classification rule. Thus, of the four Kurman and Norris criteria, confluent glandular growth and extensive papillary growth appear to be the best at differentiating potentially myoinvasive proliferations and are predictive, whereas the extensive squamous epithelium and glands embedded in fibrous stroma do not add to the predictive power of these architectural features. In another study, Norris and co-workers found that morphometrically measured epithelial cellularity best correlated with the pathologist's assignment of a case into the AH or carcinoma groups, suggesting that, in practice, complex epithelial growth is the feature experienced pathologists take most seriously in making this distinction (355).

Most proliferations in this AH/WDCA spectrum are readily placed, with practice, on one side of the line or the other (Fig. 29 and Table 12). Problems are created by those cases that straddle the line or represent variations on the AH/WDCA theme that were unanticipated by the criteria. We find the term borderline lesion useful in these circumstances. Again, taking a broader analytic view is often more helpful than prolonged staring at the curettage specimen to divine its true nature. In the vocabulary used in the AH section, it is clear that for low-risk hysterectomy patients, there is no question of not performing a hysterectomy when the endometrial lesion is borderline. The only thing at stake is rendering a possibly wrong diagnosis of malignancy, with the attendant concern that this engenders in the patient. The diagnosis of borderline lesion has the advantage of warranting a hysterectomy and tabling the issue of cancer until all the evidence is in.

Matters are more complicated for the high-penalty hysterectomy group of patients. The issue for them is whether to remove the uterus at all or to attempt reversal of the process pharmacologically. Again, the diagnosis "borderline" leaves the clinician's options open: hysterectomy or another sampling, attempted pharmacologic reversal, and resampling. In our opinion, the responsible way of handling this situation is *not* to make a dogmatic pronouncement in the face of what realistically is fairly complete ignorance about the potential of a borderline lesion, but (unpopular as if often is) to pass the uncertainty on to the clinician, who, in possession of the relevant clinical facts, is in a better position to deal with them in a more constructive and informed fashion that the pathologist.

Disintegrating Endometria Versus Endometrial Hyperplasia or Adenocarcinoma

This might seem a trivial differential diagnostic issue, but in reality it is a fairly common and often difficult problem; in rare instances, it is unresolvable and requires rebiopsy. When the stroma of benign endometria (with any of the patterns discussed earlier) disintegrates and collapses, the glands may remain intact and become closely approximated. This pattern can simulate a significant shift in the glands-to-stroma ratio in favor of glands and thus imitate the low-power appearance of hyperplasia or carcinoma. Careful attention to nuclear features usually allows for distinction of this pattern from carcinoma. Care must be taken in evaluating nuclear features, however, because degenerated nuclei may become swollen and enlarged. In menstrual endometria, a search for evidence of secretory changes in the glands, glandular apoptosis, and predecidual reaction in the stroma is often helpful (see earlier discussion).

Polypoid Fragments of Endometrium Versus Endometrial Polyp

Normal endometria, particularly secretory endometria, may have grossly polypoid areas, but they are histologically indistinguishable from surrounding nonpolypoid fragments. At the microscopic level, we require a fibrous stroma containing large, thick-walled vessels for a diagnosis of endometrial polyp.

Endometrial Polyp Versus Adenofibroma Versus Adenomyoma Versus Atypical Polypoid Adenomyoma

Most adenofibromas (AdFibs) and some adenosarcomas (see the section on mixed müllerian tumors) have a gross papillary architecture manifest microscopically either as long, epithelial-lined clefts extending into the stroma or as rounded papillae, some of which may be inserted into cystic spaces. endometrial polyps do not have this architecture (Figs. 26 and 27; compare with Figs. 73-75). Adenomyomas have a myofibromatous stroma. APAs also have smooth muscle or hybrid smooth muscle and fibrous stroma, and the glandular elements are architecturally complex and cytologically atypical (Figs. 69-72). Morules and squamous differentiation are encountered in more than 90% of APAs.

Grading of Adenocarcinoma: Grade 1 Versus Grade 2

The delimiting of endometrial carcinoma grades is as arbitrary as distinguishing AH from well-differentiated adenocarcinoma. The statistics relating grade to prognosis are summary statistics that reflect the behavior of the majority of cases that concentrate toward the centers of each of the grades; it is doubtful that those statistics would change significantly with the shifting of ambiguous cases from one side to the other of the grades 1 to 2 or 2 to 3 boundary. We are nevertheless called upon to assign an unambiguous grade to a malignancy, and the conventions for doing so have been indicated under Clinicopathologic Correlation in the section on carcinoma and in Table 10.

Grade 3 Adenocarcinoma Versus Other Neoplasms Featuring Sheet-like Proliferation of Malignant Cells

Grade 3 adenocarcinomas are, by definition, largely undifferentiated. This raises a number of differential diagnostic difficulties that are discussed under the heading of sheet-like malignant proliferations encountered in uterine curettings (see pattern 4 in Table 4).

Another technique for estimating chronological date that is sometimes employed is forward counting from the first day of the menstrual period preceding the biopsy. This method requires the assumption that the follicular phase has been 14 days long and the luteal phase will be 14 days long (i.e., it assumes an ideal cycle length of 28 days). Given the great variability in length of the follicular phase and the modest variability in length of the luteal phase in normal, fertile women, this assumption is highly unrealistic and renders this method useless.

ENDOMETRIA WITH ALTERNATIVE DIFFERENTIATED EPITHELIUM: METAPLASIAS AND SPECIAL VARIANT CARCINOMAS (214,356) (FIG. 9)

Introduction

At times, benign cells with differentiation typically encountered elsewhere in the female genital tract may be discovered in endometrial proliferations. Similarly, carcinomas arising in the endometrium may, on occasion, demonstrate differentiation found more often in neoplasms arising in other parts of the female genitalia. The concept of the extended müllerian system is a useful construct for understanding these observations (357,358). The ovarian surface "epithelium," fallopian tubes, uterus, and upper third of the vagina share a common embryologic history, and all of these structures act, in many ways, as a single extended organ system. Many of these components show similar changes during pregnancy, develop comparable epithelial metaplasias, and share a common set of differentiated neoplasms. Furthermore, several neoplasms (often of identical histologic types) may arise in different components of the müllerian system metachronously or synchronously.

Although the full range of müllerian epithelial neoplasms may develop at any site within the female genitalia, the incidence of a particular differentiated type varies from one anatomic site to another. For example, most of the surface epithelial carcinomas that arise in the ovary may also be primary in the endometrium. In the endometrium, however, endometrioid carcinomas are by far the most common type; in the ovary, endometrioid carcinomas identical to those arising in the uterus are less common than serous and mucinous types. In general, there is nothing in the intrinsic histologic characteristics of a müllerian neoplasm that pinpoints its anatomic site of origin. Papillary serous carcinoma looks much the same whether it arises in the endometrium (an infrequent occurrence) or in the ovary (a common occurrence).

These considerations have certain important implications for the histopathologist. First, clinicopathologic correlation is often required to establish the primary site of a gynecologic malignancy. In the endometrium, this is particularly true for neoplasms exhibiting mucinous (endocervical primary?) or papillary serous (ovarian primary?) differentiation. Second, the diagnosis of benign or malignant, given a particular type of differentiation, may depend on the primary site. For example, considerably more cytologic atypia, mitotic activity, and epithelial stratification is allowed in benign endometrial proliferations with mucinous areas (mucinous metaplasia) than in benign endocervical proliferations with mucinous areas. Finally, the occurrence of synchronous, primary, müllerian neoplasms at several sites in the female genital tract has important implications for staging, prognosis, and therapy.

Endometrial Epithelial Metaplasias (356)

In a variety of circumstances, benign endometrial cells may exhibit epithelial differentiation other than the well-known differentiated patterns seen in proliferative and secretory endometria. The commonly encountered alternative epithelial types ("metaplasias") are discussed here. It is important to realize that these benign alternative epithelial types may be present in association with any of the nonsecretory endometria (i.e., atrophic; weakly proliferative; disordered proliferative; hyperplastic, including AH; and endometrioid carcinoma). This is indicated in Fig. 9 (359). The clinical significance that attaches to these patterns is, as far as we know, that of the underlying associated nonsecretory pattern.

For example, patients with AH containing squamous metaplastic areas presumably have the same risk of endometrial carcinoma as those patients with hyperplasia with the same degree of cytologic atypia but uncomplicated by this differentiated feature. Benign metaplastic cells often cause diagnostic difficulties because of their unusual appearance and because they may grow in architectural arrangements also found in complex hyperplasia and in carcinoma. In particular, they may stratify (e.g., morules), or they may have cribriform patterns (e.g., ciliary metaplasia). When benign metaplastic epithelium coexists with carcinoma, the metaplastic cells do not warrant a change in the classification of the carcinoma; the classification of the carcinoma is based on the morphologic features of the malignant epithelium.

Cells with aberrant differentiation may themselves be malignant, however. In this circumstance, the term metaplasia is no longer appropriate; instead, the designation special variant carcinoma is employed. A final important differential diagnostic point: the subclassification of metaplasias into a variety of types is for descriptive and differential diagnostic purposes. Once a proliferation is determined to be a metaplasia and its degree of atypia determined, an unequivocal assignment to a particular metaplastic type is of little clinical (and probably less scientific) interest. Indeed, most metaplastic endometria are of mixed type, and it is likely that many of the patterns overlap (e.g., morules and syncytial papillary metaplasia).

Special Variant Carcinomas

The endometrium gives rise to a wide variety of differentiated carcinomas, but more than 80% are glandular neoplasms that resemble the epithelium found in endometrial hyperplasia (Table 9). Squamous or squamoid ("morular") differentiation is commonly encountered in this endometrioid or usual adenocarcinoma. Other müllerian differentiated types make up the remainder of endometrial carcinomas, the so-called special variants. Papillary serous carcinoma and clear-cell carcinoma are important because of their notorious aggressiveness. Mucinous carcinoma raises questions concerning localization, since both the cervix and the endometrium give rise to mucinous neoplasms and the treatment of carcinomas at these two sites differs. Carcinomas composed predominantly or exclusively of ciliated cells define the category of ciliated cell carcinoma and are a curiosity; however, scattered ciliated cells are frequently found in ordinary endometrioid carcinomas.

Specifics About Various Types of Differentiation

Squamous Differentiation

Squamous differentiation in the endometrium takes many forms, ranging from highly keratinized epithelia that exfoliate anucleate squames to sheet-like proliferations of cells with indistinct cytoplasmic margins, no obvious keratinization, and often a rounded contour (morules). (Figs. 44–47; Table 11) (360). Occasionally, the sheet-like morules may feature either abrupt central hyaline keratinization or a central accumulation of granular necrotic material. Sometimes morular cells are spindled. None of these cytoplasmic features in and of themselves is diagnostic of malignancy.

The nuclear features of squamous cells encountered in the endometrium range from completely bland to obviously malignant. Cytologically bland squamous elements may be asso-

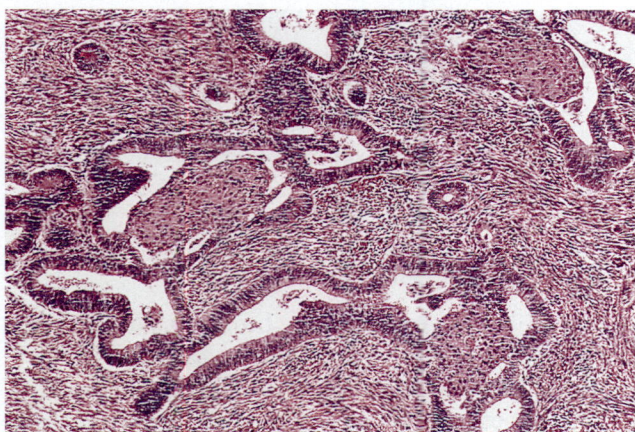

FIG. 44. Disordered proliferative endometrium with morule formation. This endometrium features widely spaced, irregularly branched and budded glands that are replaced in focal areas by rounded aggregates of squamoid cells.

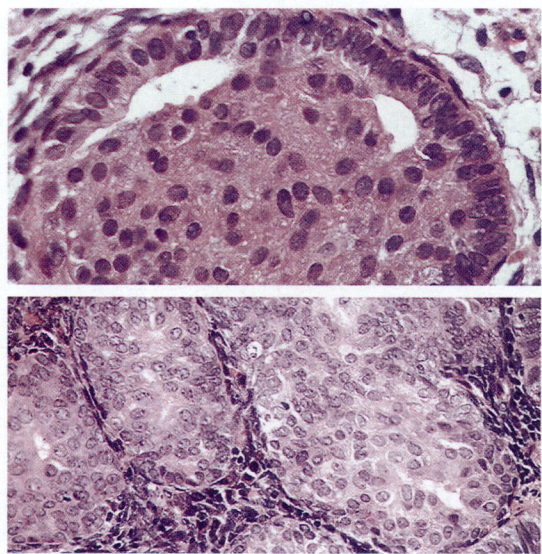

FIG. 45. Endometrial morules in areas of complex, nontypical hyperplasia. *Top:* Morules are rounded aggregates composed of sheets of cytologically bland cells with indistinct cytoplasmic margins. *Bottom:* These squamoid cells are rising from a cytologically bland, weakly proliferative epithelium.

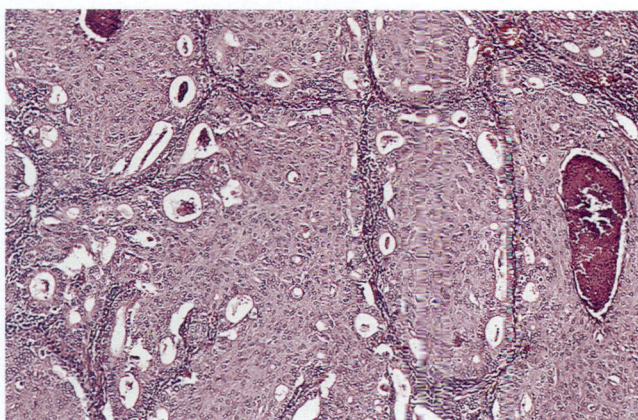

FIG. 46. Confluent morule formation with central necrosis. Morules quite frequently exhibit a peculiar type of central necrosis, which is evident in these macroglands in a polyp in what was otherwise a secretory endometrium. This pattern of necrosis is not sufficient to warrant a diagnosis of malignancy.

ciated with normal endometrial glands, hyperplasias, and glandular proliferations with the features of carcinoma. Cytologically malignant squamous elements may, on extremely rare occasions, be present in isolation (pure squamous carcinoma), but they are more often seen in association with high-grade carcinomatous glandular elements. When the squamous or morular elements lack malignant cytologic features, the prognostic and therapeutic implications of proliferations containing squamous elements are essentially those that attach to the associated glandular part of the process. That is, proliferations containing benign squamous or morular elements mixed with carcinomatous glands behave like the glandular component, whereas proliferations with identical squamous elements in a hyperplastic endometria behave like hyperplasia.

Squamous Metaplasia Associated with Benign Glandular Elements

This sort of metaplasia may be seen in association with foreign-body reactions, chemical irritants, and endometritis, but it is found most often and most extensively in hyperestrogenic states, particularly endometrial hyperplasia (361–363) (Figs. 45–47). Ichthyosis uteri refers to the complete replacement of the endometrium by benign squamous epithelium (364).

Carcinoma with Squamous Elements (365–368)

Squamous differentiation is typically encountered in endometrioid carcinomas arising in the endometrium. Two views have been taken of this phenomenon. The traditional view, which can be labeled the two-disease school, has it that endometrioid carcinomas with cytologically bland squamous elements represent one distinct disease entity (adenoacanthoma) (Fig. 47), whereas endometrioid carcinomas with cytologically malignant squamous elements (mixed adenosquamous carcinoma) represent another distinct disease entity (369–372) (Fig. 48). The squamous elements in adenosquamous carcinoma not infrequently have the appearance of large-cell nonkeratinizing carcinomas of the cervix (Figs. 48 and 49). Investigators supporting this view concede that the glandular components in the former disease are typically low grade, whereas the glandular components in the second disease are usually high grade.

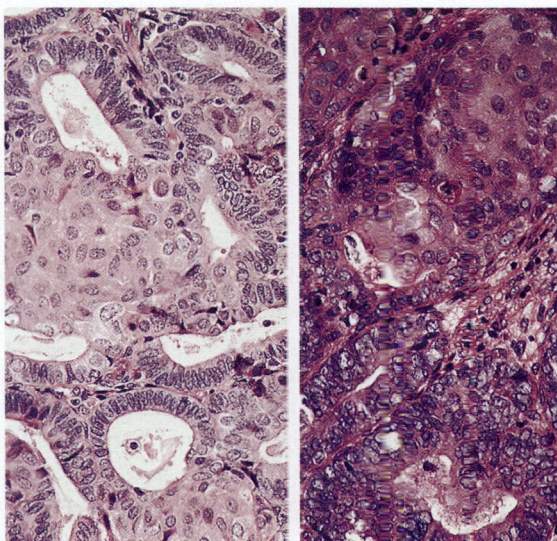

FIG. 47. Complex endometrial hyperplasia contrasted with well-differentiated adenocarcinoma, both containing morules; here they are cytologically bland morules. The distinction between hyperplasia and carcinoma is based on an evaluation of epithelium lining the glands. *Left:* The epithelium is composed of pseudostratified cytologically bland cells. *Right:* The glands are lined by cytologically malignant cells.

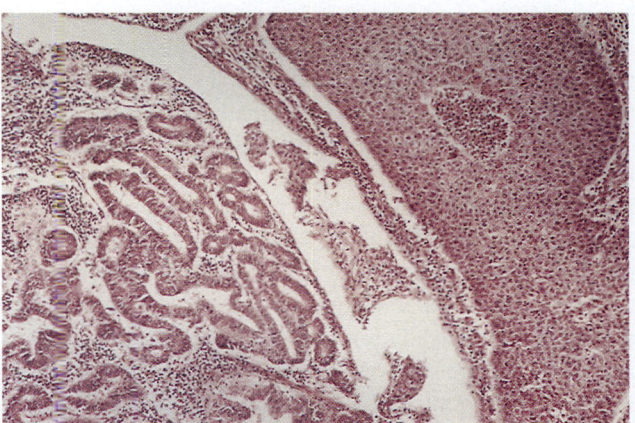

FIG. 48. Endometrial adenocarcinoma with large-cell nonkeratinizing morphologic features. In this case, the solid sheets of epithelium are reminiscent of nonkeratinizing large-cell carcinoma of the cervix. This pattern in the past has been referred to as adenosquamous carcinoma, although current classification schemes would not count this pattern as squamous differentiation.

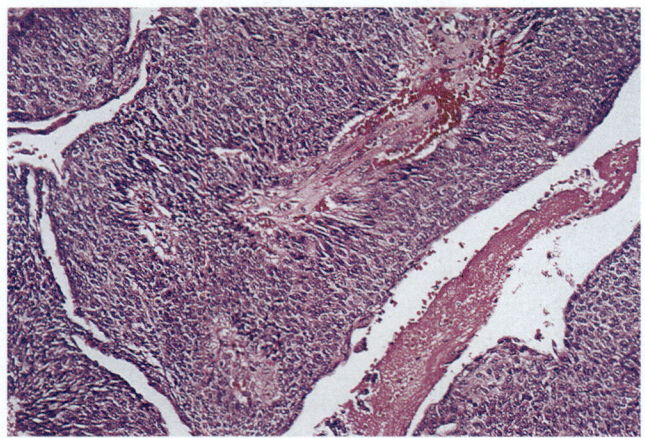

FIG. 49. Grade 3 endometrioid adenocarcinoma with large-cell nonkeratinizing morphologic characteristics. Sheets of cytologically malignant cells are interrupted by broad bands of stroma, imparting a papillary appearance. This is a higher-power view of the carcinoma illustrated in Fig. 47 and shows a pattern of differentiation that would not count as squamous.

An intermediate group of atypical adenoacanthomas with atypical, but not malignant squamous elements has been isolated by Connelly and co-workers (242); the behavior of this group is indistinguishable from that of carcinoma with bland squamous elements. Well-differentiated adenocarcinomas with bland squamous elements have a prognosis comparable to (and possibly better than) grade 1 endometrioid carcinomas without squamous elements, whereas mixed adenosquamous carcinomas are thought to be a highly aggressive malignancy comparable to (or possibly worse than) grade 3 endometrioid carcinomas without squamous elements. A differential diagnostic corollary of this view is that it is important to distinguish the sheet-like growth of grade 3 endometrioid carcinomas from adenosquamous carcinomas with large-cell nonkeratinizing areas, a task that is well nigh impossible.

The second view is that the squamous elements encountered in endometrioid carcinoma exhibit a spectrum of cytologic atypia, ranging from cytologically benign to cytologically malignant squamous proliferations and including the high-grade, large-cell nonkeratinizing type (365,373–375). Supporters of this position note that the cytologic atypia of the squamous elements more or less correlates with that of the glandular elements. They see no reason to postulate the existence of two separate diseases, and they further suggest that all of the clinically relevant information is conveyed by a simple statement of overall grade. We take the latter view; it has been supported by a large series of uniformly staged clinical stage I cases (366).

Accordingly, we do not distinguish grade 3 endometrioid carcinomas from adenosquamous carcinomas of the large-cell nonkeratinizing type. Our terminology is adenocarcinoma (specify grade) with squamous or morular metaplasia. When grade 3 adenocarcinoma with squamous or nonkeratinizing large-cell elements is present, however, it may be appropriate to point out that such neoplasms are classified by some as adenosquamous carcinoma, because clinicians are attuned to this term. In agreement with Christopherson et al., we consider glassy-cell carcinoma to be a variant of carcinoma with high-grade squamous elements (376). Carcinomas of the endometrium with squamous differentiation can be associated with a foreign body reaction on the peritoneum in the absence of metastases, apparently stemming from discharge of keratin through the fallopian tubes (334).

Differential Diagnosis

Not all endometrial proliferations with squamous elements are malignant. The differential diagnosis of bland squamous elements includes squamous metaplasia and morular metaplasia. The distinction between AH with squamous metaplasia and well-differentiated adenocarcinoma with bland squamous elements rests on an evaluation of the glandular component; the squamous component in this situation is not informative in terms of its morphologic features as to whether the proliferation is benign or malignant. Most cytologically atypical squamous proliferations of the endometrium are intimately admixed with endometrial glandular elements easily recognized as malignant. When this is not the case, the possibility of a primary squamous cell carcinoma should be considered. The recovery of pure squamous cell carcinoma in a curettage specimen always raises the possibility of a cervical primary, and suitable clinical localizing studies should be undertaken. While a handful of cases of pure squamous cell carcinoma primary in the endometrium have been reported, this is indeed a rare event (377–379). Even more of a curiosity is a verrucous carcinoma primary of the endometrium (380). On rare occasions, there may be extension of cervical carcinoma *in situ* into the uterine fundus (381,382).

Sheet-like Growth of Poorly Differentiated Carcinoma Versus Sheet-like Growth of Morules. This is an important distinction, both in deciding between benign and malignant proliferations and (particularly if one uses the FIGO grading scheme) in establishing the grade of a carcinoma. The distinction is a cytologic one. High-grade carcinomas with a sheetlike architecture of stratified cells have obvious malignant nuclear features and easily found mitotic figures. Abnormal division figures are common. In contrast, the constituent cells of morules, while they are stratified into nodules or sheets, lack malignant features, and mitotic figures are very difficult to find (Fig. 45). Central necrosis of morules is common, whether the glandular proliferation is benign or malignant (Fig. 46). When there is uncertainty as to whether the squamous elements are malignant (high grade), the glandular elements can be used for grading. Most lesions containing squamous cells that are ambiguous are low grade.

The Recovery of Abundant Bland Squamous Elements Unassociated with Glands in an Endometrial Sample. This problem occasionally arises; while carcinoma is discovered in the hysterectomy specimens of such patients more often than not, this finding by no means establishes that diagnosis. Endometria ranging from atrophic to acutely hyperplastic may be associated with large zones of squamous metaplasia or large areas of morular metaplasia.

Mucinous Differentiation (214,356)

Mucinous differentiation is relatively common in the endometrium and may be encountered in association with the entire spectrum of nonsecretory endometrial patterns. It takes many different forms. On occasion, the epithelium may be highly reminiscent of normal endocervix, and when such fragments are discovered in an endometrial curettage specimen, they may masquerade as an endocervical fragment. On other occasions, endometrial cells containing cytoplasmic mucin are arranged on delicate fibrovascular stalks. Goblet cells may be present. On still other occasions, mucin-containing cells have delicately grainy, eosinophilic to slightly basophilic cytoplasm. When mucinous differentiation is found in glands with a tubuloalveolar pattern, acute inflammatory cells are usually embedded in the pools of mucin—a useful low-power marker of mucinous differentiation. Predominantly mucinous carcinomas develop in the endometrium and sometimes resemble those found more often in the endocervix or ovary. This histologic similarity raises occasionally difficult questions of localization.

Mucinous Metaplasia

Mucinous metaplasia is most often encountered in the context of hyperestrogenic states and—in rare instances, when they are associated with an element of cervical stenosis—may produce a dramatic mucometra (Figs. 50–52) (383–386). Diffuse or focal mucinous metaplasia is typically present in endometrial polyps and is not uncommon in postmenopausal endometria, usually in association with other metaplasias.

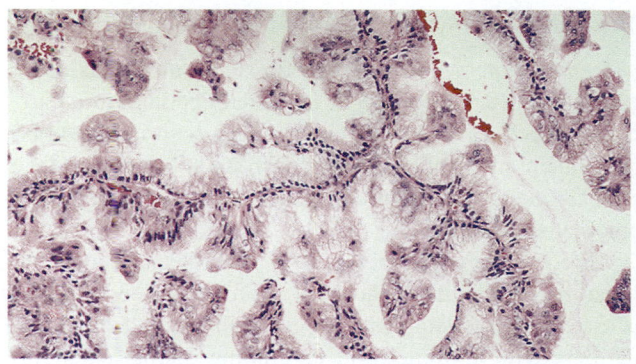
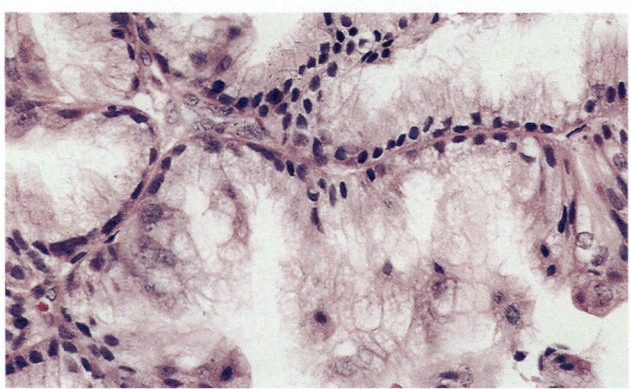

FIG. 51. Mucinous metaplasia. *Top:* A characteristic pattern of mucinous metaplasia. A delicately arborizing connective tissue scaffolding is lined by cytologically bland mucinous cells with basally situated nuclei. *Bottom:* A higher-power view of the lining cells. They are cytologically bland and have dense, uniform, inactive-appearing nuclei.

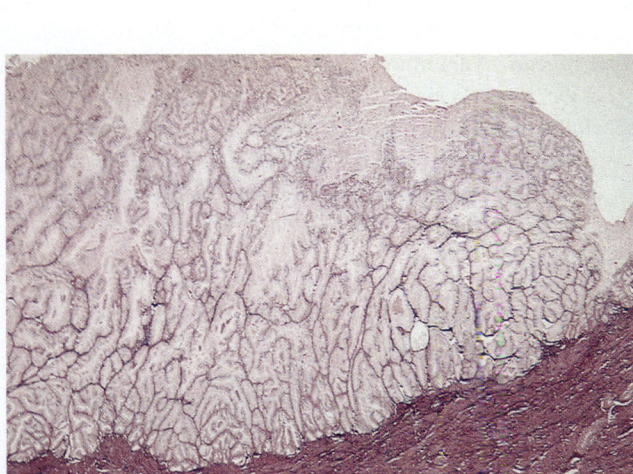

FIG. 50. Mucinous metaplasia (low power). This endometrium is composed of complex hyperplastic glands formed by cells with clear cytoplasm. The cystically dilated glands are filled with mucin, and the cytologic features of this proliferation are bland. The patient had a mucometra.

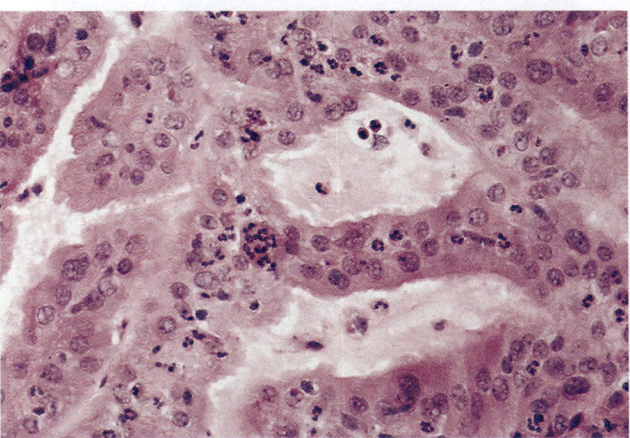

FIG. 52. Mucinous metaplasia. One characteristic of mucinous proliferations of the endometrium is their association with neutrophils. In this example, the neutrophils are present both within the mucinous epithelium and within the mucinous secretions.

Mucinous Carcinoma

Description. When searched for, focal mucinous differentiation is very common in the usual endometrioid carcinoma. Much less often, carcinoma cells with intracytoplasmic mucin are prominent and constitute more than 50% of the malignancy; in this circumstance, the term mucinous carcinoma is warranted (Fig. 53) (387–390).

Clinicopatholgic Correlation. The clinicopathologic profile of patients with mucinous carcinoma of the endometrium is essentially indistinguishable grade for grade from that of patients with endometrioid carcinoma of the usual sort; given that a patient has an endometrial primary carcinoma, the observation that it is mucin-producing is of no prognostic significance. The importance of this variant lies instead in the challenges of anatomic localization it presents when it is recovered in an endometrial sampling and in distinguishing mucinous carcinoma from complex mucinous metaplasia (see Differential Diagnosis below).

Differential Diagnosis

Atypical Mucinous Metaplasia Versus Mucinous Carcinoma. Primary mucinous endometrial carcinoma must be distinguished from mucinous metaplasia of the endometrium. The distinction is usually easy to make; when the architecture becomes complex or villoglandular, however, it can be difficult, because mucinous proliferations capable of invading the myometrium may have nuclei that are not strikingly atypical. The problems raised are essentially those discussed in connection with the separation of AH and well-differentiated adenocarcinoma (see earlier discussion). The distinction rests on evaluating both the cytologic and architectural features, and we are wary of interpreting predominantly mucinous processes with complex architecture as benign in curettage specimens. When such tissue is recovered in postmenopausal women, a hysterectomy is the best way to exclude well-differentiated mucinous carcinoma (388).

Primary Mucinous Carcinoma of the Endometrium Versus Endocervical Mucinous Carcinoma. Localization studies using differential curettage or imaging studies are sometimes required to distinguish primary endometrial from primary endocervical mucinous carcinoma (391–393). This distinction is important because the approach to therapy is quite different for carcinomas arising at each of these two sites (394). Helpful H&E features that favor an endometrial primary include associated endometrioid hyperplasia or metaplasia of the usual sort elsewhere in the endometrium (particularly hybrid mucinous endometrioid differentiation) and the presence of stromal foam cells. There are no reliable histochemical or immunohistochemical techniques to distinguish these two possibilities in an individual case, although carcinoembryonic antigen–containing neoplastic cells are more often found in primary endocervical carcinomas than in endometrioid carcinomas (395,396). In addition, vimentin and keratin coexpression in endometrial carcinomas is relatively common, while this coexpression is reported to be unusual in primary cervical adenocarcinomas; whether this pattern of staining distinguishes endocervical carcinoma from mucinous carcinoma of the endometrium is uncertain (397,398). Endometrial mucinous carcinoma may be mistaken for cervical microglandular hyperplasia in a curetting sample (399).

Primary Mucinous Carcinoma Versus Metastatic Mucinous Carcinoma. Mucinous carcinomas metastatic to the endometrium from, for example, a gastrointestinal tract primary are rare but should be given consideration (400,401). Awareness of the possibility and obtaining the relevant history usually clarify matters.

Mucinous Carcinoma Versus Cervical Microglandular Hyperplasia. Mucinous carcinomas of the endometrium on occasion mimic cervical microglandular hyperplasia. The possibility of a noncervical origin of a proliferation with this morphologic picture should be considered when fragments of epithelium with this pattern are distributed widely throughout the endometrial sample (390, 399).

Neuroendocrine Cells in Carcinomas of the Endometrium (402–408)

Argyrophilic cells are ubiquitous in the endometrium in both benign and malignant proliferations, and their presence has no clinical significance. Chromogranin immunoreactivity is present in about half of all argyrophilic cells (408,409). Rarely, a small-cell or large-cell carcinoma with neuroendocrine features arises in the endometrium (410–413). As at other sites, these are aggressive neoplasms.

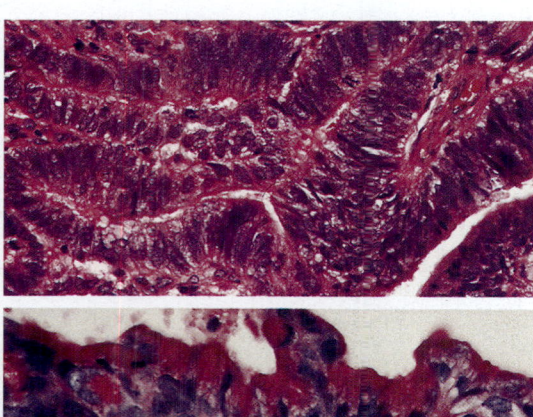
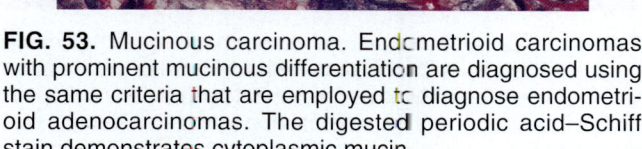

FIG. 53. Mucinous carcinoma. Endometrioid carcinomas with prominent mucinous differentiation are diagnosed using the same criteria that are employed to diagnose endometrioid adenocarcinomas. The digested periodic acid–Schiff stain demonstrates cytoplasmic mucin.

Patterns Featuring Papillary or Villoglandular Architecture

All of the proliferations listed under this heading, except syncytial papillary metaplasia, have in common a two-dimensional papillary architecture imposed by a connective tissue scaffolding. The two-dimensional papillary architecture of some of these proliferations corresponds to three-dimensional papillae ("true papillae"); others are papillary in the sense that villous adenomas appear papillary but consist three dimensionally of folia or sheets ("villous"). The two differ three dimensionally in the same way that the branches of an oak tree differ from the leaves of a cabbage; both yield papillary structures on sectioning—circular and longitudinal structures in the former and only longitudinal structures in the latter. In contrast, in syncytial papillary metaplasia it is the stratified epithelium that has the papillary architecture.

Papillary Syncytial Metaplasia (414)

This is a phenomenon that is probably closely related to morule formation and is discussed in that section. It characteristically involves the surface of the endometrium or that portion of the gland that opens onto the endometrial surface. Papillary syncytial metaplasia features a sheet-like syncytium of cytologically bland cells (Fig. 54). These cells pile up into columns in focal areas, but no fibrovascular stromal cores are present (Fig. 55). The constituent cells are cytologically bland; some nuclei may be pyknotic, however, and mitotic figures are uncommon. The sheets of cells are usually infiltrated with polymorphs. Papillary syncytial metaplasia is often found in association with endometrial breakdown and, in these instances, may represent a degenerative or reparative process as opposed to a true metaplasia (hence the term papillary syncytial change) (415).

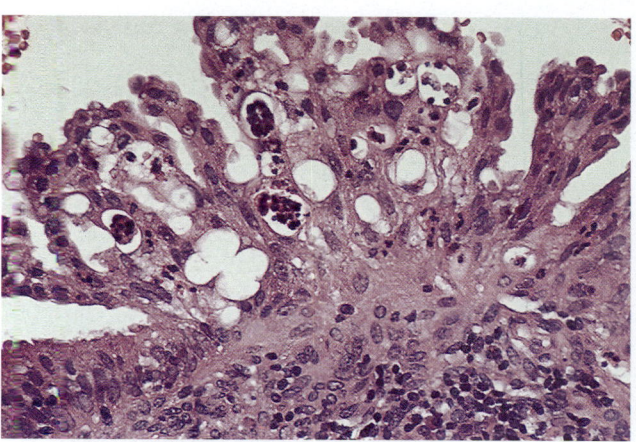

FIG. 55. Syncytial papillary metaplasia (high power). This process features cytologically bland cells arranged in a filigree pattern without discernible fibrous cores.

Benign Papillary Change

In benign papillary change, atrophic, weakly proliferative or proliferative cells without atypia line true, typically coarse connective tissue papillary cores (Figs. 56 and 57). Although this pattern is unusual and little is known about its natural history, it has no morphologic features that would suggest that it is either malignant or a cancer precursor. Care must be taken to exclude an endocervical primary, especially if the proliferation features mucinous epithelium.

Villoglandular Endometrial Hyperplasia

Not infrequently, endometrial hyperplasia has a low-power papillary configuration featuring bland, stratified columnar cells disposed over fine fibrovascular folia (villo-

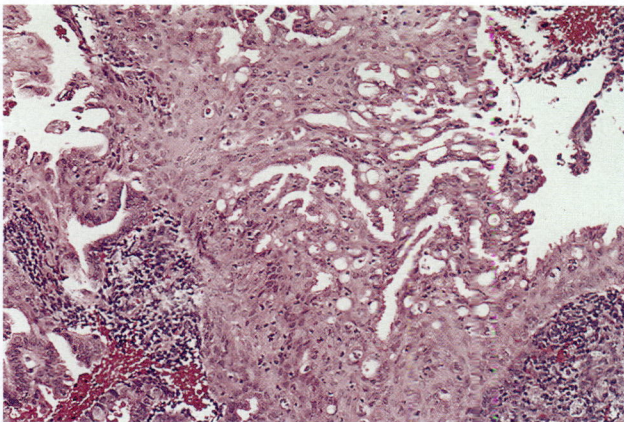

FIG. 54. Syncytial papillary metaplasia (low power). Papillary metaplasia features a sheet-like growth of epithelium reminiscent of that forming morules. In this example, the surface endometrium is covered by a filigree arrangement of cytologically bland cells with indistinct cytoplasmic margins.

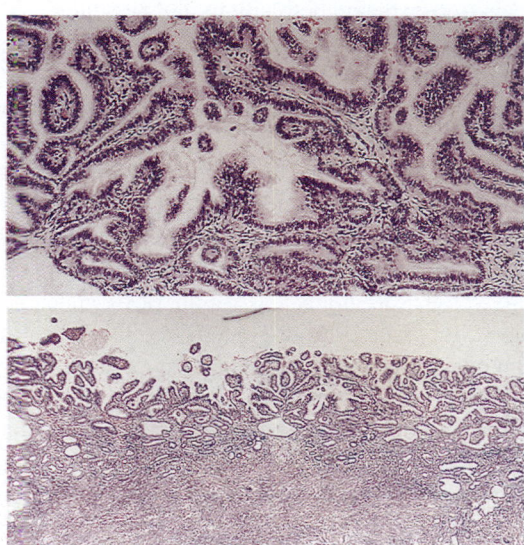

FIG. 56. Papillary change. The surface of this atrophic endometrium features a papillary proliferation. *Top:* The papillae are composed of fibrovascular stalks lined by cytologically bland, inactive nonsecretory epithelium. *Bottom:* Low-power view showing the extent of papillary change.

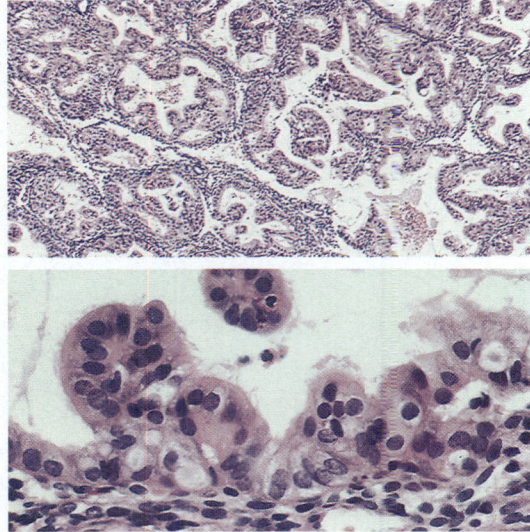

FIG. 57. Ciliated cell metaplasia with papillary change. *Top:* A pattern of simple hyperplasia with the glands thrown up in micropapillary structures. *Bottom:* The epithelium lining these papillary structures is cytologically bland and ciliated.

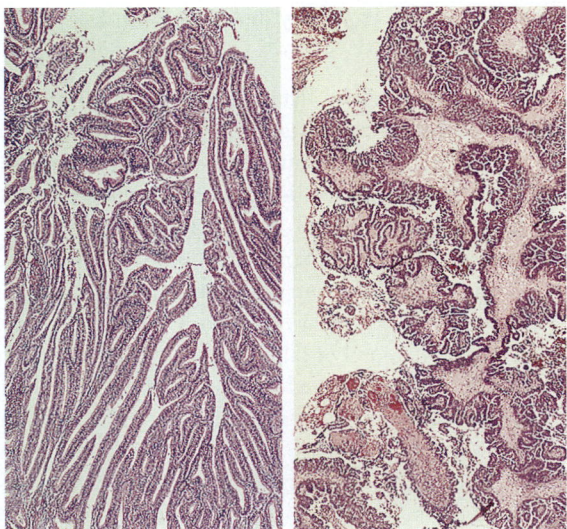

FIG. 58. Uterine papillary serous carcinoma and villoglandular carcinoma contrasted. *Right:* The typical coarse: fibrous stalks of uterine papillary serous carcinoma. The overall impression is that of serous carcinoma of the ovary. *Left:* The delicate fibrovascular stalks of villoglandular carcinoma.

glandular pattern). This configuration often blends into tubuloglandular patterns.

Villoglandular (Grade 1) Carcinoma (416–419)

WDCAs may have a low-power architecture featuring tumor cells supported by a delicate fibrovascular stroma. This pattern, labeled by us as villoglandular carcinoma, may be focal or diffuse, and it often blends imperceptibly into endometrioid carcinoma with a typical glandular pattern. It is important to note that in both villous and glandular areas, the cytologic features are low grade (see also Intermediate-grade Papillary Carcinomas). Bland squamous elements are usually encountered in villoglandular carcinoma. Some pathologists label this type of carcinoma "papillary." If this practice is adopted, then high-grade UPSC must be designated in a way that clearly distinguishes it from low-grade endometrioid carcinoma with a villoglandular pattern. This can be done by using the terminology "villoglandular—uterine papillary serous carcinoma," as we do, or by appending the modifiers low grade or high grade to the label "papillary." The unmodified label is unacceptably ambiguous.

We consider villoglandular carcinoma to be part of the spectrum of endometrioid carcinomas, and we do not classify it separately or specify it in the diagnosis line. It is important, however, to recognize that low-grade adenocarcinomas of the endometrium may have this pattern and to distinguish it from villoglandular hyperplasia and high-grade papillary carcinoma (Fig. 58). In our experience, some of the rare very well differentiated myoinvasive carcinomas that may be interpreted on sampling specimens as AH using standard criteria are villoglandular (Fig. 59) (351).

Uterine Papillary Serous Carcinoma (High-grade Papillary Carcinoma, Serous Adenocarcinoma) (416,417,420–437)

UPSC resembles ovarian serous carcinoma in its differentiated features. In the usual case, the neoplasm is composed of coarse fibrovascular stalks layered with large, highly malignant-appearing cells (Figs. 58 and 60). When these cells stratify, they may form tufts that can become detached and float freely between papillae. Tufting is a useful marker of UPSC. Nuclear pleomorphism is marked, nucleoli tend to be large and prominent, and mitotic figures are easily found.

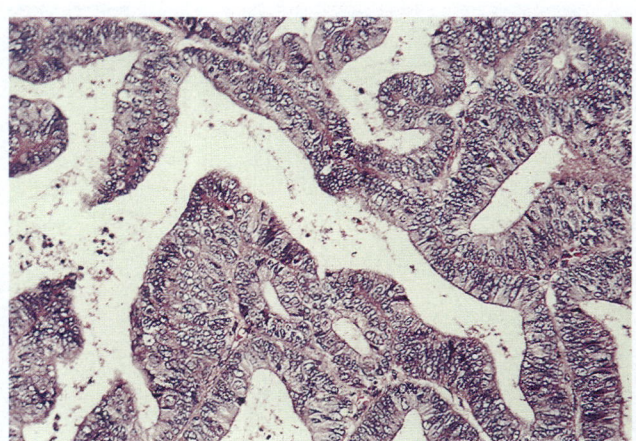

FIG. 59. Villoglandular carcinoma (well differentiated). The cells lining these delicate fibrovascular stalks are pseudostratified and have cytologic features comparable to those seen in well-differentiated adenocarcinoma.

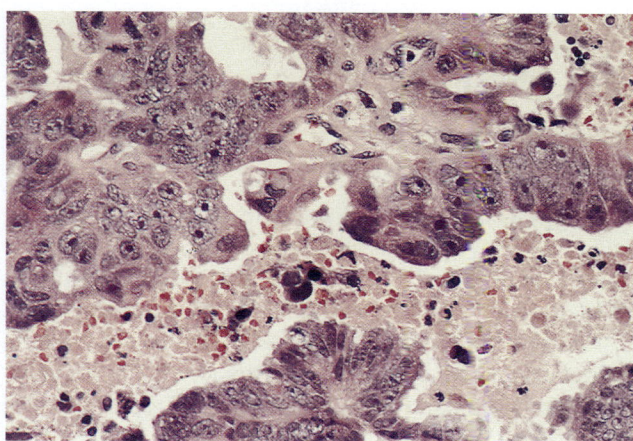

FIG. 60. Uterine papillary serous carcinoma (UPSC) (high power). A defining feature of UPSC is the presence of cells with high-grade malignant features. As illustrated here, these features include macronucleoli, multinucleated tumor giant cells, marked hyperchromatism, and nucleomegaly.

Tumor giant cells and abnormal mitotic figures are frequently encountered; in one-third of cases, psammoma bodies are present (438). Not surprisingly, UPSC is found to be aneuploid and lacks ER/PR; c-myc proto-oncogene amplification is also often present, and 90% of serous carcinomas are strongly immunoreactive for p53 (260,261,430, 439–441).

Myoinvasion is typically present at the time of diagnosis and characteristically takes the form of gaping, irregularly shaped glands producing a granulation-tissue-like response as they invade the myometrium. UPSC has a propensity for angiolymphatic invasion; at times, such invasion is so subtle that a careful search of the myometrium and serosa is required to identify the small clusters of tumor cells (or isolated psammoma bodies) within vascular spaces. Similarly, the vasculature of the cervix and ovary may be involved by UPSC without gross evidence of tumor. Myometrial and vascular invasion may be quite extensive without enlarging the uterus, and the intra-endometrial volume of the primary tumor may be small, yielding only a small number of tumor cells by curettage. Clinically unapparent peritoneal involvement is frequently discovered at the time of staging laparotomy.

On occasion, in situ UPSC cytologic changes can be found in the endometrium adjacent to UPSC. Such in situ changes may also be found in the absence of an endometrial mass, evidence of a thickened endometrium, or myometrial invasion (430,442). UPSC confined to endometrial polyps has also been reported (234). UPSC-like changes can also be found along the serosa of the uterus and fallopian tubes in conjunction with either in situ UPSC in the endometrium or an actual tumor mass. Up to 10% of clinical stage I carcinomas of the endometrium are UPSCs. As a rule, patients in whom UPSC develops are older than patients with the usual endometrioid carcinoma, they are less likely to have been on hormone replacement therapy, and it is unusual for them to have associated endometrial hyperplasia. Because the tumor cells of UPSC are easily shed and of high grade, they can often be recognized as malignant in cervical/vaginal smears, but placing the tumor clearly into the UPSC category usually requires a tissue specimen. Although UPSC accounted for approximately 10% of the surgical stage I carcinomas reviewed at Stanford, this was the histologic type in 50% of the patients who relapsed (421). Most relapses occurred within 2 years of hysterectomy.

After adjustment for stage and depth of myometrial invasion, the prognosis for patients with UPSC is significantly worse than for the combined group of patients with grades 2 and 3 endometrioid carcinomas. It has become apparent that preoperative clinical understaging is common in patients with UPSC. In one review of our experience, up to 60% of patients with clinical stage I UPSC have been found to have a higher surgical stage of disease; in fact, 50% of clinical stage I patients are promoted to surgical stage III or IV. Patients with UPSC in situ may later show signs of widespread peritoneal disease, as can patients in whom UPSC changes are confined to the serosa and fallopian tubes; molecular analyses of the p53 mutational patterns in these cases have yielded conflicting results. One study suggested that the disease is a unifocal process with early metastases (443); another concluded that at least some cases are multifocal (444).

When a diagnosis of UPSC is made on a biopsy or curettage specimen, we suggest that the surgeon perform a staging operation at the time of hysterectomy. This procedure should include careful inspection and biopsy of all the surfaces normally examined during the course of ovarian staging, in addition to lymph node sampling. Although most patients with UPSC receive some form of postoperative therapy, the effectiveness of such treatment has yet to be established.

Intermediate-grade Papillary Carcinomas

As more cases of villoglandular carcinoma and UPSC have been studied, it has become apparent that there is not complete morphologic discontinuity between low-grade villoglandular carcinoma and high-grade UPSC; instead, there are a few cases that have the features of both. Thus, as often happens, there is a morphologic spectrum bounded at one extreme by low-grade carcinoma with villoglandular growth and at the other extreme by UPSC. Scattered between these extremes are a small number of carcinomas with papillary architecture and grade 2 or grade 3 cytologic features, but the cytologic and architectural features fall short of those diagnostic of UPSC. We are unaware of any published studies of this hybrid neoplasm; the few tumors of this type with which we have experience seem to show clinical behavior intermediate between UPSC and villoglandular carcinoma. We designate them as intermediate-grade papillary carcinomas.

Differential Diagnosis

Because of the implications of a diagnosis of UPSC for prognosis and therapy, care must be taken to distinguish this neoplasm from other papillary proliferations that arise in the endometrium. This is true whether a tumor mass is present or the process is *in situ*. The main point to bear in mind is that UPSC combines papillary architecture (which has broad, often hyalinized stalks, at least in focal areas) with high-grade cytologic features, often with macronucleoli and tufting. These features serve to distinguish UPSC from other proliferations that can mimic it, such as hyperplasia with villoglandular architecture, endometrioid carcinoma with villoglandular architecture, and papillary syncytial metaplasia. Both papillary syncytial metaplasia and hyperplasia have bland cytologic characteristics, and papillary syncytial metaplasia lacks fibrovascular stromal support.

Papillary Syncytial Metaplasia and Villoglandular Hyperplasia Versus Endometrioid Adenocarcinoma with Villoglandular Architecture

Proliferations showing syncytial-like growth with small papillary-like columns of stratified cells without fibrous cores are not uncommonly encountered in the endometrium; they are clinically benign processes related to morules and squamous metaplasia (Figs. 54 and 55). These proliferations are composed of cells with small, bland nuclei with inconspicuous nucleoli. Even the low-grade villoglandular carcinomas, on the other hand, are composed of cells with at least the cytologic features found in grade 1 carcinoma. Both hyperplasia and carcinoma with villoglandular architecture share the pattern of epithelial cells arranged upon delicate fibrovascular stalks; they are distinguished by employing the architectural criteria for discriminating AH from well-differentiated adenocarcinoma (see section on hyperplasia versus carcinoma) (Fig. 29).

Villoglandular Endometrioid Carcinoma Versus Uterine Papillary Serous Carcinoma

It is usually an easy task to distinguish these two tumors because UPSC is a high-grade carcinoma featuring nucleomegaly, macronucleoli, abnormal mitotic figures, and highly abnormal chromatin, whereas villoglandular endometrioid carcinomas (VGCs) have grade 1 cytologic features (Figs. 58-60). Moreover, the stalks in UPSC tend to be broad and fibrous or hyalinized, compared with the thin fibrovascular stromal scaffolding found in VGC. Tufting and secondary papillae are generally absent in VGC. There are occasionally cases, however, that have characteristics intermediate between these two. We designate them intermediate-grade papillary carcinomas (see earlier section) and suggest treatment as for UPSC.

Carcinosarcoma Versus Uterine Papillary Serous Carcinoma

Now and then, the epithelial component of a carcinosarcoma will have UPSC features (445). The distinction between the two rests on identifying a sarcomatous component in carcinosarcomas.

Ovarian or Fallopian Tube Primary with Secondary Involvement of the Endometrium

Serous carcinomas arising primarily in the ovary or fallopian tube and involving the endometrium have an appearance identical to primary UPSC. The fact that the ovary or tube is affected may not be apparent until the time of laparotomy. Fortunately, the important fact in terms of treatment is that a high-grade serous carcinoma (site not otherwise specified) involves both ovary and uterus. The identity of the primary site is always tentative and, in general, is clinically irrelevant. Indeed, the tumors may be multifocal, as noted previously.

UPSC Versus Clear-cell Carcinoma

Clear-cell carcinoma and UPSC have in common high-grade cytologic characteristics, and clear-cell carcinomas may be focally or extensively papillary (Fig. 60; see also Fig. 68). Although typical cases of UPSC and clear-cell carcinoma are easily distinguished, a sizable minority of cases have overlapping features or consist of a mixture of both. Assignment to one or the other group in this circumstance is arbitrary and, from the point of view of clinical management, of no particular significance—both are high grade, clinically aggressive neoplasms that can spread over peritoneal surfaces.

Patterns Featuring a Prominence of Ciliated Cells

Scattered ciliated cells are normal constituents of the proliferative endometrium and are particularly prominent in the epithelium lining the endometrial surface (Fig. 61). In hy-

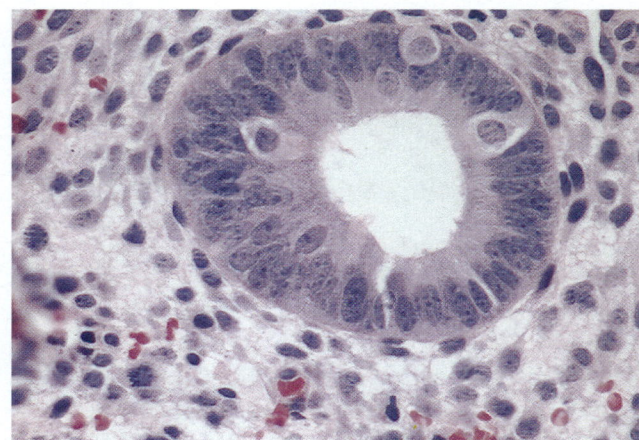

FIG. 61. Ciliated cells in a normal proliferative endometrium. This gland shows the characteristic appearance of ciliated cells in nonsecretory endometria. Some cells show luminal cilia, whereas others adjacent to the basement membrane are rounded, with vesicular nuclei, and have a grainy, eosinophilic cytoplasm. Other intermediate forms have a pear-shaped configuration.

perestrogenic states, ciliated cells sometimes become more numerous; when they become interspersed with nonciliated cells, the pattern is strikingly reminiscent of normal tubal epithelium. Ciliated cells in their normal setting deviate substantially from the "undifferentiated" proliferative cell of the normal endometrium. They have more abundant cytoplasm and rounder, larger, more vesicular nuclei ("fat nuclei") than the surrounding undifferentiated proliferative cells. They also have a tendency to stratify. The cytoplasm of ciliated cells may be clear or eosinophilic, and it sometimes contains microlumina lined by cilia producing the appearance of a cytoplasmic microcyst.

When assembled in large numbers, these cytologic peculiarities are amplified and may prompt a diagnosis of AH or carcinoma. Indeed, early illustrations of so-called carcinoma *in situ* of the endometrium depict large, nonstratified cells with rounded nuclei containing prominent nucleoli and (reportedly) eosinophilic cytoplasm. It is worth noting that the luminal borders of these cells were prominently lined by cilia. This worrisome appearance notwithstanding, the majority of endometrial proliferations that feature a prominence of ciliated cells are clinically benign. Some otherwise characteristic endometrial carcinomas contain scattered ciliated cells; rarely, a carcinoma may be composed almost entirely of malignant ciliated cells.

Ciliated Cell Prominence (Ciliated Cell Metaplasia) (214,446)

The term ciliated cell prominence (CCP) denotes a benign proliferation featuring endometrial glands lined exclusively

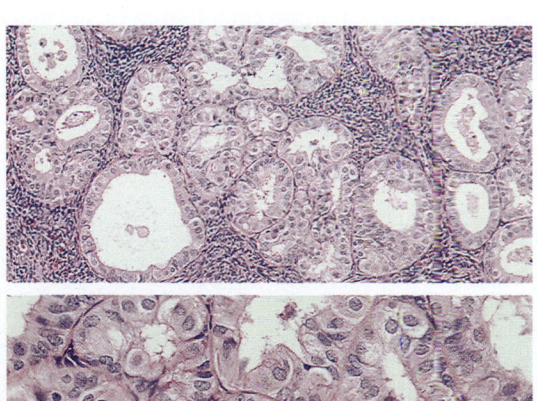

FIG. 62. Ciliated cell metaplasia involving noncomplex hyperplasia. *Top:* The low-power appearance of this proliferation is that of budded glands set within inactive, spindled stroma. *Bottom:* Pear-shaped and rounded cells with vesicular nuclei lining budded glands. The epithelium is nonstratified, and the nonciliated cells do not show features of atypical hyperplasia.

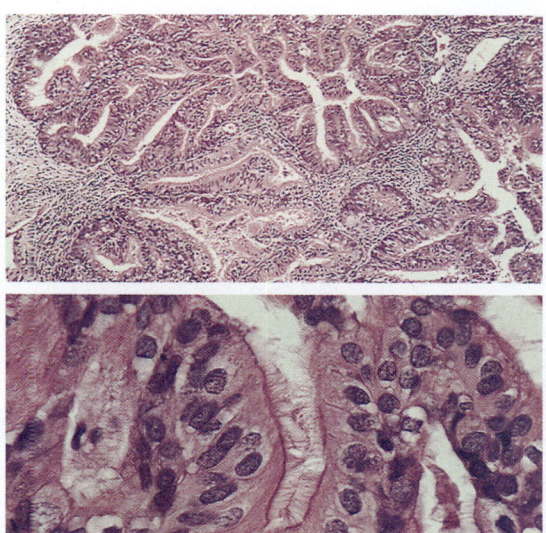

FIG. 63. Focal complex hyperplasia with ciliated cell metaplasia. *Top:* A focus of complexly budded and branched glands set within spindled stroma. *Bottom:* Fully developed ciliated cells lining these glands. Notice the prominent terminal bars and luminal cilia.

or almost exclusively by ciliated cells. Although the usual endometrium with this pattern is hyperplastic and exhibits some degree of architectural complexity, atrophic, weakly proliferative and disordered proliferative endometria may possess large numbers of ciliated cells (Fig. 62). Ciliated cells may line complexly budded glands, which, on sectioning, produce a back-to-back glandular pattern (Fig. 63). Benign ciliated cells have an enlarged nucleus, but the chromatin is delicate. When abnormal chromatin patterns are present in ciliated cells in association with easily found mitotic figures and complex architecture, the term atypical complex hyperplasia with CCP is appropriate. The combination of complex growth pattern and the baseline atypia of ciliated cells may prompt a diagnosis of carcinoma, but the eosinophilic cytoplasm of the cells and the cilia, if they are intact, alert the observer to the ciliary differentiation (Fig. 64). Moreover, the areas of glandular complexity are usually focal and small.

Ciliated Cell Carcinoma (447)

While a few scattered ciliated cells may be seen in ordinary endometrioid carcinomas, those rare carcinomas composed predominantly or almost entirely of ciliated cells are called ciliated cell carcinoma. Most of these carcinomas are grade 1 and are recognized by a combination of nuclear atypia in the range of AH to well-differentiated adenocarcinoma and an architectural pattern complex enough to meet the requirements for well-differentiated adenocarcinoma. Rarely, ciliated carcinomas with a prominent solid component are encountered; these grade 2 ciliated carcinomas strike the observer as obvious malignancies with peculiar

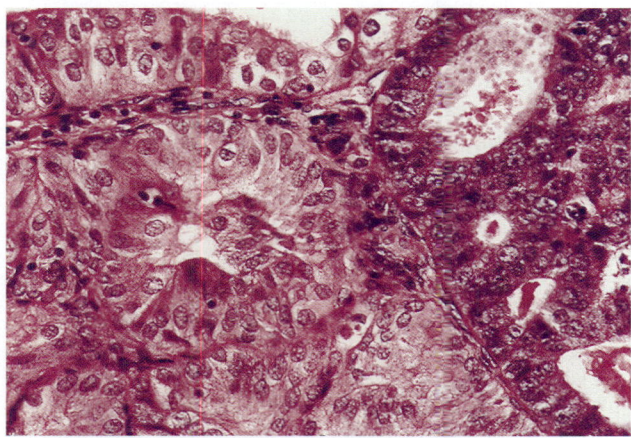

FIG. 64. Ciliated cell metaplasia adjacent to well-differentiated adenocarcinoma. The left lower portion of the photomicrograph shows ciliated cells with nucleomegaly, granular chromatin, and prominent nucleoli, while the right portion reveals adenocarcinoma. Because the metaplastic epithelium is benign, the carcinoma on the right would be designated endometrioid carcinoma.

microcystic cytoplasmic differentiation, which on closer inspection are discovered to be cilia-lined intracytoplasmic lumina.

Differential Diagnosis

Ciliated Cell Prominence in Complex Atypical Hyperplasia Versus Well-differentiated Adenocarcinoma

This differential diagnosis raises two problems. The first involves estimating the cytologic atypia of ciliated cells, if any, while the second lies in drawing the distinction between AH and WDCA—the problem discussed earlier, now in a slightly different guise (Figs. 62–64). The first problem can be approached by making a practice of searching out normal ciliated cells in benign endometria to acquire a feeling for their range of appearances. When a pure ciliated cell proliferation is composed of cells with the chromatin abnormalities seen in AH, we label the process AH with CCP.

The second problem is no more tractable in this context than it is in the usual situation. As a rule, if cilia are prominent in a proliferation, it is highly unlikely that the process will be myoinvasive or behave in a clinically malignant fashion, that is, almost all ciliated process are benign. Therefore, we take a conservative diagnostic stand and do not diagnose ciliated carcinoma until the cytologic changes are well into the range of carcinoma. There is no evidence that CCP itself is a preinvasive lesion, that is, adenocarcinoma *in situ*. CCP in the context of AH presumably carries the same risk of the subsequent development of endometrial carcinoma as the associated hyperplasia; treatment should be that appropriate for AH.

Patterns Featuring a Prominence of Clear Cells or Cells with Prominent Eosinophilic Cytoplasm But Without Visible Cilia

A variety of differentiated epithelial types in the endometrium possess clear cytoplasm. In addition to the entities discussed later herein, these types include normal secretory endometria, Arias-Stella reaction (Fig. 8), cells containing intracytoplasmic mucin (Figs. 51 and 52), and squamous or squamoid cells containing abundant glycogen—all of which have been discussed previously.

Clear-cell, Hobnail, and Eosinophilic Metaplasia (356,448)

Occasionally, benign cells in nonsecretory endometria will feature prominent clearing in the cytoplasm without histochemically demonstrable mucin or glycogen. When it is prominent, we label this change clear-cell metaplasia (Fig. 65). Rarely, endometrial cells have a nonstratified hobnail (or pear-shaped) appearance with or without clear cytoplasm (hobnail metaplasia) (Fig. 66). Another peculiar cell type periodically encountered in the endometrium has prominent cytoplasmic eosinophilia. Not infrequently, these cells are focally stratified to produce a cribriform architecture. We suspect many such cells are ciliated cells that have lost their cilia. Whether they have clear or eosinophilic cytoplasm, they lack the cytologic features of malignancy.

Secretory Endometrioid Carcinoma and Glycogen-rich Squamoid Carcinoma

Some well-differentiated endometrioid grade 1 carcinomas show a strikingly uniform cytoplasmic vacuolation reminiscent of normal early secretory endometrium (Fig. 67) (416,449,450). Such carcinomas may be detected in patients who have not received progestational agents. These neo-

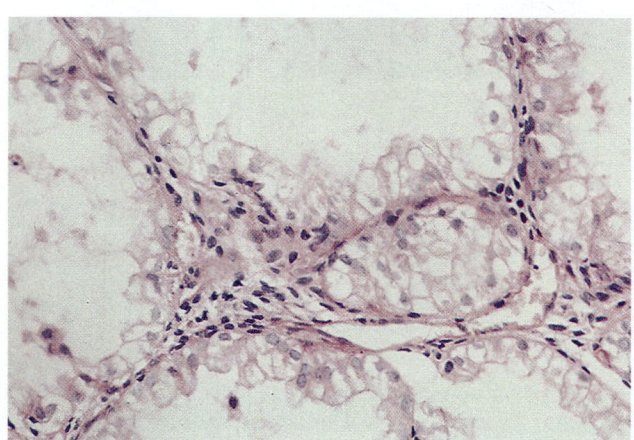

FIG. 65. Clear-cell metaplasia. The cells lining these cystically dilated, nonbudded glands have a clear cytoplasm. They feature basally situated, cytologically bland nuclei. Intracytoplasmic mucin was not seen in this case.

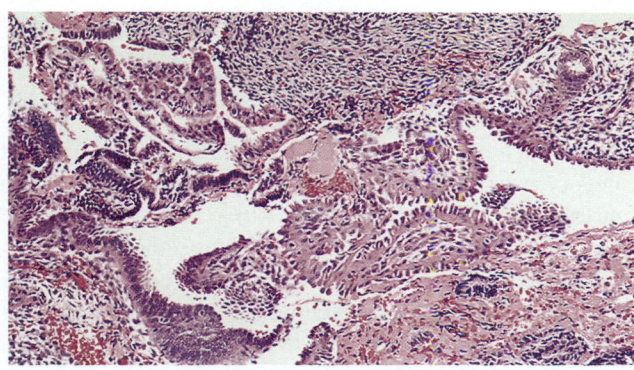

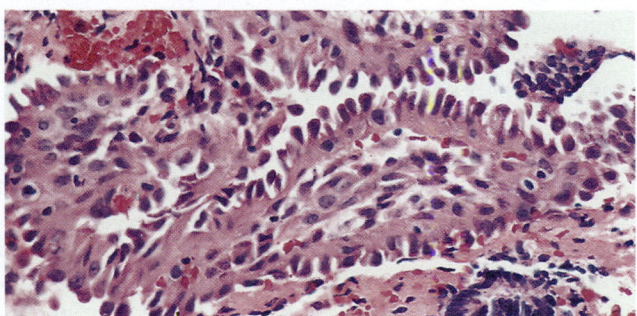

FIG. 66. Hobnail metaplasia. The surface of this inactive endometrium is lined by nonstratified cells with luminal apical blebs, imparting a hobnail appearance.

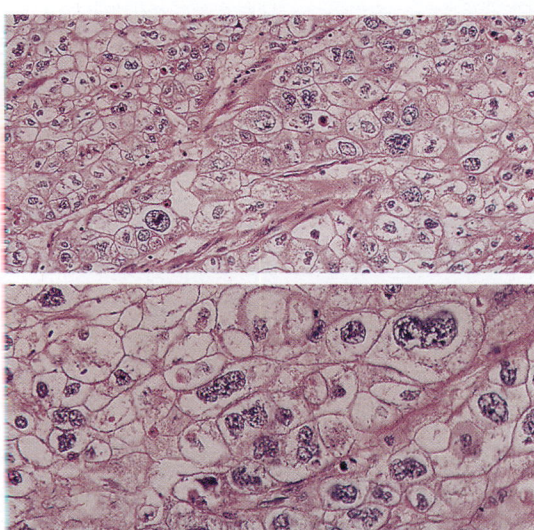

FIG. 68. Clear-cell carcinoma features a proliferation of cells with clear or eosinophilic cytoplasm, marked pleomorphism, and high-grade cytologic features. Clear-cell carcinoma may form sheets (as in this example) and papillary structures or have a tubuloglandular architecture.

plasms, which must have both the architectural and the cytologic features of carcinoma, have a prognosis essentially identical to that of grade 1 adenocarcinomas unassociated with this feature. For this reason, we consider them to be a morphologic variant of endometrioid carcinoma. From time to time, carcinomas composed of well-differentiated glandular elements and bland squamous elements will have zones of squamoid cells with markedly clear cytoplasm. On periodic acid–Schiff (PAS) preparations, these cells are usually found to contain glycogen.

Clear-cell Carcinoma (416,429,449–457)

Primary clear-cell carcinoma of the endometrium is histologically indistinguishable from clear-cell carcinoma in the ovary or in the cervicovaginal region of women exposed to diethylstilbestrol (DES). This neoplasm combines different high-grade cytologic features, characterized by enlarged, angulated nuclei with enlarged irregular nucleoli with cytoplasmic clearing (at least in focal areas) (Fig. 68). The architecture may be papillary, glandular, or sheet-like. When it is glandular, the tumor cell nuclei often protrude into the luminal space, giving rise to a hobnail or tombstone appearance. There is no known association between the development of endometrial

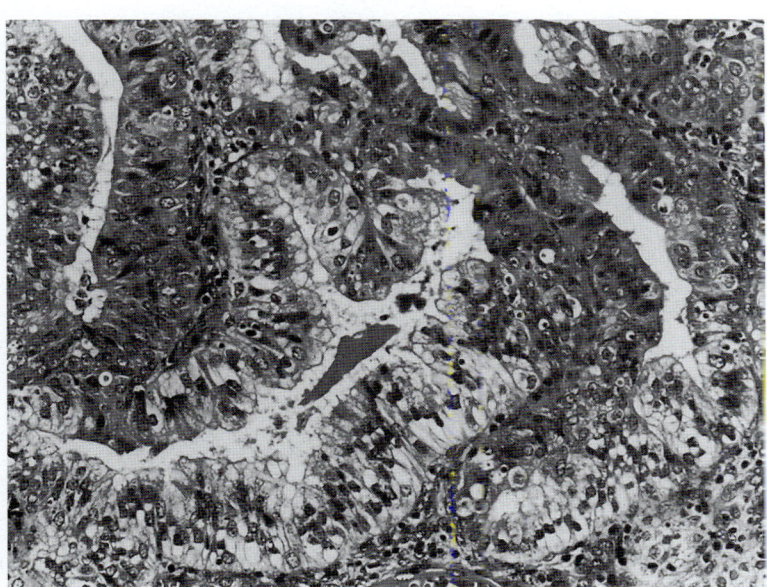

FIG. 67. Secretory carcinoma. Note the vacuolated cytoplasm and compare with Fig. 3. The vacuoles in this tumor are generally subnuclear, and therefore the pattern mimics that of an early secretory endometrium. The nuclear features of carcinoma are present, however.

clear-cell carcinoma and DES exposure. In fact, the clinical profile of patients with clear-cell carcinoma is similar to that of patients with UPSC, in that most patients are older than 60 years of age and the majority have not been taking estrogen for hormone replacement. As with UPSC, a prehysterectomy diagnosis of clear-cell carcinoma should prompt a surgical staging procedure at the time of hysterectomy. Clear-cell carcinoma and UPSC may co-exist in the same neoplasm.

Differential Diagnosis

Clear-cell Carcinoma Versus Other Proliferations Featuring Clear Cells

The distinction between secretory carcinoma and clear-cell carcinoma is a cytologic one: clear-cell carcinoma has cells with nuclei with high-grade cytologic characteristics, often protruding tombstone-like into glandular lumens (Fig. 68). On the other hand, the tumor cell nuclei in secretory carcinoma, although they are enlarged with irregular chromatin, are relatively bland and do not have a tombstone-like appearance (Fig. 67). Clear-cell carcinoma can be confused with the Arias-Stella reaction because nuclei in the latter condition can be quite large and angulated, with chromatin clearing. Attention to the clinical context and the histologic features will almost invariably serve to distinguish the two. Most patients with the Arias-Stella reaction are in the reproductive years; this change is often associated with a decidual reaction elsewhere, and, as would be expected in a secretory endometrium, glandular mitotic figures are rare or absent. Metastatic renal cell carcinoma also should be considered in the differential diagnosis of clear-cell carcinoma.

Clear-cell Carcinoma Versus Uterine Papillary Serous Carcinoma

Clear-cell areas may be encountered in UPSC; both are high-grade lesions, and the distinction between the two is of little clinical significance (Figs. 60 and 63).

Clear-cell Carcinoma: Primary Cervix Versus Primary Endometrium

Making the distinction between these two sites was more of a problem two decades ago, when cervicovaginal clear-cell carcinoma developed in rare patients exposed to DES *in utero*. Primary cervical clear-cell carcinomas are still encountered on very rare occasions and may first be found in an endometrial sampling. The localization strategy suggested in connection with mucinous carcinoma is also appropriate here.

MIXED MÜLLERIAN NEOPLASIA (458–461)

Introduction

Mixed müllerian neoplasms are biphasic epithelial-mesenchymal proliferations that exhibit a range of clinical behavior from benign (AdFib, adenomyoma, and APA) to highly malignant (carcinosarcoma). The classification of mixed müllerian neoplasms is based upon an assessment of both the epithelial and mesenchymal components; assignment of each of these components to a benign or malignant category based on morphologic characteristics results in a fourfold classification. The terms AdFib, adenomyoma, and APA are used for neoplasms with benign epithelium and benign proliferating stroma; the label adenosarcoma is used for neoplasms with benign epithelium and mitotically active or sarcomatous stroma; and the designation carcinosarcoma (malignant mixed müllerian tumor) is used for neoplasms composed of malignant epithelium and malignant stroma.

It is usual to classify all tumors containing malignant epithelium with benign stroma as carcinomas. The mesenchymal component has been regarded either as nonneoplastic fibrous scaffolding (e.g., the fibrous stromal cores of UPSC) or as a host response to the carcinoma (e.g., the granulation tissue response associated with myoinvasive carcinomas). The term carcinofibroma has been proposed for tumors in which the stroma is deemed to be neoplastic rather than reactive; however, this terminology is rarely used because determining whether stroma is reactive or a benign neoplastic proliferation is challenging at best (462,463).

Atypical Polypoid Adenomyoma and Atypical Polypoid Adenomyoma of Low Malignant Potential

Description

APA, as the name suggests, is a lesion that is biphasic and polypoid and features atypical endometrial hyperplasia (Figs. 69 and 70). Morular metaplasia is present in more than

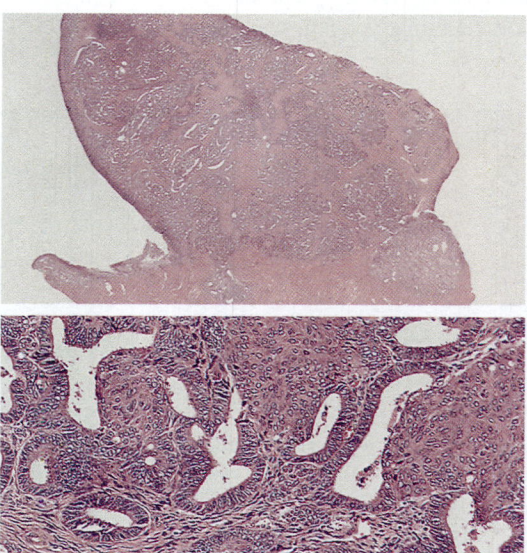

FIG. 69. Atypical polypoid adenomyoma. *Top:* The characteristic circumscribed polypoid shape of the lesion is apparent. *Bottom:* The extensive morule formation that is seen in more than 90% of these neoplasms.

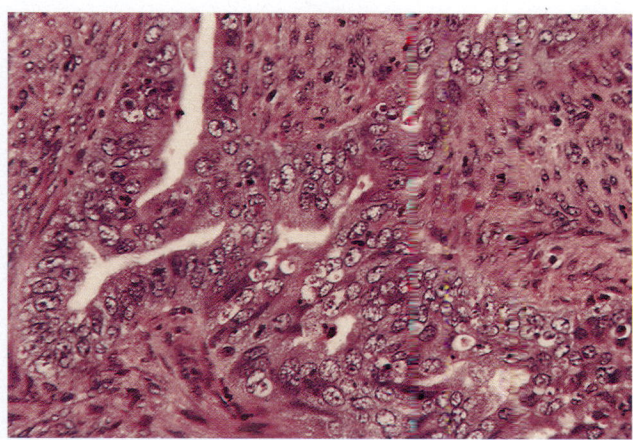

FIG. 70. Atypical polypoid adenomyoma. Higher magnification shows the bland morules and atypical cytologic features characteristic of this entity.

90% of cases (464–466). Most develop in the lower uterine segment. APA in the hysterectomy specimen is typically a sharply circumscribed lesion associated with a distinctly different endometrial proliferation elsewhere in the endometrium—not infrequently, with a normal secretory pattern. The correlate of this focalization in the intact uterus is a helpful diagnostic feature in uterine samplings; on low-power, APA is recognized by the presence of fragments of APA and fragments of normal endometrium jumbled together. Although the mesenchymal component of APA is usually described as smooth muscle, it is our experience that lesions otherwise typical of APA can have hybrid fibrous and smooth-muscle stroma (Fig. 71); infrequently, the stroma has nothing much to suggest smooth-muscle differentiation (Fig. 71) (466,467). The combination of the patient's youth, the prominent morular metaplasia, the prominent smooth-muscle or hybrid smooth-muscle and fibrous stroma, and the focal nature of the process almost always allows for recognition of APA. On occasion, the glands in an otherwise typical APA have the architectural features of well-differentiated adenocarcinoma. Because such lesions may extend into the superficial myometrium, we have suggested the label APA of low malignant potential (APA-LMP) (Fig. 72) (466).

Clinicopathologic Correlation

This localized process occurs mainly in women in the fourth and fifth decades (mean age, 38 years) and only rarely after menopause. APA has been reported in patients with Turner's syndrome, some of whom have been on estrogen replacement therapy (468). APA is a persisting or recurring, but noninvasive and nonmetastasizing process that, with rare exceptions, has not been reported to be clinically aggressive (232). APA-LMP may involve the superficial myometrium, but it has not been reported to extend beyond the uterus. Based on these observations, it seems reasonable to consider conservative treatment for the patient who wants to preserve her uterus. Indeed, one-third of patients with APA-LMP treated with something less than hysterectomy have had successful pregnancies (464,466). Because APA can persist or recur in up to half of these patients, repeated samplings may be needed to ensure that the proliferation has been eradicated. The question naturally arises as to whether APA increases the risk of a subsequent carcinoma. Although histologic progression with increasingly complex glandular architecture has been observed in recurrent APAs, this apparent histologic progression has not been associated with myometrial infiltration or any other evidence of progression to carcinoma (466). Nevertheless, long-term follow-up seems warranted if treatment is to be something less than hysterectomy—especially in patients with APA-LMP—because there may be a small risk of subsequent carcinoma associated with this approach.

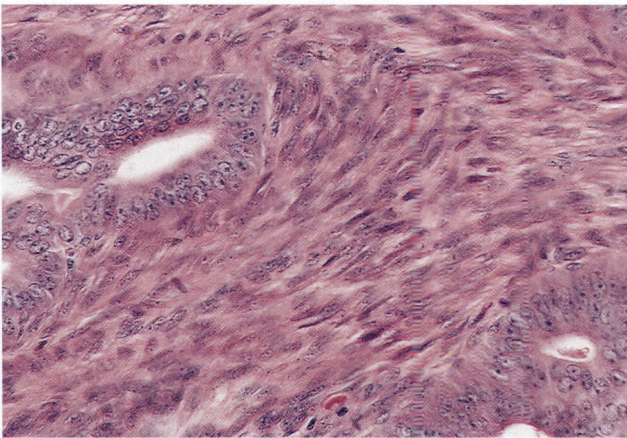

FIG. 71. Atypical polypoid adenomyoma. Smooth-muscle differentiation is characteristic of this entity, though the mesenchymal component may have a more fibrous appearance in some cases.

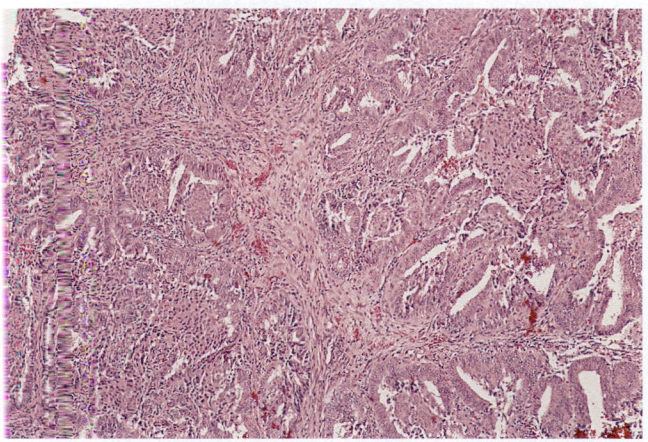

FIG. 72. Atypical polypoid adenomyoma of low malignant potential. The glands are more architecturally complex than those of atypical polypoid adenomyoma. Morular or squamous metaplasia is still prominent, but the fibromuscular stroma is compressed by the enlarged glands.

Adenofibroma, Adenosarcoma, Carcinosarcoma

In the following sections we present the clinicopathologic profiles of typical cases of the three established mixed müllerian tumors. The resemblance to fibroadenomas, phylloides tumors, and metaplastic carcinomas of the breast and to adenofibromatous lesions in the ovary is striking. An alternative view of mixed müllerian neoplasms is that these three disease entities represent concentrations of cases along what is in reality a mixed müllerian morphologic spectrum (469). This alternative view better accommodates the great heterogeneity of many of these neoplasms (i.e., mixtures of adenofibromatous, adenosarcomatous, and carcinosarcomatous areas in the same neoplasm) and the anomalous clinical behavior exhibited by some (e.g., the isolated clinically aggressive AdFib) (470).

Adenofibroma (459,471–474)

Description

AdFib mimics its namesake in the ovary in both gross and microscopic features. The neoplasm is papillary and most often sessile, and the stromal component predominates (Fig. 73–75). Its highlights, on histologic evaluation, are cytologically bland epithelium that either forms glands or is layered as surface epithelium over abundant, mitotically inactive, paucicellular, hyalinized fibrous or endometrial stroma that often takes the form of papillae. The characteristic microarchitectural details are papillary structures invaginated into cystic, epithelium-lined spaces or blunt, broad papillae lined by surface epithelium that often extends deeply into stroma. Cystic spaces are prominent. The epithelial lining may be mucinous, serous, or endometrioid (including endometrial cells with secretory activity), or it may be simple, nondescript cuboidal to columnar epithelium. Squamous metaplasia may be present. The epithelium may be all of one type or it may be mixed; occasionally, it is hyperplastic. By definition, the stroma must be bland and mitotically inactive [no more than 2 mitotic figures (mf) per 10 high-power fields (hpf) according to one definition; see Adenosarcoma), and stromal overgrowth must be absent. Usually, the stroma is paucicellular.

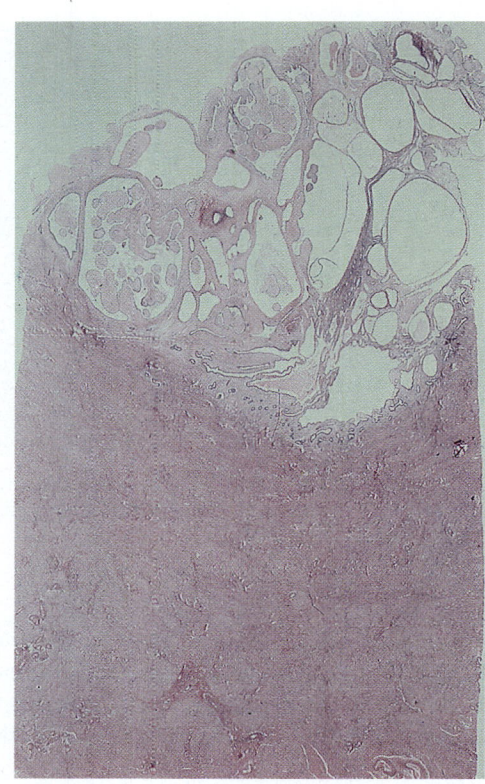

FIG. 74. This müllerian adenofibroma has an intracystic papillary architecture, a feature found in a minority of cases.

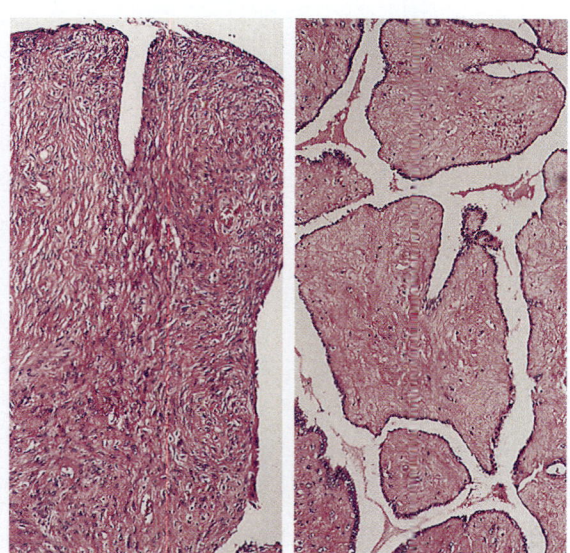

FIG. 73. Müllerian adenofibroma. This example demonstrates the cleft-like papillary architecture that is characteristic of some adenofibromas.

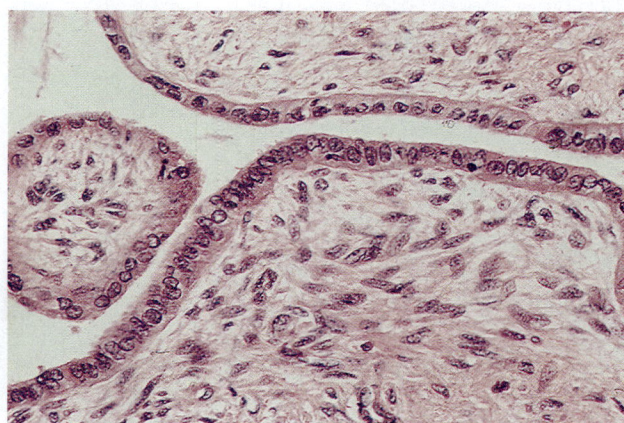

FIG. 75. Müllerian adenofibroma with bland stroma. There is no stromal condensation around the epithelium to form the cambium-like layer characteristic of adenosarcoma.

Clinicopathologic Correlation

In morphologic features, AdFib is a benign neoplasm that usually arises in the cervix or endometrium of postmenopausal women; it is almost always cured by hysterectomy. On rare occasions, however, examples have recurred within the uterus (459). Although rare cases of endocervical wall or myometrial invasion have been described, AdFib is almost always noninvasive. It is much less common than its close relative, adenosarcoma. Diagnostic difficulties arise when this neoplasm is initially seen in an endometrial sampling. In adenosarcoma (see next section), which is the chief differential diagnostic consideration in the context of AdFib, the features that best predict future behavior—that is, cellularity and mitotic activity of the stroma—vary considerably from area to area. In consequence, ruling out adenosarcoma requires, in essence, a diagnostic hysterectomy. Fortunately, uterine conservation is generally not a problem in the age group in which these two lesions most frequently occur.

Adenosarcoma (473,475–478,480,481)

Description

On gross inspection, adenosarcoma is a multicystic and sometimes fleshy neoplasm that is usually polypoid and sessile with a smooth or knobby surface, but it can be papillary. At the microscopic level, individual cases fall into two general groups. (a) The majority of cases feature uniformly distributed, often dilated glandular elements scattered throughout a cytologically bland, but at least focally cellular, stroma in a pattern similar to that seen in AdFib. The stroma is most often hypercellular around the glands (cambium layer or collar), which are lined by cells with bland nuclei (Fig. 76). Rarely, the glandular epithelium is hyperplastic but by definition cannot be cytologically malignant. (b) A minority of cases have either a morphologically malignant stroma and benign glands or a more bland, pure stromal compartment (overgrowth) in some part of the tumor (conventionally, more than 25%), associated with the mixture of benign glands and stroma characteristic of adenosarcoma elsewhere. Adenosarcomas of the first type may have the typical low-power appearance of AdFib, but they differ from that lesion in that the stroma is more cellular (particularly the cambium-layer-like cuff immediately adjacent to the epithelium) and mitotically active.

Distinguishing this pattern of adenosarcoma from AdFib is chiefly accomplished by identifying the hypercellular stroma, including the distinctive hypercellular cambium layer around the glands (a finding present in about 80% of cases), and by establishing the mitotic index (MI). Zaloudek and Norris (474) advocate 4 mf per 10 hpf as the dividing line between AdFib and adenosarcoma; Clement and Scully suggest a dividing line in the neighborhood of 2 mf per 10 hpf (459). We use the criterion of 4 mf per 10 hpf to make a diagnosis of adenosarcoma, but we consider tumors with particularly cellular stroma and/or borderline mitotic counts to be of uncertain malignant potential (UMP), particularly if subepithelial condensation is present.

Within the second group of tumors, those with stromal overgrowth have areas of "pure" stromal proliferation alternating with stroma containing scattered, enlarged, dilated, morphologically benign glandular elements. The former elements should comprise more than 25% of the tumor volume. The stroma in the areas of overgrowth may be bland or, more often, sarcomatous. Heterologous sarcoma is seen in one-fourth of adenosarcomas with stromal overgrowth; among these tumors, rhabdomyosarcoma is common (Fig. 77). The mitotic counts in tumors with stromal overgrowth are almost

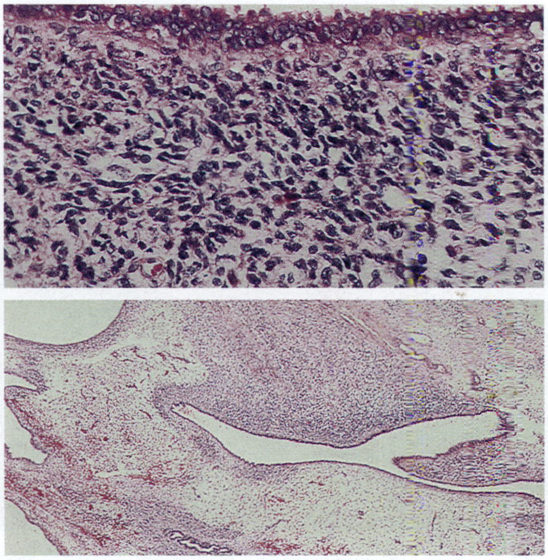

FIG. 76. Müllerian adenosarcoma. Unlike adenofibroma, the stroma is hypercellular, and the stromal cells are condensing around the cytologically benign glands.

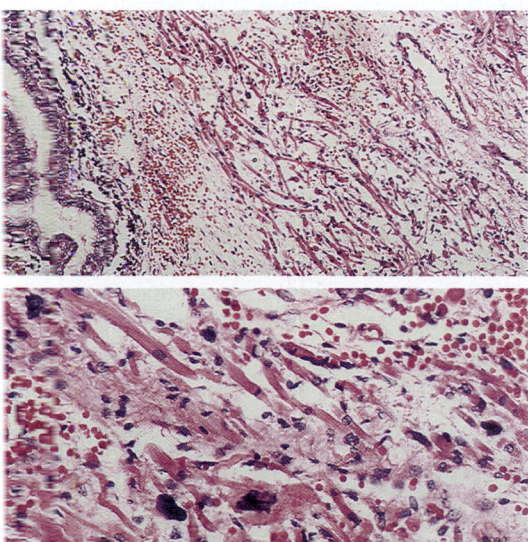

FIG. 77. Müllerian adenosarcoma. In this example, there is rhabdomyosarcomatous differentiation. When the sarcoma is high grade or when there is sarcomatous stromal overgrowth, the prognosis is adversely affected.

always well over 4 per 10 hpf. Rarely, the stromal cells in adenosarcoma arrange themselves in cord-like patterns reminiscent of the structures seen in those uterine tumors resembling ovarian sex-cord tumors and endometrial stromal tumors with epithelial elements (479).

In addition to AdFib, the differential diagnosis of adenosarcoma includes endometrial stromal sarcoma with glands. The dividing line between the two has never been set, but dilated glands with intraluminal polypoid protrusions and periglandular stromal condensation are fixtures of adenosarcoma, whereas the glands in endometrial stromal sarcoma usually are smaller and do not feature stromal condensation in intraluminal papillae. As long as the stroma is as bland as that in low-grade stromal sarcoma, the tumor will behave like low-grade stromal sarcoma. When the stroma is cytologically malignant, making the distinction from pure sarcoma depends on identifying bland neoplastic glands in some part of the tumor. In contradistinction to entrapped glands, the tumor glands of adenosarcoma are usually dilated and often irregular, and they frequently demonstrate polypoid structures that protrude into glandular lumens.

Clinicopathologic Correlation

Patients with adenosarcoma are usually postmenopausal, although this neoplasm may occur during the reproductive years. Approximately one-fourth of adenosarcomas are myoinvasive, and vascular invasion may also be present. Interestingly, myoinvasive foci, intravascular tumor, and extrauterine tumor tend to be sarcomatous rather than mixed. In the absence of stromal overgrowth, a 15% to 25% recurrence rate is seen; in the context of this finding, a recurrence rate of 45% to 70% is the rule. As a result, we label adenosarcoma with bland stroma and without stromal overgrowth as being of low malignant potential.

Most patients with adenosarcoma are cured by hysterectomy. Patients at most risk of recurrent disease are those who have high-stage tumor at the time of diagnosis, deep myoinvasion (>30% of the uterine wall), a high-grade sarcomatous component, and tumor with stromal overgrowth. Recurrent disease typically appears in the pelvis; distant metastasis from low-grade tumors is unusual, but it may develop many years after pelvic recurrence. Death from adenosarcoma is reported to result in 10% to 25% of cases; most often, the patients who die had a primary tumor that featured stromal overgrowth. Death may be delayed until many years after the initial diagnosis, particularly if the stroma is low grade.

Carcinosarcoma (Malignant Mixed Müllerian Tumor) (445,459,474,482–489)

Nomenclature

The terminology for mixed neoplasms composed of carcinoma and sarcoma is in flux. The designation malignant mixed müllerian tumor has the advantage of long entrenchment and, consequently, is the term the clinician is most likely to recognize. This observation notwithstanding, the Nomenclature Committee of the International Society of Gynecologic Pathologists has recommended that the term be replaced by carcinosarcoma, and we think this label should be adopted. The plot has been thickened by the observation that cells in the sarcomatous component of what is now officially dubbed carcinosarcoma express EMA and keratin with sufficient frequency to support the conjecture that carcinosarcomas are, in fact, metaplastic carcinomas (490–492). We think the urge to change the name yet again to reflect this interesting discovery should, in the interest of preserving the sanity of our patients and clinical colleagues, be resisted.

Description

Carcinosarcomas are almost invariably fleshy, necrotic, hemorrhagic, polypoid growths that often fill the uterine cavity (Fig. 78). Cervical and extrauterine involvement at the time of hysterectomy is common. Gross sectioning of the uterus typically reveals extensive myometrial invasion. Almost all carcinosarcomas are easily recognized as high-grade malignant neoplasms upon microscopic examination, regardless of whether the tumor is initially encountered in an endometrial sampling or a hysterectomy specimen. At the microscopic level, both the high-grade nuclear features and the biphasic pattern of this neoplasm are obvious in the typical case (Fig. 79). In many instances, however, one or the other component predominates, and differential diagnostic problems arise when this biphasic pattern is inconspicuous, particularly in endometrial samplings. The most common problem is trying to determine whether anaplastic carcinoma also contains sarcoma (see Differential Diagnosis) (Fig. 80).

The epithelial component of a carcinosarcoma may be any type of müllerian carcinoma—mucinous, squamous, endometrioid, high-grade papillary, clear cell, undifferentiated, or mixtures of these types. The endometrioid type is the most

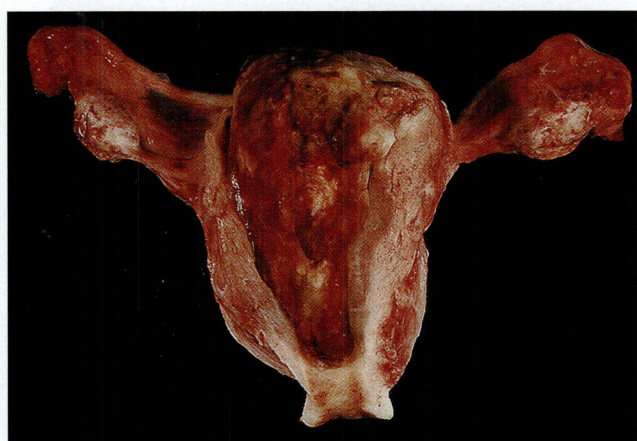

FIG. 78. Carcinosarcoma (gross features). This photograph illustrates a large, bulky, hemorrhagic, and necrotic mass filling the uterine cavity. This appearance is characteristic of carcinosarcoma.

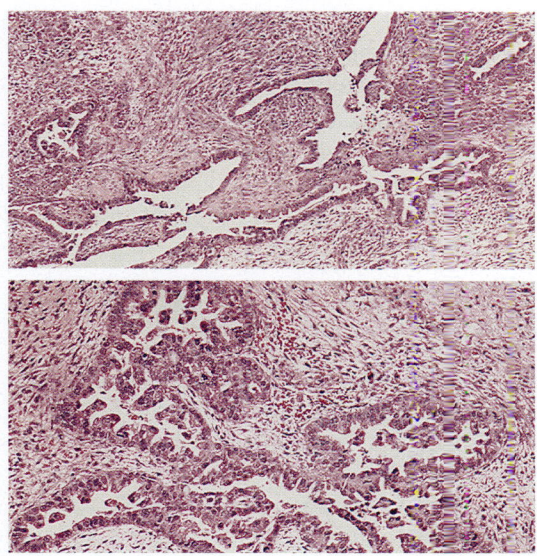

FIG. 79. Carcinosarcoma. Carcinomatous and sarcomatous differentiation is readily appreciated.

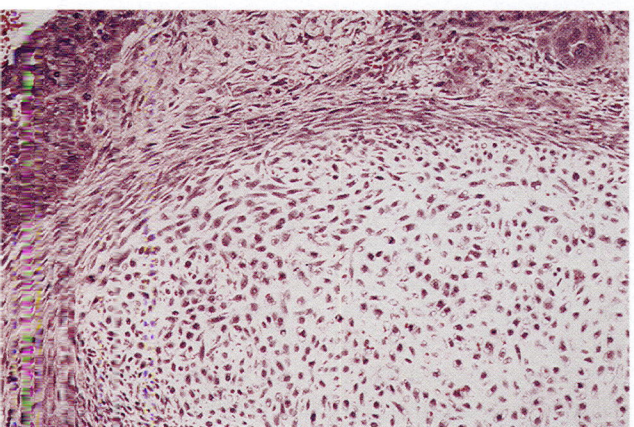

FIG. 81. Carcinosarcoma. Cartilaginous differentiation is present in this carcinosarcoma. Heterologous differentiation is helpful in identifying a sarcomatous component but is of no prognostic significance.

common. PAS-positive globules are common in carcinosarcomas. It is traditional to divide the stromal components into homologous (leiomyosarcoma, stromal sarcoma, fibrosarcoma) and heterologous (chondrosarcoma, rhabdomyosarcoma, osteosarcoma, liposarcoma) types, although there is little evidence that this ritual is clinically useful. On the other hand, identification of heterologous sarcoma is often *diagnostically* useful in singling out the tumor as carcinosarcoma rather than pure carcinoma (Figs. 81 and 82). An unusual case is the carcinosarcoma in which the carcinoma and sarcoma are both low grade. Although very few cases have been studied, these tumors appear to have low-grade behavior similar to that of low-grade adenosarcoma, so this feature should be documented.

Clinicopathologic Correlation (488,493–497)

Carcinosarcoma, with rare exceptions, is a disease of elderly menopausal women. This neoplasm sometimes has been associated with a history of radiation therapy (459). The clinical course of patients with carcinosarcoma is that of a high-grade, aggressive, malignant neoplasm. A third of patients have initial clinical evidence of extrauterine spread; in some series, as many as 40% to 50% of patients thought to have clinical manifestations of stage I disease are found to have higher stages of disease at surgery. The primary treatment is hysterectomy with surgical staging. No adjuvant therapy has been proved effective in a randomized trial by the Gynecology Oncology Group (GOG), and treatment of persistent or recurrent tumor by chemotherapy or radiation therapy practically never results in cure.

There are no consistent differences between homologous and heterologous carcinosarcomas in terms of survival. The most important prognostic features are the stage, the size of

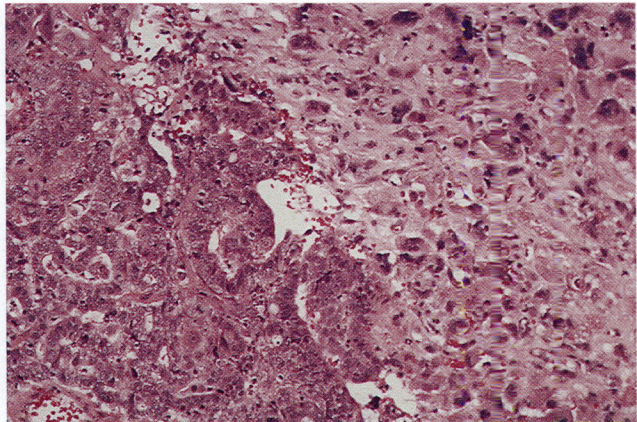

FIG. 80. Carcinosarcoma. Carcinoma is seen on the left and sarcoma on the right. As this photomicrograph demonstrates, the sarcomatous areas are often poorly differentiated and may be difficult to distinguish from undifferentiated carcinoma.

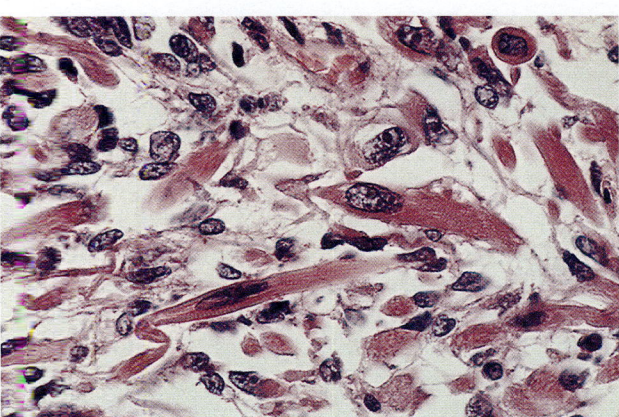

FIG. 82. Carcinosarcoma. Rhabdomyosarcomatous differentiation is common in carcinosarcomas and is a useful marker of sarcomatous differentiation.

the tumor, and the depth of myometrial invasion. For practical purposes, the only patients to achieve long-term survival are those with small tumors that are, at most, minimally myoinvasive. The converse, however, does not hold true; after extensive sectioning of the uterus, even tumors that are apparently confined to the endometrium (or to an endometrial polyp) can metastasize. The type(s) of sarcoma, the level of mitotic counts, and the grade of the sarcoma have not been shown to be significantly related to survival in large clinicopathologic series. There are conflicting reports about the significance of vascular invasion, cervical involvement, and the subtype of carcinoma. The GOG has reported that the subtype (especially serous and clear cell) and grade of the carcinomatous element are significant predictors of survival (445). We think the pathology report of a carcinosarcoma should contain information about the size and location of the tumor, the extent of myometrial invasion (if any), the status of the cervix, the presence or absence of vascular invasion, the type of carcinoma, and the status of the resection margins.

Differential Diagnosis

Endometrial Polyp Versus Adenofibroma Versus Polypoid Adenomyoma Versus Atypical Polypoid Adenomyoma

All of these tumors involve the endometrium in a conspicuously focal polypoid fashion; in addition, they have in common a prominence of their mesenchymal component. Endometrial polyp usually exhibit weak zonation, that is, centrally located, thick-walled vessels and peripherally distributed glands (Figs. 26 and 27). In contrast, AdFib, PA, and APA feature more or less uniformly distributed glands. AdFib has a papillary architecture that distinguishes it from both APA and PA (Figs. 73–75). The mesenchymal component in PA and APA is, with some exceptions, smooth muscle and fibrous, while that of AdFib is typically completely fibrous. PA and APA differ in the complexity of the architecture of the glandular component, which is complex in APA and simple in PA. In addition, APA almost always exhibits striking squamous metaplasia and morule formation (Figs. 69–71).

Atypical Polypoid Adenomyoma and Atypical Polypoid Adenomyoma of Low Malignant Potential Versus Adenocarcinoma with Bland Squamous Elements

The architectural complexity and the cytologic atypia of APA and APA-LMP are often sufficiently pronounced to raise the possibility of carcinoma, but closer examination most often establishes the presence of a prominent fibromuscular stromal component and glands that, in the usual APA, possess neither the architectural complexity nor the cytologic abnormalities of adenocarcinoma (Figs. 47 and 69–71). Because of the fibromuscular stroma, a more worrisome consideration is myoinvasive well-differentiated adenocarcinoma (Fig. 72). Set against this interpretation in APA and APA-LMP is the absence of the granulation-tissue-like host response usually associated with myoinvasive carcinoma glands, the presence of a focal lesion, and the young age of the typical patient with APA/APA-LMP. The immunohistologic properties of the stroma in APA/APA-LMP and myoinvasive well-differentiated adenocarcinoma are not sufficiently distinctive to allow for discrimination between these two processes solely on these grounds (467). Radiologic imaging studies may be useful in clarifying the issue of myoinvasion in a patient interested in preserving her fertility.

Adenofibroma Versus Adenosarcoma

When the entire uterus is available for examination, the distinction between these two tumors can usually be made using the criteria described earlier, even though there is some controversy regarding the level of mitotic activity that indicates a potential for recurrence in the absence of obviously malignant stromal cells (Figs. 73–77). This is a problem (as with AH/WDCA) whose resolution is handicapped by small numbers of cases and the indolent behavior of bland adenosarcomas. The particular solution settled upon varies from authority to authority. Zaloudek and Norris (474) present evidence to support a threshold of 4 mf per 10 hpf, whereas Clement and Scully employ the threshold of 2 mf per 10 hpf (459).

To complicate the issue, a few otherwise typical AdFibs have been reported to be myoinvasive, which means that the morphologic predictors are far from perfect (470). Since patients with either of these entities are postmenopausal in the majority of cases, the distinction is of prognostic significance only; no therapy decisions rest upon the assignment to one or the other category. When adenosarcomas are not invasive and are diagnosed as sarcoma solely on the basis of the MI, we use the modifier "of low malignant potential." In the rare circumstance of an ambiguous lesion in a woman in her reproductive years, consultation should be sought. When the stroma is obviously sarcomatous, there is no problem in assigning the case to the category of adenosarcoma.

Adenosarcoma Versus Carcinosarcoma

This distinction revolves around whether the epithelial component is malignant or benign (Figs. 76, 77, 79, and 80). Ambiguous cases are unusual, but when there is uncertainty on this point in a curettage or biopsy specimen, resolution may have to await hysterectomy. The behavior of the neoplasms can be predicted by the most anaplastic areas, although foci of malignant epithelium in what is otherwise a characteristic adenosarcoma probably predicts clinical behavior closer to adenosarcoma than to carcinosarcoma (445).

Adenosarcoma Versus Pure Sarcoma Invading Nonneoplastic Endometrium and Entrapping Glands

In adenosarcoma, the benign glands are typically distributed throughout the tumor, and they are large and cystic; in fact, they are sometimes visible on gross examination. In addition, the stroma often condenses in concentric layers around the glands to form an entrapping layer. In contrast, residual glands trapped by pure sarcoma tend to be small, are an inconspicuous focal feature, and usually are not surrounded by condensed stroma. Areas of stromal overgrowth complicate the interpretation, but in adenosarcoma the described glandular pattern is seen somewhere in the tumor.

Adenosarcoma Versus Endometrial Stromal Neoplasm with Glandular Elements

Occasionally, it becomes a problem to distinguish low-grade endometrial stromal sarcoma with glands from adenosarcoma. If epithelium is present in the former case, it usually takes the form of a very minor component of poorly circumscribed, small, tubular glands or cords of epithelial-like cells (Fig. 90). In contrast, adenosarcomas have a glandular component that is prominent, usually cystic (with intraglandular polypoid projections of stroma), and uniformly distributed throughout the tumor. As noted earlier, the stroma frequently condenses around the dilated glands (Figs. 76 and 77). Also helpful is a search for more characteristic features of low-grade endometrial stromal sarcoma, such as intravascular growth, a monomorphous population of uniform cells resembling those found in the normal proliferative endometrium, an osteoid-like collagen matrix tongue-like infiltration, and an arborizing vasculature. A rare neoplasm may have large numbers of glands embedded in a stroma that uniformly resembles proliferative phase endometrial stroma. If the classification remains uncertain after application of these differential criteria, it is worth remembering that the behavior of low-grade endometrial sarcoma and low-grade adenocarcinoma is essentially identical; thus, distinguishing between the two is not critical.

Carcinosarcoma Versus Sheet-like Proliferations of Malignant Undifferentiated Cells

This most often arises as a challenge to differential diagnosis with EMB or curettage specimens. At least two situations may be encountered. In some cases, unequivocal carcinoma is identified, but it is associated with areas of undifferentiated tumor cells that are not definitely sarcomatous; the decision then is between pure high-grade carcinoma and carcinosarcoma (Fig. 80). Immunohistochemical techniques have been used in this circumstance, but more than a few high-grade carcinomas will not react with keratin antibodies, and the cells in morphologically unequivocal sarcomatous areas may express keratin. This observation has given rise to the hypothesis that carcinosarcomas are, in fact, metaplastic carcinomas. As a result, immunohistochemical preparations, more often than not, are not reliable, and resolution of the problem must await hysterectomy (486). Sometimes the diagnosis cannot be resolved even after many sections have been taken from the hysterectomy specimen. Given this uncertain state of affairs, it is fortunate that in clinical terms very little depends on distinguishing between carcinosarcoma and anaplastic carcinoma.

The second situation involves an endometrial sample composed of sheets of undifferentiated malignant cells with neither a discernible carcinomatous component nor a sarcomatous component. Five possibilities need to be considered: pure high-grade carcinoma, pure sarcoma, lymphoma or leukemia, a carcinosarcoma in which only the undifferentiated areas have been sampled, and metastatic carcinoma (see discussion of Pattern 4).

ENDOMETRIAL STROMAL TUMORS (474,498–502)

Endometrial stromal differentiation connotes a monomorphous population of blunt, spindled to oblong cells with scanty cytoplasm and relatively small, uniform nuclei embedded in an abundant reticulin framework (Table 13). A highly characteristic feature of endometrial stromal differentiation is the delicate arborizing vasculature that sometimes features hyalinization of the arborizing vessels. In other words, the cells forming stromal tumors resemble the cells of the normal proliferative phase endometrium, and only minor deviations from this appearance are allowed. Predicting the behavior of a neoplasm with this differentiation depends

TABLE 13. *Pathologic characteristics of endometrial stromal neoplasms contrasted with the pathologic characteristics of high-grade undifferentiated uterine sarcoma*

Endometrial stromal nodule
   Histologic and cytologic features identical to low-grade stromal sarcoma
   Circumscribed with pushing margins, often small
   Fewer than ten mitoses in 10 hpf
   No lymphatic or vascular invasion
   Confined to the uterus
Low-grade endometrial stromal sarcoma
   Uniform cells that resemble proliferative phase endometrial cells, no more than slight nuclear enlargement or mild cytologic atypia, plexiform vascular pattern, hyalin often prominent
   Myometrial infiltration characterized by "tongue-like" tumor masses
   Vascular and lymphatic involvement common; grossly visible vascular intrusion giving rise to distinctive "worm-like" appearance
   May extend beyond the uterus and can metastasize
   Up to 15 normal mf/10 hpf
High-grade undifferentiated uterine sarcoma
   Cellular neoplasm with infiltrating margins, usually with extensive myometrial infiltration
   Often more than ten mitoses in 10 hpf, abnormal mitotic figures common, marked nuclear atypia, enlargement, and pleomorphism are the rule; tumor cells bear little resemblance to proliferative phase endometrial stroma and are undifferentiated
   Vascular and lymphatic invasion less often grossly visible
   Frequently extends beyond the uterus, metastases are common.

hpf, high-power field; mf, mitotic figures.

upon the stage of the tumor and on evaluation of the interface between the proliferation and the surrounding normal uterine structures (in particular, determining whether the proliferation is circumscribed or infiltrative and whether it is present within vascular spaces).

Stromal Nodule (503)

Description

The stromal nodule is a circumscribed, noninfiltrative, typically spherical mass of endometrial stromal cells without an intravascular component (Fig. 83). The cells are identical to those found in proliferative endometria or in low-grade endometrial stromal sarcoma. Mitotic figures are, in general, difficult to find, but they may be as numerous as 10 mf per 10 hpf. Microscopic stromal nodules may be completely embedded in the endometrium, but the larger nodules typically involve the myometrium (Table 13).

Clinicopathologic Correlation

Because the distinction of a stromal nodule from low-grade endometrial stromal sarcoma depends on evaluating the presence or absence of myometrial infiltration or vascular invasion, these nodules can only infrequently be reliably distinguished from low-grade stromal sarcoma in endome-

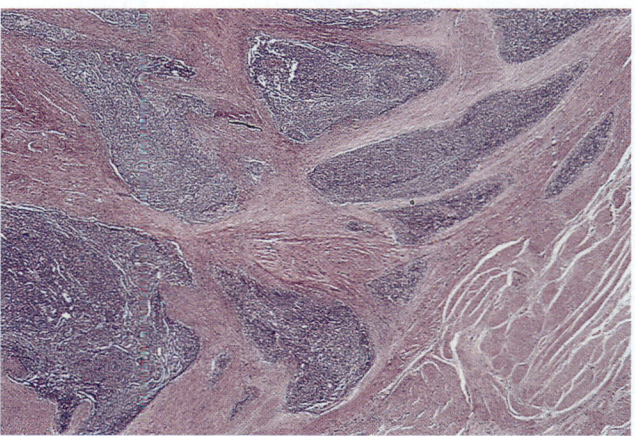

FIG. 84. Low-grade endometrial stromal sarcoma. Note the tongue-like infiltration of the myometrium characteristic of this neoplasm.

trial samplings unless fragments with vascular or myometrial invasion are recovered or unless the nodule is completely confined to the endometrium. Hysterectomy may be required to make this distinction.

Low-grade Endometrial Stromal Sarcoma (474,500–502,504–513)

Description

Low-grade stromal sarcoma, by definition, is composed of cells resembling those of the normal proliferative phase endometrium and has infiltrative margins and/or intravascular intrusion by tumor that frequently can be seen on gross inspection. Other than the infiltration and vascular intrusion, this neoplasm is indistinguishable in histologic terms from the stromal nodule (Figs. 84-89). The pattern of myometrial

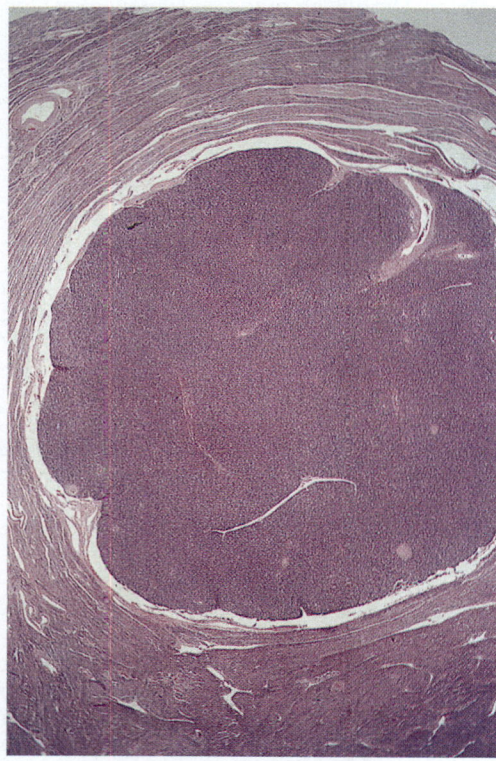

FIG. 83. Stromal nodule. A compressive, noninfiltrative margin defines this entity and serves to distinguish it from low-grade endometrial stromal sarcoma; both proliferations—stromal nodule and low-grade stromal sarcoma—have identical histologic appearances.

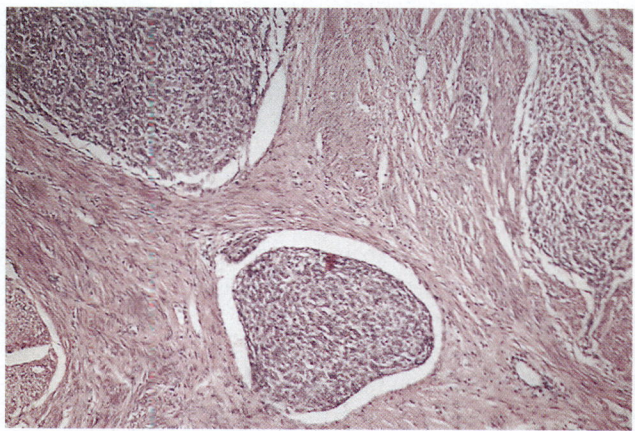

FIG. 85. Low-grade endometrial stromal sarcoma. The neoplasm is shown within the myometrium in what probably represents vascular spaces. It is often difficult to determine whether a space around a tumor nest is residual vessel or is an artifact created by the retraction of the myometrium away from tumor. From a practical point of view, it makes no difference whether the infiltration is muscular or intravascular; both are criteria of malignancy for endometrial stromal neoplasms.

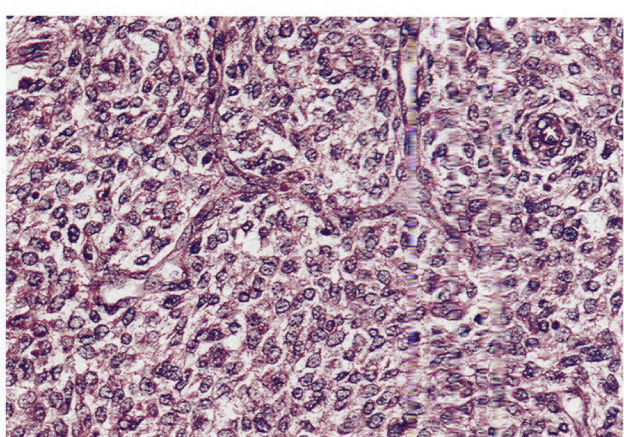

FIG. 86. Low-grade endometrial stromal sarcoma. By definition, the tumor cells must resemble the cells of normal proliferative phase endometrial stroma, that is, they must be uniform with scanty cytoplasm, as in this photomicrograph. An arborizing vascular pattern is characteristic of this neoplasm.

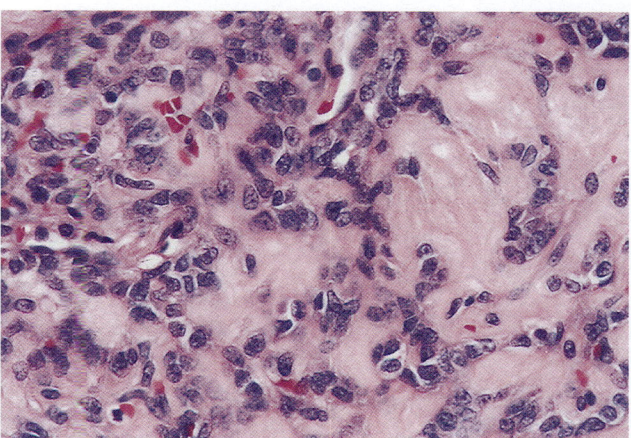

FIG. 88. Low-grade endometrial stromal sarcoma. Extensive hyalinization is seen in many endometrial stromal sarcomas. It is also seen in smooth-muscle tumors and for this reason is not helpful as a differentiating feature.

infiltration often is distinctive and consists of irregularly shaped tongues or islands of tumor cells randomly placed between bundles of smooth-muscle cells (Fig. 84). Foam cells and a decidual-like reaction may be seen. Rare cases feature foci of glands and/or tubules, and even more rarely these structures can be present throughout the tumor (514) (Fig. 90). The cells forming the glands may be keratin positive or may have the immunophenotype of smooth-muscle cells (176,513,515–518). In most low-grade endometrial sarcomas, mitotic figures are few and far between, but isolated tumors will have easily found mitotic figures.

After the publication of Norris and Taylor's classic study on endometrial stromal tumors in 1966, it was customary to divide endometrial stromal sarcomas into low- and high-grade types on the basis of mitotic counts (498). After excluding anaplastic undifferentiated sarcomas, these investigators drew the line between low-grade and high-grade stromal sarcomas at 10 mf per 10 hpf. Subsequently, Evans revived Norris and Taylor's primary division between undifferentiated endometrial sarcoma and endometrial stromal sarcoma but, based upon an analysis of 11 cases, questioned the value of stratifying the latter into low- and high-grade groups on the basis of the MI (499). Those endometrial stromal neoplasms composed of relatively bland, monomorphous, oblong to spindled cells resembling proliferative

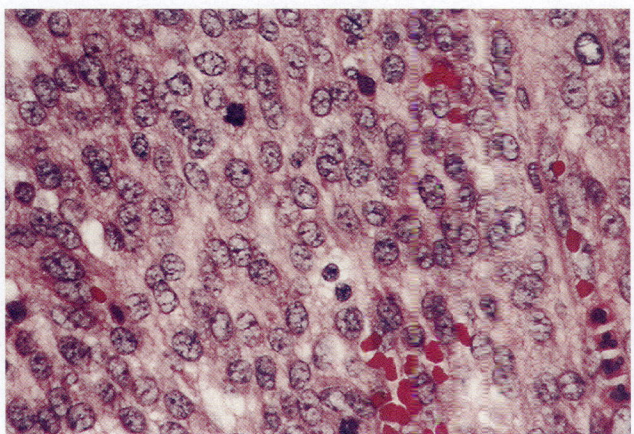

FIG. 87. Low-grade endometrial stromal sarcoma (high magnification). The uniform cells have scanty cytoplasm and uniform nuclei. Most examples of stromal sarcoma are cytologically bland and have low mitotic indexes; these features are no guarantee of a clinically benign course.

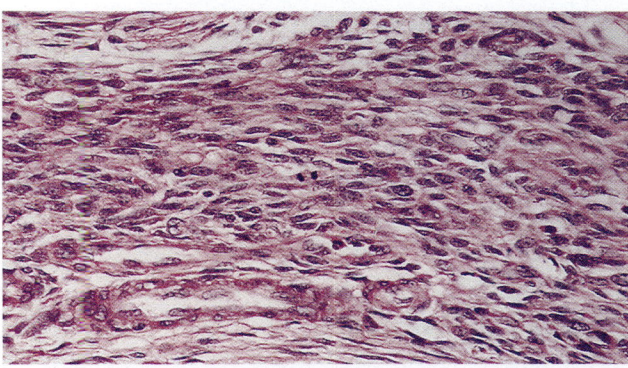

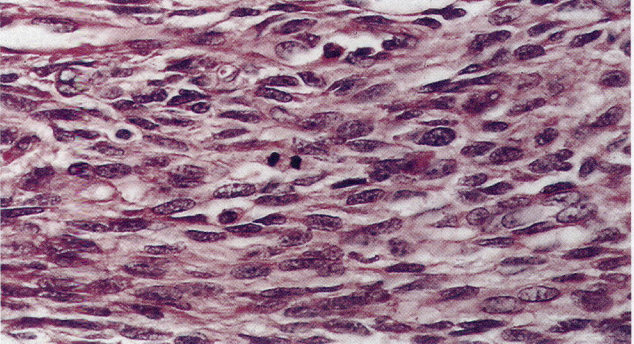

FIG. 89. Low-grade endometrial stromal sarcoma. When endometrial stromal cells take on an elongated shape, as in this photomicrograph, distinguishing them from smooth muscle becomes difficult. See text for our approach to this problem.

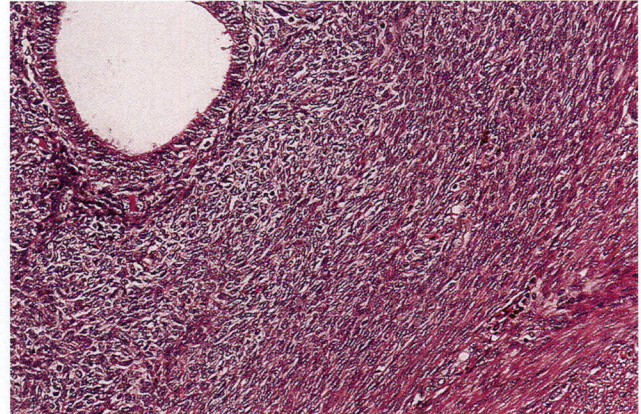

FIG. 90. Endometrial stromal sarcoma. Usually, the glands in endometrial stromal sarcoma are focal and not dilated. This feature helps distinguish them from the benign glands in müllerian adenosarcoma.

phase endometrial stromal cells, independent of the mitotic counts, are considered by Evans to be endometrial stromal sarcomas, while those lacking such features are placed in the undifferentiated endometrial sarcoma group (Table 13). The latter tumors generally are anaplastic and contain large numbers of mitotic figures, some of which may be abnormal.

The main difference between the two points of view is that Norris and Taylor concluded that stratifying neoplasms by MI is useful for tumors that both they and Evans would agree are endometrial stromal sarcomas, while Evans' data did not support this approach. A study of 93 stromal sarcomas at Stanford supports Evans' conclusions, and for this reason we do not stratify endometrial stromal sarcomas into high-grade and low-grade types (511). We continue to use the term low grade to modify the diagnosis endometrial stromal sarcoma, in order to emphasize its low-grade behavior and to avoid confusion with undifferentiated endometrial sarcoma (undifferentiated uterine sarcoma), which is high grade.

Clinicopathologic Correlation

Low-grade endometrial stromal sarcomas, including those few with a characteristic histologic pattern but with up to 15 normal mf per 10 hpf, are indolent, slowly progressing neoplasms that occur at all ages. In the Stanford series, 45% of patients with stage I disease who had both rare mitotic figures and minimal atypia experienced one or more relapses; of these patients, two (13%) died of disease at 85 and 360 months, respectively. There were no significant differences in relapse or survival rates between patients on either side of the line (10 mf/10 hpf) (511). Patients with high-stage disease fare significantly worse than those with disease confined to the uterus; high-stage patients tend to have higher MIs, and those within the high-stage group with an MI ≥10 mf per 10 hpf fare worse than those with an MI of <10.

Thus, the single most important prognostic factor appears to be the stage at presentation, while bland histologic features and low MIs are no guarantees against recurrence. The course of this disease is protracted, and recurrences and metastases are observed 20 to 30 years after the primary tumor has been removed (519,520). The cells composing endometrial stromal sarcomas possess ER/PRs, and metastatic neoplasms frequently respond to progestational therapy. The role of progesterones as adjuvant therapy is not settled (521–530). Low-grade endometrial stromal sarcomas can, on rare occasions, arise from extrauterine sites, including the ovary, vagina, and peritoneum (531–533). These tumors may also contain glands, tubules, and other epithelioid structures as well as ovarian sex-cord-like elements.

Undifferentiated Uterine Sarcoma (Undifferentiated Endometrial Stromal Sarcoma) (498,499,534)

Description

We prefer the term undifferentiated uterine sarcoma or the expression suggested by Evans, undifferentiated endometrial sarcoma, to high-grade endometrial stromal sarcoma because these anaplastic neoplasms most often bear little resemblance to proliferative phase endometrial stroma (Table 13). Undifferentiated uterine sarcoma is much less common than low-grade stromal endometrial sarcoma once one has carefully excluded leukemia, lymphoma, high-grade carcinoma, carcinosarcoma, and differentiated pure sarcomas. Undifferentiated uterine sarcomas are easily recognized as malignant and are composed of pleomorphic, undifferentiated, rounded to spindled cells with a high MI. They lack the characteristic arborizing vasculature and the areas of hyalinization characteristic of low-grade endometrial stromal sarcoma and, as Evans points out, most resemble the undifferentiated malignant stroma encountered in carcinosarcomas (Fig. 91 and Table 13) (499). All pure undifferentiated sar-

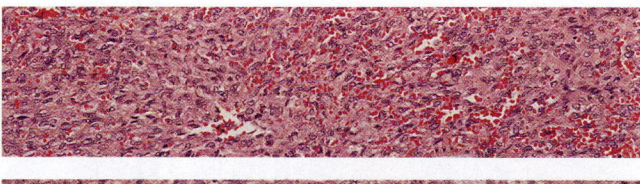
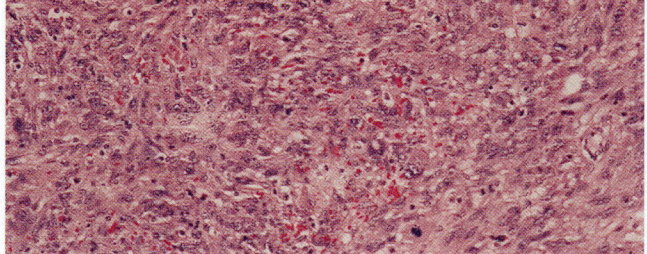

FIG. 91. Undifferentiated uterine sarcoma. Top: Undifferentiated uterine sarcomas bear little resemblance to proliferative phase endometrial stroma. They lack the arborizing vasculature of low-grade endometrial sarcomas. Bottom: Most of these neoplasms are composed of enlarged, pleomorphic cells with numerous mitotic figures.

comas of the uterus, including the giant-cell variety, can for convenience be placed in this category. Pure sarcomas containing cells differentiating along recognizable mesenchymal lines are named in a way that reflects their differentiation, that is, leiomyosarcoma, osteosarcoma, rhabdomyosarcoma, and so on.

Clinicopathologic Correlation

Undifferentiated uterine sarcomas, in sharp contrast to endometrial stromal sarcomas, behave in a highly aggressive fashion, a pattern of behavior resembling those of carcinosarcomas or pure heterologous sarcomas.

Uterine Neoplasms with Sex-cord-like Elements (459,515,517,536,537)

Description

Clement and Scully first drew attention to these unusual neoplasms in 1976 (535). The neoplastic cells that give the tumor its name are arranged in cords, hollow tubules, trabeculae, and/or sheets resembling epithelial cells, and they most often have scanty cytoplasm, indistinct cell margins, and round nuclei (Fig. 92). In some tumors, however, the constituent cells may have abundant eosinophilic or clear cytoplasm. The stroma between the epithelioid structures varies from paucicellular and fibroblastic to an appearance similar to normal proliferative endometrial stroma. Hyaline matrix may be prominent. Most tumors have pushing margins, but vascular intrusion has been observed in some cases. The cells composing the sex-cord-like areas are often inhibin positive and may express keratin (518). We include these tumors in the endometrial stromal group because of the resemblance of the constituent stromal cells to endometrial stromal cells. Moreover, glands may be present in addition to tubules and trabeculae.

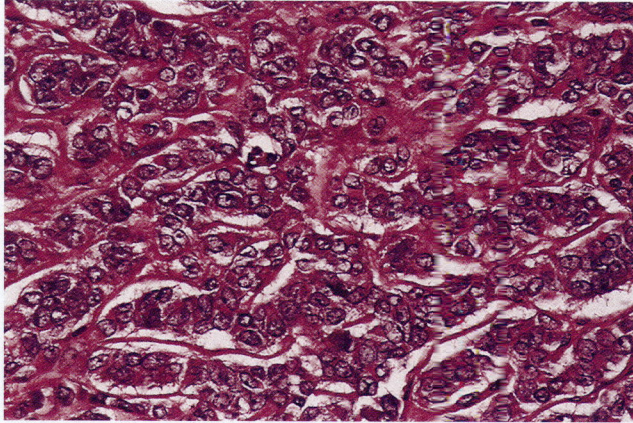

FIG. 92. Uterine tumor resembling ovarian sex-cord tumor. Endometrial stromal sarcomas sometimes have components that form tubules, trabeculae, or islands of cells. These elements may be focal or predominant or the tumor may be exclusively composed of cells arranged in such patterns.

Clinicopathologic Correlation

Most of these neoplasms are benign, but some have recurred and/or metastasized. Too few have been studied to know if there are morphologic features that would reliably predict aggressive behavior. Given the absence of data, we use the same criteria to distinguish benign from malignant sex-cord-like tumors as we do to distinguish stromal nodule from low-grade endometrial stroma sarcoma; only tumors with circumscribed borders, a low MI, and uniform cells are considered to be benign. The malignant varieties behave as do low-grade stromal sarcomas.

Differential Diagnosis

Low-grade Endometrial Stromal Sarcoma Versus Stromal Nodule

The distinction between these two can usually be made only with the entire uterus in hand and is based on the presence of infiltrating margins and/or vascular invasion in the former but not in the latter (Figs. 83–85).

Low-grade Endometrial Stromal Sarcoma Versus Adenomyosis with Sparse Glands or Non-Menstrual Endometrium Within Vessels (538,539)

Adenomyosis with sparse glands is almost always an incidental, microscopic finding in a postmenopausal woman's uterus. There is characteristically a distinctive zonal phenomenon, an atrophic version of the familiar ring of smooth-muscle hypertrophy surrounding a focus of endometrial stroma depleted of glands. Unlike the cells in endometrial stromal sarcoma, the stromal cells in this context are small and atrophic. The finding of more typical areas of adenomyosis aids in the distinction. Rarely, minute fragments of bland endometrial stroma without glands are incidentally found in spaces in a hysterectomy specimen, raising the question of low-grade stromal sarcoma within vessels. If no mass is present after a thorough search, this finding has no prognostic implication and is the nonmenstrual counterpart of menstrual endometrium within vessels, described later (see section concerning adenomyosis).

Low-grade Endometrial Stromal Sarcoma Versus Menstrual Endometrium Within Vessels

Rarely, menstrual endometrium may be found in myometrial vessels. Distinguishing it from stromal sarcoma is accomplished by noting the widespread and uniform distribution of glands admixed with cytologically bland stroma (539).

Low-grade Stromal Sarcoma Versus Lymphoma/Leukemia Versus Carcinoma

Because the constituent cells of low-grade endometrial stromal sarcoma have few discernible differentiated cytologic features (Fig. 87), identification of these tumors is mainly based on the resemblance of the constituent cells to normal proliferative endometrial stroma, the arborizing vascular pattern, the characteristic osteoid-like hyalin, and the intrusion of tumor cells into vascular spaces. When these features are muted, the diagnostic possibilities are numerous. Lymphoma and leukemia can closely mimic low-grade endometrial stromal sarcoma, and we advocate liberal use of lymphoid markers and esterase stains in any doubtful case.

Poorly differentiated carcinomas, particularly metastatic lobular carcinoma from the breast, are always a consideration when contemplating a diagnosis of low-grade endometrial stromal sarcoma (Fig. 93). PAS and keratin immunohistochemical stains are often useful, as is the clinical history. This differential diagnostic problem is complicated by the observation that the cells forming the glands or tubules in endometrial stromal tumors may express keratin as well as muscle actin and desmin (55,459,540,541). Extensive tumor within large vascular spaces is a characteristic feature of low-grade endometrial stromal sarcoma, but not the other neoplasms under consideration in this section (see later discussion of low-grade endometrial stromal sarcoma versus smooth-muscle tumor).

Low-grade Stromal Sarcoma Versus Inflammation, Fragmented Lymphoid Nodules, and Immunoblasts

Follicular center cells in lymphoid nodules and sheets of immunoblasts can come to resemble neoplastic endometrial stromal cells, particularly in endometrial biopsy specimens and curettings. Searching, on the one hand, for the characteristic endometrial stromal features discussed earlier and, on the other hand, for features of inflammatory processes, such as follicular center cells in intact lymphoid follicles, numerous plasma cells, and acute inflammatory cells, should help clarify the situation. Immunohistology is often useful in this context.

Low-grade Endometrial Stromal Sarcoma Versus Benign Smooth-muscle Tumors, Particularly Intravascular Leiomyomatosis

This problem is discussed in the introduction to the section devoted to smooth-muscle neoplasms and in Table 5. It is an important differential consideration because both benign and malignant smooth-muscle and endometrial stromal proliferations intrude into vessels and because the two types of neoplasms can closely resemble each other in histologic and immunohistochemical characteristics (Fig. 89; see also Figs. 118 and 119).

Low-grade Endometrial Sarcoma Versus High-grade Uterine Sarcoma

See the discussions concerning endometrial stromal sarcoma and undifferentiated uterine sarcoma.

Stromal Nodule and Low-grade Stromal Sarcoma Versus Sex-cord-like Tumor

By definition, stromal nodules and low-grade endometrial stromal sarcomas can contain only glands, whereas sex-cord-like tumors also contain cells arranged as tubules, trabeculae, cords, and/or sheets. Undoubtedly, there is considerable morphologic overlap, but, fortunately, the behavior of sex-cord-like tumors and endometrial stromal tumors is identical and depends on the presence or absence of infiltration, as described previously (Figs. 83, 84, and 92).

Adenofibroma and Adenosarcoma Versus Sex-cord-like Tumor

AdFib and adenosarcoma feature benign and, most often, cystically dilated glands uniformly distributed throughout the tumor, rather than the cords, trabeculae, or tubules char-

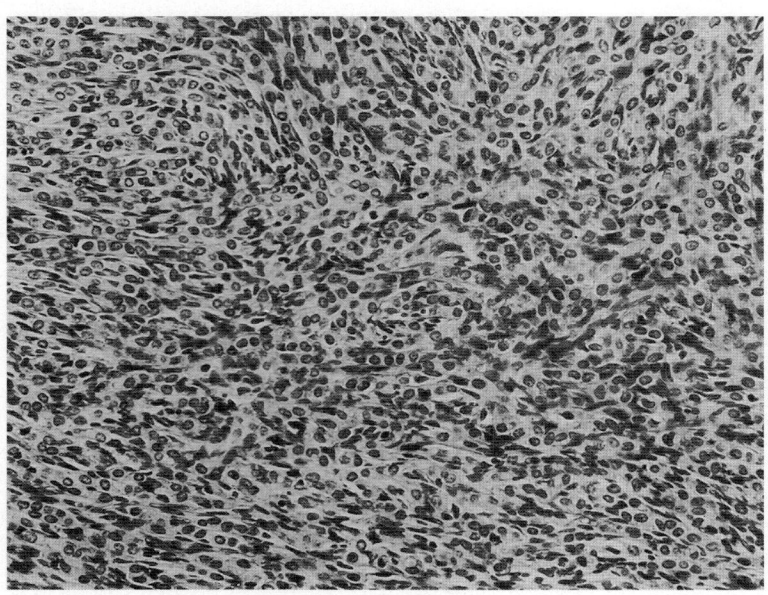

FIG. 93. Lobular carcinoma of the breast metastatic to the endometrium. The resemblance of this carcinoma to low-grade endometrial stromal sarcoma and to epithelioid smooth-muscle tumors is impressive. Whenever a diagnosis of low-grade stromal sarcoma or epithelioid smooth-muscle tumor is contemplated, the possibility of metastatic lobular carcinoma should be considered. The mimicry is heightened by the uniformity of the tumor cells, the paucity of mitotic figures, and the failure of the tumor cells to differentiate into glandular or tubular structures.

acteristic of sex-cord-like tumors. Moreover, a papillary architecture is absent in sex-cord-like tumors. In adenosarcoma, the mesenchymal component must meet the histologic or MI criterion for sarcoma, and spindled stromal cells often condense in a concentric, entrapping layer around the dilated glands (Figs. 73–77 and 92).

Endometrial Stromal Neoplasm Versus Adenosarcoma

See earlier section describing the differential diagnosis of mixed müllerian tumors.

MYOMETRIUM: NONNEOPLASTIC CONDITIONS (547–548)

Adenomyosis

Description

Endometrial tissue (glands and stroma) is considered ectopic in the uterus if it is present on the uterine serosa (endometriosis) or if it is located "excessively" deep in the myometrium (adenomyosis). The definition of "excessively" is a subject of a minor but ongoing controversy in gynecologic pathology. In clear-cut cases of adenomyosis, the uterus is grossly abnormal. When it is focal, adenomyosis mimics a leiomyoma in being a roughly spherical intramural, space-occupying lesion, but it differs from leiomyoma in that the mass cannot be shelled out easily from the surrounding uninvolved myometrium, an important point for infertility surgeons. When involvement is diffuse, the uterus is enlarged in a "globoid" fashion. In both situations the cut surface of the myometrium bulges and is coarsely trabecular; at the microscopic level, foci of basalis-type endometrial glands and stroma are delimited by hypertrophied bands of smooth muscle.

Controversy arises when no gross abnormality is present and the diagnosis is based entirely upon microscopic findings. The source of this difficulty in terms of definition is the normal irregularity of the endometrial-myometrial junction and the tendency of tangential cuts of this region to produce convincing imitations of adenomyosis. Various strategies have been offered to distinguish this situation from so-called true adenomyosis. We make the diagnosis of adenomyosis when there is definite smooth-muscle hypertrophy around foci of endometrial glands and stroma and, absent that finding, when endometrial glands and stroma lie within the outer two-thirds of the uterine wall.

Microscopic foci of adenomyosis can come to lie in vascular spaces. As long as this feature is microscopic and focal, it is harmless. The obvious problem is distinguishing these foci from gland-forming endometrial stromal sarcoma intruding into vessels. Any grossly visible mass with infiltrating margins composed of endometrial stroma and glands and gross intrusion of a stromal-glandular process into vessels should be construed as endometrial stromal sarcoma, as should extrauterine masses of endometrial stroma and glands measuring more than 2 cm. In addition, it is only the very rare stromal sarcoma that has glands distributed throughout the lesion, whereas this feature is, by definition, characteristic of adenomyosis. Borderline cases of glandular stromal processes with vascular intrusion may be encountered; we label them "adenomyosis with vascular involvement, low-grade stromal sarcoma cannot be excluded." Sometimes only fragments of endometrial stroma without glands are found in vessels. As long as there is no mass, as described here, this is considered to be a harmless form of adenomyosis in vessels.

Diffuse adenomyosis may be extensive enough to raise the question of low-grade stromal sarcoma with glands, even though it is not present in vessels. Adenomyosis does not infiltrate the myometrium in tongues, as does stromal sarcoma, and the muscular hypertrophy characteristic of adenomyosis is largely absent in stromal sarcoma. Again, it is very rare for endometrial stromal sarcoma to contain small, regular glands diffusely spread throughout the lesion.

Clinicopathologic Correlation

Patients with classic adenomyosis frequently have abnormal uterine bleeding. The clinical significance, if any, of microscopically diagnosed "pathologist's adenomyosis" is unknown, but it is undoubtedly minimal. On occasion, endometrial carcinoma may be present within foci of adenomyosis (548). It is usually accompanied by endometrial carcinoma in the uterine lining. This has the same significance as endometrial carcinoma limited to the endometrium, unless the carcinoma is invading the myometrium from the foci of adenomyosis. The difficulties in assessing whether myometrial invasion is present in this context are described in the section on endometrial carcinoma.

Changes of Pregnancy

Description

Physiologic hypertrophy and hyperplasia of the myometrium during pregnancy, as well as the characteristic trophoblastic infiltration at the implantation site, are well known. Most of the differential diagnostic difficulties presented by curettage specimens obtained during or just after gestation relate to gestational trophoblastic disease and its mimics (see chapter by Mazur and Kurman; see also the earlier section on gestational changes in the endometrium). The physiologic "chronic endometritis" that occurs during this period has been described in the section on endometritis. Clinically important postpartum bacterial infections are accompanied by the production of pus and its microscopic correlate, namely, sheets of polymorphs admixed with disintegrating endometrium.

Differential Diagnosis

The diagnosis of endometrial carcinoma or leiomyosarcoma should be considered with great trepidation in a young woman, particularly if decidua or other clues of gestation are identified. Occasionally, gestational trophoblastic disease mimics a nongestational uterine malignancy. In particular, PSTT can closely resemble leiomyosarcoma. Whenever a diagnosis of leiomyosarcoma is contemplated in a woman in her reproductive years, the possibility of PSTT should be considered.

SMOOTH-MUSCLE NEOPLASMS (TABLES 14 AND 15; FIG 94)

Introduction (460,501,502,549,550)

The majority of uterine smooth-muscle neoplasms are easily recognized as being composed of cells differentiated as smooth muscle, and the benign or malignant nature of these neoplasms is easy to evaluate. An important minority of smooth-muscle neoplasms present difficulties, however, for one or more of the following reasons: (a) they are clinically benign neoplasms with a peculiar gross appearance (Fig. 95), (b) they are clinically benign neoplasms with an unusual anatomic distribution, (c) they are clinically benign neoplasms with aberrant cytologic features, (d) they are clinically benign neoplasms with high mitotic counts, (e) they are clinically malignant but have benign morphologic features (rare), or (f) they are lesions whose smooth-muscle differentiation is not obvious.

Before evaluating the benign or malignant nature of a purported smooth-muscle proliferation in the uterus, it is imperative to ensure that the constituent cells do indeed show evidence of smooth-muscle differentiation. For most smooth-muscle tumors, this is a straightforward task because the tumor cells resemble normal myometrial cells. However, smooth-muscle cells can come to resemble epithelial cells (epithelioid smooth-muscle tumors) or endometrial stromal cells (Table 5). In the former circumstance, the blending of the epithelioid smooth-muscle cells into more obvious areas of smooth-muscle differentiation in the tumor, if such areas are present, is a good indicator that the neoplasm in question is a smooth-muscle tumor. EMA, keratin, actin, and desmin stains may be helpful, but they must be used with caution in light of the fact that smooth-muscle cells can be keratin positive and now and then can express an antigen recognized by antibodies against EMA (55,540,541). Epithelial cells are not desmin positive, however.

Smooth-muscle cells can also come to resemble endometrial stromal cells by losing much of their characteristic eosinophilic, fibrillary cytoplasm and developing closely approximated round to oblong nuclei of the type more often seen in endometrial stromal cells. At times, a trichrome stain will bring out the fibrillar brick-red cytoplasm characteristic of such altered smooth-muscle cells. Unfortunately, both smooth-muscle cells and stromal cells have been reported to express muscle actin and desmin; desmin expression by stromal cells, however, is often focal, whereas smooth-muscle cells are usually diffusely and strongly desmin positive. The weight that should be given to desmin expression in determining whether an ambiguous myometrial lesion is stromal or smooth muscle is the subject of debate, but there is an increasing tendency to classify tumors composed of desmin-positive cells as smooth muscle in type.

The distinction between a smooth-muscle tumor and an endometrial stromal tumor is of some importance, because the criteria for malignancy differ for the two tumor types. If the margins of an ambiguous lesion are pushing, the direction of differentiation makes little difference because cellular leiomyoma and stromal nodule are both benign. While infiltration of myometrium or vessels is a malignant criterion for stromal tumors, it may be found in smooth-muscle tumors that are clinically benign (55,551,552) (Table 5). Our practice

TABLE 14. *Our diagnostic strategy for uterine smooth-muscle neoplasms (based on outcome data from a study at 213 challenging smooth-muscle tumors) (549)*

Morphologic features to be evaluated (see text for definitions)
  Degree of cytologic atypic: none to mild *or* moderate to marked
  Presence or absence of coagulative tumor cell necrosis
  Mitotic index (MI)
Smooth-muscle tumors with usual differentiation
  MI <20 mf/10 hpf, *no* coagulative necrosis *no* atypia or *no more* than *mild cytologic atypia* (i.e., bland cytologic features—see text) = leiomyoma or leiomyoma with increased mitotic index (MI <5 mf/10 hpf = leiomyoma; MI ≥5 mf/10 hpf = leiomyoma with increased mitotic figures)
  MI ≥20 mf/10 hpf, no coagulative necrosis, *no* atypia or *no more* than *mild cytologic* atypia (i.e., the cytologic features must be bland—see text) = leiomyoma with increased mitotic index but experience limited
  MI <10 mf/10 hpf, no coagulative necrosis but with *diffuse moderate* to *severe* cytologic atypia = atypical leiomyoma with low risk of recurrence (1/46 failed)
  MI ≥10 mf/10 hpf, *no* coagulative necrosis but with *diffuse moderate* to *severe* cytologic atypia = leiomyosarcoma (4/10 failed)
  MI ≤10 mf/10 hpf, no coagulative necrosis but with *focal moderate* to severe cytologic atypia = leiomyoma with atypia but limited experience
  Any MI and any degree of cytologic atypia with coagulative necrosis = leiomyosarcoma (29/39 failed). Note: Most often there will be significant atypia and/or elevated mitotic counts in leiomyosarcoma in addition to the coagulative tumor cell necrosis. Be careful of the case that does not have these additional morphologic features (see text).
Smooth-muscle tumors with myxoid stroma
  MI <5 mf/10 hpf, *no* or mild atypia, no coagulative necrosis = myxoid leiomyoma
  Any MI, moderate to marked atypia with or without coagulative necrosis = myxoid leiomyosarcoma
Smooth-muscle tumor with epithelioid differentiation
  MI <5 mf/10 hpf, *no* coagulative necrosis, *no* atypia or *no more* than mild cytologic atypia = epithelioid leiomyoma (limited experience)
  MI ≥5 mf/10 hpf, *no* coagulative necrosis, none or any degree of atypia = epithelioid leiomyosarcoma (limited experience)
  Any MI and any degree of cytologic atypia *with coagulative necrosis* = epithelioid leiomyosarcoma (limited experience)

mf, mitotic figures; hpf, high-power field.

TABLE 15. *Histologic patterns of uterine smooth-muscle tumors*

Smooth-muscle tumors with usual differentiation (see definition in text)
    Usual leiomyoma and leiomyoma with increased mitotic figures (549,556,577)
        Uniform cells with elongated nuclei and often moderate amounts of sometimes fibrillar cytoplasm; sometimes the cytoplasm is sparse and difficult to discern. Nuclei may be uniformly enlarged but no more than mild pleomorphism or mild chromatin abnormalities are allowed.
        MI <5 mf/10 hpf = leiomyoma
        MI = 5–10 mf/10 hpf = leiomyoma with increased mitotic index
        MI = 10–20 mf/10 hpf = leiomyoma with increased mitotic index, but experience is limited.
    Mitotic figures must be small and normal. When hypercellular, the term cellular leiomyoma can be used but is not necessary.
    Leiomyosarcoma
        Generally, elongated cells but may be all shapes and sizes; usually moderate to severe cytologic atypia; almost always hypercellular. Uterine smooth-muscle tumors with coagulative (not hyalinizing) tumor cell necrosis are almost always leiomyosarcomas; however, tumor cell necrosis is almost invariably accompanied by an elevated mitotic index and moderate to severe atypia. Tumors with diffuse moderate to severe atypia but without coagulative tumor cell necrosis are leiomyosarcomas or atypical leiomyomas, depending on the mitotic index (see Table 4 and following table text).
Smooth-muscle tumors with unusual histological patterns
    Atypical leiomyoma with low risk of recurrence; leiomyoma with focal atypia (benign with limited experience) (485, 502, 549, 556, 557, 570–575)
        Smooth muscle tumor with either focal or diffuse moderate to severe cytologic atypia without coagulative tumor cell necrosis and an MI of <10mf/10hpf (see text for definition). Giant cells, either multinucleated or hyperlobated, and/or cells with enlarged hyperchromatic nuclei are common. Coagulative tumor cell necrosis must be absent.
    Epithelioid smooth-muscle tumors (143, 574, 582–584, 654)
        Round (epithelial-like) cells arranged in sheets and/or cords; these often blend into more elongated cells. Cytoplasm may have perinuclear clearing, or it may be clear at the periphery of the cell with a rim of eosinophilic cytoplasm around the nucleus. When the cytoplasm is totally clear, the term clear cell is appended. When tumor is composed of cells with crumpled nuclei aligned in cords often within hyalin stroma, the term plexiform tumor is used (see Table 14 and text for evaluating malignant potential of epithelioid tumors).
    Myxoid stroma (See Table 14 and text for evaluating, malignant, potential of tumors with myxoid stroma (459, 655)
    Lipoleiomyoma (592–595)
        Morphological features leiomyoma with focal to diffuse fatty differentiation
    Neurilemoma-like leiomyoma (573, 574, 596)
        Morphologic features: same as for leiomyoma, except that nuclei are palisaded, thereby causing resemblance to Verocay bodies.
    Leiomyoma with tubules or glands
        Tubules or glands found in an otherwise characteristic leiomyoma. These are rare neoplasms; most uterine mesenchymal neoplasms with such structures are endometrial stromal neoplasms or uterine tumors resembling ovarian sex-cord tumors
Unusual growth patterns
    Infiltrating leiomyoma, including leiomyomatosis (598)
        An otherwise characteristic leiomyoma with infiltrating margins. A common pattern is patches of hypercellular, benign smooth muscle throughout large areas of the myometrium (leiomyomatosis)
    Disseminated peritoneal leiomyomatosis (150, 599–605)
        Numerous small (<2.0 cm) nodules of bland, benign smooth-muscle cells, often arranged in a whorled pattern. Decidual cells are common. Pregnancy or functional ovarian tumors are commonly associated.
    Benign metastasizing leiomyoma (606–609)
        Deposits of benign smooth muscle in lymph nodes, lung, and other organs associated with a morphologically benign uterine smooth-muscle tumor. The purported metastases must be composed of bland, well-differentiated smooth muscle without anaplasia; significant pleomorphism tumor cell necrosis or abnormal mitotic figures. By definition, there can be no evidence of a smooth-muscle tumor in another organ that could conceivably be the source of the metastases. Mitotic counts are the same as for leiomyoma.
    Parasitic leiomyoma
        Uterine serosal leiomyoma that becomes detached from the uterus and derives blood supply from omentum, peritoneum, or other pelvic structures. Must have benign features (see Table 14) Very rare and must be in the pelvis, not the retroperitoneum (we have never seen one).
    Leiomyoma with vascular intrusion (610)
        Usual leiomyoma in which vascular intrusion is not visible on gross examination but is a microscopic finding within the confines of a leiomyoma.
    Intravascular leiomyomatosis (610–614)
        Grossly visible fragments of histologically benign smooth muscle extending into vascular spaces and/or microscopic extension of smooth muscle into vascular spaces outside the confines of a leiomyoma. Epithelioid cells, including clear cells and fat cells may be present. Features distinguishing it from intravascular leiomyosarcoma are the same as for distinguishing leiomyoma from leiomyosarcoma (see Table 14).

MI, mitotic index; mf, mitotic figure; hpf, high-power field.

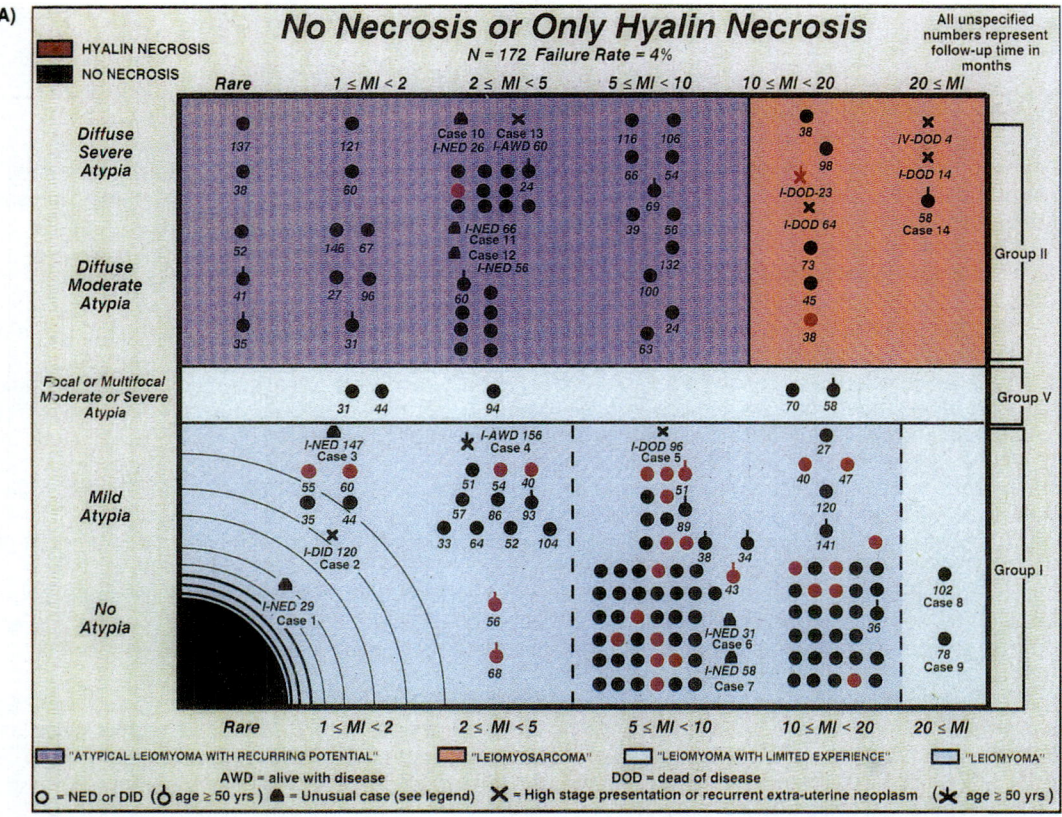
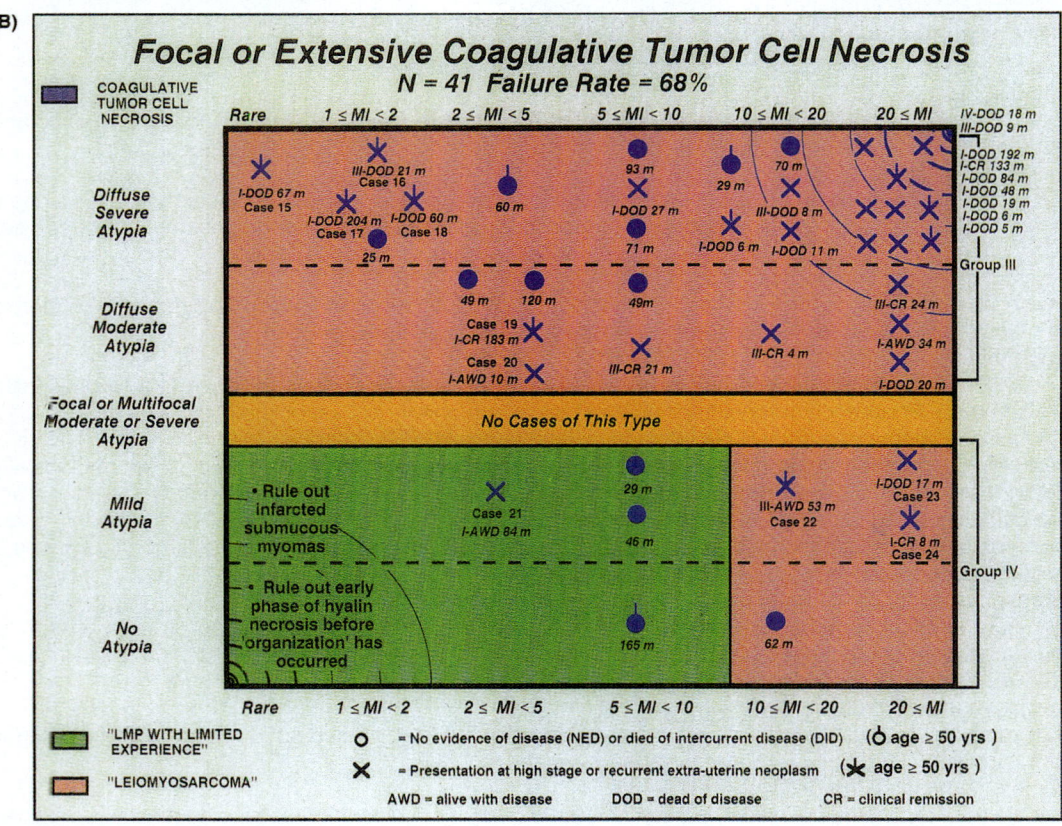

FIG. 94. A diagnostic approach for uterine smooth-muscle neoplasms exhibiting usual (standard) differentiation. Both plots depict the mitotic index along the x-axis and the degree of cytologic atypia along the y-axis. **A:** This plot sets out diagnostic labels for neoplasms that have either no coagulative tumor cell necrosis or hyaline necrosis. **B:** The diagnostic labels for neoplasms with coagulative tumor cell necrosis are depicted. MI, mitotic index; NED, no evidence of disease; DID, died of intercurrent disease; AWD, alive with disease; DOD, dead of disease; CR, clinical remission. The roman numeral next to the clinical summary indicates the surgical stage at the time of presentation; all patients represented by a circle had stage I neoplasms.

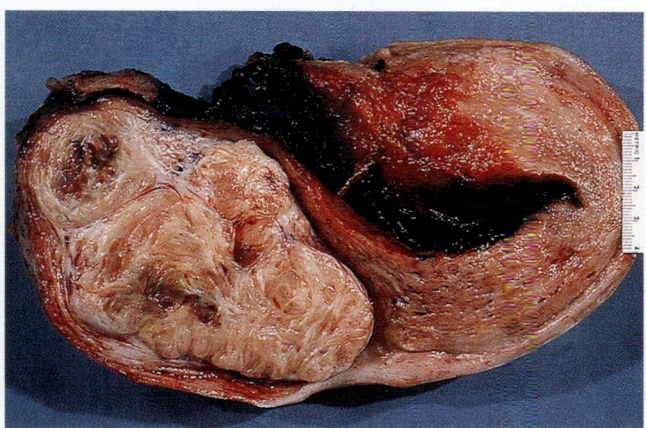

FIG. 95. Leiomyoma with areas of degeneration and old hemorrhage (gross appearance). All uterine masses that deviate from the characteristic appearance of leiomyomas such as this one should be sampled.

is to place tumors for which cellular differentiation still remains ambiguous after all reasonable maneuvers (as described above) have been tried into the endometrial stromal category for purposes of determining therapy and prognosis.

After it has been decided that a uterine tumor exhibits smooth-muscle differentiation, the next step is to review its clinical and gross features and evaluate relevant microscopic features in order to assign the tumor to a clinically meaningful category. In the past, there has been heavy reliance by most researchers on a single microscopic feature, the MI, to make this decision; in fact, at one time, all uterine smooth-muscle tumors of the "usual" type (i.e., not epithelioid or myxoid) with more than 10 mf per 10 hpf were classified as malignant, while those with a lower MI were judged to be benign. Shortly after this taxonomic practice took hold, it rather quickly became apparent that some neoplasms with an MI between 5 and 10 mf per 10 hpf behaved aggressively and that not all tumors with an MI of more than 10 behaved as clinical malignancies.

The term uncertain malignant potential was coined for the group with an MI of 5 to 9, to reflect our uncertainty about the true failure rate in this group and to indicate that our experience with neoplasms in this MI range was limited. Newer studies, including our own experience with 213 challenging uterine smooth-muscle tumors have shed new light on these problems. A common theme in all of these studies is the need for a multivariate approach to the diagnosis of uterine smooth-muscle neoplasms. We present here our approach to such diagnosis. Before we proceed, it is helpful to clarify the meaning of old terminology and introduce new terminology we have found useful.

A Vocabulary for Discussing Prognosis and Clinical Management

It is important to distinguish, on the one hand, between terms used to label clinical outcomes and, on the other hand, terms used to label groups defined on the basis of their gross and microscopic features. Histopathologic nomenclature is ambiguous in this respect. For example, "benign" is a free-floating term usefully employed in every organ system to mean, more or less, that after adequate removal of the offending lesion, the patient is cured. The same term is also employed as a morphologic label for a particular group of neoplasms all of which conform to a set of histopathologic rules or criteria. To decide if a tumor or neoplastic process is benign in the morphologic sense, one simply turns to a list of features set out in the relevant text to determine whether or not the case in hand counts as a benign example. To be sure, the specific morphologic definitions of benign that have been settled upon were fashioned by keeping one eye on clinical outcome and the other on morphologic characteristics. We sometimes make clinicopathologic terms less ambiguous by prefacing them with such clarifying descriptors as "clinically benign" and "morphologically benign."

Several observations about clinical outcome terminology are also required. Traditionally, the clinical behavior of neoplasms has been characterized dichotomously as benign or malignant, with the corollary that benign implies an absolute guarantee that the neoplasm so labeled will never behave in a clinically malignant fashion. Those tumors that are clinically malignant, then, comprise all those that are not benign. As is widely recognized, this simple-minded approach, not surprisingly, is inadequate to the task of usefully describing the wide variety of *clinical* behavior of human neoplasms observed in actual practice. Nonbenign behavior can be expressed in terms of the magnitude of the failure rate, the tempo of disease progression, the sites of failure, and the death rate, to name but a few variables.

The biologic correlate of this dichotomous clinical classification is a model that envisions malignant transformation as a kind of on/off switch at the genetic level that propagates in a clean yes/no fashion to the light microscopic level, where histopathologic diagnosis takes place. Increasingly, from a scientific point of view, this dichotomous classification does less and less justice to what is known about the biology of cancer. The following discussion focuses on three of the inadequacies of the "benign or malignant" paradigm that are particularly relevant to uterine smooth-muscle neoplasms: its unrealistic definition of the term benign, its failure to provide a useful conceptual framework for low-grade tumors, and its failure to provide a terminology to expresses degrees of confidence in a clinical prediction.

First, since every rational decision-maker knows that there are no guarantees in this life (with the exceptions of death and taxes), a more realistic rendering of "clinically benign," is something along the lines of "the failure rate after removal is sufficiently low that the prudent clinician would *act as if* the failure rate were zero." For example, uterine smooth-muscle tumors that are unremarkable in gross features and bland in histologic characteristics and that are indistinguishable from run-of-the-mill leiomyomas may very rarely metastasize to bone, lymph nodes, or the lungs. Quite sensibly, our impulse on receipt of this information is not to label all former leiomyomas as malignant but to fashion a new term —"benign metastasizing leiomyoma"—that draws attention to this phenomenon without forcing an unwarranted relabeling of leiomyomas to reflect this insignificant failure rate.

Second, the wide range of clinical behaviors that neoplasms exhibit has forced attention on the awkwardness of equating the labels "not clinically benign" and "clinically malignant." Two factors have been chiefly responsible for this focusing of our attention. (a) There exist neoplasms that are, in a number of senses, low grade. Low-grade behavior (relative to other members of the same differentiated group) may manifest itself in a number of ways, for example, by a lower failure rate, a slower tempo of disease progression, or, perhaps, a high recurrence rate but lower death rate with recurrence. (b) Then there is the fact that knowledge of this low-grade behavior not only is important for prognosis but also can be exploited to treat patients more effectively. As is well known in gynecologic oncology, the identification of "low grade" ovarian neoplasms has resulted in effective treatment strategies, the aim of which is to preserve fertility in young patients. We use the descriptor "low malignant potential" for these low-grade ovarian neoplasms.

The term we use for an analogous set of uterine smooth-muscle neoplasms is atypical leiomyoma with low risk of recurrence. The smooth-muscle tumors we include in this group are those with morphologic features that are associated with failure rate estimates that lie between 1% and 10%. Patients with such tumors could be treated with reasonable safety by myomectomy combined with careful clinical and radiologic follow-up, if they desire uterine preservation and are capable of understanding the small risk. Our experience also suggests that the neoplasms we have gathered under this heading tend to have a slower rate of progression, even if they do recur. Neoplasms with an estimated failure rate of more than 10% form the "high malignant potential" (HMP) group. Whereas a patient might reasonably opt for uterine conservation (after myomectomy) for a tumor with a less than 10% risk of recurrence, the designation HMP is used for tumors having a failure rate that overrides fertility considerations for all but the most risk-seeking patients.

The third point to be made is that groupings like "benign," "LMP," and "HMP" for purposes of clinical treatment are associated not only with a best guess of clinical outcome ("the estimated failure rate is 10% for tumors with this appearance") but also with *some measure of the reliability of that guess* (553,554). The correlate of this guess in more numeric enterprises is, of course, a confidence interval, standard deviation, or variance. Many variables, in principle, enter into an estimate of reliability. One important factor, certainly, is the number of cases of the sort under consideration that have been studied and the length of the follow-up. When the number of investigated cases is small, the morphologic predictors being used are relatively weak, and the intra- and interobserver agreement on feature evaluation is not thought to be high, we append the label "limited experience" to the best guess, to alert the clinician to this problem.

A diagnosis that might be used is "leiomyoma but limited experience." The message being conveyed with such wording is that the few cases we have seen or know about with these morphologic features have been clinically benign, but, alert to the problems of small samples, we would not be shocked if, in the fullness of time and with the acquisition of more experience, this tumor turned out to be one of LMP. Again, the diagnosis "leiomyosarcoma of HMP but limited experience" would be an appropriate way of summarizing the following clinicopathologic state of affairs. We have seen ten tumors more or less similar to the one your patient harbors, and in that group of ten the failure rate was 30%. I would not be shocked if the "true" failure rate (e.g., if there were 1,000 cases available for follow-up) was in the range bracketed by 10% and 60%. With more experience, we might discover either that this is an LMP tumor or, more likely, that we were right in judging this to be an HMP neoplasm.

Definitions of Morphologic Terms

As noted earlier, morphologic features other than the MI are powerful predictors of clinical outcome and have been incorporated into the diagnostic criteria for uterine smooth-muscle neoplasms. These features include epithelioid histologic features, myxoid stroma, cytologic atypia, and coagulative tumor cell necrosis. They are defined in the following sections.

Differentiated Cell Type

Usual smooth-muscle cells resemble normal myometrial cells in that they are elongated, with easily seen eosinophilic and sometimes fibrillar cytoplasm, and often have distinct cell membranes. These cells have a tendency to be arranged in bundles (Table 5). Epithelioid smooth-muscle cells have a round configuration, with eosinophilic to colorless cytoplasm. They may have perinuclear cytoplasmic vacuoles or a perinuclear rim of eosinophilic cytoplasm with the rest of the cytoplasm clear. When the cytoplasm is totally clear, the label clear cell is used. It is critical to distinguish the myxoid differentiation found in myxoid leiomyosarcomas from the myxoid change very often seen in "degenerating" leiomyomas (555). In myxoid leiomyosarcomas, not only is the stroma myxoid but the cells are also enlarged, with hyperchromatic nuclei, and pleomorphism is typically obvious. The usual case of myxoid leiomyosarcoma bears a striking resemblance to soft-tissue myxoid malignant fibrous histiocytoma. Both myxoid malignant fibrous histiocytoma and myxoid leiomyosarcoma are composed of cells that exhibit a range of cytologic abnormalities from bland to obviously malignant.

We think significantly atypical cells should be identified before making a diagnosis of myxoid leiomyosarcoma; in most

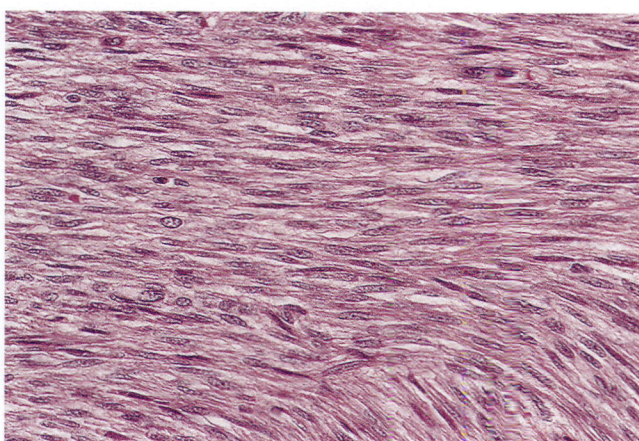

FIG. 96. Ordinary leiomyoma without cytologic atypia. Atypia is evaluated at low magnification and is based on the presence or absence of pleomorphism and hyperchromatic nuclei. In this tumor, the cells are uniform, without significant hyperchromatism; hence, there is no significant atypia.

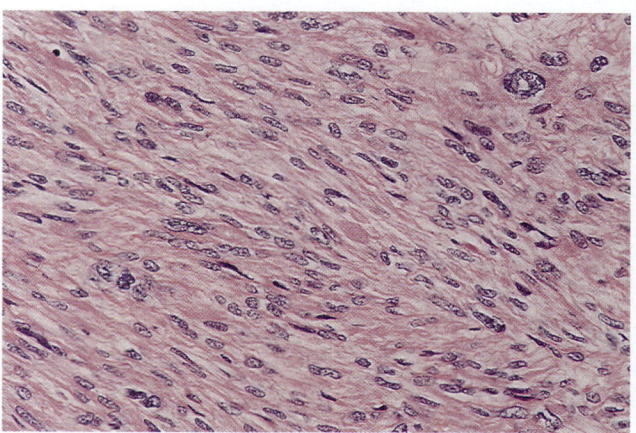

FIG. 98. Leiomyoma with rare hyperchromatic, enlarged nuclei (low power). This degree of atypia is not considered significant

cases infiltration of the myometrium is present. The MI of myxoid leiomyosarcoma, however, can be significantly less than that of the usual leiomyosarcoma. Therefore, the combination of myxoid stroma and cellular atypia must be used to recognize this neoplasm. Focal myxoid areas also can be found in an otherwise characteristic leiomyosarcoma. Leiomyomas with a myxoid stroma, on the other hand, are composed of small, bland cells without the cytologic features characteristic of myxoid leiomyosarcoma. Essentially, these are simply leiomyomas with edematous to mucoid stroma in which focal collagenation is common. They typically have thick, large-walled vessels suspended in the matrix; most often the margins are circumscribed.

Atypia (556–558)

Our study and several others have established a relationship between cytologic atypia and outcome for uterine smooth-muscle tumors. The problem, as always, is defining significant atypia in a way that is reproducible and can be communicated to others. We found that a two-tiered scheme of absent to mild atypia and moderate to severe atypia is reasonably reproducible (Figs. 96-101). Moderate to severe atypia is defined by several features. Nuclear hyperchromaticism and pleomorphism are obvious at scanning power, and cells with huge nuclei are common (Fig. 99). Enlarged and sometimes abnormal mitotic figures are a typical finding (Fig. 101). Most often, moderate to severe atypia is diffuse, but it can be focal (Fig. 102). In contrast, absent or mild atypia is characterized by uniform cells with no more than mild pleomorphism. Chromatin is usually fine to granular. The nuclei may be enlarged compared with the surrounding myometrium, but the enlargement is uniform throughout the lesion (Figs. 96 and 97). More than one or two enlarged abnormal division figures place the tumor in the group with moderate to severe atypia.

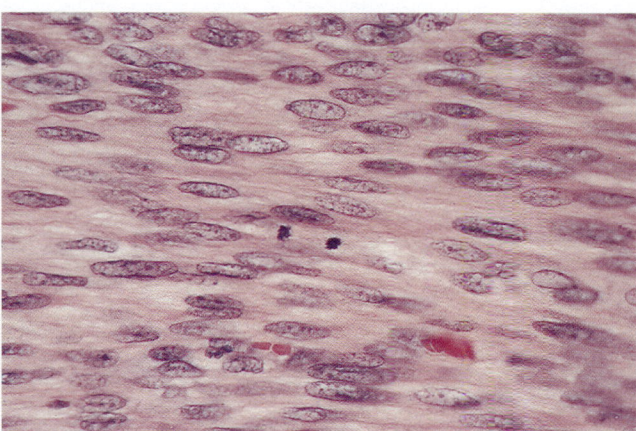

FIG. 97. Leiomyoma (high magnification). The nuclei of the cells in leiomyomas may be considerably larger than those in the surrounding myometrium, but the nuclei are uniform and most often vesicular.

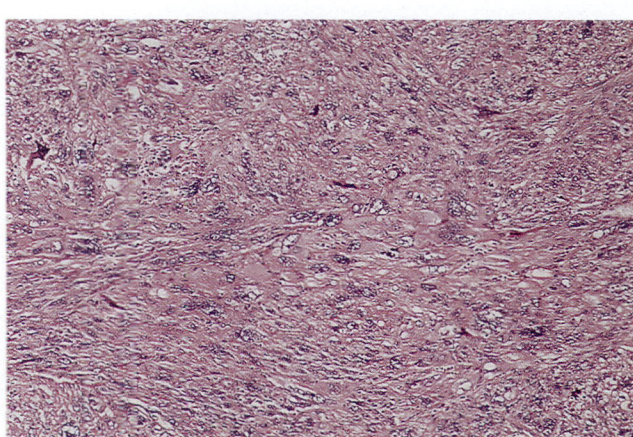

FIG. 99. Significant atypia at low magnification. The decision as to whether atypia is significant (moderate to severe) is based on low-power evaluation. In this example, there is obvious pleomorphism, and hyperchromatic nuclei can be discerned.

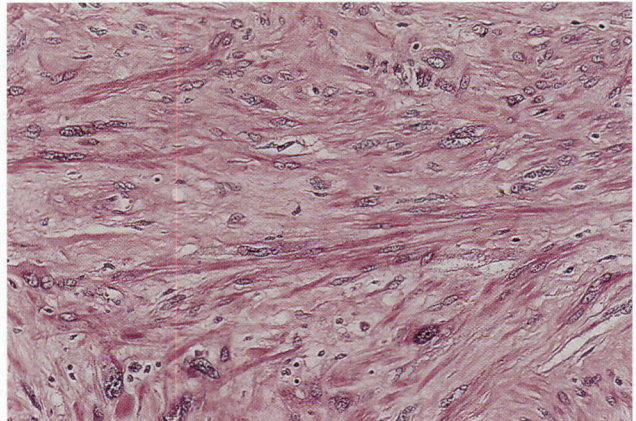

FIG. 100. Higher magnification of a smooth-muscle tumor with significant atypia. This degree of pleomorphism is at the borderline between insignificant and significant atypia.

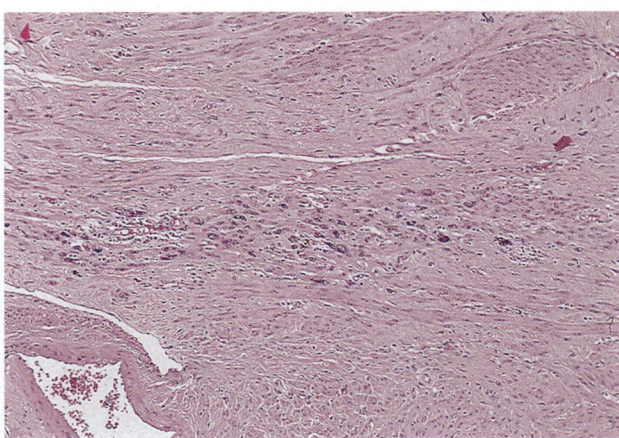

FIG. 102. Focal significant atypia. In this photomicrograph, the atypia is confined to one area, as can be discerned by the hyperchromatic, enlarged nuclei.

Mitotic Index (559,560)

The MI is based on the number of mitotic figures per 10 hpf. Only definite mitotic figures are counted (see Table 3). As will be seen later herein, compulsive counting of mitotic figures is not always necessary, depending on the presence or absence of significant atypia and/or tumor cell necrosis.

Necrosis (561–565)

In our experience, the presence or absence of necrosis and the type of necrosis are powerful predictors. We distinguish two types of necrosis in uterine smooth-muscle tumors: coagulative tumor cell necrosis and hyalinizing necrosis (Figs. 103-106). Coagulative tumor cell necrosis features an abrupt transition between necrotic cells and preserved cells (Fig. 104–106). The nuclei of the necrotic cells often retain their hematoxyphilia, and inflammatory cells are unusual. A cuff of viable cells may be seen around blood vessels. This pattern of necrosis is common in clinically malignant smooth-muscle tumors and should never be ignored. In contrast, hyalinizing necrosis exhibits a zone of usually eosinophilic collagen interposed between the dead cells and the preserved cells, a pattern reminiscent of an infarcted region being organized by granulation tissue (Fig. 103). Eosinophilic collagen matrix is characteristic, in contrast to the necrotic debris seen in tumor cell necrosis.

If dead nuclei can be discerned in areas of hyalinization, they are uniform, with often faint chromatin, compared with the nuclear hyperchromasia and pleomorphism still barely visible in tumor cell necrosis. Necrosis stemming from ulceration in submucous leiomyoma features acute inflammatory cells and a peripheral reparative process, while ghost outlines of nuclei are usually inconspicuous or absent. "Apoplectic" leiomyomas are distinguished by areas of hemorrhage, but necrosis is absent (Fig. 107). Since the advent of leuprolide therapy to shrink leiomyomata, there has been

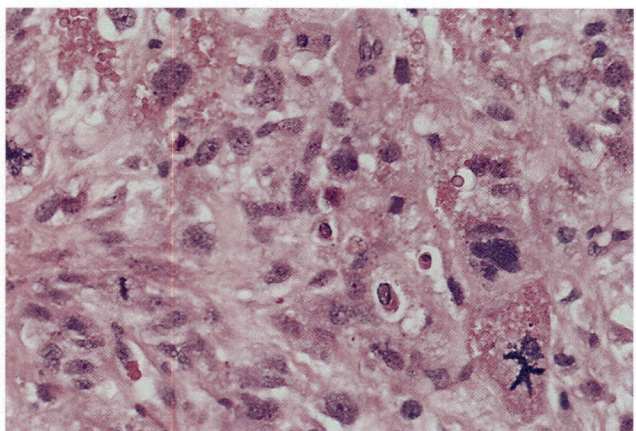

FIG. 101. Markedly atypical smooth-muscle tumor with an abnormal mitotic figure. This degree of pleomorphism and chromatic abnormality is well within the range of significant atypia. The presence of the abnormal mitotic figures suggests that this is probably leiomyosarcoma.

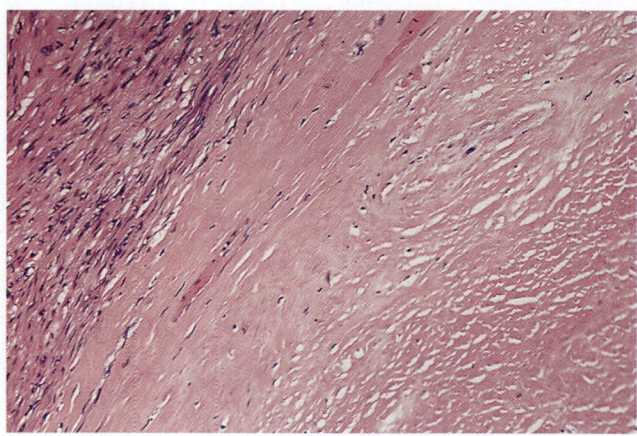

FIG. 103. Hyalinizing necrosis. There is a band of hyalinized tissue next to the viable smooth muscle, suggesting repair. The necrosis at the right does not contain discernible nuclei.

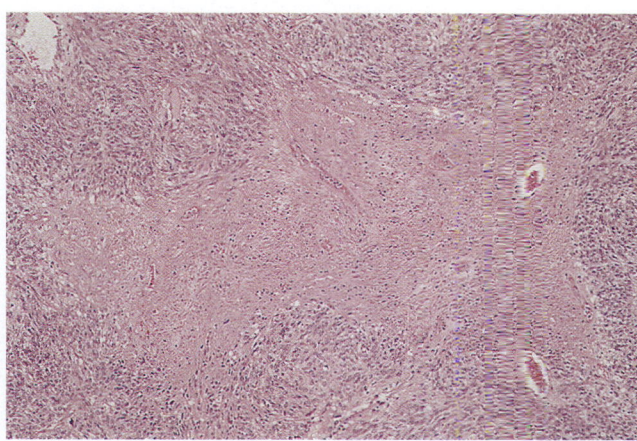

FIG. 104. Coagulative tumor cell necrosis. There is an abrupt transition between viable cells and the area of necrosis. This is one of the most useful features in identifying tumor cell necrosis.

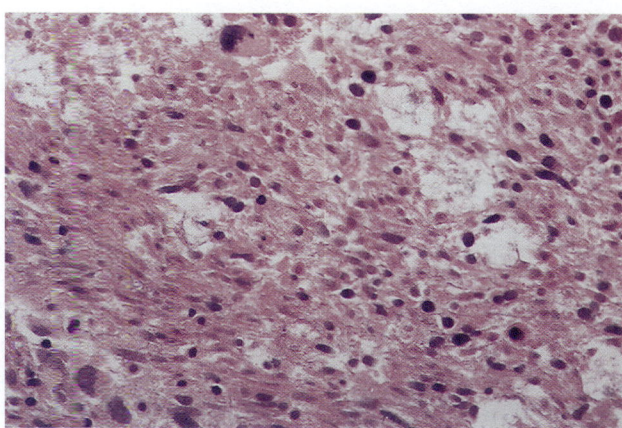

FIG. 106. Coagulative tumor cell necrosis with ghost outlines of tumor cells. Not only are the degenerating nuclei quite apparent, but there is also pleomorphism. These features help identify this as tumor cell necrosis.

controversy concerning the mechanism of shrinkage and the morphologic correlates of this process. Most investigators have not been able to detect striking differences in luprolide-treated leiomyomata compared with controls (51–54, 566,567).

Our Approach to the Diagnosis of Uterine Smooth-muscle Tumors (549)

Our approach to the diagnosis of uterine smooth-muscle tumors, outlined here, is based on our personal experience of 213 difficult cases and a review of recently published cases. These guidelines do not necessarily apply to nonuterine smooth-muscle tumors. The first step in the evaluation of a uterine smooth-muscle tumor is to be sure that the lesion in question is composed of cells demonstrating smooth-muscle differentiation. This assessment is discussed in the introduction and in Table 5. The following discussion is summarized in Tables 14 and 15.

Smooth-muscle Tumors of the Usual Sort Confined to the Uterus Without Intravascular Extension

The crucial observations to be made in this subset of tumors are to assess the presence or absence of necrosis and, if necrosis is present, to distinguish its type; to determine whether moderate to severe atypia is present; and to evaluate the MI. If the histologic appearance is that of the usual leiomyoma, with neither coagulative tumor cell necrosis nor significant atypia (as defined previously), nothing clinically useful is gained by determining the MI. The recent literature and our experience indicate that for practical diagnostic purposes, neoplasms without these two features behave in a benign fashion even if the MI is up to 20 mf per 10 hpf (but see Table 15 and later discussion under Benign Metastasizing Leiomyoma).

Although the reported experience with bland smooth-muscle neoplasms without coagulative necrosis and with mi-

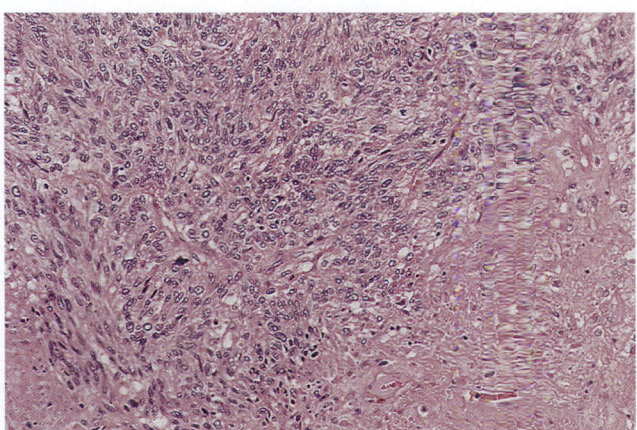

FIG. 105. Tumor cell necrosis at higher magnification. The abrupt transition between viable cells and the necrotic area can be seen.

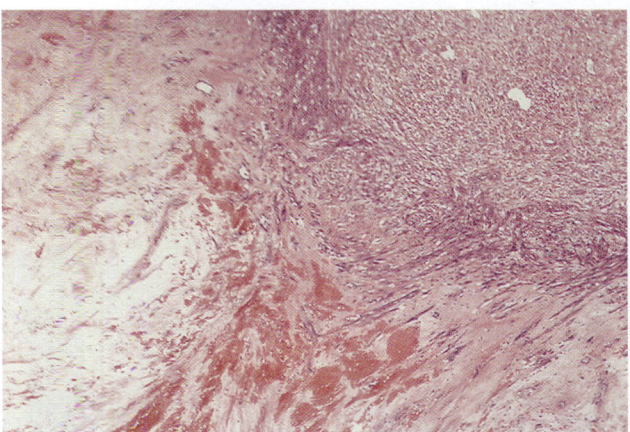

FIG. 107. Hemorrhage within a leiomyoma (apoplectic leiomyoma). Areas of hemorrhage can be found in leiomyomas, particularly in those removed from women who are pregnant or receiving hormones. Hemorrhage should not be construed as evidence of coagulative tumor cell necrosis.

totic counts ranging from 5 to 20 mf per 10 hpf is limited to approximately 200 patients, as rare tumors go, this is a substantial experience; accordingly, we think that it is appropriate to label these neoplasms as leiomyomas with increased mitotic figures. The mitotic figures should be small and normal, with no more than one or two abnormal forms in a well-sampled tumor. The same benign behavior is to be anticipated for otherwise characteristic leiomyomas that exhibit hyalin necrosis. Whereas the majority of leiomyomas contain, at most, a few normal mitotic figures, examination of grossly undistinguished and cytologically bland leiomyomas removed during the secretory phase of the menstrual cycle not infrequently turn up tumors with mitotic counts in the range of 4 to 5 normal mf per 10 hpf.

Submucous leiomyomas with surface necrosis may also contain increased numbers of cells in division near the necrosis. Even higher mitotic counts can be found in some, but not all, leiomyomas removed from women receiving progestational agents. Thus, there appear to be reasons other than neoplastic transformation for an increased MI. If low-power examination reveals significant *diffuse*, moderate to severe atypia, but no tumor cell necrosis, the mitotic counts serve to stratify the cases into two groups—atypical leiomyomas with an MI of fewer than 10 mf per 10 hpf (one of 46 failed in our group) and leiomyosarcomas with an MI of 10 or more mf per 10 hpf (four of ten failed in our group). When low-power examination reveals more than just minute foci of coagulative tumor cell necrosis (not hyalinizing necrosis—see definitions given earlier), our experience indicates that the tumor has a strong chance of behaving in a malignant fashion and should be labeled leiomyosarcoma (29 of 39 failed) if focal or diffuse, moderate to severe atypia is present—regardless of the MI. If coagulative tumor cell necrosis is evident in the absence of atypia and the presence of an MI of less than 10, the tumor should be placed in the UMP category owing to our limited experience.

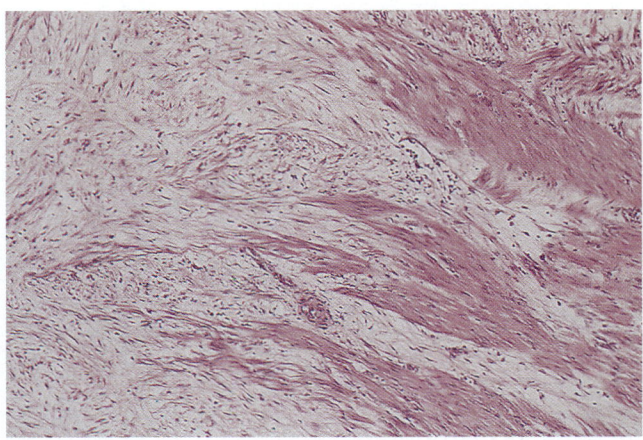

FIG. 109. Myxoid leiomyosarcoma. This myxoid neoplasm can be seen to be infiltrating the surrounding normal myometrium. Myometrial infiltration is a characteristic feature of myxoid leiomyosarcoma and should always be sought when examining a myxoid smooth-muscle neoplasm.

Myxoid Differentiation

Myxoid differentiation coupled with enlarged and atypical cells is an ominous finding (Figs. 108–110). Four of seven such uterine tumors failed in our series. Our diagnostic terminology is as follows. Benign tumors are considered to be leiomyomas with myxoid stroma. The cells are small and uniform, and there is no atypia or, at most, mild atypia; the MI is fewer than 5 mf per 10 hpf. There should be focal areas of ordinary leiomyoma. Malignant (limited experience) tumors are myxoid leiomyosarcomas. These tumors feature moderate to marked atypia with or without necrosis, with any MI. Margins are usually infiltrating.

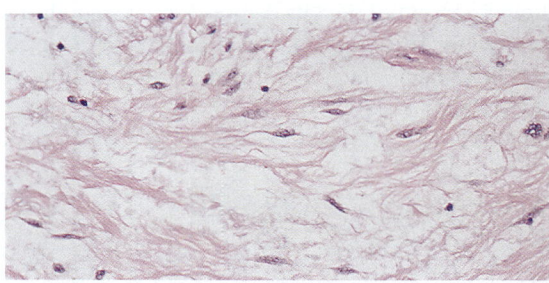
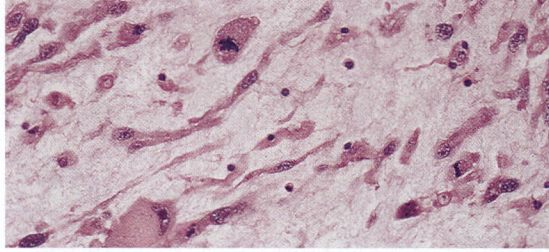

FIG. 110. Myxoid leiomyosarcoma (high magnification). *Top:* An area in which the cells are bland. Such areas can often be found in myxoid leiomyosarcoma. *Bottom:* Cytologic atypia, which should be present in almost all myxoid leiomyosarcomas, at least in focal areas.

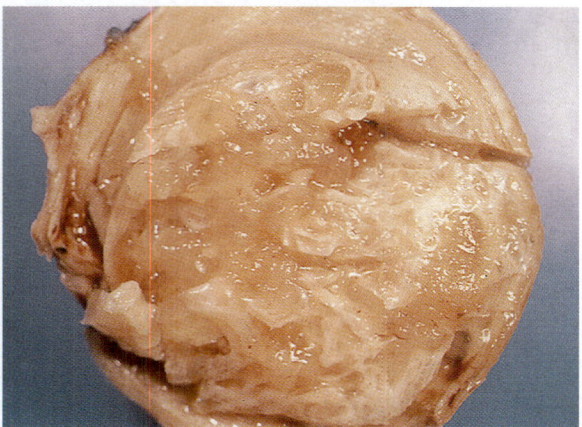

FIG. 108. Myxoid leiomyosarcoma (gross appearance). This photograph demonstrates the grossly myxoid nature of these neoplasms.

Epithelioid Differentiation

Epithelioid differentiation has been defined earlier in the chapter. Such differentiation in more than just a few foci of a uterine smooth-muscle tumor is an ominous finding, because the absence of cytologic atypia and necrosis is no guarantee of a clinically benign course when the tumor contains more than 5 mf per 10 hpf (Figs. 111 and 112). All epithelioid tumors with tumor cell necrosis in our series behaved in a malignant fashion. On the other hand, all seven epithelioid tumors in our study with an MI of less than 5, with at most minimal cytologic atypia and without necrosis, behaved benignly. The experience with epithelioid tumors as a group is limited, even when all the literature is considered. Indeed, those tumors with moderate to severe atypia without necrosis and an MI of less than 5 should be classified as UMP, because our experience is too limited to be certain about their aggressive potential.

MORPHOLOGIC TYPES OF UTERINE SMOOTH-MUSCLE TUMORS (TABLE 15)

Usual Leiomyoma (43,568)

On gross examination, the usual leiomyoma is circumscribed and white, and it has a whorled trabecular appearance on cut section. Deviations from this typical pattern are rather common and result from hypercellularity or the replacement of muscle fibers by various substances, including hyalin, collagen, blood, calcium, mucopolysaccharide, or combinations of these constitutions (569). Sampling is important in detecting leiomyosarcoma. We think that when three or fewer tumors with the characteristic white, whorled appearance of the usual leiomyoma are present in a uterus, all should be sampled. When there are more than three with this gross appearance, we randomly sample at least the three largest tumors. Any tumor that deviates from the character-

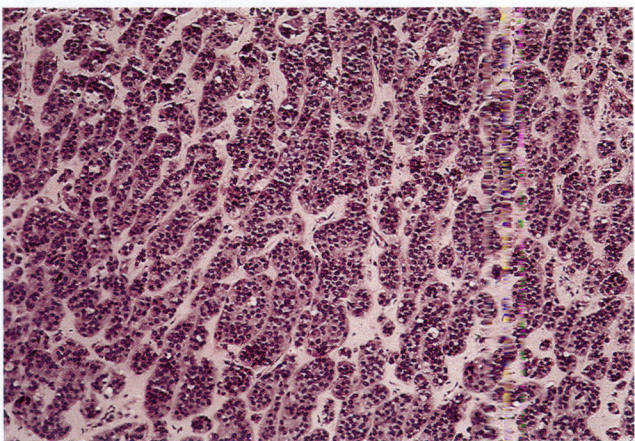

FIG. 111. Epithelioid smooth-muscle tumor of the uterus. The tumor cells have rather abundant cytoplasm and are arranged in cords, suggesting epithelium. Such tumors usually contain areas that blend with more characteristic smooth-muscle cells.

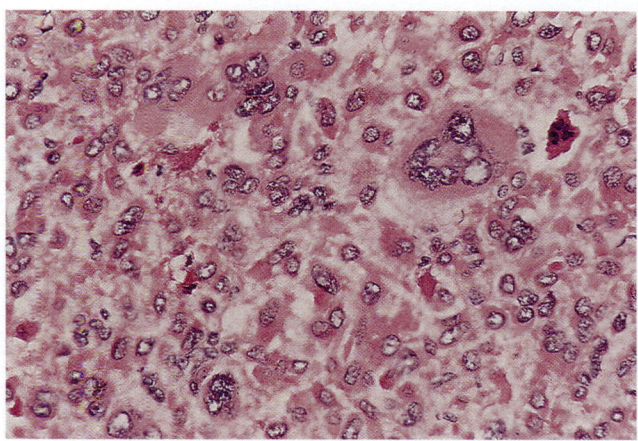

FIG. 112. Epithelioid smooth-muscle tumor with pleomorphism. This tumor contains significant atypia. Experience dictates that epithelioid smooth-muscle tumors with significant atypia behave aggressively with sufficient frequency to be considered leiomyosarcoma. This degree of atypia in epithelioid smooth-muscle neoplasms is usually accompanied by a high mitotic index and tumor cell necrosis.

istic whorled appearance expected in a leiomyoma should be sampled (Fig. 95). We believe a minimum of one section per centimeter of diameter should be taken from any smooth-muscle tumor that does not have the characteristic histologic appearance of a leiomyoma, unless the diagnosis of leiomyosarcoma is obvious on the basis of fewer sections.

At the microscopic level, the usual leiomyoma is easily recognized because the tumor cells resemble the smooth-muscle cells that form the myometrium (Fig. 96). In general, leiomyomas are more cellular, and they are composed of cells that are slightly larger than those found in the surrounding myometrium (Figs. 97 and 98). Significant variation from this pattern should be recognized, and the possibility of leiomyosarcoma, or even another tumor type, should be considered. Leiomyomas can be quite cellular, however, and they have the same clinical behavior as their less cellular components. The term cellular leiomyoma has been used for these tumors, but we know of no practical reason not to classify the cellular variants as ordinary leiomyomas.

The margins of most leiomyomas are microscopically circumscribed, but a few benign tumors will demonstrate apparent infiltration. Consequently, infiltration is not a criterion of malignancy for smooth-muscle tumors. On the other hand, most leiomyosarcomas infiltrate; in light of this fact, we evaluate the histologic features of apparently infiltrating smooth-muscle tumors very carefully. Submucous leiomyomas may well display extensive necrosis, often with acute inflammatory cells—particularly if they protrude into the endometrial cavity. Not infrequently, there will be increased mitotic activity in the tumor cells near the areas of necrosis. The coagulative tumor cell necrosis (described earlier) typical of leiomyosarcoma, however, is not associated very often with acute inflammation, and ghost outlines of cells are prominent; such cells are inconspicuous or absent in submucous necrosis. In addition, the mitotic figures seen in conjunction with inflammatory necrosis are small and normal, whereas they may be large and abnormal in leiomyosarcomas.

Hyaline necrosis is characteristic of leiomyomas; making the distinction from coagulative tumor cell necrosis is important (see definitions of morphologic features given previously). When hyalin liquifies, cysts may be produced (cystic degeneration). Myxoid and mucinous degenerations occur in leiomyomas; they are distinguished by an increase in the mucopolysaccharide content of the stroma. The result can be pools of mucinous material separating individual muscle fibers. This benign change must be differentiated from myxoid leiomyosarcoma, in which the tumor cells infiltrate the surrounding myometrium and show signs of moderate to marked pleomorphism and nucleomegaly, at least in focal areas, even though the mitotic activity may be very low (see earlier discussion of myxoid tumors). The clinical features of patients with leiomyomas, as well as the natural history of these neoplasms, are described elsewhere (502).

Differential Diagnosis

Considerations in the differential diagnosis of leiomyoma include other non-smooth-muscle neoplasms, particularly endometrial stromal tumors, and leiomyosarcoma. The former tumor is discussed in the introduction to this section and in Table 13, and the latter is discussed in the section concerning our approach to the diagnosis of uterine smooth-muscle tumors.

Leiomyoma Variants (501,502) (Table 14)

Atypical (Symplastic) Leiomyoma (485,502,556,557,570–576)

Description

The term atypical (symplastic) leiomyoma denotes those leiomyomas that contain cells meeting the criteria of moderate to severe cytologic atypia defined earlier. Most often, enlarged cells with pleomorphic nuclei can be seen at low magnification; enlarged, multinucleated giant cells may be part of this landscape. By definition, mitotic figures cannot be present in numbers in excess of 10 mf per 10 hpf, and tumor cell necrosis *must* be absent (Fig. 113). Mitotic counts higher than 10 in such a tumor indicate an HMP smooth-muscle tumor. Our diagnostic strategy for tumors with significant atypia and no tumor cell necrosis is outlined earlier and in Table 14. Smooth-muscle tumors that contain cells with diffuse moderate to severe atypia and tumor cell necrosis should be considered to be leiomyosarcoma regardless of the mitotic counts.

Highly Cellular Leiomyoma

Description

This term denotes a highly cellular, benign, smooth-muscle neoplasm that simulates low-grade stromal sarcoma (56). Large, thick-walled vessels are characteristic of the entity; these vessels are less common in stromal nodule and stromal sarcoma (Fig. 114).

Clinicopathologic Correlation

Care must be taken to consider this benign alternative when a cellular mesenchymal proliferation is recovered in an endometrial sampling. Thus, there are three questions to ask in this context. (a) What differentiation does the proliferation exhibit (smooth muscle or endometrial stromal)? (b) Under each assumption, can the criteria of malignancy be evaluated? (c) Finally, under each assumption, are the criteria of malignancy met? If a low-risk hysterectomy is contemplated, the issue is usually resolved by what amounts to a diagnostic hysterectomy. In cases of high-penalty hysterectomy, other methods should be considered (e.g., hysteroscopy, imaging studies, repeated sampling) that would clarify the situation without the need for hysterectomy. The important point is that not all cellular spindled proliferations recovered in a curettage specimen represent stromal sarcoma; the clinically innocuous cellular leiomyoma is a highly probable alternative.

Mitotically Active Leiomyoma (Leiomyoma with Increased Mitotic Index) (549,577)

Description

This term is used by us for leiomyomas that contain more than 5 *normal* mf per 10 hpf but are otherwise bland in microscopic and gross appearance and do not demonstrate tumor cell necrosis as defined earlier. It is imperative that this diagnosis *not* be used for neoplasms that exhibit moderate to severe nuclear atypia nor for those that contain abnormal mitotic figures or have zones of tumor cell necrosis.

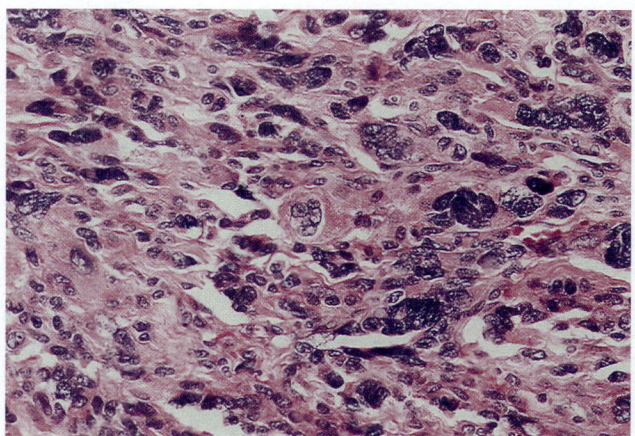

FIG. 113. Atypical leiomyoma. Although there is significant atypia, there is no tumor cell necrosis, and mitotic figures were not found. Distinguishing this tumor from leiomyosarcoma is based on the absence of tumor cell necrosis and mitotic counts less than 2 mf/10 hpf, if the atypia is diffuse. A tumor with this degree of atypia and tumor cell necrosis should be considered leiomyosarcoma.

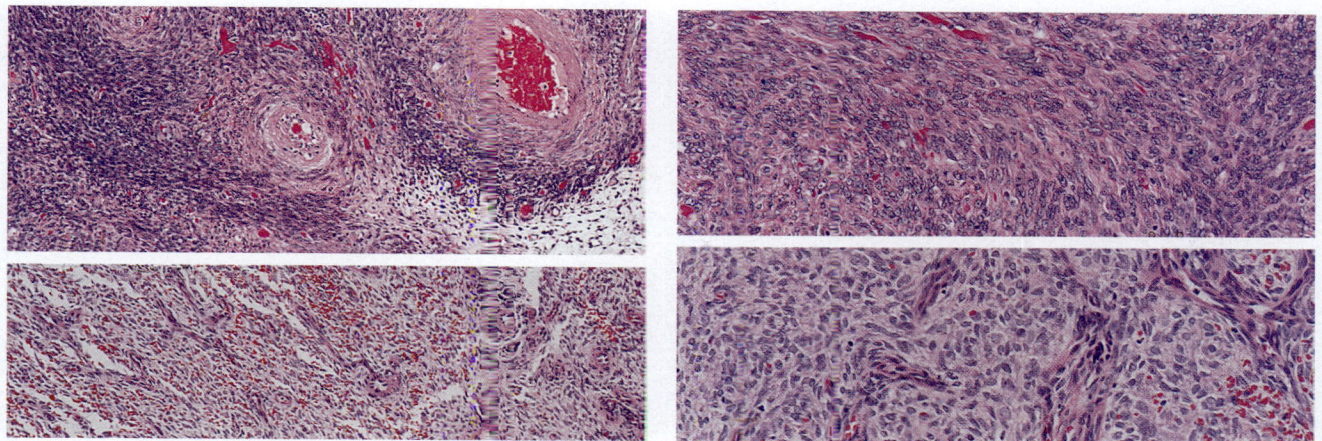

FIG. 114. Cellular leiomyoma and stromal nodule contrasted. **A:** At the top there is a cellular spindled proliferation that could represent either endometrial stromal or smooth-muscle differentiation. The presence of thick-walled vessels favors a cellular smooth-muscle neoplasm. At the bottom, in contrast, the vessels of endometrial stromal proliferations are thin walled and arborizing. **B:** The illustration shows, at the top, fascicles of spindled cells largely devoid of an arborizing vasculature, in contrast to the endometrial stromal proliferation at the bottom, in which the vasculature is prominent.

Clinicopathologic Correlation

In recent years, it has become apparent that clinically benign uterine smooth-muscle tumors may contain more than 5 and even more than 10 *normal* mf per 10 hpf (578). In our study, none of the 53 patients whose histologically bland, nonnecrotic uterine smooth-muscle tumors contained 5 to 10 mf per 10 hpf failed; likewise none of the 34 whose bland nonnecrotic tumors contained 10 to 20 normal mf per 10 hpf failed. Increased mitotic activity has been seen in submucous leiomyomas that feature inflammatory rather than coagulative necrosis as well as in the smooth-muscle tumors of patients who have been receiving progestogens or have been pregnant (569,571,579,580). Patients with none of these findings may also, on occasion, have mitotically active leiomyomas. Great care should be taken when contemplating a diagnosis of leiomyoma with increased MI, to be sure that the tumor in question is a thoroughly sectioned, completely characteristic, usual leiomyoma with no more than mild atypia and without coagulative necrosis (see previous definitions). This term should be reserved for lesions with no tumor cell necrosis in which the *only* significant deviation is an MI between 5 and 20 mf per 10 hpf. Such tumors may be cellular. If the specimen has been removed by myomectomy, it is also extremely comforting to know the lesion was easily and completely removed (shelled out) from the myometrium, rather than infiltrating it.

Epithelioid Leiomyoma (Tables 14 and 15) (143,574,581–586)

Description

The rules for evaluating the malignant potential of this uterine smooth-muscle neoplasm composed predominantly or completely of nonspindled, rounded cells with an epithelial-like appearance have been discussed earlier (see section on epithelioid differentiation). The cytoplasm of these cells may be clear or eosinophilic (Fig. 111). By definition, epithelioid leiomyomas have mitotic counts of fewer than 5 mf per 10 hpf, no more than mild atypia, and no tumor cell necrosis.

Clinicopathologic Correlation

A number of histologic patterns have been described under the heading of epithelioid leiomyoma. They include tumors composed of cells featuring perinuclear clearing, cells with peripheral cytoplasmic clearing, and cells with completely clear cytoplasm. The latter tumors have also been designated clear-cell leiomyomas (143,582,587). Plexiform tumors are sometimes included in this group; they are composed of cells with crumpled nuclei and indistinct cytoplasm arranged in cords or rows. Plexiform tumors are usually incidental findings at the endometrial myometrial junction, although they can be large or multiple (584,588). The direction of differentiation of the plexiform tumor has been the subject of controversy because the cells share features of smooth-muscle cells and endometrial stromal cells (583,589). Most ultrastructural studies suggest smooth-muscle differentiation (590,591). Keratin positivity is common, but it is associated with positive muscle markers (585).

Differential Diagnosis

On gross examination, most epithelioid leiomyomas look like smooth-muscle tumors. Distinguishing epithelioid leiomyoma from carcinoma can sometimes be a problem. The cells of epithelioid leiomyoma fail to produce convincing

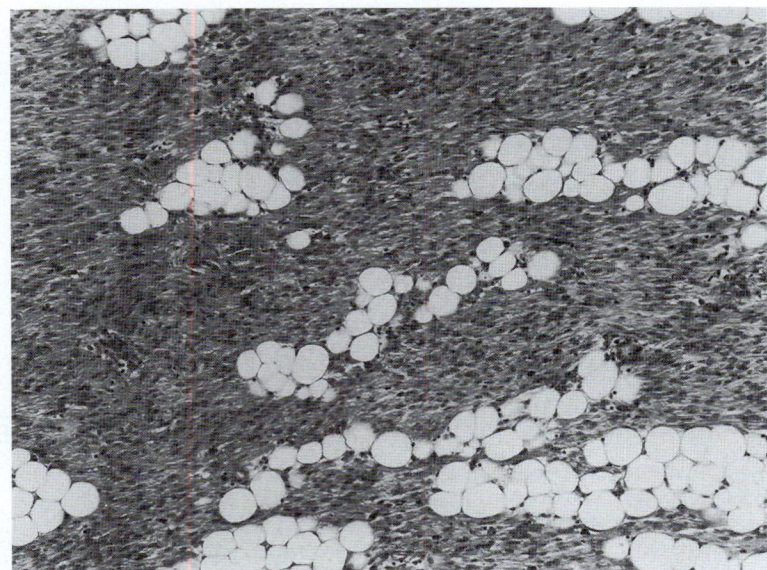

FIG. 115. Lipoleiomyoma. This uterine curiosity is easily recognized because of the fat cells interspersed among the smooth-muscle cells. The term lipoleiomyoma also includes those neoplasms that are entirely composed of benign adult fat.

glands and lack the cytologic atypia and mitotic activity of carcinoma. Immunohistochemical stains for keratin may be unreliable discriminators, since smooth-muscle cells can express keratin and EMA (585). However, it is unheard of for carcinoma cells to express desmin, and only rarely do they express muscle actin. A good strategy is to cut more H&E sections, searching for areas of more characteristic smooth-muscle differentiation within the tumor. Stromal sarcomas with epithelial structures, adenosarcomas, and AdFibs possess convincing tubular, glandular, or sex-cord-like structures.

Lipoleiomyoma (Including Uterine Lipoma) (592–595)

Description

This odd but easily recognized neoplasm is composed of an intimate admixture of mature adipocytes and smooth-muscle cells. It is mitotically inactive (Fig. 115). The term lipoleiomyoma covers a spectrum of lesions with a fat content that ranges from being a minor component in what is otherwise a leiomyoma to being a neoplasm composed entirely of mature adipocytes.

Clinicopathologic Correlation

This lesion is benign, and the only puzzle for the pathologist could be the unexpected presence of fat in a uterine tumor. Rarely, intravenous leiomyomatosis may have a fatty component (see later discussion under Intravascular [Intravenous] Leiomyomatosis and Leiomyoma with Vascular Intrusion).

Neurilemoma-like Leiomyoma (573,574,596)

Description

Uterine neoplasms composed of spindle cells, some of which exhibit neurilemoma-like palisading, are designated neurilemoma-like leiomyomas (Fig. 116). Neoplasms with this pattern are more common in the gastrointestinal tract than in the uterus.

Clinicopathologic Correlation

Most such leiomyomas are benign; however, the prognosis is based on the same mitotic and morphologic criteria used for more typical uterine smooth-muscle neoplasms.

Myxoid Leiomyoma (555,573,597)

Description

Many leiomyomas exhibiting gross degeneration on microscopic evaluation feature islands of collagenated smooth muscle set in a sea of edematous connective tissue. Large-calibered vessels are characteristically suspended in these

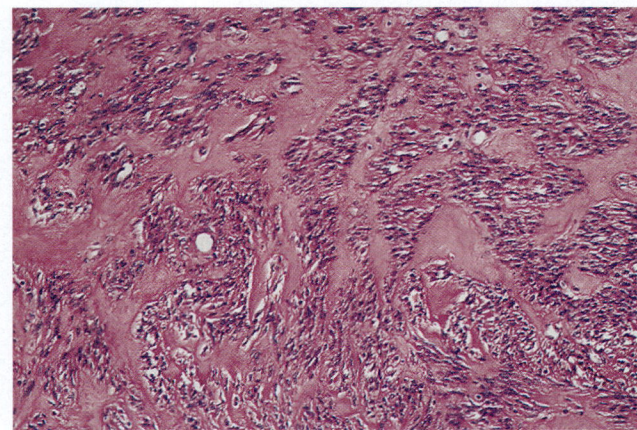

FIG. 116. Neurilemoma-like leiomyoma. A leiomyoma with extensive hyalinization, causing the nuclei to line up in register, simulating the pattern seen in schwannoma.

myxoid areas. Attention has been drawn to this completely benign and relatively common phenomenon by reports of rare, predominantly myxoid leiomyosarcomas (see earlier discussion). Now and then, a completely myxoid, paucicellular tumor whose cells do not show signs of smooth-muscle differentiation is encountered in the myometrium. As long as the cells have small and bland nuclei, do not infiltrate the myometrium, and are mitotically inactive, these tumors have a benign clinical course in our very limited experience.

Clinicopathologic Correlation

All myxoid leiomyomas are benign.

Leiomyomatosis (Infiltrating Leiomyoma) (598)

Description

Leiomyomatosis is a multinodular, diffuse proliferation of bland, mitotically inactive smooth muscle; when it is extensive, it causes the uterus to become symmetrically enlarged. At the microscopic level, the process manifests in the form of small islands of hypercellular, bland smooth muscle interspersed among areas of normally cellular smooth muscle. This results in a histologic pattern that closely mimics infiltration. Within the hypercellular nodules, smooth-muscle cells may be condensed around vessels. Because of the infiltration and the hypercellularity, leiomyosarcoma may be a diagnostic concern. We use the same diagnostic approach for leiomyomatosis as we do for ordinary smooth-muscle tumors (see earlier discussion and Table 14).

Clinicopathologic Correlation

This is a rare, benign process; the apparent infiltration and diffuse distribution should not be construed as evidence of leiomyosarcoma.

Disseminated Peritoneal Leiomyomatosis (150,599–605)

Description

This rare, benign, and probably hormone-induced lesion is characterized by multiple peritoneal nodules composed of an admixture of fibroblasts and bland smooth-muscle cells. The nodules are invariably small (less than 2 cm), and they stud the surface of the peritoneum. There may be an associated decidual reaction.

Clinicopathologic Correlation

Disseminated peritoneal leiomyomatosis (DPL) is a very rare condition that almost always occurs in young women subject to an altered hormonal mileau, usually pregnancy. Consequently, it is most often discovered incidentally at the time of caesarean section. To the surgeon, DPL may appear as metastases; the possibility of DPL should be considered whenever peritoneal nodules are encountered in a young woman, particularly if she is pregnant. Postpartum spontaneous regression is the rule.

Differential Diagnosis

Metastatic leiomyosarcoma from the uterus should demonstrate increased mitotic activity, significant cytologic atypia, and, often, tumor cell necrosis. Metastatic deposits are usually more than 2 cm in diameter. Gastrointestinal stromal tumors and leiomyosarcomas of the retroperitoneum can be bland and mitotically inactive, but they are almost always more than 2 cm in diameter. Before diagnosing DPL, it is always worthwhile knowing that there is no mass in the gastrointestinal tract or retroperitoneum.

Benign Metastasizing Leiomyoma (606–609)

Description

Women with mitotically inactive, cytologically bland, nonnecrotic uterine smooth-muscle tumors may, on very rare occasions, develop similarly benign extrauterine smooth-muscle deposits (usually in the lymph nodes or in the lungs) in the absence of a primary smooth-muscle malignancy in the gastrointestinal tract, retroperitoneum, or other nonuterine areas. Because one explanation for this phenomena is the spread of histologically benign smooth muscle from the uterine leiomyoma to distant sites, this process has been labeled benign metastasizing leiomyoma.

Clinicopathologic Correlation

The criteria for this improbable diagnosis are understandably strict, and an absolute minimal guideline is that all of the smooth-muscle tumors must have been thoroughly examined histologically and judged to be unquestionably benign in morphologic characteristics. The implication of this diagnosis is that available criteria for identifying leiomyosarcoma are inadequate to pick out those very rare uterine smooth-muscle neoplasms that are capable of involving other organs but are morphologically noninformative about this potential. This definition eliminates labeling these bland metastasizing tumors as leiomyosarcoma for eminently sensible reasons: thousands of clinically benign smooth-muscle tumors would have to be labeled malignant to anticipate the extremely rare clinically malignant tumor in this morphologic range. The "metastatic," bland smooth-muscle deposits develop most often in lymph nodes or the lung; in rare instances, the benign smooth-muscle deposits are found initially in abdominal lymph nodes and subsequently in the lungs. Because a few women with benign pulmonary smooth-muscle tumors have not had uterine tumors, some investigators believe the pulmonary process is unrelated to the presence of uterine smooth-muscle tumors; instead, they consider the lung nodules to be separate smooth-muscle proliferations. The pulmonary nodules usually progress slowly, sometimes to the point of producing pulmonary insufficiency, and they may respond to hormonal treatment.

Differential Diagnosis

The differential diagnoses are the same as for leiomyoma.

Parasitic Leiomyomas

Description

On rare occasions, leiomyomas have been reported to detach from their initial subserosa location and attach themselves to some other pelvic site. This improbable event presumably takes place through the mediation of a combination of infarction and inflammatory adhesions. A diagnosis of parasitic leiomyoma should be made with great caution, since clinically malignant smooth-muscle neoplasms arising in the retroperitoneum or gastrointestinal tract are notorious for being bland and having a low MI.

Clinicopathologic Correlation

We have never seen a convincing example of parasitic leiomyoma.

Intravascular (Intravenous) Leiomyomatosis and Leiomyoma with Vascular Intrusion (610,611,613)

Description

These terms are used to describe localized or disseminated, cytologically bland and mitotically inactive smooth muscle

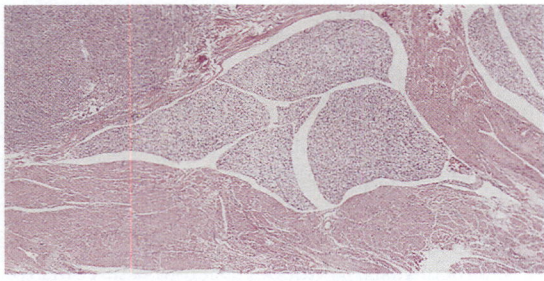
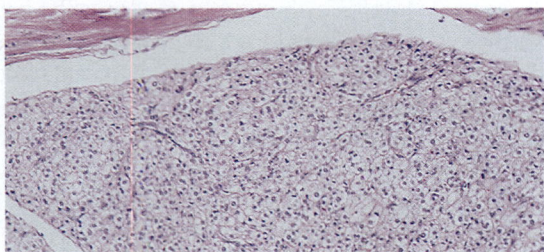

FIG. 117. Intravenous leiomyomatosis with clear cells. *Top:* Tumor cells within a vascular space. *Bottom:* The clear-cell features of the constituent cells. We evaluate the malignant potential of clear-cell tumors in the same way as we do other epithelioid smooth-muscle tumors of the uterus.

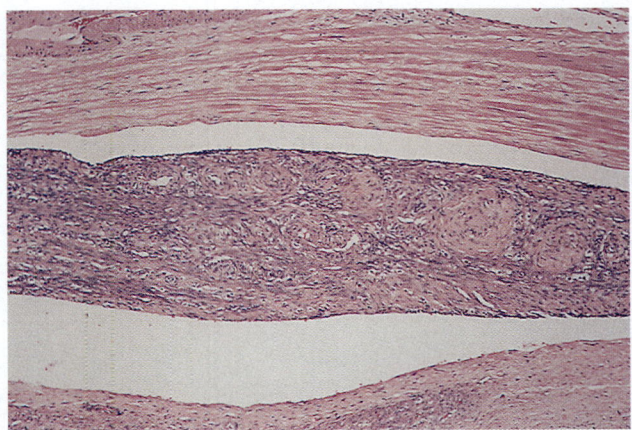

FIG. 118. Apparent intravenous leiomyomatosis. Here a plug of what appears to be neoplastic smooth muscle can be seen in a vascular space. The differential diagnosis would be intravenous leiomyomatosis or low-grade endometrial stromal sarcoma.

within vascular channels. Three situations are distinguished: a solitary, otherwise unremarkable leiomyoma associated with a microscopic focus of intravascular neoplasm within the confines of the leiomyoma; grossly visible worm-like intravascular masses of cytologically benign smooth muscle; or microscopic intrusion of benign smooth muscle into vessels outside the confines of an otherwise unremarkable leiomyoma. The first of these conditions is designated leiomyoma with vascular intrusion, while the latter two are labeled intravenous (or better, intravascular) leiomyomatosis (Fig. 117–119). Morphologic variations on the usual smooth-muscle theme (e.g., clear cells, fat, epithelioid cells, atypical cells) have been noted in intravascular leiomyomatosis (612,614).

Clinicopathologic Correlation

Leiomyomas with vascular intrusion are benign and do not recur. Microscopic intravascular leiomyomatosis (the

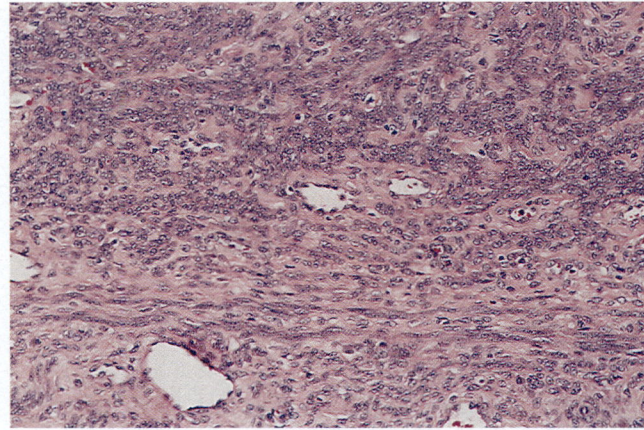

FIG. 119. Higher magnification of the preceding tumor plug (Fig. 118) indicates that the differentiation of smooth muscle from endometrial stroma is ambiguous. We consider such tumors to be of the endometrial stromal type for purposes of therapy and prognosis.

third situation described in the previous section is also, in general, a clinically benign lesion, but there exists a remote possibility of intravascular recurrence outside the uterus. Grossly visible intravascular leiomyomatosis confined to the uterus is generally cured by excising the involved organs, but occasionally it may recur within pelvic, abdominal, thoracic, or femoral vessels. It will recur more often if it has extended into extrauterine vessels at the time of hysterectomy (615,616). In rare instances, continuous extension from the uterus, through the inferior vena cava and into the heart, has been described (614,617,618). In this circumstance, the patients may be thought to have a primary cardiac neoplasm if the presence of tumor in the uterus and/or the vena cava is not noted. The definition of intravascular leiomyomatosis requires any extrauterine benign smooth muscle to remain within vascular lumens or within the chambers of the heart. The presence of morphologically benign smooth muscle within parenchymal organs excludes intravascular leiomyomatosis and raises the possibility of benign metastasizing leiomyoma or low-grade leiomyosarcoma.

Differential Diagnosis

Intravascular Leiomyomatosis Versus Low-grade Endometrial Stromal Sarcoma. In most cases, distinguishing between these two entities is straightforward and amounts to discriminating endometrial stromal differentiation from smooth-muscle differentiation (Figs. 85, 86, 118 and 119) and Table 5). In some cases, however, differentiation is ambiguous; this is not particularly surprising, given the close histogenetic and anatomic relationship of these cells (619,620). Our experience indicates that some tumors with ambiguous differentiation behave like low-grade endometrial stromal sarcoma; consequently, for purposes of treatment and prognosis, we assign cases with ambiguous differentiation to the category of low-grade endometrial stromal sarcoma.

Intravascular Leiomyomatosis Versus Leiomyosarcoma with Vascular Invasion. An MI above 5 mf per 10 hpf is distinctly unusual in intravascular leiomyomatosis, and tumor cell necrosis is not allowed. Because of the paucity of cases with an MI of about 5 that have been the subject of follow-up study, the term UMP is appropriate for cases with bland histologic features but with an MI of 5 to 15 mf per 10 hpf. Moderate to marked atypia and an MI of more than 5 in an intravascular smooth-muscle tumor is indicative of leiomyosarcoma.

Usual Leiomyosarcoma

Description

The features of almost all leiomyosarcomas deviate from the usual white, whorled macroscopic appearance of a leiomyoma, although not all grossly peculiar smooth-muscle tumors are malignant. Consequently, all uterine tumors that have deviant gross appearances must be sampled. Usual and epithelioid leiomyosarcomas are most often hemorrhagic and soft and possess the celebrated fish-flesh texture, while the myxoid variety has a mucoid consistency. The usual leiomyosarcoma most often is more than 5 cm in diameter. It is easily recognized as malignant in the vast majority of cases, and usually there is no difficulty in identifying it as a smooth-muscle neoplasm. It is common for pleomorphism to be marked, for the mitotic counts to be in the range of 15 to 30 mf per 10 hpf, and for abnormal division figures to be abundant. In addition, leiomyosarcomas rather frequently contain areas of coagulative tumor necrosis (Figs. 104-106); in fact, tumors containing areas of coagulative tumor cell necrosis behave aggressively often enough to be considered leiomyosarcoma or tumors of uncertain malignant potential, regardless of other morphologic features.

Leiomyosarcomas with coagulative necrosis almost always have other features associated with malignancy, however, such as moderate to marked atypia and increased mitotic activity (see earlier discussion); these signs should be sought in order to confirm the diagnosis (Figs. 99-101). There is a small set of leiomyosarcomas that are clearly composed of smooth-muscle cells but that are difficult to distinguish from leiomyoma because the cells are moderately to severely atypical (as defined previously) and tumor cell necrosis is not apparent. As noted earlier, the MI is used to stratify such tumors into benign and malignant categories (see Table 14). There is another small set of leiomyosarcomas that are anaplastic, with only rare tumor cells demonstrating smooth-muscle differentiation (561-565,572, 621,622).

Clinicopathologic Correlation (485,623–627) (Figs. 108–110 and 112)

Although leiomyosarcoma is among the most common of the sarcomas that arise in the uterus, it almost certainly does not evolve from "malignant degeneration" of a leiomyoma. Leiomyosarcomas are rarely associated with previous irradiation (628). Stage is the most important predictor of relapse-free survival, but there is controversy as to whether the histologic features of stage I leiomyosarcomas provide additional prognostic insight. Evans has evidence to support the size of leiomyosarcoma as a prognostic variable; those tumors that are <5 cm have a better prognosis than those that are >5 cm. The only treatment known to be effective for leiomyosarcoma is surgery, and the value of postoperative adjuvant therapy has not been established (629–631). The mean age of patients with uterine leiomyosarcoma is about 50 years; they may be found in women in the fourth decade, but leiomyosarcoma is very rare in women less than 40 years of age. The overall survival rate is 10% to 30% at 5 years.

Differential Diagnosis

Other Types of Sarcoma and Mixed Müllerian Tumors Versus High-grade Leiomyosarcoma with Difficult to Discern Smooth-muscle Differentiation. Distinguishing leiomyosarcoma from other pure sarcomas, except low-grade endometrial sarcoma (see next section), is not of great practical importance because the treatment and behavior of all high-grade uterine sarcomas are the same. Accordingly, while it is certainly reasonable to attempt to properly classify uterine sarcomas using inexpensive traditional techniques, it is uncertain whether other, more expensive techniques should be used for cases in which the direction of differentiation is in question. Carcinosarcomas have a sarcomatous stroma that can resemble leiomyosarcoma, but they also contain carcinoma. The stroma of müllerian adenosarcoma is most often fibroblastic rather than smooth muscle, and benign glands are present.

Well-differentiated Leiomyosarcoma Versus Low-grade Endometrial Stromal Sarcoma. Because the criteria for malignancy differ for smooth-muscle tumors and low-grade endometrial stromal sarcoma, an essential initial step is establishing the distinguishing features of a uterine mesenchymal tumor. Low-grade endometrial stromal sarcoma is distinguished from the benign stromal nodule on the basis of the presence or absence of infiltrating margins, independent of the number of mitotic figures. On the other hand, bland smooth-muscle neoplasms are considered benign even when they have infiltrating margins. Strategies for differentiating these tumors are presented in the introduction to this section. As noted, when in doubt about the direction of a bland uterine mesenchymal tumor's differentiation, we assign the case to the endometrial stromal group.

PURE SARCOMA OTHER THAN LEIOMYOSARCOMA AND LOW-GRADE ENDOMETRIAL STROMAL SARCOMA

For references, see the list of unusual neoplasms given in Table 16.

Description

Pure uterine sarcomas in which at least some of the tumor cells demonstrate either homologous or heterologous differentiation are classified on the basis of this differentiation, for example, chondrosarcoma, osteosarcoma, or rhabdomyosarcoma. Rarely, two types of mesenchymal differentiation are found in the same tumor; we classify such neoplasms as pure uterine sarcomas of mixed type. When the cells of a pure sarcoma do not show signs of appreciable differentiation, we place the sarcoma in the undifferentiated category. Pure undifferentiated uterine sarcoma encompasses many of the neoplasms formerly classified as high-grade endometrial stromal sarcomas (see the discussion on this subject in the section on endometrial stromal tumors). Sarcomas containing multinucleated giant cells but no other evidence of differentiation are labeled giant-cell sarcoma of the uterus.

Clinicopathologic Correlation

Setting aside low-grade endometrial stromal sarcoma, once a neoplasm has been classified as a pure uterine sarcoma, the direction of differentiation makes little difference; the treatment and prognosis are much the same for all pure uterine sarcomas. Pure sarcomas are aggressive neoplasms, and the only chance for survival is curative surgical removal.

Differential Diagnosis

Carcinosarcoma Versus Pure Sarcoma

Both carcinoma and high-grade sarcoma must be present in carcinosarcomas; however, the carcinoma may be evident only in focal areas and not in curetting specimens or poorly sampled neoplasms. Misclassifying a carcinosarcoma as a pure high-grade sarcoma is of little importance to the patient, since both tumors are treated in essentially the same way and the outcomes are similar.

Adenosarcoma Versus Pure Differentiated Sarcoma

The stroma of most adenosarcomas is low grade; however, even when the sarcoma is high grade and there is stromal overgrowth, bland, often cystically dilated glands are present somewhere in the tumor. These glands are not seen in pure sarcomas. Numerous sections of any apparently pure sarcoma should be taken to exclude the possibility stromal overgrowth in an adenosarcoma. In addition, the sarcomatous stromal cells in adenosarcomas often condense circumferentially around dilated glands. The usually diffusely distributed dilated glands and the stromal condensation help distinguish adenosarcoma from pure sarcoma infiltrating among preexisting endometrial glands.

Mesenchymal Metaplasia Versus Pure Heterologous Sarcoma

Rarely, benign bone or cartilage can be found in the uterus, and, at times, leiomyomas contain benign metaplastic bone. Mesenchymal metaplasias are distinguished from sarcoma by their fully mature and bland constituent cells—the cells do not have the malignant cytologic features found in osteosarcoma and chondrosarcoma.

Anaplastic Carcinoma Versus Lymphoma/Leukemia Versus Pure Sarcoma

Chloracetate stains, as well as immunohistochemical stains for keratins and leukocyte common antigen, may be useful in solving this differential diagnostic problem if H&E sections do not allow definitive diagnosis.

MISCELLANEOUS NEOPLASMS

Adenomatoid Tumor (Mesothelioma) (632–641)

Description

Adenomatoid mesotheliomas identical to those found in the fallopian tube may arise primarily in the uterus, usually

TABLE 16. *Unusual uterine disease processes*

Specific infections
    Actinomycosis (656)
    Bilharzia (657)
    Chlamydia (162,163,658–660)
    Coccidiomycosis (661,662)
    Cytomegalovirus (663–667)
    Enterobiasis (668,669)
    Herpes (670–672)
    Mycobacterium (673,674)
    Oxyuriasis (675)
    Papillomavirus (676)
    Toxoplasmosis (677,678)
    Tuberculosis (177–179)
Specific nonneoplastic patterns
    Asherman's syndrome of intrauterine adhesions (1–5)
    Congenital abnormalities (44,679,680)
    Calcific endometritis (681)
    Congenital intramural cysts (682)
    Eosinophilic endometritis (683)
    Giant-cell arteritis (684–687)
    Herpetic pseudo-inclusions (136)
    Histiocytic endometritis (688)
    Lymphangioleiomyomatosis (689,690)
    Lithiasis (691)
    Malacoplakia (692–694)
    Necrobiotic granulomas stemming from laser ablation of endometrium (695,696)
    Peritoneal foreign body reaction to keratin of endometrial origin (334,335)
    Pneumopolycystic endometritis (697)
    Postoperative spindle-cell nodule (698)
    Pseudolymphomatous and peculiar inflammatory lesions (699–701)
    Radiation reaction (702,703)
    Sarcoid (704–707)
    Xanthomatous endometritis (174,688,708,709)
Neoplasms
    Benign and teratomatous including fetal implants
        Brenner tumor (710)
        Fetal implants, glial implants (711–715)
        Fibroosteochondroma (716)
        Glioma (717,718)
        Hemangioma, arteriovenous malformations (719,720)
        Lipoleiomyomas, lipomas (593,594,721–723)
        Osseous and cartilagenous metaplasia (724–727)
        Heterologous tissue associated with endometrial carcinoma (728)
        Heterotopic skin (729)
        Paraganglioma and related lesions (730–732)
        Skeletal muscle or cartilagenous differentiation in leiomyomas, stromal nodule (733–736)
        Teratoma (737,738)

Malignant
    Epithelial, neuroectodermal, germ cell
        Adenoid cystic carcinoma (739)
        Endodermal sinus tumor (740,741)
        Carcinoma with giant-cell component (742)
        Primitive neuroectodermal tumor (743–746)
        Small-cell carcinoma (410–413,747,748)
        Carcinomas with trophoblastic differentiation and/or HCG secretion (749–752)
        Carcinoma with αFP production (753)
        Glassy-cell carcinoma (376,754)
        Lipid-rich clear-cell carcinoma (755)
        Squamous cell carcinoma, pure (377–379,653)
        Squamous carcinoma, spindle cell (756)
        Squamous carcinoma *in situ* (381,382)
        Sertoliform carcinoma endometrioid adenocarcinoma (96)
        Transitional cell carcinoma (757–759)
        Undifferentiated carcinoma (456)
        Verrucous carcinoma (380,760)
    Mesenchymal, mixed epithelial/mesenchymal, hematopoietic, germ cell
        Alveolar soft parts sarcoma (761–764)
        Angiosarcoma (765–767)
        Carcinofibroma (462,463)
        Carcinosarcoma
            In child (768)
            αFP production (769)
            Neuroectodermal differentiation (770)
            Small-cell carcinoma component (413)
            In endometrial polyp (233,445)
        Chondrosarcoma (771,772)
        Immature teratoma (773)
        Lipoleiomyosarcoma (774)
        Lymphoma/granulocytic sarcoma (642–647,775)
        Malignant fibrous histiocytoma (776,777)
        Osteoclastic sarcoma (778–781)
        Osteosarcoma (774,782,783)
        Rhabdomyosarcoma (774, 784–789)
        Rhabdoid tumor (790–794)
    Miscellaneous
        Wilms' tumor (795)
    Metastasis and local extension of cervical squamous carcinoma
        Metastatic carcinoma, melanoma (400,401,796–799)
        Squamous carcinoma *in situ* (381,382)
        Squamous carcinoma extension from cervix (800)

HCG, human chorionic gonadotropin; αFP, alpha-fetoprotein.

in a subserosal location near the cornua. In their gross appearance, adenomatoid mesotheliomas mimic leiomyomas, except that they are usually smaller and often yellow and less well circumscribed than leiomyomas. At the microscopic level, adenomatoid mesotheliomas consist of irregular aggregates of cuboid to flattened cells arranged in clumps, columns, or gland-like spaces interdigitating between bands of smooth muscle (Fig. 120). Cellular atypia is minimal or absent, and mitotic figures are usually sparse; in rare cases, they may be numerous. The histologic and immunohistochemical evidence to date suggests that these neoplasms differentiate along mesothelial lines.

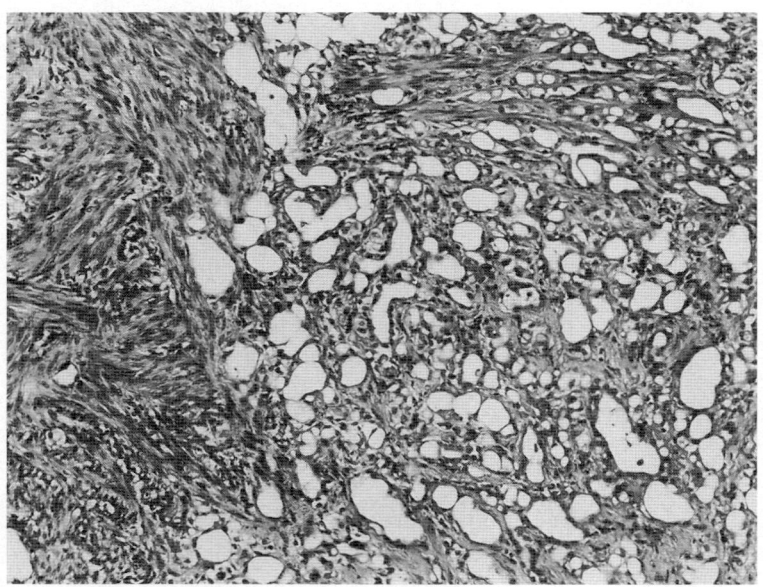

FIG. 120. Adenomatoid tumor. Numerous spaces within hyperplastic muscle make up the characteristic pattern of adenomatoid tumor. Often the spaces appear sieve-like, as in this example.

Clinicopathologic Correlation

Adenomatoid mesotheliomas develop chiefly during the reproductive years. They are usually incidental and benign findings in uteri removed for other reasons.

Differential Diagnosis

Occasionally, the gland-like spaces of adenomatoid tumors may be striking dilated, producing a pattern reminiscent of lymphangioma. The character of the cells lining the spaces and the absence of lymphocytes within the spaces should eliminate this possibility. Since both entities are benign, nothing much is at stake in this differential diagnosis. A more serious differential diagnostic possibility is invasive adenocarcinoma. Again, the cytological bland character of the cells and the absence of mitotic figures should eliminate this possibility.

Lymphoma and Leukemia (646,647)

Lymphoma and leukemia rarely involve EMB or hysterectomy specimens. Even in this unusual event, the fact that the patient has lymphoma or leukemia usually has been established. Thus, if the history is provided, the pathologist is almost never faced with recognizing lymphoma or leukemia *de novo* in a surgical specimen. This possibility must always be kept in mind, however, whenever an unusual neoplasm is encountered in the uterus. Moreover, large-cell lymphoma and granulocytic leukemia can resemble endometrial stromal sarcoma; thus, the former two conditions are always considered in the differential diagnosis of the latter tumor. A number of lymphoma mimics have been described (642–645).

RARE AND UNUSUAL DISEASES

These rare diseases are listed, with references, in Table 16.

GENERAL REFERENCES

General

Buckley CH, Fox H. *Biopsy pathology of the endometrium.* New York: Raven Press, 1989.
Clement PB, Young RH. *Tumors and tumorlike lesions of the uterine corpus and cervix.* New York: Churchill Livingstone, 1993. (*Contemporary issues in surgical pathology*, vol 19.)
Dallenbach-Hellweg G. *Histopathology of the endometrium*, 4th ed. New York: Springer-Verlag, 1987.
Kurman R, ed. *Blaustein's pathology of the female genital tract*, 4th ed. New York: Springer-Verlag, 1994.
Mazur MT, Kurman RJ. *Diagnosis of endometrial biopsies and curettings: a practical approach.* New York: Springer-Verlag, 1995.

Nonneoplastic Disease

Adashi EY, Rock JA, Rosenwaks Z. *Reproductive endocrinology, surgery, and technology.* Philadelphia: Lippincott–Raven Publishers, 1996.
Kraus FT, Damjanov I, Kaufman N, eds. *Pathology of reproductive failure.* Baltimore: Williams & Wilkins, 1991. (United States and Canadian Academy of Pathology, Inc., monograph.)
Lobo R, Mishell D, Paulson R, Shoupe D. *Mishell's textbook of infertility, contraception and reproductive endocrinology*, 4th ed. Malden, England: Blackwell Science, 1997.
Speroff L, Glass RH, Kase NG. *Clinical gynecologic endocrinology and infertility*, 5th ed. Baltimore: Williams & Wilkins, 1994.
Wentz AC, ed. *Gynecologic endocrinology and infertility for the house officer.* Baltimore: Williams & Wilkins, 1988.
Wynn R, Jollie W, eds. *Biology of the uterus*, 2nd ed. New York: Plenum Medical Book Company, 1989.
Yen SSC, Jaffe RB, eds. *Reproductive endocrinology: physiology, pathophysiology and clinical management*, 3rd ed. Philadelphia, London, Toronto: WB Saunders, 1991.

Neoplastic Disease

Burke TW, Eifel PJ, Muggia FM. Cancer of the uterine body. In: DeVita V, Hellman S, Rosenberg S, eds. *Cancer: principles and practice of oncology*, 5th ed. Philadelphia: Lippincott–Raven Publishers, 1997:1478–1499.
Coppleson M. *Gynecologic oncology: fundamental principles and clinical practice*, 2nd ed. Edinburgh: Churchill Livingstone, 1992.
DiSaia PJ, Creasman WT. *Clinical gynecologic oncology*, 5th ed. St. Louis: Mosby, 1997.

Hoskins WJ, Perez CA, Young RC. *Principles and practice of gynecologic oncology*, 2nd ed. Philadelphia: Lippincott–Raven Publishers, 1997.

Morrow CP, Curtin JP, Townsend DE. *Synopsis of gynecologic oncology*, 4th ed. New York: Churchill Livingstone, 1993.

Silverberg SG, Kurman RJ. *Tumors of the uterine corpus and gestational trophoblastic disease*. Washington, D.C.: AFIP 1992. (Rosai J, ed. *Atlas of tumor pathology*, vol x, 3rd series, fascicle 3.)

REFERENCES

1. Stillman RJ, Asarkof N. Association between mullerian duct malformations and Asherman syndrome in infertile women. *Obstet Gynecol* 1985;65:673–677.
2. Lancet M, Kessler I. A review of Asherman's syndrome, and results of modern treatment. *Int J Fertil* 1988;33:14–24.
3. Valle RF, Sciarra JJ. Intrauterine adhesions: hysteroscopic diagnosis, classification, treatment, and reproductive outcome [Comments]. *Am J Obstet Gynecol* 1988;158:1459–1470.
4. Chapman K, Chapman R. Asherman's syndrome: a review of the literature, and a husband and wife's 20-year world-wide experience. *J R Soc Med* 1990;83:576–580.
5. Schenker JG. Etiology of and therapeutic approach to synechia uteri. *Eur J Obstet Gynecol Reprod Biol* 1996;65:109–113.
6. Kaunitz AM, Masciello A, Ostrowski M, Rovira EZ. Comparison of endometrial biopsy with the endometrial Pipelle and Vabra aspirator. *J Reprod Med* 1988;33:427–431.
7. Eddowes H, Read M, Codling B. Pipelle: a more acceptable technique for outpatient endometrial biopsy. *Br J Obstet Gynaecol* 1990;97:961–962.
8. Silver MM, Miles P, Rosa C. Comparison of Novak and Pipelle endometrial biopsy instruments. *Obstet Gynecol* 1991;78:828–830.
9. Stovall TG, Ling FW, Morgan PL. A prospective, randomized comparison of the Pipelle endometrial sampling device with the Novak curette. *Am J Obstet Gynecol* 1991;5:1.
10. Fothergill DJ, Brown VA, Hill AS. Histological sampling of the endometrium: a comparison between formal curettage and the Pipelle sampler [Comments]. *Br J Obstet Gynaecol* 1992;99:779–780.
11. Jennings JC. Abnormal uterine bleeding. *Med Clin North Am* 1995;79:1357–1376.
12. Butler W. Normal and abnormal uterine bleeding. In: Rock J, Thompson J, eds. *Te Linde's operative gynecology*, 8th ed. Philadelphia: Lippincott–Raven Publishers, 1997:453–475.
13. Stock R, Kanbour A. Prehysterectomy curettage. *Obstet Gynecol* 1975;45:537–541.
14. Vuopala S. Diagnostic accuracy and clinical applicability of cytological and histological methods for investigating endometrial carcinoma. *Acta Obstet Gynecol Scand Suppl* 1977;70:1–72.
15. Grimes D. Diagnostic dilation and curettage: a reappraisal. *Am J Obstet Gynecol* 1982;142:1–6.
16. Stovall T, Solomon S, Ling F. Endometrial sampling prior to hysterectomy [published erratum appears in *Obstet Gynecol* 1989;74(1):105]. *Obstet Gynecol* 1989;73:405–409.
17. Ferry J, Farnsworth A, Webster M, Wren B. The efficacy of the Pipelle endometrial biopsy in detecting endometrial carcinoma. *Aust N Z J Obstet Gynaecol* 1993;33:76–78.
18. Ben-Baruch G, Seidman DS, Schiff E, Moran O, Menczer J. Outpatient endometrial sampling with the Pipelle curette. *Gynecol Obstet Invest* 1994;37:260–262.
19. Read MD. Outpatient endometrial assessment. *Br J Hosp Med* 1995;54:150–153.
20. Rose PG. Endometrial carcinoma. *N Engl J Med* 1996;335:640–649.
21. Brill AI. What is the role of hysteroscopy in the management of abnormal uterine bleeding? *Clin Obstet Gynecol* 1995;3:319–445.
22. Emanuel MH, Wamsteker K, Lammes FB. Is dilatation and curettage obsolete for diagnosing intrauterine disorders in premenopausal patients with persistent abnormal uterine bleeding? *Acta Obstet Gynecol Scand* 1997;76:65–68.
23. Nasri M, Coast G. Correlation of ultrasound findings and endometrial histopathology in postmenopausal women. *Br J Obstet Gynecol* 1989;96:1333–1338.
24. Granberg S, Wikland M, Karlsson B, Norstrom A, Friberg LG. Endometrial thickness as measured by endovaginal ultrasonography for identifying endometrial abnormality. *Am J Obstet Gynecol* 1991;164:47–52.
25. Goldchmit R, Katz Z, Blickstein I, Caspi B, Dgani R. The accuracy of endometrial Pipelle sampling with and without sonographic measurement of endometrial thickness [Comments]. *Obstet Gynecol* 1993;82:727–730.
26. Cacciatore B, Ramsay T, Lehtovirta P, Ylostalo P. Transvaginal sonography and hysteroscopy in postmenopausal bleeding. *Acta Obstet Gynecol Scand* 1994;73:413–416.
27. Osmers R, Volksen M, Rath W, Kuhn W. Vaginosonographic detection of endometrial cancer in postmenopausal women. *Int J Gynaecol Obstet* 1990;32:35–37.
28. Langer RD, Pierce JJ, O'Hanlan KA, et al. Transvaginal ultrasonography compared with endometrial biopsy for the detection of endometrial disease: Postmenopausal Estrogen/Progestin Interventions Trial [Comments]. *N Engl J Med* 1997;337:1792–1798.
29. Van Bogaert L, Maldague P, Staquet J. Endometrial biopsy interpretation: shortcomings and problems in current gynecologic practice. *Obstet Gynecol* 1978;51:25–28.
30. Schindler A, Schmidt G. Post-menopausal bleeding: a study of more than 1,000 cases. *Maturitas* 1980;2:269–274.
31. Dewhurst J. Postmenopausal bleeding from benign causes. *Clin Obstet Gynecol* 1983;26:769–776.
32. Rubin S. Postmenopausal bleeding: etiology, evaluation, and management. *Med Clin North Am* 1987;71:59–69.
33. Noyes R. Normal phases of the endometrium. In: Hertig A, Norris H, Abell M, eds. *The uterus*. Baltimore: Williams & Wilkins, 1973:110–135.
34. Wentz A. *Luteal phase inadequacy*, 3rd ed. Boston, Toronto: Little, Brown and Company, 1988:405–462. (Behrman S, Kistner R, Patton GJ, eds. *Progress in infertility*.)
35. Martinez AR, Voorhorst FJ, Schoemaker J. Reliability of urinary LH testing for planning of endometrial biopsies. *Eur J Obstet Gynecol Reprod Biol* 1992;43:137–142.
36. Ferenczy A. How to date the endometrial cycle. *Contemp Ob/Gyn* 1981;18:115–133.
37. Castelbaum AJ, Wheeler J, Coutifaris CB, Mastroianni LJ, Lessey BA. Timing of the endometrial biopsy may be critical for the accurate diagnosis of luteal phase deficiency [Comments]. *Fertil Steril* 1994;61:443–447.
38. Noyes R. Uniformity of secretory endometrium: study of multiple sections from 100 uteri removed at operation. *Fertil Steril* 1956;7:103–109.
39. Dockery P, Li T, Rogers A, Cooke I, Lenton E, Warren M. An examination of the variation in timed endometrial biopsies. *Hum Reprod* 1988;3:715–720.
40. Gibson M, Badger GJ, Byrn F, Lee KR, Korson R, Trainer TD. Error in histologic dating of secretory endometrium: variance component analysis. *Fertil Steril* 1991;56:242–247.
41. Wathen PI, Henderson MC, Witz CA. Abnormal uterine bleeding. *Med Clin North Am* 1995;79:329–344.
42. Chambers JT, Chambers SK. Endometrial sampling: When? Where? Why? With what? *Clin Obstet Gynecol* 1992;35:28–39.
43. Vollenhoven B, Lawrence A, Healy D. Uterine fibroids: a clinical review. *Br J Obstet Gynaecol* 1990;97:285–298.
44. Rock J. Infertility: surgical aspects. In: Yen S, Jaffe R, eds. *Reproductive endocrinology: physiology, pathophysiology and clinical management*, 3rd ed. Philadelphia: WB Saunders, 1991:710–734.
45. Dicker D, Dekel A, Orvieto R, Bar-Hava I, Peleg D, Ben-Rafael Z. The controversy of laparoscopic myomectomy. *Hum Reprod* 1996;11:935–937.
46. Donnez J, Mathieu PE, Bassil S, Smets M, Nisolle M, Berliere M. Laparoscopic myomectomy today. Fibroids: management and treatment. The state of the art. *Hum Reprod* 1996;11:1837–1840.
47. Dubuisson JB, Chapron C. Laparoscopic myomectomy today: a good technique when correctly indicated. *Hum Reprod* 1996;11:934–935.
48. Nezhat F, Seidman DS, Nezhat C, Nezhat CH. Laparoscopic myomectomy today: why, when and for whom? *Hum Reprod* 1996;11:933–934.
49. Colgan TJ, Pendergast S, Le BM. The histopathology of uterine leiomyomas following treatment with gonadotropin-releasing hormone analogues. *Hum Pathol* 1993;24:1073–1077.
50. Crow J, Gardner RL, McSweeney G, Shaw RW. Morphological changes in uterine leiomyomas treated by GnRH agonist goserelin. *Int J Gynecol Pathol* 1995;14:235–242.
51. Rutgers J, Spong CY, Sinow R, Heiner J. Leuprolide acetate treatment and myoma arterial size. *Obstet Gynecol* 1995;86:386–388.

52. Sreenan JJ, Prayson RA, Biscotti CV, Thornton MH, Easley KA, Hart WR. Histopathologic findings in 107 uterine leiomyomas treated with leuprolide acetate compared with 126 controls. *Am J Surg Pathol* 1996;20:427–432.
53. Deligdisch L, Hirschmann S, Altchek A. Pathologic changes in gonadotropin releasing hormone agonist analogue treated uterine leiomyomata. *Fertil Steril* 1997;67:837–841.
54. Demopoulos RI, Jones KY, Mittal KR, Vamvakas EC. Histology of leiomyomata in patients treated with leuprolide acetate. *Int J Gynecol Pathol* 1997;16:131–137.
55. Franquemont D, Frierson H, Mills S. An immunohistochemical study of normal endometrial stroma and endometrial stromal neoplasms: evidence for smooth muscle differentiation. *Am J Surg Pathol* 1991;15:861–870.
56. Oliva E, Young RH, Clement PB, Bhan AK, Scully RE. Cellular benign mesenchymal tumors of the uterus: a comparative morphologic and immunohistochemical analysis of 33 highly cellular leiomyomas and six endometrial stromal nodules, two frequently confused tumors. *Am J Surg Pathol* 1995;19:757–768.
57. Poropatich C, Rojas M, Silverberg SG. Polymorphonuclear leukocytes in the endometrium during the normal menstrual cycle. *Int J Gynecol Pathol* 1987;6:230–234.
58. Noyes R, Hertig A, Rock J. Dating the endometrial biopsy. *Fertil Steril* 1950;1:3–25.
59. Ferenczy A, Bertrand G, Gelfand M. Proliferation kinetics of human endometrium during the normal menstrual cycle. *Am J Obstet Gynecol* 1979;133:859–867.
60. Johannisson E, Parker R, Landgren B, Diczfalusy E. Morphometric analysis of the human endometrium in relation to peripheral hormone levels. *Fertil Steril* 1982;38:564–571.
61. Johannisson E, Landgren B, Rohr H, Diczfalusy E. Endometrial morphology and peripheral hormone levels in women with regular menstrual cycles. *Fertil Steril* 1987;48:401–408.
62. Wynn RM. The human endometrium: cyclic and gestational changes. In: Wynn R, Jollie W, eds. *Biology of the uterus*, 2nd ed. New York: Plenum Medical Book Company, 1989:289–332.
63. Li T, Dockery P, Rogers A, Cooke I. How precise is histologic dating of endometrium using the standard dating criteria? *Fertil Steril* 1989a;51:759–763.
64. Strauss JI, Gurpide E. The endometrium: regulation and dysfunction. In: Yen S, Jaffe R, eds. *Reproductive endocrinology: physiology, pathophysiology and clinical management*, 3rd ed. Philadelphia, London, Toronto: WB Saunders, 1991:309–356.
65. Hendrickson M, Kempson R. Uterus and fallopian tubes. In: Sternberg S, ed. *Histology for pathologists*. New York: Raven Press, 1992:797–834.
66. Valle RF. Hysteroscopy. *Curr Opin Obstet Gynecol* 1991;3:422–426.
67. Corson S. Operative hysteroscopy for infertility. *Clin Obstet Gynecol* 1992;35:229–241.
68. Gutmann JN. Imaging in the evaluation of female infertility. *J Reprod Med* 1992;37:54–61.
69. March CM. Hysteroscopy. *J Reprod Med* 1992;37:293–311.
70. Robertson W. A reappraisal of the endometrium in infertility. *Clin Obstet Gynaecol* 1984;11:209–226.
71. Dallenbach-Hellweg G. *Histopathology of the endometrium*, 4th ed. New York: Springer-Verlag, 1987.
72. Speroff L, Glass R, Kase N. *Clinical gynecologic endocrinology and infertility*, 4th ed. Baltimore: Williams & Wilkins, 1989.
73. Collins J. Diagnostic assessment of the ovulatory process. *Semin Reprod Endocrinol* 1990;8:145–155.
74. Pillet MC, Wu TF, Adamson GD, Subak LL, Lamb EJ. Improved prediction of postovulatory day using temperature recording, endometrial biopsy, and serum progesterone. *Fertil Steril* 1990;53:614–619.
75. McNeely MJ, Soules MR. The diagnosis of luteal phase deficiency: a critical review [Comments]. *Fertil Steril* 1988;50:1–15.
76. Landgren B, Unden A, Diczfalusy E. Hormonal profile of the cycle in 68 normally menstruating women. *Acta Endocrinol (Copenh)* 1980;94:89–98.
77. Lenton E, Sexton L. Normal variation in the length of the luteal phase of the menstrual cycle: identification of the short luteal phase. *Br J Obstet Gynecol* 1984;91:685.
78. Davis O, Berkeley A, Naus G, Cholst I, Freedman K. The incidence of luteal phase defect in normal, fertile women, determined by serial endometrial biopsies [Comments]. *Fertil Steril* 1989;51:582–586.
79. Grunfeld L, Sandler B, Fox J, Boyd C, Kaplan P, Navot D. Luteal phase deficiency after completely normal follicular and periovulatory phases. *Fertil Steril* 1989;52:919–923.
80. Li T, Rogers A, Lenton E, Dockery P, Cooke I. A comparison between two methods of chronological dating of human endometrial biopsies during the luteal phase, and their correlation with histologic dating. *Fertil Steril* 1987;48:928.
81. Li TC, Rogers AW, Dockery P, Lenton EA, Cooke ID. A new method of histologic dating of human endometrium in the luteal phase. *Fertil Steril* 1988;50:52–60.
82. Noyes R, Haman J. Accuracy of endometrial dating. *Fertil Steril* 1953;4:504–517.
83. Scott RT, Snyder RR, Strickland DM, et al. The effect of interobserver variation in dating endometrial histology on the diagnosis of luteal phase defects. *Fertil Steril* 1988;50:888–892.
84. Shoupe D, Mishell DJ, Lacarra M, et al. Correlation of endometrial maturation with four methods of estimating day of ovulation. *Obstet Gynecol* 1989;73:88–92.
85. Kim-Björklund T, Landgren BM, Hamberger L, Johannisson E. Comparative morphometric study of the endometrium, the fallopian tube, and the corpus luteum during the postovulatory phase in normally menstruating women. *Fertil Steril* 1991;56:842–850.
86. Koninckx P, Goddeeris P, Lauweryns J, de Hertogh R, Brosens I. Accuracy of endometrial biopsy dating in relation to the midcycle luteinizing hormone peak. *Fertil Steril* 1977;28:443–445.
87. Li TC, Lenton EA, Dockery P, Rogers AW, Cooke ID. The relation between daily salivary progesterone profile and endometrial development in the luteal phase of fertile and infertile women. *Br J Obstet Gynaecol* 1989;96:445–453.
88. Collins J. Diagnostic assessment of the infertile male partner. *Curr Probl Obstet Gynecol Fertil* 1987;10:173–224.
89. Davidson B, Thrasher T, Seraj I. An analysis of endometrial biopsies performed for infertility. *Fertil Steril* 1987;48:770–774.
90. Collins J. Diagnostic assessment of the infertile female partner. *Curr Probl Obstet Gynecol Fertil* 1988;11:1–42.
91. Thompson DW. The role of histologic assessment of endometrium and cytohormonal applications in the diagnosis and treatment of infertility. *Curr Opin Obstet Gynecol* 1990;2:863–868.
92. Press M, King W. Distribution of peroxidase and granulocytes in the human uterus. *Lab Invest* 1986a;54:188–203.
93. Kamat B, Isaacson P. The immunocytochemical distribution of leukocytic subpopulations in human endometrium. *Am J Pathol* 1987;127:66–73.
94. Bulmer J, Lunny D, Hagin S. Immunohistochemical characterization of stromal leucocytes in nonpregnant human endometrium. *Am J Reprod Immunol Microbiol* 1988;17:83–90.
95. Marshall R, Jones D. An immunohistochemical study of lymphoid tissue in human endometrium. *Int J Gynecol Pathol* 1988;7:225–235.
96. Radwanska E, Hammond J, Smith P. Single midluteal progesterone assay in the management of ovulatory infertility. *J Reprod Med* 1981;26:85–89.
97. Daly D, Tohan N, Doney T, Maslar I, Riddick D. The significance of lymphocytic-leukocytic infiltrates in interpreting late luteal phase endometrial biopsies. *Fertil Steril* 1982;37:786–791.
98. Wentz A. Diagnosing luteal phase inadequacy [Editorial]. *Fertil Steril* 1982;37:334–335.
99. Daly D, Walters C, Soto-Albors C, Riddick D. Endometrial biopsy during treatment of luteal phase defects is predictive of therapeutic outcome. *Fertil Steril* 1983;40:305–310.
100. Smith S, Lenton E, Landgren B, Cooke I. The short luteal phase and infertility. *Br J Obstet Gynaecol* 1984;91:1120–1122.
101. Zorn J, Cedard L, Nessman C, Savale M. Delayed endometrial maturation in women with normal progesterone levels: the dysharmonic luteal phase syndrome. *Gynecol Obstet Invest* 1984;17:157–162.
102. Cumming D, Honore L, Scott J, Williams K. The late luteal phase in infertile women: comparison of simultaneous endometrial biopsy and progesterone levels. *Fertil Steril* 1985;43:715–719.
103. Dallenbach-Hellweg G. The endometrium of infertility: a review. *Pathol Res Pract* 1984;178:527–537.
104. Jones G. The physiology of menstruation and the corpus luteum function. *Int J Fertil* 1986;31:143–147.
105. Balasch J, Vanrell J. Corpus luteum insufficiency and fertility: a matter of controversy. *Hum Reprod* 1987;2:557–567.
106. Brodie B, Wentz A. An update on the clinical relevance of luteal phase inadequacy. *Semin Reprod Endocrinol* 1989;7:138–154.

107. Soules MR, McLachlan RI, Ek M, Dahl KD, Cohen NL, Bremner WJ. Luteal phase deficiency: characterization of reproductive hormones over the menstrual cycle. *J Clin Endocrinol Metab* 1989;69:804–812.
108. Jones G. Corpus luteum: composition and function. *Fertil Steril* 1990;54:21–26.
109. Clement P. Pathology of gamete and zygote transport: cervical, endometrial, myometrial, and tubal factors in infertility. In: Kraus F, Damjanov I, Kaufman N, eds. *Pathology of reproductive failure*. Baltimore: Williams & Wilkins, 1991:140–194.
110. Cook C. Luteal-phase defect. *Clin Obstet Gynecol* 1991;34:198–210.
111. Daly DC. Current treatment strategies for luteal phase deficiency. *Clin Obstet Gynecol* 1991;34:222–231.
112. Jones GS. Luteal phase defect: a review of pathophysiology. *Curr Opin Obstet Gynecol* 1991;3:641–648.
113. Nakajima ST, Gibson M. Pathophysiology of luteal-phase deficiency in human reproduction. *Clin Obstet Gynecol* 1991;34:157–179.
114. Olive DL. The prevalence and epidemiology of luteal-phase deficiency in normal and infertile women. *Clin Obstet Gynecol* 1991;34:157–166.
115. Thornburgh I, Anderson MC. The endometrial deficient secretory phase. *Histopathology* 1997;30:11–15.
116. Ginsburg KA. Luteal phase defect: etiology, diagnosis and management. *Endocrinol Metab Clin North Am* 1992;21:85–104.
117. Benda J. Clomiphene's effect on endometrium in infertility. *Int J Gynecol Pathol* 1992;11:273–282.
118. March CM, Mishell DJ, McNeile LG. Luteal phase defect [Letter; Comment]. *Fertil Steril* 1990;53:189–190.
119. Jordan J, Craig K, Clifton DK, Soules MR. Luteal phase defect: the sensitivity and specificity of diagnostic methods in common clinical use [Comments]. *Fertil Steril* 1994;62:54–62.
120. Castelbaum AJ, Lessey BA. Corpus luteum defect "alloyed gold standard" [Letter; Comment]. *Fertil Steril* 1995;63:427–428.
121. Wentz A. Endometrial biopsy in the evaluation of infertility. *Fertil Steril* 1980;33:121–124.
122. Wentz AC, Kossoy LR, Parker RA. The impact of luteal phase inadequacy in an infertile population. *Am J Obstet Gynecol* 1990;162:937–943.
123. Li T, Dockery P, Rogers A, Cooke I. A quantitative study of endometrial development in the luteal phase: comparison between women with unexplained infertility and normal fertility. *Br J Obstet Gynaecol* 1990;97:576–582.
124. Li TC, Dockery P, Cooke ID. Endometrial development in the luteal phase of women with various types of infertility: comparison with women of normal fertility. *Hum Reprod* 1991;6:325–330.
125. Karamardian L, Grimes D. Luteal phase deficiency: effect of treatment on pregnancy rates. *Am J Obstet Gynecol* 1992;167:1391–1398.
126. Jones G. Luteal phase insufficiency. *Clin Obstet Gynecol* 1973;16:255–273.
127. Bell CD, Ostrezega E. The significance of secretory features and coincident hyperplastic changes in endometrial biopsy specimens. *Hum Pathol* 1987;18:830–838.
128. Cruz-Aquino M, Shenker L, Blaustein A. Pseudosarcoma of the endometrium. *Obstet Gynecol* 1967;29:93–96.
129. Hesla J, Kurman R, Rock J. Histologic effects of oral contraceptives on the uterine corpus and cervix. *Semin Reprod Endocrinol* 1989;7:213–219.
130. Henzl M. Contraceptive hormones and their clinical use. In: Yen S, Jaffe R, eds. *Reproductive endocrinology: physiology pathophysiology and clinical management*, 3rd ed. Philadelphia, London, Toronto: WB Saunders, 1991:807–829.
131. Leather A, Savvas M, Studd J. Endometrial histology and bleeding patterns after eight years of continuous combined estrogen and progestogen therapy in postmenopausal women. *Obstet Gynecol* 1991;78:1008–1010.
132. Byrjalsen I, Thormann L, Meinecke B, Riis B, Christiansen C. Sequential estrogen and progestogen therapy: assessment of progestational effects on the postmenopausal endometrium. *Obstet Gynecol* 1992;79:523–528.
133. Ober W. Effects of oral and intrauterine administration of contraceptives on the uterus. *Hum Pathol* 1977;8:513–527.
134. Ludwig H. The morphologic response of the human endometrium to long-term treatment with progestational agents. *Am J Obstet Gynecol* 1982;142:796–808.
135. Hertig A. Gestational hyperplasia of endometrium: a morphologic correlation of ova, endometrium, and corpora lutea during early pregnancy. *Lab Invest* 1964;13:1153–1191.
136. Mazur M, Hendrickson M, Kempson R. Optically clear nuclei: an alteration of endometrial epithelium in the presence of trophoblast. *Am J Surg Pathol* 1983;7:415–423.
137. Mazur MT, Duncan DA, Younger JB. Endometrial biopsy in the cycle of conception: histologic and lectin histochemical evaluation. *Fertil Steril* 1989;51:764–769.
138. Buxton C, Olson L. Endometrial biopsy inadvertently taken during conception cycle. *Am J Obstet Gynecol* 1969;105:702–706.
139. Wentz A, Herbert C, Maxson W, Hill G, Pittaway D. Cycle of conception endometrial biopsy. *Fertil Steril* 1986;46:196–199.
140. Herbert CM, Hill GA, Maxson WS, Wentz AC, Osteen KG. Use of a sensitive urine pregnancy test before endometrial biopsies taken in the late luteal phase. *Fertil Steril* 1990;53:162–164.
141. Kaminski PF, Lyon DS. Implications of sampling the implantation site in the endometrial biopsy for infertility. *J Reprod Med* 1990;35:208–210.
142. Kjer J, Eldon K. The diagnostic value of the Arias-Stella phenomenon. *Zentralbl Gynakol* 1982;104:753–756.
143. Mazur M, Priest J. Clear cell leiomyoma (leiomyoblastoma) of the uterus: ultrastructural observations. *Ultrastruct Pathol* 1986;10:249–255.
144. Angel E, Davis J, Nagle R. Immunohistochemical demonstration of placental hormones in the diagnosis of uterine versus ectopic pregnancy. *Am J Clin Pathol* 1985;84:705–709.
145. O'Connor D, Kurman R. Intermediate trophoblast in uterine curettings in the diagnosis of ectopic pregnancy. *Obstet Gynecol* 1988;72:665–670.
146. Arias-Stella J. Atypical endometrial changes produced by chorionic tissue. *Hum Pathol* 1972;3:450–453.
147. Silverberg S. Arias-Stella phenomenon in spontaneous and therapeutic abortion. *Am J Obstet Gynecol* 1972;112:777–780.
148. Arias-Stella J. Gestational endometrium. In: Hertig A, Norris H, Abell M, eds. *The uterus*. Baltimore: Williams & Wilkins, 1973:185–212.
149. Fienberg R, Lloyd H. The Arias-Stella reaction in early normal pregnancy: an involutional phenomenon. The ovary-placenta changeover as a possible cause. *Hum Pathol* 1974;5:183–190.
150. Clement PB, Young RH, Scully RE. Nontrophoblastic pathology of the female genital tract and peritoneum associated with pregnancy. *Semin Diagn Pathol* 1989a;6:372–406.
151. Huettner PC, Gersell DJ. Arias-Stella reaction in nonpregnant women: a clinicopathologic study of nine cases. *Int J Gynecol Pathol* 1994;13:241–247.
152. Milchgrub S, Sandstad J. Arias-Stella reaction in fallopian tube epithelium: a light and electron microscopic study with a review of the literature. *Am J Clin Pathol* 1991;95:892–895.
153. Young RH, Clement PB. Pseudoneoplastic glandular lesions of the uterine cervix. *Semin Diagn Pathol* 1991;8:234–249.
154. Cartwright PS. Diagnosis of ectopic pregnancy. *Obstet Gynecol Clin North Am* 1991;18:19–37.
155. Lientig C, Korat A, Deutch M, Brandes JM. Decidual vascular changes in early pregnancy as a marker for intrauterine pregnancy. *Am J Clin Pathol* 1988;90:284–288.
156. Ober W, Grady H. Sub-involution of the placental site. *Bull N Y Acad Med* 1961;37:713–730.
157. Andrew AC, Bulmer JN, Wells M, Morrison L, Buckley CH. Subinvolution of the uteroplacental arteries in the human placental bed. *Histopathology* 1989;15:395–405.
158. Young RH, Kurman RJ, Scully RE. Placental site nodules and plaques: a clinicopathologic analysis of 20 cases. *Am J Surg Pathol* 1990;14:1001–1009.
159. Huettner PC, Gersell DJ. Placental site nodule: a clinicopathologic study of 38 cases. *Int J Gynecol Pathol* 1994;13:191–198.
160. Genest DR, Brodsky G, Lage JA. Localized endometrial proliferations associated with pregnancy: clinical and histopathologic features of 11 cases. *Hum Pathol* 1995;26:1233–1240.
161. Johannsson E, Fournier K, Riotton G. Regeneration of the human endometrium and presence of inflammatory cells following diagnostic curettage. *Acta Obstet Gynecol Scand* 1981;60:451–457.
162. Winkler B, Reumann W, Mitao M, Gallo L, Richart R, Crum C. Chlamydial endometritis: a histological and immunohistochemical analysis. *Am J Surg Pathol* 1984;8:771–778.
163. Jones R, Mammel J, Shepard M, Fisher R. Recovery of *Chlamydia trachomatis* from the endometrium of women at risk for chlamydial infection. *Am J Obstet Gynecol* 1986;155:35–39.

164. Moyer D, Mishell DJ, Bell J. Reactions of human endometrium to the intrauterine device. I. Correlation of the endometrial histology with the bacterial environment of the uterus following short-term insertion of the IUD. *Am J Obstet Gynecol* 1970;106:799–809.
165. Moyer D, Mishell DJ. Reactions of human endometrium to the intrauterine foreign body. II. Long term effects on the endometrial histology and cytology. *Am J Obstet Gynecol* 1971;111:66–80.
166. Cadena D, Cavanzo F, Leone C, Taylor H. Chronic endometritis: a comparative clinicopathologic study. *Obstet Gynecol* 1973; 41:733–738.
167. Rotterdam H. Chronic endometritis: a clinicopathologic study. *Pathol Annu* 1978;13:209–231.
168. Greenwood S, Moran J. Chronic endometritis: morphologic and clinical observations. *Obstet Gynecol* 1981;58:176–184.
169. Buckley H. Endometrial inflammation. In: Fox H, ed. *Haines and Taylor: obstetrical and gynaecological pathology*, 4th ed. New York: Churchill Livingstone, 1995:405–420.
170. Kiviat NB, Wolner-Hanssen P, Eschenbach DA, et al. Endometrial histopathology in patients with culture-proved upper genital tract infection and laparoscopically diagnosed acute salpingitis. *Am J Surg Pathol* 1990;14:167–175.
171. Stern RA, Svoboda NS, Frank TS. Analysis of chronic endometritis for *Chlamydia trachomatis* by polymerase chain reaction. *Hum Pathol* 1996;27:1085–1088.
172. Korn AP, Bolan G, Padian N, Ohm SM, Schachter J, Landers DV. Plasma cell endometritis in women with symptomatic bacterial vaginosis. *Obstet Gynecol* 1995;85:387–390.
173. Platt L, Yonekura M, Ledger W. The role of anaerobic bacteria in postpartum endomyometritis. *Am J Obstet Gynecol* 1979;135: 814–817.
174. Barua R, Kirkland J, Petrucco O. Xanthogranulomatous endometritis: case report. *Pathology* 1978;10:161–164.
175. Dawagne M, Silverberg S. Foam cells in endometrial carcinoma: a clinicopathologic study. *Gynecol Oncol* 1982;13:67–75.
176. Ladefoged C, Lorentzen M. Xanthogranulomatous inflammation of the female genital tract [Comments]. *Histopathology* 1988; 13:541–551.
177. Nogales-Ortiz F, Tarancon I, Nogales FJ. The pathology of female genital tuberculosis: a 31-year study of 1,436 cases. *Obstet Gynecol* 1979;53:422–428.
178. Bazaz-Malik G, Maheshwari B, Lal N. Tuberculous endometritis: a clinicopathological study of 1,000 cases. *Br J Obstet Gynaecol* 1983 90:84–86.
179. Margolis K, Wranz PA, Kruger TF, Joubert JJ, Odendaal HJ. Genital tuberculosis at Tygerberg Hospital: prevalence, clinical presentation and diagnosis. *S Afr Med J* 1992;81:12–15.
180. Cowan BD, Morrison JC. Management of abnormal genital bleeding in girls and women [Comments]. *N Engl J Med* 1991;324:1710–1715.
181. Rueda RJ, Hemmings R, Falcone T, Tulandi T. Dysfunctional uterine bleeding: a reappraisal. *Curr Probl Obstet Gynecol Fertil* 1991,(May/June):70–96.
182. Awwad JT, Toth TL, Schiff I. Abnormal uterine bleeding in the perimenopause. *Int J Fertil Menopausal Stud* 1993;38:261–269.
183. Bayer SR, DeCherney AH. Clinical manifestations and treatment of dysfunctional uterine bleeding. *JAMA* 1993;269:1823–1828.
184. Galle PC, McRae MA. Abnormal uterine bleeding: finding and treating the cause. *Postgrad Med* 1993;93:73–76, 80–81.
185. Falcone T, Desjardins C, Bourque J, Granger L, Hemmings R, Quiros E. Dysfunctional uterine bleeding in adolescents. *J Reprod Med* 1994;39:761–764.
186. Speroff L, Glass R, Kase N. *Clinical gynecologic endocrinology and infertility*, 5th ed. Baltimore: Williams & Wilkins, 1994.
187. Brenner PF. Differential diagnosis of abnormal uterine bleeding. *Am J Obstet Gynecol* 1996;175:766–769.
188. Chuong CJ, Brenner PF. Management of abnormal uterine bleeding. *Am J Obstet Gynecol* 1996;175:787–792.
189. Lavin C. Dysfunctional uterine bleeding in adolescents. *Curr Opin Pediatr* 1996;8:328–332.
190. Long CA. Evaluation of patients with abnormal uterine bleeding. *Am J Obstet Gynecol* 1996;175:784–786.
191. Deligeoroglou E. Dysfunctional uterine bleeding. *Ann N Y Acad Sci* 1997;816:158–164.
192. Geller SE, Bernstein SJ, Harlow SD. The decision-making process for the treatment of abnormal uterine bleeding. *J Womens Health* 1997;6:559–567.
193. Caufriez A. Menstrual disorders in adolescence: pathophysiology and treatment. *Horm Res* 1991;36:156–159.
194. Meyer V, Malkasian G, Dockerty M, Decker D. Postmenopausal bleeding from atrophic endometrium. *Obstet Gynecol* 1971;38: 731–738.
195. Baitlon D, Hadley J. Endometrial biopsy: pathologic findings in 3,600 biopsies from selected patients. *Am J Clin Pathol* 1975;63:9–15.
196. Choo Y, Mak K, Hsu C, Wong T, Ma H. Postmenopausal uterine bleeding of nonorganic cause. *Obstet Gynecol* 1985;66:225–228.
197. Archer D, Mcintyreseltman K, Wilborn W, et al. Endometrial morphology in asymptomatic postmenopausal women. *Am J Obstet Gynecol* 1991;165:317–322.
198. Nedoss B. Dysfunctional uterine bleeding: relation of endometrial histology to outcome. *Am J Obstet Gynecol* 1971;109:103–107.
199. Speroff L, Glass RH, Kase NG. *Clinical gynecologic endocrinology and infertility*, 5th ed. Baltimore: Williams & Wilkins, Chapter 6 (Anovulation) 1994:1029.
200. Whitehead M, Townsend P, Pryse-Davies J, Ryder T, King R. Effects of estrogens and progestins on the biochemistry and morphology of the postmenopausal endometrium. *N Engl J Med* 1981;305: 1599–1605.
201. Chamlian D, Taylor H. Endometrial hyperplasia in young women. *Obstet Gynecol* 1970;36:659–666.
202. Fraser I, Baird D. Endometrial cystic glandular hyperplasia in adolescent girls. *J Obstet Gynaecol Br Commonw* 1972;79:1009–1015.
203. Welch W, Scully R. Precancerous lesions of the endometrium. *Hum Pathol* 1977;8:503–512.
204. Fox H, Buckley C. The endometrial hyperplasias and their relationship to endometrial neoplasia. *Histopathology* 1982;6:493–510.
205. Scully R. Definition of endometrial carcinoma precursors. *Clin Obstet Gynecol* 1982;25:39–48.
206. Fox H. Atypical hyperplasia and adenocarcinoma of the endometrium. In: Morrow C, Bonnar J, O'Brien T, Gibbons W, eds. *Recent clinical developments in gynecologic oncology*. New York: Raven Press, 1983:69–81.
207. Gelfand M, Ferenczy A. Advances in diagnosis and treatment of endometrial hyperplasia and carcinoma. *Compr Ther* 1983;9:12–23.
208. Winkler B, Alvarez S, Richart R, Crum C. Pitfalls in the diagnosis of endometrial neoplasia. *Obstet Gynecol* 1984;64:185–194.
209. Kraus F. High-risk and premalignant lesions of the endometrium. *Am J Surg Pathol* 1985;9(3)[Suppl]:31–40.
210. Kurman R, Kaminski P, Norris H. The behavior of endometrial hyperplasia: a long-term study of "untreated" hyperplasia in 170 patients. *Cancer* 1985;56:403–412.
211. Norris H, Connor M, Kurman R. Preinvasive lesions of the endometrium. *Clin Obstet Gynaecol* 1986;13:725–738.
212. Silverberg S. Hyperplasia and carcinoma of the endometrium. *Semin Diagn Pathol* 1988;5:135–153.
213. Ferenczy A, Gelfand M. The biologic significance of cytologic atypia in progestogen-treated endometrial hyperplasia. *Am J Obstet Gynecol* 1989;160:126–131.
214. Longacre TA, Kempson RL, Hendrickson MR. Endometrial hyperplasia, metaplasia and carcinoma. In: Fox H, ed. *Haines and Taylor: obstetrical and gynaecological pathology*, 4th ed. New York: Churchill Livingstone, 1995:421–510.
215. Hendrickson M, Kempson R. The differential diagnosis of endometrial adenocarcinoma: some viewpoints concerning a common diagnostic problem. *Pathology* 1980;12:35–61.
216. Fenoglio C, Crum C, Ferenczy A. Endometrial hyperplasia and carcinoma: Are ultrastructural, biochemical and immunocytochemical studies useful in distinguishing between them? *Pathol Res Pract* 1982;174:257–284.
217. Hendrickson M, Ross J, Kempson R. Toward the development of morphologic criteria for well-differentiated adenocarcinoma of the endometrium. *Am J Surg Pathol* 1983;7:819–838.
218. Huang S, Amparo E, Fu Y. Endometrial hyperplasia: histologic classification and behavior. *Surg Pathol* 1988;1:215–229.
219. Lee KR, Scully RE. Complex endometrial hyperplasia and carcinoma in adolescents and young women 15 to 20 years of age: a report of 10 cases. *Int J Gynecol Pathol* 1989;8:201–213.
220. Yen S. Chronic anovulation caused by peripheral endocrine disorders. In: Yen S, Jaffe R, eds. *Reproductive endocrinology: physiology, pathophysiology and clinical management*, 3rd ed. Philadelphia, London, Toronto: WB Saunders, 1991:576–630.

221. Yen S. Chronic anovulation due to CNS-hypothalamic pituitary dysfunction. In: Yen S, Jaffe R, eds. *Reproductive endocrinology: physiology, pathophysiology and clinical management*, 3rd ed. Philadelphia, London, Toronto: WB Saunders, 1991:631–684.
222. Andersson M, Storm H, Mouridsen H. Incidence of new primary cancers after adjuvant tamoxifen therapy and radiotherapy for early breast cancer. *J Natl Cancer Inst* 1991;83:1013–1017.
223. Jordan VC. The role of tamoxifen in the treatment and prevention of breast cancer. *Curr Probl Cancer* 1992;16:129–175.
224. Wolf D, Jordan V. Gynecologic complications associated with long-term adjuvant tamoxifen therapy for breast cancer. *Gynecol Oncol* 1992;45:118–128.
225. Barakat RR. Benign and hyperplastic endometrial changes associated with tamoxifen use. *Oncology (Huntingt)* 1997;11:35–37.
226. Tavassoli F, Kraus F. Endometrial lesions in uteri resected for atypical endometrial hyperplasia. *Am J Clin Pathol* 1978;70:770–779.
227. Sherman A, Brown S. The precursors of endometrial carcinoma. *Am J Obstet Gynecol* 1979;135:947–956.
228. Kistner R. Treatment of hyperplasia and carcinoma in situ of the endometrium. *Clin Obstet Gynecol* 1982;25:63–74.
229. Wentz W. Progestin therapy in lesions of the endometrium. *Semin Oncol* 1985;12:23–27.
230. Soh E, Sato K. Clinical effects of danazol on endometrial hyperplasia in menopausal and postmenopausal women. *Cancer* 1990;66:983–988.
231. Van Bogaert L-J. Clinicopathologic findings in endometrial polyps. *Obstet Gynecol* 1988;71:771–773.
232. Silverberg S, Kurman R. *Tumors of the uterine corpus and gestational trophoblastic disease*. Washington, D.C.: AFIP, 1992. (Rosai J, ed. Atlas of tumor pathology, 3rd series, fascicle 3.)
233. Barwick K, LiVolsi V. Heterologous mixed mullerian tumor confined to an endometrial polyp. *Obstet Gynecol* 1979 53:512–514.
234. Silva E, Jenkins R. Serous carcinoma in endometrial polyps. *Mod Pathol* 1990;3:120–128.
235. Pettersson B, Adami H-O, Lindgren A, Hesselius I. Endometrial polyps and hyperplasia as risk factors for endometrial carcinoma: a case-control study of curettage specimens. *Acta Obstet Gynecol Scand* 1985;64:653–659.
236. Nuovo M, Nuovo G, McCaffrey R, Levine R, Barron B, Winkler B. Endometrial polyps in postmenopausal patients receiving tamoxifen. *Int J Gynecol Pathol* 1989;8:125–131.
237. Corley D, Rowe J, Curtis M, Hogan W, Nouroff J, LiVolsi V. Postmenopausal bleeding from unusual endometrial polyps in women on chronic tamoxifen therapy. *Obstet Gynecol* 1992;79:111–16.
238. Silva EG, Tornos CS, Follen MM. Malignant neoplasms of the uterine corpus in patients treated for breast carcinoma: the effects of tamoxifen. *Int J Gynecol Pathol* 1994;13:248–258.
239. Burke TW, Tortolero LG, Malpica A, et al. Endometrial hyperplasia and endometrial cancer. *Obstet Gynecol Clin North Am* 1996;23:411–456.
240. Zaino RJ. Taking another look at endometrial adenocarcinoma [Editorial]. *Int J Gynecol Pathol* 1996;15:187–190.
241. Burke TW, Eifel PJ, Muggia FM. Cancer of the uterine body. In: DeVita V, Hellman S, Rosenberg S, eds. *Cancer: principles and practice of oncology*, 5th ed. Philadelphia: Lippincott–Raven Publishers, 1997:1478–1499.
242. Connelly P, Alberhasky R, Christopherson W. Carcinoma of the endometrium. III. Analysis of 865 cases of adenocarcinoma and adenoacanthoma. *Obstet Gynecol* 1982;59:569–575.
243. Christopherson W, Connelly P, Alberhasky R. Carcinoma of the endometrium. V. An analysis of prognosticators in patients with favorable subtypes and stage I disease. *Cancer* 1983;51:1705–1709.
244. Eifel P, Ross J, Hendrickson M, Cox R, Kempson R, Martinez A. Adenocarcinoma of the endometrium: analysis of 256 cases with disease limited to the uterine corpus. Treatment comparisons. *Cancer* 1983;52:1026–1031.
245. Creasman W, Morrow C, Bundy B, Homesley H, Graham J, Heller P. Surgical pathologic spread patterns of endometrial cancer: a Gynecologic Oncology Group study. *Cancer* 1987;60:2035–2041.
246. Fanning J, Evans M, Peters A, Samuel M, Harmon E, Bates J. Endometrial adenocarcinoma histologic subtypes: clinical and pathologic profile. *Gynecol Oncol* 1989;32:288–291.
247. Anonymous. Announcements: FIGO stages—1988 revision. *Gynecol Oncol* 1989;35:125–127.
248. Creasman W. New gynecologic cancer staging. *Obstet Gynecol* 1990;75:287–288.
249. Nielsen A, Thomsen H, Nyholm H. Evaluation of the reproducibility of the revised 1988 International Federation of Gynecology and Obstetrics Grading System of endometrial cancers with special emphasis on nuclear grading. *Cancer* 1991;68:2303–2309.
250. Sidawy MK, Silverberg SG. Endometrial carcinoma: pathologic factors of therapeutic and prognostic significance. *Pathol Annu* 1992;27:153–185.
251. Zaino RJ, Silverberg SG, Norris HJ, Bundy BN, Morrow CP, Okagaki T. The prognostic value of nuclear versus architectural grading in endometrial adenocarcinoma: a Gynecologic Oncology Group study. *Int J Gynecol Pathol* 1994;13:29–36.
252. Zaino RJ, Kurman RJ, Diana KL, Morrow CP. The utility of the revised International Federation of Gynecology and Obstetrics histologic grading of endometrial adenocarcinoma using a defined nuclear grading system: a Gynecologic Oncology Group study. *Cancer* 1995;75:81–86.
253. Aalders J, Abeler V, Kolstad P, Onsrud M. Postoperative external irradiation and prognostic parameters in stage I endometrial carcinoma: clinical and histopathologic study of 540 patients. *Obstet Gynecol* 1980;56:419–427.
254. Berek J, Hacker N, Hatch K, Young R. Uterine corpus and cervical cancer. *Curr Probl Cancer* 1988;12:61–131.
255. Mittal K, Barwick K. Diffusely infiltrating adenocarcinoma of the endometrium: a subtype with poor prognosis. *Am J Surg Pathol* 1988;12:754–758.
256. Morrow CP, Bundy BN, Kurman RJ, et al. Relationship between surgical-pathological risk factors and outcome in clinical stage I and II carcinoma of the endometrium: a Gynecologic Oncology Group study. *Gynecol Oncol* 1991;40:55–65.
257. Gal D, Recio FO, Zamurovic D. The new International Federation of Gynecology and Obstetrics surgical staging and survival rates in early endometrial carcinoma. *Cancer* 1992;69:200–202.
258. Hawwa ZM, Nahhas WA, Copenhaver EH. Postmenopausal bleeding. *Lahey Clin Found Bull* 1970;19:61–70.
259. Bokhman JV. Two pathogenetic types of endometrial carcinoma. *Gynecol Oncol* 1983;15:10–17.
260. Sherman ME, Bur ME, Kurman RJ. p53 in endometrial cancer and its putative precursors: evidence for diverse pathways of tumorigenesis. *Hum Pathol* 1995;26:1268–1274.
261. Lax SF, Kurman RJ. A dualistic model for endometrial carcinogenesis based on immunohistochemical and molecular genetic analyses. *Verh Dtsch Ges Pathol* 1997;81:228–232.
262. Pere H, Tapper J, Wahlström T, Knuutila S, Butzow R. Distinct chromosomal imbalances in uterine serous and endometrioid carcinomas. *Cancer Res* 1998;58:892–895.
263. Fearon ER, Vogelstein B. A genetic model for colorectal tumorigenesis. *Cell* 1990;61:759–767.
264. Silverberg S, Makowski E, Roche W. Endometrial carcinoma in women under 40 years of age: comparison of cases in oral contraceptive users and non-users. *Cancer* 1977;39:592–598.
265. Crissman J, Azoury R, Barnes A, Schellhas H. Endometrial carcinoma in women 40 years of age or younger. *Obstet Gynecol* 1981;57:699–704.
266. Ostor A, Adam R, Gutteridge B, Fortune D. Endometrial carcinoma in young women. *Aust N Z J Obstet Gynaecol* 1982;22:38–42.
267. Gallup DG, Stock RJ. Adenocarcinoma of the endometrium in women 40 years of age or younger. *Obstet Gynecol* 1984;64:417–420.
268. Quinn M, Kneale B, Fortune D. Endometrial carcinoma in premenopausal women: a clinicopathological study. *Gynecol Oncol* 1985;20:298–306.
269. Wilkinson E, Friedrich EJ, Mattingly R, Regali J, Garancis J. Turner's syndrome with endometrial adenocarcinoma and stilbestrol therapy. *Obstet Gynecol* 1973;42:193–200.
270. Fechner R, Kaufman R. Endometrial adenocarcinoma in Stein-Leventhal syndrome. *Cancer* 1974;34:444–452.
271. McCarroll A, Montgomery D, Harley J, McKeown E, MacHenry J. Endometrial carcinoma after cyclical oestrogen-progestogen therapy for Turner's syndrome. *Br J Obstet Gynaecol* 1975;82:421–423.
272. Wood G, Boronow R. Endometrial adenocarcinoma and the polycystic ovary syndrome. *Am J Obstet Gynecol* 1976;124:140–142.
273. McDonald T, Malkasian G, Gaffey T. Endometrial cancer associated with feminizing ovarian tumor and polycystic ovarian disease. *Obstet Gynecol* 1977;49:654–658.
274. Kim YB, Holschneider CH, Ghosh K, Nieberg RK, Montz FJ. Progestin alone as primary treatment of endometrial carcinoma in premenopausal women: report of seven cases and review of the literature. *Cancer* 1997;79:320–327.

275. Randall TC, Kurman RJ. Progestin treatment of atypical hyperplasia and well-differentiated carcinoma of the endometrium in women under age 40. *Obstet Gynecol* 1997;90:434–440.
276. Scully R. Estrogens and endometrial carcinoma. *Hum Pathol* 1977;8:481–483.
277. Robboy S, Bradley R. Changing trends and prognostic features in endometrial cancer associated with exogenous estrogen therapy. *Obstet Gynecol* 1979;54:269–277.
278. Collins J, Donner A, Allen L, Adams O. Oestrogen use and survival in endometrial cancer. *Lancet* 1980;2:961–964.
279. Silverberg S, Mullen D, Faraci J, et al. Endometrial carcinoma: clinical-pathologic comparison of cases in postmenopausal women receiving and not receiving exogenous estrogens. *Cancer* 1980;45: 3018–3026.
280. British Gynaecological Cancer Group. Oestrogen replacement and endometrial cancer: a statement by the British Gynaecological Cancer Group. *Lancet* 1981;1:1359–1360.
281. Davies J, Rosenshein N, Antunes C, Stolley P. A review of the risk factors for endometrial carcinoma. *Obstet Gynecol Surv* 1981;36: 107–116.
282. Horwitz R, Feinstein A, Vidone R, Sommers S, Robboy S. Histopathologic distinctions in the relationship of estrogens and endometrial cancer. *JAMA* 1981;246:1425–1427.
283. Smith D, Prentice R, Bauermeister D. Endometrial carcinoma: histopathology, survival, and exogenous estrogens. *Gynecol Obstet Invest* 1981;12:169–179.
284. Mahboubi E, Eyler N, Wynder E. Epidemiology of cancer of the endometrium. *Clin Obstet Gynecol* 1982;25:5–17.
285. Robboy S, Miller A, Kurman R. The pathologic features and behavior of endometrial carcinoma associated with exogenous estrogen administration. *Pathol Res Pract* 1982;174:237–256.
286. Lipsett M. Hormones, medications, and cancer. *Cancer* 1983;51: 2426–2429.
287. Bhagavan B, Parmley T, Rosenshein N, Jefferys J, Grisso J, Stolley P. Comparison of estrogen-induced hyperplasia to endometrial carcinoma. *Obstet Gynecol* 1984;64:12–15.
288. McGonigle KF, Karlan BY, Barbuto DA, Leuchter RS, Lagasse LD, Judd HL. Development of endometrial cancer in women on estrogen and progestin hormone replacement therapy. *Gynecol Oncol* 1994;55:126–132.
289. Fornander T, Rutqvist LE. Adjuvant tamoxifen and second cancers [Letter]. *Lancet* 1989;1:616.
290. Fornander T, Rutqvist LE, Cedermark B, et al. Adjuvant tamoxifen in early breast cancer: occurrence of new primary cancers. *Lancet* 1989;1:117–120.
291. Fisher B, Costantino JP, Redmond CK, Fisher ER, Wickerham DL, Cronin WM. Endometrial cancer in tamoxifen-treated breast cancer patients: findings from the National Surgical Adjuvant Breast and Bowel Project (NSABP) B-14 [Comments]. *J Natl Cancer Inst* 1994;86:527–537.
292. Rutqvist LE, Johansson H, Signomklao T, Johansson U, Fornander T, Wilking N. Adjuvant tamoxifen therapy for early stage breast cancer and second primary malignancies: Stockholm Breast Cancer Study Group [Comments]. *J Natl Cancer Inst* 1995;87:645–651.
293. Cohen I, Altaras MM, Shapira J, Tepper R, Beyth Y. Postmenopausal tamoxifen treatment and endometrial pathology. *Obstet Gynecol Surv* 1994;49:823–829.
294. Cohen I, Altaras MM, Shapira J, et al. Time-dependent effect of tamoxifen therapy on endometrial pathology in asymptomatic postmenopausal breast cancer patients. *Int J Gynecol Pathol* 1996;15: 152–157.
295. Fisher B. Commentary on endometrial cancer deaths in tamoxifen-treated breast cancer patients [Comments]. *J Clin Oncol* 1996;14: 1027–1039.
296. Cheng WF, Lin HH, Torng PL, Huang SC. Comparison of endometrial changes among symptomatic tamoxifen-treated and nontreated premenopausal and postmenopausal breast cancer patients. *Gynecol Oncol* 1997;66:233–237.
297. Berliere M, Charles A, Galant C, Donnez J. Uterine side effects of tamoxifen: a need for systematic pretreatment screening. *Obstet Gynecol* 1998;91:40–44.
298. Killackey MA, Hakes TB, Pierce VK. Endometrial adenocarcinoma in breast cancer patients receiving antiestrogens. *Cancer Treat Rep* 1985;69:237–238.
299. Malfetano JH. Tamoxifen-associated endometrial carcinoma in postmenopausal breast cancer patients [Comments]. *Gynecol Oncol* 1990;39:82–84.
300. De Muylder X, Neven P, De Somer M, Van Belle Y, Vanderick G, De Muylder E. Endometrial lesions in patients undergoing tamoxifen therapy. *Int J Gynaecol Obstet* 1991;36:127–130.
301. Gal D, Kopel S, Bashevkin M, Lebowicz J, Lev R, Tancer ML. Oncogenic potential of tamoxifen on endometria of postmenopausal women with breast cancer: preliminary report. *Gynecol Oncol* 1991;42:120–123.
302. Barakat RR, Wong G, Curtin JP, Vlamis V, Hoskins WJ. Tamoxifen use in breast cancer patients who subsequently develop corpus cancer is not associated with a higher incidence of adverse histologic features [Comments]. *Gynecol Oncol* 1994;55:164–168.
303. Mecklin JP, Jarvinen HJ. Tumor spectrum in cancer family syndrome (hereditary nonpolyposis colorectal cancer). *Cancer* 1991;68: 1109–1112.
304. Watson P, Lynch HT. Extracolonic cancer in hereditary nonpolyposis colorectal cancer. *Cancer* 1993;71:677–685.
305. Hendrickson M, Ross J, Eifel P, Cox R, Martinez A, Kempson R. Adenocarcinoma of the endometrium: analysis of 256 cases with carcinoma limited to the uterine corpus. Pathology review and analysis of prognostic variables. *Gynecol Oncol* 1982;13:373–392.
306. Piver M, Lele S, Barlow J, Blumenson L. Paraaortic lymph node evaluation in stage I endometrial carcinoma. *Obstet Gynecol* 1982; 59:97–100.
307. DiSaia PJ, Creasman WT. *Clinical gynecologic oncology*, 5th ed, vol 8. St. Louis: Mosby, 1997:657.
308. Hanson MB, van Nagell, JR Jr, Powell DE, et al. The prognostic significance of lymph-vascular space invasion in stage I endometrial cancer. *Cancer* 1985;55:1753–1757.
309. Sivridis E, Buckley C, Fox H. The prognostic significance of lymphatic vascular space invasion in endometrial adenocarcinoma. *Br J Obstet Gynaecol* 1987;94:991–994.
310. Gal D, Recio F, Zamurovic D, Tancer M. Lymph vascular space involvement: a prognostic indicator in endometrial adenocarcinoma. *Gynecol Oncol* 1991;42:142–145.
311. Ambros RA, Kurman RJ. Combined assessment of vascular and myometrial invasion as a model to predict prognosis in stage I endometrioid adenocarcinoma of the uterine corpus. *Cancer* 1992;69:1424–1431.
312. Szpak C, Creasman W, Vollmer R, Johnson W. Prognostic value of cytologic examination of peritoneal washings in patients with endometrial carcinoma. *Acta Cytol* 1981;25:640–646.
313. Lurain JR, Rumsey NK, Schink JC, Wallemark CB, Chmiel JS. Prognostic significance of positive peritoneal cytology in clinical stage I adenocarcinoma of the endometrium. *Obstet Gynecol* 1989;74: 175–179.
314. Turner DA, Gershenson DM, Atkinson N, Sneige N, Wharton AT. The prognostic significance of peritoneal cytology for stage I endometrial cancer. *Obstet Gynecol* 1989;74:775–780.
315. Grimshaw RN, Tupper WC, Fraser RC, Tompkins MG, Jeffrey JF. Prognostic value of peritoneal cytology in endometrial carcinoma. *Gynecol Oncol* 1990;36:97–100.
316. Doering D, Barnhill D, Weiser E, Burke T, Woodward J, Park R. Intraoperative evaluation of depth of myometrial invasion in stage I endometrial adenocarcinoma. *Obstet Gynecol* 1989;74:930–933.
317. Malviya V, Deppe G, Malone JJ, Sundareson A, Lawrence W. Reliability of frozen section examination in identifying poor prognostic indicators in stage I endometrial adenocarcinoma. *Gynecol Oncol* 1989;34:299–304.
318. Noumoff JS, Menzin A, Mikuta J, Lusk EJ, Morgan M, LiVolsi VA. The ability to evaluate prognostic variables on frozen section in hysterectomies performed for endometrial carcinoma. *Gynecol Oncol* 1991;42:202–208.
319. Shim JU, Rose PG, Reale FR, Soto H, Tak WK, Hunter RE. Accuracy of frozen-section diagnosis at surgery in clinical stage I and II endometrial carcinoma. *Am J Obstet Gynecol* 1992;166:1335–1338.
320. Lutz M, Underwood PJ, Kreutner AJ, Miller M. Endometrial carcinoma: a new method of classification of therapeutic and prognostic significance. *Gynecol Oncol* 1978;6:83–94.
321. Templeton A. Reporting of myometrial invasion by endometrial cancer. *Histopathology* 1982;6:733.
322. Longacre T, Hendrickson M. Diffusely infiltrative endometrial adenocarcinoma: an adenoma malignum pattern of myoinvasion. *Am J Surg Pathol* 1999 (*in press*).
323. Hall J, Young R, Nelson JJ. The prognostic significance of adenomyosis in endometrial carcinoma. *Gynecol Oncol* 1984;17:32–40.

324. Jacques S, Lawrence W. Endometrial adenocarcinoma with variable-level myometrial involvement limited to adenomyosis: a clinicopathologic study of 23 cases. Gynecol Oncol 1990;37:401–407.
325. Boronow R, Morrow C, Creasman W, et al. Surgical staging in endometrial cancer: clinical-pathologic findings of a prospective study. Obstet Gynecol 1984;63:825–832.
326. Berman M, Afridi M, Kanbour A, Ball H. Risk factors and prognosis in stage II endometrial cancer. Gynecol Oncol 1982;14:49–61.
327. Kadar N, Kohorn E, LiVolsi V, Kapp D. Histologic variants of cervical involvement by endometrial carcinoma. Obstet Gynecol 1982;59:85–92.
328. Frauenhoffer E, Zaino R, Wolff T, Whitney C. Value of endocervical curettage in the staging of endometrial carcinoma. Int J Gynecol Pathol 1987;6:195–202.
329. Caron C, Tetu B, Laberge P, Bellemare G, Raymond EE. Endocervical involvement by endometrial carcinoma on fractional curettage: a clinicopathological study of 37 cases. Mod Pathol 1991;4:644–647.
330. Choo Y, Naylor B. Multiple primary neoplasms of the ovary and uterus. Int J Gynaecol Obstet 1982;20:327–334.
331. Eifel P, Hendrickson M, Ross J, Ballon S, Martinez A, Kempson R. Simultaneous presentation of carcinoma involving the ovary and the uterine corpus. Cancer 1982;50:163–170.
332. Ulbright T, Roth L. Metastatic and independent cancers of the endometrium and ovary: a clinicopathologic study of 34 cases. Hum Pathol 1985;16:28–34.
333. Montoya F, Martin M, Schneider J, Matia JC, Rodriguez EF. Simultaneous appearance of ovarian and endometrial carcinoma: a therapeutic challenge. Eur J Gynaecol Oncol 1989;10:135–139.
334. Chen K, Kostich N, Rosai J. Peritoneal foreign body granulomas to keratin in uterine adenoacanthoma. Arch Pathol Lab Med 1978;102:174–177.
335. Kim K, Scully R. Peritoneal keratin granulomas with carcinomas of endometrium and ovary and atypical polypoid adenomyoma of endometrium: a clinicopathological analysis of 22 cases. Am J Surg Pathol 1990;14:925–932.
336. Goplerud D, Belgrad R. The importance of histologic grade in stage II endometrial carcinoma. Surg Gynecol Obstet 1979;148:406–408.
337. Kinsella T, Bloomer W, Lavin P, Knapp R. Stage II endometrial carcinoma: 10-year follow-up of combined radiation and surgical treatment. Gynecol Oncol 1980;10:290–297.
338. Burrell M, Franklin ED, Powell J. Endometrial cancer: evaluation of spread and follow-up of one hundred eighty-nine patients with stage I or stage II disease. Am J Obstet Gynecol 1982;144:181–185.
339. Berman M, Ballon S, Lagasse L, Watring W. Prognosis and treatment of endometrial cancer. Am J Obstet Gynecol 1980;136:679–688.
340. Bruckman J, Bloomer W, Marck A, Ehrmann R, Knapp R. Stage III adenocarcinoma of the endometrium: two prognostic groups. Gynecol Oncol 1980;9:12–17.
341. Figge D, Otto P, Tamimi H, Greer B. Treatment variables in the management of endometrial cancer. Am J Obstet Gynecol 1983;146:495–500.
342. DiSaia PJ, Creasman WT. Clinical gynecologic oncology, 5th ed. St. Louis: Mosby, 1997:84–93.
343. Belinson JL, Lee KR, Badger GJ, Pretorius RG, Jarrell MA. Clinical stage I adenocarcinoma of the endometrium: analysis of recurrences and the potential benefit of staging lymphadenectomy. Gynecol Oncol 1992;44:17–23.
344. Creasman W, Soper J, McCarty KJ, McCarty KS, Hinshaw W, Clarke-Pearson D. Influence of cytoplasmic steroid receptor content on prognosis of early stage endometrial carcinoma. Am J Obstet Gynecol 1985;151:922–932.
345. Liao B, Twiggs L, Leung B, Yu W, Potish R, Prem K. Cytoplasmic estrogen and progesterone receptors as prognostic parameters in primary endometrial carcinoma. Obstet Gynecol 1986;67:463–467.
346. Carcangiu ML, Chambers JT, Voynick IM, Pirro M, Schwartz PE. Immunohistochemical evaluation of estrogen and progesterone receptor content in 183 patients with endometrial carcinoma. I. Clinical and histologic correlations. Am J Clin Pathol 1990;94:247–254.
347. Chambers JT, Carcangiu ML, Voynick IM, Schwartz PE. Immunohistochemical evaluation of estrogen and progesterone receptor content in 183 patients with endometrial carcinoma. II. Correlation between biochemical and immunohistochemical methods and survival. Am J Clin Pathol 1990;94:255–260.
348. Carcangiu ML, Chambers JT. Sex steroid receptors in gynecologic neoplasms. Pathol Annu 1992;27:121–151.
349. Kurman R, Norris H. Evaluation of criteria for distinguishing atypical endometrial hyperplasia from well-differentiated carcinoma. Cancer 1982;49:2547–2559.
350. Norris H, Tavassoli F, Kurman R. Endometrial hyperplasia and carcinoma: diagnostic considerations. Am J Surg Pathol 1983;7:839–847.
351. Longacre TA, Chung MH, Jensen DN, Hendrickson MR. Proposed criteria for the diagnosis of well-differentiated endometrial carcinoma: a diagnostic test for myoinvasion. Am J Surg Pathol 1995;19:371–406.
352. Feichter G, Hoffken H, Heep J, et al. DNA-flow-cytometric measurements on the normal, atrophic, hyperplastic and neoplastic human endometrium. Virchows Arch A Pathol Anat Histopathol 1982;398:53–65.
353. Colgan T, Norris H, Foster W, Kurman R, Fox C. Predicting the outcome of endometrial hyperplasia by quantitative analysis of nuclear features using a linear discriminant function. Int J Gynecol Pathol 1983;1:347–352.
354. Thornton J, Quirke P, Wells M. Flow cytometry of normal, hyperplastic, and malignant human endometrium: a study of ploidy and proliferative indices including comparison with in vitro S-phase labeling. Am J Obstet Gynecol 1989;161:487–492.
355. Norris H, Becker R, Mikel U. A comparative morphometric and cytophotometric study of endometrial hyperplasia, atypical hyperplasia, and endometrial carcinoma. Hum Pathol 1989;20:219–223.
356. Hendrickson M, Kempson R. Endometrial epithelial metaplasias: proliferations frequently misdiagnosed as adenocarcinoma. Report of 89 cases and proposed classification. Am J Surg Pathol 1980;4:525–542.
357. Lauchlan S. The secondary müllerian system. Obstet Gynecol Surv 1972;27:133–146.
358. Lauchlan S. Metaplasias and neoplasias of müllerian epithelium. Histopathology 1984;8:543–557.
359. Andersen W, Taylor PJ, Fechner R, Pinkerton J. Endometrial metaplasia associated with endometrial adenocarcinoma. Am J Obstet Gynecol 1987;157:597–604.
360. Dutra F. Intraglandular morules of the endometrium. Am J Clin Pathol 1959;31:60–65.
361. Lane M, Dacalos E, Sobrero A, Ober W. Squamous metaplasia of the endometrium in women with an intrauterine contraceptive device: follow-up study. Am J Obstet Gynecol 1974;119:693–697.
362. Crum C, Richart R, Fenoglio C. Adenoacanthosis of endometrium: a clinicopathologic study in premenopausal women. Am J Surg Pathol 1981;5:15–20.
363. Blaustein A. Morular metaplasia misdiagnosed as adenoacanthoma in young women with polycystic ovarian disease. Am J Surg Pathol 1982;6:223–228.
364. Kucukali T, Ertoy D, Ayhan A. Ichthyosis uteri associated with a uterine squamous papilloma. Eur J Gynaecol Oncol 1996;17:37–41.
365. Silverberg S. Significance of squamous elements in carcinoma of the endometrium: a review. In: Fenoglio C, Wolfe M, eds. Progress in surgical pathology, vol 4. New York: Masson, 1982:115–136.
366. Zaino R, Kurman R. Squamous differentiation in carcinoma of the endometrium: a critical appraisal of adenoacanthoma and adenosquamous carcinoma. Semin Diagn Pathol 1988;5:154–171.
367. Zaino R, Kurman R, Herbold D, et al. The significance of squamous differentiation in endometrial carcinoma: data from a Gynecologic Oncology Group study. Cancer 1991;68:2293–2302.
368. Abeler V, Kjørstad K. Endometrial adenocarcinoma with squamous cell differentiation. Cancer 1992;69:488–495.
369. Ng A, Reagan J, Storaasli J, Wentz W. Mixed adenosquamous carcinoma of the endometrium. Am J Clin Pathol 1973;59:765–781.
370. Haqqani M, Fox H. Adenosquamous carcinoma of the endometrium. J Clin Pathol 1976;29:959–966.
371. Alberhasky R, Connelly P, Christopherson W. Carcinoma of the endometrium. IV. Mixed adenosquamous carcinoma: a clinical-pathological study of 68 cases with long-term follow-up. Am J Clin Pathol 1982;77:655–664.
372. Demopoulos R, Dubin N, Noumoff J, Blaustein A, Sommers G. Prognostic significance of squamous differentiation in stage I endometrial adenocarcinoma. Obstet Gynecol 1986;68:245–250.
373. Silverberg S, Bolin M, DeGiorgi L. Adenoacanthoma and mixed adenosquamous carcinoma of the endometrium: a clinicopathologic study. Cancer 1972;30:1307–1314.
374. Salazar O, DePapp E, Bonfiglio T, Feldstein M, Rubin P, Rudolph J. Adenosquamous carcinoma of the endometrium: an entity with an inherent poor prognosis? Cancer 1977;40:119–130.

375. Warhol M, Rice R, Pinkus G, Robboy S. Evaluation of squamous epithelium in adenoacanthoma and adenosquamous carcinoma of the endometrium: immunoperoxidase analysis of involucrin and keratin localization. *Int J Gynecol Pathol* 1984;3:82–91.
376. Christopherson W, Alberhasky R, Connelly P. Glassy cell carcinoma of the endometrium. *Hum Pathol* 1982;13:418–421.
377. Bibro M, Kapp D, LiVolsi V, Schwartz P. Squamous carcinoma of the endometrium with ultrastructural observations and review of the literature. *Gynecol Oncol* 1980;10:217–223.
378. Lifshitz S, Schauberger C, Platz C, Roberts J. Primary squamous cell carcinoma of the endometrium. *J Reprod Med* 1981;26:25–27.
379. Simon A, Kopolovic J, Beyth Y. Primary squamous cell carcinoma of the endometrium. *Gynecol Oncol* 1988;31:454–461.
380. Ryder D. Verrucous carcinoma of the endometrium: a unique neoplasm with long survival. *Obstet Gynecol* 1982;59:78S–80S.
381. Salm R. Superficial intra-uterine spread of intra-epithelial cervical carcinoma. *J Pathol* 1969;97:719–723.
382. Kanbour A, Stock R. Squamous cell carcinoma in situ of the endometrium and fallopian tube as superficial extension of invasive cervical carcinoma. *Cancer* 1978;42:570–580.
383. Honore L. Benign obstructive myxometra: report of a case. *Am J Obstet Gynecol* 1979;134:847–849.
384. Demopoulos R, Greco M. Mucinous metaplasia of the endometrium: ultrastructural and histochemical characteristics. *Int J Gynecol Pathol* 1983;1:383–390.
385. Wells M, Tiltman A. Intestinal metaplasia of the endometrium. *Histopathology* 1989;15:431–433.
386. Baird DB, Reddick RL. Extraovarian mucinous metaplasia in a patient with bilateral mucinous borderline ovarian tumors: a case report. *Int J Gynecol Pathol* 1991;10:96–103.
387. Tiltman A. Mucinous carcinoma of the endometrium. *Obstet Gynecol* 1980;55:244–247.
388. Ross J, Eifel P, Cox R, Kempson R, Hendrickson M. Primary mucinous adenocarcinoma of the endometrium. A clinicopathologic and histochemical study. *Am J Surg Pathol* 1983;7:715-729.
389. Melhem M, Tobon H. Mucinous adenocarcinoma of the endometrium: a clinico-pathological review of 18 cases. *Int J Gynecol Pathol* 1987;6:347–355.
390. Zaloudek C, Hayashi GM, Ryan IP, Powell CB, Miller TR. Microglandular adenocarcinoma of the endometrium: a form of mucinous adenocarcinoma that may be confused with microglandular hyperplasia of the cervix. *Int J Gynecol Pathol* 1997;16:52–59.
391. Hricak H, Lacey C, Schriock E, et al. Gynecologic masses: value of magnetic resonance imaging. *Am J Obstet Gynecol* 1985;153:31–37.
392. Cacciatore B, Lehtovirta P, Wahlström T, Ylostalo P. Preoperative sonographic evaluation of endometrial cancer. *Am J Obstet Gynecol* 1989;160:133–137.
393. Posniak H, Olson M, Dudiak C, et al. MR imaging of uterine carcinoma: correlation with clinical and pathologic findings. *Radiographics* 1990;10:15–27.
394. Morrow CP, Curtin JP, Townsend DE. *Synopsis of gynecologic oncology*, 4th ed, vol 12. New York: Churchill Livingstone, 1993:558.
395. Czernobilsky B, Katz Z, Lancet M, Gaton E. Endocervical-type epithelium in endometrial carcinoma: a report of 10 cases with emphasis on histochemical methods for differential diagnosis. *Am J Surg Pathol* 1980;4:481–489.
396. Cohen C, Shulman G, Budgeon L. Endocervical and endometrial adenocarcinoma: an immunoperoxidase and histochemical study. *Am J Surg Pathol* 1982;6:151–157.
397. Dabbs D, Geisinger K, Norris H. Intermediate filaments in endometrial and endocervical carcinomas: the diagnostic utility of vimentin patterns. *Am J Surg Pathol* 1986;10:568–576.
398. Azumi N, Jones M, Joyce J, et al. Endometrial and endocervical adenocarcinomas: immunohistochemical studies and differentiating markers. *Mod Pathol* 1991;4:54a(abst).
399. Young R, Scully R. Uterine carcinomas simulating microglandular hyperplasia: a report of six cases. *Am J Surg Pathol* 1992;16:1092–1097.
400. Kumar N, Hart W. Metastases to the uterine corpus from extragenital cancers: a clinicopathologic study of 63 cases. *Cancer* 1982;50:2163–2169.
401. Kumar A, Schneider V. Metastases to the uterus from extrapelvic primary tumors. *Int J Gynecol Pathol* 1983;2:134–140.
402. Ueda G, Yamasaki M, Inoue M, Kurachi K. A clinicopathologic study of endometrial carcinomas with argyrophil cells. *Gynecol Oncol* 1979;7:223–232.
403. Prade M, Gadenne C, Duvillard P, Bognel C, Charpentier P. Endometrial carcinoma with argyrophilic cells. *Hum Pathol* 1982;13:870–871.
404. Bannatyne P, Russell P, Wills E. Argyrophilia and endometrial carcinoma. *Int J Gynecol Pathol* 1983;2:235–254.
405. Aguirre P, Scully R, Wolfe H, DeLellis R. Endometrial carcinoma with argyrophil cells: a histochemical and immunohistochemical analysis. *Hum Pathol* 1984;15:210–217.
406. Scully R, Aguirre P, DeLellis R. Argyrophilia, serotonin, and peptide hormones in the female genital tract and its tumors. *Int J Gynecol Pathol* 1984;3:51–70.
407. Sivridis E, Buckley C, Fox H. Argyrophil cells in normal, hyperplastic, and neoplastic endometrium. *J Clin Pathol* 1984;37:378–381.
408. Inoue M, Delellis R, Scully R. Immunohistochemical demonstration of chromogranin in endometrial carcinomas with argyrophil cells. *Hum Pathol* 1986;17:841–847.
409. Ueda G, Nishino T, Saito J, Abe Y, Shimizu H, Tanizawa O. Detection of chromogranin in argyrophil cells of endometrial carcinoma. *Gynecol Oncol* 1987;27:159–165.
410. Olson N, Twiggs L, Sibley R. Small-cell carcinoma of the endometrium: light microscopic and ultrastructural study of a case. *Cancer* 1982;50:760–765.
411. Kumar N. Small cell carcinoma of the endometrium in a 23-year-old woman: light microscopic and ultrastructural study. *Am J Clin Pathol* 1984;81:98–101.
412. Paz R, Frigerio B, Sundblad A, Eusebi V. Small-cell (oat cell) carcinoma of the endometrium. *Arch Pathol Lab Med* 1985;109:270–272.
413. Manivel C, Wick M, Sibley R. Neuroendocrine differentiation in mullerian neoplasms: an immunohistochemical study of a "pure" endometrial small-cell carcinoma and a mixed mullerian tumor containing small-cell carcinoma. *Am J Clin Pathol* 1986;86:438–443.
414. Rorat E, Wallach R. Papillary metaplasia of the endometrium: clinical and histopathologic considerations. *Obstet Gynecol* 1984;64:90S–92S.
415. Zaman SS, Mazur MT. Endometrial papillary syncytial change: a nonspecific alteration associated with active breakdown. *Am J Clin Pathol* 1993;99:741-745.
416. Christopherson W, Alberhasky R, Connelly P. Carcinoma of the endometrium. II. Papillary adenocarcinoma: a clinical pathological study, 46 cases. *Am J Clin Pathol* 1982;77:534–540.
417. Chen J, Trost D, Wilkinson E. Endometrial papillary adenocarcinomas: two clinicopathological types. *Int J Gynecol Pathol* 1985;4:279–288.
418. O'Hanlan K, Levine P, Harbatkin D, et al. Virulence of papillary endometrial carcinoma. *Gynecol Oncol* 1990;37:112–119.
419. Ambros RA, Ballouk F, Malfetano JH, Ross JS. Significance of papillary (villoglandular) differentiation in endometrioid carcinoma of the uterus. *Am J Surg Pathol* 1994;18:569–575.
420. Lauchlan S. Tubal (serous) carcinoma of the endometrium. *Arch Pathol Lab Med* 1981;105:615–618.
421. Hendrickson M, Ross J, Eifel P, Martinez A, Kempson R. Uterine papillary serous carcinoma: a highly malignant form of endometrial adenocarcinoma. *Am J Surg Pathol* 1982;6:93–108.
422. Jeffrey J, Krepart G, Lotocki R. Papillary serous adenocarcinoma of the endometrium. *Obstet Gynecol* 1986;67:670–674.
423. Chambers J, Merino M, Kohorn E. Uterine papillary serous carcinoma. *Obstet Gynecol* 1987;69:109–113.
424. Christman J, Kapp D, Hendrickson M, Howes A, Ballon S. Therapeutic approaches to uterine papillary serous carcinoma: a preliminary report. *Gynecol Oncol* 1987;26:228–235.
425. Sutton G, Brill L, Michael H, Stehman F, Ehrlich C. Malignant papillary lesions of the endometrium. *Gynecol Oncol* 1987;27:294–304.
426. Gallion H, van Nagell, JR Jr, Powell D, et al. Stage I serous papillary carcinoma of the endometrium. *Cancer* 1989;63:2224–2228.
427. Kuebler D, Nikrui N, Bell D. Cytologic features of endometrial papillary serous carcinoma. *Acta Cytol* 1989;33:120–126.
428. Abeler V, Kjprstad K. Serous papillary carcinoma of the endometrium: a histopathological study of 22 cases. *Gynecol Oncol* 1990;39:266–271.
429. Wilson T, Podratz K, Gaffey T, Malkasian GJ, O'Brien P, Naessens JM. Evaluation of unfavorable histologic subtypes in endometrial adenocarcinoma. *Am J Obstet Gynecol* 1990;162:418–423.
430. Sherman ME, Bitterman P, Rosenshein NB, Delgado G, Kurman RJ. Uterine serous carcinoma: a morphologically diverse neoplasm with unifying clinicopathologic features. *Am J Surg Pathol* 1992;16:600–610.

431. Goff BA, Kato D, Schmidt RA, et al. Uterine papillary serous carcinoma: patterns of metastatic spread [Comment]. Gynecol Oncol 1994;54:264–268.
432. Hendrickson MR, Longacre TA, Kempson RL. Uterine papillary serous carcinoma revisited [Editorial; Comment]. Gynecol Oncol 1994;54:261–263.
433. Gitsch G, Friedlander ML, Wain GV, Hacker NL. Uterine papillary serous carcinoma. A clinical study. Cancer 1995;75:2239-2243.
434. Kato DT, Ferry JA, Goodman A, et al. Uterine papillary serous carcinoma (UPSC): a clinicopathologic study of 30 cases. Gynecol Oncol 1995;59:384–389.
435. Nordstrom B, Strang P, Lindgren A, Bergstrom L, Tribukait B. Endometrial carcinoma: the prognostic impact of papillary serous carcinoma (UPSC) in relation to nuclear grade, DNA ploidy and p53 expression. Anticancer Res 1996;16:899–904.
436. Carcangiu ML, Tan LK, Chambers JT. Stage IA uterine serous carcinoma: a study of 13 cases. Am J Surg Pathol 1997;2:1507–1514.
437. Turner BC, Knisely JP, Kacinski BM, et al. Effective treatment of stage I uterine papillary serous carcinoma with high dose-rate vaginal apex radiation (192Ir) and chemotherapy. Int J Radiat Oncol Biol Phys 1998;40:77–84.
438. Factor S. Papillary adenocarcinoma of the endometrium with psammoma bodies. Arch Pathol 1974;98:201–205.
439. Sasano H, Comerford J, Wilkinson D, Schwartz A, Garrett C. Serous papillary adenocarcinoma of the endometrium: analysis of proto-oncogene amplification, flow cytometry, estrogen and progesterone receptors, and immunohistochemistry. Cancer 1990;65:1545–1551.
440. Tashiro H, Isacson C, Levine R, Kurman RJ, Cho KR, Hedrick L. p53 gene mutations are common in uterine serous carcinoma and occur early in their pathogenesis. Am J Pathol 1997;150:177–185.
441. Tashiro H, Lax SF, Gaudin PB, Isacson C, Cho KR, Hedrick L. Microsatellite instability is uncommon in uterine serous carcinoma. Am J Pathol 1997;150:75–79.
442. Ambros RA, Sherman ME, Zahn CM, Bitterman P, Kurman RJ. Endometrial intraepithelial carcinoma: a distinctive lesion specifically associated with tumors displaying serous differentiation. Hum Pathol 1995;26:1260–1267.
443. Kupryjanczyk J, Thor AD, Beauchamp R, Forenb C, Scully RE, Yandell DW. Ovarian, peritoneal, and endometrial serous carcinoma: clonal origin of multifocal disease. Mod Pathol 1996;9:166–173.
444. Muto MG, Welch WR, Mok SC, et al. Evidence for a multifocal origin of papillary serous carcinoma of the peritoneum. Cancer Res 1995;55:490–492.
445. Silverberg S, Major F, Blessing J, et al. Carcinosarcoma (malignant mixed mesodermal tumor) of the uterus: a Gynecologic Oncology Group pathologic study of 203 cases. Int J Gynecol Pathol 1990;9:1–19.
446. Fruin A, Tighe J. Tubal metaplasia of the endometrium. J Obstet Gynaecol Br Commonw 1967;74:93–97.
447. Hendrickson M, Kempson R. Ciliated carcinoma: a variant of endometrial adenocarcinoma. A report of 10 cases. Int J Gynecol Pathol 1983;2:1–12.
448. Bergeron C, Ferenczy A. Oncocytic metaplasia in endometrial hyperplasia and carcinoma [Letter]. Int J Gynecol Pathol 1988;7:93–95.
449. Kurman R, Scully R. Clear cell carcinoma of the endometrium: an analysis of 21 cases. Cancer 1976;37:872–882.
450. Tobon H, Watkins G. Secretory adenocarcinoma of the endometrium. Int J Gynecol Pathol 1985;4:328–335.
451. Silverberg SG, De Giorgi, LS. Clear cell carcinoma of the endometrium: clinical, pathologic, and ultrastructural findings. Cancer 1973;31:1127–1140.
452. Eastwood J. Mesonephroid (clear cell) carcinoma of the ovary and endometrium: a comparative prospective clinico-pathological study and review of literature. Cancer 1978;41:1911–1928.
453. Crum CF, Fechner RE. Clear cell adenocarcinoma of the endometrium: a clinicopathologic study of 11 cases. Am J Diagn Gynecol Obstet 1979;1:261–267.
454. Photopulos G, Carney C, Edelman D, Hughes R, Fowler WJ, Walton L. Clear cell carcinoma of the endometrium. Cancer 1979;43:1448–1456.
455. Webb G, Lagios M. Clear cell carcinoma of the endometrium. Am J Obstet Gynecol 1987;156:1486–1491.
456. Abeler VM, Kjørstad KE, Nesland JM. Undifferentiated carcinoma of the endometrium: a histopathologic and clinical study of 31 cases. Cancer 1991;68:98–105.
457. Kanbour-Shakir A, Tobon H. Primary clear cell carcinoma of the endometrium: a clinicopathologist study of 20 cases. Int J Gynecol Pathol 1991;10:67–78.
458. Ober W. Uterine sarcomas: histogenesis and taxonomy. Ann N Y Acad Sci 1959;75:568–585.
459. Clement P, Scully R. Uterine tumors with mixed epithelial and mesenchymal elements. Semin Diagn Pathol 1988;5:199–222.
460. Zaloudek C, Norris H. Mesenchymal tumors of the uterus. In: Kurman R, ed. Blaustein's pathology of the female genital tract, 4th ed. New York: Springer-Verlag, 1994:487–528.
461. Ostor AG, Rollason TP. Mixed tumours of the uterus. In: Fox H, ed. Haines and Taylor: obstetrical and gynecologic pathology, 4th ed. New York: Churchill Livingstone, 1995:587–621.
462. Chen K, Vergon J. Carcinomesenchymoma of the uterus. Am J Clin Pathol 1981;75:746–748.
463. Engdahl E, Wolfhagen U. Carcinofibroma: a rare variant of mixed mullerian tumor. Acta Obstet Gynecol Scand 1988;67:85–88.
464. Mazur M. Atypical polypoid adenomyomas of the endometrium. Am J Surg Pathol 1981;5:473–482.
465. Young R, Treger T, Scully R. Atypical polypoid adenomyoma of the uterus: a report of 27 cases. Am J Clin Pathol 1986;86:139–145.
466. Longacre TA, Chung MH, Rouse RV, Hendrickson MR. Atypical polypoid adenomyofibromas (atypical polypoid adenomyomas) of the uterus: a clinicopathologic study of 55 cases. Am J Surg Pathol 1996;20:1–20.
467. Soslow RA, Chung MH, Rouse RV, Hendrickson MR, Longacre TA. Atypical polypoid adenomyofibroma (APA) versus well-differentiated endometrial carcinoma with prominent stromal matrix: an immunohistochemical study. Int J Gynecol Pathol 1996;15:209–216.
468. Clement P, Young R. Atypical polypoid adenomyoma of the uterus associated with Turner's syndrome: a report of three cases, including a review of "estrogen-associated" endometrial neoplasms and neoplasms associated with Turner's syndrome. Int J Gynecol Pathol 1987;6:104–113.
469. Ostor A, Fortune D. Benign and low grade variants of mixed mullerian tumour of the uterus. Histopathology 1980;4:369–382.
470. Clement P, Scully R. Mullerian adenofibroma of the uterus with invasion of myometrium and pelvic veins. Int J Gynecol Pathol 1990;9:363–371.
471. Vellios F, Ng A, Reagen J. Papillary adenofibroma of the uterus: a benign mesodermal mixed tumor of mullerian origin. Am J Clin Pathol 1973;60:543–551.
472. Grimalt M, Arguelles M, Ferenczy A. Papillary cystadenofibroma of endometrium: a histochemical and ultrastructural study. Cancer 1975;36:137–144.
473. Zaloudek C, Norris H. Adenofibroma and adenosarcoma of the uterus: a clinicopathologic study of 35 cases. Cancer 1981;48:354–366.
474. Zaloudek C, Norris H. Mesenchymal tumors of the uterus. In: Fenoglio C, Wolfe M, eds. Progress in surgical pathology, vol 3. New York: Masson, 1981:1–35.
475. Clement P, Scully R. Mullerian adenosarcoma of the uterus: a clinicopathologic analysis of ten cases of a distinctive type of mullerian mixed tumor. Cancer 1974;34:1138–1149.
476. Christopherson W. Mullerian adenosarcoma of the uterus [Letter]. Am J Surg Pathol 1980;4:413–414.
477. Czernobilsky B, Hohlweg-Majert P, Dallenbach-Hellweg G. Uterine adenosarcoma: a clinicopathologic study of 11 cases with a reevaluation of histologic criteria. Arch Gynecol 1983;233:281–294.
478. Clement P. Mullerian adenosarcomas of the uterus with sarcomatous overgrowth: a clinicopathological analysis of 10 cases. Am J Surg Pathol 1989;13:28–38.
479. Clement P, Scully R. Mullerian adenosarcomas of the uterus with sex cord–like elements: a clinicopathologic analysis of eight cases. Am J Clin Pathol 1989;91:664–672.
480. Clement P, Scully R. Mullerian adenosarcoma of the uterus: a clinicopathologic analysis of 100 cases with a review of the literature. Hum Pathol 1990;21:363–381.
481. Kaku T, Silverberg S, Major F, Miller A, Fetter B, Brady M. Adenosarcoma of the uterus: a Gynecologic Oncology Group clinicopathologic study of 31 cases. Int J Gynecol Pathol 1992;11:75–88.
482. Norris H, Roth E, Taylor H. Mesenchymal tumors of the uterus. II. A clinical and pathologic study of 31 mixed mesodermal tumors. Obstet Gynecol 1966;28:57–63.
483. Barwick K, LiVolsi V. Malignant mixed mullerian tumors of the uterus: a clinicopathologic assessment of 34 cases. Am J Surg Pathol 1979;3:125–135.

484. King M, Kramer E. Malignant mullerian mixed tumors of the uterus: a study of 21 cases. *Cancer* 1980;45:188–190.
485. Marchese M, Liskow A, Crum C, McCaffrey R, Frick H. Uterine sarcomas: a clinicopathologic study, 1965–1981. *Gynecol Oncol* 1984;18:299–312.
486. Geisinger K, Dabbs D, Marshall R. Malignant mixed mullerian tumors: an ultrastructural and immunohistochemical analysis with histogenetic considerations. *Cancer* 1987;59:1781–1790.
487. Auerbach H, LiVolsi V, Merino M. Malignant mixed mullerian tumors of the uterus: an immunohistochemical study. *Int J Gynecol Pathol* 1988;7:123–130.
488. Gagne E, Tetu B, Blondeau L, Raymond PE, Blais R. Morphologic prognostic factors of malignant mixed mullerian tumor of the uterus: a clinicopathologic study of 58 cases. *Mod Pathol* 1989;2:433–438.
489. Meis J, Lawrence W. The immunohistochemical profile of malignant mixed mullerian tumor: overlap with endometrial adenocarcinoma [Comments]. *Am J Clin Pathol* 1990;94:1–7.
490. Bitterman P, Chun B, Kurman R. The significance of epithelial differentiation in mixed mesodermal tumors of the uterus: a clinicopathologic and immunohistochemical study. *Am J Surg Pathol* 1990;14:317–328.
491. Costa MJ, Khan R, Judd R. Carcinoma (malignant mixed mullerian [mesodermal] tumor) of the uterus and ovary: correlation of clinical, pathologic, and immunohistochemical features in 29 cases. *Arch Pathol Lab Med* 1991;115:583–590.
492. De Brito P, Orenstein J, Silverberg S. Carcinosarcoma of the female genital tract: immunohistochemical and ultrastructural analysis of 28 cases. *Hum Pathol* 1993;24:132–142.
493. Macasaet M, Waxman M, Fruchter R, et al. Prognostic factors in malignant mesodermal (mullerian) mixed tumors of the uterus. *Gynecol Oncol* 1985;20:32–42.
494. Spanos WJ, Peters L, Oswald M. Patterns of recurrence in malignant mixed mullerian tumor of the uterus. *Cancer* 1986;57:155–159.
495. Dinh T, Slavin R, Bhagavan B, Hannigan E, Tiamson E, Yandell R. Mixed mesodermal tumors of the ovary: a clinicopathologic study of 14 cases. *Obstet Gynecol* 1988;72:409–412.
496. Nielsen S, Podratz K, Scheithauer B, O'Brien P. Clinicopathologic analysis of uterine malignant mixed mullerian tumors. *Gynecol Oncol* 1989;34:372–378.
497. Podczaski E, Woomert C, Stevens CJ, et al. Management of malignant, mixed mesodermal tumors of the uterus. *Gynecol Oncol* 1989;32:240–244.
498. Norris H, Taylor H. Mesenchymal tumors of the uterus. I. A clinical and pathological study of 53 endometrial stromal tumors. *Cancer* 1966;19:755–766.
499. Evans H. Endometrial stromal sarcoma and poorly differentiated endometrial sarcoma. *Cancer* 1982;50:2170–2182.
500. Kempson R, Hendrickson M. Pure mesenchymal neoplasms of the uterus corpus. In: Fox H, ed. *Haines and Taylor: obstetrical and gynaecological pathology*, 4th ed. Edinburgh: Churchill Livingstone, 1995:524–537.
501. Kempson R, Hendrickson M. Pure mesenchymal neoplasms of the uterine corpus: selected problems. *Semin Diagn Pathol* 1988;5:172–198.
502. Hendrickson M, Kempson R. Pure mesenchymal neoplasms of the uterus corpus. In: Fox H, ed. *Haines and Taylor: obstetrical and gynaecological pathology*, 4th ed. New York: Churchill Livingstone, 1995:538–573.
503. Tavassoli F, Norris H. Mesenchymal tumours of the uterus. VII. A clinicopathological study of 60 endometrial stromal nodules. *Histopathology* 1981;5:1–10.
504. Kempson R, Bari W. Uterine sarcomas: classification, diagnosis, and prognosis. *Hum Pathol* 1970;1:331–349.
505. Hart W, Yoonessi M. Endometrial stromatosis of the uterus. *Obstet Gynecol* 1977;49:393–403.
506. Mazur M, Askin F. Endolymphatic stromal myosis: unique presentation and ultrastructural study. *Cancer* 1978;42:2661–2667.
507. Thatcher S, Woodruff J. Uterine stromatosis: a report of 33 cases. *Obstet Gynecol* 1982;59:428–434.
508. Fekete P, Vellios F. The clinical and histologic spectrum of endometrial stromal neoplasms: a report of 41 cases. *Int J Gynecol Pathol* 1984;3:198–212.
509. Abrams J, Talcott J, Corson J. Pulmonary metastases in patients with low-grade endometrial stromal sarcoma: clinicopathologic findings with immunohistochemical characterization. *Am J Surg Pathol* 1989;13:133–140.
510. August C, Bauer K, Lurain J, Murad T. Neoplasms of endometrial stroma: histopathologic and flow cytometric analysis with clinical correlation. *Hum Pathol* 1989;20:232–237.
511. Chang K, Crabtree G, Lim-Tan S, Kempson R, Hendrickson M. Primary uterine endometrial stromal neoplasms: a clinicopathologic study of 117 cases. *Am J Surg Pathol* 1990;14:415–438.
512. Abrams J, Corson J, Gee B, Farhood A. Immunohistochemistry of endometrial stromal sarcoma (ESS). *Hum Pathol* 1991;22:224–230.
513. Lillemoe I, Perrone T, Norris H, Dehner L. Epithelial-like areas of endometrial stromal sarcomas. *Hum Pathol* 1991;115:215–219.
514. Clement P, Scully R. Endometrial stromal sarcomas of the uterus with extensive endometrioid glandular differentiation: a report of three cases that caused problems in differential diagnosis. *Int J Gynecol Path* 1992;11:163–173.
515. Fekete PS, Vellios F, Patterson BD. Uterine tumor resembling an ovarian sex-cord tumor: report of a case of an endometrial stromal tumor with foam cells and ultrastructural evidence of epithelial differentiation. *Int J Gynecol Pathol* 1985;4:378–387.
516. Sullinger J, Scully R. Uterine tumors resembling ovarian sex-cord tumors: a clinicopathologic and immunohistochemical study. *Mod Pathol* 1989;2:93a(abst).
517. Fukunaga M, Miyazawa Y, Ushigome S. Endometrial low-grade stromal sarcoma with ovarian sex cord–like differentiation: report of two cases with an immunohistochemical and flow cytometric study. *Pathol Int* 1997;47:412–415.
518. Baker RJ, Hildebrandt RH, Rouse RV, Hendrickson MR, Longacre TA. Inhibin and CD99 (MIC2) expression in uterine stromal neoplasms with sex-cord-like elements. *Mod Pathol* 1998;11:100 (abst).
519. Dail D. Pulmonary metastases of uterine stromal sarcomas: unique histologic appearance suggesting their source. *Lab Invest* 1980;42:110(abst).
520. Gloor E, Schnyder P, Cikes M, et al. Endolymphatic stromal myosis: surgical and hormonal treatment of extensive abdominal recurrence 20 years after hysterectomy. *Cancer* 1982;50:1888–1893.
521. Baker V, Walton L, Fowler WJ, Currie J. Steroid receptors in endolymphatic stromal myosis. *Obstet Gynecol* 1984;63:72S–74S.
522. Piver M, Rutledge F, Copeland L, Webster K, Blumenson L, Suh O. Uterine endolymphatic stromal myosis: a collaborative study. *Obstet Gynecol* 1984;64:173–178.
523. Sutton G, Stehman F, Michael H, Young P, Ehrlich C. Estrogen and progesterone receptors in uterine sarcomas. *Obstet Gynecol* 1986;68:709–714.
524. Katz L, Merino M, Sakamoto H, Schwartz P. Endometrial stromal sarcoma: a clinicopathologic study of 11 cases with determination of estrogen and progestin receptor levels in three tumors. *Gynecol Oncol* 1987;26:87–97.
525. De Fusco P, Gaffey TA, Malkasian GJ, Long HJ, Cha SS. Endometrial stromal sarcoma: review of Mayo Clinic experience, 1945–1980. *Gynecol Oncol* 1989;35:8–14.
526. Tosi P, Sforza V, Santopietro R. Estrogen receptor content, immunohistochemically determined by monoclonal antibodies, in endometrial stromal sarcoma. *Obstet Gynecol* 1989;73:75–78.
527. Berchuck A, Rubin S, Hoskins W, Saigo P, Pierce V, Lewis JJ. Treatment of endometrial stromal tumors. *Gynecol Oncol* 1990;36:60–65.
528. Larson B, Silfversward C, Nilsson B, Pettersson F. Endometrial stromal sarcoma of the uterus: a clinical and histopathological study. The Radiumhemmet series 1936–1981. *Eur J Obstet Gynecol Reprod Biol* 1990;35:239–249.
529. Mansi J, Ramachandra S, Wiltshaw E, Fisher C. Endometrial stromal sarcomas. *Gynecol Oncol* 1990;36:113–118.
530. Sabini G, Chumas JC, Mann WJ. Steroid hormone receptors in endometrial stromal sarcomas: a biochemical and immunohistochemical study. *Am J Clin Pathol* 1992;97:381–386.
531. Ulbright T, Kraus F. Endometrial stromal tumors of extra-uterine tissue. *Am J Clin Pathol* 1981;76:371–377.
532. Young R, Prat J, Scully R. Endometrioid stromal sarcomas of the ovary: a clinicopathologic analysis of 23 cases. *Cancer* 1984;53:1143–1155.
533. Chang KL, Crabtree GS, Lim-Tan SK, Kempson RL, Hendrickson MR. Primary extrauterine endometrial stromal neoplasms: a clinicopathologic study of 20 cases and a review of the literature. *Int J Gynecol Pathol* 1993;12:282–296.
534. Yoonessi M, Hart W. Endometrial stromal sarcomas. *Cancer* 1977;40:898–906.

650. Christopherson W, Alberhasky R, Connelly P. Carcinoma of the endometrium. I. A clinicopathologic study of clear-cell carcinoma and secretory carcinoma. *Cancer* 1982;49:1511–1523.
651. LiVolsi V. Adenocarcinoma of the endometrium with psammoma bodies. *Obstet Gynecol* 1977;50:725–728.
652. Walker A, Mills S. Serous papillary carcinoma of the endometrium: a clinicopathologic study of 11 cases. *Diagn Gynecol Obstet* 1982;4:261–267.
653. Abeler V, Kjørstad K. Endometrial squamous cell carcinoma: report of three cases and review of the literature. *Gynecol Oncol* 1990;36:321–326.
654. Buscema J, Carpenter S, Rosenshein N, Woodruff J. Epithelioid leiomyosarcoma of the uterus. *Cancer* 1986;57:1192–1196.
655. King M, Dickersin G, Scully R. Myxoid leiomyosarcoma of the uterus: a report of six cases. *Am J Surg Pathol* 1982;6:589–598.
656. Bhagavan B, Gupta P. Genital actinomycosis and intrauterine contraceptive devices: cytopathologic diagnosis and clinical significance. *Hum Pathol* 1978;9:567–578.
657. Rodriguez M, Okagaki T, Richart R. Mycotic endometritis due to *Candida*: a case report. *Obstet Gynecol* 1972;39:292–294.
658. Weström L. Gynecologic chlamydial infections. *Infection* 1982;10(Suppl):S40–S45.
659. Winkler B, Crum C. Chlamydia trachomatis infection of the female genital tract: pathogenetic and clinicopathologic correlations. *Pathol Annu* 1987;22:193–223.
660. Stamm WE. Diagnosis of *Chlamydia trachomatis* genitourinary infections. *Ann Intern Med* 1988;108:710–717.
661. Salgia K, Bhatia L, Rajashekaraiah K, Zangan M, Hariharan S, Kallick C. Coccidioidomycosis of the uterus. *South Med J* 1982;75:614–616.
662. Bylund D, Nanfro J, Marsh W Jr. Coccidioidomycosis of the female genital tract. *Arch Pathol Lab Med* 1986;110:232–235.
663. McCracken A, D'Agostino A, Brucks A, Klassen W. Acquired cytomegalovirus infection presenting as viral endometritis. *Am J Clin Pathol* 1974;61:556–560.
664. Dehner L, Askin F. Cytomegalovirus endometritis: report of a case associated with spontaneous abortion. *Obstet Gynecol* 1975;45:211–214.
665. Wenckebach G, Curry B. Cytomegalovirus infection of the female genital tract: histologic findings in three cases and review of the literature. *Arch Pathol Lab Med* 1976;100:609–612.
666. Brodman M, Deligdisch L. Cytomegalovirus endometritis in a patient with AIDS. *Mt Sinai J Med* 1986;53:673–675.
667. Frank T, Himebaugh K, Wilson M. Granulomatous endometritis associated with histologically occult cytomegalovirus in a healthy patient. *Am J Surg Pathol* 1992;16:716–720.
668. Schenken J, Tamisiea J. *Enterobium vermicularis* (pinworm) infection of the endometrium. *Am J Obstet Gynecol* 1956;72:913–914.
669. McMahon J, Connolly C, Long S, Meehan F. Enterobius granulomas of the uterus, ovary and pelvic peritoneum: two case reports. *Br J Obstet Gynaecol* 1984;91:289–290.
670. Schneider V, Behm F, Mumaw V. Ascending herpetic endometritis. *Obstet Gynecol* 1982;59:259–262.
671. Robb J, Benirschke K, Mannino F, Voland J. Intrauterine latent herpes simplex virus infection. II. Latent neonatal infection. *Hum Pathol* 1986;17:1210–1217.
672. Duncan A, Varner R, Mazur M. Uterine herpes virus infection with multifocal necrotizing endometritis. *Hum Pathol* 1989;20:1021–1024.
673. Sweet R. Genital mycoplasmas. In: Behrman S, Kistner R, Patton GJ, eds. *Progress in infertility*, 3rd ed. Boston: Little Brown and Company, 1988:47–54.
674. Khatamee MA, Sommers SC. Clinicopathologic diagnosis of mycoplasma endometritis. *Int J Fertil* 1989;34:52–55.
675. Mayayo E, Mestres M, Sarmiento J, Camblor G. Pelvic oxyuriasis. *Acta Obstet Gynecol Scand* 1986;65:805–806.
676. Venkataseshan V, Woo T. Diffuse viral papillomatosis (condyloma) of the uterine cavity. *Int J Gynecol Pathol* 1985;4:370–377.
677. Remington J, Melton M, Jacobs L. Chronic toxoplasma infection in the uterus. *J Lab Clin Med* 1960;56:879–883.
678. Stray-Pedersen B, Lorentzen-Styr A. Uterine toxoplasma infections and repeated abortions. *Am J Obstet Gynecol* 1977;128:716–721.
679. Jones HJ. Congenital anomalies of the uterus. In: Condos B, Riddick D, eds. *Pathology of infertility*. New York: Thieme 1987:29–40.
680. Golan A, Langer R, Bukovsky I, Caspi E. Congenital anomalies of the mullerian system. *Fertil Steril* 1989;51:747–755.

681. Untawale V, Gabriel J Jr, Chauhan P. Calcific endometritis. *Am J Obstet Gynecol* 1982;144:482–483.
682. Sherrick J, Vega J. Congenital intramural cysts of the uterus. *Obstet Gynecol* 1962;19:486–493.
683. Miko T, Lampe L, Thomazy V, Molnar P, Endes P. Eosinophilic endomyometritis associated with diagnostic curettage. *Int J Gynecol Pathol* 1988;7:162–172.
684. Pirozynski W. Giant-cell arteritis of the uterus: report of two cases. *Am J Clin Pathol* 1976;65:308–313.
685. Bell D, Mondschein M, Scully R. Giant cell arteritis of the female genital tract: a report of three cases. *Am J Surg Pathol* 1986;10:696–701.
686. Lombard C, Moore M, Seifer D. Diagnosis of systemic polyarteritis nodosa following total abdominal hysterectomy and bilateral salpingo-oophorectomy: a case report. *Int J Gynecol Pathol* 1986; 5:63–68.
687. Marrogi A, Gersell D, Kraus F. Localized asymptomatic giant cell arteritis of the female genital tract. *Int J Gynecol Pathol* 1991;10:51–58.
688. Buckley C, Fox H. Histiocytic endometritis. *Histopathology* 1980;4:105–110.
689. Gyure KA, Hart WR, Kennedy AW. Lymphangiomyomatosis of the uterus associated with tuberous sclerosis and malignant neoplasia of the female genital tract: a report of two cases. *Int J Gynecol Pathol* 1995;14:344–351.
690. Longacre TA, Hendrickson MR, Kapp DS, Teng NN. Lymphangioleiomyomatosis of the uterus simulating high-stage endometrial stromal sarcoma. *Gynecol Oncol* 1996;63:404–410.
691. Alpert LC, Haufrect EJ, Schwartz MR. Uterine lithiasis. *Am J Surg Pathol* 1990;14:1071–1075.
692. Thomas WJ, Sadeghieh B, Fresco R, Rubenstone A, Stepto R, Carasso B. Malacoplakia of the endometrium, a probable cause of postmenopausal bleeding. *Am J Clin Pathol* 1978;69:637–641.
693. Chen K, Hendricks E. Malacoplakia of the female genital tract. *Obstet Gynecol* 1985;65:84S–87S.
694. Kawai K, Fukuda K, Tsuchiyama H. Malacoplakia of the endometrium: an unusual case studied by electron microscopy and a review of the literature. *Acta Pathol Jpn* 1988;38:531–540.
695. Smith JH, Kennedy A, Sharp F, Reid PC, Thurrell W. Necrotising granulomas of the uterine corpus [Letter; Comment]. *J Clin Pathol* 1994;47:381–382.
696. Aqel NM. Necrobiotic granulomas of the urogenital system [Letter; Comment] *J Clin Pathol* 1995;48:185.
697. Perkins M. Pneumopolycystic endometritis. *Am J Obstet Gynecol* 1960;80:332–336.
698. Clement P. Postoperative spindle-cell nodule of the endometrium. *Arch Pathol Lab Med* 1988;112:566–568.
699. Young R, Harris N, Scully R. Lymphoma-like lesions of the lower female genital tract: a report of 16 cases. *Int J Gynecol Pathol* 1985;4:289–299.
700. Gilks C, Taylor G, Clement P. Inflammatory pseudotumor of the uterus. *Int J Gynecol Pathol* 1987;6:275–286.
701. Ferry J, Harris N, Scully R. Uterine leiomyomas with lymphoid infiltration simulating lymphoma: a report of seven cases. *Int J Gynecol Pathol* 1989;8:263–270.
702. Kraus F. Irradiation changes in the uterus. In: Norris H, Hertig A, Abell M, eds. *The uterus*. Baltimore: William & Wilkins, 1973:457–488.
703. Fajardo L. *Pathology of radiation injury*. New York: Masson, 1982:13.
704. Ho K-H. Sarcoidosis of the uterus. *Hum Pathol* 1979;10:219–222.
705. DiCarlo F Jr, DiCarlo J, Robboy S, Lyons M. Sarcoidosis of the uterus. *Arch Pathol Lab Med* 1989;113:941–943.
706. Sandvei R, Bang G. Sarcoidosis of the uterus. *Acta Obstet Gynecol Scand* 1991;70:165–167.
707. Menzin AW, You TT, Deger RB, Brooks JS, King SA. Sarcoidosis in a uterine leiomyoma. *Int J Gynaecol Obstet* 1995;48:79–84.
708. Pounder D, Iyer P. Xanthogranulomatous endometritis associated with endometrial carcinoma. *Arch Pathol Lab Med* 1985;109:73–75.
709. Russack V, Lammers R. Xanthogranulomatous endometritis: report of six cases and a proposed mechanism of development. *Arch Pathol Lab Med* 1990;114:929–932.
710. Arhelger R, Bocian J. Brenner tumor of the uterus. *Cancer* 1976;38:1741–1743.
711. Newton C, Abell M. Iatrogenic fetal implants. *Obstet Gynecol* 1972;40:686–691.
712. Tyagi S, Saxena K, Rizwi R, Langley F. Foetal remnants in the uterus and their relation to other uterine heterotopia. *Histopathology* 1979;3:339–345.

713. Roca A, Guajardo M, Estrada W. Glial polyp of the cervix and endometrium: report of a case and review of the literature. *Am J Clin Pathol* 1980;73:718–720.
714. Gronroos M, Meurman L, Kahra K. Proliferating glia and other heterotopic tissues in the uterus: fetal homografts? *Obstet Gynecol* 1983;61:261–266.
715. Brown L, Wells M. Heterotopic adipose and glial tissue in the endometrium with staining for glial fibrillary acidic protein: case report. *Br J Obstet Gynaecol* 1986;93:637–639.
716. Fukuoka M, Fujii S, Konishi I, Mori T, Parmley TH, Woodruff JD. Fibro-osteochondroma of the uterus. *Obstet Gynecol* 1987;70:517–521.
717. Young R, Kleinman G, Scully R. Glioma of the uterus: report of a case with comments on histogenesis. *Am J Surg Pathol* 1981;5:695–699.
718. Liao S, Choi B. Expression of glial fibrillary acidic protein by neoplastic cells of mullerian origin. *Virchows Arch B Cell Pathol* 1986;52:185–193.
719. Fleming H, Ostor AG, Pickel H, Fortune DW. Arteriovenous malformations of the uterus. *Obstet Gynecol* 1989;73:209–214.
720. Malhotra S, Sehgal A, Nijhawan R. Cavernous hemangioma of the uterus [Letter]. *Int J Gynaecol Obstet* 1995;51:159–160.
721. Jacobs D, Cohen H, Johnson J. Lipoleiomyomas of the uterus. *Am J Clin Pathol* 1965;44:45–51.
722. Resta L, Maiorano E, Piscitelli D, Botticella MA. Lipomatous tumors of the uterus: clinico-pathological features of 10 cases with immunocytochemical study of histogenesis. *Pathol Res Pract* 1994;190:378–383.
723. Horie Y, Ikawa S, Kadowaki K, Minagawa Y, Kigawa J, Terakawa N. Lipoadenofibroma of the uterine corpus: report of a new variant of adenofibroma (benign mullerian mixed tumor). *Arch Pathol Lab Med* 1995;119:274–276.
724. Roth E, Taylor H. Heterotopic cartilage in the uterus. *Obstet Gynecol* 1966;27:838–844.
725. Bhatia N, Hoshiko M. Uterine osseous metaplasia. *Obstet Gynecol* 1982;60:256–259.
726. Ejeckam GC, Haseeb F, Ahamad R, Azadeh B. Endometrial ossification. *Trop Geogr Med* 1991;43:314–316.
727. Shimizu M, Nakayama M. Endometrial ossification in a postmenopausal woman. *J Clin Pathol* 1997;50:171–172.
728. Nogales F, Gomez-Morales M, Raymundo C, Aguilar D. Benign heterologous tissue components associated with endometrial carcinoma. *Int J Gynecol Pathol* 1982;1:286–291.
729. Taylor R, Welch K. Heterotopic skin in the uterus: a report of an unusual case. *J Reprod Med* 1984;29:837–840.
730. Young T, Thrasher T. Nonchromaffin paraganglioma of the uterus: a case report. *Arch Pathol Lab Med* 1982;106:608–609.
731. Tavassoli F. Melanotic paraganglioma of the uterus. *Cancer* 1986;58:942–948.
732. Martin P, Pulitzer D, Reed R. Pigmented myomatous neurocristoma of the uterus [Comments]. *Arch Pathol Lab Med* 1989;113:1291–1295.
733. Martin-Reay D, Christ ML, La PR. Uterine leiomyoma with skeletal muscle differentiation: report of a case. *Am J Clin Pathol* 1991;96:344–347.
734. Terada S, Tomita Y, Nakagawa T, Akasofu K, Mizukami Y. Heterotopic striated muscle in the myometrium in a patient with myoma uteri. *Gynecol Obstet Invest* 1991;32:191–192.
735. Lloreta J, Prat J. Endometrial stromal nodule with smooth and skeletal muscle components simulating stromal sarcoma. *Int J Gynecol Pathol* 1992;11:293–298.
736. Yamadori I, Kobayashi S, Ogino T, Ohmori M, Tanaka H, Jimbo T. Uterine leiomyoma with a focus of fatty and cartilaginous differentiation. *Acta Obstet Gynecol Scand* 1993;72:307–309.
737. Nicholson G. Studies of tumour formation: polypoid teratoma of the uterus. *Guy's Hosp Rep* 1956;105:157.
738. Martin E, Scholes J, Richart R, Fenoglio C. Benign cystic teratoma of the uterus. *Am J Obstet Gynecol* 1979;135:429–431.
739. Gernow A, Ahrentsen O. Adenoid cystic carcinoma of the endometrium. *Histopathology* 1989;15:197–198.
740. Pileri S, Martinelli G, Serra L, Bazzocchi F. Endodermal sinus tumor arising in the endometrium. *Obstet Gynecol* 1980;56:391–396.
741. Joseph M, Fellows F, Hearn S. Primary endodermal sinus tumor of the endometrium: a clinicopathologic, immunocytochemical, and ultrastructural study. *Cancer* 1990;65:297–302.
742. Jones MA, Young RH, Scully RE. Endometrial adenocarcinoma with a component of giant cell carcinoma. *Int J Gynecol Pathol* 1991;10:260–270.
743. Hendrickson M, Scheithauer B. Primitive neuroectodermal tumor of the endometrium: report of two cases, one with electron microscopic observations. *Int J Gynecol Pathol* 1986;5:249–259.
744. Rose PG, O'Toole RV, Keyhani RS, Qualman S, Boutselis JG. Malignant peripheral primitive neuroectodermal tumor of the uterus. *J Surg Oncol* 1987;35:165–169.
745. Daya D, Lukka H, Clement P. Primitive neuroectodermal tumors of the uterus: a report of four cases. *Hum Pathol* 1992;23:1120–1129.
746. Fraggetta F, Magro G, Vasquez E. Primitive neuroectodermal tumour of the uterus with focal cartilaginous differentiation. *Histopathology* 1997;30:483–485.
747. Tohya T, Miyazaki K, Katabuchi H, Fujisaki S, Maeyama M. Small cell carcinoma of the endometrium associated with adenosquamous carcinoma: a light and electron microscopic study. *Gynecol Oncol* 1986;25:363–371.
748. Schmidt D. Neuroendocrine tumors of the uterus. *Verh Dtsch Ges Pathol* 1997;81:260–265.
749. Civantos F, Rywlin A. Carcinomas with trophoblastic differentiation and secretion of chorionic gonadotrophins. *Cancer* 1972;29:789–798.
750. Tsoutsoplides G. Ectopic production of human chorionic gonadotropin by a highly anaplastic adenocarcinoma of the endometrium. *Am J Obstet Gynecol* 1980;136:694–695.
751. Savage J, Subby W, Okagaki T. Adenocarcinoma of the endometrium with trophoblastic differentiation and metastases as choriocarcinoma: a case report. *Gynecol Oncol* 1987;26:257–262.
752. Pesce C, Merino MJ, Chambers JT, Nogales F. Endometrial carcinoma with trophoblastic differentiation: an aggressive form of uterine cancer. *Cancer* 1991;68:1799–1802.
753. Kubo K, Lee GH, Yamauchi K, Kitagawa T. Alpha-fetoprotein-producing papillary adenocarcinoma originating from a uterine body: a case report. *Acta Pathol Jpn* 1991;41:399–403.
754. Hachisuga T, Sugimori H, Kaku T, Matsukuma K, Tsukamoto N, Nakano H. Glassy cell carcinoma of the endometrium. *Gynecol Oncol* 1990;36:134–138.
755. Yorishima M, Hiura M, Moriwaki S, et al. Clear cell carcinoma of the endometrium with lipid-producing activity: histologic and ultrastructural study suggesting a unique neoplasm. *Int J Gynecol Pathol* 1989;8:286–295.
756. Yamashina M, Kobara T. Primary squamous cell carcinoma with its spindle cell variant in the endometrium: a case report and review of literature. *Cancer* 1986;57:340–345.
757. Chen KT. Extraovarian transitional cell carcinoma of female genital tract [Letter; Comment]. *Am J Clin Pathol* 1990;94:670–671.
758. Spiegel GW, Austin RM, Gelven PL. Transitional cell carcinoma of the endometrium. *Gynecol Oncol* 1996;60:325–330.
759. Lininger RA, Ashfaq R, Albores-Saavedra J, Tavassoli FA. Transitional cell carcinoma of the endometrium and endometrial carcinoma with transitional cell differentiation. *Cancer* 1997;79:1933–1943.
760. Hussain S. Verrucous carcinoma of the endometrium: a case report. *APMIS* 1988;96:1075–1078.
761. Gray GJ, Glick A, Kurtin P, Jones H. Alveolar soft part sarcoma of the uterus. *Hum Pathol* 1986;17:297–300.
762. Nolan N, Gaffney E. Alveolar soft part sarcoma of the uterus. *Histopathology* 1990;16:97–99.
763. Quinonez G, Paraskevas M, Diocee M, Lorimer S. Angiosarcoma of the uterus: a case report. *Am J Obstet Gynecol* 1991;164:90–92.
764. Burch DJ, Hitchcock A, Masson GM. Alveolar soft part sarcoma of the uterus: case report and review of the literature. *Gynecol Oncol* 1994;54:91–94.
765. Ongkasuwan C, Taylor J, Tang C, Prempree T. Angiosarcomas of the uterus and ovary: clinicopathologic report. *Cancer* 1982;49:1469–1475.
766. Witkin G, Askin F, Geratz J, Reddick R. Angiosarcoma of the uterus: a light microscopic, immunohistochemical, and ultrastructural study. *Int J Gynecol Pathol* 1987;6:176–184.
767. Tallini G, Price FV, Carcangiu ML. Epithelioid angiosarcoma arising in uterine leiomyomas [Comments]. *Am J Clin Pathol* 1993;100:514–518.
768. Amr S, Tavassoli F, Hassan A, Issa A, Madanat F. Mixed mesodermal tumor of the uterus in a 4-year-old girl. *Int J Gynecol Pathol* 1986;5:371–378.
769. Kawagoe K. A case of mixed mesodermal tumor of the uterus with alpha-fetoprotein production. *Jpn J Clin Oncol* 1985;15:577–583.
770. Gersell D, Duncan D, Fulling K. Malignant mixed mullerian tumor of the uterus with neuroectodermal differentiation. *Int J Gynecol Pathol* 1989;8:169–178.

771. Clement P. Chondrosarcoma of the uterus: report of a case and review of the literature. *Hum Pathol* 1978;9:726–732.
772. Kofinas A, Suarez J, Calame R, Chipeco Z. Chondrosarcoma of the uterus. *Gynecol Oncol* 1984;19:231–237.
773. Ansah-Boateng Y, Wells M, Poole D. Coexistent immature teratoma of the uterus and endometrial adenocarcinoma complicated by gliomatosis peritonei. *Gynecol Oncol* 1985;21:106–110.
774. Vakiani M, Mawad J, Talerman A. Heterologous sarcomas of the uterus. *Int J Gynecol Pathol* 1982;1:211–219.
775. Alvarez A, Ortiz JA, Sacristan F. Large B-cell lymphoma of the uterine corpus: case report with immunohistochemical and molecular study. *Gynecol Oncol* 1997;65:534–538.
776. Chou S, Fortune D, Beischer N, et al. Primary malignant fibrous histiocytoma of the uterus: ultrastructural and immunocytochemical studies of two cases. *Pathology* 1985;17:36–40.
777. Fujii S, Kanzaki H, Konishi I, Yamabe H, Okamura H, Mori T. Malignant fibrous histiocytoma of the uterus. *Gynecol Oncol* 1987;26:319–330.
778. Darby A, Papadaki L, Beilby J. An unusual leiomyosarcoma of the uterus containing osteoclast-like giant cells. *Cancer* 1975;36:495–504.
779. Kindblom L, Seidal T. Malignant giant cell tumor of the uterus: a clinico-pathologic, light- and electron-microscopic study of a case. *Acta Pathol Microbiol Scand A* 1981;89:179–184.
780. Pilon V, Parikh N, Maccera J. Malignant osteoclast-like giant cell tumor associated with a uterine leiomyosarcoma. *Gynecol Oncol* 1986;23:381–386.
781. Kawai K, Senba M, Tagawa H, Suzuki K, Matsuo T, Tsuchiyama H. Osteoclast-type giant cell tumor of the endometrium: an immunohistochemical study. *Zentralbl Allg Pathol* 1989;135:743–749.
782. Crum C, Rogers B, Andersen W. Osteosarcoma of the uterus: case report and review of the literature. *Gynecol Oncol* 1980;9:256–268.
783. Piscioli F, Govoni E, Polla E, Pusiol T, Dalri P, Antolini M. Primary osteosarcoma of the uterine corpus: report of a case and critical review of the literature. *Int J Gynaecol Obstet* 1985;23:377–385.
784. Donkers B, Kazzaz B, Meijering J. Rhabdomyosarcoma of the corpus uteri: report of two cases with review of the literature. *Am J Obstet Gynecol* 1972;114:1025–1030.
785. Hart W, Craig J. Rhabdomyosarcomas of the uterus. *Am J Clin Pathol* 1978;70:217–223.
786. Hays D, Shimada H, Raney RJ, et al. Sarcomas of the vagina and uterus: the Intergroup Rhabdomyosarcoma study. *J Pediatr Surg* 1985;20:718–724.
787. Montag T, D'ablaing G, Schlaerth J, Gaddis OJ, Morrow C. Embryonal rhabdomyosarcoma of the uterine corpus and cervix. *Gynecol Oncol* 1986;25:171–194.
788. Jacques SM, Lawrence WD, Malviya VK. Uterine mixed embryonal rhabdomyosarcoma and fetal rhabdomyoma. *Gynecol Oncol* 1993;48:272–276.
789. Chiarle R, Godio L, Fusi D, Soldati T, Palestro G. Pure alveolar rhabdomyosarcoma of the corpus uteri: description of a case with increased serum level of CA-125. *Gynecol Oncol* 1997;66:320–323.
790. Cho K, Rosenshein N, Epstein J. Malignant rhabdoid tumor of the uterus. *Int J Gynecol Pathol* 1989;8:381–387.
791. Fitko R, Brainer J, Schink JC, August CZ. Endometrial stromal sarcoma with rhabdoid differentiation [Letter; Comment]. *Int J Gynecol Pathol* 1990;9:379–382.
792. Niemann TH, Goetz SP, Benda JA, Cohen MB. Malignant rhabdoid tumor of the uterus: report of a case with findings in a cervical smear. *Diagn Cytopathol* 1994;10:54–59.
793. Hsueh S, Chang TC. Malignant rhabdoid tumor of the uterine corpus. *Gynecol Oncol* 1996;61:142–146.
794. McCluggage WG, Date A, Bharucha H, Toner PG. Endometrial stromal sarcoma with sex cord–like areas and focal rhabdoid differentiation. *Histopathology* 1996;29:369–374.
795. Bittencourt A, Britto J, Fonseca LJ. Wilms' tumor of the uterus: the first report of the literature. *Cancer* 1981;47:2496–2499.
796. Casey J, Shapiro R. Metastatic melanoma presenting as primary uterine neoplasm: a case report. *Cancer* 1974;33:729–731.
797. Wood C. Metastatic melanoma simulating a primary endometrial tumor. *Am J Obstet Gynecol* 1978;131:820–821.
798. Allenby P, Chowdhury L. Histiocytic appearance of metastatic lobular breast carcinoma. *Arch Pathol Lab Med* 1986;110:759–760.
799. Abu-Rustum NR, Curtin JP, Burt M, Jones WB. Regression of uterine low-grade smooth-muscle tumors metastatic to the lung after oophorectomy. *Obstet Gynecol* 1997;89:850–852.
800. Perez C, Camel H, Askin F, Breaux S. Endometrial extension of carcinoma of the uterine cervix: a prognostic factor that may modify staging. *Cancer* 1981;48:170–180.

CHAPTER 54

The Ovary

Robert H. Young, Philip B. Clement, and Robert E. Scully

NONNEOPLASTIC DISORDERS

Nonneoplastic lesions of the ovary may form pelvic masses and may be associated with hormonal manifestations, simulating ovarian neoplasms in clinical characteristics. These lesions can also resemble ovarian tumors at operation and even on gross pathologic examination. It is important to recognize them from the viewpoints of prognosis and therapy. Even normal ovarian structures (1) are occasionally misinterpreted as neoplasms on histologic examination. The granulosa cells of the normal follicle and normal theca externa cells typically exhibit brisk mitotic activity, which in the former case can lead to misinterpretation as neoplastic epithelial cells and in the latter case to misinterpretation as neoplastic mesenchymal cells. The granulosa cells of normal follicles can also be introduced as artifacts into tissue spaces or vascular channels during sectioning, and they may be confused with small-cell carcinoma, especially when they are shrunken or crushed. Occasionally, luteinized granulosa cells are present on the surface of the ovary as the result of follicle rupture and may be misinterpreted as mesothelial cells or, if they are numerous, even as malignant mesothelioma.

Inflammatory Disorders

Common Bacterial Infections

Pelvic inflammatory disease (PID) of bacterial origin accounts for most ovarian infections in the Western world. Ovarian involvement almost always stems from salpingitis and typically takes the form of a tubo-ovarian abscess, which is usually bilateral. With resolution of the infection, the only side effects may be tubo-ovarian fibrous adhesions; occasionally, a healed abscess is converted into a tubo-ovarian cyst, which may be considered an ovarian cystic neoplasm at operation. These inflammatory cysts may even be misdiagnosed as ovarian serous or endometrioid cystadenomas on microscopic examination. In some cases, the presence of focal inflamed tubal plicae in the lining of the cysts is an important clue to the diagnosis. Ovarian changes similar to those of polycystic ovarian disease (PCOD) have been reported in cases of tubo-ovarian inflammatory disease (2).

A unilateral or bilateral ovarian abscess without tubal involvement is much more rare than a tubo-ovarian abscess. The former is the result of direct or lymphatic spread from a nongynecologic pelvic inflammatory process (diverticulitis, appendicitis, inflammatory bowel disease, postoperative pelvic infection) or, uncommonly, of a blood-borne infection (3). Rarely, ovarian abscess develops within an endometriotic cyst (4). The external surface of an ovary harboring an abscess is often unremarkable, and the nature of the process may not be apparent until the organ is sectioned. An uncommon complication of an ovarian or tubo-ovarian abscess is rupture, typically into the peritoneal cavity with secondary peritonitis (5) and, infrequently, into an adjacent organ, such as the colon (6), bladder (7), or vagina (8), with fistula formation. From time to time, a chronic ovarian abscess eventuates in a solid, yellow, tumor-like xanthogranuloma composed of foamy histiocytes admixed with multinucleated giant cells and other chronic inflammatory cells (9). Pseudotumorous xanthogranulomatous inflammation with more diffuse involvement of the adnexa has also been described (10).

Uncommon Bacterial Infections

Pelvic actinomycosis, an uncommon disorder, is usually a complication of the use of an intrauterine device (IUD), although most cases of IUD-associated PID are nonactinomycotic (11–14). The adnexal involvement is typically unilat-

---

R. H. Young: Department of Pathology, Massachusetts General Hospital, Harvard Medical School, Boston, Massachusetts 02114.

P. B. Clement: Department of Pathology, Vancouver Hospital and Health Sciences Center, University of British Columbia, Vancouver, British Columbia V5Z 1M9, Canada.

R. E. Scully: Department of Pathology, Massachusetts General Hospital, Harvard Medical School, Boston, Massachusetts 02114.

eral (Fig. 1), with large abscesses in which actinomycotic "sulfur" granules may be visible. Microscopic examination reveals the characteristic colonies of actinomyces and a nonspecific inflammatory response composed predominantly of neutrophils, foamy histiocytes, lymphocytes, and plasma cells. The actinomyces colonies may be extremely few, necessitating extensive sampling to identify them; a fluorescent antibody stain may help in pinpointing them (15).

Ovarian involvement is present in only 10% of cases of pelvic tuberculosis and is usually the consequence of tubal disease, which is much more frequent (16). On inspection, the ovaries typically have tubal-ampullary adhesions; visible caseous lesions are rare. On histologic examination, involvement is typically confined to the ovarian cortex. Spread to the peritoneum may result in intraoperative misdiagnosis of an ovarian neoplasm with peritoneal implants (16,17). Very rare bacterial infections affecting the ovary include syphilis, leprosy, and malacoplakia; the last lesion may be related to infection by several species of bacteria (18,19).

Other Rare Infections

Ovarian schistosomiasis is relatively common in endemic areas (20). An enlarged tube and ovary, numerous fibrous adhesions between them, and scattered peritoneal nodules may be encountered at operation. A granulomatous inflammatory infiltrate, often containing eosinophils, is seen in response to *Schistosoma* ova; dense fibrosis is frequently found at later stages of the disease. Ovarian involvement by

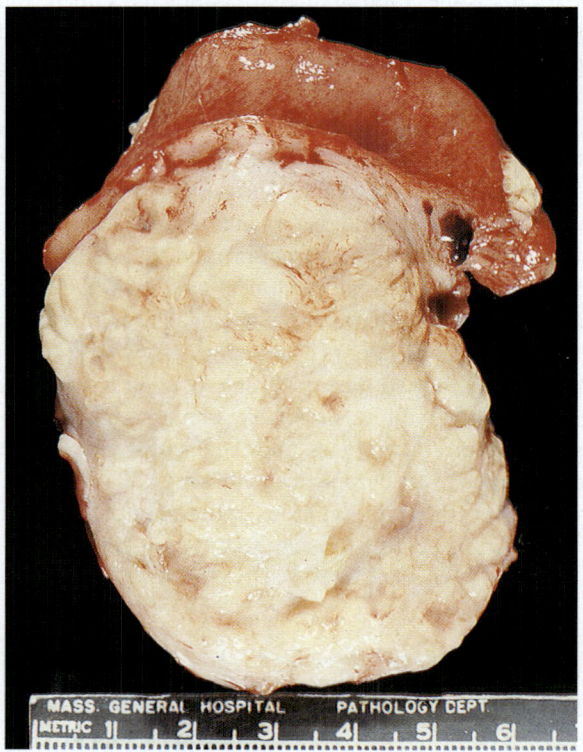

FIG. 1. Actinomycosis of ovary. The ovary is replaced by a yellow mass.

Enterobius vermicularis is usually an incidental operative finding on the ovarian surface (21). The granulomas, which typically contain eosinophils and may exhibit caseous necrosis, surround the adult female worms and ova. Rare cases of ovarian echinococcosis have been described (22).

Fungal infections of the ovary are unusual, even in patients with disseminated mycoses. Rare examples of ovarian involvement by blastomycosis, coccidioidomycosis, and aspergillosis have been described (19). Oophoritis stemming from cytomegalovirus has been an uncommon finding in immunosuppressed patients, usually at autopsy and as part of a generalized infection (23,24). Foci of superficial cortical hemorrhagic necrosis may be seen on gross inspection; microscopic examination reveals coagulative necrosis, an inflammatory response, and cytomegalic inclusion bodies within stromal and endothelial cells.

Noninfectious Granulomas

Foreign material may evoke a granulomatous reaction on the ovarian and peritoneal surfaces, mimicking metastatic carcinoma. Starch granules from surgical gloves or, less often, from starch-containing douche fluid or lubricants can evoke a foreign-body or tuberculoid granulomatous response (25). Foreign-body granulomas may also be due to talc (26), hysterosalpingographic contrast material (27), keratin from ruptured dermoid cysts or endometrial or ovarian endometrioid adenocarcinomas with squamous differentiation (28), and bowel contents (29).

Isolated noninfectious ovarian granulomas have typically developed in patients who have previously undergone ovarian operation (30–32). These granulomas are usually multiple and bilateral and have hyalinized or necrotic cores surrounded by palisading histiocytes and a fibrous pseudocapsule. In one series (32), the granulomas contained carbon pigment produced by previous operative fulguration or laser therapy.

Granulomatous oophoritis can be caused upon occasion by sarcoidosis (33) and Crohn's disease. In the case of Crohn's disease, involvement is generally the consequence of direct extension of the inflammatory process from the bowel; the ipsilateral fallopian tube is often affected as well (34). So-called cortical granulomas are common incidental microscopic lesions of unknown origin within the ovarian cortex of women in the late reproductive and postmenopausal age groups. These lesions consist of a variable admixture of epithelioid cells, lymphocytes, and multinucleated giant cells. They have no known clinical significance (19,35).

Surface Proliferative Lesions

Epithelial Inclusion Glands

Surface epithelial inclusion glands arise from cortical invaginations of surface epithelium that have lost their connection with the surface (Fig. 2). Although they are most numerous in postmenopausal women, they have also been

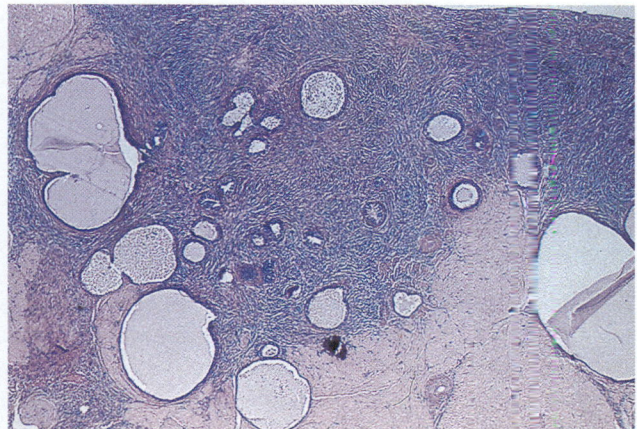

FIG. 2. Inclusion glands and cysts are numerous within the ovarian stroma.

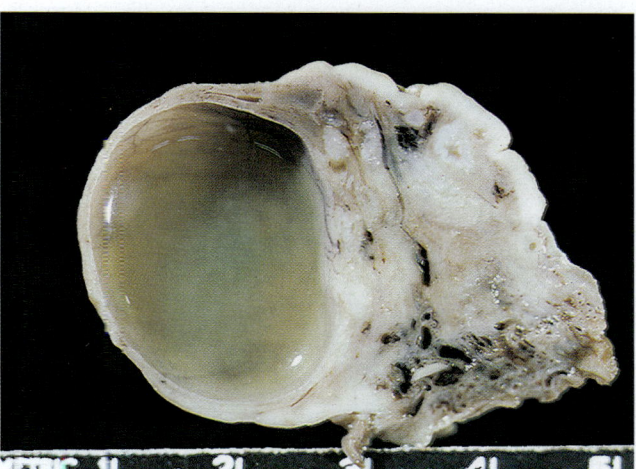

FIG. 3. Follicle cyst. The cyst is thin-walled and filled with clear fluid. (From ref. 40.)

found in fetuses, infants, and adolescents (36,37). These inclusions can measure up to 1 cm in diameter and be visible on gross inspection, but most of them are incidental microscopic findings in the form of multiple glands or cysts, scattered singly or in clusters throughout the superficial cortex (Fig. 2); less commonly, they are found in the deeper cortical or medullary stroma.

Inclusion cysts may be particularly numerous in cases of peritoneal serous borderline neoplasia. In these and other cases, they may be associated with striking numbers of psammoma bodies within them or in the adjacent stroma; they may be accompanied by surface fibrous adhesions. The inclusion cysts are typically lined by a single layer of columnar epithelium, which may be ciliated. Less often, the gland lining is a single layer of endometrioid or endocervical-type epithelium (38). An Arias-Stella-like reaction may be evident in the lining cells in pregnant patients (37). Occasionally in adults, and typically in fetal and premenarchal ovaries, the cysts have a flat or cuboidal lining. The infrequent finding of dysplastic epithelium lining the cysts supports the hypothesis that they may give rise to surface epithelial carcinomas (39). In a few instances, there is striking hydropic change of the cells lining epithelial inclusion glands, creating an appearance that can mimic that of a signet-ring-cell carcinoma (40).

Surface Stromal Proliferations

Nodular or papillary stromal projections from the ovarian surface are common incidental histologic findings in the late reproductive and postmenopausal age groups. They are composed of ovarian stroma exhibiting variable degrees of hyalinization, covered by a single layer of surface epithelium (40).

Mesothelial Proliferations

Proliferation of mesothelial cells, which are occasionally slightly atypical, may be encountered on the surface of the ovaries or periovarian adhesions. When they are present in association with an ovarian tumor, they may be misinterpreted as representing spread of the tumor (41). These proliferations are similar to those seen elsewhere on the peritoneal surfaces and are discussed in detail in Chapter 56.

Solitary Follicle Cysts

Clinical Features

Solitary (one or occasionally a few) follicle cysts are common, particularly soon after menarche and around the time of menopause (Figs. 3 and 4). They may be encountered, however, at any age, from the fetal period to 7 years after the clin-

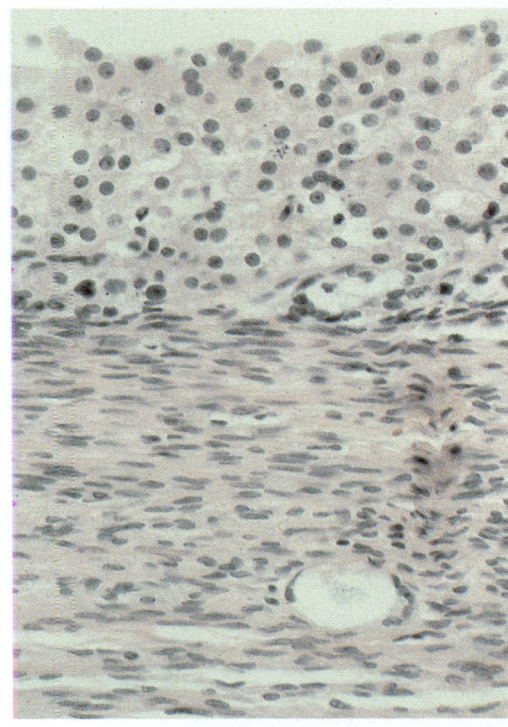

FIG. 4. Follicle cyst. The cyst is lined by luteinized cells.

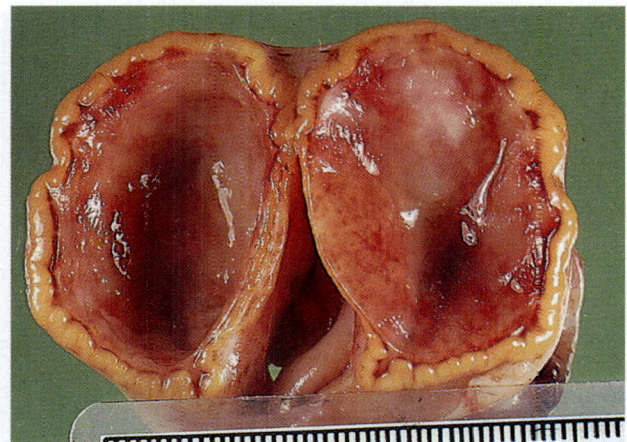

FIG. 5. Corpus luteum cyst. Note the smooth lining of the cyst and the convoluted yellow rim.

ical onset of menopause (42–46). Corpus luteum cysts (Fig. 5) usually occur during the reproductive years, but in exceptional cases they can develop after an isolated ovulation several years after the clinical onset of menopause (40). Corpora lutea have been encountered very rarely in the ovaries of newborns (47). Follicle cysts may be incidental findings or result in palpable adnexal masses or manifestations related to increased estrogen production, such as isosexual precocity (48), menstrual disturbances (44), or endometrial hyperplasia (45). An uncommon result of both follicle and corpus luteum cysts is rupture with hemoperitoneum. This complication is more apt to occur in patients who have been receiving anticoagulant therapy or have a bleeding diathesis (49). The bleeding may be massive and even fatal. A corpus luteum cyst arising in residual ovarian tissue is the most typical finding in the ovarian remnant syndrome; complications have included ureteral and intestinal obstruction (50).

The great majority of follicle cysts result from abnormal gonadotropin stimulation. In most children, however (including those with the McCune-Albright syndrome), the cysts appear to be autonomous, and the triggering mechanism is unknown. Isosexual pseudoprecocity caused by these cysts may regress spontaneously or after puncture of the cyst (51). Autonomous cysts may be single or multiple. In the McCune-Albright syndrome, they may be accompanied by corpora lutea and a potential for pregnancy and may recur after excision (52).

A rare type of solitary follicle cyst, the "large solitary luteinized follicle cyst of pregnancy and the puerperium" (LSLFCPP), is presumably related to chorionic gonadotropin stimulation (53). The patients show signs of a palpable adnexal mass or an ovarian cyst discovered during cesarean section. None of the cysts of this type reported to date have been bilateral or associated with clinical evidence of an endocrine disturbance.

Gross Features

Follicle and corpus luteum cysts are unilocular, smooth-surfaced, and thin-walled and rarely exceed 8 cm in diameter (Figs. 3 and 5). The reported examples of LSLFCPPs, however, have had a median diameter of 25 cm. Corpus luteum cysts are usually recognizable on gross examination because all or part of the wall may be yellow or convoluted (Fig. 5). The contents of follicle and corpus luteum cysts vary from serous or serosanguinous fluid to clotted blood.

Microscopic Features

Follicle cysts are lined by an inner layer of granulosa cells and an outer layer of theca interna cells; the cells in either layer may be luteinized (Fig. 4). Distinction between the two layers can be facilitated by a reticulin stain, which reveals a dense network of reticulin in the theca cell layer but few or no fibrils in the granulosa cell layer. Either layer, but more often the granulosa cell layer, may be present only focally or completely absent. The LSLFCPP has a distinctive appearance; it is lined by one to several layers of large luteinized cells that may vary markedly in size and shape (Fig. 6); it may be impossible to distinguish the granulosa cell from the theca cell component. The luteinized cells typically exhibit focal marked nuclear pleomorphism and hyperchromatism. The lining of corpus luteum cysts is composed of luteinized granulosa cells interrupted externally by wedges of smaller theca lutein cells. A prominent innermost layer of connective tissue is typically present, and portions of the cyst wall may be lined predominantly by fibrous tissue. The corpus luteum cysts associated with pregnancy typically contain hyaline bodies and, in the latter part of pregnancy, small foci of calcification. Involution of a corpus luteum cyst from time to time leads to the formation of a corpus albicans cyst.

Differential Diagnosis

Cysts otherwise similar to follicle and corpus luteum cysts but measuring less than 3 cm in diameter are generally regarded as physiologic and designated cystic follicles and cystic corpora lutea, respectively. Differentiation of LSLFCPPs from unilocular cystic granulosa cell tumors is discussed un-

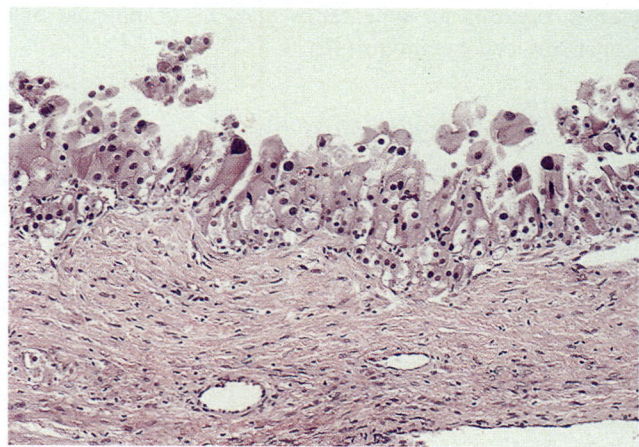

FIG. 6. Large luteinized solitary follicle cyst of pregnancy and puerperium. The lining cells are luteinized, and some have enlarged bizarre nuclei.

der the latter heading. Simple cysts have no lining or one composed of a layer of nonspecific flattened cells; some are probably of follicular origin and others of surface epithelial origin.

Hyperreactio Luteinalis

Clinical Features

Hyperreactio luteinalis, the bilateral presence of several luteinized follicle cysts, is most commonly associated with disorders of pregnancy in which there are high levels of circulating chorionic gonadotropin (hCG), such as hydatidiform mole, choriocarcinoma, fetal hydrops, and multiple gestations (54–58), but it has also been reported during otherwise normal single pregnancies (57). The disorder may become clinically apparent at any time during pregnancy or may be an incidental finding at cesarean section. Much less often, clinical manifestations arise within the first 10 days postpartum or, exceptionally, late in the puerperium. The patients usually have pain or palpable adnexal masses or both (58). In patients with hyperreactio luteinalis stemming from trophoblastic disease, cystic ovarian enlargement may be detected at the time of dilatation and curettage or during the postoperative follow-up period (59). In approximately 25% of the cases that have been unassociated with trophoblastic disease, the patient has been virilized (60). Complications include ascites, torsion, and rupture with intraabdominal bleeding. Hyperreactio luteinalis typically regresses in the postpartum period but sometimes persists for up to 6 months. An iatrogenic form of hyperreactio luteinalis, referred to as the ovarian hyperstimulation syndrome, develops in women undergoing ovulation induction, typically with follicle-stimulating hormone followed by hCG and less often with clomid alone (61,62). Patients with this disorder may also have ascites and occasionally hydrothorax of acute onset (acute Meigs' syndrome).

Pathologic Features

On gross examination, several almost invariably bilateral cysts result in moderate to massive ovarian enlargement up to 26 cm in diameter (Fig. 7); the cysts may be filled with clear or hemorrhagic fluid. One or more corpora lutea are present in patients with the ovarian hyperstimulation syndrome. Microscopic examination reveals large follicle cysts with marked luteinization of the theca interna layer and, to a lesser extent, the granulosa cell layer (Fig. 8). There is usually marked congestion and edema of the stroma, and stromal luteinization may be present as well.

Granulosa Cell Proliferations

Focal proliferations of granulosa cells that resemble small tumors of microscopic size may be encountered as an incidental finding in the ovary. Most of the reported examples have been discovered in pregnant women (53). The lesions typically develop in atretic follicles, but only a minority of the follicles are affected in a given case. Microscopic exam-

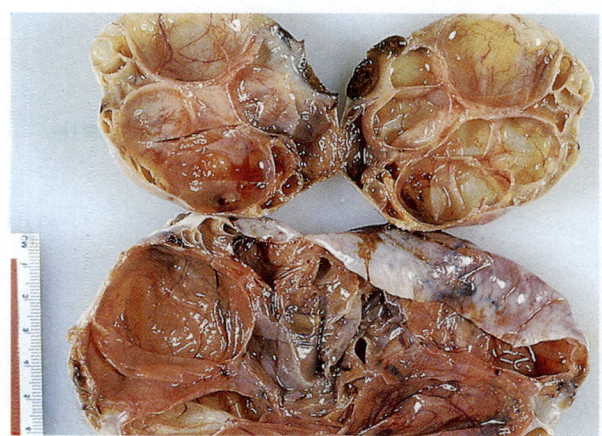

FIG. 7. Hyperreactio luteinalis. Both ovaries are replaced by several thin-walled cysts.

ination usually reveals small aggregates of granulosa cells arranged in diffuse, insular, trabecular, or microfollicular patterns (Fig. 9). The granulosa cells have the typical cytologic features of those encountered in the adult granulosa cell tumor. Rarely, they are luteinized and form nodules. A solid tubular pattern resembling a Sertoli cell tumor also has been encountered. The finding of these lesions often leads to consideration of a small neoplasm, but their usual presence in the ovary of a pregnant patient, small size, and typical multifocality suggest a nonneoplastic proliferation related to the hormonal milieu of pregnancy.

Polycystic Ovarian Disease, Stromal Hyperplasia, and Stromal Hyperthecosis

Morphologic and physiologic investigations have shown that these disorders, which may be associated with androgenic or estrogenic manifestations or both, are part of a continuum and that sharp distinctions cannot always be made among them. In spite of this overlap, it is appropriate to de-

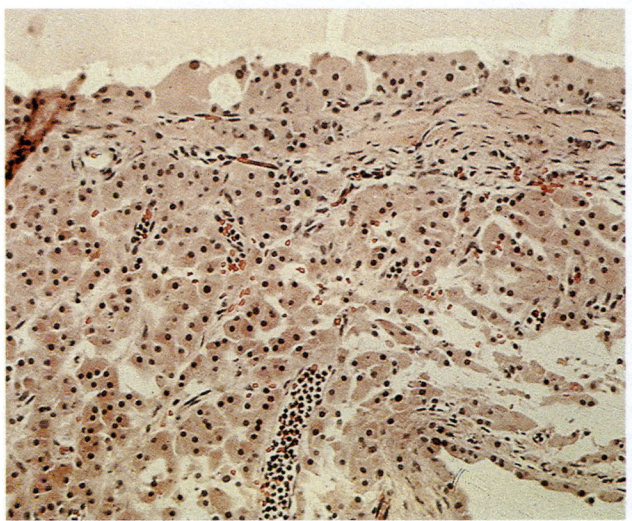

FIG. 8. Hyperreactio luteinalis. Two cysts are lined by luteinized granulosa cells; outside are thick layers of luteinized theca cells.

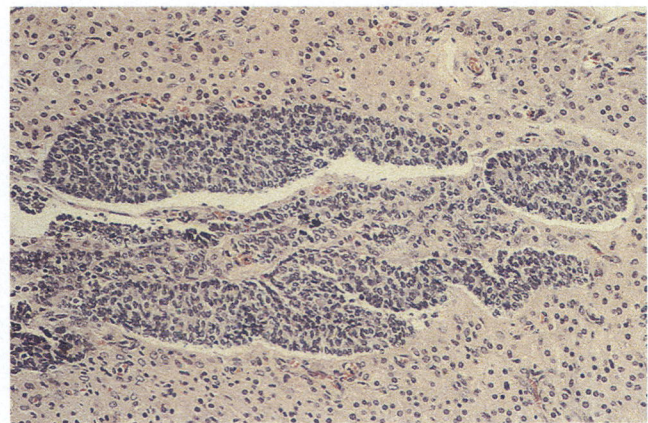

FIG. 9. Granulosa cell proliferation. Nests of granulosa cells have proliferated within an atretic follicle.

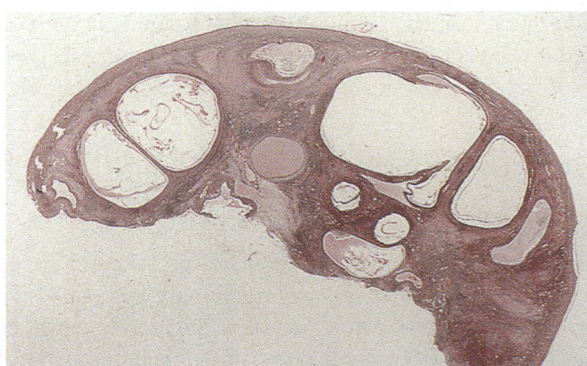

FIG. 10. Polycystic ovarian disease. Several follicle cysts are present; corpora lutea and albicantia are absent.

scribe the typical clinical and pathologic features of each separately, inasmuch as they generally differ in each category.

Polycystic Ovarian Disease (PCOD) (Stein-Leventhal Syndrome)

Clinical Features

PCOD has been estimated to affect 3.5% to 7.0% of the female population (64). The pathogenetic and endocrinologic features of the disorder are complex and have been reviewed elsewhere (65,66). Patients typically present in their third decade with a history of oligomenorrhea (rarely primary amenorrhea) or, occasionally, menometrorrhagia, accompanied by infertility and, in approximately half the cases, hirsutism; virilization is rare. The ovaries may be palpably enlarged. Examination of the endometrium may reveal a hypoactive proliferative appearance, cystic hyperplasia, atypical hyperplasia, or, in a small number of cases, adenocarcinoma that is almost always well differentiated (67,68).

Gross Features

Both ovaries are usually enlarged, but they may be of normal size. They have a white surface, with cysts less than 1 cm in diameter visible just below it. The central portion of the ovary is composed of stroma with few or no signs of ovulation, that is, corpora lutea or albicantia.

Microscopic Features

A hypocellular, fibrotic superficial cortex that resembles a fibrous capsule is evident (Figs. 10 and 11). Most of the cystic follicles contain relatively few granulosa cells but have a prominent layer of luteinized theca interna cells (follicular hyperthecosis) (Fig. 11). Maturing follicles and atretic follicles exhibiting prominent luteinization of the theca interna are twice as numerous as in normal ovaries (64,69). Although corpora lutea and albicantia are typically absent, the former have been described in up to 30% of otherwise typical cases of PCOD (69). The deeper cortical and medullary stroma is often hyperplastic and may exhibit hyperthecosis (69); if hyperthecosis is more than minor in extent, stromal hyperthecosis should also be diagnosed.

Findings similar to those of PCOD may also be seen during or shortly after puberty, in childhood hypothyroidism, and in disorders in which normal cyclic gonadotropin release is disrupted. These include late-onset congenital adrenal hyperplasia and primary hypothalamic-pituitary disorders, particularly those associated with hyperprolactinemia. Polycystic ovaries have also been described in patients after cessation of long-term use of oral contraceptives (70,71) as well as in those with periovarian adhesions (2). In the former group of patients, the disorder may have been present before the initiation of oral contraceptives in at least some cases.

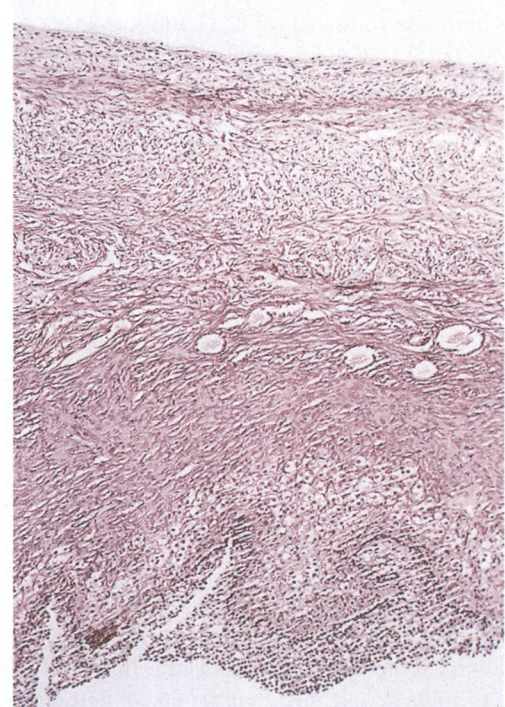

FIG. 11. Polycystic ovarian disease. Note collagenization of the outermost cortex and the thick band of luteinized theca cells around the follicle in the lower portion of the illustration.

Stromal Hyperplasia and Hyperthecosis

Proliferation of ovarian stromal cells is common in perimenopausal and early-postmenopausal women, and a sharp distinction cannot be drawn between normal stromal proliferation and so-called stromal hyperplasia (72). Nonetheless, the latter designation seems appropriate for cases in which the proliferation is of moderate to marked degree. Stromal hyperthecosis refers to the presence of luteinized stromal cells within an almost invariably hyperplastic ovarian stroma.

Clinical Features

Stromal hyperplasia is most common in patients in their sixth and seventh decades (72). It is difficult to assess the endocrine significance of stromal hyperplasia per se because no investigators have separately analyzed cases of simple hyperplasia and those in which the hyperplasia is accompanied by hyperthecosis. There is suggestive evidence, however, that stromal hyperplasia may be associated with androgen hypersecretion as well as obesity, hypertension, and disorders of glucose metabolism, although not as often or obtrusively as in cases of stromal hyperthecosis (72). Snowden et al. (73) have shown an association between stromal hyperplasia and endometrial adenocarcinoma, for which there is evidence of an estrogenic background in some cases. Androgen production by nonluteinized ovarian stromal cells is consistent with their content of oxidative enzymes, the so-called enzymatically active stromal cells (74).

Stromal hyperthecosis is usually encountered in patients in their sixth to ninth decades. It has been documented at autopsy in one-third of patients over the age of 55 years (72). In this age group, it is usually mild and without obvious clinical manifestations. Younger patients may show signs of marked virilization, obesity, hypertension, and decreased glucose tolerance (75,76). Stromal hyperthecosis (or, occasionally, PCOD) typically accompanies the HAIR-AN syndrome, which consists of hyperandrogenism (HA) insulin resistance (IR), and acanthosis nigricans (AN) (77). In many patients the clinical features of stromal hyperthecosis are less obtrusive, simulating those of PCOD. As in cases of PCOD, estrogenic manifestations such as endometrial hyperplasia or carcinoma are present in rare instances (76,78). The disorder can be familial, but these cases are unusual (79).

Gross Features

Both stromal hyperplasia and hyperthecosis may cause bilateral ovarian enlargement, with each ovary measuring up to 8 cm in diameter and mimicking ovarian neoplasia. The cut surface is homogeneous, firm, and white or yellow (Fig. 12). In premenopausal patients with hyperthecosis, sclerocystic changes similar to those seen in PCOD are usually also present (80).

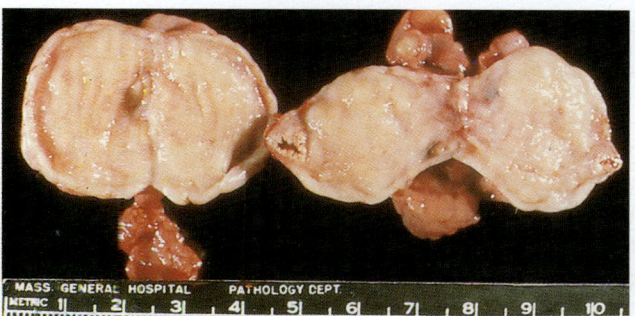

FIG. 12. Stromal hyperthecosis. Both ovaries are almost completely replaced by homogeneous yellow-white tissue.

Microscopic Features

Both the cortical and the medullary stroma may be hyperplastic. In stromal hyperthecosis, luteinized stromal cells appear singly, in small clusters (Fig. 13), or in nodules. They have abundant eosinophilic to vacuolated cytoplasm containing variable amounts of lipid and a round nucleus with a central small nucleolus. Associated ovarian findings have included small foci of metaplastic smooth muscle in the ovarian stroma (81), Leydig cell hyperplasia (82), Leydig cell tumors (82,83), and stromal luteomas (84). One of the latter was associated with the HAIR-AN syndrome (85). In patients with that syndrome, an additional microscopic finding is the presence of a hypocellular stroma exhibiting edema or fibrosis; the prominent stromal hyperplasia that is typical of stromal hyperthecosis is often absent (86).

Massive Edema and Fibromatosis

Tumor-like enlargement of one or both ovaries as the result of an accumulation of edema fluid within the ovarian stroma has been designated massive ovarian edema (87–89). Another tumor-like lesion, termed ovarian fibromatosis, has clinical and pathologic features that overlap with those of massive edema, suggesting a probable relationship between the two entities (88).

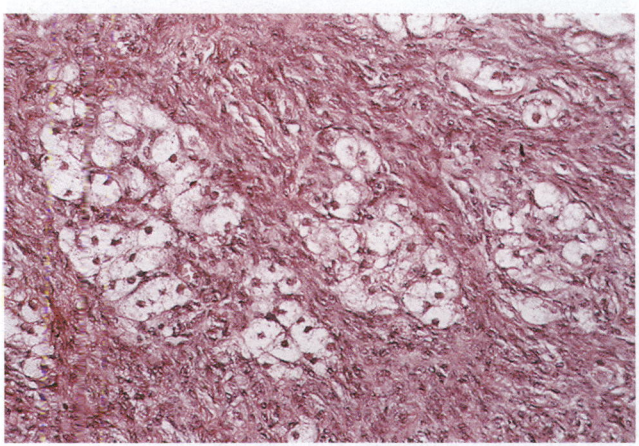

FIG. 13. Stromal hyperthecosis. Clusters of luteinized cells with vacuolated cytoplasm lie in the ovarian stroma.

Massive Edema

Clinical Features

The patients have ranged in age from 6 to 33 years, with an average of 21 years. Three-fourths of them have had abdominal or pelvic pain, which may be acute and accompanied by abdominal swelling. In the remaining patients, the clinical manifestations have been menstrual irregularities, evidence of androgen excess, or both; the plasma testosterone level has been elevated in some cases. Examination typically reveals a palpable mass. The ovarian enlargement is unilateral in about 90% of cases. Partial or complete torsion of the involved ovary has been present in at least half the cases. Isolated patients have had Meigs' syndrome.

Gross Features

The ovary is enlarged, soft, and fluctuant (Fig. 14), ranging in diameter from 5.5 to 35 cm (mean, 11.5 cm); the heaviest example weighed 2,400 g. The external surface is shiny, white, and smooth, and the cut surface is pale, homogeneous, and soft, exuding a watery fluid. The superficial cortex appears white and fibrotic. The presence of follicles, which are often cystic, within the edematous tissue distinguishes massive edema from an edematous fibroma, which displaces rather than envelops follicles, with rare exceptions, usually at their periphery.

Microscopic Features

The striking finding on low magnification is marked, diffuse stromal edema that surrounds follicles and their derivatives (Fig. 15) but typically spares the thickened, fibrotic superficial cortex. Higher magnification shows abundant pale-staining fluid, which may have a focal microcystic appearance. In nonedematous areas, the stroma may resemble normal stroma, hyperplastic stroma, or the type of stroma

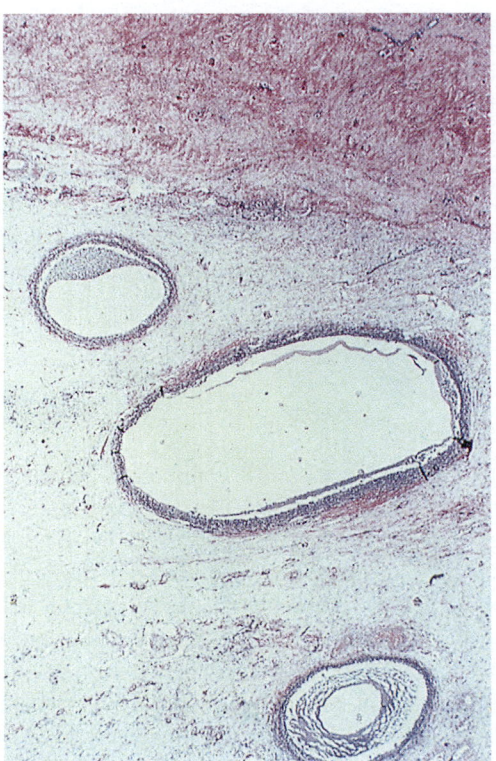

FIG. 15. Massive edema. Pale, edematous stroma surrounds several graafian follicles.

seen in ovarian fibromatosis. In approximately 40% of cases, luteinized stromal cells are present. Associated findings include vascular dilatation within the ovary and, from time to time, the mesosalpinx and rare foci of necrosis. The contralateral ovary is typically normal in appearance, but it may also be enlarged and edematous. In exceptional cases, it is not edematous but is affected by stromal hyperthecosis or appears sclerocystic.

Differential Diagnosis

Massive edema can be distinguished from ovarian neoplasms with an edematous or myxoid appearance, such as edematous fibroma, sclerosing stromal tumor, Krukenberg tumor, and the rare ovarian myxoma by the absence of characteristic features of those tumors as well as by the inclusion of follicular derivatives within the lesion.

Fibromatosis

Clinical Features

The age of the affected patients has ranged from 13 to 39 years, with an average of 25 years (88). Clinical manifestations include menstrual abnormalities, abdominal pain, and, rarely, hirsutism or virilization. An adnexal mass is usually palpable. The process is usually unilateral; in 15% of cases, the involved ovaries have undergone torsion.

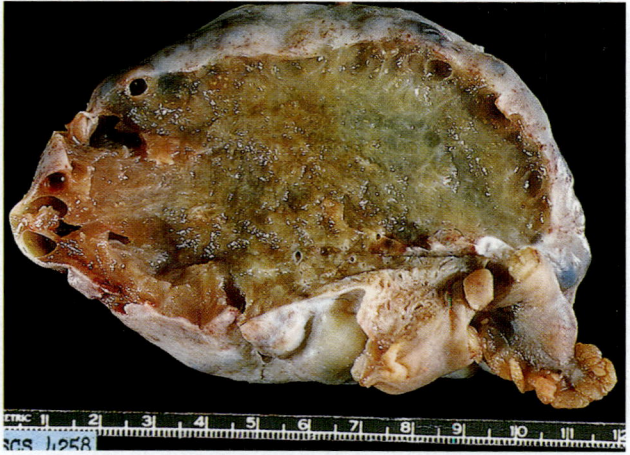

FIG. 14. Massive edema. The ovary is replaced by gelatinous tissue.

Pathologic Features

Gross examination shows ovaries 6 to 12 cm in diameter with smooth, white external surfaces. The cut surfaces are firm, white, and solid, although cystic follicles are recognizable within the lesion in one-third of cases (Fig. 16). On microscopic examination, a proliferation of spindle cells producing variable amounts of collagen is visible, with an appearance varying from moderately cellular fascicles of spindle cells with a focal storiform pattern to relatively acellular bands of dense collagen (Fig. 17) (88). The process typically surrounds normal follicle structures and produces collagenous thickening of the superficial cortex. Foci of stromal edema are present in approximately half the cases. Luteinized stromal cells and microscopic foci of sex-cord cells have been seen in a few cases.

Differential Diagnosis

Ovarian fibromatosis should be distinguished from fibroma, which usually appears in older age groups, is typically nonfunctioning, and almost never contains follicles or their derivatives. The few small aggregates of sex-cord cells in fibromatosis should not cause confusion with a sex cord–stromal tumor.

Pregnancy Luteoma

Pregnancy luteoma is characterized by tumor-like ovarian enlargement during pregnancy as the consequence of solid proliferations of luteinized cells derived from theca lutein or luteinized stromal cells (90–92). The disorder is probably related to hCG stimulation, but the rarity of pregnancy luteomas in association with trophoblastic disease and the almost exclusive occurrence of the lesions during the third trimester, when hCG levels are lower than earlier in pregnancy, indicate that this hormone is not the only factor in their development.

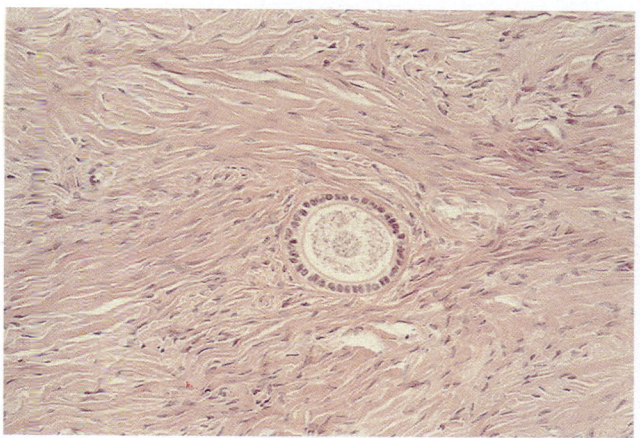

FIG. 17. Fibromatosis. Dense, hyalinized fibrous tissue has replaced the normal ovarian stroma and surrounds a primary follicle.

Clinical Features

Most patients have been in their third or fourth decades, black, and multiparous. The lesion is usually discovered incidentally at term during cesarean section or postpartum tubal ligation. Infrequently, a pelvic mass is palpable or causes obstruction of the birth canal. In approximately 25% of cases, there is hirsutism or virilization; two-thirds of female infants born to such mothers also show signs of virilism (93). Regression of the enlarged ovaries usually begins within days after delivery, and they become normal in size within several weeks.

Gross Features

The lesions range from small nodules to masses up to 20 cm in diameter, with soft, fleshy, circumscribed, brown (Fig. 18) or gray cut surfaces; foci of hemorrhage are common. They

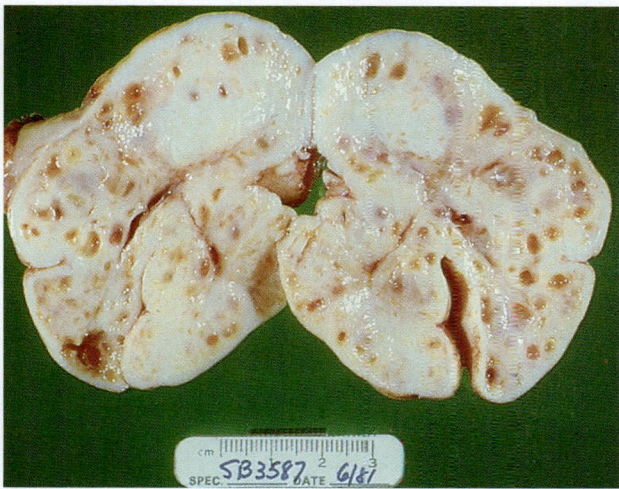

FIG. 16. Fibromatosis. The sectioned surfaces of the ovary reveal dense white tissue surrounding cystic follicles.

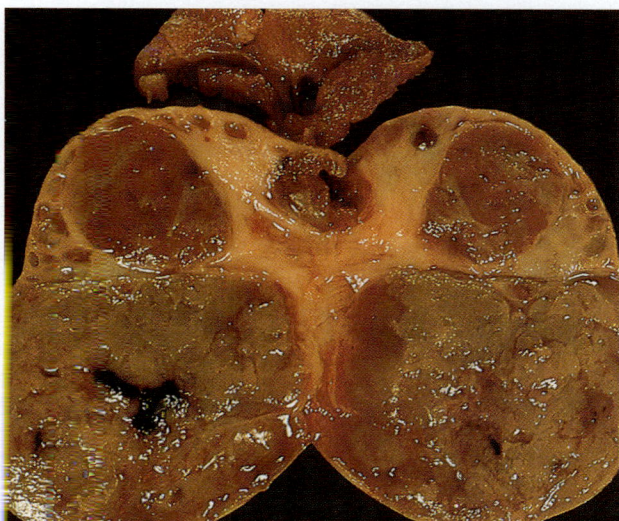

FIG. 18. Pregnancy luteoma. The sectioned surfaces of the ovary show several nodules of pale brown to red tissue.

are multiple in at least half the cases and bilateral in a third. On examination of the ovaries days to weeks postpartum, focally infarcted lesions or brown puckered scars (94) are visible.

Microscopic Features

The sharply circumscribed nodules (Fig. 19) are composed of polygonal cells intermediate in size between the luteinized granulosa and theca cells of adjacent follicles. Occasionally, the cells are arranged in cords or small clusters or surround spaces containing colloid-like material (Fig. 19). The cytoplasm is abundant, eosinophilic, and finely granular and contains little or no lipid. Less common features include focal ballooning degeneration of the cytoplasm and small numbers of intracellular hyaline droplets similar to those seen in the corpus luteum of pregnancy. The nuclei may be slightly pleomorphic and hyperchromatic; mitotic figures range up to seven per 10 high-power fields (hpf), with an average of two or three; occasionally, atypical forms are seen (91). The intercellular stroma is scanty, and reticulin fibrils surround groups of cells. Postpartum examination of the lesions shows lipid accumulation in the cells, round cell infiltration, and fibrosis (94).

Differential Diagnosis

If several bilateral nodules are present, a major difficulty in intraoperative differential diagnosis is distinguishing these lesions from metastatic carcinoma, especially Krukenberg tumor. Like the pregnancy luteoma, Krukenberg tumor can also bring about virilization if luteinization of its stroma occurs. Frozen section of a biopsy specimen or an excised nodule should establish the correct diagnosis. Although a number of lesions containing luteinized cells that arise during pregnancy may enter the differential diagnosis on microscopic examination, the gross appearance of multiple, bilateral, solid nodules is distinctive of pregnancy luteoma. Neoplasms composed in part or totally of luteinized cells, that is, those in the sex cord–stromal and steroid cell categories, are almost always unilateral and solitary. Sex cord–stromal tumors typically contain nonluteinized foci and have a denser reticulin pattern and more abundant intracellular lipid than pregnancy luteomas. Tumors in the steroid cell group that are composed entirely of lipid-poor or lipid-free steroid cells may closely resemble or be indistinguishable from pregnancy luteomas. This differential diagnosis is discussed on page 2358.

Hilus Cell Hyperplasia

Clinical Features

Hilus cell hyperplasia may be seen during pregnancy, as a result of hCG administration, and in postmenopausal women, in whom the process may be related to their high luteinizing hormone level (72,95,96). Prominent degrees of hilus cell hyperplasia were found in more than 40% of women over 70 years of age in one autopsy study (72). As-

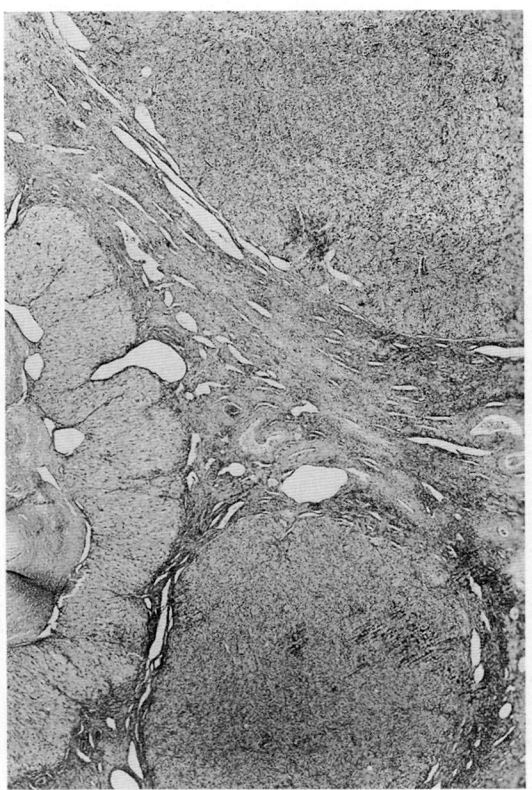
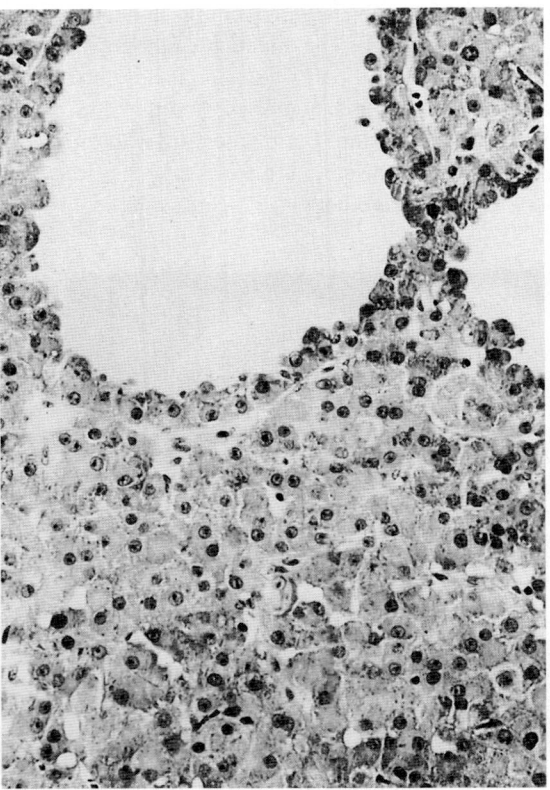

FIG. 19. Pregnancy luteoma. Two large nodules of lutein cells lie to the right of a corpus luteum (left). Note the follicle-like structures within the luteoma (right).

sessment of the role of hilus cell hyperplasia in endocrine disturbances is often complicated by the coexistence of stromal hyperthecosis, a hilus cell tumor, or both (97) but rare cases in which isolated hilus cell hyperplasia has been apparently responsible for androgenic or estrogenic manifestations have been reported. In some cases, elevated plasma testosterone levels have been documented (98).

Pathologic Features

Hilus cell hyperplasia may be grossly visible as several yellow hilar nodules, usually less than 2 mm in diameter. On microscopic examination, the hilus cells are arranged in nodular (Fig. 20) or diffuse patterns; multinucleated cells and a few mitotic figures may be seen (90,91). In elderly women, the hyperplastic hilus cells may be enlarged and have bizarre shapes and hyperchromatic nuclei (Fig. 20). Hilus cell hyperplasia may also develop adjacent to an ovarian tumor and result in endocrine, particularly androgenic, manifestations (99).

Stromal–Leydig Cell Hyperplasia

Leydig cells containing Reinke crystals have been encountered now and then within the ovarian stroma away from the hilus, usually as a focal microscopic finding in an ovary exhibiting otherwise typical stromal hyperthecosis, hilus cell hyperplasia, or a hilus cell tumor (82). Leydig cells have also been described in rare instances within the non-neoplastic stroma of a variety of ovarian neoplasms or in the ovarian stroma adjacent to an ovarian neoplasm (40,99).

Stromal Metaplasias

Decidual Reaction

Clinical Features

An ectopic decidual reaction may be confined to the ovarian stroma or be part of a more widespread decidual transformation of the submesothelial pelvic stroma (see Chapter 56). An ovarian decidual reaction is usually a response of the stromal cells to high circulating or local levels of estrogen and progesterone. The process is seen most often during pregnancy, as early as the ninth week of gestation; it is present in almost all ovaries at term (100–104). Less often, ectopic decidua is associated with trophoblastic disease, progestin treatment, an adjacent corpus luteum, an adjoining metastatic tumor, or a steroid-secreting lesion of the ovary or adrenal gland. Ovarian irradiation may be followed by a decidual reaction, possibly by increasing the sensitivity of the stromal cells to hormonal stimulation (105). Occasionally, ectopic decidua occurs within the ovaries of premenopausal and postmenopausal women without an obvious cause.

Pathologic Features

The decidual foci may be grossly visible as soft, red surface nodules, ridges, or patches (101,103), but more frequently they are incidental findings on microscopic examination. The decidual cells are typically found in the superficial cortical stroma or in surface adhesions, where they may be disposed singly, as small nodules, in sheets, or as small polypoid projections from the ovarian surface (101,106). Most of the cells are indistinguishable from eutopic decidual cells; occasionally, they mimic signet ring cells owing to a basophilic appearance of the cytoplasm, which may displace the nuclei to the periphery. Cells transitional in appearance between spindle-shaped ovarian stromal cells and fully decidualized cells are also usually present. In some cases, ultrastructural examination has revealed smooth-muscle cells (107). A rich network of distended capillaries and a sprinkling of lymphocytes are typically found within the decidual foci. Florid examples can simulate metastatic carcinoma, particularly if the decidual cells show focal cytologic atypia or have signet ring–like features. Degenerative changes within the decidua are typically seen postpartum.

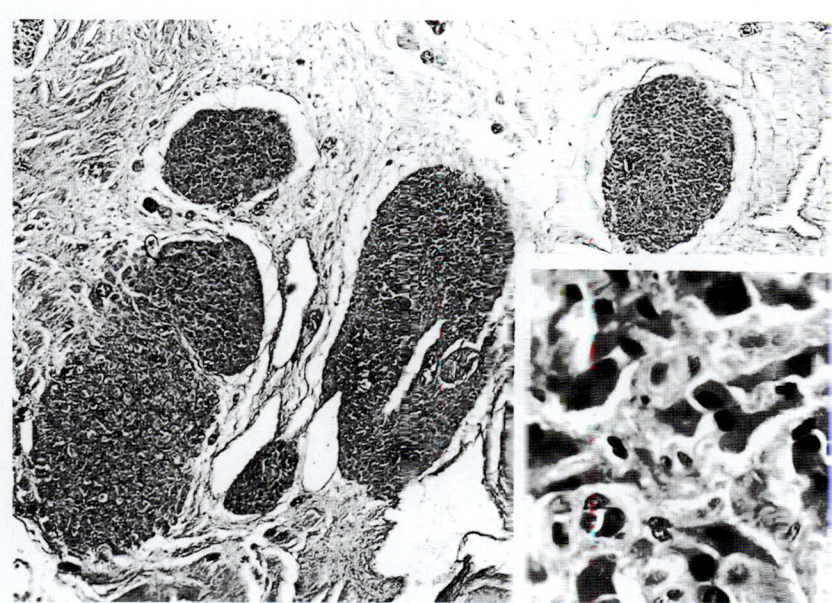

FIG. 20. Hilus cell hyperplasia. Several nodules of hilus cells are prominent in the ovarian hilus. Inset: Hilus cells of bizarre shapes with hyperchromatic nuclei. (From ref. 40.)

Other Stromal Metaplasias

Small nodules of metaplastic smooth muscle are encountered from time to time within otherwise unremarkable ovarian stroma, within the hyperplastic stroma of stromal hyperthecosis, and within the stroma surrounding nonneoplastic or neoplastic cysts. Foci of mature fat also have been described as occasional incidental findings within the superficial stroma (108). Heterotopic bone formation in the ovary in the absence of an ovarian neoplasm is rare. It typically occurs within periovarian adhesions or in the walls of endometriotic cysts; in exceptional cases, it develops within otherwise normal ovaries (109).

Disorders Causing Ovarian Failure

Premature ovarian failure is generally defined as secondary amenorrhea and infertility before the age of 35 years. If one excludes cases of gonadal maldevelopment and obvious chromosomal abnormalities as well as surgical, radiation-induced, or drug-induced ablation of ovarian function, three disorders are associated with distinctive ovarian changes in patients with premature ovarian failure: premature follicle depletion (true premature menopause), the resistant ovary syndrome, and autoimmune oophoritis. All of these disorders probably include a number of subtypes of diverse pathogenesis (110,111).

True Premature Menopause

The true premature menopause is characterized by ovaries that are typically small and resemble microscopically normal perimenopausal or postmenopausal ovaries (110–113). Some cases may be caused by relatively minor chromosomal abnormalities.

Resistant Ovary Syndrome

The resistant ovary syndrome is found in approximately 20% of patients with premature ovarian failure and is characterized by primary or secondary amenorrhea, high gonadotropin levels, and resistance to both endogenous and exogenous gonadotropins, even when administered in massive doses (114–117). The pathogenesis of the disorder is unknown, but a deficiency of follicle-stimulating hormone and luteinizing hormone (LH) receptors in the follicles, the presence of antibodies to these receptors, and a postreceptor defect have all been implicated.

The ovaries typically have a normal prepubertal or adult appearance on gross inspection. On histologic examination, there is an appropriate number of normal-appearing primordial follicles but a complete or nearly complete absence of developing follicles beyond the antral stage. Atretic follicles and signs of previous ovulation may be seen. Unusual histologic findings have included focal or diffuse hyalinization of atretic follicles in the preantral stage (117) and central calcification within atretic follicles (115). Stromal luteinization and hilus cell hyperplasia in rare instances result from a high level of luteinizing hormone and are associated with virilization (97). A histologic pattern similar to that seen in the resistant ovary syndrome may occur in the context of morbid obesity, Cushing's syndrome, and hypogonadotropic ovarian failure stemming from hypothalamic-pituitary dysfunction (19).

Autoimmune Oophoritis

At least 25 reported cases of autoimmune oophoritis have been confirmed histologically (110,111,118–121). In most of them, the patients had oligomenorrhea or amenorrhea; occasionally, symptoms related to enlarged polycystic ovaries or abnormal vaginal bleeding have been the initial manifestations (121–123). In most of these cases, and others in which ovarian biopsy has not been performed, antibodies to steroid-hormone-producing cells, including granulosa and theca cells, have been present in the serum (124–131). The ovarian failure is usually preceded or accompanied by one or more of the following disorders, most of which are thought to have an autoimmune basis: idiopathic Addison's disease, idiopathic hypoparathyroidism, hyperthyroidism, Hashimoto's disease, hypothyroidism, myasthenia gravis, juvenile-onset diabetes mellitus, juvenile rheumatoid arthritis, sicca syndrome, vitiligo, pernicious anemia, alopecia, autoimmune hemolytic anemia, idiopathic thrombocytopenia purpura, and mucocutaneous candidiasis.

On gross examination, the ovaries are usually of normal size, but they may be enlarged and polycystic (121–123). On histologic inspection, primordial follicles appear normal, but inflammatory cells begin to infiltrate the theca cell layer as it differentiates at the edge of early-maturing follicles (Fig. 21). The intensity of the infiltrate increases with the degree of follicular maturation, and as the follicles enlarge, the inflammatory cells and degenerating granulosa cells desquamate into the lumen. If corpora lutea are present, they are similarly inflamed (122). Lymphocytes and plasma cells pre-

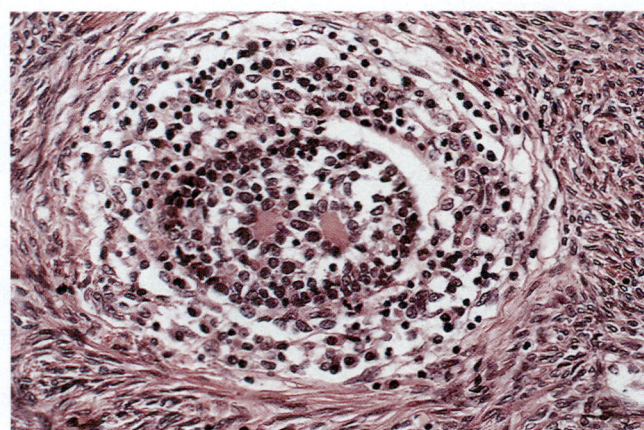

FIG. 21. Autoimmune oophoritis. Lymphocytes and plasma cells have infiltrated the theca interna layer of a preantral follicle.

dominate, but eosinophils, histiocytes, and sarcoid-like granulomas have also been described (122). Occasionally, lymphoid infiltrates have been found in the ovarian hilus, sometimes in a perineural distribution, accompanied by an absence of Leydig cells, suggesting destruction of the latter by the inflammatory process (119). In 25% of the cases in one series (122), abnormal follicles with hyalinization were encountered.

Cytotoxic Drug Effects

Cytotoxic drugs may be associated with a variety of ovarian changes, including a reduction or depletion of follicles, impaired follicular maturation, and focal or diffuse cortical fibrosis (19,111). These findings are consistent with clinical evidence of diminished ovarian endocrine function or ovarian failure in some patients. The ovarian failure is sometimes reversible after the cessation of therapy.

Radiation Effects

The ovary is among the most radiosensitive of organs, and ovarian failure occurs in most patients who receive pelvic radiation (18). Relatively low doses (500 to 600 R) are associated with complete or nearly complete disappearance of primordial and developing follicles, fibrosis of the ovarian stroma, and vascular sclerosis in more than 90% of patients. The ovarian stroma is more radioresistant than the follicles and may continue to secrete androgens after exposure.

Idiopathic Calcification

Clement and Cooney (132) described a case of extensive bilateral ovarian calcification that resulted in a stony-hard consistency of both ovaries, which were of normal size and filled with numerous spherical laminated calcific foci without accompanying epithelial cells. The cause of the calcification was not apparent.

Congenital Lesions

These very rare lesions include lobulated, accessory, and supernumerary ovaries; splenic-gonadal fusion; and adrenal cortical rests (19,40).

TUMORS

Most ovarian tumors cannot be confidently distinguished from one another on the basis of their clinical or gross characteristics. These features may provide important diagnostic clues in some cases, however, and both the clinician and the pathologist should be aware of them in formulating a differential diagnosis. One of the most important clinical features is the age of the patient. Approximately one of eight ovarian tumors in patients under 45 years of age is malignant, whereas in older women the corresponding figure is almost one of two (40,133). The single most common ovarian tumor, the dermoid cyst, is encountered at all ages, as are most of the tumors in the sex cord–stromal category. Other ovarian neoplasms, in contrast, are largely restricted to certain age groups. For example, primitive germ cell tumors are almost never encountered in women over 50 years of age. In contrast, the adult forms of germ cell cancer, usually squamous cell carcinomas arising in dermoid cysts, are typically seen in older women and increase in incidence with advancing age. Some rare primitive tumors indistinguishable from germ cell tumors, such as yolk sac tumor and choriocarcinoma, are of somatic-cell origin in older patients. Within the surface epithelial group, borderline tumors are often seen in women in their thirties and even in younger women, whereas carcinomas in this category are rare in women under 40 years of age, most of those encountered being of the mucinous type.

The stage and laterality of ovarian cancers are also clues to their nature. For example, sex cord–stromal tumors are almost always confined to one ovary. Therefore, when one is examining a tumor that is bilateral or has spread beyond the ovary one should be cautious in making a diagnosis of sex cord–stromal tumor. On the other hand, the approximately 65% rate of bilaterality of tumors that are metastatic to the ovary indicates that they should always be a diagnostic consideration when one encounters bilateral tumors, particularly if their morphologic features are not characteristic of any primary ovarian cancer and even in some situations in which they are. Nevertheless, accurate diagnosis of ovarian tumors depends primarily on a knowledge of the wide range of microscopic features they may exhibit. In the following discussion, emphasis will be placed on gross and microscopic features that are important in differential diagnosis. Immunohistochemical and ultrastructural findings will be included only when they are helpful in establishing the diagnosis. Because of space considerations, clinical manifestations including, staging (134), histogenesis, and therapy will receive relatively little comment. The classification used will be that of the World Health Organization (WHO), with slight modifications (Table 1) (135).

Surface Epithelial–Stromal Tumors

These tumors, which will be referred to as "surface epithelial" or "epithelial" tumors, account for approximately two-thirds of all ovarian neoplasms, and their malignant forms account for about 90% of ovarian cancers in the Western world (40). Most epithelial tumors are derived from the ovarian surface epithelium, which develops from the coelomic epithelium (mesothelium) that covers the embryonic gonad. The ovarian coelomic epithelium is continuous with the nearby coelomic epithelium, which penetrates the underlying mesenchyme to form the müllerian duct. This embryonic proximity is reflected in the various directions of müllerian differentiation exhibited by the surface epithelium when it undergoes neoplasia, for example, toward fallopian

TABLE 1. Classification of Ovarian Tumors and Tumor-Like Lesions

Surface epithelial–stromal tumors
  Serous tumors
    Benign
      Cystadenoma and papillary cystadenoma
      Surface papilloma
      Adenofibroma and cystadenofibroma
    Of borderline malignancy (of low malignant potential)
      Cystic tumor and papillary cystic tumor
      Surface papilloma
      Adenofibroma and cystadenofibroma
    Malignant
      Adenocarcinoma, papillary adenocarcinoma, and papillary cystadenocarcinoma
      Surface papillary adenocarcinoma
      Malignant adenofibroma and cystadenofibroma
  Mucinous tumors, endocervical-like and intestinal type
    Benign
      Cystadenoma
      Adenofibroma and cystadenofibroma
    Of borderline malignancy (of low malignant potential)
      Cystic tumor
        Variant — with intraepithelial carcinoma
      Adenofibroma and cystadenofibroma
    Malignant
      Adenocarcinoma and cystadenocarcinoma
      Malignant adenofibroma and cystadenofibroma
  Endometrioid tumors
    Benign
      Adenoma and cystadenoma
      Adenofibroma and cystadenofibroma
    Of borderline malignancy (of low malignant potential)
      Adenofibroma and cystic tumor
      Adenofibroma and cystadenofibroma
    Malignant
      Carcinoma
        Adenocarcinoma
        Adenocarcinoma with squamous differentiation
        Malignant adenofibroma and cystadenofibroma
      Endometrioid stromal sarcoma
      Malignant mesodermal (müllerian) mixed tumor, homologous and heterologous
      Mesodermal adenosarcoma
  Clear-cell tumors
    Benign
    Of borderline malignancy (of low malignant potential)
    Malignant
      Adenocarcinoma
      Malignant adenofibroma and cystadenofibroma
  Transitional cell tumors
    Brenner tumor
    Brenner tumor of borderline malignancy (proliferating)
    Malignant Brenner tumor
    Transitional cell carcinoma
  Squamous cell tumors
  Undifferentiated carcinoma
    Variants
      Small cell carcinoma, pulmonary type
      Neuroendocrine carcinoma, non-small cell type
  Mixed epithelial tumors
    Benign
    Of borderline malignancy (of low malignant potential)
    Malignant

Sex cord–stromal tumors
  Granulosa–stromal cell tumors
    Granulosa cell tumor
      Adult type
      Juvenile type
    Tumors in the thecoma-fibroma group
      Thecoma
        Typical
        Luteinized[a]
        Variant: with sclerosing peritonitis
      Fibroma-Fibrosarcoma
        Fibroma
        Cellular fibroma
        Fibrosarcoma
      Stromal tumors with minor sex cord elements
      Sclerosing stromal tumor
      Signet-ring stromal tumor
      Others
  Sertoli–stromal cell tumors (androblastomas)
    Sertoli cell tumor
    Sertoli–Leydig cell tumor
      Well-differentiated
      Of intermediate differentiation
        Variant — with heterologous elements (specify type)
      Poorly differentiated
        Variant — with heterologous elements (specify type)
      Retiform
        Variant — with heterologous elements (specify type)
      Mixed
    (Leydig cell tumor)[b]
  Gynandroblastoma
  Sex-cord tumor with annular tubules
  Unclassified
Steroid cell tumors
  Stromal luteoma
  Leydig cell tumor
    Hilus cell tumor
    Leydig cell tumor, non-hilar type
  Steroid cell tumor, not otherwise specified
Tumors of the rete ovarii
Germ cell tumors
  Dysgerminoma
    Variant — with syncytiotrophoblast cells
  Yolk sac tumor (endodermal sinus tumor)
    Variant
      Polyvesicular vitelline tumor
      Hepatoid
      Glandular
  Embryonal carcinoma
  Choriocarcinoma
  Polyembryoma
  Teratomas
    Immature
    Mature
      Solid
      Cystic
        Dermoid cyst (mature cystic teratoma)
        Dermoid cyst with secondary tumor (specify type)
      Fetiform

(continued)

TABLE 1. Continued

Germ cell tumors (cont'd)	Tumor of probable wolffian origin
Monodermal	Small-cell carcinoma, hypercalcemic type
Struma	Hepatoid carcinoma
Carcinoid	Myxoma
Insular	Gestational trophoblastic diseases
Trabecular	Soft-tissue tumors not specific to ovary and miscellaneous
Strumal	other tumors
Goblet cell	Malignant lymphomas and leukemias
Neuroectodermal tumors	Secondary (metastatic) tumors
Sebaceous tumors	Tumor-like conditions
Others	Solitary follicle cyst
Mixed germ-cell tumors	Corpus luteum cyst
Germ cell-sex cord-stromal tumors	Multiple follicle cysts (polycystic ovaries)
Gonadoblastoma	Stromal hyperplasia and hyperthecosis
Pure	Massive edema
Mixed with dysgerminoma or another form of germ cell	Fibromatosis
tumor	Pregnancy luteoma
Of nongonadoblastoma type	Multiple luteinized follicle cysts (hyperreactio luteinalis)
Tumors of rete ovarii	Large solitary follicle cyst of pregnancy and puerperium
Mesothelial tumors	Granulosa cell proliferations of pregnancy
Adenomatoid tumor	Endometriosis
Mesothelioma	Surface epithelial inclusion cysts
Tumors of uncertain cell type and miscellaneous tumors	Simple cysts
	Inflammatory lesions

[a] Tumors that resemble luteinized thecomas but in which crystals of Reinke are identified in the steroid cells are designated stromal–Leydig cell tumors.
[b] Leydig cell tumors are generally considered in the category of steroid cell tumors because of their close resemblance to other tumors in that category.

tube epithelium in serous neoplasms, endometrial epithelium in endometrioid tumors, and endocervical epithelium in mucinous neoplasms.

As a woman approaches menopause, the ovarian surface epithelium often extends into the underlying stroma to form epithelial inclusion glands, which may become cystic. This process occurs less often during reproductive life and rarely before puberty. Although epithelial tumors can arise directly from the surface epithelium and grow exophytically, they typically originate from its inclusion glands, accounting for the cystic (endophytic) nature of most of these tumors. Epithelial tumors become solid when they contain a large stromal component or when malignant cells within them proliferate to form masses.

Some subtypes of epithelial tumor that are included in the surface epithelial category may not be of surface epithelial derivation in every case. For example, rare Brenner tumors arise from the rete ovarii or are associated with a monodermal teratoma, and some mucinous tumors may be monophyletic endodermal teratomas. The evidence suggesting a germ cell origin for mucinous tumors includes a 5% rate of adjacent dermoid cyst, the common finding of mucinous glands in the walls of dermoid cysts and in other teratomas, and the lining of mucinous cystic tumors by intestinal rather than endocervical-type epithelium in at least 25% of cases. The last finding does not necessarily establish an endodermal origin of the tumor, since it may reflect only endodermal metaplasia of epithelium of mesodermal derivation. Despite these histogenetic problems, Brenner tumors and mucinous tumors are still placed in the surface epithelial category to maintain the simplicity of the classification. Careful study of epithelial tumors often reveals two or even three cell types. When one or more additional cell types account for less than 10% of the neoplasm, it is classified on the basis of its predominant cellular element; otherwise, it is designated a form of mixed epithelial tumor.

In addition to being subdivided according to cell type, epithelial tumors are subclassified according to three other criteria, two of them architectural and the third related to the degree of proliferation and nuclear features of the neoplastic cells. Some tumors, particularly those in the serous category, may be exophytic, endophytic, or both. When exophytic growth is present, the word "surface" is added to the tumor's designation, for example, "serous surface papillary carcinoma." Except for the benign Brenner tumor, which almost always has a predominant stromal component, most epithelial neoplasms of other cell types are primarily epithelial, with only a minor component derived from the ovarian stroma. When the latter tumors have a predominant stromal component, the terms adenofibroma and cystadenofibroma (if grossly visible cysts are present) are used.

A minority of epithelial tumors are intermediate between clearly benign and obviously malignant in their histologic features and clinical behavior. The International Federation of Gynecology and Obstetrics initially adopted the designation tumor of low malignant potential for such neoplasms, but the term tumor of borderline malignancy has been preferred by the WHO committee on classification and nomenclature of ovarian tumors (135). Tumors in this category are characterized by a degree of epithelial proliferation greater than that seen in benign tumors of the same cell type but an absence of "obvious" or "destructive" stromal invasion (136–147). Borderline tumors, however, may be associated with peritoneal implants, which are occasionally invasive (147–152). Also, in approximately 20% of cases of serous borderline tumor, regional lymph nodes harbor foci of what has been generally interpreted as metastatic tumor (153–156) (see later discussion). Rarely, borderline tumors metastasize distantly. The diagnosis of borderline malignancy is based on an examination of the primary tumor, however, without regard for the presence or absence of extension beyond the ovary. This diagnostic approach is justified because the survival is typically long, even in cases with extraovarian spread. Nevertheless, a few borderline tumors are fatal, often after many years.

Serous Tumors

Serous neoplasms account for 20% to 50% of all ovarian tumors, and their benign forms account for a similar proportion of benign ovarian neoplasms. Approximately 70% of serous tumors are benign, 5% to 10% are of borderline malignancy, and 20% to 25% are carcinomas. Borderline and invasive serous tumors together make up 35% to 40% of all ovarian cancers. Benign serous tumors may occur at any age, but they are most common during the fifth decade. Borderline tumors are encountered most frequently between the ages of 30 and 60 years, and carcinomas are found most often between the ages of 40 and 70 years.

Gross Features

Benign serous tumors may be endophytic (cystadenomas), exophytic (surface papillomas), or both. The serous cystadenoma is typically unilocular, but it may be multilocular and is characterized by thin-walled cyst(s) filled with watery or occasionally mucinous or hemorrhagic fluid. The cyst(s) may contain polypoid excrescences, which are firm if the stroma is dense and fibrous and soft if it is edematous. Serous cystadenomas, which are bilateral in approximately 10% of cases, can be large but only occasionally attain the huge dimensions more often reached by mucinous cystadenomas.

Serous surface papillomas appear as polypoid excrescences on the serosal surface of one or both ovaries. They are often associated with an underlying cystic component. Serous adenofibromas and cystadenofibromas are hard, white, predominantly solid fibromatous tumors, within which are small glands or cysts containing clear fluid and sometimes polypoid excrescences.

Serous cystic tumors and surface papillomas of borderline malignancy (Figs. 22 and 23) have gross features similar to those of benign serous papillary tumors, except that their

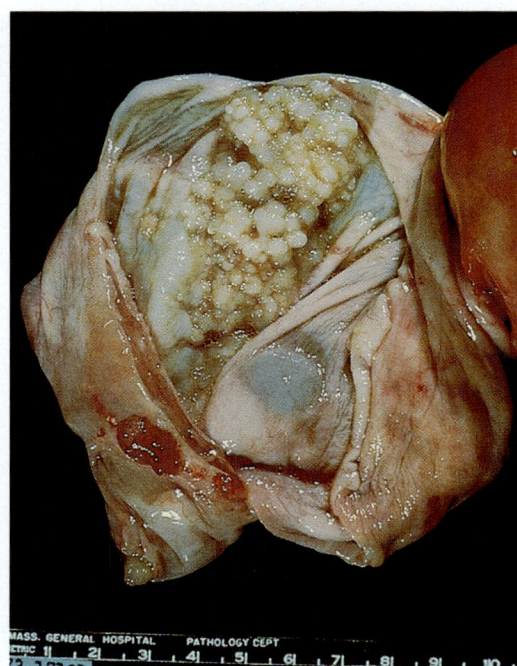

FIG. 22. Serous papillary cystadenoma of borderline malignancy. White polypoid excrescences that were soft arise from the lining of the cyst.

papillae are generally more extensive, finer, and softer. Microscopic examination is necessary to distinguish these tumors reliably. Serous borderline cystic tumors sometimes secrete thick, mucinous fluid, which should not lead to the precipitous diagnosis of mucinous tumor on gross examination. Serous borderline tumors are obviously bilateral in approximately 25% of stage I cases. In an additional 10% of cases, involvement of the opposite ovary is evident on microscopic examination; occasionally, the microscopic tumor is observed to have arisen in an epithelial inclusion cyst.

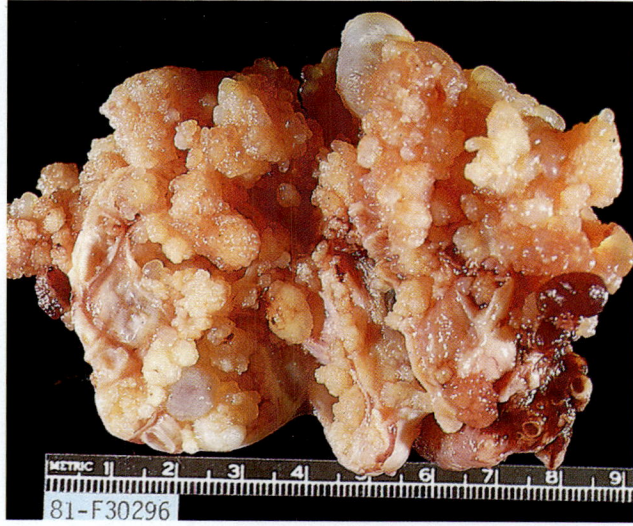

FIG. 23. Serous surface papilloma of borderline malignancy. Papillae and polypoid fronds cover most of the outer surface of the ovary.

Serous carcinomas may be predominantly cystic and papillary, entirely solid and firm, or both cystic and solid. The poorly differentiated forms lack distinctive features on gross examination, sharing with other types of ovarian carcinoma nonspecific characteristics of malignancy, such as friability, necrosis, and hemorrhage. Rarely, serous carcinomas appear in the form of surface papillary or granular deposits (Fig. 24), which may be inconspicuous or even undetectable on gross examination (serous surface carcinomas) (157). Serous carcinomas in general are bilateral in about two-thirds of cases, but only about one-third of stage I and IIa tumors involve both ovaries (40).

Microscopic Features

The cysts and papillae of benign serous tumors are typically lined by epithelium similar to that of the fallopian tube. Tumors lined entirely by nonciliated cuboidal or columnar epithelium that resembles ovarian surface epithelium are also generally classified within the serous category despite their indifferent appearance and evidence that some of them may be endometrioid rather than serous. The epithelial cells of benign serous tumors may secrete mucin, but when it is present, it is confined to the lumens of cysts and the apical portion of the cytoplasm of the lining cells. Psammoma bodies are generally inconspicuous. When papillae are found, they are composed almost entirely of stroma, which may be dense and collagenous or markedly edematous. In adenofibromas and cystadenofibromas, glands and cysts are scattered within a predominantly fibromatous stroma. Occasionally, otherwise typical benign serous tumors containing minor foci with nuclear stratification and atypia are retained in the benign category.

Serous borderline tumors are characterized by polypoid excrescences and papillae lined by atypical proliferating epithelial cells (Fig. 25). The proliferation takes the form of cellular stratification associated with small cellular papillary buds that typically emanate from the cyst lining or surface of the ovary and from larger polypoid excrescenses, usually with an arborizing pattern. The cellular buds appear to be detached from their moorings, floating off the outer surface of the tumor or into a cyst lumen, depending on whether the tumor is exophytic or endophytic (Fig. 25). The extent of the papillary cellular proliferation in serous borderline tumors varies; it is striking in a minority of cases. In some such cases filiform cellular papillae emanate from the inner or outer surface of the tumor or both, resulting in a "non-hierarchical," so-called micropapillary pattern (Fig. 26); a cribriform pattern (Fig. 27); and, rarely, a solid pattern or a combination of these patterns (147,158–160).

The neoplastic cells of serous borderline tumors typically have scanty cytoplasm, but a few cells may be bulbous with

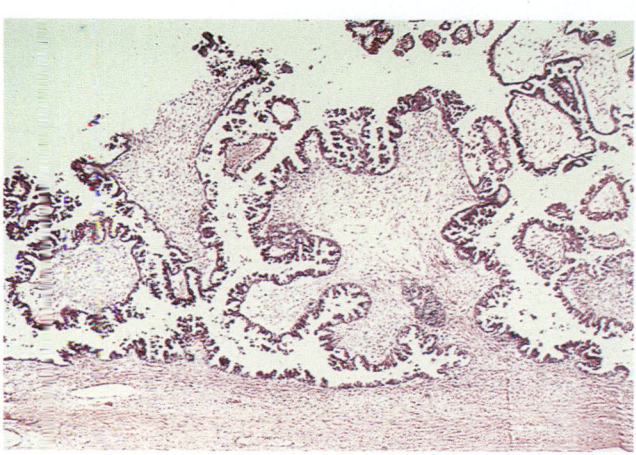

FIG. 25. Serous papillary cystadenoma of borderline malignancy. Papillae lined by stratified epithelial cells project into the lumen. Note the exuberant proliferation of small clusters of cells off the larger papillae and the absence of invasion of the stroma. (From ref. 135.)

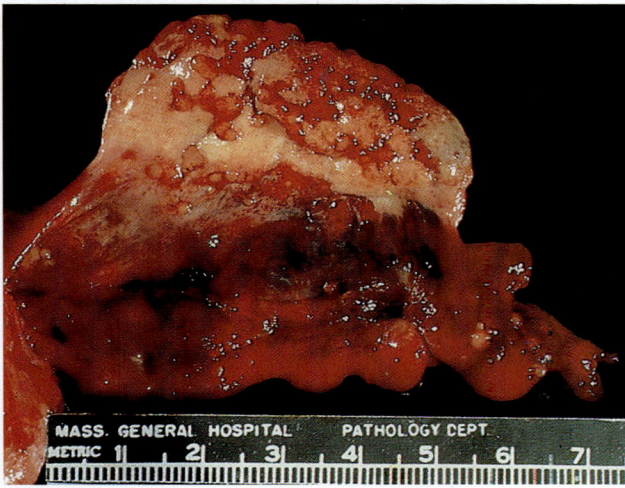

FIG. 24. Serous surface carcinoma. Small nodules with associated hemorrhage are visible on the external surface of the ovary, whose normal shape is retained.

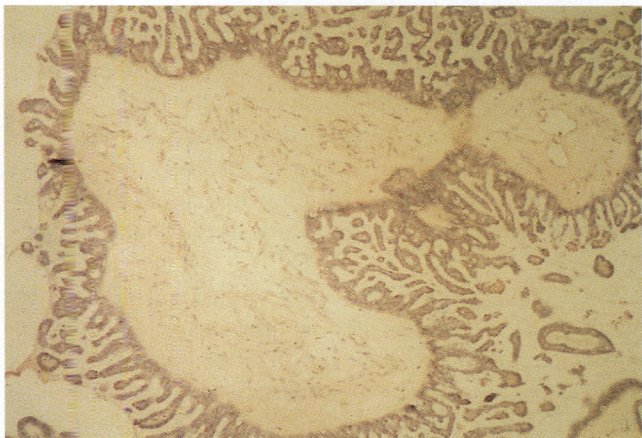

FIG. 26. Serous papillary cystadenoma of borderline malignancy. Filiform cellular papillae emanate from a large polypoid structure in a "non-hierarchical" pattern that has been referred to as micropapillary.

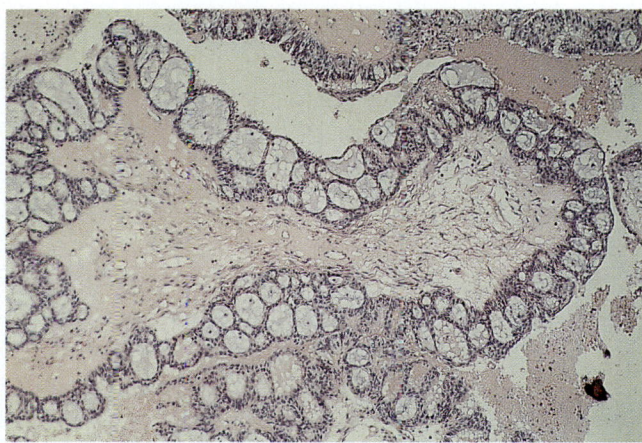

FIG. 27. Serous papillary cystadenoma of borderline malignancy. A large polypoid frond is covered by epithelium that exhibits a striking cribriform pattern.

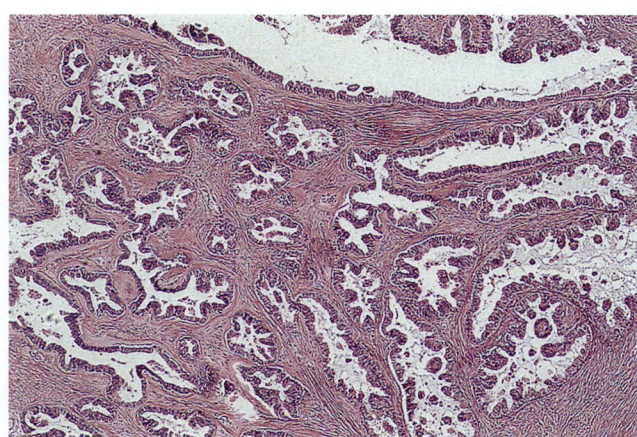

FIG. 28. Serous papillary cystadenoma of borderline malignancy. There is extensive, orderly invagination of the neoplastic glands into the stromal component of the neoplasm. The stroma is unaltered in appearance.

abundant eosinophilic cytoplasm; in rare cases, such cells predominate. Varying degrees of nuclear atypicality may be present, and mitotic figures range from few to moderate in number. Ciliated cells are characteristically present, and psammoma bodies are found in approximately one-fourth of cases. In borderline tumors that secrete thick mucin, it is largely confined to the lumen and the apical portion of the cytoplasm of epithelial cells. A minority of serous borderline tumors are adenofibromatous or cystadenofibromatous.

Although the absence of obvious stromal invasion distinguishes serous borderline tumors from carcinomas according to the WHO, some investigators (158,159) believe that noninvasive serous tumors with a micropapillary or cribriform pattern should be called carcinomas. In their experience, when such tumors are associated with peritoneal implants, the latter are invasive more often than in cases of ovarian serous borderline tumors lacking these patterns. Eichhorn and associates (160) reported a smaller increase in the rate of invasive implants associated with these unusual patterns and retained micropapillary and cribriform noninvasive tumors in the borderline category for two reasons: (a) such an approach preserves the WHO criteria and avoids chaos in the reporting of these tumors, and (b) the prognosis associated with these tumors appears to be much closer to that of the typical serous borderline tumor than to that of serous carcinoma. It is important, however, to recognize these atypical patterns and search with unusual care for invasion in both the primary tumor and its implants when they are present.

Recognizing stromal invasion in serous borderline tumors may be difficult because they are often characterized by extensive, complex glandular proliferations with or without papillae that interdigitate with the stromal component of the tumor (Fig. 28). The stroma in these areas of pseudoinvasion, however, does not differ in its appearance from areas of stroma lacking epithelial elements, and the intrastromal glands have an orderly arrangement. In contrast, the destructive stromal invasion of a carcinoma is characterized by a disorderly disposition of neoplastic glands in the stroma, typically with a desmoplastic and occasionally with a myxoid or hyaline stromal response. In some serous borderline tumors, broad areas in which glands and nests lie within a desmoplastic stroma are plastered on the surfaces of polypoid excrescences, simulating desmoplastic noninvasive peritoneal implants (see next page). This process, which has been referred to as "auto-implantation" (40), should not be confused with true stromal invasion, which is not a surface phenomenon.

In approximately 10% of serous borderline tumors, focal microinvasion of the stroma, occasionally accompanied by lymphatic invasion, is encountered in otherwise typical neoplasms (161–163). Single neoplastic cells or irregular nests or papillary clusters of cells, sometimes accompanied by psammoma bodies, are present within the stromal component (Fig. 29). In some cases, these cells have abundant eosinophilic cytoplasm. The designation of serous borderline tumor with microinvasion has arbitrarily been restricted

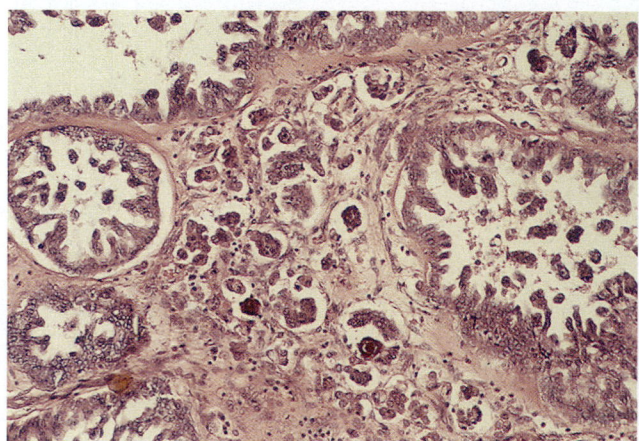

FIG. 29. Serous papillary cystadenoma of borderline malignancy with microinvasion of the stroma. Numerous small clusters of invasive carcinoma cells are present at the center.

to tumors containing one or more such foci not exceeding 3 mm in maximal linear dimension or 10 mm² in area. The prognosis in cases of microinvasion appears to be similar to that associated with borderline tumors without microinvasion. Only one of more than 40 patients with follow-up data has died of microinvasive tumor; that patient had stage III disease (156,161–163). Serous tumors, whether benign, borderline, or malignant, tend to be uniform throughout a given specimen and generally lack the intimate admixtures of benign, borderline, and malignant neoplasia that are often seen in mucinous tumors and less frequently in endometrioid and clear-cell neoplasms, but there are striking exceptions that emphasize the importance of thorough sampling, particularly of tumors with any unusual features.

Serous borderline tumors are associated with peritoneal foci of serous-type cellular proliferation in 16% to 59% of cases (150,151), more frequently when the tumor has a surface component (152). In some cases, these foci are composed of cytologically benign serous cells, which are not considered implants of the ovarian tumor and are designated endosalpingiosis. When the peritoneal lesions are formed of cells with features of borderline malignancy, they are regarded by some investigators as independently primary peritoneal tumors, exemplifying a "field change" involving extraovarian as well as ovarian mesothelium (147).

It is impossible at the present time to be certain whether peritoneal borderline lesions are true implants or independent proliferations, except in cases in which the ovarian surfaces are uninvolved or only minimally involved. Clonality studies of serous carcinomas, however, suggest that associated peritoneal involvement, at least in those cases, is metastatic (164,165), in contrast to primary peritoneal serous tumors, which are polyclonal (166). For purposes of staging and in the following discussion, serous peritoneal lesions accompanying serous borderline tumors of the ovary will be referred to as implants, except for foci of endosalpingiosis.

Peritoneal implants of serous borderline tumors have been classified as noninvasive and invasive (147–151), with the former subdivided into epithelial and desmoplastic subtypes (Figs. 30–32) (150). In epithelial noninvasive implants, papillary proliferations of atypical serous cells with at most a minimal stromal component are present on the surface of the peritoneum (Fig. 30), in smoothly contoured subperitoneal invaginations, or in invaginations between lobules of omental fat. The cytologic atypia of these implants usually approximates that in the primary ovarian tumor. Desmoplastic noninvasive implants (Fig. 31) are characterized by a predominance of reactive stroma and are layered onto the peritoneal surface, including that lining invaginations between omental fat lobules. Within these implants, small glands and papillae lined by atypical serous cells, as well as single cells and psammoma bodies, are entrapped in proliferating fibroblastic tissue (Fig. 31), which is often infiltrated by acute and chronic inflammatory cells. Necrosis, fibrin deposition, and hemorrhage are occasionally seen.

Invasive implants, in contrast, are characterized by an irregular infiltration and destruction of the underlying tissue (Fig. 32). They typically resemble grade 1 serous carcinoma. An ovarian serous tumor that is associated with invasive implants, however, is classified according to its appearance and not that of its implants. In the largest study of serous border-

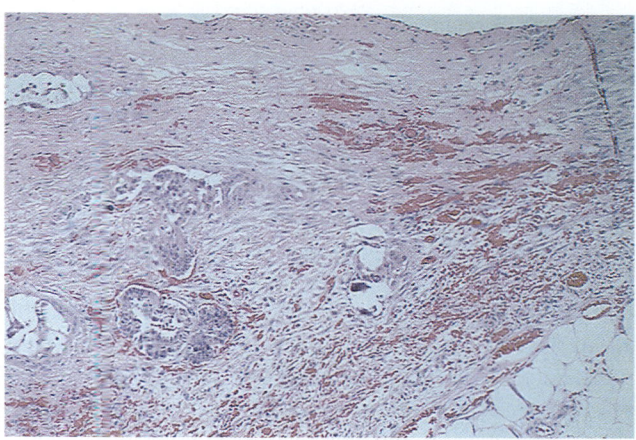

FIG. 31. Peritoneal implant of serous borderline tumor, which is noninvasive and desmoplastic.

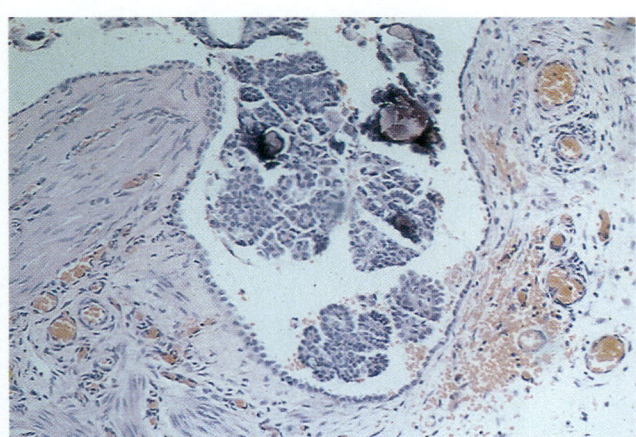

FIG. 30. Peritoneal implant of serous borderline tumor, which is noninvasive and epithelial.

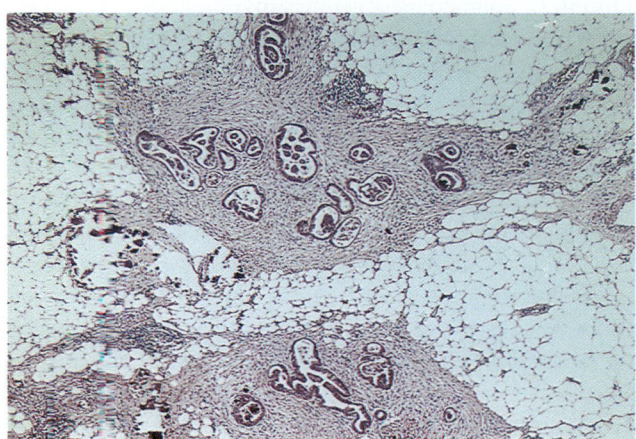

FIG. 32. Peritoneal implant of serous borderline tumor, invasive of omentum.

line tumors associated with peritoneal implants (56 cases) (150), their separation into invasive and noninvasive categories had important prognostic implications. Ninety percent of the patients with noninvasive implants followed for 4 or more years, or until death, had no progression of disease, in contrast to only 17% of those with invasive implants. Severe nuclear atypicality in the implants was also independently correlated with a poor prognosis in that study.

It must be emphasized that serous carcinomas, as well as serous borderline tumors of the ovary, can be associated with noninvasive implants, which may be desmoplastic. These implants typically have a higher degree of nuclear atypicality and contain a larger epithelial component than the noninvasive desmoplastic implants of serous borderline tumors. When the epithelial component of a desmoplastic implant occupies close to half of its area, a diagnosis of carcinoma should be strongly suspected. When it occupies a smaller area approaching that dimension, extensive sampling of peritoneal lesions available for study should be done to exclude carcinoma. The desmoplastic noninvasive implants of serous borderline tumors and carcinomas may be impossible to distinguish with certainty in some cases, but the nature of the primary tumor is usually known in such cases, lessening the importance of the interpretation of the implants.

Another confusing, relatively common association of ovarian serous borderline tumors is with the presence of atypical serous epithelium in pelvic or paraaortic lymph nodes. In some cases, the epithelium appears benign and lines glands typically located in the lymphoid tissue or capsule of the node instead of in its sinuses (so-called müllerian inclusion glands or lymph node endosalpingiosis) (167); such glands have been reported in 30% to 40% of surgically excised pelvic or paraaortic lymph nodes from patients without ovarian tumors (168). In other cases (up to 20%), the serous epithelium in the node has borderline features. A diagnosis of true metastasis is warranted if the lesion is confined to the lymph node sinuses and is composed unquestionably of epithelial cells. Reactive peritoneal mesothelial cells can travel to lymph nodes, become deposited within their sinuses, and simulate metastatic neoplastic epithelial cells (169). Immunohistochemical investigation may be necessary to distinguish these cell types (170,171). When a small focus of serous borderline tumor is confined to the lymphoid tissue or capsule of a node and is accompanied by uninvolved müllerian inclusion glands elsewhere in the node, one can confidently diagnose an independently primary borderline tumor of the lymph node. Future studies of lymph node involvement in cases of serous borderline neoplasia of the ovary must be accompanied by rigorous microscopic investigation to distinguish among these processes before the rate of true lymph node metastasis in this disease can be established. Currently available evidence suggests that the presence of lymph node involvement in cases of serous borderline neoplasia of the ovary does not adversely affect the prognosis (153–156).

Serous carcinomas exhibit obvious stromal invasion and

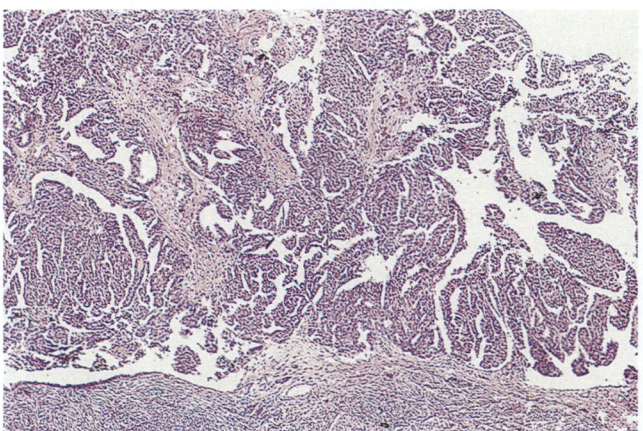

FIG. 33. Serous surface carcinoma. Note the origin of the lesion from the ovarian surface in the lower portion of the illustration. The neoplasm is characterized by many fine papillae and slit-like lumina.

are characterized by one or more of the following features: fine papillae (Fig. 33); irregular, often slit-like glandular lumens (Fig. 34); small, tight nests of tumor cells and single tumor cells growing in a dense fibrous or hyalinized stroma; glomeruloid formations; and psammoma bodies. Large areas in a serous carcinoma may lack these distinctive features and grow in the form of sheets of cells occasionally punctured by small cysts. A rare pattern of well-differentiated serous car-

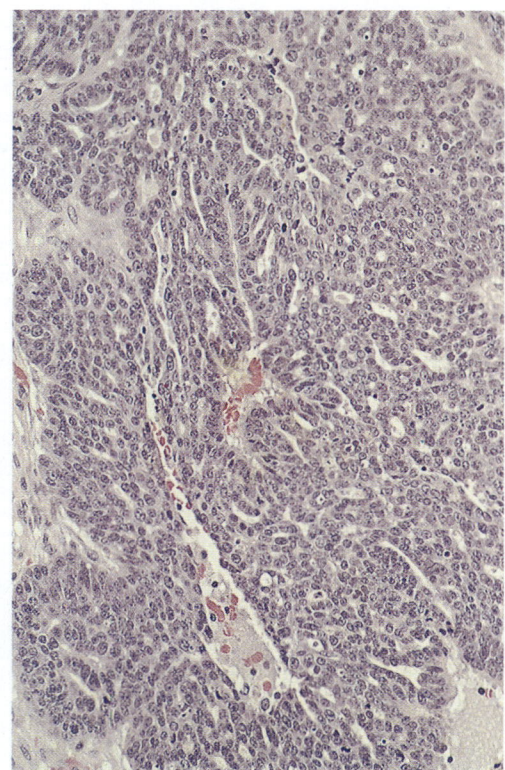

FIG. 34. Serous adenocarcinoma. Small, slit-like glandular lumina are prominent.

cinoma is characterized by papillae lined by tumor cells lying in spaces without an endothelial lining, probably created by secretion of serous fluid by the neoplastic cells. Exceptional serous carcinomas have a component resembling adenoid cystic carcinoma (172), undergo focal squamous differentiation (173), or have a reticular pattern superficially suggesting yolk sac tumor.

The designation serous is applied to most poorly differentiated ovarian carcinomas that do not have the tubular glands or squamous differentiation of endometrioid carcinoma, the conspicuous intracellular mucin of mucinous carcinoma, or the diagnostic features of some other types of epithelial cancer. When a solid pattern is the exclusive or almost exclusive feature of an ovarian carcinoma, however, it should be classified as undifferentiated unless the cytologic features suggest another cell type, such as transitional cell; serous carcinoma is often associated with a minor component of transitional cell carcinoma. They usually exhibit at least minimal invasion of the underlying or adjacent ovarian stroma if it is not effaced and are typically high grade.

The cells in most serous carcinomas have nonspecific features, and the diagnosis is usually made on the basis of one or more distinctive patterns. Rare cellular features that may cause diagnostic confusion are a focal hobnail shape, which suggests the possibility of clear-cell carcinoma, or abundant eosinophilic cytoplasm, which may suggest malignant mesothelioma, particularly if the tumor has a prominent surface component. It is usually possible to make a diagnosis in such cases on the basis of characteristic patterns of these tumors; immunohistochemical staining may also aid in distinguishing between serous and mesothelial tumors (170,171).

A rare form of low-grade serous carcinoma with a favorable prognosis is the so-called psammocarcinoma (174) (see Fig. 43, Chapter 56). This tumor, which can also be primary in the peritoneum, appears to be more similar in clinical characteristics to the serous borderline tumor than to serous carcinoma, but it differs in its microscopic features from the former in the prominence of psammoma bodies infiltrating the ovarian stroma. The four criteria recommended for the diagnosis of psammocarcinoma are invasion of the ovarian stroma or its vascular spaces (or, in extraovarian areas of involvement, invasion of any intraperitoneal tissue or its vascular spaces), no more than mild to moderate nuclear atypia, epithelial nests no more than 15 cells in their largest linear dimension, and the presence of psammoma bodies in at least 75% of the papillae or nests.

Differential Diagnosis

Serous cystadenomas may be confused with the rare rete cystadenoma (page 2358), but the latter has a hilar location, is commonly surrounded by a layer of smooth muscle or a band of hyperplastic hilus cells, typically exhibits shallow crevices along its inner surface, and is lined by cells that contain few or no cilia. In rare cases, cystic struma ovarii may simulate serous cystadenoma but contains at least a minor focus composed of recognizable thyroid follicles in the wall or the septa of the cyst (page 2367). Serous surface papillary adenofibromas should be distinguished from the relatively common tiny, warty excrescences (surface stromal proliferations) that may be encountered on the outer surface of the ovary of adult women. The latter lesions are typically multifocal and do not form a mass lesion. When a diagnosis of adenofibroma is based solely on the presence of glands lined by indifferent-appearing cuboidal cells in a predominantly fibromatous stroma, its interpretation as a serous tumor may be incorrect. The occasional association of such a tumor with endometrioid carcinoma in the same specimen suggests that the cuboidal lining cells may be endometrioid instead of serous or indifferent with a propensity to endometrioid differentiation (175).

Serous borderline tumors are only occasionally confused with other neoplasms. Their distinction from serous carcinomas and differentiation of their mucin-secreting subtype from mucinous borderline tumor have already been discussed. The difference between serous borderline tumors and retiform Sertoli–Leydig cell tumors (SLCTs) is considered under the latter heading (page 2354).

Although serous carcinoma is the epithelial cancer typically associated with papillae, other tumors in this category—particularly endometrioid and clear-cell carcinomas—may be papillary as well. The papillae in endometrioid carcinomas are more uniform, longer, broader, and more villous than the thin, generally irregular, small cellular papillae of serous carcinomas. Small tufts of cells with squamous features within the glands of some endometrioid tumors should not be misconstrued as the cellular papillae of a serous tumor. Papillae in clear-cell carcinomas are lined by hobnail or clear cells and frequently have hyalinized cores; other distinctive patterns of clear-cell carcinoma are almost always admixed with the papillary pattern. Hobnail cells seen in otherwise typical serous borderline tumors and carcinomas are almost always present only in small foci.

Although squamous differentiation in ovarian adenocarcinomas almost invariably indicates their endometrioid nature, it is seen now and then in serous carcinomas (172). Serous carcinomas may also be confused with retiform SLCTs and ependymomas; these differential diagnoses are discussed under those headings. Making the distinction between serous carcinoma and metastatic carcinoma is rarely a problem, but from time to time metastatic breast carcinoma simulates serous carcinoma. Women with breast cancer are at increased risk of ovarian carcinoma; indeed, one study (176) showed that when a patient with breast cancer has an adnexal cancer, it is more likely to be primary in the ovary than metastatic. In such cases, comparison of the morphologic features of the ovarian cancer with those of the breast cancer is usually diagnostic. If it is not, immunohistochemical staining may be helpful; positive results for gross cystic disease fluid protein-15 strongly favors metastatic breast carcinoma, and CA125 staining favors ovarian carcinoma (177–181).

Mucinous Tumors

Mucinous tumors account for about 15% of all ovarian neoplasms (133,182,183). Cystadenomas make up a higher proportion of benign ovarian tumors and account for approximately 85% of all mucinous tumors. Borderline tumors are slightly less common than carcinomas, which account for 6% to 10% of all ovarian cancers. Mucinous cystadenomas most frequently develop during the third through fifth decades; borderline and invasive tumors usually develop during the fourth through seventh decades. Mucinous tumors are more common in the first two decades than the other surface epithelial tumors (184). Mucinous ovarian tumors occur at an increased rate in patients with Peutz-Jeghers syndrome (PJS) (185). Some patients, both with and without this syndrome, have mucinous adenocarcinoma of the cervix associated with an ovarian mucinous tumor (185–187); in some cases the ovarian tumor is a metastasis.

Gross Features

Mucinous tumors tend to be the largest of all ovarian tumors. Many are 15 to 30 cm in diameter and weigh up to 4,000 g or more. Benign mucinous tumors are bilateral in less than 5% of cases; borderline and invasive forms involve both ovaries in 5% to 10% of cases. The relatively rare borderline tumors of the müllerian (endocervical) type, however, are bilateral much more often than those of the intestinal type (40% vs. 6%) (188).

Mucinous cystadenomas are usually multilocular (Fig. 35); the cysts have thin walls and are filled with thick to watery mucinous fluid. Borderline and invasive tumors commonly contain papillae and solid areas, which may be soft and mucoid or firm. Borderline tumors of the müllerian type, in contrast to the more common intestinal variant, are typically unilocular. Necrosis and hemorrhage are more common in carcinomas than borderline and benign tumors, but their occasional presence in the context of these two neoplasms may create a deceptively worrisome appearance on gross examination. Because benign, borderline, and invasive components are frequently admixed, it is important to sample mucinous tumors thoroughly.

The mucinous ovarian cystic tumors that may be present in cases of pseudomyxoma peritonei are discussed under metastatic tumors because a preponderance of evidence favors the metastatic nature of these ovarian tumors. Such cases are typically associated with appendiceal mucinous tumors. Mucinous cystadenomas and, less often, borderline tumors and carcinomas are associated with a Brenner tumor or dermoid cyst in a small proportion of cases.

Microscopic Features

The usual mucinous cystadenoma is lined by epithelium resembling endocervical epithelium, consisting of a single row of uniform, mucin-filled columnar cells with basal nuclei. Less often, the lining resembles that of the intestine, with goblet cells scattered among more numerous mucin-free cells. This type of epithelium almost always contains argyrophil cells (189), sometimes argentaffin cells, and, rarely, Paneth cells. Epithelium of the intestinal type is much more common in borderline than in benign mucinous tumors. Small papillae may project into the lumens of mucinous cystadenomas, but prominent papillarity is uncommon; infrequently, foci of squamous metaplasia are encountered. The stromal element within mucinous cystadenomas is often conspicuous but only rarely predominates to form a mucinous adenofibroma (190). Occasionally, bands of smooth muscle and plaques of calcium or bone are present in the stroma. Minor epithelial atypicality is compatible with the diagnosis of mucinous cystadenoma, but significant degrees of epithelial stratification, budding and bridging, and nuclear atypia are indicative of borderline malignancy (Fig. 36).

Borderline mucinous tumors may be of the endocervical-like (müllerian) (188) or intestinal type (191–200). Intestinal mucinous borderline tumors (IMBTs) account for approximately 85% to 90% of cases and have been studied more extensively than endocervical-like forms. The criteria for determining whether a tumor of the intestinal type is borderline or a carcinoma are the subject of controversy. Both borderline and invasive mucinous neoplasms often contain glands and cysts within a nondesmoplastic stroma that is scanty or resembles ovarian stroma or fibroma, making the detection of stromal invasion more difficult than in serous tumors. In 1973, Hart and Norris (191) suggested that in the absence of clear-cut evidence of invasion, a carcinoma should be diagnosed when the nuclei of the lining cells are stratified to four layers or more; shortly thereafter, Hart (137) proposed that a cribriform pattern or the presence of stroma-free papillae also warranted the diagnosis of carcinoma. Cumulative evidence from the literature, however, supports the inclusion of the Hart-Norris noninvasive "carcinomas" in the borderline category, since the prognosis associated with them in stage I cases appears to be almost as good as that of more typical borderline tumors without these architectural features.

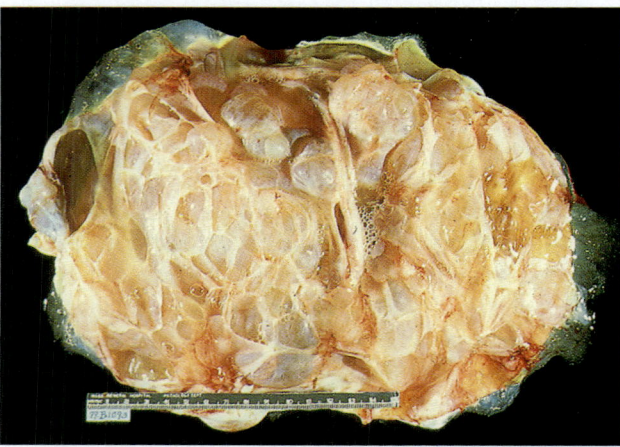

FIG. 35. Multilocular mucinous cystadenoma.

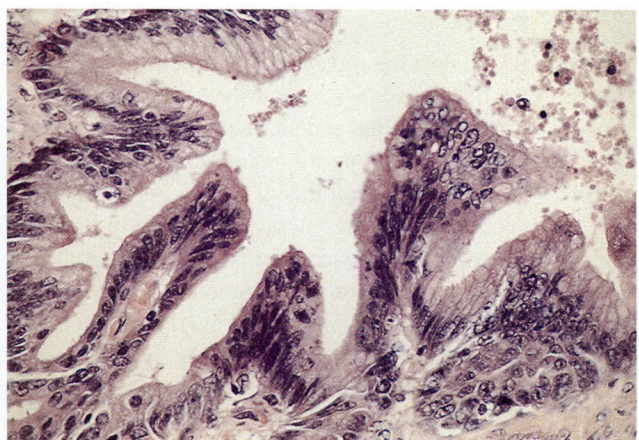

FIG. 36. Mucinous cystadenoma of borderline malignancy, intestinal type. Note the filiform papillae and nuclear stratification.

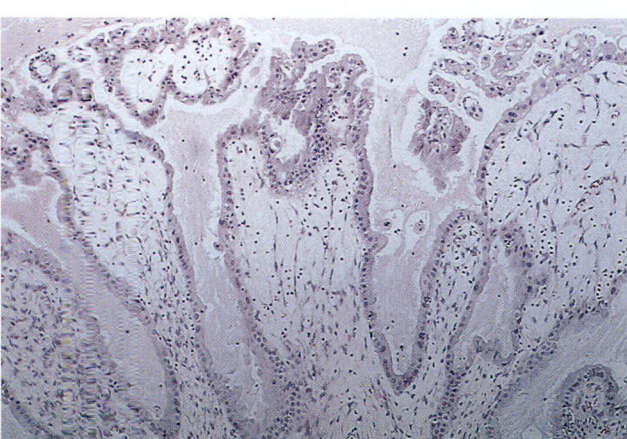

FIG. 38. Mucinous cystadenoma of borderline malignancy, endocervical type. Cellular clusters bud from edematous papillae. Note the inflammatory cell infiltrate.

Hoerl and Hart (199) now refer to the former tumors as "intraglandular carcinomas." We continue to designate them mucinous tumors of borderline malignancy, but we indicate that they constitute a variant by adding the phrase "with intraepithelial carcinoma" (Fig. 37) (40,200). It is important to distinguish these tumors from the less atypical mucinous borderline tumors of the intestinal type because they are first seen at a higher stage than the latter (192,194), require more extensive sectioning to rule out stromal invasion, and warrant further investigation because of the limited number of carefully analyzed cases reported specifically as borderline tumors with intraepithelial carcinoma.

The two major microscopic features of müllerian or endocervical-like mucinous borderline tumors (EMBTs) that differ from those of IMBTs are papillae that resemble those of serous borderline tumors in their architectural features (Fig. 38) and a lining of exclusively or predominantly endocervical-type epithelium, with rare or no goblet cells and no argyrophil cells—or, at most, only small numbers of them. In contrast, when papillae are encountered in IMBTs, they tend to be filiform (Fig. 36) and branching, without the cellular tufting typical of EMBTs. In addition, an extensive, acute inflammatory infiltrate is typically prominent in the stroma and lumens of EMBTs, in contrast to only minor degrees of inflammation in isolated IMBTs. Approximately 30% of EMBTs are accompanied by endometriosis, which is rare in association with IMBTs. Despite the occasional presence of peritoneal implants or lymph node metastasis, EMBTs have an excellent prognosis. The stratification criterion of Hart and Norris (199), which is helpful in distinguishing typical IMBTs from those with intraepithelial carcinoma, is not reliable in the distinction of EMBTs from intraepithelial carcinomas, since EMBTs may exhibit cellular stratification of up to 20 layers.

Mucinous carcinomas vary considerably in their microscopic appearance from one case to another and are usually not clearly divisible into endocervical-like and intestinal types (Fig. 39). Cysts, glands, solid masses, clusters, and individual cells may be present in various combinations. The

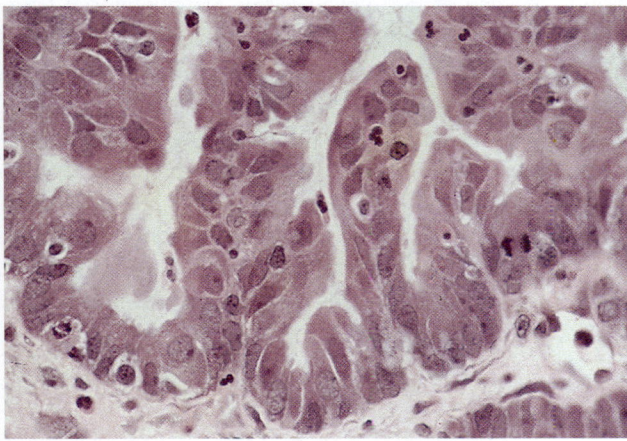

FIG. 37. Mucinous cystadenocarcinoma of borderline malignancy with intraepithelial carcinoma.

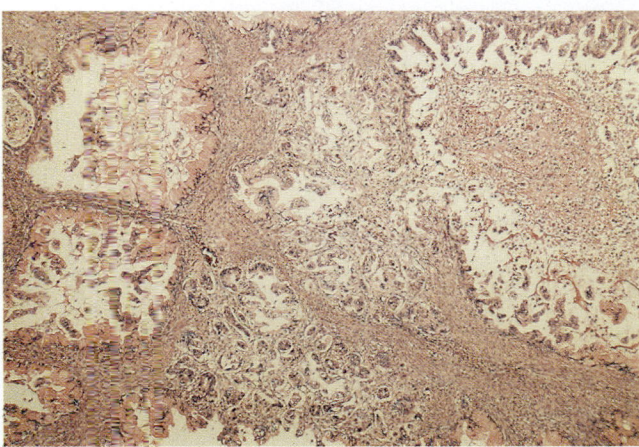

FIG. 39. Mucinous cystadenocarcinoma. There is irregular penetration of the stroma of the tumor by small clusters of carcinoma cells.

tumor cells vary from mucin-rich—resembling endocervical, intestinal goblet, or signet-ring cells—to mucin-free cells, which may be well differentiated, except for their lack of mucin, or poorly differentiated. The stroma may be desmoplastic but is often scanty or fibromatous or resembles cellular ovarian stroma.

Otherwise typical mucinous cystic tumors, whether benign, borderline, or malignant, may contain one or more solid mural nodules that differ markedly in their microscopic features from the remainder of the tumor (40,201–208). In some cases, the nodule is an anaplastic carcinoma, which may be composed of large cells with abundant cytoplasm or smaller cells with scanty cytoplasm (Fig. 40) (203,205,208). Rarely, a nodule has the features of a high-grade sarcoma, such as a fibrosarcoma (201), or a carcinosarcoma (206). Isolated nodules may be composed of benign giant cells (202) or may be leiomyomas (204,205). The most perplexing category of nodular lesions, sarcoma-like nodules, are characterized by sarcoma-like proliferations containing mixtures of atypical spindle-shaped cells, giant cells commonly of the epulis type, inflammatory cells, and histiocytes. Mitotic figures, including highly atypical forms, may be present. Cytokeratin stains may show positive cells, presumably of the neoplastic epithelial type, within the heterogeneous background.

Unlike malignant nodules, which invade the stroma and sometimes the vessels and have a less heterogeneous appearance, sarcoma-like nodules are sharply demarcated (201). There is overlap in the features of these two types of nodules, however, making evaluation of individual cases difficult. For example, some malignant nodules are well demarcated. An uneventful follow-up of patients with sarcoma-like nodules suggests a bizarre reactive process. More detailed study, including extensive immunohistochemical staining and more follow-up data, is necessary to delineate clearly the clinicopathologic features and differential diagnosis of these nodules, a number of which are probably closely related within a spectrum of tumor-host interactions.

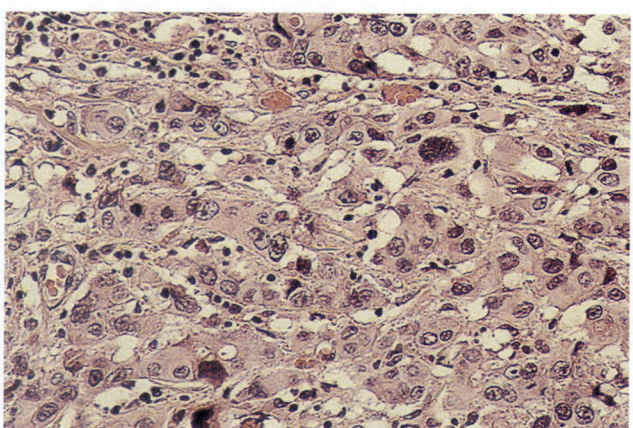

FIG. 40. Anaplastic carcinoma arising in the wall of a mucinous cystic tumor. Note the characteristic abundant cytoplasm of the tumor cells.

Differential Diagnosis

Mucinous adenocarcinomas and endometrioid adenocarcinomas may be difficult to distinguish. Although they occasionally produce abundant mucin, endometrioid carcinoma cells contain at most only minor quantities of mucin in their apical cytoplasm. Very small foci of benign-appearing endocervical-type cells may be encountered in endometrioid carcinomas, but their presence alone does not warrant a diagnosis of mucinous carcinoma. Squamous differentiation strongly favors an endometrioid over a mucinous carcinoma. Although most mucinous carcinomas of the ovary do not resemble metastatic mucinous carcinomas, which are usually from the gastrointestinal tract but occasionally from other sites, the latter tumors sometimes cause diagnostic confusion.

A microscopic criterion favoring the primary nature of mucinous adenocarcinoma on histologic examination is the usual admixture of the former with benign and borderline components. This criterion is not entirely reliable, however, since cysts lined by benign-appearing or borderline-appearing mucinous epithelium are now and then encountered within metastatic adenocarcinomas. In one series, 11% of metastatic intestinal carcinomas contained deceptively benign-appearing foci (209). Goblet cells are more common in primary mucinous carcinomas, but they are occasionally present in metastatic adenocarcinomas as well. Implants on the ovarian surface and prominent vessel invasion favor metastasis. Clinical and operative findings strongly suggestive of metastasis, such as the previous or coincidental presence of a bowel, or other (e.g. pancreatic), carcinoma, mesenteric lymph node and liver metastases, and bilaterality and multinodularity of the ovarian tumor(s), are more helpful diagnostic clues than the microscopic features of the tumor in some cases.

Endometrioid Tumors

Less than 5% of all ovarian tumors are of the endometrioid type, but endometrioid carcinomas account for up to 15% of ovarian cancers. These tumors are defined as neoplasms resembling one of the typical forms of endometrial carcinoma (adenocarcinoma, including secretory adenocarcinoma; adenocarcinoma with squamous differentiation). An origin from endometriosis, which can be verified in 5% to 10% of cases, is not required for the diagnosis. Endometriosis is not generally regarded as a neoplasm, and benign endometrioid tumors, with the exception of adenofibromas (210–212), are very rare. Endometrioid tumors of borderline malignancy are also uncommon (212–214). Endometrioid carcinomas occur mainly in the fifth decade and beyond (215–220).

Gross Features

Endometrioid adenofibromas, including those of borderline malignancy, are predominantly solid tumors (Fig. 41),

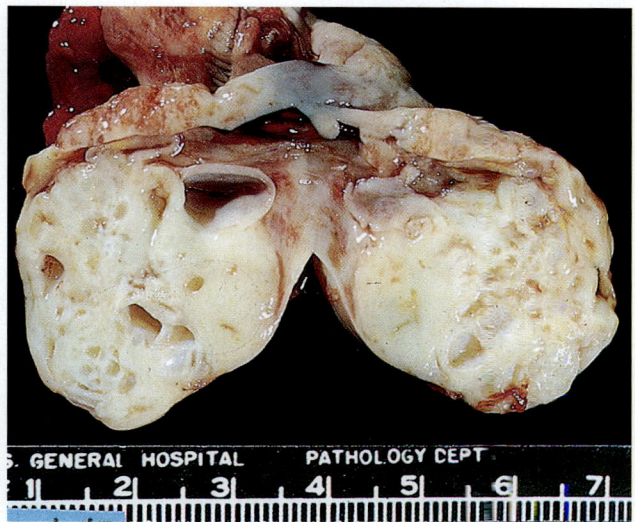

FIG. 41. Endometrioid adenofibroma. The sectioned surfaces show predominantly solid white tissue containing cysts. (From ref. 40.)

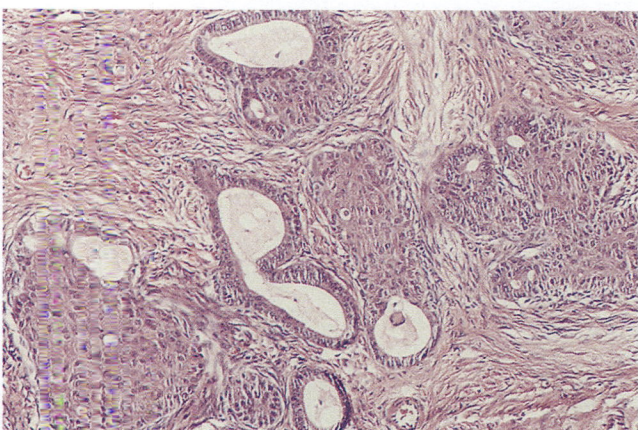

FIG. 42. Endometrioid adenoacanthofibroma. Endometrioid glands, some of which have undergone squamous differentiation, lie within a fibromatous stromal component.

which may contain varying numbers of cysts (cystadenofibromas). Endometrioid carcinomas may be cystic or solid and lack gross features that distinguish them from serous carcinomas, except for the minority that arise from an endometriotic cyst (218,219). In such cases, an otherwise typical chocolate cyst contains a polypoid growth within its lumen, often accompanied by varying degrees of invasion of its wall. Some tumors are noninvasive, and the entirely intracystic nature of the carcinoma in such cases should be recorded because of its favorable prognostic implications. Endometrioid carcinomas often have an adenofibromatous component, which may be separate from typical carcinomatous tissue or account entirely for the gross appearance of the tumor. Up to one-third of ovarian endometrioid carcinomas are accompanied by carcinoma of the uterine corpus, which usually closely resembles ovarian tumors on microscopic inspection and is most often an independent primary tumor (see page 2333).

Microscopic Features

Endometrioid tumors are characterized by tubular glands simulating to different extents those of proliferative, secretory, hyperplastic, or adenocarcinomatous endometrium. Benign forms of endometrioid neoplasia include rare lesions resembling endometrial polyps, which may arise in endometriotic cysts, and adenofibromas, some of which show focal squamous differentiation (adenoacanthofibromas) (Fig. 42) (210–212). Endometrioid tumors of borderline malignancy include the relatively rare atypical papillomas and polyps confined within endometriotic cysts (218) and endometrioid adenofibromas, in which the glandular epithelium is atypical or has an appearance of low-grade carcinoma but does not invade the stroma (210–214). Varying degrees of atypical hyperplasia within foci of endometriosis should be classified as pre-cancerous according to terminology used for similar endometrial lesions and not as neoplasms.

Endometrioid adenocarcinomas are characterized by the presence of distinctive tubular glands lined by pseudostratified, mucin-free epithelium (Fig. 43) (215–219). The glands may be cystically dilated, and villous papillae are occasionally seen within cyst lumens (Fig. 44). In one-fourth to one-third of cases, the glandular cells differentiate focally into squamous cells, which have a pattern ranging from benign-appearing round or oval morules to aggregates of obviously

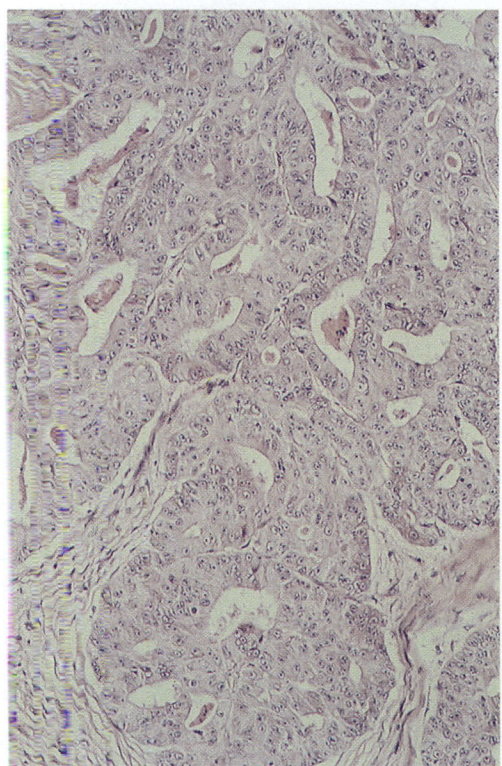

FIG. 43. Endometrioid adenocarcinoma. Tubular glands resemble those of endometrial adenocarcinoma.

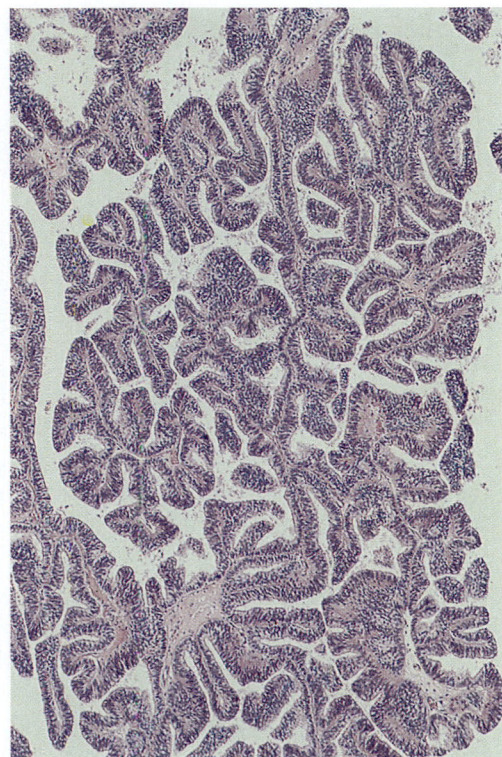

FIG. 44. Endometrioid adenocarcinoma. This neoplasm has a prominent villiform architecture.

malignant squamous cells (217). Foci of abortive squamous differentiation in the form of rounded groups of spindle-shaped cells are seen from time to time in endometrioid carcinomas and may be a helpful clue to the diagnosis in such cases (221).

Basal vacuolation similar to that seen in the 16-day secretory endometrium is occasionally observed in ovarian endometrioid carcinomas (secretory carcinomas), as it is in a small minority of endometrial adenocarcinomas. Abundant mucin secretion is sometimes encountered in endometrioid carcinomas, but typically the mucin is secreted from the surfaces of the cells or accumulates only in the uppermost portion of their cytoplasm. Rare endometrioid adenocarcinomas are of the ciliated-cell or oxyphilic type (223,224).

Endometrioid carcinomas have a variety of unusual patterns that may cause them to resemble sex cord–stromal tumors (221,225–227). Such patterns are only rarely encountered in other forms of surface epithelial cancer. Small glands (Fig. 45) and solid tubular structures may be indistinguishable from the hollow or solid tubules of a Sertoli cell or SLCT. Epithelial islands and trabeculae, particularly when punctured by microacini, may mimic the insular, trabecular, and microfollicular (Fig. 46) patterns of a granulosa cell tumor (GCT). Endometrioid carcinomas, like almost any other type of ovarian tumor, may contain luteinized cells in their stroma, and when these cells are dispersed between small glands, the resemblance of the tumor to a well-differentiated SLCT is enhanced.

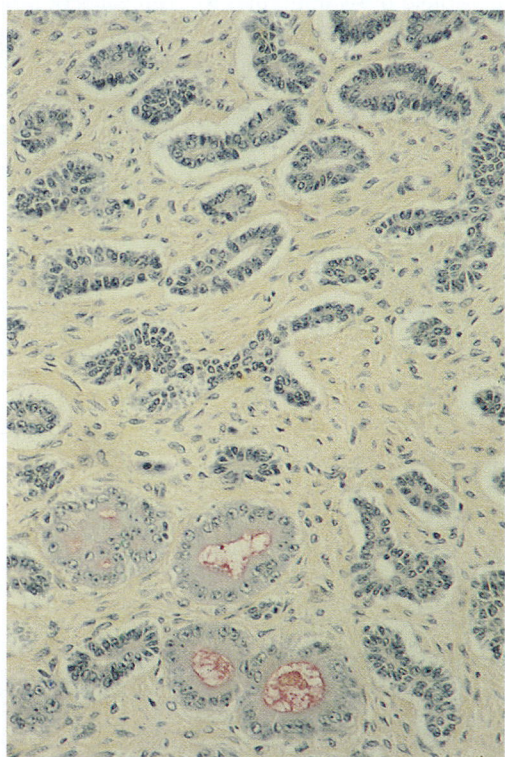

FIG. 45. Endometrioid adenocarcinoma. The small tubules resemble those of a Sertoli cell tumor. A few tubules at the bottom contain intraluminal mucin (mucicarmine stain).

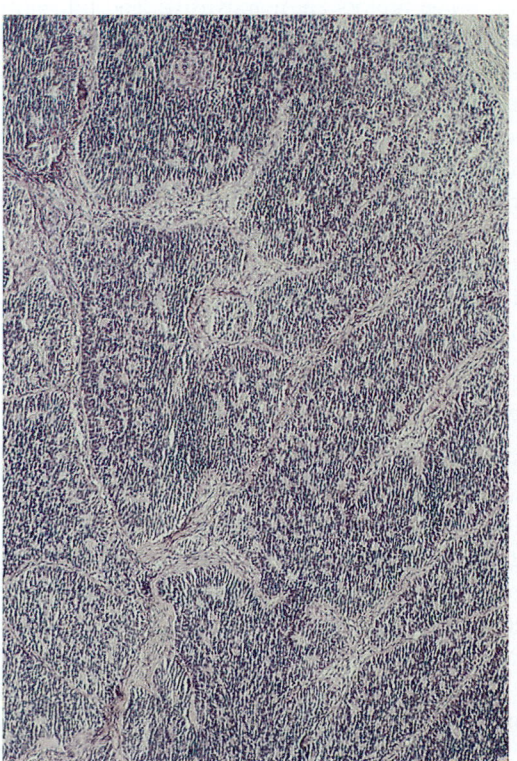

FIG. 46. Endometrioid carcinoma resembling granulosa cell tumor. Numerous small cavities simulate Call-Exner bodies.

A few endometrioid carcinomas have a focal or extensive component of spindle cells (as distinct from the rounded spindle-cell foci of abortive squamous differentiation mentioned earlier) that often merge with easily recognizable epithelial cells (Fig. 47) and usually stain immunohistochemically for markers of epithelial differentiation (222). The spindle cells should not be misinterpreted as the mesenchymal component of a carcinosarcoma. Rare endometrioid carcinomas transform focally to typical alpha-fetoprotein (AFP)-positive yolk sac tumor (228,229). The variety of unusual patterns in endometrioid carcinomas highlights the importance of sampling that is adequate to establish the nature of the tumor.

Differential Diagnosis

A major difficulty in the recognition of endometrioid carcinoma arises when poorly differentiated forms have microscopic features that merge almost imperceptibly with those of poorly differentiated serous carcinomas. This problem accounts at least in part for the differences in the reported rates of these tumors in various series of ovarian cancer cases. In questionable cases of the poorly differentiated type, it is preferable to place the tumor in the serous rather than an unclassified category. The differential diagnosis of endometrioid carcinoma and mucinous carcinoma has been discussed on page 2330.

Metastatic adenocarcinoma from the intestine is occasionally difficult to distinguish from endometrioid carcinoma (230). The lumens of glands and cysts in the former tumor are characteristically filled with eosinophilic debris containing nuclear fragments ("dirty" necrosis); this feature is usually, but not invariably, absent in the latter tumor (231). Also, the glands in metastatic intestinal carcinomas are typically lined by more poorly differentiated cells than those in endometrioid adenocarcinomas. The rare clear-cell variant of intestinal adenocarcinoma (232) can be confused with a secretory endometrioid adenocarcinoma because of the striking subnuclear clearing in the glands of both tumors. Immunohistochemistry may be helpful in difficult cases (with CK 7, CA 125, and HAM 56 positivity favoring an ovarian origin and CK20 and carcinoembryonic antigen staining favoring an intestinal origin) (232–235), although the differentiation can almost always be made with conventional clinical, gross, and routine microscopic findings.

Endometrioid carcinomas resembling sex cord–stromal tumors contain at least some glands that are larger and generally lined by less well differentiated epithelium than the tubules of a SLCT. The presence of an adenofibromatous component, squamous differentiation, or more than small amounts of intraluminal mucin excludes the diagnosis of sex cord–stromal tumor, except that mucin is usually present in the heterologous form of SLCT. The latter type of tumor, however, has other easily distinguishable features. Immunohistochemical testing may aid in a challenging case. Endometrioid carcinomas stain for epithelial membrane antigen (EMA) and CK-7 (226,227); conversely, staining for α-inhibin establishes the diagnosis of a sex-cord tumor (227). From a clinical viewpoint, SLCTs, in contrast to endometrioid tumors, typically occur in young women and often cause virilization.

Endometrioid carcinomas with prominent foci of spindle-shaped epithelial cells (222) should be differentiated from malignant mesodermal mixed tumors (MMMTs), in which the spindle cells are of the mesenchymal type. The spindle-shaped epithelial cells of endometrioid carcinomas are generally less atypical than both the epithelial and mesenchymal components of an MMMT. When tumor resembling a typical or a secretory type of endometrioid adenocarcinoma is encountered in a young woman, the possibility of an endometrioid-like YST should be considered (page 2362). Thorough sampling in search of more typical forms of yolk sac or endometrioid neoplasia and immunohistochemical staining for AFP and EMA may be indicated in order to solve this problem in differential diagnosis.

A variety of approaches have been used to determine whether concurrent endometrioid carcinomas of the ovary and endometrium are independent primary tumors or involve metastasis from one organ to the other. In addition to the clinical, gross, and histologic features of the two tumors, DNA and genetic studies have been used (40,236–238) but have yielded confusing results from one investigation to another. We rely largely on clinical, gross, and light microscopic findings to determine the probable site(s) of origin of the tumors. The additional presence of endometriosis in the ovary or of atypical endometrial hyperplasia in the uterus favors primary neoplasia at one or the other site, respectively. The prognosis in cases in which the tumor is confined to the ovary and uterus is so close to that of carcinoma restricted to one or the other organ that an independent primary origin of the two tumors in that situation appears highly probable and the prognosis appears to depend largely on the depth of invasion of the myometrium by the endometrial tumor (236).

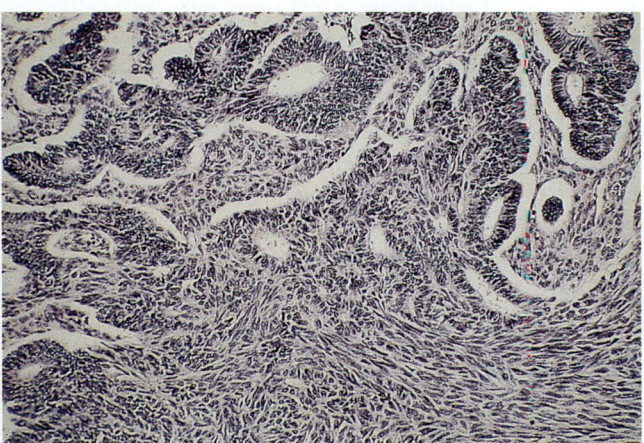

FIG. 47. Endometrioid adenocarcinoma with spindled epithelial cells.

Malignant Mesodermal Mixed Tumors

MMMTs (carcinosarcomas) of the ovary (239–242) are classified in the endometrioid category because they resemble the tumors with that designation that arise most commonly in the endometrium. Although these tumors contain epithelial and mesenchymal elements, both of which are malignant, immunohistochemical and genetic studies have supported a monoclonal origin of both components (243–245). Most MMMTs develop in postmenopausal women. At operation, there is evidence of spread beyond the ovary in more than half the cases.

Gross Features

These tumors are composed of soft to firm, yellow to brown, solid tissue, often exhibiting hemorrhage, necrosis, and cystic degeneration. They may be predominantly cystic. Occasionally, bone or cartilage is evident on palpation.

Microscopic Features

The epithelial component is usually high grade and most often resembles serous or endometrioid carcinoma, but malignant mucinous, squamous, or clear-cell elements may be encountered. The mesenchymal component may have the features of a fibrosarcoma, leiomyosarcoma, endometrioid stromal sarcoma, or nonspecific sarcoma or, in heterologous tumors, a rhabdomyosarcoma, chondrosarcoma, or osteosarcoma. Intracellular and extracellular hyaline droplets that are periodic acid–Schiff (PAS) positive may be present in the sarcomatous and sometimes in the carcinomatous component.

Differential Diagnosis

The neoplasm that is most often confused with heterologous MMMT is immature teratoma. In contrast to the former tumor, the latter is very rarely found in women older than 50 years, contains elements derived from all three germ layers, lacks a malignant component of the müllerian type, and almost always contains a prominent primitive neuroepithelial component. Finally, the cartilage in immature teratomas has an embryonic or fetal appearance, whereas in MMMTs it usually resembles the cartilage of a poorly differentiated chondrosarcoma, with marked nuclear atypicality. Heterologous Sertoli-Leydig cell tumors (SLCTs) with islands of cartilage or rhabdomyoblasts may cause diagnostic difficulty, but the finding of Leydig cells, sex-cord formations, tubules, or elements of endodermal type should facilitate the diagnosis.

Differentiation of homologous MMMT from moderately or poorly differentiated SLCT without heterologous elements is aided by finding typical foci of SLCT elsewhere in the specimen. Also, SLCTs rarely have an epithelial component that resembles müllerian-type carcinoma, except for the heterologous form that contains mucinous epithelium and the retiform subtype, which can simulate serous or endometrioid carcinomas but occurs in a much younger age group than MMMT. Finally, SLCTs often lead to virilization. In difficult cases, staining for EMA and inhibin are useful because the former is almost always evident in MMMTs but only rarely in SLCTs (226) and then in only a few Sertoli cells; inhibin staining identifies the tumor as belonging in the Sertoli–Leydig cell category (227,247–254). Endometrioid stromal sarcomas with sex cord–like differentiation can also enter the differential diagnosis of MMMT; they are better differentiated, however, and their sex cord–like elements resemble those of a sex-cord tumor rather the müllerian-epithelial component of a MMMT.

Mesodermal (Müllerian) Adenosarcomas

Mesodermal (müllerian) adenosarcomas (255–259), at least 14 cases of which have been reported (259), are characterized by a malignant stromal component that is typically homologous and a proliferating endometrioid glandular component. The glandular constituent may show a variety of types of müllerian differentiation and may be atypical, occasionally having the appearance of adenocarcinoma *in situ*. These tumors, which are often clinically aggressive (259), should be distinguished from endometrioid polyps and adenofibromas. In contrast to the stroma of endometrioid polyps, that of adenosarcomas is cellular and atypical, with characteristic collaring of the glands; in addition, large polypoid fronds typically extend into the lumens of cystic glands. Although the stroma of adenosarcomas may undergo fibromatous differentiation, it is basically of the endometrial stromal type; the resemblance to endometrial stroma is best appreciated in the periglandular cellular cuffs. In contrast, the stroma of endometrioid adenofibroma is exclusively fibromatous.

Endometrioid Stromal Sarcomas

General Features

A major problem in the diagnosis of primary endometrioid stromal sarcoma of the ovary (260–264) is its differentiation from metastatic endometrial stromal sarcoma, the sarcoma that is most frequently associated with ovarian spread (265). In one reported series of 23 sarcomas of endometrial stromal type involving the ovary (261), nine cases involved both the ovary and the uterus; in at least five of the nine cases, there was strong evidence of spread from the uterus to the ovary. In some cases of metastatic involvement of the ovary, the history of uterine neoplasm may be remote; accordingly, before the diagnosis of a primary endometrioid stromal sarcoma of the ovary is made, a careful history is required, complemented, if possible, by microscopic review of a previous hysterectomy specimen. An origin in ovarian endometriosis also establishes the primary nature of the ovarian tumor. In the cited series (261), the 14 patients without uterine disease had an average age of 52 years. Their clinical symptoms were similar to those of patients with other ovarian tumors. Only four of the 14 tumors were stage I.

Gross Features

These tumors are often large and may be solid, solid and cystic, or, rarely, predominantly cystic. The sectioned surfaces of the solid areas are usually tan to yellow and soft or firm. Foci of hemorrhage and necrosis are present in approximately one-third of the cases.

Microscopic Features

A diffuse arrangement of small cells is the most common pattern. The tongue-like extravascular and intravascular growth pattern seen in uterine tumors of the same type is rarely encountered within the ovary; it is present most often when the tumor has extended elsewhere. In almost all cases, small arteries resembling the spiral arteries of the endometrium are distributed uniformly throughout the tumor. The tumor cells are typically small and oval to spindle-shaped, usually with scanty cytoplasm. A few tumors have cells containing small to moderate amounts of pale cytoplasm. Sometimes the neoplasms have focal sex cord–like patterns (Fig. 48) similar to those encountered in a small number of uterine endometrial stromal tumors (266). Large components indistinguishable from ovarian fibroma, collections of foam cells, and hyaline plaques may be present. In almost half the cases, endometriosis is identified adjacent to the tumor, or a few focal glands of endometrioid type are evident within it (262).

Differential Diagnosis

When metastasis from the uterus has been excluded, these tumors are most frequently misinterpreted as sex cord–stromal tumors, usually granulosa cell tumor (GCT), thecoma, or fibroma. The usual advanced stage and frequent bilaterality of the endometrioid stromal sarcoma, however, argue against a diagnosis of any tumor in the sex cord–stromal category. In addition, sex cord–stromal tumors lack the characteristic cell type, the numerous small arteries, and the common association with endometriosis of endometrioid stromal sarcomas. Furthermore, GCTs do not have the individual cellular investment by reticulin fibrils that is characteristic of endometrioid stromal sarcoma. The presence of sex cord–like foci may cause further confusion with sex cord–stromal tumors (Fig. 48). Inhibin staining of almost all GCTs and SLCTs confirms their diagnosis (227,247–254). Endometrioid stromal sarcomas are distinguished from other pure ovarian sarcomas because of their characteristic cell type, vascular pattern, and typical association with endometriosis.

Clear-cell Tumors

Benign and borderline clear-cell tumors are uncommon, and almost all of them fall into the adenofibroma category (210,267). Clear-cell carcinomas account for more than 5% of all ovarian cancers; they occur most frequently between the ages of 40 and 70 years (268–274).

Gross Features

Clear-cell adenofibromas are indistinguishable on gross examination from other forms of adenofibroma, except that the presence of closely packed tiny cysts (which initially prompted the term parvilocular cystoma) (275) is suggestive of the diagnosis. Clear-cell carcinomas may be solid but are often predominantly cystic; they typically appear as a unilocular cyst containing one or more solid nodules protruding into the lumen (Fig. 49). Clear-cell carcinoma is the ovarian tumor that is most often associated with ovarian and pelvic endometriosis; it occasionally arises within an endometriotic cyst. Multilocular cysts are present less often. Variable portions of a specimen containing clear-cell carcinoma may be benign or show evidence of borderline adenofibroma. The carcinomatous tissue may have a white, yellow, or light brown color, with varying amounts of hemorrhage and necrosis (Fig. 50). Clear-cell carcinomas are rarely bilateral.

Microscopic Features

Adenofibromas of the clear-cell type contain glands and cysts lined by flat cells, flat to low cuboidal hobnail cells, typical columnar hobnail cells, or clear cells. These tumors are subdivided into benign, borderline (Fig. 51), and malignant categories according to criteria similar to those used for such tumors in the endometrioid category. Before diagnosing a benign or borderline clear-cell adenofibroma, one

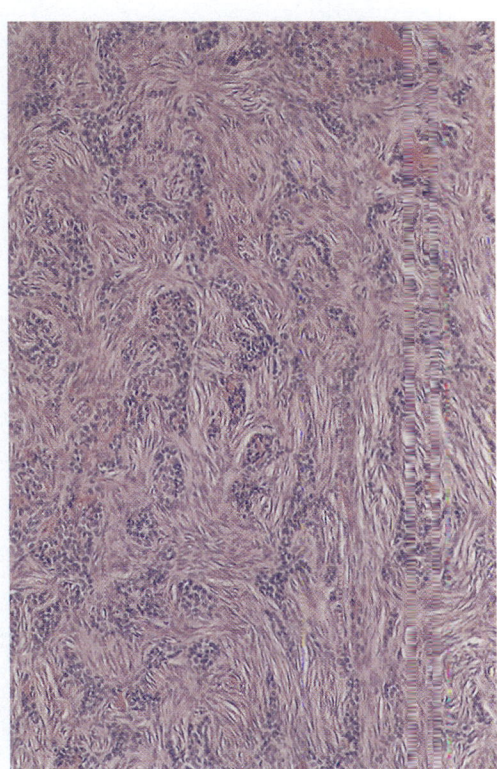

FIG. 48. Low-grade endometrioid stromal sarcoma with sex cord–like differentiation.

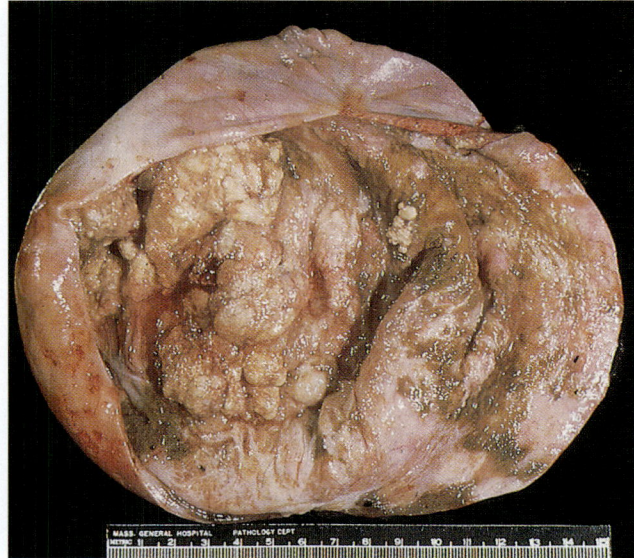

FIG. 49. Clear-cell adenocarcinoma arising in endometriotic cyst. A cauliflower-like mass of carcinoma protrudes into the lumen of the cyst, the lining of which shows brown patches.

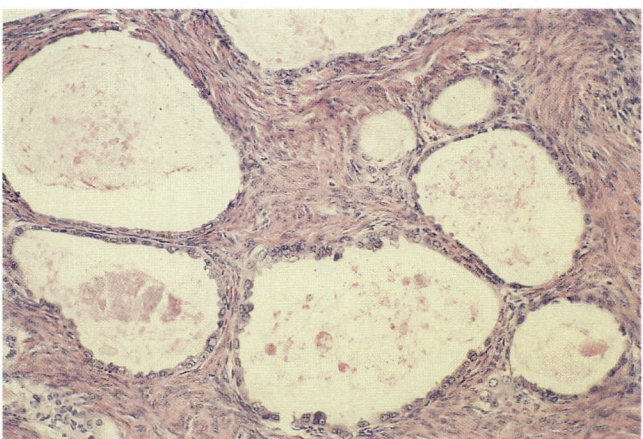

FIG. 51. Clear-cell adenofibroma of borderline malignancy. Tubules, most of them cystically dilated, are lined by atypical cells, including a few that are hobnail-like. Note the background fibromatous stroma.

should sample the specimen carefully because tumor subtypes often coexist with clear-cell carcinoma.

Clear-cell carcinoma is characterized by diffuse (Figs. 52 and 53), tubulocystic (Figs. 54 and 55), papillary (Figs. 56 and 57), and, infrequently, trabecular (Fig. 58) patterns. The most common cell types are clear (Fig. 53), hobnail (Fig. 55), and flat (Fig. 54). Clear cells can be found in almost all cases and are by far the most common cell type in tumors with a diffuse pattern. These cells are typically polyhedral, have distinct cell membranes, and contain abundant clear cytoplasm and eccentric nuclei (Fig. 53). The cytoplasm is rich in glycogen and may also contain varying amounts of lipid. Hobnail cells, which are found in most of the tumors, are characterized by prominent bulbous nuclei that protrude into the lumens of tubules and cysts (Fig. 55). Sometimes, the linings of dilated cysts become markedly flattened, producing a deceptively benign appearance. The papillae of clear-cell carcinomas are often complex and frequently contain hyalinized cores (Fig. 57).

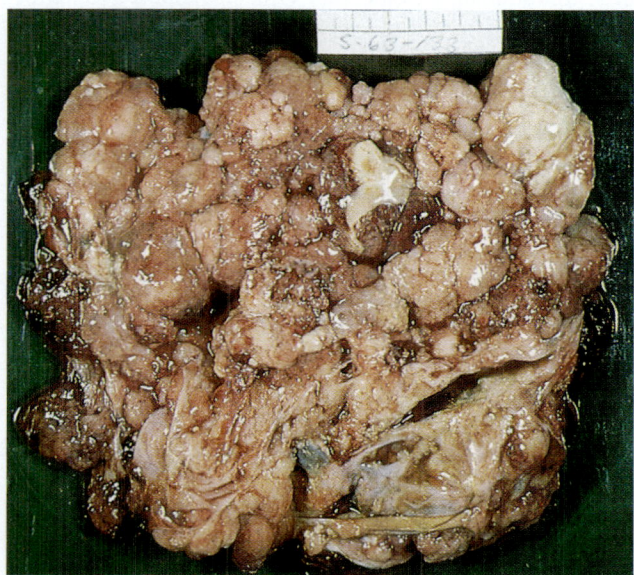

FIG. 50. Clear-cell carcinoma forms a solid tumor with cysts and necrosis.

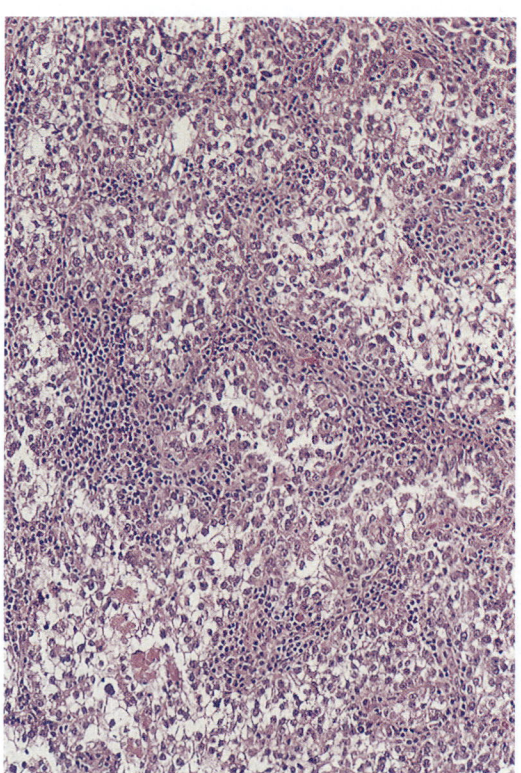

FIG. 52. Clear-cell carcinoma. The presence of a dense lymphocytic and plasmacytic infiltrate imparts a superficial resemblance to dysgerminoma on low-power examination.

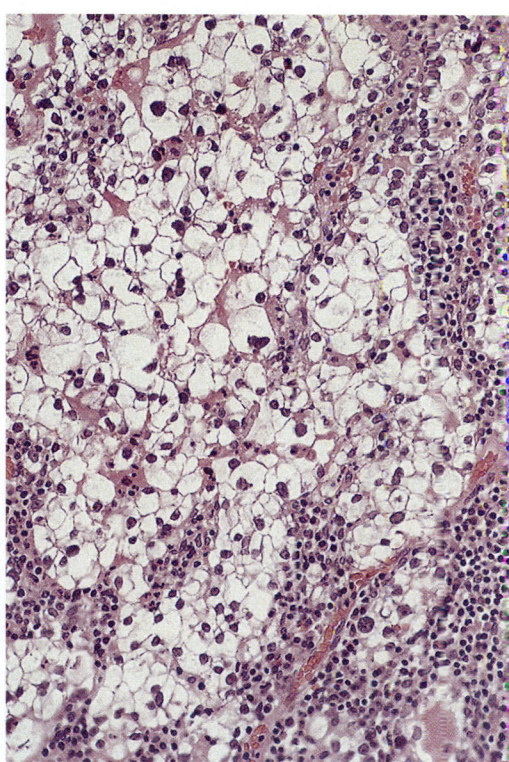

FIG. 53. Clear-cell carcinoma. Note the eccentric nuclei and abundant clear cytoplasm as well as a chronic inflammatory infiltrate.

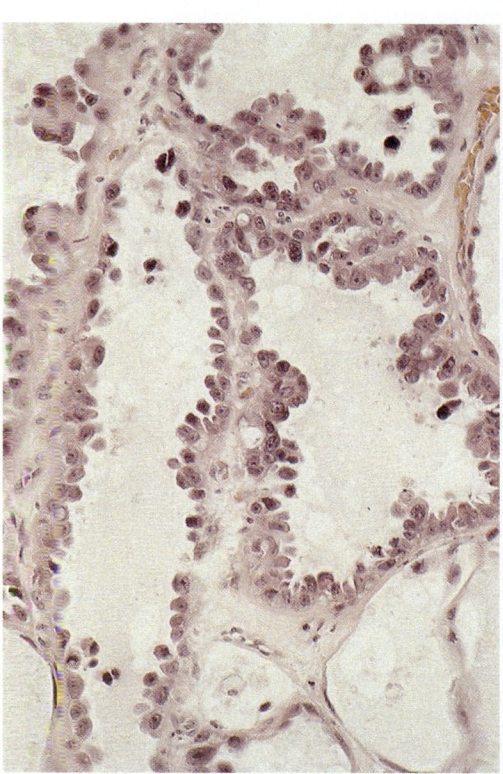

FIG. 55. Clear-cell carcinoma with a tubulocystic pattern and prominent hobnail cells.

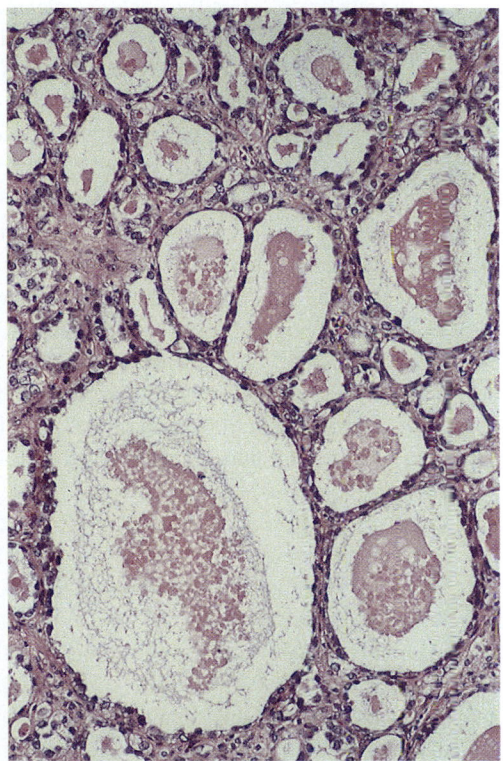

FIG. 54. Clear-cell carcinoma with tubulocystic pattern.

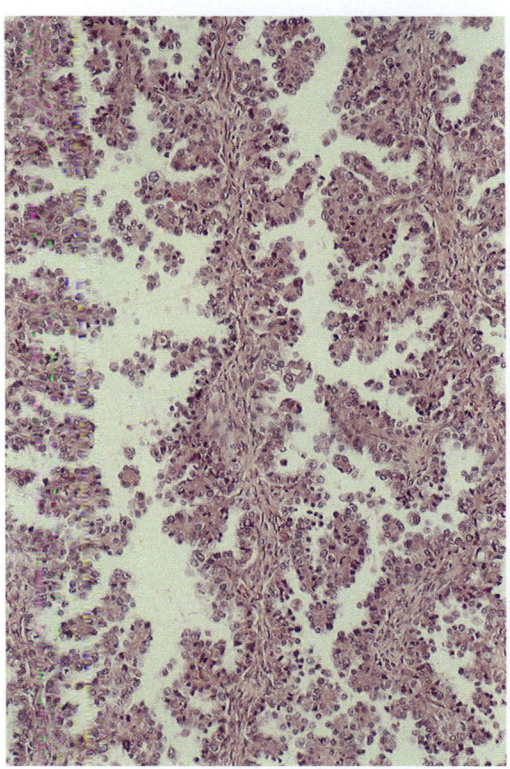

FIG. 56. Clear-cell carcinoma. Several papillae project into the lumina of tubular glands.

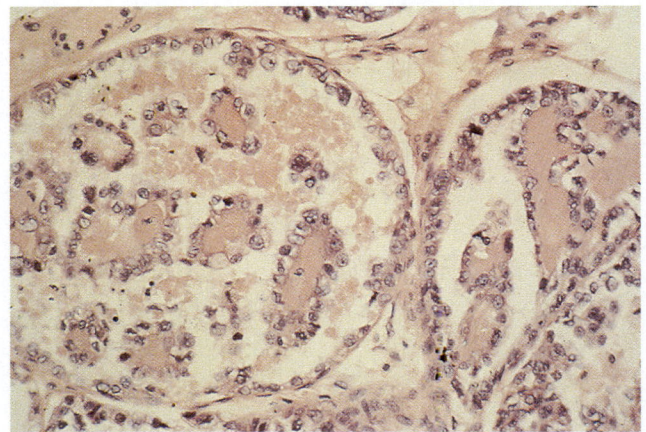

FIG. 57. Clear-cell carcinoma. Note several papillae with hyalinized eosinophilic cores, a characteristic feature of the papillae of clear-cell carcinomas.

The lumens of the tubules and cysts usually contain mucin, but, as in serous and endometrioid tumors, intracellular mucin is customarily confined to the luminal tips of the cells. An exception is the focal presence of aggregates of mucin-containing signet-ring cells, which have a bull's-eye appearance. Very rarely, these cells predominate in clear-cell carcinoma. Occasional cases of clear-cell carcinoma contain sheets, cords, or nests of cells with abundant eosinophilic cytoplasm (oxyphilic cells) (Fig. 58), which rarely are the predominant cell type (277). In exceptional cases, extensive amounts of basement membrane material occupy the stroma. Clear-cell carcinomas may contain hyaline bodies, which were present in 25% of the cases in one series (269). When the clear-cell carcinoma is poorly differentiated, many of its characteristic features are absent, and it may be difficult to distinguish from other surface epithelial carcinomas. Clear-cell carcinoma is often admixed with endometrioid carcinoma, with which it is closely related.

Differential Diagnosis

Clear-cell carcinoma is the surface epithelial cancer that is most often confused with primitive germ cell tumor—usually dysgerminoma or yolk sac tumor (YST), even though the young age of patients with either of the latter tumors provides strong evidence against a diagnosis of clear-cell carcinoma. Clear-cell carcinoma may be confused with a dysgerminoma when it has a diffuse pattern and is composed entirely of clear cells. The dysgerminoma cell is rounded with flattened edges, however, in contrast to the polyhedral cell of clear-cell carcinoma, and the nuclei in dysgerminomas are typically central and contain one to four prominent nucleoli, unlike the nuclei in clear-cell carcinomas, in which nucleoli are generally not prominent. Special staining may reveal the presence of mucin in clear-cell carcinomas, but not in dysgerminomas. Finally, at least a sprinkling of lymphocytes is almost always seen in the latter tumors. Occasional cases of clear-cell carcinoma composed exclusively of clear cells have a diffuse inflammatory cell infiltrate simulating that of dysgerminoma on low-power examination (Fig. 52), but the infiltrate typically contains plasma cells and other inflammatory cells as well as lymphocytes, in contrast to the pure or almost pure lymphocytic infiltrate of dysgerminoma.

Clear-cell carcinomas from time to time have a loose, edematous appearance, replicating the reticular pattern of a YST. The nuclei in YSTs, however, are almost always more primitive in appearance than those of clear-cell carcinoma, and the papillae are characteristically simple, containing a single central vessel and lacking a hyalinized eosinophilic core. The additional presence of other typical patterns of clear-cell carcinoma, an origin in endometriosis, or an admixture with endometrioid carcinoma may be very helpful in the diagnosis of clear-cell carcinoma, while the finding of other patterns of YST or an admixture with other forms of germ cell neoplasia establishes the diagnosis of YST. Hyaline bodies are less common in clear-cell carcinoma than in YSTs, but their presence or absence is not decisive in the differential diagnosis. The immunohistochemical finding of AFP strongly favors a diagnosis of YST, but now and then clear-cell carcinoma exhibits similar staining (277); the latter tumor is positive for Leu-M1 much more often than YST.

The rare metastatic renal cell carcinoma (278) may be indistinguishable from clear-cell carcinoma that is composed exclusively of clear cells. Clinical data, including radiologic studies, may be necessary in some cases to rule out metasta-

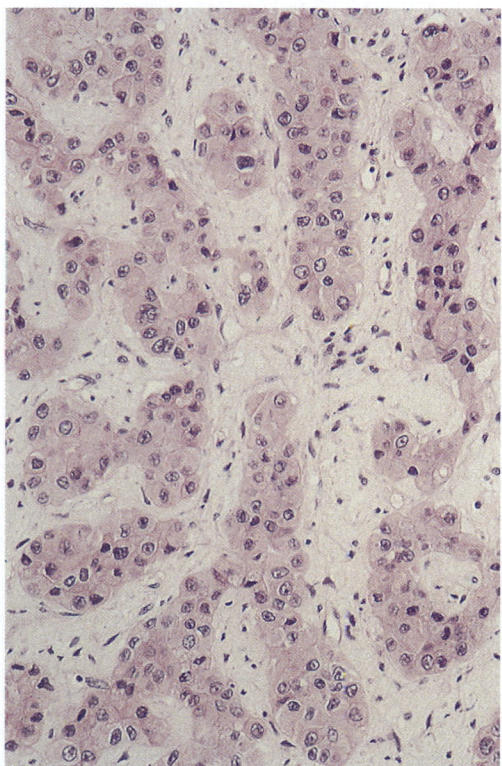

FIG. 58. Oxyphilic clear-cell carcinoma with a trabecular pattern.

sis (see page 2381). Another metastatic tumor that may enter the differential diagnosis of clear-cell carcinoma is metastatic clear-cell adenocarcinoma of the intestine (232).

Clear-cell carcinomas composed predominantly or exclusively of oxyphilic cells (277) may closely resemble steroid cell tumors and other ovarian tumors characterized by cells with abundant eosinophilic cytoplasm, such as hepatoid YST (279) and hepatoid carcinoma (280). Other patterns of clear-cell carcinoma are always present in its oxyphilic variant. The latter is not associated with endocrine manifestations related to steroid hormone production, as is the steroid cell tumor, nor does it stain for inhibin, as does the steroid cell tumor (254). Hepatoid YST develops in young women, often contains foci of more typical yolk sac neoplasia, and shows positive results for AFP. Hepatoid carcinoma occurs in an age group similar to clear-cell carcinoma, but lacks the foci of typical clear-cell carcinoma present in the oxyphilic form of that tumor; moreover, hepatoid carcinoma may contain foci of serous carcinoma (281).

Transitional Cell Tumors

Although it has been recognized for years that some poorly differentiated ovarian carcinomas resemble transitional cell carcinoma but lack an associated component of Brenner tumor (282), the entity of transitional cell carcinoma has become established only relatively recently (283–286). The current WHO classification (135) divides tumors containing malignant transitional cells into two groups: those in which there is malignant transformation of the epithelial component of a benign Brenner tumor (malignant Brenner tumors) and those in which a benign Brenner component is absent (transitional cell carcinomas).

Brenner Tumors

General Features

These tumors account for 2% to 3% of all ovarian neoplasms (287–293); less than 2% of the reported cases have been borderline (proliferative) or malignant (294–299), but the rate of borderline or malignant change in clinically detectable Brenner tumors is greater than 5% (295,296). Most of the benign neoplasms have been encountered in the fourth through eighth decades, with a peak in the late forties and early fifties. Borderline and malignant Brenner tumors occur in women who are, on average, 10 years older than those with benign tumors.

Gross Features

Benign Brenner tumors are typically small, usually less than 2 cm in diameter. They are most often incidental findings at operation or on pathologic examination (Fig. 59); approximately 6% are bilateral. Most Brenner tumors are solid; 10% to 25% appear as small, firm nodules in the wall of a mucinous cystadenoma. Occasionally they are associated with

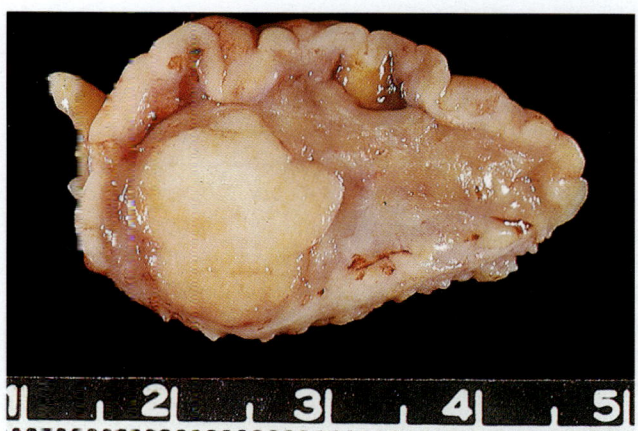

FIG. 59. Brenner tumor. A sharply demarcated, yellow-white fibromatous tumor occupies a portion of the sectioned surface of the ovary.

a dermoid cyst and rarely with carcinoid or struma ovarii (40). The benign tumors are well circumscribed, with a hard and fibromatous gray, white, or slightly yellow cut surface. Occasionally, the tissue is gritty, owing to calcific deposits, and rarely, it is massively calcified. Tiny cysts may be visible with a hand lens or the naked eye. Rare benign Brenner tumors are large and predominantly cystic. Borderline tumors are characteristically cystic and unilocular or multilocular, with cauliflower-like papillomatous masses protruding into one or more of the locules (Fig. 60). From time to time, borderline tumors are solid. Malignant Brenner tumors may be solid or cystic, with mural nodules; they have no distinctive features except that, in contrast to transitional cell carcinomas, they may resemble or have a variably sized component that resembles benign Brenner tumor.

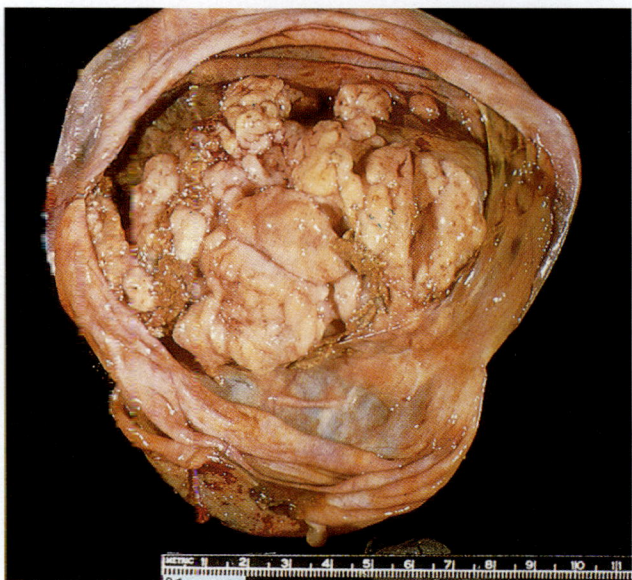

FIG. 60. Borderline Brenner tumor. A unilocular cyst contains a large polypoid mass of white tumor tissue arising from its lining.

Microscopic Features

The typical benign Brenner tumor is composed of rounded, sharply demarcated small nests of epithelial cells lying within an abundant fibromatous stroma (Fig. 61). The nests may be solid or have a central lumen that contains dense eosinophilic material or mucin. Most of the neoplastic cells are polygonal to ovoid and have pale cytoplasm and oval nuclei, some of which may have a central longitudinal groove. The cells lining the lumens range from flat to columnar, often contain mucin, and occasionally bear cilia. Cysts of varying sizes lined entirely by mucinous or transitional epithelium are sometimes encountered. The stromal component may be focally hyalinized, and calcific plaques may be present.

Borderline Brenner tumors, which some investigators prefer to designate "proliferating" (294) or "proliferative" (295) because the clinically malignant behavior of these tumors has not yet been demonstrated, are generally characterized by cysts into which protrude papillae lined by proliferating cells that are mainly of transitional cell type (Fig. 62). The lining cells resemble those of grade 1 to grade 3 papillary carcinoma of urinary tract. Mucin-containing cells may also be encountered, typically in the innermost layer of the epithelial lining. No invasion of the stroma is evident, and a benign Brenner component is also present in all cases. In malignant Brenner tumors, grade 1 to 3 nests of transitional cell carcinoma or, occasionally, squamous cell carcinoma irreg-

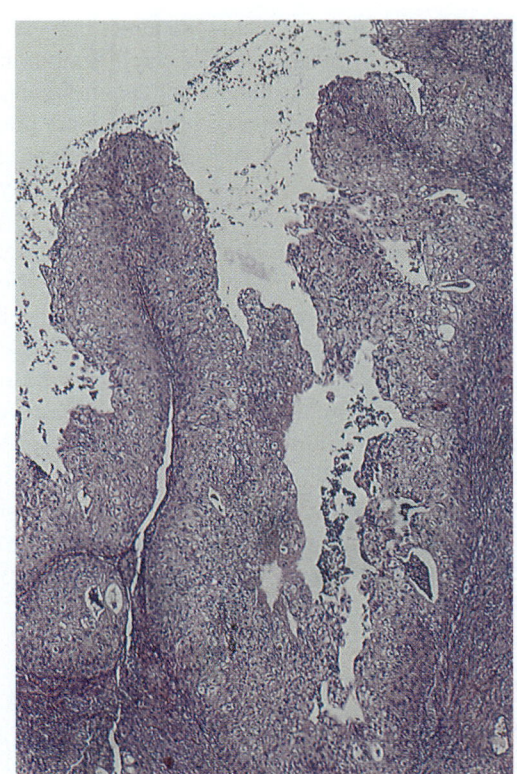

FIG. 62. Borderline Brenner tumor. Papillae lined by proliferating transitional epithelium protrude into the lumen of a cyst.

ularly infiltrate the stromal component of the tumor; the tumor cells may also line cysts (Fig. 63). Mucinous cells may be identified among the malignant transitional or squamous cells, but mucinous adenocarcinomas in association with Brenner tumors should be diagnosed as such.

The criteria for malignant Brenner tumor are the subject of controversy. Following the WHO recommendation, we require obvious stromal invasion for the diagnosis. We further divide borderline Brenner tumors into those that are composed of grade 1 malignant transitional cells, which we designate borderline tumors (without qualification), and those in

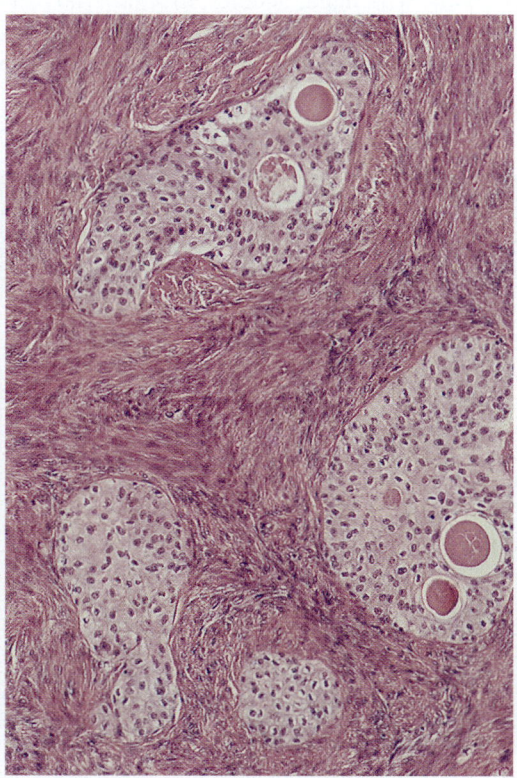

FIG. 61. Brenner tumor. Nests of transitional cells, some containing cysts, lie in a fibromatous stroma.

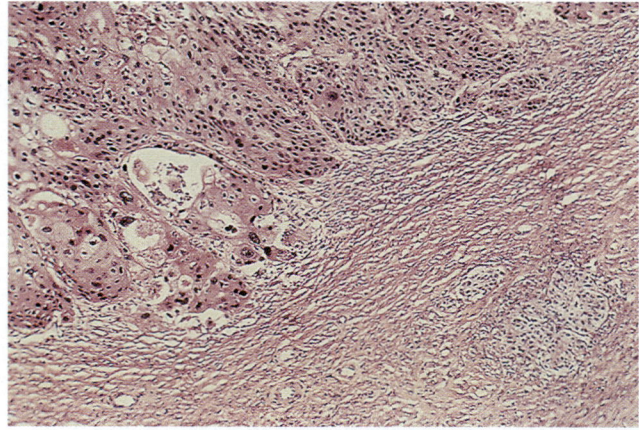

FIG. 63. Malignant Brenner tumor with squamous cell carcinoma and benign Brenner tumor.

which the transitional cells are grade 2 or 3, which we report as borderline tumors with intraepithelial carcinoma.

Transitional Cell Carcinoma

Transitional cell carcinomas do not differ in their age distribution or clinical symptoms from other types of epithelial cancer (283–286). The pure form of transitional cell carcinoma accounts for only 1% of surface epithelial carcinomas, mixed carcinomas with a predominant transitional cell component comprise 5%, and those with a minor transitional cell component make up 3% (285). The major clinical impetus for acceptance of transitional cell carcinoma as a distinct entity was provided by the M. D. Anderson Cancer Center's finding that carcinomas with a predominant component of this type of tumor respond much better to chemotherapy than most other surface epithelial cancers (284,285). Since the initial publication from that center, the results of two additional investigations from other institutions have appeared, with one failing to confirm (286) and the other supporting (300) the M. D. Anderson findings.

Transitional cell carcinomas may be solid or solid and cystic. On microscopic examination, they resemble those of the urinary tract. The cysts often have a lining of undulating papillae covered by stratified malignant transitional epithelium (Fig. 64) and focal papillae. Solid areas may consist of masses of tumor cells or, in some cases, circumscribed nests of uniformly malignant transitional cells within a fibromatous stroma, the so-called Brenner pattern of transitional cell carcinoma. Mucin droplets and, rarely, glands and small cysts containing mucin may be present.

Differential Diagnosis

Benign Brenner tumors with large mucinous cysts may be misdiagnosed as mucinous cystadenomas if the focal presence of transitional cells at the periphery of the mucinous cells is not recognized. Borderline and malignant Brenner tumors are distinguished from metastatic transitional cell carcinomas from the urinary tract by the finding of benign Brenner nests or glands or cysts lined by mucinous epithelium in the former (299). Primary transitional cell carcinoma, however, can be closely mimicked by metastatic disease. The usual clinical, gross, and microscopic criteria for differentiating primary from secondary ovarian tumors (see pages 2376–2377) are helpful in this differential diagnosis. In difficult cases immunohistochemistry may be of great help. Urinary tract tumors of this type have been shown to be reactive for CK20, in contrast to primary ovarian transitional cell carcinomas (301). A more common problem is distinguishing transitional cell carcinoma from other surface epithelial carcinomas, particularly poorly differentiated and undifferentiated forms. Such tumors have a greater tendency to grow in diffuse masses; when they have a pattern simulating that of papillary transitional cell carcinomas, it is more often due to the presence of pseudopapillae resulting from central necrosis with dropout of necrotic cellular debris.

Squamous Cell Tumors

Although squamous elements are frequently seen in endometrioid tumors and much less often in serous, mucinous, and Brenner tumors, relatively few pure squamous cell neoplasms of the ovary have been reported. A number have been epidermoid cysts (302–304). Nests of transitional epithelium were present in the walls of several of these cases (303), suggesting an origin from Walthard nests. Other epidermoid cysts have contained teratomatous foci as well as Walthard nests, however; they belong in the germ cell category of tumors (304).

Squamous cell carcinomas of the ovary (305–308) usually arise in dermoid cysts, less often from endometriosis, and rarely in Brenner tumors. In the latter two situations, the tumors can be confidently placed in the surface epithelial category of neoplasms. Approximately 24 cases of pure squamous cell carcinoma of the ovary of uncertain origin have also been described (308). In almost half of those cases, carcinoma *in situ* of the cervix was also diagnosed, raising the question of either independently primary cervical and ovarian neoplasia or metastasis to the ovary from an undiscovered focus of invasion of the cervical tumor. Squamous cell carcinoma arising in the context of endometriosis may form discrete masses protruding into the lumen or infiltrating the wall of an endometriotic cyst; in other cases, the tumor is predominantly solid or cystic without distinctive features.

Microscopic examination reveals nests of squamous cells infiltrating the stroma as well as cysts lined by malignant squamous epithelium, sometimes with polypoid intraluminal growth. The tumor cells usually have the typical appearance of those of squamous cell carcinoma, but in some cases they are spindle-shaped, resembling a sarcoma. In a study of 37 squamous cell carcinomas of the ovary, five tumors were characterized by a predominantly spindle-cell pattern (308). Other histologic patterns in that series (which is the largest

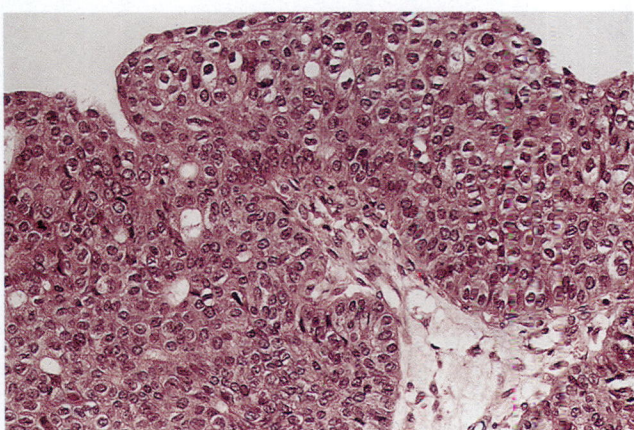

FIG. 64. Transitional cell carcinoma. A cyst is lined by undulating, transitional-type epithelium.

on this subtype of ovarian carcinoma) were papillary or polypoid, cystic, insular, diffusely infiltrative, and verruciform. In some of the cases, foci of obvious squamous differentiation were relatively inconspicuous, particularly when the tumors were high grade.

Differential Diagnosis

Generous sampling may be necessary to establish the primary nature of a squamous cell carcinoma occupying the ovary. In cases in which an ovarian origin cannot be established, it is important to exclude metastasis, particularly from the cervix (309). In very rare cases, squamous cell carcinoma *in situ* of the cervix spreads along the endometrial and tubal epithelium to the ovarian surface and may invade en route and metastasize to the ovary while remaining intraepithelial within the cervix (310). Squamous cell carcinomas of the ovary must also be distinguished from endometrioid carcinomas with extensive squamous differentiation; in such cases malignant endometrioid glands are also identifiable. Squamous cell carcinomas with a prominent spindle-cell pattern may be misdiagnosed as sarcomas if the sometimes minor foci of recognizable squamous differentiation are not appreciated. Papillary squamous cell carcinomas should be differentiated from transitional cell carcinomas, which is usually straightforward because of the presence of unequivocal squamous foci.

Mixed Epithelial Tumours

A wide variety of mixtures of epithelial cell types have been found within this category of tumors (216,271,311). Several types of mixed tumor are relatively common, including combined Brenner and mucinous cystic tumor, predominantly endocervical-like mucinous cystic tumor of borderline malignancy that also contains epithelial cell types other than mucinous types (including hobnail cells that should not lead to misdiagnosis as clear-cell carcinoma) (311), endometrioid carcinoma admixed with clear-cell carcinoma (216,271); transitional cell carcinoma associated with another type of carcinoma (284,285), and endometrioid carcinoma with a serous or undifferentiated component (312).

In cases of combined Brenner and mucinous neoplasia, we place the tumor in the mixed epithelial category if both components are recognizable on gross examination or if the minor component (Brenner tumor or pure mucinous tumor) accounts for at least 10% of the neoplasm. The finding of mucinous epithelium within Brenner epithelial nests or cysts, even if it is extensive, is not sufficient to warrant a diagnosis of mixed epithelial tumor. The presence of serous, endometrioid, or squamous elements in an otherwise pure mucinous borderline tumor of the endocervical-like type has not been shown to affect the prognosis (311). Because endometrioid and clear-cell carcinomas are associated with a similar prognosis stage for stage, a combination of the two tumors probably has little clinical significance. A component of serous or undifferentiated carcinoma in an otherwise endometrioid carcinoma greatly diminishes the survival rate (313). The significance of mixtures of transitional cell carcinoma with other forms of malignant epithelial neoplasia has already been discussed.

Undifferentiated Carcinoma

The WHO defines an undifferentiated carcinoma as one that exhibits no or only rare and minor foci of differentiation (135); others have defined it as a carcinoma over half of which lacks differentiation (313). If one uses the WHO definition, significantly less than 5% of carcinomas are undifferentiated. Most undifferentiated carcinomas do not have distinctive features, but a few unusual variants exist and are discussed later herein. The clinical features of most undifferentiated carcinomas resemble those of high-grade serous carcinomas. Approximately half the tumors are bilateral, and spread beyond the pelvis at diagnosis is common (131). The neoplastic tissue is predominantly solid and often shows areas of hemorrhage, necrosis, and cyst formation.

Microscopic Features

A variety of patterns are encountered, including diffuse masses and irregular nests and cords of epithelial cells separated by a stroma that may be desmoplastic. Psammoma bodies, glands, papillae, or mucin pools and mucin droplets may be present in very small numbers. The tumor cells can vary greatly in size and exhibit obvious malignant features (Fig. 65); tumor giant cells are often present. Rarely, undifferentiated carcinomas or undifferentiated components of specific types of epithelial tumor transform focally into choriocarcinoma (314).

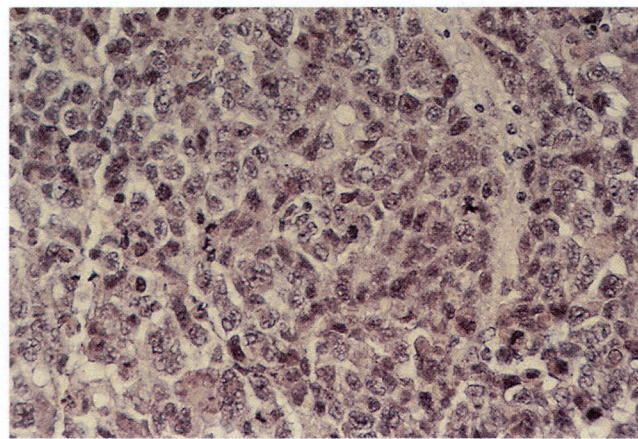

FIG. 65. Undifferentiated carcinoma. Note the nuclear pleomorphism.

Small-cell Carcinoma, Pulmonary Type

The distinctive variant of undifferentiated carcinoma that is associated with hypercalcemia in approximately two-thirds of cases and has been designated "small-cell carcinoma" (315) is discussed in detail in the section on miscellaneous tumors (page 2373), since it remains of uncertain cell lineage. Carcinomas similar in histologic features to pulmonary small-cell carcinoma also may be primary in the ovary (316). Because the nonspecific phrase small cell is appropriate for both of these neoplasms (which differ in their clinical and pathologic features), the former tumors have been referred to as "small-cell carcinomas, hypercalcemic type" and the latter as "small-cell carcinomas, pulmonary type."

Eleven of the latter tumors have been reported in women 28 to 85 years of age, who had clinical symptoms typical of ovarian cancer (316). Six tumors were unilateral, and five were bilateral; seven had spread beyond the ovary. On microscopic inspection, they were found to be composed largely of cells with the characteristic features of pulmonary small-cell carcinoma (Fig. 66). A component of endometrioid carcinoma was present in four tumors (Fig. 66); one tumor showed squamous differentiation, one was associated with a cyst lined by atypical mucinous cells, and two were focally admixed with a Brenner tumor. These findings strongly suggest a surface epithelial derivation. It is important to distinguish these tumors from small-cell carcinomas of the hypercalcemic type as well as other small-cell tumors of the ovary, both primary and metastatic.

The older age of patients with the pulmonary type of small-cell carcinoma is in marked contrast to the young age of almost all patients with ovarian small-cell carcinoma of the hypercalcemic type. Moreover, hypercalcemia, even though it occasionally accompanies pulmonary small-cell carcinoma, has not been reported in association with this type of tumor originating in the ovary. On microscopic examination, small-cell carcinomas of the pulmonary type do not contain the follicles commonly seen in hypercalcemic small-cell carcinomas or the large cells with abundant cytoplasm that are present in approximately 40% of the latter tumors. The nuclei of hypercalcemic tumors contain easily identifiable nucleoli, which vary in size, in contrast to the molded, finely stippled nuclei with inconspicuous nucleoli in the pulmonary-type of small-cell carcinoma. Flow cytometry characteristically reveals diploidy in hypercalcemic small-cell carcinoma and aneuploidy in the pulmonary type (316).

Neuroendocrine Carcinoma of the Non-small-cell Type

Eight undifferentiated ovarian cancers with neuroendocrine features on immunohistochemical or ultrastructural examination, but without the light microscopic features of small-cell carcinoma, have been reported (317). These tumors were composed of larger cells, in some cases with abundant cytoplasm, and resembled large-cell neuroendocrine carcinoma of the lung. They were also accompanied by a component of surface epithelial tumor, most often of the mucinous type; one tumor had a component of endometrioid adenocarcinoma.

Sex Cord–Stromal Tumors

These neoplasms account for approximately 6% of all ovarian tumors and for most clinically functioning ovarian tumors (318). They contain elements of sex-cord and stromal derivation in varying combinations and with differing amounts of cytologic atypia and mitotic activity (Table 1). The most common subtype of sex cord–stromal tumor is the endocrinologically inactive fibroma. The remainder most frequently exhibit differentiation toward more specific ovarian-type cells (granulosa cells and theca cells) and, less often, toward testicular-type cells (Sertoli cells and Leydig cells). A few such tumors appear to be intermediate or indifferent or contain cells of both ovarian and testicular types.

Granulosa Cell Tumors

These tumors account for approximately 1.5% of all ovarian neoplasms and for 6% of ovarian cancers (319). Approximately three-fourths are estrogenic, but rare examples, including a disproportionate number of large, thin-walled cystic tumors, are androgenic (320). Patients without endocrine symptoms are usually first seen for abdominal swelling or pain. Pain may be acute, owing to rupture and hemoperitoneum, which occurs in up to 10% of cases (321). A mass is usually palpable on pelvic or abdominal examination, but about 10% of tumors are discovered during operation for abnormal uterine bleeding or at the time of pathologic examination (322).

Two-thirds of patients are postmenopausal (323–325); less than 5% are prepubertal. Most of the tumors in children and young adults differ in pathologic characteristics from the usual tumor encountered in women over 30 years of age, and

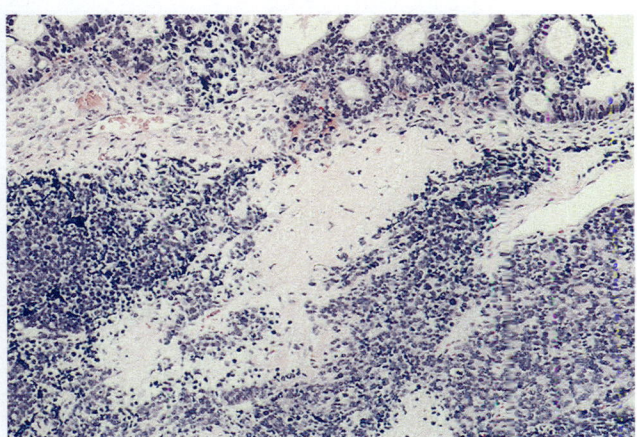

FIG. 66. Small-cell carcinoma, pulmonary type. Note the component of endometrioid glands (top).

the designations juvenile granulosa cell tumor (JGCT) and adult granulosa cell tumor (AGCT) (326) have been introduced to distinguish the two morphologic types. Occasionally, JGCTs are seen in older women, and, conversely, some AGCTs develop in children and young women. When a GCT of either type arises in prepubertal girls, it is associated with isosexual pseudoprecocity in about 75% of cases. Both forms of GCT are stage I in the great majority of cases, and less than 5% are bilateral.

Adult Granulosa Cell Tumor

Gross Features. These tumors vary greatly in size, with an average diameter of 12.5 cm (324). Their appearance varies from uniformly solid to uniformly cystic. Most often, there is a yellow to white solid component and a hemorrhagic constituent that is solid or cystic (Fig. 67). Necrosis is relatively uncommon. The cystic tumors are often thin-walled (Fig. 68), sometimes resembling serous cystadenomas (320).

Microscopic Features. Examination reveals granulosa cells usually accompanied by a stromal component of fibroblasts, theca cells, or lutein cells in various combinations. Several patterns are encountered; two or more are often present in the same specimen. The microfollicular pattern (Fig. 69) is characterized by small follicles (Call-Exner bodies) that may contain eosinophilic material with nuclear debris, hyalinized basement membrane–like material, or, very rarely, a basophilic secretion. A macrofollicular pattern of large, relatively uniform follicles resembling follicle cysts is occasionally seen. Insular and trabecular patterns appear as islands and anastomosing bands of granulosa cells, respectively. The diffuse pattern (Fig. 70) is characterized by sheets of round, oval, or slightly spindle-shaped cells, some-

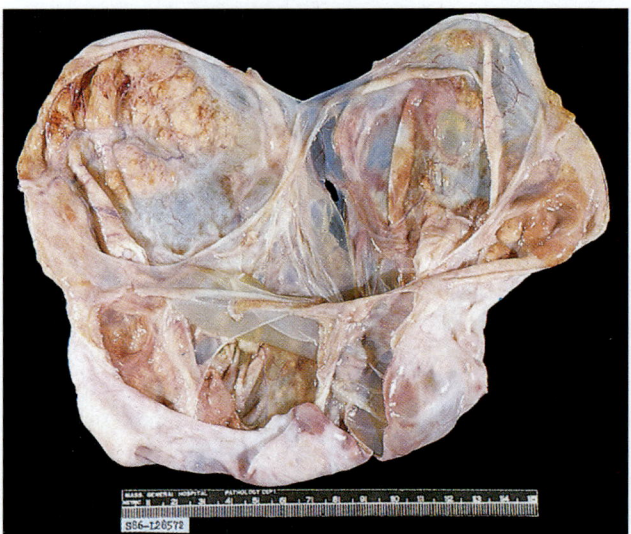

FIG. 68. Granulosa cell tumor, adult type. This multiloculated neoplasm has small foci of pink-yellow tumor tissue adherent to its lining.

times imparting a sarcomatoid appearance to the tumor. Uncommon patterns include watered-silk and gyriform. The former is characterized by parallel, thin, winding cords and the latter by a zigzag arrangement of cords. In unusual cases, true tubules with lumens and solid tubular structures are present in small numbers.

The nuclei of the granulosa cells are typically pale and round and oval or angular and are often haphazardly oriented. They are commonly grooved (Fig. 71), but the grooves may be inconspicuous, particularly in tumors with a diffuse pattern. Significant pleomorphism is usually absent, but approximately 2% of AGCTs contain cells with large, bizarre, hyperchromatic nuclei, which resemble the bizarre nuclei seen in symplastic leiomyomas (327). Mitotic activity is not often conspicuous, and the mitotic rate is two or fewer per 10 hpf in approximately three-fourths of cases (321). The cytoplasm of the granulosa cells is frequently scanty but may

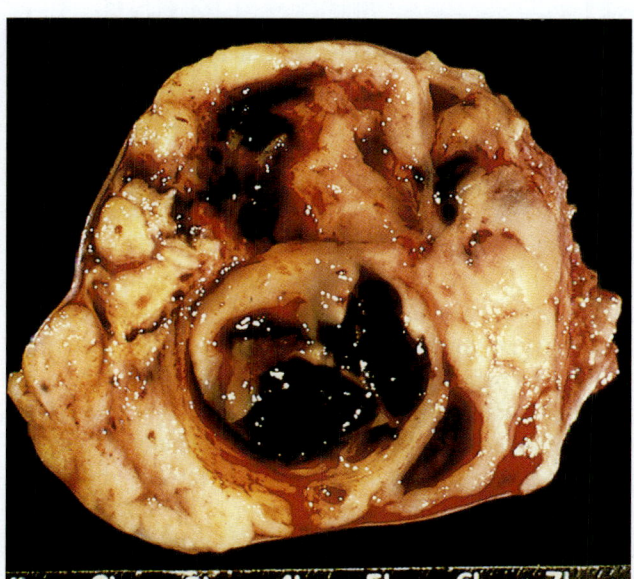

FIG. 67. Granulosa cell tumor, adult type. The neoplasm is composed of yellow-white tissue with hemorrhage, some of which is intracystic.

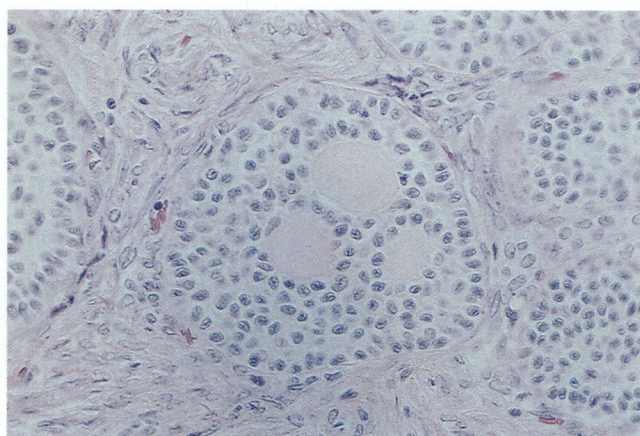

FIG. 69. Granulosa cell tumor, adult type with Call-Exner bodies.

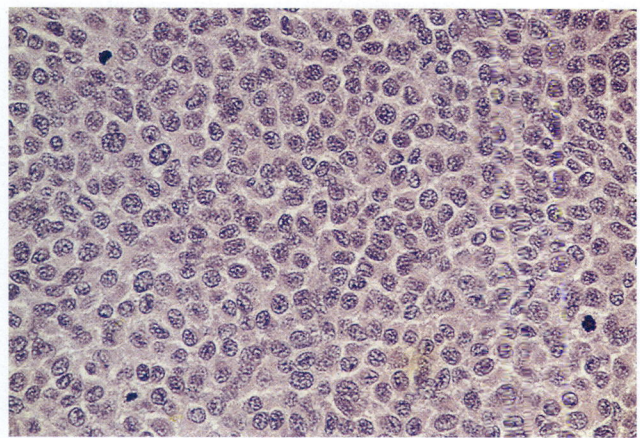

FIG. 70. Granulosa cell tumor, adult type, diffuse pattern.

be abundant and eosinophilic, resulting in a luteinized appearance. Extensive luteinization is uncommon (328). In a few tumors, the cytoplasm is abundant and pale or vacuolated. A variably thecomatous or fibromatous component is usually present and may predominate. The designation of fibroma or thecoma with minor sex-cord elements (page 2349) should be applied to those tumors whose granulosa cell component accounts for less than 10% of the tumor (329). Very rarely, the stroma of an AGCT has the appearance of a high-grade sarcoma (330) or exhibits adipose or osseous metaplasia (318).

Differential Diagnosis. Undifferentiated carcinomas and adenocarcinomas with very small, uniform glands are often misinterpreted as diffuse and microfollicular AGCTs, respectively. In contrast to AGCTs, carcinomas are bilateral in more than 25% of cases, often have spread beyond the ovary, and may be extensively necrotic on gross examination. On microscopic inspection, carcinomas, unlike AGCTs, typically have hyperchromatic, often pleomorphic nuclei (Fig. 65) with many, often atypical mitotic figures; they may also contain psammoma bodies and intracellular mucin. Stroma, when present in an undifferentiated carcinoma, is typically fibrous and often desmoplastic, in contrast to the fibrothecomatous stromal component of AGCT.

AGCTs may be difficult to distinguish from pure stromal tumors, such as thecomas, cellular fibromas, and fibrosarcomas. Reticulin stains may show abundant intercellular fibrils in these tumors, unlike the scanty reticulin of AGCTs. In some cases, the pattern of fibrils is intermediate between AGCT and typical thecoma, and the differential diagnosis may be difficult or impossible. The almost exclusively spindle-cell nature of fibromas and fibrosarcomas is rarely seen in AGCTs. Extensively luteinized AGCTs may be difficult to distinguish from steroid cell tumors, but thorough sampling usually discloses foci with the typical microscopic features of the former tumor type. Distinguishing AGCT from endometrioid tumor, carcinoid tumor, endometrioid stromal sarcoma, and small-cell carcinoma of the hypercalcemic type is discussed in the sections on those neoplasms.

The differentiation of AGCTs from tumors other than those in the sex cord–stromal category may be aided by immunohistochemical staining for inhibin, which is almost always positive in GCTs and most other sex cord–stromal tumors that have been studied to date and is typically negative, or at most weakly positive, in tumors that are not sex cord–stromal tumors (227,247–254). Furthermore, EMA and CK7, which give positive results in most surface epithelial carcinomas, stain negative in GCTs (226,227). Desmin may aid in the distinction from an epithelioid smooth muscle tumor, a rare differential diagnosis (see page 2372).

Occasionally, making the distinction between a unilocular or multilocular macrofollicular AGCT and one or more follicular cysts may be troublesome. This is particularly likely if the patient is pregnant or in the puerperium, since LSLFCPP (53) may be indistinguishable on gross inspection from a unilocular cystic AGCT (page 2310). The very large luteinized cells of LSLFCPP, some of which contain large, bizarre nuclei, differ, however, from those of unilocular AGCT which are rarely uniformly luteinized and almost never contain bizarre nuclei. In addition, the focal presence of neoplastic granulosa cells within the walls of most cystic AGCTs contrasts with their absence in follicle cysts. The distinction of GCTs from granulosa cell proliferations (63) has been discussed on page 2311.

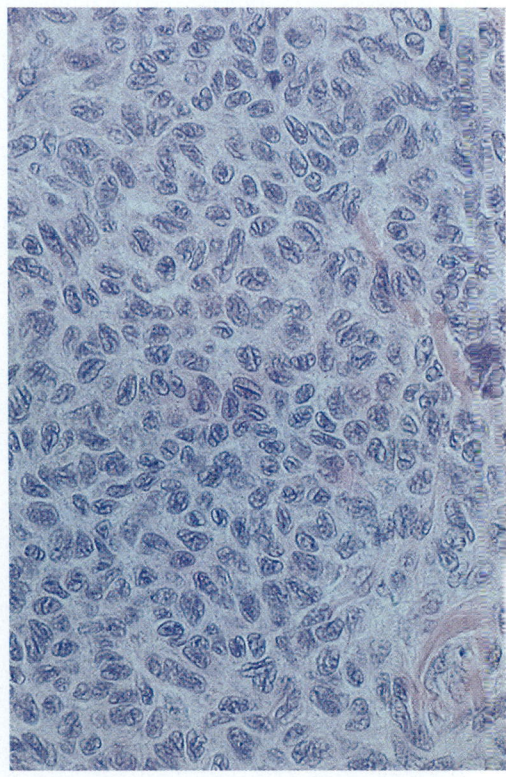

FIG. 71. Granulosa cell tumor, adult type, diffuse pattern, with prominent nuclear groves.

Juvenile Granulosa Cell Tumor

Gross Features. JGCT, like AGCT, is typically partly solid, containing cysts that may be filled with blood (Fig. 72); uniformly solid or cystic tumors also are seen. The neo-

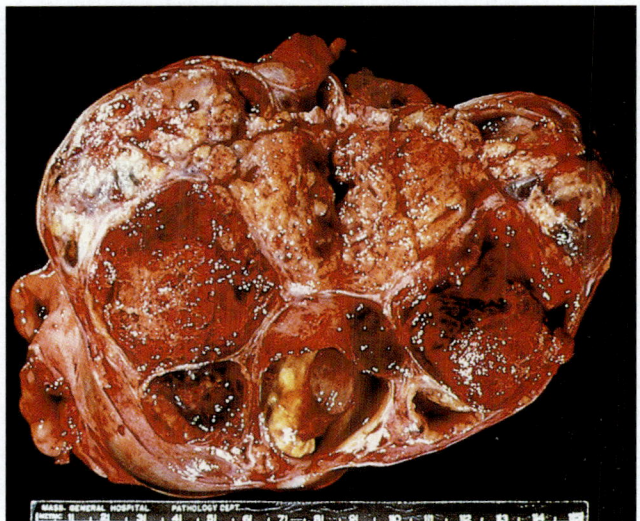

FIG. 72. Juvenile granulosa cell tumor. The sectioned surface reveals solid, lobulated tissue with areas of hemorrhage and necrosis and cyst formation.

plastic tissue may be gray, cream-colored, brown, or yellow; from time to time, large areas of necrosis or hemorrhage are present.

Microscopic Features. Sheets or nodular aggregates of neoplastic granulosa cells are usually punctured by varying numbers of irregular or round to oval follicles (Fig. 73) (326,331–333). Rare tumors have scant or no follicles. The follicles rarely attain the size of those in macrofollicular AGCTs, but they are much larger than Call-Exner bodies.

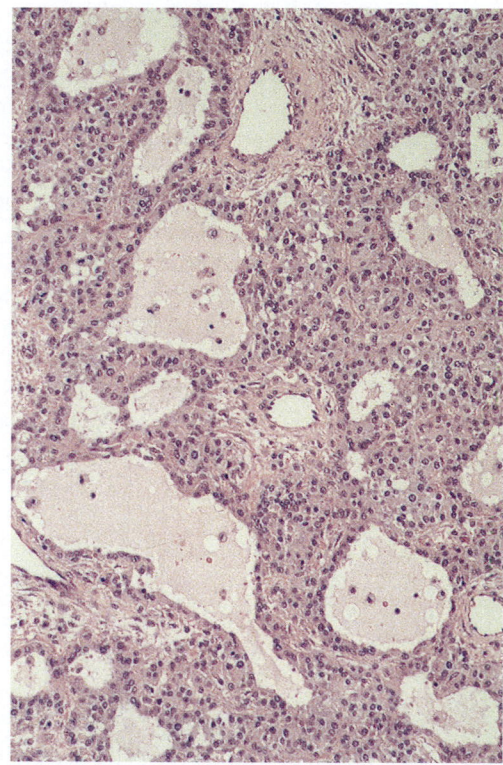

FIG. 73. Juvenile granulosa cell tumor. Follicles of varying sizes and shapes are separated by cellular areas.

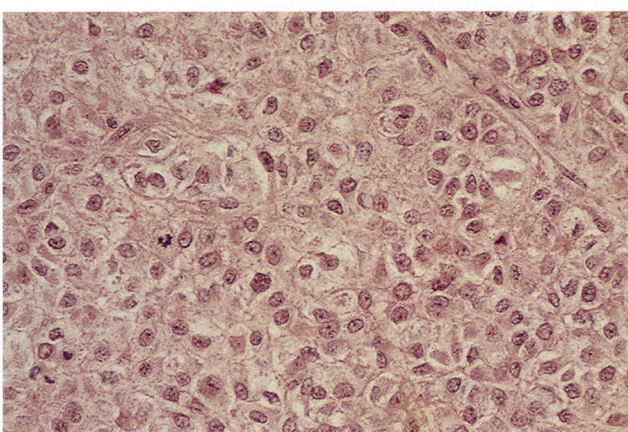

FIG. 74. Juvenile granulosa cell tumor. Note the abundant eosinophilic cytoplasm, mitotic activity, and absence of grooves in rounded, hyperchromatic nuclei.

Typically, they contain a eosinophilic or basophilic mucicarminophilic secretion. In the diffuse areas, there may be a background of basophilic, mucinous fluid. Theca cells are often present between the nodules of granulosa cells; occasionally, both cell types are arranged in a disorderly fashion and are difficult to distinguish. In some cases, the nodules of granulosa cells are solid; they may undergo hyalinization, somewhat resembling corpora albicantia.

Both the granulosa and theca cells usually have abundant eosinophilic (Fig. 74) or heavily vacuolated cytoplasm, that is, they are luteinized. The neoplastic cells have hyperchromatic, round nuclei that are only infrequently grooved. Mitotic figures, which may be atypical, are often numerous. In 10% to 15% of cases, there is marked nuclear atypia (Fig. 75) (290); in a few tumors, hobnail-like cells line the follicles. Tumors from pregnant patients may exhibit prominent edema (334). Occasionally, JGCTs are combined with SLCT of intermediate differentiation (page 2354).

Differential Diagnosis. The differential diagnosis of JGCT includes AGCT and a variety of other neoplasms. The follicles of JGCT are more irregular in size and shape than those of AGCT, and its cells are usually more extensively luteinized, with nuclei that are round and hyperchromatic

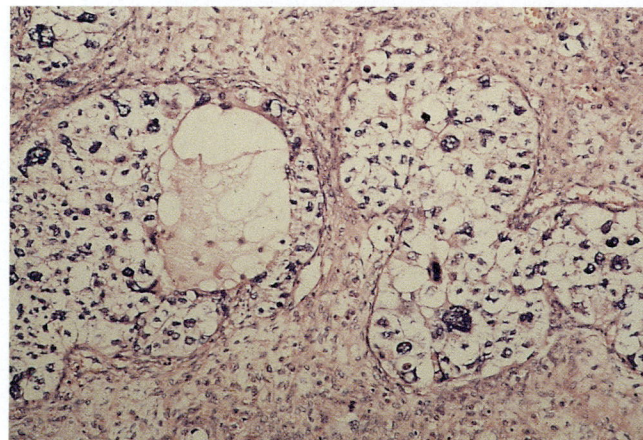

FIG. 75. Juvenile granulosa cell tumor. Note the nuclear pleomorphism.

and lack grooves. The mucicarminophilic, often basophilic follicular content in JGCT also differs from the eosinophilic basement membrane material, often accompanied by degenerating nuclei, that is present in the microfollicles of AGCTs. JGCTs are often misdiagnosed as malignant germ cell tumors. The latter tumors are more common in young women than JGCTs and are associated in isolated cases with hCG-induced isosexual pseudoprecocity. The nuclei of JGCTs are not as primitive-appearing as those of either YST or embryonal carcinoma, and the follicular pattern of JGCTs is not a feature of either of those tumors. Immunohistochemical evidence of hCG in embryonal carcinomas and choriocarcinomas and of AFP in YSTs, as well as staining of JGCTs for inhibin, may be helpful in difficult cases (254).

JGCT is sometimes misinterpreted as thecoma because of the occasional absence or rarity of follicles, the typically abundant cytoplasm of the neoplastic cells, and the occasional predominance of theca cells. Thorough sampling to demonstrate follicles as well as reticulin stains to establish the granulosa cell nature of at least some of the tumor cells are important in terms of diagnosis. Furthermore, thecomas rarely exhibit significant mitotic activity, infrequently occur before 30 years of age, and are exceptionally rare in children. A predominantly diffuse pattern in luteinized JGCT may suggest the diagnosis of steroid cell tumor, but the uniformity as well as the cytologic features of the latter tumor would be unusual for JGCT, which almost always contains more easily recognized diagnostic areas. Pregnancy luteomas sometimes contain rounded follicle-like spaces and may resemble luteinized JGCT. Its cells are uniform, however, and it is multiple and bilateral in one-half and one-third of the cases, respectively.

The only surface epithelial tumors with which JGCTs might be confused are clear-cell and undifferentiated carcinomas. The tubulocystic variant of clear-cell carcinoma is suggested when follicles in JGCTs are lined by cells resembling hobnail cells; JGCTs with high-grade nuclear atypia may suggest undifferentiated carcinoma. The absence of other patterns of clear-cell carcinoma, the young age of the patient, and the presence of follicles and of focal areas typical of JGCT provide evidence for its diagnosis. The differing results of inhibin and EMA staining can establish the diagnosis in difficult cases. Possible confusion of JGCT with small-cell carcinoma of the hypercalcemic type is discussed on page 2366.

A metastatic tumor that can simulate JGCT is malignant melanoma (335). Some tumors of this type contain follicle-like spaces, and some contain cells with abundant eosinophilic cytoplasm, closely simulating the follicular and solid patterns of JGCTs. Metastatic malignant melanoma, however, is very rare in the first two decades of life, when approximately 80% of JGCTs are encountered. Knowledge of the concurrent or previous existence of primary malignant melanoma may also be helpful. Since the previous removal of a malignant melanoma may have been remote, or the primary tumor may have regressed, however, the possibility of metastatic melanoma should be considered in the differential diagnosis of JGCT, especially when the patient is older than 20 years of age. It is more likely that the neoplasm represents metastatic melanoma if the ovarian tumor is bilateral. Differential staining for inhibin and HMB 45 should establish the diagnosis in challenging cases.

Tumors in the Thecoma-Fibroma Group

Fibroma

Fibromas typically occur in patients over 40 years of age (the average age is 48 years) (336) and are rare in children, except for those in patients with the basal cell nevus (Gorlin's) syndrome, in whom the tumors are almost always bilateral, multinodular, and calcified (337). Fibromas over 10 cm in diameter are associated with ascites in up to 40% of cases and Meigs' syndrome (ascites and pleural effusion) in about 1% (338,339).

Gross Features. Fibromas average 6 cm in diameter (336) and are typically uniformly solid, firm, white neoplasms; a few specimens are soft and edematous. Rare examples are predominantly white but have yellow foci. Hemorrhage, necrosis, calcification, and cyst formation may be seen. Cellular fibromas are apt to be larger and softer, with a much higher rate of hemorrhage and necrosis than typical fibromas (340,341).

Microscopic Features. The classic appearance is that of spindle cells resembling fibroblasts and producing collagen; a storiform pattern is often present. The cellularity varies but is not marked. Hyaline plaques may be seen, and some tumors are diffusely edematous. Cytologic atypia and mitotic activity are usually absent or minor in extent. Fibromatous tumors that contain lutein cells belong in the category of luteinized thecoma.

Differential Diagnosis. The most common problem in diagnosis is distinguishing fibroma from thecoma. Both tumors are derived from the ovarian stromal cell; because a spectrum exists between the two, any distinction is necessarily arbitrary. We place tumors in the fibroma category unless a component is characterized by cells that are large and contain abundant pale cytoplasm, which is usually, but not invariably, vacuolated and filled with lipid; such tumors are typically associated with estrogenic manifestations. Fat stains are not diagnostic because small to moderate amounts may be present in the spindle cells of a fibroma, as in many other tumors. Thecomas diagnosed on the basis of their appearance on routine staining are almost always inhibin positive; a few fibromas diagnosed on the same basis, however, are sometimes focally inhibin positive as well (254). Some authors use the term fibrothecoma for tumors in the intermediate zone between fibroma and thecoma.

Fibromatosis of the ovary (page 2314) may closely resemble fibroma. Fibromatosis, however, envelops follicles and their derivatives, in contrast to fibroma, which typically displaces them. A similar difference helps distinguish massive edema of the ovary (page 2314), which is closely related to fibromatosis from an edematous fibroma. Individual Krukenberg tumors, Brenner tumors, and carcinoid tumors may resemble fibromas on gross examination, but their diagnostic epithelial components facilitate their identification on microscopic inspection.

Fibromatous tumors are differentiated from rare smooth-muscle and nerve sheath tumors of the ovary based on standard criteria for differential diagnosis of these tumors at other sites. A storiform pattern in a fibromatous tumor of the ovary does not warrant a diagnosis of fibrous histiocytoma.

Cellular Fibroma and Fibrosarcoma

In cellular fibroma, the nuclei are closely packed and more rounded than in a typical fibroma, with an average of three or fewer mf per 10 hpf; collagen is also much less conspicuous (340). Cellular fibromas are almost always benign unless they are adherent or ruptured, but occasionally one recurs many years after surgery in the absence of adhesion or rupture. Fibrosarcomas, which typically show greater mitotic activity and moderate to marked nuclear atypia, are almost always malignant (340) and may have distinctive chromosomal changes (341).

Thecoma (Typical Form)

Typical thecomas are about one-third as common as GCTs. The great majority are associated with estrogenic manifestations (342–344). In one large study (343), 84% of the patients were postmenopausal, with a mean age of 59 years; only 10% of the women were less than 30 years of age. Because thecomas are usually smaller than GCTs, they are less likely to be palpable on pelvic examination. Only 3% are bilateral.

Gross Features. Thecomas are typically solid yellow masses (Fig. 76), although they may be predominantly white and only focally yellow. They average about 7 cm in diameter. Cystic degeneration occurs from time to time, but it is rarely conspicuous.

Microscopic Features. Large, rounded, ill-defined cells with abundant pale, often vacuolated cytoplasm, usually containing lipid, are typically present (Fig. 77). The nuclei are round to oval and pale. A fibromatous component often separates sheets and nests of theca cells. Hyaline plaques are a characteristic and sometimes conspicuous feature (Fig. 77); in some cases, there are large confluent zones of hyalin-

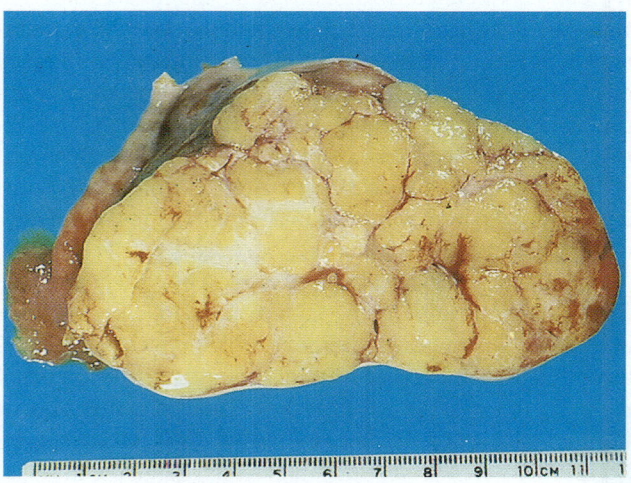

FIG. 76. Thecoma. The sectioned surface exhibits solid, lobulated, yellow tissue.

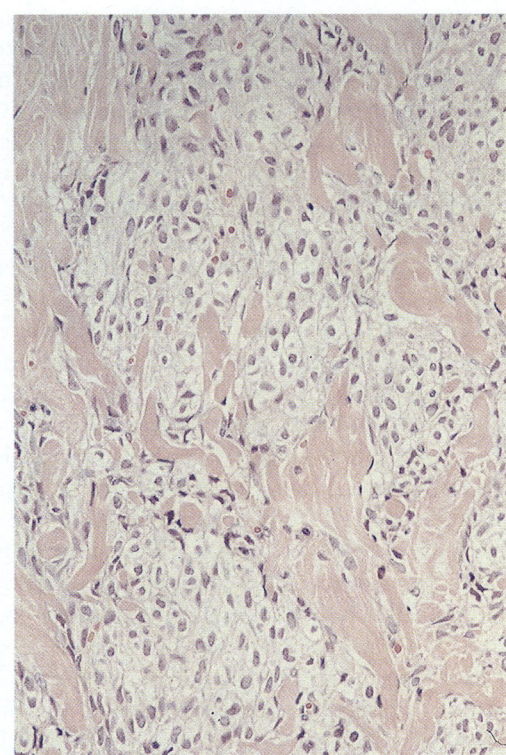

FIG. 77. Thecoma. Aggregates of rounded cells with abundant pale cytoplasm are traversed by bands of hyalinized collagen.

ization. Foci of calcification may be present. Extensive calcification has been seen in rare cases, typically in young women (344). A few thecomas exhibit mild cytologic atypia, and, now and then, bizarre nuclei are seen in otherwise typical tumors (327). Significant atypia and conspicuous mitotic activity accompanied by clinically malignant behavior are exceptional (345).

Luteinized Thecoma

This tumor has features of fibroma or typical thecoma but also contains lutein cells, found singly or in clusters or masses (Fig. 78) (346,347). Luteinized thecomas are seen in a younger age group than typical thecomas. About half of them are estrogenic, and 10% are androgenic (347). Approximately 15 cases of an unusual subtype that is associated with potentially fatal sclerosing peritonitis have been reported (348–351). This lesion is often bilateral and may enlarge the ovary irregularly, instead of forming a discrete mass, suggesting a hyperplastic rather than neoplastic process in some cases. On microscopic examination, it is seen to contain lutein cells that are smaller and less easily identified than those in the usual luteinized thecoma, and it may have areas of edema that can create a microcystic pattern (Fig. 79). Despite brisk mitotic activity in many cases there is no evidence that the lesion has the potential to metastasize. The pathogenesis of the accompanying sclerosing peritonitis remains a mystery.

Differential Diagnosis. Tumors that, on low-power examination, appear to be luteinized thecomas rarely contain

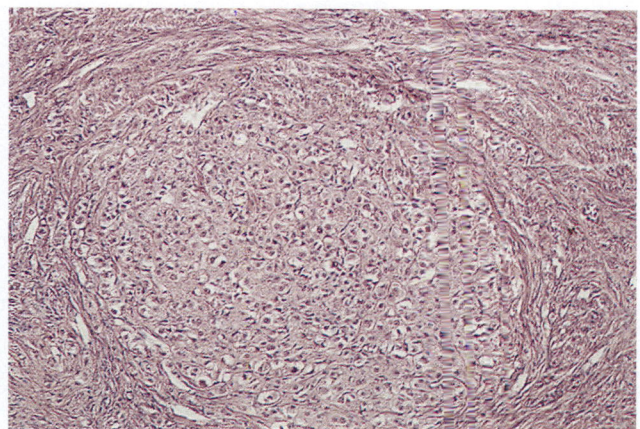

FIG. 78. Luteinized thecoma. A nodule of luteinized cells lies within a fibromatous stroma.

crystals of Reinke; such tumors have been designated stromal–Leydig cell tumors (82). When the lutein cells in a luteinized thecoma are extensive, it may simulate a steroid cell tumor, not otherwise specified, because some steroid cell tumors have a fibromatous component (352,353); in those tumors however, the fibromatous component accounts for less than 10% of the tumor. Luteinized thecomas must also be distinguished from stromal hyperthecosis. This lesion is almost always bilateral, in contrast to luteinized thecoma, and the lutein cells in stromal hyperthecosis are in the context of small hyperplastic stromal cells with minimal collagen production.

The diffuse luteinization of thecomas that may be seen in pregnant patients can lead to diagnostic confusion with pregnancy luteomas (page 2315). The latter, however, are multiple in half of the cases, contain little or no lipid, and do not have features of fibroma or thecoma. In addition, although they are hyperplastic rather than neoplastic, pregnancy luteomas usually exhibit more mitotic activity than typical luteinized thecomas.

The differential diagnosis of the peculiar luteinized thecomas associated with sclerosing peritonitis includes both nonneoplastic and neoplastic lesions. These thecomas differ from stromal hyperthecosis in the accompanying clinical features. In addition, hyperthecosis does not cause the marked ovarian enlargement (over 8 cm) that is present in some cases of luteinized thecoma. It also does not have the striking surface nodular configuration of some of the latter tumors. Moreover, in stromal hyperthecosis there is no obliteration of the underlying ovarian architecture. Finally, the stromal cells in hyperthecosis lack the mitotic activity that is often a striking feature of these luteinized thecomas. The distinctive features of luteinized thecomas, including the clinical picture, gross characteristics, and striking mitotic activity, distinguish them from massive edema or fibromatosis. Their particular characteristics also set them apart from such tumors as cellular fibromas and SSTs, which might occasionally be diagnostic considerations.

Stromal Tumors with Minor Sex-cord Elements

Predominantly fibromatous or thecomatous tumors rarely contain scattered aggregates of sex-cord derivation occupying less than 10% of the area of the tumor. Nests composed of cells resembling granulosa cells or indifferent sex cord–type cells, or tubules lined by cells resembling Sertoli cells, may be seen. The overall appearance and behavior of these tumors is more like those of a fibroma or thecoma than those of a sex-cord tumor (329).

Sclerosing Stromal Tumor

This distinctive tumor occurs at a younger average age than typical thecoma or fibroma—more than 80% of patients are less than 30 years old (40,354,355). Most patients are first seen for nonspecific symptoms related to an ovarian mass; estrogenic manifestations have been present only occasionally, and associated virilization during pregnancy is rare. All the reported tumors have been unilateral and benign.

Gross Features

A well-demarcated, predominantly solid white mass with yellow flecks is typical; areas of edema and cyst formation

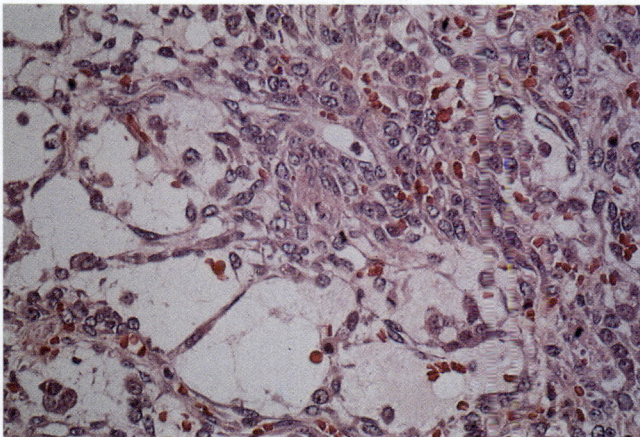

FIG. 79. Luteinized thecoma of the type associated with sclerosing peritonitis. Note the microcystic change.

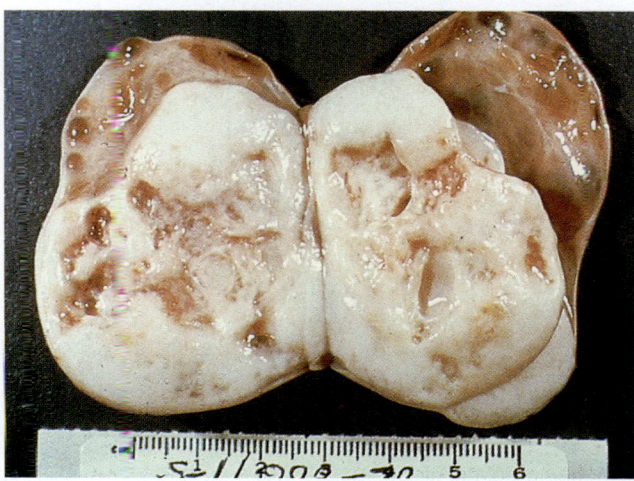

FIG. 80. Sclerosing stromal tumor. The sectioned surface of the neoplasm is white. Note cyst formation. (From ref. 40.)

are common (Fig. 80). Rare specimens are predominantly cystic. The tumors average 10 cm in diameter, ranging up to 17 cm (354).

Microscopic Features

Low-power examination usually shows ill-defined cellular pseudolobules (Fig. 81) separated by a stroma that varies from densely hyalinized to markedly edematous. Two cell types are intermingled within the nodules: spindle cells producing collagen and round to oval cells with small, dark nuclei. The latter have vacuolated cytoplasm containing lipid and suggest degenerated lutein cells (Fig. 82). In an occasional tumor, the round or oval cells have dense eosinophilic cytoplasm and large nuclei containing prominent nucleoli, characteristic of lutein cells. Mitotic figures are absent or present in only small numbers. Another distinctive feature is a network of thin-walled, often ectatic blood vessels within the nodules.

Differential Diagnosis

The heterogeneous appearance of the sclerosing stromal tumor (SST) contrasts with the relative homogeneity of fibromas and thecomas. Although fibromas may be edematous, the edema is generally diffuse rather than focal. Hyaline plaques, a conspicuous feature of many fibromas and thecomas, are rare in SSTs. The lutein cells in SSTs typically

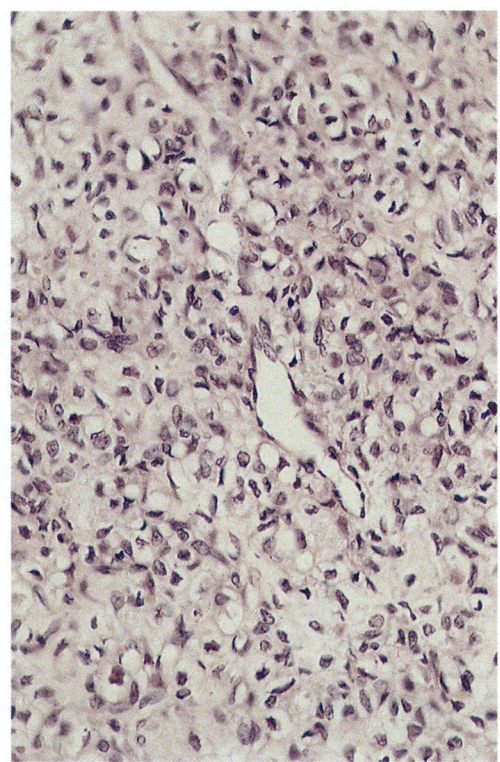

FIG. 82. Sclerosing stromal tumor. High-power view of the cellular area of the neoplasm shows a prominent component of rounded cells with clear cytoplasm. Some spindle-shaped cells are also visible.

appear degenerated, unlike their typical robust appearance in luteinized thecomas. Rarely, the vacuolated cells in SST have eccentric, compressed nuclei and simulate the signet-ring cells of Krukenberg tumor. The vacuoles in SSTs, however, contain lipid rather than mucin. The prominent vascularity in SSTs may suggest the diagnosis of hemangiopericytoma; no well-documented ovarian case of the latter tumor has been reported, however. SSTs are inhibin positive (254).

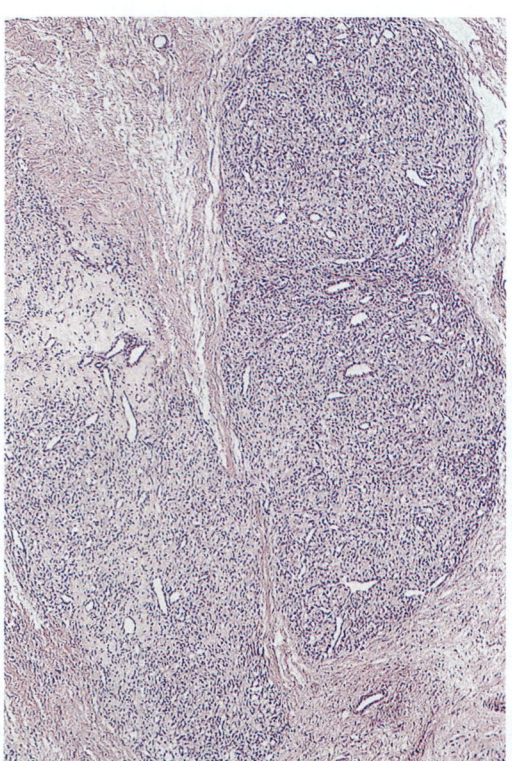

FIG. 81. Sclerosing stromal tumor. Cellular pseudolobules containing ectatic blood vessels are separated by hyalinized connective tissue.

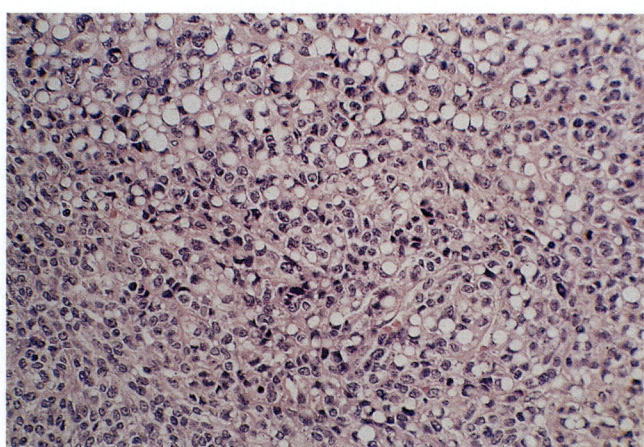

FIG. 83. Signet ring–stromal tumor.

Signet Ring–Stromal Tumor

At least five examples of this neoplasm, all occurring in adults and all nonfunctioning, have been described (356,357). They were solid or solid and cystic. On microscopic examination, spindle cells were diffusely distributed and merged almost imperceptibly with rounded cells containing eccentric nuclei and single large vacuoles resembling signet-ring cells (Fig. 83). These cells were diffusely or focally distributed. Stains for lipid and mucin showed negative results. Electron microscopic examination has shown that in some cases the vacuoles result from generalized edema of the cytoplasmic matrix, in other cases from swelling of mitochondria, and in still others from cytoplasmic pseudoinclusions of edematous extracellular matrix. An important consideration in the differential diagnosis is Krukenberg tumor, but negative mucin stains exclude that diagnosis. The signet ring–stromal tumor lacks the pseudolobulation, lipid-rich cells, and prominent vascularity of SST.

Sertoli and Sertoli–Leydig Cell Tumors

Sertoli Cell Tumors

These uncommon tumors occur at an average age of 27 years (358). Estrogenic effects have been present in two-thirds of the cases, and a few tumors, mostly of the lipid-rich type (359), have caused isosexual pseudoprecocity (358–361). Two such tumors were found in sisters with the Peutz-Jeghers syndrome (361). Almost all the tumors have been unilateral. Very rarely, Sertoli cell tumors have malignant histologic features and metastasize distantly.

Gross Features. The tumors average 9 cm in diameter and are typically uniform, solid, yellow neoplasms.

Microscopic Features. Hollow or solid tubules (Fig. 84) usually predominate and are separated by a variable amount of fibrous stroma. A diffuse or solid trabecular pattern is occasionally seen. The hollow tubules are lined by columnar to cuboidal cells with moderate amounts of pale or slightly eosinophilic cytoplasm. The solid tubules are filled with pale cells that may contain moderate to abundant lipid in the lipid-rich Sertoli cell tumor (Fig. 84) (359). Some tumors are composed of cells with abundant eosinophilic cytoplasm (362). The nuclei in Sertoli cell tumors usually lack atypical features.

Differential Diagnosis. Sertoli cell tumors should be distinguished from the rare large Sertoli cell tumors composed of uniform, solid tubules filled with immature Sertoli cells that may develop in the testes of patients with the complete form of the androgen-insensitivity syndrome (363). Such patients have a normal female habitus; primary amenorrhea; no uterus; a contralateral testis, which may be composed predominantly of cellular stroma resembling ovarian stroma; an absence of pubic and axillary hair; and a 46,XY karyotype. SLCTs are distinguished from Sertoli cell tumors by the presence in the former of more than rare Leydig cells or their spindle-cell precursors. Differentiation from low-grade en-

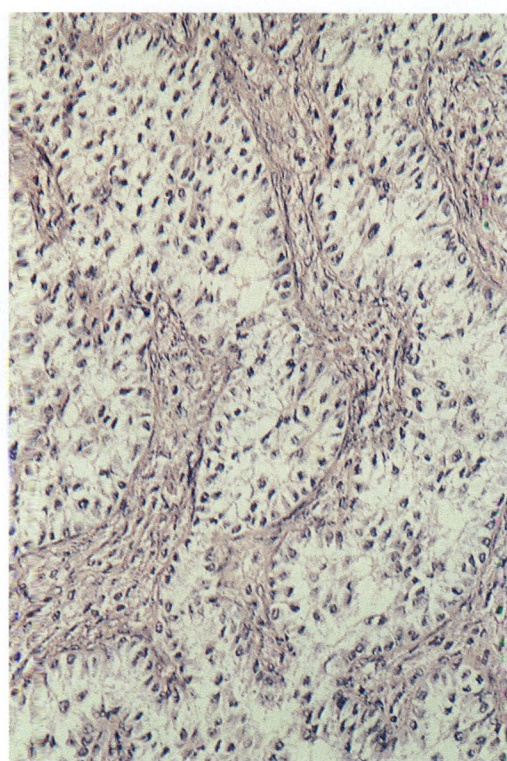

FIG. 84. Lipid-rich Sertoli cell tumor. This neoplasm has a solid tubular architecture and is composed of cells with large amounts of pale cytoplasm.

dometrioid carcinoma and Krukenberg tumor is discussed on pages 2333 and 2377. Ovarian tumors of probable wolffian origin (364) may have prominent solid tubules but almost always have other patterns, including sieve-like areas and solid areas composed of small oval or spindle cells. Rare carcinoid tumors with a solid tubular pattern are distinguished from Sertoli cell tumors by silver staining, immunohistochemical staining for neuroendocrine markers, and electron microscopic features. Sertoli cell tumors are often positive for inhibin, sometimes strongly so, but a few wolffian tumors are weakly positive in focal areas (254).

Sertoli–Leydig Cell Tumors

SLCTs account for less than 0.2% of ovarian neoplasms (365–377). Their peak occurrence is during the early reproductive years—the average age of patients is 25 years (367). Approximately half the patients show initial signs of hirsutism or virilization, but occasionally there are estrogenic manifestations. Patients without endocrine manifestations have symptoms attributable to a pelvic or abdominal mass. A few tumors have been associated with elevated serum AFP levels (369,377).

Gross Features. The diameter of SLCTs varies greatly, averaging 10 cm. Typically, they form firm, lobulated, yellow or tan, solid masses (Fig. 85) with a smooth external surface. Cysts may be conspicuous—particularly if the tumor contains heterologous elements (374,375) or has a retiform

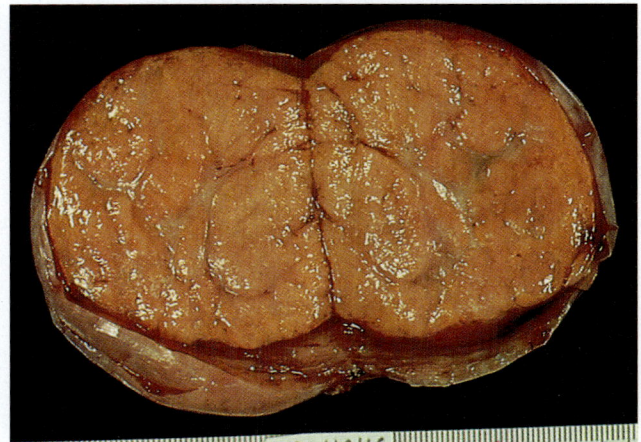

FIG. 85. Sertoli-Leydig cell tumor of intermediate differentiation. The sectioned surfaces of the neoplasm are lobulated and yellow.

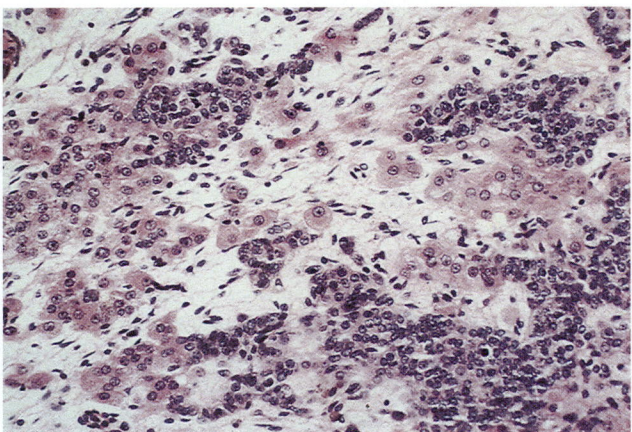

FIG. 86. Sertoli-Leydig cell tumor of intermediate differentiation. Note the clusters of immature Sertoli cells with darkly staining nuclei and islands of pale Leydig cells with abundant cytoplasm and round nuclei containing prominent nucleoli.

component (371–373)—but they are less common than in GCTs. Tumors with a prominent mucinous component may simulate mucinous cystic tumors, and those with a retiform component are often soft, "spongy," or cystic with large, edematous intraluminal polypoid excrescences simulating serous papillary tumors. Areas of hemorrhage and necrosis are uncommon, except in poorly differentiated subtypes. Only 2% of SLCTs are bilateral (367).

Microscopic Features. SLCTs have been divided into five subtypes according to the WHO classification (Table 1). Well-differentiated SLCTs (368) are composed of hollow or solid tubules similar to those in well-differentiated Sertoli cell tumors, but the stroma contains more than a minor component of cells resembling Leydig cells. Crystals of Reinke have been identified within these cells in only a minority of cases. The tubules are usually small and round to oval, but they are sometimes large and of varying shapes. They may be lined by stratified cells and, rarely, resemble the glands of low-grade endometrioid adenocarcinoma (370).

Tumors of intermediate differentiation often have a lobulated appearance on low magnification, with densely cellular areas intersected by hypocellular fibrous or edematous stroma. Within the cellular areas, cords, thick columns, nests, or, uncommonly, solid or hollow tubules are present; they are composed of cells with small, round to oval nuclei and scanty cytoplasm, suggestive of immature Sertoli cells (Figs. 86 and 87). Occasionally, these cells contain abundant pale or vacuolated cytoplasm and, infrequently, the cytoplasm is eosinophilic. The Sertoli cells are separated by varying numbers of Leydig cells and indifferent stromal cells (Figs. 86 and 87). The sex-cord and Leydig cells are often most recognizable at the periphery of the cellular lobules and near the margin of the tumor as a whole. Some tumors of intermediate differentiation contain areas composed of small spindle-shaped cells with appreciable mitotic activity. Cysts of different sizes, sometimes containing a eosinophilic secretion, may also be present and may resemble thyroid follicles. Some SLCTs have a diffuse rather than a lobular architecture. In isolated instances, SLCTs contain cells with bizarre nuclei (328). Tumors in pregnant patients in the third trimester typically show edema and large sheets of Leydig cells (334).

Poorly differentiated SLCTs are characterized by a diffuse growth of cells that are highly active mitotically and usually spindle shaped, suggesting fibrosarcoma. Less often, the cells are rounded and simulate those of undifferentiated carcinoma. Tubules and sex cord–like formations as well as Leydig cells, or the presence of more distinctive focal pat-

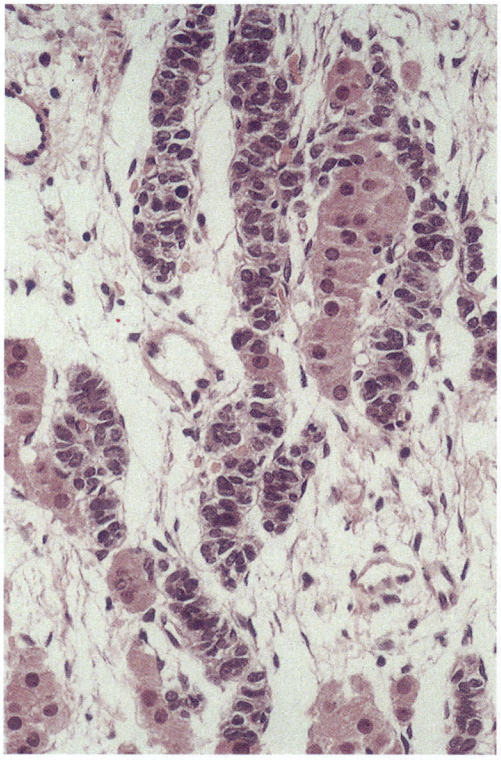

FIG. 87. Sertoli-Leydig cell tumor of intermediate differentiation. Cords of immature Sertoli cells reminiscent of the sex cords of the developing testis and clumps of larger Leydig cells are visible.

terns of Sertoli–Leydig cell neoplasia, which may be minor in extent, are necessary to establish the diagnosis.

Patterns simulating that of the rete testis and characterizing retiform tumors are found in approximately 10% of SLCTs (371–373). These tumors are seen typically in children and young women, who are 10 years younger on average than patients with other types of SLCT. The growth patterns include cysts with papillae containing fibrous cores, networks of slit-like tubules, larger tubules, and broad, elongated bands of epithelial cells. The tubules are commonly lined by one or several layers of cells with round, usually regular nuclei and scanty cytoplasm. The cores of the papillae may be small and hyalinized or large and edematous. The papillae may be simple or have a complex, branching pattern with a lining of stratified atypical cells (Fig 88); glomeruloid structures are often present. The stroma of the tumor varies from densely cellular to hyalinized or edematous. Only about 10% of these tumors are purely retiform; most of them also exhibit other patterns of SLCT.

Heterologous elements are found in about 20% of SLCTs and have been encountered only in tumors of intermediate or poor differentiation and in retiform tumors (374–377). The most common component, present in almost 90% of cases, is mucinous epithelium of gastrointestinal type (Fig. 89). It contains goblet cells in more than half the cases, argentaffin cells in one-third, and argyrophil cells in virtually all. The mucinous epithelium is usually benign, but occasionally it indicates borderline or low-grade carcinoma. In some of the tumors containing argentaffin cells, microscopic areas of carcinoid are also present (374,375). Approximately one-fourth of heterologous tumors have foci of immature skeletal muscle, cartilage, or both (376). Mesenchymal heterologous elements are usually found in tumors that have a sarcomatoid background. Very rarely, cells resembling hepatocytes or neuroectodermal elements are present (377).

Differential Diagnosis. SLCTs are difficult to distinguish from GCTs on gross inspection, except that they almost never form unilocular thin-walled cysts, rarely form multilocular thin-walled cysts, and occasionally contain a muci-

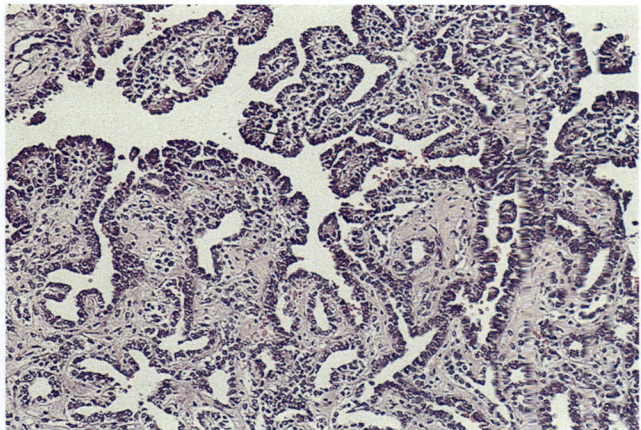

FIG. 88. Retiform Sertoli-Leydig cell tumor. Elongated tubules, papillae, and cellular stratification impart a resemblance to a malignant common epithelial neoplasm.

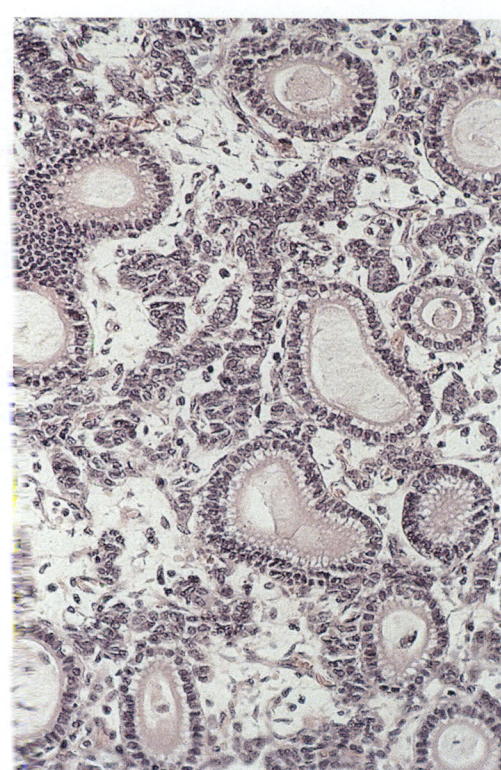

FIG. 89. Sertoli-Leydig cell tumor with heterologous elements. Mucinous glands are separated by cords and clusters of Sertoli cells.

nous cystic component. At the microscopic level, typical GCTs and SLCTs differ considerably, but characteristic features of one tumor type are often present as minor foci in the other type. The prominent tubules and discrete clusters of Leydig cells in well-differentiated SLCTs readily distinguish them from GCTs, although rare GCTs contain small numbers of well-formed tubules and, in exceptional cases, Leydig cells with crystals of Reinke (40). Similarly, isolated SCLTs contain minor aggregates of granulosa cells. The cells of GCTs are more mature in appearance than those of most SLCTs, and although nuclear grooves may be seen in Sertoli cells, they are seldom as conspicuous as they often are in GCTs. The stromal component of SLCT frequently has a sarcomatous appearance, which is rare in the stromal component of GCTs. Heterologous elements are almost diagnostic of SLCT, and a retiform pattern is not seen in GCT. A thecomatoid stroma is only infrequently present in SLCTs. Finally, the Leydig cells of SLCTs tend to cluster in small groups, whereas in GCTs, luteinized theca cells are usually not prominent and cluster much less often.

The retiform variant of SLCT may be misdiagnosed as yolk sac tumor because of the young age of the patient, but the two tumors have little in common in terms of microscopic characteristics. Pure or almost pure retiform tumors, however, may closely resemble surface epithelial tumors and have occasionally been reported as such. The papillae of retiform SLCT can simulate closely those of the serous borderline tumor and, if nuclear stratification is pronounced and glands and solid epithelial foci are present in the stroma, can simulate serous or endometrioid carcinoma. Juxtaposition of epithelium and cellular stroma in retiform SLCTs has also suggested MMMT. Confusion with the very rare primary ovarian Wilms' tumor (378) is also possible. Clinical and pathologic features, including the young age of the patient, androgenic manifestations in 20% of the cases, and the consistent finding of more typical patterns of SLCT provide clues to the diagnosis of retiform SLCT. Inhibin positivity can be very helpful in difficult cases (247–254).

Nonretiform SLCTs in a few instances are misinterpreted as primitive germ cell tumors, particularly during pregnancy, when the stromal edema may impart a loose, reticular appearance similar to that of YST. The nuclei of SLCTs are not as primitive, however, as those of YST, and the usual presence of Sertoliform tubules and the lack of staining for AFP exclude the latter diagnosis.

Heterologous SLCTs are most often misdiagnosed as teratomas but, in contrast to the latter tumors, almost never contain neuroectodermal tissue. Common constituents of teratomas, such as squamous epithelium and skin appendages, have not been reported in SLCTs. Heterologous SLCTs containing glands and cysts lined by gastrointestinal-type epithelium may be confused on gross examination with pure mucinous cystic tumors of the ovary. Although a history of virilization is much more suggestive of SLCT, mucinous tumors that stimulate the development of luteinized stromal cells may also be masculinizing. The diagnosis of heterologous SLCT rests on finding a Sertoli–Leydig cell component, which is usually of intermediate differentiation, between the glands and cysts or at the periphery of the tumor.

Since the carcinoid components of SLCTs are usually of microscopic size, it is not likely that SLCTs will be confused with carcinoid tumors of other origins. Heterologous tumors with mesenchymal elements may be mistaken for ovarian sarcomas when there are few recognizable Sertoli–Leydig cells. Before a pure ovarian sarcoma is diagnosed in a young woman with signs of virilization, heterologous SLCT should be excluded by adequate sampling. Criteria for the differentiation of SLCTs from endometrioid carcinomas, tubular Krukenberg tumors, and carcinoids are discussed under those headings.

Gynandroblastoma

Tumors interpreted as containing Sertoli–stromal cell and granulosa–stromal cell elements in varying proportions have been reported as gynandroblastoma. Because minor components of one tumor frequently occur in an otherwise typical tumor of the other type, the diagnosis of gynandroblastoma should be reserved for neoplasms containing at least 10% of the second tumor type, and both components should be well differentiated to avoid a lack of reproducibility of diagnosis. If this strict definition is used, the gynandroblastoma is exceedingly rare (379,380). When less well differentiated components—such as JGCT and SLCT of intermediate differentiation—co-exist (381), the pathologist's report is more meaningful clinically if the specific designation of each component is included in the diagnostic term.

Unclassified Sex Cord–Stromal Tumors

Approximately 5% to 10% of sex cord–stromal tumors have patterns and cell types intermediate between those of SLCTs and GCTs or unusual patterns that do not permit reproducible placement in either category (382). For example, Talerman and associates (383) have described and designated as "diffuse nonlobular androblastoma" those tumors that are characterized by a diffuse fibrothecomatous or granulosa cell–like proliferation, with minor foci of typical Sertoliform tubules in almost all cases. The few tumors of this type that we have seen differed significantly in appearance from the usual SLCT, and it may be preferable to designate such tumors as unclassified sex cord–stromal tumor, GCT with minor foci of tubular differentiation, or fibroma or thecoma with minor sex-cord elements.

Sex cord–stromal tumors from pregnant patients are particularly likely to cause problems in diagnosis. In one study of such cases, 17% were placed in the unclassified category, and others diagnosed as GCT or SLCT had large areas with an indifferent appearance (334). A major feature that led to difficulty in classification was the presence of prominent edema in the tumor, prominent luteinization in GCTs, and extensive Leydig cell maturation in SLCTs during the third trimester of pregnancy.

Sex-cord Tumor with Annular Tubules

One-third of sex-cord tumors with annular tubules (SCTATs) are associated with Peutz-Jeghers syndrome (PJS) [gastrointestinal polyposis, oral and cutaneous melanin pigmentation, and, rarely, adenoma malignum (minimal deviation adenocarcinoma) of the cervix] (384–389) and are benign. In patients with PJS, the tumor has always been an incidental finding at operation or autopsy, whereas in those without the syndrome it has been detected clinically and has pursued a malignant course in approximately one-fourth of cases (385). Estrogenic manifestations, including menstrual disturbances and isosexual precocity, are present in about 40% of patients with SCTAT, with or without PJS. An unusual number of SCTATs in patients without the syndrome have produced progesterone, sometimes associated with decidual changes in the endometrium (387).

Gross Features

The appearance differs, depending on whether the patient has PJS. In those patients with the syndrome, the tumors are typically multifocal, bilateral, focally calcified, and no more than 3 cm in diameter. Tumors from patients without PJS are almost always unilateral; usually large, solid, and yellow; and rarely calcified. Cysts are occasionally present but almost never predominate.

Microscopic Features

SCTATs are characterized by sharply circumscribed, ring-shaped tubules encircling nodules of hyalinized basement membrane–like material (Fig. 90). Simple tubules encircle single hyaline nodules; the more common complex tubules surround several nodules. The lumens of the tubules are filled with pale cytoplasm, and the nuclei are located in an antipodal arrangement along the margins of the hyaline nodules and at the periphery of the simple and complex tubules. In some areas the cells proliferate toward the centers of the tubules. Isolated tubules are elongated, as in typical Sertoli cell tumors. In the tumors associated with PJS, a few nests may be composed of cells containing large, lipid-laden vacuoles; there is often focal calcification of the tubules, which may be extensive.

In large tumors unassociated with PJS, multifocality and calcification are rare; foci of typical GCT (384), solid tubular Sertoli cell tumor, or both may be present. Because bundles of Charcot-Bottcher filaments have been found on ultrastructural examination in a few cases, some investigators regard SCTAT as a type of Sertoli cell tumor (363,386,390). On the other hand, other researchers have considered it a variant of GCT because of a prominent GCT component in some cases (384). Owing to its distinctive clinicopathologic features, it is preferable to consider SCTAT a specific subtype of sex cord–stromal tumor, with a potential for bidirectional differentiation.

Another rare sex cord–stromal tumor has been reported in two girls with PJS and isosexual pseudoprecocity (390). The unusual microscopic features included tubular differentiation, a retiform pattern, and a diffuse proliferation of cells, some of which contained abundant eosinophilic cytoplasm.

Steroid Cell Tumors

The terms lipoid cell tumor and lipid cell tumor had been used for many years to describe neoplasms composed of large, round or polyhedral cells that resemble lutein, Leydig, and adrenocortical cells (391). Although most tumors in this category contain abundant intracellular fat, approximately 25% do not, leading to the paradox of lipid-free so-called lipid cell tumors. To avoid this incongruity, the designation steroid cell tumors has been proposed (40,392). These tumors are divided into three major categories: stromal luteoma (393), Leydig cell tumor (394), and steroid cell tumor not otherwise specified (NOS) (392).

Stromal Luteoma

This designation has been applied to small steroid cell tumors that lie within the ovarian stroma and presumably arise from it. The capacity of ovarian stroma to differentiate into lutein cells is exemplified by the nonneoplastic disorder stromal hyperthecosis, which is present in areas uninvolved by tumor in more than 90% of cases of stromal luteoma (393). Microscopic nodules of lutein cells may develop in stromal hyperthecosis (nodular hyperthecosis), but the term stromal luteoma should be reserved for nodules that are at least 0.5 cm in diameter. Some large steroid cell tumors of the NOS type are undoubtedly of stromal origin, but a specific diagnosis of stromal luteoma cannot be made when the tumor is not confined within the ovarian stroma.

Approximately 20% of steroid cell tumors belong in the stromal luteoma category (393). These tumors occur over a wide age range, but they are rare in young women and usually develop after the menopause (average age, 58 years). Approximately 60% are estrogenic and 12% androgenic. Underlying stromal hyperthecosis may contribute to the associated endocrine abnormality, which is sometimes longstanding. The tumors are well circumscribed and rarely exceed 3 cm in diameter.

A mass of luteinized cells arranged diffusely or in nests and cords is characteristic. The cytoplasm is typically eosinophilic and contains relatively little lipid. Lipochrome granules are present in more than half the cases. Mitotic figures are uncommon. Approximately 20% of stromal luteomas exhibit a degenerative change seen only rarely in other steroid cell tumors, characterized by irregular spaces that may simulate glands or vessels (Fig. 91). The stroma is typically sparse, but in about 20% of cases it is focally fibrotic and hyalinized (393).

Leydig Cell Tumors

The Leydig cell nature of a steroid cell tumor can be confirmed only by the identification of cytoplasmic Reinke crystals on light or electron microscopy (394). Because only 35% to 40% of testicular Leydig cell tumors are found to contain these crystals on light microscopic examination, however, some ovarian steroid cell tumors of the NOS type are most probably Leydig cell tumors lacking crystals. Leydig cell tumors identifiable as such account for approximately 15% of steroid cell tumors.

These tumors can originate in the hilus or within the ovar-

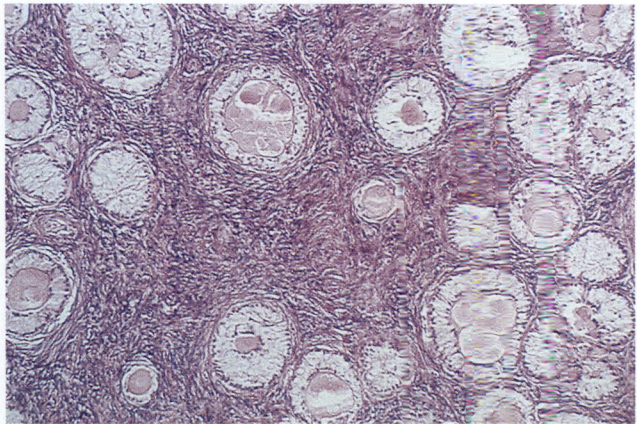

FIG. 90. Sex-cord tumor with annular tubules from a patient with Peutz-Jeghers syndrome. Simple and complex annular tubules encircle hyaline masses.

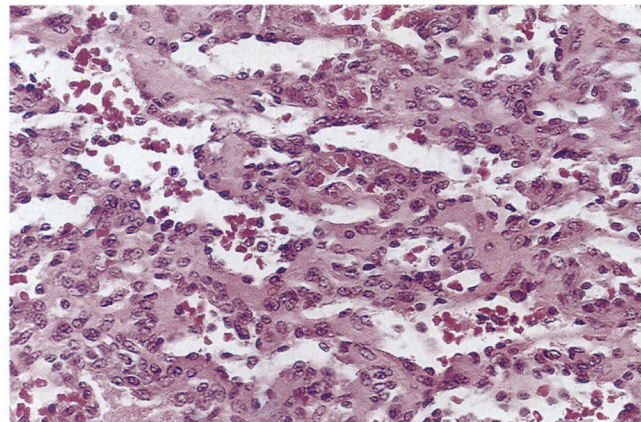

FIG. 91. Stromal luteoma. Degenerative changes have produced irregular spaces.

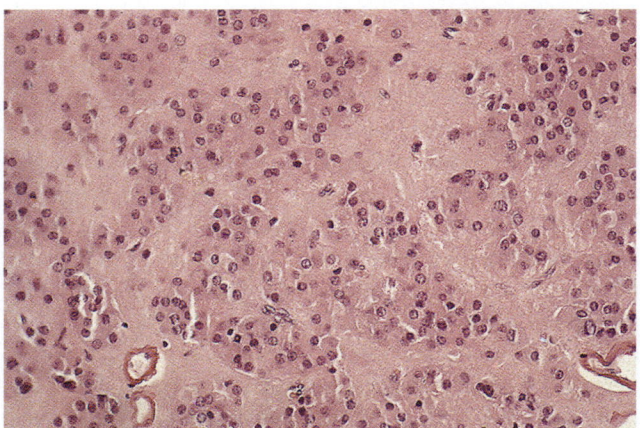

FIG. 92. Leydig cell tumor. The nuclei are aggregated, resulting in the presence of acellular eosinophilic zones.

ian stroma (Leydig cell tumor, nonhilar type) (83). Hilus cell tumors, which are more common, arise from normal hilus cells that are usually located in the hilus adjacent to nonmedullated nerve fibers. These cells have been found in 80% to 85% of normal ovaries. Only four Leydig cell tumors evolving from ovarian stromal cells have been reported (83). An ovarian stromal cell derivation for these tumors is tenable, because they lie within the ovarian stroma and because intracytoplasmic crystals of Reinke can be found in isolated instances in the steroid cells of what appear to be otherwise typical stromal hyperthecosis. In some cases, a Leydig cell tumor straddles the hilus and the medullary stroma, making it impossible to determine whether the tumor is of hilar or stromal origin. Hilus cell tumors have been diagnosed at an average age of 58 years; they cause hirsutism or virilization in 80% of patients (394). The androgenic manifestations are often milder and of longer duration than those associated with SLCTs, but they may be abrupt. Occasionally, there are estrogenic manifestations.

Gross Features

Hilus cell tumors range from 1 to 15 cm in diameter; the great majority are less than 5 cm in diameter. Almost all are unilateral. They are well circumscribed, fleshy, and brown, black, orange-red, or yellow; hemorrhagic mottling is common.

Microscopic Features

Sheets, cords, or nests of uniform rounded or polyhedral cells with large, central nuclei containing one or more prominent nucleoli are characteristic. In some areas there may be a nucleus-free perivascular zone (Fig. 92). The cytoplasm is eosinophilic and finely granular, although small cytoplasmic lipid vacuoles may be present. Lipochrome pigment is seen in varying numbers of tumor cells. Reinke crystals (Fig. 93) are present by definition, but their detection may require prolonged search. Fibrinoid degeneration of large blood vessel walls is a typical and seemingly distinctive feature. Like stromal luteomas, these tumors occasionally contain degenerative spaces that simulate blood vessels. Except for their location, the pathologic features of Leydig cell tumors of the nonhilar type are similar to those of hilus cell tumors. The almost certain diagnosis of hilus cell tumor can be made if a steroid cell tumor lacking Reinke crystals has more than one of the following features: a hilar location, a background of hilus cell hyperplasia, a close association with nonmedullated nerve fibers, a uniform nucleus-free zone around blood vessels, and fibrinoid degeneration of the vessels within the tumor.

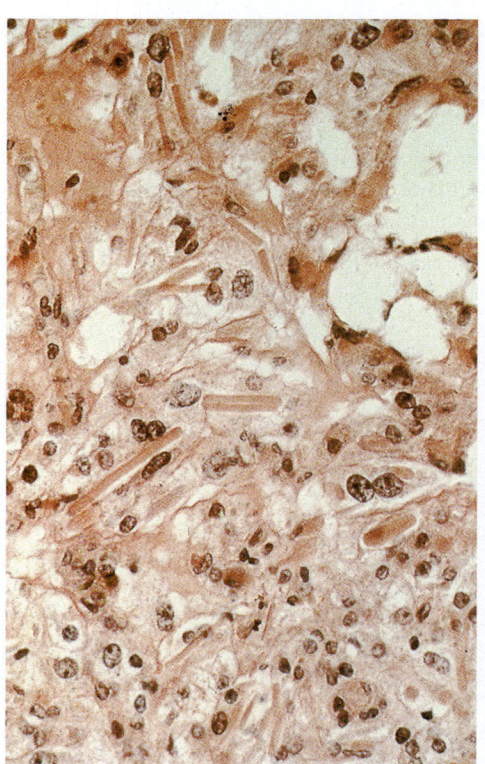

FIG. 93. Crystals of Reinke in Leydig cell tumor.

Steroid Cell Tumor, Not Otherwise Specified

Steroid cell tumors that cannot be diagnosed as stromal luteoma or Leydig cell tumor are the most common subtype, accounting for 56% of the cases in one series (392). These tumors occur at any age, with an average age of 43 years. They are most often associated with virilization (41%), but occasionally they are estrogenic or unassociated with endocrine manifestations. Rare examples in children have produced isosexual pseudoprecocity, and several tumors have resulted in Cushing's syndrome (395). The tumors are almost always unilateral and usually found at stage I.

Gross Features

On examination well-circumscribed masses that range up to 45 cm in diameter but are usually from 3–10 cm are typically evident (392). Most are yellow (Fig. 94) or orange due to abundant intracytoplasmic lipid, but they may be red to brown if they are lipid-poor or dark brown to black if they contain abundant lipochrome pigment. Necrosis, hemorrhage, and cystic degeneration are now and then observed.

Microscopic Features

Cells are arranged diffusely, in nests, or in columns separated by a rich vascular network. A minor fibromatous component and areas of hyalinization are rare. The more common type of tumor cell is polygonal and of medium to large size, with slightly granular, eosinophilic cytoplasm. A second cell type is larger with abundant spongy cytoplasm; transitions between the two cell types are usual (Fig. 95). Both cells have distinct cell membranes and central nuclei with a prominent nucleolus. Intracytoplasmic lipochrome pigment is present in about one-third of the cases (347). Nuclear atypia is generally slight or absent, but it is moderate or marked in approximately 25% of cases. The mitotic rate varies and does not clearly correlate with nuclear atypia.

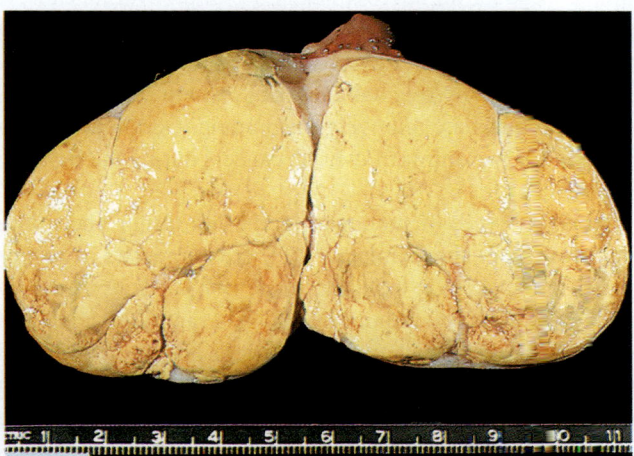

FIG. 94. Steroid cell tumor, not otherwise specified. The neoplasm has a lobulated, yellow sectioned surface. (From ref. 347.)

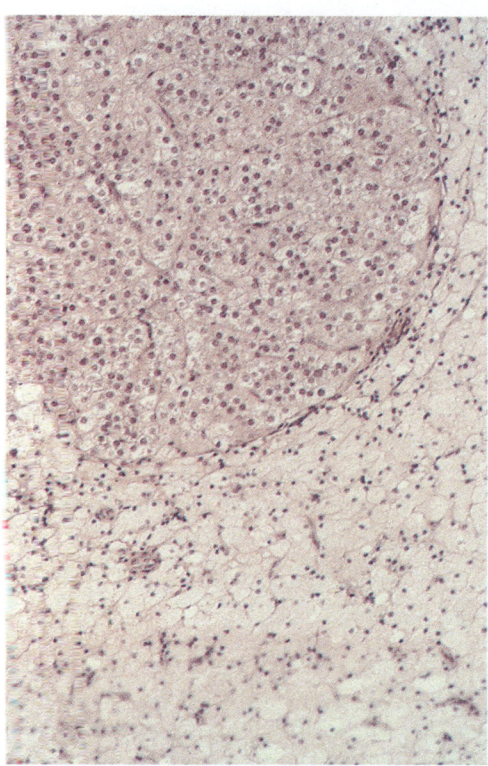

FIG. 95. Steroid cell tumor. Some of the cells have abundant dense eosinophilic cytoplasm whereas others have pale vacuolated cytoplasm.

Approximately 40% of the tumors in this category show clinical signs of malignancy (392). Although the only absolute evidence of malignancy is metastasis, a variety of clinicopathologic features correlate with malignant behavior. In one study (392), the malignant tumors occurred in patients who were on average 16 years older than those with a favorable outcome. Approximately 78% of tumors more than 7 cm in diameter were malignant, whereas smaller tumors were invariably benign (392). Approximately two-thirds of tumors with severe nuclear atypia and 80% of those with two or more mitotic figures per 10 hpf had a malignant course (392).

Differential Diagnosis

Steroid cell tumors may be confused with other neoplasms, including extensively luteinized GCT and thecoma, clear-cell carcinoma, metastatic renal cell carcinoma, and lipid-rich Sertoli cell tumor. Rare extensively luteinized GCTs and thecomas can be identified by the additional presence of nonluteinized GCT in the former and the finding of more than a minor fibrothecomatous area with abundant reticulin in the latter. Clear-cell carcinoma and metastatic renal cell carcinoma generally have glycogen-rich cytoplasm and eccentric nuclei, in contrast to the characteristic lipid-filled cytoplasm and central nuclei of lipid-rich steroid cell tumors. Oxyphilic clear-cell carcinomas exhibit, at least in focal areas, patterns characteristic of typical clear-cell carcinoma. Differentiating a lipid-rich Sertoli cell tumor with a diffuse pattern from a steroid cell tumor depends mostly on identifying areas with a tubular pattern in the former.

Pregnancy luteomas may be difficult to distinguish from lipid-free or lipid-poor steroid cell tumors developing during pregnancy. Both lesions can lead to virilization. Unlike steroid cell tumors, however, approximately one-third of pregnancy luteomas are bilateral, and one-half are multiple. The pregnancy luteoma also may contain numerous mitotic figures; in contrast, steroid cell tumors with no cytologic atypia or minimal degrees of it usually contain only rare mitotic figures. Although it may be impossible to make a certain diagnosis when a solitary nodular mass of lipid-poor steroid cells is encountered during the third trimester of pregnancy, it is presumed to be a pregnancy luteoma unless clear-cut evidence indicates otherwise.

Tumors of the Rete Ovarii

These lesions are uncommon; most of them are cystadenomas or papillary cystadenomas (396,397). Rete cystadenomas are found most often in postmenopausal women, who have nonspecific androgenic or estrogenic manifestations (99,397). Other rete tumors include small adenomas and rare carcinomas (396).

Gross Features

The cysts range up to 24 cm (average, 8.7 cm) in diameter, have a hilar location, and are either unilocular or multilocular. They typically contain clear or yellow fluid and have thin walls with smooth linings. Adenomas have usually been incidental microscopic findings, and the only rete carcinoma reported had nonspecific gross features.

Microscopic Features

The walls of rete cystadenomas are composed of fibrovascular tissue, which frequently contains fascicles of smooth muscle. The luminal surfaces characteristically have thin, shallow crevices and are lined by columnar, cuboidal, or flat cells that are only rarely ciliated (Fig. 96). Hyperplasia of hilus cells, frequently seen in the cyst wall, accounts for the virilization that is occasionally associated with these lesions. Intracystic papillae may be prominent (397). Adenomas are composed of closely packed small tubules within the ovarian hilus, some of which may be dilated and contain simple papillae. A single rete adenocarcinoma was characterized by an irregular network of branching tubules and cysts that contained papillae with fibrovascular or hyalinized cores. The tubules, cysts, and papillae were lined by obviously malignant, nonciliated cuboidal cells. There were also areas of solid growth and extensive transitional cell metaplasia.

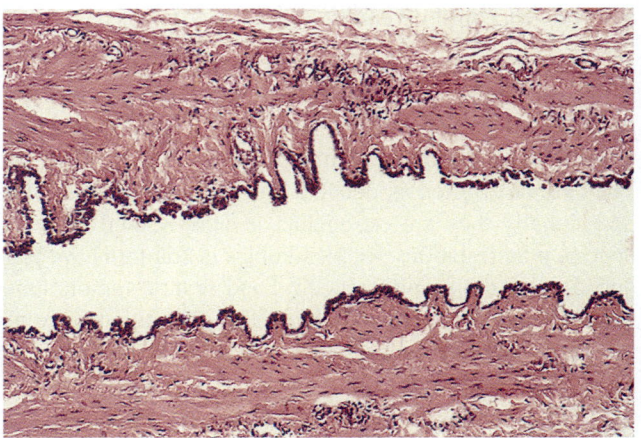

FIG. 96. Rete cyst. Note the columnar epithelial lining, the formation of crevices, and the layer of smooth muscle subjacent to the epithelium.

Differential Diagnosis

Rete cystadenomas are often misdiagnosed as serous cystadenomas; this differential diagnosis has been discussed on page 2327. Rete adenomas may be confused with female adnexal tumors of probable wolffian origin, but the latter tumors typically have patterns other than tubular or papillary that are incompatible with the diagnosis of rete tumor. The rete carcinoma (396) is distinguished from pure retiform SLCT primarily by its focal solid pattern and transitional cell metaplasia; the latter feature has been not seen in SLCTs of any type. This unique tumor also occurred in an elderly woman.

Germ Cell Tumors

Germ cell tumors account for approximately 30% of all ovarian tumors (40). Ninety-five percent of germ cell tumors are dermoid cysts (mature cystic teratomas), and most of the remainder are malignant. Dermoid cysts account for one-third of benign ovarian neoplasms, and malignant germ cell tumors account for approximately 3% of all ovarian cancers in Western countries. The rate of malignant germ cell tumors, however, is as high as 15% in countries whose populations are largely oriental and black, where surface epithelial carcinomas are relatively uncommon. Germ cell tumors account for two-thirds of ovarian cancers during the first two decades of life.

Most subtypes of malignant germ cell tumor occur in a pure form, but approximately 10% are composed of two or more subtypes. It is essential, therefore, to examine every malignant germ cell tumor carefully and sample all areas that differ in gross appearance. If the tumor proves to be mixed on microscopic examination, the relative amounts of each component should be recorded in the diagnosis. The more common category of malignant germ cell tumors comprises those with primitive or immature elements; less common are malignant tumors of the adult type, which almost always develop in dermoid cysts and are usually encountered in older women.

Dysgerminoma

Clinical Features

Dysgerminomas are the most common of the primitive germ cell tumors; they account for nearly half of such tumors, for 1% of all ovarian cancers, and for 5% to 10% of ovarian cancers in the first two decades of life (40,398–401). Eighty percent of dysgerminomas develop in women younger than 30 years of age (mean, 21 years); they are extremely rare over the age of 50 years and under the age of 5 years. Most patients have signs or symptoms related to an abdominal mass. In patients with associated gonadoblastoma, an underlying abnormality in gonadal development may dominate the clinical picture. Rare patients with dysgerminomas that elaborate hCG may experience hormonal manifestations, which are typically estrogenic (isosexual precocity, menstrual irregularities) but occasionally androgenic (402); the clinical picture can mimic that of an ectopic or intrauterine pregnancy or a hydatidiform mole (403,404).

About 65% of dysgerminomas are found at stage Ia; at higher stages, the contralateral ovary, pelvic and paraaortic lymph nodes, and/or the peritoneum are typically involved. The 5-year survival rate approaches 100% for stage I tumors. Because of the sensitivity of dysgerminomas to chemotherapy and radiation therapy, the 5-year survival rate for patients with higher-stage disease or recurrent tumors is currently more than 80%.

Gross Features

Dysgerminomas are generally solid tumors with a median diameter of 15 cm. The serosal surface is smooth or bosselated. The sectioned surfaces are typically soft, fleshy, lobulated, and cream-colored, gray, pink, or tan (Fig. 97). Areas of cystic degeneration, necrosis, and hemorrhage are occasionally present and should be sampled to exclude other types of malignant germ cell tumor, which may require different therapy. Calcification suggests the possibility of an underlying gonadoblastoma. The tumor is grossly bilateral in about 10% of the cases; in another 10%, microscopic foci of tumor are present in a grossly negative contralateral ovary.

Microscopic Features

Cells resembling primordial germ cells are arranged predominantly in diffuse, insular, or trabecular patterns (Fig. 98). The uniform, rounded tumor cells have clear to eosinophilic cytoplasm, which is almost always glycogen-rich, discrete cell membranes, and a central, large, rounded or flattened nucleus (Fig. 98), which contains one or a few prominent nucleoli. Mitotic figures are usually numerous.

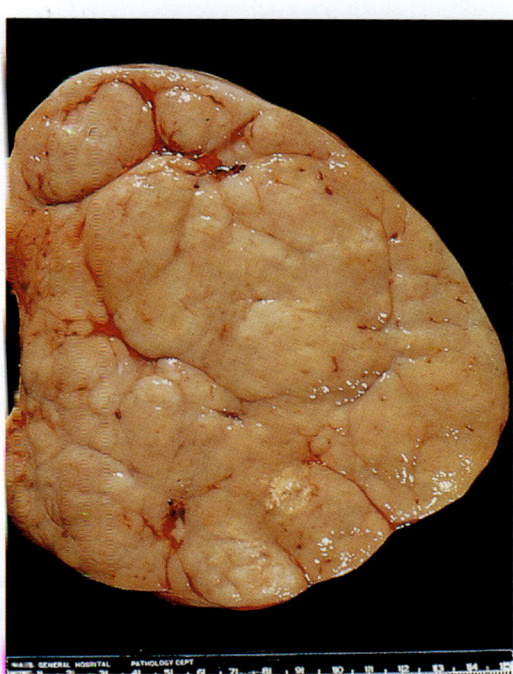

FIG. 97. Dysgerminoma. The neoplasm has a lobulated tan-white sectioned surface.

The characteristic stroma consists of thin to broad fibrous bands infiltrated by mature lymphocytes, sometimes with lymphoid follicle formation. Sarcoid-like granulomas are present in 20% of cases and now and then are confluent, sometimes almost obscuring the underlying tumor.

About 5% to 10% of dysgerminomas contain syncytiotrophoblastic giant cells (SGCs) (Fig. 99), which are immunoreactive for hCG (402–405). The serum level of hCG is frequently elevated in such cases, and there may be estrogenic or androgenic clinical manifestations (402,403). The SGCs may be intimately associated with blood-filled sinusoids, but the characteristic biphasic growth pattern of choriocarcinoma, with accompanying cytotrophoblast, is absent.

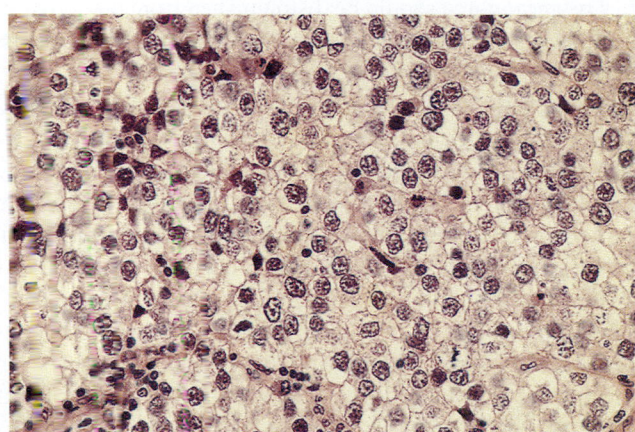

FIG. 98. Dysgerminoma. The tumor cells have clear cytoplasm and predominantly central nuclei with frequent prominent nucleoli. Note the presence of a few lymphocytes.

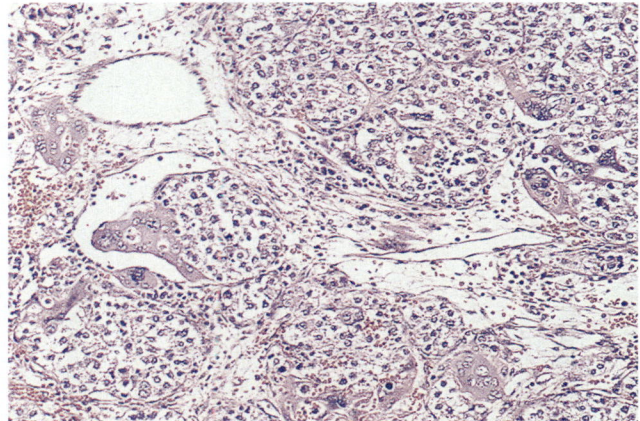

FIG. 99. Dysgerminoma with syncytiotrophoblast cells.

Extensive sampling of apparently pure dysgerminomas producing hCG is important, to exclude foci of choriocarcinoma or embryonal carcinoma. The presence of one or the other of the last two components warrants a diagnosis of mixed germ cell tumor. A few patients with pure dysgerminoma have elevated hCG levels without verifiable SGCs or admixed embryonal carcinoma or choriocarcinoma; in such cases, the dysgerminoma cells may be immunoreactive for hCG (406).

Luteinized stromal cells are occasionally present, within the stroma of the tumor or at its periphery (99,402), especially when the tumor contains syncytiotrophoblast cells; the lutein cells are the probable source of the estrogenic or androgenic manifestations that are present in some patients. Foci of calcification suggest an origin in a partly or completely obliterated gonadoblastoma (page 2371). Extensive sampling may identify residual gonadoblastoma, and the patient's karyotype may reflect an underlying disorder in gonadal development.

Differential Diagnosis

Dysgerminoma should be distinguished from other malignant germ cell tumors with possible diffuse patterns, specifically YST and embryonal carcinoma. Diffuse YST is distinguished by its greater nuclear variation, hyaline bodies, lack of stromal lymphocytes, and the presence of other characteristic patterns as well as immunoreactivity for AFP. The extremely rare pure embryonal carcinoma has nuclei that are larger, more hyperchromatic, and more pleomorphic than those of the dysgerminoma and almost always contains SGCs. The distinction of dysgerminoma from clear-cell carcinoma has been discussed on page 2338. Large-cell lymphomas may simulate dysgerminomas on gross examination and at the microscopic level, and the almost invariable sprinkling of lymphocytes in the stroma of the latter enhances their microscopic similarity. The differing nuclear features, the virtually universal absence of glycogen in lymphomas, and a variety of distinctive immunohistochemical reactions facilitate the differential diagnosis. Other tumors with solid masses of cells, such as GCT and primary or metastatic poorly differentiated carcinomas, differ on histologic inspection from dysgerminomas to the extent that they rarely present a diagnostic problem.

Yolk Sac Tumor

Clinical Features

YSTs (endodermal sinus tumors) account for approximately 20% of primitive germ cell tumors (407–423). They are almost as common as dysgerminomas in women under the age of 20 years. They occur most frequently in childhood and adolescence, at a mean age of 19 years, and are very rare over the age of 40 years. Patients show signs of abdominal pain, often of sudden onset, and a large abdominal or pelvic mass. The serum AFP level is almost always elevated before surgery; measurement of serum AFP is also useful in monitoring therapy.

YST is almost always a rapidly growing, highly malignant neoplasm; there is evidence of extraovarian spread to the peritoneum, retroperitoneal lymph nodes, or both in approximately one-third of patients. Before the use of combination chemotherapy, survival rates were poor. More recently, such treatment has achieved survival rates of more than 80% in patients with stage I disease and approximately 50% in patients with higher-stage tumors.

Gross Features

YSTs are typically large, with a median diameter of 15 cm. The external surface is usually smooth and glistening, although 25% have capsular tears from preoperative or intraoperative rupture (408). The sectioned surfaces are composed of soft, friable, yellow to gray tissue often containing cysts (Fig. 100); very rare tumors are entirely cystic (413). Extensive areas of hemorrhage and necrosis are common. A

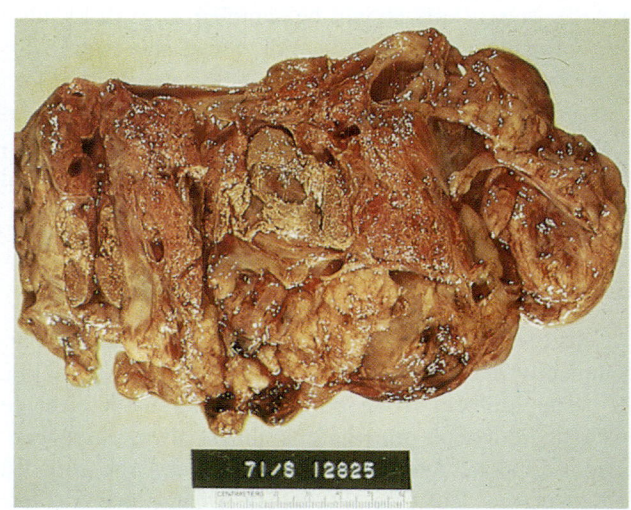

FIG. 100. Yolk sac (endodermal sinus) tumor. The neoplasm is solid and cystic with focal necrosis.

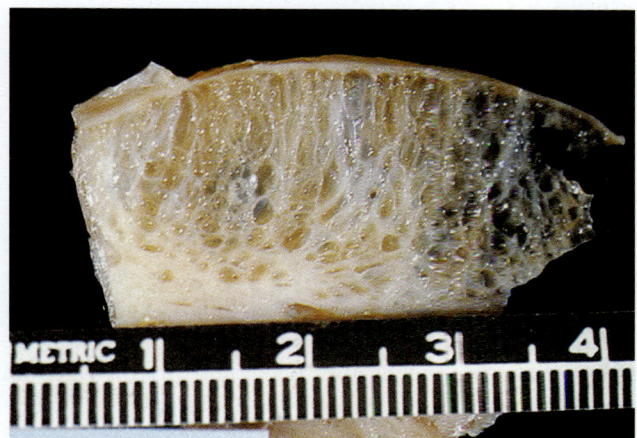

FIG. 101. Yolk sac tumor with polyvesicular vitelline pattern. Numerous small cysts with thin walls are visible.

honeycomb appearance due to the presence of many small cysts may indicate a polyvesicular vitelline variant (Fig. 101). There may be gross evidence of other germ cell components, most often a dermoid cyst. YSTs are virtually never bilateral, although a dermoid cyst is present in the contralateral ovary in approximately 10% of cases.

Microscopic Features

The most common pattern of YST is reticular (Fig. 102), characterized by a loose meshwork of spaces lined by primitive tumor cells with cytoplasm that is clear due to its glycogen and, occasionally, lipid content. The hyperchromatic, irregular, large nuclei contain prominent nucleoli; mitotic figures are numerous. In many tumors, a reticular pattern merges with a microcystic or macrocystic pattern. Schiller-Duval bodies have been reported to be present in up to 75% of the tumors in one series (408), but they are less common in our experience (40). They consist of single papillae that vary from rounded to elongated, with a connective tissue core containing a single central vessel (Fig. 103). These structures are covered by primitive columnar cells and lie in a space lined by cuboidal or flattened cells. Schiller-Duval bodies are usually distributed focally; when they are prominent, they give rise to the so-called endodermal sinus pattern. Eosinophilic, PAS-positive, diastase-resistant hyaline bodies of different sizes are present in most YSTs, most numerous in areas with a reticular or hepatoid pattern.

A variety of less common, but still characteristic patterns occur in YSTs, admixed with the reticular pattern. Rarely, these patterns predominate or occur in a pure form. The polyvesicular vitelline pattern (Fig. 104) is characterized by cysts lined by columnar, cuboidal, or flattened cells separated by a dense, spindle-cell stroma (409). The cysts may exhibit eccentric constrictions, simulating the division of the primary yolk sac vesicle into a large component lined by flat cells that resembles the vestigial portion of the embryonic yolk sac and a smaller component lined by taller epithelium that simulates the forerunner of the primitive gut and its derivatives in the embryo.

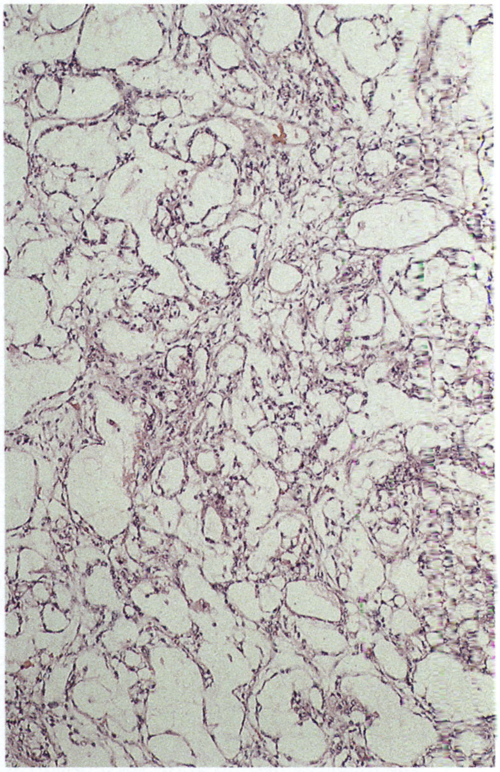

FIG. 102. Yolk sac tumor, reticular pattern.

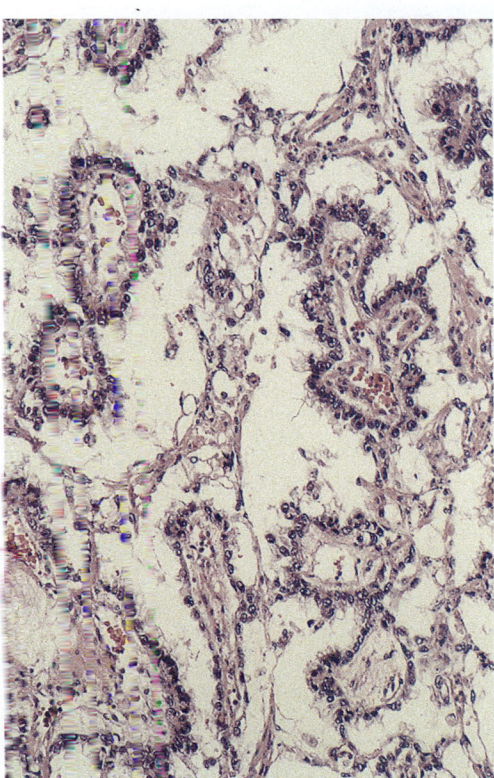

FIG. 103. Yolk sac tumor. Numerous Schiller-Duval bodies are present.

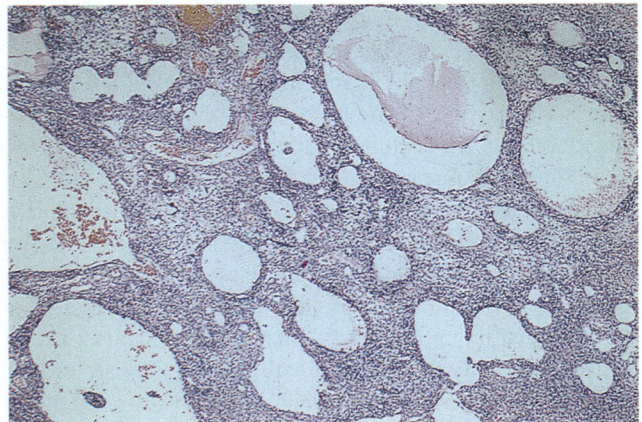

FIG. 104. Yolk sac tumor, polyvesicular vitelline pattern. The vesicles are separated by cellular mesenchyme.

The hepatoid pattern (Fig. 105) resembles hepatocellular carcinoma (279,419,420,422). It is distinguished by large polygonal cells with abundant eosinophilic cytoplasm growing in compact masses separated by thin fibrous bands. In some cases, glandular spaces filled with mucin impart a honeycomb pattern similar to that sometimes seen in hepatocellular carcinomas. In other cases, a glandular pattern predominates, and may be characterized by primitive epithelial cells forming rounded cribriform islands (412,415) or by better differentiated glands resembling those of typical or secretory endometrioid adenocarcinoma (Fig. 106). Tumors of the latter type have been designated endometrioid-like YSTs (413). One such tumor contained foci of carcinoid tumor (421). "Parietal" differentiation is identified by small extracellular accumulations of basement membrane material, typically within reticular areas (422).

Nonspecific patterns in YST include solid, papillary, and adenofibromatous. A mesenchyme-like component, made up of spindle cells with few mitoses in a myxoid, vascular background, may occur in untreated YST, but it is more common and prominent after chemotherapy (414). From time to time, YSTs contain areas of cells with large intracellular vacuoles and eccentric nuclei, creating an appearance resembling liposarcoma. Enteric-type glands are found in up to 50% of YSTs; they are lined by bland mucinous columnar cells, goblet cells, and, infrequently, Paneth cells. Rare YSTs contain small numbers of SGCs. Luteinized stromal cells, granulomatous inflammation, and erythropoietic foci are occasionally found.

Immunohistochemical findings are useful in diagnosing YST, particularly when it has an unusual histologic pattern (405). The tumor is often immunoreactive for AFP, although the staining may be focal. The contents of glands and cysts in YST with polyvesicular vitelline, hepatoid, and endometrioid-like patterns also show positive results for this antigen. Hyaline droplets usually test negative for AFP. The

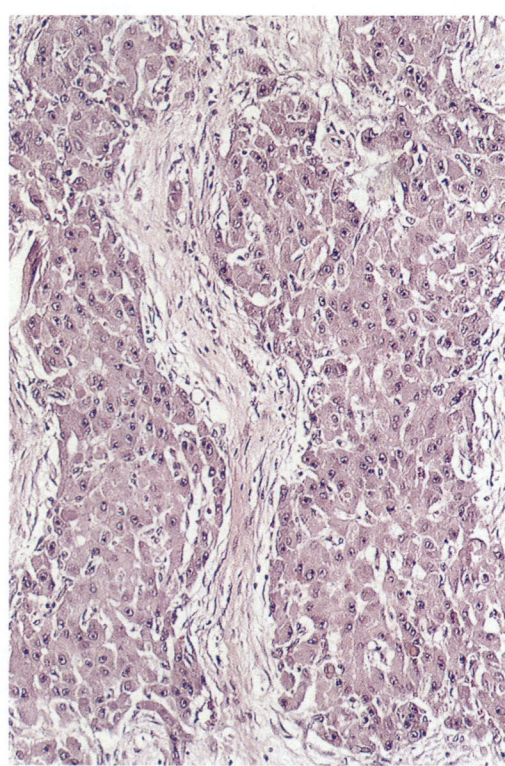

FIG. 105. Yolk sac tumor, hepatoid pattern. Trabeculae of cells with abundant eosinophilic cytoplasm impart a resemblance to hepatocellular carcinoma.

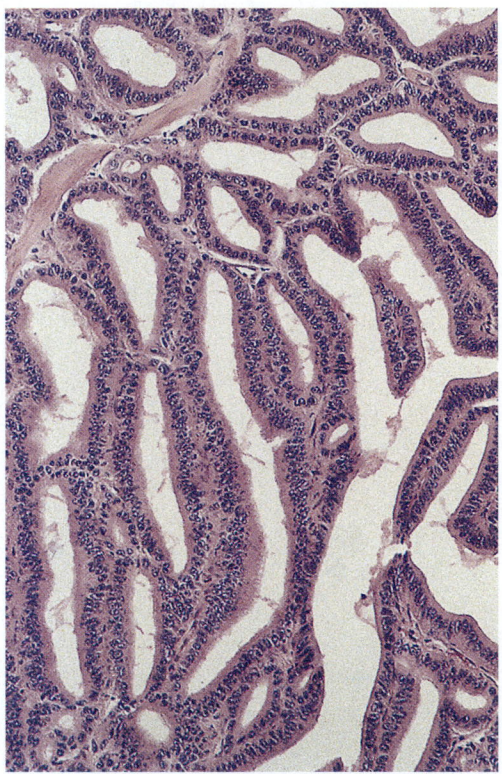

FIG. 106. Yolk sac tumor with glands resembling those of well-differentiated endometrioid carcinoma.

enteric glands and their contents are immunoreactive for carcinoembryonic antigen.

Differential Diagnosis

Clear-cell carcinoma is the tumor most often confused with YST; that differential diagnosis has been discussed on page 2338. The distinctions between endometrioid-like YSTs and endometrioid adenocarcinomas and between hepatoid YSTs and hepatoid carcinomas are discussed under those headings. Endometrioid-like YSTs should be distinguished from the rare YSTs that have been reported in association with endometrioid carcinoma (228,229).

Embryonal Carcinoma

Clinical Features

Embryonal carcinoma is very rare in the ovary, accounting for only about 3% of primitive ovarian germ cell tumors (424–426). Most patients are children or young adults with a median age of 15 years. In more than half the cases, there is isosexual pseudoprecocity, abnormal uterine bleeding, or amenorrhea. Serum hCG and AFP levels are elevated. Laparotomy reveals extraovarian spread in 40% of cases. The 5-year survival for patients with stage I disease in the only reported series was 50%, but long-term survival has been reported with chemotherapy in that series and in subsequent cases (425,426).

Gross Features

The tumors are large, with a median diameter of 17 cm. The external surface may be ruptured. The cut surfaces are predominantly solid and variegated, with white, tan-gray, and yellow soft tissue alternating with cysts containing mucoid material. Hemorrhage and necrosis are common.

Microscopic Features

The tumors are characterized by solid masses, glands, and papillae composed of or lined by large cells with amphophilic or vacuolated cytoplasm, well-defined cell membranes, and round, vesicular, often pleomorphic overlapping nuclei containing one or more prominent nucleoli. Mitotic figures are numerous. Isolated SGCs are almost always present. Some tumor cells are immunoreactive for AFP; whether such cells are AFP-reactive embryonal carcinoma cells or reflect yolk sac differentiation is the subject of controversy. Both SGCs and mononucleated cells can be positive for hCG. Enteric glands and minor foci of mature teratoma may be encountered.

Differential Diagnosis

The differences between embryonal carcinoma and dysgerminoma have been discussed on page 2350. Differentiating embryonal carcinoma from YST is based primarily on the absence of the characteristic patterns of the latter tumor. Although pure embryonal carcinoma typically contains isolated SGCs, it lacks the biphasic pattern of choriocarcinoma.

Polyembryoma

This very rare primitive germ cell tumor is characterized by a preponderance of embryoid bodies (Fig. 107), mimicking normal early embryos (428–432). Nakashima et al. (430) have pointed out that teratomatous differentiation is almost always of the endodermal type. Hepatoid differentiation was present in one case (429). Because these tumors contain trophoblast, they may be associated with high levels of hCG and related endocrine manifestations. The serum AFP level may also be elevated (428,432).

Choriocarcinoma

Ovarian choriocarcinomas account for less than 1% of primitive ovarian germ cell tumors (433,434). Choriocarcinomas that appear before puberty or that are associated with other germ cell tumor components are clearly of germ cell origin. Such tumors are found in patients under the age of 20 years, with symptoms of abdominal enlargement and pain. The serum level of hCG is elevated, leading to isosexual pseudoprecocity as well as menstrual abnormalities or androgenic changes in older patients. Most of the tumors have been fatal, although an improved prognosis has been reported with aggressive chemotherapy (434).

Pure choriocarcinomas are typically solid, hemorrhagic, and friable. On microscopic inspection, there is a biphasic pattern consisting of an intimate mixture of cytotrophoblast and syncytiotrophoblast, accompanied by hemorrhage. In certain areas, however, the tumor may have a nonspecific appearance. The syncytiotrophoblast is intensely immunoreactive for hCG. Choriocarcinoma should be distinguished from germ cell tumors containing isolated syncytiotrophoblastic

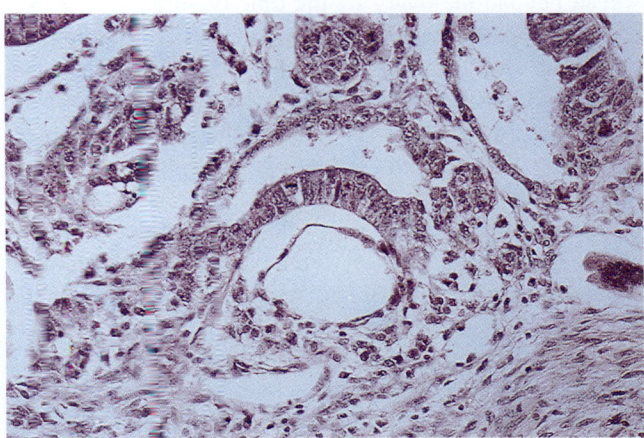

FIG. 107. Polyembryoma. The embryoid body in the center consists of a thick germ disc above which lies an amniotic cavity and below which lies a yolk sac cavity.

cells, such as embryonal carcinoma, dysgerminoma, and YST. In addition, germ cell–derived choriocarcinomas should be differentiated from primary or metastatic gestational choriocarcinomas and from the rare poorly differentiated carcinomas in older women that contain foci suggestive of or indistinguishable from choriocarcinoma and that secrete hCG (314,435).

Teratomas

The great majority of all teratomas are composed of tissues representing at least two, but usually all three embryonic layers (40). If the neoplastic tissue is uniformly mature, the tumor is termed mature teratoma (almost always a dermoid cyst); the presence of any immature tissue—with one rare exception (page 2366)—warrants a designation of immature teratoma. Occasionally, a teratoma has a large component of a single endodermal or ectodermal type of tissue or is composed exclusively of such tissue. Tumors of this type are referred to as monodermal teratomas.

Immature Teratomas

Clinical Features. Immature teratomas are the third most common of the primitive germ cell tumors, accounting for almost 20% of all cases, 1% of ovarian cancers in general, and 10% to 20% of cases encountered in the first two decades of life (436–452). They are most often found in young adults and children, at a median age of 18 years, who typically have a palpable abdominal or pelvic mass that is frequently accompanied by pain (437). Rarely, immature teratomas are found in patients who have had an ipsilateral dermoid cyst removed months to years earlier (441,446). The risk of subsequent immature teratoma developing in such patients may be slightly increased, particularly if the cyst is bilateral or has ruptured or when there are several cysts (441). Isolated patients with immature teratoma have elevated serum AFP or hCG levels (439,440).

Approximately one-third of immature teratomas have spread beyond the ovary by the time of surgery. The incidence of spread increases with higher grades of tumor. Extraovarian spread usually takes the form of peritoneal implants and less often lymphatic or hematogenous metastases. Before the use of combination chemotherapy, survival rates in patients with high-grade tumors, particularly those with high-grade implants, were poor. In contrast, 90% to 100% of patients in two recent studies who underwent combination chemotherapy, and most of whom had grade 2 or 3 tumors, achieved sustained remission (438,442). After chemotherapy, high-grade implants typically are replaced by mature tissue, necrotic tumor, fibrous tissue, or combinations of these types of tissue. Once in a while, mature tissue continues to grow (growing teratoma syndrome) requiring a second operation (447). Patients with exclusively mature peritoneal implants, which are composed of glia, almost always have a benign clinical course, even in the absence of postoperative treatment (436,449). In three cases, however, tumor resembling glioblastoma multiforme arose from peritoneal gliomatosis (452).

Gross Features. The tumors are usually large, with a median diameter of 18 cm, and form encapsulated masses with smooth, glistening outer surfaces. The tumor is ruptured in almost half the cases. The cut surfaces are predominantly solid in the great majority of cases, but small cysts containing mucinous, serous, or bloody fluid or hair are frequently present (Fig. 108). Dermoid cysts can be identified in approximately 25% of cases (441). The solid areas, which are usually composed of neural tissue, are typically soft, fleshy, and gray to pink, with focal hemorrhage and necrosis. Areas of bone and cartilage may be visible or palpable. Bilateral involvement is very rare in the absence of extraovarian spread, but the opposite ovary harbors a dermoid cyst or, less often, another benign tumor in approximately 10% of cases (441).

Microscopic Features. The immature, embryonic-type tissue varies from small foci to a predominant component and is composed primarily of neuroectodermal elements (Figs. 109 and 110). These elements consist of neuroepithelial rosettes and tubules, cellular foci of mitotically active glia, and, occasionally, small areas resembling glioblastoma multiforme or neuroblastoma. Immature or embryonal epithelium of various ectodermal and endodermal types, as well as immature cartilage and skeletal muscle, are frequently encountered. Uncommon findings include isolated SGCs, a few foci of endodermal elements (yolk sac tissue, enteric glands, hepatic tissue), and immature renal tissue.

Immature teratomas have been graded from 1 to 3 based on the amount of immature, almost always neural tissue (437). Grade 1 tumors have rare foci of embryonal neural tissue occupying less than 1 low-power (×40) field (lpf) in any slide, grade 2 tumors contain moderate quantities of embryonal neural tissue, occupying more than 1 but fewer than 4 lpfs in any slide, grade 3 tumors contain large quantities of embryonal neural tissue occupying 4 or more lpfs in any slide. A similar grading system can be applied to peritoneal

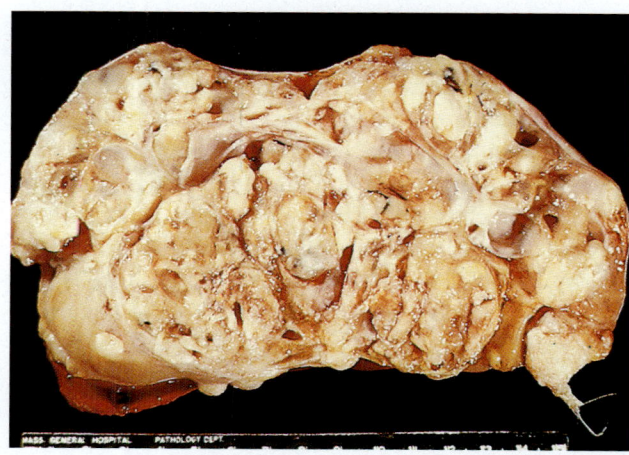

FIG. 108. Immature teratoma. The neoplasm has a solid and cystic sectioned surface.

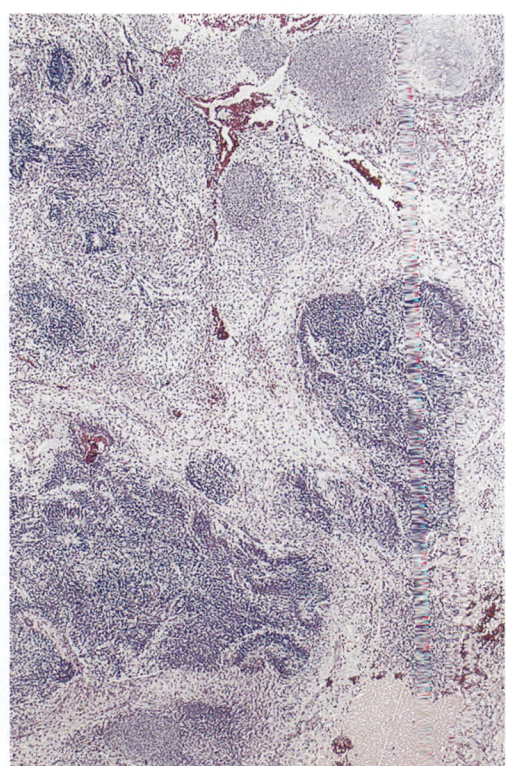

FIG. 109. Immature teratoma with immature neural tissue and nodules of cartilage.

implants. Immature teratomas or mature solid teratomas are sometimes associated with implants composed entirely of mature glial tissue, so-called peritoneal gliomatosis (Fig. 111) (436,444); occasionally, mature elements of other types are also present. These implants sometimes lie adjacent to foci of endometriosis (449,450). Pelvic and paraaortic lymph nodes rarely contain similar mature tissue (439,445).

Differential Diagnosis. The distinction between immature teratomas and mature solid teratomas is based on the identification of foci of immaturity, which may be minor in extent. Predominantly solid teratomas should, therefore, be carefully sampled to exclude such foci. Differentiation from heterologous MMMTs and primitive neuroectodermal tumors is discussed in the sections dealing with those neoplasms.

Mature Teratomas

Clinical Features. Mature teratomas, which are almost all cystic (dermoid cysts), account for approximately 25% of all ovarian tumors, 30% of benign ovarian tumors, and more than two-thirds of all ovarian tumors in patients under the age of 15 years (40). These tumors usually develop in children or women in the reproductive age group but are sometimes not detected until years after the menopause. Rare tumors are familial (453). Patients typically have initial symptoms of a pelvic mass. The tumors may undergo torsion or rupture, causing acute abdominal pain. Rupture into an adjacent organ may lead to the passage of cyst contents or the

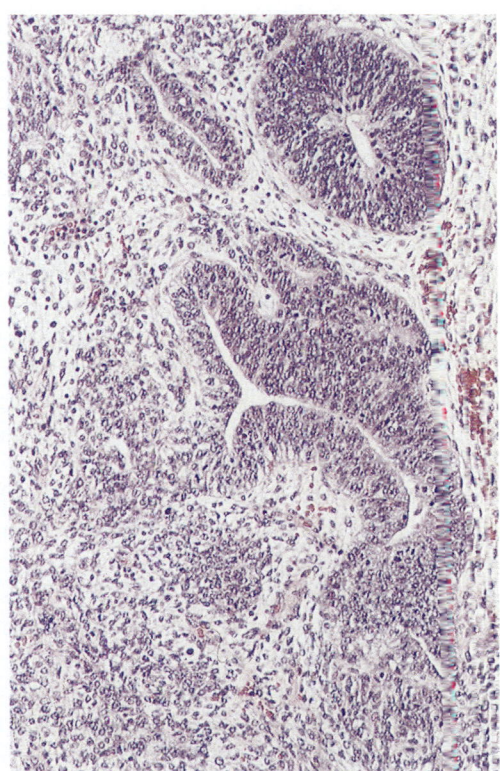

FIG. 110. Immature teratoma with immature neuroepithelial tubules.

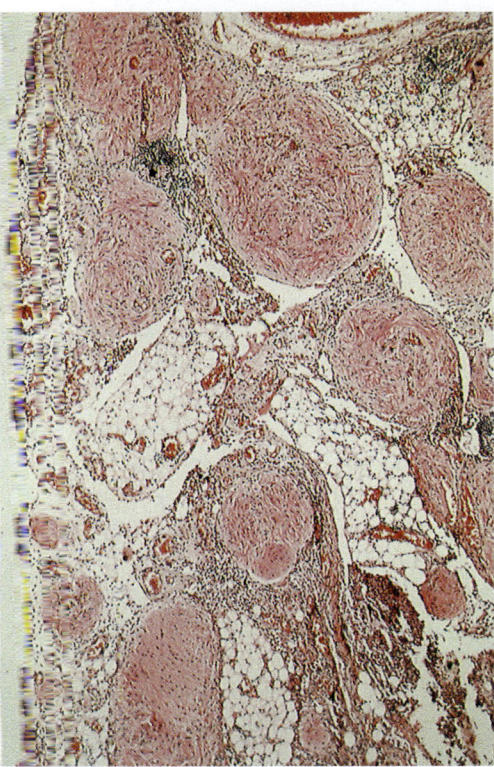

FIG. 111. Glial implants in the omentum in a patient with ovarian teratoma.

entire cyst into the urinary bladder, vagina, or rectum (454–456). Slow leakage of a dermoid cyst into the peritoneal cavity may result in foreign-body granulomas, which can mimic tumor implants or tuberculous granulomas. Rare complications include Coombs'-positive hemolytic anemia (cured by removal of the tumor) (457,458), infection, peritoneal melanosis (see Chapter 56) and the very rare development of a subsequent immature teratoma in the residual ovarian tissue (441,446). Mature solid teratomas are occasionally accompanied by mature glial implants, which are almost always associated with an excellent prognosis (436).

Mature teratomas are benign, except for the 1% to 2% that harbor adult-type cancers, most commonly squamous cell carcinoma (308,454,459). This complication should be suspected in patients over 40 years of age with tumors adherent to surrounding structures or that have areas of nodularity, mural thickening, hemorrhage, or necrosis. Patients with squamous cell carcinoma that has spread beyond the ovary, as well as those with certain rarer forms of malignant change (such as sarcoma), typically have a poor prognosis. In contrast, more than 90% of patients with squamous cell carcinoma confined to the ovary survive.

Gross Features. Mature teratomas are almost always dermoid cysts but are rarely predominantly solid. In the latter cases, the gross appearance is similar to that of immature teratoma, except that soft areas and foci of hemorrhage and necrosis are much less common. Dermoid cysts are globular or ovoid, with a white to gray external surface; most are less than 15 cm in diameter. Yellow to brown sebaceous material and hair fill one or more cysts, which are typically lined by tissue resembling skin. Single or several rounded, polypoid masses, designated mamillae or Rokitansky's protuberances and composed predominantly of fat, may protrude into the cyst lumen. Teeth are present in one-third of cases, either in the cyst wall or protruding into the cavity. Now and then, they are embedded in a rudimentary mandible or maxilla. Bone, cartilage, mucinous cysts, adipose tissue, thyroid, and brain tissue may be seen. Rarely, partially developed organs (bowel, appendix, skull, vertebrae, limb buds, external genitalia, eyes) may be present (460), or the mature teratoma may take the form of a homunculus (fetiform teratoma) (461). Approximately 12% of dermoid cysts are bilateral; infrequently, there are several in one ovary. A tumor arising within a dermoid cyst may appear as a polypoid mass, mural nodule, or mural plaque; if it is large, it may form a solid mass that partially obliterates the underlying cyst. Foci of hemorrhage and necrosis within malignant components are common.

Microscopic Features. Dermoid cysts are composed of adult and sometimes a small amount of fetal-type tissue, which usually represents all three germ layers. Ectodermal derivatives predominate in almost all cases and include epidermis, pilosebaceous structures, sweat glands, and neural tissue. The last component is most often glial, but more organized structures, such as cerebrum, cerebellum, and choroid plexus, can be present (462). Mesodermal derivatives include smooth muscle, bone, cartilage, and fat. Endodermal derivatives include respiratory and gastrointestinal structures and thyroid tissue. Rare constituents comprise retinal, pancreatic, thymic, adrenal, pituitary, renal, pulmonary, mammary, prostatic, and other tissues (463–469). Mitotic figures are absent or rare, but they may be seen in tissues in which they are normally present during late fetal or early postnatal life, such as cerebellum or developing teeth.

The various tissues are often arranged in an organoid fashion, for example, cartilage and mucinous glands may underlie respiratory epithelium, and layers of smooth muscle with intervening Auerbach's plexus may surround intestinal mucosa. Respiratory and glial tissue occasionally line portions of the cyst wall. Lipogranulomatous and fibrosing inflammatory reactive tissue may be seen in response to the escape of cyst contents into the adjacent stroma (470). Rare dermoid cysts contain tiny foci of immature tissue, which have not been reported to be associated with recurrence or the later development of immature teratoma (441).

Approximately 75% of cancers arising in dermoid cysts are invasive or, in rare cases, *in situ* squamous cell carcinomas (308). The remainder have included carcinoid, thyroid carcinoma, undifferentiated carcinoma, adenocarcinoma, sarcoma, malignant melanoma, basal cell carcinoma, primitive neuroectodermal tumors and glioblastoma multiforme, and lymphoma (454,456, 459,471–474). In exceptional cases, benign neoplasms arise in dermoid cysts, including adrenocorticotropic hormone (ACTH)– or prolactin-secreting pituitary adenomas, thyroid adenomas, and hemangiomas (40,475). When these tumors are composed of specialized tissues, such as thyroid, carcinoid, or pituitary tissue, and form a major component of the specimen, they are classified as monodermal teratomas.

Monodermal Teratomas

Struma Ovarii

Clinical features. Struma is the most common form of monodermal teratoma (40). Although thyroid tissue can be identified on microscopic inspection in up to 20% of dermoid cysts, the term struma ovarii is appropriate only when such tissue is recognizable on gross examination or occupies most or all of the tumor. The peak age of incidence is in the fifth decade; a few cases have been reported in prepubertal girls and postmenopausal women. Ascites develops in approximately one-third of patients (476), and, rarely, a Meigs' type of syndrome is present. A few examples have caused or contributed to hyperthyroidism (477).

Although 5% to 10% of strumas have been considered malignant (478–486), only a small number have been associated with extraovarian spread (bone, liver, brain, lungs, mediastinum, opposite ovary, regional lymph nodes, peritoneum). In the remaining cases, the diagnosis of malignancy has been based solely on microscopic criteria, and some tumors originally reported as malignant are now known to be the typically benign strumal carcinoid (page

2368). Once in a while, struma implants on the peritoneum as benign-appearing nodules of thyroid tissue (peritoneal strumosis) that do not affect longevity (485,486).

Gross features. The thyroid tissue is typically brown or green-brown, predominantly solid, and gelatinous. Usually, struma occurs in a pure form; less often, it is associated with a dermoid cyst or is a component of strumal carcinoid. Rare strumas are found in the wall of mucinous cystadenomas or are admixed with Brenner tumor (487). Some examples of struma ovarii appear as unilocular or multilocular cysts containing brown to green gelatinous fluid (Fig. 112) (488). Occasionally, the contralateral ovary contains a dermoid cyst or even another struma.

Microscopic features. Struma may resemble normal thyroid tissue or adenoma of the macrofollicular, microfollicular, embryonal, or mixed type. Oxyphilic, clear-cell, and solid tubular forms of thyroid adenoma have also been reported (Fig. 113) (489). Areas of "thyroiditis" are seen in isolated instances. Colloid within the follicles often contains birefringent calcium oxalate crystals and is immunoreactive for thyroglobulin. The lining of cystic struma may be overlooked as being of thyroid type in some cases, if cystic struma is not considered in the differential diagnosis (Fig. 114). Uniformly accepted microscopic criteria for malignant change in struma have not been established. A papillary pattern with typical nuclear characteristics or extraovarian spread provides the best evidence of malignancy. Most tumors that appear malignant on microscopic examination, however, pursue a benign clinical course (485).

Differential diagnosis. Cystic strumas containing gelatinous fluid can be mistaken on gross examination for mucinous cystic tumors; the green to brown color of the fluid in the former case provides strong evidence of the correct diag-

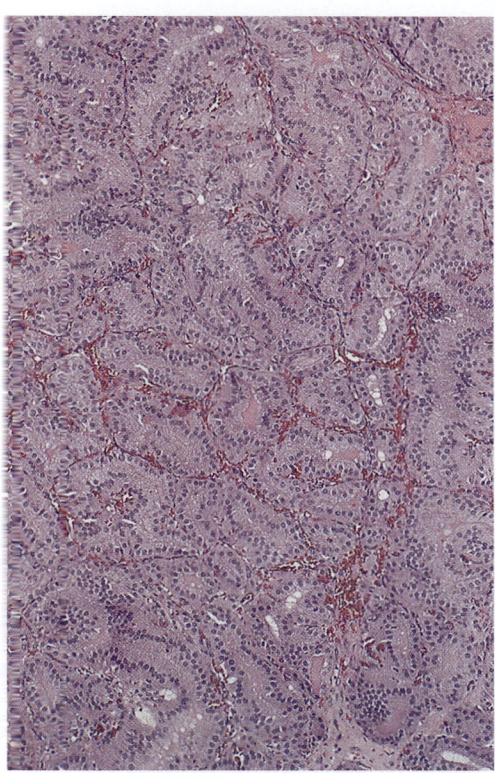

FIG. 113. Struma ovarii with solid tubular pattern simulating Sertoli cell tumor. This tumor stained for thyroglobulin.

nosis (488). In rare cases, when the struma forms a unilocular or oligolocular, thin-walled cyst containing watery fluid, it can simulate a serous cystadenoma on gross and microscopic inspection, but careful examination of the cyst wall or septa reveals at least an isolated recognizable thyroid follicle (488). Clear-cell carcinomas, endometrioid carcinomas, SLCTs, and pregnancy luteomas may contain small cysts closely resembling thyroid follicles, but other characteristic features in such tumors almost always permit their distinc-

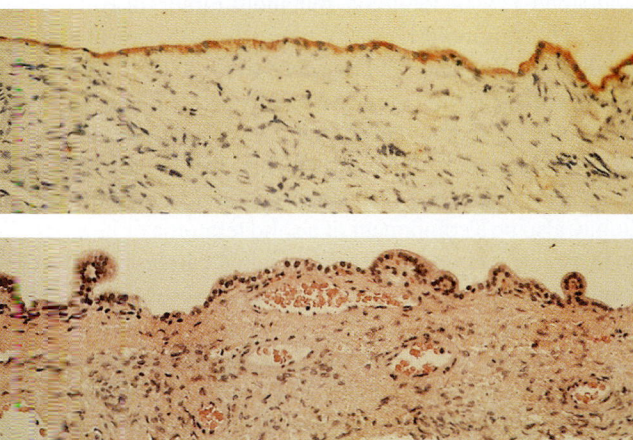

FIG. 114. Cystic struma ovarii. The bottom panel shows the cyst lining, which is not obviously lined by cells of thyroid type. The top panel shows immunoreactivity for thyroglobulin of the cyst-lining cells.

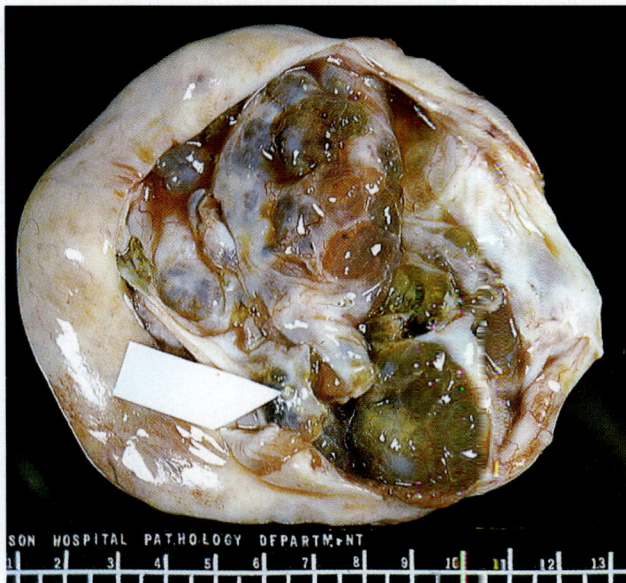

FIG. 112. Struma ovarii. A large cystic neoplasm contains multiple locules that have a brown-green color.

tion. Oxyphilic adenomas in strumas may be mistaken for other oxyphilic neoplasms, such as steroid cell tumors, and solid tubular adenomas may closely simulate Sertoli cell tumors (Fig. 113). In these and other challenging cases, the finding of true thyroid follicles and calcium oxalate crystals and immunoreactivity for thyroglobulin confirms the diagnosis of struma (Fig. 114). The differential diagnosis of struma also includes the extremely rare case of ovarian metastasis from carcinoma of the thyroid gland (490).

Carcinoids

Clinical features. Carcinoids are the second most common form of ovarian monodermal teratoma (40). They are divided into insular, trabecular, and goblet cell (mucinous) pure carcinoids and strumal carcinoids. The patients range in age from early reproductive years to postmenopausal, although those in the latter age group predominate. A pelvic mass is typically evident. Approximately one-third of insular carcinoids are accompanied by the carcinoid syndrome, which disappears after removal of the tumor (491). Infrequently, strumal carcinoid also has been associated with the syndrome. Patients with the syndrome are usually older than 50 years of age and have tumors larger than 7 cm in diameter. Other clinical findings include androgenic or estrogenic manifestations related to stromal luteinization or peripheral steroid cell proliferation (99,492), constipation (493), hyperinsulinemic hypoglycemia (494), and thyroid hyperfunction associated with strumal carcinoids (492).

These tumors are of low malignant potential—less than 5% are complicated by metastasis and death. Most of the malignant tumors have been of the insular or goblet cell type. A few patients have died of progressive carcinoid heart disease despite complete surgical removal of an insular carcinoid (491). Only two patients with strumal carcinoid have had metastatic disease (492); in one it appears to have been the struma rather than the carcinoid component that metastasized (495).

Gross features. All primary ovarian carcinoids have been unilateral, although in 15% of cases the opposite ovary has contained a cystic teratoma, mucinous tumor, or Brenner tumor. The carcinoid tissue is typically firm, tan to yellow, predominantly solid, and variably fibrous (Fig. 115). Cysts filled with clear fluid are occasionally present; now and then, the tumor is predominantly cystic. In some cases, the tumor may form a nodule that protrudes into the lumen or thickens the wall of a dermoid cyst or a mucinous cystic tumor (496); it may also be a component of a solid teratoma or be admixed with Brenner tumor or struma (strumal carcinoid). The carcinoid and struma may be identifiable on gross examination as separate components or form a single homogeneous mass.

Microscopic features. Approximately 75% of carcinoids are mixed with other teratomatous elements. Insular carcinoids resemble midgut carcinoids and are characterized by discrete cellular masses and nests (Fig. 116) separated by scanty to abundant fibrous or fibromatoid stroma (491). Small glands lined by columnar cells with copious cytoplasm often puncture the cellular islands (Fig. 116), particu-

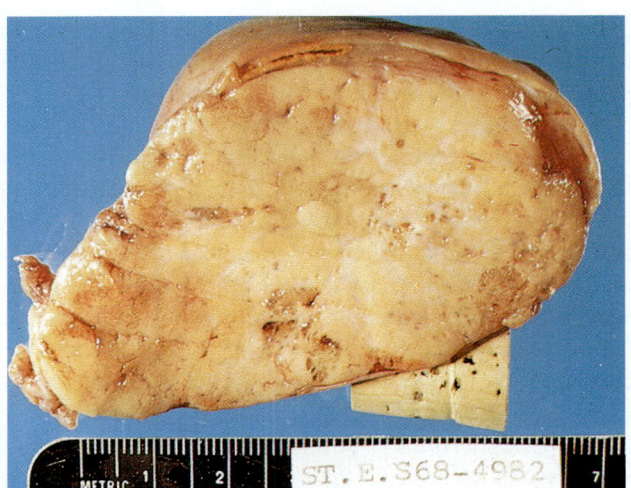

FIG. 115. Primary carcinoid tumor. The neoplasm has a tan sectioned surface.

larly at their periphery. Eosinophilic secretion, which may be calcified, is present within the lumens of the glands. The tumor cells have round, uniform nuclei containing coarse chromatin granules and rare mitotic figures. The peripheral cells of the islands and the glandular cells contain red-brown argentaffin granules, which are often visible on routine staining. An intimate relationship of the tumor to respiratory or gastrointestinal epithelium is sometimes evident.

Trabecular carcinoids resemble hindgut carcinoids and are characterized by long, wavy, parallel ribbons of cells separated by scanty to abundant fibrous stroma (497–501). The ribbons are composed of columnar cells, usually two or three cells thick, with oblong nuclei oriented perpendicular to the axis of the ribbon. The moderately abundant eosinophilic cytoplasm typically contains argyrophilic granules. The nuclei have finely dispersed chromatin and a few mitotic figures. An insular pattern is a minor feature in about 20% of cases. Associated teratomatous elements are almost always present. In rare instances, ovarian carcinoids have a spindle-cell or poorly differentiated pattern (502) or are

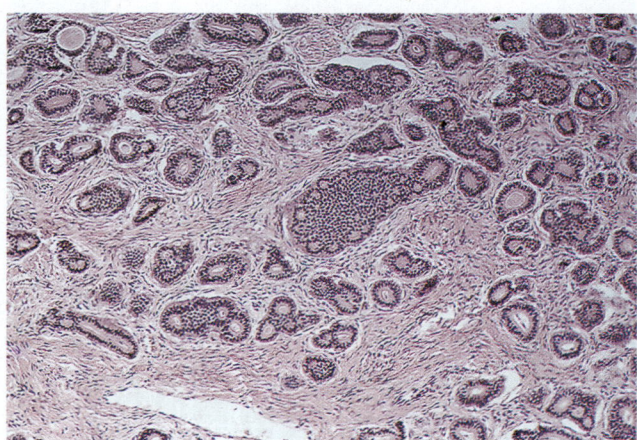

FIG. 116. Carcinoid tumor, insular pattern. Note many small acini within the nests.

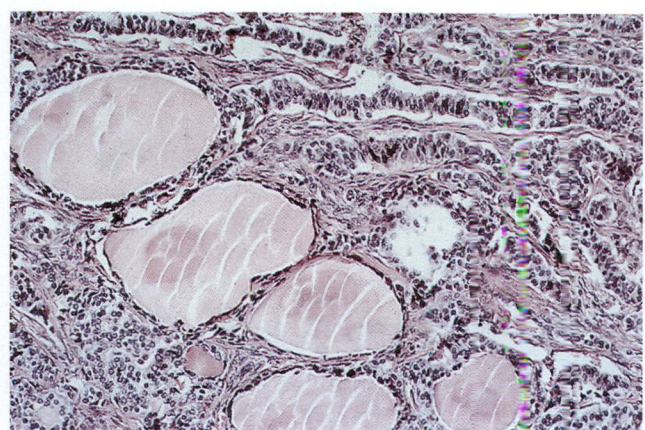

FIG. 117. Strumal carcinoid. Several trabeculae of carcinoid tumor are intimately associated with thyroid follicles.

characterized by solid tubules resembling those of a Sertoli cell tumor.

Goblet cell (mucinous) carcinoids resemble analogous appendiceal tumors (503,504). They usually occur in a pure form but may be associated with strumal carcinoid, mature teratoma, or epidermoid cyst. They consist of small nests (Fig. 118) or glands composed of or lined by goblet cells, argyrophil cells (some of which may also be argentaffin), and hybrid cells containing both mucin and granules. The nuclei are uniform, small, and round to oval. The nests and glands may lie within pools of mucin. More poorly differentiated cells, typically of the signet-ring-cell type, may invade the stroma singly, in small nests, or diffusely, mimicking Krukenberg tumor.

The components of strumal carcinoids are intimately admixed either at their interface or diffusely (Fig. 117); either component may predominate. The carcinoid is trabecular in half the cases, mixed trabecular and insular in most of the remainder, and purely insular only occasionally. The thyroid component resembles normal thyroid tissue or follicular adenoma and may contain calcium oxalate crystals. Argyrophilic granules are typically present within the cells, forming trabeculae and lining thyroid follicles (499,501). Almost half the tumors also contain argentaffin granules (492). From time to time, small glands lined by intestinal epithelium are encountered, or there is a component of goblet cell carcinoid (506). Rare strumal carcinoids contain amyloid (499). On ultrastructural examination, neuroendocrine-type granules are present within cells growing in a trabecular pattern; the follicles may be lined by similar neuroendocrine cells, thyroid epithelial cells, or a mixture of the two (500,501). Occasionally, tumors initially diagnosed as trabecular carcinoids prove to be strumal carcinoids on more extensive sampling.

Immunohistochemical findings. Serotonin has been identified in insular, strumal, and mucinous subtypes. In addition, approximately 25% of carcinoids contain peptide hormones, most often pancreatic polypeptide, glucagon, enkephalin, and somatostatin (505). Those found less often have been substance P, calcitonin, vasoactive intestinal peptide, neurotensin, beta-endorphin, and ACTH. Trabecular, strumal, and insular carcinoids were immunoreactive for at least one peptide hormone in 53%, 42%, and 7% of cases, respectively (505). Neuron-specific enolase has been verified in insular and strumal carcinoids (507), and thyroglobulin has been identified in the follicular cells and sometimes in the trabecular cells of strumal carcinoids (500,501).

Differential diagnosis. In the absence of teratomatous elements, primary carcinoid may be difficult to distinguish from metastatic carcinoid (page 2379). Evidence favoring or establishing the diagnosis of metastasis includes the definite or probable presence of a carcinoid in the gastrointestinal tract, lung, or elsewhere; extraovarian metastases; bilaterality; intraovarian growth in the form of several nodules; and persistence of the carcinoid syndrome or elevated 5-hydroxyindoleacetic acid levels in the urine after removal of the ovarian tumor. Many of these features are equally useful in differentiating primary goblet cell carcinoid with a focal signet-ring-cell pattern from Krukenberg tumor.

Despite their usually distinctive microscopic characteristics, several types of ovarian carcinoid can be confused with a number of other primary ovarian tumors, especially GCT, SLCT, and Brenner tumor. In contrast to the glands of carcinoids, the Call-Exner bodies of GCTs have irregular margins and contain watery or hyaline material and, often, shrunken nuclei. The granulosa cells surrounding a Call-Exner body lack the eosinophilic cytoplasm that separates the nuclei from the lumen of a carcinoid gland. Moreover, these cells typically have pale, grooved, haphazardly oriented nuclei instead of round, coarsely stippled nuclei. The sex cords in SLCTs of intermediate differentiation are shorter, less uniform, and more sparsely distributed than the elongated ribbons of trabecular carcinoid. In addition, several other distinctive patterns of SLCT may facilitate the diagnosis. Rare carcinoid tumors, however, form large, solid tubules closely resembling those of Sertoli cell tumor. The epithelial cells of Brenner tumors, in contrast to those of carcinoid tumors, have a distinct urothelial appearance with grooved nuclei. In addition, the glands in Brenner nests are often lined by mu-

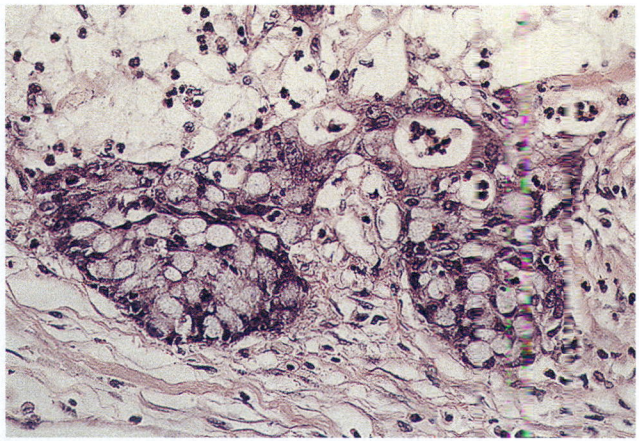

FIG. 118. Mucinous carcinoid. Small nests are composed of goblet cells and mucin-free cells that were argyrophilic.

cinous cells, unlike those of a carcinoid. Immunohistochemical staining for neuroendocrine, thyroid, and sex cord–stromal (inhibin) markers can be diagnostic in difficult cases.

Neuroectodermal Tumors

Included in this group of neoplasms are well-differentiated tumors, most often ependymomas; primitive tumors resembling primitive neuroectodermal tumors of the central nervous system, including medulloblastoma, medulloepithelioma, and neuroblastoma; and anaplastic tumors resembling glioblastoma multiforme (508–510). These tumors are encountered most often during the second to fourth decades. The initial symptoms are usually nonspecific, but upon occasion there are hormonal manifestations as a result of stromal luteinization. The tumors are typically large. Primitive and anaplastic subtypes usually appear malignant on gross examination, have often spread beyond the ovary, and usually pursue an aggressive course. Microscopic features are those of similar nervous system neoplasms. Ovarian ependymomas (Fig. 119) are associated with a favorable prognosis even with extraovarian spread.

Primitive neuroectodermal tumors may be difficult to distinguish from other small-cell malignant tumors of the ovary that develop in young women, such as small-cell carcinomas. Thorough sampling and immunohistochemical staining for glial fibrillary acidic protein are often helpful. Ependymomas may be confused with sex cord–stromal and surface epithelial tumors, but their distinctive light microscopic features, including perivascular rosettes and a few true rosettes, combined with immunohistochemical staining for glial fibrillary acidic protein should permit their recognition (510).

Sebaceous Tumors

At least nine sebaceous neoplasms, almost all of which arose in dermoid cysts, have been reported (511,512). They occurred in women with an average age of 58 years. All the women had nonspecific, mass-related symptoms, and all the tumors were unilateral. At the microscopic level, various forms of sebaceous neoplasia have been encountered, including sebaceous adenoma, basal cell carcinoma with sebaceous differentiation, and sebaceous carcinoma. Large numbers of mature, bubbly sebaceous cells in a tumor arising within a dermoid cyst should confirm the diagnosis. These tumors have had a favorable prognosis; one patient had recurrence, but no fatalities have been reported.

Rare Monodermal Teratomas

Included in this group are tumors resembling the retinal anlage tumor (513–515) and cysts lined by mature glial tissue (516,517), ependymal epithelium (518), respiratory epithelium (519), and melanotic epithelium (520). Epidermoid cysts, lined exclusively by mature squamous epithelium, may be monodermal teratomas in at least some cases (302–304). Two tumors of special interest in the monodermal category were pituitary-type adenomas, one secreting ACTH and causing Cushing's syndrome (521) and the other secreting prolactin and causing hyperprolactinemia (522). Both tumors arose in dermoid cysts.

Mixed Malignant Germ Cell Tumors

Approximately 8% of primitive ovarian germ cell tumors are mixed (523). They emphasize the importance of careful gross examination and judicious sampling for microscopic study. The prognosis for mixed germ cell tumors may depend on both the nature and the quantity of the most malignant element (523). In one study, this element did not adversely affect the prognosis unless it accounted for more than one-third of the tumor area. Such a correlation, however, was not confirmed in a later series (524). There has been one report of a unique mixed germ cell tumor that consisted predominantly of immature pancreatic tissue with islet cells, accompanied by foci of benign and malignant mucinous epithelium, dysgerminoma, YST, and immature teratoma (525).

Mixed Germ Cell–Sex Cord–Stromal Tumors

Gonadoblastoma

Clinical Features

Gonadoblastoma is a rare tumor found almost exclusively in patients with an underlying gonadal disorder; it accounts for two-thirds of gonadal tumors in women with abnormal gonadal development (40,526). Affected patients are typically children or young adults. The clinical picture may include a mass and virilization caused by the tumor as well as clinical manifestations of the underlying gonadal disorder. Because at least a portion of one gonad and, at times, both gonads are replaced by tumor, it may be possible to identify specifically the nature of the underlying gonadal abnormality. When a sexual disorder can be diagnosed, it is almost al-

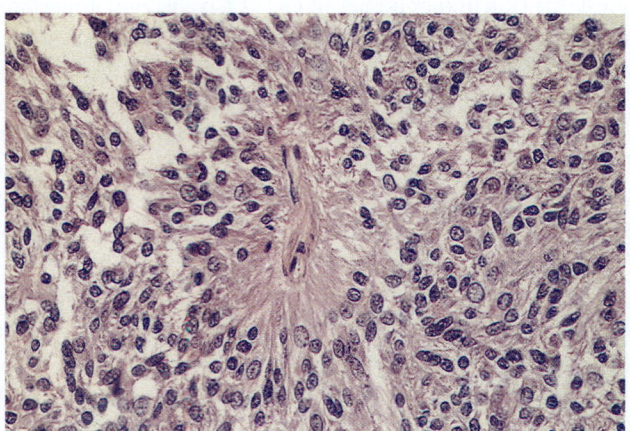

FIG. 119. Ependymoma. A perivascular pseudorosette is present in the center.

ways 46XY pure gonadal dysgenesis or mixed gonadal dysgenesis, which is often associated with a 45X,46XY karyotype and occasionally with another mosaic or a 46XY karyotype. Gonadoblastomas arise most often in phenotypic women, who usually show signs of virilization; a minority are phenotypic men with varying degrees of feminization. Very rarely, gonadoblastomas appear in otherwise normal women with a history of pregnancy (527). Gonadoblastoma without an invasive germ cell tumor component is benign. Because of the frequency with which the tumor gives rise to malignant germ cell tumor, however, it should be regarded as an *in situ* form of cancer.

Gross Features

The gross appearance varies with the size, the presence or absence of an associated malignant germ cell tumor, and the extent of calcification. The tumors may be soft and fleshy, firm and cartilaginous, flecked with calcium, or totally calcified. Their color varies from brown to yellow to gray. Pure gonadoblastomas are typically less than 8 cm in diameter, and 25% are microscopic. Those with a malignant germ cell tumor component can be much larger. Approximately one-third of gonadoblastomas are bilateral; less often, the contralateral gonad contains a malignant germ cell tumor, usually a germinoma, with no trace of underlying gonadoblastoma. The gonad in which a gonadoblastoma develops is of uncertain nature in 60%, an abdominal or inguinal testis in 20%, and a gonadal streak in 20% of the cases. Extremely rare gonadoblastomas arise in apparently normal ovaries.

Microscopic Features

Discrete cellular nests composed of an intimate mixture of germ cells and smaller epithelial cells of the sex-cord type are the cardinal histologic feature (Fig. 120) (526). The germ cells are similar to those of dysgerminoma and seminoma in

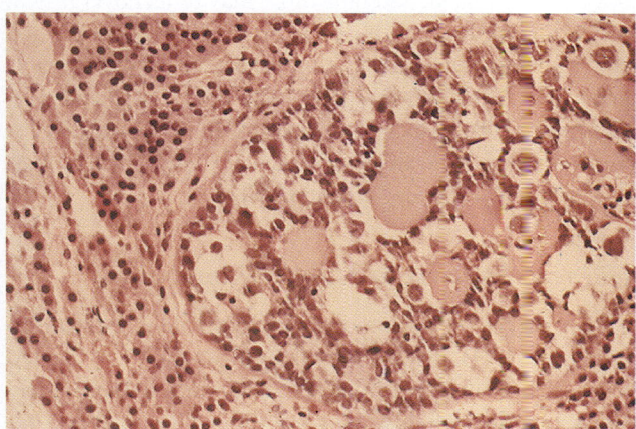

FIG. 120. Gonadoblastoma. Germ cells with abundant clear cytoplasm, smaller cells of the sex-cord type, and hyaline bodies are visible. Note lutein–Leydig cells in the stroma.

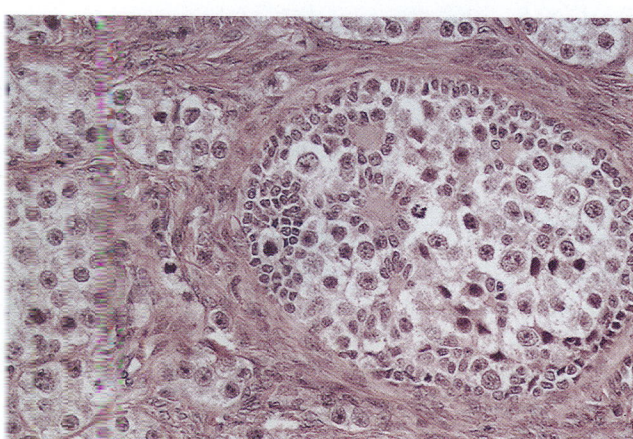

FIG. 121. Gonadoblastoma (right) associated with germinoma (left).

most cases and usually exhibit mitotic activity. In some cases, the germ cells resemble immature testicular germ cells or spermatogonia (528). The smaller, round to oval epithelial cells have pale nuclei, are mitotically inactive, and resemble most immature Sertoli cells; Charcot-Bottcher bundles of crystals have been identified in their cytoplasm. Within the discrete nests, these cells surround circular spaces filled with eosinophilic hyalinized basement membrane material, line the periphery of the nests with a central accumulation of germ cells, or surround individual germ cells. Rarely, the germ cells and sex cord–like cells have a diffuse instead of a nesting pattern. The discrete nests are separated by scanty to abundant fibrous stroma, which contains Leydig cells or luteinized cells in two-thirds of cases.

The typical histologic appearance of gonadoblastoma can be altered or obliterated by extensive deposition of basement membrane–like material; calcification, which typically forms laminated spheres and mulberry-like masses; or overgrowth by a malignant germ cell tumor, which occurs in approximately half the cases. The malignant tumor is a germinoma in 80% of cases (Fig. 121). Its extent ranges from a focus of microinvasion to massive replacement of the underlying gonadoblastoma. Less often, YST, embryonal carcinoma, choriocarcinoma, or immature teratoma develops (529,530).

Differential Diagnosis

Gonadoblastomas can be confused with pure dysgerminomas and SCTATs. Dysgerminoma or seminoma in a patient with maldeveloped gonads and a Y chromosome should raise the question of its origin in gonadoblastoma. The only clue may be a tiny focus of calcification or a rare nest of typical gonadoblastoma. SCTAT resembles gonadoblastoma in its similar growth pattern, basement membrane–like material, and calcification, but it lacks a germ cell component. Gonadoblastoma should also be distinguished from unclassified germ cell–sex cord–stromal tumors, discussed in the following section. Finally, microscopic gonadoblastoma-like structures have been found in 15% of the ovaries of normal fetuses and newborn infants (531).

Germ Cell–Sex Cord–Stromal Tumors, Nongonadoblastoma Type

This category includes all tumors that contain germ cells, sex-cord elements, and, occasionally, lutein or Leydig-type cells but lack the distinctive patterns of gonadoblastoma (532–539). Patients are usually under the age of 10 years and have normal gonadal development and a normal karyotype. Isosexual precocity and one bilateral example have been reported (537,538). Most of the tumors have been benign, but two metastasized.

The few such tumors reported have varied in their microscopic features. Sex cord–type cells and germ cells may grow diffusely, in cords simulating sex cords, or within small, solid tubules (Fig. 122). The sex cord–type cells may have a retiform pattern (534–536). The sex-cord element may be less mature than in gonadoblastoma, and the germ cells may resemble those of dysgerminoma; in other cases, they lack clear cytoplasm and have large, round nuclei without prominent nucleoli. Hyaline bodies and calcification characteristic of gonadoblastoma are very unusual. An associated dysgerminoma was found in one case.

Nonspecific Mesenchymal and Miscellaneous Other Tumors

Benign

Fibromas, the most common mesenchymal tumors of the ovary, have been discussed on page 2347. Leiomyomas account for almost 1% of benign ovarian neoplasms (540–543). They vary greatly in size (543) and are similar in histologic features to leiomyomas encountered elsewhere, including a few epithelioid forms. Immuno stains aid in establishing their diagnosis. Mitotic activity has not been shown to be diagnostic of leiomyosarcoma unless atypical features are also present (542). Too few cases have been reported with adequate follow-up data, however, to establish valid criteria for the diagnosis of malignancy. About 20 ovarian hemangiomas have been reported (40); a few have been associated with isolated hemangiomas elsewhere or generalized hemangiomatosis (544). Many have been incidental findings at autopsy. These tumors are most often situated in the medulla and hilus and are of the cavernous type; they must be distinguished from the normally numerous vessels in the ovarian medulla of older women. One or a few benign neural tumors, ganglioneuromas, lipomas, lymphangiomas, myxomas, chondromas, osteomas, and pheochromocytomas also have been found in the ovary (545). Ovarian lipomas may arise from rare foci of adipose metaplasia.

At least ten ovarian myxomas have been documented (546–550). Most of the tumors developed in reproductive-age patients with asymptomatic unilateral adnexal masses; one arose in a premenarchal girl (550). The tumors had an average diameter of 11 cm and were soft, with areas of cystic degeneration. On microscopic inspection, spindle-shaped and stellate cells are scattered on a myxoid background; a rich vascular network is often present in the tumor, but lipoblasts are absent. Small islands within the tumor may resemble ovarian fibroma or leiomyoma. In one case, there was a component of SST (547). One aneuploid tumor that exhibited mild nuclear atypia and slight mitotic activity recurred after many years, but it was positive for desmin and may have been a low-grade myxoid leiomyosarcoma (549). In addition to myxoid liposarcoma, the differential diagnosis includes other ovarian soft-tissue tumors that have myxoid change.

Sarcomas

A few pure or apparently pure sarcomas, such as fibrosarcoma (340,551–555); leiomyosarcoma, including the myxoid variant (556–558); malignant schwannoma (559); lymphangiosarcoma (545); angiosarcoma (560,561); and osteosarcoma (562–564) may arise in the ovary. Such sarcomas as rhabdomyosarcoma (565–567), chondrosarcoma (568), and osteogenic sarcoma (569) may reflect overgrowth within a complex tumor, such as MMMT, mesodermal adenosarcoma, immature teratoma, dermoid cyst, or heterologous SLCT. Isolated sarcomas have been associated with surface epithelial–stromal tumors (570,571). The microscopic features of ovarian sarcomas are analogous to their counterparts in other organs and tissues.

Malignant Lymphoma and Leukemic Involvement

The ovary contains tumor in approximately 25% of patients with non-Hodgkin's lymphoma at autopsy and in up to 50% of those with leukemia. Clinically detectable ovarian enlargement is much less common (572–576). With the exception of Burkitt's lymphoma, ovarian involvement as the initial manifestation of lymphoma or leukemia is rare. Well under 1% of extranodal lymphomas involve the ovary.

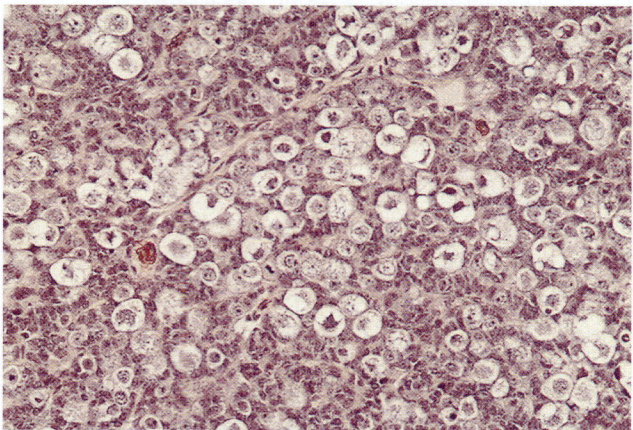

FIG. 122. Germ cell–sex cord–stromal tumor, unclassified. The tumor is composed of large, round, clear germ cells and smaller sex-cord cells with scanty cytoplasm.

Gross Features

Lymphomas and leukemic tumors typically form intact smooth or nodular masses composed of homogeneous, usually fleshy but occasionally firm tissue that is gray, pink, white, or yellow. They often measure more than 10 cm (40). Areas of hemorrhage, necrosis, and cystic degeneration may be present. About half the tumors are bilateral. In cases of granulocystic sarcoma, a green color may be a clue to the diagnosis (576).

Microscopic Features

Both diffuse and nodular growth patterns are encountered, but these patterns may be distorted and compartmentalized by stromal sclerosis, which can result in an insular or cord-like pattern (Fig. 123). The tumor cells can infiltrate ovarian follicles without destroying them, and follicle-like spaces are sometimes formed by the tumor cells themselves.

In adults, most histologic subtypes of non-Hodgkin's lymphoma, both follicular and diffuse, have been encountered. In children, the majority of the reported cases have been of the small noncleaved cell type, either of the Burkitt or non-Burkitt category. Extraovarian involvement is found at laparotomy in about two-thirds of patients with lymphoma. In exceptional cases, the ovary is the first site of relapse in children with acute lymphoblastic leukemia (577), and ovarian involvement is the first manifestation of Hodgkin's disease (578) or plasmacytoma (579).

Differential Diagnosis

Malignant lymphomas may be indistinguishable on gross examination from dysgerminomas. The former, however, have a 50% rate of bilaterality, in contrast to the 10% rate of dysgerminomas. Although these tumors may resemble each other superficially on microscopic examination, their nuclei and their immunohistochemical features are strikingly different. The single-file arrangement of lymphoma and leukemic cells may simulate metastatic carcinoma, particularly one of breast origin. Diffuse lymphoma can resemble GCT or small-cell carcinoma of the hypercalcemic type on low magnification. Numerous immunohistochemical markers are available to identify tumors as lymphomas; granulocytic sarcomas (Fig. 124) can be distinguished by chloroacetate esterase staining or, more accurately, by immunostaining for myeloperoxidase (576). The possibility of granulocytic sarcoma should be considered when evaluating cases of suspected ovarian lymphoma, since many cases of granulocytic sarcoma have been initially misinterpreted as such. It is helpful to bear in mind that granulocytic sarcoma is often seen on routine stains to be composed of cells with more finely dispersed nuclear chromatin and more abundant cytoplasm, which may be deeply eosinophilic, than lymphoma cells with nuclei of the same size (576). Definite identification of eosinophilic myelocytes may be crucial in making the diagnosis and obtaining confirmatory immunostains.

Small-cell Carcinoma, Hypercalcemic Type

This distinctive ovarian tumor (580–585) has occurred in both girls and women, 7 to 44 years of age (average, 23 years); it is the most common form of undifferentiated ovarian carcinoma in this age group. Approximately two-thirds of tumors are associated with paraendocrine hypercalcemia, accounting for half the ovarian tumors associated with that disorder. Small-cell carcinomas are almost always unilat-

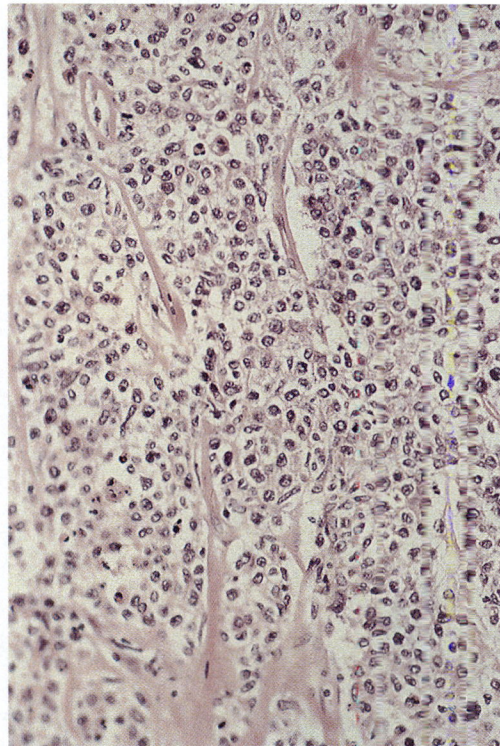

FIG. 123. Malignant lymphoma. The tumor is composed of large lymphoid cells intersected by fibrous bands.

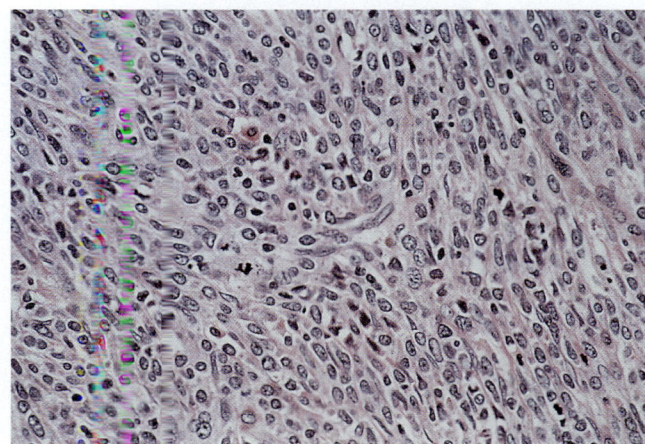

FIG. 124. Granulocytic sarcoma. There is a diffuse growth of cells whose features are apt to lead to misinterpretation as malignant lymphoma if the rare myeloid cells that are visible in the illustration are not taken into account.

eral; approximately one-third show signs of extraovarian spread at the time of laparotomy.

Gross Features

The tumors usually form large, predominantly solid, cream-colored to gray masses, often with areas of softening, necrosis, and hemorrhage. They may closely resemble ovarian lymphomas and dysgerminomas.

Microscopic Features

Diffuse sheets of small, closely packed cells with scanty cytoplasm and nuclei containing single nucleoli are typical. Mitotic figures are common. The tumor also grows as small islands, cords (Fig. 125), and trabeculae. Follicle-like structures lined by tumor cells are present in the great majority of cases (Fig. 126). These spaces typically contain eosinophilic fluid, but on occasion their content is basophilic. In approximately 40% of tumors, a varying proportion of cells contain abundant eosinophilic cytoplasm, which may have a globular, hyaline quality (Fig. 127), and large nuclei that have single prominent nucleoli. Mucinous epithelium is encountered in about 10% of cases (Fig. 128). In most cases, electron microscopy shows nonspecific epithelial features. Abundant rough endoplastic reticulum is the most characteristic finding (581,584); large cells may contain whorls of microfilaments. Dense-core granules have been reported in isolated

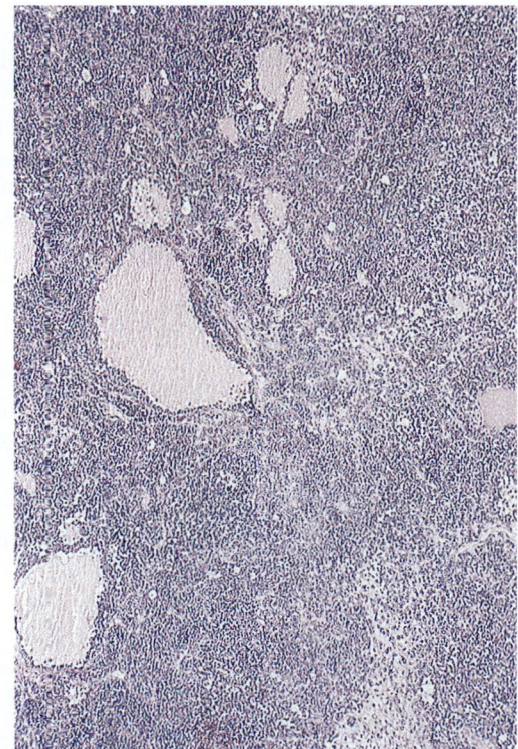

FIG. 126. Small-cell carcinoma, hypercalcemic type. Follicle formation is striking.

instances, but their identification as such and significance are questionable. The tumor cells stain variably for vimentin, cytokeratin, and EMA (582). Flow cytometry on paraffin-embedded material has shown a diploid pattern of DNA (583).

Differential Diagnosis

Small-cell carcinomas are most often misinterpreted as AGCTs or JGCTs. From a clinical viewpoint, hypercalcemia

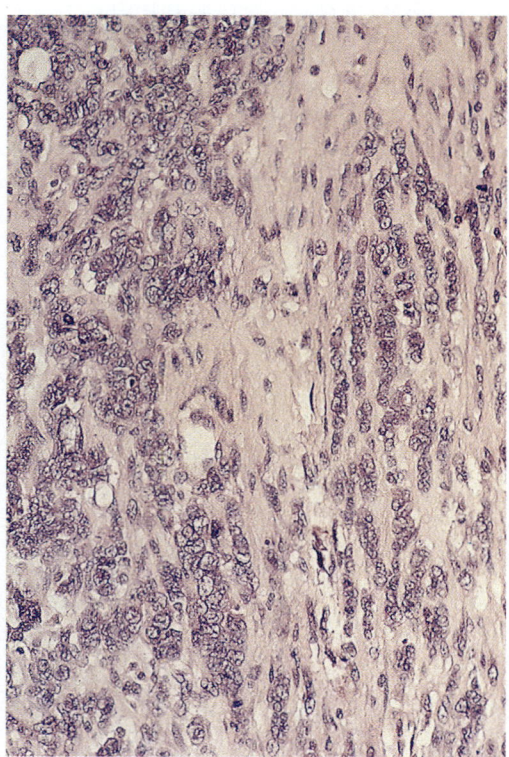

FIG. 125. Small-cell carcinoma, hypercalcemic type. The tumor cells grow in small clusters and cords.

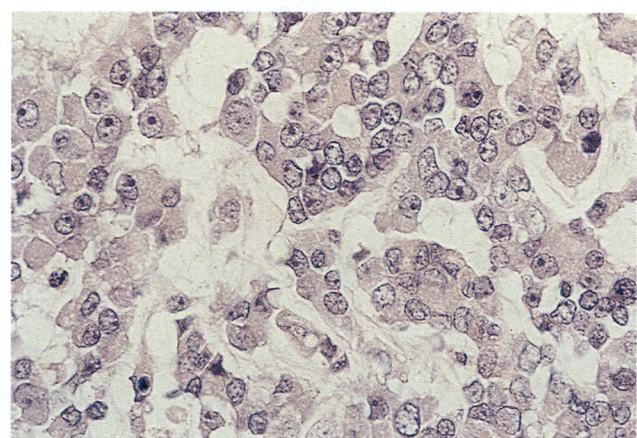

FIG. 127. Small-cell carcinoma, hypercalcemic type. This tumor contains large cells with abundant eosinophilic cytoplasm and central nuclei with prominent nucleoli.

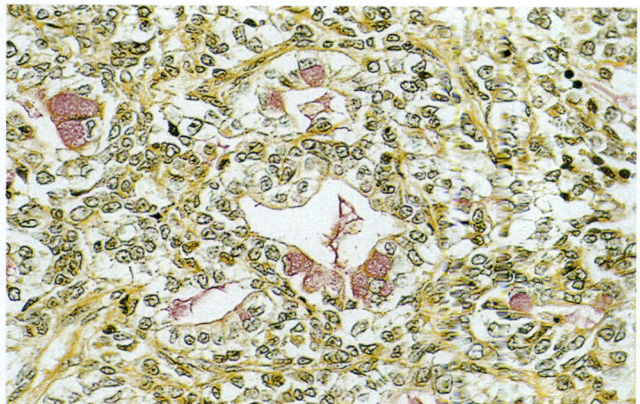

FIG. 128. Small-cell carcinoma, hypercalcemic type. A mucicarmine stain shows the presence of intracellular mucin in some of the tumor cells.

strongly favors a diagnosis of small-cell carcinoma, and evidence of estrogen excess favors a diagnosis of GCT. In addition, the rate of extraovarian spread of small-cell carcinomas is much higher than that of GCTs. The nuclei of small-cell carcinomas differ considerably from those of AGCTs—they are more hyperchromatic and mitotically active and lack grooves. The occasional predominance of large cells with abundant cytoplasm in small-cell carcinoma and the young age at which it occurs may suggest the possibility of JGCT. In addition to the differing clinical features of the two tumors, their characteristic microscopic patterns are also helpful. The follicles of JGCTs usually contain mucicarminophilic fluid, in contrast to the follicles in the great majority of small-cell carcinomas. The occasional presence of mucinous epithelium within small-cell carcinoma is inconsistent with the diagnosis of GCT. Immunohistochemical staining for inhibin and lack of staining for EMA should confirm the diagnosis of GCT. Small-cell carcinomas can also be confused with malignant lymphomas and sometimes with metastatic malignant melanoma (335) and metastatic alveolar rhabdomyosarcoma (586), but clinicopathologic features and immunohistochemical staining, if necessary, clarify these differential diagnoses.

Hepatoid Carcinoma

The designation hepatoid carcinoma has been given to a rare subtype of ovarian carcinoma resembling hepatocellular carcinoma and gastric hepatoid carcinoma (280). Six of the seven patients whose cases were reported were postmenopausal, and one was of reproductive age. Five of the seven tumors had spread beyond the ovary. Sheets, trabeculae, and cords of cells with moderate to large amounts of eosinophilic cytoplasm and round to oval central nuclei are characteristic. Varying numbers of tumor cells stain for AFP. Two tumors were admixed with serous carcinoma, strongly suggesting a surface epithelial origin (280,281).

Differential Diagnosis

This tumor must be distinguished from the rare hepatocellular carcinoma metastatic to the ovary (587) and other ovarian tumors that have cells with abundant eosinophilic cytoplasm. Clinicopathologic features must be considered in making the sometimes difficult distinction between hepatoid carcinoma and metastatic hepatocellular carcinoma. A hepatic mass suggestive of a primary neoplasm is strong evidence in favor of metastasis to the ovary, but in one case the primary liver tumor was discovered only after bilateral ovarian metastases had been resected (587).

Although bile pigment has not been described as a feature of ovarian hepatoid carcinomas, it has been documented in hepatoid carcinomas arising at other sites; for this reason its presence cannot be considered diagnostic of hepatic origin. Hepatoid YST almost always develops in young women and usually contains additional typical forms of yolk sac neoplasia. Differentiation of hepatoid carcinomas from oxyphilic clear-cell carcinomas has been discussed on page 2339. The cells of lipid-poor or lipid-free steroid cell tumors resemble those of hepatoid carcinomas. Steroid cell tumors, however, are usually associated with endocrine manifestations and would not be expected to stain for AFP; similarly, a hepatoid carcinoma would not be expected to stain for inhibin.

Tumors of Probable Wolffian Origin

Rare ovarian tumors (364,588) are identical at the microscopic level to their more common counterparts originating within the broad ligament or from the serosa of the broad ligament or the fallopian tube, which have been designated female adnexal tumors of probable wolffian origin.

Gross Features

The ovarian tumors average 12 cm in diameter, are solid or focally cystic, and are almost always stage Ia. The solid tissue varies from gray-white to tan or yellow and may be rubbery or firm.

Microscopic Features

The solid areas may be diffuse or composed of closely packed tubules. Varying amounts of fibrous stroma may result in a lobulated appearance. Cysts, which may be numerous and impart a sieve-like pattern (Fig. 129), typically contain eosinophilic secretion within their lumens. The tubules are closely packed and may be solid or hollow. In apparently diffuse areas, a tubular pattern may be unmasked by PAS or reticulin staining. The cells are oval or spindle shaped and contain scanty eosinophilic cytoplasm or pale cytoplasm in solid tubular areas. Rare tumors contain areas with poorly differentiated cells; such tumors may have a malignant behavior.

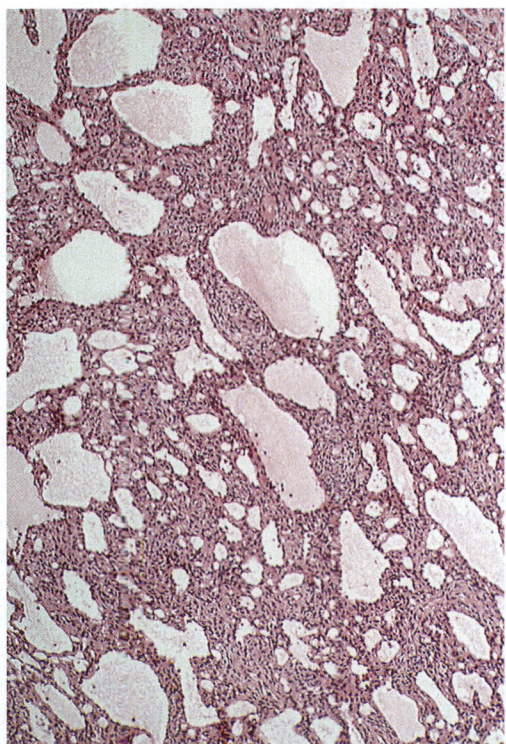

FIG. 129. Ovarian tumor of probable wolffian origin. The cysts impart a sieve-like pattern.

Differential Diagnosis

These tumors are often misinterpreted as sex cord–stromal tumors, particularly Sertoli cell tumors, because the tubules of the two tumors may be indistinguishable. The other patterns of the wolffian-type tumor are incompatible, however, with Sertoli cell tumor. In isolated cases, large hollow tubules resemble the glands of endometrioid adenocarcinoma, but other patterns of the neoplasm and the absence or scarcity of intraluminal mucin help rule out this diagnosis. Wolffian-like tumors with diffuse growth can be misinterpreted as undifferentiated carcinomas on low power, but high-power evaluation generally shows cells with bland cytologic features and few mitotic figures. Ependymomas rarely have cysts and in some areas superficially resemble wolffian tumors. Wolffian tumors are among the few ovarian tumors not of sex cord–stromal origin that can stain focally for inhibin (254); accordingly, this type of staining is not always definitive in differentiating wolffian tumors from sex-cord tumors.

Adenomatoid Tumor

This benign tumor of mesothelial origin is found on rare occasions immediately adjacent to the ovary (589). In one series of six cases, the patients ranged from 23 to 79 years of age. Four tumors were less than 1 cm, and one was 5 cm in diameter. Five tumors were predominantly hilar, with focal medullary extension. The tumors are identical at the microscopic level to their counterparts in the fallopian tube and uterus. Because of their rarity in the ovary, diagnostic errors are sometimes made. One example was initially considered to be YST because it had a focal reticular pattern and contained hyaline bodies; a lack of significant nuclear atypicality and a negative result with AFP immunostaining excluded the latter diagnosis.

Intraabdominal Desmoplastic Small Round-cell Tumor

This tumor is discussed in detail in Chapter 56. Women with this neoplasm may have prominent ovarian involvement at diagnosis, leading to diagnostic confusion with primary ovarian neoplasms. Three patients with this clinical picture were teenage girls (590); ovarian involvement was bilateral in two of them. In all the cases, there was extensive extraovarian disease at the time of operation. Since many ovarian tumors are characterized by small cells, there is a wide range of differential diagnoses. A prominent nesting pattern of small cells in a desmoplastic stroma, as well as a young age of the patient, should lead to consideration of this tumor. Immunohistochemical positivity for both cytokeratin and desmin generally establishes the diagnosis.

Malignant Mesothelioma

Ovarian involvement by peritoneal mesotheliomas is usually limited to the ovarian surface and occasionally the superficial stroma, but, rarely, the ovary is extensively involved, with a clinical picture similar to that of ovarian cancer. In one study ovarian involvement was present in ten of 13 patients with peritoneal mesothelioma (591), and, in another series, all nine malignant mesotheliomas appeared in the form of ovarian masses (591). Two of the nine tumors in the latter series were considered ovarian primary tumors because of their confinement to the ovary. The malignant mesotheliomas, whether primary or secondary, were characterized on microscopic examination by tubular, papillary, and solid patterns and relatively uniform cells with considerable eosinophilic cytoplasm. In routinely stained sections, these tumors are usually readily distinguishable from serous carcinoma by their pattern of growth and cytologic features, although histochemical or immunohistochemical stains are sometimes necessary to confirm the diagnosis (170,171).

Metastatic Tumors

Certain clinical and operative findings should alert the pathologist to the possibility of ovarian metastasis (593). These features include the previous or concurrent existence of primary tumor elsewhere and a pattern of extraovarian spread that is atypical for ovarian cancer. For example, hepatic or pulmonary metastases in the absence of extensive peritoneal spread would be unusual for ovarian cancer. Because metastases to the ovary are bilateral in two-thirds to three-fourths of cases, metastasis should be considered in the evaluation of bilateral disease, especially if the tumor is not of the serous type. About 10% to 20% of surgically encountered bilateral ovarian cancers are metastatic. Two other gross findings highly suggestive of metastasis are the presence of several nodules and involvement of the ovarian surface without generalized peritoneal spread. Single or several cysts, even when they are thin-walled, do not exclude metastasis. Prominent vascular space invasion is more typical of metastasis.

Krukenberg Tumors

Krukenberg tumors are carcinomas with a prominent component of signet-ring cells (594–597). They usually originate in the stomach. The primary tumor may be very small, escaping detection at operation or even for 5 or more years after surgery. A few Krukenberg tumors originate in the breast, other portions of the gastrointestinal tract, gallbladder, uterine cervix, and urinary bladder. Rare Krukenberg tumors may be primary, but that diagnosis should be made only if the patient has survived for 10 years or more after removal of the ovarian tumor(s) or when an exhaustive autopsy has disclosed no extraovarian primary site (598). Women with Krukenberg tumors tend to be unusually young for patients with metastatic carcinoma. Most of them are between 40 and 50 years of age, but a sizable proportion are in their twenties. The symptoms are usually nonspecific, but there may be endocrine manifestations, particularly virilization during pregnancy, as a result of stromal luteinization (40).

Gross Features. Krukenberg tumors are bilateral in 60% to 80% of cases. They are almost always solid, with a smooth or bosselated contour; they rarely contain thin-walled cysts (Fig. 130). The cut surfaces vary from firm, white to tan, and fibroma-like to red, fleshy, and gelatinous. Necrosis and hemorrhage are common.

Microscopic Features. Rounded malignant epithelial cells, many of which have a signet-ring-cell appearance, are embedded in a cellular stroma (Fig. 131). The stroma in some cases is less cellular and fibrous or edematous. The neoplastic cells are found singly or in clumps or form small

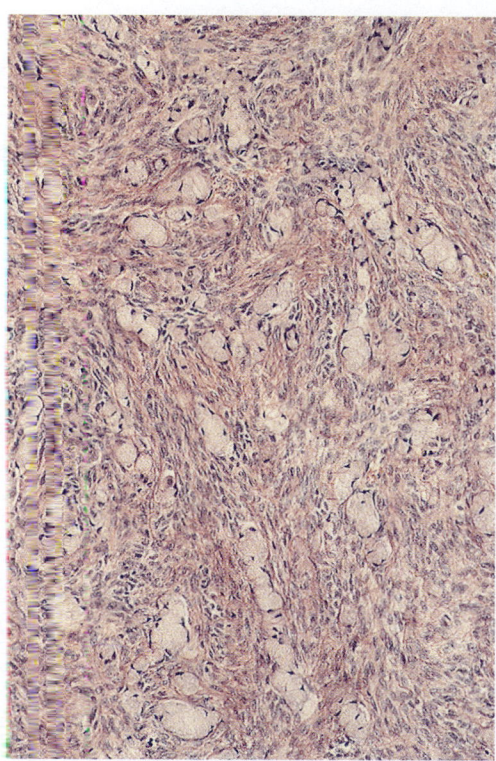

FIG. 131. Krukenberg tumor. Signet-ring cells lie within a cellular stroma.

glands; occasionally, the predominant architecture is tubular (tubular Krukenberg tumor) (Fig. 132) (599). Cysts lined by well-differentiated tumor cells resembling those of mucinous cystadenomas may be seen. Stromal pools of cell-free mucin are often present. The stromal cells are typically closely packed, plump, and spindle shaped. From time to time, the stroma is luteinized, sometimes extensively (40).

Differential Diagnosis. Krukenberg tumors must be distinguished from SLCTs and clear-cell carcinomas composed predominantly of signet-ring cells, as well as fibromas and SSTs. Confusion with SLCT occurs in the context of tubular Krukenberg tumors. The latter tumors, however, are bilateral in a large proportion of cases and are usually associated with an extraovarian primary tumor and often with other evidence of spread. Microscopic evidence of signet-ring cells is incompatible with a diagnosis of SLCT, with the very rare exception of a heterologous form containing a component of goblet cell carcinoid. In addition, the nuclei of tubular Krukenberg tumors are more atypical than those within the tubules of SLCT. Clear-cell carcinomas containing signet-ring cells have prominent components typical of clear-cell carcinoma and lack a cellular stroma; their signet-ring cells have a characteristic targetoid cytoplasm. Fibromas and SSTs do not have cells with cytoplasmic mucin amongst other differences (40).

Intestinal Carcinoma

From 2% to 10% of women with intestinal cancer have ovarian metastases during the course of their disease

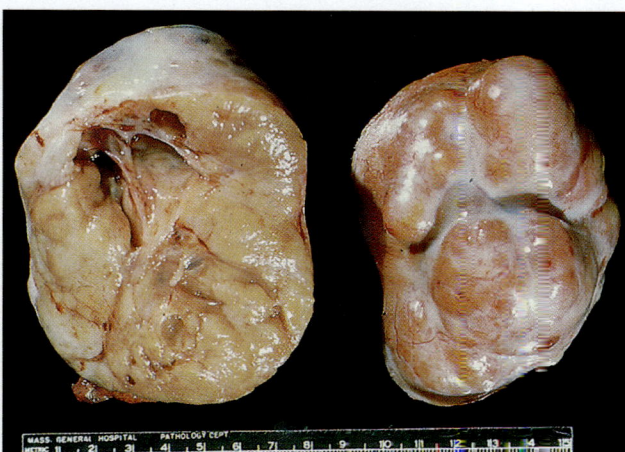

FIG. 130. Krukenberg tumor. The neoplasm has a bosselated external surface, and its sectioned surface shows lobulated, tan tissue.

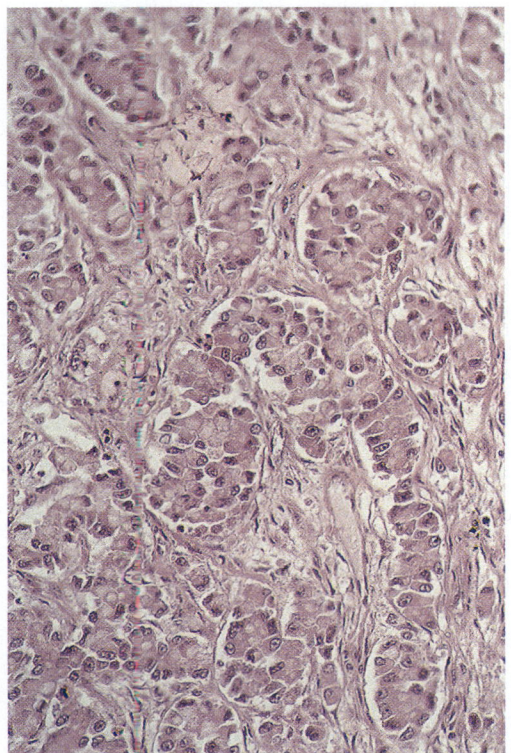

FIG. 132. Tubular Krukenberg tumor. Note signet-ring cells in many of the solid tubules.

(209,600–605). Metastasis is more likely to occur if the woman is under 40 years of age, presumably because of the greater vascularity of the ovary in that age group. The patients fall into three categories: those with an intestinal carcinoma who subsequently have ovarian metastasis (50–75% of cases), those with ovarian involvement discovered during resection of intestinal carcinoma, and those who are first diagnosed with an ovarian tumor (3–20% of cases) (603). Most intestinal metastases originate in the large intestine, but a few examples are from the small bowel.

Gross Features. Approximately two-thirds of the tumors are bilateral. Sectioning of smaller tumors generally reveals firm or soft, solid tissue, whereas larger tumors are composed of friable yellow, red, or gray tissue with cysts that contain necrotic tumor, mucinous or clear fluid, or blood. Rare examples are composed of several thin-walled cysts, resembling mucinous cystadenoma (Fig. 133).

Microscopic Features. The metastases resemble, to various extents, primary intestinal carcinomas, typically forming glands lined by poorly differentiated stratified epithelial cells lacking mucin and containing numerous mitotic figures. Necrosis is often present and can be extensive. It is often of the "dirty necrosis" type (Fig. 134), with centers of large, round aggregates composed of eosinophilic material containing abundant nuclear debris and viable glands surrounding the necrotic material in a garland arrangement (230,606). Occasionally, cystic glands lined by well-differentiated mucin-rich cells are prominent. Some tumors are colloid carcinomas. The stroma varies from negligible to abundant. It may be desmoplastic, edematous, or myxoid but often resembles ovarian stroma. Stromal lutein cells are present in about one-third of cases (607). Metastatic bowel cancers are among those most frequently associated with stromal luteinization; in such cases, steroid hormone production sometimes results in endocrine manifestations (607). The rare clear-cell adenocarcinoma of the intestine may also spread to the ovary and simulate secretory, endometrioid carcinoma or clear-cell adenocarcinoma (232).

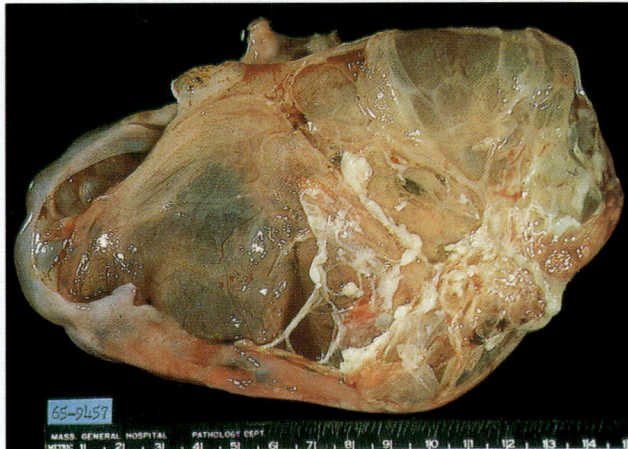

FIG. 133. Metastatic rectal carcinoma. This multicystic neoplasm simulates a mucinous cystadenoma.

Differential Diagnosis. The most difficult tumors to exclude on microscopic evaluation are primary mucinous and endometrioid carcinomas, the differential diagnoses of which have been discussed under those headings. Distinguishing metastatic intestinal clear-cell adenocarcinoma from primary clear-cell adenocarcinoma has also been covered under the latter heading.

Carcinoid Tumors

Carcinoid tumors account for approximately 2% of ovarian metastases (608). Almost all patients are older than 40

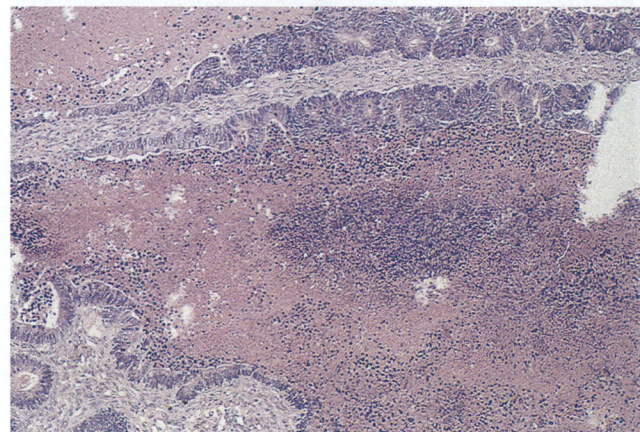

FIG. 134. Metastatic adenocarcinoma of the colon. Large masses of tumor show central "dirty" necrosis.

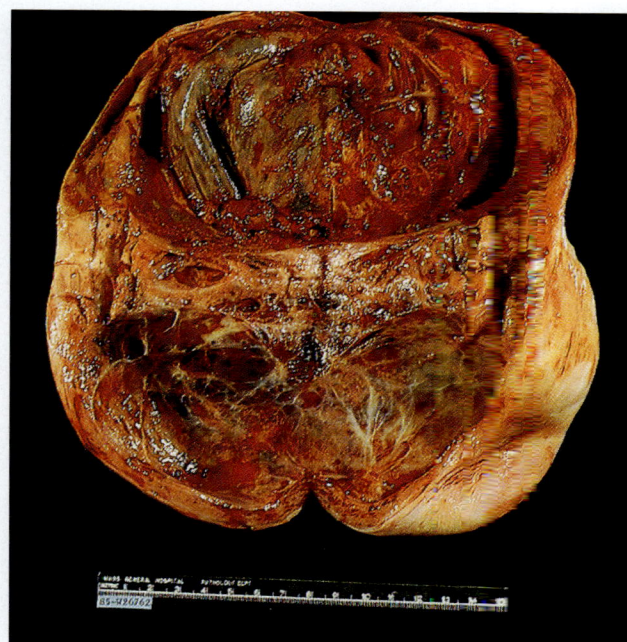

FIG. 135. Metastatic carcinoid tumor. The tumor is predominantly cystic with extensive hemorrhage.

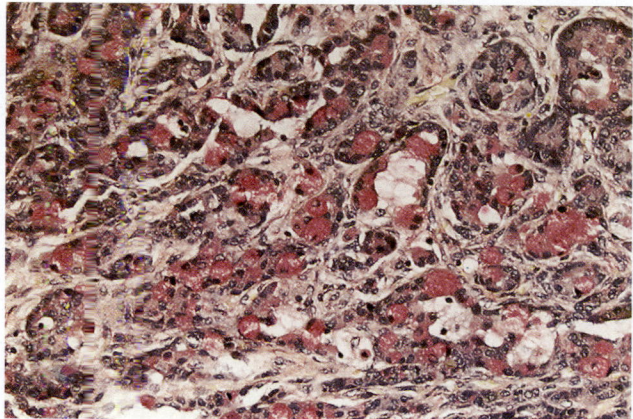

FIG. 137. Metastatic mucinous carcinoid. Note the staining of goblet cells for mucin (mucicarmine stain).

years of age; approximately half of them have the carcinoid syndrome. The ileum is usually the primary site but the cecum, jejunum, appendix, colon, stomach, pancreas, and bronchus are rare sources.

Gross Features. Metastatic carcinoids are usually bilateral. They vary in size and are solid, with smooth or bosselated serosal surfaces. Sectioning demonstrates single or confluent, firm, white or yellow nodules, which may resemble fibromas, thecomas, or Brenner tumors. The presence of numerous cysts filled with watery fluid in some cases causes the tumor to resemble a cystadenofibroma. Isolated tumors are predominantly a cystic (Fig. 135). Necrosis and hemorrhage may develop in solid tumors, and some of the cysts may contain blood.

Microscopic Features. An insular pattern is most common (Fig. 136), but trabecular and sometimes solid tubular patterns are also encountered. Small, round glands are typical; they often contain homogeneous eosinophilic secretion, which may calcify, sometimes forming psammoma bodies. Larger glands and cysts lined by one or a few layers of neoplastic cells are sometimes seen. With rare exceptions, carcinoid is the only ovarian metastatic tumor that can elicit a fibroma-like stromal proliferation, which may become extensively hyalinized. Metastatic goblet cell carcinoids have been predominantly of appendiceal origin. They are composed of rounded nests and glands that contain goblet cells and neuroendocrine cells (Figs. 137 and 138). They may also have foci resembling Krukenberg tumor and pools of mucin surrounding the glands and nests.

Differential Diagnosis. Metastatic carcinoids may be confused with primary carcinoid tumors (page 2368), GCTs, Sertoli tumors or SLCTs, Brenner tumors, adenofibromas, cystadenofibromas (benign, borderline, and malignant), and adenocarcinomas of various types. These differential diagnoses have been discussed under the relevant headings.

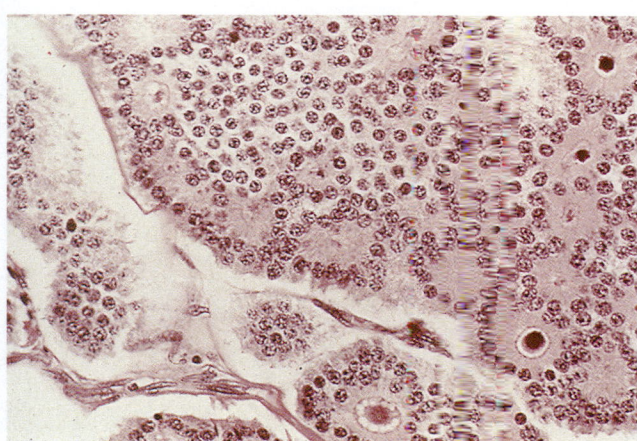

FIG. 136. Metastatic carcinoid tumor. Note round nuclei with coarse chromatin and acini containing inspissated secretion. (From ref. 135.)

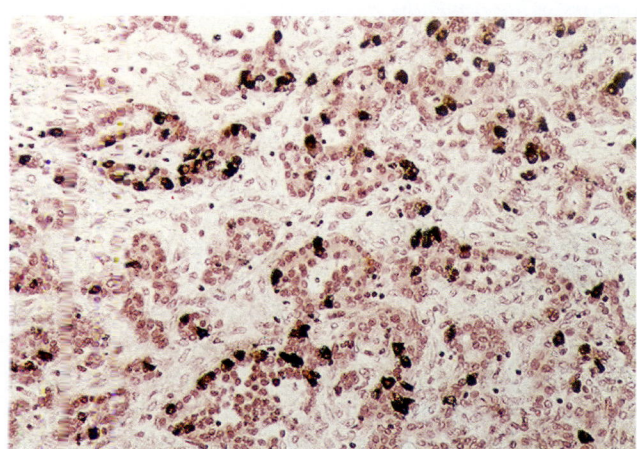

FIG. 138. Metastatic mucinous carcinoid. Note the staining of argentaffin granules (Masson-Fontana stain).

Breast Carcinoma

Approximately one-third of patients with breast cancer have ovarian metastases during the course of their disease (609,610). The involvement is bilateral in 60% to 80% of cases (611). About two-thirds of affected ovaries appear normal on gross examination (612). Only 2% to 11% of prophylactic oophorectomy specimens from patients with breast cancer contain metastases (605,613). Very rarely, metastatic breast carcinoma initially appears in the form of signs or symptoms of an ovarian tumor (614).

Gross Features. The ovaries often have irregular, nodular surfaces and typically contain firm or gritty white nodules of various sizes; cysts may be present, but only rare specimens are entirely cystic.

Microscopic Features. Lobular carcinomas, particularly those containing signet-ring cells, spread to the ovary more frequently than ductal carcinomas (615), but metastases of the latter tumor are more common because of their greater overall incidence. In many cases, a diffuse pattern is conspicuous at low magnification, but small clusters, cords, or ribbons of cells are usually apparent on high-power examination. The stroma varies from sparse to abundant; stromal luteinization is uncommon (616), in contrast to its incidence in metastatic intestinal carcinomas. Occasionally, the features are those of a Krukenberg tumor.

Differential Diagnosis. Rare, predominantly gland-forming, papillary, or poorly differentiated metastases may resemble surface epithelial carcinomas; an insular pattern may mimic that of a carcinoid tumor; and a diffuse pattern may suggest a lymphoma. Metastatic breast carcinomas have also been misinterpreted as GCTs, but the contrasting features of the neoplastic cells and especially of their nuclei, the differing patterns of growth, and the clinical findings facilitate its distinction in almost all cases. Immunohistochemical staining for gross cystic disease fluid protein 15 strongly suggests metastatic breast carcinoma over a primary ovarian carcinoma, whereas staining for CA125 favors an ovarian origin (177,181).

Tumors of the Appendix

Some metastatic appendiceal tumors have been adenocarcinomas of intestinal types, including signet-ring-cell and "colloid" types (617,618), but approximately one-fourth have been goblet cell carcinoids (619,620). The signet-ring-cell tumor metastases are generally of the Krukenberg type. Appendiceal primary tumors are often overlooked at operation because the ovarian tumors are typically much larger (618).

The association between low-grade mucinous cystic tumors of the appendix and coexisting, microscopically similar tumors of the ovary in cases of pseudomyxoma peritonei has been acknowledged for many years, but it has remained perplexing and the subject of controversy (621–628). This appendiceal lesion has been variously designated mucocele, mucinous cystadenoma, or low-grade mucinous cystadenocarcinoma. The ovarian tumors often have prominent mucinous cystadenoma-like areas, but when thoroughly sampled, they are usually found to contain foci of stratified epithelium suggestive of borderline malignancy. In this situation, pseudomyxoma peritonei, which is almost always present, has generally been attributed to the ovarian tumor, which has been considered primary and assigned an ovarian cancer stage.

Most investigators (621,625–628), however, have concluded that the appendiceal tumor is primary and the ovarian tumor(s) metastatic in the great majority of these cases. The findings supporting this conclusion are the histologic similarity of the appendiceal and ovarian tumors, the rate of bilateral ovarian involvement, the predominance of right-sided ovarian involvement when the tumor is unilateral, the usual presence of mucin and atypical mucinous cells on the ovarian surfaces, and a variety of immunohistochemical and molecular genetic findings in these cases (627,628). Although it may be difficult to distinguish ovarian tumors associated with pseudomyxoma peritonei from indisputable mucinous cystadenomas and cystadenomas of borderline malignancy in the absence of that disorder, the former tumors are much more often bilateral and may have a jelly-like consistency on gross examination; in addition, their mucinous lining cells are usually very tall, and they are always associated with pseudomyxoma ovarii (dissection of mucin, with or without tumor cells, into the stroma of the tumor).

Tumors of Pancreas and Gallbladder

Although spread of these tumors to the ovary is uncommon, even at autopsy, striking examples of clinically significant ovarian metastases have been encountered (629,630). The usual bilateral ovarian involvement is a helpful clue, since primary ovarian mucinous tumors are bilateral in less than 10% of cases. Additional features suggesting metastasis include extensive extraovarian tumor, ovarian surface implants (Fig. 139), and prominent vascular invasion within the

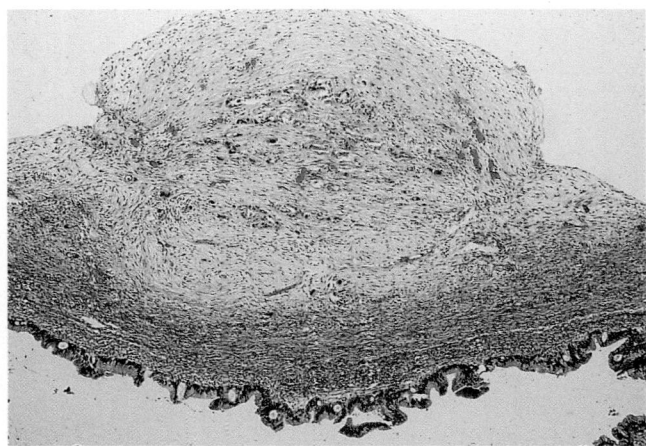

FIG. 139. Metastatic pancreatic adenocarcinoma. The cortical surface is involved by a surface implant showing infiltrating tumor cells associated with a stromal reaction that causes an elevation above the level of the adjacent cortex. Note the underlying cystic component of the metastatic cancer.

ovary. Often, the metastases contain large areas simulating borderline or benign mucinous ovarian neoplasia; less often, foci simulate endometrioid adenocarcinoma. Rare metastases from these organs are Krukenberg tumors (596).

Tumors of the Kidneys and Adrenal Glands

Despite the relative rarity of spread of renal cell carcinoma to the ovary, a few striking cases have been reported. Ten renal cell carcinomas associated with symptomatic ovarian metastases have been described (40,278). The patients were adults with an average age of 52 years. In six cases the ovarian tumor was discovered first, and in one of them, the primary renal tumor was not detected until 8 years after the ovarian tumor. The ovarian tumor in three cases was initially misdiagnosed as primary clear-cell carcinoma. The metastases ranged from 7 to 18 cm in greatest dimension; two were bilateral. Microscopic examination showed solid nests composed of clear epithelial cells or tubules lined by clear cells and containing intraluminal eosinophilic material or blood. A prominent sinusoidal vascular pattern was characteristically present. Mucin stains showed negative results. The latter two findings and the homogeneous clear-cell pattern without hobnail cells or other patterns of ovarian clear-cell carcinoma aid in recognizing these tumors as metastatic, but radiologic studies of the kidneys are necessary in some cases to make the differential diagnosis. One rhabdoid tumor of the kidney appeared as an ovarian mass before the renal neoplasm was discovered (631). Among adrenal gland tumors, neuroblastomas spread to the ovary most frequently. More than 25% are found to involve the ovary at autopsy (631,632). Rare patients are first diagnosed with ovarian metastases (631), which must be distinguished from immature teratomas with a predominant neuroblastoma component or the very rare pure primary ovarian neuroblastoma.

Tumors of the Urinary Bladder, Ureter, and Urethra

It may be difficult to distinguish between a urinary tract metastatic tumor and a borderline or malignant Brenner tumor or a primary ovarian transitional cell carcinoma (299), but immunohistochemical staining may be helpful in solving the problem (page 2341). Three signet-ring-cell carcinomas metastatic from the bladder have been Krukenberg tumors (299).

Malignant Melanoma

Ovarian involvement is often found at autopsy in patients with malignant melanoma, and clinically evident tumors are also encountered (335,633,634). In a study of 20 cases, the patients ranged in age from 21 to 60 years and usually showed signs of abdominal swelling or pain (335). Approximately half the patients also had extraovarian metastases, usually within the pelvis and upper abdomen. Five patients had no known history of cutaneous melanoma, which may have regressed spontaneously in some of them. The ovarian metastases were bilateral in nine cases and ranged up to 20 cm in greatest dimension. Most of them were not grossly pigmented. The most common microscopic appearance is that of large cells with abundant eosinophilic cytoplasm growing diffusely or in nodular aggregates. Occasionally, however, small cells with scanty cytoplasm predominate; in some cases spindle cells are present, but they rarely predominate. Growth in discrete rounded aggregates with a nevoid appearance is helpful diagnostically. A confusing feature is the presence of follicle-like spaces (Fig. 140). Nine of the tumors contained intracytoplasmic melanin pigment, and in cases studied immunohistochemically, most of the tumor cells were positive for S-100 protein and many of them for HMB-45.

Differential Diagnosis. Metastatic melanoma must be distinguished from the rare primary ovarian melanomas that arise in the wall of a dermoid cyst, sometimes accompanied by junctional activity beneath the squamous lining of the cyst. Recognition of teratomatous elements is important in establishing the primary nature of a melanoma. Most melanomas metastatic to the ovary have been primary in the skin, but some have arisen in the choroid or elsewhere.

Metastatic melanomas may closely resemble lipid-poor steroid cell tumors or pregnancy luteomas. Melanin can be misinterpreted as lipochrome pigment, which may be a feature of steroid cell tumors. Sometimes, small cells with scanty cytoplasm and nuclear grooves result in a resemblance to AGCT. In one report (634), three of ten metastatic melanomas were initially misinterpreted as sex cord–stromal tumors. The follicle-like spaces (Fig. 140) of metastatic melanoma (335) can lead to confusion with JGCT or small-cell carcinoma of the hypercalcemic type, as discussed under those headings.

Miscellaneous Other Ovarian Metastases of Nongenital Origin

Approximately 5% of women with pulmonary carcinomas are found to have ovarian metastases at autopsy (635), but symptomatic metastases are rare. Unusual metastases to the

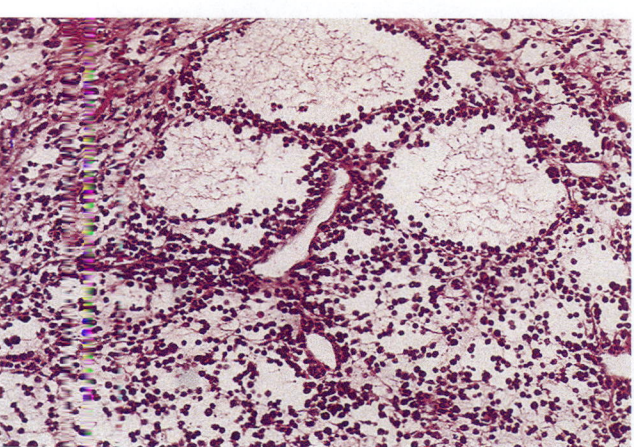

FIG. 140. Metastatic malignant melanoma. Note the follicle-like spaces.

ovary have included small-cell carcinomas from sites other than the lung (636), adenoid cystic carcinoma of salivary gland origin (593,637), alveolar and embryonal rhabdomyosarcomas (586), leiomyosarcoma, hemangiosarcoma, Ewing's sarcoma, chondrosarcoma, osteogenic sarcoma (265), and chordoma (638).

Tumors of the Uterine Corpus, Cervix, and Fallopian Tube

Endometrial Carcinoma. Ovarian involvement by endometrial carcinoma has been reported in 34% to 40% of autopsy cases (639,640) and 5% to 15% of hysterectomy specimens. The differentiation of metastatic endometrial and primary endometrioid carcinoma of the ovary has been discussed on page 2333.

Uterine Sarcomas. The differentiation of metastatic endometrial from primary endometrioid sarcoma of the ovary has been discussed on page 2334.

Cervical Carcinoma. Mucinous adenocarcinomas of the cervix appear to be associated with ovarian tumors of similar type more frequently than squamous cell carcinomas and other adenocarcinomas (185–187). In one series, 10% of cervical mucinous adenocarcinomas were accompanied by similar ovarian tumors (187). In such cases, it may be difficult to determine whether the tumors are metastatic from one organ to the other or independent primary tumors. Consideration of the criteria used in diagnosing coexistent ovarian and corpus carcinomas and in evaluating metastatic tumors in general usually allow distinctions to be made.

Less than 1% of cervical squamous cell carcinomas metastasize to the ovary (309). The occasional association of ovarian squamous cell carcinoma with squamous cell carcinoma *in situ* of the cervix suggests that in exceptional cases, invasive squamous cell carcinomas of both organs may be separate primary tumors. Cervical adenosquamous carcinoma, undifferentiated carcinoma, and transitional cell carcinoma metastatic to the ovary have also been documented (309). Cervical carcinomas of the neuroendocrine type, either small-cell carcinoma or carcinoma of the intermediate type, have also metastasized to the ovary, sometimes resulting in misdiagnosis as a primary ovarian tumor, including one example as in a small-cell carcinoma of the hypercalcemic type (309).

Trophoblastic Tumors. Up to 22% of uterine choriocarcinomas spread to the ovary (617). It may be impossible to discriminate between primary ovarian choriocarcinoma of either gestational or germ cell origin and metastasis from a uterine choriocarcinoma that has regressed. The tumor should be thoroughly sampled in an attempt to discover teratomatous elements, thus establishing a germ cell origin. Invasive hydatidiform mole and placental site trophoblastic tumor have also been found to spread to the ovary (617).

Carcinoma of the Fallopian Tube. The ovary is involved in approximately 13% of carcinomas of unquestionable tubal origin, usually by direct extension (641). Determination of whether a carcinoma affecting both organs is primary in one or the other is generally made on the basis of the gross pathologic findings. If they yield an equivocal answer, the tumor is usually considered to be a primary ovarian carcinoma because of its much greater incidence. Recent screening results, however, suggest that an ovarian origin may be too often diagnosed in that situation (642). Perhaps the term tubo-ovarian carcinoma would be more accurate in questionable cases (643). Because most tubal carcinomas resemble serous or undifferentiated carcinomas of the ovary, microscopic examination is rarely helpful in establishing a primary site. Primary mucinous and clear-cell carcinomas of the tube are rare, however, and tumors of these types involving both organs are therefore probably of ovarian origin (644).

REFERENCES

1. Clement PB. Histology of the ovary. In: Sternberg SS, ed. *Histology for pathologists*, 2nd ed. Philadelphia: Lippincott–Raven Publishers, 1997.
2. Quan A, Charles D, Craig JM. Histologic and functional consequences of periovarian adhesions. *Obstet Gynecol* 1963;22:96–101.
3. Willson JB, Black JR. Ovarian abscess. *Am J Obstet Gynecol* 1964;90:34–43.
4. Lipscomb GH, Ling FW, Photopulos GJ. Ovarian abscess arising within an endometrioma. *Obstet Gynecol* 1991;78:951–954.
5. Mickal A, Sellman AH, Beebe JL. Ruptured tuboovarian abscess. *Am J Obstet Gynecol* 1968;100:432–436.
6. Simstein NL. Colo-tubo-ovarian fistula as complication of pelvic inflammatory disease. *South J Med* 1981;74:512–513.
7. London AM, Burkman RT. Tuboovarian abscess with associated rupture with fistula formation into the urinary bladder. *Am J Obstet Gynecol* 1979;135:1113–1114.
8. Claman P, Dover M, Saginur R, Tao H, Orizaga M. Spontaneous ovarian-to-vaginal fistula: a case report. *Am J Obstet Gynecol* 1991;164:71–72.
9. Pace EH, Voet EH, Melancon JT. Xanthogranulomatous oophoritis: an inflammatory pseudotumor of the ovary. *Int J Gynecol Pathol* 1984;3:398–402.
10. Shalev E, Zuckerman H, Rizescu I. Pelvic inflammatory pseudotumor (xanthogranuloma). *Acta Obstet Gynecol Scand* 1982;61:285–286.
11. Bhagavan BS, Gupta PK. Genital actinomycosis and intrauterine contraceptive devices. *Hum Pathol* 1978;9:567–578.
12. Schmidt WA, Bedrossian CWM, Ali V, et al. Actinomycosis and intrauterine devices. *Diagn Gynecol Obstet* 1980;2:165–177.
13. Schmidt WA. IUDs, inflammation, and infection: assessment after two decades of IUD use. *Hum Pathol* 1982;13:878–881.
14. Muller-Holzner E, Ruth NR, Abfalter E, et al. IUD-associated pelvic actinomycosis: a report of five cases. *Int J Gynecol Pathol* 1995;14:70–74.
15. Pine L, Curtis EM, Brown JM. Actinomyces and the intrauterine contraceptive device: aspects of the fluorescent antibody stain. *Am J Obstet Gynecol* 1985;152:287–290.
16. Nogales-Ortiz F, Taracon I, Nogales FF. The pathology of female genital tract tuberculosis. *Obstet Gynecol* 1979;53:422–428.
17. Sutherland AM. Postmenopausal tuberculosis of the female genital tract. *Obstet Gynecol* 1982;59:54S–57S.
18. Chalvardjian A, Picard L, Shaw R, et al. Malacoplakia of the female genital tract. *Am J Obstet Gynecol* 1980;138:391–394.
19. Clement PB. Nonneoplastic lesions of the ovary. In: Kurman RJ, ed. *Blaustein's pathology of the female genital tract*, 4th ed. New York: Springer-Verlag, 1994:597–645.
20. Tiboldi T. Involvement of human and primate ovaries in schistosomiasis: a review of the literature. *Ann Soc Belg Med Trop* 1978;58:9–20.
21. McMahon JN, Connolly CE, Long SV, et al. Enterobius granulomas of the uterus, ovary and pelvic peritoneum: two case reports. *Br J Obstet Gynaecol* 1984;91:289–290.
22. Hangval H, Habibi H, Moshref A, et al. Case report of an ovarian hydatid cyst. *J Trop Med Hyg* 1979;82:34–35.

23. Subietas A, Deppisch LM, Astarloa J. Cytomegalovirus oophoritis: ovarian cortical necrosis. *Hum Pathol* 1977;8:285–292.
24. Williams DJ, Connor P, Ironside JW. Pre-menopausal cytomegalovirus oophoritis. *Histopathology* 1990;16:405–407.
25. Nissim F, Ashkenazy M, Borenstein R, et al. Tuberculoid cornstarch granulomas with caseous necrosis: a diagnostic challenge. *Arch Pathol Lab Med* 1981;105:86–88.
26. Mostofa SAM, Bargeron CB, Flower RW, et al. Foreign body granulomas in normal ovaries. *Obstet Gynecol* 1985;66:701–702.
27. Teilum G, Madsen V. Endometriosis ovarii et peritonei caused by hysterosalpingography. *Br J Obstet Gynaecol* 1950;57:10–15.
28. Kim KR, Scully RE. Peritoneal keratin granulomas with carcinomas of endometrium and ovary and atypical polypoid adenomyoma of endometrium: a clinicopathological analysis of 22 cases. *Am J Surg Pathol* 1990;14:925–932.
29. Gilks CB, Clement PB. Colo-ovarian fistula: a report of two cases. *Obstet Gynecol* 1987;69:533–537.
30. Herbold DR, Frable WJ, Kraus FT. Isolated noninfectious granuloma of the ovary. *Int J Gynecol Pathol* 1984;2:380–391.
31. Kernohan NM, Best PV, Jandial V, Kitchener HC. Palisading granuloma of the ovary. *Histopathology* 1991;19:279–280.
32. Tatum ET, Beattie JF Jr, Bryson K. Postoperative carbon pigment granuloma: a report of eight cases involving the ovary. *Hum Pathol* 1996;27:1008–1011.
33. Chalvardjian A. Sarcoidosis of the female genital tract. *Am J Obstet Gynecol* 1978;132:78–80.
34. Honore LH. Combined suppurative and noncaseating granulomatous oophoritis combined with distal ileitis (Crohn's disease). *Eur J Obstet Gynecol Reprod Biol* 1981;12:91–94.
35. Hughesdon PE. The endometrial identity of benign stromatosis of the ovary and its relation to other forms of endometriosis. *J Pathol* 1976;119:201–209.
36. Blaustein A. Surface cells and inclusion cysts in fetal ovaries. *Gynecol Oncol* 1981;12:222–233.
37. Blaustein A, Kantius M, Kaganowicz A, et al. Inclusions in ovaries of females aged day 1–30 years. *Int J Gynecol Pathol* 1982;1:145–153.
38. Mulligan RM. A survey of epithelial inclusions in the ovarian cortex of 470 patients. *J Surg Oncol* 1976;8:61–66.
39. Scully RE. Ovary. In: Henson DE, Albores-Saavedra J, eds. *The pathology of incipient neoplasia*, 2nd ed. Philadelphia: WB Saunders, 1993:283–300.
40. Scully RE, Young RH, Clement PB. Tumors of the ovary, maldeveloped gonads, fallopian tube and broad ligament. In: *Atlas of tumor pathology*, 3rd series, fascicle 23. Washington, D.C.: Armed Forces Institute of Pathology, 1998 (in press).
41. Clement PB, Young RH. Florid mesothelial hyperplasia associated with ovarian tumors: a potential source of error in tumor diagnosis and staging. *Int J Gynecol Pathol* 1993;12:51–58.
42. Brune WH, Pulaski EJ, Shuey HE. Giant ovarian cyst: report of a case in a premature infant. *N Engl J Med* 1957;257:876–878.
43. Landrum B, Ogburn PL Jr, Feinberg S, et al. Intrauterine aspiration of a large fetal ovarian cyst. *Obstet Gynecol* 1986;68:11S–14S.
44. Piver MS, Williams LJ, Marcuse PM. Influence of luteal cysts on menstrual function. *Obstet Gynecol* 1970;35:740–751.
45. Stevens ML, Plotka ED. Functional lutein cyst in a postmenopausal woman. *Obstet Gynecol* 1977;50:27S–29S.
46. Strickler RC, Kelly RW, Askin FB. Postmenopausal ovarian follicle cyst: an unusual cause of estrogen excess. *Int J Gynecol Pathol* 1984;3:318–322.
47. Miles PA, Penney LL. Corpus luteum formation in the fetus. *Obstet Gynecol* 1983;81:525–529.
48. Kosloske AM, Goldthorn JF, Kaufman E, et al. Treatment of precocious pseudopuberty associated with follicular cysts of the ovary. *Am J Dis Child* 1984;138:147–149.
49. Hallatt JG, Steele CH Jr, Snyder M. Ruptured corpus luteum with hemoperitoneum: a study of 173 surgical cases. *Am J Obstet Gynecol* 1984;149:5–9.
50. Payan HM, Gilbert EF. Mesenteric cyst–ovarian implant syndrome. *Arch Pathol Lab Med* 1987;111:282–284.
51. Monteleone JA, Monteleone PL, Danis RK. Pseudoprecocious puberty associated with isolated follicle cyst of the ovary. *J Pediatr Surg* 1973;8:949–950.
52. Danon M, Robboy SJ, Kim S, et al. Cushing's syndrome, sexual precocity and polyostotic fibrous dysplasia (Albright syndrome) in infancy. *J Pediatr* 1975;87:917–921.
53. Clement PB, Scully RE. Large solitary luteinized follicle cyst of pregnancy and puerperium. *Am J Surg Pathol* 1980;4:431–438.
54. Caspi E, Schreyer P, Bukovsky J. Ovarian lutein cysts in pregnancy. *Obstet Gynecol* 1973;42:388–398.
55. Girouard DP, Barclay DL, Collins CG. Hyperreactio luteinalis: review of the literature and report of 2 cases. *Obstet Gynecol* 1964;23:513–525.
56. Santen NA, Smith JP, Rutledge FN, et al. Plasma testosterone levels in trophoblastic disease and the effects of oophorectomy and chemotherapy. *J Clin Endocrinol Metab* 1972;34:558–561.
57. Bared DH, Gimovsky ML, Petrie RH, et al. Diagnosis and management of bilateral theca lutein cysts in a normal term pregnancy. *Diagn Gynecol Obstet* 1981;3:27–30.
58. Wajda KJ, Lucas JG, Marsh WL. Hyperreactio luteinalis: benign disorder masquerading as an ovarian neoplasm. *Arch Pathol Lab Med* 1989;113:921–925.
59. Planner RS, Abell DA, Barbaro CA, et al. Massive enlargement of the ovaries after evacuation of hydatidiform moles. *Aust N Z J Obstet Gynaecol* 1982;22:96–100.
60. Berger NG, Repke JT, Woodruff JD. Markedly elevated serum testosterone in pregnancy without fetal virilization. *Obstet Gynecol* 1984;63:260–262.
61. Haning RV Jr, Strawn EY, Nolten WE. Pathophysiology of the ovarian hyperstimulation syndrome. *Obstet Gynecol* 1985;66:220–224.
62. Golan A, Ron-el R, Herman A, Soffer Y, Weinraub Z, Caspi E. Ovarian hyperstimulation syndrome: an update review. *Obstet Gynecol Surv* 1989;44:430–440.
63. Clement PB, Young RH, Scully RE. Ovarian granulosa cell proliferations of pregnancy: a report of nine cases. *Hum Pathol* 1988;19:657–662.
64. Futterweit W. *Polycystic ovarian disease: clinical perspectives in obstetrics and gynecology*. New York: Springer Verlag, 1985.
65. Franks S. Polycystic ovary syndrome. *N Engl J Med* 1995;333:853–861.
66. Waterworth DM, Bennett ST, Gharani N, et al. Linkage and association of insulin gene VNTR regulatory polymorphism with polycystic ovary syndrome. *Lancet* 1997;349:986–990.
67. Gallup DG, Stock RJ. Adenocarcinoma of the endometrium in women 40 years of age or younger. *Obstet Gynecol* 1984;64:417–419.
68. Ramzy I, Nisker JA. Histologic study of ovaries from young women with endometrial adenocarcinoma. *Am J Clin Pathol* 1979;71:253–256.
69. Hughesdon PE. Morphology and morphogenesis of the Stein-Leventhal ovary and of so-called "hyperthecosis." *Obstet Gynecol Surv* 1982;37:59–77.
70. Plate WP. Ovarian changes after long-term oral contraception. *Acta Endocrinol* 1976;55:71–77.
71. Ryan GM, Craig J, Reid DE. Histology of the uterus and ovaries after long-term cyclic norethynodrel therapy. *Am J Obstet Gynecol* 1964;90:715–725.
72. Boss JH, Scully RE, Wegner KH, et al. Structural variations in the adult ovary: clinical significance. *Obstet Gynecol* 1965;25:747–763.
73. Snowden JA, Harkin PJR, Thornton JG, Wells M. Morphometric assessment of ovarian stromal proliferation: a clinicopathological study. *Histopathology* 1989;14:369–379.
74. Scully RE, Cohen RB. Oxidative-enzyme activity in normal and pathologic human ovaries. *Obstet Gynecol* 1964;24:667–681.
75. Braithwaite SS, Erkman-Balis B, Avila TD. Postmenopausal virilization due to ovarian stromal hyperthecosis. *J Clin Endocrinol Metab* 1978;46:295–300.
76. Maccio G, Tieu TM, Aiman J. Atypical ovarian hyperthecosis in a virilized postmenopausal woman. *Am J Clin Pathol* 1985;83:101–107.
77. Barbieri RL, Ryan KJ. Hyperandrogenism, insulin resistance, and acanthosis nigricans syndrome: a common endocrinopathy with distinct pathophysiologic features. *Am J Obstet Gynecol* 1983;147:90–101.
78. Sternberg WH, Sneeden VD, Fearl JD. A clinical and pathologic review of ovarian stromal hyperplasia and its possible relationship to common diseases of the female reproductive system. *Am J Obstet Gynecol* 1974;119:375–381.
79. Judd HL, Scully RE, Herbst AL, et al. Familial hyperthecosis: comparison of endocrinologic and histologic findings with polycystic ovarian disease. *Am J Obstet Gynecol* 1973;117:976–982.
80. Nagamari M, Lingold JC, Gomez JR, et al. Clinical and hormonal studies in hyperthecosis of the ovaries. *Fertil Steril* 1981;36:326–332.

81. Scully RE. Smooth-muscle differentiation in genital tract disorders [Editorial]. *Arch Pathol Lab Med* 1981;105:505–507.
82. Sternberg WH, Roth LM. Ovarian stromal tumors containing Leydig cells. I. Stromal-Leydig cell tumor and non-neoplastic transformation of ovarian stroma to Leydig cells. *Cancer* 1973;32:940–951.
83. Roth LM, Sternberg WH. Ovarian stromal tumors containing Leydig cells. II. Pure Leydig cell tumor, non-hilar type. *Cancer* 1973;32:952–960.
84. Scully RE. Stromal luteoma of the ovary. *Cancer* 1964;17:769–778.
85. Givens JR, Kerber IJ, Wiser WL, Anderson RN, Coleman SA, Fish SA. Remission of acanthosis nigricans associated with polycystic ovarian disease and a stromal luteoma. *J Clin Endocrinol Metab* 1974;38:347–355.
86. Dunaif A, Hoffman AR, Scully RE, et al. Clinical, biochemical, and ovarian morphologic findings in women with acanthosis nigricans and masculinization. *Obstet Gynecol* 1985;66:545–552.
87. Kalstone CE, Jaffe RB, Abell MR. Massive edema of the ovary simulating fibroma. *Obstet Gynecol* 1969;34:564–571.
88. Young RH, Scully RE. Fibromatosis and massive edema of the ovary, possibly related entities: a report of 14 cases of fibromatosis and 11 cases of massive edema. *Int J Gynecol Pathol* 1984;3:153–178.
89. Yüce K, Yücel A, Tanir M, Ayhan A, Ayhan A. Massive bilateral ovarian edema: report of 2 cases. *Eur J Gynaecol Oncol* 1998; 19:305–309.
90. Sternberg WH, Barclay DL. Luteoma of pregnancy. *Am J Obstet Gynecol* 1966;95:165–181.
91. Norris HJ, Taylor HB. Nodular theca-lutein hyperplasia of pregnancy (so-called "pregnancy luteoma"): a clinical and pathologic study of 15 cases. *Am J Clin Pathol* 1967;47:557–566.
92. Rice BF, Barclay DL, Sternberg WH. Luteoma of pregnancy. *Am J Obstet Gynecol* 1969;104:871–878.
93. Hensleigh PA, Woodruff JD. Differential maternal-fetal response to androgenizing luteoma or hyperreaction luteinalis. *Obstet Gynecol Surv* 1978;33:262–271.
94. Malinak LR, Miller GV. Bilateral multicentric ovarian luteomas of pregnancy associated with masculinization of a female infant. *Am J Obstet Gynecol* 1965;91:251–259.
95. Sternberg WH. The morphology, androgenic function, hyperplasia, and tumours of the human ovarian hilus cells. *Am J Pathol* 1949;25:493–521.
96. Sternberg WH, Segaloff A, Gaskill CJ. Influence of chorionic gonadotropin on human ovarian hilus cells (Leydig-like cells). *J Clin Endocrinol Metab* 1953;13:139–153.
97. Davidson BJ, Waisman J, Judd HL. Long-standing virilism in a woman with hyperplasia and neoplasia of ovarian lipidic cells. *Obstet Gynecol* 1981;58:753–759.
98. Meldrum DR, Frumar AM, Shamonki IM, et al. Ovarian and adrenal steroidogenesis in a virilized patient with gonadotropin-resistant ovaries and hilus cell hyperplasia. *Obstet Gynecol* 1980;56:216–221.
99. Rutgers JL, Scully RE. Functioning ovarian tumors with peripheral steroid cell proliferation: a report of twenty-four cases. *Int J Gynecol Pathol* 1986;5:319–337.
100. Bersch W, Alexy E, Heuser HP, et al. Ectopic decidua formation in the ovary (so-called deciduoma). *Virchows Arch A Pathol Anat Histopathol* 1973;360:173–177.
101. Herr JC, Heidger PM Jr, Scott JR, et al. Decidual cells in the human ovary at term. I. Incidence, gross anatomy and ultrastructural features of merocrine secretion. *Am J Anat* 1978;152:7–28.
102. Rewell RE. Extra-uterine decidua. *J Pathol* 1972;105:219–222.
103. Starup J, Visfeldt J. Ovarian morphology in early and late human pregnancy. *Acta Obstet Gynecol Scand* 1974;53:211–218.
104. Clement PB, Young RH, Scully RE. Nontrophoblastic pathology of the female genital tract and peritoneum associated with pregnancy. *Semin Diagn Pathol* 1989;6:372–406.
105. Ober WB, Grady HG, Schoenbucher AK. Ectopic ovarian decidua without pregnancy. *Am J Pathol* 1957;33:199–217.
106. Israel SL, Rubenstone A, Meranze DR. The ovary at term. I. Decidua-like reaction and surface cell proliferation. *Obstet Gynecol* 1954;3:399–407.
107. Herr JC, Platz CE, Heidger PM Jr, et al. Smooth muscle within ovarian decidual nodules: a link to leiomyomatosis peritonealis disseminata? *Obstet Gynecol* 1979;53:451–456.
108. Honore LH, O'Hara KE. Subcapsular adipocytic infiltration of the human ovary: a clinicopathological study of eight cases. *Eur J Obstet Gynecol Reprod Biol* 1980;10:13–20.
109. Shipton EA, Meares SD. Heterotopic bone formation in the ovary. *Aust N Z J Obstet Gynaecol* 1965;5:100–102.
110. Russell P, Bannatyne P, Sherman RP, et al. Premature hypergonadotropic ovarian failure: clinicopathological study of 19 cases. *Int J Gynecol Pathol* 1982;1:185–201.
111. Scully RE. Gonadal pathology of genetically determined diseases. In: Kraus FT, Damjanov I, eds. *The pathology of reproductive failure*. Baltimore: Williams and Wilkins, 1991:257–285. (International Academy of Pathology monograph no. 33).
112. Board JA, Redwine FO, Moncure CW, et al. Identification of differing etiologies of clinically diagnosed premature menopause. *Am J Obstet Gynecol* 1979;134:936–944.
113. Aiman J, Smentek C. Premature ovarian failure. *Obstet Gynecol* 1985;66:9–14.
114. Koninckx PR, Brosens IA. The "gonadotropin-resistant ovary" syndrome as a cause of secondary amenorrhea and infertility. *Fertil Steril* 1977;28:926–931.
115. Gloor E, Juillard E, Curchod A, et al. Ovarian hypoplasia with follicular calcifications. *Am J Clin Pathol* 1982;78:857–860.
116. Talbert LM, Raj MHG, Hammond MG, et al. Endocrine and immunologic studies in a patient with resistant ovary syndrome. *Fertil Steril* 1984;42:741–744.
117. Case Records of Massachusetts General Hospital. Case 46—1986. *N Engl J Med* 1986;315:1336–1343.
118. Coulam CB, Kempers RD, Randall RV. Premature ovarian failure: evidence for autoimmune function. *Fertil Steril* 1981;36:238–240.
119. Gloor E, Hurlimann J. Autoimmune oophoritis. *Am J Clin Pathol* 1984;81:105–109.
120. Sedmak DD, Hart WR, Tubbs RR. Autoimmune oophoritis: a histopathologic study of involved ovaries with immunologic characterization of the mononuclear cell infiltrate. *Int J Gynecol Pathol* 1987;6:73–81.
121. Lonsdale RN, Roberts PF, Trowell JE. Autoimmune oophoritis associated with polycystic ovaries. *Histopathology* 1991;19:77–81.
122. Bannatyne P, Russell P, Shearman RP. Autoimmune oophoritis: a clinicopathologic assessment of 12 cases. *Int J Gynecol Pathol* 1990;9:191–207.
123. Biscotti CV, Hart WR, Lucas JG. Cystic ovarian enlargement resulting from autoimmune oophoritis. *Obstet Gynecol* 1989;74:492.
124. Irvine WJ, Chan MMW, Scarth L, et al. Immunological aspects of premature ovarian failure associated with idiopathic Addison's disease. *Lancet* 1968;2:883–887.
125. Irvine WJ, Chan MMW, Scarth L. The further characterization of autoantibodies reactive with extra-adrenal steroid-producing cells in patients with adrenal disorders. *Clin Exp Immunol* 1969;4:489–503.
126. Reuhsen MDM, Blizzard RM, Garcia-Bunuel R, et al. Autoimmunity and ovarian failure. *Am J Obstet Gynecol* 1972;112:693–703.
127. Irvine WJ, Barnes EW. Addison's disease, ovarian failure and hypoparathyroidism. *Clin Endocrinol Metab* 1975;4:379–433.
128. Coulam CB, Ryan RJ. Premature menopause I. Etiology. *Am J Obstet Gynecol* 1979;133:639–643.
129. Coulam CB. The prevalence of autoimmune disorders among patients with primary ovarian failure. *Am J Reprod Immunol* 1983;4:63–66.
130. Damewood MD, Zacur HA, Hoffman GJ, et al. Circulating antiovarian antibodies in premature ovarian failure. *Obstet Gynecol* 1986;68:850–854.
131. Alper MM, Garner PR. Premature ovarian failure: its relationship to autoimmune disease. *Obstet Gynecol* 1985;66:27–30.
132. Clement PB, Cooney TP. Idiopathic multifocal calcification of the ovarian stroma. *Arch Pathol Lab Med* 1992;116:204–205.
133. Koonings PP, Campbell K, Mishell DR Jr, Grimes DA. Relative frequency of primary ovarian neoplasms: a 10-year review. *Obstet Gynecol* 1989;74:921–926.
134. Beahrs OH, Henson DE, Hutter RV, Kennedy BJ, eds. *Manual for staging of cancer*, 4th ed. Philadelphia: JB Lippincott Co, 1992.
135. Scully RE. *International histological classification of tumours: histological typing of ovarian tumours*, 2nd ed. Heidelberg: Springer-Verlag, 1998 (*in press*).
136. Taylor HC Jr. Studies in the clinical and biological evolution of adenocarcinoma of the ovary. *J Obstet Gynecol Br Commonw* 1959;66:827–842.
137. Hart WR. Ovarian epithelial tumors of borderline malignancy (carcinomas of low malignant potential). *Hum Pathol* 1977;8:541–549.
138. Katzenstein A-LA, Mazur MT, Morgan TE, Kao MS. Proliferative serous tumors of the ovary. *Am J Surg Pathol* 1978;2:339–355.

139. Russell P. The pathological assessment of ovarian neoplasms. III. The malignant "epithelial" tumors. *Pathology* 1979;11:493–532.
140. Bostwick DG, Tazelaar HD, Ballon SC, Hendrickson MR, Kempson RL. Ovarian epithelial tumors of borderline malignancy a clinical and pathologic study of 109 cases. *Cancer* 1986;58:2052–2065.
141. Bell DA, Scully RE. Clinical perspectives on borderline tumors of the ovary. In: Stenchever MA, ed. *Current topics in obstetrics and gynecology.* New York: Elsevier Science Publishing, 1991: 119–134.
142. Longacre TA, Kempson RL, Hendrickson MR. Well-differentiated serous neoplasms of the ovary. In: *State of the art reviews: pathology, surface epithelial neoplasms of the ovary,* vol. 1. Philadelphia: Hanley & Belfus, 1992:255–306.
143. DeNictolis M, Montironi R, Tommasoni S, et al. Serous borderline tumors of the ovary: a clinicopathologic, immunohistochemical, and quantitative study of 44 cases. *Cancer* 1992;70:152–160.
144. Kurman RJ, Trimble CL. The behavior of serous tumors of low malignant potential: Are they ever malignant? *Int J Gynecol Pathol* 1993;12:120–127.
145. Barnhill DR, Kurman RJ, Brady MF, et al. The behavior of stage I ovarian serous tumors of low malignant potential: a Gynecologic Oncology Group study. *Trans Am Gynecol Obstet Soc* 1995;12: 35–42.
146. Kennedy AW, Hart WR. Ovarian papillary serous tumors of low malignant potential (serous borderline tumors): a long-term follow-up study, including patients with microinvasion, lymph node metastasis, and transformation to invasive serous carcinoma. *Cancer* 1996;78:278–286.
147. Silva EG, Kurman RJ, Russell P, Scully RE. Symposium: ovarian tumors of borderline malignancy. *Int J Gynecol Pathol* 1996; 15:281–302.
148. McCaughey WTE, Kirk ME, Lester W, Dardick I. Peritoneal epithelial lesions associated with proliferative serous tumours of the ovary. *Histopathology* 1984;8:195–208.
149. Michael H, Roth LM. Invasive and noninvasive implants in ovarian serous tumors of low malignant potential. *Cancer* 1986;57: 1240–1247.
150. Bell DA, Weinstock MA, Scully RE. Peritoneal implants of ovarian serous borderline tumors: histologic features and prognosis. *Cancer* 1988;62:2212–2222.
151. Gershenson DM, Silva EG. Serous ovarian tumors of low malignant potential with peritoneal implants. *Cancer* 1990;65:578–585.
152. Segal GH, Hart WR. Ovarian serous tumors of low malignant potential (serous borderline tumors): the relationship of exophytic surface tumor to peritoneal "implants." *Am J Surg Pathol* 1992;16:577–583.
153. Rice LW, Berkowitz RS, Mark SD, Yavner DL, Lange JM. Epithelial ovarian tumors of borderline malignancy. *Gynecol Oncol* 1990;39:195–198.
154. Leake JF, Rader JS, Woodruff JD, Rosenshein NB. Retroperitoneal lymphatic involvement with epithelial ovarian tumors of low malignant potential. *Gynecol Oncol* 1991;42:124–130.
155. DiRe F, Paladini D, Fontanelli R, Feudale EA, Raspagliesi F. Surgical staging for epithelial ovarian tumors of low malignant potential. *Int J Gynecol Cancer* 1994;4:310–314.
156. Tan LK, Flynn SD, Carcangiu ML. Ovarian serous borderline tumors with lymph node involvement: clinicopathologic and DNA content study of seven cases and review of the literature. *Am J Surg Pathol* 1994;18:904–912.
157. Bell DA, Scully RE. Early de novo ovarian carcinoma: a study of fourteen cases. *Cancer* 1994;73:1859–1864.
158. Burks RT, Sherman ME, Kurman RJ. Micropapillary serous carcinoma of the ovary: a distinctive low-grade carcinoma related to serous borderline tumors. *Am J Surg Pathol* 1996;20:319–330.
159. Seidman JD, Kurman RJ. Subclassification of serous borderline tumors of the ovary into benign and malignant types: a clinicopathologic study of 65 advanced stage cases. *Am J Surg Pathol* 1996; 20:1331–1345.
160. Eichhorn JE, Bell DA, Young RH, Scully RE. Ovarian serous borderline tumors with micropapillary and cribriform patterns: a study of 40 cases and comparison with 44 cases without these patterns. *Am J Surg Pathol* 1998 (*in press*).
161. Tavassoli FA. Serous tumor of low malignant potential with early stromal invasion (serous LMP and microinvasion). *Mod Pathol* 1988;1:407–414.
162. Bell DA, Scully RE. Ovarian serous borderline tumors with stromal microinvasion: a report of 21 cases. *Hum Pathol* 1990;21:397–403.
163. Nayar R, Siriaunkgul S, Robbins KM, McGowan L, Ginzan S, Silverberg SG. Microinvasion in low malignant potential tumors of the ovary. *Hum Pathol* 1996;27:521–527.
164. Tsao SW, Mok SCH, Knapp RC, et al. Molecular genetic evidence of a unifocal origin for human serous ovarian carcinomas. *Gynecol Oncol* 1993;48:5–10.
165. Kupryjanczyk J, Thor AD, Beauchamp R, Polemba C, Scully RE, Yandell DW. Ovarian, peritoneal and endometrial serous carcinoma: p53 analysis supports a clonal origin of multifocal disease. *Mod Pathol* 1996;9:166–173.
166. Muto MG, Welch WR, Mok SCH, et al. Evidence for a multifocal origin of papillary serous carcinoma of the peritoneum. *Cancer Res* 1995;55 490–492.
167. Eadar N, Krumerman M. Possible metaplastic origin of lymph node "metastases" in serous ovarian tumor of low malignant potential (borderline serous tumor). *Gynecol Oncol* 1995;59:394–397.
168. Karp LA, Czernobilsky B. Glandular inclusions in pelvic and abdominal para-aortic lymph nodes. *Am J Clin Pathol* 1969;52:212–218.
169. Clement PB, Young RH, Oliva E, Summer HW, Scully RE. Hyperplastic mesothelial cells within abdominal lymph nodes: mimic of metastatic ovarian carcinoma and serous borderline tumors. A report of two cases associated with ovarian neoplasms. *Mod Pathol* 1996;9:879–886.
170. Khoury N, Raju U, Crissman JD, Zarbo RJ, Greenawald KA. A comparative immunohistochemical study of peritoneal and ovarian serous tumors and mesotheliomas. *Hum Pathol* 1990;21:811–819.
171. Gaffey MJ, Mills SE, Swanson PE, Zarbo RJ, Shah AR, Wick MR. Immunoreactivity for BER-EP4 in adenocarcinomas, adenomatoid tumors, and malignant mesotheliomas. *Am J Surg Pathol* 1992; 16:593–599.
172. Eichhorn JH, Scully RE. "Adenoid cystic" and basaloid carcinomas of the ovary: evidence for a surface epithelial lineage. A report of 12 cases. *Mod Pathol* 1995;8:731–740.
173. Ulbright TM, Roth LM, Sutton GP. Papillary serous carcinoma of the ovary with squamous differentiation. *Int J Gynecol Pathol* 1990;9:86–94.
174. Gilks CB, Bell DA, Scully RE. Serous psammocarcinoma of the ovary and peritoneum. *Int J Gynecol Pathol* 1990;9:110–121.
175. Hughesdon P. Benign endometrioid tumours of the ovary and the mullerian concept of ovarian epithelial tumours. *Histopathology* 1984;8:977–990.
176. Curtin JP, Barakat RR, Hoskins WF. Ovarian disease in women with breast cancer. *Obstet Gynecol* 1994;84:449–452.
177. Monteagudo C, Merino MJ, LaPorte N, Neumann RD. Value of gross cystic disease fluid protein-15 in distinguishing metastatic breast carcinoma among poorly differentiated neoplasms involving the ovary. *Hum Pathol* 1991;22:368–372.
178. Wick MR, Lillemore TJ, Copland GT, Swanson PE, Manivel JC, Kiang DT. Gross cystic disease fluid protein-15 as a marker for breast cancer: immunohistochemical analysis of 690 human neoplasms and comparison with alpha-lactalbumin. *Hum Pathol* 1989;20:281–287.
179. Loy TS, Quesenberry JT, Sharp SC. Distribution of CA 125 in adenocarcinomas: an immunohistochemical study of 481 cases. *Am J Clin Pathol* 1992;98:175–179.
180. Leake J, Woolas RP, Daniel J, Oram DH, Brown CL. Immunocytochemical and serological expression of CA 125: a clinicopathological study of 40 malignant ovarian epithelial tumours. *Histopathology* 1994;24:57–64.
181. Brown FW, Campagna LB, Dunn JK, Cagle PT. Immunohistochemical identification of tumor markers in metastatic adenocarcinoma: a diagnostic adjunct in the determination of primary site. *Am J Clin Pathol* 1997;107:12–19.
182. Bennington JL, Ferguson BR, Haber SL. Incidence and relative frequency of benign and malignant ovarian neoplasms. *Obstet Gynecol* 1968;32:627–632.
183. Cariker M, Dockerty M. Mucinous cystadenomas and mucinous cystadenocarcinomas of the ovary: a clinical and pathological study of 355 cases. *Cancer* 1954;7:302–310.
184. Lack EE, Young RH, Scully RE. Pathology of ovarian neoplasms in childhood and adolescence. *Pathol Annu* 1992;27(pt. 2):281–356.
185. Young RH, Scully RE. Mucinous ovarian tumors associated with mucinous adenocarcinomas of the cervix: a clinicopathological analysis of 15 cases. *Int J Gynecol Pathol* 1988;7:99–111.
186. LiVolsi VA, Merino MJ, Schwartz PE. Coexistent endocervical adenocarcinoma and mucinous adenocarcinoma of ovary: a clinicopathologic study of four cases. *Int J Gynecol Pathol* 1983;1:391–402.

187. Kaminski PF, Norris HJ. Coexistence of ovarian neoplasms and endocervical adenocarcinoma. *Obstet Gynecol* 1984;64:553–556.
188. Rutgers JL, Scully RE. Ovarian mullerian mucinous papillary cystadenoma of borderline malignancy: a clinicopathological analysis of 30 cases. *Cancer* 1988;61:340–348.
189. Aguirre P, Scully RE, Dayal Y, DeLellis RA. Mucinous tumors of the ovary with argyrophil cells: an immunohistochemical analysis. *Am J Surg Pathol* 1984;8:345–356.
190. Bell DA. Mucinous adenofibromas of the ovary: a report of 10 cases. *Am J Surg Pathol* 1991;15:227–232.
191. Hart WR, Norris HJ. Borderline and malignant mucinous tumors of the ovary: histologic criteria and clinical behavior. *Cancer* 1973;31:1031–1045.
192. Chaitin BA, Gershenson DM, Evans HL. Mucinous tumors of the ovary: a clinicopathologic study of 70 cases. *Cancer* 1985;55:1958–1962.
193. Sumithran E, Susil BJ, Looi LM. The prognostic significance of grading in borderline mucinous tumors of the ovary. *Hum Pathol* 1988;19:15–18.
194. Watkin W, Silva EG, Gershenson DM. Mucinous carcinoma of the ovary: pathologic prognostic factors. *Cancer* 1992;69:208–212.
195. Hendrickson MR, Kempson RL. Well-differentiated mucinous neoplasms of the ovary. In: *State of the art reviews. Pathology: surface epithelial neoplasms of the ovary.* Philadelphia: Hanley & Belfus, 1992:1–27.
196. DeNictolis M, Montironi R, Tommasoni S, et al. Benign, borderline, and well-differentiated malignant intestinal mucinous tumors of the ovary: a clinicopathologic, histochemical, immunohistochemical, and nuclear quantitative study of 57 cases. *Int J Gynecol Pathol* 1994;13:10–21.
197. Guerrieri C, Hogberg T, Wingren S, Fristedt S, Simonsen E, Boeryd B. Mucinous borderline and malignant tumors of the ovary: a clinicopathologic and DNA ploidy study of 92 cases. *Cancer* 1994;74:2329–2340.
198. Siriaunkgul S, Robbins KM, McGowan L, Silverberg SG. Ovarian mucinous tumors of low malignant potential: a clinicopathologic study of 54 tumors of intestinal and mullerian type. *Int J Gynecol Pathol* 1995;14:198–208.
199. Hoerl HD, Hart WR. Primary ovarian mucinous cystadenocarcinomas: a clinicopathologic study of 49 cases with long term follow-up. *Am J Surg Pathol* 1998;22:1449–1462.
200. Lee KR, Scully RE. Mucinous tumors of the ovary. *Mod Pathol* 1998;11:107A.
201. Prat J, Scully RE. Sarcomas in ovarian mucinous tumors: a report of two cases. *Cancer* 1979;44:1327–1331.
202. Prat J, Scully RE. Ovarian mucinous tumors with sarcoma-like mural nodules: a report of seven cases. *Cancer* 1979;44:1333–1344.
203. Prat J, Young RH, Scully RE. Ovarian mucinous tumors with foci of anaplastic carcinoma. *Cancer* 1982;50:300–304.
204. Lifschitz-Mercer B, Dgani R, Jacob N, Fogel M, Czernobilsky B. Ovarian mucinous cystadenoma with leiomyomatous mural nodule. *Int J Gynecol Pathol* 1990;9:80–85.
205. Nichols GE, Mills SE, Ulbright TM, Czernobilsky B, Roth LM. Spindle cell mural nodules in cystic ovarian mucinous tumors: a clinicopathologic and immunohistochemical study of five cases. *Am J Surg Pathol* 1991;15:1055–1062.
206. Suurmeijer AJ. Carcinosarcoma-like mural nodule in an ovarian mucinous tumor. *Histopathology* 1991;18:268–271.
207. Matias-Guiu X, Aranda I, Prat J. Immunohistochemical study of sarcoma-like mural nodules in a mucinous cystadenocarcinoma of the ovary. *Virchows Arch A Pathol Anat Histopathol* 1991;419:89–92.
208. Baergen RN, Rutgers JL. Mural nodules in common epithelial tumors of the ovary. *Int J Gynecol Pathol* 1994;13:62–72.
209. Ulbright TM, Roth LM, Stehman FB. Secondary ovarian neoplasia: a clinicopathologic study of 35 cases. *Cancer* 1984;53:1164–1174.
210. Kao GF, Norris HJ. Unusual cystadenofibromas: endometrioid, mucinous, and clear cell types. *Obstet Gynecol* 1979;54:729–736.
211. Kao GF, Norris HJ. Cystadenofibromas of the ovary with epithelial atypia. *Am J Surg Pathol* 1978;2:357–363.
212. Roth LM, Czernobilsky B, Langley FA. Ovarian endometrioid adenofibromatous and cystadenofibromatous tumors: benign, proliferating, and malignant. *Cancer* 1981;48:1838–1845.
213. Bell DA, Scully RE. Atypical and borderline endometrioid adenofibromas of the ovary. *Am J Surg Pathol* 1985;9:205–214.
214. Synder RR, Norris HJ, Tavassoli F. Endometrioid proliferative and low malignant potential tumors of the ovary: a clinicopathologic study of 46 cases. *Am J Surg Pathol* 1988;12:661–671.
215. Czernobilsky B, Silverman BB, Mikuta JJ. Endometrioid carcinoma of the ovary: a clinicopathologic study of 75 cases. *Cancer* 1970;26:1141–1152.
216. Kurman RJ, Craig JM. Endometrioid and clear cell carcinoma of the ovary. *Cancer* 1972;29:1653–1664.
217. Fu YS, Stock RJ, Reagan JW, Storaasli JP, Wentz WB. Significance of squamous components in endometrioid carcinoma of the ovary. *Cancer* 1979;44:616–621.
218. Mostoufizadeh M, Scully RE. Malignant tumors arising in endometriosis. *Clin Obstet Gynecol* 1980;23:951–963.
219. DePriest PD, Banks ER, Powell DE, et al. Endometrioid carcinoma of the ovary and endometriosis: the association in postmenopausal women. *Gynecol Oncol* 1992;47:71–75.
220. Kline RC, Wharton JT, Atkinson EN, Burke TW, Gershenson DM, Edwards CL. Endometrioid carcinoma of the ovary: retrospective review of 145 cases. *Gynecol Oncol* 1990;39:337–346.
221. Young RH, Prat J, Scully RE. Ovarian endometrioid carcinomas resembling sex cord–stromal tumors: a clinicopathologic analysis of 13 cases. *Am J Surg Pathol* 1982;6:513–522.
222. Tornos C, Silva EG, Ordonez NG, Gershenson DM, Young RH, Scully RE. Endometrioid carcinoma of the ovary with a prominent spindle-cell component, a source of diagnostic confusion: a report of 14 cases. *Am J Surg Pathol* 1995;19:1343–1353.
223. Eichhorn JH, Scully RE. Endometrioid ciliated-cell tumors of the ovary: a report of five cases. *Int J Gynecol Pathol* 1996;15:248–256.
224. Pitman MB, Young RH, Clement PB, Dickersin GR, Scully RE. Oxyphilic endometrioid carcinoma of the ovary and endometrium: a report of nine cases. *Int J Gynecol Pathol* 1994;13:290–301.
225. Roth LM, Liban E, Czernobilsky B. Ovarian endometrioid tumors mimicking Sertoli and Sertoli-Leydig cell tumors: sertoliform variant of endometrioid carcinoma. *Cancer* 1982;50:1322–1331.
226. Aguirre P, Thor AD, Scully RE. Ovarian endometrioid carcinomas resembling sex cord–stromal tumors: an immunohistochemical study. *Int J Gynecol Pathol* 1989;8:364–373.
227. Guerrieri C, Frånlund B, Malmström H, Boeryd B. Ovarian endometrioid carcinomas simulating sex cord–stromal tumors: a study using inhibin and cytokeratin 7. *Int J Gynecol Pathol* 1998;17:266–271.
228. Rutgers JL, Young RH, Scully RE. Ovarian yolk sac tumor arising from an endometrioid carcinoma. *Hum Pathol* 1987;18:1296–1299.
229. Nogales FF, Bergeron C, Carvia RE, Alvaro T, Fulwood HR. Ovarian endometrioid tumors with yolk sac tumor component, an unusual form of ovarian neoplasm: analysis of six cases. *Am J Surg Pathol* 1996;10:1056–1066.
230. Lash RH, Hart WR. Intestinal adenocarcinomas metastatic to the ovaries: a clinicopathological evaluation of 22 cases. *Am J Surg Pathol* 1987;11:114–121.
231. DeCostanzo DC, Elias JM, Chumas JC. Necrosis in 84 ovarian carcinomas: a morphologic study of primary versus metastatic colonic carcinoma with a selective immunohistochemical analysis of cytokeratin subtypes and carcinoembryonic antigen. *Int J Gynecol Pathol* 1997;16:245–249.
232. Young RH, Hart WR. Metastatic intestinal carcinomas simulating primary ovarian clear cell carcinoma and secretory endometrioid carcinoma: a clinicopathologic and immunohistochemical study of five cases. *Am J Surg Pathol* 1998;22:805–815.
233. Berezowski K, Stastny JF, Kornstein MJ. Cytokeratins 7 and 20 and carcinoembryonic antigen in ovarian and colonic carcinoma. *Mod Pathol* 1996;9:426–429.
234. Loy TS, Calaluce RD, Kenney GL. Cytokeratin immunostaining in differentiating primary ovarian carcinoma from metastatic colonic adenocarcinoma. *Mod Pathol* 1996;9:1040–1044.
235. Cheung ANY, Chiu P-M, Khoo U-S. Is immunostaining with HAM56 antibody useful in identifying ovarian origin of metastatic adenocarcinomas? *Hum Pathol* 1997;28:91–94.
236. Zaino RJ, Unger ER, Whitney C. Synchronous carcinomas of the uterine corpus and ovary. *Gynecol Oncol* 1984;19:329–335.
237. Prat J, Matias-Guiu X, Barreto J. Simultaneous carcinoma involving the endometrium and the ovary: a clinicopathologic, immunohistochemical, and DNA flow cytometric study of 18 cases. *Cancer* 1991;68:2455–2459.
238. Shenson DL, Gallion HH, Powell DE, Pieretti M. Loss of heterozygosity and genomic instability in synchronous endometrioid tumors of the ovary and endometrium. *Cancer* 1995;76:650–657.

239. Morrow CP, d'Ablaing G, Brady LW, Blessing JA, Hreshchyshyn MM. A clinical and pathologic study of 30 cases of malignant mixed mullerian epithelial and mesenchymal ovarian tumors: a gynecologic oncology group study. *Gynecol Oncol* 1984;18:278–292.
240. Dictor M. Malignant mixed mesodermal tumor of the ovary: a report of 22 cases. *Obstet Gynecol* 1985;65:720–724.
241. Terada KY, Johnson TL, Hopkins M. Roberts JA. Clinicopathologic features of ovarian mixed mesodermal tumors and carcinosarcomas. *Gynecol Oncol* 1989;32:228–232.
242. George E, Manivel JC, Dehner LP, Wick MR. Malignant mixed müllerian tumors: an immunohistochemical study of 47 cases, with histogenetic considerations and clinical correlation. *Hum Pathol* 1991;22:215–223.
243. Bitterman P, Chun B, Kurman RJ. The significance of epithelial differentiation in mixed mesodermal tumors of the uterus: a clinicopathologic and immunohistochemical study. *Am J Surg Pathol* 1990;14:317–328.
244. Mayall F, Rutty K, Campbell F, Goddard H. p53 immunostaining suggests that uterine carcinosarcomas are monoclonal. *Histopathology* 1994;24:211–214.
245. Thompson L, Chang B, Barsky SH. Monoclonal origins of malignant mixed tumors (carcinosarcomas): evidence for a divergent histogenesis. *Am J Surg Pathol* 1996;20:277–285.
246. Costa MJ, Morris RJ, Wilson R, Judd R. Utility of immunohistochemistry in distinguishing ovarian Sertoli-stromal cell tumors from carcinosarcomas. *Hum Pathol* 1992;23:787–797.
247. Flemming P, Wellmann A, Maschek HJ, et al. Monoclonal antibodies against inhibin represent key markers of adult granulosa cell tumors of the ovary even in their metastases. *Am J Surg Pathol* 1995;19:927–933.
248. Costa MJ, Ames PF, Walls J, Roth LM. Inhibin immunohistochemistry applied to ovarian neoplasms: a novel, effective diagnostic tool. *Hum Pathol* 1997;281:247–254.
249. Rishi M, Howard LN, Bratthauer GL, Tavassoli FA. Use of monoclonal antibodies against human inhibin as a marker for sex cord–stromal tumors of the ovary. *Am J Surg Pathol* 1997;21:583–589.
250. McCluggage WG, Maxwell P, Sloan JM. Immunohistochemical staining of ovarian granulosa cell tumors with monoclonal antibodies against inhibin. *Hum Pathol* 1997;28:1034–1038.
251. Stewart CJR, Jeffers MD, Kennedy A. Diagnostic value of inhibin immunoreactivity in ovarian gonadal stromal tumours and their histological mimics. *Histopathology* 1997;31:67–74.
252. Zheng W, Sung CJ, Hanna I, et al. α and β subunits of inhibin/activin as sex cord–stromal differentiation markers. *Int J Gynecol Pathol* 1997;16:263–271.
253. Riopel MA, Perlman EJ, Seidman JD, et al. Inhibin and epithelial membrane antigen immunohistochemistry assist in the diagnosis of sex cord–stromal tumors and provide clues to the histogenesis of hypercalcemic small cell carcinomas. *Int J Gynecol Pathol* 1998;17:46–53.
254. Kommoss F, Oliva E, Bhan AK, Young RH, Scully RE. Inhibin expression in ovarian tumors and tumor-like lesions: an immunohistochemical study. *Mod Pathol* 1998;11:656–664.
255. Clement PB, Scully RE. Extrauterine mesodermal (mullerian) adenosarcoma. *Am J Clin Pathol* 1978;69:276–283.
256. Roth LM, Langley FA, Fox H, Wheeler JE, Czernobilsky B. Ovarian clear cell adenofibromatous tumors: benign, of low malignant potential, and associated with invasive clear cell carcinoma. *Cancer* 1984;53:1156–1163.
257. Kao GF, Norris HJ. Benign and low grade variants of mixed mesodermal tumor (adenosarcoma) of the ovary and adnexal region. *Cancer* 1978;42:1314–1324.
258. Dellers EA, Valente PT, Edmonds PR, Balsara G. Extrauterine mixed mesodermal tumors: an immunohistochemical study. *Arch Pathol Lab Med* 1991;115:918–920.
259. Fukunaga M, Nomura K, Endo Y, Ushigome A, Aizawa S. Ovarian adenosarcoma. *Histopathology* 1997;30:283–287.
260. Silverberg SG, Fernandez FN. Endolymphatic stromal myosis of the ovary: a report of three cases and literature review. *Gynecol Oncol* 1981;12:129–138.
261. Young RH, Prat J, Scully RE. Endometrioid stromal sarcomas of the ovary: a clinicopathologic analysis of 23 cases. *Cancer* 1984;53:1143–1155.
262. Baiocchi G, Kavanagh JJ, Wharton JT. Endometrioid stromal sarcoma arising from ovarian and extraovarian endometriosis: report of two cases and review of the literature. *Gynecol Oncol* 1990;36:147–151.
263. Shiraki M, Otis CN, Powell JL. Endometrial stromal sarcoma arising from ovarian and extraovarian endometriosis: report of two cases and review of the literature. *Surg Pathol* 1991;4(4):333–343.
264. Chang KL, Crabtree GS, Lim-Tan SK, Kempson RL, Hendrickson MR. Primary extrauterine endometrial stromal neoplasms: a clinicopathologic study of 20 cases and a review of the literature. *Int J Gynecol Pathol* 1993;12:282–296.
265. Young RH, Scully RE. Sarcomas metastatic to the ovary: a report of 21 cases. *Int J Gynecol Pathol* 1990;9:231–252.
266. Clement PB, Scully RE. Uterine tumors resembling ovarian sex-cord tumors. *Am J Clin Pathol* 1976;66:512–525.
267. Bell DA, Scully RE. Benign and borderline clear cell adenofibromas of the ovary. *Cancer* 1985;56:2922–2931.
268. Sevchuk MM, Winkler-Monsanto B, Fenoglio CM, Richart RM. Clear cell carcinoma of the ovary: a clinicopathologic study with review of the literature. *Cancer* 1981;47:1344–1351.
269. Kemi PJ, Meurmann L, Gronroos M, Talerman A. Clear cell (mesonephroid) tumor of the ovary with characteristics resembling endodermal sinus tumor. *Int J Gynecol Pathol* 1982;1:95–100.
270. Kennedy AW, Biscotti CV, Hart WR, Webster KD. Ovarian clear cell adenocarcinoma. *Gynecol Oncol* 1989;32:342–349.
271. Brescia RJ, Dubin N, Demopoulos RI. Endometrioid and clear cell carcinoma of the ovary: factors affecting survival. *Int J Gynecol Pathol* 1989;8:132–138.
272. Jenison EL, Montag AG, Griffiths CT, et al. Clear cell adenocarcinoma of the ovary: a clinical analysis and comparison with serous carcinoma. *Gynecol Oncol* 1989;32:65–71.
273. Crozier MA, Copeland LJ, Silva EG, Gershenson DM, Stringer CA. Clear cell carcinoma of the ovary: a study of 59 cases. *Gynecol Oncol* 1989;35:199–203.
274. Montag AG, Jenison EL, Griffiths CT, Welch WR, Lavin PT, Knapp RC. Ovarian clear cell carcinoma: a clinicopathologic analysis of 44 cases. *Int J Gynecol Pathol* 1989;8:85–96.
275. Schiller W. Parvilocular cystoma of the ovary. *Arch Pathol* 1943;35:391–413.
276. Young RH, Scully RE. Oxyphilic clear cell carcinoma of the ovary: a report of nine cases. *Am J Surg Pathol* 1987;11:661–667.
277. Zirker TA, Silva EG, Morris M, Ordonez NG. Immunohistochemical differentiation of clear-cell carcinoma of the female genital tract and endodermal sinus tumor with the use of alpha-fetoprotein and LEU-M1. *Am J Clin Pathol* 1989;91:511–514.
278. Young RH, Hart WR. Renal cell carcinoma metastatic to the ovary: a report of three cases emphasizing possible confusion with ovarian clear cell adenocarcinoma. *Int J Gynecol Pathol* 1992;11:96–104.
279. Prat J, Bhan AK, Dickersin GR, Robboy SJ, Scully RE. Hepatoid yolk sac tumor of the ovary (endodermal sinus tumor with hepatoid differentiation): a light microscopic, ultrastructural and immunohistochemical study of seven cases. *Cancer* 1982;50:2355–2368.
280. Ishikura H, Scully RE. Hepatoid carcinoma of the ovary: a report of five cases of a newly described tumor. *Cancer* 1987;60:2775–2784.
281. Scurry JP, Brown RW, Jobling T. Combined ovarian serous papillary and hepatoid carcinoma. *Gynecol Oncol* 1996;63:138–142.
282. Hart WR. Pathology of malignant and borderline epithelial tumors of ovary. In: Coppleson M, ed. *Gynecologic oncology: fundamental principles and clinical practice*. Edinburgh: Churchill Livingstone, 1981.
283. Austin RM, Norris HJ. Malignant Brenner tumor and transitional cell carcinoma of the ovary: a comparison. *Int J Gynecol Pathol* 1987;6:29–39.
284. Robey SS, Silva EG, Gershenson DM, McLemore D, El-Naggar A, Ordonez NG. Transitional cell carcinoma in high-grade high-stage ovarian carcinoma. *Cancer* 1989;63:839–847.
285. Silva EG, Robey-Cafferty SS, Smith TL, Gershenson DM. Ovarian carcinomas with transitional cell carcinoma pattern. *Am J Clin Pathol* 1990;93:457–470.
286. Hollingsworth HC, Steinberg SM, Silverberg SG, Merino MJ. Advanced stage transitional cell carcinoma of the ovary. *Hum Pathol* 1996;27:1267–1272.
287. Jorgensen EO, Dockerty MB, Wilson RB, Welch JS. Clinicopathologic study of 53 cases of Brenner's tumors of the ovary. *Am J Obstet Gynecol* 1970;108:122–127.
288. Silverberg SG. Brenner tumor of the ovary: a clinicopathologic study of 60 tumors in 54 women. *Cancer* 1971;28:588–596.
289. Ehrlich CE, Roth LM. The Brenner tumor: a clinicopathologic study of 57 cases. *Cancer* 1971;27:332–342.

290. Fox H, Agrawal K, Langley FA. The Brenner tumour of the ovary: a clinicopathological study of 54 cases. *J Obstet Gynecol Br Commonw* 1972;79:661–665.
291. Bransilver BR, Ferenczy A, Richart RM. Brenner tumors and Walthard cell nests. *Arch Pathol* 1974;98:76–86.
292. Waxman M. Pure and mixed Brenner tumors of the ovary: clinicopathologic and histogenetic observations. *Cancer* 1979;43:1830–1839.
293. Trebeck CE, Friedlander ML, Russell P, Baird PJ. Brenner tumors of the ovary: a study of the histology, immunohistochemistry and cellular DNA content in benign, borderline and malignant ovarian tumours. *Pathology* 1987;19:241–246.
294. Roth LM, Sternberg WH. Proliferating Brenner tumors. *Cancer* 1971;27:687–693.
295. Miles PA, Norris HJ. Proliferative and malignant Brenner tumors of the ovary. *Cancer* 1972;30:174–186.
296. Hallgrimson J, Scully RE. Borderline and malignant Brenner tumours of the ovary: a report of 15 cases. *Acta Pathol Microbiol Scand (A)* 1972;80(suppl):233:56–66.
297. Roth LM, Dallenbach-Hellweg G, Czernobilsky B. Ovarian Brenner tumors. I. Metaplastic, proliferating, and of low malignant potential. *Cancer* 1985;56:582–591.
298. Roth LM, Czernobilsky B. Ovarian Brenner tumors. II. Malignant. *Cancer* 1985;56:592–501.
299. Young RH, Scully RE. Urothelial and ovarian carcinomas of identical cell types: problems in interpretation. A report of three cases and review of the literature. *Int J Gynecol Pathol* 1988;7:197–211.
300. Shimizu Y, Kamoi S, Amada S, Akiyama F, Silverberg SG. Toward the development of a universal grading system for ovarian epithelial carcinoma: testing of a proposed system in a series of 461 patients with uniform treatment and follow-up. *Cancer* 1998;82: 893–901.
301. Soslow RA, Rouse RV, Hendrickson MR, Silva EG, Longacre TA. Transitional cell neoplasms of the ovary and urinary bladder: a comparative immunohistochemical analysis. *Int J Gynecol Pathol* 1996;15:257–265.
302. Nogales FF, Silverberg SG. Epidermoid cysts of the ovary: a report of five cases with histogenetic considerations and ultrastructural findings. *Am J Obstet Gynecol* 1976;124:523–528.
303. Young RH, Prat J, Scully RE. Epidermoid cyst of the ovary: a report of three cases with comments on histogenesis. *Am J Clin Pathol* 1980;73:272–276.
304. Fan LD, Zang HY, Zhang XS. Ovarian epidermoid cyst: report of eight cases. *Int J Gynecol Pathol* 1996;15:69–71.
305. Kashimura M, Shinohara M, Hirakawa T, Kamura T, Matsukuma K. Clinicopathologic study of squamous cell carcinoma of the ovary. *Gynecol Oncol* 1989;34:75–79.
306. Sworn MJ, Jones H, Letchworth AT, Herrington CS, McGee JO. Squamous intraepithelial neoplasia in an ovarian cyst, cervical intraepithelial neoplasia and human papillomavirus. *Hum Pathol* 1995;26:344–347.
307. Mai KT, Yazdi M, Bertrand MA, LeSaux N, Cathcart L. Bilateral primary ovarian squamous cell carcinoma associated with human papilloma virus infection and vulvar and cervical intraepithelial neoplasia. *Am J Surg Pathol* 1996;20:767–772.
308. Pins MR, Young RH, Daly WJ, Scully RE. Primary squamous cell carcinoma of the ovary: a report of 37 cases. *Am J Surg Pathol* 1996;20:823–838.
309. Young RH, Gersell DJ, Roth LM, Scully RE. Ovarian metastases from cervical carcinomas other than pure adenocarcinomas: a report of 12 cases. *Cancer* 1993;71:407–418.
310. Pins MR, Young RH, Crum CP, Leach H, Scully RE. Cervical squamous carcinoma in situ with intraepithelial extension to upper genital tract and invasion of tubes and ovaries: report of a case with HPV analysis. *Int J Gynecol Pathol* 1997;16:272–278.
311. Rutgers JL, Scully RE. Ovarian mixed-epithelial papillary cystadenomas of borderline malignancy: a clinicopathological analysis. *Cancer* 1988;61:546–554.
312. Tornos C, Silva EG, Khorana SM, Burke TW. High-stage endometrioid carcinoma of the ovary: prognostic significance of pure versus mixed histologic types. *Am J Surg Pathol* 1994;18:687–693.
313. Silva EG, Tornos C, Bailey MA, Morris M. Undifferentiated carcinoma of the ovary. *Arch Pathol Lab Med* 1991;115:377–381.
314. Oliva E, Andrada E, Pezzica E, Prat J. Ovarian carcinomas with choriocarcinomatous differentiation. *Cancer* 1993;72:2441–2446.
315. Young RH, Oliva E, Scully RE. Small cell carcinoma of the ovary, hypercalcemic type: a clinicopathologic analysis of 150 cases. *Am J Surg Pathol* 1994;18:1102–1116.
316. Eichhorn JH, Young RH, Scully RE. Primary ovarian small cell carcinoma of the pulmonary type: a clinicopathologic, immunohistologic, and flow cytometric analysis of 11 cases. *Am J Surg Pathol* 1992;16:926–938.
317. Eichhorn JH, Lawrence WD, Young RH, Scully RE. Ovarian neuroendocrine carcinomas of non-small cell type associated with surface epithelial adenocarcinomas: a study of five cases and a review of the literature. *Int J Gynecol Pathol* 1996;15:303–314.
318. Young RH, Scully RE. Ovarian sex cord–stromal tumors: recent advances and current status. *Clin Obstet Gynaecol* 1984;11:93–134.
319. Hodgson JE, Dockerty MB, Mussey RD. Granulosa cell tumor of the ovary: a clinical and pathologic review of sixty-two cases. *Surg Gynecol Obstet* 1945;81:631–642.
320. Nakashima N, Young RH, Scully RE. Androgenic granulosa cell tumors of the ovary: a clinicopathologic analysis of 17 cases and review of the literature. *Arch Pathol Lab Med* 1984;108:786–791.
321. Stenwig JT, Hazekamp JT, Beecham JB. Granulosa cell tumors of the ovary: a clinicopathological study of 118 cases with long term follow-up. *Gynecol Oncol* 1979;7:136–152.
322. Fathalla MF. The occurrence of granulosa and theca tumors in clinically normal ovaries. *J Obstet Gynaec Br Commonw* 1967;74: 279–282.
323. Sjostedt S, Wahlen T. Prognosis of granulosa cell tumors. *Acta Obstet Gynecol Scand* 1961;40[Suppl 6]:3–26.
324. Fox H, Agrawal K, Langley FA. A clinicopathologic study of 92 cases of granulosa cell tumor of the ovary with special reference to the factors influencing prognosis. *Cancer* 1975;35:231–241.
325. Bjorkholm E, Silfersward C. Prognostic factors in granulosa cell tumors. *Gynecol Oncol* 1981;11:261–274.
326. Young RH, Dickersin GR, Scully RE. Juvenile granulosa cell tumor of the ovary: a clinicopathologic analysis of 125 cases. *Am J Surg Pathol* 1984;8:575–596.
327. Young RH, Scully RE. Ovarian sex cord–stromal tumors with bizarre nuclei: a clinicopathologic analysis of seventeen cases. *Int J Gynecol Pathol* 1983;1:325–335.
328. Young RH, Oliva E, Scully RE. Luteinized adult granulosa cell tumors of the ovary: a report of four cases. *Int J Gynecol Pathol* 1994;13:302–310.
329. Young RH, Scully RE. Ovarian stromal tumors with minor sex cord elements: a report of seven cases. *Int J Gynecol Pathol* 1983;2:227–234.
330. Susil BJ, Sumithran E. Sarcomatous change in granulosa cell tumor. *Hum Pathol* 1987;18:397–399.
331. Lack EE, Perez-Atayde AR, Murthy ASK, Goldstein DP, Crigler JF, Vawter GF. Granulosa theca cell tumors in premenarchal girls: a clinical and pathological study of ten cases. *Cancer* 1981;48:1846–1854.
332. Zaloudek C, Norris HJ. Granulosa tumors of the ovary in children: a clinical and pathologic study of 32 cases. *Am J Surg Pathol* 1981;6:503–512.
333. Biscotti CV, Hart WR. Juvenile granulosa cell tumors of the ovary. *Arch Pathol Lab Med* 1989;113:40–46.
334. Young RH, Dudley AG, Scully RE. Granulosa cell, Sertoli-Leydig cell and unclassified sex cord–stromal tumors associated with pregnancy: a clinicopathological analysis of thirty-six cases. *Gynecol Oncol* 1984;18:181–205.
335. Young RH, Scully RE. Malignant melanoma metastatic to the ovary: a clinicopathologic analysis of 20 cases. *Am J Surg Pathol* 1991;15:849–860.
336. Dockerty MB, Masson JC. Ovarian fibromas: a clinical and pathologic study of two hundred and eighty-three cases. *Am J Obstet Gynecol* 1944;47:741–752.
337. Gorlin RJ. Nevoid basal cell carcinoma syndrome. *Medicine* 1987;66:98–113.
338. Meigs JV. Fibroma of the ovary with ascites and hydrothorax—Meigs' syndrome. *Am J Obstet Gynecol* 1954;67:962–987.
339. Samanth KK, Black WC. Benign ovarian stromal tumors associated with free peritoneal fluid. *Am J Obstet Gynecol* 1970;107:538–545.
340. Prat J, Scully RE. Cellular fibromas and fibrosarcomas of the ovary: a comparative clinicopathologic analysis of seventeen cases. *Cancer* 1981;47:2663–2670.
341. Tsuji T, Kawauchi S, Utsunomiya T, Nagata Y, Tsuneyoshi M. Fibrosarcoma versus cellular fibroma of the ovary: a comparative study of their proliferative activity and chromosome aberrations using MIB-

1 immunostaining, DNA flow cytometry, and fluorescence in situ hybridization. *Am J Surg Pathol* 1997;21:52–59.
342. Sternberg WH, Gaskill CJ. Theca-cell tumors: with a report of twelve new cases and observations on the possible etiologic role of ovarian stromal hyperplasia. *Am J Obstet Gynecol* 1950;59:575–537.
343. Bjorkholm E, Silfversward C. Theca-cell tumors: clinical features and prognosis. *Acta Radiol Oncol Radiat Phys Biol* 1980;19:241–244.
344. Young RH, Clement PB, Scully RE. Calcified thecomas in young women: a report of four cases. *Int J Gynecol Pathol* 1988;7:343–350.
345. Waxman M, Vuletin JC, Urcuyo R, Belling CG. Ovarian low grade stromal sarcoma with thecomatous features: a critical reappraisal of the so-called "malignant thecoma." *Cancer* 1979;44:2206–2217.
346. Roth LM, Sternberg WH. Partly luteinized theca-cell tumor of the ovary. *Cancer* 1983;51:1697–1704.
347. Zhang J, Young RH, Arseneau J, Scully RE. Ovarian stromal tumors containing lutein or Leydig cells (luteinized thecomas and stromal Leydig cell tumors): a clinicopathological analysis of fifty cases. *Int J Gynecol Pathol* 1982;1:270–285.
348. Clement PB, Young RH, Hanna W, Scully RE. Sclerosing peritonitis associated with luteinized thecomas of the ovary: a clinicopathological analysis of six cases. *Am J Surg Pathol* 1994;18:1–13.
349. Iwasa Y, Minamiguchi S, Konishi I, Onodera H, Zhou J, Yamabe H. Sclerosing peritonitis associated with luteinized thecoma of the ovary. *Pathol Int* 1996;46:510–514.
350. Spiegel GW, Swiger FK. Luteinized thecoma with sclerosing peritonitis presenting as an acute abdomen. *Gynecol Oncol* 1996;61:275–281.
351. Werness BA. Luteinized thecoma with sclerosing peritonitis. *Arch Pathol Lab Med* 1996;120:303–306.
352. Hughesdon PE. Ovarian lipoid and theca cell tumors: their origins and interrelations. *Obstet Gynecol Surv* 1966;21:245–288.
353. Hughesdon PE. Lipid cell thecomas of the ovary. *Histopathology* 1983;7:681–692.
354. Chalvardjian A, Scully RE. Sclerosing stromal tumors of the ovary. *Cancer* 1973;31:664–670.
355. Gee DC, Russell P. Sclerosing stromal tumours of the ovary. *Histopathology* 1979;3:367–376.
356. Ramzy I. Signet-ring stromal tumor of ovary: histochemical, light, and electron microscopic study. *Cancer* 1976;38:166–172.
357. Dickersin GR, Young RH, Scully RE. Signet ring stromal and related tumors of the ovary. *Ultrastruct Pathol* 1995;19:401–419.
358. Young RH, Scully RE. Ovarian Sertoli cell tumors: a report of ten cases. *Int J Gynecol Pathol* 1984;2:349–363.
359. Teilum G. Homologous ovarian and testicular tumors. III. Estrogen producing Sertoli cell tumors (androblastoma tubulare lipoides) of the human testis and ovary. *J Clin Endocrinol* 1949;9:301–318.
360. Tavassoli FA, Norris H. Sertoli tumors of the ovary: a clinicopathologic study of 28 cases with ultrastructural observations. *Cancer* 1980;46:2281–2297.
361. Solh HM, Azoury RS, Najjar SS. Peutz-Jeghers syndrome associated with precocious puberty. *J Pediatr* 1983;103:593–595.
362. Ferry JA, Young RH, Engel G, Scully RE. Oxyphil Sertoli cell tumor of the ovary: a report of three cases, two in patients with the Peutz-Jeghers syndrome. *Int J Gynecol Pathol* 1994;13:259–266.
363. Rutgers JL, Scully RE. The androgen insensitivity syndrome (testicular feminization): a clinicopathologic study of 43 cases. *Int J Gynecol Pathol* 1991;10:126–144.
364. Young RH, Scully RE. Ovarian tumors of probable wolffian origin: a report of 11 cases. *Am J Surg Pathol* 1983;7:125–135.
365. Roth LM, Anderson MC, Govan ADT, Langley FA, Gowing NFC, Woodcock AS. Sertoli-Leydig cell tumors: a clinicopathologic study of 34 cases. *Cancer* 1981;48:187–197.
366. Zaloudek C, Norris HJ. Sertoli-Leydig tumors of the ovary: a clinicopathologic study of 64 intermediate and poorly differentiated neoplasms. *Am J Surg Pathol* 1984;8:405–418.
367. Young RH, Scully RE. Ovarian Sertoli-Leydig cell tumors: a clinicopathological analysis of 207 cases. *Am J Surg Pathol* 1985;9:543–569.
368. Young RH, Scully RE. Well-differentiated ovarian Sertoli-Leydig cell tumors: a clinicopathological analysis of 23 cases. *Int J Gynecol Pathol* 1984;3:277–290.
369. Gagnon S, Tetu B, Silva EG, McCaughey WTE. Frequency of α-fetoprotein production by Sertoli-Leydig cell tumors of the ovary: an immunohistochemical study of eight cases. *Mod Pathol* 1989;2:63–67.
370. Dardi LE, Miller AW, Gould VE. Sertoli-Leydig cell tumor with endometrioid differentiation. *Diagn Gynecol Obstet* 1982;4:227–234.
371. Young RH, Scully RE. Ovarian Sertoli-Leydig cell tumors with a retiform pattern: a problem in histopathologic diagnosis. A report of 25 cases. *Am J Surg Pathol* 1983;7:755–771.
372. Roth LM, Slayton RE, Brady LW, Blessing JA, Johnson G. Retiform differentiation in ovarian Sertoli-Leydig cell tumors: a clinicopathologic study of six cases from a gynecologic oncology group study. *Cancer* 1985;55:1093–1098.
373. Talerman A. Ovarian Sertoli-Leydig cell tumor (androblastoma) with retiform pattern: a clinicopathologic study. *Cancer* 1987;60:3056–3064.
374. Young RH, Prat J, Scully RE. Ovarian Sertoli-Leydig cell tumors with heterologous elements. I. Gastrointestinal epithelium and carcinoid: a clinicopathologic analysis of thirty-six cases. *Cancer* 1982;50:2448–2456.
375. Waxman M, Damjanov I, Alpert L, Sardinsky T. Composite mucinous ovarian neoplasms associated with Sertoli-Leydig and carcinoid tumors. *Cancer* 1981;47:2044–2052.
376. Prat J, Young RH, Scully RE. Ovarian Sertoli-Leydig cell tumors with heterologous elements. II. Cartilage and skeletal muscle: a clinicopathological analysis of twelve cases. *Cancer* 1982;50:2465–2475.
377. Young RH, Perez-Atayde AR, Scully RE. Ovarian Sertoli-Leydig cell tumor with retiform and heterologous components: report of a case with hepatocytic differentiation and elevated serum alpha-fetoprotein. *Am J Surg Pathol* 1984;8:709–718.
378. Sahn A, Benda JA. Primary ovarian Wilms' tumor. *Cancer* 1988;64:1460–1463.
379. Anderson MC, Rees DA. Gynandroblastoma of the ovary. *Br J Obstet Gynaecol* 1975;82:68–73.
380. Chalvardjian A, Derzko C. Gynandroblastoma: its ultrastructure. *Cancer* 1982;50:710–721.
381. McCluggage WG, Sloan JM, Murnaghan M, White R. Gynandroblastoma of ovary with juvenile granulosa component and heterologous intestinal type glands. *Histopathology* 1996;29:251–257.
382. Seidman JD. Unclassified gonadal stromal tumors: a clinicopathologic study of 32 cases. *Am J Surg Pathol* 1996;20:699–706.
383. Talerman A, Hughesdon PE, Anderson MC. Diffuse nonlobular ovarian androblastoma usually associated with feminization. *Int J Gynecol Pathol* 1982;1:155–171.
384. Hart WR, Kumar N, Crissman JD. Ovarian neoplasms resembling sex cord tumors with annular tubules. *Cancer* 1980;45:2352–2363.
385. Young RH, Welch WR, Dickersin GR, Scully RE. Ovarian sex cord tumor with annular tubules: review of 74 cases including 27 with Peutz-Jeghers syndrome and four with adenoma malignum of the cervix. *Cancer* 1982;50:1384–1402.
386. Ahn GH, Chi JG, Lee SK. Ovarian sex cord tumor with annular tubules. *Cancer* 1986;57:1066–1073.
387. Dolan J, Al-Timimi AH, Richards SM, et al. Does ovarian sex cord tumor with annular tubules produce progesterone? *J Clin Pathol* 1986;39:29–35.
388. Gustafson ML, Lee MM, Scully RE, et al. Mullerian inhibiting substance as a marker for ovarian sex-cord tumor. *N Engl J Med* 1992;326:466–471.
389. Srivasta PJ, Kenney GL, Podratz KC. Disseminated cervical adenoma malignum and bilateral ovarian sex cord tumors with annular tubules associated with Peutz-Jeghers syndrome. *Gynecol Oncol* 1994;53:256–264.
390. Young RH, Dickersin GR, Scully RE. A distinctive ovarian sex cord-stromal tumor causing sexual precocity in the Peutz-Jeghers syndrome. *Am J Surg Pathol* 1985;7:233–243.
391. Taylor HE, Norris HJ. Lipid cell tumors of the ovary. *Cancer* 1967;20:1953–1962.
392. Hayes MC, Scully RE. Ovarian steroid cell tumors, not otherwise specified (lipid cell tumors): a clinicopathological analysis of 63 cases. *Am J Surg Pathol* 1987;11:835–845.
393. Hayes MC, Scully RE. Stromal luteoma of the ovary: a clinicopathological analysis of 25 cases. *Int J Gynecol Pathol* 1987;6:313–321.
394. Paraskevas M, Scully RE. Hilus cell tumor of the ovary: a clinicopathological analysis of 12 Reinke crystal-positive and nine crystal-negative cases. *Int J Gynecol Pathol* 1989;8:299–310.
395. Young RH, Scully RE. Ovarian steroid cell tumors associated with Cushing's syndrome: a report of three cases. *Int J Gynecol Pathol* 1987;5:40–48.
396. Rutgers JL, Scully RE. Cysts (cystadenomas) and tumors of the rete ovarii. *Int J Gynecol Pathol* 1988;7:330–342.

397. Nogales FF, Carvia RE, Donne C, Campello TR, Vidal M, Martin A. Adenomas of the rete ovarii. *Hum Pathol* 1997;28:1428–1433.
398. LaPolla JP, Benda J, Vigliotti AP, et al. Dysgerminoma of the ovary. *Obstet Gynecol* 1987;69:859–867.
399. De Palo G, Lattuada A, Kenda R, et al. Germ cell tumors of the ovary: the experience of the national cancer institute of Milan. I. Dysgerminoma. *Int J Radiat Oncol Biol Phys* 1987;13:853–860.
400. Bjorkholm E, Lundell M, Gyftodimos A, Silfversward C. Dysgerminoma: the Radiumhemmet series 1927–1984. *Cancer* 1990;65:38–44.
401. Schwartz PE, Chambers SK, Chambers JT, Kohorn E, McIntosh S. Ovarian germ cell malignancies: the Yale University experience. *Gynecol Oncol* 1992;45:26–31.
402. Case Records of the Massachusetts General Hospital. Case 11—1972. *N Engl J Med* 1972;286:594–600.
403. Zaloudek CJ, Tavassoli FA, Norris HJ. Dysgerminoma with syncytiotrophoblastic giant cells: a histologically and clinically distinctive subtype of dysgerminoma. *Am J Surg Pathol* 1981;5:361–367.
404. Brettell JR, Miles PA, Herrera G, et al. Dysgerminoma with syncytiotrophoblastic giant cells presenting as a hydatidiform mole. *Gynecol Oncol* 1984;18:393–401.
405. Niehans GA, Manivel JC, Copland GT, Scheithauer BW, Wick MR. Immunohistochemistry of germ cell and trophoblastic neoplasms. *Cancer* 1988;62:1113–1123.
406. Mullin TJ, Lankerani MR. Ovarian dysgerminoma: immunocytochemical localization of human chorionic gonadotropin in the germinoma cell cytoplasm. *Obstet Gynecol* 1986;68:80S–83S.
407. Teilum G. Endodermal sinus tumors of the ovary and testis: comparative morphogenesis of the so-called mesonephroma ovarii (Schiller) and extraembryonic (yolk sac-allantoic) structures of the rat's placenta. *Cancer* 1959;12:1092–1105.
408. Kurman RJ, Norris HJ. Endodermal sinus tumor of the ovary: a clinical and pathologic analysis of 71 cases. *Cancer* 1976;38:2404–2419.
409. Nogales FF Jr, Matilla A, Nogales-Ortiz F, et al. Yolk sac tumors with pure and mixed polyvesicular vitelline patterns. *Hum Pathol* 1978;9:553–566.
410. Gershenson DM, Del Junco G, Herson J, et al. Endodermal sinus tumor of the ovary: the M. D. Anderson experience. *Obstet Gynecol* 1983;61:194–202.
411. Nakashima N, Fukatsu T, Nagasaki T, et al. The frequency and histology of hepatic tissue in germ cell tumors. *Am J Surg Pathol* 1987;11:682–692.
412. Cohen MB, Friend DS, Molnar JJ, Talerman A. Gonadal endodermal sinus (yolk sac) tumor with pure intestinal differentiation: a new histologic type. *Pathol Res Pract* 1987;182:609–616.
413. Clement PB, Young RH, Scully RE. Endometrioid-like yolk sac tumor of the ovary: a clinicopathological analysis of eight cases. *Am J Surg Pathol* 1987;11:767–778.
414. Michael H, Ulbright TM, Brodhecker CA. The pluripotential nature of the mesenchyme-like component of yolk sac tumor. *Arch Pathol Lab Med* 1989;113:1115–1119.
415. Kim CR, Hsiu JG, Given FT. Intestinal variant of ovarian endodermal sinus tumor. *Gynecol Oncol* 1989;33:379–381.
416. Kawai M, Kano T, Furuhashi Y, et al. Prognostic factors in yolk sac tumors of the ovary: a clinicopathologic analysis of 29 cases. *Cancer* 1991;67:184–192.
417. Fujita M, Inoue M, Tanizawa O, Minagawa J, Yamada T, Tani T. Retrospective review of 41 patients with endodermal sinus tumor of the ovary. *Int J Gynecol Cancer* 1993;3:329–335.
418. Nogales FF. Embryonic clues to human yolk sac tumors: a review. *Int J Gynecol Pathol* 1993;12:101–107.
419. Young RH. New and unusual aspects of ovarian germ cell tumors. *Am J Surg Pathol* 1993;17:1210–1224.
420. Young RH, Scully RE. Unusual patterns, subtypes, and differential diagnosis of gonadal yolk sac tumors. In: Nogales FF, ed. *The human yolk sac and yolk sac tumors*. Heidelberg: Springer-Verlag, 1993:309–342.
421. Dickersin GR, Oliva E, Young RH. Endometrioid-like variant of ovarian yolk sac tumor with foci of carcinoid: an ultrastructural study. *Ultrastruct Pathol* 1995;19:421–429.
422. Ulbright TM, Roth LM, Brodhecker CA. Yolk sac differentiation in germ cell tumors: a morphologic study of 50 cases with emphasis on hepatic, enteric, and parietal yolk sac features. *Am J Surg Pathol* 1986;10:151–164.
423. Santesson L, Marrubini G. Clinical and pathological survey of ovarian embryonal carcinomas, including so-called "mesonephromas" (Schiller), or "mesoblastomas" (Teilum), treated at the Radiumhemmet. *Acta Obstet Gynecol Scand* 1957;36:399–419.
424. Kurman RJ, Norris HJ. Embryonal carcinoma of the ovary: a clinicopathologic entity distinct from endodermal sinus tumor resembling embryonal carcinoma of the adult testis. *Cancer* 1976;38:2420–2433.
425. Nakakuma K, Tashiro S, Uemura K, et al. Alpha-fetoprotein and human chorionic gonadotropin in embryonal carcinoma of the ovary: an 8-year survival case. *Cancer* 1983;52:1470–1472.
426. Ueda G, Abe Y, Yoshida M, Fujiwara T. Embryonal carcinoma of the ovary: a six-year survival. *Int J Gynecol Obstet* 1990;31:287–292.
427. Manivel JC, Niehans G, Wich MR, Dehner LP. Intermediate trophoblast in germ cell neoplasms. *Am J Surg Pathol* 1987;11:693–701.
428. Takeda A, Ishizuka T, Goto T, et al. Polyembryoma of ovary producing alpha-fetoprotein and HCG: immunoperoxidase and electron microscopic study. *Cancer* 1982;14:1878–1889.
429. Prat J, Matias-Guiu X, Scully RE. Hepatic yolk sac differentiation in an ovarian polyembryoma. *Surg Pathol* 1987;2:147–150.
430. Nakashima N, Murakami S, Fukatsu T, et al. Characteristics of "embryoid body" in human gonadal germ cell tumors. *Hum Pathol* 1988;19:1144–1154.
431. King ME, Hubbell MJ, Talerman A. Mixed germ cell tumor of the ovary with a prominent polyembryoma component. *Int J Gynecol Pathol* 1991;10:88–95.
432. Chapman DC, Grover R, Schwartz PE. Conservative management of an ovarian polyembryoma. *Obstet Gynecol* 1994;83:879–882.
433. Jacobs AJ, Newland JR, Green RK. Pure choriocarcinoma of the ovary. *Obstet Gynecol Surv* 1982;37:603–609.
434. Vance RP, Geisinger KR. Pure nongestational choriocarcinoma of the ovary: report of a case. *Cancer* 1985;56:2321–2325.
435. Civantos F, Rywlin A. Carcinomas with trophoblastic differentiation and secretion of chorionic gonadotropins. *Cancer* 1972;29:789–798.
436. Robboy SJ, Scully RE. Ovarian teratoma with glial implants on the peritoneum. *Hum Pathol* 1970;1:643–653.
437. Norris HJ, Zirkin HJ, Benson WL. Immature (malignant) teratoma of the ovary: a clinical and pathological study of 58 cases. *Cancer* 1976;37:2359–2372.
438. Gershenson DM, Del Junco G, Silva EG, et al. Immature teratoma of the ovary. *Obstet Gynecol* 1986;68:624–629.
439. Perrone T, Steiner M, Dehner LP. Nodal gliomatosis and alpha-fetoprotein production: two unusual facets of grade I ovarian teratoma. *Arch Pathol Lab Med* 1986;110:975–977.
440. Perrone T, Steeper TA, Dehner LP. Alpha-fetoprotein localization in pure ovarian teratoma: an immunohistochemical study of 12 cases. *Am J Clin Pathol* 1987;88:713–717.
441. Yanai-Inbar I, Scully RE. Relation of ovarian dermoid cysts and immature teratomas: an analysis of 350 cases of immature teratoma and 10 cases of dermoid cyst with microscopic foci of immature tissue. *Int J Gynecol Pathol* 1987;6:203–212.
442. Koulos JP, Hoffman JS, Steinhoff MM. Immature teratoma of the ovary. *Gynecol Oncol* 1989;34:46–49.
443. Steeper TA, Mukai K. Solid ovarian teratomas: an immunocytochemical study of thirteen cases with clinicopathologic correlation. In: Sommers SC, Rosen PP, eds. *Pathology annual*, part 1. New York: Appleton-Century-Crofts, 1984;19:81–92.
444. Nielsen SNJ, Scheithauer BW, Gaffey TA. Gliomatosis peritonei. *Cancer* 1985;56:2499–2503.
445. Boehner JF, Gallup DG, Talledo OE, et al. Solid ovarian teratoma with neuroglial metastases to periaortic lymph nodes and omentum. *South Med J* 1987;80:649–652.
446. Anteby EY, Ron M, Revel A, Shimonovitz S, Ariel I, Hurwitz A. Germ cell tumors of the ovary arising after dermoid cyst resection: a long term follow-up study. *Obstet Gynecol* 1994;83:605–608.
447. Geisler JP, Goulet R, Foster RS, Sutton GP. Growing teratoma syndrome after chemotherapy for germ cell tumors of the ovary. *Obstet Gynecol* 1994;84:719–721.
448. Bonazzi C, Peccatori F, Colombo N, Lucchini V, Cantu MG, Mangioni C. Pure ovarian immature teratoma, a unique and curable disease: 10 years' experience of 32 prospectively treated patients. *Obstet Gynecol* 1994;84:598–604.
449. Calder CJ, Light AM, Rollason TP. Immature ovarian teratoma with mature peritoneal metastatic deposits showing glial, epithelial, and endometrioid differentiation: a case report and review of the literature. *Int J Gynecol Pathol* 1994;13:279–282.

450. Dworak O, Knopfle G, Varcmin-Schultheiss K, Meyer G. Gliomatosis peritonei with endometriosis externa. *Gynecol Oncol* 1988;29:263–266.
451. O'Connor DM, Norris HJ. The influence of grade on the outcome of stage I ovarian immature (malignant) teratoma and the reproducibility of grading. *Int J Gynecol Pathol* 1994;13:283–289.
452. Dadmanesh F, Miller DM, Swenerton KD, Clement FB. Gliomatosis peritonei with malignant transformation. *Mod Pathol* 1997;10:597–601.
453. Kim R, Bohm-Velez M. Familial ovarian dermoids. *J Ultrasound Med* 1994;13:225–228.
454. Pantoja E, Noy MA, Axtmayer RW, et al. Ovarian dermoids and their complications: comprehensive historical review. *Obstet Gynecol Surv* 1975;30:1–20.
455. Ayhan A, Aksu T, Develioglu O, Tuncer S, Ayhan A. Complications and bilaterality of mature ovarian teratomas (clinicopathological evaluation of 286 cases). *Aust N Z J Obstet Gynaecol* 1991;31:83–85.
456. Comerci JT Jr, Licciardi F, Bergh PA, Gregori C, Breen JL. Mature cystic teratoma: a clinicopathologic evaluation of 517 cases and review of the literature. *Obstet Gynecol* 1994;84:22–28.
457. Payne D, Muss HB, Homesley HD, et al. Autoimmune hemolytic anemia and ovarian dermoid cysts: case report and review of the literature. *Cancer* 1981;48:721–724.
458. Clement PB, Young RH, Scully RE. Clinical syndromes associated with tumors of the female genital tract. *Semin Diagn Pathol* 1991;8:204–233.
459. Peterson WF. Malignant degeneration of benign cystic teratomas of the ovary: a collective review of the literature. *Obstet Gynecol Surv* 1957;12:793–830.
460. Woodfield B, Katz DA, Cantrell CJ, et al. A benign cystic teratoma with gastrointestinal tract development. *Am J Clin Pathol* 1985;83:236–240.
461. Abbott TM, Hermann WJ, Scully RE. Ovarian fetiform teratoma (homunculus) in a 9-year-old girl. *Int J Gynecol Pathol* 1984;2:392–402.
462. Remadi S, Burkhardt K, Straccia AT, Pizzolato G, MacGee W. Well differentiated cerebellar tissue within a mature cystic teratoma. *Pathol Res Pract* 1998;194:371–374.
463. Akhtar M, Young I, Broady H. Anterior pituitary component in benign cystic ovarian teratomas: report of three cases. *Am J Clin Pathol* 1975;64:14–19.
464. Oi RH, Dobbs M. Lactating breast tissue in benign cystic teratoma. *Am J Obstet Gynecol* 1978;130:729–731.
465. Vadmal M, Hajdu SI. Prostatic tissue in benign cystic ovarian teratomas. *Hum Pathol* 1996;27:428–429.
466. Brumback RA, Brown BS, di Sant'Agnese A. Unique finding of prostatic tissue in a benign cystic ovarian teratoma. *Arch Pathol Lab Med* 1985;109:675–677.
467. Ulirsch RC, Goldman RL. An unusual teratoma of the ovary: neurogenic cyst with lactating breast tissue. *Obstet Gynecol* 1982;60:400–402.
468. McKeel DW Jr, Askin FB. Ectopic hypophyseal hormonal cells in benign cystic teratoma of the ovary: light microscopic histochemical dye staining and immunoperoxidase cytochemistry. *Arch Pathol Lab Med* 1978;102:122–128.
469. Sahin AA, Ro JY, Chen J, Ayala AG. Spindle cell nodule and peptic ulcer arising in a fully developed gastric wall in a mature cystic teratoma. *Arch Pathol Lab Med* 1990;114:529–531.
470. Rubin A, Papadaki L. Multicystic structures appearing in mature cystic teratoma of the ovary: an immunohistochemical and ultrastructural study. *Histopathology* 1990;17:359–363.
471. Tsukamoto N, Matsukuma K, Matsumura M, et al. Primary malignant melanoma arising in cystic teratoma of the ovary. *Gynecol Oncol* 1986;23:395–400.
472. Davis GL. Malignant melanoma arising in mature ovarian cystic teratoma (dermoid cyst): report of two cases and literature analysis. *Int J Gynecol Pathol* 1996;15:356–362.
473. Ueda G, Sato Y, Yamasaki M, et al. Malignant fibrous histiocytoma arising in a benign cystic teratoma of the ovary. *Gynecol Oncol* 1977;5:313–322.
474. Seifer DB, Weiss LM, Kempson KL. Malignant lymphoma arising within thyroid tissue in a mature cystic teratoma. *Cancer* 1986;58:2459–2461.
475. Feuerstein IM, Aronson BL, McCarthy EF. Bilateral ovarian cystic teratomata mimicking bilateral pure ovarian hemangiomata: case report. *Int J Gynecol Pathol* 1984;3:393–397.
476. Kempers RD, Dockerty MB, Hoffman DL, et al. Struma ovarii: ascitic, hyperthyroid and asymptomatic syndromes. *Ann Intern Med* 1970;72:883–893.
477. King AE, Ma JT, Wang C, Young RH. Hyperthyroidism during pregnancy due to coexistence of struma ovarii and Graves' disease. *Postgrad Med J* 1990;66:132–133.
478. Haseton PS, Kelehan P, Whittaker JS, et al. Benign and malignant struma ovarii. *Arch Pathol Lab Med* 1978;102:180–184.
479. Pardo-Mindan FJ, Vazquez JJ. Malignant struma ovarii: light and electron microscopic study. *Cancer* 1983;51:337–343.
480. Yannopoulos D, Yannopoulos K, Ossowski R. Malignant struma ovarii. In: Sommers SC, Rosen PP, eds. *Pathology annual.* New York: Appleton-Century-Crofts, 1976:403–413.
481. Zakhem A, Aftimos G, Kreidy R, Salem P. Malignant struma ovarii: report of two cases and selected review of the literature. *J Surg Oncol* 1990;43:61–65.
482. Devaney K, Snyder R, Norris HJ, Tavassoli FA. Proliferative and histologically malignant struma ovarii: a clinicopathologic study of 54 cases. *Int J Gynecol Pathol* 1993;12:333–343.
483. Rosenblum NG, LiVolsi VA, Edmonds PR, Mikuta JJ. Malignant struma ovarii. *Gynecol Oncol* 1989;32:224–227.
484. Willemse PHB, Oosterhuis JW, Aalders JG, et al. Malignant struma ovarii treated by ovariectomy, thyroidectomy, and ^{131}I administration. *Cancer* 1987;60:178–182.
485. Kragel PJ, Devaney K, Merino MJ. Struma ovarii with peritoneal implants: a case report with lectin histochemistry. *Surg Pathol* 1991;4:274–281.
486. Karseladze AI, Kulinitch SI. Peritoneal strumosis. *Pathol Res Pract* 1994;190:1086–1088.
487. Moor S, Waxman M. Mixed ovarian tumor composed of Brenner and thyroid elements. *Cancer* 1976;38:1997–2001.
488. Szyfelbein WM, Young RH, Scully RE. Cystic struma ovarii: a frequently unrecognized tumor. A report of 20 cases. *Am J Surg Pathol* 1994;18:1102–1116.
489. Szyfelbein WM, Young RH, Scully RE. Struma ovarii simulating ovarian tumors of other tumors of other types: a report of 30 cases. *Am J Surg Pathol* 1995;19:21–29.
490. Young RH, Jackson A, Wells M. Ovarian metastasis from thyroid carcinoma 12 years after partial thyroidectomy mimicking struma ovarii: report of a case. *Int J Gynecol Pathol* 1994;13:181–185.
491. Robboy SJ, Norris HJ, Scully RE. Insular carcinoid primary in the ovary: a clinicopathologic analysis of 48 cases. *Cancer* 1975;36:404–418.
492. Robboy SJ, Scully RE. Strumal carcinoid of the ovary: an analysis of 50 cases of a distinctive tumor composed of thyroid tissue and carcinoid. *Cancer* 1980;46:2019–2034.
493. Motoyama T, Katayama Y, Watanabe H, Okazaki E, Shibuya H. Functioning ovarian carcinoids induce severe constipation. *Cancer* 1992;70:513–518.
494. Ashtor MA. Strumal carcinoid of the ovary associated with hyperinsulinemic hypoglycemia and cutaneous melanosis. *Histopathology* 1995;27:463–467.
495. Armes JE, Ostör AG. A case of malignant strumal carcinoid. *Gynecol Oncol* 1993;51:419–423.
496. Robboy SJ. Insular carcinoid of ovary associated with malignant mucinous tumors. *Cancer* 1984;54:2273–2276.
497. Robboy SJ, Scully RE, Norris HJ. Primary trabecular carcinoid of the ovary. *Obstet Gynecol* 1977;49:202–207.
498. Talerman A, Evans MI. Primary trabecular carcinoid tumor of the ovary. *Cancer* 1982;50:1403–1407.
499. Dayal Y, Tashjian AH Jr, Wolfe HJ. Immunocytochemical localization of calcitonin-producing cells in a strumal carcinoid with amyloid stroma. *Cancer* 1979;43:1331–1338.
500. Stagno PA, Petras RE, Hart WR. Strumal carcinoids of the ovary: an immunohistologic and ultrastructural study. *Arch Pathol Lab Med* 1987;111:440–446.
501. Snyder RR, Tavassoli FA. Ovarian strumal carcinoid: immunohistochemical, ultrastructural, and clinicopathologic observations. *Int J Gynecol Pathol* 1986;5:187–201.
502. Czernobilsky B, Segal M, Dgani R. Primary ovarian carcinoid with marked heterogeneity of microscopic features. *Cancer* 1984;54:585–589.
503. Alenghat E, Okagaki T, Talerman A. Primary mucinous carcinoid tumor of the ovary. *Cancer* 1986;58:777–783.
504. Volpert HR, Fuller AF, Bell DA. Primary mucinous carcinoid tumor of the ovary: a case report. *Int J Gynecol Pathol* 1989;8:156–162.

505. Sorrong B, Falkmer S, Robboy SJ, et al. Neurohormonal peptides in ovarian carcinoids: an immunohistochemical study of 81 primary carcinoids and of intraovarian metastases from six mid-gut carcinoids. *Cancer* 1982;49:68–74.
506. Matias-Guiu X, Forteza J, Prat J. Mixed strumal and mucinous carcinoid tumor of the ovary. *Int J Gynecol Pathol* 1995;14:179–183.
507. Inoue M, Ueda G, Nakajima T. Immunohistochemical demonstration of neuron-specific enolase in gynecologic malignant tumors. *Cancer* 1985;55:1686–1690.
508. Aguirre P, Scully RE. Malignant neuroectodermal tumor of the ovary, a distinctive form of monodermal teratoma: report of five cases. *Am J Surg Pathol* 1982;6:283–292.
509. Kleinman GM, Young RH, Scully RE. Primary ovarian neuroectodermal tumors: a report of 25 cases. *Am J Surg Pathol* 1993;17:764–778.
510. Kleinman GM, Young RH, Scully RE. Ependymoma of the ovary: report of three cases. *Hum Pathol* 1984;15:632–638.
511. Chumas JC, Scully RE. Sebaceous tumors arising in ovarian dermoid cysts. *Int J Gynecol Pathol* 1991;10:356–363.
512. Papadopoulos AJ, Ahmed H, Pakarian FB, Caldwell CJ, McNicholas J, Raju KS. Sebaceous carcinoma arising within an ovarian cystic mature teratoma. *Int J Gynecol Cancer* 1995;5:76–79.
513. Hameed K, Burslem MRG. A melanotic ovarian neoplasm resembling the "retinal anlage" tumor. *Cancer* 1970;25:564–567.
514. Sinniah R, O'Brien FV. Pigmented progonoma in a dermoid cyst of the ovary. *J Pathol* 1973;109:357–359.
515. King ME, Mouradian JA, Micha JP, et al. Immature teratoma of the ovary with predominant malignant retinal anlage component: a parthenogenically derived tumor. *Am J Surg Pathol* 1985;9:221–231.
516. Karten G, Sher JH, Marsh MR, et al. Neurogenic cyst of the ovary: a rare form of benign cystic teratoma. *Arch Pathol* 1968;86:563–567.
517. Fogt F, Vortmeyer AO, Ahn G, et al. Neural cyst of the ovary with central nervous system microvasculature. *Histopathology* 1994;24:477–480.
518. Tiltman AJ. Ependymal cyst of the ovary. *S Afr Med J* 1985;68:424–425.
519. Clement PB, Dimmick JE. Endodermal variant of mature cystic teratoma of the ovary: report of a case. *Cancer* 1979;43:383–385.
520. Anderson MC, McDicken IW. Melanotic cyst of the ovary. *J Obstet Gynecol Brit Commonw* 1971;78:1047–1049.
521. Axiotis CA, Lippes HA, Merino MJ, et al. Corticotroph cell pituitary adenoma within an ovarian teratoma: a new cause of Cushing's syndrome. *Am J Surg Pathol* 1987;11:218–224.
522. Palmer PE, Bogojavlensky S, Bhan AK, Scully RE. Prolactinoma in wall of ovarian dermoid cyst with hyperprolactinemia: report of a case. *Obstet Gynecol* 1990;75:540–543.
523. Kurman RJ, Norris HJ. Malignant mixed germ cell tumors of the ovary: a clinical and pathologic analysis of 30 cases. *Obstet Gynecol* 1976;48:579–589.
524. Gershenson DM, Del Junco G, Copeland LJ, et al. Mixed germ cell tumors of the ovary. *Obstet Gynecol* 1984;64:200–206.
525. Ueda G, Yamasaki M, Inoue M, et al. A rare malignant ovarian mixed germ cell tumor containing pancreatic tissue with islet cells. *Int J Gynecol Pathol* 1984;3:220–231.
526. Scully RE. Gonadoblastoma: a review of 74 cases. *Cancer* 1970;25:1340–1356.
527. Nakashima K, Nagasaka T, Fukata S, et al. Ovarian gonadoblastoma with dysgerminoma in a woman with two normal children. *Hum Pathol* 1989;20:814–816.
528. Jorgensen N, Müller J, Jaubert F, Clausen OP, Skakkebaek NE. Heterogeneity of gonadoblastoma germ cells: similarities with immature germ cells, spermatogonia and testicular carcinoma in situ cells. *Histopathology* 1997;30:177–186.
529. Talerman A. Gonadoblastoma associated with embryonal carcinoma. *Obstet Gynecol* 1974;43:138–142.
530. Hart WR, Burkons DM. Germ cell neoplasms arising in gonadoblastomas. *Cancer* 1979;43:669–789.
531. Kedzia H. Gonadoblastoma: structures and background of development. *Am J Obstet Gynecol* 1983;147:81–85.
532. Talerman A. A distinctive gonadal neoplasm related to gonadoblastoma. *Cancer* 1972;30:1219–1224.
533. Talerman A, van der Harten JJ. A mixed cell–sex cord stroma tumor of the ovary associated with isosexual precocious puberty in a normal girl. *Cancer* 1977;40:889–894.
534. Tavassoli FA. A combined germ cell-gonadal stromal-epithelial tumor of the ovary. *Am J Surg Pathol* 1983;7:73–84.
535. Talerman A. A combined germ cell-gonadal stromal-epithelial tumor of the ovary or a hamartoma [Letter]. *Am J Surg Pathol* 1984;8:638–639.
536. Tokuoka S, Aoki Y, Hayaski Y, et al. A mixed germ cell-sex cord-stromal tumor of the ovary with retiform tubular structure: a case report. *Int J Gynecol Pathol* 1985;4:161–170.
537. Lacson AG, Gillis DA, Shawwa A. Malignant mixed germ cell-sex cord-stromal tumors of the ovary associated with isosexual precocious puberty. *Cancer* 1988;61:2122–2133.
538. Jacobsen GK, Braendstrup O, Talerman A. Bilateral mixed germ cell sex-cord stroma tumour in a young adult woman: case report. *APMIS Suppl* 1991;23:132–137.
539. Zuntova A, Motlik K, Horejsi J, Eckschlager T. Mixed germ cell–sex cord stromal tumor with heterologous structures. *Int J Gyncecol Pathol* 1992;11:227–233.
540. Fallahzadeh H, Dockerty MB, Lee RA. Leiomyoma of the ovary: report of five cases and review of the literature. *Am J Obstet Gynecol* 1972;113:394–398.
541. Tsalacopoulos G, Tiltman AJ. Leiomyoma of the ovary: a report of 3 cases. *S Afr Med J* 1981;59:574–575.
542. Prayson RA, Hart WR. Primary smooth-muscle tumors of the ovary: a clinicopathologic study of four leiomyomas and two mitotically active leiomyomas. *Arch Pathol Lab Med* 1992;116:1068–1071.
543. Kandalaft PL, Esteban JM. Bilateral massive ovarian leiomyomata in a young woman: a case report with review of the literature. *Mod Pathol* 1992;5:586–589.
544. Miyauchi J, Mukai M, Yamazaki K, Kosi I, Higashi S, Hori S. Bilateral ovarian hemangiomas associated with diffuse hemangioendotheliomatosis: a case report. *Acta Pathol Jpn* 1987;37:1347–1355.
545. Talerman A. Nonspecific tumors of the ovary, including mesenchymal tumors and malignant lymphoma. In: Kurman RJ, ed. *Blaustein's pathology of the female genital tract*, 4th ed. New York: Springer-Verlag, 1994:915–937.
546. Eichhorn JH, Scully RE. Ovarian myxoma: clinicopathologic and immunocytologic analysis of five cases and a review of the literature. *Int J Gynecol Pathol* 1991;10:156–169.
547. Costa MJ, Thomas W, Majmudar B, Hewan-Lowe K. Ovarian myxoma: ultrastructural and immunohistochemical findings. *Ultrastruct Pathol* 1992;16:429–438.
548. Costa MJ, Morris R, DeRose PB, Cohen C. Histologic and immunohistochemical evidence for considering ovarian myxoma as a variant of the thecoma-fibroma group of ovarian stromal tumors. *Arch Pathol Lab Med* 1993;117:802–80.
549. Tetu B, Bonenfant J. Ovarian myxoma: a study of two cases with longterm follow-up. *Am J Clin Pathol* 1991;95:340–346.
550. Pai S, Naresh KN, Desai PB, Borges AM. Ovarian myxoma in a premenarchal girl. *Gynecol Oncol* 1994;55:453–455.
551. Shakfeh SM, Woodruff JD. Primary ovarian sarcomas: report of 46 cases and review of the literature. *Obstet Gynecol Surg* 1987;42:331–349.
552. Nieminen V, von Numers C, Purola E. Primary sarcoma of the ovary. *Acta Obstet Gynecol Scand* 1969;48:423–432.
553. Kraemer BB, Silva EG, Sniege N. Fibrosarcoma of ovary: a new component in the nevoid basal-cell carcinoma syndrome. *Am J Surg Pathol* 1984;8:231–236.
554. Miles PA, Kiley KC, Mena H. Giant fibrosarcoma of the ovary. *Int J Gynecol Pathol* 1985;4:83–87.
555. Anderson B, Turner DA, Benda J. Ovarian sarcoma. *Gynecol Oncol* 1987;26:183–192.
556. Nogales FF, Ayala A, Ruiz-Avila I, Sirvent JJ. Myxoid leiomyosarcoma of the ovary: analysis of three cases. *Hum Pathol* 1991;22:1268–1273.
557. Friedman HD, Mazur MT. Primary ovarian leiomyosarcoma: an immunohistochemical and ultrastructural study. *Arch Pathol Lab Med* 1991;115:941–945.
558. Monk BJ, Nieberg R, Berek JS. Primary leiomyosarcoma of the ovary in a perimenarchal female. *Gynecol Oncol* 1993;48:389–393.
559. Stone GC, Bell DA, Fuller A, Dickersin GR, Scully RE. Malignant schwannoma of the ovary: report of a case. *Cancer* 1986;58:1575–1582.
560. Nielsen GP, Young RH, Prat J, Scully RE. Primary angiosarcoma of the ovary: a report of seven cases and review of the literature. *Int J Gynecol Pathol* 1997;16:378–382.
561. Nucci MR, Krausz T, Lifschitz-Mercer B, Chang JKC, Fletcher CDM. Angiosarcoma of the ovary: clinicopathologic and immunohisto-

562. Hirakawa T, Tsuneyoshi M, Enjoji M, Shigyo R. Ovarian sarcoma with histologic features of telangiectatic osteosarcoma of bone. *Am J Surg Pathol* 1988;12:567–572.
563. Hines JF, Compton DM, Stacy CC, Potter ME. Pure primary osteosarcoma of the ovary presenting as an extensively calcified adnexal mass: a case report and review of the literature. *Gynecol Oncol* 1990;39:259–263.
564. Sakata H, Hirahara T, Ryu A, Sawada T, Yamamoto M, Sakurai I. Primary osteosarcoma of the ovary: a case report. *Acta Pathol Jpn* 1991;41:311–317.
565. Guerard MJ, Arguelles MA, Ferenczy A. Rhabdomyosarcoma of the ovary: ultrastructural study of a case and review of the literature. *Gynecol Oncol* 1983;15:325–339.
566. Chen YF, Leung CS, Ma L. Primary embryonal rhabdomyosarcoma of the ovary in a 4-year-old girl. *Histopathology* 1989;15:303–311.
567. Nielsen GP, Young RH, Rosenberg AE, Oliva E, Prat J, Scully RE. Primary ovarian rhabdomyosarcoma: a report of 13 cases. *Int J Gynecol Pathol* 1998;17:113–119.
568. Talerman A, Auerbach WM, Van Meurs AJ. Primary chondrosarcoma of the ovary. *Histopathology* 1981;5:319–324.
569. Ngwalle KE, Hirakawa T, Tsuneyoshi M, Enjoji M. Osteosarcoma arising in a benign dermoid cyst of the ovary. *Gynecol Oncol* 1990;37:143–147.
570. Allen C, Stephens M, Williams J. Combined high grade sarcoma and serous ovarian neoplasm. *J Clin Pathol* 1992;45:263–264.
571. Tsujimura T, Kawano K. Rhabdomyosarcoma coexistent with ovarian mucinous cystadenocarcinoma: a case report. *Int J Gynecol Pathol* 1992;11:58–62.
572. Osborne BM, Robboy SJ. Lymphomas or leukemia presenting as ovarian tumors: an analysis of 42 cases. *Cancer* 1983;52:1933–1943.
573. Fox H, Langley FA, Govan AD, Hill AS, Bennett MH. Malignant lymphoma presenting as an ovarian tumour: a clinicopathological analysis of 34 cases. *Br J Obstet Gynecol* 1988;95:386–390.
574. Ferry JA, Young RH. Malignant lymphoma, pseudolymphoma, and hematopoietic disorders of the female genital tract. *Pathol Annu* 1991;26(pt. 1):227–263.
575. Monterroso V, Jaffe ES, Merino MJ, Medeiros LJ. Malignant lymphomas involving the ovary: a clinicopathologic analysis of 39 cases. *Am J Surg Pathol* 1993;17:154–170.
576. Oliva E, Ferry JA, Young RH, Prat J, Srigley JR, Scully RE. Granulocytic sarcoma of the female genital tract: a clinicopathologic study of 11 cases. *Am J Surg Pathol* 1997;27:1156–1165.
577. Cecalupo AJ, Frankel LS, Sullivan P. Pelvic and ovarian extramedullary leukemic relapse in young girls. *Cancer* 1982;50:587–593.
578. Long JP, Patchefsky AS. Primary Hodgkin's disease of the ovary: a case report. *Obstet Gynecol* 1971;38:680–682.
579. Cook HT, Boylston AE. Plasmacytoma of the ovary. *Gynecol Oncol* 1988;29:378–381.
580. Dickersin GR, Kline IW, Scully RE. Small cell carcinoma of the ovary with hypercalcemia: a report of eleven cases. *Cancer* 1982;49:186–197.
581. McMahon JT, Hart WR. Ultrastructural analysis of small cell carcinomas of the ovary. *Am J Clin Pathol* 1988;90:523–529.
582. Aguirre P, Thor AD, Scully RE. Ovarian small cell carcinoma: histogenetic considerations based on immunohistochemical and other findings. *Am J Clin Pathol* 1989;92:140–149.
583. Eichhorn JH, Bell DA, Young RH, et al. DNA content and proliferative activity in ovarian small cell carcinomas of the hypercalcemic type: implications for diagnosis, prognosis, and histogenesis. *Am J Clin Pathol* 1992;98:579–586.
584. Dickersin GR, Scully RE. An update on the electron microscopy of small cell carcinoma of the ovary with hypercalcemia. *Ultrastruct Pathol* 1993;17:411–422.
585. Young RH, Oliva E, Scully RE. Small cell carcinoma of the ovary, hypercalcemic type: a clinicopathologic analysis of 150 cases. *Am J Surg Pathol* 1994;18:1102–1116.
586. Young RH, Scully RE. Alveolar rhabdomyosarcoma metastatic to the ovary: a report of two cases and a discussion of the differential diagnosis of small cell malignant tumors of the ovary. *Cancer* 1989;64:899–904.
587. Young RH, Gersell DJ, Clement PB, Scully RE. Hepatocellular carcinoma metastatic to the ovary: a report of three cases discovered during life with discussion of the differential diagnosis of hepatoid tumor of the ovary. *Hum Pathol* 1992;23:574–580.
588. Hughesdon PE. Ovarian tumours of wolffian or allied nature: their place in ovarian oncology. *J Clin Pathol* 1982;35:526–535.
589. Young RH, Silva EG, Scully RE. Ovarian and juxtaovarian adenomatoid tumors: a report of six cases. *Int J Gynecol Pathol* 1991;10:364–371.
590. Young RH, Eichhorn JH, Dickersin GR, Scully RE. Ovarian involvement by the intra-abdominal desmoplastic small round cell tumor with divergent differentiation: a report of three cases. *Hum Pathol* 1992;23:454–464.
591. Goldblum J, Hart WR. Localized and diffuse mesotheliomas of the genital tract and peritoneum in women: a clinicopathologic study of nineteen true mesothelial neoplasms, other than adenomatoid tumors, multicystic mesotheliomas and localized fibrous tumors. *Am J Surg Pathol* 1995;19:1124–1137.
592. Clement PB, Young RH, Scully RE. Malignant mesotheliomas presenting as ovarian masses: a report of nine cases, including two primary ovarian mesotheliomas. *Am J Surg Pathol* 1996;20:1067–1080.
593. Young RH, Scully RE. Metastatic tumors in the ovary: a problem-oriented approach and review of the recent literature. *Semin Diagn Pathol* 1991;8:250–276.
594. Hale RW. Krukenberg tumor of the ovaries: a review of 81 records. *Obstet Gynecol* 1968;32:221–225.
595. Holtz F, Hart WR. Krukenberg tumors of the ovary: a clinicopathological analysis of 27 cases. *Cancer* 1982;50:2438–2447.
596. Yakushiji M, Tazaki T, Nishimura H, Kato T. Krukenberg tumors of the ovary: a clinicopathological analysis of 112 cases. *Acta Obstet Gynecol Jpn* 1987;39:479–485.
597. Wong PC, Ferenczy A, Fan L-D, McCaughey E. Krukenberg tumors of the ovary: ultrastructural, histochemical, and immunohistochemical studies of 15 cases. *Cancer* 1986;57:751–760.
598. Joshi VV. Primary Krukenberg tumor of ovary: review of literature and case report. *Cancer* 1968;22:1199–1207.
599. Bullon A, Arseneau J, Prat J, Young RH, Scully RE. Tubular Krukenberg tumor: a problem in histopathologic diagnosis. *Am J Surg Pathol* 1981;5:225–232.
600. Burt CAV. Prophylactic oophorectomy with resection of the large bowel for cancer. *Am J Surg* 1951;82:571–577.
601. Cutait R, Lesser ML, Enker WE. Prophylactic oophorectomy in surgery for large-bowel cancer. *Dis Colon Rectum* 1983;26:6–11.
602. Graffner HOL, Alm POA, Oscarson JEA. Prophylactic oophorectomy in colorectal carcinoma. *Am J Surg* 1983;146:233–235.
603. Harcourt EF, Dennis DL. Laparotomy for "ovarian tumors" in unsuspected carcinoma of the colon. *Cancer* 1968;21:1244–1246.
604. O'Brien PH, Newton BB, Metcalf JS, Rittenbury MS. Oophorectomy in women with carcinoma of the colon and rectum. *Surg Gynecol Obstet* 1981;153:827–830.
605. Johansen H. Clinical aspects of metastatic ovarian cancer of extragenital origin. *Acta Obstet Gynecol Scand* 1960;39:681–697.
606. Daya D, Nazerali K, Frank GL. Metastatic ovarian carcinoma of large intestinal origin simulating primary ovarian carcinoma: a clinicopathologic study of 25 cases. *Am J Clin Pathol* 1992;97:751–758.
607. Scully RE, Richardson GS. Luteinization of the stroma of metastatic cancer involving the ovary and its endocrine significance. *Cancer* 1961;14:827–840.
608. Robboy SJ, Scully RE, Norris HJ. Carcinoid metastatic to the ovary: a clinicopathologic analysis of 35 cases. *Cancer* 1974;33:798–811.
609. Lee YN, Hori JM. Significance of ovarian metastases in therapeutic oophorectomy for advanced breast cancer. *Cancer* 1971;27:1374–1378.
610. Gagnon Y, Tetu B. Ovarian metastases of breast carcinoma: a clinicopathologic study of 59 cases. *Cancer* 1989;64:892–898.
611. Puga FJ, Gibbs CP, Williams TJ. Castrating operations associated with metastatic lesions of the breast. *Obstet Gynecol* 1973;41:713–719.
612. Lumb G, Mackenzie DH. The incidence of metastases in adrenal glands and ovaries removed for carcinoma of the breast. *Cancer* 1959;2:521–526.
613. Erickman M, Ferreira B. Metastasis of breast carcinoma to the ovaries: incidence, significance, and relationship to survival. A preliminary study. *Grace Hosp Bull* 1967;45:44–49.
614. Young RH, Carey RW, Robboy SJ. Breast carcinoma masquerading as a primary ovarian neoplasm. *Cancer* 1981;48:210–212.
615. Harris M, Howell A, Chrissohou M, Swindell RIC, Hudson M, Sell-

wood RA. A comparison of the metastatic pattern of infiltrating lobular carcinoma and infiltrating duct carcinoma of the breast. *Br J Cancer* 1984;50:23–30.
616. Caron P, Roche H, Gorguet H, Martel P, Bennet A, Carton M. Mammary ovarian metastases with stroma cell hyperplasia and postmenopausal virilization. *Cancer* 1990;66:1221–1224.
617. Young RH, Scully RE. Metastatic tumors of the ovary. In: Kurman RJ, ed. *Blaustein's pathology of the female genital tract*, 4th ed. New York: Springer-Verlag, 1994.
618. Ronnett BM, Kurman RJ, Shmookler BM, Sugarbaker PH, Young RH. The morphologic spectrum of ovarian metastases of appendiceal adenocarcinomas: a clinicopathologic and immunohistochemical analysis of tumors often misinterpreted as primary ovarian tumors or metastatic tumors from other gastrointestinal sites. *Am J Surg Pathol* 1997;21:1144–1155.
619. Merino MJ, Edmonds P, LiVolsi V. Appendiceal carcinoma metastatic to the ovaries and mimicking primary ovarian tumors. *Int J Gynecol Pathol* 1985;4:110–120.
620. Hirschfield LS, Kahn LB, Winkler B, Bochner RZ, Gibstein AA. Adenocarcinoid of the appendix presenting as bilateral Krukenberg tumor of the ovaries. *Arch Pathol Lab Med* 1985;109:930–933.
621. Young RH, Gilks CB, Scully RE. Mucinous tumors of the appendix associated with mucinous tumors of the ovary and pseudomyxoma peritonei: a clinicopathological analysis of 22 cases supporting an origin in the appendix. *Am J Surg Pathol* 1991;15:415–429.
622. Seidman JD, Elsayed AM, Sobin LH, Tavassoli FA. Association of mucinous tumors of the ovary and appendix: a clinicopathologic study of 25 cases. *Am J Surg Pathol* 1993;17:22–34.
623. Young RH, Gilks CB, Scully RE. Letter to the Editor. *Am J Surg Pathol* 1993;17:1068–1070.
624. Seidman JD, Elsayed AM, Sobin LH, Tavassoli A. Authors reply to the editor. *Am J Surg Pathol* 1993;17:1070–1071.
625. Prayson RA, Hart WR, Petras RE. Pseudomyxoma peritonei: a clinicopathologic study of 19 cases with emphasis on site of origin and nature of associated ovarian tumors. *Am J Surg Pathol* 1994;18:591–603.
626. Ronnett BM, Kurman RJ, Zahn CM, et al. Pseudomyxoma peritonei in women: a clinicopathologic analysis of 30 cases with emphasis on site of origin, prognosis, and relationship to ovarian mucinous tumors of low malignant potential. *Hum Pathol* 1995;56:509–524.
627. Ronnett BM, Shmookler BM, Diener-West M, Sugarbaker PH, Kurman RJ. Immunohistochemical evidence supporting the appendiceal origin of pseudomyxoma peritonei in women. *Int J Gynecol Pathol* 1997;16:1–9.
628. Cuatrecasas M, Matias-Guiu X, Prat J. Synchronous mucinous tumors of the appendix and the ovary associated with pseudomyxoma peritonei: a clinicopathologic study of six cases with comparative analysis of c-Ki-ras mutations. *Am J Surg Pathol* 1996;20:739–746.
629. Young RH, Hart WR. Metastases from carcinomas of the pancreas simulating primary mucinous tumors of the ovary: a report of seven cases. *Am J Surg Pathol* 1989;13:748–756.
630. Young RH, Scully RE. Ovarian metastases from carcinoma of the gallbladder and extrahepatic bile ducts simulating primary tumors of the ovary: a report of six cases. *Int J Gynecol Pathol* 1990;9:60–72.
631. Young RH, Kozakewich HPW, Scully RE. Metastatic ovarian tumors in children: a report of 14 cases and review of the literature. *Int J Gynecol Pathol* 1993;12:8–19.
632. Meyer WH, Yu GW, Milvenan ES, Jeffs RD, Kaizer H, Leventhal BG. Ovarian involvement in neuroblastoma. *Med Pediatr Oncol* 1979;7:49–54.
633. Hameed K. Melanotic ovarian neoplasms. *Prog Clin Cancer* 1973;5:209–217.
634. Fitzgibbons PL, Martin SE, Simmons TJ. Malignant melanoma metastatic to the ovary. *Am J Surg Pathol* 1987;11:959–964.
635. Young RH, Scully RE. Ovarian metastases from cancer of the lung: problems in interpretation. A report of seven cases. *Gynecol Oncol* 1985;21:337–350.
636. Eichhorn JH, Young RH, Scully RE. Non-pulmonary small cell carcinomas of extragenital origin metastatic to the ovary: a report of seven cases. *Cancer* 1993;71:177–186.
637. Longacre TA, O'Hanlan K, Hendrickson MR. Adenoid cystic carcinoma of the submandibular gland with symptomatic ovarian metastases. *Int J Gynecol Pathol* 1996;15:349–355.
638. Zukerberg LR, Young RH. Chordoma metastatic to the ovary. *Arch Pathol Lab Med* 1990;114:208–210.
639. Bunker ML. The terminal findings in endometrial carcinoma. *Am J Obstet Gynecol* 1959;77:530–538.
640. Beck RP, Latour JPA. Necropsy reports on 36 cases of endometrial carcinoma. *Am J Obstet Gynecol* 1963;85:307–311.
641. Mazur MT, Hsueh S, Gersell DJ. Metastases to the female genital tract: analysis of 325 cases. *Cancer* 1984;53:1978–1984.
642. Woolas R, Jacobs I, Prys Davies A, et al. What is the true incidence of primary fallopian tube carcinoma? *Int J Gynecol Cancer* 1994;4:384–388.
643. Green TH, Scully RE. Tumors of the fallopian tube. *Clin Obstet Gynecol* 1962;5:886–906.
644. Alvarado-Cabrero I, Young RH, Vamvakas EC, Scully RE. Carcinoma of the fallopian tube: a clinicopathological study of 105 cases with observations on staging and prognostic factors. *Gynecol Oncol* 1998 (in press).

CHAPTER 55

The Fallopian Tube and Broad Ligament

Robert H. Young, Philip B. Clement, and Robert E. Scully

INFLAMMATORY DISEASES

Acute Salpingitis

Acute salpingitis may be secondary to sexually transmitted infection by *Neisseria gonorrhoeae*, *Chlamydia*, or *Mycoplasma*, or may result from an infection by a variety of other organisms including streptococci, staphylococci, coliform bacilli, and anaerobic bacteria, which may reach the tubes by way of the lymphatic or blood vessels, especially after an abortion or pregnancy (1–3). The tube is typically enlarged, edematous, and erythematous (Fig. 1), frequently with fibrinopurulent serosal and luminal exudate, and is often adherent to adjacent tissues, including the ovary, which may be involved as part of a tubo-ovarian abscess. Microscopic examination reveals a marked neutrophilic infiltration of the tubal plicae associated with congestion and edema. The mucosa may be ulcerated with purulent exudate in the lumen. The epithelium is often hyperplastic and may exhibit reactive atypia, occasionally resulting in an appearance that simulates that of carcinoma (see below). In occasional cases of salpingitis, chlamydial antigens have been demonstrable with immunoperoxidase staining (4).

It should be emphasized that acute inflammatory cells may be seen in the lumen and lamina propria of the tube at the time of menstruation and the puerperium (5,6), and, occasionally, to a lesser extent at other times during the menstrual cycle (7). In these cases of "physiologic salpingitis" (5–7), edema and lymphatic dilatation in the tubal plicae are usually present as well. The inflammation, which is maximal at midmenstruation, only rarely involves the muscularis, is unaccompanied by necrosis or ulceration, and is not followed by chronic inflammatory cell infiltration.

R. H. Young and R. E. Scully: Department of Pathology, Massachusetts General Hospital; Harvard Medical School, Boston, Massachusetts 02114.

P. B. Clement: Department of Pathology, Vancouver Hospital and Health Sciences Center, University of British Columbia, Vancouver, British Columbia V5Z 1M9.

Chronic Salpingitis

In chronic salpingitis, the tube is usually enlarged, distorted, and adherent to the ovary and adjacent tissues (Fig. 2). If the infection has caused adherence of the fimbriae, obliteration of the ostium may lead to a hydrosalpinx with a thin translucent wall and a content of clear fluid, or a pyosalpinx. Hydrosalpinx is typically bilateral but may be unilateral (Fig. 3). Resolution of a tubo-ovarian abscess may result in a tubo-ovarian cyst. Microscopic examination of the tube reveals shortened, blunted, and fibrotic plicae containing chronic inflammatory cells. Plical fusion typically results in the formation of pseudoglandular spaces [chronic follicular salpingitis (Fig. 4)]. In cases of hydrosalpinx only a few small plicae usually remain, and the lining epithelium is typically flattened or low cuboidal. Late stages of chronic salpingitis may result in fibrous obliteration of the lumen, typically in the cornual-isthmic region.

Granulomatous Salpingitis

Mycobacterial Causes

The most common cause of granulomatous salpingitis is infection with *Mycobacterium tuberculosis* or *Mycobacterium bovis*. Eighty to 90% of women with genital tuberculosis have tubal involvement (8), and the process is bilateral in 90% of the cases (8–10). Early or mild infection results in irregular thickening or nodularity of the wall; serosal tubercles are visible in about 20% of the cases (9). In more severe forms of tuberculous salpingitis, there may be dense tubo-ovarian adhesions, a thickened wall, an ulcerated mucosa, and a caseous luminal exudate. The ostium of the tube generally remains open, in contrast to most other forms of chronic salpingitis. On microscopic examination the characteristic feature is the presence of tuberculous granulomas, which may be caseating, within the mucosa (Figs. 5 and 6); a marked epithelial hyperplasia may simulate adenocarcinoma (Fig 5) (see below), and Schaumann bodies may be conspicuous. The muscularis shows varying degrees of

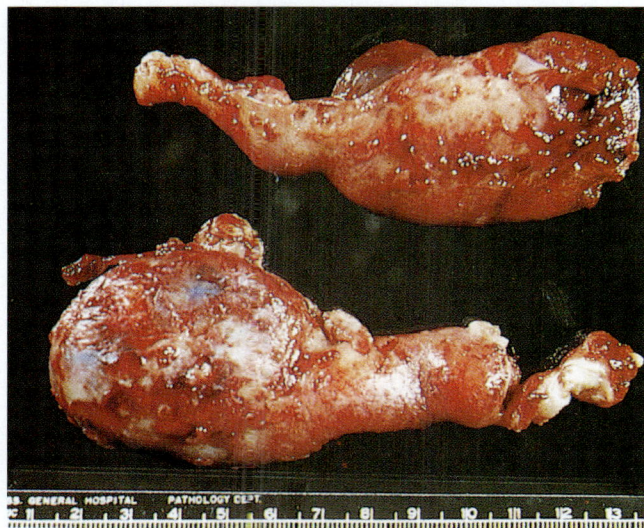

FIG. 1. Acute and chronic salpingitis. Both tubes are distended, and there is closure of the fimbriated ends, extensive congestion, and hemorrhage on the serosal surfaces.

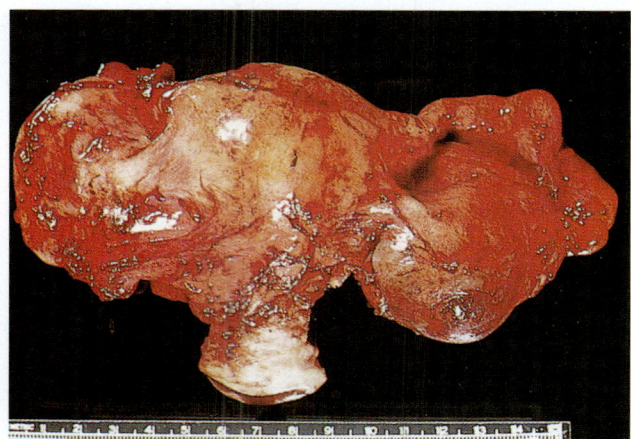

FIG. 2. Chronic salpingo-oophoritis. Both tubes and ovaries are bound down in hemorrhagic adhesions that largely obscure the tube on one side.

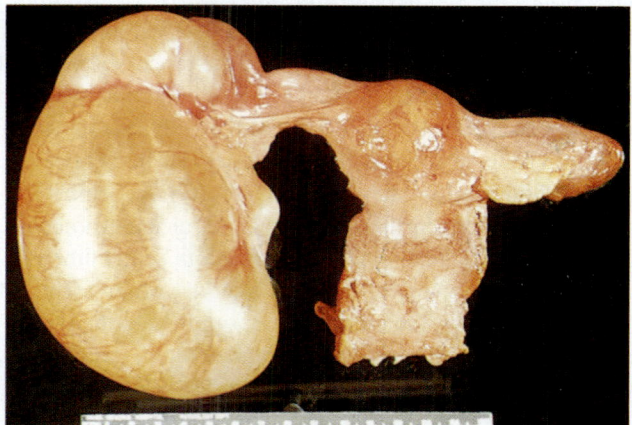

FIG. 3. Unilateral hydrosalpinx. The tube is markedly dilated and thin walled.

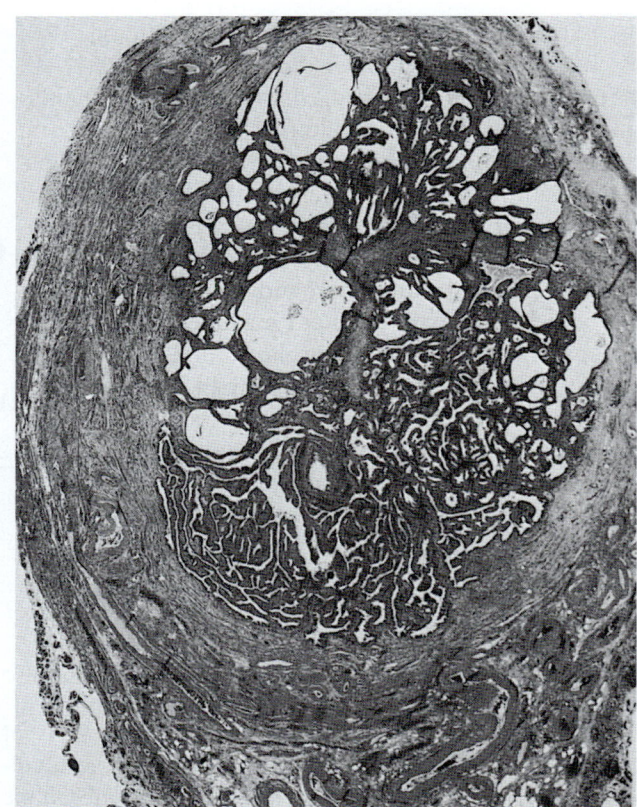

FIG. 4. Chronic follicular salpingitis. The tubal plicae are adherent to one another, and variably sized follicle-like spaces have resulted. (From ref. 10.)

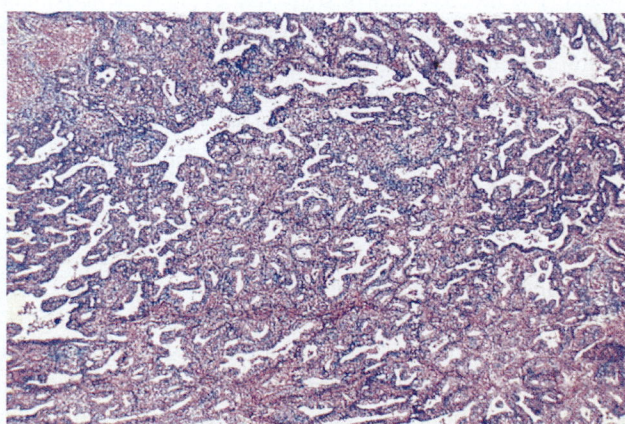

FIG. 5. Tuberculous salpingitis. The plicae contain tubercles *(upper left)* with marked epithelial hyperplasia simulating the appearance of adenocarcinoma.

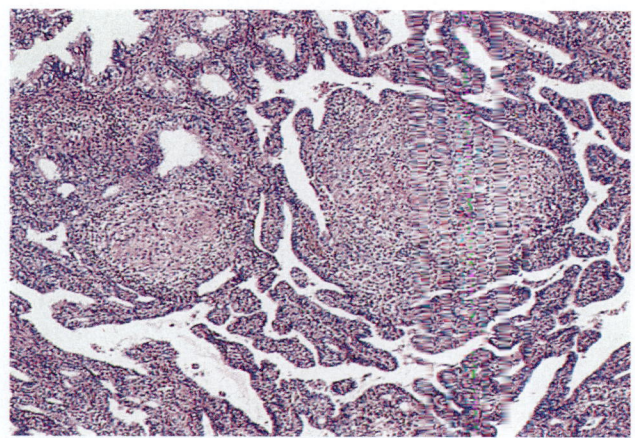

FIG. 6. Tuberculous salpingitis. Note granulomas within inflamed plicae.

chronic inflammation and fibrosis. The diagnosis should be confirmed with special stains or culture. The differential diagnosis includes very rare cases of leprous salpingitis (11).

Actinomycosis

Actinomycosis of the fallopian tube is encountered most often in patients with an intrauterine contraceptive device (12,13). The disease is bilateral in almost half the cases (12), and the ovaries are frequently also involved. Gross inspection may reveal various nonspecific manifestations of acute and chronic salpingitis, but the only specific finding is the presence of small yellow flecks (sulfur granules) within the luminal exudate. A fistulous communication with the bowel, urinary bladder, or skin may be present. Microscopic examination reveals that the diagnostic granules are composed of masses of the gram-positive filamentous bacteria surrounded by a purulent exudate; a typical granulomatous response is rare.

Fungal Infections

Fungi are rare causes of granulomatous salpingitis, with cases of blastomycosis and more commonly coccidioidomycosis reported in the American literature (14–17). Typically, a tubo-ovarian abscess or inflammatory tubo-ovarian mass is associated with tubercle-like nodules on the peritoneal surfaces. The causative organisms are generally identifiable on microscopic examination.

Parasitic Infestations

Schistosomiasis of the tube is rare in the United States but common in areas of endemic disease (18,19). *Schistosoma haematobium* is the usual agent. Grossly, the tube may exhibit nodularity or scarring due to the fibrosis elicited by the deposition of ova. Microscopically, there is a granulomatous reaction to the characteristic ova (20).

Involvement of the tube by *Enterobius vermicularis* is probably secondary to migration of the pinworm from the lower female genital tract. Infestation may cause a nodular thickening of the wall (21); seeding of the pelvic peritoneum by ova with a surrounding reaction may simulate tubercles. Fragments of the worms or their ova are surrounded by necrotic debris, an eosinophil-rich infiltrate, foreign-body giant cells, granulation tissue, and fibrous tissue. Cysticercosis of the tube has also been reported (22).

Foreign Body Salpingitis

Granulomatous salpingitis may result when irritative agents such as lubricant jellies, mineral oil, powder containing talc or starch, and radiographic contrast media are introduced into the genital tract (Fig. 7) (23–25). Grossly, the tube may have a yellow or chocolate-brown appearance, suggesting the diagnosis of endometriosis. When lipid material is the causative agent, numerous foamy histiocytes in the mucosa are characteristic. Typically, a foreign-body giant cell reaction is present and may extend to the serosa. Although so-called lipoid salpingitis usually results from the introduction of foreign material, occasional lipoid granulomas have been reported in gonococcal and tuberculous salpingitis (24). Thus, an infectious process should be excluded before attributing the lesion to foreign material.

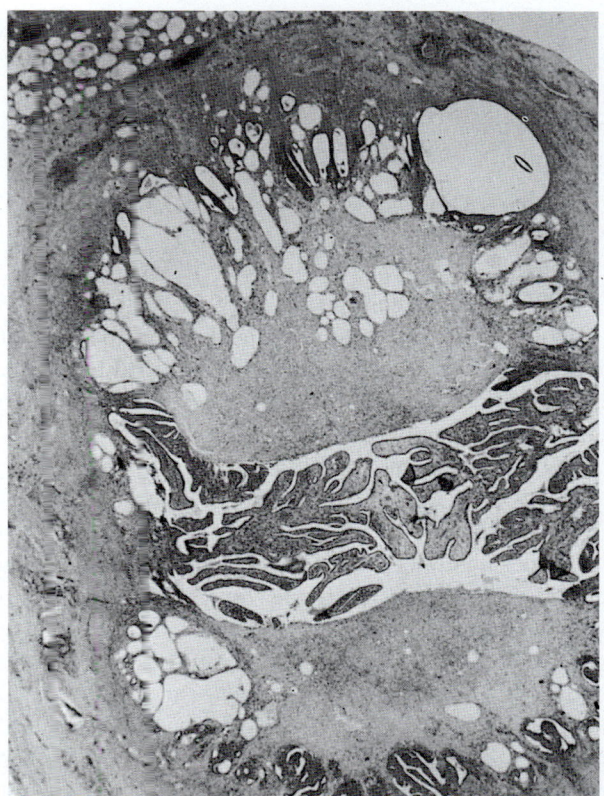

FIG. 7 Lipoid salpingitis. The lumen is markedly narrowed by a granulomatous reaction to oily contrast medium (clear spaces). (From ref. 10.)

Other Causes

Other causes of granulomatous salpingitis include involvement by Crohn's disease (26) and sarcoidosis (27,28). With regard to the distinction between sarcoidosis and tuberculosis, it should be remembered that Schaumann bodies may be seen in cases of tuberculosis. Diffuse infiltration of the endosalpinx by histiocytes can be seen in chronic pelvic inflammatory disease (xanthogranulomatous salpingitis) (29–31) and malacoplakia (32,33). Numerous pigmented histiocytes (pseudoxanthoma cells) containing lipofuscin (ceroid) may be encountered in the tubal mucosa in pelvic endometriosis (34) and after pelvic irradiation (35). Tubal palisading granulomas with central necrosis have been described secondary to tubal diathermy (36). A granulomatous reaction may also be encountered in small to medium-sized arteries in patients with giant cell arteritis (37).

Ligneous Salpingitis

Rare cases of ligneous inflammation of the female genital tract may involve the fallopian tube and may account for infertility in these patients. The lesion is characterized by amorphous eosinophilic hyaline material, and may be associated with similar involvement of other sites in the female genital tract or ligneous conjunctivitis (38).

Changes Secondary to Ligation

Following ligation, the fallopian tube may develop proximal luminal dilatation, plical attenuation with pseudopolyp formation and chronic inflammation, and plical thickening in the distal tubal segment (39). These changes become more pronounced with increasing postoperative intervals.

TUMOR-LIKE LESIONS

Amyloidosis

Involvement of the fallopian tube by amyloidosis is rare. In one unusual case, a 47-year-old woman had heavy menstrual bleeding with extensive amyloidosis of the genital organs, appendix, and omentum (40).

Salpingitis Isthmica Nodosa

Salpingitis isthmica nodosa (SIN) is of uncertain pathogenesis and may cause infertility or predispose to ectopic pregnancy. It usually occurs in young women, with a mean age of 26 years (41–44). SIN typically appears as one or more yellow-white nodular swellings up to 2 cm in diameter, usually in the tubal isthmus. It may be grossly inconspicuous. It is bilateral in approximately 85% of cases (44). Microscopically, glands lined by tubal epithelium lie within hyperplastic smooth muscle (Fig. 8). Occasionally, glands are surrounded by endometrial-type stroma or are cystically dilatated. Serial sectioning shows that the glands are diverticula that commu-

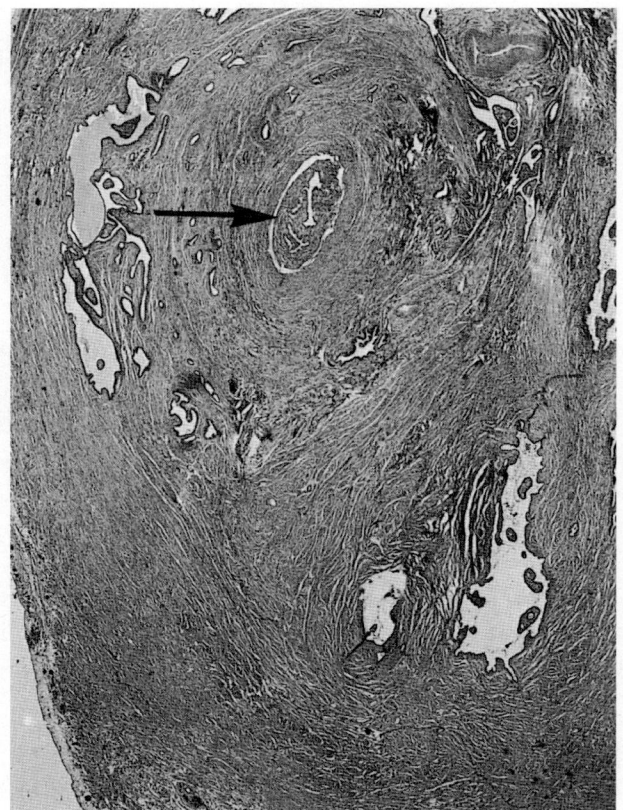

FIG. 8. Salpingitis isthmica nodosa. The tubal isthmic lumen (arrow) is surrounded by numerous small, gland-like diverticula that extend deeply into the muscularis. (From ref. 10, with permission.)

nicate with the tubal lumen. SIN should be easily distinguished from carcinoma by the regular distribution of its widely spaced glands, the lack of significant cellular atypia, and the absence of a stromal response (Fig. 9). SIN accompanied by severe tubal inflammation, however, may have a pseudocarcinomatous appearance, as described below.

Ectopic Pregnancy and Other Pregnancy-Related Lesions

In the usual tubal pregnancy there is distention of the ampullary segment of the tube (45), typically resulting in a sausage-shaped appearance with a thinned or ruptured wall and a dusky red serosa (Fig. 10). Microscopic examination may reveal fetal parts, villi that are frequently degenerative, trophoblast, and blood clot, which accounts for the marked luminal distention (46). The lamina propria shows decidual change in about one-third of the cases (45). Evidence of an underlying predisposing disorder such as chronic salpingitis, salpingitis isthmica nodosa, endometriosis, or a small tumor may be present. Rarely the hemorrhagic mass resulting from the ectopic pregnancy dissects into the broad ligament and may even extend to the contralateral adnexa (47). Tubal trophoblastic tumors (see below) (48) should be diagnosed with criteria applied to analogous uterine tumors.

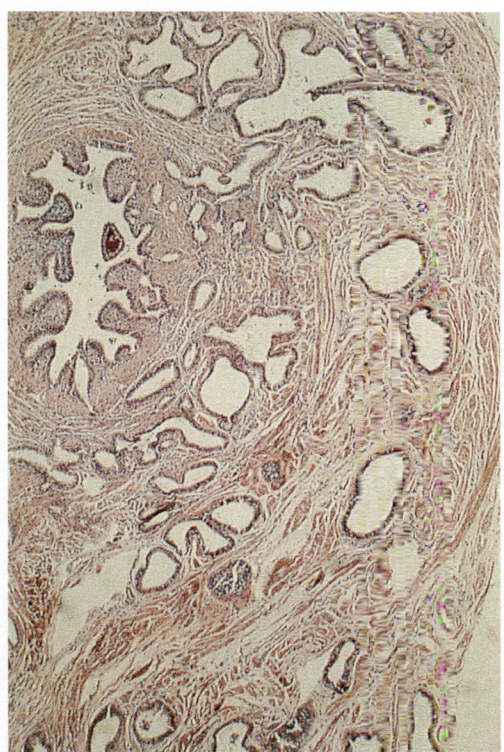

FIG. 9. Salpingitis isthmica nodosa. Gland-like structures have extended to the serosa. Note lack of any stromal reaction around the glands.

Trophoblastic tissue derived from an unsuspected ectopic pregnancy may be retained in the fallopian tubes (49,50). This tissue may form a tumor-like mass visible at laparotomy or represent an incidental histologic finding in tubal ligation or other specimens. The trophoblastic tissue usually consists of intermediate trophoblast and eosinophilic hyalinized material, often accompanied by hyalinized chorionic villi (49). In some cases the lesion takes the form of a placental site nodule (50).

Torsion

Isolated torsion of the tube is rare, but tubal torsion often accompanies torsion of the adjacent ovary. The disorder occurs in women of all ages (51,52). Most often the patient is a young woman whose ovary is the seat of a neoplasm or cyst, usually of only moderate size. In 18% of the cases, however, both the tube and ovary are otherwise normal (51). On gross inspection, the involved tube, which is right-sided in two-thirds of the cases, is swollen and typically dusky blue (51).

A rare complication of torsion is tubo-ovarian autoamputation (53–55). Such patients are found at operation to have no tube or ovary on one side. In some cases, a calcified nodule is found in the vicinity or lying free in the peritoneal cavity; microscopic examination may disclose features compatible with calcified ovarian or tubal tissue.

Prolapse

Prolapse of the fallopian tube occasionally occurs following hysterectomy, which has been performed by the vaginal route in approximately 80% of cases (56–58). On clinical examination, a lesion simulating granulation tissue is visible at the vaginal apex (see chapter 51, in which this disorder is discussed in more detail). In a unique case, the fallopian tube prolapsed into the urinary bladder, clinically mimicking a carcinoma (59).

Endometriosis

The term *endometriosis* has been applied to three distinct lesions in the fallopian tube. Most commonly, it refers to serosal or subserosal endometriotic foci associated with endometriosis elsewhere in the pelvis; the myosalpinx is not involved in most of the cases (60).

Endometrial tissue may extend directly from the uterine cornu, replacing the mucosa of the interstitial and isthmic portions of the tube in 25% and 10% of women, respectively (Fig. 11). This finding is considered to be a normal morphologic variation, although the ectopic endometrial tissue may

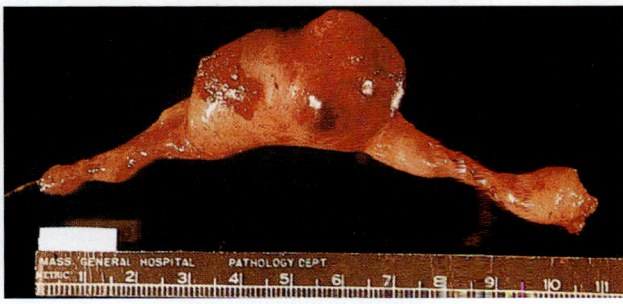

FIG. 10. Tubal pregnancy.

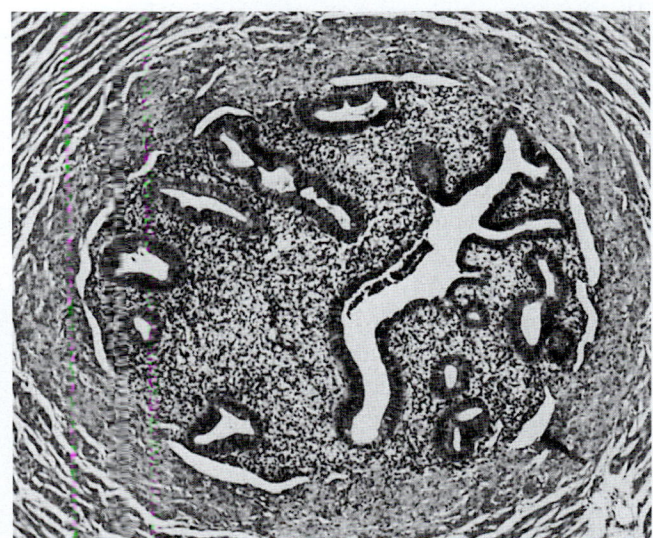

FIG. 11. Endometriosis (colonization) of the fallopian tube. The tubal lumen is occluded by endometrial glands and stroma.

give rise to intratubal polyps. The latter have been found in from 1% of hysterosalpingographic studies to 11% of hysterectomy and salpingo-oophorectomy specimens (61). The polyps may be associated with ectopic pregnancy and, particularly if bilateral, infertility. They are typically unilateral, pink to red lesions, 0.2 to 1.3 cm in diameter, with a smooth surface and a broad-based mucosal attachment. Microscopically, they consist of nonfunctioning endometrium (62–66). When ectopic endometrial tissue in the interstitial and isthmic portions of the tube causes luminal occlusion, the term *endometrial colonization* has been arbitrarily applied (67–70). The process may represent only an exaggeration of the normal variation described above; involvement may be bilateral. This lesion is said to account for 15% to 20% of cases of infertility and may be associated with tubal pregnancy.

The third type of tubal endometriosis has been designated as postsalpingectomy endometriosis (71–73). It occurs at the tip of the proximal tubal stump, typically 1 to 4 years after tubal ligation. It is closely related to, and may be associated with, salpingitis isthmica nodosa. The lesion is analogous to uterine adenomyosis, consisting of endometrial glands and stroma extending from the endosalpinx into the muscularis, and frequently to the serosal surface. Hysterosalpingography or India ink injection of a resected specimen may show tuboperitoneal fistulous tracts (74) through which postligation pregnancies may result. Postsalpingectomy endometriosis has been documented in 20% to 50% of tubes examined after ligation. The frequency of this complication is increased if electrocautery is used, if the proximal stumps are short, and if the postligation interval is long.

Walthard Nests

Nests of transitional (urothelial) epithelium referred to as Walthard nests are commonly found on the serosal surfaces of the fallopian tubes, mesosalpinx, and mesovarium (75). They are often visible grossly as one or more white to yellow nodules or cysts (Fig. 12) a few millimeters in diameter, and have occasionally been mistaken for granulomas. Histologically, they are well-circumscribed, small solid nests, cysts, or, less commonly, surface plaques that replace the normal mesothelium. The nests are composed of cytologically benign, mitotically inactive, transitional-type cells; their nuclei have fine chromatin, a prominent nuclear groove, and one or two small nucleoli. Less commonly the cells have a nonkeratinizing squamous appearance. The cysts are also lined by transitional cells, which may be flattened; inspissated eosinophilic secretion and mucin may be seen within the lumina.

Cysts

Paratubal cysts are common incidental findings (Fig. 13); rarely, they are large enough to be clinically significant. They are usually of müllerian (paramesonephric) origin, and

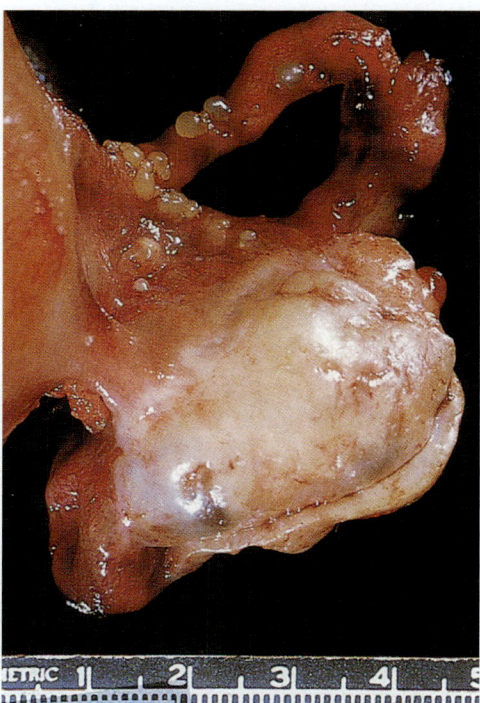

FIG. 12. Walthard nests. Small yellow cysts are present on the tubal serosa.

lined by a single layer of tubal-type ciliated epithelium (so-called hydatids of Morgagni) (76,77). Some cysts have a few plicae. They are generally attached to the fimbriated end of the tube by a pedicle. Mesonephric remnants lie in the broad ligament (78); they may be cystic but more often form small tubules lined by low columnar to cuboidal, nonciliated cells surrounded by a prominent layer of smooth muscle. Some paratubal cysts are of mesothelial origin and are lined by flattened cells with surrounding fibrous or fatty tissue.

Ectopic Tissue in Fallopian Tube and Broad Ligament

Ectopic nests of hilus cells may occur in the fallopian tube and paratubal tissue (79–81). In a thorough examination of

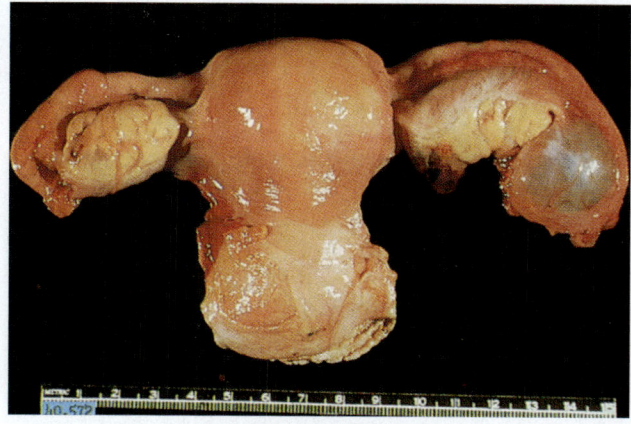

FIG. 13. Paratubal cyst.

over 2,000 fallopian tubes, Honore and O'Hara (81) found hilus cells in 0.5%. The cells were found only in the endosalpinx and paratubal connective tissue, being most common in the fimbriae. Encapsulated adrenal cortical nests have been found in the broad ligament in 23% of hysterectomy specimens (82). They typically form small yellow nodules in the infundibulopelvic ligament just beneath the peritoneum. Microscopically, all three layers of the adrenal cortex are present, but the medulla is absent. A single case of ectopic pancreas in the fallopian tube has been reported (83).

Metaplastic Lesions

The tubal epithelium rarely undergoes mucinous metaplasia (84). This may be associated with mucinous tumors of the cervix, ovary, or both, most commonly in patients with the Peutz-Jeghers syndrome (85–88). Serotonin and somatostatin have been detected immunohistochemically in the metaplastic mucinous cells, as well as within the adjacent normal-appearing epithelial cells in cases of the Peutz-Jeghers syndrome (89). In the rare transitional cell metaplasia transitional cells focally replace the tubal mucosa. These cells may be a source of tubal transitional cell carcinomas (90). Squamous metaplasia of the tubal epithelium is also seen rarely.

A rare lesion designated metaplastic papillary tumor of the fallopian tube has been encountered as an incidental microscopic finding in pregnant and postpartum women and rarely, nonpregnant women (91–93). The lesion involves only part of the circumference of the mucosa; small, rounded cysts may be present within the papillae. The epithelial cells are large, with abundant, eosinophilic cytoplasm (Fig. 14) which occasionally contains mucin, and large, oval vesicular nuclei; mitotic figures are rare. The lesion is distinguishable from primary tubal carcinoma by its microscopic size, lack of invasion, and bland-appearing or only slightly atypical nuclei. Whether this lesion is metaplastic or neoplastic is unclear, but it appears to bear a special relation to pregnancy and has been associated with an uneventful course in the small number of cases encountered to date.

Decidual transformation of the tubal stromal cells in the lamina propria may occur in pregnant patients (6), as well as in women on progestin therapy (94).

Hyperplastic and Pseudocarcinomatous Lesions

In patients with functioning ovarian tumors and excess estrogen production, epithelial hyperplasia associated with occasional mitotic figures but unaccompanied by cytologic atypia is common and may be the only pathologic evidence of estrogen excess, if the endometrium is not available for microscopic examination. More commonly, epithelial hyperplasia is an incidental microscopic finding, or is present in a tube that is the site of acute or chronic inflammation (95–101).

In one study, 18.5% of 124 unselected fallopian tubes removed surgically showed proliferative epithelial changes such as nuclear stratification and atypia (97). In half of these cases, there was an associated salpingitis. Some authors have designated examples of atypical hyperplasia unassociated with inflammation as carcinoma in situ (102), but no evidence has been presented that these lesions progress to carcinoma. Several studies, however, have shown an association of tubal hyperplasia with ovarian serous borderline tumors (98,101) or malignant tumors in the upper genital tract, although these changes are nonspecific.

Varying degrees of hyperplasia and atypia of the tubal epithelium and mesothelium may occur in response to inflammation, and may simulate an in situ or invasive adenocarcinoma (99). The hyperplastic epithelial changes include the formation of papillae and gland-like spaces (including a cribriform pattern) (Fig. 15) lined by cells with mild to moderate nuclear pleomorphism, hyperchromatism, and mitotic activity. The proliferation may involve the mucosa, muscularis, and serosa. When associated with pseudoglandular hyperplasia of the overlying mesothelial cells, which become in-

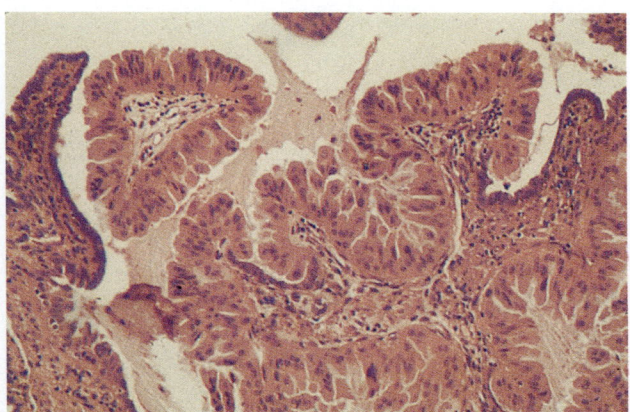

FIG. 14. Metaplastic papillary tumor. The papillae are lined by stratified cells with abundant eosinophilic cytoplasm.

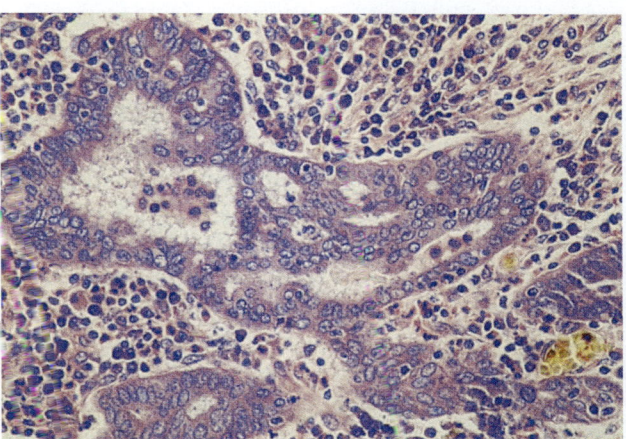

FIG. 15. Atypical epithelial hyperplasia with intraglandular bridging associated with severe chronic salpingitis.

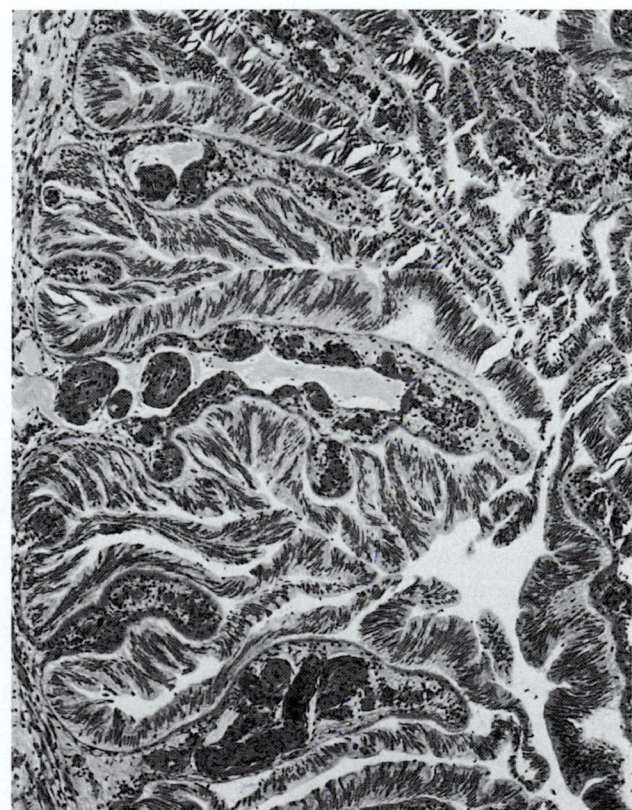

FIG. 16. Heat artifact due to cautery. The cells have a peculiar elongated appearance.

corporated within subserosal inflammatory and scar tissue, the combination of findings may lead to an erroneous interpretation of transmural carcinoma. These pseudocarcinomatous changes have long been recognized in tuberculous salpingitis (Fig. 5), but are also seen with other forms of bacterial salpingitis. A number of differences between carcinomas and pseudocarcinomatous inflammatory lesions facilitate the differential diagnosis. The great majority of carcinomas are grossly evident, are not associated with significant inflammation, and exhibit brisk mitotic activity and severe nuclear atypia. Pseudocarcinomatous changes simulating carcinoma, in contrast, are incidental microscopic findings associated with overt inflammation. If atypical mesothelial proliferation is a component of the lesion, the mesothelial cells are typically cuboidal, are often lined up in rows, and generally exhibit only mild nuclear atypia.

Heat artifact (prolonged intraoperative cautery or heating of the specimen inadvertently after surgical removal) may also simulate carcinoma by causing an appearance of marked cellular pseudostratification and dark nuclear staining (Fig. 16) (103).

The Arias-Stella reaction occurs focally in the fallopian tube in as many as 16% of patients with ectopic tubal pregnancy (104), and is rarely seen in patients with intrauterine pregnancy (105). The pregnancy-related clear cell change has also been documented rarely in the tube (106).

TUMORS

The classification used here is that of the World Health Organization with minor modification (Table 1).

Adenomatoid Tumor

The adenomatoid tumor is the most common benign tumor of the fallopian tube (107–115). It is usually an incidental finding in the myosalpinx but may compress the tubal lumen or project from the serosa. It is typically 2 cm or less in diameter and is circumscribed, firm, and gray, white, or yellow (Fig. 17); rarely it is bilateral (111). The microscopic patterns include irregular gland-like spaces that vary from elongated and slit-like to round and cystically dilated (Fig. 18), oval vacuoles, and small cords and clusters of cells. The neoplastic cells range from flattened cells sometimes confused with endothelium to large cells containing abundant eosinophilic cytoplasm. Nuclei are bland, and mitotic figures are rare. The glandular lumina and vacuoles may contain slightly basophilic fluid that is rich in hyaluronic acid. The stroma may be hyalinized and contain smooth muscle. Lymphocytes may form prominent follicles. An origin from mesothelium is now supported by most investigators, and continuity with the overlying mesothelium is occasionally seen (112). Adenomatoid tumor may be confused with other benign neoplasms, particularly lymphangiomas and leiomyomas. Careful examination of the tumor cells should permit their distinction from endothelial cells and immunoperoxidase stains for cytokeratin and with *Ulex europaeus* lectin may aid in their recognition (115). Although smooth muscle may be present in tubal adenomatoid tumors, it is rarely as prominent as in analogous uterine tumors, and the characteristic spaces of an adenomatoid tumor are not compatible with the diagnosis of a leiomyoma. Adenomatoid tumors may also be confused with cancers, such as malignant mesotheliomas and adenocarcinomas. The circumscribed gross appearance, bland cytologic findings, and mitotic inactivity characteristic of adenomatoid tumors allow distinction.

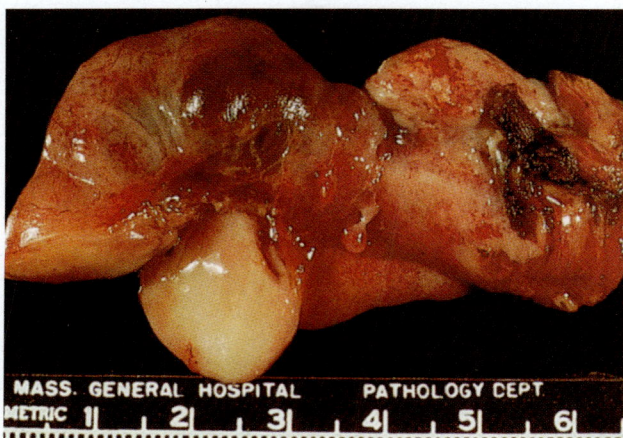

FIG. 17. Adenomatoid tumor. The tumor is well circumscribed and has a smooth, white cut surface.

TABLE 1. *World Health Organization Histologic typing of tumors of the fallopian tube (with minor modification)*

Epithelial tumors
  Benign
    Endometrioid polyp
    Papilloma
    Metaplastic papillary tumor
  Malignant
    Carcinoma *in situ*
    Serous carcinoma
    Mucinous carcinoma
    Endometrioid carcinoma
    Clear cell carcinoma
    Transitional cell carcinoma
    Squamous cell carcinoma
    Glassy cell carcinoma
    Mixed carcinoma
    Undifferentiated carcinoma
Mixed epithelial-mesenchymal tumors
  Benign
    Adenofibroma
  Malignant
    Adenosarcoma
    Malignant mullerian mixed tumor (carcinosarcoma)
Soft tissue tumors
  Benign
    Leiomyoma
    Others
  Malignant
    Leiomyosarcoma
    Others
Mesothelial tumors
  Adenomatoid tumor
Germ cell tumors
  Teratoma
    Mature
      Dermoid cyst
      Solid
    Immature
    Struma
    Carcinoid
  Others
Trophoblastic disease
  Hydatidiform mole
  Choriocarcinoma
Secondary tumors
  Carcinoma
    Squamous cell carcinoma *in situ* of cervix
    Carcinoma of cervix
    Carcinoma of endometrium
    Carcinoma of ovary
    Others
  Lymphoma and leukemia
  Others
Tumor-like lesions
  Atypical epithelial hyperplasia
  Endometrial colonization and endometriosis
  Salpingitis isthmica nodosa
  Tuberculous salpingitis
  Bacterial salpingitis
  Heat artifact
  Mesothelial hyperplasia
  Ectopic pregnancy
  Malakoplakia
  Others

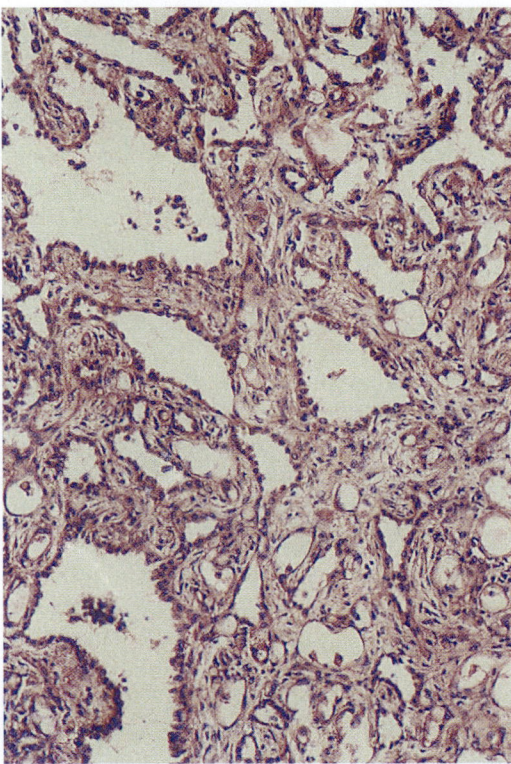

FIG. 18. Adenomatoid tumor. Small gland-like spaces and cysts are lined by cuboidal to flattened cells.

Benign Epithelial Tumors

Benign tumors of the types commonly encountered in the ovary are rare in the fallopian tube. The most common benign epithelial tumor of the tube is the endometrioid polyp. Serous adenofibromas of the tube are similar to their ovarian counterparts (116–120). Rare adenomas or cystadenomas, including two of mucinous type, papillomas, and adenomyomas have also been reported (84,121). Like carcinomas (see below) most benign epithelial tumors occur in the ampullary-infundibular regions of the tube but some, particularly serous adenofibromas, may be primary in the fimbria (Fig. 19) (122).

Epithelial Tumors of Borderline Malignancy

A few serous tumors of borderline malignancy have been primary in the fallopian tube, including its fimbriated end (122). Four tumors, three of which were associated with pseudomyxoma peritonei, have been considered examples of tubal mucinous borderline tumors (84,123). That one or more of the latter cases might have represented spread to the fallopian tube from a mucinous cystic tumor of the appendix is a possibility as the appendix was not examined microscopically in those cases. A single endometrioid adenofibroma of borderline malignancy that involved the fimbria has been documented (122).

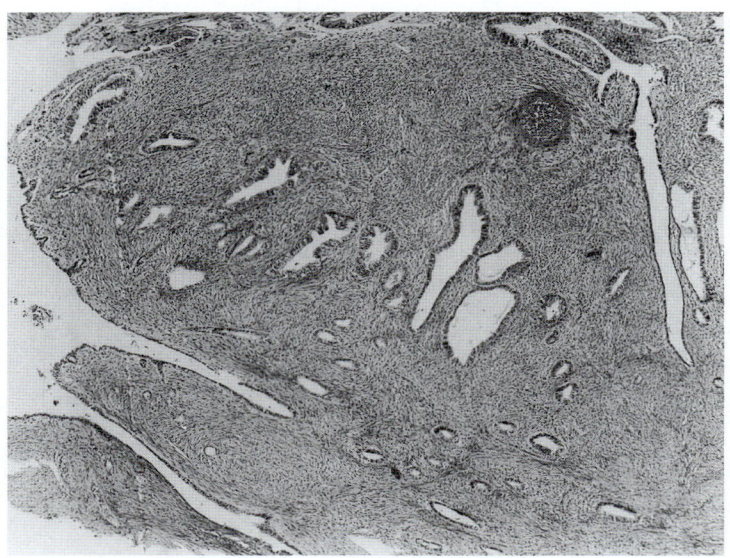

FIG. 19. Serous cystadenofibroma of fimbria.

Benign Soft Tissue Tumors

Benign soft tissue tumors may involve the fallopian tube. Leiomyomas are most common (124–129) and may undergo degenerative changes similar to those occurring in uterine smooth muscle tumors. Most tubal leiomyomas are small; they may be submucosal, intramural, or subserosal. Rarer benign tumors in this category include neurilemoma (130), angiomyolipoma (131), lipoma (132), chondroma (133), lymphangioma (134), ganglioneuroma (135), and hemangioma (136–139); the latter may result in hemoperitoneum.

Carcinoma of Fallopian Tube

Carcinoma of the fallopian tube is uncommon, accounting for only about 0.3% of gynecologic cancers (140), but this figure may be low because carcinomas of uncertain origin involving both the ovary and tube are generally classified as ovarian in view of their much higher overall frequency. In support of a higher frequency of tubal carcinoma than the figure just cited is a recent screening study using CA125 assays that detected one tubal carcinoma for every six ovarian carcinomas (141).

The distinctive presentation of intermittent, profuse, watery, clear to yellow (cholesterol-rich) vaginal discharge, accompanied by colicky abdominal pain and followed by a decrease in the size of an abdominal mass (hydrops tubae profluens) (142,143), is encountered in only a minority of the cases (under 10%) and is not pathognomonic (144). The most common symptom of tubal carcinoma, seen in two-thirds of patients, is postmenopausal bleeding. The diagnosis is usually unsuspected preoperatively. Carcinoma cells in a cytologic smear from the lower genital tract, reported in approximately 10% of cases, is strongly suggestive if no other source of malignancy is identified. In some cases, fragments of tumor are discovered in an endocervical or endometrial curettage specimen obtained as part of the investigation of postmenopausal bleeding. Most of the patients are postmenopausal with a mean age of 57 years (145–158); rare tumors occur in much younger patients, including teenagers (159).

Because primary tubal carcinoma is less common than secondary carcinoma of ovarian origin, gross as well as microscopic assessment is important in determining the primary site. When both the tube and ovary are replaced by a carcinoma compatible microscopically with an origin in either, the designation tubo-ovarian carcinoma has been applied (116). Occasionally, a noninvasive, superficially invasive, or (rarely) a borderline tubal carcinoma is associated with a similar serous tumor in the ovary. In such cases, the tumors may reflect independent primary neoplasia, rather than spread from one organ to the other (160).

Tubal carcinomas characteristically appear as fusiform swellings that may have the external appearance of a hydrosalpinx (Fig. 20) or hematosalpinx. In other cases, the tube is not appreciably enlarged, and the fimbriated end re-

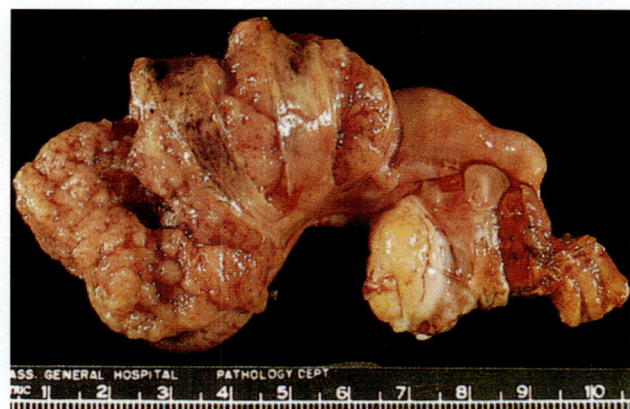

FIG. 20. Carcinoma of fallopian tube. A markedly expanded tube has been incised to disclose a friable, tan, papillary tumor.

mains open. Occasional tumors are primary in the fimbria and in our experience a fimbrial origin of a pelvic neoplasm is often initially overlooked (123). It has been recommended that tumors primarily in the fimbria be given a special stage, 1(F), in the staging system for fallopian tube carcinoma because the tumor cells are exposed directly to the peritoneal cavity even though they do not invade the tubal wall (122).

Bilaterality has been reported in 10% to 20% of cases but in our experience the figure is only about 3% (158). On opening the tube, the tumor may be extensive (Fig. 19) or it may form a solitary localized nodule (Fig. 21). Tumor varies in color from pink to tan to white, and in consistency from friable to firm. In some cases it is predominantly or entirely endophytic, and in others it is sessile, with firm, white tissue infiltrating the wall. Hemorrhage and necrosis are common, and cyst formation is occasionally seen.

Rare cases of carcinoma *in situ* of the fallopian tube have been reported, one of them after tamoxifen therapy (161). This diagnosis should be limited to flat or minimally papillary lesions that are not appreciable on gross inspection and are characterized by cells with obviously malignant nuclear features. An appearance indistinguishable from that of carcinoma *in situ* may be produced by spread of carcinoma from elsewhere, for example the ovary, to the fallopian tube.

Carcinomas of the various surface epithelial types encountered in the ovary have been reported in the fallopian tube, but there are differences in the frequency of these neoplasms in the tube as compared to the ovary. Some that are relatively common in the ovary, such as mucinous and clear cell, are exceptionally rare in the tube. On the basis of our personal experience and that in the literature, about 50% of tubal carcinomas are serous, about one-quarter endometrioid, one-fifth transitional or undifferentiated, and the remainder are of other rare epithelial cell types (158). The microscopic features are generally as seen in the ovary. Serous tumors that grow primarily into the tubal lumen may exhibit prominent papillarity (Fig. 22), whereas those that invade the

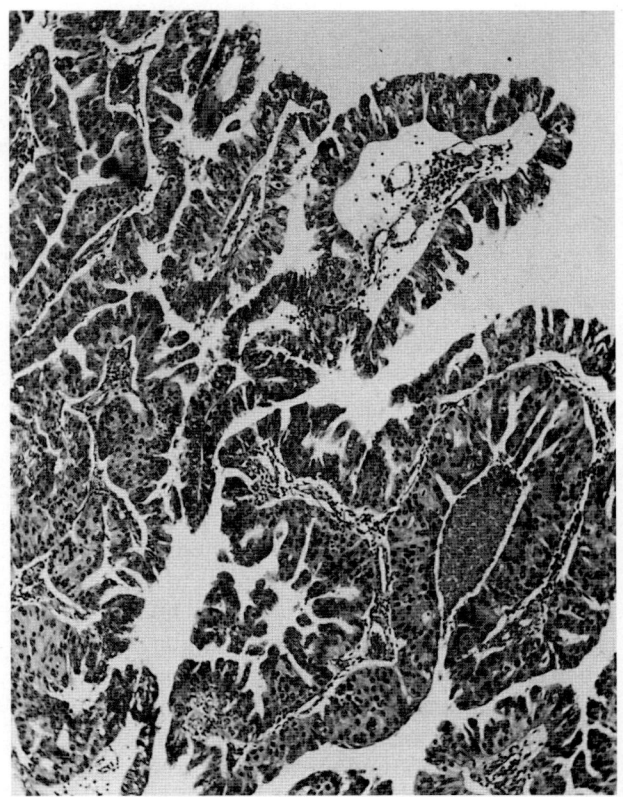

FIG. 22. Serous papillary adenocarcinoma of fallopian tube of serous type.

wall and are high grade may have a solid or alveolar pattern (Fig. 23).

It has recently been emphasized that endometrioid carcinoma is the second commonest subtype of tubal carcinoma (162), and it is a neoplasm that is important to recognize because in many cases it is a noninvasive (Fig. 24) or minimally invasive tumor and accordingly has a better prognosis than that associated with carcinoma of the tube in general.

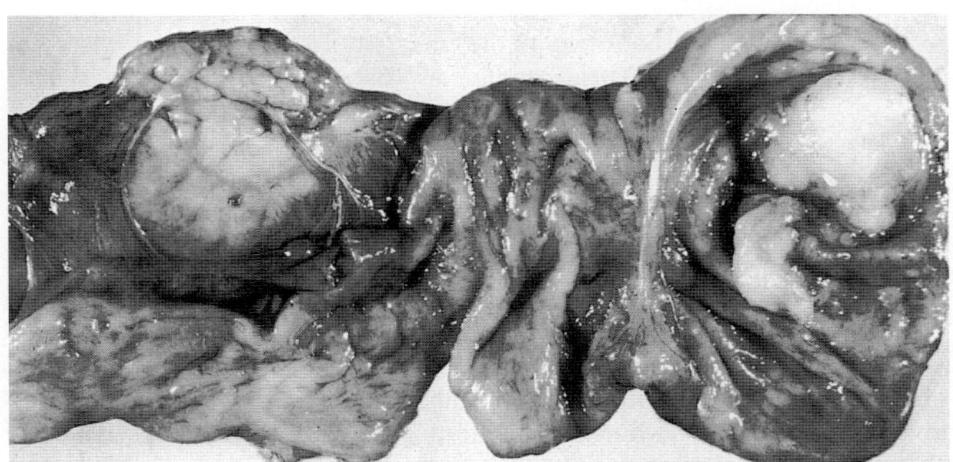

FIG. 21. Carcinoma of fallopian tube. The opened tube courses along the lower border of the left half of the specimen and occupies the entire right half, where an irregular nodule of carcinoma is seen on the mucosal surface. The ovary is visible *(upper left)*. (From ref. 116.)

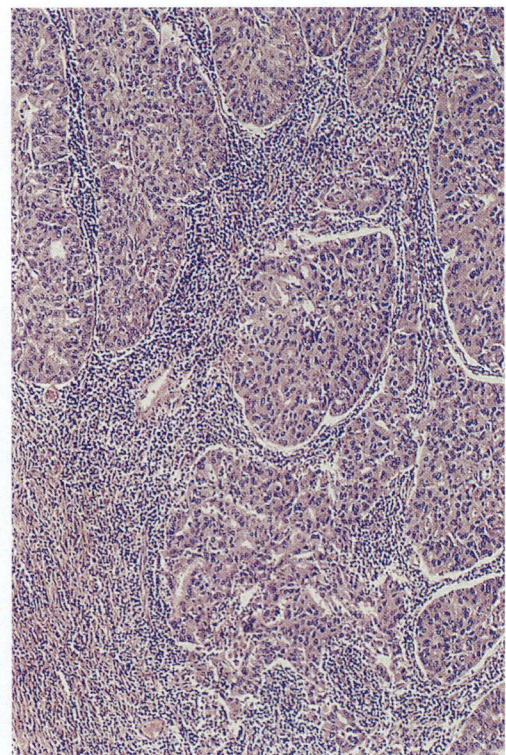

FIG. 23. Adenocarcinoma of the fallopian tube with a solid (alveolar) pattern.

Most endometrioid carcinomas of the tube resemble their endometrial counterparts, including the presence of squamous metaplasia. They may be associated with endometriosis (163). They also may contain a prominent component of spindled epithelial cells, which should not lead to their misdiagnosis as carcinosarcoma (164).

A variant of tubal endometrioid adenocarcinoma is one that superficially resembles the female adnexal tumor of probable wolffian origin (see below) (164). These tumors are characterized by a predominant pattern of small, closely packed cells punctuated by numerous glandular spaces. The latter are typically small, but occasionally are cystically dilated. Many of the glands contain a dense, colloid-like secretion (Fig. 25) that is positive with the periodic acid-Schiff stain. In the solid areas of these tumors, spindle cells that focally form concentric whorls are common. In cases of this type, small numbers of tubular glands typical of endometrioid adenocarcinoma are usually identified, facilitating diagnosis. In addition, the mitotic activity and cytologic atypia of the tumors, although variable, usually exceeds that seen in wolffian duct tumors. Finally, small amounts of intracellular mucin are often present, arguing against a wolffian nature. It should also be noted that the intraluminal location of these tumors would be exceptional for a wolffian neoplasm, which typically occurs in the broad ligament or, if attached to the tube, hangs from it on a pedicle.

As noted above, most of the remaining primary carcinomas of the tube reported are transitional cell carcinomas or undifferentiated carcinomas with a nonspecific appearance (158); only a small number or even single cases of other subtypes including clear cell carcinoma (165), squamous cell carcinoma (166), mucinous carcinoma (167), small cell undifferentiated carcinoma (158), glassy cell carcinoma (168), hepatoid carcinoma (169), and lymphoepithelioma-like carcinoma (158) are described.

Malignant Müllerian Mixed Tumor and Sarcomas

Approximately 70 malignant müllerian mixed tumors of the fallopian tube have been reported (170–173). The age distribution and clinical presentation are similar to those of tubal carcinoma. The typical gross appearance is that of a large, sometimes polypoid, mass protruding into the lumen (Fig. 26). The microscopic features and prognosis are simi-

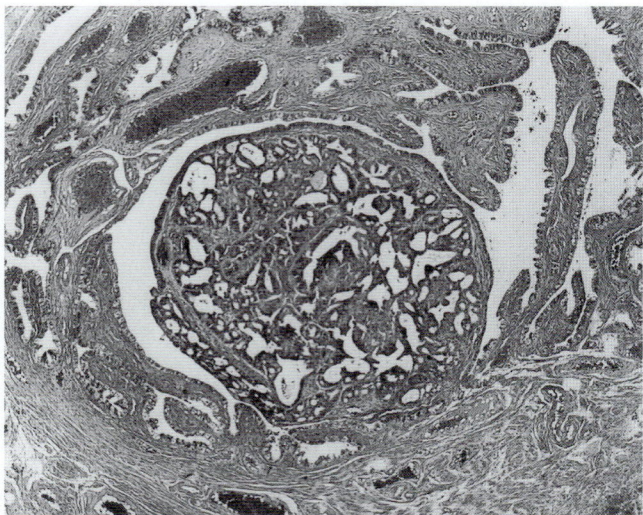

FIG. 24. Endometrioid adenocarcinoma of fallopian tube. A small tumor with typical histology protrudes into the tubal lumen.

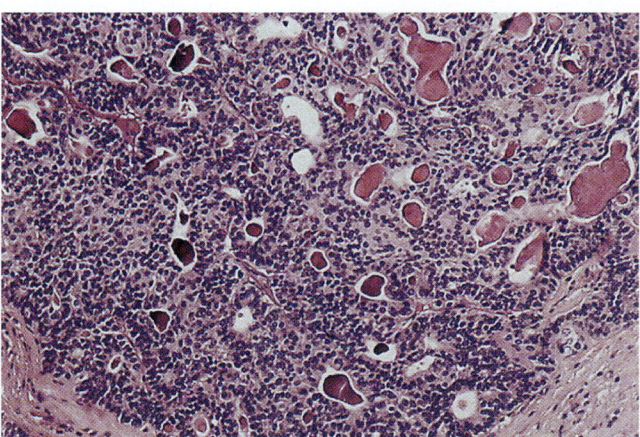

FIG. 25. Endometrioid adenocarcinoma of fallopian tube. The tumor has many small acini containing an eosinophilic colloid-like secretion. This pattern may cause confusion with a wolffian neoplasm.

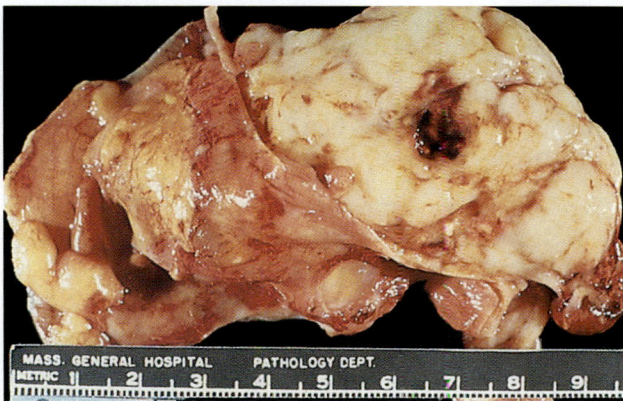

FIG. 26. Malignant müllerian mixed tumor. A markedly distended tube has been opened to disclose a large, soft, white tumor with focal hemorrhage.

lar to those of analogous tumors occurring elsewhere; both homologous and heterologous types have been encountered. The differential diagnosis includes endometrioid carcinomas with spindle cells, in which the latter cells are epithelial rather than mesenchymal, as well as immature teratomas. This differential is resolved using the criteria applicable in the ovary (see chapter by Young et al.). Occasional leiomyosarcomas of the tube and broad ligament have been reported (174) as have single examples of embryonal rhabdomyosarcoma (175) and adenosarcoma (176).

Malignant Lymphoma and Leukemia

The female genital tract is involved in approximately 40% of women who die with disseminated lymphoma (177), and the fallopian tube is affected in many of these cases. In one large series of lymphomas presenting as an ovarian mass, the tube was involved in 26% of the cases (178). Tubal involvement is less common than ovarian involvement by lymphoma and is almost always less conspicuous on gross inspection. We are not aware of a reported case of lymphoma presenting in, and apparently confined to, the fallopian tube but have recently seen a case of this type. The gross and microscopic features of tubal lymphoma are similar to those seen elsewhere. The tube may also be infiltrated in patients with leukemia (179).

Germ Cell Tumors

Approximately 50 teratomas of the tube have been reported (180). They are usually attached by a pedicle to the tubal mucosa and have ranged from 0.7 to 20 cm in diameter. Most of these tumors have been cystic and mature, but rare examples have been solid or immature (181). One solid mature teratoma contained an area of insular carcinoid (182), and two others were composed entirely of thyroid tissue (183).

Trophoblastic Disease

Hydatidiform moles and choriocarcinomas occur rarely in the fallopian tube or mesosalpinx (184–188) and may mimic an ectopic pregnancy, both clinically and grossly.

Secondary Tumors of the Fallopian Tube

In addition to relatively common involvement by ovarian borderline tumors and carcinomas, the tube may be involved by endometrial or cervical carcinoma (including *in situ* squamous carcinomas) (189), either by direct extension (190) or by way of the tubal lumen. In contrast to the ovary, the tube is involved only occasionally by metastases from an extragenital site. In a review of 149 cases of metastases to the genital tract from an extragenital site, there was only one tubal metastasis, in contrast to 113 ovarian metastases (189). In our experience, however, microscopic evidence of tubal metastases is not as rare as the above figure indicates. In two other studies, 3% (149) and 7% (191) of metastases to the tube had their origin outside the genital tract. Tubal involvement by mucinous epithelium in cases of pseudomyxoma peritonei has been noted earlier.

Female Adnexal Tumor of Probable Wolffian Origin

This tumor has been interpreted as wolffian in origin because of its location and the presence within it of patterns and cytologic features unlike those of müllerian tumors on both light and electron microscopic examination. Approximately 40 cases have now been reported (192–195). The patients have ranged from 15 to 72 years of age (mean: 47). They typically have nonspecific clinical manifestations such as abdominal pain or swelling, or have asymptomatic masses that are discovered incidentally.

Grossly, these tumors lie within the broad ligament (Fig. 27) or hang from it or from the fallopian tube by a pedicle. They average approximately 8 cm in diameter and are typically rounded masses with bosselated external surfaces (Fig. 27). Cut surfaces are solid or solid and cystic (Fig. 28). The

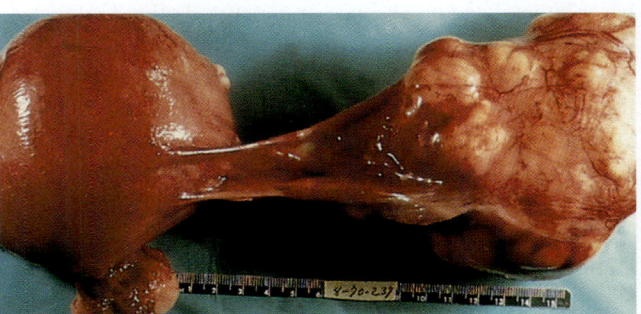

FIG. 27. Female adnexal tumor of probable wolffian origin. A bosselated solid mass is present within the leaves of the broad ligament. (From ref. 192.)

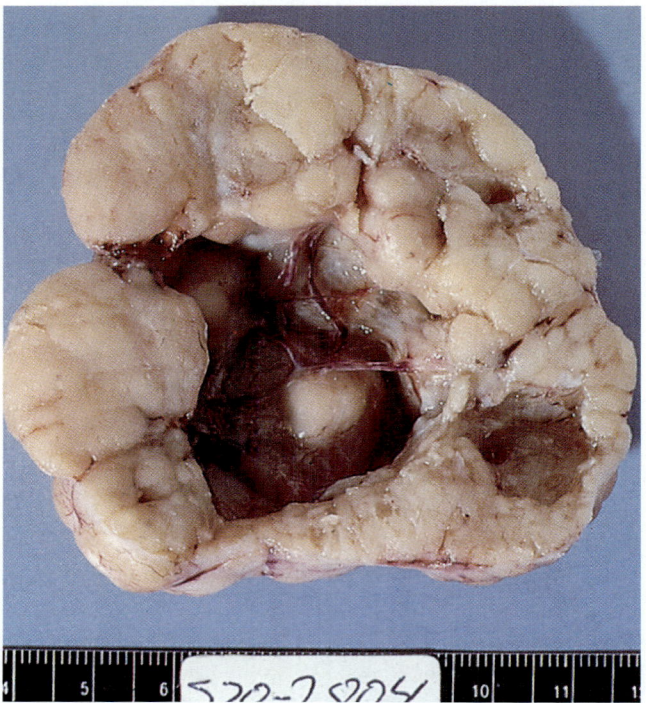

FIG. 28. Female adnexal tumor of probable wolffian origin. The sectioned surface of the tumor discloses lobulated, yellow-white tissue with cystic degeneration. (From ref. 192.)

totic figures, but others have had a bland appearance, indicating the necessity of long-term follow-up in all cases.

Serous and Other Müllerian Tumors of the Broad Ligament

Serous cystadenomas and serous cystadenomas of borderline malignancy have been reported in the broad ligament (196), typically in young women (mean age: 33 years). They have been unilateral, unilocular cysts ranging up to 13 cm in diameter. Typically, they have an ovarian-like stroma but lack ova and follicular derivatives. Local excision has been curative. One broad ligament neoplasm was a serous borderline tumor with microinvasion (197). One serous cystadenoma of the broad ligament had a Brenner tumor component and four pure Brenner tumors of the broad ligament have been recorded (198). One borderline mucinous cystadenoma primary in the broad ligament also has been described (199). One cystadenofibroma that was probably of endometrioid type was reported in a patient with von Hippel–Lindau disease (200).

Thirteen carcinomas of Müllerian type primary in the broad ligament have been reported (197,201). The patients ranged in age from 29 to 76 years (mean: 46) and usually presented with vague lower abdominal symptoms or a palpable pelvic mass, or because of an associated disorder such

solid tissue varies from gray-white to tan or yellow and is usually firm or rubbery; hemorrhage and necrosis are rare. Microscopically, diffuse, tubular, cystic, and sieve-like patterns may be seen (Fig. 29). The tubules may be solid (Fig. 30) or may contain small lumina. They are lined by cuboidal to columnar cells with scanty cytoplasm; occasional cells may contain abundant pale cytoplasm. The cysts are usually lined by flattened cells (Fig. 29). The nuclei are usually small, round to oval, and pale (Fig. 30). Some tumors have a focally prominent, hyalinized stroma or fibrous bands that separate cellular foci into lobules. When the tumor cells grow in solid sheets, they may have a mesenchymal, spindle-shaped appearance; often vacuoles similar to those encountered in adenomatoid tumors are seen. Electron microscopic examination of several tumors has shown a thick peritubular basal lamina, and an absence or paucity of cilia, Golgi complexes, secretory granules, and glycogen, features favoring a wolffian origin. Immunohistochemically, the tumors have been positive for cytokeratin (AE 1/3) but have typically been negative for epithelial membrane antigen (EMA), carcinoembryonic antigen (CEA), S-100 protein, and B72.3 (194).

Most examples of this neoplasm occurring in the broad ligament have been benign, but four malignant tumors have been reported (195) with evidence of peritoneal spread at the time of diagnosis or recurrence 6 or more years after removal of the primary tumor. Some of the clinically malignant tumors had cells with pleomorphic nuclei and numerous mi-

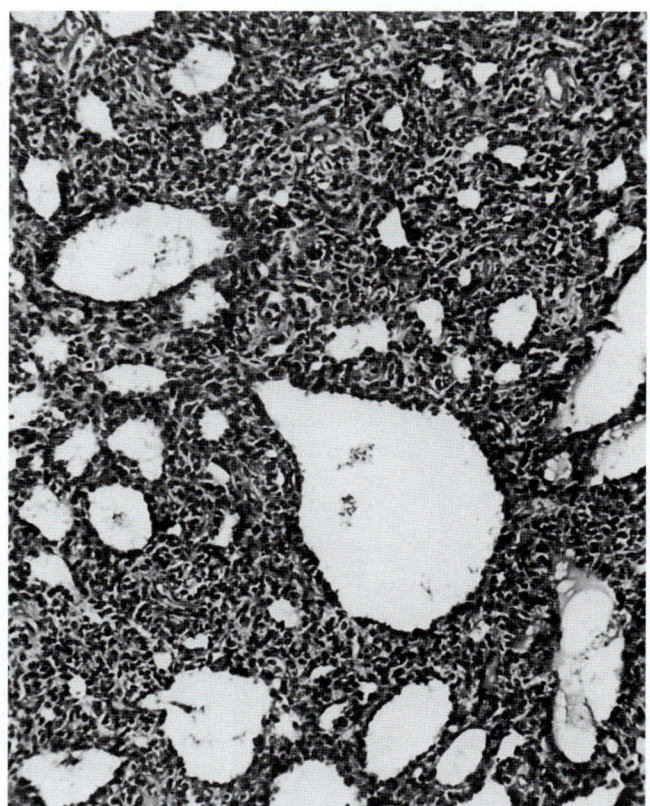

FIG. 29. Female adnexal tumor of probable wolffian origin with a sieve-like pattern.

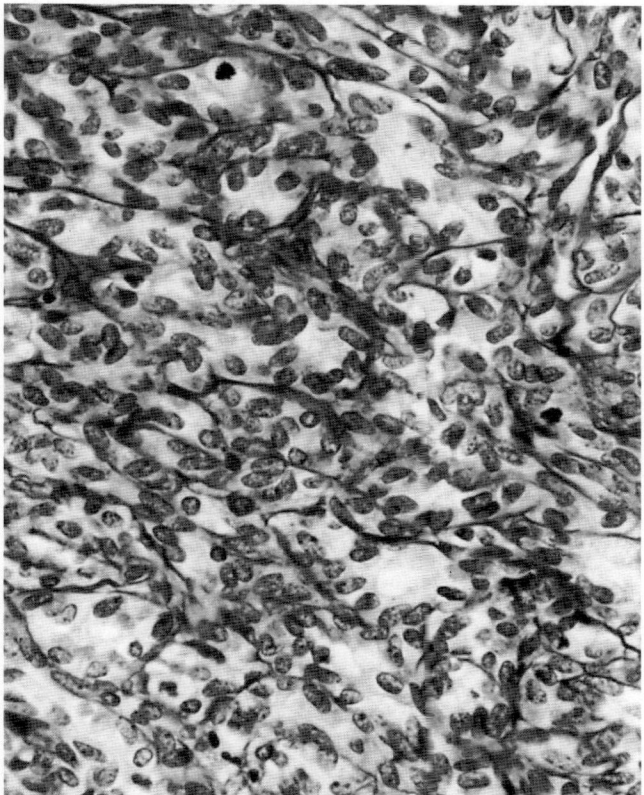

FIG. 30. Female adnexal tumor of probable wolffian origin. Closely packed solid tubules lined by cells with round to oval, uniform nuclei are present. Two mitotic FIG.s are visible. Periodic acid-Schiff stain.

as pelvic endometriosis. The tumors were up to 13 cm in greatest dimension, and were variably solid and cystic. All have been unilateral. Microscopically, there were four endometrioid carcinomas, four clear cell carcinomas, two serous carcinomas, one probable mucinous adenocarcinoma, and two papillary adenocarcinomas of undetermined cell type. An association with endometriosis was present in at least three cases, and two had apparently independent primary adenocarcinomas of the endometrium. The prognosis for these patients was favorable, with only one patient known to have developed distant metastases. The differential diagnosis in these cases is usually straightforward; obviously, spread from a primary tumor elsewhere in the genital tract should be excluded. However, involvement of the broad ligament by a metastasis in the form of a large discrete tumor is uncommon.

Soft Tissue–Type Tumors

A great variety of soft tissue tumors has been described in the broad ligament and potentially any subtype might arise there. By far the most common is the leiomyoma, which has the same spectrum of morphologic features seen in its uterine counterpart. The most common sarcoma of the broad ligament is the leiomyosarcoma with rare examples of miscellaneous other soft tissue–type sarcomas and endometrioid stromal sarcomas arising from endometriosis (202).

Rare Tumors of the Broad Ligament

Three ependymomas of the broad ligament or mesovarium have been reported in patients 13, 45, and 47 years of age (203,204). They were 1.0, 9.5, and 13 cm in largest dimension and microscopically resembled ependymomas of the central nervous system. Immunoperoxidase stains for glial fibrillary acidic protein were positive in all the cases. One tumor contained islands of cartilage. Intraabdominal spread was present at presentation in one case and tumor recurred 11 years later in a second (212).

Four patients with von Hippel–Lindau disease who had papillary cystadenomas of the broad ligament have been reported (205–207). The cystadenomas were bilateral in two cases, and, in one, the diagnosis of von Hippel–Lindau disease was established only after the broad ligament tumors had been removed (207). Microscopically, the cystadenomas were identical to the more common epididymal lesions of this type. Rare examples of ovarian-type tumors including dermoid cysts (208), yolk sac tumor (209), fibrothecoma (210), steroid cell tumors (211,212), and sex cord tumor with annular tubules (213) have also been reported in the broad ligament. Pheochromocytoma has also been primary in the broad ligament (214).

REFERENCES

1. Chow AW, Malkasian KL, Marshall JR, Guze LB. The bacteriology of acute pelvic inflammatory disease—value of cul-de-sac cultures and relative importance of gonococci and other aerobic or anaerobic bacteria. *Am J Obstet Gynecol* 1975;122:876–879.
2. Thadapalli H, Gorbach SL, Keith L. Anaerobic infections of the female genital tract: bacteriologic and therapeutic aspects. *Am J Obstet Gynecol* 1973;117:1034–1040.
3. Thompson SE, Hager WD, Wong K-H, et al. The microbiology and therapy of acute pelvic inflammatory disease in hospitalized patients. *Am J Obstet Gynecol* 1980;136:179–186.
4. Winkler B, Reumann W, Mitao M, Gallo L, Richart RM, Crum CP. Immunoperoxidase localization of chlamydial antigens in acute salpingitis. *Am J Obstet Gynecol* 1985;152:275–278.
5. Nassberg S, McKay DG, Hertig AT. Physiologic salpingitis. *Am J Obstet Gynecol* 1954;67:130–134.
6. Hellman LM. The morphology of the human fallopian tube in the early puerperium. *Am J Obstet Gynecol* 1949;57:154–163.
7. Smith HA, Greene RR. Physiologic salpingitis? *Am J Obstet Gynecol* 1956;72:174–179.
8. Schaefer G. Tuberculosis of the female genital tract. *Clin Obstet Gynecol* 1970;13:965–998.
9. Nogales-Ortiz F, Tarancon I, Nogales FF. The pathology of female genital tuberculosis. *Obstet Gynecol* 1979;53:422–428.
10. Lawrence WD, Scully RE. Pathology of the fallopian tube. In: Hunt RB, ed. *Atlas of female infertility surgery*. Chicago: Year Book Medical, 1986:11–24.
11. Bonar BE, Rabson AS. Gynecologic aspects of leprosy. *Obstet Gynecol* 1957;9:33–43.
12. Braby HH, Dougherty CM, Mickal A. Actinomycosis of the female genital tract. *Obstet Gynecol* 1964;23:580–583.
13. Paalman RJ, Dockerty MB, Mussey RD. Actinomycosis of ovaries and fallopian tubes. *Am J Obstet Gynecol* 1949;58:419–431.
14. Hamblen EC, Baker RD, Martin DS. Blastomycosis of the female reproductive tract with report of a case. *Am J Obstet Gynecol* 1935;30:345–356.

15. Murray JJ, Clark CA, Lands RH, Heim CR, Burnett LS. Reactivation blastomycosis presenting as a tuboovarian abscess. *Obstet Gynecol* 1984;64:828–830.
16. Bylund DJ, Nanfro JJ, Marsh WL Jr. Coccidioidomycosis of the female genital tract. *Arch Pathol Lab Med* 1986;110:232–235.
17. Saw EC, Smale LE, Einstein H, Huntington RW. Female genital coccidioidomycosis. *Obstet Gynecol* 1975;45:199–202.
18. Frost O. Bilharzia of the fallopian tube. *S Afr Med J* 1975;49:1201–1203.
19. Gelfand M, Ross MD, Blair DM, Weber MC. Distribution and extent of schistosomiasis in female pelvic organs with special reference to the genital tract, as determined at autopsy. *Am J Trop Med Hyg* 1971;20:846–849.
20. Arean VM. Manson's schistosomiasis of the female genital tract. *Am J Obstet Gynecol* 1956;72:1038–1053.
21. Symmers W St C. Pathology of oxyurasis. *Arch Pathol* 1950;50:475–516.
22. Abraham JL, Spore WW, Benirschke K. Cysticercosis of the fallopian tube: histology and microanalysis. *Hum Pathol* 1982;13:665.
23. Campbell JS, Nigam S, Hurtig A, Sahasrabudhe MR, Marino I. Mineral oil granulomas of the uterus and parametrium and granulomatous salpingitis with Schauman bodies and oxalate deposits. *Fertil Steril* 1964;15:278–289.
24. Elliott GB, Brody H, Elliott KA. Implications of "lipoid salpingitis." *Fertil Steril* 1965;16:541–548.
25. Rubin IC. Lipoidal granuloma in fallopian tubes localized by intrauterine diodrast injection, with special reference to the value of follow-up x-ray films. *Radiology* 1939;33:350–353.
26. Brooks JJ, Wheeler JE. Granulomatous salpingitis secondary to Crohn's disease. *Obstet Gynecol* 1977;49:31s–33s.
27. Chalvardjian A. Sarcoidosis of the female genital tract. *Am J Obstet Gynecol* 1978;132:78–80.
28. Kay S. Sarcoidosis of the fallopian tubes. Report of a case. *Br J Obstet Gynaecol* 1956;63:871–874.
29. Kunakemakorn P, Ontai G, Balin H. Pelvic inflammatory pseudotumor: a case report. *Am J Obstet Gynecol* 1976;126:286–287.
30. Shalev E, Zuckerman H, Rizescu I. Pelvic inflammatory pseudotumor (xanthogranuloma). *Acta Obstet Gynecol Scand* 1982;61:285–286.
31. McEntee GP, Coughlan M, Corrigan T, Dervan P. Pelvic inflammatory pseudotumor: problems in clinical and histological diagnosis. Case report. *Br J Obstet Gynaecol* 1985;92:1067–1069.
32. Chen KTK, Hendricks EJ. Malakoplakia of the female genital tract. *Obstet Gynecol* 1985;65:84s–87s.
33. Klempner LB, Giglio PG, Niebles A. Malacoplakia of the ovary. *Obstet Gynecol* 1987;69:537–540.
34. Clement PB, Young RH, Scully RE. Necrotic pseudoxanthomatous nodules of ovary and peritoneum in endometriosis. *Am J Surg Pathol* 1988;12:390–397.
35. Herrera GA, Riemann BEF, Greenberg HL, Miles PA. Pigmentosis tubae, a new entity: light and electron microscopic study. *Obstet Gynecol* 1983;61:80s–83s.
36. Roberts JT, Roberts GT, Maudsley RF. Indolent granulomatous necrosis in patients with previous tubal diathermy. *Am J Obstet Gynecol* 1977;129:112–113.
37. Bell DA, Mondschein M, Scully RE. Giant cell arteritis of the female genital tract. A report of three cases. *Am J Surg Pathol* 1986;10:696–701.
38. Scurry J, Planner R, Fortune DW, Lee CS, Rode J. Ligneous (pseudomembranous) inflammation of the female genital tract. A report of two cases. *J Reprod Med* 1993;38:407–412.
39. Stock RJ. Histopathologic changes in fallopian tubes subsequent to sterilization procedures. *Int J Gynecol Pathol* 1983;2:13–27.
40. Copeland W, Hawlay PC, Teteris NJ. Gynecologic amyloidosis. *Am J Obstet Gynecol* 1985;153:555–556.
41. Schenken JR, Burns EL. A study and classification of nodular lesions of the fallopian tubes. "Salpingitis isthmica nodosa." *Am J Obstet Gynecol* 1943;45:624–636.
42. Benjamin CL, Beaver DC. Pathogenesis of salpingitis isthmica nodosa. *Am J Clin Pathol* 1951;21:212–222.
43. Majmudar B, Henderson PH III, Sample E. Salpingitis isthmica nodosa: a high-risk factor for tubal pregnancy. *Obstet Gynecol* 1983;62:73–78.
44. Wrork OH, Broders AC. Adenomyosis of the fallopian tubes. *Am J Obstet Gynecol* 1942;44:412–432.
45. Pauerstein CJ, Croxatto HB, Eddy CA, Ramzy I, Walters MD. Anatomy and pathology of tubal pregnancy. *Obstet Gynecol* 1986;67:301–308.
46. Budowick M, Johnson TRB, Genadry R, Parmley TH, Woodruff JD. The histopathology of the developing tubal ectopic pregnancy. *Fertil Steril* 1980;34:169–171.
47. Case Records of the Massachusetts General Hospital (case 11-1976). *N Engl J Med* 1976;294:600–605.
48. Westerhout FC. Ruptured tubal hydatidiform mole. Report of a case. *Obstet Gynecol* 1964;23:138–139.
49. Jacques SM, Qureshi F, Ramirez NC, Lawrence WD. Retained trophoblastic tissue in fallopian tubes: a consequence of unsuspected ectopic pregnancies. *Int J Gynecol Pathol* 1997;16:219–224.
50. Nayar R, Snell J, Silverberg SG, Lage JM. Placental site nodule occurring in a fallopian tube. *Hum Pathol* 1996;27:1243–1245.
51. Hibbard LT. Adnexal torsion. *Am J Obstet Gynecol* 1985;152:456–461.
52. Schultz LR, Newton WA, Clatworthy HW. Torsion of previously normal tube and ovary in children. *N Engl J Med* 1963;268:343–346.
53. Sebastian JA, Baker RL, Cordray D. Asymptomatic infarction and separation of ovary and distal uterine tube. *Obstet Gynecol* 1973;41:531–535.
54. Nissen ED, Kent DR, Nissen SE, Feldman BM. Unilateral tuboovarian autoamputation. *J Reprod Med* 1977;19:151–153.
55. Beyth Y, Bar-On E. Tuboovarian autoamputation and infertility. *Fertil Steril* 1984;42:932–933.
56. Sapan IP, Solberg NS. Prolapse of the uterine tube after abdominal hysterectomy. *Obstet Gynecol* 1973;42:26–32.
57. Silverberg SG, Frable WJ. Prolapse of fallopian tube into vaginal vault after hysterectomy. *Arch Pathol* 1974;97:100–103.
58. Wheelock JB, Schneider V, Goplerud DR. Prolapsed fallopian tube masquerading as adenocarcinoma of the vagina in a postmenopausal woman. *Gynecol Oncol* 1985;21:369–375.
59. Anastasiades KD, Majmudar B. Prolapse of fallopian tube into urinary bladder, mimicking bladder carcinoma. *Arch Pathol Lab Med* 1983;107:613–614.
60. Sheldon RS, Wilson RB, Dockerty MB. Serosal endometriosis of fallopian tubes. *Am J Obstet Gynecol* 1967;99:882–884.
61. Lisa JR, Gioia JD, Rubin IC. Observations on the interstitial portion of the fallopian tube. *Surg Gynecol Obstet* 1954;99:159–169.
62. Rubin IC, Lisa JR, Trinidad S. Further observations on ectopic endometrium of the fallopian tube. *Surg Gynecol Obstet* 1956;103:469–474.
63. Donnez J, Casanas-Roux F, Ferin J, Thomas K. Tubal polyps, epithelial inclusions, and endometriosis after tubal sterilization. *Fertil Steril* 1984;41:564–568.
64. McLaughlin DS. Successful pregnancy outcome following removal of bilateral cornual polyps by microsurgical linear salpingotomy with the aid of the CO2 laser. *Fertil Steril* 1984;42:939–941.
65. Fernstrom I, Lagerlof B. Polyps in the intramural part of the fallopian tubes. A radiographic and clinical study. *Br J Obstet Gynaecol* 1964;71:681–691.
66. David MP, Ben-Zwi D, Langer L. Tubal intramural polyps and their relationship to infertility. *Fertil Steril* 1981;35:526–531.
67. Cioltei A, Tasca L, Titiriga L, Maakaron G, Calciu V. Nodular salpingitis and tubal endometriosis. I. Comparative clinical study. *Acta Eur Fertil* 1979;10:135–141.
68. De Brux J. The contribution of pathological anatomy to the diagnosis and prognosis of different forms of tubal sterility. *Acta Eur Fertil* 1975;6:185–195.
69. Fortier KJ, Haney AF. The pathologic spectrum of uterotubal junction obstruction. *Obstet Gynecol* 1985;65:93–98.
70. Madelenat P, De Brux J, Palmer R. L'etiologie des obstructions tubaires proximales et son role dan le pronostic des implantations. *Gynecologie* 1977;28:47–53.
71. Sampson JA. Postsalpingectomy endometriosis (endosalpingiosis). *Am J Obstet Gynecol* 1930;20:443–480.
72. Sampson JA. Pathogenesis of postsalpingectomy endometriosis in laparotomy scars. *Am J Obstet Gynecol* 1945;50:597–620.
73. Stock RJ. Postsalpingectomy endometriosis: a reassessment. *Obstet Gynecol* 1982;60:560–570.
74. Rock JA, Parmley TH, King TM, Laufe LE, Su BC. Endometriosis and the development of tuboperitoneal fistulas after tubal ligation. *Fertil Steril* 1981;35:16–20.
75. Theoh TB. The structure and development of Walthard nests. *J Pathol Bacteriol* 1953;66:433–439.

76. Gardner GH, Greene RR, Peckham BM. Normal and cystic structures of the broad ligament. *Am J Obstet Gynecol* 1948;55:917–939.
77. Samaha M, Woodruff JD. Paratubal cysts: frequency, histogenesis, and associated clinical features. *Obstet Gynecol* 1985;65:691–694.
78. Bransilver BR, Ferenczy A, Richart RM. Female genital tract remnants. An ultrastructural comparison of hydatid of Morgagni and mesonephric ducts and tubules. *Arch Pathol Lab Med* 1973;96:255–261.
79. Palomaki JF, Blair OM. Hilus cell rest of the fallopian tube. A case report. *Obstet Gynecol* 1971;37:60–62.
80. Lewis JD. Hilus-cell hyperplasia of ovaries and tubes. *Obstet Gynecol* 1964;24:728–731.
81. Honore LH, O'Hara KE. Ovarian hilus cell heterotopia. *Obstet Gynecol* 1979;53:461–464.
82. Falls JL. Accessory adrenal cortex in the broad ligament. Incidence and functional significance. *Cancer* 1955;8:143–150.
83. Mason TE, Quagliarello JR. Ectopic pancreas in the fallopian tube. Report of a first case. *Obstet Gynecol* 1976;48:70s–73s.
84. Seidman JD. Mucinous lesions of the fallopian tube. A report of 7 cases. *Am J Surg Pathol* 1994;18:1205–12.
85. Costa J. Peutz-Jeghers syndrome. Case presentation. *Obstet Gynecol* 1977;50:15s–17s.
86. Gloor E. Un cas de syndrome de Peutz-Jeghers associé à un carcinoma mammaire bilatéral, à un adenocarcinome du col uterin et à des tumeurs des cordons sexuels à tubules annelés bilaterales dans les ovaries. *Schweiz Med Wochenschr* 1978;108:717–721.
87. Berger G, Frappart L, Berger F, et al. Tubules anneles de l'ovaire, metaplasie mucipare tubaire, hyperplasie glandulo-kystique et mucipare de l'endocol et syndrome de Peutz-Jeghers. *Arch Anat Cytol Pathol* 1981;29:353–357.
88. Young RH, Scully RE. Mucinous ovarian tumors associated with mucinous adenocarcinomas of the cervix. A clinicopathological analysis of 16 cases. *Int J Gynecol Pathol* 1988;7:99–111.
89. Fetissof F, Berger G, Dubois MP, Philippe A, Lansac J, Jobard P. Female genital tract and Peutz-Jeghers syndrome: an immunohistochemical study. *Int J Gynecol Pathol* 1985;4:219–229.
90. Egan AJM, Russell P. Transitional (urothelial) cell metaplasia of the fallopian tube mucosa: morphological assessment of three cases. *Int J Gynecol Pathol* 1996;15:72–76.
91. Saffos RO, Rhatigan RM, Scully RE. Metaplastic papillary tumor of the fallopian tube—a distinctive lesion of pregnancy. *Am J Clin Pathol* 1980;74:232–236.
92. Keeney GL, Thrasher TV. Metaplastic papillary tumor of the fallopian tube: a case report with ultrastructure. *Int J Gynecol Pathol* 1988;7:86–92.
93. Bartnik J, Powell S, Moriber-Katz S, Amenta PS. Metaplastic papillary tumor of the fallopian tube. Case report, immunohistochemical features, and review of the literature. *Arch Pathol Lab Med* 1989;113:545–547.
94. Mills SE, Fechner RE. Stromal and epithelial changes in the fallopian tube following hormonal therapy. *Hum Pathol* 1980;11:583–585.
95. Dougherty CM, Cotten NM. Proliferative epithelial lesions of the uterine tube. I. Adenomatous hyperplasia. *Obstet Gynecol* 1964;24:849–854.
96. Pauerstein CJ, Woodruff JD. Cellular patterns in proliferative and anaplastic disease of the fallopian tube. *Am J Obstet Gynecol* 1966;96:486–492.
97. Moore SW, Enterline HT. Significance of proliferative epithelial lesions of the uterine tube. *Obstet Gynecol* 1975;45:385–390.
98. Robey SS, Silva EG. Epithelial hyperplasia of the fallopian tube. Its association with serous borderline tumors of the ovary. *Int J Gynecol Pathol* 1989;8:214–20.
99. Cheung AN, Young RH, Scully RE. Pseudocarcinomatous lesions of the fallopian tube associated with salpingitis. A report of 14 cases. *Am J Surg Pathol* 1994;8:1125–1130.
100. Stern J, Buscema J, Parmley T, Woodruff JD, Rosenshein NB. Atypical epithelial proliferations in the fallopian tube. *Am J Obstet Gynecol* 1981;140:309–312.
101. Yanai-Inbar I, Siriaunkgul S, Silverberg SG. Mucosal epithelial proliferation of the fallopian tube: a particular association with ovarian serous tumor of low malignant potential? *Int J Gynecol Pathol* 1995;14:107–113.
102. Ryan GM. Carcinoma in situ of the fallopian tube. *Am J Obstet Gynecol* 1962;84:198.
103. Cornog JL, Currie JL, Rubin A. Heat artifact simulating adenocarcinoma of fallopian tube. *JAMA* 1970;214:1118–1119.
104. Birch HW, Collins CG. Atypical changes of genital epithelium associated with ectopic pregnancy. *Am J Obstet Gynecol* 1961;81:1198–1208.
105. Milchgrub S, Sandstad J. Arias-Stella reaction in a fallopian tube epithelium. A light and electron microscopic study with a review of the literature. *Am J Clin Pathol* 1991;95:892–895.
106. Tziortziotis D, Bouros AC, Ziogas VS, Young RH. Clear cell hyperplasia of the fallopian tube epithelium associated with ectopic pregnancy: report of a case. *Int J Gynecol Pathol* 1997;16:79–80.
107. Evans N. Mesotheliomas of the uterine and tubal serosa and the tunica vaginalis testis. *Am J Pathol* 1943;19:461–471.
108. Golden A, Ash JE. Adenomatoid tumors of the genital tract. *Am J Pathol* 1945;21:63–73.
109. Bolton RN, Hunter WC. Adenomatoid tumors of the uterus and adnexa. Report of eleven cases. *Am J Obstet Gynecol* 1958;76:647–652.
110. Jackson JR. The histogenesis of the "adenomatoid" tumor of the genital tract. *Cancer* 1958;11:337–350.
111. Youngs LA, Taylor HB. Adenomatoid tumors of the uterus and fallopian tube. *Am J Clin Pathol* 1967;48:537–545.
112. Pauerstein CJ, Woodruff JD, Quinton SW. Developmental patterns in "adenomatoid lesions" of the fallopian tube. *Am J Obstet Gynecol* 1968;100:1000–1007.
113. Salazar H, Kanbour A, Burgess F. Ultrastructure and observations on the histogenesis of mesotheliomas "adenomatoid tumors" of the female genital tract. *Cancer* 1972;29:141–152.
114. Taxy JB, Battifora H, Oyasu R. Adenomatoid tumors: a light microscopic, histochemical, and ultrastructural study. *Cancer* 1974;34:306–316.
115. Stephenson TJ, Mills PM. Adenomatoid tumors; an immunohistochemical and ultrastructural appraisal of their histogenesis. *J Pathol* 1986;148:327–335.
116. Green TH, Scully RE. Tumors of the fallopian tube. *Clin Obstet Gynecol* 1962;5:886–906.
117. Silverman AY, Artinian B, Sabin M. Serous cystadenofibroma of the fallopian tube: a case report. *Am J Obstet Gynecol* 1978;130:593–595.
118. Kanbour AI, Burgess F, Salazar H. Intramural adenofibroma of the fallopian tube. Light and electron microscopy. *Cancer* 1973;31:1433–1439.
119. De La Fuente AA. Benign mixed mullerian tumour—adenofibroma of the fallopian tube. *Histopathology* 1982;6:661–666.
120. Chen KTK. Bilateral papillary adenofibroma of the fallopian tube. *Am J Clin Pathol* 1981;75:229–231.
121. Gisser SD. Obstructing fallopian tube papilloma. *Int J Gynecol Pathol* 1986;5:179–182.
122. Alvarado-Cabrero I, Navani SS, Young RH, Scully RE. Tumors of the fimbriated end of the fallopian tube: a clinicopathologic analysis of 20 cases, including nine carcinomas. *Int J Gynecol Pathol* 1997;16:189–196.
123. McCarthy JH, Aga R. A fallopian tube lesion of borderline malignancy associated with pseudomyxoma peritonei. *Histopathology* 1988;13:223–225.
124. Crissman JD, Handwerker D. Leiomyoma of the uterine tube: report of a case. *Am J Obstet Gynecol* 1976;126:1046.
125. Klein HZ, Smith RL. Fibromyoma of the uterine tube. *Obstet Gynecol* 1965;26:515–517.
126. Roberts CL, Marshall HK. Fibromyoma of the fallopian tube. *Am J Obstet Gynecol* 1961;82:364–366.
127. Moore OA, Waxman M, Udoffia C. Leiomyoma of the fallopian tube: a cause of tubal pregnancy. *Am J Obstet Gynecol* 1979;134:101–102.
128. Talerman A. Leiomyoma of the fallopian tube. *Int J Gynaecol Obstet* 1974;12:145–147.
129. Honore LH. Parauterine leiomyomas in women: a clinicopathologic study of 22 cases. *Eur J Obstet Gynecol Reprod Biol* 1981;11:273–279.
130. Okagaki T, Richart RM. Neurilemoma of the fallopian tube. *Am J Obstet Gynecol* 1970;106:929.
131. Katz DA, Thom D, Bogard P, Dermer MS. Angiomyolipoma of the fallopian tube. *Am J Obstet Gynecol* 1984;148:341–343.
132. Dede JA, Janovski NA. Lipoma of the uterine tube—a gynecologic rarity. *Obstet Gynecol* 1963;22:461–467.
133. Spanta R, Lawrence WD. Soft tissue chondroma of the fallopian tube. Differential diagnosis and histogenetic considerations. *Pathol Res Pract* 1995;191:174–176.
134. Sanes S, Warner R. Primary lymphangioma of the fallopian tube. *Am J Obstet Gynecol* 1939;37:316–321.

135. Weber DL, Fazzini E. Ganglioneuroma of the fallopian tube: a hitherto unreported finding. *Acta Neuropathol (Berl)* 1970;16:173–175.
136. Ebrahimi T, Okagaki T. Hemangioma of the fallopian tube. *Am J Obstet Gynecol* 1973;115:864–865.
137. Patel DR, Kawalek R, Iger J. Cavernous hemangioma of the fallopian tube. *Int Surg* 1973;58:420–421.
138. Talerman A. Haemangioma of the fallopian tube. *Br J Obstet Gynaecol* 1969;76:559–560.
139. Joglekar VM. Haemangioma of the fallopian tube. Case report. *Br J Obstet Gynaecol* 1979;86:823–825.
140. Benedet JL, White GW. Malignant tumors of fallopian tube. In: Coppleson M, ed. *Gynecologic oncology, fundamental principles and clinical practice*. Edinburgh: Churchill Livingstone, 1981:621–629.
141. Woolas R, Jacobs I, Prys Davies A, et al. What is the true incidence of primary fallopian tube carcinoma? *Int J Gynecol Cancer* 1994;4:384–388.
142. Goldman JA, Gans B, Eckerling B. Hydrops tubae profluens—a symptom in tubal carcinoma. *Obstet Gynecol* 1961;18:631–634.
143. Goldman JA, Eckerling B. Hydrops tubae profluens—a symptom in tubal carcinoma. *Obstet Gynecol* 1961;18:631–634.
144. Sedlis A. Primary carcinoma of the fallopian tube. *Obstet Gynecol Surv* 1961;16:209–226.
145. Eddy GL, Copeland LJ, Gershenson DM, Atkinson EN, Wharton JT, Rutledge FN. Fallopian tube carcinoma. *Obstet Gynecol* 1984;64:546–552.
146. Roberts JA, Lifshitz S. Primary adenocarcinoma of the fallopian tube. *Gynecol Oncol* 1982;13:301–308.
147. Kinzel GE. Primary carcinoma of the fallopian tube. *Am J Obstet Gynecol* 1976;125:816–820.
148. Schiller HM, Silverberg SG. Staging and prognosis in primary carcinoma of the fallopian tube. *Cancer* 1971;28:389–395.
149. Finn WF, Javert CT. Primary and metastatic cancer of the fallopian tube. *Cancer* 1949;2:803–814.
150. Hu CY, Taymor ML, Hertig AT. Primary carcinoma of the fallopian tube. *Am J Obstet Gynecol* 1950;59:58–67.
151. Momtazee S, Kempson RL. Primary adenocarcinoma of the fallopian tube. *Obstet Gynecol* 1968;32:649–656.
152. Benedet JL, White GW, Fairey RN, Boyes DA. Adenocarcinoma of the fallopian tube. Experience with 41 patients. *Obstet Gynecol* 1977;50:654–657.
153. Yoonessi M. Carcinoma of the fallopian tube. *Obstet Gynecol Surv* 1979;34:257–270.
154. Boutselis JG, Thompson JN. Clinical aspects of primary carcinoma of the fallopian tube. A clinical study of 14 cases. *Am J Obstet Gynecol* 1971;111:98–101.
155. Raju KS, Barker GH, Wiltshaw E. Primary carcinoma of the fallopian tube. Report of 22 cases. *Br J Obstet Gynaecol* 1981;88:1124–1129.
156. Brown MD, Kohorn EI, Kapp DS, Schwartz PE, Merino M. Fallopian tube carcinoma. *Int J Radiat Oncol Biol Phys* 1985;11:583–590.
156a.Yeung HHY, Bannatyne P, Russell P. Adenocarcinoma of the fallopian tubes: a clinicopathological study of eight cases. *Pathology* 1983;15:279–286.
157. Hellström A-C, Silfverswärd C, Nilsson B, Pettersson F. Carcinoma of the fallopian tube. A clinical and histopathologic review. The Radiumhemmet series. *Int J Gynecol Cancer* 1994;4:395–400.
158. Alvarado-Cabrero I, Young RH, Vamvakakas EC, Scully RE. Carcinoma of the fallopian tube: a clinicopathological study of 105 cases with observations on staging and prognostic factors. *Gynecol Oncol* (In press).
159. Kahn ME, Norris S. Primary carcinoma of the fallopian tubes. *Am J Obstet Gynecol* 1934;28:393–402.
160. Bannatyne P, Russell P. Early adenocarcinoma of the fallopian tubes. A case for multifocal tumorigenesis. *Diagn Gynecol Obstet* 1981;3:49–60.
161. Sonnendecker HE, Cooper K, Kalian KN. Primary fallopian tube adenocarcinoma in situ associated with adjuvant tamoxifen therapy for breast carcinoma. *Gynecol Oncol* 1994;52:402–407.
162. Navani SS, Alvarado-Cabrero I, Young RH, Scully RE. Endometrioid carcinoma of the fallopian tube: a clinicopathologic analysis of 26 cases. *Gynecol Oncol* 1996;63:371–378.
163. Gaffney EF, Cornog J. Endometrioid carcinoma of the fallopian tube arising in endometriosis. *Obstet Gynecol* 1978;52:34s–36s.
164. Daya D, Young RH, Scully RE. Endometrioid carcinoma of the fallopian tube resembling an adnexal tumor of probable wolffian origin. A report of six cases. *Int J Gynecol Pathol* 1992;11:122–130.
165. Voet RL, Lifshitz S. Primary clear cell adenocarcinoma of the fallopian tube: light microscopic and ultrastructural findings. *Int J Gynecol Pathol* 1982;1:292–298.
166. Malinak LR, Miller GV, Armstrong JT. Primary squamous cell carcinoma of the fallopian tube. *Am J Obstet Gynecol* 1966;95:1167–1168.
167. Jackson-York GL, Ramzy I. Synchronous papillary mucinous adenocarcinoma of the endocervix and fallopian tubes. *Int J Gynecol Pathol* 1992;11:63–67.
168. Herbold DR, Axelrod JH, Bobowski SJ, et al. Glassy cell carcinoma of the fallopian tube. A case report. *Int J Gynecol Pathol* 1988;7:384–390.
169. Aoyama T, Mizuno T, Andou K, Takagi T, Mizuno T, Eimoto T. a-Fetoprotein-producing (hepatoid) carcinoma of the fallopian tube. *Gynecol Oncol* 1996;63:261–266.
170. Muntz HG, Rutgers JL, Tarraza HM, Fuller AF. Carcinosarcomas and mixed mullerian tumors of the fallopian tube. *Gynecol Oncol* 1989;34:109–115.
171. Carlson JA, Ackerman BL, Wheeler JE. Malignant mixed mullerian tumor of the fallopian tube. *Cancer* 1993;71:187–192.
172. Hellstrom AC, Auer G, Silversward C, Pettersson F. Prognostic factors in malignant mixed müllerian tumor of the fallopian tube; the Radiumhemmet series 1923–1994. *Int J Gynecol Cancer* 1996;6:467–472.
173. Seraj IM, King A, Chase D. Malignant mixed mullerian tumor of the oviduct. *Gynecol Oncol* 1990;37:296–301.
174. Herbold DR, Fu YS, Silbert SW. Leiomyosarcoma of the broad ligament. A case report and literature review with follow-up. *Am J Surg Pathol* 1983;7:285–292.
175. Buchwalter CL, Jenison EL, Fromm M, Mehta VT, Hart WR. Pure embryonal rhabdomyosarcoma of the fallopian tube. *Gynecol Oncol* 1997;67:95–101.
176. Gollard R, Kosty M, Bordin G, Wax A, Lacey C. Two unusual presentations of mullerian adenosarcoma: case reports, literature review, and treatment considerations. *Gynecol Oncol* 1995; 59:412–22.
177. Rosenberg SA, Diamond HD, Jaslowitz B, Craver LF. Lymphosarcoma—a review of 1269 cases. *Medicine* 1961;40:31–84.
178. Osborne BM, Robboy SJ. Lymphomas or leukemia presenting as ovarian tumors. An analysis of 42 cases. *Cancer* 1983;52:1933–1943.
179. Cecalupo AJ, Frankel LS, Sullivan MP. Pelvic and ovarian extramedullary leukemic relapse in young girls. A report of four cases and review of the literature. *Cancer* 1982;50:587–593.
180. Horn T, Jao W, Keh PC. Benign cystic teratoma of the fallopian tube. *Arch Pathol Lab Med* 1983;107:48.
181. Sweet RL, Selinger HE, McKay DG. Malignant teratoma of the uterine tube. *Obstet Gynecol* 1975;45:553–556.
182. Scully RE. Germ cell tumors of the ovary and fallopian tube. In: *Progress in gynecology*, vol IV. New York: Grune & Stratton, 1963: 335–347.
183. Hoda SA, Huvos AG. Struma salpingis associated with struma ovarii. *Am J Surg Pathol* 1993;17:1187–1189.
184. Westerhout FC Jr. Ruptured tubal hydatidiform mole. Report of a case. *Obstet Gynecol* 1964;23:138–139.
185. Govender NSK, Goldstein DP. Metastatic tubal mole and coexisting intrauterine pregnancy. *Obstet Gynecol* 1977;49:67s–69s.
186. Ober W, Maier RC. Gestational choriocarcinoma of the fallopian tube. *Diagn Gynecol Obstet* 1982;3:213–231.
187. Kay S, Schneider V, Litt J. Choriocarcinoma of the mesosalpinx masquerading as congestive heart failure: ultrastructural observations of the tumor. *Int J Gynecol Pathol* 1983;2:72–87.
188. Dekel A, van Iddekinge B, Isaacson C, Dicker D, Feldberg D, Goldman J. Primary choriocarcinoma of the fallopian tube. Report of a case with survival and postoperative delivery. Review of the literature. *Obstet Gynecol Surv* 1986;41:142–148.
189. Mazur MT, Hsueh S, Gersell DJ. Metastases to the female genital tract. Analysis of 325 cases. *Cancer* 1984;53:1978–1984.
190. Pins MR, Young RH, Crum CP, Leach IH, Scully RE. Cervical squamous cell carcinoma in situ with intraepithelial extension to the upper genital tract and invasion of the tubes and ovaries: report of a case with human papilloma virus analysis. *Int J Gynecol Pathol* 1997;16:272–278.
191. Woodruff JD, Julian CG. Multiple malignancy in the upper genital cancer. *Am J Obstet Gynecol* 1969;103:810–819.
192. Kariminejad MH, Scully RE. Female adnexal tumor of probable wolffian origin. A distinctive pathologic entity. *Cancer* 1973;31:671–677.
193. Sivathondan Y, Salm R, Hughesdon PE, Faccini JM. Female adnexal tumour of probable wolffian origin. *J Clin Pathol* 1979;32:616–624.

194. Tavassoli FA, Andrade R, Merino M. Retiform wolffian adenoma. *Prog Surg Pathol* 1990;11:121–136.
195. Daya D. Malignant female adnexal tumor of probable wolffian origin with review of the literature. *Arch Pathol Lab Med* 1994;118:310–312.
196. Aslani M, Ahn G-H, Scully RE. Serous papillary cystadenoma of broad ligament of broad ligament: a report of 25 cases. *Int J Gynecol Pathol* 1988;7:131–138.
197. Aslani M, Scully RE. Primary carcinoma of the broad ligament. Report of four cases and review of the literature. *Cancer* 1989;64:1540–1545.
198. Pschera H, Wikström B. Extraovarian Brenner tumor coexisting with serous cystadenoma. Case report. *Gynecol Obstet Invest* 1991;31:185–187.
199. Jensen ML, Nielsen MN. Broad ligament mucinous cystadenoma of borderline malignancy. *Histopathology* 1990;16:89–103.
200. Werness BA, Guccion JG. Tumor of the broad ligament in von Hippel-Lindau disease of probable mullerian origin. *Int J Gynecol Pathol* 1997;16:282–285.
201. Altaras MM, Jaffe R, Corduba M, Holtzinger M, Bahary C. Primary paraovarian cystadenocarcinoma: clinical and management aspects and literature review. *Gynecol Oncol* 1990;38:268–272.
202. Persad V, Anderson MF. Endometrial stromal sarcoma of the broad ligament arising in the area of endometriosis in a paramesonephric cyst. Case report. *Br J Obstet Gynaecol* 1977;84:149–152.
203. Bell DA, Woodruff JM, Scully RE. Ependymoma of the broad ligament. A report of two cases. *Am J Surg Pathol* 1984;8:203–209.
204. Grody WW, Nieberg RK, Bhuta S. Ependymoma-like tumor of the mesovarium. *Arch Pathol Lab Med* 1985;109:291–293.
205. Gersell DJ, King TC. Papillary cystadenoma of the mesosalpinx in von Hippel-Lindau disease. *Am J Surg Pathol* 1988;12:145–149.
206. Funk KC, Heiken JP. Papillary cystadenoma of the broad ligament in von Hippel-Lindau disease. *Am J Radiol* 1989;153:527–528.
207. Korn WT, Schatzki SC, Disciullo AJ, Scully RE. Papillary cystadenoma of the broad ligament in von Hippel-Lindau disease. *Am J Obstet Gynecol* 1990;163:596–598.
208. Gabbay-Mor M, Ovadia Y, Neri A. Accessory ovaries with bilateral dermoid cysts. *Eur J Obstet Gynecol Reprod Biol* 1982;14:171–173.
209. Huntington RW, Bullock WK. Yolk sac tumors of extragonadal origin. *Cancer* 1970;25:1368–1376.
210. Merino MJ, LiVolsi VA, Trepeta RW. Fibrothecoma of the broad ligament. *Diagn Gynecol Obstet* 1980;2:51–54.
211. Roth LM, Davis MM, Sutton GP. Steroid cell tumor of the broad ligament arising in an accessory ovary. *Arch Pathol Lab Med* 1996;120:405–409.
212. Sasano H, Sato S, Yajima A, Akama J, Nagura H. Adrenal rest tumor of the broad ligament: case report with immunohistochemical study of steroidogenic enzymes. *Pathol Int* 1997;47:493–496.
213. Griffith LM, Carcangiu M-L. Sex cord tumor with annular tubules associated with endometriosis of the fallopian tube. *Am J Clin Pathol* 1991;96:259–262.
214. Al-Jafari MS, Panton HM, Gradwell E. Phaeochromocytoma of the broad ligament. Case report. *Br J Obstet Gynaecol* 1985;92:649–651.

CHAPTER 56

The Peritoneum

Philip B. Clement, Robert H. Young, and Robert E. Scully

INFLAMMATORY LESIONS

Acute Peritonitis

Acute diffuse peritonitis, characterized by a serosal fibrinopurulent exudate, is most commonly associated with a perforated viscus, and is usually bacterial or chemical (bile or gastric or pancreatic juice) in origin. The lipases in pancreatic juice also typically produce fat necrosis. Spontaneous bacterial peritonitis occurs most often in children and in adults who are immunocompromised or have cirrhosis of the liver (1,2). Rare infectious causes of acute peritonitis include candida (3), actinomycetes (4), and amebae (5). Recurrent attacks of acute peritonitis are an almost constant feature of familial Mediterranean fever (recurrent polyserositis; periodic disease) (6).

Granulomatous Peritonitis

A variety of infectious and noninfectious agents can cause granulomatous peritonitis. The peritoneum may be studded with nodules, which can mimic disseminated tumor at operation. The diagnosis rests on the histologic, and in some cases, microbiologic, identification of the causative agent.

Infectious Causes

Tuberculous peritonitis may be secondary to spread from a focus within the abdominopelvic cavity or be a manifestation of miliary spread (7–9). The clinical picture, including an elevated CA125 in some cases, may mimic that of disseminated ovarian carcinoma (9). The granulomas are characterized by caseous necrosis and Langhans' type giant cells; mycobacteria may be demonstrated by acid-fast stains or immunofluorescence methods. Rarely, granulomatous peritonitis is a complication of fungal infections, including histoplasmosis (10), coccidioidomycosis (11), and cryptococcosis (12), and parasitic infestations, including schistosomiasis (13), oxyuriasis (14,15), echinococcosis (4), ascariasis (16), and strongyloidiasis (17).

Noninfectious Causes

Foreign material, usually recognizable on microscopic examination, can elicit a granulomatous reaction on the peritoneum. Starch granules from surgical gloves (18–20), douche fluid (21) and lubricants (22) typically incite a granulomatous and fibrosing peritonitis; in occasional cases the inflammatory reaction may be of tuberculoid type with caseous necrosis (23). The periodic acid-Schiff (PAS)-positive starch granules exhibit a characteristic Maltese-cross configuration under polarized light. Talc was once an important cause of granulomatous and fibrosing peritonitis because of its use as a lubricant on surgical gloves (24,25), but talc-induced peritonitis has also been described more recently in drug abusers (26). Other iatrogenic causes of granulomatous peritonitis include cellulose and cotton fibers from surgical pads and drapes (27–29), hemostatic materials (30,31), and oily substances, such as hysterosalpingographic contrast medium, mineral oil, and paraffin (32–35). The last three substances are associated with a lipogranulomatous reaction.

Escaped bowel contents, including vegetable matter, food-derived starch (36), and barium sulfate (37), can produce a peritoneal foreign-body reaction. Sebaceous material and keratin from ruptured dermoid cysts typically evoke an intense granulomatous, lipogranulomatous, and fibrosing peritoneal inflammatory reaction that may mimic a neoplasm at operation (38–40). Granulomatous inflammation to keratin exfoliated from the surfaces of uterine and ovarian adenoacanthomas is discussed below (see Tumor-Like Le-

---

P. B. Clement: Department of Pathology, Vancouver Hospital and Health Sciences Center, University of British Columbia, Vancouver, British Columbia V5Z 1M9.

R. H. Young and R. E. Scully: Department of Pathology, Massachusetts General Hospital; Harvard Medical School, Boston, Massachusetts 02114.

sions). Spillage of amniotic fluid at cesarean section with its content of vernix caseosa (lanugo hair, squamous cells, keratin) and meconium (bile and pancreatic and intestinal secretions) can result in a granulomatous peritonitis (Fig. 1) (41). Meconium peritonitis, caused by bowel perforation *in utero*, can also be a problem in newborn infants; in boys, the process may involve the tunica vaginalis and result in a tumor-like scrotal mass (42–44). Calcification, rather than granulomatous inflammation, may dominate the microscopic picture. Chronic bile peritonitis may be associated with granulomatous inflammation and fibrosis; cholesterol crystals and bile pigment may be identifiable within giant cells (45). Granulomatous peritonitis also has been described secondary to Crohn's disease (46), sarcoidosis (47,48), and Whipple's disease (49). Necrotizing peritoneal granulomas have been described following diathermy ablation of endometriosis (50).

Nongranulomatous Histiocytic Lesions

The peritoneum can be occasionally involved by histiocytic infiltrates rather than discrete granulomas. Ceroid-rich histiocytes involving the peritoneum and omentum may occur secondary to endometriosis (51) or in association with a peritoneal decidual reaction (52). The differential in such cases includes peritoneal melanosis (see Tumor-Like Lesions). Nonpigmented histiocytes, sometimes admixed with smaller numbers of hyperplastic mesothelial cells, can occasionally occur as nodular aggregates on the peritoneum that may appear as small grossly visible nodules at operation (53,53a). We are aware of a histiocytic peritoneal nodule from a patient with a granulosa cell tumor in which the histiocytes were initially misinterpreted microscopically as metastatic granulosa cell tumor. Ruffolo and Suster (54) described a diffuse histiocytic proliferation of the pelvic peritoneum associated with endocervicosis. The histiocytes in histiocytic nodules can be distinguished from any admixed mesothelial cells or from pure proliferations of hyperplastic mesothelial cells by the different immunoreactivity of the two cell types (53,53a).

Mucicarminophilic histiocytosis is characterized by histiocytes that contain polyvinylpyrrolidone (PVP), a substance that has been used as a blood substitute (55). These cells can be found in many sites, both within and outside the female genital tract, including pelvic lymph nodes and the omentum. The histiocytes have vacuolated basophilic to lavender cytoplasm and an eccentric nucleus, an appearance that may suggest the diagnosis of signet-ring cell adenocarcinoma. The histiocytes are mucicarminophilic, but in contrast to neoplastic signet-ring cells, are PAS-negative; a variety of other stains are also helpful in the differential diagnosis (55). Mucicarminophilic peritoneal histiocytes potentially mimicking a signet-ring cell adenocarcinoma can also be encountered as a reaction to oxidized regenerated cellulose, a hemostatic agent (55a).

Peritoneal Fibrosis

Reactive peritoneal fibrosis, often accompanied by fibrous adhesions, is a common sequela of prior peritoneal inflammation, and a frequent complication of a surgical procedure (56). In occasional cases, it may difficult to differentiate between markedly reactive peritoneal fibrosis and a desmoplastic mesothelioma, particularly in a small biopsy specimen (57). Features favoring a diagnosis of mesothelioma include nuclear atypia, necrosis, the presence of organized patterns of collagen deposition (fascicular, storiform), and infiltration of adjacent tissues (57).

Localized hyaline plaques are a common incidental finding on the splenic capsule, and are probably related to splenic congestion (58). Fibrous thickening of the peritoneum has been described in patients with hepatic cirrhosis and ascites (59). Hyalinized silicotic nodules involving the peritoneum have been described in patients with silicosis (60).

Sclerosing peritonitis is a rare disorder characterized by a fibrous peritoneal thickening. Concato (61) described pearly white thickening of the peritoneum, either in the form of discrete plaques or continuous sheets involving the hepatic, splenic, and diaphragmatic peritoneum. More recent reports have described a similar lesion that encases the small bowel ("abdominal cocoon") causing bowel obstruction. It occurs in an idiopathic form, typically affecting adolescent girls (62,63), or it may be secondary to practolol therapy (64), chronic ambulatory peritoneal dialysis (65,66), sarcoidosis (67), the use of a peritoneovenous (LeVeen) shunt (68), and ovarian fibrothecomatous tumors or tumor-like lesions (Fig. 2) (69). In the latter situation, the peritoneal lesions may be misinterpreted intraoperatively or even on microscopic examination as metastatic tumor (69). Sclerosing peritonitis should be distinguished from peritoneal encapsulation, a congenital malformation in which an accessory peritoneal membrane encases loops of small bowel in a sac-like structure (70,71).

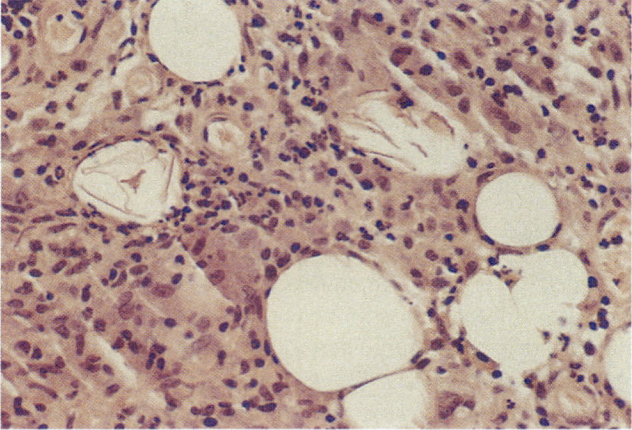

FIG. 1. Meconium peritonitis. The omentum is infiltrated with histiocytes, including foreign body-type giant cells. Note keratin debris.

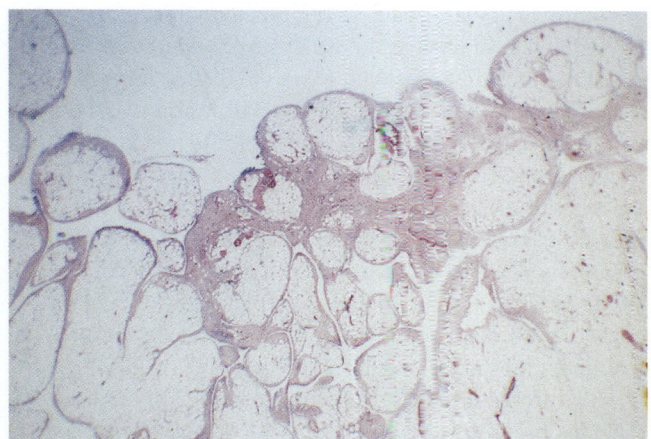

FIG. 2. Sclerosing peritonitis involving omentum in a woman with a luteinized thecoma of the ovary.

Rare Types of Peritonitis

Eosinophilic peritonitis is seen rarely in cases of eosinophilic gastroenteritis and the hypereosinophilic syndrome (72). Isolated cases of eosinophilic ascites have been associated with childhood atopy, peritoneal dialysis, vasculitis, lymphoma or metastatic carcinoma, and ruptured hydatid cysts (72). Rare cases of peritonitis may be secondary to peritoneal involvement by collagen-vascular diseases, including systemic lupus erythematosus (73) and Degos' disease (74).

TUMOR-LIKE LESIONS

Mesothelial Hyperplasia

Hyperplasia of mesothelial cells is a common response to inflammation and chronic effusions (Figs. 3–6). Hyperplastic lesions may be noted at operation as solitary or multiple small nodules, but more commonly are incidental findings on microscopic examination (57,75–77). Mesothelial hyperplasia often involves the adnexal areas in cases of chronic salpingitis and endometriosis (78), and is occasionally en-

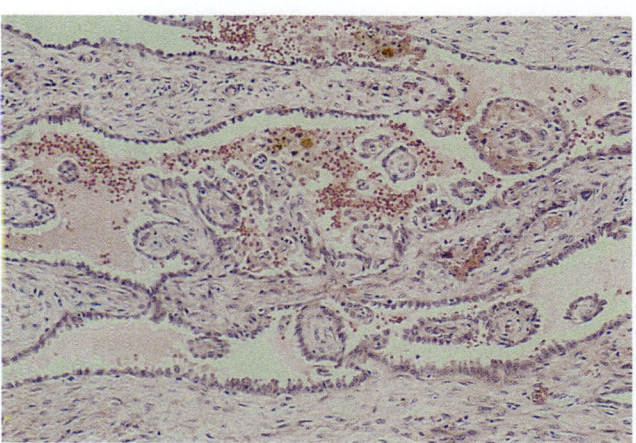

FIG. 4. Mesothelial hyperplasia. Reactive mesothelial cells line irregular spaces and stromal papillae. The stroma consists of inflamed fibrous tissue.

countered, particularly in the omentum, in association with ovarian tumors (79). Mesothelial hyperplasia can also occur on the surface of the ovary or within the superficial ovarian stroma overlying a borderline epithelial tumor and may be misinterpreted as invasive tumor (Fig. 6) (79). Mesothelial hyperplasia may be confined to a hernia sac, and in such cases may be due to trauma or incarceration (80). Hyperplastic mesothelial cells occasionally are an incidental microscopic finding within pelvic and intraabdominal lymph nodes, and in such cases are usually associated with and are probably secondary to mesothelial hyperplasia of the peritoneum (Fig. 7) (81).

In florid examples, solid, trabecular, tubular, papillary or tubulopapillary patterns (Figs. 3–6) and limited degrees of extension of the mesothelial cells into the underlying tissues may be seen. The cells are often focally disposed in linear, sometimes parallel, thin layers, separated by fibrin or fibrous tissue. When lymph nodes are involved, hyperplastic mesothelial cells typically occupy subcapsular and intranodal sinusoids (Fig. 7) (81). Hyperplastic mesothelial cells

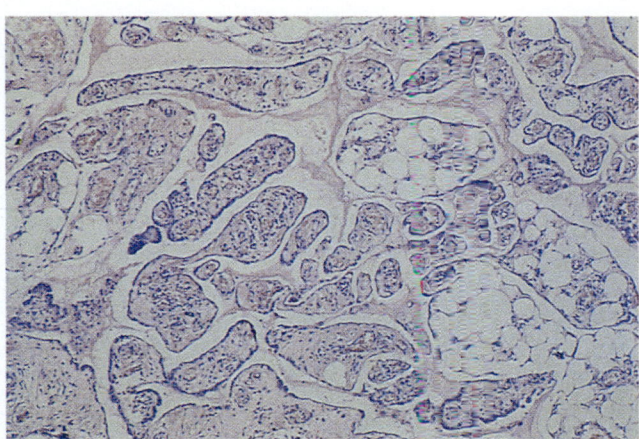

FIG. 3. Papillary mesothelial hyperplasia involving omentum.

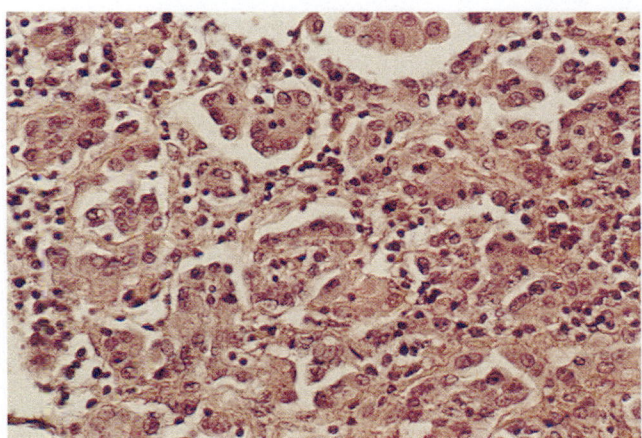

FIG. 5. Papillary mesothelial hyperplasia of pelvic peritoneum. Note admixed inflammatory cells.

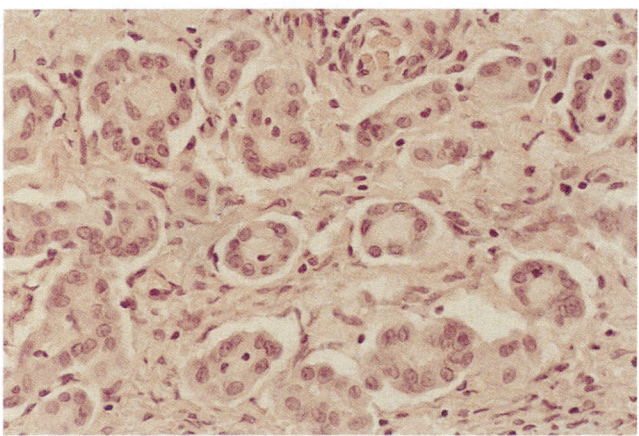

FIG. 6. Mesothelial hyperplasia in wall of ovarian müllerian mucinous tumor of borderline malignancy. Small tubules are embedded within a fibrous stroma.

may have cytoplasmic vacuoles containing acid mucin (predominantly hyaluronic acid) or, less commonly, may exhibit marked cytoplasmic clearing (57). Mild to moderate nuclear pleomorphism, mitotic figures, and occasional multinucleated cells may be seen. Psammoma bodies are encountered in occasional cases, and, rarely, eosinophilic strap-shaped cells resembling rhabdomyoblasts have been described (80).

The major differential diagnosis of mesothelial hyperplasia is with diffuse malignant mesothelioma (DMM). McCaughey and co-workers (57,82) have noted that the presence of grossly visible nodules, necrosis, conspicuous large cytoplasmic vacuoles, severe nuclear pleomorphism, and deep infiltration favor DMM over mesothelial hyperplasia. Some of these features, however, such as severe nuclear atypia, are not always present or may be present only focally within a DMM. Special techniques may facilitate the differential diagnosis. Intense cytoplasmic immunoreactivity for epithelial membrane antigen is characteristic of the cells of DMM but not hyperplastic mesothelial cells (83). Morphometry has shown that reactive mesothelial cells generally have smaller nuclei that the cells of a DMM (84), and there

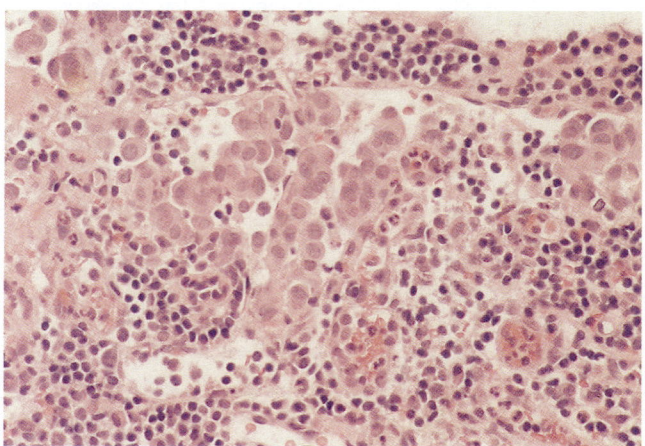

FIG. 7. Hyperplastic mesothelial cells within a sinusoid of a pelvic lymph node.

are more nucleolar organizer regions in malignant mesothelial cells than in reactive ones (85,86). Despite these differential features, in occasional cases the distinction between a hyperplastic and malignant mesothelial lesion may be difficult or impossible, particularly in a biopsy specimen. If the lesion in question is a DMM, follow-up usually reveals its nature within several months because of its typical rapid growth. In contrast, an atypical mesothelial proliferation occasionally persists for years without an apparent cause (57). An apparently benign, otherwise typical mesothelial proliferation, however, occasionally precedes the appearance of a malignant mesothelioma (57,87).

The differential diagnosis of mesothelial hyperplasia also includes borderline serous tumors of primary peritoneal or ovarian origin. Similarly, intranodal hyperplastic mesothelial cells should not be confused with nodal involvement by metastatic serous borderline tumor (SBLT) or a primary intranodal SBLT arising from intranodal endosalpingiosis (see below). Grossly visible tumor, columnar cells with or without cilia, the presence of intracellular or extracellular neutral mucin, and numerous psammoma bodies favor a serous tumor. Immunohistochemical markers for epithelial differentiation (see discussion on DMM, below) may also be of value in the differential diagnosis.

Peritoneal Inclusion Cysts

Peritoneal inclusion cysts typically occur in the peritoneal cavity of women in the reproductive age group (88–97). Rarely they occur in males and similar lesions have been described in the pleural cavity (77,98–100). Some are incidental findings at laparotomy in the form of single or multiple, small, thin-walled, translucent, unilocular cysts that may be attached or lie free in the peritoneal cavity. Occasionally they may involve the round ligament simulating an inguinal hernia (101) or occupy the superficial cortex of the spleen (96). The cysts have a smooth lining, contents that vary from yellow and watery to gelatinous, an uncomplicated histologic appearance of a single layer of typically flattened, and benign-appearing mesothelial cells, and they pose no diagnostic problems. While most of these unilocular mesothelial cysts are probably reactive in origin, some of those located in the mesocolon, mesentery of the small intestine, retroperitoneum, and splenic capsule may be developmental (95,96).

Multilocular cystic masses that may measure up to 20 cm in diameter (Fig. 8) and are lined by mesothelial cells are referred to as multilocular peritoneal inclusion cysts (MPICs), benign cystic mesotheliomas, inflammatory cysts of the peritoneum, or postoperative peritoneal cysts (88–95). MPICs are usually associated with clinical manifestations, most commonly lower abdominal pain, a palpable mass, or both. They are usually attached to pelvic organs and may simulate a cystic ovarian tumor on clinical examination, at laparotomy (93), or even on pathologic examination (102); the upper abdominal cavity, the retroperitoneum, or hernia sacs may also be involved (95). Unlike the smaller unilocular

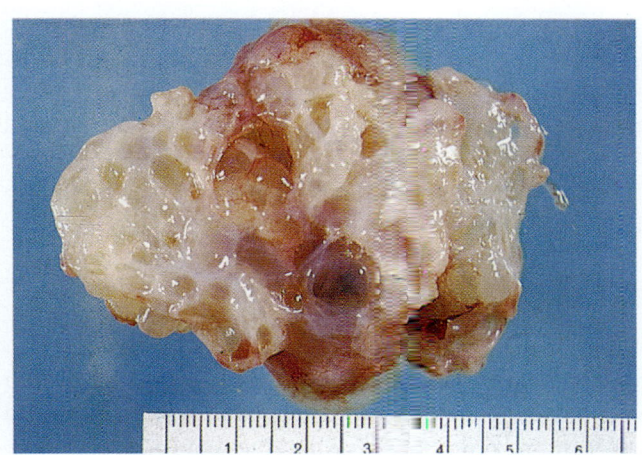

FIG. 8. Peritoneal inclusion cyst. The multilocular cystic mass consists of multiple cysts separated by fibrous tissue.

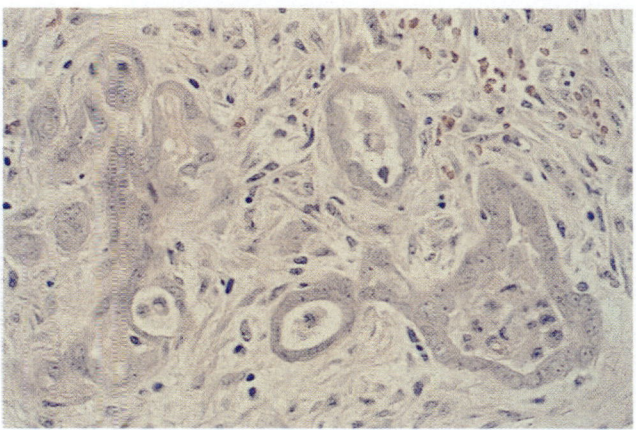

FIG. 10. Peritoneal inclusion cyst with mural mesothelial cell proliferation. Atypical mesothelial cells form small nests and gland-like structures within a cellular inflamed fibrous stroma.

cysts, the septa and walls of MPICs may contain abundant fibrous tissue. Their contents may resemble those of the unilocular cysts or be serosanguineous or bloody.

On microscopic examination, MPICs are typically lined by a single layer of flat to cuboidal, occasionally hobnail-shaped mesothelial cells with generally bland nuclear features, although a degree of reactive atypia is not infrequent (Fig. 9). The lining cells occasionally form small papillae and cribriform patterns or undergo squamous metaplasia (94,95). In some cases, mural proliferations of typical or atypical mesothelial cells arranged singly, as gland-like structures or nests (Fig. 10), or in adenomatoid tumor-like patterns may be encountered, creating an infiltrative appearance that should not be confused with a malignant tumor (93–95). Occasional vacuolated mesothelial cells in the stroma may simulate signet-ring cells (95). Intra- and extra-cellular hyaline bodies have been encountered in rare cases (97). The septa typically consist of a loose, fibrovascular connective tissue with a sparse inflammatory infiltrate. In some cases, marked acute and chronic inflammation, abundant fibrin, broad bands of granulation and fibrous tissue, and evidence of recent and remote hemorrhage may be seen in the cyst walls.

A history of a prior abdominal operation, pelvic inflammatory disease, endometriosis, or combinations thereof, was present in 84% of patients in one series (95), suggesting a role for inflammation in the pathogenesis of the cysts (95,103–105). An inflammatory pathogenesis is also supported by the occurrence of cases in which the dividing line between florid adhesions association with inflammation and a MPIC may be difficult. With one exception (100), there has been no association with asbestos exposure. Follow-up examinations have not disclosed a malignant behavior in cases that we consider MPICs, but in as many as one-half of the cases the lesions have recurred one or more times from months to many years postoperatively (95). It is likely, however, that at least some of these "recurrences" are the result of newly formed postoperative adhesions. For these reasons (while accepting that low-grade cystic mesotheliomas occur rarely, see below), we prefer the designation "multilocular peritoneal inclusion cyst" to "benign cystic mesothelioma" for such lesions, until there is convincing evidence for their neoplastic nature.

Aside from the contentious problem of their distinction from true cystic mesotheliomas (see below), MPICs are confused most often with multilocular cystic lymphangiomas (88). In contrast to MPICs, the latter typically occur in children, more frequently in boys, and are usually extrapelvic, being almost always localized to the mesentery of the small intestine, omentum, mesocolon, or retroperitoneum. Their contents may be chylous, and on histologic examination lymphoid aggregates and smooth muscle, which are rare findings in MPICs, are typically present within their walls. In problematic cases, immunohistochemical stains to distinguish between endothelial and mesothelial cells may be useful. Another lesion that merits consideration in the differential diagnosis of MPICs is the rare multicystic adenomatoid

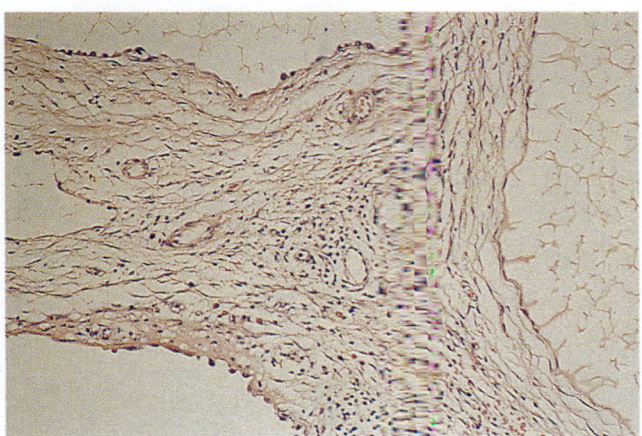

FIG. 9. Peritoneal inclusion cyst. Cystic spaces are lined by a single layer of flat to low cuboidal mesothelial cells. The stroma consists of loose fibrous tissue with a sparse chronic inflammatory cell infiltrate.

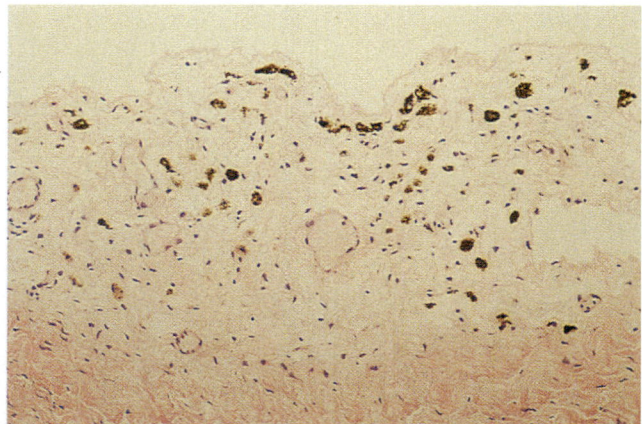

FIG. 11. Peritoneal melanosis. Melanin-laden histiocytes lie within the submesothelial connective tissue.

tumor (106,107). In contrast to MPICs, the latter typically involve the myometrium, contain foci of typical adenomatoid tumor, and lack prominent numbers of inflammatory cells. A detailed discussion of other lesions in the differential diagnosis of MPICs has recently been presented elsewhere (95).

Calcifying Fibrous Pseudotumor

This rare, likely reactive lesion is usually an incidental finding on the visceral peritoneum of the small bowel and stomach in adults (108); it can be misinterpreted intraoperatively as metastatic carcinoma. The process usually takes the form of a well-circumscribed solid mass up to 2.0 cm in diameter, often with a gritty sectioned surface. Microscopic examination reveals dense hyalinized collagen often in concentric whorls, with occasional banal-appearing fibroblasts, lymphocytes and plasma cells (which may be perivascular), and numerous psammoma bodies.

Splenosis

Splenosis, which results from implantation of splenic tissue, is typically an incidental finding at laparotomy months to years after splenectomy for traumatic rupture of the spleen (109–111). A few to innumerable, red-blue, peritoneal nodules, ranging from punctate to 7 cm in diameter, are scattered widely throughout the abdominal, and less commonly the pelvic cavity. The intraoperative appearance may mimic endometriosis, benign or malignant vascular tumors, or metastatic cancer.

Trophoblastic Implants

Implants of trophoblast on the pelvic or omental peritoneum may occur as a complication of the operative treatment of tubal pregnancy (112–114). The implants are more likely to occur in cases managed by laparoscopy (1.9% of cases) than those managed by laparotomy (0.6% of cases), and are more likely to occur after salpingotomy than salpingectomy (114). The clinical presentation in such cases includes an initial decline in the serum human chorionic gonadotropin (hCG) (associated with removal of the ectopic pregnancy) followed by a rising level, abdominal pain, and in some cases, intraabdominal hemorrhage (114). Microscopic examination of the implants reveals viable trophoblastic tissue that may include chorionic villi.

Melanosis

The four reported cases of melanosis, or melanotic pigmentation of the peritoneum, have all been associated with ovarian dermoid cysts; in two cases, the cysts had ruptured preoperatively (115–118). At laparotomy, focal or diffuse, tan to black, peritoneal staining or similarly pigmented, tumor-like nodules are encountered within the pelvis and in the omentum. Some of the cysts within the ovarian tumors exhibit pigmentation of their contents and lining. On histologic examination, the ovarian and peritoneal pigmentation consists of melanin-laden histiocytes within a fibrous stroma (Fig. 11). In at least two of the reported cases and in a third case we have encountered, gastric mucosa was prominent within an otherwise typical dermoid cyst. No obvious source for the pigment could be identified in any of the cases. These cases of benign peritoneal melanosis should be distinguished from metastatic malignant melanoma, a distinction that is straightforward because of the bland nuclear features and mitotic inactivity of the pigmented histiocytes.

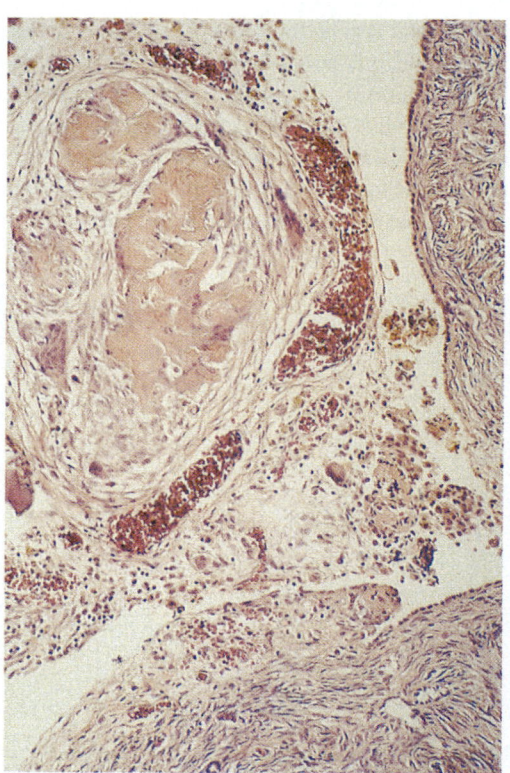

FIG. 12. Keratin granuloma on surface of ovary in a woman with an endometrial adenoacanthoma.

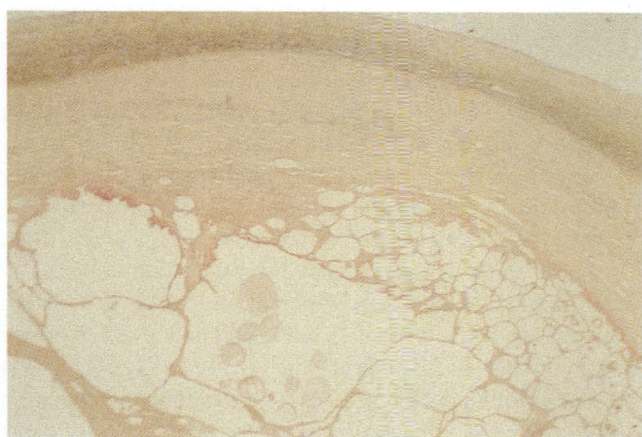

FIG. 13. Infarcted appendix epiploica.

Peritoneal Keratin Granulomas

Peritoneal granulomas that form in response to implants of keratin derived from neoplasms of the female reproductive tract may be confused with metastatic tumor (119,120). The tumors are most commonly endometrioid carcinomas with squamous differentiation originating in the endometrium or ovary, or rarely, squamous cell carcinomas of the cervix or atypical polypoid adenomyomas of the uterus (119,120). The granulomas consist of laminated deposits of keratin, sometimes with ghost squamous cells, surrounded by foreign-body giant cells and fibrous tissue (Fig. 12). Follow-up data on these patients suggest that the granulomas have no prognostic significance, although they should be thoroughly sampled by the gynecologist and carefully examined microscopically by the pathologist to exclude the presence of viable tumor. The differential diagnosis includes peritoneal granulomas in response to keratin derived from other sources, as discussed earlier in this chapter.

Infarcted Appendix Epiploica

Appendices epiploicae may undergo torsion and infarction (121,122). Subsequent calcification can result in a hard tumor-like mass that may be found attached or loose in the peritoneal cavity. In the late stages, these structures are typically composed of layers of hyalinized connective tissue surrounding a central necrotic and calcified zone in which infarcted adipose tissue in usually recognizable (Fig. 13).

MESOTHELIAL NEOPLASMS

Localized Fibrous Tumor

Localized fibrous tumors of the type that involve the pleura are extremely rare in the peritoneal cavity (Fig. 14) (123–126). Although once referred to as "fibrous mesotheliomas," they are now generally considered to originate from submesothelial fibroblasts. Their clinical and pathologic features, including strong immunoreactivity for vimentin and CD34 and negativity for cytokeratin, are similar to those of encountered in the pleura and elsewhere, and facilitate their distinction from desmoplastic mesotheliomas (123–126). Rare tumors with focal hypercellularity, marked nuclear pleomorphism, and a high mitotic rate have been interpreted as histologically malignant (126,127).

Adenomatoid Tumor

This benign tumor of mesothelial origin rarely arises from extragenital peritoneum, such as the omentum (128) or mesentery (129), but is much more commonly encountered within the male and female genital tracts, and is discussed in the chapters dealing with these subjects.

Well-Differentiated Papillary Mesothelioma

Well-differentiated papillary mesotheliomas (WDPMs) of the peritoneum are uncommon lesions; approximately 40 cases have been reported in detail (130–133). Seventy-five percent of the cases have occurred in women, who are usually of reproductive age; occasional patients are postmenopausal. WDPMs are usually an incidental finding at operation but rare cases have been associated with abdominal pain or ascites. Occasional patients, including two who were sisters, have had possible exposure to asbestos (131).

At laparotomy and on gross examination, WDPMs are solitary or multiple, and appear as gray to white, firm, papillary or nodular lesions measuring <2 cm in diameter. The omental and pelvic peritoneum is typically involved (131); several examples have also been encountered on the gastric, intestinal, or mesenteric peritoneum (130). Microscopic examination reveals fibrous papillae covered by a single layer of flattened to cuboidal mesothelial cells (Fig. 15) with occasional basal vacuoles; the nuclear features are bland and mitotic figures are rare or absent. Less commonly, the mesothelial cells are arranged in a tubulopapillary pattern, branching cords, or solid sheets (131). The stroma of some

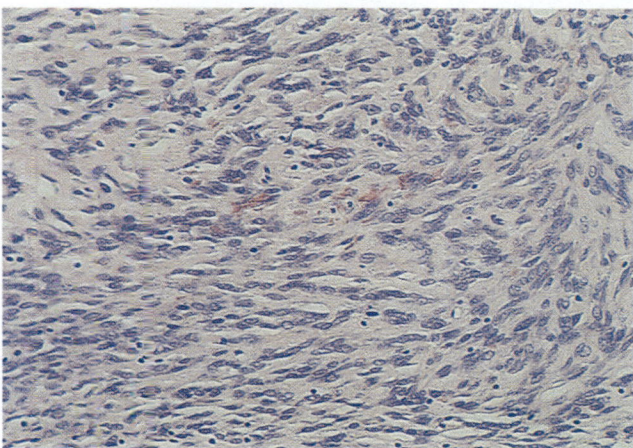

FIG. 14. Localized fibrous tumor ("fibrous mesothelioma") of the peritoneum.

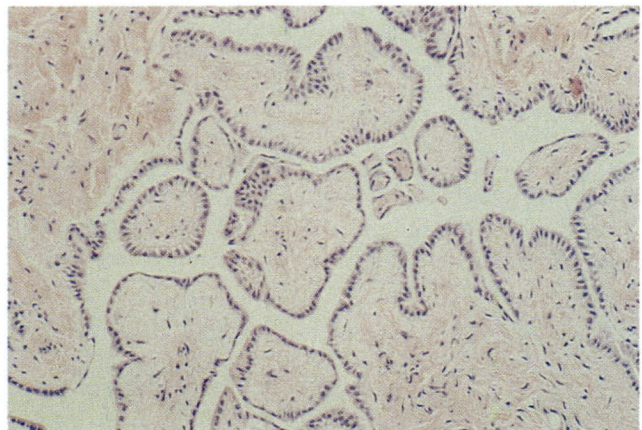

FIG. 15. Well-differentiated papillary mesothelioma. Fibrous papillae are lined by a single layer of uniform mesothelial cells.

tumors may be extensively fibrotic, and psammoma bodies are encountered in occasional cases. When multiple lesions are present, they should each be sampled histologically as some malignant mesotheliomas may focally resemble WDPMs (133). The diagnosis of WDPM should be strictly reserved for tumors with diffusely bland nuclear features.

With the exception of one case, which appeared to evolve into a diffuse malignant mesothelioma (132), follow-up studies suggest that most WDPMs are benign, although occasional examples have persisted for decades (131). Although several patients with WDPM have died, it is possible that the adjuvant therapy used in such cases was a contributory factor (131). Daya and McCaughey (131) therefore suggest that adjuvant therapy be withheld from patients with WDPM unless there is clear evidence of progression. Goldblum and Hart (133), who divided their cases of peritoneal mesotheliomas into localized (one site involved) and diffuse (more than one site involved), found that all of the diffuse tumors had at least focally malignant histologic features and that only localized lesions with uniformly benign histologic features had a predictably benign clinical course.

Low-Grade Cystic Mesotheliomas

Although we believe that most multilocular cystic mesothelial lesions are MPICs, we have seen very rare cases of what appear to be bona fide multicystic mesotheliomas. In contrast to MPICs, the cysts are lined, at least focally, by markedly atypical mesothelial cells, and the tumors may contain areas of conventional malignant mesothelioma on histologic examination (134).

Diffuse Malignant Mesothelioma

Clinical Features

Diffuse malignant mesotheliomas (DMMs) of the peritoneal cavity, being much less common than their pleural counterparts, account for only 10% to 20% of all DMMs (135–139). These tumors are particularly rare in women, in whom most malignant papillary neoplasms of the peritoneum are extraovarian papillary serous carcinomas (see Lesions of the Secondary Müllerian System, below).

The male:female ratio is ~2:1 and the patients are usually middle-aged or elderly (135–139); occasional peritoneal DMMs, however, occur in young adults and children (140–143). The patients typically present with nonspecific manifestations, including abdominal discomfort and distention, digestive disturbances, and weight loss (135–139). Some patients have had an elevated CA125 (144). Ascites is present in the majority of cases, and cytologic examination of the ascitic fluid may be diagnostic of DMM in some cases (139). The diagnosis, however, usually requires laparotomy (or laparoscopy) and biopsy. Peritoneal DMMs may rarely present within a hernia or hydrocele sac (139), as a retroperitoneal, hepatic, umbilical, intestinal, or pelvic (including ovarian) tumor (133,145–149), or as cervical or inguinal lymphadenopathy (150).

The majority of patients have a history of asbestos exposure, although this association is uncommon in females (133,149). Other potential etiologic factors include chronic inflammation, organic chemicals, nonasbestos mineral fibers, irradiation, and genetic factors (151–153). Most patients survive less than 2 years after diagnosis, although occasional long-term survivals have been reported (138,139,144,154,155). More recently, intensive chemotherapy of patients with early tumors has resulted in improved survival (156).

Pathologic Features

At laparotomy, the visceral and parietal peritoneum are diffusely thickened or extensively involved by nodules and plaques. The viscera are often encased by tumor and may be invaded, although local invasion and metastases to lymph nodes, liver, lungs, and pleura are less frequent than in association with carcinomas showing comparable degrees of peritoneal involvement (135). Significant degrees of invasion or metastatic involvement of abdominal viscera, however, may be encountered at autopsy, as exemplified by some cases with transmural invasion of bowel wall or massive replacement of the pancreas (135).

The histologic features (Figs. 16 and 17) are identical to DMMs involving the pleura, except for a possibly lower frequency of biphasic and purely sarcomatoid tumors (135). Occasional sarcomatoid and biphasic peritoneal DMMs, however, occur, including one biphasic tumor in which the sarcomatous component contained rhabdoid cells (145). A prominent inflammatory response occurs in some tumors, which may take the form of a dense lymphocytic infiltrate, granulomas, or numerous foamy, lipid-rich histiocytes (143,149,157). Rare peritoneal DMMs lack a tubulopapillary pattern and are characterized by an exclusively sheet-like pattern composed of polygonal cells with abundant

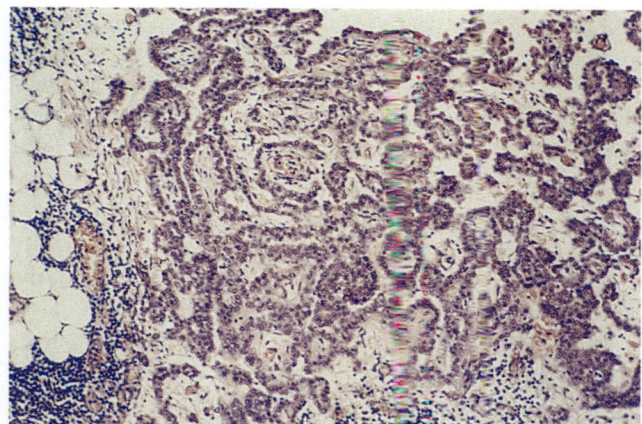

FIG. 16. Diffuse malignant mesothelioma with tubulopapillary pattern.

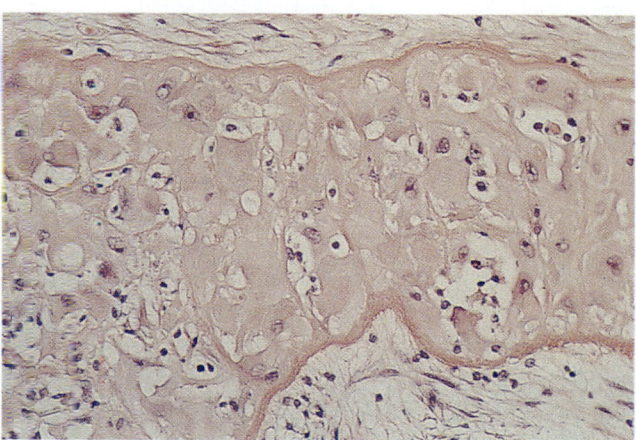

FIG. 18. Malignant peritoneal mesothelioma from a young woman. The tumor cells have abundant eosinophilic cytoplasm. This type of tumor may be misdiagnosed initially as representing ectopic decidua.

eosinophilic cytoplasm, so-called deciduoid mesotheliomas (Fig. 18) (141,142). The three such tumors that have been described all occurred in young females (13 to 24 years of age) and at least two were rapidly fatal. The immunohistochemical (see next section) and ultrastructural features of peritoneal DMMs are similar to their pleural counterparts.

Differential Diagnosis

The differential diagnosis of DMM with atypical mesothelial hyperplasia has been previously discussed (see Mesothelial Hyperplasia). The other frequently problematic lesion in the differential diagnosis is adenocarcinoma with diffuse peritoneal involvement, including metastatic adenocarcinomas, and, in women, adenocarcinomas of primary peritoneal origin (see Lesions of the Secondary Müllerian System, below). Certain patterns of DMM, such as the biphasic and the sarcomatoid, particularly when considered in conjunction with the gross characteristics of the tumor, are almost diagnostic. Tumors with a tubulopapillary pattern may present a greater problem, but such a pattern may be distinctive particularly when the lesional cells are characteristic of mesothelial cells, that is, polygonal cells with moderate amounts of eosinophilic cytoplasm. The presence of columnar cells favors a diagnosis of adenocarcinoma. Most of the primary peritoneal adenocarcinomas are of papillary serous type and are indistinguishable from primary ovarian serous carcinomas, including, in contrast to DMMs, the frequent presence of cells with bizarre nuclear features and large numbers of psammoma bodies. Deciduoid DMMs should obviously be distinguished from an ectopic decidual reaction (see Lesions of the Secondary Müllerian System). A variety of features including prominent nucleoli, mitotic activity, immunoreactivity of the lesional cells for cytokeratin, and ultrastructural findings, facilitate the diagnosis.

Histochemical and immunohistochemical stains may be helpful in the differential diagnosis with adenocarcinoma (153–169). DMMs are characterized by an absence of neutral mucins (in contrast to adenocarcinomas) and the presence of acid mucin (predominantly hyaluronic acid) within vacuoles, appreciable as alcian blue-positive, digested periodic acid-Schiff (DPAS)-negative, hyaluronidase-sensitive material (162). It should be remembered, however, that hyaluronic acid may leach from formalin-fixed tumors, resulting in false-negative staining. Also, the cell borders and stroma of DMMs may stain intensely DPAS-positive and occasional DMMs may contain small DPAS-positive cytoplasmic granules (162). Immunoreactivity for both cytokeratin (including sarcomatous DMMs) and vimentin, in addition to negative staining for a variety of antigens that include carcinoembryonic antigen (CEA), B72.3, Leu-M1, LN1, Ca19-9, S-100 protein, Ber-EP4, and placental alkaline phosphatase (PLAP), favors a diagnosis of DMM over carcinoma (162,164,167,169). Wick et al. (160) have recently found that reactivity for at least two of three epithelial markers (CEA, B72.3, Leu-M1) appear to exclude a diagnosis of mesothelioma (160).

Several studies have addressed the usefulness of immuno-

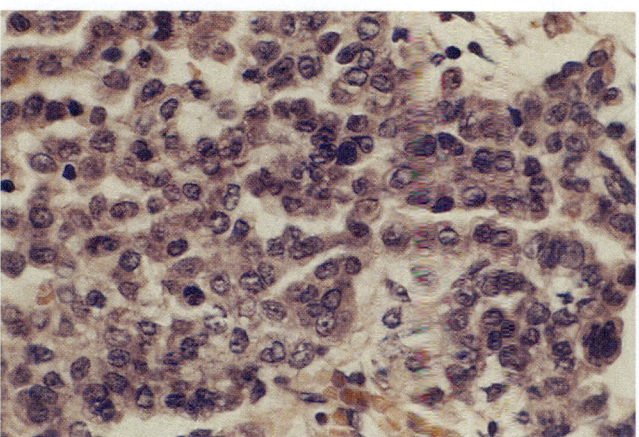

FIG. 17. Diffuse malignant mesothelioma, higher power of tumor in previous figure. The cells have malignant nuclear features.

histochemistry in the differential diagnosis of peritoneal DMMs with primary or secondary involvement of the peritoneum by papillary serous carcinoma. Bollinger et al. (158) have suggested that two profiles (S-100 and B72.3 positivity; S-100 and PLAP positivity) are seen in the majority of serous adenocarcinomas but are absent in DMMs. More recently, Ordonez (169) found that serous carcinomas but not DMMs stained with B72.3, Leu-M1, Ber-EP4, MOC-31, and CA19-9, whereas thrombomodulin stained the majority of DMMs but only rare serous carcinomas. Calretinin is another antigen that is present in almost all DMMs but absent in almost all serous carcinomas (168). It should be stressed, however, that no single immunohistochemical stain is diagnostic in the separation of DMM from adenocarcinoma, and the results of a panel of antibodies should be interpreted in conjunction with the hematoxylin and eosin (H&E) and mucin stains.

MISCELLANEOUS PRIMARY TUMORS

Intraabdominal Desmoplastic Small Round-Cell Tumor (DSRCT)

Approximately 200 examples of this tumor have been described since the initial report by Gerald and Rosai in 1989 (170–189). The tumor is of uncertain histogenesis, but its predilection for serosal surfaces suggests that it may be a primitive tumor of mesothelial origin (mesothelioblastoma) (175). Unique to DSRCTs is the fusion of the Ewing's sarcoma (EWS) gene on chromosome 22 and the Wilms' tumor gene (WT1) on chromosome 11 resulting from the chromosomal translocation [t(11;22) (p13;q12)] (183–185,188, 189). DSRCTs have a strong male predilection (M:F ratio 4:1) and are most common in adolescents and young adults [mean age 22 years in the largest series (175)]. The patients typically present with abdominal distention, pain, and a palpable abdominal, pelvic, or scrotal mass, sometimes in association with ascites. The serum neuron-specific enolase has been elevated in some cases (182). Laparotomy typically discloses a variably sized but usually large, intraabdominal mass associated with smaller peritoneal implants of similar appearance (175). Any portion of the peritoneal cavity (or less commonly the retroperitoneum) may be affected, and the tumor is frequently confined to the pelvis. In men, there may be significant involvement of the tunica vaginalis (resulting in a paratesticular mass) (171,187), and in women, the ovaries, in some cases mimicking a primary ovarian tumor (180). Rare tumors have been pleural based (189).

On gross examination, the outer aspect of the tumors, which may reach 40 cm in diameter, is smooth or bosselated, and the neoplastic tissue is firm to hard and gray-white, with foci of myxoid change and necrosis (Fig. 19). Direct invasion of intraabdominal or pelvic viscera has been noted in occasional cases (175,180). On microscopic examination, sharply circumscribed aggregates of small epithelioid cells are delimited by a cellular desmoplastic stroma (Fig. 20).

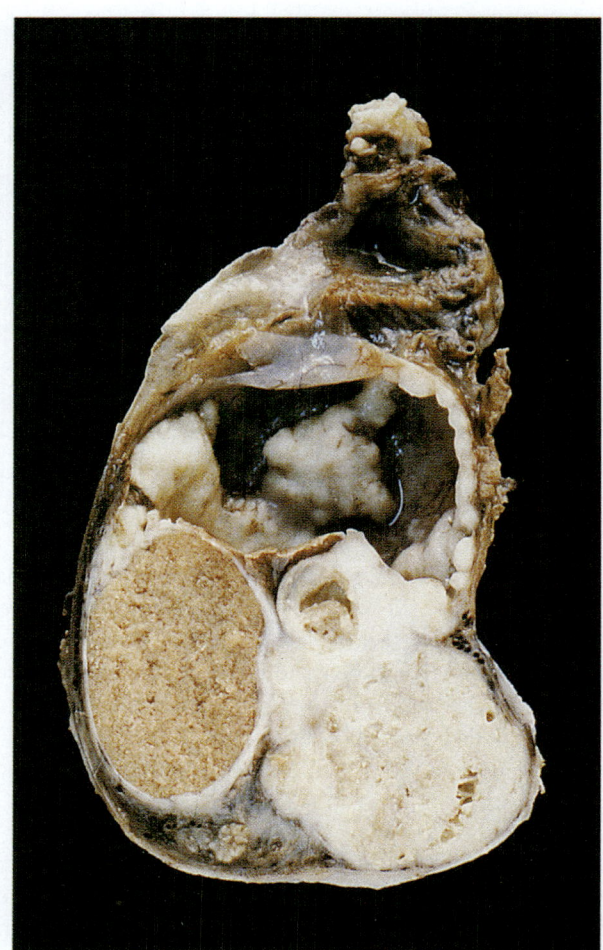

FIG. 19. Desmoplastic small round cell tumor involving tunica vaginalis. (Courtesy of Dr. Jaime Prat, Barcelona.)

The aggregates vary in size and shape from tiny clusters and slender trabeculae to rounded or irregularly shaped islands that often coalesce. Peripheral palisading of basaloid cells in some of the nests is a common feature. Central necrosis with or without calcification, or occasional spaces containing eosinophilic fluid, may be present in some of the larger islands. The tumor cells are uniform, with scanty cytoplasm, indistinct cell borders, and small to medium-sized, round, oval, or spindle-shaped hyperchromatic nuclei with clumped chromatin. The nucleoli are usually inapparent but one or more small nucleoli may be visible in some cells. Mitotic figures and single necrotic cells are numerous.

Variations in the basic pattern include foci of tumor cells with eosinophilic cytoplasmic inclusions and an eccentric nucleus, resulting in a rhabdoid appearance (Fig. 21) (175). Vacuolated cells that resemble signet-ring cells may also be seen. Features noted in occasional cases have included rosette-like or gland-like spaces, tubules or glands (sometimes with luminal mucin), minor foci of pleomorphic tumor cells, and a biphasic pattern due to a population of cells with more abundant cytoplasm admixed with the typical population of small cells (175,180). The stroma, which may be scanty in some tumors, frequently contains blood vessels

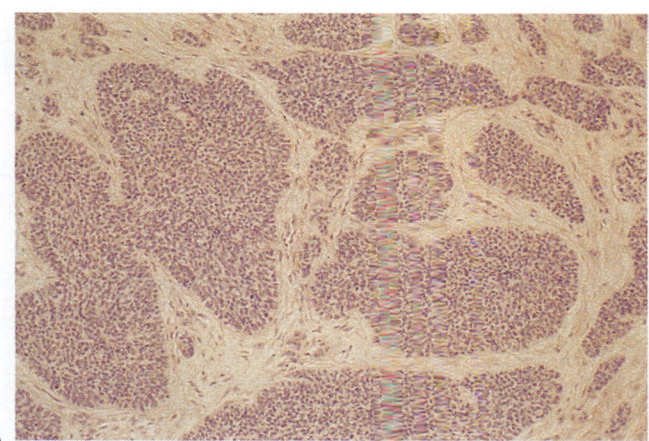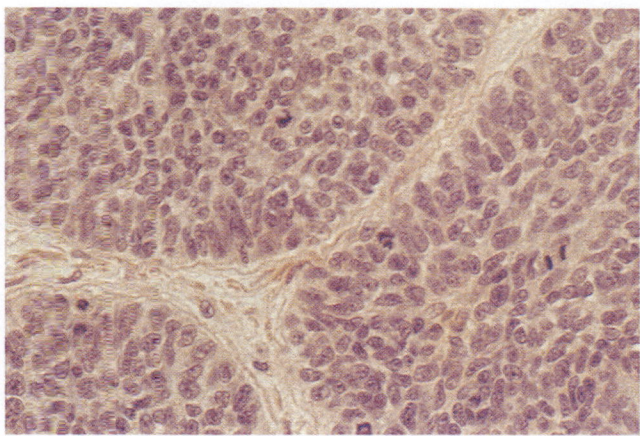

FIG. 20. A,B: Desmoplastic small round cell tumor.

with prominent endothelial and perithelial cells (175). Invasion of vascular spaces, especially lymphatics, is a common feature; lymph nodes are occasionally involved by tumor.

Special techniques, especially immunohistochemistry, indicate a multidirectional phenotype, including immunoreactivity for epithelial [low molecular weight cytokeratins, epithelial membrane antigen (EMA)], neural/neuroendocrine (NSE, Leu-7), and muscle (desmin) markers, as well as vimentin (175). Desmin and vimentin immunoreactivity is typically paranuclear and globular, and is particularly intense in cells with a rhabdoid appearance. The tumors are also typically immunoreactive with anti-WT1 antibody (188) or EWS-WT1 chimeric protein (189). The stroma is typically immunoreactive for vimentin and muscle specific actin. Ultrastructural variability suggests a range of differentiation in these tumors. Cell junctions have varied from scant and primitive to more prominent ones including intermediate, desmosomal, and tight types. Paranuclear intermediate cytoplasmic filaments have been a prominent feature in most of the cases, as has basal lamina surrounding the nests of tumor. Intraluminal microvillus-like structures, polar cell processes, microtubules, lipid droplets, glycogen, and dense-core granules have been encountered in some cases. Detection of EWS/WT1 gene fusion by reverse transcriptase-polymerase chain reaction is diagnostic (183,184,185, 189).

The DSRCTs should be distinguished from other malignant small cell tumors that may involve the peritoneum; this differential diagnosis is detailed elsewhere (175). The characteristic age of the patient, the distribution of the tumor, and its typical microscopic and immunohistochemical features should facilitate the diagnosis in most cases.

The treatment of the tumors has usually consisted of debulking and postoperative chemotherapy, irradiation, or both. The tumor is highly aggressive, with over 90% of patients dying from tumor progression. In many cases, there has been an initial partial response to chemotherapy followed by uncontrollable tumor relapse. Even in advanced stages, the bulk of the tumor tends to remain within the peritoneal cavity; extraabdominal metastases, however, have occurred in occasional patients (175).

Malignant Vascular Tumors

Four malignant peritoneal tumors of vascular origin—two epithelioid hemangioendotheliomas and two epithelioid angiosarcomas—have been recently described (190,191). The tumors were diagnosed in male and female patients who were 34 to 51 years of age; all of the tumors were fatal. The tumors had sheet-like and clustered patterns with variable degrees of vascular differentiation. Features that initially suggested the diagnosis of malignant mesothelioma included a widespread distribution, a tubulopapillary pattern, reactive and neoplastic spindle cells creating a biphasic pattern, and immunoreactivity for vimentin and variable reactivity for cytokeratin. Immunoreactivity of the tumor cells for at least two endothelial markers, a finding absent in a control group of DMMs, facilitated the diagnosis.

Inflammatory Myofibroblastic Tumor

Day et al. (192) reviewed the features of seven cases of abdominal inflammatory pseudotumor, a lesion that has also

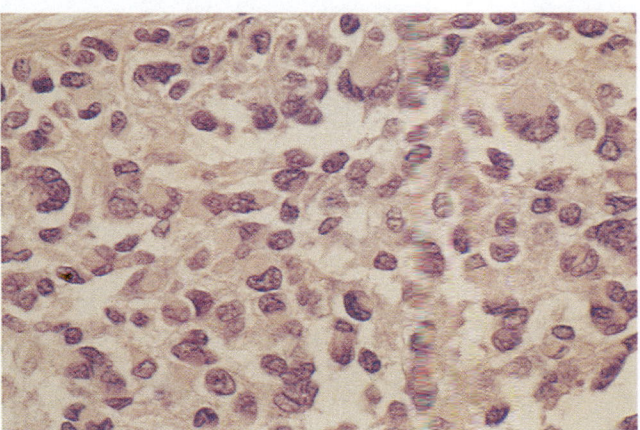

FIG. 21. Desmoplastic small round cell tumor. Note occasional cells with rhabdoid features.

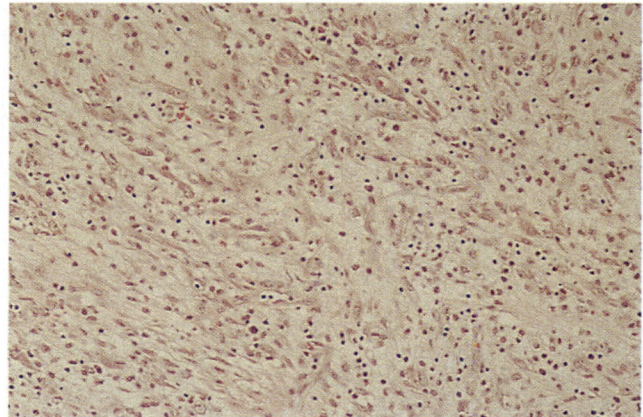

FIG. 22. Inflammatory pseudotumor ("inflammatory myofibroblastic tumor") involving peritoneum.

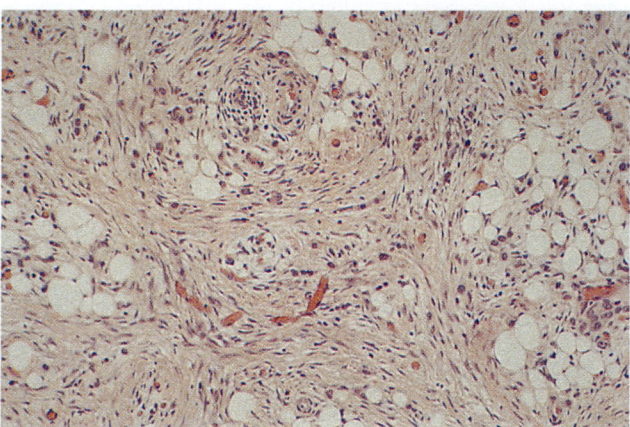

FIG. 23. Metastatic signet-ring carcinoma to the omentum. Note sparsely distributed tumor cells within an abundant fibrous stroma.

been referred to as "plasma cell granuloma" or, more recently, "inflammatory myofibroblastic tumor" (193). The abdominal lesions are typically encountered in patients younger than 20 years of age who present with an mass, fever, growth failure or weight loss, hypochromic anemia, thrombocytosis, and polyclonal hypergammaglobulinemia (192). Laparotomy typically reveals a solid mesenteric mass that on microscopic examination consists of myofibroblastic spindle cells, mature plasma cells, and small lymphocytes (Fig. 22). All of the patients have had an uneventful postoperative course with disappearance of the clinical manifestations.

Omental-Mesenteric Myxoid Hamartoma

This designation was applied by Gonzalez-Crussi et al. (194) to a lesion in infants characterized by multiple omental and mesenteric nodules composed of plump mesenchymal cells in a myxoid, vascularized stroma. The diagnosis of the referring pathologists was usually that of some type of sarcoma, but the follow-up was uneventful. It was concluded that these lesions are probably hamartomatous.

METASTATIC TUMORS

Peritoneal involvement by metastatic tumor is typically a result of seeding from a primary tumor arising within the abdomen or pelvis, most commonly the ovary. Peritoneal serous tumors in which the ovaries are normal or only minimally involved may arise directly from the peritoneum (see Lesions of the Secondary Müllerian System, below) or rarely are metastatic from a serous papillary carcinoma of the endometrium or fallopian tube. Other tumors that may be associated with peritoneal seeding include carcinomas of the breast (195,196) and gastrointestinal tract, especially the colon and stomach, and the pancreas. In such cases, the metastatic tumor may take the form of signet-ring cells widely scattered in a fibrous stroma (Figs. 23 and 24). Occasionally the signet-ring cells can have relatively bland nuclear features, resulting in a deceptively benign appearance.

Pseudomyxoma Peritonei

Peritoneal spread of a mucinous neoplasm, usually arising in the appendix, may be accompanied by mucinous ascites, so-called pseudomyxoma peritonei (197–204). The peritoneal involvement is usually multifocal, but occasionally may be confined to one area, such as a hernia sac (204). The microscopic appearance of lesions designated pseudomyxoma peritonei has included (a) free intraabdominal mucin (mucinous ascites); (b) peritoneal mucin deposits containing inflammatory and mesothelial cells and sometimes organizing capillaries and fibroblasts, but usually lacking neoplastic epithelial cells; and (c) pools of mucin, which may or may not contain neoplastic cells surrounded by dense collagenous tissue (dissecting mucin) (Fig. 25). Neoplastic cells, if present, are usually well-differentiated mucinous columnar cells of intestinal type (Fig. 25). No consensus exists as to whether all

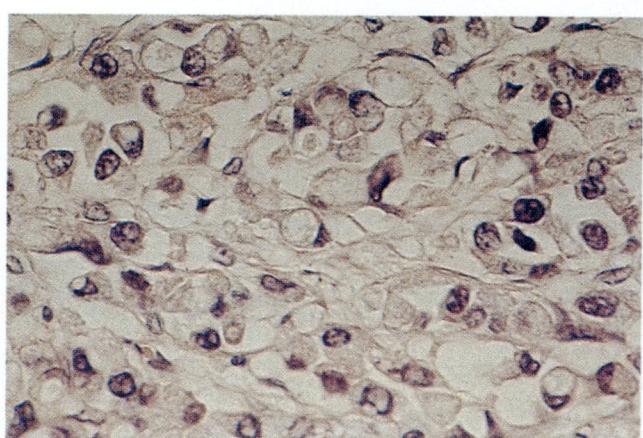

FIG. 24. Metastatic signet ring carcinoma to the omentum. Higher power view of tumor in previous figure. Typical signet-ring tumor cells are present.

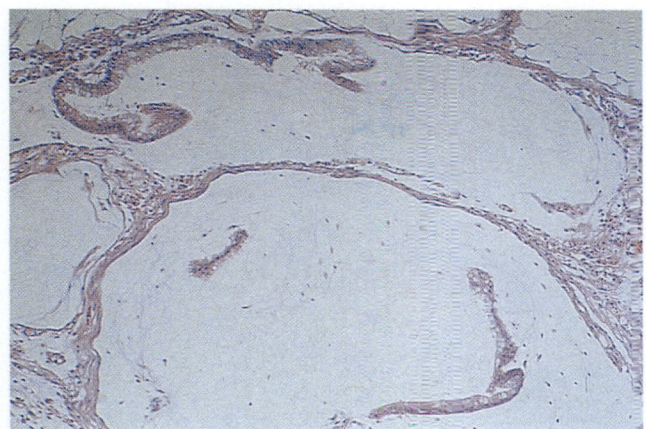

FIG. 25. Pseudomyxoma peritonei.

or only some of these collections of intraabdominal mucus warrant the designation of pseudomyxoma peritonei.

The primary tumor in the majority of cases of pseudomyxoma peritonei is a low-grade mucinous tumor of the appendix, which may be visible only microscopically, and therefore an appendectomy should be performed in all cases of pseudomyxoma peritonei. Cases of the latter not associated with an appendiceal tumor may be due to metastases from mucinous tumors elsewhere in the gastrointestinal and pancreaticobiliary tracts, from mucinous borderline tumors of the ovary, or from mucinous tumors in other sites. Most studies however, have found that the majority of cystic ovarian mucinous tumors associated with pseudomyxoma peritonei are metastatic from an appendiceal tumor (198, 201,202). Acellular mucin dissecting through the ovarian stroma ("pseudomyxoma ovarii") is often present in these cases.

It is preferable to apply the diagnosis 'pseudomyxoma peritonei" to only clinical or intraoperative findings, rather than in a pathology report. The report should include (a) an appraisal of the tumors (appendiceal, ovarian, or other) as benign, borderline, or malignant, with a notation as to the presence or absence of rupture; (b) an assessment of the peritoneal lesions as mucinous ascites (free abdominal fluid), organizing mucinous fluid, or mucin dissection with fibrosis; and (c) the presence or absence of neoplastic cells and, if present, whether they appear benign, borderline (atypical), or malignant. Cell-free peritoneal deposits in pseudomyxoma peritonei are associated with a better prognosis than deposits containing well-differentiated mucinous epithelium (201), whereas peritoneal deposits composed of carcinomatous cells are associated with a poorer prognosis than the latter (203).

LESIONS OF THE SECONDARY MÜLLERIAN SYSTEM

These lesions share an origin from the so-called secondary müllerian system, that is, the pelvic and lower abdominal mesothelium and the subjacent mesenchyme of females (205–207). The müllerian potential of this layer is consistent with its close embryonic relation to the primary müllerian system (the müllerian ducts), which arises by invagination of the coelomic epithelium. Lesions of the secondary müllerian system include those containing endometrioid, serous, and mucinous epithelium, simulating normal or neoplastic endometrial, tubal, and endocervical epithelium. The metaplastic potential of the pelvic peritoneum also includes differentiation toward cells of transitional (urothelial) type, exemplified most commonly by Walthard nests. Proliferation of the subjacent mesenchyme may accompany epithelial differentiation of the mesothelium or may give rise to a variety of pure mesenchymal lesions composed of endometrial stromal-type cells, decidua, or smooth muscle.

Endometriosis

Endometriosis is defined as the presence of endometrial tissue outside the endometrium or myometrium. Usually both epithelium and stroma are seen, but occasionally the diagnosis of endometriosis can be made when only one component is present. Etiologic, pathogenetic, and clinical aspects of endometriosis, which have been reviewed in detail elsewhere (207), are not considered here as they do not have a significant bearing on histologic interpretation. The occurrence of endometriosis in extraperitoneal sites is also discussed elsewhere (207).

Microscopic Features

Depending on their duration and their superficial or deep location in relation to the peritoneal surface, endometriotic foci may appear as punctate, red, blue, brown, or white spots or patches with either a slightly raised or puckered surface (Fig. 26) (208–210). Ecchymotic or brown areas have sometimes been described as "powder burns." The endometriotic foci are frequently associated with dense fibrous adhesions. The lesions may form nodules or cysts, or both. Rarely, pelvic peritoneal endometriosis may present as multiple, polypoid masses of soft gray tissue that fill the pelvis, simulating a malignant tumor (211–213).

Endometriotic cysts (endometriomas) most commonly involve the ovaries, where they may partially or almost completely replace the normal tissue; bilateral involvement occurs in one-third to one-half of the cases (214,215). The cysts rarely exceed 15 cm in diameter; larger examples are more likely to harbor a neoplasm. Endometriotic cysts are commonly covered by dense fibrous adhesions, which may result in fixation to adjacent structures. The cyst walls are usually thick and fibrotic, with a smooth or shaggy, brown to yellow lining (Fig. 27). The cyst contents typically consist of altered, semifluid or inspissated, chocolate-colored material (Fig. 27); rarely, the cyst is filled with watery fluid. Any solid areas in the cyst wall or intraluminal polypoid projections should be sampled histologically, as they may be cancers arising from the epithelial or stromal component of the

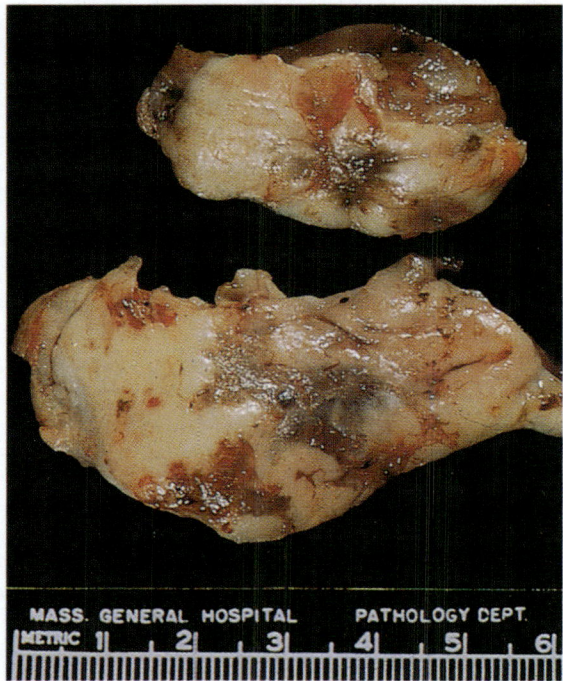

FIG. 26. Endometriosis of ovaries. Multiple hemorrhagic and pigmented foci involve the serosal surfaces. Some of the lesions have a puckered appearance.

cyst. Rare complications of endometriosis, typically during pregnancy, include rupture (usually ovarian or intestinal) producing acute abdominal symptoms (216–218) or hemorrhage from endometriotic lesions that have undergone decidual transformation (219).

Microscopic Features

The appearance of endometriotic tissue varies with the extent of its response to the normal hormonal fluctuations of the menstrual cycle and the duration of the process (Figs. 28–32). When the appearances of simultaneous samples of

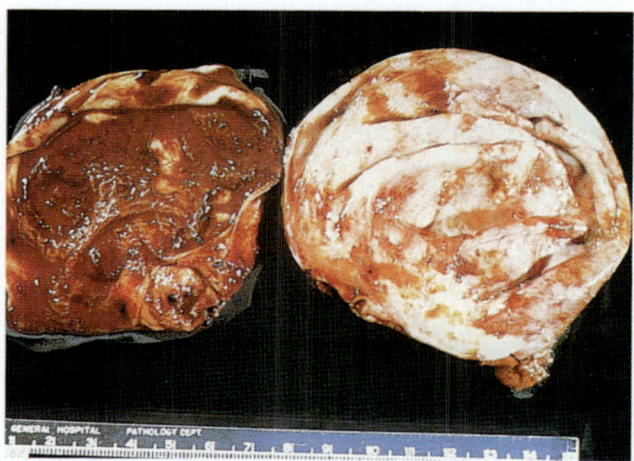

FIG. 27. Endometriotic cysts of ovaries. One of the cysts is filled with thick chocolate-colored material.

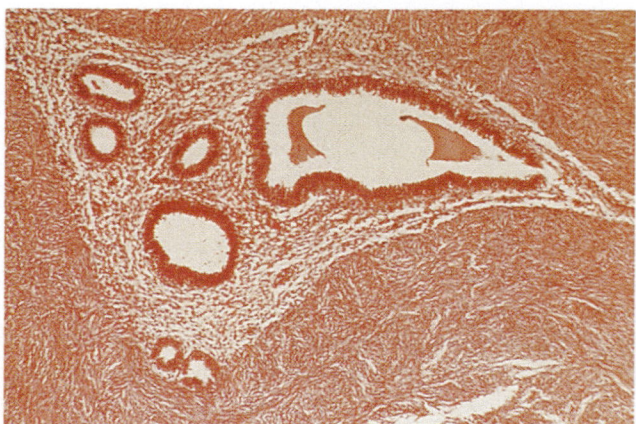

FIG. 28. Endometriosis of ovary. The endometriotic focus, composed of proliferative-type endometrial glands and stroma, is surrounded by ovarian stroma.

eutopic endometrium and endometriotic foci are compared, the latter exhibit cyclic changes in from 44% to 80% of the cases, and there is considerable variability in glandular morphology (220,221). When more than one endometriotic focus is examined in the same patient, the appearances of the specimens do not differ significantly from one to another (220). In most postmenopausal patients with endometriosis, the endometriotic tissue is atrophic with glands that are occasionally cystic and are lined by flattened epithelial cells surrounded by a dense fibrotic stroma (Fig. 30); the appearance is similar to that of simple or cystic atrophy of the endometrium (222). In a minority of cases, however, the endometriotic tissue has an active appearance, with or without the metaplastic and hyperplastic changes that are more commonly present in premenopausal women (see below).

Menstruation into endometriotic foci results in hemorrhage within the stroma and glandular lumina, as well as a secondary inflammatory response consisting predominantly of a diffuse infiltration of histiocytes. The latter typically convert the extravasated red blood cells into glycolipid and granular brown pigment, becoming so-called pseudoxanthoma cells (Figs. 31–33) (51). Most of the pigment is hemo-

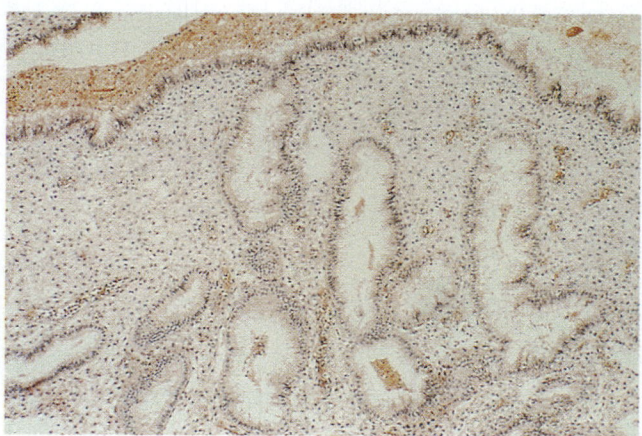

FIG. 29. Endometriosis with a secretory appearance.

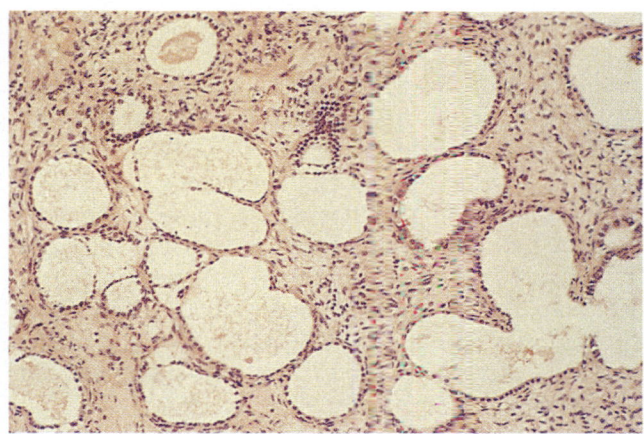

FIG. 30. Endometriosis in a postmenopausal woman. The cystic endometriotic glands are lined by flattened cells and separated by a fibrous stroma.

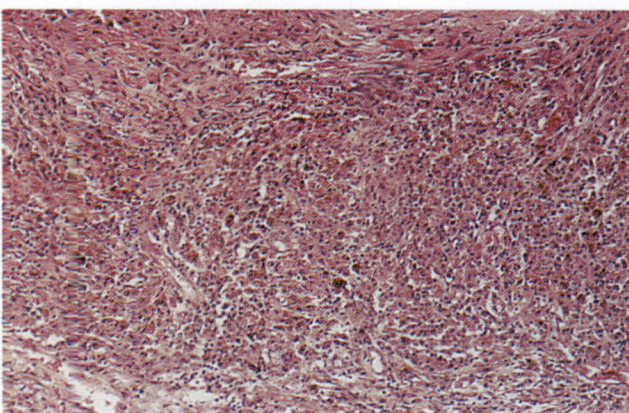

FIG. 32. Lining of endometriotic cyst. The endometriotic epithelium and stroma have been replaced by fibrous tissue and large numbers of pseudoxanthoma cells.

fuscin, and hemosiderin is typically present to a much lesser extent (51). The amount of pigment in an endometriotic lesion appears to increase with its age, and early lesions are frequently nonpigmented (209). Variable numbers of lymphocytes and smaller numbers of other inflammatory cells may be present. Large numbers of neutrophils with microabscess formation should raise the possibility of secondary bacterial infection (223).

In endometriotic cysts, the epithelial cells lining the cyst may be large and cuboidal with abundant eosinophilic cytoplasm and large atypical nuclei (Fig. 34) (224,225). The significance of such nuclear atypia is unclear. Although it may be a reactive change, these atypical cells can be aneuploid (226) or merge with borderline tumors or adenocarcinomas (227,228). In one study of women with this finding and no adjacent neoplasm, however, no endometriosis-related tumors developed during follow-up (229).

The epithelial and stromal lining of an endometriotic cyst frequently becomes attenuated, and the former may be reduced to a single layer of cuboidal cells that may retain some endometrial characteristics but that are often devoid of specific features. In such circumstances, recognition of the cyst as endometriotic may only be possible if a rim of subjacent endometrial stroma persists. Commonly, the cyst lining of endometrial epithelium and stroma is totally lost, and replaced by granulation tissue, dense fibrous tissue, and variable numbers of pseudoxanthoma cells (presumptive endometriosis) (Fig. 32). Occasionally ovarian and extraovarian endometriosis takes the form of necrotic pseudoxanthomatous nodules characterized by a central zone of necrosis surrounded by pseudoxanthoma cells, often in a palisaded arrangement, hyalinized fibrous tissue, or both (Fig. 35); typical endometriotic glands and stroma may be sparse or absent (51).

Endometriosis that involves the uterine ligaments or the walls of hollow viscera is typically associated with striking proliferation of the indigenous smooth muscle, creating an appearance similar to that of adenomyosis (Fig. 36). The endometriotic stroma itself may also undergo smooth muscle metaplasia, which is encountered most often within the walls of ovarian endometriotic cysts, but occasionally elsewhere (230–238). Extensive amounts of smooth muscle in such

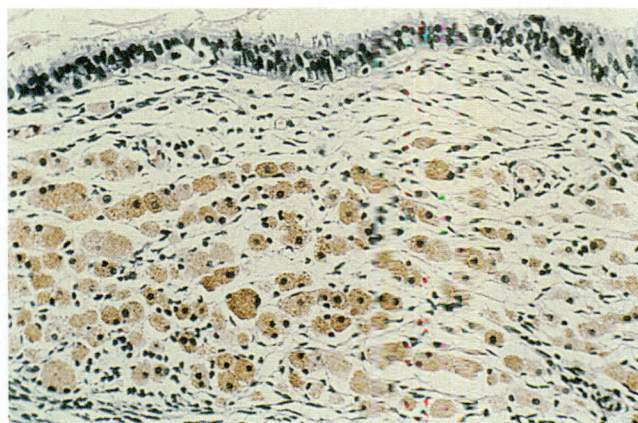

FIG. 31. Lining of endometriotic cyst. Note pigmented histiocytes (pseudoxanthoma cells) in stroma.

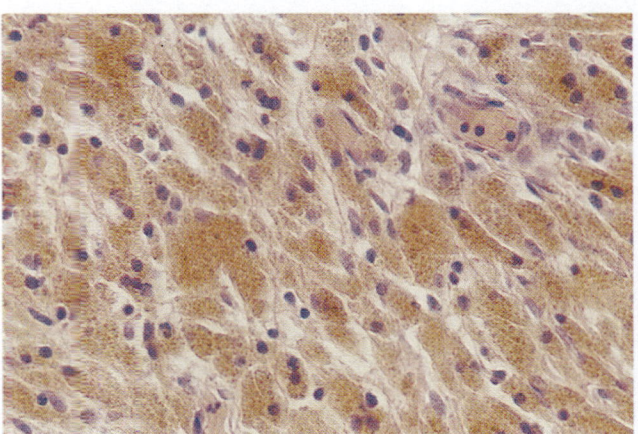

FIG. 33. Pseudoxanthoma cells. Most of the pigment in the cells is hemofuscin (ceroid), not hemosiderin.

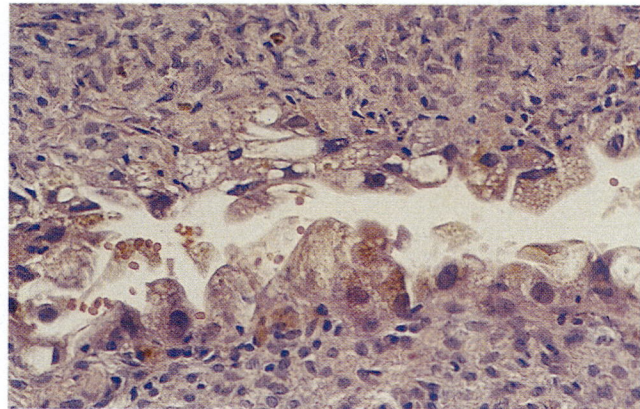

FIG. 34. Lining of endometriotic cyst. The epithelial cells have eosinophilic cytoplasm and atypical nuclei.

cases can result in endomyometriosis or uterus-like masses, which have been described within an obturator lymph node (230), the ovary (231,234,235), the broad ligament (236), the lumbosacral region (237), and, in males, the scrotum (232). In some cases, a uterus-like mass in the region of the ovary may represent a congenital malformation rather than an unusual manifestation of endometriosis (238).

Rare cases of endometriosis are characterized by an absence or rarity of glands, so-called stromal endometriosis (239); it should be noted, however, that the same term has been used in the older literature to refer to what is now designated low-grade endometrial stromal sarcoma. Stromal endometriosis is most commonly encountered in the ovary, where it is typically an incidental microscopic finding within the ovarian stroma (benign stromatosis) (240). There is usually no associated pelvic endometriosis, and the process likely represents a metaplastic response of the ovarian stromal cells. We have also encountered a disproportionate number of cases of stromal endometriosis within the uterine cervix (239). Histologic examination of the lesions showed

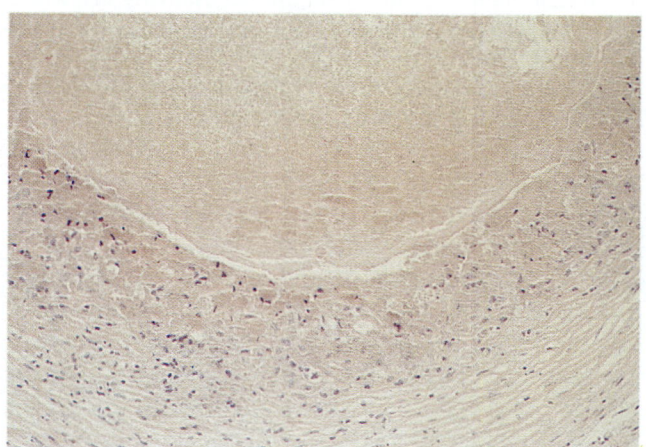

FIG. 35. Necrotic pseudoxanthomatous nodule of endometriosis. Pseudoxanthoma cells surround a central zone of necrotic debris.

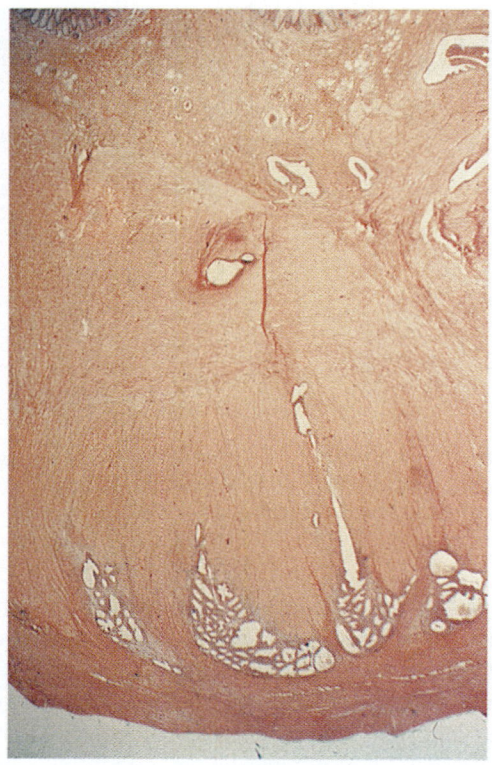

FIG. 36. Endometriosis of bowel wall. The muscularis propria is thickened by hyperplastic smooth muscle that surrounds the foci of endometriosis.

well-circumscribed foci within the superficial stroma of the cervix composed of endometrial stromal cells, small blood vessels, and extravasated erythrocytes (Fig. 37). Apart from the absence or paucity of endometrial glands, the clinical and pathologic features were similar to those of previously described cases of superficial endometriosis of the cervix.

Metaplastic changes similar to those occurring in eutopic endometrial glands have been described in endometriotic glands. These include tubal (ciliated) (205,224,241), hobnail (224), and, rarely, squamous (242) and mucinous metaplasia; the latter may be characterized by the presence of endocervical-type cells or less often, goblet cells (243,244). Rarely, endometriotic stroma may exhibit a myxoid appearance [potentially mimicking pseudomyxoma peritonei (245)], or focal ossification and calcification (246,247). Perineural (248) and vascular invasion (249) have been reported rarely in otherwise typical, benign endometriotic lesions.

A variety of hyperplastic and atypically hyperplastic changes similar to those occurring in the endometrium have been described in endometriotic glands, sometimes related to an endogenous or exogenous estrogenic stimulus (Fig. 38) (209,250–253) or more recently secondary to tamoxifen therapy (254). It is logical to conclude that such atypical changes have a malignant potential similar to those in the endometrium, as evidenced by rare cases of hyperplastic endometriosis preceding an adenocarcinoma in the same site

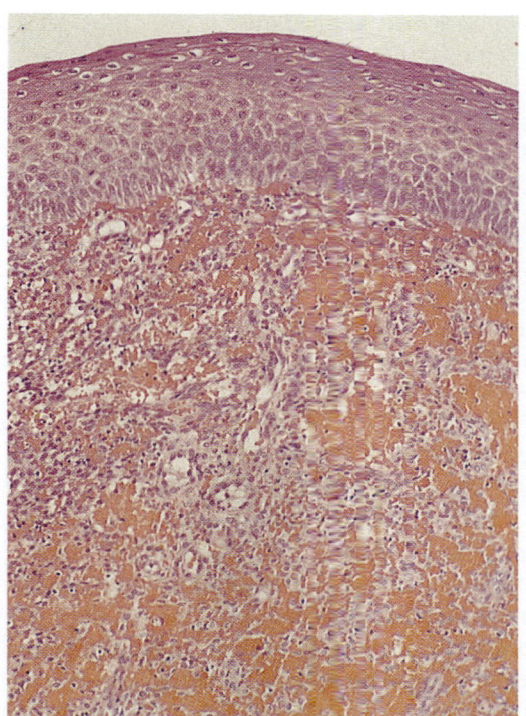

FIG. 37. Stromal endometriosis of cervix. Large numbers of erythrocytes separate the endometrial stromal cells.

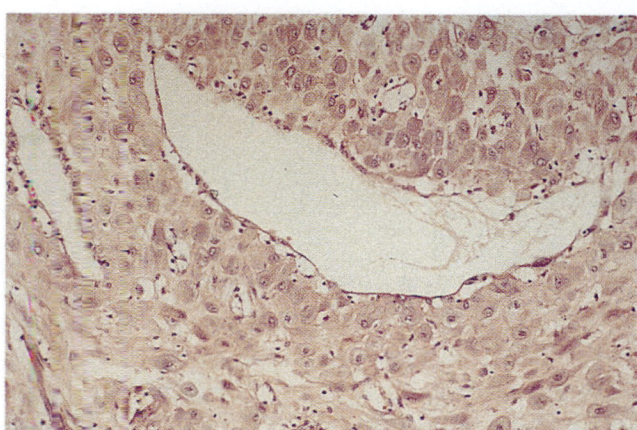

FIG. 39. Endometriosis in pregnancy. The decidualized stroma surrounds glands lined by flattened cells.

(251,253,255) or that have coexisted with carcinoma in the same specimen (256–258). Endometriotic tissue may also exhibit progestational changes (Figs 29 and 39), especially during pregnancy (Fig. 39) or progestin therapy (259). In such cases, examination reveals a decidual reaction with atrophy of the endometrial glands, which are small and lined by cuboidal or flattened epithelial cells (Fig. 39). In pregnancy, the glands rarely exhibit an Arias-Stella reaction, optically clear nuclei, or both (260,261). Necrosis of the decidual cells, foci of marked stromal edema, and infiltration by

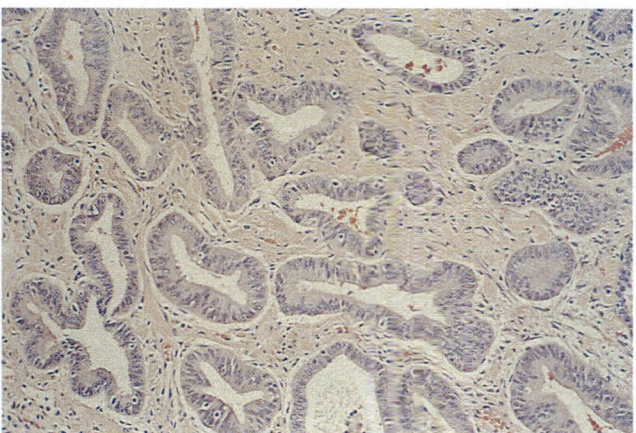

FIG. 38. Pelvic endometriosis exhibiting atypical hyperplasia in woman on estrogen replacement therapy. The endometriotic glands exhibit both architectural and cytologic atypia. Foci of well-differentiated endometrioid adenocarcinoma were found elsewhere in the specimen.

lymphocytes are additional findings in patients receiving progestational agents (259). Atrophic changes similar to those that are seen typically in the endometriotic foci of postmenopausal patients may be present in premenopausal patients treated with oral contraceptives or danazol (262–264). In one study, one-third of the endometriotic foci disappeared or were replaced by fibrous tissue after danazol therapy (264).

Associated Lesions and Differential Diagnosis

Rare examples of endometriosis have been encountered in intimate association with foci of peritoneal leiomyomatosis (265–267), glial implants of ovarian teratomas (268,269), and nodules of splenosis (270). Liesegang rings may rarely be found within the walls of endometriotic cysts (271). Endometriosis may also be accompanied by, and should be distinguished from, endosalpingiosis, which is characterized by glands lined by benign tubal-type epithelium, unassociated with endometrial stroma (see below). Necrotic pseudoxanthomatous nodules should be distinguished from other ovarian and peritoneal necrotic nodules, such as infectious granulomas and isolated palisading granulomas of the ovary (272), and as noted earlier, peritoneal granulomas related to diathermy (50). Such lesions, in addition to having characteristic features, lack the numerous pseudoxanthoma cells that are typical of endometriotic lesions.

Rare examples of recurrent or metastatic low-grade endometrial stromal sarcomas (ESSs) with benign-appearing or atypical endometrial glands may be confused with endometriosis (273). Indeed, we believe that some lesions referred to as "aggressive endometriosis" likely represent ESSs with a prominent glandular component (274). These tumors, however, contain foci of more typical ESS devoid of glands, and in some cases, prominent mitotic activity of the stromal cells, sex-cord–like elements, and prominent vascular invasion.

Neoplasms Arising from Endometriosis

A malignant tumor has been documented to arise in from 0.3% to 0.8% of cases of ovarian endometriosis, but the exact frequency of cancer originating in pelvic endometriosis is unknown because the frequency of endometriosis in the general population is unknown and because some cancers that arise in endometriosis may overgrow and obliterate the endometriosis from which the tumor arose (213,275,276). In some cases, the tumors arising in endometriosis have been preceded by prolonged unopposed estrogen replacement therapy (275,277). Two recent studies have found that a significant proportion (20–25%) of ovarian epithelial tumors are associated with endometriosis (257,258). Both studies found that ~50% of ovarian clear cell carcinomas are associated with endometriosis, and in one study (257), 42% of endometrioid carcinomas were endometriosis-related. In the latter study, the endometriosis showed atypical microscopic changes in 60% of the cases.

Approximately 75% of tumors complicating endometriosis arise within the ovary. The most common extraovarian site is the rectovaginal septum; less frequent sites include the vagina, colon and rectum, urinary bladder, and other sites in the pelvis and abdomen. Endometrioid carcinoma is the most common tumor arising within endometriosis, accounting for almost 70% of such cases (276). Direct origin of endometrioid carcinoma from endometriotic tissue has been demonstrated in as many as 24% of cases in some series (213). At least 90% of the carcinomas arising from extraovarian endometriosis have also been of endometrioid type (213,275,276). Rarely, endometrioid tumors arising in ovarian and extraovarian endometriosis may exhibit a benign or borderline adenofibromatous pattern (212,251).

Clear cell carcinoma is the second most common tumor originating in endometriosis, accounting for approximately 14% of such cases (276). In some studies, the frequency of endometriosis coexisting with clear cell carcinoma of the ovary is even higher than with endometrioid carcinoma; pelvic endometriosis has been reported in 24% to 49% of cases of ovarian clear cell carcinoma (278). A few examples of clear cell carcinoma arising within extraovarian endometriosis have also been described (275,279,280).

Rare epithelial tumors of other types arising from endometriosis include ovarian serous cystadenomas of low malignant potential (281), benign and malignant mucinous tumors (212,227,228), and squamous cell carcinomas (282,283). Endometrioid stromal sarcomas and malignant mesodermal mixed tumors, similar on microscopic examination to those arising in the uterus, may originate in ovarian and extraovarian endometriosis (244,284–286). Sixty percent of endometrial stromal sarcomas apparently arising within the ovary have been associated with ovarian endometriosis (244). Vaginal endometriosis was the probable source of one extrauterine pelvic adenosarcoma (287). Two examples of yolk sac tumor have arisen in association with endometriosis (288,289), and in one unique case, a sex cord tumor with annular tubules arose in association with serosal endometriosis of the fallopian tube (290).

Peritoneal Endometrioid Lesions Other than Endometriosis

Benign glands lined by endometrial epithelium (but lacking endometrial stroma) with the peritoneal distribution of endosalpingiosis occasionally occur (205). Some may represent foci of endometriosis in which the stromal component has undergone atrophy. Benign endometrioid peritoneal implants lacking an endometrial stromal component have also been reported in association with a borderline ovarian endometrioid tumor (278). The peritoneal lesions were interpreted as having arisen directly from the peritoneum.

A variety of extrauterine, extraovarian, pelvic, or retroperitoneal neoplasms of endometrioid type occur in the absence of demonstrable endometriosis. These tumors have generally been considered to arise directly from the mesothelium or submesothelial stroma. They have included endometrioid cystadenofibroma (291,292) and cystadenocarcinoma (293), endometrioid stromal sarcoma (294), homologous and heterologous types of malignant mesodermal mixed tumor (Fig. 40) (295), and mesodermal adenosarcoma (296–299).

Peritoneal Serous Lesions

Endosalpingiosis

Clinical Features

Endosalpingiosis refers to the presence of histologically benign glands lined by tubal-type epithelium occurring outside the confines of the fallopian tube. This disorder occurs almost exclusively in females, typically during the reproductive era, with a mean age of 29.7 years in one study (300), al-

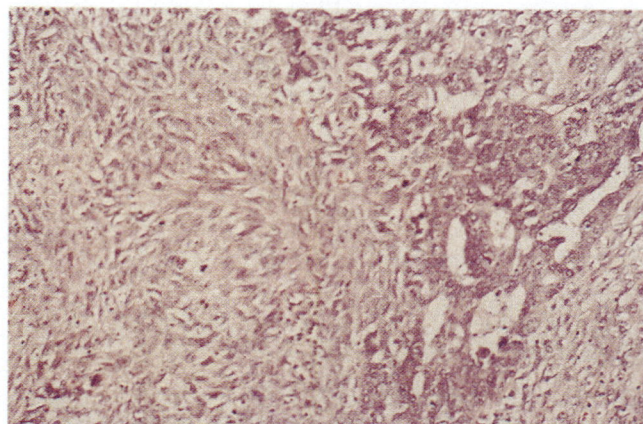

FIG. 40. Primary peritoneal malignant mixed mesodermal tumor (carcinosarcoma). No tumor was present in the uterus or ovaries.

though occasional cases have been described in postmenopausal women. Endosalpingiosis is almost always an incidental finding either at the time of operation or more commonly on microscopical examination. Zinsser and Wheeler (300) found endosalpingiosis in 12.5% of surgically removed omenta in a retrospective study, but this figure doubled when omenta were examined more thoroughly in a prospective study. Endosalpingiosis may be detected as multiple fine pelvic calcifications on x-ray examination (301) or as psammoma bodies within cul-de-sac fluid (302,303), peritoneal washings (304,305), the lumen of the fallopian tube (306), or cervical Papanicolaou smears (301,306,307).

An origin from mesothelium (the secondary müllerian system) is favored by most investigators, but the association of endosalpingiosis with chronic salpingitis implicates implantation of sloughed tubal epithelium as another histogenetic mechanism (300). A similar association with serous tumors of borderline malignancy suggests that some endosalpingiotic foci may represent tumor implants that have undergone maturation (308).

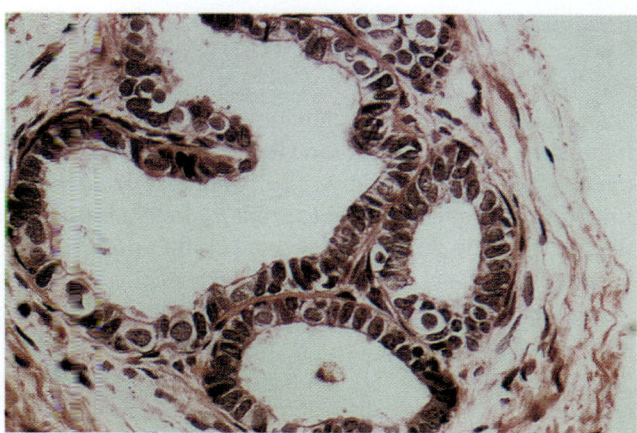

FIG. 41. Endosalpingiosis of omentum. The glands are lined by a single layer of uniform, cuboidal to columnar cells. Occasional cells have pale cytoplasm and are ciliated.

Pathologic Features

Endosalpingiosis is most commonly encountered on the pelvic peritoneum covering the uterus, fallopian tubes, ovaries, and cul-de-sac (300–302,308–311). Less frequent sites include the pelvic parietal peritoneum (309), omentum (300,301,308), bladder (311) and bowel serosa (311–313), the paraaortic area (314), and within skin, including laparotomy scars (315). Endosalpingiosis is usually inapparent at the time of operation or on gross inspection of the involved tissues, but may be visible as multiple, white to yellow, opaque or translucent, fluid-filled cysts that are usually only several millimeters in diameter (302,309–311,316,317). Rarely, however, larger cysts may be seen (318). Rare cases with extensive involvement of the walls of the urinary bladder (319) or uterus (318) have presented as multicystic tumor-like masses in these sites.

Microscopic examination reveals multiple, simple glands, often cystically dilated and lined by a single layer of epithelium resembling that of the normal fallopian tube (Fig. 41). The glands are frequently surrounded by a loose or dense connective tissue stroma that may contain a sparse mononuclear inflammatory cell infiltrate. The glands may exhibit irregular contours, crowding, and intraluminal stromal papillae (300). The three cell types of the normal fallopian tube epithelium are found in varying numbers: pale ciliated cells, secretory cells, and dark rod-like, intercalated or "peg" cells (Fig. 41) (300). The cells have prominent luminal margins, distinct borders, and basal nuclei. Focal cellular pseudostratification may be present. The nuclei have fine chromatin and delicate nuclear membranes, and typically lack significant atypia or mitotic activity (300). Psammoma bodies are frequently present within the lumina or in the adjacent stroma. Endosalpingiotic glands may rarely extend into the underlying tissues, including, as noted above, involvement of the muscularis propria of the urinary bladder, and the wall of the uterine corpus or cervix (313,318,319). In the urinary bladder, the endosalpingiotic glands are usually admixed with other benign müllerian glands (mucinous, endometrioid), so-called müllerianosis (319). Staining with the PAS method reveals a basement membrane surrounding each gland, and PAS-positive, diastase-resistant material in the apices of the lining cells and within the glandular lumina (300).

The term *atypical endosalpingiosis* refers to endosalpingiosis with cellular stratification including cellular buds, cribriform patterns, and varying degrees of cellular atypia, in the absence of an ovarian serous tumor of borderline malignancy (320). Atypical endosalpingiosis has rarely abutted (and in such cases has likely been the origin of) intranodal serous neoplasms (321).

Differential Diagnosis

Atypical endosalpingiosis merges microscopically with peritoneal serous tumors of borderline malignancy (see next section). Bell and Scully (320) use the latter term if the "lesions composed of tubal-type epithelium exhibit papillarity, tufting, or detachment of cell clusters ... even when they arise on a background of endosalpingiosis."

Endosalpingiotic glands should be differentiated from mesonephric remnants, which are common incidental microscopic findings in the region of the fallopian tube. Mesonephric tubules are typically located more deeply than endosalpingiosis and characteristically have a collar of smooth muscle under the epithelial lining, which is typically a single layer of nonciliated, low columnar to cuboidal cells (322).

Endosalpingiosis in a nonneoplastic lesion, and its presence (in the absence of residual tumor) at the time of second-look laparotomy in patients with ovarian epithelial neoplasms does not justify additional treatment (323).

Peritoneal Serous Tumors

Serous Borderline Tumors

Occasional tumors resembling ovarian serous borderline tumors are characterized by widespread extraovarian peritoneal involvement and absent or minimal ovarian surface involvement. Patients with these tumors are typically under the age of 35 years, often present with infertility, chronic pelvic or abdominal pain, small bowel obstruction secondary to fibrous adhesions associated with the neoplastic foci, or an adnexal mass (324,325). At operation, focal or miliary granules, adhesions, or both involve the peritoneum. Microscopic examination reveals superficial tumor that resembles noninvasive epithelial or desmoplastic implants of borderline serous tumors of ovarian origin (Fig. 42). Endosalpingiosis is present in >80% of the cases; 85% of patients have had no clinical evidence of persistent or progressive disease on follow-up, and most of the rest remain well after resection of recurrent tumor (324,325).

Serous Carcinomas

Most primary peritoneal serous neoplasms are high-grade invasive serous carcinomas that extensively involve the peritoneum, so-called serous surface papillary carcinomas, papillary serous carcinomas of the peritoneum, or extraovarian peritoneal serous papillary carcinoma (EPSPC) (326–352). Some EPSPCs have been diagnosed after prophylactic oophorectomy performed because of a family history of ovarian cancer (327,344).

Criteria for EPSPC proposed by the Gynecologic Oncology Group (GOG) (342) are as follows:

1. Both ovaries are either normal in size or enlarged by a benign process. In the judgment of the surgeon and the pathologist, the bulk of the tumor is in the peritoneum and the extent of tumor involvement at one or more extraovarian sites is greater than on the surface of either ovary.
2. Microscopic examination of the ovaries reveals (a) no tumor; (b) tumor confined to the surface epithelium with no evidence of cortical invasion; (c) tumor involving the ovarian surface and the underlying cortical stroma but less than 5 by 5 mm in diameter; (d) tumor less than 5×5 mm within the ovarian substance, with or without surface involvement.
3. The histologic and cytologic characteristics of the tumor are predominantly serous and similar or identical to those of ovarian serous papillary adenocarcinomas of any grade.
4. Cases in which an oophorectomy had been performed before the diagnosis of EPSPC must have one of the following: (a) a pathology report to document the absence of carcinoma in the specimen, with review of all the slides of the ovarian specimen if the oophorectomy had been performed within 5 years of the diagnosis of EPSPC; (b) if the oophorectomy had been performed more than 5 years before the diagnosis of EPSPC, the pathology report of the specimen is required, and an attempt to review the slides must be made.

The typical intraoperative appearance of a primary peritoneal serous carcinoma, with widespread, often bulky, peritoneal tumor associated with ovaries of normal size, may mimic that of a diffuse malignant mesothelioma or peritoneal carcinomatosis associated with an unknown primary tumor. EPSPCs resemble their ovarian counterparts on microscopic and immunohistochemical examination. One study, however, found the frequency of Her-2/*neu* overexpression in EPSPCs to be almost twice that present in case-matched primary ovarian adenocarcinoma (350). The distinction of EPSPCs from malignant mesothelioma has been previously discussed. EPSPCs have a prognosis similar to that of high-stage ovarian serous carcinomas.

Low-grade peritoneal serous carcinomas are much less common that their high-grade counterparts, and resemble peritoneal serous borderline tumors except for the presence of invasion, including in some cases, lymphatic invasion (352). A subset of these tumors, characterized by numerous psammoma bodies, has been referred to as psammocarcinoma (Fig. 43) (353,354). Low-grade serous carcinomas, including psammocarcinomas, are indolent tumors associated with a favorable long-term prognosis (352–354).

Rare extraovarian serous tumors take the form of localized, typically cystic masses, usually within the broad ligament (see chapter by Young et al., "Fallopian Tube and Broad Ligament") and less commonly, within the retroperitoneum. Serous papillary cystadenomas and adenofibromas, serous borderline tumors, and serous carcinomas have been described in these sites (355–363).

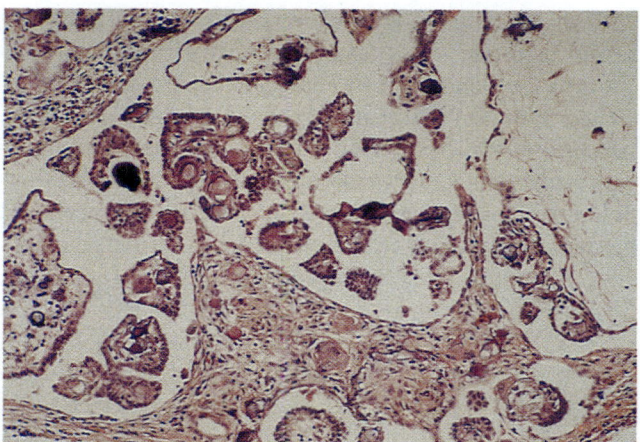

FIG. 42. Extraovarian borderline serous tumor involving the pelvic peritoneum. The ovaries were grossly unremarkable, but their serosal surfaces were involved by similar tumor on microscopic examination.

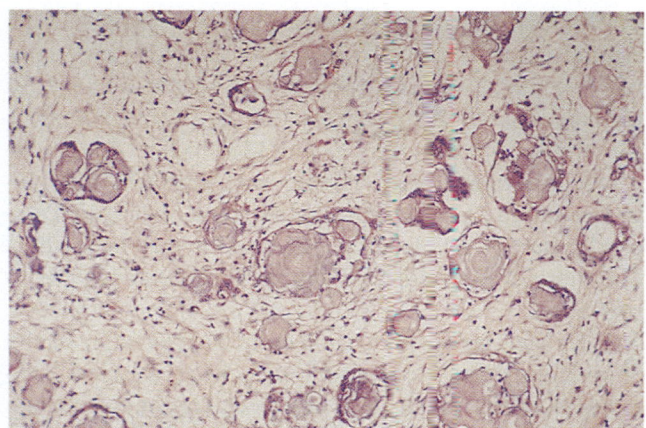

FIG. 43. Extraovarian low-grade serous carcinoma (psammocarcinoma) involving the omentum. The tumor consists almost entirely of psammoma bodies within a dense fibrous stroma. Some of the psammoma bodies are surrounded by a thin rim of neoplastic epithelial cells

Peritoneal Mucinous Lesions

Benign glands of endocervical type involving the peritoneum, so-called endocervicosis, are rare, but examples involving the posterior uterine serosa, cul-de-sac, and the urinary bladder have been documented (205,364,365). In the last site, the lesions formed tumor-like masses that involved the posterior wall or posterior dome of the bladder in women of reproductive age (364,365). Microscopically, benign endocervical-type glands were located predominantly within the smooth muscle of the muscularis propria. In several cases, the infiltrative pattern of the glands, mild epithelial atypia, and a reactive periglandular stroma, alone or in combination, resulted in an initial misdiagnosis of well-differentiated adenocarcinoma.

Mucinous neoplasms, similar to those occurring within the ovary, have been described in extraovarian sites, typically in the retroperitoneum (205,366–369); a single case has been described in the inguinal region (370). These tumors form large cystic masses that on histologic examination have resembled ovarian mucinous cystadenomas, borderline tumors, or cystadenocarcinomas; some have contained ovarian-type stroma in their walls. Although it is possible that some of these tumors originate within a supernumerary ovary, the great rarity of the latter, the absence of follicles or their derivatives within the ovarian-like stroma, and the rare occurrence of similar tumors in males, strongly support a peritoneal origin.

Peritoneal Transitional, Squamous, and Clear Cell Lesions

Nests of transitional (urothelial) epithelium referred to as Walthard nests are commonly present on the pelvic peritoneum in women of all ages, typically involving the serosal surfaces of the fallopian tubes, mesosalpinx and mesovarium (371–373). They are uncommon on the ovarian surface, but may be seen in the hilus, probably originating from the peritoneum of the mesovarium. Walthard nests, which are also seen in men, usually in the vicinity of the epididymis (374), are discussed in more detail elsewhere (see chapter 55). Rare extraovarian Brenner tumors have been encountered, most commonly in the broad ligament (see chapter 55) (375). In contrast to Walthard nests, squamous metaplasia of the peritoneum is rare; one such case has been recently described (367). Two clear cell carcinomas of apparent peritoneal origin have been recently reported. One was a localized mass within the sigmoid mesocolon (377), whereas the other diffusely involved the peritoneum (378); there was no demonstrable endometriosis in either case.

Peritoneal Decidua

Clinical and Operative Findings

An ectopic decidual reaction similar to that seen in the lamina propria of the fallopian tube, cervix, and vagina may also be seen within the submesothelial stroma of the peritoneal cavity (379–387). Frequent sites of ectopic decidua include the submesothelial stroma of the fallopian tubes, uterus and uterine ligaments, appendix and omentum, and within pelvic adhesions. Rare sites have included the serosal surfaces of the diaphragm, liver, and spleen (382,384), and the renal pelvis (383).

Submesothelial decidua is typically an incidental microscopic finding, but florid lesions may be visible at the time of cesarean section or postpartum tubal ligation as multiple, gray to white, focally hemorrhagic nodules or plaques studding the peritoneal surfaces and simulating a malignant tumor (384,385). Several cases have been associated with massive, occasionally fatal, intraperitoneal hemorrhage during the third trimester, labor, or the puerperium (385,386). Other rare clinical presentations include abdominal pain, which may simulate that of appendicitis, and hydronephrosis or hematuria secondary to renal pelvic involvement (383).

Histologic Appearance

Microscopic examination discloses submesothelial decidual cells disposed individually or arranged in nodules or plaques (Fig. 44). Smooth muscle cells, probably derived from submesothelial myofibroblasts (379), may be admixed. The decidual foci are typically vascular and contain a sprinkling of lymphocytes. Focal hemorrhagic necrosis and varying degrees of nuclear pleomorphism and hyperchromasia of the decidual cells may suggest a tumor such as a malignant mesothelioma, especially of the deciduoid type (141,142), but their bland appearance and mitotic inactivity militate against such a diagnosis. In occasional cases, some or even most of the decidual cells may contain vacuoles with basophilic mucin and an eccentric location of the nucleus, potentially suggesting metastatic signet-ring cell carcinoma. In

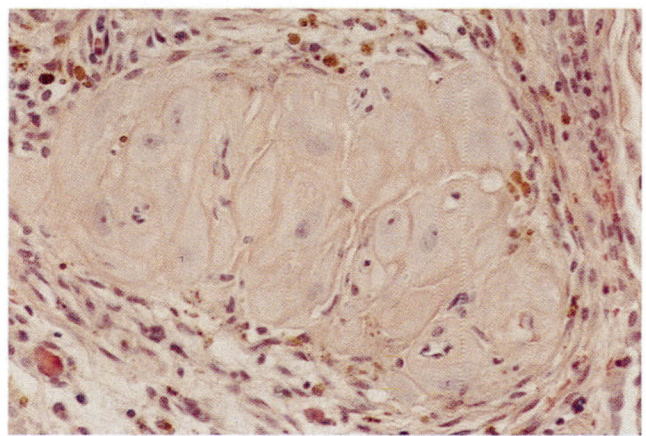

FIG. 44. Ectopic decidua within the omentum.

contrast to the cells of the latter, however, the vacuoles within the decidual cells contain acidic, rather than neutral, mucin.

Peritoneal Leiomyomatosis (see Chapter 53).

Retroperitoneal Lymph Node Lesions

Benign Glands of Müllerian Type

Clinical Features

Benign glands of müllerian type are most commonly encountered within pelvic and paraaortic lymph nodes of females (311,314,388–392), and less often in inguinal and femoral lymph nodes (393,394). Because these glands are almost always incidental microscopic findings in lymph nodes removed in cases of pelvic carcinoma, their reported frequency, which has varied from 2% to 41%, depends on the number of lymph nodes removed and the extent of the histologic sampling. Almost all of the patients have been adults, although rare examples have been reported in children (314). In males, the presence of similar glands have been recorded rarely within lymph nodes in the pelvis and abdomen (395,396), as well as the mediastinum (397). Although typically without clinical or intraoperative manifestations, rare examples of lymph nodes containing müllerian-type glands have been associated with a false-positive lymphangiogram (398), ureteral obstruction secondary to lymph node enlargement (399), or visible enlargement at the time of operation (400).

In a number of patients, intranodal glandular inclusions have been accompanied by endosalpingiosis of the peritoneum (311,314), salpingitis isthmica nodosa, or acute and chronic salpingitis (314,390,400). Other patients have had coexistent ovarian serous tumors, which have been benign or borderline tumors, or carcinomas (388,394).

Pathologic Features

On gross examination, the glands are usually not apparent, although rarely they are recognizable as cysts measuring up to a few millimeters in diameter (399,401). The glands are typically located in the periphery of the node, most commonly within its capsule or between the lymphoid follicles in the superficial cortex (Fig. 45); rarely they lie free within the subcapsular sinuses (390). In florid cases, they can be diffusely distributed throughout the lymph node (390,400). Intraglandular or periglandular psammoma bodies are commonly present. Intranodal glands may be surrounded by a thin rim of fibrous tissue or directly abut surrounding lymphoid cells.

The glands may be round and cystically dilated or exhibit an irregular contour due to infolding. They are most commonly lined by a single layer of cuboidal to columnar tubal-type epithelium, with an admixture of ciliated, secretory, and intercalated cell types (Fig. 45). With special stains, mucin can be demonstrated in the apical portion of the secretory cells and within the gland spaces (389,400). Acute and chronic inflammatory cells may be present within the lumina. The cells have a benign appearance with regular, basally oriented or pseudostratified, oval to round nuclei, fine nuclear chromatin, and occasional small nucleoli. Mitotic figures are typically absent. In rare cases, the cells exhibit varying degrees of atypia and stratification; the latter can produce an intraglandular cribriform pattern or luminal obliteration by sheets of cells (Fig. 45) (311,388,400).

Examples of intranodal glandular inclusions lined by benign endometrioid epithelium (205,391), mucinous epithelium of endocervical (391,401,402) or goblet-cell type (396), or metaplastic squamous epithelium (394,403) have been reported. Rarely, endometriotic stroma is present around the glands, warranting a diagnosis of endometriosis.

Differential Diagnosis

In most cases the distinction between glandular inclusions and metastatic adenocarcinoma is not difficult unless a primary ovarian serous tumor of low malignant potential is pre-

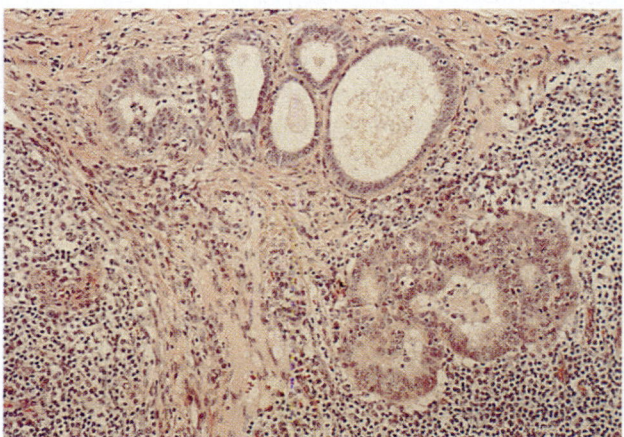

FIG. 45. Typical and atypical endosalpingiotic glands in subcapsular region of a pelvic lymph node. Four glands (*top*) in the capsule of the node are lined by a single layer of benign, ciliated columnar cells. In several other glands, the lining cells are atypical and form cribriform arrangements.

sent, in which case the distinction may be difficult or impossible. Features favoring a benign diagnosis include a capsular or interfollicular location of the glands, lining cells of multiple types including ciliated forms, a lack of significant cellular atypia and mitotic activity, periglandular basement membranes, and an absence of a desmoplastic stromal reaction. Complicating the differential diagnosis is the very rare development of borderline or frankly malignant change in müllerian glandular inclusions in lymph nodes (321, 388,404). Similarly, intranodal nests of benign squamous epithelium should not be mistaken for metastatic squamous cell carcinoma (403). Features favoring a benign diagnosis include bland cytologic features, mitotic inactivity, and, in some cases, an origin within benign glands.

Ectopic Decidua

Ectopic decidua, unassociated with endometriosis, has been described as a rare, incidental microscopic finding in paraaortic and pelvic lymph nodes, usually removed as part of a radical hysterectomy for carcinoma of the cervix in pregnant patients (381,403,405–409). A subserosal ectopic decidual reaction may be present elsewhere in the pelvis (407). In some cases, the decidual tissue has been recognized on careful macroscopic examination as tiny, gray, subcapsular nodules (407). On microscopic examination the decidual nests typically occupy the subcapsular sinus and superficial cortex (Fig. 46), although more central parts of the lymph node may also be involved. The cells appear benign, but may contain occasional bizarre, hyperchromatic nuclei, mimicking metastatic squamous cell carcinoma (407). The absence of mitotic activity, keratinization, stromal desmoplasia, and cytokeratin reactivity, should facilitate the diagnosis. Metastatic squamous cell carcinoma, however, may be present in the same node (409).

Leiomyomatosis

Rare cases of lymph node involvement by mitotically inactive, cytologically benign smooth muscle have been de-

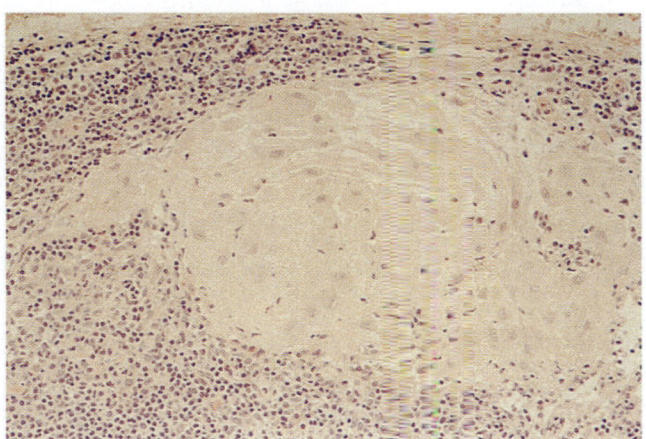

FIG. 46. Ectopic decidua in subcapsular region of a pelvic lymph node.

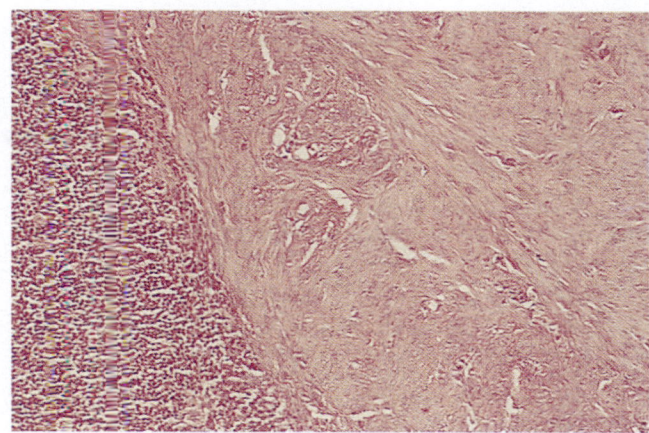

FIG. 47. Leiomyomatosis of pelvic lymph node. Islands of benign smooth muscle replace the normal nodal parenchyma.

scribed (Fig. 47) (265,410–415). Most patients have had concurrent, typical uterine leiomyomas, and less commonly, disseminated peritoneal leiomyomatosis (413), or similar nodules within the lungs (410,412). In pregnant patients, the process may merge with intranodal decidua (413). The possible histogenesis of the decidua includes an origin from entrapped subcoelomic mesenchyme (415), myofibroblastic organization of intranodal decidua (413), and lymphatic spread from uterine leiomyomas (410,411,414). The presence of benign-appearing smooth muscle in a lymph node should also bring into consideration the diagnosis of lymphangioleiomyomatosis (416,417). In this disorder, there is usually, but not invariably, associated pulmonary involvement and the lesional cells are strongly immunoreactive for HMB-45 (417). Benign intranodal smooth muscle should also be distinguished from metastatic well-differentiated leiomyosarcoma of uterine origin. Patients with the latter usually have a large uterine mass, and on histologic examination the intranodal tumor is cellular and exhibits evidence of cellular atypicality and mitotic activity.

REFERENCES

1. Targan SR, Chow AW, Guze LB. Role of anaerobic bacteria in spontaneous peritonitis of cirrhosis. Report of two cases and review of the literature. *Am J Med* 1977;62:397–403.
2. Weinstein MP, Iannini PB, Stratton CW, et al. Spontaneous bacterial peritonitis. A review of 28 cases with emphasis on improved survival and factors influencing prognosis. *Am J Med* 1978;64:592–598.
3. Bayer AS, Blumenkrantz MJ, Montgomerie JZ, et al. Candida peritonitis. Report of 22 cases and review of the English literature. *Am J Med* 1976;61:832–840.
4. Williams GT. The peritoneum. In: Morson BC, ed. *Alimentary tract. Systemic pathology*, vol 3, Symmers WSC, ed. New York: Churchill Livingstone, 1987;417–450.
5. Kapoor OP, Nathwani BN, Joshi VR. Amoebic peritonitis. A study of 73 cases. *J Trop Med Hyg* 1972;75:11–15.
6. Sohar E, Gafni J, Pras M, et al. Familial Mediterranean fever. A survey of 470 cases and review of the literature. *Am J Med* 1967;43:227–253.
7. Bastani B, Shariatzadeh MR, Dehdashti F. Tuberculous peritonitis.

Report of 30 cases and review of the literature. *Q J Med* 1985;56: 549–557.
8. Haddad FS, Ghossain A, Sarvaya E, et al. Abdominal tuberculosis. *Dis Colon Rectum* 1987;30:724–735.
9. Nistal de Paz F, Fernandez BH, Simon RP, et al. Pelvic-peritoneal tuberculosis simulating ovarian carcinoma: report of three cases with elevation of the CA 125. *Am J Gastroenterol* 1996;91:1660–1661.
10. Reddy P, Gorelick DF, Brasher CA, et al. Progressive disseminated histoplasmosis as seen in adults. *Am J Med* 1970;48:629–636.
11. Saw EC, Shields SJ, Comer TP, et al. Granulomatous peritonitis due to coccidioides immitis. *Arch Surg* 1974;108:369–371.
12. Watson NE Jr, Johnson AH. Cryptococcal peritonitis. *South Med J* 1973;66:387–388.
13. Blumberg H, Srinivasan K, Parnes IH. Peritoneal schistosomiasis simulating carcinoma. *NY State J Med* 1966;66:758–761.
14. Sjovall A, Akerman M. Peritoneal granulomas in women due to the presence of enterobius S. oxyuris vermicularis. *Acta Obst Gynecol Scand* 1968;47:361–372.
15. Dalrymple JC, Hunter JC, Ferrier A, et al. Disseminated intraperitoneal oxyuris granulomas. *Aust NZ J Obstet Gynaecol* 1986;26: 90–91.
16. Reddy CRRM, Venkateswar Rao D, Sarma ENB, et al. Granulomatous peritonitis due to ascaris lumbricoides and its ova. *J Trop Med Hyg* 1975;78:146–149.
17. Lintermans JP. Fatal peritonitis, an unusual complication of strongyloides stercoralis infestation. *Clin Pediatr* 1975;14:974–975.
18. Coder DM, Olander GA. Granulomatous peritonitis caused by starch glove powder. *Arch Surg* 1972;105:83–86.
19. Ignatius JA, Hartmann WH. The glove starch peritonitis syndrome. *Ann Surg* 1972;175:338–367.
20. Holmes EC, Eggleston JC. Starch granulomatous peritonitis. *Surgery* 1972;71:85–90.
21. Hidvegi D, Hidvegi I, Barrett J. Douche-induced pelvic peritoneal starch granuloma. *Obstet Gynecol* 1978;52:15S–18S.
22. Saxen L, Kassinen A, Saxen E. Peritoneal foreign-body reaction caused by condom emulsion. *Lancet* 1963;1:1295–1296.
23. Nissim F, Ashkenazy M, Lorenstein R, et al. Tuberculoid cornstarch granulomas with caseous necrosis. *Arch Pathol Lab Med* 1981; 105:86–88.
24. Eiseman B, Seelig MG, Womack NA. Talcum powder granuloma: a frequent and serious postoperative complication. *Ann Surg* 1947; 126:820–832.
25. Postlethwait RW, Howard HL, Schanher PW, et al. Comparison of tissue reaction to talc and modified starch glove powder. *Surgery* 1949;25:22–29.
26. Castelli MJ, Armin A, Husain A, et al. Fibrosing peritonitis in a drug abuser. *Arch Pathol Lab Med* 1985;109:767–769.
27. Tinker MA, Burdman D, Deysine M, et al. Granulomatous peritonitis due to cellulose fibers from disposable surgical fabrics. *Ann Surg* 1974;180:831–835.
28. Godleski JJ, Gabriel KL. Peritoneal responses to implanted fabrics used in operating rooms. *Surgery* 1981;90:828–834.
29. Janoff K, Wayne R, Huntwork B, et al. Foreign body reactions secondary to cellulose lint fibers. *Am J Surg* 1984;147:598–600.
30. Deger RB, LiVolsi VA, Noumoff JS. Foreign body reaction (gossypiboma) masking as recurrent ovarian cancer. *Gynecol Oncol* 1995;56:94–96.
31. Park SA, Giannattasio C, Tancer ML. Foreign body reaction to the intraperitoneal use of avitene. *Obstet Gynecol* 1981;58:664–668.
32. Norris JC, Davison TC. Peritoneal reaction to liquid petrolatum. *JAMA* 1934;103:1846–1847.
33. Teilum G, Madsen V. Endometriosis ovarii et peritonaei caused by hysterosalpingography. *Br J Obstet Gynaecol* 1950;57:10–16.
34. Marshall SF, Forse RA. Peritoneal adhesions: report of a case of paraffinoma. *Surg Clin North Am* 1952;32:903–908.
35. Grosskinsky CM, Clark RL, Wilson PA, Novotny DB. Pelvic granulomata mimicking endometriosis following the administration of oil-based contrast media for hysterosalpingography. *Obstet Gynecol* 1994;83:890–892.
36. Davies JD, Ansell ID. Food-starch granulomatous peritonitis. *J Clin Pathol* 1983;36:435–438.
37. Kay S. Tissue reaction to barium sulfate contrast medium. *Arch Pathol* 1954;57:279–284.
38. Waxman M, Boyce JG. Intraperitoneal rupture of benign cystic ovarian teratoma. *Obstet Gynecol* 1976;48:9S–13S.
39. Stuart GCE, Smith JP. Ruptured benign cystic teratomas mimicking gynecologic malignancy. *Gynecol Oncol* 1983;16:139–143.
40. Stern JL, Buscema J, Rosenshein NB, et al. Spontaneous rupture of benign cystic teratomas. *Obstet Gynecol* 1981;57:365–366.
41. George E, Leyser S, Zimmer HL, Simowitz DA, Agress RL, Nordin DD. Vernix caseosa peritonitis: an infrequent complication of cesarean section with distinctive histopathologic features. *Am J Clin Pathol* 1995;103:681–684.
42. Tibboel D, Gaillard JLJ, Molenaar JC. The importance of mesenteric vascular insufficiency in meconium peritonitis. *Hum Pathol* 1986;17:411–416.
43. Forouhar F. Meconium peritonitis. Pathology, evolution, and diagnosis. *Am J Clin Pathol* 1982;78:208–213.
44. Dehner LP, Scott D, Stocker JT. Meconium periorchitis: a clinicopathologic study of four cases with a review of the literature. *Hum Pathol* 1986;17:807–12.
45. Sanner RF Jr. Chronic idiopathic bile peritonitis. *JAMA* 1965;194: 238–240.
46. Daum F, Boley SJ, Cohen MI. Miliary Crohn's disease. *Gastroenterology* 1974;67:527–530.
47. Wong M, Rosen SW. Ascites in sarcoidosis due to peritoneal involvement. *Ann Intern Med* 1962;57:277–280.
48. Trimble EL, Saigo PE, Freeberg GW, Rubin SC, Hoskins WJ. Peritoneal sarcoidosis and elevated CA 125. *Obstet Gynecol* 1991; 78:976–977.
49. Isenberg JI, Gilbert SB, Pitcher JL. Ascites with peritoneal involvement in Whipple's disease. *Gastroenterology* 1971;60:305–310.
50. Clarke TJ, Simpson RHW. Necrotizing granulomas of peritoneum following diathermy ablation of endometriosis. *Histopathology* 1990; 16:400–402.
51. Clement PB, Young RH, Scully RE. Necrotic pseudoxanthomatous nodules of the ovary and peritoneum in endometriosis. *Am J Surg Pathol* 1988;12:390–397.
52. White J, Chan Y-F. Lipofuscinosis peritonei associated with pregnancy-related ectopic decidua. *Histopathology* 1994;25:83–85.
53. Chan JKC, Loo KT, Yau BKC, Lam SY. Nodular histiocytic/mesothelial hyperplasia: a lesion potentially mistaken for a neoplasm in transbronchial biopsy. *Am J Surg Pathol* 1997;21:658–663.
53a. Ordonez NG, Ro JY, Ayala AG. Lesions described as nodular mesothelial hyperplasia are primarily composed of histiocytes. *Am J Surg Pathol* 1998;22:285–292.
54. Ruffolo R, Suster S. Diffuse histiocytic proliferation mimicking mesothelial hyperplasia in endocervicosis of the female pelvic peritoneum. *Int J Surg Pathol* 1993;1:101–106.
55. Kuo T, Hsueh S. Mucicarminophilic histiocytosis. A polyvinylpyrrolidone (PVP) storage disease simulating signet-ring cell carcinoma. *Am J Surg Pathol* 1984;8:419–428.
55a. Kershisnik MM, Ro JY, Cannon GH, Ordonez NG, Ayala AG, Silva EG. Histiocytic reaction in pelvic peritoneum associated with oxidized regenerated cellulose. *Am J Clin Pathol* 1994;103:27–31.
56. Weibel MA, Majno G. Peritoneal adhesions and their relation to abdominal surgery. *Am J Surg* 1973;126:345–353.
57. McCaughey WTE, Al-Jabi M. Differentiation of serosal hyperplasia and neoplasia in biopsies. *Pathol Annu* 1986;21(1):271–292.
58. Wanless IR, Bernier V. Fibrous thickening of the splenic capsule. *Arch Pathol Lab Med* 1983;107:595–599.
59. Buhac I, Jarmolych J. Histology of the intestinal peritoneum in patients with cirrhosis of the liver and ascites. *Dig Dis* 1978;23:417–422.
60. Miranda RN, McMillan PN, Pricolo VE, Finkelstein SD. Peritoneal silicosis. *Arch Pathol Lab Med* 1996;120:300–302.
61. Concato L. Sulla poliomenorrhea scrofolosa o tisi delle sierose. *Gior Intern Sc Med* 1881;3:1037–1053.
62. Dehn TCB, Lucas MG, Wood RFM. Idiopathic sclerosing peritonitis. *Postgrad Med J* 1985;61:841–842.
63. Foo KT, Ng KC, Rauff A, et al. Unusual small intestinal obstruction in adolescent girls: the abdominal cocoon. *Br J Surg* 1978;65: 427–430.
64. Marshall AJ, Baddeley H, Barritt DW, et al. Practolol peritonitis. A study of 16 cases and a survey of small bowel function in patients taking beta adrenergic blockers. *Q J Med* 1977;46:135–149.
65. Bradley JA, McWhinnie DL, Hamilton DNH. Sclerosing obstructive peritonitis after continuous ambulatory peritoneal dialysis. *Lancet* 1983;2:113–114.
66. Wallace S, Sabto J, Pedersen J, Gurr FW. Peritoneal sclerosis in CAPD. *Pathology* 1992;24:4(abst).

67. Ngo Y, Messing B, Marteau P, et al. Peritoneal sarcoidosis: an unrecognized cause of sclerosing peritonitis. *Dig Dis Sci* 1992;37:1776–1780.
68. Cambria RP, Shamberger RC. Small bowel obstruction caused by the abdominal cocoon syndrome: possible association with the LeVeen shunt. *Surgery* 1984;95:501–503.
69. Clement PB, Young RH, Hanna W, Scully RE. Sclerosing peritonitis associated with luteinized thecomas of the ovary: a clinicopathological analysis of six cases. *Am J Surg Pathol* 1994;18:1–13.
70. Sayfan J, Adam YG, Reif R. Peritoneal encapsulation in childhood. Case report, embryologic analysis, and review of literature. *Am J Surg* 1979;138:725–727.
71. Sieck JO, Cowgill R, Larkworthy W. Peritoneal encapsulation and abdominal cocoon. Case report and review of the literature. *Gastroenterology* 1983;84:1597–1601.
72. Adams HW, Mainz DL. Eosinophilic ascites. A case report and review of the literature. *Dig Dis* 1977;22:40–42.
73. Metzger AL, Coyne M, Lee S, et al. In vivo LE cell formation in peritonitis due to systemic lupus erythematosus. *J Rheumatol* 1974;1:130–133.
74. Lomholt G, Hjorth N, Fischermann K. Lethal peritonitis from Degos' disease (malign and atrophic papulosis). *Acta Chir Scand* 1968;134:495–501.
75. Foyle A, Al-Jabi M, McCaughey WTE. Papillary peritoneal tumors in women. *Am J Surg Pathol* 1981;5:241–249.
76. Hansen RM, Caya JG, Clowry LJ Jr, et al. Benign mesothelial proliferation with effusion. Clinicopathologic entity that may mimic malignancy. *Am J Med* 1984;77:887–892.
77. McCaughey WTE, Kannerstein M, Churg J. *Tumors and pseudotumors of the serous membranes. Atlas of tumor pathology,* series 2, fascicle 20. Washington, DC: Armed Forces Institute of Pathology, 1985.
78. Kerner H, Gaton E, Czernobilsky B. Unusual ovarian, tubal and pelvic mesothelial inclusions in patients with endometriosis. *Histopathology* 1981;5:277–282.
79. Clement PB, Young RH. Florid mesothelial hyperplasia associated with ovarian tumors: a possible source of error in tumor diagnosis and staging. *Int J Gynecol Pathol* 1993;12:51–58.
80. Rosai J, Dehner LP. Nodular mesothelial hyperplasia in hernia sacs. A benign reactive condition stimulating a neoplastic process. *Cancer* 1975;35:165–175.
81. Clement PB, Young RH, Oliva E, Sumner HW, Scully RE. Hyperplastic mesothelial cells within abdominal lymph nodes: a mimic of metastatic ovarian carcinoma and serous borderline tumor. A report of two cases associated with ovarian neoplasms. *Mod Pathol* 1996;9:879–886.
82. Daya D, McCaughey WTE. Pathology of the peritoneum: a review of selected topics. *Semin Diagn Pathol* 1991;8:277–289.
83. Whitaker D, Shilkin KB. Diagnosis of pleural malignant mesothelioma in life—a practical approach. *J Pathol* 1984;143:147–175.
84. Kwee WS, Veldhuizen RW, Golding FP, et al. Histologic distinction between malignant mesothelioma, benign pleural lesion and carcinoma metastasis. *Virchows Arch [A]* 1982;397:287–299.
85. Ayres JG, Crocker JG, Skilbeck NQ. Differentiation of malignant from normal and reactive mesothelial cells by the argyrophil technique for nucleolar organiser region associated proteins. *Thorax* 1988;43:366–370.
86. Soosay GN, Griffiths M, Papadaki L, et al. The differential diagnosis of epithelial-type mesothelioma from adenocarcinoma and reactive mesothelial proliferation. *J Pathol* 1991;163:299–305.
87. Riddell RH, Goodman MJ, Moossa AR. Peritoneal malignant mesothelioma in a patient with recurrent peritonitis. *Cancer* 1981;48:134–139.
88. Carpenter HA, Lancaster JR, Lee RA. Multilocular cysts of the peritoneum. *Mayo Clin Proc* 1982;57:634–638.
89. Schneider V, Partridge JR, Gutierrez, et al. Benign cystic mesothelioma involving the female genital tract report of four cases. *Am J Obstet Gynecol* 1983;145:355–359.
90. Katsube Y, Mukai K, Silverberg SG. Cystic mesothelioma of the peritoneum. A report of five cases and review of the literature. *Cancer* 1982;50:1615–1622.
91. Dumke K, Schnoy N, Specht G, et al. Comparative light and electron microscopic studies of cystic and papillary tumors of the peritoneum. *Virchows Arch [A]* 1983;399:25–39.
92. Moor JH Jr, Crum CP, Chandler JC, Feldman PS. Benign cystic mesothelioma. *Cancer* 1980;45:2395–2399.
93. McFadden DE, Clement PB. Peritoneal inclusion cysts with mural mesothelial proliferation. A clinicopathological analysis of six cases. *Am J Surg Pathol* 1986;10:844–854.
94. Weiss SW, Tavassoli FA. Multicystic mesothelioma: an analysis of pathologic findings and biologic behavior in 37 cases. *Am J Surg Pathol* 1988;12:737–746.
95. Ross MJ, Welch WR, Scully RE. Multilocular peritoneal inclusion cysts (so-called cystic mesotheliomas). *Cancer* 1989;64:1336–1346.
96. Arber DA, Strickler JG, Weiss LM. Splenic mesothelial cysts mimicking lymphangiomas. *Am J Surg Pathol* 1997;21:334–338.
97. Lamovec J, Sinkovec J. Multilocular peritoneal inclusion cyst (multicystic mesothelioma) with hyaline globules. *Histopathology* 1996;28:466–469.
98. Blumberg NA, Murrary JF. Multicystic peritoneal mesothelioma. *S Afr Med J* 1981;59:85–86.
99. Sienkowski I, Russell AJ, Dilly SA, et al. Peritoneal cystic mesothelioma: an electron microscopic and immunohistochemical study of two male patients. *J Clin Pathol* 1986;39:440–445.
100. Kjellevold K, Nesland JM, Holm R, et al. Multicystic peritoneal mesothelioma. *Pathol Res Pract* 1986;181:767–771.
101. Harper GB Jr, Awbrey BJ, Thomas CG Jr, et al. Mesothelial cysts of the round ligament simulating inguinal hernia. Report of four cases and review of the literature. *Am J Surg* 1986;151:515–517.
102. Jones EG, Donovan AJ. Adenomatoid tumor of the ovary versus mesothelial reaction. *Am J Obstet Gynecol* 1965;92:694–698.
103. Dencpoulos RI, Kahn MA, Feiner HD. Epidemiology of cystic mesotheliomas. *Int J Gynecol Pathol* 1986;5:379–381.
104. Gussman D, Thickman D, Wheeler JE. Postoperative peritoneal cysts. *Obstet Gynecol* 1986;68:53S–55S.
105. Lees RF, Feldman PS, Brenbridge NAG, et al. Inflammatory cysts of the pelvic peritoneum. *Am J Roentgenol* 1978;131:633–636.
106. Iwasaki I, Yu TJ, Tamaru J, Asanuma K. A cystic adenomatoid tumor of the uterus simulating lymphangioma grossly. *Acta Pathol Jpn* 1985;35:989–993.
107. Bisset DL, Morris JA, Fox H. Giant cystic adenomatoid tumor (mesothelioma) of the uterus. *Histopathology* 1988;12:555–558.
108. Kocova L, Michal M, Sulc M, Zamecnik A. Calcifying fibrous pseudotumor of visceral peritoneum. *Histopathology* 1997;31:182–184.
109. Fleming CR, Dickson ER, Harrison EG Jr. Splenosis: autotransplantation of splenic tissue. *Am J Med* 1976;61:414–419.
110. Overton TH. Splenosis: a cause of pelvic pain. *Am J Obstet Gynecol* 1982;143:969–970.
111. Matonis LM, Luciano AA. A case of splenosis masquerading as endometriosis. *Am J Obstet Gynecol* 1995;173:971–973.
112. Thatcher SS, Grainger DA, True LD, DeCherney AH. Pelvic trophoblastic implants after laparoscopic removal of a tubal pregnancy. *Obstet Gynecol* 1989;74:514–515.
113. Reich H, De Caprio J, McGlynn F, et al. Peritoneal trophoblastic tissue implants after laparoscopic treatment of tubal ectopic pregnancy. *Fertil Steril* 1989;52:337.
114. Cartwright PS. Peritoneal trophoblastic implants after surgical management of tubal pregnancy. *J Reprod Med* 1991;36:523–524.
115. Alonso JF, Martin GM, Nisco FS, et al. Melanogenic ovarian tumors. *Am J Obstet Gynecol* 1962;84:667–676.
116. Fukushima M, Sharpe L, Okagaki T. Peritoneal melanosis secondary to a benign dermoid cyst of the ovary: a case report with ultrastructural study. *Int J Gynecol Pathol* 1984;2:403–409.
117. Lee D, Pontifex AH. Melanosis peritonei. *Am J Obstet Gynecol* 1975;122:526–527.
118. Sanin AA, Ro JY, Chen J, Ayala AG. Spindle cell nodule and peptic ulcer arising in a fully developed gastric wall in a mature cystic teratoma. *Arch Pathol Lab Med* 1990;114:529–531.
119. Chen KTK, Kostich ND, Rosai J. Peritoneal foreign body granulomas to keratin in uterine adenoacanthoma. *Arch Pathol Lab Med* 1978;102:174–177.
120. Kim K, Scully RE. Peritoneal keratin granulomas with carcinomas of endometrium and ovary and atypical polypoid adenomyoma of endometrium. *Am J Surg Pathol* 1990;14:925–932.
121. Eliott GB, Freigang B. Aseptic necrosis, calcification and separation of appendices epiploicae. *Ann Surg* 1962;155:501–505.
122. Vaorg PN, Guyot H, Moulin G, et al. Pseudotumoral organization of a twisted epiploic fringe or 'hard-boiled egg' in the peritoneal cavity. *Arch Pathol Lab Med* 1990;114:531–533.
123. Young RH, Clement PB, McCaughey ET. Solitary fibrous tumors ("fibrous mesotheliomas") of the peritoneum: a report of three cases. *Arch Pathol Lab Med* 1990;114:493–495.

124. Flint A, Weiss SW. CD-34 and keratin expression distinguishes solitary fibrous tumor (fibrous mesothelioma) of pleura from desmoplastic mesothelioma. *Hum Pathol* 1995;26:428–431.
125. Fukunaga M, Naganuma H, Nikaido T, Haruda T, Ushigome S. Extrapleural solitary fibrous tumor: a report of seven cases. *Mod Pathol* 1997;10:443–450.
126. Hanau CA, Miettinen M. Solitary fibrous tumor: histological and immunohistochemical spectrum of benign and malignant variants presenting at different sites. *Hum Pathol* 1995;26:440–449.
127. Fukunaga M, Naganuma H, Ushigome S, Endo Y, Ishikawa E. Malignant solitary fibrous tumour of the peritoneum. *Histopathology* 1996;28:463–466.
128. Hanrahan JB. A combined papillary mesothelioma and adenomatoid tumor of the omentum. Report of a case. *Cancer* 1963;16:1497–1500.
129. Craig JR, Hart WR. Extragenital adenomatoid tumor. Evidence for the mesothelial theory of origin. *Cancer* 1979;433:1678–1679.
130. Goepel JR. Benign papillary mesothelioma of peritoneum: a histological, histochemical and ultrastructural study of six cases. *Histopathology* 1981;5:21–30.
131. Daya D, McCaughey WTE. Well-differentiated papillary mesothelioma of the peritoneum. A clinicopathologic study of 22 cases. *Cancer* 1990;65:292–296.
132. Burrig K, Pfitzer P, Hort W. Well-differentiated papillary mesothelioma of the peritoneum: a borderline mesothelioma. *Virchows Archiv [A]* 1990;417:443–447.
133. Goldblum J, Hart WR. Localized and diffuse mesotheliomas of the genital tract and peritoneum in women. A clinicopathologic study of nineteen true mesothelial neoplasms, other than adenomatoid tumors, multicystic mesotheliomas, and localized fibrous tumors. *Am J Surg Pathol* 1995;19:1124–1137.
134. DeStephano DB, Wesley JR, Heidelberger KP, Hutchison RJ, Blane CE, Coran AG. Primitive cystic hepatic neoplasm of infancy with mesothelial differentiation: report of a case. *Pediatr Pathol* 1985;4:291–302.
135. Kannerstein M, Churg J. Peritoneal mesothelioma. *Hum Pathol* 1977;8:83–94.
136. Jones DEC, Silver D. Peritoneal mesotheliomas. *Surgery* 1979;86:556–560.
137. Plaus WJ. Peritoneal mesothelioma. *Arch Surg* 1988;123:763–766.
138. Piccigallo E, Jeffers LJ, Reddy R, et al. Malignant peritoneal mesothelioma. A clinical and laparoscopic study of ten cases. *Dig Dis Sci* 1988;33:633–639.
139. Asensio JA, Goldblatt P, Thomford NR. Primary malignant peritoneal mesothelioma. A report of seven cases and a review of the literature. *Arch Surg* 1990;125:1477–1481.
140. Kane MJ, Chahinian AP, Holland JF. Malignant mesothelioma in young adults. *Cancer* 1990;65:1449–1455.
141. Talerman A, Montero JR, Chilcote RR, Okagaki T. Diffuse malignant peritoneal mesothelioma in a 13-year-old girl. Report of a case and review of the literature. *Am J Surg Pathol* 1985;9:73–80.
142. Nascimento AG, Keeney GL, Fletcher CDM. Deciduoid peritoneal mesothelioma. An unusual phenotype affecting young females. *Am J Surg Pathol* 1994;18:439–445.
143. Geary WA, Mills SE, Frierson HF, Pope TL. Malignant peritoneal mesothelioma in childhood with long-term survival. *Am J Clin Pathol* 1991;95:493–498.
144. Almudevar Bercero E, Garcia-Rostan Y, Perez GMA, Garcia Bragado F, Jiminez C. Prognostic value of high serum levels of CA-125 in malignant secretory peritoneal mesotheliomas affecting young women. A case report with differential diagnosis and review of the literature. *Histopathology* 1997;31:267–273.
145. Matsukuma S, Aida S, Hata Y, Sugiura Y, Tamai S. Localized malignant peritoneal mesothelioma containing rhabdoid cells. *Pathol Internat* 1996;46:389–391.
146. Chen KTK. Malignant mesothelioma presenting as Sister Joseph's nodule. *Am J Dermatopathol* 1991;13:300–303.
147. Mayall FG, Gibbs AR. Malignant peritoneal mesothelioma giving rise to multiple intestinal polyps. *Histopathology* 1991;18:480–482.
148. Fukayama M, Takizawa T, Koike M, et al. Malignant peritoneal mesothelioma as a pelvic mass. *Acta Pathol Jpn* 1987;37:1149–1156.
149. Clement PB, Young RH, Scully RE. Malignant mesotheliomas presenting as ovarian masses. A report of nine cases, including two primary ovarian mesotheliomas. *Am J Surg Pathol* 1996;20:1067–1060.
150. Sussman J, Rosai J. Lymph node metastasis as the initial manifestation of malignant mesothelioma. Report of six cases. *Am J Surg Pathol* 1990;14:818–828.
151. Gilks B, Hegedus C, Freeman H, et al. Malignant peritoneal mesothelioma after remote abdominal radiation. *Cancer* 1988;61:2019–2021.
152. Peterson JT Jr, Greenberg SD, Bufflier PA. Non-asbestos-related malignant mesothelioma. A review. *Cancer* 1984;54:951–960.
153. Huncharek M. Genetic factors in the aetiology of malignant mesothelioma. *Eur J Cancer* 1995;31A:1741–1747.
154. Brenner J, Sordillo PP, Magill GB. Seventeen year survival in a patient with malignant peritoneal mesothelioma. *Clin Oncol* 1981;7:249–251.
155. Norman PE, Whitaker D. Nine-year survival in a case of untreated peritoneal mesothelioma. *Med J Aust* 1989;150:43–44.
156. Antman KH, Klegar KL, Pomfret EA, et al. Early peritoneal mesothelioma: a treatable malignancy. *Lancet* 1985;2:977–981.
157. Kitazawa M, Kaneko H, Toshima M, et al. Malignant peritoneal mesothelioma with massive foamy cells. *Acta Pathol Jpn* 1984;34:687–692.
158. Bollinger DJ, Wick MR, Dehner LP, et al. Peritoneal malignant mesothelioma versus serous papillary adenocarcinoma. A histochemical and immunohistochemical comparison. *Am J Surg Pathol* 1989;13:659–670.
159. Donna A, Betta P, Jones JSP. Verification of the histologic diagnosis of malignant mesothelioma in relation to the binding of an antimesothelial cell antibody. *Cancer* 1989;63:1331–1336.
160. Wick MR, Loy T, Mills SE, et al. Malignant epithelioid pleural mesothelioma versus peripheral pulmonary adenocarcinoma: a histochemical, ultrastructural, and immunohistologic study of 103 cases. *Hum Pathol* 1990;21:759–766.
161. Stirling JW, Henderson DW, Spagnolo DV, Whitaker D. Unusual granular reactivity for carcinoembryonic antigen in malignant mesothelioma (letter). *Hum Pathol* 1990;21:678–679.
162. McCaughey WTE, Colby TV, Battifora H, et al. Diagnosis of diffuse malignant mesothelioma: experience of a US/Canadian mesothelioma panel. *Mod Pathol* 1991;4:342–353.
163. Azumi N, Underhill CB, Kagan E, Sheibani K. A novel biotinylated probe specific for hyaluronate: its diagnostic value in diffuse malignant mesothelioma. *Am J Surg Pathol* 1992;16:116–121.
164. Sheibani K, Esteban JM, Bailey A, et al. Immunopathologic and molecular studies as an aid to the diagnosis of malignant mesothelioma. *Hum Pathol* 1992;23:107–116.
165. Gaffey MJ, Mills SE, Swanson PE, et al. Immunoreactivity for BER-EP4 in adenocarcinomas, adenomatoid tumors, and malignant mesotheliomas. *Am J Surg Pathol* 1992;16:593–599.
166. Hammar SP, Bockus DE, Remington FL, Rohrbach KA. Mucin-positive epithelial mesotheliomas: a histochemical, immunohistochemical, and ultrastructural comparison with mucin-producing pulmonary adenocarcinomas. *Ultrastruct Pathol* 1996;20:293–325.
167. Sheibani K, Stroup RM. Immmunopathology of malignant mesothelioma. *Pathol State of the Art Reviews* 1996;4:191–212.
168. Doglioni C, Dei Tos AP, Laurino L, et al. Calretinin: a novel immunocytochemical marker for mesothelioma. *Am J Surg Pathol* 1996;20:1037–1046.
169. Ordonez NG. Role of immunohistochemistry in distinguishing epithelial peritoneal mesotheliomas from peritoneal and ovarian serous carcinomas. *Am J Surg Pathol* 1998;22:1203–1214.
170. Gerald WL, Rosai J. Desmoplastic small cell tumor with divergent differentiation. *Pediatr Pathol* 1989;9:177–183.
171. Sesterhenn WL, Davis CJ, Mostofi FK. Undifferentiated malignant epithelial tumors involving serosal surfaces of scrotum and abdomen in young males. *J Urol* 1987;137:214a(abst).
172. Ordonez NG, Zirkin R, Bloom RE. Malignant small-cell epithelial tumor of the peritoneum coexpressing mesenchymal-type intermediate filaments. *Am J Surg Pathol* 1989;13:413–421.
173. Gonzalez-Crussi F, Crawford SE, Sun CJ. Intraabdominal desmoplastic small-cell tumors with divergent differentiation. Observations on three cases of childhood. *Am J Surg Pathol* 1990;14:633–642.
174. Variend S, Gerrard M, Norris PD, Goepel JR. Intra-abdominal neuroectodermal tumour of childhood with divergent differentiation. *Histopathology* 1991;18:45–51.
175. Gerald WL, Miller HK, Battifora H, et al. Intra-abdominal desmoplastic small round cell tumor. *Am J Surg Pathol* 1991;15:499–513.
176. Layfield LJ, Lenarsky C. Desmoplastic small cell tumors of the peritoneum coexpressing mesenchymal and epithelial markers. *Am J Clin Pathol* 1991;96:536–543.

177. Norton J, Monaghan P, Carter RL. Intra-abdominal desmoplastic small cell tumour with divergent differentiation. *Histopathology* 1991;19:560–562.
178. Prat J, Matias-Guiu X, Algaba F. Desmoplastic small round-cell tumor (letter). *Am J Surg Pathol* 1992;16 306–308.
179. Cheung NYA, Khoo US, Chan KW. Intra-abdominal desmoplastic small round-cell tumour. *Histopathology* 1992;20:531–534.
180. Young RH, Eichhorn JH, Dickersin GR, Scully RE. Ovarian involvement by the intra-abdominal desmoplastic small round cell tumor with divergent differentiation: a report of three cases. *Hum Pathol* 1992;23:454–464.
181. Ordonez NG, El-Naggar AK, Ro JY, Silva EG, Mackay B. Intra-abdominal desmoplastic small cell tumor: a light microscopic, immunocytochemical, ultrastructural, and flow cytometric study. *Hum Pathol* 1993;24:850–865.
182. Schroder S, Padberg B. Desmoplastic small-cell tumor of the peritoneum with divergent differentiation: immunocytochemical and biochemical findings (letter). *Am J Clin Pathol* 1993;99:353–354.
183. Brodie SG, Stocker SJ, Wardlaw JC, et al. EWS and WT-1 gene fusion in desmoplastic small round cell tumor of the abdomen. *Hum Pathol* 1995;26:1370–1374.
184. Argatoff LH, O'Connell JX, Mathers JA, Gilks CB, Sorenson PHB. Detection of the EWS/WT1 gene fusion by reverse transcriptase-polymerase chain reaction in the diagnosis of intra-abdominal desmoplastic small round cell tumor. *Am J Surg Pathol* 1996;20:406–412.
185. Dorsey BV, Benjamin LE, Rauscher F I, et al. Intra-abdominal desmoplastic small round-cell tumor: expansion of the pathologic profile. *Mod Pathol* 1996;9:703–709.
186. Amato RJ, Ellerhorst JA, Ayala AG. Intrabdominal desmoplastic small cell tumor. Report and discussion of five cases. *Cancer* 1996;78:845–851.
187. Cummings OW, Ulbright TM, Young RF, Del Tos AP, Fletcher CDM, Hull MT. Desmoplastic small round cell tumors of the paratesticular region. A report of six cases. *Am J Surg Pathol* 1997;21:219–225.
188. Charles AK, Moore IE, Berry PJ. Immunohistochemical detection of the Wilms' tumour gene WT1 in desmoplastic small round cell tumour. *Histopathology* 1997;30:312–214
189. Gerald W, Ladanyi M, de Alava E, et al. Clinical, pathologic and molecular spectrum of desmoplastic small round cell tumor based on review of 109 cases. *Mod Pathol* 1997;10:1 a(abst).
190. Lin BT-Y, Colby T, Gown AM, et al. Malignant vascular tumors of the serous membranes mimicking mesothelioma. A report of 14 cases. *Am J Surg Pathol* 1996;20:1431–1439.
191. Attanoos RL, Dallimore NS, Gibbs AR. Primary epithelioid haemangioendothelioma of the peritoneum: an unusual mimic of diffuse malignant mesothelioma. *Histopathology* 1997;30:375–377.
192. Day DL, Sane S, Dehner LP. Inflammatory pseudotumor of the mesentery and small intestine. *Pediatr Radiol* 1986;16:210–215.
193. Pettinato G, Manivel JC, De Rosa N, Dehner LP. Inflammatory myofibroblastic tumor (plasma cell granuloma). Clinicopathologic study of 20 cases with immunohistochemical and ultrastructural observations. *Am J Clin Pathol* 1990;94:538–545.
194. Gonzalez-Crussi F, deMello DE, Sotelo-Avila C. Omental-mesenteric myxoid hamartomas. *Am J Surg Pathol* 1983;7:567–578.
195. Merino MJ, Livolsi VA. Signet ring carcinoma of the female breast: a clinicopathologic analysis of 24 cases. *Cancer* 1981;48:1830–1837.
196. Abu-Rustum NR, Aghajanian CA, Venkatraman ES, Feroz F, Barakat RR. Metastatic breast carcinoma to the abdomen and pelvis. *Gynecol Oncol* 1997;66:41–44.
197. Michael H, Sutton G, Roth LM. Ovarian carcinoma with extracellular mucin production: reassessment of "pseudomyxoma ovarii et peritonei." *Int J Gynecol Pathol* 1987;6:298–312
198. Young RH, Gilks CB, Scully RE. Mucinous tumors of the appendix associated with mucinous tumors of the ovary and pseudomyxoma peritonei. A clinicopathological analysis of 22 cases supporting an origin in the appendix. *Am J Surg Pathol* 1991;5:415–429.
199. Seidman JD, Elsayed AM, Sobin LH, Tavassoli FA. Association of mucinous tumors of the ovary and appendix. A clinicopathologic study of 25 cases. *Am J Surg Pathol* 1993;17 22–34
200. Costa MJ. Pseudomyxoma peritonei. Histologic predictors of patient survival. *Arch Pathol Lab Med* 1994;118:1215–1219.
201. Prayson RA, Hart WR, Petras RE. Pseudomyxoma peritonei. A clinicopathologic study of 19 cases with emphasis on site of origin and nature of associated ovarian tumors. *Am J Surg Pathol* 1994;18:591–603.
202. Rennett BM, Kurman RJ, Zahn CM, et al. Pseudomyxoma peritonei in women: a clinicopathologic analysis of 30 cases with emphasis on site of origin, prognosis, and relationship to ovarian mucinous tumors of low malignant potential. *Hum Pathol* 1995;56:509–524.
203. Rennett BM, Zahn CM, Kurman RJ, Kass ME, Sugarbaker PH, Shmookler BM. Disseminated peritoneal adenomucinosis and peritoneal mucinous carcinomatosis. A clinicopathologic analysis of 109 cases with emphasis on distinguishing pathologic features, site of origin, prognosis, and relationship to "pseudomyxoma peritonei." *Am J Surg Pathol* 1995;19:1390–1408.
204. Young RH, Rosenberg AE, Clement PB. Mucin deposits presenting within inguinal hernia sacs: a presenting finding of low grade mucinous cystic tumors of the appendix. A report of two cases and review of the literature. *Mod Pathol* 1997;10:1228–1232.
205. Lauchlan SC. The secondary müllerian system. *Obstet Gynecol Surv* 1972;27:133–146.
206. Ober WB, Black MB. Neoplasms of the subcoelomic mesenchyme. *Arch Pathol Lab Med* 1955;59:698–705.
207. Clement PB. Endometriosis, lesions of the secondary müllerian system, and pelvic mesothelial proliferations. In: Kurman RJ, ed. *Blaustein's pathology of the female genital tract*. New York: Springer-Verlag, 1994:647–703.
208. Fox H, Buckley CH. Current concepts of endometriosis. *Clin Obstet Gynaecol* 1984;11:279–287.
209. Jansen RPS, Russell P. Nonpigmented endometriosis: clinical, laparoscopic, and pathological definition. *Am J Obstet Gynecol* 1986;155:1154–1159.
210. Dmowski WP. Pitfalls in clinical, laparoscopic and histologic diagnosis of endometriosis. *Acta Obstet Gynecol Scand Suppl* 1984;123:61–66.
211. Cantor JO, Fenoglio CM, Richart RM. A case of extensive abdominal endometriosis. *Am J Obstet Gynecol* 1979;134:846–847.
212. Scully RE, Richardson GS, Barlow JF. The development of malignancy in endometriosis. *Clin Obstet Gynecol* 1966;9:384–411.
213. Mostoufizadeh M, Scully RE. Malignant tumors arising in endometriosis. *Clin Obstet Gynecol* 1980;23:951–963.
214. Dmowski WP, Radwanska E. Current concepts on pathology, histogenesis and etiology of endometriosis. *Acta Obstet Gynecol Scand Suppl* 1984;123:29–33.
215. Egger H, Weigmann P. Clinical and surgical aspects of ovarian endometriotic cysts. *Arch Gynecol* 1982;233:37–45.
216. Floberg J, Backdahl M, Silfersward C, Thomassen PA. Postpartum perforation of the colon due to endometriosis. *Acta Obstet Gynecol Scand* 1984;63:183–184.
217. Anderson M, Edmond RM. Rupture of an endometriotic cyst in late pregnancy. *Br J Obstet Gynaecol* 1974;81:907–908.
218. Rosman F, D'Ablaing III G, Marrs RP. Pregnancy complicated by ruptured endometrioma. *Obstet Gynecol* 1983;62:519–521.
219. Rogers WS, Seckinger DL. Decidual tissue as a cause of intrabdominal hemorrhage during labor. *Obstet Gynecol* 1965;25:391–397.
220. Bergvist A, Ljungberg O, Myhre E. Human endometrium and endometriotic tissue obtained simultaneously: a comparative histological study. *Int J Gynecol Pathol* 1984;3:135–145.
221. Metzger DA, Olive DL, Haney AF. Limited hormonal responsiveness of ectopic endometrium: histologic correlation with intrauterine endometrium. *Hum Pathol* 1988;19:1417–1424.
222. Kempers RD, Dockerty MB, Hunt AB, et al. Significant postmenopausal endometriosis. *Surg Gynecol Obstet* 1960;111:348–356.
223. Lipscomb GH, Ling FW, Photopulos GJ. Ovarian abscess arising within an endometrioma. *Obstet Gynecol* 1991;78:951–954.
224. Czernobilsky B, Morris WJ. A histologic study of ovarian endometriosis with emphasis on hyperplastic and atypical changes. *Obstet Gynecol* 1979;53:318–323.
225. Schuger L, Simon A, Okon E. Cytomegaly in benign ovarian cysts. *Arch Pathol Lab Med* 1986;110:928–929.
226. Balouk F, Ross JS, Wolf BC. Ovarian endometriotic cysts. An analysis of cytologic atypia and DNA ploidy patterns. *Am J Clin Pathol* 1994;102:415–419.
227. Rutgers JL, Scully RE. Ovarian müllerian mucinous papillary cystadenomas of borderline malignancy. A clinicopathological analysis. *Cancer* 1988;61:340–348.
228. Rutgers JL, Scully RE. Ovarian mixed-epithelial papillary cystadeno-

228. mas of borderline malignancy of müllerian type. A clinicopathological analysis. *Cancer* 1988;61:546–554.
229. Seidman JD. Prognostic importance of hyperplasia and atypia in endometriosis. *Int J Gynecol Pathol* 1996;15:1–9.
230. Rohlfing MB, Kao KJ, Woodard BH. Endomyometriosis: possible association with leiomyomatosis disseminata and endometriosis (letter). *Arch Pathol Lab Med* 1981;105:556–557.
231. Cozzutto C. Uterus-like mass replacing ovary. Report of a new entity. *Arch Pathol Lab Med* 1981;105:508–511.
232. Scully RE. Smooth-muscle differentiation in genital tract disorders (editorial). *Arch Pathol Lab Med* 1981;105:505–507.
233. McDougal RA, Roth LM. Ovarian adenomyoma associated with an endometriotic cyst. *South Med J* 1986;79:640–642.
234. Pueblitz-Peredo S, Luevano-Flores E, Rincon-Taracena R, Ochoa-Carrillo FJ. Uteruslike mass of the ovary: endomyometriosis or congenital malformation? A case with a discussion of histogenesis. *Arch Pathol Lab Med* 1985;109:361–364.
235. Rahilly MA, Al-Nafusi A. Uterus-like mass of the ovary associated with endometrioid carcinoma. *Histopathology* 1991;18:549–551.
236. Chalmers JA. Mulleroma—a rare cause of dysmenorrhoea. *Br J Obstet Gynaecol* 1961;68:762–764.
237. Kurman RJ, Funk RL, Kirshenbaum AH. Spina bifida with associated choristoma of müllerian origin. *J Pathol* 1969;99:324–327.
238. Rosai J. Uteruslike mass replacing ovary (letter). *Arch Pathol Lab Med* 1982;106:364.
239. Clement PB, Young RH, Scully RE. Stromal endometriosis of the uterine cervix. A variant of endometriosis that may simulate a sarcoma. *Am J Surg Pathol* 1990;14:449–455.
240. Hughesdon PE. The endometrial identity of benign stromatosis of the ovary and its relation to other forms of endometriosis. *J Pathol* 1976;119:201–209.
241. Lauchlan SC. The cytology of endometriosis. *Am J Obstet Gynecol* 1966;94:533–535.
242. von Numers C. Observations on metaplastic changes in the germinal epithelium of the ovary and on the aetiology of ovarian endometriosis. *Acta Obstet Gynecol Scand* 1965;44:107–116.
243. Leiman G, Naylor G. Mucinous metaplasia in scar endometriosis. Diagnosis by aspiration cytology. *Diagn Cytopathol* 1985;1:153–156.
244. Young RH, Prat J, Scully RE. Endometrioid stromal sarcomas of the ovary. A clinicopathologic analysis of 23 cases. *Cancer* 1984;53:1143–1155.
245. Clement PB, Granai CO, Young RH, Scully RE. Endometriosis with myxoid change: a case simulating pseudomyxoma peritonei. *Am J Surg Pathol* 1994;18:849–853.
246. Gerbie AB, Greene RR, Reis RA. Heteroplastic bone and cartilage in the female genital tract. *Obstet Gynecol* 1958;11:573–578.
247. Shipton EA, Meares SD. Heterotopic bone formation in the ovary. *Aust N Z J Obstet Gynaecol* 1965;5:100–102.
248. Roth LM. Endometriosis with perineural involvement. *Am J Clin Pathol* 1973;59:807–809.
249. Abdel-Shahid RB, Beresford JM, Curry RH. Endometriosis of the ureter with vascular involvement. *Obstet Gynecol* 1974;43:113–117.
250. Kapadia SB, Russak RR, O'Donnell WF, Harris RN, Lecky JW. Postmenopausal ureteral endometriosis with atypical adenomatous hyperplasia following hysterectomy, bilateral oophorectomy, and long-term estrogen therapy. *Obstet Gynecol* 1984;64:60S–63S.
251. Granai CO, Walters MD, Safaii H, et al. Malignant transformation of vaginal endometriosis. *Obstet Gynecol* 1984;64:592–595.
252. Ray J, Conger M, Ireland K. Ureteral obstruction in postmenopausal woman with endometriosis. *Urology* 1985;26:577–578.
253. Young EE, Gamble CN. Primary adenocarcinoma of the rectovaginal septum arising from endometriosis. Report of a case. *Cancer* 1969;24:597–601.
254. Buckley CH. Tamoxifen and endometriosis. Case report. *Br J Obstet Gynaecol* 1990;97:645–646.
255. Moll UM, Chumas JC, Chalas E, Mann WJ. Ovarian carcinoma arising in atypical endometriosis. *Obstet Gynecol* 1990;75:537–539.
256. LaGrenade A, Silverberg SG. Ovarian tumors associated with atypical endometriosis. *Hum Pathol* 1988;19:1080–1084.
257. Fukunaga M, Nomura K, Ishikawa E, Ushigome S. Ovarian atypical endometriosis: its close association with malignant epithelial tumors. *Histopathology* 1997;30:249–255.
258. Toki T, Fujii S, Silverberg SG. A clinicopathologic study of the association of endometriosis and carcinoma of the ovary using a scoring system. *Int J Gynecol Cancer* 1996;6:68–75.
259. Kistner RW. Current status of the hormonal treatment of endometriosis. *Clin Obstet Gynecol* 1966;9:271–292.
260. Moller NE. The Arias-Stella phenomenon in endometriosis. *Acta Obstet Gynecol Scand* 1959;38:271–274.
261. Sobel HJ, Marquet E, Schwarz R, et al. Optically clear endometrial nuclei. *Ultrastruct Pathol* 1984;6:229–231.
262. Fechner RE. The surgical pathology of the reproductive system and breast during oral contraceptive therapy. *Pathol Annu* 1971:6:299–319.
263. Pedersen H, Rank F. Morphology of endometriosis before and during treatment with danazol. *Acta Obstet Gynecol Scand Suppl* 1984;123:13–14.
264. Schweppe KW, Wynn RM. Endocrine dependency of endometriosis: an ultrastructural study. *Eur J Obstet Gynecol Reprod Biol* 1984;17:193–208.
265. Horie A, Ishii N, Matsumoto M, et al. Leiomyomatosis in the pelvic lymph node and peritoneum. *Acta Pathol Jpn* 1984;34:813–819.
266. Kaplan C, Benirschke K, Johnson KC. Leiomyomatosis peritonealis disseminata with endometrium. *Obstet Gynecol* 1980;55:119–122.
267. Kuo T, London SN, Dinh TV. Endometriosis occurring in leiomyomatosis peritonealis disseminata. Ultrastructural study and histogenetic consideration. *Am J Surg Pathol* 1980;4:197–204.
268. Albukerk JN, Berlin M, Palladino VC, et al. Endometriosis in peritoneal gliomatosis (letter). *Arch Pathol Lab Med* 1979;103:98–99.
269. Bassler R, Theele CH, Labach H. Nodular and tumorlike gliomatosis peritonei with endometriosis caused by a mature ovarian teratoma. *Pathol Res Pract* 1982;175:392–403.
270. Sinder C, Dochat GR, Wentsler NE. Splenoendometriosis. *Am J Obstet Gynecol* 1965;92:883–884.
271. Clement PB, Young RH, Scully RE. Liesegang rings in endometriosis. A report of three cases. *Int J Gynecol Pathol* 1989;8:271–276.
272. Herbold DR, Frable WJ, Kraus FT. Isolated noninfectious granuloma of the ovary. *Int J Gynecol Pathol* 1984;2:380–391.
273. Clement PB, Scully RE. Endometrial stromal sarcomas of the uterus with extensive endometrioid glandular differentiation. A report of three cases that caused problems in differential diagnosis. *Int J Gynecol Pathol* 1992;11:163–173.
274. Kempson RL, Hendrickson MR. Pure mesenchymal neoplasms of the uterine corpus. In: Fox H, ed. *Haines and Taylor Obstetrical and Gynaecological Pathology*. New York: Churchill Livingstone, 1987:426.
275. Brooks JJ, Wheeler JE. Malignancy arising in extragonadal endometriosis. A case report and summary of the world literature. *Cancer* 1977;40:3065–3073.
276. Heaps JM, Nieberg RK, Berek JS. Malignant neoplasms arising in endometriosis. *Obstet Gynecol* 1990;75:1023–1028.
277. Reimnitz C, Brand E, Nieberg RK, et al. Malignancy arising in endometriosis associated with unopposed estrogen replacement. *Obstet Gynecol* 1988;71:444–447.
278. Russell P. The pathological assessment of ovarian neoplasms. II. The proliferating "epithelial" tumours. *Pathology* 1979;11:251–282.
279. Hitti IF, Glasberg SS, Lubicz S. Clear cell carcinoma arising in extraovarian endometriosis: report of three cases and review of the literature. *Gynecol Oncol* 1990;39:314–320.
280. Ahn GH, Scully RE. Clear cell carcinoma of the inguinal region arising from endometriosis. *Cancer* 1991;67:116–120.
281. Gray LA, Barnes ML. Relation of endometriosis to ovarian carcinoma. *Am Surg* 1965;31:798–806.
282. Lele SB, Piver S, Barlow JJ, et al. Squamous cell carcinoma arising in ovarian endometriosis. *Gynecol Oncol* 1978;6:290–293.
283. Naresh KN, Ahuja VK, Rao CR, et al. Squamous cell carcinoma arising in endometriosis of the ovary. *J Clin Pathol* 1991;44:958–959.
284. Shiraki M, Otis CN, Powell JL. Endometrial stromal sarcoma arising from ovarian and extraovarian endometriosis—report of two cases and review of the literature. *Surg Pathol* 1991;4:333–343.
285. Chumas JC, Thanning L, Mann WJ. Malignant mixed müllerian tumor arising in extragenital endometriosis: report of a case and review of the literature. *Gynecol Oncol* 1986;23:227–233.
286. Cooper P. Mixed mesodermal tumour and clear cell carcinoma arising in ovarian endometriosis. *Cancer* 1978;42:2827–2831.
287. Mahoney AD, Waisman J, Zeldis LJ. Adenomyoma. A precursor of extrauterine müllerian adenosarcoma? *Arch Pathol Lab Med* 1977;101:579–584.
288. Lankerani MR, Aubrey RW, Reid JD. Endometriosis of the colon with mixed "germ cell" tumor. *Am J Clin Pathol* 1982;78:555–559.

289. Rutgers JL, Young RH, Scully RE. Ovarian yolk sac tumor arising from an endometrioid carcinoma. *Hum Pathol* 1987;18:1296–1299.
290. Griffith LM, Carcangiu M. Sex cord tumor with annular tubules associated with endometriosis of the fallopian tube. *Am J Clin Pathol* 1991;96:259–262.
291. Hafiz MA, Toker C. Multicentric ovarian and extraovarian cystadenofibroma. *Obstet Gynecol* 1986;68:94S–9 S
292. Ortega I, Nogales F, Gonzalez-Campora R, et al. Extragenital endometrioid cystadenofibroma. *Acta Obstet Gynecol Scand* 1982;61:283–284.
293. Clark JE, Wood H, Jaffurs WJ, et al. Endometrioid-type cystadenocarcinoma arising in the mesosalpinx. *Obstet Gynecol* 1979;54:656–658.
294. Chang KL, Crabtree GS, Lim-Tan SK, Kempor RL, Hendrickson MR. Primary extrauterine endometrial stromal neoplasms: a clinicopathologic study of 20 cases and a review of the literature. *Int J Gynecol Pathol* 1993;12:282–296.
295. Mira JL, Fenoglio-Preiser CM, Husseinzadeh N. Malignant mixed müllerian tumor of the extraovarian secondary müllerian system. Report of two cases and review of the English literature. *Arch Pathol Lab Med* 1995;119:1044–1049.
296. Bard ES, Bard DS, Vargas-Cortes F. Extrauterine müllerian adenosarcoma; a clinicopathologic report of a case with distant metastases and review of the literature. *Gynecol Oncol* 1987;26:251–274.
297. Clement PB, Scully RE. Extrauterine mesodermal (müllerian) adenosarcoma. A clinicopathologic analysis of five cases. *Am J Clin Pathol* 1978;69:276–283.
298. Russell P, Slavutin L, Laverty CR, et al. Extrauterine mesodermal (müllerian) adenosarcoma. A case report. *Pathology* 1979;11:557–560.
299. Kerner H, Lichtig C, Beck D. Extrauterine müllerian adenosarcoma of the peritoneal mesothelium: a clinicopathologic and electron microscopic study. *Obstet Gynecol* 1989;73:510–513.
300. Zinsser KR, Wheeler JE. Endosalpingiosis in the omentum. A study of autopsy and surgical material. *Am J Surg Pathol* 1982;6:109–117.
301. Tutschka BG, Lauchlan SC. Endosalpingiosis. *Obstet Gynecol* 1980;55:57S–60S.
302. Holmes MD, Levin HS, Ballard LA. Endosalpingiosis. *Cleve Clin Q* 1981;48:345–352.
303. Kern WH. Benign papillary structures with psammoma bodies in culdocentesis fluid. *Acta Cytol* 1969;13:178–180.
304. Sidaway MK, Silverberg SG. Endosalpingiosis in female peritoneal washings: a diagnostic pitfall. *Int J Gynecol Pathol* 1987;6:340–346.
305. Sneige M, Fernandez T, Copeland LJ, et al. Müllerian inclusions in peritoneal washings. *Acta Cytol* 1986;30:271–276.
306. Hallman KB, Nahhas WA, Connolly PJ. Endosalpingiosis as a source of psammoma bodies in a Papanicolaou smear. A case report. *J Reprod Med* 1991;36:675–678.
307. Kern SB. Prevalence of psammoma bodies in Papanicolaou-stained cervicovaginal smears. *Acta Cytol* 1991;35:81–88.
308. McCaughey WTE, Kirk ME, Lester W, et al. Peritoneal epithelial lesions associated with proliferative serous tumours of the ovary. *Histopathology* 1984;8:195–208.
309. Burmeister RE, Fechner RE, Franklin RR. Endosalpingiosis of the peritoneum. *Obstet Gynecol* 1969;34:310–318.
310. Bryce RL, Barbatis C, Charnock M. Endosalpingiosis in pregnancy. Case report. *Br J Obstet Gynaecol* 1982;89:135–138.
311. Chen KTK. Benign glandular inclusions of the peritoneum and periaortic lymph nodes. *Diagn Gynecol Obstet* 1981;3:265–268.
312. Dallenbach-Hellweg G. Atypical endosalpingiosis a case report with consideration of the differential diagnosis of glandular subperitoneal inclusions. *Pathol Res Pract* 1987;182:180–182.
313. Cajigas A, Axiotis CA. Endosalpingiosis of the vermiform appendix. *Int J Gynecol Pathol* 1990;9:291–295.
314. Shen SC, Bansal M, Purrazzella R, et al. Benign glandular inclusions in lymph nodes, endosalpingiosis, and salpingitis isthmica nodosa in a young girl with clear cell adenocarcinoma of the cervix. *Am J Surg Pathol* 1983;7:293–300.
315. Dore N, Landry M, Cadotte M, et al. Cutaneous endosalpingiosis. *Arch Dermatol* 1980;116:909–912.
316. Sinykin MB. Endosalpingiosis. *Minn Med* 1960;43:759–761.
317. Schuldenfrei R, Janovski NA. Disseminated endosalpingiosis associated with bilateral papillary serous cystadenocarcinoma of the ovaries. A case report. *Am J Obstet Gynecol* 1962;84:382–389.
318. Clement PB, Young RH. Tumor-like manifestations of florid cystic endosalpingiosis: a report of four cases including the first reported cases of mural endosalpingiosis of the uterus. *Am J Surg Pathol* (In press).
319. Young RH, Clement PB. Müllerianosis of the urinary bladder. *Mod Pathol* 1996;9:731–737.
320. Bell DA, Scully RE. Benign and borderline serous lesions of the peritoneum in women. *Pathol Annu* 1989;24(2):1–25.
321. Prade M, Spatz A, Bentley R, Duvillard P, Bognel C, Robboy SJ. Borderline and malignant serous tumor arising in pelvic lymph nodes: evidence of origin in benign glandular inclusions. *Int J Gynecol Pathol* 1995;14:87–91.
322. Bransilver BR, Ferenczy A, Richart RM. Female genital tract remnants. An ultrastructural comparison of hydatid of Morgagni and mesonephric ducts and tubules. *Arch Pathol Lab Med* 1973;96:255–261.
323. Copeland LJ, Silva EG, Gershenson DM, et al. The significance of müllerian inclusions found at second-look laparotomy in patients with epithelial ovarian neoplasms. *Obstet Gynecol* 1988;71:763–770.
324. Bell DA, Scully RE. Serous borderline tumors of the peritoneum. *Am J Surg Pathol* 1990;14:230–239.
325. Biscotti CV, Hart WR. Peritoneal serous micropapillomatosis of low malignant potential (serous borderline tumors of the peritoneum). A clinicopathologic study of 17 cases. *Am J Surg Pathol* 1992;16:467–475.
326. Gooneratne S, Sassone M, Blaustein A, et al. Serous surface papillary carcinoma of the ovary: a clinicopathologic study of 16 cases. *Int J Gynecol Pathol* 1982;1:258–269.
327. Tobacman JK, Tucker MA, Kase R, Greene MH, Costa J, Fraumeni JF Jr. Intra-abdominal carcinomatosis after prophylactic oophorectomy in ovarian-cancer-prone families. *Lancet* 1982;2:795–797.
328. Hochster H, Wernz JC, Muggia FM. Intra-abdominal carcinomatosis with histologically normal ovaries. *Cancer Treat Rep* 1984;68:921–922.
329. August CZ, Murad TM, Newton M. Multiple focal extraovarian serous carcinoma. *Int J Gynecol Pathol* 1985;4:11–23.
330. White PF, Merino MJ, Barwick KW. Serous surface papillary carcinoma of the ovary: a clinical, pathologic, ultrastructural, and immunohistochemical study of 11 cases. *Pathol Annu* 1985;20(1):403–418.
331. Mills SE, Andersen WA, Fechner RE, Austin MB. Serous surface papillary carcinoma. A clinicopathologic study of 10 cases and comparison with stage III-IV ovarian serous carcinoma. *Am J Surg Pathol* 1988;12:827–834.
332. Dalrymple JC, Bannatyne P, Russell P, et al. Extraovarian peritoneal serous papillary carcinoma. A clinicopathologic study of 31 cases. *Cancer* 1989;64:110–115.
333. Feuer GA, Shevchuk M, Calanog A. Normal-sized ovary carcinoma syndrome. *Obstet Gynecol* 1989;73:786–792.
334. Raju U, Fine G, Greenawald KA, Ohorodnik JM. Primary papillary serous neoplasia of the peritoneum: a clinicopathologic and ultrastructural study of eight cases. *Hum Pathol* 1989;20:426–436.
335. Rutledge ML, Silva EG, McLemore D, El-Naggar A. Serous surface carcinoma of the ovary and peritoneum. A flow cytometric study. *Pathol Annu* 1989;24(2):227–235.
336. Wick MR, Mills SE, Dehner LP, Bollinger DJ, Fechner RE. Serous papillary carcinomas arising from the peritoneum and ovaries. A clinicopathologic and immunohistochemical comparison. *Int J Gynecol Pathol* 1989;8:179–188.
337. Fromm G, Gershenson DM, Silva EG. Papillary serous carcinoma of the peritoneum. *Obstet Gynecol* 1990;75:89–95.
338. Khoury N, Raju U, Crissman JD, Zarbo RJ, Greenawald KA. A comparative immunohistochemical study of peritoneal and ovarian serous tumors, and mesotheliomas. *Hum Pathol* 1990;21:811–819.
339. Ransom DT, Shreyaskumar RP, Keeney GL, Malkasian GD, Edmonson JH. Papillary serous carcinoma of the peritoneum. A review of 33 cases treated with platin-based chemotherapy. *Cancer* 1990;66:1091–1094.
340. Truong LD, Maccato ML, Awalt H, et al. Serous surface carcinoma of the peritoneum: a clinicopathologic study of 22 cases. *Hum Pathol* 1990;21:99–110.
341. Altaras MM, Aviram R, Cohen I, et al. Primary peritoneal papillary serous adenocarcinoma: clinical and management aspects. *Gynecol Oncol* 1991;40:230–236.
342. Bloss JD, Liao S, Buller RE, et al. Extraovarian peritoneal serous papillary carcinoma: a case-control retrospective comparison to papillary adenocarcinoma of the ovary. *Gynecol Oncol* 1993;50:347–351.

343. Killackey MA, Davis AR. Papillary serous carcinoma of the peritoneal surface: matched-case comparison with papillary serous ovarian carcinoma. *Gynecol Oncol* 1993;51:171–174.
344. Piver MS, Jishi MF, Tsukada Y, Nava G. Primary peritoneal carcinoma after prophylactic oophorectomy in women with a family history of ovarian cancer. A report of the Gilda Radner familial ovarian cancer registry. *Cancer* 1993;71:2751–2755.
345. Fowler JM, Nieberg RK, Schooler TA, Berek JS. Peritoneal adenocarcinoma (serous) of müllerian type: a subgroup of women presenting with peritoneal carcinomatosis. *Int J Gynecol Cancer* 1994;4:43–51.
346. Mullhollan TJ, Silva EG, Tornos C, Guerrieri C, Fromm G, Gershenson D. Ovarian involvement by serous surface papillary carcinoma. *Int J Gynecol Pathol* 1994;13:120–126.
347. Rothacker D, Mobius G. Varieties of serous surface papillary carcinoma of the peritoneum in Northern Germany: a thirty-year autopsy study. *Int J Gynecol Pathol* 1995;14:310–318.
348. Zhou J, Iwasa Y, Konishi I, et al. Papillary serous carcinoma of the peritoneum in women. A clinicopathologic and immunohistochemical study. *Cancer* 1995;76:429–436.
349. Ben-Baruch G, Sivan E, Moran O, Rizel S, Menczer J, Seidman DS. Primary peritoneal serous papillary carcinoma: a study of 25 cases and comparison with stage III-IV ovarian papillary serous carcinoma. *Gynecol Oncol* 1996;60:393–396.
350. Kowalski LD, Kanbour AI, Price FV, et al. A case-matched molecular comparison of extraovarian versus primary ovarian adenocarcinoma. *Cancer* 1997;79:1587–1594.
351. Moll UM, Valea F, Chumas J. Role of p53 alteration in primary peritoneal carcinoma. *Int J Gynecol Pathol* 1997;16:156–162.
352. Weir MM, Bell DA, Young RH. Grade 1 peritoneal serous carcinomas: a report of 14 cases and comparison with 7 peritoneal serous psammocarcinomas and 19 peritoneal serous borderline tumors. *Am J Surg Pathol* 1998;22:849–862.
353. McCaughey WTE, Schryer MJP, Lin X, et al. Extraovarian pelvic serous tumor with marked calcification. *Arch Pathol Lab Med* 1986;110:78–80.
354. Gilks CB, Bell DA, Scully RE. Serous psammocarcinoma of the ovary and peritoneum. *Int J Gynecol Pathol* 1990;9:110–121.
355. Genadry R, Parmley T, Woodruff JD. The origin and clinical behavior of the parovarian tumor. *Am J Obstet Gynecol* 1977;129:873–879.
356. Honore LH, Nickerson KG. Papillary serous cystadenoma arising in a paramesonephric cyst of the parovarium. *Am J Obstet Gynecol* 1976;125:870–871.
357. Kanbour A, Salazar H, Stock R. Papillary cystadenoma originating in hydatid cyst of morgagni: clinicopathologic study and observations on histogenesis. *Lab Invest* 1978;38:350(abst).
358. Steinberg L, Rothman L, Drey NW. Müllerian cyst of the retroperitoneum. *Am J Obstet Gynecol* 1970;107:963–964.
359. Czernobilsky B, Lancet M. Broad ligament adenocarcinoma of müllerian origin. *Obstet Gynecol* 1972;40:238–242.
360. Aslani M, Ahn G, Scully RE. Serous papillary cystadenoma of borderline malignancy of broad ligament. *Int J Gynecol Pathol* 1988;7:131–138.
361. Aslani M, Scully RE. Primary carcinoma of the broad ligament. Report of four cases and review of the literature. *Cancer* 1989;64:1540–1545.
362. Ulbright TM, Morley DJ, Roth LM, et al. Papillary serous carcinoma of the retroperitoneum. *Am J Clin Pathol* 1983;79:633–637.
363. de Peralta MN, Delahoussaye PM, Tornos CS, Silva EG. Benign retroperitoneal cysts of müllerian type: a clinicopathologic study of three cases and review of the literature. *Int J Gynecol Pathol* 1994;13:273–278.
364. Clement PB, Young RH. Endocervicosis of the urinary bladder: a report of six cases of a benign müllerian lesion that may mimic adenocarcinoma. *Am J Surg Pathol* 1992;16:533–542.
365. Nazeer T, Ro JY, Tornos C, Ordonez NG, Ayala AG. Endocervical-type glands in the urinary bladder: a clinicopathologic study of six cases. *Hum Pathol* 1996;27:816–820.
366. Banerjee R, Gough J. Cystic mucinous tumours of the mesentery and retroperitoneum: report of three cases. *Histopathology* 1988;12:527–532.
367. Pennell TC, Gusdon JP Jr. Retroperitoneal mucinous cystadenoma. *Am J Obstet Gynecol* 1989;160:1229–1231.
368. Pearl ML, Valea F, Chumas J, Chalas E. Primary retroperitoneal mucinous cystadenocarcinoma of low malignant potential: a case report and literature review. *Gynecol Oncol* 1996;61:150–152.
369. Lee I-W, Ching K-C, Pang M, Ho T-H. Two cases of primary retroperitoneal mucinous cystadenocarcinoma. *Gynecol Oncol* 1996;63:145–150.
370. Sun CJ, Toker C, Masi JD, et al. Primary low grade adenocarcinoma occurring in the inguinal region. *Cancer* 1979;44:340–345.
371. Bransilver BR, Ferenczy A, Richart RM. Brenner tumors and Walthard cell nests. *Arch Pathol Lab Med* 1974;98:76–86.
372. Roth LM. The Brenner tumor and the Walthard cell nest. An electron microscopic study. *Lab Invest* 1974;31:15–23.
373. Teoh TB. The structure and development of Walthard nests. *J Pathol* 1953;66:433–439.
374. Sundarasivarao D. The müllerian vestiges and benign epithelial tumours of the epididymis. *J Pathol Bacteriol* 1953;66:417–432.
375. Hampton HL, Huffman HT, Meeks GR. Extraovarian Brenner tumor. *Obstet Gynecol* 1992;79:844–846.
376. Schatz JE, Colgan TJ. Squamous metaplasia of the peritoneum. *Arch Pathol Lab Med* 1991;115:397–398.
377. Evans H, Yates WA, Palmer WE, et al. Clear cell carcinoma of the sigmoid mesocolon: a tumor of the secondary müllerian system. *Am J Obstet Gynecol* 1990;162:161–163.
378. Lee KR, Verma U, Belinson J. Primary clear cell carcinoma of the peritoneum. *Gynecol Oncol* 1991;41:259–262.
379. Herr JC, Platz CE, Heidger PM Jr, et al. Smooth muscle within ovarian decidual nodules: a link to leiomyomatosis peritonealis disseminata? *Obstet Gynecol* 1979;53:451–456.
380. Ober WB, Grady HG, Schoenbucher AK. Ectopic ovarian decidua without pregnancy. *Am J Pathol* 1957;33:199–214.
381. Zaytsev P, Taxy JB. Pregnancy-associated ectopic decidua. *Am J Surg Pathol* 1987;11:526–530.
382. Harbitz HF. Ectopic decidua. *Acta Path Microbiol Scand Suppl* 1936;26:16–20.
383. Bettinger HF. Ectopic decidua in renal pelvis. *J Pathol Bacteriol* 1947;5:686–687.
384. O'Sullivan D, Heffernan CK. Deciduosis peritonei in pregnancy. Report of two cases. *Br J Obstet Gynaecol* 1960;67:1013–1016.
385. Kwan D, Pang LSC. Deciduosis peritonei. *Br J Obstet Gynaecol* 1964;71:804–806.
386. Richter MA, Choudhry A, Barton JJ, et al. Bleeding ectopic decidua as a cause of intraabdominal hemorrhage. A case report. *J Reprod Med* 1983;28:430–432.
387. Buttner A, Bassler R, Theele C. Pregnancy-associated extopic decidua (deciduosis) of the greater omentum. An analysis of 60 biopsies with cases of fibrosing deciduosis and leiomyomatosis peritonealis dissimenata. *Pathol Res Pract* 1993;189:352–359.
388. Ehrmann RL, Federschneider JM, Knapp RC. Distinguishing lymph node metastases from benign glandular inclusions in low-grade ovarian carcinoma. *Am J Obstet Gynecol* 1980;136:737–746.
389. Karp LA, Czernobilsky B. Glandular inclusions in pelvic and abdominal para-aortic lymph nodes. *Am J Clin Pathol* 1969;52:212–218.
390. Kheir SM, Mann WJ, Wilkerson JA. Glandular inclusions in lymph nodes. The problem of extensive involvement and relationship to salpingitis. *Am J Surg Pathol* 1981;5:353–359.
391. Russell P, Laverty CR. Benign 'müllerian' rests in pelvic lymph node. *Pathology* 1980;12:129–130.
392. Schnurr RC, Delgado G, Chun B. Benign glandular inclusions in para-aortic lymph nodes in women undergoing lymphadenectomies. *Am J Obstet Gynecol* 1978;130:813–816.
393. Silton RM. More glandular inclusions (letter). *Am J Surg Pathol* 1979;3:285–286.
394. Schneider V. Benign glandular lymph node inclusions. *Diagn Gynecol Obstet* 1980;2:313–320.
395. Huntrakoon M. Benign glandular inclusions in the abdominal lymph nodes of a man. *Hum Pathol* 1985;16:644–646.
396. Tazelaar HD, Vareska G. Benign glandular inclusions. *Hum Pathol* 1986;17:100–101.
397. Longo S. Benign lymph node inclusions. *Hum Pathol* 1976;7:349–354.
398. Schneider V, Walsh JW, Goplerud DR. Benign glandular inclusions in para-aortic lymph nodes: a cause for false positive lymphangiography. *Am J Obstet Gynecol* 1980;138:350–352.
399. Weir JH, Janovski NA. Paramesonephric lymph-node inclusions—a cause of obstructive uropathy. *Obstet Gynecol* 1963;21:363–367.
400. Kempson RL. Consultation Case. *Am J Surg Pathol* 1978;2:321–325.

401. Ferguson BR, Bennington JL, Haber SL. Histochemistry of mucosubstances and histology of mixed müllerian pelvic lymph node glandular inclusions. Evidence for histogenesis by müllerian metaplasia of coelomic epithelium. *Obstet Gynecol* 1969;33:617–625.
402. Baird DB, Reddick RL. Extraovarian mucinous metaplasia in a patient with bilateral mucinous borderline ovarian tumors: a case report. *Int J Gynecol Pathol* 1991;10:96–103.
403. Mills SE. Decidua and squamous metaplasia in abdominopelvic lymph nodes. *Int J Gynecol Pathol* 1983;2:209–215.
404. Koss LG. Miniature adenoacanthoma arising in an obturator lymph node. Report of a case. *Cancer* 1963;16:1369–1372.
405. Ashraf M, Boyd CB, Beresford WA. Ectopic decidual reaction in para-aortic and pelvic lymph nodes in the presence of cervical squamous cell carcinoma during pregnancy. *J Surg Oncol* 1984;26:6–8.
406. Burnett RA, Millan D. Decidual change in pelvic lymph nodes: a source of possible diagnostic error. *Histopathology* 1986;10:1089–1092.
407. Covell LM, Disciullo AJ, Knapp RC. Decidual change in pelvic lymph nodes in the presence of cervical squamous cell carcinoma during pregnancy. *Am J Obstet Gynecol* 1977;127:674–676.
408. Yoonessi M, Satchindanand SK, Ortinez CC, et al. Benign glandular elements and decidual reaction in retroperitoneal lymph nodes. *J Surg Oncol* 1982;19:81–86.
409. Cobb CJ. Ectopic decidua and metastatic squamous carcinoma: presentation in a single pelvic lymph node. *J Surg Oncol* 1988;38:126–129.
410. Boyce CR, Buddhdev HN. Pregnancy complicated by metastasizing leiomyoma of the uterus. *Obstet Gynecol* 1973;42:252–258.
411. Abell MR, Littler ER. Benign metastasizing uterine leiomyoma. Multiple lymph nodal metastases. *Cancer* 1975;36:2206–2213.
412. Cramer SF, Meyer JS, Kraner JF, et al. Metastasizing leiomyoma of the uterus. S-phase fraction, estrogen receptor, and ultrastructure. *Cancer* 1980;45:932–937.
413. Hsu YK, Rosenshein NB, Parmley TH, et al. Leiomyomatosis in pelvic lymph nodes. *Obstet Gynecol* 1981;57:91S–93S.
414. Idelson MG, Davids AM. Metastasis of uterine fibroleiomyomata. *Obstet Gynecol* 1963;21:78–85.
415. Rigaud C, Bogomoletz WV. Leiomyomatosis in pelvic lymph node. (Letter) *Arch Pathol Lab Med* 1983;107:153–154.
416. Bhattacharyya AK, Balogh K. Retroperitoneal lymphangioleiomyomatosis. A 36-year benign course in a postmenopausal woman. *Cancer* 1985;56:1144–1146.
417. Gyure KA, Hart WR, Kennedy AW. Lymphangiomyomatosis of the uterus associated with tuberous sclerosis and malignant neoplasia of the female genital tract: a report of two cases. *Int J Gynecol Pathol* 1995;14:344–351.

Subject Index

Subject Index

A
Abdominal cocooning, 1398, 2416
Aberrant immunoreactivity, 138–139
Abetalipoproteinemia, malabsorption in, 1359
Abruptio placentae, 2088
Abscess(es)
 brain, 399–400, 460
 Brodie's, 260, 283
 hepatic, 1557, 1558
 tubo-ovarian, 2307
Acanthamoeba, keratitis due to, 982
Acantholysis, 5
 intraepidermal bullae with, 18–23
 intraepidermal bullae without, 18
 subcorneal bullae with, 17–18
 subcorneal bullae without, 17
Acantholytic dermatosis, transient, 21
Acanthoma
 clear cell, 50
 large-cell, 53
 pilar sheath, 64
 spectacle-frame, 952–953
Acanthosis, 5
 glycogenic, of esophagus, 1304
 prurigoform, 16–17
 verrucous, 17
Acanthosis nigricans, 25
Achalasia, 1295
Achlorhydria, 1502
Acid maltase deficiency, 125
Acid mucin, in prostate carcinoma, 1913
Acidophil body, 1510
Acidophilic wings, of pituitary, 495
Acidophil stem cell adenoma, of pituitary, 498, 500, 511–512
Acinar cell(s), pancreatic
 altered, 1470–1471
 normal, 1473
Acinar cell carcinoma, of pancreas, 1484–1486
Acinar cell cystadenocarcinoma, of pancreas, 1491
Acini, of breast, 325, 327
Acinic cell carcinoma, of salivary glands, 865–866
Acinic cell tumor, of bronchus, 1099
Acinous cell carcinoma, of larynx, 940

Acne rosacea, 33
Acoustic neuroma, 447, 969–971
Acquired immunodeficiency syndrome (AIDS). *See also* Human immunodeficiency virus (HIV)
 bone marrow in, 656–658
 cholecystitis in, 1639–1641
 CNS lesions in, 401–404
 dementia in, 402
 ears in, 958
 gastritis in, 1324–1325
 intestinal biopsy in, 1370–1374
 liver in, 1546–1547
 lung biopsy in, 1056–1059
 myocardial lesions in, 1220–1221
 spleen in, 781
 testis in, 1962
Acrodermatitis enteropathica, 1359–1360
Acrospiroma, 59, 60, 61, 64
Acrotrichium, 4
ACTH. *See* Adrenocorticotropic hormone (ACTH)
Actin, in pulmonary neoplasms, 1109, 1110
Actinic keratosis, 51–53
 bowenoid, 54
Actinic lentigo, 97, 99
Actinomycosis
 of fallopian tube, 2397
 pelvic, 2307–2308
Adamantinoma, 292–293, 303
Adamantinomatous craniopharyngioma, 516–519
Addison's disease, 594, 595
Adenitis, viral, 723
Adenoacanthofibroma, endometrioid, 2331
Adenoacanthomas, colorectal, 1439
Adenocarcinoid tumor, appendiceal, 1445–1446
Adenocarcinoma
 anal, 1678–1679
 appendiceal, 1444–1445
 basal cell, 860–861
 bile duct, 1597, 1663–1664
 bladder, 1873–1874
 cervical. *See under* Cervical carcinoma
 colorectal, 1431, 1436–1437, 1439
 of ear

 inner, 971–972
 middle, 967
 endometrial. *See* Endometrial adenocarcinoma
 esophageal, 1299, 1301–1303
 of fallopian tube, 2405
 of gallbladder, 1651–1653
 gastric, 1330
 of liver, 1586, 1587
 of lung. *See under* Pulmonary neoplasms
 bronchial gland cell type of, 1086
 ovarian. *See* Ovarian tumors, carcinoma
 pancreatic, 1477–1484
 microglandular, 1496–1497
 of pleura, pseudomesotheliomatous, 1139–1141
 prostate. *See* Prostate cancer
 of rete testis, 2014–2015
 of salivary glands, 869
 mucin-producing, 869
 polymorphous low-grade, 869–870
 sinonasal, 898–900
 of small intestine, 1436
 of thymus, 1179
 of vagina, 2141–2142
 of vulva, 2129
Adenofibroma(s)
 endometrial, 2245, 2260–2261, 2264, 2270–2271
 of ovary, 2330–2331
 metanephric (nephrogenic), 1811–1812
 in children, 1850
 of ovary, 2335–2336
 papillary, of cervix, 2194
Adenohypophysial neuronal choristomas, 521
Adenoid basal carcinoma, of cervix, 2194
Adenoid cystic carcinoma
 of breast, 357
 of cervix, 2194
 of ear, 957
 of lacrimal gland, 1001
 of larynx, 940
 of prostate, 1934
 pulmonary, 1098–1099
 of salivary glands, 867–869
 sinonasal, 898

Adenoid squamous cell carcinoma, of
vulva, 2128
Adenoma(s)
ACTH, 512, 514
adrenal cortical, 598–600
appendiceal, 1442
bile duct, 1597, 1599
of bladder, 1861–1862
of breast
  ductal, 344, 371–372
  lactating, 365
  pleomorphic, 372
  tubular, 364
of colon, 1381–1382
of ear
  external, 955
  middle, 963–965
of esophagus, 1296
of extrahepatic bile ducts, 1661
of gallbladder, 1646, 1649
gastric, 1328–1329
hepatocellular, 1515, 1564–1567
intestinal, 1424–1436
  biopsy specimen of, 1430–1431
  and cancer, 1425–1427, 1431
  flat, 1418, 1428–1430, 1435–1436
  malignant, 1432
  pathology of, 1427–1428
  prevalence of, 1425
  with pseudoinvasion/misplaced
    epithelium, 1432–1434
  serrated, 1415–1416
  tubular, 1427–1428
  villous, 1427–1428
of lacrimal gland, pleomorphic, 1001
of larynx, 939–940
of lungs, 1072–1073
metanephric, 1811–1812
  in children, 1850
nephrogenic, 1861–1862
of nipple, 370–371
  syringomatous, 371
papillary eccrine, 63
parathyroid, 565–567
  atypical, 568
  with stromal component, 568–569
  and thyroid carcinoma, 536
Pick's, 1946, 1947
pituitary. See Pituitary adenoma(s)
of prostate, basal cell, 1933
salivary gland
  basal cell, 860–861
  canalicular, 860
  carcinoma arising in, 870–872
  clear-cell, 860
  glycogen-rich, 860
  monomorphic, 859–860
  pleomorphic, 857–859
  sebaceous, 863
sebaceous, 61, 63
thyroid

C-cell, 550
follicular, 544–545
Hürthle cell, 547–548, 560
hyalinizing trabecular, 545
papillary, 542
paraganglioma-like, 545
tubular apocrine, 63
vestibular gland, 2117
Adenoma malignum, of cervix,
  2187–2188
Adenomatoid tumor(s)
adrenal, 606
of fallopian tube, 2402
odontogenic, 844
of ovary, 2376
of peritoneum, 2421
of testis, 2018–2019
of uterus, 2288–2290
Adenomatosis, nipple, 63
Adenomatous hyperplasia
of rete testis, 2014
of salivary glands, 855
Adenomatous polyposis, familial, 1418,
  1434
Adenomatous polyposis syndromes, 1418,
  1434–1436
Adenomyoepithelial adenosis, 373
Adenomyoepithelioma, of breast, 373
Adenomyoma
endometrial, 2245, 2258–2259, 2264
of small bowel, 1360
Adenomyomatosis, of gallbladder, 1639,
  1646
Adenomyomatous hyperplasia, of
  gallbladder, 1639, 1646
Adenomyosis, of myometrium, 2271
Adenopathy
reactive, 715–730
  causing architectural effacement,
    726–730
  with follicular hyperplasia, 715–722
  with interfollicular hyperplasia,
    722–726
  sinus histiocytosis with massive,
    724–726
Adenosarcoma
cervical, 2195–2196
endometrial, 2261–2262, 2264–2265,
  2270–2271
of ovary, 2334
Adenosine monophosphate (AMP)
  deaminase deficiency, 126
Adenosis
of breast, 328, 329, 330–334
  adenomyoepithelial, 373
  apocrine, 329, 331
  blunt duct, 329, 330
  microglandular, 332, 333–334
  nodular, 331
  sclerosing, 330–331, 332
  secretory, 334

simple, 330
tubular, 333
vaginal, 2133–2135
Adenosis tumor, of breast, 331
Adenosquamous carcinoma
of breast, 359–360
of cervix, 2193–2194
of endometrium, 2240, 2247–2249,
  2264
of esophagus, 1299, 1304
of lung, 1095
of oral cavity, 831–834
of pancreas, 1480–1481
of penis, 2056
of prostate, 1930
of thymus, 1178–1179
Adenovirus
colitis due to, 1371
hepatitis due to, 1515, 1535–1536
Adenylate deaminase deficiency, 126
Adipose tissue lesions, 166
Adnexal tumors
female, of probable wolffian origin,
  2407–2408
of skin, 59–60
Adrenal cortex, development, anatomy,
  and physiology of, 589–591
Adrenal cortical adenomas, 598–600
Adrenal cortical carcinoma, 600–605
Adrenal cortical hormone synthesis,
  defects in, 1965
Adrenal cortical hyperplasia, 595–597
Adrenal cortical nodules, 600
Adrenal cortical rests, 1948
Adrenal cysts, 605
Adrenal cytomegaly, 593
Adrenal glands, 589–619
adenomatoid tumors of, 606
aplasia of, 592
carcinosarcoma of, 608
congenital anomalies and
  developmental disorders of,
  592–594
connective tissue tumors of, 606–607
in Conn's syndrome, 599–600
in Cushing's syndrome, 595–596,
  598–599
development, anatomy, and physiology
  of, 589–591
dysembryonic neoplasms of, 608
ectopic, 592
heterotopic, 592
hyperfunctional states of, 595–598
hypofunctional states of, 594–595
lymphoma of, 607–608
malignant melanoma of, 608
metastases to, 607
myelolipoma of, 605
oncocytic tumors of, 605–606
ovarian thecal metaplasia of, 606
union (fusion) of, 592

Adrenal gland tumors, ovarian metastases of, 2381
Adrenal hemorrhage, 594
Adrenal hyperplasia, congenital, 593–594
Adrenal hypoplasia, 592–593
Adrenal insufficiency, 594–595
Adrenal medulla
 development, anatomy, and physiology of, 591
 ganglioneuroblastoma of, 608–613
 ganglioneuroma of, 613–614
 neuroblastoma of, 608–613
 neuroendocrine cells and neoplasms of, 484
 pheochromocytoma of, 614–618
  composite, 616–617, 635–636
  familial, 617–618, 637
  malignant, 617
 tumors of, 608–618
Adrenal medullary hyperplasia, 618–619
Adrenal pseudocysts, 605
Adrenocortical disease, primary pigmented nodular, 597–598
Adrenocorticotropic hormone (ACTH)
 ectopic production of, 596
 pancreatic tumors producing, 1501
 plasma concentration of, 590
Adrenocorticotropic hormone (ACTH) adenomas, 512, 514
Adrenogenital syndromes, 600
 congenital, 593–594
Adrenoleukodystrophy, 465
Adrenomyeloneuropathy, 593
Adriamycin cardiomyopathy, 1212
Adventitial cystic disease, 1277
Adventitial dermis, 4
AFP (alpha fetoprotein), in hepatocellular carcinoma, 1576
Aganglionosis, zonal, 1391
Aging, blood vessels with, 1253, 1254
Agminate nevi, 99
AIDS. See Acquired immunodeficiency syndrome (AIDS)
AIDS dementia complex, 402
Alagille's syndrome, 1518–1519
Albright's syndrome, 302
Albumin, in hepatocellular carcinoma, 1583, 1584
Alcohol, and oral squamous cell carcinoma, 810
Alcoholic cardiomyopathy, 1212
Alcoholic hepatitis, 1511, 1529–1530
 steato-, 1515
Aldosterone
 regulation of secretion of, 590–591
 urinary concentration of, 590
Alkylating agents, effect on testis of, 1958
Allergic bronchopulmonary aspergillosis, 1024–1025
Allergic contact dermatitis, 6–7
Allergic granulomatosis of Churg and Strauss, 29
Allergic granulomatous prostatitis, 1898
Allergic vasculitis, 28
Alopecia mucinosa, 33–34
Alpha *1*-antitrypsin, in liver, 1515
Alpha *1*-antitrypsin deficiency
 liver in, 1519–1521
 panniculitis due to, 39
Alpha chain disease, 691
Alpha fetoprotein (AFP), in hepatocellular carcinoma, 1576
Alport's syndrome, 1734–1736, 1776
Alternating fascicle pattern, 169
Aluminum toxicity, 244, 250
Alveolar damage, diffuse, 1018–1021
Alveolar proteinosis, pulmonary, 1053–1054
Alveolar rhabdomyosarcoma, 172–174
Alveolar soft part sarcoma, 190–191
Alveolitis, extrinsic allergic, 1021–1023
Alzheimer's disease, 392, 393, 463–464
Amebiasis, intestinal, 1385
Amebic abscesses, hepatic, 1557, 1558
Ameloblastic carcinoma, 847
Ameloblastic fibroma, 843
Ameloblastic fibrosarcoma, 848
Ameloblastoma, 842–843
 malignant, 847
Amianthoid fibers, intranodal hemorrhagic spindle-cell tumor with, 729–730
Amine precursor uptake and decarboxylation (APUD) cell concept, 483, 625
Amine precursor uptake and decarboxylation (APUD)omas, 2176
Amiodarone, thyroid abnormalities due to, 534
Amnionitis, 2095, 2096, 2097, 2100–2103
Amnion nodosum, 2092
AMP (adenosine monophosphate) deaminase deficiency, 126
Amyloid angiopathy, 407, 1270
Amyloid deposits
 adrenal insufficiency due to, 594
 of eyelids, 990
Amyloidoma, of CNS, 455
Amyloidosis
 of bladder, 1859
 of cornea, familial subepithelial, 980
 diffuse septal, 1056
 of fallopian tube, 2398
 gastrointestinal involvement in, 1339–1340, 1391
 lichen, 37
 of liver, 1513, 1543, 1544
 macular, 37
 nodular
  intraparenchymal, 1056
  of skin, 37
 primary, 691
 prostatic, 1898
 pulmonary, 1056
 renal, 1741–1742, 1777
 restrictive cardiomyopathy due to, 1218–1220
 of skin, 37
 of testes, 1950
 of thyroid, 534–535
 tracheobronchial, 1056
Amylopectin, in liver, 1515
Amylopectinosis, 1519, 1520, 1521
Anal. See also under Anus
Anal canal
 embryology of, 1671
 intraepithelial neoplasia of, 1677
 normal anatomy of, 1671–1673
Anal columns, 1671
Anal fissures, 1674
Anal fistulas, 1674
Analgesic nephropathy, 1759–1760
Anal sinuses, 1671
Anal tags, 1673
Anal transitional zone, 1671, 1672
 surface epithelial carcinomas of, 1674–1678
Anal valves, 1671
Anaplastic carcinoma
 of pancreas, 1486–1487
 of salivary gland, 873
 thyroid, 552–553, 562
Anaplastic large-cell lymphoma, 758–759
ANCAs (antineutrophil cytoplasmic autoantibodies), in pauciimmune crescentic and necrotizing glomerulonephritis, 1713
Androgen insensitivity syndrome, 1965–1967
 and germ cell tumors, 1978
Androgen therapy, in transsexuals, 377
Anemia
 aplastic, 653
 megaloblastic, intestines in, 1352
 pernicious, osteoarthritis in, 225–227
 refractory, 662
Anetoderma, 25
Aneurysm(s), 1256–1258
 aortic, 1256–1257
 berry, 1256
 coronary artery, 1237
 myocardial, 1224–1225
 pseudo-, 1256
  myocardial, 1225
Aneurysmal bone cyst, 300–301
 sinonasal, 914–915
 solid, 301
Angiitis
 cerebral, 407
 granulomatous, of CNS, 407, 1260, 1262, 1265–1266
 lymphocytic, benign, 1037
 pulmonary, 1040–1046

Angioblastic meningioma, 441
　of sellar region, 518
Angioblastoma, of Nakagawa, 176
Angioblastomatosis, myxoid, 295
Angiocentric lymphoma, 74, 889, 907–908
Angiodysplasia, 1274–1276
Angioendothelioma, malignant, 1101
Angiofibroma, 153–154
　cellular, 154
　giant cell, 154
　nasopharyngeal, 908–909
　of vulva, 2121
Angiofollicular lymphoid hyperplasia, 721–722
Angiofollicular lymphoid hyperplasia (AFLH), 1159
Angioimmunoblastic lymphadenopathy, 685
　with dysproteinemia, 726–727, 782
Angioimmunoblastic T-cell lymphoma, 757
Angioimmunoproliferative lesion, 1036
Angiokeratomas, of vulva, 2119
Angioleiomyoma, 69
Angiolipoma, 166
　cellular, 150
Angiolymphoid hyperplasia, with eosinophilia, 71, 176
Angiomas
　of breast, 368
　cavernous, 407, 408
　of gastrointestinal tract, 1458
　intramuscular, 166
　littoral cell, 798
　of orbit, 998–999
Angiomatoid malignant fibrous histiocytoma, 165
Angiomatosis
　bacillary, 69–70, 177
　　lymph nodes in, 729
　　spleen in, 792
　intramuscular, 174
　intravascular, 71
Angiomatous meningioma, 441–442
Angiomyofibroblastoma, 152, 155
　paratesticular, 2021
　of vulva, 2121
Angiomyolipoma, 166
　of liver, 1586, 1612
　renal, 1812–1816
Angiomyomas, 169
Angiomyxoid lesions, 155–156
Angiomyxoma, 152
　aggressive, 155
　　paratesticular, 2021
　　of urinary tract, 1882
　　of vulva, 2120–2121
　superficial, 155
Angiopathy, amyloid, 1270
Angioplasty, 1271, 1272–1273
Angiosarcoma

　adrenal, 607
　of bone, 294–295
　of breast, 368–369
　　radiation-induced, 369
　cardiac, 1241
　cutaneous, 72–73
　of liver, 1586, 1607–1609, 1610
　of peritoneum, epithelioid, 2425
　pseudo-, 71
　pulmonary, 1047
　sinonasal, 910–911
　soft tissue, 179–181
　of spleen, 798–799
Ankylosing spondylitis, aorta in, 1258
Anogenital glands, 2111
Anorchia, 1947
Antiandrogen therapy, of prostatic carcinoma, 1925–1926
Antibiotic-associated colitis, 1365
Antiglomerular basement membrane (anti-GBM) disease, 1714–1715
Antimesothelial antibodies, 1133–1135
Antineutrophil cytoplasmic autoantibodies (ANCAs), in pauciimmune crescentic and necrotizing glomerulonephritis, 1713
Antrochoanal polyps, 891
Anus, 1671–1680. See also under Anal
　carcinoid tumors of, 1679
　carcinoma of
　　adeno-, 1678–1679
　　basal cell, 1680
　　pathologic features of, 1675–1676
　　precursor lesions of, 1677–1678
　　prognostic features of, 1676–1677
　　small-cell (neuroendocrine), 1679
　　squamous-cell, 1675
　　surface epithelial, 1674–1678
　congenital abnormalities of, 1673
　Crohn's disease of, 1674
　embryology of, 1671
　fissures and fistulas of, 1674
　hemorrhoids of, 1673
　melanoma of, 1679–1680
　normal anatomy of, 1671–1673
　Paget's disease of, 1680
　polyps of
　　fibroepithelial, 1673
　　inflammatory cloacogenic, 1673–1674
　　lymphoid, 1674
　skin around, 1680
Aortic aneurysms, 1256–1257
Aortic coarctation, 1244
Aortic ectasia, 1258
Aortic insufficiency, 1226–1227
Aorticopulmonary paragangliomas, 629, 1184
Aortic regurgitation, 1226–1227
Aortic stenosis, 1225–1226
　supravalvular, 1244

Aortic valve, normal, 1225
Aortic valvular disease, 1225–1227
Aphalalia, 2038
Aplasia
　adrenal gland, 592
　germinal cell, 1952–1953, 1956–1957
Aplastic anemia, 653
Apocrine adenoma, tubular, 63
Apocrine adenosis, 329, 331
Apocrine carcinoma, 358
　in situ, 341
Apocrine glands, 5
Apocrine metaplasia, 329
Apoptosis, 5, 410
Appendicitis, 1395
Appendix
　developmental abnormalities of, 1394–1395
　inflammatory conditions of, 1395
　neoplasms of, 1442–1446
　　ovarian metastases of, 2380
　neuroma of, 1395
　normal histology of, 1394
　specimen processing for, 1394
Appendix epiploica, infarcted, 2421
APUD (amine precursor uptake and decarboxylation) cell concept, 483, 625
APUDomas, 2176
Arachnoid nodule, pulmonary, 1101
Argyrophilic carcinoma
　of breast, 357–358
　in situ, 341
　of cervix, 2176
Argyrophilic plaques, 463–464
Arias-Stella reaction, 2182, 2220, 2221
Arrector pili muscles, 4
Arterial thrombosis, 1270–1271
Arteriohepatic dysplasia, 1518–1519
Arteriovenous malformations (AVMs), 1274
　of CNS, 407–408
Arteritis
　cranial (giant cell, temporal), 1258, 1260, 1262–1264, 1265
　Takayasu's, 1258, 1260, 1262, 1264–1265
Arthritis
　due to avascular necrosis, 229–230
　due to calcium pyrophosphate crystal deposition disease, 231–232
　general features of, 223–224
　gouty, 230–231
　due to Hoffa's disease, 227
　due to hydroxyapatite deposition, 232
　osteo-, 224–227
　rheumatoid, 228–229
　due to sarcoidosis, 234
　septic, 233–234
　suppurative, 233
Arthropod-bite reaction, 27

Asbestosis, 1015
Asbestos-related mesothelioma, 1120
Aseptic necrosis, of femoral head, 308
Askin's tumor, 195
Aspergillosis
    allergic bronchopulmonary, 1024–1025
    of liver, 1536
    sinonasal, 886
Astler-Coller classification, for colorectal carcinoma, 1440
Astroblastoma, 411, 419
Astrocytic neoplasms, granular cell, 419–420
Astrocytoma(s), 411, 415–420
    anaplastic, 411, 418
    cerebellar, 417
    cystic, 416, 460
    diffuse, 417–418
    fibrillary, 418
    gemistocytic, 411, 418–419
    giant cell, 411
    low-grade, 417–418
    pilocytic, 411, 416–417
    subependymal giant cell, 419
Atheroembolic disease, renal, 1764
Atherosclerosis, 1235–1237, 1253–1254
    aneurysms due to, 1256
Atopic dermatitis, 7
Atrioventricular node, cystic tumor (mesothelioma) of, 1240
Atrophic lichen planus, 10
Atrophic vaginitis, 2136
Atrophie blanche, 29
Atrophy
    benign prostatic, 1905–1906
    cervical, 2166
    endometrial, 2223–2224, 2241–2242
    muscular, 115–116
        infantile spinal, 127
Auricle
    malformations of, 949
    petrified, 951
Autoimmune enteropathy, 1355
Autoimmune gastritis, 1319
Autoimmune hepatitis, 1511, 1512, 1542–1543, 1547, 1548
Autoimmune oophoritis, 2318–2319
Autoimmune thyroid disease, 531–534, 536
Autonomic nerve tumors, gastrointestinal, 1338
Avascular necrosis, 229–230
AVMs (arteriovenous malformations), 1274
    of CNS, 407–408
Axillary lymph nodes, metastases of breast carcinoma to, 362–363
Azzopardi phenomenon, 490

B

B72.3, in mesothelioma, 1133
Bacillary angiomatosis, 69–70, 177
    lymph nodes in, 729
    spleen in, 792
Bacteroides fragilis, chorioamnionitis due to, 2102
Baker's cyst, 241
Balanitis
    gangrenous, 2041
    Zoon's, 2041–2042
Balanitis circumscripta plasmacellularis, 2041–2042
Balanitis xerotica obliterans, 2041
Balanoposthitis, 2038–2039
Balantidiasis, intestinal, 1385
Balloon cells, in gastroesophageal reflux disease, 1286–1287
BALT lymphoma, 1032–1035
Banff classification, 1772
Barium granuloma, 1394
Barrett's esophagus, 1290–1295
    defined, 1290–1291
    diagnosis of, 1292–1293
    dysplasia in, 1293–1295
    other premalignant markers in, 1295
    pathologic features of, 1291–1292
Barrett's mucosa, 1291
Bartholin's duct cyst, 2114
Bartholin's glands, 2111
    carcinoma of, 2129
Basal cell adenoma
    of prostate, 1933
    of salivary gland, 860–861
Basal cell carcinoma (BCC), 57–58
    anal, 1680
    of ear, 954
    of eyelid, 991
    nevoid, 55, 839
    of penis, 2057–2058
    of prostate, 1933–1934
    of vulva, 2129
Basal cell hyperplasia, of prostate, 1933–1934
Basal cell layer, 4
Basaloid squamous cell carcinoma
    of esophagus, 1299, 1301
    of larynx, 940
    of mediastinum, 1170, 1176
    of oral cavity, 834–835
    of penis, 2051
    of vulva, 2125–2126
Basaloid squamous intraepithelial lesions, of penis, 2043–2045
Basaloid tumors, of cutaneous adnexa, 61
Basement membrane, 4
B-cell leukemia
    chronic lymphocytic, 670–673, 738–741
        spleen in, 782–784
    prolymphocytic, 673
B-cell lymphoma(s), 737–751
    biology of, 737–738
    Burkitt's, 739, 750–751
    classification of, 737
    cutaneous, 74–75
    differential diagnosis of, 739
    diffuse large, 739, 746–749
    follicular center, 739, 743–745
    of intestines, 1454
    intravascular, 749
    of liver, 1618
    lymphoplasmacytoid, 739, 741
    mantle cell, 739, 741–742
    microvillous, 749–750
    nodal marginal zone, 739, 745–746
    primary effusion, 749
    primary mediastinal (thymic), 748–749
    small lymphocytic, 738–741
    of spleen, 787–789
    T-cell-rich, 75, 749
B-cell neoplasms, 670–676
Becker muscular dystrophy, 121
Beckwith-Wiedemann syndrome, 593
Bednar tumors, 66
Behçet's syndrome
    gastrointestinal manifestations of, 1383
    of vulva, 2119
Bellini duct carcinoma, 1803–1805
Bence Jones cast nephropathy, 1751–1752
Benign prostatic hypertrophy (BPH), 1893–1895
Ber-EP4, in mesothelioma, 1131
Berger's disease, 1730–1733, 1776
Berry aneurysm, 1256
Beryllium granulomas, 31
BG-8, in mesothelioma, 1131–1133
Bicuspid valves, 1225
Bile
    in hepatocellular carcinoma, 1582
    pigmentation of, 1514
Bile duct(s)
    aberrant, 1630
    adenoma of, 1597, 1599
    cysts of, 1656–1657
    extrahepatic, 1655–1666
        benign tumors of, 1661
        carcinoma of, 1657, 1658, 1661–1666
        congenital anomalies of, 1656–1657
        embryonal rhabdomyosarcoma of, 1666
        malignant tumors of, 1661–1666
        metastases to, 1666
        normal anatomy and histology of, 1655–1656
        obstruction of, 1642
        in sclerosing cholangitis, 1657–1661
        specimen processing for, 1655–1656
    hamartoma of, 1519, 1597, 1598–1599
    interlobular, 1510
    intrahepatic
        benign tumors and tumor-like lesions of, 1597, 1598–1599
        malignant tumors of, 1599–1602
        metastases to, 1602

Bile duct(s) *(contd.)*
  reactive proliferation of, 1597, 1599
  vanishing, 1545, 1546
Biliary atresia, 1516–1519
  extrahepatic, 1656
Biliary cirrhosis, primary, 1511, 1512, 1513, 1527–1528, 1547, 1548
Biliary colic, 1632
Biliary cystadenocarcinoma, 1557, 1561–1562
Biliary cystadenoma, 1557, 1561–1562
Biliary fistulas, 1635
Biliary glycoprotein I, in mesothelioma, 1130
Biliary tract, neuroendocrine cells and neoplasms of, 484
Biliary tract disease, liver in, 1512, 1524–1528
Biloma, 1561
Biopsy
  bone, 264–265
  bone marrow, 651–652
  brain, 391–393
  breast
    categories of specimens from, 319–322
    frozen section from, 319–320
    localization, 322–324
    needle, 320–321
    open, 321
    pathology report for, 325
  bronchial
    of adenocarcinoma, 1089
    of large-cell carcinoma, 1094
    of small-cell carcinoma, 1083
  endometrial, 2203–2204
  endomyocardial, 1209–1210
  esophageal, 1284
  gastrointestinal
    in AIDS patients, 1370–1374
    mucosal, 1312
  liver, 1509–1510
    absence of normal structures in, 1516
    "nearly normal," 1516
    for tumor diagnosis, 1555–1557
  lung, 1011–1012, 1069–1071
    in immunocompromised host, 1056–1059
  muscle, 109–120
  of pancreas, 1473–1474
  of prostate, 1901
  renal, 1702–1703
  skin, 3–4
  of small intestine, 1349
  testicular, 1956–1958
Birbeck granules, 1028
Bizarre parosteal osteochondromatous proliferation, 309
Bladder, 1853–1886
  adenoma of, 1861–1862
  aggressive angiomyxoma of, 1882

amyloidosis of, 1859
anatomy of, 1853–1854
benign mesenchymal neoplasms of, 1882
carcinoid tumors of, 1882
carcinoma of. *See* Bladder carcinoma
carcinosarcoma of, 1876–1878
condyloma of, 1862–1863
diverticula of, 1859–1860
endometriosis of, 1858
hematologic neoplasms of, 1882
inflammatory disorders of, 1854–1858
inflammatory pseudosarcomatous lesions of, 1863–1864
inverted papilloma of, 1862
lymphoepithelioma of, 1878
malakoplakia of, 1858–1859
melanoma of, 1882
metaplasia of, 1860–1862
neuroendocrine neoplasms of, 490
papillary tumors of, 1868–1871
paraganglioma of, 636, 1882
plasma cell granuloma of, 1856
reactive proliferative changes of, 1860
sarcomas of, 1881–1882
Bladder carcinoma, 1864–1879
  adeno-, 1873–1874
  blood group-related antigens in, 1885–1886
  chorio-, 1878
  classification of, 1864–1865
  cytology of, 1882–1884
  epidemiology of, 1864
  flow cytometry of, 1884–1885
  genetics and molecular genetics of, 1886
  in situ, 1871–1872, 1883
  lymphoepithelioma form of, 1878
  neuroendocrine, 1875–1876
  ovarian metastases of, 2381
  papillary lesions and, 1868–1871
  sarcomatoid (spindle cell, giant cell), 1876–1878
  signet-ring cell, 1874
  small cell, 1875–1876
  squamous cell, 1873
  staging of, 1865–1867
  transitional cell, 1867–1868
    nested, 1878
  urachal, 1874–1875
  verrucous, 1873
Blastema
  aplastic, 1687
  nodular, 1687
Blastoma, pulmonary, 1099–1100
Blood group antigens, in bladder cancer, 1885–1886
Blood vessels
  with aging, 1253, 1254
  diseases of. *See* Vascular disease
  normal, 1253

prosthetic, 1271, 1274
tumors of, 1277
Blue nevus
  cellular, 96
  common, 96
  prostatic, 1899
Blue rubber bleb nevus syndrome, intestinal involvement in, 1387
Blunt cell adenosis, of breast, 329, 330
B-lymphoblastic leukemia, 751
B-lymphoblastic lymphoma, 751
Bohn's nodules, 836
Bombesin, 485
Bone(s)
  examination of, 243–245
  fracture of, 255–257
  tissue structure of, 243
  woven (immature), 245
Bone cysts, 300–302
Bone disease(s)
  due to abnormal formation of organic matrix, 248–249
  due to abnormal mineralization, 249–250
  chronic multifocal osteomyelitis, 260
  due to hypoparathyroidism, 251–252
  hypophosphatasia, 250
  metabolic, 245–255
  due to metal toxicity, 250
  myositis ossificans circumscripta, 258
  neoplastic. *See* Bone tumor(s)
  nonneoplastic, 243–260
  osteogenesis imperfecta, 248–249
  osteomalacia, 249–250
  osteopetrosis, 254–255
  osteoporosis, 253–254
  Paget's disease, 252–253
  posttraumatic, 255–259
  pyogenic osteomyelitis, 259–260
  reactive periostitis, 259
  rickets, 249–250
Bone formation, 244–245
Bone infarction, 257–258, 308
Bone infection, 259–260
Bone marrow, 651–699
  in AIDS, 656–658
  in angioimmunoblastic lymphadenopathy, 685
  atrophy of, 655
  B-cell neoplasms of, 670–676
  biopsy of, 651–652
  cellularity of, 653–656
  in Gaucher disease, 692
  granulomas of, 656, 685
  in heavy chain disease, 690–691
  hematopoiesis in, 652–653
  histiocytic proliferations of, 691–695
  in histiocytosis
    Langerhans cell, 693
    malignant, 695
  histology of, 652–653

hypercellular, 653–654
hypocellular, 653
in immunoglobulin deposition diseases, 691
immunosecretory disorders of, 685–691
in infection-associated hemophagocytic syndrome, 693–695
inflammatory disorders of, 656–658
in leukemia
  acute, 659–662
  chronic myeloid, 663–664
  hairy cell, 674–676
  large granular lymphocyte, 677
lymphocyte progenitor cells in, 684–685
lymphoid neoplasms of, 667–670
  reactive, 683–684
in lymphoma
  Burkitt's, 676
  follicular cell, 674
  histiocytic, 695
  Hodgkin's, 680–683
  mantle cell, 674
  marginal zone, 674–676
  non-Hodgkin's, 667–670, 679–680
  T-cell, 676–680
lymphoma-like lesions of, 683–685
in lymphoproliferative disorders, 667–670
  T-cell, 676–680
in mast cell disease, 665–667
metabolic diseases of, 699
metastatic tumors of, 695–699
in monoclonal gammopathy of undetermined significance, 689
in mycosis fungoides, 678
in myelodysplastic syndrome, 662–663
in myelofibrosis
  chronic idiopathic, 664–665
  reactive, 656
myeloproliferative disorders of, 663–667
necrosis of, 655–656, 696
in Niemann-Pick disease, 692
in plasma cell myeloma, 686–689
in plasmacytomas, 689
in polycythemia vera, 664
in Sézary syndrome, 678
in storage histiocyte disorders, 691–693
in thrombocythemia, 664
in Waldenström's macroglobulinemia, 690
Bone marrow transplant, 654–655
Bone resorption, 247
  abnormal, 251–255
Bone tumor(s), 263–309
  adamantinoma, 293–294
  biopsy of, 264–265
  vs. bizarre parosteal osteochondromatous proliferation, 309
  vs. bone cysts, 300–302

vs. bone infarct, 308
vs. chest wall hamartoma, 307
chondroblastoma, 274–275
chondroid, 271–281
  benign, 271–276
  malignant, 276–281
chondroma, 272–274
chondrosarcoma, 276–281
chordoma, 297–298
classification of, 263–264
conditions simulating, 299–309
vs. congenital fibromatosis, 308
Ewing's tumor, 269–271
fibrohistiocytic, 295–296
fibroma
  chondromyxoid, 275–276
  desmoplastic, 296
fibrosarcoma, 296–297
fibrous, 296–297
vs. fibrous dysplasia and osteofibrous dysplasia, 302–303
fibrous histiocytoma, 295–296
vs. fracture callus, 304
giant cell, 291–292
grading and staging of, 265–266
hemangioendothelioma, 294–295
hemangiopericytoma, 295
vs. hyperparathyroidism, 307
vs. Langerhans' cell histiocytosis, 306
lipogenic, 299
lipoma, 299
liposarcoma, 299
lymphoma, 267–269
vs. mastocytosis, 307
vs. metaphyseal fibrous defects, 304
vs. metastatic carcinoma, 299–300
myeloma, 266–267
vs. myositis ossificans, 305
neural, 299–300
neurilemoma, 299–300
vs. neuropathic joint, 308
notochordal, 297–298
osteoblastoma, 283
osteochondroma, 271–272
osteogenic, 281–291
  benign, 281–283
  malignant, 283–291
osteoma, 283
  osteoid, 281–283
vs. osteomyelitis, 305
osteosarcoma, 283–291
vs. Paget's disease, 306
sarcoma
  Paget's, 286
  postradiation, 286
vs. sinus histiocytosis with massive lymphadenopathy, 309
small cell neoplasms, 266–271
specimen handling for, 265
vs. subungual exostosis and subungual keratoacanthoma, 308

vs. synovial chondromatosis, 307–308
vascular, 294–295
Bony spurs, 223
BOOP (bronchiolitis obliterans organizing pneumonia), 1025
Borrelia burgdorferi, 399
Botryoid rhabdomyosarcoma, 172
Bovine spongiform encephalopathy, 406
Bowel. *See also* Intestine(s)
  brown, 1389
  defunctionalized, 1377
Bowenoid actinic keratosis, 54
Bowenoid papulosis, 54, 55
  of penis, 2045–2046
  of vulva, 2124
Bowen's disease, 54, 55
  vs. Paget's disease of nipple, 360
BPH (benign prostatic hypertrophy), 1893–1895
Brain, 389–466
  abscess of, 399–400
  acquired immunodeficiency syndrome of, 401–404
  biopsy of, 391–393
  cerebritis of, 397–399
  cerebrovascular diseases of, 406–408
  clinical and radiographic perspective on, 394–395
  clinical history of, 389–390
  Creutzfeldt-Jakob disease of, 404–405
  cysts of, 459–463
  dementia of, 463–464
  demyelination of, 464–465
  encephalitis of, 400–401
  epilepsy of, 465–466
  frozen sections of, 391, 479
  hemorrhage of, 406–407
  hereditary prion diseases of, 405–406
  histochemical stains for, 394, 479–480
  infectious diseases of, 397–406
  Lyme disease of, 399
  macroscopic specimen interpretation for, 395
  "mad cow" disease of, 405
  meningitis of, 397–399
  neuroborreliosis of, 399
  neurocysticercosis of, 398
  progressive multifocal leukoencephalopathy of, 403–404
  reactive changes of, 395–397
  sarcoidosis of, 398–399
  spongiform encephalopathies of, 404–406
  surgical specimens from, 390–394
  terms and abbreviations used for, 389
  therapeutic resection of, 393–394
  tuberculosis of, 398
  tumors of. *See* Brain tumor(s)
  vascular malformation of, 407–408
  Whipple's disease of, 399
Brainerd diarrhea, 1368

Brain tumor(s), 408–459
  amyloidoma, 455
  astrocytomas, 415–420
  carcinoma, 456–458
  in children, 408, 409
  chondroma and chondrosarcoma, 446
  chordoma, 445
  choroid plexus epithelial, 432–433
  craniopharyngioma, 456
  desmoplastic small cell, 456
  dysembryoplastic neuroepithelial, 431
  ependymoblastoma, 424–425
  ependymomas, 420–424
  gangliocytoma, 430–431
  ganglioglioma, 430–431, 432
  ganglioneuroblastoma, 432
  germ cell, 450–452
  glioblastoma multiforme, 427–429
  gliomas, 410–429
    with epithelial metaplasia, 429
    margins of, 410–415
    radiation-induced, 429
  gliomatosis cerebri, 418
  gliosarcoma, 429
  hemangioblastoma, 455–456
  hemangiopericytoma, 444–445
  hematopoietic and lymphoid, 452–455
  histiocytosis, 454–455
  leukemia, 454
  lipoma, 455
  lymphoma, 452–454
  malignant potential of, 408
  medulloblastoma, 434–438
  medulloepithelioma, 438
  medullomyoblastoma, 437
  melanocytic, 458–459
  meningioma, 438–445
  metastatic, 456–459
  nerve sheath, 447–449
  neurilemoma, 447–448
  neurinoma, 447–448
  neurocytoma, 431–432
  neuroendocrine, 449–450
  neurofibroma, 448
  neuronal, 429–432
  oligoastrocytoma, 426
  oligodendroglioma, 425–426
  paraganglioma, 449
  pineal cell, 433–434
  pituitary adenoma, 449–450
  polar spongioblastoma, 438
  primitive neuroectodermal, 437
  proliferative capacity of, 408–410
  relative frequency of, 408, 409
  rhabdoid, atypical, 438
  sarcomas, 446–447
  schwannoma, 447–448
  teratoid, atypical, 438
  teratoma, 451
  undifferentiated and multipotential, 434–438

Breast(s), 319–379
  adenoma of
    ductal, 344, 371–372
    lactating, 365
    nipple, 370–371
    pleomorphic, 372
    tubular, 364
  adenomyoepithelioma of, 373
  adenosis of, 328, 329, 330–334
  androgen therapy effect on, 377
  angioma of, 368
  angiosarcoma of, 368–369
  benign tumors of, 367–368
  biopsy of
    localization, 322–324
    needle, 320–321
    open, 321
  carcinoid tumor of, 357–358
  carcinoma of. See Breast carcinoma
  collagenous spherulosis of, 378–379
  cystosarcoma phyllodes of, 366–367
  cysts of, 329, 330
  diabetic mastopathy of, 375–376
  duct ectasia of, 375
  fat necrosis of, 374
  fibroadenolipoma of, 377
  fibroadenoma of, 363–364
    cellular intracanalicular, 366–367
    giant, 364
    juvenile, 365
  fibrocystic change of, 328–329
  foreign body reaction of, 374
  frozen section of, 319–320
  galactocele of, 378
  granulation tissue polyp of, 345
  gynecomastia of, 376
  hamartoma of, 377
  hemopoietic tumors of, 369
  hormone receptors in, 324–325
  hyperplasia of
    atypical, 335–336
      lobular, 330, 347
    epithelial, 329, 334–336
    fibroadenomatoid, 364
    intraductal, 334–335
    lobular epithelial, 347
    papillary duct, 377
    pseudoangiomatous, 377–378
  hypertrophy of, juvenile, virginal, or physiologic, 377
  inflammatory lesions of, 373–376
  lactational change in, 327
  lactiferous duct fistula of, 374
  leiomyoma of, 368
  lipoma of, 367
  lymphocytic lobulitis of, 375–376
  lymphoma of, 369
  macromastia of, in pregnancy, 377
  magnetic resonance imaging of, 324
  mammography of, 322–323
  mastitis of
    chronic granulomatous (perilobular), 374–375
    periductal, 375
  mesenchymal tumors of, 367
  metaplastic epithelial change of, 329–330
  metastases to, 362
  microdochectomy of, 321–322
  mucocele-like lesions of, 378
  myofibroblastoma of, 373
  neurilemoma of, 368
  neuroendocrine neoplasms of, 488
  neurofibroma of, 368
  normal, 325–328
  papillary lesions of, 344–347
  papilloma of, 329, 344–346
  papillomatosis of, juvenile, 377
  pathology report for, 325
  periductal stromal tumor of, 366–367
  phyllodes tumor of, 366–367
  postmastectomy lymphangiosarcoma of, 369
  pseudolymphoma of, 369–370
  radial scar of, 331–333
  Rosai-Dorfman lesion of, 370
  sarcoma of, 368
    radiation-induced, 369
  specimens of
    categories of, 319–322
    mastectomy, 322
    processing of, 319
  specimen x-ray of, 322–324
  Stewart-Treves syndrome of, 369
  stromal giant cells of, 379
  ultrasound of, 324
Breast carcinoma
  benign breast disease and risk of, 348–349
  benign lesions that mimic, 328
  chemotherapy changes in, 361
  classification of, 349–350
  histologic grading of, 352
  infiltrating, 349–360
    adenoid cystic, 357
    apocrine, 358
    argyrophil, 357–358
    cribriform, 356–357
    ductal, 350–352
    juvenile, 358
    lobular, 352–354
    low grade adenosquamous, 359–360
    matrix-producing, 359
    medullary, 354–355
    metaplastic, 358–359
    mucinous (colloid, mucoid, gelatinous), 355–356
    myoblastoid, 360
    with neuroendocrine differentiation, 357–358
    papillary, 357
    pseudosarcomatous, 358–359

sarcomatoid, 358–359
secretory, 358
signet ring cell, 358
spindle cell, 359
squamous cell, 359
tubular, 332, 356, 371
inflammatory, 360
in situ
  clinical significance of, 348–349
  ductal, 336–344
    apocrine, 341
    biological markers for, 343
    cancerization of lobules in, 342, 348
    classification of, 336–338
    clinging, 340–341
    clinical significance of, 349
    comedo, 338–339
    cystic hypersecretory, 341
    vs. epithelial hyperplasia, 335, 343–344
    high-grade, 338–339
    intermediate-grade, 340
    intermediately differentiated, 340
    low-grade, 339–340
    neuroendocrine (argyrophilic), 341
    papillary, 344, 346–347
    poorly differentiated, 338–339
    prognostic index for, 343
    signet ring cell, 341
    surgical margins for, 342–343
    well-differentiated, 339–340
  lobular (intralobular), 347–348
in males, 361
metastatic, 362–363
  to ovaries, 2380
due to Paget's disease of nipple, 360–361
prognostic markers for, 352
prostatic, 1925
radiation changes in, 361–362
Breast disease, benign, 328–329
  and risk of carcinoma, 348–349
Breast tissue
  electron microscopy of, 325
  general guidelines for histopathologic interpretation of, 328
  gross examination of, 319, 320
  histochemistry of, 325
  immunohistochemistry of, 325, 326
  special stains for, 325
  subgross examination of, 324
Brenner tumors, 2339–2341
Broad ligament
  ectopic tissue in, 2400–2401
  rare tumors of, 2409
  serous and other müllerian tumors of, 2408–2409
  soft tissue-type tumors of, 2409
Brodie's abscess, 260, 283

Bromodeoxyuridine, as marker of cellular proliferation, 409
Bronchi
  neoplasms of. *See* Pulmonary neoplasms
  segmental anatomy of, 1069, 1070
Bronchial biopsy
  of adenocarcinoma, 1089
  of large-cell carcinoma, 1094
  of small-cell carcinoma, 1083
Bronchial gland carcinomas, 1098–1099
Bronchiolitis, 1017
Bronchiolitis obliterans, 1022, 1024, 1026–1027
Bronchiolitis obliterans organizing pneumonia (BOOP), 1025
Bronchitis-bronchiolitis, follicular, 1031
Bronchocentric granulomatosis, 1025–1026
Bronchogenic cysts, 1151–1152
Bronchopulmonary tree, neuroendocrine cells and neoplasms of, 484
Brown bowel syndrome, 1389
Brown tumors, 251, 252
Brunner's gland(s), 1349
  hyperplasia of, 1360–1361
Brunner's gland nodule, 1361
Brunn's nests, 1860
Buccal mucosa, squamous cell carcinoma of, 825
Buck's fascia, 2037
Budd-Chiari syndrome, liver in, 1511, 1514, 1529, 1538
Buerger's disease, 1262, 1266
Bulla(e), 5
  intraepidermal
    with acantholysis, 18–23
    without acantholysis, 18
  subcorneal
    with acantholysis, 17–18
    without acantholysis, 17
  subepidermal
    with inflammation, 23–24
    without inflammation, 24
Bullous diseases, 17–23
Bullous impetigo, 17–18
Bullous pemphigoid, 23
Burkitt's lymphoma, 676, 739, 750–751
  of intestines, 1454
  of mediastinum, 1160
Bursitis, 241

C

C1q nephropathy, 1719, 1776
N-Cadherin, in mesothelioma, 1135
Caisson's disease, 258
Calcification
  of placenta, 2098
  prostatic, 1898
Calcifying aponeurotic fibroma, 154
Calcifying cyst, odontogenic, 839

Calcifying epithelial odontogenic tumor, 843–844
Calcifying fibrous pseudotumor, of peritoneum, 2420
Calcinosis cutis, 37–38
Calciphylaxis, 37–38
Calcium carbonate stones, 1633
Calcium deficiency, osteomalacia due to, 249–250
Calcium hydroxyapatite deposition, 232
Calcium pyrophosphate crystal deposition disease, 231–232
Calculi, prostatic, 1898
Callus, fracture, 256–257, 304
Calretinin, in mesothelioma, 1135
Calymmatobacterium granulomatis, 2039, 2115
Cambium layer, 172, 173
Canalicular adenoma, 860
Canal of Nuck, cyst of, 2113
Cancerization, of lobules, 342, 348
Candidiasis
  esophagitis due to, 1288
  of liver, 1536
  of vagina, 2136
  of vulva, 2117
Capillariasis, 1359
Capillaritis, 28
Capillary hemangioblastoma, of CNS, 455–456
Capillary hemangioma
  of gingiva, 807
  lobular, 69, 174
  sinonasal, 909–910
  of orbit, 998
Capillary-lymphatic space invasion, by cervical carcinoma, 2171–2172
Capillary telangiectasia, of CNS, 407, 408
Cap polyps, inflammatory, 1423
Capsular drop, 1777
Carbohydrate storage diseases, 125–126
Carcinoembryonic antigen (CEA)
  in hepatocellular carcinoma, 1582, 1583
  in mesothelioma, 1125–1126, 1130–1131
  in pulmonary neoplasms, 1109
Carcinoid tumors, 483, 486–491
  of anus, 1679
  appendiceal, 1445
  of breast, 357–358, 488
  of gallbladder, 1655
  of intestine, 1446–1448
  of larynx, 487–488
  of lung, 1082–1083, 1095–1097
  of mediastinum, 1169, 1182–1183, 1190, 1198–1199
  of middle ear, 964–965
  of ovary, 488–489, 2368–2370, 2378–2379
  of prostate, 488, 1928
  renal, 1809–1810

Carcinoid tumors *(contd.)*
  of skin, 487
  spindle cell thymic, 1194
  testicular, 488–489, 2000–2001
  thymic, 486–487, 1182–1183, 1190, 1198–1199
    spindle cell, 1194
  of urinary bladder, 490
  of urinary tract, 1882
  of uterine cervix, 489–490
Carcinoma
  adrenal cortical, 600–605
  ameloblastic, 847
  of anus, 1674–1679, 1680
  basal cell. *See* Basal cell carcinoma (BCC)
  bile duct, 1657, 1658, 1661–1666
  of bladder. *See* Bladder carcinoma
  breast. *See* Breast carcinoma
  cervical. *See* Cervical carcinoma
  choroid plexus, 412, 433
  clear cell. *See* Clear cell carcinoma
  of CNS, 412, 456–458
    desmoplastic, 413
    embryonal, 412, 452
    small cell, 414
  colorectal, 1436–1442
  of conjunctiva, 985–986
  of ear, 954
    adeno-, 967, 971–972
    adenoid cystic, 957
    basal cell, 954
    mucoepidermoid, 957
    squamous cell, 954–955, 967
    verrucous, 954–955
  endometrial. *See* Endometrial adenocarcinoma
  esophageal, 1297–1304
  of fallopian tube, 2404–2406
    pseudo-, 2401–2402
  of gallbladder, 1647–1648, 1650–1654
  gastric, 1330–1334
  hepatocellular. *See* Hepatocellular carcinoma
  of kidneys
    collecting duct, 1803–1805
    medullary, 1805–1806
    renal cell, 1785–1799
  lacrimal sac, 1002
  of larynx, 931–941
  lung. *See under* Pulmonary neoplasms
  Merkel cell, 59
  metastatic. *See* Metastases
  mucinous. *See* Mucinous carcinoma
  mucoepidermoid, 833, 866–867
  myoepithelial, 864–865
  neuroendocrine, 59, 450, 485–491
  odontogenic, 847–848
  of oral cavity, 831–834
    spindle-cell, 828–831
    verrucous, 824–828
  of ovary. *See under* Ovarian tumors
  pancreatic, 1477–1487
  papillary. *See* Papillary carcinoma
  parathyroid, 567–568
  of penis, 2046–2057
  peritoneal serous, 2434
  pituitary, 515–516
  prostate. *See* Prostate cancer
  renal cell, 1785–1799
  of renal pelvis, 1879
  of rete testis, 2014–2015
  salivary duct, 872–873
  of salivary glands. *See* Salivary glands, carcinoma of
  sarcomatoid. *See* Sarcomatoid carcinoma
  sebaceous cell, of eyelid, 991–992
  of seminal vesicles, 1935–1936
  showing thymus-like differentiation, 1196
  signet ring cell. *See* Signet ring cell carcinoma
  sinonasal
    adeno-, 898–900
    small-cell undifferentiated (oat cell), 902
    squamous cell, 895–898
    undifferentiated, 903
  small-cell. *See* Small-cell carcinoma
  of soft tissue, 193
  spindle cell. *See* Spindle cell carcinoma
  squamous cell. *See* Squamous cell carcinoma (SCC)
  sweat gland, 60, 65
  of testis
    chorio-, 1995–1997
    embryonal, 1985–1990
  thymic
    primary, 1176–1180, 1199
    sarcomatoid, 1192–1194
  thyroglossal duct, 557–558
  thyroid. *See* Thyroid carcinoma
  transitional cell. *See* Transitional cell carcinoma
  of ureter, 1879
  of urethra, 1880–1881
  of urothelial tract. *See under* Urothelial tract
  verrucous. *See* Verrucous carcinoma
  vulvar, 2125–2129
Carcinoma *in situ* (CIS), 53–55, 336
  of bladder, 1871–1872, 1883
  of bronchi and lungs, 1073–1074
  cervical, 2184–2186
  ductal. *See* Ductal carcinoma *in situ* (DCIS)
  oral, 812–814
  of penis, 2043–2045
Carcinosarcoma
  of adrenal glands, 608
  of bladder, 1876–1878
  colorectal, 1439
  cutaneous, 58
  endometrial, 2254, 2262–2264, 2265
  of lung, 1099–1100
  of oral cavity, 830
  of ovary, 2334
  of prostate, 1935
Cardiac devices, 1244
Cardiac disease. *See* Heart disease
Cardiac glands, 1283–1284
  in Barrett's esophagus, 1292, 1293
Cardiac mucosa inflammation, in gastroesophageal reflux disease, 1288
Cardiac myxoma, 1238–1240, 1277
Cardiac transplantation, 1222–1224
Cardiac tumors, 1237–1241
Cardiomyopathy(ies), 1210–1215
  adriamycin, 1212
  in AIDS, 1220–1221
  alcoholic, 1212
  congestive (dilated), 1211–1215
  defined, 1210
  familial, 1211
  hypertrophic, 1210–1211
  due to metabolic, storage, and endocrine disorders, 1212–1215
  peripartum, 1211–1212
  restrictive, 1218–1222
Carditis, 1319–1320
Carney's syndrome, 145, 1338
Carnitine deficiency, 126
Carnitine palmityltransferase (CPT) deficiency, 126
Caroli's disease, 1557, 1560
Caroli's syndrome, 1557, 1560
Carotid bodies, 626–627
Carotid body paragangliomas, 628
  familial, 636–637
  with other endocrine disorders, 637
Cartilage
  diseases of, 33–41
  injury to, 223
  regeneration of, 223
Cartilaginous tumors, of larynx, 942
Caruncles
  of eye, 988
  urethral, 1856
Castleman's disease
  lymph nodes in, 721–722
  mediastinum in, 1159, 1198
  spleen in, 781
Cataract, 992–993
Catecholamines
  biosynthesis and metabolism of, 591
  levels of urinary, 592
Cat-scratch disease, 719
Cauda equina region, paraganglioma of, 643–644
Cavernous angioma, of CNS, 407, 408
Cavernous hemangioma

adrenal, 606–607
of liver, 1603–1605
of orbit, 998
CBD (common bile duct), 1655
C cell(s), 531
C-cell adenoma, 550
C-cell hyperplasia, 551–552
C-cell lesions, 548–552
CD. *See* Crohn's disease (CD)
CD15, in mesothelioma, 1133
CD30+ lymphoma, 75–76
CD31, as marker for soft tissue tumors, 139–140
CD34, as marker for soft tissue tumors, 139
CD44H, in mesothelioma, 1135
CD57, as marker for soft tissue tumors, 142
CD68, as marker for soft tissue tumors, 140
CD146 antibody, 2075
CEA. *See* Carcinoembryonic antigen (CEA)
Celiac sprue, 1350–1352
Cell coupling, 245
Cellular angiofibroma, 154
Cellular angiolipoma, 150
Cellular blue nevus, 96
Cellular fibroma, of ovary, 2348
Cellular hemangioma, 175
Cellular intracanalicular fibroadenoma, breast, 366–367
Cellular myxoid liposarcoma, 167, 169
Cellular proliferation, markers of, 409
Cellular schwannoma, 185
Cellulitis, of penis, 2039
Cemental dysplasia, periapical, 845–846
Cementifying fibroma, 846
Cementoblastoma, 846–847
Cementoma, 845–847
  gigantiform, 847
Cemento-ossifying fibroma, sinonasal, 915–916
Central core disease, 122
Central nervous system (CNS), 389–466
  abscess of, 399–400
  cerebrovascular diseases of, 406–408
  clinical and radiographic perspective on, 394–395
  clinical history of, 389–390
  cysts of, 459–463
  dementia of, 463–464
  demyelination of, 464–465
  epilepsy of, 465–466
  granulomatous angiitis of, 1260, 1262, 1265–1266
  hemorrhage of, 406–407
  histochemical stains for, 394
  infectious diseases of, 397–406
    acquired immunodeficiency syndrome of, 401–404

  cerebritis of, 397–399
  Creutzfeldt-Jakob disease of, 404–405
  encephalitis of, 400–401
  hereditary prion diseases of, 405–406
  "mad cow" disease of, 405
  meningitis of, 397–399
  progressive multifocal leukoencephalopathy of, 403–404
  spongiform encephalopathies of, 404–406
  reactive changes of, 395–397
  specimens from
    categories of, 390–394
    macroscopic, 395
  terms and abbreviations used for, 389
  tumors of. *See* Brain tumor(s)
  vascular malformation of, 407–408
Central stromal crystalline dystrophy, 980
Centronuclear myopathy, 112, 123
Cerebellopontine angle, tumors of, 971–972
Cerebral angiitis, 407
Cerebral vasculitis, 407
Cerebritis, 396, 397–399
Cerebromeningeal hemophagocytic lymphohistiocytosis, 401
Cerebrospinal fluid, in middle ear, 968–969
Cerebrovascular diseases, 406–408
Ceroid histiocytosis, of spleen, 792–793
Ceroidosis, 1388, 1389
Ceruminoma, 955
Cervical carcinoma
  adeno-, 2184–2193
    classification of, 2187
    clear cell, 2191
    early invasion by, 2186
    endocervical-type, 2187
    endometrioid, 2190–2191
    epidemiology of, 2186
    in situ, 2184–2186
    mesonephric, 2193
    metastatic, 2194–2196
    minimal deviation, 2187–2188
    mixed, 2194
    ovarian metastases of, 2382
    serous papillary, 2191–2192
    with small cell undifferentiated carcinoma, 2194
    symptoms of, 2186–2187
    villoglandular papillary, 2188–2190
  adenoid basal, 2194
  adenoid cystic, 2194
  adenosquamous, 2193–2194
  argyrophilic, 2176
  capillary-lymphatic space invasion by, 2171–2172
  condylomatous, 2174–2176
  glassy cell, 2194

  lymphoepithelioma-like, 2177
  neuroendocrine, 2176
  oat cell, 2176
  papillary, 2174
  poorly differentiated, 2176
  sarcomatoid, 2177
  small cell undifferentiated, 2176–2177
    with adenocarcinoma, 2194
  spindle cell, 2177
  squamous cell, 2172–2176
    microinvasive, 2168–2172
  staging of, 2172–2173
  undifferentiated, 2176–2177
  verrucous, 2174
Cervical intraepithelial neoplasia (CIN), 2155–2168
  with atrophy, 2166
  classification of, 2157–2163
  diagnostic criteria for, 2157
  differential diagnosis of, 2163–2164
  high-grade, 2159–2160, 2161, 2164–2165
  histologic variations in presentation of, 2160–2163
  with immature metaplastic-type differentiation, 2163, 2166
  keratinizing, 2161
  low-grade, 2158–2159, 2160, 2163–2164
  nonepithelial alterations, 2166–2168
  papillary immature, 2161–2163
  pathogenesis of, 2156–2157
  postmenopausal squamous atypia in, 2164
  due to radiation effect, 2166
  reactive/reparative epithelial changes in, 2163–2164, 2165–2166
  vaginal papillomatosis in, 2163
Cervical lymph nodes, metastasis from oral squamous cell carcinoma to, 814
Cervicitis, 2155
Cervix, 2155–2197
  adenoma malignum of, 2187–2188
  Arias-Stella reaction of, 2182
  atrophy of, 2166
  atypical oxyphilic metaplasia of, 2182–2184
  benign glandular lesions of, 2177
  carcinoma of. *See* Cervical carcinoma
  condylomata of, 2156–2157, 2174
  endocervicitis of, 2180–2182
  endometriosis of, 2180
  glandular atypia of, 2182–2184
  glandular dysplasia of, 2184
  glandular hyperplasia of
    diffuse laminar, 2177–2178
    mesonephric, 2179–2180
    micro-, 2178–2179
  inflammations of, 2155
  intraepithelial neoplasia of. *See* Cervical intraepithelial neoplasia (CIN)

Cervix *(contd.)*
    leiomyomas of, 2196
    lymphomas of, 2197
    müllerian papilloma of, 2182
    nabothian cysts of, 2177
    neuroendocrine neoplasms of, 489–490
    papillary neoplasms of, 2174
    polyps of
        endocervical, 2177
        of endometrial origin, 2196
        fibroepithelial, 2196
    sarcomas of, 2196–2197
    soft tissue neoplasms of
        benign, 2196
        malignant, 2196–2197
    tubuloendometrial metaplasia of, 2180
    tunnel clusters of, 2177
Chagas' disease, myocarditis due to, 1216–1217
Chalazion, 988
Chancre
    hard, 2039
    soft, 2040
Chancroid
    of penis, 2040
    of vulva, 2115
Charcot-Böttcher crystals, 1943, 1944
Charcot-Bouchard aneurysms, 1256
Charcot's joint, 223–224, 227, 308
CHD (common hepatic duct), 1655
Chemodectoma
    of middle ear, 965–967
    of neck, 628
    pulmonary, 1101
Chemotherapy
    breast changes due to, 361
    effect on intestines of, 1352, 1392–1393
    effect on testis of, 1958
    gastritis due to, 1323
    for testicular germ cell tumors, 2003–2004
Chest wall hamartoma, 307
Children
    bone marrow metastases in, 697
    breast carcinoma in, 358
    fibrous proliferations in, 154
    pancreatic neoplasms in, 1493–1494
    renal neoplasms in, 1825–1851
        carcinoma, 1849–1850
        clear cell sarcoma, 1842–1847
        differential diagnosis of, 1828, 1829
        lymphoma, 1851
        mesoblastic nephroma, 1839–1842
        metanephric adenofibroma and metanephric adenoma, 1850
        ossifying tumor, 1850
        primitive neuroepithelial tumor, 1850
        rhabdoid tumor, 1847–1849
        specimen handling for, 1825–1826
        staging of, 1826–1828
        Wilms' tumor (nephroblastoma), 1829–1839
Chlamydia trachomatis
    cervicitis due to, 2155
    chorioamnionitis due to, 2102
    of penis, 2039–2040
    of vulva, 2115
Chloroma, 1187
Cholangiocarcinoma, 1661
    hepatic, 1593
    intrahepatic, 1599–1602
Cholangitis, 1524
    ascending, 1524, 1525, 1526
    sclerosing, 1512, 1526–1527, 1547, 1548, 1657–1661
Cholecystitis, 1635–1642
    acute, 1635–1636
    AIDS-related, 1639–1641
    chronic, 1636–1639
    eosinophilic, 1641
    gangrenous, 1636
    lymphocytic, 1642
    xanthogranulomatous, 1641–1642
Cholecystitis glandularis proliferans, 1639
Choledochal cysts, 1656–1657
Choledocholithiasis, 1634–1635, 1636
Cholelithiasis, 1631–1635
Cholestasis, 1514
    gallbladder in, 1642
    of sepsis, 1536
Cholesteatoma
    of inner ear, 972
    of middle ear, 961–963
    sinonasal, 890
Cholesterol emboli, 1764
Cholesterol granuloma, of ear, 959, 972
Cholesterolosis, 1631
Cholesterol polyps, of gallbladder, 1646, 1648
Cholesterol stones, 1633–1634
Chondroblastic osteosarcoma, 278, 280, 284–285
Chondroblastoma, 274–275, 276
Chondrocalcinosis, 231–232
Chondrodermatitis nodularis chronica helicis, 34, 952
Chondroid chordoma, 298
Chondroid lipoma, 166
Chondroid syringoma, 63
Chondroid tumors, 271–281
    benign, 271–276
    malignant, 276–281
Chondroma, 272–274
    of CNS, 446
    extraskeletal, 189
    of larynx, 942
    periosteal, 273–274
Chondromalacia, idiopathic cystic, of ear, 953
Chondromatosis
    secondary, 238
    synovial, 237–238, 307–308
Chondromatous hamartoma, of lung, 1103
Chondromyxoid fibroma, 275–276
Chondrosarcoma, 273, 276–281
    clear cell, 279
    of CNS, 446
    conventional, 276–277
    dedifferentiated, 278, 279–280
    extraskeletal, 189–190
    grading of, 277–278
    of larynx, 942
    mesenchymal, 281
        sinonasal, 916–917
    myxoid, 152
    periosteal, 279
    secondary, 278–279
Chordoma, 161, 297–298, 412, 445
    chondroid, 298
    of mediastinum, 1195
    of sellar region, 518
    sinonasal, 917
Chorioamnionitis, 2095, 2096, 2097, 2100–2103
Chorioangiosis, 2105–2106
Choriocarcinoma
    of CNS, 413, 421, 451–452, 458
    endometrial, 2221
    gestational, 2076–2080
    of mediastinum, 1182
    ovarian, 2363–2364
    testicular, 1995–1997
    of urothelial tract, 1878
Choristoma
    adenohypophysial neuronal, 521
    of conjunctiva, 984
    of middle ear, 963
Choroid, 994–996
Choroid plexus
    carcinoma of, 412, 433
    epithelial tumors of, 432–433
    meningioma of, 442
    papilloma of, 412, 433
Chromaffin cells, 591
Chromogranin, 484
Chromogranin A, in neuroendocrine tumors, 1106
Chromophil adenoma, renal, 1796
Chromophil renal cell carcinoma, 1792–1796, 1805
    in children, 1839
Chromophobe renal cell carcinoma, 1796–1799, 1803
Chronic lymphocytic leukemia (CLL)
    B-cell, 670–673, 738–741
    immunoblastic transformation of, 673
    mixed cell type, 670
    spleen in, 782–784
    T-cell, 677
    transformation of, 670–673
Chronic lymphoproliferative disorders (CLPDs), B-cell, 670–673

Chronic myeloid leukemia (CML), 663–664, 794–795
Chronological dates, 2211
Churg-Strauss syndrome
 allergic angiitis and granulomatosis of, 1045–1046
 nasal polyps in, 889
 small vessel vasculitis in, 1260
Cicatricial pemphigoid, 23
 ocular, 984
Ciliary body, 994–996
Ciliated cell carcinoma, of endometrium, 2255–2256
Ciliated cell metaplasia, of endometrium, 2255, 2256
Ciliated cell prominence, of endometrium, 2255, 2256
Ciliated metaplasia, of stomach, 1314
CIN. See Cervical intraepithelial neoplasia (CIN)
Cirrhosis, 1513, 1540–1542
 primary biliary, 1511, 1512, 1513, 1527–1528, 1547, 1548
Cisplatin, effect on testis of, 1958
CJD (Creutzfeldt-Jakob disease), 392, 393, 404–405, 463
Clear cell acanthoma, 50
Clear cell adenocarcinoma, of vagina, 2141–2142
Clear cell adenoma, 860
Clear cell carcinoma
 of cervix, 2191
 of endometrium, 2221, 2254, 2257–2258
 hepatocellular, 1580–1581
 of liver, 1586
 of ovary, 2335–2339
 of pancreas, 1497
 renal, 1787–1791
 of salivary gland, 873
 of thymus, 1179
Clear cell chondrosarcoma, 279
Clear cell lesions, peritoneal, 2435
Clear cell meningioma, 442
Clear cell metaplasia
 of breast, 329
 of endometrium, 2256
Clear cell sarcoma, 191, 193–194
 of kidney, 1842–1847, 1849
Clear cell tumor
 of ovary, 2335–2339
 pulmonary, 1101
 of thyroid, 556–557
Clitoris, congenital anomalies of, 2113
CLL. See Chronic lymphocytic leukemia (CLL)
Cloquet's lymph node, 2111–2112
Clostridium difficile, pseudomembranous colitis due to, 1365
CML (chronic myeloid leukemia), 663–664, 794–795

CMV. See Cytomegalovirus (CMV)
CNS. See Central nervous system (CNS)
Cocaine abuse, myocarditis due to, 1218
Codman's triangle, 284
Colic, biliary, 1632
Colitis
 active, 1362–1364
  diffuse, 1362–1363
  focal, 1363–1364
 in AIDS patients, 1371–1374
 antibiotic-associated, 1365
 bacterial, 1364
 chronic, 1361–1362
 collagenous, 1366–1368
 diversion, 1377
 eosinophilic, 1368
 hemorrhagic, 1364–1365
 indeterminate, 1375–1376
 infectious, 1363, 1364–1366
 ischemic, 1369, 1376, 1382–1384
 lymphocytic, 1366–1368
 microscopic, 1366
 pseudomembranous, 1365, 1383
 ulcerative. See Ulcerative colitis (UC)
 viral, 1365
Colitis cystica profunda, 1369–1370
Collagen, dermal, alterations of, 34–35
Collagenous colitis, 1366–1368
Collagenous fibroma, 153
Collagenous spherulosis, of breast, 378–379
Collagenous sprue, 1355
Collagen vascular disease
 myocardial lesions in, 1218
 thyroid fibrosis due to, 535
Collecting duct carcinoma, 1803–1805
Colloid bodies, 5, 9
Colloid cyst, 460–461
Colon
 adenoma of, 1425
 biopsy of, 1361
 carcinoma of. See Colorectal carcinoma
 cathartic, 1388, 1389
 dysplasia of, 1379–1382
 normal histology of, 1361
 stromal tumors of, 1456
Colonopathy, fibrosing, 1394
Colony-stimulating factors (CSFs), 655
Colorectal carcinoma, 1436–1442
 adeno-, 1431, 1436–1437, 1439
  mucinous, 1437
 adenomas and, 1425–1427, 1431
 adenosquamous, 1439
 biologic markers of, 1442
 hereditary nonpolyposis, 1440
 inflammatory bowel disease and, 1379–1382
 intramucosal, 1431
 invasive vs. in situ, 1431
 of large intestine and rectum, 1436–1439

 of ovary, 2377–2378
 pathology of, 1436
 prognostic indicators in, 1441–1442
 small cell, 1437–1439
 small early flat, 1439
 specimen handling for, 1441
 squamous, 1439
 staging of, 1440–1441
 of stomach, 1330, 1331
 undifferentiated, 1439, 1442, 1443
 unusual forms of, 1439
Colorectal mucosal prolapse syndromes, 1369–1370
Colostomies, 1379
Columella, 885
Columnar cell metaplasia, of breast, 329
Columns of Morgagni, 1671
Comedo ductal carcinoma *in situ*, 338–339
Common bile duct (CBD), 1655
Common blue nevus, 96
Common hepatic duct (CHD), 1655
Common variable immunodeficiency disease (CVID), intestines in, 1355
Complete maturation arrest, 1951–1952, 1956
Condyloma acuminatum, 49
 with cervical carcinoma, 2174–2176
 of cervix, 2156–2157, 2174
 giant cell, 2059–2061
 of penis, 2040–2041
 of urothelial tract, 1862–1863
 of vagina, 2136
 of vulva, 2116–2117
Condyloma latum
 of penis, 2039
 of vulva, 2114
Condylomatous carcinoma, of penis, 2051
Congenital adrenal hyperplasia, defects in adrenal cortical hormone synthesis with, 1965
Congenital fiber-type disproportion, 123
Congenital hepatic fibrosis, 1519, 1557, 1560
Congestive cardiomyopathy, 1211–1215
Congestive heart failure, liver in, 1511, 1514
Conjunctiva, 983–988
 cysts of, 984
 developmental abnormalities of, 983–984
 inflammation of, 984–985
 lymphoid tumors of, 987
 neoplasms of, 985–986
 pinguecula of, 988
 pterygium of, 988
Conjunctivitis, 984–985
 ligneous, 984
Connective tissue matrix, abnormal formation of, 248–249
Connective tissue nevi, 60–61

Connective tissue tumors, 60–67
  adrenal, 606–607
Conn's syndrome, 595, 599–600
Constipation, severe idiopathic, 1389
Contact dermatitis
  allergic, 6–7
  irritant, 7
Contraction artifact, 112
Conus elasticus, 926
Copper-binding protein, in hepatocellular carcinoma, 1582, 1583
Corbus's disease, 2041
Cores, in muscle biopsy, 117–118
Cornea, 977–983
  bullous keratopathy of, 979
  calcific bank keratopathy of, 978
  chronic actinic (climatic droplet) keratopathy of, 978–979
  epithelial ingrowth of, 983
  evaluation of, 977–978
  keratitis due to infection of, 981–983
  keratoconus of, 979
  neoplasms of, 983
  nonspecific responses of, 978
  pannus of, 978
  rheumatoid arthritis of, 983
Corneal dystrophies, 979–981
Corneal grafts, 978
Coronal sulcus, 2035
Coronary artery aneurysms, 1237
Coronary artery bypass grafts, 1237, 1273
Coronary vascular disease, 1235–1237
Corpora cavernosa, 2037
Corpus luteum cysts, 2310–2311
Cortical adenomas, 598–600
Cortical carcinoma, 600–605
Cortical hyperplasia, 595–597
Cortical irregularities, of femur, 304
Cortical nodules, 600
Corticotroph cell, 497
Corticotroph cell adenoma, 498, 501, 512–514
  silent, 498, 512, 513–514
Corticotropin-releasing hormone, ectopic production of, 596
Cortisol, plasma and urinary concentrations of, 590
Corynebacterium minutissimum, 2115
Cowden's disease, 1418, 1419
  gastric polyps in, 1326
Cowper's glands, 1907
CPT (carnitine palmityltransferase) deficiency, 126
Cranial arteritis, 1258, 1260, 1262–1264, 1265
Craniofacial bones, giant-cell tumors of, 914
Craniopharyngioma, 412, 456
  adamantinomatous, 516–519
  cystic, 461

  papillary, 519
  sinonasal, 905
Creutzfeldt-Jakob disease (CJD), 392, 393, 404–405, 463
Cribriform carcinoma, of breast, 356–357
Cribriform plate, 885
Critical care myopathy, 127
Crohn's disease (CD), 1374–1375, 1376
  of anus, 1674
  of appendix, 1395
  biopsy specimen in, 1363
  dysplasia and cancer in, 1382
  of esophagus, 1290
  of liver, 1513, 1543
  polyps in, 1420
  of stomach, 1320
  of vulva, 2120
Crohn's enteritis, 1375, 1376
Crohn's vasculitis, 1375
Cronkite-Canada syndrome, 1328, 1418, 1424
Crooke's hyaline change, 512
Crust, 5
Cryoglobulinemic glomerulonephritis, 1739–1741, 1776–1777
Crypt hyperplasia, 1350–1352
Crypt hypoplasia, 1352–1353
Cryptorchidism, 1945–1947
  and germ cell tumors, 1947, 1978
Cryptosporidiosis
  of gallbladder, 1640
  gastritis due to, 1324
  intestinal, in AIDS patients, 1372–1373
Crystalloids, in prostate carcinoma, 1913
CSFs (colony-stimulating factors), 655
Cushing's syndrome, 595–596, 598–599
  pituitary adenoma in, 498, 512
Cutaneous appendage neoplasms, of vulva, 2133
Cutaneous ciliated cyst, 62
Cutaneous diseases. *See* Skin disease(s)
Cutaneous gout, 38–39
Cutaneous neural tumors, 67–68
Cutaneous T-cell lymphoma, 75–76
  vs. chronic spongiotic dermatitis, 17
  vs. spongiotic dermatitis, 6
Cutaneous tumors. *See* Skin tumor(s)
Cutaneous vascular calciphylaxis, 38
CVID (common variable immunodeficiency disease), intestines in, 1355
Cycle days, 2211
Cyclophosphamide
  effect on testis of, 1958
  hemorrhagic cystitis due to, 1856–1858
Cyclospora cayetanensis, 1374
Cyclosporin nephrotoxicity, 1772–1774
Cylindroma, 61
  of ear, 956
  of salivary glands, 867
Cyst(s)

  adrenal, 605
  ameloblastoma, 843
  aneurysmal bone, sinonasal, 914–915
  Baker's, 241
  bile duct, 1656–1657
  bone, 300–302
  breast, 329, 330
  bronchogenic, 1151–1152
  calcifying, 839
  choledochal, 1656–1657
  of CNS, 459–463
  colloid, 460–461
  of conjunctiva, 984
  corpus luteum, 2310–2311
  of cutaneous adnexa, 62
  cutaneous ciliated, 62
  of degenerative joint disease, 302
  dentigerous, 836
  dermoid, 62
    of CNS, 461
    of conjunctiva, 984
    epibulbar, 984
    of eyelid, 990–991
    of orbit, 996–998
    ovarian, 2365–2366
    of retrorectal space, 1391–1392
    of testis, 1999
  endometriotic, 2427–2428, 2429, 2430
  enteric, 1152–1153
  enterogenous, 461, 462, 1391
  ependymal, 460, 461
  epidermoid
    of bone, 302
    of CNS, 461–462
    of inner ear, 972
    of retrorectal space, 1391–1392
    of testis, 2012–2013
    of vulva, 2113
  epididymal, 1960
  eruption, 838
  esophageal, 1304
  of eyelid, 990–991
    sudoriferous, 990
  fissural, 840–842
  ganglion, 302
  Gartner's duct, 2114, 2137
  gingival, 836
  glandular, 839–840
  glial, 459–460
  globulomaxillary, 841–842
  Gorlin, 839
  hepatic, 1557–1563
  inclusion
    of conjunctiva, 984
    of eyelid, 990
    of ovary, 2309
    peritoneal, 2418–2420
  infundibular, 62
  of jaw, 835–842
  kerato-, 838–839
  lateral periodontal, 836

median palatine, 841
median raphe, 2038
mediastinal, 1149–1156
meningeal, 460, 462–463
mucous retention and extravasation, 35
nabothian, 2177
nasolabial (nasoalveolar), 841
nasopalatine, 841
neuroepithelial, 460
in nevoid basal cell carcinoma syndrome, 839
odontogenic, 835–840, 842
ovarian
    dermoid, 2365–2366
    inclusion, 2309
    in polycystic ovarian disease, 2312
    solitary follicle, 2309–2311
pancreatic, 1487–1488
    lymphoepithelial, 1492
paradental, 836
parathyroid, 568, 1149–1151
paratubal, 2400
penile, 2038
periapical, 835–836
pericardial, 1152
pineal, 460
placental, 2092–2093
prostatic, 1898–1899
pseudo-
    adrenal, 605
    of ear, 953
    hepatic, 1557, 1561
    pancreatic, 1488, 1493
radicular, 835–836
Rathke's cleft, 519
renal, 1686–1689, 1692–1696, 1767
residual, 836
retrorectal, 1391–1392
salivary, 854–855
seminal vesicle, 1935
sinonasal, 890
of spleen, 797
of stomach, 1313
testicular, 1959
third pharyngeal pouch, 1150
thymic, 1149–1151
trichilemmal, 62
vaginal, 2137
vellus hair, 62
vulvar, 2113–2114
X-cell, 2092–2093
Cystadenocarcinoma
    biliary, 1557, 1561–1562
    of ovary, 2328–2330
    of pancreas
        acinar cell, 1491
        mucinous, 1488–1490, 1493
Cystadenoma(s)
    appendiceal, 1442
    biliary, 1557, 1561–1562
    of broad ligament, 2409

of ovary
    mucinous, 2328
    rete, 2358
    serous papillary, 2322–2325, 2327
papillary, of testis, 2019
seminal vesicle, 1935
Cystic dysplasia, of rete testis, 2014
Cystic fibrosis
    fibrosing colonopathy in, 1394
    liver in, 1513, 1520, 1521, 1522
    nasal polyps in, 891
Cystic hamartoma, retrorectal, 1391–1392
Cystic hygromas, 1153
Cystic hyperplasia, of breast, 341
Cystic hypersecretory ductal carcinoma *in situ*, 341
Cystic meningoceles, 1153
Cystic mesotheliomas, of peritoneum, 2422
Cystic neoplasms
    of atrioventricular node, 1240
    pancreatic, 1488–1493
Cystic nephroma, 1807
    in children, 1834–1835
Cystic seminomas, 1155–1156, 1198
Cystic teratomas, mediastinal, 1153–1155, 1198
Cystic thymomas, 1155–1156
Cystinosis, 1761
Cystitis, 1854–1858
    eosinophilic, 1855
    follicular, 1855–1856
    hemorrhagic, 1856–1858
    iatrogenic, 1856
    interstitial, 1855
    polypoid, 1855
    radiation, 1856
    schistosomal, 1855
    tuberculous, 1854–1855
Cystitis cystica, 1860
Cystitis glandularis, 1860, 1861
Cystosarcoma phyllodes, of breast, 366–367
Cytokeratin
    in hepatocellular carcinoma, 1583, 1584
    as marker for soft tissue tumors, 143
    in pulmonary neoplasms, 1109
Cytokines, in chorioamnionitis, 2101
Cytomegalovirus (CMV)
    adrenal insufficiency due to, 594
    in AIDS
        of CNS, 402
        intestinal, 1371
        pulmonary, 1058
    of endocervical glands, 2182
    esophagitis due to, 1289
    of gallbladder, 1640–1641
    gastritis due to, 1324
    hepatitis due to, 1515, 1534
Cytoplasmic pale bodies, in fibrolamellar hepatocellular carcinoma, 1591

Cytosine arabinoside, effect on testis of, 1958
Cytotoxic drug effects, on ovary, 2319
Cytotrophoblasts, 2067
    vacuolated, 2068

D

Dacryoadenitis, 1000
Dacryoliths, 1002
D&C (dilatation and curettage), 2203
Dandy-Walker malformation, 1689
Darier's disease, 21
DBCP (1,2-dibromo-3 chloropropane), effect on testis of, 1958
DCIS. *See* Ductal carcinoma *in situ* (DCIS)
Decidua
    ovarian, 2317
    peritoneal, 2435–2436, 2437
Dedifferentiation, 289
    of chondrosarcoma, 278, 279–280
    of malignant fibrous histiocytoma, 165–166
Defunctionalized bowel, 1377
Degenerative joint disease, cysts of, 302
Dehydroepiandrosterone, plasma and urinary concentrations of, 590
Delta agent, 1534
Dementia, 392, 393, 463–464
    AIDS, 402
    with Lewy bodies, 464
Demodicosis, of eyelids, 989
Demyelination, 392, 464–465
Dendritic cell sarcomas, 763–764
Denervating diseases, 127
Dense deposit disease, 1709, 1775
Dental lamina, 805
Dentigerous cysts, 836
de Quervain's disease, 531
Dermal deposits, alterations of, 34–35
Dermal hypoplasia, focal, 810
Dermal inflammatory cell infiltrates, diffuse, 29–30
Dermal inflammatory patterns, 26–27
Dermatitis
    atopic, 7
    contact
        allergic, 6–7
        irritant, 7
    granulomatous, 31–33
    lichenoid interface, 9–10
    neuro-, 16–17
    pigmented purpuric lichenoid, of Gougerot and Blum, 28
    psoriasiform, 8
    seborrheic, 7
    spongiotic, 6
        acute and subacute, 6–9
        chronic, 16–17
    stasis, 8
    vacuolar interface, 10–14

Dermatitis herpetiformis, 23–24
  intestines in, 1353
Dermatofibroma. See Fibrous histiocytoma
Dermatofibrosarcoma protuberans, 66–67, 160
Dermatomyositis, 12, 114, 124
Dermatopathic lymphadenopathy, 724
Dermatopathology. See Skin disease(s)
Dermatophytosis, 7
Dermatosis
  acute febrile neutrophilic, 29
  progressive pigmentary, of Schamberg, 28
  subcorneal pustular, 17
  transient acantholytic, 21
Dermis, 4, 5
  "normal," 24–25
Dermoid cyst(s), 62
  of CNS, 461
  of conjunctiva, 984
  epibulbar, 984
  of eyelid, 990–991
  of orbit, 996–998
  ovarian, 2365–2366
  of retrorectal space, 1391–1392
  of testis, 1999
Dermolipomas, of conjunctiva, 984
DES (diethylstilbestrol), in utero exposure to, vaginal abnormalities due to, 2133–2135
Desmin, as marker for soft tissue tumors, 141
Desmin storage myopathy, 123–124
Desmoids, periosteal, 304
Desmoid-type fibromatosis, of mediastinum, 1166–1167
Desmoplastic fibroblastoma, 153
Desmoplastic fibroma, 296
Desmoplastic infantile ganglioglioma, 432
Desmoplastic small cell tumor, of brain, 456
Desmoplastic small round cell tumor, 195
  intraabdominal, 2424–2425
  of ovary, 2376
  of testis, 2017–2018
Desmoplastic supratentorial neuroepithelial tumor of infancy, 419
Desquamative inflammatory vaginitis, 2136
Desquamative interstitial pneumonia, 1015–1018
Diabetes mellitus
  gastroparesis due to, 1340
  liver in, 1543
  mastopathy in, 375–376
  nephropathy in, 1727–1730, 1776
  peripheral neuropathy of, 225–227
  vascular disease in, 1253, 1254, 1255, 1256

Dialysis, of kidney, 1765–1767
Diarrhea
  Brainerd, 1368
  watery, 1502
1,2-Dibromo-3 chloropropane (DBCP), effect on testis of, 1958
Diethylstilbestrol (DES), in utero exposure to, vaginal abnormalities due to, 2133–2135
Dieulafoy's malformation, 1276, 1339
Digital fibrokeratoma, 62
Digital fibroma, of childhood, recurrent, 65
Dilatation and curettage (D&C), 2203
Diphalalia, 2038
Diphenylhydantoin, thyroiditis due to, 533
Dirofilariasis, 1045
Disc herniation, 239–240
Discoid lupus erythematosus (DLE), 10–12
Dissecting aneurysm, 1256, 1257
Dissecting resorption, 247
Distal myopathy, 122
Diversion colitis, 1377
Diverticular polyps, 1423
Diverticulosis
  jejunal, 1389
  pseudo-, of esophagus, 1304
Diverticulum(a)
  of bladder, 1859–1860
  esophageal, 1305
  of gallbladder, 1630, 1639
  intestinal, 1384–1386
    inflammatory bowel disease and, 1377
    small, 1391
    Meckel's, 1391
DLE (discoid lupus erythematosus), 10–12
Donor-transmitted nephrosclerosis, 1774
Dowager's hump, 253
Drug effects
  gastritis due to, 1323
  liver disease due to, 1511–1516, 1528–1529, 1547, 1548
  lymphadenopathy due to, 727
  myocarditis due to, 1217–1218
  on testis, 1955–1956, 1958
  thyroiditis due to, 533–534
Drug eruption
  fixed, 14
  lichenoid, 10
DUB (dysfunctional uterine bleeding), 2223
Duchenne muscular dystrophy, 120–121
Ductal adenoma, 344, 371–372
Ductal carcinoma, infiltrating, 350–352
Ductal carcinoma in situ (DCIS), 336–344
  apocrine, 341
  biological markers for, 343
  cancerization of lobules in, 342, 348
  classification of, 336–338

  clinging, 340–341
  clinical significance of, 349
  comedo, 338–339
  cystic hypersecretory, 341
  vs. epithelial hyperplasia, 335, 343–344
  high-grade, 338–339
  intermediate-grade, 340
  intermediately differentiated, 340
  low-grade, 339–340
  neuroendocrine (argyrophilic), 341
  papillary, 344, 346–347
  poorly differentiated, 338–339
  prognostic index for, 343
  signet ring cell, 341
  surgical margins for, 342–343
  well-differentiated, 339–340
Ductal epithelial hyperplasia, 334–335
Duct ectasia, 375
Dukes' classification, of rectal carcinoma, 1440
Duodenitis, 1354–1355
Duodenum
  carcinoids of, 1447–1448
  stromal tumors of, 1456
Duplication cysts, of retrorectal space, 1391–1392
Dysembryonic neoplasms, of adrenal glands, 608
Dysembryoplastic neuroepithelial tumor, 431
Dysfunctional uterine bleeding (DUB), 2223
Dysgenetic male pseudohermaphroditism, 1967
Dysgerminomas, 2359–2360
Dyshidrosis, 7
Dyskeratoma, warty, 62
Dyskeratosis, 5
Dysplasia
  of bone, 302–303
  of bronchi and lungs, 1073–1074
  of cervix gland, 2184
  of colon, 1379–1382
  esophageal
    in Barrett's esophagus, 1293–1295
    squamous, 1300
  of gallbladder, 1643, 1645–1648
  intestinal neuronal, 1390–1391
  of larynx, 929–931
  monostotic, 957
  of oral cavity, 812–814
  osteofibrous, 293, 303
  periapical cemental, 845–846
  renal, 1686–1689
  of rete testis, 2014
  sinonasal, 915–916
  squamous
    of esophagus, 1300
    of oral cavity, 812–814
    of stomach, 1333–1334
  thymic, 1161

Dysplastic gangliocytoma, of cerebellum, 431
Dysplastic nevus, 101–102
Dysproteinemia, angioimmunoblastic lymphadenopathy with, 726–727
Dystrophin, 121
Dystrophy, vulvar, 2121–2123

E

Ear, 949–972
  external, 949–958
    adenoid cystic carcinoma of, 957
    adenoma (ceruminoma) of, 955
    basal cell carcinoma of, 954
    benign fibroosseous lesion of, 957
    chondrodermatitis nodularis chronic helicis of, 952
    cylindroma of, 956
    epithelioid hemangioma of, 953
    exostosis of, 957–958
    gout of, 951
    hair granuloma of, 950
    idiopathic cystic chondromalacia (pseudocysts) of, 953
    Kaposi's sarcoma of, 958
    keloid of, 953
    keratin implantation granuloma of, 950–951
    keratosis obturans of, 950–951
    Kimura's disease of, 953
    Langerhans' cell histiocytosis of, 953
    malakoplakia of, 952
    malformations of, 949
    malignant external otitis of, 949
    malignant lymphoma of, 958
    melanotic neoplasms of, 957
    mucoepidermoid carcinoma of, 957
    ochronosis of, 951
    osteoma of, 957–958
    petrified auricle of, 951
    relapsing polychondritis of, 950
    rhabdomyosarcoma of, 958
    spectacle-frame acanthoma (granuloma fissuratum) of, 952–953
    squamous cell carcinoma of, 954–955
    starch granuloma of, 949
    syringocystadenoma papilliferum of, 955
    xanthoma associated with hyperlipoproteinemia of, 951
  inner, 969–972
    acoustic neuroma of, 969–971
    adenocarcinoma of, 971–972
    cholesteatoma (epidermoid cyst) of, 972
    cholesterol granuloma of, 972
    lipoma of, 971
    metastases to, 972
    neurofibromatosis 2 of, 970–971
    vestibular schwannoma of, 969–970
  middle, 958–969
    adenoma of, 963–965
    carcinoid tumor of, 964–965
    cholesteatoma of, 961–963
    cholesterol granuloma of, 959
    choristomas of, 963
    congenital stapes fixation of, 968–969
    glial masses of, 963
    jugulotympanic paraganglioma of, 965–967
    meningioma of, 965
    metastases to, 967
    neoplasms of, 960–967
    osteogenesis imperfecta of, 969
    otitis media of, 958–960
    otosclerosis of, 967–968
    papillary adenocarcinoma of, 967
    sarcoid of, 960
    squamous cell carcinoma of, 967
    tympanosclerosis of, 959–960
Eaton-Lambert syndrome, 127
EBV (Epstein-Barr virus)
  hepatitis due to, 1534, 1536
  leiomyosarcoma and, 171
Eccrine adenoma, papillary, 63
Eccrine glands, 5
Eccrine poroma, 61
Echinococcosis, hepatic, 1557, 1558–1559
Ecthyma, of vulva, 2115
Ectochordosis physaliphora, 297
Ectopic hormone production, 486
Ectopic pregnancy, 2398–2399
Eczema
  endogenous, 7
  nummular, 7
Eczematid-like purpura of Doucase and Kapetanakis, 28
Edema, of ovary, massive, 2314
Ehlers-Danlos syndrome, intestinal involvement in, 1387
Elastofibroma, 154
Electron microscopy
  of breast tissue, 325
  of renal tissue, 1703–1704
Emboli, cholesterol, 1764
Embryoma, diffuse, of testis, 2002
Embryonal carcinoma
  of CNS, 412, 452
  of mediastinum, 1181
  of ovary, 2363
  of testis, 1985–1990
Embryonal rhabdomyosarcoma, 172
  of cervix, 2195
  of extrahepatic bile ducts, 1665, 1666
  of vagina, 2142–2143
Emphysematous vaginitis, 2136–2137
Empty sella syndrome, 522–523
Encephalitis, 396, 400–401
  herpes simplex virus, 392, 400
  HIV, 401
Encephalitozoon intestinalis, in AIDS patients, 1373–1374
Encephalomyelitis, postinfectious, 400–401
Encephalopathies, spongiform, 404–406
Enchondroma, 272–273
Endarterectomy, 1271–1272
Endocarditis, 1230–1233
  infective, 1231–1232
  nonbacterial thrombotic, 1232–1233
  rheumatic, 1232
  with systemic lupus erythematosus, 1232
Endocervical glands
  atypia of, 2182–2184
  dysplasia of, 2184
  hyperplasia of
    diffuse laminar, 2177–2178
    mesonephric, 2179–2180
    micro-, 2178–2179
  tuboendometrial metaplasia of, 2180
Endocervical-like mucinous borderline tumors, 2329
Endocervical polyps, 2177
Endocervical-type adenocarcinoma, 2187
Endocervicitis, 2180–2182
Endocervicosis, 2435
Endocrine cells, in nonendocrine tumors, 491–492
Endocrine neoplasms
  gastric, 1334–1335
  of pancreas, 1497–1501
Endocrine therapy, of prostatic carcinoma, 1925–1926
Endodermal sinus tumor
  of CNS, 412, 452
  of mediastinum, 1181
  of ovary, 2360–2363
  of vagina, 2142
  of vulva, 2129–2130
Endometrial adenocarcinoma, 2230–2258
  architectural patterns for, 2231, 2232–2233
  atypical hyperplasia and, 2229
  cervix in, 2238–2239
  ciliated cell, 2255–2256
  classification of, 2231
  clear-cell, 2221, 2254, 2257–2258
  clinicopathologic correlation of, 2234–2236
  differential diagnosis of, 2241–2245
  endometrioid, 2230–2241
  estrogen therapy and, 2236
  extrauterine, 2239
  general description of, 2230–2234
  glycogen-rich squamoid, 2256–2257
  metastatic, 2270
  mucinous, 2250
  myoinvasive, 2236–2238
  neuroendocrine cells in, 2250
  ovarian metastases of, 2382

Endometrial adenocarcinoma *(contd.)*
  papillary serous, 2252–2254
  secretory, 2218–2219, 2256–2257
  with squamous elements, 2240, 2247–2249, 2264
  staging and grading of, 2231–2234, 2235, 2236, 2239–2241, 2245
  usual type of, 2230–2241
  variants of, 2246–2258
  villoglandular, 2252, 2254
  well-differentiated, 2239–2241
Endometrial biopsy, 2203–2204
Endometrial colonization, 2400
Endometrial dating, 2211–2214
Endometrioid adenocarcinoma
  of cervix, 2190–2191
  of fallopian tube, 2405–2406
  of ovary, 2331–2333
  of uterine corpus, 2230–2241
Endometrioid tumors
  of ovary, 2330–2333
  peritoneal, 2432
Endometriomas, 2427–2428
Endometriosis, 2427–2431
  cervical, 2180
  of colon and rectum, 1459–1460
  defined, 2427
  differential diagnosis of, 2431
  of fallopian tube, 2399–2400
  lesions associated with, 2431
  macroscopic features of, 2427–2428
  microscopic features of, 2428–2431
  neoplasms arising from, 2432
  postsalpingectomy, 2400
  in pregnancy, 2431
  stromal, 2430, 2431
  of urothelial tract, 1858
  vaginal, 2137
    and carcinoma, 2142
  of vulva, 2114
Endometriotic cysts, 2427–2428, 2429, 2430
Endometritis, 2221–2222
Endometrium, 2210–2271
  adenocarcinoma of. *See* Endometrial adenocarcinoma
  adenofibroma of, 2245, 2260–2261, 2264, 2270–2271
  adenomyoma of, atypical polypoid, 2245, 2258–2259, 2264
  adenosarcoma of, 2261–2262, 2264–2265, 2270–2271
  with alternative differentiated epithelium, 2245–2258
  atrophic, 2223–2224, 2241–2242
  carcinosarcoma of, 2254, 2262–2264, 2265
  choriocarcinoma of, 2221
  ciliated cell patterns in, 2254–2256
  disintegrating, 2210, 2244
  endometrioid, 2223
  epithelial cell vacuolation of, 2216–2217
  gestational, 2219–2221
  glands-to-stroma ratio of, 2206
  glandular features of, 2206
  hemorrhage of, 2217
  hyperplasia of, 2226–2230, 2242–2244
    atypical, 2226–2230, 2242–2244, 2256
    villoglandular, 2251–2252, 2254
  inactive, 2223–2224, 2241–2242
  infections of, 2221–2222
  inflammation of, 2210, 2221–2222
  interval, 2214–2215, 2216
  menstrual, 2215–2216
  metaplasia of
    ciliated cell, 2255, 2256
    clear-cell, hobnail, and eosinophilic, 2256–2258
    epithelial, 2245–2246
    mucinous, 2249, 2250
    papillary syncytial, 2251, 2254
  mixed müllerian neoplasia of, 2258–2265
  morular differentiation of, 2246–2249
  mucinous differentiation of, 2249–2250
  necrosis of, 2210, 2221–2222
  nonsecretory patterns of, 2222–2245
  in normal menstrual cycle, 2210–2217
  out-of-phase, 2217–2218
  papillary or villoglandular architecture in, 2251–2254
  pattern diagnosis for, 2205–2210
  polyps of, 2230, 2244–2245, 2264
  proliferative
    disordered, 2224–2226, 2242
    normal, 2214, 2216
    weakly, 2223–2224, 2241–2242
  samples of, 2203–2204
  sarcoma of
    pure, 2264–2265, 2288
    stromal, 2266–2270, 2288, 2334–2335, 2431
    undifferentiated, 2268–2269
  secretory, 2215, 2216
    abnormal patterns of, 2217–2219
  sheetlike proliferations of, 2210, 2245, 2265
  spindle-cell proliferations of, 2208–2209
  squamous (squamoid, morular) differentiation of, 2246–2249
  stromal features of, 2206
  stromal tumors of, 2265–2271
    nodules, 2265, 2266, 2269, 2270
    sarcomas, 2265, 2266–2270, 2334–2335, 2431
    with sex-cord-like elements, 2269, 2270–2271
  vasculature of, 2206–2208
Endomyocardial biopsy, 1209–1210
Endophthalmitis, 976
Endosalpingiosis, 2432–2433
  lymph node, 2326
Endothelial dystrophy, congenital hereditary, 980
Endothelialitis, 1544–1545
Endothelial markers, for soft tissue tumors, 139–140
Endothelial tumors, malignant, 178–181
Endovascular stenting, 1271
Endovasculopathy, hemorrhagic, of placenta, 2098
End-stage renal disease (ESRD), 1765–1767
Entamoeba histolytica, in AIDS patients, 1371
Enteric cysts, 1152–1153
Enteritis, Crohn's, 1375, 1376
Enterobius vermicularis
  of appendix, 1395
  of fallopian tube, 2397
Enterocolitis
  AIDS-related, 1374
  lymphocytic, 1352
  necrotizing, 1383
  neutropenic, 1383
  pseudomembranous, 1365, 1383
  radiation, 1383
Enterocytozoon bieneusi, in AIDS patients, 1373–1374
Enterogenous cysts, 461, 462, 1391
Enteropathy
  autoimmune, 1355
  familial, 1352–1353
  gluten-sensitive, 1350–1352
  tufting, 1360
Enteropathy-associated T cell lymphoma, 1350, 1450–1453
Eosinophil(s), intraepithelial, in gastroesophageal reflux disease, 1287
Eosinophilia
  angiolymphoid hyperplasia with, 71, 176
  pulmonary, 1023–1026
  tropical, 1023
Eosinophilia/myalgia syndrome, 145, 153
Eosinophilic cholecystitis, 1641
Eosinophilic colitis, 1368
Eosinophilic cystitis, 1855
Eosinophilic esophagitis, 1290
Eosinophilic fasciitis, 145, 153
Eosinophilic gastritis, 1321
Eosinophilic gastroenteritis, 1357
Eosinophilic granuloma
  of bone, 306, 693
  of pituitary, 522
  pulmonary involvement in, 1028–1030
Eosinophilic metaplasia, of endometrium, 2256

Eosinophilic peritonitis, 2417
Eosinophilic pleuritis, 1030
Eosinophilic pustular folliculitis, 34
Ependymal cyst, 460, 461
Ependymoblastoma, 414, 424–425
Ependymoma(s), 411, 413, 420–424
  anaplastic, 411, 424
  of broad ligament, 2409
  clear cell, 423
  epithelioid, 422
  low-grade, 422–423
  malignant, 413, 424
  myxopapillary, 413, 423–424
  papillary, 422
  tanycytic, 411, 423
Ephelis, of conjunctiva, 986
Epibulbar dermoids, 984
Epidermal inclusion cyst
  of eyelid, 990
  vaginal, 2137
Epidermal inflammatory patterns, 6–17
  erythema multiforme, 14–16
  lichenoid interface dermatitis, 9–10
  spongiotic dermatitis, 6–9, 16–17
  vacuolar interface dermatitis, 10–14
  verrucous acanthosis, 16
Epidermal nevus, 49
Epidermal tumors, 49–59
Epidermis, 4
  "normal," 24–25
Epidermodysplasia verruciformis, 55
Epidermoid cyst
  of bone, 302
  of CNS, 461–462
  of inner ear, 972
  of retrorectal space, 1391–1392
  of testis, 2012–2013
  of vulva, 2113
Epidermolysis, 5
Epidermolysis bullosa, 24
Epidermolytic hyperkeratosis, 22–23, 52–53
Epidermotropism, 6
Epididymal tumors, 1974, 2018–2020
Epididymis, 1959–1960
Epididymitis, 1959–1960
Epiglottic cancer, 933–934
Epiglottis, 925
Epilepsy, 392, 465–466
Epiphrenic diverticula, 1305
Epiploic appendices, infarcted, 1394
Epispadias, 2038
Epithelial hyperplasia
  of breast, 329, 334–336
    vs. ductal carcinoma in situ, 335, 343–344
  in gastroesophageal reflux disease, 1285
  of oral cavity, 810
Epithelial inclusion glands, of ovary, 2308–2309
Epithelial markers
  for mesothelioma, 1129–1133
  for soft tissue tumors, 143
Epithelial membrane antigen, as marker for soft tissue tumors, 143
Epithelial metaplasia
  of breast, 329–330
  of endometrium, 2245–2246
  glioblastoma and gliosarcoma with, 429
Epithelial misplacement, intestinal, 1432–1434
Epithelial myoepithelial carcinoma, of salivary glands, 864–865
Epithelial tumors, of fallopian tube, 2403
Epithelioid angiosarcomas, of peritoneum, 2425
Epithelioid hemangioendothelioma, 73, 178–179
  of bile ducts, 1602
  of liver, 1602, 1608, 1609–1611
  of lungs, 1101
  of mediastinum, 1195
  of peritoneum, 2425
Epithelioid hemangioma, 175–176
  of ear, 953
Epithelioid leiomyoma, 170
  of uterus, 2273, 2283–2284
Epithelioid leiomyosarcoma, of mediastinum, 1189, 1190
Epithelioid sarcoma, 191
Epithelioid smooth-muscle tumor, of uterus, 2281
Epithelioid trophoblastic tumor, 2082–2085
Epithelioid tumor, of stomach, 1338
Epithelioma
  sebaceous, 61, 63
  of vagina, 2138
Epitheliosis, of breast, 329, 334
Epstein-Barr virus (EBV)
  hepatitis due to, 1534, 1536
  leiomyosarcoma and, 171
Epstein's pearls, 836
Epulis, fibroid, 807
Erlenmeyer flask deformity, 254
Erosion, 5
Eruption cysts, 838
Erysipelas, of vulva, 2115
Erythema, gyrate (figurate), 26
Erythema annulare centrifugum, 26
Erythema chronicum migrans, 26
Erythema elevatum diutinum, 28–29
Erythema gyratum repens, 26
Erythema induratum, 39
Erythema multiforme, 15
Erythema nodosum, 39
Erythema toxicum neonatorum, 18
Erythrasma, 2115
Erythroleukoplakia, 812
Erythroplakia, 812
Erythropoietic protoporphyria, liver in, 1520, 1523
Escherichia coli, enterohemorrhagic, 1364–1365
  in AIDS patients, 1372
Esophageal atresia, 1304
Esophageal carcinoma, 1297–1304
  adeno-, 1299, 1301–1303
  adenosquamous, 1299, 1304
  Barrett's esophagus and, 1293–1295
  basaloid, 1299, 1301
  differential diagnosis of, 1299
  mucoepidermoid, 1304
  pathologic evaluation of, 1297
  sarcomatoid, 1299, 1300–1301
  in situ, 1300
  small cell, 1299, 1303–1304
  squamous cell, 1298–1301
  TNM staging of, 1297, 1298
  verrucous, 1299, 1301
Esophageal cysts, 1304
Esophageal diverticula, 1305
Esophageal stenosis, 1304
Esophageal webs and rings, 1304–1305
Esophagitis, 1285–1290
  active, 1285
  acute, 1285
  Candida, 1288
  corrosive, 1290
  due to Crohn's disease, 1290
  cytomegalovirus, 1289
  eosinophilic, 1290
  due to gastroesophageal reflux disease, 1285–1288
  due to graft-versus-host disease, 1290
  herpes, 1288–1289
  histologic clues to etiology of, 1285
  HIV, 1290
  infectious, 1288–1290
  irradiation, 1290
  pill-induced, 1290
  reflux, 1285–1288
  due to skin disorders, 1290
Esophagus, 1283–1305
  achalasia of, 1295
  adenoma of, 1296
  Barrett's (columnar epithelium-lined), 1290–1295
    defined, 1290–1291
    diagnosis of, 1292–1293
    dysplasia in, 1293–1295
    other premalignant markers in, 1295
    pathologic features of, 1291–1292
  benign tumors of, 1295–1297
  carcinoma of. See Esophageal carcinoma
  dysplasia of
    in Barrett's esophagus, 1293–1295
    squamous, 1300
  glycogenic acanthosis of, 1304
  granular cell tumor of, 1297
  leiomyoma of, 1296
  leiomyomatosis of, 1295

Esophagus *(contd.)*
  lymphoma of, 1304
  malignant melanoma of, 1299, 1304
  metastases to, 1304
  muscular hypertrophy of, 1295
  neuromuscular disorders of, 1295
  normal features of, 1283–1284
  polypoid tumors of, 1296–1297
  sarcoma of, 1304
  specimen handling for, 1284
  squamous papilloma of, 1296
  systemic sclerosis of, 1295
ESRD (end-stage renal disease), 1765–1767
Essential thrombocythemia, 664
Esthesioneuroblastoma, of sellar region, 518
Estrogen therapy
  effect on testis of, 1955–1956, 1958
  and endometrial carcinoma, 2236
Ewing's sarcoma
  of bone, 263, 269–271
  vs. neuroblastoma, 611
  soft tissue, 194–195
Excurrent duct obstruction, 1953–1955, 1960
Exocytosis, 5, 6
Exostosis
  of ear, 957–958
  subungual, 308
External auditory meatus, atresia of, 949
Extrahepatic bile duct(s), 1655–1666
  benign tumors of, 1661
  carcinoma of, 1661–1666
  congenital anomalies of, 1656–1657
  embryonal rhabdomyosarcoma of, 1666
  malignant tumors of, 1661–1666
  metastases to, 1666
  normal anatomy and histology of, 1655–1656
  obstruction of, gallbladder in, 1642
  in sclerosing cholangitis, 1657–1661
  specimen processing for, 1655–1656
Extrahepatic biliary atresia, 1516–1518, 1656
Extraosseous plasmacytoma of mediastinum, 1188–1189, 1190
Extraovarian peritoneal serous papillary carcinoma, 2434
Extrinsic allergic alveolitis, 1021–1023
Extrusion, of nucleus pulposus, 239
Eye(s), 975–1002
  caruncle of, 988
  choroid of, 994–996
  ciliary body of, 994–996
  conjunctiva of, 983–988
    cysts of, 984
    developmental abnormalities of, 983–984
    inflammation of, 984–985
    lymphoid tumors of, 987
    neoplasms of, 985–986
    pinguecula of, 988
    pterygium of, 988
  cornea of, 977–983
    bullous keratopathy of, 979
    calcific bank keratopathy of, 978
    chronic actinic (climatic droplet) keratopathy of, 978–979
    dystrophies of, 979–981
    evaluation of, 977–978
    grafts to, 978
    keratitis due to infection of, 981–983
    keratoconus of, 979
    neoplasms of, 983
    nonspecific responses of, 978
    pannus of, 978
    rheumatoid arthritis of, 983
  globe of, 975–977
    foreign bodies in, 975–976
    glaucoma of, 977
    inflammation of, 976
    phthisis bulbi of, 976
    trauma to, 975
  iris of, 994–996
  lacrimal drainage apparatus of, 1001–1002
  lacrimal gland of, 1000–1001
  lens of, 992–993
  optic nerve of, 999–1000
  orbit of, 996–999
    developmental anomalies of, 996–998
    inflammation of, 998
    mucoceles of, 998
    tumors of, 998–999
  retina of, 993–994
  sclera of, 983
Eyelid(s), 988–992
  amyloid deposits of, 990
  chalazion of, 988
  cysts of, 990–991
  hordeolum (stye) of, 989
  mites of, 989
  molluscum contagiosum of, 989
  nematodes of, 990
  neoplasms of, 991–992
  pyogenic granuloma of, 988
  sarcoidosis of, 989
  verruca vulgaris of, 989

F

Fabry's disease, cardiomyopathy due to, 1213–1214
Face, fibrous papule of, 61–62
Factor VIII-related antigen, as marker for soft tissue tumors, 140
Factor XIIIa, as marker for soft tissue tumors, 140–141
Fallopian tube(s), 2395–2408
  amyloidosis of, 2398
  cysts of, 2400
  ectopic pregnancy of, 2398–2399
  ectopic tissue in, 2400–2401
  endometriosis of, 2399–2400
  hyperplastic lesions of, 2401–2402
  inflammatory diseases of, 2395–2398
  ligation of, changes secondary to, 2398
  metaplastic lesions of, 2401
  prolapse of, 2137, 2399
  pseudocarcinomatous lesions of, 2401–2402
  torsion of, 2399
  tumor-like lesions of, 2398–2402
  tumors of, 2402–2409
    adenomatoid, 2402
    benign epithelial, 2403
    benign soft tissue, 2404
    carcinoma, 2404–2406
      ovarian metastases of, 2382
    classification of, 2403
    epithelial, of borderline malignancy, 2403
    female adnexal, of probable wolffian origin, 2407–2408
    germ cell, 2407
    lymphoma and leukemia, 2407
    malignant Müllerian mixed, 2406–2407
    metaplastic papillary, 2401
    sarcomas, 2406–2407
    secondary, 2407
    trophoblastic, 2407
  Walthard nests of, 2400
Familial adenomatous polyposis, 1418, 1434
  attenuated, 1435
Familial enteropathy, 1352–1353
Familial hypocalciuric hypercalcemia, 569
Familial polyposis coli, 1418
Fasciitis
  eosinophilic, 145, 153
  necrotizing, of vulva, 2115
  nodular, 145–147
  of nasopharynx, 912
  proliferative, 147
Fascioscapulohumeral dystrophy, 121
Fat necrosis
  of breast, 374
  pancreatic, 40–41
  subcutaneous, of newborn, 40
Fatty changes, of liver, 1515, 1543, 1547, 1548
Fatty infiltration, of muscle, 115
Fatty tumors, of liver, 1612
Female adnexal tumor, of probable wolffian origin, 2407–2408
Feminization, 595, 600
Femoral head, aseptic necrosis of, 308
Femur, cortical irregularities of, 304
Fetal nucleated red blood cells, 2105
Fiber(s), muscle. *See* Muscle fibers
Fiber-osteoid, 301
Fiber-type disproportion, congenital, 123

Fibroadenolipoma, of breast, 377
Fibroadenoma, of breast, 363–364
   cellular intracanalicular, 366–367
   giant, 364
   juvenile, 365
Fibroadenomatoid hyperplasia, of breast, 364
Fibroblastic meningioma, 411, 440
Fibroblastic osteosarcoma, 284
Fibroblastic tumors, of larynx, 942
Fibroblastoma
   desmoplastic, 153
   giant-cell, 160
Fibrocystic change, 328–329
Fibroelastomas, papillary, cardiac, 1240
Fibroepithelial polyp
   of anus, 1673
   of cervix, 2196
   of gingiva, 807
   of vagina, 2137–2138
   of vulva, 2117
Fibrogenic proliferations, of mediastinum, 1165–1167
Fibrohistiocytic markers, for soft tissue tumors, 140–141
Fibrohistiocytic proliferation, of vagina, 2139
Fibrohistiocytic tumor, plexiform, 159–160
Fibrohistiocytic tumors
   of bone, 295–296
   of soft tissue, 159–160
Fibroid epulis, 807
Fibroid polyps, inflammatory
   of intestines, 1423–1424
   of stomach, 1327–1328
Fibrokeratoma, acquired (digital), 62
Fibrolamellar hepatocellular carcinoma, 1589–1593
Fibrolipoma, of vulva, 2119
Fibroma(s)
   ameloblastic, 843
   of bone, 264, 304
   calcifying aponeurotic, 154
   cementifying, 846
   chondromyxoid, 275–276
   collagenous, 153
   desmoplastic, 296
   digital, of childhood, 65
   of gonadal stromal origin, 2009
   of larynx, 942
   medullary, 1816–1817
   nonossifying, 304
   nuchal, 153
   odontogenic, 845
   ossifying
      of ear, 957
      of long bones, 302
      peripheral, 807
      sinonasal, 915–916
   of ovary, 2347–2348

   sinonasal, 911, 915–916
   soft tissue, 153
   of testis, 2009, 2016
Fibromatosis, 155–156
   congenital, 308
   desmoid-type, of mediastinum, 1166–1167
   infantile digital, 154
   juvenile hyaline, 154
   of larynx, 942
   of mesentery or retroperitoneum, 1397
   of ovary, 2314–2315
   sinonasal, 911
Fibromatosis colli, 154
Fibromyxoid sarcoma, low-grade, 158
Fibromyxoid tumors
   ossifying, 157
   pseudosarcomatous, 148
Fibroosseous lesions
   of ear, 957
   sinonasal, 915–916
Fibrosarcoma
   ameloblastic, 848
   of bone, 296–297
   of CNS, 411
   inflammatory, 158
   of larynx, 942
   of liver, 1615
   of ovary, 2348
   sclerosing epithelioid, 158–159
   sinonasal, 912
   of soft tissue, 157–159
   well-differentiated, 158
Fibrosing colonopathy, in cystic fibrosis, 1394
Fibrosing mediastinitis, 1167–1168
Fibrosing thyroid lesions, 534–535
Fibrosis
   CNS, 411
   of liver, 1513
   meningeal, 397
   of muscle, 115
   peritoneal, 2416
   pleural, 1118–1119
   pulmonary, 1012–1015
   retroperitoneal, 153, 1396, 1397–1398
Fibrous defects
   cortical, 304
   metaphyseal, 304
Fibrous dysplasia
   of bone, 302–303
   monostotic, 957
   sinonasal, 915–916
Fibrous hamartoma of infancy, 154
Fibrous histiocytoma
   benign
      of bone, 295
      cutaneous, 62–65
      of larynx, 942
      soft tissue, 159
   malignant

      angiomatoid, 165
      of bone, 295–296
      of CNS, 411
      as final common pathway, 165–166
      giant-cell type, 163–165
      inflammatory, 165
      of larynx, 942
      of liver, 1615
      myxoid, 152, 163
      natural history by subtype of, 161
      soft tissue, 160–166
      storiform/pleomorphic, 162–163
      superficial, 67, 162
   of mediastinum, 1161–1162
   of orbit, 999
   sinonasal, 912
Fibrous hyperplasia, of gingiva, 807
Fibrous obliteration, of appendix, 1395
Fibrous papule, of face, 61–62
Fibrous polyps, atypical, 151
Fibrous tumors
   of bone, 296–297
   of peritoneum, 2421
   soft-tissue, 152–154
   solitary
      of mediastinum, 1165–1166
      of pleura, 1119–1120
      renal, 1817
      sinonasal, 911–912
      of soft tissue, 156
Fibroxanthoma, atypical, 67, 159, 162
Figurate erythemas, 26
Fine needle aspiration
   of bone, 264–265
   of breast tissue, 320–321
   of hepatocellular carcinoma, 1584–1585
   of liver, 1555–1556
   of lymph nodes, 711
   of paragangliomas, 637–639
   of thyroid, 558–563
Fish-mouth appearance, 254
Fissural cysts, of jaw, 840–842
Fistulas, biliary, 1635
Fixed drug eruption, 14
Flail leaflet, 1229
Fleck dystrophy, 980
Florid papillomatosis, of nipple, 370–371
Flow cytometry, of bladder cancer, 1884–1885
Focal nodular hyperplasia (FNH), 1513, 1565, 1567–1569
Follicle cysts, of ovary, 2309–2311
Follicle-stimulating hormone (FSH) deficiency, in males, 1955
Follicular adenoma, of thyroid, 544–545
Follicular bronchitis-bronchiolitis, 1031
Follicular carcinoma, of thyroid, 546–547
Follicular center lymphoma, 75, 674, 739, 743–745
Follicular cystitis, 1855–1856

Follicular dendritic cell sarcoma, 763–764
Follicular hyperplasia
  of lymph nodes, 744
  of spleen, 780–781
Follicular lymphoma, of spleen, 786–787
Follicular mucinosis, 33–34
Follicular thyroid nodules, 544–548, 559–560
Folliculitis
  bacterial and fungal, 33
  eosinophilic pustular, 34
  multifocal granulomatous, 531
  of vulva, 2115
Foreign bodies
  in eye, 975–976
  granulomas due to, 31–32
Foreign body reaction, of breast, 374
Foreign body salpingitis, 2397
Foreskin, 2035
  carcinoma of, 2057
Fournier's gangrene, 2039
Fox-Fordyce disease, 2114
Fracture(s), 255–257
  avulsion, 256
  comminuted, 256
  compound, 256
  fatigue, 256
  insufficiency, 304
  stress, 256
Fracture callus, 256–257, 304
Fragile X syndrome, 1956
Freckle, of conjunctiva, 986
Freezing artifact, 111–112
Frenulum, 2035
Frozen sections
  of bone, 264
  of brain, 391, 479
  of breast tissue, 319–320
  of lung, 1071
  of muscle, 110, 115–116
  of soft tissue tumors, 135
  of thyroid, 558
Fructose intolerance, hereditary, liver in, 1520
FSH (follicle-stimulating hormone) deficiency, in males, 1955
Fuchs' endothelial dystrophy, 979–980
Fundic gland polyp, 1327
Fungal infections
  of brain, 398
  of fallopian tube, 2397
  folliculitis due to, 33
  of liver, 1536–1537
  of ovary, 2308
  of penis, 2039
  sinonasal, 886–887
Funisitis, necrotizing, 2102–2103
Fusobacterium amnionitis, 2101
Fusospirochetal gingivitis, 807

G

GAGs (glycosaminoglycans), in mesothelioma, 1125–1126
Galactocele, 378
Galactosemia, liver in, 1520
Gallbladder, 1629–1655
  adenomas of, 1646, 1649
  adenomyomatous hyperplasia of, 1639, 1646
  agenesis of, 1631
  benign tumors of, 1649–1650
  carcinoid tumors of, 1655
  carcinoma of, 1647–1648, 1650–1654
    ovarian metastases of, 2380–2381
  cholecystitis of, 1635–1642
    acute, 1635–1636
    AIDS-related, 1639–1641
    chronic, 1636–1639
    eosinophilic, 1641
    gangrenous, 1636
    lymphocytic, 1642
    xanthogranulomatous, 1641–1642
  cholelithiasis of, 1631–1635
  cholesterolosis of, 1631
  in chronic cholestatic disorders, 1642
  congenital abnormalities of, 1630–1631
  diverticular disease of, 1630, 1639
  dysplasia of, 1643, 1645–1648
  in extrahepatic bile duct obstruction, 1642
  heterotopias of, 1631
  hydrops of, 1635
  hypoplastic, 1631
  melanoma of, 1655
  metaplasia of, 1643, 1645, 1647–1648
  metastases to, 1655
  mucocele of, 1635
  multiseptate, 1630
  normal anatomy and histology of, 1629–1630
  papillary hyperplasia of, 1643–1645, 1647–1648
  polyps of, 1645, 1646, 1648–1649
  sarcomas of, 1654–1655
  specimen processing for, 1630
  strawberry, 1632
  vasculitis of, 1642–1643
Gallbladder sludge, 1632
Gallstone(s), 1631–1635
Gallstone ileus, 1635
Gamma chain disease, 690–691
Gamma-enolase, 484
Gangliocytic paraganglioma, 643
  of gastrointestinal tract, 1458–1459
Gangliocytoma, 430–431
  of cerebellum, 431
  of sellar region, 520–521
Ganglioglioma, 430–431
  anaplastic, 430–431
  desmoplastic infantile, 432
Ganglion, 240–241

Ganglion cell tumors, 411, 413, 429–432
Ganglion cyst, 302
Ganglioneuroblastoma
  adrenal, 608–613
  of CNS, 432
  of mediastinum, 1172
Ganglioneuroma
  adrenal, 610, 613–614
  intestinal, 1418, 1419–1420
  mediastinal, 1164–1165
Gangrene, Fournier's, 2039
Gangrenous balanitis, 2041
Gardnerella vaginalis, 2135
Gardner's syndrome, 1418, 1435
Gastrectomy, stomach after, 1325–1326
Gastric antral vascular ectasia, 1339
Gastric atrophy, 1315
Gastric dysplasia, 1333–1334
Gastric erosion, 1316–1317
Gastric mucosa
  biopsy specimens of, 1312
  enlarged folds of, 1329–1330
  normal appearances of, 1311
Gastrinoma, 1500
Gastrin-releasing peptide, 485
Gastritis, 1315–1325
  active, 1317
  acute erosive, 1316–1317
  atrophic, 1315
    multifocal, 1318–1319
  autoimmune, 1319
  chemical, 1322
  chemotherapy, 1323
  chronic nonspecific, 1315
  classification of, 1315–1316
  due to cryptosporidium, 1324
  due to cytomegalovirus, 1324
  from drug therapy, 1323
  emphysematous, 1317
  eosinophilic, 1321
  follicular, 1317
  granulomatous, 1320–1321
  Helicobacter, 1317–1318, 1325
  due to herpes simplex virus, 1324
  in immunosuppressed patients, 1324–1325
  ischemic, 1323
  lymphocytic, 1321–1322
  due to *Mycobacterium avium-intracellulare*, 1324
  polypoid cystic (polypoid hypertrophic), 1327
  radiation, 1322–1323
  reflux, 1322
  superficial, 1315
  suppurative (phlegmonous), 1317–1318
Gastritis cystica polyposa, 1327
Gastroenteritis
  eosinophilic, 1357
  infectious, 1353–1354

Gastroesophageal junction, 1284, 1292–1293
  adenocarcinoma of, 1303
Gastroesophageal reflux disease (GERD), 1285–1288
Gastrointestinal autonomic nerve tumor, 1457
Gastrointestinal stromal tumors, 1337–1339, 1454–1457
Gastrointestinal tract. See also Intestines
  hemorrhagic necrosis of, 1383
  multiple lymphomatous polyposis of, 1453–1454
  neuroendocrine cells and neoplasms of, 484
Gastroparesis, due to diabetes mellitus, 1340
Gastropathy
  hypertrophic hypersecretory, 1329
  reactive, 1322
Gaucher's disease
  bone marrow in, 692
  liver in, 1520, 1522
  spleen in, 793–794
GBM (glomerular basement membrane, thinnings of, 1733, 1776
G-CSF (granulocyte-colony-stimulating factor), 655
Gelatinous drop-like dystrophy, 980
Gemistocytes, 418–419
Genitalia, ambiguous, 2112
Genital warts. See Condyloma acuminatum
GERD (gastroesophageal reflux disease), 1285–1288
Germ cell tumors
  of CNS, 450–452
  of fallopian tube, 2407
  hepatic, 1557, 1562–1563
  of mediastinum
    cystic, 1153–1156
    malignant, 1181–1182, 1190
    prognosis for, 1198
  of ovary, 2358–2370
    carcinoid, 2368–2370
    choriocarcinoma, 2363–2364
    dysgerminomas, 2359–2360
    embryonal carcinoma, 2363
    mixed malignant, 2370
    neuroectodermal, 2370
    polyembryoma, 2363
    sebaceous, 2370
    struma ovarii, 2366–2368
    teratomas, 2364–2370
    yolk sac, 2360–2363
  of seminal vesicles, 1936
  of testis, 1974–2004
    biopsy of, 1957
    carcinoid, 2000–2001
    choriocarcinoma, 1995–1997
    classification of, 1974–1976
    cryptorchidism and, 1947
    diffuse embryoma, 2002
    embryonal carcinoma, 1985–1990
    epidemiology of, 1977–1979
    histogenesis of, 1976–1977
    intratubular, 1979–1980
    mixed, 2001–2002
    polyembryoma, 2002
    postchemotherapy resections of, 2003–2004
    primitive neuroectodermal, 2001
    regression of, 2002–2003
    seminoma, 1980–1983, 1986
      spermatocytic, 1983–1985, 1986
    teratoma, 1997–2000
    trophoblastic, 1995–1997
      placental-site, 1997
    yolk sac, 1990–1995
Germinal cell aplasia, 1952–1953, 1956–1957
Germinal centers, progressive transformation of, 732
Germinoma
  of CNS, 413, 450–451
  of sellar region, 518
Gestational trophoblastic disease, 2067–2085
  choriocarcinoma, 2076–2080
  classification of, 2068
  epithelioid trophoblastic tumor, 2082–2085
  exaggerated placental site, 2074–2075
  hydatidiform mole, 2069–2074
    complete, 2069–2071
    invasive, 2073–2074
    partial, 2071–2073
  placental-site nodule, 2075–2076
  placental-site trophoblastic tumor, 2074, 2080–2082
  trophoblast during normal gestation and, 2067–2069
GH. See Growth hormone (GH)
Giant cell angiofibroma, 154
Giant cell arteritis, 1258, 1260, 1262–1264, 1265
Giant cell carcinoma
  of bladder, 1876–1878
  hepatocellular, 1580
Giant-cell fibroblastoma, 160
Giant cell granuloma
  of gingiva, 807–808
  of pituitary, 522
  sinonasal, 914–915
Giant cell interstitial pneumonia, 1017
Giant cell malignant fibrous histiocytoma, 163–165
Giant cell tumor
  of bone, 291–292
  of craniofacial bones, 914
  of larynx, 944
  of tendon sheath, 182
Giant condyloma, 2059–2061
Giardiasis, 1358
  in AIDS patients, 1371
Gingiva, 805
  cysts of, 836
  fibroid epulis of, 807
  inflammatory papillary hyperplasia of, 808–809
  peripheral giant-cell granuloma of, 807–808
  pyogenic granuloma of, 807
  squamous cell carcinoma of, 824
Gingivitis, 805–809
  acute necrotizing (fusospirochetal), 807
Gitter cells, 412
Glandular atypia, of cervix, 2182–2184
Glandular cyst, odontogenic, 839–840
Glandular dysplasia, endocervical, 2184
Glandular hyperplasia, of cervix
  diffuse laminar, 2177–2178
  mesonephric, 2179–2180
  micro-, 2178–2179
Glandular tumors, of cutaneous adnexa, 63
Glans corona, 2035
Glans penis, 2035
Glassy cell carcinoma, of cervix, 2194
Glaucoma, 977
Gleason grading system, 1902–1905, 1920–1921
Glial cyst, 459–460
Glial heterotopia, sinonasal, 905
Glial masses, of middle ear, 963
Glioblastoma multiforme, 411, 413, 427–429
Glioma(s), 410–429
  astrocytomas, 415–420
  ependymoblastoma, 424–425
  ependymomas, 420–424
  glioblastoma multiforme, 427–429
  gliomatosis cerebri, 418
  gliosarcoma, 429
  malignancy-associated, 429
  margins of, 396
  oligoastrocytoma, 426
  oligodendroglioma, 425–426
  optic nerve, 999
  sinonasal, 905
  tumor margins of, 410–415
Gliomatosis, peritoneal, 2365
Gliomatosis cerebri, 418
Gliosarcoma, 411, 413, 429
Gliosis, 395–396
  cavitary, 460
  glioma vs., 412–414
Globe, 975–977
  foreign bodies in, 975–976
  glaucoma of, 977
  inflammation of, 976
  phthisis bulbi of, 976
  trauma to, 975
Globulomaxillary cyst, 841–842

Glomangiosarcoma, 178
Glomerular basement membrane (GBM), thinnings of, 1733, 1776
Glomerular capillaries, acellular closure of, 1736–1745, 1776–1777
Glomerular capillary wall lesions, 1716–1730
Glomerular disease
  with acellular closure of glomerular capillaries, 1736–1745, 1776–1777
  approach to diagnosis of, 1701, 1702
  generalizations about, 1704–1705
  with isolated hematuria, 1730–1736, 1776
  with nephritic syndrome, 1705–1716
  nonglomerulonephritic, 1716–1730
  pattern recognition in, 1701, 1702, 1775
  in rheumatoid arthritis, 1749
  specific patterns in, 1775–1777
  in systemic lupus erythematosus, 1745–1749, 1777
Glomerular tip lesion, 1717
Glomerulocystic kidney disease, 1694, 1696
Glomeruloid bodies, in yolk sac tumor, 1991
Glomerulonephritis, 1705–1716
  crescentic, 1709–1715, 1775–1776
    immune complex, 1714
    pauciimmune, 1712–1714
  cryoglobulinemic, 1739–1741, 1776–1777
  diffuse extracapillary proliferative, 1709–1715, 1775–1776
  diffuse intracapillary proliferative, 1705–1706, 1775
  fibrillary, 1742–1745, 1777
  focal, 1714–1715
  hypercellular (true, proliferative), 1705–1716
  immunotactoid, 1742–1745, 1777
  membranoproliferative, 1706–1709, 1775
  membranous, 1724–1727, 1776
  mesangiocapillary, 1706–1708, 1775
  with nephrotic syndrome, 1705–1716
  pattern recognition in, 1775
  postinfectious (poststreptococcal), 1705–1706, 1775
  rapidly progressive, 1709–1715, 1775–1776
  specific patterns in, 1775–1777
Glomerulonephropathy, membranous, 1724–1727, 1776
Glomerulopathy
  collapsing, 1723–1724, 1776
  immunotactoid, 1742–1745, 1777
  nonamyloidotic fibrillary, 1742–1745, 1777
  transplant, 1771–1772

Glomerulosclerosis, 1713, 1717, 1719–1723, 1776
  diabetic, 1727–1730, 1776
Glomerulus(i)
  normal, 1701, 1702
  obsolescent, 1711, 1712
  terminology for, 1777–1778
Glomus coccygeum, 644
Glomus tumor, 68–69, 178
  of middle ear, 965–967
  of vulva, 2119
Glottic cancer, 931–933
Glucagonoma, 15, 1500–1501
"Glue-ear," 959
Gluten-sensitive enteropathy, 1350–1352
Glycogen, in mesothelioma, 1125
Glycogenic acanthosis, of esophagus, 1304
Glycogen nuclei, in liver, 1515
Glycogenosis
  type II, 125
  type V, 125
  type VII, 125–126
Glycogen-rich adenoma, 860
Glycogen storage disease, liver in, 1519, 1520
Glycoprotein adenoma, 514
Glycosaminoglycans (GAGs), in mesothelioma, 1125–1126
GM2 gangliosidosis, liver in, 1520
GM-CSF (granulocyte-monocyte-colony-stimulating factor), 655
Goblet cell carcinoid tumor, appendiceal, 1445–1446
Goiter
  diffuse toxic, 533
  nodular, 544, 559
  toxic nodular, 533, 543
Goltz-Gorlin syndrome, 810
Gonad(s), streak, 1967
Gonadal dysgenesis
  and germ cell tumors, 1978
  mixed, 1964–1965, 1967–1968
  pure, 1967
Gonadoblastoma
  of ovary, 2370–2372
  of testis, 1967–1968, 2010–2011
Gonadotroph cell, 497
Gonadotroph cell adenoma, 499, 514
Gonadotropin deficiency, 1955–1956
Gonorrhea
  suppurative arthritis due to, 233
  of vulva, 2114–2115
Goodpasture's syndrome, 1046–1047
Gorhan's disease, 294
Gorlin cyst, 839
Gout
  cutaneous, 38–39
  of ear, 951
  joint disease in, 230–231
  nephropathy of, 1761
  pseudo-, 232

Graft-*versus*-host disease (GVHD)
  esophagitis due to, 1290
  gastric, 1324–1325
  intestines in, 1368–1369
  of liver, 1512, 1544–1546
Granular cell astrocytic neoplasms, 419–420
Granular cell schwannoma, 185
Granular cell tumor
  of esophagus, 1297
  of extrahepatic bile ducts, 1661
  of larynx, 929
  of pituitary, 518, 519–520
  of soft tissue, 191–192
  of vulva, 2119
Granular corneal dystrophy, 980, 981
Granulation tissue, in vagina, 2137
Granulation tissue polyp, of breast, 345
Granulocyte-colony-stimulating factor (G-CSF), 655
Granulocyte-monocyte-colony-stimulating factor (GM-CSF), 655
Granulocytic leukemia, 663–664
Granulocytic sarcoma
  mediastinal, 1187–1188, 1190–1191
  of testis, 2012
Granuloma(s)
  of bladder, 1856
  of bone, 306
  of bone marrow, 656, 685
    eosinophilic, 693
  CNS, 411
  of ear
    cholesterol, 959, 972
    external, 949–951, 952–953
    hair, 950
    inner, 972
    keratin implantation, 950–951
    middle, 959
    starch, 949
  eosinophilic
    of bone, 306
    of bone marrow, 693
    of pituitary, 522
    pulmonary, 1028–1030
  due to foreign materials, 31–32
  giant-cell
    of gingiva, 807–808
    of pituitary, 522
    sinonasal, 914–915
  of gingiva, 807–808
  hyalinizing, pulmonary, 1037–1038
  infectious, 31
  intestinal, barium, 1394
  of larynx, 926–927
    plasma cell, 944
  lethal midline, 887–889
  of liver, 1510–1514, 1547–1548
  ovarian, 2308
  peritoneal, 2420, 2421
    plasma cell, 2425–2426

of pituitary, 522
plasma cell
  of bladder, 1856
  of larynx, 944
  peritoneal, 2425–2426
  pulmonary, 1038–1040
posttransurethral resection, 1897–1898
pulmonary
  eosinophilic, 1028–1030
  hyalinizing, 1037–1038
  plasma cell, 1038–1040
pyogenic, 69, 174
  of eyelid, 988
  of gingiva, 807
sinonasal, 889–890
Granuloma annulare, 32
Granuloma fissuratum, 952–953
Granuloma inguinale
  of penis, 2039
  of vulva, 2115
Granulomatosis
  bronchocentric, 1025–1026
  Churg-Strauss, 29, 1045–1046
  hepatic, 1513
  lymphocytic, 1037
  lymphomatoid, 29, 75
    pulmonary, 1035–1037
  necrotizing sarcoidal, 1040, 1043–1044
  pulmonary, 1040–1046
    lymphomatoid, 1035–1037
  Wegener's
    of lung, 1040–1043
    of orbit, 998
    of penis, 2042
    sinonasal, 888–889
    of skin, 29
    vasculitis due to, 1260, 1267
Granulomatous angiitis, 407, 1260, 1262, 1265–1266
Granulomatous dermatitis, 31–33
Granulomatous gastritis, 1320–1321
Granulomatous inflammation
  of eye, 976
  of muscle, 115
Granulomatous myositis, idiopathic, 115
Granulomatous peritonitis, 2415–2416
Granulomatous prostatitis
  allergic, 1898
  nonspecific, 1896–1897
Granulomatous salpingitis, 2395–2398
Granulomatous vasculitis, 29
Granulosa cell proliferations, of ovary, 2311
Granulosa cell tumors
  of ovary, 2343–2347, 2353
  of testis, 2009
Graves' disease, 543
Ground glass cells, in liver, 1515
Growth hormone (GH) cell adenomas, 500, 509–510

Growth hormone (GH) cell-prolactin (PRL) cell adenoma, 498, 500, 511
Growth hormone (GH) excess, pituitary adenoma due to, 512
Growth hormone (GH)-producing adenomas, 509–512
Gruber-Frantz tumor, 1495–1496
Gummas, 2039
GVHD. See Graft-*versus*-host disease (GVHD)
Gynandroblastoma, 2354
Gynecomastia, 376
Gyrate erythemas, 26

H

Haemophilus ducreyi, 2115
Haemophilus influenzae, chorioamnionitis due to, 2102
Hair bulb, 4
Hair follicles, 4
  diseases of, 33–41
Hair granuloma, of ear, 950
Hair matrix, 4
Hairy cell leukemia, 674–676, 751
  liver in, 1620
  spleen in, 795–796
Halo nevus, 92
Hamartoma
  bile duct, 1519, 1597, 1598–1599
  of breast, 377
  chest wall, 307
  cystic
    renal, 1806–1807
    retrorectal, 1391–1392
  fibrous, of infancy, 154
  mesenchymal, of liver, 1557, 1563, 1614
  myoepithelial, of small bowel, 1360
  omental-mesenteric myxoid, 2426
  of parathyroid, 568–569
  pulmonary, 1103
  respiratory epithelial adenomatoid, 895
  splenic, 797
Hamartomatous polyps, intestinal, 1418, 1419
  inverted, 1432–1434
Hand-Schüller-Christian disease, 306, 693
  pituitary in, 522
Hanseman cells, 1759
Hartmann's pouch, 1629
Hashimoto's thyroiditis, 532, 559
  fibrosing variant of, 533
Hassal-Henle bodies, 979
HAV (hepatitis A virus), 1531
Haversian canal, 247
Haversian systems, 247–248
HBME-1, in mesothelioma, 1134
HBV (hepatitis B virus), 1531, 1532–1534
HCV (hepatitis C virus), 1531, 1532–1534
Heart disease, 1209–1244
  in AIDS, 1220–1221

cardiomyopathies, 1210–1215
  restrictive, 1218–1222
collagen vascular, 1218
coronary vascular, 1235–1237
devices used for, 1244
endomyocardial biopsy for, 1209–1210
ischemic, 1224–1225
myocarditis, 1215–1218
of pericardium, 1241–1244
prosthetic valves for, 1233–1235
sarcoidosis, 1218
tumors, 1237–1241
valvular, 1225–1233
Heart transplantation, 1222–1224
Heavy chain disease, 690–691
Heck's disease, 810
Helicobacter gastritis, 1317–1318, 1325
Helminth infection, of liver, 1537
Hemangioblastic meningioma, 441
Hemangioblastoma, 411, 412, 455–456, 460
Hemangioendothelioma
  of bone, 294–295
  epithelioid
    cutaneous, 73
    of liver, 1602, 1608, 1609–1611
    of mediastinum, 1195
    of peritoneum, 2425
    pulmonary, 1101
    soft tissue, 178–179
  infantile, of liver, 1605–1606
  kaposiform, 178
  pseudomesotheliomatous, 1141–1142
  retiform, 179
  of salivary gland, 874
  spindle-cell, 73, 176
Hemangioendotheliosarcoma, of bone, 294–295
Hemangioma(s), 174–177
  acquired tufted, 70
  of bone, 294
  capillary
    lobular, 69, 174
      of gingiva, 807
      sinonasal, 909–910
    of orbit, 998
  cardiac, 1241
  cavernous
    adrenal, 606–607
    of liver, 1603–1605
    of orbit, 998
  cellular (juvenile), 175
  epithelioid, 175–176
  of ear, 953
  glomeruloid, 70–71
  histiocytoid, 71
  intestinal, 1387
  intramuscular, 166
  of larynx, 943
  of liver, 1603–1605
  microvenular, 70, 176

Hemangioma(s) *(contd.)*
  perilobular, 368
  pulmonary sclerosing, 1101–1102
  renal, 1817
  of salivary glands, 873–874
  sinonasal, 910
  sinusoidal, 176–177
  spindle-cell, 176
  of spleen, 798
  targetoid hemosiderotic (hobnail), 177
  of vulva, 2119
Hemangiomatosis, pulmonary capillary, 1051
Hemangiopericytic meningioma, 421, 444–445
Hemangiopericytoma, 181
  of bone, 295
  of CNS, 414, 444–445
  of mediastinum, 1161–1162
  of orbit, 999
  renal, 1817, 1818
  of salivary gland, 874
  of sellar region, 518
  sinonasal, 910
Hematogones, 684–685
Hematologic neoplasms
  of prostate, 1934–1935
  of urinary tract, 1882
Hematoma, subdural, 406
Hematopoiesis, 652–653
  extramedullary, 1511, 1512, 1516
Hematopoietic neoplasms
  of CNS, 452–455
  of thyroid, 555
Hematuria, 1777
  benign recurrent (benign familial essential, benign persistent), 1733, 1776
  isolated, glomerular disease with, 1730–1736, 1776
Hemochromatosis, 1221–1222, 1523
  cardiomyopathy due to, 1213
Hemolytic-uremic syndrome (HUS), 1736–1739, 1774
Hemophagocytic syndrome, 724
  virus-associated, 693–695, 1536
Hemorrhage
  brain, 396, 406–407
  intervillous, 2098
  meningeal, 406–407
  pulmonary, 1046–1047
  subarachnoid, 406
Hemorrhagic colitis syndrome, 1364–1365
Hemorrhagic cystitis, 1856–1858
Hemorrhagic endovasculopathy, of placenta, 2098
Hemorrhagic necrosis, of gastrointestinal tract, 1383
Hemorrhoids, 1673
Hemosiderin, intravillous, 2098
Hemosiderosis
  idiopathic pulmonary, 1047
  secondary, 1522, 1523
Hemosiderotic synovitis, 237
Henoch-Schönlein purpura, 1260, 1261, 1267, 1730–1733
Hepatic artery obstruction, 1538
Hepatic fibrosis, 1513
  congenital, 1519, 1692
Hepatic iron index, 1522
Hepatic portoenterostomy, 1516
Hepatic venous outflow obstruction, 1511, 1513, 1514
Hepatitis
  alcoholic, 1511, 1529–1530
  autoimmune, 1511, 1512, 1542–1543, 1547, 1548
  bacterial, 1536
  fungal, 1536–1537
  helminth, 1537
  medication-induced, 1511
  neonatal, 1516
  protozoal, 1537
  Q fever, 1537
  steato-, 1515, 1543, 1547, 1548
  "surgical," 1511
  viral, 1530–1536
    acute, 1530–1532
    chronic, 1532–1534, 1547, 1548
    due to cytomegalovirus, 1534
    delta agent in, 1534
    differential diagnosis of, 1534–1535
    due to Epstein-Barr virus, 1534
    in immunocompromised host, 1535–1536
    infiltrate in, 1511, 1512, 1531
    necrosis in, 1531, 1532, 1533
Hepatitis A virus (HAV), 1531
Hepatitis B virus (HBV), 1531, 1532–1534
Hepatitis C virus (HCV), 1531, 1532–1534
Hepatoblastoma, 1593–1598
  clinical features of, 1593–1594
  differential diagnosis of, 1595, 1596
  pathologic features of, 1594–1596
  staging of, 1597
  treatment, outcome, and prognostic factors for, 1597–1598
Hepatocellular adenoma, 1515, 1564–1567
Hepatocellular carcinoma, 1575–1593
  advanced, 1577–1585
  vs. benign tumors, 1565, 1585–1588
  biopsy for, 1556
  borderline nodules and, 1573–1575
  clinical findings in, 1576
  cytologic appearance and variants of, 1579–1581
  cytoplasmic deposits in, 1581–1584
  differential diagnosis of, 1565, 1585–1588
  DNA analysis and molecular biology of, 1585
  epidemiology of, 1575
  fatty change in, 1515
  fibrolamellar, 1589–1593
  fine needle aspiration of, 1584–1585
  vs. hepatoblastoma, 1595
  histologic grading of, 1578–1579
  histologic patterns in, 1579
  immunohistochemistry of, 1581–1584
  large-cell change and, 1585
  macroscopic features of, 1577–1578
  microscopic features of, 1578–1579
  pathogenesis of, 1575–1576
  small, 1576–1577
  staging of, 1577, 1578
  treatment, outcome, and prognostic factors for, 1588–1589
Hepatocellular carcinoma-cholangiocarcinoma, 1593
Hepatocellular necrosis, 1510, 1511
Hepatocellular proliferative disease, nonneoplastic, 1538–1540
Hepatocellular tumors, benign and borderline, 1563–1575
Hepatocytes, large-cell change of, 1585
Hepatoid carcinoma, of ovary, 2375
Hepatolithiasis, 1634–1635
Hepatoportal sclerosis, 1516, 1538
Hepatorenal disease, polycystic, 1519
Hepatotoxicity, 1511–1516, 1528–1529
HepPar-1, 1583
Herald patch, 7
Hereditary flat adenoma syndrome, 1418, 1435–1436
Hereditary hemorrhagic telangiectasia, intestinal involvement in, 1387
Hereditary mixed polyposis syndrome, 1418
Hereditary nonpolyposis colon cancer, 1440
Hermaphroditism, 1968
  pseudo-
    female, 2112
    male, 1964–1968
Herniated disc, 239–240
Hernia uteri inguinale, 1964
Herpes gestationis, 23
Herpes simplex virus (HSV), 21–22
  of cervix, 2155
  encephalitis due to, 392, 400
  esophagitis due to, 1288–1289
  gastritis due to, 1324
  hepatitis due to, 1515, 1535–1536
  keratitis due to, 982–983
  of penis, 2040
  of rectum and anus, 1371
  of vulva, 2116
Herpesvirus, of endocervical glands, 2182
Herpes zoster infection, 21–22
Herring bodies, 497

Heterotopias, of stomach, 1312–1313
Heterotopic ossification, 305
Hidradenitis suppurativa, of vulva, 2115
Hidroadenoma papilliferum, 63, 2132
Hidrocystoma, 62
   of eyelid, 990
Hilar cysts, multiple, of liver, 1557, 1560–1561
Hilus cell hyperplasia, of ovary, 2316–2317
Hirschsprung's disease, 1388, 1390, 1391
   anus in, 1673
Histiocytic lymphoma, 695
Histiocytic medullary reticulosis, of lymph nodes, 762–763
Histiocytic necrotizing lymphadenitis, 718
Histiocytic neoplasms
   of lymph nodes, 761–764
   of peritoneum, 2416
Histiocytic proliferation
   in bone marrow, 691–695
   in spleen, 792–794
Histiocytoma, fibrous. *See* Fibrous histiocytoma
Histiocytosis
   ceroid (sea-blue), 792–793
   of CNS, 411, 454–455
   Langerhans. *See* Histiocytosis X
   lipid, 792–794
   malignant
      bone marrow in, 695
      lymph nodes in, 762–763
      small bowel in, 1357
      spleen in, 794
   mucicarminophilic, 2416
   regressing atypical, 162
   sinus, with massive lymphadenopathy, 309, 724–726
Histiocytosis X
   of bone, 306, 693
   of ear, 958
   of liver, 1618–1620
   of lymph nodes, 763
   of pituitary, 522
   of spleen, 794
Histoplasma, liver infection with, 1536
HIV. *See* Human immunodeficiency virus (HIV)
Hives, 27
HMFG-2, in mesothelioma, 1133
HNK-1, 485
Hobnail hemangioma, 177
Hobnail metaplasia, of endometrium, 2256
Hodgkin's disease, 730–737
   bone in, 269
   bone marrow in, 680–683
   classification of, 730–731
   clinical features of, 731
   diagnosis of, 730
   differential diagnosis of, 682–683, 713–714

hepatic involvement in, 1618, 1619
lymphocyte-depleted, 731, 736–737
lymphocyte-predominant, 713–714, 731–733
mediastinal
   large-cell, 1186–1187, 1190–1191
   mixed-cellularity, 1192
   prognosis for, 1198
mixed-cellularity, 731, 734–736
   mediastinal, 1192
nodular-sclerosing, 713–714, 731, 733–734
   mediastinal, 1186–1187
vs. non-Hodgkin's lymphoma, 714
pathologic features of, 731–737
posttreatment biopsies in, 682
Reed-Sternberg cells in, 730
spleen in, 789–790
syncytial, 1186–1187, 1190–1191
Hofbauer cells, 2105, 2106
Hoffa's disease, 227
Honeycomb lung, 1018
Hordeolum, 989
Hormone production, ectopic, 486
Hormone receptors, in breast, 324–325
Hormone therapy, of prostatic carcinoma, 1925–1926
Howship's lacunae, 247
HPV. *See* Human papillomavirus (HPV)
HSV. *See* Herpes simplex virus (HSV)
Human immunodeficiency virus (HIV). *See also* Acquired immunodeficiency syndrome (AIDS)
   bone marrow in, 656–658
   CNS lesions in, 401–404
   esophagitis in, 1290
   lymph nodes in, 719–721
   mycobacterial spindle-cell pseudotumor with, 728–729
   myositis due to, 125
   nephropathy with, 1723–1724, 1776
Human papillomavirus (HPV)
   and anal canal intraepithelial neoplasia, 1677
   and cervical cancer, 2156–2157
   in oral papilloma, 809
   of penis, 2040–2041, 2057
   vulvar infection with, 2116–2117
Humoral hypercalcemia of malignancy, 569
Hunner's ulcer, 1855
Hurler's disease, 1522
Hürthle cell lesions, 547–548, 560
HUS (hemolytic-uremic syndrome), 1736–1739, 1774
Hyalin, Mallory's
   in hepatocellular carcinoma, 1582–1583
   in liver, 1515, 1529–1530
Hyaline droplets, in nephrotic syndrome, 1717, 1778

Hyaline fibers, 113
Hyaline globules
   in hepatocellular carcinoma, 1582
   in paragangliomas, 636
Hyalinizing clear-cell carcinoma, of salivary gland, 873
Hyalinizing granuloma, pulmonary, 1037–1038
Hyalinizing spindle-cell tumor, with giant rosettes, 158
Hyalinizing trabecular adenoma, of thyroid, 545
Hyalinosis, 1777
Hydatidiform mole, 2069–2074
   complete, 2069–2071
   invasive, 2073–2074
   partial, 2071–2073
Hydatidosis, hepatic, 1557, 1558–1559
Hydrocele, of tunica albuginea, 2015
Hydronephrosis, congenital, 1689–1690
Hydropic degeneration, 5
Hydrops, of gallbladder, 1635
Hydrosalpinx, 2395, 2396
Hydroxyapatite deposition, 232
21-Hydroxylase deficiency, 593
Hygromas, cystic, 1153
Hymen, congenital anomalies of, 2113
Hymenal cyst, 2113
Hyoid bone, 925–926
Hyperaldosteronism, cortical hyperplasia due to, 597
Hypercalcemia
   familial hypocalciuric, 569
   humoral, of malignancy, 569
   ovarian small-cell carcinoma with, 2373–2375
Hyperganglionosis, 1390–1391
Hypergastrinemia, 1502
Hyperkeratosis, 5
   epidermolytic, 22–23, 52–53
Hyperlipoproteinemia, xanthoma with, of ear, 951
Hypernephroma, 1785
   sarcomatoid, 296
Hyperosteoidosis, 246
Hyperparathyroidism, 244
   abnormal bone resorption due to, 251–252
   bone disease due to, 307
   ectopic, 570
   primary, 565–568
   secondary, 570
Hyperplaseogenous polyps, of stomach, 1326–1327
Hyperplasia
   adenomatous
      of rete testis, 2014
      of salivary glands, 855
   adenomyomatous, of gallbladder, 1639, 1646
   adrenal

Hyperplasia, adrenal *(contd.)*
   congenital, 593–594
   cortical, 595–597
   medullary, 618–619
 angiofollicular, 721–722
   of mediastinum, 1159
 angiolymphoid, with eosinophilia, 71, 176
 of breast
   atypical, 335–336
     ductal, 335–336, 344
     lobular, 330, 347
   epithelial, 329, 334–336
     vs. ductal carcinoma *in situ,* 335, 343–344
     lobular, 347
   fibroadenomatoid, 364
   intraductal, 334–335
   papillary duct, 377
   pseudoangiomatous, 377–378
 of Brunner's glands, 1360–1361
 C-cell, 551–552
 of cervix gland
   diffuse laminar, 2177–2178
   mesonephric, 2179–2180
   micro-, 2178–2179
 of conjunctiva, 987
 endometrial, 2226–2230, 2242–2244
   atypical, 2226–2230, 2242–2244, 2256
   villoglandular, 2251–2252, 2254
 endothelial, 151
 of extrahepatic bile ducts, 1664
 of fallopian tube, 2401–2402
 of gallbladder
   adenomyomatous, 1639, 1646
   papillary, 1643–1645, 1647–1648
 in gastroesophageal reflux disease, 1286
 of gingiva, 807
 of intestines, crypt, 1350–1352
 of lacrimal gland, 1001
 of liver, focal nodular, 1513, 1565, 1567–1569
 of lymph nodes, 744
   follicular, 715–722
   interfollicular, 722–726
   lymphoid
     angiofollicular, 1159
     of lacrimal gland, 1001
     of mediastinum, 1158
     of orbit, 999
     reactive, of conjunctiva, 987
     sinonasal, 906
 of mediastinum
   angiofollicular, 1159
   lymphoid, 1158
 micronodular pneumocyte, 1053
 of oral cavity, 810
   papillary, 808–809
   pseudoepitheliomatous, 825
 of orbit, 999
 of ovary
   hilus cell, 2316–2317
   stromal, 2313
   stromal-Leydig cell, 2317
 of pancreas, 1482
 of pancreatic ducts, 1471–1472
 papillary
   of extrahepatic bile ducts, 1664
   of gallbladder, 1643–1645
   of oral cavity, 808–809
   of pancreas, 1482
   of penis, 2043
   of peritoneum, 2417–2418
   of thyroid, 542
   of tonsils, 810
 of parathyroid, 567
 of penis, 2038, 2042–2043
   papillary, 2043
   pseudoepitheliomatous, 2043
   squamous, 2042–2043
 of peritoneum, 2417–2418
 pleural, 1118
 of prostate, 1933–1934
 pseudoepitheliomatous, 5
   of oral cavity, 825
   of penis, 2043
 of rete testis, 2014
 of salivary glands, 855
 sebaceous, 63
 of spleen, 780–782
 squamous cell
   of penis, 2042–2043
   of vulva, 2122–2123
 of thyroid, 542
 of tonsils, 810
 verrucous, 49–50
 of vulva, 2122–2123
Hyperplastic polyps
 of appendix, 1442
 of intestines, 1413–1415
 of stomach, 1326–1327
Hyperreactio luteinalis, 2311
Hypersensitivity myocarditis, 1217–1218
Hypersensitivity pneumonitis, 1021–1023
Hypertension
 benign
   arteriosclerosis in, 1255
   vascular changes in, 1762
 defined, 1762
 histologic changes in, 1253, 1254, 1255
 malignant
   necrosis in, 1255
   nephrosclerosis in, 1763
 primary plexogenic, 1048–1049
 pulmonary, 1047–1051
Hypertensive renal disease, 1761–1763
Hyperthecosis, of ovary, stromal, 2313
Hyperthyroidism, 543
 autoimmune, 543
 central, 543
 nodular thyroid disease and, 543
 painless thyroiditis with, 533
Hypertrophic cardiomyopathy, 1210–1211
Hypertrophic intracranial pachymeningitis, 397
Hypertrophic pyloric stenosis, 1313–1314
Hypertrophic scar, 35
Hypertrophy
 benign prostatic, 1893–1895
 of esophagus, 1295
 muscle, 115–116
Hypoepiglottic ligament, 926
Hypoganglionosis, 1390
Hypoglycemia, hyperinsulinemic, 1501–1502
Hypokalemia, 1502
Hypophosphatasia, 250
Hypophosphatemia, osteomalacia due to, 250
Hypophysis, neuroendocrine cells and neoplasms of, 484
Hypophysitis, lymphocytic, 522
Hypoplasia
 adrenal, 592–593
 dermal, 810
 of gallbladder, 1631
 of intestines, crypt, 1352–1353
 of penis, 2038
 renal, 1685–1686
Hypospadias, 2038
Hypospermatogenesis, 1951
Hysterectomy
 for endometrial hyperplasia, 2229–2230
 specimens from, 2204

I

IBD. *See* Inflammatory bowel disease (IBD)
Ichthyosis, 25
Ichthyosis vulgaris, 25
IgA nephropathy, 1730–1733, 1776
IgM nephropathy, 1718–1719
Ileal reservoirs, 1377–1379
Ileitis
 postcolectomy, 1379
 prestomal, 1379
Ileocecal syndrome, 1383
Ileostomies, 1379
Ileum, stromal tumors of, 1456
Ileus, gallstone, 1635
Immune-mediated myopathies, 124–125
Immune thrombocytopenic purpura, 781, 782
Immunoblastic lymphadenopathy, 685, 726–727
Immunocholangitis, 1513
Immunocompromised host
 liver in, 1511
 lung biopsy in, 1056–1059
 meningitis in, 398
 viral hepatitis in, 1535–1536
Immunocytoma, 741

cutaneous, 75
of spleen, 784
Immunodeficiency syndrome(s)
  acquired. See Acquired immunodeficiency syndrome (AIDS)
  intestines in, 1355–1356
Immunofluorescence, of renal tissue, 1773
Immunoglobulin deposition diseases, 691
Immunohistochemistry
  of breast tissue, 325, 326
  of prostatic carcinoma, 1926–1927
Immunoproliferative small-intestinal disease, 1449–1450
Immunoreactivity, aberrant, 138–139
Immunosecretory disorders, of bone marrow, 685–692
Immunosuppressed patients, gastritis in, 1324–1325
Impetigo
  bullous, 17–18
  of vulva, 2115
Implantation site, 2166–2168
Implantation site reaction, 2220–2221
Inclusion body myositis, 114, 124–125
Inclusion body sarcoma, 192
Inclusion cysts
  of conjunctiva, 984
  of eyelid, 990
  of ovary, 2309
  peritoneal, 2418–2420
Infancy, fibrous hamartoma of, 154
Infantile digital fibromatosis, 154
Infantile hemangioendothelioma, 1605–1606
Infantile myofibromatosis, 154
Infantile spinal muscular atrophy, 127
Infarction
  bone, 257–258, 308
  maternal floor, 2093–2094
  placental, 2093, 2097–2098
Infection-associated hemophagocytic syndrome, 693–695
Infectious diseases
  of bone, 259–260
  of central nervous system, 397–406
  of testis, 1960–1963
Infectious granulomas, 31
Infectious mononucleosis
  lymph nodes in, 723
  spleen in, 791–792
Infertility
  endometrial biopsy for, 2203–2204, 2211–2214
  luteal phase defect and, 2211–2212, 2217–2218
  male, 1950–1955
Inflammatory bowel disease (IBD)
  and carcinoma, 1379–1382
  and diverticular disease, 1377
  dysplasia in, 1379–1382
  idiopathic, 1374
  lesions associated with surgical procedures for, 1377–1379
  polyps in, 1420
  types of, 1374–1377
Inflammatory carcinoma, of breast, 360
Inflammatory conditions
  of bone marrow, 656–658
  of breast, 373–376
  of conjunctiva, 984–985
  of eye, 976
  of fallopian tubes, 2395–2398
  of larynx, 926–927
  of mesentery and retroperitoneum, 1395–1398
  of orbit, 998
  of ovary, 2307–2308
  of pancreas, 1474–1477
  of peritoneum, 2415–2417
  of pituitary, 522–525
  sinonasal, 886–890
Inflammatory malignant fibrous histiocytoma, 165
Inflammatory myofibroblastic tumor
  of intestines, 1397
  of liver, 1612–1613
  of mediastinum, 1167–1168
  of peritoneum, 2425–2426
Inflammatory myopathies, 114–115, 124–125
Inflammatory papillary hyperplasia, 808–809
Inflammatory polyps
  cloacogenic, 1673–1674
  of intestines, 1420–1424
  of stomach, 1327–1328
Inflammatory pseudotumor
  of bladder, 1856, 1863–1864
  of intestines, 1397
  of liver, 1612–1613
  of lymph nodes, 728
  of orbit, 998
  of peritoneum, 2425–2426
  pulmonary, 1102–1103
  soft tissue, 155
  of spleen, 799
Inflammatory skin disease(s), 3–41
  bullous and pustular, 17–25
  dermal, 26–27
  epidermal, 6–17
  erythema multiforme, 14–16
  of hair follicles and cartilage, 33–41
  lichenoid interface dermatitis, 9–10
  specimen preparation for, 3–4
  spongiotic dermatitis, 6–9, 16–17
  terminology for, 5
  vacuolar interface dermatitis, 10–14
  vasculitis and vasculopathy, 28–33
  verrucous acanthosis, 16
Infundibular cyst, 62
Insulinoma, 1500
Interdigitating dendritic cell sarcoma, 764
Intermediate filaments, in mesothelioma, 1127–1129
Internalization, nuclear, 112
Internal mammary artery grafting, 1271, 1273
Intersex syndromes, 1963–1968
  and germ cell tumors, 1978
Interstitial cystitis, 1855
Interstitial fibrosis
  diffuse, 1012–1015
  of testis, 1953
Interstitial pneumonia
  acute, 1020
  desquamative, 1015–1018
  giant-cell, 1017
  lymphocytic, 1031–1032
  nonspecific, 1018
  unusual, 1012–1015
Intervertebral disc, herniated, 239–240
Intervillositis, 2097
Intervillous hemorrhage, 2098
Intervillous thrombi, 2093
Intestinal biopsy, in AIDS patients, 1370–1374
Intestinal metaplasia, 1314–1315
Intestinal metaplastic epithelium, of Barrett's esophagus, 1291, 1292, 1293
Intestinal motility, 1387–1391
Intestinal mucinous borderline tumors, 2328, 2329
Intestinal mucosa
  flat, 1350, 1351
  prolapse of, 1423
Intestinal neuronal dysplasia, 1390–1391
Intestinal polyps, 1413–1436
  hamartomatous, 1419
  hyperplastic, 1413–1415
  inflammatory, 1420–1423
    fibroid, 1423–1424
    secondary to mucosal prolapse, 1423
  juvenile, 1420
  lymphoid, 1424
  mixed hyperplastic/adenomatous, 1415–1416
  neoplastic, 1424–1436
  nonneoplastic, 1413–1415
  Peutz-Jeghers, 1416–1419
  of small bowel, 1360–1361
Intestine(s), 1349–1398. See also Colon; Small intestine
  in abetalipoproteinemia, 1359
  in acquired immunodeficiency syndrome, 1370–1374
  in acrodermatitis enteropathica, 1359–1360
  adenomas of, 1424–1436
    biopsy specimen of, 1430–1431
    and cancer, 1425–1427, 1431
    flat, 1418, 1428–1430, 1435–1436

Intestine(s), adenomas of *(contd.)*
    malignant, 1432
    pathology of, 1427–1428
    prevalence of, 1425
    with pseudoinvasion/misplaced
        epithelium, 1432–1434
    serrated, 1415–1416
    tubular, 1427–1428
    villous, 1427–1428
  in autoimmune enteropathy, 1355
  bacterial infections of, 1384
  carcinoid tumors of, 1446–1448
  carcinoma of. *See also* Colorectal
    carcinoma
    of ovary, 2377–2378
    of stomach, 1330, 1331
  chemotherapy effect on, 1352,
    1392–1393
  in dermatitis herpetiformis, 1353
  developmental abnormalities of,
    1391–1392
  diverticular disease of, 1384–1386
  duodenitis of, 1354–1355
  duplication of, 1391
  endometriosis of, 1459–1460
  in eosinophilic gastroenteritis, 1357
  gangliocytic paraganglioma of,
    1458–1459
  ganglioneuroma of, 1418, 1419–1420
  in immunodeficiency syndromes,
    1355–1356
  in infectious gastroenteritis, 1353–1354
  inflammatory disease of, 1361–1370,
    1374–1382
  ischemic disease of, 1382–1384
  in kwashiorkor, 1352
  lipoma of, 1459
  lymphangiectasia of, 1359
  in lymphocytic enterocolitis, 1352
  lymphoma of, 1443, 1449–1454
    T-cell, 1357
  malabsorption by, 1349–1360
  malakoplakia of, 1460
  in marasmus, 1352
  in mastocytosis, 1354
  in megaloblastic anemia, 1352
  mesenchymal tumors of, 1443
  metastases to, 1443, 1460–1461
  microvillus inclusion disease of,
    1352–1353
  neuroendocrine tumors of, 1446–1448
  neurogenic tumors of, 1457–1458
  nodules of, 1360–1361
  nonneoplastic tumors of, 1394
  parasitic infections of, 1358–1359, 1385
  peptic ulcer disease of, 1354–1355
  pneumatosis cystoides intestinalis of,
    1392
  in protein allergies, 1352
  pseudo-obstruction of, 1387–1391
  radiation effect on, 1352, 1392–1393
  in sprue
    celiac, 1350–1352
    collagenous, 1355
    tropical, 1353
  stasis syndromes of, 1354
  stromal tumors of, 1454–1457
  in Torkelson syndrome, 1355
  in tufting enteropathy, 1360
  in ulcerative jejunoileitis, 1357
  undifferentiated neoplasms of, 1442,
    1443
  vascular lesions of, 1386–1387, 1458
  in Waldenström's macroglobulinemia,
    1359
  in Whipple's disease, 1356
  in Zollinger-Ellison syndrome, 1354
Intraabdominal desmoplastic small round-
    cell tumor, 2424–2425
  of ovary, 2376
Intracystic papillary carcinoma, 346–347
Intracytoplasmic sperm infection, 1956,
    1957
Intraductal cholangiocarcinoma, 1601
Intraductal hyperplasia, 334–335
Intraductal papillary-mucinous neoplasms,
    1482–1483, 1493
Intraepidermal bullae, with acantholysis,
    18–23
Intrahepatic bile ducts
  benign tumors and tumor-like lesions
    of, 1597, 1598–1599
  malignant tumors of, 1599–1602
Intrahepatic cholangiocarcinoma,
    1599–1602
Intralobar nephrogenic rests, 1835, 1836
Intralobular carcinoma, 347–348
Intramuscular angioma, 166
Intramuscular angiomatosis, 174
Intramuscular hemangiomas, 166
Intranodal hemorrhagic spindle-cell tumor
    with amianthoid fibers, 157,
    729–730
Intratubular germ cell neoplasia,
    1976–1977, 1978, 1979–1980
Intravascular lymphoma, 749
Intravascular lymphomatosis, 74
Intravascular papillary endothelial
    hyperplasia, 71
Intravascular sclerosing bronchoalveolar
    tumor, 1100–1101
Intravenous drug abusers, lung lesions in,
    1051
Intravillous hemosiderin, 2098
Inverted papillomas, of urothelial tract,
    1862
Involucrum, 260
Iodide
  thyroid carcinoma due to, 536
  thyroiditis due to, 533
Iris, 994–996
Iron
  hepatocellular, 1522
  pigmentation of, 1513
Iron deposition, in thyroid, 535
Irradiation effect. *See* Radiation therapy
Irritant contact dermatitis, 7
Ischemic bowel disease, 1369, 1376,
    1382–1384
  vs. Crohn's disease, 1376
Ischemic myocardial disease, 1224–1225
Islet-cell tumors, 1497–1501
Islets of Langerhans
  in aging, 1472–1473
  anatomy of, 1469
Isospora belli, intestinal, in AIDS patients,
    1373

J

Jaw
  cysts of, 835–842
  structures of, 805, 806
Jejunal diverticulosis, 1389
Jejunoileitis, ulcerative, 1357
Jejunum, stromal tumors of, 1456
Joint disease(s), 223–241
  avascular necrosis, 229–230
  bursitis, 241
  calcium pyrophosphate crystal
    deposition, 231–232
  disc herniation, 239–240
  ganglion, 240–241
  general features of, 223–224
  gout, 230–231
  Hoffa's (synovial lipomatosis), 227
  hydroxyapatite deposition, 232
  meniscal tears, 238–239
  Morton's neuroma, 241
  neuropathic, 223–224, 227, 308
  osteoarthritis, 224–227
  osteochondritis dissecans, 238
  pigmented villonodular synovitis,
    236–237
  primary synovial chondromatosis,
    237–238
  in response to artificial joint implants,
    234–236
  rheumatoid arthritis, 228–229
  in sarcoidosis, 234
  septic arthritis, 233–234
  in tuberculosis, 234
Joint implants, artificial, tissue response
    to, 234–236
Jugulotympanic paraganglioma, 628,
    965–967
Juvenile carcinoma, of breast, 358
Juvenile epithelial dystrophy, 980
Juvenile fibroadenoma, 365
Juvenile granulosa cell tumors, 2345–2347
Juvenile hemangioma, 175
Juvenile hyaline fibromatosis, 154
Juvenile papillomatosis, 377
Juvenile polyps

of intestines, 1418, 1420
of stomach, 1326
Juvenile xanthogranuloma, 65–66
Juxtaglomerular cell tumor, 1807–1809

K

Kallmann's syndrome, 1955
Kaposiform hemangioendothelioma, 178
Kaposi's sarcoma (KS)
  cutaneous, 72
  of ear, 958
  in gastrointestinal tract, 1374
  of gastrointestinal tract, 1458
  of liver, 1609, 1612
  of lymph node, 728
  soft tissue, 182
Kasabach-Merritt syndrome, 145
Kawasaki disease, 1260, 1261, 1266–1267
Kearns-Sayre syndrome, 126
Keloids, 35, 153
  of ear, 953
Keratin(s)
  in mesothelioma, 1127–1129
  wet, 517
Keratin granulomas, 31
  of ear, 950–951
  peritoneal, 2420, 2421
Keratinizing squamous cell carcinoma
  of thymus, 1177–1178
  of vulva, 2125–2126
Keratinizing squamous intraepithelial lesions, of cervix, 2161
Keratinocytes, 4
Keratinocytic lesions, preinvasive, 50–51
Keratitis, due to organisms, 981–982
Keratoacanthoma
  cutaneous, 55–57
  of oral cavity, 825
  subungual, 308
  of vulva, 2117
Keratoconus, 979
Keratocyst, odontogenic, 838–839
Keratopathy
  bullous, 979
  calcific band, 978
  chronic actinic (climatic droplet), 978–979
Keratosis
  actinic (senile, solar), 51–53
    bowenoid, 54
  lichenoid, 53
  seborrheic, 49–50
    of vulva, 2117
Keratosis follicularis, 21
Keratosis obturans, of ear, 950–951
Ki-67, as marker of cellular proliferation, 409
Ki-67 index, 2074–2075
Kidney(s)
  Ask-Upmark, 1691
  developmental abnormalities of, 1685–1696
  dialysis of, 1765–1767
  duplex, 1688
  dwarf or doll's, 1686
  dysplastic, 1686–1689
  enlargement of, 1690
  glomerular cysts of, 1696
  glomeruli of, 1777–1778
  glomerulocystic, 1694, 1696
  hydronephritic, 1689–1690
  hypoplastic, 1685–1686
  multicystic, 1686–1688
  myeloma, 1751–1752
  neoplasms of. See Renal neoplasms
  polycystic disease of, 1692–1695
  segmental atrophy of, 1691
  shock, 1752
  terminology for, 1777–1778
  transplantation of. See Renal transplantation
  in tuberous sclerosis, 1695–1696
  tubulointerstitium of, 1778
  unirenicular or unipapillary, 1686
  vascular lesions of, 1761–1765
  vasculature of, 1778
  in von Hippel-Lindau disease, 1696
Kidney disease. See Renal disease
Kikuchi-Fujimoto disease, 718
Kimmelstiel-Wilson nodule, 1728
Kimura's disease
  of ear, 953
  of lymph nodes, 718–719
  of skin, 71
Klatskin tumors, 1663
Klinefelter's syndrome, 1953
Klippel-Trenaunay-Weber syndrome, intestinal involvement in, 1387
Krukenberg tumors, of ovary, 2377
KS. See Kaposi's sarcoma (KS)
Kwashiorkor, 1352

L

Labeling index, 409
Labia, congenital anomalies of, 2113
Lacrimal drainage apparatus, 1001–1002
Lacrimal gland, 1000–1001
Lacrimal sac, 1001–1002
Lactating adenoma, 365
Lactiferous duct fistula, 374
Lactoferrin, in pulmonary neoplasms, 1109
Lactotroph cell, 497
Lactotrophic adenoma, 498
Lamellar ichthyosis, 25
Langerhans cell(s), 4
Langerhans cell histiocytosis
  of bone, 306, 693
  of ear, 958
  of liver, 1618–1620
  of lymph nodes, 763
  of pituitary, 522
  of spleen, 794
Large-cell acanthoma, 53
Large-cell calcifying Sertoli cell tumor, 2008
Large-cell carcinoma, of lung, 1092–1095
Large-cell change, of hepatocytes, 1585
Large-cell lymphoma, of spleen, 787–789
Large-cell non-Hodgkin's lymphoma, of mediastinum, 1185–1186, 1190–1191, 1198
Large-duct obstruction, 1516, 1524–1526
Large granular lymphocyte leukemia, 677, 796–797
Large intestine. See Colon
Large polygonal-cell neoplasms, of mediastinum, 1176–1187
  differential diagnosis of, 1190–1191
Larynx, 925–944
  anatomy of, 925–926
  atypia, dysplasia, and carcinoma of, 929–931
  basaloid carcinoma of, 940
  carcinoma of, 931–941
    acinous cell, 940
    adenoid cystic, 940
    atypia, dysplasia, and, 929–931
    metastatic, 941
    mucoepidermoid, 940
    neuroendocrine, 940–941
    small-cell (oat cell), 941
    squamous cell, 931–939
      glottic, 931–933
      histologic appearance of, 936–938
      incidence of, 931
      with spindle cell elements, 939
      staging of, 931
      supraglottic, 933–935
      transglottic, 936
      verrucous, 938–939
  cartilaginous tumors of, 942
  chondromas of, 942
  chondrosarcomas of, 942
  epithelial neoplasms of, 927–929
  fibroblastic tumors of, 942
  giant-cell tumor of, 944
  granular cell tumor (myoblastoma) of, 929
  granulomas of, 926–927
  hemangiomas of, 943
  inflammatory lesions of, 926–927
  leiomyoma of, 943
  lipoma of, 943
  liposarcoma of, 943
  lymphoid neoplasms of, 943–944
  mesenchymal tumors of, 941–944
  nerve sheath tumors of, 943
  neuroendocrine neoplasms of, 487–488
  papillomas of, 927–929
  paraganglioma of, 629, 940
  plasma cell granuloma of, 944

Larynx *(contd.)*
  pleomorphic adenomas (benign mixed tumors) of, 939–940
  polyp (nodule) of, 927, 943
  rhabdomyomas of, 942
  rhabdomyosarcoma of, 942–943
  salivary gland-like tumors of, 939–940
  skeletal muscle tumors of, 942–943
  synovial sarcoma of, 943
  vascular neoplasms of, 943
Lattice corneal dystrophy, 980–981
Legionnaire's disease, 1058
Leiomyoblastoma, 170
Leiomyoma(s)
  of breast, 368
  cervical, 2194
  of esophagus, 1296
  of larynx, 943
  of ovary, 2372
  renal, 1816
  of soft tissue, 169–170
    bizarre, 150
    epithelioid, 170
  uterine, 2281–2287
    apoplectic, 2278, 2279
    atypical (symplastic), 2273, 2276, 2282
    benign metastasizing, 2273, 2285–2286
    epithelioid, 2273, 2283–2284
    highly cellular, 2282
    infiltrating, 2273, 2285
    lipo-, 2273, 2284
    mitotically active, 2282–2283
    myxoid, 2284–2285
    neurilemoma-like, 2273, 2284
    parasitic, 2273, 2286
    with tubules or glands, 2273
    usual type of, 2281–2282
    with vascular intrusion, 2273, 2286–2287
  of vagina, 2138–2139
  vascular, 69, 169
  of vulva, 2119
Leiomyomatosis
  of esophagus, 1295
  of peritoneum, 2437
  uterine, 2273, 2285
    disseminated peritoneal, 2273, 2285
    intravascular (intravenous), 2270, 2273, 2286–2287
Leiomyomatous rhabdomyosarcoma, 172
Leiomyosarcoma
  and Epstein-Barr virus, 171
  of liver, 1615
  of mediastinum, epithelioid, 1189, 1190
  of prostate, 1933
  renal, 1816
  of soft tissue, 170–171
  of urothelial tract, 1881
  uterine, 2273, 2280, 2287–2288
  of vulva, 2119
Lennert's lymphoma, 787
Lens, 992–993
  prosthetic intraocular, 993
Lentiginous hyperplasia, 89
Lentiginous melanocytic nevus, 98
Lentiginous melanoma, acral, 104
Lentiginous melanosis, of penis, 2042
Lentigo, 97
  solar (actinic), 52, 97, 99
  of vulva, 2117–2118
Lentigo maligna, 104
Leprosy
  sinonasal, 887
  testis in, 1961
Lethal midline granuloma, 887–889
Letterer-Siwe disease
  bone in, 306
  bone marrow in, 693
  pituitary in, 522
Leu-7
  as marker for soft tissue tumors, 142
  as neuroendocrine marker, 485
  in pulmonary neoplasms, 1107–1108
Leukemia(s)
  acute, 659–662
    lymphoblastic, 659–662
    myeloid, 659–661
  B-cell
    chronic lymphocytic, 670–673, 738–741
    prolymphocytic, 673
  B-lymphoblastic, 751
    precursor, 670, 751
  of breast, 369
  chronic lymphocytic
    B-cell, 670–673, 738–741
    immunoblastic transformation of, 673
    mixed cell type, 670
    spleen in, 782–784
    T-cell, 677
    transformation of, 670–673
  chronic myeloid, 663–664, 794–795
  of CNS, 454
  of fallopian tube, 2407
  granulocytic, 663–664, 794–795
  hairy cell
    bone marrow in, 674–676
    lymph nodes in, 751
    spleen in, 795–796
  large granular cell, 677, 796–797
  of liver, 1511, 1512, 1617–1620
  lymph nodes in, 766
  lymphoblastic, acute, 659–662
  lymphocytic, chronic
    B-cell, 670–673, 738–741
    immunoblastic transformation of, 673
    mixed cell type, 670
    spleen in, 782–784
    T-cell, 677
    transformation of, 670–673
  metastatic, 1461
  myeloid
    acute, 659–661
    chronic, 663–664, 794–795
  natural killer cell, 796–797
  of ovary, 2372–2373
  plasma cell, 689
  precursor B-lymphoblastic, 670, 751
  precursor T-lymphoblastic, 677
  prolymphocytic
    B-cell, 673
    spleen in, 790
    T-cell, 677
  of prostate, 1935
  renal involvement in, 1818
  spleen in, 782–784, 790, 794–797
  T-cell
    adult, 759–760
    chronic lymphocytic, 677
    prolymphocytic, 677
  of testis, 1957, 2012
  T-lymphoblastic, precursor, 677
  of uterus, 2269–2270, 2290
Leukemic infiltrates, 78
Leukemic reticuloendotheliosis, 751
Leukocytoclasia, 5
Leukocytoclastic vasculitis, 28–29
Leukodystrophy, 593
Leukoencephalopathy
  HIV, 401
  progressive multifocal, 392, 403–404
Leukoplakia, 811–812, 825–827
  speckled, 812
Leu-M1, in mesothelioma, 1133
Leydig cell(s), 1943, 1944
Leydig cell hyperplasia, of ovary, 2317
Leydig cell tumor
  of ovary, 2355–2356
  of testis, 2004–2006
LH (luteinizing hormone) deficiency, in males, 1955
Lhermitte-Duclos disease, 431
LH (luteinizing hormone) surge, 2211, 2212
Lichen amyloidosis, 37
Lichen aureus, 28
Lichenification, 5
Lichen nitidus, 10
Lichenoid dermatitis, pigmented purpuric, of Gougerot and Blum, 28
Lichenoid drug eruption, 10
Lichenoid interface change, 5
Lichenoid interface dermatitis, 9–10
Lichenoid keratosis, 53
Lichen planopilaris, 10
Lichen planus, 10
Lichen sclerosus et atrophicus, 36–37
  of vulva, 2121–2122
Lichen simplex chronicus, 16–17
  of vulva, 2122
Lichen striatus, 8

Light chain deposition disease
　bone marrow in, 691
　kidneys in, 1750–1751
　restrictive cardiomyopathy due to, 1330
Light eruption, polymorphous, 26
Ligneous salpingitis, 2398
Limb-girdle dystrophy, 121–122
Lingual thyroid, 529, 557
Lip, squamous cell carcinoma of, 823
Lipid granulomas, bone marrow, 656
Lipid histiocytoses, of spleen, 792–794
Lipid islands, of stomach, 1313
Lipidosis, 30–31
　sphingomyelin cholesterol, 692
Lipid storage diseases, 126
Lipoadenoma, of parathyroid, 568–569
Lipoblastoma, 149–150
Lipofuscin, pigmentation of, 1513
Lipogenic tumors, of bone, 299
Lipogranulomas, of liver, 1513
Lipoid cell tumors, of ovary, 2355–2358
Lipoid nephrosis, 1716–1718, 1776
Lipoid salpingitis, 2397
Lipoleiomyoma, 2273, 2284
Lipoma
　of bone, 299
　of breast, 367
　chondroid, 166
　of CNS, 455
　of inner ear, 971
　intestinal, 1459
　of larynx, 943
　mediastinal, 1162
　pleomorphic, 149
　pseudo-, hepatic, 1612
　renal, 1816
　of salivary gland, 874
　soft tissue, 166
　spindle-cell, 148–149
　uterine, 2273, 2284
　of vulva, 2119
Lipomatosis
　pseudo-, of intestines, 1392
　synovial, 227
Lipomatous tumor, atypical, 166–167
Liposarcoma, 161, 166–169
　of bone, 299
　of larynx, 943
　myxoid, 152, 167–169
　　cellular (round-cell), 167, 169
　　pleomorphic (dedifferentiated), 167, 169
　renal, 1816
　well-differentiated, 166–167
Liquefaction degeneration, 5
Littoral cell angiomas, 798
Liver
　abscesses of, 1557, 1558
　acidophil body of, 1510
　in acquired immunodeficiency syndrome, 1546–1547

　adenoma of, 1515, 1564–1567
　in alpha 1-antitrypsin deficiency, 1519–1521
　amyloidosis of, 1513, 1587, 1588
　angiomyolipoma of, 1586, 1612
　angiosarcoma of, 1586, 1607–1609, 1610
　autoimmune hepatitis of, 1511, 1512, 1542–1543
　bacterial infections of, 1511, 1513, 1536
　ballooning degeneration of, 1510
　benign and borderline tumors of, 1563–1575
　biopsy of, 1509–1510
　　absence of normal structures in, 1516
　　"nearly normal," 1516
　　for tumor diagnosis, 1555–1557
　carcinoma of
　　adeno-, 1586, 1587
　　cholangio-, 1593
　　clear-cell, 1586
　　hepatocellular. *See* Hepatocellular carcinoma
　　lobular lymphocytic infiltrate in, 1511
　　sclerosing, 1593
　　squamous cell, 1586
　cirrhosis of, 1513, 1540–1542
　congestion of, 1514
　in Crohn's disease, 1513
　in cystic fibrosis, 1513, 1520, 1521, 1522
　cystic masses of, 1557–1563
　developmental anomalies of, 1516–1519
　fatty changes of, 1515, 1543, 1547, 1548
　fatty tumors of, 1612
　fibrosarcoma and malignant fibrous histiocytoma of, 1615
　fibrosis of, 1513
　　congenital, 1519, 1557, 1560
　focal nodular hyperplasia of, 1513, 1565, 1567–1569
　foreign material in, 1513
　fungal infections of, 1511, 1513, 1536–1537
　germ cell tumors of, 1557, 1562–1563
　graft-*versus*-host disease of, 1512, 1544–1546
　granulomas of, 1510–1514, 1547–1548
　helminth infections of, 1537
　hemangioendothelioma of
　　epithelioid, 1602, 1608, 1609–1611
　　infantile, 1605–1606
　hemangioma of, 1603–1605
　hemorrhage of, 1514
　hepatitis of
　　peliosis, 1514, 1529, 1538, 1606
　　"surgical," 1511
　　viral, 1511, 1512, 1530–1536

　hepatoblastoma of, 1593–1598
　heterotopic tumors of, 1616
　in immunocompromised host, 1511
　inflammatory myofibroblastic tumor of, 1612–1613
　intracellular "inclusions" of, 1515
　ischemia of, 1511
　Kaposi's sarcoma of, 1609, 1612
　leiomyosarcoma of, 1615
　leukemia of, 1511, 1512, 1617–1620
　lipogranulomas of, 1513
　lobular inflammation of, 1510, 1511
　lymphangioma of, 1605
　lymphoma of, 1511, 1512, 1615–1616, 1617–1620
　masses of, 1553–1557
　　biopsy of, 1555–1556
　　classification of, 1553, 1554
　　histologic findings adjacent to, 1556–1557
　　intraoperative consultation for, 1555
　　prevalence of, 1553, 1555
　　specimen handling for, 1553–1555
　in mastocytosis, 1619, 1620
　melanoma of, 1586, 1588
　mesenchymal hamartoma of, 1557, 1563, 1614
　metastases to, 1586, 1587, 1616–1617
　mycobacterial infection of, 1513
　necrosis of, 1510, 1511
　neuroendocrine tumors of, 484, 1586, 1588, 1592–1593, 1602–1603
　nodular regenerative hyperplasia of, 1514, 1516, 1538–1540, 1565, 1569–1571
　nodules of
　　borderline (dysplastic), 1571–1575
　　macroregenerative, 1571–1575
　　solitary (fibrosing) necrotic, 1613
　parasitic infestation of, 1512
　partial nodular transformation of, 1539, 1540
　pigments in, 1514
　portal inflammation of, 1510, 1512
　protozoal infections of, 1537
　pseudolipoma of, 1612
　Q fever of, 1537
　Reye's syndrome of, 1543
　rhabdomyosarcoma of, 1614, 1615
　rickettsial infection of, 1513
　sarcoidosis of, 1513
　sarcoma of, 1586, 1613–1615
　sclerosis of, 1513
　in sepsis, 1511, 1514
　in syphilis, 1513
　in systemic disease, 1543–1544
　teratomas of, 1557, 1562–1563
　transplantation of, 1512, 1544–1546, 1588–1589
　trauma to, 1511
　unusual cells in, 1516

Liver *(contd.)*
  vascular disorders of, 1537–1538
  vascular tumors of
    benign, 1603–1606
    malignant, 1606–1612
  viral infections of, 1511, 1513
  in Wilson's disease, 1512, 1515, 1522–1524
Liver cell dysplasia, 1585
Liver disease, 1509–1548
  alcoholic, 1511, 1529–1530
  definition of terms for, 1510
  differential diagnosis of, 1510–1514
    common problems in, 1547–1548
  histologic chronic, 1547
  laboratory studies in, 1514–1516
  medication-induced, 1511–1516, 1528–1529, 1547, 1548
  metabolic, 1513, 1515, 1516, 1519–1524
  nonneoplastic hepatocellular proliferative, 1538–1540
  obstructive, 1524–1526
  polycystic, 1557, 1560
  of uncertain etiology, 1542–1543
Lobular capillary hemangioma, 69, 174
  of gingiva, 807
  sinonasal, 909–910
Lobular carcinoma
  infiltrating, 352–354
  in situ, 347–348
Lobular hyperplasia, of breast
  atypical, 330, 347
  epithelial, 347
Lobular neoplasia, of breast, 347–348
Lobular panniculitis, 39
Lobule(s), 325, 327
  cancerization of, 342, 348
  residual lactating, 327
Lobulitis, lymphocytic, 375–376
Löffler's syndrome
  lungs in, 1023
  restrictive cardiomyopathy due to, 1220
Long bones, ossifying fibroma of, 302
Loose bodies, 224
LPD (luteal phase defect), 2211–2212, 2217–2218
Lumpectomy, 321
Lung(s)
  honeycomb, 1018
  neoplasms of. *See* Pulmonary neoplasms
  nonneoplastic disease of. *See* Pulmonary disease
  patterns of injury to, 1011, 1012
  segmental anatomy of, 1069, 1070
Lung biopsy, 1011–1012, 1069–1071
  in immunocompromised host, 1056–1059
Lung tumors. *See* Pulmonary neoplasms
Lupus erythematosus

discoid, 10–12
systemic. *See* Systemic lupus erythematosus (SLE)
Lupus nephritis, 1745–1749, 1777
Lupus panniculitis, 41
Lupus pernio, 31
Lupus profundus, 41
Lushka ducts, 1630
Luteal phase defect (LPD), 2211–2212, 2217–2218
Luteinized thecoma, 2348–2349
Luteinizing hormone (LH) deficiency, in males, 1955
Luteinizing hormone (LH) surge, 2211, 2212
Luteoma
  pregnancy, 2315–2316, 2358
  stromal, 2355
Lyme disease, of brain, 399
Lymphadenitis, histiocytic necrotizing, 718
Lymphadenoma, sebaceous, 863
Lymphadenopathy
  angioimmunoblastic, 685
    with dysproteinemia, 726–727, 782
  dermatopathic, 724
  due to drug reactions, 727
  immunoblastic, 685, 726–727
  reactive, 715–730
    causing architectural effacement, 726–730
    with follicular hyperplasia, 715–722
    with interfollicular hyperplasia, 722–726
  sinus histiocytosis with massive, 309
Lymphangiectasis
  intestinal, 1359
  of vulva, 2119
Lymphangioleiomyomatosis, pulmonary, 1052–1053
Lymphangioma
  hepatic, 1605
  of mediastinum, 1153
  of orbit, 998–999
  pancreatic, 1492
  of salivary glands, 874
  soft tissue, 71
  of spleen, 798
  of vulva, 2119
Lymphangiomyoma, 178
Lymphangiomyomatosis
  pulmonary, 1052–1053
  soft tissue, 178
Lymphangiosarcoma, postmastectomy, 369
Lymphatics, 1271
Lymphatic tracking, 1033
Lymphedema, 1271
Lymph node(s), 709–766
  in angiofollicular hyperplasia, 721–722
  in angioimmunoblastic lymphadenopathy with

dysproteinemia, 726–727
axillary, metastases of breast carcinoma to, 362–363
in bacillary angiomatosis, 729
in B-cell chronic lymphocytic leukemia, 738–741
in B-cell lymphoma, 737–751
  diffuse large, 739, 746–749
  follicular center, 739, 743–745
  intravascular, 749
  lymphoplasmacytoid, 739, 741
  mantle cell, 739, 741–742
  microvillous, 749–750
  nodal marginal zone, 739, 745–746
  primary effusion, 749
  primary mediastinal (thymic), 748–749
  small lymphocytic, 738–741
  T-cell-rich, 749
in Burkitt's lymphoma, 739, 750–751
carcinoma of, 715
in Castleman's disease, 721–722
in cat-scratch disease, 719
classification of diseases of, 711–712
in dendritic cell sarcomas, 763–764
in dermatopathic lymphadenopathy, 724
differential diagnosis of diseases of, 712–715
examination of, 709–711
in hemophagocytic syndrome, 724
in histiocytic necrotizing lymphadenitis, 718
histiocytic neoplasms of, 715, 761–764
in HIV infection, 719–721
in Hodgkin's disease, 730–737
  vs. other lymphomas, 713–715
in immunoblastic lymphadenopathy, 726–727
in immunocytoma, 741
infarction of, 728
in infectious mononucleosis, 723
inflammatory pseudotumor of, 728
intramammary, 328
Kaposi's sarcoma of, 728
in Kikuchi-Fujimoto disease, 718
in Kimura's disease, 718–719
leukemic involvement of, 715, 766
metastases to, 764–765
  from adenosquamous carcinoma, 1095
  from oral squamous cell carcinoma, 814–815
  from prostatic carcinoma, 1920, 1925
  from thyroid carcinoma, 538–539
mycobacterial spindle-cell pseudotumor of, 728–729
in mycosis fungoides, 760
in natural killer cell lymphoma, 751–753, 760–761
in palisaded myofibroblastoma, 729–730

penile, 2037–2038
in phenytoin reaction, 727
plasmacytoma of, 751
in posttransplant proliferative disorders, 723–724
reactive adenopathy of, 715–730
reactive states *vs.* neoplastic diseases of, 712–713
retroperitoneal, lesions of, 2436–2437
in rheumatoid arthritis, 715–716
in Rosai-Dorfman disease, 724–726
in sarcoidosis, 727–728
in Sézary syndrome, 760
in sinus histiocytosis with massive adenopathy, 724–726
in Sjögren's syndrome, 717
spindle-cell lesions of, 728
in Still's disease, adult-onset, 717
in syphilis, 719
in systemic lupus erythematosus, 717–718
in T-cell lymphoma, 751–761
    adult, 759–760
    anaplastic large-cell, 758–759
    angioimmunoblastic, 757
    lymphoblastic, 753–754
    peripheral, 754–756
    precursor, 753–754
    primary extranodal, 760–763
thyroid tissue in, 530
in toxoplasmosis, 719
vascular transformation of sinuses of, 729
vasoproliferative lesions of, 728
in viral adenitis, 723
in Whipple's disease, 722–723
Lymph node endosalpingiosis, 2326
Lymphoblastic lymphoma, of mediastinum, 1159–1160, 1174–1175
Lymphocyte(s), intraepithelial, in gastroesophageal reflux disease, 1287
Lymphocyte-depleted Hodgkin's disease, 731, 736–737
Lymphocyte-predominant Hodgkin's disease, 713–714, 731–733
Lymphocyte-predominant thymoma, 1158–1161
Lymphocyte progenitor cells, increased, 684–685
Lymphocytic aggregates, 683
Lymphocytic angiitis and granulomatosis, benign, 1037
Lymphocytic colitis, 1366–1368
Lymphocytic enterocolitis, 1352
Lymphocytic gastritis, 1321–1322
Lymphocytic hypophysitis, 522
Lymphocytic interstitial pneumonia, 1031–1032
Lymphocytic lesions, of thyroid, 555

Lymphocytic leukemia, chronic
    B-cell, 670–673, 738–741
    immunoblastic transformation of, 673
    mixed cell type, 670
    spleen in, 782–784
    T-cell, 677
    transformation of, 670–673
Lymphocytic lobulitis, 375–376
Lymphocytic vasculitis, 29
Lymphoepithelial cysts, pancreatic, 1492
Lymphoepithelial lesion
    pulmonary, 1034
    salivary gland
        benign, 855–856
        malignant, 856–857
Lymphoepithelioma
    nasopharyngeal, 897
    salivary gland, 856
    of urothelial tract, 1878
Lymphoepithelioma-like carcinoma
    of cervix, 2177
    of mediastinum, 1192
    of thymus, 1178, 1180
Lymphogranuloma venereum, of penis, 2039–2040
Lymphohistiocytosis, cerebromeningeal hemophagocytic, 401
Lymphoid hyperplasia
    angiofollicular, 1159
    of lacrimal gland, 1001
    of mediastinum, 1158
    of orbit, 999
    reactive, of conjunctiva, 987
    sinonasal, 906
Lymphoid infiltrates, pulmonary, 1030–1032
Lymphoid lesions, reactive, 683–684
Lymphoid neoplasms
    of bone marrow, 667–670
    classification of, 711–712
    of CNS, 452–455
    cutaneous, 73–79
    differential diagnosis of, 712–715
    of larynx, 943–944
Lymphoid polyps
    of anus, 1674
    intestinal, 1424
Lymphoma(s)
    of adrenal glands, 607–608
    in AIDS, 658
    angiocentric
        cutaneous, 74
        sinonasal, 889, 907–908
    BALT, 1032–1035
    B-cell, 737–751
        biology of, 737–738
        Burkitt's, 739, 750–751
        classification of, 737
        cutaneous, 74–75
        differential diagnosis of, 739
        diffuse large, 739, 746–749

        follicular center, 739, 743–745
        of intestines, 1454
        intravascular, 749
        of liver, 1618
        lymphoplasmacytoid, 739, 741
        mantle cell, 739, 741–742
        microvillous, 749–750
        nodal marginal zone, 739, 745–746
        primary effusion, 749
        primary mediastinal (thymic), 748–749
        small lymphocytic, 738–741
        of spleen, 787–789
        T-cell-rich, 75, 749
    B-lymphoblastic, 751
        precursor, 670, 751
    of bone, 267–269, 296
    of breast, 369
    Burkitt's, 676, 739, 750–751
        of intestines, 1454
        of mediastinum, 1160
    cardiac, 1241
    CD30+, 75–76
    of cervix, 2196
    of CNS, 396, 414, 452–454
    of conjunctiva, 987
    cutaneous, 27, 73–76
    cutaneous T-cell, *vs.* spongiotic dermatitis, 6, 17
    differential diagnosis of, 161
    of ear, 958
    esophageal, 1304
    of fallopian tube, 2407
    follicular center, 75, 674, 739, 743–745
        of spleen, 786–787
    gastric, 1335–1337
    hepatic, 1511, 1512, 1615–1616, 1617–1620
    histiocytic, 695
    Hodgkin's. *See* Hodgkin's disease
    intestinal, 1443, 1449–1454
    intravascular, 749
    of lacrimal gland, 1001
    of larynx, 943
    Lennert's, 787
    of liver, 1618
    lymphoplasmacytoid, 673, 739, 741
        of spleen, 784
    mantle cell, 674, 739, 741–742
        of spleen, 784–785
    mantle zone, 75
    marginal zone, 739, 745–746
        of spleen, 674–676, 785–786
    of mediastinum, 1159–1161, 1190
        B-cell, 748–749
        lymphoblastic, 1159–1160, 1174–1175
        small-cell malignant, 1174–1175
    mucosa-associated lymphoid tissue (MALT)
        of intestine, 1449–1450

Lymphoma(s), mucosa-associated
        lymphoid tissue (MALT) (contd.)
    of mediastinum, 1160–1161,
        1174–1175
    of stomach, 1335–1337
  natural killer cell, 751–753, 760–761
    sinonasal, 907–908
  vs. neuroblastoma, 611
  non-Hodgkin's, 667–670
    blood involvement by, 680
    low-grade, 670
    posttherapy, 679
  of orbit, 999
  of ovary, 2372–2373
  of pancreas, 1503
  of prostate, 1934–1935
  pseudo-, 74
    of breast, 369–370
    pulmonary, 1032
    sinonasal, 906
  pulmonary, 1032–1035
  renal, 1818
    in children, 1851
  salivary gland, 874–875
  of sellar region, 518
  sinonasal, 906, 907–908
  small lymphocytic, 673, 738–741
    of spleen, 782–784
  of spleen, 782–790
    follicular, 786–787
    large-cell, 787–789
    lymphoplasmacytoid, 784
    mantle cell, 784–785
    marginal zone, 674–676, 785–786
    small lymphocytic, 782–784
    with villous lymphocytes, 786
  T-cell, 74, 75–76, 676–680, 751–761
    adult, 679, 759–760
    anaplastic large-cell, 758–759
    angioimmunoblastic, 757
    cutaneous, 6, 17
    enteropathy-associated, 1357
    of intestines, 1454
    of liver, 1618
    lymphoblastic, 753–754
    peripheral, 78, 678–679, 754–756
    precursor, 753–754
    primary extranodal, 760–763
    sinonasal, 907–908
    of spleen, 787–789
  testicular, 2011–2012
  thyroid, 555, 562
  T-lymphoblastic, precursor, 677
  of uterus, 2269–2270, 2290
  vaginal, 2142
  of vulva, 2130
Lymphoma-like lesions, 683–685
Lymphomatoid granulomatosis
  cutaneous, 29, 75
  pulmonary, 1035–1037
Lymphomatoid papulosis, 12–14, 75–76

Lymphomatosis, intravascular, 74
Lymphomatous polyposis, multiple, of
        gastrointestinal tract, 1453–1454
Lymphoplasmacytoid lymphoma, 673,
        739, 741
  of spleen, 784
Lymphoproliferative disorders
  chronic, 667–670
    B-cell, 670–673
  posttransplant, 723–724, 1769,
        1774–1775
  T-cell, 676–680

M

Macroglobulinemia, Waldenström's
  bone marrow in, 690
  intestinal involvement in, 1359
  spleen in, 784
Macromastia, in pregnancy, 377
Macroorchidism, 1956
Macrophages, brain, 396–397
Macroregenerative nodules, 1571–1575
Macular amyloidosis, 37
Macular corneal dystrophy, 980
Macule, 5
"Mad cow" disease, 406
Maffucci's syndrome, 274
MAIC, See Mycobacterium avium-
        intracellulare (MAIC)
Malabsorption, 1349–1360
  due to abetalipoproteinemia, 1359
  due to acrodermatitis enteropathica,
        1359–1360
  due to autoimmune enteropathy, 1355
  due to celiac sprue, 1350–1352
  due to chemotherapy effect, 1352,
        1392–1393
  due to collagenous sprue, 1355
  due to dermatitis herpetiformis, 1353
  due to duodenitis, 1354–1355
  due to enteropathy-associated T-cell
        lymphoma, 1357
  due to eosinophilic gastroenteritis, 1357
  due to immunodeficiency syndromes,
        1355–1356
  due to infectious gastroenteritis,
        1353–1354
  due to kwashiorkor, 1352
  due to lymphangiectasia, 1359
  due to lymphocytic enterocolitis, 1352
  due to marasmus, 1352
  due to mastocytosis, 1354
  due to megaloblastic anemia, 1352
  due to microvillus inclusion disease,
        1352–1353
  due to parasitic infestations, 1358–1359
  due to peptic ulcer disease, 1354–1355
  due to protein allergies, 1352
  due to radiation, 1352, 1392–1393
  due to stasis syndromes, 1354
  due to Torkelson syndrome, 1355

  due to tropical sprue, 1353
  due to tufting enteropathy, 1360
  due to ulcerative jejunoileitis, 1357
  due to Waldenström's
        macroglobulinemia, 1359
  due to Whipple's disease, 1356
  due to Zollinger-Ellison syndrome,
        1354
Malakoplakia
  of bladder, 1858–1859
  of ear, 952
  intestinal, 1460
  of prostate, 1898
  pulmonary, 1030
  renal, 1759
  of testis, 1963
Male(s)
  breast carcinoma in, 361
  gynecomastia in, 376
Male infertility, 1950–1955
Male pseudohermaphroditism, 1964–1968
Malignant melanoma. See Melanoma
Mallory's hyalin
  in hepatocellular carcinoma, 1582–1583
  in liver, 1515, 1529–1530
MALTomas
  of intestine, 1449–1450
  of mediastinum, 1160–1161, 1174–1175
  of stomach, 1335–1337
Mammary carcinoma. See Breast
        carcinoma
Mammary lobules, 325, 327
  cancerization of, 342, 348
  carcinoma of
    infiltrating, 352–354
    in situ, 347–348
  hyperplasia of
    atypical, 330, 347
    epithelial, 347
  neoplasia of, 347–348
  residual lactating, 327
Mammography, 322–323
Mammosomatotroph cell adenoma, 498,
        500, 511
Mantle cell lymphoma, 674, 739, 741–742
  of spleen, 784–785
Mantle zone lymphoma, 75
Marasmus, 1352
Marfan disease, aorta in, 1258
Marginal zone lymphoma, 674–676
  of spleen, 785–786
Masculinization, 2112
Mast cell disease, 307, 665–667
Mast cell infiltrates, 78–79
Mastectomy specimens, 322
Mastitis
  chronic granulomatous (perilobular),
        374–375
  periductal, 375
Mastocytosis, 307
  cutaneous, 78–79

intestines in, 1354
liver in, 1619, 1620
systemic, 797
Mastopathy, indurative, 331–333
Maternal floor infarction, 2093–2094
Matrix-producing carcinoma, of breast, 359
Maturation arrest, 1951–1952, 1956
Maxilla, structures of, 805, 806
Maxillary tuberosity, 805
McArdle's disease, 125
M cells, 1361
Meatus urethralis, 2035
Meckel's diverticulum, 1391
Meckel syndrome, 1689
Meconium aspiration syndrome, 2104
Meconium periorchitis, 2015
Meconium staining, 2091, 2104–2105
Median palatine cysts, 841
Median raphe cysts, 2038
Mediastinitis, sclerosing (fibrosing), 1167–1168
Mediastinum, 1147–1199
  benign mesenchymal neoplasms of, 1162–1167
  carcinoid tumor of, 1169, 1182–1183, 1190, 1198–1199
    spindle cell thymic, 1194
  carcinoma of
    basaloid squamous cell, 1170, 1175
    lymphoepithelioma-like, 1192
    neuroendocrine
      large-cell, 1182–1183
      prognosis for, 1198–1199
      small-cell, 1168–1170, 1175–1176, 1199
    oat cell, 1168–1170, 1175
    parathyroid, 1180–1181, 1190, 1199
    thymic
      primary, 1176–1180, 1199
      sarcomatoid, 1192–1194
  Castleman's disease of, 1159, 1198
  chordoma of, 1195
  clinical features of lesions of, 1147–1148
  cystic lesions of, 1149–1156
    bronchogenic, 1151–1152
    differential diagnosis of, 1156
    enteric, 1152–1153
    parathyroid, 1149–1151
    pericardial, 1152
    thymic, 1149–1151
  ectopic lesions of, 1196
  fibrogenic proliferations of, 1165–1167
  fibrous histiocytoma of, 1161–1162
  ganglioneuromas of, 1164–1165
  germ cell tumors of
    cystic, 1153–1156
    malignant, 1181–1182, 1190
    prognosis for, 1198

granulocytic sarcoma of, 1187–1188, 1190–1191
gross features of lesions of, 1148–1149
hemangioendothelioma of, epithelioid, 1195
hemangiopericytoma of, 1161–1162
Hodgkin's disease of
  large-cell, 1186–1187, 1190–1191
  mixed cellularity, 1192
  prognosis for, 1198
hygromas of, 1153
inflammatory myofibroblastic tumors of, 1167–1168
large polygonal-cell neoplasms of, 1176–1187
  differential diagnosis of, 1190–1191
leiomyosarcoma of, epithelioid, 1189, 1190
lipomas of, 1162
lymphangiomas of, 1153
lymphoid hyperplasia of, 1158
lymphoma of, 1159–1161, 1190
  lymphoblastic, 1159–1160, 1174–1175
  non-Hodgkin's
    large-cell, 1185–1186, 1190–1191, 1198
    mixed large- and small-cell, 1191
    small-cell, 1159–1161, 1174–1175
  small-cell malignant, 1174–1175
melanoma of, 1190, 1199
meningoceles of, 1153
mesothelioma of, malignant
  epithelioid, 1189
  sarcomatoid, 1194
metastases to, 1176, 1189–1190, 1199
mixed large- and small-cell malignant tumors of, 1191–1192
myofibroblastic proliferations of, 1165–1167
nerve sheath tumors of, 1162–1164
neuroblastoma of, 1170–1172, 1175
paragangliomas of, 1184–1185, 1190, 1199
plasmacytoma of, extraosseous, 1188–1189, 1190
pleomorphic neoplasms of, malignant, 1192–1194
primitive neuroectodermal tumor of, 1172–1173, 1175
prognostic features of neoplasms of, 1196–1199
rhabdomyosarcoma of, 1173–1174, 1175
seminomas of, 1181, 1182, 1198
  cystic, 1155–1156
small-cell neoplasms of, 1168–1176
  differential diagnosis of, 1175–1176
spindle cell neoplasms of, malignant, 1192–1194
teratomas of, 1153–1155, 1198

thymic dysplasia of, 1161
thymic yolk sac tumor of, sarcomatoid, 1194
thymolipomas of, 1162
thymoliposarcoma of, 1195
thymomas of, 1156–1162
  cystic, 1155–1156
  epithelial spindle-cell, 1161–1162
  lymphocyte-predominant, 1158–1161
  microscopic, 1161
  prognostic features of, 1196–1198
Medication effects. See Drug effects
Medullary carcinoma
  of breast, with lymphoid stroma, 354–355
  renal, 1805–1806
    in children, 1849, 1850
Medullary cells, 591
Medullary fibroma, 1816–1817
Medullary thyroid carcinoma, 549–551, 561–562
Medulloblastoma, 414, 434–438
  desmoplastic, 413, 437
  lipomatous, 437–438
Medulloepithelioma, 412, 438
  optic nerve, 1000
Medullomyoblastoma, 414, 437
Meesman's dystrophy, 980
Megacolon, aganglionic, 1390
Megakaryocytes, in liver, 1516
Megaloblastic anemia, intestines in, 1352
Melanoacanthoma, 97
Melanocytes, 4, 89–90, 484
  epithelioid, 91
Melanocytic lesions, 89–105
  benign, 89–100
  of CNS, 458–459
  of conjunctiva, 986
  malignant, 100–105
  of prostate, 1899
  of vagina, 2137
  of vulva, 2117
Melanocytic nevus
  acquired, 91–93
  congenital, 93, 99–100
  of ear, 957
  lentiginous, 98
  with pigment elimination, 100
  recurrent, 98
  regressing, 98–99
  traumatized, 100
Melanocytosis
  congenital ocular, 986
  dermal, 96–97
  oculodermal, 986
Melanoma, 100–105
  acral lentiginous, 104
  of adrenal glands, 608
  anal, 1679–1680
  benign juvenile, 93–95
  borderline and minimal deviation, 17

Melanoma *(contd.)*
  CNS, 411, 412, 413, 457, 458–459
  conjunctival, 986
  differential diagnosis of, 161
  dysplastic nevus and, 101–102
  of esophagus, 1299, 1304
  of eyelid, 992
  of gallbladder, 1655
  histologic and cytologic characteristics of, 100–101
  histologic forms of, 102–104
  intraocular, 994–996
  lentigo maligna form of, 104
  of liver, 1586, 1588
  of mediastinum, 1190, 1199
  metastatic, 1460–1461
  NIH Consensus recommendations on pathology reporting for, 104–105
  nodular, 103–104
  of ovary, 2347, 2381
  vs. Paget's disease of nipple, 360
  of penis, 2057
  pulmonary, 1101
  radial growth phase, 102–103
  sinonasal, 903–904
  in situ, 55
  of soft parts, 194
  spindle-cell, 133
  superficial spreading, 103–104
  of urinary tract, 1882
  vaginal, 2142
  vertical growth phase, 103
  vulvar, 2130
Melanophagocytes, 9
Melanosis
  lentiginous, of penis, 2042
  peritoneal, 2420
  primary acquired, 986
Melanosis coli, 1389
Melanosis duodeni, pseudo-, 1349
Melanotic neuroectodermal tumor, of testis, 2019–2020
MELAS (myopathy, encephalopathy, lactic acidosis, stroke) syndrome, 126
Mel-CAM antibody, 2075
Meltzer-Lyon test, 1635
Membranoproliferative glomerulonephritis, 1706–1709, 1775
Membranous fat necrosis, of breast, 374
Ménétrier's disease, 1329–1330
Meningeal cyst, 460, 462–463
Meningeal fibrosis, 397
Meningeal hemorrhage, 406–407
Meningeal tumors, 438–447
Meningioma(s), 412, 421, 438–445
  aggressive, 442–444
  anaplastic (malignant), 421, 444
  angioblastic, 441
    of sellar region, 518
  angiomatous, 441–442
  atypical, 442–444
  choroid, 442
  clear cell, 442
  fibroblastic (fibrous), 440
  fibroelastic (fibrous), 411
  hemangioblastic, 441–442
  hemangiopericytic, 421, 444–445
  meningotheliomatous (syncytial), 440
  of middle ear, 965
  optic nerve, 1000
  papillary, 444
  psammomatous, 438, 441
  pulmonary, 1101
  rhabdoid, 442
  of sellar region, 518
  sinonasal, 905–906
  transitional (mixed), 413, 440
Meningitis, 397–399
  lymphocytic, 402
Meningoceles, cystic, 1153
Meningotheliomatous meningioma, 440
Meniscal tears, 238–239
Menopause, premature, 2318
Menstrual cycle, endometrium in, 2210–2217
MEN syndromes. *See* Multiple endocrine neoplasia (MEN) syndrome
Merkel cell(s), 484, 487
Merkel cell carcinoma, 59
MERRF (myoclonus epilepsy with ragged red fibers) syndrome, 126
Mesangial hypercellularity, 1777
Mesangial interposition, 1777
Mesangial sclerosis, nodular, 1777
Mesangiocapillary glomerulonephritis, 1706–1708, 1775
Mesangiolysis, 1777
Mesenchymal chondrosarcoma, 281
  sinonasal, 916–917
Mesenchymal hamartoma, of liver, 1557, 1563, 1614
Mesenchymal polyps, of esophagus, 1296–1297
Mesenchymal tumors
  of breast, 367
  of intestines, 1443
  of kidney, 1817–1818
  of larynx, 941–944
  of orbit, 999
  of prostate, 1932–1933
  of testis, 2013
  of urinary tract, 1882
Mesenchymoma, 190
Mesenteritis, idiopathic retractile (sclerosing), 1396–1397
Mesentery, inflammatory lesions of, 1395–1398
Mesoblastic nephroma
  adult, 1806–1807
  in children, 1839–1842
Mesodermal adenosarcomas, of ovary, 2334
Mesodermal mixed tumors, of ovary, 2334
Mesonephric adenocarcinoma, of cervix, 2193
Mesonephric cyst, 2114
  vaginal, 2137
Mesonephric hyperplasia, of cervix, 2179–2180
Mesonephric papilloma, of vagina, 2138
Mesonephric remnants, 2135
Mesothelial hyperplasia
  of peritoneum, 2417–2418
  of pleura, 1118
Mesothelial neoplasms, of peritoneum, 2421–2424
Mesothelioma
  ancillary diagnostic procedures for, 1124–1133
  antimesothelial antibodies in, 1133–1135
  of atrioventricular node, 1240
  B72.3 in, 1133
  Ber-EP4 in, 1131
  BG-8 in, 1131–1133
  biphasic, 1124
  calretinin in, 1135
  carcinoembryonic antigen in, 1125–1126, 1130–1131
  CD44H in, 1135
  classification of, 1121–1124
  clinical features of, 1121
  cystic, 2422
  cytologic diagnosis of, 1135–1137
  desmoplastic, 1129, 1138–1139
  electron microscopy of, 1126
  epithelial, 1121, 1122, 1137–1138, 1189
  epithelial markers for, 1129–1133
  etiology, incidence, and histogenesis of, 1120–1121
  fibrous, 1122–1123, 1138, 2421
  glycogen in, 1125
  glycosaminoglycans in, 1125–1126
  HBME-1 in, 1134
  histochemistry of, 1125
  histologic features and differential diagnosis of, 1123–1124
  HMFG-2 in, 1133
  illustrative cases of, 1137–1142
  immunohistochemistry of, 1126–1133
  in situ, 1118
  intermediate filaments in, 1127–1129
  keratins in, 1127–1129
  Leu-M1 (CD15) in, 1133
  localized epithelial, 1119
  malignant, 1120–1139
    of peritoneum, 2418, 2422–2424
  of mediastinum
    epithelioid, 1189
    sarcomatoid, 1194
  mixed, 1124

mucins in, 1125
N-cadherin in, 1135
of ovary, 2376
papillary, 2421–2422
pathologic findings in, 1121
of peritoneum
    diffuse malignant, 2418, 2422–2424
    fibrous, 2421
    low-grade cystic, 2422
    well-differentiated papillary, 2421–2422
pulmonary, 1092
sarcomatous, 1122–1123, 1138, 119–
of testis, 2016
thrombomodulin in, 1134
of uterus, 2288–2290
vimentin in, 1129
Mesothelium
defined, 1117
regeneration of, 1117–1118
Metabolic disease(s)
of bone, 245–255, 699
of kidney, 1760–1761
of liver, 1513, 1515, 1516, 1519–1524
neuromuscular, 125–126
of stomach, 1339–1340
Metal toxicity, 244, 250
Metanephric adenofibroma, 1811–1812
in children, 1850
Metanephric adenoma, 1811–1812
in children, 1850
Metaphyseal fibrous defects, 304
Metaplasia
of bladder, 1860–1862
of breast, 329–330
of cervix
    immature squamous, 2163, 2166
    papillary immature, 2161–2163
of CNS, glioblastoma and gliosarcoma with, 429
of endocervical glands
    atypical oxyphilic, 2182–2184
    tuboendometrial, 2180
endometrial
    ciliated cell, 2255, 2256
    clear-cell, hobnail, and eosinophilic 2256–2258
    epithelial, 2245–2246
    mucinous, 2249, 2250
    papillary syncytial, 2251, 2254
of fallopian tube, 2401
of gallbladder, 1643, 1645, 1647–1648
intestinal, 1314–1315
    of Barrett's esophagus, 1291, 1292, 1293
of kidney, 1847
of ovary, stomal, 2317–2318
of pancreas, 1314
of pancreatic ducts, 1471–1472
of prostate, mucinous, 1899
pyloric gland

of gallbladder, 1645
of pancreas, 1472
of stomach, 1314
    pseudo-, 1311
sialo-, 855, 890
of spleen, 795
squamous
    of breast, 329–330
    of cervix, 2163, 2166
    of stomach, 1311, 1314–1315
    ciliated, 1314
of urothelium, 1860–1862
Metaplastic carcinoma, of breast, 358–359
Metastases
adrenal, 607
from benign mixed tumors of salivary gland, 859
to bile ducts, 1602
to bone, 296, 299–300
to bone marrow, 695–699
to brain, 456–458
within breast, 362
from breast carcinoma, 362–363
cardiac, 1241
to cervix, 2194–2196
to ear
    inner, 972
    middle, 967
to esophagus, 1304
to extrahepatic bile duct, 1666
to eyelids, 992
to fallopian tube, 2407
to gallbladder, 1655
intestinal, 1443, 1460–1461
to larynx, 941
to liver, 1543, 1586, 1587, 1616–1617
to lung, 1092, 1103–1104
lymph node, 764–765
    from adenosquamous carcinoma, 1095
    from oral squamous cell carcinoma, 814–815
    from prostatic carcinoma, 1920, 1925
    from thyroid carcinoma, 538–539
to mediastinum, 1176, 1189–1190, 1199
to optic nerve, 1000
of oral squamous cell carcinoma, 814–815
from osteosarcoma, 285–286
to ovary, 2376–2382
to pancreas, 1503
from paragangliomas, 643
to penis, 2059
peritoneal, 2426–2427
to pituitary, 518, 521–522
from prostatic carcinoma, 1920, 1925
to salivary glands, 875
to spleen, 799
to testis, 2013–2014
to thyroid, 556, 557, 562
of thyroid carcinoma, 538–539

to vagina, 2143
to vulva, 2130
Methotrexate, effect on testis of, 1958
Methyl methacrylate, in joint prostheses, 235–236
Meyenberg complex, 1519
MIB-1, as marker of cellular proliferation, 409
MIC2, as marker for soft tissue tumors, 142
Michaelis-Gutmann bodies, 1030, 1759
Microabscess, 5
Microaneurysms, 1256
Microangiopathy, thrombotic, 1736–1739, 1770, 1776
Microcalcification, of breast tissue, 323
Microcystic, map dot, and fingerprint dystrophy, 980
Microdochectomy, 321–322
Microgemistocytes, 425
Microglandular adenocarcinoma, of pancreas, 1496–1497
Microglandular adenosis, of breast, 332, 333–334
Microglandular hyperplasia, of cervix, 2178–2179
Microinvasive carcinoma, of cervix, 2168–2172
Micrometastases, of breast carcinoma, 362
Micronodular pneumocyte hyperplasia, 1053
Microsporidia
of gallbladder, 1640–1641
intestinal, in AIDS patients, 1373–1374
Microvenular hemangioma, 176
Microvillous lymphoma, 749–750
Microvillus inclusion disease, 1352–1353
Midfacial necrotizing lesion, 887–889
Midline destructive disease, idiopathic, 889
"Milk lines," and vulvar lesions, 2120
Mineralization, abnormal, 249–250
Mineral oil granulomas, 31
Minicore disease, 123
Minimal change disease, 1716–1718, 1776
Minimal change nephrotic syndrome, 1716–1718, 1776
Minimal deviation melanoma, 105
Mirizzi's syndrome, 1633
Mites, of eyelids, 989
Mitochondria, giant, in liver, 1515
Mitochondrial myopathies, 118–119, 126
Mitotic index, of uterine smooth-muscle neoplasms, 2278, 2282–2283
Mitral regurgitation, 1228–1229, 1230
Mitral stenosis, 1228
Mitral valve
myxomatous, 1229
normal, 1227–1228
Mitral valve prolapse, 1229
Mitral valvular disease, 1227–1230

Mixed gonadal dysgenesis, 1964–1965, 1967–1968
Mixed tumors
  of appendix, 1446
  of lacrimal gland, 1001
  of larynx, 939–940
  of mediastinum, 1191–1192
  müllerian, 2258–2265
  of ovary, 2370–2372
  of salivary glands
    benign, 857–859
    malignant, 870–872
  of testis
    germ cell, 2001–2002
    germ cell–sex cord-stromal, 2010–2011
    sex cord-stromal, 2009–2010
  vaginal, 2138
  of vulva, 2132–2133
Mole, 91–93
  changing, 98
  hydatidiform, 2069–2074
    complete, 2069–2071
    invasive, 2073–2074
    partial, 2071–2073
Molluscum contagiosum, 49
  of eyelids, 989
  of penis, 2040
  of vulva, 2117
Mondor's phlebitis, 2042
Mongolian spot, 96
Monoclonal antibodies, in pulmonary neoplasms, 1107–1108
Monoclonal gammopathy-associated renal diseases, 1750–1752
Monoclonal gammopathy of undetermined significance, 689
Monoclonal immunoglobulin deposition diseases, 691
Mononucleosis, infectious
  lymph nodes in, 723
  spleen in, 791–792
Montgomery's tubercles, 327
Morphea, 36
Morton's neuroma, 241
Morular differentiation, of endometrium, 2246–2249
Mouth. *See* Oral cavity
MS (multiple sclerosis), 465
Mucha-Habermann disease, 12–14
Mu chain disease, 691
Mucicarminophilic histiocytosis, 2416
Mucin(s), in mesothelioma, 1125
Mucinosis, follicular, 33–34
Mucinous adenocarcinoma
  of breast, 355–356
  colorectal, 1437
  of endometrium, 2250
  of ovary, 2328–2330
  of pancreas, 1481–1482
  of prostate, 1927–1928

Mucinous cystadenocarcinoma, of pancreas, 1488–1490, 1493
Mucinous cystic neoplasms, of pancreas, 1488–1490, 1493
Mucinous differentiation, of endometrium, 2249–2250
Mucinous lesions, peritoneal, 2435
Mucinous metaplasia, of endometrium, 2249, 2250
Mucinous tumors
  of appendix, 1442–1444
  of ovary, 2328–2330
Mucin-producing adenocarcinoma, 869
Muciphages, 1361
Mucocele
  of appendix, 1442
  of gallbladder, 1635
  of orbit, 998
  of salivary gland, 854
  sinonasal, 890
Mucocele-like lesions, of breast, 378
Mucoepidermoid carcinoma, 833
  of conjunctiva, 985
  of ear, 957
  of esophagus, 1299, 1304
  of larynx, 940
  pulmonary, 1098, 1099
  of salivary glands, 866–867
  of thymus, 1178
  of thyroid, 556
Mucoid wedge, of pituitary, 495
Mucopolysaccharidosis, liver in, 1519, 1520
Mucor, liver infection with, 1536–1537
Mucormycosis, sinonasal, 886
Mucosa-associated lymphoid tissue (MALT) lymphomas (MALTomas)
  of intestine, 1449–1450
  of mediastinum, 1160–1161, 1174–1175
  of stomach, 1335–1337
Mucosal erosion/ulceration, in gastroesophageal reflux disease, 1287–1288
Mucosal prolapse syndromes, 1369–1370
Mucous cysts
  retention and extravasation, of salivary gland, 854
  vaginal, 2137
  vulvar, 2113–2114
Muir Torre syndrome, 1418, 1436
Müllerian adenofibroma, 2245, 2260–2261, 2264, 2270–2271
Müllerian adenosarcoma
  of ovary, 2334
  of uterine corpus, 2261–2262, 2264–2265, 2270–2271
Müllerian duct, persistent, 1964–1965
Müllerian inclusion glands, 2326
Müllerian papilloma, 2182
Müllerian system, lesions of secondary, 2427–2437

Müllerian tumors
  of broad ligament, 2408–2409
  mixed
    of fallopian tube, 2406–2407
    of uterine corpus, 2258–2265
Multicore disease, 123
Multicystic dysplasia kidney, 1686–1688
Multidirectional differentiation, of neoplasms, 491–492
Multiple endocrine neoplasia (MEN) syndromes, 486
  familial pheochromocytoma with, 617–618
  familial sympathoadrenal paragangliomas in, 637
  parathyroid in, 568
Multiple myeloma, 267
Multiple sclerosis (MS), 465
Mumps, effect on testes of, 1961–1962
Munro's microabscess, 8
Muscle(s)
  normal, 110–111
  reactions to injury of, 112
  red *vs.* white, 111
Muscle biopsy, 109–120
  artifacts in, 111–112
  atrophy in, 115–116
  changes in histochemical profile in, 115–120
  clinical information from, 109
  collection and preparation for, 109–110
  contraindications to, 109, 110
  cores in, 117–118
  fatty infiltration in, 115
  fiber necrosis in, 113
  fiber regeneration in, 114
  fiber shape in, 116
  fiber splitting in, 116–117
  fibrosis in, 115
  frozen sections of, 110, 115–116
  of general reactions to injury, 112
  hyaline fibers in, 113
  hypertrophy in, 115–116
  inflammation in, 114–115
  interpretation of, 110–120
  mitochondrial abnormalities in, 118–119
  mottled fibers in, 117
  nemaline rods in, 118
  of normal muscle, 110–111
  nuclear changes in, 112–113
  planning and procedures for, 109–110
  ring fibers in, 113
  routine paraffin sections of, 110, 112–115
  targets in, 117–118
  type grouping in, 116
  vacuolar change in, 119–120
Muscle fibers
  hyaline, 113
  mottled, 117

SUBJECT INDEX / I-43

necrotic, 113
ragged red, 118–119, 126
regenerating, 114
ring, 113
shape of, 116
size of, 110–111
splitting of, 116–117
target, 117–118
typing of, 111
Muscle markers, for soft tissue tumors, 141–142
Muscle-specific actin, as marker for soft tissue tumors, 141
Muscular atrophy, 115–116
infantile spinal, 127
Muscular dystrophies, 120–124
Muscular hypertrophy, 115–116
of esophagus, 1295
Myasthenia gravis, 127
Mycobacterial infection
of liver, 1513
of middle ear, 960
of testis, 1961
Mycobacterial pseudotumor
of lung, 1039–1040
of lymph nodes, 728–729
Mycobacterial salpingitis, 2395–2397
Mycobacterium avium-intracellulare (MAIC)
in AIDS
intestinal, 1371–1372
pulmonary, 1057–1058
gastritis due to, 1324
in small bowel, 1356
Mycoplasma, chorioamnionitis due to, 2101
Mycosis fungoides, 76–78, 678
of lymph nodes, 760–761
Mycotic aneurysms, 1256
Mycotoxicosis, pulmonary, 1023
Myelinoclastic diffuse sclerosis, 465
Myelodysplastic syndrome, 662–663
Myelofibrosis, 696
chronic idiopathic, with myeloid metaplasia, 664–665
reactive, 656
Myeloid metaplasia
chronic idiopathic myelofibrosis with, 664–665
of spleen, 795
Myelolipoma, adrenal, 605
Myeloma, 266–267
indolent, 689
multiple, 267, 686–689
nonsecretory, 689
osteosclerotic, 689
plasma cell, 686–689
of sellar region, 518
smoldering, 689
Myeloma cast nephropathy, 1751–1752
Myeloma kidney, 1751–1752

Myeloproliferative disorders
chronic, 663–667
liver in, 1543
Myelosclerosis, malignant, 665
Myoadenylate deaminase deficiency, 126
Myoblastoid carcinoma, of breast, 360
Myoblastomas, of larynx, 929
Myocardial biopsy, 1209–1210
Myocardial disease(s), 1209–1225
in AIDS, 1220–1221
cardiomyopathies, 1210–1215
restrictive, 1218–1222
collagen vascular, 1218
endomyocardial biopsy for, 1209–1210
ischemic, 1224–1225
myocarditis, 1215–1218
sarcoidosis, 1218
Myocardial infarction, 1224
Myocarditis, 1215–1218
bacterial, 1215–1216
drug-induced, 1217–1218
hypersensitivity, 1217–1218
idiopathic (viral), 1215
infectious, 1215–1217
parasitic, 1216–1217
toxic, 1218
Myocardium, normal histology of, 1209
Myoclonus epilepsy with ragged red fibers (MERRF) syndrome, 126
Myocyte, 110
MyoD1, as marker for soft tissue tumors, 142
Myoepithelial carcinoma, of salivary glands, 864
Myoepithelial hamartoma, of small bowel, 1360
Myoepithelioma, of salivary glands, 863
Myofibroblastic proliferations, of mediastinum, 1165–1167
Myofibroblastic tumors, 155
inflammatory
intestinal, 1397
of mediastinum, 1167–1168
of peritoneum, 2425–2426
Myofibroblastoma, 157
of breast, 373
palisaded, 729–730
Myofibromatosis, infantile, 154, 308
Myofibrosarcoma, 158
Myogenin, as marker for soft tissue tumors, 142
Myoglandular polyps, inflammatory, 1423
Myoglobin, as marker for soft tissue tumors, 141
Myomectomy specimens, 2204–2205
Myometrium, 2271–2272
Myopathy(ies)
centronuclear, 112, 123
congenital, 122
critical care, 127
desmin storage, 123–124

distal, 122
inflammatory and immune-mediated, 114–115, 124–125
mitochondrial, 118–119, 126
myotubular, 123
nemaline, 118, 123
Myopathy, encephalopathy, lactic acidosis, stroke (MELAS) syndrome, 126
Myopericytomas, 181
Myophosphorylase deficiency, 125
Myositis
HIV, 125
idiopathic granulomatous, 115
inclusion body, 114, 124–125
proliferative, 147
viral, 125
Myositis ossificans, 152, 305
Myositis ossificans circumscripta, 258
Myospherulosis, sinonasal, 890
Myotonic muscular dystrophy, 122
Myotubular myopathy, 123
Myxedema, 37
Myxofibrosarcoma, 152, 158, 163
Myxoid angioblastomatosis, 295
Myxoid chondrosarcoma, 152
Myxoid leiomyoma, 2273, 2284–2285
Myxoid leiomyosarcoma, 2280
Myxoid liposarcoma, 152, 167–169
cellular, 167, 169
Myxoid malignant fibrous histiocytoma, 152, 163
Myxoma
cardiac, 1238–1240, 1277
nerve sheath, 68
ovarian, 2372
sinonasal, 916
soft tissue, 151–152
Myxoma peritonei, pseudo-, 2426–2427
Myxomatous valve, 1229

N

Nabothian cysts, 2177
Nasal cavity and nasopharynx, 885–917
anatomy of, 885–886
aneurysmal bone cyst of, 914–915
angiofibroma of, 908–909
carcinoma of
adeno-, 898–900
sinonasal undifferentiated, 903
small-cell undifferentiated (oat cell), 902
squamous cell, 895–898
chordoma of, 917
cysts of, 890
displaced neural lesions of, 904–906
fibrous and fibrohistiocytic lesions of, 911–912
fungal infections of, 886–887
giant-cell granuloma of, 914–915
granulomatous reactions of, 889–890
hemangiopericytoma of, 910

Nasal cavity and nasopharynx *(contd.)*
   inflammatory lesions of, 886–890
   leprosy of, 887
   lobular capillary hemangioma of, 909–910
   lymphoid hyperplasia (pseudolymphoma) of, 906
   lymphoma of, 906
      angiocentric (T-natural killer cell), 907–908
   malignant melanoma of, 903–904
   mesenchymal chondrosarcoma of, 916–917
   midfacial necrotizing lesion of, 887–889
   mucocele of, 890
   myospherulosis of, 890
   myxoma of, 916
   necrotizing sialometaplasia of, 890
   neuroblastoma of, 900–902
   osseous tumors of, 914–917
   paraganglioma of, 904
   plasmacytoma of, 907
   polyps of, 890–892
   rhabdomyomas of, 912
   rhabdomyosarcoma of, 912–914
   rhinoscleroma of, 887
   sarcoidosis of, 889
   squamous and schneiderian papillomas of, 892–895
   teratocarcinosarcoma of, 914
   tuberculosis of, 887
   vascular lesions of, 908–911
Nasal polyps, 890–892
Nasal septum, 885
NASH (nonalcoholic steatohepatitis), 1515, 1543
Nasoalveolar cyst, 841
Nasolabial cyst, 841
Nasopalatine cyst, 841
Natural killer (NK) cell leukemia, 796–797
Natural killer (NK) cell lymphoma, 751–753, 760–761
   sinonasal, 907–908
NCA (nonspecific cross-reacting antigen), in mesothelioma, 1130
N-cadherin, in mesothelioma, 1135
N-CAM (neural cell adhesion molecule), in pulmonary neoplasms, 1106
Necrobiosis, 32
Necrobiosis lipoidica, 32–33
Necrolysis, toxic epidermal, 15
Necrosis
   acute tubular, 1752–1754
   aseptic, of femoral head, 308
   avascular, 229–230
   of endometrium, 2210
   of gastrointestinal tract, 1383
   in hepatitis, 1531, 1532, 1533
   hepatocellular, 1510, 1511
   subchondral, 229–230
   of umbilical artery, meconium-induced, 2104–2105
   in uterine smooth-muscle neoplasms, 2278–2279
Necrotizing enterocolitis, 1383
Necrotizing fasciitis, of vulva, 2115
Necrotizing funisitis, 2102–2103
Necrotizing sarcoidal granulomatosis, 1040, 1043–1044
Necrotizing vasculitis, 28
Neisseria gonorrhoeae, 2114–2115, 2135
Nelson's syndrome, 1948
   pituitary adenoma in, 498, 512–513
Nemaline myopathy, 118, 123
Nemaline rods, 118
Nematodes, of eyelids, 990
Neonate
   hemochromatosis of, 1522
   necrotizing enterocolitis of, 1383
   subcutaneous fat necrosis of, 40
Nephritic syndrome
   defined, 1701, 1777
   glomerular diseases with, 1705–1716
Nephritis
   acute infectious tubulointerstitial, 1754–1755
   acute interstitial, 1755–1757
   chronic interstitial, 1757–1759
   diffuse suppurative, 1754–1755
   hereditary (familial), 1734–1736, 1776
   lupus, 1745–1749, 1777
Nephroblastoma, 1829–1839
   in adults, 1812
   anaplastic nuclear changes in, 1832–1834
   blastemal patterns in, 1830–1831, 1839
   clear cell sarcoma *vs.,* 1846
   clinical features of, 1829
   cystic variants of, 1834–1835
   differential diagnosis of, 1838–1839
   epithelial patterns in, 1831, 1839
   gross features of, 1829–1830
   metaplastic neoplasia *vs.,* 1842
   microscopic features of, 1830–1832
   multicentric, 1829, 1830
   nephrogenic rests and nephroblastomatosis with, 1835–1838
   rhabdoid tumor of kidney *vs.,* 1849
   stromal patterns in, 1831–1832, 1839
   teratoid, 1832, 1839
   therapy effect on, 1832
   triphasic, 1830, 1838–1839
   ultrastructural and immunohistochemical studies of, 1832
Nephroblastomatosis, 1835–1838
Nephrocalcinosis, 1760
Nephrogenic adenofibroma, 1811–1812
   in children, 1850
Nephrogenic adenoma, 1861–1862
Nephrogenic rests, 1835–1838
Nephroma
   cystic, 1807
      in children, 1834–1835
   mesoblastic
      adult, 1806–1807
      in children, 1839–1842
Nephromegaly, congenital, 1690
Nephronophthisis, familial juvenile, 1694
Nephropathy
   analgesic, 1759–1760
   C1q, 1719, 1776
   diabetic, 1727–1730, 1776
   hereditary (familial), 1734–1736, 1776
   human immunodeficiency virus-associated, 1723–1724, 1776
   hyperuricemic (urate), 1761
   IgA, 1730–1733, 1776
   IgM, 1718–1719
   membranous, 1724–1727, 1776
   myeloma (Bence Jones) cast, 1751–1752
   reflux, 1688, 1689, 1757–1759
   of systemic lupus erythematosus, 1745–1749, 1777
   thin basement membrane, 1733, 1776
Nephrosclerosis
   arterial and arteriolar (benign), 1761–1763
   donor-transmitted, 1774
   malignant, 1763
Nephrosis, lipoid, 1716–1718, 1776
Nephrotic syndrome
   defined, 1701, 1777
   diffuse mesangial hypercellularity in, 1718
   focal global glomerulosclerosis in, 1723
   glomerular capillary wall lesions leading to, 1716–1730
   glomerular mesangial IgM deposition in, 1718–1719
   minimal change, 1716–1718, 1776
Nephrotoxicity, cyclosporin, 1772–1774
Nerve sheath tumors
   of CNS, 447–449
   cutaneous myxoma, 68
   of larynx, 943
   of mediastinum, 1162–1164
   peripheral, 185–188
   of salivary gland, 874
Nesidioblastosis, 1502
Nesidiodysplasia, 1502
Nested proliferation, 89
Neural cell adhesion molecule (N-CAM), in pulmonary neoplasms, 1106
Neural markers, for soft tissue tumors, 142
Neural tumors
   of bone, 298–299
   of CNS, 429–432

of skin, 67–68
of vulva, 2119
Neurilemoma
    of bone, 298–299
    of breast, 368
    of CNS, 447–448
    of larynx, 943
    of mediastinum, 1163–1164
    of salivary gland, 874
    soft tissue, 185
Neurilemoma-like leiomyoma, of uterus, 2273, 2284
Neurinoma, 447–448
Neuroblastoma
    adrenal, 608–613
    of bone, 270
    of CNS, 414, 432
    of mediastinum, 1170–1172, 1175
    olfactory, 900–902
Neuroborreliosis, 399
Neurocysticercosis, 398
Neurocytoma, central, 411, 431–432
Neurodermatitis, 16–17
Neuroectodermal tumor
    melanotic, of testis, 2019–2020
    of ovary, 2370
    primitive
        of CNS, 414, 437
        of mediastinum, 1172–1173, 1175
        renal, 1810–1811
            in children, 1850
        soft tissue, 194–195
        of testis, 2001
Neuroendocrine carcinoma
    of anus, 1679
    of bladder, 1875–1876
    of breast, 341
    of cervix, 2176
        and adenocarcinoma, 2194
    of CNS, 450
    cutaneous, 59
    of mediastinum
        large-cell, 1182–1183
        prognosis for, 1198–1199
        small-cell, 1168–1170, 1175–1176, 1199
    of ovary, 2343
    of salivary gland, 873
Neuroendocrine cells, 483–484
    in situ hybridization and polymerase chain reaction of, 486
    ultrastructural characteristics of, 485–486
Neuroendocrine differentiation, neoplasms with, 491–492
Neuroendocrine markers, 484–485
Neuroendocrine neoplasms, 483–484, 486–491
    of breast, 357–358, 488
    of CNS, 449–450
    of intestine, 1446–1448

of larynx, 487–488, 940–941
of liver, 1586, 1588, 1592–1593, 1602–1603
multidirectional differentiation of, 491–492
of ovary and testes, 488–489
of prostate, 488, 1928–1929
renal, 1809–1811
in situ hybridization and polymerase chain reaction of, 486
of skin, 487
of thymus, 486–487
ultrastructural characteristics of, 485–486
of urinary bladder, 490
of uterine cervix, 489–490
Neuroendocrine system, 483–492
    diffuse or dispersed, evolution of concept of, 483
    ectopic hormone production by, 486
    multiple endocrine neoplasia syndromes of, 486
    regulatory peptides and amines of, 485
    sympathoadrenal, 632–633
Neuroepithelial cyst, 460
Neuroepithelial tumor, dysembryoplastic, 431
Neurofibrillary tangles, 464
Neurofibroma
    of breast, 368
    of CNS, 411, 448
    cutaneous, 68
    of larynx, 943
    mediastinal, 1164
    of salivary gland, 874
    soft tissue, 185–186
    vulvar, 2119
Neurofibromatosis (NF), 186–187
    of inner ear, 970–971
Neurogenic tumors, of intestines, 1457–1458
Neuroma
    acoustic, 447, 969–971
    appendiceal, 1395
    cutaneous, 68
    Morton's, 241
Neuromuscular diseases, 120–127
    carbohydrate storage, 125–126
    critical care myopathy, 127
    denervating, 127
    inflammatory and immune-mediated, 124–125
    lipid storage, 126
    metabolic, 125–126
    muscle biopsy in, 109–120
    muscular dystrophies, 120–124
    of neuromuscular junction, 127
Neuromuscular junction disorders, 127
Neuron-specific enolase (NSE), 484
    in small-cell carcinoma, 1105
Neuropathic joint, 223–224, 227, 308

Neurothekeoma, 68
Neutrophilic dermatosis, acute febrile, 29
Neutrophilic vascular reactions, 29–30
Neutrophilic venulitis, 28
Neutrophil infiltration, in gastroesophageal reflux disease, 1287
Nevocellular nevi, of conjunctiva, 986
Nevoid basal cell carcinoma syndrome, 55, 839
Nevus(i)
    agminate, 99
    blue
        cellular, 96
        common, 96
        of prostate, 1899
    combined, 97
    compound, 91
    connective tissue, 60–61
    dermal, 91
    dysplastic, 101–102
    epidermal, 49
    halo, 92
    of Ito, 96–97
    junctional, 91
    melanocytic
        acquired, 91–93
        congenital, 91, 99–100
        lentiginous, 98
        with pigment elimination, 100
        recurrent, 98
        regressing, 98–99
        traumatized, 100
    nevocellular, of conjunctiva, 986
    organoid, 49
    of Ota, 96–97, 986
    pigmented spindle cell, 95
    spindle and epithelial cell, 93–95
    Spitz, 93–95
    of vulva, 2117–2118
Nevus cell
    intraepidermal (type A), 91
    lymphocyte-like (type B), 91
    neural (type C), 91–92
Nevus sebaceous of Jadassohn, 49
Nevus spilus, 99
Newborn. See Neonate
Next menstrual period (NMP), 2211
NF (neurofibromatosis), 186–187
    of inner ear, 970–971
NFA-1 (normal fecal antigen), in mesothelioma, 1130
NHL. See Non-Hodgkin's lymphoma (NHL)
Niemann-Pick disease, 692
    liver in, 1520
Nil disease, 1716–1718, 1776
Nil lesion, 24–25
Nipple
    adenoma of, 370–371
        syringomatous, 371

Nipple *(contd.)*
  adenomatosis of, 63
  florid papillomatosis of, 370–371
  Paget's disease of, 360–361
Nipple discharge, 321–322
NK (natural killer) cell leukemia, 796–797
NK (natural killer) cell lymphoma, 751–753, 760–761
  sinonasal, 907–908
NMP (next menstrual period), 2211
Nodal marginal zone B-cell lymphoma, 739, 745–746
Nodular adenosis, of breast, 331
Nodular amyloidosis, 37
Nodular and diffuse fibrous proliferation, of testis, 2015–2016
Nodular blastema, 1687
Nodular fasciitis, 145–147
  of nasopharynx, 912
Nodular goiter, 544, 559
  toxic, 533, 543
Nodular melanoma, 103–104
Nodular mesangial sclerosis, 1777
Nodular regenerative hyperplasia, 1514, 1516, 1538–1540, 1565, 1569–1571
Nodular-sclerosing Hodgkin's disease, 713–714, 731, 733–734
  of mediastinum, 1186–1187
Nodular tenosynovitis, 182
Nodular vasculitis, 39
Nodule(s), 5
  adrenal cortical, 600
  endometrial stromal, 2265, 2266, 2269, 2270
  of genitourinary tract, postoperative, 148
  Kimmelstiel-Wilson, 1728
  of larynx, 927, 943
  of liver
    macroregenerative and borderline (dysplastic), 1571–1575
    solitary (fibrosing) necrotic, 1613
  placental-site, 2075–2076, 2221
  rheumatoid, 33, 229
  of small bowel, 1360–1361
  spindle cell
    postoperative
      of genitourinary tract, 1863–1864
      of soft tissue, 148
    of vagina, 2139
  subepidermal calcified, 38
  thyroid. *See* Thyroid nodules
Nonalcoholic steatohepatitis (NASH), 1515, 1543
Non-Hodgkin's lymphoma (NHL)
  blood involvement by, 680
  of bone marrow, 667–670
  vs. Hodgkin's disease, 714
  low-grade, 670
  of mediastinum
    large-cell, 1185–1186, 1190–1191, 1198
    mixed large- and small-cell, 1191
    small-cell, 1159–1161, 1174–1175
  posttherapy, 679
Nonspecific cross-reacting antigen (NCA), in mesothelioma, 1130
Nonsteroidal anti-inflammatory drugs (NSAIDs), gastritis due to, 1323
Normal fecal antigen (NFA-I), in mesothelioma, 1130
Nose. *See* Nasal cavity and nasopharynx
Notochordal tumors, 297–298
NSE (neuron-specific enolase), 484
  in small-cell carcinoma, 1105
Nuchal fibroma, 153
Nuclear changes, in muscle biopsy, 112–113
Nucleated red blood cells, fetal, 2105
Nucleolar organizer regions (NORs), 409–410
Nucleus pulposus, 239
Null-cell adenoma, 499, 501, 514–515
Nummular eczema, 7

O
Oat cell carcinoma
  of cervix, 2176
  of larynx, 941
  of mediastinum, 1168–1170, 1175
  sinonasal, 902
Ochronosis, of ear, 951
Oculopharyngeal muscular dystrophy, 122
Odontogenic carcinoma, 847–848
Odontogenic cysts, 835–840
  calcifying (Gorlin), 839
  carcinoma arising in, 842
  dentigerous, 836
  eruption, 838
  gingival, 836
  glandular, 839–840
  keratocysts, 838–839
  lateral periodontal, 836
  in nevoid basal cell carcinoma syndrome, 839
  paradental, 836
  periapical (radicular), 835–836
  residual, 836
Odontogenic tumors, 842–847
  adenomatoid, 844
  ameloblastic fibroma, 843
  ameloblastoma, 842–843
  calcifying epithelial (Pindborg), 843–844
  cementoma, 845–847
  fibroma, 845
  odontomas, 847
  squamous, 844–845
  unicystic ameloblastoma cyst, 843
Odontomas, 847
Ofuji's disease, 34
OKT-9, in pulmonary neoplasms, 1107–1108
Olfactory mucosa, 885
Olfactory neuroblastoma, 900–902
Oligoastrocytoma, 413, 426
  anaplastic, 413
Oligodendroglioma, 412, 425–426
  anaplastic (malignant), 412, 426
Oligomeganephronia, 1685
Ollier's disease, 274
Omental-mesenteric myxoid hamartoma, 2426
Oncocytic carcinoma
  hepatocellular, 1581
  of pancreas, 1497
Oncocytoma
  adrenal, 605–606
  pituitary, 501
  renal, 1799–1803
  of salivary gland, 862–863
Oncocytosis
  renal, 1800–1802
  of salivary glands, 855
Onion skinning, 1778
Oophoritis
  autoimmune, 2318–2319
  bacterial, 2307–2308
  granulomatous, 2308
Opportunistic infections, in AIDS, 402
Optic nerve, 999–1000
Oral cavity
  papilloma of, 809–810
  squamous cell carcinoma of, 810–835
    adenosquamous, 831–834
    basaloid, 834–835
    distant metastasis of, 818
    epidemiology of, 810
    etiology of, 810–811
    multiple primary, 814
    papillary, 828
    precursors to, 811–812
    prognostic indicators for, 818–819
    regional lymph node metastasis of, 817–818
    resection margins in, 819–820
    site-specific considerations for, 820–824
    in situ, 812–814
    spindle-cell, 828–831
    squamous dysplasia and, 812–814
    staging of, 816–817
    unusual variants of, 824–835
    verrucous, 824–828
Ora serrata, 1284
Orbit, 996–999
  developmental anomalies of, 996–998
  inflammation of, 998
  mucoceles of, 998
  tumors of, 998–999
Orchiectomy, 1973–1974
Orchitis, 1960–1963

nonspecific granulomatous, 1962–1963
Organic matrix, abnormal formation of, 248–249
Oropharynx, squamous cell carcinoma of, 825
Orthokeratosis, 5
Osgood-Schlatter's disease, 256
Os penis, 2038
Osseous tumors, sinonasal, 914–917
Ossification, heterotopic, 305
Ossifying fibroma
  of ear, 957
  of long bones, 302
  sinonasal, 915–916
Ossifying fibromyxoid tumor, 157
Ossifying renal tumor of infancy, 1850
Osteitis fibrosa cystica, 251
Osteoarthritis, 224–227
Osteoblast(s), 245
Osteoblastoma, 283
  aggressive, 283
  malignant, 283
  osteosarcoma resembling, 283
  pseudomalignant, 283
Osteocartilaginous lesions, 189–190
Osteochondritis dissecans, 238
Osteochondroma, 271–272
Osteochondromatous proliferation, bizarre parosteal, 309
Osteoclasts, 247
Osteocytes, 245
Osteofibrous dysplasia, 293, 303
Osteogenesis imperfecta, 248–249
  of middle ear, 969
Osteogenic tumors, 281–291
  benign, 281–283
  malignant, 283–291
Osteoid, 246
  fiber-, 301
Osteoid osteoma, 243, 281–283
Osteoma, 283
  of ear, 957–958
  extraskeletal, 189
  osteoid, 243, 281–283
  sinonasal, 916
Osteomalacia, 244, 246–247, 249–250
Osteomyelitis
  vs. bone neoplasms, 305
  carcinoma in, 305
  chronic multifocal, 260
  pyogenic, 259–260
    of vertebral column, 233–234
Osteonecrosis, 229–230
Osteons, 247–248
Osteopenia, 253
Osteopetrosis, 254–255
Osteophytes, 223
Osteoporosis, 244, 253–254
  transient migratory, 254
Osteosarcoma, 283–291
  chondroblastic, 278, 280, 284–285

conventional, 283–286
extraosseous, 190
fibroblastic, 284
low-grade, 287–288
Paget's, 286
parosteal, 288–289
periosteal, 289
postradiation, 286
resembling osteoblastoma, 283
sinonasal, 916
small cell, 288
surface, 288–291
telangiectatic, 286–287
Osteosclerotic myeloma, 267, 689
Otitis, malignant external, 949
Otitis media, 958–960
Otosclerosis, of middle ear, 967–968
Ovarian failure, 2318–2319
Ovarian thecal metaplasia, 606
Ovarian tumors, 2319–2382
  adenomatoid, 2376
  adenosarcomas, mesodermal (Müllerian), 2334
  Brenner, 2339–2341
  carcinoid, 2368–2370, 2378–2379
  carcinoma
    chorio-, 2363–2364
    clear-cell, 2335–2339
    embryonal, 2363
    endometrioid, 2330–2333
    hepatoid, 2375
    mucinous, 2328–2330
    neuroendocrine, 2343
    serous, 2323, 2326–2327
    small-cell
      hypercalcemic, 2373–2375
      pulmonary type, 2343
    squamous cell, 2341–2342
    transitional cell, 2341
    undifferentiated, 2342
  carcinosarcomas, 2334
  classification of, 2320–2321
  clear-cell, 2335–2339
  dermoid cysts, 2365–2366
  dysgerminoma, 2359–2360
  endodermal sinus, 2360–2363
  endometrioid, 2330–2333
  fibroma, 2347–2348
  fibrosarcoma, 2348
  germ cell, 2358–2370
  gonadoblastoma, 2370–2372
  granulosa cell, 2343–2347, 2353
  gynandroblastoma, 2354
  intraabdominal desmoplastic small round-cell, 2376
  Krukenberg, 2377
  leiomyomas, 2372
  leukemia, 2372–2373
  Leydig cell, 2355–2356
  lipoid cell, 2355–2358
  luteoma

  pregnancy, 2315–2316, 2358
  stromal, 2355
  lymphoma, 2372–2373
  melanoma, 2347, 2381
  mesenchymal, 2372
  mesodermal
    adenosarcoma, 2334
    malignant mixed, 2334
  mesothelioma, malignant, 2376
  metastatic, 2376–2382
  mixed
    epithelial, 2342
    germ cell-sex cord-stromal, 2370–2372
  mucinous, 2328–2330
  Müllerian, 2334
  myxomas, 2372
  neuroectodermal, 2370
  neuroendocrine, 488–489
  polyembryoma, 2363
  of rete ovarii, 2358
  sarcomas
    endometrioid stromal, 2334–2335
    pure, 2372
  sebaceous, 2370
  serous, 2322–2327
  Sertoli cell, 2351
  Sertoli-Leydig cell, 2351–2354
  sex-cord-stromal, 2343–2355
    with annular tubules, 2354–2355
    unclassified, 2354
  signet ring-stromal, 2350–2351
  squamous cell, 2341–2342
  steroid cell, 2355–2358
  stromal
    with minor sex-cord elements, 2349
    sclerosing, 2349–2350
  struma ovarii, 2366–2368
  surface epithelial-stromal, 2319–2322
  teratomas, 2364–2370
    immature, 2364–2365
    mature, 2365–2366
    monodermal, 2366–2370
  thecoma, 2348–2349
  transitional cell, 2339–2341
  of wolffian origin, 2375–2376
  yolk sac, 2338, 2360–2363
Ovarian-type epithelial tumors, of testis, 2016–2017
Ovary(ies), 2307–2382
  bacterial infections of, 2307–2308
  calcification of, 2319
  congenital lesions of, 2319
  decidual reaction of, 2317
  endometriosis of, 2428
  endometriotic cysts of, 2427–2428, 2429, 2430
  epithelial inclusion glands of, 2308–2309
  fibromatosis of, 2314–2315
  follicle cysts of, 2309–2311

Ovary(ies) *(contd.)*
　granulomas of, 2308
　granulosa cell proliferations of, 2311
　hilus cell hyperplasia of, 2316–2317
　hyperreactio luteinalis of, 2311
　inflammatory disorders of, 2307–2308
　massive edema of, 2314
　polycystic disease of, 2312
　resistant, 2318
　Stein-Leventhal syndrome of, 2312
　stromal hyperplasia and hyperthecosis of, 2313
　stromal-Leydig cell hyperplasia of, 2317
　stromal metaplasias of, 2317–2318
　surface proliferative lesions of, 2308–2309
　tumors of. *See* Ovarian tumors
Ovotestis, 1968
Ovulation, 2211–2214
Oxalosis
　bone marrow in, 692
　renal, 1760–1761

P

Pachymeningitis, hypertrophic intracranial, 397
Pacinian corpuscle, hyperplastic, 1394
Pagetoid proliferation, 89
Pagetoid reticulosis, 78
Paget's disease
　of anus, 1680
　of bone, 244, 252–253, 306
　differential diagnosis of, 55
　of nipple, 360–361
　of vulva, 2130–2132
Paget's sarcoma, 286
Palate
　papillomatosis of, 808–809
　squamous cell carcinoma of, 825
Palisaded myofibroblastoma, 157, 729–730
Panbronchiolitis, diffuse, 1027
Pancreas, 1469–1503
　acinar metaplasia of, 1314
　in aging, 1470–1473
　anatomy of, 1469
　annular, 1469
　anomalies of, 1469–1470
　atypical papillary hyperplasia of, 1482
　biopsy of, 1473–1474
　carcinoma of. *See* Pancreatic carcinoma
　cystic neoplasms of, 1488–1493
　cysts of, 1487–1488
　　lymphoepithelial, 1492
　diagnostic techniques for, 1473–1474
　ectopic, 1312–1313
　endocrine neoplasms of, 1497–1501
　fat necrosis of, 40–41
　Gruber-Frantz tumor of, 1495
　heterotopia of, 1360

　heterotopic, 1470
　in hypergastrinemia, 1502
　in hyperinsulinemic hypoglycemia, 1501–1502
　in hypokalemia, 1502
　inflammatory conditions of, 1474–1477, 1478
　inflammatory pseudotumor of, 1503
　intraductal papillary-mucinous neoplasms of, 1482–1483, 1493
　islet-cell tumors of, 1497–1501
　lymphangiomas of, 1492
　lymphomas of, 1503
　metastases to, 1503
　minor abnormalities of, 1470–1473
　mixed exocrine-endocrine neoplasms of, 1495
　neoplasms of indeterminate type of, 1493–1497
　normal cells of, 1473–1474
　pseudocysts of, 1488, 1493
　serous neoplasms of, 1490–1491, 1493
　solid-cystic-papillary epithelial neoplasm of, 1495–1496
　transplantation of, 1474
　watery diarrhea-achlorhydria syndrome of, 1502
Pancreas divisum, 1470
Pancreatic carcinoma, 1477–1487
　acinar cell, 1484–1486
　anaplastic (pleomorphic, sarcomatoid, undifferentiated), 1486–1487
　clear cell, 1497
　ductal, 1477–1484
　　clinical features of, 1477
　　cytologic features of, 1479–1480
　　differential diagnosis of, 1483–1484
　　pathologic features of, 1477–1479
　　premalignant conditions and, 1482–1483
　　uncommon types of, 1480–1482
　microglandular, 1496–1497
　oncocytic, 1497
　ovarian metastases of, 2380–2381
　small cell, 1487
Pancreatic ducts, 1469
　atrophy of, 1484
　carcinoma of. *See* Pancreatic carcinoma, ductal
　dilatation of, 1471, 1484
　hyperplasia and metaplasia of, 1471–1472
Pancreatic islet cells, 484
Pancreatitis
　acute, 1474–1475
　chronic, 1475–1477
　　vs. ductal adenocarcinoma, 1477, 1478, 1483–1484
Pancreatoblastoma, 1493–1494
Pancytopenia, 653
Panencephalitis, subacute sclerosing, 401

Panniculitis, 39
　alpha *1*-antitrypsin deficiency, 39
　factitial, 41
　lobular, 39
　lupus, 41
　physical, 41
　septal, 39
Pannus
　of cornea, 978
　of joint, 228
Panophthalmitis, 976
Papanicolaou smear, 2157
Papillary adenocarcinoma
　of cervix
　　serous, 2191–2192
　　villoglandular, 2188–2190
　of middle ear, 967
　of pancreas, 1482
Papillary adenofibroma, of cervix, 2194
Papillary adenoma
　renal, 1796
　of thyroid, 542
Papillary carcinoma
　of breast
　　infiltrating, 357
　　intracystic, 346–347
　　intraduct, 344, 346–347
　of penis, 2055
　of thyroid, 534, 535–542
　　columnar cell variant of, 541
　　diffuse sclerosis variant of, 541–542, 556
　　encapsulated variant of, 542
　　etiology of, 535–536
　　fine needle aspirate specimens of, 561
　　flow cytometry of, 539
　　follicular variant of, 540
　　immunohistochemistry of, 539
　　occult, 540
　　and parathyroid adenomas, 536
　　pathology of, 536–539
　　pink cell variant of, 541
　　prognostic factors in, 539–540
　　solid variant of, 542
　　subtypes of, 540–542
　　tall cell variant of, 540–541
　　ultrastructure of, 539
Papillary craniopharyngioma, 519
Papillary cystadenoma
　of broad ligament, 2409
　of ovary, 2322–2325, 2327
　of testis, 2019
Papillary cystadenoma lymphomatosum, 861–862
Papillary dermis, 4
Papillary duct hyperplasia, 377
Papillary eccrine adenoma, 63
Papillary endocervicitis, 2180
Papillary endothelial hyperplasia, 151
Papillary fibroelastomas, cardiac, 1240

Papillary hidradenoma, 63
  of vulva, 2132
Papillary hyperplasia
  of extrahepatic bile ducts, 1664
  of gallbladder, 1643–1645
  of oral cavity, 808–809
  of pancreas, 1482
  of penis, 2043
  of peritoneum, 2417–2418
  of thyroid, 542
  of tonsils, 810
Papillary immature metaplasia,
    of cervix, 2161–2163
Papillary meningioma, 444
Papillary mesothelioma, of peritoneum,
    2421–2422
Papillary-mucinous neoplasms,
    intraductal, 1482–1483, 1493
Papillary neoplasms
  of bladder, 1868–1871
  of breast, 344–347
  of cervix, 2174
Papillary renal cell carcinoma,
    1792–1796, 1805
  in children, 1839
Papillary serous carcinoma, uterine,
    2252–2254
Papillary squamous cell carcinoma,
    of oral cavity, 828
Papillary syncytial metaplasia, of
    endometrium, 2251, 2254
Papillary syringoma, 63
Papilloma(s)
  of breast, 329, 344–346
    atypical hyperplasia within, 346
    multiple, 345–346
    solitary benign intraduct,
      344–345
  choroid plexus, 412, 433
  of conjunctiva, 985
  of esophagus, 1296
  lacrimal sac, 1002
  of larynx, 927–929
  of lungs, 1072
  Müllerian, 2182
  oral, 809–810, 825
  of ovary, 2322
  sinonasal, 892–895
  squamous
    of conjunctiva, 985
    of esophagus, 1296
    of oral cavity, 825
  of urothelial tract, 1862
  of vagina, 2138
Papillomatosis, 5, 17
  of breast, 329, 334
    juvenile, 377
  of glans corona, 2042
  of nipple, 370–371
  palatal, 808–809
  vaginal, 2163

Papulosis
  bowenoid, 54, 55
    of penis, 2045–2046
    of vulva, 2124
  lymphomatoid, 12–14, 75–76
Paracrine regulation, 483, 485
Paradental cysts, 836
Paraffinomas, 2042
Paraffin sections, of muscle biopsy,
    110, 112–115
Paraganglia, of head and neck region,
    625–628
Paraganglioma(s), 625–644
  aorticopulmonary, 629, 1184
  carotid body, 628
  of cauda equina region, 643–644
  of CNS, 412, 449
  cytology and fine-needle aspiration
    of, 637–639
  differential diagnosis of, 161
  DNA content of, 642
  electron microscopic features of, 639
  extraadrenal, 634–636
  gangliocytic, 643
    of gastrointestinal tract, 1458–1459
  of head and neck region, 628–632
  immunohistochemistry of, 639–642
  intraadrenal, 614–618
  jugulotympanic, 628, 965–967
  laryngeal, 629, 940
  malignant, 642–643
  mediastinal, 1184–1185, 1190, 1199
  multicentric and familial
    occurrence of, 636–637
  and other endocrine disorders, 637
  paravertebral, 1184
  pulmonary, 1101
  sinonasal, 904
  sympathoadrenal, 634–636
    familial, 637
  of urinary tract, 1882
  vagal, 628–629
Paraganglioma-like adenoma,
    of thyroid, 545
Paraganglion, 484
Parakeratosis, 5
Paranasal sinuses
  anatomy of, 885
  carcinoma of, 903
    adeno-, 898–900
    small-cell (oat cell), 902
    squamous cell, 895–896
  displaced neural lesions in, 904–906
  fibrous and fibrohistiocytic lesions of,
    911–912
  fungal infections of, 886–887
  lymphoplasmacytic proliferations in,
    906–908
  malignant melanoma of, 903–904
  mucocele of, 890
  necrotizing sialometaplasia of, 890

  polyps of, 890–892
  rhabdomyosarcoma of, 912–914
  squamous and schneiderian papillomas
    of, 892–895
  teratocarcinosarcoma of, 914
  tuberculosis of, 887
Paraneurons, 483
Parapsoriasis-poikiloderma complex, 77
Parasitic infections
  of brain, 398
  of fallopian tube, 2397
  of intestines, 1358–1359, 1385
  myocarditis due to, 1216–1217
Paratesticular tumors, 1974, 2020–2021
Parathyroid, 563–571
  adenomas of, 565–567
    atypical, 568
    with stromal component, 568–569
    and thyroid carcinoma, 536
  anatomy and histology of, 563–565
  carcinoma of, 567–568
    of mediastinum, 1180–1181,
      1190, 1199
  clonality of, 570–571
  cysts of, 568, 1149–1151
  cytology of, 570
  diseases of, 565
  embryology of, 563
  in familial hypocalciuric
    hypercalcemia, 570
  flow cytometry of, 570
  genetic studies of, 571
  hamartoma of, 568–569
  humoral hypercalcemia of malignancy
    of, 570
  in hyperparathyroidism
    ectopic, 570
    primary, 565–568
    secondary, 570
  hyperplasia of, 567
  intraoperative assessment of, 569–570
  lipoadenoma of, 568–569
  in multiple endocrine neoplasia
    syndromes, 568
  neuroendocrine cells and
    neoplasms of, 484
  proliferative markers of, 570
Parathyromatosis, 569
Paraurethral cyst, 2113
Paravertebral paragangliomas, 1184
Parosteal osteochondromatous
    proliferation, bizarre, 309
Parosteal osteosarcoma, 288–289
Parotid gland. See Salivary glands
Parvovirus B19 infection, in AIDS, 658
Patch, 5
PCNA (proliferating cell nuclear antigen)
  in CNS neoplasms, 409
  in pulmonary neoplasms, 1108, 1109
PCR (polymerase chain reaction), of
    lymph nodes, 710

Pediatrics. See Children
Peliosis hepatis, 1514, 1529, 1538, 1606
Pelvic inflammatory disease (PID),
    ovarian infection in, 2307
Pemphigoid
    bullous, 23
    cicatricial, 23
        ocular, 984
Pemphigus
    benign familial, 21
    paraneoplastic, 20
Pemphigus erythematosus, 18–20
Pemphigus foliaceus, 18–20
Pemphigus vegitans, 20
Pemphigus vulgaris, 20
Penile intraepithelial neoplasia,
    2043–2045
Penile shaft, 2037
Penis, 2035–2061
    agenesis of, 2038
    anatomy of, 2035–2038
    anomalies of, 2038
    balanitis circumscripta plasmacellularis
        of, 2041–2042
    balanitis xerotica obliterans of, 2041
    bowenoid papulosis of, 2045–2046
    carcinoma of, 2046–2057
        adenosquamous, 2056
        basal cell, 2057–2058
        basaloid, 2051
        classification of, 2046–2056
        condylomatous, 2051
        epidemiology of, 2046
        growth patterns of, 2046–2048
        histologic subtypes of, 2048–2056
        and human papillomavirus, 2057
        infiltrating, 2049–2051
        in situ, 2043–2045
        multicentric, 2047–2048
        papillary, 2055
        prognosis for, 2056–2057
        sarcomatoid, 2055–2056
        superficial spreading, 2046
        usual type of, 2049–2051
        verruciform, 2047, 2051
        verrucous, 2053–2054
        vertical growth, 2046–2047
        warty, 2051
    cellulitis of, 2039
    concealed, 2038
    condylomas of, 2040–2041
        giant, 2059–2061
    cysts of, 2038
    dermatologic conditions of, 2042
    duplication of, 2038
    Fournier's gangrene of, 2039
    gangrenous balanitis of, 2041
    hypoplasia and hyperplasia of, 2038
    infectious diseases of, 2038–2041
    inflammation of, 2038–2041
    lateral curvature of, 2038
    lentiginous melanosis of, 2042
    melanomas of, 2057
    metastases to, 2059
    Mondor's phlebitis of, 2042
    papillomatosis of glans corona of, 2042
    paraffinomas of, 2042
    Peyronie's disease of, 2042
    phimosis of, 2041
    precancerous lesions of, 2043–2045
    rare neoplasms of, 2057–2059
    sexually transmitted infections of,
        2039–2041
    soft tissue tumors of, 2058
    squamous hyperplasia of, 2042–2043
    Tancho's nodules of, 2042
    torsion of, 2038
    tuberculosis of, 2039
    verruciform xanthoma of, 2042
    webbed, 2038
    Wegener's granulomatosis of, 2042
Peptic ulcer disease, 1325, 1354–1355
Percutaneous transluminal coronary
    angioplasty (PTCA), 1272–1273
Perianal skin, 1680
Periapical cemental dysplasia, 845–846
Periapical cysts, 835–836
Peribiliary gland cysts, 1557, 1560–1561
Peribursitis, proliferative, 148
Pericardial cysts, 1152
Pericardial neoplasms and masses,
    1242–1244
Pericarditis, 1241–1242
Pericardium, normal, 1241
Pericholangitis, 1527
Periductal stromal tumor, of breast,
    366–367
Perilobar nephrogenic rests, 1835, 1836
Perilobular hemangiomas, 368
Perineurial cell tumor, 186
Periodontal cysts, lateral, 836
Periodontitis, 807
Periorchitis
    chronic proliferative, 2015–2016
    meconium, 2015
Periosteal chondroma, 273–274
Periosteal chondrosarcoma, 279
Periosteal desmoids, 304
Periosteal osteosarcoma, 289
Periostitis, reactive, 259
Peripheral nerve sheath tumors, 185–188
    of salivary gland, 874
Peripheral neuroectodermal tumor, 270
Peripheral T-cell lymphoma, 78, 678–679,
    754–756
Peritoneal gliomatosis, 2365
Peritoneal implants, of serous borderline
    tumors of ovary, 2325–2326
Peritoneal leiomyomatosis, disseminated,
    2273, 2285
Peritoneum, 2415–2437
    adenomatoid tumor of, 2421
    calcifying fibrous pseudotumor of,
        2421
    carcinoma of, serous, 2434
    clear cell lesions of, 2435
    decidua of, 2435–2436, 2437
    endometrioid lesions of, 2432
    endometriosis of, 2427–2432
    endosalpingiosis of, 2432–2433
    fibrosis of, 2416
    histiocytic lesions of, 2416
    inclusion cysts of, 2418–2420
    infarcted appendix epiploica of, 2421
    inflammatory lesions of, 2415–2417
    inflammatory myofibroblastic tumor of,
        2425–2426
    intraabdominal desmoplastic small
        round-cell tumor of, 2424–2425
    keratin granulomas of, 2421
    leiomyomatosis of, 2437
    localized fibrous tumor of, 2421
    lymph node lesions of, 2436–2437
    melanosis of, 2420
    mesothelial hyperplasia of, 2417–2418
    mesothelial neoplasms of, 2421–2424
    mesothelioma of
        diffuse malignant, 2418, 2422–2424
        fibrous, 2421
        low-grade cystic, 2422
        well-differentiated papillary,
            2421–2422
    metastatic tumors of, 2426–2427
    mucinous lesions of, 2435
    omental-mesenteric myxoid hamartoma
        of, 2426
    primary tumors of, 2424–2426
    pseudomyxoma of, 2426–2427
    secondary Müllerian system lesions of,
        2427–2437
    serous tumors of, 2434
    splenosis of, 2420
    squamous cell lesions of, 2435
    transitional cell lesions of, 2435
    trophoblastic implants in, 2420
    tumor-like lesions of, 2417–2421
    vascular tumors of, malignant, 2425
Peritonitis, 2415–2417
    acute, 2415
    eosinophilic, 2417
    granulomatous, 2415–2416
    meconium, 2416
    rare types of, 2417
    sclerosing, 1398, 2416
    tuberculous, 2415
Peritonitis fibroplastica encapsulatum, 1398
Perivascular inflammation, of CNS, 397
Perivascular inflammatory cell infiltrates,
    26–27
Perivillositis, 2097
Perlman syndrome, 1690
Persistent müllerian duct syndrome,
    1964–1965

Peutz-Jeghers syndrome
  gastric polyps in, 1326
  intestinal polyps in, 1416–1419
Peyronie's disease, 2042
PFK (phosphofructokinase) deficiency, 125–126
Phenytoin, lymphadenopathy due to, 727
Pheochromocytoma, adrenal, 614–618
  composite, 616–617, 635–636
  familial, 617–618, 637
  malignant, 617
  pseudo-, 614
Phimosis, 2041
Phlebectasia, 1387
Phlebitis
  of gallbladder, 1643
  Mondor's, 2042
Phosphofructokinase (PFK) deficiency, 125–126
Phospholipase A2, in chorioamnionitis, 2101
Phthisis bulbi, 976
Phycomycosis, sinonasal, 886
Phyllodes tumor
  of breast, 366–367
  of prostate, 1932
  of seminal vesicles, 1936
Phyrigian cap, 1630
Pick's adenoma, 1946, 1947
Pick's disease, 464
PID (pelvic inflammatory disease), ovarian infection in, 2307
Pigment(s), in thyroid, 535
Pigmented purpuras, 28
Pigmented purpuric lichenoid dermatitis of Gougerot and Blum, 28
Pigmented spindle cell nevus, 95
Pigmented villonodular synovitis, 182, 236–237
Pigment incontinence, 9
Pigment stones, 1634
Pilar sheath acanthoma, 64
Pilar tumor, of vulva, 2117
Pilomatricoma, 61, 62
Pilonidal cyst, vulvar, 2113
PIN (prostatic intraepithelial neoplasia), 1914–1917
Pindborg tumor, 843–844
Pineal cell tumors, 433–434
Pineal cyst, 460
Pineoblastoma, 414, 434
Pineocytoma, 411, 434
Pinguecula, 988
Pinworm, of appendix, 1395
Pituitary, 495–525
  adenomas of. *See* Pituitary adenoma(s)
  anterior lobe of, 495
  carcinoma of, 515–516
  giant-cell granuloma of, 522
  granular cell tumor of, 519–520
  hyperplasia of, 516

inflammatory disorders of, 522–525
Langerhans histiocytosis of, 524
lymphocytic hypophysitis of, 522
metastases to, 518, 521–522
nonadenomatous lesions of, 516–522
normal, 495–497
oncocytoma of, 501
posterior lobe of, 497
Rathke's cleft cyst of, 519
sarcoidosis of, 522
Pituitary adenoma(s), 495, 497–515
  acidophil stem cell, 498, 500, 511–512
  ACTH, 512
  classification of, 502–503
  clinical characteristics of, 498–499
  vs. CNS lesions, 412, 449–450
  corticotroph cell, 498, 501, 512–514
    silent, 498, 512, 513–514
  in Cushing's disease, 498, 512
  differential diagnosis of, 518
  diffuse, 503
  due to extrapituitary disease
    with adrenocorticotropic hormone excess, 514
    with growth hormone excess, 512
  glycoprotein, 514
  gonadotroph cell, 499, 514
  growth hormone cell, 500, 509–510
  growth hormone-producing, 509–512
  invasive, 515
  lactotrophic, 498
  mammosomatotroph cell, 498, 500, 511
  massive, 503
  mixed growth hormone cell-prolactin cell, 498, 500, 511
  multiple, 497
  in Nelson's syndrome, 498, 512–513
  with neuronal metaplasia, 521
  null-cell, 499, 501, 514–515
  pathology of, 498–499, 503–504
  plurihormonal, 499, 501, 511
  prolactin cell, 500, 506–509
  silent, subtype III, 499, 501, 515
  sinonasal, 904–905
  somatotrophic, 498
  specimen handling for, 504–506
  thyrotroph cell, 499, 501, 514
  ultrastructural features of, 500–501
  undifferentiated-cell, 514–515
Pituitary apoplexy, 504
Pituitary stone, 506
Pityriasis lichenoides chronica, 12–14
Pityriasis lichenoides et varioliformis acuta, 12–14
Pityriasis rosea, 7
Pityriasis rubra pilaris, 9
Placenta, 2087–2107
  calcification of, 2098
  chorangiosis of, 2105–2106
  chorioamnionitis of, 2095, 2096, 2097, 2100–2103

circummarginate, 2092
circumvallate, 2092
cysts of, 2092–2093
edema of, 2090
extrachorial, 2091–2092
fetal nucleated red blood cells in, 2105
gross abnormalities of, 2089–2095
hemorrhagic endovasculopathy of, 2098
indications for examination of, 2087, 2088
infarcts and intervillous thrombi of, 2093–2094, 2097–2098
infectious diseases of, 2100–2104
insertion of extraplacental membranes into, 2091–2092
intervillositis and perivillositis, 2097
intervillous hemorrhage of, 2098
intravillous hemosiderin in, 2098
ischemic changes of, 2093–2094, 2097–2098
meconium staining of, 2091, 2104–2105
microscopic pathology of, 2095–2098
in multiple pregnancy, 2098–2100
necrotizing funisitis of, 2102–2103
normal development of, 2089
sample accession, storage, processing, and artifacts for, 2087–2089
shape of, 2090–2091
surface color of, 2091
surface lesions of, 2092
in surgical pathology, 2100
in twin transfusion syndrome, 2099–2100
umbilical cord abnormalities of, 2094–2095
vascular abnormalities of, 2106–2107
villitis of, 2097, 2103–2104
villous dysmaturity of, 2105
weight and size of, 2089–2090
Placenta accreta, 2091
Placental implantation site, 2166–2168
Placental separation, premature, 2088
Placental site
  exaggerated, 2074–2075
  subinvolution of, 2221
Placental-site nodules, 2075–2076, 2221
Placental-site trophoblastic tumor, 2074, 2080–2082, 2221
  of testis, 1997
Placenta previa, 2095
Plaques, 5
  pleural, 1118–1119
Plasma cell granuloma, 155
  of bladder, 1856
  of larynx, 944
  of peritoneum, 2425–2426
  pulmonary, 1038–1040
Plasma cell leukemia, 689
Plasma cell myeloma, 686–689

Plasmacytoma
  of bone, 267, 689
  of larynx, 944
  of lymph nodes, 751
  of mediastinum, extraosseous, 1188–1189, 1190
  pulmonary, 1101
  renal, 1818
  of sellar region, 518
  sinonasal, 907
  of spleen, 784
  of testis, 2012
Pleomorphic adenoma, of breast, 372
Pleura, 1117–1142
  benign tumors of, 1119–1120
  fibrosis (plaque) of, 1118–1119
  malignant mesothelioma of. See Mesothelioma
  mesothelial hyperplasia of, 1118
  regeneration of mesothelium of, 1117–1118
Pleuritis, eosinophilic, 1030
Plexiform fibrohistiocytic tumor, 159–160
Plurihormonal adenomas, 499, 501, 511
PNET. See Primitive neuroectodermal tumor (PNET)
Pneumatosis cystoides intestinalis, 1392
Pneumoconiosis, 1015
Pneumocystis carinii, in AIDS, 1057
Pneumonia
  bronchiolitis obliterans organizing, 1025
  eosinophilic, chronic, 1023–1024
  interstitial
    acute, 1020
    desquamative, 1015–1018
    giant-cell, 1017
    lymphocytic, 1031–1032
    nonspecific, 1018
    unusual, 1012–1015
  Pneumocystis carinii, 1057
  unusual interstitial, 1012–1015
Pneumonitis, hypersensitivity, 1021–1023
PODs (postovulatory days), 2211, 2213
POEMS syndrome, 689
Polyangiitis, microscopic, 1260
Polyarteritis nodosa
  of gallbladder, 1642
  inflammatory myopathy in, 115
  vasculitis in, 1260, 1267
Polychondritis, relapsing, 950
Polycystic hepatorenal disease, 1519
Polycystic kidney disease, 1557, 1560, 1692–1695
Polycystic liver disease, 1557, 1560
Polycystic ovarian disease, 2312
Polycythemia vera, 664
Polyembryoma
  of ovary, 2363
  of testis, 2002
Polyethylene, in joint prostheses, 235

Polymerase chain reaction (PCR), of lymph nodes, 710
Polymorphous light eruption, 26
Polymyositis, 114, 124
Polyorchism, 1947
Polyp(s)
  anal, 1673–1674
  appendiceal, 1442
  of breast, 345
  cervical, 2177, 2194
    fibroepithelial, 2196
  defined, 1413
  endocervical, 2177
  endometrial, 2230, 2244–2245, 2264
  esophageal, 1296–1297
  fibroepithelial, 807
    of cervix, 2196
    of vulva, 2117
  fibrous, atypical, 151
  of gallbladder, 1645, 1646, 1648–1649
  gastric, 1326–1329
  granulation tissue, of breast, 345
  intestinal, 1413–1436
    hamartomatous, 1419
    inverted, 1432–1434
    hyperplastic, 1413–1415
    inflammatory, 1420–1423
      fibroid, 1423–1424
      secondary to mucosal prolapse, 1423
    juvenile, 1418, 1420
    lymphoid, 1424
    mixed hyperplastic/adenomatous, 1415–1416
    neoplastic, 1424–1436
    nonneoplastic, 1413–1415
    Peutz-Jeghers, 1416–1419
  nasal, 890–892
  of small bowel, 1360–1361
  urethral, 1879–1880, 1934
  vaginal, 2137–2138
  vocal cord, 927, 943
  of vulva, 2117
Polypoid adenomyoma, of endometrium, 2245, 2258–2259, 2264
Polypoid cystitis, 1855
Polypoid mucosal prolapse, of stomach, 1327
Polypoid xanthogranulomatous pseudotumor, of vagina, 2136
Polyposis, multiple lymphomatous, of gastrointestinal tract, 1453–1454
Polyposis coli, familial, 1418, 1434
Polyposis syndromes, intestinal, 1418, 1434–1436
Poroma, eccrine, 61
Porphyria cutanea tarda, 24
  liver in, 1520
Portal vein obstruction, 1514, 1538
Posterior polymorphous dystrophy, 980
Postmastectomy lymphangiosarcoma, 369

Postmenopausal squamous atypia, 2164
Postovulatory days (PODs), 2211, 2213
Postradiation sarcoma, 286
Posttransplant lymphoproliferative disorder, 723–724, 1769, 1774–1775
Potter sequence, 1692
Pouchitis, 1377–1379
PRAD 1 oncogene, 570
Preauricular sinus, 949
Pregnancy
  ectopic, 2398–2399
  endometriosis in, 2431
  endometrium during, 2219–2221
  fatty liver of, 1515, 1543–1544
  large luteinized follicle cyst of, 2310
  macromastia in, 377
  molar, 2069–2074
  multiple, placenta in, 2098–2100
  myometrium during, 2271–2272
Pregnancy luteoma, 2315–2316, 2358
Premature ovarian failure, 2318–2319
Primitive neuroectodermal tumor (PNET)
  of CNS, 414, 437
  of kidney, 1810–1811
    in children, 1850
  of mediastinum, 1172–1173, 1175
  of soft tissue, 194–195
  of testis, 2001
Prion(s), 404
Prion diseases, hereditary, 405–406
Proconvertases, 485
Proctitis
  allergic, 1368
  ulcerative (follicular), 1376–1377
Proctosigmoiditis, mucosal, 1376–1377
Progestogen effect, 2219
Progressive multifocal leukoencephalopathy, 392, 403–404
Progressive pigmentary dermatosis of Schamberg, 28
Progressive systemic sclerosis, intestinal involvement in, 1387
Prolactin cell adenoma, 500, 506–509
Prolactinoma, 500, 506–509
Proliferating cell nuclear antigen (PCNA)
  in CNS neoplasms, 409
  in pulmonary neoplasms, 1108, 1109
Proliferative fasciitis, 147
Proliferative myositis, 147
Proliferative peribursitis, 148
Prolymphocytic leukemia
  B-cell, 673
  spleen in, 790
  T-cell, 677
Prostate, 1893–1936
  adenosis of, 1911–1914
  amyloid of, 1898
  anatomy and histology of, 1893
  basal cell hyperplasia of, 1933–1934

benign nonneoplastic lesions of, 1898–1899
biopsy of, 1901
calculi and calcification of, 1898
cancer of. See Prostate cancer
cribriforming lesions of, 1917
cysts of, 1898–1899
hematologic lesions of, 1934–1935
infections of, 1895–1896
inflammatory conditions of, 1896–1898
leukemia of, 1935
lymphomas of, 1934–1935
malakoplakia of, 1898
melanocytic lesions of, 1899
neuroendocrine neoplasms of, 488
posttransurethral resection granulomas of, 1897–1898
Roman bridge and cribriform formation of, 1917
urethral polyps of, 1934
Prostate cancer, 1899–1934
  acid mucin in, 1913
  adenoid cystic, 1934
  vs. adenosis, 1911–1914
  atrophic, 1905–1906
  basal cell, 1933–1934
  vs. benign cribriform lesions, 1917
  benign glands in, 1907–1909
  carcinosarcomas, 1935
  clinical presentation of, 1900–1902
  clinical stages T1a and T1b, 1923–1924
  clinical stage T1c, 1924–1925
  clinical stage T2b (palpable), 1917–1923
  clinical stage T3, 1925
  collagenous nodules (mucinous fibroplasia) in, 1910
  crystalloids in, 1913
  ductal, 1929–1930
  endocrine therapy of, 1925–1926
  extent of cancer on biopsy for, 1905
  extraprostatic extension (capsular penetration) of, 1918–1920
  glomerulations in, 1910
  grading system for, 1902–1905, 1920–1921
  vs. hepatocellular carcinoma, 1586
  immunohistochemical techniques in, 1926–1927
  incidence of, 1899–1900
  location of tumor in, 1918
  lymph node metastases of, 1920
  margins of resection in, 1921–1923
  mesenchymal, 1932–1933
  metastatic, 1460, 1920, 1925
  microscopic diagnosis of, 1905–1914
  mucinous, 1927–1928
  needle biopsy of, 1906–1911, 1913, 1924–1925
  with neuroendocrine differentiation, 1928–1929
  new techniques and biomarkers for, 1935
  overdiagnosis of, 1905–1907
  with perineural invasion, 1909–1910
  ploidy of, 1923
  progression after radical prostatectomy of, 1918
  prostatic intraepithelial neoplasia and, 1914–1917
  radiation therapy of, 1926
  radical prostatectomy specimen in, 1917–1918
  sarcomas, 1932–1933
  seminal vesicle invasion by, 1920
  vs. seminal vesicles, 1906–1907
  squamous, 1930
  staging system for, 1900
  transitional cell, 1930–1931
  transurethral resection of, 1911–1912, 1923–1924
  tumor volume in, 1923
  under diagnosis of, 1907–1909, 1910–1911
  vascular invasion by, 1923
  with xanthomatous cytoplasm, 1909
Prostatectomy, radical
  grade from, 1920–1921
  margins of resection in, 1921–1923
  ploidy and, 1923
  progression after, 1918
  specimens from, 1917–1918
  for stages T1a and T1b disease, 1924
  tumor volume in, 1923
  vascular invasion in, 1923
Prostate-specific acid phosphatase (PSAP), 1901, 1926–1927
Prostate-specific antigen (PSA), 1901, 1926–1927
Prostatic atrophy, benign, 1905–1906
Prostatic duct adenocarcinoma, 1929–1930
Prostatic hypertrophy, benign, 1893–1895
Prostatic intraepithelial neoplasia (PIN), 1914–1917
Prostatic urethral polyps, 1880
Prostatitis
  allergic granulomatous, 1898
  bacterial, 1895
  mycotic, 1895
  nonspecific granulomatous, 1896–1897
  tuberculous, 1895–1896
Prosthetic valves, 1233–1235
Prosthetic vessels, 1271, 1274
Protein allergies, malabsorption due to, 1352
Protoporphyria, erythropoietic, liver in, 1520, 1523
Protozoal infection, of liver, 1537
Prurigoform acanthosis, 16–17
Prurigo nodularis, 16–17
PSA (prostate-specific antigen), 1901, 1926–1927
Psammocarcinoma, 2434, 2435
Psammoma bodies, in thyroid carcinoma, 537–538
Psammomatous meningioma, 438, 441
PSAP (prostate-specific acid phosphatase), 1901, 1926–1927
Pseudoaneurysms, 1256
  myocardial, 1225
Pseudoangiomatous hyperplasia, of breast, 377–378
Pseudoangiosarcoma, 71
Pseudocapsule, 266
Pseudocarcinoma, of fallopian tube, 2401–2402
Pseudocysts
  adrenal, 605
  of ear, 953
  hepatic, 1557, 1561
  pancreatic, 1488, 1493
Pseudodiverticulosis, of esophagus, 1304
Pseudoepitheliomatous hyperplasia, 5
  of oral cavity, 825
  of penis, 2043
Pseudogout, 232
Pseudohermaphroditism
  female, 2112
  male, 1964–1968
Pseudoinvasion, adenoma with, 1432–1434
Pseudolipoma, hepatic, 1612
Pseudolipomatosis, of intestines, 1392
Pseudolymphoma, 74
  of breast, 369–370
  pulmonary, 1032
  sinonasal, 906
Pseudomelanosis duodeni, 1349
Pseudomembranous colitis, 1365, 1383
Pseudomesotheliomatous adenocarcinoma, 1139–1141
Pseudomesotheliomatous hemangioendothelioma, 1141–1142
Pseudomyxoma peritonei, 2426–2427
Pseudopheochromocytoma, 614
Pseudopyloric metaplasia, 1311
Pseudosarcomas, 132–133, 145–152
Pseudosarcomatous carcinoma, of breast, 358–359
Pseudosarcomatous fibromyxoid tumors, 148
Pseudosarcomatous lesions, of bladder, 1863–1864
Pseudotumor
  calcifying fibrous, of peritoneum, 2420
  inflammatory
    of bladder, 1856, 1863–1864
    of intestines, 1397
    of liver, 1612–1613
    of lymph nodes, 728

Pseudotumor, inflammatory (contd.)
  of orbit, 998
  of peritoneum, 2425–2426
  pulmonary, 1102–1103
Pseudoxanthoma elasticum, 1387
Psoriasiform dermatitis, 8
Psoriasis, pustular, 8
Psoriasis vulgaris, 8
PTCA (percutaneous transluminal coronary angioplasty), 1272–1273
Pterygium, 988
Puberty, male, 1955
Pulmonary disease, 1011–1059
  alveolar proteinosis, 1053–1054
  amyloidosis, 1056
  angiitis and granulomatosis, 1040–1046
  bronchiolitis obliterans, 1026–1027
  capillary hemangiomatosis, 1051
  desquamative interstitial pneumonia, 1015–1018
  diffuse alveolar damage, 1018–1021
  diffuse interstitial fibrosis, 1012–1015
  eosinophilic granuloma, 1028–1030
  eosinophilic reactions, 1023–1026
  extrinsic allergic alveolitis, 1021–1023
  hemorrhage, 1046–1047
  hemosiderosis, 1047
  honeycomb lung, 1018
  hyalinizing granuloma, 1037–1038
  hypersensitivity pneumonitis, 1021–1023
  hypertension, 1047–1051
  lymphangiomyomatosis, 1052–1053
  lymphocytic infiltrations, 1030–1037
  mycotoxicosis, 1023
  plasma cell granuloma, 1038–1040
  sarcoidosis, 1054–1056
  veno-occlusive, 1049–1051
Pulmonary neoplasms, 1069–1110
  adenocarcinoma, 1084–1092
    biologic behavior of, 1090
    biopsy interpretation in, 1089
    bronchial gland cell type of, 1086
    bronchial surface cell type of, 1085
    Clara cell type of, 1086–1087
    cytologic classification of, 1084–1089
    fetal lung type of, 1089
    function of, 1090–1091
    goblet cell type of, 1085–1086
    malignant progression of, 1090
    vs. mesothelioma, 1092
    metastatic, 1092
    mixed (indeterminate) cell type of, 1089
    prognostic factors for, 1089–1090
    subtyping of, 1091–1092
    type II alveolar epithelial cell type of, 1087–1088
  adenosquamous carcinoma, 1095
  amine and peptide hormones in, 1104–1105
  arachnoid nodule, 1101
  benign clear cell tumor, 1101
  benign epithelial, 1072–1073
  blastoma, 1099–1100
  bronchial gland carcinomas, 1098–1099
  carcinoid tumors, 1082–1083, 1095–1097
  carcinoma in situ, 1073–1074
  carcinosarcoma, 1099–1100
  chemodectoma, 1101
  cytokeratin in, 1109
  dysplasia, 1073–1074
  enzymes in, 1105–1106
  epidermal tumor, 1100
  hamartoma, 1103
  histologic classification of, 1072, 1114–1115
  immunohistochemistry of malignant, 1104–1110
  inflammatory pseudotumor, 1102–1103
  intravascular sclerosing bronchoalveolar tumor, 1100–1101
  large-cell carcinoma, 1092–1095
    biologic behavior of, 1094–1095
    gross features of, 1092–1093
    histologic features of, 1093
    interpretation of bronchial biopsy specimens in, 1094
    ultrastructural and immunohistochemical characteristics of, 1093–1094
  materials for diagnosis of, 1069–1071
  melanoma, 1101
  meningioma, 1101
  metastases, 1092, 1103–1104
  monoclonal antibodies in, 1107–1108
  neural cell adhesion molecule in, 1106
  oncogenes and antioncogenes in, 1109–1110
  paraganglioma, 1101
  pathology report on resection of, 1071–1072
  plasmacytoma, 1101
  proliferating or DNA-synthesizing cells in, 1109
  sclerosing hemangioma, 1101–1102
  small-cell carcinoma, 1078–1084
    vs. atypical carcinoid, 1082–1083
    clinical aspects of, 1083–1084
    histologic classification of, 1082
    interpretation of bronchial biopsy specimens in, 1083
    morphologic variation in, 1079–1082
  squamous cell carcinoma, 1074–1078
    biologic behavior of, 1078
    early, 1075–1077
    gross features of, 1074–1077
    histologic characteristics of, 1077–1078
    sugar chains in, 1108–1109
    surfactant apoprotein in, 1107
    survival rate with, 1078
    tumorlet, 1103
    vimentin in, 1106
Pulmonary-renal syndrome, 1715
Pulmonic valvular disease, 1230
Purpura(s), 28
  Henoch-Schönlein (anaphylactoid), 1260, 1261, 1267, 1730–1733
  immune thrombocytopenic, 781, 782
  pigmented, 28
  thrombotic thrombocytopenic, 781, 1736–1739
Purpura annularis telangiectodes of Majocchi, 28
Pustular diseases, 17–23
Pustular psoriasis, 8
Pustule, 5
Pyelitis, 1856
Pyelonephritis
  acute, 1754–1755
  chronic, 1757–1759
  xanthogranulomatous, 1758
Pyloric gland metaplasia
  of gallbladder, 1645
  of stomach, 1314
    pseudo-, 1311
  of pancreas, 1472
Pyloric stenosis, hypertrophic, 1313–1314
Pyoderma gangrenosum, 29–30
Pyogenic abscesses, hepatic, 1557, 1558
Pyogenic granuloma, 69, 174
  of eyelid, 988
  of gingiva, 807
Pyogenic osteomyelitis, 233–234
Pyriform sinus, 926
  cancer of, 936

Q
Q fever, 1537

R
Radial growth phase melanoma, 102–103
Radial scar, 331–333
Radiation exposure
  effect on testis of, 1958–1959
  thyroid carcinoma due to, 536
Radiation therapy
  astrocytomas or glioblasomas due to, 429
  breast changes due to, 361–362
  cystitis due to, 1856
  effect on cervix of, 2166
  effect on endocervical glands of, 2182
  effect on intestines of, 1352, 1392–1393
  effect on ovary of, 2319
  effect on testis of, 1959
  effect on thyroid of, 534
  effect on vulva of, 2119
  enterocolitis due to, 1383

esophagitis due to, 1290
gastritis due to, 1322–1323
for prostatic carcinoma, 1926
sarcoma after
   of bone, 286
   of breast, 369
   soft tissue, 196
vascular disease due to, 1269–1270
Radicular cysts, 835–836
Ragged red fibers, 118–119, 126
Ranula, 854
Rathke's cleft cyst, 519
Reactive adenopathy, 715–730
  causing architectural effacement, 726–730
  with follicular hyperplasia, 715–722
  with interfollicular hyperplasia, 722–726
Reactive hyperplasia
  of conjunctiva, 987
  of spleen, 780–782
Reactive lymphoid lesions, 683–684
Reactive myelofibrosis, 656
Reactive periostitis, 259
Reactive/reparative epithelial changes, of cervix, 2163–2164, 2165–2166
Rectum
  carcinoids of, 1448
  carcinoma of. *See* Colorectal carcinoma
  stromal tumors of, 1456
  ulcers of, 1369–1370
Red blood cells, fetal nucleated, 2105
Reed-Sternberg cells, 680, 681, 713, 730
Reflux, gastroesophageal, 1285–1288
Reflux esophagitis, 1285
Reflux nephropathy, 1688, 1689, 1757–1759
Reinke's crystals, 1943, 1944
Reis-Bucklers' dystrophy, 980
Reiter's syndrome, of vulva, 2119
Renal artery dysplasia, 1276–1277
Renal artery stenosis, 1763–1764
Renal biopsy, 1702–1703
Renal cell carcinoma, 1785–1799
  in children, 1839, 1849–1850
  chromophobe, 1796–1799, 1803
  clinical features of, 1788
  conventional (clear cell), 1787–1791
  differential diagnosis of, 1790–1791
  epidemiology of, 1785–1786
  grading and staging of, 1786–1787
  gross features of, 1788–1789
  microscopic features of, 1789–1790
  multilocular cystic, 1792
  outcome for, 1791
  ovarian metastases of, 2381
  papillary (chromophil), 1792–1796, 1805
    in children, 1839
  Xp11.2, 1849–1850
Renal dialysis, 1765–1767

Renal disease, 1701–1778
  with acellular closure of glomerular capillaries, 1736–1745, 1776–1777
  algorithm for diagnosis of, 1701, 1702
  Alport's syndrome, 1734–1736, 1776
  amyloidosis, 1741–1742, 1777
  analgesic nephropathy, 1759–1760
  antiglomerular basement membrane disease, 1714–1715
  atheroembolic, 1764
  Bence Jones cast nephropathy, 1751–1752
  Berger's disease, 1730–1733, 1776
  C1q nephropathy, 1719, 1776
  cholesterol emboli, 1764
  classification of, 1701, 1775–1777
  collapsing glomerulopathy, 1723–1724, 1776
  cystic, 1686–1689, 1692–1696
    acquired, 1767
  cystinosis, 1761
  dense deposit, 1709, 1775
  diabetic nephropathy, 1727–1730, 1776
  electron microscopy of, 1703–1704
  end-stage, 1765–1767
  focal sclerosis, 1713, 1717, 1719–1723, 1776
  generalizations about, 1704–1705
  glomerular capillary wall lesions, 1716–1730, 1776
  glomerulocystic, 1694, 1696
  glomerulonephritis, 1705–1716
    crescentic, 1709–1715, 1775–1776
      immune complex, 1714
      pauciimmune, 1712–1714
    cryoglobulinemic, 1739–1741, 1776–1777
    diffuse extracapillary proliferative, 1709–1715, 1775–1776
    diffuse intracapillary proliferative, 1705–1706, 1775
    fibrillary, 1742–1745, 1777
    focal, 1714–1715
    hypercellular (true, proliferative), 1705–1716
    immunotactoid, 1742–1745, 1777
    membranoproliferative, 1706–1709, 1775
    membranous, 1724–1727, 1776
    mesangiocapillary, 1706–1708, 1775
    with nephrotic syndrome, 1705–1716
    pattern recognition in, 1775
    postinfectious (poststreptococcal), 1705–1706, 1775
    rapidly progressive, 1709–1715, 1775–1776
    specific patterns in, 1775–1777
  glomerulosclerosis, focal segmental, 1713, 1717, 1719–1723, 1776
  gout, 1761
  with hematuria, 1730–1736, 1776

Henoch-Schönlein (anaphylactoid) purpura, 1730–1733
hereditary nephritis, 1734–1736
human immunodeficiency virus-associated nephropathy, 1723–1724, 1776
hypertensive, 1761–1763
hyperuricemic nephropathy, 1761
IgA nephropathy, 1730–1733, 1776
IgM nephropathy, 1718–1719
immunofluorescence of, 1703
immunotactoid glomerulopathy, 1742–1745, 1777
light chain deposition, 1750–1751
lipoid nephrosis, 1716–1718, 1776
malakoplakia, 1759
membranous nephropathy, 1724–1727
metabolic disorders, 1760–1761
minimal change, 1716–1718, 1776
monoclonal gammopathy-associated, 1750–1752
myeloma cast nephropathy, 1751–1752
with nephritic syndrome, 1705–1716
nephritis
  acute infectious tubulointerstitial, 1734–1736
  acute interstitial, 1755–1757
  chronic interstitial, 1757–1761
  diffuse suppurative, 1734–1736
  hereditary (familial), 1734–1736, 1776
nephrocalcinosis, 1760
nephrosclerosis
  arterial and arteriolar (benign), 1761–1763
  malignant, 1763
nephrotic syndrome
  diffuse mesangial hypercellularity in, 1718, 1776
  focal global glomerulosclerosis in, 1723
  glomerular capillary wall lesions leading to, 1716–1730
  glomerular mesangial IgM deposition in, 1718–1719
  glomerulonephritis with, 1705–1716
  minimal change, 1716–1718, 1776
nil, 1716–1718, 1776
nonamyloidotic fibrillary glomerulopathy, 1742–1745
nonamyloidotic monoclonal immunoglobulin deposition, 1750–1751
oxalosis, 1760–1761
pattern recognition in, 1775
polycystic, 1557, 1560, 1692–1695
pulmonary-renal syndrome, 1715
pyelonephritis
  acute, 1754–1755
  chronic, 1757–1759
reflux nephropathy, 1757–1759

Renal disease *(contd.)*
  renal artery stenosis, 1763–1764
  review of, 1775–1777
  in rheumatoid arthritis, 1749
  specific patterns in, 1775–1777
  in systemic lupus erythematosus, 1745–1749, 1777
  terminology for, 1777–1778
  thin basement membrane, 1733, 1776
  thrombotic microangiopathy, 1736–1739, 1770, 1776
  tissue sampling and preparation in, 1702–1703
  tuberculosis, 1759
  tubular necrosis, acute, 1752–1754
  tubulointerstitial, 1752–1761
  vascular, 1761–1765
  vasculitis, 1764–1765
Renal dysplasia, 1686–1689
Renal failure, acute, 1752–1754
Renal hypoplasia, 1685–1686
Renal neoplasms
  adenofibroma, 1811–1812
    in children, 1850
  adenoma
    metanephric, 1811–1812
      in children, 1850
    papillary (chromophil), 1796
  angiomyolipoma, 1812–1816
  carcinoid tumor, 1809–1810
  carcinoma
    collecting duct, 1803–1805
    medullary, 1805–1806
      in children, 1849, 1850
    renal cell, 1785–1799
      in children, 1839, 1849–1850
  classification of, 1785, 1786
  clear cell sarcoma, 1842–1847, 1849
  epidemiology of, 1785–1786
  grading and staging of, 1786–1787
    in children, 1826–1828
  hamartoma, cystic (leiomyomatous), 1806–1807
  hemangioma, 1817
  hemangiopericytoma, 1817
  hematologic, 1818
  juxtaglomerular cell tumor, 1807–1809
  leiomyoma, 1816
  leiomyosarcoma, 1816
  leukemia, 1818
  lipoma, 1816
  liposarcoma, 1816
  lymphoma, 1818
    in children, 1851
  medullary fibroma, 1816–1817
  mesenchymal, 1817–1818
  metaplastic, 1847
  nephroblastoma, 1812
  nephroma
    cystic, 1807
    mesoblastic, 1806–1807
    in children, 1839–1842
  oncocytoma, 1799–1803
  ossifying, 1850
  pediatric, 1825–1851
    carcinoma, 1849–1850
    clear cell sarcoma, 1842–1847
    differential diagnosis of, 1828, 1829
    lymphoma, 1851
    mesoblastic nephroma, 1839–1842
    metanephric adenofibroma and metanephric adenoma, 1850
    ossifying tumor, 1850
    primitive neuroepithelial tumor, 1850
    rhabdoid tumor, 1847–1849
    specimen handling for, 1825–1826
    staging of, 1826–1828
    Wilms' tumor (nephroblastoma), 1829–1839
  peripheral nerve sheath, 1817
  plasmacytoma, 1818
  primitive neuroectodermal, 1810–1811
    in children, 1850
  rhabdoid, 1847–1849
  rhabdomyosarcomas, 1817–1818
  solid and cystic biphasic, 1806–1807
  solitary fibrous, 1817
  Wilms' tumor, 1812
Renal pelvis, carcinoma of, 1879
Renal segmental atrophy, 1691
Renal sinus, 1826–1828
Renal transplantation, 1767–1775
  cyclosporin nephrotoxicity in, 1772–1774
  FK506 toxicity in, 1774
  lymphoproliferative disorders after, 1774–1775
  rejection of
    acute interstitial (cellular), 1768–1770
    acute vascular (humoral), 1770–1771
    Banff classification of, 1772
    chronic, 1771–1772, 1774
    hyperacute, 1767–1768
Renal tubular dysgenesis, 1690–1691
Renomedullary interstitial cell tumor, 1816–1817
Residual cysts, 836
Resistant ovary syndrome, 2318
Resorption bays, 247
Resorption droplets, 1717, 1778
Respiratory epithelial adenomatoid hamartoma, 895
Restrictive cardiomyopathy, 1218–1222
Retention cysts, of prostate, 1899
Retention polyps, of stomach, 1326
Rete ovarii, tumors of, 2358
Rete ridges, 4
Rete testis, 1959
  tumors of, 1974, 2014–2015
Reticular dermis, 4
Reticuloendotheliosis, leukemic, 751
Reticulosis
  histiocytic medullary, 762–763
  pagetoid, 78
Retiform hemangioendothelioma, 179
Retina, 993–994
Retinoblastoma, 993–994
Retinoblastoma gene, 570
Retrodifferentiation, of malignant fibrous histiocytoma, 165–166
Retroperitoneal fibrosis, 153, 1396, 1397–1398
Retroperitoneal lymph node lesions, 2436–2437
Retroperitoneum, inflammatory lesions of, 1395–1398
Retrorectal space, developmental cysts of, 1391–1392
Reye's syndrome, 1543
Rhabdoid meningioma, 442
Rhabdoid sarcoma, 191, 192
Rhabdoid tumor
  of CNS, 438
  of kidney, 1847–1849
  of soft tissue, 192
Rhabdomyoma
  of larynx, 942
  sinonasal, 912
  soft tissue
    adult, 171
    fetal and genital, 150–151
  vaginal, 2139
Rhabdomyosarcoma, 161, 171–174
  alveolar, 172–174
  botryoid, 172
  of CNS, 414
  of ear, 958
  embryonal, 172
    of cervix, 2195
    of extrahepatic bile ducts, 1665, 1666
    of vagina, 2142–2143
  of larynx, 942–943
  leiomyomatous, 172
  of liver, 1614, 1615
  of mediastinum, 1173–1174, 1175
  vs. neuroblastoma, 611
  new classification of, 174
  of orbit, 999
  paratesticular, 1986, 2020–2021
  pleomorphic, 174
  of prostate, 1933
  renal, 1817–1818
  sinonasal, 912–914
  spindle-cell, 172
  of urothelial tract, 1881
Rheumatic endocarditis, 1232
Rheumatic fever, 1261
Rheumatoid arthritis, 228–229
  cornea in, 983
  inflammatory myopathy in, 115
  lung disease in, 1044–1045
  lymph nodes in, 715–716

renal disease in, 1749
Rheumatoid disease
  aorta in, 1258
  vasculitis in, 1268
Rheumatoid nodules, 33, 229
Rhinoscleroma, 887
Rhinosporidiosis, 886
Richter's syndrome
  bone marrow in, 673
  splenic, 784
Rickets, 249–250
Rickettsial infection, of liver, 1513
Riedel's thyroiditis, 534
Rimmed vacuole, 119–120
Ring fibers, 113
Ringworm, 7
Rokitansky-Aschoff sinuses, 1630, 1639
Rosai-Dorfman lesion, 370
Rosenmüller's lymph node, 2111–2112
Rosenthal fibers, 416–417
Rosettes, 420–422
Round-cell liposarcoma, 167, 169
Rushton bodies, 835
Russell bodies, 228, 741

S

S-100 protein, as marker for soft tissue tumors, 142
Saliva, 853
Salivary duct carcinoma, 872–873
Salivary gland(s), 853–875
  adenoma of
    basal cell, 860–861
    monomorphic, 859–860
    pleomorphic, 857–859
    sebaceous, 863
  benign lymphoepithelial lesion of, 855–856
  carcinoma of
    actinic cell, 865–866
    adeno-, 869
      basal cell, 860–861
      polymorphous low-grade, 869–870
    adenoid cystic, 867–869
    anaplastic small-cell, 873
    hyalinizing clear-cell, 873
    mucoepidermoid, 866–867
    myoepithelial, 864–865
    neuroendocrine, 873
    sebaceous of, 863
  cysts of, 854–855
  embryology of, 853
  hemangioendothelioma of, 874
  hemangiomas of, 873–874
  hemangiopericytoma of, 874
  histology of, 853
  lipoma of, 874
  lymphadenoma of, 863
  lymphangioma of, 874
  lymphoepithelial lesion of, malignant, 856–857
  lymphoma of, malignant, 874–875
  metastatic tumors to, 875
  mixed tumors of
    benign, 857–859
    malignant, 870–872
    metastasizing, 859
  myoepithelioma of, 863
  neoplasms of, 857–875
  nerve sheath tumor of, benign peripheral, 874
  noninflammatory conditions of, 855
  oncocytoma of, 862–863
  papillary cystadenoma lymphomatosum of, 861–862
  sarcomas of, 874
  in Sjögren's syndrome, 855–856
  Warthin's tumor of, 861–862
Salivary gland-like tumors
  of larynx, 939–940
  of sella, 521
Salmonellosis, intestinal, 1384
Salpingectomy, endometriosis after, 2400
Salpingitis, 2395–2398
  acute, 2395
  chronic, 2395
  follicular, 2395, 2396
  foreign body, 2397
  granulomatous, 2395–2398
  ligneous, 2398
  lipoid, 2397
  tuberculous, 2395–2397
Salpingitis isthmica nodosa, 2398
Sarcoglycans, 121–122
Sarcoidosis
  arthritis due to, 234
  of brain, 398–399
  cutaneous, 31
  of eyelids, 989
  gastric, 1320–1321
  of lacrimal gland, 1000
  of liver, 1513
  lymph nodes in, 727–728
  of middle ear, 960
  muscle in, 115
  of myocardium, 1218
  ocular, 984
  of pituitary, 522
  pulmonary, 1054–1056
  sinonasal, 889
Sarcolemmal nuclei, 110
Sarcoma(s)
  by age group, 172
  alveolar soft part, 190–191
  angio-. See Angiosarcoma
  of brain, 446–447
  of breast, 368
    radiation-induced, 369
  cardiac, 1241
  categories of, 133–134
  of cervix, 2194–2195
  chondro-. See Chondrosarcoma
  clear cell
    of kidney, 1842–1847, 1849
    soft tissue, 191, 193–194
  cytogenetics in, 136
  dendritic cell, 763–764
  DNA ploidy of, 144–145
  endometrial
    pure, 2264–2265, 2288
    stromal, 2266–2270, 2288, 2431
    undifferentiated, 2268–2269
  epithelioid, 191, 192–193, 1101
  esophageal, 1304
  Ewing's
    of bone, 263, 269–271
    vs. neuroblastoma, 611
    soft tissue, 194–195
  of fallopian tube, 2406–2407
  fibro-. See Fibrosarcoma
  fibromyxoid, 158
  of gallbladder, 1654–1655
  grading of, 144
  hepatic, 1586, 1613–1615
  histogenesis of, 134, 136–139
  inclusion body, 192
  Kaposi's. See Kaposi's sarcoma (KS)
  of kidney, 1842–1847, 1849
  of larynx, 943
  leiomyo-. See Leiomyosarcoma
  lipo-. See Liposarcoma
  mediastinal, granulocytic, 1187–1188, 1190–1191
  origin and etiology of, 134
  osteo-. See Osteosarcoma
  of ovary
    endometrioid stromal, 2334–2335
    pure, 2372
  Paget's, 286
  postradiation, 196, 286
  prognostic factors for, 135, 143, 144–145
  of prostate, 1932–1933
  pseudo-, 132–133, 145–152
  renal, 1816
  rhabdoid, 191, 192
  rhabdomyo-. See Rhabdomyosarcoma
  of salivary gland, 874
  of seminal vesicles, 1936
  staging of, 144
  of stomach, 1338
  syndromes of, 145
  synovial, 181, 182–183
  of testis, granulocytic, 2012
  therapy for, 136
  thyroid, 554
  tumors mimicking, 132–133, 145–152
  of urothelial tract, 1881–1882
  vaginal, 2142–2143
  vulvar, 2130
Sarcoma botryoides, sinonasal, 913
Sarcomatoid carcinoma
  of bladder, 1876–1878

Sarcomatoid carcinoma *(contd.)*
　of breast, 358–359
　of cervix, 2177
　of esophagus, 1299, 1300–1301
　hepatocellular, 1581
　metastatic, 296, 299–300
　of pancreas, 1486–1487
　of penis, 2055–2056
　thymic, 1192–1194
Sarcomatoid hypernephroma, 296
Sarcomatoid mediastinal malignant mesothelioma, 1194
Sarcomatoid thymic yolk sac tumor, 1194
Scabies, 17
　of penis, 2039
Scale, 5
Scale crust, 5
Scar, 35
SCC. *See* Squamous cell carcinoma (SCC)
Schiller-Duval bodies, 1991, 2361
Schistosomiasis
　cystitis due to, 1855
　of fallopian tube, 2397
　intestinal, 1385
　ovarian, 2308
Schneiderian membrane, 885
Schneiderian papillomas, 892–895
Schnyder's corneal dystrophy, 980
Schwannoma(s)
　of CNS, 411, 447–448
　cutaneous, 68
　intestinal, 1457–1458
　of larynx, 943
　of salivary gland, 874
　of soft tissue, 185
　of stomach, 1338
　vestibular, 969–970
Scirrhous tumors, 351
Sclera, 983
Scleredema, 37
Sclerema neonatorum, 40
Scleroderma, 36
　of esophagus, 1295
　pulmonary disease in, 1014
　vascular disease in, 1268–1269
Scleroelastic scar, 331–333
Sclerosing adenosis
　of breast, 330–331, 332
　of prostate, 1913, 1914
Sclerosing cholangitis, 1512, 1526–1527, 1547, 1548, 1657–1661
Sclerosing epithelioid fibrosarcoma, 158–159
Sclerosing hemangioma, pulmonary, 1101–1102
Sclerosing hepatic carcinoma, 1593
Sclerosing hyaline necrosis, 1530
Sclerosing lesion, of breast, 331–333
Sclerosing mediastinitis, 1167–1168
Sclerosing peritonitis, 1398

Sclerosing stromal tumor, of ovary, 2349–2350
Scrapie, 406
Sea-blue histiocytosis, 792–793
Sebaceous adenoma, 61, 63, 863
Sebaceous cell carcinoma
　of eyelid, 991–992
　of salivary gland, 863
Sebaceous epithelioma, 61, 63
Sebaceous gland hyperplasia, of vulva, 2117
Sebaceous hyperplasia, 63
Sebaceous lymphadenoma, 863
Sebaceous tumors
　cutaneous, 64
　of ovary, 2370
Seborrheic dermatitis, 7
Seborrheic keratosis, 49–50
　of vulva, 2117
Secretogranin, 484
Secretory adenosis, of breast, 334
Secretory carcinoma
　of breast, 358
　endometrioid, 2256–2257
Segmental subchondral infarction, 229–230
Seizures, 465–466
Sella, empty, 522–523
Sellar region tumors, 516–522. *See also* Pituitary; Pituitary adenoma(s)
Seminal vesicles
　carcinoma of, 1935–1936
　cystadenomas of, 1935
　cysts of, 1935
　germ-cell tumors of, 1936
　invasion by prostatic carcinoma of, 1920
　phyllodes tumors of, 1936
　vs. prostatic adenocarcinoma, 1906–1907
　sarcomas of, 1936
Seminiferous tubules, 1943
Seminoma, 1980–1983, 1986
　cystic, 1155–1156
　of mediastinum, 1181, 1182, 1198
　spermatocytic, 1983–1985, 1986
Senile keratosis, 51–53
Sepsis, liver in, 1511, 1514, 1536
Septal panniculitis, 39
Septic arthritis, 233–234
Sequestration, of intervertebral disc, 239
Serotonin-producing tumors, of pancreas, 1501
Serous carcinoma
　of cervix, 2191–2192
　of fallopian tube, 2405
　peritoneal, 2434
Serous tumors
　of broad ligament, 2408–2409
　of ovary, 2322–2327
　of pancreas, 1490–1491, 1493

　　peritoneal, 2434
Serrated adenoma, intestinal, 1415–1416
Sertoli cells, 1943–1944
Sertoli cell tumors
　of ovary, 2351
　of testis, 2006–2008
Sertoli-Leydig cell tumors
　of ovary, 2351–2354
　of testis, 2008–2009
SETTLE (spindle cell epithelial tumors with thymus-like differentiation), 1196
Sex-cord-like elements, uterine neoplasms with, 2269, 2270–2271
Sex cord-stromal tumors
　of ovary, 2343–2355
　　with annular tubules, 2354–2355
　　unclassified, 2354
　of testis, 1974, 2004–2010
Sex-cord tumors with annular tubules, 2354–2355
Sex-determining region Y, 1944
Sézary syndrome
　bone marrow in, 678
　lymph nodes in, 760–761
　skin in, 77–78
Shingles, 21–22
Shock kidney, 1752
Sialometaplasia, necrotizing, 855, 890
Signet ring cell carcinoma
　of bladder, 1874
　of breast, 358
　　ductal *in situ*, 341
　of prostate, 1928
Signet ring-stromal tumor, of ovary, 2350–2351
Silica granulomas, 31
Silicone breast implants, 374
Silicone rubber, in joint prostheses, 236
Singer's node, 927, 943
Sinuses
　of Morgagni, 1671
　paranasal. *See* Paranasal sinuses
　vascular transformation of, 177–178
Sinus histiocytosis, with massive lymphadenopathy
　bone in, 309
　liver in, 1536
　lymph nodes in, 724–726
Sinusoidal hemangioma, 176–177
Sipple syndrome
　familial sympathoadrenal paragangliomas in, 637
　parathyroid in, 568
Sjögren's syndrome
　lymph nodes in, 717
　salivary glands in, 855–856
Skene's duct cyst, 2113
Skene's glands, 2111
Skenoid fibers, 1455
Skin, normal histology of, 4–5

Skin biopsy, 3–4
Skin disease(s)
  bullous and pustular, 17–25
  of cartilage, 33–41
  erythema multiforme, 14–16
  of hair follicles, 33–41
  inflammatory, 6–33
    dermal, 26–27
    epidermal, 6–17
  lichenoid interface dermatitis, 9–10
  nonneoplastic, 3–41
  specimen preparation for, 3–4
  spongiotic dermatitis, 6–9, 16–17
  terminology for, 5
  vacuolar interface dermatitis, 10–14
  vasculitis and vasculopathy, 28–33
  verrucous acanthosis, 16
  of vulva, 2118–2119
Skin tumors
  adnexal, 59–60
  of connective tissue, 60–67
  epidermal, 49–59
  of lymphoid tissues, 73–79
  melanocytic, 89–105
    benign, 89–100
    malignant, 100–105
  neural, 67–68
  neuroendocrine, 487
  nonmelanocytic, 49–79
  vascular, 68–73
SLE. See Systemic lupus erythematosus (SLE)
Small-cell carcinoma
  of anus, 1679
  of bladder, 1875–1876
  of cervix, 2176–2177
    and adenocarcinoma, 2194
  of CNS, 414
  colorectal, 1437–1439
  of esophagus, 1299, 1303–1304
  of larynx, 941
  of lung, 1078–1084
    vs. atypical carcinoid, 1082–1083
    clinical aspects of, 1083–1084
    histologic classification of, 1082
    interpretation of bronchial biopsy specimens in, 1083
    morphologic variation in, 1079–1082
  neuroendocrine, of mediastinum, 1168–1170, 1175–1176, 1199
  of ovary
    hypercalcemic, 2373–2375
    pulmonary type, 2343
  of pancreas, 1487
  of prostate, 1928–1929
  of salivary gland, 873
  sinonasal, 902
Small-cell malignant lymphomas, of mediastinum, 1174–1175
Small-cell neoplasms
  of bone, 266–271

  of mediastinum, 1168–1176
    differential diagnosis of, 1175–1176
Small-cell osteosarcoma, 288
Small intestine. See also Intestine(s)
  in abetalipoproteinemia, 1359
  in acrodermatitis enteropathica, 1359–1360
  adenoma of, 1425
  in autoimmune enteropathy, 1355
  biopsy specimen of, 1349
  carcinoids of, 1448
  in celiac sprue, 1350–1352
  chemotherapy effect on, 1352, 1392–1393
  in collagenous sprue, 1355
  in dermatitis herpetiformis, 1353
  diverticula of, 1391
  duodenitis of, 1354–1355
  in enteropathy-associated T-cell lymphoma, 1357
  in eosinophilic gastroenteritis, 1357
  in immunodeficiency syndromes, 1355–1356
  immunoproliferative disease of, 1449–1450
  in infectious gastroenteritis, 1353–1354
  in kwashiorkor, 1352
  lymphangiectasia of, 1359
  in lymphocytic enterocolitis, 1352
  lymphomas of, 1449
  malabsorption by, 1349–1360
  in marasmus, 1352
  in mastocytosis, 1354
  in megaloblastic anemia, 1352
  microvillus inclusion disease of, 1352–1353
  normal histology of, 1349–1350
  parasitic infestations of, 1358–1359
  patterns of abnormal architecture of, 1350–1360
  peptic ulcer disease of, 1354–1355
  polyps and nodules of, 1360–1361
  in protein allergies, 1352
  radiation effect on, 1352, 1392–1393
  stasis syndromes of, 1354
  in Torkelson syndrome, 1355
  transplantation and rejection of, 1393–1394
  in tropical sprue, 1353
  in tufting enteropathy, 1360
  in ulcerative jejunoileitis, 1357
  in Waldenström's macroglobulinemia, 1359
  in Whipple's disease, 1356
  in Zollinger-Ellison syndrome, 1354
Small lymphocytic lymphoma, 673, 738–741
  of spleen, 782–784
Small noncleaved cell lymphoma, of mediastinum, 1174–1175
Small-vessel disease, of brain, 407

Smoker's granules, 1017
Smoldering myeloma, 689
Smooth muscle actin, as marker for soft tissue tumors, 141–142
Smooth muscle neoplasms
  soft tissue, 161, 169–171
  uterine, 2272–2288
    atypia in, 2277
    diagnostic strategy for, 2272–2275, 2279–2281
    differential diagnosis of, 2270, 2272–2275
    epithelioid differentiation of, 2281
    histologic patterns of, 2273
    leiomyomas, 2273, 2281–2287
    leiomyosarcoma, 2273, 2280, 2287–2288
    mitotic index of, 2278, 2282–2283
    morphologic features of, 2276–2279
    myxoid differentiation of, 2280
    necrosis in, 2278–2279
    prognosis and clinical management of, 2275–2279
    of usual sort, 2273, 2279–2280
Sneddon-Wilkinson disease, 17
Soft tissue tumors, 131–196
  of adipose tissue, 166
  angiomyxoid, 155–157
  aspiration biopsy cytology of, 135
  of broad ligament, 2409
  carcinoma, 193
  of cervix, 2196–2197
  consultation for, 135
  electron microscopy of, 143
  excisional biopsy of, 136
  of fallopian tube, 2404
  fibrohistiocytic, 159–160
  fibrosarcomas, 157–159
  fibrous, 152–154
  frozen section of, 135
  hemangiopericytoma, 181
  histogenesis of, 134, 136–139
  immunohistochemistry of, 137–139, 143
  liposarcoma, 166–169
  malignant endothelial, 178–181
  malignant fibrous histiocytoma, 160–166
  malignant granular cell, 191–195
  margins of, 135
  markers for, 137, 138, 139–143
  melanoma, 194
  mesenchymoma, 190
  mimicking sarcomas, 132–133, 145–152
  molecular diagnosis of, 137
  myofibroblastomas, 157
  needle and incisional biopsy of, 135–136
  osteocartilaginous, 189–190
  pathology report on, 135

Soft tissue tumors (contd.)
   of penis, 2058
   of peripheral nerve sheath, 185–188
   philosophical approach to diagnosis of, 131–132
   prognostic factors for, 135, 143, 144–145
   of prostate, 1932–1933
   pseudosarcomas, 132–133, 145–152
   sarcomas. See Sarcoma(s)
   of smooth muscle, 169–171
   of striated muscle, 171–174
   of synovial origin, 182–183
   tissue sections of, 134–135
   vacuolated, 161, 169
   vascular, 174–178
Solar keratosis, 51–53
Solar lentigo, 52, 97, 99
Solid-cystic-papillary epithelial neoplasm, of pancreas, 1495–1496
Solitary fibrous tumors
   of mediastinum, 1165–1166
   of pleura, 1119–1120
   renal, 1817
   sinonasal, 911–912
   of soft tissue, 156
Solitary rectal ulcer syndrome, 1369–1370
Somatostatin-producing tumors, of pancreas, 1501
Somatotroph cell, 497
Somatotrophic adenoma, 498
Speckled, cloudy dystrophy, 980
Spectacle-frame acanthoma, 952–953
Spermatic cord
   torsion of, 1948–1949
   tumors of, 1974, 2020–2021
Spermatocytic seminoma, 1983–1985, 1986
Spermatogenesis
   hypo-, 1951
   normal, 1944, 1951
Spherulosis, collagenous, of breast, 378–379
Sphingomyelin cholesterol lipidosis, 692
Spider cells, 171
Spindle cell carcinoma
   of bladder, 1876–1878
   of breast, 359
   of cervix, 2177
   of conjunctiva, 986
   hepatocellular, 1581
   of oral cavity, 828–831
   of soft tissue, 133
   of vulva, 2128
Spindle cell epithelial tumors with thymus-like differentiation (SETTLE), 1196
Spindle cell epithelioma, of vagina, 2138
Spindle cell hemangioendothelioma, 73
Spindle cell hemangioma, 176
Spindle cell lipoma, 148–149

Spindle cell melanoma, 133
Spindle cell nevus, 93–95
   pigmented, 95
Spindle cell nodules
   postoperative
     of genitourinary tract, 1863–1864
     of soft tissue, 148
   of vagina, 2139
Spindle cell pseudotumor, mycobacterial, 728–729
Spindle cell rhabdomyosarcoma, 172
Spindle cell tumors
   of endometrium, 2208
   gastric, 1337–1338
   hyalinizing, with giant rosettes, 158
   intranodal hemorrhagic, 729–730
   of lymph node, 728
   of mediastinum, malignant, 1192–1194
   of vulva, 2121
Spiradenoma, 61
Spiral valve of Heister, 1629
Spirochetosis, intestinal, 1371
Spitz nevus, 93–95
Spleen, 779–799
   in acute septic splenitis, 792
   in bacillary angiomatosis, 792
   congestion of, 790–791
   cysts of, 797
   developmental lesions of, 797
   hamartomas of, 797
   histiocytic proliferations of, 792–794
   in Hodgkin's disease, 789–790
   immunocytoma of, 784
   in infectious mononucleosis, 791–792
   inflammatory pseudotumor of, 799
   in leukemia
     B-cell chronic lymphocytic, 782–784
     chronic myeloid, 794–795
     hairy cell, 795–796
     large granular lymphocyte, 796–797
     prolymphocytic, 790
   lymphoma of
     follicular, 786–787
     large-cell, 787–789
     lymphoplasmacytoid, 784
     malignant, 782–790
     mantle cell, 784–785
     marginal zone, 785–786
     small lymphocytic, 782–784
     with villous lymphocytes, 786
   metastases to, 799
   myeloid metaplasia of, 795
   nonhematopoietic tumors of, 797–799
   plasmacytomas of, 784
   processing specimens of, 779–780
   reactive follicular hyperplasia of, 780–781
   reactive nonfollicular hyperplasia of, 781–782
   red pulp disorders of, 790–799
   in systemic mastocytosis, 797

   vascular neoplasms of, 797–799
   white pulp disorders of, 780–790
Splenic-gonadal fusion, 1947–1948, 2015
Splenitis, acute septic, 792
Splenosis, of peritoneum, 2420
Spondylitis, ankylosing, aorta in, 1258
Spondylosis deformans, 239
Spongiform encephalopathies, 404–406
Spongiform pustule of Kogoj, 8
Spongioblastoma, polar, 411, 438
Spongiosis, 5, 6
Spongiotic dermatitis, 6
   acute and subacute, 6–9
   chronic, 16–17
Sprue
   celiac (nontropical), 1350–1352
   collagenous, 1355
   tropical, 1353
Squamoid tumors, of cutaneous adnexa, 64
Squamous atypia, postmenopausal, 2164
Squamous cell carcinoma (SCC), 58
   anal, 1675–1678
   of bladder, 1873
   of breast, 359
   of cervix, 2172–2176
     microinvasive, 2168–2172
   colorectal, 1439
   of conjunctiva, 985
   of ear
     middle, 967
     outer, 954–955
   of esophagus, 1298–1301
   of eyelid, 991
   vs. keratoacanthoma, 57
   of larynx, 931–939
   of liver, 1586
   of mediastinum, basaloid, 1170, 1176
   of nasopharynx, 896–898
   of nose and paranasal sinuses, 895–896
   oral, 810–835
     adenosquamous, 831–834
     basaloid, 834–835
     of buccal mucosa, 825
     distant metastasis of, 818
     epidemiology of, 810
     etiology of, 810–811
     of floor of mouth, 824
     of gingiva, 824
     in situ, 812–814
     of lip, 823
     multiple primary, 814
     of oropharynx, 825
     of palate, 825
     papillary, 828
     precursors to, 811–812
     prognostic indicators for, 818–819
     regional lymph node metastasis of, 817–818
     resection margins in, 819–820

site-specific considerations for, 820–824
spindle-cell, 828–831
squamous dysplasia and, 812–814
staging of, 816–817
of tongue, 823–824
of tonsil, 825–826
unusual variants of, 824–835
verrucous, 824–828
of ovary, 2341–2342
of penis, 2046–2057
of prostate, 1930
pulmonary, 1074–1078
biologic behavior of, 1078
early, 1075–1077
gross features of, 1074–1077
histologic characteristics of, 1077–1078
of thymus, 1177–1178
of vagina, 2140–2141
of vulva, 2125–2129
Squamous cell tumors
of ovary, 2341–2342
peritoneal, 2435
of thyroid, 538, 555–556
Squamous differentiation, of endometrium, 2246–2249
Squamous dysplasia
of esophagus, 1300
of oral cavity, 812–814
Squamous elements, endometrial carcinoma with, 2240, 2247–2249, 2264
Squamous hyperplasia
of penis, 2042–2043
of vulva, 2122–2123
Squamous intraepithelial lesions
of cervix, 2157–2168
with atrophy, 2166
classification of, 2157–2163
differential diagnosis of, 2163–2164
high-grade, 2159–2160, 2161, 2164–2165
histologic variations in presentation of, 2160–2163
with immature metaplastic-type differentiation, 2163, 2166
keratinizing, 2161
low-grade, 2158–2159, 2160, 2163–2164
nonepithelial alterations, 2166–2168
papillary immature, 2161–2163
postmenopausal squamous atypia in, 2164
due to radiation effect, 2166
reactive/reparative epithelial changes in, 2163–2164, 2165–2166
vaginal papillomatosis in, 2163
of penis, 2043–2045
of vulva, 2122, 2123–2125
Squamous metaplasia

of breast, 329–330
of cervix, 2163, 2166
Squamous odontogenic tumor, 844–845
Squamous papilloma
of conjunctiva, 985
of esophagus, 1296
of oral cavity, 825
sinonasal, 892–895
Stalk section effect, 504, 506
Stapes, congenital fixation of, 968–969
Staphylococcal scalded skin syndrome, vs. toxic epidermal necrolysis, 15
Starch granules, 32
Starch granuloma, of ear, 949
Stasis dermatitis, 8
Stasis syndromes, of small intestine, 1354
Steatocystoma, 62
Steatohepatitis, 1515, 1543, 1547, 1548
Stein-Leventhal syndrome, 2312
Stellate scar, 331–333
Stercoral ulcer, 1383
Stereotactic biopsy, of brain, 391–393
Steroid cell tumors, of ovary, 2355–2358
Steroid hormones, plasma and urinary concentrations of, 590
Stevens-Johnson syndrome, 15
Stewart-Treves syndrome, 369
Still's disease, adult onset, lymph nodes in, 717
Stomach, 1311–1340
adenoma of, 1328–1329
autonomic nerve tumors of, 1338
biopsy specimen handling for, 1312
carcinoma of, 1330–1334
carditis of, 1319–1320
in Cowden disease, 1326
Crohn's disease of, 1320
in Cronkhite-Canada syndrome, 1328
cysts of, 1313
duplications of, 1313
dysplasia of, 1333–1334
endocrine tumors of, 1334–1335
enlarged mucosal folds of, 1329–1330
epithelioid tumors of, 1338
gastritis of, 1315–1325
graft-versus-host disease of, 1324–1325
heterotopias of, 1312–1313
hypertrophic hypersecretory gastropathy of, 1329
hypertrophic pyloric stenosis of, 1313–1314
inflammatory conditions of, 1315–1325
lymphomas of, 1335–1337
Ménétrier's disease of, 1329–1330
metabolic diseases involving, 1339–1340
metaplasia of, 1311, 1314–1315
normal appearances of, 1311–1312
peptic ulcer disease of, 1325
in Peutz-Jeghers syndrome, 1326
polypoid mucosal prolapse of, 1327

polyps of, 1326–1329
postgastrectomy, 1325–1326
reactive gastropathy of, 1322
sarcoidosis of, 1320–1321
sarcomas of, 1338
spindle cell tumors of, 1337–1338
stromal tumors of, 1337–1339
subnuclear vacuolated cells of, 1314
syphilis of, 1320
vascular lesions of, 1339
watermelon, 1339
xanthelasma of, 1313
in Zollinger-Ellison syndrome, 1329
Stomal polypoid hyperplasia, of stomach, 1327
Stomatitis, ulcerative (Vincent's), 807
Storage histiocyte disorders, 691–693
Stratum basale, 4
Stratum corneum, 4
Stratum granulosum, 4
Stratum lucidum, 4
Stratum malpighii, 4
Stratum spinosum, 4
Streak gonads, 1967
Streptococcal glomerulonephritis, 1705–1706, 1775
Stress, 243
Striated muscle lesions, 171–174
Stromal endometriosis, 2430, 2431
Stromal giant cells, of breast, 379
Stromal hyperplasia, of ovary, 2313
Stromal hyperthecosis, of ovary, 2313
Stromal-Leydig cell hyperplasia, of ovary, 2317
Stromal luteoma, 2355
Stromal metaplasias, of ovary, 2317–2318
Stromal nodules, endometrial, 2265, 2266, 2269, 2270
Stromal polyps, of vagina, 2137–2138
Stromal sarcomas
of cervix, 2195
endometrial, 2265, 2266–2270, 2288, 2431
endometrioid, of ovary, 2334–2335
Stromal tumors
endometrial, 2265–2271
gastric, 1337–1339
periductal, 366–367
Strongyloidiasis, 1358–1359
Struma ovarii, 2366–2368
Sturge-Weber disease, 407
Stye, 989
Subacute sclerosing panencephalitis, 401
Subarachnoid hemorrhage, 406
Subchondral necrosis, 229–230
Subcorneal bullae
with acantholysis, 17–18
without acantholysis, 17
Subcorneal pustular dermatosis, 17
Subcutaneous fat necrosis, of newborn, 40
Subcutis, 4

Subdural hematoma, 406
Subependymoma, 411, 423
Subepidermal bullae
  with inflammation, 23–24
  without inflammation, 24
Subepidermal calcified nodule, 38
Subungual exostosis, 308
Subungual keratoacanthoma, 308
Sudoriferous cysts, of eyelid, 990
Sugar tumor, of lungs, 1101
Superficial glands, 1283–1284
Superficial spreading melanoma, 103–104
Superficial squamous cell carcinoma
  of esophagus, 1300
  of vulva, 2127
Supraglottic cancer, 933–935
Surfactant apoprotein, in pulmonary neoplasms, 1107
Sweat gland carcinomas, 60, 65
Sweet's syndrome, 29
Sydney system, for gastritis, 1315–1316
Sympathoadrenal neuroendocrine system, 632–633
Synaptophysin, 484–485
Syncytial meningioma, 440
Syncytiotrophoblast, 2067
Synovial chondromatosis, 237–238, 307–308
Synovial lesions, 182–183
Synovial lipomatosis, 227
Synovial sarcoma
  of larynx, 943
  of soft tissue, 181, 182–183
Synovitis
  hemosiderotic, 237
  pigmented villonodular, 182, 236–237
Syphilis
  aorta in, 1257, 1258
  arthritis due to, 233
  liver in, 1513
  lymph nodes in, 719
  penis in, 2039
  secondary, 16
  of stomach, 1320
  testis in, 1962
  of vagina, 2135
  of vulva, 2114
Syringocystadenoma papilliferum, of ear, 955
Syringoma, 63
  chondroid, 63
  papillary, 63
  of vulva, 2133
Syrinx, wall of, 459–460
Systemic connective tissue diseases, inflammatory myopathy in, 114–115
Systemic lupus erythematosus (SLE)
  endocarditis with, 1232
  inflammatory myopathy in, 115
  lymph nodes in, 717–718
  myocardial lesions in, 1218
  nephropathies of, 1745–1749, 1777
  skin in, 10–12
  small-vessel disease of brain in, 407
  vasculitis in, 1268
Systemic sclerosis, of esophagus, 1295

T

Tabes dorsalis, osteoarthritis in, 225–227
Tailgut cysts, 1391–1392
Takayasu's disease, 1258, 1260, 1262, 1264–1265
Talc granulomas, 32
Tamoxifen, and endometrial carcinoma, 2236
Tancho's nodules, 2042
Target fibers, 117–118
Targetoid(s), 117–118
Targetoid hemosiderotic hemangioma, 177
Tarui disease, 125–126
Tattoo pigment granulomas, 31
T-cell leukemia
  adult, 679, 759–760
  chronic lymphocytic, 677
T-cell lymphoma(s), 676–680, 751–761
  adult, 679, 759–760
  anaplastic large-cell, 758–759
  angioimmunoblastic, 757
  cutaneous, 6, 17
  enteropathy-associated, 1357, 1450–1453
  of intestines, 1454
  of liver, 1618
  lymphoblastic, 753–754
  peripheral, 78, 678–679, 754–756
  precursor, 753–754
  primary extranodal, 760–763
  sinonasal, 907–908
  soft tissue, 74, 75–76
  of spleen, 787–789
T-cell prolymphocytic leukemia, 677
T-cell-rich B-cell lymphoma, 75, 749
Teeth, and anatomy of jaw, 805
Telangiectasia
  capillary, of CNS, 407, 408
  hereditary hemorrhagic, intestinal involvement in, 1387
Telangiectatic osteosarcoma, 286–287
Temporal arteritis, 1258, 1260, 1262–1264, 1265
Temporal bone, tumors of apex of petrous, 971–972
Tendon sheath
  fibroma of, 153
  giant-cell tumor of, 182
Tenosynovitis, nodular, 182
Teratocarcinosarcoma, sinonasal, 914
Teratoid/rhabdoid tumor, atypical, 438
Teratoma(s)
  of CNS, 413, 451
  of fallopian tube, 2407
  hepatic, 1557, 1562–1563
  mediastinal, 1153–1155, 1198
    immature, 1154
  ovarian, 2364–2370
    immature, 2364–2365
    mature, 2365–2366
    monodermal, 2366–2370
  testicular, 1997–2000
  thyroid, 557
Terminal duct lobular unit, 325, 327, 328
Testicular feminization, 1965–1967
  and germ cell tumors, 1978
Testicular regression syndrome (TRS), 1947, 1965
Testicular sperm extraction, 1956, 1957
Testicular-splenic fusion, 1947–1948, 2015
Testicular tumors, 1973–2021
  adenocarcinoma, 2014–2015
  adenomatoid, 2018–2019
  adenomatous hyperplasia, 2014
  aggressive angiomyxoma, 2021
  angiomyofibroblastoma, 2021
  carcinoid, 2000–2001
  choriocarcinoma, 1995–1997
  classification of, 1973, 1974, 1976
  cystic dysplasia, 2014
  cysts, 1959
    dermoid, 1999
    epidermoid, 2012–2013
  desmoplastic small round cell, 2017–2018
  diffuse embryoma, 2002
  embryonal carcinoma, 1985–1990
  epididymal, 1974, 2018–2020
  fibromas, 2009, 2016
  germ cell, 1974–2004
    biopsy of, 1957
    classification of, 1974–1976
    cryptorchidism and, 1947
    epidemiology of, 1977–1979
    histogenesis of, 1976–1977
    intratubular, 1976–1977, 1978, 1979–1980
    mixed, 2001–2002
    postchemotherapy resections of, 2003–2004
    regression of, 2002–2003
  gonadoblastoma, 2010–2011
  granulocytic sarcoma, 2012
  granulosa cell, 2009
  gross examination of, 1973–1974
  hydrocele, 2015
  leukemia, 2012
  Leydig cell, 2004–2006
  lymphomas, 2011–2012
  meconium periorchitis, 2015
  melanotic neuroectodermal, 2019–2020
  mesenchymal, 2013
  mesothelioma, 2016
  metastatic, 2013–2014

mixed germ cell-sex cord-stromal, 1974, 2010–2011
neuroendocrine, 489
nodular and diffuse fibrous proliferation, 2015–2016
ovarian-type epithelial, 2016–2017
papillary cystadenoma, 2019
para-, 1974, 2020–2021
of "passenger" and non-Leydig interstitial cells, 1974, 2011–2014
plasmacytoma, 2012
polyembryoma, 2002
primitive neuroectodermal, 2001
prostatic carcinoma, 1925
of rete testis, 1974, 2014–2015
rhabdomyosarcoma, 1986, 2020–2021
seminoma, 1980–1983, 1986
  spermatocytic, 1983–1985, 1986
Sertoli cell, 2006–2008
Sertoli-Leydig cell, 2008–2009
sex cord-stromal, 1974, 2004–2010
of spermatic cord, 1974, 2020–2021
splenic-gonadal fusion, 1947–1948, 2015
staging of, 1974, 1975
teratoma, 1997–2000
trophoblastic, 1995–1997
  placental-site, 1997
of tunica albuginea, 1974, 2015–2018
yolk sac, 1990–1995
Testis(es), 1943–1968
  adrenal cortical rests in, 1948
  in AIDS, 1962
  amyloidosis of, 1950
  anatomy and physiology of, 1943–1944, 1973
  in androgen insensitivity syndrome, 1965–1967
  anorchid, 1947
  bell-clapper abnormality of, 1948
  biopsy of, 1956–1958
  congenital abnormalities of, 1945–1948
  in congenital adrenal hyperplasia, 1965
  cryptorchid, 1945–1947
  development of, 1944–1945, 1963
  drug effect on, 1958
  embryology of, 1944–1945
  enlargement of, 1956
  epididymis of, 1959–1960
  excurrent duct obstruction of, 1953–1955
  in germinal cell aplasia, 1952–1953
  in gonadal dysgenesis, 1967–1968
  in gonadotropin deficiency, 1955–1956
  in hermaphroditism, 1968
  in hypospermatogenesis, 1951
  infectious disease of, 1960–1963
  in infertility, 1950–1955
  in intersex syndromes, 1963–1968
  karyotypic abnormalities of, 1953
  in Klinefelter's syndrome, 1953
  in leprosy, 1961
  malakoplakia of, 1963
  maturation arrest of, 1951–1952
  in mumps, 1961–1962
  in nonspecific granulomatous orchitis, 1962–1963
  in persistent müllerian duct syndrome, 1964–1965
  in pseudohermaphroditism, 1964–1968
  radiation effect on, 1958–1959
  regression of, 1947, 1965
  in spermatogenesis, 1951
  in syphilis, 1962
  torsion and infarction of, 1948–1949
  in tuberculosis, 1961
  tubular sclerosis and interstitial fibrosis of, 1953
  tumors of. See Testicular tumors
  undescended, 1945–1947
  varicocele of, 1949–1950
  vasculitis of, 1950
Testis-determining factor, 1944
Thecoma, of ovary, 2348–2349
Thin basement membrane disease, 1733, 1776
Third pharyngeal pouch cyst, 1150
Third ventricle, colloid cyst of, 460–461
Thrombi, intervillous, 2093
Thromboangiitis obliterans, 1262, 1266
Thrombocythemia, essential, 664
Thrombocytopenic purpura
  immune, 781, 782
  thrombotic, 781, 1736–1739
Thrombomodulin, in mesothelioma, 1134
Thrombotic microangiopathy, 1736–1739, 1770, 1776
Thrombotic pulmonary hypertension, 1049
Thrombotic thrombocytopenic purpura, 781, 1736–1739
Thymic dysplasia, 1161
Thymolipoma, 1162
Thymoliposarcoma, 1195
Thymomas, 1156–1162
  classification of, 1156–1157
  cystic, 1155–1156
  epithelial spindle-cell, 1161–1162
  lymphocyte-predominant, 1158–1161
  microscopic, 1161
  organoid, 1158
  prognostic features of, 1158, 1196–1198
  staging system for, 1197
  of thyroid, 557
Thymus
  B-cell lymphoma of, 748–749
  carcinoid tumors of, 1182–1183, 1190, 1198–1199
    spindle cell, 1194
  carcinomas of
    primary, 1176–1180, 1199
    sarcomatoid, 1192–1194
  cysts of, 1149–1151
  neuroendocrine neoplasms of, 486–487
  yolk sac tumor of, sarcomatoid, 1194
Thymus-like differentiation
  carcinomas showing, 1196
  spindle cell epithelial tumors with, 1196
Thyroepiglottic ligament, 926
Thyroglossal duct(s), thyroid tissue in, 529
Thyroglossal duct carcinoma, 557–558
Thyroglottic ligament, 926
Thyroid, 529–563
  amyloidosis of, 534–535
  anatomy of, 530–531
  autoimmune disease of, 531–534, 536
  carcinoma of. See Thyroid carcinoma
  C-cell lesions of, 548–552
  C-cell of, 484
  clear cell tumors of, 556–557
  developmental anomalies of, 529–530
  development of, 529
  diffuse enlargements of, 531
  fibrosing lesions of, 534–535
  fine needle aspiration of, 558–563
  follicular adenoma of, 544–545
  follicular neoplasms of, 542–543, 544–548, 559–560
  frozen section diagnosis for, 558
  goiter of
    diffuse toxic, 533
    nodular, 544, 559
    toxic nodular, 533, 543
  Graves' disease of, 543
  hematopoietic lesions of, 555
  Hürthle cell lesions of, 547–548, 560
  inborn errors of metabolism of, 543
  iron deposition in, 535
  lingual, 529, 557
  lymphocytic lesions of, 555
  lymphoma of, 555, 562
  maldescent of, 529
  metastases to, 556, 557, 562
  multifocal granulomatous folliculitis of, 531
  pigments in, 535
  radiation fibrosis of, 534
  sarcoma of, 554
  squamous cell lesions of, 538, 555–556
  teratomas of, 557
Thyroid carcinoma
  anaplastic, 552–553, 562
  follicular, 546–547
  insular, 552
  intratracheal and intralaryngeal, 558
  medullary, 549–551, 561–562
  mucoepidermoid, 556
  papillary, 534, 535–542
    columnar cell variant of, 541
    diffuse sclerosis variant of, 541–542, 556
    encapsulated variant of, 542
    etiology of, 535–536
    fine needle aspirate specimens of, 561

Thyroid carcinoma, papillary *(contd.)*
    flow cytometry of, 539
    follicular variant of, 540
    immunohistochemistry of, 539
    occult, 540
    and parathyroid adenomas, 536
    pathology of, 536–539
    pink cell variant of, 541
    prognostic factors in, 539–540
    solid variant of, 542
    subtypes of, 540–542
    tall cell variant of, 540–541
    ultrastructure of, 539
  poorly differentiated, 552
  small cell, 553
  squamous cell, 556
Thyroiditis, 531
  acute, 531
  autoimmune, 531–534, 559
  chronic lymphocytic, 532–533, 559
  drug-associated, 533–534
  focal nonspecific, 533
  granulomatous subacute, 531
  Hashimoto's, 532, 559
    fibrosing variant of, 533
  invasive fibrous, 534
  ligneous, 534
  lymphocytic, 533
    juvenile, 533
  nonsuppurative, 531
  painless, with hyperthyroidism, 533
  palpation, 531
  Reidel's, 534
Thyroid nodules
  fine needle aspiration and management of, 563
  follicular, 542–543, 544–548, 559–560
  due to hyperthyroidism, 543
  due to inborn errors of metabolism, 543
  due to papillary carcinoma, 535–542
  due to papillary hyperplasia, 542
  toxic, 543
  in toxic nodular goiter, 533, 543
Thyrotroph cell, 497
Thyrotroph cell adenoma, 499, 501, 514
Tinea capitis, 7
Tinea corporis, 7
Tinea cruris, 7
  of vulva, 2117
Tinea faciale, 7
Tinea manuum, 7
Tinea pedis, 7
Tissue-core biopsy, of breast tissue, 320–321
Tobacco, and oral squamous cell carcinoma, 810
Tongue, squamous cell carcinoma of, 823–824
Tonsils
  papillary lymphoid hyperplasia of, 810
  squamous cell carcinoma of, 825–826

Tophi
  cutaneous, 38–39
  of ear, 951
  of joints, 231
Torkelson syndrome, 1355
Toxic epidermal necrolysis, 15
Toxic myocarditis, 1218
Toxic shock syndrome, 2135–2136
Toxoplasmosis
  CNS, 392
    in AIDS, 402
  lymph nodes in, 719
  pulmonary, in AIDS, 1058
Tracheobronchial amyloidosis, 1056
Transglottic cancer, 936
Transitional cell carcinoma
  of bladder, 1867–1868
    nested, 1878
  of ovary, 2341
  of prostate, 1930–1931
Transitional cell tumors
  of ovary, 2339–2341
  peritoneal, 2435
Transitional meningioma, 413, 440
Transplantation
  cardiac, 1222–1224
  liver, 1512, 1544–1546, 1588–1589
  lymphoproliferative disorders after, 723–724
  of pancreas, 1474
  renal, 1767–1775
    glomerulopathy after, 1771–1772
  small bowel, 1393–1394
Transsexuals, androgen therapy in, 377
Transurethral resection of the prostate (TURP)
  adenocarcinoma *vs.* adenoma in, 1911–1912
  granulomas after, 1897–1898
  prostatic carcinoma detected on, 1923–1924
Traumatic inclusion cysts, of vulva, 2113
Trench mouth, 807
Trephine biopsy, 651–652
Treponema pallidum, 2114
Trichilemmal cyst, 62
Trichilemmoma, 64
  proliferating, 60, 64
Trichoepithelioma, 61
Trichofolliculoma, 60, 61, 62
Trichomonas vaginalis, 2136
Trichuriasis, intestinal, 1385
Tricuspid valvular disease, 1230
Tropheryma whippelii, 1356
Trophoblast(s), during normal gestation, 2067–2069
Trophoblastic disease
  classification of, 2068
  of fallopian tube, 2407
  gestational, 2067–2085
    choriocarcinoma, 2076–2080

    exaggerated placental site, 2074–2075
    hydatidiform mole, 2069–2074
      complete, 2069–2071
      invasive, 2073–2074
      partial, 2071–2073
    placental-site nodule, 2075–2076
Trophoblastic implants, in peritoneum, 2420
Trophoblastic tumors
  epithelioid, 2082–2085
  ovarian metastases of, 2382
  placental-site, 2074, 2080–2082, 2221
  of testis, 1995–1997
Tropical eosinophilia, 1023
Tropical sprue, 1353
Tryptophan ingestion, and eosinophilia/myalgia syndrome, 145, 153
Tubal ligation, changes secondary to, 2398
Tubal pregnancy, 2398–2399
Tubal prolapse, 2137
Tuberculosis
  adrenal insufficiency due to, 594
  of bones and joints, 234
  of brain, 398
  cystitis due to, 1854–1855
  intestinal, 1376, 1384
  of middle ear, 960
  pelvic, 2308
  of penis, 2039
  peritonitis due to, 2415
  prostatitis due to, 1895–1896
  renal, 1759
  salpingitis due to, 2395–2397
  sinonasal, 887
  testis in, 1961
  of vulva, 2115
Tuberous sclerosis, renal involvement in, 1695–1696
Tuboendometrial metaplasia, of endocervical glands, 2180
Tubo-ovarian abscess, 2307
Tubo-ovarian autoamputation, 2399
Tubular adenoma
  apocrine, 63
  of breast, 364
Tubular adenosis, of breast, 332, 333
Tubular atrophy, 1778
Tubular carcinoma, of breast, 332, 356, 371
Tubular congeries, 1947
Tubular necrosis, acute, 1752–1754
Tubular protein resorption droplets, 1717, 1778
Tubular sclerosis, of testis, 1953
Tubulitis, 1755, 1778
Tubuloalveolar mucus-secreting glands, 1629
Tubulointerstitial diseases, 1752–1761
Tubulointerstitium, terminology for, 1778

Tufted hemangioma, 176
Tufting enteropathy, 1360
Tumefactive fibroinflammatory lesions, 153
Tumoral calcinosis, 232
Tumorlet, pulmonary, 1103
Tumorlette, of pituitary adenoma, 503
Tumor margin, of glioma, 410–415
Tunica albuginea, tumors of, 1974, 2015–2018
Tunnel clusters, 2177
Turcot's syndrome, 1418, 1435
Turner's syndrome, intestinal involvement in, 1387
TURP. See Transurethral resection of the prostate (TURP)
Twin transfusion syndrome, 2099–2100
Tylectomy, 321
Tympanosclerosis, 959–960
Tyndall effect, 100
Typhlitis, 1383
Tyrosinemia, liver in, 1519, 1520

U

Ulcer(s)
  cutaneous, 5
  Hunner's, 1855
  peptic, 1325, 1354–1355
  rectal, 1369–1370
  stercoral, 1383
Ulcerative colitis (UC), 1374–1375, 1376
  and carcinoma, 1379–1382
  chronic (quiescent), 1361–1362
  diffuse active, 1362–1363
  polyps in, 1420
  resolving, 1363
Ulcerative jejunoileitis, 1357
Ulcerative proctitis, 1376–1377
Ulcerative stomatitis, 807
Umbilical artery
  meconium-induced necrosis of, 2104–2105
  single, 2095
Umbilical cord abnormalities, 2094–2095
Urachal carcinoma, 1874–1875
Urate nephropathy, 1761
Ureaplasma urealyticum, chorioamnionitis due to, 2101
Ureter
  carcinoma of, 1879
  endometriosis of, 1858
Ureteritis, 1856
Urethra
  carcinoma of, 1880–1881
  caruncles of, 1856
  penile, 2037
  polyps of, 1879–1880, 1934
Urethral valves, 1856
Urethritis, 1856
Urinary bladder. See Bladder
Urothelial tract, 1853–1886
  adenoma of, 1861–1862
  aggressive angiomyxoma of, 1882
  amyloidosis of, 1859
  anatomy of, 1853–1854
  benign mesenchymal neoplasms of, 1882
  carcinoid tumors of, 1882
  carcinoma of, 1864–1879
    adeno-, 1873–1874
    blood group-related antigens of, 1885–1886
    chorio-, 1878
    classification of, 1864–1865
    cytology of, 1882–1884
    differential diagnosis of, 1805
    epidemiology of, 1864
    flow cytometry of, 1884–1885
    genetics and molecular genetics of, 1886
    in situ, 1871–1872, 1883
    lymphoepithelioma form of, 1878
    neuroendocrine, 1875–1876
    ovarian metastases of, 2381
    papillary lesions and, 1868–1871
    renal pelvis and ureteral, 1879
    sarcomatoid (spindle cell, giant cell), 1876–1878
    signet-ring cell, 1874
    small cell, 1875–1876
    squamous cell, 1873
    staging of, 1865–1867
    transitional cell, 1867–1868
      nested, 1878
    urachal, 1874–1875
    urethral, 1880–1881
    verrucous, 1873
  carcinosarcoma of, 1876–1878
  choriocarcinoma of, 1878
  condyloma of, 1862–1863
  diverticula of, 1859–1860
  endometriosis of, 1858
  hematologic neoplasms of, 1882
  inflammatory disorders of, 1854–1858
  inflammatory pseudosarcomatous lesions of, 1863–1864
  inverted papilloma of, 1862
  lymphoepithelioma of, 1878
  malakoplakia of, 1858–1859
  melanoma of, 1882
  metaplasia of, 1860–1862
  papillary tumors of, 1868–1871
  paragangliomas of, 1882
  plasma cell granuloma of, 1856
  polyps of, 1879–1880
  reactive proliferative changes of, 1860
  sarcomas of, 1881–1882
Urticaria, 27
Uterine bleeding, dysfunctional, 2223
Uterine cervix. See Cervix
Uterine corpus, 2203–2290
  adenomatoid tumor of, 2288–2290
  differential diagnosis of gross findings in, 2205
  endometrium of. See Endometrium
  lipoma of, 2273, 2284
  lymphoma/leukemia of, 2269–2270, 2290
  mesothelioma of, 2288–2290
  mitotic activity in, 2205, 2206, 2282–2283
  myometrium of, 2271–2272
  papillary serous carcinoma of, 2252–2254
  pattern diagnosis for, 2205–2210
  smooth-muscle neoplasms of, 2272–2288
    atypia in, 2277
    diagnostic strategy for, 2272–2275, 2279–2281
    differential diagnosis of, 2270, 2272–2275
    epithelioid differentiation of, 2281
    histologic patterns of, 2273
    leiomyomas, 2273, 2281–2287
    leiomyosarcoma, 2273, 2287–2288
    mitotic index of, 2278, 2282–2283
    morphologic features of, 2276–2279
    myxoid differentiation of, 2280
    necrosis in, 2278–2279
    prognosis and clinical management of, 2275–2279
    of usual sort, 2273, 2279–2280
  specimens from, 2203–2205
  unusual disease processes of, 2289
Utricle cysts, of prostate, 1898–1899
Uveal tumors, 994–996
Uveitis, sympathetic, 994

V

Vacuolar change, in muscle, 119–120
Vacuolar interface change, 5
Vacuolar interface dermatitis, 10–14
Vacuole(s)
  artifactual, 111–112
  rimmed, 119–120
Vagal paragangliomas, 628–629
Vagina, 2133–2143
  adenocarcinoma of, 2141–2142
  adenosis of, 2133–2135
  agenesis of, 2133
  anatomy of, 2133
  benign conditions of, 2136–2139
  congenital anomalies of, 2133–2135
  cysts of, 2137
  embryonal rhabdomyosarcoma of, 2142–2143
  endodermal sinus tumor of, 2142
  infectious diseases of, 2135–2136
  lymphoma of, 2142
  malignant neoplasms of, 2140–2143
  melanoma of, 2142
  mesonephric papilloma of, 2138

Vagina *(contd.)*
  mesonephric remnants in, 2135
  metastases to, 2143
  mixed tumor of, 2138
  papillomatosis of, and squamous
      intraepithelial lesions, 2163
  polypoid xanthogranulomatous
      pseudotumor of, 2136
  premalignant conditions of, 2139–2140
  rhabdomyoma of, 2139
  sarcomas of, 2142–2143
  spindle cell nodule of, 2139
  squamous cell carcinoma of, 2140–2141
  stromal polyps of, 2137–2138
  in toxic shock syndrome, 2135–2136
  verrucous carcinoma of, 2141
Vaginal intraepithelial neoplasia (VAIN),
    2139–2140
Vaginitis
  atrophic, 2136
  bacterial, 2135–2136
  candidal, 2136
  desquamative inflammatory, 2136
  emphysematous, 2136–2137
  noninfectious causes of, 2137
Vaginosis, bacterial, 2135
VAIN (vaginal intraepithelial neoplasia),
    2139–2140
Valves
  bicuspid, 1225
  floppy, 1229
  myxomatous, 1229
  native, 1225
  prolapsed, 1229
  prosthetic, 1233–1235
Valvular disease, 1225–1233
  aortic, 1225–1227
  due to endocarditis, 1230–1233
  mitral, 1227–1230
  postinflammatory, 1225–1226
  pulmonic, 1230
  right-sided, 1230–1233
  tricuspid, 1230
Vanishing bile duct syndrome, 1545, 1546
Varicella, 21
Varicella zoster, in liver, 1515
Varicocele, 1949–1950
Vascular dementia, multiinfarct, 464
Vascular dilatation, in gastroesophageal
    reflux disease, 1287
Vascular disease, 1253–1277
  amyloid angiopathy, 1270
  aneurysms, 1256–1258
  arterial and venous thrombosis,
      1270–1271
  atherosclerosis, 1253–1254
  in children, 1261
  of CNS, 407–408
  cutaneous, 28–33
  in diabetes, 1253, 1254, 1255, 1256
  in hypertension, 1253, 1254, 1255

  inflammatory, 1259–1268
  of intestinal tract, 1386–1387
  of kidneys, 1761–1765
  of liver, 1537–1538
  malformations and dysplasias,
      1274–1277
  of placenta, 2106–2107
  radiation-induced, 1269–1270
  in rheumatologic disorders,
      1268–1269
  sinonasal, 908–911
  of stomach, 1339
  of vulva, 2119
Vascular ectasia, of right colon, 1386
Vascular leiomyoma, 69, 169
Vascular structure
  with aging, 1253, 1254
  normal, 1253
Vascular surgery, 1271–1274
Vascular transformation, of sinuses,
    177–178
Vascular tumors, 1277
  of bone, 294–295
  of intestines, 1458
  of larynx, 943
  of peritoneum, 2425
  of skin, 68–73
  of soft tissue, 161, 174–178
  of spleen, 797–799
Vasculitis, 1259–1268
  allergic, 28
  cerebral, 407
  in children, 1261
  Crohn's, 1375
  cutaneous, 28–33
    leukocytoclastic, 1260
  defined, 1259
  of gallbladder, 1642–1643
  granulomatous, 29
  histopathologic diagnosis of, 1259–1260
  immunopathology of, 1260–1261
  isolated, 1268
  large- and medium-vessel, 1260,
      1261–1267
  leukocytoclastic, 28–29
    cutaneous, 1260
  lymphocytic, 29
  necrotizing, 28
  nodular, 39
  reactive changes *vs.*, 1259
  renal, 1764–1765
  small-vessel, 1260, 1267
  of testes, 1950
Vasculopathy. *See* Vascular disease
Vas deferens, agenesis of, 1954
Vasitis nodosum, 1954
Vasoactive intestinal peptide, pancreatic
    tumors producing, 1501
Vasoproliferative lesions, of lymph node,
    728
Vasovasotomy, 1954

Vein bypass grafting, 1271
Vellus hair cyst, 62
Veno-occlusive disease
  of liver, 1511, 1514, 1529, 1538
  pulmonary, 1049–1051
Venous malformation, of CNS, 407, 408
Venous thrombosis, 1270–1271
Venulitis, neutrophilic, 28
Vermiform appendix, 1394–1395
  developmental abnormalities of,
      1394–1395
  inflammatory conditions of, 1395
  neoplasms of, 1442–1446
    ovarian metastases of, 2380
  neuroma of, 1395
  normal histology of, 1394
  specimen processing for, 1394
Verocay bodies, 448
Verruca plana, 49
Verruca plantaris, 49
Verruca vulgaris, 17, 49
  of eyelids, 989
Verruciform carcinoma, of penis, 2047,
    2051
Verruciform xanthoma
  of penis, 2042
  of vulva, 2117
Verrucous acanthosis, 17
Verrucous carcinoma
  of cervix, 2174
  cutaneous, 58–59
  of ear, 954–955
  of esophagus, 1299, 1301
  of larynx, 938–939
  of nasal cavity, 896
  of oral cavity, 824–828
  of penis, 2053–2054
  of urothelial tract, 1873
  of vagina, 2141
  of vulva, 2128–2129
Verrucous hyperplasia, 49–50
Vertebral column, pyogenic osteomyelitis
    of, 233–234
Vertebral compression fractures, 253
Vertical growth phase melanoma, 103
Verumontanum mucosal gland
    hyperplasia, 1907
Vesicle, 5
Vestibular gland adenoma, 2117
Vestibular schwannoma, 969–970
Vestibulitis syndrome, vulvar, 2118
Villitis, 2097, 2103–2104
  diffuse, 2105
Villoglandular carcinoma, of
    endometrium, 2252, 2254
Villoglandular hyperplasia, of
    endometrium, 2251–2252, 2254
Villoglandular papillary adenocarcinoma,
    of cervix, 2188–2190
Villous dysmaturity, 2105
Villous edema, 2089

Villous lymphocytes, splenic lymphoma
with, 786
Villus(i), intestinal, 1349
abnormalities of
severe, 1350–1352
variable, 1350, 1352–1360
Vimentin
as marker for soft tissue tumors, 138
in mesothelioma, 1129
in pulmonary neoplasms, 1106
VIN (vulvar intraepithelial neoplasia),
2122, 2123–2125
Vincent's disease, 807
Viral adenitis, 723
Viral-associated hemophagocytic
syndrome, 1536
Viral hepatitis, 1530–1536
Viral myocarditis, 1215
Viral myositis, 125
Virilization, 595, 600, 2112
Visceral myopathies, 1388–1389
Visceral neuropathies, 1388, 1389
Vitamin D deficiency osteomalacia, 244,
246–247, 249–250
Vitiligo, 24–25
Vocal cord polyp, 927, 943
Vocal cords. See Larynx
Vocal ligament, 926
von Hippel-Lindau disease
familial pheochromocytoma with,
617–618
renal cysts in, 1696
von Meyenburg's complex, 1597,
1598–1599
von Recklinghausen's disease, 186
familial pheochromocytoma with,
617–618
Vulva, 2111–2133
adenocarcinoma of, 2129
aggressive angiomyxoma,
angiomyofibroblastoma, and
angiofibroma of, 2120–2121
Bartholin's gland carcinoma of, 2129
basal cell carcinoma of, 2129
benign lesions of, 2117–2120
bowenoid papulosis of, 2123
candidiasis of, 2117
in chancroid, 2115
in chlamydia, 2115
condyloma acuminatum of, 2116–2117
congenital anomalies of, 2112–2113
Crohn's disease of, 2120
cutaneous appendage neoplasms of,
2133
cysts of, 2113–2114
dermatologic conditions of, 2118–2119
dystrophy of, 2121–2123
endodermal sinus tumor of, 2129–2130
endometriosis of, 2114
in erythrasma, 2115
Fox-Fordyce disease of, 2114

in gonorrhea, 2114–2115
in granuloma inguinale, 2115
herpes simplex of, 2116
hidradenitis suppurativa of, 2115
hidradenoma papilliferum of, 2132
infectious diseases of, 2114–2117
leiomyomas of, 2119
lichen sclerosis of, 2121–2122
lymphomas of, 2130
malignant neoplasms of, 2125–2130
melanoma of, 2130
metastases to, 2130
"milk lines" and lesions of, 2120
mixed tumors of, 2132–2133
molluscum contagiosum of, 2117
necrotizing fasciitis of, 2115
normal anatomy and histology of,
2111–2112
Paget's disease of, 2130–2132
sarcomas of, 2130
specimens from, 2112
squamous cell carcinoma of, 2125–2129
squamous intraepithelial neoplasia of,
2122, 2123–2125
in syphilis, 2114
syringomas of, 2132–2133
tinea cruris of, 2117
tuberculosis of, 2115
vascular lesions of, 2119
verrucous carcinoma of, 2128–2129
vestibulitis syndrome of, 2118
Vulvar intraepithelial neoplasia (VIN),
2122, 2123–2125

W
Waldenström's macroglobulinemia
bone marrow in, 690
intestinal involvement in, 1359
spleen in, 784
Walthard nests, 2400
of peritoneum, 2435
Wart(s)
common, 17
genital. See Condyloma acuminatum
Warthin's tumor, 861–862
Warty carcinoma. See Verrucous
carcinoma
Warty dyskeratoma, 62
Warty squamous intraepithelial lesion, of
penis, 2045
Waterhouse-Friderichsen syndrome, 594,
595
Watermelon stomach, 1339
Watery diarrhea-achlorhydria syndrome,
1502
Weber-Christian disease, 1397
Wegener's granulomatosis
of lung, 1040–1043
of orbit, 998
of penis, 2042
of skin, 29

vasculitis due to, 1260, 1267
Wermer's syndrome, parathyroid in, 568
Wet keratin, 517
Whipple's disease
of brain, 399
gastric granulomas in, 1320
intestines in, 1356
lymph nodes in, 722–723
mesentery and retroperitoneum
in, 1396
Wiedemann-Beckwith syndrome, 1690
Wilms' tumor, 1829–1839
in adults, 1812
anaplastic nuclear changes in,
1832–1834
blastemal patterns in, 1830–1831,
1839
clear cell sarcoma vs., 1846
clinical features of, 1829
cystic variants of, 1834–1835
differential diagnosis of, 1838–1839
epithelial patterns in, 1831, 1839
gross features of, 1829–1830
metaplastic neoplasia vs., 1842
microscopic features of, 1830–1832
multicentric, 1829, 1830
nephrogenic rests and
nephroblastomatosis with,
1835–1838
rhabdoid tumor of kidney vs., 1849
stromal patterns in, 1831–1832, 1839
teratoid, 1832, 1839
therapy effect on, 1832
triphasic, 1830, 1838–1839
ultrastructural and
immunohistochemical studies of,
1832
Wilson's disease, 1512, 1515, 1522–1524,
1547, 1548
Winkler's disease, 952
Wolffian cyst, 2114
Wolffian origin
female adnexal tumor of, 2407–2408
ovarian tumors of, 2375–2376
Wolman disease, liver in, 1520
Woodworkers, nasal adenocarcinoma in,
899

X
Xanthelasma
cutaneous, 30–31
of stomach, 1313
Xanthoastrocytoma, pleomorphic,
411, 419
Xanthogranuloma
of CNS, 412
juvenile, 65–66, 162
Xanthogranulomatous cholecystitis,
1641–1642
Xanthogranulomatous pyelonephritis,
1758

Xanthoma
  cutaneous, 30–31
  of ear, 951
  of prostate, 1899
  of stomach, 1313
  verruciform
    of penis, 2042
    of vulva, 2117
Xanthoma elasticum, pseudo-, 1387
X-cell cysts, 2092–2093

X-linked ichthyosis, 25

Y

Yersiniosis, intestinal, 1384
Yolk sac carcinomas, of mediastinum, 1181
Yolk sac tumor
  of ovary, 2338, 2360–2363
  sarcomatoid thymic, 1194
  of testis, 1990–1995

Z

Zellweger syndrome, liver in, 1519, 1520
Zenker's diverticula, 1305
Zirconium granulomas, 31
Z-line, 1284
Zollinger-Ellison syndrome
  small intestine in, 1354
  stomach in, 1329
Zonation effect, 145
Zoon's balanitis, 2041–2042

17450

```
RD              Diagnostic surgical
57                 pathology.
.D53
1999
v.2
                                    36602
$349.00
```

DATE			